WEINER'S PAIN MANAGEMENT

A Practical Guide for Clinicians

SEVENTH EDITION

WEINER'S PAIN MANAGEMENT

A Practical Guide for Clinicians

SEVENTH EDITION

Edited by

Mark V. Boswell
B. Eliot Cole

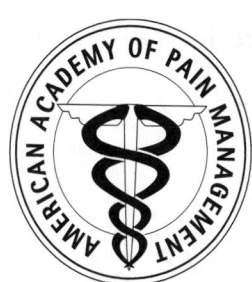

AMERICAN ACADEMY OF PAIN MANAGEMENT

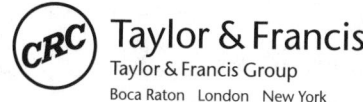

Taylor & Francis
Taylor & Francis Group
Boca Raton London New York

A CRC title, part of the Taylor & Francis imprint, a member of the
Taylor & Francis Group, the academic division of T&F Informa plc.

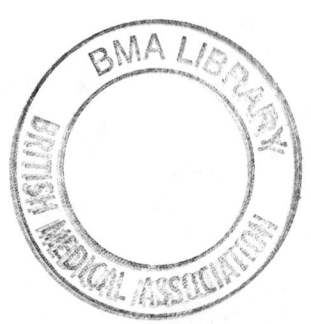

Published in 2006 by
CRC Press
Taylor & Francis Group
6000 Broken Sound Parkway NW, Suite 300
Boca Raton, FL 33487-2742

Library of Congress Cataloging-in-Publication Data

Weiner's pain management : a practical guide for clinicians.-- 7th ed. / edited by Mark V. Boswell, B. Eliot Cole.
   p. ; cm.
   Rev. ed. of: Pain management / editor, Richard S. Weiner. 6th ed. c2002.
  Includes bibliographical references and index.
  ISBN 0-8493-2262-6 (alk. paper)
   1. Pain--Treatment. 2. Analgesia. [DNLM: 1. Pain--therapy. 2. Pain--diagnosis. 3. Patient Care Management. WL 704 W423p 2005] I. Title: Pain management. II. Boswell, Mark V. III. Cole, B. Eliot. IV. Weiner, Richard S., Ph. D. V. Pain management.

RB127.P33233 2005
616'.0472--dc22   2004065101

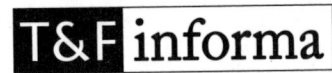

Taylor & Francis Group is the Academic Division of T&F Informa plc.

Visit the Taylor & Francis Web site at
http://www.taylorandfrancis.com

and the CRC Press Web site at
http://www.crcpress.com

Dedication to Richard S. Weiner, PhD

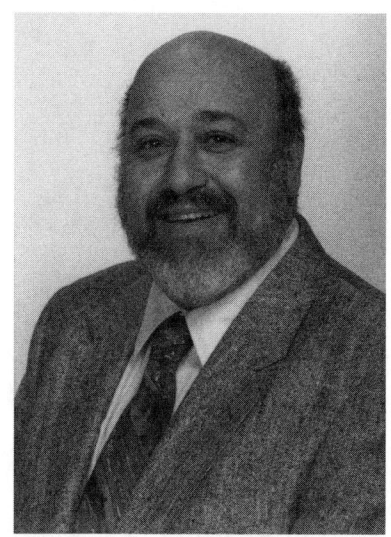

While standing upon the shoulders of giants helped advances to occur, the genius of Richard S. Weiner, PhD was that he could see the finished puzzle within the constituent pieces. He took pre-existing parts and ideas that others had over-looked, pulled them together in altered ways and created new results. He created harmony from the chaos others perceived. He did more than talk about the developing field of pain management; he walked the walk and co-founded the American Academy of Pain Management with Kathryn A. Weiner, PhD. Together, the Weiners created a new organization that finally met the needs of its pain practitioner members through pain-related education, practitioner cre-dentialing, pain program accreditation, outcome measurement, and many other offerings. Bringing together leaders in the field of pain management to create the American Academy of Pain Management's textbook, *Pain Management: A Practical Guide for Clinicians,* was one of his greatest accomplishments and was a continuing source of pride for Richard. Revising six editions became his commitment to the advancement of the pain management profession.

For Richard editing each edition of the textbook was a challenging process that required more than a year of preparation. Richard weathered this process six times in 12 years to make certain that the American Academy of Pain Manage-ment's textbook was clinically useful, current, and the best source for multidisciplinary information about the assessment, evaluation, and treatment of pain. For Richard, this was his labor of love and he gave his very best to this process.

Many might say that authoring textbooks is just too much work. It is far more effort than most people would ever willingly take upon themselves. Richard never saw the textbook as too much work for himself. He looked forward to the revision process and the updating of the chapters with each new edition. He enthusiastically called authors, new and old alike, to talk with them about their submissions, suggested points to discuss, and then called up others to tell them about what he had learned in the new chapters when he received them. No matter how many hours or how many authors were involved, he treated each of the authors with consideration, excitement, and respect. He asked of the authors more than some knew that they had within themselves, but always knew what they could accomplish if properly motivated. Richard was the consummate manager, who not only managed ideas, but the people bringing the ideas to fruition.

Knowing that he was quite seriously ill in 2001, Richard began to consider future goals for the American Academy of Pain Management. He knew that in another couple of years the seventh edition of the textbook would need to be written to maintain the currency associated with the book. In his own amazing way, and in his attempt to find goodness and humor even in the worst of circumstances, he speculated that he wouldn't have to edit any more textbooks if he didn't respond to his anti-cancer therapies. He even tried to cheer up those who were so concerned about him by telling us that the chemotherapy was easier than editing the textbook. He helped to identify the principal editor for the seventh edition of the textbook before his death in May 2002.

Practitioners fortunate enough to have personally known Richard, continue to mourn his passing. His hundreds of personal friends and members of his immediate family remember all that he gave to our evolving profession. Always the gentleman in his dealings with others, he shall best be remembered as the man who gathered together the many disciplines that constitute the modern field of pain management to improve the treatment of pain for so many unfortunate sufferers he never met. He never wanted special recognition, but wanted the profession to mature and to see the "mainstreaming" of pain management services.

We miss Richard. Not a day goes by when we do not think about something he said to one of us, some lesson he taught us, or some opportunity he created for all of us who now follow in his footsteps. Few men pass through our lives and have as significant an impact as he did for each of us personally and for so many of our colleagues. While his life was far too short, his accomplishments more than filled his lifetime and left a permanent legacy for all of us. It is only fitting that this *Seventh Edition* be dedicated to the outstanding work and life of Dr. Richard S. Weiner.

Mark V. Boswell, MD, PhD and B. Eliot Cole, MD, MPA

Contents

SECTION II Discipline-Specific Approaches

Alfred V. Anderson, MD, DC, Section Editor

SECTION III Common Pain Problems

David Glick, DC, Section Editor

SECTION IV   *Diagnostic Tests and Evaluations*
A. Elizabeth Ansel, RN, Section Editor

SECTION V   *Behavioral Approaches*
Nelson H. Hendler, MD, MS, Section Editor

SECTION VI   *Pharmacotherapy*
Robert B. Supernaw, PharmD, Section Editor

SECTION VII   *Procedures and Techniques*
Laxmaiah Manchikanti, MD, Section Editor

SECTION XI   Legal and Ethical Considerations
B. Eliot Cole, MD, MPA, Section Editor

SECTION XII   Beliefs, Religion, and Spirituality
Richard H. Cox, MD, PhD, DMin, Section Editor

Preface

PLEASE READ THIS PREFACE!

Few people ever bother to read the preface of a textbook, much less the preface of a book on the subject of pain management. This completely revised Seventh Edition is the most comprehensive rewrite of *Pain Management: A Practical Guide for Clinicians.* Unlike the previous six editions, every attempt has been made to offer evidence-based, clinically relevant information. This book is intended for pain practitioners and busy practitioners from other disciplines trying to provide relief for those suffering with pain.

Uniquely, the book unfolds the "story" of pain and its management just as those suffering present themselves to clinicians for help. Major perspectives and challenges are initially identified, leading to an appreciation of the various disciplines providing care. Common pain problems and diagnostic methods used in pain management next give "flesh" to the skeletal story. Treatment options unfold from least invasive to most invasive as we explore behavioral approaches, pharmacotherapy, procedural techniques and the integrative options. The needs of special populations, along with the legal aspects of care, belief systems and spiritual matters, and practice issues finally complete the book.

While no textbook is completely able to cover the entirety of a subject, the intent of this book is to give any reader the "fast take" on pain-related information needed for the next patient, the upcoming examination, or to satisfy some academic question. This book intends to be the "first and last" source for most clinicians needing to know something about pain management. The book has ample references to guide future self-inquiry, allowing readers to know the original source work and independently reach conclusions about the material presented.

The American Academy of Pain Management's textbook remains a work in continuous development. As the Seventh Edition becomes available, budgeting and planning begin anew for the eighth edition to follow in five years. No one holds all of the truth, and the leadership of the Academy expects that in years to come this book will continue to evolve from one editor to the next, always fresh and current in its presentation, and true to the original charge given to each of us practicing in pain management by our late, founding Executive Director, Richard S. Weiner, PhD.

Please enjoy the material included within these pages. Make note of areas that were covered superficially and need more detail. Be willing to help your colleagues "push the envelope" in future editions by writing chapters, providing peer review, and offering suggestions for continuous improvement.

About the Editors

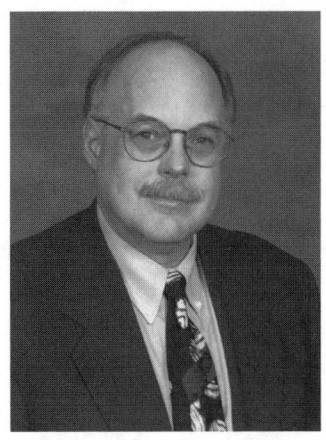

Mark V. Boswell, MD, PhD is chief of pain medicine, director of the Pain Medicine Fellowship Program, and associate professor of anesthesiology at Case Western Reserve University in Cleveland, Ohio. Trained in interventional pain management, medical acupuncture and end-of-life care, Dr. Boswell has been actively involved in clinical pain management, pain-related research, and academic medicine for more than 15 years. Dr. Boswell is editor-in-chief for *Pain Physician*, the official publication for the American Society of Interventional Pain Physicians (ASIPP).

Dr. Boswell earned his PhD in experimental pathology and MD from Case Western Reserve University. He completed an anesthesia residency after a categorical surgical internship, a research fellowship in neuroscience, and additional training in interventional pain management. Dr. Boswell was named the Outstanding Clinical Teacher in Anesthesiology in 1992 from CWRU School of Medicine and received the Outstanding Educational Achievement Award from ASIPP in 2004.

Dr. Boswell was vice-chair of the School of Medicine of CWRU, serves on numerous committees at University Hospitals of Cleveland, including pharmacy and therapeutics, QualChoice Medical Policy and the Rehabilitative Services Advisory Committee. He is a frequent presenter at local, national and international meetings, an accomplished author, and committed member of his community, family, and church.

Dr. Richard S. Weiner personally asked Dr. Boswell to serve as the principal editor for the Seventh Edition of the American Academy of Pain Management's textbook. Under Dr. Boswell's editorial leadership the Seventh Edition has been revised entirely to embrace the evidence basis for pain diagnosis and management. Dr. Boswell has introduced many new sections and made this edition the most diverse in the disciplines involved, the most comprehensive in scope of practice, and the most clinically relevant.

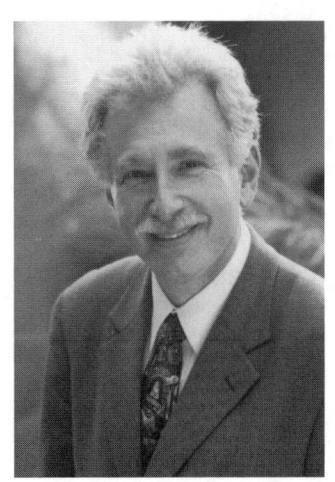

Dr. B. Eliot Cole earned his undergraduate degree in bacteriology from the University of California, his medical doctorate from Wake Forest University School of Medicine, and his master's in public administration from the University of Nevada, Las Vegas. He performed residencies in psychiatry and neurology at North Carolina Baptist Hospital, and completed an anesthesia-based fellowship in pain management at the University of California, Los Angeles, Center for Health Sciences. The American Psychiatric Association awarded Dr. Cole Fellow status in 1995 and Distinguished Fellow status in 2002.

Dr. Cole has been active in pain management since 1985, as a pain management fellow, a clinician, and as an active member of many pain-related organizations. He served on the American Academy of Pain Management's Board of Advisors, Board of Directors, numerous committees, was the organization's President from January 1, 1994 until December 31, 1995, and was the Interim Executive Director from March 1 until December 31, 1998.

Currently, Dr. Cole is a consultant in pain management for the Hawaii Permanente Medical Group and for the American Academy of Pain Management, serves as the Executive Director for the American Society of Pain Educators, and vice-president for medical and scientific affairs for Aventine HealthSciences. Dr. Cole is the program dean for pain studies at the University of Integrated Studies. Dr. Cole enjoys lecturing and writing about pain management, care of the terminally ill, medical policy-making, and ethical issues.

Acknowledgments

The Editors wish to sincerely thank the people who directly and indirectly helped with the development of the seventh edition of this book. Without the help of all these people, and many others not formally mentioned, it would not exist. In addition to thanking every single author, the Editors especially want to thank and recognize the extraordinary efforts of:

Alfred Anderson, MD, DC
A. Elizabeth Ansel, RN
Lois Baker
Robert A. Bonakdar, MD
Barbara Boswell, RN
Kathleen Broglio, APN-Rx
Richard H. Cox, MD, PhD, DMin
Erika Dery
David Glick, DC
Nelson H. Hendler, MD, MS
Laxmaiah Manchikanti, MD
Barbara Ellen Norwitz
Kathryn Padgett, PhD
Thomas J. Romano, MD, PhD
Steve Siwek, MD
Robert B. Supernaw, PharmD
Mimi Williams

Section Editors

Section 1
Perspectives of Pain
Mark V. Boswell, MD, PhD

Section 2
Discipline Specific Approaches
Alfred V. Anderson, MD, DC

Section 3
Common Pain Problems
David Glick, DC

Section 4
Diagnostic Tests and Evaluations
A. Elizabeth Ansel, RN

Section 5
Behavioral Approaches
Nelson H. Hendler, MD, MS

Section 6
Pharmacotherapy
Robert B. Supernaw, PharmD

Section 7
Procedures and Techniques
Laxmaiah Manchikanti, MD

Section 8
Integrative and Complementary Approaches
Robert A. Bonakdar, MD

Section 9
Electrical and Magnetic Therapies
Mark V. Boswell, MD, PhD

Section 10
Special Populations
Thomas J. Romano, MD, PhD

Section 11
Legal and Ethical Considerations
B. Eliot Cole, MD, MPA

Section 12
Beliefs, Religion and Spirituality
Richard H. Cox, MD, PhD, DMin

Section 13
Practice Issues
Steven Siwek, MD

List of Contributors

Salahadin Abdi, MD, PhD
Clinical Professor of Anesthesiology
Chief, Pain Medicine
University of Miami School of Medicine
Miami, Florida

Harry Adelson, ND
Private Practice
Docere Clinics
Salt Lake City, Utah
and
Board of Directors
American Association of Naturopathic Physicians

Christine L. Algren, RN, MSN, EdD
Clinical Associate Professor
Vanderbilt University School of Nursing
Nashville, Tennessee

John T. Algren, MD, FAAP
Pediatric Anesthesiologist
Vanderbilt Children's Hospital
Nashville, Tennessee
and
Professor, Anesthesiology & Pediatrics
Vice-Chairman for Educational Affairs
Department of Anesthesiology
Vanderbilt University Medical Center
Nashville, Tennessee

Terry Altilio, LMSW
Social Work Coordinator
Department of Pain Medicine and Palliative Care
Beth Israel Medical Center
New York, New York

Lori T. Andersen, EdD, OTR/L, FAOTA
Associate Professor, Occupational Therapy
Nova Southeastern University
Ft. Lauderdale, Florida

Alfred V. Anderson, MD, DC
Medical Director
Pain Assessment and Rehabilitation Center
Minneapolis, Minnesota

Frank Andrasik, PhD
Senior Research Scientist, Professor of Psychology
Institute for Human and Machine Cognition
University of West Florida
Pensacola, Florida

A. Elixabeth Ansel, RN
Pain Net Education, Inc.
Columbus, Ohio

Visanthi Arumugam, MD
Assistant Professor
Elmhurst Hospital Center
Mt. Sinai School of Medicine
New York, New York

Robert L. Barkin, PharmD, MBA, FCP, DAAPM
Associate Professor
Rush University Medical Center Faculty
Anesthesiology, Family Medicine, Pharmacology,
Rush Pain Center
Chicago, Illinois
North Shore Pain Center
Skokie, Illinois

Stacie J. Barkin, MEd, MA, PsyD, Candidate, National Board of Certified Counselors
Chicago, Illinois

Rev. Randol G. Batson, BS
Director
Mission and Spiritual Care
The Methodist Hospitals
Gary, Indiana

Samira Kanaan Beckwith, CHE, LCSW
Hope Hospice
Ft. Myers, Florida

Kelly Black, MD
Private Practice
Arizona Sports Medicine Consultants
Scottsdale, Arizona

Kacie Blalock, MS, CRC
Department of Rehabilitation Psychology and Special
  Education
University of Wisconsin
Madison, Wisconsin

Hal Blatman, MD
Private Practice
Cincinnati, Ohio

Elena N. Bodnar, MD
Electrical Trauma Research Program
Departments of Surgery, Medicine and Anatomy
University of Chicago
Chicago, Illinois

Jennifer Bolen, JD
Assistant U.S. Attorney
USDOJ, Eastern District of Tennessee
The J. Bolen Group, LLC,
Knoxville, Tennessee

Robert A. Bonakdar, MD
Director of Pain Management
Scripps Center for Integrative Medicine
La Jolla, California

Mark V. Boswell, MD, PhD
Director, Anesthesia Pain Service
Associate Professor of Anesthesiology,
University Hospitals of Cleveland and Case Western
  Reserve University School of Medicine
Cleveland, Ohio

David E. Bresler, PhD, LAc
The Bresler Center
Malibu, California

Jill Broderick, MS, OTR/L
Private Practice
Morristown, New Jersey

Christopher R. Brown, DDS, MPS
Private Practice
Versailles, Indiana

Kathleen Sitley Brown, PhD
Director, Pain Rehabilitation Program
Department of Psychology
Tripler Army Medical Center
Honolulu, Hawaii

Jan M. Burte, PhD, MS Psychopharm, DAAPM
Adjunct Professor,
Nova Southeastern University
Miami, Florida
Private Practice
Boca Raton, Florida

Suzanne Young Bushfield, PhD, MSW
Assistant Professor of Social Work
Arizona State University West
Phoenix, Arizona

C. Stephen Byrum, PhD
The Byrum Consulting Group
Signal Mt., Tennessee

Alexandra Campbell, PhD
Director, Pain Program Accreditation and Outcomes
  Measurement
American Academy of Pain Management
Sonora, California

Claudia E. Campbell, RN, BSN
LDS Hospital Intermountain Health Care
Salt Lake City, Utah

Stacy Carter, PhD
James A. Haley Veterans Affairs Hospital
Tampa, Florida

Denise Catalano, MS, CRC, Doctoral Student
Department of Rehabilitation Psychology and Special
  Education
University of Wisconsin
Madison, Wisconsin

Fong Chan, PhD, CRC
Professor
Department of Rehabilitation Psychology and Special
  Education
University of Wisconsin
Madison, Wisconsin

David Chapman, MD, MS
Adjunct Faculty
Midwestern University School of Osteopathic Medicine
Private Practice
Arizona Sports Medicine Consultants
Phoenix, Arizona

Frank Chessa, PhD
Assistant Professor, Philosophy
Bates College
Lewiston, Maine

Michael E. Clark, PhD
Clinical Director
Chronic Pain Rehabilitation Program
and
Associate Professor
University of South Florida and University of South
  Florida Medical School
Tampa, Florida

Daniel J. Clauw, MD
Professor of Medicine
Assistant Dean for Clinical and Translational Research
Director, Chronic Pain and Fatigue Research Center
Director, Center for the Advancement of Clinical
  Research
The University of Michigan
Ann Arbor, Michigan

B. Eliot Cole, MD, MPA
Program Dean
University of Integrated Studies
Sonora, California
and
Executive Director
American Society of Pain Educators
Montclair, New Jersey
and
Consultant
American Academy of Pain Management
Sonora, California
and
Consultant
Hawaii Permanente Medical Group
Honolulu, Hawaii

Paola M. Conte, PhD
Staff Psychologist
The David Center for Children's Pain and Palliative
  Care
Hackensack University Medical Center
Hackensack, New Jersey

Richard H. Cox, MD, PhD, DMin
Provost
Colorado School of Professional Psychology
Colorado Springs, Colorado

Jason DaCosta, MD
Department of Anesthesiology
University Hospitals of Cleveland and Case Western
  Reserve University School of Medicine
Cleveland, Ohio

Lorie T. DeCarvalho, PhD
National Center for PTSD
Department of Veterans Affairs
White River Junction, Vermont

Timothy R. Deer, MD
Medical Director
The Center for Pain Relief
and
Clinical Faculty
The West Virginia University School of Medicine
Charleston, West Virginia

Richard Derby, MD
Clinical Associate Professor
Stanford University
and
Private Practice
Spinal Diagnostics and Treatment Center
Daly City, California

W. John Diamond, MD
Private Practice
Intermedica LLC
Reno, Nevada

Jan Dommerholt, PT, MPS, FAAPM
Pain & Rehabilitation Medicine
Bethesda, Maryland

Lenore B. Duensing, MEd
Director of Communications and Outreach
American Pain Foundation
Baltimore, Maryland

Elmer E. Dunbar, MD
Pain Control Network P.S.C.
Louisville, Kentucky

John Duncan, PhD
Clinical Assistant Professor
Department of Psychiatry
University of Oklahoma Health Sciences Center
Norman, Oklahoma

Joe Durant, BA, NCTMB
Private Practice
Coastal Neurological Institute
Brunswick, Georgia

Stefan Engström, PhD
Department of Neurology
Vanderbilt University Medical Center
Nashville, Tennessee

Betty Lou Ervin-Cox, PhD, PsyD
Dean of Students, Professor
Colorado School of Professional Psychology
Colorado Springs, Colorado

Kathleen U. Farmer-Cady, PsyD
Private Practice
Headache Care Center,
Springfield, Missouri

Roger B. Fillingim, PhD
Associate Professor
University of Florida College of Dentistry
Gainesville, Florida

David Fishbain, MD, DFAPA
Professor of Psychiatry and Adjunct Professor of
  Neurological Surgery and Anesthesiology,
University of Miami School of Medicine
The Rosomoff Miami Pain Center,
Miami Beach, Florida

R. Michael Gallagher, DO, FACOFP
Director
University Headache Center
and
Professor and Dean
University of Medicine and Dentistry of New Jersey
School of Osteopathic Medicine
Stratford, New Jersey

Robert J. Gatchel, PhD, ABPP
The Eugene McDermott Center for Pain Management
The University of Texas Southwestern Medical Center at
  Dallas
Dallas, Texas

Robert D. Gerwin, MD
Assistant Professor of Neurology,
Johns Hopkins University
Bethesda, Maryland

Paula Gilchrist, DPM, PT
Private Practice
Pittsburgh, Pennsylvania
and
President
Board of Directors
American Academy of Pain Management (2004–2005)
Sonora, California

James Giordano, PhD
Senior Scholar
Center for Clinical Bioethics
Georgetown University
Washington, D.C.

Ronald J. Gironda, PhD
James A. Haley Veterans Affairs Hospital
  Counseling Center
and
University of South Florida
Tampa, Florida

David M. Glick, DC
Private Practice
Richmond, Virginia

Gerald Q. Greenfield, Jr., MD, FACS, FICS
Private Practice
The San Antonio Orthopaedic Group
San Antonio, Texas

Rainier Guiang, MD
Department of Anesthesiology
University Hospitals of Cleveland
Case Western Reserve University School of Medicine
Cleveland, Ohio

Hans Hansen, MD
Medical Director
The Pain Relief Centers
Conover, North Carolina

Richard E. Harris, PhD
University of Michigan School of Medicine
Ann Arbor, Michigan

Barbara A. Hastie, PhD
Research Assistant Professor
University of Florida College of Dentistry
Gainesville, Florida

Stephen R. Hays, MD, FAAP
Assistant Professor
Anesthesiology & Pediatrics
Vanderbilt University Medical Center
and
Director, Pediatric Pain Services
Vanderbilt Children's Hospital
Nashville, Tennessee

Nelson H. Hendler, MD, MS
Assistant Professor of Neurosurgery
Johns Hopkins University School of Medicine
Clinical Director
Mensana Clinic
Stevenson, Maryland

Alan R. Hirsch, MD
Assistant Professor
Departments of Neurology and Psychiatry
Rush Presbyterian St. Luke's Medical Center
Chicago, Illinois

Gregory L. Holmquist, PharmD, BCOP
Pain and Palliative Care Pharmacist
Seattle, Washington
and
Palliative Care Strategies
Bothell, Washington

Carin V. Hopps, MD
Assistant Professor of Urology
Medical College of Ohio
Toledo, Ohio

Candace Howe, MD
Resident, Department of Obstetrics and Gynecology
David Geffen School of Medicine at UCLA
University of California–Los Angeles
Los Angeles, California

Max Ito, PhD, OTR/L
Assistant Professor of Occupational Therapy
Nova Southeastern University
Ft. Lauderdale, Florida

Arcangelo M. Iusco, MD
Assistant Professor
Rush Medical College
and
Attending Anesthesiologist
Rush University Medical Center
and
North Shore Pain Center
Skokie, Illinois

Jeffrey W. Janata, PhD
Assistant Professor of Psychiatry
University Hospitals of Cleveland and Case Western
  Reserve University School of Medicine
Cleveland, Ohio

Gary W. Jay, MD, DAAPM
Senior Program Medical Scientist
Schwarz Pharma
Research Triangle Park, North Carolina

Art Jordan, MD
Medical Director
Pain Management Center
Carolina Health Specialists
Myrtle Beach, South Carolina

Ajay R. Kashi, BDS
Biomedical Materials Engineering Sciences
Alfred University
Alfred, New York

Pam Kasyan-Itzkowitz, MS, OTR/L, CHT
Assistant Professor of Occupational Therapy
Nova Southeastern University
Ft. Lauderdale, Florida

Anne Marie Kelly, RN, BC, BSN
Pain Management Educator and Consultant
Catholic Memorial Home
Fall River, Massachusetts

Nancy Kishino, OTR, CBE
West Coast Spine Restoration Center
Riverside, California

**Barbara L. Kornblau, JD, OT/L, FAOTA, DAAPM,
  CCM, CDMS**
Professor, Occupational Therapy
Nova Southeastern University
Ft. Lauderdale, Florida
and
Private Practice
Miami, Florida

Pamela F. Kozey, CMTPT, BEd
Private Practice
Rehoboth Beach, Deleware

Grace M. Kuo, PharmD
Assistant Professor
Department of Family and Community Medicine
Baylor College of Medicine
and
Program Director, Southern Primary-Care Urban
  Research Network
and
President, Consultant Pharmacist of Med Info Service,
  Inc.
Houston, Texas

Sean R. Lacey, MD
Assistant Professor
Division of Gastroenterology
Case Western Reserve University and University Hospitals
  of Cleveland
Cleveland, Ohio

James S. Lapcevic, DO, PhD, JD, FCLM
Private Practice
Harmony Medical Center
Black Lick, Pennsylvania

W David Leak, MD
President, PainNet Inc.
Columbus, Ohio

Bruce Y. Lee, MD
Physician–Scientist Fellow
University of Pennsylvania Health System
Philadelphia, Pennsylvania

Eun-Jeong Lee, MA, Doctoral Student
Department of Rehabilitation Psychology and Special
  Education
University of Wisconsin
Madison, Wisconsin

Gloria K. Lee, PhD
Assistant Professor of Rehabilitation Counseling
Department of Counseling, School and Educational
  Psychology
State University of New York at Buffalo
Buffalo, New York

Raphael C. Lee, MD, ScD, PhD, FACS
Electrical Trauma Research Program
Departments of Surgery, Medicine and Anatomy
University of Chicago
Chicago, Illinois

Raphael J. Leo, MD, FAPM
Assistant Professor
Department of Psychiatry
State University of New York at Buffalo
Erie County Medical Center
Buffalo, New York

Felix S. Linetsky, MD
Assistant Professor
Department of Anesthesiology
University of South Florida
Tampa, Florida
and
Clinical Associate Professor
Department of Osteopathic Principles
Nova Southeastern College of Osteopathic Medicine
and
Private Practice
Orthopaedic Medicine and Pain Treatment
Palm Harbor, Florida

Ross E. Lipton, MD
Director
Electrophysiology Laboratory
Avicenna Spine & Joint Institute
Salt Lake City, Utah

Michael Loes, MD
Director
Arizona Pain Institute
Phoenix, Arizona

David R. Longmire, MD
Clinical Assistant Professor,
Department of Internal Medicine
University of Alabama School of Medicine–Huntsville
  Program
Huntsville, Alabama

Leland Lou, MD
The Eugene McDermott Center for Pain Management
The University of Texas Southwestern Medical Center
  at Dallas
Dallas, Texas

Laxmaiah Manchikanti, MD
Medical Director
Pain Management Center of Paducah
Paducah, Kentucky

Rick Marinelli, ND MAcOM
Private Practice,
Natural Medicine Clinic
Portland, Oregon

Lynne Matallana
Director, National Fibromyalgia Association
Orange, California

Richard S. Materson, MD
Clinical Professor
Physical Medicine and Rehabilitation
University of Texas and Baylor College of Medicine
Houston, Texas

Michael J. McLean, MD
Department of Neurology
Vanderbilt University Medical Center
Nashville, Tennessee

Rafael Miguel, MD
Professor of Anesthesiology
Director of Pain Management Fellowship Program
University of South Florida
Tampa, Florida
and
Chief, Anesthesiology Service
H. Lee Moffit Cancer Center & Research Institute
Tampa, Florida

Michael J. Nelson, DC
Associate Clinician
Pain Assessment and Rehabilitation Center
Minneapolis, Minnesota

Andrew B. Newberg, MD
Professor of Radiology and Psychiatry
University of Pennsylvania Health System
Philadelphia, Pennsylvania

Anh L. Ngo, MD, MBA
Department of Anesthesiology
University Hospitals of Cleveland
Case Western Reserve University School of Medicine
Cleveland, Ohio

Siegfried Othmer, PhD
The EEG Institute of the Brain
Othmer Foundation
Woodland Hills, California

Susan Othmer, BA, BCIAC
The EEG Institute of the Brain
Othmer Foundation
Woodland Hills, California

John Peppin, DO, FACP
Private Practice
Iowa Pain Management Clinic
Des Moines, Iowa

Bruce A. Piszel, MD
Assistant Professor in Anesthesiology and Physical
  Medicine and Rehabilitation
Department of Anesthesiology
University Hospitals of Cleveland and Case Western
  Reserve University School of Medicine,
Cleveland, Ohio

Maurice Policar, MD
Assistant Professor
Elmhurst Hospital Center
Mt. Sinai School of Medicine
New York, New York

Andrea J. Rapkin, MD
Professor
Department of Obstetrics and Gynecology
David Geffen School of Medicine at UCLA
University of California–Los Angeles
Los Angeles, California

Margie Rodriguez LeSage, LMSW, PhD
Assistant Professor
School of Social Work
Michigan State University
East Lansing, Michigan

Katherine E. Rojahn, MD
Electrical Trauma Research Program
Departments of Surgery, Medicine and Anatomy
University of Chicago
Chicago, Illinois

Thomas Romano, MD, PhD
Private Practice
Martins Ferry, Ohio

Ethan Russo, MD
Missoula, Montana

Lloyd Saberski, MD
Department of Medicine, Yale-New Haven Hospital
Advanced Diagnostic Pain Treatment Centers
Yale-New Haven Health at Long Wharf
New Haven, Connecticut

Hossein Sadeghi-Nejad, MD
Associate Professor of Urology
UMDNJ New Jersey Medical School
and
Chief of Urology
NJ Veterans Affairs Hospitals
and
Director
Center for Male Reproductive Medicine
Hackensack University Medical Center
Hackensack, New Jersey

Subrata Saha, PhD
Professor of Biomaterials, Biomedical Materials
  Engineering Sciences
Alfred University
Alfred, New York

Michael E. Schatman, PhD
Pinnacle Health Rehab Options
Harrisburg, Pennsylvania

David Schultz, MD
Medical Director
Medical Advanced Pain Specialists
Minneapolis, Minnesota

Allan D. Seftel, MD
Associate Professor of Urology and Reproductive Biology
Department of Urology
Case Western Reserve University and University Hospitals
  of Cleveland
Cleveland VA Medical Center
Cleveland, Ohio

Gabriel E. Sella, MD, MPH, MSc, PhD (HC)
Private Practice
Ohio Valley Disability Institute
Martins Ferry, Ohio

Nancy Shaw, CMTPT, MS
Myofascial Pain Treatment Center
Springfield, Virginia

Vijay Singh, MD
Medical Director
Pain Diagnostics Associates
Niagara, Wisconsin

Steven Siwek, MD
Medical Director
The Pain Center of Arizona
Phoenix, Arizona

Michael Stanton-Hicks, MD
Vice Chairman, Division of Anesthesia
Professor
Cleveland Clinic Lerner College of Medicine at CWRU
Department of Pain Management
Cleveland, Ohio

Milan P. Stojanovic, MD
Director
Interventional Pain Program
Massachusetts General Hospital
Boston, Massachusetts
and
Assistant Professor in Anesthesia
Harvard Medical School
Cambridge, Massachusetts

Robert B. Supernaw, PharmD
Professor and Dean
Wingate University School of Pharmacy
Wingate, North Carolina

Myrna C. Tashner, EdD
State of Iowa, DDSB
Unity Center of Dynamic Living
Urbandale, Iowa

Andrea M. Trescot, MD
Medical Director
The Pain Center
Orange Park, Florida

Dana Ullman, MPH
Director
Homeopathic Educational Services
Berkeley, California

Clayton A. Varga, MD
Clinical Assistant Professor of Medicine
UCLA School of Medicine
Los Angeles, California
and
Pasadena Rehabilitation Institute
Pasadena, California

Bradley D. Vilims, MD
Private Practice
Interventional Pain Physician
Colorado Pain Specialist
Greenwood Village, Colorado

Gary A. Walco, PhD
Professor of Pediatrics
University of Medicine and Dentistry of New Jersey,
New Jersey Medical School
and
Director
The David Center for Children's Pain and Palliative Care
Hackensack University Medical Center
Hackensack, New Jersey

Steven D. Waldman, MD, JD
Medical Director, The Headache & Pain Center
Clinical Professor of Anesthesiology
University of Missouri–Kansas City School of Medicine
Kansas City, Missouri

Tom Watson, DPT, MEd, PhD, DAAPM
Private Practice
Escondido, California

Charles Wellman, MD
Medical Director
Hospice of the Western Reserve University and Case
  Western Reserve University School of Medicine
Cleveland, Ohio

James E. Williams, OMD, LAc, AP, FAAIM
Private Practice
and
formerly East West College of Natural Medicine
Sarasota, Florida

James W. Woessner, MD, PhD
Private Practice
Honolulu, Hawaii

B. Berthold Wolff, PhD
Professor
New York University School of Medicine
New York, New York
and
Founding president of the American Pain Society

Anthony T. Yeung, MD
Arizona Institute for Minimally Invasive Spine Care
Phoenix, Arizona
and
Voluntary Associate Clinical Professor
University of California San Diego
La Jolla, CA

Christopher A. Yeung, MD
Arizona Institute for Minimally Invasive Spine Care
Phoenix, Arizona
and
Voluntary Clinical Instructor
University of California San Diego
La Jolla, California

Robert W. Young, Jr., PhD
Director of Psychology
Florida Pain & Rehabilitation Institute
Holiday, Florida

Section I

Perspectives of Pain

Mark V. Boswell, MD, PhD, Section Editor

1

A Brief History of Pain from a Personal Perspective

B. Berthold Wolff, PhD

Pain — The Fifth Vital Sign? Pain is a natural phenomenon of all humankind. Yet, until recently, it has been a sadly neglected field of behavior and medicine. In 1958, when I started to study human pain behavior, I was amazed to find how little knowledge of pain and its treatment was available. At that time, most clinicians believed that "real" pain had an underlying physical or physiological basis. Therefore, treating this underlying cause by appropriate therapeutic methods would cure or at least control the basic problem and the patient's pain would be alleviated. Should the patient continue to complain of pain following "successful" treatment, except for malignancies, the patient was often told "it is all in your head" — or worse he would be called a malingerer. Actually, this may still occur occasionally.

In the 1950s, there existed no gate control theory, no real understanding of endogenous morphine-like substances (endorphins), no awareness of differences between acute and chronic (intractable) pain, and there was no generally accepted definition of pain. There also existed no national, international, or regional pain associations.

The ancient philosophers, such as Plato and Aristotle, placed pain together with pleasure among the passions of the soul. In his 1939 review, Dallenbach suggested that Aristotle's great influence on Western scientific thought delayed the recognition of pain as a sensation for almost two thousand years. Eventually, however, the 19th century permitted much research into the neurophysiological basis of pain. In 1884, both Blix and Goldscheider, independently of each other, finally established that pain was a sensation by demonstrating specific pain points in the skin.

In contrast, however, some other physiologists and psychologists believed that pain resulted from "overstimulation" of receptors (Wundt, 1874). Thus, at the end of the 19th century, three different "pain" theories co-existed. The old emotional (pain–pleasure) theory and two neurophysiological theories, the "specificity" theory (i.e., pain-specific receptors/fibers) and the "intensivity" theory (i.e., too much stimulation).

The early 20th century saw a shift toward specificity theory, such as Sherrington (1906), indicating that there are specific nerve endings for pain. Zotterman (1959) observed that in several "classical" experiments during the 1930s pain was apparently subserved by A-delta and C fibers. The faster-conducting A-delta fibers yield sharp and well-localized pain, whereas the slower C fibers yield dull and poorly localized pain sensations. This type of information led Lewis (1942; Lewis & Kellgren, 1939) to postulate the existence of two separate sensory pain systems, one transmitting pain from the skin and the other from deeper and visceral tissues. However, subsequent work by others, especially that of the Oxford group of anatomists (Weddell, Sinclair, & Feindel, 1948), indicated that the differences observed by Lewis, suggesting a two-pain system, could also be adequately explained in terms of pattern and density of innervation, which differ between skin and deeper tissue. Our own early work in my laboratory (Jarvik & Wolff, 1962; Wolff & Jarvik, 1961) demonstrated that two different pain responses could be elicited from the same tissue locus (gluteus medius muscle) and also tended to refute Lewis's two-pain systems theory. Further work by the Oxford group (Feindel, Weddell, & Sinclair,

1948) suggested that pain sensation may depend upon central analysis of space–time pattern of neural activity.

Eventually, this type of research led to the important gate theory of pain, published by Melzack and Wall in 1965, which revolutionized the field of human pain mechanisms. Simply stated, the gate theory postulated a "gating" mechanism that controlled the feedback of fast-conducting fibers from the central nervous system to advancing slower-conducting fibers either inhibiting or allowing progress through the "gate." Thus, a central nervous system analysis is required allowing both physiological and psychological influences. Four decades have passed since the introduction of the gate theory and like all good science, progress has been made and the theory further modified. However, this chapter is not concerned with current concepts but with a historical background from my personal perspective.

It is relevant at this point to mention an interesting problem. While our knowledge of pain and pain mechanisms has significantly increased during the 20th and early 21st centuries, we still lack a generally accepted definition of pain. A century ago, Sherrington (1906, p. 229) defined pain as "the psychical adjunct of an imperative protective reflex." Nearly all 20th-century pain researchers disagree with his definition, but they have eschewed defining pain themselves (Beecher, 1959). More recently, Merskey and Bogduk (1994) for the International Association for the Study of Pain defined pain as an "unpleasant sensory and emotional experience associated with actual or potential tissue damage or described in terms of such damage" (p. 210). This definition, while passable, is in my opinion not completely adequate. Many years ago, I had the pleasure of personally discussing the problem of an adequate definition of pain with Dr. Harold Merskey and I applaud his courage and persistence in eventually coming up with a definition.

There are several problems. Pain, while almost always unpleasant, is not necessarily so. Occasionally, one pain may serve as a relief for another pain (e.g., counter-irritation). In an experimental study, we have observed that white noise is generally reported as more aversive than pain (Wolff et al, 1976). Another problem is that it is often difficult to communicate pain to others because we may lack appropriate words and may thus resort to analogy. This problem has recently been highlighted in a review by Schott. (2004). Both clinically and in the laboratory, pain tends to be defined operationally, such as withdrawal from a noxious stimulus, the patient or subject saying "pain," marking a point along a line, relaxing tense muscles. However, pain defined in this manner can strictly speaking only refer to the specific situation rather than act as an absolute. Consequently, it is yet premature to define pain in absolute terms.

My own work started in 1958, while I was a member of the New York University Rheumatic Diseases Study Group. Specifically the question was raised whether it is possible to (1) measure a patient's pain level objectively and (2) predict a given patient's ability to tolerate (clinical) pain during physical rehabilitation and postoperative exercises of an operated joint. Obviously, with that background and at that time, the emphasis was on deep somatic arthritic pain rather than on cutaneous or visceral pain. Consequently, I chose to utilize a strictly psychophysical approach to devise a technique and measure the patient's pain response. Pain threshold determinations had been made by earlier investigators, such as von Frey (1897), on the skin, culminating in the "heroic" studies of Hardy, Wolff, and Goodell (1952), who used themselves as guinea pigs to measure pain threshold and pain discrimination with radiant heat on the skin. They developed the Dol scale of pain and introduced the radiant heat dolorimeter. Their work can be regarded as the first major psychophysical study of human pain. However, at that time, less psychophysical information existed for deep somatic tissues.

Kellgren (1937–38, 1938) had published some studies on muscle pain although his work was not strictly as psychophysical as that of Hardy et al. However, Kellgren's studies served as a beginning for our own deep somatic pain research. After experimenting with several different body loci, we chose the gluteus medius muscle as the most suitable site (Wolff et al, 1961). We developed a single-blind psychophysical technique permitting the insertion of 32 hypodermic needles in rosette fashion through eight anesthetized blebs of the overlying skin. The muscle was stimulated at each different needle point with 0.2 ml of sterile iso-, hyper-, or hypotonic saline in randomized fashion and a lower and upper pain threshold was measured (Jarvik & Wolff, 1962; Wolff & Jarvik, 1951). We were able to demonstrate, as briefly mentioned previously, that the same body locus could produce two different pain responses, namely, well-localized, sharp pain intensity of short duration (from hypotonic saline and water) and a diffuse, dull ache after a relatively long interval of onset and long duration. This technique, while of scientific value, is rather cumbersome to be used routinely in a pain center. Therefore, few other studies had been published on human muscle pain until the 1980s (Capra & Ra, 2004).

Numerous studies involving experimentally induced pain in humans have been done during the second half of the 20th and the start of the 21st centuries. Different types of noxious stimuli have been employed, such as electrical, mechanical, thermal, and chemical. In the laboratory, attempts are usually made to have the noxious stimulus simulate clinical pain of some kind or other and then to investigate whatever parameter is relevant to the purpose of the experiment. In the mid-20th century a major stumbling block for experimentally induced pain studies in humans was the criticism that such laboratory pain was artificial and bore no resemblance to "real" (pathological) clinical pain, especially in terms of the emotional/psychological components of clinical pain, which were lacking in the experimental model. Dr. Henry K. Beecher (1959) of Harvard was one of the chief critics of experimental human pain and for years carried on a (published) dispute with the Cornell group of Hardy et al. on the latters' dolorimetric work with humans. At that time, Beecher was an important figure with great influence in the pain arena and clinical pharmacology, who, in my opinion, had a major negative impact on human laboratory pain work. Eventually, Beecher changed his mind and announced that he and Smith et al. (1966) had developed an experimental method — the submaximum effort tourniquet technique — which had validity for clinical pain and could be used to study analgesic agents. Consequently, with Beecher's "blessing," experimental human pain studies became "respectable" again.

In our own work with experimentally induced pain in humans, we focused on several pain response parameters and not only on the pain threshold. In psychophysical terms, the latter is the point at which pain is first reported 50% of the time; i.e., it is really a measure of minimal pain. We applied experimental procedures that also allowed us to collect reports of maximal pain tolerated by the subject — the pain tolerance level. (There is some confusion in the literature about terms such as *pain tolerance*, but we use this term to denote the upper threshold). A third parameter, which we called pain sensitivity range (PSR) is the difference between the pain threshold and the pain tolerance, i.e., pain tolerance – pain threshold = PSR. A fourth response parameter is the just-noticeable-difference between successive levels of stimulus intensity.

Hardy et al.'s Dol scale is based on these just-noticeable differences. In a number of experimental studies in our laboratory using several different pain-induction techniques, we were able to demonstrate that the pain tolerance is the most sensitive parameter for analgesic assays with both mild and potent drugs, such as aspirin and morphine; i.e., it is a valid tool (Wolff et al, 1969). Some investigators have used yet another response parameter, namely, the drug request point, i.e., the stimulus intensity level at which the subjects would have requested a pain killer, had it been clinical pain. Single dose, as well as cross-over designs, have been used in these experimental studies. While the latter are statistically more powerful than single-dose designs, they suffer from an interaction effect, such as order of presentation or expectancy. In recent years, experimental pain in humans has been used less frequently for drug (analgesic) studies but animal models are still widely used.

The important contribution of Dr. W. Crawford Clark (1969) should be mentioned at this point, as he was the first to introduce signal detection theory or sensory decision theory (SDT) to the field of human pain studies in 1969. Clark's approach originally was based on Swets's work (1961) who publicized SDT in 1961. SDT was devel-

oped to detect a weak signal above background noise and essentially challenged the sensory threshold of classical psychophysics. In turn, Clark criticized the classical pain threshold as being contaminated by both sensory and judgmental components, while SDT permits separation. SDT caused considerable excitement among many pain researchers resulting in numerous publications, both pro and con. I reviewed this area (Wolff, 1978) discussing classical as well as "new" psychophysical parameters.

In human pain studies, both clinical and experimental, differences in pain behavior have been observed between and within various groups. Frequently, observed differences have been ascribed to ethnic differences, Afro-American, Irish, Scandinavian, Jewish, etc. Unfortunately, such "ethnic" differences have implied "racial" (a dirty word) or "genetic" differences for some authors and are eschewed politically. A good and brief review has been published by Morris (2001) in which he questions the scientific validity of so-called ethnicity. Many years before this publication, I also was interested in ethnocultural factors of pain and published a review with an anthropologist (Wolff & Langley, 1968). On the basis of our own studies, as well as those of several other investigators, it is my belief that pain behavior and pain responses are largely learned responses, molded by many variables, especially sociocultural, and that so-called "ethnic" differences simply reflect such learned behavior. Consequently, it is possible to modify such response under appropriate conditions (Horland & Wolff, 1973). This is not to deny that physiological and genetic differences may exist, but more evidence is required. Within homogeneous groups, age and gender differences are often observed, but again how much is learned and how much (if any) is genetic? We have also noted apparent lateral dominance differences in the same individual. The nondominant side appears to be more sensitive to noxious stimuli than the dominant side, but the latter is more discriminative (Wolff et al., 1965).

In recent decades ethical considerations have played an increasingly important role in experimental and clinical pain studies — both human and animal. Strict standards have been set by both institutional and governmental bodies to guard the rights of animal and human subjects, and funded investigations require approval from various "independent" and "impartial" committees. This is most laudable in spite of greater "red tape." In the "old" days, many investigators paid little heed for the suffering of conscious animals being experimented upon. Now, the animal must be able to escape (avoid, terminate) the noxious stimulus. In laboratory human pain studies, it was considered appropriate for the experimenter to be his or her own first guinea pig, such as Hardy et al. in their radiant heat work, previously mentioned. In my personal experience, I was my first guinea pig when we tested various muscles for the hypertonic saline method. I well remember hobbling around for a few days after we used the gastrocnemius muscle and obviously decided against this muscle. The ethical problem in general is that the experimenter is not the best judge of noxious procedures to be "inflicted" on human volunteers. Historically, the famous Dahlem Konferenzen sponsored a symposium on "Pain and Society" in November 1979 in Berlin to which I was privileged to be invited and selected to be the rapporteur of a small group of other invited pain mavens, including Drs. Ronald Melzack, Hans Kosterlitz, Sir Michael Bond, Kenneth Craig, Giancarlo Carli, Jane Dum, Hartmund Brinkhus, and Wei-ming Tu. In terms of ethics, our group recommended that the Golden Rule, which states, "Therefore all things whatsoever ye would that man should do to you, do ye even so to them," should be amended to "Do not do unto others what you would not have done to yourself, and do not do unto others what they would not have done unto themselves" (Wolff et al, 1980). It is only 25 years ago that such a statement had to be made, which may surprise many current pain specialists. Another major ethical problem in clinical studies is the use of placebo when there is pathology. A "good" experimental study with a new or untested treatment, e.g., an analgesic drug, should be double-blind and include placebo. Yet, if the experimental modality is therapeutically effective, what ethical right is there not to use it with the placebo group?

Historically, two animal techniques for measuring pain have been standard procedures in analgesic assays, namely, the Eddy hot plate method and the radiant heat tail flick method. In the former, the pain response is measured when the mouse lifts its hind paw and in the latter when the rat flicks its tail. In human experimental pain studies both verbal and nonverbal (e.g., withdrawal) responses are used. What about clinical pain? Obviously, both verbal (e.g., "I am in pain," "Ouch!") and nonverbal (e.g., wincing, rubbing, tensing) responses have been observed and are in daily use by the practitioner. However, for human analgesic studies, two methods have become standard, namely, a numerical rating scale (NRS) or the visual analogue scale (VAS). The former requires the patient to state his or her pain level along a numerical scale, usually from 5 to 10 points. Incidentally, many investigators consider a larger scale (e.g., 10 points) to be more accurate and discriminative than shorter ones. However, scaling has several inherent errors well known to psychophysicists, such as clustering, and therefore, a shorter (say, 5 points) scale may often be more valid because it is easier for the patient to do the ratings. The VAS has become very popular. I remember its being introduced into the field of human pain by Dr. E. C. Huskisson in 1974. It consists of a straight line, generally horizontal and 10 cm in length. One end represents no pain and the other the most extreme pain. The patient is requested to mark a point along the line to represent his or her pain level. An unmarked rather than a graded line tends to be more valid for human analgesic assays. There are many other measures of human pain, such as questionnaires, among which the McGill pain questionnaire is probably the best known.

The discovery of morphine-like opiates in the brain in the 1970s was another major advance in the second half of the 20th century. Endorphins, as these endogenous opiates were named, have been studied extensively since that time. A number of investigators in different laboratories across the Western world pursued this line of chemical investigation making it difficult to pinpoint the originator. Many of us in the pain field felt that this work deserved a Nobel prize, but perhaps there were too many researchers. The endorphins are involved in various aspects of analgesia and a variety of receptors have been identified. Pharmaceutical companies have and are studying a variety of potential drugs that may act upon such receptors or modify related chemical processes to produce better analgesics.

The use of opiates, such as morphine, for clinical pain has been practiced for a long time. They have been used for immediate postoperative acute pain as well as for palliative care in cancer patients. However, morphine or other opiates were not considered suitable for long-term treatment of nonmalignant intractable pain. In the mid-20th century, when I first started to study pain, many physicians were afraid to prescribe adequate doses of morphine for patients for fear they would become addicted. In fact, this fear also permeated the nursing profession and occasionally a nurse would question a doctor's prescription of morphine. In other words, patients were frequently undermedicated as far as opiates were concerned. Yet, the irony is that undermedication can still produce addiction under certain circumstances. Fortunately, in recent years, pain practitioners have attempted to change this medical attitude and insist that if morphine or other opiates are prescribed, it should be done in adequate doses to relieve pain properly.

A newer question relates to the use of opiates for long-term care of nonmalignant chronic pain. Some pain specialists advocate the use of opiates for such patients, claiming good results. However, other practitioners have seriously questioned such an approach. I like to mention aspirin at this point. This non-narcotic, nonsteroidal, anti-inflammatory drug has been around since the late 19th century. It has serious side effects; it can certainly burn holes in tissue because it is an acid and can cause Reye's syndrome in children. Yet, in spite of that, aspirin is an effective analgesic for many pain conditions. Acetaminophen is now used more frequently and tends to replace aspirin in pain management.

Historically, it is worth mentioning amitriptyline, a tricyclic antidepressant, which has been used by psychiatrists for a very long time to treat depression. In the 1960s and 1970s, several clinicians experimented with various psychotropic drugs including amitriptyline to control pain.

Amitriptyline in low doses appeared to have analgesic effects. Originally, many psychiatrists criticized pain physicians for using such low doses for pain management, well below the generally recommended doses for depression. In fact, I know some psychiatrists who refered to such low doses as producing nothing else but a placebo effect. It took several years for the analgesic effect of amitriptyline to be "officially" recognized, although many clinicians still prescribe the higher psychiatric doses rather than the lower analgesic doses. Other tricyclics for pain relief have also been studied and are used frequently. The American Pain Society publishes a short guide on "Principles of Analgesic Use in the Treatment of Acute Pain and Cancer Pain," at the time of writing already in its fifth edition, which is very useful for the practicing clinician.

I indicated at the beginning of this chapter that in the mid-20th century, we lacked knowledge in several areas. As stated before, at the time, pain was generally regarded as what we now call acute. Dr. John J. Bonica was one of the first to stress that acute and chronic pain must be differentiated. He termed chronic pain as a malefic state and said that it makes no sense to talk about "benign" chronic pain to separate it from cancer pain. While it may now seem obvious to classify pain into three major groups, namely, acute, cancer (or malignant), and chronic (or intractable) nonmalignant, it is Bonica who must be credited for promoting such distinctions. Many pain mavens call Bonica the "father of chronic pain," although I am not sure if he really would have liked that title. Recent and current research on pain based on neurophysiological and chemical investigations has demonstrated the plasticity of the brain and neural circuits involved in pain behavior. However, the above classification still has practical value.

I have always stressed the importance of communication both within and between professions for clinical practice and research. Initially, I worked in the field of arthritis and rheumatology and learned about the important contributions of nurses, physical therapists, orthopedic surgeons, and other health professionals in addition, of course, to the rheumatologists. In 1965, I was privileged to become a charter member and later president of the now-called Association of Rheumatology Health Professionals, joining forces with the rheumatologists in the American College of Rheumatology. As the name implies, the association brings together professionals from many fields working in arthritis and the rheumatic diseases. I considered this to be a good example for pain professionals. In 1964, just before the creation of the Association of Rheumatology Health Professionals, my colleague Dr. Thomas Kantor and I invited several pain "specialists" of whom we knew and who worked within a radius of about 100 miles from New York City to come to monthly luncheon sessions at New York University School of Medicine in order to network. We thus formed the New York Pain Group. It was disappointing, however, that only about 30

individuals, who were actively engaged in pain management and research, participated. Therefore, after 4 years of seeing each other, we stopped these meetings. It must be noted that at that time in the 1960s, there was still little interest in pain and the above group essentially comprised all then-active pain investigators in the greater New York City area. It was also a really interdisciplinary group with neurosurgeons, nurses, psychologists, physiatrists, rheumatologists, neurologists, statisticians, and others.

It was with great interest that I learned in 1973, that Dr. Bonica had invited many pain investigators to a meeting in Issaquah, Seattle, which eventually led to the formation of the International Association for the Study of Pain (IASP). This was indeed a very courageous and highly significant endeavor by Bonica to bring together pain clinicians and researchers from all across the world to exchange knowledge and communicate with each other. The first International Congress of IASP was held in Florence, Italy, in 1975 and was highly successful; other congresses are now held every 3 years in different countries. The IASP also publishes a journal, *Pain*, originally under the editorship of Dr. Patrick Wall, which has become the most influential scientific journal in the field of pain.

Stimulated by Bonica's success in forming an international pain organization, I decided to review what had originally been the New York Pain Group, especially after receiving enthusiastic support from many colleagues in the greater New York City area. Therefore, in 1974, I started the New York Pain Society, which almost immediately became the New England Pain Association following strong urging from Bonica. Rapidly thereafter, we enlarged to become the North-Eastern Pain Association and, as such, supported the IASP as one of its first chapters. Concurrently, the West Coast pain scientists formed the Western Pain Association and also joined the IASP as a chapter. In view of the steadily increasing interest in pain across the United States, both American societies enlarged, the Western including states west of the Rockies while the Eastern included states east of the Rockies. The latter again changed its formal name to Eastern Pain Association and has been functioning as such ever since.

In view of the rapidly rising interest in pain, I continued to feel that we should have a national pain organization in the United States in addition to the regional societies, a view shared by many of my Eastern colleagues. We considered it important that we have support for such a national U.S. organization from our Western U.S. colleagues as well as from the IASP. In 1975, during the First International IASP Congress, Dr. Pierre L. LeRoy and I discussed this issue with Dr. Bonica. The latter was concerned that an American pain organization might overshadow the IASP both financially and numerically and recommended that we wait some time until the IASP became a stronger organization. However, the success of the IASP, as well as the need to have a national society that could represent pain scientists nationally rather than regionally, encouraged me to form a national U.S. pain organization. Therefore, I started informal discussions with Dr. Bonica, mainly by telephone, and we had Dr. Arthur F. Battista and Dr. B. Raymond Fink negotiate on our behalf — successfully. Thus, with Dr. Bonica's support, a national society could be started in the United States. In 1977, a meeting was arranged in Chicago to which Dr. Bonica and I invited 12 participants each, representing various interests. This meeting successfully supported the idea of a national organization and the American Association for the Study of Pain, shortly thereafter changed to the American Pain Society (APS), was formed, and I was elected as its first president. The Eastern and Western groups became chapters of the APS, which now has several regional chapters.

The APS has steadily grown and is representative of U.S. pain clinicians and researchers. The APS is truly multidisciplinary and includes all professions involved with pain. In view of its multidisciplinary structure, I decided that it could not have "trade union" functions but had to be predominantly scientific and educational. However, some physicians felt pain medicine had become important and that there should be a new specialty (or subspecialty) and eventually this led to the formation of the American Academy of Pain Medicine (AAPM). Fortunately, this did not pose a threat to the aims and goals of the APS. Furthermore, other professions can have pain specialists with their own guidelines within their profession. There always has been and still is concern that the APS is too scientific and research oriented and fails to cater to the practicing clinician while at the same time basic scientists often complain that the APS is too clinical. It is difficult to satisfy both views.

Because the APS gives no certificates or diplomas for proficiency in pain control, Dr. Richard Weiner years ago decided that there should be an organization to do so. Dr. Weiner had discussions with APS Board Members, including myself, and realized that this could not be a function for the APS. He thus formed the American Academy of Pain Management — the other AAPM — which focuses on the practicing health professional, provides education, and awards credentials of proficiency. It has now become one of the major pain organizations in the United States.

In this chapter, I have rambled along various historical paths often associated with my own functions and role. It is thus a little autobiographical although I hope not too boring. Detailed histories of pain may be found in other publications. Here I have cursorily reviewed the historical background leading up to the Melzack and Wall gate theory of pain and focused on the mid- and second half of the 20th century. In my opinion, the gate theory and the discovery and role of endorphins were the two most significant scientific contributions to pain in the latter half of the 20th century. Clinically, the realization that pain is a specialty of its own and requires a multidisciplinary as well as multimodel approach should be regarded as another significant contribution. Associated with both the clinical and scientific contributions has been the much greater interest in pain, its mechanism, and management. Better communication and networking, largely due to the formations of regional, national, and international pain societies followed by the publications of several pain-oriented journals, have also contributed to our constantly increasing better understanding of pain — now often regarded as the Fifth Vital Sign.

REFERENCES

Beecher, H. K. (1959). *Measurement of subjective responses: Quantitative effects of drugs*. New York: Oxford University Press.

Blix, M. (1884). Experimentelle Beiträge zur Lösung der Frage über die Speifische Energie der Hautherven. *Zeitschrift für Biologie, 20,* 141.

Capra, N., & Ro, J. Y. (2004). Human and animal experimental models of acute and chronic muscle pain: Intramuscular analgesic injections. *Pain, 110,* 3.

Clark, W. C. (1969). Sensory-decision theory analysis of the placebo effect on the criterion for pain and thermal sensitivity (d'). *Journal of Abnormal Psychology, 74,* 363.

Dallenbach, K. N. (1939). Pain: History and present status. *American Journal of Psychology, 52,* 331.

Feindel, W. H., Weddell, G., & Sinclair, D. C. (1948). Pain sensibility in deep somatic structures. *Journal of Neurology, Neurosurgery, and Psychiatry, 11,* 113.

Goldscheider, A. (1884). Die Specifische Energie der Gefühlsnerven der Haut, *Monatsschrift für Prakt. Darmat., 31,* 283.

Hardy, J. D., Wolff, H. G., & Goodell, H. (1952). *Pain sensations and reactions*. Baltimore: Williams & Wilkins.

Horland, A. A., & Wolff, B.B. (1973). Effect of suggestion upon experimental pain. *Journal of Abnormal Psychology, 81,* 39.

Huskisson, E. C. (1974). Measurement of pain. *Lancet, 21,* 127.

Jarvik, M. E., & Wolff, B. B. (1962). Differences between deep pain responses to hypertonic and hypotonic saline solutions. *Journal of Applied Physiology, 17,* 841.

Kellgren, J. H. (1937–38). Observations on referred pain arising from muscle. *Clinical Science, 3,* 175.

Kellgren, J. H. (1938). A preliminary account of referred pain arising from muscle, *British Medical Journal, 1,* 325.

Lewis, T. (1942). *Pain*. New York: Macmillan.

Lewis, T., & Kellgren, J. H. (1939). Observations relating to referred pain, visceromotor reflexes and other associated phenomena. *Clinical Science, 4,* 47.

Melzack, R., & Wall, P. D. (1965). Pain mechanisms: A new theory. *Science, 150,* 971.

Merskey, H., & Bogduk, N. (1994). *Classification of chronic pain: Description of chronic pain syndromes and definitions of pain terms* (2nd ed.). Seattle: IASP Press.

Morris, D. B. (2001). Ethnicity and pain. *Pain — Clinical Updates, International Association for the Study of Pain, 9,* 1.

Schott, G. D. (2004). Communicating the experience of pain: The role of analogy. *Pain, 108,* 209.

Sherrington, C. (1906). *The integrative action of the nervous system.* Cambridge: Cambridge University Press (Reprint 1948).

Smith, G. M. et al. (1966). An experimental pain method sensitive to morphine in man. The submaximum effort tourniquet technique. *Journal of Pharmacology and Experimental Therapeutics, 154,* 324.

Swets, J. A. (1961). Is there a sensory threshold? *Science, 134,* 168.

von Frey, M. (1897). Untersuchungen Über dis Sinnesfunctionen der menschlichen Haut: Druckempfindung und Schmerz. *Abhandlungen Gesammelten Wissenschaften, 40,* 175.

Weddell, G., Sinclair, D. C., & Feindel, W. H. (1948). An anatomical basis for alterations in quality of pain sensitivity. *Journal of Neurophysiology, 11,* 99.

Wolff, B. B. (1978). Behavioral measurement of human pain. In R. A. Sternback (Ed.). *The psychology of pain* (p. 129). New York: Raven Press.

Wolff, B. B. et al. (1961). Quantitative measures of deep somatic pain: preliminary study with hypertonic saline. *Clinical Science, 20,* 345.

Wolff, B. B. et al. (1969). Response of experimental pain to analgesic drugs: III. Codeine, aspirin, amobarbital and placebo. *Clinical Pharmacology and Therapeutics, 10,* 217.

Wolff, B. B. et al. (1980). Evolution of expression of pain (acute and chronic): Group report. In H. W. Kosterilitz, & L. Y. Terenius (Eds.). *Pain and society* (p. 81). Weinheim: Dahlem Konferenzen, Verlag Chemie.

Wolff, B. B., & Jarvik, M. E. (1961) A quantitative measure of deep somatic pain. *Arthritis & Rheumatism, 4,* 126 (abstract).

Wolff, B. B., & Langley, S. (1968). Cultural factors and the response to pain: A review. *American Anthropologist, 70,* 494.

Wolff, B. B., Cohen, P., & Greene, C. T. (1976). Behavioral mechanisms of human pain: Effects of expectancy, magnitude and type of cross-model stimulation. In J. J. Bonica, & D. Albe-Fessard (Eds.). *Advances in pain research and therapy* (Vol. 1, p. 327). New York: Raven Press.

Wolff, B. B., Krasnegor, N. A., & Farr, R. S. (1965). Effect of suggestion upon experimental pain response parameters. *Perceptual and Motor Skills, 21,* 675.

Wundt, W. (1874). *Grundzüge der Physiologischen Psychologie.* Leipzig: W. Engelmann.

Zotterman, Y. (1959). The peripheral nervous mechanism of pain: A brief review. In *Pain and itch: Nervous mechanisms* (p. 15). Boston: Little Brown.

2

Fibromyalgia: Patient Beliefs and Expectations

Lynne Matallana

Yes, when I see a healthcare professional, I am a fibromyalgia "patient," but more importantly I am a human being — a living, breathing, feeling person who must face, on a daily basis, a constellation of distressing symptoms that cause both physical and mental anguish. Like millions of others with fibromyalgia, not only do I have to live with the consequences and challenges that its chronic symptoms cause, I have to live with the fact that there are many people who give no credence to my condition, dismissing my suffering because they don't understand it or don't want to get involved with those of us who are seen as "difficult patients who constantly complain."

Ten years ago I believed that if you became sick, all you had to do was go to a doctor, get a diagnosis, be given the appropriate treatment, and within time (hopefully not a long period of time) you would feel better and your life would return to normal. Yes, a naive concept, but one that had been my experience. We live in a world that possesses more scientific medical knowledge than ever before. We place physicians on pedestals as they transplant hearts, cure cancers, and remove brain tumors. These acts are truly incredible, almost incomprehensible feats of accomplishment. So when only a few days after having had surgery for endometriosis I started to experience a variety of disturbing symptoms, including widespread body pain, unrelenting fatigue, migraine headaches, and the inability to easily organize my thoughts, I felt certain that a visit to my doctor would solve the problems. Instead, it marked the beginning of my passage into a new life. A journey that would mean learning to live well despite chronic pain, one of the most desperate of human conditions, yet one that still in many ways remains challenging and mysterious to the medical community.

Although it took me some time to come to accept the fact that doctors don't possess a magic wand to make pain disappear and that my expectations of their "God-like" ability to cure me was not only unfair but silly, I couldn't accept their conclusion that there was nothing wrong with me and that there was nothing that could be done to help. Was there truly no hope for my future? Although even at times I questioned my sanity, wondering if my pain was "real," I believed that no matter what the cause of my suffering, I deserved to be treated with respect as a human being and that my experience could not and should not just be dismissed because others didn't understand it. My pain didn't fit into their reality, but my pain was very much my constant reality.

When I first became ill scientific *proof* of my condition lagged behind my state of misery, but I believed that *I* shouldn't be seen as a pariah, a nuisance to the medical community and valueless to humanity. However, that is how I felt. I wanted and needed help, so that I could regain my worth and continue to contribute to society. Pain is not new, so how could the medical community not accept my pain as real or help treat it as something that truly existed? Was I naïve to also think that a physician should be *compassionate* to my distress no matter what the illness? Was it simply because the *type* of pain that I experienced did not yet have evidence of organic pathology, unlike pain from a broken limb or a cancerous growth, that made it unworthy of concern? Without empirical evidence, my pain was invisible to everyone except me. And my frustration with the situation made me frantic, and I turned into that "difficult and constantly complaining patient." I hated what I had become. I hated the looks of frustration on the faces of my family and doctors. I felt like the little baby who cries and cries, trying to let others know that there is something wrong, but no one can figure out the reason for the screams. I couldn't imagine a life where I was supposed to just quietly disappear. Like the women of my grandmother's generation whose complaints were dismissed as one of those "middle-age women's things," which left them retreating to their beds for days, weeks, and years at a time. I valued life too much not to fight for a life of quality, despite fibromyalgia. I tried to be understanding of the frustrations that everyone around me was feeling. I felt guilt because *I* had caused them distress and yet angry that they couldn't take away my pain.

I remember as a child the first time I looked through a microscope and a drop of water from a pond turned into a world of small invisible creatures that hadn't existed in my reality a few seconds earlier. Even though my fibromyalgia pain weighed me down with frustration, fear, disillusionment, guilt, and even anger, I wanted to fight the temptation to believe the cluster of preconceived negative assumptions that were attached to *my* illness. I wasn't crazy, I wasn't just stressed, I wasn't lazy, or just a negative person. Why was I supposed to suffer because of other people's ignorance and lack of acceptance? Of course it was easier to just turn away than to try to make sense out of something that didn't fit into the way the medical community *currently* looked at and accepted things. But we *can't* be reluctant to look through the microscope and discover new truths, to recognize that we can't *see* everything easily, so we must take a closer look, refusing to turn a blind eye, especially when it involves a large community of people who are truly suffering.

Unlike most patients with fibromyalgia who do not have the circumstances that allow them the opportunity to keep searching for answers, I had the emotional and financial support that allowed me to continue to seek out help. Although there were times that I began to lose faith, my pain urged me on, a constant reminder that there was no room for self-doubt. My pain was real and it wasn't something that could be ignored. It wasn't just the medical community that had left me feeling stranded and isolated; it was friends, employers, and society who questioned my pain and fatigue. Even the media talked about a *new* illness that was thought to affect people who were "lazy and out of physical condition." What had I done that was deserving of *abandonment and judgment*? I kept telling myself — I did nothing wrong. This was an *illness*, not a punishment. So there had to be answers and there had to be people out there who *did* care. I just had to find them.

Unfortunately, today and even more so ten years ago, knowledgeable physicians on fibromyalgia are rare. Thirty-seven doctors and two years later, I found my compassionate, open-minded, knowledgeable doctor. I came to understand that my quality of life was going to be influenced by our doctor–patient relationship. I realized that it was going to take time to build this relationship and that we both had to make a commitment to working hard and doing our part as *a team*. I couldn't have expectations

that my doctor was going to cure me, and my doctor couldn't expect me to not share my suffering with him. I trusted him to keep me informed of the most recent treatment options available to people with fibromyalgia, and he trusted me to try to keep a positive attitude and to be willing to take his medical advice while making personal life-style changes that would help improve my overall symptoms. We both made a commitment — he to treating and encouraging me to the best of his ability, and I to being a pro-active patient, implementing a multidisciplinary self-management plan, working to achieve both physical and mental balance. Even though much of the "responsibility" did fall on me, the patient, his willingness to diligently keep up with new research findings that led to the implementation of new treatment options encouraged me and resulted in treatments (both pharmacological and alternative) that helped reduce my symptoms.

When asked, most individuals with fibromyalgia express above all else the need to feel "normal" and understood. Living with an "invisible" illness can strip away people's self-confidence and make them feel isolated and alone. All need and feel better when they receive validation, whether it is for what they have accomplished, what they think, or what they feel. When you are told that what you are feeling is not real, it is like being told that *you and your feelings* have no value. We as individuals need our lives to have value, a purpose, without which we feel cast out, alone, and even abnormal. Pain that is not validated causes one to feel guilt, fear, and hopelessness, which in turn can even become disillusionment and depression. Referring to fibromyalgia as being a "waste basket" diagnosis alludes to the fact that the diagnosis has no value, again discrediting and belittling the personal experience. It is evident that even before pursuing efforts to reduce their symptoms, people with fibromyalgia can greatly benefit from acts of compassion, acceptance, and the gift of hope.

In pain states that are caused by injury, the treatment protocol is to treat the injury, thereby eliminating the problem that is causing the pain. However, fibromyalgia is a condition of central sensitization and neuroendocrine dysfunction, so the pain experience becomes chronic. For a person living with constant pain it is an ongoing challenge to find ways to achieve a better quality of life. The actions taken and avenues pursued by a person with fibromyalgia are based specifically on the chronic nature and idiosyncrasy of the syndrome. Each individual's personality affects the way in which he or she approaches the problem. With the lack of reliable treatment options, the individual can feel that there is nothing available to help and can become depressed and withdrawn, while others spend hours searching for solutions, becoming overwhelmed with a countless selection of unreliable treatments touted to "cure" or help relieve symptoms. Desperation can sometimes outweigh common sense and one can become compulsive in the attempt to find relief. Those of us who were once independent and self-sufficient can find ourselves needy and desperate for others to concentrate only on our dilemma, at times not even recognizing that our neediness can actually push others away.

In that fibromyalgia is a syndrome of multiple symptoms and overlapping conditions, the extent of the complaints can seem questionable to those on the "outside," and patients often find themselves trying to explain, as well as understand, a myriad of ever-changing ailments. One day you'll be suffering with a burning pain sensation all over your body and the next day you'll experience cognitive dysfunction, dizziness, and anxiety. Then you'll find yourself gaining confidence as things slowly start getting better, and then the next day you'll be experiencing nagging unrelenting pain that seems to come from nowhere. Living in a world where we look at things in relationship to cause and effect, people with fibromyalgia can become disheartened by the inability to find this type of relationship when it comes to their pain and symptoms.

Overanalysis of the situation can lead to nothing but confusion, and therefore, it is important to realize that with our current limited understanding of central sensitization, it is often impossible to predict a cause/effect relationship when it comes to symptoms. In those situations where one can identify a "trigger" for a specific symptom, a small sense of control can emerge, helping one to better self-manage the condition. However, when one expects a certain reaction, for example, spending several days in bed in order to relieve pain and exhaustion, and that result does not occur, the sense of control becomes elusive and the ensuing frustration is not surprising.

It is important to realize that our "cause and effect" expectations are based on our existing experiences and knowledge of the reactions of a healthy body or one with a specific disease or trauma. But in the case of fibromyalgia, we are learning that the problem is "system failure," or in other words, symptoms that are caused by disordered sensory processing at a central level. For a person experiencing "pain amplification," the existing cause-and-effect "rules" do not apply. It is only with additional research that we will be able to assist the person with fibromyalgia by better understanding the cause(s) of this illness. We as patients will experience more control over symptoms when we come to understand the new relationship of cause and effect, which produces fibromyalgia symptoms.

It is at this point that one realizes yet another challenge confronting those of us living with fibromyalgia. Not only must we adapt to living with disruptive, disabling symptoms for which there is often little relief, but we must also live with an illness that produces symptoms that don't "react" like our preconceived expectations. Besides the physical pain that must be endured, this lack of control

and resulting feelings of abnormality cause extreme emotional suffering. Until we understand the cause(s) of the "system breakdown," and we can find ways to correct that problem, patients must find ways to feel a sense of control over their illness through limited existing avenues — usually consisting of options that involve extensive self-motivation and patience. In the past, the focus has been on the patient's learning to accept and live with the pain (and other symptoms) through means of counseling, cognitive behavioral therapy, biofeedback, etc. These are excellent ways to deal with the situation, but they are not solving the actual problem so as to eliminate the symptoms. For years patients have had to learn ways to adapt and adjust to their illness rather than have options that will "fix" them. Today, there are more options available to help people with fibromyalgia cope with their symptoms. But the continuous waxing and waning cycle still robs certain individuals of the freedom to plan daily activities and move forward with their life.

Fibromyalgia obviously affects the patient in numerous ways, but it must be pointed out that fibromyalgia also affects the lives of all who share the patient's life. As with any chronic illness, individuals find themselves in roles that they are not comfortable with or even refuse to accept. Spouses and family members must become caregivers, employers are asked to make work accommodations, physicians are asked to treat patients with exceptional needs, and friends are relied upon to provide support and assistance. When one or more of these people decide that they cannot or will not accept the responsibilities that go along with their new role in their relationship with this person, more emotional trauma ensues. Often fibromyalgia can make a person dependent on others for various aspects of their livelihood. When an individual becomes chronically ill there are people around that person who will not be able to cope and will remove themselves from the situation. In the case of a person who is chronically ill with fibromyalgia, an "invisible illness" that is difficult at best to understand and doesn't have the "credibility" of other chronic illnesses, the chances of disassociation become even greater. Living with fibromyalgia all alone is something that far too many people have to face.

Fibromyalgia is not just a problem that affects a specific group of people. It is a health condition that touches the lives of millions and millions of people every day. The negative implications of this illness are far reaching and must be given the attention necessary to ensure that we will find the answers that will allow us to eliminate the suffering caused by this disorder. Education is the key to providing a future that guarantees hope for those who live with fibromyalgia. As a patient, I can live with an illness that causes pain, but as a person, I can't live with the knowledge that others have dismissed this pain and find it unworthy of their concern and acceptance.

3

The Neuroscience of Pain and Analgesia

James Giordano, PhD

By definition, pain is a noxious sensation that evokes perceptions of dysphoria and illness. The linkage of sensory phenomena with cognitive processes is important to the strong avoidant motor reflexes, autonomic events, and emotional responses that are co-terminal with both the pain experience and its expectation (Cazzullo & Gala, 1987). The scientific perspective has evolved to characterize pain as a heterogeneous entity that may be classified by temporal (i.e., acute, chronic), mechanistic (i.e., nociceptive, inflammatory, neuropathic), and phenomenologic (i.e., eudynia, maldynia) factors. Far from being mutually exclusive, these classifications are both overlapping and interactive and can be useful when elucidating the qualitative, quantitative, and pathologic variables that contribute to a particular clinical pain syndrome (Woolf & Max, 2001). The neural substrates that are involved in processing noxious input contribute to both the sensation and cognitive–emotional phenomena of pain.

NOCICEPTORS

The first step in the nociceptive sensory pathway is the transduction of noxious thermal, mechanical, or chemical stimuli to a relevant neural electrophysiologic signal. In cutaneous, muscle, and visceral tissues, free nerve endings of nocisponsive primary afferents are responsible for this transduction step. Cationic channels on free nerve endings respond to noxious stimuli directly and to evoked changes in the innervated tissues.

Two nonselective cation channels, molecularly similar to vanilloid receptor-1 and vanilloid receptor-like protein 1, are responsive to noxious heat (>45°C) and thermal sensitization (Davis, 2000). A related cation channel, the cold- and menthol-receptor-1 (CMR1/transient receptor potential M8) is responsive to noxious cold (8 to 25°C) and menthol (McKemy, Neuhausser, & Julius, 2002). In both cases, thermal change produces an ungating of the channel(s) to induce cationic flux.

Noxious mechanical input (i.e., compression, shear, tensile distortion) is subserved by a nonspecific cation channel that is gated by mechanical linkage to bridging elements of the free nerve ending membrane and the matrix of surrounding tissue (Mannsfeldt, Carroll, Stucky, & Lewin, 1999). Transduction occurs as these stimuli distort the mechanical field of the neural membrane, transforming channel configuration and producing an inward Na^+, K^+, or Ca^{2+} current. The receptor potential for free nerve endings appears to be a graded response, with time- and intensity-dependence of the membrane polarity. Once the conductance threshold for Na^+ is achieved, activation of voltage-gated Na^+ channels occurs, leading to a propagation of the depolarization along the membrane of the primary nociceptor. As well, the influx of both Na^+ and Ca^{2+} elevates the concentration of intracellular Ca^{2+} that activates a variety of intracellular signaling systems capable of producing short- and long-term changes in neuronal function (and perhaps microstructure; *vide infra*).

In addition to the direct action of noxious stimuli upon nociceptors, high-intensity input may incur local tissue disruption or membrane damage to evoke the release of fatty acids and free ions from cell membranes. The enzyme phospholipase-A2 catalyzes free membrane fatty acids to produce the omega-6, arachidonic acid, that then serves as the initiative substrate for (latent) induction of the isoenzyme cyclooxygenase 2 (COX-2) to induce the inflammatory cascade, subsequently mediated by the for-

TABLE 3.1
Algogenic Substances/Stimuli and Substrates Mediating Effects

Algogenic stimulus	Substrate(s)	Effect(s)
H^+ ion	VR1 receptor	Na^+, Ca^{2+} influx
Protons	Acid-sensitive ion channel (ASIC)	Na^+ influx
Noxious heat >45°C (and capsaicin)	VR1, VRL-1 receptor proteins	Na^+, K^+, Ca^{2+} influx
Noxious cold 8–25°C (and menthol)	CMR1/trpM8	Na^+, K^+, Ca^{2+} influx
Mechanical distortion	Nonselective cation channel	Na^+, K^+, Ca^{2+} influx
BDNF	Trk-B receptor	MAPK activation–transcription effects
Prostaglandin-E_2	Prostanoid receptor	Metabotropic activation of protein kinase
Serotonin	5-HT_3 receptor	Na^+ influx
		NK-1 receptor sensitization
		NO production
Adenosine (or ATP)	A_2 purinoreceptor	Sensitization of Na^+ channels
Glutamate	AMPA receptor	Na^+ influx
	NMDA receptor (GluR)	Ca^{2+} influx
	mGlu receptor	Phospholipase-C-induced rise in intracellular Ca^{2+}
		Protein kinase-C phosphorylation/sensitization of trk-B
Bradykinin	Bradykinin B_2 receptor	Cationic influx

mation of biologically active prostaglandins, most specifically prostaglandin synthase–generated prostaglandin-E2. Prostaglandin-E2 acts upon the free endings of nociceptors to produce a receptor-mediated increase in adenyl cyclase to elevate cyclic adenosine monophosphate (cAMP) and engage specific protein kinases. Protein kinase A and C can phosphorylate membrane proteins to affect the sensitivity of prostanoid, kinin, or amine receptors as well as increase the sensitivity and/or modify the configurational state of ion channels (McClesky & Gold, 1999). Such changes can produce a leftward shift in nociceptor membrane thresholds, which can sensitize the affected primary afferents to subsequent stimulation by increasing the number and frequency of nociceptor depolarizations produced by both noxious stimuli (e.g., contributing to hyperpathic responses) and perhaps innocuous stimuli (i.e., allodynia; Gold, Levine, & Correa, 1998; Ji, Kohno, Moore, & Woolf, 2003). Table 3.1 presents an overview of noxious stimuli and the substrates that transduce their neural activity.

Subsequent to transduction, the nociceptive signal is conducted from free nerve endings in the periphery (or viscera) along the membrane of primary nociceptive afferents via depolarization induced by sodium influx subserved by $Na_v1.8$ and $Na_v1.9$ subtypes of Na^+ channels, that are specific to nociceptor membranes (Amaya et al., 2000). There are two types of primary nociceptive afferents, A-delta and C-fibers. These subtend distinct types of noxious input (e.g., thermal, mechanical, polymodal) and are strongly contributory to the differing subjective sensory qualities of fast (i.e., "first") and

slow (i.e., "second") pain, respectively (Ochoa & Torebjork, 1981).

PRIMARY AFFERENTS

A-Delta Fibers

These fibers are small, thinly myelinated neurons, 1 to 5 μm in diameter, with conduction velocities in the range of 5 to 30 m/s. The rapid rate of conduction is responsible for the initial sensation of pain, "first pain," typically described as sharp, localized, and well defined. A-delta fibers have small receptive fields and are relatively modality specific. This latter quality is a function of specific, high-threshold ion channels on the free endings of A-delta afferents that are differentially activated by distinct high-intensity thermal or mechanical input (Julius & Basbaum, 2001). A-delta thermosponsive fibers respond to extremes of temperature. One population is activated by noxious heat, with an initial response threshold in the range of 40 to 45°C. Response function increases directly, although not necessarily linearly, as a consequence of temperature elevation, with maximal responses occurring at temperatures of 46 to 53°C. These responses subserve both the rapid, demonstrably painful response to an initial presentation of noxious heat and the ability to quickly discriminate extent of thermal pain as a function of heat intensity. A second population, high threshold cold afferents, responds to cold temperatures at or below a threshold of approximately 8°C, with increasing cold sensitivity to temperatures less than 25°C (Price & Dubner, 1977; see Table 3.1).

A-delta mechanoreceptive afferents are activated by high-intensity mechanical stimulation (deep pressure, stab, pinch, stretch), although these fibers may be sensitized by, and become secondarily responsive to, noxious heat. Unlike A-delta thermal afferents, sensitized A-delta mechanoreceptive afferents respond to suprathreshold heat (usually in excess of 50 to 55°C) and/or repetitive presentation of noxious heat, rather to a singular exposure to a heat stimulus at or above the nociceptive threshold (Kumazawa & Perl, 1976). The sensitization of this second population of nociceptive A-delta afferents may contribute to the hyperalgesia observed following heat and mild to moderate burn injury.

C-Fibers

C-fibers are small, unmyelinated afferents with broader receptive fields than A-delta fibers. C-fiber diameters range from 0.25 to 1.5 μm, and the absence of myelin leads to slower conductance velocities that vary from 0.5 to 2 m/s. This slower conductance together with the broad receptor fields subserve clinical "second pain," a diffuse, poorly localized burning, throbbing, or gnawing sensation that follows and that is temporally and qualitatively distinct from the initial sensation of "first pain" (Torebjork, 1974). Numerically, C-fibers constitute the majority of primary nociceptive afferent innervation of cutaneous tissue. C-fibers are polymodal, and can be activated by thermal, mechanical, and chemical stimuli. This latter quality reflects the direct engagement of C-fibers by specific chemicals that perfuse the neuronal microenvironment of C-fiber free endings following cellular disruption. Free H^+ ion (i.e., lowered pH), protons, and adenosine triphosphate (ATP) are all capable of activating C-fibers. H^+ acts by sensitizing the VR1 vanilloid receptor (that is also responsive to noxious heat) and enhancing Na^+ and Ca^{2+} influx (Caterina et al. 1999). Protons stimulate C-fibers by acting at an acid-sensitive ion channel to evoke an inward Na^+ current (Waldman & Lazdunsky, 1998). Adenosine, liberated from ATP by hydrolysis, binds to an A_2 purinoreceptor, to sensitize Na^+ channel excitation (Gold, 1999; see Table 3.1).

In addition to responding to noxious (thermal, mechanical, and chemical) stimuli, C-fiber polymodal afferents may be sensitized by substrates of the inflammatory cascade (e.g., prostaglandin-E2, bradykinin) that are released following thermal or mechanical insult (Gold et al., 1998; Levine & Reichling, 1999). Once sensitized, these C-fibers can be activated by certain types of nonnoxious, low-intensity stimulation. This may account for the persistent second pain and hyperalgesia that occurs following burn injury or other inflammatory states (Rowbotham & Fields, 1996). In this light, C-fibers may contribute to multiple sensations from a painful region.

C-fibers also innervate muscle tissue, localized to the intrafibril matrix, tendons, and areas surrounding the vascular walls (Iggo, 1974). C-fiber muscle afferents are polymodal and are responsible for the nociceptive response to intense mechanical stimulation (Jones, Newham, Obletter, & Giamberardino, 1987) that produces numerous substances as a consequence of both aerobic and anaerobic metabolism. C-fibers innervating muscular tissues are activated by H^+ ions as a constituent of the acidic postmetabolic environment (Mills, Newham, & Edwards, 1982) as well as end products of inflammation due to exercise-induced micro- or macrotraumatic insult (including bradykinin, histamine, and 5-HT; Vecchiet, Giamberardino, & Marini, 1987), mechanical distention of microedema (Newham & Jones, 1985), and heat (Mense, 1977). Although not directly activated by muscular contraction or the stretch reflex, intramuscular C-fibers can be sensitized (under ischemic conditions) to respond to even small myofibril contraction and may respond vigorously to excessive stretch (Vecchiet et al., 1987). It appears that ischemia yields an increased concentration of free adenosine that acts at A_2 purinoreceptors to produce G protein–mediated modulation of Na^+ channel thresholds (Gold, 1999). This sensitization helps to explain the diffusely painful response to both passive and active movement of over-exerted, traumatized, or ischemic skeletal muscle.

Visceral Primary Nociceptive Afferents

Numerous stimuli are capable of producing visceral pain (see Gebhart, 1995, for review). Distention, compression, and chemical and tactile irritation of several visceral structures have all been shown to elicit distinct and quantifiable pain responses in humans (Willis, 1985), that are often accompanied by reports of localized somatic and cutaneous pain. The diversity of response to various types of noxious stimuli suggests the presence of afferents with polymodal qualities. Taken with the diffuse, poorly localized quality that often accompanies visceral pain, such findings implicate the involvement of C-fiber-type innervation (Dubner, 1985; Gebhart, 1995). C-fiber-type afferents innervate several visceral structures, even though studies have also demonstrated presence of A-delta fibers with polymodal sensitivity, particularly in the testes and structures surrounding the heart (Paintal, 1972; Uchida & Murao, 1974). As well, a small, unmyelinated J fiber has been identified in the parenchyma of the lung (Paintal, 1972). J fibers have structural properties, receptive fields, and conductance velocities similar to C-fibers and respond to high-intensity mechanical changes in lung volume (i.e., distention and compression), inflammation, and exogenous chemical irritants (e.g., acidic and basic substances; Coleridge, Coleridge, & Luck, 1965).

TABLE 3.2
Physiologic and Neurochemical Properties of Primary Afferent Nociceptors

Type	Stimulus	Anatomy	Diameter	Conduction/Properties	Chemistry
A-delta fiber	High threshold Mechanical Thermal (>45°C) (<20°C) Mixed-sensitized	Free endings Myelinated Punctate fields	1–5 μm	10–30 m/s Fast; First pain; Well localized	Glutamate Substance-P CGRP (?) VIP Postsynaptic activation of AMPA receptors Short-term NK-1 receptor activation
C-fiber	High threshold Polymodal Thermal Mechanical Chemical	Free endings Unmyelinated Diffuse receptive fields	0.5–1.5 μm	0.5–2 m/s Slow; Second pain; Chronic; Poorly localized; Sensitized	Glutamate Substance-P CGRP Postsynaptic activation of NMDA, Glu receptors Potentiated NK-1 receptor activation May induce neural plasticity

Nociceptive afferent innervation of visceral structures has several characteristics that are markedly distinct from those in cutaneous and muscle tissues. First, nociceptive afferent innervation of the viscera is relatively sparse, with considerable diffusion at projection sites at second-order neurons within the spinal dorsal horn (Cervero & Iggo, 1980). Thus, nociceptive input from the viscera may not evoke strong, well-localized volleys of excitation capable of spatially or temporally summating at spinal relays. Second, the nature of visceral afferents is such that sensitization by chemical mediators and/or sympathetic activity (see below) appears to be required for their sustained firing. Given the sparse distribution of these fibers throughout the viscera and the diffuse connections with nociceptive units of the spinal cord, it appears that this sustained firing is responsible for the activation of second-order spinal afferents and, ultimately, the transmission of visceral nociceptive signals. The perception of visceral nociception is vague, becoming more intense (and better localized) as increased painful activity in the innervated structure(s) sensitizes the involved afferents (Dubner, 1985). Third, nociceptive afferent innervation of the viscera is often structurally co-localized with sympathetic afferent (and perhaps efferent) neurons. Noxious stimulation from the viscera can lead to concurrent excitation of both visceral nociceptive afferents and sympathetic innervation, capable of producing retrograde sympathetic outflow and sympathetically maintained regional hyperalgesia and altered autonomic tone. However, such sympathetic alterations are not exclusive to visceral pain; sympathetic effects are strongly contributory to the constellation of nociceptive, vasomotor, and sudomotor features of complex regional pain syndromes (CRPS) that can affect somatic innervation, as well. In such cases, excessive stimulation of sympathetic axons or endings (either by ephaptic transmission from adjacent nociceptive afferents or directly by peripheral tissue insult) can induce increased synthesis of high-affinity adrenoceptors, thereby perpetuating the cycle of peripheral adrenergic sensitivity, sympathetically-maintained pain, and alterations in peripheral autonomic regulation (Campbell, Meyer, & Raja, 1992, for an overview). Last, visceral nociceptive afferents are often anatomically integrated with somato-cutaneous nociceptive afferents within dorsal root ganglia or within the aggregate of primary afferent synaptic fields at second-order afferents of the spinal cord (Willis, 1985). Reciprocal sensitization within the dorsal root ganglion and the overlap of second-order receptive fields for both visceral and somato-cutaneous input subserve the somatic referred component that is characteristic of much of visceral pain. It is clinically relevant to understand the convergence of visceral and somato-cutaneous afferents when attempting to predict involvement of visceral structures in patterns of referred somatic pain.

PROJECTIONS TO THE SPINAL DORSAL HORN

Although a small number of nociceptive afferents synapse within the ventral spinal cord, the vast majority of somato-cutaneous and visceral nociceptive primary afferent fibers project to defined areas of the superficial dorsal horn (Gobel, 1976). This area has been anatomically distinguished into discrete zones, the laminae of Rexed. The laminae are numbered consecutively from dorsal to ventral regions (Rexed, 1952). Both A-delta and C-fibers terminate on specific populations of second-order spinal neurons in laminae I, II, IIa, and V that are the origin of the ascending spinal pathways critical to pain transmission. Specifically, A-delta fibers terminate in laminae I, II, and to a lesser extent, IIa (Gobel, 1976), while C-fibers project to laminae II, IIa, and V (Torebjork, 1974). The anatomic, physiologic, and neurochemical properties of primary nociceptive afferents are presented in Table 3.2.

Neurochemistry of Primary Afferent Pain Transmission

The principal neurochemical mediator at the synaptic cleft between primary afferent nociceptors and dorsal horn cells is glutamate. Postsynaptically, glutamate is capable of binding to two types of discrete receptors (Woolf, 2004). The first, the AMPA (alpha-amino-3-hydroxy-5-methyl-isoxazole-4 propionic acid) receptor, appears to be the initial or first molecular target for glutamate binding. Glutamate-induced AMPA receptor activation evokes a ligand-gated sodium current in postsynaptic second-order neurons of the dorsal horn that produces a rapid depolarization. AMPA receptor-mediated depolarization modulates glutamate-induced activation of the second class of receptor, the N-methyl-D-aspartate (NMDA) receptor, by allosteric modulation of magnesium binding to a shared or cooperative domain of the NMDA receptors. With persistent AMPA receptor activation, the rise in intracellular sodium displaces a magnesium "gate" from the NMDA receptor, thereby increasing its sensitivity or releasing it from an inaccessible configuration to actively bind glutamate (Woolf & Salter, 2000).

There are two types of NMDA receptor: a fast-on, slow-off, ionotropic, Ca^{2+} channel site (GluR) that subserves a durable calcium influx and a metabotropic, G protein–coupled receptor (mGluR). Of the eight identified mGluR sites, three are positively coupled to phospholipase-C (PLC). In nociceptive neurons, one type of mGluR engages PLC to induce inositol triphosphate (IP3) to release calcium from intracellular stores. These effects elevate the level of intracellular calcium; this activates a Ca^{2+}-sensitive protein kinase-C (PKC) to phosphorylate serine and threonine residues in the submembrane pool of NMDA and AMPA receptors, thereby inducing post-translational changes that subsequently increase the number and sensitivity of these receptors (Luo et al., 2001; South et al., 2003). Metabotropic glutamate receptors can also act through intracellular diacylglycerol (DAG) to activate PKC to phosphorylate the tyrosine kinase-B (trkB) receptor for brain-derived neurotrophic factor (BDNF; Kerr et al., 1999). BDNF, a secretory protein, is produced and released by primary nociceptive afferents (McMahon & Bennett, 1999). The action of BDNF at postsynaptic trk-receptors initiates mitogen-activated protein kinase (MAPK) capable of affecting gene transcription (Friedman & Greene, 1999).

Taken together, these glutamate-dependent reactions may be responsible for the sensitization of second-order afferents to input from nociceptors. There is further evidence to suggest that prolonged activation of newly synthesized NMDA receptors may instigate PKC-mediated activation of transcription factors to affect genomic elements to facilitate ongoing alteration of cell membrane components (e.g., sensitized ion channels, additional upregulated receptors) and produce durable changes in second-order nociceptive afferent function (Stubhaug, Breivik, Eide, Kreunen, & Foss, 1997).

While brief, suprathreshold primary nociceptor activity causes the release of glutamate, prolonged and/or intense C-fiber activation induces the release of the undecapeptide tachykinin, substance-P (Cao et al., 1998). Initially, substance-P binds postsynaptically to neurokinin-2 (NK-2) receptors on second-order dorsal horn neurons. However, with more prolonged excitation, substance-P also binds to NK-1 receptors to activate G protein–mediated, metabotropic, slow onset, durable shifts in membrane potential (Woolf, 2004). The continued activation of NK-1 receptors induces DAG-dependent activation of protein kinase (A and C) to phosphorylate NMDA receptors, leading to enhanced intracellular calcium levels (Thompson, Dray, & Urban, 1994). Latent (i.e., 30 to 60 min) calcium-mediated phosphorylation of transcription elements stimulates production of the early-phase proto-oncogenes, *c-fos, c-jun,* and *Krox-24* (Jin et al., 2003; Lanteri-Minet, Isnardon, de Pommery, & Menetreu, 1993). The induction of these proto-oncogenes produces protein products that both act as metabolic regulatory units and produce late-gene effects that may be responsible for transcribing and translating novel (and perhaps aberrant) proteins involved in functional and microstructural remodeling of second-order neurons that are actively processing chronic pain (Jin, Zhuang, Woolf, & Ji, 2003). According to Doubell, Mannior, & Woolf (1999) such remodeling characteristically results in a reduced firing threshold, increases in durability and frequency of response, expansion of the functional postsynaptic region (i.e., the receptive field), and a suppression of inhibitory potentials (subserved by both downregulation of receptors for inhibitory transmitters and a loss of inhibitory synapses). These processes are similar to long-term potentiative (LTP) and depressive (LTD) mechanisms, respectively, and it is likely that they play a role in central sensitization and directly contribute to neuropathic pain syndromes (Ji et al., 2003; Randic, Jiang, & Cerne, 1993).

Additionally, sensitized primary afferents are capable of antidromic or retrograde release of neurochemical mediators of the inflammatory response (Fitzgerald, 1989). Substance-P provokes degranulation of mast cells in peripheral tissue leading to the release of several potent vasoactive and proinflammatory mediators including histamine and serotonin (Holsapple, Schnur, & Yin, 1980). Substance-P may also act directly as a vasodilator. In addition to antidromic release of substance-P, primary afferent nociceptors release calcitonin gene-related peptide (CGRP) from terminal branches to affect distal peripheral (and/or visceral) tissues. CGRP activates the enzyme NO (nitric oxide) synthase from

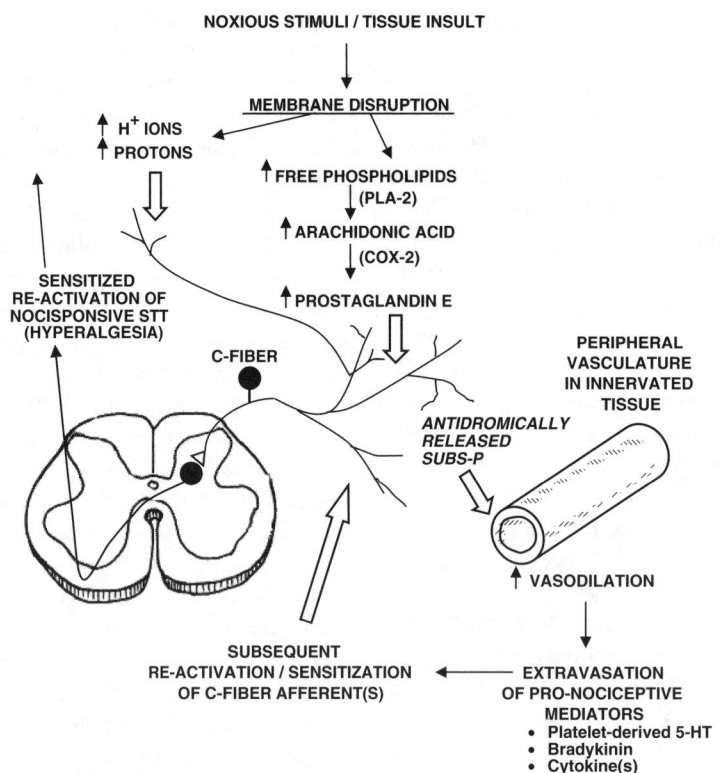

FIGURE 3.1 Schematic depiction of mechanisms subserving inflammatory pain and subsequent neurogenic inflammation. Although noxious stimuli (e.g., heat, high-intensity mechanical stress, and/or chemical irritants) can act directly at nonselective cationic channels on free nerve endings, such stimuli can also disrupt membrane integrity and evoke the formation of prostaglandin-E_2 (via initiation of the arachidonic acid cascade) and liberation of H^+ ion and protons. These substances induce depolarization of C-fibers, causing both an orthodromic and antidromic release of substance-P. Antidromically released substance-P acts as a vasodilatory agent, both directly and through nitric oxide–mediated mechanisms. Extravasation of blood-borne substances (e.g., 5-HT, bradykinin, cytokines) stimulate and/or sensitize C-fibers, perpetuating both nociception and inflammation. PLA-2: phospholipase-A2; COX-2: cyclo-oxygenase-2.

the vascular endothelium leading to an increase production of NO and ultimately vasodilatation. Taken together, the effects of histamine, mast cell–derived serotonin, substance-P, and CGRP produce potent peripheral vasodilatory effects that lead to extravasation of chemical mediators that both propagate the neurogenic inflammatory response and are directly pro-nocisponsive (Figure 3.1). These include vasoactive intestinal peptide (VIP), bradykinin, and platelet-derived serotonin (Gupta & Bhide, 1979; Handwerker, 1976). Of particular interest is the effect of rising concentrations of serotonin in extravascular tissue from mast cells and degranulated platelets. As peripheral serotonin concentrations rise, serotonin 5-HT_3 receptors on terminals of C-fiber primary afferents are engaged to produce a rapid Na^+ influx, depolarizing C-fibers and leading to continuity of this cycle (Giordano & Dyche, 1989; Sufka, Schomburg, & Giordano, 1992). Additionally, locally concentrated free serotonin appears to sensitize both 5-HT_3 and NK-1 receptors on C-fiber afferents, thereby increasing subsequent responsivity to serotonin and substance-P (Giordano & Gerstmann, 2004).

SECOND-ORDER AFFERENTS

The dorsal horn of the spinal cord is a critical site for the convergence and neural processing of nociceptive information from peripheral primary afferent fibers. A-delta and C-fibers form synaptic connections on wide dynamic range (WDR) and nociceptive-specific (NS) neurons within the spinal cord whose functional properties contribute to both spatial and temporal transformations of the afferent input. As depicted in Figure 3.2, the majority of these second-order neurons aggregate in the dorsal horn, project contralaterally, and ascend within the anterolateral quadrant(s) as the spinothalamic tract (STT) to sites within the brainstem, midbrain, and thalamus. The unique physiologic characteristics of WDR and NS neurons encode specific qualities of intensity, modality, and localization to the nociceptive signal that is transmitted to supraspinal targets.

WIDE DYNAMIC RANGE NEURONS

WDR neurons are localized with highest concentrations in laminae I, II, V, and VI, with greatest numbers found

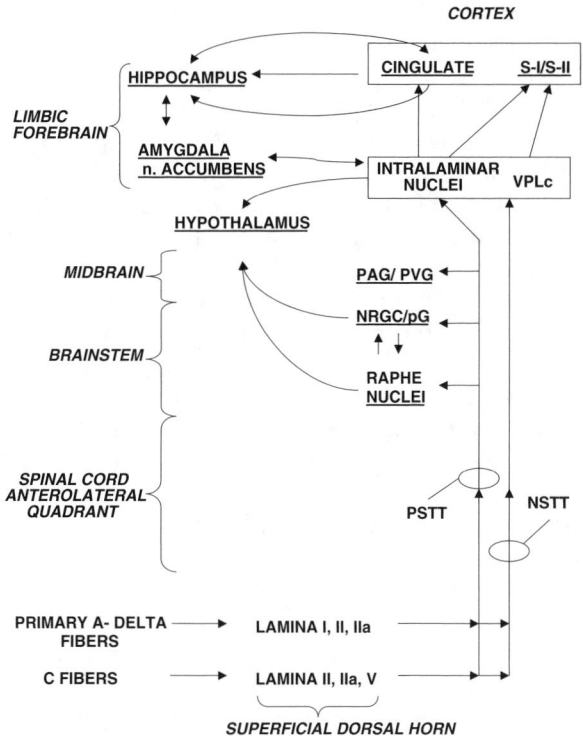

FIGURE 3.2 Diagrammatic depiction of afferent pathways subserving nociception. Primary afferent (A-delta and C) fibers synapse upon second-order neurons in the superficial laminae of the dorsal horn. These units decussate and ascend in the contralateral anterolateral column as the spinothalamic tract(s). The NSTT is a relatively direct pathway that projects to the VPLc nucleus of the thalamus. Thalamo-cortical projections from VPLc are predominantly to S-I, subserving stimulus discriminatory functions. The PSTT comprises the spinoreticular pathway, which projects to monoaminergic nuclei of the brainstem, and the spinotectal pathway that projects to the midbrain PAG. The PSTT projects to thalamic intralaminar, medial, and latero-dorsal nuclei. Connections among the brainstem, intralaminar nuclei, and hypothalamus mediate autonomic and neuroendocrine responses to nociceptive input. Projections from the intralaminar nuclei to the cingulate and from the cingulate bilaterally to S-II and the hippocampus are involved in associative and evaluative domains of pain processing. Refer to text for further description of afferent processing of pain sensation and cognition. NRGC: nucleus reticularis gigantocellularis; NRpG: nucleus reticularis paragigantocellularis; NSTT: neospinothalamic tract; PSTT: paleo-spinothalamic tract; PAG/PVG: periaqueductal/periventricular gray; S-I/S-II: somatosensory cortices I and II; VPLc: ventroposterior laterocaudal nucleus of the thalamus.

in the latter levels. Although WDR neurons receive input from low-threshold cutaneous mechanoreceptor afferents (A-beta type), they are also a site of convergence for both A-delta and C-fiber nociceptive afferents. WDR neurons that are driven by nociceptive input are hierarchically organized within the dorsal horn, with the majority of primary A-delta and C-fiber afferent input occurring in

laminae V (Maixner, Dubner, Bushnell, Kenshalo, & Oliveras, 1986). The size and responsivity of WDR neuron receptive fields increases progressively from laminae I to V: WDR units in laminae I and II have smaller receptive fields that are sensitive to gentle mechanical stimuli; those of laminae V have larger, overlapping receptive fields with graded sensitivities containing small, discrete regions excited by non-nociceptive input and broad regions that are maximally sensitive to high-threshold nociceptive stimulation (Mayer, Price, & Becker, 1975).

WDR neurons are not individually sensitive to specific types of stimuli. Rather, individual WDR neurons, based on response properties within their receptive fields, function to discriminate stimulus intensity. Increases in stimulus intensity activate coexistent areas of receptive fields of numerous WDR neurons. This pattern of engagement would involve slight differences in temporal activation, with individual WDR responses becoming phase shifted. The activation of greater numbers of WDR neurons by high-intensity nociceptive stimuli would therefore result in both spatial and temporal summation of these responses (Hayes, Price, & Dubner, 1979).

NOCICEPTIVE-SPECIFIC NEURONS

In contrast to the anatomical distribution of WDR neurons, NS neurons are found in highest concentrations in laminae I and II, with lesser numbers in laminae V (Dubner & Bennett, 1983). NS neurons receive excitatory input from A-delta fibers and polymodal C-fiber afferents. Generally, NS neurons have small, non-overlapping receptive fields with a well-defined, center-surround organization. The central region is maximally excited by high-intensity stimuli, while the outer region is differentially excited by frequency-based repetitive stimulation. This outer region may be inhibited by non-noxious input. The homogeneity of input from nocisponsive primary afferents and the small size and nociceptive selectivity of their receptive fields provide evidence that NS neurons appear to function in localization, and perhaps qualitative discrimination of particular types of noxious input (i.e., noxious pressure and heat; Willis, 1979).

Although painful sensations and responses can be evoked by WDR neuron excitation alone, both WDR and NS activity appears to be necessary for the constellation of spatial and temporal qualities ascribed to pain (Mayer et al., 1975). This becomes apparent when the convergent inputs of A-delta and C-fibers upon WDR and NS neurons are considered. The unique properties of the primary afferents and the second-order neurons essentially "assemble" the neurologic pain signal. For example, the sensation of first-pain as punctate, well localized, and temporally well defined is a function of the response characteristics of both rapidly conducting A-delta primary afferents and their excitation of WDR and NS neurons. In contrast, second-pain, a more diffuse, long-lasting nociceptive sensation that follows the initial stimulus, is the result of the threshold, firing, and conduction properties of C-fibers sustained by local tissue damage and/or chemical change, as well as patterns of temporal and spatial summation of C-fiber inputs by WDR and NS neurons (Mayer et al., 1975; Price & Dubner, 1977). Both WDR and NS neurons are capable of after-responses that persist as a consequence of the number and frequency of nociceptive afferent volleys (Willis, 1979), factors that are related to nociceptive stimulus intensity and continuity.

The anatomic and physiologic properties of second-order afferents also subserve the phenomenon of referred pain. As previously discussed, primary afferent innervation of visceral and deep muscular structures is organized so that these fibers converge upon WDR and NS neurons that also receive input from primary nociceptive (and non-nociceptive) afferents from specific somato-cutaneous regions (Selzer & Spencer, 1969). The convergence of visceral and cutaneous afferents from a given somatotome upon second-order WDR and NS neurons underlies patterns of referred pain. Thus, sensory information from the viscera is often subjectively interpreted as afferent information from a cutaneous structure within the corresponding somatotome.

SPINOTHALAMIC TRACT(S)

The majority of WDR and NS neurons project contralaterally within the spinal cord and ascend within the anterolateral quadrant, forming the spinothalamic tract(s) (STT). A minority of fibers remain ipsilateral and ascend outside of the STT within the ventrolateral white matter to supraspinal sites that correspond to the contralateral anterolateral quadrant projections (Appelbaum et al., 1975). Anatomically, axons from second-order neurons in the superficial dorsal horn (laminae I and II) are segregated from those of deeper laminae (lamina V). This provides anatomical separation between the neospinothalamic (NSTT) and paleo-spinothalalmic (PSTT) tracts. While both the NSTT and PSTT may be considered "labeled-lines" for the transmission of pain signals, the differential localization of NS neurons to laminae I and II, in contrast to a greater abundance of WDR neurons in lamina V, subserves functional distinctions in the type of nociceptive information that is transmitted in these pathways (Giesler, Yezierski, Gerhart, & Willis, 1981).

The NSTT projects directly to the ventroposterior lateral (VPL) nuclei of the thalamus and is composed predominately of NS neurons from lamina I and II (Kenshalo et al., 1980). WDR neurons are in smaller numbers within these laminae, and they comprise only a minority of NSTT fibers. NS neurons receive almost completely homogeneous input from A-delta and high-threshold polymodal C-fiber afferents, and encode stimulus localization and

modality. Therefore, the main role of the NSTT appears to involve transmission of these signal qualities to the thalamus (Price, Hayes, Ruda, & Dubner, 1978).

The PSTT is composed of axons from second-order neurons arising in lamina IIa and V of the spinal cord. WDR neurons constitute the majority of cells from this lamina, with only a smaller number of NS neurons contributing to the axonal pool of the PSTT (Appelbaum, Beall, Foreman, & Willis, 1975). Heterogeneous input to lamina V WDR neurons from both nocisponsive and non-nocisponsive primary afferents contributes to the transmission of some non-nociceptive signals along the PSTT. WDR neurons of lamina V also send axons ipsilaterally to ascend within the dorsal column medial lemniscal tract (Boivie, 1980; refer to Figure 3.7 later in the chapter). This latter pathway is responsible for the transmission of light touch, vibration, and other low-threshold stimuli. Given the role of lamina V WDR neurons to encode noxious stimulus intensities, the co-localized transmission of both nociceptive and non-nociceptive afferent information within the PSTT appears to serve a stimulus discriminatory function (Price & Dubner, 1977). This is further supported by the properties of PSTT WDR neurons to accumulate strong after-responses following nociceptive input. Such after-responses override weaker impulses evoked by non-nociceptive afferent stimuli and produce temporally summated volleys within the PSTT. These events are correlated to, and appear to subserve, the qualities and subjective characteristics of second-pain.

Unlike the NSTT, the PSTT is not a direct thalamic pathway. PSTT fibers project to several supraspinal sites that are involved in (nociceptive) sensory processing and that exert pain modulatory control. The PSTT is divided into spinoreticular, spinotectal, and ultimately spinothalamic projections. Spinoreticular pathways project to areas of the brainstem reticular formation. These include the raphe nuclei of the rostro-ventral medulla and the nuclei reticularis gigantocellularis (NRGC) and paragigantocellularis (NRpG) of the caudal pons (Basbaum & Fields, 1978).

Spinotectal projections terminate within the tectum and periaqueductal gray (PAG) region of the midbrain (Beitz, 1982). The spinoreticular and spinotectal circuits function in centrifugal pain control, and ascending neurons from these sites serve as relays between spinal pathways and higher centers that mediate the cognitive and affective dimensions of pain. Of particular note are defined tracts from the reticular formation to several regions of the limbic forebrain, and a reciprocal neuraxis involving the PAG, periventricular gray region (PVG), hypothalamus, and brainstem (Guilbaud, Bernard, & Besson, 1994). Thalamic projections of the PSTT differ from those of the NSTT; PSTT fibers project diffusely to the thalamus, with terminations at the intralaminar nuclei (Ralston, 1984), the centro-median parafascicular complex, and the laterodorsal and the mediodorsal nuclei (Mancia et al., 1987). (Refer to Figure 3.2 and Figure 3.6, later in the chapter).

BRAINSTEM NOCICEPTIVE NEURAXES

As depicted in Figure 3.2, PSTT neurons differentially project to specific sites within the brainstem. Some stimulus-specificity exists in PSTT activation of raphe and/or NRGC/NRpG neurons. Input from NS and/or WDR units excited by thermosponsive primary afferents appears to evoke greater excitation of raphe circuitry, while WDR and NS neurons driven by mechanosponsive input elicit somewhat greater activation of the NRGC/NRpG (Giordano & Barr, 1988; Kuraishi, Hirota, Satoh, & Takagi, 1985). Both circuits are apparently engaged by chemosponsive or polymodal C-fiber afferent activation of WDR or NS neurons. It has been suggested that such stimulus specificity is maintained at the midbrain level and may be involved in the differential activation of PAG-raphe or PAG-NRGC centrifugal analgesic systems (as described further in this chapter). Whether these distinctions actually subserve modality specificity or reflect differential activation based upon stimulus intensity remains speculative (Craig, 2003). Of note is the existence of specific cells that respond differentially to PSTT input. One group of brainstem cells, "on" cells, depolarizes in response to PSTT input driven by noxious stimulation. These cells appear to augment transmission of pain via facilitation of spinal afferent output. Another group, the "off" cells, hyperpolarizes upon PSTT activation and reduces nociceptive transmission along spinally originating PSTT pathways (Heinricher, Morgan, Tortorici, & Fields, 1994). The net actions of these cells appears to augment or suppress the pain signal and may play a role in frequency-dependent or intensity-dependent encoding for given types of noxious stimuli. Additionally, PSTT excitation of "on" cells activates hypothalamic, cingulate, insular, and septal systems involved in pain-related aversive and arousal responses (Kalivas & Barnes, 1993).

MIDBRAIN NOCICEPTIVE MECHANISMS

There is anatomical evidence to demonstrate that PSTT fibers project to the midbrain PAG both directly and through interneuronal pathways from the reticular formation. The PAG is somatotopically and perhaps stimulus-specifically organized. Somatotopic organization corresponds to the ascending hierarchy of PSTT afferents from progressively rostral somatotomes: the posterior PAG receives input from PSTT fibers of the caudal spinal cord while the anterior PAG receives PSTT projections from more rostral regions.

Stimulus-specific organization of the PAG seems to be a function of characteristics of populations of PSTT

WDR or NS neurons that are selectively excited by mechanical, thermal, or polymodal primary afferents. While it is difficult to determine whether absolute stimulus-specific organization exists, it is likely that regions of the PAG respond to somatotopic innervation of the periphery and would thus be maximally excited by input from a particular modality or intensity.

Although the function of the PAG in centrifugal pain control is clear, the role of the PAG in afferent processing of the nociceptive signal remains more enigmatic. Pathways exist between the PAG and hypothalamus and several structures of the forebrain, including the septal nuclei and amygdala (see Figure 3.2). Stimulation of the PAG or fibers within this pathway elicits an array of arousal and behavioral activation responses that have distinct aversive or frightening emotional content (Cailliet, 1993). Such responses have significant conditioning potential, primarily by activating "upstream" neuraxes involving the mammillo-thalamic tract, anterior thalamic nucleus, and subsequent involvement of the cingulatum and ultimately the hippocampus (Ploghaus et al., 1999). It is not completely understood whether the PAG can evoke these responses alone or acts in concert with the reticular system, cingulate gyrus, insula, and frontal cortex.

THE THALAMUS

The NSTT and PSTT project to different regions within the thalamus. NSTT neurons project to a caudal area of the ventroposterior lateral nucleus (VPLc). Nociceptive inputs from the NSTT are arranged in columnar zones that are somatotopically organized. Thalamic neurons within these zones retain many response characteristics of WDR and NS units. Thalamic wide-range neurons have center-surround receptive fields with distinct, small areas sensitive to low-threshold excitation and a broad area that is excited by high-threshold nociceptive input. Thalamic NS neurons, like their spinothalamic counterparts, have smaller receptive fields that are excited by high-intensity mechanical or thermal input (see Albe-Fessard, Condes-Lara, Sanderson, & Levante, 1983, for review).

Both WDR and NS neurons of the VPLc summate responses as a function of stimulus frequency and intensity (Gerhart, Yezierski, Fang, & Willis, 1983). Slow temporal and spatial summation is accompanied by a prolonged firing phase that exceeds the actual noxious stimulus and primary and secondary afferent discharges. It is probable the temporal aspects of pain *perception* reflect serial processing of afferent information from the peripheral to the thalamic levels, with progressive extension of after-discharges along the pathway (and perhaps subsequently to cortical sites; see below). It is tempting to speculate that such effects may "match" sensory, arousal, and environmental cues in establishing conditioned responses to circumstances surrounding painful stimuli.

The PSTT projects to the intralaminar thalamic nuclei, the dorsal nucleus centralis lateralis, and medialis dorsalis (see Figure 3.6). Most of the neurons within these thalamic areas are of the wide range type, sensitive to both nociceptive and non-nociceptive activation and with extensive overlapping input from cutaneous and visceral innervation (Curry, 1972; Dong, Ryu, & Wagman, 1978). These units do not have the adaptive properties of neurons of the VPLc; intralaminar neurons summate responses, but response patterns do not reflect direct spatial or temporal transformation of increments in stimulus frequency or intensity (Guilbaud, Caille, Besson, & Benelli, 1977). Unlike neurons of the VPLc, intralaminar neurons appear to be arranged in a "looser" somatotopic pattern and project diffusely to S-II, as well as the anterior and posterior cingulate gyrus regions of the cortex, and a reciprocal pathway to the amygdala has been described (Burton & Jones, 1976; see Figure 3.6). The response patterns of individual intralaminar neurons, together with their anatomic distribution to cortical and amygdalar projections, suggest that PSTT-intralaminar thalamic pathways act to engage these systems in behavioral activation, aversive-emotional, and nocifensive responses.

CORTICAL PROJECTIONS

Neurons from the NSTT project to the VPLc of the thalamus; thalamo-cortical fibers from this region terminate in S-I (and to a lesser extent S-II areas) of the somatosensory cortex. Thalamo-cortical fibers from the intralaminar, lateral, and medial dorsal nuclei, driven by the PSTT, project more diffusely, with a smaller number terminating in S-I, while the majority project bilaterally to S-II (Figure 3.6) (Albe-Fessard, 1983). The somatotopic organization of the thalamus is preserved in S-I and to some extent S-II; nociceptive input contributes to distinct regions of somatosensory activation within the cortex (i.e., the sensory "homunculus," the spatial representation of bodily structures across the cortical sensory field).

Somatosensory cortical regions are arranged in vertical dominance columns in which hierarchical processing of afferent input occurs. Only a small percentage of nociceptive input constitutes each given cortical column (Kaas, 1993). Nociceptive thalamo-cortical input is differentially distributed within each column. Superficial cortical layers receive thalamic input from non-nociceptive pathways, while WDR- and NS-activated inputs are concentrated throughout the deeper cortical layers (Kaas, 1993). Thus, for any given bodily region represented in a cortical column there is an array of non-noxious information (relayed through medial lemniscal tracts) and nociceptive information (relayed through the STTs) that creates the "depiction" of sensations that determine the subjective sensory experience (Ralston & Ralston, 1994). The integrity of the pain signal and unique qualities of its duration and intensity are a function of additive transformation of afferent volleys from primary nociceptors through multiple processing ultimately terminating in cortical neurons. The slow adaptation, long after-discharges, and highly modifiable spatial and temporal summation of cortical S-I and S-II neurons contribute to the subjective, temporospatial, discriminative dimensions of pain sensation (Mayer et al., 1975).

As depicted in Figure 3.6, there are projections from S-II to the anterior cingulate via the insula and to the posterior cingulate through a direct, reciprocal pathway (Vogt, Finch, & Olson, 1992). The role of the anterior cingulum in pain sensation and pain-related behavioral responses is well documented (Devinsky, Morrell, & Vogt, 1995), such that the superior, anterior cingulate is commonly referred to as the nociceptive cingulate area (NCA). Anterior cingulate–hypothalamic projections mediate components of neuroendocrine and autonomic responses to pain sensation (Bromm & Desmedt, 1995). The involvement of the hypothalamus is initiative in engaging multiple, non-opioid, hormonally mediated forms of pain modulation (Bodnar, Kelly, Steiner, & Glusman, 1978; Lewis, Cannon, Stapleton, & Liebeskind, 1980; Lewis, Chudler, Cannon, & Liebeskind, 1981; see Watkins & Mayer, 1982, for review). Diagrammatic depiction of putative hormonal mechanisms of pain modulation is shown in Figure 3.3. Additionally, Losel et al. (2003) suggest that the nongenomic action of steroid hormones on neurotransmitter receptors may be a mechanism that alters hypothalamic function to affect the activity of other supratentorial structures. This may subserve distinctions in pain presentation and responses that occur in various neuroendocrine (and perhaps psychiatric) states (e.g., premenstrual disorder, depression; Kalin & Dawson, 1986).

Efferent connections that project from the anterior cingulate to the caudate, putamen, and nucleus accumbens mediate motor responses to pain (Kalivas & Barnes, 1993) and may be involved in repetitive and/or stereotypical behaviors observed in (chronic) pain states. Afferent pathways from the hippocampus via the subicular complex and entorrhinal cortex (together with efferent input from the posterior cingulum) mediate cognitive and memory-based aspects of pain (Vogt et al., 1992).

Afferent and efferent connections exist between the posterior cingulate, the lateral dorsal thalamic nucleus, and the amygdala. As well, the posterior cingulum receives efferent input from the inferior temporal, mediotemporal, and inferior parietal cortices. These pathways appear to subserve the higher cognitive-emotional dimension of pain sensation (Bromm, 2001). The anatomy of these pathways well illustrates that the subjective experience of pain may vary according to myriad combinations of extero- and, perhaps, interoceptive circumstances for each individual.

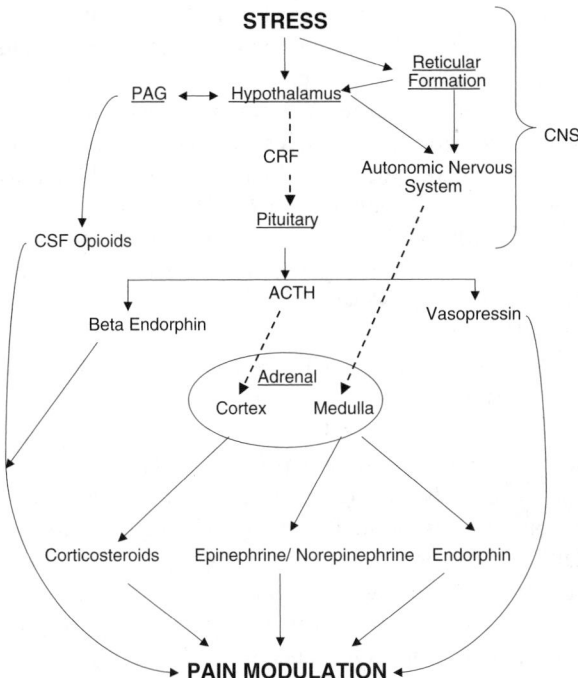

STRESS

FIGURE 3.3 Representation of certain stress-induced analgesic mechanisms. Exogenous stress can engage the reticular system and hypothalamus to heighten the activity of the autonomic nervous system. As well, hypothalamic involvement in the stress response can engage the hypothalamic–pituitary–adrenal axis. Together, these mechanisms synergistically lead to a systemic increase in glucocorticoid and epinephrine/norepinephrine level(s). The pituitary, adrenal medulla, and midbrain periaqueductal grey region (PAG) release opioids, which act on populations of opioid receptors in the central nervous system (CNS) and periphery. These opioid and non-opioid pain modulatory systems can be engaged together or distinctly, dependent upon the type, intensity, and duration of the provocative stress(or). It is interesting to note that prolonged or acute disturbance of this system may be contributory to altered patterns of pain modulation and an alteration in pain sensitivity (see text for details). ACTH: adrenocorticotropic hormone; CRF: corticotropin releasing factor; CSF: cerebrospinal fluid.

The assemblage of sensory input together with memory, emotional response(s), and cognitive state creates conscious experience of pain that contributes to its perception. However, there is a considerable philosophical debate whether pain can be completely defined as a perception (Wikler, 1979). The complexity and strongly subjective nature of pain strengthen the hypothesis that the hierarchical neural processing that expands the sensory signal into an aggregate of combined awareness of internal state, circumstances surrounding the event, and memory and emotional components that impart contextual "meaning" to the experience qualifies pain as a discrete event of consciousness. This becomes significant in light of the involvement of nonsensory central nervous system structures in nociceptive processing. Thus, it may be that the

experience of pain represents both a conscious interpretation of the sensory experience caused by activation of neural pathways and an epiphenomena of higher-order consciousness resulting from the change in brain state.

PAIN MODULATING SYSTEMS

INTRASPINAL PAIN MODULATION

Pain modulation can occur through the activation of local circuits within the spinal dorsal horn. Interneurons that receive collateral projections from primary A-delta and C-fibers are found in laminae I, II, and V. These interneurons form reciprocal synapses upon primary afferent(s) and, in certain cases, second-order WDR and NS neurons. The majority of such interneuronal connections are found within a given horizontal section of the spinal cord, although Willis and Coggeshall (1991) have shown that some interneurons have terminal fields that are trans-segmental. Pharmacologic and electrophysiologic evidence has demonstrated that these interneurons are inhibitory; many produce and release the inhibitory transmitter gamma amino butyric acid (GABA), as well as the opioid peptides dynorphin and leu- and/or met-enkephalin (Fields, Heinricher, & Mason, 1991). Acting at postsynaptic $GABA_B$ receptors on primary and second-order afferents, GABA induces a chloride ion flux to produce hyperpolarization. Dynorphin binds post-synaptically with kappa-opioid receptors (Corbett et al., 1982). There is some heterogeneity in kappa receptor populations; however, most found in the spinal cord are negatively coupled to N-type calcium ionic channels. Dynorphin binding at these kappa sites on primary or second-order afferents closes the calcium channel, thereby producing a hyperpolarizing inhibitory current, essentially "tuning down" or "shutting off" the transmission of nociceptive information along this neuraxis (Han & Xie, 1982). In contrast, leu- and met-enkephalin act at delta, and to a lesser extent mu opioid, receptors to engage G protein–mediated kinases to phosphorylate and open K^+ channels, enhancing K^+ influx and producing graded hyperpolarization (Duggan & North, 1983). Recently, endogenous cannabinoids, including anandamide and 2-arachadoylglycerol, have been shown to exert spinal anti-nociceptive effects by acting at type-1 cannabinoid (CB1) receptors in the dorsal root ganglion and superficial spinal cord (Hohmann & Herkenham, 1999; Pertwee, 2001; Rice, 2001). Cannabinoid CB1 receptors are also expressed in cortical and subcortical brain regions where anandamide (and exogenous *cannabis sativa* and 9-tetrahydrocannabinol) exerts pain modulatory effects, as well (Rice, 2001).

This local circuit inhibition modulates firing of primary A-delta and C-fibers afferents; a particular frequency pattern of primary afferent firing may excite populations of local interneurons to exert recurrent inhibition. Simi-

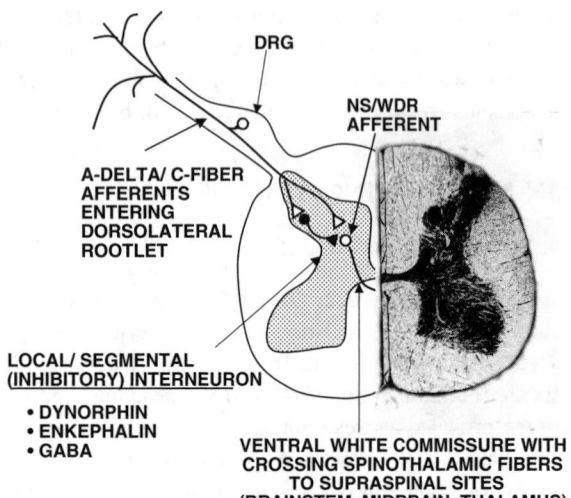

FIGURE 3.4 Local/segmental inhibition producing pain modulation within the dorsal horn of the spinal cord. A-delta and C-fibers synapse upon interneurons that release dynorphin, enkephalin, or gamma amino butyric acid (GABA) to postsynaptically suppress/modulate the activity of second-order nociceptive specific neurons (NS) and wide dynamic range neurons (WDR) afferents. As well, the endogenous cannabinoid anandamide may act at specific cannabinoid (CB1) receptors to inhibit nociceptive transmission within the dorsal root ganglion and superficial dorsal horn (not illustrated). The level of local spinal inhibition may be dependent on the spatial and frequency intensity of incoming nociceptive afferent volleys. Increased primary afferent activity is capable of overcoming local inhibition. As well, these spinal inhibitory interneurons can be driven by descending bulbospinal activation. Complete description of these mechanisms appears in text. (*Note*: Not to scale.)

larly, primary afferent activity may evoke local spinal inhibition of certain populations of second-order WDR and NS neurons to limit the "gain" of mild nociceptive input (Figure 3.4).

BULBOSPINAL PAIN MODULATION

Projections from the (P)STT synapse upon neurons in the rostro-ventral medulla and ventromedial pons (Basbaum & Fields, 1978). In the rostro-ventral medulla, the projection fields include neurons of the raphe nuclei, including the nuclei raphe alatus, dorsalis, and raphe lateralis. These sites are combined when referring to the nucleus raphe magnus (NRM). In the caudal pons, the PSTT projects specifically to the subcerulear nuclear group, consisting of the nucleus reticularis gigantocellularis, nucleus reticularis paragigantocellularis, and the nucleus paragigantocellularis lateralis (NpGL). These sites are often referred to as the reticular magnocellular nuclei (RMC). The NRM and RMC also receive efferent input from the PAG as well as this afferent input from the PSTT. Both neuraxes are capable, either alone or in concert, of exciting NRM or RMC neurons to elicit centrifugal or bulbospinal pain

modulation, respectively (see Fields & Basbaum, 1999, for review). Mixed inhibitory and excitatory connections between these groups of brainstem nuclei exist (Stamford, 1995); this inter-brainstem inhibition appears to determine the relative participation of NRM, RMC, or both groups in bulbospinal analgesia. Moderate levels of activity within the RMC inhibit the NRM. In contrast, higher levels of RMC activity excite certain NRM neurons. The NRM maintains tonic modulation of the RMS, and phasic, "burst" activity of NRM cells can engage activity within the RMC (Fields, 2000).

As previously discussed, two distinct subtypes of neurons exist throughout the rostral medulla. These are referred to as "on" or "off" cells, with reference to their electrophysiologic response patterns to noxious afferent input. "On" cells become active with noxious afferent stimulation and appear to potentiate afferent transmission. "Off" cells become quiescent in response to afferent noxious input, and the lack of facilitatory input to the spinal cord decreases the frequency and duration of nociceptive transmission. "On" cells suppress "off" cells; thus, once sensitized, "on" cells can potentiate nociception by driving volleys of transmission within the spinal cord. Opioid projections from the PAG inhibit the activity of "on" cells, and thereby eliminate their capacity for facilitating the pain signal and also disinhibit "off" cells to exert an analgesic effect (Fields & Basbaum, 1999; Heinricher et al., 1994.)

Axonal projections from the NRM and RMC descend in the dorsolateral funiculi (DLF) of the spinal cord and terminate in dense synaptic fields within laminae I, II, and V of the dorsal horn (Basbaum & Fields, 1979). Synaptic connections within these layers involve polysynaptic circuits of multiple spinal interneurons, as well as monosynaptic contacts with WDR, NS, and primary afferent neurons. Spinal interneurons receiving efferent projections from the brainstem synapse on WDR and NS second-order neurons as well as the terminals of primary afferent fibers. As previously described, these interneurons are neurochemically heterogeneous, releasing the inhibitory transmitters GABA, enkephalin, dynorphin, and/or anandamide. These interneuronal contacts provide selective, multifocal inhibition of specific groups of nociceptive afferents.

Synaptic connections between bulbospinal and WDR, NS, and perhaps primary afferent neurons exist in laminae I, II, and V (Fields et al., 1991). A single fiber from the brainstem may synapse on several second-order afferents within a given lamina. The differential projection of NRM or RMC terminals onto discrete populations of mechanosponsive, thermosponsive, or polymodally driven WDR and NS neurons in laminae I, II, and V further suggests that some stimulus or modality specificity may exist in the analgesic axis that originates from these brainstem nuclei (Abbott & Melzack, 1982; Giordano & Barr, 1988; Kuraishi, Harada, Aratani, Satoh, & Takagi, 1983; Kuraishi et al., 1985).

Midbrain Pain Modulation

There is considerable evidence to show that the midbrain PAG is a principal site for endogenous pain control. Efferent projections from the cingulate gyrus, limbic forebrain structures, and hypothalamus are capable of exciting opioid (i.e., endorphinergic, enkephalinergic, and orphaninergic) neurons of the PAG, as do inputs from the PSTT (Fields & Basbaum, 1999). The PAG exerts pain modulation by centrifugal inhibition of the spinal second-order afferents that comprise the PSTT and NSTT. This effect primarily involves disinhibition of bulbospinal projections from the NRM and NRGC/NRpG (Fields, Bry, & Hentall, 1983). Defined pathways from the PAG to the raphe nuclei and NRGC/NRpG are activated by high-threshold, high-frequency afferent volleys from the PSTT. Mechanical, thermal, or polymodal nocisponsive units of the PSTT appear to differentially stimulate discrete areas of the PAG to activate the raphe nuclei, NRGC/NRpG, or both (Fields et al., 1983; Fields & Basbaum, 1999). It is not fully understood whether selective PAG engagement of raphe-spinal or NRGC/NRpG spinal neuraxes is dependent on the modality, frequency, or intensity of the evoking afferent input (Abbott & Melzack, 1982; Giordano & Barr, 1988; Kuraishi et al., 1985).

The former system involves a release of opioids from the PAG that enhances the output of serotonergic cells of the raphe nuclei, thereby causing an increased turnover and release of serotonin in pathways that descend in the dorsal lateral funiculi (Fields & Anderson, 1978). These serotonergic fibers synapse heterogeneously in lamina I, II, and V, where serotonin may postsynaptically bind to heterogeneous populations of serotonin ($5-HT_1$, $5-HT_2$) receptors on processes of primary and/or second-order nociceptive neurons (LeBars, 1988, see also Fields & Basbaum, 1999, for review). As well, serotonin may bind to postsynpatic $5-HT_3$ receptors on an interneuron pool in several laminae of the dorsal horn to evoke the release of the inhibitory transmitters GABA, dynorphin, and enkephalin to produce graded inhibition of second-order pain transmitting afferents (Giordano, 1991). PAG-NRGC connections involve a release of opioids from the periaqueductal gray that suppress GABAergic interneurons, thereby disinhibiting noradrenergic neurons of the reticular formation (whose axons similarly descend in the dorsal lateral funiculi) to evoke a release of norepinephrine in lamina II and V. Norepinephrine binds to postsynaptic $alpha_2$ receptors on primary (and perhaps second-order) neurons to produce a graded hyperpolarizing inhibitory current, thereby "toning down" these neurons and producing a reductive modulation of volleys from nociceptive primary and second-order afferents (Dostrovsky, Shah, & Gray, 1983; Dubuisson & Wall, 1980).

The described connections between the PAG and brainstem are polysynaptic, involving pools of both excitatory glutaminergic and inhibitory GABAergic interneuronal relays. Tonic glutaminergic excitation of the brainstem produces low-level modulation of STT volleys and appears to have a "band-pass filtering" effect upon the nature and extent of low-level noxious sensory input that is transmitted to higher centers (Behbehani & Fields, 1979; Fields & Basbaum, 1999). In contrast, spatially or temporally summated high-frequency volleys from PSTT cells activate opioid systems of the PAG that suppress the tonic activity of inhibitory GABAergic interneurons that terminate upon descending neurons of the RMC and/or NRM (Dostrovsky et al., 1983). This suppression of tonic inhibition releases (i.e., disinhibits) the brainstem, thereby facilitating descending inhibition of nociceptive afferent transmission within the spinal cord. Such "volume control" is a function of the nature of the afferent nociceptive stimulus, the extent of PAG activation of PSTT (and perhaps cortical, hypothalamic, and mesolimbic) neurons, and the relative degree of excitation or inhibition of specific neural circuits to the brainstem. Thus, the PAG can discriminably recruit (or suppress) bulbospinal substrates whose net output determines the extent and properties of centrifugal pain modulation (Figure 3.5). These subcortical pain modulatory systems are summarized in Table 3.3.

Cortical Inhibitory Processing

The pathways through which cortical pain modulation occurs are presented in Figure 3.6. Neurons of the sensory cortex are capable of inhibitory control over the thalamo-cortical units of STT origin that project to them (although cortico-thalamic inhibition can also occur over neurons of the medial lemniscal tract that are non-nocisponsive). The extent of inhibition appears to vary with frequency and intensity of thalamo-cortical input. For nociceptive input that is both rapidly temporally and spatially summating, there is a greater level of inhibition (Guilbaud et al., 1994). Sensory cortical inhibition involves "normalization" or "stabilization" of afferent volleys. This compensates for differences in response characteristics between thalamic and cortical neurons and ultimately enhances the input–response function of thalamically driven, nociceptive cortical inputs. In this way, a more direct transformation of the incoming sensory signal is generated without oversummation. Cortical neurons can also excite both thalamo-cortical fibers and STT units directly. This inhibition and excitation serves a modulatory role over afferent information that affects cortical circuitry. Thus, cortical neurons can discriminately amplify or reduce the extent of nociceptive input (Sawamoto et al., 2000). Such modifications strengthen the signal-to-noise ratio of particular afferent volleys and facilitate discrimination of sensory input. This alternate excitation/inhibition may also subserve changes in the nociceptive sensorium as a consequence of levels of cortical activity (e.g., sleep, hypnosis, biofeedback), and

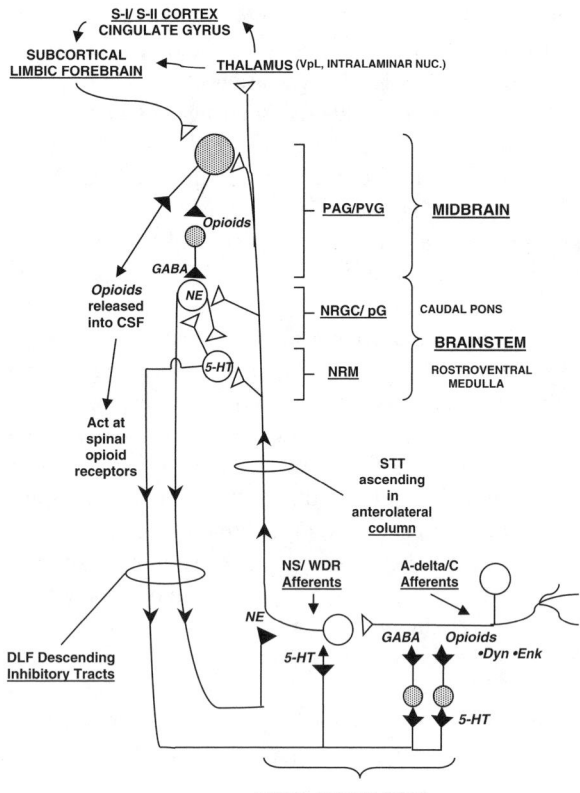

FIGURE 3.5 Representation of pathways involved in bulbospinal and centrifugal analgesia. Afferent volleys from the STT can activate 5-HT and/or NE systems of the brainstem and cause the release of these monoamines within the dorsal horn. Postsynaptically, 5-HT can directly inhibit the activity of nociceptive afferents and may act by stimulating inhibitory interneurons within the superficial cord to (indirectly) suppress nociceptive afferent output. NE acts directly to inhibit the firing of nociceptive afferents. Both 5-HT and NE systems can be engaged by the release of opioids from the PAG (through suppression of GABAergic inhibition of bulbospinal output). Opioids are also released into the cerebral spinal fluid and act at spinal opioid receptors to produce antinociception. Descending influences from the limbic forebrain can also stimulate the PAG. A complete description of brainstem and midbrain pain modulatory systems is provided in the text. Excitatory synapses are depicted by open endings/icons. Inhibitory synapses/neurons are depicted by shaded icons. CB1: cannabinoid-1 receptor; CSF: cerebrospinal fluid; Dyn: dynorphin; DLF: dorsolateral funiculus; Enk: enkephalin; GABA: gamma amino butyric acid; 5-HT: serotonin; NE: norepinephrine; NRM: nucleus raphe magnus; NRGC/pG: nucleus reticularis gigantocellularis/paragigantocellularis; NS: nociceptive specific neurons; NUC: nucleus; PAG/PVG: periaqueductal/periventricular gray; STT: spinothalamic tract; VpL: ventroposterior lateral nucleus of the thalamus; WDR: wide dynamic range neurons.

may be contributory to the elicitation of pain by cognitive expectation or anticipation (Fields, 2000).

It is of interest to note that changes in higher-order consciousness (i.e., cognitive changes) can alter the appre-

ciation, extent, or contextual "value" of sensory phenomena. While the pain-modulatory role of acute sympathetic arousal has long been known (Pribram & McGuinness, 1975), more recent studies have revealed that events that engage cortical and limbic areas to produce alterations of first- and second-order consciousness may have significant pain suppressive effects as well (Hugdahl, 1996; Lou et al., 1999). The long-held "placebo response" is better described as a patient-centered response, in which the participation in some event (e.g., relaxation, types of patient–clinician interaction, meditation, prayer) induces neurochemical change(s) in reticular and mesolimbic/cortical areas (d'Aquili & Newberg, 1993; Levine, Gordon, & Fields, 1978; Saver & Rabin, 1997). Such changes can affect neuraxes to alter nociceptive processing, as well as other physiological events (e.g., immune function, autonomic tone; Amanzio & Benedetti, 1999; Petrovic, Kalso, Petersson, & Ingvar, 2002). This concomitantly activates higher-order consciousness to interpret the interoceptive state (and its effects) and circumstantially "frame" this interpretation relative to environmental, behavioral, and cognitive events that are temporally antecedent and/or coincident. The pairing of these phenomena can have profound conditioning effects. In this way, such inductive events (and awareness of their biological effects) assume both salutogenic value to the patient and "noetic" value that is rich in subjective interpretation of the event itself (Giordano & Engebretson, 2004; Newberg, Tashner, both in this volume).

DORSAL COLUMNAR PAIN MODULATION

Low-threshold mechanosponsive dorsal column afferents, driven by A-beta mechanoreceptors, also exert modulatory influence over WDR and NS neurons that make up the STT. Interneurons in laminae IIa, III, and IV with synaptic fields linking the dorsal columns and STT evoke brief inhibitory postsynaptic potentials (IPSPs) in STT cells following dorsal column excitation by low intensity mechanical stimuli (Lee, Chung, & Willis, 1985). These IPSPs persist after termination of the low-intensity stimulus and cause a short-lasting, rightward shift in both the time- and threshold-based stimulus response function of the affected WDR and NS cells within the STT. In other words, low-level mechanical stimulation of the dorsal column tract is capable of "overriding" or "de-sensitizing" WDR and NS activity within the STT. As well, the dorsal column projects to the nuclei cuneatus and gracilis of the medulla, and as the medial lemniscal pathway, decussates to terminate in the VPL of the thalamus (Willis, 1985; Figure 3.7).

Continuous, low-level phasic or high-frequency repetitive stimulation of the medical lemniscal pathway can produce selective activity within the VPL that can suppress STT-induced input(s) and reduce thalamo-cortical transmission of nociceptive information (Campbell, 1982; Sweet & Wepsic, 1968; Willis, 1985). These phenomena

TABLE 3.3
Physiologic and Pharmacologic Properties of Selected Pain Modulating Systems

System	Anatomy	Chemistry	Physiology/Properties
Intraspinal Segmental	Interneurons, laminae II, V Synaptic contact with recurrent processes of A-delta fibers	Opioid Dynorphin Leu/met-enkephalin GABA Anandamide	Acts upon κ-receptors Acts upon δ (and perhaps μ) receptors Acts upon GABA$_B$ receptors: potentiates chloride flux hyperpolarization Acts upon CB1 receptors
Bulbospinal NRM	Descending fibers from NRM of medulla Fibers descend via DLF Mono- and polysynaptic contacts with primary and second-order units of dorsal horn Synapse upon interneurons	5-HT	Acts on postsynaptic 5-HT$_{1b}$ receptors on (presynaptic) primary afferents and (postsynaptic) second-order neurons Hyperpolarizing; inhibitory Acts on postsynaptic 5-HT$_3$ receptors on GABA and opioid spinal interneurons; excitatory; evokes release of inhibitory modulators
RMC	Descending fibers from NRCG/NRpG of pons Fibers descend via DLF Mono- and polysynaptic contacts with primary and second-order afferents of dorsal horn	NE	Acts on postsynaptic α$_2$ receptors on (presynaptic) afferents and second-order afferents Graded hyperpolarization, inhibitory
Midbrain PAG PVG	Multilevel connections: inputs from hypothalamus, limbic system, cortex Activated by STT Polysynaptic contact with brainstem to disinhibit centrifugal modulatory systems	Opioid Leu/met-enkephalin Endorphin Orphanin	Acts on μ and δ sites Acts on μ-receptor subtypes Some direct opioid release into CSF Graded slow hyperpolarization; inhibitory

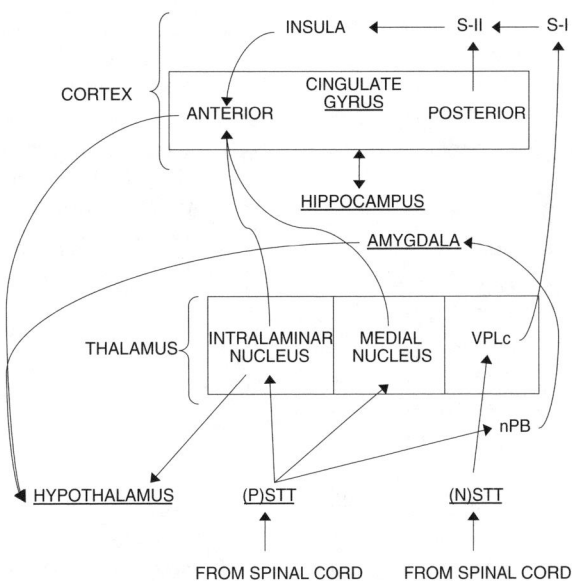

FIGURE 3.6 Schematic diagram of projections from the spinothalamic tract and thalamus to higher centers mediating the emotional, executive, and cognitive dimensions of pain processing. As described in the text, the PSTT diffusely projects to the intralaminar and medial nuclei of the thalamus. Projections from these nuclei to the anterior cingulum subserve emotive aspects of pain. The anterior cingulum also receives input from the posterior cingulum and S-II associative cortex, both via the insula. Reciprocal connections exist between the cingulum and hippocampus. The integrative role of the cingulate gyrus becomes evident in light of these pathways. The PSTT engages the amygdala via the parabrachial nucleus. Hypothalamic activation by the PSTT occurs both through this pathway and by a PSTT-intralaminar nuclei neuraxis. This neural circuit is involved in activational and arousal dimensions of pain. The NSTT projects to the VPLc thalamic nucleus, from where thalamo-cortical pathways project to both S-I and S-II. This pathway is primarily involved with sensory discriminative aspects of the pain signal. However, the interaction of S-I and S-II, and the contribution of S-II input to the cingulate (via the insula) play a synergistic role in cognitive–emotional dimensions of pain consciousness. nPB: parabrachial nucleus; (N)STT: neospinothalamic tract; (P)STT: paleospinothalamic tract; S-I/S-II: primary and associative somatosensory cortex; VPLc: caudal ventroposterior lateral nucleus of the thalamus.

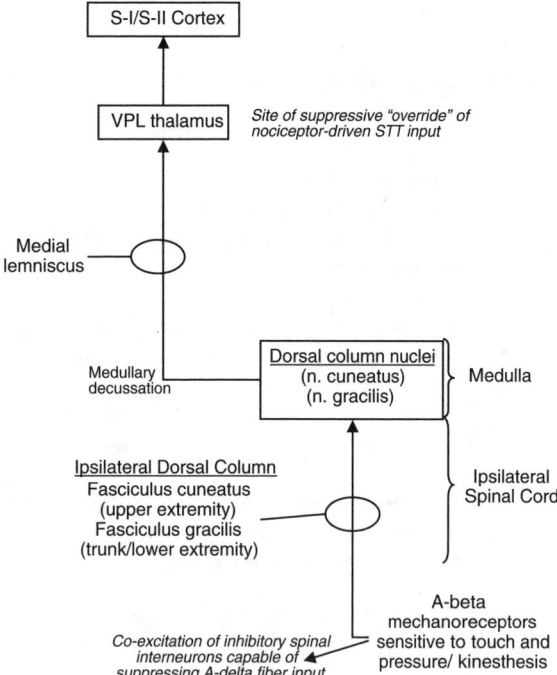

FIGURE 3.7 Schematic depiction of the dorsal column/medial lemniscal pathway and its role in pain modulation. As described in text, A-beta mechanoreceptors can excite inhibitory neurons within the dorsal horn to suppress low-level A-delta nociceptive fiber activity. As well, A-beta mechanoreceptor input can stimulate medial lemniscal pathways from the dorsal column nuclei. Lemniscal projections to the VPL nucleus of the thalamus can modulate coterminal nociceptive input from the STT.

subserve the clinical efficacy of dorsal column electro-stimulation (DCS) and help to explain the somewhat beneficial effect of rubbing a painful area. The effects of dorsal column stimulation, however, seem to be relatively temporally limited in circumstances of long-standing, durable, or progressively increasing pain. With continued A-delta and C-fiber activity, the function (and perhaps microstructural architectural re-modeling) of the STT and/or supraspinal nociceptive neuraxes enhances the transmission of the pain signal, thereby overcoming the viability of spinal or thalamic suppression by dorsal column input (Erickson & Long, 1983). Augmented dorsal column stimulation is then required to regain suppression over STT input, and clinically there appears to be an asymptotic (i.e., ceiling or plateau) pattern to the relative efficacy of serially incremented DCS against progressive neuropathic pain.

SUMMARY

The anatomical and physiologic systems that subserve pain and analgesia are complex. Heterogeneous populations of neurons from the periphery, through the spinal cord, brainstem, thalamus, and ultimately cortical and limbic systems, with discrete neurochemical and physiological properties all contribute to the amalgam of sensations and the cognitive phenomena known as pain. By understanding the structure and function of this system, we may develop enhanced therapeutic approaches for chronic pain that target these substrates more effectively and selectively, thereby reducing deleterious side effects while facilitating an enhanced quality of life.

ACKNOWLEDGMENTS

The author wishes to acknowledge the untiring, cheerful technical and graphic artistic assistance of Sherry Loveless in preparation of this manuscript. As well, the author is appreciative of ongoing collaborative and intellectual exchanges with Drs. Tom Schultea, Robert Barkin, B. Eliot Cole, Philipp Lippe, Pierre LeRoy, and Scott Raven.

This chapter is dedicated to the memory and work of Dr. Richard Weiner: a mentor, supporter, colleague, and friend.

REFERENCES

Abbott, F., & Melzack, R. (1982). Brainstem lesions dissociate neural mechanisms of morphine analgesia in different kinds of pain. *Brain Research, 251,* 149–155.

Albe-Fessard, D. (1983). A possible role for the lateral and medial system of somatic projection of pain appreciation. *Brain Research, 253,* 221–256.

Albe-Fessard, D., Condes-Lara, M., Sanderson, P., & Levante, A. (1983). Tentative explanation of the special role played by the areas of paleospinothalamic projection in patients with deafferentation pain syndromes. In L. Kruger, & J. C. Liebeskind (Eds.), *Advances in pain research and therapy* (Vol. 6, pp. 167–182). New York: Raven Press.

Albe-Fessard, D., Levante, A., & Rokyta, R. (1971). Cortical projections of cat medial thalamic cells. *International Journal of Neuroscience, 1,* 317–338.

Amanzio, M., & Benedetti, F. (1999). Neuropharmacological dissection of placebo analgesia: Expectation-activated opioid systems versus conditioning-activated specific subsystems. *Journal of Neuroscience, 19,* 484–494.

Amaya, F., Decosterd, I., Samad, T. A., et al. (2000). Diversity of expression of the sensory neuron-specific TTX-resistant voltage-gated sodium ion channels SNS and SNS2. *Molecular and Cellular Neuroscience, 15,* 331–342.

Appelbaum, A. E., Beall, J. B., Foreman, R. D., & Willis, W. D. (1975). Organization and receptive fields of primate spinothalamic tract neurons. *Journal of Neurophysiology, 38,* 572–586.

Basbaum, A. I., & Fields, H. L. (1978). Endogenous pain control mechanisms: Review and hypothesis. *Annals of Neurology, 4,* 451.

Basbaum, A. I., & Fields, H. L. (1979). The origin of descending pathways in the dorsolateral funiculus of the spinal cord of the cat and rat: further studies of the anatomy of pain modulation. *Journal of Comparative Neurology, 187,* 513.

Behbehani, M., & Fields, H. L. (1979). Evidence that an excitatory connection between the PAG and NRM mediates stimulation-produced analgesia. *Brain Research, 170,* 85–93.

Beitz, A. (1982). The organization of afferent projections to the midbrain periaqueductal grey of the rat. *Journal of Neuroscience, 7,* 133–159.

Bodnar, R. J., Kelly, D. D., Steiner, S. S., & Glusman, M. (1978). Stress-produced analgesia and morphine-produced analgesia: lack of cross-tolerance. *Pharmacology, Biochemistry, and Behavior, 8,* 661–666.

Boivie, J. (1980). Anatomical observation on the dorsal column nuclei, their thalamic projection and the cytoarchitecture of some somatosensory thalamic nuclei in the monkey. *Journal of Comparative Neurology, 178,* 17–48.

Bromm, B. (2001). Brain images of pain. *News in Physiological Sciences, 16,* 244–249.

Bromm, B., & Desmedt, J. (1995). *Pain and the brain: From nociception to cognition.* New York: Raven Press.

Burton, H., & Jones, E. G. (1976). The posterior thalamic region and its cortical projection in new world and old world monkeys. *Journal of Comparative Neurology, 168,* 249–302.

Cailliet, R. (1993). *Pain: Mechanisms and management* (pp. 1–49). Philadelphia: F. A. Davis.

Campbell, J. N. (1982). Examination of the possible mechanisms by which stimulation of the spinal cord in man relieves pain. *Applied Neurophysiology, 44,* 181.

Campbell, J. N., Meyer, R. A., & Raja, S. N. (1992). Is nociceptor activation by alpha-1 adrenoceptors the culprit in sympathetically-maintained pain? *American Pain Society Journal, 1*(1), 3–11.

Cao, Y. Q., Mantyh, P. W., Carlson, E. J., et al. (1998). Primary afferent tachykinins are required to experience moderate to intense pain. *Nature, 392,* 390–394.

Caterina, M. J., Rosen, T. A., Tominaga, M., et al. (1999). A capsaicin-receptor homologue with a high threshold for noxious heat. *Nature, 398,* 436–441.

Cazzullo, C. L., & Gala, C. (1987). Cognitive and emotional aspects of pain. In M. Tiengo, J. Eccles, A. C. Cuello, & D. Ottoson (Eds.), *Advances in pain research and therapy* (Vol. 10, pp. 255–264). New York: Raven Press.

Cervero, F., & Iggo, A. (1980). The substantia gelatinosa of the spinal cord: A critical review. *Brain, 103,* 717–772.

Coleridge, H. M., Coleridge, J. C. G., & Luck, J. C. (1965). Pulmonary afferent fibres of small diameter stimulated by capsaicin and by hyperinflation of the lungs. *Journal of Physiology, 179,* 248–262.

Corbett, A., Patterson, S., McKnight, A., et al. (1982). Dynorphin (1-8) and (1-9) are ligands for the kappa subtype of opiate receptor. *Nature, 299,* 79–81.

Craig, A. D. (2003). Pain mechanisms: labeled lines versus convergence in central processing. *Annual Review of Neuroscience, 26,* 1–30.

Curry, M. J. (1972). The exteroceptive properties of neurones in the somatic part of the posterior group (PO). *Brain Research, 44,* 439–462.

d'Aquili, E.G., & Newberg, A. B. (1993). Limnality, trance and unitary states in ritual and meditation. *Studia Liturgica, 23,* 2–34.

d'Aquili, E. G., & Newberg, A. B. (2000). The neuropsychology of aesthetic, spiritual and mystical states. *Zygon, 35,* 39–52.

Davis, K. D. (2000). The neural circuitry of pain explored with functional MRI. *Neurology Research, 22*(3), 313–317.

Devinsky, O., Morrell, M. J., & Vogt, B. A. (1995). Contributions of the anterior cingulate cortex to behavior. *Brain, 118,* 279–306.

Dong, W. K., Ryu, H., & Wagman, I. H. (1978). Nociceptive responses of neurons in medial thalamus and their relationship to spinothalamic pathways. *Journal of Neurophysiology, 41,* 1592–1613.

Dostrovsky, J., Shah, Y., & Gray, B. (1983). Descending inhibitory influences from the PAG, NRM and adjacent reticular formation. Effects on medullary dorsal horn nociceptive and non-nociceptive neurons. *Journal of Neurophysiology, 49,* 948–968.

Doubell, T. P., Mannion, R., & Woolf, C. J. (1999). The dorsal horn: State-dependent sensory processing, plasticity and the generation of pain. In P. D. Wall, & R. Melzack (Eds.), *Textbook of pain* (4th ed., pp. 165–182). Edinburgh: Churchill-Livingstone.

Dubner, R. (1985). Specialization in nociceptive pathways: Sensory discrimination, sensory modulation and neural connectivity. In H. L. Fields et al. (Eds.), *Advances in pain research and therapy* (Vol. 9, pp. 111–137). New York: Raven Press.

Dubner, R., & Bennett, G. J. (1983). Spinal and trigeminal mechanisms of nociception. *Annual Review of Neuroscience, 6,* 381–418.

Dubuisson, P., & Wall, P. (1980). Descending influences on receptive fields and activity of single units recorded in laminae I, II and III of cat spinal cord. *Brain Research, 199,* 283–298.

Duggan, A., & North, R. A. (1983). Electrophysiology of opioids. *Pharmacology Review, 35,* 219–281.

Erickson, D. L., & Long, D. M. (1983). Ten-year follow-up of dorsal column stimulation. In J. J. Bonica, U. Lindblom, & A. Iggo (Eds.), *Advances in pain research and therapy* (Vol. 5, pp. 583–589). New York: Raven Press.

Fields, H. L. (2000). Pain modulation: expectation, opioid analgesia and virtual pain. *Progress in Brain Research, 122,* 245–253.

Fields, H. L., & Anderson, S. D. (1978) Evidence that raphespinal neurons mediate opiate and midbrain-stimulation induced analgesias. *Pain, 5,* 333–349.

Fields, H. L., & Basbaum, A. I. (1999). Central nervous system mechanisms of pain modulation. In P. D. Wall, & R. Melzack (Eds.), *Textbook of pain* (4th ed., pp. 309–330). Edinburgh: Churchill-Livingstone.

Fields, H. L., Bry, J., & Hentall, I. (1983). The activity of neurons in the rostral medulla of the rat during withdrawal from noxious heat. *Journal of Neuroscience, 3,* 2545–2552.

Fields, H. L., Heinricher, M. M., & Mason, P. (1991). Neurotransmitters in nociceptive modulatory circuits. *Annual Review of Neuroscience, 14,* 219–245.

Fitzgerald, M. (1989). Arthritis and the nervous system. *Trends in Neuroscience, 12,* 86–87.

Friedman, W. J., & Greene, L. A. (1999). Neurotrophin signaling via Trks and p75. *Experimental Cell Research, 253,* 131–142.

Gebhart, G. F. (1995). Visceral pain. In G. F. Gebhart (Ed.). *Progress in pain research and management* (Vol. 5). Seattle: IASP Press.

Gerhart, K. D., Yezierski, R. P., Fang, Z. R., & Willis, W. D. (1983). Inhibition of primate spinothalamic tract neurons by stimulation in ventral posterior lateral (VPLc) thalamic nucleus: Possible mechanisms. *Journal of Neurophysiology, 49,* 406–423.

Giesler, G. J., Yezierski, R. P., Gerhart, K. D., & Willis, W. D. (1981). Spinothalamic tract neurons that project to medial and/or lateral thalamic nuclei: Evidence for a physiologically novel population of spinal cord neurons. *Journal of Neurophysiology, 46,* 1285–1308.

Giordano, J. (1991). Analgesic profile of centrally administered 2-methylserotonin against acute pain in rats. *European Journal of Pharmacology, 199,* 233–236.

Giordano, J., & Barr, G. A. (1988). Possible role of spinal 5-HT in mu- and kappa opioid receptor-mediated analgesia in the developing rat. *Developmental Brain Research, 33,* 121–127.

Giordano, J., & Dyche, J. (1989). Differential analgesic actions of serotonin 5-HT3 receptor antagonists in the mouse. *Neuropharmacology, 28,* 423–426.

Giordano, J., & Engebretson, J. (2004). The neuroscience of spiritual experiences: Basis for a new epistemology. *ISSEEM Abstracts, 2.*

Giordano, J, & Gerstmann, H. (2004). Patterns of serotonin- and 2-methylserotonin-induced pain may reflect 5-HT3 receptor sensitization. *European Journal of Pharmacology, 483,* 267–269.

Gobel, S. (1976). Principles of organization in the substantia gelatinosa layer of the spinal trigeminal nucleus. In J. J. Bonica, & D. Albe-Fessard (Eds.), *Advances in pain research and therapy* (Vol. 1, pp. 165–185). New York: Raven Press.

Gold, M. S. (1999). Tetrodotoxin-resistant Na$^+$ currents and inflammatory hyperalgesia. *Proceedings of the National Academy of Sciences of the United States of America, 96,* 7645–7649.

Gold, M. S., Levine, J. D., & Correa, A. M. (1998). Modulation of TTX-R Ina by PKC and PKA and their role in PGE2-induced sensitization of rat sensory neurons *in vitro. Journal of Neuroscience, 18,* 10345–10355.

Guilbaud, G., Caille, D., Besson, J. M., & Benelli, G. (1977). Single unit activities in ventral posterior and posterior group thalamic nuclei during nociceptive and non-nociceptive stimulation in the cat. *Archives Italiennes de Biologie, 115,* 38–56.

Guilbaud, G., Bernard, J.F., & Besson, J.M. (1994). Brain areas involved in nociception and pain. In P. D. Wall, & R. Melzack (Eds.), *Textbook of pain* (4th ed., pp. 113–128). Edinburgh: Churchill-Livingstone.

Gupta, R. M., & Bhide, M. B. (1979). Role of 5-HT in acute inflammation and anaphylaxis. *Indian Journal of Medical Research, 69,* 657–658.

Han, J., & Xie, C. (1982). Dynorphin: Potent analgesic effects in the spinal cord of the rat. *Life Sciences, 31,* 1781–1784.

Handwerker, H. O. (1976). The influences of algogenic substances serotonin and bradykinin on the discharge of unmyelinated cutaneous fibers identified as nociceptors. In J. Bonica, & D. Albe-Fessard (Eds.), *Advances in pain research and therapy* (Vol. 1, pp. 41–46). New York: Raven Press.

Hayes, R. L., Price, D. D., & Dubner, R. (1979). Behavioral and physiological studies of sensory coding and modulation of trigeminal nociceptive input. In J. J. Bonica, J. C. Liebeskind, & D. Albe-Fessard (Eds.), *Advances in pain research and therapy* (Vol. 3, pp. 219–243). New York: Raven Press.

Heinricher, M. M., Morgan, M. M., Tortorici, V., and Fields, H. L. (1994). Disinhibition of off-cells and antinociception produced by an opioid action within the rostral ventromedial medulla. *Neuroscience, 63,* 279–288.

Hohmann, A. G., & Herkenham, M. (1999). Localization of central cannabinoid CB1 receptor messenger RNA in neuronal subpopulations of rat dorsal ganglia: A double-label *in situ* hybridization study. *Neuroscience, 90,* 923–931.

Holsapple, M. P., Schnur, M., & Yin, G. K. (1980). Pharmacologic modulation of edema mediated by prostaglandin, serotonin and histamine. *Agents & Actions, 10,* 368–373.

Hugdahl, K. (1996). Cognitive influences on human autonomic nervous system function. *Current Opinion in Neurobiology, 6,* 252–258.

Iggo, A. (1974). Cutaneous receptors. In J. I. Hubbard (Ed.), *The peripheral nervous system* (pp. 374–404). New York: Plenum Press.

Ji, R.R., Kohno, T., Moore, K. A., & Woolf, C. J. (2003). Central sensitization and LTP: Do pain and memory share similar mechanisms? *Trends in Neuroscience, 26,* 696–705.

Jin, S. X., Zhuang, Z. Y., Woolf, C. J., & Ji, R. R. (2003). P38 mitogen-activated protein kinase is activated after a spinal nerve ligation in spinal cord microglia and dorsal root ganglion neurons and contributes to the generation of neuropathic pain. *Journal of Neuroscience, 23,* 4017–4022.

Jones, D. A., Newham, D. J., Obletter, G., & Giamberardino M. A. (1987). Nature of exercise-induced muscle pain. In M. Tiengo, J. Eccles, A. C. Cuello, & D. Ottoson (Eds.), *Advances in pain research and therapy* (Vol. 10, pp. 207–218). New York: Raven Press.

Julius. D., & Basbaum, A. I. (2001). Molecular mechanisms of nociception. *Nature, 413,* 203–210.

Kaas, J. H. (1993). Functional organization of the somatosensory cortex in primates. *Annals of Anatomy, 175,* 509–518.

Kalin, N. H., & Dawson, G. (1986). Neuroendocrine dysfunction in depression: hypothalamic-anterior pituitary systems. *Trends in Neuroscience, 9,* 261–266.

Kalivas, P. W., & Barnes, C. D. (1993). *Limbic motor circuits and neuropsychiatry.* Boca Raton, FL: CRC Press.

Kenshalo, D. R., Giesler, C. J., Leonard, R. B., & Willis, W. D. (1980). Responses of neurons in primate ventral posterior lateral nucleus to noxious stimuli. *Journal of Neurophysiology, 43*, 1594–1614.

Kerr, B. J., Bradbury, E. J., Bennett, D. L., et al. (1999). Brain-derived neurotrophic factor modulates nociceptive sensory inputs and NMDA-evoked responses in the rat spinal cord. *Journal of Neuroscience, 19*, 5138–5148.

Kumazawa, T, & Perl, E. R. (1976). Differential excitation of dorsal horn marginal and substantia gelatinosa neurons by primary afferent units with fine (A-delta and C) fibers. In Y. Zotterman (Ed.), *Sensory functions of the skin in primates with special reference to man* (pp. 67–89). Oxford: Pergamon Press.

Kuraishi, Y., Harada, Y., Aratani, S., Satoh, M., & Takagi, H. (1983). Separate involvement of spinal noradrenergic and serotonergic systems in morphine analgesia: differences in mechanical and thermal algesic tests. *Brain Research, 273*, 245–249.

Kuraishi, Y., Hirota, N., Satoh, M., & Takagi, H. (1985). Antinociceptive effects of intrathecal opiates, NE and 5-Ht in rats: Mechanical and thermal algesic tests. *Brain Research, 326*, 168–171.

Lanteri-Minet, M., Isnardon, P., dePommery, J., & Menetrey, D. (1993). Spinal and hindbrain structures involved in visceroreception and visceronociception as revealed by the expression of Fos, Jun and Krox-24 proteins. *Neuroscience, 55*, 735–753.

LeBars, D. (1998). Serotonin and pain. In N. N. Osborne, & M. Hamon (Eds.), *Neuronal serotonin* (pp. 171–226). New York: Wiley.

Lee, K. H., Chung, J. M., & Willis, W. D. (1985). Transcutaneous nerve stimulation inhibits spinothalamic tract cells. In H. L. Fields, et al. (Eds.), *Advances in pain research and therapy* (Vol. 9, pp. 203–210). New York: Raven Press.

Levine, J. D., Gordon, N. C., & Fields, H. L. (1978). The mechanism of placebo analgesia. *Lancet, 2*, 654–657.

Levine, J. D., & Reichling, D. B. (1999). Peripheral mechanisms of inflammatory pain. In P. D. Wall, & R. Melzack (Eds.), *Textbook of pain* (4th ed., pp. 59–84). Edinburgh: Churchill-Livingstone.

Lewis, J. W., Cannon, J. T., Stapleton, J. M., and Liebeskind, J. C. (1980). Stress activates endogenous pain-inhibitory systems: Opioid and non-opioid mechanisms. *Proceedings of the Western. Pharmacology Society, 23*, 85–88.

Lewis, J. W., Chudler, E. H., Cannon, J. T., & Liebeskind, J. C. (1981). Hypophysectomy differentially affects morphine and stress analgesia. *Proceedings of the Western. Pharmacology Society, 24*, 323–326.

Losel, R. M., Falkenstein, E., Feuring, M., Schultz, A., Tillmann, H.-C., Rossol-Haseroth, K., & Wehling, M. (2003). Nongenomic steroid action: Controversies, questions and answers. *Physiology Review, 83*, 965–1016.

Lou, H. C., Kjaer, T. W., Friberg, L., Wildschiodtz, G., Holm, S., & Nowak, M. (1999). A 15O-H$_2$O PET study of meditation and the resting state of normal consciousness. *Human Brain Mapping, 7*, 98–105.

Luo, Z. D., Chaplan, S. R., Higuera, E. S., Sorkin, L. S., Staudermann, K. A., Williams, M. E., et al. (2001). Upregulation of dorsal root ganglion (alpha)-2-(delta) calcium channel subunit and its correlation with allodynia in spinal nerve-injured rats. *Journal of Neuroscience, 21*, 1868–1875.

Maixner, W., Dubner, R., Bushnell, M. C., Kenshalo, D. R., & Oliveras, J. L. (1986). Wide dynamic range dorsal horn neurons participate in the encoding process by which monkeys perceive the intensity of noxious heat stimuli. *Brain Research, 374*, 385–388.

Mancia, M., Mariotti, M., Caraceni, A., et al. (1987). Center median-parafascicular thalamic complex and mediodorsal nucleus unitary responses to noxious stimuli and their conditioning by limbic and mesencephalic stimulations. In M. Tiengo, J. Eccles, A. C. Cuello, & D. Ottoson (Eds.), *Advances in pain research and therapy* (Vol. 10, pp. 17–30). New York: Raven Press.

Mannsfeldt, A. G., Carroll, P., Stucky, C. L., & Lewin, G. R. (1999). Stomatin, a MEC-2-like protein is expressed by mammalian sensory neurons. *Molecular and Cellular Neuroscience, 13*, 391–404.

Mayer, D. J., Price, D. D., & Becker, D. P. (1975). Neurophysiological characterization of the anterolateral spinal cord neurons contributing to pain perception in man. *Pain, 1*, 51–58.

McClesky, E. W., & Gold, M. S. (1999). Ion channels of nociception. *Annual Review of Physiology, 61*, 835–856.

McKemy, D. D., Neuhausser, W. M., and Julus, D. (2002). Identification of a cold receptor reveals a general role for TRP channels in thermosensation. *Nature, 416*, 52–58.

McMahon, S. B., & Bennett, D. L. (1999). Trophic factors and pain. In P. D. Wall, & R. Melzack (Eds.). *Textbook of pain* (4th ed., pp. 105–128). Edinburgh: Churchill-Livingstone.

Mense, S. (1977). Muscular nociceptors. *Journal of Physiology, 73*, 233–240.

Mills, K. R., Newham, D. J., & Edwards, R. H. T. (1982). Force, contraction frequency and energy metabolism as determinants of ischemic muscle pain. *Pain, 14*, 149–154.

Newham, D. J., & Jones, D. A. (1985). Intramuscular pressure in the painful human biceps. *Clinical Science, 69*, 27P.

Ochoa, J., & Torebjork, H. E. (1981). Pain from skin and muscle. *Pain*, Suppl. 1, 87.

Paintal, A. S. (1969). Mechanism of stimulation of type-J pulmonary receptors. *Journal of Physiology, 203*, 511–532.

Paintal, A. S. (1972). Cardiovascular receptors. In *Handbook of sensory physiology*, I: *Enteroceptors* (Vol. 3, pp. 1–45). Heidelberg: Springer Verlag.

Pertwee, R. G. (2001). Cannabinoid receptors and pain. *Progress in Neurobiology, 63*, 569–611.

Petrovic, P., Kalso, E., Petersson, K. M., & Ingvar, M. (2002). Placebo and opioid analgesia- imaging a shared neuronal network. *Science, 295*, 1737–1740.

Ploghaus, A., Tracey, I., & Gati, J. S., et al. (1999). Dissociating pain from its anticipation in the human brain. *Science, 284*, 1979–1981.

Pribram, K. H., & McGuinness, D. (1975). Arousal, activation and effort in the control of attention. *Psychology Review, 82*, 116–149.

Price, D. D., & Dubner, R. (1977). Neurons that subserve the sensory-discrimination aspects of pain. *Pain*, *3*, 307–338.

Price, D. D., Hayes, R. L., Ruda, M., & Dubner, R. (1978). Spatial and temporal transformations of input to the spinothalamic tract neurons and their relation to the somatic sensations. *Journal of Neurophysiology, 41*, 933–947.

Ralston, H. J. (1984). The fine structure of the ventrobasal thalamus of the monkey and the cat. *Brain Research*, 356, 228–241.

Ralston, H. J., & Ralston, D. D. (1994). Medial lemniscal and spinal projections to the Macaque thalamus: An electron microscopic study of differing GABAergic circuitry serving thalamic somatosensory mechanisms. *Journal of Neuroscience, 14*, 1485–1502.

Randic, M., Jiang, M. C., & Cerne, R. (1993). Long-term potentiation and long-term depression of primary afferent neurotransmission in the rat spinal cord. *Journal of Neuroscience, 13*, 5228–5241.

Rexed, B. (1952). The cytoarchitectonic organization of the spinal cord of the cat. *Journal of Comparative Neurology, 96*, 415–495.

Rice, A. S. C. (2001). Cannabinoids and pain. *Current Opinion in Investigative Drugs, 2*, 399–414.

Rowbotham, M. C., & Fields, H. L. (1996). The relationship of pain, allodynia and thermal sensation in post-herpetic neuralgia. *Brain, 119*(Pt. 2), 347–354.

Saver, J. L., & Rabin, J. (1997). The neural substrates of religious experience. *Journal of Neuropsychiatry and Clinical Neurosciences, 9*, 498–510.

Sawamoto, N., Honda, M., Okada, T., et al. (2000). Expectation of pain enhances responses to non-painful somatosensory stimulation in the anterior cingulate cortex and parietal operculum/posterior insula: An event related functional magnetic resonance imaging study. *Journal of Neuroscience, 20*, 7438–7445.

Selzer, M., & Spencer, W. A. (1969). Convergence of visceral and cutaneous afferent pathways in the lumbar spinal cord. *Brain Research, 14*, 331–348.

South, S. M., Kohno, T., Kaspar, B. K., Hegarty, D., Vissel, B., Drake, C. T., et al. (2003). A conditional deletion of the NR1 subunit of the NMDA receptor in adult spinal cord dorsal horn reduces NMDA currents and injury-induced pain. *Journal of Neuroscience, 23*, 5031–5040.

Stamford, J. A. (1995). Descending control of pain. *British Journal of Anaesthesia, 75*, 217–227.

Stubhaug, A., Breivik, H., Eide, P. K., Kreunen, M., & Foss, A. (1997). Mapping of punctate hyperalgesia around a surgical incision demonstrates that ketamine is a powerful suppressor of central sensitization to pain following surgery. *Acta Anaesthesiologica Scandinavica*, 41, 1124–1132, 1997.

Sufka, K. J., Schomburg, F. M., & Giordano, J. (1992). Receptor mediation of 5-HT-induced inflammation and nociception in rats. *Pharmacology, Biochemistry, and Behavior, 41*(1), 53–55.

Sweet, W. H., & Wepsic, J. G. (1968). Treatment of chronic pain by stimulation of primary afferent neurons. *Transactions of the American Neurological Association, 93*, 103.

Thompson, S. W. N., Dray, A., & Urban, L. (1994). Injury-induced plasticity of spinal reflex activity: NK-1 neurokinin receptor activation and enhanced A- and C-fiber mediated responses in the rat spinal cord in vitro. *Journal of Neuroscience, 14*, 3672–3687.

Torebjork, H. E. (1974). Afferent C-units responding to mechanical, thermal and chemical stimuli in human non-glabrous skin. *Acta Physiologica Scandinavica, 92*, 374.

Uchida, Y., & Murao, S. (1974). Bradykinin-induced excitation of afferent cardiac sympathetic C-fibers. *Japanese Heart Journal, 15*, 84–91.

Vecchiet, L., Giamberardino, M. A., & Marini, I. (1987). Immediate muscular pain from physical activity. In M. Tiengo, J. Eccles, A. C. Cuello, & D. Ottoson (Eds.), *Advances in pain research and therapy* (Vol. 10, pp. 193–206). New York: Raven Press.

Vogt, B. A., Finch, D. M., & Olson C. R. (1992). Functional homogeneity in the cingulate cortex: The anterior executive and posterior evaluative regions. *Cerebral Cortex, 2*, 435–443, 1992.

Waldmann, R., & Lazdunski, M. (1998). H+-gated cation channels: neuronal acid sensors in the NaC/DEG family of ion channels. *Current Opinion in Neurobiology, 8*, 418–424.

Watkins, L. R., & Mayer, D. J. (1982). The organization of endogenous opiate and nonopiate pain control systems. *Science, 216*, 1185–1192.

Wikler, D. (1979). Pain and the senses. In *Brain and mind: Ciba Foundation Symposium 69* (pp. 315–322). Amsterdam: Exerpta Medica.

Willis, W. D. (1979). Physiology of the dorsal horn and spinal cord pathways related tom pain. In R. F. Beers, & E. G. Bassett (Eds.), *Mechanisms of pain and analgesia compounds* (pp. 143–156). New York: Raven Press.

Willis, W. D. (1985). *The pain system*. Basel: Karger.

Willis, W. D., & Coggeshall, R. E. (1991). *Sensory mechanisms of the spinal cord*. New York: Plenum Press.

Woolf, C. J. (2004). Pain: Moving from symptom control toward mechanism-specific pharmacologic management. *Annals of Internal Medicine, 140*, 441–451.

Woolf, C. J., & Max, M. B. (2001). Mechanism-based pain diagnosis: issues for analgesic drug development. *Anesthesiology, 95*, 241–249.

Woolf, C. J., & Salter, M. W. (2000). Neuronal plasticity: Increasing the gain in pain. *Science, 288*, 1765–1769.

4

Overview of Pain: Classification and Concepts

James W. Woessner, MD, PhD

Pain is generally described as an unpleasant sensation. Pain, as a concept and symptom, is discussed and described throughout professional and lay medical literature. Pain is the reason for initial contact with any physician for the vast majority of medical problems, e.g., abdominal pain, chest pain, limb pain, low back pain. As such, pain *condition* classification is very sophisticated and advanced, as demonstrated by the IASP Chronic Pain Classification system (Merskey & Bogduk, 1994) and others (Derasari, 2000; Waldman, 2003).

The foundation for the history of physiological pain (mechanism) classification essentially started with Descartes (Melzack & Wall, 1965) in the 17th century but has not been framed in these terms until recently (Thienhaus & Cole, 1998, 2001). The history of pain condition classification is synonymous with the history of pain in humankind.

Only recently have physician neuroscientists and medical doctors begun to focus on pain mechanisms that are the foundation for understanding pain conditions and, therefore, for pain classification (Dallel & Voisin, 2001). This effort should proceed rapidly because much information is already available. However, this progression is hindered by the difficulties of transferring scientific knowledge to medical practice.

The main reason to classify (i.e., label or name) clinical presentations of symptoms centered around pain is to facilitate communication between patient and doctor for better pain care outcomes. The goal of therapy is to reduce suffering and increase function, which is the overriding purpose for practicing pain management and is at the core of this textbook and of medicine itself (Fields & Martin, 2001).

THE PRESENT STATE OF PAIN THEORY AND THOUGHT

Pain is described in a myriad of ways:

- In temporal terms: chronic pain, subacute pain, and acute pain
- In characterizations: intermittent pain, intractable pain, lancinating pain, referred pain, burning pain, and dull pain
- In medical diagnoses: phantom pain, cancer pain, vascular pain, arthritic pain, nerve pain, muscle pain, fibromyalgia, myofascial pain, sympathetically maintained pain, and complex regional pain syndrome
- In mechanistic/etiologic terms: neuropathic and nociceptive pain
- In anatomic perceptional terms: headache, back pain, neck pain, facial pain, limb pain, abdominal pain, etc.
- In source or origin terms: central pain as originating in the spinal cord or brain, or peripheral pain
- In psychiatric/psychogenic terms: psychosomatic ("all-in-the-head") pain, etc.

Caudill (1995) analyzed pain from different angles to emphasize its complexity:

- Biologically — Serves as a signal that the body has been harmed.

- Psychologically — Is experienced as emotional suffering.
- Behaviorally — Alters the way a person moves and acts.
- Cognitively — Calls for thinking about its meaning, its cause, and possible remedies.
- Spiritually — Serves as a reminder of mortality.
- Culturally — Tests a people's fortitude or forces their submission.

DSM-IV-TR PAIN DISORDERS

Pain Disorders are coded for their medical conditions in the *DSM-IV-TR* (American Psychiatric Association, 2000; First and Pincus, 2000) as follows:

307.80 Pain Disorder Associated with Psychological Factors
307.89 Pain Disorder Associated with Both Psychological Factors and a General Pain Condition

Elsewhere, the *DSM-IV-TR* (First & Pincus, 2000) attributes neural dysfunction to pain. Again, these are only descriptive categories and do not provide insight into underlying pain mechanism. Suffering, or the affective component, is not separated.

PAIN CLASSIFICATION CHARACTERISTICS

Pain has been classified by anatomic location, body system, duration, severity, frequency, and etiology (Cole, 2002). Merskey and Bogduk (1994) have done a prodigious job of compiling numerous pain conditions, basically all pain conditions mentioned in modern medical literature. Refer to Table 4.1 for a summary of the characteristics of this and other current systems of pain classification.

To add complexity, many factors, such as culture, personality, psychosocial stressors, nutritional status, and other disease states, can be involved to influence the degree of perceived pain and to confound understanding of the causal factors of the pain.

Healthcare professionals and the general public tend to think of location first for most pain classification systems. Waldman (2002, 2003) did so in listing and describing many locations for both common and uncommon pain conditions.

The simplest traditional categorization of pain has been "acute" and "chronic." Acute pain is usually just a result of the stimulation of a normally functioning pain detection system and serves to allow us to avoid or minimize tissue damage. Chronic pain merely means that pain is perceived over a long period of time, which is often arbitrarily set at 3 to 6 months.

However, while the chronology of pain has further subdivided pains basically into "acute" and "chronic," there is a mechanistic relationship, i.e., acute pain is simple nociceptive pain and chronic pain is a complex mix of pathologies along the neural pathways. Dr. Lippe (1998) has suggested the useful terms, *eudynia* (good pain) and *maldynia* (bad pain). As a generalization, many would describe eudynia as acute, and maldynia as chronic, although actual, individual cases tend to be more complex in both cases.

"Biopsychosocial" considerations are one step up from the "traditional" classification. The "pathogenetic"

TABLE 4.1
Pain Classification Systems

Categories	I	II	III	IV	V
Traditional	Acute	Subacute	Chronic		
Biopsychosocial	Acute	Recurrent acute	Cancer related	Chronic nonmalignant	
Pathogenetic	Primary	Secondary	TX. Effect (chemotherapy, tissue trauma, edema, etc.)		
ICD-9[a]	Disease process	Pain location	Secondary		
Dickerson (special case adapted by Brookoff, 2000, who elaborates the various subtypes)	Neuropathic	Inflammatory	Long-term		
IASP[b,c]	Region	System	Chronology	Intensity	Etiology

Note: The "traditional" classification scheme addresses chronology, location, and gross mechanisms.

[a] International Classification of Diseases, 9th edition.

[b] International Association for the Study of Pain.

[c] Merkey & Bogduk, 1994.

TX = therapy; Effect = therapy effect.

system grossly indicates the cause, primary or secondary, as major disease classifications. Inflammatory and long-term designations can involve both nociceptive and neuropathic pain. The IASP system provides a more detailed description of the pain, but fails to approach the cause, except generally in Etiology; the IASP definition of pain avoids linking pain to a specific stimulus.

The biopsychosocial model includes four categories: acute, recurrent acute, cancer-related, and chronic non-malignant pain. The first two categories deal with timing issues; the latter two categories speak to whether cancer is involved. Although useful in incorporating the issue of suffering, we suggest that these categories bear little relationship to mechanisms of pain. Except, perhaps, for vascular headaches, identifying the location of the pain is not necessary to basic understanding. The basic pain mechanisms are the same — whether for arm, leg, abdominal, or ear pain. Further, we think that the mechanisms of pain and pain pathways are the same, whether or not cancer is involved.

The most advanced concepts are expressed by Craig (2002), who states that pain is just one manifestation of the mind–body homeostasis system. From the patient's point of view, the spectrum of pain control spans temporary treatments (usually pharmaceutical) in suppressing pain to permanent remission or cure of underlying pathology/disease.

Obviously, these are all very useful concepts; but, are still generally academic in nature and do not provide much practical help to a physician. Concepts of pain pathophysiology, and thus classification, are abundantly available in the scientific and medical literatures. There is a need to refine and clarify all of this information and apply it as simply as possible to the treatment of pain in the physician's office.

PAIN AND SUFFERING

Pain is an unpleasant sensation appreciated as suffering. Most of the present pain classification systems actually include suffering as an essential part of the pain condition described. If suffering is removed, then, theoretically, pain can occur without suffering and would then logically seldom come to medical attention.

Suffering, as a separate life experience, may remain in the psychopsychiatric realm and not be objectively measurable for some time. There is an implied linkage between pain and suffering, which we disconnect here.

PAIN IS A MICROSCOPIC EVENT

Certainly, the first step is to understand that nociceptive pain is not a psychological event; it is a microscopic physical, chemical, or thermal event.

Acute, noxious stimulation of nociceptive pain (detecting something at the pain nerve ending), which may also precede neuropathic pain (hypersensitive transmission pathways), occurs at microscopic pain nerve endings as a signal that something is wrong, physically, chemically, or thermally. The neurotransmitters across synapses and endogenous and exogenous neurotoxic substances are microscopic. The upstream normally functioning peripheral and central neurons are microscopic. Then, neuropathic pain is, by definition, pathology of neurons. Because neurons are microscopic, peripherally or centrally, neuropathic pain can be likewise nothing but a "microscopic" event.

The presence of macroscopic pathology may or may not explain local pain, nociceptively or neuropathically. Macroscopic pathology, in other words, is not necessary, and may even be unrelated, for pain to occur or pain to be perceived. However, many patients and clinicians seek macroscopic pathology as *the* explanation for pain and suffering, e.g., most low back pain patients think of a "slipped disc" first, even though at least 85% of low back pain is nonspecific and, indeed, microscopic.

Functional MRI (Coghill et al., 1994) or PET scans (Iadarola et al., 1995) can show characteristic areas of activation in response to noxious stimuli in both nociceptive and neuropathic pan states. While not yet used in daily clinical practice, this information illustrates that pain is measurable in that it cuases physiological brain phenomena akin to "perception." Suffering is likely to be manifested in different patterns, sometimes with the areas activated by pain, and sometimes without the coincidence of pain. Thus, there are some cases that theoretically could have pain without suffering. Lepers have no pain and no direct suffering (Brand, 1993).

PAIN MECHANISMS

It has been known in medical science for decades that evolutionarily advanced somatic A-delta fibers and primitive sympathetic C-fibers transmit pain signals under specific circumstances. In addition to transmitting cold information, the A-delta fibers also transmit thermal and mechanical pain information relatively quickly and with precise locational information to the central nervous system. The C-fibers, on the other hand, transmit thermal and mechanical pain information relatively slowly and rather imprecisely to the central nervous system, i.e., warm pain and achy/burning pain are seen by the central nervous system as "through fogged glass."

Perception may be defined as the localization and quantification by the central nervous system of signals from the A-delta and C-fiber pain pathways. Present pain *condition* classification systems are helpful, but these classification systems are complex and do not seem to be organized to provide the practicing physician with handles

TABLE 4.2
Peripheral Nerve Fiber Types/Characteristics

Class\Units	Stimuli/Function	Perception	Conduction Velocity (m/s)	Diameter (microns)	Myelinated
A-alpha fibers	Motor contraction Efferent transmission	None direct	30–85	12–22	Yes
A-beta fibers	Vibration, pressure Afferent transmission	Vibration, pressure	30–70	5–12	Yes
A-delta fibers*	Cold sensation, pain Fast pain, localized touch Afferent transmission	Cold sensation, pain Localized touch	5–30	1–5	Yes
C-fibers**	Hot sensation, pain Slow pain, generalized touch Afferent transmission	Hot sensation and pain Generalized touch	0.5–2.0	0.3–1.3	No

Note: Based on Haines, 1997; Cousins & Bridenbaugh, 1998; Ganong, 2003.

* Spinal laminas I and V.
** Spinal laminas I and II.
*** C-fibers can still be clumped and embedded in other nonconducting tissue.

that can help the physician more effectively treat those patients presenting with pain — particularly chronic pain. Medical doctors depend on knowledge of the pathophysiology, or at least a diagnosis, to decide on treatment. Thus, to maximize likelihood of a correct and effective treatment and a positive outcome, physicians need to understand where and what the pain mechanism is and how the pain is perceived.

A relatively recent trend has been to look at basic mechanisms of pain (Dallel & Voisin, 2001). By doing so, we are seeking to look one level deeper at the underlying mechanisms so treatment can be facilitated. Dallel and Voisin (2001) recognize the need for a clear roadmap: "Once pain-generating mechanisms are known, it becomes possible to establish the appropriate treatment of pain." We suggest that refining these concepts is a giant step in the right direction and propose to present a simple, clear pathophysiologically based classification model. We contend that pain treatment should primarily focus on reversing pathologic mechanisms that cause the pain in the first place.

Any one or combination of the microscopic mechanisms can contribute to pain: nerve pain ending/"sensor" stimulation, neural "wire" misfiring, and central nervous system/"perceptron" dysfunction (Woessner, 2002a).

RELEVANT NEUROANATOMY AND NEUROPHYSIOLOGY

It appears that the locational patterns of disease, including neuropathology, and the mixture of these mechanisms that are dynamic over time make understanding the basic neuroanatomy and neurophysiology important.

Nerves, or neurons, are long tubes of protoplasm (rather than a series of sausage links), which may, or may not, be surrounded by poorly conducting myelin (insulation). Nerves generally come in various sizes and characteristics and have numerous branches to other neurons. Neurons interact/communicate via numerous electrical (gap junction) and chemical synapses. There are motor (efferent) neurons, which primarily carry signals from the brain to muscles, and sensory (afferent) neurons, which primarily carry signals from the periphery to the brain.

The primary focus for investigation by pain practitioners should be the small sensory nerves, which carry unpleasant signals to the brain that may or may not be perceived by the brain. Descartes depicted a noxious stimulus causing information to flow along a pain pathway to the brain that is then perceived as pain in his famous illustration of a boy's foot touching the edge of a fire (as in Melzack & Wall, 1965). Characteristics of nerve fibers, including classification and conduction velocities, are listed in Table 4.2.

There are three types of fibers that carry pain signals to the brain — A-beta, A-delta, and C-fibers. The first two are evolutionarily modern fibers that are myelinated (insulated) and carry nerve impulses rapidly to the cortical regions of the brain (Haines, 1997).

Neural signals are conveyed by sodium and potassium ions moving out and into neurons via voltage-gated channels in specific patterns to form a relatively slow (see Table 4.2; not 186,000 mi/sec) moving wave of information to, from, and within the central nervous system. These voltage-gated channels are concentrated in "holes" in the myelin (nodes of Ranvier) of the somatic nerves (A fibers), but are more evenly distributed in the more primitive, unmyelinated nerve fibers (C-fibers).

In the absence of neural wire damage, there is a continuum across various numbers of synapses (switching stations) from the source or place of stimulation to the site of perception. At the distal end of sensory nerves, there are various types of nerve endings. When it comes to pain nerves, those endings are so-called "free" nerve endings. At the proximal end are the perceptor areas of the brain (Haines, 1997).

The A-beta fibers are probably reserved for deep, lancinating pain; certainly these carry vibratory signals. The A-delta fibers are somatic, myelinated fibers that have primary connections to the cortical regions of the brain. These fibers convey sharp, lancinating, easily localized pain signals; these pain sensations usually pass quickly unless constant or recurrent stimulation occurs.

Then, a more generalized, burning/aching pain sensation is perceived in the brain. This latter pain takes longer to pass. The C-fibers are relatively primitive and are not covered by myelin and conduct rather slowly to the subcortical part of the brain (Haines, 1997). Thus, when one experiences a paper cut, one quickly appreciates a "zing" followed by a "burning" pain. You know exactly where the "zing" comes from (A-delta pain pathways), but the brain "sees" the burning pain through "fogged glass" (C-fiber pain pathways).

Now that we know generally how these small nerves work, we need to know where these nerve endings and small pain nerves reside. Our standard anatomy books often do not depict or describe these networks of nerves. Dr. Fishman (2000), an insightful pain doctor, has described in his book entitled *The War on Pain* that these nerve fibers cover and line most of the tissue plane surfaces throughout the body.

HOW PAIN IS MEASURED

If pain is separated from suffering, it is easy to understand that pain is then measurable physiologically. As indicated in Table 4.2, neurophysiologists have assigned identifiable physiological functions to different nerve types. As with large-fiber functional testing, the small fibers, i.e., the A-delta and C-fibers, can be tested electrically and thermally. Measurement of small pain fiber function by preferred frequency transmission measurements (= current perception threshold [CPT]) has been clinically available for more than ten years. Thermal testing is as old as neurology itself; the basic physical examination includes qualitative testing with the handle of a reflex hammer as is for comparative cold sensation and heated for comparative warm sensation. In the laboratory, neuroscientists have been able to quantify thermal nerve, i.e., A-delta and C-fiber, function for decades. Machines are available now to test the function of pain nerve pathways in clinical settings. Testing pain

nerves thus provides valuable information for diagnosis, and more effective treatment (Woessner, 2002b).

Imaging of pain perception has also been accomplished with transcranial magnetic stimulation (Gale, 2004), positron emission tomography (PET) (Iadarola, et al., 1995), single photon emission computed tomography (SPECT), functional magnetic resonance imaging (fMRI) (Coghill, et al., 1999) and near infrared spectroscopy techniques (NIRS) (Cope, 2000). "Research in diagnostic imaging of neuronal activity is … endemic at many academic medical centers. … The ability to map transmission of pain and other disorders not only to block but to alter and reprogram neurotransmission is now a very active and ever-changing research area (Cope, 2000)."

An interesting question arises from this research: Can a human being perceive pain without suffering? My clinical experience indicates that this is exactly so. Most clinicians, indeed, do understand that patients suffer for a variety of reasons. Thus, what medicine really needs is Suffering Relief Specialists rather than Pain Medicine Specialists per se. With the proper mindset, a pain specialist should be able to tackle the broader, and sometimes separate, issue of suffering. Thus, measuring and understanding physiological pain and comparing the results to perceived pain allow the clinician to more precisely treat "pain patients."

PROPOSED PHYSIOLOGICAL PAIN MODEL

This physiological pain model (Woessner, 2002a) focuses on underlying causative mechanisms, as opposed to the pain condition classification systems listed in Table 4.1. To review terms, nociceptive pain is merely normal functioning of the neural sensor/wire/perception system. This system serves useful purposes in alerting the brain to bodily injury. Neuropathic and central pain, however, is a manifestation of true dysfunction and can be the "disease" itself.

If we consider a bundle of axons, neuropraxia, axonotmesis, and neurotmesis represent points along a complex continuum of damage to axons and nerves. The three possibilities for individual axons are normal function, hyperfunction (hyperesthesia, hyperalgesia, hyperpathia, and allodynia), and hypofunction (hypoesthesia, hypoalgesia, and conduction block). Hyperfunction can also be thought of as sensitization or irritation. The ultimate hypofunction is axon death without regrowth. Free nerve endings can also be sensitized or irritated, which is considered here to be in the neuropathic category.

Understanding neurophysiology of pain pathways is helpful. Further, we propose that all pain can be understood by considering problems of stimulation of sensors, conduction along nerves, and/or perception in the spinal cord and brain. The perception then may involve feedback, either positive or negative (i.e., release or not of native painkiller, e.g., endorphins). If negative, the result is, by and large, a dysfunction that conceptually could stand alone.

Haines (1997) describes an electronic schematic of the nerve cell membrane and forms the basis of concepts discussed below. A key concept is that the neural pain system follows basic electrochemical principles.

The analogy of the neural net in complex electrical circuitry seems to be an accurate one. The pain sensors (free nerve endings) are relatively simple. The wires (peripheral nerves) are even simpler. The central nervous system is incredibly complex. We are discovering that the spinal cord is not just a transmission device; complex interactions can occur here also. Finally, the complexity of the brain is difficult to imagine with millions of neurons and billions of synapses (Haines, 1997).

Stimulation of the sensors is nociceptive or eudynia. Malfunction of the wires and perceptron is neuropathic. Note that neuropathic pain is divided into central and peripheral parts of the pain nervous system because, while relatively little is known about either, these two parts of the pain pathways are clearly distinguished from each other.

Essentially no pain condition is unifactorial. For the actual pain conditions that the practicing physician encounters, it is useful to assess the pain using a conceptual framework. This approach is useful as a tool in assessing an individual patient's pain and deciding on treatment within the conceptual pain model.

STIMULATION OF PAIN SENSORS (NOCICEPTION)

Normal stimulation of pain sensors is the "good" pain described in *The Gift Nobody Wants* (Brand, 1993). It is termed "eudynia" in that the free nerve endings of pain pathways are working perfectly and normally — giving good information to the body and brain that tissue is being damaged — or is about to be damaged — and that the body needs to do something about it. Impact on mechano(noci)ceptors, heat or cold stimulation of thermo(noci)-ceptors, or caustic chemicals on chemo(noci)ceptors start the process of perception of pain. In other words, this type of pain is based on mechanical, thermal, and/or chemical stimulation of normally functioning pain nerves; nerves that detect pain as a signal indicating impending or active tissue damage.

MISFIRING OF WIRES (NEUROGENIC OR NEUROPATHIC PAIN)

During the normal transmission of neural signals to the central nervous system, any damage to the neural pathway itself may manifest itself analogously to "static" in radio transmissions. This neural "static" alters the neural signal and is then perceived as pain. Nerves can be damaged just as any soft tissue, in which these nerves occur, can be damaged. Neuropathic pain, therefore, is a result of damaged and malfunctioning wires/nerve fibers. One can also conceive of similar damage to nerve fibers in the central nervous system. As long as those fibers are not the end of the pathway, the phenomenon is the same. Damaged nerve fibers follow a course of anatomic and physiologic change involving irritation (hyperactivity) and dysfunction/death (hypoactivity) (Iadarola et al., 1995). Upon nerve death, of course, signals can no longer be transmitted along the neural pathway.

Mechanisms of hypersensitive or pain neuropathology include "rapid repriming" of sodium channels or "electrical bursting in pain signaling neurons." These sodium channels are specific to the "spinal sensory neurons" (Waxman, 2001, p. 382). Waxman et al. (2001) provide significant detail of this mechanism without indicating the nerve type; we assume that a similar mechanism works for both the A-delta and C-fiber pain nerves and, at least, is related to local microscopic mechanical and chemical occurrences.

DYSFUNCTION OF PERCEPTION (CENTRAL PAIN)

The most complex, and very difficult to study, part of the pain pathway(s) is in the central nervous system and occurs at the end of the neural pathway, where these signals are interpreted. Perception and consequences can occur in the dorsal horn. If central neurons malfunction in any part of the pain perception pathway, one possible consequence is that the brain perceives "pain." The environment of the central nervous system can also play a part. This complex system can be considered together to be a *perceptron* (Woessner, 2002a). This word has been chosen to convey the true complexity and computer-like nature of these central nervous system phenomena. If the "perception" is the cause of the perceived pain, this pain pathology can also be called central neurogenic pain.

ANTINOCICEPTIVE DYSFUNCTION

The human body possesses antipain (antinociception) systems including endorphins, enkephalins, etc. that are utilized as natural pain killers and neural feedback modulation to reduce perception of pain and the quantity of pain signals arriving at the "perceptron." In normal function, the human body releases these painkillers to modulate or mollify pain. At the very least, if these chemicals are not released or do not arrive at the affected receptors, the perceptrons will appreciate pain or greater pain, in the presence of pain signals (Craig, 2002).

Pain experts have also recognized that pain is nociceptive and/or neuropathic (Abrams, 2000), which are commonly thought to be equivalent to "acute" and "chronic," respectively. The difficulty is that most acute and chronic pain conditions are a combination of both nociceptive and neuropathic pain, which can and do change over time. An acutely damaged nerve can result in acute neuropathic pain, and chronic arthritis can result in a chronic recurrent nociceptive pain.

Antinociceptive dysfunction (Brookoff, 2000) occurs in the perceptron (brain and/or spinal cord) and can worsen both nociceptive and neuropathic pains; antinociceptive pain, in other words, is dysfunction of the natural pain modulation system (Heinricher, 2002). Then, externally delivered painkillers are antinociceptive, as well.

Then, there are natural pain modulations that can malfunction resulting in more pain (hyperalgesia) or even pain without a noxious stimulus (allodynia). In this physiological manner, pain can be better understood. Each possible mechanism is dynamic in anatomical location, along pain pathways, and over time; each mechanism is individual and unique according to the underlying pain condition.

COMPLEX PAIN FROM A MIXTURE OF MECHANISMS

Over time and with the presence of widespread and/or severe causal factors, more than one aspect of the pain perception system may be malfunctioning at the same time. For example, it is common for patients to develop pain in a limb due to trauma that injures small pain fibers in addition to the other soft tissue. One can have stump pain along with phantom pain, possibly not coincidentally. Central sensitization can develop over time in a patient with ongoing peripheral disease. Dysfunctional efferent reflexes or reactions can change the physical and chemical environment of pain sensors, which then causes nociceptive pain as in complex regional pain syndrome (CRPS).

REFERRED PAIN AND NONTENDER SYNDROMES

Likewise, clinicians should be aware of pain perceived in body areas that are not tender on palpation. In other words, referred pain is pain that is perceived separately from the true pain generator and was first discussed in publications by Sturge (1883), Ross (1887), and others (Bonica and Loesser, 2001; Coda & Bonica, 2001). Local acute pain is relatively easy to understand, and physicians usually appreciate radicular pain, which is one type of referred pain. The concept of referred pain can be difficult for clinicians and patients alike.

Physicians strive to achieve the best possible understanding of pain conditions and try to find an acceptable label or diagnosis, even for conditions and presentations that are uncommon and/or difficult to understand. As the patient's presentation becomes more complex and as pain conditions become more chronic, physiologically legitimate presentations may not be understood.

Understanding referred pain requires specialized and diverse knowledge along with wide clinical experience. Suggesting that complaints are "non-anatomic" or "non-physiologic" may very well be a clear indication of the diagnostician's ignorance rather than a negative reflection on the motives of the patient. Individual variations in the presenting pain patterns complicate interpretation. Even well-known and classic pain patterns may be difficult to diagnose in the face of complex disease and multiple causes of pain. There are other complex, and poorly understood, pain conditions defined below.

REFERRED PAIN MECHANISMS

Kosek and Hansson (2003) have specifically found that "referred pain is most likely a consequence of misinterpretation of the origin of input from the stimulated focal pain area, due to excitation of neurons somewhere along the neuraxis with projected fields in the referred pain area … [this] suggests that the divergence of the input is not reciprocally arranged."

The best-known referred pain patterns may originate from viscera and myofascial trigger points. Each type is presented below. Other pain syndromes, with different names, however, also fall within this general category with the broad definition given above, where the pain is perceived at a site separate from the pathology.

Ombregt et al. (2003) have provided more precise principles limiting and defining referred pain:

1. Radicular pain is directly related to spinal segments.
2. The perceived pain site and causative pathology are usually on same side of midline.
3. The main pain is usually felt deeply.
4. The referred pain is referred distally within a dermatome, but not necessarily throughout that dermatome.
5. Referred pain may be contiguous with or may be separated from pathology.

The author proposes a sixth principle (Woessner, 2003): that the site of perceived pain is not tender, whereas the site of pathology is tender. Central pain phenomena do not necessarily fit completely within these general principles, but it is still useful to understand the similarities.

Selzer and Spencer (1969) suggest five underlying mechanisms involved with referred pain:

1. "Convergence-Projection" describes one neuron receiving impulses from two sources; i.e., peripheral neurons, resulting in the central path-

ways not being able to distinguish between the sources (Ruch, 1960).

2. "Peripheral Branching of Primary Afferent Nociceptors" involves the fact that single neurons are very long narrow tubes that may have various branches that come from different peripheral sources, again making it impossible for central pain pathways to distinguish the source.

3. "Convergence-Facilitation" is ephatic transmission that occurs where nerves from two different body areas are in close proximity and results in signals from the viscera being transmitted along an associated spinothalamic tract to be perceived in the brain as coming from various skin areas (originally proposed by Ruch, 1960).

4. "Sympathetic Nervous System Activity," which is suggested to restrict blood flow to an area causing pain in that area or by releasing substances that sensitize nerve endings in the area of perceived pain such that hyperesthesia or allodynia occurs. Except as illustrated elsewhere, this possibility does not make much sense.

5. "Convergence or Image Projection at the Supraspinal Level" describes ephaptic transmission in central locations rather than at the dorsal root, or some similar mechanism to be perceived as being pain in one area while the stimulation comes from another.

There are, of course, other possibilities and/or contributing factors to referred pain:

1. Note that when nerve root pathology affects only the nerve root surface pain nerves, we expect local pain to be perceived and local tenderness to be elicited. For more severe pathology that extends physically as pressure and chemically to the pain nerves inside the nerve root, we expect that the brain would perceive the pain more distal to nontender locations in the feet or hands, understood as "radicular" pain. This mechanism is likely for all non-central syndromes considered here.

2. Mistransmission or ephatic transmission solely in the central nerve system, as in the phantom pain phenomenon discussed in the labeled section below.

3. The embryologic relationship of the internal organs to spinal levels, which is then directly related to sympathetic chain levels. The importance of the embryologic levels must reflect organization in the central nervous system. In addition, the main nerve fiber type of the sympathetic nerve system is the C-fiber, the primitive, unmyelinated pain fiber, emphasizing that ontogeny follows phylogeny.

4. Along these pathways, neuropathic pain can also be referred and, in some cases, may indicate that the nerve is "trying" to normalize, to heal. Certainly, dead neurons do not transmit pain signals or any other impulse.

5. Central pain syndromes could very easily fit into the same category as phantom pain. Deafferent pain syndrome is consistent with "total body amputation" from the head/brain and represents a pain syndrome without nerve impulses of any sort coming from the periphery. In other words, the pathology or dysfunction is in the neurons of the central nervous system, but not necessarily just in the brain.

6. Wide dynamic range (WDR) neurons and interneurons of the spinal cord represent neuropathic dysfunction that could by specific, complex mechanisms end with the perception of pain where there is no pathology; the pathology, in this case, is in the spinal cord.

7. Sympathetic chain pathology is the same as the spinal cord pathology. We may eventually identify WDR neurons of the sympathetic chains; we will probably come up with a different name.

8. Patchy brain modulation of pain, i.e., antinociception, could well leave the brain appreciating pain where there is no pain with or without a reason, i.e., nerve impulses of any kind coming from elsewhere.

Certainly, more than one or all of these phenomena could occur together to form the various widespread and complex pain problems that a physician must manage and try to cure.

EMBRYOLOGY AND REFERRED PAIN

Various authors (Marcus, 1998; Ombregt et al., 2003) discuss the embryologic basis for referred pain. Certainly, the referred pain mechanisms must have a relationship to nerve pathways and networks. These pathways and networks are geometrically and positionally related to where the precursor structures occurred in early ontogenic stages and how these structures migrate during growth and maturation. Thus, referred pain patterns have an evolutionarily ancient (phylogenic) and developmentally individual relationship (ontogenic) to dermatomes, myotomes, sclerotomes, viscerotomes, etc. Central pathway and network pathology can probably be understood in the same way.

FACTORS CAUSING REFERRED PAIN

Ombregt et al. (2003) described factors that predispose to referred pain. Stronger central and/or proximal deep (vs. superficial) stimuli more likely cause the perception of pain beyond the pathology. Sclerotomal referred pain is more likely than myotomal referred pain, and much more likely than bone pain. This order of occurrence may be generally inversely related to intensity and pain-related dysfunction.

Marcus (1998) adds and states differently that "tenacious" pain stimulation is more likely to be referred; superficial pain is more likely to be localizable (less likely referred), deep (excluding bone) is more likely referred; soft tissue referred pain is less localizable, i.e., more likely referred; and distal pathology is more localizable than proximal.

VISCEROTOMES

Visceral referred pain is probably the most widely recognized, while still being the least understood of all the referred pain patterns. Head (1893) noted disturbances of sensation arising from visceral disorders. Cousins (1987) refers to these patterns as "viscerotomes." Lingappa and Farey (2000), in fact, describe "referred pain" as "the phenomenon in which injury to internal organs causes pain that localizes, in part, to surface structures or other organs clearly distinct from the site of primary injury. Typically, the pain is referred to other structures that have the same embryonic origin" (pp. 798). There are established patterns of referred pain from internal organs. Drewes et al. (2003) have provided a detailed description of the various referred visceral pain distributes, providing basic information to understand the complexities of viscerotomes.

Ephatic transmission is analogous to electrical shorting out. Via these shorts, "many different afferent sensory nociceptive neurons synapse with the same ascending fibers in the spinal cord," which causes the brain to mistake the origin of the pain signals; in other words, the pain feels like it is coming for some typical locations on the skin or nearby subcutaneous tissues and possibly deeper structures, rather than the actual internal organ from which the pain signals are coming (Lingappa & Farey, 2000, pp. 798–799). These scientists also suggest that the brain generally will have more recent memory of surface/subcutaneous pain and will "ignore" deep pain until an inciting event occurs.

With A-delta pain fiber involvement, a skin injury is easily locatable. Visceral pain is difficult for the human brain to locate because the pain is "referred" to the skin and involves sympathetic C-fibers, which subserve poorly localized pain.

Angina pectoris is well known to cause left arm pain, alerting to the possibility of impending myocardial infarc-

tion. Abdominal pain that becomes rapidly generalized implies perforation and leakage of fluid into the peritoneal cavity, irritating the parietal peritoneum. Biliary pain can radiate to the right inferior scapula. Pancreatic and abdominal aneurismal pain may radiate to the back. Ureteral colic classically is referred to the groin and thigh (Haist & Robbins, 2002).

The areas of the body to which visceral pain is referred are described in narrative rather in schematics. Note that we expect that each patient will display variations on these generalizations. Word descriptions may actually represent reality better than the various published schematics because each viscerotome schematic is different and inconsistent, with individuals and populations being unique and different to some degree.

COMMON PAIN RADIATION PATTERNS (WOESSNER, 2003)

Lungs: Pain is referred in a collar-like band completely around the neck from about C6 to T3 levels.

Diaphragm: Pain is referred in a pattern similar to the lungs.

Heart: Pain can be referred to around the mouth, but is more commonly referred over the left chest and contiguously down the anterior left arm and directly to the mid-back between the scapulae from T4 to T7.

Gallbladder: Pain is referred to superior and lateral right shoulder, offset superior similar in size and circular shape to the superficial distribution of the axillary nerve.

Liver: Pain is referred in a similar pattern to the heart, but only on the right hemi-body.

Stomach: Pain is referred just to the right of midline in the epigastric area and to the mid-back, just below the referred angina from T7 to T9.

Ovaries: Pain is referred to the skin area immediately over the ovaries anteriorly and directly posteriorly, but more lateral.

Appendix: Pain is referred to the umbilicus and then to McBurney's point in the right hypogastric area when parietal peritoneum becomes inflamed.

Kidneys: Pain is referred to the skin area somewhat below the kidneys, posteriorly only, and medial to the posterior referred ovarian pain; there is also an area half way down the right lateral thigh, the right chest just to the right of the lower sternum.

Ureters: Pain is referred to an anterior band across the pelvis, including the groin and the genitals, but not extending to the back.

Bladder: Pain is referred to a continuous area encompassing the sacrum from S2 down to the upper medial thighs.

RADICULAR PAIN

Radicular pain originates at the nerve root, cervical, thoracic, lumbar, or sacral, and typically radiates or is referred along a dermatome. Dermatomal pain suggests nerve root involvement from a herniated disc or other physical or chemical irritation at the nerve root exiting from the spinal canal.

Consistent with the definition, there can be various pathologies at the nerve roots, which include (1) nerve root compression from a herniated disc, (2) foraminal stenosis from bone spurs or arthritis irritating the nerve root, (3) nerve root pressure from mass lesions, (4) chemical changes at the nerve roots secondary to diabetes, (5) scarring from previous spinal surgery or chronic disc pathology, and (6) all other nerve root injuries. The radiating component is technically "referred pain." This type of "referred pain" is not a nociceptive process; it is neuropathic, even if momentary. Pain with such a specific distribution seems unlikely to even be central.

Thinking of the distribution of pain nerves in the cross section of a nerve root is instructive. If the pathology is minor, the pain on this surface of the nerve root is most affecting, and thus local pain is appreciate (Woessner, 2002a). With more compression the pain nerve pathways/axons deeper in the nerve root are affected and "fool" the brain into thinking that the pain is located more distal toward the limb involved.

OVERLAPPING DISTRIBUTIONS

The nerves that innervate dermatomes interdigitate at the borders to some extent, making the boundary edges fuzzy. In addition, the sensory distributions, which characterize and define dermatomes, may not be identical to the pain patterns. Therefore, exact determinations of pain perception distributions are not "cut and dried" (Bonica & Loeser, 2001).

REFERRED MUSCULAR PAIN

Referred muscle pain in voluntary muscles is most often accompanied by secondary hyperalgesia and hypotrophic changes. A schematic of these referral distributions is shown in *Bonica's Management of Pain* (Coda & Bonica, 2001).

"Myotomal" pain involves problems with the fascial tissue planes that surround muscle groups. While "myotomal" may not be the correct description, when muscles were injected with hypertonic saline, which is an experimental substance known to produce pain, mapped patterns of referred pain emerged (Coda & Bonica, 2001). While we would expect that these would be the same referred

pain patterns as myofascial trigger points, gross inspections reveal no clear congruence or overlap.

SCLEROTOMES

Pain referred from tendinous and/or ligamentous interfaces with bone surfaces has no specific, well-recognized name (Hackett, 1958). Sclerotomes are pain referral patterns from sites of enthesopathy, i.e., pathology of the collagenous attachments (tendons, ligaments, cartilage, etc.) to bones generated by inflammation (Bonica & Loeser, 2001).

DURAL PAIN PATTERNS

Bogduk (2003) has recognized that the spinal dura is innervated. Cailliet (1988) has further shown that the dura is innervated by sympathetic C-fibers. Ombregt et al. (2003) and Butler (1991) have postulated that certain pain perception patterns occur when the pain nerves on the dura are stimulated.

Certainly, these diffuse patterns do not even vaguely resemble dermatomal distributions. They are much more widespread than the limited zones of referred trigger point pain. For instance, dural nerves stimulated by scar tissue in the lumbar region may result in perceived pain and discomfort throughout the legs.

Kernig's and Brudzinski's signs, i.e., the meningeal signs (Gerard & Kleinfield, 1993), are reminiscent of this same phenomenon. By definition, these are consistent with meningeal irritation, i.e., dural irritation, where A-delta and C-fiber pain nerve endings occur, anteriorly and laterally (Cailliet, 1988).

THERMATOMES

There are thermal patterns of pain, which are probably related to the distribution of sympathetic C-fibers nerves and with sympathetic chain pathway components, without shorting, crossing over, emphatically to the A-delta fiber pathways.

Hooshmand (2000) has coined the word *thermatomes* to describe referred pain patterns related to the circulatory distribution of sympathetic C-fiber nerves. These relatively amorphous distributions are consistent with the observation that these C-fiber nerve pathways end up seeing pain "through fogged glass."

If we think of the possible evolutionary origin of the sympathetic chains, which in lower animals transmit all efferent and afferent nerve impulses, those pathways should be able to reestablish transmission pathways in compensation, much like collateral circulation.

FACIAL REFERRAL PATTERNS

Pain referral patterns in the innervation of the face and anterior neck are not completely appreciated by healthcare professionals.

Guyton & Hall (2000, pp. 558–560) show that:

Nasal sinus and eye aches radiate to a wide area around the eyes from below the nose and up to mid-fore.

Cerebral vault aches occur frontally to parietally at the ear.

Brainstem and cerebellar vault aches occur from the ear through the entire occiput.

PHANTOM PAIN (WOESSNER, 2003)

Phantom sensations and pain are well-described phenomena, which means that the brain perceives the existence of a body part, from which no nerve impulses could possibly be emanating.

In a sense, phantom pain is the ultimate "referred pain." Perceived pain location is obviously not where the pain is originating because there cannot be peripheral pain nerve stimulation. Stump and neuroma pains are separate pain phenomena and are not referred pain, and therefore, these pains are not phantom pain. There is surprising confusion about these, i.e., stump and neuroma pains versus phantom pain.

REFERRED PAIN DUE TO HEALING PAIN NERVES

Healing nerves and tissue cause pain by the following:

1. Inflammation is part of the healing process; the natural chemicals involved are caustic to pain nerve endings. The treatment dilemma here is if you stop the pain with anti-inflammatory medications, do you not also stop the healing?

2. Consequent muscle spasms occur. Spasm or cramping muscles change, usually decrease circulation; ischemia causes pain by causing a caustic microenvironment around nerve endings. In addition, the spasm/cramping muscles are causing pressure on the A-delta and C-fibers that occur in the myofascial tissue planes.

3. Improper healing of any tissue can reasonably contort it and cause pain and dysfunction; such nociceptive pain is caused by pressure on and/or caustic chemical environment around the nerve endings; neuropathic pain would come from the changed neuroanatomy, thus changed neurophysiology, and also from the changes in the chemical microenvironment.

HOW, IN THE END, DOES PAIN AND REFERRED PAIN CLASSIFICATION HELP?

For nociceptive pain, the primary goal is to resolve ("cure") or remove the stimulant, i.e., the causative pathology, while covering up the pain. For neuropathic pain, the goal is to stop the irritation and promote rebuilding the damaged nerves or normalization of their function. For central pain, the goal is to employ techniques to change the central nervous system neural environment. For antinociceptive pain, the goal is to normalize pain perception and reestablish natural painkiller production and function.

The ultimate approach for effectively treating pain is individualizing and balancing the various approaches for optimal results in complex chronic pain cases. By understanding the underlying mechanisms, physicians clearly have a better chance of effectively serving their patients with better pain relief. Suffering is probably the most difficult part of pain to quantify and treat. However, it is expected that suffering will improve as we improve our abilities to treat pain.

SUMMARY

Pain classification depends on the understanding of pain mechanisms. The more we know about these mechanisms, the more likely we are to apply the appropriate terms to the pain conditions that we see in our clinics. We cannot abandon the time-honored names that we are using.

Basically, there are two categories, i.e., nociceptive and neuropathic pain. Eudynia and maldynia, respectively, may actually be more useful terms because the accepted terminology may be limited by the historical processes involved in pain (condition) classification. Accurate consideration of these basic concepts should be applied to every pain condition encountered by the practitioner in order to plan appropriate treatment of the pain.

Referred pain is neuropathologic, i.e., not nociceptive. Referred pain is important because it may have diagnostic value. Referred pain adds another layer of complexity to the process of making a diagnosis. Making the diagnosis by artfully and systematically combining the findings obtained from the clinical history and physical examination allows the clinician to formulate a coherent treatment plan.

REFERENCES

Abram, S. E. (1985). Pain pathways and mechanisms. *Seminars in Anesthesia, 4,* 267–279.

American Psychiatric Association. (2000). Pain disorder. *Diagnostic and statistical manual of mental disorders: DSM-IV-TR.* (4th ed., text revision, pp. 498–503). Washington, DC: American Psychiatric Association.

Bogduk, N. (2003). Neck pain and whiplash. In T. S. Jensen et al. *Clinical pain management: Chronic pain* (pp. 505–507). London: Arnold Publishers.

Bonica, J. J. & Loeser, J. D. (2001). Applied anatomy relevant to pain. In J. D. Loeser et al. (Eds.), *Bonica's management of pain* (3rd ed., pp. 196–221). Philadelphia: Lippincott/Williams & Wilkins.

Brand, P. (1993). *The gift nobody wants*. New York: HarperCollins.

Brookoff, D. (2000). Chronic pain: 1. A new disease? Hospital Practice. McGraw-Hill [online]. Available: http://www.hosppract.com/issues/2000/07/brook.htm. Retrieved September 22, 2004.

Butler, D. S. (1991). *Mobilisation of the nervous system*. New York: Churchill Livingstone.

Cailliet, R. (1988). *Low back pain syndrome. Pain series* (4th ed.). Philadelphia: F.A. Davis.

Caudill, M. A. (1995). *Managing pain before it manages you*. New York: Guilford Press.

Chado, H. N. (1995). The current perception threshold evaluation of sensory nerve function in pain management. *Pain Digest, 5*, 127–134.

Coda, B. A., and Bonica, J. J. (2001). General considerations of acute pain. In J. D. Loeser et al. (Eds.), *Bonica's management of pain* (3rd ed., pp. 222–240). Philadelphia: Lippincott/Williams & Wilkins.

Coghill, R. C., McHaffie, J. G., & Yen, Y. (in press). Neural correlates of inter-individual differences in the subjective experience of pain. *Proceedings of the National Academy of Sciences*.

Coghill, R. C., Sang, C. N., Maisog, J. M., & Iadarola, M. J. (1999). Pain intensity processing within the human brain: A bilateral, distributed mechanism. Journal of Neurophysiology, 82, 1934–1943.

Coghill, R. C., Talbot, J. D., Evans, A. C., Meyer, E., Gjedde, A., Bushnell, M. C., & Duncan, G. H. (1994). Distributed processing of pain and vibration by the human brain. *Journal of Neuroscience, 14* (7), 4095–4108.

Cole, B. E. (2002). Pain management: Classifying, understanding, and treating pain. *Hospital Physician, 38*(6), 23–30.

Cope, D. K. (2000). Pain medicine in the year 2020. Available at http://www.asahq.org/Newsletters/2000/11_00/cope.htm#cope.

Cousins, M. J. (1987). Visceral pain. In S. Andersson et al. (Eds.), *Chronic non-cancer pain: Assessment and practical management*. Lancaster: MTP Press.

Cousins, M. J., & Bridenbaugh, P. O. (Eds.). (1998). Neural blockade. In *Clinical anesthesia and management of pain* (3rd ed.). Philadelphia: Lippincott-Raven.

Craig, A. D. (2002). Specificity and integration in central pain pathways. *Abstracts, 10th World Congress on Pain* (p. 124). Seattle: IASP Press.

Dallel, R., & Voisin, D. (2001). Towards a pain treatment based on the identification of the pain-generating mechanisms? *European Neurology, 45*, 128–132.

Derasari, M. D. (2000). Taxonomy of pain syndromes: Classification of chronic pain syndromes. In P. P. Raj (Ed.), *Practical management of pain* (3rd ed., pp. 10–16). St. Louis, MO: Mosby.

Drewes, A. M. et al. (2003). Gut pain and hyperalgesia induced by capsaicin: a human experimental model. *Pain, 104*, 333–341.

Fields, H. L., & Martin, J. B. (2001). Pain. In E. Braunwald et al. (Eds.), *Harrison's principles of internal medicine* (15th ed., pp. 55–60). New York: McGraw-Hill.

First, M. B., & Pincus, H. A. (2000). *Diagnostic and statistical manual of mental disorders (DSM-IV-TR)* (4th ed.). Washington, DC: American Psychiatric Association.

Fishman, S. (2000). *The war on pain: How breakthroughs in the new field of pain medicine are turning the tide against suffering*. New York: HarperCollins.

Gale, K. (2004). Transcranial magnetic stimulation: Can identify neurogenic pain. *Journal of Neurology, Neurosurgery and Psychiatry, 75*, 612–616.

Ganong, W. F. (2003). Excitable tissue: Nerve. In W. F. Ganong (Ed.), *Review of medical physiology* (21st ed., pp. 143–148). New York: Lange Medical Books.

Gerard, J. A., & Kleinfield, S. L. (1993). *Orthopedic testing: A rational approach to diagnosis*. New York: Churchill Livingstone.

Guyton, A. C., & Hall, J. E. (Eds.), (2000). *Textbook of medical physiology* (10th ed.). Philadelphia: W.B. Saunders.

Hackett, G. S. (1958). *Ligament and tendon relaxation (skeletal disability) treated by prolotherapy (fibro-osseous proliferation)* (3rd ed.). Springfield, IL: Charles C Thomas.

Haines, D. E. (1997). *Fundamental neuroscience*. New York: Churchill Livingstone.

Haist, S. A., & Robbins, J. B. (2002). *Internal medicine on call, 3ʳᵈ ed*. New York: Lange Medical Books/McGraw Hill.

Head, H. (1893). On disturbances of sensation with especial reference to the pain of visceral disease. *Brain, 16*, 1–133.

Heinricher, M. M. (2002). Central nervous system mechanisms in pain modulation. In K. J. Burchiel (Ed.), *Surgical management of pain* (pp. 65–75). New York: Thieme.

Hooshmand, H. (2000). *Chronic pain: Reflex sympathetic dystrophy, prevention and management*. Boca Raton, FL: CRC Press.

Iadarola, M. J., Max, M. B., Berman, K. F., Byas-Smith, M. G., Coghill, R. C., Gracely, R. H, & Bennett, G. J. (1995). Unilateral decrease in thalamic activity observed with positron emission tomography in patients with chronic neuropathic pain. *Pain, 63*, 55–64.

Kosek, E., & Hansson, P. (2003). Perceptual integration of intramuscular electrical stimulation in the focal and the referred pain area in healthy humans. *Pain, 105*, 125–131.

Lingappa, F., & Farey, K. (2000). *Physiological medicine*. New York: McGraw-Hill.

Lippe, P. (1998). An apologia in defense of pain medicine. *Clinical Journal of Pain*, 14, 189–190.

Marcus, A. (1998). *Musculoskeletal disorders: Healing methods from Chinese medicine, orthopaedic medicine and osteopathy*. Berkeley, CA: North Atlantic Books.

Melzack, R., & Wall, P. D. (1965). Pain mechanisms: A new theory. *Science, 150*, 971.

Merskey, H., & Bogduk, N. (Eds.). (1994). *Classification of chronic pain: Descriptions of chronic pain syndromes and definitions of pain terms* (2nd ed.). Seattle: IASP Press.

Ombregt, L. et al. (2003). *A system of orthopaedic medicine* (2nd ed.). Philadelphia: Churchill Livingstone.

Puckett, C. D. (2002). *The international classification of diseases, 9th ed*. The educational annotation of ECD-9-CM (Vols. 1, 2, 3). Reno, NV: Channel Publishing.

Ross, J. (1887). Segmental distribution of sensory disorders. *Brain, 10*, 333–361.

Ruch, T. C. (1960). Pathophysiology of pain. In T. C. Ruch,, & J. F. Fulton (Eds.), *Medical physiology and biophysics* (pp. 350–368). Philadelphia: W.B. Saunders.

Selzer, M., & Spencer, W. A. (1969). Convergence of visceral and cutaneous afferent pathways in the lumbar spinal cord. *Brain Research, 14*(2), 331–348.

Sturge, W. A. (1883). Phenomena of angina pectoris, and their bearing upon the theory of counterirritation. *Brain, 5*, 492–510.

Thienhaus, O., & Cole, B. E. (1998). The classification of pain. In Weiner, R. S. (Ed.), *Pain management: A practical guide for clinicians* (5th ed., pp. 19–26). Boca Raton, FL: CRC Press.

Thienhaus, O., & Cole, B. E. (2001). The classification of pain. In R. S. Weiner (Ed.), *Pain management: A practical guide for clinicians* (6th ed., pp. 27–36). Boca Raton, FL: CRC Press.

Waldman, S. D. (2002). *Atlas of common pain syndromes.* Philadelphia: W.B. Saunders.

Waldman, S. D. (2003). *Atlas of uncommon pain syndromes.* Philadelphia: W.B. Saunders.

Waxman, S. G. (2001). *Form and function in the brain and spinal cord: Perspectives of a neurologist.* Cambridge, MA: MIT Press.

Waxman, S. G. et al. (2001). Sodium channels and pain. In S. G. Waxman (Ed.), *Form and function in the brain and spinal cord: Perspectives of a neurologist* (pp. 421–431). Cambridge, MA: MIT Press.

Woessner, J. (2002a). A conceptual model of pain. *Practical Pain Management, 2*(5), 8–16, 37.

Woessner, J. (2002b). A conceptual model of pain: Measurement and diagnosis. *Practical Pain Management, 2*(6), 27–35.

Woessner, J. (2003). Referred pain vs. origin of pain pathology. *Practical pain management, 3*(5), 8–19.

5

Culture and Pain

Margie Rodríguez Le Sage, LMSW, PhD

INTRODUCTION

The growing attention that is given to understanding the influence of culture on pain stems from a number of factors that go beyond intellectual curiosity. Growing public interest in the treatment and palliation of pain, advanced technology to manage symptoms, and an increasingly diverse consumer base all combine to prompt culturally mediated issues of whether to relieve pain, for whom, with whom, how, when, and under what circumstances. The national commitment to eliminate disparity in health care outcomes along with the fact that most persons suffering health inequity are culturally and linguistically distinct compels further understanding of the relationship between culture and pain. As evidenced by emerging research, policies, and professional statements on diversity and pain, it is clear that scholars, policy makers, and clinicians are hopeful that advancing understanding of how culture informs pain experiences will contribute to optimal pain-related interventions.

The complexity of both concepts, culture and pain, has encouraged variable interpretations. Although pain is considered systemic, context dependent, multidimensional (e.g., biological, cognitive, emotional, social, and spiritual) and substantially affected by personal values and cultural traditions (Morris, 1998), culture implies an ongoing multilayered dynamic process of accepted ways of seeing, experiencing, interpreting, and expressing experiences affected by social processes and historical epoch (Moore, 1994; Shore, 1996). Models that attempt to explain pain relationship to culture generally assert that (1) pain is more than a simple neurological response to physiological injury and disease; (2) pain has mental-emotional, cultural, spiritual, and historical dimensions;

(3) pain can be influenced by personal values and spirituality as well as multiple layers of context including cultural traditions and social dislocation or disharmony; (4) pain is subjective and can only be defined by the individual; and (5) pain can be partly fabricated out of imagined lives and possible social exigencies (Bates, 1987; Glucklich, 2001; Jackson, 1994; Kleinman, 1994; Melzack & Wall,1983; Moore, 1994; Shore, 1996).

In line with current discussions that resist "ethnizing" culture, that is, limiting culture to ethnicity alone, a broader definition offered by the Office of Minority Health (Meadows, 2001, p. 1) is used here: *Culture* refers to integrated patterns of human behavior that include the language, thoughts, communications, actions, customs, beliefs, values, and institutions of racial, ethnic, religious, and social groups. A related concept, *cultural and linguistic competence*, refers to a set of congruent behaviors, attitudes, and policies that come together in a system, in an agency, or among professionals that enables effective work in cross-cultural situations. In turn, *competence* implies having the capacity to function effectively as an individual and an organization within the context of the cultural beliefs, behaviors, and needs presented by consumers and their communities (Meadows, 2000, p. 1).

The focus of this chapter is not to review the broad and complex topic of culture and pain or the accumulated findings on how culture influences pain, as that would require a book of several thousand pages, even for the parsimonious writer. Instead, this chapter focuses on addressing topics that are elementary yet important to current discussions of culture and pain, particularly in terms of appropriate and just responses to pain across cultures and linguistic traditions. This chapter encourages a broader understanding of culture and pain by briefly addressing current thinking in the analysis of culture and pain and select challenges encountered when attempting to understand culture. Potential areas for cross-cultural tension are considered in this chapter, as is research that points to disparate outcomes on pain relief across socio-cultural groups. Other topics addressed in this chapter are the importance of language when addressing culture and pain, standards for cultural and linguistic competence, and multilevel cultural and linguistic competencies that can help anticipate, mitigate, and perhaps prevent cross-cultural tension. Finally, the chapter concludes by considering challenges and opportunities to advance the effectiveness and equity in the treatment or care of pain across cultures. The choice of topics is driven by two notions: (1) better understanding of culture in an increasingly culturally and linguistically diverse world contributes to appropriate and just clinical outcomes; and (2) equity in the treatment of pain requires multilevel cultural and linguistic competencies. While the discussion in this chapter points to classic and current sources, it does not represent the extant literature that addresses culture and pain.

TOWARD A BROADER UNDERSTANDING OF CULTURE OF PAIN

Our understanding of culture and pain has advanced steadily over the last 52 years since Zborowski's classic work (1952) opened the study of pain to cultural comparisons, now regarded superficial in theory and method (see Delvecchio Good, Brodwin, Good, & Kleinman, 1994, p. 2). Our current level of analysis of culture and pain has moved beyond cultural comparisons and explorations of how meaning shapes pain experiences to one that addresses pain as a deeply personal feature of lived experience of individuals in the context of their social world and historical era. Individuals experiencing pain are not regarded as passive to the potential influence that culture can have on their perception and response to pain, but are seen as active in mediating (i.e., accepting, rejecting, modifying) cultural messages and other levels of social context that may or may not be within their control (Janes, 1999). In addition, current thinking on the influence of culture and pain considers all clinical encounters as cross-cultural, relational, and affected by imbalances of power. The multiplicity of factors, including personal values and cultural traditions that influence the attitudes about, perceptions of, and responses to pain take on special significance in clinical settings where pain becomes an interpersonal experience between the consumer and clinician and where therapeutic control is vested in the clinician (Farber Post, Blustein, Gordon, & Dubler, 1996). Current understanding of culture and pain has rediscovered the relationship between culture and voluntary pain. Current thinking

reminds us that the experience of pain, whether observed through the athlete who endures, the person who elects to undergo tattoos, the woman who elects child birth without analgesics, can signify something other than disintegration (Glucklich, 2001). Finally, current thinking does not limit culture to ethnicity but considers it to emerge from other sociocultural categories such as age, gender, religion, ablement, sexual orientation, race, national origin, linguistic tradition, and socioeconomic status.

Our broader and deeper understanding of culture and pain has encouraged developments that are certain to enhance the treatment and palliation of pain. This broader understanding of culture and pain discourages the temptation to overassign importance to cultural descriptions of groups, particularly those that are elevated above person, time, and situation and void of culture-bound information on sociocultural categories across the diversity spectrum. Current emphasis on the distinctive intimate experience of pain-in-context prompts clinicians and their sponsoring institutions to acquire multilevel competencies to best understand personal cultures and serve persons-in-their-pain experience. The renewed attention to voluntary pain and the premise that pain can be regarded a good thing that can enable a sense of belonging or connectedness challenges clinicians to think and prepare broadly to respond competently to diversity. Current thinking on culture and power that interact in clinical encounters to produce disparate outcomes has advanced commitment to explore the sources of inequity in pain relief. The emphasis that current thinking places on the complexity of culture in relationship to pain encourages clinical and scholarly engagement across disciplines, interdisciplinary rather than multidisciplinary, to more holistically and appropriately respond to pain.

Despite the advances made in our understanding of culture and pain, this field of study is in an early stage of development. Routes, patterns, and end points of cultural influence are considered complex and to reflect the multifaceted exchanges between culture and individual pain-related cognition, emotion, behavior, and spirit remains a challenge. Deeper understanding of what culture and pain mean and the processes that shape their meaning remain in development. The recent commitment by at least 15 National Institutes of Health (NIH, 2001) to support research on the social and cultural dimensions of health communicates the importance of advancing our understanding of culture and counters the tendency to use the term superficially and mechanically. While better information on how culture influences pain is being obtained, applying what is known can help allay cross-cultural misunderstandings. The following section discusses select aspects of culture that are known to challenge our grasp of its nature and influence.

CHALLENGES IN UNDERSTANDING CULTURE

A number of factors can make our understanding of cultural influences on pain particularly challenging. Understanding some of these factors permits a more accurate understanding of cultural diversity that guards against blind spots in our assessment and response to cultural difference. First, there are a great many cultures and within each single general culture, except for certain minority religious or ethnic groups (Yazar & Littlewood, 2001), there is substantial intracultural of variation, often related to other subcultural categories such as gender, age, religion, race, ablement, national origin, linguistic tradition, sexual orientation, and socioeconomic location (Miller & Eskin, 2001). The value that a specific Latina places on pain, for instance, may not be entirely a function of her ethnicity, but related to the cultural underpinnings of her religion and age, as well as the cultural construction of womanhood that assigns meaning to some of her pain. In contrast, this Latina woman's sister, who is agnostic, 10 years younger, resentful of culturally mediated messages of womanhood, and relatively removed from her Latina origins, considers all pain dehumanizing and requiring relief.

Second, due to its dynamic nature, culture changes across time. For example, discourse on the history of pain reminds us that pain lost much value after anesthetics were invented and applied in the 20th century (Cusick, 2003; Glucklich, 2001; Morris, 1991). In most general terms, this cultural shift transformed pain into a medical problem, of physical matter, and one devoid of meaning and function, thus relegating voluntary pain to deviant status.

Third, cultures intersect and persons acculturate. Defined as a multidimensional, multidirectional, developmental, interactive, and adaptive process of cultural adjustments experienced by individuals (Cuellar, Arnold, & Maldonado, 1995; Padilla & Perez, 2003) and groups (Berry, 1997; Berry & Sam, 1996), acculturation blurs cultural boundaries and creates variants of all aspects of culture. Individuals, particularly if presented with alternate forms of viewing phenomena, may reject, accept, or adapt culturally mediated messages related to pain (Johansen, 2002), not always in a definable pattern.

Once pain is suffered, it may be experienced differently by the same individual over time. For instance, a Mexican laborer who migrates from a small village in Mexico to the United States confronts an assessment of his pain that is contrary to his own. While in his native village his pain is regarded as a necessary part of living and spiritual transformation, in migration he experiences a society where pain is considered something that should be avoided. This can lead to a transformation of the pain experience, from necessary and meaningful to unnecessary and even destructive. Johansen (2002) shows, from her study of pain associated with infibulation among

Somali immigrants in Norway, that the contexts in which pain is originally suffered and subsequently remembered can affect the pain experience and its management. The implication is that not everyone from every culture group conforms all the time to a set of expected behaviors or beliefs, particularly in the face of acculturation. Cultural stereotyping (e.g., assuming that a person of Chinese heritage is stoic about pain) can contribute to inaccurate assessment and treatment of pain.

Fourth, not all behaviors are culturally based. For instance, a First Nations person who remains nonverbal during a clinical interview may not be signaling a cultural or linguistic tendency, but rather his or her resistance to the clinician's poor interviewing skills. Responses related to overwhelming pain may be void of culture as well. Intolerable pain with its mortifying character, referred to as "unmaking" of the world (Scarry, 1985), is considered a noncultural or even an anticultural experience (Jackson, 1994). The "unmaking" or counterpoint to culture that insurmountable pain may evoke is said to be due to the duration, intensity, and meaninglessness of the experience. Developing competencies to skillfully engage and interview for accurate assessment and corroboration across cultures and linguistic traditions guards against inaccurately assigning cultural significance to behavior.

Finally, in the midst of deterritorialization, the character of modernity whereby ethnic groups and communities, among other social formations, operate according to principles that transcend territorial boundaries and identities (Appadurai, 1991), it is increasingly hard to make specific local cultural assignments. Appadurai suggests that in our deterritorialized world, intertwined by the effects of media, technology, migration, tourism, and global markets, individuals belonging to what were once circumscribed local communities now are invited to imagine and envision alternative lives. Given this aspect of our postmodern world, Appadurai (1991) posits that the notion of symbolic pain may become more extraordinary both for the observer and participants. Among the many implications of Appadurai's forecast, greater cultural variation will require more attention to skillful assessment of personal cultures during clinical encounters. *Personal culture* has been defined by Pack-Brown and Braun Williams (2003) as the "organized, dynamic totality of an individual's identity ... comprised of historical, political, and economic dimensions, including religion, work experience, parental status, sexual orientation, gender and so forth" (pp. 230–231).

Understanding culture and its relationship to pain assumes special significance in clinical settings where pain becomes an interpersonal and cross-cultural experience between the consumer and clinician. The culture of Western medicine, prominent and powerful in clinical settings, provides the principal basis for the cross-cultural nature of clinical encounters. The following section briefly discusses medicine as a culture and potential areas in which cross-cultural tension can arise.

WESTERN MEDICINE AS CULTURE AND POTENTIAL CROSS-CULTURAL TENSION

Most clinical encounters responding to pain can be expected to be cross-cultural and thereby hold the potential for cross-cultural tension. This assertion is more obvious if Western medicine is viewed as the prevalent culture operating in clinical encounters and one that is at odds with those of consumers. Cultures of health care providers, growing in number as many cross national boundaries to fill labor shortages, operate in clinical encounters as well. This section briefly discusses medicine as culture and potential cross-cultural tension as it relates to culture-bound principles.

While some of Western medicine's core values, metaphors, beliefs, attitudes, and themes are not found problematic by some persons, particularly those receiving Western medical training and indoctrination, they may be considered challenging, if not threatening, by persons who are ill and in pain. Persons in pain, feeling highly dependent on others and in-the-present with their pain, may have difficulty accepting medicine's value orientation, which favors activity, mastery over nature, individualism, and future mindedness (see Stein, 1990, for an ethnographical account of American medicine). The potential for tension between clinicians and consumers is appreciated further when key components of Western medicine's world view are considered:

> (1) the "basic sciences": anatomy, physiology, biochemistry; microbiology, pathology; (2) the belief that medical science is and should be based upon rational, scientific, dispassionate, objective, professional judgment; (3) the belief that disease and its attendant suffering are ultimately to be understood in terms of pathological entities, organic in nature, and that treatment optimally consists of a technological procedure or interventions that results in a cure; (4) the belief that medical knowledge and skills are best organized by creating specialties around "organ systems." (Stein, 1990, p. xiv)

Comparing medicine's worldview with that of other groups, particularly those who encounter a disproportionate burden of inequity in the treatment and care of pain, demonstrates that the potential for cross-cultural conflict is substantial. Western medicine's tendency to distinguish illness into distinct mental and physical spheres can lead to conflict with individuals who integrate mind and body with social and natural universes (Ulusahin, Basaglu, & Paykel, 1994). Moreover, the holistic system that is frequently associated with an integrated system of prevention and healing that attributes psychological distress to physical imbalance and conversely assigns the cause of physical illness to spirits or the evil eye challenges Western medicine's world view (Avila with Parker, 2000; Mirdal, 1985). Similarly, religious medicine across cultures that are grounded in beliefs that pain can be spirit-imposed and that the sacred word or touch can lead to healing (Glucklich, 2001; Littlewood and Dein, 1995) is in direct contrast to Western medicine's worldview. Medicine's worldview as outlined is even at odds with the widely held understanding that pain is a subjective experience influenced by multiple factors that fall outside the basic sciences.

The potential for cross-cultural tension is compounded when values and beliefs that surface in clinical encounters involve major philosophical commitment to what is "good" and what is "bad." For this reason, the potential for cross-cultural tension is considered in relationship to select ethical principles that operate in clinical settings, namely, in decision making. The principles that are considered here include those that hold the most potential for generating cross-cultural tension: autonomy, beneficence, nonmaleficence, and fidelity (for discussion on ethics across cultures, see Braun, Pietsch, & Blanchette, 2000; Farber Post, Blustein, Gordon, & Dubler, 1996; Pack-Brown & Braun Williams, 2003).

AUTONOMY

Autonomy is a central principle in Western cultures that reflects the core values of individual rights, independence, and self-control (Zaner, 1988). Autonomy receives widespread support publicly, administratively, and legally, yet can be at odds with individuals who are family and group oriented. There is growing evidence that a number of groups, distinguished by age, gender, and ethnicity, prefer alternate models of decision making, models that subscribe to communitarian or hierarchical standards. Autonomy in these groups may be shared with their "families" or transferred to others, including clinicians who may be viewed as holding the knowledge and power needed to make the best decisions. Family-centered models of making decisions have found support in a number of studies (Blackhall, Murphy, Frank, Michel, & Azen, 1995; Morrison, Zayas, Mulvihill, Baskin, & Meier, 1998).

An associated cultural script, that of filial responsibility (Berger, 1998), which refers to the expectation that family members are expected to assist in some manner, may also come into conflict with the principle of autonomy and those who support it. Filial responsibility can cue family members to assist the patient in self-care functions that clinicians desire the patient to do on his or her own. Patients and families who prefer to be together for protective, instrumental, or supportive purposes can be regarded as disruptive and interfering by clinicians who endorse autonomy. Culturally competent clinicians addressing the relief of pain not only assess the patient's and family's moral basis for making decisions, they assess the role that the family assumes in the treatment and care of pain.

BENEFICENCE AND NONMALEFICENCE

While beneficence refers to the principle to do good, nonmaleficence refers to the principle to cause no harm. Because notions of what constitutes "good" and "harm" are value driven and culturally bound, we can expect certain interventions considered "beneficial" by Western standards to be viewed as harmful by some culturally distinct groups. Instances of conflict between varying perspectives of what is "good" and "not harmful" to the consumer system (patient and family) often underlie consumer choice not to take prescribed pain medication or to resist treatment altogether. The clinical challenge is to establish a working relationship built on trust and to rely on strong foundational interviewing skills to accurately assess consumer perceptions of "goodness" and "harm," as well as the basis for their choice to reject treatment. Much research has been committed to examine differing perceptions of what is regarded as "good" and "harmful" treatment (Carrese & Rhodes, 1995; for interesting and detailed account of cross-cultural conflict between Hmong consumers and Western medicine, see Fadiman, 1997).

FIDELITY, VERACITY, OR TRUTH-TELLING

A perceived fundamental duty of clinicians in Western medicine contexts to disclose information of medical status supports values related to self-determination and informed consent (Zaner, 1988). The culture-bound value of "accepting" diagnoses and prognoses, which requires full disclosure of medical status, has encouraged unflinching disclosure by clinicians. Direct disclosure can engender conflict with culturally distinct groups whose members may consider disclosure as inflicting unnecessary pain, such as Latinos (Blackhall et al., 1995), Hmong (Fadiman, 1997), Navajos (Caresse & Rhodes, 1995; McCabe, 1998), and Japanese (Kalish & Reynolds, 1976). Cultural competency calls for accurately assessing consumers' moral code on disclosure (e.g., who determines whether to disclose "truth," when is it shared, who shares it, with whom is it shared, how is it shared, and how much is shared?), in a timely manner. An institutional-level competency related to truth-telling encourages policies that dually protect a consumer's right to determine his or her own moral code on disclosure and the institution's need to guard against potential charges of negligence to disclose.

Attention to the interrelational, cross-cultural, and tension-prone nature of clinical encounters can help anticipate, mitigate, and prevent consumer–clinician conflicts. More importantly, attention to potential cultural misun-

derstanding and misuse of therapeutic control can help avert inequity in clinical outcomes. The following section summarizes research that addresses inequity in pain relief.

DISPARATE PAIN RELIEF OUTCOMES ACROSS SOCIOCULTURAL GROUPS

A growing body of literature that addresses potential inequity in clinical outcomes related to pain has been evolving and providing evidence that group-based differences, associated with culture, are related to pain-related clinical outcomes. Although this body of literature uses language and ethnicity to reference culture and ignores gender and age as cultural subcategories, its findings are worthwhile noting. A caveat when interpreting these studies is that factors that could help explain disparate outcomes are unknown (e.g., pain attitudes and perceptions, understanding and expectations of treatment, and the nature of patient–clinician interaction).

Select findings from this body of scholarship show that disparities in the treatment of pain by sociocultural categories are not due to chance alone and are evident in fracture treatment (Jones, Johnson, & McNinch, 1996; Todd, Deaton, D'Adamo, & Goe, 2000; Todd, Lee, & Hoffman, 1994; Todd, Samaroo, & Hoffman, 1993), postoperative pain following limb fracture (Ng, Dimsdale, Shragg, & Deutch, 1996), cancer pain (Bernabei et al., 1998; Cleeland, Gonin, Baez, Loehrer, & Pandya, 1997), migraine, and back pain (Tamayo-Sarver, Hinze, Cydulka, & Baker, 2004) and for persons in long-term facilities (Won et al., 1999).

In a particularly notable series of studies, Todd and associates (Todd et al., 1993, 1994, 2000) demonstrated that African Americans and Latinos were significantly less likely to receive analgesia in emergency departments for isolated bone fractures than were Whites, even though physicians rated patients' pain as similar in severity. Findings from a larger-scale study using 1997–1999 National Hospital Ambulatory Medical Care Surveys and involving a substantial sample size ($N = 67,487$) did not show differential administration of analgesics for long-bone fractures in emergency departments, yet revealed that Black patients with back pain and migraines were less likely to receive opioids in comparison with their White counterparts (Tamayo-Sarver et al., 2004). Relevant research suggests that not only may physicians have more negative perceptions of minority patients, but opioids may raise physician concerns that the patient may be seeking opioids in order to satisfy addiction or to sell them (van Ryn & Burke, 2000). Another study that did not find potentially unjust medication patterns for long-bone fractures in an emergency department suggests that hospitals serving larger ethnic minority populations may be best prepared to address cultural and linguistic difference (Karpman, Del Mar, & Bay, 1997.)

In a study that examined analgesic administration with patients treated surgically for limb fracture (Ng et al., 1996), significant differences by ethnicity in analgesic administration were found. Based on data gathered from chart reviews, the researchers found that while White patients received 22 mg/day of morphine equivalents, their Black and Hispanic counterparts received 16 and 13 mg/day, respectively. The researchers (Ng et al., 1996) suggest that patient–provider interaction during clinical encounters may partly explain differences in analgesic administration.

Findings from studies that focus on cancer-related pain are equally noteworthy. One study reported that 65% of the patients referred to as minority did not receive guideline-recommended analgesic prescriptions for their cancer-related pain compared with 50% of nonminority patients (Cleeland et al., 1997), with Latino patients at primary risk. Another study reported that older persons of ethnic minority groups who have cancer were at risk of receiving less medication or even no medication for daily pain (Bernabei et al., 1998).

Disparity according to age has been reported as well. In one study that examined analgesic administration with patients with fractures, it was found that persons aged 70 and older received less medication and had to wait longer than patients aged 20 to 50 (Jones et al., 1996). A study involving nursing home residents reported that persons older than 85 years, males, or members of non-European White group were less likely to receive pain medication even when pain was acknowledged in the patients (Won et al., 1999). Pain Management Index scores in a study that examined outcomes of pain management and predictors of patient satisfaction in hospitalized Latino patients reporting pain revealed less effective pain management with older persons (McNeill, Sherwood, Starck, & Nieto, 2001).

Disparity in pain management has also been found to vary according to gender. In a study that assessed pain management across groups (Breitbart, Rosenfeld, Passik, McDonald, Thaler, & Portenoy, 1996), it was found that besides patients with less education and those with histories of drug abuse, women were most likely to be undertreated. In another study, women were given analgesics less often and sedatives more often than men by physicians and nurses because they were seen more emotionally labile and prone to exaggerating pain symptoms (Calderone, 1999).

Inequity in pain relief at the community level has been documented as well. A study that examined the distribution of pain medication in neighborhoods (Morrison, Wallenstein, Natale, Senzel, & Huang, 2000) reported that only 26% of pharmacies in predominantly ethnic minority neighborhoods in comparison with their European American counterparts had sufficient opioid analgesics for someone with severe pain.

Although research examining group-based inequality in the treatment and care of pain is at an early stage of development, findings show that disparate outcomes in pain relief are widespread. The commitment to eliminate inequity in pain treatment outcomes directs our attention to multilevel approaches that can contribute to this goal. The following section briefly addresses the importance of language to the topic of culture and pain and provides resources that support efforts to advance cultural and linguistic competency.

THE IMPORTANCE OF LANGUAGE TO CULTURE AND PAIN

Although it has been proposed that pain is uniquely private, subjective, and beyond the construction of language (Daniel, 1991; Scarry, 1985), prevalent discourse on the topic of pain and culture asserts that pain indeed has language (Asad, 2000; Fabrega & Tyma, 1976; Glucklich, 2001; Jackson, 1994), albeit sometimes muted, silenced, and redirected such as through somatization. The function of language to label and communicate bodily sensations and meaning (Villaruel, 1995), besides delivering messages of empathy and hope, points to the need to give language its scientific and clinical due.

While researchers are called to test communication approaches designed to effectively engage linguistically distinct persons affected with pain, clinicians are called to understand culturally and linguistically distinct consumers who use different gestures and terms, even in English, to convey aspects of their pain experience. Both verbal and nonverbal messages need to be accurately interpreted in order to best respond to the pain experience. In turn, the terminology and communication approaches that are used with consumers and their families must be chosen carefully (Salimbene, 2000), even if they are English speaking. Moreover, the clinician is expected to communicate to the consumer what she or he has understood.

Attention to language is particularly warranted given the expanding linguistic diversity across the world and the disparate health care outcomes that are attributed to linguistic difference. Today, as documented by the U.S. Census Bureau (2000), more than 4.6 million people in the United States report not speaking English as their primary language, and more than 21 million report speaking English less than "very well." More astounding is the U.S. Census report that more than 300 languages are spoken in the United States. Persons who report having limited English proficiency are less likely to have a regular source of primary care (Kirkman-Liff & Mondragon, 1991; Weinick & Krauss, 2001); to undergo surgery, such as cholecystectomy (Diehl, Westwick, Badgett, Sugarek, &

Todd, 1993); and to receive preventive care (Woloshin, Schwartz, Katz, & Welch, 1997) and more likely to experience medical errors (Ghandi, Burstin, Cook et al., 1998). Moreover, persons who report having limited English proficiency report less satisfaction with the care they receive (Carrasquillo, Orav, Brennan, & Burstin, 1999; Morales, Cunningham, Brown, Honghu, & Hays, 1999). Ample evidence suggests that failure to address language and cultural issues can result in inferior quality of care, adverse outcomes, and increased health care costs (Baker, Parker, Williams, Coates, & Pitkin, 1996; Flores, Abreu, Olivar, & Kastner, 1998; Flores, Abreu, Schwartz, & Hill, 2000; Harsham, 1984).

Both federal and state laws mandate that health care organizations provide appropriate linguistic access for consumers with limited English language skills. (*Note:* While current reference to consumers who have limited English language skills is *limited English proficient [LEP] patients*, this author prefers to "place consumers first," followed by the descriptive phrase to avoid risk of labeling. The ideal would be to let consumers communicate their preference for how they would like to be categorized.) Accreditation agencies such as the Joint Commission on the Accreditation of Health Care Organizations (JCAHO) and the National Committee on Quality Assurance (NCQA) set standards and monitor compliance in language services, in addition to other health care services. The Office of Civil Rights' (OCR) "Policy Guidance on the Prohibition Against National Origin Discrimination as It Affects Persons With Limited English Proficiency," which applies to part of Title VI of the 1964 Civil Rights Act, aims to ensure equity in critical health and social services to persons with limited English language skills (Ross, 2001). Signed in August 2000, the OCR policy guidance outlines the legal responsibilities of providers who receive federal financial assistance from Health and Human Services (HHS) including:

- Develop a plan for providing written materials in languages other than English
- Establish policies and procedures for identifying and assessing language needs of the individual provider and its client population
- Provide a range of oral language assistance options, appropriate to each facilities circumstances
- Provide notice to persons with limited English language skills of the right to free language assistance
- Provide staff training and program monitoring (Ross, 2001, p. 2)

There are a number of resources available for clinicians and sponsoring institutions that need support in providing linguistic and cultural competent treatment of care:

the Department of Health and Human Services (DHHS) Office of Minority Health (OMH; http:www.omhr.gov); American Translators Association (http://www.ata-net.org); National Center for Cultural Competence (http://gucdc.georgetown.edu); Office for Civil Rights (http://www.hhs.gov/ocr); the American Medical Association's Cultural Competence Compendium (http://www.ama-assn.org/ama/pub/category/3066.html); and Cross Cultural Health Care Program (http://www.xculture.org) to list a few. The National Council on Interpreting in Health Care (NCIHC; http://www.ncihc.org), a multidisciplinary organization dedicated to promoting cultural and linguistic competent care in the interest of health care equity, provides a number of valuable Web site resources including working papers that are relevant to linguistic competence, an evaluation tool to assist organizations in assessing their linguistic needs, and links to related Web sites.

The challenge of arriving at approaches that can most appropriately assess and treat pain across cultures and linguistic traditions demands an array of multilevel competencies in various domains including knowledge, skills, and values. While the notion of achieving a *set of competencies* that permits effective work across cultures is commonly regarded as *cultural competency*, the terms are variously defined and designated (Boyle & Springer, 2001). The assortment of definitions of cultural competency and standards for cultural competency that have been drafted, while begging for uniformity, attest to the importance placed on improving outcomes and eliminating inequity in health care. (The terms *competence* and *cultural and linguistic competence* are defined earlier in this chapter.)

STANDARDS AND APPROACHES FOR MULTILEVEL CULTURAL AND LINGUISTIC COMPETENCIES

Most literature on cultural and linguistic competence primarily focuses on conceptual exploration and neglects the assessment of the theorized structure and outcome of cultural and linguistic competency. There is little evidence available on what cultural and linguistic competencies, applied when and in what fashion, work best. There is less information available on what training or background best conditions specific cultural and linguistic competencies.

Despite the limited direction that scholarship provides in the training, measurement, and clinical application of cultural and linguistic competencies, many human service and health care settings seem to be ambitiously working toward cultural and linguistic competency. Approaches and guidelines for cultural and linguistic competency, largely based on practice, observation and wisdom, have emerged in rapid fashion and are too many to reference here. This section briefly discusses national standards for cultural and linguistic competency and outlines select multilevel competencies.

STANDARDS FOR CULTURAL AND LINGUISTIC COMPETENCY

The first set of national *Standards for Cultural and Linguistic Competence* in health care delivery, released recently by the OMH (Ross, 2001) of the U.S. DHHS, as a result of the its Cultural and Linguistic Competence Standards and Research Agenda Project, represents an important step toward a more uniform and comprehensive approach to culturally and linguistically appropriate services (CLAS). The 14 standards are based on an analytical review of key laws, regulations, contracts, and competence standards and measures used by federal and state agencies and national organizations. The standards' aims are not only to ensure that services are more responsive to the individual needs of all consumers; the standards aim for health care providers, policy makers, and others in the health care community to create accountability within their organizations for providing equitable, quality services (Ross, 2001).

Evolution of instrumentation to measure and assess the status of cultural-linguistic competency has been slow but is gaining momentum (see Boyle & Springer, 2001, for discussion of well-known measures). As mentioned previously, the NCIHC offers a multilevel process by which health care organizations can evaluate their existing structure and capacity for providing linguistically and culturally appropriate care and accessibility. In a report entitled, *Cultural Competency Methodological and Data Strategies to Assess the Quality of Services in Mental Health Systems of Care: A Project to Select and Benchmark Performance Measures of Cultural Competency,* produced by the New York Office of Mental Health, the Nathan Kline Institute for Psychiatric Research, and Center for the Study of Issues in Public Mental Health (2002), a conceptual framework that explains multilevel pathways toward cultural competency, operationalization of all concepts, and data sources for each measure proposed is offered.

MULTILEVEL CULTURAL AND LINGUISTIC COMPETENCIES

A number of approaches or guidelines to help advance cultural and linguistic competencies in health care have been offered (Bakker, 1995; Flores et al., 2000; Galanti, 1997; Hizar, Shearer, & Giger, 1997; Koenig & Gates-Williams, 1995; Purnell & Paulanka, 1998; Salimbene, 2000; Spector, 2000) and are too many to fully enumerate here. While these guidelines are designated for specific health care settings, consumers, or health statuses, most are similar in that they propose multilevel competencies in the domains of knowledge, skills, and values. Most guidelines are relevant across cultures, settings, and health

or illness focus. This section focuses on summarizing eight competencies that are considered basic for cultural and linguistic competent care. Among the many competencies that have been proposed as important, Table 5.1 provides added information on the competencies that are considered basic by this author:

- Understand self in relationship to others
- Understand culture
- Value cultural beliefs and diversity
- Establish and sustain working relationships
- Recognize linguistic complexity
- Facilitate learning between providers and consumer communities
- Involve community in defining and assessing needs
- Professionalize staff hiring and training
- Institutionalize cultural and linguistic competency

Kleinman's often-quoted set of eight questions (Kleinman, 1988; Kleinman, Eisenberg, & Good, 1978), which is designed to elicit a person's explanatory model for his or her illness, is regarded as a useful guide by many person-centered clinicians who view consumers as experts of their lived-with-pain experience. The questions when addressed and adapted skillfully can be considered a classic approach to cultural competency that holds currency in modernity: (1) What do you call your problem [pain]? (2) What do you think caused your problem [pain]? (3) Why do you think it started when it did? (4) What do you think the sickness [pain] does? How does it work? (5) How severe is the sickness [pain]? Will it have a long or short course? (6) What kind of treatment do you think you should receive? What are the most important results you hope to receive with this treatment? (7) What are the chief problems [and benefits] the illness [pain] has caused? (8) What do you fear most about the [pain]?

CONCLUSION

The moral imperative to treat or palliate pain effectively and appropriately faces the challenge of adjusting to an increasingly diverse consumer base that is not only culturally and linguistically distinct, but subject to a disproportionate burden of disparate outcomes, including inadequate pain treatment. Our commitment to optimally respond to pain and to achieve equity in doing so requires a combination of sustained efforts. Further research on what culture and pain mean as well as on the routes and patterns of cultural influence on pain can provide needed information to improve not only the treatment and care of pain but also its prevention, when appropriate. While efforts to advance cultural and linguistic competency in the treatment and care of pain need continued philosoph-

TABLE 5.1
Approaches to Culturally and Linguistically Competent Care

Understand self in relationship to others
    Become aware of our own cultural background
    Know how our cultural heritage affects our definitions of normality and abnormality
    Recognize the stereotypes and preconceived notions that we hold of others
    Understand how we socially impact others
    Recognize the limits of our competencies and expertise
Understand culture
    Acquire broad knowledge of cultural and subcultural groups
    Regard potential culture-specific information as tentative insight and not an "end point" to understanding
    Understand how subcultural categories based on shared attributes and shared life experiences contribute to a person's "personal culture"
    Recognize the challenges present in understanding culture
    Acquire practical, experience-based knowledge about the community being served (e.g., Chinese teaspoons are generally larger than American ones)
Value cultural beliefs and diversity
    Respect cultural orientation, including beliefs of moral goodness
    Acknowledge decision-making preferences
    Avoid assuming anything
    Avoid making judgments
    Avoid the "golden rule"
    Trust that pain is whatever the consumer says it is
    Communicate acceptance
    Incorporate consumers' models of care with treatment plan
Establish and sustain working relationships
    Develop and use communication and facilitative skills (e.g., empathy, genuineness, warmth) to build trust, accurately assess, corroborate clinical observations, and negotiate conflicts
    Appropriately and accurately assess background, decision-making preferences, and culturally mediated beliefs, theories, and practices related to health, illness, pain, suffering, healing, caring, treatment types, health care providers, families
    Operate from strengths' perspective
    Regard consumer as expert and having the best understanding of the pain, what has helped, what has not helped, and what is likely to help
    Evaluate what beliefs would interfere with your treatment plan
    Effectively explain culture and orientations from which you are operating
    Be conservative in relating news or in providing details of potential complications
    Encourage procedures that affirm consumers' values (e.g., have larger conference rooms and waiting areas for consumers who value family)
    Avoid a treatment plan that conflicts with person's beliefs and lifestyle
    Selectively align treatment strategy with consumer's beliefs
Recognize linguistic complexity
    Recognize the linguistic variation within a cultural group
    Recognize the cultural variation within a language group

TABLE 5.1 (Continued)
Approaches to Culturally and Linguistically Competent Care

    Recognize the variation in literacy levels in all language groups
    Distinguish between translation, interpretation, and medical interpretation
    Receive training to enhance linguistic capacities and increase knowledge of cultural practices
    Contract with telephone interpreter services
    Screen all materials for cultural and linguistic appropriateness
Facilitate learning between providers and consumer communities
    Regard individuals and communities as experts
    Create and sustain "learning loops" between health care providers and consumer communities
    Partner professionals and consumers when providing professional training
Involve community in defining and assessing needs
    Enlist community members in governing boards
    Involve community members in community advisory boards, patient panels, task forces, or neighborhood meetings
    Sponsor community-based research and integrate results into program design
    Affirm that understanding gained from community-based research belongs to communities
Professionalize staff hiring and training
    Establish specific hiring qualifications and mandated training requirements in cultural and linguistic competence
    Develop and provide comprehensive and replicable training curricula
    Allocate funding and time for staff training
Institutionalize cultural and linguistic competency
    Integrate cultural/linguistic competence into all aspects of planning
    Make funding for staffing and training for cultural/linguistic competence sustainable
    Design cultural/linguistic competence activities that can be replicated and developed
    Create procedures that help disclose cultural preferences
    Apply knowledge of cultural beliefs to program areas

ical and administrative support, they will benefit the most by evidence-based direction. Scholarship must be encouraged to develop the methods and analytical tools necessary to best assess the structure and outcomes of cultural and linguistic competency, and must examine these in relationship to consumer, provider, treatment, and organizational characteristics. The development of curricula that emphasize the cultural influence on the pain experience and the examination of what training approaches work best will need continued support if quality and equity in our clinical responses to pain are to be achieved. Workers in relevant disciplines, particularly those who are underutilized in the treatment and palliation of pain, such as social workers, spiritual care providers, and music therapists, need to creatively and, at times, aggressively carve out their niche in research, clinical, and training contexts that aim for appropriate and effective pain care and equity in clinical outcomes. Finally and perhaps most importantly, just and effective clinical responses to pain across cultures are more likely to occur if consumer communities exercise their strengths and power to advise and govern the institutions that serve them.

REFERENCES

Appadurai, A. (1991). Notes and queries for a transnational anthropology. In R. G. Fox (Ed.), *Recapturing anthropology: Working in the present* (pp. 191–210), Santa Fe, NM: School of American Research Press.

Asad, T. (2000). Agency and pain: An exploration. *Culture and Religion, 1,* 29–60.

Avila, E., with Parker, J. (2000). *Woman who glows in the dark: A curandera reveals traditional Aztec secrets of physical and spiritual health.* New York: Tarcher/Putnam.

Baker, D. W., Parker, R. M., Williams, M. V., Coates, W. C., & Pitkin, K. (1996). Use and effectiveness of interpreters in an emergency department. *Journal of American Medical Association, 275,* 783–788.

Bakker, L. (1995). Communicating across cultures. *Nursing, 25*(1), 79–80.

Bates, M. S. (1987). Ethnicity and pain: A biocultural model. *Social Science and Medicine, 24,* 47–50.

Berger, J. T. (1998). Culture and ethnicity in clinical care. *Archives of Internal Medicine, 158,* 2085–2090.

Bernabei, R. Gambassi, G., Lapane, K., Landi, F., Gatsonis, C., Dunlop, R., et al. (1998). Management of pain in elderly patients with cancer. SAGE Study Group. Systematic Assessment of Geriatric Drug Use via Epidemiology. *Journal of the American Medical Association, 279,* 1877–1882.

Berry, J. W. (1997). Immigration, acculturation, and adaptation. *Applied Psychology: An International Review, 46*(1), 5–33.

Berry, J. W., & Sam, D. L. (1996). Acculturation and adaptation. In J. W. Berry, M. A. Segall, & C. Kagitubasi (Eds.), *Handbook of cross-cultural psychology: Social behaviors and application* (Vol. 3, pp. 291–326). Boston: Allyn & Bacon.

Blackhall, L. J., Murphy, S. T., Frank, G., Michel, V., & Azen, S. (1995). Ethnicity and attitudes toward patient autonomy. *Journal of the American Medical Association, 274,* 820–825.

Boyle, D. P., & Springer, A. (2001). Toward a cultural competence measure for social work and specific populations. *Journal of Ethnicity and Cultural Diversity in Social Work, 9,* 53–71.

Braun, K. L., Pietsch, J. H., & Blanchette, P. L. (Eds.). (2000). *Cultural issues in end-of-life decision-making.* Thousand Oaks, CA: Sage.

Breitbart, W., Rosenfeld, B. D., Passik, S. C, McDonald, M.V., Thaler, H., & Portenoy, R. K. (1996). The undertreatment of pain in ambulatory AIDS patients. *Pain, 65,* 243–249.

Calderone, K.L. (1999). The influence of gender on the frequency of pain and sedative medication administered to post-operative patients. *Sex Roles, 23*(11/12), 713–725.

Carrasquillo, O., Orav, E. J., Brennan, T. A., & Burstin, H. R. (1999). Impact of language barriers on patient satisfaction in an emergency department. *Journal of General Internal Medicine, 4,* 82–87.

Carrese, J., & Rhodes, L. A. (1995). Western bioethics on the Navajo Reservation: Benefit or harm? *Journal of the American Medical Association, 274,* 826–829.

Cleeland, C. S., Gonin, R., Baez, L., Loehrer, P., & Pandya, K. J. (1997). Pain and treatment of pain in minority patients with cancer: The Eastern Cooperative Oncology Group Minority Outpatient Pain Study. *Annals of Internal Medicine, 127,* 813–816.

Cuellar, I., Arnold, B., & Maldonado, R. (1995). Acculturation Rating Scale for Mexican Americans. II: A revision of the original ARSMA Scale. *Hispanic Journal Behavioral Science, 17,* 275–304.

Cusick, J. (2003, October). Spirituality and voluntary pain. *American Pain Society Bulletin, 13*(5). Retrieved from http://www.ampainsoc.org/pub/bulletin/sep03/path1.htm

Daniel, E. V. (1991). *Charred lullabies. Chapters in an anthropology of violence.* Princeton, NJ: Princeton University Press.

Delvecchio Good, M., Brodwin, P. E., Good, B. J., & Kleinman, A. (Eds.). (1994). *Pain as human experience: An anthropological perspective.* Berkeley, CA: University of California Press.

Diehl, A. K., Westwick, T. J., Badgett, R. G., Sugarek, N. J., & Todd, K. H. (1993). Clinical and sociocultural determinants of gallstone treatment. *American Journal of the Medical Sciences, 305*(6), 383–386.

Fabrega, H., & Tyma, S. (1976). Language and cultural influence in the description of pain. *British Journal of Medical Psychology, 49,* 323–337.

Fadiman, A. (1997). *The spirit catches you and then you fall down.* New York: Farrar, Straus, & Giroux.

Farber Post, L., Blustein, J., Gordon, E., & Dubler, N. N. (1996). Pain: Ethics, culture, and informed consent. *Journal of Law, Medicine, & Ethics, 24,* 1–16. Retrieved from http://www.painandthelaw.org/aslme_content/24-4c/post.pdf.

Ferrell, B. R. (1995). When culture clashes with pain control, *Nursing, 25*(5): 90.

Flores, G., Abreu, M., Olivar, M., & Kastner, B. (1998). Access barriers to health care for Latino children. *Archives of Pediatric and Adolescent Medicine, 152,* 1119–1125.

Flores, G., Abreu, M., Schwartz, I., & Hill, M. (2000). The importance of language and culture in pediatric care: Case studies from the Latino community. *Journal of Pediatrics, 137,* 842–848.

Galanti G. (1997). *Caring for patients from different cultures.* Philadelphia: University of Pennsylvania Press.

Ghandi, J. K., Burstin, H. R., Cook, E. F., et al. (1998). Drug complications. *Journal of General Internal Medicine, 15,* 149–154.

Glucklich, A. (2001). *Sacred pain: Hurting the body for the sake of the soul.* Oxford: Oxford University Press.

Harsham, P. A. (1984). A misinterpreted word worth $71 million. *Medical Economics*, June, 289–292.

Hizar, D. R, Shearer, R., & Giger, J. N. (1997). Pain and the culturally diverse patient. *Today's Surgical Nurse, 19*(6), 36–39.

Jackson, J. (1994). Chronic pain and the tension between the body as subject and object. In T. J. Csordas (Ed.), *Embodiment and experience: The existential ground of culture and self* (pp. 201–228). Cambridge: Cambridge University Press.

Janes, C. R. (1999). Imagined lives, suffering, and the work of culture: The embodied discourses of conflict in modern Tibet. *Medical Anthropology Quarterly, 13*(4), 391–412.

Johansen, R. E. B. (2002). Pain as a counterpart to culture: Toward an analysis of pain associated with infibulation among Somali immigrants in Norway. *Medical Anthropology Quarterly, 16*(3), 312–340.

Jones, J. S., Johnson, K., & McNinch, M. (1996). Age as a risk factor for inadequate emergency department analgesia. *American Journal of Emergency Medicine, 14*, 157–160.

Kalish, R. A., & Reynolds, D. K. (1976). *Death and ethnicity: A psychocultural study.* Los Angeles, CA: University of Southern California Press.

Karpman, R. R., Del Mar, N., & Bay, C. (1997). Analgesia for emergency centers' orthopaedic patients. *Clinical Orthopaedics and Related Research, 334*, 270–275.

Kirkman-Liff, B., & Mondragon. (1991). Language of interview: Relevance for research of Southwest Hispanics. *American Journal of Public Health, 81*, 1399–1404.

Kleinman, A. (1988). *The illness narratives: Suffering, healing, and the human condition.* New York: Basic Books.

Kleinman, A. (1994). Pain and resistance: The delegitimation and relegitimation of local worlds. In M. Delvecchio Good, P. E. Brodwin, B. J. Good, & A. Kleinman (Eds.), *Pain as human experience: An anthropological perspective* (pp. 169–197). Berkeley, CA: University of California Press.

Kleinman, A., Eisenberg, L., & Good, B. (1978). Cultural, illness and care-clinical lessons from anthropologic and cross-cultural research. *Annals of Internal Medicine, 88*, 251–258.

Koenig, J., & Gates-Williams, B. A. (1995). Understanding cultural difference in caring for dying patients. *Western Journal of Medicine, 163*(3), 244–249.

Koopman, C., Eisenthal, S., & Stoeckle, J. D. (1984). Ethnicity in the reported pain, emotional distress and requests of medical outpatients, *Social Science and Medicine, 18*, 487–490.

Krieger, N. (1994). Epidemiology and the web of causation: Has anyone seen the spider? *Social Science and Medicine, 39*, 887–903.

Krongrad. A., Perczek, R. E., Burke, M. A., Granville, L. J., Lai, H., & Lai, S. (1997). Reliability of Spanish translations of select urological quality of life instruments. *Journal of Urology, 158*, 493–496.

Kumasaka, L. & Miles, A. (1996). My pain is God's will. *American Journal of Nursing, 96*(6), 45–47.

Lambert, W. E., Libman, E., & Poser, E. G. (1960). The effect of increased salience of a membership group on pain tolerance. *Journal of Personality, 28*, 350–357.

Littlewood, R., & Dein, S. (1995). The effectiveness of words. *Culture, Medicine and Psychiatry, 19*, 339–383.

McCabe, M. (1998). Patient Self-Determination Act: A Native American (Navajo) perspective. *Cambridge Quarterly of Healthcare Ethics, 3,* 419–421.

McNeill, J. A., Sherwood, G. D., Starck, P. L., & Nieto, B. (2001). Pain management outcomes for hospitalized Hispanic patients. *Pain Management Nursing, 2*(1), 25–36.

Meadows, M. (2000, January). Moving towards consensus on cultural competency in health care. *Closing the Gap*, pp. 1–2.

Melzack, R., & Wall, P. G. (1983). *The challenge of pain.* New York: Basic Books.

Miller, M., & Eskin, E. (2001). Improving patient compliance. *Minority Health Today, 2*(2), 54–56.

Mirdal, G. M. (1985). The conditions of tightness: The somatic complaints of Turkish women. *Acta Psychiatrica Scandinavica, 71*, 287–296.

Moore, H. L. (1994). *A passion for difference.* Cambridge: Polity Press.

Morales, L. S., Cunningham, W. E., Brown, J. A., Honghu, L., & Hays, R. D. (1999). Are Latinos less satisfied with communication by health care providers? *Journal of General Internal Medicine, 14*, 409–407.

Morris, D. R. (1991). *The culture of pain.* Berkeley, CA: University of California Press.

Morris, D. R. (1998). *Illness and culture in the postmodern age.* Berkeley, CA: University of California Press.

Morrison, R. S., Zayas, L. H., Mulvihill, M., Baskin, S. A., & Meier, D. E. (1998). Barriers to completion of health care proxies: An examination of ethnic differences. *Archives of Internal Medicine, 158*, 2493–2497.

Morrison, R. S., Wallenstein, S., Natale, D. K., Senzel, R. S., & Huang, L. L. (2000). "We don't carry that" — failure of pharmacies in predominantly nonwhite neighborhoods to stock opioid analgesics. *New England Journal of Medicine, 342*, 1023–1026.

National Institutes of Health. (2001, December). *NIH guide: Social and cultural dimensions of health* (Program Announcement) [Online]. Retrieved from http://grants2.nih.gov/grants/guide/pa-files/PA-02-043.html.

New York State Office of Mental Health, Nathan Kline Institute for Psychiatric Research, & Center for the Study of Issues in Public Mental Health. (2002, August). *Cultural competency methodological and data strategies to assess the quality of services in mental health systems of care: A project to select and benchmark performance measures of cultural competency.* New York: Author.

Ng, B., Dimsdale, J.E., Shragg, P., & Deutch, R. (1996). Ethnic differences in analgesic consumption for postoperative pain. *Psychosomatic Medicine, 58*, 125–129.

Pack-Brown, S. P., & Braun Williams, C. (2003). *Ethics in a multicultural context.* Thousand Oaks, CA: Sage.

Padilla, A. M., & Perez, W. (2003). Acculturation, social identity, and social cognition: A new perspective. *Hispanic Journal of Behavioral Sciences, 25*(1), 35–55.

Purnell, L. D., & Paulanka, B. J. (Eds.). (1998). *Transcultural health care: A culturally competent approach.* Philadelphia: F.A. Davis.

Ross, H. (2001, February/March). Office of Minority Health publishes final standards for cultural and linguistic competence. *Closing the Gap*, pp. 1–2, 10.

Salimbene, S. (2000). *What language does your patient hurt in? A practical guide to culturally competent patient care.* Amherst, MA: Diversity Resources.

Scarry, E. (1985). *The body in pain: The making and unmaking of worlds.* New York: Oxford University Press.

Shore, B. (1996). *Culture in mind: Cognition, culture, and the problem of meaning.* New York: Oxford University Press.

Spector, R. E. (2000). *Cultural diversity in health & illness* (5th ed.), Englewood Cliffs, NJ: Prentice-Hall Health.

Stein, H.J. (1990). *American medicine as culture.* Boulder, CO: Westview Press.

Tamayo-Sarver, J. H., Hinze, S. W., Cydulka, R. K., & Baker, W. (2004). Racial and ethnic disparities in emergency in emergency department analgesic prescription. *American Journal of Public Health, 93*(12), 2067–2073.

Todd, K. H., Deaton, C., D'Adamo, A. P., & Goe, L. (2000). Ethnicity and analgesic practice. *Annals of Emergency Medicine, 35,* 11–16.

Todd, K. H., Lee, T., & Hoffman, J. R. (1994). The effect of ethnicity on physician estimates of pain severity inpatients with isolated extremity trauma. *Journal of the American Medical Association, 271,* 924–928.

Todd, K. H., Samaroo, N., & Hoffman, J. R. (1993). Ethnicity as a risk factor for inadequate emergency department analgesia. *Journal of the American Medical Association, 269,* 1537–1539.

Ulusahin, A., Basaglu, M., & Paykel, E. S. (1994). A cross-cultural comparative of depressive symptoms in British and Turkish clinical samples. *Social Psychiatry and Psychiatric Epidemiology, 29,* 31–39.

U.S. Census Bureau. (2000). *DP-2. Profile of selected social characteristics: 2000.* Retrieved from http:/factfinder.census.gov.

van Ryn, M., & Burke, J. (2000). The effect of patient race and socio-economic status of physicians' perceptions of patients. *Social Science and Medicine, 50,* 813–828.

Villaruel, A. (1995). Mexican-American cultural meanings, expressions, self care and dependent-care actions associated with experiences with pain. *Research in Nursing Health, 18,* 427–436.

Weinick, R. M., & Krauss, N. A. (2001). Racial and ethnic differences in children's access to care. *American Journal of Public Health, 90,* 1771–1774.

Woloshin, S., Schwartz, L. M., Katz, S. J., & Welch, H. G. (1997). Is language a barrier to the use of preventive services? *Journal of General Internal Medicine, 12,* 472–477.

Won, A., Lapane, K., Gambassi, G., Bernabei, R., Mor, V., & Lipsitz, L. A. (1999). Correlates and management of nonmalignant pain in the nursing home. *Journal of the American Geriatrics Society, 47,* 936–942.

Yazar, J., & Littlewood, R. (2001). Against over-interpretation: The understanding of pain amongst Turkish and Kurdish speaker in London. *The International Journal of Social Psychiatry, 47*(2), 20–33.

Zaner, R. M. (1988). *Ethics and the clinical encounter.* Englewood Cliffs, NJ: Prentice-Hall.

Zborowski, M. (1952). Cultural components in responses to pain. *Journal of Social Issues, 4,* 16–30.

Zola, I. K. (1982). *Missing pieces: A chronicle of living with a disability.* Philadelphia: Temple University Press.

6

Pain and the Family

Suzanne Young Bushfield, PhD, MSW

INTRODUCTION AND OVERVIEW OF CONCEPTUAL FRAMEWORK

Individuals construct their world of meaning in many ways and within many contexts. Pain is a powerful organizing force; living with pain becomes a central element in shaping the lives and stories of families. To be successful in mediating the experience of pain, practitioners must pay attention to the context in which the pain occurs. As Jerome Bruner (1990) argued, "interpretive meanings are very sensitive to context" (p. 24). Pain is essentially experienced subjectively, and despite attempts to address one's experience of pain objectively, the subjective reality expands beyond the individual's physical condition to include the psychological, sociocultural, and spiritual self. Helping, for the person experiencing pain, may also need to extend beyond the physical and most certainly to family and community. Pain, more than other symptoms, has a powerful potential for negatively affecting one's quality of life. The complexity of the pain experience may require a complex set of interventions and approaches that considers the knowledge, attitudes, beliefs, and practices present in the family, as well as in the larger sociopolitical context in which pain resides.

"Person, environment, and time interact dynamically" (Hutchison, 2003, p. 17). This multidimensional model for understanding human behavior recognizes that effective practice requires attention that is balanced between the uniqueness of the individual in his or her situation and the general knowledge of patterns, derived from theory and empirical research (Meyer, 1993). This tension between the objective reality and the subjective experience seems to characterize the "place" in which the person experiencing pain resides. Incorporating a multidimensional approach to understanding the person in pain

demands that we acknowledge the paradox of the person as both free and constrained, and of family and social life as both cohesive and conflicted. This perspective accepts both consistencies and contradictions and will be used to examine the influence of theories of human behavior on direct interventions targeted at the management of pain. A critical review of the evidence of the effectiveness of diverse approaches is expected to yield a greater variety of options, some of which might "fit" the diverse and unique experiences of the person experiencing the common impacts of pain, within a family context.

THE FAMILY DEFINES PAIN

WHAT IS THE FAMILY

The family, two or more people who love and care for each other, is essentially a system with attitudinal, behavioral, and communicational rules; reciprocal roles; and boundaries. "Every event within a family is multiply-determined by all the various forces operating within that system" (Andrae, 1996, p. 606). Families, whether intact or not, retain their primary influence in people's lives. Families revolve around themes and patterns that may be multigenerational, and horizontal as well as vertical (Bowen, 1978; Brown, 1991; Carter & McGoldrick, 1989). Family members must maintain both separateness from and connectedness to families. Major disruptions in the family life cycle always have an impact on its members. These basic principles related to families are important in understanding the role of the family when one of its members is experiencing pain. Early experiences, family traditions and beliefs, ascribed roles, and reciprocal encounters are all essential features of the pain experience within families.

While medicine may categorize pain according to biological, psychological, or idiopathic sources, most pain sufferers become focused on a quest for relief from the pain. Organizing one's life around pain restructures families so pervasively that often, by the time patients present for comprehensive pain management, new patterns of communication, roles, and structures have replaced the family environment that existed before pain became the central organizing feature. The relationships and transactions within the family are shaped by the pain, which becomes the proximal, contingent, and immediate environment (Saleeby, 2004). Acknowledging the importance of family, as well as the reciprocity within family systems, Northen (1994) indicated that "an illness or disability seriously influences the functioning of the family and the functioning of the family seriously influences the course of the patient's rehabilitation" (p. 168). The pervasiveness of family influences on pain is demonstrated in a variety of ways. There is evidence that family support is an important factor in the rehabilitation of chronic pain (Jamison & Virts, 1990), while family enmeshment and rigidity (Liebman, Honig, & Berger, 1976) have been associated with intractable pain. Pain has been called a "metaphor for family dysfunction" (Wynn, Shields, & Sirkin, 1992, p. 3), and chronic pain results in significant structural, communication, role and rule changes within the family system (Marcus, 1986).

WHAT IS PAIN

Webster defines pain as "**a**: usually localized physical suffering associated with bodily disorder (as a disease or injury); *also*: a basic bodily sensation induced by a noxious stimulus, received by naked nerve endings, characterized by physical discomfort (as pricking, throbbing, or aching), and typically leading to evasive action; and **b**: acute mental or emotional distress or suffering" (Merriam-Webster, 1991, p. 846). Pain becomes "chronic" when it has been in existence for 6 months and is recognized for its debilitating psychological and social effects (Snelling, 1990). Pain sufferers have very concrete needs, but their lives have been characterized by "a sense of loss of self" (Kelley & Clifford, 1997, p. 276). Just as pain becomes primary in its sufferer's world, it also becomes central in the family's world. There are significant personal and social costs associated with pain: loneliness, isolation, withdrawal and avoidance, anxiety, depression, fear, lack of trust, impaired sexual relationships, loss of productivity, strained marital and family relationships, overuse or misuse of medical care, addiction, and the development of a pain identity (Kelley & Clifford, 1997).

WHAT IS SUFFERING

The distinction between pain and its companion, suffering, has been explored (Van Hooft, 1998). Mirriam-Webster

(1991) describes *suffering* as: "Deep and poignant distress; a profound and disturbing crisis and threat to one's sense of being that exceeds the bodily sensation is characteristic of suffering" (p. 1179). Recognizing the reality of suffering as larger, more systemic, and more profound than pain allows the practitioner to understand the need for a comprehensive approach to the larger family system, in order to relieve suffering. The practitioner would be well advised to approach the patient and family with competency regarding the diverse cultural and linguistic constructs of pain and suffering. Cultural competence carries requirements of both organizations and personnel to value diversity and manage and adapt to the cultural contexts of the individuals and communities served (Goode, Jones, & Mason, 2002).

INFLUENCE OF THEORETICAL MODELS AND IMPLIED TREATMENT STRATEGIES

There is a rich range of theories found to have significant utility in contemporary practice (Andrae, 1996). This "theoretical plurality" can be both an asset and a hindrance to the practitioner. In the absence of practice-based evidence, theories may prevent us from recognizing alternative explanations. This overview of theoretical models and the treatment strategies for pain that they imply assumes that individuals, families, dyads, groups, and communities turn to professionals for treatment that is ethical, accountable, value sensitive, and effective (Andrae, 1996). Therefore, interventions for which there is a strong theoretical basis, and for which there is sufficient evidence of efficacy, are the primary focus.

EGO PSYCHOLOGY

Ego psychology is built around concepts of ego functions, defenses, ego mastery and adaptation, and object relations (Goldstein, 1996). Pain research based on principles from ego psychology has identified a number of significant contributing factors to the perception and experience of chronic pain, including a history of childhood abuse and family dysfunction (Mersky & Boyd, 1978), physical and emotional abuse (Engel, 1959; Violon, 1980), and increased dependency and the resulting attitudes of caregivers (Berry & Ward, 1995). Effective interventions focus on helping the patient to understand the pain experience and providing short term, ego supportive counseling (Roy, 1981).

While this perspective may imply a focus on the family in terms of reworking family-of-origin issues and addressing current family functioning, its focus is primarily the inner life. There are limitations of the strategies derived from ego psychology due to the reliance on insight for change, and the impact from pathologizing of the person in pain. In addition, negative attitudes toward the patient may further contribute systemically to the patient's existing damaged sense of self and ability of the patient to feel empowered to control or manage his or her pain. There is further evidence that these negative attitudes are disproportionately experienced by women, minorities, and those for whom power and access to medical care are further limited by societal power structures (Lee, 1994).

BEHAVIORAL APPROACHES

Pain is normally viewed as a warning signal that something is not right; when it persists as chronic pain, it may be influenced by operant mechanisms (Skinner, 1988). The behavioral approach assumes that when pain responses, such as grimacing, complaining, sighing, and moaning, are systematically followed by favorable consequences, such as sympathy, attention, and avoidance of unpleasant tasks, the pain behavior is reinforced and maintained (Hudgens, 1977; Marcus, 1986). The negative role of the spouse in maintaining and perpetuating chronic pain receives considerable focus in this model.

The contingency management approach (Bonica, 1990; Fordyce, 1990) to pain management is widely accepted, and many distinguished pain management programs are derived from this model. Approaches address the patient's self-talk, reframing the situation to promote cognitive restructuring, changing contingencies (reinforcers) within the family, and enlisting family as part of the treatment strategy. The goal of treatment is to help the patient return to normal functioning without pain medications, or with reduced reliance on medication. Pain behaviors are ignored; appropriate activity and interactions are reinforced with attention and praise. The approach may result in the patient learning to live a normal life by ignoring the pain. Changing family interactions and responses to pain is reframed as constructive caring, and the role of the worker in this model is to teach patients with pain and their families to eliminate the subject of chronic pain from their family system interactions (Hudgens, 1977).

Success in this model is highly dependent on several factors: (1) a supportive family amenable to retraining, (2) a patient able to learn new skills, and (3) available community supports to maintain changes (Hudgens, 1977; Marcus, 1986). The behavioral model acknowledges the impact of knowledge and attitudes on pain (Brockopp, Warden, Colclough, & Brockopp, 1996) and may include effective nonpharmacological strategies such as relaxation, imagery, and distraction (Korcz, 2003).

"Family oriented" treatment in this model places a significant focus on modifying the family response behaviors to pain, as an aspect of contingency management. However, manipulation of the environment sometimes requires collusion on the part of the family and may certainly interrupt or change the delicate balance of reciprocity within families. Acknowledging the interconnectedness of systems, it is important to recognize that the unintended consequences of behavioral manipulation may precipitate other, equally intractable problems within the family. The behavioral approach may further fail to recognize the significant attitudinal barriers from health care professionals and others regarding pain, addiction, and the harmful effects of pain medication (Korcz, 2003).

STRENGTHS AND EMPOWERMENT PERSPECTIVES

The empowerment approach makes connections between social and economic justice and individual pain and suffering (Lee, 1996). Drawing from theories on strengths (Saleeby, 1997), empowerment (Gutierrez, Parsons, & Cox, 1998), resilience (Fraser, 1997), hardiness (Kobasa, 1979), and solution-focused philosophies (De Jong & Miller, 1995), these models suggest how people overcome and resist the effects of adversity (McMillen, 1999). While there may be benefits from adversity (McMillen, 1999; Tedeschi & Calhoun, 1995), people with few coping skills, children, and those with low socioeconomic status may be less able to benefit from adversity. Pain management, in this paradigm, will address the strengths of the patient and family through a comprehensive assessment and holistic approach that acknowledges the interdependence and transactional nature of the person in his or her environment (Germain, 1991).

A strengths and empowerment perspective acknowledges the powerlessness that comes from the pathologizing of pain (either physical or psychological), versus the empowerment that derives from a validation of the experience of suffering and its impact on the individual and family. The empowerment process resides in the person, not the helper (Lee, 1996). This model assumes a biopsychosociocultural-spiritual approach to understanding the pain experience and may incorporate a variety of both active and passive techniques for pain management, including relaxation, imagery, distraction, reframing, cognitive reappraisal, patient education, patient involvement, psychotherapy, peer support, and pastoral counseling. Incorporating a humanistic perspective, this model recognizes that living with pain is a life course that calls into question meaning and suffering. People often cope with suffering and pain by seeking and finding meaning (Frankl, 1962). For many people, spirituality is a source of hope in the midst of despair (Puchalski, 2002).

The strengths and empowerment paradigm suggests a holistic approach to pain management and the family, and may include providing additional support and attention to the suffering, in order to assist the sufferer in making sense of his or her world. In contrast to behavioral approaches, exploring the person's historical experiences of pain, the sick role, and care giving and care receiving within the context of the family is both welcomed and advised. There is evidence that the patient experiencing chronic pain needs validation and understanding, both from the health care team and from family and friends (Kelley & Clifford,

1997). This need exists concurrently with concrete needs and the need for very specific coping skills. The REEP model proposed by McMillen (1999) recommends a process of reflecting, encouraging, exploring, and planning benefit, which may assist pain sufferers in constructing changes needed to facilitate recovery and growth.

Professionals addressing pain using the strengths perspective may need to focus on the experience of vulnerable populations and the need for empowerment and advocacy in the processes of accessing resources for pain management (Mendenhall, 2003), recognizing the losses experienced with chronic pain, validating the patient's struggles for survival, and formulating a plan of action to enhance a sense of control over pain, relationships, and lives (Macdonald, 2000). The practice focus in this model may include individual and family empowerment counseling, advocacy, and organization of sufferers into viable advocacy groups to influence research, policy and program construction (Glajchen & Blum, 1995).

INTERLOCKING, INTERCONNECTING, INTERINFLUENCING ASPECTS OF PAIN

A multidisciplinary team approach is necessary to maximize the potential for effectively addressing the biological components of pain both pharmaceutically and with other medical aspects; the psychological components of pain, taking multidimensional perspectives into account; the sociocultural context of pain for the person in his or her family and environment; and the spiritual components of pain, especially the meaning of pain and suffering to the individual and family. Evidence of health system inflexibility, lack of role definitions in health care, cultural and attitudinal barriers, and knowledge deficits in pain management among health care professionals all suggest that approaches must be interlocking and interconnecting with respect to direct service, education, advocacy, and research (Glajchen & Blum, 1995).

FUTURE DIRECTIONS FOR PAIN AND THE FAMILY

As the field of pain management undergoes rapid changes and development of new techniques, drugs, and intervention strategies, it is necessary for practitioners who focus on pain relief to stay current. In addition, understanding the rapid social changes affecting the family and roles within families may suggest successful approaches to pain management in the context of family. Research trials in recent years have included attention to the efficacy of alternative medicine and complementary approaches. As evidence is established for new resources, practitioners will need to disseminate this information and knowledge so that patients and families are better able to make use

of new discoveries. The study of alternative approaches, including acupuncture, massage, touch, meditation, and prayer, combined with new developments in genetics, scanning, and understanding of the neurobiology of pain and addiction, may yield entirely new approaches to pain management. In addition, greater recognition of the role of the larger community and social supports for the family may offer additional resources in managing chronic pain (Subramanian, 1991).

Policies that recognize the unique needs of women, children, minorities, and disadvantaged groups may address some of the contextual issues in which pain resides. How society responds to pain and those seeking relief is closely tied with ethical and policy issues. Continued research will need to incorporate an understanding of how social justice influences care for those experiencing pain.

The power of expectation, meaning, possibility, and intentionality may be one of the "next frontiers" in pain management. Support and acceptance of alternative resources, "what works," and the sharing and validating of these personal experiences and stories often provides pain sufferers and their families with necessary relief.

Recognizing the true anatomy of pain and suffering may need to include hope. "Cross cultural practitioners consistently report that hope is an important curative factor in all cultures and societies. The more one has hope about the power or potential for help in the healing relationship or healing process, the greater the chance that the healing process will be effective" (Harper & Lantz, 1996, p. 10).

REFERENCES

Andrae, D. (1996). Systems theory and social work treatment. In F. Turner (Ed.), *Social work treatment* (pp. 601–616). New York: The Free Press.

Berry, P., & Ward, S. (1995). Barriers to pain management in hospice: A study of family caregivers. *The Hospice Journal, 10*(4). 19–33.

Bonica, J. J. (1990). Multidisciplinary/interdisciplinary pain programs. In J. J. Bonica (Ed.), *The management of pain* (pp. 197–208). Philadelphia, PA: Lea & Febiger.

Bowen, M. (1978). *Family therapy in clinical practice.* New York: Aronson.

Brockopp, D., Warden, S., Colclough, G., & Brockopp, G. (1996). Elderly hospice patients' perspective on pain management. *The Hospice Journal, 11*(3), 41–53.

Brown, F. (1991). *Reweaving the family tapestry* (pp. 3–21). New York: W.W. Norton.

Bruner, J. (1990). *Acts of meaning.* Cambridge, MA: Harvard University Press.

Carter, B., & McGoldrick, M. (1989). *The changing family life-cycle: A framework for family therapy* (pp. 3–28). Boston, MA: Allyn & Bacon.

De Jong, P., & Miller, S. D. (1995). How to interview for client strengths. *Social Work, 40*, 729–736.

Engel, G. (1959). Psychogenic pain and the pain prone patient. *American Journal of Medicine, 26*, 899–918.

Fordyce, W. (1990). Contingency management. In J. Bonica (Ed.), *The management of pain* (pp. 1702–1709). Philadelphia, PA: Lea & Febiger.

Frankl, V. (1962). *Man's search for meaning: An introduction to logotherapy* (p. 176). Boston: Beacon Press.

Fraser, M. (Ed.). (1997). *Risk and resilience in childhood: An ecological perspective* (pp. 1–33). Washington, DC: NASW Press.

Germain, C. (1991). *Human behavior in the social environment* (p. 88). New York: Columbia University Press.

Glajchen, Y., & Blum, D. (1995). Cancer pain management and the role of social work: Barriers and interventions. *Health and Social Work, 20*(3), 200–207.

Goldstein, E. (1996). Ego psychology theory. In Turner, F. (Ed.), *Social work treatment* (pp. 191–217). New York: The Free Press.

Goode, T., Jones, W., & Mason, J. (2002, Winter). A guide to planning and implementing cultural competence. *National Center for Cultural Competence*, Georgetown University, pp. 1–8.

Gutierrez, L. M., Parsons, R. J., & Cox, E. O. (Eds.). (1998). *Empowerment in social work practice: A sourcebook* (pp. 3–15). Pacific Grove, CA: Brooks-Cole.

Harper, K., & Lantz, J. (1996). *Cross-cultural practice: Social work with diverse populations* (pp. 6–20). Chicago: Lyceum.

Hudgens, A. (1977). The social worker's role in a behavioral management approach to chronic pain. *Social Work in Health Care, 3*(2), 149–157.

Hutchison, E. (2003). *Dimensions of human behavior: Person in environment*. Thousand Oaks, CA: Sage.

Jamison, R., & Virts, K. (1990). The influence of family support on chronic pain. *Behavioral Research Therapy 28*(4), 283–287.

Kelley, P., & Clifford, P. (1997). Coping with chronic pain: Assessing narrative approaches. *Social Work, 42*, 266–277.

Kobasa, S. C. (1979). Stressful life events, personality and health: An inquiry into hardiness. *Journal of Personality and Social Psychology, 37*, 1–11.

Korcz, I. R. (2003). Oncology social workers perceived barriers to cancer pain and the relationship to the functional assessment of pain and non-pharmacological strategies. *Social Work Abstracts, 39*(2), 851.

Lee, J. (1994). *The empowerment approach to social work practice*. New York: Columbia University Press.

Lee, J. (1996). The empowerment approach to social work practice. In F. Turner (Ed.), *Social work treatment* (pp. 218–249). New York: The Free Press.

Liebman, R., Honig, P., & Berger, H. (1976). An integrated treatment program for psychogenic pain. *Family Process, 15*, 397–405.

Macdonald, J. (2000). A deconstructive turn in chronic pain treatment: A redefined role for social work. *Health and Social Work, 25*(1), 51–57.

Marcus, M. (1986). Chronic pain: A social work view. *The Social Worker-Travailleur Social, 54*(2), 60–63.

McMillen, J. C. (1999). Better for it: How people benefit from adversity. *Social Work, 44*(5), 455–467.

Mendenhall, M. (2003). Psychosocial aspects of pain management: A conceptual framework for social workers on pain management teams. *Social Work in Health Care, 36*(4), 35–51.

Merriam-Webster. (1991). *Webster's ninth new collegiate dictionary*. Springfield, MA: Merriam-Webster.

Mersky, H., & Boyd, D. (1978). Emotional adjustment and chronic pain. *Pain, 5*, 173–178.

Meyer, C. (1993). *Assessment in social work practice* (p. 10). New York: Columbia University Press.

Northen, H. (1994). *Clinical social work* (2nd ed.). New York: Columbia University Press.

Puchalski, C. (2002). Spirituality and end of life care. In A. M. Berger, R. K. Portenoy, & D. E. Weissman (Eds.), *Principles and practice of palliative care and supportive oncology* (2nd ed., pp. 799–812). Philadelphia: Lippincott/Williams & Wilkins.

Roy, R. (1981). Social work and chronic pain. *Health and Social Work, 6*(3), 61–65.

Saleeby, D. (1997). *The strengths perspective in social work practice* (pp. 3–19). New York: Longman.

Saleeby, D. (2004). The power of place: Another look at the environment. *Families in Society, 55*(1), 1–16.

Skinner, B. F. (1988). The operant side of behavior therapy. *Journal of Behavior Therapy and Experimental Psychiatry, 19*, 171–179.

Snelling, J. (1990). The role of the family in relation to chronic pain. *Journal of Advanced Nursing, 15*(7), 771–776.

Subramanian, K. (1991). The multidimensional impact of chronic pain on the spouse: A pilot study. *Social Work in Health Care, 15*(3), 47–62.

Tedeschi, R., & Calhoun, L. (1995). *Trauma & transformation: Growing in the aftermath of suffering* (pp. 77–91). Thousand Oaks, CA: Sage.

Turner, F. (1996). *Social work treatment* (pp. 1–17). New York: The Free Press.

Van Hooft, S. (1998). The meanings of suffering. *Hastings Center Report, 28*(5), 13–19.

Violon, A. (1980). The onset of facial pain: A psychological study. *Psychotherapy and Psychosomatics, 34*, 11–16.

Wynn, L. C., Shields, C. G., & Sirkin, M. I. (1992). Illness, family theory, and family therapy: Conceptual issues. *Family Process, 31*(1), 3–18.

7

Sex, Gender, and Pain: Clinical and Experimental Findings

Roger B. Fillingim, PhD, and Barbara A. Hastie, PhD

INTRODUCTION

DEFINITION OF SEX AND GENDER

In recent years, burgeoning evidence indicates sex and gender differences in pain in both clinical and experimental settings. In order to discuss these findings, it is helpful to understand the distinction between "sex" and "gender." Specifically, *sex* refers to biological substrates that clearly distinguish an organism as "male" or "female" in terms of their genetic composition including chromosomes (XX for females and XY for males), hormones, anatomy, and the subsequent development of secondary physical characteristics, which place the organisms in the category "female" or "male" (Frable, 1997; Hughes, 2003; Pollad & Hyatt, 1999; Wizemann & Pardue, 2001). Gender refers to the way in which an individual is defined based on socioculturally shaped behaviors and traits (such as femininity and masculinity) that are an amalgam of the psychological, social, and cultural factors that influence it (Pollard & Hyatt, 1999; Robinson et al., 2000; Wizemann & Pardue, 2001). Other theorists define gender as "the structured set of gendered personal identities that results when the individual takes the social construction of gender and the biological 'facts' of sex and incorporates them into an overall self-concept." (Ashmore, 1990; Pollard & Hyatt, 1999; Robinson et al., 2000; Wizemann & Pardue, 2001). It is important to recognize that gender roles are sculpted by both biological and social factors. Indeed, the relevance of social learning and its effect on sex differences in pain modulation have been presented from a neurobiological perspective (Choleris & Kavaliers, 1999).

Historically, before the 1970s, the term *gender* was glaringly absent from biomedical research literature (Ashmore, 1990; Choleris & Kavaliers, 1999; Greenberger, 2001; Pollard & Hyatt, 1999; Robinson et al., 2000; Wizemann & Pardue, 2001). In the 1970s, the movement toward equality of genders downplayed any differences either inadvertently or, in some cases, by conducting research in strictly uni-gender samples. Noting the grave inequalities in treatment as well as overrepresentation of one gender with certain pain conditions, there has been a movement in the past decade not only to study sex and gender differences but also to create models of testing and understanding the nature and origins of such differences.

Thus, in contrast to gender, it is important to highlight that the term "sex" is used exclusively for nonhuman animal investigation, as it is practically impossible to operationalize gender roles in nonhumans. Conversely, in human pain research, it is entirely possible for both sex and gender to contribute to the individual's experience of pain. Fillingim and Maixner (1995) previously proposed an interactive model of pain that encapsulated neurobiological, physiologic, hormonal, and genetic factors that dynamically and interchangeably influenced and were affected by psychological (affective), cognitive, and sociocultural factors (e.g., social learning, gender role, etc).

Thus, whereas the study of sex differences in pain may be more straightforward in nonhumans, it is extraordinarily complex in humans because it seems to be a dynamic and fluid interplay of both sex and gender. Thus, it is critical to make the distinction between sex and gender and to study their mutual, yet varying, influences on a person experiencing pain. The influence of sex versus gender is not a philosophical principle, but an empirical question, particularly with regard to health outcomes. Moreover, it is important to note the distinctions since not only can gender aspects affect expression of pain as well as the interpretation of biological traits, and the experience of pain, but also sex-related biological characteristics can contribute to, diminish, or amplify gender differences in pain.

INTEREST IN SEX, GENDER, AND PAIN

Interest in sex, gender, and pain has proliferated in the past decade. This amplified interest has been accompanied (and perhaps driven) by increased federal funding for research on this topic. This proliferation of research likely reflects the growing attention to the issue of gender in the laypublic (e.g., Mars and Venus), but also is fueled by novel findings documenting important sex differences in the neurobiology of pain in preclinical investigations. This has sparked concerted efforts to conduct translational research to the human dimension (e.g., Mogil et al. (175)). These efforts have been coupled with resurgence in clinical attention to sex and gender differences, such that clinical scientists have applied the preclinical and experimental findings to gender and sex differences in clinical treatment and outcome. Yet, despite this remarkable growth in the spectrum of research on sex and gender differences in pain, it is still a relatively nascent field of exploration.

The purpose of this chapter is to review the literature regarding sex, gender, and pain. This includes results of community surveys, epidemiological investigations, and clinical research in specific pain conditions that have addressed the issue of gender-related differences in pain. In addition, findings from human laboratory research and nonhuman animal studies are also presented. Potential mechanisms underlying sex and gender differences in pain are discussed, and important future directions for research on sex, gender, and pain are proposed.

SEX, GENDER, AND CLINICAL PAIN

COMMUNITY SURVEYS

As early as 1985, one of the first community surveys on pain in the United States was conducted. The Nuprin Pain Report was a national survey conducted on a random sample of 1254 adults. It was the first nationwide survey to provide quantitative data on pain prevalence and severity, demographic characteristics of pain sufferers; how people cope with pain; the relationship between pain and stress; the relationship between pain and health locus of control scales; use of medical and other professionals in the treatment of pain; the relationship between pain and different lifestyles and behavior patterns; and the impact of pain on work and other activities (Sternbach, 1986; Taylor & Curran, 1985). Gender was essentially a demographic variable (50.2% male; 49.8% female) and women were divided into "homemakers" and "working mothers" and men had the designation of executives, floor trader, professional/managerial/proprietor, sales/service, skilled and unskilled labor (Taylor & Curran, 1985).

Results from the survey showed that compared with men, women reported more headaches and were more affected than men in their daily activities by headache-related pain. The Nuprin Report also found that women experienced backaches, joint pains, and stomach pains slightly more than men (Taylor & Curran, 1985). Subsequently, the American Pain Foundation conducted surveys in various states to determine the extent to which pain affects the average citizen. Their findings revealed that more than 55% of the general population in different states experienced pain in the moderate to severe range and more than 40% face some kind of chronic pain condition and women seemed to outnumber men in each of the types of pain (American Pain Foundation, 2002). Other community surveys have revealed similar findings such that in general U.S. populations, women tended to report higher prevalence of several types of pain (Riley et al., 1998; Scudds & Robertson, 1998; Verhaak et al., 1998; Von Korff et al. 1988), and additional data suggest that these sex differences are most robust in middle age (LeResche, 1997; Riley & Gilbert, 2001; Verhaak et al., 1998; Von Korff et al. 1988). Specifically, women are more likely than men to experience recurrent headache disorders in each type except cluster headache (Holroyd & Lipchik, 2000; Lipton et al., 2001; Schwarts et al., 1998; Stewart et al., 1992). Women are also reported to have greater frequency than men in experiencing joint pain, abdominal pain, including irritable bowel syndrome, fibromyalgia, oral pain, specifically temporomandibular disorder (TMD), and low back pain (Barsky et al., 2001; Buckwalter & Lappin, 2000; Chang & Heitkemper, 2002; Drangsholt & LeResche, 1999; Wolfe et al.,. 1995; Wolfe et al., 1995).

In other population-based surveys, compared to men, women reported greater frequency of pain-related symptoms across multiple age groups (Buckwalter & Lappin, 2000; Croft et al., 2001; LeResche, 1999; Unruh, 1996). Furthermore, compared to men in the general population, women experienced more disruption, distress, and disability from pain (Affleck et al., 1999; Keefe et al., 2000; Leveille et al., 2000; Sandanger et al., 2000; Soares & Jablonska, 2004). In addition, other investigators found women to report more frequent use of analgesics (Eggen, 1993; Isacson & Bingefors, 2002). However, some researchers have reported increased disability among men compared to women with conditions such as low back pain in middle adulthood (Kostova & Koleva, 2001; Walsh et al., 1992).

Cultural influences on sex differences in pain are only beginning to be addressed. Thus, community surveys in cultures other than those represented in American and Western European countries are few in number. Consequently, it is acknowledged that pain experiences and expression may vary by cultures and gender-related issues such as social roles may play a part in differences displayed (Costa et al., 2001). The notion of cultural factors influencing responses to accident-related pain and subsequent development of chronic pain conditions has been briefly explored. Accident victims from Eastern European countries do not appear to report the chronic pain-related symptoms to the extent that are reported in many Western societies, including the United States (Ferrari et al., 1999; Obelieniene et al., 1999). There is evidence that coping styles, environment and other psychosocial factors across and within countries may influence recovery and pain conditions (Buitenhuis et al., 2003; Ferrari et al., 2003; Maraste et al., 2003; Miettinen et al., 2002); whether gender contributes to these sociocultural differences in pain expression has not been determined. Thus, in epidemiological studies, sex differences in pain report emerge across multiple countries and in various pain conditions; however, the extent to which these differences are due to sex differences in pain reporting versus sex differences in the experience of pain is not known (Vallerand, 1995).

EPIDEMIOLOGICAL FINDINGS

Considerable data on sex differences in pain prevalence and incidence arose inadvertently from population studies that were focused on specific diseases and pain as a secondary aspect of such health conditions (Gordis, 1988; LeResche, 1999; Unruh, 1996). When discussing gender-related differences, it is important to consider the three salient theoretical perspectives from an epidemiological perspective that include population, developmental, and ecological views (LeResche, 1999). Briefly, the population view espouses that to understand pain conditions fully, they must be examined from general populations and not just from those in treatment centers (e.g., with preexisting pain conditions). The second view, the developmental approach, asserts that it is critical to investigate pain across the lifespan since factors that influence risk may change with age and the prevalence may vary between genders at different points in the life cycle. The ecological perspective of epidemiological research promotes that any disease is a product of a combination of disease agents (e.g., genetics/biological), characteristics of the host (e.g., psychological), and the environment (e.g., social), which is highly consistent with the biopsychosocial model of pain (LeResche, 2000).

Epidemiological findings related to pain have identified several common recurrent pain conditions that differ in frequency among women and men. These include headache, migraine, facial/oral pain, musculoskeletal pain, back pain, and abdominal pain (Crombie et al., 1999; LeResche, 2000; Unruh, 1996). It should be noted that the findings discussed below come predominantly from investigations conducted in North America or Western Europe. These results must be interpreted in light of the possibility that the sex differences in the prevalence of pain may vary depending on geographic region as well as sociocultural and ethnic factors.

One of the advantages of epidemiological studies in pain is that the findings can lend explanation to magnitude of differences observed as well as risk factors in gender-specific prevalence. This is especially useful because several recent reviews of gender-related differences in pain have revealed that women have higher prevalence of pain in many different conditions and across several settings (Barsky et al., 2001; Berkley, 1997; Fillingim & Maixner, 1995; Unruh, 1996). Epidemiological research adds specificity in that women are more likely than men to report temporary or chronic pain, and it tends to be more severe, more frequent, and of longer duration than men (Andersson et al., 1993; Blyth et al., 2001; Crombie et al., 1999; Taylor & Curran, 1985; Unruh, 1996). A brief description of the most prevalent pain conditions will ensue. For a more in-depth analysis of these issues, the reader is referred to the publication by the International Association for the Study of Pain, *Epidemiology of Pain* (Crombie et al., 1999).

Back Pain. Some evidence suggests that back pain is more common among females than males (Balague et al., 1999; Hartvigsen et al., 2003); however, other data suggest minimal sex differences in the prevalence of back pain (Croft et al., 1999; Leboeuf-Yde & Kyvik, 1998; LeResche, 2000; Wedderkopp et al., 2001). Nevertheless, what is conclusive is that back pain is variable across the lifespan with changing levels of debilitation depending on the etiology and other factors often not addressed in epidemiological studies. Moreover, factors other than gender, such as genetics, occupation, socioeconomic issues, and cultural influences, may represent more important predictors of back pain (Croft et al., 1999; Leboeuf-Yde, 2004; LeResche, 2000).

Headache and Migraine. Investigations predominantly in the United States and Western Europe have reported higher rates of headaches in women than men with the exception of cluster headache (Holroyd & Lipchik, 2000; Lipton et al., 2002; Schwartz et al., 1998; Stewart et al., 1992). However, studies from myriad worldwide populations have provided some conflicting evidence, depending on the population in question (Scher, Stewart, & Lipton, 1999). A comprehensive overview of national and international studies is addressed in-depth in the International Association for the Study of Pain's (IASP) Publication entitled *Epidemiology of Pain* (Scher et al., 1999). Despite some discrepancies between studies in prevalence, based on 29 epidemiological studies, investigators report that the prevalence of headache in men appears as a flat slope across the lifespan, while in women, it appears flat until reproductive age, where there is an increase, and then a significant drop after age 60 (Scher et al., 1999). LeResche (2000) reports that in a lifetime, 60% of males and 75 to 80% of females will report experiencing headache at some point, although in women it tends to decrease with age. Thus, what is typically not contested is that even when the prevalence curves take similar shape, women tend to experience headaches in much greater number, frequency, duration, they tend to be more debilitated by them, and the female:male ratio seems to be most marked in migraines (Celentano et al., 1992; LeResche, 2000).

Abdominal Pain. Population-based studies of gastrointestinal functional-related abdominal pain have revealed a higher frequency and severity in women than men across all ages (Adelman et al., 1995; Agreus et al., 1994; Chang & Heitkemper, 2002; LeResche, 2000; Mayer et al., 1999). Moreover, the prevalence in both genders seems to be steady until the age of 40, at which time, there is a trend to decline (Unruh, 1996). However, no gender differences in onset of abdominal pain were reported in one large prospective epidemiologic investigation (Halder et al., 2002).

Joint Pain/Fibromyalgia. Women are at greater risk for joint pain and fibromyalgia/chronic widespread pain compared to men. In accordance with diagnostic criteria from the American College of Rheumatology, population studies report that women are at greater risk and have higher prevalence for both joint pain and fibromyalgia (Buckwalter & Lappin, 2000; Gran, 2003; Wolfe et al., 1995). Women and girls also report more painful sites, more intense pain, and more frequent pain (Anderson et al., 1993; Hasvold & Johnsen, 1993; White, Speechley, Harth, & Ostbye, 1999). Interestingly, the prevalence curves for men and women are similar, with an increase until approximately age 65, then a slight decrease between 65 and 74 years of age, and a gradual increase after that (LeResche, 2000; Macfarlane, 1999).

Orofacial Pain/TMD. Most epidemiological studies on orofacial pain/TMD report that women have higher prevalence as well as more pain and tenderness in jaw muscles and temporomandibular joint, and other researchers have found increased sensitivity and decreased pain tolerance and threshold in women with such disorders (Sallfors et al., 2003; Wahlund, 2003). Notably, the prevalence seems to increase sharply for females during adolescence (Pilley et al., 1992; Sallfors et al., 2003). Peak prevalence for both sexes is typically between the ages of 40 and 50 years old, (Goulet et al., 1995; Macfarlane et al., 2001; Von Korff et al., 1988) and these findings seemed to be consistent in other Western countries (Sipila et al., 2001; Wahlund, 2003). There are limited studies addressing gender-related differences in adolescents although the

same trend seems to emerge with girls reporting increased prevalence, and more pain and symptoms compared to boys (List et al., 1999; Wahlund, 2003).

These epidemiological findings offer strong evidence that in contrast to men, women are more likely to report pain at multiple body sites and they tend to be more at risk for developing certain chronic pain disorders such as TMD, fibromyalgia, irritable bowel syndrome, migraine headache, and other forms of musculoskeletal pain (LeResche, 1999; Unruh, 1996). It is important to highlight that most of these epidemiological data address adults, although a number of studies have found similar trends in children and adolescents with a higher prevalence and severity in girls compared to boys (Haugland et al., 2001; McGrath, 1999). Despite the absence of information regarding potential cultural influences, these data offer compelling evidence that women are at greater risk for developing several chronic pain conditions compared to men. Whether the *severity* of pain in clinical settings differs in women and men is now discussed.

SEX DIFFERENCES IN CLINICAL PAIN SEVERITY

Sex differences have been investigated in the acute clinical pain setting. For example, women reported greater pain than men following oral surgery as well as orthopedic and other surgical procedures (Averbuch & Katzper, 2000; Taenzer et al., 2000). Women have also reported higher pain ratings in acute cancer-related pain (Cepeda et al., 2003), procedural pain such as colonoscopy (Froehlich et al., 1997); and conditions presented in emergency rooms (Boccardi & Verde, 2003). A recent review article addressed the issue of gender-related risk in developing post-whiplash-related chronic pain condition(s) following acute injury and females were at increased risk given their initial presentation of more severe pain in the acute stage (Scholten-Peeters et al., 2003). These data highlight the importance of possible gender-correlated complications in the acute pain stage particularly that high initial pain intensity is often an important predictor for delayed functional recovery, which is consistent with the involvement of central centralization in the development of — or transition to — a chronic pain condition.

Additionally, research into gender-related differences in children's pain is a growing area of investigation. Despite the need for more empirical evidence, some studies have found that girls tended to report more pain than boys from venipuncture (Goodenough et al., 1997, 1999); although other investigators have found no sex differences among children undergoing certain medical procedures (Lander et al., 1989, 1990). To date, few investigators have examined any gender-related influences on pediatric procedural pain and more research is needed to identify such differences.

As reviewed above, there are clear gender differences in the prevalence of several chronic pain disorders; however, the evidence supporting differences in the severity of pain-related symptoms within chronic pain populations is less compelling. For example, among individuals with pain that limited their activity, women reported more frequent pain, greater pain-related affective symptoms, and higher pain-related disability compared to men (Mullersdorf & Soderback, 2000). Women reported higher levels of arthritis pain and disability than men (Affleck et al., 1999; Keefe et al., 2000), and at the time of total hip arthroplasty women reported higher levels of pain and disability than men (Holtzman et al., 2002). Similarly, pain among patients with multiple sclerosis was more frequent and severe among women (Warnell, 1991). Also, in a heterogeneous chronic pain population recruited from a multidisciplinary pain clinic, women had higher pain severity than men (Fillingim et al., 2003). However, other investigators have reported minimal sex differences in pain severity in heterogeneous chronic pain populations (Edwards et al., 2003; Robinson et al., 1998; Turk & Okifuji, 1999). Also, no sex differences in measures of clinical pain, experimental pain sensitivity, psychological/personality factors or illness behaviors were reported among patients with pain due to TMD (Bush et al., 1993). A recent study found that men had higher levels of pain and poorer pain-related adjustment in a sample of patients seeking treatment primarily for myofascial pain in a multidisciplinary clinic (Marcus, 2003). Taken together, these findings suggest that sex differences in the severity of pain-related symptoms are inconsistent among patients with chronic pain in clinical settings. This lack of differences could reflect the selection bias introduced by the decision to seek treatment.

SEX DIFFERENCES IN RESPONSES TO NOXIOUS EXPERIMENTAL STIMULI

Overall, the literature reviewed above indicates that women experience greater clinical pain than men. While multiple factors inevitably determine these sex differences in clinical pain, we have previously proposed that enhanced pain sensitivity among women may be an important contributor (Fillingim & Maixner, 1995). Before reviewing the experimental literature on sex differences in pain perception, a brief discussion of experimental pain methods will be provided. Multiple noxious stimuli are used in examining laboratory pain responses, and they differ along important dimensions, including temporal and spatial qualities, anatomical site stimulated, specificity of afferent fibers stimulated, and whether the evoked pain mimics clinical pain. Thermal and mechanical stimuli are the most commonly used methods, due to their ease of administration and convenience. It is important to recog-

nize that when multiple pain assays are conducted in the same subjects, correlations across pain stimuli are generally low (Janal et al., 1994; Lautenbacher & Rollman, 1993). Thus, different stimulation method(s) can yield discrepant results; therefore, using multiple stimulation methods that differ along important dimensions often will be most informative.

In addition to the varieties of noxious stimuli available, the methods for assessing pain-related responses must also be considered. Pain threshold (i.e., the minimum amount of stimulation required to produce a pain) and pain tolerance (the maximum amount of stimulation an individual is willing to endure) are common measures. While these responses are intuitively appealing and quantitative, they are unidimensional in nature, which makes it difficult to disentangle the behavioral, affective/motivational, and sensory components of the responses. Numerous scaling methods are available for determining perceptual responses to noxious stimuli, such as numerical rating scales, visual analog scales, and multiple item scale (e.g., the McGill Pain Questionnaire). These methods offer the advantages of permitting assessment of multiple pain dimensions and determining responses to stimuli dispersed throughout the noxious range (e.g., stimulus–response functions). A complete discussion of pain assessment methods is beyond the scope of this chapter, but the interested reader can find more detailed information elsewhere (Arendt-Nielsen & Lautenbacher, 2004; Jensen Karoly, 2001).

Numerous studies have investigated sex differences in responses to experimentally-induced pain, and both qualitative (Berkley, 1997; Berkley & Holdcroft, 1999; Fillingim, 2000; Fillingim & Maixner, 1995) and quantitative (Riley et al., 1998) reviews of this literature are available. To summarize the findings of these reviews, women display lower pain threshold and tolerance and generally report higher ratings of experimental pain compared to men. A meta-analysis revealed that the effects sizes for sex differences in pain threshold and tolerance were moderate, and the magnitude of the sex difference varies across pain stimuli (Riley et al., 1998). The least consistent results emerged from measures of thermal pain sensitivity.

Since the publication of these reviews, additional data addressing sex differences in experimental pain responses have been reported. For example, we (Fillingim et al., 1998) previously reported that, relative to men, women displayed greater temporal summation of thermal pain, and these findings have since been replicated and extended. Specifically, Robinson et al. (2004) reported greater temporal summation of thermal pain among women and that psychological factors, including anxiety and willingness to report pain, partially mediated this sex difference. Also, Sarlani and Greenspan (2002) reported greater temporal summation of mechanical pain among women than men. Cairns and colleagues (Cairns et al.,

2001; Svensson et al., 2003) reported that injection of glutamate into the masseter muscle produced higher peak pain, longer lasting pain, and a greater area of pain among women compared to men, consistent with their finding that glutamate injection evoked significantly greater muscle afferent activity among female compared to male rats.

These findings from humans are supported to some degree by findings from nonhuman animals. Several investigators have reported greater behavioral responses to laboratory pain stimuli among female compared to male rodents (e.g., (Barrett et al., 2002, 2003; Terner et al., 2003); also for reviews see (Berkley, 1997; Bodnar et al., 1998)), while others report no such differences (Kayser et al., 1996; Mogil et al., 1993). In a particularly large study, which included 8000 observations of thermal nociceptive responses in mice, females exhibited enhanced sensitivity relative to males (Chesler et al., 2002). In contrast, studies of nonhuman primates suggest greater nociceptive responses in males than females. As a whole, nonhuman animal findings seem to show less-consistent and smaller-magnitude sex differences in basal nociceptive sensitivity compared to the human literature. This is likely related to multiple factors, such as genetics, differences between nociceptive assays used in nonhumans and humans, and greater involvement of psychological factors in humans, which are discussed in more detail below.

SEX DIFFERENCES IN RESPONSES TO ANALGESIC MEDICATIONS

In addition to basal pain sensitivity, sex-related influences on responses to analgesic drugs have been reported. The antinociceptive effects of several pharmacologic agents in animals have been found to be sex dependent. Specifically, male rats exhibit greater analgesic responses to both μ and opioid agonists (Bodnar et al., 1988; Cicero et al., 1996; Cicero et al., 1996, 1997; Craft, 2003a, 2003b; Islam et al., 1993; Kepler et al., 1989; Kepler et al., 1991; Kest et al., 2000; Kiefel et al., 1992). Sex differences in morphine-induced analgesia occur following either systemic or central intracerebroventricular administration (Berglund & Simpkins, 1988; Bodnar et al., 1988).

In contrast to these findings from rodents, Miaskowski and Levine (1999) reviewed studies of patient-controlled analgesia after surgery and found that in more than half of the studies women consumed significantly less opioid medication than men; however, analgesic responses were not directly assessed in most of these studies. Additional clinical investigations that assessed both pain and opioid consumption provide contradictory findings. For example, a large study recently demonstrated that women consumed substantially less opioid medication postoperatively and females had similar or lower postsurgical pain ratings than males (Chia et al., 2002). In contrast, Gordon and col-

leagues (1995) reported no sex differences in the analgesic effects of morphine administered after oral surgery. Likewise, Kaiko et al. (1983) reported no sex differences in morphine analgesia in a large sample of patients with chronic cancer pain. More recently, Cepeda and Carr (2003) found that women required 30% more morphine than men to achieve comparable levels of postoperative analgesia. In another series of studies examining analgesic responses to -agonist-antagonists using an oral surgery model, women showed greater analgesic responses to pentazocine and more prolonged analgesia to nalbuphine and butorphanol (Gear et al., 1996) compared to men. Also, low-dose nalbuphine (5 mg) increased pain ratings in men but not women, while higher doses (10 and 20 mg) produced analgesia of longer duration in women than men (Gear et al., 1999). More recently, among 94 patients (45 F, 49 M) presenting to the emergency department with trauma-related pain, butorphanol produced greater pain relief than morphine for women, and there was a trend toward greater morphine analgesia in men than in women (Miller & Ernst, 2004). Taken together, these clinical findings suggest more robust analgesic responses to -agonist-antagonist medications among women, but sex differences in μ-opioid analgesia are less consistent.

Sex differences in responses to opioids have also been investigated with experimental pain models. Sarton and colleagues (Sarton et al., 2000) examined morphine analgesia among 10 healthy women and 10 healthy men using an electrical pain model. Women showed greater analgesic potency but slower onset and offset of analgesia. These authors had previously reported greater morphine-induced respiratory depression among women than men (Dahan et al., 1998; Sarton et al., 1999). More recently, they reported no sex differences in analgesic responses to morphine-6-glucuronide, an active metabolite of morphine (Romberg et al., 2004). Zacny (2002) reported that the μ-opioid agonists morphine, meperidine, and hydromorphone produced greater analgesic responses among women than men using cold pressor pain, but no sex differences in analgesia emerged for pressure pain. Using a substantially larger sample size than previous investigators (41 F, 38 M), we recently reported that there were no sex differences in pentazocine analgesia for pressure, thermal, and ischemic pain (Fillingim et al., 2004). Thus, evidence from laboratory studies suggests that women may experience greater μ-opioid analgesia for some pain assays than men, and the only experimental study of a -agonist-antagonist found no sex difference in analgesic responses.

The evidence reviewed above presents an inconsistent picture of sex differences in pain and analgesic responses, since the presence, direction, and magnitude of the differences reported seem to vary across pain assays and patient populations. It is also important to note that these findings refer to quantitative sex differences; i.e., do women and men differ in the amount of pain or analgesia that they display? Of potentially greater importance are qualitative sex differences in pain and analgesia; i.e., do certain factors (e.g., genetics) moderate pain and analgesic responses differently in women versus men? Such differences are particularly compelling as they may indicate sex-specific mechanisms underlying individual differences in pain and analgesia.

MECHANISMS UNDERLYING SEX DIFFERENCES IN PAIN

Before discussing the mechanisms underlying sex differences in pain responses, some general interpretive issues should be noted. First, an individual's sex (i.e., male vs. female) is not the cause of the observed group differences; rather, sex represents a convenient grouping variable that is a surrogate for potentially clinically and scientifically important biological and psychosocial factors. Second, there are two types of sex differences that should be considered, quantitative and qualitative differences. Quantitative sex differences refer to whether women and men differ in the amount of pain or analgesia that they display, and these are the most common conceptualization of sex differences. Of potentially greater importance are qualitative sex differences in pain and analgesia, which relates to whether certain factors (e.g., genetics, anxiety) influence pain-related responses differently in women versus men. Such differences are particularly compelling as they may indicate sex-specific mechanisms underlying individual differences in pain. Thus, the following discussion of mechanisms underlying sex differences in pain is relevant to both quantitative and qualitative differences.

It is important to recognize that sex differences in pain are inevitably mediated by multiple biopsychosocial factors, including basic biological mechanisms such as genetic and hormonal influences as well as sex differences in the functioning of pain modulatory systems. In addition, psychosocial factors represent important mediators of sex differences in pain responses. Examples include cognitive/affective variables (e.g., pain coping, mood, expectancies), gender role influences, and family history. While these mechanisms are frequently described as either psychosocial or biological, this conceptualization is artificial and is based more on the level of analysis than on the actual mechanism of action. For instance, sex differences in expression of pain are often attributed to the effects of stereotypic sex roles, which is typically viewed as a psychosocial issue. However, we must remember that there are neurophysiological correlates of masculine versus feminine sex roles, which may be related to differences in nociceptive processing. Thus, the "psychosocial" and "biological" mechanisms mediating sex differences in pain responses could refer to the same fundamental processes described at different levels of analysis.

Several "biological" processes have been proposed to explain sex differences in both clinical and experimental pain responses. Considerable evidence suggests that gonadal hormones are important. The clinical symptoms of several pain disorders vary across the menstrual cycle (Anderberg et al., 1999; Heitkemper & Jarrett, 1992; Keenan & Lindamer, 1992; LeResche et al., 2003), and exogenous hormone use has been associated with increased risk for or severity of clinical pain (Brynhildsen et al., 1998; LeResche et al., 1997; Musgrave et al., 2001; Wise et al., 2000). Similarly, responses to experimentally induced pain vary across the menstrual cycle in healthy women (Fillingim & Ness, 2000; Riley et al., 1999), and postmenopausal women taking hormone replacement show enhanced sensitivity to thermal pain compared to age-matched women not on hormone replacement (Fillingim & Edwards, 2001). Sex differences in analgesia may also be influenced by both organizational (i.e., long-term developmental influences) and activational (acute, receptor-mediated) effects of sex hormones (Cicero et al., 2002). A review by Fillingim and Ness (2000) concluded that, among female animals, high estrogen levels were associated with diminished opioid analgesia, which suggests activational effects of estrogen on antinociceptive responses. Cicero and colleagues (2002) found that neonatal but not adult castration significantly decreased morphine analgesia in male rats, and neonatal testosterone treatment enhanced morphine analgesia in females. Likewise, neonatal castration in males reduced the analgesia produced by morphine injected into the ventrolateral periaqueductal gray (vlPAG), while neonatal testosterone in females increased vlPAG morphine analgesia (Krzanowska et al., 2002). Thus, opioid antinociception is influenced by both activational and organizational effects of gonadal steroids. However, hormonal effects may depend on which opioid receptor subtype is activated, as it has been reported that estrogen-attenuated analgesia for μ- but not κ-opioid agonists (Sandner-Kiesling & Eisenah, 2002). To date, limited information is available regarding hormonal effects on analgesic responses in humans.

In addition to the influence of sex hormones, endogenous pain inhibitory systems may function differently in females and males. Male rodents exhibit more robust stress-induced analgesia (SIA) than females (see Berkley, 1997; Sternberg & Liebeskind, 1995 for reviews), and SIA appears to be mediated by different neurochemical mechanisms in females and males (Kavaliers & Choleris, 1997; Mogil et al., 1993). Recent findings from humans demonstrated that tonic experimental muscle pain produced a greater decrease in μ-opioid receptor availability in several brain regions among men compared to women, apparently due to increased pain-induced binding of endogenous ligand to the receptor (Zubieta et al., 2002). This suggests that the μ-opioid system may differentially modulate pain in women and men.

Genetic factors may contribute to sex differences in pain. Indeed, substantial evidence from nonhuman animals suggests that both basal nociceptive sensitivity and antinociceptive responses to drugs show significant heritability (Lariviere et al., 2002; Mogil et al., 1999a, 1999b; Mogil, 1999). Of particular relevance to the current topic are findings that sex differences in basal nociceptive sensitivity and opioid analgesia are dependent on the strain of rodent tested (Barrett et al., 2002; Cook et al., 2000; Mogil et al., 2000; Mogil et al., 2003; Terner et al., 2003). However, there is limited evidence of genetic influences on pain sensitivity and analgesic responses in humans. Pressure pain threshold was assessed in monozygotic and dizygotic twins and showed a heritability of only 10% (Macgregor et al., 1997). In contrast, recent studies suggest significant associations between single nucleotide polymorphisms (SNPs) of specific genes and experimental pain responses. One group of investigators reported heritability estimates of 22 to 46% across three pain modalities and a SNP of the δ-opioid receptor gene (*OPRD1*) was associated with thermal pain responses among men but not women (Kim et al., 2003), consistent with the results of a previous linkage mapping study in mice (Mogil et al., 1997). Zubieta and colleagues (2003) reported that an SNP of the catechol-*O*-methyltransferase gene (COMT) was marginally associated with pain report and significantly associated with pain-induced brain μ-opioid receptor binding. It was recently demonstrated that genotype at the melacocortin-1-receptor gene was associated with analgesic responses to pentazocine among women but not men (Mogil et al., 2003). These findings from both rodents and humans indicate that genetic factors are associated with pain responses, and some of these associations are sex-dependent.

In addition to these multiple "biological" factors, numerous "psychosocial" variables also contribute to sex differences in pain responses. For example, the greater levels of depression and anxiety reported by women may be associated with increased clinical pain (Kroenke & Spitzer, 1998; Moldin et al., 1993; Rajala et al., 1995), as well as enhanced experimental pain sensitivity (Cornwall & Donderi, 1988; Graffenried et al., 1978). The association of negative affect to pain may be sex related, as several investigators have reported a stronger relationship between emotional distress and pain-related symptomatology among men than women (Edwards et al., 2003; Edwards et al., 2000; McCracken & Houle, 2000; Riley et al., 2001). Relatedly, we previously reported that anxiety was more strongly associated with experimental pain sensitivity among men than women (Fillingim et al., 1996). Taken together, this evidence indicates a stronger association between psychological distress and enhanced pain responses among men.

Cognitive variables may also contribute to sex differences in pain. For instance, numerous studies have reported sex differences in cognitive and behavioral coping strategies, with women reporting higher levels of many forms of pain coping (Affleck et al., 1999; Keefe et al., 2000; Mercado et al., 2000; Osman et al., 2000; Unruh et al., 1999). Keefe et al. (2000) reported that catastrophizing mediated the higher levels of pain and disability reported by women compared to men with osteoarthritis. Another potentially important cognitive factor is self-efficacy, which predicts improved adjustment to chronic pain (Jensen et al., 1999; Jensen & Karoly, 1991), decreased procedural pain (Kashikar-Zuck et al., 1997), and lower sensitivity to experimental pain (Keefe et al., 1997). Both women and men report that men are better able than women to tolerate pain (Robinson et al., 2001), and a greater perceived ability to tolerate and control pain has been related to lower pain sensitivity among women but not men (Fillingim et al., 1996).

Stereotypic gender roles may also contribute to sex differences in pain. Among men, masculinity has been associated with higher pain thresholds (Otto & Dougher, 1985), and one study found that men but not women reported less pain to an attractive opposite-sex experimenter than to a same-sex experimenter (Levine & De Simone, 1991). Importantly, while two studies have demonstrated that sex roles are associated with experimental pain responses, in neither study did sex role measures account for the gender difference in pain (Myers et al., 2001; Otto & Dougher, 1985). In an experiment that manipulated gender role expectations, Robinson, Gagnon, Riley, & Price (2003) found that sex differences in pain responses disappeared when subjects were given gender-specific expectations regarding pain tolerance. Thus, in the laboratory setting, gender role expectancies may contribute to sex differences in pain responses; however, little information is available regarding the association of gender roles to clinical pain.

Familial factors may contribute to sex differences in pain. Several chronic pain conditions are characterized by familial aggregation, including fibromyalgia (Buskila et al., 1996; Buskila & Neumann, 1997; Pellegrino et al., 1989), headache (Aromaa et al., 2000; Ehde et al., 1991; Messinger et al., 1991; Ottman et al., 1993; Schrader et al., 1996; Turkat et al., 1984), irritable bowel syndrome (Kalantar, Locke, Zinsmeister, Beighley, & Talley, 2003; Kalantar et al., 2003), and low back pain (Balague, Troussier, & Salminen, 1999). Moreover, in community studies, individuals reporting a family history of pain have increased pain complaints (Edwards et al., 1985; Koutantji et al., 1998; Lester et al., 1994; Sternbach, 1986). The association between family history and pain may differ across sexes, as reported that familial pain history predicted pain complaints more strongly among women than men (Edwards et al., 1985). Also, an association between family pain history and enhanced experimental pain sensitivity has been reported among women but not men

(Fillingim et al., 2000; Neumann & Buskila, 1997). Whether this stronger association between familial factors and pain responses among women is due to social learning or genetic factors has yet to be determined.

Thus, multiple biopsychosocial factors contribute to sex differences in clinical and experimental pain responses. The biopsychosocial model of pain suggests that biological, psychological, and sociocultural factors interact to influence pain responses. Additional research is needed to elucidate these interactions in the context of sex differences in pain.

CONCLUSIONS AND FUTURE DIRECTIONS

The literature reviewed above clearly demonstrates that pain is characterized by both quantitative and qualitative sex differences. Multiple factors contribute to sex differences in pain responses, including those traditionally referred to as "biological" (e.g., genetics, hormones, pain modulatory systems) and "psychological" (e.g., cognitive/affective variables, social roles, family history). A major challenge for the future will be translating these findings into clinical practice. An example of this might be sex-related treatment tailoring. It seems plausible that sex differences in analgesic responses may ultimately lead to the development of sex-specific medications and/or dosing regimens. Similarly, some evidence indicates sex differences in the outcomes of nonpharmacologic treatment for pain. For example, women but not men showed significant benefit following multidisciplinary treatment for back pain (Jensen et al., 2001) and pain due to TMD (Krogstad et al., 1996). Moreover, the predictors of treatment outcomes have differed for women and men in some studies (Burns et al., 1998; Edwards et al., 2003). Therefore, in the future it may be possible to tailor interdisciplinary pain treatment by sex to optimize treatment outcomes.

Another important issue is that clinicians and scientists should be educated regarding the existence and nature of sex differences in pain. Increasing our awareness of these differences should help reduce gender-related biases, which can adversely influence treatment decisions. Indeed, some findings indicate that women presenting with chest pain were less likely than men to receive both invasive and non-invasive cardiac procedures (Roger et al., 2000). Although multiple reasons could produce these differences in medical decisions, we must avoid minimizing women's pain reports based on the assumption that women are overreporting or exaggerating symptoms, since it could just as well be true that men are underreporting (Barsky et al., 2001).

In summary, based on considerable basic and clinical pain research, we can now state the obvious with confidence, women and men are different. Women report more frequent and/or more severe clinical pain and display enhanced perceptual responses to experimentally-induced pain. In addition, responses to analgesic medications have shown sex differences, although the results are somewhat inconsistent across studies. Multiple biopsychosocial factors contribute to sex differences in pain, and continued research to further characterize the nature of sex differences in pain will inform pain treatment for patients of both sexes.

ACKNOWLEDGMENTS

This material is the result of work supported with resources and the use of facilities at the Malcom Randall VA Medical Center, Gainesville, FL. This work was supported by NIH Grants NS41670 and NS42754 and the NIH/NCMHD Loan Repayment Program.

REFERENCES

Adelman, A. M., Revicki, D. A., Magaziner, J., & Hebel, R. (1995). Abdominal pain in an HMO. *Family Medicine, 27*(5), 321–325.

Affleck, G., Tennen, H., Keefe, F. J., Lefebvre, J. C., Kashikar-Zuck, S., Wright, K., et al. (1995). Everyday life with osteoarthritis or rheumatoid arthritis: Independent effects of disease and gender on daily pain, mood, and coping. *Pain, 83*(3), 601–609.

Agreus, L., Svardsudd, K., Nyren, O., & Tibblin, G. (1994). The epidemiology of abdominal symptoms: prevalence and demographic characteristics in a Swedish adult population. A report from the Abdominal Symptom Study. *Scandinavian Journal of Gastroenterology, 29*(2), 102–109.

American Pain Foundation. (2002). *Survey of pain in the United States.* Baltimore: Mason-Dixon Polling & Research.

Anderberg, U. M., Marteinsdottir, I., Hallman, J., Ekselius, L., & Backstrom, T. (1999). Symptom perception in relation to hormonal status in female fibromyalgia syndrome patients. *Journal of Musculoskeletal Pain, 7,* 21–38.

Andersson, H. I., Ejlertsson, G., Leden, I., & Rosenberg, C. (1993). Chronic pain in a geographically defined general population: Studies of differences in age, gender, social class, and pain localization. *Clinical Journal of Pain, 9,* 174–182.

Andersson, H. I., Ejlertsson, G., Leden, I., & Schersten, B. (1999). Impact of chronic pain on health care seeking, self care, and medication. Results from a population-based Swedish study. *Journal of Epidemiology and Community Health, 53*(8), 503–509.

Arendt-Nielsen, L., & Lautenbacher, S. (2004). Assessment of pain perception. In S. Lautenbacher, & R. B. Fillingim (Eds.). New York: Kluwer Academic.

Aromaa, M., Sillanpaa, M., Rautava, P., & Helenius, H. (2000). Pain experience of children with headache and their families: A controlled study. *Pediatrics, 106*(2 Pt 1), 270–275.

Ashmore, R. (1990). Sex, gender and the individual. In L. Pervin (Ed.), *Handbook of personality: Theory and research* (pp. 486–526). New York: Guilford.

Averbuch, M., & Katzper, M. (2000). A search for sex differences in response to analgesia. *Archives of Internal Medicine, 160*(22), 3424–3428.

Averbuch, M., & Katzper, M. (2001). Gender and the placebo analgesic effect in acute pain. *Clinical Pharmacology and Therapeutics, 70*(3), 287–291.

Balague, F., Troussier, B., & Salminen, J. J. (1999). Non-specific low back pain in children and adolescents: Risk factors. *European Spine Journal, 8*(6), 429–438.

Barrett, A. C., Cook, C. D., Terner, J. M., Roach, E. L., Syvanthong, C., & Picker, M. J. (2002). Sex and rat strain determine sensitivity to kappa opioid-induced antinociception. *Psychopharmacology* (Berlin), *160*(2), 170–181.

Barrett, A. C., Smith, E. S., & Picker, M. J. (2003). Capsaicin-induced hyperalgesia and {micro}-opioid-induced antihyperalgesia in male and female fischer 344 rats. *Journal of Pharmacology and Experimental Therapeutics, 307*(1), 237–245.

Barrett, A., Smith, E., & Picker, M. (2002). Sex-related differences in mechanical nociception and antinociception produced by mu- and kappa-opioid receptor agonists in rats. *European Journal of Pharmacology, 452*(2), 163.

Barsky, A. J., Peekna, H. M., & Borus, J. F. (2001). Somatic symptom reporting in women and men. *Journal of General Internal Medicine, 16*(4), 266–275.

Berglund, L. A., & Simpkins, J. W. (1988). Alterations in brain opiate receptor mechanisms on proestrous afternoon. *Neuroendocrinology, 48*, 394–400.

Berkley, K. J. (1997). Sex differences in pain. *Behavioral and Brain Sciences, 20*, 371–380.

Berkley, K. J., & Holdcroft, A. (1999). Sex and gender differences in pain. In P. D. Wall & R. Melzack (Eds.), *Textbook of pain* (4th ed., pp. 951–965). Edinburgh: Churchill-Livingstone.

Blyth, F. M., March, L. M., Brnabic, A. J., Jorm, L. R., Williamson, M., & Cousins, M. J. (2001). Chronic pain in Australia: A prevalence study. *Pain, 89*(2–3), 127–134.

Boccardi, L., & Verde, M. (2003). Gender differences in the clinical presentation to the emergency department for chest pain. *Italian Heart Journal, 4*(6), 371–373.

Bodnar, R. J., Romero, M. T., & Kramer, E. (1988). Organismic variables and pain inhibition: roles of gender and aging. *Brain. Research Bulletin, 21*, 947–953.

Brynhildsen, J. O., Bjors, E., Skarsgard, C., & Hammar, M. L. (1998). Is hormone replacement therapy a risk factor for low back pain among postmenopausal women? *Spine, 23*(7), 809–813.

Buckwalter, J. A., & Lappin, D. R. (2000). The disproportionate impact of chronic arthralgia and arthritis among women. *Clinical Orthopedics, 372*, 159–168.

Buitenhuis, J., Spanjer, J., & Fidler, V. (2003). Recovery from acute whiplash: The role of coping styles. *Spine, 28*(9), 896–901.

Burns, J. W., Johnson, B. J., Devine, J., Mahoney, N., & Pawl, R. (1998). Anger management style and the prediction of treatment outcome among male and female chronic pain patients. *Behaviour Research & Therapy, 36*(11), 1051–1062.

Bush, F. M., Harkins, S. W., Harrington, W. G., & Price, D. D. (1993). Analysis of gender effects on pain perception and symptom presentation in temporomandibular joint pain. *Pain, 53*, 73–80.

Buskila, D., & Neumann, L. (1997). Fibromyalgia syndrome (FM) and nonarticular tenderness in relatives of patients with FM. *Journal of Rheumatology, 24*(5), 941–944.

Buskila, D., Neumann, L., Hazanov, I., & Carmi, R. (1996). Familial aggregation in the fibromyalgia syndrome. *Seminars in Arthritis & Rheumatism, 26*(3), 605–611.

Cairns, B. E., Hu, J. W., Arendt-Nielsen, L., Sessle, B. J., & Svensson, P. (2001). Sex-related differences in human pain and rat afferent discharge evoked by injection of glutamate into the masseter muscle. *Journal of Neurophysiology, 86*(2), 782–791.

Celentano, D. D., Stewart, W. F., Lipton, R. B., & Reed, M. L. (1992). Medication use and disability among migraineurs: A national probability sample survey. *Headache, 32*(5), 223–228.

Cepeda, M. S., & Carr, D. B. (2003). Women experience more pain and require more morphine than men to achieve a similar degree of analgesia. *Anesth. Analg.* 2003, *97* (5), 1464–1468.

Cepeda, M. S., Africano, J. M., Polo, R., Alcala, R., & Carr, D. B. (2003). Agreement between percentage pain reductions calculated from numeric rating scores of pain intensity and those reported by patients with acute or cancer pain. *Pain, 106*(3), 439–442.

Chang, L., & Heitkemper, M. M. (2002). Gender differences in irritable bowel syndrome. *Gastroenterology, 123*(5), 1686–1701.

Chesler, E. J., Wilson, S. G., Lariviere, W. R., Rodriguez-Zas, S. L., & Mogil, J. S. (2002). Identification and ranking of genetic and laboratory environment factors influencing a behavioral trait, thermal nociception, via computational analysis of a large data archive. *Neuroscience and Biobehavioral Review, 26*(8), 907–923.

Chia, Y. Y., Chow, L. H., Hung, C. C., Liu, K., Ger, L. P., & Wang, P. N. (2002). Gender and pain upon movement are associated with the requirements for postoperative patient-controlled iv analgesia: A prospective survey of 2,298 Chinese patients. *Canadian Journal of Anaesthesiology, 49*(3), 249–255.

Choleris, E., & Kavaliers, M. (1999). Social learning in animals: sex differences and neurobiological analysis. *Pharmacology, Biochemistry and Behavior, 64*(4), 767–776.

Cicero, T. J., Nock, B., & Meyer, E. R. (1996). Gender-related differences in the antinociceptive properties of morphine. *Journal of Pharmacology & Experimental Therapeutics, 279*(2), 767–773.

Cicero, T. J., Nock, B., & Meyer, E. R. (1997). Sex-related differences in morphine's antinociceptive activity: relationship to serum and brain morphine concentrations. *Journal of Pharmacology & Experimental Therapeutics, 282*(2), 939–944.

Cicero, T. J., Nock, B., O'Connor, L., & Meyer, E. R. (2002). Role of steroids in sex differences in morphine-induced analgesia: Activational and organizational effects. *Journal of Pharmacology and Experimental Therapeutics, 300*(2), 695–701.

Cook, C. D., Barrett, A. C., Roach, E. L., Bowman, J. R., & Picker, M. J. (2000). Sex-related differences in the antinociceptive effects of opioids: importance of rat genotype, nociceptive stimulus intensity, and efficacy at the mu opioid receptor. *Psychopharmacology* (Berlin), *150*(4), 430–442.

Cornwall, A., & Donderi, D. C. (1988). The effect of experimentally induced anxiety on the experience of pressure pain. *Pain, 35,* 105–113.

Costa, P. T., Jr., Terracciano, A., & McCrae, R. R. (2001). Gender differences in personality traits across cultures: robust and surprising findings. *Journal of Personality and Social Psychology, 81*(2), 322–331.

Coulthard, P., Pleuvry, B. J., Dobson, M., & Price, M. (2000). Behavioural measurement of postoperative pain after oral surgery. *British Journal of Oral and Maxillofacial Surgery, 38*(2), 127–131.

Craft, R. M. (2003a). Sex differences in drug- and non-drug-induced analgesia. *Life Sciences, 72*(24), 2675–2688.

Craft, R. M. (2003b). Sex differences in opioid analgesia: From mouse to man. *Clinical Journal of Pain, 19,* 175–186.

Croft, P. R., Lewis, M., Papageorgiou, A. C., Thomas, E., Jayson, M. I., Macfarlane, G. J., & Silman, A. J. (2001). Risk factors for neck pain: A longitudinal study in the general population. *Pain, 93*(3), 317–325.

Croft, P. R., Papageorgiou, A. C., Ferry, S., Thomas, E., Jayson, M. I., & Silman, A. J. (1995). Psychologic distress and low back pain. Evidence from a prospective study in the general population. *Spine, 20*(24), 2731–2737.

Croft, P. R., Papageorgiou, A. C., Thomas, E., Macfarlane, G. J., & Silman, A. J. (1999). Short-term physical risk factors for new episodes of low back pain. Prospective evidence from the South Manchester Back Pain Study. *Spine, 24*(15), 1556–1561.

Crombie, I. K., Croft, P. R., Linton, S. J., LeResche, L., & Von Korff, M. E. (1999). *Epidemiology of pain.* Seattle: IASP Press.

Dahan, A., Sarton, E., Teppema, L., & Olievier, C. (1998). Sex-related differences in the influence of morphine on ventilatory control in humans. *Anesthesiology, 88*(4), 903–913.

Drangsholt, M., & LeResche, L. (1999). Temporomandibular disorder pain. In I. K. Crombie, P. R. Croft, S. J. Linton, L. LeResche, & M. Von Korff (Eds.), *Epidemiology of pain* (pp. 203–233). Seattle: IASP Press.

Edwards, P. W., Zeichner, A., Kuczmierczyk, A. R., & Boczkowski, J. (1985). Familial pain models: The relationship between family history of pain and current pain experience. *Pain, 21,* 379–384.

Edwards, R. R., Augustson, E., & Fillingim, R. B. (2000). Sex-specific effects of pain-related anxiety on adjustment to chronic pain. *Clinical Journal of Pain, 16,* 46–53.

Edwards, R. R., Augustson, E., & Fillingim, R. B. (2003). Differential relationships between anxiety and treatment-associated pain reduction among male and female chronic pain patients. *Clinical Journal of Pain, 19,* 208–216.

Eggen, A. E. (1993). The Tromso Study: Frequency and predicting factors of analgesic drug use in a free-living population (12–56 years). *Journal of Clinical Epidemiology, 46,* 1297–1304.

Ehde, D. M., Holm, J. E., & Metzger, D. L. (1991). The role of family structure, functioning, and pain modeling in headache. *Headache, 31*(1), 35–40.

Ferrari, R., Constantoyannis, C., & Papadakis, N. (2003). Laypersons' expectation of the sequelae of whiplash injury: A cross-cultural comparative study between Canada and Greece. *Medical Science Monitor, 9*(3), CR120–CR124.

Ferrari, R., Schrader, H., & Obelieniene, D. (1999). Prevalence of temporomandibular disorders associated with whiplash injury in Lithuania. *Oral Surgery, Oral Medicine, Oral Pathology, Oral Radiology and Endodontics, 87*(6), 653–657.

Fillingim, R. B. (2000). Sex, gender and pain: women and men really are different. *Current Review of Pain, 4,* 24–30.

Fillingim, R. B., & Edwards, R. R. (2001). The association of hormone replacement therapy with experimental pain responses in postmenopausal women. *Pain, 92,* 229–234.

Fillingim, R. B., & Maixner, W. (1995). Gender differences in the responses to noxious stimuli. *Pain Forum, 4*(4), 209–221.

Fillingim, R. B., & Ness, T. J. (2000). Sex-related hormonal influences on pain and analgesic responses. *Neuroscience and Biobehavioral Reviews, 24,* 485–501.

Fillingim, R. B., Doleys, D. M., Edwards, R. R., & Lowery, D. (2003). Clinical characteristics of chronic back pain as a function of gender and oral opioid use. *Spine, 28*(2), 143–150.

Fillingim, R. B., Edwards, R. R., & Powell, T. (2000). Sex-dependent effects of reported familial pain history on clinical and experimental pain responses. *Pain, 86,* 87–94.

Fillingim, R. B., Keefe, F. J., Light, K. C., Booker, D. K., & Maixner, W. (1996). The influence of gender and psychological factors on pain perception. *Journal of Gender Cult. Health, 1,* 21–36.

Fillingim, R. B., Maixner, W., Kincaid, S., & Silva, S. (1998). Sex differences in temporal summation but not sensory-discriminative processing of thermal pain. *Pain, 75*(1), 121–127.

Fillingim, R. B., Ness, T. J., Glover, T. L., Campbell, C. M., Price, D. D., & Staud, R. (2004). Experimental pain models reveal no sex differences in pentazocine analgesia in humans. *Anesthesiology, 100,* 1263–1270.

Frable, D. E. (1997). Gender, racial, ethnic, sexual, and class identities. *Annual Review of Psychology, 48,* 139–62, 139–162.

Froehlich, F., Thorens, J., Schwizer, W., Preisig, M., Kohler, M., Hays, R. D. et al. (1997). Sedation and analgesia for colonoscopy: patient tolerance, pain, and cardiorespiratory parameters. *Gastrointestinal Endoscopy, 45*(1), 1–9.

Gear, R. W., Miaskowski, C., Gordon, N. C., Paul, S. M., Heller, P. H., & Levine, J. D. (1996). Kappa-opioids produce significantly greater analgesia in women than in men (see comments). *Nature Medicine, 2*(11), 1248–1250.

Gear, R. W., Miaskowski, C., Gordon, N. C., Paul, S. M., Heller, P. H., & Levine, J. D. (1999). The kappa opioid nalbuphine produces gender- and dose-dependent analgesia and antianalgesia in patients with postoperative pain. *Pain, 83*(2), 339–345.

Goodenough, B., Kampel, L., Champion, G. D., Laubreaux, L., Nicholas, M. K., Ziegler, J. B., & McInerney, M. (1997). An investigation of the placebo effect and age-related factors in the report of needle pain from venipuncture in children. *Pain, 72*(3), 383–391.

Goodenough, B., Thomas, W., Champion, G. D., Perrott, D., Taplin, J. E., von Baeyer, C. L., & Ziegler, J. B. (1999). Unravelling age effects and sex differences in needle pain: Ratings of sensory intensity and unpleasantness of venipuncture pain by children and their parents. *Pain, 80*(1–2), 179–190.

Gordis, L. (1988). Challenges to epidemiology in the next decade. *American Journal of Epidemiology, 128*(1), 1–9.

Gordon, N. C., Gear, R. W., Heller, P. H., Paul, S., Miaskowski, C., & Levine, J. D. (1995). Enhancement of morphine analgesia by the GABAB agonist baclofen. *Neuroscience, 69*(2), 345–349.

Goulet, J. P., Lavigne, G. J., & Lund, J. P. (1995). Jaw pain prevalence among French-speaking Canadians in Quebec and related symptoms of temporomandibular disorders. *Journal of Dental Research, 74*(11), 1738–1744.

Graffenried, B. V., Adler, R., Abt, K., Nuesch, E., & Spiegel, R. (1978). The influence of anxiety and pain sensitivity on experimental pain in man. *Pain, 4*, 253–263.

Gran, J. T. (2003). The epidemiology of chronic generalized musculoskeletal pain. *Best Practice & Research in Clinical Rheumatology, 17*(4), 547–561.

Greenberger, P. (2001). Women, men, and pain. *Journal of Womens Health and Gender-Based Medicine, 10*(4), 309–310.

Halder, S. L., McBeth, J., Silman, A. J., Thompson, D. G., & Macfarlane, G. J. (2002). Psychosocial risk factors for the onset of abdominal pain. Results from a large prospective population-based study. *International Journal of Epidemiology, 31*(6), 1219–1225.

Hartvigsen, J., Christensen, K., & Frederiksen, H. (2003). Back pain remains a common symptom in old age. A population-based study of 4486 Danish twins aged 70–102. *European Spine Journal, 12*(5), 528–534.

Hasvold, T., & Johnsen, R. (1993). Headache and neck or shoulder pain—frequent and disabling complaints in the general population. *Scandinavian Journal of Primary Health Care, 11*(3), 219–224.

Haugland, S., Wold, B., Stevenson, J., Aaroe, L. E., & Woynarowska, B. (2001). Subjective health complaints in adolescence. A cross-national comparison of prevalence and dimensionality. *European Journal of Public Health, 11*(1), 4–10.

Heitkemper, M. M., & Jarrett, M. (1992). Pattern of gastrointestinal and somatic symptoms across the menstrual cycle. *Gastroenterology, 102*(2), 505–513.

Holroyd, K. A., & Lipchik, G. L. (2000) Sex differences in recurrent headache disorders: Overview and significance. In R. B. Fillingim (Ed.), *Sex, gender, and pain* (pp. 251–279). Seattle: IASP Press.

Holtzman, J., Saleh, K., & Kane, R. (2002). Gender differences in functional status and pain in a Medicare population undergoing elective total hip arthroplasty. *Medical Care, 40*(6), 461–470.

Hughes, R. N. (2003). The categorisation of male and female laboratory animals in terms of "gender." *Brain Research Bulletin, 60*(3), 189–190.

Isacson, D., & Bingefors, K. (2002). Epidemiology of analgesic use: A gender perspective. *European Journal of Anaesthesiology Supplement, 26*, 5–15.

Islam, A. K., Beczkowska, I. W., & Bodnar, R. J. (1993). Interactions among aging, gender, and gonadectomy effects upon naloxone hypophagia in rats. *Physiology and Behavior, 54*, 981–992.

Janal, M. N., Glusman, M., Kuhl, J. P., & Clark, W. C. (1994). On the absence of correlation between responses to noxious heat, cold, electrical and ischemic stimulation. *Pain, 58*, 403–411.

Jensen, I. B., Bergstrom, G., Ljungquist, T., Bodin, L., & Nygren, A. L. (2001). A randomized controlled component analysis of a behavioral medicine rehabilitation program for chronic spinal pain: Are the effects dependent on gender? *Pain, 91*(1–2), 65–78.

Jensen, M. P., & Karoly, P. (1991). Control beliefs, coping efforts, and adjustment to chronic pain. *Journal of Consulting and Clinical Psychology, 59*, 431–438.

Jensen, M. P., & Karoly, P. (2001). Self-report scales and procedures for assessing pain in adults. In D. C. Turk & R. Melzack (Eds.), *Handbook of pain assessment* (pp. 15–34). New York: Guilford Press.

Jensen, M. P., Turner, J. A., Romano, J. M., & Karoly, P. (1991). Coping with chronic pain: A critical review of the literature. *Pain, 47*(3), 249–283.

Kaiko, R. F., Wallenstein, S. L., Rogers, A. G., & Houde, R. W. (1983). Sources of variation in analgesic responses in cancer patients with chronic pain receiving morphine. *Pain, 15*(2), 191–200.

Kalantar, J. S., Locke, G. R., III, Talley, N. J., Zinsmeister, A. R., Fett, S. L., & Melton, L. J., III. (2003). Is irritable bowel syndrome more likely to be persistent in those with relatives who suffer from gastrointestinal symptoms? A population-based study at three time points. *Alimentary Pharmacology and Therapeutics, 17*(11), 1389–1397.

Kalantar, J. S., Locke, G. R., Zinsmeister, A. R., Beighley, C. M., & Talley, N. J. (2003). Familial aggregation of irritable bowel syndrome: a prospective study. *Gut, 52*(12), 1703–1707.

Kalkman, C. J., Visser, K., Moen, J., Bonsel, G. J., Grobbee, D. E., & Moons, K. G. (2003). Preoperative prediction of severe postoperative pain. *Pain*, *105*(3), 415–423.

Kashikar-Zuck, S., Keefe, F. J., Kornguth, P., Beaupre, P., Holzberg, A., & Delong, D. (1997). Pain coping and the pain experience during mammography: A preliminary study. *Pain*, *73*(2), 165–172.

Kavaliers, M., & Choleris, E. (1997). Sex differences in *N*-methyl-D-aspartate involvement in kappa opioid and non-opioid predator-induced analgesia in mice. *Brain Research*, *768*(1–2), 30–36.

Kayser, V., Berkley, K. J., Keita, H., Gautron, M., & Guilbaud, G. (1996). Estrous and sex variations in vocalization thresholds to hindpaw and tail pressure stimulation in the rat. *Brain Research*, *742*(1–2), 352–354.

Keefe, F. J., Lefebvre, J. C., Egert, J. R., Affleck, G., Sullivan, M. J., & Caldwell, D. S. (2000). The relationship of gender to pain, pain behavior, and disability in osteoarthritis patients: The role of catastrophizing. *Pain*, *87*(3), 325–334.

Keefe, F. J., Lefebvre, J. C., Maixner, W., Salley, A. N. J., & Caldwell, D. S. (1997). Self-efficacy for arthritis pain: Relationship to perception of thermal laboratory pain stimuli. *Arthritis Care & Research*, *10* (3), 177–184.

Keenan, P. A., & Lindamer, L. A. (1992). Non-migraine headache across the menstrual cycle in women with and without premenstrual syndrome. *Cephalalgia*, *12*(6), 356–359.

Kepler, K. L., Kest, B., Kiefel, J. M., Cooper, M. L., & Bodnar, R. J. (1989). Roles of gender, gonadectomy and estrous phase in the analgesic effects of intracerebroventricular morphine in rats. *Pharmacology, Biochemistry, and Behavior*, *34*, 119–127.

Kepler, K. L., Standifer, K. M., Paul, D., Kest, B., Pasternak, G. W., & Bodnar, R. J. (1991). Gender effects and central opioid analgesia. *Pain*, *45*, 87–94.

Kest, B., Sarton, E., & Dahan, A. (2000). Gender differences in opioid-mediated analgesia: animal and human studies. *Anesthesiology*, *93*(2), 539–547.

Kiefel, J. M., & Bodnar, R. J. (1992). Roles of gender and gonadectomy in pilocarpine and clonidine analgesia in rats. *Pharmacology, Biochemistry, and Behavior*, *41*, 153–158.

Kim, H., Neubert, J. K., Iadarola, M. J., San Miguelle, A., Goldman, D., & Dionne, R. A. (2003). Genetic influence on pain sensitivity in humans: Evidence of heritability related to single nucleotide polymorphism (SNP) in opioid receptor genes. In J. O. Dostrovsky, D. B. Carr, & M. Koltzenburg (Eds.), *Proceedings of the 10th World Congress on Pain* (pp. 513–520). Seattle: IASP Press.

Kostova, V., & Koleva, M. (2001). Back disorders (low back pain, cervicobrachial and lumbosacral radicular syndromes) and some related risk factors. *Journal of Neurological Science*, *192*(1–2), 17–25.

Koutantji, M., Pearce, S. A., & Oakley, D. A. (1998). The relationship between gender and family history of pain with current pain experience and awareness of pain in others. *Pain*, *77*(1), 25–31.

Kroenke, K., & Spitzer, R. L. (1998). Gender differences in the reporting of physical and somatoform symptoms. *Psychosomatic Medicine*, *60*(2), 150–155.

Krogstad, B. S., Jokstad, A., Dahl, B. L., & Vassend, O. (1996). The reporting of pain, somatic complaints, and anxiety in a group of patients with TMD before and 2 years after treatment: Sex differences. *Journal of Orofacial Pain*, *10*(3), 263–269.

Krzanowska, E. K., Ogawa, S., Pfaff, D. W., & Bodnar, R. J. (2002). Reversal of sex differences in morphine analgesia elicited from the ventrolateral periaqueductal gray in rats by neonatal hormone manipulations. *Brain Research*, *929*(1), 1–9.

Lander, J., Fowler-Kerry, S., & Hargreaves, A. (1989). Gender effects in pain perception. *Perceptual and Motor Skills*, *68*, 1088–1090.

Lander, J., Fowler-Kerry, S., & Hill, A. (1990). Comparison of pain perceptions among males and females. *Canadian Journal of Nursing Research*, *22*, 39–49.

Lariviere, W. R., Wilson, S. G., Laughlin, T. M., Kokayeff, A., West, E. E., Adhikari, S. M. et al. (2002). Heritability of nociception. III. Genetic relationships among commonly used assays of nociception and hypersensitivity. *Pain*, *97*(1–2), 75–86.

Lautenbacher, S., & Rollman, G. B. (1993). Sex differences in responsiveness to painful and non-painful stimuli are dependent upon the stimulation method. *Pain*, *53*, 255–264.

Leboeuf-Yde, C. (2004). Back pain — Individual and genetic factors. *Journal of Electromyography and Kinesiology*, *14*(1), 129–133.

Leboeuf-Yde, C., & Kyvik, K. O. (1998). At what age does low back pain become a common problem? A study of 29,424 individuals aged 12–41 years. *Spine*, *23*(2), 228–234.

LeResche, L. (1997). Epidemiology of temporomandibular disorders: Implications for the investigation of etiologic factors. *Critical Reviews in Oral Biology & Medicine*, *8*(3), 291–305.

LeResche, L. (1999). Gender considerations in the epidemiology of chronic pain. In I. K. Crombie (Ed.), *Epidemiology of pain* (pp. 43–52). Seattle: IASP Press.

LeResche, L. (2000). Epidemiologic perspectives on sex differences in pain. In R. B. Fillingim (Ed.), *Sex, gender, and pain* (pp. 233–249). Seattle: IASP Press.

LeResche, L., Mancl, L., Sherman, J. J., Gandara, B., & Dworkin, S. F. (2003). Changes in temporomandibular pain and other symptoms across the menstrual cycle. *Pain*, *106*(3), 253–261.

LeResche, L., Saunders, K., Von Korff, M. R., Barlow, W., & Dworkin, S. F. (1997). Use of exogenous hormones and risk of temporomandibular disorder pain. *Pain*, *69*(1–2), 153–160.

Lester, N., Lefebvre, J. C., & Keefe, F. J. (1994). Pain in young adults: I. Relationship to gender and family pain history. *Clinical Journal of Pain*, *10*, 282–289.

Leveille, S. G., Resnick, H. E., & Balfour, J. (2000). Gender differences in disability: Evidence and underlying reasons. *Aging* (Milano), *12*(2), 106–112.

Levine, F. M., & De Simone, L. L. (1991). The effects of experimenter gender on pain report in male and female subjects. *Pain, 44*, 69–72.

Lipton, R. B., Scher, A. I., Kolodner, K., Liberman, J., Steiner, T. J., & Stewart, W. F. (2002). Migraine in the United States: Epidemiology and patterns of health care use. *Neurology, 58*(6), 885–894.

Lipton, R. B., Stewart, W. F., Diamond, S., Diamond, M. L., & Reed, M. (2001). Prevalence and burden of migraine in the United States: Data from the American Migraine Study II. *Headache, 41*(7), 646–657.

List, T., Wahlund, K., Wenneberg, B., & Dworkin, S. F. (1999). TMD in children and adolescents: Prevalence of pain, gender differences, and perceived treatment need. *Journal of Orofacial Pain, 13*(1), 9–20.

Macfarlane, G. J. (1999). Fibromyalgia and chronic widespread pain. In I. K. Crombie (Ed.), *Epidemiology of pain* (pp. 113–123). Seattle: IASP Press.

Macfarlane, T. V., Gray, R. J. M., Kincey, J., & Worthington, H. V. (2001). Factors associated with the temporomandibular disorder, pain dysfunction syndrome (PDS): Manchester case-control study. *Oral Diseases, 7*(6), 321–330.

Macgregor, A. J., Griffiths, G. O., Baker, J., & Spector, T. D. (1997). Determinants of pressure pain threshold in adult twins: evidence that shared environmental influences predominate. *Pain, 73*(2), 253–257.

Maraste, P., Persson, U., & Berntman, M. (2003). Long-term follow-up and consequences for severe road traffic injuries-treatment costs and health impairment in Sweden in the 1960s and the 1990s. *Health Policy, 66*(2), 147–158.

Marcus, D. A. (2003). Gender differences in chronic pain in a treatment-seeking population. *Journal of Gender Specific Medicine, 6*(4), 19–24.

Mayer, E. A., Naliboff, B., Lee, O., Munakata, J., & Chang, L. (1999). Review article: Gender-related differences in functional gastrointestinal disorders. *Alimentary Pharmacology & Therapeutics, 13*(Suppl. 2), 65–69.

McCracken, L. M., & Houle, T. (2000). Sex-specific and general roles of pain-related anxiety in adjustment to chronic pain: A reply to Edwards et al. *Clinical Journal of Pain, 16*(3), 275–276.

McGrath, P. A. (1999). Chronic pain in children. In I. K. Crombie (Ed.), *Epidemiology of pain* (pp. 81–101). Seattle: IASP Press.

Mercado, A. C., Carroll, L. J., Cassidy, J. D., & Cote, P. (2000). Coping with neck and low back pain in the general population. *Health Psychology, 19*(4), 333–338.

Messinger, H. B., Spierings, E. L., Vincent, A. J., & Lebbink, J. (1991). Headache and family history. *Cephalalgia, 11*(1), 13–18.

Miaskowski, C., & Levine, J. D. (1999). Does opioid analgesia show a gender preference for females? *Pain Forum, 8*(1), 34–44.

Miettinen, T., Lindgren, K. A., Airaksinen, O., & Leino, E. (2002). Whiplash injuries in Finland: A prospective 1-year follow-up study. *Clinical and Experimental Rheumatology, 20*(3), 399–402.

Miller, P. L., & Ernst, A. A. (2004). Sex differences in analgesia: a randomized trial of mu versus kappa opioid agonists. *Southern Medical Journal, 97*(1), 35–41.

Mogil, J. S. (1999). The genetic mediation of individual differences in sensitivity to pain and its inhibition. *Proceedings of the National Academy of Sciences of the United States of America, 96*(14), 7744–7751.

Mogil, J. S., Chesler, E. J., Wilson, S. G., Juraska, J. M., & Sternberg, W. F. (2000). Sex differences in thermal nociception and morphine antinociception in rodents depend on genotype. *Neuroscience and Biobehavioral Review, 24*(3), 375–389.

Mogil, J. S., Richards, S. P., O'Toole, L. A., Helms, M. L., Mitchell, S. R., & Belknap, J. K. (1997). Genetic sensitivity to hot-plate nociception in DBA/2J and C57BL/6J inbred mouse strains: Possible sex-specific mediation by delta2-opioid receptors. *Pain, 70*(2–3), 267–277.

Mogil, J. S., Sternberg, W. F., Kest, B., Marek, P., & Liebeskind, J. C. (1993). Sex differences in the antagonism of stress-induced analgesia: effects of gonadectomy and estrogen replacement. *Pain, 53*, 17–25.

Mogil, J. S., Wilson, S. G., Bon, K., Lee, S. E., Chung, K., Raber, P., et al. (1999a). Heritability of nociception I. Responses of 11 inbred mouse strains on 12 measures of nociception. *Pain, 80*(1–2), 67–82.

Mogil, J. S., Wilson, S. G., Bon, K., Lee, S. E., Chung, K., Raber, P., et al. (1999b). Heritability of nociception II. Types of nociception revealed by genetic correlation analysis. *Pain, 80*(1–2), 83–93.

Mogil, J. S., Wilson, S. G., Chesler, E. J., Rankin, A. L., Nemmani, K. V., Lariviere, W. R., et al. (2003). The melanocortin-1 receptor gene mediates female-specific mechanisms of analgesia in mice and humans. *Proceedings of the National Academy of Sciences of the United States of America, 100*, 4867–4872.

Moldin, S. O., Scheftner, W. A., Rice, J. P., Nelson, E., Knesevich, M. A., & Akiskal, H. (1993). Association between major depressive disorder and physical illness. *Psychological Medicine X, 23*, 755–761.

Morin, C., Lund, J. P., Villarroel, T., Clokie, C. M., & Feine, J. S. (2000). Differences between the sexes in post-surgical pain. *Pain, 85*(1–2), 79–85.

Mullersdorf, M., & Soderback, I. (2000). The actual state of the effects, treatment and incidence of disabling pain in a gender perspective — A Swedish study. *Disability and Rehabilitation, 22*(18), 840–854.

Musgrave, D. S., Vogt, M. T., Nevitt, M. C., & Cauley, J. A. (2001). Back problems among postmenopausal women taking estrogen replacement therapy. *Spine, 26*, 1606–1612.

Myers, C. D., Robinson, M. E., Riley, J. L., III, & Sheffield, D. (2001). Sex, gender, and blood pressure: Contributions to experimental pain report. *Psychosomatic Medicine, 63*(4), 545–550.

Neumann, L., & Buskila, D. (1997). Quality of life and physical functioning of relatives of fibromyalgia patients. *Seminars in Arthritis & Rheumatism, 26*(6), 834–839.

Obelieniene, D., Schrader, H., Bovim, G., Miseviciene, I., & Sand, T. (1999). Pain after whiplash: A prospective controlled inception cohort study. *Journal of Neurology, Neurosurgery, and Psychiatry, 66*(3), 279–283.

Osman, A., Barrios, F. X., Gutierrez, P. M., Kopper, B. A., Merrifield, T., & Grittmann, L. (2000). The Pain Catastrophizing Scale: Further psychometric evaluation with adult samples. *Journal of Behavioral Medicine, 23*(4), 351–365.

Ottman, R., Hong, S., & Lipton, R. B. (1993). Validity of family history data on severe headache and migraine. *Neurology, 43*(10), 1954–1960.

Otto, M. W., & Dougher, M. J. (1985). Sex differences and personality factors in responsivity to pain. *Perceptual and Motor Skills, 61*, 383–390.

Pellegrino, M. J., Waylonis, G. W., & Sommer, A. (1989). Familial occurrence of primary fibromyalgia (see comments). *Archives of Physical Medicine & Rehabilitation, 70*(1), 61–63.

Pilley, J. R., Mohlin, B., Shaw, W. C., & Kingdon, A. (1992). A survey of craniomandibular disorders in 800 15-year-olds. A follow-up study of children with malocclusion. *European Journal of Orthodontics, 14*(2), 152–161.

Pollard, T. M., & Hyatt, S. B. (1999). *Sex, gender and health.* London: Cambridge University Press.

Rajala, U., Keinanen-Kiukaanniemi, S., Uusimaki, A., & Kivela, S. L. (1995). Musculoskeletal pains and depression in a middle-aged Finnish population. *Pain, 61*(3), 451–457.

Riley, J. L. I., Robinson, M. E., Wise, E. A., & Price, D. D. (1999). A meta-analytic review of pain perception across the menstrual cycle. *Pain, 81*, 225–235.

Riley, J. L., Gilbert, G. H., & Heft, M. W. (1998). Orofacial pain symptom prevalence: selective sex differences in the elderly? *Pain, 76*(1–2), 97–104.

Riley, J. L., III, & Gilbert, G. H. (2001). Orofacial pain symptoms: An interaction between age and sex. *Pain, 90*(3), 245–256.

Riley, J. L., III, Robinson, M. E., Wade, J. B., Myers, C. D., & Price, D. D. (2001). Sex differences in negative emotional responses to chronic pain. *Journal of Pain, 2*, 354–359.

Riley, J. L., Robinson, M. E., Wise, E. A., Myers, C. D., & Fillingim, R. B. (1998). Sex differences in the perception of noxious experimental stimuli: A meta-analysis. *Pain, 74*, 181–187.

Robinson, M. E., Gagnon, C. M., Riley, J. L., III, & Price, D. D. (2003). Altering gender role expectations: effects on pain tolerance, pain threshold, and pain ratings. *Journal of Pain, 4*(5), 284–288.

Robinson, M. E., Riley, J. L., III, & Myers, C. D. (2000). Psychosocial contributions to sex-related differences in pain responses. In R. B. Fillingim (Ed.), *Sex, gender, and pain* (pp. 41–68). Seattle: IASP Press: Seattle.

Robinson, M. E., Riley, J. L., III, Myers, C. D., Papas, R. K., Wise, E. A., Waxenberg, L. A., & Fillingim, R. B. (2001). Gender role expectations of pain: Relationship to sex differences in pain. *Journal of Pain, 2*, 251–257.

Robinson, M. E., Wise, E. A., & Riley, J. L. I. (1998). Sex differences in clinical pain: A multi-sample study. *Journal of Clinical Psychology in Medical Settings, 5*, 413–423.

Robinson, M. E., Wise, E. A., Gagnon, C., Fillingim, R. B., & Price, D. D. (2004). Influences of gender role and anxiety on sex differences in temporal summation of pain. *Journal of Pain, 5*, 77–82.

Roger, V. L., Farkouh, M. E., Weston, S. A., Reeder, G. S., Jacobsen, S. J., Zinsmeister, A. R., et al. (2000). Sex differences in evaluation and outcome of unstable angina. *Journal of the American Medical Association, 283*(5), 646–652.

Romberg, R., Olofsen, E., Sarton, E., den Hartigh, J., Taschner, P. E., & Dahan, A. (2004). Pharmacokinetic-pharmacodynamic modeling of morphine-6-glucuronide-induced analgesia in healthy volunteers: Absence of sex differences. *Anesthesiology, 100*(1), 120–133.

Sallfors, C., Hallberg, L. R., & Fasth, A. (2003). Gender and age differences in pain, coping and health status among children with chronic arthritis. *Clinical and Experimental Rheumatology, 21*(6), 785–793.

Sandanger, I., Nygard, J. F., Brage, S., & Tellnes, G. (2000). Relation between health problems and sickness absence: Gender and age differences — A comparison of low-back pain, psychiatric disorders, and injuries. *Scandinavian Journal of Public Health, 28*(4), 244–252.

Sandner-Kiesling, A., & Eisenach, J. C. (2002). Estrogen reduces efficacy of (mu)- but not (kappa)-opioid agonist inhibition in response to uterine cervical distension. *Anesthesiology, 96*(2), 375–379.

Sarlani, E., & Greenspan, J. D. (2002). Gender differences in temporal summation of mechanically evoked pain. *Pain, 97*(1–2), 163–169.

Sarton, E., Olofsen, E., Romberg, R., den Hartigh, J., Kest, B., Nieuwenhuijs, D. et al. (2000). Sex differences in morphine analgesia: An experimental study in healthy volunteers. *Anesthesiology, 93*(5), 1245–1254.

Sarton, E., Teppema, L., & Dahan, A. (1999). Sex differences in morphine induced ventilatory depression reside in the peripheral chemoreflex loop. *Anesthesiology, 90*, 1329–1338.

Savedra, M. C., Holzemer, W. L., Tesler, M. D., & Wilkie, D. J. (1993). Assessment of postoperation pain in children and adolescents using the adolescent pediatric pain tool. *Nursing Research, 42*(1), 5–9.

Scher, A. I., Stewart, W. F., & Lipton, R. B. (1999). Migraine and headache: A meta-analytic approach. In I. K. Crombie (Ed.), *Epidemiology of pain* (pp. 159–170). Seattle: IASP Press.

Scholten-Peeters, G. G., Verhagen, A. P., Bekkering, G. E., van der Windt, D. A., Barnsley, L., Oostendorp, R. A., & Hendriks, E. J. (2003). Prognostic factors of whiplash-associated disorders: A systematic review of prospective cohort studies. *Pain, 104*(1–2), 303–322.

Schrader, H., Obelieniene, D., Bovim, G., Surkiene, D., Mickeviciene, D., Miseviciene, I., & Sand, T. (1996). Natural evolution of late whiplash syndrome outside the medicolegal context [see comments]. *Lancet, 347*(9010), 1207–1211.

Schwartz, B. S., Stewart, W. F., Simon, D., & Lipton, R. B. (1998). Epidemiology of tension-type headache. *Journal of the American Medical Association, 279*(5), 381–383.

Scudds, R. J., & Robertson, J. M. (1998). Empirical evidence of the association between the presence of musculoskeletal pain and physical disability in community-dwelling senior citizens. *Pain, 75*(2–3), 229–235.

Sipila, K., Veijola, J., Jokelainen, J., Jarvelin, M. R., Oikarinen, K. S., Raustia, A. M., & Joukamaa, M. (2001). Association between symptoms of temporomandibular disorders and depression: An epidemiological study of the Northern Finland 1966 Birth Cohort. *Cranio, 19*(3), 183–187.

Soares, J. J., & Jablonska, B. (2004). Psychosocial experiences among primary care patients with and without musculoskeletal pain. *European Journal of Pain, 8*(1), 79–89.

Sternbach, R. A. (1986). Survey of pain in the United States: The Nuprin Pain Report. *Clinical Journal of Pain, 2*, 49–53.

Sternberg, W. F., & Liebeskind, J. C. (1995). The analgesic response to stress: genetic and gender considerations. *European Journal of Anaesthesiology — Supplement, 10*, 14–17.

Stewart, W. F., Lipton, R. B., Celentano, D. D., & Reed, M. L. (1992). Prevalence of migraine headache in the United States. Relation to age, income, race, and other sociodemographic factors. *Journal of the American Medical Association, 267*(1), 64–69.

Svensson, P., Cairns, B. E., Wang, K., Hu, J. W., Graven-Nielsen, T., Arendt-Nielsen, L., & Sessle, B. J. (2003). Glutamate-evoked pain and mechanical allodynia in the human masseter muscle. *Pain, 10* (3), 221–227.

Taenzer, A. H., Clark, C., & Curry, C. S. (2000). Gender affects report of pain and function after arthroscopic anterior cruciate ligament reconstruction. *Anesthesiology, 93*(3), 670–675.

Taylor, H., & Curran, N. M. (1985). *The Nuprin pain report.* New York: Louis Harris & Associates.

Terner, J. M., Lomas, L. M., Smith, E. S., Barrett, A. C., & Picker, M. J. (2003). Pharmacogenetic analysis of sex differences in opioid antinociception in rats. *Pain, 106*(3), 381–391.

Turk, D. C., & Okifuji, A. (1999). Does sex make a difference in the prescription of treatments and the adaptation to chronic pain by cancer and non-cancer patients? *Pain, 82*(2), 139–148.

Turkat, I. D., Kuczmierczyk, A. R., & Adams, H. E. (1984). An investigation of the aetiology of chronic headache. The role of headache models. *British Journal of Psychiatry, 145*, 665–666.

Unruh, A. M. (1996). Gender variations in clinical pain experience. *Pain, 65*(2–3), 123–167.

Unruh, A. M., Ritchie, J., & Merskey, H. (1999). Does gender affect appraisal of pain and pain coping strategies? *Clinical Journal of Pain, 15*(1), 31–40.

Vallerand, A. H. (1995). Gender differences in pain. *Image — The Journal of Nursing Scholarship, 27*(3), 235–237.

Verhaak, P. F., Kerssens, J. J., Dekker, J., Sorbi, M. J., & Bensing, J. M. (1998). Prevalence of chronic benign pain disorder among adults: A review of the literature. *Pain, 77*(3), 231–239.

Von Korff, M., Dworkin, S. G., LeResche, L., & Krueger, A. (1998). An epidemiologic comparison of pain complaints. *Pain, 32*, 33–40.

Wahlund, K. (2003). Temporomandibular disorders in adolescents. Epidemiological and methodological studies and a randomized controlled trial. *Swedish Dental Journal Supplement*, (164), 2–64.

Walsh, K., Cruddas, M., & Coggon, D. (1992). Low back pain in eight areas of Britain. *Journal of Epidemiology and Community Health, 46*(3), 227–230.

Warnell, P. (1991). The pain experience of a multiple sclerosis population: A descriptive study. *Axone, 13*(1), 26–28.

Wedderkopp, N., Leboeuf-Yde, C., Andersen, L. B., Froberg, K., & Hansen, H. S. (2001). Back pain reporting pattern in a Danish population-based sample of children and adolescents. *Spine, 26*(17), 1879–1883.

White, K. P., Speechley, M., Harth, M., & Ostbye, T. (1999). The London Fibromyalgia Epidemiology Study: The prevalence of fibromyalgia syndrome in London, Ontario. *Journal of Rheumatology, 26*(7), 1570–1576.

Wise, E. A., Riley, J. L. I., & Robinson, M. E. (2000). Clinical pain perception and hormone replacement therapy in post-menopausal females experiencing orofacial pain. *Clinical Journal of Pain, 16*, 121–126.

Wizemann, T. M., & Pardue, M. L. E. (2001). *Exploring the biological contributions to human health: Does sex matter?* Washington, DC: National Academy Press.

Wolfe, F., Ross, K., Anderson, J., & Russell, I. J. (1995). Aspects of fibromyalgia in the general population: Sex, pain threshold, and fibromyalgia symptoms. *Journal of Rheumatology, 22*(1), 151–156.

Wolfe, F., Ross, K., Anderson, J., Russell, I. J., & Hebert, L. (1995). The prevalence and characteristics of fibromyalgia in the general population. *Arthritis & Rheumatism, 38*(1), 19–28.

Zacny, J. P. (2002). Gender differences in opioid analgesia in human volunteers: Cold pressor and mechanical pain (CPDD abstract). *NIDA Research Monograph, 182*, 22–23.

Zubieta, J. K., Heitzeg, M. M., Smith, Y. R., Bueller, J. A., Xu, K., Xu, Y. et al. (2003). COMT val158met genotype affects mu-opioid neurotransmitter responses to a pain stressor. *Science, 299*(5610), 1240–1243.

Zubieta, J. K., Smith, Y. R., Bueller, J. A., Xu, Y., Kilbourn, M. R., Jewett, D. M. et al. (2002). Mu-opioid receptor-mediated antinociceptive responses differ in men and women. *Journal of Neuroscience, 22*(12), 5100–5107.

8

Racial and Ethnic Issues in Chronic Pain Management: Challenges and Perspectives

Michael E. Schatman, PhD

INTRODUCTION

One of the greatest obstacles to the effective treatment of chronic pain is the temptation of clinicians to explain it solely in terms of physiological mechanisms. Without recognizing the complex interaction between pathophysiology and psychosocial factors, chronic pain cannot be adequately understood and, accordingly, cannot be adequately treated. Since the pioneering work of Chapman and Jones, (1944) and Zborowski (1952), numerous researchers have examined racial and ethnic influences on patients' perceptions and responses to acute and chronic pain experience. The findings of a myriad of studies on group differences in pain experience and response are mixed, which may be due, to a certain extent, to methodological issues. While additional research on racial and ethnic differences in the experience and meaning of pain may be useful, the possibility exists that findings will only marginally affect the quality of treatment minorities with chronic pain receive. Of greater importance, perhaps, is how diverse racial and ethnic groups' views of pain, health care providers, medications, and the medical system as a whole along with physician and medical system variables affect their access to the treatment that is likely to meet their specific needs.

A review of the literature suggests that some of the disparity in findings on racial and ethnic issues in chronic pain management relates to inconsistencies in operational definitions of race and ethnicity. *Race* refers to differences in major groups of people based on ancestry and physical characteristics, while *ethnicity* refers to distinctions based on behavior and culture as well as on biological and physical differences (Edwards et al., 2001).

It is also important to specify an operational definition of "chronic pain," as this is another issue regarding which considerable disagreement exists. While certain clinicians and investigators view chronicity as based on the duration of symptoms, others consider chronic pain to be defined by the amount of dysfunction it causes across a wide range of dimensions of one's life. For purposes of consistency, the International Association for the Study of Pain (IASP) definition of chronic pain as that persisting "beyond normal tissue healing time, which is assumed to be 3 months" (IASP, 1986) is used in this chapter. Both malignant and nonmalignant chronic pain are discussed.

PAIN PERCEPTION

Most of the research on racial and ethnic differences in pain experience has focused on acute pain, with much of this research involving experimental rather than clinical pain. However, a number of investigators have examined intergroup variance in the perception of chronic pain severity (Ang et al., 2003; Bates & Edwards, 1992; Bates et al., 1993; Bates et al., 1995; Garron & Leavitt, 1979; Gaston-Johansson et al., 1990; Green et al., 2003a; Greenwald, 1991; Jordon et al., 1998; Kramer et al., 2002a, b; Kramer et al., 2002; Lawlis et al., 1984; Lipton & Marbach, 1984; McCracken et al., 2001; Plesh et al., 2002; Riley et al., 2002) with mixed results. For example, while Edwards et al. (2001), Green et al. (2003a), and McCracken et al. (2001) each found that African American patients seeking treatment for chronic pain reported higher pain severity than did their Caucasian counterparts,

Ang et al. (2003), Jordan et al. (1998), and Riley et al. (2002) found no interracial differences in pain intensity in their studies, and Plesh et al. (2002) found interracial differences in pain intensity only at certain body locations. While several studies (Bates & Edwards, 1992; Bates et al., 1995; Lawlis et al., 1984) have indicated that Hispanics suffering from chronic pain report higher levels of pain severity than non-Hispanic Caucasians, it has been suggested that problems with relatively simple conceptual models and the use of univariate statistical approaches limit the meaning of these findings (Edwards & Keefe, 2000; Lipton & Marbach,1984).

Medical research often considers Hispanics a homogeneous group, with insufficient attention paid to the considerable differences between various Hispanic cultures. Keefe (1982) noted, for example, large differences between foreign-born versus American-born Mexican Americans in terms of help-seeking behavior. Similar differences are likely to exist between Puerto Rican patients with chronic pain who were born in Puerto Rico versus those born in the mainland United States, based on levels of acculturation. Comparing Puerto Ricans with Mexican Americans in their experiences of chronic pain, to take the issue yet further, should be done only with extreme caution. These same issues are likely to exist in considering the literature examining chronic pain experience among African Americans. In an excellent editorial, Edwards and Keefe (2000) noted that the meaning of pain for an individual who has recently emigrated from the Caribbean may differ greatly from that of an African American whose fourth-generation status has resulted in a different experience of acculturation. Bates and Edwards (1992) noted that "ethnic stereotyping is as dangerous as inattention to cultural variables." As the tendency for researchers of differences between races in chronic pain experience has clearly been toward ethnic stereotyping, the meaning and value of the body of existing literature in this area are questionable. More sophisticated and thoughtful research on racial and ethnic differences in the chronic pain experience would potentially be beneficial.

RESPONSE TO CHRONIC PAIN

A related area of investigation that has received considerable attention has been differences between racial and ethnic groups in terms of emotional and behavioral responses to chronic pain. Again, studies examining emotional and behavioral adaptation to chronic pain have yielded mixed results (Ang et al., 2002; Bates & Edwards, 1992; Bates et al., 1995; Brena et al., 1990; Gatchel et al., 1995; Green et al., 2003a; Greenwald, 1991; Ibrahim et al., 2003; Jordon et al., 1998; Li & Moore, 1998; McCracken et al., 2001; Riley et al., 2002; Sanders et al., 1992). However, a review of the literature suggests that the findings on racial and ethnic differences in response

to pain are more consistent than are those on intergroup differences in pain perception. For example, African American patients with chronic pain were found to display less adaptive coping strategies (Ang et al., 2002; Jordon et al., 1998), to demonstrate higher levels of physical and psychological disability (Green et al., 2003a, b; McCracken et al., 2001), and to be more avoidant of physical activity (McCracken et al., 2001) than were Caucasian patients with chronic pain. Non-Caucasians were found to be more likely to be classified as "disabled" 6 months following acute back injuries than were Caucasians (Gatchel et al., 1995). Two studies (Bates & Edwards, 1992; Bates & Rankin-Hill, 1994) have suggested that Puerto Rican patients with chronic pain reported more psychological distress and higher degrees of interference with physical activities than non-Hispanic Caucasians, with these findings attributed to differences in locus of control. While the studies implicating locus of control as responsible for differences in behavioral and emotional responses to chronic pain have compared Puerto Ricans with Anglo-Americans, external locus of control has been related to maladaptive responses to illness among African Americans as well (Bell et al., 1995; Wilson et al., 1994). Issues of locus of control are addressed later in this chapter. It should be noted, however, that the studies that suggest that Caucasians' emotional and behavioral adjustment to chronic pain is superior to those of racial and ethnic minority patients with pain may have been reliant on independent variables that were not necessarily culturally sensitive.

Two studies on cross-cultural differences in response to chronic pain should be mentioned by virtue of their blatant problems with ethnic stereotyping. Brena et al. (1990) determined that Japanese patients with chronic low back pain were less impaired psychologically, socially, vocationally, and avocationally than were American patients with low back pain. In a study of "Chronic Low Back Pain Patients Around the World," Sanders et al. (1992) compared levels of chronic low back pain–related self-perceived dysfunction in samples of American, Japanese, Mexican, Colombian, Italian, and New Zealander sufferers of chronic low back pain. The authors concluded that "there were important cross-cultural differences in chronic low back pain patients' self-perceived level of dysfunction, with the American patients clearly the most dysfunctional." They attributed the differences that they found to potential explanations including a number of sociocultural factors and differences in emotional and cognitive functioning. Unfortunately, the authors of both of these studies failed to state what constitutes being an American. Given that the American population is likely the most heterogeneous in the world, the findings of these studies tell us little of meaning regarding differences between groups in pain-related self-perception of chronic low back pain disability. Brena et al. (1990) noted that their findings may have been due to the stoicism and ethnic homogeneity of Japanese culture, making pain-related impairment less acceptable than it is in the "liberal, permissive, and pluralistic American society." However, the validity of this statement is limited due to a lack of information regarding the specific composition of the American sample.

DIFFERENCES IN THE TREATMENT OF MINORITIES VERSUS NONMINORITIES WITH CHRONIC PAIN

In general, racial and ethnic minorities have been determined not to have the same access to medical treatment and other health services as do the non-Hispanic Caucasian population, with African Americans at particular risk for underservice (Mayberry et al., 2000). As discussed above, the mixed results of research on racial and ethnic differences in pain perception do not support drawing particularly meaningful conclusions, and investigations of intergroup differences in emotional and behavioral response to pain suggest that African American and Hispanic patients may respond less favorably to chronic pain than do non-Hispanic Caucasians. However, these bodies of literature provide little insight into the disparity in treatment of chronic pain that is received by minorities as opposed to nonminority groups in the United States. The existence of this disparity is well documented in the literature, in which numerous studies on racial and ethnic differences in both acute and chronic pain treatment can be found. It appears likely that the results of many of the investigations that suggest that minorities are at higher risk for the ineffective treatment of acute pain may generalize to the treatment of chronic pain as well.

While results of several studies (Ducharme & Barber, 1995; Selbst & Clark, 1990; Wilson & Pendleton, 1989) have indicated that the inadequate prescribing of analgesics for patients in pain in emergency rooms is common, it appears that racial and ethnic minorities who present at emergency departments are at even greater risk for oligoanalgesia, despite similar levels of pain complaints (Todd et al., 1993; Todd et al., 2000). Todd and his colleagues (1993) found that 55% of Hispanics received no analgesic for long bone fractures, while no analgesic was provided for only 26% of non-Hispanic Caucasians with identical diagnoses. Of note are the results of a 1994 companion study (Todd, Lee, & Hoffman, 1994) to Todd et al.'s original work, in which no difference between physicians' assessments of pain between Caucasian and Hispanic patients was identified. Accordingly, physician error in assessment of pain levels could not account for the identified disparity in the administration of analgesics between Hispanics and non-Hispanic Caucasians. Similarly, African American patients with extremity fractures were at

66% greater risk for receiving no analgesic from an emergency medicine department than were Caucasians (Todd et al., 2000).

Ng and colleagues (1996a, b) published results of two studies that examined differences in the treatment of postoperative pain between Caucasians and racial/ethnic minorities. These investigations were conducted to assess whether the findings of Todd and colleagues (1993, 1994) would generalize from the emergency room to the postoperative setting. In both studies, Caucasian patients were provided with higher doses of analgesics than were racial or ethnic minority patients. Ng et al. (Ng et al., 1996a) acknowledged that their results could not determine whether this disparity was due to the attitudes and behaviors of the patients, of the medical staff, or some combination of the two. As is the case with the aforementioned studies on racial and ethnic differences in emergency room treatment of fractures, the results of the studies by Ng and colleagues (1996a, b) become more striking in light of a study that indicated that white patients reported *less* postoperative pain than did African Americans or Hispanics (Faucett et al., 1994).

Although the body of literature on racial and ethnic differences in the treatment of acute pain is limited, studies on such differences in the treatment of cancer pain are somewhat more abundant. Overall, the literature suggests that minority patients with cancer are more likely to be faced with oligoanalgesia than are Caucasian cancer patients. In an early study of racial and ethnic disparities in the treatment of cancer pain, Cleeland et al. (1997) compared medication practices of oncology clinics that treated primarily African Americans and Hispanics with those treating more heterogeneous patient populations. The authors determined that while 42% of all recurrent or metastatic cancer patients were undermedicated, those seen in centers that treated predominantly minorities were three times more likely than were patients treated elsewhere to report inadequate pain management. In a follow-up study, Cleeland and his colleagues (1997) determined that 65% of minority patients suffering from recurrent or metatstatic cancer did not receive Pain Management Index–recommended analgesic prescriptions, as compared with only 50% of nonminority patients. Hispanic cancer patients in this study were found to be more inadequately medicated for their pain than were African American patients, which is particularly intriguing given the results of an investigation that determined that Hispanic cancer patients reported higher levels of pain and lower quality of life than did non-Hispanic Caucasian or African American cancer patients (Juarez et al., 1999). Consistent with these results are findings that elderly minority cancer patients were statistically more likely to receive no analgesia than were elderly nonminority patients, with African Americans being 63% more likely to be untreated for their cancer pain than were non-Hispanic Caucasians (Bernabei et al., 1998).

Although a number of studies of racial and ethic disparities in the treatment of acute pain and cancer pain have been published, there are relatively few studies examining disparities in treatment between racial/ethnic minorities and nonminorities who suffer from benign chronic pain conditions. In an extensive review of racial and ethnic disparities in access to medical care, Mayberry et al. (2000) concluded, "the literature shows that racial and ethnic minorities frequently do not have the same access to medical treatment and other health services as the majority white population," and that this difference is particularly true for African Americans. While Mayberry and his colleagues reviewed the literature on racial disparities in the treatment of cancer, they did not include benign pain conditions in their review.

Among the published studies of racial and ethnic disparities in the treatment of chronic pain, the majority appear to relate to issues of *access* to services. Access to services appears to be related to a combination of patient variables, communication issues, physician issues, and social system variables, all of which contribute to suboptimal outcomes for too many minority patients with chronic pain. These variables and their impact on access to appropriate medical care for chronic pain conditions are the focus of the remainder of this chapter.

PATIENT VARIABLES

As mentioned earlier in this chapter, the findings of studies of differences between racial and ethnic groups in their perceptions of chronic pain have been mixed and therefore nonconclusive. Accordingly, these differences, if they do exist, are unlikely to adequately explain racial and ethnic disparities in access to chronic pain management services. However, as the research appears to suggest the existence of racial and ethnic group differences in emotional and behavioral responses to chronic pain, these differences merit investigation as a possible explanation for disparities in access to appropriate services.

The literature suggests that differences between racial and ethnic minorities' patterns of seeking medical assistance in dealing with chronic pain are rooted deeply within their cultures. This appears to be particularly true of Hispanic sufferers of chronic pain, although intraethnic differences may exist. Perhaps the most prolific investigators of Hispanic/Caucasian differences in chronic pain experience and response have been Bates and her colleagues (Bates & Edwards, 1992; Bates, Edwards, & Anderson, 1993; Bates & Rankin-Hill, 1994; Bates et al., 1995; Bates, Rank-Hill, & Sanchez-Ayendez, 1997). Bates and Edwards (1992), Bates, Edwards, & Anderson (1993), and Bates and Rankin-Hill (1994) determined that locus of control style is an important predictor of chronic pain

experience, affecting not only the subjective experience of pain severity, but also behavioral, psychological, and attitudinal responses. The Latino cultural tradition is one that emphasizes external locus of control, viewing reality as something that cannot be manipulated or transformed by the individual. This worldview, suggest Bates and Edwards (1992), is one that is accepted as realistic by Hispanic researchers, despite the tendency of Caucasian researchers to see external locus of control as reflective of a passive and pessimistic attitude. Bates and Rankin-Hill (1994) determined that patients with external locus of control were more likely to have sought immediate medical care upon the onset of their pain symptoms. However, their study did not indicate that locus of control style affected patients' likelihood of seeking and/or continuing to pursue medical care once a pain condition had become chronic. A review of the literature suggests that the relationship between a patient's locus of control style and willingness to seek treatment for *chronic* pain has yet to be investigated. This topic certainly merits exploration, particularly given the identified tendency of Hispanics to manifest external health locus of control (Sugarek et al., 1988; Aruffo et al., 1993; Spaulding, 1995).

Bates and Rankin-Hill (1994) suggest that among patients with chronic pain, an internal locus of control is beneficial in that it helps patients regain the perception of control over their lives and their pain. However, if an external locus of control is actually associated with seeking medical attention upon the onset of pain symptoms, is an external locus of control style necessarily maladaptive? A study by Gatchel and colleagues (2003) identified patients with acute low back pain determined to be at risk for developing chronic low back pain. Those who received early medical intervention fared better on a wide range of work, heath care utilization, medication use, and self-report of pain variables at 1-year follow-up than did those patients who did *not* receive early medical treatment. Their results were consistent with those of earlier studies (Epker et al., 1999; Gatchel et al., 1995; Jordon et al., 1998; Linton et al., 1993; Schultz et al., 2002). While Hispanics' tendencies toward external locus of control may indeed result in suboptimal emotional and behavioral responses to chronic pain, in terms of access to medical services, this culturally ingrained tendency may actually serve the function of helping avoid the development of chronicity. Further investigation is required to determine whether Hispanics' external locus of control styles actually do result in passivity and pessimism, as such attitudes could theoretically result in hopelessness and thereby serve to prevent Hispanic chronic pain sufferers from seeking access to potentially beneficial medical treatment.

It should be noted that intracultural variation in help-seeking behavior may relate to differences in access to treatment for chronic pain among Hispanics, although no such specific study appears in the literature. Keefe (1982), however, noted that foreign-born Mexican Americans are less likely to seek help from doctors than are native-born Mexican Americans. The author suggested that this distinction is likely to relate to socioeconomic status, level of acculturation, intensity of religious affiliation, the presence of a strong social support network, and familiarity with available services. While Keefe's study pertained specifically to mental health issues, it seems plausible that her results may be generalized to the seeking of treatment of other conditions, including chronic pain.

Without regard to locus of control style, Hispanics may choose to seek medical treatment for their chronic pain less frequently than do non-Hispanic Caucasians because of their tendency to rely on family and friends for assistance prior to or rather than seeking outside help. Bates and Edwards (1992) found that Hispanic sufferers of chronic pain were significantly more likely to consult friends and family for advice regarding their pain than were other ethnic groups in their study. Additionally, there exists a tradition in Hispanic culture to rely on *espiritismo* (faith healing), which may serve as a substitute for seeking mainstream medical care for chronic pain. While this possibility has not been formally investigated, Ruiz and Langrod (1976) identified a culturally accepted belief system in faith healing in a Hispanic urban ghetto. However, Lipton and Marbach (1984) noted that the levels to which pain sufferers rely on home remedies and spiritist healers are likely to be subject to intra-ethnic variation based on degree of assimilation into American society and acculturation of medical norms.

Hispanics in the United States are not the only racial or ethnic group likely to demonstrate lower levels of formal help-seeking for their chronic pain, choosing to rely on spiritual approaches instead. Jordan et al. (1998) determined that African American women were more likely to engage in "praying and hoping" as a primary strategy for dealing with chronic pain than were Caucasian women in their study. The authors noted that African Americans' greater use of praying/hoping was consistent with their emphases on church, prayer, and religion within their community, which has been supported elsewhere in the literature (Arcury, 1996; Bill-Harvey et al., 1989; Coulton et al., 1990; Cronan et al., 1993; Jacobson, 1987; Mutran, 1985). Ang et al. (2002) determined that African Americans were less than half as likely as Caucasians to consider arthroplasty as a treatment option for their severe arthritis, identifying African Americans' belief in the "helpfulness of prayer" as an important explanatory variable for this disparity.

Another patient variable that may explain, to some degree, undertreatment of chronic pain among African Americans is the relationship between their pain experience and perceived quality of life. In two studies by Ibrahim and colleagues (Ibrahim et al., 2002, 2003), negative correlations between pain quality variables and global quality of life ratings were identified among Caucasians suffering from osteoarthritis, but not among their African American counterparts. While neither of these studies directly examined the relationship between race and the perceived overall impact of chronic pain on seeking medical intervention, the possibility exists that African Americans are more likely to consider their pain as less meaningful than are Caucasians within the frequently unfortunate socioeconomic context of their lives. A number of studies (Fiscella & Franks, 1997; Fuhrer et al., 1993; Myers et al., 2002; Vermom et al., 1982) have suggested that African Americans are more likely than Caucasians to experience hopelessness in general, and it is plausible that this phenomenon can explain their decision to be reticent to seek aggressive treatment for their chronic pain. Studies have suggested that Hispanics in the United States are also more likely to evidence hopelessness than are Caucasians, and may actually manifest greater hopelessness than do African Americans (Fuhrer et al., 1993; Garcia & Marks, 1989; Kemp et al., 1999; Myers et al., 2002; Vermom et al., 1982). Accordingly, generalized hopelessness may serve as an explanation for Hispanics' reticence to seek chronic pain treatment as well. Research in this area could be useful in terms of designing psychosocial interventions for racial and ethnic minority chronic pain sufferers manifesting high levels of hopelessness.

The involvement of psychologists in interdisciplinary (and some multidisciplinary) treatment programs for chronic pain may provide yet another explanation for racial and ethnic minorities' reduced likelihood of seeking chronic pain management services. The literature suggests that African Americans are less likely to seek mental health services than are Caucasians (Alvidrez, 1999; Bristow & Patten, 2002; Diala et al., 2000; Padgett et al., 1994; Snowden, 1999; Wells et al., 2001), that African Americans view mental health services as not being particularly useful (Snell & Thomas, 1998), and that African Americans have more negative expectations of mental health services than Caucasians (Richardson, 2001). Hispanics have been found to be less likely to seek mental health services than non-Hispanic Caucasians (Alegria et al., 2002; Alvidrez, 1999; Greenberg & Rosenheck, 2003; Padgett et al., 1994; Pumariega et al., 1998; Starrett et al., 1992; Wells et al., 2001) and to be more likely to drop out of counseling prematurely (Cheung & Snowden, 1990). Some of the Hispanics' discomfort with mental health services is certainly likely to relate to issues of communication secondary to language barriers, which will be addressed later in this chapter. The possibility that racial and ethnic minorities suffering from chronic pain avoid appropriate treatment due to an aversion toward mental health services is particularly distressing given the findings that suggest that African Americans with chronic pain demonstrate less adaptive coping strategies, evidence higher levels of psychological disability, and are more avoidant of physical activity than Caucasian patients with chronic pain (Ang et al., 2002; Edwards et al., 2001; Green et al., 2003a; Jordon et al., 1998; McCracken et al., 2001;). Similarly, the strong need for psychological services in the treatment of Hispanic patients with chronic pain is supported by research that suggests that they reported higher levels of psychological distress and interference with physical activities than did non-Hispanic Caucasians with chronic pain (Bates & Edwards, 1992; Bates & Rankin-Hill, 1994). If the proponents of the aforementioned theory that Hispanics' external locus of control is detrimental to coping with chronic pain are accurate, psychologists may be particularly important in their treatment in terms of providing them with cognitive behavioral intervention, including biofeedback training. Such treatment has been found to be effective in increasing internal health locus of control among patients suffering from chronic pain and illness (Gruber et al., 1988; Mizner et al., 1988; Rybarczyk et al., 2001).

Another patient-related factor that may have an impact on access to appropriate treatment for chronic pain among racial and ethnic minorities is trust of medical professionals and the medical system in general. This factor, however, is likely to be influenced by communication issues as well as medical and social system variables, which are addressed in greater detail later in this chapter. Despite the existence of a body of literature indicating that racial and ethnic minorities trust physicians and the medical system less than do Caucasians (Doescher et al., 2000; Corbie-Smith et al., 2002; Boulware et al., 2003), there is a paucity of research on issues of trust of the medical establishment among minorities suffering from chronic pain. Lipton and Marbach (1984) determined that African American patients presenting for treatment at a facial pain clinic were significantly more skeptical regarding what they believed their physicians could do to help them as compared with Caucasian patients. Otherwise, no investigations of this type appear in the literature, and additional research is merited.

COMMUNICATION ISSUES

Related to trust issues is communication between minority patients with chronic pain and the providers of pain management services. This is obviously a physician/medical staff issue as well as a patient variable. Language barriers can certainly exist in the treatment of chronic pain, as is the case with all medical treatment. Hispanic patients who are not conversant in English are at risk of simply not understanding physicians who are non-Spanish speaking, and they are similarly likely to have problems conveying the physical, emotional, and behavioral aspects of their pain conditions to their physicians. The hope is that the rapidly growing Hispanic population and the increasing number of Spanish-speaking health care providers in the United States will progressively reduce the magnitude of this issue. The importance of physician–patient communication in cases of chronic pain can be evidenced through the results of a study by Lacroix et al. (1990), who determined that patients with chronic low back pain who had a strong understanding of their condition were statistically more likely to return to work during the course of the study than were patients with a poor understanding of their condition.

Bates et al. (1997) suggest that due to a lack of understanding of the views and values of ethnic minority patients with chronic pain by clinicians, these patients are likely to experience higher levels of treatment-related distress. Accordingly, minority patients with chronic pain are more likely to avoid medical services and are at greater risk for dropping out of treatment. Goldberg and Remy-St. Louis (1998) emphasize the importance of nonminority clinicians making a conceptual shift to understand the meaning of pain to the minority patient, as failing to do so adversely affects the credibility of the health care professional, thereby rendering treatment ineffective.

Davidhizar et al. (1997) postulate that ethnically and culturally diverse patients with pain demonstrate their pain either stoically or emotively. These two divergent response styles are determined, to a great extent, by the cultural traditions which specify the rules of conduct and conformity regarding the expression of pain. When dealing with nonminority health care professionals, both of these response styles can be problematic, as nonminority providers have the expectation that pain will be expressed neither in an overly stoic nor in an overly emotive fashion, but rather in a manner consistent with their own styles of communication. Bates et al. (1995) state that Puerto Ricans and Anglo-Americans appear to perceive and experience chronic pain differently, and that the difference is neither positive nor negative in itself. While the emotive expression of chronic pain among Puerto Ricans is considered normal and acceptable to Puerto Rican patients and medical professionals, non-Hispanic clinicians are likely to interpret the Puerto Ricans' emotive style as indicative of their inability to cope appropriately with chronic pain. The authors noted that Puerto Rican health care providers considered the patients' open display of what Anglo providers would consider excessive pain behavior to be normal and appropriate. Despite significant differences in style of expression of pain, Bates et al. (1995) did not find any differences between their Puerto Rican and non-Hispanic Caucasian groups in terms of interference with work, social, or family activities. In a study of 372 patients with chronic pain from six different ethnic groups that was conducted in New England, Bates and Edwards (1992) found that the Hispanic group's self-reported expression of pain was higher than that of the non-Hispanic Caucasian groups. While the authors did not mention the response to the Hispanics' emotive expression of pain by the clinicians who were involved in this study, it is unlikely that they considered the Hispanics' pain behavior "normal and acceptable" as had the Puerto Rican medical professionals in the Bates et al. study (1995). As Anglo health care providers are likely either directly or indirectly to express their expectations regarding "appropriate" expression of pain to Hispanic patients (and may do so in a perceivably judgmental manner), Hispanics suffering from chronic pain may feel misunderstood and alienated and, accordingly, may choose not to seek or to withdraw from treatment that could potentially benefit them.

Although a number of investigators have addressed the impact of the emotive style of Hispanic patients with chronic pain, less has been written regarding the impact of the stoic style. Kramer et al. (2002a, b) studied pain-related beliefs and the manner in which symptoms are communicated among Native Americans suffering from chronic arthritis joint pain. In both studies, the authors determined that Native Americans suffering from chronic pain tended to voice subtle pain complaints, used vague verbal descriptions for their pain, and accordingly, may have understated serious symptoms. The investigators reported that while most of these Native American pain sufferers eventually sought medical attention, the under-recognition of the severity of their symptoms resulted in suboptimal treatment as opposed to appropriate multidisciplinary care (Kramer et al., 2002b). A strength of both of these studies was the drawing of their samples from an urban area in which more than 200 different Native American tribes were represented, thereby enhancing the generalizability of their results.

A surprising paucity of research on chronic pain among Asians is evident, particularly given the rapid growth rate of the population within the United States. Salimbene (2000) emphasizes the importance of taking Asians' traditions of stoicism into consideration when providing medical services to these minority groups. The author notes the strong Buddhist and Taoist emphases in their teachings regarding stoicism, behavioral reserve, and suppression of negative thoughts and complaints. Lee et al. (1997) notes that Asians are more passive in their relationships with health care providers than are Caucasians and that they will rarely admit ignorance or ask questions regarding their care. While no literature on Asian-Americans' access to chronic pain management services has been published up to this point, Brown (1987) determined that higher levels of stoicism among Vietnamese Americans limited their utilization of the mental health care system. Stoicism among Asian Americans appears to be supported in the acute pain literature, as the results of a number of studies (Carnie & Perks, 1984; Carragee et al., 1999; Houghton et al., 1992; Houghton et al., 1993; Streltzer & Wade, 1981) have indicated that Asians require

and/or request substantially lower dosages of opioids than Caucasians post-operatively.

In a review, Lee et al. (1997) noted that although ethnic differences in the pharmacokinetics of opioids may exist, results of such studies have been mixed and have not demonstrated clinical significance. Accordingly, it appears likely that differences in requests for narcotic analgesics between Caucasians and Asians relate to the Asians' stoicism. Based on these studies, the possibility that Asian Americans are at risk for not seeking appropriate treatment for chronic pain conditions certainly should be considered. However, once again it is important to avoid stereotyping. As the pain experiences and emotional and behavioral responses to chronic pain may differ drastically between Mexican Americans and Puerto Ricans, it cannot be assumed that all Asian Americans will evidence the same levels of stoicism in regard to their chronic pain. Despite certain cultural similarities, the meaning of pain to a third-generation Japanese American is likely to be very different from that of a Vietnamese refugee whose level of acculturation is still minimal and whose history of privation due to living in the midst of a war for many years has dramatically altered his or her view of life in general.

Peripherally related to stoicism as a variable that may be related to the undertreatment of chronic pain is fear of dependence on or addiction to narcotic analgesics. Anderson et al. (2002) found that more than 90% of African Americans and 76% of Hispanics in their sample of cancer patients expressed belief that they should not be reliant on pain medications. The majority of patients in both of these groups expressed concerns regarding addiction and developing tolerance to opioids. Of the Hispanic patients, 65% reported that they were concerned regarding their families' reactions to their use of pain medications. Hispanics have been found to be particularly concerned regarding their utilization of narcotic analgesics due to a fear of becoming addicted or developing tolerance (Cleeland et al., 1997; Juarez et al., 1999). Nemoto and colleagues (1999) identified an Asian cultural construct of fear of addiction. While Caucasians suffering from chronic pain also often fear that they will become addicted to or dependent on opioids, the limited literature available suggests that this fear may be more pronounced among certain racial and cultural groups, potentially resulting in their undertreatment. Several studies (Lin & Ward, 1995; Ward & Hernandez, 1994; Ward et al., 1993) that examined fear of addiction and tolerance to opioids among cancer patients of different ethnic backgrounds have suggested that these concerns are strongest among lower socioeconomic status patients. Given the strong negative correlation between racial/ethnic minority status and socioeconomic status (U.S. Bureau of the Census, 2001), however, minority chronic pain sufferers are at greater risk

for undermedication due to fears of addiction and tolerance to narcotic analgesics.

HEALTH CARE AND SOCIAL SYSTEM VARIABLES

Mayberry et al. (2000) provided a comprehensive review
of racial and ethnic differences in access to medical care.
Their conclusion that racial and ethnic minorities, particularly African Americans, do not have the same access to
health services is consistent with their thesis of pervasive
racism in the American health care system. In *any* society,
individual health care providers are not immune to the
risk of discriminatory behavior. Mayberry and colleagues
(2000) wrote, "The history of medical care in the United
States is replete with discriminatory practices that denied
ethnic minorities access to services based on skin color.
Thus, the medical system of the past is correctly described
as a racist institution, and the legacy of racism should not
be minimized. Clearly, the patient's race, but specifically
skin color, influence decision making, whether it is overt
prejudice or subconscious perceptions" (pp. 134–135).
However, Mayberry and colleagues also wrote, "The lack
of SES (socioeconomic status) indicators in the study of
racial and ethnic differences in health care is a common
refrain among researchers" (p. 117). The importance of
taking socioeconomic status into account in studies of
racial and ethnic differences in health care can be fully
appreciated through Mayberry et al.'s finding, "In some
cases, when important variables [among which they
include SES, describing it as the "most important" explanatory variable] are controlled, racial and ethnic disparities
are reduced and may even disappear under certain circumstances" (2000, p. 112). The authors reviewed evidence
of racial and ethnic inequities in the treatment of a number
of health conditions, including heart disease and stroke,
cancer, diabetes, HIV/AIDS, mental disease, and children's health issues. Little was mentioned in the article
regarding chronic pain. Mayberry and colleagues (2000)
did not specify whether they believed that the racism in
health care in the United States is consciously or unconsciously motivated.

Mayberry et al.'s (2000) findings suggest that despite
the existence of a number of studies that indicate that
racial and ethnic minority chronic pain sufferers are at
greater risk than Caucasians for being undertreated, it is
difficult to specifically attribute this disparity in treatment
to health care providers themselves. Given the numerous
variables that can contribute to unequal treatment, methodological problems are likely to result in confounded
findings. Investigators have tended to rely on the use of
medical vignettes as a research approach for determining
whether medical professionals treat chronic pain differently based on race and ethnicity. Chibnall and Tait (1999)
present vignettes to nonphysician medical center employees in which ethnicity, the presence of litigation, and the
strength of medical evidence were varied. Each participant
was asked to evaluate the "patient's" pain, disability, and
emotional distress; to attribute causality for the patient's
pain and disability; and to rate the patient's veracity and
the extent to which the patient evoked sympathy from the
participant. While interaction effects were identified, the
study did not yield any main effects associated with ethnicity. The authors express surprise regarding the lack of
a unique effect of patient ethnicity on either attributions
or symptom evaluation, and suggest that their ethnicity
manipulation may have been too obvious to the participants. Therein lies a significant weakness of this type of
vignette study. In another vignette study, Weisse et al.
(2001) found interaction effects but no main effects of
race on primary care physicians' willingness to prescribe
narcotic analgesics for pain associated with kidney stones
or acute back pain. Weisse et al. (2003) also used vignette
methodology in a study of internists' pain management
practices in cases of renal colic and persistent back pain.
Again, no main effects for patient race were found, despite
the identification of interaction effects.

Given the aforementioned weaknesses of vignette
studies, the results of the investigations by Chibnall and
Tait (1999) and Weisse et al. (2001, 2003) should not be
taken to suggest that health care provider bias against
racial and ethnic minorities in their chronic pain management practices does not exist. As mentioned above, a lack
of an appropriate methodology for assessing provider bias
in treating patients with chronic pain limits the confidence
with which one can attribute racial and ethnic differences
in chronic pain management services to racism. Perhaps
the strongest suggestion of health care providers discriminating in their chronic pain management practices relies
on extrapolation from the companion studies by Todd et
al. (1993, 2000) mentioned earlier in this chapter in which
Hispanics received less analgesia than non-Hispanic Caucasians for acute long bone fracture pain, despite a lack
of difference in assessments of pain severity between the
two groups by physicians. Todd and colleagues (1994)
suggest that this finding of discrepant treatment could be
explained by a "straightforward bias by physicians who
are equally aware of pain in both ethnic groups, but less
interested in treating it when patients are Hispanic" (p.
928). However, the body of literature as a whole suggests
that if health care providers are actually providing inferior
levels of chronic pain management services to racially and
ethnically diverse minorities due to actual prejudice, the
empirical evidence for such a disparity is weak.

What, then, can potentially explain the findings of
inferior access to chronic pain management services to
which racial and ethnic minorities appear to be subjected?
As mentioned earlier in this chapter, the negative relationship between racial/ethnic minority status and socioeco-

nomic status has been well established (U.S. Bureau of the Census, 2001). In addition to the numerous patient variables that were mentioned earlier in this chapter, it appears that the lower socioeconomic status of racial and ethnic minorities rather than minority status itself is responsible for much of the limited access to chronic pain management that underserved minorities experience.

There exists a substantial body of literature that suggests that low socioeconomic status, independent of race and ethnicity, is positively related to underservice in medicine in general (Becker & Newsom, 2003; Franks & Fiscella, 2002; Krzyzanowska et al., 2003; Merzel & Moon-Howard, 2002; Newacheck et al., 2003a, b; Omalley et al., 2001; Ozminkowski et al., 1998; Scarinci et al., 2001). A Norwegian study (Brekke et al., 2002) in which race was not considered determined that socioeconomic status related negatively to severity of musculoskeletal pain, higher levels of pain-related physical disability, mental distress, and low life satisfaction. Most recently, Portenoy and his colleagues (2004) utilized survey methodology to assess racial and ethnic differences in pain experience between Caucasians, African Americans, and Hispanics in the United States. They found that a composite variable identified as "disabling pain" was negatively associated with socioeconomic status, although not with racial and ethnic minority status once they had controlled for socioeconomic factors. While a review of the literature indicates a lack of investigations of the specific relationship between socioeconomic status and access to appropriate treatment for chronic pain, some of the studies that have examined the relationship between racial and ethnic minority status and access to services suggest that socioeconomic factors are heavily implicated in the identified disparities.

Escalante et al. (2000) determined that recipients of hip replacements for severe arthritis were less likely to be Hispanic than of other races and ethnicities. The authors cited low socioeconomic status as one of the reasons for this underrepresentation. Similarly, Ang et al. (2003) determined that despite similar self-reported degrees of pain and dysfunction secondary to joint involvement in cases of osteoarthritis, Caucasians were significantly more likely than African Americans to undergo hip and knee replacement surgery. The authors noted that the underlying reasons for this ethnic variation are likely to be "multifactorial" and may include issues of insurance coverage. Hootman et al. (2002) determined that African Americans and Caucasians had the same number of ambulatory medical care visits for arthritis and other rheumatic conditions, but that African Americans were more likely to be seen in emergency rooms and hospital outpatient centers as opposed to private physicians' offices. The authors included insurance coverage and level of socioeconomic resources among the reasons for this disparity. In a study of cancer pain in Puerto Rico, Ward and Hernandez (1994)

attribute the use of inadequate analgesia to misconceptions regarding their utilization. The authors suggest, however, that these misconceptions were likely to relate to their subjects' low socioeconomic status rather than to their Hispanic ethnicity itself. Cleeland et al. (1994, 1997) determined that cancer patients treated in community clinical oncology programs that treated primarily minority patients were more likely to receive inadequate analgesia than were patients treated in centers that did not treat primarily minorities. The authors fail to mention the possibility that socioeconomic differences rather than racial and ethnic issues may have caused the identified disparity. Finally, a study by Payne et al. (2003) determined that African Americans suffering from breast cancer underuse hospices and palliative care relative to the general population. The authors note, however, that African Americans may find hospice care inaccessible for economic reasons.

One of the most intriguing studies of racial and ethnic minority difficulties with access to appropriate pain management services examined their relative lack of access to strong prescription narcotic analgesics. Morrison and colleagues (2000) determined that only 25% of pharmacies in minority neighborhoods in New York City carried supplies of narcotic analgesics sufficient to treat severe pain, as opposed to 72% of pharmacies in predominantly non-Hispanic Caucasian neighborhoods. Reasons for inadequate opioid supplies reported by surveyed pharmacists included a lack of demand for certain drugs, concern regarding disposal, fear of fraud and illicit narcotic use that could result in Drug Enforcement Administration investigations, fear of robbery, and problems with reimbursement by health plans and Medicaid. Surprisingly, Morrison and colleagues (2000) make no reference whatsoever to the socioeconomic status of the inhabitants of the "minority areas" in which pharmacies were surveyed. New York City's segregation is certainly as socioeconomically based as racially and ethnically based. Areas such as the South Bronx and Harlem, whose populations are composed almost entirely of racial and ethnic minorities, are among the most poverty-stricken urban areas in the nation. Studies of availability of narcotic analgesics in impoverished areas of the country which are inhabited by non-Hispanic Caucasians would help determine whether the issue of access to opioids is related to racial/ethnic or to socioeconomic factors.

While there have not been any studies published on the relationship among racial/ethnic minority status, access to chronic pain management services, and ability to pay for these services, a review of related literature may, in part, explain disparities in access. Minorities have been found to be significantly less likely to purchase health insurance, even after adjustments for income and wealth have been made (Saver & Doescher, 2000). Lillie-Blanton et al. (2000) determined that minority Americans were more concerned about health care's cost than about other issues of access to medical services. Income has been determined to be a more significant predictor of lack of health insurance coverage than is race, although racial and ethnic minorities were found to be overrepresented in the low income group (Shi, 2001). Recently, Callahan and Cooper (2004) determined that the socioeconomic variable of lack of formal education was a substantially greater predictor of a lack of health care insurance than was racial/ethnic minority status. As a group, these studies suggest that racial and ethnic minorities are more likely than non-Hispanic Caucasians to be without health care insurance, but that this lack of coverage is related to socioeconomic status and the perceived value of health insurance rather than to racial and ethnic minority status per se.

Chronic pain management services can be costly, particularly when provided in a multidisciplinary or interdisciplinary fashion. A study by Marketdata Enterprises (1995) determined the average cost of pain rehabilitation programs to be $8,100.00. This type of treatment, however, has been found to be considerably more cost-effective than any other options (Turk, 1996). The average cost of multidisciplinary chronic pain management services at present has not been assessed in the literature, but is likely to be greater than the average cost of such services at the time of the Marketdata Enterprises study due to dramatic increases in the cost of health care services in general. Regardless, it is unlikely that many patients are able and willing to pay for multidisciplinary chronic pain management services out of pocket. Accordingly, the frequent lack of adequate health care insurance among racial and ethnic minorities is likely to result in limited access to appropriate treatment of their chronic pain. Racial and ethnic minorities are overrepresented on the Medicaid rolls (Mills & Bhandari 2003). As many practitioners and for-profit chronic pain treatment centers are unwilling to accept Medicaid for their services, racial and ethnic minorities are again at greater risk for lack of access to appropriate treatment. It should be noted, however, that the insurance-related lack of access to the best possible chronic pain management services is a *socioeconomic* rather than a *racial/ethnic* variable.

CONCLUSIONS

The question of why racially and ethnically diverse minorities suffering from chronic pain are underserved in the United States is certainly a complex one. However, in reviewing the literature on patient variables, communication issues, health care provider issues, and social system variables, it appears that deeply ingrained cultural patterns of seeking access to chronic pain management services and the dual health care system based primarily upon socioeconomic status are most strongly implicated in this disparity. While some of the identified racial and ethnic inequity in access to chronic pain management services

may relate to issues within the medical and social systems independent of socioeconomic status, there exists no empirical evidence that would suggest that minorities are underserved due to overt prejudice. Nevertheless, specific instances in which racial and ethnic minorities suffering from chronic pain are undertreated based on prejudice certainly occur, as they do in other service areas within American society.

Because completely eradicating overt prejudice in medicine is unlikely, it is important that health care providers make an effort to do everything possible to overcome the impact of the patient variables that cause racial and ethnic disparities in access to chronic pain management services, as well as consciously monitoring themselves against inadvertent minority stereotyping. The key to providing more equitable access to chronic pain management services is appropriate education of both minority chronic pain sufferers and the pain management specialists who have the potential to ease their suffering. While revamping the American health care system to assure that socioeconomic factors do not affect access to quality care would be a noble undertaking, the complexities of doing so within a larger system characterized by such pervasive inequalities between social classes would be overwhelming.

Educating members of racial and ethnic minorities who suffer from chronic pain may represent a difficult undertaking, as issues of trust of the Caucasian majority-dominated medical establishment are likely to impede such efforts. Some of the patient variables (e.g., racial and ethnic minority reliance upon the family and prayer) discussed earlier in this chapter that may potentially limit access to chronic pain management services are so deeply and pervasively culturally ingrained that extreme caution would need to be taken not to risk further alienation of racial and ethnic minority members. Rather than making what are likely to be futile efforts to educate racial and ethnic minority patients with chronic pain regarding the "superiority" of the standard biomedical approaches, it would perhaps behoove health care providers to accept minorities' emphases on family and prayer. In addition to building trust, acceptance of complementary and alternative medicine *in conjunction with traditional biomedical approaches* appears to be clinically reasonable based on empirical support. Hunt et al. (2000) found that Mexican American patients with diabetes who very actively used alternative treatments such as prayer also tended to be very active using traditional biomedical methods. Ni et al. (2002) studied a sample of more than 30,000 U.S. adults, finding that people who used methods such as prayer, spiritual healing, and herbal medicine were more likely to have customary health care providers and to have visited a physician during the previous year than were those who did not use complementary and alternative medicine.

To deal with the sense of hopelessness that likely makes members of racial and ethnic minorities reluctant to seek treatment for their chronic pain, psychoeducational counseling may be beneficial. As mentioned earlier in this study, racial and ethnic minorities are less likely to seek psychological counseling than are non-Hispanic Caucasians, likely due to issues of communication and perceived benefit as well as finances. As proportionally more racial and ethnic minorities are being trained in mental health service provision (National Science Foundation, 2003), the hope exists that communication issues will become less problematic, thereby enticing minority patients to accept counseling within the context of their chronic pain treatment. Additionally, studies suggest that nurses can be effective providers of counseling services in the comprehensive treatment of chronic pain (Wells-Federman et al., 2002; Olason, 2004).

In terms of educating health care providers regarding the treatment of racial and ethnic minorities suffering from chronic pain, an article by Bates and colleagues (1997) on the effects of the cultural context of health care on the treatment of chronic pain offers clinicians some excellent ideas for maximizing patient response. The authors noted that medical professionals in Puerto Rico maintained different norms for patients' pain behaviors than did health care providers in the mainland United States, who expected more stoicism by patients. Pain behavior, when observed by Anglo health care providers, was viewed not as indicative of severe pain but rather as a sign that the patient was "overly emotional." Accordingly, Hispanic patients who demonstrated pain behavior in the presence of Anglo health care providers were not given any consideration for prompt treatment. Thus, the Hispanic chronic pain patients being treated in the mainland United States were at risk for feeling alienated by health care practitioners likely to have been seen as uninvolved and incapable of empathy, with little chance of a working alliance developing.

Bates et al. (1997) noted that cultural differences in the doctor–patient relationship exist. The authors suggested that the relationships between patients with chronic pain and their physicians in Puerto Rico were less formal and more personal than in the mainland United States. In Puerto Rico, a greater emphasis is placed on spending significant amounts of time with patients and listening to them express their concerns, fears, anger, and frustrations. Visits to patients' homes by their physicians are not uncommon. Patient-centered medical practice emphasizing empathy has been linked to improved compliance and more positive medical outcomes (Comstock et al., 1982; Scopp, 2000; Sullivan et al., 2000; van Dulmen & Bensing, 2002). Based on the research of Bates and colleagues (1997), the importance of placing more emphasis on the practitioner–patient relationship when treating Puerto Ricans with chronic pain should not be understated. Research on the importance of empathetic, patient-centered approaches in the treatment

of other racial and ethnic minorities suffering from chronic pain would also be useful.

A final difference between health care providers in Puerto Rico and those on the mainland who work with patients with chronic pain that should be mentioned is that providers in Puerto Rico function as patient advocates and counselors as well as biomedical pain practitioners (Bates et al., 1997). The authors reported that Puerto Rican physicians counseled patients with chronic pain on social and economic problems associated with their disabilities, served as patient advocates in medicolegal matters, and even served the role of vocational counselors. While no mention was made of treatment of chronic pain in Puerto Rico through a truly interdisciplinary team, the numerous roles that physicians played in patients' recoveries provided chronic pain sufferers with the benefits of interdisciplinary treatment. While multidisciplinary and interdisciplinary chronic pain management programs may include physicians, psychologists, social workers, and vocational counselors, Bates et al. (1997) described the pain physician in Puerto Rico as encompassing all of these roles. The practice of the pain physician in Puerto Rico is the antithesis of that of the pain physician in the mainland United States in terms of accessibility and scope of practice. It is accordingly not surprising that Puerto Rican patients in the mainland United States, along with other racial and ethnic minorities, do not possess the level of trust that Bates et al. (1997) described of patients with chronic pain in their article. The authors stated: "As long as the cultural backgrounds of both patients and providers are ignored in assessment and treatment programs, expensive treatments will remain primarily ineffective. Long-term investment in educating health care providers in personal cultural self-awareness, awareness of the culture of biomedicine, and in cultural relativity may lead to more effective care and treatment, and ultimately save money and reduce human suffering" (p. 1445).

THE FUTURE

Cultural awareness training is finally becoming a part of the training curricula for health care providers in the United States (Donini-Lenhoff & Hedrick, 2000). Nevertheless, racial and ethnic minorities are likely to continue to be underserved for many years to come, as changes in training, attitudes of practitioners and minority patients, and socioeconomically based issues of access to appropriate pain management are likely to occur only very gradually. A study by Anderson et al. in 2000 provided a modicum of optimism, as the authors found that only 30% of African American and Hispanic cancer patients in the study were receiving inadequate analgesics, as compared to 65% of minority patients with cancer in a study that the group had conducted only 3 years earlier (Cleeland et al., 1997). Anderson and colleagues (2000) identified a change they hope will be perpetuated. However, if this is to occur, racial and ethnic minority patients, health care providers, and the medical and social systems will all need to contribute by demonstrating initiative and flexibility.

REFERENCES

Alegria, M., et al. (2002). Mental health care for Latinos: Inequalities in use of specialty mental health services among Latinos, African Americans, and non-Latino Whites. *Psychiatric Services, 53,* 1547–1555.

Alvidrez, J. (1999). Ethnic variations in mental health attitudes and service use among low-income African American, Latina, and European American young women. *Community Mental Health Journal, 35,* 515–530.

Anderson, K. O., et al. (2000). Minority cancer patients and their providers. *Cancer, 88,* 1929–1938.

Anderson, K. O., et al. (2002). Cancer pain management among underserved minority outpatients. *Cancer, 94,* 2295–2304.

Ang, D. C. et al. (2002). Ethnic differences in the perception of prayer and consideration of joint arthroplasty. *Medical Care, 40,* 471–476.

Ang, D. C. et al. (2003). Is there a difference in the perception of symptoms between African Americans and Whites with osteoarthritis? *Journal of Rheumatology, 30,* 1305–1310.

Arcury, T. A. (1996). Gender and ethnic differences in alternative and conventional arthritis remedy use among community-dwelling rural adults with arthritis. *Arthritis Care and Research, 9,* 384–390.

Aruffo, J. F., et al. (1993). AIDS knowledge in minorities: Significance of locus of control. *American Journal of Preventive Medicine, 9,* 15–20.

Bates, M. S., & Edwards, W. T. (1992). Ethnic variations in the chronic pain experience. *Ethnicity and Disease, 2,* 63–83.

Bates, M. S., & Rankin-Hill, L. (1994). Control, culture and chronic pain. *Social Science and Medicine, 5,* 629–645.

Bates, M.S., Edwards, W.T., & Anderson, K.O. (1993). Ethnocultural influences on variation in chronic pain perception. *Pain, 52,* 101–112.

Bates, M. S., Rankin-Hill, L., & Sanchez-Ayendez, M. (1997). The effects of cultural context of health care on treatment of and response to chronic pain and illness. *Social Science and Medicine, 45,* 1433–1447.

Bates, M. S. et al. (1995). A cross-cultural comparison of adaptation to chronic pain among Anglo-Americans and native Puerto Ricans. *Medical Anthropology, 16,* 141–173.

Becker, G., & Newsom, E. (2003). Socioeconomic status and dissatisfaction with health care among chronically ill African Americans. *American Journal of Public Health, 93,* 742–748.

Bell, R. A., Summerson, J. H., & Konen, J. C. (1995). Racial differences in psychosocial variables among adults with non-insulin-dependent diabetes mellitus. *Behavioral Medicine, 21,* 69–73.

Bernabei, R., et al. (1998). Management of pain in elderly patients with cancer. *Journal of the American Medical Association, 279,* 1877–1882.

Bill-Harvey, D., et al. (1989). Methods used by urban, low-income minorities to care for their arthritis. *Arthritis Care and Research, 2,* 60–64.

Boulware, L. E., et al. (2003). Race and trust in the health care system. *Public Health Reports, 118,* 358–365.

Brekke, M., Hjortdahl, P., & Kvien, T. K. (2002). Severity of musculoskeletal pain: Relations to socioeconomic inequality. *Social Science and Medicine, 54,* 221–228.

Brena, S.F., Sanders, S. H., & Motoyama, H. (1990). American and Japanese low back pain patients: Cross-cultural similarities and differences. *Clinical Journal of Pain, 6,* 118–124.

Bristow, K., & Patten, S. (2002). Treatment-seeking rates and associated mediating factors among individuals with depression. *Canadian Journal of Psychiatry, 47,* 660–665.

Brown, F. (1987). Counseling Vietnamese refuges: The new challenge. *International Journal for the Advancement of Counseling, 10,* 259–268.

Callahan, S. T., & Cooper, W. O. (2004). Gender and uninsurance among young adults in the United States. *Pediatrics, 113,* 291–297.

Carnie, J. C., & Perks, D. (1984). The pattern of postoperative analgesic administration in non-English speaking Asian women following cesarean section. *Annals of the Royal College of Surgeons of England, 66,* 365–366.

Carragee, E. J., et al. (1999). Pain control and cultural norms and expectations after closed femoral shaft fractures. *The American Journal of Orthopedics, 28,* 97–102.

Chapman, W. P., & Jones, C. M. (1944). Variations in cutaneous and visceral pain sensitivity in normal subjects. *Journal of Clinical Investigation, 23,* 81–91.

Cheung, F. K. & Snowden, L. R. (1990). Community mental health and ethnic minority populations. *Community Mental Health Journal, 26,* 277–291.

Chibnall, J. T., & Tait, R. C. (1999). Social and medical influences on attributions and evaluations of chronic pain. *Psychology & Health, 14,* 719–729.

Cleeland, C. S., et al. (1994). Pain and its treatment in outpatients with metastatic cancer. *New England Journal of Medicine, 330,* 592–596.

Cleeland, C. S., et al. (1997). Pain and treatment of pain in minority patients with cancer. *Annals of Internal Medicine, 127,* 813–816.

Comstock, L. M., et al. (1982). Physician behaviors that correlate with patient satisfaction. *Journal of Medical Education, 57,* 105–112.

Corbie-Smith, G., Thomas, S. B., & St. George, D. M. (2002). Distrust, race, and research. *Archives of Internal Medicine, 162,* 2458–2463.

Coulton, C. J., et al., (1990). Ethnicity, self-care, and use of medical care among the elderly with joint symptoms, *Arthritis Care and Research, 3,* 19–28.

Cronan, T. A., Kaplan, R. M., & Kozin, F. (1993). Factors affecting unprescribed remedy use among people with self-reported arthritis, *Arthritis Care and Research, 6,* 149–155.

Davidhizar, R., Dowd, S., & Giger, J. N. (1997). Cultural differences in pain management. *Radiologic Technology, 68*, 345–348.

Diala, C., et al. (2000). Racial differences in attitudes toward professional mental health care and in the use of services. *American Journal of Orthopsychiatry, 70*, 455–464.

Doescher, M. P., et al. (2000). Racial and ethnic disparities in perceptions of physician style and trust. *Archives of Family Medicine, 9*, 1156–1163.

Donini-Lenhoff, F.G. & Hedrick, H.L. (2000). Increasing awareness and implementation of cultural competence principles in health professions education. *Journal of Allied Health, 29*, 241–245.

Ducharme, J., & Barber, C. (1995). A prospective blinded study on emergency pain assessment and therapy. *Journal of Emergency Medicine, 13*, 571–575.

Edwards, C., & Keefe, F. (2000). New directions in research on pain and ethnicity: A comment on Riley, Wade, Myers, Sheffield, Pappas, and Price (2002). *Pain, 100*, 211–212.

Edwards, R. R. et al. (2001). Ethnic differences in pain tolerance: Clinical implications in a chronic pain population. *Psychosomatic Medicine, 63*, 316–323.

Epker, J., Gatchel, R. J., & Ellis, E. (1999). A model for predicting chronic TMD: Practical application in clinical settings. *Journal of the American Dental Association, 130*, 1470–1475.

Escalante, A., et al. (2000). Recipients of hip replacement for arthritis are less likely to be Hispanic, independent of access to health care and socioeconomic status. *Arthritis & Rheumatism, 43*, 390–399.

Faucett, J., Gordon, N., & Levine, J. (1994). Differences in postoperative pain severity among four ethnic groups. *Journal of Pain Symptom and Management, 9*, 383–389.

Fiscella, K., & Franks, P. (1997). Does psychological distress contribute to racial and socioeconomic disparities in mortality? *Social Science & Medicine, 45*, 1805–1809.

Franks, P., & Fiscella, K. (2002). Effect of patient socioeconomic status on physician profiles for prevention, disease management, and diagnostic testing costs. *Medical Care, 40*, 717–724.

Fuhrer, M. J., et al. (1993). Depressive symptomatology in persons with spinal cord injury who reside in the community. *Archives of Physical Medicine and Rehabilitation, 74*, 255–260.

Garcia, M., & Marks, G. (1989). Depressive symptomatology among Mexican-American adults: An examination with the CES-D Scale. *Psychiatry Research, 27*, 137–148.

Garron, D. C., & Leavitt, F. (1979). Demographic and affective covariates of pain. *Psychosomatic Medicine, 41*, 525–535.

Gaston-Johansson, F. et al. (1990). Similarities in pain descriptions of four different ethnic-cultural groups. *Journal of Pain and Symptom Management, 5*, 94–100.

Gatchel, R. J., et al. (2003). Treatment- and cost-effectiveness of early intervention for acute low back pain patients: A one-year prospective study. *Journal of Occupational Rehabilitation, 13*, 1–9.

Gatchel, R. J., Polatin, P. B., & Kinney, R. K. (1995). Predicting outcome of chronic back pain using clinical predictors of psychopathology: A prospective analysis. *Health Psychology, 14*, 415–420.

Goldberg, M. A., & Remy-St. Louis, G. (1998). Understanding and treating pain in ethnically diverse populations, *Journal of Clinical Psychology in Medical Settings, 5*, 343–356.

Green, C. R. et al. (2003a). Race and chronic pain: A comparative study of young Black and White Americans presenting for management. *Journal of Pain, 4*, 176–183.

Green, C. R., et al. (2003b). The unequal burden of pain: Confronting racial and ethnic disparities in pain. *Pain Medicine, 4*, 277–294.

Greenberg, G. A., & Rosenheck, R. A. (2003). Change in mental health service delivery among Blacks, Whites, and Hispanics in the Department of Veterans Affairs. *Administration and Policy in Mental Health, 31*, 31–43.

Greenwald, H. P. (1991). Interethnic differences in pain perception. *Pain, 44*, 157–163.

Gruber, B. L., et al. (1988). Immune system and psychological changes in metastatic cancer patients using relaxation and guided imagery: A pilot study. *Scandinavian Journal of Behaviour Therapy, 17*, 25–46.

Hootman, J. M., Helmick, C. G., & Schappert, S. M. (2002). Magnitude and characteristics of arthritis and other rheumatic conditions on ambulatory medical care visits, United States, 1997. *Arthritis & Rheumatism, 47*, 571–581.

Houghton, I. T., et al. (1992). Inter-ethnic differences in postoperative pethidine requirements. *Anaesthesia and Intensive Care, 20*, 52–55.

Houghton, I. T., et al. (1993). Suxamethonium myalgia: An ethnic comparison with and without pancuronium pretreatment. *Anaesthesia, 48*, 377–381.

Hunt, L. M., Arar, N. H., & Akana, L. L. (2000). Herbs, prayer and insulin. Use of medical and alternative treatments by a group of Mexican American diabetes patients. *Journal of Family Practice, 49*, 216–223.

Ibrahim, S. A., et al. (2002). Differences in expectations of outcome mediate African American/White patient differences in "willingness" to consider joint replacement. *Arthritis & Rheumatism., 46*, 2429–2435.

Ibrahim, S. A., et al. (2003). Older patients' perceptions of quality of chronic knee or hip pain: Differences by ethnicity and relationship to clinical variables. *Journal of Gerontology: Medical Sciences, 58*, M472–477, 2003.

International Association for the Study of Pain. (1986). Classification of chronic pain. *Pain*, Suppl. 3, S1–S226.

Jacobson, D. S. (1987). The cultural context of social support and support networks. *Medical Anthropology Quarterly, 1*, 42–67.

Jordan, M. S., Lumley, M. A., & Leisen, J. C. (1998). The relationships of cognitive coping and pain control beliefs to pain and adjustment among African American and Caucasian women with rheumatoid arthritis. *Arthritis Care and Research, 11*, 80–88.

Juarez, G., Ferrell, B., & Borneman, T. (1999). Cultural considerations in education for cancer pain management. *Journal of Cancer Education, 14*, 168–173.

Keefe, S. E. (1982). Help-seeking behavior among foreign-born and native-born Mexican Americans. *Social Science and Medicine, 16*, 1467–1472.

Kemp, B., Krause, J. S., & Adkins, R. (1999). Depression among African Americans, Latinos, and Caucasians with spinal cord injury: An exploratory study. *Rehabilitation Psychology, 44*, 235–247.

Kramer, B. J., Harker, J. O., & Wong, A. L. (2002a). Arthritis beliefs and self-care in an urban American Indian population. *Arthritis & Rheumatism, 47*, 588–594.

Kramer, B. J., Harker, J. O., & Wong, A. L. (2002b). Descriptions of joint pain by American Indians: Comparison of inflammatory and non-inflammatory arthritis. *Arthritis and Rheumatism, 47*, 149–154.

Krzyzanowska, M. K., Weeks, J. C., & Earle, C. C. (2003). Treatment of locally advanced pancreatic cancer in the real world: Population-based practices and effectiveness. *Journal of Clinical Oncology, 21*, 3409–3414.

Lacroix, J. M., et al. (1990). Low-back pain: Factors of value in predicting outcome. *Spine, 15*, 495–499.

Lawlis, G. F. et al. (1984). Ethnic and sex differences in response to clinical and induced pain in chronic spinal pain patients. *Spine, 9*, 751–754.

Lee, A., Gin, T., & Oh, T. E. (1997). Opioid requirements and responses in Asians. *Anaesthesia and Intensive Care, 25*, 665–670.

Li, L., & Moore, D. (1998). Acceptance of disability and its correlates. *Journal of Social Psychology, 138*, 13–25.

Lillie-Blanton, M., et al. (2000). Race, ethnicity, and the health care system: Public perceptions and experiences. *Medical Care Research and Review, 57*(Suppl. 1), 218–235.

Lin, C., & Ward, S. (1995). Patient-related barriers to cancer pain management in Taiwan. *Cancer Nursing, 18*, 16–22.

Linton, S. J., Hellsing, A. L., & Andersson, D. (1993). A controlled study of the effects of early intervention on acute musculoskeletal pain problems. *Pain, 54*, 353–359.

Lipton, J. A., & Marbach, J. J. (1984). Ethnicity and pain experience. *Social Science and Medicine, 19*, 1279–1298.

Marketdata Enterprises. (1995). *Chronic pain management programs: A market analysis.* Valley Stream, NY: Author.

Mayberry, R. M., Mili, F., & Ofili, E. (2000). Racial and ethnic differences in access to medical care. *Medical Care Research and Review, 57*(Suppl. 1), 108–145.

McCracken, L. M. et al. (2001). A comparison of Blacks and Whites seeking treatment for chronic pain. *Clinical Journal of Pain, 17*, 249–255, 2001.

Merzel, C., & Moon-Howard, J. (2002). Access to health services in an urban community: Does source of care make a difference? *Journal of Urban Health, 79*, 186–199.

Mills, R. J., & Bhandari, S. (2003). Health insurance coverage in the United States: 2002. In *Current population reports.* Washington, DC: U.S. Census Bureau.

Mizner, D., Thomas, M., & Billings, R. (1988). Cognitive changes of migraineurs receiving biofeedback training. *Headache, 28*, 339–343.

Morrison, R. S., et al. (2000) "We don't carry that" — Failure of pharmacies in predominantly nonwhite neighborhoods to stock opioid analgesics. *New England Journal of Medicine, 342*, 1023–1026.

Mutran, E. (1985). Intergenerational family support among Blacks and Whites: Response to culture or to socioeconomic differences. *Journal of Gerontology, 40*, 382–389.

Myers, H. F., et al. (2002). Ethnic differences in clinical presentation of depression in adult women. *Cultural Diversity and Ethnic Minority Psychology, 8*, 138–156.

National Science Foundation Division of Science Resources Statistics. (2003). *Science and engineering doctoral awards: 2002* (NSF 04-303). Arlington, VA: NSF.

Nemoto, T., et al. (1999). Drug use behaviors among Asian drug users in San Francisco. *Addictive Behaviors, 24*, 823–838.

Newacheck, P. W., et al. (2003a). Disparities in adolescent health and health care: Does socioeconomic status matter? *Health Services Research, 38*, 1235–1252.

Newacheck, P. W., et al. (2003b). Disparities in the prevalence of disability between black and white children. *Archives of Pediatrics & Adolescent Medicine, 157*, 244–248.

Ng, B., et al. (1996a). The effect of ethnicity on prescriptions for patient-controlled analgesia for post-operative pain. *Pain, 66*, 9–12.

Ng, B., et al. (1996b). Ethnic differences in analgesic consumption for postoperative pain. *Psychosomatic Medicine, 58*, 125–129.

Ni, H., Simile, C., & Hardy, A. M. (2002). Utilization of complementary and alternative medicine by United States adults: Results from the 1999 national health interview survey. *Medical Care, 40*, 353–358.

O'Malley, M. S., et al. (2001). The association of race/ethnicity, socioeconomic status, and physician recommendation for mammography: Who gets the message about breast cancer screening? *American Journal of Public Health, 91*, 49–54.

Olason, M. (2004). Outcome of an interdisciplinary pain management program in a rehabilitation clinic. *Work, 22*, 9–15.

Ozminkowski, R. J., et al. (1998). What if socioeconomics made no difference? Access to a cadaver kidney transplant as an example. *Medical Care, 36*, 1398–1406.

Padgett, D. K., et al. (1994). Women and outpatient mental health services: Use by Black, Hispanic, and White women in a national insured population. *Journal of Mental Health Administration, 21*, 347–360.

Payne, R., Medina, E., & Hampton, J. W. (2003). Quality of life concerns in patients with breast cancer. *Cancer, 97*(Suppl. 1), 311–317.

Plesh, O., Crawford, P. B., & Gansky, S. A. (2002). Chronic pain in a biracial population of young women. *Pain, 99*, 515–523.

Portenoy, R. K., et al. (2004). Population-based survey of pain in the United States: Differences among White, African American and Hispanic subjects. *Journal of Pain, 5*, 317–328.

Pumariega, A. J., et al. (1998). Utilization of mental health services in a tri-ethnic sample of adolescents. *Community Mental Health Journal, 34*, 145–156.

Richardson, L. A. (2001). Seeking and obtaining mental health services: What do parents expect? *Archives of Psychiatric Nursing, 15*, 223–231.

Riley, J. L. et al. (2002). Racial/ethnic differences in the experience of chronic pain. *Pain, 100*, 291–298.

Ruiz, P., & Langrod, J. (1976). Psychiatry and folk healing: A dichotomy? *American Journal of Psychiatry, 133*, 95–97.

Rybarczyk, B., et al. (2001). A classroom mind/body wellness intervention for older adults with chronic illness: Comparing immediate and 1-year benefits. *Behavioral Medicine, 27*, 15–27.

Salimbene, S. (2000). *What language does your patient hurt in? A practical guide to culturally competent care.* Amherst, MA: Diversity Resources, Inc.

Sanders, S. H., et al. (1992). Chronic low back pain patients around the world: Cross-cultural similarities and differences. *Clinical Journal of Pain, 8*, 317–323.

Saver, B. G., & Doescher, M. P. (2000). To buy, or not to buy: Factors associated with the purchase of nongroup, private health insurance. *Medical Care, 38*, 141–151.

Scarinci, I. C. et al. (2001). Socioeconomic status, ethnicity, and health care access among young and healthy women. *Ethnicity and Disease, 11*, 60–71.

Schultz, I. Z., et al. (2002). Biopsychosocial multivariate predictive model of occupational low back disability. *Spine, 27*, 2720–2725.

Scopp, A. (2000). Clear communication skills with headache patients. *Headache Quarterly, 11*, 269–274.

Selbst, S. M., & Clark, M. (1990). Analgesic use in the emergency department. *Annals of Emergency Medicine, 19*, 1010–1013.

Shi, L. (2001). The convergence of vulnerable characteristics and health insurance in the US. *Social Science and Medicine, 53*, 519–529.

Snell, C. L., & Thomas, J. S. (1998). Young African American males: Promoting psychological and social well-being. *Journal of Human Behavior in the Social Environment, 1*, 125–136.

Snowden, L. (1999). African American service use for mental health problems. *Journal of Community Psychology, 27*, 303–313.

Spaulding, A. D. (1995). Racial minorities and other high-risk groups with HIV and AIDS at increased risk for psychological adjustment problems in association with health locus of control orientation. *Social Work in Health Care, 21*, 81–114.

Starrett, R. A., Rogers, D., & Decker, J. T. (1992). The self-reliance behavior of the Hispanic elderly in comparison to their use of formal mental health helping networks. *Clinical Gerontology, 11*, 157–169.

Streltzer, J., & Wade, T. C. (1981). The influence of cultural group on the undertreatment of postoperative pain. *Psychosomatic Medicine, 43*, 397–403.

Sugarek, N. J., Deyo, R. A., & Holmes, B. C. (1988). Locus of control and beliefs about cancer in a multi-ethnic clinic population. *Oncology Nursing Forum, 15*, 481–486.

Sullivan, L. M., et al. (2000). The doctor–patient relationship and HIV-infected patients' satisfaction with primary care physicians. *Journal of General Internal Medicine, 15*, 462–469.

Todd, K. H., Lee, T., & Hoffman, J. R. (1994). The effect of ethnicity on physician estimates of pain severity in patients with isolated extremity trauma. *Journal of the American Medical Association, 271*, 925–928.

Todd, K. H., Samaroo, N., & Hoffman, J. R. (1993). Ethnicity as a risk factor for inadequate emergency room analgesia. *Journal of the American Medical Association, 269*, 1537–1539.

Todd, K. H., et al. (2000). Ethnicity and analgesic practice. *Annals of Emergency Medicine, 35*, 11–16.

Turk, D. C. (1996). Efficacy of multidisciplinary pain clinics in the treatment of chronic pain. In M. J. Cohen & J. N. Campbell (Eds.), *Pain treatment centers at a crossroads: A practical and conceptual reappraisal* (pp. 257–273). Seattle: IASP Press.

U.S. Bureau of the Census. (2001). *Statistical abstract of the United States: 2000.* Washington, DC: U.S. Government Printing Office.

van Dulmen, A. M., & Bensing, J. M. (2002). Health promoting effects of the physician–patient encounter. *Psychology, Health & Medicine, 7*, 289–300.

Vermom, S. V., Roberts, R. E., & Lee, E. S. (1982). Response tendencies, ethnicity, and depression scores. *American Journal of Epidemiology, 116*, 482–495.

Ward, S. E. & Hernandez, L. (1994). Patient-related barriers to management of cancer pain in Puerto Rico. *Pain, 58*, 233–238.

Ward, S. E., et al. (1993). Patient-related barriers to management of cancer pain. *Pain, 52*, 319–324.

Weisse, C. S., et al. (2001). Do gender and race affect decisions about pain management? *Journal of General Internal Medicine, 16*, 211–217.

Weisse, C. S., Sorum, P. C., & Dominguez, R. E. (2003). The influence of gender and race on physicians' pain management decisions. *Journal of Pain, 4*, 505–510.

Wells, K., et al. (2001). Ethnic disparities in unmet need for alcoholism, drug abuse, and mental health care. *American Journal of Psychiatry, 158*, 2027–2032.

Wells-Federman, C., Arnstein, P., & Caudill, M. (2002). Nurse-led pain management program: Effect on self-efficacy, pain intensity, pain-related disability, and depressive symptoms in chronic pain patients. *Pain Management Nursing, 3*, 131–140.

Wilson, D. K., et al. (1994). Race and sex differences in health locus of control beliefs and cardiovascular reactivity. *Journal of Pediatric Psychology, 19*, 769–778, 1994.

Wilson, J. E., & Pendleton, J. M. (1989). Oligoanalgesia in the emergency department. *American Journal of Emergency Medicine, 7*, 660–662.

Zborowski, M. (1952). Cultural components in responses to pain. *Journal of Social Issues, 8*, 16–30.

9

Assuring the Quality of Pain Services: Assessing Outcomes

Michael E. Clark, PhD, Ronald J. Gironda, PhD, and Stacey Carter, PhD

INTRODUCTION

Quality assurance (QA) refers to the program of steps necessary to maximize customers' confidence in the reliability and utility of a product. Within health care systems, maintaining and improving quality typically involves a multitude of procedures, mechanisms, and interventions designed to evaluate health care services, identify and remove barriers to care, and enhance outcomes. QA is an *active* process that focuses on implementing change within organizations or systems within organizations. It is this focus on change that differentiates QA from other health care system structures that use more passive approaches in an attempt to change *responses* to the system, rather than changing the system itself.

Among the many components required for effective QA, whether applied to health care programs in general or specifically to pain services, assessing and monitoring outcomes is perhaps the most important. Outcomes assessment drives the QA process. It provides the means for identifying areas that need improvement, and directs efforts to change. It must be global enough to be sensitive to a range of potential service delivery problems, yet specific enough to suggest possible causes and solutions. Like QA, outcomes assessment is an ongoing process rather than a static event and requires constant maintenance, revision, and "fine tuning."

Within health care settings, outcomes assessment is a multipart process that involves "the systematic collection and analysis of information that is used to evaluate the efficacy of an intervention" (Clark & Gironda, 2002, p. 995). To be *systematic* data must be collected in a con-

sistent and repetitive manner using identical or very similar outcomes measures or instruments. The resulting data then undergo *analysis,* which refers to the process of summarizing and interpreting the data to identify any meaningful trends. Although many settings excel in collecting data, the process of analysis often is neglected or underutilized. Data that are collected but not analyzed do not fulfill the spirit of outcomes measurement nor do they contribute to QA.

In the following sections we discuss the rationale underlying the use of outcomes measures in health care settings focusing on pain-related issues. Next we offer a brief review of instruments used to assess pain outcomes focusing first on the consumer of services and second on the service delivery system. We then talk about the processes of selecting appropriate outcomes domains and applying them in clinical practice. Last, we close with some impressions and general recommendations as applied to efforts to enhance the quality of pain services provided in health care settings.

IMPORTANCE OF OUTCOMES MEASUREMENT IN CLINICAL CARE SETTINGS

The emphasis on measuring the quality of pain treatment services has intensified in the past 15 years and is exemplified by the fact that Congress declared the first decade of the 21st century as the Decade of Pain Control and Research (Joint Commission on Accreditation of Healthcare Organizations [JCAHO], 2003). Improving pain management practices is a primary component of health care's humanitarian mission, and interest in the application of QA processes to pain began following recognition that pain often is undertreated and managed inappropriately (American Pain Society Quality of Care Committee, 1995; JCAHO, 2003). This recognition spawned several movements to enhance the availability and quality of pain treatment, initially in medical settings and eventually in all patient populations. Subsequently, guidelines for pain treatment have been developed (Agency for Health Care Policy and Research, 1992, 1994; Clinical Practice Working Group [CPWG], 2003), which provide a consensus-based model of care against which health care settings can compare their own services.

Recent regulatory initiatives and legal precedents have increased the demand for quality pain care. Both health care organizations and physicians have been held financially liable for inadequate pain management (Lande & Loeser, 2001). Many states have codified statutes and regulations addressing multiple aspects of pain management (for a complete review of state pain policies see the Pain and Policies Study Group website, University of Wisconsin Comprehensive Cancer Center; http://www.medsch.wisc.edu/painpolicy/). Additionally, recommendations specific to certain treatment methods have been developed, such as the joint Department of Veterans Affairs/Department of Defense guidelines for the use of opioids for pain treatment (http://www.oqp.med.va.gov/cpg/cot/ot_base.htm; CPWG, 2003).

Changes in health care accreditation standards also are responsible for increased attention to assuring quality pain management services. For example, the Rehabilitation Accreditation Commission (CARF) has been a leader of these efforts by developing elaborate outcomes standards for pain treatment programs (1999). The American Academy of Pain Management (AAPM) began its voluntary pain program accreditation service in 1992, initially requiring participating programs to submit data to the National Pain Data Bank for benchmarking and quality assurance (AAPM, 2001). In 2001, the Joint Commission of Accreditation of Healthcare Organizations (JCAHO) incorporated pain management and assessment into its survey and accreditation process for all organizations providing direct care (Gordon et al., 2002; JCAHO, 2001). These standards build on earlier guidelines developed by the Agency for Healthcare Research and Quality (AHRQ) and the American Pain Society (APS) outlining responsibilities for improving outcomes in pain management. However, unlike these voluntary guidelines, JCAHO standards are required — health care institutions must demonstrate compliance by their pain management programs, including evidence of ongoing quality monitoring.

In addition to complying with regulatory issues and accreditation requirements, establishing routine assessment practices for the provision of pain services allows for the collection of research data to validate treatment

efficacy and to establish evidence-based standards of care (Gordon & Dahl, 2004). Pain management guidelines have been developed for different patient populations (pediatric, adult, geriatric), types of pain (acute or chronic), and conditions or procedures (low back pain, postoperative pain, cancer pain; see JCAHO, 2003, for a list of pain management guidelines).

Not only is the measurement of pain services warranted to promote clinical effectiveness, it is also advantageous from a cost-effectiveness standpoint (Turk, Loeser, & Monarch, 2002). In the age of managed care, resources for health care are limited. The use of outcome data provides a managed care organization (MCO) an evaluative tool to assist in determining which products to make available to their patients. Indeed, MCO medical directors have indicated that the likelihood of a disease program's being funded is increased by providing evidence of clinical data supporting its effectiveness (Lande & Loeser, 2001).

Finally, and perhaps most importantly, outcomes data should be integrated into the clinical decision-making process in order to improve the quality of pain treatment services provided. This is true not only for day to day patient contact, but at a systemic level as well. While this may sound daunting, this is a routine component of practitioner care. At the most basic level, all revisions in patient care stem from evaluations of treatment outcome. As an example, consider an individual presenting to a provider with chronic noncancer pain. Initially, a trial of nonsteroidal anti-inflammatories (NSAIDs) may be initiated. At the next visit, effectiveness of the NSAIDs in relieving pain and improving function will be assessed. Depending on the results of that assessment of treatment outcome, the NSAIDs may be continued unchanged, revised, or discontinued. If they are discontinued, other pharmaceuticals (e.g., opioids) or interventions (e.g., physical therapy, nerve blocks) may be considered instead. In this example, the practitioner assessed the patient's pretreatment symptom report, administered an appropriate treatment, and then assessed post-treatment symptoms. These assessments guided the provider's decision-making process and allowed for treatment modifications as clinically necessary.

The same process can be incorporated into a larger pain treatment delivery system. For instance, in a multidisciplinary pain treatment program, pretreatment measures can be collected at the time of admission into the program. Review of the results of these same measures administered at the time of discharge provides information regarding the effectiveness of the program in changing targeted domains and suggests avenues for modifying the treatment regimen to enhance outcome. In other words, there exists a continuous feedback loop providing the health care provider with quantitative information to guide subsequent treatment decisions. Figure 9.1 depicts this

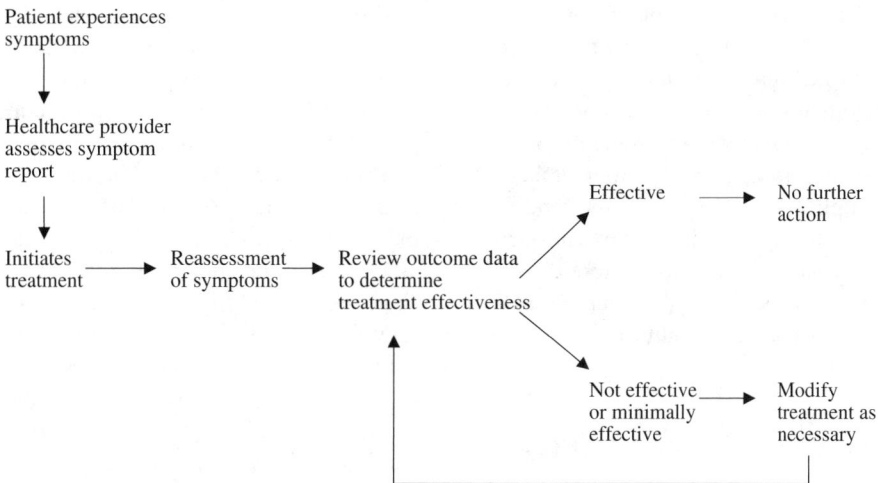

FIGURE 9.1 Clinical decision-making process.

decision-making process. With this said, however, it is important to note that assumptions regarding causation most often are based only on correlational data (i.e., changes in quality are correlated with the interventions for change employed) and, therefore, provide neither confirmation nor rejection of any hypothesized causative link. Other known or unknown factors also could account for the observed changes, particularly in settings where multiple interventions or events may have transpired between the initial assessment and the post-intervention assessment. Therefore, multiple episodes of data collection are preferred as they facilitate the identification of trends in the data that may be more reliable indicators of intervention-related change.

SELECTING RELEVANT OUTCOMES DOMAINS

Selecting appropriate outcomes measures is the key to developing a meaningful outcomes monitoring system. Two factors should be considered as part of the outcomes selection process (Clark & Gironda, 2002):

1. Pain outcomes focus (patient focused or process focused)
2. Practice setting

Pain Outcomes Focus

Patient-focused outcomes measures concentrate on changes in individuals' pain experience following interventions. To quantify change, measures must be administered at least twice (before and after treatment). For treatments spanning lengthy time intervals, repeated administrations (e.g., every month) may provide a more detailed picture of change.

Patient-focused measures often are used to evaluate a single patient's response to treatment. When they are used collectively to evaluate a specific treatment intervention or program of interventions, they serve as aggregate outcomes measures. The most common patient-focused outcome measure is pain intensity. Other measures might include pain-related interference, emotional distress, or physical capacities.

Process-focused measures concentrate on the pain service delivery system and usually are components of performance improvement activities. In some cases measures may be collected only once, but more often they will be collected repeatedly over time to evaluate trends in the measures or to assess the impact of a system intervention.

Results may be used to evaluate how well the pain service delivery system is meeting facility goals, regulatory statutes, or accreditation body (e.g., JCAHO) standards. Common measures include pain clinic waiting times, adequacy of pain assessment and treatment documentation, or compliance with patient pain education standards.

Practice Setting

Practice setting refers to attributes of the pain service delivery environment. Pain treatments may range from minimally complex (e.g., medication management) to highly technical (e.g., dorsal column stimulator implants).

In general, pain service settings that require minimal resources and use uncomplicated treatments may not warrant elaborate, expensive, and time-consuming outcomes measurement practices when less complex approaches would suffice. In contrast, more complex treatment settings requiring greater resource investment or patient risk may want to use broader, multidomain outcomes measures to assess change in a variety of pain experience areas.

The rationale underlying this variation in outcomes approach is twofold. First, from a cost–benefit perspective, when resource investment is greater, such as in complex pain treatment settings, it is reasonable to expect that outcomes should be improved. Utilization of more comprehensive outcomes measures that assess function in a greater range of domains may provide evidence of a greater range of treatment-related improvements. Second, complex pain treatment settings are likely to treat individuals with more complicated and severe pain conditions and increased pain-related dysfunction that extends across multiple domains of function. Therefore, more elaborate measures of outcomes may be needed to accurately reflect both the extent of pain-related disability and the degree of improvement attained.

ASSESSING DOMAINS OF PAIN OUTCOMES

The assessment of pain treatment outcomes is multifaceted, and the selection of appropriate measures is dependent on the objectives of outcomes measurement. Patient-focused outcomes approaches are concerned primarily with treatment-related changes in patients' pain experience. Service delivery outcomes approaches focus on monitoring and enhancing pain service delivery systems. These two approaches should not be considered mutually exclusive; more elaborate outcomes systems may include aspects of each.

PATIENT DOMAINS

Current standards for chronic pain treatment are based on biopsychosocial conceptualizations of chronic pain as a complex, multidimensional phenomenon with diverse etiologic and sustaining factors (Turk & Flor, 1999). Consistent across biopsychosocial perspectives is the underlying assumption that the chronic pain experience is a result of a dynamic interaction among biological, psychological, behavioral, and social factors that shape the individual's response to physical perturbations (Turk & Flor, 1999). Accordingly, recommendations for comprehensive treatment target multiple domains of patient functioning including the physical, perceptual, behavioral, and psychosocial status of the individual. Reflecting this multidimensional approach to conceptualization and treatment, current guidelines for pain outcomes assessment mandate the measurement of treatment-related change within each major domain of an individual's chronic pain experience (Rehabilitation Accreditation Commission, 2002).

The discussion that follows considers each of the domains of patient functioning that we believe to be an important aspect of the pain experience. While not all of these patient-centered domains are likely to be directly targeted by any single treatment approach, changes may be observed in any of these areas following even the most focused interventions due to the interrelationships among these domains. Where appropriate we have suggestions for measures that may be used to assess outcomes in each

of these domains. However, it should be noted that only those measures that have been validated with pain patient samples and were judged by the authors to have some utility for outcomes assessment were included in this discussion. Criteria for inclusion in this review were (1) evidence of acceptable reliability, (2) data supporting instrument validity, (3) prior use as a pain outcomes instrument, and (4) high utility for pain outcomes assessment, as judged by the authors. If such measures are not available, suggestions for alternative assessment strategies are provided. The domains assessed by the instruments that are reviewed are presented in Table 9.1. Absent from this review are several well-validated measures, such as the Coping Strategies Questionnaire (CSQ; Rosensteil & Keefe, 1983), which tap important aspects of the pain experience and have been widely used in pain research, but lack significant evidence of utility for general pain outcomes assessment. For the reader who is interested in a wider range of pain measures, more comprehensive reviews may be found elsewhere (Bradely, Haile, & Jaworski, 1992; Jensen & Karoly, 2001; Tait, Pollard, Margolis, Duckro, & Krause, 1987).

Pain Intensity

While practitioners may not agree on the relative importance of pain reduction as a treatment objective, pain intensity is clearly an essential outcomes assessment domain from most perspectives. Fundamentally, the sensory experience of pain is a subjective aversive phenomenon that is unique to each individual, and as such, it is difficult to describe and quantify objectively. Fortunately, several easy-to-administer, psychometrically sound scales have been developed to assess this domain of the pain experience. There are three broad categories of commonly used pain intensity measures: the Visual Analog Scale (VAS), Numeric Rating Scale (NRS), and Verbal Rating Scale (VRS). The VAS and NRS typically consist of a single item requiring patients to quantify the intensity of their "current," "usual," "least," or "worst" pain. Empirical evidence suggests that the combination of "least" and "usual" pain ratings provides the best estimate of actual pain intensity, while "least" may be the single most accurate predictor (Jensen, Turner, Turner, & Romano, 1996). However, for practical purposes clinicians can have confidence in the choice of a single VAS or NRS rating of "usual" pain, which appears to provide a reasonably valid estimate of actual pain. Interestingly, "current" and "worst" pain ratings were found to have a weaker relationship with actual pain intensity (Jensen et al., 1996).

A reliable and well-validated form of the VAS is a 10-cm line anchored with the phrases "no pain" and "worst possible pain" or "excruciating pain." Patients are instructed to bisect the line at the point that best represents their level of pain, and the score is simply the length of

TABLE 9.1
Domains of Outcome Assessed by Self-Report Measures

Measure (Items)	Pain Intensity	Pain Interference	Emotional Distress	Fear	Employment	Utilization	Satisfaction
NRS/VAS (1)	X	—	—	—	—	—	—
MPQ (20)	X	—	—	—	—	—	—
PDI (7)	—	X	—	—	—	—	—
SIP (136)	—	X	—	—	—	—	—
ODQ (10)	—	X	—	—	—	—	—
BDI (21)	—	—	X	—	—	—	—
CES-D (20)	—	—	X	—	—	—	—
STAI (40)	—	—	X	—	—	—	—
PASS (40)	—	—	—	X	—	—	—
TS (17)	—	—	—	X	—	—	—
BPI (32)	X	X	X	—	—	—	—
POQ (45)	X	X	X	X	X	X	X
MPI (52)	X	X	X	—	—	—	—
POP (23)	X	X	X	X	—	—	—

Note: NRS/VAS = Numeric Rating Scale/Visual Analog Scale; MPQ = McGill Pain Questionnaire; PDI = Pain Disability Index; SIP = Sickness Impact Profile; ODQ = Oswestry Disability Questionnaire; BDI = Beck Depression Inventory; CES-D = Center for Epidemiologic Studies — Depression Scale; STAI = State-Trait Anxiety Inventory; PASS = Pain Anxiety Symptoms Scale; TS = Tampa Scale; BPI = Brief Pain Inventory; POQ = Pain Outcomes Questionnaire; MPI = Multidimensional Pain Inventory; POP = Pain Outcomes Profile.

the segment to that point. The VAS has been found to be valid and sensitive to changes in acute, cancer, and chronic pain (Breivik, Bjornsson, & Skovlund, 2000; De Conno et al., 1994; Hutten, Hermens, & Zilvold, 2001; Jensen & Linton, 1993; Ogon, Krismer, Soellner, Kantner-Rumplmair, & Lampe, 1996), and it yields ratio level data (Jensen, Turner, & Romano, 1992). Although comparisons of horizontal and vertical line orientations yield mixed results, using the VAS horizontally may provide slightly higher sensitivity (Jensen, Turner, Romano, & Fisher, 1999; Ogon et al., 1996; Stratford, Binkley, Riddle, & Guyatt, 1998).

The NRS consists of a numeric range from 0 to 10 or 100 with anchors similar to those of the VAS, which can be administered in oral or written form. Individuals are asked to quantify their pain levels by choosing a single number from the 11- or 101-point scale. The NRS has been found to have good psychometric characteristics (Jensen et al., 1999) and to be sensitive to changes in acute, cancer, and chronic pain (De Conno et al., 1994; Paice & Cohen, 1997). The data provided by the NRS can be treated as ratio level (Jensen & Karoly, 1992).

Verbal rating scales typically consist of a list or lists of pain descriptors that are rank-ordered along a continuum of severity. Patients are asked to select the most appropriate descriptor or set of descriptors, and a score is assigned based on the rank(s) of the chosen word(s) (Jensen & Karoly, 1992). The McGill Pain Questionnaire (MPQ; Melzack, 1975a) is a well-validated, widely used VRS that consists of 20 lists of descriptors of the sensory,

affective, and evaluative dimensions of pain (Melzack, 1975b). The standard scoring procedure yields a Pain Rating Index (PRI) for each of the three subscales listed above, although in practice these subscales are often summed to create a single PRI. The PRI has been shown to be sensitive to change and valid for use among acute, cancer, and chronic populations (Davis, 1989; Lowe, Walker, & MacCallum, 1991; Sist, Florio, Miner, Lema, & Zevon, 1998). However, as is true of other verbal scales, it only yields ordinal level data as questions have been raised about the assumption of equidistance between ranked descriptors (Choiniere & Amsel, 1996). Additionally, support for the tripartite structure of the MPQ is mixed, and factor analyses generally reveal significant overlap between factors (Donaldson, 1995; Holroyd et al., 1992; Turk, Rudy, & Salovey, 1985).

Another verbal pain scale, often used in analgesic research, is a 0 to 3 categorical scale with 0 corresponding to "no pain," 1 to "mild pain," 2 to "moderate pain," and 3 to "severe pain." While there is evidence for the validity of this approach when used to differentiate between categories of pain intensity (Jensen & Karoly, 2001), this ranked-score approach often is treated as if it represented an interval scale where differences between any successive rankings are assumed to be equal. This may result in misleading estimates of changes in pain intensity and is therefore best reserved for use only as a descriptive scale.

Practical considerations suggest that the VAS or the NRS may be preferred to the MPQ or other verbal scales for the clinical assessment of pain intensity as they provide psychometrically superior data that are relatively easy to collect and score. When ease of administration and scoring are of greatest concern, the 11-point NRS may be the best choice. In contrast, when greater measurement precision is desirable, the advantage goes to the VAS or to the 101-point NRS.

Pain Interference

A central goal of pain intervention is to reduce the extent to which pain impairs physical activity, emotional functioning, and psychosocial role fulfillment. The term *pain interference* has been used to define this broad construct, which taps patients' perceptions of the degree to which pain disrupts physical and emotional functioning. Measures of pain interference should not be confused with instruments that simply quantify functional status without attempting to account for the role of pain in the reported impairment. This difference is illustrated by the contrast between the Sickness Impart Profile (SIP) psychosocial scale, which measures the extent of emotional and social difficulties that are attributed to the pain condition, and the Beck Depression Inventory (BDI; Beck, 1987), which assesses depressive symptomatology without concern for etiology.

The Pain Disability Index (PDI; Pollard, 1984) is a seven-item measure of pain interference in physical and psychosocial role performance. The PDI has good internal consistency ($\alpha = 0.87$; Tait et al., 1987) and 1-week test–retest reliability (intraclass $r = 0.91$; Gronblad et al., 1993), and it has been shown to effectively discriminate groups of pain patients with varying levels of disability (Tait, Chibnall, & Krause, 1990). The measure appears to be sensitive to change (Strong, Ashton, & Large, 1994), and it is valid for use with patients with chronic and postoperative pain (Pollard, 1984). Factor analysis supports the classification of the PDI as a unidimensional measure of pain interference (Tait et al., 1990). The PDI has practical appeal as a brief, easy-to-use, and psychometrically sound measure of general pain interference when less comprehensive assessment of pain-related disability is adequate.

The SIP is a widely used, 136-item measure of perceived impairment (Brown, 1995; Williams, 1988) with high test–retest reliability (0.92) and internal consistency (0.94; Bergner, Bobbitt, Carter, et al., 1981). The SIP administration instructions were altered by Turner and Clancy (1988) to reflect pain-related impairment rather than general physical impairment. The 14 SIP subscales assess pain interference across a wide range of functioning, and they are combined to form the physical, psychosocial, and total scales. The SIP scales have been found to possess good concurrent validity in patients with chronic pain and cancer pain (Beckham, Burker, Lytle, Feldman, & Costakis, 1997; Watson & Graydon, 1989), and they are sen-

sitive to change resulting from multidisciplinary inpatient treatment for chronic pain (Jensen, Strom, Turner, & Romano, 1992). From a practical standpoint, the main weaknesses of the SIP are its length and the relative difficulty of scoring the inventory. In addition, individuals with pain may find many SIP items to be less face valid and relevant to their condition than those of measures developed specifically to tap pain-related disability. Nevertheless, the SIP remains the "gold standard" for detailed assessment of self-reported pain interference.

The Oswestry Disability Questionnaire (ODQ) is a 10-item questionnaire assessing pain and pain-related limitations in daily activities (Fairbank, Couper, Davies, & O'Brien, 1980). Testees choose one of six response options for each item, and scores are summed across items. The ODQ has evidenced adequate stability (Davidson & Keating, 2002) and internal consistency (Hsieh, Phillips, Adams, & Pope, 1992), as well as discriminative validity (Leclaire, Blier, Fortin, & Proulx, 1997) and sensitivity to change (Davidson & Keating, 2002). ODQ item content suggests that it may be most useful for patients with more severe limitations or disability (Baker, Pynsent, & Fairbank, 1989).

Emotional Distress

Emotional distress is highly prevalent among individuals with pain, and it is a core feature of most chronic pain syndromes. Not only does emotional distress often exacerbate a pain condition, but it may also have a significant impact on treatment outcomes regardless of whether it is addressed clinically or not. Accordingly, treatment standards recognize the importance of incorporating the treatment of concurrent anxiety and depression into the intervention approach. Presented here are measures of emotional distress that, although not pain specific, are widely used in pain intervention outcomes assessment. These measures were selected based on their brevity, convenience, and general acceptance among pain researchers for outcomes assessment.

The BDI is a 21-item measure of depressive symptomatology (Beck, 1987). This widely used instrument has been shown to have adequate psychometric properties (Beck, Steer, & Garbin, 1988), and it is sensitive to change resulting from multidisciplinary pain clinic treatment (Kleinke, 1991). The BDI discriminates well between patients with chronic pain with and without depression (Geisser, Roth, & Robinson, 1997). However, researchers have raised questions about the appropriateness of using the BDI to detect depression among patients with pain (Williams & Richardson, 1993). Several BDI items contain somatic content (e.g., sleep disturbance, fatigability, and somatic preoccupation) that is confounded with commonly observed symptoms of chronic pain syndromes, and several studies have suggested that patients with pain may produce higher scores on these items as a function of their pain-related physical symptomatology (Plumb & Holland, 1977; Wesley, Gatchel, Gorofalo, & Polatin, 1999). While this may limit total score comparisons with nonpain populations, removal of the somatic items has not been found to improve the accuracy of the measure for discriminating depressed from nondepressed patients with chronic pain (Geisser et al., 1997). Consequently, clinicians may choose to use the BDI for treatment outcomes, although accurate classification of depressive symptomatology may require higher cutoffs.

An alternative measure of depression favored by some researchers for pain outcomes is the 20-item Center for Epidemiologic Studies Depression Scale (CES-D; Radloff, 1977). The CES-D has high internal reliability ($\alpha = 0.85$) in normal populations and good concurrent validity in chronic and cancer pain populations (Beckham et al., 1997; Radloff, 1977). The CES-D may be more sensitive to change than the BDI (Turk & Okifuji, 1994). Normed on a normal population, the CES-D suffers from many of the same limitations as the BDI, potentially producing a high number of false positives among patients with chronic pain and cancer pain. However, like the BDI, the CES-D has been shown to discriminate between patients with chronic pain with and without depression, and removal of somatic items did not appreciably improve accuracy (Geisser et al., 1997; Turk & Okifuji, 1994). Nonetheless, higher cutoffs should be used in pain populations.

The impact of anxiety on pain treatment outcome has not been studied as extensively as that of depression. However, the existing evidence suggests a high concordance between pain and anxiety (Polatin, Kinney, Gatchel, Lillo, & Mayer, 1993), and the need to address these symptoms in comprehensive pain intervention is well recognized. The State-Trait Anxiety Inventory (STAI) is a 40-item self-report inventory of state and trait anxiety that possesses adequate psychometric properties (Spielberger, 1983) and is widely used for pain outcomes measurement. The STAI is sensitive to change (Mongini, Defilippi, & Negro, 1997) and is an adequate choice for the clinician wishing to quantify levels of both acute anxiety and the more stable tendency to perceive one's environment as threatening.

Pain-Related Fear

Recently, researchers have begun to focus on the role of pain-specific emotional distress in the experience of pain. Emerging data indicate that pain-specific emotional distress, particularly pain-related fear, may play a more important role than general levels of affective disturbance in the development and maintenance of pain-related physical disability (McCracken, Faber, & Janeck, 1998). The construct of pain-related fear may be defined broadly as the fear of pain and the avoidance of behaviors that are anticipated to produce painful sensation or injury.

Although no evidence currently exists linking levels of pain-related fear to treatment outcome, the available data suggest that pain-related fear may seriously compromise an individual's willingness to initiate and persist in the degree of physical reactivation and restoration that is essential to reversing the progression of pain-related disability. Accordingly, clinicians and researchers are beginning to pay more attention to the role of pain-related fear in pain treatment outcome.

Of the few available measures of pain-related fear, the Pain Anxiety Symptoms Scale (PASS; McCracken, Zayfert, & Gross, 1992) and the Tampa Scale (TS; Kori, Miller, & Todd, 1990) are the most promising. The PASS is the longer of the two measures, with 40 items assessing cognitive and pain-related physiological anxiety symptoms, escape and avoidance responses, and fearful appraisal of pain (McCracken et al., 1992). The four PASS subscales have good internal consistency (McCracken, Zayfert, & Gross, 1993), and the total score has good predictive validity and appears to be adequate for outcomes assessment (McCracken et al., 1998). Scores on the PASS have been found to predict self-reported pain severity, disability, pain behavior, and range of motion on straight leg raise (McCracken, Gross, Aikens, & Carnrike, 1996; McCracken, Gross, Sorg, & Edmands, 1993). In addition, pain patients classified as "dysfunctional" by the Multidimensional Pain Inventory (MPI; Kerns, Turk, & Rudy, 1985) were more likely to produce high scores on the PASS than those classified as "interpersonally distressed" or as "adaptive copers" (Asmundson, Norton, & Allerdings, 1997).

Perhaps a better measure of the pain-related anxiety is the TS, a 17-item instrument developed to assess kinesiophobia, or the fear of movement and activity due to concerns about injury or reinjury (Kori et al., 1990). Although limited, recent evidence suggests that the TS may possess greater predictive validity than the PASS and other measures of pain-related fear. The TS has been found to be a superior predictor of a range of pain symptoms and behaviors, even after controlling for known confounding factors such as pain intensity and duration, gender, and negative emotionality. For example, the TS was an incrementally valid predictor of self-reported disability and behavioral performance during a lifting task after controlling for pain onset, lower extremity radicular pain, and pain intensity, while the PASS was not (Crombez, Vlaeyen, Heuts, & Lysens, 1999). In addition, the TS has been found to be a superior predictor of disability as compared with pain intensity, biomedical signs and symptoms, and negative emotionality (Crombez et al., 1999; Vlaeyen et al., 1999). Although there are no data on the ability of either the TS or the PASS to capture treatment-related change, either measure may be appropriate. However, given its superior predictive validity and shorter length, the TS appears to be the instrument of choice for assessing treatment-induced changes in pain-related fear.

Activity Level

Individuals with pain conditions often exhibit a pattern of gradually declining physical activity. In many cases, activity is associated with the experience of discomfort or the potential for reinjury and, therefore, is generally avoided. The resulting deconditioning increases the probability that activity will be experienced as aversive or harmful. In this manner, inactivity is reinforced and becomes an entrenched behavioral pattern. Accordingly, physical reactivation is a central component of most multidisciplinary treatment approaches, and most outcomes batteries include a measure of activity level. Unfortunately, most measures of activity rely on patient self-report, which may be subject to considerable biases stemming from such factors as differences in self-perceived effort expenditure, secondary gain factors, or inaccuracy in retrospective reporting. In response to this measurement issue, some pain experts have begun to consider the potential utility of actigraphy as a means to capture treatment-related changes in physical activity. Currently, there are at least two commercially available actigraphs that promise to provide an objective measure of this important outcomes domain. Both devices are wrist-worn and provide an unobtrusive method of recording ongoing activity counts over a period of up to 30 days. While very little literature documenting the use of these devices for pain treatment outcomes currently exists, interest in the pain research community is growing and likely to produce support for this approach within the next few years.

Physical Capacities

In contrast to functional capacities, little empirical or theoretical attention has been devoted to consideration of the role of physical capacities in pain-related disability. However, the importance of this construct, which refers to an individual's theoretical peak physical capabilities, is evident in the focus of many treatment programs on improving physical status variables such as strength, endurance, and range of motion. Unfortunately, the lack of agreement between self-report and actual physical capacities (Clark, 1996; Deyo, 1988) has complicated outcomes measurement leading many pain practitioners and researchers to suggest that objective physical capacity measures may serve as better indicators of treatment-related changes in this domain. At present there are no "gold standard" objective outcomes measures of pain-related physical capacity, although a variety of methods have been employed in attempts to quantify changes in the physical abilities of individuals with pain. Standardization of assessment methods is lacking, and practitioner ratings of function remain very popular despite numerous studies demonstrating their poor reliability. Although there are a few commercial systems that may eventually provide adequate validation data, they are very expensive and time intensive, limiting their utility for clinical settings. The best-supported performance measures, which tend to be less resource intensive, are the dual inclinometer method of assessing changes in trunk range of motion (Engelberg, 1993; Keeley et al., 1986; Mayer, Kishino, Keeley, Mayer, & Mooney, 1985) and the use of hand dynameters to evaluate upper extremity strength (Mathiowetz, Rennells, & Donahoe, 1985; Mathiowetz, Weber, Volland, & Kashman, 1984). In settings where rapid assessment is necessary, current alternatives appear limited to goniometer measures or practitioner ratings until alternative approaches are developed and validated.

Employment Status

Employment status is a key functional outcomes variable that is commonly used to evaluate the global success of chronic noncancer pain treatment programs. In fact, many treatment outcomes guidelines, such as those promulgated by CARF (Rehabilitation Accreditation Commission, 2002), mandate the use of work status as an outcomes indicator. Similarly, changes in disability status may be an important measure of the overall clinical impact of the intervention approach. Unlike most other outcomes domains discussed here, standardized measures are not required to assess changes in employment status. Current employment and disability status can be collected as part of pre- and post-treatment interviews, most commonly as a categorical variable in which the participant is characterized as being employed full-time, part-time, or not at all. An alternative approach may be to quantify the extent to which a person was gainfully employed and at work during a given period of time. Also important are changes in disability status that affect an individual's eligibility for employment, coded categorically as having a claim pending or not. Finally, for retirees or persons already established as being disabled, an increase in avocational activities may be an appropriate measure of pain treatment success as measured by volunteer work, increases in household chores or activities around the home, initiation of hobbies, or other changes consistent with general productiveness.

Relationship Outcomes

Central to current biopsychosocial conceptualizations of pain is the role of interpersonal relationships, particularly those with immediate family members. Interpersonal relationships may promote the development and maintenance of chronic pain conditions, and family involvement in the treatment process has long been recognized as an important predictor of outcome. Current treatment standards call for active significant other participation in treatment through activities such as family education, shared goal setting, and compliance support. Measurement of the effectiveness of these intervention components will depend in part on the specific aspects of the social context that are addressed clinically. Although providers may want to include general measures of family functioning such as the Dyadic Adjustment Scale (Spanier, 1976), pain-specific and behaviorally focused measures may be most useful. One option is the Significant Others Response scale of the West Haven-Yale Multidimensional Pain Inventory (Kerns et al., 1985). Also important to assess may be satisfaction with sexual intimacy in the dyadic relationship. Unfortunately, there are few standardized measures of many aspects of relationship functioning (such as sexual intimacy) that are posited to have an impact on chronic pain disability, and therefore, providers must rely on nonspecific measures validated in other populations. Interested readers are referred to Jacob and Kerns (2001) for a comprehensive review of the available measures in this area.

Health Care Utilization

Individuals with chronic pain utilize health care resources at higher rates than those without pain (Gironda, Clark, Neugaard, & Nelson, 2004). From a patient-focused outcomes perspective, excessive use of health care resources may be conceptualized as reflecting sick role behavior, and therefore, utilization variables may serve as useful indices of functional status. Reduced reliance on provider intervention may indicate a reduction of symptomatology or a shift on the part of the patient to a more self-reliant proactive role in pain management. Patient-focused health care outcomes variables may range from simple counts of medical contacts for pain over a given period of time to quantification of the socioeconomic costs to the patient for the identified visits.

Patient Satisfaction

Satisfaction with treatment is a key outcome domain that may have significant implications for patient behavior and treatment success. Treatments that meet patients' expectations are more likely to facilitate a working therapeutic relationship and engender compliance (Aharony & Strasser, 1993; Carr-Hill, 1992). However, measurement of treatment satisfaction is hindered by widely varying conceptualization and by patients' difficulty in separating their satisfaction with pain management from their satisfaction with other aspects of care (e.g., relationships with the health care providers). One of the only treatment satisfaction measures to be developed specifically for use with patients with chronic pain is the Pain Treatment Satisfaction scale (PTS). This five-item scale, which consists of items from the National Pain Data Bank comprehensive outcomes measurement system (AAPM, 2000), is included in the post-treatment version of the Pain Outcomes Questionnaire (POQ) and can also be used as a

stand-alone measure. The PTS scale has been demonstrated to have good internal consistency ($\alpha = 0.83$ to 0.90) and good concurrent and predictive validity (Clark, Gironda, & Young, 2003). As such, the PTS offers an easy-to-administer, pain-specific, and effective alternative to the generic satisfaction measures commonly relied upon by pain providers.

Drug-Related Problems

A drug related problem (DRP) is any undesirable event that involves some aspect of the patient's drug therapy and has the potential to negatively affect outcome. DRPs may include not taking or receiving the needed drug, taking or receiving the wrong drug, taking or receiving too little or too much of the correct drug, or experiencing an adverse drug reaction including drug–drug or drug–food interactions. Unfortunately, there are no widely available tools or standards for monitoring of DRPs. Providers who are interested in tracking DRPs should develop a coding and recording system that captures the types of problems described above and can be incorporated into standard assessment and documentation practices. Aggregate counts of DRPs may be tracked over time to provide a measure of the safety of prescribing practices. A root cause analysis or similar technique should be employed to refine, correct, or discontinue provider practices if the number of DRPs exceeds a predetermined threshold for a given period of time. DRP thresholds should vary according to the severity of the associated consequences (e.g., a brief medication-induced hypertensive episode vs. a medication-related death).

Multidimensional Measures

The preceding discussion has focused on unidimensional instruments, each of which measures a single pain outcomes domain. Unidimensional pain outcomes instruments generally are readily available, inexpensive, and necessitate minimal administration training time. Additionally, they are an efficient means of collecting data when only a limited number of outcomes domains are to be assessed. However, to assess multidomain pain treatment outcomes using unidimensional measures, it is necessary to assemble a battery of individual instruments. Because instrument selection is likely to vary across settings, the idiosyncratic nature of these batteries often restricts or prevents comparisons between local outcomes data and community benchmarked data. In addition, some of these instruments are quite lengthy and may include items that are not directly relevant to pain. Thus, while unidimensional measures may be the most efficient means of collecting pain data for one or two selected pain outcomes domains, the use of many unidimensional measures to cover all key chronic pain outcomes domains may decrease the utility of the obtained data while increasing staff and patient burden. In response to the limitations associated with batteries of unidimensional instruments, a few *multidimensional* pain outcomes tools have been developed. Three of these are discussed below.

Brief Pain Inventory

The Brief Pain Inventory (BPI; Cleeland & Ryan, 1994) is a 32-item instrument developed to assess pain history, pain intensity, perceived recent response to medication/treatment, and pain interference. The BPI is well validated among patients with cancer and chronic disease (e.g., osteoarthritis) pain (Clark & Gironda, 2002), and it has been translated into several languages. Factor analytic studies consistently have revealed the two-factors of pain severity and pain interference in physical functioning across samples and language versions (Caraceni et al., 1996; Radbruch et al., 1999; Saxena, Mendoza, & Cleeland, 1999; Wang, Mendoza, Gao, & Cleeland, 1996). However, empirical data are limited mostly to cancer and chronic disease samples, and little is known about the sensitivity to change or psychometric properties of the instrument when used with chronic pain populations.

Multidimensional Pain Inventory

The MPI, formerly the West Haven-Yale Multidimensional Pain Inventory, is a popular pain measure that was developed to facilitate the comprehensive assessment of patients with chronic pain (Kerns et al., 1985). Designed to be used in conjunction with behavioral and psychophysiological measures, the 52 items comprise 12 subscales that are dispersed across three sections: (1) pain intensity, pain interference, dissatisfaction with current functioning, appraisal of support form others, perceived life control, and affective distress; (2) punishing, solicitous, and distracting responses from significant others to displays of pain behaviors; and (3) frequency of the performance of household chores, outdoor work, activities away from home, and social activities (Kerns et al., 1985). Kerns and colleagues (1985) showed that the 12 subscales possess good internal consistency (α = 0.70 to 0.90) and acceptable 2-week test–retest reliability (r = 0.62 to 0.91). Adequate levels of unique variance and concurrent validity have been demonstrated for most scales (Kerns et al., 1985). The MPI appears to be sensitive to change, but the utility of specific subscales may vary across levels of adaptation and functioning (Strategier, Chwalisz, Altmaier, Russell, & Lehmann, 1997).

In addition to the measurement of treatment outcomes, the MPI has been used to classify patients with chronic pain to identify major treatment needs. Cluster analyses have yielded a three-group typology of patients with chronic pain consisting of dysfunctional, interpersonally distressed, and adaptive copers or minimizers categories (Turk & Rudy, 1990). Clinicians may find this typology useful for purposes such as planning pain treatment or testing the effectiveness of different interventions or intervention components across MPI groups of patients.

Pain Outcomes Questionnaire

The POQ is a pain outcomes package consisting of intake, post-treatment, and follow-up questionnaires. The POQ, which was originally based on the National Pain Data Bank questionnaires (AAPM, 2000), was developed specifically to assess treatment outcomes and therefore encompasses the key domains of functioning for comprehensive outcomes measurement. The outcomes package allows the clinician to track changes in pain intensity, pain interference, emotional distress, activity impairment, pain-related fear, vocational functioning, treatment satisfaction, perceived improvement, and medical resource utilization from intake through follow-up, obviating the need to use more than one measure (Clark et al., 2003). The POQ contains six core subscales which assess pain intensity, pain-interference in activities of daily living (ADLs) and mobility, negative affect, vitality impairment, and pain-related fear. The subscales possess excellent generalizability (r = 0.78 to 0.93) and acceptable 7- to 14-day test–retest reliability (r = 0.63 to 0.89). In addition, the subscales have good convergent and discriminant validity, and they are sensitive to change. Finally, confirmatory factor analyses have verified the multidimensional structure of the subscales (Clark et al., 2003). A similar but less comprehensive outcomes tool is the Pain Outcomes Profile (AAPM, 2003), which is published by the American Academy of Pain Management. It contains all of the POQ core scale items but does not assess employment status, medical utilization, or treatment satisfaction.

Advantages and Disadvantages of Multidimensional Measures

Multidimensional pain outcomes measures have several advantages relative to unidimensional measures. Because these instruments were specifically designed for pain populations, they often contain fewer total items than combinations of corresponding unidimensional measures and tend to be better integrated. Additionally, as the instruments are uniform, results can be compared across treatment settings or geographic regions, which may assist in the eventual development of universal pain outcomes benchmarks. Disadvantages of the multidimensional measures are that they may be more difficult to obtain, may require additional administration or scoring training as well as more data entry and management time, are more costly in some cases, and may not cover all of the key chronic pain outcomes domains. Nevertheless, when assessing multiple domains of outcomes in clinical settings, multidimensional measures generally are more practical.

HEALTH CARE SYSTEM DOMAINS

The preceding discussion provides an overview of the key domains of *patient* functioning that may be incorporated into an outcomes assessment system. While patient-focused assessment is critical to selecting, delivering, and refining intervention practices that produce improved patient functioning, measurement of health care system outcomes domains also provides important indices of the utility and effectiveness of pain treatment. Also called process outcomes dimensions or "service delivery outcomes" (Clark & Gironda, 2002, p. 998), these domains are the focus of efforts to monitor and improve pain service delivery systems. Typically, health care system outcomes procedures are part of facility performance improvement and accreditation activities. Unlike most patient-focused domains, health care system outcomes are not tracked using standardized measures, but rather involve monitoring aspects of service delivery or patient documentation by reviewing medical and facility records. The following discussion outlines important domains of health care system outcomes, including pain care delivery, pain care costs, and staff competency.

Pain Care Delivery

Pain care delivery outcomes encompass a range of service provision variables including pain screening and assessment procedures, clinic waiting times, patient education, the occurrence of pain-related events, and treatment effectiveness.

Pain Screening and Assessment

The foundation of effective pain treatment is thorough and reliable assessment of pain. Unfortunately, despite JCAHO standards mandating that pain be assessed in all patients, routine pain assessment is not consistently practiced across general health care settings, an omission that often results in the undertreatment of pain (American Pain Society, 1999). Evaluation of pain assessment practices is only possible when the medical records fully document the completed assessment process. It is important to note that pain intensity scores alone do not constitute a comprehensive assessment. Pain assessment should include documentation of the effects of pain on a broad range of life functions (Clark et al., 2003). Measures of pain assessment compliance may simply be the percentage of cases that evidence appropriate pain assessment documentation.

Waiting Times

Prompt access to pain treatment is an implicit corollary of current pain treatment standards. Assessment of waiting time may assess the period between the following sets of events: clinic referral and first available appointment, scheduled clinic appointment time and the time the patient actually is seen, initiation of a pain medica-

tion order and the administration of the pain medication (inpatient setting), and the patient's pain medication request and the time the medication is dispensed (inpatient setting). In some settings at least a portion of these data will be available in computerized medical record systems. However, it is likely that most facilities will need to develop specific monitors to record the relevant waiting periods.

Patient Education

Active patient and family participation in the treatment process is perhaps most successfully promoted through education regarding the experience of pain and the importance of effective pain management. Accordingly, patient and family education is considered an essential component of successful pain management programs. As with other health care systems outcomes domains, documentation of patient education should be available in the medical record. Another strategy may be to survey patients and their families regarding the nature and extent of pain education that they received.

Pain-Related Adverse Events

A pain-related adverse event may be defined as any event associated with the pain experience that negatively affects or has the potential to negatively affect the patient's well-being or probability of benefiting from treatment. Examples of common pain-related adverse events include (1) falls that result in injury, reinjury, or the reinforcement of pain-related fear of activity and (2) misuse of an opioid analgesic. Once again, careful documentation of all occurrences of pain-related adverse events is essential to evaluate clinical practices. Systematic tracking of these adverse event episodes over time may facilitate the identification of risk factors that exist within the pain service delivery system.

Treatment Effectiveness

From a health care systems outcomes perspective, treatment effectiveness evaluation differs from the patient-focused approach presented above in that the unit of measurement is not the individual patient but rather the system of clinical service provision. Appropriate units of measurement may include a provider, a group of providers, a group of clinics, etc., while the common goal is to assess the general effectiveness of the defined clinical delivery system for a group of patients treated during a given period of time. This type of evaluation is at the heart of PI efforts and may be as simple as reporting aggregate data collected as a component of the patient-focused outcomes process. An example of this approach is the evaluation of treatment-related pain intensity changes for all patients treated in a multiprovider clinic during a three-month period.

Pain Care Costs

It is estimated that direct and indirect costs associated with chronic noncancer pain exceed $125 billion yearly (Okifuji, Turk, & Kalauokalani, 1999). As mentioned previously, in this environment of soaring health care expenditures, treatment practices that do not demonstrate cost-effectiveness will no longer be economically viable as third-party payers and policy makers shift limited resources to proven intervention strategies. In a general sense, cost-effectiveness is based on a comparison of the benefits derived from receiving pain management services in relation to costs associated with those services. Important but often neglected in this discussion is the issue of cost-offset, which refers to the delayed benefits of an intervention that can be operationalized as reductions in health care costs that are reasonably believed to be attributable to the pain treatment. To conduct a cost-effectiveness evaluation, a system for capturing health care utilization and patient benefits must be developed. Monetary values must be assigned to the various types of services and patient outcomes within each category to allow estimation of the relative economic impact of patient benefits and health care expenses. If a common criterion of success is defined (e.g., return to work), costs associated with a variety of interventions can be compared (see Straus, 2002, and Turk et al., 2002, for specific examples).

Staff Competency

Staff competency in pain treatments maximizes the probability of the appropriate selection and delivery of effective interventions and minimizes the likelihood of the occurrence of pain-related adverse events. Ongoing training and education in both general and discipline-specific pain management are essential to cultivating staff competency. Routine testing of staff following completion of education or training experiences may be used to demonstrate that team members possess a criterion level of pain knowledge relevant the patient population being served. An example of this approach can be found in the work of McCaffery and Pasero (1999) who have developed and validated a test of nurses' pain knowledge and attitudes. Alternatively, changes in pain treatment approaches following focused educational experiences may be used as measures of increased pain competency.

IMPLEMENTING AN OUTCOMES-DRIVEN MODEL OF PAIN CARE

The process of designing a pain outcomes methodology consists of a series of discrete steps and requires that factors relevant to the outcomes system development pro-

cess, such as those described above, be considered carefully. In the following we provide an outline of our suggested approach to this endeavor in the hope that it will assist the reader through this process.

IDENTIFY OUTCOMES OBJECTIVES

The first step in developing a pain outcomes measurement system consists of identifying the goals, objectives, and scope of the outcomes program.

- Identify the basis for establishing the pain outcomes strategy. It may be a new hospital policy, legal opinion, or accreditation standard. Familiarity with the underlying rationale may make it easier to enlist administrative and staff support.
- Determine whether the outcomes objectives primarily focus on pain treatment issues or on the efficiency of pain service delivery. This distinction will have important implications for the eventual selection of outcomes measures.
- Define the scope of the outcomes plan. Are all available pain treatments to be included, or will only selected treatments be monitored? Does the plan cover every type of pain (acute, cancer, and chronic), or is it limited to only one or two?
- Choose which types of service settings will be included. Is it limited to outpatient areas, inpatient units, or specialty pain clinics? Are all providers working in the defined areas participating, or only some?
- Decide whether the outcomes data collection will be ongoing or limited to a preselected time interval.

IDENTIFY ADMINISTRATIVE SUPPORTS AND LIMITATIONS

Without sufficient administrative support, efforts to develop a pain outcomes system will fail. Staff will resent the added responsibilities in the absence of increased staff or concrete rewards. Presumably the basis for developing the pain outcomes system (JCAHO standards, insurer recommendations) will enhance administrative interest in the effort.

- Meet with the appropriate administrative representative to discuss anticipated costs and needed resources, citing any relevant local policies, local or national regulations, professional practice guidelines, or local competitors' outcomes practices and marketing data.
- Define the administrative limits (funds, positions) that are operative.

- Negotiate an agreement regarding support for the necessary resources.

SELECT THE RELEVANT OUTCOMES DOMAINS

Decisions regarding which pain outcomes domains to include often involve compromises between available resources and outcomes objectives. Resources may be limited, and outcomes efforts may be too ambitious. Collecting data for outcomes domains that are not central to the outcomes program objectives is a waste of staff resources and patient time.

- Select the relevant outcomes domains according to the focus of the outcomes program (treatment effects or service delivery), type of pain population involved (acute, cancer, or chronic), and setting.
- Avoid adding outcomes domains that are not directly relevant to the outcomes objectives. Additional domains may be added later if objectives change.
- Review any applicable guidelines, standards, or policies to ensure that all needed domains are included.

SELECT OR DESIGN THE NEEDED OUTCOMES MEASURES

Selecting Patient Outcomes Measures

If the objectives of the outcomes program involve evaluating the effects of pain treatment, it is likely that suitable pain outcomes instruments will be available for use. This will avoid the difficulties associated with designing and validating a new instrument and will minimize delays in implementing the outcomes programs.

- Identify potential instruments that assess the outcomes domains of interest (Table 9.1 may be helpful when matching outcomes instruments to outcomes domains).
- Investigate the reported reliabilities and review the validation data available for the identified instruments.
- Review any available data concerning reading level requirements, and determine whether those requirements are consistent with the target population's reading abilities.
- Attend to instrument length, administration and scoring requirements, and costs so as to maximize value and minimize resource demands.
- Determine whether the instruments are available in other languages if this is desirable given the characteristics of the target population.
- Choose the instrument or battery of instruments to use based on the above information.

Designing Service Delivery Outcomes Measures

As indicated previously, service delivery outcomes measures generally are not available in the form of validated outcomes instruments. In fact, with the exception of generic customer satisfaction measures, pain service delivery measures typically need to be designed locally. Fortunately, these measures are relatively simplistic. Usually they involve tracking whether required pain documentation is present or whether designated pain services were provided in an efficient and timely fashion. Thus, designing appropriate service measures may involve no more than developing pain-specific chart review forms or simple customer feedback tools.

- Identify the specific service delivery outcomes questions of interest.
- Design the necessary outcomes tools (e.g., chart review forms, customer satisfaction surveys).
- If patient surveys or questionnaires are involved, evaluate item wording, specificity, and reading level to meet the target population's abilities.

DEVELOP PROCEDURES NEEDED FOR IMPLEMENTATION

Once the scope of the outcomes project has been defined and the outcomes measures have been selected, specific procedures for implementing the outcomes system must be developed.

- Determine how the pain patients targeted for the study will be identified.
- Identify the roles, responsibilities, and training needs of all involved staff.
- Develop a timeframe for implementing all aspects of the outcomes system.
- Decide on a sampling strategy (i.e., randomly sample from among all possible data sources or attempt to collect data from every source during the data collection phase) depending on the sample size desired and the projected timeframe.

DESIGN AND PREPARE THE OUTCOMES DATABASE

Preparation of the outcomes database prior to implementation of data collection requires the review of every outcomes item or measure as well as all data entry and organization issues. Often this process yields valuable information that may streamline data collection and data management procedures.

- Decide what database and data analysis tools will be used.
- Design the necessary records storage and retrieval tools and conduct a "dry run" of data entry to identify any data collection problems.

- Make certain that the confidentiality of any patient information is maintained by discarding identifying information or by using elaborate coding or encryption strategies.
- Develop a data analysis plan in advance of data collection efforts.

COLLECT THE OUTCOMES

- Provide training in outcomes measure administration and data collection routines to relevant staff.
- Test the data collection procedures using only a few patients (treatment outcomes project) or records (service delivery project) prior to full-scale implementation.
- Arrange for backup coverage for the individuals collecting the data in the event of unexpected absences.
- Periodically review the workflow and data collection procedures to identify and troubleshoot any problem areas.

ANALYZE, TREND, AND REPORT THE DATA

Unfortunately, it is common to find that elaborate outcomes data have been collected at significant expense but then have been virtually ignored! Outcomes data analysis and trending is the cornerstone of an effective outcomes program. Analysis involves more than "eyeballing" the data. Although the level of statistical analysis will vary depending on the objectives of the outcomes plan and the psychometric sophistication of the staff involved, at the very least, it will be necessary to statistically summarize the data in a way that directly addresses the outcomes questions of interest. Ongoing review of the results by key personnel is critical and is mandated by some regulatory or accrediting bodies.

- For an ongoing outcomes program, establish a timeframe for systematically reviewing and reporting on the obtained data (monthly, quarterly, semiannually, or annually).
- Develop a report "template" that provides summary data regarding the outcomes questions and use that same template for each reporting period in order to allow comparisons over time.
- If performance improvement actions are instituted prior to or during a data collection period, note the nature of the changes implemented, along with the date, in the database so that the effects of the changes can be evaluated.
- After each reporting period, review data from all prior periods in concert with the current

results in order to identify trends of change in the data.
- Provide each staff person involved in the project with copies of the analysis report and schedule a meeting after each data collection period for review and discussion of the data and any identified trends.
- Design and complete a brief version of the analysis report for distribution to key administrators to help maintain their support for the project.
- Use the obtained data to explore any additional outcomes questions or to investigate observed trends in the data.
- Implement treatment protocol changes based on the identified trends. Changes should be introduced sequentially in order to allow the effects of each change to be evaluated separately.
- Review the outcomes data following each change in treatment protocol and decide whether to accept or reject the change.

CONCLUSIONS

The assessment of treatment outcomes is a necessary component of health care delivery and a key indicator of the quality of care delivered. In past years, evaluations of the effectiveness of pain interventions typically were based on providers' queries regarding treatment-related changes collected at patients' follow-up visits. Today, as a result of the demands of regulatory, accreditation, and advisory bodies, this informal outcomes assessment process no longer suffices. Instead, the focus is turning to the systematic collection and analysis of reliable data using validated measures. Indeed, the recent development of JCAHO pain standards and the growing national interest in pain issues have already had a profound effect on outcomes assessment within the pain management field. Outcomes measures now have become a standard component of pain treatment practices both for an individual practitioner and for health care systems. Given today's trends, it appears as if the importance of consistently monitoring, analyzing, and documenting the effects of pain treatment will continue to increase.

In this chapter we have attempted to summarize and briefly explore some of the key issues related to pain outcomes measurement endeavors. We also discussed the rationale underlying the use of outcomes measures in health care settings, focusing on pain-related issues, and provided a brief review of instruments and methods used to assess pain outcomes focusing first on the consumer of services and second on the health care delivery system. Last, we offered a method for designing and implementing appropriate outcomes measures in clinical practice settings. In recognition of the wide variety of pain practitioner settings and outcomes objectives, we tried to maintain a generalist's approach to the topic. In this regard, we may have sacrificed precision to enhance utility. Nevertheless, it is our hope that the information we have provided will be of value to clinicians seeking to implement procedures to evaluate the effectiveness of their pain treatment interventions.

AUTHOR NOTE

This work was supported in part by the James A. Haley Veterans Affairs Hospital and the Department of Veterans' Affairs Rehabilitation Research & Development Grant O3283R awarded to the first author and Department of Veterans' Affairs Rehabilitation Research & Development Career Development Award/Eastern Paralyzed Veterans Association Scholar Award B2744V awarded to the second author. The views expressed herein are solely the authors' and do not represent those of the Department of Veterans Affairs, the University of South Florida, or the Eastern Paralyzed Veterans Association.

REFERENCES

Agency for Health Care Policy and Research. (1992). *Acute pain management: Operative or medical procedures and trauma. Clinical practice guideline* (No. 92-0032). Washington, DC: U.S. Department of Health and Human Services.

Agency for Health Care Policy and Research. (1994). *Clinical practice guideline for the management of cancer pain* (No. 94-0592). Washington, DC: U.S. Department of Health and Human Services.

Aharony, L., & Strasser, S. (1993). Patient satisfaction: What we know about and what we still need to explore. *Medical Care Review, 50*, 49–79.

American Academy of Pain Management. (2000). *The National Pain Data Bank — Department of Veterans Affairs version 2*. Sonora, CA: AAPM.

American Academy of Pain Management. (2001). *Pain program accreditation manual*. Sonora, CA: AAPM.

American Academy of Pain Management. (2003). *Pain outcomes profile*. Sonora, CA: AAPM.

American Pain Society. (1999). *Principles of analgesic use in the treatment of acute pain and cancer pain* (4th ed.). Glenview, IL: Author.

American Pain Society Quality of Care Committee. (1995). Quality improvement guidelines for the treatment of acute pain and cancer pain. *Journal of the American Medical Association, 274*, 1874–1880.

Asmundson, G. J. G., Norton, G. R., & Allerdings, M. D. (1997). Fear and avoidance in dysfunctional chronic back pain patients. *Pain, 69*, 231–236.

Baker, C. D., Pynsent, P. B., & Fairbank, J. C. T. (1989). The Oswestry Disability Index revisited: Its reliability, repeatability, and validity, and a comparison with the St. Thomas's Disability Index. In M. O. Roland & J. R. Jenner (Eds.). *Back pain: New approaches to education and rehabilitation* (pp. 174–186). Manchester, England: Manchester University Press.

Beck, A. T. (1987). *Beck Depression Inventory*. San Antonio, TX: The Psychological Corporation.

Beck, A. T., Steer, R. A., & Garbin, M. G. (1988). Psychometric properties of the Beck Depression Inventory: Twenty-five years of evaluation. *Clinical Psychology Review*, 77–100.

Beckham, J. C., Burker, E. J., Lytle, B. L., Feldman, M. E., & Costakis, M. J. (1997). Self-efficacy and adjustment in cancer patients: A preliminary report. *Behavior Medicine, 23*, 138–142.

Bergner, M. Bobbitt, R. A., Carter, W. B., & Gilson, B. S. (1981). The Sickness Impact Profile: Development and final revision of a health status measure. *Medical Care, 19*, 787–805.

Bradely, L. A., Haile, J. M., & Jaworski, T. M. (1992). Assessment of psychological status using interview and self-interview instruments. In D. C. Turk & R. Melzack (Eds.). *Handbook of pain assessment* (pp. 193–213). New York: Guilford Press.

Breivik, E. K., Bjornsson, G. A., & Skovlund, E. (2000). A comparison of pain rating scales by sampling from clinical trial data. *Clinical Journal of Pain, 16*, 22–28.

Brown, D. (1995). Quality assessment and improvement activities should be incorporated into our pain practices. *Pain Forum, 4*, 48–56.

Caraceni, A., Mendoza, T. R., Mencaglia, E., Baratella, C., Edwards, K., Forjaz, M. J., et al. (1996). A validation study of an Italian version of the Brief Pain Inventory (Breve Questionario per la Valutazione del Dolore). *Pain, 65*, 87–92.

CARF. (1999). The Rehabilitation Accreditation Commission, *2000 medical rehabilitation standards manual* (pp. 46–66). Tucson, AZ: CARF The Rehabilitation Commission.

Carr-Hill, R. A. (1992). The measurement of patient satisfaction. *Journal of Public Health Medicine, 14*, 236–249.

Choiniere, M., & Amsel, R. (1996). A visual analogue thermometer for measuring pain intensity. *Journal of Pain and Symptom Management, 11*, 299–311.

Clark, M. E. (1996). MMPI-2 Negative Treatment Indicators Content and Content Component Scales: Clinical correlates and outcome prediction for men with chronic pain. *Psychological Assessment, 8*, 32–38.

Clark, M. E., & Gironda, R. J. (2002). Practical utility of outcome measurement. In R. S. Weiner (Ed.), *Pain management: A practical guide for clinicians* (6th ed., pp. 995–1010). Boca Raton, FL: CRC Press.

Clark, M. E., Gironda, R. J., & Young, R. W. (2003). Development and validation of the Pain Outcomes Questionnaire-VA. *Journal of Rehabilitation Research and Development, 40*, 381–396.

Cleeland, C. S., & Ryan, K. M. (1994). Pain assessment: Global use of the Brief Pain Inventory. *Annals Academy of Medicine Singapore, 23*, 129–138.

Clinical Practice Working Group, Veterans Health Administration, Department of Veterans Affairs and Health Affairs, Department of Defense (2003). *Management of opioid therapy for chronic pain* (10Q-CGP/OT-03). Washington, DC: Office of Quality and Performance.

Crombez, G., Vlaeyen, J. W., Heuts, P. H., & Lysens, R. (1999). Pain-related fear is more disabling than pain itself: Evidence on the role of pain-related fear in chronic back pain disability. *Pain, 80*, 329–339.

Davidson, M., & Keating, J. L. (2002). A comparison of five low back disability questionnaires: Reliability and responsiveness. *Physical Therapy, 82*(1), 8–24.

Davis, G. C. (1989). The clinical assessment of chronic pain in rheumatic disease: Evaluating the use of two instruments. *Journal of Advanced Nursing, 14*, 397–402.

De Conno, F., Caraceni, A., Gamba, A., Mariani, L., Abbattista, A., Brunelli, C., et al. (1994). Pain measurement in cancer patients: A comparison of six methods. *Pain, 57*, 161–166.

Deyo, R. A. (1988). Measuring the functional status of patients with low back pain. *Archives of Physical Medicine Rehabilitation, 69*, 1044–1053.

Donaldson, G. W. (1995). The factorial structure and stability of the McGill Pain Questionnaire in patients experiencing oral mucositis following bone marrow transplantation. *Pain, 62*, 101–109.

Engelberg, A. (Ed.). (1993). *American Medical Association guide to the evaluation of permanent impairment* (3rd ed.). Chicago: American Medical Association.

Fairbank, J. C., Couper, J., Davies, J. B., & O'Brien, J. P. (1980). The Oswestry low back pain disability questionnaire. *Physiotherapy, 66*, 271–273.

Geisser, M. E., Roth, R. S., & Robinson, M. E. (1997). Assessing depression among persons with chronic pain using the Center for Epidemiological Studies-Depression Scale and the Beck Depression Inventory: A comparative analysis. *Clinical Journal of Pain, 13*, 163–170.

Gironda, R. J., Clark, M. E., Neugaard, B., & Nelson, A. (2004). Upper limb pain in a national sample of veterans with paraplegia. *Journal of Spinal Cord Medicine, 27*, 1–8.

Gordon, D. B., & Dahl, J. L. (2004). Quality improvement challenges in pain management. *Pain, 107*, 1–4.

Gordon, D. B., Pellino, T. A., Miaskowski, C., McNeill, J. A., Paice, J. A., Laferriere, D., et al. (2002). A 10-year review of quality improvement monitoring in pain management: Recommendations for standardized outcome measures. *Pain Management Nursing, 3*, 116–130.

Gronblad, M., Hupli, M., Wennerstrand, P., Jarvinen, E., Lukinmaa, A., Kouri, J. P., et al. (1993). Intercorrelation and test-retest reliability of the Pain Disability Index (PDI) and the Oswestry Disability Questionnaire (ODQ) and their correlation with pain intensity in low back pain patients. *Clinical Journal of Pain, 9*, 189–195.

Holroyd, K. A., Holm, J. E., Keefe, F. J., Turner, J. A., Bradley, L. A., Murphy, W. D., et al. (1992). A multi-center evaluation of the McGill Pain Questionnaire: Results from more than 1700 chronic pain patients. *Pain, 48*, 301–311.

Hsieh, C. Y., Phillips, R. B., Adams, A. H., & Pope, M. H. (1992). Functional outcomes of low back pain: Comparison of four treatment groups in a randomized controlled trial. *Journal of Manipulative Physiological Therapy, 15*(1), 4–9.

Hutten, M. M., Hermens, H. J., & Zilvold, G. (2001). Differences in treatment outcome between subgroups of patients with chronic low back pain using lumbar dynamometry and psychological aspects. *Clinical Rehabilitation, 15*(5), 479–488.

Jacob, M., & Kerns, R. D. (2001). Assessment of the psychosocial context of the experience of chronic pain. In D. C. Turk & R. Melzack (Eds.), *Handbook of pain assessment* (2nd ed., pp. 362–384). New York: Guilford Press.

Jensen, I. B., & Linton, S. J. (1993). Coping Strategies Questionnaire (CSQ): Reliability of the Swedish version of the CSQ. *Scandinavian Journal of Behaviour Therapy, 22*, 139–145.

Jensen, M. P., & Karoly, P. (1992). Self-report scales and procedures for assessing pain in adults. In D. C. Turk & R. Melzack (Eds.), *Handbook of pain assessment* (pp. 135–151). New York: Guilford Press.

Jensen, M. P., & Karoly, P. (2001). Self-report scales and procedures for assessing pain in adults. D. C. Turk & R. Melzack (Eds.), *Handbook of pain assessment* (2nd ed., pp. 15–34). New York: Guilford Press.

Jensen, M. P., Strom, S. E., Turner, J. A., & Romano, J. M. (1992). Validity of the Sickness Impact Profile Roland scale as a measure of dysfunction in chronic pain patients. *Pain, 50*, 157–162.

Jensen, M. P., Turner, J. A., & Romano, J. M. (1992). Chronic pain coping measures: Individual vs. composite scores. *Pain, 51*, 273–280.

Jensen, M. P., Turner, J. A., Romano, J. M., & Fisher, L. D. (1999). Comparative reliability and validity of chronic pain intensity measures. *Pain, 83*, 157–162.

Jensen, M. P., Turner, L. R., Turner, J. A., & Romano, J. M. (1996). The use of multiple-item scales for pain intensity measurement in chronic pain patients. *Pain, 67*, 35–40.

Joint Commission on Accreditation of Healthcare Organizations. (2001). *Comprehensive hospital accreditation manual.* Oakbrook Terrace, IL: Author.

Joint Commission on Accreditation of Healthcare Organizations. (2003). *Improving the quality of pain management through measurement and action.* Oakbrook Terrace, IL: Author.

Keeley, J., Mayer, T. G., Cox, R., Gatchel, R. J., Smith, J., & Mooney, V. (1986). Quantification of lumbar function. Part 5: Reliability of range-of-motion measures in the sagittal plane and an *in vivo* torso rotation measurement technique. *Spine, 11*(1), 31–35.

Kerns, R. D., Turk, D. C., & Rudy, T. E. (1985). The West Haven-Yale Multidimensional Pain Inventory (WHYMPI). *Pain, 23*, 345–356.

Kleinke, C. L. (1991). How chronic pain patients cope with depression: Relation to treatment outcome in a multidisciplinary pain clinic. *Rehabilitation Psychology, 36*, 207–218.

Kori, S. H., Miller, R. P., & Todd, D. D. (1990). Kinesiophobia: A new view of chronic pain behavior. *Pain Management, 3*, 35–43.

Lande, S. D., & Loeser, J. D. (2001). The future of pain management in managed care. *Managed Care Interface, 14*, 69–75.

Leclaire, R., Blier, F., Fortin, L., & Proulx, R. (1997). A cross-sectional study comparing the Oswestry and Roland-Morris Functional Disability scales in two populations of patients with low back pain of different levels of severity. *Spine, 22*(1), 68–71.

Lowe, N. K., Walker, S. N., & MacCallum, R. C. (1991). Confirming the theoretical structure of the McGill Pain Questionnaire in acute clinical pain. *Pain, 46*, 53–60.

Mathiowetz, V., Rennells, C., & Donahoe, L. (1985). Effect of elbow position on grip and key pinch strength. *Journal of Hand Surgery* [America], *10*, 694–697.

Mathiowetz, V., Weber, K., Volland, G., & Kashman, N. (1984). Reliability and validity of grip and pinch strength evaluations. *Journal of Hand Surgery* [America], *9*, 222–226.

Mayer, T., Kishino, N., Keeley, J., Mayer, S., & Mooney, V. (1985). Using physical measurements to assess low back pain. *Journal of Musculoskeletal Medicine, 2*, 44–59.

McCaffery, M., & Pasero, C. (1999). *Pain: Clinical manual* (2nd ed.). St. Louis, MO: Mosby.

McCracken, L. M., Faber, S. D., & Janeck, A. S. (1998). Pain-related anxiety predicts non-specific physical complaints in persons with chronic pain. *Behaviour Research and Therapy, 36*, 621–630.

McCracken, L. M., Gross, R. T., Aikens, J., & Carnrike, C. L. M., Jr. (1996). The assessment of anxiety and fear in persons with chronic pain: A comparison of instruments. *Behaviour Research and Therapy, 34*, 927–933.

McCracken, L. M., Gross, R. T., Sorg, P. J., & Edmands, T. A. (1993). Prediction of pain in patients with chronic low back pain: Effects of inaccurate prediction and pain-related anxiety. *Behaviour Research and Therapy, 31*, 647–652.

McCracken, L. M., Zayfert, C., & Gross, R. T. (1992). The Pain Anxiety Symptoms Scale: Development and validation of a scale to measure fear of pain. *Pain, 50*, 67–73.

McCracken, L. M., Zayfert, C., & Gross, R. T. (1993). The Pain Anxiety Symptom Scale (PASS): A multimodal measure for pain specific anxiety symptoms. *Behavior Therapist, 16*, 183–184.

Melzack, R. (1975a). The McGill Pain Questionnaire. In R. Melzack (Ed.), *Pain measurement and assessment* (pp. 41–47). New York: Raven Press.

Melzack, R. (1975b). The McGill Pain Questionnaire: Major properties and scoring methods. *Pain, 1*, 277–299.

Mongini, F., Defilippi, N., & Negro, C. (1997). Chronic daily headache. A clinical and psychological profile before and after treatment. *Headache, 37*, 83–87.

Ogon, M., Krismer, M., Soellner, W., Kantner-Rumplmair, W., & Lampe, A. (1996). Chronic low back pain measurement with visual analogue scales in different settings. *Pain, 64*, 425–428.

Okifuji, A., Turk, D. C., & Kalauokalani, D. (1999). Clinical outcome and economic evaluation of multidisciplinary pain centers. In A. R. Block, E. F. Kremer, & E. Fernandez (Eds.), *Handbook of pain syndromes: Biopsychosocial perspectives* (pp. 77–98). Mahwah, NJ: Lawrence Erlbaum.

Paice, J. A., & Cohen, F. L. (1997). Validity of a verbally administered numeric rating scale to measure cancer pain intensity. *Cancer Nursing, 20*(2), 88–93.

Pain and Policies Study Group, University of Wisconsin Comprehensive Cancer Center (n.d.) Retrieved March 20, 2004, from http://www.medsch.wisc.edu/painpolicy/.

Plumb, M., & Holland, J. (1977). Comparative studies of psychological function in patients with advanced cancer. I: Self-reported depressive symptoms. *Psychosomatic Medicine, 39*, 264–276.

Polatin, P. B., Kinney, R. K., Gatchel, R. J., Lillo, E., & Mayer, T. G. (1993). Psychiatric illness and chronic low-back pain. The mind and the spine — Which goes first? *Spine, 18*(1), 66–71.

Pollard, C. A. (1984). Preliminary validity study of the pain disability index. *Perceptual and Motor Skills, 59*, 974.

Radbruch, L., Loick, G., Kiencke, P., Lindena, G., Sabatowski, R., Grond, S., et al. (1999). Validation of the German version of the Brief Pain Inventory. *Journal of Pain Symptom Management, 18*(3), 180–187.

Radloff, L. S. (1977). The CES-D Scale: A self-report depression scale for research in the general population. *Applied Psychological Measurement, 1*, 385–401.

Rehabilitation Accreditation Commission. (2002). *Standards manual: Medical rehabilitation* (rev. ed.). Tucson, AZ: Author.

Rosensteil, A. K., & Keefe, F. J. (1983). The use of coping strategies in chronic low back pain patients: Relationship to patient characteristics and current adjustment. *Pain, 17*, 33–44.

Saxena, A., Mendoza, T., & Cleeland, C. S. (1999). The assessment of cancer pain in north India: The validation of the Hindi Brief Pain Inventory — BPI-H. *Journal of Pain and Symptom Management, 17*(1), 27–41.

Sist, T. C., Florio, G. A., Miner, M. F., Lema, M. J., & Zevon, M. A. (1998). The relationship between depression and pain language in cancer and chronic non-cancer pain patients. *Journal of Pain and Symptom Management, 15*, 350–358.

Spanier, G. B. (1976). Measuring dyadic adjustment: New scales for assessing the quality of marriage and similar dyads. *Journal of Marriage and the Family, 38*, 15–28.

Spielberger, C. D. (1983). Manual for the State–Trait Anxiety Inventory (STAI). Palo Alto, CA: Consulting Psychologists Press.

Strategier, L. D., Chwalisz, K., Altmaier, E. M., Russell, D. W., & Lehmann, T. R. (1997). Multidimensional assessment of chronic low back pain: Predicting treatment outcomes. *Journal of Clinical Psychology in Medical Settings, 4*, 91–110.

Stratford, P. W., Binkley, J. M., Riddle, D. L., & Guyatt, G. H. (1998). Sensitivity to change of the Roland-Morris Back Pain Questionnaire: Part 1. *Physical Therapy, 78*, 1186–1196.

Straus, B. N. (2002). Chronic pain of spinal origin: The costs of intervention. *Spine, 27*(22), 2614–2619.

Strong, J., Ashton, R., & Large, R. G. (1994). Function and the patient with chronic low back pain. *Clinical Journal of Pain, 10*(3), 191–196.

Tait, R. C., Chibnall, J. T., & Krause, S. (1990). The Pain Disability Index: Psychometric properties. *Pain, 40,* 171–182.

Tait, R. C., Pollard, C. A., Margolis, R. B., Duckro, P. N., & Krause, S. J. (1987). The Pain Disability Index: Psychometric and validity data. *Archives of Physical Medicine and Rehabilitation, 68,* 438–441.

Turk, D. C., & Flor, H. (1999). Chronic pain: A biobehavioral perspective. In R. J. Gatchel, & D. C. Turk (Eds.), *Psychosocial factors in pain: Critical perspectives* (pp. 18–34). New York: Guilford Press.

Turk, D. C., & Okifuji, A. (1994). Detecting depression in chronic pain patients: Adequacy of self-reports. *Behaviour Research and Therapy, 32,* 9–16.

Turk, D. C., & Rudy, T. E. (1990). The robustness of an empirically derived taxonomy of chronic pain patients. *Pain, 43,* 27–35.

Turk, D. C., Loeser, J. D., & Monarch, E. S. (2002). Chronic pain: Purposes and costs of interdisciplinary pain rehabilitation programs. *The Economics of Neuroscience, 4,* 64–69.

Turk, D. C., Rudy, T. E., & Salovey, P. (1985). The McGill Pain Questionnaire reconsidered: Confirming the factor structure and examining appropriate uses. *Pain, 21,* 385–397.

Turner, J. A. &. Clancy, C. S. (1988). Comparison of operant behavioral and cognitive-behavioral group treatment for chronic low back pain. *Journal of Clinical and Consulting Psychology, 56,* 261–266.

Vlaeyen, J. W., Seelen, H. A., Peters, M., de Jong, P., Aretz, E., Beisiegel, E., et al. (1999). Fear of movement/(re)injury and muscular reactivity in chronic low back pain patients: An experimental investigation. *Pain, 82,* 297–304.

Wang, X. S., Mendoza, T. R., Gao, S. Z., & Cleeland, C. S. (1996). The Chinese version of the Brief Pain Inventory (BPI-C): Its development and use in a study of cancer pain. *Pain, 67,* 407–416.

Watson, J. H., & Graydon, J. E. (1989). Sickness Impact Profile: A measure of dysfunction with chronic pain patients. *Journal of Pain and Symptom Management, 4,* 152–156.

Wesley, A. L., Gatchel, R. J., Gorofalo, J. P., & Polatin, P. B. (1999). Toward more accurate use of the Beck Depression Inventory with chronic back pain patients. *Clinical Journal of Pain, 15,* 117–121.

Williams, A. C., & Richardson, P. H. (1993). What does the BDI measure in chronic pain? *Pain, 55,* 259–266.

Williams, R. C. (1988). Toward a set of reliable and valid measures for chronic pain assessment and outcome research. *Pain, 35,* 239–251.

10

Chronic Pain and Addiction

David A. Fishbain, MD, FAPA

INTRODUCTION

There are a number of reasons pain clinicians have been historically interested in the area of addiction. At first, chronic pain clinicians had the clinical impression that pain treatment outcome was influenced by addiction issues (Fishbain et al., 1992b). As such, the mantra in the 1980s and the early 1990s was that chronic pain patients (CPPs) should be detoxified from opioids and that placement on opioids leads to addiction. This position radically changed in the late 1980s when publications began to appear claiming success in treating intractable CPPs with chronic opioid analgesic treatment (COAT) without the development of significant addiction (Portenoy, 1989; Portenoy & Foley, 1986). The COAT literature has increased and now contains a significant number of randomized controlled trials. They have recently been the subjects of a meta-analysis (Graven et al., 2000). Findings of this meta-analysis were that patients with nociceptive and neuropathic chronic pain may benefit from COAT, while this positive effect was less clear for patients with chronic idiopathic pain. Thus, because of the clinical interest in COAT as a way of helping intractable CPPs, addiction has become a hot topic within the pain literature.

This interest in COAT and the associated addiction issue has also been influenced by a number of other developments, which have occurred at the same time. First, a significant literature developed that spoke to the chronic undertreatment of pain by health care professionals (Bendtsen et al., 1999). Second, research studies reported that some physicians were prejudiced against the use of opioids (opiophobia) because of fears of iatrogenic addiction (Bendtsen et al., 1999; Weinstein et al, 2000). Third, in the late 1990s, because of the chronic undertreatment

of pain, state licensing boards began to develop policies that supported appropriate opioid prescribing rather than policies that hindered opioid prescribing. Fourth, in the early 2000s, Joint Commission on Accreditation of Health Organizations (JCAHO) incorporated the adequate treatment of pain as a patient right. Fifth, in the early 1990s, drug technology developed a number of controlled-release opioids, which were touted as controlling pain in a more effective manner than the immediate-acting opioids.

At the present time, COAT is mired in controversy. Clinicians who do not accept the current evidence for COAT efficacy still use the addiction issue as an argument against COAT. At the same time, clinicians who use COAT note that there appear to be addiction difficulties with some patients. Thus, at the present time, the issue of addiction is of intense interest to the pain clinician.

As the reader is aware, there are numerous books on the subject of addiction and its treatment. As such, the purpose of this chapter is not to review this literature, but to familiarize the pain clinician with addiction problems and issues that would be relevant to his or her pain practice. Thus, this chapter reviews the most recent research in reference to the following: substance abuse terminology definitions, identification of psychoactive substance use–related disorders or addiction, prevalence of addiction within CPPs, methods for diagnosing addiction in CPPs, risk of addiction in CPPs on opioid exposure, risk of re-addiction in addicts with chronic pain on opioid exposure, diversion, aberrant drug-taking behaviors as indicators of addiction, pseudo-addiction, psychiatric comorbidities in CPPs with addiction, use of short-acting opioids versus long-acting opioids for COAT, opioid treatment agreements, opioids and driving, legal issues in addiction and chronic pain, and opioid detoxification methods in addicts and non-addicts. As can be seen, this chapter deals mainly with opioids and addresses other drugs of abuse, such as cocaine and cannabinoids, only peripherally. The reader is referred to addiction textbooks for in-depth discussion of the addiction issues relating to these drugs.

SUBSTANCE ABUSE TERMINOLOGY DEFINITIONS

Unfortunately, before we proceed to the addiction research relevant to chronic pain treatment, we need to address a major problem that has served as a confounder to much of this work. This is the confusion over substance abuse terminology (Fishbain et al., 1992b). Historically, there was little agreement between researchers on terms such as drug abuse, psychological dependence, drug dependence, and drug addiction (Rinaldi et al., 1988). Addiction initially meant a habit; however, in 1957 the World Health Organization (WHO) defined addiction as follows: a state or period of chronic intoxication characterized by (1) an overpowering desire or need or compulsion to continue taking the drug and to obtain it by any means; (2) tendency to increase dose; (3) a psychic (psychological) and generally physical dependence on the effects of the drug; and (4) detrimental effect on the individual and/or society (Fishbain et al., 1992b).

Because it was noted that some individuals could be physically dependent on a drug without compulsive use, and vice versa, the WHO then decided to use "dependence" as its crucial variable. Therefore, in 1964 the WHO defined drug dependence as "a state of psychic or physical dependence, or both, on a drug arising in a person following administration of that drug on a periodic or continuous basis." Around that time Rinaldi et al. (1988) performed a four-state Delphi survey of substance abuse experts to "achieve greater clarity and uniformity" for substance abuse definitions. These experts reached the consensus on 50 substance abuse terms. Seven definitions important to this article are taken from this list and presented in Table 10.3: Drug abuse, tolerance, physical dependence, psychological dependence, drug addiction, drug dependence, and drug withdrawal syndrome. It is to be noted that in the definition of drug addiction (Table 10.3), compulsive drug use is a central concept agreed upon by the experts. In addition, the following important concepts are to be noted in reference to the seven definitions in Table 10.3: they are distinct concepts in themselves and they should not be used interchangeably, physical and psychological dependence are encompassed within drug dependence, psychological dependence is distinct from tolerance and physical dependence, and tolerance and physical dependence develop on parallel time courses, but the rate of development of tolerance varies greatly between individuals (Rinaldi et al., 1988).

Psychological dependence is a behavior pattern characterized by continued craving for the substance and does not occur in every patient exposed to the substance. Compulsive drug-seeking behavior leading to overwhelming involvement in drug use and obtaining drugs is a manifestation of this craving. It is interesting to note that in some individuals compulsive drug-seeking behavior can occur before true physical dependence develops (Portenoy, 1989). These other points also apply to the interrelationship between these various concepts: one can be physically dependent without being drug addicted; one can be drug addicted without being physically dependent or drug tolerant; those who are drug addicted are likely to be physically dependent; not all drugs produce physical dependence, psychological dependence, and tolerance, with some drugs producing one manifestation only; and drug-addicted patients who are physically dependent are usually drug tolerant (Ludwig, 1980). Newman (1983) has therefore proposed that addiction needs to be redefined. He has concluded that narcotic addiction can be viewed as an "atypical response to exposure to opioids characterized by a tendency toward progressively greater consumption of the drug and a persistent disposition to relapse to drug use when abstinence has been achieved and physical dependence reversed." He then defined addiction as an "atypical behavioral pattern of drug use characterized by overwhelming involvement with the use of the drug (compulsive use), the securing of its supply, tendency toward progressive drug intake (loss of control) and the high tendency to relapse after drug withdrawal, and reversal of physical dependence."

The American Psychiatric Association (2000) incorporates some of these concepts into its diagnosis of substance dependence (Table 10.1). Unfortunately, there is difficulty in applying these criteria to CPPs for a diagnosis of addiction. For example, of seven criteria (of which three are required to fulfill this diagnosis), one relates to tolerance (criterion 1) and one to withdrawal (criterion 2). If patients with chronic pain are on significant opioids, they are invariably tolerant to opioids and manifest withdrawal when removed from opioids. Thus, these two criteria could lead to over-inclusiveness for this diagnosis in CPPs. In addition, criteria 3 and 4 (Table 10.1) can simply relate to the need to control pain. Thus, four of seven criteria may lead to over-inclusiveness in the application of this diagnosis to the patient with chronic pain.

Because of this confusion over the addiction concept and difficulties with its diagnostic application in CPPs, the American Academy of Pain Medicine, the American Pain Society, and the American Society for Addiction Medicine approved the following definition for addiction (American Academy of Pain Medicine, 2001). "Addiction is a primary, chronic, neurobiologic disease with genetic, psychosocial, and environmental factors influencing its development and manifestations. It is characterized by behaviors that include

TABLE 10.1
Criteria for a Diagnosis of Substance Dependence (DSM-IV)

Substance Dependence

A maladaptive pattern of substance use, leading to clinically significant impairment or distress, as manifested by the occurrence of three (or more) of the following during the same 12-month period:

1. Tolerance, as defined by either of the following:
   a. A need for markedly increased amounts of a substance to achieve intoxication or a desired effect
   b. Markedly diminished effect with continued use of the same amount of a substance
2. Withdrawal, as manifested by either of the following:
   a. Symptoms characteristic of withdrawal from a substance
   b. The ability to take a substance or one closely related to it, to relieve or avoid withdrawal symptoms
3. A need to take a substance in larger amounts or over a longer period than intended
4. A persistent desire to take a substance in larger amounts or over a longer period than intended
5. A great deal of time spent in activities necessary to obtain a substance (e.g., visits to multiple doctors or driving long distances), to use a substance (e.g., chain-smoking), or to recover from its effects
6. Abandonment of or absence from important social, occupational, or recreational activities because of substance use
7. Continued substance use despite knowledge of having a persistent or recurrent physical or psychological problem that is likely to have been caused or exacerbated by the substance (e.g., continued cocaine use despite recognition of cocaine-induced depression or continued drinking despite recognition that an ulcer is made worse by alcohol consumption)

Source: Adapted from American Psychiatric Association (2000).

one or more of the following: impaired control over drug use, compulsive use, continued use despite harm, and craving." No diagnostic criteria, however, were proposed. As such, the pain clinician has the option of diagnosing addiction, using the *Diagnostic and Statistical Manual of Mental Disorders* (DSM-IV) criteria (Table 10.1), keeping in mind the criteria confounders described above, or using the above American Pain Society definition. This definition is defined by five Cs: *chronicity,* impaired *control, compulsive* use, *continued* use despite harm, and *craving.* Of these, chronicity, impaired control, and continued use despite harm could also be a manifestation of seeking pain relief. As such, this definition does not shed light on the issue of the difficulty of making an addiction diagnosis in the context of chronic pain. Support for the above comes from a recent study (Elander et al., 2003) with patients with sickle cell disease. Here researchers assessed DSM-IV symptoms of substance dependence and abuse and applied the DSM-IV criteria to differentiate between pain-related symptoms and nonpain-related symptoms. Pain-related symptoms were more fre-

quent, accounting for 88% of all symptoms reported. When pain-related symptoms were included in arriving at a diagnosis, 31% of the sample met DSM-IV criteria for substance dependence versus only 2% when only the nonpain-related symptoms were used to meet criteria.

IDENTIFICATION OF PSYCHOACTIVE SUBSTANCE USE–RELATED DISORDERS OR ADDICTION IN CPPs

Because of the above discussion, the identification of addiction is a complex problem. Complicating this problem is the fact that some patients inaccurately report the use of prescribed medications or fail to report the use of nonprescribed medications or medication prescribed by other physicians, or fail to report the use of illicit drugs (Berndt et al., 1993; Fishbain et al., 1998a; Katz & Fanciullo, 2002). Thus, the use of external sources of information can be helpful. This can include an interview with the spouse, a review of medical records, and the input of prescription monitoring programs. In addition, testing of biological materials (urine) can be extremely helpful. This will be dealt with in its own section below. Because of the problem of inaccurate patient reports, the detection of addiction begins with a high index of suspicion, first trying to identify addiction risk factors (Table 10.2) and then

TABLE 10.2
Addiction Risk Factors

- Biological parent who abuses drugs
- Biological parent who has an antisocial personality
- Lower socioeconomic status
- Child of a divorce home and/or single-parent home
- Behavioral problems as a child
- Comorbid depression, alcohol abuse, antisocial personality disorder, anxiety disorder
- Current dysfunctional or enabling family system (drug abuse in a family)
- Regular contact with high risk people (drug-using friends) or involvement with high-risk activities (regular time spent in a bar)
- Smoking
- Gambling
- Impulsivity
- Multiple physical traumas
- Behaviors with compulsive, addictive quality
- High neuroticism, high extraversion
- Antisocial behaviors (arrests, fighting, early drunkenness, truancy, difficulty with school)
- Use of illicit drugs
- Belief of needing some substance to feel "normal"
- Positive response if asked if use of drugs/alcohol contributed to a problem for them

Source: Adapted from Nedejkovic, Wasan, & Jamison (2002); Robinson, Gatchel, Polatin et al. (2001).

TABLE 10.3
Substance Abuse Terminology Definitions

Term	Definition
(Drug) addiction	A chronic disorder characterized by the compulsive use of a substance resulting in physical, psychological, or social harm to the user and continued use despite that harm
(Drug) dependence	A generic term that relates to physical or psychological dependence, or both; it is characteristic for each pharmacological class of psychoactive drugs; impaired control over drug-taking behavior is implied
Drug abuse	Any use of drugs that causes physical, psychological, economic, legal, or social harm to the individual user or to others affected by the drug user's behavior
Physical dependence	A physiological state of adaptation to a drug or alcohol, usually characterized by the development of tolerance to drug effects and the emergence of a withdrawal syndrome during prolonged abstinence
Psychological dependence	The emotional state of craving a drug either for its positive effect or to avoid negative effects associated with its absence
Tolerance	Physiological adaptation to the effect of drugs, so as to diminish effects with constant dosages or to maintain the intensity and duration of effects through increased dosage
Drug withdrawal syndrome	The onset of a predictable constellation of signs and symptoms involving altered activity of the central nervous system after the abrupt discontinuation of or rapid decrease in dosage of a drug

Source: Adapted from Rinaldi, R. C. et al., 1988

TABLE 10.4
Suggestive Behavioral Patterns for Suspicion for Drug Abuse

- Cigarette smoking
- Absenteeism
- Marital discord
- Driving problems
- Financial difficulties
- Suicide attempt history
- Child abuse history
- Use of stimulants
- Frequent accidents and falls
- Blackouts
- Memory loss

TABLE 10.5
Suggestive Physical Findings for Suspicion for Drug Abuse

- Evidence of current intoxication (sleepiness, nodding)
- Spider angiomata
- Hepatomegaly
- Red facies
- Liver palms
- Salivary gland enlargement
- Cigarette burns
- Unexplained bruises/frequent falls
- Diabetes/blood pressure/ulcers not responsive to treatment
- Inflamed/eroded nasal septum
- Dilated pupils
- Track marks/injection sites
- Gunshot/knife wounds
- Poor hygiene
- Nutritional deficits
- Frequent hospitalizations
- Alcohol withdrawal signs (flushing/hyperreflexia, elevated blood pressure and pulse, tremors)
- Opioid withdrawal signs (mydriasis, sweating/irritability/rhinorrhea)

TABLE 10.6
Suggestive Laboratory Findings for Suspicion for Drug Abuse

- Abnormal liver function tests
- Elevated MCV over 95
- Hypophosphatemia
- Hyperlipidemia.
- High carbohydrate-deficient transferrin
- MCH high
- Anemia
- Positive urinalysis for illicit drugs
- Positive for HIV
- Positive for hepatitis B or C

MCV = mean corpuscular volume; MCH = mean corpuscular hemoglobin.

looking for suggestive behavioral patterns (Table 10.4). This is then followed by a search for suggestive physical findings (Table 10.5). In addition, certain laboratory tests (Table 10.6) can provide clues. There are also a number of pencil and paper tests designed to identify drug/alcohol abuse/dependence: the Michigan Alcoholism Screening Test (MAST; Katz & Fanciullo, 2002; Pokornyet al., 1972), CAGE (Steinweg & Worth, 1993), Alcohol Use Disorders Identification Consumption Test (AUDIT-C; Bush et al., 1998), Benzodiazepine Dependence questionnaire (Baillie & Mattick, 1996), the Drug Abuse Screening Test (DAST; Skinner, 1982), the Self-Administered Alcohol Screen Test (Bailey et al., 2002), and the Addiction Severity Index (Savage, 2002). However, to the author's knowledge, none of these tests taps the concept of addiction described above and will not arrive at such a diagnosis. These tests will define the patient at risk for addiction if that patient answers the questions honestly. In addition, these tools have been developed for use with alcoholics and/or street addicts. There have been no large clinical trials confirming the validity of these tests with patients given opioids for pain (Nedejkovic et al., 2002). For details and descriptions of these tests, the reader is referred to addiction textbooks.

There are a number of addiction tools that are in the process of development specifically designed for use in medical patients. The first of these is the Screening Instrument for Substance Abuse Potential (SISAP). This five-item screen helps the clinician categorize patients for lower or higher risk of abusing prescribed opioids. The five SISAP questions are as follows:

1. If you drink alcohol, how many drinks do you have on a typical day?
2. How many drinks do you have in a typical week?
3. Have you used marijuana or hashish in the past year?
4. Have you ever smoked cigarettes?
5. What is your age?

The SISAP has been shown to have a low clinical false-negative rate when tested against the database of a large ($N = 11,634$) Canadian epidemiological survey of alcohol and drug abuse (Coambs & Jarry, 1996). It has not been prospectively tested in a chronic pain population. The SISAP is designed to pick up a high percentage of alcohol or polydrug abusers. As such, it has a high false-positive rate (18%). According to the SISAP, caution should be used in prescribing opioids for the following patients:

1. Men who exceed four drinks per day or 16 drinks per week
2. Women who exceed three drinks per day or 12 drinks per week
3. A patient who admits to marijuana or hashish use in the past year. (It is recreational use of cannabis for euphoric effect that is of concern. The use of tetrahydrocannabinol, THC, derivatives to treat pain is still very controversial. Clinicians should exercise caution in recommending opioid therapy to a patient who is using cannabinoids regularly.)
4. A patient under 40 who smokes.

The second tool in development that may be relevant to CPPs is called the Screening Tool for Addiction Risk (STAR; Li et al., 2001). This is a 14-item tool that has been shown to differentiate CPPs from CPPs with a history of drug addiction on three items: prior treatment in a drug rehabilitation facility, nicotine use, and feelings of excessive nicotine use. Prior treatment in a drug facility had a 93% positive prediction value for addiction. However, it is to be noted that predictive validity was not tested here.

What is interesting here is that both the SISAP and STAR associate nicotine use with addiction risk.

If the above tools have not been developed specifically for CPPs, should the pain clinician utilize these tools in evaluating CPPs? It is the author's opinion for medicolegal reasons that the use of such tests is indicated if a clinician wishes to enlist a CPP into COAT treatment. The reasons for this are discussed below. Two other issues are important to COAT: addiction fear and detoxification fear. Recently, a number of authors have tapped the concept of addiction fear as a reason for noncompliance with COAT. Greer et al. (2001) noted addiction fear in 10.8% of patients undergoing orthopedic procedures. Patients with neuropathic pain have also been noted to voice this fear; 31.8% (Bailey et al., 2002) have expressed such a fear. Outside of potential noncompliance issues to COAT emanating from such a fear, it is likely that this group of patients would not be at risk for addiction unless it contained patients who had previous addiction and were now abstinent. To date, there has not been a questionnaire developed to tap this fear. There has, however, been a tool developed to tap the fear of detoxification. The Detoxification Fear Survey Schedule (DFSS; Ling et al., 1987) is a tool designed to quantify fear of detoxification. As pain patients are often detoxified from narcotics, such a tool could be a useful instrument to target a problem seen in some pain patients.

THE PREVALENCE OF ADDICTION WITHIN CHRONIC PAIN PATIENTS

In an early structured review, Fishbain et al. (1992b), reviewed studies relating to the prevalence of addiction within CPPs. They reported that different authors used different addiction definitions and criteria, making the data suspect. However, overall the prevalence percentages for drug abuse/drug dependence/drug addiction for patients with chronic pain were in the range of 3.2 to 18.9%. They caution that the results did not tap the concept of addiction and that the prevalence of addiction was likely to be at the middle of this range (Fishbain et al., 1992b). Since this review there have been a significant number of other studies that have directly or indirectly explored this issue. Hoffman et al. (1995a) found an addiction rate of 23.4%. Chabal et al. (1997) found an addiction rate of 34%, and Kouyanau et al., (1997) found a rate of 12%. There has also been one report of a chronic pain population at a Veterans Administration (VA) facility and a primary care setting. Here Reid et al., (2002) reported that prescription opioid abuse behavior was recorded for 24% of the VA patients and 31% of the primary care patients. As "opioid abusive behavior" does not necessarily translate into addiction (discussed below), one does not know how to interpret these results.

TABLE 10.7
Prevalence of Various Psychoactive Substance-Related Disorders within CPPs

Psychoactive Substance-Related Disorders	Prevalence within CPPs, %	More Common than General Population	Discrepancies between Authors
Current alcohol abuse/dependence	2–10.6 (Fishbain, Goldberg, Meager, & Rosomoff, 1986; Hoffmann, Olofsson, Salen et al., 1995; Katon, Egan, & Millder, 1985; Rafil, Haller, & Poklis, 1990)	No	Yes
Current drug dependence (opioids, barbiturates, sedative, cannabinoids)	5.2–34 (Skinner, 1982; Evans, 1981; Fishbain, Goldberg, Meager, & Rosomoff, 1986; Hoffmann, Olofsson, Salen et al., 1995; Katon, Egan, & Millder, 1985; Medina & Diamond, 1997; Rafil, Haller, & Poklis, 1990; Portenoy & Foley, 1986)	Probably	Yes
Current illicit drug abuse (cocaine cannabinoids, speed)	6.41–12.5 (Fishbain et al., 1998a; Evans, 1981; Rafil, Haller, & Poklis, 1990)	Probably	Yes
Total current alcohol and other drug dependence	14.9–23.4 (Fishbain, Goldberg, Meager, & Rosomoff, 1986; Hoffman, Olofsson, Salen et al., 1995; Magni, Caldieron, & Regatti-Luchini, 1990)	Probably	Yes

In addition, there have been two studies using urine toxicologies for prevalence of illicit drug use in patients with chronic pain. In the first study Fishbain et al. (1998a) reported that 8.4% of the patients had illicit drugs in their urine, while Raffi et al. (1990) reported a rate of 12.5%. Because illicit drug use has a high correlation with a predisposition to addiction in patients with chronic pain (Sees & Clark, 1993), these figures probably represent the lower end in the range for prevalence of addiction. Table 10.7 summarizes these studies in reference to various sub-categories of drug abuse/dependence.

Although the above studies attempted to develop prevalence percentages for substance use disorders, none of them used control groups. A study by Brown et al.(1996) compared rates for substance use among patients with chronic pain attending a family medicine clinic with patients attending for other reasons. There was no statistical difference in prevalence between the two groups. Thus, it is possible that prevalence for drug addiction in patients with chronic pain is no greater than in other settings. This statement is even more relevant if one considers that the above drug addiction data were reported from tertiary facilities where patients with chronic pain have more significant problems. Overall, these data indicate that the prevalence of addiction may not be too much different from the general population. However, these data are limited by the problems with the definition and diagnosis of addiction.

These figures should also be viewed in the context of the prevalence rate for addiction in the United States. This has been estimated to be from 3 to 16% for alcoholism (Savage, 1993) and from 5 to 6% for other forms of substance abuse (Portenoy, 1993). Prevalence rates for alcoholism are much greater in hospitals. Here the rates

have been reported to be 25% for medical services, 19% for neurology, and 23% for general surgery (Savage, 1993). Comparison of these prevalence rates to CPP reported prevalence rates indicates that CPP addiction prevalence rates are not necessarily greater than would be expected from general population data.

Another indirect line of evidence for/against addiction in CPPs is that of opioid use related to the presence of pain. Theoretically, opioid users with chronic pain should have higher levels of pain versus non-opioid users with chronic pain. If they do not, then they are using these drugs for addiction reasons. There have been two studies that have addressed this issue. In the first study, Ciccone et al. (2000) compared chronic pain opioid users and non-opioid users about to enter a pain management clinic for predictor variables. Opioid users were more likely to be physically disabled, be depressed, and report higher levels of pain and in more locations (Ciccone et al., 2000). Conversely, comparison of CPPs utilizing opioids long term versus only anti-inflammatories found that age, depression, personality disorder, and a history of substance abuse predicted opioid use with 79% being correctly classified (Breckenridge & Clark, 2003). Pain intensity did not predict opioid use (Breckenridge & Clark, 2003). It is to be noted that these two studies are not exactly comparable, as the second study used CPPs already selected for COAT. However, the latter study indicates that within this population, there were patients who had a history of substance abuse and that this predicted being on opioids.

The above section can then be summarized as follows: (1) addiction is found within CPPs; (2) at the present time prevalence percentages can be presented only as ranges due to disagreements between researchers; (3) at the present time it is unclear if these ranges are greater than

TABLE 10.8
Development of Craving on Exposure to Opioids in Volunteers (Non-drug Abusing)

Author, Year	Type of Population	No. of Patients Exposed	Percent with Craving
Zacny, 2003	Non-drug-abusing volunteer	18, acutely exposed to 6 sessions (oxycodone, morphine, lorazepam [placebo active])	Liking and wanting ratings no different from placebo after 24 h

that of the general population; and (4) some of the evidence indicates that these ranges may not be greater than for the general population.

ADDICTION GENETICS, RISK OF ADDICTION ON OPIOID EXPOSURE AND RISK OF RE-ADDICTION ON OPIOID EXPOSURE IN PATIENTS WITH A HISTORY OF ADDICTIVE DISEASE

Researchers working in the area of addiction have for years noted that many individuals are self-exposed to alcohol and drugs of abuse and many continue to use alcohol or illicit drugs on occasional or even on a regular basis yet only some individuals go on to develop specific addictions. This indicates that there may be a genetic predisposition in some individuals to developing addiction. Further evidence comes from family, twin, and adoption studies, which establishes the heritability of alcoholism with heterogeneity of inheritance patterns in alcohol abuse disorders and in part for other substance abuse disorders (Anthenelli et al., 1997; Kreek, 2002; Nurnberger et al., 2001). Recently, it has been postulated that an inherited neurotransmitter deficiency in the D_2 receptor makes people vulnerable to addictions and compulsions, such as alcoholism, smoking, cocaine addiction, and attention deficit hyperactivity disorder (Goldman, 1996). This has been called "the reward deficiency syndrome"(Goldman, 1996). Thus, it is likely that, on a biogenetic basis, some individuals have a greater risk than others of developing addiction on exposure to intoxicating substances (Anthenelli & Schuckett, 1997). As such, exposure of individuals with this predisposition to opioids could precipitate addiction. Similar exposure to opioids of those recovering from addictive disease could also precipitate the reemergence of addictive disease. In addition, cross-vulnerability to developing addiction to a variety of substances has been documented (Regier et al., 1984). This suggests that individuals with one addiction, for example, nicotine or alcoholism, may be at higher risk than the general public for developing addiction to other substances, for example, therapeutically prescribed opioids. Because of the above genetic vulnerability to addiction in some patients, there has been significant concern in the medical and pain lit-

erature on the development of addiction on exposure to opioids. Studies addressing this issue have been summarized in Table 10.8, Table 10.9, and Table 10.10. Table 10.8 presents a unique study performed with non-drug-abusing volunteers acutely exposed to opioids. Here, liking/wanting ratings, a measure of craving, were no different from placebo. The results of this study would then be in accord with the genetics of addiction discussed above.

The second table (Table 10.9) is divided into three sections: studies addressing general medical patients; studies addressing patients with chronic noncancer pain; and one study addressing epidemiological opioid exposure evidence. The following observations can be made from the data in Table 10.9: (1) In medical populations, the frequency of addiction on opioid exposure is almost nil. (2) In patients with chronic noncancer pain exposed to opioids, researchers report a range of addiction development from 0 to 17.3%. The studies reporting higher percentages (17.3%, Tennant et al., 1988; 9.2%, Lu et al., 1988) used aberrant drug-related behaviors (discussed below) as a means of diagnosing addiction. This may create many false positive cases. (3) A major epidemiological study (Joranson et al., 2000) demonstrated that although nationally opioid use increased, abuse cases decreased.

Overall, these data indicate that some clinicians do see addiction development with opioid exposure in patients with chronic noncancer pain, but most clinicians report low percentages for this problem.

The benzodiazepine drugs are also routinely used with CPPs. As such, there has also been concern over addiction development on exposure to these drugs. Table 10.10 highlights the one available study that has addressed this issue in a medical population. The frequency of addiction was low at 1.6%.

Use of illicit drugs is a good measure of potential addiction. Table 10.11 addresses this issue. Here CPPs exposed to opioids in a COAT treatment were subjected to urine toxicology screens. The range of urine positive for illicit drugs was from a low of 7.5% to a high of 23.1%. These data indicate that a significant percentage of CPPs *with* substance abuse problems are being placed on COAT. These substance abuse problems are likely preexistent to the COAT treatment.

TABLE 10.9
Development of Alleged Addiction on Exposure to Opioids in Medical Populations

Author, Year	Type of Population	No. of Patients Exposed	Percent with Abuse/Addiction Exposure
	Studies Addressing General Medical Patients		
Porter & Jick, 1980	Hospital General	11,882	0.03%
Perry & Heidrich, 1982	Burns	?	0%
Medina & Diamond, 1977	Headaches	2,369	0.13%
Chapman & Hill, 1989	Cancer	?	Insignificant
Cicero et al., 1999	Medical population exposed to Tramadol, a very weak opioid	757,558	0.001 to 0.002% (975 of the abuse cases had previous history of substance abuse)
	Studies of Patients with Chronic Noncancer Pain		
Moulin et al., 1996	Chronic noncancer pain	46	8.7%
Milligan et al., 2001	Chronic noncancer pain	301	1%
Dellemijn et al., 1998	Neuropathic pain	30	0%
Broaughton et al., 1999	Cancer and chronic noncancer pain	101	2%
Cowan et al., 2001	Chronic noncancer pain	36	0%
Burchman & Pagel, 1995	Chronic noncancer pain patients maintained on opioids	81	2.5% developed aberrant drug-related behavior (tried to fill prescriptions at other pharmacies)
Schaffer-Vargas et al., 1999	Chronic noncancer pain	30	0%
Doguong-Cantagrel et al., 1991	Chronic noncancer pain	91	1.1%
Cowan, 2003	Chronic noncancer pain	104	2.8%
Taub, 1982	Chronic noncancer pain	313	4.1% (presented management problems of which 61.5% had previous substance abuse)
Tennant & Uelman, 1983	Chronic noncancer pain	22	0%
France et al., 1984	Chronic noncancer pain	16	0%
Urban et al., 1986	Neuropathic pain	5	0%
Tennant et al., 1988	Chronic noncancer pain	52	17% (abuse behaviors)
Portenoy & Foley, 1986	Chronic noncancer pain	38	5.3%
Portenoy, 1989	Chronic noncancer pain	20	0%
Zenz, 1992	Chronic noncancer pain including neuropathic	100	9%
Lu et al., 1988	Chronic noncancer pain	76	9.2% (escalated their dosages)
Jamison, 1998	Chronic noncancer pain	36	2.7%
Kell, 1992	Chronic noncancer pain	16	0%
	Study of Epidemiological Opioid Exposure Evidence		
Joranson et al., 2000	Nationally representative sample of hospital emergency department admissions resulting from drug abuse	Medical use in grams per 1,000,000 population and mentions of drug abuse as percent of population	From 1990 to 1996 there was a 59% increase in use of morphine and a 6.6% increase in mentions per year of opioid abuse, but the proportion of mentions of opioid abuse relative to total drug abuse mentions decreased from 5.1 to 3.8%

A number of researchers (Collins & Streltzer, 2003; Nedejkovic et al., 2002; Sees & Clark, 1993; Weaver & Schnoll, 2002) have indicated that a previous history of addiction should not be an exclusion criteria for opioid treatment for pain. These patients with a history of addiction should be treated the same for their pain as other pain patients. At issue, however, is whether these patients develop re-addiction when exposed to opioids. Only two studies have addressed this issue and they are presented in Table 10.12. These studies report 0 to 45% and speak to a completely different experience. Both studies have low patient numbers. As such, it can only be concluded that re-addiction can occur on opioid exposure, but this issue requires much research.

TABLE 10.10
Development of Alleged Addiction on Exposure to Benzodiazepines in Medicaid Populations

Author, Year	Type of Population	No. of Patients Exposed	Percent with Escalation (as a measure of abuse/addiction exposure)
Soumerai, 2003	New Jersey Medicaid beneficiaries who received benzodiazepines for at least 2 years (low-income women with children, elderly, those receiving aid for permanently and totally disabled)	2,440	1.6% (occurred in those receiving lorazepam, on antidepressants, pharmacy hoppers [filling a prescription for the same benzodiazepine at two different pharmacies within 7 days])

TABLE 10.11
Development of Alleged Addiction on Exposure to Opioid as Identified by Drug Toxicology

Author, Year	Type of Population	No. of Patients Exposed	Percent with Abuse/Addiction Exposure
Vaglienti, 2003	Chronic noncancer pain maintained on opioids	186	23.1% had (+) urine for illicit drugs (4.8% cocaine, 18.2% THC)
Katz et al., 2003	Chronic noncancer pain maintained on opioids	122	21.3% had (+) urine for illicit drugs 13.9% had (+) urine for nonprescribed controlled drugs 13.9% had an aberrant drug-related behavior
Passik, Schreiber, Kirsch et al., 2000	Combined cancer, HIV, and chronic noncancer patients maintained on opioids	111	50% had evidence of illicit drug, a prescription medication not ordered or alcohol; note that this was a patient sample
Belgrade, 2001	Chronic noncancer patients	93	30% had some pain on noncompliant urine screen 6.5% refused urine toxicology 7.5% had illicit drugs 12.9% had unauthorized opioids 7.5% did not have expected opioid (no opioids)
Fishbain et al., 0000	Chronic non-cancer pain patients	226	11.8% did not have expected opioid
Fancullo et al., 0000	Chronic non-cancer pain patients maintained on opioids	78 of which 15 had a history of substance abuse.	3.9% positive for cocaine 20% positive for cannabinoids 7.7% positive for alcohol Approximately 33% negative for prescribed drug.

TABLE 10.12
Development of Alleged Re-Addiction on Exposure to Opioids in Addicts

Author, Year	Type of Population	No. of Patients Exposed	Percent with Abuse/Addiction Exposure
Dunbar & Katz, 1996	Substance abusers with chronic noncancer pain	20	45%
Collins & Stretzler, 2003	Substance abusers with chronic noncancer pain	4	0%

Collins & Streltzer (2003) have presented possible protective factors for re-addiction on opioid exposure, and a number of authors (Collins & Streltzer, 2003; Nedejkovic et al., 2002; Weaver & Schnoll, 2002) have attempted to develop measures to be taken to reduce re-addiction in addicts on opioid exposure. These concepts are outlined in Table 10.13 and Table 10.14. Close attention should be paid to Table 10.14, as it is the opinion of these authors that CPPs with a history of addiction can be offered COAT, but that the informed consent of these patients and monitoring should be extra stringent versus COAT patients.

TABLE 10.13

Protective Factors for Re-Addiction for Substance Abusers Exposed to Opioids for Chronic Noncancer Pain

- Prior history of alcohol dependence *alone*
- Active participation in alcoholics anonymous
- Presence of family support
- Absence of opioid treatment at entry

Source: Adapted from Dunbar, S. A. & Katz, N. P. (1996).

TABLE 10.14

Measures to Be Taken to Reduce the Risk of Relapse to Addiction in Addicts with Chronic Noncancer Pain Exposed to Opioids

- Obtain and document informed consent for risk of addiction with opioid exposure
- Consult with addiction specialist before beginning opioid exposure
- Document appropriateness/need for opioid treatment
- Encourage patient to participate in 12-step program
- Involve social support for patient (e.g., significant other) in the treatment
- Avoid rapidly peaking medications (Gardner, 1997; Kreek & Koob, 1998)
- Require frequent visits with weekly prescription
- Require one physician
- Require one pharmacy
- Ask patients to bring medications left over each visit
- Require random urines for toxicology
- Require treatment agreement
- Include measures/ways of medication compliance, e.g., written medication schedules

Source: Adapted from Collins & Stretzler, 2003; Nedejkovic, Wasan, & Jamison, 2002; Weaver & Schnoll, 2002.

The above discussion indicates that some pain researchers believe that at this time addiction or a history of addictive disease should not be considered an absolute contraindication to COAT. However, some authors have indicated that some patient characteristics may be predictive of poor response to COAT (Table 10.15). In addition, some authors have tried to develop exclusion/inclusion criteria for COAT (Table 10.16). Note that in Table 10.16, to be a candidate for COAT, a CPP should have intractable chronic pain and be a failure in other treatment. A history of addiction is a relatively exclusionary criterion.

ABERRANT DRUG-RELATED BEHAVIORS

In 1992, Jaffee described a group of drug-related behaviors, which he thought could be operationally used to diagnose/define addiction. These behaviors are presented

TABLE 10.15

Red Flags or Potential Contraindications to Chronic Opioid Analgesic Therapy

- Excessive pain intensity (10/10)
- Extreme ratings of emotional distress
- Poor coping
- Use of multiple pain descriptions
- Poor perceived social support
- Multiple pain sites
- Poor employment history
- Long-term reliance on health professionals

Source: Adapted from Nedejkovic, Wasan, & Jamison, 2002.

TABLE 10.16

Guidelines for Chronic Opioid Analgesic Therapy in Patients with Chronic Noncancer Pain

A. Inclusion Criteria (both required)
- Chronic pain (intractable)
- Failure of all other reasonable attempts at analgesia

B. Potential Exclusion Criteria (relative)
- History of substance abuse
- Chaotic home environment
- Severe character pathology

Source: Adapted from Portenoy, 1990.

in Table 10.17 and appear to represent behaviors that are sociopathic/antisocial in reference to drug use. The short list of eight behaviors developed by Jaffee (1992) was expanded to 18 behaviors by Portenoy (1994) from his own clinical experience with CPPs maintained on opioids (Table 10.17). Since then, these behaviors have been ranked by pain clinicians in order of severity (Passik, Kirsh et al., 2002). In addition, the frequency of some of these behaviors within CPPs on COAT has also been recorded (Table 10.17). A number of observations can be made from Table 10.17: (1) Clinicians consider sociopathic behavior, such as selling prescription drugs, stealing/borrowing drugs from others, injecting oral formulations, as very serious. (2) In general the more sociopathic behaviors are not frequently found in COAT patients. (3) The most frequent behaviors are aggressive complaining about need for more drug (18.2%) and requesting specific drugs (10.2%). These frequencies fall in range of those reported by Katz et al. (2003). It is to be noted that these figures may not represent or be indicative of addiction, as indicated below. (4) However, it is to be noted that 1.9% of the COAT patients admitted to concurrent use of alcohol or illicit drugs. This again indicates that within this population there may be a CPP subpopulation with significant addiction problems. Based on another study

TABLE 10.17
Representative Aberrant Drug-Related Behaviors

Probably More Predictive

- Selling prescription drugs (**1**)*
- Prescription forgery (**2**)*
- Stealing or "borrowing" drugs from others (**5**)*
- Injecting oral formulations (**3**) (1.5%)*
- Obtaining prescription drugs from nonmedical sources (**6**)*
- Concurrent abuse of alcohol or illicit drugs (**4**) (1.9%)*
- Multiple dose escalations or other noncompliance with therapy despite warnings (**8**) (13.3%)*
- Multiple episodes of prescription "loss"*
- Repeatedly seeking prescriptions from other clinicians or from emergency rooms without informing prescriber, or after warnings to desist (**7**) (5.6%)
- Evidence of deterioration in the ability to function at work, in the family, or socially that appears to be related to drug use (1.8%)
- Repeated resistance to changes in therapy despite clear evidence of adverse physical or psychological effects from the drug

Probably Less Predictive

- Aggressive complaining about the need for more drug (**9**) (18.2%)
- Drug hoarding during periods of reduced symptoms (**11**) (1.1%)
- Requesting specific drugs (10.2%)
- Openly acquiring similar drugs from other medical sources
- Unsanctioned dose escalation or other noncompliance with therapy on one or two occasions (**12**)
- Unapproved use of the drug to treat another symptom (**10**)
- Reporting psychic effects not intended by the clinician
- Resistance to a change in therapy associated with "tolerable" adverse effects with expressions of anxiety related to the return of severe symptoms

Notes: Percentages represent the frequencies of these aberrant behaviors found in 388 CPPs treated with chronic opioid analgesic therapy (Passik et al., 2002b). Numbers 1–12 represent the relative ranking of these 52 aberrant behaviors by clinicians.

* Aberrant drug related behaviors identified by Jaffe (1992) as predictive of addiction.

TABLE 10.18
Differential Diagnosis of Aberrant Drug-Taking Behaviors

Addiction

Pseudo-addiction

Other psychiatric diagnoses as a reason for inability to comply with treatment

- Encephalopathy
- Borderline personality disorder
- Depression
- Anxiety

Criminal intent (diversion)

Self-medication of mood, sleep, trauma (flashbacks), and other distress

Source: Adapted from Kirsh et al., 2002; Savage, 2002.

TABLE 10.19
Hints for the Possibility That an Established CPP on COAT Is Addicted[97]

- Unwillingness to taper opioids when other treatments are offered
- No relief from any other modality except opioids
- Preference for short-acting versus long-acting opioids

Source: Adapted from Goldman, 1993.

(Kirsh et al., 2002) these results would need to be put into appropriate context. Kirsh et al. (2002) found that current aberrant drug-related behaviors were seldom reported by CPPs, but attitude items revealed that patients would consider engaging in aberrant drug-related behaviors or would possibly excuse them in others if pain or symptom management were inadequate (Passik et al., 2000). Thus, in interpreting the presence of aberrant drug-related behaviors, the clinician needs to keep in mind that these behaviors are indicative of the differential diagnosis presented in Table 10.18.

What, then, do aberrant drug-related behaviors represent and what is their clinical utility? At the present time it is unclear whether these behaviors are indicative of or represent addiction. It is also unclear which of these behaviors are more closely related to addiction, although the more sociopathic behaviors may be more closely aligned with addiction. Finally, aberrant drug-related behaviors can best be used as a red flag during COAT treatment. Once noted by the clinician, they should trigger a search for a reason for the behavior noted according to the differential diagnosis described in Table 10.18.

If the clinician eliminates all other possibilities besides that of addiction as the reason for the aberrant drug-related behaviors, then he or she may wish to search for other hints for addiction in the patient in question (Table 10.19). There is one item in Table 10.19 that requires comment: preference for short-acting opioids versus long-acting opioids. There is some research on this issue that could potentially be clinically useful. Because short-acting opioids are thought to be associated with euphoria, transition to long-acting opioids could be a test for addiction. Some authors have therefore suggested that patients resistant to moving to long-acting opioids from short-acting opioids could have addiction issues. Raggi (2001) reported on 100 CPPs whom they attempted to switch to long-acting opioids from short-acting opioids. They reported that 28% resisted leaving the short-acting opioids and suggested that these patients could have been seeking the euphoria associated with this drug group. However, it is to be noted that there are a number of potential differential diagnoses besides that of addiction that could be the reason(s) for the resistance/refusal to move to long-acting opioids. This differential list is presented in Table 10.20.

TABLE 10.20
Differential Diagnosis for Those Chronic Pain Patients Who Resist/Refuse Transfer to Long-Acting Opioids

- Fear of increased pain
- Actual poor pain relief (i.e., breakthrough pain)
- Fear of loss of control over pain
- Fear of a loss of a coping strategy for pain
- Addiction

TABLE 10.21
Procedures to Follow if and when the Pain Clinician Suspects Addiction in a COAT CPP

- Obtain collateral information
- Reduce prescription interval
- Use pill counts
- Review patient agreement (discussed below) with patient and invoke relevant sanctions
- Do blood/urine toxicology
- Consider referring patient to addiction medicine and/or facility
- Document actions taken

Source: Adapted from Goldman, 1993.

A final issue here relates to what the pain clinician should do if he or she continues to harbor a significant suspicion that the patient is becoming addicted. Table 10.21 outlines the necessary options.

PSEUDO-ADDICTION

As noted above, pseudo-addiction is within the differential diagnosis of aberrant drug-related behaviors. As such, this concept can be understood only within the context of aberrant drug-related behaviors. Pseudo-addiction is operationally defined as aberrant drug-related behaviors that make the patient with chronic pain look like an addict. However, these behaviors stop if opioid doses are increased and pain improves (Weissman & Haddox, 1989). This indicates that the aberrant drug-related behaviors were actually a search for relief, i.e., pseudo-addiction. However, it is to be noted that there is little specific evidence for the concept of pseudo-addiction. This concept originated from one case report (Weissman & Haddox, 1989). Outside of one large-scale study reported as an abstract (McCarberg & Laskin, 2001), no studies of pseudo-addiction exist. In this last study of 500,000 patients, 316 were identified as problem opioid patients. Most of these patients, however, appeared to be pseudo-addicts. There is also some collateral evidence for the pseudo-addiction concept. Arthritic rats appeared to self-administer opioids at rates required to control their pain,

TABLE 10.22
Alleged Distinctions between Pseudo-Addiction and Addiction in Patients with Chronic Pain

Variable	Pseudo-Addicted	Addicted
Escalation of dose	Will stop escalating dose when pain controlled and may even decrease dose	Will continue escalating
Euphoria	Will not try to achieve euphoria	Will try to reach euphoria
Signs of intoxication (e.g., sedation, confusion)	No	Yes
Focus on side effects	Yes	No
Focus on consequences of side effects	Yes	No
Follow recommendations for other forms of treatment	Yes	No

rather than for the rewarding effects of the drug (Colpaert et al., 2001). This indicates that the two behaviors may also be separated in humans.

It is almost impossible to differentiate a patient with chronic pain with addiction who escalates the dose of mediation to obtain euphoria from a non-addicted patient with undertreated pain because both will exhibit aberrant drug-related behaviors (Weaver & Schnoll, 2002). The best approach for the physician is to provide more pain medications and to observe the patient for aberrant drug-related behaviors (Weaver & Schnoll, 2002) and some of the characteristics listed in Table 10.22. Although the pseudo-addiction concept lacks significant scientific support and it is unclear how clinically relevant in is, it has nevertheless become widely accepted within the pain physician community. As such, this concept has now become a focus in some medicolegal cases. Thus, pain clinicians who do COAT treatment, or who are planning to, should be aware of this concept and address it in their patient notes.

Finally, it is to be noted that there is also a differential diagnosis for pseudo-addiction that relates to inadequate pain management. This differential diagnosis is presented in Table 10.23.

COAT TREATMENT AGREEMENTS

The concept of a Treatment Agreement for COAT was first developed by Burchman and Pagel (1995). The alleged benefits of such an agreement have now been outlined in the literature (Biller & Caudill, 1999; Bolen,

TABLE 10.23
Differential Diagnosis of Pseudo-Addiction

Inadequate pain management secondary to

- Progressive pathology
- Tolerance development
- Stable conditions, but suboptimal analgesia
- Development of opioid-induced hyperalgesia (discussed below)

2003; Burchman and Pagel, 1995; Doleys & Rickman, 2003; Fishman & Kreis, 2002) and are now thought to be the following: a constructive element for a physician–patient partnership; a motivational tool for both sides to reflect on their expectations and responsibilities; a demonstration that the decision to use opioids was seriously considered by all parties involved; an informed consent tool; a tool that allows the physician to break confidentiality to call a pharmacy, etc.; indirect protection of the physician from the fear of inappropriate investigation by regulatory authorities by establishing strict guidelines under which opioids will be administered; protection of the physician against subsequent medicolegal problems because of the informed consent aspects. Because most of the state licensing boards require written treatment plans for patients on COAT, the COAT treatment agreement can substitute for the treatment plan. It is to be noted that the COAT treatment agreements have been recommended for use by legal experts in the field (Bolen, 2003). Bolen pointed out that the Federation of State Medical Boards Model Guidelines in the use of controlled substances to treat pain contemplate the use of written treatment agreements with patients with pain who have a history of or present a problem with substance abuse. These experts suggest that the COAT treatment agreement should contain the elements outlined in Table 10.24. Finally, it is to be noted that the ability of COAT treatment agreements to prevent prescription abuse has not been established in the literature (Biller & Caudill, 1999). As such, the physician using these agreements should not expect to be free of patients who may abuse opioids.

DIVERSION AND THE DRUG ENFORCEMENT AGENCY

Diversion is the use of a controlled substance for other than its intended medical use. Commonly, industry drugs are diverted to street use because their quality control makes them desirable and safe. Sources of diversion (and the legal agency responsible for that diversion) are presented in Table 10.25. A number of observations are to be noted in reference to this table. At the present time, the largest sources are patient-modified prescriptions and sale of drugs to addicts by patients. This table also confronts

TABLE 10.24
Elements to Be Included in a COAT Treatment Agreement

- Details of what the service physician will provide
- The condition or diagnosis necessitating the use of controlled substances (COAT)
- Goal of COAT, e.g., pain relief, increased function
- Risks of COAT (informed consent)
- Risks of off-label drugs, if those are to be prescribed
- Alternatives to COAT or that there are no alternatives (what reason) or that patient refused alternatives
- A list of compliance measures to be used (one pharmacy, one doctor for prescribing, pill counts, urine/serum random toxicologies, calling other pharmacists, etc.)
- Circumstances under which the agreement would be terminated and patient tapered off COAT (e.g., no decrease in pain, tolerance, no increase in function, escalation)
- An explanation of what would be considered noncompliance leading to agreement termination and referral to an addiction specialist and/or addiction program

TABLE 10.25
Sources of Diversion

- Health care professional, self-use (State Licensing Board)
- Illegitimate prescriptions:
  - Nonpatient prescription forgeries (police)
  - Patient-modified prescriptions (police)
  - Prescription obtained by illegitimate patients via doctor shopping (police)
- Drug burglary/robbery (FBI)
- Employee theft of drugs or scripts (police)
- Sale of drugs to addicts by legitimate patients (police)
- Illegal sales of prescriptions or drugs by health care professionals or pharmacies (DEA)

a general misconception of physicians who believe that the Drug Enforcement Agency (DEA) monitors any and all types of diversions. As noted in this table, the DEA is interested only in illegal sales of prescriptions of drugs by health care professionals. Thus, unless the physician is participating in such an activity, he or she is unlikely to come in contact with the DEA.

The DEA is governed by the Controlled Substance Act. As such, "it is the position of the DEA that controlled substances should be prescribed, dispensed or administered when there is a legitimate medical use" (*Physician Manual*, 1990). Therefore, the DEA cannot hold a physician criminally responsible for prescribing in the "usual course of medical practice." The DEA will send its agents into the offices of physicians whom it suspects are working outside of the "usual course of medical practice" in order to obtain controlled substances (buys). Here, the agent will look for physician–patient contact, an examination, a diag-

TABLE 10.26
Red Flags for Identifying Illegitimate Patients

Be suspicious of anyone who presents with characteristics below

- Without a family member
- Wanting appointment at end of office hours/arriving end of office hours (presents when regular physicians cannot be reached)
- As a cash-paying patient
- Insisting on being seen immediately (in a hurry)
- Not interested in having a physical examination or tests
- Unwilling to give permission for old medical records
- No physician referral
- Claims old medical records are lost
- Unwilling/unable to give names of past health care professionals
- Claims out of town and lost prescription, forgotten to pack medication, or claims it was stolen
- Has no interest in referral, wants prescription now
- Shows unusual knowledge of controlled substances
- Requests specific drug or unwilling to try any other
- Claims allergies to non-opioid analgesics
- No visible means of support except welfare/disability
- Frequent address change

Source: Adapted from Goldman, 1993; Tennant, Herman, Silliman, & Reinking, 2002.

nosis, and a prescription to meet the needs of that diagnosis. Physicians not fulfilling these criteria in the "buy" may be charged.

There are ways for physicians to protect themselves against diversion that relates to illegitimate prescriptions: always designate number of refills, even if none; use serialized, duplicate copy–resistant prescriptions; and write alpha and numeric quantity, dosage, and strength. There are also a number of signs (red flags) that may signal an illegitimate patient. These are designated in Table 10.26.

The final type of diversion that relates to physicians is that of the sale of drugs to addicts by legitimate patients. Little is known about this type of diversion except that it is claimed to be common. This type of diversion is extremely difficult to identify. To the author's knowledge, there are currently only two red flags for the possibility of this type of diversion: (1) the urine/blood toxicology screen does not contain the expected opioid or (2) the serum value of the opioids is much below what would be expected according to the patient's current dosage. As discussed under blood/urine toxicology procedures (below), a negative urine/blood toxicology does represent a differential diagnosis. As such, the patient with this type of result cannot be automatically considered to be diverting. In reference to serum values being below expected, patients do differ genetically in their opioid metabolism (Heiskanen et al., 2000). Thus, this result is also not an absolute proof of diversion.

URINE TOXICOLOGY MONITORING IN COAT AS A MEANS FOR MONITORING FOR ADDICTION

Previous research (Belgrade et al., 2001; Fishbain et al., 1998a; Joranson et al., 2000; Katz et al., 2003; Passik et al., 2000; Rafil et al., 1990; Vaglienti et al., 2003) has shown that urine toxicology studies can provide valuable information in CPPs as to their opioid and illicit drug use status. Thus, urine toxicology studies can play an important role in determining suitability for COAT and COAT adherence monitoring. However, before trying to interpret urine toxicology results, the pain clinician should understand the limits (Fishman et al., 2000) of the information provided by urine toxicology. These are outlined below.

Urine assays yield qualitative results only (positive or negative). Testing of opioid in urine is generally of two types: a screening method and a confirmatory test. Confirmatory testing may provide specific identification of individual opioid agents. Morphine, codeine, oxycodone, oxymorphone, hydrocodone, hydromorphone, heroin, methadone, and meperidine are routinely tested for in these screens. Limitations of the urine toxicology screen are the following: (1) A negative screen can rule out only opioids that are detectable. For example, it will not rule out fentanyl, buprenorphine, butorphanol, nalbuphine, and pentazocine, which are not routinely tested for in opioid screens. (2) An opioid may be present in the urine, but the detection limit of that screen may be set above the concentration of the drug in urine, thus resulting in a false-negative result. (3) Poppy seed ingestion may lead to a false-positive opioid screen. (4) Some opioids, such as oxycodone, may be less detectable than others (morphine, codeine) at therapeutic dosages, resulting in a false-negative screen. (5) Because confirmatory tests are usually limited to a certain number of opioids, not all positive determinations on a screening method will go on to be recorded as a positive test, thus leading to a false-negative result. (6) The period of detection for opioids in urine is 1 to 3 days after ingestion; however, this time period is dependent on the physiology of the individual and his or her current physiological status, e.g., hydration. Thus, there is significant individual variation in opioid clearance, which can lead to either a false-positive or false-negative result.

In general, the pain clinician can expect two types of urine toxicology results. The first of these is the unexpected substance (Table 10.27). In this situation, one would see either an illicit drug or unexpected opioid. The differential diagnosis for each of these situations is then presented in Table 10.27. The second type of urine toxicology result is that of the expected substance not being present in urine (Table 10.28). This situation was first noted by Fishbain et al. (1998a) who reported that 11.8% of the patients claiming to be taking a drug did not have evidence of that drug by urine toxicology. Since then, two

TABLE 10.27
Differential Diagnosis of Unexpected Substance in Urine

A. Illicit Drug
- Drug abuse
- Addiction
- Non-adherence to treatment agreement

B. Unexpected Opioid
- Addiction
- Non-adherence to treatment agreement
- Pseudo-addiction
- Forgetfulness/carelessness
- Use of medications for other symptoms (sleep, anxiety, depression)
- False-positive test

TABLE 10.28
Differential Diagnosis of Expected Substance (Opioid) Not Present

A. Opioid Left Over
- False-negative test
- Fear of side effects
- Forgetfulness/carelessness
- Lack of education regarding medication regimen
- Fear of social stigma
- Fear of pain episodes (hoarding drug)
- Nonbelief in drug therapy
- Medication costs
- Religious/moral beliefs

B. Opioid Not Left Over
- False-negative test
- Addiction
- Diversion
- Medication costs
- Pseudo-addiction
- Use of opioids for other symptoms (sleep, anxiety, depression)
- Non-adherence to treatment agreement

other researchers have reported on this problem in COAT patients. Belgrade et al. (2001) reported that 7.5% of his patients did not have the expected opioid in urine, while Fancullo (Joranson et al., 2000) reported that 33% of his patients did not have the expected opioid or drug in their urine. The differential diagnosis for this situation is presented in Table 10.28. It is suggested in this table that if this situation occurs, the pain clinician should ask the patient to bring in any left-over pills. The differential diagnosis in Table 10.28 is then subdivided into patients who do and do not have opioids left over. It is to be noted that if no opioids are left over, diversion is within the differential diagnosis.

The differential diagnoses lists presented in Table 10.27 and Table 10.28 are important because they point

out one major problem with urine toxicology testing. The results of the urine toxicology will not make a diagnosis of addiction or diversion, but only potentially lead to the suspicion of these problems. However, patients on COAT with urine toxicologies positive for illicit drugs are likely to have substance abuse problems and are therefore at high risk for addiction.

DO LONG-ACTING OPIOIDS HAVE LESS ADDICTION POTENTIAL?

As discussed in the introduction, the development of the technology of long-acting opioids such as controlled-release morphine, oxycodone, and fentanyl has had a significant impact on the growth and popularity of COAT. Recently, these drugs have been recommended by the European Federation of Chapters of the International Association for the Study of Pain as the drugs of choice for COAT in the treatment of chronic noncancer pain (Kalso et al., 2003). This recommendation was not based on the fact that the long-acting opioids have equal efficacy for effective pain control versus short-acting opioids (Chou et al., 2003), but on the theory that there may be less addiction risk and less tolerance development on exposure to long-acting opioids versus short-acting ones. The addiction part of this theory is based on the observation that as a general rule, opiate abusers cue in on the rate "rush" (Savage, 1999) onset in the central nervous system. This "rush" explains the popularity of lipid-soluble substances such as heroin, Dilaudid (Palladone), or fentanyl, and the lower abusability of substances such as morphine or methadone, which have slower onset. It appears that duration of action is less important than the intensity of the euphoria and the rapidity of the "rush." If the duration of the agent is too short, however, substance abusers will re-dose frequently, because the physiological components of pain continue to sustain nociceptive input. This, coupled with the fact that the patients prefer to evaluate their substances by the "rush," results in the frequent re-dosing seen when substance opiate abusers are given ready access to their medications. This is seen in situations in which patients are given patient-controlled analgesia (PCA) devices in a perioperative situation. If, however, the prescribed dosing scheduling is too long, allowing for the central nervous system levels to fall below the pain threshold, "roller coasting" can result. This is seen when brief periods of analgesia are coupled with periods of breakthrough pain. If given the opportunity, these patients may not only increase the number of doses they use (to cover painful periods), but increase the doses at each interval to increase the intensity of the euphoria.

The controlled-release opioids, because of the controlled-release aspect, have less of a tendency to create the "rush." At the same time, because of their extended activity, these agents prevent "roller coasting." In reference to tolerance development, it has been noted that as a general rule, the shorter the duration of activity of the drug, the more frequent the dosing interval necessary, the more rapid the development of tolerance.

Is there any evidence for this theory? There is one study performed with 130 drug abusers (Brookoff, 1993). In this survey study, 85% of these patients reported having tried controlled-release opioids and of these 60% reported that they were of little or no use to them (Brookoff, 1993). The reported street price of the drugs at that time seemed also to reflect this preference. The street price of controlled-release morphine was 1/16 that of hydromorphone, 1/6 that of meperidine, and 1/9 that of immediate-release morphine (Brookoff, 1993).

Since that time, drug abusers have developed methods of circumventing the controlled-release opioid delivery systems. As such, the street value of controlled-release morphine, oxycodone, and fentanyl has increased. The increase in the street price when the delivery system was compromised is indirect evidence that long-acting agents have less attraction to drug abusers. The fact the controlled release delivery system can be compromised does not decrease the theoretical potential value of these drugs. If used correctly, these drugs may lead to less addiction and slower tolerance development. However, this area requires further study.

OPIOIDS AND DRIVING

Most drugs that affect the central nervous system have the potential to impair driving (Fishbain et al., 1999). Because opioids are psychotropic central nervous system depressing drugs, there has been disagreement on the part of medical practitioners regarding whether patients taking opioids chronically and on a consistent dose schedule can drive safely and should be allowed to drive (Fishbain et al., 1999). In the United Kingdom, a medical commission on Accident Prevention, Medical Aspects of Fitness to Drive has stated, "the more powerful narcotic analgesics, such as morphine, produce marked sedation and patients requiring them should not drive." This opinion has, however been challenged by a number of researchers who cite evidence that patients taking stable doses of opioids may drive and work safely (Fishbain et al., 1999). This controversy grew in importance with the wide acceptance of COAT utilizing controlled-release opioids for cancer pain and chronic nonmalignant benign pain. Because potential instructions to stop driving to a patient using opioids essentially dooms the patient to a life of disability, the answer to this controversy has widespread implications for the patient and the medical practitioner. There is concern for what is best for the patient but also medicolegal concerns if a CPP on COAT is advised to drive and has a

motor vehicle accident (MVA). Fishbain et al. (1999, 2003) in two evidence-based structured reviews attempted to summarize the literature on driving and opioids in order to make some recommendations to COAT pain practitioners. In the first review Fishbain et al. (1999) reviewed the scientific evidence for the involvement of opioids in intoxicated driving, MVA fatalities, and MVAs. The results of this structured evidence-based review indicated that there was consistent epidemiological type B evidence that opioids probably were not associated with intoxicated driving, MVA fatalities, and certainly not associated with MVAs. In the second review, Fishbain et al. (2003) reviewed the scientific evidence for the following issues: opioids affecting psychomotor abilities of COAT patients; effect of *new/additional doses* of opioids in psychomotor abilities of COAT patients; if COAT patients are more likely to have more convictions for motor vehicle violations and MVA; and if coat patients demonstrate driving impairments as measured in driving simulators and off/on road driving? The results of this review (Fishbain et al., 2003) were as follows: (1) There was moderate, generally consistent evidence for no impairment of psychomotor abilities of opioid-maintained patients. (2) There was inconclusive evidence on multiple studies for no impairment on cognitive function of opioid-maintained patients. (3) There was strong consistent evidence on multiple studies for no impairment of psychomotor abilities immediately after being given doses of opioids. (4) There was strong consistent evidence for no greater incidence in motor vehicle violations/motor vehicle accidents versus comparable controls of opioid-maintained patients. (5) There was consistent evidence for no impairment as measured in driving simulators off/on road driving of opioid-maintained patients. Based on the above results, it was concluded that the majority of reviewed studies appeared to indicate that opioids do not impair driving-related skills in opioid-dependent/tolerant patients. This evidence was consistent in four of five research areas investigated, but inconclusive in one.

Based on the above results of these two reviews, Fishbain et al. (2003) recommended an approach to the driving problem that utilizes the above data, but also puts the responsibility for the driving decision onto the patient. The specifics of this recommended approach are outlined below.

First, the patients placed on COAT should be advised of the current status of this research. Second, they should be advised that whether they do/do not drive should be based on this information, but that it is their own personal decision. Third, they should be advised that if they choose to drive, they should follow the following rules:

1. After beginning opioid treatment or after a dose increase, they should not drive for 4 to 5 days.
2. They should not drive if they ever feel sedated.

3. They should report sedation/unsteadiness/cognitive decline immediately to the pain clinician so that reduction in dosage can be initiated.

4. Under no circumstances should they use alcohol or illicit drugs such as cannabinoids and drive.

5. They should avoid taking any over-the-counter antihistamines.

6. They should not make any changes in their medication regimens without consulting with the pain clinician.

For the situation where the pain clinician is requested to complete paperwork in which questions are asked about the patient's driving ability, the same type of approach is recommended. The pain clinician should report the current status of this research in the paperwork. In addition, the physician should report whether he or she has noted any opioid side effects, which may interfere with driving, or the absence of these. However, if a specific question relating to whether the patient can/cannot drive is encountered, that question should be marked unknown. As an explanation, the physician should state that he or she does not have knowledge of the patient's ability to drive, as that can only be determined in a driving simulator and/or on-road/off-road driving tests.

It is to be noted that the above recommendations apply to COAT patients who do not use illicit drugs. As most MVAs involving opioids usually involve the concomitant use of alcohol and other drugs, pain clinicians may not wish to make these recommendations to COAT patients whom they know have addictive disease.

ADDICTION IN CPPs AND ASSOCIATED PSYCHIATRIC COMORBIDITIES

Feinstein (1970) developed the concept of *comorbidity.* He defined this term as "any distinct clinical entity that has existed or that may occur during the clinical course of a patient who has the index disease under study." Comorbidity is important for two reasons. First, the presence of an additional disease can complicate, interfere with, or make the treatment of the index disease more difficult, making the prognosis worse (Merikangas & Gelernter, 1990). Second, in medical research and especially outcome research, failure to classify and analyze comorbid diseases may create misleading medical statistics and may cause spurious comparisons during the planning and evaluation of patient treatment (Merikangas & Gelernter, 1990). For these reasons, in the past few years there has been an explosion in the number of psychiatric studies exploring comorbidity.

Five large categories of comorbidities have been studied in psychiatric patients (Fishbain, 1999; Fishbain et al., 1998b): comorbidities between psychiatric disorders on Axis I of the DSM-IV (4th ed.); comorbidities between psychiatric disorders on Axis I and Axis II (personality disorders) of the DSM-IV; comorbidities between psychoactive substance use disorders of Axis I and other psychiatric disorders on Axis I of the DSM-IV; comorbidities between all psychiatric disorders and other medical nonpsychiatric disorders; and comorbidities within psychoactive use disorders only. Of relevance to this chapter are comorbidities relating to addiction. It has been found in psychiatric patients that patients with psychoactive use disorders usually have significant other psychiatric comorbidities on Axis I, with the most common disorders depression and anxiety. For the addictions, there is also significant comorbidity with Axis II. Generally patients with addictions will demonstrate a personality disorder. Finally, patients with one addiction will generally manifest comorbid additional addictions. For example, opioid dependence can be associated with nicotine dependence, cannabinoid abuse, alcohol dependence; i.e., there is comorbidity between substance use disorders.

It is interesting, but sad, that little work has been done on delineating whether the same types of comorbidities as described above are found in CPPs. In an early DSM psychiatric diagnosis study, Fishbain et al. (1986) found that the majority of their CPPs had more than one diagnosis on Axis I: 58.4% of the men and 61.4% of the women. Thus, comorbidities between Axis I diagnoses should be frequently encountered in CPPs. In a follow-up study, Fishbain et al. (1998c), looking at this problem, found that some affective and personality disorder diagnoses were more commonly found in CPPs who had a psychoactive substance abuse disorder diagnosis versus those who did not. This study then demonstrated that CPPs with psychoactive substance abuse diagnoses have the same pattern of comorbidity as psychiatric patients.

There have also been some interesting recent additional studies that may be clinically useful on the subject of addiction comorbidity. In a case control study (Haddox et al., 2003), it was reported that CPPs with unexplained symptoms were as likely as CPPs without those symptoms to have problems in regard to medication abuse/dependence. The question of whether CPPs with unexplained symptoms are seeking drugs is often raised. As such, this is often used as a rationale for not placing these CPPs on COAT. This study then should partially alleviate this concern. Haddox et al. (2003) recently reported on a forensic review study of overdose deaths allegedly related to oxycodone or controlled-release oxycodone. They found that of 919 deaths, 96.7% involved more than one drug, i.e., multiple addictions. Thus, individuals with multiple addictions may be at greater risk for overdose deaths. The above information on addiction and psychiatric comorbidity can be used clinically and this is the reason it is presented. First, the identification of any kind of addictive disease, e.g., opioid dependence, should trigger a search for associated psychiatric comorbidity, associated psychoactive use disorders, or associated Axis II disorders. And, second, the presence of any significant psychiatric disorder, e.g., severe depression, should trigger a search for possible associated addiction.

ADDICTION IN CPPS AND DRUG/ALCOHOL DETOXIFICATION

As pointed out above, there may be some evidence that some CPPs on COAT will display aberrant drug-related behaviors and as such may require opioid detoxification and addiction treatment. Fishbain et al. have written a number of papers and chapters on opioid (Fishbain et al., 1993) and other drug (Fishbain, 1993; Fishbain, 2002b; Fishbain et al., 1992) detoxification protocols in CPPs. However, at issue is whether CPPs with physician-perceived drug problems are best treated at multidisciplinary pain treatment facilities or drug and alcohol treatment facilities. There is no evidence in the literature that CPPs would do better if they underwent detoxification and treatment at drug and alcohol treatment facilities versus pain treatment facilities (Fishbain et al., 1986). In fact, one study (Tennant & Rawson, 1982) indicated that CPPs would do better if they undergo detoxification in pain treatment facilities. In this study from a drug treatment facility, no patient initially perceived that chronic pain due to a medical condition would be an impediment to withdrawal from opioids. However, pain masked by opioids emerged during detoxification and proved to be an insurmountable barrier to total opioid withdrawal in the majority of CPPs (Tennant & Rawson, 1982). This study speaks to the potential advantage of CPPs undergoing detoxification at multidisciplinary pain treatment facilities, where simultaneous pain treatment is also available. There are also two studies (Currie et al., 2003; Khatami et al., 1979) that looked at multidisciplinary pain facility outcome for CPPs with addiction. Both studies reported favorable treatment outcomes in terms of opioid use, with one study (Currie et al., 2003) reporting that one half of patients were opioid free at 12 months. It is also to be noted that Fishbain et al. (1995, 1997) have recommended that drug abuse/dependence/addiction is one of a set of criteria that can be used to select CPPs for multidisciplinary pain facility referral (Fishbain et al., 1995, 1997). As such, physician perception of drug problems in CPPs can then be an indication for a multidisciplinary pain treatment facility referral.

There may also be one other reason for opioid detoxification in CPPs if COAT appears to be failing. This is the development of hyperalgesia, which is thought to be secondary to tolerance and desensitization of opioid receptors (Broder & Taub, 1978). Here, pain sensitivity actually increases (Collins & Streltzer, 2003). There are actually some clinical data (Broder & Taub, 1978; Savage, 1993) that indicate that in some CPPs, pain improved with detoxification from opioids. Thus, failure of COAT in CPPs secondary to hyperalgesia could be another indication for multidisciplinary pain facility detoxification.

LEGAL ISSUES IN ADDICTION AND CHRONIC PAIN TREATMENT

Recently, because of the medical malpractice crisis, there has been significant interest in pain medicine forensics (Bolen, 2003; Fishbain, 2002a). Substance abuse/addiction in CPPs has been recognized as an area with medicolegal risk. Thus, the purpose of this section is to alert the pain clinician to issues that have already generated malpractice claims and issues that are at high risk for generating malpractice claims if not correctly documented. It is to be noted that malpractice claims are generated when there is an adverse outcome, which the medical expert in that area claims is related to a physician action, which is deemed "below the standard of medical care in the community." Thus, if a treatment agreement might have prevented an adverse action and the treatment agreement is the standard, but was not done, the physician may be held liable. Hence, it is important for the pain clinician working with patients who are at risk for addiction to be aware of these potential standards. Table 10.29 has been developed to reflect this concept. It lists both issues that have already been raised as potential standards and those that have generated malpractice claims and or potential standards that one day may generate a malpractice claim. A large part of this table shows actual standards that have been recommended by state regulatory agencies.

CONCLUSIONS

At the present time, the research area of chronic pain/addiction is in a state of flux and is developing. It is evolving into a coherent body of knowledge that at this time has some clinical utility. However, much work remains to be done.

TABLE 10.29
Potential "Standards" in COAT Treatment That Have Already Generated Malpractice Claims or May Do So in the Future

Failure of Potential Standard	Preventive Response
Failure to document COAT according to elements recommended by State Practice Guidelines for COAT	
A. Appropriate indicators	A diagnosis of intractable chronic pain
B. Document history physical examination, physical impact on pain, psychological impact of pain, and potential for substance abuse	
C. Treatment plan	Can be satisfied via treatment agreement
D. Risk/benefit discussion (informed consent)	Can be satisfied via treatment agreement
E. At each visit should document (1) pain status, (2) function status, (3) side effects, and (4) lack or presence of aberrant drug-related behaviors	
Nonrecognition of possible pseudo-addiction (Fishbain, 2002)	Document if you think the patient is demonstrating pseudo-addiction if he or she demonstrates aberrant drug-related behaviors
Lack of knowledge of methods of rotation to methadone (Fishbain, 2002)	Follow only recommended rotation schedules
Failure to ask and document part of present substance abuse/addiction history	Reason why some addiction schedules should be used
Failure to act on substance abuse/addiction information when doing COAT (Bolen, 2003)	Document actions taken or reasons for not taking actions (Table 10.21)
Failure to act on diversion suspicion	If you document diversion suspicion, call police
Failure to document that you have informed consent for reemergence of addiction in patients with a history of opioid dependence/abuse before placing on COAT (Bolen, 2003)	Should include discussion of potential for physical dependence, tolerance, side effects, cognitive effects, risk of addiction, testosterone problems, driving issues, etc.
If placing patients with previous addiction on opioids, failure to document protective factors and measures taken to prevent re-addiction	Document
Failure to document aberrant drug-related behaviors and why what action is taken	If no action taken, document why
Placing a patient on COAT without a treatment agreement	Document why you did not think treatment agreement was necessary
Failure to use urine toxicology when indicated	Document why urine toxicology was not necessary
Failure to provide informed consent on driving issue	Document
Failure to refer a COAT patient for detoxification when indicated	Document reason why not referred

REFERENCES

American Academy of Pain Medicine, American Pain Society, and American Society of Addiction Medicine. (2001). *Definitions related to the use of opioids for the treatment of pain.* Glenview, IL: Author.

American Psychiatric Association. (2000). *Diagnostic and statistical manual of mental disorders* (4th ed., text rev.). Washington, DC: APA.

Anthenelli, R., & Schuckett, A. (1997). Genetics. In J. Lowinson, P. Ruiz, R. Millman, & J. Langrod (Eds.), *Substance abuse* (pp. 41–50). Philadelphia: Williams & Wilkins.

Bailey, G. I., Weaver, D. F., & Houlden, R. L. (2002). Patients' attitudes and prior treatments in neuropathic pain: A pilot study. *Pain Research & Management, 7*(4), 199–203.

Baillie, A. J., & Mattick, R. P. (1996). The benzodiazepine dependence questionnaire: Development, reliability and validity. *British Journal of Psychology, 96*, 276–281.

Belgrade, M. J., Ismail, M., Yoon, M., & Panopoulos, G. (2001). Non-complaint drug screens during opioid maintenance analgesia for chronic non-malignant pain (Abstract No. 787, p. 42). American Pain Society meeting, San Diego.

Bendtsen, P., Hensing, G., Ebeling, C., & Schedin, A. (1999). What are the qualities of dilemmas experienced when prescribing opioids in general practice? *Pain, 82*, 89–96.

Berndt, S., Maier, C., & Schutz, H. W. (1993). Polymedication and medication compliance in patients with chronic non-malignant pain. *Pain, 52*, 331–339.

Biller, N., & Caudill, M. (1999). Commentary: Contracts, opioids, and the management of chronic nonmalignant pain. *Ethic Rounds, 17*(2), 144–145.

Bolen, J. (2003). Legal expert discusses Rush Limbaugh incident, related issues. *Pain Medicine News, 1*(6), 3.

Bolen, J. (2003, May/June). 18 suggestions to minimize drug diversion in your practice. *Pain Medicine News, 1*(6), 18.

Breckenridge, J., & Clark, J.D. (2003). Patient characteristics associated with opioid versus nonsteroidal anti-inflammatory drug management of chronic low back pain. *Journal of Pain, 4*(6), 344–350.

Broaghton, A. N., Gordon, D. N., & Miller, A. J. (1999). Long term tolerability of CR oxycodone (OxyContin® tablets) in 101 patients treated for 12 months (Abstract No. 269, p. 339). 9th World Congress on Pain.

Brodner, R. A., & Taub, A. (1978). Chronic pain exacerbated by long term narcotic use in patients with non-malignant disease: Clinical syndrome and treatment. *Mount Sinai Journal of Medicine, 45*, 233–237.

Brookoff, D. (1993). Abuse potential of various opioid medications. *Journal of General Internal Medicine, 8*, 688–690.

Brown, R. L., Patterson, J. J., Rounds, L. A., & Papasouliotis, S. A. (1996). Substance abuse among patients with chronic back pain. *Journal of Family Practice, 43*(2), 152–160.

Burchman, S. L., & Pagel, P. S. (1995). Implementation of a formal treatment agreement for outpatient management of chronic nonmalignant pain with opioid analgesics. *Journal of Pain and Symptom Management, 10*(7), 556–563.

Bush, K., et al. (1998). The AUDIT alcohol consumption questions (AUDIT-C): An effective, brief screening test for problem drinking. *Archives of Internal Medicine, 158*, 1789–1795.

Chabal, C., Erjavec, M. K., Jacobson, L., et al. (1997). Prescription opiate abuse in chronic pain patients: Criteria, incidence and predictors. *Clinical Journal of Pain, 13*(2), 150–155.

Chapman, C. R., & Hill, H. F. (1989). Prolonged morphine self-administration and addiction liability: Evaluation of two theories in a bone marrow transplant unit. *Cancer, 63*, 1636–1644.

Chou, R., Clark, E., & Helfand, M. (2003). Comparative efficacy and safety of long-acting oral opioids for chronic non-cancer pain: A systematic review. *Journal of Pain and Symptom Management, 26*(5), 1026–1048.

Ciccone, D. S., Just, N., Bandilla, E. B., Reimer, E., Ilbeigi, M. S., Wu, W. (2000). Psychological correlates of opioid us in patients with chronic nonmalignant pain: A preliminary test of the downhill spiral hypothesis. *Journal of Pain & Symptom Management, 20*(3), 180–192.

Cicero, T. J., Adams, H. E., Geller, A., Inciardi, J. A., Muñoz, A., Schnoll, S. H., et al. (1999). A postmarketing surveillance program to monitor Ultram® (tramadol hydrochloride) abuse in the United States. *Drug and Alcohol Dependence, 57*, 7–22.

Coambs, R. B., & Jarry, J. L. (1996). The SISAP: a new screening instrument for identifying potential opioid abusers in the management of chronic nonmalignant pain in general medical practice. *Pain Research & Management, 1*(3), 155–162.

Collins, E. D., & Streltzer, J. (2003). Should opioid analgesics be used in the management of chronic pain in opiate addicts? *American Journal on Addictions, 12*, 93–100.

Colpaert, F. C., Tarayre, J. P., Alliaga, M., et al. (2001). Opiate self-administration as a measure of chronic nociceptive pain in arthritic rats. *Pain, 91*(1–2), 33–45.

Cowan, D. T., Wilson-Barnett, J., Griffiths, P., & Allan, L. (2003). A survey of chronic noncancer pain patients prescribed opioid analgesics. *Pain Medicine, 4*(4), 340–351.

Cowan, D., Allan, L., Libretto, S., & Griffiths, P. (2001). Opioid drugs: A comparative survey of therapeutic and "street" use. *Pain Medicine, 2*(3), 193–203.

Currie, S. R., Hodgins, D. C., Crabtree, A., Jacobi, J., & Armstrong, S. (2003). Outcome from integrated pain management treatment for recovering substance abusers. *Journal of Pain, 4*(2), 91–100.

Dellemijn, P. L., van Duijn, H., & Vanneste, J. A. (1998). Prolonged treatment with transdermal fentanyl in neuropathic pain. *Journal of Pain and Symptom Management, 16*(4), 220–229.

Doleys, D. M., & Rickman, L. (2003). Other benefits of an opioid "agreement" [comment]. *Journal of Pain and Symptom Management, 25*(5), 402–403.

Doguong-Cantagrel, N., Magnuson, S., & Wallace, M. (1991). Tolerability and efficacy of opioids in chronic nonmaligmant pain. American Pain Society Meeting, A722, 129.

Dunbar, S. A., & Katz, N. P. (1996). Chronic opioid therapy or nonmalignant pain in patients with a history of substance abuse: Report of 20 cases. *Journal of Pain and Symptom Management, 11*(3), 163–171.

Elander, J., Lusher, J., Bevan, D., & Telfer, P. (2003). Pain management and symptoms of substance dependence among patients with sickle cell disease. *Social Science and Medicine, 57*(9), 1683–1696.

Evans, P. J. D. (1981). Narcotic addiction in patients with chronic pain. *Anaesthesia, 36*, 597–602.

Feinstein, A. (1970). The pre-therapeutic classification of comorbidity in chronic disease. *Journal of Chronic Diseases, 23*, 455.

Fishbain, D. A. (1993). Drug detoxification protocols. In C. D. Tollison, & R. S. Kunkel (Eds.). *Headache diagnosis & treatment* (Chapter 40, pp 327–346). Baltimore: Williams & Wilkins.

Fishbain, D. A. (1999). Approaches to treatment decisions for psychiatric comorbidity in the management of the chronic pain patient. *Medical Clinics of North America, 88*(3), 737–757.

Fishbain, D. A. (2002a). Medico-legal rounds: medico-legal issues and breaches of "standards of medical care" in opioid tapering for alleged opioid addiction. *Pain Medicine, 3*(2), 135–142.

Fishbain, D. A. (2002b). Opiate, hypnosedative, alcohol and nicotine detoxification protocols. In C. D. Tollison, J. R. Satterwaite, & J. W. Tollison (Eds.). *Practical pain management* (3rd ed., pp. 314–329). Philadelphia: Lippincott/Williams & Wilkins.

Fishbain, D. A., Cutler, R. B., Cole, B., Lewis, J., Rosomoff, R. S., & Rosomoff, H. L. (2003). Medico-legal rounds: Medico-legal issues and alleged breaches of "Standards of Medical Care" in opioid rotation to methadone: A case report. *Pain Medicine, 4*(2), 195–201.

Fishbain, D. A., Cutler, R. B., Rosomoff, H. L., & Rosomoff, R. S. (1997). Pain facilities: A review of their effectiveness and referral selection criteria. *Current Review of Pain, 1*, 107–115.

Fishbain, D. A., Cutler, R. B., Rosomoff, H. L., & Rosomoff, R. S. (1998c). Comorbid psychiatric disorders in chronic pain patients with psychoactive substance use disorders. *The Pain Clinic, 11*(2), 79–87.

Fishbain, D. A., Cutler, R. B., Rosomoff, H. L., & Rosomoff, R. S. (1998b). Comorbidity between psychiatric disorders and chronic pain. *Current Review of Pain, 2*, 1–10.

Fishbain, D. A., Cutler, R. B., Rosomoff, H. L., & Rosomoff, R. S. (1998a). Validity of self-reported drug use in chronic pain patients. *Clinical Journal of Pain, 15*(3), 184–191.

Fishbain, D. A., Cutler, R. B., Rosomoff, H. L., & Rosomoff RS. (1999). Can patients taking opioids drive safely? A structured evidence-based review. *Journal of Pain & Palliative Care Pharmacotherapy, 16*(1), 9–28.

Fishbain, D. A., Cutler, R. B., Rosomoff, H. L., & Rosomoff, R. S. (2003). Are opioid-dependent/tolerant patients impaired in driving-related skills? A structured evidence-based review. *Journal of Pain and Symptom Management, 25*(6), 559–577.

Fishbain, D. A., Goldberg, M., Meager, B. R., & Rosomoff, H. (1986). Male and female chronic pain patients categorized by DSM-III psychiatric diagnostic criteria. *Pain, 26*, 181–197.

Fishbain, D. A., Rosomoff, H. L., & Rosomoff, R. S. (1992a). Detoxification of nonopiate drugs in the chronic pain setting and clonidine opiate detoxification. *Clinical Journal of Pain, 8*, 191–203.

Fishbain, D. A., Rosomoff, H. L., & Rosomoff, R. S. (1992b). Drug abuse, dependence, and addiction in chronic pain patients. *Clinical Journal of Pain, 8*, 77–85.

Fishbain, D. A., Rosomoff, H. L., Rosomoff, R. S., & Cutler, R. B. (1993). Opiate detoxification protocols, a clinical manual. *Annals of Clinical Psychiatry, 3*(1), 53–65.

Fishbain, D. A., Rosomoff, H. L., Rosomoff, R. S., & Cutler, R. B. (1995). Types of pain treatment facilities and referral selection criteria, a review. *Archives of Family Medicine, 4*, 58–66.

Fishman, S. M., & Kreis, P. G. The opioid contract. *Clinical Journal of Pain, 18*(Suppl. 4), S70–S75.

Fishman, S., Wilsey, B., Yang, J., Reisfield, G., Bandman, T., & Borsook, D. (2000). Adherence monitoring and drug surveillance in chronic opioid therapy. *Journal of Pain and Symptom Management, 20*(4), 293–305.

France, R. D., Urban, B. J., & Keefe, F. J. (1984). Long-term use of narcotic analgesics in chronic pain. *Social Science and Medicine, 19*, 1379–1382.

Gardner, E. (1997). Brain reward mechanisms. In J. Lowinson, P. Luiz, R. Millman, & J. Langrod (Eds.). *Substance abuse* (3rd ed.). Baltimore: Williams & Wilkins.

Goldman, B. (1993). Use and abuse of opioid analgesics in chronic pain. *Canadian Family Physician, 131*, 151–158.

Goldman, D. (1996, April 5). Genetic variation linked to addiction prone. *Clinical Psychiatry News*.

Graven, S., de Vet, H., van Kleef, M., & Weber, W. (2000). *Proceedings of the 9th world congress on pain, progress in pain research and management, 16*, 965–972.

Greer, S., Dalton, J., Carlson, J., & Youngblood, R. (2001). Surgical patients' fear of addiction to pain medication: the effect of an educational program for clinicians. *Clinical Journal of Pain, 17*, 157–164.

Haddox, J. D., Cone, E. J., Fant, R. V., Rohay, J. M., Caplan, Y. H., Ballina, M., et al. (2003). Oxycodone involvement in deaths from drug abuse using a DAWN-based classification system (Abstract No. 29, p. 70). American Academy Pain Medicine annual meeting, Chicago.

Heiskanen, T. E., Ruesmaki, P. M., Seppala, T. A., & Kalso, E. A. (2000). Morphine or oxycodone in cancer pain? *Acta Oncologica, 39*(8), 941–947.

Hoffmann, N. G., Olofsson, O., Salen, B., & Wickstrom, L. (1995a). Prevalence of abuse and dependency in chronic pain patients. *International Journal of Addiction, 30*(8), 919–927.

Hoffmann, N. G., Olofsson, O., Salen, B., et al. (1995b). Prevalence of abuse and dependency in chronic pain patients. *International Journal of Addiction, 30*, 919–927.

Jaffee, J. (1992). Opiates: Clinical aspects. In J. Lowenson, P. Ruiz, & R. Mullman (Eds.). *Substance abuse: A comprehensive text* (pp. 186–194). Baltimore: Williams & Wilkins.

Jamison, R. N., Raymond, S. A., & Slowsby, E. A. (1998). Opioid therapy for chronic noncancer back pain; a randomized prospective study. *Spine, 23*, 2591–2600.

Joranson, D. E., Ryan, K. M., Gilson, A. M., & Dahl, J. L. (2000). Trends in medical use and abuse of opioid analgesics. *Journal of the American Medical Association, 283*(13), 1710–1714.

Katon, W., Egan, K., & Millder, D. (1985). Chronic pain: Lifetime psychiatric diagnoses and family history. *American Journal of Psychiatry, 142*, 1156–1160.

Katz, N. P., Sherburne, S., Beach, M., Rose, R. J., Vielguth, J., Bradley, J., & Fanciullo, G. J. (2003). Behavioral monitoring and urine toxicology testing in patients receiving long-term opioid therapy. *Anesthesia & Analgesia, 97*(4)1097–1102.

Katz, N., & Fanciullo, G. J. (2002). Role of urine toxicology testing in the management of chronic opioid therapy. *Clinical Journal of Pain, 18*(Suppl. 4), S76–S82.

Kell, M. (1992). Long-term methadone maintenance for intractable nonmalignant pain. *American Journal of Pain Management, 4*, 10–16.

Khatami, M., Woody, G., & O'Brien, C. (1979). Chronic pain and narcotic addiction: A multitherapeutic approach — A pilot study. *Comprehensive Psychiatry, 20*(1), 55–60.

Kirsh, K. L., Whitcomb, L. A., Donaghy, K., & Passik, S. (2002). Abuse and addiction issues in medically ill patients with pain: Attempts at clarification of terms and empirical study. *Clinical Journal of Pain, 18*, S52–S60.

Kouyanou, K., Pither, C. E., & Wessely, S. (1997). Medication misuse, abuse and dependence in chronic pain patients. *Journal of Psychosomatic Research, 43*(5), 497–504.

Kreek, M. J. (2002, June 7). Some people come equipped with addiction fighting gene. *Psychiatric News*, p. 16.

Kreek, M., & Koob, G. F. (1998). Drug dependence: Stress and dysregulation of brain reward pathways. *Drug and Alcohol Dependence, 51*, 21–47.

Li, V., Katragadda, R., Mehrotra, D., Mosuro, Y., & Friedman, R. (2001). Pain and addiction: Screening patients at risk. *Pain Medicine, 2*(3).

Ling, W., McLellan, T., & Woody, G. E. (1987). Assessing pathological detoxification fear among methadone maintenance patients: The DFSS. *Clinical Journal of Pain, 43*, 528–539.

Lu, C., Urban, B., & France, R. D. (1988). Long-term use of narcotic analgesics in chronic pain. *Social Science and Medicine, 19*, 1379–1382.

Ludwig, A. M. (1980). *Principles of clinical psychiatry.* New York: Free Press.

Magni, G., Caldieron, C., & Regatti-Luchini, S. (1990). Chronic musculoskeletal pain and depressive symptoms in the general population: An analysis of the First National Health and Nutrition Examination Survey data. *Pain, 43*, 299–307.

McCarberg, B. H., & Laskin, M. (2001). Opioid tracking in a managed care environment (Abstract 788). American Pain Society 20th Annual Scientific Meeting, Phoenix, April 19–22.

Medina, J. L., & Diamond, S. (1977). Drug dependency in patients with chronic headache. *Headache, 17*, 12–14.

Merikangas, K. R., & Gelernter, C. S. (1990). Comorbidity for alcoholism and depression. *Psychiatric Clinics of North America, 13*(4), 613–631.

Milligan, K., Lanteri-Minet, M., Borchert, K., Helmers, H., Royden, D., Hans-Georg, K., et al. (2001). Evaluation of long-term efficacy and safety of transdermal fentanyl in the treatment of chronic noncancer pain. *Journal of Pain, 2*(4), 197–204.

Moulin, D. E., Lezzi, A., Amireh, R., Sharpe, W., Boyd, D., & Merskey, H. (1996). Randomised trial of oral morphine for chronic non-cancer pain. *Lancet, 347*, 143–147.

Nedejkovic, S. S., Wasan, A., & Jamison, R. N. (2002). Assessment of efficacy of long-term opioid therapy in pain patients with substance abuse potential. *Clinical Journal of Pain, 18*, S39–S51.

Newman, R. G. (1983). The need to redefine "addiction." *New England Journal of Medicine, 18*, 1096–1098.

Nurnberger, J. I., Foroud, T., Flury, L., Su, J., Meyer, E. T., Kuolung, H., et al. (2001). Evidence for a locus on chromosome 1 that influences vulnerability to alcoholism and affective disorder. *American Journal of Psychiatry, 158*, 718–724.

Passik, S. D., Kirsh, K. L., McDonald, M. V., Ahn, S., Russak, S. M., Martin, L., et al. (2000). A pilot survey of aberrant drug-taking attitudes and behaviors in samples of cancer and AIDS patients. *Journal of Pain and Symptom Management, 19*(4), 274–286.

Passik, S. D., Kirsh, K. L., Whitcomb, L., Dickerson, P. K., & Theobald, D. E. (2002). Pain clinicians' ranking of aberrant drug-taking behaviors. *Journal of Pain & Palliative Care Pharmacotherapy, 16*(4), 39–49.

Passik, S. D., Schreiber, J., Kirsch, K. L., et al. (2000). A chart review of the ordering or urine toxicology screens in a cancer center: Do they influence pain management? *Journal of Pain and Symptom Management, 19*, 40–44.

Passik, S. D., Whitcomb, L., Kirsh, K., Ciesla, G., Kleinman, L., Vallow, S., & Portenoy, R. (2002). An assessment and documentation tool for chronic nonmalignant pain in patients treated with opioids. Paper presented at the International Conference of Pain & Chemical Dependency, New York, June 6–8.

Perry, S., & Heidrich, G. (1982). Management of pain during debridement: A survey of US burn units. *Pain, 13*, 267–280.

Physician manual: An information outline of the controlled substance/act. (1990, March). p. 21.

Pokorny, A. D., Miller, B. A., & Kaplan, H. B. (1972). Testing for alcoholics. The brief MAST: A shortened version of the Michigan Alcoholism Test. *American Journal of Psychiatry, 129*, 342–345.

Portenoy, R. (1989). Opioid therapy in the management of chronic back pain. In C. D. Tollison (Ed.), *Interdisciplinary rehabilitation of low back pain* (pp. 137–157). Baltimore: Williams & Wilkins.

Portenoy, R. K. (1990). Chronic opioid therapy in nonmalignant pain. *Journal of Pain and Symptom Management, 5*(S1), S46–S62.

Portenoy, R. K. (1993). Opioid therapy for chronic nonmalignant pain: A review of the critical issues. *Journal of Pain & Symptom Management, 11*(4), 203–217.

Portenoy, R. K. (1994). Opioid therapy for chronic nonmalignant pain; current status. In H. L. Fields, & J. C. Liebeskind (Eds.), *Progress in pain research and management* (Vol. 1). *Pharmacological approaches to the treatment of chronic pain: New concepts and critical issues.* Seattle: IASP Press.

Portenoy, R. K., & Foley, K. (1986). Chronic use of opioid analgesics in non-malignant pain: Report of 38 cases. *Pain, 25*, 171–186.

Porter, J., & Jick, H. (1980). Addiction rare in patients treated with narcotics. *New England Journal of Medicine, 302*, 123.

Raffi, A., Haller, D., & Poklis, A. (1990). Incidence of recreational drug use among chronic pain clinic patients (Abstract 33). Presented at the American Pain Society Ninth Annual Meeting.

Raggi, R. P. (2001). Methadone therapy compliance as a clinical measurement of chemical dependency (A6618, p. 5). Presented at American Pain Society meeting, San Diego.

Regier, D., Meyers, J. K., & Kramer, M. (1984). The ninth epidemiological catchment area study. *Archives of General Psychology, 41*, 934–958.

Reid, M. C., Engles-Horton, L. L., Weber, M. B., et al. (2002). Use of opioid medications for chronic noncancer pain syndromes in primary care. *Journal of General Internal Medicine, 17*(3), 173–179.

Rinaldi, R. C., Steindler, E. M., Wilford, B. B., & Goodwin, D. (1988). Clarification and standardization of substance abuse terminology. *Journal of the American Medical Association, 259*, 557–562.

Robinson, R. C., Gatchel, R. J., Polatin, P., Deschner, M., Noe, C., & Noor, G. (2001). Screening for problematic prescription opioid use. *Clinical Journal of Pain, 17*, 220–228.

Savage, S. R. (1993). Addiction in the treatment of pain: significance, recognition, and management. *Journal of Pain & Symptom Management, 8*(5), 265–278.

Savage, S. R. (1999). Opioid use in the management of chronic pain. *Chronic Pain, 83*(3), 761–787.

Savage, S. R. (2002). Assessment for addiction in pain-treatment settings. *Clinical Journal of Pain, 18*, 528–538.

Schaffer-Vargas, G., Schaffer, S., Mejia, A., & Fernandez, C. (1999). Opioid for non-malignant pain experience of Venezuelan center (Abstract No. 289, p. 345). 9th World Congress on Pain.

Sees, K. L., & Clark, H. W. (1993). Opioid use in the treatment of chronic pain; assessment of addiction. *Journal of Pain & Symptom Management, 8*(5), 257–264.

Skinner, H. A. (1982). The drug abuse screening test. *Addictive Behaviors, 7*, 363–371.

Soumerai, S. B. (2003). Long-term benzodiazepine use: Dosage escalation fears misplaced? *Psychiatric Services, 54*, 1006–1011.

Steinweg, D. L., & Worth, H. (1993). Alcoholism: Keys to the CAGE. *Addictive Behaviors, 18*, 520–523.

Taub, A. (1982). Opioid analgesics in the treatment of chronic intractable pain of nonneoplastic origin. In L. M. Kitahata (Ed.), *Narcotic analgesics in anesthesiology* (pp. 199–208). Baltimore: Williams & Wilkins.

Tennant, F. S., & Rawson, R. A. (1982). Outpatient treatment of prescription opioid dependence: comparison of two methods. *Archives of Internal Medicine, 142*, 1845–1847.

Tennant, F. S., Jr., & Uelman, G. F. (1983). Narcotic maintenance for chronic pain: Medical and legal guidelines. *Postgraduate Medicine, 73*, 81–94.

Tennant, F. S., Jr., Robinson, D., Sagherian, A., & Seecof, R. (1988, January/February). Chronic opioid treatment of intractable, non-malignant pain. *Pain Management*, pp. 18–36.

Tennant, F., Herman, L., Silliman, L., & Reinking, J. (2002, November/December). Identifying pain-drug abusers and addicts. *Practical Pain Management*, pp. 21–26.

Urban, B. J., France, R. D., Steinberger, E. K., Scott, D. L., & Maltbie, A. A. (1986). Long-term use of narcotic/antidepressant medication in the management of phantom limb pain. *Pain, 24*, 191–196.

Vaglienti, R. M., Huber, S. J., Noel, K. R., & Johnstone, R. E. (2003). Misuse of prescribed controlled substances defined by urinalysis. *West Virginia Medical Journal, 99*(2), 67–70.

Weaver, M. F., & Schnoll, S. H. (2002). Opioid treatment of chronic pain in patients with addiction. *Journal of Pain & Palliative Care Pharmacotherapy, 16*(3), 5–26.

Weinstein, S. M., Laux, L. F., Thornby, J. I., Lorimor, R. J., Hill, C. S., Thorpe, D. M., & Merrill, J. M. (2000). Physicians' attitudes toward pain and the use of opioid analgesics: Results of a survey from the Texas cancer pain initiative. *Southern Medical Journal, 93*(5), 479–487.

Weissman, D. H., & Haddox, J. D. (1989). Opioid pseudoaddiction — An iatrogenic syndrome. *Pain, 36*(3), 363–366.

Zacny, J. (2003, April). Abuse liability of oxycodone nil at acute doses. *Clinical Psychiatry News*, p. 63.

Zenz, M., Strumpf, M., & Tryba, M. (1992). Long-term oral opioid therapy in patients with chronic nonmalignant pain. *Journal of Pain and Symptom Management, 7*(2), 69–77.

11

Opioid Therapy for Chronic Noncancer Pain: Cautions, Concerns, Misconceptions, and Potential Myths

Michael E. Clark, PhD, Robert W. Young, Jr., PhD, and B. Eliot Cole, MD, MPA

INTRODUCTION

In the last decade there has been a substantial increase in the use of opioids for the treatment of chronic noncancer pain. In 1999, approximately 11% of individuals experiencing back or neck pain consumed opioid analgesics (Luo et al., 2004). Clark (2002) found that among U.S. military veterans, 44% of the individuals with chronic noncancer pain (CNCP) were receiving opioid analgesics. Sales of opioids in the United States have increased dramatically, with opioid analgesic revenues increasing 18% between 2001 and 2002, and 136% from 1998 (Savage, 2002). This increase in opioid usage parallels the success of national efforts to make opioid analgesics more available to individuals with cancer pain and terminal illnesses, coupled with changes in the accreditation standards for health care organizations (Joint Commission on Accreditation of Healthcare Organizations [JCAHO], 2000), recommendations by the Federation of State Medical Boards of the United States (FSMBUS, 1998), public statements by leading pain organizations and regulatory agencies (American Pain Society and American Academy of Pain Medicine, 1996; American Pain Society, American Academy of Pain Medicine, and American Society of Addiction Medicine, 2001, 2004), medical board actions (*OR Medical Board v Paul Bilder*, 1999, 2003), and civil suits (*Bergman v Chin*, 2001 and *Tomlinson v Whitney*, 2003) for the undertreatment of cancer-related pain. By the end of the 1990s and the beginning of the new millennium

the "perfect storm" conditions existed to make long-term administration of opioid analgesics an acceptable part of the overall management of pain for hundreds of thousands of Americans. Yet, the routine use of opioid therapy (OT) in the treatment of chronic noncancer pain remains a controversial and contentious issue. The increasing abuse of opioids by people with and without long-term pain has resulted in growing national concern and even prosecution of practitioners deemed to have been lax in their prescribing practices. Proponents and opponents for OT now abound, often substituting their unique fervor for scientific evidence.

Empirical data clearly indicate that there are numerous disadvantages and even dangers associated with opioid use. In this chapter we review some of these less-publicized data in order to heighten practitioners' awareness of these issues and to promote informed and balanced clinical decision making. Those now prescribing OT for their patients should note, however, that we do not offer an exhaustive review of all documented untoward effects of OT. For example, we do not address the multitude of common, less serious, and potentially controllable adverse effects associated with opioid use that are listed in standard pharmaceutical textbooks and product information sheets. Instead, we focus on considerations and effects with which practitioners may be less familiar and on opioid-related issues where misinformation likely abounds. Our primary purpose in writing this chapter is to address clinical issues associated with chronic daily consumption of opioid analgesics rather than their occasional short-term use as might be used in acute pain interventions.

In the following pages we present eight major concerns relating to the use of OT for the treatment of CNCP, and within each area we cite empirical data supporting our concerns. Following each concern we present recommendations for practitioners based on the available data and a conservative practice model. While these recommendations are not codified into laws, regulations, or rules in all cases, they are nevertheless our best attempt to present a framework for the therapeutic management of CNCP. We acknowledge that our beliefs, cautions, and recommendations may be just as controversial as the current drive to use OT.

CONCERNS ASSOCIATED WITH OT FOR CHRONIC, NONCANCER PAIN

NO PUBLISHED DATA FROM RANDOMIZED CONTROLLED TRIALS INDICATING THAT OT RESULTS IN LONG-TERM PAIN RELIEF FOR INDIVIDUALS WITH CNCP

Consistent with clinical guidelines evidentiary rules, randomized, double-blinded, controlled studies (RCTs) are the standard for evaluating the effectiveness of treatment interventions (Nedeljkovic, Wasan, & Jamison, 2002). RCTs minimize error and maximize estimates of specific pharmaceutical effects by requiring, at a minimum, random subject assignment, no subject or experimenter knowledge as to which group they are in (i.e., "double blinded"), and comparisons between the experimental group and one or more control groups. Control groups may represent other pharmaceutical agents, current "standard of care" practices, alternative dosing approaches, or active or inactive placebo treatments.

In identifying studies for consideration in this section, we limited our literature searches to randomized, double-blinded, controlled studies of OT with individuals with CNCP. Furthermore, because our interest was in long-term OT, we limited our search to studies using oral opioids. Searches were conducted using Medline, PubMed, PsychInfo, and Google (a popular Internet search engine), and we also consulted the reference sections of published CNCP clinical guidelines. We operationalized "long-term" as trials of at least 6 months in length. Although one could argue that because OT for CNCP may last years or even decades, long-term opioid RCTs should span periods of at least several years, given the impracticality of such lengthy trials we elected to use a more practical definition.

OT and the RCT Literature

Consistent with other reports (Ballantyne & Mao, 2003; Harden, 2002), we were unable to locate any studies meeting our RCT and long-term criteria despite decades of OT research. To date, randomized, double-blinded, RCT stud-

ies have all been relatively brief (generally only weeks). The lack of long-term opioid RCT data is particularly surprising given that a number of well-known pain professionals and researchers have called for such research for well over a decade (Turk & Brody, 1991).

Given the lack of long-term studies, we next searched the literature for RCT studies of any length that met our selection criteria. A total of 18 studies were identified and form the foundation of evidence supporting short-term opioid effectiveness. Each study then was examined in detail. In evaluating these studies it is important to note that many break study blinds after relatively short time periods, although data collection may continue. In such investigations only the blinded portion of the study was considered as part of the actual RCT.

A summary of these 18 studies is presented in Table 11.1. As is evident in the table, RCT periods have been uniformly brief, with none exceeding 9 weeks. The average RCT period over all tabled studies was only 3.74 weeks. Thus, estimates of long-term OT effectiveness rely solely on the effectiveness data reported in these relatively brief RCT studies. Additionally, our detailed examination of these studies yielded evidence of a host of methodological limitations and procedural problems, some of which are serious enough to jeopardize conclusions that OT is effective even in the short term. The most significant of these methodological problems are listed below.

High RCT Termination Rates

RCT studies of OT with CNCP have identified subject termination rates of up to 53% (Roth et al., 2000). Dropout rates for the RCT studies included in this review are presented in Table 11.1. To provide a better estimate of "real-world" effectiveness, when a placebo-controlled parallel groups design (i.e., two experimental groups, one of which is administered placebo and the other an opioid analgesic) was employed, rates were computed only for the opioid conditions of the tabled studies. Termination rates for crossover studies (i.e., all subjects experience all experimental conditions), in contrast, were based on both the opioid and the placebo periods. Although there is considerable variation in these rates, as indicated in Table 11.1, on the average approximately one third of participants dropped out of these short-term studies. These high subject termination rates probably reflect, at least in part, the frequent adverse effects associated with OT. Adverse effects occur on the average in about 50% of subjects, although rates in excess of 90% have been observed (Hale et al., 1999). Even though most adverse effects can be successfully managed, they complicate treatment and may lead to reduced compliance or potential opioid termination. Individuals who terminate OT represent real-world treatment failures, and it is reasonable to expect that the number of individuals dropping out of OT in clinical settings over longer time periods is even higher than dropout

TABLE 11.1
RCT Duration, Sample Size, and Dropout Rates in OT Studies

Study	RCT duration	No. enrolled in opioid arm(s)	No. completing opioid trial	Type of placebo	Opioid drop-out rate(s)
Arkinstall et al., 1995	1 week	46	30	Inactive	35%
Caldwell et al., 1999*	4 weeks	112	35	Inactive	69%
Caldwell et al., 2002	4 weeks	222	134	Inactive	40%
Hale et al., 1999*	2 weeks	57	44	None	37%
Huse et al., 2001	4 weeks	12	12	Inactive	0%
Kjaersgaard-Anderson et al., 1990	4 weeks	83	40	None	52%
Maier et al., 2002	2 weeks	49	37	Inactive	25%
Morley-Forster et al., 2003	20 days	19	11	Inactive	42%
Moulin et al., 1996*	9 weeks	61	43	Active	30%
Muller et al., 1998	2 weeks	55	54	None	2%
Mullican & Lacey, 2001	4 weeks	462	369	None	20%
Peloso et al., 2000	4 weeks	51	31	Inactive	39%
Roth et al., 2000	2 weeks	88	45	Inactive	51%
Rowbotham et al., 2003	8 weeks	81	59	None	27%
Sindrup et al., 1999	4 weeks	48	34	Inactive	29%
Thurel et al., 1991	2 weeks	50	41	None	18%
Watson & Babul, 1998	4 weeks	50	38	Inactive	24%
Watson et al., 2003	8 weeks	45	24	Active	47%
Means	3.74 weeks	85	58		33%

* Dropout rate includes dropouts during the titration period in these studies.

rates reported for short-term RCTs. In fact, Cowan and colleagues (2003) found that among 104 patients with CNCP treated at a pain clinic in England over an average of 14 months, 86.5% reported at least temporary cessation of their treatment, while 65% ceased OT permanently. Thus, while on the average about one third of participants drop out of short-term opioid RCTs, long-term clinical treatment probably results in higher rates of termination and, subsequently, higher failure rates.

One way to correct for high rates of treatment termination is to conduct *intent to treat* analyses. These corrective procedures include treatment dropouts in overall clinical trial efficacy calculations (Dworkin et al., 2001). Although the criteria and strategies for conducting these analyses vary (Dworkin et al., 2001), in general they provide a more realistic estimate of the overall effectiveness of the treatment. When studies fail to conduct such analyses, but experience significant subject dropout over the course of the trial, effectiveness likely will be exaggerated. Of the 18 RCT studies listed in Table 11.1, only 5 included intent to treat analyses in their methodologies, and the intent is even less common in non-RCT clinical studies. As a result, overall impressions of the efficacy of OT for the treatment of CNCP likely are overestimated.

Small Sample Sizes

Sample sizes employed in RCT studies of OT, with a few exceptions, have been small. As illustrated in Table 11.1,

50% of the tabled studies had fewer than 40 subjects complete the opioid trials, and 2 of the 18 studies reported fewer than 15 completers. As a result, associated findings may be less reliable and may be influenced greatly by characteristics of the participants (e.g., sex, race, age). The impact of small sample sizes is magnified by the practice of consolidating multiple pain types within studies. When sample size is small and one or more types of pain are over- or underrepresented, OT effects may be underestimated or overestimated if those pain conditions are differentially responsive to opioids. These sources of variation limit the generalizability of the results of smaller studies to CNCP populations beyond the research study subject pool.

Limited Reproducibility of Results

One of the foundations of the scientific method is reproducibility of results. Related to this requirement, studies must provide sufficient information concerning the procedures and measures employed to allow others to undertake replication of the investigation. A corollary of this principle implies that measures used in the study should be validated and generally available to other researchers. Furthermore, to compare results across studies of a similar nature (e.g., CNCP OT studies), core dependent variables should be similar to measures used in other investigations, and comparisons of effects (e.g., placebo vs. an active agent) should be comparable. Unfortunately, among the

18 tabled RCT studies, the majority failed to meet one or more of these standards. Four studies provided an incomplete or unclear methodology, five did not report changes in pain from baseline values, and eight relied on nonstandard pain intensity measures or used derivative measures that preclude direct comparisons with other studies.

Use of Opioid Rescue Medications

Controlled trials, whether contrasting the effects of opioids versus placebos, other active pharmaceuticals, or alternative methods of care, are conducted to evaluate the utility of specific analgesics. However, 4 of the 18 core RCT studies allowed the use of opioid rescue medications during treatment. This introduces another treatment variable into the study and prevents attributions of changes in pain intensity or pain-related functioning solely to the opioid agent(s) used in the treatment group(s).

Ineffective Blinding Procedures

In any controlled study, but particularly in placebo-controlled studies, effective blinding of the subjects and investigators is of critical importance. If subjects or experimenters are able to guess which group is the active treatment group, systematic biases may be introduced into the results particularly when subjective measures such as pain intensity, mood, or perceived impairment are used. As indicated in Table 11.1, the vast majority of RCT placebo studies examining the effectiveness of OT for treating CNCP have used *inactive placebos* as a comparison treatment. Inactive placebos may not be an appropriate control group as their inert nature may aid participants in identifying which group they are in and thereby jeopardize the study's blind assignment (Dworkin et al., 2001). They are particularly problematic in crossover studies where subjects have been exposed to both the active and inactive treatments and therefore may be better able to identify active agents based on adverse effects as well as any pain relief actions. The use of opioid rescue medications also may contribute to blinding problems in inactive placebo studies as subjects' use of the opioids may be accompanied by internal sensations that are not experienced after taking the inactive placebo.

The potential impact of this issue is evident when considering the results of the minority of studies that have assessed the integrity of their blinding procedures. To accomplish this, investigators typically ask subjects to indicate which treatment arm they were involved in (in parallel studies) or which condition included the active agent (in crossover studies). This method provides a means of estimating the success of the blinding. The results of these assessments raise questions concerning the reliability of the blinding procedures used in these core OT studies. For example, Huse and colleagues (2001) reported that the majority of study patients and all of the study physicians in their investigation comparing morphine sulfate with inactive placebo were able to correctly identify the opioid treatment. Maier and colleagues (2002), in a comparison of the effectiveness of sustained-release morphine and inactive placebo, reported that *93% of the subjects* identified correctly their involvement in the morphine arm of the study, along with 87% of the physicians and 89% of the psychologists. Attal (2000), in an opioid infusion RCT not presented in Table 11.1, reported somewhat better blind maintenance in that only 7 of 15 subjects accurately identified the opioid treatment group, while 6 were unsure and 2 believed the inactive placebo represented the active agent. Nevertheless, in this same study the examiner correctly identified the opioid treatment group in 10 of 15 cases and inaccurately identified the placebo treatment as the active condition in only 1 case. Overall, these results call into question the success of blinding procedures used in inactive placebo RCTs. Subjects or experimenters who are aware of their actual treatment condition may introduce bias in dependent measures consistent with their underlying beliefs concerning opioid effects.

One potential solution to this problem of ineffective blinding involves the use of an *active placebo* as the opioid comparison group. An active placebo is a pharmaceutical selected based on similarities between its adverse effects profile and that of the opioid under study. If ineffective blinding due to the use of inactive placebos occurs, one would expect to find increased pain reduction when appropriate active placebos are employed. In the CNCP OT literature we could identify only two studies that used an active placebo (benztropine). In the first study (Moulin et al., 1996), the authors found that following the opioid to placebo crossover, the pain intensity scores of active placebo subjects actually were *lower* than those of opioid subjects (see Figure 11.1, weeks 15 through 20), suggesting that either their crossover procedures failed or that morphine was no more effective than the active placebo in reducing pain. The fact that Moulin and colleagues also systematically assessed the integrity of their blinding procedures and reported that 47.8% of subjects and 67.4% of investigators correctly identified treatment with morphine suggested that the blind was only partially successful. In the second study (Watson et al., 2003), which examined opioid efficacy with neuropathic pain, the active placebo subjects experienced substantially less pain reduction than the opioid group. However, when they assessed the integrity of their blinding procedure, they found that 88% of their subjects and investigators correctly identified the opioid condition. Thus, in this case the blind clearly was not maintained despite the use of a placebo with an adverse effects profile similar to the opioid analgesic, and the advantage of opioid over placebo that they reported may have reflected subject and experimenter bias. They also commented on the special difficulties maintaining study blinds in crossover trials, even when active placebos are used, due to subject and experimenter exposure to both conditions.

The failure of opioid RCT double-blinding procedures may account for the relatively low levels of pain reduction associated with inactive placebos. We examined this possibility by averaging mean pain reductions from baseline for inactive placebo subjects in the nine studies where such data either were reported or could be computed from values presented in tables or figures. The average pain reduction associated with placebos over these studies was 10.4%, which is substantially smaller than the more typical 25 to 30% placebo effect observed in subjective measures used in other pharmaceutical agent studies (de Craen et al., 2000; Rickels & Schweizer, 1998). We then calculated the mean inactive placebo pain reduction for the two studies where the blinds were severely compromised (Huse et al., 2001; Maier et al., 2002) and compared it with the mean reduction found in the third inactive placebo study that was only partially compromised (Attal, 2000). As expected, the placebo effect for the seriously compromised studies (10.2%) was substantially smaller than the size found in the partially compromised study (24%). Although the latter study was evaluating the efficacy of opioid infusion rather than oral agents, the results are at least suggestive that blinding success may affect placebo success.

It is clear that RCT OT studies that fail to maintain subject and experimenter blinds are subject to biases that potentially invalidate their results. In the opioid RCT literature, all five of the studies that have examined the integrity of their blinds reported evidence suggestive of at least partial blind failure. This occurred even when active placebos were used. Blinding difficulties likely are maximized in crossover studies where participants have the opportunity to experience both experimental conditions (usually a placebo and an opioid treatment). *Ideally, all RCT studies should systematically assess the integrity of their blinding procedures and use data only from subjects and experimenters who are unable to differentiate (i.e., either they are incorrect or they are unable to decide) between the placebo and the opioid condition.* Although this would necessitate an increased sample size, it would provide some degree of assurance that subject and experimenter bias is minimized and that differences observed between an opioids and a placebo, or between an opioid and an alternative pain medication, reflect a real difference in efficacy. Use of appropriate active placebos either alone or in combination with a nonsteroidal anti-inflammatory drug (NSAID) in these experiments might enhance the reliability of experimental blinds and more accurately identify the pain reduction advantages specific to opioids. Until such studies are conducted, current data suggest that the findings from all opioid RCT studies conducted thus far are subject to question and that more attention needs to be devoted to this potential confound.

Longer-Term Opioid Studies

Generally, studies that do not meet the double-blinded, placebo-controlled, RCT standards have reported more favorable, longer-term OT outcomes. For example, Jamison, Raymond, Slawsby, Nedeljkovic, and Katz (1998), in a randomized but nondouble-blinded study of individuals with back pain, reported that OT was associated with decreased pain and improved mood (but not activity) when compared with naproxen during 16 weeks of treatment. Schofferman (1999), in a noncontrolled study, reported reduced pain and enhanced self-reported functioning in a sample in 21 of 33 individuals with chronic pain treated with a 6- to 12-week opioid trial. After 1-year of opioid maintenance therapy, the 21 responders continued to report reduced pain and improved function.

Several of the opioid RCT studies reported results for open-label extensions of their original investigation. Caldwell and associates (2002) treated 131 subjects with osteoarthritis pain completing the RCT component of their study with an opioid over 36 weeks and reported sustained pain reduction on the order of 10 to 15%. Huse and colleagues (2001) followed 9 of their original 12 patients with phantom limb pain who remained on morphine following conclusion of the RCT over a period of 12 months. They reported significant and sustained pain reduction (relative to baseline) for subjects. Roth et al. (2000) enrolled 106 patients with osteoarthritis in an open-label, 6-month extension of their original study of oxycodone and reported good long-term pain relief.

Although the results of all of these longer-term studies reported support for the efficacy of OT, their value is limited by their susceptibility to a variety of confounding effects. Indeed, placebo effects alone can exceed 32% in opioid studies (Clegg et al., 1996), indicating that data from nonplacebo-controlled studies must be interpreted accordingly. When coupled with biases that may exist in nonblinded studies (Dworkin et al., 2001), additional caution is indicated when interpreting the results from these less rigorously controlled investigations.

In summary, there remains no well-controlled, empirically sound evidence supporting the long-term effectiveness of OT for CNCP. Studies meeting clinical guidelines' evidentiary standards for strong support (i.e., double-blinded RCT studies) have not to date extended beyond 9 weeks, and all suffer from a variety of methodological weaknesses, chief of which is questionable integrity of their double-blind conditions. There continues to be a strong need for longer duration, randomized, double-blinded, placebo-controlled studies of OT that extend at least 6 to 12 months and include systematic assessment of the integrity of the study blinds. Although such a lengthy blinded trial poses substantial challenges, without such data we cannot be certain that OT works for the long term, nor can we discriminate between good and poor OT candidates. In the interim we suggest that practitioners approach decisions regarding the use of OT for CNCP cautiously, in a manner similar to other unproven but potentially helpful interventions.

Associated Practitioner Recommendations

- Evaluate every patient's response to prior treatments and reserve OT for those individuals with moderate to severe pain who have failed alternative treatments. This is consistent with the World Health Organization's (WHO, 1990) analgesic ladder, which has received almost universal acceptance. Individuals with less severe pain, those with promising responses to other treatments, or those unable to tolerate past OT interventions might be better managed using alternative (non-opioid) means.

- Refer individuals who have not participated in rehabilitation-oriented treatments to appropriate rehabilitation providers if they are available prior to initiation of OT. Strong evidence exists that alternative interventions such as physical therapy (Cheng et al., 2002; Dias, Dias, & Ramos, 2003; Fransen, Crosbie, & Edmonds, 2001; Jull et al., 2002), cognitive-behavioral therapy (Guzman et al., 2002; van Tulder et al., 2000), and comprehensive multidisciplinary pain treatment approaches incorporating psychosocial, physical, and pharmacological interventions (Turk & Okifuji, 1998; Weir et al., 1992) are effective in managing a variety of pain conditions.

- When pain is not effectively managed by non-OT approaches, or when alternatives are not available due to patient circumstances, consider initiation of OT. When possible, use it in combination with other treatments that have demonstrated effectiveness in the treatment of chronic pain, such as exercise (Frost et al., 1998; Moffett et al., 1999) or relaxation training (Stetter & Kupper, 2002). Before initiating OT, establish with patients what outcomes (decreased pain intensity, enhanced performance of activities of daily living, or improved quality of life) will be used to determine OT success (Cole, 2002).

WHEN TOLERATED, SUCCESSFUL OT FOR CNCP RESULTS IN ONLY MODEST REDUCTIONS IN PAIN INTENSITY

A second concern regarding opioid therapy relates to the degree of pain relief attained, in that even successful opioid therapy for chronic noncancer pain results in only modest reductions in pain intensity. Table 11.2 presents the mean pain reduction (i.e., change from baseline values) reported in opioid RCTs. Note that 4 of the 18 opioid RCT studies did not provide sufficient information to compute or estimate changes in pain from baseline values. For the remaining studies, pain relief percentages presented in Table 11.2 were those reported in the text or, when not reported, were computed from study tables or estimated from study figures.

As illustrated in Table 11.2, there is wide variation in the amount of pain reduction achieved in the tabled OT studies. Individual responses to OT may range from no improvement, or even intensification of pain, to total relief. In fact, in published studies up to 38% of patients undergoing an OT trial fail to report any benefit (Harden, 2002). Examination of Table 11.2 reveals that for the 14 randomized opioid trials where relief rates were reported or could be computed, the weighted average pain relief attained was 30%, which is similar to the 32% weighted average relief reported by Turk, Loeser, and Monarch (2002) in their review of eight partially overlapping OT studies. In evaluating changes in pain attributable solely to opioid analgesics, this 30% average pain relief must be compared with the 10% average pain relief we found in response to inactive placebos. The resulting 20% average benefit of opioids relative to placebos, when considered in light of recent data regarding the clinical significance of the magnitude of pain relief (Cepeda et al., 2003) among postsurgical patients, equates with patient reports of "minimal improvement." Moreover, if the 28% pain reduction experienced by active placebo subjects reported by Watson and colleagues (2003) represents the "true" placebo effect, there would be little difference between the pain relief associated with opioids and that linked to active placebos. Furthermore, consider that these pain relief estimates for OT are only for those who complete treatment. Individuals who drop out of treatment may well experience less relief, but this lower level of efficacy will not be reflected in data derived from only those who complete an OT trial.

Reported rates of opioid-related pain relief also must be considered with respect the reduced efficacy of opioids over time. In general, we know that the magnitude of pain reduction associated with stable-dose OT decreases with increasing duration of use due to the development of tolerance (Ballantyne & Mao, 2003). Tolerance refers to the need to escalate opioid doses over time to obtain constant analgesic effects. Tolerance frequently occurs in response to OT, and studies that allow dose titration over longer trial periods typically report dose escalation (Maier et al., 2002; Peloso et al., 2000). The 22-week-long study by Moulin and associates (1996) is a good example of this effect, as tolerance clearly is evident by week 5 of the study (see their figure 1, p. 143). Therefore, short-duration opioid efficacy studies may overestimate the amount of pain relief associated with fixed opioid doses continued

TABLE 11.2
Mean Pain Relief Attained in the OT Arm of RCT Studies

Study	Sample	Pain Relief
Arkinstall et al., 1995	30 PHN patients	26%
Caldwell et al., 1999	35 OA patients[1]	43%
Caldwell et al., 2002	184 OA patients	18%
Hale et al., 1999	47 CBP patients	50%[1]
Huse et al., 2001	12 CNP patients	30%
Kjaersgaard-Anderson et al., 1990	40 OA patients	17%[2]
Maier et al., 2002	49 M-NP & NOC	33%
Morley-Forster et al., 2003	11 M-NP	10%
Peloso et al., 2000	31 OA patients	55%[3]
Roth et al., 2000	20 OA patients	21%[4]
	25 OA patients	38%[5]
Rowbotham et al., 2003	29 M-P&CNP patients	43%[6]
	30 M-P&CNP patients	22%[7]
Sindrup et al., 1999	34 PNP patients	31%[8]
Thurel et al., 1991	20 LBP patients	33%[9]
	21 LBP patients	35%[10]
Watson et al., 2003	24 DN patients	67%[11]
Weighted mean pain relief		30%

Note: PHN = Postherpetic neuralgia; OA = osteoarthritis; M-NP = mixed neuropathic pain; M-P & CNP = mixed peripheral and central neuropathic pain; NOC = nociceptive pain; PNP = polyneuropathic pain; LSP = lumbar spine pain; CBP = cervicobrachial pain; DN = diabetic neuropathy; LBP = low back pain.

[1] Reduction in daily pain intensity averaged across controlled release and immediate release oxycodone groups.

[2] Reduction in "all week pain" from baseline obtained over the 4-week treatment period and computed from Kjaersgaard-Anderson et al., 1990, Table 111.

[3] Reduction in average weekly pain intensity.

[4] Reduction in pain intensity from baseline for the low-dosage group (10 mg OxyContin capsule) from Roth et al., 2000, Figure 2.

[5] Reduction in pain intensity from baseline for the high-dosage group (20 mg OxyContin capsule) from Roth et al., 2000, Figure 2.

[6] Reduction in pain intensity from baseline for the high-dosage levorphanol group (.75 mg) from Rowbotham et al., 2003, Figure 2.

[7] Reduction in pain intensity from baseline for the low-dosage levorphanol group (.15 mg) from Rowbotham et al., 2003, Figure 2.

[8] Reduction in daily pain rating from baseline for the Tramadol group from Sindrup et al., 1999, Table 2.

[9] Reduction in pain intensity occurring between day 8 and day 15 of the treatment period for patients in the paracetamol-dextropropoxyphene group from Thurel et al., 1991, Table 2.

[10] Reduction in pain intensity occurring between day 8 and day 15 of the treatment period for patients in the paracetamol-codeine group from Thurel et al., 1991, Table 2.

[11] Reduction in pain intensity corresponding to the evaluable patients presented in Watson et al., 2003, Table 2 rather than the patients who actually completed the study.

over longer time intervals. Although the obvious clinical solution to this is to escalate the dose, there are no long-term studies that have tracked the amount of opioid increase needed to maintain stable pain reductions over long time intervals. Whether opioid tolerance plateaus, continues indefinitely, accelerates, or decelerates during long-term OT is unknown, nor can we predict which individuals may be more likely to experience it. Future research examining the mechanisms associated with the development of tolerance also needs to attend to its temporal patterns and long-term treatment implications.

Thus, opioid therapy alone rarely is a solution for CNCP complaints. Individuals who tolerate opioid therapy likely do experience short-term pain reduction on the order of 20% greater than that associated with inactive placebos, but the clinical meaningfulness of this degree of relief appears to be questionable. Additionally, it is likely that similar degrees of pain reduction will not be sustained over longer time intervals due to the effects of tolerance or other mediators of opioid response, and that actual placebo effects likely are larger than generally observed due to biases introduced by double blinding failures.

Associated Practitioner Recommendations

- Assess for changes in average pain intensity following initiation of opioid therapy and routinely reassess pain intensity throughout treatment.
- Monitor and address all adverse effects.
- Titrate therapy to provide maximum pain relief with a minimum of adverse effects.
- Discontinue the opioids if pain is unchanged or increases following dose escalations, if necessary dose escalations exceed prudent practice, or if adverse effects cannot be managed adequately.

OPIOID THERAPY HAS NOT BEEN SHOWN TO IMPROVE DAILY FUNCTIONING CONSISTENTLY EVEN WHEN PAIN INTENSITY IS REDUCED

Unlike cancer pain where the focus tends to be more on palliation, in cases of noncancer pain our primary goal most often is rehabilitation (Harden, 2002). Rehabilitation, in this context, includes not only physical capabilities and performance, but also emotional, social, and work-related functioning, and necessitates multidimensional outcomes assessment (Clark & Gironda, 2002).

Opioids and Functional Improvement

Although there are a few exceptions, initial claims that OT enhances daily functioning have not been substantiated. For example, Caldwell and colleagues (2002) evaluated changes in pain intensity, sleep, and physical function on the part of 295 individuals with osteoarthritis treated with controlled-release morphine (Avinza® or MS Contin®) or inactive placebo during a 4-week randomized trial. Improvements in sleep and reductions in pain from baseline were greater for participants receiving the controlled-release morphine products relative to the placebo group. However, no significant differences between groups emerged for the physical function measure. Huse and colleagues (2001) compared the effects of morphine sulfate to an inactive placebo in a study of 12 patients with phantom limb pain. They reported that individuals treated with morphine sulfate experienced reduced pain when compared with the placebo group. However, the attained pain reduction was unrelated to scores on measures of mood, coping, catastrophizing, or social support

and interaction. Kjaersgaard-Andersen and colleagues (1990) noted improved pain control in patients with osteoarthritis of the hip in response to codeine coupled with acetaminophen, compared with acetaminophen alone, during the first week of an OT trial that was subsequently closed due to high rates of adverse effects. However, no differences in disability or psychological measures were observed. Moulin and colleagues (1996) used an active placebo (benztropine) in their crossover study of 61 individuals with CNCP of mixed etiology treated with morphine. Despite reporting that that morphine elicited reduced pain intensity prior to crossover and led to greater pain intensity reductions from baseline following crossover, they found no significant differences between the treatment conditions in measures of mood, pain disability, or self-perceived pain-related impairment and no changes from baseline values. Sator-Katzenschlager and colleagues (2003), in a large-scale study of 477 consenting consecutive mixed pain referrals (including cancer pain) to a university pain center, used a range of interventions to reduce pain while assessing a wide range of additional outcomes. The majority of patients (63%) were treated with opioids either alone or in combination with adjuvant medications. The authors found significantly reduced pain from baseline levels through a 1-year treatment and follow-up period, along with improvement in self-reported pain avoidance and "cognitive control." However, no changes in emotional status, as measured by the Profile of Mood States (POMS), or activity from pretreatment levels were found, except for an *increase* in the POMS anger measure from pretreatment to post-treatment for men. Watson and Babul (1998) used the POMS and the Beck Depression Inventory (BDI) to assess mood changes in 50 patients with postherpetic neuralgia treated with either OxyContin or inactive placebo. Although they reported significant differences in pain intensity and in an investigator rating of disability between the OxyContin and placebo subjects, no differences in any of the POMS six mood scores or the BDI were obtained.

Not all opioid studies have failed to find evidence of functional improvement, however. For example, Arkinstall and colleagues (1995) reported improved Pain Disability Index (i.e., impairment) scores on the part of 30 patients with CNCP of varied etiology treated with 7 days of controlled-release codeine compared with 7 days of inactive placebo. Maier and associates (2002) treated 49 individuals with morphine and an inactive placebo in a randomized, double-blinded study. They reported that OT was associated with significant reductions in pain, along with improved "mood" and sleep. However, depression (which apparently was not considered to be a mood variable) and exercise endurance did not change. Peloso and colleagues (2000), in a double-blind RCT, reported improved self-ratings of physical function on the part of patients with osteoarthritis treated with controlled-release codeine compared with inactive placebo. Finally, Roth et al. (2000) reported improved pain, mood, and sleep in subjects receiving 14 days of treatment with 20-mg controlled-release oxycodone compared with inactive placebo, although significant changes were not found in measures of work, activity, walking ability, or relations with others. Haythornthwaite and associates (1998) examined emotional and cognitive changes in 19 individuals receiving long-term OT for CNCP. They found that individuals treated with long-acting opioids, when compared with "usual care" subjects, reported reduced pain, hostility, and anxiety but not depression. Although the authors interpreted the results as support for a link between long-acting OT and improved "mood," the "usual care" comparison group also was undergoing OT (albeit with short-term agents) for chronic pain during the study. Therefore, the author's findings regarding reduced hostility and anxiety may reflect the impact of factors other than OT and do not lend support to relationships between OT and functional improvement.

Opioids and Functional Decline

Overall, the results do not consistently support presumptions that reduced pain intensity secondary to successful OT leads to general functional improvement. Depression in particular appears to be least responsive to OT. And most studies reporting positive effects on at least one functional measure failed to find significant associations for other similar variables. In fact, there is evidence that functioning may *decline* among some patients treated with opioids. This has been called the *Downward Spiral Hypothesis* (Schofferman, 1999; Turner et al., 1982). Although the concept has been disputed (Ciccone et al., 2000), there is clear evidence that at least in some cases, functional decline is associated with the initiation of opioid therapy. This decline includes increased pain (Brodner & Taub, 1978; Taylor et al., 1980), reduced activity levels (Fillingim et al., 2003; Turner et al., 1982), increased depression (Fillingim et al., 2003; Finlayson et al., 1986; Jarvik et al., 1981; Sproule et al., 1999), and cognitive or motor impairment or decline (Allen et al., 2003; Bruera et al., 1989; Sjogren et al., 2000).

In recent years, the potential for OT-related cognitive decline has received increasing attention due, in part, to concerns about liability stemming from motor vehicle or machinery accidents on the part of individuals consuming opioid analgesics for pain. Overall, the literature has been markedly inconsistent, with some studies reporting potential decrements in function, particularly psychomotor speed, that were related to opioid ingestion (Allen et al., 2003; Bruera et al., 1989; Jarvik et al., 1981), while others failed to find such associations (Lorenz, Beck, & Bromm, 1997; Sabatowski et al., 2003). In the best review and integration of this topic, Chapman, Byas-Smith, and Reed

(2002) concluded that OT-related cognitive impairment, to the extent that it occurs, likely is maximized during the first days of opioid intake and declines thereafter. Unfortunately, attempts to specify direct opioid effects in these studies are complicated by a variety of confounding factors, the most prominent of which is that pain itself appears to negatively affect cognitive functioning (Vainio et al., 1995). Furthermore, it is not clear that poor performance in neuropsychological tests predicts accident proneness. Simulation studies provide a more direct method to compare effects in this area. One preliminary report of comparisons of 17 patients with chronic pain treated with OT, 13 non-opioid patients, and 49 matched pain-free controls failed to detect consistent differences in performance on simulated driving tasks (Chapman, 2001). Clearly more research is needed in this area to clarify potential relationships between OT and accident risks or other hazards. The current, limited data suggest that if there are such risks, they may be most problematic at the outset of OT and may decline thereafter.

Thus, although there are inconsistencies with respect to the specific components of the downward spiral and no data as to its prevalence among CNCP patients treated with long-term OT, substantial evidence is available to support the presence of such effects among at least some individuals. Among all CPS symptoms, depression appears to be the least likely to improve in response to OT.

In conclusion, to date the preponderance of empirical data have failed to link OT-related declines in pain intensity to enhanced function. Although there is variability in some of the results, particularly with respect to cognitive function, there is little question that physical function and pain-related coping do not necessarily improve. Data also indicate that affective changes, particularly in depression, are the least responsive to successful OT and that some individuals may exhibit a decline in function following opioid initiation. Furthermore, one must consider that almost all of the blinded, placebo-controlled OT studies assessing functional changes utilized inactive placebos with little or no assessment of the integrity of their subject blinds. This approach enhances the probability of obtaining results supporting OT-related functional improvement due to subject and experimenter biases.

Associated Practitioner Recommendations

- When initiating OT, caution patients to avoid operating vehicles or engaging in activities that might endanger themselves or others due to slowed reaction times or reduced psychomotor speed for a *minimum* of 1 week and for several days after dose escalations. Note that data are mixed regarding more persistent cognitive effects and that a conservative approach would suggest extending the period of danger.

- Routinely assess for changes in physical, cognitive, and emotional functioning following initiation of opioid therapy.
- If depression is present, be aware that even successful OT is unlikely to enhance mood and, if appropriate, consider referral to a mental health professional for treatment.
- Consider cessation of opioid therapy if pain increases or function declines.

SOME INDIVIDUALS WITH CNCP AND SUBSTANTIAL PSYCHOSOCIAL IMPAIRMENT (I.E., PATIENTS WITH CHRONIC PAIN SYNDROMES), TREATED WITH OT ACHIEVE GREATER PAIN REDUCTION AND FUNCTIONAL IMPROVEMENT FOLLOWING CESSATION OF OPIOIDS DURING MULTIDISCIPLINARY TREATMENT

Chronic pain syndromes (CPS) involve significant dysfunction across a broad spectrum of areas that typically include pain, pain-related impairment, and depression (Klapow et al., 1993) among others. Often these patients have undergone years of opioid and other treatment for their pain problems with no lasting benefit. Very little information is available concerning the rates of CPS. Although Klapow et al. found that approximately 25% of their sample of patients with chronic low back pain exhibited signs of a CPS, this issue has not been addressed directly in the literature since then. Some indirect information about these rates can be considered based on the frequency of depression, which is a hallmark symptom of a CPS, among individuals with chronic pain. For some individuals, depression is intricately linked with the experience of pain (Elliott, Renier, & Palcher, 2003), increases proportionally with increases in pain intensity (Currie & Wang, 2004), appears to potentiate the degree of pain-related disability (Currie & Wang, 2004; Ericsson et al., 2002b), and independently predicts the onset of significant back or neck pain (Carroll, Cassidy, & Cote, 2004) as well as disability status (Ericsson et al., 2002). Reid, Guo, Towle, Kerns, and Concato (2002) found that between 44 and 54% of their two independent samples of individuals with mixed chronic pain had a diagnosis of depression entered in their medical records, while Elliott et al. (2003) reported a 52% prevalence rate for depression among 242 participants in a multidisciplinary chronic pain treatment program. Thus, the high rates of depression found among individuals with chronic pain suggest that Klapow and colleagues' (1993) estimate of a 25% CPS prevalence rate likely is an underestimate. In fact, the best available evidence suggests that CPS prevalence rates fall in the 40% range (Gironda, 2004). In any event, it is clear that a significant proportion of individuals with chronic pain exhibit the broader range of dysfunction associated with CPS.

To date there have been no studies examining the short-term or long-term effectiveness of OT specifically for indi-

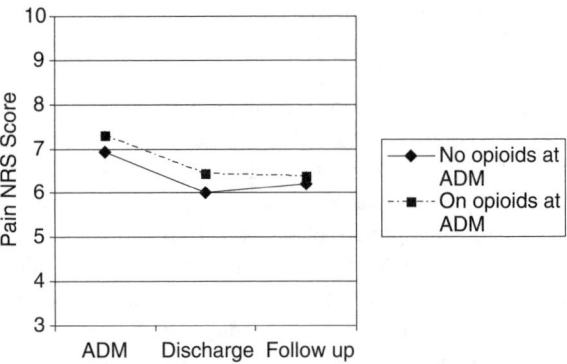

FIGURE 11.1 Mean numeric pain scores by opioid status at program admission.

viduals with a CPS. However, there now is some recent evidence that individuals with a CPS treated with OT improve after *cessation* of opioids (Clark & Gironda, 2001). In this study, 108 patients with mixed chronic pain diagnoses underwent multidisciplinary pain treatment in an 18-day, inpatient, Rehabilitation Accreditation Commission (CARF)-accredited pain program in the southeastern United States. All individuals receiving OT at admission underwent a gradual cessation of opioids during the first 7 to 10 days of treatment. Treatment emphasized physical restoration and improved pain management skills, and included a strong cognitive-behavioral focus. Multiple outcomes domain measures were administered at admission, at discharge, and at a 90-day follow up assessment.

Figure 11.1 presents the mean pain intensity scores obtained from program participants based on an 11-point numeric pain scale assessing average pain in the last week. The dotted line in the graph represents 36 patients who were taking daily opioids at admission, while the solid line reflects means for 72 patients who were not taking opioids at admission. All participants were opioid free at discharge and the 3-month follow up.

As illustrated in Figure 11.1, individuals receiving daily opioids at admission exhibited significant and equivalent reductions in pain intensity during treatment that were maintained at follow-up despite the cessation of opioids. Although pain intensity declined significantly from admission to discharge and follow up, there were no significant differences in mean pain scores between the two groups at any of the time points. Although one could hypothesize that the lack of significant differences in pain intensity at admission might have reflected the pain amelioration effects of OT, in such a case opioid cessation during treatment should have resulted in higher pain scores for these individuals at discharge and at follow up. The lack of pain intensity differences across all time points instead suggests that opioids were not contributing to pain reduction in these individuals. Thus, opioid cessation had no effect on participants' pain levels.

The ineffectiveness of opioids in this study was not confined to changes in pain intensity. Almost identical patterns were observed for measures of pain interference in activities of daily living and mobility, activity and strength, and negative affect. In each case, both groups of participants demonstrated significant and equivalent improvements in function, and there were no significant differences between the opioid and non-opioid groups at any of the three time points.

The data described above are tentative, and at present we are replicating the results in a larger sample incorporating additional measures. However, these initial results are consistent with clinician observations concerning the lack of OT-related improvement among individuals with symptoms of a CPS (Harden, 2002; Schofferman, 1993).

In summary, it is our contention that individuals with CNCP and a concurrent CPS are less likely to benefit from OT. For these individuals, the current pain treatment literature suggests that approaches incorporating a range of interventions delivered in a multidisciplinary treatment setting may provide the best outcomes at the least expense (Turk et al., 2002).

Associated Practitioner Recommendations

- Complete a comprehensive pain assessment prior to initiation of OT. A comprehensive assessment should include, at a minimum, measures of mood, pain-related impairment, physical status, social functioning, and pain intensity.
- When significant psychosocial impairment (e.g., depression, anxiety, family problems, work difficulties) is suspected or observed, consider referral to an appropriate pain specialist to determine if a CPS is present.
- If a moderate to severe CPS is confirmed, a multidisciplinary pain clinic referral should be considered, particularly when there is evidence of a poor prior response to OT.
- When either a multidisciplinary pain clinic is not available or referral is not indicated, inclusion of an active, restorative treatment component, such as physical therapy and/or a monitored and paced exercise program, may enhance outcomes (Harris & Susman 2002; Iversen, Fossel, & Katz, 2003; Liddle, Baxter, & Gracey, 2004).

RATES OF OPIOID MISUSE (I.E., OPIOID ABUSE, OPIOID NON-ADHERENCE, OR OPIOID ADDICTION) AMONG INDIVIDUALS TREATED WITH OT ARE SIGNIFICANT

Concerns about opiate use permeate our society today. Individuals with chronic pain fear becoming "addicted" or "drugged" and may refuse opioid analgesics as a result

(Gilron & Bailey, 2003). Practitioners may be reluctant to prescribe opioids (Morley-Forster et al., 2003; Potter et al., 2001), in part due to concerns about addiction (Bendtsen et al., 1999). Yet many pain specialists minimize these risks of opioid analgesic use (Aronoff, 2000; Passik & Weinreb, 2000), even among individuals with a history of substance abuse or dependence (Compton, Athanasos, & Elashoff, 2003; Currie et al., 2003), while others voice concerns related to its use (Ballantyne & Mao, 2003; Harden, 2002; Zuniga, 1998).

OPIOIDS, ADDICTION, AND MISUSE

Some of the disparity in practitioner opinions regarding the abuse potential of opioid analgesics may stem from differences in defining opioid abuse. Many pain professionals equate abuse with true addiction, or the compulsive need for and use of a habit-forming substance that is characterized by tolerance and by physiological withdrawal symptoms. True addiction to opioid analgesics appears to be relatively infrequent among individuals with CNCP. For example, Cowan and colleagues (2003) found a 2.8% addiction rate in their survey of 104 patients with chronic pain treated with OT. Kouyanou, Pither, and Wessely (1997) reported that 6.4% of 125 individuals with CNCP treated at pain clinics in London met the criteria for active substance dependence. However, practitioners' concerns may be broader and encompass not just opioid addiction, but also other patterns of opioid misuse. These include patterns such as opioid overuse, diversion, sharing, use with illicit drugs or alcohol, or use for nonpain-related purposes (e.g., sleep; anxiety reduction), all of which constitute risks to the patient or to society but do not necessarily meet the criteria for true addiction.

When patterns of inappropriate opioid use are considered together, data from chronic pain studies suggest that the rates of opioid misuse in this population are far from trivial. For example, when cases of opioid misuse, nonadherence, or addiction were considered together, Turk et al. (2002) reported a mean rate of opioid misuse of 18.4% across 13 opioid studies. Others have found even higher rates of misuse. Reid and colleagues (2002a) retrospectively examined the medical records of 98 randomly selected individuals with long-standing chronic pain treated with at least 6 months of OT in two primary care (VA and urban, hospital-based) settings. They reported that 24% of VA and 31% of non-VA primary care sample patients had documented evidence of prescription opioid abuse in their medical records. When they examined predictors of this recorded opioid abuse, the best predictor was a past history of a substance abuse disorder, followed by younger age. Chabal and associates (1997) developed an opioid abuse checklist based on accepted diagnostic criteria and administered the instrument to 76 pain clinic participants undergoing OT. They reported that 34% of the patients in OT met one of the abuse criteria, and 27.6% met three or more of the criteria. Kouyanou and colleagues (1997) reported that 83% of their subjects taking medications were potentially misusing them. Ackerman and associates (2003) compared self-reported opioid medication use with manufacturer recommendations of use among 690 individuals with chronic pain and found that patient's utilization varied significantly from what was recommended. Katz and colleagues (2003) tested urine samples of 122 CNCP clinic patients and compared the results with medical record documentation of five behaviors associated with misuse. They found that 21% of the patients had positive toxicology screen results alone (illicit substances, nonprescribed controlled medications, or alcohol), 14% had documented behaviors consistent with misuse in the absence of positive urine screens, and 8% presented with both signs. Thus, almost one half of substance-misusing patients demonstrated toxicological evidence of substance abuse or misuse in the absence of recorded abuse behaviors. Saper and colleagues (2004) reported on the 3- to 8-year outcome of 160 patients receiving daily scheduled opioids for intractable head pain (an open-label adjunct to an overall management program including many behavioral approaches). They noted that 70 patients used OT for at least 3 years, but only 26% of the 160 patients had pain relief greater than 50%. Furthermore, problem drug behaviors (dose variations, lost prescriptions, obtaining medication from more than one prescriber) were seen in 50% of the patients leading the authors to appropriately conclude, "the relative low percentage of patients with demonstrated efficacy and unexpectedly high prevalence of misuse have clinical relevance" (p. 1692).

Misuse also includes episodes of opioid intoxication resulting in death. Opioid-induced deaths may occur due to an unintentional overdose of opioid-addicted individuals or from intentional suicide. Unlike some other countries, the overall rates of opioid analgesic–related deaths are unknown in the United States due to the absence of national tracking methods. However, some data have been reported linking specific opioid agents with an increased number of deaths. Foremost among these are the much-publicized reports of increasing OxyContin overdoses (Schulte & McVicar, 2002). However, frequent overdoses of other selected opioid analgesics also have been reported. For example, the Drug Enforcement Agency (DEA) reported that emergency room visits due to hydrocodone overdose increased 48% between 1998 and 2001 (Mathews & Fields, 2003) leading to a recent proposal to reclassify the drug from a Schedule III to a Schedule II controlled substance. Another Schedule III opioid (propoxyphene) was found to be the most common method of drug-related death from presumed suicide and was second only to gunshot wounds as the cause of death by suspected intentional causes among outpatients at a southeastern medical facility over a 2-year period (Maudlin, 2004).

Overall, although the actual risk of death associated with opioid analgesic abuse undoubtedly is small, there are indications that heightened risks may be associated with certain opioid agents, suggesting that practitioners may need to exercise increased caution when these analgesics are prescribed.

Thus, available data suggest that opioid abuse, opioid nonadherence, or opioid addiction among individuals with CNCP treated with opioid analgesics occurs with a relatively high frequency. Of course, not every instance of misuse necessarily should lead to the cessation of OT. Nevertheless, the reported frequencies suggest that practitioners need to remain sensitive to the potential for misuse of opioids or the use of other substances that may negatively affect OT.

Associated Practitioner Recommendations

- Monitor every patient undergoing OT for signs of misuse, non-adherence, and addiction. The addition of periodic toxicology screens may enhance detection of abuse or misuse.
- Signs of potential misuse or non-adherence may include unusual or noncompliant usage patterns, self-reported loss or accidental destruction of prescriptions or analgesics, elaborate explanations of why adherence was not possible, and strong preferences for specific substances that are frequently abused, among others. Assume that when explanations are not clear or do not make sense either some critical information is missing or there is some type of misrepresentation occurring (Cole, 2003).
- When behavioral signs alone suggest misuse, non-adherence, or addiction, or if opioid diversion is suspected, consider observed sample collection and repeat toxicology testing.
- If misuse is identified, address safety issues (e.g., diversion, intentional or unintentional overdose) immediately; consider cessation and notifying authorities.
- If OT is terminated, monitor and treat potential withdrawal.

INITIATION AND CESSATION OF OT HAS BEEN LINKED TO THE DEVELOPMENT OF HYPERALGESIA IN HUMANS

Hyperalgesia refers to the subjective experience of increased pain that is defined by a reduced pain threshold or reduced pain tolerance. Hyperalgesia differs from opioid-related tolerance in that the latter focuses on the need for increasing opioid dosages to maintain the same degree of pain reduction.

Hyperalgesia has been found to occur following opioid administration and initially was linked to relatively rapid escalation of opioids as might occur postsurgically. However, more recently it has been documented following stable and long-term opioid use (Arner, Rawal, & Gustafsson, 1988; Ossipov et al., 2003) and during methadone maintenance therapy (Doverty et al., 2001a, 2001b). In the last several years evidence of the development of hyperalgesia in response to the *withdrawal* of opioids has also been reported (Angst et al., 2003; Compton et al., 2003; Hood, Curry, & Eisenach, 2003), even following short-term opioid infusion (Angst et al., 2003). In fact, in one study a single administration of an opioid led to rapid and large (on the order of 70%) decrease in pain threshold and pain tolerance, when compared with pre-opioid administration levels, among non-opioid-dependent males (Compton et al., 2003). This was one of the first studies using human subjects that provided experimental support for the existence of a pain *sensitization* system that can be triggered by either opioid administration or withdrawal. Interestingly, in one study the hyperalgesic effects were much stronger for hydromorphone than for morphine sulfate (Compton et al., 2003), suggesting that substance-specific differences may exist.

The development of hyperalgesia has been hypothesized to be a form of neurotoxicity associated with the accumulation of opioid metabolites (Pereira, 1997), variations in opioid receptor concentrations (Wilson, 2001), or activation of descending rostral ventromedial medulla mechanisms that facilitate pain (Ossipov et al., 2003). While the exact mechanism responsible for this opioid effect remains unknown and is no doubt complex, its existence is problematic from a pain treatment perspective and poses a paradox to practitioners. That is, attempts to relieve pain via opioid administration may, for some individuals, actually provoke increased pain, as may opioid cessation following even very brief opioid exposure.

At present, we do not know how frequently opioid-induced hyperalgesia develops. In the past its incidence was presumed to be low. However, the recent reports of opioid withdrawal-induced hyperalgesia suggest that it may be more common than initially recognized. Certainly one could hypothesize that opioid-induced hyperalgesia may account for a portion of the numerous dropouts from RCT studies and clinic-based opioid trials. Additionally, it is quite possible that the opioid tolerance frequently observed in clinical trials and patient treatment may in actuality represent hyperalgesia. Indeed, it is widely viewed that they share the same or a similar mechanism (Ossipov et al., 2003), and in the absence of pain threshold or pain tolerance testing, it would be virtually impossible to distinguish between them during patient treatment as both would lead to decreased effectiveness and dose escalation. In any event, the potential for developing increased pain following brief or extended opioid administration or cessation clearly exists and needs to be considered by pain practitioners.

Associated Practitioner Recommendations

- Prior to initiating OT, evaluate the patient's history of opioid analgesic use and assess for past episodes of opioid-induced hyperalgesia. If evidence of potential hyperalgesic experiences exists, proceed cautiously. Consider the utility of administering a test dose and observing for subsequent increases in pain intensity.
- Until more information regarding the incidence of hyperalgesia under different OT protocols is known, assess each patient treated with OT for evidence of hyperalgesia during each clinical contact regardless of the duration of the individual's ongoing opioid use.
- Evidence of hyperalgesia (but not tolerance) may indicate that OT cessation is indicated. Attempts to "treat" hyperalgesia with escalating opioid doses, as is employed when responding to opioid tolerance issues, may be counterproductive. At present the value of rotating to an alternative opioid agent in the hope of avoiding hyperalgesic responses is unknown.
- When opioids are discontinued, following either short-term or long-term OT, assess for symptoms of hyperalgesia and treat accordingly.

ACCUMULATING EVIDENCE INDICATES STRONG LINKS BETWEEN ORAL OR INTRATHECAL OPIOID ADMINISTRATION AND RAPID ONSET HYPOGONADISM AND SEXUAL DYSFUNCTION AMONG BOTH MEN AND WOMEN WITH CHRONIC PAIN

To date, five studies have examined the effects of opioid administration on hypogonadism among humans. The results of all five have been remarkably consistent among both men and women using both oral and intrathecal administration routes. A summary of the results of these studies is presented in Table 11.3.

Abs et al. (2000) compared hormonal levels in 29 men and 44 women with CNCP undergoing long-term intrathecal treatment with morphine with those of 20 non-opioid control subjects with similar pain conditions. Self-reported decreased libido or impotency was found in 96% (23/24) of the men and in 69% (22/32) of the women receiving intrathecal opioids. In addition, all 21 premenopausal women experienced either amenorrhea or an irregular menstrual cycle, with ovulation occurring in only one case. A similar pattern of findings was reported by Finch and colleagues (2000) in their comparison of 29 patients (10 men and 19 women) receiving intrathecal opioids as treatment for CNCP with 20 control subjects with pain but not receiving opioids. Testosterone levels in the males receiving opioid therapy were below normal and were significantly lower than levels in the male controls. Of the

TABLE 11.3
Incidence of OT-Associated Hypogonadism

Study	OT type	Rates	Comments
Abs et al. (2000)	Intrathecal	>86% (M)	Decreased Libido:
73 P (29 M, 44 F)	(M = 26.6 months)	100% (W)	96% Men
20 C (11 M, 9 F)			69% Women
Daniell (2002)	Oral	89%	Dose-related testosterone reduction: 87% reported sexual
54 P (males)	(range = <1 year–>10 years)		dysfunction
27 C (males)			
Finch et al. (2000)	Intrathecal	90% (M)	Decreased Libido:
30 P (11 M, 19 F)	(.02–8 years, median = 2.5 years)	75–90%(F)	60% Men
20 C (10 M, 10 F)			100% Women (premenopausal)
			Reduced testosterone (M)
			Reduced FSH and LH (F, postmenopausal)
Rajagopal et al. (2003)	Oral(minimum 12 months)	90%	Low Sexual Desire Inventory scores compared to healthy adults
20 P (males)			
Roberts et al. (2002)	Intrathecal	–74% 1 week	Testosterone levels measured
10 P (males)	(1–12 weeks)	–64% 4 weeks	Prospective study
		–48% 12 weeks	

P = patients; C = controls.

10 male subjects, 6 reported reduced libido with 4 of these subjects also reporting impotence. Reduced libido dating from the onset of opioid therapy was also reported by all 7 premenopausal women, although their median serum testosterone levels were within normal limits. In the postmenopausal women, testosterone levels were significantly lower than in the non-opioid controls although their sexual interest had fallen even prior to opioid treatment. In another study, Daniell (2002) assessed testosterone and hormones related to testosterone production in 54 male subjects receiving various forms of oral opioid therapy for CNCP. In contrast to control subjects, average hormone levels were significantly lower (in a dose-dependent manner) in the opioid group. Of the 45 men that reported normal erectile function prior to the beginning of the study, 39 reported severe erectile dysfunction or diminished libido after initiating opioid therapy.

Rajagopal and associates (2003) found reduced testosterone levels in 18 of 20 male patients with cancer-related chronic pain who had been receiving opioid therapy for at least 1 year. Compared with healthy controls, these subjects also reported significantly reduced sexual desire scores as measured by the Sexual Desire Inventory (Spector & Carey, 1990). In the only prospective study (Roberts et al., 2002) measuring the effects of opioid therapy on serum testosterone levels in 10 male subjects with CNCP, serum testosterone levels were measured prior to the onset of intrathecal opioid therapy and again after 1, 4, and 12 weeks of intrathecal infusion. Compared with baseline, serum testosterone was reduced by 74% after week 1, 64% after week 4, and 48% after week 12. Although the majority of the subjects reported poor libido and abnormal erec-

tile function at baseline, sexual dysfunction increased during the course of the study resulting in an absence of sexual activity in all 10 of the subjects after 12 weeks of OT.

Although none of the studies included comparisons between opioid and active or inactive placebo groups, the consistency of the results clearly implies causal links between initiation of OT and subsequent development of hypogonadism. Overall the studies suggest (1) there is a strong association between administration of opioids and subsequent signs of hypogonadism; (2) the gonadatrophic hormone changes occur rapidly following opioid administration; (3) there is some evidence that the association is dose related; (4) it affects the vast majority of individuals consuming opioids; and (5) gonadatrophic hormone changes correlate highly with reports of reduced libido or sexual dysfunction.

Additional research is needed to delineate both the degree and persistence of opioid-induced hypogonadism for individuals treated with long-term OT. For the present, symptoms of unexplained hypogonadism that appear to parallel OT initiation should be investigated fully.

Associated Practitioner Recommendations

- Evaluate patients for changes in sexual function following OT initiation and, if indicated, assess gonadatrophic hormone levels.
- If hypogonadism is confirmed, educate the patient and spouse or partner, if available, concerning its effects.
- Discuss the available options for treatment along with the potential adverse effects of the

treatments with the patient and partner, if available. Initiate treatment of the hypogonadism (e.g., hormonal therapy) or consider cessation of OT based on the results of this discussion.

EMOTIONAL DISTRESS AND OTHER PSYCHOSOCIAL VARIABLES ARE BETTER PREDICTORS OF WHETHER AN INDIVIDUAL WITH CHRONIC PAIN WILL BE PRESCRIBED OPIOIDS THAN IS PAIN INTENSITY OR OTHER PHYSICAL STATUS VARIABLES

Decisions regarding who should or should not receive OT for chronic pain are a complicated matter incorporating numerous patient, practitioner, and pain condition variables. Nevertheless, there is a consensus among practitioners, consistent with the WHO analgesic ladder, that opioid analgesics should be considered only for those with moderate to severe pain.

One implication of this position is that pain intensity should be positively associated with decisions to prescribe opioids for chronic pain. Yet the great preponderance of empirical data fails to find such a relationship between pain intensity and opioid use. For example, Turk and Okifuji (1997) compared 81 patients with chronic pain at a pain treatment center who were currently taking opioids for CNCP with 110 patients at the same center who were not taking opioids on a variety of measures. Turk and Okifuji found no differences between the groups on demographic, pain duration, pain onset, pain location, physical findings, or pain intensity variables. In fact, the only variables that differentiated between groups were those of number of pain behaviors, degree of functional limitation, and affective distress. For all of these variables, patients receiving opioids demonstrated significantly greater dysfunction. When the predictive value of all designated variables was investigated using logistic regression techniques, only pain behaviors emerged as a significant predictor of opioid use.

Breckenridge and Clark (2003) retrospectively examined patient and pharmacy records of 200 veterans with back pain receiving either NSAIDs ($n = 100$) or opioids ($n = 100$) for their pain. Again, they found no relationship between reported pain intensity and opioid use. Instead, logistic regression analyses revealed that individuals undergoing OT were approximately 5 times more likely to have a substance abuse disorder, 8 times more likely to experience depression, and more than 18 times more likely to have a diagnosed personality disorder than were veterans treated with NSAIDs. Clark (2002) found that 21% of his randomly selected medical clinic sample of U.S. military veterans with CNCP treated with opioid analgesics had documentation of a substance abuse history. Fillingim and colleagues (2003), in a study utilizing 240 individuals with back or neck pain evaluated at a multidisciplinary pain center, found significant positive associations between self-reported disability and dysfunction and opioid use for both men and women, and no relationship between pain intensity and opioid use. Interestingly, affective distress was positively associated with opioid use in men and negatively related in women. Similar findings noting the lack of relationships between pain intensity and/or physical findings and opioid use have been reported by Clark and Gironda (2001). Only one study has found the expected positive relationship between pain intensity and opioid use (Ciccone et al., 2000). However, consistent with the above findings, these authors also noted significant and positive associations between disability measures, activity impairment, and self-reported depression and opioid use.

Explanations proffered to account for these findings tend to cluster around the potential impact of patient behaviors on practitioner prescribing practices (Turk & Okifuji, 1997). In such a view, individuals exhibiting signs of increased physical or emotional distress, as well as those who persist in their efforts to obtain opioids, may be more successful than less dramatic or assertive individuals (i.e., the "squeaky wheel syndrome"). Indeed, the potential for patient pain behaviors to influence medical decisions is not unique to opioid prescribing alone, having been demonstrated with respect to back surgery decisions previously (Waddell et al., 1984). In this regard, pain behaviors may serve as one of a host of variables that influence practitioners' prescribing decisions (Turk & Okifuji, 1997).

An alternative explanation of these results might counter that pain intensity/opioid use relationships may be difficult to detect because in all of the above studies individuals were using opioids at the time measures were collected. Therefore, one might hypothesize that the pain-reduction effects of OT attenuated the size of the observed relationship between pain and opioid use, whereas if measures were administered *prior* to any practitioner decision whether to use opioids, significant associations might have emerged. Nevertheless, this would not explain reports noting the lack of relationship between physical examination variables or diagnostic test results and opioid use. An additional issue is that all subjects in the above studies were undergoing evaluation or treatment at specialty pain treatment sites. Given established differences between these patients and patients treated in other medical settings such as primary care (Crook, Weir, & Tunks, 1989), it may be that patients treated in other medical settings may demonstrate the expected pain intensity–opioid use relationship. Ultimately, clarification of the relationship between pain intensity or physical findings and opioid prescribing likely will await completion of one or more prospective studies that can manipulate or quantify intensity of pain behaviors and physical findings before therapeutic decisions are rendered. However, in the interim practitioners should be aware of the empirical findings thus far.

In summary, research to date has failed to find consistent relationships between pain intensity or physical findings and opioid use. Instead, the preponderance of the data has identified a range of psychosocial factors that predict opioid use. These include pain behaviors, affective distress, self-perceptions of functional limitations or pain-related impairment, active substance abuse, and presence of a personality disorder. The latter two associations are the most surprising in that substance abuse and personality disorders are potential *contraindications* for OT.

Associated Practitioner Recommendations

- Consistent with WHO recommendations, consider opioid therapy only for refractory chronic pain of moderate or severe intensity.

- Evaluate emotional distress as well as pain intensity. For individuals exhibiting significant depression, initiate a mental health referral for evaluation and treatment *prior* to deciding whether an opioid trial is indicated.

- When dramatic pain behaviors are present, proceed cautiously, and consider the possibility of other explanations for the patient's presentation including secondary gain, presence of a personality disorder, or substance abuse/misuse. If the above cannot be ruled out, refer to a mental health or substance abuse professional for assistance.

CONCLUSIONS

Empirical data indicate that the prescription of opioid analgesics is one of the most frequent interventions employed for the treatment of CNCP (Fillingim et al., 2003; Morley-Forster et al., 2003; Turk & Okifuji, 1997). Yet at present the effectiveness of long-term OT remains unsubstantiated. No long-term studies of OT efficacy have been reported despite widespread recognition of the need for such investigations. As a result, support for OT effectiveness stems from a series of short-term opioid studies. Primary among these are 18 RCTs that constitute the foundation for claims of the efficacy of OT in the treatment of CNCP. Yet, a close examination of this core of studies leads to a myriad of concerns regarding study design and the resulting findings. These concerns include the following:

1. brief (i.e., less than 6 weeks) RCT durations (15 of 18 studies);

2. high (greater than 20%) subject dropout rates (14 of 18 studies);

3. relatively small (fewer than 40 subjects completing the opioid trial) sample sizes (9 of 18 studies);

4. lack of intent-to-treat analyses (13 of 18 studies);

5. incomplete or unclear methodology (4 of 18 studies);

6. failure to report pain changes from baseline (5 of 18 studies);

7. reliance on nonstandard pain intensity measures or use of derivative measures that preclude comparisons with the results of other studies (8 of 18 studies);

8. use of opioid rescue medications during controlled trials (4 of 18 studies);

9. use of inactive rather than active placebos (10 of 12 studies); and

10. failure to assess the integrity of blinding procedures when placebos were used (9 of 13 studies).

This last methodological concern alone is sufficient to question the results of the RCT OT literature, in that the few investigators that have assessed the integrity of study blinds in both active and inactive placebo studies generally have found that the majority of subjects and providers are aware of which group or crossover period utilized opioids.

Future research evaluating OT effectiveness needs to address the many problems cited above. Although there are a variety of obstacles to conducting long-term (i.e., 6 months or more), reliable, RCT studies of opioid effectiveness, they remain the best way of determining the utility of OT in the treatment of CNCP. Additionally, there are a number of methodological improvements that could be made in shorter-term studies that would enhance the validity and value of the findings. Studies incorporating parallel treatment arms (rather than crossover designs); active placebo comparison groups; intent-to-treat analyses; validated measures of pain intensity, mood, pain interference, and disability; quantification of changes in pain from baseline as well as differences in pain intensity between experimental and control groups; and most importantly, routine and systematic assessment of the integrity of the blinding procedures are needed to redress the methodological shortcomings that plague the current OT research literature. In addition, long-term studies that may not meet the rigors of RCT methodologies, but that examine the longitudinal effects of OT on pain intensity and daily function while monitoring dropout rates and misuse, would provide needed information concerning the "real-world" utility of opioid analgesics in the treatment of CNCP.

Even if the methodological weaknesses characteristic of the opioid RCT research core are overlooked there remains much to question regarding OT effectiveness. The pain reduction associated with short-term OT, averaged over all studies we reviewed and irrespective of potential placebo effects, was only 30%, which, although significant, clearly suggests that OT should be used in conjunction with other empirically supported treatment strategies. Nor has successful (defined by reduced pain intensity) OT been linked to improved function in studies incorporating such measures, particularly in the realms of depression and disability. In fact, the function of some individuals with CNCP appears to *decline* when treated with OT (Schofferman, 1999; Turner et al., 1982), and discontinuing OT for individuals with CPS has been linked with improved function and pain (Clark & Gironda, 2001). This argues strongly for increasing emphasis on multidisciplinary pain treatment approaches and for further research assessing relationships between CPS and OT effectiveness.

Another concern with respect to OT raised in this chapter pertains to provider decisions to prescribe opioid analgesics. We have seen that pain intensity and physical status variables are poor predictors of who will receive OT. In fact, rarely has pain intensity been associated with opioid analgesic use. Although relatively little research has focused on this issue, what information we do have indicates that *psychological* factors predominate. That is, individuals exhibiting more pronounced pain behaviors, affective distress, or perceived pain-related impairment are more likely to receive opioids (Turk & Okifuji, 1997). Indeed, those with substance abuse and personality disorder histories are overrepresented among individuals receiving OT (Breckenridge & Clark, 2003). If future research establishes the effectiveness of OT for the treatment of CNCP, concomitant efforts to target individuals experiencing higher levels of pain and lower levels of psychopathology as the recipients of OT would be beneficial.

Opioid analgesic use also has been linked with a variety of serious complications beyond the assortment of adverse effects with which practitioners are most familiar. Both opioid initiation and cessation have been demonstrated to elicit hyperalgesia even following very short-term exposure (Angst et al., 2003; Compton et al., 2003; Hood et al., 2003). The mechanisms underlying the pain sensitization effects associated with hyperalgesia also may mediate opioid tolerance (Ossipov et al., 2003). In fact, it is possible that tolerance may reflect undetected hyperalgesia. Integration or differentiation of these mechanisms depends in part on including pain threshold and pain tolerance tests in future RCT studies of opioid analgesic effectiveness. OT also has been causally linked to rapid onset hypogonadism in both men and women (Abs et al., 2000; Roberts et al., 2002). Although other factors undoubtedly contribute (e.g., depression), this link may explain in large part the strong association between chronic pain and reduced sexual interest or performance. Efforts to identify the long-term consequences of potential treatments for opioid-induced hypogonadism clearly are needed. In the interim, both OT candidates and their sexual partners need to be educated regarding these effects if they are to participate in informed decision making. Finally, when rates of addiction, abuse, and non-adherence are considered together, approximately one quarter of individuals with CNCP treated with OT in primary care settings have exhibited signs of misuse (Reid et al., 2002a). Furthermore, selected opioid agents (hydromorphone, oxycodone, and propoxyphene) have been linked with more frequent overdoses and potential death. Improved methods for identifying links between specific opioid agents and risks of abuse are needed, as is research focusing on predictors of opioid analgesic misuse.

The opioid-related concerns discussed in this chapter are not exhaustive by any means. Other issues have been identified in the recent pain literature, but were not included based on their preliminary nature. These include possible racial barriers to opioid access (Tamayo-Sarver et al., 2003), opioid mediation of some aspects of anger expression (Bruehl et al., 2002; Bruehl, 2003), and the potential immunosuppressive effects of opioid analgesics (Alonzo & Bayer, 2002; Sacerdote et al., 2000) that actually may benefit individuals with selected immune system disorders such as rheumatoid arthritis. Only additional research will determine the salience of these concerns and the degree that providers will need to consider them in decisions to use OT.

We recognize that OT will continue to be used to treat CNCP and that there undoubtedly are individuals benefiting from this form of treatment. However, based on the current status of the OT literature, we believe that providers considering the use of opioid analgesics need to proceed cautiously. Data from a variety of empirical studies indicate that OT can be detrimental and that the overall effectiveness of OT for the treatment of CNCP has not been adequately demonstrated. Furthermore, while we can identify with some degree of confidence the characteristics of individuals who are poor candidates for OT, no reliable empirical data exist identifying the characteristics of individuals who are good candidates for OT. In the absence of this information, we have provided some recommendations for OT use based on the existing opioid literature to promote informed and balanced clinical decision making. These recommendations, however, do not supplant the urgent need for continued and expanded OT research, which must form the basis for the safe and effective utilization of opioids in the treatment of CNCP.

REFERENCES

Abs, R., Verhelst, J., Maeyaert, J., Van Buyten, J. P., Opsomer, F., Adriaensen, H., et al. (2000). Endocrine consequences of long-term intrathecal administration of opioids. *Journal of Clinical Endocrinology and Metabolism, 85*(6), 2215–2222.

Ackerman, S. J., Mordin, M., Reblando, J., Xu, X., Schein, J., Vallow, S., & Brennan, M. (2003). Patient-reported utilization patterns of fentanyl transdermal system and oxycodone hydrochloride controlled-release among patients with chronic nonmalignant pain [see comment]. *Journal of Managed Care Pharmacy, 9*(3), 223–231.

Allen, G. J., Hartl, T. L., Duffany, S., Smith, S. F., VanHeest, J. L., Anderson, J. M., et al. (2003). Cognitive and motor function after administration of hydrocodone bitartrate plus ibuprofen, ibuprofen alone, or placebo in healthy subjects with exercise-induced muscle damage: A randomized, repeated-dose, placebo-controlled study. *Psychopharmacology, 166*(3), 228–233.

Alonzo, N. C., & Bayer, B. M. (2002). Opioids, immunology, and host defenses of intravenous drug abusers. *Infectious Disease Clinics of North America, 16*(3), 553–569.

American Academy of Pain Medicine and the America Pain. (1996). The Use of Opioids for the Treatment of Chronic Pain: A Consensus Statement. http://www.ampainsoc. org/advocacy/opioids.htm, accessed on 4/4/05.

American Academy of Pain Medicine, the American Pain Society and the American Society of Addiction Medicine Consensus Document. (2001). Definitions Related to the Use of Opioids for the Treatment of Pain. http://www. asam.org/ppol/paindef.htm, accessed 4/4/05.

American Academy of Pain Medicine, the American Pain Society, and the American Society of Addiction Medicine. (2004). Public Policy Statement on the Rights and Responsibilities of Healthcare Professionals in the Use of Opioids for the Treatment of Pain: A Consensus Document. http://www.ampainsoc.org/advocacy/rights.htm, accessed on 4/4/05.

Angst, M. S., Koppert, W., Pahl, I., Clark, D. J., & Schmelz, M. (2003). Short-term infusion of the mu-opioid agonist remifentanil in humans causes hyperalgesia during withdrawal. *Pain, 106*(1–2), 49–57.

Arkinstall, W., Sandler, A., Goughnour, B., Babul, N., Harsanyi, Z., & Darke, A. C. (1995). Efficacy of controlled-release codeine in chronic non-malignant pain: A randomized, placebo-controlled clinical trial. *Pain, 62*(2), 169–178.

Arner, S., Rawal, N., & Gustafsson, L. L. (1988). Clinical experience of long-term treatment with epidural and intrathecal opioids — A nationwide survey. *Acta Anaesthesiology Scandinavia, 32*(3), 253–259.

Aronoff, G. M. (2000). Opioids in chronic pain management: Is there a significant risk of addiction? *Current Reviews of Pain, 4*(2), 112–121.

Attal, N. (2000). Chronic neuropathic pain: Mechanisms and treatment. *Clinical Journal of Pain, 16*(3 Suppl.), S118–S130.

Ballantyne, J. C., & Mao, J. (2003). Opioid therapy for chronic pain. *New England Journal of Medicine, 349*(20), 1943–1953.

Bendtsen, P., Hensing, G., Ebeling, C., & Schedin, A. (1999). What are the qualities of dilemmas experienced when prescribing opioids in general practice? *Pain, 82*(1), 89–96.

Breckenridge, J., & Clark, J. D. (2003). Patient characteristics associated with opioid versus nonsteroidal anti-inflammatory drug management of chronic low back pain. *Journal of Pain, 4*(6), 344–350.

Brodner, R. A., & Taub, A. (1978). Chronic pain exacerbated by long-term narcotic use in patients with nonmalignant disease: Clinical syndrome and treatment. *Mount Sinai Journal of Medicine, 45*(2), 233–237.

Bruehl, S., Burns, J. W., Chung, O. Y., Ward, P., & Johnson, B. (2002). Anger and pain sensitivity in chronic low back pain patients and pain-free controls: The role of endogenous opioids. *Pain, 99*(1–2), 223–233.

Bruehl, S., Chung, O. Y., Burns, J. W., & Biridepalli, S. (2003). The association between anger expression and chronic pain intensity: Evidence for partial mediation by endogenous opioid dysfunction. *Pain, 106*(3), 317–324.

Bruera, E., Macmillan, K., Hanson, J., & MacDonald, R.N. (1989). The cognitive effects of the administration of narcotic analgesics in patients with cancer pain. *Pain, 39*(1), 13–16.

Caldwell, J. R., Hale, M. E., Boyd, R. E., Hague, J. M., Iwan, T., Shi, M. et al. (1999). Treatment of osteoarthritis pain with controlled release oxycodone or fixed combination oxycedone plus acetaminophen added to nonsteroidal antiinflammatory drugs: A double blind, randomized, multicenter, placebo controlled trial. *Journal of Rheumatology, 26*, 862–869.

Caldwell, J. R., Rapoport, R. J., Davis, J. C., Offenberg, H. L., Marker, H. W., Roth, S. H. et al. (2002). Efficacy and safety of a once-daily morphine formulation in chronic, moderate-to-severe osteoarthritis pain: Results from a randomized, placebo-controlled, double-blind trial and an open-label extension trial. *Journal of Pain Symptom Management, 23*(4), 278–291.

Carroll, L. J., Cassidy, J. D., & Cote, P. (2004). Depression as a risk factor for onset of an episode of troublesome neck and low back pain. *Pain, 107*(1–2), 134–139.

Cepeda, M. S., Africano, J. M., Polo, R., Alcala, R., & Carr, D. B. (2003). What decline in pain intensity is meaningful to patients with acute pain? *Pain, 105*(1–2), 151–157.

Chabal, C., Erjavec, M. K., Jacobson, L., Mariano, A., & Chaney, E. (1997). Prescription opiate abuse in chronic pain patients: clinical criteria, incidence, and predictors. *Clinical Journal of Pain, 13*(2), 150–155.

Chapman, S. (2001). The effects of opioids on driving ability in patients with chronic pain. *The APS Bulletin, 11*(1), 1, 5, 9.

Chapman, S. L., Byas-Smith, M. G., & Reed, B. A. (2002). Effects of intermediate- and long-term use of opioids on cognition in patients with chronic pain. *Clinical Journal of Pain, 18*(Suppl. 4), S83–S90.

Cheng, M. S., Amick, B. C. III, Watkins, M. P., & Rhea, C. D. (2002). Employer, physical therapist, and employee outcomes in the management of work-related upper extremity disorders. *Journal of Occupational Rehabilitation, 12*(4), 257–267.

Ciccone, D. S., Just, N., Bandilla, E. B., Reimer, E., Ilbeigi, M. S., & Wu, W. (2000). Psychological correlates of opioid use in patients with chronic nonmalignant pain: A preliminary test of the downhill spiral hypothesis. *Journal of Pain Symptom Manage, 20*(3), 180–192.

Clark, J. D. (2002). Chronic pain prevalence and analgesic prescribing in a general medical population. *Journal of Pain Symptom Manage, 23*(2), 131–137.

Clark, M. E., & Gironda, R. J. (2001). Opioid cessation and chronic pain treatment outcomes. *Opioids and chronic pain: Is more less?* Symposium conducted at the 20th Annual Meeting of the American Pain Society.

Clark, M. E., & Gironda, R. J. (2002). Practical utility of outcome measurement. R. S. Weiner (Ed.), *Pain management: A practical guide for clinicians* (6th ed., pp. 995–1010). Boca Raton, FL: CRC Press.

Clegg, D. O., Reda, D. J., Weisman, M. H., Blackburn, W. D., Cush, J. J., Cannon, G. W. et al. (1996). Comparison of sulfasalazine and placebo in the treatment of ankylosing spondylitis. A Department of Veterans Affairs Cooperative Study. *Arthritis and Rheumatism, 39*(12), 2004–2012.

Cole, B. E. (2002). Prescribing opioids, relieving patient suffering and staying out of personal trouble with regulators. *The Pain Practitioner, 12*(3), 5–8.

Cole, B. E. (2003). Prescriber's update. *The Pain Practitioner, 12*(2), 4–6.

Compton, P., Athanasos, P., & Elashoff, D. (2003). Withdrawal hyperalgesia after acute opioid physical dependence in nonaddicted humans: A preliminary study. *Journal of Pain, 4*(9), 511–9.

Cowan, D. T., Wilson-Barnett, J., Griffiths, P., & Allan, L. G. (2003). A survey of chronic noncancer pain patients prescribed opioid analgesics. *Pain Medicine, 4*(4), 340–51.

Crook, J., Weir, R., & Tunks, E. (1989). An epidemiological follow-up survey of persistent pain sufferers in a group family practice and specialty pain clinic. *Pain, 36*(1), 49–61.

Currie, S. R., Hodgins, D. C., Crabtree, A., Jacobi, J., & Armstrong, S. (2003). Outcome from integrated pain management treatment for recovering substance abusers. *Journal of Pain, 4*(2), 91–100.

Currie, S. R., & Wang, J. (2004). Chronic back pain and major depression in the general Canadian population. *Pain, 107*(1–2), 54–60.

Daniell, H. W. (2002). Narcotic-induced hypogonadism during therapy for heroin addiction. *Journal of Addictive Diseases, 21*(4), 47–53.

de Craen, A. J., Tijssen, J. G., de Gans, J., & Kleijnen, J. (2000). Placebo effect in the acute treatment of migraine: subcutaneous placebos are better than oral placebos. *Journal of Neurology, 247*(3), 183–188.

Dias, R. C., Dias, J. M., & Ramos, L. R. (2003). Impact of an exercise and walking protocol on quality of life for elderly people with OA of the knee. *Physiotherapy Research International, 8*(3), 121–130.

Doverty, M., Somogyi, A. A., White, J. M., Bochner, F., Beare, C. H., Menelaou, A., & Ling, W. (2001a). Methadone maintenance patients are cross-tolerant to the antinociceptive effects of morphine. *Pain, 93*(2), 155–163.

Doverty, M., White, J. M., Somogyi, A. A., Bochner, F., Ali, R., & Ling, W. (2001b). Hyperalgesic responses in methadone maintenance patients. *Pain, 90*(1–2), 91–96.

Dworkin, R. H., Nagasako, E. M., Hetzel, R. D., & Farrar, J. T. (2001). Assessment of pain and pain-related quality of life in clinical trials. In D. C. Turk & R. Melzack (Eds.), *Handbook of pain assessment* (2nd ed., pp. 693–706). New York: Guilford Press.

Elliott, T. E., Renier, C. M., & Palcher, J. A. (2003). Chronic pain, depression, and quality of life: Correlations and predictive value of the SF-36. *Pain Medicine, 4*(4), 331–339.

Ericsson, M., Poston, W. S., Linder, J., Taylor, J. E., Haddock, C. K., & Foreyt, J. P. (2002). Depression predicts disability in long-term chronic pain patients. *Disability and Rehabilitation, 24*(6), 334–340.

The Federation of State Medical Boards of the United States, Inc. (FSMBUS) (1998, 2004). Model guidelines for the use of controlled substances for the treatment of pain (originally adopted May 2, 1998 and revised on May 4, 2004). Retrieved August 29, 2004, from http://fsmb.org/policy documents and white papers/2004_model_pain_policy.asp.

Fillingim, R. B., Doleys, D. M., Edwards, R. R., & Lowery, D. (2003). Clinical characteristics of chronic back pain as a function of gender and oral opioid use. *Spine, 28*(2), 143–150.

Finch, P. M., Roberts, L. J., Price, L., Hadlow, N. C., & Pullan, P. T. (2000). Hypogonadism in patients treated with intrathecal morphine. *Clinical Journal of Pain, 16*(3), 251–254.

Finlayson, R. E., Maruta, T., Morse, R. M., Swenson, W. M., & Martin, M. A. (1986). Substance dependence and chronic pain: profile of 50 patients treated in an alcohol and drug dependence unit. *Pain, 26*(2), 167–174.

Fransen, M., Crosbie, J., & Edmonds, J. (2001). Physical therapy is effective for patients with osteoarthritis of the knee: A randomized controlled clinical trial. *Journal of Rheumatology, 28*(1), 156–164.

Frost, H., Lamb, S. E., Moffett, J. A. K., Fairbank, J. C. T., & Moser, J. S. (1998). A fitness programme for patients with chronic low back pain: 2-year follow-up of a randomised controlled trial. *Pain, 75*(2–3), 273–279.

Gilron, I., & Bailey, J. M. (2003). Trends in opioid use for chronic neuropathic pain: a survey of patients pursuing enrollment in clinical trials. *Canadian Journal of Anaesthesiology, 50*(1), 42–47.

Gironda, R. J. (2004). The development and treatment of chronic pain syndromes. Symposium presented at the West Palm Beach Veterans Hospital Pain Week.

Guzman, J., Esmail, R., Karjalainen, K., Malmivaara, A., Irvin, E., & Bombardier, C. (2002). Multidisciplinary bio-psycho-social rehabilitation for chronic low back pain. *Cochrane Database of Systematic Reviews,* (1), CD000963.

Hale, M. E., Fleischmann, R., Salzman, R., Wild, J., Iwan, T., Swanton, R. E. et al. (1999). Efficacy and safety of controlled-release versus immediate-release oxycodone: Randomized, double-blind evaluation in patients with chronic back pain. *Clinical Journal of Pain, 15*(3), 179–183.

Harden, R.N. (2002). Chronic opioid therapy: Another reappraisal. *APS Bulletin, 12*(1), 1, 8–12.

Harris, G. R. & Susman, J. L. (2002). Managing musculoskeletal complaints with rehabilitation therapy: Summary of the Philadelphia Panel evidence-based clinical practice guidelines on musculoskeletal rehabilitation interventions. *Journal of Family Practice, 51,* 1042–1046.

Haythornthwaite, J. A., Menefee, L. A., Quatrano-Piacentini, A. L., & Pappagallo, M. (1998). Outcome of chronic opioid therapy for non-cancer pain. *Journal of Pain Symptom Management, 15*(3), 185–194.

Hood, D. D., Curry, R., & Eisenach, J. C. (2003). Intravenous remifentanil produces withdrawal hyperalgesia in volunteers with capsaicin-induced hyperalgesia. *Anesthesia & Analgesia, 97*(3), 810–815.

Huse, E., Larbig, W., Flor, H., & Birbaumer, N. (2001). The effect of opioids on phantom limb pain and cortical reorganization. *Pain, 90*(1–2), 47–55.

Iversen, M. D., Fossel, A. H., & Katz, J. N. (2003). Enhancing function in older adults with chronic low back pain: A pilot study of endurance training. *Archives of Physical Medicine and Rehabilitation, 84*(9), 1324–1331.

Jamison, R. N., Raymond, S. A., Slawsby, E. A., Nedeljkovic, S. S., & Katz, N. P. (1998). Opioid therapy for chronic noncancer back pain: A randomized prospective study. *Spine, 23*(23), 2591–2600.

Jarvik, L. F., Simpson, J. H., Guthrie, D., & Liston, E. H. (1981). Morphine, experimental pain, and psychological reactions. *Psychopharmacology, 75*(2), 124–131.

Joint Commission on Accreditation of Healthcare Organizations. (2000). *Background on the Development of the Joint Commission Standards on Pain Management*. Retrieved September 21, 2004 at http://www.jcaho.org/news+room/health+care+issues/pain.htm.

Jull, G., Trott, P., Potter, H., Zito, G., Niere, K., Shirley, D. et al. (2002). A randomized controlled trial of exercise and manipulative therapy for cervicogenic headache. *Spine, 27*(17), 1835–1843; discussion 1843.

Katz, N. P., Sherburne, S., Beach, M., Rose, R.J., Vielguth, J., Bradley, J., & Fanciullo, G. J. (2003). Behavioral monitoring and urine toxicology testing in patients receiving long-term opioid therapy. *Anesthesia & Analgesia, 97*(4), 1097–1102.

Kjaersgaard-Andersen, P., Nafei, A., Skov, O., Madsen, F., Andersen, H. M., Kroner, K. et al. (1990). Codeine plus paracetamol versus paracetamol in longer-term treatment of chronic pain due to osteoarthritis of the hip: A randomised, double-blind, multi-centre study. *Pain, 43*(3), 309–318.

Klapow, J. C., Slater, M. A., Patterson, T. L., Doctor, J. N., Atkinson, J. H., & Garfin, S. R. (1993). An empirical evaluation of multidimensional clinical outcome in chronic low back pain patients. *Pain, 55*(1), 107–118.

Kouyanou, K., Pither, C. E., & Wessely, S. (1997). Medication misuse, abuse and dependence in chronic pain patients. *Journal of Psychosomatic Research, 43*(5), 497–504.

Liddle, S. D., Baxter, G. D., & Gracey, J. H. (2004). Exercise and chronic low back pain: What works? *Pain, 107*(1–2), 176–190.

Lorenz, J., Beck, H., & Bromm, B. (1997). Cognitive performance, mood and experimental pain before and during morphine-induced analgesia in patients with chronic non-malignant pain. *Pain, 73*(3), 369–375.

Luo, X., Pietrobon, R., & Hey, L. (2004). Patterns and trends of opioid use among individuals with back pain in the U.S. *Spine, 29*, 884–890.

Maier, C., Hildebrandt, J., Klinger, R., Henrich-Eberl, C., & Lindena, G. (2002). Morphine responsiveness, efficacy and tolerability in patients with chronic non-tumor associated pain — results of a double-blind placebo-controlled trial (MONTAS). *Pain, 97*(3), 223–233.

Mathews, A. W., & Fields, G. (2003, December 3). Federal agencies seek to curb abuse of potent painkillers. *Wall Street Journal*.

Maudlin, K. (2004). A surprise trend in suicides: Were they accidental? *Federal Practitioner, 21*(1), 47–49, 58–60.

Moffett, J. K., Torgerson, D., Bell-Syer, S., Jackson, D., Llewlyn-Phillips, H., Farrin, A., & Barber, J. (1999). Randomised controlled trial of exercise for low back pain: Clinical outcomes, costs, and preferences. *British Medical Journal, 319*(7205), 279–283.

Morley-Forster, P. K., Clark, A. J., Speechley, M., & Moulin, D. E. (2003). Attitudes toward opioid use for chronic pain: A Canadian physician survey. *Pain Research Management, 8*(4), 189–194.

Moulin, D. E., Iezzi, A., Amireh, R., Sharpe, W. K., Boyd, D., & Merskey, H. (1996). Randomised trial of oral morphine for chronic non-cancer pain. *Lancet, 347*(8995), 143–147.

Muller, F. O., Odendaal, C. L., Muller, F. O., Raubenheimer, J., Middle, M. V., & Kummer, M. (1998). Comparison of the efficacy and tolerability of a paracetramol/codeine fixed-dose combination with tramadol in patients with refractory chronic back pain. *Arzneimettel-Forschung/Drug Research, 48*, 675–679.

Nedeljkovic, S. S., Wasan, A., & Jamison, R. N. (2002). Assessment of efficacy of long-term opioid therapy in pain patients with substance abuse potential. *Clinical Journal of Pain, 18*(4 Suppl.), S39–S51.

Ossipov, M. H., Lai, J., Vanderah, T. W., & Porreca, F. (2003). Induction of pain facilitation by sustained opioid exposure: Relationship to opioid antinociceptive tolerance. [Review]. *Life Sciences, 73*(6), 783–800.

Passik, S. D., & Weinreb, H.J. (2000). Managing chronic non-malignant pain: Overcoming obstacles to the use of opioids. *Advances in Therapy, 17*(2), 70–83.

Peloso, P. M., Bellamy, N., Bensen, W., Thomson, G. T., Harsanyi, Z., Babul, N., & Darke, A. C. (2000). Double blind randomized placebo control trial of controlled release codeine in the treatment of osteoarthritis of the hip or knee. *Journal of Rheumatology, 27*(3), 764–771.

Pereira, J. (1997). Emerging neuropsychiatric toxicities of opioids. *Journal of Pharmaceutical Care in Pain & Symptom Control, 5*(4), 3–29.

Potter, M., Schafer, S., Gonzalez-Mendez, E., Gjeltema, K., Lopez, A., Wu, J., Pedrin, R. et al. (2001). Opioids for chronic nonmalignant pain: Attitudes and practices of primary care physicians in the UCSF/Stanford Collaborative Research Network. University of California, San Francisco. *Journal of Family Practice, 50*(2), 145–51.

Rajagopal, A., Vassilopoulou-Sellin, R., Palmer, J. L., Kaur, G., & Bruera, E. (2003). Hypogonadism and sexual dysfunction in male cancer survivors receiving chronic opioid therapy. *Journal of Pain Symptom Management, 26*(5), 1055–1061.

Reid, M. C., Engles-Horton, L. L., Weber, M. B., Kerns, R. D., Rogers, E. L., & O'Connor, P. G. (2002a). Use of opioid medications for chronic noncancer pain syndromes in primary care. *Journal of General Internal Medicine, 17*(3), 173–179.

Reid, M. C., Guo, Z., Towle, V. R., Kerns, R. D., & Concato, J. (2002b). Pain-related disability among older male veterans receiving primary care. *Journal of Gerontology Series A: Biological Sciences and Medical Sciences, 57*(11), M727–M732.

Rickels, K., & Schweizer, E. (1998). Panic disorder: Long-term pharmacotherapy and discontinuation. *Journal of Clinical Psychopharmacology, 18*(6 Suppl. 2), 12S–18S.

Roberts, L. J., Finch, P. M., Pullan, P. T., Bhagat, C. I., & Price, L. M. (2002). Sex hormone suppression by intrathecal opioids: A prospective study. *Clinical Journal of Pain, 18*(3), 144–148.

Roth, S. H., Fleischmann, R. M., Burch, F. X., Dietz, F., Bockow, B., Rapoport, R. J. et al. (2000). Around-the-clock, controlled-release oxycodone therapy for osteoarthritis-related pain: Placebo-controlled trial and long-term evaluation. *Archives of Internal Medicine, 160*(6), 853–860.

Rowbotham, M. C., Twilling, L., Davies, P. S., Reisner, L., Taylor, K., & Mohr, D. (2003). Oral opioid therapy for chronic peripheral and central neuropathic pain. *New England Journal of Medicine, 348,* 1223–1232.

Sabatowski, R., Schwalen, S., Rettig, K., Herberg, K. W., Kasper, S. M., & Radbruch, L. (2003). Driving ability under long-term treatment with transdermal fentanyl. *Journal of Pain Symptom Management*, 25(1), 38–47.

Sacerdote, P., Bianchi, M., Gaspani, L., Manfredi, B., Maucione, A., Terno, G. et al. (2000). The effects of tramadol and morphine on immune responses and pain after surgery in cancer patients. *Anesthesia & Analgesia, 90*(6), 1411–1414.

Saper, J. R., Lake, A. E., Hamel, R. L., Lutz, T. E., Branca, B., Sims, D. B., & Kroll, M. M (2004). Daily scheduled opioids for intractable head pain: Long-term observations of a treatment program. *Neurology, 62,* 1687–1694.

Sator-Katzenschlager, S. M., Schiesser, A. W., Kozek-Langenecker, S. A., Benetka, G., Langer, G., & Kress, H. G. (2003). Does pain relief improve pain behavior and mood in chronic pain patients? *Anesthesia & Analgesia, 97*(3), 791–797.

Savage, S. R. (2002). Assessment for addiction in pain-treatment settings. *Clinical Journal of Pain, 18*(4 Suppl.), S28–S38.

Schofferman, J. (1993). Long-term use of opioid analgesics for the treatment of chronic pain of nonmalignant origin. *Journal of Pain and Symptom Management, 8*(5), 279–288.

Schofferman, J. (1999). Long-term opioid analgesic therapy for severe refractory lumbar spine pain. *Clinical Journal of Pain, 15*(2), 136–140.

Schulte, F., & McVicar, N. (2002, May). Rx for death: Patients in pain overdosing in alarming numbers. *Sun-Sentinel,* p. 1A.

Sindrup, S. H., Madsen, C., Brosen, K., & Jensen, T. S. (1999). The effect of tramadol in painful polyneuropathy in relation to serum drug and metabolite levels. *Clinical Pharmacology and Therapeutics, 66,* 636–641.

Sjogren, P., Olsen, A. K., Thomsen, A. B., & Dalberg, J. (2000). Neuropsychological performance in cancer patients: The role of oral opioids, pain and performance status. *Pain, 86*(3), 237–245.

Spector, I. P., & Carey, M. P. (1990). Incidence and prevalence of the sexual dysfunctions: a critical review of the empirical literature. *Archives of Sexual Behavior, 19*(4), 389–408.

Sproule, B. A., Busto, U. E., Somer, G., Romach, M. K., & Sellers, E. M. (1999). Characteristics of dependent and nondependent regular users of codeine. *Journal of Clinical Psychopharmacology, 19*(4), 367–372.

Stetter, F., & Kupper, S. (2002). Autogenic training: A meta-analysis of clinical outcome studies. *Applied Psychophysiology & Biofeedback, 27*(1), 45–98.

Tamayo-Sarver, J. H., Hinze, S. W., Cydulka, R. K., & Baker, D. W. (2003). Racial and ethnic disparities in emergency department analgesic prescription. *American Journal of Public Health, 93*(12), 2067–2073.

Taylor, C. B., Zlutnick, S. I., Corley, M. J., & Flora, J. (1980). The effects of detoxification, relaxation, and brief supportive therapy on chronic pain. *Pain, 8*(3), 319–329.

Thurel, C., Bardin, T., & Boccard, E. (1991). Analgesic efficacy of an association of 500-mg paracetamol plus 30-mg codeine versus 400-mg paracetamol plus 30-mg dextropropoxyphene in repeated doses for chronic lower back pain. *Current Therapeutic Research, 50*(4), 463–473.

Turk, D. C., & Brody, M. C. (1991). Chronic opioid therapy for persistent noncancer pain: Panacea or oxymoron? *APS Bulletin, 1*(1), 1, 4–7.

Turk, D. C., Loeser, J. D., & Monarch, E. S. (2002). Chronic pain: Purposes and costs of interdisciplinary pain rehabilitation programs. *Economics of Neuroscience: T.E.N., 4,* 64–69.

Turk, D. C., & Okifuji, A. (1997). What factors affect physicians' decisions to prescribe opioids for chronic noncancer pain patients? *Clinical Journal of Pain, 13*(4), 330–336.

Turk, D. C., & Okifuji, A. (1998). Efficacy of multidisciplinary pain centers: Antidote for anecdotes. *Balliere's Clinical Anesthesiology, 12,* 103–119.

Turner, J. A., Calsyn, D. A., Fordyce, W. E., & Ready, L. B. (1982). Drug utilization patterns in chronic pain patients. *Pain, 12,* 357–363.

Vainio, A., Ollila, J., Matikainen, E., Rosenberg, P., & Kalso, E. (1995). Driving ability in cancer patients receiving long-term morphine analgesia. *Lancet, 346*(8976), 667–670.

van Tulder, M. W., Ostelo, R., Vlaeyen, J. W., Linton, S. J., Morley, S. J., & Assendelft, W. J. (2000). Behavioral treatment for chronic low back pain: A systematic review within the framework of the Cochrane Back Review Group. *Spine, 25*(20), 2688–2699.

Waddell, G., Main, C. J., Morris, E. W., Di Paola, M., & Gray, I. C. (1984). Chronic low-back pain, psychologic distress, and illness behavior. *Spine, 9*(2), 209–213.

Watson, C. P., & Babul, N. (1998). Efficacy of oxycodone in neuropathic pain: A randomized trial in postherpetic neuralgia. *Neurology, 50*(6), 1837–1841.

Watson, C. P., Moulin, D., Watt-Watson, J., Gordon, A., & Eisenhoffer, J. (2003). Controlled-release oxycodone relieves neuropathic pain: A randomized controlled trial in painful diabetic neuropathy. *Pain, 105*(1–2), 71–78.

Weir, R., Browne, G. B., Tunks, E., Gafni, A., & Roberts, J. (1992). A profile of users of specialty pain clinic services: predictors of use and cost estimates. *Journal of Clinical Epidemiology, 45*(12), 1399–1415.

Wilson, G. R. (2001) *Morphine hyperalgesia: A case report.* Retrieved April 12, 2004 at http://www.dcmsonline.org/jax-medicine/2001journals/May2001/morphine.htm.

World Health Organization. (1990). *Cancer pain relief and palliative care. Report of a WHO expert committee* [World Health Organization Technical Report Series, 804]. Geneva, Switzerland: World Health Organization.

Zuniga, J. R. (1998). The use of nonopioid drugs in management of chronic orofacial pain. *Journal of Oral and Maxillofacial Surgery, 56*(9), 1075–1080.

Section II

Discipline-Specific Approaches

Alfred V. Anderson, MD, DC, Section Editor

12

The Role of Nursing in Pain Management

Claudia E. Campbell, RN, BSN

INTRODUCTION

The role of the nurse, historically and currently, is solidly centered in the direct care of the patient. (Zerwekh & Claborn, 2003). When Pellino et al. (2002) completed a role delineation study for the American Society of Pain Management Nursing in 2001, it came as no surprise that survey respondents indicated assessment, monitoring, and evaluation of pain were nurses' most common activities while caring for patients in pain. In spite of the similarity in nursing activities, nurses practice in a variety of settings including clinics, offices, hospitals, surgical centers, extended-care facilities, hospices, businesses, schools, and patients' homes, to name a few (Pellino et al., 2002). Nurses may be engaged primarily in critical care, oncology, rehabilitation, home care, supportive or administrative roles, or any of the endless variety of specialized nursing practices. In most patient care settings, nurses are the members of the multidisciplinary team to spend the most time with the patient (McCaffery et al., 2000). Regardless of the practice setting or specialty, improvement in the provision of pain management services is dependent on the involvement of nurses with necessary clinical skills and a commitment toward relieving pain.

Nursing roles are numerous and complex, so it is difficult to reduce these to a single written description sufficiently detailed to describe the impact a skilled and caring nurse has on any patient's life. Instead, the goal for this chapter is to provide readers with insight into the practice of nursing as part of the multidisciplinary team. This chapter investigates the nursing role in patient education, pain assessment, analgesic interventions, assessment of the patient's response to pain management interventions, and documentation. In addition, it explores the

nurse's role in collegial communication, patient safety, professional and community education, quality improvement, advocacy, and ethics. It also discusses nurses practicing in expanded roles.

ASSESSMENT OF PAIN

The importance of pain assessment was identified as a necessary first step in improving the effectiveness of pain management. In 1992 and again in 1994, the Agency for Health Care Policy and Research (AHCPR) published guidelines for the treatment of acute pain and cancer pain. In 1999, the Joint Commission on the Accreditation of Healthcare Organizations (JCAHO) released its standards on pain management. The JCAHO standards include a call for health care organizations to recognize the right of the patient to have his or her pain routinely assessed (JCAHO, 2001). A thorough assessment of pain is multidimensional and far more complex than simply obtaining the patient's self report of pain intensity. Patient communication about the nature and severity of pain and the impact this pain has on function and quality of life takes a skilled interviewer with sufficient time to develop the trust needed to facilitate eliciting detailed information. Although assessment of pain is the responsibility of all disciplines, nurses practicing in most settings have greater opportunities to establish this type of relationship with the patient than do the other members of the multidisciplinary team. The nurse's skill in obtaining a complete pain history will determine the quality of information made available to the other members of the team for use in decision making as the pain management regimen is determined.

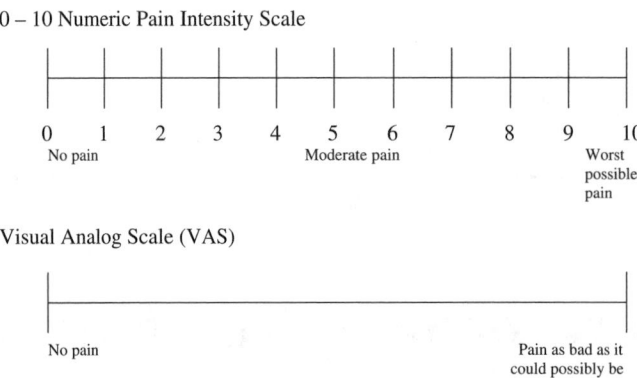

FIGURE 12.1 Pain intensity scales. From *Acute Pain Management: Operative Medical Procedures and Trauma. Clinical Practice Guideline No. 1*, by Acute Pain Management Guideline Panel (1992, February). AHCPR Publication No. 92-0032. Rockville, MD: Agency for Health Care Policy and Research.

Nurses encourage patients to share details about the character, onset, location, duration, exacerbation, and radiation of the pain and how pain influences daily functionality and quality of life. During the interview process, it is imperative to know what worked previously, what never worked, medications that were used to alleviate pain, and if any nonmedication strategies were successful. As nurses conduct assessment interviews with patients, concerns and questions are noted, and communicative ability is determined. Barriers (e.g., language or culture), when identified, require special accommodations and considerations for comprehensive treatment planning.

The patient's self-report is the single most reliable indicator of the existence and intensity of pain (AHCPR, 1992). Determining the patient's perception of pain intensity, the nurse uses one of a variety of assessment tools such as the numeric rating scale or the visual analog scale (Figure 12.1).

Tools for pain intensity rating are only as useful as patients' ability to understand and use them. Nursing communication skills ensure that patients understand the use of chosen pain assessment instruments. Nurses use pain intensity rating scales appropriate to patients' cognitive ability and language skills. Patients are asked to report pain intensity ratings without undue influence from others. The McGill Pain Questionnaire (MPQ) measures affective pain experience components in addition to pain intensity, supplementing data obtained during the nursing interview (Melzack, 1995). Using assessment tools, nurses determine pain intensity scores for the least and most intense pain levels. Patients identify whether there is breakthrough pain and, if so, what pain intensity scores occur.

A final component for pain assessment is the determination of pain intensity goals. Goals are made with consideration for acceptable levels of pain relief and ability to function (referred to as comfort and function goals). Because patients may have difficulty determining precise comfort and function goals, nurses are often in the best position to spend the time necessary to assist them in setting realistic goals and expectations for pain relief and functionality (Vallerand, 2003). Noncommunicative patients present special challenges when assessing pain, and they are at greater risk for having their pain undermanaged than are communicative patients (American Pain Society [APS], 2003). Assessment tools specifically designed to measure pain behaviors (grimacing, crying, wincing, guarding with movement, or irritability) are particularly helpful, and with other nursing assessment skills, even noncommunicative patients can be evaluated. At the end of the assessment, nurses establish expectations regarding the frequency of pain reassessment and give patients permission to report changes in pain intensity occurring between assessments, reducing patients' concerns about bothering nurses with their pain complaints.

INTERVENTIONS TO TREAT PAIN

Nurses play a crucial role in the treatment of pain using pharmacological and nonmedication therapies. Whether they are assessing a patient for pain control or compliance with the treatment plan; reviewing a prescription; obtaining, delivering, or administering medications; or initiating a nonmedication therapy, nurses are vital to ensuring a safe and effective outcome for the patient.

PHARMACOLOGICAL TREATMENT

Nurses are the team members spending the most time with patients exploring side-effect experiences and the effectiveness of pain relief from analgesics. This specific information is passed to other team members to determine individual patient variations (Vallerand, 2003). Nurses routinely administer medications to patients for the first time, so are responsible for ensuring that medications ordered are appropriate. Range orders for analgesics, unless specifically addressed in policy, require nurses to select the dose to administer and the interval of administration. Once administered, nurses' understanding of the onset of analgesia and expected duration of action, as well as potential side effects, guide nursing reassessment and subsequent administration of additional doses. These responsibilities underscore the need for collegial relationships with prescribers.

Increased numbers of opioid formulations along with a growing mainstream acceptance of pain management principles have increased the complexity of pain management decisions that nurses must make. Although more complex decision making is necessary, appropriate pain management orders reduce the need to advocate with reluctant team members. To function fully in the nursing role, a basic understanding of opioids is no longer sufficient. Nurses now must understand not only the mechanism of action of the various opioids, their rate of absorption, and the variety of routes of delivery, but also the impact of clinically significant metabolites in specific patient conditions. It is not enough to understand the timing of basic oral absorption. Opioids are now available in a variety of formulations allowing for administration of a specific formulation to relieve pain associated with a specific situation such as procedures or breakthrough pain or for around-the-clock coverage of persistent pain. This requires the nurse to understand the differences between formulations as the nurse times the administration of the opioid to achieve the best pain relief for each specific situation. Use of patient-controlled analgesia (PCA) to deliver opioids, which has become widely accepted, requires the nurse to have additional understanding of PCA and the ability to program and troubleshoot the PCA infusion devices accurately. The ability to assess side effects and determine the patient's pattern of PCA doses requested as opposed to the number of doses delivered will determine the success of PCA.

Nonopioid analgesics, such as acetaminophen and nonsteroidal anti-inflammatory drugs (NSAIDs), should be included in any analgesic regimen unless contraindicated (APS, 2003). The recommended dosages and intervals for administration of acetaminophen (APAP) and NSAIDs are more concrete than are those for opioids, so it is easier to verify the appropriateness of these agents by consulting pharmaceutical reference books. However, side effects for these medications are significant, and nurses must understand potential risks involved with administration of these medications. Nurses often administer acetaminophen for its antipyretic and analgesia effects, leading to possible overdose and hepatotoxicity if more than 4000 mg is administered within 24 h. When nurses administer acetaminophen, previous doses, including those given in combination with an opioid, must be accounted for so that the total amount of acetaminophen does not exceed the recommended daily dosage. When administering NSAIDs and coxibs, it is a nursing responsibility to screen for conditions, such as renal sufficiency, that make administration of NSAIDs or coxibs inappropriate. Even after therapy has started, nurses must continually monitor the medication's impact and potential organ system insult from the medication prescribed (e.g., the effect of an NSAID or coxib on renal function can be significant for patients who have hypotension or hypovolemia; APS, 2003). These conditions must be identified as soon as possible, and frequently it is nurses who are in the position to first identify these conditions and notify appropriate providers so the therapy may be discontinued.

Adjuvant medications, by definition, are medications whose primary indication is not the treatment of pain, but that do provide analgesia in certain conditions (Portenoy & McCaffery, 1999; Gordon, 2003). Nurses are faced with orders to administer "pain medications" that they recognize as common treatments for conditions such as seizures or depression. Nurses' understanding of these medications and their specific role in pain relief is essential. Patients require support and encouragement through a slow introduction and titration of these medications. Often it is necessary to try several different adjuvant medications before patients are able to report adequate pain relief.

INTERVENTIONAL PAIN MANAGEMENT TECHNIQUES

Nerve blocks, epidural steroid injections, electrical stimulation, and infusion of spinal opioids are interventional techniques used by pain management specialists to prevent chronic pain from occurring and to address complex pain when it occurs. The nurse assists with invasive pain procedures by completing the admission history and assessment, and by preparing patients physically and emotionally. Patient education addressing procedures reduces anxiety and encourages cooperation with postprocedural instructions. During procedures, nurses assist with patient positioning for comfort and safety, administration, and monitoring of sedation, and they provide conscious patients with information regarding progress. Nurses are knowledgeable about relevant anatomy and physiology associated with procedures and medications that are used. Nurses are able to anticipate problems and assist with emergency management. Nurses are able to monitor patient recovery and provide discharge instructions (Raj & Johnston, 2002).

NONMEDICATION TREATMENTS

Analgesic medications are the foundation for acute and cancer pain management regardless of patients' ages (APS, 2003). Regardless of the source or duration for pain, there are many nonmedication interventions that are additionally beneficial for pain management and are commonly used as adjuvants (Snyder & Wieland, 2003). Using these interventions for chronic pain allows patients to be active participants in controlling their pain rather than only relying on medications or provider initiated pain therapies (Arnstein, 2003).

Because little evidence supports that using these interventions provide analgesia, nurses must avoid using these in a singular approach. Instead, nurses must utilize all tools at hand, including easily understood and implemented nonmedication interventions with carefully crafted analgesic plans designed to provide the most effective levels of multidimensional pain relief and functionality (McCaffery & Pasero, 1999). Nonmedication treatments are used as the sole method of pain management when patients feel pain relief from these nonmedication treatments is adequate (Dalton & Coyne, 2003).

Prior to initiating nonmedication interventions, nurses assess patients' physical and emotional readiness for participation and then select interventions that are most likely to be successfully implemented. Nurses caring for patients experiencing acute pain may find that interventions that require focused attention are less practical than simple, passive interventions that do not tax patients' limited energy. Patients with chronic pain rely on their nurses to introduce them to interventions that help them to improve coping and reduce their focus on pain. Nurses can influence patients' pain through skillful application of appropriate nonmedication interventions and should be watchful for opportunities to introduce these interventions to their patients. Additionally, nurses collaborate with other interdisciplinary team members to ensure that patients are given opportunities to participate in various nonmedication interventions.

Nurses should recognize that patients' responses to nonmedication treatments are greatly dependent on patients' interest in participating with this intervention. Nonmedication interventions can be as simple as using a reassuring voice, gentle touch, or applying ice to a painful area, or as complex as assisting patients in mastering biofeedback. Physical interventions may be used to reduce swelling, muscular tension, or spasms. Interventions involving focused attention help reduce anxiety or sleeplessness (Table 12.1).

REASSESSMENT OF PAIN AND PAIN TREATMENTS

Assessment of the effectiveness and safety of the analgesic regimen is an ongoing responsibility entrusted to nurses. Just as nurses are the team members most likely to administer analgesics to patients for the first time, nurses are present when medications peak in effect for the first time. Nursing assessment includes a reassessment of patients' pain intensity, level of sedation, respiratory status, and other analgesic side effects. Assessments occur routinely and frequently until analgesic routines stabilize and responses become predictable. Failure to appreciate

---

TABLE 12.1
Examples of Nondrug Interventions

- Physical
    - Ice
    - Heat
    - Positioning
    - Massage
    - Exercise
    - Electric stimulation
- Emotional
    - Education
    - Distraction
    - Relaxation exercises
    - Music
    - Imagery
    - Meditation
    - Prayer

Note: Adapted from AHCPR, 1994; McCaffery & Pasero, 1999; and Arnstein, 2003.

---

nurses' role in reassessing patients due to poor staffing patterns or lack of nursing education increases the potential that sedation and respiratory depression go unrecognized and lead to serious complications (e.g., respiratory arrest and death).

Nurses use the same assessment tools to reassess their patients' pain intensity and to encourage familiarity with the tools. The consistent use of pain intensity tools provides accurate trending of patients' response to analgesic regimens. Just as with initial pain assessments, nurses encourage patients to rate their pain at its least and most intense, and to identify episodes of breakthrough pain and associated intensity. Once assessments of patients' pain intensity are completed, nurses use this information to determine the timing of subsequent medication or nonmedication interventions. Patients may need increased or decreased dosage of their analgesics, rotation to other agents, or other routes of delivery. Nurses determine changes to analgesic regimens and implement changes within established range orders for analgesics or advocate with prescribers for new orders.

The nursing assessment for common analgesic side effects includes respiratory status, level of sedation, pruritus, nausea, vomiting, and urinary retention. Careful attention to recognition and management of side effects when initiating new medications often determines patients' willingness to permit sufficient time to establish these regimens. The extreme variability in patients' responses to the first few doses of opioid medications makes it impossible to determine an initial dosage that is safe for every patient (APS, 2003). For this reason, administration of opioid analgesics necessitates nursing assessments for patient's levels of sedation and respiratory status. These assessments are essential for safe analgesia, and prescribers count on nurses' assessment skills when prescribing medications. Nurses prompt recognition of sedation as an indicator of impending respiratory depression, and monitoring for these changes may lead to reductions in dosage or frequency of opioids. When the respiratory status of patients becomes compromised, nurses respond with emergent administration of reversing agents to restore adequate respirations and then frequently reassess patients for continued stability.

PATIENT AND FAMILY EDUCATOR

Patients and their family members rely on the nurse to coach them through the often complex and confusing details of their pain management plan. Even the concept of "as-needed" analgesic regimens commonly prescribed for acute pain can be overwhelming for patients and families. The potential for treatment failure due to frustration and eventually noncompliance increases when patients do not understand their analgesic treatment plans and what they are suppose to do to take their medications properly.

The multidisciplinary team depends on nurses to evaluate the patient's and his or her family's ability to learn and their level of comprehension after teaching is given. Nursing assessments of patients and family members for learning barriers (e.g., anxiety, fear, and speaking languages different from those of the treatment team members) allow tailored education to meet individual patient's needs. With patients' level of understanding determined, nurses use ongoing communication with patients and their families to provide additional education.

Nurses are "interpreters" for patients and family members when they do not understand instructions given by other health care providers or team members. Introduction or reinforcement of new concepts such as the use of pain intensity rating scales, establishing a comfort and function goal, and the difference between persistent pain and breakthrough pain are often necessary before patients are able to actively participate in conversations regarding pain assessment and management. Terms describing different formulations of analgesics such as "long-acting" and "short-acting" should be presented simply and in the patient's own language whenever possible. Nurses provide patients and family members with clear instructions to report changes in the intensity of pain, when to request or use additional analgesics, how to report analgesic side effects, and whether the quality of the overall pain management regimen is facilitating recovery or improving quality of life. Nurses address misconceptions patients have about potential tolerance, dependence, or addiction to opioid analgesics with sensitivity and expertise. When needed, nurses utilize written instructions, pain diaries, and graphic representations to enhance patient understanding. Nurses commonly develop educational pamphlets, fact sheets, videos, and other materials to assist with patient and family teaching.

Use of multimodal balanced approaches to pain management are most effective in achieving adequate analgesia. However, the complexity of using multiple medications and nonmedication interventions for pain management may be difficult for patients and family members to grasp. Miaskowski et al. (2001) interviewed patients with cancer and found that the decisions patients must make regarding pain medications are more complex than those decisions required when taking an antihypertensive on a routine basis. Patients should be educated beyond the basic instructions of medication, dose, and timing to ensure development of adequate self-care skills (Schumacher et al., 2002). Lack of sufficient understanding may lead to medication errors, unnecessary medication side effects, and noncompliance with the pain management interventions. The nursing role in educating patients and their family regarding analgesic treatment plans is vital to the success and safety of pain management. Nurses are expert resources for patients and their families in vulnerable periods of care such as initiation of analgesic treatment plans or during transitions from one analgesic to another or from one route of administration to another. Principles of analgesic absorption, onset of analgesia, and expected duration of action are explained to patients and family members in simple and easily understood terms supported by written instructions. When patients are taking long-acting opioids for persistent pain relief and using short-acting opioids for breakthrough pain episodes, nurses provide coaching and encouragement so patients understand when each opioid should be taken and how to achieve the best pain relief.

Use of high-technology analgesic therapies such as intravenous, epidural, or intrathecal infusion requires additional education and support from nurses to ensure patients understand goals of treatment. When analgesics are delivered using the PCA button technology, the nursing role in education for patients is critical. Patients need to be instructed to use the PCA button properly and have a clear understanding that they should not allow anyone to push the PCA button for them due to potential ramifications should someone "assist" them.

Nurses teach about the concept of medication synergy when patients are taking adjuvant medications in combination with opioids. Often nurses initiate nonmedication interventions and provide support as patients learn and develop skills in the use of these treatments. Ongoing education and support, with answers to questions, are the hallmarks of the nursing role when patients face uncertain outcomes in their pharmacological treatment. As patients and their family members become more familiar with treatment regimens and timing of analgesics, consumption of these medications and the quality of analgesia are optimized. Patients become increasingly independent, more likely to be compliant with the analgesic regimens, and less likely to make errors.

When patients are ready for discharge from one setting to another, discharge instructions regarding pain management are given in writing and then are reviewed verbally with patients and family members. Nurses are the members of multidisciplinary teams responsible for instructing patients prior to discharge. Nurses summarize written instructions of all team members and review them together with patients. Written and detailed instructions regarding the analgesic regimen including medications, dosages, intervals for administration, and when the next dosage should be taken are reviewed for accuracy and then provided to patients. Pain diaries may be helpful to assist patients and family members to continue an organized system of tracking and timing medication administration (Schumacher et al., 2002). Nurses are generally the last members of multidisciplinary teams to review all discharge instructions with patients and ensure that patients have adequate understanding. Additional information is provided where necessary prior to patients' discharges (AHCPR, 1992).

DOCUMENTATION

Nurses' documentation when reviewed by other team members becomes the core of the interdisciplinary team's communication process. This documentation is useful in quality improvement and risk management activities. Accrediting organizations, such as the JCAHO, review nursing documentation to determine organizational compliance with required standards and institutional policies.

Nurses are vital team members, functioning as coordinators of care and facilitators of multidisciplinary team communication (St. Marie, 2003). While other disciplines, out of necessity, spend only a limited amount of time with patients and write focused notes in medical records, in most care situations nurses interact with patients multiple times during the day, permitting more specific information regarding all aspects of patients' conditions and care to be elicited. Accurate and ongoing nursing documentation of patients' assessments of pain and its side effects provides a continuous treatment record that facilitates identification of trends and assists with decision making regarding future interventions. Nursing documentation is central to the multidisciplinary team's communication. Other team members use the nurses' 24-h record of the total amount of opioids administered when calculating equianalgesic doses in the process of transitioning patients from one delivery route to another or when rotating to alternative opioids. Decisions to increase opioid doses are based on documented trends of increasing episodes of breakthrough pain and reductions in function as pain influences patients' desire to engage in daily activities. In nurses' notes, other team members find the details of the hours and days of

patients' hospitalizations or identify trends over the final weeks and months in the lives of hospice patients.

There has been a significant change in the way nurses document as health care organizations move from pen and paper to electronic medical records (EMRs). Data collected by nurses in EMRs are easily and almost immediately available to all members of the health care team for use in decision making. Electronic data are more easily used in activities such as quality improvement measurement and research. Nurses are establishing themselves as leaders in medical informatics, using their unique perspective to design documentation and data collection programs suited to the flow of the work nurses perform. These programs are becoming increasingly dynamic and are able to prompt documentation of vital assessments including pain assessments and routine pain intensity scores. Infusion pumps used to deliver pain management therapies are undergoing a technology revolution, and soon infusion pumps will be designed to interface with the EMR allowing for frequent and routine downloading of data such as medication infusion rates, changes in dosage settings, and the total amount of medication delivered to the patient. The companies that manufacture these devices recognize the value of having nurses consult as they create safer and more efficient technology.

FACILITATOR OF COLLEGIAL RELATIONSHIPS AMONG MEMBERS OF THE MULTIDISCIPLINARY TEAM

Optimal pain management is best accomplished through interdisciplinary efforts (AHCPR, 1992; Loeser, 2001). The very nature of multidisciplinary care results in fragmentation as patients interact with team members regarding specific aspects of their pain management and plan of care. Nurses are vital multidisciplinary team members facilitating continuity and cohesiveness by coordinating communication between patients and team members. This collegial relationship between nurses and other team members is vital for pain management to be safe and effective. The relationship that exists between colleagues is built on trust and respect for each other's skills and expertise (Zerwekh & Claborn, 2003).

GUARDIAN OF PATIENT SAFETY

Nurses are guardians of patient safety, and their diligence in this role prevents negative outcomes related to pain management. Nurses safely administer medications at bedsides. When medications are administered, nurses check that the right drug is being given in the ordered dose, that they are using the correct route and time, and that the medication is being administered to the correct patient by checking two separate patient identifiers.

Reducing medical error and increasing reporting of errors has become a focus of the media, consumers of health care, health care organizations, and the organizations that provide hospital accreditation (AHA et al., 2002; JCAHO, 2001). Because nurses routinely administer many medications in their practice, they are the team members most likely to make a medication administration error. Nurses must be especially alert to avoid common errors such as those made when administering short-acting and long-acting formulations of the same opioid or when programming PCA infusion devices for intravenous, epidural, or intrathecal infusions. Nurses have sufficient knowledge to identify when prescriptions are erroneous or potentially dangerous. Because of their role in medication administration, nurses have a unique understanding of processes that are difficult or prone to error and are in positions to be valuable resources on the risk assessment team of health care systems working to improve the safety of pain management within their facilities.

QUALITY IMPROVEMENT

Quality improvement activities focused on institutional pain management processes have become prevalent since the 1999 release of the JCAHO standards on pain management. Because quality improvement efforts are best accomplished through an organized multidisciplinary approach, institutions are encouraged to form a standing multidisciplinary committee with the authority to make decisions regarding pain management processes. Nurses are recognized as valuable members and are often designated as leaders of these quality improvement teams. As is the case with other aspects of pain management, nurses are in unique positions to understand a broad range of problematic processes and readily identify barriers. These nurses should be well respected by their peers and members of the health care team and identified as change leaders in their areas of practice. Regardless of the composition of the committee's membership, there should always be representation from nursing (Pasero et al., 1999).

Outdated and tradition-based practices of managing pain are often deeply ingrained within organizations. In addition to institutional quality improvement activities, nurses are also involved in specific pain management improvement activities that are designed to reduce tradition and encourage appropriate pain management practices in their individual work areas. Nurses are often on teams that design treatment algorithms, protocols, and care pathways that improve the pain care that patients receive.

ETHICS AND ADVOCACY

The nurse's role in ethics and advocacy related to pain management is critical. Opportunities to recognize and manage ethical dilemmas and to actively advocate on

TABLE 12.2
American Society of Pain Management Nursing Position Statements

- Use of Placebos for Pain Management (1996)
- End of Life Care (1998)
- Assisted Suicide (1998)
- Neonatal Circumcision Pain Relief (2001)
- Pain Management in Patients with Addictive Disease (2002)
- Use of "As-Needed" Range Orders for Opioid Analgesics in the Management of Acute Pain (2004)

Note: Full position statements available at www.aspmn.org.

behalf of the patient present challenges for even the most passionate and experienced nurse. In spite of the challenges, nurses are speaking out in greater numbers and focusing their attention on the conflicts they face as a result of their unique relationship with patients and their role within the health care team (Zerwekh & Claborn, 2003). The American Society of Pain Management Nursing (ASPMN) is a national nursing organization that has taken an active and public advocacy role in pain management issues. ASPMN has issued position statements on a variety of issues (Table 12.2) with the goal of educating and guiding nurses as they face difficult ethical dilemmas in pain management and encouraging them to recognize these dilemmas as opportunities for advocacy.

The *International Council of Nurses Code for Nurses* and the American Nurses Association (ANA) *Code of Ethics*, developed by nurses, provide professional direction for nurses facing ethical decisions and outline desirable behaviors in the nurse–patient relationship. Nurses are responsible for the basic ethical principles of autonomy, beneficence, nonmaleficence, justice, veracity, and fidelity (ANA, 2001).

The patient's right to autonomy requires nurses and other members of health care teams to respect patients as unique individuals. They must respect patients' reports of pain and rights to accept or refuse analgesic medications, treatments, or procedures. Ensuring that patients provide informed consent prior to interventional pain treatments or procedures often requires the full efforts of health care teams. Nurses assist patients and families to review pertinent information they have received so that informed consent can be given based on whether the interventional pain treatment will enhance or detract from patients' quality of life (St. Marie, 2003).

Beneficence is the duty to actively do good for patients, while nonmaleficence calls upon nurses to accept the duty to prevent or avoid doing harm whether intentional or unintentional. There is a critical balance between these two principles when treating pain, and disagreements between health care team members regarding what constitutes adequate analgesia are often core ethical dilemmas. In many of these instances, patients rely on nurses to be their advocates (Benner, 2003). Nurses advocate persistently and aggressively to ensure patients suffering with pain have the right to justice (pain relief): pain management services provided fairly and equally regardless of age, sex, ethnicity, socioeconomic status, and many other variables. Nurses have the responsibility as members of health care teams to assist patients in accessing expert pain care and ensuring that medications ordered to treat pain are accessible and affordable for patients. Nurses are reaching out to insurance providers and elected state officials advocating for reform and legislation with the goal of improving access to pain management specialists and appropriate pain medications for patients who are suffering. Legislative leaders increasingly recognize nurses as reliable advocates for improved pain management in local and national policy.

To develop trusting relationships between patients and health care teams there is a duty to tell the truth and avoid deception. It is the role of nurses to ensure that patients are presented with truthful information regarding their care, and this is the ethical rule of veracity. The use of placebos for pain management without patients' consent is in direct violation of this principle. In its position statement, *Use of Placebos for Pain Management*, ASPMN points out that the use of placebos requires deception and that as an organization it opposes the use of placebos to determine whether patients really are in pain or in place of legitimate analgesics for pain relief (ASPMN, 1996). When placebos are used, it should only occur with patients' informed consent, as in pharmaceutical trials. Unfortunately, nurses find themselves in the position of either participating in unethical administration of placebos or standing as an advocate for uninformed patients even if it means standing in opposition of the desires of prescribers. Nurses play a vital role in developing institutional policies regarding the use of placebos.

Patients depend on nurses to fairly and truthfully represent how pain management care will be provided and to follow through with the plans of care with fidelity. Nurses must master the challenge of weaving pain management interventions into the care they provide with careful attention to ensure that interventions are not delayed or missed. In turn, nurses and other members of the health care team have expectations regarding the actions of patients. Communication regarding these expectations is outlined in pain management agreements between patients and health care team members. Adherence to these pain management agreements facilitates the development of relationships built on fidelity.

NURSE EXPERT IN AN EXPANDED ROLE

Nurses who have developed an expertise in pain management are found in a variety of roles and settings, but share a common goal and passion for improving of pain management practices and relieving the suffering of patients with pain. Whether primarily practicing at patients' bedsides as resources, case managers, clinical educators, specialists, independent practitioners, anesthesia providers, or managers of organized pain management services, nurses' expertise is valued by the multidisciplinary team.

THE PAIN RESOURCE NURSE

The science of pain management is relatively new, and nurses are now putting pain management beliefs of the past aside, to base their practices on evidence rather than tradition. Even so, many nurses today enter their profession without sufficient preparation in the science of pain management. Most patients they care for as novice nurses have pain. Fortunate patients and novice nurses have as a resource bedside nurses who are experts in pain management. The need to mentor nurses while they gain expertise is paramount in the efforts to change the culture of pain management. The City of Hope National Medical Center in Duarte, California, began the first Pain Resource Nurse (PRN) program designed to train the bedside nurse to function in the role of an expert resource and mentor for other nurses (Ferrell et al., 1993). Pain resource nurses are specially trained in the concepts of pain management. As experts, pain resource nurses assist other nurses to develop skills in all aspects of pain management including pain assessment, pharmacology and equianalgesia; treatment of analgesic side effects; and the use of high-technology pain management modalities. In addition to mentoring other nurses, pain resource nurses are active participants and change leaders for the improvement of pain management within the institutions and/or in the care setting where they work.

CASE MANAGER

Case management nurses have the primary function of assisting patients and multidisciplinary teams with a focus on cost containment through the provision of quality care. Whether this is accomplished using care pathways or through careful attention to the multidisciplinary plan of care, case management nurses with expertise in pain management act as valuable resources and coordinators of care (Jerin, 2002). Patients who have a complicated course of illness and recovery often require a level of care coordination that requires more time than is realistically available to the bedside nurse. Nurse case managers provide this expanded level of care with expert knowledge of insurance plans, referral information, and pain management specialists available in the geographical region. Case management nurses who have expert pain management skills recognize that the cost and availability of analgesics must be considered when initiating an analgesic regimen because many insurance plans limit the reimbursement or restrict access to certain analgesics (Gordon, 2003). Patients who do not have sufficient prescription coverage may find the financial burden of purchasing analgesics intolerable. In addition to encouraging multidisciplinary teams to use affordable analgesic choices in analgesic regimens, case management nurses function as patients' links to many pharmaceutical companies that provide patient assistance programs. These programs are often accessible based on need or financial criteria (Vallerand, 2003).

Patients who have complex acute pain or who are facing the challenge of chronic pain may benefit from receiving pain management care from pain management specialists. Patients may feel overwhelmed or inadequately prepared to undertake the task of identifying and selecting their pain management specialist to provide ongoing pain care. Case management nurses assist patients by providing listings of pain management specialists in the patient's locale. In some geographical locations pain management specialists are not readily available. As an alternative, case management nurses may assist patients in finding primary care physicians or independent nurse practitioners recognized as good pain managers who are willing to provide ongoing care.

CLINICAL NURSE SPECIALIST AND EDUCATOR

Nurses functioning in roles of clinical nurse specialists (CNS) or educators are vital to support the ongoing learning of student nurses and nurses practicing at the bedside. Generally prepared with a master's degree or doctoral degree in nursing, CNSs and educators are recognized experts in the practice of nursing. As faculty members, nurses are responsible for developing curricula and conducting the education of the adult learner in the professional practice of nursing. In a position to influence curricula throughout all phases of the nurses' training, educators are responsible for ensuring that student nurses are schooled in the appropriate principles and practices of pain management. CNSs function primarily in health care institutional settings. The rapid changes and advancements in the science of pain management make it difficult for practicing nurses to assimilate new practices into the busy pace of everyday work without educational offerings and supportive mentoring that CNSs provide. Nurses in CNS roles are often responsible for developing and reviewing algorithms or protocols and directing quality improvement activities. CNSs and educators conduct ongoing review of current health care literature, participate in or direct nursing research, and contribute to the body of literature through publication. CNSs and educators who are passionate regarding the central role that nurses play in the success of pain management can be

remarkable and positive forces in improving the quality of pain management nursing.

ADVANCE PRACTICE NURSES

Nurse Practitioner and Certified Registered Nurse Anesthetist are advanced practice roles in which nurses functions with greater autonomy in a supervised or collaborative relationship with physicians. Rather than collaborating with physicians for orders prior to initiating changes in the pain management plan, advanced practice nurses collaborate with physicians when determining diagnoses and treatment plans, but maintain independent decision-making authority (Brown & Draye, 2003). Although the role of advanced practice nurses was first described in the 1960s, it is not unusual for these nurses today to find that the jobs they are considering may not have well-defined descriptions and roles. Nurses are embracing these challenges and opportunities that come with defining their advanced practice roles. Advanced practice nurses in many states are able to obtain prescriptive privileges for controlled substances. Prescriptive practice allows these nurses to fill a much-needed role in settings and locations where access to pain management specialists or health care providers with pain management expertise is limited. The role of advanced practice nurses has improved access to services for patients and specifically for patients in vulnerable populations such as minorities, those with low incomes, and the uninsured (Brown & Draye, 2003). Advanced practice nurses may specialize in pain management and fill roles within an interventional pain management clinic or multidisciplinary pain management center.

RESEARCHER

The National Institute of Nursing Research (NINR) encourages nursing research to focus on building nursing knowledge for the improvement of care to patients. The organizational mission statement calls for nursing research to establish a scientific basis for the care of individuals across the life span including all aspects of care from recovery to end of life (NINR, 2001). There are many unanswered questions in the practice of pain management, and nurses need to be involved in research regarding the physical, psychological, social, and financial impact and outcomes related to interventional pain management technologies (St. Marie, 2003). Nurses in pain management often fill the roles of primary investigators or co-investigators for pain management studies in addition to enrolling participants and gathering data. The rapid expansion of the science of pain management provides opportunities for nurses to be contributors to the future knowledge that will define nursing practice in pain management.

Pain Management Specialist

Nurses who specialize in pain management often are members of acute or chronic inpatient pain services and serve as staff for interventional pain clinics or multidisciplinary pain management programs, in addition to a variety of other settings where the focus is on the management of complex pain conditions. Pain management nurses combine the skills encompassed in the roles of the bedside nurse, pain resource nurse, case manager, clinical specialist, educator, and researcher into one demanding role. Expert skills in the assessment of pain in complex patient situations utilizing multiple tools and methods are necessary to ensure that pain complaints are recognized and appropriately treated. In addition, skills such as an in-depth understanding of analgesic medications, equianalgesia, and drug–drug interactions are essential. Pain management nurses provide routine assessments and oversight of the nursing care for patients, ensuring patient safety and providing support to the greater nursing staff when advanced pain management technologies are used, such as intravenous PCAs, epidural or intrathecal infusions utilizing external or implanted infusion pumps, and spinal cord stimulators. In turn, the nursing staff depends on the expertise of pain management nurses to assist when identifying unusual analgesic side effects and complications associated with pain treatments. Pain management nurses provide expertise as educators and mentors for nursing staff. There is beginning evidence to suggest that the expertise of a pain management nurse in health care settings and the nursing staff's interactions with a pain management team have a positive influence on the knowledge and beliefs of the nursing staff (Mackintosh & Bowles, 2000). Pain management nurses are generally well respected for a willingness to educate and mentor those just joining the specialty as well as those who express disdain regarding the principles of effective pain management. Indeed, within the specialty of pain management, nurses are among the most respected and recognized educators and advocates. Pain management nurses, who are editors of professional publications and members of editorial boards, author many case studies, journal articles, reports of research studies, and reference books.

SUMMARY

Although nurses practice in a variety of specialties and settings and provide patient care in collaboration with many different professions, nurses' skills are unique to the health care team and central to the optimal delivery of appropriate pain management care. Nurses more commonly hold master's and doctoral degrees and capably perform in advanced practice roles. As leaders, nurses stand out in roles that establish long-range plans influencing the delivery of health care and directly providing needed services that bring relief to those in pain. From the provision of proper patient assessments to decision making at the bedside to establishment of treatment efficacy, nurses are the frontline soldiers in the army of health care providers that battle against pain.

REFERENCES

Agency for Health Care Policy and Research (AHCPR). (1992). Clinical practice guidelines for Acute pain management in adults: Operative or medical procedures and trauma (Publication No. 92-0032). Rockville, MD: Author.

Agency for Health Care Policy and Research (AHCPR). (1994). Clinical practice guidelines for management of cancer pain. (Publication No. 94-0592). Rockville, MD: Author.

American Hospital Association, Health Research & Educational Trust, and the Institute for Safe Medication Practices. (2002) Pathways for medication safety. Retrieved from www.medpathways.info.

American Nurses Association. (2001). Code for nurses with interpretive statements. Kansas City, MO: Author.

American Pain Society (APS). (2003). Principles of analgesic use in the treatment of acute pain and cancer pain, 5th ed. Glenview, IL: Author.

American Society of Pain Management Nursing. (2004). Use of placebos for pain management. position statements. Retrieved September 24, 2004 from www.aspmn.org/html/positionstmts.htm.

Arnstein, P. (2003). Comprehensive analysis and management of chronic pain. *Nursing Clinics of North America, 38*, 403–417.

Benner, P. (2003). Enhancing patient advocacy and social ethics. *American Journal of Critical Care, 12*(4), 374–375.

Brown, M. A., & Draye, M.A. (2003). Experiences of pioneer nurse practitioners in establishing advanced practice roles. *Journal of Nursing Scholarship, 35*(4), 391–397.

Dalton, J. A., & Coyne, P. (2003). Cognitive-behavioral therapy: Tailored to the individual. *Nursing Clinics of North America, 38,* 465–476.

Ferrell, B. R., Grant, M., Richey, K. J., Ropchan, R., & Rivera, L. M. (1993). The pain resource nurse training program: A unique approach to pain management. *Journal of Pain Symptom Management, 8*, 549–556.

Gordon, D. B. (2003) Nonopioid and adjuvant analgesics in chronic pain management: Strategies for effective use. *Nursing Clinics of North America, 38*, 447–464.

Jerin, L. (2002). Care delivery models for pain management. In B. St. Marie (Ed.), *Core curriculum for pain management nursing*. St. Louis, MO: W.B. Saunders.

Joint Commission on Accreditation of Healthcare Organizations. Pain: Current understanding of assessment, management, and treatments. Retrieved September 21, 2000 from http://www.jcaho.org/news+room/health+care+issues/pain+mono_npc.pdf.

Loeser, J. D. (2001). Multidisciplinary pain programs. In J. D. Loeser, S. H. Butler, C. R. Chapman, & D. C. Turk (Eds.), *Bonica's management of pain*, (3rd ed., pp. 255–264). Philadelphia, PA: Lippincott Williams & Wilkins.

Mackintosh, C., & Bowles, S. (2000). The effect of an acute pain service on nurses' knowledge and beliefs about post-operative pain. *Journal of Clinical Nursing, 9*(1), 119–126.

McCaffery, M., Ferrell, B. R., & Pasero, C. (2000). Nurses' personal opinions about patients' pain and their effect on recorded assessments and titration of opioid doses. *Pain Management Nursing, 1*(3), 70–87.

McCaffery, M., & Pasero, C. (1999). *Pain: Clinical manual*, 2nd ed. St. Louis: Mosby.

Melzack, R. (1975). The McGill Pain Questionnaire: Major properties and scoring methods. *Pain, 1*(3), 277–299.

Miaskowski, C., Dodd, M. J., West, C., Paul, S. M., Tripathy, D., Koo, P., & Schumacher, K. (2001). Lack of adherence with the analgesic regimen: A significant barrier to effective cancer pain management. *Journal of Clinical Oncology, 19*(23), 4275–4279.

National Institute of Nursing Research. Mission Statement. (2001, June 17). Retrieved September 24, 2004 at http://ninr.nih.gov/ninr/research/diversity/mission.html.

Pasero, C. Gordon, D. B., McCaffery, M., & Ferrell, B. R. (1999). Building institutional commitment to improving pain management. In M. McCaffery & C. Pasero (Eds.), *Pain: Clinical manual* (pp. 711–744). St. Louis: Mosby.

Pellino, T. A., Willens, J., Polomano, R. C., & Heye, M. (2002). The American Society of Pain Management Nurses practice analysis: Role delineation study. *Pain Management Nursing, 3*(1), 2–15).

Portenoy, R. K. & McCaffery, M. (1999). Adjuvant analgesics. In M. McCaffery, & C. Pasero, (Eds.), *Pain: Clinical manual* (pp. 302). St. Louis, MO: Mosby, Inc.

Raj, P. P., & Johnston, M. (2002). Organization and function of the nerve block facility. In P. P. Raj (Ed.). *Textbook of regional anesthesia* (p. 148). Orlando, FL: Churchill Livingston.

Schumacher, K. L, Koresawa, S., West, C., Dodd, M., Paul, S. M., Tripathy, D. et al. (2002). The usefulness of a daily pain management diary for outpatients with cancer-related pain. *Oncology Nursing Forum, 29*(9), 1304–1313.

Snyder, M., & Wieland, J. (2003). Complementary and alternative therapies: What is their place in the management of chronic pain? *Nursing Clinics of North America, 38*, 495–508.

St. Marie, B. (2003). The complex pain patient: Interventional treatment and nursing issues. *Nursing Clinics of North America, 38*, 539–554.

Vallerand, A. H. (2003). The use of long-acting opioids in chronic pain management. *Nursing Clinics of North America, 38*, 435–445.

Zerwekh, J., & Claborn, J. (2003). *Nursing today: Transition and trends* (pp. 38–39, 45, 396). St. Louis: Saunders.

13

Allopathic Specialties

B. Eliot Cole, MD, MPA

INTRODUCTION

Allopathic medicine is the health care practice combating disease through the use of treatments producing effects different from those produced by the disease, producing a second condition that is antagonistic to the first (Arizona Medical Board, 2004). Allopathic physicians, as doctors of medicine (M.D.s), routinely do physical examinations to be able to diagnose, prevent, and treat illnesses, injuries, and other disorders, often using highly technical procedures. Allopathic physicians, as medical doctors, are not just one homogeneous group that provides the same services to all patients, but a large group of extensively educated practitioners who have initially trained in the common areas of medical science and primary medical specialties before pursuing different specialty areas of interest. Physicians working in pain management/medicine serve as valuable members of treatment teams providing multidisciplinary care for those in pain and work to prevent, remove, or control pain through the provision of unique, often highly specialized skills and therapeutics. This chapter describes for non-allopathic pain practitioners the background and training of allopathic physicians. It identifies the specialty implications for managing pain and the range of pain-related services provided by these different types of practitioners.

BECOMING A PRACTICING ALLOPATHIC PHYSICIAN

Formal education and training requirements for allopathic physicians are among the most demanding of any occupation (Bureau of Labor Statistics [BLS], 2004). To be eligible for admission to an allopathic medical school in the United States one must generally complete a 4-year undergraduate college-degree program (granting a B.A. or B.S.) with a strong emphasis on the basic sciences (American Medical Association [AMA], 2000). Entrance requirements for most American medical schools include completion of course work in biology, mathematics, chemistry, physics, and English, so the traditional "premedical" education minimally covers these areas. To keep the undergraduate experience well rounded, studying humanities and the social sciences is strongly encouraged, as the "ideal physician" understands how society works and is able to communicate and write well (American Association of Medical Colleges [AAMC], 2004a). Those wishing to apply to medical school must possess grade point averages (GPAs) well above the mean and score well on the Medical College Admission Test (MCAT), which analyzes knowledge of the basic sciences, reading and writing abilities, and overall problem-solving skills.

Having the right personality to be an allopathic physician usually requires caring deeply about other people, their problems, and their pain(s); enjoying helping people with medical skills and knowledge; enjoying the process of learning and gaining new understanding; and being interested in how the human body functions (AAMC, 2004b). Key factors affecting acceptance to medical school include completion of required undergraduate courses, GPA, score on the MCAT, extracurricular activities, letters of recommendation, and interviews with medical school faculty members. Only half of those applying to U.S. medical schools are accepted (AAMC, 2004a).

The usual 4-year medical education leading to the M.D. degree consists of preclinical and clinical training. Preclinical education involves the mastery of many basic medical sciences: anatomy, biochemistry, embryology, histology, human behavior, microbiology, pathology, physiology, pharmacology, and more. Until medical students are able to demonstrate mastery with these areas during their first 2 years of medical school, they are generally not permitted to have significant clinical contact beyond learning how to perform thorough medical histories and physicals. During their second 2 years of clinical training, allopathic students learn about the "primary care" specialties of family medicine, internal medicine, obstetrics and gynecology, pediatrics, and surgery (general and specialized), plus a few other core specialties (e.g., neurology and psychiatry) by actually working with patients under the continuous supervision of resident and attending physicians. While the education is not all-inclusive in scope, allopathic students have wide exposure to the breadth of medical practice during their 4 years of medical education and leave medical school with one or more identified interest areas.

Immediately upon completing their medical education newly graduated medical doctors serve at least 1 year of postgraduate training, commonly referred to as "internship" or postgraduate year 1 (PGY-1), putting their textbook knowledge and rudimentary clinical skills into actual clinical practice by assuming progressively greater roles in the care of patients assigned to them. Physicians are usually eligible for medical licensure after completion of an internship.

Medical licensure is always necessary for allopathic physicians to practice medicine and provide direct patient care. This licensure is unique to a jurisdiction; usually a state within the United States requires passage of a licensure examination reviewing the basic medical sciences and clinical specialties, background checks, and in some states, even letters of reference from current in-state license holders. While temporary or training licensure is available without much difficulty and required for those in training programs, unrestricted medical licensure usually requires some specified period of postgraduate training and passage of an examination. Many allopathic physicians become fully licensed during their training years, once they have completed the minimum training necessary for licensure and have passed their examinations. This may allow them to continue their own residency training while beginning to work part of the time as practicing physicians ("moonlighting").

Those planning to specialize in one or more of the major disciplines of medical practice continue their professional education by performing residency training for 2 to 6 additional years, PGY-2 to 7 (American Board of Medical Specialties [ABMS], 2002; AMA, 2000). To obtain independent licensure necessary to practice medicine, resident physicians generally remain under initially continuous direct and then increasingly indirect supervision from fully licensed senior educator physicians (attending physicians) who have already completed their training and are usually "board eligible" or fully board certified.

For many physicians, becoming knowledgeable about one of the major disciplines of medicine (family practice, internal medicine, pediatrics, neurology, obstetrics and gynecology, psychiatry, and surgery) is not enough, so they continue their training into areas of subspecialization within the larger specialties by spending additional time, usually 1 to 3 years, in fellowship programs (ABMS, 2002; AMA, 2000). Having completed 4 years of college, 4 years of medical school, 3 to 7 years in residency training, and 1 to 3 years in fellowship (12 to 18 years in training), allopathic physicians are eligible for medical licensure and voluntary specialty and subspecialty certification.

Becoming voluntarily certified or subspecialty certified requires completion of an approved residency and/or fellowship training program, having an unrestricted medical license, submission of an application to the appropriate specialty board describing the scope of training received, and then successfully passing a written examination, oral examination (15 of the 24 boards), or both (ABMS, 2002). Only those allopathic physicians who have taken and passed their board certification or subspecialty certification examinations are permitted to describe themselves as being "board certified" in the United States. Those claiming to be "board eligible" have completed only their training, but have not yet passed their certification examination(s).

MEDICAL SPECIALTIES AND CERTIFICATION PROCESSES

In the United States, the primary overall certifying body for most allopathic physicians is the American Board of Medical Specialties (ABMS). There are 24 specialty constituent boards within the ABMS that provide certification in 36 general medical specialties and an additional 88 subspecialty fields (ABMS, 2002; AMA, 2000). In the past, certifications were given for the lifetime of practitioners passing the examination(s). Certifications and subspecialty certifications are now time-limited, requiring renewal (recertification) about every 6 to 10 years (ABMS, 2002).

General medical specialties include the core clinical areas of medicine: family and internal medicine, pediatrics, neurology, obstetrics and gynecology, psychiatry, and surgery. Today, the certifying medical specialties include allergy and immunology, anesthesiology, colon and rectal surgery, dermatology, emergency medicine, family practice, internal medicine, neurological surgery, neurology, nuclear medicine, obstetrics and gynecology, ophthalmology, orthopedic surgery, otolaryngology, pathology, pediatrics, physical medicine and rehabilitation, plastic surgery, preventative medicine, psychiatry, radiology, surgery, thoracic surgery, and urology. Certified practitioners in these specialties are given certificates bearing the name of the granting authority, the "American Board of" and the name of the specialty.

Subspecialty certification, available to allopathic physicians after becoming certified in one of the major medical specialties, requires additional training and competency beyond that necessary for initially becoming specialty certified and requires passing another examination in the subspecialty area (e.g., addiction psychiatry, child neurology or psychiatry, endocrinology, gastroenterology, hematology and oncology, infectious disease, nephrology, pain medicine, pulmonary medicine, or rheumatology). Those achieving certified subspecialty status have reached the zenith in their professions, with few other honors considered more prestigious.

Certified allopathic physicians often refer to themselves as "Diplomates" of their boarding organization when they become certified, or simply "Boarded." Those using the term "Fellows" are board-certified physicians belonging to a professional society (e.g., American College of Surgery, American College of Obstetrics and Gynecology), requiring board certification for full membership, that is dedicated to furthering standards, practice, and professional and public education within individual medical specialties (ABMS, 2002). Being a "Fellow" is another way of recognizing distinguished specialty physicians, and this frequently is abbreviated as "F" plus the initials of their professional organization (i.e., F.A.C.P. for Fellow, American College of Physicians; F.A.C.S. for Fellow, American College of Surgeons; F.A.C.O.G. for Fellow, American College of Obstetrics and Gynecology).

The declared purpose of certification, according to the ABMS (2002) is to "provide assurance to the public that a certified medical specialist has successfully completed an approved educational program and an evaluation, including an examination process designed to assess the knowledge, experience and skills requisite to the provision of high quality patient care in that specialty" (p. 4). Certification does not directly establish how physicians clinically practice but is an independent "check" of allopathic physicians. In fact, certification is much like obtaining a commercial driver's license; it establishes that the holder of certification knows some prospectively agreed upon minimal set of data, which exceeds the minimum required for medical licensure, while never entirely establishing the breadth of the certificant's knowledge. However, not having certification prevents one from practicing some aspects of medicine, just as not having the specialized driver's license makes it illegal to operate a commercial vehicle.

In general, allopathic physicians after completing their training continue to work long, irregular hours; almost one third of physicians worked 60 or more hours a week in 2002 (BLS, 2004). Because of the tremendous costs associated with starting medical practice, most new allopathic physicians work as salaried employees of group medical practices, clinics, hospitals, or health networks before considering solo practice (BLS, 2004).

In the past decade it has been possible for allopathic physicians in certain specialties (anesthesiology, neurology, physical medicine and rehabilitation, and psychiatry) to obtain subspecialty certification in pain medicine from the same ABMS boards that initially credentialed them. The first boarding organization to subspecialty certify its members was the American Board of Anesthesiology (ABA, 2004) in 1993. The American Board of Psychiatry and Neurology (ABPN, 2004) and the American Board of Physical Medicine and Rehabilitation (ABPMR, 2004) added subspecialty certification for their constituent members in 2000, allowing their members to take the ABA subspecialty examination. All three of these boarding organizations initially offered a "grandfathering" practice option for establishing eligibility to take the examination during the first 4 years, before mandating completion of an Accreditation Council for Graduate Medical Education (ACGME, 2004) approved fellowship in pain medicine.

In addition to the ABMS route described above, two other credentialing options exist. Allopathic and osteopathic physicians completing allopathic residency programs leading to certification by an ABMS board are able to take the pain medicine certifying examination given by the American Board of Pain Medicine (a self-designated, voluntary credentialing organization not recognized by the ABMS) (American Board of Pain Medicine, 2004). Allopath physicians are allowed to take the American Academy of Pain Management's (a self-designated, voluntary credentialing organization not recognized by the ABMS) credentialing examination in multidisciplinary pain management after 2 years of clinical experience working with patients in pain with or without prior ABMS certification (American Academy of Pain Management, 2004).

THE ROLE OF MEDICAL SPECIALISTS IN PAIN MANAGEMENT

ALLERGY AND IMMUNOLOGY

Allergist-immunologists are trained (2 years in a fellowship) in disorders of the immune system. They are particularly knowledgeable about adverse reactions to food, insect stings, medications; asthma; eczema; immune deficiency disorders; and problems related to autoimmune disease, organ transplantation, and malignancies of the immune system. Some allergist–immunologists also are additionally trained in rheumatology or pulmonology (ABMS, 2002). Pain disorders associated with disorders of the immune system often require the collaboration of allergist–immunologists with pain practitioners.

ANESTHESIOLOGY

Anesthesiologists are trained (4 years in a residency) to provide pain relief and maintenance, or restoration, of a stable condition during and immediately following an operation or an obstetric or diagnostic procedure (ABMS, 2002). Beyond these duties, anesthesiologists diagnose and treat acute, persistent noncancer and cancer pain problems. Those practitioners with particular interest in pain medicine often provide specialized "blocks" for patients in pain (described in the Invasive Procedures section of this book).

COLON AND RECTAL SURGERY

Colon and rectal surgeons are trained (6 years of residency and fellowship) to diagnose and treat diseases of the intestinal tract, colon, rectum, anal canal, and perianal area by medical and surgical means. They also deal with other organs and tissues involved in the digestive process. These surgeons typically manage painful conditions such as hemorrhoids, fissures, abscesses, and fistulae, along with disorders of the intestine and colon. Colon and rectal surgeons perform endoscopic procedures to diagnose and treat cancer, polyps, and inflammatory conditions (ABMS, 2002).

DERMATOLOGY

Dermatologists are trained (4 years of residency) to diagnose and treat people with benign and cancer-related disorders of the skin, mouth, external genitalia, hair, and nails, as well as many sexually transmitted diseases. These physicians are experienced in the management of skin cancer, moles, tumors of the skin, contact dermatitis, and the skin manifestations of systemic and infectious diseases (ABMS, 2002). While not primary physicians for the management of pain per se, they are involved in the management of patients with painful skin conditions and do recognize the dermatological manifestations of serious underlying medical conditions.

EMERGENCY MEDICINE

Emergency physicians are trained (3 years in residency) to focus on the immediate decision making and action needed to prevent death or any further disability in the prehospital and hospital settings. These physicians are trained to recognize, evaluate, treat, stabilize, and make dispositional decisions for patients with acute illnesses and injuries (ABMS, 2002). They are the "frontline" practitioners for patients in pain both at the beginning of the process and often for months to years as chronic pain develops.

FAMILY PRACTICE

Family physicians are trained (3 years in residency) to address the total health care of the individual and the family, and to diagnose and treat a wide variety of ailments in patients of all ages. Special emphasis is placed on prevention and primary care of entire families by using consultations and community resources when necessary (ABMS, 2002). Many patients with painful disorders obtain their ongoing medications from these physicians.

INTERNAL MEDICINE

Internists train (3 years of residency) to provide long term, comprehensive medical care for adolescents, adults, and the elderly. They are particularly skilled in the diagnosis of cancer, infections, and diseases of major organ systems and have an understanding of disease prevention, wellness, substance abuse, and other issues (ABMS, 2002). Like family physicians, internists commonly follow patients with painful disorders, providing medication renewals and coordinating care with different specialists, and are frequently trained themselves in many different subspecialties (cardiology, endocrinology, gastroenterology, geriatrics, hematology, infectious disease, oncology, nephrology, pulmonology, rheumatology, and sports medicine).

MEDICAL GENETICS

Medical geneticists are trained (2 or 4 years of residency) in the diagnosis and therapeutic procedures for patients with genetically linked diseases. They are often involved in screening programs for inborn errors of metabolism, hemoglobinopathies, chromosomal abnormalities, and neural tube defects (ABMS, 2002). Painful disorders that are hereditary in nature may necessitate the involvement of medical geneticists for family planning purposes.

NEUROLOGICAL SURGERY

Neurosurgeons provide operative and nonsurgical management of disorders of the central, peripheral, and autonomic nervous systems; evaluate and treat processes modifying the function of the nervous system; and manage pain. Their training (7 years of residency) enables them to treat all of the structures of the nervous system and the supporting structures and vascular supply (ABMS, 2002). These are the physicians who perform surgical therapies (decompressive or destructive in nature) for the management of pain arising from the structures and surrounding tissues of the nervous system. Many neurosurgeons are involved with the implantation of medication delivery systems (pumps) and stimulators used for the management of intractable pain.

NEUROLOGY

Neurologists train for 4 years of residency to diagnose and treat all types of disease or impairment of the brain, spinal cord, peripheral nerves, muscles, autonomic nervous system, and the vascular supply to these structures (ABMS,

2002). They do not perform surgical procedures, but do perform a variety of diagnostic (EEG, EMG, NCV, SSEP) and therapeutic (lumbar puncture, nerve blocks) procedures. Some neurologists now subspecialize in pain medicine and take the same examination as anesthesiologists. As they are well trained in the use of anticonvulsants and other adjuvant medications, many have a particular interest in the management of neuropathic pain.

NUCLEAR MEDICINE

Nuclear medicine physicians are trained (3-year residency) to employ the properties of radioactive atoms and molecules in the diagnosis and treatment of disease. They are able to detect disease as it changes the function and metabolism of normal cells, tissues, and organs (ABMS, 2002). Many of their approaches are used in the treatment of cancer, so patients with malignancy-related pain often have some of their care provided by these practitioners. Additionally, these specialists have considerable knowledge about the effects of radiation exposure, fundamentals of physics, and principles of operation for radiation detection and imaging systems.

OBSTETRICS AND GYNECOLOGY

Obstetrician/gynecologists specialize in the medical and surgical care of the female reproductive system and associated disorders. They are commonly the primary care physicians for women (ABMS, 2002). They are best trained (4 years in residency and 2 years in clinical practice before certification) to manage pain-related disorders of the pelvic area for women and to work collaboratively with other medical specialists.

OPHTHALMOLOGY

Ophthalmologists provide comprehensive eye and vision care, and are medically trained (4 years of residency) to diagnose, monitor, and medically or surgically treat ocular and visual disorders. They also address problems affecting the component structures, eyelids, orbits, and visual pathways (ABMS, 2002). They are best able to address many of the painful conditions involving the eyes, periocular structures, and surrounding structures.

ORTHOPEDIC SURGERY

Orthopedists are trained (5 years of residency) to preserve, investigate, and restore the form and function of the extremities, spine, and associated structures by medical, surgical, and physical means. They are typically involved in the care of those with musculoskeletal problems, deformities, injuries, and degenerative disorders of the spine, hands, feet, knees, hips, shoulders, and elbows (ABMS,

2002). They provide care for acute and chronic painful conditions when bones, joints, and muscles are implicated.

OTOLARYNGOLOGY

Otolaryngologists (ear, nose, and throat, ENT) are surgeons caring for disorders of the ears, nose, and throat; respiratory, and upper alimentary systems; and related structures of the head and neck. They are trained (5 year-residency) to diagnose and provide medical and/or surgical therapy. Many focus on hearing- and voice-related conditions (ABMS, 2002), so may provide the decompressive surgical techniques needed for 8th cranial nerve tumors and other painful conditions of the ears or throat. They are inevitably involved in the care of people suffering from cancers of the head and neck. Working collaboratively with anesthesiologists and specialists in medical and radiation oncology, ENTs manage the pain experienced by their patients and continue to provide them with analgesic medications as part of ongoing postoperative care and monitoring.

PATHOLOGY

Pathologists are trained (5-year residency) to address the causes and nature of disease through the application of the biologic, chemical, and physical sciences. Pathologists use microscopic examination of tissue specimens, cells, body fluids, and secretions to diagnose, evaluate, and monitor diseases (ABMS, 2002). While rarely directly involved in the treatment of those in pain, pathologists provide much needed diagnostic services and help to define broadly the care necessary for many patients.

PEDIATRICS

Pediatricians train (3 years of residency) to care for the physical, emotional, and social health of children from birth into young adulthood. They are able to provide preventative care, diagnosis, and treatment of acute and chronic illnesses (ABMS, 2002). Their focus of care addresses the biopsychosocial and environmental influences on developing children. Children with painful disorders are usually first evaluated and managed by pediatricians; pediatricians are the primary care practitioners for many children. Numerous subspecialties within pediatrics include cardiology, critical care, endocrinology, neonatology, neurology, psychiatry, sports medicine, and others.

PHYSICAL MEDICINE AND REHABILITATION

Physical medicine and rehabilitation (PM&R) physicians (physiatrists) are concerned with the diagnosis, evaluation, and management of patients who have been injured or are physically disabled. These physicians are trained (4 year-residency) to address the needs of those having maladies involving the musculoskeletal system, sports-related injuries, and other painful conditions. They provide the primary direction for rehabilitative programs helping patients with neurological trauma and diseases of the spine, spinal cord, and brain (head injury and stroke). Increasingly, these physicians are becoming more involved in pain management to assist patients obtain maximal restoration of physical, psychological, social, and vocational function. They are well versed in the use of therapeutic exercise, prosthetics, orthotics, and other physical modalities (ABMS, 2002). They are able to take the subspecialty examination in pain medicine given by the ABMS after becoming certified in PM&R.

PLASTIC SURGERY

Plastic surgeons repair, reconstruct, or replace physical defects involving skin, musculoskeletal system, facial structures, hand and extremities, and other areas. They have special training (5 to 7 years of residency training) in the design of grafts, flaps, free tissue transfers, replantation, and use of implantable materials (ABMS, 2002). While not directly managing patients in pain, situations that cause pain (cancer, injuries, and other diseases) are commonly addressed by plastic surgery.

PREVENTIVE MEDICINE

Preventive medicine physicians address the health of individuals and defined populations to protect, promote, and maintain health and well-being (3-year residency). They work to prevent disease, disability, and premature death. These physicians may also be specialists in public health, occupational medicine, aerospace medicine, and undersea and hyperbaric medicine (ABMS, 2002). While not direct providers of pain management services, they may be the best trained to identify potentially dangerous situations that could cause painful illnesses and injuries if not addressed.

PSYCHIATRY

Psychiatrists prevent, diagnose, and treat mental, addictive, and emotional disorders after completing a 4-year residency. They understand the biopsychosocial components of illness and are prepared to treat the whole person. These physicians order and interpret laboratory tests, prescribe medications, and intervene with patients and their families coping with stress, crises, and issues in living (ABMS, 2002). They are increasingly involved in the care of patients with chronic painful disorders and are now able to take the ABMS subspecialty examination in pain medicine. Many are also subspecialists in addiction medicine, geriatric psychiatry, and neurophysiology.

RADIOLOGY

Radiologists use a variety of imaging modalities and radiological methods to diagnose and treat illnesses. Some focus primarily on diagnostic methods while others provide radiation therapy. After 4 years of residency, some radiologists subspecialize in neuroradiology, nuclear radiology, and vascular and interventional radiology (ABMS, 2002). Many patients with pain have their diagnostic and therapeutic procedures performed by radiologists.

GENERAL SURGERY

General surgeons are trained (5 years of residency) to manage many different surgical conditions involving virtually any part of the body. They establish diagnoses and provide pre-, peri-, and post-operative care for patients having surgery. Many provide overall care for the victims of trauma, perform a range of diagnostic techniques, and coordinate care with subspecialty surgeons (ABMS, 2002). Patients with pain often are, or have been, treated by surgeons before their referral to pain management practitioners.

THORACIC SURGERY

Thoracic surgeons train (7 to 8 years of residency) to manage surgical conditions within the chest. They address coronary artery disease; cancer of the lung, esophagus, and chest wall; and abnormalities of the trachea, great vessels, and heart, as well as many other conditions (ABMS, 2002). These specialists working in collaboration with other physicians may be involved in all aspects of pain management from initial diagnostic evaluation to definitive surgical treatment and, by doing so, bring much relief for those with painful conditions involving the organs and structure of the chest.

UROLOGY

Urologists train (5 years of residency) to manage benign and cancer-related medical and surgical conditions of the genitourinary system. They provide comprehensive evaluation of urinary and reproductive systems and their contiguous structures (ABMS, 2002). Pelvic pain, pain involving the genitourinary system, and conditions involving the adrenal gland often lead to urological referral.

CONCLUSION

While allopathic physicians are not the only pain practitioners, they are commonly involved in all phases of care for those suffering from painful disorders. Allopaths represent a heterogeneous group of health care providers, offering a wide array of diagnostic and therapeutic options for the management of pain. Working within allopathic medicine, they are able to offer treatments including oral medications, surgery, rehabilitative measures, and more. Working beyond allopathic medicine per se, allopathic physicians as members of multidisciplinary treatment teams are able to complement the wonderful efforts of many different types of pain practitioners and bring relief from suffering for those in pain.

REFERENCES

Accreditation Council for Graduate Medical Education (ACGME). (2004). Retrieved September 21, 2004 from http://www.acgme.org/about/ about.asp.

American Academy of Pain Management (AAPM). (2004). *Credentialing brochure*. Retrieved September 21, 2004 from http://www.aapainmanagement.org/members/Credentialing.php.

American Association of Medical Colleges (AAMC). (2004a). *Getting into medical school*. Retrieved April 3, 2004 from http://www.aamc.org/students/ considering/gettingin.htm.

American Association of Medical Colleges (AAMC). (2004b). *Making the Decision*. Retrieved April 3, 2004 from http://www.aamc.org/students/ considering/decision.htm.

American Board of Anesthesiology (ABA). (2004). *Subspecialty examinations*. Retrieved September 21, 2004 from http://www.abanes.org/examination/ exam_subspecialty.html.

American Board of Medical Specialties (ABMS). (2002). *Which medical specialist for you?* Retrieved April 3, 2004 from http://www.abms.org/ Downloads/which%20Med%20Spec.pdf.

American Board of Pain Medicine (ABPM). (2004). *Certification exam information*. Retrieved September 21, 2004 from http://www.abpm.org/certinfo.htm.

American Board of Physical Medicine & Rehabilitation (ABPMR). (2004). *Subspecialty certification*. Retrieved September 21, 2004 from http://www.abpmr.org/certification/subspecialty.html.

American Board of Psychiatry & Neurology (ABPN). (2004). *Certification*. Retrieved September 21, 2004 from http://www.abpn.com/certification/painmanagement.html.

American Medical Association (AMA). (2000). Your doctor's education, *JAMA,* September 6, 2000. Retrieved April 2, 2994 from http://www.ama-assn.org/ama/pub/category/2320.html.

Arizona Medical Board. (2004). *What does allopathic medicine mean?* Retrieved April 2, 2004 from http://www.bomex.org/faq/misc_faq.asp.

Bureau of Labor Statistics (BLS). (2004*). Occupational outlook handbook, 2004–05 edition*. Bulletin 2540. Retrieved April 2, 2004 from http://www.bls.gov/oco/print/ocos074.htm.

14

Pain Management in Dentistry

Christopher R. Brown, DDS, MPS

It is unfortunate that one of the most common sensations known to humanity is also one of the least understood. Besides love, throughout history there has been no other motivator stronger than pain. Pain can change one's life in an instant, completely turning the direction of an individual's course and those with whom he or she comes into contact. Pain, or the avoidance thereof, whether physical, psychological, or emotional, motivates every living entity from humanity to single cell organisms.

In 1979, the International Association for the Study of Pain set forth the following working definition of pain: "An unpleasant sensory and emotional experience associated with actual or potential tissue damage, or described in terms of such damage" (Wall & Melzack, 1984, p. 1). Dental pain has always held special loathing in all known civilizations. All ancient cultures had theories of dental pain origin and proposed treatments often linked with religious ceremony. It was not until the times of Henry VIII in England that practitioners began to emerge whose practices were limited to removing teeth — a truely rudimentary form of pain management.

In 1840, the first true dental college was opened in Baltimore, ushering in the modern era of dentistry and raising the level of dentistry beyond basic exodontia and expanded into other aspects of dental treatment (Glenner, Davis, & Burns, 1990). In 1997 the American Dental Association (ADA) House of Delegates adopted the following definition of Dentistry:

> Dentistry is defined as the evaluation, diagnosis, prevention and/or treatment (non-surgical, surgical or related procedures) of diseases, disorders and/or conditions of the oral cavity, maxillofacial area and/or adjacent and associated structures and their impact on the human body; provided by a dentist, within the scope of his/her education, training and experience, in accordance with the ethics of the profession and applicable law.

In spite of its late start into a specialized field of medicine, dentistry often took the lead in many aspects of pain management beyond that of the teeth and periodontium. In fact, a dentist's, Dr. Horace Wells, demonstration of nitrous oxide in 1845 helped lead the way in analgesia and anesthesia in the field of medicine (Glenner et al., 1990).

As a result of relentless dedication from the dental profession, dentistry has emerged as a true science for the control of one of the most common sources of pain known to humanity since time began — the toothache. People in all modern societies learn from childhood if there is pain in the mouth, a dentist should be initially consulted as, to borrow a current term, the "primary care physician."

In fact, dentistry has developed the reputation few other professions can claim. In the public mind, dentists are the sole practitioners to seek first for dental pain. Other aspects of the healing arts do not have the distinction of this reputation. Back pain, for example, which is probably the second most common source of pain in the United States, provides a list of possibilities for treatment from which a patient must initially choose. The result is an often confusing, confrontational system that produces high costs and uncoordinated care. The dentist, as a portal of entry physician, provides quick, cost-effective pain relief in a logical, coordinated manner. The lines of distinction between general dentists and associated specialties have been proven to work consistently.

A doctor of dental surgery (D.D.S.) or a doctor of dental medicine (D.M.D.) indicates the degree awarded upon graduation from a dental school to become a general dentist. There is no difference between the two degrees per se, only a reflection of the prerogative of the individual schools. Both degrees use the same curriculum requirements set by the ADA's Commission on Dental Accreditation. Generally, 3 or more years of undergraduate education plus 4 years of dental education are required for either degree. State licensing boards must be successfully completed according to state laws (ADA, 2004a).

Dental specialties that require additional training have been organized and recognized by the American Dental Association and approved by the Council on Dental Education and Licensure (ADA, 2004b).

Dental Public Health: Dental public health is the science and art of preventing and controlling dental diseases and promoting dental health through organized community efforts. It is that form of dental practice that serves the community rather than the individual as a patient. It is concerned with the dental health education of the public, with applied dental research, and with the administration of group dental care programs as well as the prevention and control of dental diseases on a community basis. (Adopted May 1976)

Endodontics: Endodontics is the branch of dentistry concerned with the morphology, physiology, and pathology of the human dental pulp and periradicular tissues. Its study and practice encompasses the basic and clinical sciences including biology of the normal pulp, the etiology, diagnosis, prevention, and treatment of diseases and injuries of the pulp and associated periradicular conditions (Adopted December 1983)

Oral and Maxillofacial Radiology: Oral and maxillofacial radiology is the specialty of dentistry and discipline of radiology concerned with the production and interpretation of images and data produced by all modalities of radiant energy that are used for the diagnosis and management of diseases, disorders, and conditions of the oral and maxillofacial region. (Adopted April 2001)

Oral and Maxillofacial Surgery: Oral and maxillofacial surgery is the specialty of dentistry that includes the diagnosis and surgical and adjunctive treatment of diseases, injuries, and defects involving both the functional and aesthetic aspects of the hard and soft tissues of the oral and maxillofacial region. (Adopted October 1990)

Orthodontics and Dentofacial Orthopedics: Orthodontics and dentofacial orthopedics is the dental specialty that includes the diagnosis, prevention, interception, and correction of malocclusion, as well as neuromuscular and skeletal abnormalities of the developing or mature orofacial structures. (Adopted April 2003)

Pediatric Dentistry: Pediatric dentistry is an age-defined specialty that provides both primary and comprehensive preventive and therapeutic oral health care for infants and children through adolescence, including those with special health care needs. (Adopted 1995)

Periodontics: Periodontics is the specialty of dentistry that encompasses the prevention, diagnosis, rehabilitation, and maintenance of the supporting and surrounding tissues of the teeth or their substitutes and the maintenance of the health, function, and aesthetics of these structures and tissues. (Adopted December 1992)

Prosthodontics: Prosthodontics is the dental specialty for diagnosis, treatment planning, rehabilitation, and maintenance of the oral function, comfort, appearance, and health of patients with clinical conditions associated with missing or deficient teeth and/or oral and maxillofacial tissues using biocompatible substitutes (Adopted April 2003).

Dentists unfortunately still carry the label of being the causation of pain more often than being true healers. On any given day, one can find difficult situations being referred to by individuals or the media as "as bad as a root canal" or "as painful as going to the dentist." This is in spite of the fact dentistry has made tremendous strides in minimizing or alleviating the pain involved in many dental procedures.

Within those stereotypes, however, are opportunities for dentists to provide care that sets individual practices beyond what is expected by the public. The technical aspect of dentistry when properly performed may be little appreciated by most patients. One of the true tests of a "good" dentist in the public eye is whether the patient feels any pain as a result of procedures. Often the patient's co-workers (or classmates) have already heightened a patient's apprehension with horror stories from their own past dental experiences raising the level of anxiety, and, in the truest sense, lowering the expectations of what level the care deliverer can perform. Many patients expect dentistry to hurt, being convinced that it is the norm for our profession. Delivering careful, pain-free procedures actually surprises and delights patients. Modern dental techniques allow properly trained dentists to do so on a predicable bases. Often anticipation of a painful procedure that turns out to be nonpainful can lead to acceptance of preventive care, which is the best form of pain management.

The costs dentists charge patients for pain management is not the true cost to society. Dental fees are minuscule when considering the actual costs involved. For every dollar spent in the office, there are hours of lost time in industrial production, hours of lost sleep, a reduction in the overall work force, and mistakes made at work that have to be corrected. The staggering costs to society for dental pain could be measured in the billions of dollars when all factors are considered.

Even though dentistry has led the way in cost-effective pain management and preventive care, there is still an almost unlimited number of easily preventable, painful dental problems occurring every day in the United States. For example, diseases of the periodontium are estimated to affect more than 90% of the adult American population.

That presents a need of epidemic proportions. Dental practitioners have to be well skilled in the diagnosis, treatment, and prevention of periodontal disease. Along with successful treatment comes the need for knowledge of pain control. Whether periodontal therapy is surgical or nonsurgical, patients need to have proper advice for pain control, or treatment may not be successful due to incompletion or noncompliance on the patient's part. The finest clinical procedures meet ultimate failure if the patient does not follow the dentist's proper advice. As much as we think our patients are motivated on a higher plane of thought, the truth is many still judge clinical management of periodontal disease by how much the therapy hurts them. With such an overwhelming percentage of the population affected by this problem, the knowledge of proper preoperative and postoperative pain management becomes a vital part of a successful practice.

Tied into the complexity of dental pain management are problems associated with dysfunction of the temporomandibular joints. TMJ dysfunction, or what is now currently referred to as TMD, is estimated to affect more than 25% of the American population (Zarb, Carlsson, Sessle, & Mohl, 1995). While this broad statement encompasses everything from sore mastication muscles to advanced degenerative joint disease, it is safe to say TMD in one form or another is a commonly occurring disorder. The role of the dentist in the treatment of TMD pain is vital. Dentists are the only health care providers capable of providing an adequate differential diagnosis based on proper education and clinical skills. No other profession has the training to evaluate factors such as occlusion, mandibular position, biomechanical forces, and parafunctional habits as various etiologies of the resulting facial pain. The complexity of pain control in this patient population is often exacerbated by both the acute and chronic nature of the pain complaints. The management of acute pain may present the initial challenge, but diagnosing the perpetuating factors that affect the chronicity may prove to be the ultimate key to successful clinical pain management.

Because of the multifactorial nature of TMD, dentists may be placed in the position of either a primary care physician or a team member with other health care providers. This presents situations in which dentists must become comfortable in communicating with other professional practitioners. These opportunities allow for professional growth and understanding between professions, providing a more thorough continuity of care for the pain patient. Continuity of care, or what is commonly called "teamwork," is often lacking in acute and chronic pain treatment. The dental model of care has long established itself as being effective and successful.

The dental model of care inherently gives dentists the ability to treat TMD/facial pain from their individual level of skill. While the treatment of TMD is not a recognized specialty within the American Dental Association, there are many dentists who have chosen to limit their practice to the diagnosis and treatment of these collective disorders. The education system is now established to allow dentists to pursue advancement of their clinical skills to the level they desire. Courses are now available, through universities and other organizations that train dentists, in the diagnosis and advanced treatment of muscular trigger points, various diagnostic and therapeutic nerve blocks, computer-aided adjunctive diagnostics, radiology, pharmacology, and physical supportive medicine.

Along with advanced training come opportunities to provide pain management beyond the traditional concepts of dentistry allowing dentists to function as true oral physicians. Dentists who wish to pursue this aspect of pain management can often provide the needed link between medicine and dentistry offering a unique perspective to pain control, resulting in cost-effective successful treatment.

The advent of third-party managed care has dictated a new catchphrase: "outcomes measurement." Outcomes measurement is nothing new to dentistry in the traditional sense. The treatments provided, such as crowns, bridges, and fillings, are usually judged against true measurable outcomes. There are certain criteria that need to be met for clinical success. The parameters are measured by treating dentists, patients, and third-party providers.

As dentists move into the realm of less measurable entities, such as pain management, new paradigms must be established if the profession is to prove viable as a cost-effective avenue of health care delivery. Within those paradigms, outcomes measurement must be used. The concept of using a ruler and fingertip palpation as the "gold standard" of measurement and verification is no longer acceptable if the dental profession is to advance. Objective standards and measurements must be adopted and routinely used, or a dentist's role in pain management erodes and delegates to the role of technician.

The American Academy of Pain Management, the largest pain management organization in the world with more than 5000 members, has a computerized outcomes measurement system in place that fits the needs of modern dental pain practitioners. The use of standardized intake and outcome formats allows offices that practice pain management to compare all aspects of their programs with other participating practices throughout the nation. The tracking system allows not only comparisons within the dental profession, but with other disciplines as well. In other words, the cost-effectiveness of alleviation of headaches via "dental" procedures can be compared with medical, chiropractic, physical therapy, etc. The parameters measured are consistent within the various disciplines. This is the only program that measures the total true outcomes, which are pain alleviation, cost, and individual dental versus medical components.

A conference in Bethesda, MD, sponsored by the National Institutes of Health and the National Institute of

Dental Research decried the lack of measurable outcomes available to determine the effectiveness of pain management procedures commonly used by dentists and challenged the profession to respond. As a result, several major dental groups formed "The Alliance of TMD Practitioners" to help coordinate the various dental special interest groups that have formed over ideology. A representative from each dental group has been invited to become a member to help form cohesive leadership beyond each individual member's group focus. The alliance provides an entity that allows for dissemination of information without prejudice to all member organizations.

For dentistry to compete in the new cost-effective atmosphere of today's society, high standards must be met. Dentistry has been extremely effective in cost containment when compared with allopathic medicine. With the expansion of dentistry into aspects of pain management beyond teeth and their supporting structures, the challenges of the future lie not only in its scope of treatment but also within the realm of multidisciplinary diagnosis and treatment. The term *multidisciplinary* indicates all aspects of the dental profession and its various specialties as well as all aspects of the healing arts. The unique training and abilities make dentistry a viable partner in the alleviation of one of humankind's pain and suffering.

REFERENCES

American Dental Association Web Site. Oral health topics A–Z dental definitions. (2004a). http://www.ada.org/public/topics/dds_dmd.asp.

American Dental Association Web Site. (2004b). Definitions of special areas of dental practice. Retrieved November 17, 2004 from http://www.org/prof/ed/specialties/definitions.asp#special.

Glenner, R., Davis, A., & Burns, S. (1990). *The american dentist.* Missoula, MT: Pictorial Histories Publishing Co.

Wall, P., & Melzack, R. (1984). *Textbook of pain* (p. 1). Edinburgh: Churchill Livingstone.

Zarb, G., Carlsson, G., Sessle, B., & Mohl, N. (1995). *Temporomandibular joint and masticatory muscle disorders* (pp. 159–169). St. Louis: Mosby.

15

Podiatric Medicine and the Painful Heel

Paula Gilchrist, DPM, PT

PODIATRIC MEDICINE

What is a doctor of podiatric medicine? By strict definition, a podiatrist is a medical specialist who functions specifically to diagnose and treat a variety of maladies, illnesses, and problems as they are manifest in the lower extremity, especially at the foot and ankle complex. Surgically, depending on individual residency training, board certifications, and state licensure laws, the podiatrist can operate on the ankle and the foot to repair and or remove bony and soft tissue structures. Fixation devices, bone grafts, and amputations are well within the skill and training of the podiatrist. There is no medical practitioner who is better trained in lower extremity anatomy, pathology, and biomechanics than the doctor of podiatric medicine.

There are two questions of interest. How does one become a podiatrist? Exactly what academic, clinical, and residency training does a podiatrist have? There are many course requirements for medical, dental, osteopathic, and podiatry schools. Ironically, the mandatory prerequisite courses needed for entrance to any of these schools are academically similar. From 90 to 135 college course hours are needed. Great emphasis is placed on the sciences. The curriculum includes 12 credits of biology with laboratory, 12 credits of inorganic chemistry with laboratory, 12 credits of organic chemistry with laboratory, 12 credits of physics with laboratory, 9 credits of English, and 6 credits of mathematics, which are the minimal course requirements. On occasion, a school may require an introductory-level course in anatomy and physiology. Generally, applications to the schools of podiatric medicine are made in the second term of the third year of college or in the fall of the fourth year. The Medical College Admission Test (MCAT) or the Graduate Record Examination (GRE) serves as the entrance exam for admission to podiatry school. Applicants to the schools of podiatric medicine also go through the process of entrance interviews. This can be done on a one-to one basis or with a committee interview.

Once accepted to a podiatric program, the student now begins to enjoy an intense curriculum of academic and clinical medicine. Most schools of podiatric medicine will award the doctorate degree (Doctor of Podiatric Medicine or D.P.M.) in 4 years. There are some schools that couple the doctor of podiatric medicine with a doctor of philosophy in certain preapproved areas. Overall, whether the curriculum is that of traditional coursework or problem-based education, the basic subject matter must be presented. Core curriculum is used in all seven U.S. schools of podiatric medicine (Temple School of Podiatric Medicine; Ohio College of Podiatric Medicine; Scholl College of Podiatric Medicine; New York College of Podiatric Medicine; Barry School of Podiatric Medicine; Des Moines College of Podiatric Medicine; and California College of Podiatric Medicine). This curriculum is quite similar to that used in medical schools. In fact, several schools of podiatric medicine actually share the faculty of adjoining medical schools.

The following discussion is a representation of the curriculum used in shape and form in all the schools of podiatric medicine; individual program modifications certainly do occur. During the first year's first term, course work includes gross anatomy (including dissection), histology, biochemistry, podiatric medicine, and introduction to general medicine. During the first year's second term, lower extremity anatomy (with laboratory), neuroanatomy and physiology, microbiology and immunology, physical diagnosis, and biomechanics are covered.

189

In the second year's first term, microbiology, infectious disease pathology, pharmacology and therapeutics, biomechanics and physical medicine, physical diagnosis, and rehabilitation medicine are taught. The second year's second term is generally reserved for intense courses in general and podiatric radiology, pathology and case studies, pharmacology and therapeutics, and podiatric medicine and skills of podiatric medicine.

At the completion of the second year of study, the student must take Part I of the National Board Exam. A passing grade on this examination is necessary before clinical studies can continue.

During the third year of study, clinical rotations are introduced and the student must complete studies in business administration, general medicine, sports medicine, traumatology, and podiatric surgery. In the first term of the third year, the student takes coursework in public health, jurisprudence, neurology, dermatology, and podopediatrics.

The fourth year of podiatric study is entirely clinical in nature. A total of 24 weeks of clinical externships and rotations in podiatric medicine and surgery rotations are possible at the Ohio College of Podiatric Medicine; 20 are mandatory and 4 are optional. These can be scheduled at the school clinics as well as with outside individual practitioners and surgery centers. There is also an 8-week rotation required in physical medicine and diagnosis. Podiatrists are skilled in the use of ophthalmoscopes, stethoscopes, and other medical instruments. An oral exam and a written cumulative exam are common requirements for graduation from schools of podiatric medicine. This is in addition to individual course requirements.

During the time of this fourth year of study, the student is also heavily engaged in applying and interviewing for residencies. The postdoctorate training is heavily responsible for practice formation in future years. Certified podiatric residencies are approved by the Council on Podiatric Medical Education.

In podiatric medicine, there are generally three types of residencies available. These are in the areas of podiatric medicine, podiatric surgery, and podiatric orthopedics. The terms of the residencies mostly range from 1 to 3 years in length. For those students who are fortunate to be accepted into surgical training, it is quite common to work with well-trained orthopedic surgeons after the hospital rotations in general medicine, anesthesia, dermatology, rheumatology, emergency medicine, and ophthalmology are completed.

At the completion of all formal training, the student must then sit for state licensure examinations. States can have a reciprocity agreement for licensure, but most states require a candidate to be tested in the state where practicing as a skilled podiatrist is a possibility. Once licensure is granted, the doctor of podiatric medicine must consider board certification. Many insurance companies require board certification or board eligibility status before pay-

ment for services duly rendered is considered. In the field of podiatry, there are many certifications. The Council on Podiatric Medical Education approves some board certifications, though not all. Examples of podiatric certification boards are surgery, podiatric medicine, risk management, acupuncture, and orthopedics and wound care. These certifications are not multidisciplinary, as is the credentialing given by the American Academy of Pain Management.

The next step in the career of the podiatrist is to become very familiar with licensure requirements of the state. After obtaining malpractice insurance, the podiatrist must attend continuing education seminars in order to keep the license active. A fixed number of continuing education credits per year set by the licensure board of each state is required. Failure to comply with this requirement will result in suspension of the license to practice podiatry.

Now the fun of practice really does begin. Podiatrists have the flexibility and training to take the practice in any of many directions. Memberships in many professional organizations are possible. Occasional networking and association with colleagues occur. The American Academy of Pain Management has a wealth of information in the membership of the academy alone. Sports medicine, pain management, general practice, dance consultant, acupuncture, biomechanics, surgery, dermatology, podopediatrics, and rheumatology are just a few of the areas in which a well-trained and dedicated podiatrist will have no problems finding a niche. Sometimes the real problem is in the attempt to narrow the scope of the practice. Yes, it does take years of training, sleepless nights, and thousands in school loans, but the benefits outweigh the problems. The satisfaction outweighs the risks.

HEEL PAIN

By way of example, let me tell you about a typical podiatric problem and how it is addressed. Heel pain (calcaneal pain) is one of the most common foot problems presenting to the clinical practitioner. In 1999, more than 2 million doctor visits were involved with the treatment of heel pain. Age is not a discriminating factor. Heel pain can occur in any age group, but is most frequently found from the age of 8 to 80 years of age. Heel pain is noted in women, men. and children. It is responsible for loss of workdays, loss of school days, and loss of income.

Disability from heel pain can be short term and mild to long term and fully debilitating. Problems with the heel can be associated with activity change (so-called weekend warrior), increase in weight, and change of shoe gear. Poor preparation for activity, such as running without stretching or improper shoe gear, can result in injury to many body areas, but especially to weight-bearing structures such as the heel. Foot type (pronated or supinated foot) as well as atrophy and distortion of the infracalcaneal fat pad and the presence of muscle spasm can contribute to heel pain.

In 2002, a MedLine search produced more than 12,000 "hits" with questions on heel pain. These questions ranged from the definition of heel pain, to causes, treatments, and support groups. In 2001, a news release from a survey undertaken by the American Podiatric Medical Association suggested that heel pain was present in epidemic proportions (www.apma.org).

Care for heel pain can range from the most conservative to the most radical. A myriad of treatments exist. Treatments such as rest, ice compression, elevation, medication (oral anti-inflammatories, oral steroids, vitamin therapy), steroid injections, orthotics, physical therapy modalities, exercise for strength and flexibility, massage therapy, myofascial therapy, acupuncture, acupressure, splinting, strapping, and casts are but a few of the conservative care measures. Steroid creams, magnets, and anti-inflammatory creams have also been used. Extracorporeal shock wave therapy (ESWT) is now finding a place in nonsurgical care for the treatment of infracalcaneal heel pain. Radical care, generally reserved for the most resistant of cases, does include surgical measures. Plantar fasciotomy, plantar fasciectomy, exostectomy, bursectomy, calanceal osteotomy, neurolysis and lysis of adhesions, and tendon rebalancing, shortening, and lengthening are all within the surgical realm of possibility.

Practitioners from many areas of traditional medicine and complementary care medicine treat heel pain. We all have our niche. Medical physicians tend to give medication for pain and inflammation. Podiatrists offer use of medication, orthotics for foot and joint balancing, strapping, splinting, casting, injections, and surgery. Osteopaths offer medication and bony adjustment (such as for a short leg). Chiropractors offer spinal alignments. Acupuncturists and acupressurists offer pain-blocking care. Therapists such as physical, massage, and others offer deep soft tissue relief, myofascial care, scar reduction, flexibility, and body awareness. All have similar goals: reduction of pain and inflammation and increase of normal function. There is no single line of treatment and no simple rate of cure for patients who experience heel pain.

Infectious processes as well as systemic diseases can cause heel pain. Diseases such as gout, rheumatoid arthritis, psoriatic arthritis HLA-B27 disorders, and Reiter's syndrome can cause heel pain. However, for the purpose of this discussion, the following pathologies are reviewed:

1. Plantar fasciitis
2. Heel spur syndrome
3. Haglund deformity
4. Retrocalcaneal exostosis/Achilles tendon calcification
5. Achilles tendonitis
6. Tarsal tunnel syndrome
7. Flexor hallucis longus tendonitis

For an anatomical review of the foot as well as thorough illustrations, the reader is advised to consult a standard anatomy text. *Gray's Anatomy* and *Grant's Anatomy* are excellent and clear sources for review. There are 26 mostly irregularly shaped bones in the adult human foot. This amounts to one fourth of the bones found in the entire human body. The foot itself is divided as follows:

Three bony sections:
  1. Rearfoot: Consisting of talus and calcaneus
  2. Midfoot: Consisting of navicular, cuboid, and cuneiform bones 1, 2, 3
  3. Forefoot: Consisting of metatarsals 1, 2, 3, 4, 5
Five proximal phalanges
Four middle phalanges (hallux or great toe does not have a middle phalanx)
Five distal phalanges

The sesamoid bones found under the area of the first metatarsal are not part of the foot proper

In terms of the foot musculature, there are four distinct layers of plantar muscles. The layers ranging from superficial (plantar) to deep (dorsal) are:

First Layer: Abductor digiti quinti, flexor digitorum brevis, abductor hallucis
Second Layer: Tendon of flexor hallucis longus, tendon of flexor digitorum longus, four lumbricales, and the quadratus plantae
Third Layer: Adductor hallucis, flexor hallucis brevis, flexor digiti minimi brevis
Fourth Layer: Three plantar and four dorsal interossei (the tendon of the peroneus longus muscle and the tendon of the posterior tibialis muscle in the posterior half of the foot are close to this fourth layer)

The plantar fascia, often discussed as an inflamed area in heel pain, consists of three separate compartments: medial fascia (encompasses abductor hallucis muscle), central fascia (encompasses flexor digitorum brevis), and the lateral fascia (encompasses abductor digiti minimi). The medial fascia, which has a very broad band, is often implicated in cases of plantar fasciitis. The attachment of the fascia onto the anterior medial calcaneal tubercle takes a great deal of pressure when standing and walking. The configuration of the calcaneus itself is partially responsible for this problem.

The tarsal tunnel, located on the medial side of the ankle, is often implicated in impingement syndromes that can cause heel pain. The tarsal tunnel has four distinct canals that have the laciniate ligament (flexor retinaculum) as the roof and two septa that form the borders of the canal.

Canal 1: Contains tibialis posterior muscle (primary function is to assist in plantar flexion and inversion of the foot)

Canal 2: Contains flexor digitorum longus muscle (assists in bending of the toes)

Canal 3: Contains posterior tibial nerve (L4, L5, S1, S2, and S3 nerve roots) plus the posterior tibial artery and vein

Canal 4: Contains flexor hallucis longus muscle (responsible for flexion of the great toe and assists in the push-off phase of gait; this muscle also assists in deceleration of forward motion of the tibia in a stance phase limb)

These four soft tissue canals are prevented from bowstringing (bulging out) during standing and walking by the flexor retinaculum (laciniate ligament). The medial calcaneal nerve, a branch from the posterior tibial nerve, is noted to pierce through the retinaculum and give sensory innervation to the medial side of the heel.

PLANTAR FASCIITIS

Plantar fasciitis may perhaps be the most common heel problem presenting to the clinician. It is often associated with repetitive stress injuries and is not usually the result of direct trauma. It is a soft tissue problem that can be present for years, to some degree, before the patient seeks any type of treatment. Heel spurs can be present on radiograph without symptoms of plantar fasciitis. In fact, endoscopic plantar fasciotomy serves to relieve traction at the anterior medial calcaneal tubercle by severing fascial attachments. Spur, if present, is generally not removed. The lateral attachments of the plantar fascia remain intact.

Poststatic dyskinesia is often noted. Pain occurs with great intensity when the patient arises from a resting posture or sleep. Inflamed soft tissues and muscles are tight after rest. Weight bearing stretches these areas and pain results. Pain is noted to diminish with activity. As the course of the day progresses, so does the pain. Still, the greatest pain is noted after rest.

Inflammation can be detected at any area of the fascia. It is most commonly noted at the medial calcaneal tubercle attachments of the fascia onto the calcaneus. This bony prominence serves as the point of origin of the anatomic medial band of the plantar fascia and the abductor hallucis, flexor digitorum brevis, and abductor digiti minimi muscles. Pain is generally elicited with deep palpation in front of the medial calcaneal tubercle. Pain is also greatest at the push-off phase of gait when the already inflamed fascia is stressed and is stretched as the forefoot begins to accept more body weight and the propulsive phase of gait begins.

It is important to remember that the plantar fascia assists in maintaining the arch height of the foot; it connects the rearfoot to the forefoot. With pathology present, the medial longitudinal arch of the foot can lower. Passive toe extension with the ankle in full dorsiflexion and the knee in extension can elicit pain at the heel.

Pain from plantar fasciitis can be noted to increase when there is a decrease in the flexibility of the gastro-soleus (triceps surae) complex at the calf area. The gastrocnemius muscle assists in plantar flexion of the foot and in knee flexion; the soleus muscle assists in plantar flexion of the foot. The triceps surae sends a plantar attachment under the heel and into the plantar fascia. However, remember that when the plantar fascia is stretched, inversion of the heel occurs to a slight degree. Peroneal muscles (evertors of the foot) can be involved. These muscles are working harder to perform their function. As a result, it is easy to note that evaluation cannot always be contained to the heel itself. Soft tissue attachments to the heel and around the heel must be assessed.

One method to assess for calf tightness is to apply a heel lift (on the painful foot) that does not compress to less than 1/2 to 1 in. If the plantar heel pain eases, then calf tightness must be addressed in the process of eliminating heel pain. If calf tightness is noted, it is best to stretch the Achilles tendon bilaterally. The stretch should be done with the subtalar joint of the foot in neutral position. This helps to maximize the stretch of the Achilles tendon. The stretches should be done with static holds, without bouncing. If heel lifts are needed, then the lifts should be worn in both shoes to reduce the risk of back pain until the flexibility of the gastro-soleus complex is restored. When bouncing instead of static stretching is done during exercise, shortening of the gastro-soleus muscle area is apt to occur. This shortening may cause a secondary Achilles tendonitis.

Plantar fasciitis can occur in either a supinated (cavus high-arch-type; Figure 15.1) foot or in a pronated (planus low-arch-type; Figure 15.2) foot. In pronation, the foot is noted to be quite flexible. This position is sometimes referred to as "a loose bag of bones." A cavus-type foot is inherently more rigid, an excellent propulsive foot. The cavus-type foot may require extra cushioning for relief of pain. The planus-type foot (Figure 15.2) may require only a heel lift. Note that a hint for balancing the foot is to assess the foot in neutral, that is, to assess the foot with the subtalar joint in neutral and the midtarsal joint in pronation. Either foot type can respond nicely with the use of a mechanically balanced custom-made orthotic device that controls subtalar joint motion (Figure 15.3).

In the early stages of treatment, a foot strapping to lock the first ray and transfer pressure away from the fascia and onto the tendons and toes may help relieve heel pain. It is not uncommon to find scar tissue formation on the medial side of the heel due to repetitive stress and an unbalanced foot. Lateral shift and atrophy of the infracalcaneal fat pad can occur. A heel cup may eliminate lateral shift and a heel lift may assist in cushioning. Scar tissue may be eradicated with deep soft tissue massage and fascial release therapy.

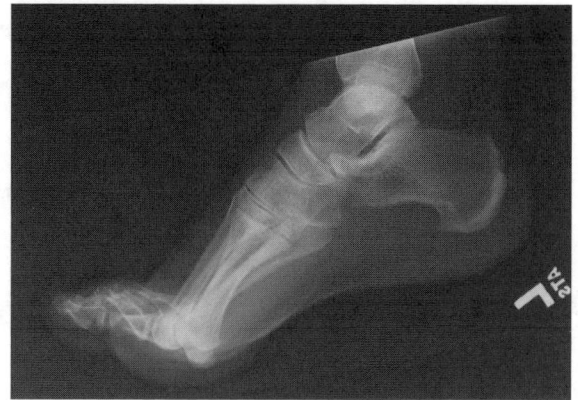

FIGURE 15.1 Supinated foot with high arch.

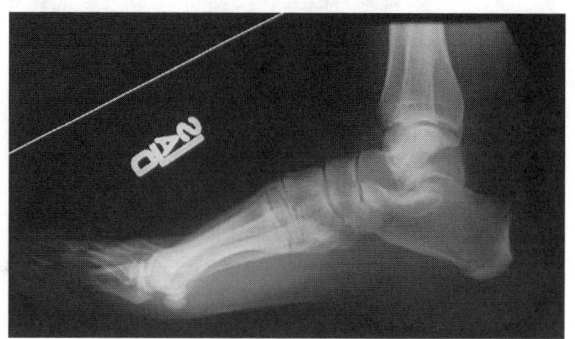

FIGURE 15.2 Pronated foot with low arch.

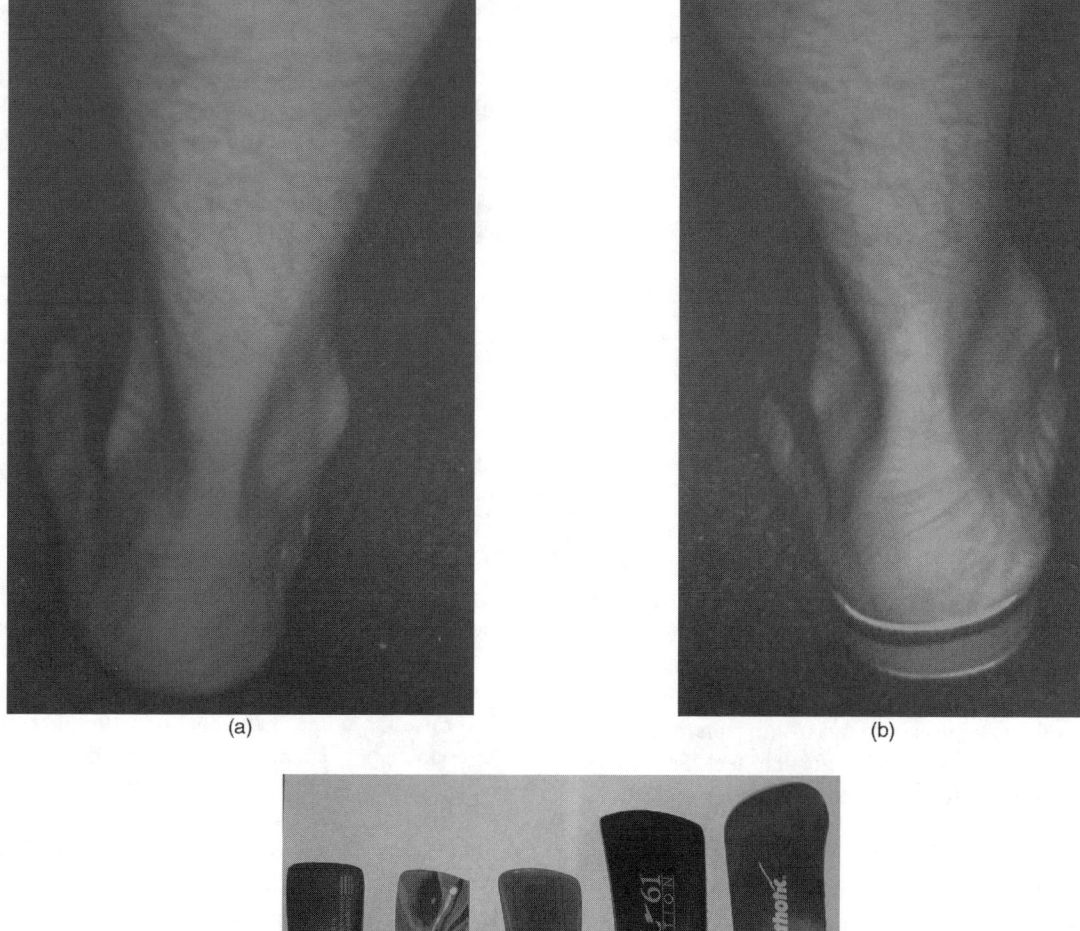

(a)

(b)

(c)

FIGURE 15.3 Orthotics: biomechanical devices made to balance the subtalar joint and control motion. (a) Low-arch foot prior to orthotic care; (b) low-arch foot with orthotic care; (c) various orthotic devices.

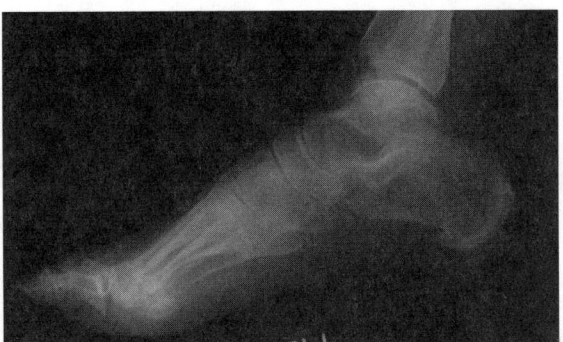

FIGURE 15.4 Infracalcaneal heel spur, traction type spur located anterior to the medial calcaneal tubercle.

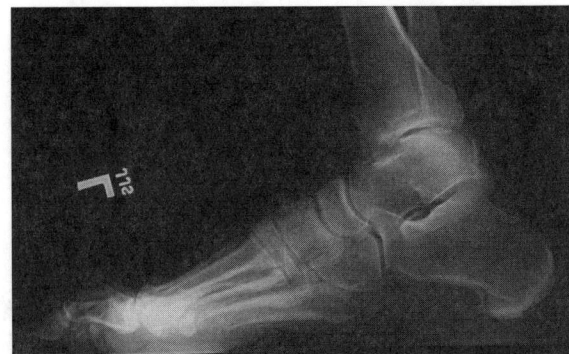

FIGURE 15.5 Haglund deformity. Note enlargement of the posterosuperior aspect of the calcaneus.

HEEL SPUR SYNDROME

Infracalcaneal heel pain (heel spur syndrome) can occur if plantar fasciitis progresses and microtears of the proximal fascia occur at the attachment areas to the heel. Low-grade periostitis occurs along with thickening in the area of trauma. Edema and fibroblastic inflammatory cell infiltration can also occur. Periosteal calcification occurs near fascial and tendonous attachments. The infracalcaneal heel spur forms in this manner (Figure 15.4). A "traction" type of spur from excessive pulling of the soft tissue is noted on lateral radiograph of the foot.

Lateral, oblique, and calcaneal axial radiographs of the foot are helpful to assess heel pain. However, for infracalcaneal spurs, the lateral view often yields the most information as to type and extent of spur. Direct bony alignment of the foot can also be evaluated with radiographs. Weight-bearing radiographs in angle and base of gait are preferable.

Pain presentation is very similar to that of plantar fasciitis. Etiology can be overuse or excess weight in a pronated or a supinated foot type. Conservative treatment is the same as in plantar fasciitis. The physical therapy modalities of iontophoresis, phonophoresis, and electrical stimulation may be of great help to reduce inflammation. Special attention to the thickness and placement of the infracalcaneal fat pad is needed to assist in pain relief. This fat pad acts as a shock absorber for the heel. Soft shoes with a long medial counter for cushioning and shock absorption may be helpful. Medial longitudinal arch support may also assist in easing inflammation. Note that not all infracalcaneal heel spurs are symptomatic. Occasionally, if the foot is well compensated, an infracalcaneal heel spur can be an incidental finding on radiographic examination.

HAGLUND DEFORMITY

Synonyms for Haglund deformity include pump bump (from female high-heel shoes) and retrocalcaneal bursitis. This bony problem (Figure 15.5) located on the lateral side of the heel is often confused with Achilles tendonitis

or bursitis. This condition can occur in patients with a prominent posterosuperior aspect of the calcaneus who wear tight or rigid counter shoes. Instability of the rearfoot can be noted.

The counter refers to that part of the shoe that "cups the heel" and gives the foot stability inside the shoe. The lateral foot radiograph helps to assess the Haglund deformity. In this entity, the counter of the shoe rubs the heel and causes pain and further enlargement of the posterosuperior aspect of the calcaneus. Clinically, the examiner should view the posterior aspect of the heels from behind and with the patient standing. The bulge is quite evident and is seen lateral to the insertion of the Achilles tendon.

Pain symptoms are generally reported as dull aching at the posterior aspect of the heel, lateral to the attachment of the Achilles tendon. The pain is greatest when the foot is dorsiflexed. A possible etiology for this pain is the pinching of the retrocalcaneal bursal sac between the Achilles tendon and the calcaneus. An adventitious (not an anatomically correct) bursal sac can form at the superficial surface of the Achilles tendon. This can further enhance pain.

Conservative care for this problem includes rest, trigger point therapy, soft heel lifts, soft counter shoes, and nonsteroidal anti-inflammatory drugs (NSAIDs). Open-back shoes can be used. Heel lifts of 1/2 to 3/8 in. are used to raise the point of the heel irritation just superior to the counter of the shoe. Ice massage may be of help. If conservative care fails, then removal of the inflamed bursal sac and partial calcaneal exostectomy may be required. Some clinicians may advocate steroid injection into the bursal sac only; however, this must be done with great caution and skill. If steroid is inadvertently placed into the Achilles tendon, spontaneous rupture of the tendon can occur.

RETROCALCANEAL EXOSTOSIS/ACHILLES TENDON CALCIFICATION

In this malady, heel spur or calcification is noted at the insertion of the Achilles tendon onto the posterior aspect

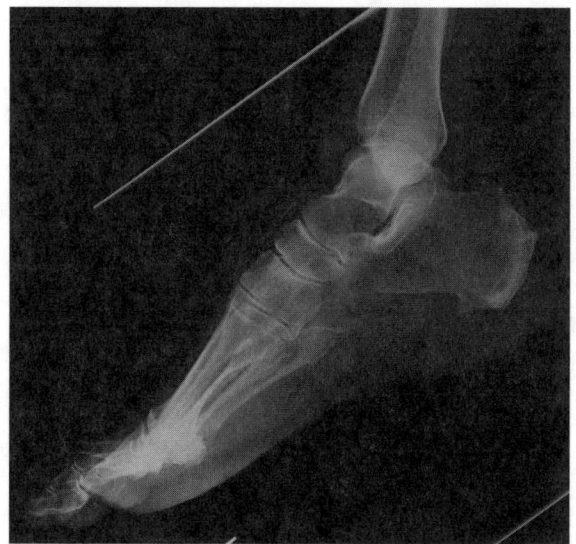

FIGURE 15.6 Retrocalcaneal exostosis. Note the spur formation at the superior aspect of the calcaneus.

of the calcaneus or within the tendon itself (Figure 15.6). This problem can be isolated or can be found in combination with retrocalcaneal bursitis or Achilles tendonitis. The Achilles tendon itself can become thick and wide; lateral radiographs reveal calcification in the calcaneal attachment of the Achilles tendon.

Pain symptoms include dull aching, especially near the insertion of the Achilles tendon onto the heel. Pain frequently occurs in the patient who is involved in athletics or dancing activities. Range of motion of the ankle is altered. Slightly less dorsiflexion of the involved ankle can be noted due to bony block caused by the exostosis. Crepitation of the Achilles tendon can occur due to chronic inflammatory and fibrous deposition throughout the tendon.

Conservative care consists of rest and modalities. Great emphasis is placed on stretches for the triceps surae. The use of ice can decrease edema as well as poststatic dyskinesia. Surgical exostectomy can require splitting of the Achilles tendon or detaching the Achilles tendon from the calcaneus in an attempt to gain exposure of the spur. The muscle does tend to lose strength with this radical approach.

ACHILLES TENDONITIS

Tendon disabilities can be caused by irritation around a tendon sheath (paratenosynovitis), pathology of the sheath itself (tenosynovitis), lesions between the sheath and the tendon (such as lipoma or xanthoma), and lesions within the sheath itself (tenosynovitis). Peritendonitis is a term used to describe inflammation of a tendon with or without a sheath. The Achilles tendon, which is the largest and strongest tendon in the body, is surrounded by a paratenon.

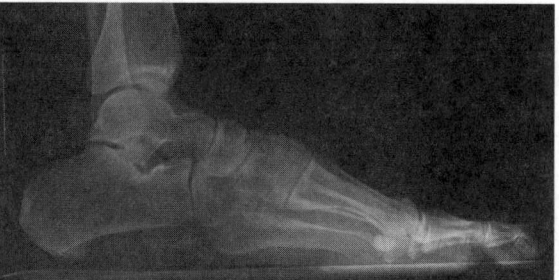

FIGURE 15.7 Achilles tendonitis. Note the swelling of the Achilles tendon.

Tendons, in general, receive blood supply from four areas: muscles, bone, paratenon, and mesotenon. The Achilles tendon has little supply from bone or muscle; much of the blood supply and hence nourishment is via the paratenon. Tendonitis is an inflammation of the tendon itself. It is generally caused from repetitive stress experienced by athletes, dancers, and jumpers. Tendonitis crepitans can be noted due to chronic inflammation of the area. Some practitioners describe this as the sound of crackling in the tendon itself.

Achilles tendonitis (Figure 15.7) is generally noted to be posterior on the heel with the greatest tenderness noted approximately 3 cm proximal to the insertion of the Achilles tendon onto the heel. Pain is noted with dorsiflexion of the ankle due to tension on the heel cord (Achilles tendon) itself. The patient may not be able to unilaterally rise up and down on the toes. Tenderness can be associated with swelling, redness, and thickening of the tendon. In dancers, pain can be noted in the propulsion off the foot, as well as during landing. During landing the triceps surae also act as a decelerator of foot motion.

Treatment consists of longer warm-ups, heel lifts, flexibility training, cross-fiber massage, modalities, NSAID medication, and possible foot strapping. Stretching is the key to care. The patient should stretch with the foot in multiple positions, both weight bearing and nonweight bearing.

TARSAL TUNNEL SYNDROME

The tarsal tunnel is located on the medial side of the ankle. The roof of the tunnel consists of the laciniate ligament (flexor retinaculum). There are four distinct canals in the tarsal tunnel, which are formed by two individual septa. The contents of the canals are posterior tibialis tendon, flexor digitorum longus tendon, posterior tibial nerve artery and vein, and flexor hallucis longus tendon. Tarsal tunnel syndrome is generally the compression or entrapment of the posterior tibial nerve as it courses under the laciniate ligament. The posterior tibial nerve divides into the medial and lateral plantar nerve and is responsible for great areas of sensory innervation in the foot. As a result, patients may not be able to pinpoint the source of heel pain. Patients may only be able to describe the pain in general, such as inferior to the medial malleolus.

Pain with this syndrome is generally of gradual onset and is described as aching, burning, and unremitting. The triad of pain, paresthesia, and numbness are not uncommon with nerve injury. Pain is noted with weight bearing and non-weight bearing. Pain can begin in the posterior aspect of the heel and continue forward to just below the medial malleolus and onto the toes. A positive Tinel (pain radiation to the toes) or Vallieux sign (pain radiation to the calf) can be noted with percussion and compression of the posterior tibial nerve as it courses around the medial malleolus. Causes for tarsal tunnel syndrome include the pronated (flat) foot that is decompensated, hypertrophy of the abductor hallucis longus muscle (causing nerve pressure), cysts of the nerve itself, or a poorly applied cast that incorporates the foot. An electromyogram may help to establish the diagnosis. Differential diagnoses include plantar fasciitis, medial calcaneal neuroma, digital plantar nerve entrapment, vascular disease, and lumbosacral radiculopathy.

Conservative care of this lesion can include a medial longitudinal arch support, strapping, and control of the subtalar joint with a custom-made biomechanical orthotic device. The goal is to control pronation and relieve stress from the medial heel structures. Medication and steroid injection can help when pathology is diagnosed early.

FLEXOR HALLUCIS LONGUS TENDONITIS

The flexor hallucis longus muscle assists in plantar flexion of the great toe. During the push-off phase of gait, the muscle locks the proximal phalanx of the great toe and assists in ease of weight distribution. This muscle helps accelerate the forward motion of the tibia onto a weight-bearing foot. When tendonitis occurs here, it is generally the result of a mechanical disturbance. Overuse is a common etiology. The patient will complain of discomfort in the sole of the foot.

Tendon pain is not generally noted with passive stretch or dorsiflexion of the great toe. Pain is noted with local pressure and palpation at the point of pathology. On examination, the flexor hallucis longus tendon stands out when the toe is passively dorsiflexed (Figure 15.8). Pain can occur the length of the tendon, but is more commonly noted at the proximal portion of the tendon. Tenderness is detected more superficially and distal to the area where heel spur tenderness is expected. The medial calcaneal tubercle is generally not tender.

Treatment for this lesion consists of soft sole shoes, modalities, and massage. A transverse arch band may also help. Tendon injection with steroid is questionable and may cause tendon rupture (Figure 15.9).

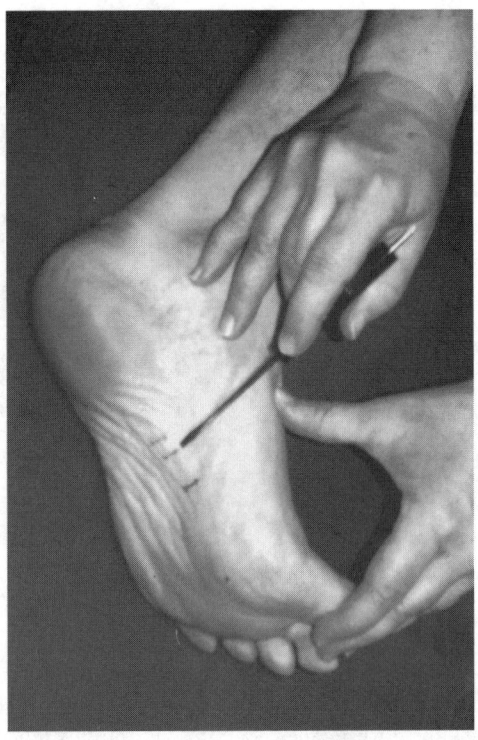

FIGURE 15.8 Flexor hallucis longus tendonitis. Note the bulge of the flexor hallucis longus.

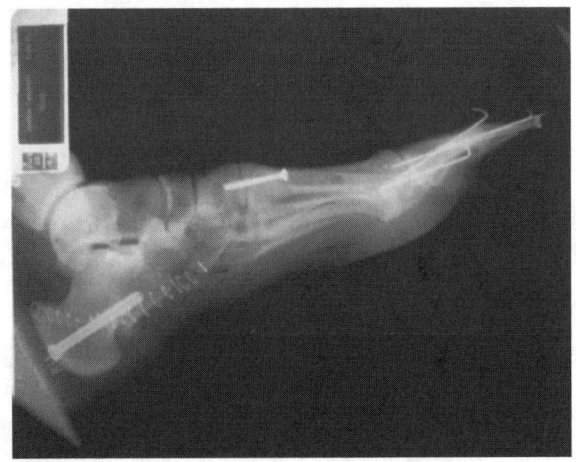

FIGURE 15.9 Did somebody mention heel pain?

SUMMARY

A final comment concerning the practice of podiatric medicine is in order. It is not uncommon to see "an older student" attend a school of podiatric medicine. Some students are looking for an adjunct to a current career, and some are looking for a new career. Some students are searching for more independence in their work experience. Some feel a need for individual and independent job satisfaction. Podiatric medicine offers all of this. If interested, each of the seven schools has a well-designed Web site for information.

As for the role of the podiatrist, heel pain is a common malady treated by many types of practitioners. It is hoped that this chapter has provided the opportunity for one to gain new insight exploring the differential diagnosis of heel pain. Once the accurate diagnosis has been made, it is necessary to follow with appropriate care. Given the potential for overlap in clinical presentation and diagnosis, reevaluation of the etiology of the pain is always a consideration, especially if the patient is not responding as expected.

BIBLIOGRAPHY

Anderson, J., E. (1978). *Grant's atlas of anatomy* (7th ed., pp. 4–122). Baltimore: Williams & Wilkins.

Barrett, S., & O'Malley, R. (1999). Plantar fasciitis and other causes of heel pain. *American Family Physician, 59*(8) 2200–2206.

Barry, N. N., & McGuire, J. L (1996). Overuse syndrome in adult athletes. *Musculoskeletal Medicine, 22*(3) 515–530.

Bateman, J. E. (1982). The adult heel. In M. H. Jahss (Ed.), Disorders of the foot. (764–775). Philadelphia, PA: WB Saunders.

Baxter, D. E. (1994). The heel in sport. *Clinical Sports Medicine, 13*, 683–693).

Biel, A. (2001). *Trail guide to the body* (2nd ed., pp. 275–320). Boulder, CO: Books of Discovery.

Cimino, W. R. (1990). Tarsal tunnel syndrome: Review of the literature. *Foot and Ankle, 11*, 47–52.

Cornwall, M.W., & McPoil, TG. (1999). Plantar fasciitis: Etiology and treatment. *Journal of Orthopedic and Sports Physical Therapy, 29*(12), 756–760.

Gudeman, D. S., Eisele, S. A., Heidt, R. S., Colosimo, A. J., & Stroupe, A. L. (1997). Treatment of plantar fasciitis by iontophoresis of 0.4% dexamethasone. *American Journal of Sports Medicine, 25*, 12–16.

Hoppenfeld, S. (1982). Physical examination of the foot by complaints. In M. H. Jahss (Ed)., *Disorders of the foot* (Vol. I, 103–107). Philadelphia: W. B. Saunders Co.

Luther, L. (1991). Soft tissue trauma of the hindfoot. In G. J. Sammarco (Eds), *Foot and ankle manual* (pp. 116–125). Malvern, PA: Lea and Febiger.

Malay, D. S., & Duggar, G. E. (1992). Heel surgery. In E. D. McGlamry, A. S. Banks, & M. S. Downey (Eds.), *Comprehensive textbook of foot surgery* (2nd ed., Vol. 1, pp. 431–455). Philadelphia: Williams and Wilkins.

Netter, F. H. (1989) Atlas of human anatomy, CIBA – Geigy Corporation (pp. 491–504).

Pfeffer, G. P. (1995). Plantar heel pain. In D. E. Baxter (Ed.), *The foot and ankle in sport* (pp. 195–205). St. Louis, MO: Mosby-Yearbook.

Root, M. L., Orien, W. P., & Weed, J. H. et al. (1977). Normal and abnormal function of the foot. In Clinical Biomechanics Corp., *Clinical Biomechanics* (Vol. 2). Los Angeles: Clinical Biomechanics Corp.

Scioli, M. (1994). Achilles tendonitis. *Orthopedic Clinics of North America, 25*, 177.

Van Wyngarden, T. M. (1997). The painful foot. Part II: Common rearfoot deformities. *American Family Physician, 55*(6), 2207–2212.

16

Chronic Spinal Pain: Mechanisms and a Role for Spinal Manual Medical Approaches to Therapy and Management

*James Giordano, PhD, Alfred V. Anderson, MD, DC, and
Michael J. Nelson, DC*

INTRODUCTION

Pain is a major public health problem in the United States; 50 million Americans are partially or totally disabled from intractable pain. According to the American Pain Society, approximately 45% of all Americans seek care for persistent pain at some point in their lives. Back pain syndromes substantively contribute to the overall epidemiologic prevalence and fiscal gravity of pain disorders. As the leading cause of occupational disability in Americans below the age of 45 (Borenstein, 1998), the economic toll of back pain exceeds $16 billion in costs dedicated to therapeutic and/or management intervention (Burton & Erg, 1997). A significant issue is the progression of acute and subacute back pain to a condition of chronicity. Chronic back pain involves physiologic, psychologic, and sociocultural variables that exacerbate the scope of its effects and complicate both the clinical picture and amenability to intervention. Although an in-depth discussion of pain taxonomy, thoroughly detailed elsewhere in this text, is beyond the scope of the present chapter, it is important to note that persistent (back) pain can be perpetuated through numerous factors and can lead to maldynia (Table 16.1). Maldynic spinal pain involves heterogeneous mechanisms of peripheral and central sensitization, frequently produces a cognitive constellation in excess of apparent organic pathology, and increases the need for (and often the paradoxical inefficacy of) multidisciplinary management approaches.

Chronic and maldynic spinal pain may be underevaluated and/or inadequately treated. Such disparity can lead to patients' frustration that reflects dissonance with patients' subjective suffering, models of spinal pain diagnosis and treatment, and clinicians' capacity to evaluate provocative mechanisms objectively and apply appropriate, case-based therapeutic intervention(s). This chapter is dedicated to a mechanistic depiction of spinal pain and its therapeutic management utilizing manual/manipulative procedures. It must be understood that the technical application of these procedures is possible across both allopathic (physical medicine and rehabilitation) and nonallopathic (osteopathic, chiropractic, and physical therapeutic) disciplines. Part I reviews substrates producing spinal pain relevant to spinal manual medicine (SMM); Part II presents an overview of SMM (across disciplines of use) from a clinical and research perspective.

PART I

INNERVATION OF SPINAL STRUCTURES

Fibers from the dorsal and ventral horns converge into roots that conjoin upon exiting the intervertebral foramina (IVF) into the common spinal nerves. These nerves are contained in dural sleeves that attach to the rim of the IVF. Beyond this point, spinal nerves bifurcate into dorsal and ventral rami containing both sensory and motor fibers. The

TABLE 16.1
Categories of Pain

Eudynia

Acute/subacute
Nociceptive
Type I/Type II pain
Somatosensory

Qualities

A-delta > C-fiber mediated
Dependent on defined peripheral organic lesion
Punctate
Stimulus based
Resolves consequential to stimulus reduction

Maldynia

Chronic/complex
Neuropathic/neurogenic
Type III pain
Consciousness based (cognitive)

Qualities

Sensitization of afferent neuraxis
Frequently independent of peripheral organic lesion
Diffuse
Bioculturally influenced
Irresolute

TABLE 16.2
Grades of Radial Fissures in Internal Disc Disruption

Grade "0"	No disruption evident in the anulus fibrous
Grade "1"	Disruption extends into inner third of the anulus fibrosus
Grade "2"	Disruption extends as far as inner two thirds of the anulus
Grade "3"	Disruption extends into outer third of the anulus fibrosus. May spread circumferentially between the lamellae of collagen

dorsal ramus divides into the medial branch that innervates the capsular and intra-articular areas of the zygapophyseal (ZP) joints, the interspinous ligaments, and the mutifidi muscles (Wyke, 1987). The lateral branch of the dorsal ramus innervates the iliocostalis and longissimi muscles in the lumbar region, and courses through these muscles to become the cutaneous cluneal nerve(s) (Edgar & Ghadially, 1976).

The ventral ramus is the source of the recurrent meningeal (sinuvertebral) nerve, which is joined by the gray ramus communicantes of the sympathetic chain to innervate the posterior longitudinal ligament, periosteum of the posterior zone of the vertebral bodies, anterior dura, epidural and basivertebral vessels, and posterolateral annulus fibrosus (Porterfield & DeRosa, 1991). Fibers of the ventral ramus directly innervate the lateral aspect of the annulus of the intervertebral discs (Bogduk, 1983). This innervation is summarized in Table 16.2.

MECHANISMS OF SPINAL PAIN

Spinal Pain Generators

Numerous anatomical structures are capable of directly or indirectly producing spinal pain. According to Bogduk (1992), an anatomical structure can be a locus of spinal pain providing it satisfies four essential criteria. First, the structure must be innervated with both receptors and fibers capable of transducing and conducting nociceptive impulses. Second, the activation of these fibers either specifically or together with concomitant input from related structures should produce pain that reflects the clinical picture. Third, these structures must be shown to be vulnerable to insult and/or trauma that can initiate and perpetuate a relevant pain syndrome. Last, strong correlation should exist between clinically identified pain syndromes and the involvement of these underlying substrates. These last two points may be somewhat problematic in light of known mechanisms of peripheral and central sensitization that may lead to activation of the afferent nociceptive neuraxis despite the absence or resolution of a provocative anatomical cause (Giordano, Chapter 3, this volume; Woolf, 2000). The following structures meet Bogduk's criteria and are thus capable of at least initiating the nociceptive process (that may lead to sensitization and maldynia).

Vertebrae

The periosteum of the vertebral bodies and arches are innervated by unmyelinated nerve fibers derived from the plexi of the anterior and posterior longitudinal ligaments. These plexi also innervate the articular capsule, aponeuroses, deep paravertebral fascia, and tendons (Groen et al., 1990; Jackson et al., 1966; Wyke, 1970). These nerves penetrate the vertebral body and innervate both the vasculature and the cancellous bone (Hirsch et al., 1963). Thus, both the vertebral periosteum and bone itself may be sensitive to inflammation, mechanical distention, and therefore, pain. As well, intraosseous hypertension can dilate the penetrant blood vessels of the vertebrae stimulating perivascular nerves and evoking pain (Arnoldi, 1972, 1976).

The vertebral periosteal elements are sources of pain secondary to two biomechanical conditions. Principal among these is spondylolysis, a fatigue fracture of the pars inter-articularis (O'Neill & Micheli, 1989) that can be acutely painful and be a source of chronic afferent sensitization. The chronic condition is the result of postfracture fibrous scarring with proliferation of nociceptive free nerve endings that are reactive to, and sensitized by, biochemical substrates of the inflammatory cascade and may directly induce neurogenic inflammation and pain (Schneiderman et al., 1995). Additionally, Bogduk (1997) suggests that bilateral pars fracture produces pain due to the action of the multifidi muscles pulling upon the loose, fractured pars segments, creating displacement and excessive mechanoreceptor activation within the related zygapophyseal joint(s).

Vertebral spinous processes, particularly those of the lumbar vertebrae, are susceptible to Baastrup's disease (Baastrup, 1933) in which spinal hyperextension leads to anterior (longitudinal) ligamentous laxity and compression of the interspinous ligament(s), and allows contact of the spinous processes of adjacent vertebrae. This can inflame the involved ligaments, cause periostitis of the contacting spinous processes, and produce pain (Jackson et al., 1966; Rhalmi et al., 1993).

Zygapophyseal Joints

The fibrous capsules of the zygapophyseal (ZP), or facet joints, are extensively innervated by unmyelinated fibers derived from the medial branches of the dorsal rami (Bogduk et al., 1982, Jackson et al., 1966) and meet proposed criteria for generating spinal pain (Bogduk, 1997). Diagnostic studies have confirmed the contribution of ZP joint pain to the epidemiologic prevalence of chronic back pain (Schwarzer et al., 1994, 1995a, 1995b). The ZP joints are susceptible to numerous pathologies such as osteoarthritis (Lewin, 1964; Magora & Schwartz, 1976), rheumatoid arthritis (Lawrence et al., 1964; Sims-Williams et al., 1977), and epiphyseal disintegration of the articular processes (King, 1955). It should be noted, however, that ZP osteoarthrosis is frequently asymptomatic for pain (Magora & Schwartz, 1976), but may incur biomechanical effects in other spinal structures that are the actual source of pain generation.

Traumatic insult to the ZP joints can produce pain. Hyperextension can result in impaction of the articular processes causing disruption of the joint capsule, inflammation, and activation of nociceptive afferents (Yang & King, 1984). Similarly, capsular disruption leading to tears, avulsion, or fracture–avulsion can be caused by rotary and/or rotation–compression torque–stress at the ZP joint (Farfan, 1985; Farfan et al., 1970; Sullivan & Farfan, 1975).

The meniscus of the ZP joint is susceptible to distortion during flexion-extension articulations (Bogduk & Engel, 1984; Bogduk & Jull, 1985). Hypothetically, mechanical entrapment of the fibro-adipose meniscus, which has been overstretched during flexion and buckled within the joint space during postural normalization/extension, could activate nociceptive fibers directly (via mechanical disruption or inflammation) or indirectly by disrupting the biomechanics of ZP joint stability and provoking compensatory muscular spasm. Additionally, it has been proposed that avulsion of articular cartilage can interfere with ZP meniscus function, disrupt ZP biomechanics during flexion/extension, and physically distend the joint capsule (Bogduk & Jull, 1985). This would pro-duce localized inflammation, biomechanical ZP joint aberration, and pain.

The Intervertebral Discs

The intervertebral discs are innervated by a plexus of nerve fibers that weaves within the outer (loose) connective tissue of the annulus fibrosus and is continuous with the innervation of the vertebral periosteum (Hirsch et al., 1963; Roofe, 1940; Yoshizawa et al., 1980). The innervated outer portion of the annulus (known as the ligamentous region) is normally shielded from mechanical loading and chemical stimuli occurring within the central nuclear zone by the structural and functional arrangement of the inner component of the annulus fibrosus (known as the nuclear envelope region; Bogduk, 1997). Four pathologies of the disc are considered to be principally provocative for pain. These are disc degradation/internal disruption, nuclear herniation, torsional-load injury, and discitis.

Internal disc degradation involves progressive change of the matrix of the nucleus pulposus. A number of etiologic possibilities may lead to degradation. One hypothesis is that fracture of the discal-vertebral endplate may induce an autoimmune inflammatory response (Bogduk, 1991; McCall et al., 1985; McCarron et al., 1987); however, there are equivocal arguments against this possibility (Gronblad et al., 1994; Olmarker et al., 1989). It is more probable that endplate fractures directly disrupt the biochemical equilibrium of the nuclear matrix, lower nuclear pH, and engage metalloproteinases to incur disc degradation (Maroudas et al., 1975; Melrose & Ghosh, 1988). The endplate fracture itself is frequently asymptomatic and often spontaneously heals. Furthermore, degradation of the nucleus is often limited. However, if nuclear metabolic changes (due to age, nutritional status, or disease) have begun to occur, proteolysis can disrupt the water-binding and cohesive ability of the nucleus to maintain and respond to load pressures. This transfers load forces abnormally through successive layers of the annulus. Such loads can exceed the stress/strain dynamics of annular fibers and induce tears of the annulus (Scott et al., 1994; Skaggs et al., 1994; Stokes, 1987). In this condition, the internal arrangement of the disc is deranged by radial fissures (Bogduk, 1991). Such fissures are graded to characterize the degree of penetration through successive architectural layers of the annulus (Sachs et al., 1987). This grading system is provided in Table 16.3.

With progressive internal disc disruption, annular fissures may extend through the periphery of the annulus and lead to frank disc herniation. As the fissure advances to the outer layers of the annulus, chemo-inflammatory substances (e.g. phospholipase-A_2, prostaglandin E_2, adenosine-ATP, hydrogen ion, enzymes, and cytokines released from locally infiltrating inflammatory cells) may stimulate chemoresponsive C-fiber afferents in the annular perimeter (Elves et al., 1975; Jaffray & O'Brien, 1986; Olmarker et

TABLE 16.3
Possible Sites of Spinal Pain Generation

Structure	Innervation
Zygapophyseal joints	Medial branch, dorsal ramus
Periosteum of vertebral arch	Medial branch, dorsal ramus
Spinous and transverse ligaments	Medial branch, dorsal ramus
Ligamentum flavum	Medial branch, dorsal ramus
Deep paraspinal musculature	Medial branch, dorsal ramus
Intermediate and superficial musculature	Lateral branch, dorsal ramus
Skin	Lateral branch, dorsal ramus (cuneal nerve)
Periosteum of posterior vertebral body	Recurrent meningeal nerve
Posterior anulus fibrosus of disc	Recurrent meningeal nerve
Internal and basivertebral veins	Recurrent meningeal nerve
Anterior dura mater	Recurrent meningeal nerve
Posterior longitudinal ligament	Recurrent meningeal nerve
Anterior/lateral anulus fibrosus	Sympathetic trunk and gray ramus
Anterior longitudinal ligament	Sympathetic trunk and gray ramus

al., 1995). Alternatively, distention of the outer fibers of the disc, both by extrusive nuclear material and by increased pressure under load, evoked by structural disruption of the inner architecture of the nuclear envelope, are capable of activating high-threshold mechanoresponsive A-delta and polymodal C-fibers (Crock, 1986). Thus, a grade-3 disc disruption may or may not be painful, depending on the relevant involvement of nociceptive fibers in outer disc layers. Frank herniation can produce local spinal pain without radicular signs or symptoms or may advance to radicular presentation if the herniation is significant enough to compress or inflame the nerve roots. In addition, nerve endings in the dura and epidural adipose tissues may be activated by inflammatory substances released by the degenerative or herniated disc (Melmon et al., 1967; Nachemson, 1969; Zvaifler, 1973). Thus, disc degeneration and herniation may sensitize the innervation of adjacent spinal structures and produce pain and hyperalgesia.

Age-related changes, primarily in the biochemistry of the nucleus pulposus, can lead to loss of the discs' functional capacity to bear and distribute load forces, thereby increasing pathologic diatheses in older patients. With age, a progressive shift to anaerobic metabolism results in decreased synthesis and concentration of proteoglycans (Scott et al., 1994; Sedowfia et al., 1982), change in collagen content (Buckwalter, 1995), and loss of elastic fibers (Johnson et al., 1985) within the nucleus and nuclear envelope. These changes result in decreased water-binding capacity of the nucleus (Hirsch et al., 1953), diminished resiliency, and an increased capacity for deformation and pathologic distortion (Vernon-Roberts & Pirie, 1977). In contrast to previous reports suggesting that loss of discal height is a cardinal feature of age-induced pathology

(Lawrence, 1969), in actuality there is an approximate 10% increase in the height of most intervertebral discs with age (Twomey & Taylor, 1985). The decrease in the imbibitive capacity of the disc appears to be a more significant contribution to pathology of the subchondral bone of the vertebral bodies (Twomey & Taylor, 1983). These changes may contribute to endplate failure, advancing the process of intervertebral disc degradation as described above (White & Panjabi, 1978). Such synergistic changes in the disc and vertebral body may be responsible, at least in part, for an increase in spinal pathology and pain in the geriatric population. Co-morbid disease (e.g., osteo- and rheumatoid arthritis, osteopenia, Paget's disease of bone) also contributes to this clinical scenario in the aged, and can predispose these patients to discal injury as described below (*vide infra*).

Torsional–rotational injury of the disc occurs when it is stressed in lateral shear beyond its rotary limit when in flexion (Farfan, 1985; Farfan & Sullivan, 1967; Pearcy, 1990). The stress forces are greatest where the annular lamellae are maximally curved and where the most torsional strain is incurred (Bogduk, 1997). This tends to occur in the posterolateral area of discs with concave posterior surfaces, while circumferential distortion (annular tears) occurs posteriorly in discs with convex posterior surfaces (Farfan et al., 1972). In torsional injury, the circumferential tear involves the superficial, ligamentous layers of the annulus, which is innervated and therefore provocative for pain (during flexion and rotation; Farfan, 1985). The nucleus pulposus or nuclear envelope fibers are not affected per se; however, it is possible that torsion–rotation injury can occur (perhaps with higher frequency) in circumstances where the outer annulus is pre-stressed due to existing grade 2 or 3 circumferential fissures.

Discitis is a relatively rare, inflammatory condition caused by microbial infection subsequent to medically invasive procedures (e.g., discography). The infection and inflammation is limited to the disc and is evoked by the direct action of pro-inflammatory and pro-nociresponsive substances (e.g., cytokines, hydrogen ion, adenosine, histamine) on nociceptive small fiber afferents (Guyer, et al., 1988).

Dura and Nerve Roots

Dura mater is innervated by a plexus of unmyelinated nerve fibers from the recurrent meningeal (sinuvertebral) nerve. Innervation is greater in the anterior areas of the dural sac and root sleeves than in the posterior dural sac and epidural adipose (Edgar & Nundy, 1964; Groen et al., 1988). Inflammation of the dura has been shown to elicit both back pain and peripheralized, referred somatic pain (Bogduk, 1997; Walton, 1977). Inflammation of the dural sleeve subsequent to disc herniation can also occur as a consequence of chemical activation of dural nociceptive afferents by components of the extrusive nucleus pulposus

(McCarron et al., 1987). Disc herniation has been proposed as a mechanism through which inflammatory fibrosis can produce adhesions that tether the dura and evoke high-threshold mechanical stimulation and pain (Spencer et al., 1983). The phenomenon of peripheralization, in which there is a spread of perceived pain to a distal somatic structure from focal spinal insult, has been reported as a consequence of dural pathology (see Aina et al., 2004, for review). Pathologic involvement of the dura or the dural sleeve may produce this centrifugally, referred type of pain due to convergent inputs of sinuvertebral and somatic pain afferents within the dorsal horn. This process involves the co-terminal activation of second-order afferents producing a dermatomal referral pattern that may be independent of, or co-morbid with, specific radiculopathy (Merskey & Bogduk, 1994).

Bogduk (1997) explicitly contends that radiculopathy, a decrement in neural conduction caused by axonal compression and/or ischemia, characteristically causes weakness, but not uniformly pain. In contrast, radicular pain may arise from sequelae of radiculopathy or may be an independent event evoked by irritation of a spinal nerve or its root (Merskey & Bogduk, 1994). The most likely mechanism of radicular pain involves chronic inflammation following exposure to nuclear material and compressive ischemic activation of neurovascular nociceptive afferents (Franson et al., 1992; Saal et al., 1990). Leakage of phospholipase-A_2 can provoke significant inflammatory responses leading to radiculitis, edema of the nerve roots, immunocyte activation, and radicular/perineural fibrosis (Cooper et al., 1995; Olmarker et al., 1989, 1993). The fibers of the sinuvertebral nerve can become sensitized, leading to subsequent mechanical hyperalgesia produced by movement of the dural sleeve and nerve roots during even normal articulation of the spine.

Muscles

The muscles of the spine are extensively innervated; the majority of the deep paraspinal musculature is innervated by the medial branch of the dorsal rami. Intermediate and superficial musculature is innervated by the lateral branch of the dorsal rami and the intertransverse muscles are innervated by the dorsal and ventral rami (Bogduk et al., 1982; Cave, 1937). The spinal musculature can evoke both focal back pain and somatic, referred pain (Bogduk, 1997) as a consequence of micro/macrotrauma (strain/sprain), compensatory spasm, and myofascial trigger points.

Microtrauma and/or macrotrauma to superficial and intermediate muscles of the spine can produce local hyperemia, and the extravasation of pro-algesic substances that activate both A-delta and C-fiber afferents in these tissues (Newham, Jones, Ghosh et al., 1988; Vecchiet et al., 1983). Local hyperemia disrupts endomysial circulation and leads to accumulation of metabolic end products, reactive oxidative species, and disrupted ATP metabolism

(Bogduk, 1997). These biochemical factors have been shown both to directly stimulate afferent nociceptive fibers and to produce subsequent sensitization such that normal eccentric loading and contraction may evoke firing of high-threshold mechanoreceptors to produce pain (Newham et al., 1988). While these variables appear to be a cause of acute and subacute back pain, their role in the instigation and maintenance of chronic pain is less clearly defined (Garrett et al., 1989).

The pathophysiology of muscle spasm contributory to, and reciprocal with, back pain is somewhat controversial (Bogduk, 1992; Roland, 1986). The neuromechanical basis of spinal muscular spasm has been proposed and discussed relative to articular disorders of the spine (Porterfield & DeRosa, 1991). Briefly, afferent input (from fibers innervating spinal structures, spinal musculature, or both) can feedforward to influence firing rate and patterns of motor units involved in the maintenance of spinal stability, postural architecture, and/or biomechanical articulation. Volleys of afferent input are capable of generating aberrant activation of motor neurons driving the spinal musculature, and produce abnormal increases in spinal muscle tone and/or contractility (Roland, 1986). Bogduk (1997) states that these contractile differences may represent a transitory hyperreflexia. It remains unclear whether spasm is a consequence *of* chronic back pain, a contributory variable *to* chronic back pain, or both, dependent on circumstance.

The seminal work of Travell and Simons has described the etiology, pathology, and effects of myofascial trigger points in detail (see Travell & Rinzler, 1952, and Simons & Travell, 1981, for early reviews). It has been suggested that ZP joint pathology and activation of spinal nociceptive afferents may incur changes in efferent motor output. This can evoke both compensatory postures and articulations capable of affecting the physiology of the spinal and paraspinal musculature and producing trigger points (Schimek & Schimek, 1984; Simons, 1988), most specifically in the multifidi, longissimi, iliocostalis, and quadratus lumborum (Sola & Kuitert, 1954; Travell & Rinzler, 1952).

Ligaments

The paraspinal ligaments (anterior and posterior longitudinal ligaments, ligamentum flavum, interspinous, and iliolumbar ligaments) are differentially innervated by free nerve endings (Jackson et al., 1966; Wyke, 1970). However, these ligaments do not uniformly meet Bogduk's criteria for sites of pain generation and, therefore, must be considered individually regarding their possible role in spinal pain. The anterior longitudinal ligament is innervated by fibers from the sympathetic branches and gray rami communicantes, while the sinuvertebral nerves innervate the posterior longitudinal ligament (Groen, Balijet, & Drukker, 1990; Pederson et al., 1956). The longitudinal ligaments are structurally conjoined to the outer ligamentous layer of the annulus of the intervertebral discs (Bogduk, 1997). The elastic nature of the ligaments and their responses along the stress–strain curve of (even excessive) spinal movement makes it improbable that they are a primary source of spinal pain. Rather, discogenic pain, as described above, may activate common afferents that innervate both the annulus and its overlying longitudinal ligaments such that, if sensitized, these afferents could discharge in response to mechanical input from the ligament (Bogduk, 1997).

The ligamentum flavum is only sparsely innervated and may actually lack afferent innervation in some regions (Yahia & Newman, 1989). As well, the highly elastic composition of the flaval ligament and its biomechanical tensile range do not render it easily vulnerable to traumatic injury (Bogduk, 1997; Kirby et al., 1989). The interspinous ligaments are considerably innervated by the medial branches of the dorsal rami (Yahia & Newman, 1989). Rissanen (1960) has shown that interspinous ligaments can degenerate and atrophy with age, increasing their vulnerability to biomechanical creep, distortion, and micro- or macrotears with spinal flexion. However, local anesthetic perfusion of interspinous ligaments was only modestly effective in reducing back pain in patients showing focal midline sensitivity upon postural flexion, suggestive of interspinous ligament pathology (Wilk, 1995). It is more reasonable to assume that degenerative laxity of the interspinous ligaments increases the vulnerability of other spinal structures (paraspinal muscles, intervertebral discs), recognized as viable pain generators, to injury.

The iliolumbar ligament is diffusely innervated by fibers of the dorsal and, to some extent, ventral rami (Bogduk, 1997). It is not well known whether this ligament fulfills the criteria for generating spinal pain in that it is difficult to clinically isolate, (anatomically) lying within the multifidi and erector spinae (Bogduk, 1997); is differentially developed across age groups and individual adults (Luk et al., 1986); and may functionally affect and be reciprocally affected by both the deep and intermediate musculature of the spine and the lower lumbar and lumbosacral joints (Collee et al., 1991; Ingpen & Burry, 1970). Macintosh and Bogduk (1986) maintain that the lumbar intramuscular aponeurosis, which forms a common tendonous attachment for the tendon of the lumbar longissimus to the posterior superior iliac spine (PSIS), may be the principal pain generator during lumbar flexion, rotation, and lateral bending. Thus, it seems that ligamentous pathology is only minimally contributory to primary spinal pain, but may exacerbate existing pathologies in other structures to produce postures and articulations that recruit these substrates to be nociceptive.

In sum, despite some disparity in the literature, it appears that pain arising from deep spinal structures (e.g., vertebral bodies, ZP joints, intervertebral discs, ligaments) is capable of affecting motor output to the spinal muscu-

lature (putatively causing physiologic dysfunction and perhaps pain) and that primary pathology of the spinal muscles may be a source of pain. In either case, increased activity of mechanoreceptor afferents within spinal muscle tissue contributes to sensitization of second-order nociceptive neurons within the dorsal horn that may result in the phenomenon of maldynia. It has also been proposed that normalizing the tone of these mechanoreceptor populations may help to restore vertebral muscular activity, stabilize existing compensatory biomechanics, and perhaps induce specific pain modulatory mechanisms. At least hypothetically, mechanoreceptor-mediated feedforward and feedback axes appear to play a role in the maintenance of spinal biomechanics, pain generation, and pain modulation along a continuum of effect(s) from functionality to pathology.

Pain Pathways

Irrespective of what structures generate nociceptive input in the spine, this afferent information is conducted along A-delta and C-fibers that enter the dorsal horn of the spinal cord. The transduction, conduction, and transmission of pain and the anatomy of the nociceptive and analgesic pathways are discussed in considerable detail elsewhere in this volume. Briefly summarized, primary nociceptive afferents synapse upon both nociceptive specific (NS) and wide-dynamic range (WDR) neurons in laminae I, II, IIa, and V of the superficial dorsal horn. Significant modulation of the nociceptive signal is possible within the dorsal horn, and low- to moderate-level nociceptive afferent input is attenuated by spinal interneuronal mechanisms involving GABAergic, glycinergic, opioid (dynorphin, enkephalin), nitric oxidergic, and anadamidergic inhibition.

Second-order afferents aggregate in the dorsal horn, and the majority of these fibers decussate within the cord and ascend contralaterally as the (paleo- and neo-) spinothalamic tracts within the anterolateral column. The paleospinothalamic tract projects to the brainstem reticular formation (i.e., the spinoreticular subtract), with specific projections to the serotonergic raphe nuclei of the rostroventral medulla and the noradrenergic reticulomagnocellular nuclei of the caudal pons. As well, paleospinothalamic fibers project to the opioid-rich, mesencephalic periaqueductal gray (PAG) and periventricular gray (PVG) regions (i.e., the spinotectal subtract). These brainstem structures may be activated singularly or in synergy to evoke bulbospinal and centrifugal analgesia, respectively. Paleospinothalamic neurons ascend to project somewhat diffusely within several thalamic nuclei, which subserve distinct qualitative and quantitative components of the nociceptive signal, and which activate cortical and subcortical limbic structures to engage affective dimensions of pain. In contrast, the neospinothalamic tract projects directly to the ventroposterior lateral (VPL) nucleus of the thalamus, an area involved in the somatotopic localization and intensity discriminative features of the pain signal(s). Thalamolimbic and thalamocortical pathways engage neuroanatomical regions including the cingulate, frontal and temporal cortices, amygdala, hippocampus, and hypothalamus, which subserve the cognitive, expectational, emotional, and perceptual aspects of pain. Cortical and limbic regions may also activate the PAG/PVG to facilitate "top-down" mechanisms of pain control that are co-terminal with, and contingent upon, specific expectational, emotional, or cognitive states (see Giordano, Chapter 3, this volume, for review). A basic overview of these pathways is schematically depicted by Figure 16.1.

Factors Affecting Spinal Pain: Sociocultural Influences

The complexity of the algesic neuraxis and the interactive involvement of several structures subserving cognition, memory, and emotion reveal that "pain" is phenomenologically greater than the somatosensation of nociception. Furthermore, patients are persons and do not live in sociocultural vacuums. As persons, they are embodiments of the ongoing interaction between genotype and phenotype and the influences of the time, environment(s), and cultures in which they live. This is compounded by the pre- and/or co-morbidity of disease; any or all of these variables can affect the biological, psychological, and behavioral extent to which the persistent somatosensory occurrence of nociception may progress to the multicomponential *illness* of maldynia. The ontology of pain, in general, and back pain specifically must account for the relative roles these variables contribute to the patients' pain experience.

Scarry (1985) states that chronic pain deconstructs patients' (and perhaps families' and social cohorts') lives. This can certainly be true of back pain, and the classic triad of the "3-D pain patient," *d*isabled, *d*ependent (upon medicalization, remuneration, and others) and *d*epressed, is a common entity in the offices of primary and specialty care providers and pain management centers. The reciprocal relationship between depression and pain is well known and well understood. Although somewhat beyond the scope of this chapter, suffice it to state that neurochemical mechanisms of chronic pain can be directly contributory to the pathogenesis of depressive illness, particularly among patients in whom there is a defined predisposition or pre-morbidity (Williamson & Schulz; 1992). The circumstantial disability of chronic pain can also precipitate depressive symptoms (Williams & Schulz, 1988), and the pain experience has been shown to be greater in patients with depressive co-morbidity (Herr et al., 1993). Of course, there are patients that exacerbate symptoms in order to achieve sec-

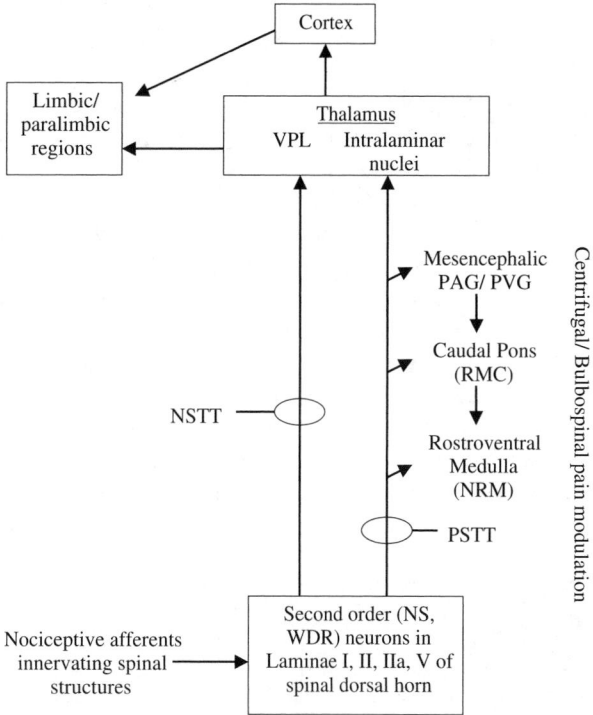

FIGURE 16.1 Schematic diagram of afferent pain-transmitting and efferent pain-modulating systems. A-delta and/or C-fibers innervating spinal pain-generating structures project to the superficial dorsal horn and form synaptic contact with NS and WDR neurons. Considerable modulation of the afferent signal occurs by local and segmental inhibition within the cord (not shown). Axons of NS and WDR neurons decussate and ascend in the anterolateral columns as the paleo-and neospinothalamic tracts. The differential projections of these spinothalamic pathways are illustrated. PSTT activation of mesencephalic and/or midbrain substrates can engage descending inhibitory control (centrifugal-bulbospinal analgesia). Thalamic projections to somatosensory cortex mediate sensory components of pain. Activation of S-II, cingulated, limbic, and paralimbic regions subserves cognitive, emotional and expectational aspects of pain. (Details in text.) Abbreviations: NRM: nucleus raphe magnus; NS: nociceptive-specific neurons; NSTT: neospinothalamic tract; PAG-PVG: periaqueductal/periventricular gray region; PSTT: paleospinothalamic tract; RMC: reticular magnocellular nuclei; VPL: ventroposterior lateral nucleus; WDR: wide dynamic range.

ondary or tertiary gain, and such behaviors often reflect ongoing psychological enfranchisement with, and expression of, distress. (At worst, symptomatic overexpression for the achievement of secondary gain may reflect malingering and fall within the medicolegal purview).

However, this pattern is not universal and Carron et al. (1985), Raspe et al. (2004), Smith and co-workers (2004), and others have shown significant cultural and community-based distinctions in the perception of, behaviors, responses to, and acknowledgment of back pain. Socioeconomic status (SES) may influence a number of variables relevant to patients' presentation and experience of back pain (Smith et al., 2001a, b; Thomas et al., 1999). Most obviously, SES is a strong determinant of access to health care, the absence or paucity of which could lead to progressive exacerbation of subacute pain to a more chronic, sensitized condition. Yet, this is not uniformly the case, and there is evidence that characteristics of hardiness, locus of control, and social cohesiveness can strongly contribute to low prevalence of back pain, even in lower SES communities (Thomas et al., 1999). Interestingly, one of the strongest contributory variables to pain is the notion of cultural pain-permissivity or a social expectation for both pain exacerbation and its expression (Mechanic, 1986; Smith et al., 2004). This appears to be particularly true among individuals with pre-morbid disease, pain, or both, for whom the sociocultural effect seems to perpetuate and augment both pain and treatment expectations (Raspe et al., 2004; Smith et al., 2004).

Hadler (2004) posits that sociocultural influence on illness is a component of the process of medicalization (see also Morris, 1998). This may well be true for maldynic back pain: while socioculturally acknowledging its existence, it remains something of a diagnostic and therapeutic enigma and thereby creates considerable discord in the social relationship between the medical community and persons who have become "patients."

This latter point speaks to Scarry's second tenet that chronic pain defies language (Scarry, 1985). There is not an effective semantic for pain, and back pain, by its complex, multifocal nature, emphatically reinforces this issue. The clinical semiotics of pain assessment often fails to convey objective value to the first-person experience of pain, leading to dissonance and frustration between patient and clinician. Many pain patients may overexpress their pain in an effort to convey the first-person impact of suffering across domains of their existence and in an attempt to recruit subjective pathos and objective unity with their clinician(s). For the clinician, understanding these dynamic variables is essential, and assessment of the patient with chronic back pain may require the development of semiotics for symptoms that are meaningful to both patients and clinicians. Equally important, however, is the establishment of semiotics that are resonant *across* medical disciplines that are based on mechanistic evaluation of the biologic, psychologic, and social factors contributing to the back pain specific to individual patients. Scarry's perceptivity of the linguistic defiance of pain may be well illustrated by the relative discord between clinical disciplines in defining and "naming" the locus and nature of the spinal lesion or dysfunction that is provocative for pain. A more uniform, mechanism-based terminology might allow for improved interdisciplinary heuristics and facilitate enhanced cooperativity of back pain care in a progressively pluralist medical society.

PART II

Spinal Manual Medicine

As addressed elsewhere in this volume, there are numerous approaches and techniques to treat and manage chronic back pain. When examining the overall therapeutic armamentarium against maldynic spinal pain, it is important to consider the relevant specificity (and therefore the relative efficacy) of these approaches, whether used alone or in combination. Paradigmatically, it is best to take a mechanistic approach to the pathology, a patient-centered approach to its manifestations, and a combined or integrative approach to care and management. While the majority of studies suggest that acute and subacute back pain regularly resolves with stabilizing exercise, short-term rest, and conservative use of nonsteroidal anti-inflammatory agents (Cady et al., 1979; Nachemson, 1983; Waddell, 1987), chronic back pain may require more extensive therapeutics or management. Diagnosis is critical, and it is important to reiterate that evaluation of underlying pathology may not be identical to identification of pain generators that might be responsive to intervention. Often, a defined organic cause of pain is non-identifiable. Therefore, it is vital to address pain from a mechanistic viewpoint and engage in therapeutic approaches that effectively target these mechanisms. There is a significant body of literature to demonstrate the efficacy of anesthesiologic procedures in cases where ongoing pain is contributory to the cycle of dysfunction and neural sensitization. As well, prudent use of systemically administered anti-inflammatory and low-grade analgesic agents has utility in diminishing central or peripheral sensitization. In cases of defined orthopedic or neurologic instability, surgical approaches may be warranted; however, there is some controversy regarding the use of surgical intervention for patients who do not present with progressive neurological signs and symptoms.

The source of chronic spinal pain may be due to aberrant and hypertonic musculature, ZP joint dysfunction, and symptomatic disc extrusion without frank herniation. The former two conditions are obviously amenable to spinal manual medicine (SMM), and there is evidence to support that SMM may produce force-relevant distraction of vertebral segments in patients with disc extrusion, allowing for resumption of annular architecture and producing symptomatic resolution (Browning, 1988). Interestingly, there is also evidence to suggest that SMM may produce a more global, nonspecific analgesia (*vide infra*), although the mechanism(s) for such effects remain speculative.

Spinal manipulation is a historically old therapeutic tradition. Ancient writings and depictions display manipulation as a part of the healing practices used in widespread locations and cultures throughout the Old World and Eurasia. In the 1800s, spinal manipulation "re-emerged" as part of folk healing traditions in Europe and the United States. At the turn of the century in the midwestern United States, two practitioner-level healing professions developed that relied on spinal manipulation as a primary means of treatment. Palmer and Still, the founders of the chiropractic and osteopathic professions, respectively, differed in their beliefs of the therapeutic effects and processes of spinal manipulation, but both acknowledged and promoted the beneficial role that spinal manipulation played in the health and restorative well-being of patients.

Despite the castigating climate fostered by the Flexner report, these professions survived through the 20th century and have established distinct niches within the post-modern medical community. While osteopathic medicine has become more assimilative to and integrated within the allopathic model, an expanding examination and progressive acceptance of chiropractic is becoming evident as a consequence of medicosocial and political support for application(s) in broader scope of public health care. Yet, it should be noted that spinal manipulation was not the sole domain of the chiropractic and osteopathic professions during the 20th century. Considerable work in the application, utilization, and refinement of various forms of SMM was conducted by Mennell, Cyriax, Paget, and many others, and types of SMM are components of physical therapy and physical medicine.

Basic Mechanics of SMM

Spinal manual techniques essentially involve both soft tissue and hard tissue (i.e., joint relevant) components. The longitudinal work of Triano and colleagues (Triano, 1989, 1991, 1992, 2001; Triano & Gudavalli, 1990; Triano & Luttges, 1985; Triano & Schultz, 1997; Triano et al., 1997a, b; Triano et al., 2002) has shown that the mobilization component primarily effects elastic soft tissue elements while the low-amplitude impulse (i.e., manipulation) component predominantly effects spinal joints. It is unclear whether these components function individually or synergistically to effect spinal substrates. Application of manual techniques can involve moving a tissue or joint through its passive range of movement. This may engage the tissue to its elastic barrier and thereby activate mechanoreceptors beyond the physiologic limit incurred during active motion. This mobilizing phase is of obvious utility in instances of a defined muscular pain focus (e.g., spasm, trigger points, hypertonicity), which may incur restrictive barriers to movement or posture and produce compensatory motor recruitment and resultant alteration in biomechanics (Beal, 1953; Bourdillon & Day 1982). Mobilization techniques are characteristically applied with low velocity, engage a minimal thrust or impulse, and are frequently used as the basis of osteopathic SMM (DiGiovanna & Schiowitz, 1991; Lamax, 1975; Stiles, 1975).

Extending the application of manual force beyond the passive range into what is known as the paraphysiologic space moves the tissue to approach its anatomic barrier, reflecting the osseous contours of the joint and the ligamentous and tendonous end-range (Sandoz, 1976). The restrictive barriers within this range may include spinal/paraspinal muscular hypertonicity and mechanical impediments of the ZP joints (Giles, 1986). Although somewhat simplistic, and certainly not reflective of practice philosophy, the major distinctions between osteopathic and chiropractic SMM involve the principal use of mobilizing versus manipulative techniques, respectively. It should be noted that the specificity of one form of SMM as compared with another may be a function of the mechanism and substrates of pain generation and/or the ability of a particular technique to engage local or nonlocal pain alleviating or modulating mechanisms.

The osseous and soft tissue components of the spine may be conceptualized as a combined mass-damped and elastic biomechanical system (Gudavalli & Triano, 1999; Triano, 2001). The mobilizing phase of SMM engages soft tissue mechanoreceptors, while the peak velocity, impulse-manipulative phase engages joint-space mechanoreceptors (Triano, 2001). Although contradictory viewpoints exist, the cavitation caused by biophysical gas-phase shifts within the ZP joint synovial fluid appears to be generally an artifact of the velocity movement and not responsible for mechanoreceptor activation or mechanical restoration of the ZP meniscus (D. Meyers, & J. Giordano, unpublished observation). A variety of conceptual and practical systems of SMM have been developed and implemented. These use non-impulse mobilization as well as a number of impulse based approaches that employ variable velocities and distinctions in the biomechanics of tissue contact (Haldeman et al., 1992). Examples of these are provided in Table 16.4.

Spinal manual medicine is predominantly used against musculoskeletal conditions in which the major constellation of features are biomechanical and the principal symptoms are reciprocal pain and dysfunction. Within this treatment category the majority of SMM is employed against low back pain (Chapman-Smith, 2000). Studies examining the efficacy of SMM against chronic (noncervical) back pain have yielded somewhat varied results. A recent systematic review by Bronfort, Haas, and colleagues (2004) assessed the efficacy of manipulation and mobilization for both acute and chronic back (as well as neck) pain. The study focused on multinational randomized clinical trials (RCTs) published through 2002. The authors concluded that moderate evidence exists to support the efficacy of manipulation and/or mobilization and that both forms of SMM afford pain outcomes that are superior to placebo and at least equivalent to combined physical and pharmacotherapy. An earlier study illustrated generally effective trends but noted conflicting evidence regarding the effects

TABLE 16.4
Manipulative/Adjustive Techniques

Manual Articular Manipulative and Adjustive Procedures
  Specific Contact Thrust Procedures
    High-velocity thrust
    High-velocity thrust with recoil
    Low-velocity thrust
  Nonspecific Contact Thrust Procedures
  Manual Force, Mechanically Assisted Procedures
    Drop-tables and terminal point adjustive thrust
    Flexion-distraction table adjustment
    Pelvic block adjusting
  Mechanical Force, Manually Assisted Procedures
    Fixed stylus, compression wave adjustment
    Moving stylus instrument adjustment
Manual Non-Articular Manipulative and Adjustive Procedures
Manual Reflex and Muscle Relaxation Procedures
  Neurologic reflex technique
  Myofascial ischemic compression procedures
  Miscellaneous soft-tissue techniques
Chiropractic Technique Systems

Full-Spine High-Velocity Techniques	**Lumbo-Pelvic Techniques**
Diversified	Cox flexion-distraction
Gonstead	Leander
Thompson terminal point	Logan Basic
Pierce-Stillwagon	
Pettibon	

  Miscellaneous/Instrument Adjustment
    Sacro-occipital technique
    Activator

Note: Adapted from Chapman-Smith, 2000.

of manipulation versus placebo (van Tulder, 2001). Weiner and Ernst (2004) reviewed the literature addressing spinal manipulation (and other complementary and alternative approaches to persistent musculoskeletal pain) and drew attention to the similarity of outcomes between manipulative treatment and placebo (i.e., sham SMM) groups. These authors also expressed concern regarding safety issues relevant to adverse effects after SMM, although the majority of adverse effects cited were consequential to cervical manipulation (see also Ernst, 2002; Ernst & Harkness, 2001). Cagnie et al. (2004) report that while minor adverse effects were frequent the predominance of these were related to cervical SMM, with lesser effects observed for other spinal regions. As well, this study raised contention that direct correlation of effects of (noncervical) SMM might be difficult to ascertain as other treatments were frequently co-administered. Jonas (2000) emphasized that while serious adverse effects of SMM are rare, such adverse sequelae can occur and strategies for identification of pre-existing risk factors and guidelines for specific application of SMM need to be developed to reduce this risk potential.

Whether attempting to illustrate trends of efficacy or incidence of risk, a uniform advocacy is for further out-

comes-based and mechanism-oriented research. Giordano et al. (2002, 2003) have discussed the need to develop and expand complementary medical research as a means to facilitate medical integration that maximizes utilization and efficiency within a public health model. However, the methodology of such research may be equally as important as its focus. While the RCT remains the *sine qua non* of biomedical research, its application beyond the disease-centered and/or pharmaceutical model may have some limitations (Jonas, 2002). Relevant to this, an important recurrent issue is what constitutes a sham treatment for SMM. This has been addressed by Triano et al. (1997a, b) and Triano and colleagues (Gudavalli & Triano, 1999; Rogers & Triano, 2003). Important considerations are the biomechanical parameters necessary to constitute SMM. In other words, what forces are required for therapeutic effect(s), and what are the nature and mechanisms of those effects? This becomes crucial when attempting to discern significant clinical outcomes produced by "real" SMM versus placebo. The question has been raised whether SMM may represent a nonspecific treatment or "placating" effect (Chapman-Smith, 2000). Refutation of such nonspecific effects was fortified by reports of distinct physiologic events induced by SMM including overall analgesia, altered muscle tone, and change in immunocyte activity (Brennan et al., 1994; Terrett & Vernon, 1984; Vernon et al., 1990). We posit that such effects may reflect a cascade of "top-down" mechanisms similar to those seen in other therapeutic approaches that are capable of eliciting a patient-centered response (Stefano et al., 2001). These putative pathways are depicted in Figure 16.2.

Such patient-centered responses are also referred to as the placebo response and involve discriminable neural and extra-neural mechanisms capable of affecting pain sensation, pain perception, cognitive state, and endocrine and immunologic processes (Lazar et al., 2000; Spiro, 1997; Stefano et al., 2001). The occurrence of such outcomes and mechanisms does not discount the therapeutic efficacy of a treatment that engages them; to the contrary, there is a building body of evidence to suggest that such mechanisms underlie diverse therapeutic approaches (Benson, 1996; Fields & Price, 1997). It may be that particular forms of SMM engage peripheral substrates to activate central neuraxes that produce both specific pain modulatory, physiologic, and salutary responses (refer to Figure 16.2). As knowledge of the network hierarchical properties of brain–body systems becomes increasingly well understood, the expanding epistemic framework allows for a more thorough evaluation of such "bottom-up"/"top down" (i.e., body–brain/mind–body) mechanisms. However, to effectively move in this direction, it is critical that academic and clinical institutions abandon political and parochial dogmatism that could restrict the ongoing reevaluation of scientific knowledge and impede progress (Flanagan & Giordano, 2002). Taken together,

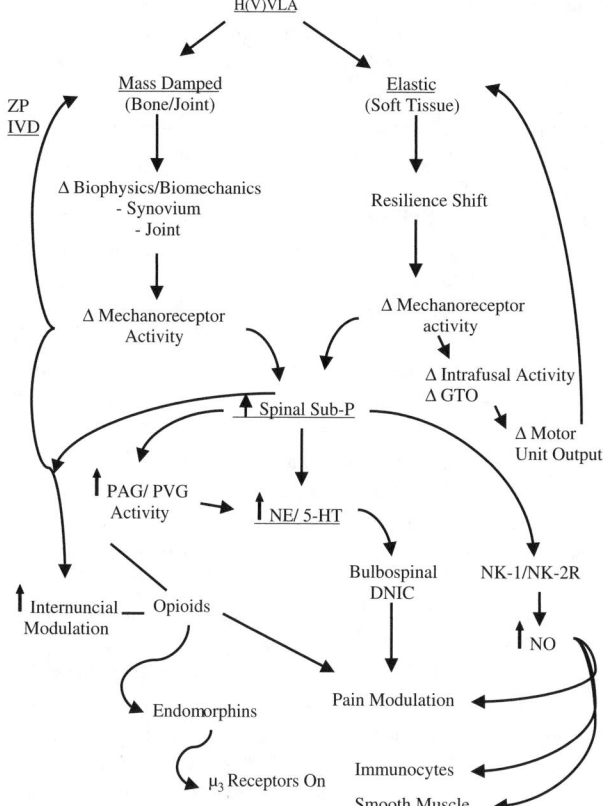

FIGURE 16.2 Diagrammatic representation of putative mechanisms of pain modulation and physiologic responses evoked/induced by manual therapeutics of spinal substrates. High- or variable-velocity, low-amplitude manual force may affect both mass-damped and elastic spinal components. Respective changes in the biophysics or biomechanics of these structures affect mechanoreceptor activity to produce local mechanical effects and evoke an intraspinal substance-P pulse. Such afferent mechanoreceptor input and the resultant substance-P pulse may engage supraspinal mechanisms to induce centrifugal pain modulation. As well, substance-P may act locally within the cord to engage interneuronal afferent modulation via opioid and/or nitric oxidergic mechanisms. Systemic effects of opioids may include immunocyte and smooth myocyte modulation. This tentative diagram is representational of existing data and hypotheses and therefore remains a speculative model. (Refer to text for details and reference citations). Abbreviations: DNIC: descending noxious inhibitory control; GTO: Golgi tendon organs; H(V)VLA: high (or variable) velocity, low-amplitude manual force; 5-HT: 5-hydroxytriptamine, serotonin; IVD: intervertebral discs; NE: norepinephrine; NK-1/NK-2R: neurokinin-1 or -2 receptors; NO: nitric oxide; PAG/PVG: periaqueductal/periventricular gray regions; ZP: zygapophyseal joints; μ_3: refers to an opioid receptor.

epistemic, philosophic, and technologic developments become viable tools to more stringently define the effects, limitations, risks, and applicable benefits of SMM. However, it is also important that this research not be limited in scope to a single evidence domain, such as the RCT.

Future research needs to be conducted that uses rigorous mixed-methods to assess both qualitative and quantitative outcomes of SMM, and that affords new applications for existing strategies and develops new and novel methodologies to investigate mechanisms that subserve these more broadly defined outcomes.

ACKNOWLEDGMENTS

The authors are grateful to Sherry Loveless for outstanding technical, administrative, and graphical support on this manuscript.

REFERENCES

Aina, A., May, S., & Clare, H. (2004). The centralization phenomenon of spinal symptoms — A systematic review. *Manual Therapy, 9*, 134–143

Arnoldi, C. C. (1972). Intravertebral pressures in patients with lumbar pain. *Acta Orthopaedica Scandinavica, 43*, 109–117

Arnoldi, C. C. (1976). Intraosseous hypertension: A possible cause of low-back pain? *Clinical Orthopaedics, 115*, 30–34.

Baastrup, C. I. (1933). Proc. Spin. Vert. Lumb. und einige zwischen diesen leigende Gelenkbildungen mit pathologischen Prozessen in dieser Region. *Fortschritte auf den Gebiete der Rontgenstrahlen, 48*, 430–435.

Beal, M. C. (1953). Motion sense. *Journal. American Osteopathic Assocociation, 53* (3), 151–153.

Benson, H. (1996). *Timeless healing.* New York: Scribner.

Bogduk, N. (1983). The innervation of the lumbar spine. *Spine, 8*, 286–293

Bogduk, N. (1991). The lumbar disc and low back pain. *Neurosurgery Clinics of North America, 2*, 791–806.

Bogduk, N. (1992). Sources of low back pain. In M. I. V. Jayson (Ed.), *The lumbar spine and back pain.* Edinburgh: Churchill Livingstone.

Bogduk, N. (1997). *Clinical anatomy of the lumbar spine and sacrum,* 3rd ed. Edinburgh: Churchill Livingstone.

Bogduk, N., & Engel, R. (1984). The menisci of the lumbar zygapophyseal joints. A review of their anatomy and clinical significance. *Spine, 9*, 454–460.

Bogduk, N., & Jull, G. (1985). The theoretical pathology of acute locked back: A basis for manipulative therapy. *Man and Medicine, 1*, 78–82.

Bogduk, N., Wilson, A. S., & Tynan, W. (1982). The human lumbar dorsal rami. *Journal of Anatomy, 134*, 383–397.

Borenstein, D. G. (1998). Management of neck pain: A primary care approach. *Hospital Practices,* 147–160.

Bourdillon, J. F., & Day, E. A. (1982). *Spinal manipulation,* 4th ed. London: William Heinemann Medical Books.

Brennan, P. C., Graham, M. A., Triano, J. J., Hondras, M. A., & Anderson, R. J. (1994). Lymphocyte profiles in patients with chronic low back pain enrolled in a clinical trial. *Journal of Manipulative and Physiological Therapeutics, 17*(4), 219–227.

Bronfort, G, Haas, M, Evans, R.L, Bouter, (2004) L M. Efficacy of spinal manipulation and mobilization for low back pain and neck pain: a systematic review and best evidence synthesis. *Spine Journal, 4*(3), 335–356.

Browning, J.E. (1988) Chiropractic distractive decompression in the treatment of pelvic pain and organic dysfunction in patients with evidence of lower sacral nerve root compression. *Journal of Manipulative and Physiological Therapeutics, 11* 437–442.

Buckwalter, J. A. (1995). Spine update. Aging and degeneration of the human intervertebral disc. *Spine, 20*, 1307–1314.

Burton, A. K., & Erg, E. (1997). Back injury and work loss. Biomechanical and psychosocial influences. *Spine, 1*, 22(21), 2575–2580.

Cady, L., Bischoff, D., & O'Connel., E. (1979). Strength and fitness and subsequent back injuries in firefighters. *Occupational Medicine, 21*, 269.

Cagnie, B., Vinck, E., Beernaert, A., & Cambier, D. (2004). How common are side effects of spinal manipulation and can these side effects be predicted? *Manual Therapy, 9*, 151–156.

Carron, H., DeGood, D. E, & Tait, R. A (1985). Comparison of low back pain patients in the United States and Zealand: psychosocial and economic factors affecting severity of disability. *Pain, 21*(1), 77–89.

Cave, A. J. E. (1937). The innervation and morphology of the cervical intertransverse muscles. *Journal of Anatomy, 71*, 497–515.

Chapman-Smith, D. (2000). *The chiropractic profession.* West Des Moines, IA: NCMIC Group Inc.

Collee, G., Dijkmans, A. C., Vandenbroucke, J. P., & Cats, A. (1991). Iliac crest pain syndrome in low back pain: frequency and features. *Journal of Rheumatology, 18*, 1064–1067

Cooper, R. G., Freemont, A. J., Hoyland, J. A., Jenkins, J. P. R., West, C. G.H., Illingworth, K. J. et al. (1995). Herniated intervertebral disc-associated periradicular fibrosis and vascular abnormalities occur without inflammatory cell infiltration. *Spine, 20*, 591–598

Crock, H. V. (1986). Internal disc disruption: Achallenge to disc prolapse 50 years on. *Spine, 11*, 650–653.

DiGiovanna, E. L., & Schiowitz, S. (1991). *An osteopathic approach to diagnosis and treatment.* Philadelphia: JB Lippincott.

Edgar, M. A., & Ghadially, J. A. (1976). Innervation of the lumbar spine. *Clinical Orthopaedics, 115*, 35–41.

Edgar, M. A., & Nundy, S. (1964). Innervation of the spinal dura mater. *Journal of Neurology, Neurosurgery, and Psychiatry, 29*, 530–534.

Elves, M.W ., Bucknill, T., & Sullivan, M. F. (1975). *In vitro* inhibition of leucocyte migration in patients with intervertebral disc lesions. *Orthopedic Clinics of North America, 6*, 599–65.

Ernst, E.(2002). Manipulation of the cervical spine: A systematic review of case reports of serious adverse events 1995–2001. *Medical Journal of Australia, 176*, 376–380.

Ernst, E., & Harkness, E. F. (2001). Spinal manipulation: A systematic review of sham-controlled double-blind randomized clinical trials. *Journal of Pain and Symptom Management, 24*, 879–889.

Farfan, H. F. (1985). The use of mechanical etiology to determine the efficacy of active intervention in single joint intervertebral joint problems. *Spine, 10*, 350–358.

Farfan, H. F., & Sullivan, J. D. (1967). The relation of facet orientation to intervertebral disc failure. *Canadian Journal of Surgery, 10*, 179–185.

Farfan, H. F., Cossette, J. W, Robertson, G. H., Wells, R. V., & Kraus, H. (1970). The effects of torsion on the lumbar intervertebral joints: The role of torsion in the production of disc degeneration. *Journal of Bone and Joint Surgery, 52A*, 468–497.

Farfan, H. F., Huberdeau, R. M., & Dubow, H. I. (1972). Lumbar intervertebral disc degeneration. The influence of geometrical features on the pattern of disc degeneration – A post mortem study. *Journal of Bone and Joint Surgery, 54A*, 492–510.

Fields, H., & Price, D. D. (1997). Toward a neurobiology of placebo analgesia. In A. Harrington (Ed.), *The placebo effect: An interdiscipline exploration.* Cambridge, MA: Harvard University Press.

Flanagan, J., & Giordano, J. (2002). The role of the institution in developing the next generation chiropractor: clinician and researcher. *Journal of Manipulative Physiological Therapeutics, 25*(3), 193–196.

Franson, R. C, Saal, J. S., & Saal, J. A.(1992). Human disc phospholipase A2 is inflammatory. *Spine, 17*, S129–S132.

Garrett, W., Anderson, G., & Richardson, W. (1989). Muscle: future directions. In J. W. Frymoyer & S. L. Gordon (Eds.), *New perspectives on low back pain.* Park Ridge: American Academy of Orthopaedic Surgeons.

Giles, L. G. F., Taylor, J. R., & Cockson, A. (1986). Human zygapophyseal joint synovial folds. *Acta Anatomica, 126*, 110–114.

Giordano, J., Boatwright, D., Stapleton, S., & Huff, L. (2002). Blending the boundaries: Steps toward an integration of complementary and alternative medicine into mainstream practice. *Journal of Alternative and Complementary Medicine, 8*(6), 897–906.

Giordano, J., Garcia, M. K., Boatwright, D., & Klein, K. (2003). Complementary and alternative medicine in mainstream public health: A role for research in fostering integration. *Journal of Alternative and Complementary Medicine, 9*(3), 441–445.

Groen, G., Balijet, B., & Drukker, J. (1988). The innervation of the spinal dura mater: Anatomy and clinical implications. *Acta Neurchirurigica, 92*, 39–46.

Groen, G., Balijet, B., & Drukker, J. (1990). The nerves and nerve plexuses of the human vertebral column. *American Journal of Anatomy, 188*, 282–296.

Gronblad, M., Virri, J., Tolonen, J., Seitsalo, S., Kaapa, E., Kankare, J. et al. (1994). A controlled immunohistochemical study of inflammatory cells in disc herniation tissue. *Spine, 19*, 2744–2751.

Gudavalli, M. R., & Triano J. J. (1999). An analytic model of lumbar motion segment in flexion. *Journal of Manipulative Physiological Therapeutics, 22*(4), 201–208.

Guyer, R. D, Collier, R., Stith, W. J., Ohnmeiss. D. D., Hochschuller, S.H., Rashbaum, R.F. et al. (1988). Discitis after discography. *Spine, 13*, 1352–1354.

Hadler, N. M. (2004). Point of view. *Spine, 29*, 1021.

Haldeman, S., Chapman-Smith, D., & Peterson, D. M. (1992). (Eds) *Guidelines for chiropractic quality assurance and practice parameters.* Gaithersburg MD: Aspen.

Herr, K. A., Mobily, P. R., & Smith, C. (1993). Depression and the experience of chronic back pain: A study of related variables and age differences. *Clinical Journal of Pain, 9*, 104–114.

Hirsch, C., Inglemark, B., & Miller, M. (1963). The anatomical basis for lowback pain. *Acta Orthopaedica Scandinavica, 33*, 1.

Hirsch, C., Paulson, S., Sylven, B., & Snellman, O. (1953). Biophysical and physiological investigation on cartilage and other mesenchymal tissues: Characteristics of human nuclei pulposi during aging. *Acta Orthopaedica Scandinavica, 22,* 175–183.

Ingpen, M. L., & Burry, H. C. (1970). A lumbo-sacral strain syndrome. *Annals of Physical Medicine, 10*, 270–274.

Jackson, H. C., Winkelmann, R. K., & Bickel, W. H. (1966). Nerve endings in the human lumbar spinal column and related structures. *Journal of Bone Surgery, 48A*, 1272–1281.

Jaffray, D., & O'Brien, J. P. (1986). Isolated intervertebral disc resorption: A source of mechanical and inflammatory back pain? *Spine, 11*, 397–401.

Johnson, E. F., Berryman, H., Mitchell, R., & Wood, W. B. (1985). Elastic fibres in the anulus fibrosus of the human lumbar intervertebral disc. A preliminary report. *Journal of Anatomy, 143*, 57–63.

Jonas, W. B. Foreword in Chapman-Smith, D. (2000). *The chiropractic profession.* West Des Moines, IA: MCMIC Group.

Jonas, W. B. (2002). Evidence, ethics and the evaluation of global medicine. In D. Callahan (Ed.), *The role of complementary and alternative medicine, accommodating pluralism.* Washington, DC: Georgetown University Press.

King, A. B. (1955). Back pain due to loose facets of the lower lumbar vertebrae. *Bulletin. Johns Hopkins Hospital, 97*, 271–283.

Kirby, M. C., Sikoryn, T. A., Hukins, D. W. L., & Aspden, R. M. (1989). Structure and mechanical properties of the longitudinal ligaments and ligamentum flavum of the spine. *Journal of Biomedical Engineering, 11*, 192–196.

Lamax, E. (1975). Manipulative therapy: A historical perspective from ancient times to the modern era. In M. Goldstein (Ed.), *The research status of spinal manipulative therapy.* Bethesda, MD: National Institute of Neurological and Communicative Disorders and Stroke, Monograph, 15.

Lawrence, J. S., Sharp, J., Ball, J., & Bier, F. (1964, May). Rheumatoid arthritis of the lumbar spine. *Annals of the Rheumatic Diseases, 23*, 205–217.

Lawrence, J. S. (1969). Disc degeneration, its frequency and relationship to symptoms. *Annals of the Rheumatic Diseases, 28*, 121–138.

Lazar, S. W., Bush, G., Gollub, R. L, Fricchione, G. L, Khalsa, G., & Benson, H. (2000). Functional brain mapping of the relaxation response and meditation. *Neuroreport, 11*(7), 1581–1585.

Lewin, T. (1964). Osteoarthritis in lumbar synovial joints. *Acta Orthopaedica Scandinavica* (Suppl) *73*, 1–112.

Luk, K. D. K., Ho, H. C., & Leong, J. C. Y. (1986). The iliolumbar ligament. A study of its anatomy, development and clinical significance. *Journal of Bone and Joint Surgery, 68B*, 197–200.

Macintosh, J. E., & Bogduk, N. (1986). The morphology of the lumbar erector spinae. *Spine, 12*, 658–668.

Magora, A., & Schwartz, A. (1976). Relation between the low back pain syndrome and x-ray findings. Degenerative osteoarthritis. *Scandinavian Journal of Rehabilitation Medicine, 8*, 115–125.

Maroudas, A., Nachemson, A., Stockwell, R., & Urban, J., (1975). Some factors involved in the nutrition of the intervertebral disc. *Journal of Anatomy, 120*, 113–30.

McCall, I. W., Park, W. M., O'Brien, J. P., & Seal, V. (1985). Acute traumatic intraosseous disc herniation. *Spine, 10*, 134–137.

McCarron, R. F., Wimpee, M. W., Hudkins, P. G., & Laros, G. S. (1987). The inflammatory effect of the nucleus pulposis: A possible element in the pathogenesis of lowback pain. *Spine, 12*, 760.

Mechanic, D. (1986). The concept of illness behaviour. *Journal of Chronic Diseases, 15*, 189–194.

Melmon, K. L., Webster, M. E., Goldfinger, S. E., & Seegmiller, J. E. (1967). The presence of a kinin in inflammatory synovial effusion from arthritides of varying etiologies. *Arthritis and Rheumatism, 10*(1), 13–20.

Melrose, J., & Ghosh, P. (1988). The noncollagenous proteins of the intervertebral disc. In P. Ghosh (Ed.), *The biology of the intervertebral disc* (Vol. 1), Boca Raton: CRC Press.

Merskey, H., & Bogduk, N. (Eds.). (1994). Classification of chronic pain. *Descriptions of chronic pain syndromes and definitions of pain terms,* 2nd ed. Seattle: IASP Press.

Morris, D. (1998). *Illness and culture in the postmodern age.* Berkeley: University of California Press.

Nachemson, A. (1969). Intradiscal measurements of pH in patients with lumbar rhizopathies. *Acta Orthopaedica Scandinavica, 40*, 23–42.

Nachemson, A. (1983). Work for all. For those with low back pain as well. *Clinical Orthopaedics, 179*, 77–85.

Newham, D. J., Jones, D. A., Ghosh, G., & Aurora, P. (1988). Muscle fatigue and pain after eccentric contractions at long and short length. *Clinical Science (London), 74*(5), 553–557.

O'Neill, D. B., & Micheli, L. J. (1989). Postoperative radiographic evidence for fatigue fracture as the etiology in spondylolysis. *Spine, 14*, 1342–1355.

Olmarker, K., Rydevik, B., & Holm, S. (1989). Edema formation in spinal nerve roots induced by experimental, graded compression. *Spine, 14*, 311, 336.

Olmarker, K., Rydevik, B., & Nordborg, C. (1993). Autologous nucleus pulposus induces neurophysiologic and histologic changes in porcine cauda equina nerve roots. *Spine, 18*, 1425–1432.

Olmarker, K., Blomquist, J., Stromberg, J., Nannmark, U., Thomsen, P., & Rydevik, B. (1995). Inflammatogenic properties of nucleus pulposus. *Spine, 20*, 665–669.

Pearcy, M. J. (1990). Inferred strains in the intervertebral discs during physiological movements. *Journal of Man and Medicine, 5*, 68–71.

Pederson, H. E., Blunck, C. F. J., & Gardner, E. (1956). The anatomy of lumbosacral posterior rami and meningeal branches of spinal nerves (sinu-vertebral nerves): With an experimental study of their function. *Journal of Bone and Joint Surgery, 38A*, 377–391.

Porterfield, J., & DeRosa, C. (1991). *Mechanical low back pain. Perspectives in functional anatomy.* Philadelphia: W.B Saunders Company.

Raspe, H., Matthis, C., Croft, P., O'Neil, T. et al. (2004). Variation in back pain between countries. The example of Britain and Germany. *Spine, 29*(9).

Rhalmi, S., Yahia, L., Newman, N., & Isler, M. (1993). Immunohistochemical study of nerves in lumbar spine ligaments. *Spine, 18*, 264–267.

Rissanen, P. M. (1960). The surgical anatomy and pathology of the supraspinous and interspinous ligaments of the lumbar spine with special reference to ligament ruptures. *Acta Orthopaedica Scandinavica* (Suppl) *46*, 1–100.

Rogers, C. M., & Triano, J. J. (2003). Biomechanical measure validation for spinal manipulation in clinical settings. *Journal of Manipulated and Physiological Therapeutics, 26*(9), 539–548.

Roland, M. O. (1986). A critical review of the evidence for a pain-spasm-pain cycle in spinal disorders. *Clinical Biomechanics, 1*, 102–109.

Roofe, P. G. (1940). Innervation of annulus fibrosus and posterior longitudinal ligament. *Archives in Neurology and Psychiatry, 44*, 100–103.

Saal, J. S., Franson, R. C., Dobrow, R., Saal, J. A., White, A. H., & Goldthwaite, N. (1990). High levels of inflammatory phospholipase A2 activity in lumbar disc herniations. *Spine, 15*, 674–678.

Sachs, B. L., Vanharanta, H., Spivey, M. A., Guyer, R. D., Videman, T., Rashbaum, R. F. et al. (1987). Dallas discogram description: A new classification of CT/ discography in low-back disorders. *Spine, 12*, 287–294.

Sandoz, R. (1976). Some physical mechanisms and effects of spinal adjustments. *Annals of the Swiss Chiropractic Association, 6*, 91–141.

Scarry, E. (1985). *The body in pain. The making and unmaking of the world.* Oxford: Oxford University Press.

Schimek, J. J., & Schimek, F. (1984). Letter to the editor. *Pain, 20*, 307–310.

Schneiderman, G. A., McLain, R. F., Hambly, M. F., & Nielson, S. L. (1995). The pars defect as a pain source: A histological study. *Spine, 20*, 1761–1764.

Schwarzer, A. C., Aprill, C. N., Derby, R., Fortin, J., Kine, G., & Bogduk, N. (1994). The relative contributions of the disc and zygapophyseal joint in chronic low back pain *Spine, 19*, 801–806.

Schwarzer, A. C., Wang, S., Bogduk, N., McNaught, P. J., & Laurent, R. (1995a). Prevalence and clinical features of lumbar zygapophyseal joint pain: A study in an Australian population with chronic low back pain. *Annals of Rheumatic Diseases, 54*, 100–106.

Schwarzer, A. C., Wang, S., O'Driscoll, D., Harrington, T., Bogduk, N., & Laurent, T. (1995b). The ability of computed tomography to identify a painful zygapophyseal joint in patients with chronic low back pain. *Spine, 20*, 907–912

Scott, J. E., Bosworth, T. R., Cribb, A. M., & Taylor, J. R. (1994). The chemical morphology of age-related changes in human chemical morphology of age-related changes in human intervertebral disc glycosaminoglycans from cervical, thoracic and lumbar nucleus pulposus and anulus fibrosus. *Journal of Anatomy, 184*, 73–82.

Sedowfia, K. A., Tomlinson, I. W., Weiss, J. B., Hilton, R. C., & Jayson, M. I. V. (1982). Collagenolytic enzyme systems in human intervertebral disc. *Spine, 7*, 213–222.

Simons, D. G. (1988). Myofascial pain syndromes: Where are we? Where are we going? *Archives of Physical Medicine and Rehabilitation, 69*, 207–212.

Simons, D. G., & Travell, J. (1981). Myofascial trigger points, a possible explanation (letter). *Pain, 10*, 106–109.

Sims-Williams, H., Jason, M. I. V., & Baddeley, H. (1977). Rheumatoid involvement of the lumbar spine. *Annals of the Rheumatic Diseases. 36*, 524–531.

Skaggs, D. L., Weidenbaum, M., Iatridis, J. C., Ratcliffe, A., & Mow, V. C. (1994). Regional variation in tensile properties and biomechanical composition of the human lumbar anulus fibrosus. *Spine, 19*, 1310–319.

Smith, B. H., Elliott, A. M., Hannaford, P. C., Chambers, W. A., & Cairns-Smith, W. (2004). Factors related to the onset and persistence of chronic back pain in the community: results from a general population follow-up study. *Spine, 29*, 1032–1040.

Smith, B. H., Elliott, A. M., Chambers, W.A. et al. (2001a). The impact of chronic pain in the community. *Family Practice, 18*, 292–299.

Smith, B. H., Penny, K. I., Elliott, A. M. et al. (2001b). The level of expressed need: A measure of help-seeking behaviour for chronic pain in the community. *European Journal of Pain, 5*, 257–266.

Sola, A. E., & Kuitert, J. H. (1954). Quadratus lumborum myofasciitis. *Northwest Medicine, 53*, 1003–1005.

Spencer, D. L., Irwin, G. S., & Miller, J. A. A. (1983). Anatomy and significance of fixation of the lumbosacral nerve roots in sciatica. *Spine, 8*, 672.

Spiro, H. (1997). Clinical reflections on the placebo phenomenon. In A. Harrington (Ed.), *The placebo effect: An interdisciplinary exploration.* Cambridge, MA: Harvard University Press.

Stefano, G. B., Fricchione, G. L., Slingsby, B. T., & Benson, H. (2001). The placebo effect and relaxation response: Neural processes and their coupling to constitutive nitric oxide. *Brain Research Reviews, 35*(1), 1–19.

Stiles, E. G. (1975). Manipulative techniques: Four approaches. *Osteopathic Medicine, 1*, 27–30.

Stokes, I. A. F. (1987). Surface strain on human intervertebral discs. *Journal of Orthopaedic Research, 5*, 348–355.

Sullivan, J. D., & Farfan, H. F. (1975). The crumpled neural arch. *Orthopedic Clinics of North America, 6,* 199–213.

Terrett, C., & Vernon, H. (1984). Manipulation and pain tolerance. A controlled study of the effect of spinal manipulation on paraspinal cutaneous pain tolerance levels. *American Journal of Physical Medicine, 63*(5), 217–225.

Thomas, E., Silman, A. J., Croft, P. R. et al. (1999). Predicting who develops chronic low back pain in primary care: A prospective study. *British Medical Journal, 318,* 1662–1667.

Travell, J., & Rinzler, S. H. (1952). The myofascial genesis of pain. *Postgraduate Medicine, 11,* 425–434.

Triano, J. J., & Luttges, M. (1985). Myoelectric paraspinal response to spinal loads: Potential for monitoring low back pain. *Journal of Manipulative and Physiological Therapeutics, 8*(3), 137–145.

Triano, J. (1989). Skin accelerometer displacement and relative bone movement of adjacent vertebrae in response to chiropractic percussion thrusts. *Journal of Manipulative and Physiological Therapeutics, 12*(5), 406–411.

Triano, J., & Gudavalli, M. R. (1990). The physics of spinal manipulation. Part I. The myth of F = ma.. *Journal of Manipulative and Physiological Therapeutics, 13*(9), 550–552.

Triano, J. J. (1991). The physics of spinal manipulation. Part I. The myth of F – ma. *Journal of Manipulative and Physiological Therapeutics, 12* (5), 406–411.

Triano, J. J. (1992). Studies on the biomechanical effect of a spinal adjustment. *Journal of Manipulative and Physiological Therapeutics, 15*(1), 71-75.

Triano, J. J., McGregor, M., & Skogsbergh, D. R. (1997). Use of chiropractic manipulation in lumbar rehabilitation. *Journal of Rehabilitation Research and Development, 34*(4), 394–404.

Triano, J. J., Rogers, C. M., Combs, S., Potts, D., & Sorrels, K. (2002). Developing skilled performance of lumbar spine manipulation. *Journal of Manipulative and Physiological Therapeutics, 25*(6), 353–361.

Triano, J., & Schultz, A. B. (1997). Loads transmitted during lumbosacral spinal manipulative therapy. *Spine, 22*(17), 1955–1964.

Triano, J. J. (2001). Biomechanics of spinal manipulative therapy. *Spine Journal, 1*(2), 121–130.

Twomey, L. T., & Taylor, J. R. (1983). Sagittal movements of the human lumbar vertebral column: A quantitative study of the role of the posterior vertebral elements. *Archives of Physical Medicine and Rehabilitation, 64,* 322–325.

Twomey, L. T., & Taylor, J. R. (1985). Age changes in lumbar intervertebral discs. *Acta Orthopaedica Scandinavica, 56,* 496–499.

van Tulder, M. W. (2001). Treatment of low back pain: Myths and facts. *Schmerz, 15*(6), 499–503.

Vecchiet, L., Marini, I., & Feroldi, P. (1983). Muscular pain caused by isometric contraction: evaluation of pain through visual analog scale. *Clinical Therapeutics, 5*(5), 504–508.

Vernon, H. T., Aker, P. et al. (1990). Pressure pain threshold evaluation of the effect of spinal manipulation in the treatment of chronic neck pain: A pilot study. *Journal of Manipulative and Physiological Therapeutics, 13,* 13–16.

Vernon-Roberts, B., & Pirie, C. J. (1977). Degenerative changes in the intervertebral discs of the lumbar spine and their sequelae. *Rheumatology and Rehabilitation, 16,* 13–21.

Waddell, G. (1987). Failures of disc surgery and repeat surgery. *Acta Orthopaedica Belggica, 53*(2), 300–302.

Walton, J. N. (Ed.) (1977). *Brain's diseases of the nervous system,* 8th ed. Oxford: Oxford University Press.

Weiner, D., & Ernst, E. (2004). Complementary and alternative approaches to the treatment of persistent musculoskeletal pain. *Clinical Journal of Pain, 20*(4), 244–255.

White, A. A., & Panjabi, M. M. (1978). *Clinical biomechanics of the spine.* Philadelphia: Lippincott.

Wilk, V. (1995). Pain arising from the interspinous and supraspinous ligaments. *Australasian Musculoskeletal Medicine, 1,* 21–31.

Williams, A. K., & Schulz, R. (1988). Association of pain and physical dependency with depression in physically ill middle- aged and elderly. *Physical Therapy, 68,* 1226–1230.

Williamson, G. M., & Schulz, R. (1992). Pain, activity restriction, and symptoms of depression among community-residing adults. *Journal of Gerontology, 47,* 367–372.

Woolf, C. J. (2000). Pain. *Neurobiology of Disease, 7*(5) 504–510.

Wyke, B. (1970). The neurologic basis for thoracic spinal pain. *Rheumatology and Physical Medicine, 10*(7), 356–367.

Wyke, B. (1987). The neurology of low-back pain. In M. I. V. Jayson (Ed.), *The lumbar spine and back pain,* 2nd ed. Tunbridge Wells: Pitman.

Yahia, L. H., & Newman, N. A. (1989). A light and electron microscopic study of spinal ligament innervation. *Z mikroskop anat Forsch Leipzig 103,* 664–674.

Yang, K. H., & King, H. I. (1984). Mechanisms of facet load transmission as a hypothesis for low-back pain. *Spine, 9,* 557–565.

Yoshizawa, H., O'Brien, J. P., Thomas-Smith, W., & Trumper, M. (1980). The neuropathology of intervertebral discs removed for low-back pain. *Journal of Pathology, 132,* 95–104.

Zvaifler, N. J. (1973). The immunopathology of joint inflammation in rheumatoid arthritis. *Advances in Immunology, 16,* 265–336.

17

Occupational Therapy

Lori T. Andersen, EdD, OTR/L, FAOTA, Barbara L. Kornblau, JD, OT/L, FAOTA, DAAPM, and Jill Broderick, MS, OTR/L

OCCUPATIONAL THERAPY HELPS PEOPLE PARTICIPATE IN THEIR LIVES

Occupational therapists play a significant role on the pain management team as the members who look at how pain affects one's everyday life and one's ability to participate in the important everyday task of life or "occupations." Pain treatment teams benefit from the occupational therapist's contribution regarding how the individual functions in the everyday activities of his or her life. Occupational therapy is so named because the term *occupation* refers to "everything people do to occupy themselves, including looking after themselves (self-care), enjoying life (leisure), and contributing to the social and economic fabric of their communities (productivity or work)" (Law, Polatajko, Baptiste, & Townsend, 1997).

Pain can hinder participation in life roles and associated activities. For example, Phyllis had to give up her job as a computer operator due to severe neck pain, which also compromised her role as a homemaker. Jane is not able to hold her new grandchild due to severe arthritic pain in both her shoulders. George is unable to bend at the waist to tie his shoes due to a work injury, which left him with chronic low back pain. Occupational therapy can help people like Phyllis, Jane, and George resume their life roles and daily activities or, in other words, regain their ability to participate in life.

Occupational therapists must graduate from an accredited academic occupational therapy program, pass a national certification examination, and meet requirements of individual states for licensure or certification. Occupational therapists have a minimum of a bachelor's degree in occupational therapy. Some have master's or doctoral degrees in occupational therapy.

ROLE OF OCCUPATIONAL THERAPY IN PAIN MANAGEMENT

An essential aspect of occupational therapy is in the creation of a therapeutic milieu during both evaluation and treatment of the client. This includes creating a subtle shift in the client's expectations from being "treated" to a process in which he or she must actively participate in occupational therapy intervention. Occupational therapy is not a "passive" therapy, but rather a "doing" therapy, actively involving the client. All intervention actively involves clients performing, responding, and using feedback from the process to enhance positive change in behavior as it pertains to their perceptions, cognition, or ability to perform tasks in various environments or contexts. In this chapter, a case study illustrates how occupational therapy intervenes with clients experiencing pain to enable them to participate in their life roles and daily activities.

CASE STUDY

John Smith was living the American Dream. He was working for the power company as a power line installer and repairer. He was earning a good salary, so Mary, his wife of 15 years, no longer had to work. She could stay at home to care for their two children, one boy (age 7) and one girl (age 4). For the first 6 years of their marriage, John attended school and then worked various jobs with electrical contractors. Mary worked as a receptionist to help make ends meet. When John landed the job with the power company, they realized their dream of buying a house and starting a family.

The new house had plenty of room for family "additions" and was perfect for entertaining their close-knit family and friends. A dedicated family man, John coached his son's Little League team. He recently built an outdoor "club house/doll house" for his daughter using his woodworking skills. To him, woodworking was a relaxing occupation — one that he valued and helped define him. John used his computer to search for and draw up plans for his construction projects. He was planning to build a new wood deck on his house when he was injured on the job.

John hurt his back when a heavy toolbox started to fall off a slow moving company truck. Reaching out to try to prevent the toolbox from falling, he twisted his back and was thrown to the ground. John was hospitalized for a few days with severe back pain and then sent home. He was unable to return to work.

John's doctor referred him to therapy with the goal of returning to work. He started attending therapy every day, but he feared reinjuring himself and he feared what might happen when he returned to work. He knew he wouldn't be able to climb poles or pick up the heavy tools and supplies and he didn't have the flexibility in his back to get into "tight" areas. He soon quit attending therapy sessions.

John was still experiencing severe, chronic back pain 6 months later. He was having difficulty with some of the simplest tasks — rolling and moving in bed, getting in and out of the bathtub, bathing and dressing himself, including tying his shoes. Because of the pain he experienced while bathing and dressing, he dreaded these tasks, and usually delayed his morning routine or even avoided it for the day. His appearance suffered. John was uncomfortable in most any position — sitting, standing, or lying. When standing or walking he would often try to brace himself to minimize the pain by using his extended arms on a table or countertop. His movements were painful and awkward. He tried to avoid reaching for or picking up anything, restricting his participation in many daily living tasks. The pain made it difficult to sleep at night. He was tired constantly. The lack of sleep made him cranky and contributed to family arguments. Unable to sit for more than 20 minutes at a time without discomfort, John avoided trips in the car and trips in airplanes. Family outings and vacations were compromised. Friends and family came less frequently to visit. His plans for the wood deck, and many pleasurable afternoons with his family, came to a halt. He had to quit his volunteer work as coach of his son's Little League team. His son did not understand why.

As John was not able to go back to work, he collected worker's compensation. He filed suit against the toolbox manufacturer for wrongful injury from a defective product. His worker's compensation case and his third-party action dragged on through the administrative process and the courts. Eventually, the family's financial situation suffered and Mary had to go back to work to make ends meet. While it was a difficult adjustment to become the "breadwinner," she was happy to get out to the house as her relationship with John had suffered. John now became the "homemaker," reversing roles with Mary, albeit on a limited basis. Because of the pain, he was not able to perform all the chores that Mary did, such as meal preparation, housekeeping, shopping, and driving the children to various activities, not to mention the handyman activities he used to do. This further strained the marriage and family life. Mary felt overworked and resentful. The children didn't understand why their father was acting differently toward them. John felt useless, depressed, and hopeless. The American Dream had become a nightmare, and he didn't know what to do about it.

The devastating effects of pain are quite evident in this case study. Not only is pain a physical problem, but pain also restricts an individual's participation in various life roles and activities, what one wants to do and what one needs to do. For example, in the case of John Smith, participation in his roles as "husband," "father," "worker," "productive member of society," "volunteer" (Little League coach), "friend," and "family member" had been restricted. Participation in daily living tasks such as simple self-care, household management, parenting, work, and hobbies was also restricted. John not only suffered physically, but financially and psychologically as well. The effects of pain reached beyond the individual to affect the entire family and social system of the individual.

OCCUPATIONAL THERAPY EVALUATION

Occupational therapists look at the person, the tasks he or she must perform, and the environment in which performance occurs to determine if the factors involved in the person, task, and environment will support participation. To do this, the occupational therapist works in collaboration with the client to identify the client's everyday roles and the environments in which the client needs to function. The occupational therapist also analyzes the tasks or activities in which the client wants and needs to participate.

The evaluation process in occupational therapy is a two-step, client-centered, collaborative process (American Occupational Therapy Association, 2002). During the first step, the occupational therapist develops an occupational profile by looking at the client's needs, problems, and concerns about how he or she performs desired and expected daily activities. In the second step, the occupational therapist evaluates the client's abilities in all areas of occupational performance — activities of daily living (ADL), instrumental activities of daily living (IADL), education, work, play, leisure, and social participation (American Occupational Therapy Association, 2002). The occupational therapist may use interviews, observations, informal testing, and formal testing such as functional capacities evaluations, the Canadian Occupational Performance Measure (a client-centered measure of self-perception of abilities), and various pain scale measures.

The John Smith case study example illustrates this part of the evaluation process. Using a client-centered approach, the therapist would determine why John is seeking occupational therapy services. What is John's occupational history — his values, interests, and meaningful occupations? What are John's priorities and expected outcomes? Does he want to improve his occupational performance? Does he want to prevent further injuries? Does he want to improve his quality of life? Does John see the need to change his roles or adapt to his new situation?

A significant factor that often interferes with performance and participation is the role change that often accompanies chronic pain. A perfect example of this role change happened to John. After finding himself unable to work for more than 6 months and his family in severe financial trouble, his wife returned to work and he took on the roles of "homemaker" and "mom." The occupational therapist will also find that some of John's life roles have been disrupted. He no longer is able to participate with his son's Little League or other hobbies, his social participation with friends has declined, and his family life has suffered.

During the second step, the occupational therapist assesses the client's occupational performance using various assessment tools. What areas of occupation can John perform successfully? Which ones cause John problems or put him at risk for reinjury? During this step, the occupational therapist focuses on occupational performance issues and looks at factors that might support performance or hinder performance. This step of the evaluation includes looking at motor skills, process skills, and client factors or abilities (American Occupational Therapy Association, 2002). In John's case, as in many other cases of clients experiencing chronic pain, pain is one of the factors that can hinder performance and limit flexibility, strength, and endurance. John fatigues quickly, has difficulty lifting and carrying items, and has difficulty with simple tasks such as tying his shoes and rolling over in bed. Also in John's case, as with many others, the depression that accompanies chronic pain can hinder performance, affecting motivation and self-esteem. Inadequate coping skills, stress, medication side effects, and sleep disturbance that accompany chronic pain can also hinder performance.

From the onset of occupational therapy intervention, goals for discharge are discussed. The client must start to develop an image of participating and reengaging in former or new roles. Again, the collaborative process is at work as client and occupational therapist identify what the client hopes to accomplish in occupational therapy. Together they develop long-term and short-term goals to lead the client back into activities and roles. An orga-

nized and sequential process is devised using clear behavioral objectives that serve as an unstated contract about expectations of performance for the client and therapeutic outcomes.

OCCUPATIONAL THERAPY INTERVENTIONS

Occupational therapy intervention generally focuses on "changing" the person, adapting the task, adapting the environment, or helping to redesign lifestyle to facilitate a person's participation in life roles and activities.

CREATING A "CHANGE" IN THE PERSON

Bearing witness to the client's pain is a critical part in the development of the therapeutic relationship in occupational therapy. The client with pain often experiences a great deal of grief and loss. Many times the process of identifying the impact of occupational performance problems during the evaluation crystallizes clients' awareness regarding their inability to perform as they did before their accident or injury. The occupational therapist's ability to validate clients' experience and frustrations helps clients to develop more realistic perspectives on their functional status while fostering a respectful and trusting relationship. For many clients, past encounters with the medical community resulted in failure to alleviate pain or improve status and inadvertently may have contributed to greater feelings of helplessness. The occupational therapist can play a pivotal role in changing the client's perspective from acceptance of the helplessness characteristic of the sick role to active participation required in other life roles. Centering treatment on "occupation" (as defined by everyday activities and organized by role choices), acknowledging loss, and the use of a collaborative approach in occupational therapy sends a powerful message to clients that they are entering into a dynamic phase of managing their chronic pain and returning to function.

Such is the case with John, who terminated therapy as he feared reinjury. His life spun out of control. The occupational therapist will establish a respectful and trustful relationship, giving him control and actively involving him through use of occupations and goals important to him.

Client Education — Modifying the Perception of Disability

The initial assessment provides a reference point regarding clients' perceptions of disability as well as functional status as they pertain to occupation. The occupational therapist is challenged to provide methods to alter this perception and enhance motivation as well as participation in daily activity. Maladaptive behavioral responses such as fear of movement (due to fear of exacerbating pain), posturing, expectations of failure, anxiety, and related stress responses serve as barriers to progress. Client education directed at breaking down these barriers is used to help the client regain control and enhance motivation in all areas of performance.

Energizing Sense of Control

Client education involves teaching individuals that there are many different ways to be successful. Whether the occupational therapist chooses to use a restorative approach or teach skills to compensate for functional loss by using an alternative method to perform a task or adapt tasks and/or environment, all modes seek to create the client's ability to accomplish tasks. Problem-solving techniques and new skills provided in occupational therapy add to the client's belief that he or she has options and can effect change. There are many skills the occupational therapist can help a client to develop:

- Altering perception of function/loss
- Time management skills
- Organization skills
- Habit exploration/modification
- Role modification/role balance
- Use of relaxation techniques (diaphragmatic breathing, visualization, imagery, biofeedback)
- Use of proper body mechanics
- Incorporation of ergonomics
- Improving functional capacities
- Incorporating energy conservation techniques
- Pacing skills
- Assertive communication

Martensson, Marklund, & Fridlund (1999) found that a rehabilitation program focusing on developing ego-strength, awareness of resources for pain control, education on body functions, relaxation techniques, and ergonomics increased clients' self-confidence. These clients were able to manage symptoms of pain, they were less fearful of pain, and they returned to previous activities with fewer pain complaints (Martensson et al., 1999). The belief in the ability to be successful as well as feeling confident about using new skills adds to the client's motivation to participate in occupational therapy and pursue therapeutic goals both in the clinic and in the home environment. The therapist and the client explore these skills during the occupational therapy process. The question of improving function becomes less about what the person can do but rather how he or she can do it.

Another core aspect of client education for the client with chronic pain is providing an understanding of behavioral changes that happen during the course of coping with chronic pain. Client education about specific aspects of a diagnosis appears less useful than developing an aware-ness of how people react to pain and develop subsequent stress-related responses (Rogers, Shaer, & Herzig, 1984). Educating clients about pain behaviors such as bracing, holding maladaptive postures, and reducing active movement in an attempt to limit pain helps break the pain cycle from becoming a downward spiral of further loss of physical capacity and function. Occupational therapy education provides information about these areas via use of body awareness activities such as videotaping movement or using photography during functional tasks and biofeedback to demonstrate faulty movement patterns. Posture and body mechanics instruction is provided and applied to daily activity with an emphasis on restoring movement and function while using motor patterns that reduce the likelihood of further injury, strain, or exacerbating pain. Studies show that education in good body mechanics during lifting can change behavior, improving lifting styles and incorporating good body mechanics (Lieber, Rudy, & Boston, 2000; McCauley, 1990). Clients are taught they have options regarding how to use their bodies and often gain a greater sense of confidence with movement.

To enhance perception of control, occupational therapy also provides education regarding techniques to improve self-regulation, in particular to reduce stress and pain-related symptoms. Relaxation training, using diaphragmatic breathing, body scans, visualization, imagery, and shifting attention (Fehmi, in press), can be taught in the clinic to reduce excessive autonomic nervous system output that contributes to excess muscle tension and feelings of anxiety. Occupational therapy intervention considers lifestyle factors that contribute to stress alongside relaxation training to focus on establishing a healthy balance between work (including self-care and home care initially then branching to other work-related roles), rest, and leisure.

Clients learn to take a wider view of the pain experience, looking into premorbid and current behavioral patterns that may influence stress and pain. All these factors effect arousal of the central nervous system. The concept of self-regulation can be expanded to include the choices people make in lifestyle and balanced activity — factors also considered in fostering "wellness." Certainly occupational therapy seeks to address many goals — from increased function to resuming roles to a life lived well.

Making Use of Feedback

Inherent in the process of engagement and collaboration is the use of feedback. The occupational therapist may initially provide feedback about changes in perception regarding stress, pain behaviors, goal choices, etc., but eventually encourages clients to start to use information about control of symptoms and function on their own. For example, using electromyographic (EMG) biofeedback may initially help clients reduce muscle tension and/or bracing patterns. Over time, clients learn to increase body awareness to know they are tensing muscles and can then alter that behavior. For example, the occupational therapist observes John's posture and notes he is shifting his weight to the right, flexing his trunk to the right side, holding the torso forward, and flexing the neck toward the right shoulder. The occupational therapist determines he is creating additional muscle imbalance with this posture and tensing of muscles, which is likely to create additional pain over the time. John may not even realize that he favors his left side. However, using EMG biofeedback, John can learn to gradually correct this posture and reduce excessive muscle tone in numerous muscle groups involved in holding this position. The reduction in muscle tension and regained symmetry may help to reduce overall levels of pain.

Pain itself can be used as feedback to the person who has returned to many activities but starts to "overdo" participation and flares up symptoms. Clients may use pain as feedback and decide to pace their participation in activity so they can remain active but include short rest breaks when they feel fatigued. The use of various types of feedback, particularly during routine daily activities demonstrates the integration of therapeutic concepts and provides the impetus to facilitate change, return to function, and regain a sense of self-confidence.

ADAPTING THE ACTIVITY

Modification of an activity is an intervention approach used by occupational therapists (American Occupational Therapy Association, 2002). Working closely with the client, the occupational therapist analyzes the demands and component parts of activities the client wants and needs to do. By analyzing the activity and taking into consideration client preferences, an occupational therapist identifies various ways to modify or adapt an activity. Participation in an activity in spite of a limitation in body function or structure is the focus of the modification or adaptation. The occupational therapist may recommend doing the activity in a different way, such as incorporating good body mechanics, joint protection techniques, or energy conservation techniques into the activity. The occupational therapist may also recommend using a tool or an adaptive device that protects joints, saves energy, or minimizes pain during an activity.

Use of an adaptive device helps to break the pain cycle and helps the client regain functional abilities. The occupational therapist evaluates which adaptive devices the client will benefit from, assists the client to obtain these devices, and educates the client in the use of the devices.

For example, a "reacher" is a tool that extends one's reach when grabbing/picking up items. It eliminates the need to bend to the floor or to reach up over head if trunk flexibility or reaching ability is limited because of pain.

Use of this tool minimizes stress on the spine. John can use a reacher to extend his reach to put his pants on over his feet or to reach up overhead in the kitchen to get a food item. A sock aid and a long-handled bath brush are other adaptive aids that are used to extend reach for lower extremity dressing and bathing, respectively, minimizing stress on the spine. Other examples of adaptive aids are the long-handled shoe horn and elastic shoelaces, which eliminate the need for reaching to tie shoes. Properly adjusted, the elastic shoelaces create slip-on shoes that John could put his feet into with the help of the long-handled shoe horn.

Pain limits energy and participation in activity. One study found that clients with pain report temporal imbalances in activities, activities require more effort, and clients become stressed and tense because of the pain (Mullersdorf, 2002). Clients can often learn to be sensitive to the different aspects of their pain and use this information to modify activities and facilitate participation (Peolsson, Hyden, & Larsson, 2000). Use of energy conservation techniques enables a client to complete all daily living tasks within his or her energy reserve or pain limit. The occupational therapist works with a client to determine in which activities the client wants and needs to participate. The occupational therapist analyzes the activities and assists the client to plan his or her daily or weekly activities to distribute high-energy and/or physically demanding activities throughout the day or week.

For example, John may distribute his morning self-care activities throughout the morning. He might take a shower and wrap himself in a terry cloth robe to dry, modifying how the activity is done. This would eliminate the task of using a towel and bending to reach all areas of his body, also eliminating stress on the spine. John could rest while eating his breakfast and dress himself after breakfast. The energy conservation technique of sitting on a chair or a stool while performing grooming activities such as shaving and brushing his teeth will also protect his back by minimizing pain from standing and bending forward over the sink.

In another example, John may be able to complete high-energy or physically demanding tasks such as a household repair or woodworking activity on one day and play catch with his son on another day. To enable John to play catch with his son, the activity could be modified by having John sit in a chair that facilitates good postural alignment. This would minimize stress on his spine. Facilitating return to his occupational role of being a father and coach, it could also help improve the skills of his son and son's teammates who would have to be more accurate in their throwing.

Other energy conservation techniques include using equipment that minimizes energy output. This equipment frequently protects the joints of the body as well. Use of a rolling cart will help John to transport items that he needs to use for various activities such as transporting tools for handyman repairs. He will avoid lifting and carrying items, limiting stress on the spine while participating in activities.

When modifying or adapting any activity, it is important that the person practice the activity in the new way so it becomes habit and routine. Ensuring that the new method of performing the task becomes routine or habit assists the client to resume normal activities and normal occupational roles.

MODIFYING THE ENVIRONMENT

Modification of the environment is another intervention strategy used by occupational therapists. Activity priorities are again determined by the client. The occupational therapist analyzes each activity and the environment in which the activities take place to determine if environmental modifications will facilitate the client's participation. Environmental modifications, as with activity modifications, may assist in saving energy, protecting joints, and minimizing pain.

Organizing one's work area so that it is easy to gather tools and materials for a task saves energy and minimizes stress on the spine. Items used together should be stored together. Most frequently used items should be stored in an easy-to-reach location that does not require bending or reaching overhead — generally around waist to shoulder height. For example, shoes can be placed in a shoe bag over a closet door between waist and shoulder level. This concept can be applied to certain tools and supplies John might use for handyman activities. These tools and supplies should be stored in a location, around waist level, so that John is able to reach them without bending. If used frequently, tools and supplies, such as drills, miter saws, may also remain setup, saving energy from setup and restoration each time.

In John's case, consideration may need to be given to the height of work surfaces to encourage proper musculoskeletal alignment. Analysis of activities and activity demands will help determine appropriate height of work surfaces. Changing the height of work surfaces may be accomplished by placing blocks under a table to raise the height or perhaps providing a chair or stool to position the client at the appropriate work height. Provision of the chair or stool saves energy as well. The work area can also be set up so items are within easy reach while working, thereby avoiding bending and stress on the spine.

Setting up John's computer workstation to support musculoskeletal alignment is another example of adapting the environment to prevent and/or reduce pain. The workstation chair should be designed to provide support for John's lower back while positioning the head neck and trunk in line with each other, to support his elbows and position his forearms in line with his wrists, and be adjust-

able so his feet are flat on the floor. The top of the monitor should be around eye level (Occupational Safety and Health Administration, 2004). It is also important to ensure that other aspects of the environment, lighting, temperature, noise minimize stress on the person using the workstation.

LIFE STYLE REDESIGN

Clients who experience pain show deficits in their occupational performance from role changes, barriers to their performance, and difficulties adapting to their lives. In addition to changes to the environment, which can facilitate performance and participation, changes in the daily tasks one performs or in one's lifestyle make a difference in one's health and one's ability to participate in life activities.

Clients experiencing pain often find themselves lacking in the daily meaningful activity in which they had participated. For example, John believes he can no longer participate in woodworking, a significant preinjury meaningful activity. He finds himself unable to coach his son's Little League. He has adopted the role of "homemaker." The lack of meaningful activities in his life and the role changes put John's pain in the forefront and allow his pain to take over his life.

Research shows that incorporating meaningful activities into daily routines in one's life promotes heath, well-being, and participation in life. In occupational therapy we refer to this as "lifestyle redesign." Lifestyle redesign is an occupational therapy intervention process that provides clients with strategies to control their own lives by adopting daily routines of meaningful activities to promote health, well-being, and participation in life. Lifestyle redesign has proved successful in a variety of treatment contexts (Clark et al., 1997; Luebben, 2000).

Lifestyle redesign structures a person's day with meaningful activities that remove barriers to performance. For clients who experience chronic pain, barriers that require removal include pain, stress, lack of coping skills, the belief that one's pain prevents participation in life's activities, and others. Lifestyle redesign takes a collaborative effort between the occupational therapist and the client. Together they find activities that are meaningful to the client and can thus break down the barriers to participation. People participating in purposeful activities have longer tolerance for pain than those participating in nonpurposeful activities (Heck, 1988). Participation in meaningful tasks helps to break the pain cycle and get people back to "doing."

Some of the activities clients with pain need to incorporate into their routine include activities and strategies that relieve symptoms associated with chronic pain. These activities need to become an integral part of the daily routine activities in one's life — not just a "therapy experience." Some of these activities one might include in lifestyle redesign for individuals with chronic pain include aquatic therapy, Tai Chi, and yoga.

Aquatic Therapy

Aquatic therapy takes advantage of the buoyancy and resistive properties of water, and the soothing properties of heat to promote increased movement with decreased pain. Water walking, water dancing, or other water exercises incorporated into one's daily routine can increase one's participation in life while increasing pain-free movement and decreasing pain. Research has shown the benefits of aquatic therapy for individuals with fibromyalgia, osteoarthritis, rheumatoid arthritis, low back pain, and a variety of musculoskeletal disorders (Hall et al., 1996; Konlian, 1999; Mannerkorpi, Ahlmen, & Ekdahl, 2002; McNeal, 1999; Prins & Cutner, 1999; Sim & Adams, 2002; Wyatt et al., 2001. These studies show benefits that include increases in range of motion, pain-free movement, self-esteem, and endurance; improved sleep; and decreased pain, stress, and symptoms of depression. Occupational therapy intervention incorporates aquatics into one's daily routine, not merely for the sake of exercise but to facilitate an overall, big-picture lifestyle redesign.

Tai Chi

Tai Chi is a centuries-old form of exercise that combines slow, gentle, coordinated movements with focused deep breathing and relaxation. Tai Chi is usually done in a group setting. Occupational therapists recommend incorporating Tai Chi into one's daily routines as part of the lifestyle redesign process for clients experiencing chronic pain. Although most of the studies to date have used small sample sizes, these studies have shown that regular Tai Chi decreases the pain intensity scores in older adults with chronic arthritis pain (Adler et al., 2000), decreases perception of joint pain and stiffness and perceived difficulties in physical functioning in older woman with osteoarthritis (Song et al., 2003), and achieves significant improvement in symptom control and health-related quality of life in individuals with fibromyalgia (Taggart et al., 2003). Although these and several other studies support Tai Chi's role in improving quality of life and decreasing pain, Wang, Cellet, and Lau's (2004) recent systematic review of 47 studies of Tai Chi's effect on health outcomes in people with chronic conditions suggests that more rigorous studies are needed to properly evaluate the effects of Tai Chi on health.

Incorporating Tai Chi into one's daily routine contributes to one's lifestyle redesign by giving clients experiencing chronic pain a starting point to participate in mild, relaxing exercises in a social environment. Decreasing pain and other symptoms, combined with increased participation, can give meaning to clients such as John who have not been able to participate in any of their normal everyday activities. This may be the first step to establishing new routines of everyday life.

Yoga

Yoga is a centuries-old mind–body–spirit intervention practiced though different methodologies, which all, to some degree, focus on movement, postures, concentration, consciousness, healthy lifestyle, and controlled breathing. Yoga can occupy a significant role in the lives of individuals experiencing chronic pain by decreasing pain symptoms and thus increasing the ability to participate in normal routine activities.

Research shows that yoga can contribute to the relief of pain-related symptoms in a number of contexts. In one study, clients with osteoarthritis in their hands reported a decrease in pain during activity and an increase in finger range of motion following a regularly scheduled course of yoga intervention (Garfinkel et al., 1994). Garfinkel and colleagues (1998) found that individuals with carpal tunnel syndrome experienced, among other things, a reduction in pain and an increase in grip strength following a regular series of yoga-based intervention. Researchers report that individuals with chronic pain from migraines, osteoarthritis, neck pain, and other sources, who participated in regularly scheduled yoga classes all reported some improvement. The improvement was measured by clients' reports of a decrease in the use of pain medication, decreased levels of anxiety, and an increase in the ability to participate in everyday activities at home (Linz, 2004; Martin, 2001).

While these studies look promising and a plethora of anecdotal reporting exists to back up those findings, as with the Tai Chi research, more rigorous research is needed to further support yoga's efficacy with clients in pain. A systematic review of more than 300 articles on the potential health benefits of yoga reports that while preliminary evidence shows yoga may be beneficial when used in conjunction with traditional treatment interventions for, among other conditions, stress, anxiety disorder, and depression, further research is needed in better-designed studies with larger samples of participants (Harvard Medical School, 2003).

If clients experiencing chronic pain find yoga helpful to their symptom control, it can be a meaningful activity to incorporate into a lifestyle redesign program as a step back toward the goal of participation. Participation in yoga, Tai Chi, and aquatics also functions to begin a role change back to a participating individual in society as part of the lifestyle redesign process.

SUMMARY

Occupational therapy's focus — to ensure a match between the person, environment, and occupation (task) — relies on interventions that can change the person and modify the task or environment so people can participate in their life roles and activities. Occupational therapy plays a vital role in the pain management team, to bridge the gap between individuals identifying themselves as people in pain and as participating members of society.

BIBLIOGRAPHY

American Occupational Therapy Association. (2002). Occupational therapy practice framework: Domain and process. *American Journal of Occupational Therapy, 56,* 609.

Adler, P. et al. (2000). The effects of Tai Chi on older adults with chronic arthritis pain. *Journal of Nursing Scholarship, 32*(4), 377.

Clark, F. et al. (1997). Occupational therapy for independent-living older adults: A randomized controlled trial. *JAMA, 278*(16), 1321.

Fehmi, L. (in press). Attention to attention. In J. Kamiya et al. (Eds.). *Applied neurophysiology and brain biofeedback.* Trevose, PA: Future Health, Inc. Available online at http://www.futurehealth.org/eegbook.htm

Garfinkel, M.S. et al. (1994). Evaluation of a yoga based regimen for treatment of osteoarthritis of the hands. *Journal of Rheumatology, 21*(12), 2341.

Garfinkel, M.S. et al. (1998). Yoga-based intervention for carpal tunnel syndrome: A randomized trial. *Journal of the American Medical Association, 280*(18), 1601.

Hall, J. et al. (1996). A randomized and controlled trial of hydrotherapy in rheumatoid arthritis. *Arthritis Care Research, 9*(3), 206.

Harvard Medical School (2003). Yoga 2003, Aetna Intelihealth. Retrieved March 28, 2004, from http://www.intelihealth.com/IH/ihtPrint/WSIHW000/8513/408/358876.html?d=dmtContent&hide=t&k=basePrint.

Heck, S. A. (1988). The effect of purposeful activity on pain tolerance. *American Journal of Occupational Therapy, 42,* 577.

Konlian, C. (1999). Aquatic therapy: Making a wave in the treatment of low back injuries. *Orthopedic Nursing, 18*(1), 11.

Law, M., Polatajko, H., Baptiste, S., & Townsend, E. (1997) Core concepts in occupational therapy. In E. Townsend, et al. (Eds.), *Enabling occupation: An OT perspective* (pp. 29–56). Ottawa, Ontario: Canadian Association of Occupational Therapists.

Lieber, S. J., Rudy, T. E., & Boston, J. R. (2000). Effects of body mechanics training on performance of repetitive lifting. *American Journal of Occupational Therapy, 54,* 166.

Linz, D. (2004). Healthy for life – Yoga for your pain. Retrieved March 28, 2004 from http://wchstv.com/newsroom/healthyforlife/1863.shtml.

Luebben, A.J. (2000). Worksite modification and lifestyle redesign: A quick fix. RESNA. Retrieved March 28, 2004, from http://www.resna.org/ProfResources/Publications/Proceedings/2000/EnvAccom/QuickFix.php.

Mannerkorpi, K., Ahlmen, M., & Ekdahl, C. (2002). Six and 24-month follow-up of pool exercise therapy and education for patients with fibromyalgia. *Scandanavian Journal of Rheumatology, 31*(5), 306.

Martensson, L., Marklund, B., & Fridlund, B. (1999) Evaluation of a biopsychosocial rehabilitation programme in primary healthcare for chronic pain patients. *Scandinavian Journal of Occupational Therapy, 6,* 157.

Martin, S. (2001, Sept.–Oct.). Easing the pain: managing chronic ailments. *Psychology Today.* Retrieved March 28, 2004, from http://www.findarticles.com/cf_dls/m1175/5_34/82261888/p1/article.jhtml

McCauley, M. (1990). The effect of body mechanics instruction on work performance among young workers. *American Journal of Occupational Therapy, 42,* 402.

McNeal, R. L. (1999). Aquatic therapy for patients with rheumatic disease, *Rheumatic Disease Clinics in North America, 16*(4), 915.

Mullersdorf, M., (2002). Needs and problems related to occupational therapy as perceived by adult Swedes with long-term pain. *Scandinavian Journal of Occupational Therapy, 9,* 79.

Occupational Safety and Health Administration. (2004). *Computer workstations.* Washington, DC: Author. Retrieved March 28, 2004, from http://www.osha.gov/SLTC/etools/computerworkstations/index.html

Peolsson, M., Hyden, L.-C., & Larsson, U. S. (2000). Living with chronic pain. *Scandinavian Journal of Occupational Therapy, 7,* 114.

Prins, J. & Cutner, D. (1999). Aquatic therapy in the rehabilitation of athletic injuries. *Clinical Sports Medicine, 18*(2), 477.

Rogers, S., Shuer, J., & Herzig, S. (1984). The use of biofeedback techniques in occupational therapy in persons with chronic pain. *Occupational Therapy in Health Care, 3*(1), 103.

Sim, J., & Adams, N. (2002). Systematic review of randomized controlled trials of nonpharmacological interventions for fibromyalgia. *Clinical Journal of Pain, 18*(5), 324.

Song, R. et al. (2003). Effects of Tai Chi exercise on pain, balance, muscle strength, and perceived difficulties in physical functioning in older women with osteoarthritis: A randomized clinical trial. *Journal of Rheumatology, 30,* 2039.

Taggart, H.M. et al. (2003). Effects of Tai Chi on fibromyalgia symptoms and health-related quality of life. *Orthopedic Nursing, 22*(5), 353.

Wang, C., Cellet, J.P., & Lau, J. (2004). The effect of Tai Chi on health outcomes in patients with chronic conditions: A systematic review. *Archives of Internal Medicine, 164*(5), 493.

Wyatt, F. B. et al. (2001). The effects of aquatic and traditional exercise programs on persons with knee osteoarthritis, *Journal of Strength Cond. Res., 15*(3), 337.

18

Physical Therapy and Pain Management

Tom Watson, DPT MEd, PhD, DAAPM

INTRODUCTION

Physical therapy intervention dates to the ancient Greeks, ancient Egyptians, Chinese, and Romans, who used heat, sunlight, electric eels, massage therapy, and manipulation. Physical therapy today utilizes physical agents including modalities such as heat or cold, electricity, light, magnets, ultrasound, traction, manual therapies such as manipulation or mobilization, and therapeutic exercises. Pain management is always a team approach and coordination among medical doctors, physical therapists, chiropractors, psychologists, pharmacists, and other health care practitioners is of primary importance for the patient to reach an optimal level of function with adequate pain resolution or control.

Physical therapy today consists of proper evaluation and examination of the body's musculoskeletal and neurological systems. This will include a history, a review of related diagnostic interventions such as x-ray and laboratory, and a structured examination of range of motion, strength, sensory integrity, gait, locomotion, balance, joint mobility and function, posture, and location of pain in order to identify the tissue in lesion. Low back pain is the most frequent diagnosis seen by physical therapists. Part of this chapter is directed toward low back pain.

Following a thorough evaluation and examination, therapeutic interventions are based on the findings or the tissue(s) in lesion. Therapeutic interventions consist of alleviating the impairments, functional limitations, or pain and improving motion, function, and life activities. These interventions include but are not limited to physical agents; electrotherapeutic modalities; manual therapy techniques including manipulation, mobilization, and soft tissue massage; therapeutic exercise including strengthening–coordination–function, activities of daily living, use of proper body mechanics, self-care/home program and pain management techniques, instruction in adaptive devices such as orthotics or prosthetics, and instruction in prevention of further injury or pain.

To treat pain, one must understand the process of pain. Various modalities and procedures are used to inhibit or alleviate pain based on the category of pain and the type of nerve fiber transmitting the nociceptive information. Pain, according to the IASP (International Association for the Study of Pain), is "an unpleasant sensory or emotional experience associated with actual or potential tissue damage and described in terms of such damage." Pain is the primary reason for visits to a clinician, according to Watson (1995a). Pain always evokes a sensory or emotional response. When pain occurs, suffering and pain behaviors follow. Pain is classified in three categories: (1) acute: lasting 4 to 6 weeks; (2) subacute: lasting 6-weeks to 6 months; and (3) chronic: 6 months or symptoms lasting longer than the anticipated time for recovery. The brain records pain experiences in the thalamus, sensory cortex, and limbic system. Pain is transmitted to the brain through the neurological process of nociception. Nociception occurs when tissue is damaged and chemical or endogenous agents are released. These agents include bradykinins, serotonin, cytokines, protons, sensory neuropeptides, and arachidonic acids that include leukotrienes and prostaglandins. Special nerve endings or type IV mechanoreceptors, i.e., free nerve endings, absorb these chemicals and transfer the information to the spinal cord. The main nociceptor acting nerves are A-beta fibers, which are thickly myelinated, mostly sensory, and 10% transmit pain; A-delta fibers, which are thinly myelinated and transmit sharp/lancinating pain; and C-fibers, which are nonmyelinated fibers usually associated with dull or chronic pain. Pain transmission enters the spinal cord via the dorsal horn. Information from nociceptor fibers is transferred through the dorsal horn to one of six lamina or levels. Information from A-delta fibers terminates in lamina V and I, C-fibers terminate in lamina II, and A-beta fibers terminate in lamina III, IV, and VI. There are exceptions and crossovers that occur. Pain information ascends through the spinal thalamic tract or Lissaurs track and terminates in the thalamus, somatosensory cortex, limbic system, midbrain, hypothalamus, or thalamic nuclei. These areas of the brain respond, causing a pain memory, a response, and/or a pain behavior. In other words, the patient will respond to the pain based on past history and react according to the type and severity of the pain.

Developing a treatment intervention must begin with identification of the problem, the needs of the patient, and the outcome goals for the patient. An appropriate evaluation procedure to identify the tissue in lesion, according to Cyriax (1982), is the first step in physical therapy pain management. This will allow for proper selection of the manual therapy techniques, exercise protocols, modalities, and patient education intervention that are necessary.

EVALUATION

The Ola Grimsby Institute (OGI, 1998a) developed the "diagnostic pyramid" for the purpose of identifying a "tissue in lesion" and arriving at the proper treatment format (Figure 18.1). The proper flow of this pyramid requires that all the suspect tissues be provoked to reproduce the symptoms, thereby eliminating normal tissue and arriving at the pathology. Cyriax (1982) originally described this concept. The top of the pyramid lists 13 different tissue types and the vertical column represents 12 evaluation categories of this pyramid allowing examination of all tissues available to a physical therapist. Therapists can begin with very basic observation and questioning, and then use hands-on techniques to examine the tissue involved. Active range of motion tests all anatomical structures. Passive range of motion tests structures such as nervous, ligaments, capsules, bursa, bone, blood vessels, and connective tissue. When examining muscles and tendons, Cyriax stated that when active and passive motion is restricted or painful in opposite directions, this indicates contractile or muscle tissue as the tissue in lesion. When active and passive motions are restricted and/or painful in the same direction, there is an arthrogenic or joint tissue lesion. The pyramid examines strength, palpation, joint play, and neurological testing, and concludes with specific laboratory, electrophysiological, and radiological results. Cyriax goes on to state provoked (aggravated) tissue minus normal (healthy) tissue equals pathological tissue. Pathological tissue (the tissue causing the problem) minus

contraindications (treatments not allowed) equals the treatment approach. The treatment is based on the information obtained through the diagnostic pyramid and directed specifically to the tissues identified in the evaluation. Another advantage to using evaluation procedures is to assess both the patient and the referring clinician in arriving at an appropriate to diagnoses.

There are times that physical symptoms will be manifested by tissues or conditions other than orthopedic, musculoskeletal, or neurological. Symptoms of sciatica, for example, may be caused by intermittent claudication, dissecting aneurysms, neoplastic conditions, osteoporosis, congenital conditions, or genital–urinary disorders. The experienced physical therapist may also assist in identifying certain psychological syndromes, as described by Martelli, Zasler, Nicholson, Pickett, and May (2002), such as factious disorders, somatoform disorders, hypochondriasis, or conversion disorders. Furthermore, Waddell signs such as overreaction, widespread hypersensitivity, axial loading sign, rotation sign, and differences between straight leg raise from sitting to supine should be identified. Other non-organic signs may be found during examination/history, including lower extremities giving way, no pain-free episodes in the past year, treatment intolerance, and frequent number of hospital admissions for the same condition.

After evaluating and analyzing the entire intake information including physical findings, psychological findings, laboratory, x-ray and other testing, the physical therapist can develop an appropriate treatment program. This treatment program may include modalities, manual therapy, therapeutic exercise intervention including a home exercise program, self-pain management techniques, instruction in adaptive devices, patient education regarding present condition, and injury prevention.

Pain can be treated by physical therapy with various uses of modalities, manual therapies, therapeutic exercises, and assisted devices. High-intensity afferent stimulation will cause pain inhibition. Manipulation causes a fast stretch in collagen tissue resulting in a response in the basilar neuron; GABA inhibits NMDA, directly affecting the gamma loop leading to the muscle spindle resulting in inhibition of pain and muscle tension. Slow stretch deforms collagen and also inhibits pain but not muscle tension. Electrical stimulation at 110 to 140 Hz is a very powerful high-intensity afferent stimulation. Other high-intensity afferent stimulators include alcohol, pain, Baroque music, and having sex (OGI, 1998).

MODALITIES

The majority of modalities including heat, cold, ultrasound, traction, galvanic stimulation, interferential current, and transcutaneous electrical nerve stimulation (TENS) are for pain management. A few modalities such

Facility:

Patient:

Medical Diagnosis:

Date:

Therapist:

Summation of Tissue(s) in Lesion	SKIN	SUB-CUTANEOUS	LIGAMENT FASCIA	MUSCLE TENDON	JOINT CAPSULE	BURSA	JOINT CARTL	JOINT ENTRAP	NERVE	DISC	BONE	VASCULAR
X-RAY/LAB MR/CAT/EMG	144	145	146	147	148	149	150	151	152	153	154	155
SEGMENTAL PLAY	131	132	133	134	135	136	137	138	139	140	141	142
JOINT PLAY	118	119	120	121	122 — extremity	123	124	125 — blocked	126	127	128	129
SPECIAL TESTS	105	106	107	108	109	110	111	112	113	114	115	116
NEURO TESTS	92	93	94	95	96	97	98	99	100	101	102	103
PALPATION	79	80	81	82	83	84	85	86	87	88	89	90
RESISTED MOTION	66	67	68	69	70 — Spine	71	72	73	74	75	76	77
PASSIVE MOTION	53	54	55	56	57	58	59	60	61	62	63	64
ACTIVE MOTION	40	41	42	43	44	45	46	47	48	49	50	51
STRUCTURAL INSPECTION	27	28	29	30	31	32	33	34	35	36	37	38
HISTORY INTERVIEW	14	15	16	17	18	19	20	21	22	23	24	25
INITIAL OBSERVATION	1	2	3	4	5	6	7	8	9	10	11	12

KEY

+	Positive means indicative of the tissue
X	Eliminated
O	More testing (or clarifying tests) required

?	Test (information) does not determine the tissue
—	It is not indicative of the tissue
(shaded)	Test does not apply to the ELIMINATION of tissue
(blank)	Tissue eliminated or confirmed by this block

FIGURE 18.1 The Diagnostic Pyramid. From Ola Grimsby Institute, "Diagnostic Pyramid. General Principles of Evaluation," 1998, *Orthopedic Manual Therapy, 630*, p. 7. Reprinted with permission.

as microcurrent stimulation, sympathetic therapy systems (STS), and laser therapy may have therapeutic value.

The use of heat dates to the ancient Greeks and Romans, who used hot rocks, hot water, open fires, hot sand or oils, or the sun. Therapeutic heat includes radiant heat — sun, open fires, glowing coals, or metals — and agents conductive of heat — hot water, thermal springs, and heated agents (oils, sands, grains). The ancient Greeks believed sweating was very helpful as it caused body poisons to run out through the pores of the skin. Therapeutic cold agents include ice and chemical freezing agents such as ethyl chloride. Both are high-intensity afferents and will inhibit pain in as little as 5 minutes. Various sources recommend not using either heat or cold for more than 5 minutes as it may cause tissue damage, damage collagen fibers, or increase edema as the body tries to either cool or warm itself. There currently is insufficient evidence to support or refute the previous statement.

ULTRASOUND

Ultrasound is a type of therapeutic heat generated by sound waves. A deep heating effect occurs by the transmission of sound waves through a coupling medium into the tissues. A meta-analysis published in the journal *Pain* (Gam, 1995), "Ultrasound Therapy in Musculoskeletal Disorders: A Meta-Analysis," reviewed 293 papers published since 1950, and none showed evidence of pain relief achieved by ultrasound versus a sham. The article concluded that the use of ultrasound treatment for musculoskeletal disorders is based at empirical experience, lacking firm evidence and well-designed controlled studies. The journal *Physical Therapy* published two articles on ultrasound by Baker et al. (2001a, 2001b). "A Review of Therapeutic Ultrasound: Effectiveness Studies" evaluated 35 randomized controlled studies published between 1975 and 1999 using ultrasound for treating people with pain, musculoskeletal injuries, and soft tissue lesions. Of the studies, 10 were judged to have acceptable trial methods. Of those, 2 trials suggested therapeutic ultrasound is more effective in treating some clinical problems (carpal tunnel syndrome or calcific tendonitis) than placebo ultrasound, and 8 trials suggested it was not effective in treating clinical problems. This article concluded, "there's little evidence that active therapeutic ultrasound is more effective than placebo ultrasound for treating people with pain, musculoskeletal injuries, or promoting soft tissue healing" (Baker et al., 2001a). The second article, "A Review of Therapeutic Ultrasound: Biophysical Effects" (Baker et al., 2001b), examined the literature regarding the physical effects of therapeutic ultrasound and whether these effects might be considered sufficient to provide a biological reason for the use of ultrasound for the people with pain or soft tissue injury. The article

concluded, "there is currently insufficient biophysical evidence to provide scientific foundation for the clinical use of therapeutic ultrasound for the treatment of people with pain or soft tissue injury."

INTERFERENTIAL CURRENT

The Austrian physicist Nemec developed interference current therapy (IFC). Two electrical currents, each with a different frequency, 4000 and 4100 Hz, are applied to the skin through surface electrodes and an interference pattern is established at the intersection of the two currents. (Fernando, 2002.)

Other frequencies of greater than 2000 Hz and less than 10,000 Hz with a sweep range of 0 to 200 Hz are now being used. The skin's resistance (ohms) to electricity significantly drops at 2000 Hz. The theory is that although frequencies greater than 2000 Hz and less than 10,000 are classified as "medium frequencies" and have no direct therapeutic effect on the body, medium frequencies appear to penetrate deeper into the tissues and carry the lower-frequency current (0 to 200 Hz) theoretically causing a greater impact on A-delta fibers and stimulating endorphin release, resulting in significant pain reduction. The result of this interference pattern is that the targeted tissue receives a net frequency of 0 to 200 Hz of low-frequency current. The main advantage of this type of current is that lower-intensity output is required. Also, this low-frequency current produces superficial muscle contractions and tends to depolarize the muscle membrane to a great extent. Moreover, motor nerves and sensory nerves are more readily depolarized at lower frequencies. Therefore, deep stimulation of muscle and nerve is possible by the selective application of IFC using from 1 to 200 Hz.

At frequencies of 0 to 10 Hz, motor nerves are readily depolarized and muscle contractions initiated. This frequency can be used for muscle contraction, muscle relaxation, muscle strengthening, and muscle reeducation. Also, smooth muscles surrounding blood vessels reportedly respond well to stimulation at these lower levels. IFC also allows the therapist to effectively reduce and treat edema in acute conditions, and pain relief is possible from frequencies of 110 to 140 Hz. The specific features of interference current are no polar effects, as pure sinusoidal current is used; stimulation of cell division; increased adenosine released through depolarization of the cell membrane leading to adenosine triphosphate; improved microcirculation due to increased adenosine release; and ATP splitting, which results in an increase of free phosphate ions beneficial for mineralization (Fernando, 2002). Interferential current is effective for a temporary decrease of pain and may be used as a home unit for pain management. There are no significant long-term outcomes.

TRANSCUTANEOUS ELECTRICAL NERVE STIMULATION

In 46 A.D., Scribonius Largus described the use of the torpedo fish, an electric eel, to control pain. This was the beginning of the technique of electrical stimulation for the relief of pain. TENS uses electrodes to stimulate the skin in the treatment of acute and chronic pain conditions. In 1967, Drs. Shealy and Mortimer (1970) developed a dorsal column stimulator for surgical implantation in patients with chronic intractable pain. At the time, they used TENS as a screening device for their patients. Eventually, they eliminated the surgery because they found that the screening process alone brought relief. At that point, TENS, as an alternative method of pain management, became a reality. In addition, Drs. Melzack and Wall's Control Therapy of Pain Perception convinced the medical community of the benefits of electrical neuromodulation of pain. The physiological basis for the treatment is the stimulation of large myelinated afferent fibers, a-delta fibers, which at the level of the spinal cord tend to block the passage of painful impulses carried by smaller unmyelinated afferent fibers – c fibers. (Fernando, 2002.)

There is no consistent information to demonstrate that TENS "cures" anything. It can be highly effective in managing pain with patients suffering from chronic orthopedic or neurological pain. It does not appear to be effective in managing pain of fibromyalgia or neuropathies. It should not be used transcranially.

HIGH VOLTAGE GALVANIC STIMULATION

High voltage galvanic stimulation is based on positive and negative polarity. The primary function has been for reduction of edema and pain management. Interstitial fluid accumulation, edema, is mostly negatively charged fluids. By placing a negative electrode over the area of edema and a positive electrode proximal or distal to the edema site, electronic stimulation can disperse some of the negatively charged fluids from the site of edema. It can also temporarily inhibit pain.

MICROCURRENT STIMULATION

Joseph M. Mercola, D.O., and Daniel L. Kirsch, Ph.D., D.A.A.P.M., coined the term "microcurrent electrical therapy" (MET) to define a new form of electronic intervention using biocompatible waveforms as opposed to previous uses of electrical therapy as an application of force (Mercola & Kirsch, 1995).

Microcurrent stimulation is based on the Arendt–Schultz physics principle of low-intensity stimulation's causing profound biophysical response. This device works on the cellular level using milliamp current. It appears to be highly effective through research with peripheral neuropathies and post-operative pain (Kirsch & Smith, 2000).

Cranial electrical stimulation (CES), also a type of microcurrent, has been researched and proved effective in reducing chronic headaches and improving serotonin levels. It was initially used for the treatment of patients with closed-head injuries. It can prevent or abort migraine headaches (Brotman, 1989) and significantly decreases the pain of fibromyalgia. Patients with depression, insomnia, chronic pain, chronic headaches, and fibromyalgia have reported increased energy and a feeling of well-being. It may also have an effect on the pain neural matrix in the cerebral cortex. The device is applied through ear clips or on the scalp (Kirsch & Smith, 2000).

SYMPATHETIC THERAPY SYSTEMS

Sympathetic therapy systems (STS) was developed and patented by Dr. Donald Rhodes, a pain specialist in Corpus Christi, TX, in August 2000. This device was marketed and distributed by Dynatronics and has been approved by the FDA for use in "symptomatic relief of chronic intractable pain and/or management approach post traumatic or post surgical pain." This device uses medium-frequency current to affect the sympathetic system by treating the pain systemically rather than locally. Guido (2001, 2002) studied the effects of STS patients with peripheral neuropathy. He reported 80% of 20 patients reported an overall improvement in their quality of life and sleep and 40% reduced their medications. These patients had previously not responded to other therapeutic interventions. This chapter's author has used the STS on more than 150 patients with fibromyalgia, chronic intractable headaches, and peripheral neuropathies. The majority of patients have reported significantly decreased pain, decreased medication usage, and improved functional ability. This device did not appear to work with diabetic neuropathy.

LOW-POWER LASER

LASER is an acronym for Light Amplification by Stimulated Emission of Radiation. Laser therapy dates to the 1950s when it was first used in Europe for the reduction of pain and inflammation. There was inadequate and insufficient evidence to support its continued use; however, empirical evidence seemed to support its function. Laser therapy, like microcurrent stimulation, is also based on the Arendt–Schultz physics principle of low-intensity stimulation's causing profound biophysical response and supports the theory that less energy rather than more causes the body cells to exhibit a greater physiological response. The laser works on a photobiostimulation principle. Laser output is measured in nanometers. It was called cold, soft, or low-level laser therapy when used during the 1970s to the 1990s. The helium neon laser, 632.8 nm, and the gallium aluminum arsenide laser, 810 nm, were used for superficial wound healing and acute and chronic pain with or without inflammation. The gallium arsenide or infrared laser, at 904 nm, was used for deep pain and deep wound healing, scar tissue, and calcium deposits. Either laser could be used for auricular therapy or on body acupuncture points. Low-power cold laser technology appears to reduce inflammation, improve range of motion, engage proprioception, and integrate locomotive process. There are no actual contraindications to cold laser therapy. Relative contraindications include pregnancy, malignant melanoma, or general illness. Direct radiation in the eyes must be avoided as this can cause damage to the retina (Watson, 1995). Laser therapy appears to decrease swelling and acute traumatic soft tissue injury conditions (Oschman, 2004).

MAGNETIC THERAPY

Magnetic therapy has been used for thousands of years for treating acute and chronic pain. Many professional football teams, golfers, and other athletes utilize various forms of magnetic chairs, belts, and treatment devices. Magnetic therapy is also useful in treating animals in pain as it emits a subsensory sensation. It is covered in much greater detail in Chapter 84 of this book.

PHONOPHORESIS

Phonophoresis is the process of driving medication into the subcutaneous tissue using ultrasound. The studies done have been poor and limited, and had minimal controls. Anecdotal responses, however, are good (Watson, 1995). The medications listed as used included corticosteroids, salicylates, nonsteroidal anti-inflammatory drugs (NSAIDs), DMSO, Manitol, insulin, anesthetics, vitamins, antibiotics, and antispasmodics.

IONTOPHORESIS

Iontophoresis is the process of electrically transmitting ions through the skin into the underlying tissues through the cellular membranes. The process is based on the principle that like charges repel like charges. A positive current will drive positive ions and negative currents will drive negative ions into the body through the cellular membranes. Knowledge of the chemical solutions being driven in and the tissues being treated is absolutely necessary. All types of extremity and trunk myofascial pain, strains, inflammatory orthopedic pain, and neuritis can respond to iontophoresis. The following chemicals are indicated for these conditions: dexamethasone for inflammatory conditions, magnesium as a muscle relaxant, acetic acid for calcium deposits, sodium chloride to soften scars, copper sulfate for fungal infections, salicylates for edema and pain reduction, lidocaine and marcaine for painful bursitis

or neuritis, and zinc to assist with wound healing. Iontophoresis is also used in dermatology, otorhinolaryngology, ophthalmology, and on the spinal cord.

Iontophoresis is the introduction of medicinal ions through the skin into the tissue using direct electrical current (Garzione, 1968). It is used to deliver a locally high concentration of the drug with little systemic side effects, as the hepatic first pass elimination is bypassed. The concept, simply put, is that like poles repel. The charged ion is repelled into the tissue by the same pole of the direct current stimulator. In 1908, Leduc conducted an experiment putting two rabbits in series with the same direct current so the current had to pass through both rabbits. The first rabbit was connected by the positive electrode soaked in strychnine sulfate with the current leaving by the negative electrode soaked in plain water. The second rabbit was connected to the positive pole soaked with water and by the negative pole soaked with potassium cyanide. The first rabbit was seized by tetanic contractions, indicative of strychnine poisoning, and the second rabbit died rapidly with symptoms of cyanide poisoning. The two animals were replaced with two new rabbits and the current flow was reversed. Neither animal was harmed, as the ions were not repelled by the opposite charge (Banga & Chien, 1998; Garzione, 1968).

Studies using radiolabeled tracers have shown that 3 to 32% of the drug is delivered by iontophoresis (Glass, 1980; Zunkel et al., 1959). The most common drug studied is dexamethasone. Studies have shown that this drug can be phoresed into the tissue and is effective in reducing symptoms (Li et al., 1996; Nirschl et al., 2003). There are more than 200 case reports of using iontophoresis with alternative ions, but there is little double-blind, placebo-controlled evidence that these other ions are efficacious.

The drug must be in an ionized state, have a charge or be able to have a charge introduced on it by pH manipulation, be soluble in water for good ion formation, and be soluble in fat for good tissue penetration and permeability (Garzione, 1968).

The advantages of iontophoresis or phonophoresis are there are no needles, medication stays locally versus systemic, the stomach and liver are bypassed, the medication is not degraded or absorbed, and the chances of overdosing are greatly reduced.

EVIDENCE-BASED MODALITIES EFFECTIVENESS

The effectiveness of modalities must be based on evidence. Therapeutic exercise programs and massage are addressed later in this chapter. Evidence-based practice for the treatment of low back pain is of growing concern in the field of rehabilitation. Low back pain is a leading cause of workers' compensation claims in the United States and Canada. It is estimated that 60 to 90% of the adult population will experience low back pain and 30%

of all low back pain will become chronic. A special article entitled, "Philadelphia Panel Evidence-Based Clinical Practice Guidelines (EBCPG) in Selected Rehabilitation Intervention for Low Back Pain" (Scalzitti, 2001) was published in *Physical Therapy*. The correct management of low back pain is extremely relevant to outcome. This panel evaluated random control studies, observation studies as defined by the Cochrane Collaboration, and literature review using meta-analysis. The results were compared with the Québec Task Force on spinal disorders (QTF) and the Agency for Health-Care Policy and Research (AHCPR).

Multiple interventions were used by a variety of clinicians for treatment of low back pain. The Philadelphia Panel evaluated nine interventions for the treatment of low back pain: thermotherapy, therapeutic exercise, therapeutic massage, electromyographic (EMG) feedback, mechanical traction, ultrasound, TENS, electrical stimulation, and combined rehabilitation intervention. The practitioners responding included family physicians, orthopedic physicians, physical therapists, members of the American College of Rheumatology, physiatrists, and neurologists. The purpose of the article was to describe EBCPGs developed by the panel for rehabilitation intervention of low back pain and in acute low back pain and in subacute low back pain. Strengthening exercises in flexion and extension were effective in subacute, chronic, and postoperative low back pain. Mechanical traction, ultrasound, and EMG biofeedback demonstrated no consistent clinical outcomes with acute, subacute, chronic, or postoperative patients with low back pain. There was insufficient evidence for or against therapeutic massage, electrical stimulation, or combining rehabilitation interventions.

The QTF and *British Medical Journal* recommended therapeutic massage based on clinical practitioners' preferences and not on contributed clinical trial results. The article cited unpublished studies suggesting therapeutic massage may have a clinical therapeutic benefit. The lack of well-designed and controlled random studies limited the assessment of the effectiveness of the rehabilitation of patients with low back pain. EBCPGs support the use of therapeutic exercise in acute, chronic, subacute, and postoperative low back pain, and continuation of normal activities in acute low back pain. There is at present a lack of evidence to support the use of other modality interventions.

Modalities can be very effective in managing pain but are predominantly ineffective in resolving or curing pain.

MANUAL THERAPY

The evaluation process determines the tissue lesion or what structure needs treatment. Manual therapy techniques including massage, mobilization, and manipulation

are highly effective in reducing pain, muscle guarding, and producing increased range of motion. The evaluation will determine whether there is a hypermobility or a hypomobility of a joint and the amount of tension in the muscles surrounding the joint. Hypermobilities, or excessive motion, in a spinal or extremity joint are effectively treated with stabilization exercises and are addressed later in this chapter. Hypomobility, or restricted motion, at a spinal or extremity joint is effectively treated with manual therapy. Manual therapy philosophies include Mennell's — there is a pathological condition or joint disease; osteopathic structure governs function according to Cyriax — all pain has an anatomical source and with correct diagnosis and treatment directed at the cause a positive outcome will occur. The majority of information covered is a combination of osteopathic and Cyriax philosophies.

Dorland's Medical Dictionary (1965) defines manipulation as "skillful or dexterous treatment by the hand and in physical therapy, the forceful pressure/movement of a joint within or beyond its active limit of motion" (p. 873). Manipulation and mobilization date back to Hippocrates in 460 b.c. Basmajian documented "laying on of hands" in the Old Testament of the Bible as described by Harris (1993) in "History and Development of Manipulation and Mobilization." Hippocrates advocated several types of manipulation, including single force thrust, prolonged pressure by sitting on the patient, shaking movement, and a foot being applied to the bony prominence. The Turks advocated manipulation during traction as recorded in a textbook of the renaissance era.

Other writings from Arabia, China, Germany, and France list various forms of manipulation from the 17th and 18th centuries. Ambrose Pare, during that same era, introduced the terms "subluxation of the spine" (Harris, 1993, p. 14). Andrew Taylor Still introduced osteopathic manipulation in the late 1800s. He believed diseases were due to abnormal bony situations. Bonesetters were prominent in Mexico and famous for "stamping or trampling" techniques that are still practiced today. Sarah Mapps, also known as Crazy Sally or Cross Eyed Sally, was in high demand in London during the early 1700s for her "bone setting ability" (Harris, 1993, p. 10).

James Cyriax, a famous orthopedic surgeon in the 1900s, defines manipulation as "a method of treatment that consists of different sorts of passive movement performed by the hand in a definitive manner for prescribed purpose" (Harris, 1993, p. 14). The main reason was for correction of internal derangement. He believed a displaced fragment could be moved and the disc could be "sucked up" by distraction. He disagreed with osteopathic techniques and advocated manipulation to be done by physical therapists. Cyriax further states, "for thousands of years manipulation treatment for low back pain has been common practice, Hippocrates straightened kyphosis, Galen replaced outward dislocated vertebrae, and Pare wrote about subluxation of the spine" (Harris, p. 14). He further states, "bone setters replaced out of place bones, osteopaths treated the osteopathic lesion, orthopedic surgeons manipulated the sacroiliac (SI) joint, chiropractors replaced subluxed vertebrae, and neurologist have stretched the sciatic nerve" (Harris, 1993, p. 13). There has been success met by all clinicians performing these techniques. Cyriax concludes, "clearly the mechanism has been a fragment of disc that has become dislocated and put back into place, a protruding disk sucked up, a jammed or blocked joint was unlocked, or a nerve root was shifted off a prolapsed disc" (Harris, 1993, p. 13). He referred his patients to physical therapy for heat treatment, massage, and exercise. Orthopedists and physical therapists complement each other in dealing with all types of soft tissue lesions.

There are various types of manipulation and mobilization as described by Nyberg (1993) in *Rationale for Manual Therapies*. The basis for doing manipulation or mobilization is detection of motion impairment or a biomechanical problem of spinal movement. This biomechanical problem may be hypomobility (restricted motion) or hypermobility (excessive motion). Each produces motion around a nonphysiological axis. There is ambiguity and no clear definition among health care practitioners on the term "manipulation." It may be a vigorous high-speed maneuver to reduce displacement resulting in a pop or crack or gentle motion to improve range of motion and soft tissue extensibility. Nyberg (1993) lists nine types of manipulation:

1. General (original)–specific
2. Localized
3. Indirect–direct
4. Noncontact–contact
5. Soft tissue–joint mobilization (nonthrust)–manipulation (thrust)
6. Application
Graded oscillation	Under anesthesia
Progressive loading	General
Sustained loading	Specific
7. Mobilization
   Joint mobilization
   Soft tissue therapy
   Soft tissue mobilization
   Myofascial release
8. Neuromuscular therapy
   Proprioception neuromuscular facilitation
   Muscle energy
9. Positional release therapies
   Strain/counterstrain
   Functional or active
   Assisted motion therapy

A general spinal manipulation involves a load applied to more than one joint or spinal segment with pressure transmitted to a number of joint/segments that have been determined to be hypomobile. Specific spinal manipulation is force applied to one segment or spinal joint and minimal force transmission through an involved spinal segment. Direct manipulation is a force applied in the direction of motion restriction or barrier. Indirect manipulation involves movement in the opposite direction of motion restriction. Contact manipulation requires hand or finger placement on the involved area or spinal segment, which may include spinous process, laminae, facet joints, or transverse processes. Noncontact manipulation involves hand or finger placement away from the spinal segment or area in lesion (also known as Maignes treatment). Noncontact manipulation may be used because an area is too painful or because additional leverage is needed to achieve a soft tissue or joint release. Soft tissue therapy does not involve high-velocity motion and therefore is defined as soft tissue mobilization myofascial release.

Graded oscillation is a form of cyclic loading whereby alternating pressure, off and on, is delivered at different parts of the available range with either small- or large-amplitude motions in the beginning, middle, or end of range. Progressive loading mobilization involves a series of short-amplitude, spring-type pressure applications. Sustained loading is continuous, uninterrupted pressure where the force may remain at the same intensity or increase or decrease depending on the patient reaction.

Joint mobilization is nonthrust manipulation and the pressure varies from gentle to vigorous, but is imparted slowly as opposed to thrust or high-velocity manipulation. Soft tissue therapy involves manual contact, pressure, or movements primarily to myofascial tissues. It is defined as manual manipulation of soft tissue administered for the purpose of producing effects of the nervous, muscular, lymph, and circulatory systems. The techniques involve classical massage, connective tissue massage, Rolfing, acupressure, and soft tissue stretching. Myofascial release is a form of soft tissue therapy based on a reflexive responsive that reduces tissue tension.

Proprioceptive neuromuscular facilitation, developed by Kabat and Knott (Nyberg, 1993, p. 33), is a method of promoting or hastening the response of the neuromuscular mechanism through stimulation of proprioceptors. Muscle energy is a form of manipulative treatment using active muscle contraction and varying intensities from a precisely controlled position in the specific direction against a distinctly executed counterforce. Neuromuscular motion disorders are the basis for the use of positional release therapies. Improper neuromuscular mechanisms are responsible for establishing and maintaining joint motion abnormality.

The two types of positional release therapies are strain/counterstrain and a functional technique known as active assisted therapy. Strain/counterstrain, developed by Jones (Ward, 1993), is the passive placement of the body in the position of greatest comfort to reduce pain. Pain relief is achieved by the reduction of continuing inappropriate proprioceptive activity that maintains the motion dysfunction and is carried out away from the motion restriction or in the direction of motion ease and comfort. Positional therapy or active assisted motion therapy is performed by the patient and is based on the fact that motion response is the result of a demand placed on the body and that demand causes a response from each motion segment.

The criteria for manipulation are based on the assessment, type of dysfunction, and the patient's attitude. Minimal manipulation is indicated for acute conditions. Subacute, settled, or chronic conditions respond to nonthrust and sustained loading to increase joint range of motion. There is little overall evidence to validate one type as more effective for any specific dysfunction. The therapist must be aware of the restricted motion and the direction of restriction or hypermobility, control the force or amplitude of the technique, be aware of the tissue recruitment, and expect specific tissue response to the techniques performed.

The application of specific manual therapy can be partly determined by the type of mechanoreceptors located in the specific regions to be treated. Type I and type II receptors are located throughout the body. Type I mechanoreceptors are slow adapting and can be used to inhibit pain. They are predominately at the neck, hip, and shoulder region. They respond to slow collagen stretching. Collagen stretching assists in increasing range of motion and reducing pain. Type II mechanoreceptors are fast adapting, and predominate in the lumbar spine, hand, foot, and temperomandibular joint (TMJ). Oscillation techniques assist in lubrication of a joint and in pain reduction. Either of these techniques, oscillation or collagen stretch, can be applied at any of the spinal or extremity joints. (OGI, 1998b) The ultimate goal of joint mobilization/manipulation techniques is to lower the threshold of activity at a joint or muscle via dorsal horn inhibition. EMG studies demonstrated that following manipulation/mobilization increased active range of motion and decreased muscle tone and following massage/stretching demonstrated increased range of motion but increased EMG activity.

There is evidence that specific mobility testing of the spine will reveal loss of functional mobility or hypomobility and increased mobility or hypermobility. Fritz's (2004) research suggests that hypomobilities respond better to manipulation/mobilization and hypermobilities respond more to stabilization exercises. Furthermore, Jewell (2004) suggests that patients with sciatica will achieve a greater therapeutic benefit when receiving joint mobility treatments or general exercises as compared with other interventions according to his research.

RISK FACTORS

How effective is spinal manipulation therapy (SMT)? Powell, Hanigan, and Olivero's (1993) article in neuro-

surgery online, "A Risk/Benefit Analysis of Spinal Manipulation Therapy for Relief of Lumbar or Cervical Pain," attempts to answer that question. SMT is performed on more than 12 million Americans each year. The authors reviewed 140 cases in the literature and determined six risk factors associated with complications of SMT. The risk factors were misdiagnosis, failure to recognize the onset or progression of neurological symptoms or signs, improper technique, SMT performed in the presence of coagulation disorders, herniated nucleus pulposus (HNP), and manipulation of the cervical spine. Most of the clinical trials reviewed had flaws, but the data suggested that SMT demonstrated consistent effectiveness as an alternative treatment for adults with acute low back pain. SMT, according to the authors, has not been shown to be superior to other conservative methods or provide long-term benefits. The risk/benefit analysis for SMT is acceptably low for adults with low back pain of less than 1-week duration. The ratio, however, was unacceptably high for patients with radicular symptoms or signs associated with prolapsed disc or with neck pain.

The evidence supports the use of spinal manipulation for low back pain. Some patients do not respond to manipulation of the low back. Fritz, Whitman, Flynn, Wainner, and Childs's (2004) study published in *Physical Therapy* included 75 patients with nonradicular low back pain. Of the patients, 20 (28%) did not improve with manipulation. The study identified six variables for a nonresponse to manipulation: longer symptom duration, having symptoms in the buttocks or leg, absence of lumbar hypomobility, less hip rotation range of motion, less discrepancy in left-to-right hip internal rotation range of motion, and a negative Gaenslen's sign. Utilizing appropriate evaluation techniques will ensure a greater positive outcome when administering manual therapy.

SOFT TISSUE MASSAGE

How does massage therapy or soft tissue mobilization (STM) work? Grodin and Cantu (1993) describe the history, physiology of soft tissue mobilization, scar tissue formation, and the effects of massage. The term "soft tissue massage" includes myofascial release, muscle energy, traditional massage, Rolfing, and movement therapies such as Feldenkrais, Traegering, and proprioceptive neuromuscular facilitation (PNF). STM rationale is based on the structure and function of soft tissue, taking into account the histology, biomechanics, and gross morphology. Histologically, the body has five types of connective tissue and compounds including ordinary connective tissue, blood cells, cartilage, adipose tissue, and bone. STM is directed at ordinary connective tissue, superficial and deep fascia sheaths, nerve and muscle sheaths, supporting framework of internal organs, aponeurosis, ligaments, joint capsules, periosteum, and tendons.

The most abundant cell in connective tissue is collagen. Type 1 collagen, of 19 types of collagen, is found in ordinary connective tissue. Also found in connective tissue are glycosamino-glycans and water (Grondin & Cantu, 1993), which serve as a mechanical barrier for foreign matter, acts as a medium for diffusion of nutrients and waste products, provides lubrication, and maintains space between collagen fibers. The ground substance is composed of glycosaminoglycans (GAG) and water. Studies performed on animals have shown the deleterious effects of immobilization on soft tissue structures. Analysis of the cells and chemical components reported changes in water content and no significant loss of collagen in connective tissue immobilized less than 9 weeks. There was a 30 to 40% loss of GAG, primarily in hyaluronic acid. The loss of GAG theoretically results in approximation of adjacent collagen fibers and/or increase in abnormal cross-linking. Normal collagen has a half-life of 300 to 500 days, and GAG has a half-life of 1.7 to 7 days. There were demonstrated actual increases in cross-link formation of fibers after 9 weeks of immobilization. The consequence of cross-linking was decreased tissue pliability. Decreased tissue pliability was the result of fatty infiltration and increased microscopic cross-linking.

Movement is the primary factor in maintaining homeostasis between collagen synthesis and tissue degradation. Normal mechanical pressures on tissue promote biological activation for alignment of fibroblast and muscle cells in the line of stress. This also helps maintain normal biochemical activity in connective tissue. Movement inhibits contractures by facilitating proteoglycan synthesis that maintains lubrication and space between collagen fibers. When trauma or injury occurs, scar tissue formation may result. Scar tissue formation occurs in four phases. In the *inflammatory phase,* which begins immediately and lasts 24 to 48 hours, blood clotting occurs and macrophages rush to sites to breed, clean, and prevent infection. Immobilization is important in this phase to prevent further damage. The *granulation phase* results in increased vascularization for removing necrotic tissue and providing nutrition. The time varies depending on the tissue damage and extent of trauma. The *fibroblastic phase* results in collagen and ground substance increases; collagen is laid down in an irregular pattern, and the collagen has weak hydrogen bonds. During the *maturation phase,* lasting 3 to 8 weeks, the collagen shrinks, matures, and solidifies.

The collagen can absorb more stress and significant tissue remodeling can occur with proper mobilization and therapeutic techniques if stresses are applied appropriately in the line of stress. If nothing is done or if treatment is not appropriate, then there is significant loss of tissue extensibility, scar tissue may form, and abnormal alignment of collagen fibers occurs. Massage or soft tissue mobilization can be used during the maturation phase, and

has an effect on circulation, blood flow, cutaneous temperature, and morphology of blood vessels.

There are several types of STM. The connective tissue massage or Bindegewebmassage, described by Dicke in the 1920s (Grondin & Cantu, 1993), involved stroking a hypersensitive area until it was warm and superficial circulation reappeared. This became known as the visceral somatic response. Hoffa massage (traditional effleurage and petrissage) consists of upward stroking or gliding over the muscle in the direction of the muscle fibers. Rolfing involves manual manipulation of myofascia in order to "balance the body in the gravitational field." It focuses on the different aspects of positional integrity. Other soft tissue work included movement approaches such as PNF and Feldenkrais.

The best approach is based on the condition being treated. Hypermobility responds to stabilization and an autonomic approach. Hypomobility responds to soft tissue mobilization. Menell (cited in Grondin & Cantu, 1993) states there are only two effects of any type of massage: reflexive and mechanical. Movement or mobilization rehydrates connective tissue, stimulates ground substance production, aides in collagen fiber orientation, and breaks up fatty adhesions. Mobilization causes plastic deformation of the connective tissue resulting in improved extensibility, lengthening, and mobility. The histological changes produced mechanically by myofascial manipulation are decreased muscle tone and increased extensibility. The patient is ready for postural reeducation and therapeutic exercises following intervention of STM/mobilization. STM is contraindicated over tissues in the state of acute inflammation and should be avoided over hypermobile or unstable spinal segments such as in spondylolisthesis.

NEURAL MOBILIZATION

David Butler (Grondin & Cantu, 1993) introduced the concept of neural mobilization in 1989. There is at present inadequate and inconsistent validity and efficacy in the literature to substantiate this technique. These mobilization techniques are directed at peripheral nerves and utilize stretching exercises, gliding exercises, or both. There is minimal indication that neural mobilization may provide some relief of symptoms for mechanical allodynia of the hand (Kietrys, 2003). Anecdotal responses are encouraging, but lack scientific validity.

OTHER TYPES OF MANUAL THERAPY

There are other types of manual therapy beyond the scope of this chapter which are addressed more thoroughly in other chapters of this book. ASTYM (advanced soft tissue therapy) system, for example, utilizes various mechanical tools and applies specific pressure to certain body areas to stimulate fibroblast recruitment and activation, guiding and aligning the healing of collagen, decreasing pain, and producing stronger healthier tissue.

IMMOBILIZATION

Prolonged immobilization and bed rest have a devastating effect on all body systems. Immobilization of patients in pain should be avoided. Early movement and motion utilizing manual therapy techniques and structured exercise are important in reducing the morbidity of patients in pain. Morris (1999), in the *British Journal of Therapy and Rehabilitation*, outlined the effects of immobilization on the musculoskeletal system. Prolonged immobilization or bed rest affects muscle, bone, cartilage, connective tissue, joint capsule/synovial membrane, ligaments, and tendon structures.

Muscle tissue suffers from disuse atrophy and a 10% loss of strength can occur within 1 week. Disuse atrophy affects antagonistic or slow-twitch muscle fiber. There is a decrease in protein synthesis and a decrease in the size of muscle fibers. Immobilization in a shortened position will lead to overall loss of muscle length and a loss of sarcomeres. Immobilization in a lengthened position will add length to sarcomeres. This can lead to an imbalance of agonist and antagonist. The research, described by Morris (1999), has shown that early controlled mobilization improved the quality and rate of repair of damaged muscle tissue.

Disuse osteoporosis, or bone loss, begins within days of immobilization and is measured by increased urine calcium levels in patients on prolonged bed rest. The bone loss is a result of decreased loading on bone. Cartilage becomes weaker and can deteriorate rapidly as the result of the loss of GAG and waste from the collagen matrix. This degeneration results from loss of motion and loss of loading on the cartilage. Further cartilage damage may occur due to impairment of nutrition to the cartilage. Cartilage changes due to immobilization can occur within a few weeks and the damage is largely irreversible.

Periarticular connective tissue, including joint capsule, ligaments, and tendon, loses water and GAG during immobilization. There is an increase in collagen synthesis and degradation results in more immature collagen, with a change in the overall collagen mass. When there are no stresses placed on immobilized immature collagen, its overall structure is weaker, the fibers are randomly laid down, and more cross-linkage occurs. Adhesions form that can lead to contractures as a result of increased cross-linking of collagen.

Joint capsule immobilization leads to capsular contracture, thickening and shortening on the flexed side, lengthening and thinning on the extended side, and loss of GAG and water. This leads to stiffness of the joint, hypertrophy of the synovial membrane, and increased potential for adhesions between the synovial membrane and cartilage.

Ligaments undergo marked atrophy, loss of tension strength, and weakness at insertion sites as a result of immobilization. Full recovery of strength in immobilized ligaments can require more than a year. Tendon and ligament immobilizations are very similar. Recovery of strength in tendons requires several months. Tendon repair recovery is improved by early controlled mobilization.

Immobilization affects quality and quantity of life, as the musculoskeletal system does not respond well to immobilization. The end result is the deterioration and weakness of the body's tissue. Recovery is a slow process and care must be taken during activity and exercise to avoid further tissue damage.

THERAPEUTIC EXERCISE

Therapeutic exercise programs are aimed at reducing pain and increasing stability. Programs begin with exercises aimed at increasing circulation into a muscle, improving endurance, and facilitating coordination so motion occurs around a normal physiological axis, and increasing strength and power.

SCIENTIFIC THERAPEUTIC EXERCISE PROGRESSIONS

The Ola Grimsby Institute (1998c) introduced the concept of Scientific Therapeutic Exercise Progressions (STEP). The concept is that each patient benefits most fully from an exercise plan individually tailored to the pathology and the tissue tolerance of the particular individual. This program provides the optimal exercise progressions each patient requires at every level of rehabilitation. It is divided into three phases:

Phase 1. This is the pain free-phase that focuses on coordination, mobility, and stability around a physiological axis throughout the range of motion. The emphasis here is reducing pain, reducing symptoms, and increasing circulation. This is normally the subacute stage. There is minimal resistance, range, and repetition.

Phase 2. This is the restoration of function phase that focuses on increasing tissue tolerance to levels corresponding to the demands of activities of daily living and restoring function. The methods employed will consist of increasing one or more of the following: strength, endurance, range of motion, speed, weight-bearing capability, and coordination. It is estimated that it will take 5,000 to 6,000 repetitions to regain the former coordination of the tonic or phasic muscles in a joint system following an injury.

The principle of overload, which states that habitually overloading a system will cause it to respond and adapt, is utilized in phase 2. The Holten diagram displays the relationship between the number of repetitions until fatigue and a percentage of the "resistant maximal" (RM) used in each repetition. This is valid for either isotonic or isometric exercises. RM describes the resistance a group of muscles is capable of overcoming in one repetition. Endurance, according to the Holten curve, is defined as the functional quality that increases with more than 30 repetitions or using less than 60% of 1 RM. Coordination, as used in STEP, is defined as "the contraction and relaxation of muscles in a specific consecutive order and with a specific magnitude to produce movement around those axes of motion that are best suited for a specific function" (Ola Grimsby Institute, 1998). Coordination therefore refers to the quality of motion. The three criteria used in testing for one 1 RM are fatigue, pain in either the primary or secondary site of pathology, and loss of coordination in the required motion. Testing and training are not done in the same session.

There are three types of muscle contraction. Concentric contraction occurs when a muscle shortens and generates tension. Mechanical work is positive because the movement is in the same direction as the tension and joint movement. Eccentric work occurs when a muscle lengthens as a result of a force external to the muscle stretching. Mechanical work is negative because the net muscle movement is in the opposite direction of the muscles force. Isometric work occurs when the muscle neither lengthens nor shortens and produces tension. The greatest contractile tension in a muscle occurs in the length–tension curve. In concentric contraction the muscle is weakest at its beginning length of tension (actively insufficient), strongest 20% into its length to 20% past its mid-length, and weakest at the end of range.

Factors affecting the length–tension relationship are histological, biomechanical, and neurophysiological. Histological factors occur as a result of minimal overlap of a sarcomere's actin and myosin filaments at full extension, which allows for the production of very little tension in a muscle or at the end of range when no more overlap can occur. This is considered active insufficiency. Biomechanical factors are described as the motion of the lever where the angle of the tension insertion into the bone directs where the greatest contractile force from the muscle is produced. When the muscular forces are perpendicular to the lever arm, such as the biceps to the forearm, the greatest muscle force will be generated. The neurophysiology of joint mechanical receptors influences muscle facilitation around a joint. Type I mechanical receptors facilitate tonic muscle and type II facilitate phasic muscle. The beginning range of collagen tension is the only range of tension where both types of mechanoreceptors fire; type II fires in mid-range, and type I fires at the end of range. The beginning range of collagen tension in clinical terms is the resting or loose-packed position. This is the only range where both type I and type II mechanoreceptors fire together to facilitate the greatest amount of both tonic and phasic fibers.

The important component of STEP is to utilize collagenous tension specifically to recruit and facilitate muscle fibers. The pulley system is recommended in the STEP program as acceleration and deceleration can be controlled. Speed and resistance remain consistent with pulleys throughout the range of contraction for fiber recruitment and physiological coordination. Both concentric and eccentric contractions occur during pulley exercises. The lower extremities will not strengthen as consistently eccentrically as the upper extremities will. Eccentric exercises produce hypertrophy of a muscle, venous flow, and removal of waste products between contractions. Concentric exercise will increase capillary density, and 75% of metabolic activity in a muscle occurs during the concentric phase.

Phase 3. This phase involves combining concentric and eccentric contractions such as in PNF patterns to finalize strengthening and coordination. The patients are pain free and are preparing to return to their preinjury levels of activity or sports participation at this time.

BALL THERAPY

There is no single treatment that is successful in treating low back pain. One possible approach is the Swedish gym ball for rehabilitating spinal dysfunction as described by Irion (1992). Lumbar stabilization techniques, including balance, strengthening, and proprioceptive activities, as performed with a 55- to 65-cm Swedish ball, can be part of a comprehensive program in patients with low back pain and dysfunction. The gym ball allows the patients to develop proper and pain-free movement patterns. The goals of lumbar stabilization and the gym ball are to promote healing and develop appropriate movement patterns.

Treatment progression is divided into the acute phase, lasting 2 to 3 days, and the training phase, lasting through the remainder of the rehabilitation program. The initial exercises include abdominal isometrics and gluteal sets, which give the patient instruction in proper lumbo pelvic motion. Education in safe movement patterns is the goal of the training phase. Appropriate exercise equipment for improving flexibility, endurance, and strengthening is left to the therapists' discretion. The training phase progresses to dynamic lumbar stabilization using the gym ball for improving balance, coordination, strength, and stability. Correction of muscle imbalance, controlled motion, and good posture are implemented in this phase. The techniques used with the gym ball promote smooth, coordinated movement patterns and maintain correct, appropriate lumbo pelvic alignment, resulting in good movement patterns and postural control.

To use the gym ball, patients must find a functional position of the spine, described as the most stable and asymptomatic position for the task at hand. Patients are trained to stay in this midrange of lumbo pelvic motion, also known as a neutral position. However, variation may occur based on the underlying pathology. Conditions such as spinal stenosis or spondylolisthesis may prevent patients from assuming this mid-range pain-free position. Dynamic stabilization is a complex neuromuscular skill in which a more neutral spine position is maintained by continuous fine adjustments in muscle tension in response to fluctuating loads. The patient must master the functional position and lumbar stability before starting a gym ball program. The gym ball must not reproduce the pattern that initially brought the patient in for treatment. The intensity of the program should be to the point of fatigue, almost losing control of the quality of moment or functional position, but not actually losing control. Quality of movement is more important than quantity of movement.

Indications for the gym ball program include general poor conditioning, improper posture/body mechanics, psychomotor conditions, sacroiliac dysfunction, post-lumbar laminectomy, degenerative disc disease, post-spinal fusion, herniated or bulging disc, thoracic strain, cervical pathologies, spinal stenosis, and spondylolisthesis. Relative contraindications include pulmonary dysfunction, cardiac problems, hypertension, and obesity. The exercises are performed sitting or lying on the ball. Increasing the length of lever arm while on the ball results in the progression of exercise. Patients move arms and/or legs in traditional movements, working agonist and antagonistic muscles in alternating motions while maintaining the functional position of the spine. The motions are begun in the sagittal and coronal planes and progress to oblique and torsional patterns. The measurable outcome is to regain appropriate movement patterns.

PILATES

Pilates exercise programs are based on Joseph Pilates's training techniques developed in the 1920s. These programs can be used for general conditioning and fitness or recovery from orthopedic injury or trauma of surgery. There is no current evidence-based information on Pilates programs. Pilates has become increasingly popular and is used by many physical therapists. Pilates developed specific principles and performing specific active stretching movements that include breath, awareness, concentration, balance, centering, control, flowing motion, and precision. The emphasis of these exercises is directed at the trunk and abdomen for stability. There is also extremity motion that helps to facilitate active stretching. Therapeutic exercise programs must be supervised and directed by a qualified therapist (Lombardo, 2003).

OTHER FORMS OF THERAPEUTIC EXERCISE

Other forms of exercise that may help reduce pain include Feldenkrais, yoga, and plyometric training. Yoga, very simplified, involves placing the body in specific nonpainful positions and meditating. It is spiritually "getting in touch with yourself" or some other focus such as Jesus or other god. It is not pure mysticism. Plyometric training is used to train the eccentric activity for lengthening contraction of a muscle's action. Although it places a greater strain on the tendons and ligaments, it may be beneficial in reducing pain and facilitating endurance, motion, and strength.

HOME PROGRAMS

Home programs are a vital part of the treatment schedule of any patient with pain. A home program should include instructions of do's and don'ts for body mechanics, lifting, sitting, lying down, and any kind of activities of daily living. For example, a patient with low back pain standing at a sink or ironing might benefit from using a footstool to rest one foot on and alleviate pressure on the low back. Home exercise programs are used for lubrication of joints, increasing range of motion, reducing pain, and reducing muscle tension. The patients must be actively instructed in the exercises, given a copy of the exercises with the appropriate dosage, and told to stop the exercises if their pain increases or they feel tired.

ADAPTIVE EQUIPMENT

Physical therapists are in a unique position to provide many adaptive devices for patients to use at home. These devices may be felt inserts for shoes; instruction in using braces or supports on lower extremities, backs, or upper extremities; supports for sleeping at night to position the body in a more comfortable position; instruction in the use of walking devices such as canes, walkers, crutches, and home pain management devices such as TENS, STS, CES, IFC, or EGS (electro-galvanic stimulation) units, in short, any kind of device that will help patients function more normally and reduce their pain.

PREPARATION FOR COURT TESTIMONY

Physical therapists may be called to testify in a court of law or provide depositions for patients who are suffering from pain and are seeking financial compensation (Watson, 1995). The purpose of court testimony as a physical therapist may be as a treating therapist, expert witness, or defendant. A *treating therapist* will be asked to present evaluation findings, treatment administered, and outcome of the treatment program. The documentation of all findings and treatments will be thoroughly scrutinized in court. The therapist should not answer opinion questions or speculate on other outcomes. The *expert witness* is a consultant qualified to address pain conditions and treatment programs. Testimony should be based on evaluation findings and treatment administered, audiovisuals and models, KISS (keep it simple, silly), and the therapist must be prepared to give an opinion. The therapist must be relaxed, compassionate, and noncombative even when assaulted by an opposing attorney. The *defendant physical therapist* is in court as a result of malpractice. The best course of action to not become a defendant physical therapist is prevention, having good communication and clear documentation, being professional and cautious when working with the opposite sex, and receiving informed consent from a patient. Always get an attorney and listen to the attorney's advice.

INDICATIONS FOR PHYSICAL THERAPY

Physical therapy is indicated for the major types of acute and chronic pain. Acute pain may include sprains or strains, postsurgical or post-traumatic events, acute-onset headaches without neurological complications, and orthopedically caused pain. The treatments utilized here include heat or cold, electrotherapy to manage pain or reduce swelling, manual therapies, and pain-free exercises. Chronic pain conditions such as failed back or neck surgeries, fibromyalgia, chronic headache syndromes, and general chronic pain syndromes may also be managed and/or sometimes treated with various modalities: TENS, manual therapies, and pain-free exercises. Certain types of chronic pain such as cancer pain, chronic headaches, and peripheral neuropathies may respond to laser therapy, microcurrent therapy, or STS therapy.

CONCLUSIONS

Physical therapy is a skill and an art using the head, hands, and heart. The head learns the anatomy, physiology, pain symptoms, and what evidence-based outcomes various types of modalities, exercises, and manual therapies produce. The hands apply the modalities, the manual therapies, and exercises. The heart supplies the empathy and the understanding that patients with pain need more than just modalities and exercise. Patients with pain need someone to lay hands on them, talk to, and listen, someone who cares. Physical therapists who treat patients with pain must have very big hearts.

Remember: "Pain does not have to be a way of life."

REFERENCES

Agnew, L. R. C., Aviado, D. M., Brody, J. I., & Burrow, W. (1965). *Dorlands medical dictionary* (24th ed.). Philadelphia, PA: W. B. Saunders.

Banga, A. K., & Chien, Y. W. (1998). Iontophoretic delivery of drugs: Fundamentals, developments and biomedical applications. *Journal of Controlled Release, 7,* 1–24.

Brotman, P. (1989). Low intensity transcranial electrical stimulation improves the efficacy of thermal biofeedback and quieting reflex in the treatment of classical migraine headache. *American Journal of Electromedicine, 6*(5), 121–123.

Fernando, C. (2002). Physical therapy and pain management. In R. S. Weiner (Ed.), *Pain management: A practical guide for clinicians* (6th ed., pp. 739–746). Boca Raton, FL: CRC Press.

Fritz, J. M., Whitman, J. M., Flynn, T. W., Wainner, R. S., & Childs, J. D. (2004). Factors related to the inability of individuals with low back pain to improve with a spinal manipulation. *Physical Therapy, 84*(4), 173–189

Gam, A. N. (1995). Ultrasound therapy in musculoskeletal disorders, *Pain.*

Garzione, J. (1968). Iontophoresis. In A. L. Watkins (Ed.), *A manual of electrotherapy* (3rd ed.). Philadelphia, PA: Lea and Febiger.

Glass, J. M. (1980). The quantity and distribution of radio labeled dexamethasone delivered to tissue by iontophoresis. *International Journal of Dermatology, 19*(9), 519–525.

Grodin, A., & Cantu, R. (1993). Soft tissue mobilization. In J. Basmajian, (Ed.), *Rational manual therapies* (pp. 199–219). Baltimore: Williams and Wilkins.

Guido, E. H. (2001, April). Effects of sympathetic therapy and chronic pain in peripheral neuropathy subjects. *Abnormal Peripheral Neuropathies.*

Guido, E.H. (2002). Effects of sympathetic therapy on chronic pain in peripheral neuropathy subjects. *American Journal of Pain Management, 12,* 1.

Harris, J. D. (1993). History and development of manipulation and mobilization. In J. Basmajian & R. Nyberg (Eds.), *Rational manual therapies* (pp. 7–22). Baltimore: Williams and Wilkins.

Irion, J. (1992). Use of the gym ball in rehabilitation of spinal dysfunction. *Orthopaedic Physical Therapy Clinics of North America, Exercise Technology, 1,* 375–398.

Jewell, D. V. (2004). Mobilization exercises increase the likelihood of meaningful improvement disability and patients with sciatica. *Journal of Orthopaedic and Sports Physical Therapy, 34*(1).

Kietrys, D. M. (2003). Neural mobilization: An appraisal of the evidence regarding validity and efficacy. *Orthopaedic Physical Therapy Practice, 15*(4), 18–19.

Kirsch, D., & Smith R. (2000). The use of cranial electrotherapy stimulation in the management of chronic pain: A review. *Neuro Rehabilitation, 14,* 85–94.

Li, L. C, et al. (1996). The efficacy of dexamethasone iontophoresis for the treatment of rheumatoid arthritic knees: A pilot study. *Arth. Care and Research, 9*(2), 126–132.

Lombardo, L. (2003, October). Therapy or exercise? Using Pilates for healing and for fitness can mean 2 different things. *Advance for Physical Therapist and PT Assistants, 22,* 12–13.

Martelli, M., Zasler, N., Nicholson, K., Pickett, T., & May, R. (2002). Assessing the veracity of pain complaints and associated disability. In R. S. Weiner (Ed.), *Pain management: A practical guide for clinicians* (6th ed., pp. 789–793). Boca Raton, FL: CRC Press.

Mercola, J. M., & Kirsch, D. L. (1995). The basis of microcurrent electrical therapy (MET) and conventional medical practice. *Journal of Advancement in Medicine, 8*(2), 102–120.

Morris, J. (1999). The effect of immobilization on the musculoskeletal system. *British Journal of Therapy and Rehabilitation.* Retrieved from http://www.markallen group.com.

Nirschl, R. P. et al. (2003). Iontophoretic administration of dexamethasone sodium phosphate for acute epicondylitis: A randomized, double-blinded, placebo-controlled study. *American Journal of Sports Medicine, 31*(2), 189–195.

Nyberg, R. (1993). Manipulation: Definition, types, application. In J. Basmajian, & R. Nyberg (Eds.), *Rational manual therapies* (pp. 21–24). Baltimore: Williams and Wilkins.

Ola Grimsby Institute (1998b). Evidence based manual therapy of the spine. *Orthopaedic Manual Therapy, Course Curriculum.*

Ola Grimsby Institute. (1998a). Diagnostic pyramid. General principles of evaluation. *Orthopaedic Manual Therapy, Course Curriculum, 630,* 7.

Ola Grimsby Institute. (1998c). STEP: Scientific therapeutic exercise progressions. *Orthopaedic Manual Therapy, Course Curriculum, 705,* 7–23.

Powell, F., Hanigan, W., & Olivero, W. (1993). A risk/benefit analysis of spinal manipulation therapy for relief of lumbar or cervical pain. *Neurosurgery Online.com., 3,* 73–74.

Robertson, V., & Baker, K. (2001a). A review of therapeutic ultrasound: Biophysical effects, *Physical Therapy,* July.

Robertson, V., & Baker, K. (2001b). A review of therapeutic ultrasound: Effectiveness studies, *Physical Therapy,* July.

Scalzitti, D. A. (2001). Philadelphia panel evidenced-based clinical practice guidelines (EBCPG) on selected rehabilitation interventions for low back pain. *Physical Therapy, 81,* 1641–1674.

Ward, R. C. (1993). Myofascial release concepts. In J. Basmajian & R. Nyberg (Eds.), *Rational manual therapies* (pp. 223–242). Baltimore: Williams and Wilkins.

Watson, T. (1995). Physiology of pain. *Orthopaedic Physical Therapy Clinics of North America. Pain Management, 4,* 423–442.

Zunkel, H. T. et al. (1959, May). Iontophoresis studies with a radioactive tracer. *Archives of Physical Medicine and Rehabilitation,* 193–196.

19

Social Work

Terry Altilio, LMSW

INTRODUCTION

Since the late 1970s, social work experts have been articulating and encouraging a role for the profession in the complex and rich specialty of pain management (Altilio, 2004; Hamilton, 1967; Holden et al., 1999; Hudgens, 1977; Kelley & Clifford, 1997; O'Neill, 2003; Roy, 1985a; Subramanian, 1991a, 1991b, 1994; Subramanian & Rose, 1988a). In many respects the profession has reflected the attitudes of the larger society as well as the field of health care wherein the treatment of pain has been viewed as a choice rather than an essential responsibility mandated by ethical principles such as beneficence and respect for the dignity of persons. Social workers practice in a range of settings, including hospitals, nursing homes, facilities for senior centers, hospices, correctional facilities, chemical dependency programs, mental health facilities, social service agencies, and private offices, providing extensive opportunity to advocate for, and promote and provide competent, compassionate pain management. This opportunity creates a mandate that clinicians become knowledgeable of the myriad issues that inform pain-related experiences. Social work authors have encouraged this potential for professional contribution and advocacy as it easily evolves both from our presence in multiple settings and from historical traditions and values such as commitment to vulnerable populations, social justice, and respect for the worth and dignity of the individual. An assessment of the person in the environment, which might include social, economic, cultural, and spiritual aspects of his or her experience, is fundamental to social work practice. These values infuse the profession's approach to clinical care, research, and policy work, and they have become increasingly important as the care of persons with pain has moved beyond the medical model to a multidimensional focus and most currently beyond the clinical relationship to the political, regulatory, and legislative arenas.

SOCIAL WORK AND PAIN MANAGEMENT: A UNIQUE FIT

The management of pain is often a shared responsibility — shared with patients and families, shared between disciplines. The care is enriched when disciplines come together bringing their unique perspectives, knowledge, and values. Social workers bring a worldview that is based in the belief and value that a *"person in environment"* perspective is the essence of comprehensive assessment and that the engagement process *"starts where the client is"* (Hamilton, 1967). These key social work values are also embedded in the treatment principles that pain is a multidimensional experience and that competent and compassionate care begins with a belief in the patient's report of pain. Acceptance of the patient's report, his or her language and metaphors, implies acceptance of the person and the perception of his or her experience; this is the basis of a beginning trusting and therapeutic relationship. The ongoing exchange, assessment, and expertise of the clinicians adds richness and depth to that report — expands and informs the multidimensional work that is often indicated and necessary. Identification of strengths is basic to the clinical and problem-solving approach of social work. This emphasis on strengths and competence is often key to assisting people who have been overwhelmed by pain to recover their voice, restore self-esteem, maximize their abilities, and create avenues of hopefulness and meaning in their lives. The unique heritage of social work creates an expectation of holistic assessment and interventions which may range from the practical to the clinical to policy aspects of the pain experience.

The social work profession has a rich tradition and commitment to social justice, advocacy, and empowerment. These values are relevant to any discussion of the underserved person with pain and to the many barriers that limit access to adequate management of pain. The identification of barriers can be viewed as the beginning of the systemic diagnostic assessment that guides interventions whether they are on an individual, family, system, or policy level. The increasing presence of social work practitioners in advocacy organizations such as the American Pain Foundation, Alliance of Cancer Pain Initiatives, and many state pain initiatives speaks to the emerging recognition that the undertreatment of pain is the shared responsibility of many disciplines. Our commitment to self-determination, empowerment, and social justice mandates that the profession respond not only at the clinical level but also on the policy, political, and institutional level (O'Neill, 2003). The policy and regulatory focus of social work in the area of pain is most celebrated in the efforts of David Joranson, who has worked for decades to study and improve the national and international regulatory environment surrounding the use of opioids and the management of pain. The merging of social work values with key issues and principles of pain management is striking, and it informs the advocacy efforts of many social work clinicians who challenge their peers to become knowledgeable and expert, and to expand the presence of the profession in the field.

A HISTORICAL REVIEW

In 1981, Golden and Steiner published "Unique Needs of People with Chronic Pain" in the *Journal of Health and Social Work*. Reflective of the unique professional perspective, the authors discussed the individual, societal, and professional response to a multidimensional health problem that was cloaked in stigma. The article was intended to make practitioners "aware of the prevalence and nature of chronic pain so that their subjective and even unconscious relationship to this condition takes on new form and meaning" (p. 47). The authors noted increased patient vulnerability by virtue of minority or poverty status and/or gender as well as the potential for cultural variation in the pain experience. In addition to the societal and financial impact, chronic pain was described as a hidden epidemic often accompanied by threats to autonomy and competence, positive identity, and meaningful social relationships. Clinicians were challenged to recognize that social values and professional attitudes can create and reinforce isolation and stigma of chronic pain sufferers. The proposed factors that contributed to the social reluctance to accept the phenomena and prevalence of chronic pain

included the absence of methods to measure and prove pain and the inability to understand the cause, compounded by the fact that cures are elusive, reflecting and reinforcing feelings of practitioner incompetence.

Although the first pain clinic was established in 1961, many persons with chronic pain continued to receive care through local health and welfare agencies, reinforcing the need for social work clinicians to establish specialized skills to assist persons with pain. Suggested roles included therapist/teacher, broker/advocate; all were based on a therapeutic alliance intended to foster the restoration and enhancement of autonomy and competence. Therapist and teacher tasks included increasing the ability to describe, partialize, and manage the pain experience within the context of maintaining role function, minimizing strain in relationships, enhancing the environment to nourish and facilitate, and increasing coping skills. Advocate and broker roles involved a guide and liaison function driven by problem identification and focused on accessing available and needed resources and developing a plan to create a responsive treatment system (Golden & Steiner, 1981). The roles of advocate and broker, while important in 1981, are crucial today when health care systems have become more complex, inaccessible, and challenging for patients, families, and many clinicians as well.

Additionally, in 1981, Roy described the global nature of the psychosocial effects of chronic pain and suggested that the complex and multidimensional factors that infuse the chronic pain experience are a natural fit with a profession that incorporates comprehensive assessment of emotional, family, social, and environmental issues. A social work assessment is intended to identify relevant etiologic data, determine the effect of pain on psychological and social functioning, understand coping style, and create a diagnostic formulation to be used with medical input for the development of a treatment plan. Roy (1981) maintains, "the essential element — and the special if not unique focus that social work can bring to bear upon an assessment of a patient with chronic pain — is the understanding of the person-environment paradigm in all its complications" (p. 56). In chronic pain this may include such complicated and interconnected issues as a feeling of failure after numerous investigations and interventions, a sense of not being believed, and misunderstood when clinicians introduce the concept that psychological issues may impact the pain experience.

Precise exploration of roles, function, and the multiple aspects of family structure and dynamics is followed by a developmental history, which often informs the comprehensive understanding and the formulation of a treatment plan based on the individual, family, conflicts, and sociocultural factors. Suggested therapeutic interventions include client-centered, short-term educational and problem-solving approaches that foster coping and adaptation, improved family relationships, resumption of roles, restoration of autonomy, and diminishment of maladaptive pain behaviors. While acknowledging the absence of outcome data on specific treatment strategies, Roy (1981) reinforces the importance of the social work perspective of addressing social, psychological, and environmental dimensions of the chronic pain experience and sees the integration of social work clinicians into multidisciplinary pain centers as an opportunity for the profession to both challenge traditional methods and demonstrate efficacy.

In 1986, Marcus proposed a social work view of chronic pain based in systems theory, which complemented team perspectives and integrated data from relevant frames of reference to provide a context and map that served to guide assessment and target interventions. In an effort to capture a visual representation of the complexity of interacting factors that contribute to the chronic pain experience, Marcus created a model that included pain, limitations and consequent emotional response, the reactions of others (including health care professionals), psychosocial stresses, and financial issues, as well as a comprehensive exploration of the personality, attitudes, culture, roles, and health status of the person with pain. The systems map allowed for assessment of the individual in relation to each variable providing an overview of factors influencing the pain experience. The modality validated pain as a problem in itself and as a "part" of the individual's reality, which has social and emotional impact. Treatment involved engaging the patient in active participation to reduce the disabling effects of pain and to enhance control, coping, and ego functioning. Interventions might include exploration and adaptation of role, education, problem solving, relaxation training, family interventions, and alleviation of external stresses through patient empowerment or systems negotiation (Marcus, 1986).

During the 1980s these generic articles providing overviews of the social work role were accompanied by an eclectic group of publications in social work journals and included pain in the dying (Milner, 1980); incest and pelvic pain (Caldirola et al., 1983; Gross, Doerr, Caldirola, Guzinski et al., 1981); burn pain (Weinberg & Miller, 1983); headache (Roy, 1984); disability, pain, and narcissism (Rousso, 1985); pain and marital difficulties (Roy, 1985a); family and chronic pain (Roy, 1985b); chronic pain, depression, and elderly people (Roy, 1986); chronic pain and cognitive behavioral group intervention (Rose & Feldman, 1986; Subramanian, 1994; Subramanian & Rose, 1988a, 1988b); pediatric end-of-life care (Price, 1989); and end-of-life symptom management as a contributing factor to social work job satisfaction (Parry & Smith, 1987).

In 1996, Sieppert surveyed 212 medical social workers in Canada, addressing their attitudes toward and knowledge of chronic pain by combining focus group and survey techniques. Subramanian's social work publications in the late 1980s and early 1990s encouraged clinicians to transfer an ecological systems model to the assess-

ment of personal, psychological, social, and situational factors that infuse the experience of pain. Social workers were providing services in many settings other than pain clinics, which created the potential to have an impact on chronic pain in a large population both clinically and through research (Rose & Feldman, 1986; Subramanian & Rose, 1988b; Subramanian, 1987, 1991a, 1991b). Sieppert's investigations explored preparedness of medical social work to maximize these opportunities.

Sieppert's study supported Subramanian's view that social workers were becoming more visible participants on pain teams, as 40 of 47 organizations that maintained chronic pain programs employed social workers, implying that their skills and theoretical perspectives were valued. Only three respondents identified chronic pain as their primary focus, indicating that the profession was just beginning to explore pain as an area of interest. Findings from this study indicated that medical social workers recognized the importance of chronic pain treatment and the significance of this work to their own professional practice. They confirmed the need for training and expansion of their practice to the field of pain, and the underlying themes pointed to the value of social work in the area of advocacy and in assessment and intervention in psychosocial issues and family disruption. This study suggested that the highly positive orientation toward nonmedical treatment of pain and social work involvement in chronic pain services was not matched by the knowledge base of medical social workers, a discrepancy that must be addressed from the individual practitioner level as well as the level of social work education.

Practitioners have the capacity to explore independently the extensive literature, and educators must assume responsibility for developing pain-related training (Sieppert, 1996). The need for education of social workers is consistent with and sadly reflective of the need for pain management education and training of our nursing and physician colleagues.

During this same decade, the role, responsibility, and scope of social work practice in the management of cancer pain was being articulated in the writing of Loscalzo and Amendola (1990). Psychosocial and cognitive behavioral interventions were recommended as adjuncts to medical management, which might include pharmacologic, surgical, anesthetic, and radiologic interventions. The multidimensional, practical, problem-solving orientation of social work was at the core of a comprehensive, humane approach to meeting the practical, psychological, and emotional needs of oncology patients and their families who were coping with pain (Loscalzo & Amendola, 1990). The oncology literature had identified numerous barriers to the adequate management of cancer pain, and Glajchen, Blum, and Calder (1995) extended the advocacy and clinical focus of social work to the prevention of unnecessary pain and to overcoming barriers through direct service, education, advocacy, and research. Direct service roles included facilitating communication; assessing strengths, resources, and limitations; providing psychological support; and developing problem-solving approaches that extend beyond the medical model to the environmental realities of the patient/family experience. Education of patients and families might take place with individuals, in psychoeducational groups, and workshops and might include interdisciplinary discussion of specific patient family issues or discharge planning needs.

Advocacy is a shared responsibility with pain management colleagues and for social workers; the scope often goes beyond the patient and family to multiple systems such as organizations, policy arenas, and insurers. Also included is the empowering of patients and their families to act as their own advocates. Clinicians themselves are encouraged to pursue research both to enhance quality of life for patients and families and to advocate for the profession by developing a literature supportive of social work practice (Glajchen, Blum, & Calder, 1995).

During the 1990s in addition to generic articles exploring the expanding areas of practice, social work literature included research directed toward quality of life in patients with back problems (Claiborne et al., 1999) as well as psychosocial problems in urban and poor children with sickle cell anemia (Barbarin, Whitten & Bonds, 1994), sickle cell group intervention (Butler & Beltran, 1993), pediatric migraine (Gilbert, 1999), long-term breast cancer survivors (Polinsky, 1994), chronic illness in a therapist (Elliott, 1996), childhood sex abuse and chronic back pain (Pecukonis, 1996), narrative approaches in treatment of patients with fibromyalgia (Kelley & Clifford, 1997), the impact of a virtual environment on pain and anxiety (Holden et al., 1999), cognitive behavioral interventions (Loscalzo & Jacobsen, 1990), and COPE problem solving in pain-related problems (Loscalzo & Bucher, 1999).

Current literature addressing generic issues and the role of social work in pain management reflects the recognition of the complexity and multidimensional issues surrounding the clinical, social, economic, and policy aspects of pain. MacDonald (2000) in the article, "A Deconstructive Turn in Chronic Pain Treatment: A Redefined Role for Social Work" challenges the diagnostic and treatment processes applied to patients whose pain is described as idiopathic. Writing as an educator, social worker, and chronic pain sufferer, she suggests a reevaluation of a treatment approach that focuses on the management of behaviors and attempts to reestablish well behaviors through the withdrawal of reinforcing influences. The author applies a process of "deconstruction" to the contingency management model, taking "apart socially constructed categories as a way of seeing how a particular world view is constructed" (Ristock & Pennel, 1996, p. 114). Using the word *sufferer* is intentional and is chosen to identify the "chronic pain patients' existence — their

physical, emotional and spiritual struggle" (MacDonald, 2000, p. 52). The contingency management model is challenged first in the area of criteria for application.

MacDonald suggests that professional judgment of excess behaviors is an effort to gauge an unmeasurable pain experience against operationally defined behavior. The supposition that chronic pain sufferers experience "gains" through their experience of pain contradicts the language of sufferers who speak of multiple losses. Social workers and health care professionals are encouraged to "listen to the voices of sufferers" to recognize their losses, validate their struggle, and create a plan to assist in rebuilding a sense of control. The withdrawal of reinforcing behaviors by staff and/or family runs the risk of alienating sufferers and increasing isolation, a potential outcome that obviates the goal of supporting and building families. The contingency model is also challenged as an approach that demands compliance, seeks out discrepancies in sufferer's behaviors, and thus contradicts relationships built on trust and active involvement.

MacDonald reinforces the traditional values of social work, including social, political, and economic distribution of resources and power and the promotion of the self-determination, dignity, and worth of all people. She suggests that these values create both a mandate and an opportunity to engage some of the inherent conflicts and challenges in delivery of care to chronic pain sufferers. Practice suggestions include nonhierarchical modalities of individual and family empowerment counseling, advocacy, organization of sufferers, research, and program construction (MacDonald, 2000).

A paper by Mendenhall (2003) provides a framework for social workers that conceptualizes barriers to pain management as misinformed personal beliefs of health care providers, undeveloped and inadequate industry policies, and dysfunctional social mores rather than a lack of adequate science. These barriers, when framed as psychological, social, and cultural elements, become a focus for social work intervention. A review of the literature concerning vulnerable populations, barriers, and social policy explores how the inclusion of social work perspectives creates options for overcoming barriers. Empowerment practice principles are offered as a framework to expand the effectiveness of multidisciplinary efforts to improve access to pain relief. The author invites social work clinicians to participate with colleagues to create effective policy to influence psychological, social, and cultural barriers with particular attention to the most vulnerable populations. Social policy aspects, including the Joint Commission on Accreditation of Healthcare Organizations (JCAHO) standards, federal regulations, and issues related to assisted suicide, are discussed, weaving in the important concerns emanating from the use of controlled substances and the impact of media and legislation on the use of medications for management of pain. A thorough review of empowerment theory sets the framework for integrating the core values of social justice, integrity, competence, and service to guide the profession's participation in the multidimensional issues of pain management. For example, social justice relates to identifying and advocating for those who receive differential care and to accepting responsibility for working toward solutions. Integrity requires social workers to define proactively their role in management of pain motivated by the well-known implications of untreated pain in the lives of patients and their families. Competence demands that clinicians practice within an area of expertise and expand their knowledge base as needs arise. The value of service is both to the patient and to institution and may be reflected in multidimensional approaches to increasing the status and adequacy of pain management. In summary, Mendenhall challenges the social work profession to view pain and its psychological, quality of life, financial, regulatory, and social policy aspects as well within the mission of social work as articulated in the 1999 *Code of Ethics*, "enhance human well being and help meet the basic needs of all people, with particular attention to the needs and empowerment of people who are vulnerable, oppressed and living in poverty" (National Association of Social Workers, 1999, p. 1).

Over the past 4 years, the social work literature has expanded to reflect the multidimensional nature of the pain experience and the eclectic focus of the profession. Glajchen (2003) has written of the delayed recognition within the health care system of the effects on family caregivers who assist persons coping with cancer pain. The fact that the impacts of pain extend beyond the individual to family and caregivers and into the social, psychological, spiritual, and social realms reinforces the need for clinicians to extend their assessment and interventions beyond the patient. Recommended treatment strategies focus both on enhancing coping skills as well as professional interventions that reflect the responsibility of clinicians to engage the family in decisions and planning and to support, validate, and educate (Glajchen, 2003). Otis-Green and colleagues (2002) describe an integrated psychosocial spiritual model for cancer pain management, which involves the collaborative effort of multiple oncology mental health professionals to assess from their unique perspective and create a comprehensive treatment plan to optimize effective, holistic pain management. The emerging emphasis on palliative and end-of-life care has fostered a growing literature and educational programs that include pain and symptom management as an expected social work competency (Otis-Green et al., 2002). Postgraduate educational programs, fellowships, and Web-based learning modules have included pain and symptom management as an essential part of the curriculum.

In addition to the clinical aspect of end-of-life care, Roff (2001) in an article, "Analyzing End-of-Life Care

Legislation: A Social Work Perspective," advocated the need for social workers to have a clear understanding of the political and social climate as well as the policy proposals that are designed to respond to end-of-life challenges, one of which is unrelieved pain. To that end, she discusses frameworks for evaluating the adequacy of legislation and applies it to the Pain Relief Promotion Act, the Conquering Pain Act, and the Advance Planning and Compassionate Care Act. The expectation that clinicians become informed and involved in the policy aspects of pain is a recognition that the experience of the patients and families is profoundly influenced by the social and political environment in which they find themselves and that holistic care requires involvement and attention on multiple levels.

WHO ARE SOCIAL WORKERS, WHAT DO THEY DO, AND HOW DO THEY DO IT?

The Substance Abuse and Mental Health Services Administration (2000) reported that professional social workers are the largest group of mental health providers. In 1998, it was estimated that there were 190,000 clinically trained social workers. About 600,000 people hold social work degrees at the bachelor's, master's, and doctoral levels http://www.socialworkers.org/pressroom/features/general/profession.asp. Social work has the same educational challenges as our colleagues in medicine and nursing — to infuse generalist curriculum with knowledge about pain as a multidimensional issue that affects the individual, family, and larger society; to create programs to train specialists; and to increase the number of ongoing continuing education opportunities. With that said, social workers approach problems from a biopsychosocial perspective seeking to understand not only pain but also the setting in which the person functions and lives. To that end, we will join patients and colleagues to understand

- Who the patient is
- What values, beliefs, hopes, goals, and history informs their experiences and perceptions
- The impact and meaning of pain in their lives and the lives of others
- The reciprocal relationship between biological, psychological, cultural, spiritual, social, economic, family, caregiver, social system, and political aspects of the person's experience

We will listen for

- Strengths, resources, areas of competence
- Metaphoric communication

- Language that diminishes the other and reflects sufferer and/or clinician helplessness and hopelessness such as "failed" and "noncompliant"
- Opportunities to empower and restore some small semblance of control or purpose

We will intervene, in collaboration with colleagues, from a recognition that pain, medications, and various adaptations such as filing for disability or using a walker have symbolic significance and ramifications in multiple areas such as self-image, role definition, and family structure. Interventions might include

- Psychodynamic therapy, family counseling, cognitive behavioral techniques, problem solving
- Individual, family, group modalities
- Education, advocacy, and negotiation of systems
- Resource finding or development, networking
- Practical needs
- Discharge planning and referral

SUMMARY

The enhancement and extension of social work professional presence into the clinical, advocacy, research, and policy aspects of pain management is a natural outgrowth of the values, skills, and perspectives that are at the core of the profession. We are in the valuable position of being employed in many settings beyond the health care system and have the consequent responsibility to ensure that our practitioners recognize and maximize the opportunity to intervene with pain-related issues. It is the respectful thing to do.

REFERENCES

Altilio, T. (2004). Pain and symptom management: An essential role for social workers. In J. Berzoff & P. Silverman (Eds.), *Living with dying.* New York: Columbia University Press.

Barbarin, O. A., Whitten, C.F., & Bonds, S. M. (1994). Estimating rates of psychosocial problems in urban and poor children with sickle cell anemia. *Health and Social Work* *19*(2), 112–119.

Butler, D. J., & Beltran, L. R. (1993). Functions of an adult sickle cell group: Education, task orientation and support. *Health and Social Work, 18*(1), 49–55.

Caldirola, D. et al. (1983). Incest and pelvic pain: The social worker as part of a research team. *Health and Social Work, 8*(4), 309–319.

Claiborne, N. et al. (1999). Measuring quality of life in back patients: Comparison of Health Status Questionnaire 2.0 and Quality of Life Inventory. *Social Work in Health Care, 28*(3), 77–94.

Elliott, C. M. (1996). Through the glass darkly; chronic illness in the therapist. *Clinical Social Work Journal, 24*(1), 21–34.

Gilbert, M. C. (1999). Coping with pediatric migraine. *Social Work in Health Care, 28*(3), 21–34.

Glajchen, M. (2003). Role of family caregivers in cancer pain management. In R. K. Portenoy & E. Bruera (Eds.), *Cancer pain.* Cambridge, U.K.: Cambridge University Press.

Glajchen, M., Blum, D., & Calder, K. (1995). Cancer pain management and the role of social work: Barriers and interventions. *Health and Social Work, 20* (3), 200–206.

Golden, J. M., & Steiner, J. R. (1981). Unique needs of people with chronic pain. *Health and Social Work, 6*(3), 47–53.

Gross, R. J., Doerr, H., Caldiorala, D., Guzinski, G.M. et al., (1981). Borderline syndrome and incest in chronic pelvic pain patients. *International Journal of Psychiatry in Medicine, 10*(1), 79–96.

Hamilton, G. (1967). *Theory and practice of social casework.* New York: Columbia University Press, chap. 1.

Holden, G. et al. (1999). Evaluating the effects of a virtual environment (STARBRIGHT World) with hospitalized children. *Research on Social Work Practice, 9*(3), 365–382.

Hudgens, A. (1977). The social worker's role in a behavioral management approach to chronic pain. *Social Work in Health Care, 3,* 149–157, 1977.

Kelley, P., & Clifford, P. (1997). Coping with chronic pain: Assessing narrative approaches. *Social Work, 42*(3), 266–277.

Loscalzo, M., & Amendola, J. (1990). Psychosocial and behavioral management of cancer pain – The social work contribution. In K. M. Foley, J. J. Bonica, & V. Ventafridda (Eds.), *Advances in pain research and therapy.* (Vol. 16, pp. 429–442). New York: Raven Press.

Loscalzo, M., & Bucher, J. A. (1999). The COPE model: Its clinical usefulness in solving pain-related problems. *Journal of Psychosocial Oncology, 16*(3/4), 93–117.

Loscalzo, M. & Jacobsen, P. B. (1990). Practical behavioral approaches to the effective management of pain and distress. *Journal of Psychosocial Oncology, 8*(2/3), 139–169.

MacDonald, J. E. (2000). A deconstructive turn in chronic pain treatment – A redefined role for social work. *Health and Social Work, 25*(1), 51–57.

Marcus, M. (1986). Chronic pain – A social work view. *The Social Worker-Le-Travailleur-Social, 54*(2), 60–63.

Mendenhall, M. (2003). Psychosocial aspects of pain management: A conceptual framework for social workers on pain management teams. *Social Work in Health Care, 36*(4), 35–51.

Milner, C. J. (1980). Compassionate care for the dying person. *Health and Social Work, 5*(2), 5–10.

National Association of Social Workers (1999). *Code of Ethics.* Washington D.C.: National Association of Social Workers.

O'Neill, J.V. (2003). Pain: not only a health care problem. *NASW NEWS,* September.

Otis-Green, S. et al. (2002). An integrated psychosocial-spiritual model for cancer pain management. *Cancer Practice*, *10*, S58–S65.

Parry, J. K., & Smith M. J. (1987). A study of social worker's job satisfaction as based on an optimal model of care for the terminally ill. *Journal of Social Service Research*, *11*(1), 39–58.

Pecukonis, E. V. (1996). Childhood sexual abuse in women with chronic intractable back pain. *Social Work in Health Care*, *23*(3), 1–16.

Polinsky, M.L. (1994). Functional status of long-term breast cancer survivors: Demonstrating chronicity. *Health and Social* Work, *19*(3), 165–173.

Price, K. (1989). Quality of life for terminally ill children. *Social Work*, *34*(1), 53–54.

Ristock, J., & Pennell, J. (1996). *Community research as empowerment: Feminist links, postmodern interruptions*. Toronto: Oxford University Press.

Roff, S. (2001). Analyzing end of life care legislation: A social work perspective. *Social Work in Health Care, 33*(1), 51–68.

Rose, S. D., & Feldman, R. A. (1986, Fall). Research in social group work, *Social Work with Groups*, *9*(3).

Rousso, H. (1985). The relationship between physical disability and narcissism: A critique of the literature. *Clinical Social Work Journal*, *13*(1), 5–17.

Roy, R. (1981). Social work and chronic pain. *Health and Social Work*, *6*(3), 54–62.

Roy, R. (1984). Psychosocial assessment of chronic headache. *Health and Social Work*, *9*(4), 284–293.

Roy, R. (1985a). Chronic pain and marital difficulties. *Health and Social Work*, *10*(3), 199–107.

Roy, R. (1985b, Winter). The family and chronic pain. *International Journal of Family Therapy*, *7*(4).

Roy, R. A. (1986, Winter). Psychosocial perspective on chronic pain and depression in the elderly. *Social Work in Health Care*, *12*(2), 27–36.

Sieppert, J. D. (1996). Attitudes toward and knowledge of chronic pain – A survey of medical social workers. *Health and Social Work*, *21*(2), 130–122.

Subramanian, K. (1987). Group training for the management of chronic pain in interpersonal situations. *Social Work with Groups*, *9*, 55–57.

Subramanian, K. (1991a). The multidimensional impact of chronic pain on the spouse: A pilot study. *Social Work in Health Care*, *15*, 47–62.

Subramanian, K. (1991b). Structured group work for the management of chronic pain: An experimental investigation. *Research on Social Work Practice*, *4*, 32–45.

Subramanian, K. (1994). Long-term follow-up of a structured group treatment for the management of chronic pain. *Research on Social Work Practice*, *4*, 208–223.

Subramanian, K., & Rose, S. D. (1988a, Winter). Pain management treatment: A 2-year follow-up study. *Social Work Research and Abstracts*, *24*(4), 2–3.

Subramanian, K., & Rose, S. D., (1988b, Winter). Social work and the treatment of chronic pain. *Health and Social Work*, *13*(1), 49–60,

Substance Abuse and Mental Health Services Administration. (2002). Mental health, United States, 2000. Retrieved from http://www.mentalhealth.samhsa.gov/publications/allpubs/SMA01-3537/default.asp.

Weinberg, N., & Miller, N.J. (1983). Burn care: A social work perspective. *Health and Social Work*, *8*(2), 97–105.

20

Vocational Rehabilitation

Fong Chan, PhD, CRC, Gloria K. Lee, PhD, Kacie Blalock, MS, CRC,
Denise E. Catalano, MS, CRC, and Eun-Jeong Lee, MA

Work is considered therapeutic and essential for both the physiological survival and psychological well-being of people in contemporary societies (Chan et al., 1997; Dawes, Lofquist, & Weiss, 1968; Perrone, Perrone, Chan, & Thomas, 2000). Recognizing the importance of work, vocational rehabilitation professionals have consistently advocated for work as a fundamental human right of people with disabilities (Rubin & Roessler, 1995; Wright, 1980). Thus, the primary goal of vocational rehabilitation is to assist individuals with disabilities gain or regain their independence through employment or some form of meaningful activity (Parker & Szymanski, 1998; Rubin & Roessler, 1995). Several major vocational rehabilitation systems have been established to help people with disabilities achieve their employment goals, including, most notably, the state–federal vocational rehabilitation program and the private sector rehabilitation system.

Vocational intervention is also considered appropriate in medical rehabilitation programs (Chan, Parker, Lynch, & Johnson, 1986). However, Fawber and Wachter (1987) argued that traditional vocational rehabilitation, which typically occurs at the end of the treatment continuum, is insufficient for effecting successful job placement for persons with chronic illness and disability. Rather, they proposed a treatment-oriented placement process that seeks to distribute responsibility for vocational rehabilitation outcomes among all interdisciplinary team members throughout the entire treatment continuum. The important benefit of aggressive vocational rehabilitation programming within the overall operation of any treatment program is its capacity to provide direction, focus, and meaning to other therapies or services. Vocational rehabilitation

is therefore best regarded as a "pull factor" (i.e., providing direction and meaning) and, as such, is distinguished from other "push factor" therapies (i.e., those from which the hope is the client will become independent) (McMahon & Fraser, 1988). The probability of successful vocational outcome is enhanced when all therapies can be related to work and when work can be related to therapy. McMahon and Fraser provided specific suggestions regarding how interdisciplinary team members might approach their respective duties to maximize the level and stability of ultimate job placement.

The interplay between vocational adjustment and psychological adjustment is well documented in the rehabilitation and counseling literature (Perrone et al., 2000). Without any doubt, vocational rehabilitation can play an important role in enhancing psychosocial and vocational outcomes of people with disabilities including people with chronic pain. Hence, it is imperative for health care professionals who work with patients with pain in rehabilitation to become familiar with the philosophies, processes, and systems of vocational rehabilitation in order to incorporate return-to-work as one of the major rehabilitation goals for their clients and to utilize vocational rehabilitation as major treatment resources.

The purpose of this chapter is to (1) provide an overview of the state–federal vocational rehabilitation program, the private sector rehabilitation system, and the rehabilitation processes associated with these systems; (2) review best practices and outcomes of vocational rehabilitation within the context of evidence-based practice; and (3) discuss qualifications of vocational rehabilitation professionals in a multidisciplinary rehabilitation team.

VOCATIONAL REHABILITATION SYSTEMS

State–Federal Vocational Rehabilitation Program

The state–federal vocational rehabilitation program was established on a federal level in 1920, with the passage of the Smith–Fess Act (Public Law [PL] 66-236). This rehabilitation legislation offered grants-in-aid to state vocational rehabilitation agencies to provide vocational services to people with physical disabilities. The Vocational Rehabilitation Amendments of 1943 (PL 78-113), referred to as the Barden-LaFollette Act, extended state vocational rehabilitation services from serving only people who had physical disabilities as their primary disabilities to services for people with mental retardation and mental illness (Parker & Szymanski, 1998). Currently, vocational rehabilitation is defined by the 1998 Amendments to the Rehabilitation Act as a comprehensive sequence of services, mutually planned by the consumer and rehabilitation counselor, to maximize employability, independence, and integration and participation of people with disabilities in the workplace and the community.

Prior to 1973, the rehabilitation philosophy of the state–federal vocational rehabilitation program could be described as an economic-return philosophy. The emphasis was on returning as many people with disabilities to work as possible and at a minimal cost in order to demonstrate the cost-effectiveness of vocational rehabilitation programs. Therefore, the priority was to serve people with mild and moderate disabilities. With the passage of the 1973 Rehabilitation Act Amendments emphasizing services to people with *severe* disabilities, the philosophy of rehabilitation has evolved from an economic-return philosophy to a disability-rights philosophy — that is, working and living independently and assertively in the community is considered a civil right of people with disabilities. As expected, consumerism and empowerment become central to the vocational rehabilitation process in the state–federal program in recent years.

Rehabilitation counselors have the direct service responsibilities for working with people with disabilities in the rehabilitation process and are central to the success of the state–federal vocational rehabilitation program. Specifically, rehabilitation counseling has been described as a process where the counselor works collaboratively with the client to understand existing problems, barriers, and potentials to facilitate the client's effective use of personal and environmental resources for career, personal, social, and community adjustment following disability (Parker & Szymanski, 1998). In carrying out this multifaceted process, rehabilitation counselors must be prepared to assist individuals in adapting to the environment, change environments to accommodate the needs of the individual, and work toward the full participation of individuals in all aspects of society, with a particular focus on independent living and work (Jenkins, Patterson, & Szymanski, 1998).

To be eligible for services, an applicant for vocational rehabilitation services must (1) have a physical or mental impairment, which for such individual constitutes or results in a substantial impediment to employment, and (2) be able to benefit in terms of an employment outcome from vocational rehabilitation services. In addition, because of limited financial resources, vocational rehabilitation programs in their respective states are required to develop "order of selection" plans to prioritize services for people with disabilities (e.g., people with several significant functional limitations requiring multiple services over an extended period of time may receive the highest priority for services, while people with less severe disabilities may be placed on a waiting list). Currently, the federal government provides for 78.7% of the budget for state-run vocational rehabilitation programs, which translates roughly into about $2 billion in federal grants, matched by $645 million in state and local funds. Because of the federal reporting requirements, state-run vocational rehabilitation programs all follow a fairly standard rehabilitation process:

- Eligibility determination
- Rehabilitation plan development
- Service provision
- Job placement

During the eligibility determination phase, the focus of rehabilitation services is on diagnoses. Typically, a vocational rehabilitation client will be referred to diagnostic services such as general and specialty medical examinations, psychological evaluation, and vocational evaluation. The purpose of these diagnostic examinations is to determine functional limitations related to disability; to identify psychosocial, educational, and economic factors that might interact with disabilities to impede ability to work and live independently; to identify the strengths of the client; to develop appropriate vocational goals; and to identify services needed to achieve the client's immediate objectives and long-term vocational rehabilitation goals. During the service provision stage, the majority of the services provided to people with disabilities include restoration of physical function (e.g., surgery, prosthesis, or assistive technology); restoration of mental function (e.g., psychotherapy); academic, business, or vocational training; personal or vocational adjustment training; employment counseling; and job placement and job referral (Spitznagel, 2002).

As mentioned, the interplay between vocational adjustment and psychological adjustment is well documented in the rehabilitation and counseling psychology literature (Perrone et al., 2000). Rehabilitation health professionals working with clients with chronic pain condition should consider state-run vocational rehabilitation program as a potential resource for referral, especially if the client is interested in vocational assessment and counseling, vocational training, and job placement. State-run vocational rehabilitation programs are particularly appropriate for clients with limited financial means.

WORKERS' COMPENSATION AND INSURANCE BENEFITS SYSTEMS

The impetus for private sector rehabilitation (also known as proprietary rehabilitation and insurance rehabilitation) can be traced to the skyrocketing cost of workers' compensation in the 1970s (Chan & Leahy, 1999; Shaw, McMahon, Chan, Taylor, & Wood, 1997). Private sector rehabilitation grew in response to the demand for vocational rehabilitation services by workers' compensation insurance carriers (Matkin, 1995). Federal legislation also promoted the growth of private sector case management services. The 1970 Federal Occupational and Safety Health Act (OSHA) (PL 91-596) required the development of a National Commission on State Workmen's Compensation Laws. This commission issued a report in 1972 with 84 recommendations for improvement of the workers' compensation system, including recommendations related to vocational rehabilitation (Parker & Szymanski, 1998). The report suggested that not enough was being done to help injured workers to return to work and acknowledged the apparent problems in attempting to have the state–federal rehabilitation system serve the workers' compensation caseload (Matkin, 1995). It recommended the creation of specific rehabilitation units with medical/rehabilitation divisions. Funding for vocational rehabilitation was paid by employers, which resulted in many states enacting mandatory rehabilitation programs (Jenkins et al., 1998). By 1976, 27 states had developed some type of vocational rehabilitation program and, during the late 1970s and early 1980s, many more enacted mandatory provision of vocational rehabilitation within their workers' compensation laws. As a result, fewer and fewer workers' compensation and insurance benefits programs relied solely on the public rehabilitation program to return their claimants to work. The primary goal of private sector rehabilitation services is an early return to work and to minimize loss of earnings capacity by the injured worker to help mitigate insurer and employer losses. Since the 1970s, rehabilitation nurses and rehabilitation counselors have been hired in increasing numbers to provide medical and vocational case management services to workers' compensation recipients. As expected, the majority of injured workers served in private sector rehabilitation reported injuries to the head, neck, back, trunk, and the extremities, with back injuries appearing to be most prevalent, consisting of at least 50% of the workers' compensation cases (Davidson, 1994).

1. Return to work: same job, same employer
2. Return to work: same job modified, same employer
3. Return to work: different job (capitalizing on transferable skills), same employer
4. Return to work: same job, different employer
5. Return to work: same job modified, different employer
6. Return to work: different job (capitalizing on transferable skills), different employer
7. Return to work: different job with re-training, same or different employer
8. Return to work: self-employment

FIGURE 20.1 The return-to-work hierarchy. Adapted from R.E. Matkin (1995) in Foundations of the rehabilitation process, 4th ed. Austin, TX: Pro-Ed.

Historically, the vocational rehabilitation process within the context of the workers' compensation system is similar to the federal–state vocational rehabilitation process of eligibility determination, rehabilitation planning, treatment/intervention, and job placement. Vocational rehabilitation is defined as the array of services designed to facilitate and ease the return to work (Berkowitz, 1990). Typical services include, but are not limited to, vocational training, general skills upgrading, refresher courses, career counseling, on-the-job training program, job search, and consultation with employers for job accommodation and modification. It generally follows a path of least resistance and, inherently, minimal cost to the employer, while seeking to return the injured worker to preinjury vocational functioning. The return-to-work philosophy in private rehabilitation differs somewhat from the federal–state vocational rehabilitation program in that it is based on an economic model and not a human rights model. The optimal outcome for workers' compensation rehabilitation is to return the injured worker to his or her former employment capacity and not his or her optimal potential. The return-to-work hierarchy in private rehabilitation is presented in Figure 20.1.

After several decades of explosive growth, private sector rehabilitation has now witnessed a reduction in the use of vocational rehabilitation services in workers' compensation due to lack of concrete evidence for its efficacy (Berkowitz & Berkowtiz, 1991; Habeck, Kress, Scully, & Kirchner, 1994). As pointed out by Habeck (1996), the fundamental problem for this less than successful experiment of private sector rehabilitation is precisely due to the traditional vocational rehabilitation process it follows. Unfortunately, services from rehabilitation professionals most often are brought to bear after the critical, early period of intervention has passed, and the barriers to rehabilitation posed by time delay, litigation, and the demotivating effects of disincentives have occurred. Vocational rehabilitation in work disability is most often used as a "last-ditch effort" after all other attempts have failed. The rehabilitation process is typically controlled by third parties and removed from the worksite, and the essential relationship between employer and the employee in the rehabilitation process has been lost. In addition, the weakening of the work injury programs can be attributed to the failure of the rehabilitation counseling profession to carefully document justifications for rehabilitation services and the lack of empirical data to justify vocational rehabilitation (Chan et al., 2001; Currier, Chan, Berven, Habeck, & Taylor, 2001).

Disability management, a proactive work rehabilitation approach, is now touted as an alternative service paradigm to the reactive traditional individual-focused service approach in private sector rehabilitation. Akabas, Gates, and Galvin (1992) define disability management as follows:

> A workplace prevention and remedial strategy that seeks to prevent disability from occurring or, lacking that, to intervene early following the onset of disability, using coordinated, cost-conscious, quality rehabilitation service that reflects an organizational commitment to continued employment of those experiencing functional work limitations. (p. 2)

From the onset, employer commitment and involvement in disability prevention and management are considered central to the success of disability management. According to Habeck (1996), the practice of disability management can be differentiated from traditional private-sector vocational rehabilitation in terms of the ability of disability management specialists to (1) provide early intervention and return-to-work programming at the onset of injury or illness, (2) provide services at the workplace to a greater extent, and (3) maintain a proactive employer–employee focus. In response to the need to diversify private sector rehabilitation services, private rehabilitation specialists are beginning to change their practice approach to embrace the proactive approach of disability management in workers' compensation.

The evolvement of disability management practice can be best demonstrated within the 24-hour care (integrated benefits systems) framework of the managed care movement (Lui, Chan, Kowk, & Thorson, 1999). In general, 24-hour care means an employee is covered around-the-clock under a managed care package, whether or not an accident or illness is job related (Knight, 1997). Knight suggested group health (HMO) and workers' compensation carriers have much to learn from each other. She cited back injury as an example of how the same injury may be approached very differently by the two benefit systems. For example, rehabilitation professionals in workers' compensation benefit systems often recommend more frequent therapy and move aggressively to other methods, whereas group health practice stays with a treatment for a much longer time. She believes that return-to-work techniques would also help group health contain costs. In addition, the use of a single provider to treat an employee's occu-

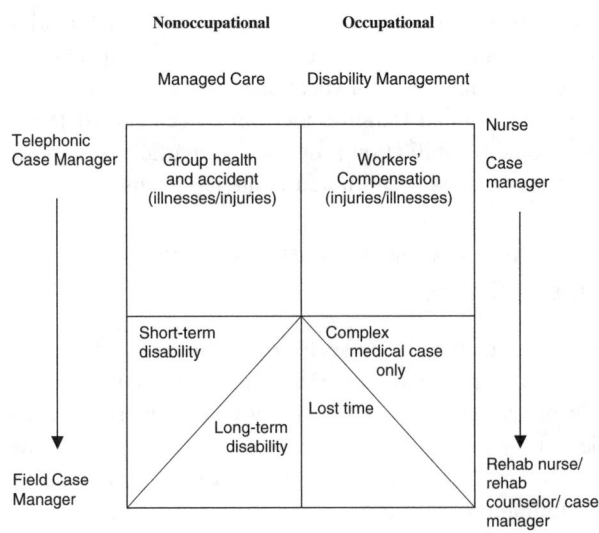

FIGURE 20.2 Case management interventions in an integrated health care system. From *Health Care and Disability Case Management* (p. 106), edited by F. Chan and M. Leahy, 1999, Lake Zurich, IL: Vocational Consultants Press. Reprinted with permission.

pational and non-occupational injuries would prevent duplicate claims and services.

Lui et al. (1999) provides a framework for conceptualizing health care and disability case management services that includes vocational rehabilitation counselors within an integrated health care system. Figure 20.2 depicts the relationship between occupational and non-occupational injuries/illnesses, the roles of vocational rehabilitation counselors in the intervention process, and a continuum of health care and disability case management interventions.

Under this model, a 24-hour care plan could benefit from both the advent of case management interventions developed for managed care (group health) and disability management (workers' compensation). At the highest level, the concern of the employers is the physical and mental health of their employees. Case management interventions at this level include wellness programs, health education, stress management training, and employee assistance programs to foster a healthy life style. Safety education and the design of an ergonomically sound workplace can help prevent work-related injuries. Case managers with a rehabilitation counseling, nursing, occupational therapy, or physical therapy background could be responsible for handling these prevention activities. A rehabilitation case manager who is also a certified rehabilitation counselor or a licensed professional counselor could also provide in-house vocational and psychosocial adjustment counseling.

Case management interventions at the time of illnesses and injuries would focus on *early* medical intervention and conflict resolution to avoid an adversarial relationship between the employee and the employer. Early intervention requires the cultivation of easy access to a network of quality providers such as rehabilitation counselors, who understand occupational health and return-to-work issues. Telephonic medical case management would be appropriate for most situations; the resulting compressed timeframe in medical management would reduce the number of cases that become lost-time cases. However, field-based case management may be required for catastrophic injuries or complicated medical cases (e.g., chronic pain). Examples of cases considered to be catastrophic include amputations, traumatic head injury, spinal cord injuries, severe burns, multiple factures, and crushing injuries. Other indicators that a field-based case manager/rehabilitation counselor intervention may be needed include when:

- The physician reports that the injured worker is unlikely to return to his or her former job
- The physician labels the period of disability as indefinite
- There is prolonged physical therapy
- There is prolonged excessive chiropractic treatment
- The physician cannot offer a specific treatment plan
- The medical diagnosis or prognosis is unclear
- Medical complications develop in addition to injury
- There are coexisting medical problems (e.g., epilepsy)
- The employee is unhappy with the treatment program, fails to follow the treatment plan, or seeks a second medical opinion
- Experimental, alternative, or otherwise unsubstantiated medical procedures are included in the treatment plan
- There is a psychiatric reaction to the injury or condition (e.g., depression)

Nursing case managers would be responsible for this level of care. For cases of severe injuries/illnesses resulting in disabilities (short/long-term disability or lost time), intensive medical case management would be required to ensure optimal medical rehabilitation. At the same time, the use of rehabilitation counselors to promote early *safe* returns to work may be extremely important. As soon as the client is medically stable and the functional capacity of the person can be accurately predicted, a vocational rehabilitation counselor would be assigned to conduct a functional job analysis, identify job accommodation needs, determine transitional alternative duties, and provide disability adjustment counseling to help the client cope with his or her disabling conditions. The goal is to help the client return safely to his or her previous level of employment as soon as possible. If unfeasible, the goal would be to help identify alternative job placement and/or retraining needs. In addition, the rehabilitation case manager would be involved in training job supervisors and co-workers regarding the on-the-job support needs of the disabled worker.

Recently, McMahon et al. (2000) documented a phenomenon of the progression of disability benefits (PODB). They defined PODB as the migration of workers with work-limiting disabilities as they move through a system of economic disability benefits resulting in their ultimate placement into the Social Security Disability Insurance (SSDI) system. An effective way to control the growth of the SSDI enrollees is to initiate programs that would reduce the flow of new persons onto these rolls. In this context, one could argue that health care and disability case management could be construed as one form of "service intervention." The Social Security Administration is currently exploring innovative ways (e.g., the ticket-to-work initiatives) to return SSDI recipients to gainful employment. It is clear that rehabilitation counselors can play a significant role in providing upstream services such as disability prevention, disability management, disruption of PODB, and downstream services such as vocational rehabilitation services for recipients of short-term disability, long-term disability, and SSDI benefits.

Vocational rehabilitation counselors in the private sector also play a significant role in forensic rehabilitation as vocational experts. Rehabilitation counselors can be retained to assess the preinjury work capacity/earning capacity and post-injury work capacity/earning capacity of clients as well as the life care planning needs of clients in workers' compensation, medical malpractice, third-party liability, and other personal injury litigations. The vocational expert plays a vital role in the hearing process by presenting evidence on behalf of either the plaintiff (injured worker) or the defendant (insurer, employer) (Lynch, Lynch, & Beck, 1992; Matkin, 1995; Weed & Field, 1994). This "forensic" role of the vocational case manager is becoming more common although recent legislative and policy initiatives have sought to diminish this litigious environment.

EVIDENCE SUPPORTING THE EFFECTIVENESS OF VOCATIONAL REHABILITATION

Evidence-based practice can be defined as a total process beginning with knowing what clinical questions to ask, how to find the best practice, and how to critically appraise the evidence for validity and applicability to the particular care situation (Chronister, Cardoso, Lee, Chan, & Leahy, 2005). The best evidence then must be applied by a clinician with expertise in considering the patient's unique values and needs. The final aspect of the process is evaluation of the effectiveness of care and the continual improvement of the process. Ottenbacher and Maas (1999) indicate that the "best evidence" for evidence-based practice is derived from a series of research study results that form an empirical consensus regarding the effectiveness of a specific treatment approach. Within the field of medicine, with its positivist scientific methods tradition, the "gold standard" for scientific evidence is randomized clinical trials, and the method of choice for determining the cumulative evidence of the effectiveness of a treatment is meta-analysis. Holm (2000) and Gray (1997) describe a hierarchy of levels of evidence from which professionals can formulate an empirical consensus and determine "best evidence" regarding the effectiveness of a treatment approach:

- Level 1 evidence is defined as strong evidence from at least one systematic review of multiple well-designed randomized controlled trials.
- Level 2 evidence is defined as strong evidence from at least one properly designed randomized controlled trial of appropriate size.
- Level 3 evidence is defined as evidence from well-designed trials without randomization, single group pre–post, cohort, time series, or matched case-controlled studies.
- Level 4 evidence is defined as evidence from well-designed non-experimental studies from more than one center or research group.
- Level 5 evidence is defined as opinions of respected authorities, based on clinical evidence, descriptive studies, or reports of expert committees.

EVIDENCE FOR THE FEDERAL–STATE VOCATIONAL REHABILITATION PROGRAM

As discussed, vocational rehabilitation services typically include several of the following: diagnostic evaluation, medical restoration, personal adjustment training, independent living training, job readiness training, vocational training, and job placement. The use of experimental research to validate the effectiveness of vocational rehabilitation is, unfortunately, uncommon due to the complex and holistic nature of the rehabilitation process (Johnston, Stineman, & Velozo, 1997). Contemporary vocational rehabilitation intervention encompasses a broad scope of services, spans along the medical–vocational rehabilitation continuum from acute care to community based services, and is provided through an array of disciplines (e.g., nursing, social work, and rehabilitation counseling) for individuals with diverse and complex impairments and disabilities. The process typically involves a range of personal and environmental processes and the interactions thereof, making it difficult to determine what aspects of

service delivery contribute to what outcomes (Johnston et al., 1997). Bolton (2004) contends that it would be virtually impossible to design and implement a randomized study to examine the overall effect of state-run vocational rehabilitation programs because clients who are eligible for services must be served and clients who are placed on waiting lists according to "order of selection" criteria are clients with less severe disabilities and therefore are very different from clients who receive vocational rehabilitation services immediately.

Conversely, counseling is a central, integrative activity that serves to unify the rehabilitation service delivery process. Within this context, there does exist a variety of *indirect* Level 1 evidence that suggests that the counseling context of rehabilitation service provision results in benefits to clients. Literally hundreds of experimental studies of the efficacy of counseling have been reported in the research literature during the past 50 years. The initial meta-analysis of these investigations concluded that clients benefit considerably from the various types of psychotherapeutic and counseling interventions (Smith & Glass, 1977; Smith, Glass, & Miller, 1980; Wampold, 2001). In a meta-analysis of 475 controlled outcome studies, Smith et al. (1980) demonstrated an average effect size of .85 standard deviation on the outcome measure of the treatment over the control group, indicating that the typical client receiving counseling was better off than 80% of those untreated but in need of counseling.

Additionally, the working relationship between the client and counselor, which is most often referred to in the literature as the "working alliance," has gained overwhelmingly strong empirical support as a primary influence on rehabilitation and counseling outcomes. Working alliance can be defined as (1) the client's affective relationship with the therapist, (2) the client's motivation and ability to accomplish work collaboratively with the therapist, (3) the therapist's empathic responding to and involvement with the client, and (4) client and therapist agreement about the goals and tasks of therapy.

In a meta-analysis involving thousands of studies designed to investigate the efficacy of counseling interventions on client outcomes, Wampold (2001) determined that it is common factors such as working alliance, empathic listening, and goal setting that underlie all psychotherapeutic approaches that affect outcomes, not techniques associated with specific theoretical orientations. He found that at least 70% of psychotherapeutic effects are due to common factors, 8% are due to specific factors (i.e., different theoretical orientations/techniques), and the remaining 22% was partially attributed to individual client differences. In a review of extant meta-analyses related specifically to the efficacy of working alliance, Horvath (1994) found a "robust relationship" between working alliance and positive counseling outcomes, with an average effect size of $r = .26$. Working alliance is especially conducive to active participation between clients and counselors in the rehabilitation process (Chan et al., 1997). Schelat (2001) surveyed 255 state vocational rehabilitation (VR) clients who were closed successfully or unsuccessfully in 1998 and found that all factors of working alliance (i.e., goal, task, and bond) are predictive of rehabilitation outcomes, with high scores strongly predictive of successful outcomes. Lustig, Strauser, Rice, and Rucker (2002) examined survey data of 2,732 VR clients during fiscal year 2000 and found that (1) employed clients had a stronger working alliance than unemployed clients ($d =$ .73; large effect), (2) a stronger working alliance was related to a more positive client perception of future employment prospects ($r = .51$; large effect), and (3) a stronger working alliance was related to employed rehabilitation clients' satisfaction with their current jobs ($r = .15$; small effect). Donnell, Lustig, and Strauser (2004) surveyed 305 individuals with mental illness and also found working alliance to be related to employment outcomes and job satisfaction. The results of these rehabilitation studies suggest that the working alliance may be an important aspect of vocational rehabilitation services that can lead to positive rehabilitation outcomes.

Promoting self-efficacy is another important aspect of vocational rehabilitation. Although skills training is frequently used to promote the self-efficacy of individuals with severe and persistent mental illness and alcohol and other drug abuse problems, the concept of skills training in the areas of social skills, coping skills, general life skills, and specific job skills is also applicable to individuals with other disabilities. Bolton and Akridge (1995) conducted a meta-analysis of skills training interventions for people with disabilities in vocational rehabilitation and found that outcome measures resulted in an estimated true effect size of +.93, suggesting substantial benefit to the typical participant.

In psychiatric rehabilitation, numerous narrative reviews indicated that skills training using behavioral methods is effective in teaching a variety of social and living skills to persons with mental health problems. Benton and Schroeder (1990), in a meta-analysis of the efficacy of social skills training for individuals with schizophrenia, found that 69% of the people receiving social skills training were better off than people without social skills training. People with alcohol dependence receiving social skills training and coping skills training also were found to maintain a higher number of abstinent days than people without such training (Drummond & Glautier, 1994; Eriksen, Bjornstad, & Gotestam, 1986; Hester & Miller, 2003). Hester and Miller indicate that the social and coping skills training approach is the most efficacious treatment in substance abuse rehabilitation.

Although it is not possible to conduct randomized clinical trials for state-run vocational rehabilitation services as an independent variable, the state–federal voca-

tional rehabilitation program is required by the Rehabilitation Act to conduct ongoing research to demonstrate the effectiveness of rehabilitation interventions on employment outcomes of people with disabilities. There is ample Levels 3 and 4 evidence that vocational rehabilitation is an effective intervention to enhance the employment outcomes of people with disabilities. For example, during fiscal 1995, state-run vocational rehabilitation programs provided services to 1.3 million people with disabilities (Kaye, 1998). In that year, 350,700 clients exited the system after receiving services. Of those who exited the system, 210,000 clients (60%) were considered to have been rehabilitated, and people with orthopedic impairments represented the largest group (21%) of successful cases. The 60% employment rate is significantly higher than the 33% employment rate for people with disabilities in the general population. Industrial (26%) or services jobs (25%) represented the most common job placement outcomes (Kaye, 1998). Dean, Dolan, and Schmidt (1999) conducted an independent study to examine the cost-effectiveness of the federal–state vocational rehabilitation program, using a quasi-experimental research design and found that vocational rehabilitation returns roughly $2.50 for each dollar spent. The Rehabilitation Service Administration (RSA) that administers the state–federal vocational rehabilitation program has reported to the Congress that every dollar spent on vocational rehabilitation to return people with disabilities to gainful employment generates $18.00 in tax payment to the government. Recently, RSA conducted a longitudinal study, using a random sample of 8,500 clients, to examine the effectiveness of vocational rehabilitation services (Research Triangle Institute, 2002). Clients of vocational rehabilitation services in the RSA study indicated the following:

- Their counselors were interested and concerned about their needs (70%) and were willing to listen to their ideas and suggestions (75%).
- They were given sufficient choice in the selection of their vocational goals (75%) and were satisfied with their goals (76%).
- Vocational rehabilitation services had helped them become employed (61%), and they obtained the job they wanted as a result of vocational rehabilitation services (63%).

PRIVATE SECTOR REHABILITATION

There is a paucity of outcomes research in private sector rehabilitation; no randomized clinical trail studies were found for private sector rehabilitation. Johnson, Chan, and Questad (1987) found that severity of disability, presence of an attorney, number of previous back injury claims, and lifting restrictions are strong predictors of case expenditures. Faimon, Hester, Decelles, and Gaddis (1987) reported the following 10 variables to be significant in predicting return-to-work status of clients with long-term disability claims: type of financial support received due to the disability, level of education, percentage of wage replacement of the predisability earnings, predisability occupation, type of disability, type of predisability employer group, gender, age, population density of area of residence, and marital status. Lam, Bose, and Geist (1989) examined all 216 workers' compensation case file closures (from 1983 through 1987) of a proprietary rehabilitation company and found that the most frequent medical diagnosis was low-back pain (54%). The rehabilitation rate of the company was 61%, with 36% of the clients returned to work with the same employer after rehabilitation and 25% to a new employer. Preinjury physical demands of the job and the residual physical capacity of the client were found to be the two most important factors differentiating the employed and unemployed groups.

Zaidman and Clifton (cited in Davidson, 1994) examined the long-term effectiveness of workers' compensation rehabilitation in Minnesota. Results of their study indicated that at the time of program completion, 69% of workers in the study returned to work with an average wage of $360 per week (93% of the average preinjury wage). Of the remaining 31% who did not return to work, one third settled the cases and about two thirds eventually returned to work. Zaidman and Clifton indicated that early intervention significantly increased the probability of returning to work; an acceleration of the intervention by 6 months raised the likelihood of retuning to work by two percent. They attributed two factors, older age (older than 40 years) and living in rural areas, as the main reasons for unsuccessful rehabilitation.

There are some empirical evidences that disability management is effective in controlling costs in work injury programs (Daiker, 1995; Lui, 1993; Tabak, 1995). Habeck, Leahy, Hunt, Chan, and Welch (1991) found that an organization's workers' compensation experience may be affected by organizational factors and behaviors that can be controlled or influenced. Further, Habeck et al. (1991) found that reduced incidence of work injury was associated with certain employer behaviors that emphasized safety and prevention. They found a lower incidence of workers' compensation claims in organizations that were more actively involved in safety, in the prevention and management of work injuries/disabilities, and in open and participatory relationships with employees. In a subsequent study of a larger random sample of employers, Habeck and colleagues (Habeck, Hunt, & VanTol, 1998; Habeck, Scully, VanTol, & Hunt, 1998) found fewer incidents that resulted in lost workdays and a lower incidence of total lost workdays and workers' compensation claims in organizations that were more diligent and thorough in their safety efforts. These employers devoted management time and resources to support prevention, to provide a proactive approach to return to work beginning as early as possible and involving all the parties in the process toward accommodation, and to create a work climate that values people.

UNUM Insurance Company of America, a leading provider of disability insurance, employee benefits, long-term care, and retirement products, works with high-risk employers at the organization level to implement disability management programs. These programs include prevention activities such as job restructuring, ergonomic engineering, and job safety training and early intervention such as stay-at-work services and other vocational rehabilitation intervention for injured worker receiving short-term disability or long-term disability benefits. A cost–benefit formula is applied based on the cost of services, the cost of providing present and future benefits, and employer and employee benefits. Using this formula, UNUM has calculated that for every dollar expended, there is a return in the range of $5 to $7 (Hunt, Habeck, Owens, & Vandergoot, 1996). Similarly, United Health Care, one of the largest health maintenance organizations with more than 2.7 million enrollees, using an integrated disability management service approach, also reported a five-to-one return on investment, supporting the benefits of disability management services in private sector rehabilitation (Hunt et al., 1996).

VOCATIONAL REHABILITATION OF INDIVIDUALS WITH CHRONIC PAIN

There has been limited research conducted to determine the effect of vocational interventions on the rehabilitation outcomes of chronic pain patients. Allaire, Li, and LaValley (2003) conducted a randomized controlled trial study to study the effectiveness of vocational rehabilitation for patients with rheumatic diseases. The researchers found that at 48-month follow-up, 97 of 122 (80%) participants in the vocational rehabilitation intervention group remained employed with no job loss, as compared with 72 of 120 people (60%) in the control group. They concluded that early intervention is the key to the successful outcomes, as vocational rehabilitation intervention is more effective for individuals who are at risk of losing their jobs but less effective for individuals who had already lost their jobs.

Multidisciplinary pain treatment programs have been popular to treat chronic pain disability when other methods have failed. Loeser, Seres, and Newman (1990) report an exemplary 3-week, structured, outpatient program, staffed by an attending physician and psychologist, physical and occupational therapists, pharmacists, nurses, and vocational rehabilitation counselors. The program has a strong, operant-behavioral focus where pain behaviors are not reinforced by staff, while coping and competency behaviors are reinforced. Patients are taught about chronic pain disability and rehabilitation, and about increasing their competency and perceived self-efficacy to cope with pain and the rehabilitation process through the cognitive-behavioral and psychoeducational components of the program. Aerobic exercise and strength-training, using quotas, are key components as well. Family members and/or significant others are required to participate to ensure that the environment to which the patient returns is modified. Vocational rehabilitation is frequently a significant component.

Aronoff, McAlary, Witkower, and Berdell (1988) also indicate that a multidisciplinary approach of chronic pain management involves specialists from various professions to modify pain and drug-seeking behavior and to interrupt the disability process as desirable. Aronoff et al. (1988) conducted a systematic review of various multidisciplinary pain treatment programs and reported return-to-work rates of these programs ranging from 50 to 100%. They found that vocational rehabilitation is an integrated component in many of these multidisciplinary pain programs. Vocational rehabilitation services provided by these programs typically include work hardening, job search, job placement, and job accommodations and modifications.

Recently, Turk (2002) reviewed the clinical effectiveness and cost-effectiveness of various medical and rehabilitation treatment programs for individuals with chronic pain. Some of the common treatment modalities include pharmacology, surgery, spinal cord stimulators, implantable drug delivery systems, and pain rehabilitation programs. He found that none of the single mentioned treatment modalities has a significant effect on the elimination of pain. However, multidisciplinary pain rehabilitation programs do provide comparable reduction in pain, in addition to having a significant improvement in other outcome measures such as decreased use of medication, decreased health care utilization, increased functional activities, increased rate of return to work, and higher closure of disability claims. In terms of vocational outcomes, Turk (2002) indicated that the return-to-work rates of patients participating in multidisciplinary pain rehabilitation programs ranged from 48 to 65%, as compared with other treatment modalities such as lumbar surgery (20%) and implanted medication delivery (5 to 31%). Turk (2002) remarked that most individuals who have been out of the workforce for a long period of time tend to have difficulty finding jobs due to the lack of updated vocational training, job search, and development skills and can therefore readily benefit from vocational rehabilitation interventions.

QUALIFICATIONS OF VOCATIONAL REHABILITATION PROFESSIONALS

As mentioned, rehabilitation counselors are central to the delivery of vocational rehabilitation services. Since 1967, rehabilitation counselor roles and functions studies have been conducted on a regular basis, with several receiving support from the Commission on Rehabilitation Counselor Certification (CRCC) and the Council on Rehabilitation Education (CORE) (Leahy, Chan, & Saunders, 2003; Leahy, Shapson, & Wright, 1987; Leahy, Szymanski, & Linkowski, 1993). Leahy et al. (2003) conducted the most recent roles and functions study, which involved a survey of a large random sample of certified rehabilitation counselors. This study examined the perceived importance of major job functions and knowledge domains that underlie contemporary rehabilitation counseling practice and credentialing. Results revealed seven major job functions as central to the professional practice of rehabilitation counseling in today's practice environment: (1) vocational counseling and consultation, (2) counseling interventions, (3) community-based rehabilitation service activities, (4) case management, (5) applied research, (6) assessment, and (7) professional advocacy.

The vocational counseling and consultation function was composed of four subfactors: (1) job development and placement, (2) career counseling, (3) employer consultation, and (4) vocational planning and assessment. The tasks associated with counseling interventions were organized into three subfactors: (1) providing individual, group, and family counseling; (2) building consumer–counselor working relationships; and (3) helping consumers cope with specific psychosocial issues related to disabilities. The community-based rehabilitation service function represents activities that involve such tasks as (1) researching resources and funding available in the community for consumers, (2) advocating for consumers and their families, (3) benefits counseling, (4) and marketing rehabilitation services to the community. The case management function involves such activities as (1) obtaining written reports regarding client progress, (2) developing rapport/referral network with physicians and other rehabilitation health professionals, (3) reporting to referral sources regarding progress of cases, and (4) making financial decisions for caseload management. The applied research function focuses primarily on applying research skills to evidence-based professional practice (e.g., reviewing clinical rehabilitation literature on a given topic or case problem). The assessment function represents assessment activities such as selecting and administering standardized tests and conducting ecological assessment. Finally, the professional advocacy function involves applying disability-related policy and legislation to daily rehabilitation practices. On a daily basis, the most frequently performed tasks fall under the functional domains of case management, professional advocacy, and counseling, followed by vocational consultation, assessment, utilization of community-based services, and applied research (for evidence-based practice).

Roles, functions, and knowledge validation research has been used to guide the development of graduate curriculum in rehabilitation counseling. Currently, there are

90 graduate programs in rehabilitation counseling accredited by the National Council on Rehabilitation Education. In addition, roles and functions studies have been used to develop national examinations for the certification of rehabilitation counselors with the certified rehabilitation counselor credential considered the "gold standard" for vocational rehabilitation professionals. The Certified Rehabilitation Counselor (CRC) credentialing process was the first, and considered to be the best, established certification mechanism in the counseling and rehabilitation professions within the United States (Leahy & Holt, 1993). The CRCC was officially incorporated in January 1974 to conduct certification activities on a nationwide basis. Since that time, more than 23,000 qualified professionals have participated in the certification process. Today, more than 14,000 CRCs are practicing in the United States and in several other countries (Shaw, Leahy, & Chan, 2005).

The primary purpose of certification is to provide assurance to rehabilitation counseling clients that services will be provided in a manner that meets the national standards of quality. Such standards are also considered by the profession to be in the best interest of the client (Leahy & Holt, 1993). To guide these standards, the CRCC established a Code of Professional Ethics for Rehabilitation Counselors, which delineates exemplary rehabilitation counseling as being a service that is client centered, is sensitive to an array of disabilities, is vocationally inclusive, encourages a collaborative and multidisciplinary focus, and is defined within the context of an established profession (Tarvydas, Peterson, & Michaelson, 2005). In addition to the CRC credential, many rehabilitation counselors hold related credentials such as the certified case manager (CCM), which has a strong focus on medical case management, or the certified disability management specialist (CDMS), which emphasizes vocational case management. The latter replaced the certified insurance rehabilitation specialist (CIRS) credential (Tarvydas et al., 2005).

There is good empirical evidence to support that counselors with a master's degree in rehabilitation counseling (the minimum requirement for a CRC) have better rehabilitation outcomes (Cook & Bolton, 1992; Szymanski, 1991; Szymanski & Danek, 1992; Szymanski & Parker, 1989). Szymanski and colleagues investigated the relationship of rehabilitation counselor education and experience to client outcomes in Arkansas, Maryland, New York, and Wisconsin. They found that counselors with master's degrees in rehabilitation counseling (or closely related fields) produce better outcomes for clients with severe disabilities as compared with counselors without such educational preparation. Frain, Ferrin, Wampold, and Rosenthal (2004) conducted a meta-analysis of rehabilitation outcome studies done between 1980 and 2004. They found a small educational effect of $d_+ = .20$, indicating that the average client who is served by a counselor with a master's degree in rehabilitation counseling is better off than 58% of those in the control group who are treated by a counselor without a master's degree in rehabilitation counseling. While the effect size of education is small, this is above and beyond the effect of interventions provided as part of the vocational rehabilitation process.

SUMMARY

There is some empirical evidence to support the efficacy, clinical utility, and cost-effectiveness of vocational rehabilitation in returning people with chronic illnesses or disabilities to competitive employment. Research reporting the cost-effectiveness ratios of public and private sector rehabilitation programs varies considerably, ranging from approximately a 3-to-1 ratio to an 18-to-1 ratio. Central to the delivery of vocational rehabilitation services is the rehabilitation counselor, with moderate support found for counselors with graduate training in rehabilitation counseling being more effective than counselors without degrees in rehabilitation counseling. There is strong empirical evidence to support the efficacy of certain components of the counseling process including working alliance and skills training. There is a paucity of research, however, addressing the efficacy of vocational rehabilitation for people with chronic pain. Yet, a high percentage of clients served by the public and private sector rehabilitation systems are reported to have orthopedic or back injuries indicating that vocational rehabilitation interventions might be useful for people with chronic pain. Nevertheless, programmatic outcome research conducted specifically to determine the effect of vocational rehabilitation on the psychosocial and vocational outcomes of people with chronic pain is warranted.

In closing, vocational rehabilitation services have been found to be underused and their values unappreciated in the treatment of patients with pain (Straaton & Fine, 1997). However, vocational rehabilitation represents a highly desirable alternative to a "work disability." Vocational rehabilitation can help prevent or minimize potentially devastating personal consequences of a work disability that often culminated in the loss of employment, reduce excessive dependence on other persons and health and social service agencies, and save enormous amounts of taxpayer and third-party money. For these reasons, rehabilitation health professionals need to be more knowledgeable and efficient in the early identification and referral of patients with pain to vocational rehabilitation.

REFERENCES

Akabas, S. H., Gates, L. B., & Galvin, D. E. (1992). *Disability management: A complete system to reduce costs, increase productivity, meet employee needs, and ensure legal compliance.* New York: AMACOM.

Allaire, S. H., Li, W., & LaValley, M. P. (2003). Reduction of job loss in persons with rheumatic diseases receiving vocational rehabilitation. *Arthritis & Rheumatism, 48*(11), 3212–3218.

Aronoff, G. M., McAlary, P. W., Witkower, A., & Berdell, M. S. (1988). Pain treatment programs: Do they return workers to the workplace? *Occupational Medicine, 3*(1), 123–136.

Berkowitz, M. (1990). *Returning injured workers to employment: An international perspective.* Geneva, Switzerland: World Health Organization/International Labor Office.

Berkowitz, M., & Berkowitz, E. (1991). Rehabilitation in the work injury program. *Rehabilitation Counseling Bulletin, 34*, 182–196.

Bolton, B. (2004). Counseling and rehabilitation outcomes. In F. Chan, N. L. Berven, K. R. Thomas (Eds.), *Counseling theories and techniques for rehabilitation health professionals* (pp. 444–465). New York: Springer.

Bolton, B., & Akridge, R. A. (1995). A meta-analysis of skills training programs for rehabilitation clients. *Rehabilitation Counseling Bulletin, 38*, 262–273.

Benton, M. K., & Schroeder, H. E. (1990). Social skills training with schizophrenia: A meta-analysis evaluation. *Journal of Consulting and Clinical Psychology, 58*, 741–747.

Chan, F., & Leahy, M. (1999). *Healthcare and disability case management.* Lake Zurich, IL: Vocational Consultants Press.

Chan, F., Lui, J., Rosenthal, D., Pruett, S., & Ferrin, J.M. (2002). Managed care and rehabilitation counseling. *Journal of Rehabilitation Administration, 26*(2), 85–97.

Chan, F., Parker, H. J., Lynch, R. T., & Johnson, K. (1986). Social standing of rehabilitation counselors in medical settings. *Rehabilitation Counseling Bulletin, 29*, 205–208.

Chan, F., Reid, C., Roldan, G., Kaskel, L., Rahimi, M., & Mpofu, E. (1997). Vocational assessment and evaluation of people with disabilities. *Physical Medicine and Rehabilitation Clinics of North America, 8*(2), 311–325.

Chan, F., Taylor, D., Currier, K., C.H. Chan, Wood, C., & Lui, J. (2001). Disability management practitioners: A work behavior analysis. *Journal of Vocational Rehabilitation, 5*(1), 47–56.

Chronister, J.A., Cardoso, E., Lee, G. K., Chan, F., & Leahy, M. (2005). Evidence-based practice in case management. In F. Chan, M. Leahy,, & J. Saunders (Eds.), *Case management for rehabilitation health professionals.* Osage Beach, MO: Aspen Professional Services.

Cook, D.W., & Bolton, B. (1992). Rehabilitation counselor education and case performance: An independent replication. *Rehabilitation Counseling Bulletin, 36*, 37–43.

Currier, F., Chan, F., Berven, N., Habeck, R., & Taylor, D. (2001). Job functions and knowledge domains for disability management practice: A Delphi study. *Rehabilitation Counseling Bulletin, 44*, 133–143.

Daiker, B. (1995). Managed care in workers' compensation. *AAOHN Journal, 43*, 422–427.

Davidson, C. J. (1994). Vocational rehabilitation services in workers' compensation programs. Evaluating research model effectiveness. *Benefits Quarterly, 10*(4), 49–57.

Dawes, R., Lofquist, L., & Weiss, D. (1968). *A theory of work adjustment* (rev. ed.). Minneapolis: Minnesota Studies in Vocational Rehabilitation, XXIII, Industrial Relations Center, University of Minnesota.

Dean, D. H., Dolan, R. C., & Schmidt, R. M. (1999). Evaluating the vocational rehabilitation program using longitudinal data. Evidence for quasi-experimental research design. *Evaluation Review, 23*(2), 162–189.

Donnell, C., Lustig, D., & Strauser, D. (2004). Working alliance: Rehabilitation outcomes for persons with severe mental illness. *Journal of Rehabilitation, 70*(2), 12–18.

Drummond, D. C., & Glautier, S. (1994). A controlled trial of cue exposure treatment in alcohol dependence. *Journal of Consulting and Clinical Psychology, 62*, 809–817.

Eriksen, L., Bjornstad, S., & Gotestam, K. G. (1986). Social skills training in groups for alcoholic: One-year treatment outcomes for group and individuals. *Addictive Behavior, 11*, 309–329.

Faimon, G. R., Hester, E. J., Decelles, P. G., & Gaddis, E. L. (1987). Return to work potential: Identification by the Menninger RTW Scale and by rehabilitation professionals. *Journal of Job Placement, 3*(2), 21–28.

Fawber, H. L., & Wachter, J. F. (1987). Job placement as a treatment component of the vocational rehabilitation process. *Journal of Head Trauma Rehabilitation, 2*, 27–33.

Frain, M., Ferrin, M., Wampold, B., & Rosenthal, D. A. (submitted). Rehabilitation counselor training: A meta-analysis of rehabilitation outcomes based on educational levels of the counselor.

Gray, J. A. M. (1997). *Evidence-based healthcare: How to make health policy and management decisions.* New York: Churchill Livingston.

Habeck, R.V. (1996). Differentiating disability management and rehabilitation. *National Association of Rehabilitation Professionals in the Private Sector Journal, 11*(2), 8–20.

Habeck, R.V., Kress, M., Scully, S. M., & Kirchner, K. (1994). Determining the significance of the disability management movement for rehabilitation counselor education. *Rehabilitation Education, 8*, 195–240.

Habeck, R.V., Leahy, M.J., Hunt, H.A., Chan, F., & Welch, E.M. (1991). Employer factors related to worker's compensation claims and disability management. *Rehabilitation Counseling Bulletin, 34*(3), 210–226.

Habeck, R. V., Scully S. M., VanTol, B., & Hunt, H. A. (1998). Successful employer strategies for preventing and managing disability. *Rehabilitation Counseling Bulletin, 42*(2), 144–162.

Hester, R. K., & Miller, W. R. (2003). *Handbook of alcoholism treatment approaches: Effective alternatives.* Boston: Allyn & Bacon.

Holm, M. B. (2000). Our mandate for the new millennium: Evidence-based practice. *American Journal of Occupational Therapy, 54,* 575–585.

Horvath, A. (1994). Research on the alliance. In A. Horvath & L. Greenberg (Eds.), *The working alliance: Theory, research, and practice* (pp. 259–286). New York: Wiley.

Hunt, H.A., Habeck, R.V., Owens, P., & Vandergoot, D. (1996). Disability and work. Lessons from the private sector. In J. L. Mashaw, V. Reon, R. V. Burkhauser, & M. Berkowitz (Eds.), *Disability, work, and cash benefits* (pp. 245–270). Kalamazoo, MI: Upjohn Institute for Employment Research.

Jenkins W., Patterson, J., & Szymanski E. M. (1998). Philosophical, historical, and legislative aspects of the rehabilitation counseling profession. In R. M. Parker & E. M. Szymanski (Eds.), *Rehabilitation counseling. Basics and beyond* (3rd ed., pp. 1–40). Austin, TX: Pro-Ed.

Johnson, K. L., Chan, F., & Questad, K. (1987). Statistical prediction in proprietary rehabilitation. *Rehabilitation Counseling Bulletin, 30,* 130–135.

Johnston, M. V., Stineman, M., & Velozo, C. A. (1997). Outcome research in medical rehabilitation. Foundations from the past and directions for the future. In M. J. Fuhrer (Ed.). *Assessing medical rehabilitation practices. The promise of outcomes research.* Baltimore: Paul H. Brookes.

Kaye, H. S. (1998, March). Vocational rehabilitation in the United States. *Disability Statistics Abstract, 20,* 1–4.

Knight, H. (1997). 24-hour care today. *The Case Manager, 8*(1), 39–42.

Lam, C. S., Bose, J. L., & Geist, G. O. (1989). Employment outcomes of private rehabilitation clients. *Rehabilitation Counseling Bulletin, 32,* 300–311.

Leahy, M., Chan, F., & Saunders, J. (2003). A work behavior analysis of contemporary rehabilitation counseling practices. *Rehabilitation Counseling Bulletin. 46,* 66–81.

Leahy, M. J., & Holt, E. (1993). Certification in rehabilitation counseling: History and process. *Rehabilitation Counseling Bulletin, 37,* 71–80.

Leahy, M. J., Shapson, P. R., & Wright, G. N. (1987). Rehabilitation counselor competencies by role and setting. *Rehabilitation Counseling Bulletin, 31,* 94–106.

Leahy, M., Szymanski, E., & Linkowski, D. (1993). Knowledge importance in rehabilitation counseling. *Rehabilitation Counseling Bulletin, 37,* 130–145.

Loeser, J., Seres, J., & Newman, R. (1990). Interdisciplinary multimodal management of chronic pain. In J. J. Bonica, C. R. Chapman, W. E. Fordyce, & J. D. Loeser (Eds.), *The management of pain in clinical practice* (pp. 2107–2120). Baltimore: Williams and Wilkins.

Lui, J. (1993). Trends and innovations in private sector rehabilitation for the 21st century. In E. Perlman & C. E. Hansen (Eds.), *Private sector rehabilitation: Trends and issues for the 21st century* (pp. 47–50). Alexandria, VA: National Rehabilitation Association.

Lui, J., Chan, F., Kwok, J., & Thorson, R. (1999). Managed care concepts in the delivery of case management services. In F. Chan & M. Leahy (Eds.), *Health care and disability case management* (pp. 91–120). Lake Zurich, IL: Vocational Consultants Press.

Lustig, D., Strauser, D., Rice, D., & Rucker, T. (2002). The relationship between working alliance and rehabilitation outcomes. *Rehabilitation Counseling Bulletin, 46,* 25–33.

Lynch, R. K., Lynch, R. T., & Beck, R. (1992). Rehabilitation counseling in the private sector. In R. M. Parker, & E. M. Szymanski (Eds.), *Rehabilitation counseling: Basics and beyond* (2nd ed., pp. 73–101). Austin, TX: Pro-ed.

Matkin, R. E. (1995). Private sector rehabilitation. In S. E. Rubin, & R. T. Roessler (Eds.), *Foundations of the vocational rehabilitation process* (4th ed., pp. 375–398). Austin, TX: Pro-Ed.

McMahon, B. T., & Fraser, R. T. (1988). Basic issues and trends in head injury rehabilitation. In S. E. Rubin & N. Rubin, (Eds) *Contemporary issues in rehabilitation counseling* (pp. 197–216). Austin, TX: Paul Brookes.

McMahon, B. T., Danczyk-Hawley, C. E., Reid, C., Flynn, B. S., Habeck, R.V., Kregel, J., & Owens, P. (2000). The progression of disability benefits. *Journal of Vocational Rehabilitation, 15,* 3–15.

Ottenbacher, K.J., & Maas, F. (1999). How to detect effects: Statistical power and evidence-based practice in occupational therapy research. *American Journal of Occupational Therapy, 53*(2), 181–188.

Parker, R. M. & Szymanski, E. M. (1998). *Rehabilitation counseling. Basics and beyond* (3rd ed.). Austin, TX: Pro-Ed.

Perrone, K.M., Perrone, P.A., Chan, F., & Thomas, K.R. (2000). Assessing efficacy and importance of career counseling competencies. *Career Development Quarterly, 48,* 212–225.

Research Triangle Institute International. (2002). Longitudinal Study of the Vocational Rehabilitation Program. Report 1: How Consumer Characteristics Affect Access to, Receipt of, and Outcomes of VR Services. Raleigh, NC: Author.

Rubin, S. E., & Roessler, R. T. (1995). *Foundations of the vocational rehabilitation process* (4th ed.) Austin, TX: Pro-Ed.

Schelat, R. K. (2001). The predictive capacity of the working alliance in vocational rehabilitation outcomes. *Dissertation Abstract, 61*(7-B), 3553.

Shaw, L., Leahy, M., & Chan, F. (2005). Case management: Historical foundations and current trends. In F. Chan, M. Leahy, & J. Saunders (Eds.), *Case management for rehabilitation health professionals* (pp. 3–27). Osage Beach, MO: Aspen Professional Services.

Shaw, L., McMahon, B.T., Chan, F., Taylor, D., & Wood, C. (1997). Survey of CORE accredited programs in rehabilitation counseling regarding private-sector case management. *Journal of Rehabilitation, 63*(2), 46–51.

Spitznagel, R. J. (2002). State/federal vocational rehabilitation program. In J. D. Andrew & C. W. Faubion (Eds.), *Rehabilitation services: An introduction for the human services professionals* (pp. 55–89). Osage Beach, MO: Aspen Professional Services.

Smith, M. L., & Glass, S. V. (1977). Meta-analysis of psychotherapy outcomes studies. *American Psychologist, 32,* 752–760.

Smith, M. L., Glass, S. V., & Miller, T. I. (1980). *The benefits of psychotherapy.* Baltimore: The Johns Hopkins University Press.

Straaton, K. V., & Fine, P. R. (1997). Addressing work disability through vocational rehabilitation services. *Bulletin on the Rheumatic Disease, 46*(3), 1–3.

Szymanski, E.M. (1991). The relationship of level of rehabilitation counselor education to rehabilitation client outcome in the Wisconsin Division of Vocational Rehabilitation. *Rehabilitation Counseling Bulletin, 35*, 23–37.

Szymanski, E. M., & Danek, M..M. (1992). The relationship of rehabilitation counselor education to rehabilitation client outcome: A replication and extension. *Journal of Rehabilitation, 58*(1), 49–56.

Szymanski, E. M., & Parker, R. M. (1989). Relationship of rehabilitation client outcome to level of rehabilitation counselor education, *Journal of Rehabilitation, 54*(4), 32–36.

Tabak, M. H. (1995, February). Merging managed care and workers' compensation. *Risk Management*, 16–19.

Tarvydas, V., Peterson, D., & Michaelson, S. D. (2005). Clinical decision-making and ethical issues in case management. In F. Chan, M. Leahy, & J. Saunders (Eds.), *Case management for rehabilitation health professionals* (pp. 144–175). Osage Beach, MO: Aspen Professional Services.

Turk, D. C. (2002). Clinical effectiveness and cost-effectiveness of treatments for patients with chronic pain. *The Clinical Journal of Pain, 18*, 355–365.

Wampold, B. (2001). *The great psychotherapy debate.* Mahwah, NJ: Lawrence Erlbaum Associates.

Weed, R.O., & Field, T.F. (1994). *Rehabilitation consultant's handbook* (rev. ed.). Athens, GA: Elliott & Fitzpatrick, Inc.

Wright, G. N. (1980). *Total rehabilitation.* Boston: Little Brown.

21

The Pharmacist Role in Pain Management

Gregory L. Holmquist, PharmD, BCOP

INTRODUCTION

Surveys of public opinion have consistently ranked pharmacy as a highly respected profession. In general, pharmacists are respected for their knowledge, integrity, compassion, ability to provide "down-to-earth" relevant information about medications, and overall friendly, courteous demeanor. In an outpatient setting, pharmacists often represent the last professional seen by a patient prior to implementing a medical treatment. Having the last interaction affords an opportunity to prevent problems overlooked by other health care professionals. As opposed to the respect shown to the pharmacy profession by many, pharmacists may be viewed by some as obstructionists. Waiting in long lines to pick up expensive medications, for which the insurance company will not authorize coverage, may lead to patient frustration. Frustration intensifies if the prescription is not ready or if the prescriber does not authorize the refill. Patients who perceive that a "drug" is the only answer or the chief solution to their condition may view the pharmacist as a roadblock to successful procurement of their "miracle." Unfortunately, in many of these circumstances, the pharmacist is the one who is blamed as the responsible party.

The dichotomy of viewpoints of the pharmacy profession is most likely related to the perception of the role of the pharmacist. Pharmacy is both a business and a profession. For the most part, the "business" of pharmacy encompasses retail and wholesale aspects of marketing and selling medications (both over-the-counter and prescription products), ancillary products (including everything from sun-tanning lotions to condoms), and a variety of products unrelated to the medical world (e.g., greeting cards, candy, and books). The business side of pharmacy includes large and small chain stores, community pharmacies, pharmaceutical companies, wholesalers, and others. The "profession" of pharmacy, usually referred to as "clinical pharmacy," can take place in any of the aforementioned business models. Clinical pharmacy is a broad term that usually refers to pharmacist's involvement in assuring that medications are handled, stored, and dispensed in the safest, most efficacious, and most clinically sound manner and that drug-related problems are minimized. Another term often used to describe the clinical activities of pharmacists is "pharmaceutical care." The American Pharmaceutical Association defines *pharmaceutical care* as patient-centered, outcome-oriented pharmacy practice. Pharmaceutical care is designed to promote health, prevent disease, and assess, monitor, initiate, and modify medication use to assure that drug therapy regimens are safe and effective.[1] Activities pertinent to the provision of pharmaceutical care include prevention of drug-related problems through review of medication regimens, medical records, and charts of outpatients, nursing home residents, and hospitalized patients; consultation with members of the health care team to assist in the design of clinically efficacious and cost-effective drug regimens; education of the lay public and health care providers on the appropriate use of medications and methods to prevent the occurrence of adverse effects; design and oversight of drug research; and numerous other clinical interventions that ultimately serve to enhance the medical care of patients. Both the "business" and the "profession" of pharmacy have changed dramatically in the past century[2] (Table 21.1). This has led to a consequent change in the practice of pharmacy and the role of pharmacists.

Fulfilling the pharmacy needs of the more than 50 million persons in the United States who suffer from pain

TABLE 21.1
The Changing Role of Pharmacy

Time Period	Key Practice Points
Late 1800s	• Independently owned stores predominated
	• Most owners of pharmacies never attended pharmacy schools; training occurred through apprenticeship
	• Common name for owner was "druggist"
	• Main job was selling patent medicines and supervising the sale of sodas, candy, and cigars, with prescription drug business secondary
	• Most prescriptions were mixtures of opium, ipecac, quinine, iron, digitalis, belladonna
	• Hospital pharmacists only in the largest and most established institutions
Early 1900s	• Food and Drugs Act passed in 1906
	• Harrison Narcotic Act passed in 1914
	• First requirement for pharmacy school diploma for licensure in New York in 1905
	• During prohibition pharmacies handled prescriptions for medicinal alcohol; hospitals hired pharmacists to provide inventory control and safeguard of medicinal alcohol supplies
	• Drugstore soda fountains replaced taverns as social gathering places during prohibition (1920–1933)
	• Hospital pharmacists made effort to differentiate themselves from community pharmacists via associations
	• American Association of Colleges of Pharmacy (AACP) adopted a 4-year bachelor's degree as the national requirement (1928)
Mid-1900s	• Pharmacists the only medical professionals exempted from service in World War II
	• Supreme Court ruled that FDA could enforce its designation of prescription-only status for certain medications (1948)
	• Durham–Humphrey Amendment to the Food, Drug and Cosmetic Act resulted in removing almost all discretionary latitude of pharmacists in determining prescription versus nonprescription status
	• Mass manufacturing reduces need for pharmacist to compound prescriptions leading to the era of "count and pour"
	• American Pharmaceutical Association (APhA) (1952) code of ethics for pharmacists delineates pharmacist role as "safeguarding the preparation, compounding and dispensing of drugs and the storage and handling of drugs and medical supplies"; the pharmacist is instructed to "not discuss the therapeutic effects or composition of a prescription with a patient" but instead to send the patient to the physician for such discussions
	• In addition to numerous penicillin derivatives, introduction of numerous new medications in the 1950s that influence the outcomes of diseases (warfarin, chlorpromazine, methotrexate, reserpine, tolbutamide, hydrochlorothiazide, hydrocortisone, and imipramine)
	• Five-year degree instituted as the norm for pharmacists (1960)
Late 1900s	• Clinical pharmacy role emphasized at Hilton Head conference (1985)
	• Model of pharmaceutical care established that defines the role of pharmacists to identify and prevent drug-related problems
	• State and federal laws allow for expanding the role of pharmacy technicians to free pharmacist time for clinical interventions
	• Omnibus Budget Reconciliation Act of 1990 (OBRA '90) recognized pharmacists as professionals whose expertise can be effectively utilized to promote rational outcomes from drug therapy
	• Institution of automated prescription filling machines separates the pharmacist farther from the "count and pour" functions
	• Doctor of Pharmacy degree (Pharm.D.) established as the national requirement for pharmacists
	• Most states mandate that pharmacists provide education (counseling) to patients receiving new prescriptions

Note: Adapted from Higby, G. J. (1997). *American Journal of Health-System Pharmacy, 54,* 1805.

can be complex, challenging, and time-consuming. Most patients with chronic pain syndromes will at some point in their life require palliation with multiple medications including simple analgesics (acetaminophen, aspirin, nonsteroidal anti-inflammatory drugs [NSAIDS]), adjuvant agents (antidepressants, anticonvulsants, local anesthetics, N-methyl-D-aspartate [NMDA], receptor antagonists, muscle relaxants, topical agents, etc.), and opioids. Furthermore, patients with pain conditions often require the prescribing (and endless refilling) of large quantities of multiple medications for a myriad of associated symptoms such as insomnia, depression, anxiety, and muscle spasms. Guidelines and expert opinion[3-24] suggest that medications should not be used as a sole strategy in the comprehensive

management of pain syndromes, nor should they be viewed as "quick fixes." Unfortunately, many patients with pain syndromes have inflated, and often unrealistic, expectations for the chief purpose of medications. Pharmacists must recognize that there are many opportunities to affect the care of these patients, both positively and negatively, as well as to play a fundamental role in reinforcing key messages regarding the role of medications for pain.

Despite reports of pain-focused pharmaceutical care services, [25-29] studies of practicing pharmacists have generally shown an inadequate level of knowledge about the therapeutics of pain management[30] and the laws and regulations governing the use of opioid analgesics[31]. Before discussing the potential positive roles of the pharmacist in pain management, it is vital to present a brief discussion of one key area in which the pharmacist can be a barrier to effective pain management. This area is the conflict in the pharmacists' perceived roles in advocating for strong pain medications (i.e., opioids) versus their stewardship of controlled substances. For example, from the patient perspective, it seems that some pharmacists are excessively suspicious of them and their motivations for having pain or "wanting" a pain medication, excessively worried about "addiction," and excessively nervous about dispensing a prescription for anything other than small quantities of widely recognized pain medications. The patient is often scrutinized in a suspicious manner whenever a prescription for a pain medication is presented.

Granted, an appropriate role of the pharmacist is to ascertain the safety, validity, and clinical appropriateness of prescribed medication(s). However, suspicions may be exaggerated for certain pain medications, the number of refills listed, the perceived legality of the prescription, and among other things, the number of pills prescribed (perhaps pharmacists wondering to themselves, "Was it supposed to be 100 tablets or was that '10' changed to a '100' by the patient by the addition of a '0'?"). Furthermore, without adequate clinical information relating to the patient's pain condition, the pharmacist may become nervous about the patient taking the medication on a "regular basis." Counseling the patient, the pharmacist may erroneously state, "Only take this medication when and IF you have pain" (giving the subliminal message, "These 100 pills better last a lifetime!"). Pharmacists who focus their role toward being "drug police" versus being patient advocates also increase the reluctance of physicians to prescribe pain medications. Using the drug police mentality, pharmacists sometimes turn their suspicions to the prescriber, (perhaps muttering to themselves, "Wow, that doc sure does prescribe a lot of pain meds!").

Practitioners who were once willing to provide pharmacological interventions become frustrated with justifying the validity of pain medication prescriptions to this type of pharmacist. Pharmacists who do not possess an in-depth understanding of up-to-date pain management principles and current controlled substances policies may compound the problem further. Drawing the wrong conclusion, the pharmacist may consider that the chronic use of certain pain medication prescriptions (e.g., opioids) is "poor practice," "marginally legal," or "not in the patient's best interest." Ultimately, the pharmacist who envisions his or her role more in the realm of drug police may deem it necessary to interrogate the physician regarding the validity of the prescription, may make skeptical, condescending comments to patients regarding their intent for use of the medication(s), or may even go so far as to report the physician to the medical board or Drug Enforcement Agency. Obviously, these actions are time-consuming and costly to the prescriber, are intimidating and unsettling to the patient, and do not further the goals of care.

While the above discussion may give the appearance that the pharmacist's role in managing pain is mainly counterproductive, it is the author's opinion that the majority of pharmacists provide a benefit to the interdisciplinary team approach. The remainder of this chapter highlights key roles for pharmacists in pain management, from both the "business" and the "professional" side of pharmacy.

Americans spend more than $75 billion per year on prescription and nonprescription drugs. Problems associated with improper use of medications are illustrated by the following:

- Improper use of prescription medicines due to lack of knowledge costs the economy an estimated $20 billion to $100 billion per year.[1]
- American businesses lose an estimated 20 million workdays per year due to incorrect use of medicines.[1]
- The failure to have prescriptions dispensed and/or renewed has resulted in an estimated cost of $8.5 billion for increased hospital admissions and physician visits — nearly 1% of the country's total health care expenditures.[1]
- Documented records indicate that medication errors are responsible for more than 7,000 deaths annually[32]
- An FDA review found that there were more than 56,000 emergency room visits a year due to acetaminophen overdoses, about a quarter of them unintentional. Additionally, it found that there were about 100 deaths annually associated with acetaminophen.[33]
- Conservative estimates from U.S. data suggest that on an annual basis more than 100,000 people are hospitalized for gastrointestinal bleeds secondary to NSAIDS and, of those, 16,500 die.[34]
- In 2001, of 22,242 poisoning deaths in the United States, 14,078 (63%) were unintentional. In an analysis of 11 states, the substances associated most frequently with unintentional and undetermined poisoning deaths were cocaine (15%), alcohol (8%), heroin (7%), antidepressants (5%), benzodiazepines (5%), and methadone (5%). Nonspecific categories, such as "other opioids" (e.g., codeine, morphine, oxycodone, and hydrocodone), "other synthetic narcotics," "other and unspecified narcotics," and "other and unspecified drugs, medicaments, and biological substances" accounted for approximately half of all the documented substances associated with unintentional and undetermined poisoning deaths.[35]

- In an unpublished study, two out of three terminally ill persons experiencing moderate to severe pain refused additional pain treatment. The top reason patients with cancer refused additional pain treatment was fear of addiction.

EDUCATION

All the above and other problems could perhaps be influenced by one of the most important and influential roles of the pharmacist: education. Patient and family education is a vital component of the pharmacist's professional and ethical duty. A position statement by the American Society of Health System Pharmacists affirms, "Pharmacists can contribute to positive outcomes by educating and counseling patients to prepare and motivate them to follow the pharmacotherapeutic regimens and monitoring plans."[36] The general broad-based goals of patient education surrounding pain medications are to ensure that the patient fully understands (1) the role of the medication for their pain syndrome; (2) the potential benefits, risks, and side effects; (3) what action to take should a side effect occur; (4) how to properly use, store, and if needed, dispose of the medication; (5) potential drug–drug interactions with current therapies, newly prescribed medications, and any subsequently purchased over-the-counter medications; (6) action to take in the event a dose is missed; (7) the availability or lack of refills and the process to obtain refill authorizations; and (8) techniques for self-monitoring of drug therapy. And, of course, the pharmasist needs to answer any questions the patient might have.

In addition to broad-based educational objectives, there are specific pain medication–related teaching opportunities that the pharmacist is the ideal professional to address. First, prior to implementation of any pharmacological intervention, pharmacists can assist patients to clearly understand key concepts regarding the appropriate role for analgesics and adjunctive medications in the overall treatment plan. Second, because many patients have fears of taking medications in general and these fears are often magnified with opioid analgesics, pharmacists can be key to allaying unwarranted fears. Key discussion/education topics to meet these two specific areas include teachings on physical dependence versus addiction risks, tolerance concerns, medication agreements (also referred to as "medication contracts"), "trial-and-error" approach to adjuvant medications, benefits versus risks of simple analgesics, role of maintenance opioid therapy and adjuvant medications, pharmacological rationale of short-acting versus long-acting time-release opioids, role of topical therapies, and nonpharmacological alternatives. The fear of addiction is so engrained in the minds of patients and families that it often becomes the greatest barrier to the willingness of patients and family members to administer these medications, even when pain is at a high level during the final weeks, days, and hours of life. A frank and open discussion between the pharmacist and the patient/family will not just allay fears, but will increase the likelihood of proactive pain management.

The pharmacist can also be a valuable asset in reinforcing key concepts and messages conveyed by other members of the pain team. When a patient hears a message consistently repeated by various respected health professionals, the message can become a powerful influence to changing behaviors that ultimately will improve the functioning and care of the patient. For example, many patients with chronic pain have inflated views of the role of a medication for improving their pain and functioning. Some patients may opt out of lifestyle modifications, physical therapy, and rehabilitation programs if they can "just take a pill to feel better." This erroneous mentality, a very passive approach, can lead patients to becoming more dysfunctional over time. Passive activities (taking medications, massage therapies, etc.) may provide a certain level of comfort, but they often do not improve the functionality of the patient over the course of time. A chief strategy of many pain clinics is to assist patients improve their functioning by establishing exercise, physical therapy, socialization, and recreational goals, and then, over a period of time, having the patient incrementally increase activities in these areas. From a behavioral viewpoint, it is suggested that therapies that divert the patient's attention from their pain are more likely to improve function, and vice versa.[37] The pharmacist, by reinforcing the message that "medications are only one part of the strategy to deal with chronic pain" and emphasizing "the need to engage in active strategies (e.g., regular exercise, weight loss, physical therapy)" can assist in balancing the patient's perceptions and behaviors regarding the use of pain medications. This ultimately will improve patient adherence to a comprehensive interdisciplinary plan, resulting in improvements in functioning and pain. Examples of key messages that pharmacists can reinforce are summarized in Table 21.2.

The members of the pain team or hospice team, including the physician, psychologist, nurse, physical therapist, physiatrist, social worker, and others, look to the pharmacist as the definitive source of medication information. Providing education to these professionals affords an opportunity to positively affect the use of medications to manage pain. Today's graduating pharmacist has undergone 6 years of college and graduate education to attain the Doctor of Pharmacy degree. Additionally, after graduation, many pharmacists attend 1- or 2-year general or specialty residencies and/or fellowships. The training the pharmacist receives not only focuses on drug knowledge, but also includes courses on literature evaluation, research methodology, biostatistics, pathophysiology of diseases, and much more. The advanced training adapts the pharmacist well to the role of providing education to the other

TABLE 21.2
"Key Messages" to Patients with Pain Regarding Medications

Message

1. The pain team uses many methods to help control your pain. Medications may or may not be the best method for your pain condition.
2. Medications alone typically are not able to totally relieve your pain. Based upon the type of pain you have, we may use medications other than opioids (narcotics) to help control your pain.
3. In order for the pain team to obtain the most effective pain control for your condition it is important that you help us monitor your level of comfort, sleep, exercise, and activities by keeping a daily diary. Bring this diary with you to each doctor appointment.
4. Many of the medications we use to help control your pain take several weeks to work. You must continue taking the medications as directed in order for the pain team to know if this medication will work for you. Also, report any bothersome side effects to your doctor.
5. If it is decided that the use of an opioid (narcotic) is the best choice for your pain condition, it is important that you follow all directions exactly. Having to take opioids (narcotics) for pain does not mean that you automatically will become an "addict."
6. Medications more commonly used to treat depression or seizures can be effective in certain pain conditions. Using one of these medications for your pain condition does not necessarily mean that we think you are depressed or that the pain is only in your mind.
7. Because pain conditions change over periods of time, we may need to change medications, increase the dose of your current medication, and/or attempt to decrease the amount of pain medication you are taking.
8. The right dose of a pain medication is the lowest dose that works.
9. Constipation is one of the most frequent side effects of pain medications. The pain of constipation can sometimes be worse than the pain we are treating with the medications. It is important that you take stool softeners and mild laxatives prescribed by your physician. The goal is to have one bowel movement every day or every other day.
10. Taking medications other than those prescribed by your physician can cause serious side effects. Let the pain team know of all medications you are taking (including those medications you buy over-the-counter).
11. Anxiety can be caused by pain as well as cause more pain. However, it is best not to use medications to control anxiety.
12. Taking too much over-the-counter pain relievers such as acetaminophen (Tylenol) or ibuprofen (Advil, Motrin) or naproxen (Alleve) can be harmful to your kidneys and liver. Let your doctor or pharmacist know if you plan on using any of these medications.

health care providers on the team. Education can occur as one-on-one consults, formal lectures, informal in-services, continuing education articles, written and oral summaries of published studies, formulary reviews, written educational materials for patients, treatment algorithms, and a host of other activities that add value to the care of the patient with pain. The use of medications, especially opioids, for managing pain can be a controversial issue. Pharmacists lend credibility to medication decisions by factual analysis of studies. Evidenced-based decisions are becoming a hallmark of good medical practice. Pharmacists are well trained to quickly review the medical literature, offer a science-based critique, and distill key points of the literature into a clinically sound recommendation.

Finally, advocacy represents an indirect, but very important educational opportunity. Patient advocacy uses the knowledge and compassion of a pharmacist to informally educate practitioners. Because of the inherent trust in pharmacists, patients will often disclose information to a pharmacist that would not be shared with other members of the health care team. Advocacy is an active role in which the pharmacist, in listening to the patient or in reviewing the medication record, uses his or her extensive drug knowledge to compassionately encourage and persuade a practitioner to prescribe a needed medication or discontinue an unneeded or side-effect-prone medication. Advocacy centers on the patient's palliative care needs and uses good communications skills to educate the practitioner, allay myths and fears, and instill a confidence in the pre-

scriber that the care of the patient will be improved if the pharmacist's recommendation is implemented.

COLLABORATION

Collaborative drug therapy affords an opportunity for the pharmacist to work directly with the physician and others to design regimens that are safe and clinically effective. The team approach is designed to maximize the patient's quality of life, reduce the frequency of avoidable drug-related problems, and improve the overall benefits of medications. Collaboration puts the patient at the center of a team that includes a pharmacist, a physician, and other health care professionals. It includes basic dispensing functions, drug information services, the solving of patient-related and medication-related problems, and decision making regarding drug prescribing and monitoring and drug regimen adjustments.[38] While there are no published studies suggesting direct measurable benefits of collaboration in the area of pain management, several studies have assessed pharmacist participation in drug therapy decisions in a variety of settings, including pharmacy-based disease management and on hospital rounds.[39,40,41] In these and other published studies, pharmacist collaboration in drug therapy has been deemed successful, leading to improved patient care and safety and lowered medical costs.

Physicians collaborating with pharmacists regarding complex pain management cases have an opportunity to simplify drug therapy choices, minimize the risk of drug-related problems, and co-develop unique medication regimens. Patients with chronic pain or those who are terminally ill with end-of-life pain often are receiving multiple medications. Patients with pain are at higher risk for drug interactions and adverse effects, as they often require the simultaneous administration of multiple medications for pain, other symptoms, and underlying conditions not related to pain, yet all are often vital to the overall care of the patient. Collaboration implies that the pharmacist will provide recommendations to the physician regarding several aspects of therapy, including (1) selection of new medications that will not interact with current medications; (2) discontinuance of medications that are ineffective or that have a high risk of interacting with current medications deemed as essential; (3) dose reduction or dose increase of interacting drugs to avoid toxicities and maintain maximal efficacy; (4) route selection and information on how to administer medications via unique routes (e.g., inhalation therapy, buccal absorption, transdermal delivery) to ensure adequate serum levels and clinical efficacy; and (5) information on third- or fourth-line options, when other evidence-based, standard-of-care options have failed to improve the quality of life of the patient with pain. The pharmacist is skilled and adept in reviewing complex medication scenarios and making recommendations for modifications not just to simplify the administration of the medication regimen, but also to minimize adverse effects and drug interactions. Collaboration with a pharmacist can greatly assist the physician who has exhausted "standard" options.

DRUG SAFETY

Medications have the power to heal and the power to cause tremendous harm. For the patient with pain, the goal of any medication is to improve the overall quality of life more than the side effects of the medication diminishing it. Many patients with chronic pain and cancer pain will require the use of multiple medications for years, potentially decades, and perhaps even the rest of their lives. Given the longevity of medication use, patients with pain are at risk for serious adverse events. Given the multiple medications prescribed, they are at risk for drug–drug interactions. The pharmacist is in a unique position to be a guardian of drug safety. The pharmacist is mandated by law to maintain comprehensive medication profiles for every patient. Because most medication profiles are computerized, it is a simple process to examine for patterns of dangerous drug use. Additionally, most pharmacies have computerized prescription entry systems that are programmed to readily identify serious and potentially serious drug interactions.

A key example suggestive of how pharmacists can use information from medication profiles to improve drug safety in patients with pain relates to acetaminophen toxicity. Many patients are unaware of the risk of developing hepatotoxicity from the consumption of excessive doses of acetaminophen products or from the combination of chronic alcohol consumption and acetaminophen. Many patients with pain are also unaware that trade name analgesic combination products such as Vicodin®, Lortab®, Norco®, Lorcet®, Tylox® contain large amounts of acetaminophen. Furthermore, patients often do not make the connection between the common brand name of acetaminophen (Tylenol®) and the warnings given by the pain team regarding not to exceed the maximal daily doses of acetaminophen. The pharmacist, via computerized patient profiles, can easily review months and years of medication use, readily compute the average daily amount of acetaminophen (from all sources) that the patient is consuming, and instantly determine if the patient is at risk for acetaminophen-induced toxicity. Collaboration with the physician to develop a treatment plan to reduce average daily acetaminophen consumption can prevent 1 of the 100 plus deaths associated annually with this commonly used analgesic.

Another key drug safety measure that pharmacists can influence includes recognition and differentiation between patient behaviors that are typical of drug abuse, diversion, or addiction versus those of untreated pain. While the vast majority of patients who use opioids for pain do so in a manner consistent with the directions prescribed by the physician and only a small percentage of patients receiving opioids for pain become iatrogenically addicted, pharmacists have an ethical obligation to ensure that all drugs are used in the safest possible manner and only for the medical condition prescribed. There is a fine balance that a pharmacist must walk between being compassionate and being duped.

Pharmacists should not overbalance their perceived duty as drug police with their duty to ensure that patients are respected, believed, and given the dignity that everyone deserves. Pharmacists should be outspoken on both the negative aspects of drug abuse and the shortcomings of poor pain management. Pharmacists understand the pharmacological basis for "physical dependence" and that it is not to be equated with "addiction." Pharmacists understand how "tolerance" influences drug dosing. Patients who are erroneously labeled "drug seekers," when in fact they have a legitimate pain that is not being managed, are often denied prescriptions for opioid analgesics or have received very limited quantities. Patients denied appropriate analgesics often desperately consume excessive dosages of over-the-counter analgesics (including alcohol), which can lead to serious adverse effects.

Other drug safety activities performed by pharmacists include verifying medication dosages and correcting errors; interpreting and confirming poorly legible or illegible handwritten prescriptions; ensuring appropriate use of medication delivery systems; calculating and verifying opioid dose conversions, reviewing medication profiles for medications that might be contraindicated due to patient specific factors (e.g., age, renal dysfunction, allergies); recommending therapies to counteract the adverse effects of analgesics; ensuring the integrity of sterile products for intravenous, intrathecal, or epidural use; and correcting erroneous and mythical pain management information that patients receive from uninformed health care practitioners, fearful family members, and unscrupulous Internet sites.

COMPOUNDING

In the 1930s and 1940s, pharmacists compounded about 60% of all medications. During the 1950s and 1960s, as more drugs were mass-produced, compounding declined. Beginning in the 1980s, compounding began to reemerge as a way to meet specific patient needs. Today, according to the Professional Compounding Centers of America, some 43,000 prescriptions — about 1% of all prescriptions — are compounded each day. A "compounded medication" is a customized medication prepared by a pharmacist according to a doctor's specifications to meet an individual patient need. Compounded medications can be specialized preparations for oral, sublingual, transdermal, topical, intravenous, subcutaneous, intra-articular, inhalation, and spinal use. Conventional medicine has usually accepted the idea that some patients are not good candidates for mass-produced drugs. They may be allergic to preservatives or dyes in the drugs or sensitive to standard drug strengths. In these cases, a compounding pharmacist can prepare a drug to alter its strength, eliminate the allergens, or make it more digestible or palatable. A compounding pharmacist can also put a drug in a form that does not have to be taken orally, thus avoiding systemic side effects.

The advantages of a compounded medication can be significant. Many medications used for pain and palliative treatment are commercially available in only oral or parenteral formulations and in standard strengths. For a patients with chronic pain, having a product that can be prepared for a topical application may mean lack of systemic side effects. For end-of-life patients who are unable to swallow, having a product compounded into a buccal, transdermal, or rectal formulation may allow a family member or the patients to continue to administer medications at home, thereby allowing them to live their final days, weeks, or months in the comfort of their home setting.

There are risks associated with the use of compounded medications when they are prepared without the specialized services of a pharmacist trained in the compounding process. Infections and deaths can occur if preparations of parenteral therapies occur without the use of appropriate equipment and sterile techniques. Efficacy can be compromised or toxicities can occur if products are compounded without rigid quality control standards. In spite of numerous anecdotal reports and cases suggesting efficacy of compounded topical analgesics such as gabapentin, dextromethorphan, and amitriptyline, there is a lack of controlled trials demonstrating clear benefits, appropriate application techniques, or approved dosages. Pharmacists can assist in providing recommendations for the use of topical products and direct physicians to products that have support in the literature to suggest efficacy.

DISPENSING, STOCKING, FILLING

Over the past 20 years the role of pharmacists has evolved to one that spends less time with "product" and more time with the patient. While the expanded role of technicians and advancements in technology have freed the pharmacist from many of the duties traditionally associated with the "count, lick, and pour" role, the pharmacist is still a critical link in the chain of drug distribution to the patient. To dispense opioid analgesics, pharmacists must comply with the requirements of federal and state drug, pharmacy, and controlled substances laws. Federal and state laws mandate that the pharmacist is responsible for the inventorying and accountability of all scheduled (controlled) substances. Most patients with pain will be prescribed some form of a controlled substance and the pharmacist is key in ensuring that all legal requirements are fulfilled with the filling and dispensing of the product. Beyond what the law allows, pharmacists have little discretion in refill authorization, telephone/fax prescriptions, emergency authorizations, etc. The pharmacist serves a role as "gatekeeper" who must determine whether dispensing a prescription order will serve a legitimate medical purpose and be in the usual course of professional practice.

The pharmacist's role in inventory control also has potential ramifications for patients with pain. Studies suggest that if pharmacies do not stock certain controlled substances, it is often due to fear of robbery. In 1986, Kanner and Portenoy[42] reported that 29% of pharmacies randomly sampled in New York City did not stock Schedule II opioid analgesics because of a fear of being robbed; only 3% stocked oral morphine. In 1989, Kanner and Cooper[43] found that 38% of a national sample of pharmacies stocked oral morphine. Those that did not stock the drug indicated that the reasons were a lack of prescription demand and fear of robbery. The results from these two studies generally mirror those from surveys of pharmacies in other states, such as New Mexico (1992)[44] and South Carolina (1993),[45] and from a 2000 survey of New York City pharmacies.[46] Pharmacists play a pivotal role in ensuring patient access to controlled substances.

The pharmacist who dispenses medications is in the unique position of being the last health care professional to have contact with the patient prior to the administration of the medication. Patient fears and concerns are often expressed and the pharmacist has one last opportunity to dispel myths and allay unwarranted fears. Ascertaining the patient's level of understanding of therapy decisions can also occur at this time. Finally, the dispensing pharmacist has an opportunity to recommend any appropriate over-the-counter medications (e.g., laxatives, analgesics) that might benefit the patient.

PAIN TEAMS, HOSPICE CARE, AND SPECIALIZED PHARMACIES

Pharmacists are increasingly well recognized for their critical role on multidisciplinary pain management teams across a variety of health care settings. Depending on the setting, pain management teams consist of a combination of disciplines such as physicians, nurses, physical and occupational therapists, psychologists, social workers, chaplains, nursing assistants, and pharmacists. The pharmacist role on chronic pain teams includes a combination of many of the roles discussed earlier in this chapter (e.g., education of patient, family, and pain team members; advocacy for appropriate drug therapies; collaboration with team members; assurance of drug safety; decisions on the role of compounded medicines; and occasionally, drug-dispensing duties). As a member of the pain team, the role of the pharmacist is formalized, and recommendations are dictated and transcribed into the medical record. Having a pharmacist on the pain team ensures that medication decisions are evidence-based. As a member of a pain team, the pharmacist usually has additional responsibilities for broad-based clinical activities such as developing, or co-developing with medical leadership, treatment algorithms; writing formulary drug reviews and monographs; and organizing patient-centered medication education. These activities increase the odds that a consistent medical plan will be in place for patients and strengthen patient perceptions and compliance with pain team therapy recommendations.

Hospices, similar to pain clinics/teams, employ the pharmacist for his or her skill in designing clinically effective and cost-effective therapy regimens for patients with pain and other end-of-life symptoms. The roles of a pharmacist in hospices are similar to many of those on the pain team with two exceptions. As part of the hospice team the pharmacist will not just focus on pain, but will provide recommendations on managing a variety of other symptoms common to patients during their terminal phase (e.g., breathlessness, edema, itching, nausea, cachexia, delirium, myoclonus). The other variation in the role of the pharmacist on the hospice team is the great focus on palliation of symptoms versus improvement of functioning in the patient with chronic pain. Granted, a chief goal in the care of a hospice patient is to maintain or improve functioning whenever possible, and it is accepted that the means to obtain both palliation and functional improvement can be similar. However, in the care of the hospice patient the overriding goal of care is palliation, and often this means a more aggressive approach with the use of strong opioids. Pharmacists use their expertise not only to advocate for aggressive palliation of pain and other end-of-life symptoms, but also to provide the information for how to do so in a safe manner.

Finally, with specialization occurring in many areas of pharmacy practice (e.g., oncology, cardiology, psychotherapeutics, nuclear medicinals, and others), it makes sense for specialized practices in pain management. One area of specialization that is occurring in the area of pain management is the use of electronic prescribing systems (eR_X) in concert with specialized pain management pharmacies. Coupled with the risks and complexities of prescribing medications for patients with chronic pain syndromes, there are reasonable expectations that the use of eR_X could provide favorable benefits to pain specialists and other practitioners who prescribe large numbers of analgesic medications.

Some eR_X system benefits in this setting could reasonably include improving clinical decisions and time efficiencies for assessing, treating, and monitoring patients with pain; reducing physician liabilities; eliminating prescription fraud; and providing meticulous prescribing record documentation to meet and exceed that required by regulatory agencies. Currently, most eR_X systems utilize a laptop computer or wireless, electronic prescription writing and transmitting device such as a handheld computer or a PDA. Many of the systems have been designed to be user friendly, secure, Health Insurance Portability and Accountability Act (HIPAA) compliant, and able to provide complete medication prescribing and utilization documentation. eR_X hardware devices eliminate the need for traditional prescription pads by incorporating software that offers numerous functions for managing patient records and enhancing medical office productivity.

The electronic system eliminates the potential of handwriting errors and the risk of prescription counterfeiting. Unlike an ordinary prescription pad, the handheld prescription unit directly transmits the dispensing order to the pharmacy, which checks for frequency of use and/or potential misuse by the patient. Most systems allow the physician to select from the self-contained list of applicable medications after entering an authorization code for the medication. The device, by eliminating the need for a handwritten prescription, avoids prescription loss, alteration, copying, and forgery. Coded access to the prescription unit ensures that if the physician misplaces the unit or leaves it unattended, it is useless to another party and cannot be utilized to transmit prescriptions falsely.

When the patient arrives at the pharmacy, the prescription is often ready, in advance of patient arrival, minimizing lengthy waits. Other benefits to some eR_X systems include (1) the electronic screening of new prescriptions against the patient's profile to prevent adverse drug events related to dosage errors, known allergies, and drug–drug interactions, and to minimize errors with look-alike and sound-alike names; and (2) the provision of monthly activity reports, which among other things, identifies those patients who have failed to pick up their prescriptions. One key value-added service offered by some of the eR$_X$ systems is a "Refill Management Service." This service reduces physician office phone calls and associated frustrations because of the involvement of pharmacy staff proactively reviewing electronic patient medication records and telephoning patients several days prior to the anticipated refill date. Some systems allow patients a choice of coming in to pick up new and refilled prescription(s) or having the prescription(s) home-delivered via the U.S. mail service or via a bonded courier. Physicians who prefer to authorize refill prescriptions at an office visit discover the convenience and time saved by renewing medications via a few mouse clicks on the electronic device, instead of manually recopying multiple medications on paper prescriptions.

FINAL THOUGHTS

Indeed, the pharmacist has an important role in pain management. The right drug, at the right dose, administered to the right patient, monitored for appropriate outcomes, may afford tremendous functional improvement for a patient with pain. The pharmacist, as the "drug expert" can influence the patient's perspective on the medication, and whether or not he or she will comply. The pharmacist can positively influence the prescriber's selection of a medication, dosage, or route, thereby improving the benefit-to-risk ratio. In our search to improve the quality of life in our patients we must remember that we have many options, of which medications are but one option. The pharmacist is the ideal professional to assist the physician and other health team members, as well as the patient and family members, in developing the best medication plan for improving the lives of pain patients.

Medications are not perfect. The decision to use a medication or not can be an emotional decision for both the professional and the patient. Many patients blame themselves or are blamed by others for having pain and for having an ulterior motive for wanting a medication. In our search to improve the quality of life in our patients, we must remember that medications themselves have no inherent morality. It is the inappropriate use of medications, or lack of use, that oftentimes is the essence of the morality of medicines. Ultimately, the pharmacist's role in pain management comes down to one phrase: "to ensure that medications are used appropriately."

REFERENCES

1. American Pharmaceutical Association. (2004). The pharmacy profession: Transitioning from prescription provider to health care manager. American Pharmaceutical Association. Retrieved April 15, 2004 from http://www.pharmacyandyou.org/about/pharmcarefacts.html.
2. Higby, G. J. (1997). American pharmacy in the twentieth century. *American Journal Health-System Pharmacy, 54,* 1805.
3. Portenoy, R. K. (1997). Opioid therapy for chronic non-malignant pain: A review of the critical issues. *Journal of Pain Symptom Management, 11,* 203.
4. Federation of State Medical Boards of the United States, Inc. (1998). *Model guidelines for the use of controlled substances for the treatment of pain.* Euless TX: Author.
5. American Geriatric Society. (1998). Clinical practice guidelines: The management of chronic pain in older persons. *Journal of the American Geriatric Society, 46,* 635.
6. Graziotte, P. J., & Goucke C. R. (1997). The use of oral opioids in patients with chronic non-cancer pain. Management strategies, *Medical Journal of Australia,167,* 30.
7. Andersen, S., & Leikersfeldt, G. (1996). Management of chronic non-malignant pain. *British Journal of Clinical Practice, 50,* 324.
8. Marcus, D. A. (2000). Treatment of nonmalignant chronic pain. *American Family Physician, 61,* 1331.
9. Stacey, B. R. (1996). Effective management of chronic pain. The analgesic dilemma. *Postgraduate Medicine, 100,* 281.
10. Katz, W. A., Approach to the management of nonmalignant pain. *American Journal of Medicine, 101*(Suppl 1A), 54S.
11. Godfrey, R. G. (1996). A guide to the understanding and use of tricyclic antidepressants in the overall management of fibromyalgia and other chronic pain syndromes. *Archives of Internal Medicine, 156,* 1047.
12. Leland, J.Y., (1999). Chronic pain: Primary care treatment of the older patient. *Geriatrics, 54,* 23.
13. Smith, B. H., Hopton, J. L., & Chambers, W. A. (1999). Chronic pain in primary care. *Family Practice, 16,* 475.
14. Bannwarth, B. (1999). Risk-benefit assessment of opioids in chronic noncancer pain. *Drug Safety, 21,* 283.
15. Pappagallo, M., & Heinberg, L. J. (1997). Ethical issues in the management of chronic nonmalignant pain. *Seminars in Neurology, 17,* 203.
16. Parrott, T. (1999). Using opioid analgesics to manage chronic noncancer pain in primary care. *Journal of the American Board of Family Practitioners, 12,* 293.
17. Savage, S. R. (1999). Opioid use in the management of chronic pain., *Medical Clinics of North America, 83,* 761.
18. Chapman, C.R., & Dunbar, P. J. (1998). Measurement in pain therapy: Is pain relief really the endpoint? *Current Opinion in Anaesthesiology, 11,* 533.
19. Schneider, J.P. (1998). Management of chronic noncancer pain: A guide to appropriate use of opioids. *Journal of Care and Management, 4,* 10.

20. Gasser, V., & Peluso, R. (1997, September). Managing chronic, non-malignant pain. *American Druggist*, 74.

21. Portenoy, R. K. (1994). Opioid therapy for chronic non-malignant pain: Current status. In H. L. Fields & J. C. Liebeskind (Eds.). *Progress in pain research and management* (pp. 247–287). Seattle: IASP Press.

22. American Medical Directors Association. (1999). *Chronic pain management in the long-term care setting. Clinical practice guidelines.* Columbia, MD: American Medical Directors Association.

23. Lister, B. J. (1996). Dilemmas in the treatment of chronic pain. *American Journal of Medicine, 101*(Suppl 1A), 2S.

24. Katz, W. A. (1998). The needs of a patient in pain. *American Journal of Medicine, 105*(Suppl 1B), 2S.

25. Ernst, M. E., Doucette, W. R., Dedhiya, S. D. et al. (2001). Use of point-of-service health status assessments by community pharmacists to identify and resolve drug-related problems in patients with musculoskeletal disorders. *Pharmacotherapy.*, 21, 988.

26. Lothian, S. T., Fotis, M. A., von Gunten, C. F. et al. (1999). Cancer pain management through a pharmacist-based analgesic dosing service. *American Journal of Health System Pharmacy, 56*, 1119.

27. Malone, D. C., Carter, B. L., Billups, S. J., et al. (2001) Can clinical pharmacists affect SF-36 scores in veterans at high risk for medication-related problems? *Medical Care, 39*, 113.

28. Ratka, A. (2002). The role of a pharmacist in ambulatory cancer pain management. *Current Pain Headache Report,* 1911.

29. Lipman, A. G., & Berry, J. I. (1995). Pharmaceutical care of terminally ill patients. *Journal of Pharmaceutical Care in Pain and Symptom Control, 3*, 31.

30. Krisk, S. E., Lindley, C. M., & Bennett, M. (1994). Pharmacy-perceived barriers to cancer pain control: Results of the North Carolina Cancer Pain Initiative Pharmacist Survey. *Annals of Pharmcotherapy, 28*, 857.

32. Phillips, D. P., Christenfeld, N., & Glynn, L. M. (1998). Increase in US medication-error deaths between 1983 and 1993. *Lancet, 351*, 643.

32. Joranson, D. E., & Gilson, A. M. (2001). Pharmacists' knowledge of and attitudes toward opioid pain medications in relation to federal and state policies. *Journal of the American Pharmaceutical Association, 41*, 213.

33. FDA. Retrieved April 15, 2004 from www.fda.gov. .

34. Wolfe, M., Lichtenstein, D., & Singh, G. (1999). Gastrointestinal toxicity of nonsteroidal anti-inflammatory drugs. *New England Journal of Medicine, 340*, 1888.

35. Unintentional and undetermined poisoning deaths – 11 states, 1990–2001. (2004, March 26). *MMWR Weekly, 53*(11); 233–238. Retrieved April 15, 2004 from http://www.cdc.gov/mmwr/preview/mmwrhtml/mm5311a2.htm.

36. American Society of Health System Pharamcists. ASHP guidelines on pharmacist-conducted patient education and counseling. Retrieved April 15, 2004 from http://www.ashp.org/bestpractices/medtherapy/Medication%20Therapy%20&%20Patient%20Care%20Org.%20&%20Deliv.%20of%20Serv.%20Guide.%20Pharm.%20Con.%20Pat.%20Ed.pdf.

37. Fordyce, W. (1992). Opioids, pain and behavioral outcomes. *American Pain Society Journal, 1*, 282.

38. Carmichael, J. M., O'Connell, M. B., Devine, B. et al. (1997). Collaborative drug therapy management by pharmacists. American College of Clinical Pharmacy. *Pharmacotherapy, 17*, 1050.

39. Alliance for Pharmaceutical Care. Partners to Improve Health Outcomes. Evidence of the value of the pharmacist. Alliance for Pharmaceutical Care. Partners to Improve Health Outcomes. Retrieved April 15, 2004 from www.accp.com/position/paper6.pdf.

40. McMullin, S. T., Hennenfent, J. A., Ritchie, D. J. et al. (1999). A prospective, randomized trial to assess the cost impact of pharmacist-initiated interventions, *Archives of Internal Medicine, 159*, 2306.

41. Leap, L. I., Cullen, D. J., Clapp, M. D. et al. (1999). Pharmacist participation on physician rounds and adverse drug events in the intensive care unit. *Journal of the American Medical Association, 282*, 267.

42. anner, R. M., & Portenoy, R. K. (1986). Unavailability of narcotic analgesics for ambulatory cancer patients in New York City. *Journal of Pain and Symptom Management, 1*, 87.

43. Kanner, R. M., & Cooper, E. S. (1989). Availability of narcotic analgesics for ambulatory patients with pain. In C. S. Hill, Jr. & W. S. Fields (Eds.) *Advances in pain research and therapy, Volume II* (pp. 191–195). New York, NY: Raven Press.

44. Holdsworth, M.T., & Raisch, D. W. (1992). Availability of narcotics and pharmacists' attitudes toward narcotic prescriptions for cancer patients, *Annnals of Pharmacotherapy, 26*, 321.

45. Rabon, P. G., Linette, D. C., Gonzales, M. F. et al. (1993). Limited availability of medications for cancer patients. *Southern Medical Journal, 86*, 914.

46. Morrison, R. S., Wallenstein, S., Natale, D. K. et al. (2002). "We don't carry that": Failure of pharmacies in predominantly nonwhite neighborhoods to stock opioid analgesics. *New England Journal of Medicine, 342*, 1023.

22

The Role of the Chaplain

Rev. Mr. Randol G. Batson, BS

It was the summer of 1986 and Ruth was dying, her body ravaged by malignancy. The pain seemed intractable, but for the chemical agent that transported her conscious mind to a precious state of relief somewhere between reverie and restless slumber. Brief interludes of clarity that had become increasingly less frequent were angry, bitter, and demanding.

During their presence in the home of the daughter who cared for Ruth, the hospice team observed many strange dynamics that appeared to be a way of life for the patient and her adult children. Ruth's two sons and one daughter were perceived as cold, indifferent people, yet each, in his or her own way, appeared possessive of the others.

One afternoon when Ruth seemed to be experiencing a more conscious episode, the chaplain asked what in her memory was the source of her intense pain. As though she had awaited that invitation for 43 years, Ruth slowly unraveled her story.

It was World War II and she was the young bride of a U.S. Navy flyer who in 4 short years of marriage had given her three hungry mouths to feed and mountains of diapers to wash. The stresses were many, and all too frequently erupted into a private battlefield on the homefront. One Sunday afternoon Ruth and her husband were engaged in yet another angry confrontation when he was required to leave for a scheduled training maneuver.

Frustrated at being left alone again with three demanding babies and feeling cheated over the issue that remained unresolved, Ruth shouted after her husband, I wish you were dead! Can you imagine the rest of the story? There was an apparent mechanical failure, the plane went down, and the young husband was killed. Believing she had set his fate, Ruth turned her guilt inward to self and a bitter,

undemonstrative, controlling mother raised three angry, undemonstrative, controlling children.

It was the first time in 43 years that Ruth had shared the depth of her pain with another human being, and in the catharsis there was a release of tears that had been bottled up beyond her remembrance. The chaplain helped Ruth find forgiveness for herself and reconnect with the tenderness of the love she had shared so briefly with her husband. The next time her three children gathered at their mother's bedside, they found a stranger who, for the first time in many years, reached out to touch them tenderly. Even amidst the physical pain that screamed from Ruth's body, her face displayed a softer demeanor, her voice free of its characteristic harshness. Ruth drew her children closer to her and repeated the dark secret she had revealed to the chaplain. Slowly, haltingly, she omitted no detail, punctuating each revelation with her tears. Before she finished her children too were crying. Ruth told them for the first time in their collective memory that she loved them, and she asked forgiveness for the many ways she had formed their lives by her own negativity. They responded with expressions of love and forgiveness toward her, and toward one another. There were embraces, positive affirmations, and more tears.

Within a week the hospice medical director discerned that Ruth was overmedicated for pain, and her morphine was reduced. It appeared as though the pain in her body had retreated as the festering boil in her memory continued to heal.

There was consensus among the hospice team that Ruth had been healed. That she died 2 weeks later seemed almost insignificant. Most people with cancer of the pancreas and liver do, after all, die from the disease process. More certainly, all people die sooner or later. Unlike many, however, Ruth died with peace of mind. She found forgiveness of self that enabled her to accept the forgiveness of God, whoever or whatever she perceived God to be. She died with hope and with a sense of completion that gave rebirth to her children, thereby empowering them to release some of their own painful, emotional baggage and live with greater joy.

Ruth's story and the somewhat dramatic conclusion of her life pose certain questions, which many clinicians and researchers are no longer content to ignore. What was the complex relationship between her painful memories, replete with unforgiveness and self-condemnation, and the pain that a terminal disease process expressed in her body? Was it coincidence, or did the emotional catharsis and spiritual healing at the end of her life have any direct bearing on the ability of clinical caregivers to manage her pain effectively and yet maximize for herself and her family the quality of her final days? What is spirituality and spiritual care? Of what consequence is such an ethereal dimension to medical science?

These questions prompt many more, and the answers often seem beyond empirical evidence. In the past 30 years, however, medical scientists with strong interest in the spiritual dimensions of life have increasingly dared to ask such questions and to seek answers within the scope of clinical trial. Although still only comprising a small percentage of total research, such trials and/or considerations have become so common, and the interest in spiritual possibilities so universal, that it is no longer extraordinary to find them reported in the most mainstream medical journals, including *Journal of the American Medical Association, Southern Medical Journal, New England Journal of Medicine,* and *American Journal of Psychiatry.* Many medical scientists now understand that each human person is a total entity, a very complex communion of various dimensions, physical and nonphysical, compounded by psychological, familial, and social history; that among those is a component commonly called "spiritual" that has the power to profoundly affect the rest, a component that may even be a foundation block of total health. From the interest in possibility and evidence has risen an annual continuum of seminars, workshops, and conferences such as Harvard Medical School's *Spirituality and Healing in Medicine.* Those possibilities have also become a major focus of the work of such prestigious entities as the National Institute for Healthcare Research founded by the late David B. Larson, M.D., M.S.P.H., and the John Templeton Foundation.

It is important to establish that this discussion is not an effort to verify or support the existence of deity or divinity — God — as it were. Larry Dossey, M.D., a leader in the new frontier of spiritual consciousness in medicine and author of *New York Times* bestsellers, which include *Healing Words: The Power of Prayer and the Practice of Medicine* (Harper, San Francisco, 1993) and *Reinventing*

Medicine: Beyond Mind–Body to a New Era of Healing (Harper, San Francisco, 1999), asserts that to try to prove the existence of God is like nailing Jell-O® to a wall. Nor is this an attempt to further any religious agenda, although it may not be possible to consider comprehensively spirituality and the role of the chaplain without acknowledging religion, and religious practices, as a component of the spiritual dimension. That may be especially true because a preponderance of clinical research in spirituality and medicine has surrounded the religious identity and practices of test subjects.

Rather, this chapter is intended to raise consciousness of spiritual reality and the power it holds over health and wellness, pain management, healing, ease, and disease. Dale Matthews, M.D., F.A.C.P., of Georgetown University School of Medicine and coauthors (1993) of *The Faith Factor: An Annotated Bibliography of Clinical Research on Spiritual Studies* estimate that about 75% of spirituality studies have confirmed health benefits.

It is now regarded by many that all people have spiritual needs. It may even be possible that the most abject atheist has spiritual needs. Why? How? Because an inherent need for meaning, and to experience purpose in life, seems to be universal. Even the most seemingly negative demonstrate a basic need to give and receive love. This need seems present at birth, regardless of how it may be masked or pushed from consciousness by the psychosocial circumstances of this world. Forgiveness is widely believed to be a universal need, and avenues to transcendence appear likewise to be needed by people of every land and culture. Clifford C. Kuhn, M.D., of the Division of Behavioral Medicine at the University of Louisville School of Medicine, who advocates a spiritual inventory of the medically ill patient, defines spirituality as those capacities that enable a human being to rise above or transcend any experience at hand (Kuhn, 1988). In the case of the previously discussed hospice patient, forgiveness appears to have enabled Ruth to rise above, to transcend, the pain of cancer and the certainty of her impending death.

SPIRITUALITY: WHAT IS IT?

How do we define spirituality? Definition may be as elusive as the dimension itself. Many have found enlightenment, however, in a demonstration used by Marcia Baumert, F.S.P.A. (pers. commun.), a chaplain at Genesis Medical Center in Davenport, Iowa. When teaching about spirituality, Sister Marcia places a wide-mouth jar before her group and says, "This is Charlie." She then adds stones sufficient to fill the jar to the top and explains that the stones represent Charlie's total physical composition, DNA to organs, bones to skin, hair, and even eye color. She asks the question, "Is this all there is of Charlie?" The audience usually responds "No" with total acclamation.

Sister Marcia then adds small pebbles to the jar, explaining that they represent Charlie's mental capacities. When the jar will hold no more pebbles, she asks, "Is this all there is to Charlie?" Most will still respond "No." Sister Marcia then pours sand into the jar, carefully filling it and shaking the sand down into the empty space between the pebbles and the larger stones. She explains that the sand represents the psychosocial composition of Charlie's life, including all that is retained in Charlie's memory bank, conscious and unconscious. At the completion of that phase of the demonstration many in the room will deliver an affirmative response to Sister Marcia's inquiry as to whether that's all there is of Charlie. She then takes a pitcher of water from under the table and pours the water into the jar. The audience watches with interest and amazement to see how much water Charlie can hold. When the jar is filled to the top, Sister Marcia explains that the water represents Charlie's spirituality, and she invites them to observe the way the water changes the total context of the other ingredients. There are color changes, the pebbles and sand move and settle in ways that they seemed unable to do before. The water creates the appearance of mortar, as though it were a bonding agent for the other components. Sister Marcia invites her audience to observe that there is no place within the jar, Charlie, not affected by the water, and she explains that as the true nature of spirituality.

The word *spirituality* derives from *spiritus*, a Latin root that means "breath of life," and has historically been understood mainly within the context of religion. In the latter half of the 20th century, however, there arose a consciousness of spirituality as broader and more comprehensive than organized religion, integral to all people whether or not they recognize it, and irrespective of their identity with deity or religion. For many, religion is merely a piece of the pie, and the size of that piece corresponds to the importance that person places upon religion. For others, religion is the total pie. Determination of which position is more accurate may be as elusive as Dr. Dossey's image of nailing Jell-O to the wall. For the purpose of this discussion it really doesn't matter. What does matter is that health care providers — physicians, nurses, and all other members of the interdisciplinary care group — recognize that every patient may have a spiritual composition with the power to influence his or her total health. Often understood as energy, even as electric energy, spirituality can be our friend or our enemy, depending on the care with which it is respected, channeled, and used. That possibility should be of prime concern to all who practice healing arts and science.

RELATIONSHIP

My 25 years experience in spiritual health care has given me the consciousness that spirituality is, to a great extent, about relationship — the relationship of each person to self, to God or Higher Power, to family, to society. It is about one's relationship to the macrocosm of life. The personal experience shared by so many spiritual health care providers, e.g., chaplains, is now supported by studies that in various ways affirm or indicate the possibility that these "relationship factors" may have a role in some disease processes, and in healing. Excellent collections of such studies are to be found in *Scientific Research on Spirituality and Health: A Consensus Report,* edited by David B. Larson, M.D., M.S.P.H.; James P Swyers, M.A.; and Michael E. McCullough, Ph.D. (1997) as well as in *The Faith Factor: An Annotated Bibliography of Clinical Research on Spiritual Subjects* (Mathews, Lawson, & Barry, 1993).

Returning to Sister Marcia's, demonstration, if there were within the jar "Charlie" any area where the water did not flow, Charlie would not be totally integrated. That one dry pocket within the jar would be "out of relationship" with the rest of its components, and would have power to affect the total context of the other ingredients. Charlie would be out of balance, out of relationship. The same would be true of spirituality. If we cannot prove that it is so, we can also not prove that it is not so. The possibility evidenced by Ruth's story and countless similar cases experienced daily by multidisciplinary caregivers offers powerful motivation for physicians to seek a spiritual assessment of their patients, and to integrate spiritual care into their total care continuum.

SPIRITUAL PAIN

With the emergence of a consciousness for the critical role of spirituality in total health has come consideration of a phenomenon called spiritual pain. Like spirituality, spiritual pain may not lend itself easily to definition. If, however, spirituality is, as I have come to understand, about relationships, it would follow that spiritual pain is a manifestation of broken relationships. Surely we've all known its symptoms: a hollow feeling in the pit of the stomach, or a tight sensation, even nonphysical pain, in the heart region of the chest. It can be reflected in chronic anger, in bitterness, or in negativity. It can express as a fearful, mistrusting attitude, and it may be present in acute loneliness or depression. Tears, fatigue, and nonverbal body language can represent spiritual pain. It is irrefutable that such symptoms may have their basis in clinical psychosis and can often be treated with medical interventions. Clinical examples such as Ruth, however, suggest that many may be the sole result of spiritual pain or a combination of spiritual pain and clinical psychosis. Dare we even to ask ourselves the ages-old question, "Which came first, the chicken or the egg?"

Spiritual pain is beyond the scope of traditional medical interventions, save for mood-altering drugs, which serve as a Band-Aid® rather than a cure, and it is healed only in the reestablishment of healthy relationship. The outcome of spiritual healing may be renewed self-esteem, forgiveness, peace of mind, the infusion of joy, reconnection to love, and the return of hope, meaning, and purpose. It may be characterized by renewed faith consciousness, the courage to endure challenge and to reach for victory. There can be renewed vitality and a resurgence of energy.

A contemporary supposition yet unproven, perhaps beyond proof, but held by many clinicians to be worthy of consideration is that spiritual pain can be a precursor to physical pain. Certainly, it would have seemed so in Ruth's case. When her spiritual pain was relieved, i.e., when she found the healing of memories that facilitated forgiveness and the restoration of her relationship to self, to her family, and to her deceased husband, the physical pain quotient generated naturally by the ravages of her physical disease process was reduced. She required less pain medication to be comfortable. She was more lucid and was thereby able to enjoy a greater quality of life for the remainder of her days.

WHY SPIRITUAL CARE?

Recognition of the power of the spiritual dimension and the importance of spiritual care is of vital importance to health care providers because it can be a complementary tool or therapy that is useful for most patients, regardless of their faith consciousness or religious practice. That the vast body of clinical studies on spirituality to date surround religion and people of faith can be viewed as both negative and positive. The danger is that they may reinforce the consciousness that spiritual needs are always religious in nature and spiritual care is always religious care. Because religion does not fit for some people, patients and caregivers alike, there is a risk that such understandings may result in the deprivation of therapeutic opportunity.

Amidst the ethereal, however, religious practices do provide some concrete basis for comparison. Were we to attempt to nail fruit Jell-O to the wall, it would at least be possible to spear a piece of fruit as the Jell-O dropped away. Perhaps the fruit within the Jell-O is a valid metaphor for religion within spirituality. People of faith do provide a basis for measurement and comparison to those without faith or religious practice. The studies increase annually, and their effect is being profoundly felt in Western medicine. In 1993, only 3 of the 123 colleges of medicine in the United States offered courses on spirituality and spiritual care. According to Dr. Larry Dossey (1998), that number had grown to 50 in 1999, and in 2003 Dr. Dossey believed the number to be greater than 90. At a collaborative conference in Dallas, Texas in September, 2000, the Association of American Medical Schools and the National Institute for Healthcare Research sought ways to more effectively integrate spiritual care into academic medical curricula.

A PATIENT MANDATE

Beside the existence of clinical indications for spiritual care, personal beliefs and practices of a majority of patients would seem to mandate the attention of health care professionals.

A 1990 Gallup study found Americans to be a highly religious people:

- 96% reported belief in God
- 75% claimed to pray at least once a day
- 58% said, "religion is very important in my life"
- 43% claimed to have attended worship services within the past week

One national poll of 1,000 adults found that 63% wanted their physicians to talk to them about spiritual health, but that only 10% reported their physicians having done so (McNichol, 1996.) In another national poll, 82% of 1,004 adults reported belief in the power of prayer, and 64% said physicians should pray with patients who so request (Wallis, 1996). According to a statement of the late Elisabeth Targ, M.D., quoted in the *Western Journal of Medicine,* December 1998, "Eighty-two percent of Americans believe in the healing power of prayer. Research indicates that they may be right" (Sicher et al., 1998).

Doubly blessed, perhaps, are patients who want such care and are so fortunate as to have a physician able and willing to participate. With the increasing body of evidence in favor of spiritual care, together with professional dialogue, it would seem that many physicians are now entering into spiritual "communion" with their patients in more visible and discernable ways. For others, however, it just does not fit — even for many who embrace personal spiritual or religious practices. Nor should that be subject to judgment. My own perspective throughout many years of spiritual health care, however, is that all caregivers should be spiritual caregivers. The key is consciousness. It is of critical importance that even those without religious identity be clearly conscious of the role that the previously named "relationship factors" may play in sickness and health, and that they be mindful and respectful of the importance that many, perhaps most, patients place upon spirituality.

Some, physicians and chaplains alike, argue that spiritual care should be left to the professional spiritual caregivers, the chaplains, that there are too many inherent risks for physicians to wear "chaplains' collars." While there may be credibility to that position, there are surely many personal variables, which will not be considered here. The bottom line should again be the consciousness of all physicians to consider spiritual factors and, at the very least, to make an appropriate referral to the chaplain who is equipped to do a spiritual assessment and to work together with the physician in providing the highest possible level of total care for the patient.

Chaplains are privileged caregivers within the hospital environment in that they have freedom to move among patients at will, without medical orders. That is due in part to the historical role of the chaplain as a religious minister whose activities were governed by patient preference. It is also influenced by the fact that spiritual care is not currently, and never has been, a chargeable service. Therein, a double-edge sword exists. Non-requirement for a medical order has given autonomy to the chaplain, and has afforded opportunity for spontaneous relationships and "ah-ha" moments, which have led to meaningful outcomes. It has, however, enabled the presence of some chaplains whose skills and practices were not equal to professional standards, while failing to develop avenues of communication between chaplains and physicians.

Until 30 years ago it was not at all uncommon for hospital chaplains merely to be ordained ministers or members of religious orders. Completion of an accredited continuum of clinical pastoral education, including internship, is now the standard to which most health care institutions aspire. Professional organizations such as the Association of Professional Chaplains, the National Association of Catholic Chaplains, and the National Association of Jewish Chaplains establish high standards of clinical practice for professional accreditation and require continuing education for renewal of credentials. As spiritual care becomes more broadly accepted as a valid component of total care, institutional providers are more commonly requiring that their chaplains be certified professionals. While most accrediting organizations require that certified chaplains receive and maintain ecclesiastical endorsement, membership now comprises both ordained persons and laity, male and female. The quality of professional spiritual care has been greatly enhanced by the expanded playing field of acceptable candidates, and it has helped spiritual care to move beyond the "box" of traditional religion to a model that is more compatible with all patients and members of the multidisciplinary care team.

A professional chaplain puts aside his or her personal agenda. Rather, the patient's needs and the patient's agenda are the primary focus of the chaplain's work. A skillful chaplain may "invite" the patient to opportunities that result in the opening of pathways to memory and doorways to spiritual consciousness. It is the patient, however, who leads, and the patient who determines the direction and the outcome of the intervention. Beyond the right to accept or reject the care of a physician, an institution, or a particular intervention, the chaplain as facilitator may well represent the patient's greatest opportunity for personal autonomy in allopathic care.

The evolution of health care into the age of controlled reimbursements, preferred provider organizations, and health maintenance organizations has affected the operation and practice of many providers. Chaplains, like professionals in all other disciplines, have been affected by the ensuing changes. It is now a rare institution that can afford to maintain a spiritual care staff sufficient to routinely see all new admits and follow them to discharge. Chaplains must often triage patients and rely upon referrals from other caregivers. Nursing rounds and discharge planning conferences are avenues through which patients are routinely identified for spiritual intervention.

Some of the best opportunities I have known, and the ones that enabled me to facilitate the most positive outcomes, are those that have come from physicians, either by way of a personal contact or through a referral in the patient medical record. In my experience as a hospice chaplain, it was the norm to receive personal communication about patients and specific requests for spiritual care from the hospice medical director. Within the hospital setting, my experience has found such referrals to be outside the norm. Nonetheless, they seem to occur with greater frequency each year. When a physician and a chaplain take the time to develop a relationship of trust, and communicate together in the patient's behalf, insightful opportunities for total healing are often found.

I remember a patient several years ago who was what hospital staff called a "frequent flyer." A fine-looking and healthy-appearing man in his early 70s, he presented every few months with heart symptoms that his cardiologist seemed unable to manage effectively at home. While his pathology was supported by clinical evidence, his cardiologist was nonetheless stumped by his apparent inability to effectively control symptoms that normally respond well to medical intervention. While visiting the patient at the time of one of his hospitalizations, I engaged him in a "walk down memory lane." During that time together I learned that his mother had died when he was about 7 years old. His father worked out of town and, rather than take his son along or arrange for him to stay in the home of family members or friends, had placed him in one of the old-time state orphanages. For the remainder of his childhood he rarely saw his father. In a lucky year his father would show up once, maybe twice, for a brief visit as though he were making a courtesy call to a hospitalized acquaintance. There were no special remembrances at Christmas or birthdays. The patient spoke of understanding that times were hard. It was during the years of the Great Depression, and as a father and grandfather himself, he had come to accept that his father might have done the best he thought he could at the time. Still his eyes brimmed with tears when he recalled those years of loneliness, and the feeling of disconnection from the two people who had been the foundation of his life and his security.

Later that day I chanced to see his cardiologist, with whom I had a friendly but casual relationship, and I asked him if he could spare me a couple of minutes to share an insight I had gained about his patient. We sat together in a charting area at the nurse station and I began to relate to him what I had learned. Imagine my surprise and personal satisfaction when, after relating the story of the patient's unhappy childhood, the physician exclaimed enthusiastically, "A broken heart! What a metaphor that is for the physical malady I am trying to treat." Excitedly, we developed a plan whereby I would work with the patient to help him find healing for his painful memory and to access forgiveness for his father. The success of such a plan was contingent on the patient's willingness to participate. He was, and he did, with an observable outcome. His damaged physical heart was, of course, not mended. His doctor and I presumed, however, that his broken spiritual heart found the healing it needed because his condition became manageable by the medical means the physician could provide. He enjoyed a life of renewed quality, and he was no longer a "frequent flyer" at the hospital. As pleasing an outcome for me personally was that the physician and I developed a much more collegial relationship, and we found ourselves working together often to effect better patient outcomes.

In-depth spiritual care can be a great deal like peeling an onion. Human beings are such incredibly complex lifeforms, and who and what we are is governed by so many factors beyond genetic predisposition, that there are may be layers upon layers to be peeled away in order to effect spiritual healing sufficient to influence physical outcomes.

How well I remember Elizabeth, a swollen, patheticlooking woman with unkempt gray hair and sad eyes. Yet, the stage photograph that she always brought with her to the hospital depicted a vibrant, slender, dark-haired beauty in a flowing taffeta gown. Elizabeth had been an opera star of no small renown. The only child of foreign-born parents of modest means, she had climbed the ladder to success by her own wit, talent, and sheer determination. She had sung at many of the more famous opera houses of the world, including New York City's Metropolitan, and she was intimate with people whose names were household words in America. Her parents took little pride in show business "nonsense," however. Aging with poor health, frightened, and alone, they begged her to come home and settle down where she could be near them in their declining years. Succumbing to their pressure, Elizabeth put her career on hold and came home with the intent to return to the stage after her parents had died. She declined many opportunities during the years when her parents lived longer than expected and, ultimately, the exciting life she had known became history.

Hungry for a life beyond the mundane responsibility of caring for sickly parents, Elizabeth found companionship in George, an uninteresting accountant some years her senior. She married George and he shared the responsibility of caring for her parents during their few remaining years. Elizabeth and George had one daughter, Sylvia, a materially indulged child who, as an adult, presented as

self-centered and resentful. When Sylvia was 10 years old, Elizabeth developed a close friendship with Joyce, a sweetly assertive woman. The friendship soon encompassed an inordinate quantity of Elizabeth's time, at the expense of George and Sylvia. Elizabeth and Joyce began to call themselves "sisters," and after a couple of years Joyce moved into Elizabeth and George's home and became "Aunt Joyce" to Sylvia. As the bond between the "sisters" grew stronger, the space between Elizabeth and George became a chasm. Ultimately, by mutual agreement of husband and wife, a room at the rear of the large home was made suitable for George. He lived somewhat the life of a boarder in his own home and died prematurely.

After George's death Elizabeth's own health declined. Her joints began to swell and ache, symptomatic of osteoarthritis, and she developed a litany of ailments considered by her physician to be somatic in nature. Among those, an asthmatic condition became chronic and, together with the osteoarthritis, limited her mobility. She became sedentary, obese, and frightened. Deprived of sleep, unable to breathe easily, and wracked with pain, Elizabeth started using prescription sleep aids at night, and later during the daytime. A self-generating cycle seemed to have been set into motion.

As chaplain of the unit where Elizabeth was hospitalized for several days out of every month, I had developed a relationship with her, and with Joyce, who was faithfully at her side from early morning until visiting hours ended in the evening. They were women who professed Christian faith, and they always seemed encouraged by a visit and a prayer. It was difficult, however, to accomplish anything at a deeper level with Elizabeth because Joyce was always present, often assuming the responsibility of Elizabeth's spokesperson. I had heard the story of her life more times than one, but I had the sense there was some deep spiritual pain, which influenced Elizabeth's current condition — a source too "sacred" to attempt to access in Joyce's presence.

One day I determined to work a swing shift, which caused me to be at the hospital after visiting hours were over and Joyce had gone home. I went to Elizabeth's room and engaged her in conversation during which I gently invited her down memory lane, into her relationship with George. I had already secured Elizabeth's trust through my previous ministry to her. The time was apparently right, and it was a place where she was ready to go. It soon became apparent that Elizabeth was burdened by guilt for the way she had replaced George in his own home and in their marriage. She wept with remorse that she had not had the opportunity to tell George that she truly did love him, and that she was sorry for the ways she failed him.

Moved by Spirit from within, I suggested to Elizabeth that there was a way in which she could communicate the things she needed to say to George, and the stage was set for an elementary Gestalt intervention. I helped her get up, and positioned her in the bedside recliner. I then moved a guest chair and seated myself opposite her, knees to knees. I invited Elizabeth to close her eyes as I led her into a short relaxation exercise. I then suggested to her that through the power of the Holy Spirit, in which she professed faith, she could speak to George. I told her that I was George's surrogate. She should say to me whatever things she needed to say to him, and George would hear.

Elizabeth slowly began to speak just as though she were talking to George. Before long, her words poured forth in sobs, a waterfall of tears cascading down her swollen face. She told George that she was haunted by the memory of how she had hurt him and Sylvia, and that she was filled with grief. She told him that she did love him more than she realized at the time, and that she was most appreciative of the many ways he had been such a good husband and father. Acknowledging that she was not worthy of forgiveness, she asked him nonetheless to find it in his heart to forgive her.

When Elizabeth's words ceased and she became calmer, I spoke as though I were George. I told her that from where I lived in Eternity I had the ability to see circumstances clearly. I told her that I understood the things that motivated her to make choices that had caused me to be so disappointed, and that with all my heart I forgave her. Acknowledging that it takes two to fail as well as to succeed, I asked her forgiveness for all the ways in which I had failed her, and I professed my continued love for her. I also assured her that I was waiting for her, and that she could talk to me whenever she needed, just the same way she prayed to God. Reaching forth, I wrapped my arms tightly around Elizabeth, and she enfolded hers about me. She wept softly on my shoulder as she might have done with her husband in younger, happier days.

There was a remarkable change in Elizabeth by the next day. She had rested well. There was about her a discernable energy shift. She seemed almost serene and happy. On the following day she was discharged, never to reenter the hospital. Joyce phoned me early one morning after 5 weeks had passed and sobbed that Elizabeth had not awakened that morning. I was asked to do the funeral, which required a 2-hour drive to the cemetery where Elizabeth's parents and George were buried. Joyce rode alone with me, and she spoke of her wonder at the change in her companion during the weeks preceding her death. Elizabeth's attitude had become more as it was in the beginning of their friendship. She was peaceful and relaxed. She also seemed to have been healthier. The medications that her physician prescribed were more effective at controlling Elizabeth's pain. She breathed more comfortably and she slept without assistance. Elizabeth's improvement had, in fact, been so dramatic that Joyce was totally stunned to find that she had died during her sleep. I don't recall whether I suggested that her newly found peace of mind might have enabled Elizabeth to release the attitudes and self-judgment that bound her to a life of misery, and go to wherever it was her spirit was being called.

SECURITY IN THE PRESENCE OF THE UNKNOWN

How unfortunate it is that the ones whom patients trust so implicitly, physicians and nurses who may even be responsible for the sustenance or preservation of life itself, must often be the ones who cause pain and suffering in order to accomplish or seek the outcome the patient desires. The most sensitive and compassionate caregivers must sometimes use implements, tools, and treatments that are uncomfortable, painful, and often very fearsome to their patients. The chaplain can represent a nonthreatening, caring presence to whom the patient can cling for temporary strength and comfort, especially if that chaplain has had an opportunity to develop a nurturing relationship with the patient.

It was in my first year as a hospital chaplain that I met George, a rugged, outdoors kind of man who, in his early 70s, still took great delight in his hunting and fishing trips, and pride in the large garden that he maintained for his wife at their rural retirement home. The progression of diabetes, however, resulted in a pedal wound that ultimately required amputation of his foot. Rugged as he was, George was a man of deep Christian faith and he bonded to me through the prayer and supportive presence I provided to him. Regrettably, the stump wound did not heal and the decision was made to amputate again, further up the leg. Before George was discharged, it became apparent that there was infection present in the second stump and, among the various procedures used to facilitate healing, a decision was made to lance the stump and clean out the infected substance that had collected inside. The procedure was to be accomplished in George's hospital bed, under local anesthesia. He was terrified and tearful, and was reticent to sign consent for the procedure. When I attempted to reassure him that the minor surgery was essential to his recovery, and that the physician would be as gentle with him as possible, he determined that he would only consent if I would be with him throughout.

The medical team welcomed the support and I was positioned in surgical gown at the patient's head where I could hold his hands firmly and speak words of encouragement. George's unit nurse was present, touching him and providing compassionate reassurance. However, she was also the one who gave him injections and, according to the nature of her duty, did a variety of invasive things to him. In my role as chaplain I was the only one who was totally nonthreatening, and therefore represented the security he needed for that occasion. Ultimately, George did recover and it was always a source of tremendous joy whenever he stopped by the hospital to see me, walking on the prosthesis, which enabled him still to hunt and fish.

The chaplain's ability to provide security is also evidenced in my experience with Alma, a patient with severe coronary occlusions. At nearly 80 years old, Alma was a strong-appearing, physically attractive lady who, until the appearance of heart symptoms, had enjoyed a vital and productive life. Two cardiologists and a surgeon had, however, discerned that without multiple bypass surgery she was in danger of a major event that could end her life or render her a cardiac invalid. Alma was terrified. She had never previously been hospitalized, and the thought of having her chest invaded was overwhelmingly fearsome for her. When, after two consults, the surgeon was unable to reach verbal consent for the surgery to be scheduled, he asked her if she was a person who prayed. "Oh, yes," she responded, and then bore to him a firm testimony of what an important role faith played in her life. The surgeon was one with whom I had a collegial relationship, and whose patients I had often attended to provide prayer support during surgery, and so he asked her whether it would help her to know that a chaplain could be present in the room, praying for her safety and for the medical team throughout the surgery. Alma expressed interest in that possibility, and the surgeon wrote a referral to me.

After a very brief intervention, including prayer, Alma agreed that she would consent to the surgery with the assurance that I would provide on-location prayer support. I continued to pray with Alma for each of the next 2 days before the date of her surgery, and in pre-op holding on the morning of the big day. When it was time for her to be transported to the surgical suite, I helped push the gurney and I held her hand while the anesthesiologist put her to sleep. Then I took my place on a stool against the wall at the foot of the operating table and assumed an attitude of prayer for a very long time. There were complications, and what was expected to be 4 to 6 hours became 11 hours before Alma was moved to the Surgical Intensive Care Unit. The surgery was successful, however, and after a reasonable period of recovery, she was discharged to home. I followed Alma closely during the remainder of her hospitalization and maintained telephone contact with her for several weeks during her continued recovery at home. During that time she declared often that she would not have consented to the surgery without the security that there was a chaplain nearby who was praying continually for her safety and for the entire team in whose hands she had placed her life.

A CHAPLAIN TO SELF

Little evidence is more credible than that which we have, ourselves, experienced. So it was with me when I had spinal surgery in 1997. A congenital structural defect had, with advancing age, progressed to a condition that limited the quality of my life. I had for more than 2 years consumed maximum daily quantities of nonsteroidal anti-inflammatory drugs, and I used a cane to stand straight and to decrease the orthopedic stress that resulted in pain, which spiraled downward through my pelvis and my right leg whenever I walked or stood in one place. After extensive physical therapy and thorough neurological work-ups, I accepted the recommendation of a neurosurgeon who believed that vertebras L-4, L-5, and S-1 should be fused, and rods should be inserted to reinforce my lower spine. That surgery was totally successful, and my comfort level and personal stamina during the post-operative period and throughout my recovery were so dramatic as to amaze the surgeon and the entire care team.

I believe it noteworthy that as a spiritual care provider I consider the condition of my own spiritual health to be above average. I have no fear of death. My consciousness of self as a spiritual being, one who dwells in a physical "vehicle" during this life experience on planet Earth, frees me from any fear over what will happen to me whenever this vehicle, my body, can no longer sustain me. I know that I will just separate out of it, and that I will be as alive, more conscious perhaps, than before. While I prefer to remain with my family and friends in this Earth experience which I so enjoy, I live daily with confidence that whenever the phenomenon called death comes to me, it is okay. Having worked in hospitals for over 25 years, I trust medical procedures and the professionals who accomplish them. More than that, I trust God who is my constant and most intimate companion. I always expect the best for myself, and even though outcomes are not always as I desired them or designed them, the delivery of my higher good seems always evident. Armed with a positive attitude formed of faith and confidence, and supported by a prayer army — family and friends — I went to the operating room with no more anxiety than if I were taking an exciting journey. There was no expectation of any outcome less than total success and happiness.

When awakened in post-op, my first consciousness was a wave of nausea, feeling that I needed to vomit. That sensation could not have lasted more than 10 seconds, and it was the totality of my difficult symptoms following surgery. I was taken back to my room around 12:30 P.M., bright eyed and laughing. My wife and friends who waited could not believe it. Three shifts of nurses who thought I should sleep could not believe it either. I received visitors, talked on the telephone, and watched television continually until I finally closed my eyes to sleep sometime around 2:00 A.M. on the next day. For the first 24 to 48 hours after surgery I was given injections for pain. Those were soon discontinued, however, because, they simply weren't needed. The injections were changed to oxycodone that I took only in the late afternoon and evening when I experienced an unpleasant but tolerable sensation in my pelvic girdle and legs. On a scale of 1 to 10, it probably never escalated higher than a 4, even without the drug.

I was out of bed and walking with the physical therapist on the morning after surgery, and on the fourth day I was discharged to home. My wife's anxiety over how I was going to ascend the stairs to our second-floor bedroom was replaced with astonishment when I simply walked up, changed into lounging pajamas, and got onto the bed. The oral oxycodone was flushed down the toilet within about 3 days after returning home. I found the consciousness-numbing effect of the medication to be far less tolerable than the mild afternoon and evening discomfort in my hips and legs, and within only about 10 days following surgery there was no longer any remaining sensation of pain. The incision itself, a "centipede" that ran from the center of my back to the top of my buttocks, was never more than slightly sore.

It is undeniable that as an employee of the medical center where my surgery was performed, I was the recipient of the best care available. Further, my anesthesiologist and neurosurgeon were recognized as the "A Team." I bless them for their good work on my behalf. Nor can we ignore the truth that every person is unique, each with a different pain threshold and with his or her own capacities to heal. Regardless, I know at the very core of my being that the condition of my spiritual health was instrumental in effecting the pain-free outcome that I experienced from such an invasive surgery. I have repeatedly seen evidence just as dramatic with patients who endured surgical procedures as radical as cardiothoracic and intracranial. As evidenced through the personal experience of spiritual caregivers the world over, and by the increasing body of clinical research, robust spiritual health disposes the patient to the most successful outcomes, and quality spiritual care enhances the efficacy of the medical interventions provided.

YOUR COLLEAGUE, THE CHAPLAIN

How often it seems that those things most obvious are the ones we overlook. Patients regularly receive referrals from one physician to another for specialized care. Likewise, doctors consistently utilize the skills of physical therapists, occupational therapists, psychologists, nutritionists, and social workers, to effect the most positive outcomes for their patients. It is still the exception, however, when a physician actually makes a referral to the chaplain. Old habits and old attitudes die slowly and hard. Far too often the chaplain is viewed as only the religious practitioner, the nice person who comes to pray or read scripture, or to encourage or "save souls." That model may be as archaic as the "country doctor" who rode the circuit from home to home and practiced out of a black bag. While there are still chaplains whose consciousness limits them to religious endeavors, or whose practice is exclusive and

self-serving, they are no longer well received within the mainstream of professional, spiritual health care. Despite the good they do, such practitioners may continue to feed attitudes that have for so long polarized science and religion, medical practice and spiritual care.

The few case studies considered in this chapter evidence the resource that the chaplain can represent to physicians who are willing to leave no stone unturned in affecting the greatest outcomes for their patients. We don't always understand, and may never understand, the true nature of the spiritual dimension and the power it holds over sickness and health, life and death. But if personal experience does not lend credibility, these examples, nonetheless, demonstrate the incredible value and potential of sound spiritual care that is now evidenced clinically at an annually increasing rate. Even those who attribute such outcomes to the placebo effect would be remiss to deny the value of placebo when the desired end is reached.

HOPE: A SPIRITUAL PLACEBO

In his book *The Anatomy of Hope: How People Prevail in the Face of Illness* (2004), author Jerome Groopman evidences the understanding of many scientists and health care professionals that the placebo effect is hope in action. He calls hope "the very heart of healing," and he asserts, "For those who have hope, it may help some to live longer, and it will help all to live better."

Throughout recorded history the power of hope has been evidenced by the ability of individuals to survive and to emerge victorious over the most insurmountable of difficulties. In our own age, survivors of death camps such as Auschwitz, prisoners of war, and persons subject to unthinkable economic, cultural, and political oppression have credited hope as the lifeline that enabled them to survive. Spiritually conscious health care providers are continuous observers of the mystery of hope. What enables an actively dying patient, even though comatose, to survive until the last or most important person arrives? How do some patients survive long after the ravages of a disease process medically allow? Why do some patients totally overcome or recover from injuries or diseases that offer no possibility of survival? The answers to such questions would again seem as attainable as "nailing Jell-O to the wall." But again the questions emerges, "So what?" Some things we may never prove, but they are no less worthy of consideration or acceptance. The evidence is clear that hope has power beyond our ability to define or to quantify. Whether it is placebo may be a non-issue so long as its outcome is positive and meaningful to the patient or family.

With people living longer, many well remember the days still glorified on the video screen when the physician was truly the "hope bearer" by his or her ability to come to the home with that wonderful little black bag of miracles. "Doc" had time to sit by the bedside of a critically ill patient throughout the night, or to sit at the kitchen table and have pie and coffee with the family, sharing their burden, supporting them in their fear. With population growth, urban expansion, specialization, the evolution of society, and the control that third-party payers maintain over health care providers, such practices are now limited, if not virtually impossible for even the most spiritually conscious and caring physicians. Change is not without benefit, however. Today's health care chaplain is for many a hope-bearer and an extension of the physician. When partnered with a chaplain or a spiritual care team, physicians can devote their time and energy to the specialized demands of clinical patient care with confidence that their patients have a present resource to help them find hope where hope can be found.

A COAT OF MANY COLORS

Not just a resource for patients and physicians, professional chaplains interface closely with patient families, multidisciplinary members of the health care team, volunteers, and community members who are significant to the patient, or who can provide support in whatever challenges the patient may face. For patients whose life meaning and hope are founded in faith or religious practices, chaplains can represent the power, which is there to be found. When called to be religious practitioners, professional chaplains seek appropriate ways to transcend dogma and the boundaries that are often present in religion and denomination. The chaplain's job is never to proselytize nor to define truth. Rather, the chaplain provides the presence that the patient needs, or facilitates the patient's connection to the faith leader who can. Conversely, the chaplain reinforces the institution's duty to protect patients from visitors who represent religious agendas contrary to the patient's wishes.

The professional chaplain's services also extend to non-religious needs of patients, families, visitors, physicians, volunteers, and other members of the multidisciplinary team. Common activities and responsibilities may include

- Spiritual assessment
- Spiritual risk screening
- Patient advocacy
- Crisis intervention and critical incident stress management
- Grief support
- Facilitation of advance directives
- Facilitation of organ/tissue donation
- Resource referral
- Facilitation of communication
- Conflict resolution

- Participation in patient care conferences and medical rounds
- Participation in multidisciplinary/interdisciplinary education
- Participation in bioethics consults and institutional review boards
- Staff support for both professional and personal crises
- Institutional support during times of organizational crisis or transition
- Implementation of the organizational mission

Having provided spiritual support and crisis intervention over the years to physicians, nurses, and a variety of staff persons, from housekeepers to administrators, dealing with issues ranging from personal grief to suicidal ideation, I have always considered one of the most vital roles of the chaplain to be that of keeping the rest of the team spiritually healthy.

A fairly common practice among bedside caregivers has for many years been to call the chaplain when all else fails or whenever things seem to be getting too out of control. Although flawed, that line of thinking has nonetheless given chaplains many opportunities to prove their worth, if in no other way than to provide a calm presence in the eye of the storm. As clinical consciousness for the value of spiritual care increases, however, chaplains are regarded more consistently as vital members of the care team, and their professional intervention is sought more proactively. Many physicians now include a spiritual assessment in their total care continuum. It is becoming increasingly more common for physicians to work collaboratively with chaplains in their dedicated efforts to accomplish desirable and lasting outcomes for their patients. Medical educators and practitioners of renown such as Larry Dossey, M.D., a Diplomate in the American Board of Internal Medicine; Harold G. Koenig, M.D, of Duke University; Christina Puchalski, M.D., of George Washington University; Herbert Benson, M.D., of Harvard University; Dale Matthews, M.D., of Georgetown University; and the late David B. Larson, M.D., of Duke University are but a few who have gained international recognition for their individual and collaborative efforts to bring spiritual consciousness to academic medicine. Together with countless others, they serve the cause of total care by being, themselves, spiritual caregivers and by espousing and utilizing the tremendous resource present in the professional chaplain.

REFERENCES

Byrd, R. C. (1998). Positive therapeutic effects of intercessory prayer in a coronary care unit population, *Southern Medical Journal, 81*(7), 826.

Dossey, L (1998). *Validating spiritual care through clinical research.* Seminar of Mayo Medical Center Dept. of Continuing Education, Rochester, MN, 1998.

Gallup, Jr., G. H. (1990). *Religion in America.* Princeton, NJ: Princeton Religious Research Center.

Harvard Medical School Department of Continuing Education and The Mind/Body Medical Institute (1995, 1996). *Spirituality and healing in medicine.* Conference of Harvard Medical School Department of Continuing Education and The Mind/Body Medical Institute, Deaconess Hospital, Boston, MA.

Groopman, J. (2004). *The anatomy of hope: How people prevail in the face of illness.* New York: Random House.

Kuhn, C. C. (1988). *Ryandic, 6*(2).

Larson, D. B., Swyers, J. P., & McCullough, M. E. (1997). *Scientific research on spirituality and health.* Rockville, MD: National Institute for Healthcare Research.

Mathews, D. A., Larson, D. B., & Barry, C. P. (1993). *The faith factor: An annotated bibliography of clinical research on spiritual subjects.* Rockville, MD. National Institute for Healthcare Research.

McNichol, T. (1996, April 5–7). The new faith in medicine. *USA Weekend,* 4.

Puchalski, C. M., & Larson, D. B. (1998). Developing curricula in spirituality and medicine. *Academic Medicine, 73*(9).

Sicher, F. et al. (1998). A randomized double-blind study of the effect of distant healing in a population with advanced AIDS. *Western Journal of Medicine, 169,* 356–363.

Wallis, C. (1996, June 24). Faith and healing. *Time,* 62.

Section III

Common Pain Problems

David Glick, DC, Section Editor

23

Acute Pain Management

Anh L. Ngo, MD, MBA, and Rainier Guiang, MD

INTRODUCTION

Acute pain serves as a warning system of potential or actual injury. It allows a person to sense when the body is physically threatened and to modify behavior to avoid further tissue damage. This evolutionary advantage is clear when one compares people who have impaired pain sensation with normal individuals. Those with congenital abnormalities, such as a lack of C nociceptive fibers, or acquired conditions such as diabetic peripheral neuropathy sustain more traumatic injuries.

Pain caused by surgical intervention or medical procedures, however, is maladaptive and does not serve any useful purpose. In fact, poorly treated pain is detrimental to several bodily systems, including immunomodulation, stress hormone levels, sympathetic tone, and the cardiovascular system (Ashburn & Ready, 2001; Carr et al. 1992; Max & Payne, 1999; Ready, 2000). Thus, while it is harmful to eliminate all pain when it serves its natural protective purpose, it is compassionate and medically appropriate to treat acute and postsurgical pain.

The Agency for Health Care Policy and Research released clinical practice guidelines in 1992, which set the standard for pain management for surgery and trauma (Carr et al. 1992). The American Society of Anesthesiologists formulated practice guidelines for acute pain management in the perioperative setting in 1995 (Ready et al. 1995). Protocols for acute pain management services in hospitals are available (Ashburn & Ready, 2001; Macintyre & Ready, 2001; Ready, 2000; Sinatra, 1998).

In 2001, the Joint Commission on Accreditation of Healthcare Organizations (JCAHO) published pain management standards for health care facilities (JCAHO, 2001). As providers became more aware of the standards,

in 2003, JCAHO provided follow-up recommendations for improving the quality of pain management through performance measures and suggestions for action (JCAHO, 2003). Health care facilities must now recognize the right of patients for timely assessment and management of pain. This process includes identifying inadequately treated pain during the initial assessment of patients and during subsequent reassessments. Patient, patient family, and caregiver education is central to the process as well.

Acute pain in the medical setting may be due to surgery, accidental injury, or exacerbation of a chronic medical condition. Examples include surgical incisions with attendant injury to skin, muscles, bones, and joints; distension of hollow abdominal or pelvic organs; and irritation of pleura or peritoneum. Acute pain may also be an exacerbation of a chronic condition, such as sickle cell crisis, gallstones, migraine headache, herpes zoster, ischemic tissue pain, and cancer. Regardless of the cause, acute pain is harmful to homeostasis and increases the risk of complications.

Untreated pain has negative effects on organ systems and the healing process. Pain can increase risk to problems such as myocardial infarction, congestive heart failure, and infection. Acute pain incites the body's reflex responses for a hypermetabolic state by increasing catecholamine and cortisol levels — which heighten protein catabolism, gluconeogenesis, lypolysis, and hypercoagulability. Pain can also stimulate the cardiovascular system causing hypertension, tachycardia, increased cardiac workload, and a higher cardiac oxygen demand. These physiologic changes place the patient at risk for perioperative ischemia, myocardial infarction, and stroke, particularly if the patient is elderly or has cerebral or coronary

285

artery disease. Pain also depresses the immune system, increasing the susceptibility of postoperative infections for patients (Sinatra, 1998).

Acute pain after upper abdominal or thoracic surgical procedures can lead to an increased risk of respiratory complications. Guarding and splinting in this area results in a decrease in vital capacity, tidal volume, and functional residual capacity while it increases respiratory rate. The result is an inability to effectively clear bronchial secretions leading to atelectasis, pneumonia, and respiratory failure. Effective pain control improves respiratory function in the postoperative patient, leads to earlier ambulation after surgery, and decreases the risk of deep vein thromboses and pulmonary emboli.

While there are many medical consequences for a patient after injury or surgery, acute pain also affects the institution of medical practice. Pain can cause increases in health care expenditures with prolonged hospital stays and increased pain-related visits. Therefore, prudent evaluation, identification, and treatment of acute pain are vital for the health of patients and the medical system.

EVALUATION OF THE PATIENT IN PAIN

Unfortunately, to date there is no objective test that can measure the severity of a patient's pain. Vital signs such as heart rate, blood pressure, and respiratory rate have been shown to be inconsistent with the subjective severity of pain. To infer severity, the verbal or visual analog scale has become widely accepted in modern medical practice. The scale ranges from 0 to 10, where "0" indicates no pain while a value of "10" indicates the worst pain imaginable. Prior to asking patients to assign a value, it is important to orient them to what characteristics define a score of 10. Examples of a 10 score could be equated to having a surgical incision without any anesthesia or described in terms of pain so severe they would be unable to tolerate it. Patients who can perform their activities of daily living or sleep soundly at night are unlikely to have pain levels of 9 or 10. These designations are reserved for patients who are in excruciating pain. Once determined, the pain score should be documented in the medical record and used to gauge the efficacy of future treatments.

Effective pain management strikes a balance between achieving adequate pain control and minimizing the potential physiological side effects associated with the chosen modality of treatment. A patient receiving a therapeutic dose of morphine may have significant pain reduction, but also develop sedation and, rarely, clinically significant respiratory depression. It is always safer to start with lower doses of pain medications and then titrate the dose to an acceptable level of pain control rather than be too aggressive and have to give a reversal agent. The goal of complete pain relief is rarely necessary and sometimes unreasonable. Recall that the sensation of pain is a pro-

tective mechanism and to completely inhibit this could mask other underlying pathology that may need to be addressed. A reasonable goal for pain reduction is to a level of 4 or less on the verbal or visual analog scale or to a level at which the patient can comfortably tolerate the pain without adverse side effects.

HISTORY AND PHYSICAL EXAMINATION

A detailed history and physical examination with special consideration of the pain history is the initial step in assessing the patient. The pain history should include inquiries into the characteristics of the pain, including location, quality (sharp, dull, aching, throbbing, burning, lancinating, etc.), duration, and factors that exacerbate or relieve it. The past medical and surgical history should pay special attention to disorders such as respiratory, renal, and liver disease, which may affect the choice of treatment modality. Current infection, coagulation disorders, or spine disease may contraindicate neuraxial (epidural or intrathecal) or regional modes of treatment. Tolerance from chronic pain medication use or a history of alcohol or illicit drug abuse must also be considered when determining an appropriate starting dose of pain medication. A patient's prior response to surgery and subsequent postoperative recovery course may give the provider insight into the patient's threshold for pain and the expected response to different pain treatment modalities.

The physical examination should start with an assessment of the patient's vital signs. In the acute postoperative setting, this may include blood pressure, heart rate, respiratory rate and peripheral oxygen saturation (pulse oximetry). Hypertension, tachycardia, and tachypnea may be objective signs of uncontrolled pain whereas a low respiratory rate, change in mental status, and hypotension may indicate respiratory depression from opioids. An observation regarding the patient's general appearance and condition should be documented. A patient found sleeping comfortably but reporting a pain score of 10 may indicate either a misunderstanding of the pain score or drug-seeking behavior. A focused, systematic physical exam should include an evaluation of mental status; auscultation of the heart, lungs, and abdomen; and gentle palpation of painful areas. In the postoperative setting, examination of the intravenous line and epidural catheter must also be documented as they are common sources of pain other than the primary surgical site. Thorough documentation of the initial history, physical, and pain score and then again with each subsequent patient encounter is the key to gauging the progress of a treatment plan objectively.

When acting on behalf of the primary (requesting) service, the consulting service (such as the pain service) should verify that all recommendations are documented in the medical chart and communicated directly to the primary service to avoid any confusion or misunderstandings. Patients should be involved in the decision-making process regarding the pain management plan. For hospitalized patients, the pain service may follow the patient on a daily basis and adjust the treatment plan as necessary.

BASIC ACUTE PAIN MANAGEMENT STRATEGIES

The provider must first determine the severity of the pain (mild, moderate, or severe), choose an analgesic, and finally determine the optimal route of administration. There are several routes available to deliver pain medications: enterally, administered via the alimentary tract, or parenterally, administered by means other than the alimentary tract. Enteral administration involves the oral, sublingual, or rectal route whereas the parenteral route includes intravenous, epidural, intrathecal, subcutaneous or transcutaneous, and intramuscular administration. The choice of modality depends on the patient's condition, the availability of easy intravenous access, and the presence of a functioning gastrointestinal tract. Although technically easy to administer, intramuscular injections have fallen out of favor with many physicians for two reasons. First, intramuscular drug uptake is variable, and second, patients generally do not like receiving injections.

MILD TO MODERATE PAIN

Nonsteroidal anti-inflammatory drugs (NSAIDs) and acetaminophen are first-line medications for the patient in mild to moderate pain. The choice of which agent to start with depends on the existence of comorbidities, such as renal disease or bleeding diatheses in the case of NSAIDs or liver disease in the case of acetaminophen. Currently, there is only one NSAID, ketorolac, available for intravenous administration. Approval of a parenteral COX 2 selective drug, paracoxib, is anticipated in the near future. Failure to achieve adequate pain control with near maximal doses of these medications warrants the addition of an opioid.

Opioid medications differ from NSAIDs in that opioids do not have a strict ceiling dose; further dosage increase will provide incrementally more pain relief. In contrast, NSAIDs have a clear ceiling dose. Once exceeded, additional drug will not provide more analgesia, but will increase the risk of drug-induced side effects. Note that the concept of a "weak" opioid does not have much pharmacologic support and often simply means that the particular drug is combined with acetaminophen or NSAID. In such cases, using a weak opioid limits the amount of actual opioid that can be delivered, without potentially providing too much acetaminophen. Table 23.1

TABLE 23.1
NSAIDs: Dosing Data for Adult Patients

Drug	Usual Adult Dose	Comments
		Oral NSAIDs
Acetaminophen	650–975 mg q 4 hr	Acetaminophen lacks the peripheral anti-inflammatory activity of other NSAIDs; maximum dose of 4 g per day; may be contraindicated with alcohol use
Aspirin	650–975 mg q 4 hr	The standard against which other NSAIDs are compared; inhibits platelet aggregation; may cause postoperative bleeding
Celecoxib	100 QD to BID	COX 2 selective NSAID with improved platelet and GI profile
Diflunisal	1000 mg initial dose followed by 500 mg q 12 hr	Equivalent in strength to codeine 60 mg plus acetaminophen; fewer platelet effects than aspirin
Ibuprofen	400 mg q 4–6 hr	Available as several brand names and as generic; also available as oral suspension
Naproxen	500 mg initial dose followed by 250 mg q 6–8 hr	Also available as oral liquid
Naproxen sodium	550 mg initial dose followed by 275 mg q 6–8 hr	Sodium salt may have faster therapeutic effect
Salsalate	500 mg q 4 hr	May have minimal anti-platelet activity
Valdecoxib	10 to 20 mg q day	COX-2 selective NSAID
		Parenteral NSAID
Ketorolac tromethamine	30 or 60 mg i.m./i.v. initial dose followed by 15 or 30 mg q 6 hr Oral dose following IM dosage: 10 mg q 6–8 hr	Use not to exceed 5 days

Note: Modified and updated from *Acute Pain Management: Operative or Medical Procedures and Trauma.* Clinical Practice Guideline. Rockville, MD: Agency for Health Care Policy and Research, 1992.

QD = per day; BID = twice a day.

TABLE 23.2
Opioids: Dosing Data for Adult Patients

	Approximate Equianalgesic Doses		Recommended Starting Dose (adults weighing more than 50 kg)	
	Oral	Parenteral	Oral	Parenteral
Opioid Agonist Drug				
Morphine	30 mg q 3–4 hr	10 mg q 3–4 hr	30 mg q 3–4 hr	10 mg q 3–4 hr
Codeine	130 mg q 3–4 hr	75 mg q 3–4 hr	60 mg q 3–4 hr	60 mg q 2 hr (IM/SQ)
Hydromorphone	7.5 mg q 3–4 hr	1.5 mg q 3–4 hr	6 mg q 3–4 hr	1.5 mg q 3–4 hr
Hydrocodone (with acetaminophen)	30 mg q 3–4 hr	Not available	10 mg q 3–4 hr	Not available
Meperidine[a]	300 mg q 2–3 hr	100 mg q 3 hr	Not recommended	100 mg q 3 hr
Oxycodone	15–20 mg q 3–4 hr	Not available	10 mg q 3–4 hr	Not available

[a] Also see warnings with meperidine, listed in Table 23.3.

Note: The oral to parenteral ratio of morphine with chronic dosing is 3:1. The oral:parenteral ratio for hydromorphone is 5:1. These are only approximate doses, and clinical use of these tables demands caution. Doses should be titrated to effect. Modified and updated from *Acute Pain Management: Operative or Medical Procedures and Trauma*. Clinical Practice Guideline. Rockville, MD: Agency for Health Care Policy and Research, 1992.

displays the starting and maximum doses of NSAIDs and acetaminophen. Table 23.2 shows equianalgesic doses of opioids compared with morphine. NSAIDs and opioids are discussed in greater detail in Chapters 53 and 54, respectively.

MODERATE TO SEVERE PAIN

Patients who undergo major surgeries (cardiothoracic or open abdominal procedures) or procedures associated with intense postoperative pain (knee replacements) may require greater amounts of analgesics or more sophisticated analgesic delivery methods. For patients in severe pain, the intravenous administration of an opioid is usually the treatment of choice. An adequate intravenous dose of an opioid leads to rapid pain relief because a therapeutic blood level of drug is quickly achieved; this is facilitated by avoidance of the first pass effect in the liver.

Morphine, hydromorphone, and fentanyl are pure opioid agonists, available in oral and intravenous formulations. Pure opioid agonists, in contrast to partial agonists (and NSAIDs), have no theoretical dosage "ceiling effect." In theory, pure agonists can be titrated to pain relief without risk of end organ toxicity. However, one must keep in mind that all opioids are associated with dose-dependent side effects such as respiratory depression, sedation, and constipation. The actual dosage ceiling reached depends on the patient, clinical situation, patient monitoring (e.g., in the intensive care unit (ICU), and the physician's comfort with the analgesic protocol. Failure to achieve adequate analgesia for acute, nociceptive pain with a single opioid may be due to inadequate dosing, inappropriate frequency of administration, or onset of unwanted side effects, which prevents further titration.

Once pain control is achieved, pain levels should decrease over the first few postoperative or post-injury days, and the use of sustained-release opioids (e.g., MS Contin®, Oramorph®, OxyContin®, and Duragesic®) typically is not necessary or indicated. Although controlled-release preparations may be appropriate for patients who were on a stable opioid dose prior to the current episode of acute pain, the use of controlled-release analgesics is predicated on the need for a stable, around-the-clock dosage. The appropriate dose may be difficult to predict in a given patient, particularly in the acute pain or postsurgical situation.

ADVANCED PAIN MANAGEMENT STRATEGIES

Patient controlled analgesia (PCA) employs an electronic, programmable pump that delivers on patient demand a preset amount of pain medication, usually by the intravenous route (Macintyre & Ready, 2001). The health care provider generally must program a bolus dose, demand dose, lockout interval, hourly (or 4-hourly) maximum dose, and an optional basal rate. The bolus dose is the initial loading dose given to achieve a therapeutic level of medication. The demand dose is the dose that will be self-administered each time the patient pushes the button. The lockout interval is the time that must elapse before the patient will be allowed another dose on demand. The hourly maximum dose is the programmed total amount of drug that theoretically may be delivered within the given time period. The basal rate is an optional programmed hourly background infusion of opioid. An example of a typical regimen for hydromorphone would be the following: Demand dose 0.2 mg, lockout interval 10 minutes, hourly maximum 1.2 mg, basal rate 0 mg/h. See Table

TABLE 23.3
PCA Settings for Commonly Used Opioids

	Morphine	Hydromorphone	Meperidine	Fentanyl
Concentration	1 mg/ml	0.2 mg/ml	10 mg/ml	20 µg/ml
Demand Dose	1 mg	0.2 mg	10 mg	20 µg
Lockout interval	10 min	10 min	10 min	8 min
Basal Rate/hr	1 mg	0.2 mg	10 mg	20 mcg/hr
Hourly limit	7 mg	1.4 mg	70 mg	100 mcg

Note: Meperidine should not be used in patients with renal insufficiency, or for longer than 48 hours. The total 24-hour dose of meperidine should not exceed 600 mg in the average adult. Meperidine is not a first-line drug, but may have a role for patients who are allergic to or have excessive nausea with morphine-based products. Morphine metabolites accumulate with renal insufficiency. Remember that morphine is not dialyzable. Hydromorphone is generally considered to be safe for patients with poor renal function, as is fentanyl. However, metabolites may accumulate that cause central nervous system problems. Patients with concomitant hepatic dysfunction will have unpredictable responses to opioids because of prolonged metabolism.

23.3 for commonly used opioids and PCA settings. Not all patients are candidates for PCA.

The theory behind PCA is simple. When the patient experiences pain, he or she pushes the button, pain medication is delivered, and the patient experiences an increment of pain relief. If the increment of relief is inadequate, the patient pushes the button again and will receive an additional dose of medication, as long as the lockout interval, in this case 10 minutes, has elapsed since initially pushing the button. If less than 10 minutes has lapsed, the patient will not receive the additional dose. If the pain is inadequately controlled with the current settings, the provider can review the history of attempts and injections, which is electronically stored by the pump. A high ratio of attempts to injections can indicate an inadequate demand dose, a lockout interval that is too long, or an inadequate understanding by the patient of how to use the pump. For instance, a patient who does not understand that a few minutes are required from the time the button is pressed to the onset of pain relief may press the button multiple times in rapid succession.

The PCA has a built-in safety mechanism that safeguards the patient from unwanted respiratory depression. If the demand dose causes unwanted sedation, the patient falls asleep and is rendered incapable of pushing the button again until the sedation wears off.

It is important to note that sedation may herald the development of clinically significant respiratory depression. Dosing should be reduced to allow any sedative effects to wear off. Adequate oxygenation should be verified by pulse oximetry. Use of a sedation scale is suggested (0 = fully awake; 1 = mildly drowsy; 2 = frequently drowsy but easy to awaken; 3 = somnolent and difficult to arouse; S = sleeping). A score of 2 warrants turning off any basal infusion and reducing the demand dose, typi-

cally by 50%. A score of 3 requires further intervention, possibly including the use of a reversal agent such as naloxone (carefully titrated to vital signs, oxygen saturation, and respiratory function). The goal of PCA therapy is to provide adequate pain relief, with pain scores generally less than 4 of 10 and sedation scores less than 2.

The addition of the optional basal infusion renders the inherent safety mechanism of PCA less effective, because the background infusion, by definition, is not under the patient's control. This extra amount of analgesic may be sufficient to cause sedation and increases the risk of respiratory depression. Patients with basal infusions should be monitored more frequently for signs of sedation or respiratory depression. In our institution, we do not routinely add basal infusions, except on the first night following surgery, unless there is a demonstrated need to provide the basal infusion. Use with elderly patients is not recommended.

On occasion, well-intentioned family members, fearing that the patient is experiencing pain, will push the button for the patient. This also defeats the PCA concept and may increase the risk of respiratory depression. Family members must be made of aware of this danger and instructed not to administer analgesic doses for the patient.

Any opioid available in an intravenous formulation can be used with a PCA device. However, fentanyl and meperidine warrant special mention. Fentanyl is an opioid analgesic with potency 50 to 80 times greater than that of morphine. Because of its high potency, risk of diversion, rapid onset of effect, and the fact that most physicians are not familiar with fentanyl, its use on the general medical floors is discouraged, unless appropriate expertise with the drug is available.

On the other hand, fentanyl is commonly used in the operating rooms by experienced anesthesiologists and in the intensive care units for patients on continuous monitors, and in some postoperative settings, fentanyl may be considered a drug of choice. Advantages of fentanyl include its rapid onset and lack of active metabolites that are excreted by the kidney. Provided that liver function is normal, fentanyl will not accumulate with renal insufficiency.

Meperidine has fallen out of favor in many hospitals because of potential toxicity associated with its metabolite, normeperidine, which is renally excreted and can accumulate in plasma, even with normal renal function. Normeperidine has been shown to lower seizure thresholds and cause myoclonus, even following therapeutic doses of meperidine. Nonetheless, meperidine usage remains widespread, despite its poor image. Although meperidine may be appropriate for patients who become nauseated with morphine derivatives (e.g., morphine, oxycodone, and hydromorphone), or for patients with true allergies to morphine derivatives, it can no longer be considered a first-line drug. In any case, meperidine should not be given in doses greater than 600 mg in a 24-hour period for the average adult and should not be administered for more than 48 hours, even with normal renal or central nervous system function (Max & Payne, 1999).

Providing patients with dosing independence, within programmed parameters, is one of the best features of PCA. When patients are placed on staff-dependent administration of pain medication, there may be a delay in response due to staffing levels and demands from other patients, often delaying pain relief. PCA has the advantage of allowing the patient to control the frequency of opioid administration without the time delay of having to ask the nursing staff or physician for another dose of analgesic. This efficiency leads to greater patient satisfaction as well as removing the burden of following a fixed dosing schedule by the nursing staff.

EPIDURAL INFUSIONS

An epidural catheter can be used to provide intraoperative regional anesthesia and postoperative analgesia (Liu, Allen, & Olsson, 1998; Narinder, 2000). Intraoperatively, the epidural is dosed with various concentrations of preservative free local anesthetics such as lidocaine, chlorprocaine, bupivacaine, or ropivacaine, which results in a dense sensory blockade and varying degrees of motor blockade, depending on the agent used. In some cases the epidural may be the sole modality of intraoperative anesthesia. However, in the postoperative period, the presence of motor blockade can be considered detrimental by delaying early ambulation and compromising respiratory function. Fortunately, dilute formulations of local anesthetics, combinations of local anesthetics and opioids, or opioid infusions alone can be safely infused, providing analgesia without delaying recovery time. Formulations and doses

used for epidural infusions at University Hospitals of Cleveland are listed in Table 23.4 and Table 23.5.

The mechanisms of action of epidural local anesthetics and epidural opioids are different (Narinder, 2000). Epidural local anesthetics act primarily on the spinal nerve roots in closest proximity to the epidural catheter tip and lose effectiveness as the medication spreads. Local anesthetic epidural infusions produce segmental analgesia. Therefore, the catheter tip should be positioned at the spinal dermatome closest to the level of the incision to take full advantage of the technique, which allows the smallest infusion rate and reduces the risk of lower extremity weakness and hypotension.

On the other hand, epidural opioids act on receptor-mediated sites in the spinal cord dorsal horn and supraspinal brain sites. The degree of distal spread is determined by the opioid's hydrophilic or hydrophobic properties. Hydrophilic opioids such as morphine and hydromorphone tend to spread rostrally, whereas the lipophilic, hydrophobic opioid fentanyl tends to act locally at the dorsal horn of the spinal cord, closer to the site of injection. However, the high lipid solubility of fentanyl enhances its systemic absorption. Indeed, the analgesic effect of epidurally administered fentanyl is due in part to systemic action at supraspinal sites.

Epidural opioids are particularly effective in thoracic and upper abdominal surgeries where the infusions can provide excellent postoperative pain relief that is titratable to a patient's pain level. When combined, epidural local anesthetics and opioids can have additive effects.

Meta-analysis indicates that regardless of the choice of opioid or local anesthetic or whether the epidural catheter is placed in the thoracic or lumbar spine, epidural analgesia is superior to parenteral opioid administration (Block et al., 2003). Moreover, with appropriate monitoring, the technique is safely administered on hospitals wards.

TABLE 23.4

Standard Epidural Infusion Mixtures Used at University Hospitals of Cleveland

Name	Mixture
Bupivacaine/Hydromorphone	Bupivacaine (0.1%) Hydromorphone (0.01 mg/ml) 4–6 ml/hr
Morphine	Morphine (0.05 mg/ml) 4–8 ml/hr
Bupivacaine	Bupivacaine (0.1%) 4–6 ml/hr

Note: Hydromorphone is used more often than morphine. User preference or side effects, such as nausea, may suggest use of the alternate opioid.

TABLE 23.5
Examples of Epidural Infusions Used, Depending on the Surgery and Spinal Level of Epidural Catheter Insertion

Surgery	Epidural Catheter Insertion Level	Infusion Type
Thoracotomy	T5–T10	Bupivacaine/hydromorphone at 4–8 ml/hr
Upper abdominal procedure	T8–T12	Bupivacaine/hydromorphone at 4–8 ml/hr
Abdominal hysterectomy	T12–L1	Bupivacaine/hydromorphone at 4–8 ml/hr
Knee replacement	L3–L4	Bupivacaine at 4–8 ml/hr plus i.v. PCA

Note: See Table 23.4 for components of the infusions. These are approximate infusion rates, titrated to effect. In our institution, patients with total joint replacements have their epidural catheters removed the day after surgery, because all are started on coumadin the night of surgery; postoperative analgesia is continued with intravenous PCA.

A recent advance in epidural pain management is the use of patient controlled epidural analgesia (PCEA). As with intravenous PCA, patients have the ability to receive demand doses of epidural analgesics (opioids and/or local anesthetics) in addition to the normal basal rate. In one study, the use of PCEA with bupivacaine and fentanyl demonstrated better analgesia over standard epidural infusions and higher patient satisfaction, a lower incidence of side effects, and reduced overall costs (Liu & Benzon, 2000; Liu et al., 1998).

Epidural infusions are wonderful when they work. However, these too occasionally fail, but the failure rate is generally less than about 15%. Inadequate pain relief may be caused by improper catheter placement, migration of the epidural catheter out of the epidural space, or an extended delay between epidural dosing in the operating room and starting of the epidural infusion in the recovery area. Therefore, it is recommended that the epidural infusion be started as soon as the patient arrives in the recovery area. Generally, epidural catheters can be used safely up to 1 week, provided that catheter placement employed sterile technique and there is proper ongoing daily care of the catheter. Not all patients are appropriate candidates for epidural infusions. Specific factors to consider include patient preference, coagulation profile, and the presence of infection systemically or at the site of proposed catheter insertion.

COMMON CLINICAL SCENARIOS

THE POST ANESTHESIA CARE UNIT

The Post Anesthesia Care Unit (PACU), also known as the postsurgical recovery area, is by definition an intensive care unit. This unit is staffed by physicians and highly skilled nurses in ratios similar to those of an intensive care unit and is therefore able to deliver a level of care higher than what is available on the wards. Predetermined criteria such as hemodynamic stability and adequate pain control must be achieved prior to transfer to other patient care areas or discharge from the hospital. As all patients are monitored with blood pressure, telemetry, and pulse oximetry recording, the PACU is the safest place to initiate a pain treatment regimen. On the floors, review of the PACU records, including opioid requirements and response to treatment, can be a useful guide to determine which medications and dosages to use.

Upon the patient's arrival in the PACU, a systematic chart and operative course review should be performed with special attention to identifying patients with difficult airways and postextubation respiratory complications. The presence of these problems should warrant conservative dosing of opioids. Identification of preexisting pain syndromes and review of medication requirements may provide insight into future pain requirements. A focused physical exam should be performed and pre- and posttreatment pain scores documented. An example of opioid starting doses for an otherwise healthy adult patient could be morphine 2 to 5 mg i.v. every 15 minutes, hydromorphone 0.2 to 0.5 mg i.v. every 10 minutes, or fentanyl 25 to 50 μg i.v. every 5 minutes, and titrated until adequate pain control is achieved. Opioid naïve and elderly patients should receive smaller doses of intravenous opioids, allowing an appropriate interval for the onset of relief to take place before redosing. This approach will minimize the risk of unnecessary sedation and respiratory depression. In the absence of active bleeding, risk of bleeding, or renal disease, NSAIDs can reduce the requirements for opioids and the risk of sedation or respiratory depression.

THE HOSPITAL FLOOR

With the exception of the PACU, the floor will be the most common place where hospitalized patients may need acute pain management. Whether admitted for surgical recovery, from the emergency department, or directly from a physician's office, these patients require the same thorough assessment, detailed workup, and formulation of a course of action as previously described. For postoperative pain, where the source of pain is easily identified, simple titration of intravenous opioids through PRN orders and frequent assessments or, better yet, through PCA is usually a good course of action.

Patients admitted from the emergency department or directly from physicians' offices, where the etiology of pain is less certain, require a higher level of assessment and vigilance when starting a pain regimen. Patients who present for acute exacerbations of chronic diseases, such as a sickle cell crisis, pancreatitis, or cancer pain, may already be taking opioids chronically as outpatients. In such cases, the dose of opioids taken as an outpatient must be factored in to avoid starting an opioid at a dose too low to provide adequate analgesia. One may consider calculating the outpatient hourly dose-equivalent, and delivering an equianalgesic, parenteral dose via a PCA by basal infusion. In addition, an appropriate demand dose for breakthrough pain should be allowed. This approach requires extensive experience with PCA and in calculating conversion doses. Close monitoring is required, although the ICU setting may not be necessary.

Once the patient's analgesic requirement has been established or medical condition has stabilized, one must consider the possibility that the patient may require long-term pain therapy, such as for cancer-related pain. Unfortunately, logistical problems and lack of appropriate monitoring may make PCA impractical for general home use. On the other hand, home PCA commonly is used for patients with intractable pain due to cancer.

The conversion of intravenous to oral doses of opioids is mandatory and may be facilitated by using conversion tables or conversion calculators. However, these should only be used as guidelines, because marked variability with the final dose and dosing intervals is the rule rather than the exception.

The Outpatient Clinic

Most often, NSAIDs and acetaminophen prescribed in moderate doses are appropriate for outpatient pain management, given the low probability of life-threatening side effects. Fixed-combination opioids taken in conservative doses for short-term therapy can safely be prescribed. When starting a fixed-combination drug, such as hydrocodone and acetaminophen, the patient should be advised not to operate heavy machinery or drive until the response to the new medication is determined. Noncancer pain requiring larger dosages of opioids or cancer pain refractory to aggressive therapy should be reevaluated for other causes of pain and a referral to a pain management specialist for possible interventional therapy should be considered.

Acute or poorly controlled chronic pain may be a reason for consulting with the pain service. In the outpatient clinic, after initial evaluation, the provider must decide if the patient's medical condition and pain can be controlled on an outpatient-basis or if a higher level of care and monitoring is necessary, which would require admission to the hospital. If hospital admission is required, PCA is a convenient, efficient method of achieving rapid pain relief.

Patients with Cancer Pain

The diagnosis of advanced or metastatic cancer carries special significance to the pain practitioner due to its chronic nature and frequent poor prognosis. The psychological and emotional implications to the patient family can contribute to the modulation and perception of pain. It is common and expected that a patient with active cancer will eventually present with new pain complaints. Often these acute pain exacerbations are secondary to progression of the cancer to other areas of the body, pain from cancer treatments (surgical, chemotherapy), or the development of tolerance to the current pain regimen.

When the pain is severe and debilitating, inpatient admission and aggressive intravenous pain management is warranted while the cause of the exacerbation is determined. In the postoperative setting, if the patient with cancer has been on chronic opioids, standard postoperative doses may be inadequate to achieve pain control. As with all patients on chronic opioids, stool softeners and stimulant laxatives should be prescribed to avoid constipation, which is a common source of pain and discomfort.

Patients Who Abuse Opioids

When patients who abuse drugs present with acute pain, the practitioner's reflex is to call for a pain management consultation to avoid dealing with the patient and his or her abuse or addiction problem. The frustration involved with potential secondary gain issues, the fear of being unable to control the patient's pain without large doses of opioids, the fear of causing a patient to relapse into drug abuse behavior, and frank worries about deception and criminal activity may prompt physicians to label such patients as "difficult." The acute pain setting is probably not the ideal forum for preaching the virtues of drug rehabilitation. All patients suffering from acute pain arising from demonstrable injury deserve the same consideration and access to pain relief as patients who do not abuse drugs. Although avoiding the use of opioids might be ideal is this instance, certain situations, such as acute trauma or postoperative pain, may require the use of opioids. In the case of the recovered abuser, the alternative to the need for opioids may be as simple as placing an epidural catheter for postoperative pain control. For those with ongoing abuse, opioid tolerance represents the main obstacle to achieving satisfactory pain control. Here, the question is not which drug to use, but how much. There is no place for the use of partial agonists or agonist/antagonists such as nalbuphine or pentazocine in this situation, as the antagonist properties of these drugs may induce withdrawal symptoms.

The initial evaluation of patients currently using illicit drugs involves obtaining an accurate history of prior and current drug use and the nature of the current pain. Identification of drugs used, frequency of use, and response should be documented. This requires a frank, honest discussion with the patient and description of consequences resulting from deception.

It may be impossible to accurately convert a street drug of unknown purity such as heroin to an equianalgesic dose of pharmaceutically pure opioid. However, analgesics tables provide a starting point for further dosage titration. Intravenous PRN or PCA dosing, while titrating the analgesic to patient comfort, may be used to rapidly establish the patient's opioid requirement. PCA dosing with a basal rate will help ensure against accidental underdosing and subsequent withdrawal symptoms.

The PCA pump with its opioid-filled syringe in close proximity to the patient may invite drug abusers to attempt to administer doses manually by manipulating the syringe or pump apparatus. It should be made clear that such behavior will result in the discontinuance of the PCA. Once the acute pain is under control, it is beneficial to seek the advice of Psychiatry or Addiction Medicine when formulating a long-term plan for possible drug rehabilitation.

PATIENTS TAKING CHRONIC OPIOIDS

The approach to treatment of acute pain in patients on long-term opioids is similar to that of patients who abuse opioids. However, the conversion calculation is more precise, because an accurate history of which opioid was used is readily available. Depending on the nature of the acute pain, whether surgical or traumatic, these patients will require their normal daily dose of opioid as well as an additional dose to cover the new acute pain.

The first step is to determine the outpatient dose of opioid and convert that to an equianalgesic hourly dose of parenteral opioid, to be delivered by hourly basal infusion with the PCA device. The demand dose may be calculated as approximately equal to the hourly basal infusion rate. The demand dose should be carefully titrated with the goal of relieving the new acute pain. Subsequently, the 24-hour total amount of opioid given can then be used to calculate a basal infusion that more closely matches the patient's ongoing needs and requires less reliance on the demand dose. Another approach would be to augment judicious opioid use with NSAIDs or acetaminophen, with the goal of minimizing the increase in total opioid requirement. In all cases, assessment and reassessment are keys to providing safe, effective dose conversions and satisfactory pain relief.

For patients on chronic, high-dose opioids (e.g., oral morphine of more than 90 mg per day), epidural analgesia with a local anesthetic and/or opioid for postoperative pain control must be augmented with supplemental oral or parenteral opioids to prevent withdrawal symptoms. Withdrawal can occur even with epidural opioids.

Withdrawal can be avoided by providing at least one third of the usual daily dose of opioid, in divided doses, given every 4 hours or so. Signs of withdrawal include restlessness, irritability, hypertension, and tachycardia, so the clinician must be prepared to adjust the opioid dose as needed to treat withdrawal symptoms.

PATIENTS WITH RENAL OR LIVER DISEASE

When choosing an analgesic, drug metabolism and excretion must be considered, given the prevalence of renal and hepatic disease in the general population. NSAIDs, as previously mentioned, can worsen renal disease and are contraindicated in patients with renal insufficiency. Acetaminophen may be contraindicated in patients with hepatic disease due to the formation of hepatotoxic metabolites. Opioids are metabolized in the liver, some to pharmacologically active compounds excreted via the kidneys.

Morphine is metabolized to morphine-6-glucuronide, which is more potent than morphine, but more hydrophilic and less able to cross the blood–brain barrier. Meperidine is metabolized to normeperidine, which can cause seizure activity, not reversible by naloxone. Both morphine-6-glucuronide and normeperidine are excreted by the kidneys and will accumulate with renal insufficiency. Therefore, both morphine and meperidine are contraindicated in renal insufficiency. In the presence of renal disease, hydromorphone and fentanyl are excellent choices given their lack of active metabolites. Note should be made that epidural catheter placement may seem to offer an advantage, but must be balanced against the potential risk of coagulopathy often seen in such patients.

GERIATRIC PATIENTS

In the last decade, much interest has grown in the field of geriatrics due to the ever-increasing size of the elderly population in Western countries. Physiologically, elderly patients differ from young adults by having less body water, lean muscle mass, and increased body fat. The cardiac, respiratory, and renal systems may begin to show signs of compromise. Elderly patients have a higher incidence of systemic diseases, which also tend to be at later stages of progression. On occasion, these systemic impairments may pose a barrier to effective pain relief. For example, cognitive impairment as with Alzheimer's dementia may eliminate the possibility of using a PCA.

Cognitive problems may make assessment of pain difficult, and the clinician must be patient and flexible. Use of faces-based pain scales may be helpful if the patient cannot comprehend a numerical pain scale.

Geriatric patients tend to metabolize pain medications less efficiently, which can lead to a greater incidence of side effects such as sedation, respiratory depression, and constipation. Opioid dosing should be decreased by at least 50% of the usual dose that would be given to a young adult; as with younger patients, titration to the desired analgesic effect is the best strategy to minimize the risk of injury, particularly in frail patients.

SUMMARY

The art and science of pain management need not be overly difficult, but they require attention to detail. With awareness that a patient is in pain and knowledge of methods that provide effective treatment, pain management often becomes a straightforward endeavor. However, the clinician must have a commitment to providing good medical care, possess a basic understanding of analgesic pharmacology, and be willing to utilize adequate analgesics to achieve satisfactory pain relief.

Untreated pain can have clinically significant consequences. However, patients have a right to effective pain management, and it is not necessary to invoke the risk of physiologic consequences to justify good pain management.

The key to successful pain management is assessment and reassessment. For most patients, pharmacologic methods are the mainstay for treating acute pain. NSAIDs are effective for mild to moderate pain, and can have significant opioid-sparing effects as well. For moderate to severe pain, oral or parenteral opioids or more specialized techniques, such as epidural infusions, may be indicated.

For hospitalized patients, more advanced techniques can provide excellent pain relief, even after major surgery. Although oral opioids may be effective if the patient can take medications by mouth, PCA is safe and effective and allows rapid titration of intravenous opioids for pain relief. Epidural infusions provide superior postsurgical pain relief, particularly when opioids are combined with local anesthetics and the catheter is positioned at a dermatomal level near the incision.

Certain patient populations warrant special consideration, particularly geriatric patients, patients with renal or hepatic insufficiency, patients on chronic opioids, and those with acute pain due to cancer. Patients who currently abuse opioids can be a particular challenge, but satisfactory pain control can be achieved with appropriate titration of opioids, and with epidural infusions in selected patients.

For all patients, the appropriate course of action is based on the history and physical examination, repeated pain assessments, proper patient education, and participation of the patient in the decision-making process. It is also important to remember that pain management is a team effort, particularly in the hospital setting and for patients with complicated medical problems.

Although occasionally labor intensive, the ability to provide good pain management remains one of the exemplary skills of modern medicine. Competent pain management also remains a rewarding professional experience for the clinician.

REFERENCES

Agency for Health Care Policy and Research. (1992). *Acute Pain Management: Operative or Medical Procedures and Trauma.* Clinical practice guideline. Rockville, MD: author.

Ashburn, M. A., & Ready, L. B. (2001). Postoperative pain. In Loeser, J. D. (Ed.), *Bonica's management of pain, 3rd edition* (pp. 765–779). Philadelphia: Lippincott Williams and Wilkins.

Block, B. M., Liu, S. S., Rowlingson, A. J., Cowan, A. R., Cowan, J. A., Jr., & Wu, C. L. (2003). Efficacy of postoperative epidural analgesia: A meta-analysis. *Journal of the American Medical Association, 290:* 2455–2463.

Carr, D. B. et al. (1992). *Clinical practice guideline: Acute pain management: Operative or medical procedures and trauma.* Rockville, MD: Agency for Health Care Policy and Research, U.S. Department of Health and Human Services.

Joint Commission on Accreditation of Healthcare Organizations. (2001). Pain: Current Understanding of Assessment, Management, and Treatments. Retrieved September 21, 2004, from http://www.jcaho.org/ news+room/health+ care+issues/pain+mono_npc.pdf.

Joint Commission on Accreditation of Healthcare Organizations. (2003). Improving the Quality of Pain Management Through Measurement and Action. Retrieved September 21, 2004 from http://www. jcaho.org/news+room/health +care+issues/pain+mono_ jc.pdf.

Joint Commission on Accreditation of Healthcare Organizations (2001). Background on the Development of the Joint Commission Standards on Pain Management. Retrieved September 21, 2004, from http://www.jcaho.org/news+ room/health+care+issues/pain.htm.

Liu, S. S., Allen, H., & Olsson, G. (1998). Patient-controlled epidural analgesia with bupivicaine and fentanyl on hospital wards: Prospective experience with 1,030 surgical patients. *Anesthesiology, 87,* 688–695.

Liu, S. S., & Benzon, H. T. (2000). Outcomes and complications of acute pain management. In P. P. Raj (Ed.), *Practical management of pain, 3rd edition* (pp. 871–889). St. Louis: Mosby, Inc.

Macintyre, P. E., & Ready, L. B. (2001). *Acute pain management. A practical guide, 2nd edition.* London: WB Saunders.

Max, M. B., & Payne, R. (1999). *Principles of analgesic use in the treatment of acute pain and cancer pain, 4th edition,* Glenwood, IL: American Pain Society.

Narinder, R. (2000). Spinal opioids for acute pain management. In P. P. Raj (Ed.), *Practical management of pain, 3rd edition* (pp. 689–709). St. Louis: Mosby, Inc.

Ready, L. B. (2000). Acute perioperative pain. In R. D. Miller (Ed.), *Anesthesia, 5th edition*. Philadelphia, PA: Churchill Livingstone.

Ready, L. B. et al. (1995). Practice guidelines for acute pain management in the perioperative setting: A report by the American Society of Anesthesiologists task force on pain management, acute pain section. *Anesthesiology, 82*, 1071.

Sinatra, R. S. (1998). Acute pain management and acute pain services. In M. J. Cousins, & P. O. Bridenbaugh (Eds.), *Neural blockade in clinical anesthesia and management of pain, 3rd edition* (pp. 793–835). Philadelphia: Lippincott-Raven.

24

Neuropathic Pain

David R. Longmire, MD, Gary W. Jay, MD, DAAPM, and Mark V. Boswell, MD, PhD

INTRODUCTION

In presenting this chapter the authors' original purpose was to offer a review of established *concepts* of neuropathic pain, supplemented by discussion of current practices related to its assessment and management. These goals notwithstanding, reports of more than a century of medical observation and research have demonstrated that neuropathic pain is much more than a concept or a single disorder. It is instead an evolving collection of established clinical and experimental conditions, all of which share the perpetuation of pain symptoms or pain-related behavior created by injury to neural tissue other than that involved with simple nociception (Bennett, 1994; Fields, 1987).

Although neuropathic pain has been operationally defined as an abnormal pain state that arises from a damaged peripheral nervous system (PNS) or central nervous system (CNS) (Merskey & Bogduk, 1994), there is evidence to suggest that several disease states within this category have active residual involvement of nociceptors at the site of the original injury, creating a mixed nociceptive–neuropathic pattern. As well, several painful disorders categorized as neuropathic are created or maintained by aberrant neural communication involving autonomic nervous system pathways that are not considered to be purely peripheral or central. These include complex regional pain syndromes (CRPS) Type I and II (reflex sympathetic dystrophy and causalgia, respectively) and sympathetically maintained pain (SMP) (Dworkin et al., 2003; Jay, 1996).

DIAGNOSTIC EVALUATION OF NEUROPATHIC PAIN

There exist two lines of thought relative to the clinical diagnosis of pain syndromes of this type. One suggests that because the symptom characteristics of neuropathic pain are not pathognomonic for the condition, their lack of specificity makes the diagnosis difficult to reach (Boswell et al., 2001). Another provides evidence to support certain symptom characteristics as strong indicators of neuropathic pain (Krause & Backonja, 2003). Regardless of which attitude is correct, the pain practitioner hoping to differentiate neuropathic from non-neuropathic disorders must begin, as always, with the clinical history.

MEDICAL PAIN HISTORY

The style of medical history which has been modified for the specific documentation of pain has been described in detail elsewhere (Longmire, 1991a, 1996). Within that system the clinician acquires patient information regarding at least eight aspects of the pain problem: A mnemonic often used to ensure that completeness of data collection regarding each characteristic is PQRST, in which P = provocative, palliative factors; Q = quality, R = region (of onset), radiation, and referred pain; S = severity, and T = timing. Of these characteristics, those that are most commonly considered in the diagnosis of neuropathic pain are quality (burning, shooting, tingling, sharp, or shock-like), timing (continuous or intermittent/paroxysmal), and provocative (stimulus-evoked or stimulus-independent) (Bennett, 1994). While verbal reports of the regional (spatial) distribution may be helpful in determining the relationship of pain to specific neurological syndromes, the use of a standardized Pain Drawing Instrument is preferred for documentation. One tragic error made by clinicians in the past is the dismissal of pain as being organic simply because it did not resemble an anatomic or dermatomal distribution. In fact, many neuropathic pains, which are maintained or mediated through autonomic pathways, may follow a pattern of sympathetic sclerotomes or blocks of pain referred from deep muscular or visceral afferent reflexes.

In recording pain severity or intensity, it is important to document the patient's subjective report using standardized scales such as a verbal Numeric Rating Scale (NRS-11) or nonverbal Visual Analogue Scale. Even more important is to avoid the cardinal sin of confusing results of a verbal and visual scale by reporting: "the patient stated that his/her Visual Analogue Score was 6 out of 10." For patients with multifocal neuropathic pain or mixed neuropathic/myofascial pain, a verbal scale is preferred, as it can be used easily to record intensity *for each region*, not just the peak or average pain. Finally, it has been suggested that this mnemonic should be changed to add the letter O, for *other* (associated) symptoms, such as loss of sensation or nonpainful paresthesias or dysesthesia occurring in the same general area as the pain.

PHYSICAL EXAMINATION OF PATIENTS WITH NEUROPATHIC PAIN

In general, all major parts of the physical examination are important for adequate determination of the presence of local disease, which may cause pain (Longmire, 1991b, 1996). Patients in whom the *symptom* characteristics suggest neurological origin may also demonstrate regional abnormalities of motor or reflex functions. However, the portions of the examination that are most relevant to the evaluation of neuropathic pain are those related to sensory dysfunction, such as hypoesthesia, hyperesthesia, hyperalgesia, and allodynia (Dworkin et al., 2003; Fields, 1987; Krause & Backonja, 2003; Longmire, 1991b).

There are three important aspects in performing the sensory examination in patients with neuropathic pain: (1) it must be remembered that the information obtained is still subjective, (2) stimulation with different modalities may create a mixed or uninterpretable response pattern, and (3) there may also be hypoesthesia or even areas of total anesthesia in the middle of areas that the patient describes as being so painful. The severity of a pain condition can be related to the size of a painful area, but the intensity is independent, no matter how large or small the territory.

INTEGRATION OF HISTORY/PHYSICAL DATA FOR NEUROPATHIC PAIN EVALUATION

It is evident from the preceding paragraphs that the duration and complexity of the clinical evaluation of human neuropathic pain is very dependent on the patient's ability to tolerate long and potentially uncomfortable procedures. For screening purposes, however, different methods have been developed to provide a combination of individual components of the history and physical examination. The simpler and more direct methods are exemplified by Galer and Jensen (1997) and Krause and Backonja (2003). A Neuropathic Pain Questionnaire has been developed: demonstrates burning pain, shooting pain, numbness, electric pain, tingling pain, squeezing pain, freezing pain, and significant sensitivity to touch. Analysis of the elements reveals that the three most valuable features are the symptoms of numbness, tingling pain, and the mixed response of symptoms/signs expressed as increased pain due to touch on physical examination.

LABORATORY, RADIOLOGIC, AND ELECTRODIAGNOSTIC ASSESSMENT

Once the history, physical findings, and neuropathic pain questionnaire have yielded sufficient evidence to support the potential presence of neuropathic pain, specific biochemical, structural, and neurophysiological tests may be applied to confirm or eliminate certain disorders from the differential diagnosis.

Laboratory evaluation is necessary to determine the presence of hematologic, chemical, or pathological processes with a high potential for causing or contributing to the pain (Kennedy, 1996; Kennedy & Longmire, 1992). Such tests are also used to monitor (1) systemic response to treatment because there are often effects on renal and hepatic function and (2) serum levels of primary analgesics and certain adjuvant medications such as anticonvulsants. DNA and other specific biochemical tests for neuropathic pain disorders that have a familial tendency or pattern of inheritance can be helpful for genetic counseling, but they are not often ordered in primary care pain practice. Similarly, direct and electron microscopic assessments of nerve tissue obtained at biopsy are only used selectively for the definitive pathological diagnosis of certain illnesses such as neuropathy.

Radiologic evaluation (Leak, 1992) provides valuable information about the presence or absence of structural lesions compressing or invading tissues of the brain, brainstem, spine, spinal cord, root, plexus, or nerve. Certain specialized tests are known to be helpful in the diagnostic assessment of specific conditions, e.g., triple-phase contrast bone scan as a tertiary way of testing for CRPS Type I/RSD.

Electroneurodiagnostic tests are helpful in localizing structural lesions or regional dysfunction in many disorders of the nervous system, not just those related to neuropathic pain. However, common procedures such as electroencephalography and electromyography/nerve conduction studies to the medical assessment of painful conditions of brain and the spinal cord, root, and nerve, respectively, are known to be helpful in confirming and localizing many neurological illnesses presenting with pain (Longmire, 1993). For painful disorders such as CRPS types I and II and SMP, a wide range of electrophysiological tests of sympathetic sudomotor function can be found (Longmire et al., 1996) including selective tissue conductance assessment of the skin over painful and nonpainful regions (Longmire & Parris, 1991; Longmire & Woodley, 1993).

NEUROPATHIC PAIN SYNDROMES

In primary care as well as many types of specialty practice, the term *neuropathic pain* has been most often thought of as simply meaning painful peripheral neuropathy, as commonly occurs in severe diabetes mellitus. This association may have developed based on the high incidence of diabetes and the bilateral, distal distribution of other symptoms (sensory loss) and signs (reduced temperature, circulatory compromise) commonly seen in this illness. In general clinical practice, the pains of well-known neurological disorders such as those created by herpes zoster and inflammatory involvement of the trigeminal nerves are more likely to be thought of as focal neuralgias, rather than neuropathic pain. Similarly, the pain created by local compression of nerve roots is considered to represent just one aspect of a radiculopathy rather than being part of a neuropathic pain syndrome. Even when contralateral pain is created by unilateral thalamic or other deep hemispheric infarctions, the symptoms are first thought to represent a specific (central post-stroke) syndrome, rather than being part of a more general (neuropathic) pain category.

In addition to those syndromes mentioned in the preceding paragraph, there are several common conditions known to be associated with severe, persistent neuropathic pain (Scadding, 1992).

NEUROPATHIC PAIN DISORDERS BY ETIOLOGY

In theory, almost any of the pathological processes known to create damage or dysfunction to neural tissue can be considered as potential causes for neuropathic pain. Viral/bacterial, aseptic inflammation, pressure due to neoplasm or other structural lesions, degenerative, ischemia, autoimmune, toxic, traumatic, endocrine/metabolic mechanisms have all been implicated in the production of pain (Kennedy, 1996; Kennedy & Longmire, 1992; Longmire, 1996; Table 24.1).

TABLE 24.1
Common Causes of Neuropathic Pain

Polyneuropathy
    Diabetes (insulin-dependent and non-insulin-dependent)
    Alcoholism
    Human immunodeficiency virus
    Hypothyroidism
    Renal failure
    Chemotherapy (vincristine, cisplatinum, paclitaxel, metronidazole)
    Anti-HIV drugs
    B_{12} and folate deficiencies
Mononeuropathy
    Entrapment syndromes
    Traumatic injury
    Diabetes
    Vasculitis
Plexopathy
    Diabetes
    Avulsion
    Tumor
Root syndromes and radiculopathy
    Compressive lesions
    Inflammatory
    Diabetes
Post-herpetic neuralgia
Trigeminal neuralgia
Phantom limb pain
RSD/causalgia/CRPS

Note: Modified from B. S. Galer, *Neurology, 45*(Suppl. 9), pp. S17–S25, 1995.

INITIAL SYMPTOM MANAGEMENT

There is some disagreement about which treatment approaches (pharmacologic or interventional) represent the best and worst chances for symptom control. Nevertheless, the mainstay of treatment of neuropathic pain is pharmacologic. Effective regimens often require multiple medications. Attempts at monotherapy with standard analgesics including opioids tend to be less effective because neuropathic pain is often resistant to medications of that type (Arner & Meyerson, 1988; Dellemijn, 1999; Portenoy, Foley, & Inturrisi, 1990).

Neuropathic pain may be treated with some success using adjuvant analgesics, i.e., medications not traditionally considered to be pain relievers (Hegarty & Portenoy, 1994). Adjuvant analgesics, such as tricyclic antidepressants and anticonvulsants, do not have strong antinociceptive analgesic properties in experimental or clinical studies, but have been shown to be helpful in neuropathic pain states (McQuay et al., 1996; Swerdlow, 1984). In addition, the possible effectiveness of opioids for neuropathic pain should not be overlooked, although doses may be considerably higher than typical antinociceptive doses.

The clinician should also keep in mind that successful management of chronic pain often requires treating neuropathic pain as well as pain associated with tissue injury, because both conditions may coexist and interact to maintain the painful condition. Chronic pain syndromes are often a product of integrated nociceptive and neuropathic mechanisms and, as such, require consideration of both types for any pain lasting greater than 3 to 6 months.

MECHANISTIC BASIS OF NEUROPATHIC PAIN MANAGEMENT

Management of neuropathic pain is a complicated endeavor and often is frustrating to patient and physician alike. This stems from our relatively poor understanding of mechanisms and the limited efficacy of currently available analgesics. Therapeutic approaches vary greatly among physicians reflecting the paucity of randomized clinical trials, particularly those comparing different drug regimens.

Given our current level of understanding of neuropathic pain mechanisms and the limitations of available drugs, nonpharmacological methods may be as effective as pharmacological approaches. Recalcitrant chronic pain syndromes warrant an interdisciplinary approach, which may include attempts to treat the underlying disease (e.g., causes of the peripheral neuropathy) as well as formulation of a rational approach to medications, interventions such as nerve blocks, and psychological and physical therapies.

It is often helpful to consider the various medications useful for neuropathic pain in terms of their traditional pharmacological indications (e.g., anticonvulsants and antidepressants). However, it is necessary to keep in mind that all these drugs have incompletely understood mechanisms of action, and the drug categories are more conventional than mechanistic.

From a practical standpoint, medications remain the pillar of pain management strategies, despite their limitations. From a conceptual standpoint, adjuvant analgesic drugs may be categorized into two broad classes, membrane-stabilizing agents and medications that enhance inhibitory mechanisms in the dorsal horn. This classification system may provide a simple framework with which to approach therapy; however, it should be kept in mind that most of these drugs have multiple mechanisms of action, and their effects may often overlap. Given the limitations of our current drugs, pain management often becomes an exercise in polypharmacy, where the clinician uses multiple medications to target different symptoms. This strategy may optimize the chances for success, but complicates management issues when side effects develop.

MECHANISMS OF ACTION

Membrane-stabilizing agents include local anesthetics such as lidocaine and some anticonvulsant drugs, including car-

bamazepine, phenytoin, and valproic acid (Tanelian & Victory, 1995). Their molecular mechanism of action involves blockade of frequency- and voltage-dependent sodium channels on damaged or regenerating neuronal membranes (Devor, 1994, 1995). It appears that minimal doses of suppressive drugs may inhibit ectopic discharges without interfering with normal neuronal function. It is also possible that the sodium channel targets are atypical and not involved in normal neuronal conduction. Although the evidence is less substantial, corticosteroids also appear to have effects on membrane conductance (Castillo et al., 1996; Devor, Govrin-Lippmann, & Raber, 1985). In addition, tricyclic antidepressants, such as amitriptyline, have effects on sodium channels (Pancrazio et al., 1998), an action that is distinct from their effects on the reuptake of serotonin and norepinephrine. The latter are traditionally thought to be responsible for their effects on depression and pain.

Conventional wisdom maintains that the adjuvant analgesics, particularly the tricyclic antidepressants and clonazepam and baclofen, modulate inhibitory mechanisms in the spinal cord and brain. Inhibitory pathways descend from the periaqueductal gray, reticular formation, and nucleus raphe magnus in the dorsolateral funiculus to the dorsal horn. These pathways mediate antinociception by adrenergic, serotonergic, GABAergic (γ-amino butyric acid), and opioid mechanisms (Yaksh, 1979). Although the putative mechanisms are complex and poorly understood, serotonergic effects are mediated in part by action on GABAergic interneurons (Alhaider, Lei, & Wilcox, 1991). For example, facilitory effects of large myelinated afferent fibers may be suppressed by tonic GABAergic activity, removal of which results in allodynia (Yaksh & Malmberg, 1994).

As noted earlier, tricyclic antidepressants alter monoamine transmitter activity at neuronal synapses by blocking presynaptic reuptake of norepinephrine and serotonin, thereby modulating descending inhibitory spinal pathways. However, additional mechanisms include effects on membranes, interaction with NMDA activity (Eisenach & Gebhart, 1995), and sodium channel blockade (Pancrazio et al., 1998).

It is crucial that psychosocial and emotional factors be explored because there is a high comorbidity of depression and anxiety disorders in patients with chronic pain. Moreover, given the similarities between the pharmacology of mood and depression and pain transmission (e.g., serotonin and norepinephrine), patients with concomitant systemic illness and stress may be at risk for depression and development of an abnormal chronic pain state. Pharmacological management of depression may improve neuropathic pain by addressing overlapping but distinct mechanisms.

ABLATIVE PROCEDURES

After multiple medication trials in which there has been minimal therapeutic benefit and perhaps significant drug-related side effects, patients may believe that they have little recourse but to undergo invasive, ablative procedures in attempts to relieve their pain. Specific treatment modalities aimed at the underlying pathophysiology are usually not possible in most neuropathies, particularly with chronic sensory polyneuropathies. In general, ablative procedures are not warranted because of the high probability of long-term worsening of pain. Except for patients with advanced cancer-related pain, nerve ablation is likely to provide only temporary benefit, leaving the patient with sensory and perhaps motor deficits. Exceptions to this phenomenon appear to be ablation of sympathetic fibers, visceral plexi, and medial branch nerve blocks, which denervate painful facet joints in the spine. In cases of nerve entrapment, where ongoing nerve compression is likely to be responsible for pain, neurolysis or transposition of the nerve may provide benefit, as long as pain is not due to irreversible underlying nerve damage. In all cases of neuropathic pain, even when neuropathy is evident, it is appropriate from time to time to reevaluate the presumed etiology of the neurological problem.

When a medication trial proves to be ineffective, a multidimensional or interdisciplinary approach should be considered. Again, this includes an attempt to treat the underlying disease, as well as specific pharmacological, psychological, and physical therapy interventions. The outcome measure for successful treatment should include increased activity as well as decreased subjective pain ratings and improved patient satisfaction. The treatment goal in chronic neuropathic pain is different from that in acute pain. In the usual acute pain setting, the goal is nearly complete relief of pain, to allow recovery of normal function during the healing process. With chronic neuropathic pain, limitations of current analgesics usually make complete pain relief a very unrealistic goal. Therefore, attention to increasing function and comfort and treating associated problems, such as depression, become paramount. Reducing dependence on opioid medications may or may not be an important goal. The objectives to consider with chronic opioid therapy include determining whether nonopioid approaches have been tried, whether the pain syndrome is opioid responsive, and whether the patient demonstrates appropriate improvement in function, without undue side effects or evidence of abuse of medications.

Nonpharmacological approaches to treating neuropathic pain include the use of a TENS (transcutaneous electrical nerve stimulation) unit although relief may be poor when burning pain is a prominent complaint. This may be explained by the fact that burning pain is a C-fiber-mediated sensation, whereas TENS units probably modulate large fiber input into the dorsal horn.

Spinal cord stimulation may be efficacious for chronic pain, including neuropathic pain (North et al., 1993) and complex regional pain syndrome/reflex sympathetic dys-

trophy (Kemler et al., 2000). Mechanisms involved are poorly understood, which reflects current understanding of neuropathic pain states in general. However, central effects may include alteration in dorsal horn processing and transmission in the tract of Lissauer (Iacono, Guthkelch, & Boswell, 1992) and suppression of sympathetic outflow from the intermediolateral gray column of the spinal cord. The latter effect may explain improved peripheral blood flow in patients with chronic peripheral vascular insufficiency. The Craig PENS (percutaneous neural stimulation) technique, a novel application of electroacupuncture, has been shown effective in herpes zoster, diabetic peripheral neuropathy, and sciatica (Ahmed et al., 1998; Ghoname et al., 1999; Hamza et al., 2000).

Available evidence indicates that nonpharmacological approaches such as TENS and Craig PENS can provide an initial rational therapeutic strategy and may obviate the need for potentially toxic medications, improve the effectiveness of current analgesic regimens, or reduce the amount of medications required. Spinal cord stimulation still tends to be a treatment of last resort, although judicious use earlier in the course of treatment is probably warranted in carefully selected patients. Considering the current high cost of medication, alternative approaches, if efficacious, may prove to be cost effective.

A peculiar property of the nervous system is its plasticity. Damage to nerves often results in alteration or amplification of the signal encoded by the nerve. For example, peripheral nerve ablation, performed with good therapeutic intentions, may result in a pain syndrome that is worse than the one originally being treated. When dealing with the nervous system, "shooting the messenger" (the nerve) often intensifies and distorts the message. The new pain syndrome may be more severe and associated with allodynia, hyperalgesia, and spontaneous and paroxysmal pain, all in the presence of mild to moderate cutaneous numbness. This complex of signs and symptoms is paradoxical to the patient and confusing to the clinician, but quite typical of neuropathic pain.

MECHANISTIC APPROACH TO THE SELECTION OF TREATMENT

When standard therapies are found to be only partially effective in controlling symptoms, it is often helpful to select other medications or interventions based on the compatibility of the mechanisms of the illness and the treatment being considered (Goli, 2002). For example, it has become popular to contrast neuropathic pain with typical post-injury, nociceptive pain. Nociceptive pain, typically thought to indicate a properly functioning nervous system, is considered physiological because it results from activation of nociceptors, specialized nerve endings that respond to high-threshold noxious stimuli and generally serve a protective function. In contrast, neuropathic pain may be thought of as pathophysiological because it arises from a damaged PNS or CNS and provides no obvious protective benefit (Bennett, 1994; Tanelian & Victory, 1995).

On the other hand, pain associated with peripheral neuropathy may be maintained by sustained peripheral nociceptive input (Gracely, Lynch, & Bennett, 1992). Strong nociceptive input often produces central sensitization, an abnormal pain amplification process in the CNS. Therefore, the definitional borders of neuropathic pain are becoming more diffuse, not more distinct, as we gain a better understanding of the remarkable plasticity of the nervous system and its close association with the various tissues that it innervates.

Neuropathic pain may be classified as stimulus-evoked or stimulus-independent pain. Stimulus-evoked pain can result from stimulation of nervi nervorum present in connective tissue surrounding otherwise intact nerves. Painful stimuli that activate nociceptors around nerves include inflammation and tissue injury from tumor or trauma (Woolf & Mannion, 1999).

Stimulus-independent neuropathic pain may result from damage to afferent sensory fibers in the PNS or CNS. In this case, ongoing inflammation is usually absent. Days to months after peripheral nerve injury, persistent abnormal primary afferent activity from the periphery may arise from hypersensitive nerve terminals or nerves (Price, Mao, & Mayer, 1994).

PATHOPHYSIOLOGIC PROCESSES SUBSERVING NEUROPATHIC PAIN

As one might expect, there is substantial evidence that abnormal nerve activity is an important mechanism underlying the spontaneous pain typical of neuropathic pain states (Devor, 1994, 1995; Tanelian & Victory, 1995). It is hypothesized that sites of ectopic foci develop on injured or regenerating nerves in the periphery; at the level of the nociceptor, neuromas, or segments of injured nerves; at the dorsal root ganglion; and in the dorsal horn of the spinal cord. Indeed, after nerve transection, increased sensitivity occurs, followed in a few days by spontaneous activity. These abnormal ectopic foci may be thought of as spontaneous pain generators, resulting in paroxysmal and spontaneous pain.

Precise pathophysiology is unclear, but pharmacological evidence suggests that ectopic activity is due to an increased number of sodium channels or, more likely, to an abnormal subtype of sodium channel, resulting in unstable sodium channel activity (Chaplan, 2000). Pharmacological evidence supporting this hypothesis is the effectiveness of local anesthetics and some anticonvulsants (sodium channel-blocking drugs) in neuropathic

pain. These drugs presumably produce frequency- and voltage-dependent blockade of sodium channels on damaged neurons (Devor, 1995). The abnormal sodium channel involved in neuropathic pain states may be a tetrodotoxin-insensitive subtype, found only in neural tissue (Novakovic et al., 1998). Accumulation of atypical as well as tetrodotoxin-sensitive sodium channels (responsible for normal nerve conduction) may explain the often inadequate therapeutic benefit of current sodium channel-blocking drugs.

Work in animal models demonstrates that voltage-dependent calcium channels may also be important in modulating neuropathic transmission. Unfortunately, the currently available calcium channel blockers are cardioselective and are not particularly effective in neuropathic pain. There appear to be at least six calcium channel subtypes, and studies with novel N-type calcium channel blockers are promising in animals (Chaplan, 2000). Preliminary studies with conotoxin (SNX-111) are positive although the drug must be administered intrathecally.

Gabapentin, a novel anticonvulsant, appears to bind to the a2d subunit of a voltage-dependent calcium channel. Work by Chaplan (2000) and colleagues demonstrates that messenger RNA and protein for the a2d subunit are increased more than 10-fold in dorsal root ganglia following nerve injury, but are not changed after other forms of tissue injury. Blockade of a retrograde signal from the injury site (which may involve nerve growth factor) prevents upregulation of the a2d subunit. Chaplan points out that the a2d subunit does not seem to play a role in normal channel kinetics but may effect calcium channel assembly and insertion into the neuronal membrane. Thus, the subunit may act as a drug-binding site and secondarily modify channel kinetics.

COMPLEX REGIONAL PAIN SYNDROMES AS NEUROPATHIC PAIN

Following peripheral nerve injury, concomitant alternations may be evident in dorsal root ganglia, including transmitter changes and increased density of sympathetic nerve terminals (McLachlan et al., 1993). Tyrosine hydroxylase positive cell terminals that produce norepinephrine migrate from vessels supplying the dorsal root ganglion to nerve ganglion cells following sciatic nerve injury. The dorsal root ganglia then express a-adrenergic receptors. This may be a putative link between peripheral tissue injury, nerve injury, and sympathetically maintained pain states, such as reflex sympathetic dystrophy and causalgia (CRPS Type I and II, respectively). In the periphery, sprouting nerve terminals may exhibit sensitivity to prostaglandins, cytokines, and catecholamines. These kinds of changes further increase the complexity of the neuropathic pain picture and blur the distinctions between nociceptive and neuropathic pain.

It should be noted that not all stimulus-independent pain is mediated by spontaneous activity in primary sensory neurons. Loss of normal inhibitory mechanisms, whether segmental, supraspinal, or both, may also cause neuropathic pain (Woolf & Mannion, 1999). After deafferentation injury, particularly following loss of C-fibers, arborization of Ab fibers into the substantia gelatinosa of the dorsal horn may result in central sensitization and allodynia (Woolf, Shortland, & Coggeshall, 1992). Available evidence supports the contention that tactile allodynia is mediated by large myelinated Ab afferents with input that is modulated at supraspinal sites in the dorsal columns (Ossipov et al., 2000).

This may explain why TENS and spinal cord stimulation, which produce a low-threshold, tingling sensation, characteristic of large fiber afferent activation, may be effective in chronic pain states, particularly neuropathic pain. Tactile allodynia should be differentiated from thermal allodynia, which appears to be mediated by nonmyelinated C-fibers and amplified by pathological spinal dynorphin.

STIMULUS-EVOKED NEUROPATHIC PAIN AND OPIOID ANALGESICS

Various studies suggest that stimulus-evoked neuropathic pain is more sensitive to opioids than stimulus-independent pain (Dellemijn, 1999). Opioid responsiveness may be maintained in some forms of stimulus-evoked pain because opioid receptors in the substantia gelatinosa are preserved. On the other hand, segmental loss of presynaptic central opioid receptors occurs following injury or loss of C-fibers, typically seen after deafferentation injury. However, the magnitude of receptor loss is minimal and largely segmental, and only partly explains the diminished opioid-responsiveness characteristic of neuropathic pain (Ossipov et al., 2000).

Supraspinal facilitative mechanisms may also be involved in maintenance of neuropathic pain and opioid resistance. Evidence suggests that sustained afferent drive induces facilitation of spinal cord pain transmission involving a descending pathway from the rostroventral medial medulla (RVM) (Ossipov et al., 2000). Tonic facilitation may involve supraspinal cholesystokinin (CCK), traditionally thought of as a visceral hormone that regulates emptying of the gallbladder. CCK antagonists injected into the RVM in animals reverse tactile and thermal allodynia produced by spinal nerve ligation (Kovelowski et al., 2000). Mechanistically, these antiopioid and pronociceptive actions may occur at spinal and supraspinal sites. Spinal CCK may antagonize opioid effects at the level of the primary afferent terminal in the spinal cord. Both CCK and opioids colocalize on primary nociceptive afferent neurons in the dorsal horn. In addition, CCK may act on supraspinal opioid-dependent pathways in the RVM to reduce opioid responsiveness and, thus, impair descending inhibition, an important mechanism involved in opioid pain relief. Ultimately, CCK antagonists may prove useful for treating neuropathic pain states.

The phenomenon of reduced opioid responsiveness in neuropathic pain has prompted extensive studies in animals, particularly the effects of intrathecal opioids on pain associated with thermal and tactile stimulation. The similarities between opioid tolerance and neuropathic pain are also an area of active study (Vanderah et al., 2000). It is well known that N-methyl-D-aspartate (NMDA) antagonists appear to minimize the development of opioid tolerance. Spinal dynorphin may be a common link between NMDA, central sensitization, and reduced opioid responsiveness. Following spinal nerve ligation, dynorphin levels in the spinal cord increase, suggesting that dynorphin may act as a pronociception mediator (Ossipov et al., 2000).

Although, under certain circumstances, dynorphin appears to have analgesic properties, it is becoming increasingly clear that dynorphin also has nonopioid, antianalgesic properties. Antiserum to dynorphin blocks thermal hyperalgesia after nerve injury in rats. Moreover, antiserum to dynorphin or MK801, an NMDA antagonist, restores normal spinal morphine analgesia following spinal nerve ligation. Furthermore, both agents restore morphine synergy between the brain and spinal cord (Ossipov et al., 2000), which is required for the full clinical analgesic effects of morphine. Therefore, current evidence suggests that the pain-promoting effect of dynorphin is mediated by the NMDA receptor. Although the full clinical ramifications of dynorphin are far from understood, it is clear that sustained nociceptive drive from the periphery maintains elevated levels of spinal dynorphin, which, in turn, may have toxic effects on the spinal cord. Thus, reducing sustained peripheral nociceptive input into the spinal (i.e., pain relief) may be an important way to reduce the incidence of neuropathic pain (Caudle & Mannes, 2000).

Currently, NMDA antagonists, such as ketamine, have only limited indications because of significant side effects. Ultimately, however, medications like NMDA antagonists may become available that can reduce the effects of pathological spinal dynorphin.

CENTRAL POST-STROKE PAIN

Central post-stoke pain (CPSP) was originally thought to be "thalamic" pain, as described by Dejerine and Roussy (1906), although it was described even earlier in 1883 (Greiff, 1883). Dejerine and Roussy (1906) characterized their eponymous thalamic pain syndrome as including hemiplegia; hemiataxia and hemiastereognosis; difficulties with both superficial and deep sensation; persistent, paroxysmal, typically intolerable pain; and choreoathetoid movements.

The reported incidence of CPSP varies widely from 2% (Bowsher, 1993) to 8% (Anderson et al., 1995) of patients suffering and to 25% (MacGowan et al., 1997) in patients with lateral medullary infarctions (Wallenberg's syndrome).

The onset of the pain may be immediate or delayed for months to years (Bowsher, 1995; Holmgren et al., 1990; Leijon et al., 1989). The pain may encompass a large part of the contralateral body, but it may also involve only a small area. The pain attributes include dysesthesias, spontaneous or evoked, and burning.

Sensory abnormalities are also associated with CPSP. These may include altered sensory processing, whereby warm and cold stimulation applied to the skin may be perceived as paresthesias or dysesthesias rather than cold or warm (Anderson et al., 1995). Allodynia is found (Bowsher, 1996; Wessel et al., 1994) in 55 to 70% of patients. Hyperalgesia and dysesthesia are also frequently seen (Mersky, 1986).

Locations of the lesions inducing the CPSP are definitively referable to the spinothalamo-cortical tract/pathway, typically associated with abnormal evoked sensations in the peripherally affected area (Andersen et al., 1995; Boivie, 1994; Jensen & Lenz, 1995). There are at least three thalamic regions, which directly or indirectly, receive spinothalamic projections that appear to be involved in the development of CPSP: the ventroposterior thalamus, including the posteriorly and inferiorly located nuclei bordering on that region; the reticular nucleus; and the medial intralaminar region. It is the ventroposterior thalamic region that is proposed to be most significantly involved in central pain (Boivie, 1992; Jones, 1992; Lenz, 1992). It should also be noted that cerebrovascular lesions located above the diencephalon, i.e., in the parietal lobe, may also induce CPSP (Boivie, 1994; Sandy, 1985; Wessel et al., 1994).

Sympathetic dysfunction has also been felt to play a role in central pain secondary to signs of abnormal sympathetic activity: edema, hypohydrosis, trophic skin changes, changes in skin color, and decreased skin temperature (Bowsher, 1996; Riddoch, 1938). It is also noted that some or many of these changes may be secondary to "movement allodynia" (Bowsher, 1995), which makes the patient keep the affected limb motionless.

Reports of CPSP associated with abnormal "epileptiform" activities in thalamic cells may be involved with central pain (Gorecki et al., 1989; Hirato et al., 1994; Yamashiro et al., 1991). This would also indicate that some aspects of the problem may be secondary to cortical involvement, as epileptiform discharges typically are associated with that region.

Treatment of the CPSP is difficult and may include antidepressants, anticonvulsants, antiarrhythmics, analgesics, and nonmedication treatment including TENS, dorsal column stimulation, and deep brain stimulation (DBS).

One undesirable effect of repetitive DBS is the reduction of the seizure threshold, known as kindling. One of the authors (Longmire) is aware of a patient whose pain was only partially reduced with the original stimulus parameters of DBS. In an attempt to improve pain control, that individual used the external controller to increase the amount of stimulation above the amount by the attending neurosurgeon. After several days of this maneuver, the patient suffered a first-ever focal onset, secondarily generalized seizure. To the authors' knowledge, this patient may represent the first case of self-induced kindling of seizures in a human patient using DBS for pain control. Other treatments include sympathetic blockade, as well as surgical interventions, including cordotomy, dorsal root entry zone lesions, thalamotomy, or cortical and subcortical ablation (Awerbuch, 1990; Bowsher & Nurmikko,1996; Davidoff et al., 1987; Edgar et al., 1993; Ekbom, 1966; Kastrup et al., 1987; Leijon & Boivie 1989a, 1989b, 1989c; Loh et al., 1981; Nashold & Bullitt, 1981; Portenoy, Foley et al., 1990; Siegfried, 1983; Siegfried & Demierre, 1984; Swerdlow, 1986; Tasker, 1990; Tasker et al., 1991).

ANTICONVULSANTS

Anticonvulsants are useful for trigeminal neuralgia, postherpetic neuralgia, diabetic neuropathy, and central pain (Hegarty & Portenoy, 1994; Swerdlow, 1984). Although anticonvulsants have traditionally been thought of as most useful for lancinating pain, they may also relieve burning dysesthesias. Chemically, anticonvulsants are a diverse group of drugs, are typically highly protein bound, and undergo extensive hepatic metabolism. Carbamazepine has a long history of use for neuropathic pain, particularly trigeminal neuralgia. Trigeminal neuralgia is an U.S. Food and Drug Administration (FDA)-approved indication for the drug. Carbamazepine is chemically related to the tricyclic antidepressant imipramine, has a slow and erratic absorption, and may produce numerous side effects, including sedation, nausea, vomiting, and hepatic enzyme induction. In 10% of patients, transient leukopenia and thrombocytopenia may occur, and in 2% of patients, hematologic changes can be persistent, requiring stopping the drug (Hart & Easton, 1982; Sobotka, Alexander, & Cook, 1990; Tohen et al., 1995). Aplastic anemia is the most severe complication associated with carbamazepine, which may occur in 1:200,000 patients. Although requirements for hematologic monitoring remain debatable, a complete blood cell count, hepatic enzymes, blood urea nitrogen, and creatinine are recommended at baseline; and these are checked again at 2, 4, and 6 weeks, and every 6 months thereafter. Carbamazepine levels should be drawn every 6 months and after changing the dose to monitor for toxic levels and verify that the drug is within the therapeutic range (4 to 12 mg/cc).

Patients with low pretreatment white blood cell (WBC) counts are at increased risk of developing leukopenia (WBC < 3000/mm^3). Because toxicity is entirely unpredictable, it is important to instruct patients to recognize clinical signs and symptoms of hematologic toxicity, such as infections, fatigue, ecchymosis, and abnormal bleeding, and to notify the physician if they develop. To improve compliance, carbamazepine should be started at a low dose (e.g., 50 mg twice daily) and increased over several weeks to a therapeutic level (200 to 300 mg four times a day). When a therapeutic dosage is achieved, a controlled-release preparation may provide more stable blood levels and enhance patient compliance.

Oxcarbazepine, a metabolite of carbamazepine, may be safer from the standpoint of potential hepatic toxicity and bone marrow depression. However, the potential for hyponatremia requires monitoring of serum sodium levels.

Phenytoin also has well-known sodium channel-blocking effects and is useful for neuropathic pain (Swerdlow, 1984). However, it is less effective than carbamazepine for trigeminal neuralgia (Blom, 1962). We have also noted that neuropathic pain caused by structural lesions causing nerve or root compression can paradoxically increase when phenytoin is administered. Phenytoin has a slow and variable oral absorption, some of which is dependent on gastrointestinal motility and transit time. Toxicity includes CNS effects and cardiac conduction abnormalities. Side effects are common and include hirsuitism, gastrointestinal and hematologic effects, and gingival hyperplasia (Brodie & Dichter, 1996). Allergies to phenytoin are common, and may involve skin, liver, and bone marrow. Phenytoin doses in the range of 100 mg two or three times a day may be helpful for neuropathic pain; therapeutic blood levels are in the range of 10 to 20 mg/ml. There are numerous potential drug interactions, including induction of cytochrome P450 enzymes, which may accelerate the metabolism of other drugs. Because of side effects and toxicity, phenytoin is not a first-line drug for neuropathic pain.

Valproic acid appears to interact with sodium channels but may also alter GABA metabolism. The principal FDA approved use of valproic acid is for the prophylaxis of migraine headache (Matthew et al., 1995). Potential toxicity includes hepatic injury and thrombocytopenia, particularly in children on multiple antiepileptic medications, although valproic acid is generally considered safe for adults.

Divalproex sodium is better tolerated than valproic acid. The recommended starting dose is 250 mg twice daily, although some patients may benefit from doses up to 1000 mg/day. As a prophylactic drug, valproic acid can reduce the frequency of migraine attacks by about 50% (Matthew et al., 1995). Although there is little published information on the efficacy of valproic acid for neuropathic pain syndromes, based on its mechanism of action it may be useful alone or in combination with other adjuvant drugs.

Clonazepam may be useful for radiculopathic pain and neuropathic pain of a lancinating character. Clonazepam enhances dorsal horn inhibition by a GABAergic mechanism. The drug has a long half-life (18 to 50 h), which reduces the risk of inducing an abstinence syndrome on abrupt withdrawal. The major side effects of clonazepam include sedation and cognitive dysfunction, especially in elderly people. Although the risk of organ toxicity is minimal, some clinicians recommend periodic complete blood count (CBC) and liver function tests for monitoring. Starting doses of 0.5 to 1.0 mg at bedtime are appropriate to reduce the incidence of daytime sedation.

Gabapentin is a popular anticonvulsant for neuropathic pain. Gabapentin was released for use in the United States in 1994, for the treatment of adults with partial epilepsy. Almost immediately after its release, physicians began to use gabapentin for various neuropathic pain disorders, such as diabetic peripheral neuropathy and postherpetic neuralgia. The structural similarity of gabapentin to GABA suggested that the drug might be useful for neuropathic pain. Although tricyclic antidepressants have been proved clinically effective for neuropathic pain for years, they often fail to provide adequate pain relief or they cause unacceptable side effects. Therefore, when gabapentin became available, its benign side-effect profile quickly made it very popular among physicians. Although initial enthusiasm for the drug was based largely on word of mouth, anecdotal published reports, and discussions at clinical meetings, animal studies have substantiated the efficacy of gabapentin in various types of neuropathic pain. Over time, a growing consensus concerning the usefulness of gabapentin has emerged.

It is clear that gabapentin is not a direct GABA agonist, although indirect effects on GABA metabolism or action may occur. A leading hypothesis suggests that gabapentin interacts with a novel receptor on a voltage-activated calcium channel (Chaplan, 2000; Taylor et al., 1998). Inhibition of voltage-gated sodium channel activity (such as occurs with classical anticonvulsants, e.g., phenytoin and carbamazepine) and amino acid transport, which alters neurotransmitter synthesis, may also occur. Although gabapentin is not an NMDA antagonist, there is evidence that gabapentin interacts with the glycine site on the NMDA receptor (Jun & Yaksh, 1998).

Ligation of rat spinal nerves L5 and L6 (the Chung model) produces characteristic pain behaviors, including allodynia, which are typical of neuropathic pain. Chapman et al. (1998) demonstrated that gabapentin reduces pain in the Chung model. Gabapentin appears to act primarily in the CNS, in contrast to amitriptyline, which seems to act centrally and peripherally (Abdi, Lee, & Chung, 1998). Gabapentin also is effective in reducing pain behavior in the second phase of the formalin test, a model of central sensitization and neuropathic pain (Shimoyama et al., 1997a). Gabapentin reduces spinally mediated hyperalgesia seen after sustained nociceptive afferent input caused by peripheral tissue injury. Gabapentin also enhances spinal morphine analgesia in the rat tail-flick test, a laboratory model of nociceptive pain (Shimoyama et al., 1997b).

Gabapentin is effective in reducing painful dysesthesias and improving quality of life scores in patients with painful diabetic peripheral neuropathy (Backonja et al., 1998). Of patients randomized to receive gabapentin, 56% achieved a daily dosage of 3600 mg divided into three doses per day. The average magnitude of the analgesic response was modest, with a 24% reduction in intensity at the completion of the study compared with controls. Side effects were common. Dizziness and somnolence occurred in about 25% of patients, and confusion occurred in 8% of patients.

Morello et al. (1999) compared gabapentin with amitriptyline for diabetic neuropathy and found both equally effective. Although gabapentin probably has fewer contraindications than tricyclic antidepressants, it is considerably more expensive.

Post-herpetic neuralgia (PHN) is another difficult neuropathic syndrome. PHN affects approximately 10 to 15% of patients who develop herpes zoster and is a particularly painful syndrome associated with lancinating pain and burning dysesthesias. The incidence of PHN is age related, with up to 50% of patients older than 60 years of age developing persistent pain after a bout of herpes zoster. Pain relief usually requires pharmacological therapy. Unfortunately, most medications are not very effective. For example, only about one half of patients obtain adequate relief with antidepressants.

Rowbotham et al. (1998) evaluated the efficacy of gabapentin for the treatment of PHN. Of patients taking gabapentin, 65% achieved a daily dosage of 3600 mg. Although the average magnitude of pain reduction with gabapentin was modest, with approximately a 30% reduction in pain compared with controls, statistically pain reduction was highly significant. In addition, gabapentin improved sleep parameters and quality of life scores. Adverse effects that occurred more commonly in the gabapentin group included somnolence (27%), dizziness (24%), ataxia, peripheral edema, and infection (7 to 10%). Based on the data of Rowbotham and colleagues, it is reasonable to consider gabapentin as first-line therapy for post-herpetic neuralgia. Gabapentin probably is at least as effective as antidepressants, with fewer contraindications. Gabapentin may be used as monotherapy or add-on treatment.

Although gabapentin can theoretically be started at 300 mg three times a day with most patients, it has been the clinical experience of one of the authors (Longmire) that giving lower initial doses (100 mg) and gently escalating the drug to a schedule of four times a day (three times a day with meals and again at bedtime) has improved compliance. Use of the bedtime dose may assist with sleep and reduces nocturnal pain. In addition, this reduces the risk of patients stopping the drug because of side effects, before a therapeutic dose (i.e., 25 mg per kg per day) is achieved. In our experience the gentlest schedule involves starting with a bedtime dose of 100 mg for 2 days. The daily dose is then increased to 100 mg twice a day with breakfast and supper or breakfast and at bedtime, for 2 days. Thereafter, the dose can be increased to three times a day with meals and at bedtime. Further titration every 3 to 7 days can be continued until pain relief, side effects, or a maximum daily dose in the range of 2400 to 3600 mg/day is reached. An instruction sheet for the patients is helpful in clarifying the dosage schedule.

Gabapentin is generally well tolerated, even in the geriatric population, and has a safer side-effect profile than tricyclic antidepressants. In the PHN study, the majority of patients were titrated to 3600 mg/day, and the median patient age was 73 years. The kidneys excrete gabapentin, and the dosage must be reduced for patients with renal insufficiency (Beydoun et al., 1995). Table 24.2 presents various adjuvant analgesics for neuropathic pain.

ANTIDEPRESSANTS

Tricyclic antidepressants have been used for years for the management of neuropathic pain syndromes, including diabetic neuropathy, postherpetic neuralgia, and migraine headache (Max, 1994; McQuay et al., 1996; Onghena & van Houdenhove, 1992). However, pain relief is often modest and accompanied by side effects. Controlled studies indicate that approximately one third of patients will obtain more than 50% pain relief, one third will have minor adverse reactions, and 4% will discontinue the antidepressant because of major side effects (McQuay et al., 1996). Fortunately, some patients obtain excellent pain relief.

Because comparisons between tricyclic antidepressants have not shown great differences in efficacy (Max, 1994; McQuay et al., 1996), the choice of which antidepressant to use often depends on the side-effect profile of a given drug. For example, when a patient is having difficulty sleeping because of pain, a more sedating drug, such as amitriptyline, may be indicated. On the other hand, desipramine, which is less sedating, may be better tolerated in elderly patients.

The tricyclic antidepressants are generally highly protein bound with large volumes of distribution and long elimination half-lives. They undergo extensive hepatic first-pass metabolism and typically have active metabo-

TABLE 24.2
Adjuvant Analgesics for Neuropathic Pain

Drug Class	Mechanism of Drug Action
Anticonvulsants	
Carbamazepine	Sodium channel blockade
Carbatrol	
Trileptal	
Topiramate	
Lamotrigine	
Levotiracetam	
Phenytoin	Sodium channel blockade
Valproic acid	Sodium channel blockade
Gabapentin	Calcium channel binding
Clonazepam	GABAergic mechanism
Antidepressants	
Amitriptyline	As a group, norepinephrine and serotonin reuptake effects, possible NMDA effects, and sodium channel blockade
Nortriptyline	
Imipramine	
Desipramine	
Fluoxetine	Serotonin selective effects
Paroxetine	Serotonin selective effects
Venlafaxine	Mixed serotonin/norepinephrine uptake inhibitor (and opioid receptor binding effects)
Duloxetine	Mixed serotonin/norepinephrine uptake inhibitor
Antiarrhythmics	
Lidocaine	As a group sodium channel-blocking effects
Mexiletine	
EMLA cream	
Miscellaneous	
Corticosteroids	Anti-inflammatory and membrane stabilizing effects
Baclofen	GABA-B agonist
Capsaicin	Vanilloid agonist and C-fiber neurotoxin

lites. Although effective doses may be lower than typically used for depression, this is often not the case. Patients must be warned of potential side effects including sedation, cognitive changes, and orthostatic hypotension from a-adrenergic blockade. Anticholinergic side effects are common and include constipation, urinary retention, and exacerbation of glaucoma. Antihistaminic effects may cause sedation. Because of their long half-lives, these drugs may be given as a single bedtime dose. To minimize side effects, small doses (e.g., 10 to 25 mg) are used initially and increased over several weeks to a therapeutic dose, generally in the range of 50 to 150 mg/day. An electrocardiogram (ECG) is recommended if there is a history of cardiac disease. ECG changes such as QRS widening, PR and QT prolongation, and T wave flattening can be induced by these agents. Tricyclic antidepressants may have quinidine-like actions, consistent with their sodium channel-blocking effects, particularly in patients with underlying ischemic cardiac disease or arrhythmias (Glassman et al., 1993). Because abrupt discontinuation of antidepressants may precipitate withdrawal symptoms, such as insomnia, restlessness, and vivid dreams, a gradual taper over 5 to 10 days is recommended. Occasional blood levels are recommended, as well as CBC and hepatic studies to monitor for organ toxicity.

Amitriptyline is a tertiary amine that inhibits norepinephrine and serotonin reuptake equally (American Medical Association, 1993). Amitriptyline is probably the most commonly used tricyclic agent for neuropathic pain. Amitriptyline also is the most sedating of the tricyclic antidepressants and has the most potent anticholinergic effects. A starting dose of 25 mg at bedtime is recommended.

Amitriptyline is metabolized into nortriptyline, a secondary amine with twice as much inhibition of norepinephrine reuptake, compared with serotonin. Nortriptyline is less sedating than amitriptyline with fewer anticholinergic side effects. A starting dose of 10 mg at bedtime is generally well tolerated.

Imipramine is a tertiary amine with equal inhibition of norepinephrine and serotonin uptake. This drug is moderately sedating and has average anticholinergic effects. The suggested starting dose is 25 mg at bedtime. Because of unpredictable metabolism, occasional blood levels are suggested. Imipramine is metabolized to a secondary amine, desipramine, which is a much more selective inhibitor of norepinephrine uptake. Desipramine is less sedating and has fewer anticholinergic effects than imipramine or amitriptyline, is at least as effective for pain control, and is better tolerated by elderly patients.

Compared with tricyclic agents, serotonin selective reuptake inhibitors (SSRIs) for neuropathic pain have been relatively disappointing. In addition, they are more expensive than the older generic agents. Nonetheless, at relatively high doses (e.g., 60 mg), paroxetine is effective for diabetic neuropathy (Sindrup et al., 1990). Fluoxetine may also be useful in the treatment of rheumatic pain conditions, many of which have neuropathic components (Rani et al., 1996). SSRIs are better tolerated than tricyclic antidepressants and should be considered as first-line drugs in patients with concomitant depression. In this group they may serve double duty.

Venlafaxine is a novel phentylethylamine antidepressant that is chemically distinct from the older tricyclic antidepressants and the serotonin selective uptake inhibitors. Although venlafaxine blocks serotonin and norepinephrine reuptake, its analgesic actions may be mediated by both an opioid mechanism and adrenergic effects (Shcreiber et al., 1999). The drug may be at least as well tolerated as tricyclic agents and more effective for pain than standard doses of serotonin-selective drugs. Indeed, an initial report suggests that venlafaxine is effective for neuropathic pain (Galer, 1995). Venlafaxine should be started at one half of a 37.5 mg tablet twice daily and titrated weekly to a maximum of 75 mg, taken twice a day. Nausea appears to be the most common side effect.

Recently, clinical trials have demonstrated that several selective serotonin and norepinephrine reuptake inhibitors in the same class as venlafaxine, including milnacipran and duloxetine, are effective in relieving neuropathic pain. This class of antidepressants is as effective as the tricyclic antidepressants, and much better tolerated from a side-effect profile (Briley, 2004) Clinical trials comparing duloxetine at 60 mg per day against placebo, during 9-week randomized, double-blind trials, demonstrated that duloxetine-treated patients had significantly greater improvement in overall pain, back pain, and shoulder pain. About half of the improvements were independent of the benefit noted for depression (Fava et al., 2004). The most common side effects with duloxetine tend to be nausea, somnolence, dizziness, decreased appetite, and constipation.

The FDA recently approved duloxetine (Cymbalta®) for pain treatment of pain caused by diabetic peripheral neuropathy. Currently, this is the only FDA-approved treatment for this painful diabetic peripheral neuropathy. The magnitude of the response appears to be modest, with about 50% of patients noting 30% pain relief; approximately 30% of patients taking placebo obtained this amount of relief. However, this additional treatment option is welcome, given the fact that tricyclic antidepressants have significant side effects and SSRIs have not proven to be efficacious, except perhaps at high doses.

ANTIARRHYTHMICS

Antiarrhythmics block ectopic neuronal activity at central and peripheral sites (Chabal et al., 1992). Lidocaine, mexiletine, and phenytoin (type I antiarrhythmics) stabilize neural membranes by sodium channel blockade. Lidocaine suppresses spontaneous impulse generation on injured nerve segments, dorsal root ganglia, and dorsal horn wide-dynamic range neurons (Abram & Yaksh, 1994; Sotgiu et al., 1992). Lidocaine infusions have been used to predict the response of a given neuropathic pain disorder to antiarrhythmic therapy (Burchiel & Chabal, 1995). Lidocaine may be effective at subanesthetic doses, and following nerve blocks, analgesia may outlast conduction block for days or weeks (Burchiel & Chabal, 1995; Chaplan et al., 1995; Jaffe & Rowe, 1995). It has been reported that patients with PNS injury experience better pain relief than those with central pain syndromes (Galer et al., 1993). If a trial infusion of lidocaine is effective, a trial of oral mexiletine is worth considering.

Prior to starting mexiletine, a baseline electrocardiogram is recommended to determine if the patient has underlying ischemic heart disease. Dosages may be increased from 150 to 250 mg three times a day over several days. Taking the medication with food may minimize gastric side effects, which are common and a major reason for discontinuing the drug. Other side effects of mexiletine are nervous system effects such as tremor and diplopia. Once on a stable dose, a serum level should be obtained (the therapeutic range is between 0.5 and 2.0 mg/ml).

TOPICAL PREPARATIONS OF LOCAL ANESTHETICS

Topical preparations of local anesthetics may be effective for neuropathic pain when there is localized allodynia or hypersensitivity. Topical blockade of small- and large-fiber nerve endings should reduce mechanical and thermal allodynia. A topical lidocaine patch (Lidoderm 5% lidocaine) has become available, which can be applied to painful areas in shingles (herpes zoster) and in more chronic forms of neuropathic pain such as diabetic neuropathy or the ischemic neuropathies created by prolonged peripheral vascular insufficiency. Up to three patches may be applied at one time to the painful area. The patches can be worn for up to 12 hours a day. However, the treating physician must ensure that the patient understands that chronic forms of neuropathic pain may require a longer therapeutic trial, e.g., 30 days, before optimal symptomatic control can be determined. In patients with diabetic neuropathy, the addition of topical lidocaine patches to exogenous GABAergic oral agents may provide further improvement of symptom control.

A topical cream, eutectic mixture of local anesthetic (EMLA cream), a mixture of lidocaine and prilocaine, may also be useful for cutaneous pain. The cream may be applied three or four times a day to the painful area.

CORTICOSTEROIDS

Corticosteroids are clearly useful for neuropathic pain, particularly in stimulus-evoked pain such as lumbar radiculopathy. The anti-inflammatory effects of corticosteroids are well known, which may partly explain their efficacy for pain. When administered epidurally for treatment of discogenic radiculopathy, corticosteroids inhibit phospholipase A_2 activity and suppress the perineural inflammatory response caused by leakage of disk material around the painful nerve root (Saal et al., 1990). However, corticosteroids also act as membrane stabilizers by suppressing ectopic neural discharges (Castillo et al., 1996; Devor et al., 1985). Therefore, some of the pain-relieving action of corticosteroids may be due to a lidocaine-like effect.

Depot forms of corticosteroids injected around injured nerves provide pain relief and reduce pain associated with entrapment syndromes. Corticosteroids are also effective if given orally or systemically. In cancer pain syndromes, steroids such as dexamethasone may be first-line therapy for neuropathic pain. The potential side effects of corticosteroids are well known and may be seen whether medication is given orally, systemically, or epidurally.

BACLOFEN

Baclofen is useful for trigeminal neuralgia and other types of neuropathic pain (Fromm et al., 1984), particularly as an add-on drug. Baclofen is a GABA-B agonist and is presumed to hyperpolarize inhibitory neurons in the spinal cord (Yaksh & Malmberg, 1994), thereby reducing pain. This GABA effect appears to be similar to benzodiazepines, such as clonazepam. Side effects of baclofen can be significant and include sedation, confusion, nausea, vomiting, and weakness, especially in elderly patients. A typical starting dose is 5 mg three times a day. Thereafter, the drug can be increased slowly to 20 mg four times a day. Abrupt cessation may precipitate withdrawal with hallucinations, anxiety, and tachycardia. The drug is excreted by the kidneys and the dosage must be reduced in renal insufficiency.

CAPSAICIN

Capsaicin is a C-fiber-specific neurotoxin and is one of the components of hot peppers that produces a burning sensation on contact with mucous membranes. Topical preparations are available over the counter and are widely used for chronic pain syndromes. Capsaicin is a vanilloid receptor agonist and activates ion channels on C-fibers that are thermotransducers of noxious heat (>43°C) (Caternia et al., 1997). With repeated application in sufficient quantities, capsaicin can inactivate primary afferent nociceptors. For patients with pain due to sensitized nociceptors, capsaicin may be effective if the patients can tolerate the pain induced by the medication. The drug causes intense burning, which may abate with repeated applications and gradual inactivation of the nociceptors. However, in patients with tactile allodynia, which is probably mediated by large fibers, capsaicin may not be as effective. Capsaicin extracts are available commercially as topical preparations, containing 0.025 and 0.075% and should be applied to the painful area three to five times a day. The preparation may be better tolerated if it is used after application of a topical local anesthetic cream.

SUMMARY AND RECOMMENDATIONS

Neuropathic pain is a common cause of chronic pain and tends to be resistant to usual doses of traditional analgesic medications. Three classic examples of neuropathic pain include trigeminal neuralgia, post-herpetic neuralgia, and diabetic neuropathy. Neuropathic pain is often described as lancinating or burning in nature. Both types of pain may be present at the same time, often accompanied by allodynia.

Neuropathic pain may be manageable with one or more adjuvant analgesic drugs, often prescribed as part of a comprehensive treatment plan. From a theoretical point of view, it may be helpful to categorize adjuvant analgesics into two broad classes of drugs: those that act as membrane-stabilizing agents and those that enhance dorsal horn inhibition. Membrane-stabilizing drugs may act by blocking sodium and calcium channels on damaged neural membranes. Medications that enhance dorsal horn inhibition appear to act by augmenting spinal biogenic amine and GABAergic mechanisms. From a clinical standpoint, given the paucity of our understanding of neuropathic pain mechanisms and how the medications actually work, it is probably more useful to classify adjuvant drugs according to their traditional therapeutic indications (e.g., antidepressants and anticonvulsants). This point of view is strengthened by the fact that most drugs appear to have multiple mechanisms and sites of action, making further subclassification arbitrary and probably inaccurate.

Anticonvulsants, particularly carbamazepine (and more recently gabapentin), are useful for neuropathic pain. Although conventional wisdom suggests that anticonvulsants may be most effective for lancinating pain, anticonvulsants also are useful for burning dysesthesias. The mechanism of action of gabapentin is poorly understood, but the drug has been demonstrated to bind to a novel voltage-dependent calcium channel receptor. Gabapentin reduces the pain due to diabetic peripheral neuropathy and post-herpetic neuralgia. The overall safety record with gabapentin is good, making it an attractive alternative to carbamazepine and tricyclic antidepressants, particularly for elderly patients.

Clonazepam is another option and also poses minimal risk from the standpoint of organ toxicity. Clonazepam may be useful for radicular pain and pain associated with tumors, such as plexopathy. In addition, clonazepam may be used to supplement other adjuvant drugs. When given at bedtime, the mild sedating effect of clonazepam can be helpful for patients who have difficulty sleeping because of pain.

Antidepressants have been used effectively for years in the management of multiple pain syndromes, including diabetic neuropathy, post-herpetic neuralgia, rheumatoid arthritis, osteoarthritis, migraine headache, low back pain, and fibromyalgia. However, pain relief is often modest and accompanied by side effects. Studies indicate that only one third of patients obtain more than 50% pain reduction. However, some patients obtain dramatic pain relief.

The choice of which antidepressant to use for neuropathic pain often depends on the particular side effect profile of a given drug, as comparisons of individual tricyclic antidepressants have not shown great differences in efficacy. When a patient is having difficulty sleeping

because of pain, a more sedating drug, such as amitriptyline, is appropriate. On the other hand, desipramine,
which is considerably less sedating and has fewer anticholinergic effects, may be much better tolerated in
elderly patients.

SSRIs for neuropathic pain have been disappointing,
although paroxetine at relatively high doses is useful for
diabetic neuropathy. Fluoxetine may be useful in the treatment of rheumatic pain conditions, many of which have
neuropathic components. As with the tricyclic agents, the
SSRIs are probably interchangeable. However, SSRIs are
better tolerated than tricyclics and may be extremely
effective in treating patients with chronic pain and concomitant depression.

It remains unclear whether anticonvulsants or antidepressants should be first-line therapy for neuropathic pain.
Similar results have been obtained with both, and current
evidence concerning drug efficacy does not support the
use of one drug over another. In many cases, selection of
a particular drug may depend more on expected side
effects (e.g., sedation) or the clinician's experience with
the drug, than on theoretical considerations about mechanisms of drug action. It must be remembered that treatment of neuropathic pain remains largely empirical. In
addition, for maximum analgesic benefit, more than one
drug may be necessary. Until more effective medications
become available, polypharmacy will remain the rule
instead of the exception. This is probably understandable,
given the multiple mechanisms involved in the pathophysiology of neuropathic pain.

In general, for neuropathic pain either gabapentin or
amitriptyline (or a similar tricyclic antidepressant) should
be first-line therapy. When considering issues such as time
to effective analgesic action and toxicity, gabapentin is
more attractive. Gabapentin often is our first choice, followed by a tricyclic antidepressant, such as nortriptyline.
Both drugs must be started slowly and titrated to effect,
perhaps to rather high levels, for full benefit. However,
tricyclics have many potential side effects that must be
considered, particularly anticholinergic and cardiac interactions and organ toxicity. Clearly, gabapentin is a safer
drug, but may cause sedation or dysphoria in some patients.
Occasionally, patients complain of weight gain and non-
pitting edema. Until recently, other disadvantages of gabapentin included its cost (approximately 10 times the cost
of a generic tricyclic antidepressant at usual starting doses)
and the need to take the drug three or four times a day.
Keep in mind that the dosage of gabapentin must be
reduced appropriately for patients with renal insufficiency.

Recently, the FDA approved duloxetine, a selective
serotonin norephinephrine reuptake inhibitor, for the treatment of painful peripheral diabetic neuropathy. Although
clinical experience is not yet widespread with duloxetine
for this indication, this is the only FDA-approved drug for
painful diabetic peripheral neuropathy.

When an appropriate medication trial has been ineffective, an interdisciplinary approach should be considered. Reducing dependence on opioid medications may or
may not be a primary goal, depending on whether the pain
syndrome is opioid responsive, the patient is demonstrating appropriate improvements in function, and there are
not undue side effects or evidence of drug abuse.

Current evidence indicates that nonpharmacological
approaches may be reasonable, may obviate or reduce the
need for potentially toxic medications, and may improve
the effectiveness of analgesic regimens. Spinal cord stimulation may reduce pain in selected patients. Less invasive
techniques, including TENS units and percutaneous nerve
stimulation, are also beneficial.

The goals of providing medical care for patients with
neuropathic pain are often directed by changes in the
quality, intensity, timing, and regional distribution of the
patients' symptoms, rather than objective signs or test
results of the underlying etiology.

When considering those limitations it is helpful to
target specific symptoms, for example, burning pain with
tricyclic antidepressants and sharp, shooting pain with
anticonvulsants. However, from a practical standpoint,
pharmacological choices are often based on physician
experience and comfort with the safety and efficacy profiles of a given drug. Moreover, the high cost of new drugs
for which no generic yet exists may make older tricyclic
antidepressants, such as amitriptyline, the only cost-
effective alternative for some patients. Until more effective drugs become available, the pharmacological
approach remains largely one of trial and error. In the
meantime, nonpharmacological strategies may assume a
larger role in clinical practice.

The authors agree that effective management of neuropathic pain requires patience and persistence on the part
of the clinician and the patient. The ability of some
patients to accept incomplete pain relief during many therapeutic trials, simply with the hope that an optimal treatment may be determined, provides an example of courage
that should be emulated by all health care givers. When a
patient's internal strengths flag due to protracted suffering,
physicians should be prepared to treat, or arrange consultative treatment for, the anxiety and depression that often
accompany prolonged pain illness.

REFERENCES

Abdi, S., Lee, D. H., & Chung, J. M. (1998). The anti-allodynic
    effects of amitriptyline, gabapentin, and lidocaine in a
    rat model of neuropathic pain. *Anesthesia and Analge-
    sia, 87,* 1360–1366.
Abram, S. E. & Yaksh, T. L. (1994). Systemic lidocaine blocks
    nerve injury-induced hyperalgesia and nociceptor-
    driven spinal sensitization in the rat. *Anesthesiology, 80,*
    383–391.

Ahmed, H. E., Craig, W. F., White, P. F., et al. (1998). Percutaneous electrical nerve stimulation: An alternative to antiviral drugs for acute herpes zoster. *Anesthesia and Analgesia, 87*, 1–4.

Alhaider, A. A., Lei, S. Z., & Wilcox, G. L. (1991). Spinal 5-HT3 receptor-mediated antinociception: Possible release of GABA. *Journal of Neuroscience, 11*, 1881–1888.

American Medical Association. (1993). Drugs used in mood disorders. *AMA Drug Evaluations Annual* (pp. 277–306). Chicago: American Medical Association.

Andersen, G., Vestergaard, K., Ingeman-Neilsen, M., & Jensen, T. S. (1995). The incidence of central post-stroke pain. *Pain, 61*, 187–193.

Arner, S., & Meyerson, B. A. (1988). Lack of analgesic effect of opioids on neuropathic and idiopathic forms of pain. *Pain, 33*, 11–23.

Awerbuch, A. (1990). Treatment of thalamic pain syndrome with Mexilitene. *Annals of Neurology, 28*, 233.

Backonja, M. M., Beydoun, A., Edwards, K. R., Schwartz, S. J., Fonseca, V., Hes, M. et al. (1998). Gabapentin for the symptomatic treatment of painful neuropathy in patients with diabetes mellitus. A randomized controlled trial. *Journal of the American Medical Association, 280*, 1831–1836.

Bennett, G. J. (1994). Neuropathic pain. In P. D. Wall & R. Melzack (Eds.), *Textbook of pain, 3rd ed.* (pp. 201–224). Edinburgh: Churchill Livingstone.

Beydoun, A., Uthman, B. M., & Sackellares, J. C. (1995). Gabapentin: Pharmacokinetics, efficacy, and safety. *Clinical Neuropharmacology, 18*, 469–481.

Blom, S. (1962). Trigeminal neuralgia: Its treatment with a new anticonvulsant drug (G-32883). *Lancet, 1*, 839–840.

Boivie, J. (1992). Hyperalgesia and allodynia in patients with CNS lesions. In W. D. J. Willis (Ed.), *Hyperalgesia and Allodynia* (pp. 363–373). New York: Raven.

Boivie, J. (1994) Central pain. In P. D. Wall, & R. Melzack (Eds.).*Textbook of pain, 3rd ed.* (pp. 871–902). Edinburgh: Churchill Livingstone.

Boswell, M. V., Rosenberg, S. K., & Chelimsky, T. C. (2001), Neuropathic pain: Mechanisms and management. In R.S. Weiner, (Ed.). *Pain management: A practical guide for clinicians, 6th edition* (pp. 181–194). Boca Raton, FL: CRC Press.

Bowsher, D. (1993). Sensory consequences of stroke [Letter]. *Lancet, 341*, 156.

Bowsher, D. (1995). The management of central post-stroke pain [Review]. *Postgraduate Medicine Journal, 71*, 598–604.

Bowsher, D. (1996). Central pain: Clinical and physiological characteristics. *Journal of Neurology, Neurosurgery, and Psychiatry, 61*, 62–69.

Bowsher, D., & Nurmikko, T. (1996). Central post-stroke pain drug treatment options. *Disease Management, 5*, 160–165

Briley, M. (2004). Clinical experience with dual action antidepressants in different chronic pain syndromes. *Human Psychopharmacology, 19*, S2

Brodie, M. J., & Dichter, M. A. (1996). Antiepileptic drugs. *New England Journal of Medicine, 334*, 168–175.

Burchiel K. J., & Chabal C. (1995). A role for systemic lidocaine challenge in the classification of neuropathic pains. *Pain Forum, 4*, 81–82.

Castillo, J., Curley, J., Hotz, J., Uezono, M., Tigner, J., Chasin, M. et al. (1996). Glucocorticoids prolong rat sciatic nerve blockade *in vivo* from bupivacaine microspheres. *Anesthesiology, 85*, 1157–1166.

Caternia, M. J., Schumacher, M. A., Tominga, M. et al. (1997). The capsaicin receptor: A heat-activated ion channel in the pain pathway. *Nature, 389*, 816–824.

Caudle, R. M., & Mannes, A. J. (2000). Dynorphin, friend or foe? *Pain, 87*, 235–239.

Chabal, C., Jacobson, L., Mariano, A., Chaney, E., & Britell, C. W. (1992). The use of oral mexiletine for the treatment of pain after peripheral nerve injury. *Anesthesiology, 76*, 513–517.

Chaplan, S. R. (2000). Neuropathic pain: Role of voltage-dependent calcium channels. *Regional Anesthesia and Pain Medicine, 25*, 283–285.

Chaplan, S. R., Flemming, B.W., Shafer, S. L., & Yaksh, T. L. (1995). Prolonged alleviation of tactile allodynia by intravenous lidocaine in neuropathic rats. *Anesthesiology, 83*, 775–785.

Chapman, V., Suzuki, R., Chamarette, H. L. C., Rygh, L. J., & Dickenson, A. H. (1998). Effects of systemic carbamazepine and gabapentin on spinal neuronal responses in spinal nerve ligated rats. *Pain, 75*, 261–272.

Davidoff, G., Guarrachini, M., Roth, E, Sliwa, J., & Yarkony, G. (1987). Trazodone hydrochloride in the treatment of dysesthetic pain in traumatic myelopathy: A randomized, double blind, placebo-controlled study. *Pain, 29*, 151–161.

Dejerine, J., & Roussy, G. (1906). Le syndrome thalamique. *Revue Neurologique, 14*, 52–532.

Dellemijn, P. (1999). Are opioids effective in relieving neuropathic pain? *Pain, 80*, 453–462.

Devor, M. (1994). The pathophysiology of damaged peripheral nerves. In P. D. Wall, & R. Melzack (Eds.), *Textbook of pain* (3rd ed., pp. 79–100). Edinburgh: Churchill Livingstone.

Devor, M. (1995). Neurobiological basis for selectivity of sodium channel blockers in neuropathic pain. *Pain Forum, 4*, 83–86.

Devor, M., Govrin-Lippmann, R., & Raber, P. (1985). Corticosteroids suppress ectopic neural discharge originating in experimental neuromas. *Pain, 22*, 127–137.

Dworkin, R. W., Backonja, M., Rowbotham, M. C., Allen, R. A., Argoff, C. R., Bennett, G. J. et al. (2003). Advances in neuropathic pain. *Archives of Neurology, 60*, 1524–1534.

Edgar, R. E., Best, L. G., Quail, P. A., & Obert, A. D. (1993). Computer-assisted DREZ microcoagulation: Posttraumatic spinal deafferentation pain. *Journal of Spinal Disease, 6*, 48–56.

Eisenach, J. C., & Gebhart, G. F. (1995). Intrathecal amitriptyline acts as an N-methyl-D-aspartate receptor antagonist in the presence of inflammatory hyperalgesia in rats. *Anesthesiology, 83*, 1046–1054.

Ekbom, K. (1966). Tegretol, a new therapy of tabetic lightning pains. *Acta Medica Scandinavica, 179*, 251–252.

Fava, M. et al. (2004). The effect of duloxetine on painful physical symptoms in depressed patients: Do improvements in these symptoms result in higher remission rates? *Journal of Clinical Psychology, 65*, 521.

Fields, H. L. (1987). Painful dysfunction of the nervous system. In H. L. Fields (Ed.),, *Pain* (pp. 133–167). New York: McGraw-Hill Book Company.

Fromm, G. H., Terrence, C. F., & Chattha, A.S. (1984). Baclofen in the treatment of trigeminal neuralgia: Double-blind study and long-term follow-up. *Annals of Neurology, 15*, 240–244.

Galer, B. S. (1995). Neuropathic pain of peripheral origin: Advances in pharmacologic treatment. *Neurology, 45* (Suppl. 9), S17–S25.

Galer, B. S. & Jensen, M. P. (1997). Development and preliminary validation of a pain measure specific to neuropathic pain: The neuropathic pain scale. *Neurology, 48*, 332–338.

Galer, B. S., Miller, K. V., & Rowbotham, M. C. (1993). Response to intravenous lidocaine infusion differs based on clinical diagnosis and site of nervous system injury. *Neurology, 43*, 1233–1235.

Ghoname, E. A., White, P. F., Ahmed, H. E., Hamza, A., Craig, W. F., & Noe, C. E. (1999). Percutaneous electrical nerve stimulation: An alternative to TENS in the management of sciatica. *Pain, 83*, 193–199.

Glassman, A., Roose, S., & Bigger, J. (1993). The safety of tricyclic antidepressants in cardiac patients. Risk-benefit reconsidered. *Journal of the American Medical Association, 269*, 2673–2677.

Goli, V. (2002). *A mechanistic approach to the treatment of neuropathic pain: Symposium.* San Antonio, TX: Dannemiller Foundation.

Gorecki, J., Hirayama, T., Dostrovsky, J. O. et al. (1989). Thalamic stimulation and recording in patients with deafferentation and central pain. *Stereotactic and Functional Neurosurgery, 52,* 120–126.

Gracely, R. H., Lynch, S. A., & Bennett, G. J. (1992). Painful neuropathy: Altered central processing, maintained dynamically by peripheral input. *Pain, 51*, 175–194.

Greiff, N. (1883). Zur localization der hemichorea. *Archiv fur der Psychologie and Nervenkrankheiten, 14*, 598.

Hamza, M. A., White, P. F., Craig, W. F., Ghoname, E. S. et al. (2000). Percutaneous electrical nerve stimulation: A novel analgesic therapy for diabetic neuropathic pain. *Diabetes Care, 23*, 365–370.

Hart, R. G., & Easton, J. D. (1982). Carbamazepine and hematological monitoring. *Annals of Neurology, 11*, 309–312.

Hegarty, A., & Portenoy, R. K. (1994). Pharmacotherapy of neuropathic pain. *Seminars in Neurology, 14*, 213–224.

Hirato, M., Watanabe, K., Takahashi, A. et al. (1994). Pathophysiology of central (thalamic) pain: Combined change of sensory thalamus with cerebral cortex around central sulcus. *Stereotactic and Functional Neurosurgery, 62*, 300–303.

Holmgren, H., Leijon, G., Boivie, J. et al. (1990). Central post-stroke pain — Somatosensory evoked potentials in relation to location of the lesion and sensory signs. *Pain, 40*, 43–52.

Iacono, R. P., Guthkelch, A. N., & Boswell, M. V. (1992). Dorsal root entry zone stimulation for deafferentation pain. *Stereotactic and Functional Neurosurgery, 59*, 56–61.

Jaffe, R. A., & Rowe, M. A. (1995). Subanesthetic concentrations of lidocaine selectively inhibit a nociceptive response in the isolated rat spinal cord. *Pain, 60*, 167–174.

Jay, G. W. (1996). The autonomic nervous system. In P. P. Raj (Ed.), *Pain medicine: A comprehensive review* (pp. 461–464). St. Louis: Mosby.

Jensen, T. S., & Lenz, F. A. (1995). Central post-stroke pain: A challenge for the scientist and the clinician [Editorial]. *Pain, 61*, 62–69.

Jones, E. G. (1992). Thalamus and pain. *APS Journal, 1*, 58–61.

Jun, J. H., & Yaksh, T. L. (1998). The effect of intrathecal gabapentin and 3-isobutyl gamma-aminobutyric acid on the hyperalgesia observed after thermal injury in the rat. *Anesthesia and Analgesia, 86*, 348–354.

Kastrup, J., Petersen, P., Dejgard, A., Angelo, H. R., & Hilsted, J. (1987). Intravenous lidocaine infusion — A new treatment of chronic painful diabetic neuropathy? *Pain, 28*, 69–75.

Kemler, M. A., Barendse, G. A. M, van Kleef, M., de Vet, H. C. W., Rijks, C. P. M., Furnee, C. A. et al. (2000). Spinal cord stimulation in patients with chronic reflex sympathetic dystrophy. *New England Journal of Medicine, 343*, 618–624.

Kennedy, L. D. (1996). Laboratory investigations. In P. P. Raj (Ed.). *Pain medicine, A comprehensive review* (pp. 47–54). St. Louis: Mosby.

Kennedy, L. D. & Longmire D. R. (1992). Medical/laboratory evaluation of pain patients. *Pain Digest, 1*(4), 306–312.

Kovelowski, C. J., Ossipov, M. H., Sun, H., Malan, T. P., & Porecca, F. (2000). Supraspinal cholecystokinin may drive tonic descending facilitation mechanisms to maintain neuropathic pain in the rat. *Pain, 87*, 265–273.

Krause, S. J. & Backonja, M.-M. (2003). Development of a neuropathic pain questionnaire. *The Clinical Journal of Pain, 1,* 306–314

Leak, W. D. (1992). Radiological assessment of the pain patient. *Pain Digest, 1*(3), 218–224.

Leijon, G., & Boivie, J. (1989a). Central post-stroke pain - A controlled trial of amitriptyline and carbamazepine. *Pain, 36*, 27–36.

Leijon, G., & Boivie, J. (1989b). Treatment of neurogenic pain with antidepressants. *Nordisk Psykiatrisk Tidsskrift, 43* (Suppl 20), 83–87.

Leijon, G., & Boivie, J. (1989c). Central post-stroke pain - The effect of high and low frequency TENS. *Pain, 38*, 187–191.

Leijon, G., Boivie, J., & Johansson, I. (1989). Central post-stroke pain — Neurological symptoms and pain characteristics. *Pain, 36*, 13–25.

Lenz, F. A., (1992). Ascending modulation of thalamic function and pain: Experimental and clinical data. In F. Sicuteri (Ed.), *Advances in pain research and therapy* (pp. 177–196). New York: Raven.

Loh, L., Nathan, P. W., & Schott, G. D. (1981). Pain due to lesions of central nervous system removed by sympathetic block. *British Medical Journal, 282*, 1026–1028.

Longmire, D. R. (1991a), The medical pain history. *Pain Digest, 1*(1), 9–34.

Longmire, D. R. (1991b). The Physical Examination: Methods and application in the clinical evaluation of pain. *Pain Digest, 1*(2), 136–143.

Longmire, D. R. (1993). Electrodiagnostic studies in the assessment of painful disorders. *Pain Digest, 1*, 2-16.

Longmire, D. R. (1996). Evaluation of the pain patient. In P. P. Raj, (Ed.). *Pain medicine, A comprehensive review* (pp. 26–34). St. Louis: Mosby.

Longmire, D. R., & Parris, W. C. V. (1991). Selective tissue conductance in the assessment of sympathetically mediated pain. In W. C. V. Parris (Ed.). *Contemporary issues in chronic pain* (pp. 147–160). Boston: Kluwer Academic Press.

Longmire, D. R., & Woodley, W. E. (1993). Clinical neurophysiology of pain-related sympathetic sudomotor dysfunction. Tutorial 11. *Pain Digest, 3*, 202–209.

Longmire, D. R., Stanton-Hicks, M., Ranieri, T. A., Woodley, W. E., & Leak, W. D. (1996). Laboratory methods used in the diagnosis of sudomotor dysfunction and complex regional pain syndromes: A critical review. *Pain Digest, 6*, 21–29.

MacGowan, D. J., Janal, M. N., Clark, W. C. et al. (1997). Central poststroke pain and Wallenberg's lateral medullary infarction: Frequency, character and determinants in 63 patients. *Neurology, 49*, 120–125.

Matthew, N. T., Saper, J. R., Silberstein, S. D., Rankin, L., Markley, H. G., Solomon, S. et al. (1995). Migraine prophylaxis with divalproex. *Archives of Neurology, 52*, 281–286.

Max, M. (1994). Antidepressants as analgesics. In H. L. Fields, & J. C. Liebeskind (Eds.). *Pharmacological approaches to the treatment of chronic pain: New concepts and critical issues. Progress in pain research and management* (vol. 1, pp. 229–246). Seattle: IASP Press.

McLachlan, E. M., Janig, W., Devor, M., & Michaelis, M. (1993). Peripheral nerve injury triggers noradrenergic sprouting within dorsal root ganglia. *Nature, 363*, 543–546.

McQuay, H. J., Tamer, M., Nye, B. A., Carroll, D., Wife, P. J., & Moore, R. A. (1996). A systematic review of antidepressants in neuropathic pain. *Pain, 68*, 217–227.

Merskey, H. H. & Bogduk, N. (1994). *Classification of chronic pain: Descriptions of chronic pain syndromes and definitions of pain terms* (2nd ed., pp. 212–213). Seattle: IASP Press.

Mersky, H. H., Lindblom, U., Mumford, J. M., & Nathan, P. W. (1986): Pain terms: A current note with definitions and notes on usage. *Pain* (Suppl. 3), 216–221.

Morello, C. M., Leckband, S. G., Stoner, C. P., Moorhouse, D. F., & Sahagian, G.A. (1999). Randomized double-blind study comparing the efficacy of gabapentin with amitriptyline on diabetic peripheral neuropathy. *Archives of Internal Medicine, 159*, 1931–1937.

Nashold, B. S., & Bullitt, E. (1981) Dorsal root entry zone lesions to control central pain in paraplegics. *Journal of Neurosurgery, 55*, 414–419.

North, R. B., Kidd, D. H., Zahurak, M., James, C. S., & Long, D. M. (1993). Spinal cord stimulation for chronic, intractable pain: Experience over two decades. *Neurosurgery, 32*, 383–394.

Novakovic, S. D., Tzoumaka, E., McGivern, J. G. et al. (1998). Distribution of the tetrodotoxin-resistant sodium channel PN3 in rat sensory neurons in normal and neuropathic conditions. *Journal of Neuroscience, 18*, 2174–2187.

Onghena, P., & van Houdenhove, B. (1992). Antidepressant-induced analgesia in chronic non-malignant pain: A meta-analysis of 39 placebo controlled studies. *Pain, 49*, 205–220.

Ossipov, M. H., Lai, J., Malan, T. P., & Porreca, F. (2000). Spinal and supraspinal mechanisms of neuropathic pain. *Annals. New York Academy of Sciences, 909*, 12–24.

Pancrazio, J. J., Kamatchi, G. L., Roscoe, A. K., & Lynch, C., III. (1998). Inhibition of neuronal Na+ channels by antidepressant drugs. *Journal of Pharmacology and Experimental Therapeutics, 284*, 208–214.

Portenoy, R. K., Foley, K. M., & Inturrisi, C. E. (1990). The nature of opioid responsive-ness and its implications for neuropathic pain: New hypotheses derived from studies of opioid infusions. *Pain, 43*, 272–286.

Price, D. D., Mao, J., & Mayer, D. J. (1994). Central neural mechanisms of normal and abnormal pain states. In H. L. Fields, & J. C. Liebeskind (Eds.). *Pharmacological approaches to the treatment of chronic pain: New concepts and critical issues. Progress in pain research and management* (vol. 1, pp. 61–84). Seattle: IASP Press.

Rani, P. U., Naidu, M. U. R., Prasad, V. B. N., Rao, T. R. K., & Shobha, J. C. (1996). An evaluation of antidepressants in rheumatic pain conditions. *Anesthesia and Analgesia, 83*, 371–375.

Riddoch, G. (1938). The clinical features of central pain. *Lancet, 234*, 1093–1098, 1150–1056, 1205–1209.

Rowbotham, M., Harden, N., Stacey, B., Bernstein, P., & Magnus-Miller, L. (1998). Gabapentin for the treatment of postherpetic neuralgia. A randomized controlled trial. *Journal of the American Medical Association, 280*, 1837–1842.

Saal, J. S., Franson, R. C., Dobrow, R., Saal, J. A., White, A. H., & Goldthwaite, N. (1990). High levels of inflammatory phospholipase A2 activity in lumbar disc herniations. *Spine, 15*, 674–678.

Sandy, R. (1985). Spontaneous pain, hyperpathia and wasting of the hand due to parietal lobe haemorrhage. *European Neurology, 24*, 1–3.

Scadding, J. W. (1992). Neuropathic pain. In A. K. Asbury, G. M. McKhann, & W. I. McDonald (Eds.), *Diseases of the nervous system: Clinical neurobiology* (2nd ed., pp. 858–872). Philadelphia: Harcourt Brace Jovanovich, WB Saunders Company.

Schreiber, S., Backer, M. M., & Pick, C. G. (1999). The antinociceptive effect of venlafaxine in mice is mediated through opioid and adrenergic mechanisms. *Neuroscience Letters, 273*, 85–88.

Siegfried, J. (1983). Long term results of electrical stimulation in the treatment of pain my means of implanted electrodes. In C. Rizzi, & T. A. Visentin (Eds.). *Pain therapy* (pp. 463–475). Amsterdam: Elsevier.

Siegfried, J., & Demierre, B. (1984). Thalamic electrostimulation in the treatment of thalamic pain syndrome. *Pain* (Suppl. 2), 116.

Shimoyama, N., Shimoyama, M., Davis, A. M., Inturrisi, C. E., & Elliott, K. J. (1997a). Spinal gabapentin is antinociceptive in the rat formalin test. *Neuroscience Letters, 222,* 65–67.

Shimoyama, M., Shimoyama, N., Inturrisi, C. E., & Elliott, K. J. (1997b). Gabapentin enhances the antinociceptive effects of spinal morphine in the rat tail-flick test. *Pain, 72,* 375–382.

Sindrup, S. H., Gram, L. F., Brosen, K., Eshj, O., & Morgensen, E. F. (1990). The selective serotonin reuptake inhibitor paroxetine is effective in the treatment of diabetic neuropathy symptoms. *Pain, 42,* 135–144.

Sobotka, J. L., Alexander, B., & Cook, B. L. (1990). A review of carbamazepine's hematologic reactions and monitoring recommendations. *DICP. The Annals of Pharmacotherapy, 24,* 1214–1219.

Sotgiu, M. L., Lacerenza, M., & Marchettini, P. (1992). Effect of systemic lidocaine on dorsal horn neuron hyperactivity following chronic peripheral nerve injury in rats. *Somatosensory and Motor Research, 9,* 227–233.

Swerdlow, M. (1984). Anticonvulsant drugs and chronic pain. *Clinical Neuropharmacology, 7,* 51–82.

Swerdlow, M. (1986). Anticonvulsants in the therapy of neuralgic pain. *The Pain Clinic, 1,* 9–19.

Tanelian, D. L., & Victory, R. A. (1995). Sodium channel-blocking agents. Their use in neuropathic pain conditions. *Pain Forum, 4,* 75–80.

Tasker, R. (1990). Pain resulting from central nervous system pathology (central pain). In J. J. Bonica (Ed.), *The management of pain* (pp. 264–280). Philadelphia: Lea and Febiger.

Tasker, R., de Carvalho, G., & Dostrovsky, J. O. (1991). The history of central pain syndromes, with observations concerning pathophysiology and treatment. In K. L. Casey (Ed.), *Pain and central nervous disease: The central pain syndromes* (pp. 31–58). New York: Raven.

Taylor, C. P., Gee, N. S., Su, T. Z., Kocsis, J. D., Welty, D. F., Brown, J. P. et al. (1998). A summary of mechanistic hypotheses of gabapentin pharmacology. *Epilepsy Research, 29,* 233–249.

Tohen, M., Castillo, J., Baldessarin, R. J., Zarate, C., & Kando, J. C. (1995). Blood dyscrasias with carbamazepine and valproate: A pharmacoepidemiological study of 2,228 patients at risk. *American Journal of Psychiatry, 152,* 413–418.

Vanderah, T. W., Gardell, L. R., Burgess, S. H., et al. (2000). Dynorphin promotes abnormal pain and spinal opioid antinociceptive tolerance. *Journal of Neuroscience, 20,* 7074–7079.

Wessel, K., Vieregge, P., Kessler, C., & Kompf, D. (1994). Thalamic stroke: Correlation of clinical symptoms, somatosensory evoked potentials and CT findings. *Acta Neurologica Scandinavica, 90,* 167–173.

Woolf, C. J., & Mannion, R. J. (1999). Neuropathic pain: Aetiology, symptoms, mechanisms, and management. *Lancet, 353,* 1959–1964.

Woolf, C. J., Shortland, P., & Coggeshall, R. E. (1992). Peripheral nerve injury triggers central sprouting of myelinated afferents. *Nature, 355,* 75–77.

Yamashiro, K., Iwayama, K, Kurihara, M. et al. (1991). Neurones with epileptiform discharge in the central nervous system and chronic pain: Experimental and clinical investigations. *Acta Neurochirurgica. Supplementum* (Wien) *52,* 130–132.

Yaksh, T. L. (1979). Direct evidence that spinal serotonin and noradrenaline terminals mediate the spinal antinociceptive effects of morphine in the periaqueductal gray. *Brain Research, 160,* 180–185.

Yaksh, T. L, & Malmberg, A. B. (1994). Central pharmacology of nociceptive transmission. In P. D. Wall & R. Melzack (Eds.), *Textbook of pain* (3rd ed., pp. 165–200). Edinburgh: Churchill Livingstone.

25

Primary Headache Disorders

R. Michael Gallagher, DO, FACOFP

INTRODUCTION

Headache disorders are an exceedingly common patient complaint and have been described throughout recorded medical history. Symptoms of head pain were noted as early as 7000 B.C. (Lyons & Petrucelli, 1978), and Neolithic trepanned skulls suggest the extreme measures once taken to relieve head pain that was attributed to evil spirits (Venzmer, 1972). Currently, the National Headache Foundation reports that more than 45 million Americans have chronic, recurring headaches. Each year, U.S. businesses lose billions of dollars to absenteeism and medical expenses caused by headache, and headache sufferers spend in excess of $4 billion on nonprescription analgesics (National Headache Foundation, 2000). Headache is responsible for approximately 10 million physician consultations per year (Linet & Stewart, 1987), and it is the fourth most common reason for emergency room visits in the United States (McCaig & Burt, 2003).

Although the last two decades of the 20th century produced significant advances in our understanding of headache, the precise pathophysiology of the primary headache disorders remains unknown. For many years, primary headaches were classified symptomatically, as either vascular headaches (migraine and cluster) or nonvascular headaches (tension-type). Technological advances in the 1980s allowed researchers to see for the first time that changes in cerebral blood flow during headache episodes, particularly in migraine, did not occur exclusively in areas defined by vascular boundaries.

In 1988, the International Headache Society (IHS) published a classification system for headache disorders (Headache Classification Committee of the International Headache Society [HCCIHS], 1988). Although the clas-

sification was designed to help diagnose patients for clinical trials, the IHS criteria reflect international expert consensus, and unlike earlier headache diagnostic criteria, they outline the specific characteristics necessary to confirm and to exclude a broad range of headache disorders (Friedman, Finley, & Graham, 1962). According to the IHS, most chronic or recurring head pain can be classified as one of the "primary headache disorders": tension-type, migraine, or cluster. Each of these headache types, as the descriptor suggests, can occur without the presence of a known underlying disorder. The IHS system classifies all other types of headache as "secondary headache disorders," as they can always be attributed to one of hundreds of indirect causes of head pain (e.g., fever, trauma, subarachnoid hemorrhage, medication). This chapter reviews the diagnosis and treatment of primary headache disorders and cervicogenic headache.

PRIMARY HEADACHE DISORDER MANAGEMENT — OVERALL APPROACH

The vast majority of patients with headache can be successfully treated. When therapy is successful, the management of headache can be extremely rewarding for the patient and for the physician. However, headache treatment sometimes is time-consuming and difficult. When it does not succeed, or if it succeeds only partially, the challenge can quickly become frustrating. Help for headache sufferers rests with the empathetic, knowledgeable medical professional who is willing to establish an honest partnership that aims at relieving symptoms, restoring function, and reducing disability, not toward "curing" the "problem." In many cases, a clinician's ability to educate patients will be key; all headache patients should clearly understand the goals of their treatment plans. Unfortunately, many patients with headache seek medical attention during severe attacks, which demand immediate attention and prevent the complete evaluation necessary to make an accurate diagnosis. The most productive time for assessment is when the patient is headache-free or not so debilitated as to interfere with a complete history taking and examination. After the diagnosis is made, the clinician and patient can develop a realistic, achievable treatment plan.

There are two main elements of headache treatment. *Abortive treatment* aims at relief once a headache attack has begun, and *prophylactic treatment* is used to prevent or reduce the likelihood of headache episodes before they occur. Abortive treatment is used in patients whose headaches are infrequent and for those headaches that break through in spite of prophylactic therapy. When headaches are frequent or unresponsive to abortive medication, prophylactic measures should be taken. Many clinicians begin prophylaxis when a patient has more than three severe headache attacks per month, but this can vary from patient to patient.

Whether preventive or abortive therapy is indicated, management should follow a definite plan incorporating the clinician and the patient into a team that works actively to reduce the frequency and/or severity of headaches. All medicating and treatment modalities should be selected based on efficacy, patient tolerability, and adherence to recommended safety guidelines. Impressions and physical findings should be completely explained to the patient at whatever level and pace necessary to ensure complete understanding. The headache condition should also be explained, emphasizing the fact that the disorder is real, not imagined, and that it is controllable, not curable. Once a plan is developed, follow up and continuing care are important elements in a successful outcome.

TENSION-TYPE HEADACHE

In the 1988 IHS classification of headache, a headache type once known as "muscle contraction headache" was renamed "tension-type headache" (TTH) (HCCIHS, 1988). Traditionally, it was believed that TTH was caused by sustained muscle contraction of the neck, jaw, scalp, and facial muscles. It has since been learned, however, that the sustained contraction of pericranial muscles associated with TTH may occur as an epiphenomenon to possible central disturbances, not as a primary process. Alterations in the levels of serotonin (5-HT), substance P (SP), and neuropeptide Y in the serum or platelets have been shown in patients affected by TTH, leading to speculation that these neurotransmitters are involved in the genesis and modulation of pain in the condition (Ferrari, 1993; Gallai, Sarchielli, Trequattrini et al., 1994; Nakano, Shimomura, Takahashi, & Ikawa, 1993; Rolf, Wiele, &

Brune, 1981; Schoenen, 1990; Shukla et al., 1987; Takeshima, Shimomura, & Takahashi, 1987). Without definitive evidence of central activity, however, the cause of TTH remains unknown.

TTH is the most common type of headache and is considered to have episodic (ETTH) and chronic (CTTH) variations. One-year period prevalence estimates using the IHS criteria indicate that as large a percentage as 93% of the general population has at least one tension-type headache per year, although some investigators have found ETTH rates as low as 14.3% (Rasmussen et al., 1991; Lavados & Tenhamm, 1997). CTTH sufferers (more than 180 headache attacks per year) are far less common than ETTH sufferers; the highest 1-year period prevalence ever recorded for CTTH was 8.1% (Tekle et al., 1995).

Both ETTH and CTTH are characterized by intermittent or persisting bilateral pain, often described as a squeezing pressure or a tight band around the head. Some patients experience pain in the temporal or occipital regions, the forehead, or the vertex. The location of symptoms can vary from attack to attack, and associated tightness of the neck and shoulders is common. Unlike migraine, TTH is neither preceded by prodromal symptoms, nor are TTH episodes typically associated with nausea or vomiting. The intensity of pain in TTH varies widely, but it is not usually incapacitating. TTH can last from hours to days and, in some cases, persist for months. The IHS diagnostic criteria for ETTH and CTTH are listed in Table 25.1 (HCCIHS, 1988).

PRECIPITATING FACTORS

TTH frequently occurs during periods of stress or emotional upset. Some patients with CTTH may display evidence of anxiousness as well as poor coping and adaptation skills. If headaches are frequent or near daily, depression may be involved and should be considered, even in the absence of obvious signs, such as mood changes, crying spells, or loss of appetite. Organic processes may also be involved in the precipitation of TTH. When the cause is organic rather than psychogenic, the pain may also be resistant to usual treatment modalities. Organic causes can be numerous, but the more commonly encountered in clinical practice include degenerative joint disease of the cervical spine, head or neck trauma, temporomandibular joint dysfunction, or ankylosing spondylitis (see Cervicogenic Headache, p. 325).

TREATMENT

ETTH can be resolved with nonpharmacologic measures, analgesics, muscle relaxants, or some combination of these modalities. Nonpharmacologic options for TTH include manipulation, massage, exercise, cold or warm packs, stress avoidance, and relaxation techniques (Table

---

TABLE 25.1
IHS Diagnostic Criteria for Episodic Tension-Type Headache

A. At least 10 previous headache episodes fulfilling criteria B to D listed below. Number of days with such headache <180/year (<15/month).

B. Headache lasting from 30 minutes to 7 days

C. At least two of the following pain characteristics:
   - Pressing/tightening (non-pulsating) quality
   - Mild or moderate intensity (may inhibit, but does not prohibit activities)
   - Bilateral location
   - No aggravation by walking stairs or similar routine physical activity

D. Both of the following:
   - No nausea or vomiting (anorexia may occur)
   - Photophobia and phonophobia are absent, or one but not the other is present

E. At least one of the following:
   - History, physical, and neurological examinations do not suggest one of the disorders listed in groups 5 to 11
   - History and/or physical and/or neurological examinations do suggest such disorder, but it is ruled out by appropriate investigations
   - Such disorder is present, but tension-type headache does not occur for the first time in close temporal relation to the disorder

Source: Data from Headache Classification Committee of the International Headache Society, *Cephalgia, 8*(7), 1–96, 1988.

25.2) (Stevens, 1993). When these approaches do not provide adequate relief, simple analgesics, such as acetaminophen (APAP), aspirin (ASA), or nonsteroidal anti-inflammatory drugs (NSAIDs), often will relieve the symptoms of ETTH. If simple analgesics fail, caffeinated combination analgesics often will provide effective relief. In TTH studies, it has been shown that it takes about 40% more of a simple analgesic to equal the analgesic potency

---

TABLE 25.2
Nonpharmacologic Management of Headache

- Topical heat or cold packs
- Topical analgesic balms
- Respite from stressors
- Stress-reduction education
- Relaxation techniques (including biofeedback, hypnotherapy, vacation)
- Regular exercise
- Physical therapy
- Massage therapy
- Manipulative therapy

Source: Data from Stevens, M. B., *American Family Physician, 47,* 799–805, 1993.

---

of the simple analgesic plus caffeine (Laska et al., 1984; Migliardi et al., 1994). If a prescription is required to provide adequate relief, some patients with ETTH will benefit from the combination of isometheptene, APAP, and dichloralphenazone. Other options include the alpha-agonist tizanidine, ASA combined with the muscle relaxants orphenadrine or carisoprodol, or APAP added to chlorzoxazone. In some patients, the symptoms of TTH can be extremely severe and require potentially addictive analgesic combination drugs containing butalbital or an opioid. These drugs provide analgesia and reduce the anxiety often associated with pain (Table 25.3). As with any potentially addicting drug, however, the amount prescribed should be limited and patients should understand that daily or near-daily use must be avoided.

Patients with CTTH require a different approach. Prescribing the stronger analgesics in this patient subset greatly enhances the risk of abuse. Prophylactic treatment may be needed for patients with CTTH or for those whose attacks are caused by organic abnormalities. Pharmacological treatment of CTTH can include the judicious use of sedatives or muscle relaxants, but most patients who respond do so only temporarily, and the risk of habituation is significant when these medications are used daily or near daily.

The NSAIDs and antidepressants appear to be the most useful in preventing TTH (Gallagher & Freitag, 1987b). Most patients with CTTH who improve with NSAID treatment will do so in 2 to 3 weeks. Side effects of the NSAIDs include fluid retention, nausea, diarrhea, dizziness, and gastric and duodenal irritation. Renal function monitoring should be done periodically to avoid renal injury in patients who take NSAIDs regularly. Bedtime tricylic antidepressants (TCA) or serotonin reuptake inhibitor antidepressants (SSRI) may also be effective in reducing the frequency of CTTH pain. Therapeutic response can take as long as 4 weeks. The TCA regimen should begin with a low dose and will be gradually titrated to the individual patient's needs. Side effects vary depending on the agent and the patient, but they most frequently include drowsiness, postural hypotension, weight gain, constipation, and dry mouth.

Nonpharmacologic options for CTTH include manual manipulation and soft tissue massage techniques to the scalp, cervical, or thoracic areas, stress management, and muscle tension–reducing biofeedback. Consider psychotherapeutic interventions for patients whose headaches are related to significant emotional conflict or are refractory to treatment. Choices can range from supportive to long term and may involve the family physician, psychiatrist, or psychologist.

MIGRAINE

An estimated 28 million Americans, about 18% of women and 6% of men, suffer from migraine (Stewart et al.,

TABLE 25.3
Selected Medications for Tension-Type Headache

Drug	Brand Name	Dose
Aspirin	Bayer/Bufferin/Ecotrin	650–1,000 mg
Acetaminophen	Tylenol	500–1,000 mg
Aspirin/acetaminophen/caffeine	Excedrin	2 tablets
Ibuprofen	Advil/Motrin	400 mg
Naproxen	Aleve/Naprosyn	225–550 mg
Carisoprodol/aspirin	Soma compound	2 tablets
Carisoprodol	SOMA	1 tablet
Chlorzoxazone	Parafon Forte	1 tablet
Butalbital/aspirin/caffeine	Fiorinal	1 tablet
Butalbital/acetaminophen/caffeine	Fioricet/Esgic/Repan	1 tablet
Flurbiprofen	Ansaid	50–100 mg
Isometheptene/dichloralphenazone/acetaminophen	Midrin/Duradrin	2 capsules at onset followed by 1 tablet hourly prn (up to 5)
Ketoprofen	Orudis	12.5–25 mg
Metaxalone	Skelaxin	2 tablets
Orphenadrine/aspirin/caffeine	Norgesic	2 tablets
	Norgesic Forte	1 tablet
Rofecoxib	Vioxx	25 mg
Tizanidine	Zanaflex	2–4 mg
Tramadol/acetaminophen	Ultrocet	1 tablet

2000). This chronic, neurologic disorder is characterized by periodically recurring attacks of head pain that are accompanied by gastrointestinal, visual, and auditory disturbances. Although the intensity and severity of attacks tend to vary throughout the migraine population, as well as within the same migraineur over a series of episodes, estimates suggest that pain and disability are mild in approximately 5 to 15% of attacks, moderate to severe in 60 to 70% of attacks, and incapacitating in 25 to 35% of attacks (Stewart, Schecter, & Lipton, 1994). The disorder occurs most frequently among persons aged 25 to 55, concentrating its burden on those who are typically in their most productive years (Stewart et al., 1992). Patients with migraine consistently report lower mental, physical, and social well-being than do unaffected controls (Lipton et al., 2000; Terwindt et al., 2000).

According to the IHS, migraine is "an idiopathic, recurring headache disorder manifesting in attacks lasting 4 to 72 hours. Typical characteristics of headache are unilateral location, pulsating quality, moderate to severe intensity, aggravation by routine physical activity, and association with nausea, photo-, and phonophobia" (HCCIHS, 1988). Migraine rarely occurs on a daily basis; typical frequency is one to four per month. In some patients, the migraine may occur once yearly or as often as 15 to 20 times per month.

Migraine pain typically affects one side of the head, can switch sides, or can become generalized. Many patients report that their pain localizes around or behind the eye, or in the frontotemporal area. The pain may radi-

ate toward the occiput or upper neck during an attack. The shoulder and lower portion of the neck also may be involved. In some cases, the pain radiates to the face.

A number of associated symptoms can accompany the pain of an acute attack. Nausea or vomiting, in addition to either photophobia or phonophobia, is required for the diagnosis of migraine. However, dizziness, lightheadedness, irritability, blurred or double vision, anorexia, constipation, diarrhea, chills, tremors, cold extremities, ataxia, dysarthria, and fluid retention may also be present. Some patients may experience lethargy and fatigue for several days following an attack. The occasional patient will report being especially mentally alert and agile during the early stages of the migraine attack.

A prodrome or aura often precedes migraine attacks. Aura symptoms are usually visual, typically start just before the acute headache, and continue for less than 1 hour. Aural symptoms include scotomata, teichopsia, fortification spectra, photopsia, paresthesias, visual and auditory hallucinations, hemianopsia, and metamorphopsia (Diamond, 1997). Despite the absence of visual and other prodromal characteristics, sufferers of migraine without aura have also described premonitions of impending migraine attacks. These symptoms are usually vague and can occur from 2 to 72 hours before an attack. The list of painless warnings includes hunger, anorexia, drowsiness, depression, food cravings, irritability, tension, restlessness, talkativeness, excess energy, and euphoria. Table 25.4 lists the complete IHS criteria for migraine with aura and migraine without aura.

TABLE 25.4
IHS Diagnostic Criteria for Migraine without Aura and Migraine with Aura

Migraine without Aura

A. At least five attacks fulfilling criteria B to D

B. Attack lasts 4 to 72 hours (untreated or unsuccessfully treated)

C. Attack has at least two of the following characteristics:
   - Unilateral location
   - Pulsating quality
   - Moderate or severe intensity (inhibits or prohibits daily activities)
   - Aggravation by walking stairs or similar routine physical activity

D. During attack at least one of the following:
   - Nausea and/or vomiting
   - Photophobia and phonophobia

E. At least one of the following:
   - History, physical. and neurological examinations do not suggest a secondary disorder
   - History and/or physical and/or neurological examinations do suggest such disorder, but it is ruled out by appropriate investigations
   - Such disorder is present, but migraine attacks do not occur for the first time in close temporal relation to the disorder

Migraine with Aura

A. At least two attacks fulfilling B

B. At least three of the following four characteristics:
   - One or more fully reversible aura symptoms indicating focal cerebral cortical and/or brainstem dysfunction
   - At least one aura symptom developing gradually over more than 4 minutes or two or more symptoms occur in succession
   - No aura symptom lasting more than 60 minutes; if more than one aura symptom present, accepted duration is proportionally increased
   - Headache following aura with a free interval of less than 60 minutes (it may also begin before or simultaneously with the aura)

C. At least one of the following:
   - History, physical, and neurological examinations do not suggest a secondary disorder
   - History and/or physical and/or neurological examinations do suggest such disorder, but it is ruled out by appropriate investigations
   - Such disorder is present, but migraine attacks do not occur for the first time in close temporal relation to the disorder

Source: Data from Headache Classification Committee of the International Headache Society, *Cephalgia, 8*(7), 1–96, 1988.

PRECIPITATING FACTORS

Certain factors, known as "triggers," can play a precipitating role in the onset of migraine attacks. Migraine triggers are categorized as physiological, psychological, or external stimuli. Although they are highly individualized, some of the most common migraine triggers appear in Table 25.5.

Foods long have been implicated in triggering migraine attacks. The more commonly reported by patients are fats, dairy products, various fruits and vegetables, artificial sweeteners, food additives, and salt. Many medications can precipitate headache as a side effect, but more often the headaches are described as pressure-like and not typical of migraine. These medications are voluminous and it should be kept in mind that individual sensitivities are highly variable (Table 25.6).

Physiological Factors

Migraine sufferers can be particularly sensitive to changes in eating and sleeping patterns. Fasting or missing a meal is a known headache trigger and patients with migraine should be encouraged to maintain a regular meal schedule. Sleep irregularities also precipitate a migraine and attacks that occur on weekends, holidays, or during vacations have been linked to oversleeping (Wilkinson, 1986). To avoid "weekend" or oversleep headaches, patients should be instructed to go to bed when they are tired and to arise at the same time each day. Lack of sleep and fatigue may also provoke an acute migraine attack.

A relationship between the menstrual cycle and migraine attacks is well documented and partially accounts for the higher prevalence of migraine in women. Among female migraineurs, 60 to 70% note a menstrual link to their migraine attacks, with severe attacks occurring immediately before, during, or after their menses (Diamond, 1997). Many sufferers will report a remission of migraine after the first trimester of pregnancy or see an improvement or complete remission of their headaches after menopause (Honkasalo et al., 1993). Oral contraceptives should be used judiciously in patients with migraine, as these drugs have long been known to increase the frequency, severity, duration, and complications of migraine (Whitty, Hockaday, & Whitty, 1966). Also, hormone replacement therapy (HRT) should be avoided in postmenopausal migraineurs, as these hormones can exacerbate or restart migraine attacks. However, side effects and headaches have been reduced in some with the patch delivery system or the use of continuous or low-dose estrogen.

The link between diet and migraine varies with the individual patient. The amines, including tyramine and phenylethylamine, nitrates, monosodium glutamate (MSG), and alcohol have all been implicated as triggers. Tyramine is found in aged cheese, pickled foods, freshbaked yeast breads, and marinated foods. Another amine, phenylethylamine, is contained in chocolate, which is thought to precipitate attacks in many. The nitrates, which promote vasodilation, are found in cured meats. Many processed and Chinese foods contain MSG, which has been associated with headache. Alcohol has both central and direct vasodilating properties, and in some patients, migraine attacks can be precipitated, especially with red

TABLE 25.5
Recognized Migraine Triggers

Physiological	Psychological	External
Fasting, changes in eating patterns	Stress (external or unconsciously created)	Allergies
Over- or undersleeping	Post-stress "let down"	Loud noises
Exercise	Repressed hostility	Smoke
Cold/iced beverages	Depression	Strong odors
Ice cream	Fear	Bright or flickering lights
Food triggers (see Table 25.6)	Anger	Barometric pressure changes
Drugs (more common):		Sunglare
Danazol		Altitude changes
Diclofenac		Weather changes
Estrogen		Airline flights
H_2 receptor blockers		
Hydralazine		
Indomethacin		
Niacin		
Nicotinic acid		
Nifedipine		
Nitrates		
Nitrofurantoin		
Nitroglycerin		
Reserpine		

wine. Other possible triggers for migraine include caffeine, nicotine, ice cream, hypoglycemia, allergy, and monoamine oxidase inhibitors (MAOIs). Migraineurs who are sensitive to dietary triggers should be instructed to avoid the substances to which they are susceptible whenever possible.

Psychological Factors

Stress probably is the most readily identified psychological trigger of an acute migraine attack. However, many patients with migraine will remain headache-free during a severely stressful period only to experience a severe headache when the stress has resolved. Depression, fear, anger, anxiety, and repressed hostility may also be associated with migraine. Although avoiding stress is difficult, reducing stress is not, and instruction on coping methods may be beneficial for "psychologically overloaded" patients. Other psychological triggers may require additional counseling, treatment, or both.

External Stimuli

Some patients with migraine will describe a relationship between their headaches and weather. Rapid changes in barometric pressure as well as extreme variations in weather have been shown to provoke a migraine attack in certain patients (Diamond et al., 1989). During or subsequent to travel to an area with an altitude substantially different from the patient's norm (i.e., the mountains for those who live at sea level, and vice versa), a patient may report an increase in headache frequency. A diuretic, such as acetazolamide, used on the day of a flight may help to prevent these headaches. Other external migraine triggers include bright or flashing lights, loud noises, and strong odors (such as smoke, perfume, or cleaning fluids).

TREATMENT

With a confirmed diagnosis of migraine, the clinician and patient should begin to devise a treatment plan that accounts for the practical realities of the patient's lifestyle. Migraine treatment plans usually involve some combination of behavioral change (avoiding triggers, increasing exercise, and relaxation) and pharmaceutical and nonpharmaceutical pain management approaches (prophylactic or abortive medications, manipulation and massage, cold compresses, warm baths). Determining the relative value of these strategies for each patient will shape the course of both acute and long-term therapy.

Behavioral changes and nonmedicinal treatments can be valuable, particularly in patients with frequent or severe migraine attacks. Most treatment plans incorporate behavioral modification in the form of avoiding foods, beverages, or situations that trigger attacks; each patient will be unique in this regard. Similarly, the use of cold compresses, warm baths, or massage for migraine should be governed by the nature of the individual's disorder.

If medication is a part of the treatment plan, the selection can be tailored to the patient's needs. Before

TABLE 25.6
Migraine Food Triggers

Beverages	Dairy
Alcoholic	Aged and processed cheese
Caffeine (limit to 2 cups/day)	Yogurt (limit to 1/2 cup/day)
Chocolate milk	
Buttermilk	**Baked Goods**
	Fresh baked breads
Meat/Fish	Sourdough
Pickled herring	
Chicken livers	**Vegetables**
Sausage	Fava beans
Salami	Lima beans
Pepperoni	Navy beans
Bologna	Peapods
Frankfurters	Sauerkraut
Marinated meats	Onions
Aged, canned, or cured meats	
	Desserts
Fruits	Chocolate
Canned figs	
Raisins	**Other**
Papaya	Soy sauce
Passion fruit	MSG
Avocado	Meat tenderizer
Bananas	Seasoning salt
Red plums	Canned soups
Citrus fruits (limit to 1/2 cup/day)	TV dinners
	Garlic
	Yeast extracts

Note: Extracted from the National Headache Foundation Headache Diet, Chicago, IL.

recommending or prescribing any medication for migraine, however, it is crucial to determine all remedies the patient may have already tried before consulting, as detailed information in this area may reveal important therapeutic limitations and opportunities. Familiarity with the wide range of options for migraine pharmaco-therapy can increase the likelihood of meeting an individual patient's needs.

Standard Migraine Medications

Pharmacological therapy is most often the main compo-nent in migraine therapy. There are three broad categories of pharmacologic treatment of migraine: prophylactic, abortive, and symptomatic. If migraine attacks occur four or more times per month, or if attacks are incapacitating, many clinicians consider prophylactic therapy. If a patient has four or fewer migraine attacks per month, abortive treatment alone may be indicated. However, the clinician should determine the appropriateness of prophylaxis. When acute pain does not respond to abortive measures, symptomatic therapy can be employed as a backup.

Prophylactic Treatment

Preventive medications can be a part of a comprehensive plan, which may include behavior modification, diet coun-seling, exercise, stretching, or biofeedback. The goal of prophylaxis is to prevent the onset of migraine attacks, limit their frequency, or limit their severity. The decision about which medication or class of medications to use generally depends on comorbidities and interactions with concomitant medications. Beta-blockers, for example, could be used in patients with hypertension but are con-traindicated in those with asthma; a patient with depres-sion taking an SSRI should not take an MAOI for migraine because of dangerous interactions. Drugs currently approved for long-term use in migraine prophylaxis include propranolol, timolol, methysergide, divalproex sodium, and topiramate.

Propranolol, an adrenergic blocker, one of the most frequently used drugs in the prophylactic therapy of migraine, must be given carefully in patients with coro-nary heart disease and thyrotoxicosis. It may exacerbate coronary ischemia and can produce unstable angina or even myocardial infarction (Diamond, 1997). Propranolol is contraindicated in patients with asthma, chronic obstructive lung disease, congestive heart failure, or arte-rioventricular conduction disturbances. In some patients, administration may cause depression, nightmares, leth-argy, fatigue, sexual dysfunction, and weight gain. Patients being treated with insulin or oral hypoglycemia drugs, or patients taking MAOIs, should avoid propranolol use. Pro-pranolol is administered from 60 to 240 mg per day in a simple, long-acting dosage or in divided doses. Timolol is another beta-blocker that carries an FDA indication for migraine. It is an alternative to propranolol and can be taken in doses of 5 to 30 mg per day. Other beta-blockers, such as nadolol, atenolol, and metoprolol, have been used with varying degrees of success.

The alpha-agonist clonidine may be useful for migraineurs who are sensitive to cheeses and other foods containing tyramine (Diamond, 1997). Side effects are usually mild and include drowsiness, dry mouth, consti-pation, orthostatic hypertension, depression, and occa-sional disturbances of ejaculation.

Divalproex sodium is FDA approved for migraine pre-vention and is particularly useful in migraineurs with epi-leptic seizures, bipolar disorder, and possibly head trauma (Rapoport & Adelman, 1998). An extended-release for-mulation of divalproex, which produces less fluctuation in plasma concentrations than the standard therapy, is also available. The recommended starting dose for the extended-release formulation is 500 mg daily and can be increased to 1000 mg daily. Divalproex sodium should be avoided in any patient with a history of hepatitis or abnor-mal liver function; it is contraindicated in pregnancy, as it is associated with neural tube defects. Divalproex sodium can be combined with tricyclic antidepressants or other medications in patients whose headaches are difficult to control (Gallagher, Mueller, & Freitag, 2002).

Methysergide is closely related to ergotamine and promotes serotonin inhibition and mild vasoconstriction. This agent is usually prescribed in doses of 2 mg three times daily and should not be used for more than 4 to 6 consecutive months, after which a 1-month hiatus is required before resuming therapy. Upon initiation of therapy, some patients experience transient mental confusion, nausea, vomiting, muscle cramps or aches, and insomnia. If the symptoms persist for more than 3 days or the patient develops evidence of peripheral vasoconstriction, claudication, or angina, the medication should be stopped. Methysergide is contraindicated in patients with peripheral vascular or cardiovascular disease, hypertension, active ulcer, cardiac vascular disease, hepatic or renal dysfunction, fibrotic conditions, or pregnancy. Approved by the FDA for migraine prophylaxis, the drug's sustained use is contraindicated because of the potential for cardiopulmonary and retroperitoneal fibrosis (Diamond, 1997). During the treatment period, the patient should be examined at regular intervals to detect the possible development of fibrotic conditions, murmurs, or pulse deficits. Some clinicians employ continuous methysergide therapy and monitor for fibrosis with computed tomographic (CT) scanning of the abdomen.

Topiramate, a polysaccharide anticonvulsant with several mechanisms of action, has also been assessed in various clinical studies for prevention of migraine. The average daily dose varies from 50 to 200 mg per day and its effectiveness has been demonstrated (Biandes et al., 2004; Gallagher et al., 2002; Kruzs & Scott, 1999; Silberstein, Neto, Schmitt et al., 2004). Transient paresthesias are common, and an unusual side effect of topiramate is that it may cause some patients to lose weight during a course of therapy. With a positive efficacy and tolerability profile, topiramate appears to be a promising option for patients with frequent migraine.

Abortive Treatment

Abortive medications indicated in the treatment of migraine include both over-the-counter (OTC) and prescription agents. These include ibuprofen and APAP/aspirin/caffeine as well as a range of prescription-only medications, including ismotheptane, ergotamine preparations, naproxen sodium, rofecoxib, dihydroergotamine (DHE), and the 5HT1b-1d receptor agonists (triptans). Selected abortive agents are reviewed below.

Over the counter: Multiple studies of ibuprofen and the combination APAP/aspirin/caffeine have demonstrated efficacy superior to placebo in treating migraine and its symptoms (Codispoti et al., 2001; Lipton et al., 1998). The OTC medications are well tolerated, effective (espe-

cially when taken early in the attack), and rarely cause serious side effects.

Ergotamine preparations: The utility of these medications in arresting migraine attacks is due to their ability to counteract the dilation of small cerebral arteries and arterioles, primarily the branches of the external carotid artery. Nausea and lethargy are common side effects of the ergotamine preparations. Ergotamine tartrate use should be limited and not repeated for at least 4 days to avoid the possibility of ergotamine rebound headache, characterized by a self-sustaining cycle of daily or near daily migraine headaches coupled with the urge to take ergotamine to relieve symptonms (Gallagher, 1983). Ergotamine and its derivatives should be avoided in elderly and in pregnant patients. Dihydroergotamine, which was developed as an improvement over ergotamine tartrate, is highly effective and has a better safety profile. It is available in parenteral and nasal formulations. The nasal spray is more convenient and tolerable, has a low recurrence rate, and resolves migraine attacks in up to 70% of patients (Gallagher, 1996).

Nonsteroidal anti-inflammatory drugs: NSAIDs have been shown to be superior to placebo and equivalent to other reference drugs in the abortive treatment of migraine (Pradalier, Clapin, & Dry, 1988). Nonprescription formulations of ibuprofen have also been approved for the treatment of acute migraine. Although fewer side effects are reported with NSAIDs than with ergotamine and triptans, gastrointestinal, renal, and hepatic risks linked with NSAIDs are possible (Rapoport & Adelman, 1998). The COX-2 rofecoxib (unavailable in the U.S. market) has demonstrated effectiveness and causes fewer GI side effects than other fast-acting NSAIDs (Silberstein et al., 2004).

Isometheptene: This sympathomimetic with vasoconstrictive effects is found in combination with acetaminophen 325 mg and dichloralphenazone 100 mg. The combination can be effective in migraine without aura. It is taken orally, two capsules at onset headache and one each hour thereafter, to a maximum of five capsules in 1 day. Side effects include drowsiness and nausea, and it is contraindicated in patients with uncontrolled hypertension, with renal disease, or those taking MAO inhibitors.

5-HT (5-hydroxytryptamine) agonists: The serotonin agonists triptans became a mainstay of acute migraine headache treatment in the 1990s and now are the treatment of choice of most clinicians. Their therapeutic effects are thought to be the result of activation of the $5HT_{1B-1D}$ receptors. Three mechanisms of action have been proposed: cranial vasoconstriction, peripheral neuronal inhibition, and an inhibition of transmission through second-order neurons of the trigeminocervical complex, all of which inhibit the effects of activated nociceptive trigeminal afferents (Goadsby, 2000; Goadsby, Lipton, & Ferreri, 2002; Humphrey et al., 1990; Moskowitz & Cutrer, 1993). The

TABLE 25.7
Triptans

Medication	Brand Name	Form	Dosage	Half-Life	Recurrence Range
Sumatriptan	Imitrex	Oral tab	50, 100 mg	2 h	35–47%
		Nasal spray	5, 20 mg		
		Subcutaneous injection	6 mg		
Zolmitriptan	Zomig	Oral tab	2.5, 5 mg	2.5–3 h	22–37%
		Melt tab	2.5, 5 mg		
		Nasal spray	5 mg		
Naratriptan	Amerge	Oral tab	1, 2.5 mg	6 h	17–28%
Rizatriptan	Maxalt	Oral tab	5, 10 mg	2 h	35–47%
		Melt tab	5, 10 mg		
Almotriptan	Axert	Oral tab	6.25, 12.5 mg	3.5 h	18–30%
Frovatriptan	Frova	Oral tab	2.5 mg	25 h	7–25%
Eletriptan	Relpax	Oral tab	20, 40, 80[a] mg	5 h	6–34%

[a] 80 mg not available in United States.

migraine drugs marketed as "next generation" agents are similar to sumatriptan. As of this writing, there are seven additional triptans: zolmitriptan, naratriptan, rizatriptan, almotriptan, elitriptan, frovatriptan, and eletriptan.

The onset of action, duration of action, recurrence of headache, and tolerability vary with the triptan. Side effects tend to be a little greater with the more rapidly absorbed triptans, and the recurrence rate of headache tends to be less with the longer-acting triptans. Individual tolerability and efficacy can vary with the patient and a trial with different triptans may be necessary in some sufferers.

Reports of clinical experience with the approved triptans suggest that while they all are effective, response is highly individualized. Various attempts have been made to analyze and compare the triptans. Frietag and co-workers (2000), in a retrospective study of clinical experiences with naratriptan, rizatriptan, and zolmitriptan, concluded that all were highly effective, and they observed that no clear differences between them would distinguish one agent as "the best." A study by Ferrari et al. (2001) using a meta-analysis of 53 clinical trials comparing efficacy, recurrence, and duration of action was completed in 2001. Efforts were made to adjust for differences in protocols and placebo response, but there was not a clear agreement by specialists on its validity and usefulness. A limited number of clinical trials compared zolmitriptan with sumatriptan, rizatriptan with zolmitriptan, eletriptan with sumatriptan, almotriptan with sumatriptan, and so on (Diener, Pascual, & Vega, 2000; Gallagher, Dennish, Spierings, & Chitra, 2000; Sandrinia et al., 2002; Spierings et al., 2001) (Table 25.7).

The triptans initially were recommended for the treatment of moderate to severe migraine attacks. Clinical trials were conducted with traditional protocols and patients were instructed to treat only when migraine symptoms were well established. However, efficacy rates on average remained well under 70%. Consequently, the later view of specialists changed to treat sufferers at the onset of attacks. Recent studies have shown that early treatment results in more rapid efficacy rates, often within 2 hours of treatment (Carpay et al., 2004; Matthew, 2003).

As a class of drugs, the triptans are contraindicated in patients with ischemic heart disease, uncontrolled hypertension, and cerebrovascular disease. Triptans exert physiologic activity primarily in the cranial circulation, but can affect the coronary circulation to a much lesser degree. To date, there has been substantial human exposure to triptans and clinically significant myocardial ischemia or infarctions are rare (Goadsby et al., 2002; Mueller, Gallagher, & Ciervo, 1996; Ottevanger et al., 1994; Welsch et al., 2001). Chest pain following triptan use is a troubling side effect that occurs in a small percentage of patients.

Recurrence of headache within 24 hours, following initial relief, is a concern with migraineurs being treated with abortive medications. The recurrent headache results in the patient's needing to take additional medication and in some cases results in medication overuse. Recurrence appears to be influenced by pharmokinetics and pharmacological properties of the triptans. The triptans with the longer half-life and 5HT1-b receptor potency, such as frovatriptan, naratriptan, and eletriptan, tend to have the lower recurrence rates (Geraud, Keywood, & Senard, 2003). Some sufferers who experience longer migraine attacks or women who experience menstrual migraine frequently benefit from the longer-half-life triptans.

Sumatriptan was the first triptan to be widely used for the acute treatment of migraine headache. Because its availability predated other triptans, sumatriptan often is used as the comparator drug in head-to-head trials for the later-released triptans. Absorption is rapid and its elimination half-life is 2 hours. It is available in multiple forms including subcutaneous injection (6 mg), a rapid release oral table (50 mg, 100 mg), and nasal spray (5 and 20 mg). The subcutaneous injection tends to produce a rapid and effective response, but duration of action can be brief and a repeat dose is frequently required. The oral and nasal forms are effective, more convenient, and generally better tolerated.

Zolmitriptan was the second triptan to become available. It has a relatively rapid onset of action and an elimination half-life of 2.5 to 3 hours. Zolmitriptan demonstrates a favorable consistency rate among patients, especially when a second dose is used (Tepper et al., 1999). It is available in oral tablets (2.5 mg, 5 mg), melt tab (2.5, 5 mg), and nasal spray (5 mg).

Naratriptan was the first of the longer-acting triptans and is available in 1 and 2.5 mg tablets. Its elimination half-life is 6 hours and its onset of action is gradual. Patient tolerability is good and it often is used in sufferers with slow-onset and longer-duration migraine attacks. Natatriptan frequently is used in menstrually related migraine and can be helpful in "mini-prophylaxis" during the vulnerable period of time (Newman et al., 2001).

Rizatriptan has a rapid onset of action and an elimination half-life of 2 hours. It has a favorable one dose, 2-hour pain-free response without recurrence (Pascual et al., 2000). Rizatriptan is available in oral tablets (5, 10 mg) and melt tablet (5, 10 mg) with 10 mg being the usual starting dose. Patients who are concomitantly taking propranolol should be advised to take a lesser dose, 5 mg, because of increased rizatriptan plasma levels with propranolol use.

Almotriptan is an oral triptan with a broad T_{max} range of 1.4 to 3.8 hours. It has an elimination half-life of 3.5 hours, and its efficacy, tolerability, and recurrence profiles are favorable. Almotriptan is available in oral tablets (6.25, 12.5 mg) with 12.5 mg being the recommended dose. Unusual for this triptan is its incidence of chest pain side effects that are similar to placebo (Dahlof et al., 2001).

Frovatriptan is a relatively new triptan with a long duration of action. It has a 25-hour elimination half-life and a favorable headache recurrence rate (Ryan et al., 2002). Frovatriptan is well tolerated and is available in 2.5 mg oral tablets. Because of its long duration of action, it is frequently used in menstrual migraine and in patients who suffer with prolonged attacks.

Eletriptan is the most recent triptan to be released. It has a rapid onset of action with a relatively longer duration of action. Its elimination half-life is 5 hours. Eletriptan is available in oral tablets (20, 40 mg in the U.S., and an additional 80 mg elsewhere). It has been shown to be well tolerated and frequently effective in patients who have not responded to other treatment (Farkkila et al., 2003).

Approximately two thirds of patients report neck symptoms during migraine attacks (Blau & MacGregor, 1993). Stiffness and pain of muscles of the neck can be a part of premonitory symptoms or part of the headache phase of migraine (Waelkens, 1985). Physiotherapy, massage, or soft tissue osteopathic or chiropractic manipulative treatment can be of help in aborting or reducing symptoms of the attack in these patients, especially when used with medication (Astin & Ernst, 2002). Local anesthetic or saline infiltration injections into painful neck muscles can relieve migraine in some patients (Tfelt-Hansen, Louis, & Olesen, 1981).

Symptomatic Treatment

Symptomatic treatment for pain is indicated for patients with migraine whose abortive medications have failed or in patients who experience severe pain early in the migraine attack. Symptomatic agents are sometimes referred to as "rescue medications." Transnasal butorphanol, a nasal preparation, is one of the more useful drugs in patients with infrequent attacks. Pain relief has been demonstrated as early as within 15 minutes (Goldstein, Marek, & Winner, 1998), and the nasal formulation is particularly convenient for patients who are suffering from nausea or vomiting. Other options for rescue therapy include injectable NSAIDs, butalbital combinations, opioids, opioid-like agents, and other combination compounds. Because of their overuse potential and the possibility of rebound headache (overuse headache), proper prescribing precautions must be observed when using symptomatic medications (Limmroth et al., 2002).

INTRACTABLE MIGRAINE

Episodic migraine may become incessant and refractory to standard care (Matthew, Reuveni, & Perez, 1987). For many of these patients, drug dependence is a factor; for others, disabling headaches continue, unabated, seemingly indefinitely. For such patients, clinicians should be aware of several approaches to the management of intractable migraine. DHE, administered in a protocol developed by Raskin (1986), can produce a headache-free state in 90% of patients with intractable migraine within 2 days. Metoclopramide or antinauseants are used adjunctively with DHE to suppress accompanying symptoms (Ramaswamy & Bapna, 1987). Alternative treatments for intractable migraine include parenteral steroids such as dexamethasone, ketorolac (30 to 60 mg intramuscularly or intravenously), chlorpromazine (0.1 mg/kg intravenously every 6 to 8 hours), or naratriptan (2.5 mg twice daily for a limited period of time) (Gallagher, 1986; Gallager & Mueller, 2003; Newman, 2000).

CLUSTER HEADACHE

Cluster headache is a devastatingly severe type of recurrent vascular headache. It sometimes is referred to as histaminic cephalalgia, histaminic headache, Horton's cephalalgia, Horton's headache, Horton's syndrome, or migrainous neuralgia. Its clinical constellation of symptoms with the characteristic patient behavioral tendencies during attacks should make it easy to recognize and distinguish from migraine or tension-type headache. Of the recurrent headache syndromes, it is probably the most distressing and brutal to the afflicted.

A cluster attack is characterized by severe unilateral pain, often described as a burning, boring, or stabbing sensation in the area of the eye, temple, or forehead with radiation to the jaw, ear, or neck. During attacks, sufferers often pace or become extremely active, similar to patients experiencing renal colic. Frequently associated with the pain are ipsilateral lacrimation, eye injection, rhinorrhea, congestion, facial droop, or sweating of the face. The pain usually builds quickly over several minutes and lasts approximately 30 to 90 minutes in most sufferers.

Cluster headache attacks can occur numerous times daily, sometimes at the same hour each day. Early morning awakening with headache two to three hours after retiring is common. In its typical form, episodic cluster, the headaches cluster or group for periods of weeks to months and mysteriously disappear for months to years, thus the name "cluster headache." In its chronic form, which affects approximately 10 to 15% of sufferers, the headaches continue to occur indefinitely, affording the patients few headache-free days (Ekbom & Olivarius, 1971). The IHS criteria for cluster headache are shown in Table 25.8.

The typical onset of cluster headache is in the third or fourth decade of life, although cluster attacks have been reported from childhood to the late 60s (Heyck, 1981). Unlike migraine, cluster headache is more prevalent in men; its gender ratio favors men by 5:1. The etiology remains poorly understood. However, it has been proposed that vasomotor, hypothalamic, or neurohormonal disturbances may be involved (Kudrow, 1983; Moskowitz, 1984; Saper, 1983).

Unlike migraine, diet does not seem to precipitate cluster, although an occasional patient will report that chocolate can be a factor. The one exception, however, is the consumption of alcohol during cluster periods. Many cluster patients are heavy smokers, former smokers, and alcohol drinkers. During remission periods when patients are not on preventive medications, alcohol appears to have no provoking effect.

TREATMENT

The preferred approach to the treatment of cluster headache patients is prophylactic. The tremendous pain and relatively short but frequent attacks makes symptomatic treatment less practical and often ineffective. Appropriate pharmacological prophylactic regimens can reduce the frequency and severity of attacks in most patients. When treating patients with cluster headache, the benefits of

---

TABLE 25.8

IHS Diagnostic Criteria for Cluster Headache

A. At least five attacks fulfilling B to D

B. Severe unilateral orbital, supraorbital, and/or temporal pain lasting 15 to 180 minutes untreated

C. Headache is associated with at least one of the following signs that have to be present on the pain-side:
   1. Conjunctival injection
   2. Lacrimation
   3. Nasal congestion
   4. Rhinorrhea
   5. Forehead and facial sweating
   6. Miosis
   7. Ptosis
   8. Eyelid edema

D. Frequency of attacks: from one every other day to eight per day

E. At least one of the following:
   - History, physical, and neurological examinations do not suggest a secondary disorder
   - History and/or physical and/or neurological examinations do suggest such disorder, but it is ruled out by appropriate investigations
   - Such disorder is present, but cluster headache does not occur for the first time in close temporal relation to the disorder

Source: Data from Headache Classification Committee of the International Headache Society, *Cephalgia, 8*(7), 1–96, 1988.

---

therapy should be weighed against the hazards of taking medication. Patients should be monitored closely, as some of the medications prescribed in treatment can potentially cause problems. Ergotamine and DHE preparations, methysergide, calcium channel blockers, corticosteroids, and lithium are commonly used. Other agents, such as cyproheptadine, indomethacin, chlorpromazine, antidepressants, doxepin, and ergonovine, have been used with limited success.

For patients with cluster headache, ergotamine tartrate is administered orally in divided doses throughout the day and will often limit the severity and frequency of cluster attacks. The daily dose should be kept as low as possible (1 to 2 mg daily), and additional ergotamine for breakthrough headaches should not be permitted. Individual tolerance and sensitivity vary greatly, and patients should be followed closely for untoward reactions and complications.

Methysergide, an ergotamine derivative, also may be used to treat patients with cluster headache. It is administered orally in divided doses not to exceed 8 mg per day. If being used in patients with the chronic form, a drug holiday after 4 to 6 months of use is recommended (see Migraine Prophylactic Treatment).

Corticosteroids, alone or in combination with methysergide, are frequently effective for difficult patients. Their mechanism of action is not completely understood, but it is thought to involve suppression of hormonal mechanisms. This treatment is more suited for patients with episodic cluster headache, as its long-term use could be hazardous. However, because of the extreme distress and suffering of some patients with chronic cluster headache, corticosteroids can provide temporary relief while other prophylactic drugs are being introduced.

Prednisone or triamcinolone is commonly prescribed, although others are effective. The steroids are given in divided doses that must be titrated to the individual. The average daily starting dose is 60 mg of prednisone or 16 mg of triamcinolone. The medication is then tapered over 2 to 4 weeks with adherence to usual steroid precautions. Side effects include fluid retention, weight gain, gastrointestinal disturbances, lethargy, and Cushing's syndrome. Contraindications are hypertension, diabetes, peptic ulcer disease, infection, active immunization, or pregnancy.

Calcium channel blocking drugs have been helpful to many patients, especially those with the chronic form of cluster. It is believed that they alter smooth muscle tone of cerebral arteries by interfering with calcium ion function (Gallagher & Freitag, 1987a). Verapamil generally is well tolerated and more frequently used. It has been suggested as a first-line pharmacologic treatment for the prevention of cluster headache, although weeks of therapy may be required before control of the condition is established (Saper, 2000). It is given in divided doses with an average daily dosage of 360 to 480 mg per day. The most frequent side effects with verapamil are constipation and fluid retention. Verapamil is contraindicated in hypotension, cardiac conduction disease, and significant renal or hepatic disease. Other calcium channel blockers sometimes used are nifedipine (40 to 280 mg per day) and nimodipine (30 to 60 mg per day).

Lithium carbonate is reported to be effective in reducing frequency and severity of attacks in the treatment of patients suffering with the chronic form of cluster headache. Its mechanism of action has been debated, but it may involve its effect on cyclic changes in serotonin and histamine or electrical conductivity in the central nervous system (Diamond & Dalessio, 1980; Gallagher & Freitag, 1987a). It is administered orally in divided doses with a daily dosage of 600 to 1200 mg. Serum lithium level monitoring is necessary to avoid toxicity. Effective therapeutic ranges vary greatly, but generally should not exceed 1.2 meq/liter. NSAIDs and thiazide derivatives should be used with caution; when used concomitantly, these agents will raise the potential risks of toxicity. Side effects include fatigue, tremor, sleep disturbances, diarrhea, decreased thyroid function, goiter, and fluid retention. Lithium is contraindicated in the presence of significant renal or cardiovascular disease.

Abortive therapy for cluster patients is of limited effectiveness because of the relatively brief headaches and the time necessary for medication absorption. Few non-pharmacologic measures are helpful to patients with cluster headache. However, the complete abstinence from alcohol during cluster periods is imperative. Drinking alcohol, without question, will interfere with prophylactic therapy. Reducing cigarette smoking and caffeine consumption, as well as avoiding of daytime napping, may benefit some patients (Diamond & Dalessio, 1980; Gallagher & Freitag, 1987a). The inhalation of oxygen during a cluster attack is a relatively safe and effective treatment and, in the majority of sufferers, will abort attacks within 12 minutes (Kudrow, 1981). Oxygen is administered at a rate of 7 liters per minute by facial mask at the onset of attack and continued for up to 15 minutes. The main drawback to the use of oxygen is the cumbersome equipment, which makes it difficult to transport for patients whose attacks are unpredictable.

For patients who experience longer headaches and those who are not sufficiently controlled by preventive medication, abortive medication may be needed. This generally is limited to a triptan, ergotamine, or analgesics. The injectable, nasal, or faster-acting triptans, sublingual or injectable ergotamine, and nasal or injectable DHE can be administered early in the attack. This may give relief to some, while simply delaying the completion of the headache attack in others. The usual triptan, ergotamine, and DHE precautions must be observed, which limit the amount that can be taken and the number of headaches that can be treated. Analgesics and sedatives are of limited help, but they aid certain patients psychologically and reduce the anxiety associated with cluster attacks. Unmonitored use of these medications should be avoided, as potential habituation or toxicity can develop.

MIXED HEADACHE SYNDROME AND CHRONIC DAILY HEADACHE

Many patients with headache experience more than one distinct headache type, with pain-free periods between attacks. However, there is a group of patients who experience intermittent migraine attacks superimposed on a daily or near daily, less-intense headache similar to that of TTH. This pattern is characteristic of the mixed vascular headache syndrome. The patient with mixed headache syndrome is one of the more difficult to manage.

The patient with daily headache will, in many cases, have a long history of evaluations and failed therapeutic attempts. Such patients' constant fear of the daily or near-daily headaches worsening will sometimes lead to self-treatment and excessive medication use. The frequent use of any immediate-relief medication for head pain can cause rebound headache, which perpetuates the problem and often renders other treatments ineffective until the immediate-relief medications are discontinued (Kudrow, 1982). Psychogenic factors, such as chronic stress, anxiety, burnout, or depression, are often present and further contribute to the ongoing problem.

The patient–doctor relationship is critical in the management of patients with mixed headache. A definite, comprehensive treatment plan that addresses each element of the patient's problem must be developed and supervised by a single physician. The patient must be educated as to the nature of his or her headaches and how each aspect of treatment is expected to contribute to the control of the headaches. Once a plan is begun, continuity of care with regular follow-up visits is vital.

The treatment of the chronic daily or mixed headache syndrome usually will require prophylactic medications in addition to "tailored" nonpharmacologic measures such as diet, exercise, stretching, stress reduction, biofeedback, social adjustments, and counseling. Patients experiencing only a chronic daily dull headache usually will do best with a single nightly dose of a tricyclic antidepressant such as amitriptyline or nortriptyline. Other patients who experience coexisting tension-type and migraine headaches will require that each individual component be treated with its own appropriate therapy. The management of tension-type and migraine headache has been described earlier in this chapter. Patients who do not respond to outpatient therapy or who are unable to withdraw from frequent analgesic or ergotamine use may benefit from hospitalization at dedicated in-patient, tertiary care facilities (Diamond, Freitag, & Maliszewski, 1986).

CERVICOGENIC HEADACHE

Physicians and patients anecdotally have associated neck symptoms with headaches for a long period of time. Identifying the specific association among neck pathology, neck symptoms, and specific headache types has presented more of a challenge. In fact, some experts believe that more questions on this topic have been raised than the availability of acceptable and reliable answers. Adding to the complexity of this issue is the relatively high percentage of atypical headache that specialists encounter (i.e., atypical migraine, cluster, or tension-type headache.) Regardless, it is clear that the neck–headache association does exist and should become a part of the evaluation and treatment of headache sufferers.

Diagnosis

The definition of "cervicogenic headache" or "headache associated with neck disorders" has varied with specialty group, society, or association. In general, it can be defined as headache originating from muscular, articular, osseous, neurologic, or vascular structures of the neck. The headache frequently is unilateral, starting in the neck and becoming protracted. Some sufferers experience restricted ranges of motion of the neck, ipsilateral shoulder and arm pain, and on occasion, photo/phonophobia similar to migraine. Different areas of the cervical spine can be involved and many causes can be attributed to its symptoms (Sjaastad, 1997). Most specialists consider cervicogenic headache to be a syndrome and not a disease.

The IHS includes radiological evidence of movement abnormalities, abnormal posture, congenital abnormalities, bone fractures, tumors, rheumatoid arthritis, or distinct cervical pathology. However, the sensitivity of radiological studies in determining headache cause has been questioned (Fredriksen et al., 1989; Pfaffenrah et al., 1988). The Cervicogenic Headache International Study group of 1998 includes diagnostic anesthetic blockade as confirmatory evidence, but again, the confirmation of a diagnosis by therapeutic procedure can be questioned (Sjaastad, Fredriksen, & Pfaffenrath, 1998). Nerve blocks relieve pain locally or along the distribution of the anesthetized nerve and may not identify the origin of pain.

The varied criteria used to differentiate cervicogenic headache as a distinct entity rather than a precipitant of migraine or other types of headache account for a widely variable prevalence. Complicating the matter further is the reporting of cervicogenic headache in patients who suffer with concomitant migraine without aura and/or other distinct headache disorders. The reported prevalence varies greatly from 0.4% to as high as 42% in a population of headache sufferers older than age 50 (Leone, D'Amico et al., 1995; Olesen, 1990; Pearce, 1995; Pfaffneath & Kaube, 1990). Regardless, cervicogenic headache is an entity that deserves adequate attention of those clinicians evaluating and treating patients with headache.

Cervicogenic headache can occur after whiplash and neck or head injury, and has been reported or mentioned in various manuscripts. In one study of 222 patients with whiplash headache treated in an emergency department, 8% were diagnosed with cervicogenic headache (Drottning, Staff, & Sjaastad, 2002). Even minor trauma can be enough to unmask an underlying neck problem, which results in neck pain or cervicogenic headache (Wilson, 1991). Falling outside the cervicogenic headache criteria are those patients whose cervical pathology exacerbates primary headache disorders (Mueller, 2003).

Unilateral migraine without aura and cervicogenic headache share similar symptoms that can pose a diagnostic challenge for the clinician. This may account for varying outcomes when patients with similar symptoms are treated with the same regimen. In addition, as migraine sufferers age, attacks precipitated by the neck tend to increase. For this reason, a carefully made diagnosis is critical for the patient to receive optimum treatment and relief.

Pathophysiology

The neck is replete with pain-sensitive structures, which include muscles, bony attachments, nerve roots, arteries, dural matter, joints, intervertebral ligaments, and periosteum of vertebral bodies. Although little is known about the nerve supply of the atlanto-occipital (C0, C1) articulation, the upper cervical segments (C1 to C3) converge with trigeminal sensory fibers in the trigeminocervical nucleus in the upper cervical spinal cord (Bogduk, 1992; Edmeads, 1988; Wilson, 1991). Many clinicians believe that cervicogenic headaches originate from this area. However, other areas of the neck can be involved and the lower cervical segments also may cause radiating pain to the neck, shoulder, or arm.

Direct stimulation of the dura can occur by way of a dura–muscular band that connects the posterior spinal dura matter to the rectus capitus posterior minor muscle at the atlanto-occipital (C0, C1) junction (Hack et al., 1995). Consequently, it is presumed that torsion strain injuries or repetitive muscle contraction of the upper neck can more directly precipitate pain and headache.

Neck strain, injury, or chronic muscle spasm of the scalp, neck, or shoulders may result in heightened muscle sensitivity similar to the allodynia proposed in migraine (Bendtsen, 2000; Burstein, Cutrer, & Yarnitsky, 2000). Consequently, a lowered pain threshold may contribute to greater headache and associated symptoms.

TREATMENT

Patients who suffer with cervicogenic headache may have experienced pain for an extended period of time and frequently present a significant challenge to the clinician. The most successful treatment usually is comprehensive and can involve medication, physical therapy, manipulation, exercise, behavior modification, counseling, nerve blocks, nerve stimulation, radiofrequency, and in some cases, surgical intervention. The correct diagnosis, an individualized treatment plan, and a motivated patient afford the best chance of relief.

In many cases, the patient suffering with cervicogenic headache has taken a multitude of medications or has been subjected to various interventional procedures. This, of itself, adds another complexity for the clinician. These patients frequently are frustrated and, because they may have taken a particular medication in the past, may challenge the clinician on the selection of a pharmacologic regimen. This is when it is an absolute necessity to achieve "buy-in" and an understanding of the patient for the comprehensive treatment plan. The medication or medications in combination with other physical interventions or psychosocial therapies often are the difference between success and failure.

In some cases, the clinician may discover that the patient is taking excessive analgesics (prescription and OTC) and/or tranquilizers to relieve symptoms. As with other headache treatment, previously described, the daily or near daily use of analgesics, especially those containing caffeine can cause rebounding (Limmroth et al.,

2002). Successful treatment rarely is achieved until the offending medications are withdrawn.

PHARMACOLOGIC TREATMENT

Pharmacologic treatment of cervicogenic headache can include medications used in other headache disorders, such as anti-inflammatory drugs, muscle relaxants, analgesics, antinauseants, antiepileptics, and antidepressants. It is unusual that one medication alone will be adequate to effectively control cervicogenic headache. Combinations of medications in patients, who are appropriately screened, often are most useful, e.g., NSAIDs with muscle relaxants. Also, the clinician should be cognizant that the perception of pain differs from patient to patient. The patient's state of mind and expectation as well as pain modulation activity of the brain can influence treatment outcome (Naider, Ramesh, Anuradha et al., 1991).

The NSAIDs can be of significant value in a treatment regimen. From aspirin to the COX-2 inhibitors, there is a wide array and selection, which can be individualized for the patient, taking into account tolerability, onset, and duration of action. Regardless of the medication used, all NSAIDs are not equally effective in every patient and an alternative may be necessary. In some situations when there is severe inflammation, the temporary and judicious use of steroids can be considered.

The central-acting muscle relaxants can be helpful, especially when there is spasm or disruption of normal muscle tone. These agents have effects on higher brain centers and have analgesic as well as anxiolytic effects (Gallagher, 2002).

Baclofen, chlorphenesin, carbamate, chlorzoxazone, metaxalone, methocarbamol, orphenadrine, or tizanidine can be used in the usual doses. Diazepam is a benzodiazepine with significant anxiolytic, hyponotic, and sedative effects as well as muscle relaxation. Although other benzodiazepines are used, diazepam tends to be preferred because of its rapid primary and secondary peak levels, 1 hour and 6 to 12 hours, respectively. However, caution should be used because of tolerance and dependency possibilities with a benzodiazepine. Cyclobenzaprine is similar to the tricyclic antidepressants with like actions and adverse effects. It is preferred by some specialists because of its long duration of action and its psychotherapeutic and antidepressant effects. Evening doses can minimize its sedative effects.

The tricyclic antidepressants (TCA) and like drugs historically have been used for a multitude of pain and headache disorders. Relief has been reported in migraine and TTH, neuritic conditions, chronic pain, myofascial syndrome, fibromyalgia, and "unexplained physical symptoms and symptom" syndromes (Cormeck, Ziegler, & Hassanein, 1976; Diamond & Baltes, 1971; Gallagher, 2002; O'Malley, Jacson, Santoro et al., 1999). The TCAs were derived from neuroleptics and their psychotherapeutic effects seem to enhance improvement in patients with emotional and depression overlay.

Amitriptyline is considered the basic TCA, but others can be substituted with equal benefit. Side effects can be numerous, especially its anticholinergic and sedative effects. Imipramine, nortriptyline, maprotiline, desipramine, or doxepin also can be prescribed. In general, starting with a low dose in the evening and titrating to tolerability and efficacy is recommended. Protriptyline is nonsedating and is rarely given at night because of its strong anticholinergic effects.

In numerous studies, the anticonvulsants have demonstrated effectiveness in various types of headache and neck pain (Gallagher, 2002). An understanding of their exact mode of action is unclear. However, similar neurophysiologic mechanisms have been suggested for both pain and epilepsy and the anticonvulsants have shown usefulness in the treatment of head pain (Naider et al., 1991). Divalproex sodium and topiramate are more commonly used and frequently in combination with NSAIDs or muscle relaxants. Other anticonvulsants such as gabapentin, carbamazepine, felbamate, and phenytoin are utilized to a lesser degree. Divalproex sodium is indicated by the FDA for the treatment of migraine headache and various studies have demonstrated the effectiveness of topiramate. These medications have been discussed earlier in the chapter.

PHYSICAL MANAGEMENT

The muscles of the neck are prone to spasm from a multitude of causes. The necessary muscle tone of the neck is maintained by complex neurological mechanisms. Biologic disturbances, injuries, or physical abnormalities can interfere and cause sustained spasm of the neck, scalp, and shoulder muscles, which contributes to the headache.

The restoration of normal physiologic function and tone of the muscles of the neck and scalp is important in treating sufferers with head pain of neck origin. Appropriate physical therapeutic modalities such as heat, cold, ultrasound, or massage, tailored to the patient as part of a comprehensive program, can be of value (Vernon, McDermaid, & Hagino, 1999). In some patients, immobilization of the neck may be necessary, but should be limited in duration and followed by stretching and muscle strengthening exercises. In all cases, however, care should be given to the physical evaluation to ensure that discomfort to the patient does not aggravate the pain and symptoms.

Acupressure, acupuncture, transcutaneous nerve stimulation (TENS), and local muscle or facet join injections are sometimes utilized with varying degrees of success. Cervical epidural steroid injections are not commonly used, but can be considered in selected patients, with clear pathology within the vertebral canal, which is accessible to an epidural injection (Wilson, 1991).

Manipulative treatment properly administered by an osteopathic physician or chiropractor can be of help. Slow-paced progression of manipulation beginning with gentle stretching of muscle and manual cervical traction, later followed by muscle energy and strain/counterstrain techniques when appropriate, is more effective. Too aggressive or improperly administered manual treatments can result in more pain for the patient (Biondi, 2000). Therefore, frequent evaluations with appropriate modifications to the physical program are necessary.

Radiofrequency lesioning to decrease the nociceptive input from various areas of the cervical spine has been reported to be of help. However, the number of cases reported is few, and recurrence of symptoms can be common. Also, the degree of headache and the diagnosis of cervicogenic headache are not always clear. However, it appears that radiofrequency treatment shows promise for the future if standardization of trials and/or treated patients can be established (Mehta & Sluijter, 1995; Vankleef et al., 1993).

Surgical intervention is considered only when patients are nonresponsive to medical and physical modalities. Risks and benefit should be balanced and the patient should completely understand all aspects of a surgical alternative; only the rare patient may present with grossly apparent physical pathology of the neck requiring surgery. The majority of patients will be less clear.

Surgical procedures more commonly include ganglionectomy, ventral decompression, and dorsal laminectomy and laminoplasty. A review of 102 carefully selected patients who were surgically treated showed an 80% improvement of pain (Jensen, 2000).

REFERENCES

Astin, J. A., & Ernst, E. (2002). The effectiveness of spinal manipulation for the treatment of headache disorders: A systematic review of randomized clinical trials. *Cephalalgia, 22*, 617–623.

Bendtsen, L. (2000). Central sensitization in tension-type headache-possible pathophysiological mechanisms. *Cephalalgia, 20*(5), 456–508.

Biandes, J. L. et al. (2004). Topiramate for migraine prevention. *Journal of the American Medical Association, 291*, 965–973.

Biondi, D. (2000). Cervicogenic headache: Mechanisms evaluations, and treatment strategies. *Journal of the American Osteopathic Association, 100*(9), 7–14.

Blau, J. N., & MacGregor, M. B. (1993). Migraine and the neck. *Headache, 34*, 88–90.

Bogduk, N. (1992). The anatomical basis for cervicogenic headache. *Journal of Manipulative Physiological Therapy, 15*, 67–70.

Burstein, R., Cutrer, M. F., & Yarnitsky, D. (2000). The development of cutaneous allodynia of spinal and supraspinal neurons in migraine. *Brain, 123*, 1703–1709.

Carpay, H. et al. (2004). Efficacy of a new formulation of sumatriptan tablets when administered early in a migraine attack. *Proceedings of the National Headache Foundation's Headache Research Summit.*

Codispoti, J. R. et al. (2001). Efficacy of nonprescription doses of ibuprofen for treating migraine headache: A randomized controlled trial. *Headache, 41,* 665–679.

Cormeck, J., Ziegler, D., & Hassanein, R. (1976). Amitriptyline in the prophylaxis of migraine. Effectiveness and relationship of migraines and antidepressant effect. *Neurology, 26,* 121–127.

Dahlof, C. et al. (2001). Dose finding, placebo-controlled study of oral almotriptan in the acute treatment of migraine. *Neurology, 57,* 1811–1817.

Diamond, S. (1997). Recommendations for primary care providers: Diagnosis and treatment of migraine. *Headache Quarterly, 8*(Suppl.), 6–14.

Diamond, S., & Baltes, B. (1971). Chronic tension headache-treated with amitriptyline – a double-blind study. *Headache, 111,* 110–116.

Diamond, S., & Dalessio, D. (1980). *Practicing physician's approach to headache* (2nd ed.). Baltimore: Williams & Wilkins.

Diamond, S., Freitag, F., & Maliszewski, M. (1986). In-patient treatment of headache: Long-term results. *Headache, 26,* 189–197.

Diamond, S. et al. (1989). The effects of weather on migraine frequency. *Headache, 29,* 322.

Diener, H. C., Pascual, J., & Vega, P. (2000). Comparison of rizatriptan 10 mg versus zolmitriptan 2.5 in migraine (Poster). *Headache Quarterly, 11,* 51–52.

Drottning, P., Staff, P., & Sjaastad, O. (2002). Cervicogenic headache after whiplash injury. *Cephalalgia, 22*(3), 165–171.

Edmeads, J. (1988). The cervical spine and headache. *Neurology, 38,* 1874–1878.

Ekbom, K., & Olivarius, B. (1971). Chronic migrainous neuralgia: Diagnosis and therapeutic agents. *Headache, 11,* 97–101.

Farkkila, M. et al. (2003). Eletriptan for the treatment of migraine in patients with previous poor response or tolerance to oral sumatriptan. *Cephalalgia, 12*(6), 463–471.

Ferrari, M. D. (1993). Biochemistry of tension-type headache. In J. Olesen & J. Schoenen (Eds.), *Tension-type headache: Classification, mechanisms, and treatment* (pp. 115–126). New York: Raven Press.

Ferrari, M. D. et al. (2001). Oral triptans (serotonin $5HT_{1B/1D}$ agonists) in acute migraine treatment: A meta-analysis of 53 trials. *Lancet, 358,* 1668–1675.

Fredriksen, T. A., et al. (1989). Cervicogenic headache. Radiological investigation concerning head/neck. *Cephalalgia, 9,* 139–146.

Freitag, F. G. et al. (2000). The new treatments in migraine: First year clinical experience. *Headache Quarterly, 11,* 33–36.

Friedman, A. P., Finley, K. H., & Graham, J.R. (1962). Classification of headache. *Archives of Neurology, 6,* 173–176.

Gallagher, R. M. (1983). Ergotamine withdrawal causing rebound headache. *Journal American Osteopathic Association, 82*(9), 677.

Gallagher, R. M. (1986). Emergency treatment of intractable migraine headache. *Headache, 26,* 74–75.

Gallagher, R. M. (1996). Acute treatment of migraine with dihydroergotamine nasal spray. *Archives of Neurology, 53,* 1285–1291.

Gallagher, R. M. (2002). Anticonvulsant and muscle relaxants. In C. Tollison, J. Satterthwaite, & J. Tollison (Eds.). *Practical pain management* (pp. 278–287). Philadelphia: Lippincott Williams Wilkins.

Gallagher, R. M., & Freitag, F. (1987a). Cluster headache: Diagnosis and treatment. *Journal of Osteopathic Medicine, 1,* 10–18.

Gallagher, R. M., & Freitag, F. (1987b). Muscle contraction headache: Diagnosis and treatment. *Journal of Osteopathic Medicine, 1*(6), 8–17.

Gallagher, R. M., & Mueller, L. (2003). Managing intractable migraine with naratriptan. *Headache, 43,* 991–993.

Gallagher, R. M., Dennish, G., Spierings, E. L. H., & Chitra, R. (2000). A comparative trial of zolmitriptan and sumatriptan for the acute oral treatment of migraine. *Headache, 40,* 119–128.

Gallagher, R. M., Mueller, L. L., & Freitag, F. G. (2002). Divalproex sodium in the treatment of migraine and cluster headaches. *Journal. American Osteopathic Association, 102*(2), 92–94.

Gallai, V., Sarchielli P., Trequattrini, A. et al. (1994). Neuropeptide Y in juvenile migraine and tension-type headache. *Headache, 34,* 35–40.

Geraud, G., Keywood, C., & Senard, J. M. (2003). Migraine headache recurrence: Relationship to clinical pharmacological and pharmacokinetic properties of triptans. *Headache, 43,* 376–388.

Goadsby, P. J. (2000). The pharmacology of headache. *Progress in Neurobiology, 62,* 509–525.

Goadsby, P. J., Lipton, R. B., & Ferrari, M. D. (2002). Migraine: Current understanding and treatment. *New England Journal of Medicine, 346*(4), 257–270.

Goldstein, J., Marek, J. G., & Winner, P. (1998). Comparison of butorphanol nasal spray and Fiorinal with codeine in the treatment of migraine. *Headache, 38,* 516–522.

Hack, G. O. et al. (1995). Anatomic relationship between rectus capitus posterior minor muscle and dura matter. *Spine, 20,* 2484–2486.

Headache Classification Committee of the International Headache Society. (1988). Classification of the diagnostic criteria for headache disorders, cranial neuralgias, and facial pain. *Cephalalgia, 8*(Suppl. 7), 1–96.

Heyck, H. (1981). *Headache and facial pain.* Chicago: Yearbook of Medical Publishers.

Honkasalo, M. L. et al. (1993). A population-based survey of headache and migraine in 22,809 adults. *Headache, 33,* 403–412.

Humphrey, P. P. A. et al. (1990). Serotonin and migraine. *Annals. New York Academy of Sciences, 600,* 587–598.

Jensen, J. (2000). Surgical treatment of non-responsive cervicogenic headache. *Clinical and Experimental Rheumatology, 18*(Suppl. 19), 567–570.

Kruzs, J. C., & Scott, V. (1999). Topiramate in the treatment of chronic migraine and other headaches. *Headache, 39,* 363.

Kudrow, L. (1981). Response of cluster headache to oxygen inhalation. *Headache, 21,* 1–4.

Kudrow, L. (1982). Paradoxical effects of frequent analygesic use. *Advances in Neurology, 33,* 335–341.

Kudrow, L. (1983). Cluster headache. *Neurologic Clinics, 1,* 370.

Laska, E. M. et al. (1984). Caffeine as an analgesic adjuvant. *Journal of the American Medical Association, 251,* 1711–1718.

Lavados, P. M., & Tenhamm, E. (1997). Epidemiology of migraine headache in Santiago, Chile: A prevalence study. *Cephalalgia, 17,* 770–777.

Leone, M., D'Amico, D. et al. (1995). Possible identification of cervicogenic headache among migraine cases: An analysis of 374 patients. *Headache, 35,* 461–464.

Limmroth, V., et al. (2002). Features of medication overuse headache following overuse of different acute headache drugs. *Neurology, 59,* 101 –1014.

Linet, M. S., &Stewart, W. F. The epidemiology of migraine headache. In J. N. Blau (Ed.), *Migraine: Clinical and research aspects* (p. 451). Baltimore, MD: The Johns Hopkins University Press.

Lipton, R. B. et al. (1998). Efficacy and safety of the nonprescription combination of acetaminophen, aspirin, and caffeine in alleviating headache pain of an acute migraine attack: Three double-blind, randomized, placebo-controlled trials. *Archives of Neurology, 55,* 210–217.

Lipton, R. B. et al. (2000). Migraine, quality of life, and depression: A population-based case-control study. *Neurology, 55,* 629–635.

Lyons, A. S., & Petrucelli, R. J. (1978). *Medicine: An illustrated history* (p. 27). New York: Harry N. Abrams.

Mathew, N. T., Reuveni, U., & Perez, F. (1987). Transformed or evolutive migraine. *Headache, 27,* 102–106.

Matthew, N. T. (2003). Early intervention with almotriptan improves sustained pain-free response in acute migraine. *Headache, 43*(10), 1075–1079.

McCaig, L. F., & Burt, C. W. (2003, June 4,5). National hospital ambulatory medical care survey. Emergency department sumary. *Advanced Data from Vital and Health Statistics,* 335.

Mehta, M., & Sluijter, M. (1995). Radiofrequency nerve blockade in pain therapy. *International Journal of Pain Therapy, 5,* 89–99.

Migliardi, J. R. et al. (1994). Caffeine as an analgesic adjuvant in tension headache. *Clinical Pharmacology and Therapeutics, 56*(5), 76–86.

Moskowitz, M. (1984). The neurobiology of vascular head pain. *Annals of Neurology, 16,* 157–168.

Moskowitz, M. A., & Cutrer, M. (1993). Sumatriptan: A receptor-targeted treatment for migraine. *Annual Review of Medicine, 44,* 145–154.

Mueller, L. (2003, April). Cervicogenic headache: A diagnostic and therapeutic dilemma. *Headache and Pain,* 29–37.

Mueller, L., Gallagher, R. M., & Ciervo, C. A. (1996). Vasospasm-induced myocardial infarction with sumatriptan. *Headache, 36,* 329–331.

Naider, M., Ramesh, K., Anuradha, R. et al. (1991). Evaluations of phenytoin in rheumatoid arthritis: An open study. *Drugs under Experimental and Clinical Research, 17,* 71–275.

Nakano, T., Shimomura, T., Takahashi, K., & Ikawa, S. (1993). Platelet substance P and 5-hydroxytryptamine in migraine and tension-type headache. *Headache, 33,* 528–532.

National Headache Foundation web site. *NHF Headache Facts.* Retrieved October, 2000 from http://www.headaches.org.

Newman, L. C. (2001, November). Inpatient treatment strategies for intractable headache [Abstract]. Scottsdale Headache Symposium, American Headache Society.

Newman, L. et al. (2001). Naratriptan as short-term prophylaxis of menstrually associated migraine: A randomized, double-blind, placebo-controller study, *Headache, 41,* 241–256.

Olesen, J. (1990). *Classification and diagnostic criteria for headache disorders, cranial neuralgias and facial pain.* Copenhagen: International Headache Society.

O'Malley, P., Jackson, J., Santoro, J. et al. (1999). Antidepressant therapy for unexplained symptoms and symptom syndromes. *Journal of Family Practice, 48*(12), 980–990.

Ottevanger, J. P. et al. (1994). Adverse reactions attributed to sumatriptan. A postmarketing study in general practice. *European Journal of Clinical Pharmacology, 47,* 305–309.

Pascual, J. et al. (2000). Prospective study on triptan tablet consumption per attack in Spain [Abstract]. *Cephalalgia, 20,* 411–412.

Pearce, J. (1995). Cervicogenic headache: A personal view. *Cephalalgia, 15,* 463–469.

Pfaffeneath, V., & Kaube, H. (1990). Diagnosis of cervicogenic headache. *Functional Neurology, 5,* 159–164.

Pfaffenrah, V. et al. (1988). Cervicogenic headache: Results of computer-based measurements of cervical spine mobility in 15 patients. *Cephalalgia, 8,* 45–48.

Pradalier, A., Clapin, A., & Dry, J. (1988). Treatment review: Nonsteroidal anti-inflammatory drugs in treatment and long-term prevention of migraine attacks. *Headache, 28,* 550–557.

Ramaswamy, S., & Bapna, J. S. (1987). Antagonism of morphine tolerance and dependence by metoclopramide. *Life Sciences, 40,* 807–810.

Rapoport, A., & Adelman, J. (1998). Cost of migraine management: A pharmacologic overview. *American Journal of Managed Care, 4*(4), 531–545.

Raskin, N. H. (1986). Repetitive intravenous dihydroergotamine as therapy for intractable migraine. *Neurology, 36,* 995–997.

Rasmussen, B. K. et al. (1991). Epidemiology of headache in a general population – A prevalence study. *Journal of Clinical Epidemiology, 44,* 1147–1157.

Rolf, L. H., Wiele, G., & Brune, G. G. (1981). 5-Hydroxytryptamine in platelets of patients with muscle contraction headache. *Headache, 21,* 10–11.

Ryan, R. et al. (2002). Clinical efficacy of frovatriptan: Placebo-controlled studies. *Headache, 42*(Suppl. 2), S84–S92.

Sandrinia, G. et al. (2002). Eletriptan vs. sumatriptan. A double blind, placebo controlled, multiple migraine attack study, *Neurology, 59*, 1210–1217.

Saper, J. (1983). *Headache disorders: Current concepts and treatment strategies* (pp. 76–77). Boston: John Wright-PSG, Inc.

Saper, J. (2000, November 4). Cluster headache [Abstract]. Scottsdale Headache Symposium, American Headache Society.

Schoenen, J. (1990). Tension-type headache: Pathophysiologic evidence for a disturbance of "limbic" pathways to the brain stem [Abstract]. *Headache, 30*, 314–315.

Shukla, R. et al. (1987). Serotonin in tension headache. *Journal of Neurology, Neurosurgery and Psychiatry, 50*, 1682–1684.

Silberstein, S. D., Neto, W., Schmitt, J. et al. (2004). Topiramate in migraine prevention. *Archives of Neurology, 61*, 490–495.

Silberstein, S. et al. (2004). Randomized placebo-controlled trial of rofecoxib in the acute treatment of migraine. *Neurology, 62*, 1552–1557.

Sjaastad, O. (1997). Cervicogenic headache. *Functional Neurology, 12*(1), 305–317

Sjaastad, O., & Fredriksen, T. A., & Pfaffenrath V. (1998). Cervicogenic headache: Diagnostic criteria. *Headache, 38*, 442–445.

Spierings, E. L. et al. (2001). Oral almotriptan vs. oral sumatriptan in the abortive treatment of migraine. *Archives of Neurology, 58*, 944–950.

Stevens, M. B. (1993). Tension-type headaches. *American Family Physician, 47*, 799–805.

Stewart, W. F., Schecter, A., & Lipton, R.B. (1994). Migraine heterogeneity: disability, pain intensity, and attack frequency and duration. *Neurology, 44*, S24–S29.

Stewart, W. F. et al. (1992). Prevalence of migraine in the United States: Relation to age, income, race, and other sociodemographic factors. *Journal of the American Medical Association, 287*, 64–69.

Stewart, W. F. et al. (2000, February). American Migraine Study II. Diamond Headache Clinic Research and Education Foundation Annual Meeting, Palm Springs, CA.

Takeshima, T., Shimomura, T., & Takahashi, K. (1987). Platelet activation in muscle contraction headache and migraine. *Cephalalgia, 7*, 239–243.

Tekle, H. R. et al. (1995). Migraine, chronic tension-type headache, and cluster headache in an Ethiopian rural community. *Cephalalgia, 15*, 482–488.

Tepper, S. J. et al. (1999). A long-term study to maximize migraine relief with Zomig. *Current Medical Research and Opinion, 15*, 254–271.

Terwindt, G. M. et al. (2000). The impact of migraine on quality of life in the general population: The GEM study. *Neurology, 55*, 624–629.

Tfelt-Hansen, P., Louis, I., & Olesen, J. (1981). Prevalence and significance of muscle tenderness during common migraine attacks. *Headache, 21*, 49–54.

Vankleef, M. et al. (1993). Effects and side effects of a radiofrequency lesion of the dorsal root ganglion in patients with cervical pain syndrome. *Pain, 52*, 49–53.

Venzmer, G. (1972). *Five thousand years of medicine* (p. 19). New York: Taplinger Publishing.

Vernon, H., McDermaid, C., & Hagino, C. (1999). Systematic review of randomized clinical trials of complementary/alternative therapies in the treatment of tension-type and cervicogenic headache. *Journal of Alternative and Complementary Medicine, 7*, 142–155.

Waelkens, J. (1985). Warning symptoms in migraines: characteristic and therapeutic implications. *Cephalalgia, l5*, 223–228.

Welsch, K. M. A. et al. (2001). Tolerability of sumatriptan: clinical trials and post-marketing experience. *Cephalalgia, 21*, 164–165.

Whitty, C. M. W., Hockaday, J. M., & Whitty, M. M. (1966). The effect of oral contraceptives on migraine. *Lancet, 1*, 856.

Wilkinson, M. (1986). Clinical features of migraine. In F. C. Rose (Ed.), *Handbook of clinical neurology: Headache* (Vol. 4, pp. 117–133). Amsterdam: Elsevier.

Wilson, P. (1991). Chronic neck pain and cervicogenic headache. *Clinical Journal of Pain, 7*(1), 5–11.

26

Post-Traumatic Headache: Diagnosis, Pathophysiology, and Treatment

Gary W. Jay, MD, DAAPM

INTRODUCTION

Post-traumatic headache (PTHA) is a poorly understood disorder. There are 2 million traumatic brain injuries (TBI) each year, 500,000 of which are serious enough to need hospitalization (Brown, Fann, & Grant, 1994). Another study indicates that PTHA affects more than 2 million Americans each year (Cady & Farmer, 1998).

Patients with PTHA range from 30 to 80% of patients who have had a mild head injury (Elkind, 1992). Chronic PTHA (see below) is associated with increased headache frequency and disability compared with nontraumatic headache (Marcus, 2003).

The International Classification of Diseases (ICD-10) classification system is based on criteria that primarily concern the temporal relationship as well as pathogenicity between the relationship of PTHA and trauma, and ignore the clinical features of the PTHA (World Health Organization, 1997). These criteria state that the headache onset must occur within 2 weeks of the traumatic event or the patient's return to consciousness. However, post-traumatic cluster headache, for example, typically does not fit this time course. Furthermore, the ICD-10 criteria for acute or chronic PTHA require one of the following: loss of consciousness, a period of antrograde amnesia of at least 10 minutes, or abnormal neurological examination/neurodiagnostic testing. The ICD-10 criteria find that acute PTHA resolves in 8 weeks, while chronic PTHA lasts longer than 8 weeks. This is in counterdistinction to the International Headache Society (IHS) criteria (Headache Classification Committee of the International Headache Society [HCCIHS], 1988).

These criteria are contrary to the most commonly accepted criteria, those of the Brain Injury Special Interest Group of the American Congress of Rehabilitation Medicine (Kay, Harrington et al., 1993), which states that minor traumatic brain injury (MTBI) is a "traumatically induced physiological disruption of brain function" (p. 86) associated with at least one of the following: any period of loss of consciousness; any memory loss for events just before or after the accident; any alteration in mental state at the time of the accident, such as feeling dazed, disoriented, or confused; and focal neurological deficits, which may or may not be transient. Most importantly, there is no necessity of direct head trauma to meet the diagnosis.

Nosological problems abound, such as the synonymous use of various terminology — concussion, minor traumatic brain injury, postconcussion syndrome/disorder, and post-trauma syndrome. For a number of specific reasons, it is felt that the postconcussion syndrome, which affects multiple organ systems, should be differentiated from MTBI (Jay, 2000). Patients with PTHA do not, by definition as well as clinically, have to have a coexisting MTBI.

PTHA may occur alone or as part of the postconcussion syndrome. Post-traumatic headache has been classified by the IHS as associated with head trauma and as acute (resolving within 8 weeks after injury) or chronic (lasting longer than 8 weeks). The IHS divides PTHAs into disorders associated with (1) significant head trauma and/or confirmatory signs or (2) minor head trauma with no confirmatory signs. It states that significant head trauma is defined by loss of consciousness, post-traumatic amnesia lasting longer than 10 minutes, or abnormalities in at least two of the following: neurologic evaluations, skull radiograph, neuroimaging, evoked potentials, spinal fluid evaluation, vestibular functioning, or neuropsychological testing. The IHS has determined that headache must occur less than 14 days after injury or after a patient regains consciousness (HCCIHS, 1988).

There is an inverse relationship between the occurrence of PTHA and the degree of traumatic brain injury. One study found chronic daily PTHA in 80% of patients ($N = 54$) with a MTBI and 11% had no headache. In patients with moderate to severe TBI ($N = 23$), 27% had chronic daily PTHA, 68% had no headache (Couch & Bearss, 2001). A number of other authors also found that PTHA was the most common symptom after MTBI as well as the most common part of the postconcussion syndrome (Martelli, Grayson, & Zasler, 1999; Packard & Ham, 1994; Uomoto & Esselman, 1993).

By some definitions, headache after head trauma can be "postconcussive," if the patient has had a period of unconsciousness, or "post-traumatic," if there was no associated loss of consciousness (LOC). Furthermore, studies note that patients with MTBI who had no LOC developed headaches that were more intractable to treatment (Yagamuchi, 1992).

The trauma inducing PTHA has been noted in one study to be less than half (45%) secondary to motor vehicle accidents, 30% from falls, 20% from accidents at work or play (Jennet & Frankowski, 1990). Typically, the neurological examination is negative, so these patients' complaints are considered inconsequential, unless the patients are in litigation, when other possibly incorrect assumptions about the patients' PTHA may be made.

Post MTBI or "whiplash" headaches are one of neurotraumatology's most prominent problems. One study found of 112 patients who experienced whiplash or an acceleration/deceleration injury, 42 (37%) had post-traumatic tension-type headaches, 30 patients (27%) had post-traumatic migraine headache, 20 patients (18%) had cervicogenic headache, and 20 patients (18%) had headaches that do not fit specific primary headache criterion; 93% of 104 patients had neck pain with their headaches (Radanov, Di Stefano, & Augustiny, 2001).

Another study (Keidel & Diener, 1997) found that whiplash injury and minor head trauma are followed by PTHA in about 90% of patients. PTHA secondary to whiplash injury was noted to be located occipitally in 67% of patients, with dull, pressing, or dragging characteristics in 77%. Post-traumatic tension-type headache was most common and was found in 85% of patients. Of patients with PTHA after minor head trauma or whiplash injury, 80% had remission of their headaches within 6 months. Chronic PTHA lasting at least 4 years was found in 20% of patients.

PTHA has been found to have great variation in both nature and severity. In another study, 78% of 297 patients

had either continuous or intermittent headache secondary to MTBI (Jacobsen, 1963).

A German study found that 80% of patients who had a whiplash injury recovered within a few months, while 15 to 20% developed "late whiplash injury syndrome" with many complaints of the cervico-cephalic syndrome, including PTHA, vertigo, instability, nausea, tinnitus, and hearing loss (Claussen & Claussen, 1995).

As previously noted, many clinicians view PTHA, by definition, as persisting 2 months or longer; this includes the IHS criteria. This may be considered an arbitrary timeframe as the definition of chronic pain is different, being pain persisting for 3 to 6 months. Some studies indicate PTHA patients improve or change over 6 months and then plateau. One felt that 6 months was a better time period for chronicity, as it was more consistent with the chronic pain literature (Packard & Ham, 1993b). Other estimates of persistence for 6 months or more are as high as 44% (Martelli et al., 1999).

PTHAs can be classified as part of the PTHA syndrome, part of the postconcussive syndrome, or by themselves, as an independent medical problem, which may be secondary to an MTBI or whiplash injury or a part of the postconcussive syndrome (Packard, Weaver, & Ham, 1993). If the latter, it may be associated with depression, irritability, decreased memory, fatigue, dizziness, decreased concentration, and tinnitus (Alberti, Sarchielli, Mazzotta, & Gallai, 2001). The postconcussive syndrome is associated with decreased cognitive functioning, impairment of rapid processing of information, decreased attention and short term memory (Elkind, 1992; Jay, 2000).

The pathophysiology of chronic PTHA (CPTHA) has biological, psychological, and sociological aspects. Post-traumatic tension-type headache is the most common form of PTHA, but exacerbation of migraine-like headaches also occurs (Jay, 2000; Solomon, 2001).

It is important to note two aspects of CPTHA with respect to its association with the postconcussive syndrome. First, it is very important to treat the headache problem prior to beginning to treat the cognitive deficits associated with an MTBI. Second, these patients react differently to treatment (Jay, 2000). MTBI patients with PTHA or pain frequently also have attentional deficits as well as psychological distress, both of which can coexist with chronic headache/pain alone. It is therefore important to determine all coexisting diagnoses early on and to factor these problems into the design of treatment for headache and/or pain (Jay, 2000; Uomoto & Esselman, 1993).

It is also important to note that after a structural lesion has been ruled out, treatment of PTHA is very similar to treatment of the primary headaches, vascular and tension-type (Solomon, 2001).

A closed-head injury with brain concussion or contusion is the most frequent type of head injury in children. Headache is a major complaint of early and late postinjury periods. Of 100 children (3 to 14 years of age), 83% had headache after cerebral concussion/contusion: 56% had acute PTHA; 27% had CPTHA, tension-type; 3% had post-traumatic migraine; 21% had headache lasting the entire year of observation (Lemka, 1999).

In another study of children 3.3 to 14.9 years of age (mean 11.2) who were followed for 5 to 29 months (average 12.5), 5 patients had post-traumatic migraine, 13 patients had post-traumatic tension-type headache, and 3 children had mixed headache. Tension-type headache was more common in children with chronic PTHA than those with no history of head injury (Callaghan & Abu Arafeh, 2001).

Sakas, Whittaker, Whitwell, & Singounas (1997) felt that children who experience neurological deterioration after trivial head injury without focal structural abnormalities (i.e., headache, confusion, vomiting, hemiparesis, cortical blindness, and seizures) may have an "unstable trigeminovascular reflex" that is activated by craniofacial trauma. They note that head trauma may be associated with noncongestive cerebral hyperemia. They further propose that head trauma activates the trigeminal nerve endings in the face, scalp, dura, or cortex and, via a reflex, causes vasodilatation and cerebral hyperemia.

Briefly, the basic pathophysiological elements found in an MTBI may include axonal shearing; marked increases in the excitotoxic neurotransmitters including acetylcholine and glutamate; a lack of the cohesiveness of the blood–brain-barrier, which becomes "porous" for 8 to 24 hours or more; and possible changes in the hemodynamics of the brain (Jay, 2000).

The most important aspect to keep in mind is that the "type" of PTHA must be accurately diagnosed so that appropriate treatment can be prescribed.

Typically, PTHA is noted after acceleration/deceleration injuries (whiplash) in up to 90% of patients who experience MTBI (Keidel & Diener, 1997). These headaches can be determined to be post-traumatic tension-type, migraine, cluster, or possibly, cervicogenic. Aside from motor vehicle injuries, PTHAs may be secondary to work related injuries, slip and fall injuries, and violent altercations. These headaches are frequently part of the postconcussive syndrome, which refers to the above noted signs and symptoms that may follow a blow to the head or an acceleration/deceleration injury, but which may or may not induce an MTBI.

Acute post-traumatic tension-type headache, the most frequently diagnosed PTHA (defined as 15 headache days or fewer a month), may last up to 3 to 6 months; after that it becomes "chronic." The IHS has determined that 15 headache days or more a month defines chronic headache (HCCIHS, 1988). General pain management principles place pain as chronic after 3 to 6 months, after physiological healing has occurred. Up to 80% of patients with PTHA will have their pain remit within 6 months, leaving an estimated 20% of patients with chronic PTHA, which may last years in many cases.

A simple concussion may also be associated with PTHA, as well as, in the extremes, vegetative and even psychotic difficulties (Kojadinovic, Momcilovic, Popovic et al.,1998; Muller, 1974).

PTHA may also be associated with dizziness, irritability, and decreased concentration, even without the additional finding of a minor traumatic brain injury. Patients with chronic PTHA frequently present significant difficulties for the typical general practitioner, as well as the neurological specialist. This may be especially true if there is evidence of *de novo* migraine or cluster headache.

Because of the emotional/affective aspects that most frequently accompany PTHA, including depression and anxiety disorders as well as problems with anger, the affective component of PTHA may contribute to the patients' perception of the degree to which their PTHAs are disabling (Duckro, Chibnall, & Tomazic, 1995; Fordyce, Roueche, & Prigatano, 1982). Patients with PTHA may also meet the diagnostic criteria from the DMS-IV for post-traumatic stress disorder and, thus, require additional appropriate treatment (Hickling, Blanchard, Schwartz et al., 1992).

Clinically, it has been noted that patients with PTHA who also have a MTBI may have additional treatment-related problems. It may be difficult to establish the presence of an MTBI via neuropsychological testing as long as the PTHAs persist, as the headache pain generally makes such evaluations more difficult for the patient and may have a true negative effect on the testing itself, making the differential diagnosis more difficult (Duckro et al., 1995; Jay, 2000). Other reports indicate that there is little if any problem with a patient with MTBI performing a neuropsychological evaluation while he or she is having significant PTHA (Lake, Branca, Lutz, & Saper, 1999), but clinically this appears to be quite unrealistic.

Medicolegally, PTHA is a common problem, as the patient does not "look" ill and may have few if any abnormalities on examination. In depositions, or in court, a physician is frequently asked to explain why such a significant problem was found after a relatively minor "rear-end" automobile accident or slip and fall. Why, it is asked, do professional football players, for example, not have a high incidence of PTHA and/or MTBI? The answer is simple, and based on two things — physical conditioning and the fact that when they play, these people are always very prepared and always anticipate the possibility of physical contact or trauma. This differentiates them from the vast majority of people who are not even close to being in optimal physical condition and who are injured unexpectedly, before they are even aware of the impending trauma, and are therefore unable to physically prepare themselves for a trauma by, for example, bracing themselves against the headrest before their car is struck from behind.

A great deal of research has shown that when the head is free, rather than confined, it is more susceptible to the effects of an acceleration/deceleration injury. Six decades ago, it was shown in cats that less force was required to produce concussion when the head was free to move, as compared with when it was fixed or confined in place (Denny-Brown & Russell, 1941). The concept of "whiplash," essentially a legal term, medically known as acceleration/deceleration, is very important, as it involves a multitude of medical aspects. When an acceleration/deceleration injury occurs (most frequently from a rear-end automobile accident), the physical or gravitational forces of a massive object such as a car striking another automobile are passed onto the most fragile and movable object not firmly secured in the automobile that was struck: the passenger. Even when the passenger is wearing a seat belt, the head — the ball at the end of a tether (the neck) — is first thrown forward and then backwards, when the tether can reach no farther and snaps back. If the head is turned at the moment of impact, the rotational forces are also very important, particularly in the etiology of a traumatic brain injury.

PTHA encompasses a number of different diagnostic entities. Specific diagnosis is needed for appropriate treatment. These diagnoses include

Post-traumatic migraine headache
Post-traumatic cluster headache
Post-traumatic tension-type headache
Temperomandibular joint (TMJ) related headache
Neuropathic pain syndromes
Cervicogenic headache

POST-TRAUMATIC MIGRAINE

Trauma may be one of the triggers of migraine, and in some cases it may be the predominant or even the sole precipitating event in the onset of migraine (Solomon, 1998). Trauma may trigger the first attack of migraine in a susceptible patient; biochemical along with epidemiological studies/factors have implicated trauma as the main etiological factor in the onset of new migraine (Solomon, 1998).

Whiplash, with or without MTBI, may decrease an individual's migraine threshold as well as exacerbate an episodic migraine pattern, which was previously under good control (Jennet & Frankowski, 1990).

Post-traumatic migraine, which may begin *de novo*, without a previous personal or family history of migraine, may have neurochemical similarities with MTBI, although they are not always found together. These may include increased extracellular potassium and intracellular sodium, calcium, and chloride; serotonergic changes;

decreases in magnesium; excessive release of excitatory amino acids; changes in catecholamine and endogenous opioid tonus; decreased glucose utilization; changes in neuropeptides and abnormalities in nitric oxide formation and function (Jay, 1999; Packard & Ham, 1997). Packard & Ham (1997) hypothesized that the presence of similar changes suggested PTHA associated with MTBI and migraine may share a common headache pathway.

Migraine, including post-traumatic migraine, may be associated with a number of neurological symptoms or phenomena. These may include transient global amnesia, vestibular dysfunction, visual and auditory changes, and possibly, an increased incidence of seizures (Buchholz & Reich, 1996; Jay, 1999; Leisman, 1990).

The trigeminovascular system is of great import in migraine (Jay, 1999). In some children who develop post-traumatic neurological deterioration without focal lesions after minor head trauma, there may be an association with an "unstable trigeminovascular reflex," which induces the release of perivascular vasodilatory peptides that can contribute to cerebral hyperemia (Sakas et al., 1997).

Transient global amnesia (TGA) was initially attributed to bilateral temporal lobe seizure phenomena, but more recently it has been attributed to migraine by some (Jay, 1999), and thought to be a totally separate disorder by others, possibly due to a different form of paroxysmal disorder in the brainstem (Schmidtke & Ehmsen, 1998). TGA in the pediatric population is still felt to be secondary to ischemia of the temporobasal structures induced by an MTBI and associated with a migrainous diathesis (Vohanka & Zouhar, 1988).

PTHA, including migraine, is commonly associated with children, adolescents, and teens who play football and frequently goes unreported (Sallis & Jones, 2000). Any degree of postconcussion headache in high school athletes a week postinjury is likely associated with an incomplete recovery postconcussion (Collins, Field, Iverson et al., 2003).

Caution is needed when returning high school athletes to the playing field after a concussion. On-field mental status changes appear to have some prognostic utility and should be taken into account when making return-to-play decisions after concussion. Athletes who show on-field mental status changes for more than 5 minutes have longer-lasting postconcussion symptoms and memory decline (Lovell, Collins, Iverson et al., 2003).

"Roller coaster" migraine is also seen, following many short but fairly significant brain insults delivered during a roller coaster ride, and may be an important factor in triggering a patient's post-traumatic migraine headache (McBeath & Nanda, 2000).

Migraine equivalents, transient neurological symptomatology not associated with headache, are not uncommon; proper diagnosis is more difficult to the generalist, as well as the neurologist. In some, possibly more susceptible individuals, minor, even trivial, head trauma can induce a migraine equivalent known as "footballer's migraine" as well as "post-traumatic cortical blindness." This particular migraine equivalent is certainly rare, but transient total blindness may certainly be cause to call for a total, "full court press" workup (Harrison & Walls, 1990).

Other, more common forms of transient neurological disturbances associated with migraine are brainstem symptoms including vestibular difficulties, such as dizziness, disequilibrium, vertigo, and motion intolerance. These symptoms may also present as a migraine equivalent, between migraine headache episodes or instead of the cephalic pain. Vertigo as a migraine equivalent may occur in about 25% of patients with migraine, with the diagnosis made, typically, by history of familial migraine, as all testing is usually negative. Migraine can also mimic Meniere's disease, with "vestibular Meniere's disease" more frequently, but still not commonly, associated with migraine (Baloh, 1997; Harker & Rassekh, 1988). Also, one should not forget the cervical causes of vertigo and dizziness, secondary to post-traumatic cervical and/or myofascial pathophysiology.

There is also a question of the possible relationship between post-traumatic migraine and post-traumatic benign encephalopathy. The latter, in children, may be associated with cortical blindness, brainstem disturbances, and seizure, lasting from 5 minutes to 48 hours (Vohanka & Zouhar, 1990).

A significant question then arises. Post-traumatic vertigo or dizziness is a very frequent accompaniment to MTBI. It may be secondary to peripheral, labyrinthine disturbance, brainstem disturbance secondary to trauma, or it may be a migraine equivalent. The importance of this differential is most significant, possibly, when treatment is attempted.

As noted, trauma may induce the first migraine attack in a possibly susceptible patient or increase the frequency and possibly the severity of preexisting migraine. The etiology of these changes may be secondary to neuronal and/or axonal abnormalities secondary to trauma as well as post-traumatic involvement of the trigeminovascular system.

Prophylactic treatment is typically with valproic acid, an anticonvulsant medication. The use of beta-blockers such as propranolol may also be useful, but this may have significant side effects. The same is true for verapamil. The use of a triptan for abortive care is well tolerated if used appropriately.

Cluster headache has also been seen secondary to head trauma, again possibly secondary to neuronal and/or axonal injury. The incidence ranges from 6 to 10% (Duckro, Greenberg, Schultz et al., 1992; Packard & Ham, 1997). Many times, this is seen as a primary chronic, rather than episodic, form of cluster or cluster-like headache. Clinically, this is one of the rarest forms of PTHA seen.

Treatment, abortive or prophylactic, has been dealt with elsewhere (Jay, 1999).

POST-TRAUMATIC TENSION-TYPE HEADACHE

Post-traumatic tension-type headache (PTTHA; with or without secondary analgesic rebound headache) is probably the most common primary headache disorder found after trauma. Diagnostically, and clinically, this entity appears to be almost if not totally identical to acute and chronic tension-type headache without a traumatic etiology.

The diagnostic criteria of tension-type headache, according to the IHS (HCCIHS, 1988) describes episodic tension-type headache as being recurrent headache occurring fewer than 15 days a month, lasting from 30 minutes to 7 days. The pain characteristics include two of four of the following: pain with a pressing/tightening (nonpulsating) quality; pain that is mild to moderate in intensity and may inhibit, but not prohibit, activities; pain that is always bilateral; and pain that is not aggravated by walking stairs or doing other routine physical activity. These criteria also state that both of the following are true: no nausea or vomiting, but anorexia may occur, and photophobia and phonophobia are absent, or one but not the other is present. All other organic diagnoses must be ruled out first, as well as other primary headache diagnoses, including migraine and cluster headache.

In PTTHA, like non-post-traumatic tension-type headache, the pain is typically described as aching or pressure like, "like there's a vice around my head." The pain has also been described as feeling like a tight band around the head. The pain is typically bilateral, although it may be unilateral. It may include various areas, some or all of the following: occipito-nuchal, bifrontal, bitemporal, suboccipital, at the vertex (crown) of the head; the pain may also extend into the neck and shoulders.

The pain intensity may wax and wane depending on a number of factors including movement, activity level, stress, and others. Even in PTTHA, emotional/psychological aspects may increase pain. There is a female preponderance.

Unlike patients with migraine headache, patients with PTTHA may carry on with their activities. Most take some form of analgesic, frequently on a daily basis. Without question, patients with PTTHA may also have migraine, post-traumatic or otherwise.

The patient with chronic PTTHA has headache 15 or more days a month. This is also a diagnostic exercise, as most frequently, nosologically, PTTHA may be one of several headache diagnoses all of which are part of a chronic daily headache differential, which would include analgesic rebound headache, at a minimum.

The patient with PTTHA frequently has headache daily or every other day. The headache is typically there when patients awaken and remains until they go to sleep.

The intensity of the pain varies, decreasing for several hours after analgesics are taken.

The majority of patients with PTTHA, if seen early on, will have associated pericranial muscle spasm or pain, while others will not, yet still complain of pain.

Patients with PTTHA will also endure elements of depression and anxiety. There is a "chicken and egg" aspect to this, in terms of which problem comes first. In many cases, central neurochemical changes begin concurrently with the injury and manifest as both pain and affective disturbances (see below).

Nosologically, post-traumatic headache is incident to trauma. Some problems may be noted in making this diagnosis: the patient may not experience direct trauma to the head, but have an acceleration/deceleration injury (whiplash); there may not be significant physical findings on examination (conversely, there may be physical findings that are missed unless a good musculoskeletal examination is done); secondary to the lack of profound physical findings, the patient may be labeled with a psychogenic diagnosis, or worse, with the term *malingering*.

When one understands the pathophysiology of the problem, specifically PTTHA, it should be understood that the history and physical examination must be done quite specifically, not with "one size fits all diagnoses." Knowing what questions to ask and what, on occasion, can be fairly subtle physical findings to look for on examination are obviously important.

PATHOPHYSIOLOGY OF PTTHA

The typical PTTHA begins post-acceleration/deceleration injury, which most frequently occurs during a motor vehicle accident. A slip and fall accident as well as a sports-related injury or a violent altercation can be the initiating event.

As described above, the head and the neck, likened to a ball on a chain, is flung forward and backward from acceleration/deceleration forces, frequently without direct trauma to the head, or following direct trauma to the head. However it occurs, the physical forces involved will cause the cervical and shoulder musculature, at a minimum, to be suddenly stretched and sustain both microtears and strain/trauma as well as endure a reflex muscle contraction after the sudden stretching. It is obviously important to understand the myofascial pain syndrome.

Pathological changes in the musculoskeletal system may initiate, modulate, or perpetuate PTTHA. Episodic and chronic PTTHA are, at least at first, secondary to a muscle-induced pain syndrome that is typically associated with the aforementioned myofascial pain syndrome (MPS).

The central nervous system controls muscle tone via systems that influence the gamma efferent neurons in the anterior horn cells of the spinal cord, which act on the alpha motor neurons supplying muscle spindles. The Renshaw cells, apparently via the inhibitory neurotransmitter gamma aminobutyric acid (GABA), will influence this synaptic system. There is also supraspinal control from cortical, subcortical, and limbic afferent and efferent systems. Physiological and emotional inputs interact in the maintenance or flux of muscle tone. Adverse influences from both localized or regional myofascial nociception, with or without limbic (affective) stimulation, may produce significant muscle spasm, which, if prolonged, will become tonic with the additional aspects of increased anxiety or a maintained muscle contraction-pain cycle (Diamond & Dalessio, 1980; Speed, 1983). This helps to differentiate acute versus chronic PTTHA, to a degree.

Tonic or continued post-traumatic muscle contraction may induce hypoxia via compression of small blood vessels. Ischemia, the accumulation of pain-producing metabolites (bradykinin, lactic acid, serotonin, prostaglandins, etc.), may increase and potentiate muscle pain and reactive spasm. These nociception-enhancing or algetic chemicals may stimulate central mechanisms that through continued stimulation, may induce continued reactive muscle spasm/contraction and maintenance of the myogenic nociceptive cycle (Dorpat & Holmes, 1955; Hong, Kniffki, & Schmidt, 1978; Perl, Markle, & Katz, 1934).

Changes in peripheral blood flow in muscle seen in patients with chronic tension-type headache appear to be secondary to disturbances in the regulation of peripheral mechanisms due to central sensitization. Muscle pain in tension-type headache may be secondary to microtrauma of muscle fibers and tendonous insertions, accentuated by the accumulation of algetic metabolites: serotonin, bradykinin, and potassium ions effectively stimulate skeletal muscle nociceptors (Mense, 1993). When combinations of endogenous substances (serotonin, bradykinin, prostaglandin E_2, histamine) were slowly infused into the trapezius muscles of patients with episodic tension-type headache, they developed significantly more pain and muscle tenderness than healthy controls (Mork, Ashina, Bendtsen et al., 2003).

Although PTHA may include migraine, some of Moskowitz and Cutrer's work (1993) may be pertinent here. They have shown that when stimulated antidromically, the trigeminal nerve can release vasoactive/algetic peptides such as substance P, neurokinin A, bradykinin, neuropeptides Y, vasoactive intestinal peptide, and calcitonin-gene-related peptide from its afferent nerves, which innervate vascular structures. This can initiate a sterile inflammation that will lower the pain threshold, causing exacerbations in pain from typically benign behavior such as movement of the head. (This is *not* allodynia.) It is conceivable that such a disruption of the trigeminal system may possibly help determine neurogenic pain in some patients who may be susceptible to migraine and who develop PTHA.

As discussed below, the myofascial aspects of tension-type headache are clinically identical to those of PTTHA, with the significant difference in diagnoses being the etiology — post-traumatic or otherwise.

The MPS was, for a long while, ignored in the pathophysiology of headache of any type. Some researchers found a causal relationship between muscle spasm and headache (Martin & Mathews, 1978; Rodbard, 1970; Sakuta, 1990), while others have felt that muscle spasm associated with headache is an epiphenomenona, not the etiology of headache (Haynes, Cuevas, & Gannon, 1982; Philips, 1978; Philips & Hunter, 1982; Riley, 1983; Robinson, 1980; Simons, Day, Goodell, & Wolff, 1943), but a reflexive response. Other authors have indicated that muscle activity/spasm or increased tone may be more pronounced in migraine than in tension-type headaches (Bakal & Kaganov, 1977; Cohen, 1978).

Unfortunately, this research, which was obtained via electromyographic (EMG) studies, appears to be problematic, as the various authors evaluated different groups of muscles in different types of patients, many of whom had poorly defined diagnoses (Anderson & Franks, 1981; Bakal & Kaganov, 1977; Martin & Mathews, 1978; Pozniak-Patewicz, 1976). Other authors defined chronic tension-type headache as an entity with or without associated pericranial muscle disorder. The concept of muscle fatigue was not taken into consideration; metabolically spent muscles may become relatively flaccid, losing aspects of increased tonus or spasm.

Also of interest is the fact that the vast majority of research deals with tension-type headache, not PTTHA; in spite of identical physical/clinical findings as well as historical findings, all are essentially the same, except for the presence of initiating trauma.

One study found a positive correlation between pericranial muscle tenderness and headache intensity, with the former felt to be a source of nociception (Langemark & Olesen, 1987; Shoenen, Pasqua, & Sianard-Gainko, 1991). Another study (Langemark, Jensen, Jensen, & Olesen, 1989) found that pressure pain thresholds in patients with chronic tension-type headache were highly dependent on myofascial factors. This study indicated that the generally lower pain thresholds in patients with chronic tension-type headache suggested a dysmodulation of central nociception. A lower pain threshold in patients with chronic tension-type headache, when compared with normal volunteers, was also noted (Bendtsen, Jensen, & Olesen, 1996a; Borgeat, Hade, Elie, & Larouche, 1984). Findings of decreased pressure pain and tolerance thresholds indicate the presence of allodynia (pain elicited by non-painful stimuli) and hyperalgesia (increased sensitivity to painful stimuli), in patients with chronic tension-type headache. That patients with chronic tension-type headache are hypersensitive to different types of stimuli applied at both cephalic and extracephalic regions would

indicate that the pain sensitivity in the central nervous system is increased in the supraspinal regions.

Scalp muscle tenderness and sensitivity to pain in both patients with migraine and patients with tension-type headache were measured in another study, and the author indicated that the pathophysiology of tension-type headache may involve a diffuse disruption of central pain-modulating mechanism (Drummond, 1987). Lower pain thresholds were also found in patients diagnosed with myofascial pain syndromes, including lower back pain (Malow, Grimm, & Olsen, 1980; Yang, Richlin, Brand, Wagner, & Clark, 1985).

It should be noted that the diagnoses in the majority of research papers include tension-type headache (TTHA), but whether they were associated with trauma is typically not indicated.

Both patients with PTTHA and with chronic tension-type headache frequently have a stereotypic posture, with their shoulders raised and their heads flexed forward. This tightly held posture, or muscular splinting, is effective in preventing unconscious head movement that may induce pain. The continued splinting, by maintaining tonic muscle contraction, also works to increase myogenic nociception and perpetuate this cycle.

The pericranial muscles are innervated by sensory fibers in nerves from the second or third cervical roots and in the trigeminal nerve (Langemark & Jensen, 1988). The functions of these muscles contribute to the maintenance of posture and the stabilization of the head, as well as withdrawal and protection of the head. These factors contribute to the myofascial aspects of both TTHA and PTTHA.

Muscle fatigue occurs, both metabolic and neurochemical in nature, and typically follows prolonged or tonic muscle spasm. It may be secondary to "sympatheticopenia" or the depletion of epinephrine and norepinephrine (NEP), the peripheral sympathetic transmitters (Cailliet, 1993). The muscle spindle is directly affected by the sympathetic nervous system via these neurotransmitters, particularly NEP. Prolonged and sustained peripheral sympathetic activity may lead to depletion of NEP at the synaptic receptors. Continued afferent sympathetic input from myogenic nociception, at least in part from buildup through ischemia of nociceptive metabolites, may result in sympatheticopenia (Cailliet, 1993; Jay, 1996). There are also significant sympathetic aspects of myofascial pain (Jay, 1995b).

The sympathetic nervous system also interacts with the trigeminal system and may act as an activating entity. Sympathetic fibers from the stellate ganglia innervate the cranial and cervical structures. These fibers extend rostrally and form a large nerve plexus behind the origin of the vertebral artery and superiorly, with the cervical ganglia lying on the capitus longus muscle behind the carotid sheath at the base of the skull. Sympathetic fibers supply the carotid, basilar, and cerebellar circulatory vessels. Sympathetic fibers in the carotid sheath interconnect with the caudate nucleus of the trigeminal nerve, providing interactions between the two systems (Shealy, 1995). Autonomic fibers surrounding the carotid do appear to be involved in the induction of significant pain in patients with cluster headache (Jay, 2001).

Tenderness of the cervical, thoracic, and lumbar paravertebral muscles is also positively correlated with pericranial muscle tenderness (Langemark, Olesen, Poulsen, & Bech, 1988). It has also been noted that the contraction of shoulder and cervical muscles as well as emotional arousal contributes to tension-type headache (Murphy & Lehrer, 1990). These issues are significant factors in PTTHA.

Three mechanisms of muscle pain are thought to be relevant to acute, but more often chronic, tension-type headache, which has the same physiological stigmata of PTTHA, in that myogenic nociception may be induced by (1) low-grade inflammation associated with the release of algetic, or pain-inducing substances, rather than signs of acute inflammation; (2) short- or long-lasting relative ischemia; and (3) tearing of ligaments and tendons secondary to abnormal sustained muscle tension (Langemark & Jensen, 1988). These factors do not take into consideration the possibly more significant initial trauma from acceleration/deceleration injuries, slip and fall accidents, and other reasons for direct or indirect head trauma that induces muscle trauma, primarily or secondarily.

Increased myofascial pain sensitivity in tension-type headache may be secondary to activation or sensitization of peripheral nociceptors, most probably from a combination of mechanisms.

Myofascial Pain Syndrome

Travell and Rinzler (1952) identified the contribution of musculoskeletal factors in the etiology of acute and chronic tension-type headache. They demonstrated that there are consistent patterns of referred pain from trigger points within specific muscle and defined perpetuating factors that convert acute myofascial pain into a chronic pain syndrome (Travell & Simons, 1983).

The myofascial pain syndrome is a localized or regional pain problem associated with small zones of hypersensitivity within skeletal muscle called trigger points. With palpation of these points, pain is referred to adjacent or even distant sites. Trigger points in the head, neck, and upper back may elicit headache, as well as tinnitus, vertigo, and lacrimation, all features noted in patients with PTTHA as well as chronic tension-type headache (Jay, 1995a; see Figure 26.1 through Figure 26.8).

Trigger points may be active, with consistently reproducible pain on palpation, or latent, with no clinically associated complaints of pain, but with associated muscle dysfunction. Trigger points may shift between active and latent states. Clinically, continuous myogenic nociception from active trigger points appears to be a prime instigator of the central

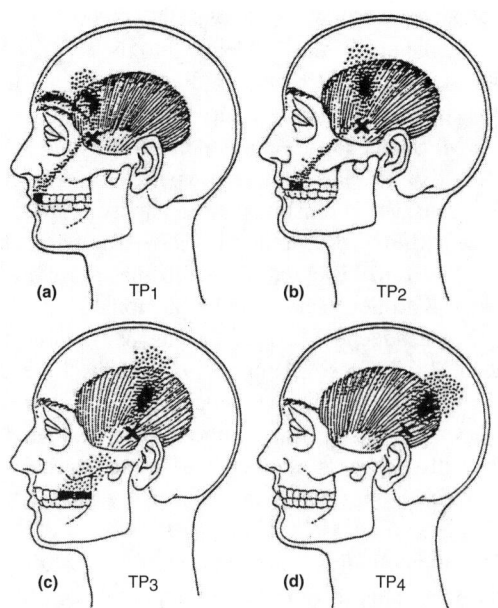

FIGURE 26.1 Referred pain patterns from trigger points in the left temporalis muscle. Dark areas show essential zones; spillover zones are stippled. (a) Anterior "spokes" of pain arising form the anterior fibers, trigger point 1 region. (b) and (c) Middle spokes, trigger point 2 and 3 regions. (d) Posterior supra-auricular spoke, trigger point 4 region. From Jay, G. W., 1995a. In *Treating the Headache Patient* (pp. 211–233), R. K. Cady & A. W. Fox (Eds.). New York: Marcel Decker. Reprinted with permission.

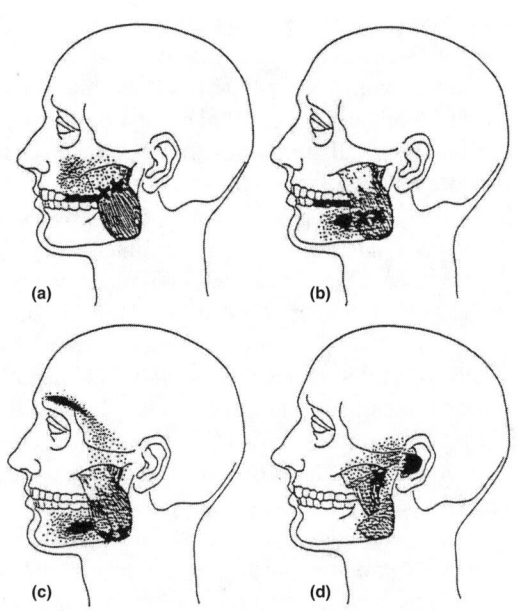

FIGURE 26.2 Each (x) indicates a trigger point in various parts of the masseter muscle. Dark areas show essential zones; spillover zones are stippled. (a) Superficial layer, upper portion. (b) Superficial layer, mid-belly. (c) Superficial layer, lower portion. (d) Deep layer, upper part, just below the temporomandibular joint. From Jay, G. W., 1995a. In *Treating the Headache Patient* (pp. 211–233), R. K. Cady & A. W. Fox (Eds.). New York: Marcel Decker. Reprinted with permission.

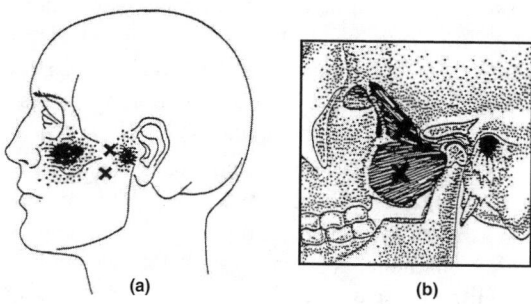

FIGURE 26.3 Referred pain pattern (a) of trigger points (x) in the left lateral psterygoid muscle (b). From Jay, G. W. 1995a. In *Treating the Headache Patient* (pp. 211–233), R. K. Cady & A. W. Fox (Eds.). New York: Marcel Decker. Reprinted with permission.

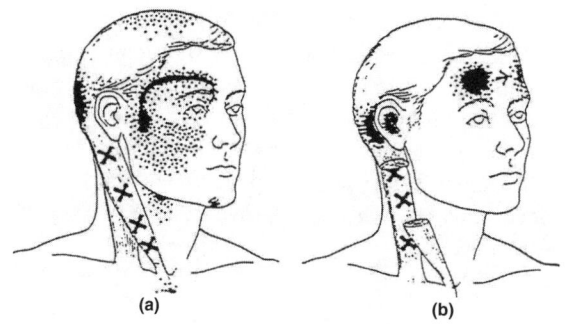

FIGURE 26.4 Referred pain patterns with location of corresponding trigger points (x) in the right sternocleidomastoid muscle. Dark areas show essential zones; spillover zones are stippled. (a) The sternal (superficial) division; (b) the clavicular (deep) division. From Jay, G. W. 1995a. In *Treating the Headache Patient* (pp. 211–233), R. K. Cady & A. W. Fox (Eds.). New York: Marcel Decker. Reprinted with permission.

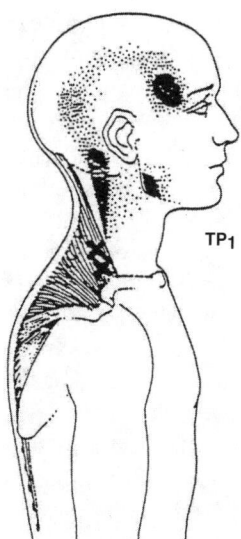

FIGURE 26.5 Referred pain pattern and location of trigger point (x) in theupper trapezius muscle. Dark areas show essential zones; spillover zones are stippled. From Jay, G. W. 1995a. In *Treating the Headache Patient* (pp. 211–233), R. K. Cady & A. W. Fox (Eds.). New York: Marcel Decker. Reprinted with permission.

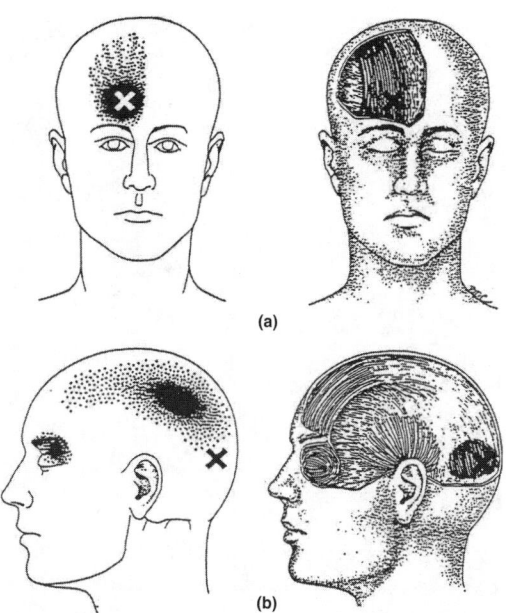

FIGURE 26.6 Pain patterns (shaded areas) referred from trigger point (x) in the occipitofrontalis muscle, commonly associated with unilateral, supraorbital, or ocular headache. (a) Right frontalis belly; (b) left occipitalis belly. From Jay, G. W. 1995a. In *Treating the Headache Patient* (pp. 211–233), R. K. Cady & A. W. Fox (Eds.). New York: Marcel Decker. Reprinted with permission.

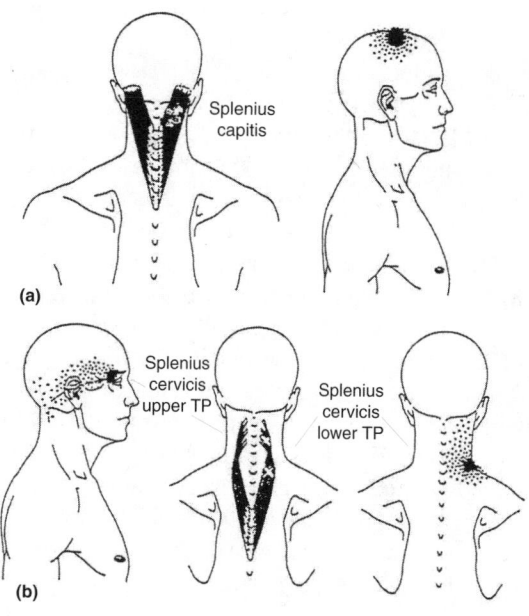

FIGURE 26.7 Trigger points (x) and referred pain patterns (shaded areas) for the right splenius capitis and splenius cervicis muscles. (a) Splenius capitis trigger point that overlies the occipital triangle; (b) left, the upper splenius cervicis trigger point (TP) refers pain to the orbit. The dashed arrow represents pain shooting from the inside of the head to the back or pain shooting from the inside of the head to the back of the eye. Right, another site of pain referral. From Jay, G. W. 1994. In *Treating the Headache Patient* (pp. 211–233), R. K. Cady & A. W. Fox (Eds.). New York: Marcel Decker. Reprinted with permission.

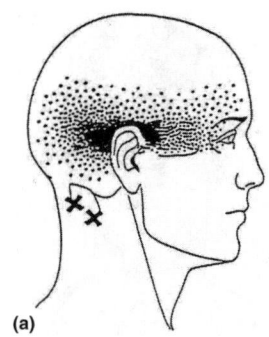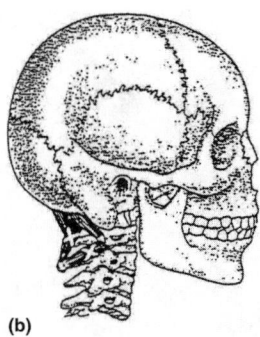

(a)   (b)

FIGURE 26.8 Referred pain pattern (shaded area) of trigger points (x) in the right suboccipital muscles (b). From Jay, G. W. 1995a. In *Treating the Headache Patient* (pp. 211–233), R. K. Cady & A. W. Fox (Eds.). New York: Marcel Decker. Reprinted with permission.

neurochemical nociceptive dysmodulation found in patients with chronic tension-type headache as well as PTTHA.

Increased stiffness, weakness, and fatigue as well as a decreased range of motion are typically found in muscles in which trigger points are identified. These muscles may be shortened, with increased pain perceived on stretching. Patients may protect these muscles by adapting poor posture with sustained contraction, as noted above (Fricton, 1990; Langemark & Jesnen, 1988). The resulting muscular restrictions may perpetuate existing trigger points and aid in the development of others.

Other authors (Fricton, Kroening, Haley, & Siegart, 1985) found that a large percentage of patients suffering from an MPS of the head and neck were found to have significant postural problems, with forward head tilt and rounded shoulders, as well as poor standing and sitting postures, all findings frequently seen in both patients with chronic tension-type headache as well as those with PTTHA.

MPS of the head and neck, via myofascial trigger point referred pain, may mimic other conditions, including migraine headache, TMJ dysfunction, sinusitis, and cervical neuralgias, as well as various otological problems including tinnitus, ear pain, and dizziness (Fricton, 1990).

The onset of an acute, single-muscle MPS may be associated with trauma, such as an acceleration/deceleration injury, a slip and fall, or even a direct blow. It may also come on insidiously, for example, in patients who work multiple hours typing or at the computer.

The MPS may show a spontaneous regression to a latent status, with continued muscular dysfunction, but with significant diminution of the initial pain complaints. In other patients, the MPS may "metastasize" and involve associated musculature, becoming regional, or even involving multiple muscular regions.

OTHER CLINICAL ASPECTS

After the onset of chronic PTTHA (CPTTHA), emotional/psychological factors including stress, anxiety, and depression may become important in the maintenance or perpetuation of the headache. This is frequently seen in the patients with the postconcussive syndrome. Patients with MTBI have other significant emotional stigmas that contribute to this headache diathesis.

A major difficulty in the literature is that determinations of depression, anxiety, and other affective components to the PTTHA are found to occur in patients with CPTTHA. Without premorbid psychological analyses, it is very difficult to state with any certainty whether these patients were depressed or anxious prior to the onset of their headache problems. It is therefore possible that the neurochemical changes associated with CPTTHA, such as probable central serotonergic dysfunction, initiate depression as a response to these pain-induced neurochemical changes (see below).

Some authors have noted that the "conversion V" found in the hypochondriasis, depression, and hysteria scales of the Minnesota Multiphasic Personality Inventory is a marker for chronic TTHA as well as PTTHA; however, similar responses are found in patients with chronic non-headache pain (Jay, Grove, & Grove, 1987; Kudrow, 1986; Martin & Rome, 1967).

ASSOCIATED SLEEP DISORDERS

There appears to be an important relationship among sleep, headache, and the muscle-pain syndromes. Central biogenic amines, particularly serotonin and norepinephrine, are important to sleep physiology as well as to the central pain-modulating systems. Both human and animal research indicates that central serotonin metabolism plays a role in pain modulation, affective states, and the regulation of non-REM (rapid eye movement) sleep (Goldenberg, 1990).

A high incidence of sleep difficulties has been found in patients with chronic tension-type headache (Mathew, Glaze, & Frost, 1985). Different sleep disorders appear to be associated with different headache entities. CTTHA and CPTTHA appear to be similar if not identical. Migraine has been found to occur in association with REM sleep, as well as have an association with excessive stage 3, 4, and REM sleep (Shahota & Dexter, 1990). Chronic TTHA has been found to be associated with frequent awakenings and decreased slow wave sleep, as well as an alpha-wave intrusion into stage 4 sleep (Drake, Pakalnis, Andrews, & Bogner, 1990).

Moldofsky, Scariabrick, England et al. (1975) noted a disturbance in stage 4 sleep to be the first laboratory-based abnormality found in fibromyalgia. They induced a similar alpha non-REM pattern of alpha-wave intrusion in delta (stage 4) sleep in normal subjects by stage 4 sleep deprivation. These subjects developed musculoskeletal pain and affective changes comparable with those seen in patients with fibromyalgia. Small doses of serotonergic tricyclic antidepressant medications, which reduced the alpha intrusions into stage 4 sleep, were used to ameliorate the symptoms.

Alpha-wave intrusions into deep sleep have also been found in patients with other chronic pain syndromes, including rheumatoid arthritis (Goldenberg, 1989). The alpha non-REM disturbance has also been seen in asymptomatic people as well as in those who experience severe emotional stress, such as combat veterans (Goldenberg, 1990). In the latter group, the veterans with this sleep disorder also complained of chronic headaches, diffuse pain, and emotional distress.

Sleep disturbance is also associated with increased pain severity. As noted above, patients with chronic headache seem to have a higher incidence of sleep abnormalities than do normal, pain-free subjects. Etiological aspects of chronic headache may be linked to sleep abnormalities as an initiating event or as the result of the underlying pathologically dysmodulated neurochemical factors inducing a sleep disorder.

OTHER POSSIBLE ASSOCIATED FACTORS

There are several possible mechanical etiologies of chronic PTTHA. First is cervical spondylosis, which is defined as a degenerative disease affecting intervertebral discs and apophyseal joints of the cervical spine. While several authors indicate a possible correlation between cervical spondylosis and TTHA and PTTHA (Harrison & Walls, 1990; Jay, 1999; Packard & Ham, 1997), others conclude the contrary (Iansek, Heywood, Karnaghan, & Nalla, 1987), suggesting that the basis of existing headache is secondary to muscle contraction and/or central neurochemical dysmodulation.

Cervicogenic headache, from referred pain perceived in any region of the head that was referred by a primary source in the musculoskeletal tissues innervated by cervical nerves, is a second suggestive diagnosis. It is discussed in detail below.

Last, the dental literature has been most active in reporting a possible correlation between TMJ dysfunction and tension-type headache, including PTTHA (Forsell, 1985; Mikail & Rosen, 1980). The relationship appears to be dependent mainly on tenderness of the masticatory muscles, which may have other etiologies and induce TMJ dysfunction, when it exists, on a secondary basis (Magnusson & Carlsson, 1978a, 1978b; Philips & Hunter, 1982). Clinically, in the presence of direct trauma to the TMJ, the incidence of anatomical dysfunction is increased.

NEUROPHYSIOLOGICAL CHANGES

Fewer than 50% of patients with PTTHA complain of mild associated autonomic symptoms such as lack of appetite, hyperirritability, dizziness, and increased light sensitivity (photophobia) (Olesen, 1988). Notably, some of these symptoms may be secondary to autonomic changes associated with active myofascial trigger points located in the head and neck.

While muscle contraction and tenderness may be interpreted as primary symptoms of PTTHA, EMG activity, and muscle tenderness increase, in some studies more often during migraine than tension-type headache (Cohen, 1978; Olesen, 1978; Tfelt-Hansen, Lous, & Olesen, 1981).

In research comparing patients with TTHA with patients with common migraine exposed to auditory stimulation, patients with TTHA showed a lower heart-rate reactivity than patients with migraine (Ellertsen, Norby, & Sjaastad, 1987). It was shown that patients with TTHA exhibited the greatest cardiovascular arousal during headache (Haynes, 1981). In another study (Bakal and Kaganov, 1977), both patients with migraine and patients with TTHA had decreased pulse velocity. In a psychophysiological comparison of migraine and tension-type headache, it was found that patients with migraine are vasodilated and patients with TTHA are vasoconstricted both during and between headache episodes (Cohen, 1978). During another study, administration of ergotamine tartrate, a vasoconstrictor, increased the pain of tension-type headache, while amyl nitrate, a vasodilator, yielded only transient pain relief (Tunis & Wolff, 1954).

Greater sympathetic arousal was found in patients with tension-type headache as compared with controls (Murphy & Lehrer, 1990). Another study reported both patients with TTHA and patients with migraine demonstrated cardiovascular sympathetic hypofunction, indicated by low basal levels of NEP, as well as orthostatic hypotension (Mikamo, Takeshima, & Takahashi, 1989). It has been suggested that patients with TTHA have phasic hypersympathetic activity, while migraineurs do not differ from controls during psychogalvanic response testing (Covelli & Ferrannini, 1987).

Evidence of pupillary sympathetic hypofunction and subtle anisocoria has been found in both patients with tension-type headache and patients with migraine (Takeshima, Takao, & Takahaishi, 1987). It was suggested that this may have reflected a central bioaminergic system dysfunction. Another study suggested a pupillary sympathetic system imbalance in patients with CTTHA, who showed asymmetric mydriasis after tyramine instillation and in the physiologic pupillary tests (Shimomura & Takahashi, 1986). Oculomotor dysfunction in the amplitude and number of corrective saccades during testing of patients with TTHA has also been found (Rosenhall, Johansson, & Orndahl, 1987).

The oculocephalic sympathetic functions were evaluated in five patients with PTHA (Khurana, 1995). Thermoregulatory sweat testing and biochemical papillary responses were evaluated. Four patients who had experienced a "whiplash" injury were found to have bilateral sympathetic dysfunction, while one patient who had trauma to the forehead had unilateral sympathetic dysfunction. The biochemical papillary responses were diagnostic soon after the initial post-traumatic injury, while the thermoregulatory sweat test was found to be abnormal up to 56 months postinjury. The author also noted that the oculocephalic sympathetic dysfunction may induce head pain by an effect on cephalic pain via its effects on the trigeminovascular system.

Drummond (1986) has reported increased photophobia in patients with TTHA as compared with controls. He hypothesized that changes in central neurotransmitter modulation may induce increased sensitivity or hyperexcitability-induced photophobia.

Episodic platelet abnormalities with associated serotonergic dysfunction have been well documented in migraine (D'Andrea, Toldeo, Cortelazzo, & Milone, 1982; Hanington, Jones, Amess, & Wachowicz, 1981). Nonepisodic decreased platelet serotonin in patients with chronic tension-type headache has also been documented (Rolf, Wiele, & Brune, 1981).

Patients with PTHA have been found to have decreased regional cerebral blood flow, with regional and hemispheric asymmetries, which supports an organic etiology for chronic PTHA (Gilkey, Ramadan, Aurora, & Welch, 1997).

The P300 event-related potential was found to be useful in evaluating cognitive problems in patients with the postconcussive syndrome with associated PTHA. Abnormal P300 latency was found to be associated with decrements in cognition, in spite of the lack of detectable lesions found on neuroimaging, indicating that functional impairment of specific cerebral areas can occur in patients with associated PTHA, cognitive deficits, and abnormal P300 latencies only (Alberti et al., 2001).

Another group looked at the changes in auditory evoked potentials in patients with postconcussive syndrome that included PTHA. Consistent abnormalities were noted which could reflect post-traumatic disturbances in the presumed subcortical middle latency auditory evoked potential generators, or in the frontal or temporal cortical structures that would modulate them (Drake, Weate, & Newell, 1996).

Brainstem-mediated antinociceptive inhibitory reflexes of the temporalis muscles, using the latencies and durations of the early and late exteroceptive suppression (ES1 and ES2), were evaluated. Abnormalities of the trigeminal inhibitory temporalis reflex was felt to be based on a transient dysfunction of the brainstem-mediated reflex circuit specifically of the late polysynaptic pathways, with the reflex abnormalities considered to be correlates of the post-traumatic cervico-cephalic pain syndrome, which pointed to alterations in central pain control in patients with acute PTHA secondary to whiplash injury (Keidel, Rieschke, Juptner, & Diener, 1994; Keidel, Rieschke, Stude et al., 2001).

Again, it must be reiterated that the single differentiating aspect between chronic TTHA and chronic PTTHA is the historical factor of some form of trauma. Findings on examination and treatment techniques and methodology are the same, with the same outcomes in both entities, if done appropriately. The research noted above does not differentiate patients with TTHA from those with PTTHA. Clinically and diagnostically there are few, if any, differences.

NEUROANATOMY AND NEUROCHEMISTRY

The central modulation of pain appears to originate in the brainstem and involves at least two systems. The "descending" inhibitory analgesia system appears to regulate the "gating" mechanisms of the spinal cord. This system includes the midbrain periaquaductal gray region, the medial medullary raphe nuclei, and the adjacent reticular formation, as well as dorsal horn neurons in the spinal cord (Basbaum & Fields, 1984). The "ascending" pain modulation system originates in the midbrain and is projected to the thalamus (Andersen & Dafny, 1983). Both systems utilize biogenic amines, opioid peptides, and nonopioid peptides (Andersen & Dafny, 1983; Basbaum & Fields, 1984; Raskin, 1988b).

The ascending system appears to show more relevance to headache disorders. This system has projections from the brainstem to the medial thalamus, which include large numbers of serotonergic and opiate receptors. The midbrain dorsal raphe nucleus, a serotonergic nucleus, projects to the medial thalamus and is associated with pain perception. Serotonergic projections to the forebrain are implicated in the regulation of the sleep cycle, mood changes, pain perception, and the hypothalamic regulation of hormone release (Raskin, 1988).

The endogenous opiate system (EOS) within the central nervous system may act as a nociceptive "rheostat" or "algostat," setting pain modulation to a specific level. As this level changes, an individual's pain tolerance may also change. Fluctuations in pain intensity may be interpreted as secondary to fluctuations in the function of antinociceptive pathways (Fields, 1988; Wall, 1988). Headache, along with other "non-organic" central pain problems, is thought to be the most common expression of impairment of the antinociceptive systems (Sicuteri, 1982).

The EOS modulates the neurovegetative triad of pain, depression, and autonomic disturbances that are found in only two conditions: chronic tension-type headache (posttraumatic or otherwise) and acute morphine abstinence (Sicuteri, 1982). The EOS is also implicated as primary protagonist in idiopathic headadche (Sicuteri, 1982; Sicuteri, Spillantini, & Fanciullacci, 1985). Reduced plasma concentrations of beta-endorphin have been found in patients with idiopathic headache, including those with chronic (and post-traumatic) tension-type headache

(Facchinetti & Genazzani, 1988; Genazzani, Nappi, Gacchinetti et al., 1984; Mosnaim, Diamond, Wolf et al., 1989; Nappi, Gacchinetti, Legnante et al., 1982).

A primary relationship also exists between the EOS and the biogenic amine systems that are intrinsic to both the pathophysiology of pain modulation and its treatment. Clinical and neuropharmacological information indicates that dysmodulated serotonergic neurotransmission probably generates chronic headache and head pain. It has also been noted that the ordinary, acute, or periodic headache may be the "noise" of serotonergic neurotransmission (Raskin, 1988).

Decreased levels of serotonin (Giacovazzo, Bernoni, Di Sabato, & Martelletti, 1990; Rolf et al., 1981; Shimomura & Takahashi, 1990) (with good indications of an impairment of serotonergic metabolism in patients with chronic tension-type headache), substance P, an excitatory neuropeptide (Almay, Johansson, von Knorring et al., 1988; Pernow, 1983), and plasma norepinephrine (Takeshima, Takao, Urakami et al., 1989) are found in patients with chronic tension-type headache. The last is also indicative of peripheral sympathetic hypofunction, which may participate in the etiology or maintenance of central opioid dysfunction (Nappi et al., 1982). Platelet GABA levels are significantly increased in patients with chronic tension-type headache. This may also act as a balance mechanism to deal with neuronal hyperexcitability and be associated with depression (Kowa, Shimomura, & Takahashi, 1992).

The opioid receptor mechanisms appear to be very susceptible to desensitization, or the development of tolerance. In patients with chronic tension-type headache, opioid receptor hypersensitivity is marked, secondary to the chronically diminished secretion of neurotransmitters. This "empty neuron syndrome" may involve both autonomic and nociceptive afferent systems, as well as being latent, subpathological, or pathological with spontaneous manifestations (Sicuteri, Nicolodi, & Fusco, 1988).

The EOS modulates the activity of monoaminergic neurons. A chronic EOS deficiency can provoke transmitter leakage, of both opioid and bioaminergic neurotransmitters, and lead to neuronal exhaustion and "emptying," as well as compensatory effector cell hypersensitivity. The poor release of neurotransmitter along with cell/receptor hypersensitivity appears to be the most important phenomenon of the hypoendorphin syndromes. It has also been concluded that chronic tension-type headache, and clinically PTTHA, may result from dysmodulation of nociceptive impulses, with associated sensitized receptors (Langemark et al., 1989).

Central factors may also be responsible for increased myofascial pain and sensitivity in patients with PTTHA. These central factors may include sensitization of second-order neurons in the spinal cord dorsal horn and trigeminal nucleus along with sensitization of supraspinal neurons and decreased descending antinociceptive activity from supraspinal neuronal systems (Bendtsen, 2000).

Chronic tension-type headache, including the chronic post-traumatic tension-type headache, may be, along with other chronic idiopathic headache, a "pain disease" directly linked to central dysmodulation of the nociceptive and antinociceptive systems, either latent or pathological in nature. Research indicates that at least two arms of the main endogenous antinociceptive systems, the EOS and the serotonergic systems, are involved in the pathogenesis of chronic tension-type headache. Clinical diagnosis and treatment of PTTHA demonstrate identical findings. This problem appears to be progressive, and the dysfunctions may result from neuronal exhaustion secondary to continuous activation of these systems (Facchinetti & Genazzani, 1988; Sicuteri et al., 1988).

PATHOPHYSIOLOGY

Looking at the upper portion of Figure 26.1, most of the basics have been mentioned: Continuous peripheral stimulation from myofascial nociceptive input from an MPS, with or without trigger points, may effectively trigger a change in the central pain "rheostat" associated with nociceptive input, secondary to the continuous need for pain-modulating antinociceptive neurotransmitters. This increased myofascial pain sensitivity may be secondary to activation or sensitization of peripheral nociceptors. The affective aspects of pain, including depression, anxiety, and fear, are secondary to changes in neurotransmitters such as serotonin and norepinephrine and directly influence myofascial nociception, as well as further reinforce central neurochemical changes.

After between 4 to 6 and 12 weeks or so, changes in the central nervous system's central modulation of nociception can occur. Secondary to continuous peripheral nociceptive stimulation, in association with affective changes, the central modulating mechanisms will assume a primary rather than a secondary or reactive role in pain perception, as well as antinociception, shifting the initiating aspects of pain perception from the peripheral regions to the central nervous system.

As noted earlier, patients with chronic tension-type headache show lower pressure pain tolerance than normal controls which indicates that the central nervous system is sensitized at the level of the spinal cord dorsal horn and trigeminal nucleus (Bendtsen, 2000; Bendtsen, Jensen, & Olesen, 1996b). Sensitivity in muscle (Bendtsen, 2003) as well as the skin is also noted, and the latter may indicate an expansion of receptive fields and convergence secondary to central sensitization.

This intrinsic shift may make innocuous stimuli more aggravating to the pain-modulating systems, the "irritable everything syndrome." The already dysmodulated internal feedback mechanisms may react until central neurochemical mechanisms dominate, secondary to neurotransmitter exhaustion, and receptor hypersensitivity and abnormal biogenic amine metabolism/exhaustion occur. These neurochemical changes may induce and/or exacerbate a sleep disorder (serotonergic in nature, from the nucleus raphe magnus), which by itself can perpetuate the central neurochemical dysmodulation, which is primarily responsible for chronic tension-type headache.

Chronic post-traumatic tension-type headache, whether or not it is associated with an MTBI, has the same pathophysiological mechanisms. In the presence of an MTBI, other significant pathophysiological changes occur, which can potentiate or exacerbate the mechanisms described above.

In the face of dysmodulated neurochemical systems found in chronic tension-type headache, add direct myofascial trauma as an initiating event. The effects of diffuse axonal injury from MTBI, which also affects the neurochemistry of the brain as neuronal degeneration and death occurs, can exacerbate the neurotransmitter pathophysiology. This may also explain the initiation of *de novo* migraine, as brainstem trigeminovascular mechanisms may obviously be affected. Finally, excitotoxic injury, which leads to cell death from the over-exuberant production of acetylcholine and glutamate, also may induce significant neuropathological "holes" in the primary neurotransmitter systems and exacerbate the headache pathophysiology.

Affective changes follow, with the additional problem of possible cognitive changes resulting from MTBI. The cognitive changes may make treatment of PTTHA more difficult.

PTTHA is the most common sequela of an MTBI. It may also be associated with iatrogenic analgesic abuse. Before treatment or even diagnosis of cognitive deficits is attempted, inappropriate medications must be stopped and the headache ameliorated. Most commonly, for this to be done, the patient must be treated using an interdisciplinary headache treatment protocol. Please see the *Headache Handbook: Diagnosis and Treatment* for the details of this protocol (Jay, 1999).

The neurochemical factors leading to the perpetuation of PTTHA appear to be further and more complexly involved than in chronic tension-type headache without associated MTBI. Treatment is most appropriately and cost-effectively performed in an interdisciplinary headache rehabilitation program. Tricyclic medications, GABAnergic medications, and nonsteroidal anti-inflammatory drugs (NSAIDs) are appropriate, while narcotics, Dilantin, barbiturates, and early-generation benzodiazepines are not.

It is worth noting that patients with MTBI who complain of headache do not appear to perceive their headache pain the same way as patients with headache without MTBI. These patients know that they have headaches. On a scale of 0 (no pain) to 10 (worst pain imaginable),

individual patients, when first seen, will give high numbers, e.g., 7 to 10, which is correlated to pathophysiological myofascial findings, including decreased cervical range of motion, muscle spasm, active trigger points, and more. As they go through treatment, they will regain appropriate physical functioning: normal cervical range of motion, amelioration of spasm and trigger points, etc, with a marked associated improvement of function. The patients' affect will be brighter, they will smile, have fewer if any pain behaviors, and resume doing the physical things they enjoy.

Yet, when asked, they will continue to state that their headache pain is at the same level of 7 to 10 as when they were first seen. Whether they are perseverating or are just unable to give an accurate subjective pain level (probable frontal lobe involvement), their stated pain levels may not change very much at all. Therefore, they must be evaluated on improvements in function, not by self-reported subjective decrements in headache pain levels.

EVALUATION AND TREATMENT OF PTTHA

As Olesen (1991) also noted, the expression of headache is the sum of the input into the trigeminal system, with vascular, sympathetic, myofascial, and central factors all possibly contributing to the clinical picture of headache. It is up to the clinician to try to determine how much each aspect contributes to the clinical picture — only then can an appropriate treatment paradigm be determined.

In attempting to acquire this information, the medical evaluation includes a very detailed history, which must include the facts, as the patient remembers them, of the initiating trauma; preexisting headache; a very detailed headache history including the location, intensity, frequency, duration of the headache; the pain attributes (very important); associated symptoms such as nausea and vomiting; and factors that increase or decrease the headache pain. A thorough medication history is necessary, typically asking specifically about over-the-counter analgesic medications, which can also produce analgesic rebound headache.

At least the mini-mental status evaluation should be performed, with testing of the patient's short- and long-term memory, mental acuity, and the presence of behavioral changes. It may be necessary to speak with the patient's family to determine some of these changes, as pain may cause the patient to focus on things other than a possible loss of cognitive functioning.

An evaluation of the patient's psychological status should be done, including screens for depression (and all three neurovegetative aspects: sleep, appetite, and libido), as well as personality changes, motivational changes, and ability to continue working. Again, it may be necessary to speak with family members or even co-workers to determine what is happening. Laboratory tests are typically not helpful. Neuroimaging will most frequently have been done after the injury. The general physical examination, neurological examination, and musculoskeletal examinations follow.

The neurological examination of patients with migraine is, in the absence of complicated aura, negative. The examination of the patient with cluster headache may yield signs of a partial Horner's syndrome. The examination of the patient with PTTHA may yield a great deal of information.

Typically, the neurological examination is negative. It's the musculoskeletal evaluation that will provide the facts. Begin by observing the patient's shoulders. In the vast majority of cases, there is an asymmetry of the acromioclavicular joints, with one higher than the other secondary to greater ipsilateral muscle spasm. The large muscles should be carefully palpated for both general tenderness and the presence of trigger points. These include the trapezius muscles, the deltoids, the scalenes, the rhomboids, the levaeter scapulae, and all associated muscles, including the pericranial musculature. Pay careful attention to the sternocleidomastoid muscles, particularly in patients complaining of dizziness and tinnitus. Palpate the bioccipital and bitemporal insertions. Look for true pericranial muscle tenderness, as well as masseter pain or tenderness. Observe the patient open the mouth: look for the amount of space between the teeth and see if the jaw deviates. Perform the passive as well as active cervical range of motion. Observe the patient's head: is it flexed forward? Is it tilted to one side? What about the shoulders: are they rounded? Rolled forward? Evaluate the presence and degree of muscle spasm found in the paravertebral muscles over the entire length of the spine. If the patient is a chronic tension-type headache sufferer, post-traumatic or otherwise, or if there is a complaint of upper extremity or hand numbness, perform an axillary stretch maneuver as well as the Adson's maneuver to evaluate for a myogenic thoracic outlet syndrome. And these are just the basics.

Until you know what you are dealing with physiologically, it is impossible to determine an appropriate treatment plan. Once you know, and are positive about your diagnosis reached by the history and physical/neurological examination, you can begin to formulate a treatment plan.

Treatment of Acute PTTHA

The medical management of acute or episodic PTTHA is relatively simple. Remember that the older nomenclature titled these headaches as "acute muscle contraction headache" or "tension headache." This form of headache is the most common, as previously indicated, accounting for up to 80% of all non-organic types of headache. It has been estimated that greater than 90% of Americans experience an acute tension-type headache, with or without predis-

posing trauma, at some time. The majority of these headaches are self-treated with over-the-counter medications and therefore never come to the attention of a physician. This indicates that the statistics are probably low, in that a fairly large number go unnoticed by physicians.

The greatest problem in the treatment of acute PTTHA is the avoidance of the development of analgesic rebound headache, which can easily occur if a patient is overmedicated. This is one step into the development of chronic or daily PTTHA.

Physicians should be particularly familiar with the various types of medications that can be used for patients complaining of acute PTTHA. The old adage that less is better certainly applies here. Many patients deal with the pain and discomfort by taking two aspirin and relaxing. Exercise is useful, as is a simple glass of wine, on an occasional basis. Any type of relaxation that distracts patients from their headache is useful.

Dealing with the medication management, physicians have a more than ample supply from which to choose. It may therefore be tempting to overtreat a minor headache with medications that have a significant risk of dependency. The simple analgesics are easily chosen by the patient, if not the physician. They are inexpensive and easy to get. They include aspirin and acetaminophen. Like the other NSAIDs, aspirin appears to work by inhibiting the synthesis of prostaglandin by blocking the action of cyclooxygenase, an enzyme that enables the conversion of arachidonic acid to prostaglandin to occur. Remember that prostaglandins are synthesized from cellular membrane phospholipids after activation or injury and sensitize pain receptors.

Aspirin, the prototypical NSAID, has anti-inflammatory and antipyretic properties, along with its pain-relieving properties. The recommended adult dose for treatment of acute PTTHA is 650 mg every 6 hours. Taking the aspirin with milk or food may decrease gastric irritation. Aspirin can also double bleeding time for 4 to 7 days after taking 650 mg. Peak blood levels are found after 45 minutes. The plasma half-life is 2 to 3 hours.

Acetaminophen usage is common. It provides about the same amount of analgesia as aspirin, but does not have the gastrointestinal side effects. That acetaminophen may work by inhibition of prostaglandin synthesis in the central nervous system has been suggested. It has much weaker anti-inflammatory activity than aspirin. Peak plasma levels occur between 30 and 60 minutes. Its plasma half-life is 2 to 4 hours.

Ibuprofen, an NSAID, is also available over the counter in doses of 200 mg per tablet. It can cause significant gastrointestinal distress. It has a half-life of 2 to 4 hours, with peak plasma levels attained in 1 to 2 hours. The adult dosage is 200 to 400 mg every 4 to 6 hours, with a maximum of 1200 mg per day.

These medications are frequently sold in combination with other drugs such as caffeine, which exerts no specific analgesic effects, but may potentiate the analgesic effects of aspirin and acetaminophen. There are aspirin–caffeine combination drugs (Anacin®) and aspirin, acetaminophen, and caffeine combinations (Excedrin Extra-Strength®, Excedrin Migraine®, and Vanquish®). The recommended dosage is two tablets every 6 hours as needed.

The biggest problem is that taking aspirin, acetaminophen, or combination tablets daily or even every other day for a week or more (possibly less) can induce the problem of analgesic rebound headache (which is discussed below).

As with birth control pills, when you ask patients what medications they are taking, they may forget that the birth control pill or aspirin or acetaminophen are medications, and forget to tell you, or even be too embarrassed to tell you because they are taking a large number of pills each day, so you must be certain to ask specifically.

There are a number of NSAIDs that are prescribed. Because of the variability in their efficacy, pharmacokinetics, and side effects, patients may need to be tried on more than one, sequentially, not in combination, to determine the best one for them.

The NSAIDs work, as noted before, by interfering with the action of cyclooxygenase in the synthesis of prostaglandins. Gastrointestinal side effects are common in up to 15 to 20% of patients and may include epigastric pain, nausea, heartburn, and abdominal discomfort. A history of gastrointestinal bleeding or ulcerations should indicate that great caution must be used if these medications are used at all. The most frequently prescribed NSAIDs include

Naproxen sodium (Anaprox®), which reaches peak plasma levels in 1 to 2 hours and has a mean half-life of 13 hours. It can be taken at 275 or 550 mg every 6 to 8 hours, with a top dosage of 1375 mg per day. Remember that this NSAID is useful in treating hormonally related migraine.

Ibuprofen (Motrin®) is prescribed in dosages of 100 and 800 mg per tablet. The suggested dosage for mild to moderate pain is 400 mg every 4 to 6 hours as needed.

Ketoprofen (Orudis®) is a cyclooxygenase inhibitor, but also stabilizes lysosomal membranes and possibly antagonizes the actions of bradykinin. Its peak plasma level is reached in 1 to 2 hours, and it has a 2-hour plasma half live. It is now over the counter (12.5 mg tablets), but is best used at 50 to 75 mg capsules. The recommended daily dosage is 150 to 300 mg a day in three or four divided doses. Gastrointestinal side effects are generally mild. Care should be taken when given to a patient with impaired renal function.

Keterolac tromethamine (Toradol®) can be given orally or parentally for moderate to severe acute headache pain. Peak plasma levels occur after intramuscular injection in about 50 minutes. Its analgesic effect is considered to be roughly equivalent to a 10 mg dose of intramuscular (IM) morphine. The typical injectable dose is 60 mg. Because of its potentially significant hepatic/renal side effects, the FDA has stated that Toradol should be given orally, after an IM injection of 60 mg, at 10 mg, every 8 hours, for a maximum of 5 days.

The COX-2 inhibitors (celecoxib and rofecoxib) are nonsteroidal anti-inflammatory agents that also have analgesic properties without, for most patients, the typical gastrointestinal problems associated with NSAIDs. They appear to work by inhibiting prostaglandin synthesis, via inhibition of cyclooxygenase-2, which corresponds to its improved gastrointestinal side-effect profile, while not affecting the cyclooxygenase-1 isozyme responsible for its anti-inflammatory functions. Celecoxib may be taken twice a day, 100 to 200 mg, while rofecoxib is taken once a day, at dosages ranging from 12.5 to 50 mg. The third Cox-2 inhibitor, valdecoxib, is utilized at dosages of 10 to 20 mg a day. Rofecoxib was withdrawn from use at the end of 2004 secondary to apparent cardiovascular problems. The fate of valdecoxib and celecoxib remains to be seen.

Muscle relaxants are given for acute tension-type headache by some clinicians. They are probably best utilized during the first 3 weeks postinjury-related headache. They are useful in patients with significant muscle spasm and pain, which may be seen in acute PTTHA, but which is not usually seen with an episodic tension-type headache. They are used appropriately after the development of muscle spasm after injury such as a slip and fall, motor vehicle accident, work and athletic injuries, or overstretching.

These medications work via the development of a therapeutic plasma level. Their exact mechanism of action is unknown, but they do not directly affect striated muscle, the myoneural junction, or motor nerves. They produce relaxation by depressing the central nerve pathways, possibly through their effects on higher central nervous system centers, which modifies the central perception of pain without affecting the peripheral pain reflexes or motor activity.

Carisoprodol (Soma®) is a central nervous system depressant that metabolizes into a barbiturate, which makes it both addictive and particularly inappropriate to use for patients with pain from muscle spasm in addition to MTBI. It acts as a sedative and it is thought to depress polysynaptic transmission in interneuronal pools at the supraspinal level in the brainstem reticular formation. It is short lived, with peak plasma levels in 1 to 2 hours and a 4 to 6 hour half-life. Dosage is 350 mg every 6 to 8 hours. It should not be mixed with other central nervous system depressants. It is also marketed in two other combined forms (with aspirin as Soma Compound) and with codeine, for additional analgesic effects.

Chlorzoxazone (Parafon Forte DSC®) is a centrally acting muscle relaxant with fewer sedative properties. It inhibits the reflex arcs involved in producing and maintaining muscle spasm at the level of the spinal cord and subcortical areas of the brain. It reaches it peak plasma level in 3 to 4 hours, and its duration of action is 3 to 4 hours. It is well tolerated, and side effects are uncommon. Dosage is 500 mg three times a day.

Metaxalone (Skelaxin®) is a centrally acting skeletal muscle relaxant that is chemically related to mephenaxalone, a mild tranquilizer. It is thought to induce muscle relaxation via central nervous system depression. Onset of action is about 1 hour, with peak blood levels in 2 hours, and duration of action is 4 to 6 hours. The recommended dose is 2,400 to 3,200 mg a day in divided doses (tablets are 400 mg each). It should be used carefully in patients with impaired liver function and should not be used at all in patients with significant renal or liver disease as well as those with a history of drug-induced anemias. Side effects include nausea, vomiting, gastrointestinal upset, drowsiness, dizziness, headache, nervousness, and irritability, as well as rash or pruritis. Jaundice and hemolytic anemia are rare.

Methocarbamol (Robaxin®) is a centrally acting skeletal muscle relaxant. It may inhibit nerve transmission in the internuncial neurons of the spinal cord. It has a 30-minute onset of action. Peak levels are found in about 2 hours, and its duration of action is 4 to 6 hours. It comes as 500 and 750 mg tablets. Tablets containing methocarbamol and aspirin (Robaxisal) are also available. The recommended dose of Robaxin is 750 mg three times a day. As with all of these medications, it should be taken for 7 to 10 days. It is well tolerated, with initial side effects, which resolve over time, including lightheadedness, dizziness, vertigo, headache, rash, gastrointestinal upset, nasal congestion, fever, blurred vision, urticaria, and mild muscular incoordination. In situations of severe, seemingly intractable muscle spasm, Robaxin may be given intravenously in doses of about 1 g every 8 to 12 hours.

Orphenedrine citrate (Norflex®, Norgesic®) is a centrally acting skeletal muscle relaxant with anticholinergic properties thought to work by blocking neuronal circuits, the hyperactivity of which may be implicated in hypertonia and spasm. It is available in injectable and oral formulations. The IM dose of Norflex is 2 mg, while the intravenous dosage is 60 mg in aqueous solution. The oral formulation (Norflex) is given in 100 mg tablets, 1 tablet every 12 hours. Norgesic is a combination form, including caffeine and aspirin, and should be given 1 or 2 tablets every 6 to 8 hours. Norgesic Forte, a stronger combination,

is given 1/2 to 1 tablet every 6 to 8 hours. Because of its anticholinergic effects, it should be contraindicated in patients with glaucoma, prostatic enlargement, or bladder outlet obstruction. Its major side effects are also secondary to its anticholinergic properties and include tachycardia, palpitations, urinary retention, nausea, vomiting, dizziness, constipation, and drowsiness. It may also cause confusion, excitation, hallucinations, and syncope.

Many of these medications are given in combination with other drugs, including barbiturates (butalbital and meprobamate) and narcotics (codeine, oxycodone, propoxyphene, etc.). This is probably not a good idea, as the barbiturates and narcotics can easily help develop patient dependence.

A good combination used by the author is methocarbamol 750 mg three times a day for 10 days in patients with significant spasm, accompanied by ketoprofen, 75 mg, every 6 to 8 hours as needed, with food as needed. For the acute PTTHA, 1 tablet of each taken together every 6 to 8 hours for two to three doses works very well.

For patients with extreme pain on an acute basis, the use of tramadol hydrochloride (50 to 100 mg every 4 to 6 hours) may be helpful. This medication appears to bind to the opioid receptors as well as inhibit reuptake of serotonin and norepinephrine. Other patients may need an opioid such as codeine or hydrocodone. These medications should be given for up to 7 to 10 days, if necessary. One published rule of thumb notes that immediate-relief analgesic medication of any kind should be taken no more than 2 days a week.

Again, narcotic medications should not be used, if they can be avoided, for the patient with acute TTHA, as the risk of dependence, as well as analgesic rebound headache, is too great.

It may be appropriate to include a short course of physical therapy for patients with significant myofascial findings on an acute basis.

Remember, too, that simple acute PTTHA is a problem that the headache specialists are rarely called in to see. It is the patient's family physician or chiropractor who most frequently sees this problem.

One of the most important treatments is most often forgotten — simply educating the patient regarding what exactly is going on. Patients need explanations of what is causing their pain and what is being done to help them as well as how a particular medication or treatment helps their particular problem. This is even more important for patients with chronic PTHA.

Medication Management of Chronic PTTHA

The medication treatment of choice is the tricyclic antidepressants (TCAs) or the specific serotonergic reuptake inhibitors (SSRIs).

The TCA medication of choice is amitriptyline, a sedating tricyclic antidepressant. As all of the tricyclics, it works in the synapse to decrease reuptake of serotonin and (depending on the individual medication) NEP. Amitriptyline, unlike the other TCAs, also works to repair the damage in stage 4 sleep architecture. It is the most sedating tricyclic. The typical dosage is between 10 and 50 mg at night. The author has found it rare to need more than 20 or 30 mg at night.

Amitriptyline appears to have prophylactic treatment ability secondary to its blockade of serotonin and noradrenergic reuptake in the central nervous system. It has been noted that amitriptyline may also act as an *N*-methyl-D-aspartate (NMDA) receptor antagonist (Watanabe, Saito, & Abe, 1993). The analgesic effects of amitriptyline may result from this ability (Eisenach & Gebhart, 1995). NMDA receptor activation is prominently involved in the development of sensitization of the spinal cord dorsal horn, which appears to be found in chronic tension-type headache patients, particularly if the hypothesis of central sensitization in these patients is correct, as this clinical fact could indicate.

Treatment with amitriptyline may also be associated with a reduction of myofascial tenderness, probably secondary to segmental reduction of central sensitization along with peripheral antinociceptive activity (Bendtsen & Jensen, 2000).

Doxepin® is also a very good tricyclic. Anticholinergic side effects such as sedation are reduced (but not by much) when compared with amitriptyline. It does *not* work on the sleep architecture. It is used at the same dosage levels of amitriptyline. Notice that the tricyclics are not used in their antidepressant dosages, anywhere from 100 to 350 mg a day. Even though the doses are low, their effectiveness in the treatment of chronic PTTHA is present.

The SSRIs include Prozac®, Paxil®, and Zoloft®. These medications are not typically sedating (although for some patients they may be), and with the exclusion of those patients, they are energizing. They should be given in the morning. Prozac and Paxil should start at 10 to 20 mg a day, and they can be increased to 60 to 80 mg. Zoloft should be given at 25 to 50 mg in the morning, up to 150 mg in divided doses. The doses should be divided, giving one when the patient arises in the morning (around 7:00 A.M.) and one at noon. Explain to the patients that taking these medications later than noon can, in many cases, give them problems sleeping.

One can also safely combine 10 to 40 mg of Prozac or Paxil, or 50 mg of Zoloft, with a small dose of amitriptyline or doxepin (10 to 30 mg) at night. Inappropriate dosages of these two forms of medications can, rarely, induce the serotonin syndrome. There are other excellent antidepressants such as Wellbutrin®, Serzone®, and Effexor®. These should be considered as needed. Do not combine these medications with the MAO inhibitors.

Another excellent medication is Clonazepam®, a fifth-generation form of benzodiazepine. It is GABAnergic in effect. It works at the level of the internuncial neurons of the spinal cord to enhance muscle relaxation. It helps, a bit, with anxiolysis. It has a side effect of sedation. In doses of 4 to 12 mg a day, it works as an anticonvulsant. At smaller doses, 0.5 to 1 mg given at night, it is very useful in the treatment of patients with chronic tension-type headache. The sedation lasts for a shorter time than the sedation from tricyclics, and this in itself is useful.

If the acute use of muscle relaxant medications is not enough to end the problem, Tizanidine® is a good choice of medication after the first 3 weeks or so have elapsed and the patient is still exhibiting painful neuromuscular spasm. Tizanidine is an alpha$_2$ noradrenergic agonist (Coward, Davies, Herrling, & Rudeberg, 1984; Sayers, Burki, & Eichenberger, 1980). It has supraspinal effects by inhibiting the facilitation of spinal reflex transmission by the descending noradrenergic pathways, as it decreases firing of the noradrenergic locus ceruleus (Palmeri & Wiesendanger, 1990). It acts presynaptically in the spinal cord inducing a polysynaptic reduction in released excitatory transmitters (Davies, Johnson, & Lovering, 1983). It also decreases hyperexcitability of the muscle without acting on the neuromuscular junctions or muscle fibers (Wagstaff, Koch, Hirst, Bryson, & von Wartburg, 1989). Short acting, its maximum plasma concentrations are reached within 1 to 2 hours (Wagstaff & Bryson, 1997. It has a large first-pass metabolism, with a half-life of 2.1 to 4.2 hours (*Professional's handbook of drug therapy for pain*, 2001). Dosages should be slowly increased, starting at 1 to 2 mg at night and slowly increasing to 20 to 24 mg. Maximum dosage is 36 mg in divided dosages, typically found in patients who need an antimyotonic. Interestingly, this medication appears to decrease muscle pain while providing its antimyotonic effects.

In the opinion of this author, treating patients with chronic PTTHA with tricyclics, physical therapy, psychotherapy, etc. will not work if the patient is taking daily or four times a week analgesic medications of any type! In the presence of analgesic rebound headache, nothing will show long-lasting effectiveness until the chronic analgesics are stopped. More information regarding appropriate use of medications can be obtained from any clinical pharmacology text (*Professional's handbook of drug therapy for pain*, 2001). Nonmedication treatments may include biofeedback-assisted relaxation (Ham & Packard, 1996), as well as a trial of percutaneous electrical nerve stimulation (Ahmed, White, Craig et al., 2000).

Cost-Effective Treatment of Chronic PTTHA

Treatment of CPTTHA is best accomplished via an interdisciplinary rehabilitation approach, the main purpose of which is *not* to "teach the patient to live with the headache," but to properly diagnose and effectively ameliorate or stop the patient's headache.

Drug detoxification is the necessary first step, whether the patient is overutilizing simple, over-the-counter analgesics or narcotics or barbiturates. Chronic daily analgesics appear to prevent appropriate functioning of the EOS (via negative neurochemical feedback loops) and other associated antinociceptive systems, inducing analgesic rebound headaches, which are secondary problems from the medications that induce headache secondary to purely neurochemical/neurophysiological changes. Vascular rebound headaches from overutilization of vasoconstrictors may also occur and must be stopped before other treatment is applied. Clinically, an effective way to detoxify patients with CTTHA is with the repetitive DHE-45 protocol described by Raskin (1988b). Concurrently, prophylactic medications should be started. The use of prophylactic medications, as well as physical therapy and other treatments given while a patient is enduring analgesic rebound headaches, is an ineffectual waste of time and money.

One study of 34 patients with PTHA and the postconcussion syndrome found that the repetitive use of DHE-45 and metaclopramide induced improvement in headache in 85% of patients, improved memory in 94%, improved sleep in 94%, and decreased dizziness in 88% (McBeath & Nanda, 1994). Many of the postconcussive syndrome improvements may have been secondary to the diminution of headache pain.

Another small study found the use of subcutaneous sumatritptan (6 mg) to be useful when treating PTHA that is refractory to other medication treatment (Gawel, Rothbart, & Jacobs, 1993).

The use of divalproex sodium was found to be a safe, effective treatment for patients with persistent chronic daily PTHA in a study that did not differentiate migraine from nonmigrainous PTHA (Packard, 2000). Sodium valproate is a good anticonvulsant choice for the patient with TBI as it does not produce any further cognitive decline, unlike Dilantin®, Phenobarbital®, or Neurontin® (Jay, 2000).

After detoxification, an outpatient interdisciplinary headache rehabilitation program using neuropharmacological therapy (to restore neurochemical homeostasis), physical therapy (Jay, Brunson, & Branson, 1989), psychotherapy, and stress management (including biofeedback-enhanced neuromuscular re-education and muscle relaxation) is the most time- and cost-effective treatment. Optimal psychotherapy or physical therapy regimens by themselves will not resolve myofascial difficulties or depression if the affective, sleep, and central nervous system neurochemical dysmodulation affecting them is not concurrently and appropriately treated. The interdisciplinary treatment paradigm also enables fine-tuning of diag-

nosis and possible determination of a secondary or "hidden" etiology for a patient's headaches.

In patients with recalcitrant soft tissue pain problems the use of botulinum toxin A or B to decrease muscle spasm and pain has increased significantly (Argoff, 2002; Gobel, Heinze, Heinze-Kuhnk, & Jost, 2001). However, several randomized, placebo-controlled studies do not support the effectiveness of botulinum toxin in the treatment of headache (Gobel, Lindner, Krack et al., 1999; Smuts, Baker, Smuts et al., 1999). In one randomized study (Rollnik, Tanneberger, Schubert et al., 2000) no improvement of primary or secondary pain end points was found after 6 weeks. Similar findings were reported in a study of episodic tension-type headache (Eros & Doric, 2002). More recent abstracts presented at the American Headache Society meeting in 2002 touted more successful results; however, few patients were noted to have CPTHA (Ashina, Lassen, Bendtsen et al., 1999; Miller, 2002; Troost, 2002).

Future use of nitric oxide synthase inhibitors may also promise to bring headache relief (Basbaum & Fields, 1984; Keidel et al., 2001). These studies indicate that the locus for nociception for CPHTA is found in the brainstem, not the peripheral nervous system.

Nitric oxide (NO) is found in the nociceptive neurons in the trigeminal nucleus caudalis and possibly higher in the central nervous system (Ashima, Lassen, et al., 1999). Inhibition of nitric oxide synthase (NOS), which enables the generation of NO, decreases central sensitization in animal models of continuous pain. In a clinical investigation of an NOS inhibitor, both headache and pericranial myofascial tenderness and hardness in patients with chronic tension-type headache were diminished (Ashina, Bendtsen, Jensen et al., 1999; Ashima, Lassen et al., 1999). This study supports the theory that central sensitization is involved in the pathophysiology of chronic tension-type headache.

The use of the interdisciplinary pain management paradigm to treat these patients also enables early goal-setting and continued education throughout the evaluation and treatment process.

Failure to treat the patient with chronic PTTHA with an interdisciplinary, whole-person approach (Figure 26.9) is responsible for multiple treatment failures as well as monetary waste, as long-term response — headache remediation — is most often not achieved.

OTHER ASPECTS OF POST-TRAUMATIC HEADACHE

An initial trauma may involve soft tissue injury to the scalp or face, which may be followed by an entrapment of a sensory nerve, or the sensory nerve may have been cut via laceration during the trauma. The entrapment may

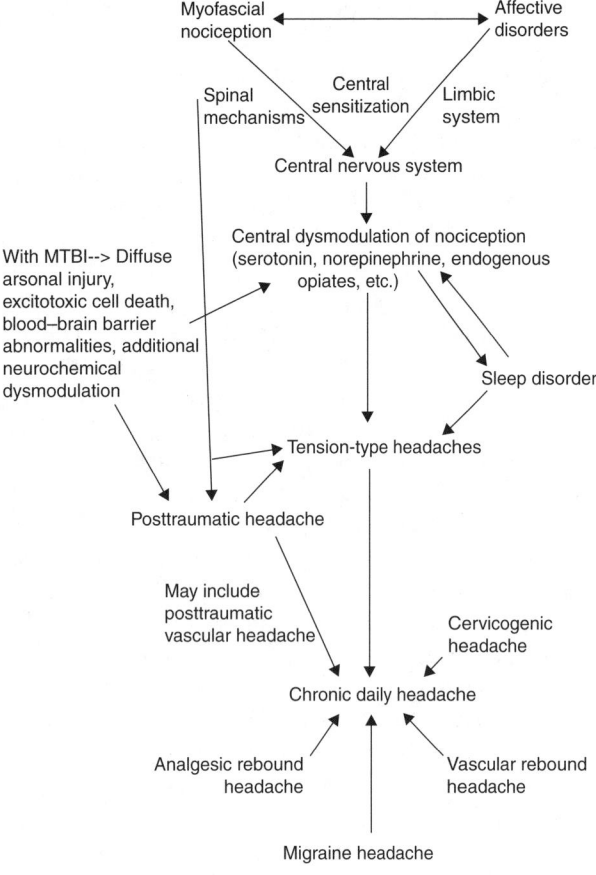

FIGURE 26.9 Headache diatheses found in posttraumatic headache patients.

also occur during suturing of a laceration. Such entrapments may induce nerve, or neuropathic, pain. This is easily differentiated from other primary headache types. The pain is constant, burning, and relegated to the sensory distribution of the affected nerve. Anticonvulsant medications such as carbamazepine are best for the first-line treatment. Neurontin has been used, but it has different, possibly more significant, side effects in some patients, particularly in those with a concurrent MTBI. In some cases, neurolytic procedures such as radiofrequency coagulation or cryo-ablation may be necessary. Both are good procedures, but have varying durations of benefit, most typically between 6 to 12 months.

Without question, injuries to the cervical spine and the superficial and deep structures of the neck (muscles, ligaments, bone, discs, or nerve roots) may occur. Cervical pain from trigger points in spasmed musculature as well as from cervical joint dysfunction may be referred to the head.

If the post-traumatic pain is suboccipital with lancinating, electrical-like shooting pain attributes, secondary to involvement of the occipital neurovascular bundle (the occipital nerve, artery, and vein), or secondary to prolonged muscle spasm/contraction or excessive vascular

dilatation impinging on the greater occipital nerve of Arnold, this pain is known as occipital neuralgia. It is always in the C_2 distribution at the back of the head. Indomethacin may be an effective treatment for this problem. Steroidal injections may also be utilized. Neuroablative procedures should be performed only when all other treatment has failed.

Preexisting arthritis or discogenic disease may also be exacerbated by the initial trauma. An appropriate neurological evaluation will help with these entities.

The dysautonomic cephalalgia of Vijayan (1977) is associated with injury to the anterior aspect of the carotid sheath. The headache is severe and unilateral, in the frontotemporal area, and associated with ipsilateral hyperhidrosis and dilatation of the ipsilateral pupil. The role of sympathetic nervous system dysfunction, while it may remain controversial, is shown in many studies, as noted above. Also, the signs and symptoms are, of course, similar to cluster headache.

Zasler (1999) also published an interesting case demonstrating late or delayed PTHA secondary to post-traumatic tension pneumocephalus.

CERVICOGENIC HEADACHE

Just as the community of headache specialty physicians was rather hesitant to accept that the musculature played any role in tension-type headache, post-traumatic or otherwise, the idea that headache can arise from the structures of the neck still has many detractors.

Dwyer, Aprill, and Bogduk (1990) utilized fluoroscopic control to stimulate joints at segments C_{2-3} to C_{6-7} by distending the joint capsule with injections of contrast medium. They were able to show that each joint produced a clinically distinguishable, characteristic pattern of referred pain that enabled the construction of pain charts to be used in determining the segmental location of symptomatic joints in patients presenting with cervical zygapophyseal pain.

The diagnostic criteria for cervicogenic headache (CGHA) have been noted by several authors to differ a bit. Bogduk, Corrigan, Kelley et al. (1985) defined them as referred pain perceived in any region of the head, which was referred by a primary nociceptive source in the musculoskeletal tissues innervated by cervical nerves. Clinical features include pain that is not lancinating, and is dull or aching but could be throbbing, located in the occipital, parietal, temporal, frontal, or orbital regions, unilaterally or bilaterally. There is some indication of cervical spine abnormality such as neck pain, tenderness, impaired cervical motion, aggravation of the headache by neck movements, or a history of cervical trauma.

Bogduk and co-authors' (1985) diagnostic criteria included identification by clinical examination or by imaging of the cervical sources of pain found, by valid antecedent studies, to be reliably associated with the head pain. Their criteria also include complete relief of the head pain seen after controlled local anesthetic blockade of one or more cervical nerves or structures innervated by cervical nerves.

The North American Cervicogenic Headache Society determined that CGHA is essentially referred pain noted in any region of the head, caused by primary nociceptive sources in the musculoskeletal tissues that are innervated by the cervical nerves (Sjaastad, Fredriksen, Pfaffenrath, 1990). The pain of CGHA begins in the occipitonuchal region and is typically secondary to an abnormality within the region of the occiput to C_3 that results from trauma or prolonged postural/functional strain (Sjasstad et al., 1990).

Sjaastad et al. (1990) also weighed in with specific criteria. They noted that CGHA are one sided, but could also be bilateral, "unilaterally on two sides." The duration of a headache or exacerbation ranges from several hours to several weeks. Initially, the headache may be episodic, but can later become chronic-fluctuating. Symptoms and signs are referrable to the neck, and include decreased range of cervical motion and mechanical precipitation of attacks, and autonomic symptoms such as nausea and photophobia are not marked, if present. A positive response to appropriate anesthetic blockade is considered essential.

Sjaastad et al. (1990) noted several major criteria:

1. Symptoms and signs of cervical involvement:
   a. Provocation of an irradiating head pain similar to the spontaneously occurring one:
      i. By neck movement and/or sustained awkward head positioning, and/or
      ii. By external pressure over the upper neck or head on the side ipsilateral to the pain
   b. Restriction of cervical range of motion
   c. Ipsilateral neck, shoulder, or arm pain of a vague, nonradicular nature or, on occasion, sharp arm pain in a radicular region

Symptoms and signs 1a to 1c are listed in "order of importance." One or more of these must be present for the term cervicogenic headache to be used. Point 1a is itself a sufficient criterion, but 1b and 1c are not. Point 2 is a necessary additional point.

2. Confirmation by diagnostic anesthetic blocks
3. Unilateral pain which does not shift from side to side
4. Pain characteristics:
   a. Nonthrobbing pain, usually beginning in the neck
   b. Episodes of varying duration
   c. Fluctuating, continuous pain

5. Other characteristics of some importance:
   a. Marginal or no effect from treatment with indomethacin
   b. Marginal or no effect from treatment with triptans or ergots
   c. Female preponderance
   d. History of head or neck trauma

None of the single points under 4 or 5 is essential.

6. Other descriptions of less importance — various headache-related phenomena that are rarely present, and of only mild to moderate severity when present:
   a. Nausea
   b. Photo- and phonophobia
   c. Dizziness
   d. Blurred vision ipsilateral to the pain
   e. Difficulty with swallowing
   f. Fluid around the eye epsilateral to the pain

The anatomical basis of CGHA is thought to be secondary to convergence in the trigeminocervical nucleus between nociceptive afferents from the field of the trigeminal nerve and the receptive fields of the first three cervical nerves. Headache appears to be secondary to structural problems in regions innervated by C_1 to C_3. These regions include the muscles, joints, and ligaments of the upper three cervical segments, as well as the dura mater of the spinal cord and the posterior cranial fossa and the vertebral artery (Bogduk, 1992).

Other anatomical causation has been identified and includes

1. Disrupted and/or ruptured cervical discs with irritation of the sympathetic sinu-vertebral nerves (in the disc) and nerve roots by mechanical and chemical means at single or multiple levels
2. Irritation of the articular branches to the cervical zygapophyseal joints derived from the medial branches of the cervical dorsal rami
3. Irritation of the peripheral branches and unmyelinated nerve structures to the muscle attachments at the spinous process of C_2 supplied by the C_2 and C_3 nerve roots; this includes the rectus capitis posterior, major obliquus capitis inferior major, semispinalis cervicis multifidus, semispinalis capitis major, and rectus capitis posterior minor, and interspinal muscles at C_{1-2} and C_{2-3}
4. Pain from the end fibers of the greater tertiary occipital and sympathetic nerve structures with its C-fibers including the periosteum and suboccipital musculature (semispinalis capitis, rec-

tus capitis posterior minor and major, trapezius, and occipitalis) (Blume, 1997)

The treatment of CGHA begins with diagnostic anesthetic blocks that are typically mixed with long-acting steroids such as hydrocortisone. This should temporarily relieve the CGHA for hours to days. If pain relief lasts for weeks to months, blocks should be repeated.

Once a specific targeted joint or disc is identified, the latter with discography if needed, a number of procedures have been used for treatment of CGHA:

1. Neurolysis of the C_2 nerve root via decompressive surgery (Poletti, 1983) as well as partial denervation of the suboccipital and paraspinal musculature (Pikus & Phillips, 1995)
2. Radiofrequency lesions to the muscle attachments of the spinous process at C_2 (Blume, Kakolewski, Richardson, & Rojas, 1982; Rogal, 1995)
3. Radiofrequency neurotomy of the sinu-vertebral nerves to the upper cervical disc, as well as to the outer layer of the C_3 or C_4 nerve root (Sluijter, 1990)
4. Radiofrequency denaturation of the occipital nerve (Blume, 1976; Blume et al., 1981; Blume & Ungar-Sargon, 1986)
5. Radiofrequency denaturation of the C_2 medial rami (Rogal, 1986)
6. Cervical discectomy and fusion
7. C_2 ganglionectomy (Jansen & Spoerri, 1985)

The last procedure is not often performed, while there remain proponents of radiofrequency lesioning versus the "old" cervical discectomy and fusion.

It is imperative to differentiate CGHA from both migraine headache and PTTHA, as the treatments are completely different. Unfortunately, the literature in general argues the question of cervicogenic headache, although not the idea that headache may be associated with cervical pathology. It should be noted that the International Association for the Study of Pain has recognized cervicogenic headache as a pain syndrome (Zwart, 1997). The criteria use neck mobility as the major indicator of this diagnosis, but both tension-type headache and migraine have associated decrements in cervical mobility.

The different criteria for the diagnosis of CGHA make other previously recognized primary headache sufferers fall into a diagnostic hole. There appears to be too much overlap in the varying diagnoses. Likewise, patients with the diagnosis of CGHA may also fall into other diagnostic categories or even multiple diagnostic categories (Leone, D'Amico, Grazzi et al., 1998; Pfaffenrath & Kaube, 1990; Sjaastad, Bovim, & Stovner, 1992; Treleaven, Jull, & Atkinson, 1994).

Not to be forgotten is the fact that the diagnosis specifically may follow an acceleration/deceleration injury or other cervical trauma (Obelieniene, Bovim, Schrader et al., 1998; Treleaven et al., 1994). This makes it imperative to consider the diagnosis of CGHA in patients with PTHA who do not show improvement following appropriate treatment for other diagnosed headache diatheses. On the other hand, clinically, CGHA appears to be found in less than 3 to 5% of the PTTHA population. If a patient with PTHA also has an MTBI, the level of difficulty in making the diagnosis and treating that patient increases dramatically.

Psychological factors exist; the neurochemical aspects of depression and anxiety, for instance, are well known. In the presence of an MTBI, they become more difficult to tease out and deal with, as the patients may be dealing with pain as well as changes in cognition and behavior, including frontal lobe difficulties such as increased irritability and labile emotionality.

LEGAL ASPECTS

It appears, to this author, seems a sad commentary that a section dealing with "legal aspects" is even needed in a medical textbook chapter. But it is.

There is no set, established method used in determining an impairment rating for PTHA. The *AMA Guides to the Evaluation of Permanent Impairment*, 5th edition (Cocciarella & Andersson, 2001) now allows a "pain" impairment, but it is not particularly specific to PTHA and behavioral aspects are important. Packard and Ham (1993a) developed a mnemonic to do this: IMPAIRMENT: for Intensity, Medication use, Physical signs/symptoms, Adjustment, Incapacitation, Recreation, Miscellaneous activity of daily living, Employment, Number (frequency), and Time (duration of attacks). Each is scored from 0 to 2 points, with three physician modifiers, including motivation for treatment, overexaggeration, or overconcern and degree of legal interest. Unfortunately, their methodology has not been taken into wide use.

Another major problem facing patients and their treating physicians is the question of medicolegal disability secondary to the PTHA syndrome, with or without the question of MTBI. Patients whose injuries involved a skull fracture, subdural hematoma, or severe lacerations and whose gray matter is leaking out of their ears *may* not have a problem in regard to disability. Unfortunately, for patients and their physicians, insurance problems do exist, beginning with obtaining approval to treat a PTHA syndrome.

Some insurance companies deny that there is such a thing as an MTBI or PTHAs. They have a number of paid consultants to assure the legal system that this is so. They will try to prevent clinicians from even becoming involved with treating these patients by refusing to pay them for treatment. *It does not matter* how devastating a patient's symptoms are; the patient will still face a difficult and totally unjustified legal battle just to get treatment approved, never mind the question of disability compensation.

It is interesting (but medically expected) that the vast majority of patients with PTHA, particularly those with headaches as part of a postconcussion syndrome, present the same way. This is pertinent, as the legal concern is typically that the patient complaining of significant PTHA is either lying or malingering. They are for real and are expressing the same symptomatology from the same causation (head trauma or acceleration/deceleration injuries). This is just like patients with chicken pox who initially present, clinically, in the same way.

Then there is the *M* word — malingering. This is associated with the idea that settlement of litigation is all that is needed to put a stop to the PTHA syndrome. This is also a favorite theme of the insurance companies. True malingering is almost as rare as hens' teeth. There are published studies that demonstrate that legal settlement has nothing to do with the patients' symptoms ending or encouraging them to return to work (Cicerone, 1992; Elkind, 1989; Evans, 1992; Merskey & Woodford, 1972).

Chronic PTHAs, with or without the other aspects of the postconcussion syndrome, are extremely common after head trauma as well as after an acceleration/deceleration injury. These patients are very consistent in their presentations as well as in their descriptions of their symptoms and sequelae. This consistency is strong evidence that their problems are organic in nature and produced by the trauma.

Most patients with PTHA will have their headache resolve if they are given appropriate medical treatment. About 15 to 20% will have prolonged difficulties. Correct diagnosis and treatment in the majority of cases should decrease this percentage.

REFERENCES

Ahmed, H. E., White, P. F., Craig, W. F., et al. (2000). Use of percutaneous electrical nerve stimulation (PENS) in the short-term management of headache. *Headache, 40*(4), 311–315.

Alberti, A., Sarchielli, P., Mazzotta, G., & Gallai, V. (2001). Event-related potentials in posttraumatic headache. *Headache, 41*(6), 579–585.

Almay, B. G. L., Johansson, F., von Knorring, L. et al. (1988). Substance P in CSF of patients with chronic pain syndromes. *Pain, 33*, 3.

Andersen, E., & Dafny, N. (1983). An ascending serotonergic pain modulation pathway from the dorsal raphe nucleus to the parafascicularis nucleus of the thalamus. *Brain Research, 269*, 57.

Anderson, C. D., & Franks, R. D. (1981). Migraine and tension headache: Is there a physiological difference? *Headache, 21*, 63.

Argoff, C. (2002). Successful treatment of chronic daily headache with Myobloc. Poster presented at the 21st Annual Scientific Meeting of the American Pain Society, Baltimore, MD, March 14–17.

Ashina, M., Bendtsen, L., Jensen, R., et al. (1999). Possible mechanisms of action of nitric oxide synthase inhibitors in chronic tension-type headache. *Brain, 122*, 1629.

Ashina, M., Lassen, L. H., Bendtsen, L. et al. (1999). Effect of inhibition of nitric oxide synthase on chronic tension-type headache: A randomized crossover trial. *Lancet, 353*, 287.

Bakal, D. A., & Kaganov, J. A. (1977). Muscle contraction and migraine headache: Psychophysiologic comparison. *Headache, 17*, 208.

Baloh, R. W. (1997). Neurotology of migraine. *Headache, 37*, 615–621.

Basbaum, A. I., & Fields, H. L. (1984). Endogenous pain control systems: Brainstem spinal pathways and endorphin circuitry. *Annual Review of Neuroscience, 7*, 309.

Bendtsen, L. (2000). Central sensitization in tension-type headache: Possible pathophysiologic mechanisms. *Cephalalgia, 20*, 486–508.

Bendtsen, L. (2003). Central and peripheral sensitization in tension-type headache. *Current Headache Reports, 2*, 460–465.

Bendtsen, L., & Jensen, R. (2000). Amitriptyline reduces myofascial tenderness in patients with chronic tension-type headache. *Cephalalgia, 20*, 603–610.

Bendtsen, L., Jensen, R., & Olesen, J. (1996a). Decreased pain detection and tolerance thresholds in chronic tension-type headache. *Archives of Neurology, 53*, 373–376.

Bendtsen, L., Jensen, R., & Olesen, J. (1996b). Qualitatively altered nociception in chronic myofascial pain. *Pain, 65*, 259–264.

Blume, H. G. (1976). Radiofrequency denaturation in occipital pain: A new approach in 114 cases. *Advanced Brain Research Therapy, 1*, 691–698.

Blume, H. G. (1997). Diagnosis and treatment modalities of cervicogenic headaches. *Head and Neck Pain, Newsletter of the Cervicogenic Headache International Study Group, 4*, 1–2.

Blume, H. G., & Ungar-Sargon, J. (1986). Neurosurgical treatment of persistent occipital myalgia-neuralgia syndrome. *Journal of Cranio-Mandibular Practice, 4*, 65–73.

Blume, H. G., Kakolewski, J. W., Richardson, R. R., & Rojas, C. H. (1981). Selective percutaneous radiofrequency thermodenervation of pain fibers in the treatment of occipital neuralgia: Results in 450 cases. *Journal of Neurological and Orthopedic Surgery, 2*, 261–268.

Blume, H. G., Kakolewski, J. W., Richardson, R. R., & Rojas, C. H. (1982). Radiofrequency denaturation in occipital pain: Results in 450 cases. *Applied Neurophysiology, 45*, 543–548.

Bogduk, N. (1992). The anatomical basis for cervicogenic headache. *Journal of Manipulative and Physiological Therapeutics, 15*, 67–70.

Bogduk, N., Corrigan, B., Kelly, R. et al. (1985). Cervical headache. *Medical Journal of Australia, 143*, 202–207.

Borgeat, F., Hade, B., Elie, R., & Larouche, L. M. (1984). Effects of voluntary muscle tension increases in tension headache. *Headache, 24,* 199.

Brown, S. J., Fann, S. R., & Grant, I. (1994). Postconcussional disorder: Time to acknowledge a common source of neurobehavioral comorbidity. *Journal of Neuropsychiatry and Clinical Neuroscience, 6,* 15–22.

Buchholz, D. W., & Reich, S. G. (1996). The menagerie of migraine. *Seminars in Neurology, 16,* 83–93.

Cady, R. K., & Farmer, K. (1998). Posttraumatic headache. In R. E. Windsor & D. M. Lox (Eds.), *Soft tissue injuries: Diagnosis and treatment* (pp. 207–224). Philadelphia: Hanley & Belfus.

Cailliet, R. (1993). *Pain: Mechanisms and management* (p. 83). Philadelphia: F.A. Davis.

Callaghan, M., & Abu Arafeh, I. (2001). Chronic posttraumatic headache in children and adolescents. *Developmental Medicine and Child Neurology, 43*(12), 819–822.

Cicerone, K. D. (1992). Psychological management of postconcussive disorders. *Physical Medicine and Rehabilitation State of the Art Reviews, 6,* 129–141.

Claussen, C. F., & Claussen, E. (1995). Neurootological contributions to the diagnostic follow-up after whiplash injuries. *Acta Otolaryngologica. 520*(Suppl Pt 1), 53–56.

Cocchiarella, L., & Andersson, G. B. J. (2001). *AMA guides to the evaluation of permanent impairment.* Atlanta, GA: American Medical Association Press.

Cohen, M. J. (1978). Psychophysiological studies of headache: Is there similarity between migraine and muscle contraction headaches? *Headache, 18,* 189.

Collins, M. W., Field, M., Iverson, G. et al. (2003). Relationship between postconcussion headache and neuropsychological test performance in high school athletes. *American Journal of Sports, 31*(2), 168–173.

Couch, J.R., & Bearss, C. (2001). Chronic daily headache in the posttrauma syndrome: Relation to extent of head injury. *Headache, 41*(6), 559–564.

Covelli, V., & Ferrannini, E. (1987). Neurophysiologic findings in headache patients. Psychogalvanic reflex investigation in migraineurs and tension headache patients. *Acta Neurologica, 9,* 354.

Coward, D. M., Davies, J., Herrling, P., & Rudeberg, C. (1984). *Pharmacological properties of tizanidine (DS 103-282)* (pp. 61–71). New York: Springer-Verlag.

D'Andrea, G., Toledo, M., Cortelazzo, S., & Milone, F. F. (1982). Platelet activity in migraine. *Headache, 22,* 207.

Davies, J., Johnson, S. E., & Lovering, R. (1983). Inhibition by DS 103-282 of D-(^{3}H)aspartate release from spinal cord slices. *British Journal of Pharmacology, 78,* 2P.

Denny-Brown, D., & Russell, W. R. (1941). Experimental cerebral concussion. *Brain, 64,* 93.

Diamond, S., & Dalessio, D. J. (1980). *The practicing physicians approach to headache* (3rd ed.). Baltimore: Williams and Wilkins.

Dorpat, T. L., & Holmes, T. H. (1955). Mechanisms of skeletal muscle pain and fatigue. *Archives of Neurology and Psychiatry, 74,* 628.

Drake, M. E., Pakalnis, A., Andrews, J. M., & Bogner, J. F. (1990). Nocturnal sleep recording with cassette EEG in chronic headaches. *Headache, 30,* 600.

Drake, M. E., Weate, S. J., & Newell, S. A. (1996). Auditory evoked potentials in postconcussive syndrome. *Electromyography and Clinical Neurophysiology, 36*(8), 457–462.

Drummond, P. D. (1986). A quantitative assessment of photophobia in migraine and tension headache. *Headache, 26,* 465.

Drummond, P. D. (1987). Scalp tenderness and sensitivity to pain in migraine and tension headache. *Headache, 27,* 45.

Duckro, P. N., Greenberg, M., Schultz, K. T. et al. (1992). Clinical factors of chronic post-traumatic headache. *Headache Quarterly, 3,* 295–308.

Duckro, P. N., Chibnall, J. T., & Tomazic, T. J. (1995). Anger, depression, and disability: A path analysis of relationships in a sample of chronic posttraumatic headache patients. *Headache, 35*(1), 7–9.

Dwyer, A., Aprill, C., & Bogduk, N. (1990). Cervical zygapophyseal joint pain patterns I: A study in normal volunteers. *Spine, 15,* 453–457.

Eisenach, J. C., & Gebhart, G. F. (1995). Intrathecal amitriptyline acts as an N-methyl-D-aspartate receptor antagonist in the presence of inflammatory hyperalgesia in rats. *Anesthesiology, 83,* 1046–1054.

Elkind, A. H. (1989). Headache and facial pain associated with head injury. *Otolaryngologic Clinics of North America, 22,* 1251–1271.

Elkind, A. H. (1992). Posttraumatic headache. In S. Diamond & D. J. Dalessio (Eds.), *The practicing physician's approach to headache* (5th ed., pp. 146–161). Baltimore: Williams & Wilkins.

Ellertsen, B., Norby, H., & Sjaastad, O. (1987). Psychophysiological response patterns in tension headache: Effects of tricyclic antidepressants. *Cephalalgia, 7,* 55.

Eros, E. J., & Doric, D. W. (2002). The effects of botulinum toxin-type A on disability in episodic and chronic migraine [Abstract]. Presented at the American Headache Society Meeting, Seattle, WA, June 21–June 23.

Evans, R. W. (1992). The postconcussion syndrome and the sequelae of mild head injury. *Neurologic Clinics, 10,* 815–847.

Facchinetti, F., & Genazzani, A.R. (1988). Opioids in cerebrospinal fluid and blood of headache sufferers. In J. Elesen & L. Edvinsson (Eds.). *Basic mechanisms of headache* (p. 261). Amsterdam: Elsevier Science.

Fields, H. L. (1988). Sources of variability in the sensation of pain. *Pain, 33,* 195.

Fordyce, C. J., Roueche, J. R., & Prigatano, G. P. (1982). Enhanced emotional reactions in chronic head trauma patients. *Journal of Neurology, Neurosurgery and Psychiatry, 46,* 621–624.

Forsell, H. (1985). Mandibular dysfunction and headache. *Proceedings. Finnish Dental Society of Washington, Supplement II, 81,* 591.

Fricton, J. R. (1990). Myofascial pain syndrome. In J. R. Fricton & E. Awad (Eds.), *Advances in pain research and therapy.* (vol. 17, p. 107). New York: Raven Press.

Fricton, J. R., Kroening, R., Haley, D., & Siegart, R. (1985). Myofascial pain syndrome of the head and neck: A review of clinical characteristics of 164 patients. *Oral Surgery, 60*, 615.

Gawel, M. G., Rothbart, P., & Jacobs, H. (1993). Subcutaneous sumatriptan in the treatment of acute episodes of post-traumatic headache. *Headache, 33*(2), 96–97.

Genazzani, A. R., Nappi, G., Gacchinetti, F. et al. (1984). Progressive impairment of CSF B-EP levels in migraine sufferers. *Pain, 18*, 127.

Giacovazzo, M., Bernoni, R. M., Di Sabato, F., & Martelletti, P. (1990). Impairment of 5HT binding to lymphocytes and monocytes from tension-type headache patients. *Headache, 30*, 20.

Gilkey, S. J., Ramadan, N. M., Aurora, T. K., & Welch, K. M. (1997). Cerebral blood flow in chronic posttraumatic headache. *Headache, 37*(9), 583–587.

Gobel, H., Heinze, A., Heinze-Kuhnk, A., & Jost, W. H. (2001). Evidence-based medicine: Botulinum toxin A in migraine and tension-type headache. *Journal of Neurology, 248*(Suppl 1), 34–38.

Gobel, H., Lindner, V., Krack, P. et al. (1999). Treatment of chronic tension-type headache with botulinum toxin. *Cephalalgia, 19*, 455.

Goldenberg, D. L. (1989). Diagnostic and therapeutic challenges of fibromyalgia. *Hospital Practice, 9*, 39.

Goldenberg, D. L. (1990). Fibromyalgia and chronic fatigue syndrome: Are they the same? *Journal of Musculoskeletal Medicine, 7*, 19.

Ham, L. P., & Packard, R. C. (1996). A retrospective, follow-up study of biofeedback-assisted relaxation therapy in patients with posttraumatic headache. *Biofeedback and Self-Regulation, 21*(2), 93–104.

Hanington, E., Jones, R. J., Amess, J. A. L., & Wachowicz, B. (1981). Migraine: A platelet disorder. *Lancet, ii*, 720.

Harker, L. A., & Rassekh, C. (1988). Migraine equivalent as a cause of episodic vertigo. *Laryngoscope, 98*, 160–164.

Harrison, D. W., & Walls, R. M. (1990). Blindness following minor head trauma in children: A report of two cases with a review of the literature. *Journal of Emergency Medicine, 8*, 21–24.

Haynes, S. N. (1981). Muscle contraction headache – A psychophysiological perspective. In S. N. Haynes & L. R. Gannon (Eds.), *Psychosomatic disorders: A psychophysiological approach to etiology and treatment*. New York: Praeger Press.

Haynes, S. N., Cuevas, J., & Gannon, L. R. (1982). The psychophysiological etiology of muscle-contraction headache. *Headache, 22*, 122.

Headache Classification Committee of the International Headache Society. (1988). Classification and diagnostic criteria for headache disorders, cranial neuralgias and facial pain. *Cephalalgia, 8*(Suppl 7), 1–96.

Hickling, E. J., Blanchard, E. B., Schwartz, S. P. et al. (1992). Headaches and motor vehicle accidents: Results of the psychological treatment of post-traumatic headache. *Headache Quarterly, 3*, 285–289.

Hong, S., Kniffki, K., & Schmidt, R. (1978). Pain abstracts. *Second World Congress on Pain 1*, 58.

Iansek, R., Heywood, J., Karnaghan, J., & Nalla, J. I. (1987). Cervical spondylosis and headaches. *Clinical and Experimental Neurology, 23e*, 175.

Jacobsen, S. A. (1963). *The posttraumatic syndrome following head injury* (pp. 63–65). Springfield, IL: Charles C Thomas.

Jansen, J., & Spoerri, O. (1985). Atypical retro-orbital pain and headache due to compression of upper cervical roots. In V. Pfaffenrath, P. O. Lundberg, & O. Sjaastad (Eds.), *Updating in headache* (pp. 14–16). Berlin: Springer-Verlag.

Jay, G. W. (1995a). Chronic daily headache and myofascial pain syndromes: Pathophysiology and treatment. In R. K. Cady & A. W. Fox (Eds.), *Treating the headache patient* (pp. 211–233). New York: Marcel Decker.

Jay, G. W. (1995b). Sympathetic aspects of myofascial pain. *Pain Digest, 5*, 192–194.

Jay, G. W. (1996). The autonomic nervous system: Anatomy and pharmacology. In P. Raj (Ed.), *Pain medicine – A comprehensive review* (pp. 461–465). St. Louis: Mosby.

Jay, G. W. (1999). *Headache handbook: Diagnosis and treatment* (pp. 17–32). Boca Raton, FL: CRC Press.

Jay, G. W. (2000). *Minor traumatic brain injury handbook: Diagnosis and treatment*. Boca Raton, FL: CRC Press.

Jay, G. W. (2003). Cluster headache. In A. O'Daly (Ed.), *Encyclopedia of life sciences*. London: Elsevier.

Jay, G. W., Brunson, J., & Branson, S. J. (1989).The effectiveness of physical therapy in the treatment of chronic daily headaches. *Headache, 29*, 156.

Jay, G. W., Grove, R. N., & Grove, K. S. (1987). Differentiation of chronic headache from non-headache pain patients using the Millon Clinical Multiaxial Inventory (MCMI). *Headache, 27*, 124.

Jennet, B., & Frankowski, R. F. (1990). The epidemiology of head injury. In R. Braakman (Ed.), *Handbook of clinical neurology* (p. 116). New York: Elsevier.

Kay, T., Harrington, D. E. et al. (1993). Definition of mild traumatic brain injury. *Journal of Head Trauma Rehabilitation 8*(3), 86.

Keidel, M., & Diener, H.C. (1997). Posttraumatic headache. *Nervenarzt, 68*(10), 769–777.

Keidel, M., Rieschke, P., Juptner, M., & Diener, H. C. (1994). Pathological jaw opening reflex after whiplash injury. *Nervenarzt, 65*(4), 241–249.

Keidel, M., Rieschke, P., Stude, P. et al. (2001). Antinociceptive reflex alteration in acute posttraumatic headache following whiplash injury. *Pain, 92*(3), 319–326.

Khurana, R. K. (1995). Oculocephalic sympathetic dysfunction in posttraumatic headaches. *Headache, 35*(10), 614–620.

Koch, P., Hirst, D. R., & von Wartburg, B. R. (1989). Biological fate of sirdalud in animals and man. *Xenobiotica, 19*, 1255–1265.

Kojadinovic, Z., Momcilovic, A., Popovic, L. et al. (1998). Brain concussion — A minor craniocerebral injury. *Medicinski Pregled, 51*, 165–168.

Kowa, H., Shimomura, T., & Takahashi, K. (1992). Platelet gamma-amino butyric acid levels in migraine and tension-type headache. *Headache, 32*, 229.

Kudrow, L. (1986). Muscle contraction headaches. In F. C. Rose (Ed.), *Handbook of clinical neurology* (vol. 48, p. 343). Amsterdam: Elsevier Science Publishing.

Lake, A. E., Branca, B., Lutz, T. E., & Saper, J. R. (1999). Headache level during neuropsychological testing and test performance in patients with chronic posttraumatic headache. *Journal of Head Trauma Rehabilitation, 14*(1), 70–80.

Langemark, M., & Jensen, K. (1988). Myofascial mechanisms of pain. In J. Olesen & L. Edvinsson (Eds.). *Basic mechanisms of headache* (p. 321). Amsterdam: Elsevier Science Publishers B.V.

Langemark, M., & Olesen, J. (1987). Pericranial tenderness in tension headache. A blind controlled study. *Cephalalgia, 7,* 249.

Langemark, M., Jensen, K., Jensen, T. S., & Olesen, J. (1989). Pressure pain thresholds and thermal nociceptive thresholds in chronic tension-type headache. *Pain, 38,* 203.

Langemark, M., Olesen, J., Poulsen, D. P., & Bech, P. (1988). Clinical characterization of patients with chronic tension headache. *Headache, 28,* 590.

Leisman, G. (1990). Lateralized effects of migraine and ANS seizures after closed head injury. *International Journal of Neuroscience, 54,* 63–82.

Lemka, M. (1999). Headache as the consequence of brain concussion and contusion in closed head injuries in children. *Journal of Neurology Neurochir Poland, 33*(Suppl 5), 37–48.

Leone, M., D'Amico, D., Grazzi, L. et al. (1998). Cervicogenic headache: A critical review of the current diagnostic criteria. *Pain, 78,* 1–5.

Lovell, M. R., Collins, M. W., Iverson, G.L. et al. (2003). Recovery from mild concussion in high school athletes. *Journal of Neurosurgery, 98*(2), 296–301.

Magnusson, T., & Carlsson, G. E. (1978a). Comparison between two groups of patients in respect to headache and mandibular dysfunction. *Swedish Dental Journal, 2,* 85.

Magnusson, T., & Carlsson, G. E. (1978b). Recurrent headaches in relation to temporomandibular joint pain-dysfunction. *Acta Odontologica Scandanivica, 36,* 333.

Malow, R. M., Grimm, L., & Olsen, R. E. (1980). Differences in pain perception between myofascial pain dysfunction and normal subjects: A signal detection analysis. *Journal of Psychosomatic Research, 24,* 303.

Marcus, D. A. (2003). Disability and chronic posttraumatic headache. *Headache, 43*(2), 117–121.

Martelli, M. F., Grayson, R. L, & Zasler, N. D. (1999). Posttraumatic headache: Neuropsychological and psychological effects and treatment implications. *Journal of Head Trauma Rehabilitation, 14*(1), 49–69.

Martin, M. J., & Rome, H. P. (1967). Muscle contraction headache: Therapeutic aspects. *Research and Clinical Studies in Headache 1,* 205.

Martin, P. R., & Mathews, A. M. (1978). Tension headaches: Psychophysiological investigation and treatment. *Journal of Psychosomatic Research, 22,* 389.

Mathew, N. T., Glaze, D., & Frost, J. (1985). Sleep apnea and other sleep abnormalities in primary headache disorders. In C. Rose (Ed.). *Migraine. Proceedings of the 5th International Migraine Symposium, London, 1984* (p. 40). Basel: Karger.

McBeath, J. G., & Nanda, A. (1994). Use of dihydroergotamine in patients with postconcussion syndrome. *Headache, 4,* 34(3), 148–151.

McBeath, J. G., & Nanda, A. (2000). Roller coaster migraine: An underreported injury? *Headache, 40*(9), 745–747.

Mense, S. (1993). Nociception from skeletal muscle in relation to clinical muscle pain. *Pain, 54,* 241–289.

Merskey, H., & Woodford, J. M. (1972). Psychiatric sequelae after minor head injury. *Brain, 95,* 521–528.

Mikail, M., & Rosen, H. (1980). History and etiology of myofascial pain-dysfunction syndrome. *Journal of Prosthetic Dentistry, 44,* 438.

Mikamo, K., Takeshima, T., & Takahashi, K. (1989). Cardiovascular sympathetic hypofunction in muscle contraction headache and migraine. *Headache, 29,* 86.

Miller, T. (2002). Retrospective cohort analysis of 48 chronic headache patients treated with botulinum toxin-type A (Botox) in a combination fixed injection site and follow-the-pain protocol [Abstract]. Presented at the American Headache Society Meeting, Seattle, WA, June 21–June 23.

Moldofsky, H., Scariabrick, P., England, R. et. al. (1975). Musculoskeletal symptoms and non-REM sleep disturbances in patients with fibrositis syndrome and healthy subjects. *Psychosomatic Medicine, 37,* 341.

Mork, H., Ashina, M., Bendtsen, L. et al. (2003). Induction of prolonged tenderness in patients with tension-type headache by means of a new experimental model of myofascial pain. *European Journal of Neurology, 10,* 249–256.

Moskowitz, M. A., & Cutrer, F. M. (1993). Sumatriptan: A receptor-targeted treatment for migraine. *Annual Review of Medicine, 44,* 145–154.

Mosnaim, A D., Diamond, S., Wolf, M. E. et al. (1989). Endogenous opioid-like peptides in headache: An overview. *Headache, 29,* 368.

Muller, G. E. (1974). Atypical early posttraumatic syndromes. *Acta Neurologica Belgica, 74,* 163–181.

Murphy, A. I., & Lehrer, P. M. (1990). Headache versus non-headache state: A study of electrophysiological and affective changes during muscle contraction headache. *Behavioral Medicine, 16,* 23.

Nappi, G., Gacchinetti, G., Legnante, G. et al. (1982). Impairment of the central and peripheral opioid system in headache. Paper presented at the Fourth International Migraine Trust Symposium, London.

Obelieniene, D., Bovim, G., Schrader, H. et al. (1998). Headache after whiplash: A historical cohort study outside the medico-legal context. *Cephalalgia, 18,* 559–564.

Olesen, J. (1978). Some clinical features of the acute migraine attack. An analysis of 750 patients. *Headache, 18,* 268.

Olesen, J. (1988). Clinical characterization of tension headache. In J. Olesen & L. Edvinsson (Eds.), *Basic mechanisms of headache* (p. 9). Amsterdam: Elsevier Science.

Olesen, J. (1991). Clinical and pathophysiologic observations in migraine and tension-type headache explained by integration of vascular, supraspinal and myofascial inputs. *Pain, 46,* 125–132.

Packard, R., & Ham, L. P. (1994). Posttraumatic headache. *Journal of Neuropsychiatry and Clinical Neuroscience, 6*(3), 229–236.

Packard, R. C. (2000). Treatment of chronic daily posttraumatic headache with divalproex sodium. *Headache, 40*(9), 736–739.

Packard, R. C., & Ham, L. P. (1993a). Impairment ratings for posttraumatic headache. *Headache, 33*(7), 359–364.

Packard, R.C., & Ham, L. P. (1993b). Posttraumatic headache: determining chronicity. *Headache, 33*(3), 133–134.

Packard, R. C., & Ham, L. P. (1997). Pathogenesis of posttraumatic headache and migraine: A common headache pathway? *Headache, 37,* 42–52.

Packard, R. C., Weaver, R., & Ham, L.P. (1993). Cognitive symptoms in patients with posttraumatic headache. *Headache, 33*(7), 365–368.

Palmeri, A., & Wiesendanger, M. (1990). Concomitant depression of locus coeruleus neurons and of flexor reflexes by an alpha$_2$-adrenergic agonist in rats: A possible mechanism for an alpha$_2$-mediated muscle relaxation. *Neuroscience, 34,* 177–187.

Perl, S., Markle, P., & Katz, L. N. (1934). Factors involved in the production of skeletal muscle pain. *Archives of Internal Medicine, 53,* 814.

Pernow, B. (1983). Substance P. *Pharmacological Reviews, 35,* 85.

Pfaffenrath, V., & Kaube, H. (1990). Diagnostics of cervicogenic headache. *Functional Neurology, 5,* 159–164.

Philips, C. (1978). Tension headache: Theoretical problems. *Behaviour Research and Therapy, 16,* 249.

Philips, C., & Hunter, M. S. (1982). A psychophysiological investigation of tension headache. *Headache, 22,* 173.

Pikus, H., & Phillips, J. (1995). Characteristics of patients successfully treated for cervicogenic headache by surgical decompression of the second cervical nerve root. *Headache, 35,* 621–629.

Poletti, C. E. (1983). Proposed operation for occipital neuralgia: C2 and C3 root decompression. *Neurosurgery, 12,* 221–224.

Pozniak-Patewicz, E. (1976). Cephalgic spasm of head and neck muscles. *Headache, 15,* 261.

Professional's handbook of drug therapy for pain. (2001). Springhouse, Pennsylvania: Springhouse.

Radanov, B. P., Di Stefano, G., & Augustiny, K. F. (2001). Symptomatic approach to posttraumatic headache and its possible implications for treatment. *European Spine Journal, 10*(5), 403–407.

Raskin, N. H. (1988a). On the origin of head pain. *Headache, 28,* 254.

Raskin, N. H.(1988b). *Headache* (2nd ed.). New York: Churchill Livingstone.

Riley, T. L. (1983). Muscle-contraction headache. *Neurologic Clinics, 1,* 489.

Robinson, C. A. (1980). Cervical spondylosis and muscle contraction headaches. In D. J. Dalessio (Ed.), *Wolff's headache and other head pain* (4th ed., p. 362). New York: Oxford University Press.

Rodbard, S. (1970). Pain associated with muscle contraction. *Headache, 10,* 105.

Rogal, O. J. (1986). Successful treatment for head, facial and neck pain. *The TMJ Dental Trauma Center, 1,* 3–10.

Rogal, O. J. (1995). Rhizotomy procedures about the face and neck for headaches. Paper presented at the North American Cervicogenic Headache Conference, Toronto, Canada, September.

Rolf, L. H., Wiele, G., & Brune, G. G. (1981). 5-hydroxytryptamine in platelets of patients with muscle contraction headache. *Headache, 21,* 10.

Rollnik, J. D. Tanneberger, O., Schubert, M. et al. (2000). Treatment of tension-type headache with botulinum toxin-type A: A double-blind, placebo-controlled study. *Headache, 40,* 300.

Rosenhall, U., Johansson, G., & Orndahl, G. (1987). Eye motility dysfunction in patients with chronic muscular pain and dysesthesia. *Scandinavian Journal of Rehabilitation Medicine, 19,* 139.

Sakas, D. E., Whittaker, K. W., Whitwell, H. L., & Singounas, E. G. (1997). Syndromes of posttraumatic neurological deterioration in children with no focal lesions revealed by cerebral imaging: Evidence for a trigeminovascular pathophysiology. *Neurosurgery, 41*(3), 661–667.

Sakuta, M. (1990). Significance of flexed posture and neck instability as a cause of chronic muscle contraction headache. *Rinsho Shinkeigato, 30,* 254.

Sallis, R. E., & Jones, K. (2000). Prevalence of headaches in football players. *Medicine and Science in Sports and Exercise, 32*(11), 1820–1824.

Sayers, A. C., Burki, H. R., & Eichenberger, E. (1980). The pharmacology of 5-chloro-4-(2-imidazolin-2gamma-1-amino)-2,1,3-benzothiadiazole (DS 103 282), a novel myotonic agent. *Arzneimittelforschung, 30,* 793–803.

Schmidtke, K., & Ehmsen, L. (1998). Transient global amnesia and migraine. A case control study. *European Neurology, 40,* 9–14.

Shahota, P. K., & Dexter, J. D. S. (1990). Sleep and headache syndromes: A clinical review. *Headache, 30,* 80.

Shealy, C. N. (1995). Spinally mediated headache. In R. K. Cady & A. W. Fox (Eds.), *Treating the headache patient* (pp. 235–256). New York, Marcel Dekker.

Shimomura, T., & Takahashi, K. (1986). Pupillary functional asymmetry in patients with muscle contraction headache. *Cephalalgia, 6,* 141.

Shimomura, T., & Takahashi, K. (1990). Alteration of platelet serotonin in patients with chronic tension-type headache during cold pressor test. *Headache, 30,* 581.

Shoenen, J., Pasqua, V. D., & Sianard-Gainko, J. (1991). Multiple clinical and paraclinical analyses of chronic tension-type headache associated or unassociated with disorder of the pericranial muscles. *Cephalalgia, 11,* 135.

Sicuteri, F. (1982). Natural opioids in migraine. In M. Critchley, A. P. Friedman, S. Gorini et al. (Eds.), *Advances in neurology* (vol. 33, p. 65). New York: Raven Press.

Sicuteri, F., Nicolodi, M., & Fusco, B. M. (1988). Abnormal sensitivity to neurotransmitter agonists, antagonists and neurotransmitter releasers. In J. Olesen & L. Edvinsson (Eds.), *Basic mechanisms of headache* (p. 275). Amsterdam: Elsevier Science.

Sicuteri, F., Spillantini, M.G., & Fanciullacci, M. (1985). "Enkephalinase" in migraine and opiate addiction. In C. Rose (Ed.), *Migraine: Proceedings of the Fifth International Migraine Symposium* (p. 86). Basel: S. Karger.

Simons, D. J., Day, E., Goodell, H., & Wolff, H. G. (1943). Experimental studies on headache: Muscles of the scalp and neck as sources of pain. *Associated Research on Nervous and Mental Disorders Proceedings, 23,* 228.

Sjaastad, O., Bovim, G., & Stovner, L. J. (1992). Laterality of pain and other migraine criteria in common migraine. A comparison with cervicogenic headache. *Functional Neurology, 7,* 289–294.

Sjaastad, O., Fredriksen, T. A., & Pfaffenrath, V. (1990). Cervicogenic headache diagnostic criterion. *Headache, 30,* 725–726.

Sluijter, M. E. (1990). Radiofrequency lesions in the treatment of cervical pain syndromes. *Procedure Technique Series* (pp. 2–19). Holland: Radionics.

Smuts, J. A., Baker, M. K., Smuts, H. M. et al. (1999). Botulinum toxin-type A as prophylactic treatment in chronic tension-type headache. *Cephalalgia, 19,* 454.

Solomon, S. (1998). John Graham Senior Clinicians Award Lecture. Posttraumatic migraine. *Headache, 38*(10), 772–778.

Solomon, S. (2001). Posttraumatic headache. *Medical Clinics of North America, 85*(4), 987–996.

Speed, W. G. (1983). Muscle contraction headaches. In J. R. Saper (Ed.), *Headache disorders* (p. 115). Boston: John Wright.

Takeshima, T., Takao, Y. U., Urakami, K. et al. (1989). Muscle contraction headache and migraine. Platelet activation and plasma norepinephrine during the cold pressor test. *Cephalalgia, 9,* 7.

Takeshima, T., Takao, Y., & Takahashi, K. (1987). Pupillary sympathetic hypofunction and asymmetry in muscle contraction headache. *Cephalalgia, 7,* 257.

Tfelt-Hansen, P., Lous, I., & Olesen, J. (1981). Prevalence and significance of muscle tenderness during common migraine attack. *Headache, 21,* 49.

Travell, J., & Rinzler, S. H. (1952). The myofascial genesis of pain. *Postgraduate Medicine, 11,* 425–434.

Travell, J. G., & Simons, D. G. (1983). *Myofascial pain and dysfunction: The trigger point manual.* Baltimore, Williams and Wilkins.

Treleaven, J., Jull, G., & Atkinson, L. (1994). Cervical musculoskeletal dysfunction in post-concussional headache. *Cephalalgia, 14,* 273–279.

Troost, B. (2002). Botulinum toxin-type A (Botox, Allergan, Irvine, CA) therapy for intractable headaches [Abstract]. Presented at the American Headache Society Meeting, Seattle, WA, June 21–June 23.

Tunis, M. M., & Wolff, H. G. (1954). Studies on headache: cranial artery vasoconstriction and muscle contraction headache. *Archives of Neurology and Psychiatry 71,* 425.

Uomoto, J. M., & Esselman, P. C. (1993). Traumatic brain injury and chronic pain: Differential types and rates by head injury severity. *Archives of Physical Medicine and Rehabilitation, 74*(1), 61–64.

Vijayan, N. (1977). A new post-traumatic headache syndrome. *Headache, 17,* 19–22.

Vohanka, S., & Zouhar, A. (1990). Benign posttraumatic encephalopathy. *Activitas Nervosa Superior (Praha), 32,* 179–183.

Vohanka, S., & Zouhar, A. (1988). Transient global amnesia after mild head injury in childhood. *Activitas Nervosa Superior (Praha), 30,* 68–74.

Wagstaff, A. J., & Bryson, H. (1997). Tizanidine: A review of its pharmacology, clinical efficacy and tolerability in the management of spasticity associated with cerebral and spinal disorders. *Drugs, 53,* 435–452.

Wall, P. D. (1988). Stability and instability of central pain mechanisms. In R. Dubner & M. R. Bond (Eds.), *Proceedings of the Fifth World Conference on Pain* (p. 13). Amsterdam: Elsevier Science.

Watanabe, Y., Saito, H., & Abe, K. (1993). Tricyclic antidepressants block NMDA receptor-mediated synaptic responses and induction of long-term potentiation in rat hippocampal slices. *Neuropharmacology, 32,* 479–486.

World Health Organization. (1997) ICD-10 Guide for headaches. *Cephalalgia, 17,* S19.

Yagamuchi, M. (1992). Incidence of headache and severity of head injury. *Headache, 32,* 427–431.

Yang, J. C., Richlin, D., Brand, L., Wagner, J., & Clark, W. C. (1985). Thermal sensory decision theory indices and pain threshold in chronic pain patients and healthy volunteers. *Psychological Medicine, 47,* 461.

Zasler, N. D. (1999). Posttraumatic tension pneumocephalus. *Journal of Head Trauma Rehabilitation, 14*(1), 81–84.

Zwart, J. A. (1997). Neck mobility in different headache disorders. *Headache, 37,* 6–11.

27

Temporomandibular Joint Dysfunction

Christopher R. Brown, DDS, MPS

INTRODUCTION

The art and science of the diagnosis and management of temporomandibular joint (TMJ) dysfunction has come a long way since its humble beginnings in the 1920s. Since then, many treatment philosophies have come and gone. Often patients have been bounced from one treatment discipline to another, leaving them feeling rejected, ignored, and depressed, with little effective resolution of their pain. There have been many attempts to find the "solution" to this baffling problem in both dentistry and medicine. The truth of the matter is there is not a single solution to TMJ dysfunction because it is not a single entity; rather, it is a group of problems from different etiologies lumped under one broad and often generic diagnosis. The most effective way to help patients suffering from head, neck, and facial pain, collectively called TMJ dysfunction, is for all practitioners of the arts to work together to achieve an accurate diagnosis and resulting management. The technology, knowledge, and training exist to bring all professions together to assist in the alleviation of head, neck, and facial pain.

The abbreviation TMJ is a very misused term. It is commonly used descriptively both as human anatomy and also erroneously as a diagnostic entity. The term TMJ used correctly describes only the temporomandibular joints, which are diarthroidal joints connecting the mandible to the skull. When delineating a dysfunction of the TMJs, the term TMD is the more accepted term, "D" referring to the dysfunction of the TMJs. The term TMD is in and of itself a very vague diagnosis. In fact, TMD does not indicate a single diagnostic entity but rather a collection of symptoms affecting or arising from the TMJs, the muscles of mastication, and/or contiguous soft and hard tissue

entities. This accounts for much confusion within the professional community of all disciplines that diagnose and treat facial pain. TMD is often used to describe collectively anything from sore muscles of the face from cheering too hard at a ballgame all the way to advanced degenerative joint disease. As a result, many patients, clinicians, and third-party payers have found themselves in a virtual no man's land of confusion.

The occurrence of TMD symptoms will vary according to epidemiological studies (Kaplan & Assael, 1991). Symptomatically, it has been conservatively estimated that more than 10 million people in the United States suffer from symptoms attributed to TMD. Up to 75% of nonpatient populations have at least one sign of TMJ dysfunction. Approximately 33% of these have at least one painful symptom in the face or TMJs. While reports may differ somewhat among epidemiological estimations, TMD sufferers are most commonly females (a ratio of 5 to 1) between the ages of 15 and 45 years (Cady & Fox, 1995). It is a real problem that costs the United States billions of dollars in health care and lost days of productivity.

Historically, Costen in 1934 first addressed this entity by hypothesizing that lost vertical dimension in the facial structures was the main source of symptomatology (Bell, 1982). As a result, the idea of "opening the bite" through various forms of dental reconstruction became the chief pathway to problem solving; hence, the field of TMJ fell into dentistry and the role of occlusion as the dominant etiological factor was conceptualized. Dentistry, as a leader in TMD treatment, began a strict focus in the role of occlusion and alterations of mandibular position to reduce or eliminate facial pain. Unfortunately, the treatment approach for TMD has often been as if it was a single disease entity. The search has been for an answer to a very complex problem that often requires multiple treatment modalities and interdisciplinary approaches. Although there have been concerted efforts to discover the cure for TMD, logic would dictate that the first approach, as in any disease entity, should be to achieve an accurate working differential diagnosis. Through the decades following Costen's initial approach, scientific constructs have begun to emerge. Dentistry along with a multidisciplinary approach has begun to find workable solutions for TMJ/facial pain resolution.

ANATOMY

Functionally, the TMJs involve the articulation of the mandibular condyles in the temporal bones. The fossae are the concavities hosting the mandibular condyles and the eminentiae are the bony convexities anterior to the fossae. The articulating surfaces of the temporal bones consist of concave, thin bony surfaces or fossae, and convex, thick bony surfaces or eminentiae. In addition, the TMJs include soft tissue structures including the articulating discs (menisci), retrodistal tissues, joint capsules, and synovium. The discs medially and laterally insert at the medial and lateral poles of the condyles. Anteriorly, the discs are continuous with the superior belly of the lateral pterygoid muscles. The temporomandibular capsule is a dense fibrous tissue sheet enclosing each joint in a 360° fashion with its insertion lines at the neck of the condyle below and at the temporal bone above. The upper and lower compartments of the TMJs have a synovial lining, which appears to have a highly active immunologic ability to produce antibodies, and collagenase type materials, which help to protect and ensure the continuity of the synovial fluid. The TMJs, while considered synovial joints, actually have a number of attributes that distinguish themselves from other synovial joints in the human body. The TM joints' articulating surfaces are covered by fibrocartilage rather than hyaline. They are actually divided into upper and lower compartments by a fibrous meniscus (disc), the purpose of which is to help facilitate the motions of both rotation and translation. TMJs are the only joints in the human body that must work in harmony with another joint during function and dysfunction. A dysfunctional joint often will create an equal and opposite force on the contralateral joint (e.g., hypomovement on the left can produce hyperfunction on the right). The function of the TMJs can be influenced by masticatory muscles, supportive structures of the joints, teeth, and parafunctional activities.

The anatomy of TMJs provides both rotational and translational movement. The TMJs are actually formed by the mandibular condyles fitting into the glenoid fossae of the temporal bones. The condyle and glenoid fossae are separated by a fibrous cartilage disc (meniscus), which divides the joint into the upper and lower chambers. The articular portion of the disc, which is composed of connective tissue, is devoid of any nerves or vessels. The posterior attachment of the disc, however, is richly vascularized and innervated. The disc itself is attached to the condyle both medially and laterally by collateral ligaments that permit both rotational and translational movement of the disc/condyle complex during opening and closing of the mouth. Rotational movement occurs between the condyle and the surface of the disc during early opening, while translation takes place in the space between the superior surface of the disc and the glenoid fossa. Synovial fluid provides lubrication to the joint and acts as a medium for transporting nutrients and waste products to and from the articular surfaces. The joint surface cartilage and the attached structures allow for an almost frictionless articulation while transmitting compressive forces uniformly to the subchondral bone (Bumann & Lotzmann, 2002).

SUPPORTING MUSCULATURE

Mandibular movement and stability are assisted by a series of skeletal muscles. The primary masticatory muscles include the masseter, medial pterygoid, temporalis, digastric, and lateral pterygoid muscles, which are further divided into the inferior and superior belly. All muscles collectively account for mandibular motion and provide stabilization for the condyle/disc during function. Musculoskeletal disturbances of the entire body are the leading cause of disability in people in their working years (Mense & Simons, 2001). A majority of collective symptomatic orofacial pain complaints are musculoskeletal in nature which may lead to TMJ articular dysfunction. Muscle pain complaints often include myofascial trigger points and resulting skeletal unit restriction.

INNERVATION AND VASCULAR SUPPLY

The innervation of the TMJs and supporting structures is primarily supplied by the trigeminal and facial nerves. The trigeminal nerve (cranial nerve V) provides both sensory and motor innervation and, hence, is the primary nerve that supplies the TMJs themselves. Sensory fibers of the trigeminal nerve extend to synapses in the trigeminal spinal nucleus of the brainstem. The trigeminal nerve is divided into three branches: the ophthalmic, maxillary, and mandibular. The mandibular nerve provides sensory and/or motor branches to the medial and lateral pterygoid muscles, temporalis, masseter, and TMJs via the auriculotemporal nerve, which while passing behind the TMJs, emerges distal to the condyle, then traverses into the temporal area. It also supplies sensory perception to the tongue and the lower teeth. The TMJs primary nerve supplies arise from the auriculotemporal nerve posteriorly, the masseteric nerve medially, and the posterior deep temporal nerve laterally. While the facial nerve (cranial nerve

VII) does not directly supply the TMJs per se, it does provide motor and sensory functions to associated musculature and supporting structures including the orbicularis oculi and the anterior two thirds of the tongue. Afferent information from sensory receptors produces stimuli causing both concurrent muscular contraction and inhibition resulting in antagonistic inhibition. This myotatic reflex helps protect the masticatory from sudden stretching of the muscles. Golgi tendon organs protect against muscle overcontraction by inhibition stimulation directly to the affected muscles (Okeson, 1989). The result is a complex control system allowing for both protection and function. The arterial supply to the TMJs originates from the superficial temporal artery (posterior to the joint), the posterior auricular artery, the deep auricular artery, the lateral-pterygoid pedicle, and the masseteric artery; the last three are branches of the maxillary artery.

CLASSIFICATION OF TM DISORDERS

A classification system for TM disorders, as originally presented by Bell (1989), is presented in Table 27.1. This system is more accurately a categorization of orofacial pain etiologies, rather than TMD alone, and suggests correctly that TMD is actually a continuum of disorders rather than a single clinical entity.

SYMPTOMOLOGY

The symptoms involved with TMD are often varied and at first may seem unrelated. An old catchphrase for TMD was "the great imposter." This moniker was given because of the diversity of symptoms that may be attributed to other conditions as well. Any or all of the following may be as a result of TMD: (1) TMJ noise (popping, clicking, grinding, crepitation), (2) mandibular trismus or the inability to open the mouth uniformly (can be measured in lack of opening or deviation of the mandible from the midline), (3) pain in or approximating the TMJs, (4) headaches (bilateral, unilateral, occipital, frontal, that may be exacerbated by chewing or stress), (5) neck aches, (6) inability to properly fit the maxillary and mandibular teeth together (this may be perceived by the patient as "not a normal bite"), (7) facial pain on chewing (located around the TMJs or perceived by the patient as a headache, earache), (8) tinnitus, (9) earache (bilateral, unilateral, in the absence of ear pathology), (10) excessive ear wax (usually found in conjunction with chronic retrodistal inflammation and posterior displacement of the condyle), (11) photosensitivity, (12) dysphagia, (13) palpable masticatory muscle trigger points, and (14) myalgia (generalized in the head and neck or focalized in the masticatory muscles).

The severity of these symptoms may range from annoying to debilitating. They also may fluctuate with

TABLE 27.1
Classification of TM Disorders

I. Physical (non-neurogenic) Origins of Pain
   A. Superficial somatic pain
      1. Cutaneous
      2. Mucogingival
   B. Deep somatic pain
      1. Musculoskeletal pain
         a. Muscle pain
            i. Protective splinting
            ii. Myofascial trigger point pain
            iii. Muscle spasm pain
            iv. Muscle inflammation pain
         b. Temporomandibular joint pain
            i. Disc attachment pain
            ii. Retrodistal pain
            iii. Capsular pain
            iv. Arthritic pain
         c. Osseous and periosteal pain
         d. Soft connective tissue pain
         e. Periodontal dental pain
      2. Visceral pain
         a. Pulpal dental pain
         b. Vascular pain
II. Neurogenic Pain
   A. Neuropathic
      1. Traumatic neuroma
      2. Paroxysmal neuralgia
         a. Idiopathic neuralgia
         b. Symptomatic neuralgia
      3. Neuritic neuralgia
         a. Peripheral neuritis
         b. Herpes zoster
         c. Post-herpetic neuralgia
   B. Deafferentation pain
      1. Sympathetically maintained pain syndromes
      2. Anesthesia dolorosa
      3. Phantom pain
III. Psychogenic Origins of Pain
   A. Chronic facial pain
   B. Psychoneurotic pain
      1. Conversion hysteria
      2. Delusional pain

time. It is not unusual for patients to go through a period of quiescence. As in any nonmalignant pain entity, fluctuations of intensity and duration are to be expected.

WHY DO THE TMJs MAKE NOISE?

The TMJs "pop," "click," and/or "crunch" for a variety of reasons. The most common clinical situation is a displacement of the disc(s) to the anterior/medial with a resulting distalization of the condylar head(s) within the glenoid fossae. These conditions result in the classic "popping" of the TMJ(s). A chronic displacement of the disc(s), especially in women, may lead to degeneration of the condylar head(s), distortion of the disc(s), and total dysfunction of the TMJ(s) resulting in pain. As this degeneration progresses, the noises emitted by the TMJs may change to crepitation as a result of a roughening of the articulating surfaces or soft tissue articular breakdown. Along with this degeneration often comes restriction of mandibular range of motion, loss of function, and an increase in pain. In certain individuals, ischemic necrosis of the condylar heads may exacerbate the situation.

Anatomical variations, such as aberrations of the condylar heads, discs, capsular lining, retrodistal tissues, and articulating surfaces, that are nonpathological, may cause the TMJs to make noise. Various types of arthritic conditions that lead to articular surface degeneration can also contribute as in any synovial joint. Growths or foreign bodies present within the TMJs, although rare, must be ruled out in the presence of TMJ noise. A careful analysis of the individual patient must be accomplished to determine if the joint noises are pathologic, contributory to pain, or circumstantial. A cursory examination can be accomplished by fingertip palpation, auscultation by stethoscope, or Doppler. Achieving a definitive diagnosis may require the use of computer-aided diagnostics including joint vibrational analysis, EMGs, MRIs, and a combination of radiographs.

ETIOLOGIES OF TMD PAIN

The most common origin of TMD-type pain is musculoskeletal and its various subsets. Other etiologies can include neurological, vascular, cartilage, bone, and dental. Aside from anatomically specific functional disorders, the TMJs are subject to the same pathology that affects other synovial joints such as various kinds of arthritis, synovitis, hyperuricemia, neoplasia, and fibrosis (Bell, 1982). Patients may have pain from multiple sources producing similar symptoms all of which may need to be addressed for effective pain management (Raj, 2003).

TMD and orofacial pain cannot be approached as a unique entity from the rest of the body in which the laws of human physiology and physics do not apply. Although there are several factors that make the TMJs anatomically and functionally unique, their form, function, and physiology are very similar to other synovial joints. When making clinical assessments of TMJ dysfunction and resulting orofacial pain, keep in mind the principles of treating other joints. This concept will help guide an accurate differential diagnosis. There are no other joints in the body for which there has been such a zealous search for a solution for pain and dysfunction. The answer is actually simple, in a roundabout way. There is not a single answer to the entity known as TMD. It is without a doubt multifactorial in nature, both symptomatically and etiologically. For suc-

cessful resolution, clinicians from various disciplines must work together.

Any malady with multiple etiologies and various precipitating factors does not accommodate the scientific model desired for clinical study. Close scrutiny of clinical studies to measure and delineate pain involving humans and their idiosyncrasies results in scientific flaws when compared with laboratory controlled tests. The best that can be accomplished is a blend of academia, clinical study, and common sense. While trends can be followed and measured, epidemiological studies must be estimated and weighed in conjunction with unique individual factors to achieve a full understanding of the pain entity.

THE ROLE OF OCCLUSION

The importance of occlusion in the etiology of TMD is controversial. Occlusion, from an epidemiology standpoint, does not as a whole play a dominant role in TMD. Occlusal factors should be considered, although as possible contributing factors, when developing a differential diagnosis on an individual basis (McNeill, 1993). Occlusal factors may place the patient at a higher risk for dysfunctions and parafunctional activities, which may result in orofacial pain. Occlusion may play a major role in a given individual and his or her painful state. Another person suffering from similar symptoms may not have occlusion as an etiology. The treating doctor, however, must have a thorough understanding of occlusion to help provide a differential diagnosis. Malocclusion, like all other variables, may be a subset of pain etiologies that needs to be understood and analyzed. The kinematics of the stomatognathic system requires harmony of all components for normal pain-free function. Any aspect of the system at any give time may dominate causing dysfunction with resulting pain. Therefore, a multidisciplinary approach usually yields the best clinical results.

TRAUMA

Trauma is one of the most common etiologies of TMD. In fact, it has been estimated that trauma accounts for the majority of TMDs (McNeill, 1993). According to Shankland, 1998), it is estimated that 44 to 99% of all TMJ problems are a result of trauma.

Direct trauma to the mandible, depending on the pulse duration and force vectors, is capable of injuring the TMJs. This can be in the form of soft tissue damage or bony involvement. There is no such thing as a pure direct blow except under strict laboratory conditions. Resulting injuries may depend on the position of the head on an *X/Y* axis, the position of the mandible at the time of impact, the angle of the blow, the amount of soft tissue to absorb the blow, the modulus of elasticity of the individual's tissue under those particular circumstances, etc. Even under the banner of "direct trauma," all these factors lead to other forces often thought of as indirect such as shear, torsion, compression, and tension. While injury categories are certainly evident and can be theoretically delineated, each person's physical response to trauma is unique. Keep in mind the term *direct* is descriptive as to the point of impact only and to the tissue precisely affected and not to the total injury component. Every *direct* injury has a facet of *indirect* as well.

Soft tissue injuries to the TMJs can be the result of direct blows to the mandible. The categories of these injuries are considered the result of "crush" type forces. Because of the nature of the anatomy, there are various soft tissue components (menisci, cartilage, blood vessels, etc.) juxtapositioned between bony surfaces, the condylar head, the superior articulating surface of the bony socket, and the distal and medial aspects of the socket. When a condyle is forced beyond its physiological range either anteriorly or posteriorly, especially in rapid motion, the chance of a crush-type injury exists. The result is a disruption of the joint surfaces and supporting tissues on both a cellular and macrolevel. Hemarthrosis may result, leading not only to an acute situation, but also to a synovitis that contributes to inflammation of the affected surfaced resulting in long-term articular degeneration and possible degenerative joint disease.

Direct blows to the mandible or TMJs causing immediate soft tissue damage usually result in a rapid onset of symptoms. This is a generalization and must be ascertained with each patient's unique situation. It is not uncommon for the victim to feel a change in occlusion, noticing their teeth do not match together normally, soon after the traumatic event. If the meniscus/menisci are anteriorly displaced but within the physiologic range of motion of the condylar head, the injury may be accompanied by popping or clicking of the TMJs due to displacement of the menisci. This may be unilateral or bilateral. If unilateral, this noise may be accompanied by trismus or deviation of the mandible to the side of the disc displacement. This is in essence a hypomobility/subluxation of the affected TMJ. By nature, the contralateral side results in hypermobility with a deviation of the mandible away from the joint. Another possibility as a result of a direct blow, if there is an influx of fluid into the affected joint, the void left by a displaced disc may be filled by fluid volume resulting in no noticeable joint noise. This lack of joint noise can often lead to a misdiagnosing of TMJ injuries and to a lag time or what is commonly referred to as "latency period" before effective treatment can be initiated.

In some cases, the force and pulse duration is such that the disc is displaced beyond the physiologic range of motion of the condylar head resulting in a disc displacement that is not "recaptured" during motion. The result is a severely injured TMJ that does not make noise, unaffected mandibular range of motion, and little if any deviation of the mandible. This is a particularly difficult injury to diagnose initially due to the lack of overt clinical symptoms. The clinician must be astute and soft tissue injuries must be considered as a result of direct blows to the mandible. A one-time examination may not be sufficient to develop a true diagnosis. The patient should be seen on a 2-week, 6-week, and up to 6-month follow-up to determine if function is altered and a micro/cellular level injury has led to an alteration in system function.

A form of direct impact to the face that is becoming more prevalent is air bag inflations. While there is no question that air bags save lives, it has also been indicated that passengers who do not wear their seat belts and those who sit so close to the air bags that they receive the full force of inflation may actually have a greater chance of injury in low-speed collisions (Hollowell & Stucki, 1974). Careful review of crash test films indicates that often the dummies contacting the air bags lead with their chins. Because of the dummies' construction, the forces to the TMJs have not been measured, but dentists across the nation are reporting patients with broken teeth, facial abrasions, facial bone fractures, and TMJ disc displacements as a result of impacts with air bags. As a rule of thumb, when you have a patient who has been involved in a motor vehicle accident with sufficient force to inflate an air bag, suspect a TMJ injury.

INDIRECT TRAUMA

Think of the head, neck, and mandible in the form of a free body diagram, each a separate entity held together by various soft tissue components. In a direct blow to the mandible, for instance, there is a point of impact at which blunt trauma (crush) can occur. If there is enough force, the mandible is moved along a vector line until it contacts another bony component (the skull). The force transmitted moves the skull along the same vector that will ultimately cause movement of the neck as well. Along and between the bony interfaces and interconnections lie various soft tissues, which absorb the shock and are subjected to these forces.

In an indirect injury to the TMJs from acceleration injury (whiplash) in a rear-end motor vehicle accident (REMVA), the dynamics and chain of events change, but the results are similar. In a REMVA, the auto actually moves out from under the occupant. The first movement is the relative forward motion of the torso followed by movement of the neck occurring within 0.1 to 0.2 seconds. There is a lag time of skull movement during this motion. The skull moves both translationally for a brief period of time and in an arch around the movement of the neck (rotational). Considering the component of a free body diagram, there is also a lag time regarding mandibular movement when comparing the mandible to the skull and the cervical column. This movement is also both translational and rotational by nature of the anatomy. This lag time forces the soft tissues to absorb the energy involved while going from standing still (zero acceleration) to multidirectional movement. If the soft tissues did not absorb this movement the skull and mandible would disarticulate. The time period of energy transfer is so short that there is often movement of the head, neck, and TMJs before the Golgi tendon organs have time to fire the muscle bundles for resistance, resulting in muscular damage on either a microlevel, macrolevel, or both (Foust et al, 1974; Schneider et al., 1975). Once this absorption has been completed and the various body components are in motion, yet at different vectors, the movement is interrupted by the neck and torso contacting the seat or head rest. There comes a brief moment when all rearward movement is stopped with multidirectional compressive forces on the "shock absorbers," which are the soft tissues. The whole process is begun again in reverse with the skull leading the way arching around the neck and mandible, producing large compressive and shear forces on the supporting soft tissues as the body goes through the rebound stage of deceleration.

There are aspects of indirect trauma in acceleration injuries in which the victim did not hit his or her head that warrant attention. The first is *contact among the mandible, skull, and cervical spine*. The only thing that actually stops bone striking bone is the soft tissue components. The amount of forces involved is influenced greatly by the acceleration of the various body parts both in unison and relatively with each other. $F = M \times A$ (F = force, M = mass, A = acceleration). The second is *the neck and skull striking the head rest*. It has been indicated that head rests are often not designed properly to stop cervical injuries (Anonymous, 1995). The resulting forces in some instances may in fact be magnified, resulting in added forces to the neck. The third is *the chin hitting the chest during the ride down or deceleration phase*. It has been suggested that striking the chin on the chest reduces the forces on the cervical spine (Mertz & Patrick, 1967). The law of conservation of energy, however, dictates that the forces must go somewhere. They are not dissipated. The resulting stresses on the mandible and, therefore, the TMJs may increase as a result. Last, due to the shortness of the force duration and confusion and disorientation of the occupants, the patient's history regarding this brief period is not always reliable. The actual time of impact is very short, averaging between .1 and .2 seconds. The victim's recollection may or may not be accurate. The actual resulting injuries to the body are a more significant indication of trauma.

Many chronic TMJ disorders may not be readily apparent at the initial injury and may be temporally removed from the development of symptoms (Raj, 1996). It is not uncommon for a latency period to exist between the traumatic event and the dysfunction and pain in the TMJs and soft tissue supporting structures. This relatively asymptomatic period of time can extend from 3 to 6 months. Because acceleration-induced TMD, by nature of human anatomy and REMVAs, are commonly associated with cervical injuries (Talley & Ousley, 1994), the focus on the cervical injuries, as well as the pain, often takes precedence over injuries to the TMJs. Cervical soft tissue injuries produce such similar symptoms that the two are often confused early in treatment. There is a direct connection between the trigeminal nerves that help mediate noxious stimuli and the motor movements of various structures of the TMJs, and the occipital nerves originating in the cervical spine. Anatomical dissections indicate direct anastomization of these two supposedly separate nervous components (Baburr, 1989; Cox & Cocks, 1979). A change in function of the musculature of the masticatory system via the occipital nerves and the trigeminal system may result, leading to a delayed onset of TMD symptoms without initial direct damage to the TMJs. Damage to the TMJs and their supporting structures can also occur on a cellular level and may take time to cause systemic changes that are perceived by the patient as pain. Microdamage in the human body may lead to macrodamage that leads to dysfunction. This process may take months to complete depending on which level damage has occurred and whether healing has taken place.

Resulting injuries can initiate a repetitive strain syndrome. As a result of trauma, the occlusal surfaces of the teeth may be the only component of the masticatory system that has not been altered. The unchanged occlusion takes over the masticatory system's dominant role causing a tug of war among edematous soft tissues of the TMJs themselves, dysfunctional muscles, damaged ligaments, strained capsules, and the teeth. This discrepancy may surface clinically as bruxism, exacerbating an already compromised functional ability. The result is a scenario not unlike other repetitive strain syndromes that result from biochemical insults, cellular breakdown, and eventually system breakdown as a function of repetitive dysfunction and time. Misdiagnosis is probably one of the leading causes of delay of treatment onset. People are often advised that the pain will go away and to wait. NSAIDs, muscle relaxants, and rest, while appropriate initially, may not be efficacious for a given patient. If pain and dysfunction persists then further evaluation and treatment is in order. The development of a good working relationship with dentists specifically trained in the diagnosis and treatment of TMD in a multidisciplinary team approach is extremely important for successful diagnosis and treatment.

PSYCHOGENIC ORIGINS

The exact role of emotional problems such as stress, anxiety, and depression in patients with TMD is uncertain. Diamond and Delessio (1980) report a phenomenon of "depression headache," which is a somatic characterization of depression. It has been suggested that almost any psychiatric disorder predisposes patients to tension-type headaches. Too often patients with clearly discernible signs of TMD have been diagnosed as having somatization of emotional disorders resulting in pain. The variability of pain complaints associated with frequent maladaptive behavioral psychosocial sequelae often leads clinicians to diagnose TMD problems as purely psychogenic. Having a good working relationship with a skilled dentist can prove vital in achieving an accurate diagnosis from which to initiate treatment. In many cases, chronic muscle spasm of the masticatory and cervical muscles results in a vague diagnosis of "tension" type headaches. After months of pain, the patient's serotonin level can become depleted resulting in clinical depression. This is sometimes coupled with many visits to multiple doctors all with no diagnosis, direction, or hope of recovery. Before a patient is relegated to the category of psychosomatic disorders or somatization, clinically demonstrable signs of TMD should be pursued by a dentist specifically trained in the diagnosis and management of TMD.

SLEEP DISTURBANCES

Sleep deprivation often accompanies chronic pain. The patient's situation can become a "chicken or egg" dilemma. It is known that the interruption of stage IV — deep restorative sleep — is common in patients with chronic pain (Cady & Fox, 1995). There are times sleep disturbances are initiated by an acute episode such as trauma or surgery and, when perpetuated, result in chronic sleep deprivation (Cady & Fox, 1995). On the front line of defense in treating TMD is to make sure the patient is sleeping well. There should be a differentiation between a lack of sleep due to pain and a true sleeping disorder, which may require the attention of a physician concentrating in the area of sleep disorders and deprivation.

TREATMENT OPTIONS

Traditionally, TMD treatment is divided into two phases. Phase I is the segment of treatment that includes all techniques designed for pain reduction, tissue healing, and restoring the TMJs to a state of quiescence. Phase II is the segment of treatment that corrects any discrepancies between the mandibular position, the teeth, and the supporting structures that is often thought of as the dental aspect of TMD treatment.

PHASE I

There is, of course, not one sole treatment mode that will help alleviate dysfunction of TMJs or the resulting pain. As in any problem, there are multiple ways to address issues and achieve clinical success. As a rule of thumb, a conservative approach should be used initially. Physical modalities such as moist heat, ice massage, rest, and a soft food diet should be attempted as a first line of defense. A mild exercise regimen may augment healing and reduction of symptoms. NSAIDs, muscle relaxants, and analgesics should be used as adjuncts for a limited period of time. Narcotics should be prescribed with caution due to the potential for both physical and/or emotional attenuation. As in any chronic pain condition, tricyclic antidepressants have been found efficacious both for the inhibition of serotonin uptake and as an adjunct for sleep.

If symptoms do not resolve rapidly, then an intraoral orthotic designed to relax the musculature and reduce intra- and extra-capsular inflammation should be employed. Pharmacological support as previously mentioned can help in pain reduction. Physical therapy modalities in conjunction with a guided rehabilitation program will help restore the patient to proper form and function. Other supportive care can be furnished by speech pathologists, occupational therapists, dietitians, massage therapists, and biofeedback programs.

Surgical intervention should be used with caution. Often arthrocentesis or arthroscopy is preferred over a full open joint procedure. There are times, due to severe degenerative joint disease, that more complex surgeries or variations of joint reconstruction may be needed. These, however, are rare, and careful case selection is tantamount to assuring success. Physical therapy rehabilitation is a must following any type of surgical intervention. The regimen must be carefully designed to restore the affected areas to proper physiologic function allowing for maximum medical improvement.

PHASE II

There are times restoring TMJs to proper form and function requires alterations in the dentition. Several methods can be used in combination for this purpose. These methods almost never should be attempted when the patient is in an active state of pain but rather should be used as a finishing technique only after Phase I has been successful (Shankland, 2001). In most instances pain is a soft tissue phenomenon. Hard tissue landmarks, as indicated by x-rays, do not dictate a "pain-free" position for the patient. Categorically you cannot look at x-rays, casts of the teeth, or other hard tissue diagnostics alone and predict within the realm of human physiologic function where a pain-free stomatognathic position should be. Drawing these conclusions is often erroneous and indicates a possible misunderstanding of pain etiology. Not everyone needs perfect occlusion or aesthetically pleasing teeth to live a pain-free life. The object of TMD treatment should be the resolution of the patient's pain, not the restoration of the dentition to as perfect a position as possible unless dictated

TABLE 27.2
Common Methods of Phase II Finishing Techniques

1. *Equilibration.* This is a technique in which the enamel surfaces of the teeth are altered by the use of dental handpiece to restore proper occlusal alignment with the TMJs and their supporting structures.
2. *Crown and Bridge: Prosthetics.* Missing or broken teeth often need to be restored to provide maximum stomatognathic support during function. There are a variety of devices that fall into this category all of which aim for the same result. The required prosthesis is dictated by patient's need and desire.
3. *Orthodontics.* This technique is best used when there is a resulting discrepancy between the maxillary and mandibular position or the patient's teeth have had limited restorative work. This finishing technique can be quite effective when properly utilized.
4. *Use of an appliance/orthotic on an as-needed basis.* There are times when this is the most conservative and logical approach to a chronic problem. The use of this technique should be infrequent, however, and after all other physical means are exhausted. Long-term use of an orthotic can cause problems with the teeth and periodontium. There is also the chance of dental compensation with the orthotic yielding an acquired malocclusion or mandibular reposturing.
5. *Orthognathic surgery.* Surgical techniques should be used judiciously. Great care must be taken to guide the patient to as pain free a state as possible before any reconstructive surgery should be attempted. Rarely is surgery an initial treatment.

by the patient's specific needs. A lot of people are in chronic pain with perfect occlusion, and many with terrible occlusion and compromised stomatognathic function are pain-free. A proper diagnosis and clinical stabilization will help determine the need for Phase II treatment. Methods for Phase II finishing techniques are shown in Table 27.2.

THE TWO-MINUTE TMJ EXAM

Initial screening for TMD does not have to be complicated. Table 27.3 delineates some simple procedures that will help provide an indication if there is a need for a dental consultation to rule out TMD as a contributing factor to the patient's pain complaints.

MULTIDISCIPLINARY PAIN TREATMENT

Because TMD is often a manifestation of multiple precipitating factors, management requires cooperation between many health care professionals. A review of the signs and symptoms often associated with TMD brings to mind many clinical possibilities that need to be considered when determining a proper diagnosis. No one profession can dominate all care when it comes to chronic pain. The artificial delineation of practice parameters as dictated by licensure and custom is artificial indeed when it comes to the management of pain.

TABLE 27.3
The Two-Minute TMJ Exam

1. *Maximum mouth opening.* Look for limitations or deviations
   a. Normal is approximately the width of three fingers without pain
   b. Mandibular opening should be relatively straight without deviation
2. *Joint noise.* Healthy TMJs should be virtually silent both to you the clinician and the patient
   a. Popping, clicking, or grinding in one or both of the TMJs in the presence of facial pain, headaches, or neck aches
   b. This can be by patient report, manual palpation of the TMJs, or using a stethoscope
3. *Pain upon muscle palpation.* Facial muscles in healthy conditions are not tender to touch
   a. Masseters
   b. Temporalis
   c. Intraoral muscles
4. Otological exam
   a. Excessive earwax bilaterally or unilaterally in the absence of obvious pathology
   b. Pain in the external auditory canals distal to the TMJs upon insertion of the otoscope in the absence of obvious pathology

The key to success in the management of the patients with facial pain is to understand the limitations of one's own abilities and to appreciate the talents and skills of other professions. While one profession may be the primary provider in any given situation, the manifestation of the various symptoms of the patients with TMD in all probability will require a true team effort. Although many patients can present a challenge for treatment, one of the benefits to the practitioner is the opportunity to communicate with fellow professionals outside his or her chosen discipline. Discussion with others can produce exciting opportunities for learning and sharpening each other's diagnostic skills. Unfortunately, without these opportunities various disciplines of the healing arts go without communication resulting in a misunderstanding of each other's abilities. The modern age of information availability and transfer are converging the once rigid walls between professions, resulting in a better, more rounded approach to management of the patient with TMD/chronic head, neck, and facial pain.

COMMON CONCERNS ABOUT TMD

Determining if a patient's headache complaints are related to a dysfunction of the TMJs: Obvious indications may include popping noises, inability to open his or her mouth, pain in the TMJs upon chewing, etc. There are frequently more insidious indications as well. Remember the TMJs and their supporting structures may produce symptoms anywhere along the trigeminal nerve tract, making the diagnosis difficult at times.

TMJ problems and mouthpiece use: While an orthotic (appliance) is necessary in many situations, localized inflammation sometimes may be handled conservatively by NSAIDs, muscle relaxants, exercise, and physical therapy. As with any other functional orthotic, the design is dictated by the patient's needs. Often they are used to keep the mandibular condyles from pressing into the edematous retro-discal lamina, which is richly innervated. Decompressing of the joint mechanism is often necessary to help break the spasm–pain–spasm cycle reducing pain and dysfunction. In addition, orthotics can also be used strictly for myositis, myalgia, muscular imbalance, or repositioning the mandible on a temporary or permanent basis.

TMJs that pop and click: A proper diagnosis is necessary to determine if TMJ noises are contributing to the patient's pain. TMJ noises are one of many symptoms that indicate pathology but are not pathognomotic for pathology that needs to be treated.

TMJ patients and headaches: Many times the temporalis, masseters, lateral pterygoids, and various neck muscles are all under tension. A TMJ headache is often a skeletal muscle contraction headache. Across the board, 80% of all headaches are of the muscle contraction variety. A chronic dysfunction of the TMJs may result in chronic muscle tension.

TMJ therapy: The length of time needed will vary greatly according to the type of problem as well as its chronicity. Obviously, a muscle sprain will respond more quickly than a joint with rheumatoid arthritis. Unfortunately, all conditions of this nature are erroneously placed under the label of *TMJ* and should be more accurately differentially diagnosed.

Prevalence of TMJ: Women outnumber men about eight to one except for victims of automobile accidents, where the ratios tend to be more equal. Women also suffer about the same ratio for every other joint injury. They seek care more often than men in about those same numbers for other afflictions. The reasons are thought to be structural, hormonal, and societal.

TMJ pain caused by depression: Depression may play a major role in some cases of facial pain but does not lead to a true dysfunction of the TMJs. Chronic pain from any source often leads to depression due to depletion of serotonin and other neurotransmitters. Remember, many TMJ sufferers have been labeled as malingering due to improper or misdiagnoses and have been suffering for years. Chronic pain may take on a familial setting exacerbating feelings of guilt, inadequacy, and depression.

Curing TMJ: As in any condition, without proper diagnosis, there can be no cure. Many acute injuries to the TMJs, if caught early, will respond rapidly to conservative care, often within days or weeks. Even patients with chronic conditions can be successfully managed with proper treatment. Conservative care of chronic degenerative TMJ often yields a positive response using procedures from physical medicine such as those previously mentioned.

Proper time for a dental consultation: A properly trained dentist should be thought of as a partner in the management of head, neck, and facial pain. Dentistry and other disciplines do not compete with each other. The more each profession understands the other, the more comfortable each will feel in asking for opinions. As a rule of thumb, if a patients with headache/facial pain does not respond to a medicinal treatment regimen, then a consultation with a dentist should be in order. All fields of pain management working together often yield a synergism resulting in good clinical results and satisfied patients.

Dental referrals for TMJ: Many dentists, due to the complexity and time needed to treat these types of patients, choose not to treat patients with TMD. On the other hand, some dentists choose to concentrate their practices in this field and have spent much time in continuing education and specialized training. Typically, a well-trained dentist should look at teeth as a component in the pain cycle and not always as the sole entity. The way the bite fits together may or may not be an issue in the patient's head, neck, or facial pain, and the dentist should have the proper training to be able to differentiate. A treating dentist should also have the mind-set of a "team" approach so that proper treatment reciprocation is present.

REFERENCES

Anonymous. (1995, September). Insurance Institute for Highway Safety Status Report, *30*(8), 6, 7.

Baburr, L. (1989). Occipital neuralgia alias C2-3 radiculopathy. *The Journal of Neurological and Orthopedic Medicine and Surgery, 10*(2), 133.

Bell, W. (1982). *Temporomandibular disorders — Classification, diagnosis, management* (2nd ed., p. 177). Chicago: Year Book Medical Publishers

Bell, W. (1989). *Orofacial pains — Classification, diagnosis, management yearbook* (pp. 100–101). Chicago: Year Book Medical Publishers.

Bumann, A., & Lotzmann, U. (2002). *TMJ disorders and orofacial pain: The role of dentistry in a multidisciplinary diagnostic approach* (p. 19). Stuttgart: Thieme.

Cady, R., & Fox, A. (1995). *Treating the headache patient* (pp. 219–259). New York: Dekker, Inc.

Cox, C., & Cocks, G. (1979, January). Occipital neuralgia. *Journal of the Medical Association of the State of Alabama,* 25.

Diamond, S., & Dalessio, D. J. *The practicing physician's approach to headache* (3rd ed., pp. 99–108). Baltimore: Williams and Wilkins.

Foust, D. R., et al. (1974). Cervical range of motion and Dynamic response and strength of cervical muscle. *SAE Transactions, 4*(82), SAE Paper No. 730975, Reprinted November 1974 and 1973.

Hollowell, W. P., & Stucki, S. L. (1974). Improving Occupant Protection Systems in Frontal Crashes. SAE International Congress & Exposition 1996, Detroit. SAE Paper No. 960665.

Kaplan, A., & Assael, L. (1991). *Temporomandibular disorders: Diagnosis and treatment*. Philadelphia: W.B. Saunders.

McNeill, C. (1993). *Temporomandibular disorders: Guidelines for classification, assessment and management*. Chicago: Quintessence Books.

Mense, S., & Simons, D. (2001). *Muscle pain: Understanding its nature, diagnosis, and treatment*. Philadelphia: Lippincott Williams, and Wilkins.

Mertz, H. J. Jr., & Patrick L. M. (1967). Investigation of the kinematics and kinetics of whiplash. *Proceedings, 11th Stapp Car Crash Conference*, SAE 670919, Detroit MI, Society of Automotive Engineers.

Okeson, J. (1989). *Management of temporomandibular disorders and occlusion* (2nd ed.). Philadelphia: The C.V. Mosby Company.

Raj, P. (1996). *Pain medicine: A comprehensive review*. St. Louis: C.V. Mosby.

Raj, P. (2003). *Pain medicine: A comprehensive review* (2nd ed.). Philadelphia: C.V. Mosby.

Schneider, L. W. et al. (1975). Biomechanical properties of the human neck in lateral flexion. *Proceedings of the Nineteenth Stapp Car Crash Conference*, November 17–19, San Diego. Society of Automotive Engineers. SAE Paper No. 751156.

Shankland, W. (1998). *TMJ: Its many faces* (2nd ed.). Columbus, OH: Anadem Publishing.

Shankland, W. (2001). *Face the pain: The challenge of facial pain*. Columbus, OH: Aomega Publishing Co.

Talley, R., & Ousley, L. (1994, November). Cervical trauma as an etiology of TMD, Literature Review. The American Academy of Head, Neck and Facial Pain.

28

Abdominal Pain

Sean R. Lacey, MD

INTRODUCTION

Pain originating from the abdominal region can challenge even the best clinician. As with any patient symptom, it is of utmost importance to obtain a detailed history. Unlike other regions of the body, many different organ systems can give rise to abdominal symptoms. Pain originating from the gastrointestinal tract and its solid organ constituents is the focus of this chapter. Other potential causes of abdominal pain including vascular, gynecological, and renal sources should be considered although they are not the subjects of this chapter.

When first evaluating a patient with abdominal pain, it is extremely important to establish a timeline of events. In doing so, the clinician will separate acute from chronic pain and constant from intermittent pain. It will allow the physician to focus on the pain for which the patient is seeking consultation. Extracting the location or locations of pain and whether the pain has changed in location over time can elucidate the physician and allow for a more focused exam. If the pain seems to radiate to other regions, this can also give helpful information. Also, the association of new symptoms other than pain can narrow the differential diagnosis for the origin of pain. Such symptoms may include, but not be limited to, nausea, vomiting, diarrhea, constipation, bloating, intestinal bleeding, weight loss, early satiety, dysuria, dysparunia, and fever. The association of symptoms with eating, fasting, or how they change with flatus or bowel movements can also assist in providing additional information to arrive at a correct diagnosis.

The physical examination is an extremely valuable tool to use in cases where abdominal pain is present. Usually, the sequence of events used during the exam includes inspection first; followed by auscultation, palpation, and percussion. Inspection and palpation are the most useful, however. Many of the organs of the abdominal cavity are palpable even under normal circumstances, and therefore, knowing and appreciating the normal abdomen are essential. When the normal abdominal structures are well known, it will be much easier to recognize the "abnormal" abdomen. When palpating the abdomen, first identify where the painful region or regions are located by asking the patient, then examine that area *last*. This will allow for a more through exam by keeping the patient comfortable and preventing involuntary contractions of the abdominal musculature.

It may be easiest to separate the contents of the abdomen into solid and viscous structures. Solid structures are often appreciated during the physical exam and include the liver, spleen, pancreas, kidneys, uterus, and ovaries. Hollow organs such as stomach, intestines, urinary bladder, and gallbladder are generally not well appreciated, but may be palpable and appreciated if involved in a neoplastic process or if they are distended by air/gas.

In the performance of the physical exam it is important to follow a general routine so that a thorough exam is employed. However, depending on the clinical circumstance, an astute diagnostician will occasionally employ other techniques to confirm/refute suspicions. The most common way of examining the abdomen is to have the patient lie in a supine position. Flexing the knees will often take tension from rectus muscles of the anterior abdominal wall and allow for a more successful experience during palpation. In conveying and recording the exam findings, it is important to identify the location or topography of the abdomen. This is illustrated in Figure 28.1. The most commonly used system divides

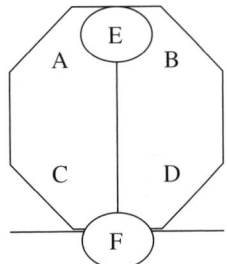

FIGURE 28.1 Topographical regions of the abdomen. A = right upper quadrant; B = left upper quadrant; C = right lower quadrant; D = left lower quadrant; E = epigastric; F = suprapubic.

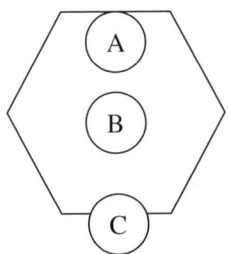

FIGURE 28.2 Locations of visceral pain and organs often associated with each region. A = epigastrium: stomach, duodenum, liver, biliary tree pancreas; B = periumbilical: small intestine, appendix, right colon; C = suprapubic: transverse/left colon, rectum, gynecological.

the abdomen into four quadrants with their intersection through the umbilicus. More specific regions have been described as either periumbilical or epigastric in location. Making the distinction about location is important in following the clinical course of the patient and conveying the findings to other colleagues. A simple diagram such as that illustrated in the figure with the area of pain shaded can be very helpful in following such patients with chronic symptoms.

Throughout the years, many physical exam maneuvers and findings have been associated with clinical conditions. Although many of the signs and symptoms elicited during the physical exam are lacking specificity and sensitivity and have not undergone rigorous scientific testing, it is important to mention them. In modern-day medicine, the clinical suspicion of a condition has been augmented by confirmatory testing, including serology and diagnostic imaging (i.e., magnetic resonance imaging, computed tomography, and ultrasound). Included in Table 28.1 are common signs elicited during the physical examination and the clinical condition(s) often associated with each.

Pain can be visceral, somatic, or referred. Visceral nociceptors are most sensitive to stretch and these stretch receptors are located in the muscular layers of the hollow viscera between the muscularis mucosa and submucosa and in the serosa of solid organs (Leek, 1972). This type of pain is generally not well localized and patients will often give a very vague description of their discomfort. Nerves that transmit these signals originate from multiple segments and can be mechanoreceptors or nocireceptors, among others. These nerves are nonmyelinated and give rise to symptoms that are diffuse and poorly localized, typically described as achy, gnawing, burning, or cramping. Somatic pain tends to be much better localized and may be easier for patients to describe. Nerves are often myelinated. Irritated areas that may give rise to somatic pain include the abdominal wall, parietal peritoneum, or diaphragm. Referred pain is located in the same dermatome as the source for the pain, but is perceived in a distant location. Pain is often well localized and therefore does resemble somatic pain in its characteristics (Figure 28.2).

TABLE 28.1
Common Physical Exam Signs and Associated Conditions

Physical Signs	Examination Findings	Clinical Condition(S)
Caput medusa	Engorged veins extending out from the umbilicus	Portal vein thrombosis, vena cava obstruction
Cullen's sign	Blue discoloration around the umbilicus	Hemoperitoneum
Grey Turner's sign	Discoloration of skin of lower abdomen and/or flanks; color may vary red/blue/purple	Hemorrhagic pancreatitis, bowel infarction
Borborygmus	Intestinal sounds heard without the assistance of a stethoscope associated with abdominal pain and visible peristalsis	Partial or complete intestinal obstruction
Rebound tenderness	Pain resulting from rapid withdrawal of depressed fingertips	Peritoneal inflammation; perforated viscous
Murphy's sign	Cessation of inspiration in mid-breath secondary to pain when gallbladder comes in contact with examining fingers in RUQ	Cholecystitis

TABLE 28.2
Causes of Acute Abdomen Pain According to Pain Quality and Onset

Pain Type	Possible Condition
Excruciating, acute onset over seconds	Heart attack, perforated ulcer, ruptured aneurysm, biliary or renal colic
Rapid, severe and constant over minutes	Acute pancreatitis, mesenteric ischemia/infarction, complete bowel obstruction
Gradual onset/steady over hours	Acute cholecystitis, diverticulitis, appendicitis
Intermittent/colicky pain over hours	Early pancreatitis/bowel obstruction

TABLE 28.3
Causes of Ascites Based on SAAG Measurement

SAAG ≥ 1.1 g/dl	SAAG < 1.1 g/dl
Cardiac ascites	Chylous acities
Cirrhosis	Peritoneal carcinomatosis
Hepatic failure	Infection, tuberculosis, chlymydia
Alcoholic hepatitis	Biliary ascites
Massive liver involvement with tumor	Pancreatic ascites
Budd-Chiari syndrome	Bowel perforation
Hepatocellular carcinoma	Peritonitis from connective tissues diseases
Portal vein thrombosis	
Myxedema	
Acute fatty liver of pregnancy	
VOD (venoocclusive disease)	

The evaluation of the acute abdomen must take into consideration many factors, but most important is that of whether surgery is needed. Generally, acute abdominal pain is described as sudden in onset and present for less than 24 hours. In the setting of a perforated viscous, the emergent need for surgery may be a lifesaving measure. Careful attention should be paid to the characteristics of abdominal pain and the progression of current symptoms. Although this detailed history does not always allow the correct diagnosis to be made, certainly some conditions are associated with common symptoms and the clinical suspicion will be higher for that particular entity.

Table 28.2 depicts common causes of the acute abdomen and the typical characteristics associated with each.

PAIN FROM FLUID

Collections of fluid outside the intestinal lumen are generally considered abnormal. However, a small accumulation of fluid in the cul-de-sac in female patients can be a nonspecific finding. Ascites is never normal. Fluid in the peritoneal cavity usually does not cause pain unless there is a significant amount of fluid, called "tense ascites." In this circumstance, the abdomen is distended and pressure is exerted on the abdominal wall as well as on the intra-abdominal contents. Relief can be achieved by decompressing the distended abdomen with paracentesis or diuretic therapy. If the fluid is infected, the peritoneum can become inflamed leading to pain. Spontaneous bacterial peritonitis (SBP) should always be suspected in patients with ascites, but only 50% of patients with SBP will complain of abdominal pain (O'Grady, Lake, & Howdle, 2000). SBP is a condition where the ascitic fluid is infected, but a source cannot be identified. A significant proportion of hospitalized patients with ascites, 10 to 30%, may have or develop SBP (Yu & Hu, 2001; Jaffe, Chung, & Friedman, 1996). Patients with a low ascitic protein content are at higher risk for the development of SBP and those with a prior history of SBP have a 70% chance of

a recurrent episode (Garcia-Tsao, 2001). Mortality rates have dropped significantly given the prompt recognition of the infection and appropriate therapy; however, inpatient mortality still approaches 20% and the 2-year survival rate is 30% after a documented case of SBP (Garcia-Tsao, 2001).

The diagnosis of SBP is made by examination of the ascitic fluid. If the leukocyte count exceeds 250 cells/mm^3 or ascitic fluid culture is positive, SBP is confirmed (Guarner & Runyon, 1995). Solely relying on a positive culture is not sufficient, as many patients, up to 40%, will exhibit culture negative SBP (Yu & Hu, 2001). In the past, ascites was evaluated using the terms *transudative* or *exudative*. This terminology has been largely replaced by the determination of the serum-ascites albumin gradient (SAAG). The determination of the SAAG can be accomplished by measuring the serum and ascites albumin concentrations at the same time and subtracting the ascitic fluid albumin concentration from the serum albumin concentration. This is highly accurate in predicting ascites from portal hypertension (Runyon, 1998). The differential diagnosis of ascites based on SAAG is listed in Table 28.3 (Runyon, 1998).

LIVER AND BILIARY PAIN

Conditions that affect the liver often will go unnoticed by the patient. It is only when the liver capsule expands that pain is generally perceived. Therefore, most any condition that causes liver enlargement will produce pain. Pain will also generally be more intense if the capsule expands at a rapid rate. The number of conditions that can lead to liver enlargement is quite extensive and is beyond the scope of this chapter. Common conditions that are recognized to cause rapid liver enlargement are acute hepatitis, alcoholic hepatitis, and space-occupying lesions such as metastatic and primary liver neoplasms.

Pain originating from the gallbladder classically presents as a positive Murphy's sign, but this is generally only appreciated in acute cholecystitis, a condition that occurs when the cystic duct becomes blocked. Pain is usually in the right upper quadrant and radiates to the right scapula and is associated with nausea and vomiting. Fever is usually also present along with leukocytosis. Symptoms of biliary colic are also very similar to those of cholecystitis; however; the pain symptoms generally subside after several hours, whereas pain from cholecystitis can persist longer until more definite therapy is begun (i.e., antibiotics, cholecystectomy, etc.). Last, cholangitis, an infection of the bile ducts, can have similar presenting signs/symptoms. This infection generally produces significantly high fevers, chills, rigors, and abnormal liver enzyme values. Jaundice will often accompany this infection. The cornerstone of therapy involves systemic antibiotics and prompt decompression of the biliary tree. This is usually accomplished via endoscopic retrograde cholagiopancreatography or percutaneous transhepatic catheter drainage.

IRRITABLE BOWEL SYNDROME

Irritable bowel syndrome (IBS) is an extremely common condition and has been prevalent for many years. Physicians and other health care professionals historically have thought that it was a condition brought on by psychiatric problems and that it was "in the patient's head." Although there has been no definite connection between psychological disorders and IBS, there does seem to be a higher incidence of comorbid psychiatric conditions (Olden, 2002). Referral centers have reported that patients seeking consultation have a high percentage (54 to 94%) of already recognized coexisting psychiatric disorders such as anxiety or depression (Olden, 2002; Thompson, 2002). Sexual abuse has also been seen more commonly in patients suffering from IBS (Michell & Drossman, 1987). It is not clear if there is a cause–effect relationship between psychiatric disorders and IBS, but it does seem to influence which patients are more apt to seek medical attention for IBS symptoms and it may also influence symptom severity and outcome (Michell & Drossman, 1987).

In more recent years, IBS has finally received much-needed attention. Significant research into the cause of this disorder has led to new discoveries to explain symptoms and subsequently to new therapies. The impact that IBS has on North America is astounding. Approximately, 15% of the adult population is affected by the symptoms of IBS, two thirds of which are female (American College of Gastroenterology, 2002; Brandt et al., 2002). In one study of 1,597 patients with IBS, 57% reported daily symptoms, 25% reported weekly symptoms, and 50% of respondents had experienced symptoms for longer than 10 years (Schmulson & Chang, 1999). Additionally, symptoms interfered with work where 12% stopped work-

TABLE 28.4
Diagnosing Irritable Bowel Syndrome; ROME II Criteria

1. Patient has had abdominal pain or discomfort for at least 12 weeks over the past 12 months. Pain does not need to occur in consecutive weeks.
2. Abdominal pain or discomfort has two of the following three features:
   a. Relief with defecation
   b. Onset associated with an alteration in bowel movement frequency
   c. Onset associated with an alteration in stool appearance/form
3. Nine symptoms supporting the diagnosis of IBS
   a. Fewer than three bowel movements per week
   b. More than three bowel movements per day
   c. Hard or lumpy stools
   d. Loose or watery stools
   e. Straining during bowel movements
   f. Urgency
   g. Feeling of incomplete evacuation
   h. Passing mucus during bowel movement
   i. Abdominal fullness, bloating, or swelling

ing and 47% had missed days at work secondary to their symptoms (Schmulson & Chang, 1999). IBS symptoms also can interfere with leisure activities, diet, and social relationships in a negative way, thus leading to impaired quality of life (Schmulson & Chang, 1999; Whitehead, Palsson, & Jones, 2002). The financial impact is also significant. Because there are no objective biochemical markers, anatomical defects, or physical exam findings that are clearly linked to IBS, the diagnosis is made by the constellation of symptoms and the presenting characteristics a patient possesses (Brandt et al., 2002: Hungin et al., 2002).

IBS is a multisymptom complex that is manifested by alteration in bowel habit frequency, stool consistency, and associated abdominal discomfort (pain, cramping, bloating, etc.). In an effort to help define the characteristics for IBS and ultimately to establish a "common ground" to study this disorder, specific diagnostic criteria have been developed by the Multinational Working Teams to Develop Diagnostic Criteria for Functional Gastrointestinal Disorders (International Foundation for Functional Gastrointestinal Disorders, 2002). The resultant ROME II criteria are very helpful in arriving at an accurate diagnosis of IBS (Table 28.4).

Patients who present other signs or symptoms, sometime called "red flags," which may represent diseases mimicking IBS, may require additional testing. Red flags may include, but not be limited to, occult positive stool, overt gastrointestinal bleeding, weight loss, vomiting, anemia, fever, family history of celiac disease, intestinal cancers, or inflammatory bowel disease.

The treatments of IBS are generally focused around alleviating the predominant symptoms. In other words, if

TABLE 28.5
Commonly Used Treatments/Medications for the Management of IBS

Drug Class	Dosage	Side Effects	Intended Use
Antispasmodics			
Dicyclomine	10–40 mg qid	Sedation, dry eyes and mouth, urinary retention, constipation	Improve abdominal pain/bloating
Hyoscyamine	0.125–0.25 mg tid–qid	Same as dicyclomine	Improve abdominal pain/bloating
Bulking Agents			
Fiber	20–35 g/day	Bloating/gas	Improve constipation
Antidiarrheals			
Loperamide	2–4 mg qid, max of 16 mg/24 hrs	Nausea/constipation, dry mouth/abdominal pain	Improve diarrhea
Diphenoxylate	5 mg tid–qid	Constipation, abdominal pain	Improve diarrhea
Atropine	—	Nausea, anorexia	—
Cholestyramine	4 g qd–q12h	Gas, may affect absorption of other drugs	Bile resin binder
Opiates	Variable	Sedation/constipation, addiction potential	—
Laxatives			
Lactulose	10–20 g qd–bid	Bloating/gas/cramping	Improve constipation
Polyethylene glycol	17 g/day	Bloating/gas/diarrhea	Improve constipation
Tricyclic Antidepressants			
Amitriptyline	10–100 mg qhs	Dry mouth/eyes, sedation, constipation	Improve diarrhea/pain
Imipramine	10–100 mg qhs	Same as amitriptyline	Improve diarrhea/pain
SSRIs			
Sertraline	Variable	Sexual dysfunction	Improve pain
Fluoxetine	—	Sedation, fatigue, weight gain	—
5-HT$_3$ Antagonist			
Alosetron	1 mg qd × 4 wks, if tolerated 1 mg bid	Ischemic colitis, constipation	Improve diarrhea, pain, and bloating
5-HT$_4$ Agonist			
Tegaserod	6 mg bid × 12 wks	Diarrhea, headache, ischemic colitis	Improve constipation, pain, bloating

a patient is constipated with hard/lumpy stools, then the treatment would be to soften the bowel movement and increase frequency of bowel habits. Traditional therapies have been the use of antispasmatics, laxatives, antidiarrheal agents, and fiber. Table 28.5 presents a list of drugs that are commonly used, including doses and potential side effects.

Only recently have new therapeutic agents been developed and FDA-approved for the treatment of IBS. It is known that serotonin receptors are very plentiful in the intestinal tract. Binding to these receptors is important in the regulation of motility and secretion of the bowel. Cortisol, acetylcholine, histamine, and serotonin are some of the more important hormones currently under investigation for the understanding of IBS.

Serotonin has become a focus of interest because of the rich concentration of this substance in the intestinal tract; in fact, nearly 95% of this hormone is found within the enterochormafin cells of the intestine. Of note are the

drugs alosetron HCl (Lotronex™; Glaxo-SmithKline) and tergasarod (Zelnorm®; Novartis). Alosetron, a 5-HT$_3$ receptor antagonist, gained FDA approval for the treatment of diarrhea-predominant IBS (IBS-D); however, it was voluntarily removed from the market secondary to potential adverse events thought to possibly be caused by the drug in November 2000. Some of the adverse events include ischemic colitis and constipation. After additional consideration, the FDA approved the use of alosetron in June 2002 under a restricted prescribing program. As of this writing, only women with severe IBS-D who have failed other traditional therapies are eligible for treatment. Patients and physicians are required to sign an agreement form and special stickers are required to prescribe the medicine. Initial dosage of alosetron is 1 mg daily for 4 weeks which can be increased to a maximum of 1 mg twice daily if it is tolerated. If no symptom improvement is achieved after 4 weeks of treatment at the maximum dose, it is then advised to discontinue alosetron and seek alternative management options. Alosetron has not only been shown to decrease the number of bowel movements, but perhaps just as important, it has also been demonstrated that it has some efficacy in relieving global symptoms of IBS and therefore improving quality of life (Lievre, 2002). For more information regarding the educational materials for Lotronex or to enroll in the prescribing program, call 888-825-5249 or visit www.lotronex.com.

Tegaserod was released in July 2002 and is FDA-approved for the treatment of constipation-predominant IBS (IBS-C). Tegaserod is a 5-HT$_4$ receptor agonist, which is involved in the peristaltic action of the gut (Lacy, 2002). Large randomized controlled studies have been done using tegaserod and have demonstrated significant global symptom improvement (pain, bloating) in addition to relieving constipation problems. Nearly two thirds of women studied had improvement or resolution of IBS-C related symptoms (Brandt et al., 2002; Lacy, 2002; Muller-Lissner et al., 2001; Prather et al., 2000). At the current time, tegaserod is approved only for use in women, but studies showing efficacy in men with IBS-C are currently in progress. In April 2004, Novartis, makers of Zelnorm, released a statement warning physicians of the dangers of diarrhea that can be induced by the medication and rare case reports of ischemic colitis. All potential serious adverse events are to be reported to the FDA MEDWATCH program.

INFLAMMATORY BOWEL DISEASE

Crohn's disease (CD) and ulcerative colitis (UC) are idiopathic intestinal inflammatory disorders that are lifelong. Both diseases are associated with abdominal pain, among other symptoms, including gastrointestinal bleeding, diarrhea, fistula, abscess, weight loss, anemia, and increased prevalence of intestinal cancer, especially of the colon when it is involved. Both diseases are associated with relapses resulting in high morbidity and have a negative impact on quality of life (Cohen, 2002). The goal of treatment of these chronic illnesses is to control symptoms effectively, to prevent complications as a result of the disease, and to avoid adverse reactions related to available treatment. Although the etiology is not completely understood, several mechanisms are important in the development and manifestation of inflammatory bowel disease (IBD) and include genetic as well as environmental factors. The therapies available continue to evolve and currently involve conventional therapy in addition to biologic and anti-tumor necrosis factor-alpha (TNF-alpha) agents. It is hoped that a cure will be discovered, but for the 1 to 2 million plus patients with IBD in North America (Crohn's & Colitis Foundation of America, Inc., 2004), symptomatic control offers the best opportunity for improved quality of living.

CD is a lifelong illness that can be diagnosed at any time; however, it is most often diagnosed in the second to third decades. CD can affect any part of the digestive tract with the ileum and cecum the most commonly affected. Symptoms that often accompany active CD include abdominal pain, fever, and diarrhea. Intestinal bleeding is also seen, but less often. One cardinal feature that distinguishes CD from UC is transmural inflammation of the intestinal lumen. This inflammatory process makes patients with CD more prone to fistula, abscess, and perforation. In fact, nearly 35% of patients with CD will develop fistulae (Schwartz et al., 2002). Other systemic manifestations of CD include malnutrition, osteoporosis, arthritis, uveitis, and nephrolithiasis. Once diagnosed and appropriately managed, remission is often achieved. Unfortunately, 47% of individuals will experience a relapse within the first year (Moum et al., 1997) and nearly 50% of patients with CD will undergo surgery within a decade of being diagnosed with the illness (Mekhijan et al., 1979).

The management of CD is composed of conventional agents (i.e., corticosteroids, aminosalicylates, and antibiotics) and newer therapies to be discussed. Corticosteroids are very good at inducing remission rapidly with success rates of 60 to 92% (Malchow et al, 1984; Modigliani et al., 1990; Summers et al., 1979). Clinical symptoms may also be improved with steroid use, but there remains endoscopic evidence of active inflammation despite the use of steroids (Yang & Lichtenstein, 2002). The chronic long-term use of steroids is not very effective in maintaining remission and has a high likelihood of causing side effects. Table 28.6 lists the common side effects seen with chronic corticosteroid usage.

In an effort to reduce the side effects of corticosteroids, a newer second-generation steroid agent was developed, budesonide. It has low systemic bioavailability due to its high first-pass hepatic metabolism. It is able to induce remission relative effectively at a rate of 52 to 69% (Campieri et al., 1997; Greenber et al., 1996; Retgeerts et al., 1994; Thomsen et al., 1998). Unfortunately, it also is not able to achieve long-term maintenance of remission, and relapse rates are similar in those patients using placebo compared with budesonide 6 mg daily (Ferguson et al., 1998; Greenberg et al., 1994; Lofberg et al, 1996).

TABLE 28.6
Side Effects Associated with Corticosteroid Use in the Treatment of Crohn's Disease

Dermatological	Acne, hirsutism, striae, telengiectasia
Endocrine	Adrenal suppression, diabetes
Ophthalmologic	Cataracts, glaucoma, retinal hemorrhage
Musculoskeletal	Weakness, osteoporosis
Metabolic	Hyperlipidemia, fluid retention, electrolyte abnormality
Infectious	Increased risk of infection
Psychiatric	Insomnia, anxiety, psychosis, depression

Immune system–modulating agents have also been implemented to help maintain remission, but are not efficacious in inducing remission. 6-Mercaptopurine (6-MP) and azathioprine (AZ) have been used for many years as a way to diminish the need to use steroids and have therefore been called steroid-sparing agents. Although they are generally thought to be safer for chronic use than corticosteroids, the use of 6-MP and AZ requires continuous monitoring. One of the biggest limitations of their use is the slow onset of action. In patients who do respond favorably to these medications, the effect may not occur for 3 to 6 months after initiation of the medication. Also there are known side effects of 6-MP and AZ that include nausea, abnormal liver enzymes, pancreatitis, and allergic reactions. Bone marrow suppression can also occur and may be more profound in patients with diminished/absent thiopurine methyltransferase (TPMT) enzyme activity, a problem seen in 11% of the general population. As a consequence, it has been suggested to measure complete blood counts weekly upon initiation of therapy for the first month, biweekly for the next month, and then monthly to every 3 months thereafter. As a way to reduce potential toxicities related to their use, some have proposed the measurement of TPMT activity prior to commencing therapy; however, a consensus has not been reached regarding this routine practice. Approximately 45% of patients maintained on AZ were able to sustain remission compared with 7% tapered to placebo (Candy et al., 1995). The accepted doses for 6-MP and AZ are 1.5 and 2.5 mg/kg/day, respectively.

Methotrexates (MTX), cyclosporine A, mycophenolate mofetil, and tacrolimus have also been used as immunomodulators. The most data exist for the use of MTX for the induction/maintenance of remission; however, all of these agents are generally reserved for those who have failed other more conventional therapies.

Aminosalicylates have also been long used to help intestinal inflammation related to UC and CD. The exact mechanism of action for these drugs is not known, but several theories have been proposed. It is thought that this class of drugs may influence and downregulate the production of proinflammatory cytokines (TNF-alpha, interleukin-1, and nuclear factor kappa B). They may also affect oxygen free radical production and lymphocyte/monocyte activity (Lichtenstein, 2003). Several different aminosalicylate agents have been developed (Table 28.7) and are generally well tolerated, but all can have a paradoxical effect of making IBD symptoms worse. Should this happen, the medication should be discontinued. Formulations of the 5-aminosalicylate (5-ASA), the active portion of the medicine, are designed to be released in the lumenal intestinal tract at different locations. Most of the formulations are meant to release 5-ASA in the distal ileum/colon, but Pentasa® (mesalamine; Proctor and Gamble) can be delivered to the proximal small bowel

TABLE 28.7
5-ASA Agents Available and Recommended Doses

Sulfasalazine	500 mg tablets	2–6 g/day
Mesalamine		
Pentasa	250 mg capsules	2–4g/day
Asacol	400 mg tablets	2–4.8 g/day
Suppository	500 mg	0.5–1 g/day
Enema	4 g	2–4 g/day
Olsalazine	250 mg capsules	1.5–3 g/day
Balsalazide	750 mg capsule	2–6 g/day

also. Topical mesalamine in the form of suppositories and enemas is also available to treat the rectum and distal colon, respectively.

The presence of bacteria in the bowel may be partially responsible for the inflammation seen in IBD. Clinical and experimental data have shown a delay in recurrence of CD follow surgery if the fecal stream is diverted. Also, bacteria have been shown in the wall of the intestine and within mesenteric lymph nodes. Although the exact mechanism by which bacteria exert their effect is not well understood, the use of antibiotics to alter the bacterial makeup/concentration has been part of the treatment of active IBD (Stein & Lichtenstein, 2001). Metronidazole and ciprofloxacin have been used most extensively for the treatment of active IBD, especially when the colon is involved. The accepted dose of metronidazole is 10 to 20 mg/kg/day and for ciprofloxacin is 1 g/day.

Ciprofloxacin is better tolerated, with up to 90% of patients reporting a metallic taste with the use of metronidazole. Antibiotics have also been particularly helpful in management of perianal CD. Information regarding the long-term efficacy in the management of remission as maintenance therapy using antibiotics is lacking.

Tremendous enthusiasm has emerged with the discovery and use of newer biological agents in controlling inflammation of the bowel, in particular the use of infliximab for the treatment of CD. Infliximab is a chimeric IgG monoclonal antibody directed against TNF-alpha. In binding to TNF-alpha, it can make the biological activity of this proinflammatory cytokine inactive. Infliximab has been used to treat CD with modest success rates. The use of infliximab at a dose of 5 mg/kg has been shown to allow complete response of fistulizing disease in 33% of patients and partial response in an additional 30.8%. Those with inflammatory and fistulizing disease had a 69% complete response and 15.5% partial response (Ricart et al., 2001). Infliximab for the treatment of UC is currently under investigation.

It remains hopeful that other biological agents will be helpful in managing IBD. Modulators of cytokine production, cellular adhesion, and bacterial activity may be the best agents to offer long-term control of inflammatory activity. As these agents and others are tested, the future treatments may be much different than what are currently offered, which by many standards, is suboptimal in the management of this difficult disease.

REFERENCES

American College of Gastroenterology Functional Gastrointestinal Disorders Task Force. (2002). Evidence-based position statement on the management of irritable bowel syndrome in North America. *American Journal of Gastroenterology, 97,* S1–S5.

Brandt, L. J., et al. (2002). Systematic review on the management of irritable bowel syndrome in North America. *American Journal of Gastroenterology, 97,* S7–S26.

Campieri, M. et al. (1997). Oral budesonide is as effective as oral prednisolone in active Crohn's disease. The Global Budesonide Study Group. *Gut, 41,* 209–214.

Candy, S. et al. (1995). A controlled double blind study of azathioprine in the management of Crohn's disease. *Gut, 37,* 674–678.

Cohen, R. D. (2002). The quality of life in patients with Crohn's disease. *Alimentary Pharmacology and Therapeutics, 16,* 1603–1609.

Crohn's & Colitis Foundation of America, Inc. www.ccfa.org. Accessed on 9/25/2004.

Ferguson, A. et al. (1998). Oral budesonide as maintenance therapy in Crohn's disease — results of a twelve month study. Global Budesonide Study Group. *Alimentary Pharmacology and Therapeutics, 12,* 175–183.

Garcia-Tsao, G. (2001). Current management of the complications of cirrhosis and portal hypertension. *Gastroenterology, 120,* 726–748.

Greenberg, G. R, et al. (1994). Oral budesonide for active Crohn's disease: Canadian Inflammatory Bowel Disease Study Group. *New England Journal of Medicine, 331,* 836–841.

Greenberg, G. R. et al. (1996). Oral budesonide as maintenance treatment for Crohn's disease: A placebo controlled, dose ranging study: Canadian Inflammatory Bowel Disease Study Group. *Gastroenterology, 110,* 45–51.

Guarner, C., & Runyon, B.A. (1995). Spontaneous bacterial peritonitis: Pathogenesis, diagnosis and management. *Gastroenterologist, 3,* 311–328.

Hungin, A. P. S., et al. (2002). Irritable bowel syndrome: prevalence and impact in the USA — the truth in IBS Survey. *American Journal of Gastroenterology, 97,* S280–281.

International Foundation for Functional Gastrointestinal Disorders. (2002, August). IBS in the Real World Survey. 1–19.

Jaffe, D. L., Chung, R. T., & Friedman, L. S. (1996). Management of portal hypertension and its complications. *Medical Clinics of North America, 80,* 1021–1034.

Lacy, B. E. (2002). Tegaserod: A new 5-HT4 agonist. *Journal of Clinical Gastroenterology, 34,* 27–33.

Leek, B. (1972). Abdominal visceral receptors. In E. Neil (Ed.), *Enteroceptors: Handbook of sensory physiology* (vol. 3). New York: Springer-Verlag.

Lichtenstein, G. (2003). *Inflammatory bowel disease.* Thorofare, NJ: Slack Inc.

Lievre, M. (2002). Alosetron for irritable bowel syndrome. *British Medical Journal, 325,* 555–556.

Lofberg, R. et al. (1996). Budesonide prolongs time to relapse in ileal and ileocaecal Crohn's disease: A placebo controlled one-year study. *Gut, 39,* 82–86.

Malchow, H. et al. (1984). European Cooperative Crohn's Disease Study (ECCDS): Results of drug treatment. *Gastroenterology, 86,* 249–266.

Mekhijan, H. S. et al. (1979). National Cooperative Crohn's Disease Study: Factors determining recurrence of Crohn's disease after surgery. *Gastroenterology, 77,* 907–913.

Michell, C. M. & Drossman, D. A. (1987). Survey of the AGA membership relating to patients with functional gastrointestinal disorders. *Gastroenterology, 92,* 1282–1284.

Modigliani, R. et al. (1990). Clinical, biological, and endoscopic picture of attacks of Crohn's disease. Evolution of prednisolone. *Gastroenterology, 98,* 811–818.

Moum, B. et al. (1997). Clinical course during the first year after diagnosis in ulcerative colitis and Crohn's disease. Results of a large prospective population-based study in southeastern Norway, 1990–93. *Scandinavian Journal of Gastroenterology, 32,* 1005–1012.

Muller-Lissner, S. et al. (2001). Tegaserod, a 5-HT4 receptor partial agonist, relieves symptoms in irritable bowel syndrome patients with abdominal pain, bloating, and constipation. *Alimentary Pharmacology and Therapeutics, 15,* 1655–1666.

O'Grady, J., Lake, J., & Howdle, P. (2000). *Comprehensive clinical hepatology.* London, OH: Mosby.

Olden, K. W. (2002). Diagnosis of irritable bowel syndrome. *Gastroenterology, 122,* 1701–1714.

Prather, C. M. et al. (2000). Tegaserod accelerates orocecal transit in patients with constipation predominant irritable bowel syndrome. *Gastroenterology, 118,* 463–468.

Retgeerts, P. et al. (1994). A comparison of budesonide with prednisolone for active Crohn's disease. *New England Journal of Medicine, 331,* 842–845.

Ricart, E. et al. (2001). Infliximab for Crohn's disease in clinical practice at the Mayo Clinic: The first 100 patients. *American Journal of Gastroenterology, 96,* 722–729.

Runyon, B.A. (1998). Ascites and SBP. In M.H. Sleisenger et al. (Eds.), *Sleisenger and Fordtran's gastrointestinal and liver disease* (6th ed., pp. 1310–1333). Philadelphia: W.B. Saunders.

Schmulson, M. W. & Chang, L. (1999). Diagnostic approach to the patient with irritable bowel syndrome. *American Journal of Medicine, 107,* S20–S26.

Schwartz, D. A. et al. (2002). The natural history of fistulizing Crohn's disease in Olmsted County, Minnesota. *Gastroenterology, 122,* 875–880.

Stein, R. B., & Lichtenstein, G.R. (2001). Medical therapy for Crohn's disease: State of the art. *Surgical Clinics of North America, 81(1),* 71–101.

Summers, R. W. et al. (1979). National Cooperative Crohn's Disease Study: Results of drug treatment. *Gastroenterology, 77,* 847–869.

Thompson, W. G. (2002). The treatment of irritable bowel syndrome. *Alimentary Pharmacology and Therapeutics, 16,* 1395–1406.

Thomsen, O. O. et al. (1998). A comparison of budesonide and mesalamine for active Crohn's disease: International Budesonide–Mesalamine Study Group. *New England Journal of Medicine, 339,* 370–374.

Whitehead, W. E., Palsson, O., & Jones, K. R. (2002). Systematic review of the comorbidity of irritable bowel syndrome with other disorders: What are the causes and implications? *Gastroenterology, 122,* 1140–1156.

Yang, Y. X., & Lichtenstein, G. R. (2002). Corticosteroids in Crohn's disease. *American Journal of Gastroenterology, 97,* 803–823.

Yu, A. S., & Hu, K. Q. (2001). Management of ascites. *Clinics in Liver Disease, 5,* 541–568.

29

Fundamental Concepts in the Diagnosis of Low Back Pain

Bruce A. Piszel, MD

EPIDEMIOLOGY AND RISK FACTORS FOR LOW BACK PAIN

It has been estimated that episodic low back pain is frequent or persistent in 15% of the U.S. population, with a lifetime prevalence of 65 to 80% (Manchikanti, Singh, & Saini, 2002). In addition, approximately 8% of the entire working population will become disabled in any given year, contributing to 40% of all lost workdays. Regarding cost estimates in relation to morbidity and mortality of occupational injury or illness, direct costs total $65 billion, with indirect costs approaching $106 billion.

Low back pain is the most common cause of chronic illness irrespective of gender in adults younger than 65 years of age, and the second most common in adults older than 65 years of age (Nachemson, Waddell, & Norlund, 2000). Low back pain–associated disability continues to rise with approximately 10 million lost workdays per year in 1955 and 105 million in 1995 (a 10.5-fold increase). The annual incidence of low back pain from all causes is about 60% (Lawrence, Helmick, & Arnelt, 1998). Frequent or persistent low back pain occurs in about 15% of the population during the course of a year. Herniated discs are associated with radicular symptoms in about 2% of patients. In contrast, only about 25% of episodes of low back pain are associated with sciatica (Borenstein, Wiesel, & Boden, 2004). Other causes of low back pain include osteoarthritis (15%) and fibromyalgia (2%).

There has been much debate about the correlation between potential risk factors and the actual development of low back pain (Manchikanti & Fellows, 2002). These risk factors are listed in Table 29.1. Low back pain continues to be an important clinical, social, economic, and public health problem affecting the United States and the world. Risk factors are many, but none is convincingly causal.

The specific causes of low back pain are diverse and vary with age. Common causes of low back pain are listed in Table 29.2. Radiculopathy due to herniated disc may be more common in younger patients, whereas radiculopathy in patients older than 50 years of age may be associated with degenerative changes of the spine, which reflects the age-related incidence of disk herniation. Indeed, disc herniation may be uncommon in patients younger than 25 years or older than 60 years of age (McCormick, 2000). The majority of patients are male, often with a history of trauma.

It is important to note that back pain may result from nonspinal causes, such as pancreatitis and aortic aneurysms that refer pain to the back. Common causes of pain referred to the low back are shown in Table 29.3. Metastatic tumors involving the spine become more common with advancing age, particularly tumors of lung, breast, and prostate (Table 29.4). Although relatively uncommon, infections of the spine account for about 1:20,000 hospital admissions per year (Miller & Jubelt, 2000).

The more common causes of low back pain are discussed in this chapter:

- Erector spinae muscular strain
- Radiculopathy
- Central canal stenosis

TABLE 29.1
Potential Risk Factors of Low Back Pain

Physical Factors	Individual Factors	Habits	Psychosocial Factors
Occupational	Genetic make up	Smoking	Marital
Heavy physical work	Age	Exercise	Social
Static work postures	Gender	Posture	Psychological
Bending, twisting, and lifting	Height	Physical activity	History of back pain
Vibration	Weight	Alcohol consumption	Family history
	Kyphosis		Work environment
	Scoliosis		Job dissatisfaction
	Leg length discrepancy		

TABLE 29.2
Causes of Low Back Pain

- Facet (zygapophyseal) joint
- Sacroiliac joint
- Trochanteric bursitis
- Fibromyalgia and other muscular causes
- Ligamentous injury
- Spondylolisthesis
- Herniated nucleus pulposis
- Discogenic (from a degenerated disc not causing radicular symptoms)
- Osteoarthritis and/or spondylosis (degenerative spine disease)
- Spinal stenosis (associated with neurogenic claudication or radiculopathy)
- Osteoporosis/fracture producing axial back pain and/or radiculopathy
- Rheumatoid diseases, particularly involving the cervical spine
- Osteomyelitis/discitis (bacterial and fungal infections)

TABLE 29.3
Common Nonspinal Causes of Low Back Pain

- Pancreatitis
- Pancreatic cancer
- Kidney stones
- Aortic aneurysm
- Retroperitoneal processes (e.g., psoas abscess)

TABLE 29.4
Common Malignancies Causing Low Back Pain

- Metastatic tumors
  - Lung cancer
  - Breast cancer
  - Prostate cancer
- Multiple myeloma (primary spinal tumor)

Note: Malignancies due to metastatic tumor involving the spine are a common cause of back pain in older patients, particularly those with a previous history of cancer.

- Arthritic changes of the facet (zygapophyseal) joint
- Piriformis syndrome
- Metastatic lesions of the vertebrae from a primary cancer
- Sacroiliac joint pain
- Arachnoiditis
- Secondary gain and/or drug-seeking behavior

ERECTOR SPINAE MUSCULAR STRAIN

The erector spinae muscle group is named anatomically from lateral to medial: iliocostalis, longissimus, and spinalis. Muscle strain is a common presenting problem when dealing with low back pain. (Remember, muscles strain; ligaments sprain.) It often occurs with overexertion by the patient involved in sports, incorrect posture the patient assumes when lifting heavy objects, or through repetitive movements either with extension alone or through a combination of extension and rotation as is involved in snow shoveling.

Muscular strains are categorized as first-degree, second-degree, and third-degree strains. First-degree strains are minor and indicate muscular injury at the microscopic level. Second-degree strains (moderate strain) involve a partial tear of the muscle(s) involved, and a third-degree strain is a complete tear of the muscle.

Low back pain from a strain is usually localized to the muscles involved and does not radiate down the thigh or leg as would be seen with a radiculopathy. There tends to be localized tenderness to palpation due to the development of trigger points, possibly in conjunction with muscular spasm. Symptoms can be reproduced with extension of the erector spinae group along with truncal rotation.

RADICULOPATHY

Radiculopathy may be defined as an abnormality of the spinal nerve root that may result in numbness or weakness, depending on whether afferent or efferent nerve fibers are involved. Causes of radiculopathy include mechanical compression and vascular compromise of the root. Radiculopathy per se does not imply that the injured nerve root is painful. On the other hand, radicular pain implies irritation of a spinal nerve root, rather than root compression. Possible causes of root irritation include leakage of inflammatory material from a damaged disc onto the nerve root. Patients may present with radicular pain radiating in a dermatomal pattern, without obvious nerve root compression on magnetic resonance imaging (MRI) or neurologic deficit. Some patients will have both radiculopathy and radicular pain.

The spinal nerve root injury usually begins proximal to the dorsal root ganglion, due to compression of the involved nerve root or inflammatory changes caused by the herniated disc. The proximal location of the abnormality decreases the sensitivity of electromyographic (EMG) studies because muscles of the lower extremity are supplied by more than one spinal nerve level. Therefore, a negative EMG, in and of itself, does not rule out a radiculopathy.

The structural causes of radiculopathy include protrusion or frank rupture of an intervertebral disc, inflammation due to material derived from the herniated disc, intervertebral foraminal stenosis, osteophytes, and rarely, infection. Narrowing of the intervertebral foramen may be due to trauma and degeneration. Slippage of one vertebral body on another may result in nerve root entrapment and radicular symptoms. Spondylolisthesis occurs when one vertebra moves either anteriorly or posteriorly (anterolisthesis or retrolisthesis, respectively) and may be congenital, associated with spondylolysis (fracture of the pars interarticularis), or acquired, related to degenerative changes.

The symptoms of lumbar radiculopathy and radicular pain are common and fairly characteristic. The patient may have low back pain with numbness or paresthesias that radiate in a dermatomal pattern, characteristically below the knee. The L5 or S1 nerve roots are most often involved.

Upon examination, decreased sensation, motor weakness, changes in reflexes, and muscle spasms may be present. In an acutely ruptured disk, having the patient perform a Valsalva maneuver may reproduce the patient's symptoms.

An L4 radiculopathy may specifically depress the patellar reflex, cause weakness of the leg extensors or ankle muscle dorsiflexors, and radiate to the medial aspect of the foot. An L5 radiculopathy may present with weakness of the extensor hallicus longus and with pain referred to the dorsum of the foot. An S1 radiculopathy may present with gastrocnemius weakness, Achilles tendon reflex abnormalities, and pain that radiates to the lateral aspect of the foot.

Keep in mind the differential diagnosis of anterior and posterior tarsal tunnel syndrome (anterior represents compression of the deep peroneal nerve, and posterior the compression of the posterior tibial nerve at the ankle) that may mimic radicular pain and radiculopathy. In addition, just because a patient presents with pain in the back and leg does not in and of itself secure the diagnosis of a radiculopathy. If the patient has a history of coronary artery disease, cerebrovascular disease, or any other vasculopathy, it is appropriate to assess the popliteal, dorsalis pedis, and posterior tibial pulses as part of the physical examination. Pain that involves the lower extremities, with ambulation, suggests ischemia (vascular claudication) of the muscles of the legs. Absent pulses on examination warrant Doppler studies to evaluate adequacy of blood flow to the legs. On the other hand, back pain that occurs with the patient standing, but not walking, suggests a spinal etiology.

Given the fact that the differential diagnosis of low back pain includes arthritides and infection, depending on the patient's presentation, appropriate laboratory studies may include a complete blood count, erythrocyte sedimentation rate, C-reactive protein, antinuclear antibody, and HLA-B27.

CENTRAL CANAL STENOSIS

Central canal stenosis may be due to a bulging or herniated disc, spondylolisthesis, arthropathy of the zygopophyseal (facet) joints, and pathology of the interlaminar ligaments. This process classically presents with neurogenic claudication; however, in the early stage of the disease, the patient may be asymptomatic. The patient will present with leg or calf pain while standing or walking that does not improve with rest (differentiating this from vascular claudication, which does improve with rest) but will improve with forward flexion of the lumbar spine, even while standing. For example, a patient may experience relief of symptoms while leaning over a shopping cart at the grocery store or walking up stairs, both involving forward flexion of the lumbar spine. Pain may worsen when walking down stairs, which requires extension of the lumbar spine. Additional findings may include altered reflexes, motor weakness, and the presence of numbness or paresthesias. However, the neurologic exam may be normal when the patient is seated and asymptomatic. Also, the clinician should inquire about the presence of urinary or fecal incontinence and saddle anesthesia (frank numbness of the perineum), as these, in addition to motor weakness, could indicate the presence of a cauda equina syndrome, which is an indication for surgical decompression of the spine.

FACET (ZYGAPOPHYSEAL) SYNDROME

The facet (zygapophyseal) joint is a synovial diarthrodial joint that receives its innervation from the medial branches of the posterior primary division. Facet joint pain may be caused by arthritic changes to the joint itself, due to osteoarthritis or rheumatoid arthritis; however, in many instances, the etiology is unknown. Degeneration of the facet joints may be worsened with loss of intervertebral disc height, resulting in the facets becoming weight-bearing joints.

The patient typically presents with low back pain reproducible with palpation lateral to the spinous processes, along with extension of the spine or truncal rotation. The patient's pain typically does not radiate inferiorly and does not involve paresthesias. The incidence of facet-mediated pain is quite common, accounting for symptoms in at least a third of patients with low back pain (Manchikanti, Singh, & Saini, 2001).

PIRIFORMIS SYNDROME

Piriformis syndrome should be considered when formulating a differential diagnosis for lumbar radiculopathy. The underlying mechanism presumably involves an entrapment neuropathy of the sciatic nerve (which divides distally into the tibial and common peroneal nerves) between the piriformis muscle superiorly and the inferior gemellus inferiorly. In some patients, the symptoms may be more severe because the sciatic nerve pierces the piriformis muscle (may occur in 12% of the population). Patients may present with weakness, numbness or paresthesias, and pain in a sciatic nerve distribution. An effective way to differentiate sciatic nerve entrapment from lumbosacral radiculopathy is to palpate the piriformis (located between the sacrum and greater trochanter of the femur) to assess if point tenderness is present. Piriformis syndrome may demonstrate point tenderness, whereas radiculopathy does not present with such focal signs on examination. Also, internal rotation of the femur, which stretches the piriformis muscle, may aggravate pain.

METASTATIC CANCER INVOLVING THE SPINE

Low back pain due to metastasis needs to be considered in patients with unremitting back pain, particularly in patients with a history of cancer. Bone pain can involve both nociceptive and neuropathic elements. The nociceptive mechanisms involve bone destruction from osteoblastic and osteolytic lesions. Neuropathic pain may result from tumor invasion of the spinal nerve, which may also involve a nociceptive process. Tumors that commonly metastasize to the spine are listed in Table 29.3.

In older men, prostate cancer needs to considered, because of the relatively high lifetime prevalence of prostate cancer. As previously mentioned, metastatic spread occurs from the prostate to the lumbar vertebrae via Batson's venous plexus. On examination, there may be point tenderness over the spinous processes and lamina. Also, there may be pain to percussion with a reflex hammer.

SACROILIAC JOINT PAIN

Sacroiliac joint pain can be caused by osteoarthritis, rheumatoid arthritis, ligamentous strain due to poor posture while lifting, and collagen vascular diseases. The patient typically presents with pain around the sacroiliac joint with radiation to the buttock, groin, and possibly the posterior thigh, generally without radiation below the knee. Also, those with reproducible symptoms on palpation over the sacroiliac joint should have a plain radiograph taken to exclude overt pathology, such as tumor. Again, when collagen vascular diseases are suspected (the patient may present with systemic complaints), a rheumatologic panel is necessary.

ARACHNOIDITIS

Pain from arachnoiditis occurs as a result of inflammation of the arachnoid membrane surrounding the spinal rootlets. Although the exact etiology of arachnoiditis is still unclear, a number of possible causes have been implicated. These include infection, intrathecal administration of medications, disc herniation, and as a complication of thickening and scarring of roots following myelography.

The patient with arachnoiditis may present with burning, radiating pain (the pattern of symptoms depending on the nerve root affected), altered reflexes, numbness or paresthesias, frank motor weakness, or bowel and bladder abnormalities.

FEIGNING OF SYMPTOMS

The clinician will at some point encounter a patient suspected of exaggerating symptoms due to drug-seeking behavior or for acquiring disability payments. In 1980, Waddell (Waddell, McCulloch, Kummel, & Venner, 1980) presented a list of signs that may help distinguish patients with non-organic back pain from those with pain more likely to be associated with structural causes. Known as Waddell's signs, these criteria remain in common use:

- Pain in lumbar region with superficial palpation
- Nonpainful palpation of a previously painful area with distraction
- Non-anatomic pain distribution; for example, pain that radiates from the lumbar spine inferiorly and superiorly to the ear
- Overreaction to provocative tests
- Reproducibility of low back pain symptoms when rotating the trunk with the center of rotation below the lumbar spine; the area of the body that is rotating is the hips, knees, and ankles

Each item present is given one point. A score of 0 to 2 is considered to be within normal limits. A score greater than 2 should alert the physician to the possibility of non-organic pain that requires further investigation.

If a patient presents with hip flexor weakness that the clinician believes is due to poor effort on the part of the patient, the physician can lay the patient supine and perform a Hoover's maneuver. The physician lifts the patient's lower extremities by cupping the calcaneus with the palmar aspect of the hand. Then, the patient is asked to lift the symptomatic leg first, and then the other leg. If the patient is not giving a full effort, the physician will not feel the patient pushing down with the opposite lower extremity.

There are patients who present with histories or symptoms that should alert the physician to the possibility of drug-seeking behavior. These include

- History of multiple physician visits for pain without any clear diagnosis
- History of opioid prescriptions without any clear diagnosis or specific workup
- Multiple opioid allergies except "the one" that relieves the patient's pain
- Pain complaints in non-anatomic distributions as indicated on the dermatome drawing
- Admission by the patient of acquiring opioids without a physician's prescription because none of the other physicians understands or can diagnose his or her pain, requiring the patient to self-medicate

It is the responsibility of the doctor to bring up the subject of drug abuse and addiction, and if the patient admits to having a problem, an addiction medicine consult is indicated. Long-term opioid therapy may be appropriate for the management of low back pain, but the risks and potential benefits are a matter of increasing controversy.

LOW BACK PAIN HISTORY

The clinician should have the patient complete a specific pain history:

- The patient should complete a pain drawing indicating areas of pain with a red pencil and areas of numbness or paresthesias with a blue-colored pencil. Figure 29.1 is a dermatomal drawing used by the pain clinic at University Hospitals of Cleveland.
- On a scale of 1–10, the patient should quantify the pain (when interviewing the patient, it is helpful to give an example of "ten out of ten" pain).
- Where is the pain localized?

- Does the pain radiate, and to what part of the body?
- Is the pain accompanied by numbness?
- What exacerbates the pain and what improves it?
- Pain characterization (is it sharp, dull, electric-like)?
- Does the pain interfere with the patient's sleep (initiation or maintenance)?
- Does the pain affect the patient's mood?
- Does the pain interfere with the patient's activities of daily living?
- Is there a periodicity to the pain (worse in the morning, afternoon, or evening)?
- Was there an inciting event?
- Is the pain work related?
- Is the patient currently involved in litigation?
- Is the pain worsening?
- Is there a history of a psychiatric illness?
- Previous workup for pain?
- Medication allergies and all current medications
- Past medical history
- Past surgical history
- Social history
- Family history

RADIOGRAPHIC STUDIES

Plain radiography is frequently the first imaging study ordered because it is the most widely available and the least expensive modality to image the lumbar spine. Plain films can provide information on acute and chronic changes. In the acute setting, a radiograph is the most expedient tool to demonstrate a fracture. Chronic changes such as bone spurs, intervertebral disc height collapse, vacuum disc phenomenon, and endplate remodeling can also be seen. Malalignment of bony structures such as vertebral bodies, pedicles, and zygopophyseal joints provides evidence of spondylolysis, spondylolisthesis, scoliosis, and kyphosis.

Assessing the integrity of the osseous structures can identify bony destruction and erosive changes from malignancy, infection, spondyloarthropathies, and metabolic diseases. It is widely believed that routine radiographs of the lumbar spine are of limited value in the workup and treatment of acute nontraumatic low back pain. This may be true for low back pain without radicular symptoms, in the acute nontraumatic setting. However, there are specific factors that necessitate the ordering of plain films:

- Age over 50
- Neuromotor deficits
- Unexplained weight loss
- Suspicion of ankylosing spondylitis
- Drug or alcohol abuse

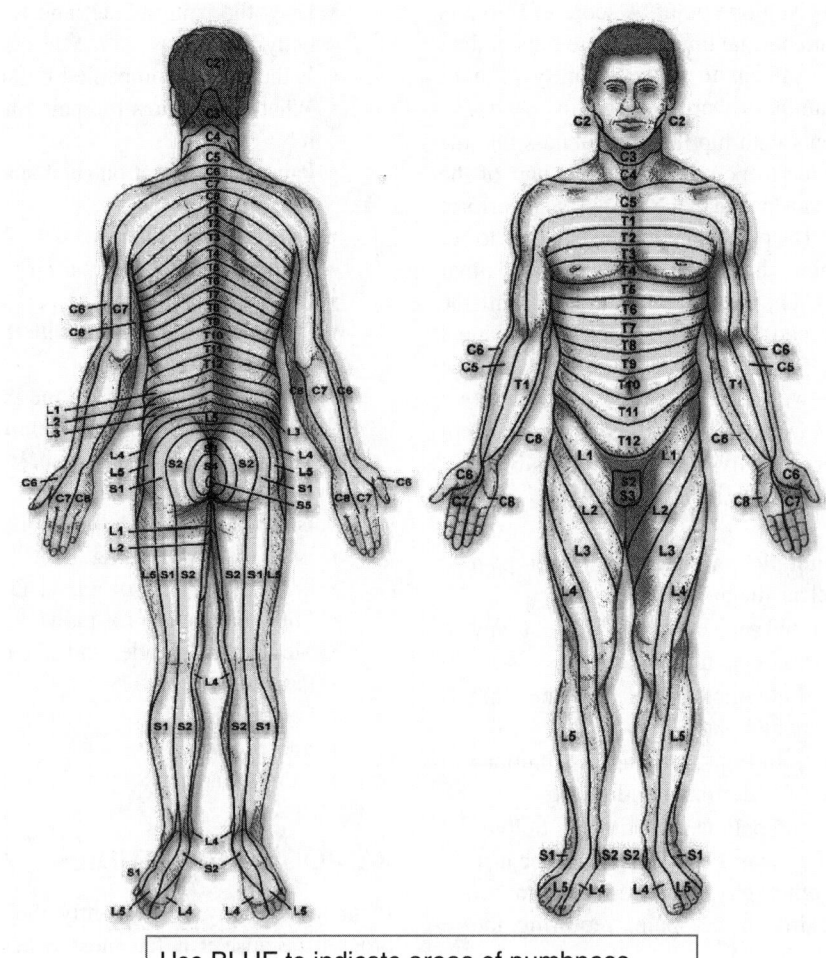

Use BLUE to indicate areas of numbness
Use RED to indicate areas of pain

FIGURE 29.1 Pain drawing. Patient uses colored pencils to indicate painful areas and numbness.

- Cancer history
- Corticosteroid use
- Fever
- Impending litigation
- Low back pain and neurologic compromise of unclear etiology

Although the majority of patients have resolution of low back pain over 4 to 6 weeks, as many as 10% will continue to have back pain longer than 6 weeks, despite conservative management. In this group of patients with subacute low back pain, radiographs are recommended. It is worth remembering that plain radiographs can assess the spine dynamically rather that statically and identify degenerative changes, fractures, and tumors.

COMPUTED TOMOGRAPHY

Computed tomography (CT) provides the most detailed osseous images. In the lumbar spine, CT is used primarily to evaluate bony anatomy, particularly the spinal canal and cortical bone integrity. CT can be performed more quickly than an MRI, making it an ideal test to assess the spinal column following major trauma. Other indications include patients unable to undergo an MRI because of weight, claustrophobia, and the presence of ferromagnetic shrapnel, aneurismal clips, or some implantable devices. CT scans are relatively contraindicated in pregnancy and surgical fusion with instrumentation (the metal hardware creates scatter resulting in artifact often severely limiting the usefulness of the images).

MAGNETIC RESONANCE IMAGING

This imaging modality is used clinically to provide superior and detailed soft tissue images. The soft tissue imagery evaluates water density within different types of tissues. Intra- and extrathecal neural elements, epidural space, spinal ligaments, paraspinal soft tissues, disc morphology, and alignment can be evaluated. When used with gadolinium contrast, MRI provides unparalleled visualization of intramedullary diseases such as myelomalacia, syrinx, neoplasms, demyelination, intradural, and extradural tumors and spinal infections. Furthermore, it can differentiate between recurrent and retained disc herniation and scar tissue.

About 30% of asymptomatic people have MRI evidence of a disc protrusion (asymmetric disc bulge extending beyond the interspace (Jenson, Brant-Zawadski, & Obuchowski, 1994). For those over 50 years of age, two thirds of individuals show disc abnormalities, compared with about one third of individuals younger than 30 years. Although a large proportion of asymptomatic patients may have abnormalities on MRI, the study is useful when evaluating patients with focal neurologic findings accompanying radicular symptoms, in addition to back pain.

The physics of image generation during an MRI is complicated and beyond the scope of this chapter. Essentially, an external magnet polarizes the hydrogen protons in water molecules and a specific radiofrequency is pulsed into the body. Depending on the number of mobile hydrogen ions intrinsic in the tissue, different images will be generated. The three primary spins sequences are longitudinal relaxation time (T1), transverse relaxation time (T2), and proton density. T1-weighted images are best to evaluate fat-rich tissues such as bone marrow. An evolving hemorrhage and other high-protein fluid collections can also be evaluated. T2-weighted images emphasize extracellular water, such as cerebrospinal fluid, fluid collections, cysts, and abscesses.

Necrotic tissue, neoplasm, and the intervertebral disc are examples of tissues that have high signal intensity on T2-weighted images. Proton density–weighted images are best used to evaluate spinal ligaments and zygapophyseal joint morphology.

When compared with CT, MRI is more sensitive for providing radiologic evidence of lumbar discogenic disease because it provides better information on the soft tissues before disc contours change. These alterations include annular tears and disc desiccation.

Both CT and MRI are adept at identifying a disc herniation. A focal protrusion is a disc herniation where there is an annular contour abnormality. But the displaced nuclear material is still contained within the outer wall of the annulus. In contrast, a disc extrusion is present when nuclear material is found beyond the outer wall of the annulus, suggesting a tear of the annulus. It can be contained by the posterior longitudinal ligament (known as a subligamentous extrusion). CT is not as sensitive as MRI in differentiating this type of abnormality. Also, an MRI is the best means to identify disc degeneration associated with stenosis.

MRI is the imaging modality of choice in patients who have undergone prior disc surgery. MRI has difficulty discriminating posterior disc margins from postoperative changes. After 6 months of surgery, MRI with gadolinium is recommended. In this case, the MRI is useful in evaluating the degree of neural encroachment from soft tissues, such as the ligamentum flavum, disc, and facet joint capsule.

MRI is superior to plain films and CT scans for imaging tumors of the lumbar spine. If tumor or infection is suspected, gadolinium is used because it enhances neovascularized proliferating tissue, inflammatory processes, and necrotic tissue.

The imaging study ordered should be based on the patient's history and clinical examination, with due consideration of the structures that need to be visualized. Although MRI and CT can identify abnormalities, no imaging study can ascertain whether an abnormality is painful.

ELECTRODIAGNOSIS

If a patient presents with a radiculopathy that includes muscle weakness and sensory changes, EMG may be a helpful tool to determine if the lesion exists centrally or peripheral to the spinal nerve root. This is especially true after a diagnostic block fails to improve a patient's symptoms. EMG interpretations are complex and are usually performed by an experienced rehabilitation physician or neurologist. However, a physician treating pain should be familiar with some of the muscles and nerves that are tested during a routine radiculopathy screen.

Although an EMG usually includes nerve conduction velocity (NCV) testing, the overall test is typically referred to as an EMG. The motor portion of the NCV typically evaluates the following nerves (Preston & Shapiro, 1998):

- Peroneal nerve: extensor digitorum brevis, and tibialis anterior
- Tibial nerve: abductor hallicus brevis and abductor digiti quinti pedis

The sensory portion of the NCV will include sural and superficial nerves and, occasionally, the saphenous and the lateral and medial plantar nerves

Suggested muscles to be sampled in the EMG proper for a suspected lumbosacral radiculopathy include:

- Tibialis anterior (L4–L5)
- Medial gastrocnemius (S1–S2)
- Flexor digitorum longus (L5–S1)
- Extensor digitorum brevis (L5–S1)
- Vastus lateralis (L2–L4)
- Gluteus medius (L5–S1)
- Mid and low lumbar paraspinals (L4–S1)

The EMG results will help guide the treatment options with regard to location of the lesion (peripheral vs. centrally located) and whether a surgical consultation is warranted.

BASICS OF THE PHYSICAL EXAMINATION FOR LOW BACK PAIN

The initial examination should be comprehensive, in that low back provocative tests should be used, in addition to tests that examine the hip and pelvis. This is especially true if the lumbar tests fail to reproduce symptoms. A good place to start is to ask the patient to demonstrate active range of motion of the lumbar spine in the following planes: extension, flexion, right and left lateral flexion, and finally, right and left rotation. It is a good idea to demonstrate these maneuvers first and stand close to the patient during the movements, in case the patient loses balance. Also, instruct the patient to stop the maneuver whenever pain is experienced.

While the patient is standing, ask the patient to walk on the heels and toes, while nearby or holding the patient's hands to accurately assess the strength of the plantar flexors and dorsiflexors.

The primary plantar flexors of the ankle include the following:

- Peroneus longus and brevis: innervated by the superficial peroneal nerve (S1)
- Gastrocnemius and soleus: innervated by the tibial nerve (S1 and S2)
- Flexor hallicus longus: innervated by the tibial nerve (L5)
- Flexor digitorum longus: innervated by the tibial nerve (L5)
- Tibialis posterior: innervated by the tibial nerve (L5)

The primary dorsiflexors of the ankle include

- Tibialis anterior: innervated by the deep peroneal nerve (L4 and L5)
- Extensor hallicus longus: innervated by the deep peroneal nerve (L5)
- Extensor digitorum longus: innervated by the deep peroneal nerve (L5)

If these muscles (ankle dorsiflexors and plantar flexors) are tested while the patient is seated or supine, the physician will not get an accurate assessment of the muscle strength because these muscles are quite powerful, as they carry the weight of the entire body.

Muscle strength is classified using the following scale:

5/5 Normal muscle strength
4/5 Muscle strength slightly decreased from normal
3/5 Muscle strength greater than gravity (antigravity that gives way quite easily to the slightest pressure)

2/5 Muscle strength not able to overcome gravity, but movement of the joint takes place with gravity eliminated; e.g., if bicep flexion strength is less than a grade of three, lift the elbow up and see if the joint moves in the horizontal plane
1/5 The examiner is able to see the muscle contracting; however, there is no joint movement
0/5 No muscle contraction seen (flaccid paralysis)

With the patient seated on the examination table, assess muscular strength of the hip flexors and knee flexion strength. The muscles involved in these movements and their innervations are as follows:

- Hip flexors: Iliopsoas: innervated by the femoral nerve (L1,2,3). Note that the rectus femoris is also involved in flexion of the hip.
- Hip adduction: Adductor longus: innervated by the obturator nerve (L2,3,4). Note that the adductor magnus, brevis, pectineus, and gracilis are also involved in adduction.
- Hip abduction: Gluteus medius: innervated by the superior gluteal nerve (L5). Note the gluteus minimus also plays a role in this movement.
- Knee extension: Quadriceps: innervated by the femoral nerve (L2,3,4).
- Knee flexion: Hamstrings (made up of the semimembranosis, semitendinosis, and biceps femoris): innervated by the tibial nerve (L5–S1).

With the patient seated, test the deep tendon reflexes of the lower and upper extremities. These include the following:

- Biceps reflex: (C5)
- Triceps reflex: (C7)
- Patellar reflex: (L4)
- Hamstring reflex: (L5)
- Achilles tendon reflex: (S1)

In the seated position, the paraspinal musculature can be palpated, looking for spasm and trigger points. Finally, tapping the reflex hammer over the spinous processes to evaluate for the presence of bony pain or tenderness.

There are extensive formally named clinical maneuvers to assess the low back, many overlapping. The straight leg raise (SLR) test is used to assess for the presence of nerve root irritation, which would support the diagnosis of radiculopathy. The examiner raises the leg on the symptomatic side until the patient complains of pain, noting the approximate point when the pain begins as well as whether the pain is localized to the back or radiates into the extremity. If radiating pain is elicited, the examiner lowers the leg slightly and, while dorsiflexing the foot (Braggard's test), determines whether the radiating pain is replicated. The examiner can also extend the great toe (Sicard's test), both maneuvers indicative of positive root tension signs. If the initial test is negative, the examiner can increase the tension on the sciatic nerve by performing the same maneuvers. Many examiners should note the approximate angle of hip flexion assuming 0° to 35° typically causes pain due to extradural involvement, 30° to 70° from disc pathology, and 70° to 90° indicates lumbar joint pain. Alternatively, the examiner places one hand under the patient while palpating the lumbosacral spine, so as to help better differentiate the location of the pain (Goldwaith's test). In the case of unilateral pain, the asymptomatic side is then tested. If the patient experiences pain on the symptomatic side while raising the asymptomatic lower extremity, it could indicate a disc protrusion medial to the nerve root on the symptomatic side (Fajersztajn's test, also called a contralateral or well leg SLR test). Elevating the patient's legs together, and asking the patient to hold the legs up or having the patient raise both legs together several inches above the table (leg-lowering or Milgram's test) are both signs of increasing intrathecal pressure, often associated with nerve root compression, such as a disc herniation. The prudent examiner will often alter the examination based on the examination findings to even better help differentiate or confirm the suspected cause of the patient's pain.

With the patient remaining in the supine position, the passive range of motion of both hips is assessed by flexing the hips to the end range of motion and then moving the hips in an arc laterally and returning the lower extremity to the original position onto the examining table.

Now, the examiner asks the patient to roll over into the prone position. The examiner can assess the hip extensor strength, sacroiliac joint, and tender zygopophyseal joints. The examiner can locate the sacroiliac joint by starting at the superior aspect of the gluteal crease and palpating at an angle up to the point where the superior articular process contacts the inferior articular process of the fifth lumbar vertebrae. A provocative test that can be performed to reproduce pain from the sacroiliac joint is the Yeoman's test. This is performed by flexing the leg and grasping the ankle with both hands and lifting the leg and thigh, which puts maximal stress on the joint. Palpate the facet joints that lie on either side of the spinous processes.

The piriformis muscle should be examined with the asymptomatic side down and the hip and knee flexed. This stretches the muscle and makes palpation more likely to reproduce symptoms. The piriformis is located between the sacrum and greater trochanter. If point tenderness is elicited over the piriformis with or without radiation of pain distally, the piriformis may be the pain generator.

SUMMARY

The diagnosis of low back pain can be difficult due to large number of possible etiologies involved. It is incum-bent on the clinician to obtain a complete and thorough history, addressing questions specific to the patient's complaints and mitigating factors.

The hallmark of a thorough examination includes the reproducibility of symptoms, as there may be poor correlation between radiographic abnormalities and symptoms. Of equal importance is making sure that the patient's complaints are not due to a potentially life-threatening condition, such as prostate cancer that has metastasized to the lumbar spine. Also, it is important to address the issue of the patient who may be feigning symptoms for secondary gain or the patient who demonstrates drug-seeking behavior.

Although the list of potential diagnoses is long, muscular strain, degenerative changes in the spine producing facet-mediated and discogenic pain, and radiculopathy are commonly seen in the clinic. The most important service a physician can do for the patient is to clearly delineate a differential diagnosis. This will help narrow the list of possible causes to a more specific diagnosis, upon which definitive treatment can be planned. It is also important to remember that there are common nonspinal causes of pain that must be considered when evaluating patients with back pain.

Diagnostic studies may help identify pain generators in the spine that are amenable to specific therapeutic interventions. The role of interventional pain management is considered in detail in Section VII of this textbook.

REFERENCES

Borenstein, D. G., Wiesel, S. W., & Boden, S. D. (2004). Epidemiology of neck and low back pain. In D. G. Borenstein, S. W. Wiesel, & S. D. Boden (Eds.), *Low back and neck pain* (3rd ed., pp. 37–58). Philadelphia: Saunders.

Jensen, M. C. et al. (1994). Magnetic resonance imaging of the lumbar spine in people without back pain. *New England Journal of Medicine, 331*, 69–73

Lawrence, R. C., Helmick, C. G., & Arnett, F. C. (1998). Estimates of the prevalence of arthritis and selected musculoskeletal disorders in the United States. *Arthritis Rheumatism, 41*, 778–799.

Manchikanti, L., & Fellows, B. (2002). Risk factors of low back pain. In L. Manchikanti, C. W. Slipman, & B. Fellows (Eds.), *Low back pain diagnosis and treatment* (p. 22). Paducah: ASIPP Publishing, American Society of Interventional Pain Physicians.

Manchikanti, L., Singh, V., & Saini, B. (2002). Epidemiology of low back pain. In L. Manchikanti, C. W. Slipman, & B. Fellows (Eds.) *Low back pain diagnosis and treatment* (pp. 3–20). Paducah, KY: ASIPP Publishing.

Manchikanti, L., Singh, V., & Saini, B. (2001). Evaluation of the relative contributions of various structures in chronic low back pain. *Pain Physician, 4*, 308–316.

McCormick, P. C. (2000). Intervertebral discs and radiculopathy. In L. P. Rowland (Ed.). *Merritt's neurology* (10th ed., pp. 424–430). Philadelphia: Lippincott Williams and Wilkins.

Miller, J. R., & Jubelt, B. (2000). Bacterial infections. In L. P. Rowland (Ed.), *Merritt's neurology* (10th ed., pp. 103–126). Philadelphia: Lippincott Williams and Wilkins.

Nachemson, A. L., Waddell, G., & Norlund, A. L. (2000). Epidemiology of neck and low back pain. In A. L. Nachemson (Ed.). *Neck and back pain: The scientific evidence of causes, diagnosis, and treatment* (pp. 165–187). Philadelphia: Lippincott Williams and Wilkins.

Preston, D. C., & Shapiro, B. E. (1998). *Electromyography and neuromuscular disorders: Clinical electrophysiologic correlations.* Boston, MA: Butterworth-Heinemann.

Waddell, G., McCulloch, J. A., Kummel, E., & Venner, R. M. (1980). Nonorganic physical signs in low-back pain. *Spine, 5,* 117–25.

30

Chronic Pelvic Pain

Andrea J. Rapkin, MD, and Candace Howe, MD

INTRODUCTION

Chronic pelvic pain is, by definition, pain that persists for more than 6 months. In its various forms, chronic pelvic pain affects an estimated 12 to 15% of women in the United States, accounting for more than $881 million spent each year on outpatient visits (Mathias et al., 1996). It is one of the most common but taxing problems in gynecologic practice. Even after a thorough workup, the etiology may remain obscure, and the relationship between certain types of pathology and the pain response may be inconsistent and often inexplicable. In the patient who has no obvious pathology, it may be tempting to remove pelvic structures for their physiological variations. Approximately 12% of all hysterectomies are performed for pelvic pain and 30% of patients who present to pain clinics have already had a hysterectomy (Chamberlain & La Ferla, 1987; Reiter, 1990b).

The purpose of this chapter is to outline the anatomy and physiology of pelvic pain and to explore the differential diagnosis and management of chronic pelvic pain, including the role of medication, surgery, psychotherapy, and the multidisciplinary pain management.

NEUROANATOMY AND NEUROPHYSIOLOGY OF PELVIC PAIN

The pelvic viscera receive afferent innervation by way of the autonomic nerve trunks (Kumazawa, 1986). The major neural pathways for visceral pain from the female pelvic organs travel with the sympathetic nerve bundles and have cell bodies in a thoracolumbar distribution. Sensory afferents that travel with the parasympathetic (sacral) fibers are probably of secondary importance for pain transmission from the pelvic organs. These latter nerves have their cell bodies in the sacral dorsal root ganglia (Kumazawa, 1986). The innervation of the female pelvic viscera and somatic structures is depicted in Figure 30.1 and Table 30.1. The transmission of painful stimuli from the pelvic organs relies on an intact lumbosacral autonomic nervous system (Cervero & Tattersall, 1986). However, the sacral autonomics are crucial for urination, defecation, and reflex regulation of the reproductive organs (Kumazawa, 1986). The role of the sacral autonomics in the genesis of pelvic pain is likely but remains to be delineated. A large proportion of the sacral afferents from the colon and urinary bladder are usually silent. Only 5% of colon afferents and 2.5% of bladder afferents can be activated by mechanical distension. A proportion of the nonmechanosensitive unmyelinated sacral afferents are chemosensitive and can develop *de nouveau* mechano-sensitivity (Janig et al., 1993). These usually "silent" fibers may be activated by and sensitized by inflammation or unusually strong mechanical stimulation and may play a role in pelvic pain of urinary tract or gastrointestinal etiology and theoretically from the internal reproductive organs as well.

The cell bodies of the afferent axons from the pelvic organs are located in the dorsal (sensory) ganglia of the spinal nerves (Fields, 1987). Before entering the spinal gray matter of the dorsal horn, branches of these afferent axons may extend for two or more segments beyond the level at which the original axons entered the cord. Much of neuronal modulation occurs in the dorsal horn. Evidence from animal studies indicates that supraspinal factors interact at the level of the dorsal horn to modulate the sensory perception of pain from the pelvic viscera (Berkley & Hubscher, 1995; De Groat, 1994).

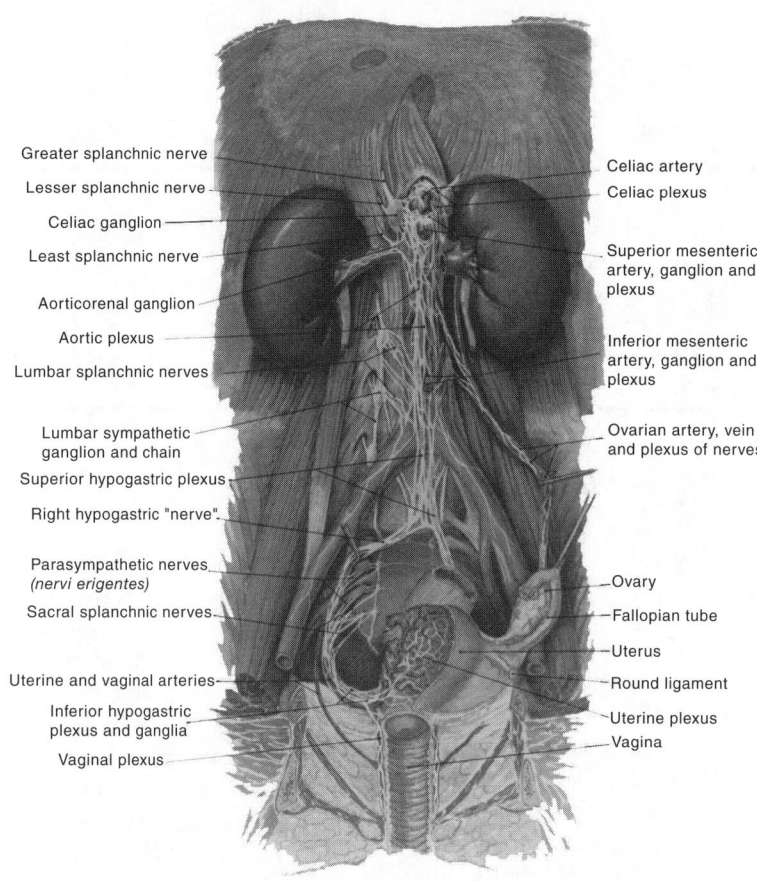

FIGURE 30.1 The innervation of the female pelvic viscera.

TABLE 30.1
Innervation of the Female Pelvis

Organ	Spinal Segments	Nerves
Abdominal wall	T12–L1	Iliohypogastric, ilioinguinal, genitofemoral
Lower abdominal wall, anterior vulva, urethra, and clitoris	L1–L2	Ilioinguinal, genitofemoral
Lower back	L1–L2	
Pelvic floor, anus, perineum, and lower vagina	S2–S4	Pudendal, inguinal, genitofemoral, posterofemoral cutaneous
Upper vagina, cervix, uterine corpus, inner third of fallopian tube, broad ligament, upper bladder, terminal ileum, and terminal large bowel	T11–L2 S2–S4	Thoracolumbar autonomics (sympathetics) via hypogastric plexus; sacral autonomics (parasympathetics) via pelvic nerve
Ovaries, outer two thirds of fallopian tubes, and upper ureter	T9–T10	Thoracic autonomics (sympathetics) via renal and aortic plexus and celiac and mesenteric ganglia, aortic and superior mesenteric plexuses

The dorsal horn is an important site of modulation of afferent input (Cervero & Tattersall, 1986). The second-order neurons are subjected to excitatory and/or inhibitory interactions. For example, if a visceral structure and a cutaneous (somatic) structure transmitting to the same second-order neuron in the dorsal horn are stimulated simultaneously, the second-order neuron response may be greater than either the cutaneous or the visceral stimulus would evoke on its own. These viscero-somatic neurons tend to have larger receptive fields than the somatic neurons. There are also many more somatic second-order neurons than there are viscero-somatic neurons (Cervero & Tattersall, 1986). Both of these facts may account for the vague, poorly localizable quality of visceral pelvic pain.

The concept of neuromodulation has proved promising as a partial explanation for the persistence of chronic pelvic pain. Prolonged severe acute pain unrelieved for more than 24 hours induces neuroplastic changes via excessive and prolonged stimulation of N-methyl-D-aspartate (NMDA) receptors and increase nerve irritability, among other mechanisms. This irritability creates an allodynia and hyperalgesia (Doggweiler-Wiygul, 2001). In addition to afferent conduction due to noxious stimuli there is damage to local tissue by antidromic conduction. Neurogenic inflammation can become pathogenic such as in disorders like asthma, migraines, endometriosis, and arthritis (Wesselmann, 2001). This may prove important in the development of new medical treatment for chronic pelvic pain, which could be directed at prolonged neurogenic inflammation, visceral, and referred hyperalgesia.

The neurophysiology of pain transmission from the viscera (internal organs such as bowel, bladder, rectum, uterus, ovaries, and fallopian tubes) differs from that of somatic structures (cutaneous elements, fascia, muscles, parietal peritoneum, mesentery, external genitalia, anus, urethra). Nociceptors receive pain evoked at somatic nerves, whereas a plentitude of nonspecific receptors receive pain induced in the viscera (Berkley, 1994; Cervero, 1994). Visceral pain, in contrast to somatic pain, is usually deep, difficult to localize, and frequently associated with various autonomic reflexes such as restlessness, nausea, vomiting, and diaphoresis (Procacci et al., 1986). Early surgical studies performed under local anesthesia have shown that cutting, crushing, or burning the bowel, for example, evokes no pain, whereas distension of muscular organs or hollow viscera, stretching of the capsule of solid organs, hypoxia or necrosis of viscera, production of algesic (pain producing) substances, rapid compression of ligaments or vessels, and inflammation may cause severe pain. In contrast, cutting or crushing a somatic structure produces exquisite pain that is well localized (Procacci et al., 1986). Well-localized abdominal wall or pelvic floor pain in patients with chronic pelvic pain is likely secondary to referred hyperalgesia, myofascial pain/trigger points, or nerve entrapment. Familiarity

with the anatomy of somatic structures delineating the pelvis is therefore important (McDonald & Rapkin, 2001).

PERIPHERAL CAUSES OF CHRONIC PELVIC PAIN

ADHESIONS

The differential diagnosis of the peripheral component of pelvic pain is listed in Table 30.2. Laparoscopic studies for the evaluation of chronic pelvic pain would suggest that adhesions play a prominent role. However, when these studies were performed, nongynecologic sources of pelvic pain such as abdominal wall or pelvic floor myofascial pain or neuropathy, irritable bowel syndrome, and interstitial cystitis were often not excluded prior to laparoscopy. Adhesions were present in 16 to 44% of the patients undergoing laparoscopy for chronic pelvic pain (depending on the series) (Kresch et al., 1984; Liston et al., 1972; Lundberg et al., 1973; Rapkin, 1986; Renaer, 1981). Do adhesions actually cause pelvic pain? Of 100 patients Kresch laparoscoped for chronic pelvic pain, 38% had adhesions and 10% had bowel adhesions. However, of 50 asymptomatic patients undergoing laparoscopy for sterilization, only 12% had adhesions and only 2% exhibited adhesions involving the bowel. These differences were highly significant (Kresch et al., 1984). Keltz et al. (1995) in a combined retrospective/prospective study found colon to side-wall adhesions in a higher proportion of patients (93 vs. 13%) with pelvic pain than the control group (sterilization).

In comparison, Rapkin (1986) noted that many infertility patients with severe adhesions had no pain and compared the results of laparoscopies performed on two groups of patients—the first group complained of chronic pelvic pain and the second group had infertility, without complaints of pain. When evaluating both the site and density of adhesions, it was notable that there were no significant differences between the group with chronic pelvic pain and asymptomatic patients in the infertility group. The results of this study question the role of pelvic adhesions as a common cause of chronic pelvic pain.

If adhesions cause pain, then lysis of adhesions should relieve pain. A prospective noncontrolled, nonrandomized study of lysis of adhesions did not show significantly lower postoperative pain ratings (Steege & Scott, 1991). However, *post hoc* analysis consisting of separation of the subjects into those with and without psychosocial dysfunction revealed a significant improvement in pain scores in the group without psychosocial dysfunction. An early prospective randomized study of adhesiolysis revealed no differences in the pain scores between the groups (adhesiolysis vs. no adhesiolysis). Again, *post hoc* analysis of the data suggested there was a significant improvement (although only on two of the three methods of pain assess-

TABLE 30.2
Peripheral Causes of Chronic Pelvic Pain

Gynecologic
    Noncyclic
    Adhesions
    Endometriosis
    Salpingo-oophoritis
    Acute
    Subacute
    Ovarian remnant syndrome
    Pelvic congestion syndrome (varicosities)
    Ovarian neoplasms
    Pelvic relaxation
    Cyclic
    Primary dysmenorrhea
    Secondary dysmenorrhea
    Imperforate hymen
    Transverse vaginal septum
    Cervical stenosis
    Uterine anomalies (congenital malformation, bicornuate uterus, blind
        uterine horn)
    Intrauterine synechiae (Asherman's syndrome)
    Endometrial polyps
    Uterine leiomyoma
    Adenomyosis
    Pelvic congestion syndrome (varicosities)
    Endometriosis
    Atypical cyclic
    Endometriosis
    Adenomyosis
    Ovarian remnant syndrome
    Chronic functional cyst formation
Gastrointestinal
    Irritable bowel syndrome
    Ulcerative colitis
    Granulomatous colitis (Crohn's disease)
    Carcinoma
    Infectious diarrhea
    Recurrent partial small bowel obstruction
    Diverticulitis
    Hernia
    Abdominal angina
    Recurrent appendiceal colic
Genitourinary
    Recurrent or relapsing cystourethritis
    Urethral syndrome
    Interstitial cystitis
    Ureteral diverticuli or polyps
    Carcinoma of the bladder
    Ureteral obstruction
    Pelvic kidney
Neurologic
    Nerve entrapment syndrome
    Neuroma
    Trigger points
Musculoskeletal
    Low back pain syndrome
    Congenital anomalies

TABLE 30.2 (Continued)
Peripheral Causes of Chronic Pelvic Pain

    Scoliosis and kyphosis
    Spondylolysis
    Spondylolisthesis
    Spinal injuries
    Inflammation
    Tumors
    Osteoporosis
    Degenerative changes
    Coccydynia
    Myofascial syndrome
    Fibromyalgia
Systemic
    Acute intermittent porphyria
    Abdominal migraine
    Systemic lupus erythematosus
    Lymphoma
    Neurofibromatosis

ment) in pain scores in the subgroup of patients with dense vascular adhesions involving small bowel (Peters et al., 1991). A more recent prospective randomized controlled multicenter trial concluded that although laparoscopic adhesiolysis relieves chronic abdominal pain, it is not more beneficial than diagnostic laparoscopy alone (Swank et al., 2003). In addition, they remind the reader of the 10 to 25% of bowel injuries that occur during laparoscopic adhesiolysis for pain (Chapron et al., 1999; Swank et al., 2002) and the risk of bleeding or bladder and ureteral injury. As many as 20 to 90% of adhesions reform or form *de nouveau* after an adhesiolysis procedure. A review from the Cochrane database concluded that the outcome was no different in women who had had adhesiolysis of minor to moderate adhesions than in women who had not undergone surgery (Stones & Mountfield, 2004). The authors did, however, comment that there may be a possible benefit for patients with severe adhesions based on a small subgroup with significant benefits seen after adhesiolysis.

Advances using a 3-mm laparoscope have enabled development of "conscious pain mapping" whereby patients under local anesthesia and conscious sedation guide in determining which adhesions are those associated with pain (Palter, 1999). An observational pain mapping study of 50 women under local anesthesia demonstrated that 62% of the patients had pelvic adhesions found at the time of laparoscopy, but only 25 of these cases reported adhesions that exhibited tenderness to manipulation (Almeida & Val-Gallas, 1997). In a series by Howard (2003a), 7 of 21 patients with adhesions had focal dramatic tenderness upon manipulation of their adhesions. Although adhesions may be prevalent in patients with chronic pelvic pain, these adhesions may or may not be the cause of pain. Tenderness elicited by probing or traction during pain mapping may very well be simply a hyperalgesic central response to a mechanical stimulus. It is this truth that makes it difficult to ascertain whether the source of pain identified is in fact responsible for the patients' pain and makes the value of directed pain mapping questionable. No studies to date have noted improved outcome with pain mapping and guided laparoscopic management.

Investigators have proposed the routine use of barrier agents for the prevention of adhesion formation to reduce the chances of pelvic pain and infertility in the future. A Cochrane review of evidence-based studies found that the absorbable adhesion barrier Interceed reduces the incidence of adhesion formation, both new formation and reformation, at laparoscopy and laparotomy, but there are insufficient data to support its use to improve pregnancy rates (Farquhar et al., 2003). In addition, Gore-Tex may be superior to Interceed in preventing adhesions, but its usefulness is limited by the need for suturing and later removal (Farquhar et al., 2003). These barriers, of course, would not prevent adhesions due to causes such as pelvic inflammatory disease and endometriosis.

ENDOMETRIOSIS

Another "peripheral" cause of chronic pelvic pain is endometriosis. The actual incidence of endometriosis is unknown because many individuals undoubtedly have endometriosis without sufficient symptomatology to warrant surgical intervention. It seems that the incidence of endometriosis is increasing. However, this apparent increase in prevalence may be a reflection of the more liberal use of laparoscopy and of the recognition of atypical forms of endometriosis. Endometriosis is noted in patients undergoing laparoscopy for chronic pelvic pain in anywhere from 5 to 37% of the cases (Kresch et al., 1984; Liston et al., 1972; Lundberg, Wall, & Mathers, 1973).

The diagnosis of endometriosis is usually made in the thirties or forties; however, it has been noted to be a prominent diagnosis in adolescents and women in their twenties who are evaluated for chronic pelvic pain (Chatman & Ward, 1982). In fact, endometriosis has been suggested by one study to be the etiology in up to 70% of adolescents with chronic pelvic pain unresponsive to medical treatment (Probst & Laufer, 1999).

The most common symptoms of endometriosis are dysmenorrhea, dyspareunia, infertility, and abnormal uterine bleeding, usually from a secretory endometrium (Kitchen, 1985). Three criteria have been proposed to indicate endometriosis as the cause of pelvic pain (Hurd, 1998). These criteria are that the pain should be cyclic, worsening before and during menses; that endometriosis must be diagnosed surgically, and finally that appropriate medical or surgical treatment should result in prolonged pain relief. The first requirement, that the pain be cyclic,

exacerbated before and during menses, is thought to occur as a result of endometrial implants in the pelvis that are hormonally responsive. Dysmenorrhea may be so prolonged that the patient may complain of what seems like acyclic, continuous pain; beginning 7 to 10 days before the onset of the menstrual period and persisting until 1 week or so after the bleeding has ceased. The patient often describes pressure-like pain and aching in the lower abdomen, back, and rectum. There may be radiation of pain into the vagina, thighs, or perineum.

Dyspareunia is common when the disease involves the cul-de-sac (pouch of Douglas), uterosacral ligaments, or rectovaginal septum directly, or may also be related to referred hyperalgesia to the vagina. Pain with defecation (dyschezia) may also be present even in patients without direct bowel wall involvement. These symptoms may be due to endometrial implants near the rectum. Urinary urgency, frequency, and bladder pain may also be associated with urinary tract involvement. If these urinary symptoms are present, the physician should also be aware that interstitial cystitis may be the cause and this should be ruled out as described later.

Because endometriosis may be present in unusual locations, the manifestations of endometriosis are protean (Kitchen, 1985). Usually the previously noted common symptoms and signs are present, but, rarely, patients may complain of rectal bleeding, symptoms similar to bowel obstruction, suprapubic pain, and/or urinary symptoms (such as frequency, dysuria, or hematuria). If ureteral involvement is present, there may be flank pain, backache, or hypertension. Signs and symptoms of an acute abdomen occur infrequently and are usually related to rupture of an endometrioma or bowel obstruction.

Examination of patients with endometriosis may reveal tenderness and nodularity on the rectovaginal examination of the uterosacral ligaments and posterior cul-de-sac (Kitchen, 1985). Progressive disease results in findings of obliteration and fibrosis of the cul-de-sac, and fixed retroversion of the uterus. Enlarged ovaries (endometriomas) with decreased mobility may be noted.

The second criterion is that endometriosis be diagnosed surgically (Hurd, 1998). Laparoscopy is necessary for definitive diagnosis of endometriosis although the diagnosis may be suggested by history and pelvic examination. Evidence of powder burns, red or blue spots, and nearby puckering of the peritoneal surface is almost 100% specific for endometriosis, although laparoscopically directed biopsy is optimal (Vercellini et al., 1991). Ultrasound is not diagnostic and cannot differentiate an endometrioma from a benign or malignant ovarian neoplasm, and scattered small implants are not detectable by ultrasound. Magnetic resonance imaging (MRI) has been suggested as being useful for the detection of endometriotic lesions and endometriomas, especially when using a fat-saturated MRI, which can pick up lesions that are less than 5 mm 50% of the time (Takahashi et al., 1996). Laboratory studies are usually not specific. CA-125 and erythrocyte sedimentation rate (ESR) can be elevated in women with endometriosis.

Currently research is being more and more focused on possible markers for endometriosis. The difficulty with encountering a reliable marker is lack of specificity. Initially CA-125 and ESR, as above, were looked at but were found to be elevated in multiple processes that could be occurring besides endometriosis. A current marker of interest is aromatase P450 (the enzyme that converts androstenedione and testosterone to estrone), which is expressed in eutopic endometrium of women with endometriosis, but not in disease-free controls (Kitawaki et al., 1997; Nobel et al., 1996). Expression of aromatase P450 is independent of the timing of the menstrual cycle and has a sensitivity of 91% and a specificity of 100% according to Kitawaki et al. (1999). Other authors have found that the sensitivity and specificity is closer to 82% and 59%, respectively, and therefore it is not a viable marker for clinical use (Dheenadayalu et al., 2002). In addition other serum markers such as soluble intercellular adhesions molecules-1, placental protein-14 (glycodelin), and antiendometrial and anticarbonic anhydrase antibodies yield the same poor specificity (Brosens et al., 2003; Somigliana, 2002). Finally, new possibilities on the horizon are leptin levels and interleukin-6 because their proinflammatory and neoangiogenic actions may promote endometriosis and therefore be useful markers (Vigano et al., 2002).

The final criterion is that appropriate medical or surgical treatment of endometriosis should result in prolonged pain relief (Hurd, 1998). Endometriosis can be treated with nonsteroidal anti-inflammatory drugs (NSAIDs) for pain control along with hormonal agents such as androgenic hormones (Danocrine®), progestins (oral or injectable), estrogen–progestin combinations, or gonadotropin-releasing hormone agonists (GnRH-a) to create pseudomenopause and to atrophy ectopic endometrial implants (Rice, 2002). An expert consensus panel recently published recommendations for therapy in *Fertility and Sterility* (Gambone et al., 2002). According to these experts the first-line medical treatment should begin with a trial of NSAIDs with or without combined estrogen–progestin formulations (Gambone et al., 2002; Rice, 2002; Rouff & Lema, 2003). Estrogen–progestin combinations have been established as first-line agents for many years and recently many new forms in addition to oral contraceptives such as the combined estrogen–progestin contraceptive patch and ring are available. A new generation of NSAIDs, which inhibit cyclooxygenase-2 (COX-2), are as effective at treating dysmenorrhea as ibuprofen or naproxen and they have a much lower risk of causing gastric ulceration and inhibiting platelet function (Katz, 2002; Morrison et al., 1999; Ormrod et al., 2002; Rouff

& Lema, 2003; Scott & Lamb, 1999; Weaver, 2001). The disadvantage of COX-2 over COX-1 inhibitors is a much higher cost. If this therapy fails, then second-line therapy consists of either a 3-month trial of full-dose danazol, GnRH-a or a progestin such as medroxyprogesterone acetate (MPA).

Progestins induce decidualization and decrease the proliferation of endometriotic tissues. Medroxyprogesterone acetate in a 50 mg oral daily dose has been found to be just as effective at reducing pelvic pain as danazol, as danazol and an oral contraceptive, and as compared with a GnRH-a in randomized trials, although the effects regress after 6 to 12 months (Fedele et al., 1989; Vercellini et al., 1993; Walton & Batra, 1992). A *Cochrane Review* article recently concluded that both continuous progestins and antiprogestins (mifepristone, RU-486) are effective in the treatment of painful symptoms of endometriosis. Progestins given in the luteal phase have not been shown to be effective (Prentice et al., 2003). Mifepristone, 50 to 100 mg/day, was shown to decrease pain scores and induce amenorrhea without hypoestrogenism in small, open-label, cohort studies (Kettel et al., 1996). Progestin side effects include weight gain, breast atrophy, hot flushes, and hirsutism (Rice, 2002).

Danazol is a synthetic androgen that inhibits endometrial stimulation and growth resulting in atrophy by inhibiting pituitary gonadotropin release and ovarian steroid synthesis. Many randomized controlled studies (RCTs) have shown that it is more effective at relieving pain over placebo in laparoscopically diagnosed endometriosis (Kauppila et al., 1988; Telimaa et al., 1987, 1990; Telimaa et al., 1987). Danazol, although effective, has many intolerable side effects such as hirsutism, acne, and voice deepening.

GnRH-a are also very commonly used and effective in the treatment of endometriotic pain. There are many formulations available such as buserelin and nafarelin, which are given via an intranasal route; leuprolide depot, which is given intramuscularly; and leuprolide and goserelin, which are given subcutaneously (Rice, 2002). GnRH-a reduce proliferation by inhibiting pituitary pulsatile release of GnRH and therefore the positive drive for ovaries to produce endometrial growth-enhancing estrogen. GnRH has been extensively studied alone and in comparison with other agents. Depot leuprolide acetate (3.75 mg/month) was shown in one RCT of 100 women to cause a significant decrease in dysmenorrhea, pelvic pain, and tenderness as compared with a control group (Ling & Pelvic Pain Study Group, 1999). This study also reported the benefit, efficacy, and safety of medical treatment with depot leuprolide before laparoscopy based on empirical, clinical diagnosis. GnRH-a re-treatment for recurrent endometriotic symptoms after effective 3 to 6 months prior GnRH-a use has been found to positively affect symptom severity (Hornstein et al., 1997a).

If a GnRH-a is used, a hormonal add-back therapy, such as norethindrone acetate with or without estrogen, prevents long-term hypoestrogenic side effects such as bone loss and vasomotor symptoms (Hornstein et al., 1998). Surrey and Judd (1992) showed in a study containing 19 patients receiving GnRH-a with either norethindrone (10 mg/day orally) or norethindrone (2.5 mg/day) along with a cyclic bisphosphonate (etidronate, 400 mg/day orally) for 48 weeks that pain symptoms, extent of disease, and vasomotor symptoms were all suppressed, but that bone density was unchanged (no significant difference).

If side effects or risks prevent medical therapy or if there is a finding of an adnexal mass or infertility, then surgical evaluation should be considered. Laparoscopic electrosurgery, laser surgery, or laparotomy with resection or ablation of disease often is reserved for treatment of severe endometriosis. A prospective cohort study on patients with stage III to IV endometriosis found that 87.7% of the patients were satisfied or very satisfied with the results of their ablative laparoscopic surgery at 12 months postoperatively and that no surgical complications had occurred (Jones & Sutton, 2003). Laparoscopic surgical resection may have a place in patients with minimal to moderate endometriosis. In a prospective randomized double-blinded study of 63 women with minimal to moderate endometriosis subjected to laser laparoscopy 62% of the women noted improvement in pain after 6 months and, at the time of the 1-year follow-up, there was continued improvement in 90% of the initial responders (Sutton et al., 1997). After review of the literature one can conclude that in comparison with expectant treatment, there is a significant amount of pain relief at 6 months after surgery with laser laparoscopic surgery for minimal, mild, and moderate endometriosis (Jacobson et al., 2003).

Of note, laparoscopic pain mapping of endometriotic lesions and directed obliteration have been attempted. In a study by Howard (2003a), patients who underwent directed destruction of their endometriotic lesions had no better outcomes of pain relief than a historical control group undergoing laparoscopy prior to the introduction of laparoscopic pain mapping.

Very commonly, after conservative surgical therapy, adjunctive medical therapy is given. This, however, is controversial and in a study by Bianchi et al. (1999) danazol was given for 3 months in 77 women with moderate-to-severe disease and they reported that it did not significantly improve pelvic pain or short-term reproductive outcomes. On the other hand, G. Morgante (1999) found that 6 months of 100 mg/day of Danazol resulted in significantly ($P < 0.01$) lower pain scores than in the control group and that there were no significant differences between the two groups' estrogen concentrations, bone mineral density, or side effects. Another study compared patients who received ablative therapy and 6 months of postoperative GnRH-a with patients who were treated with

excision alone and found that at the end of 2 years 60% of the GnRH-a group was pain free and only 23% of the untreated group was still pain free (Winkel, 1999). The conclusion one can draw on review of the available studies is that short courses of treatment (3 months) do not delay recurrence of endometriosis-associated pain but longer courses of 6 months do, lasting up to 12 months post-treatment (Bianchi et al., 1999; Busacca et al., 2001; Hornstein et al., 1997b, 1998; Parazzini et al., 1994; Telimaa et al., 1987; Vercellini et al., 1999).

Patients who do not desire fertility may opt for radical surgery for endometriosis, which consists of a total abdominal hysterectomy with bilateral salpingo-oophorectomy as well as removal of any residual gastrointestinal (GI), genitourinary (GU), or peritoneal disease. It should be noted that patients with endometriosis, who have failed hormonal or conservative surgical therapy, may still benefit from the pain management approach (Rapkin & Kames, 1987). At least 30% of patients with recurrent pain after treatment of endometriosis did not have residual disease at the time of repeat laparoscopy.

There are many new treatments on the horizon, most of which are based on altering the factors that stimulate the immune system, cytokine secretion, and growth factors involved in the pathology of endometriosis. Tumor necrosis factor alpha, an activator of macrophages, has been found to be an important modulator of immune system responses, endometrial cell turnover, and cell adhesion (Sidell et al., 2003). Studies of pentoxifylline, an anti-tumor necrosis factor agent, in animals have shown regression of implants and reversal of surgically induced endometriosis-associated infertility (D'Hooghe, 2003; Nothnick, Curry, & Vernon, 1994; Steinleitner et al., 1991). In addition, a small pilot study in humans recently showed a benefit in the treatment of infertility with the use of pentoxifylline (Balasch et al., 1997). Aromatase (as described earlier), another factor in the growth of endometriosis, converts steroids such as testosterone and androstenedione to estrogens such as estradiol and estrone (Bulun, 1999; Fang et al., 2002). Normal endometrium does not express aromatase, but endometriotic implants do (Fang et al., 2002). Animal model studies have shown near total resolution of endometriotic nodules with the use of aromatase inhibitors and these inhibitors are felt to be the preferred treatment for the rare postmenopausal women with recurrent endometriosis (D'Hooghe, 2003; Fang et al., 2002; Somigliana et al., 2003; Takayama et al., 1998; Vigano et al., 2003). GnRH antagonists (e.g., cetrorelix) are now being studied. One author reported that 15 of 15 patients receiving 3 mg of cetrorelix subcutaneously once a week over 8 weeks remained symptom free (including mood changes, hot flushes, loss of libido, vaginal dryness, and other symptoms) and 9 of 15 patients who showed a mean stage III disease on diagnostic laparotomy pretreatment had a 60% regression to a stage II after treatment

(Kupker et al., 2002). Finally, estrogen antagonists (selective estrogen receptor modulators) such as raloxifene are showing promising results at controlling endometriotic lesion growth in recent studies (Somigliana et al., 2003; Vigano et al., 2003).

Endometriosis is a common finding in reproductive-age women, but it is clear in many women with chronic pelvic pain and endometriosis that the latter may not be the cause of the pain and may be only a contributing or associated factor. A response to medical management may also suggest a different underlying pathology since gastrointestinal, urological, and other gynecological processes can improve with therapies used to treat endometriosis. There is no significant correlation between the amount of disease and pain severity although higher-stage disease tends to be associated with a greater prevalence and increased intensity of pain. Additionally, there is no correlation between location of pain and site of endometriotic lesions and as many as 30 to 50% of patients regardless of stage have no pain (Fukaya et al., 1993). However, deeply infiltrating lesions, particularly of the uterosacral ligaments, are strongly associated with pain (Cornillie et al., 1990). Vaginal and uterosacral endometriosis has been associated with complaints of deep dyspareunia probably due to neural invasion in the region of the uterine nerve and the inferior hypogastric nerve (Vercellini et al., 1996).

Clinically, it is possible to determine whether there is a relationship between pain and endometriosis in a specific patient because of the hormonal sensitivity of the disease and the potential to surgically cure disease. Clearly, pain that does not respond to adequate surgical and medical management of endometriosis should be reevaluated for another source of pain as the cause or for the possibility of central sensitization as a major contributory factor. As discussed earlier, neuroplastic changes induced by persistent inflammation and nociceptive input from endometriotic tissue implants may lead to central sensitization. This could account for persistence of pain after medical or surgical ablation. A recent psychophysiological study demonstrated central sensitization in the responses to an experimental pain stimulus in women with endometriosis (Bajaj et al., 2003).

PELVIC CONGESTION

The concept of autonomic nervous system dysfunction leading to a vascular disorder affecting the uterine and ovarian veins was proposed in 1954 and has been resurrected over the last decade (Hobbs, 1976; Perry, 2001; Taylor, 1954). Patients in Taylor's work typically complained of secondary dysmenorrhea, low back pain, dyspareunia, infertility, and menorrhagia. Their pain was usually bilateral, lower pelvic in distribution, and exacerbated with the menstrual period. Two thirds of the patients also complained of nervous tension, chronic fatigue, breast tenderness, and spastic colon, as well as symptoms similar to the premenstrual syndrome. On exam, patients manifested tenderness over the uterus. The cervix and the fundus of the uterus were often bulky and the ovaries often enlarged with multiple functional cysts. The parametria, especially the uterosacral ligaments, were noted to be tender and indurated.

Beard and co-authors (1984) performed the only blinded study of venograms in patients with chronic pelvic pain. Larger mean ovarian vein diameters, delayed disappearance of contrast medium, and ovarian plexus congestion were present in a significantly greater proportion of women with chronic pelvic pain without pathology than those with pathology or controls. In support of pelvic congestion as a true entity in the spectrum of causes of pelvic pain, Foong et al. (2002) in a prospective, controlled longitudinal study using Beard's criteria for diagnosis of pelvic congestion found systemic microvascular dysfunction due to neutrophil-mediated increases in postcapillary resistance measurements. Diagnostic means other than venograms include transvaginal ultrasound, which may reveal uterine enlargement, thickened endometrium, cystic ovaries, and dilated pelvic veins, or more recently for more detailed visualization of structures, MRI (Adams et al., 1990; Gupta & McCarthy, 1994; Stones et al., 1990).

It was noted that nearly all patients with pelvic congestion were of reproductive age, and therefore hormonal suppression consisting of a hypoestrogenic environment was considered as a mode of treatment. Medroxyprogesterone acetate (MPA) given in doses of 30 mg daily for 3 months was administered in a randomized, placebo-controlled treatment trial for women with chronic pelvic pain with pelvic congestion (abnormal venograms) (Farquhar et al., 1989). A study of 84 subjects included four separate groups: MPA alone, MPA and psychotherapy, placebo plus psychotherapy, and placebo alone. MPA was significantly more effective after the 3-month treatment period than psychotherapy or placebo. Patients reported a 50% reduction in pain in the MPA group and 33% reduction in pain score after receiving placebo. However, pain returned in the MPA group after stopping treatment but did not return in the placebo group. Psychotherapy did not reduce pain in the short term, but there was a positive interaction between MPA and psychotherapy 9 months after the treatment was concluded. However, 9 months post-treatment, improvement was reported irrespective of the treatment group. This response coupled with a strong placebo response reaffirms central factors in this condition. It also suggests that hormonal suppression with MPA or GnRH agonists with or without low-dose estrogen and progestin hormone add-back may be therapeutic. A prospective randomized trial looking at efficiency of goserelin acetate versus MPA using pelvic venogram scores and subjective symptomatic resolution (including anxiety, depressive states, and sexual functioning) found that 1 year after 6 months of treatments goserelin was superior to MPA (Soysal et al., 2001).

A few small noncontrolled studies have assessed the more invasive technique of transcatheter embolotherapy of the ovarian and internal iliac veins to treat pelvic congestion, with results revealing good short-term success (Capasso et al., 1997; Chung & Huh, 2003; Pieri et al., 2003; Sichlau et al., 1994; Tarazov et al., 1997). Long-term efficacy remains to be evaluated (Venbruz & Lambert, 1999).

SALPINGO-OOPHORITIS

Salpingo-oophoritis can cause chronic pelvic pain, although patients usually present with symptoms and signs of acute or subacute infection before the pain becomes chronic. More commonly, a patient will present with frequent recurrent infections. Sweet and Gibbs (1985) proposed criteria for making the diagnosis of salpingitis on clinical grounds. Patients should have a history of lower abdominal pain as well as lower abdominal tenderness (with or without rebound), cervical motion tenderness, and adnexal tenderness. In addition, they must have one of the following: temperature greater than 38°C, leukocytosis (greater than 10,500 white blood cells per cubic millimeter), culdocentesis fluid containing white cells and bacteria on Gram stain, presence of an inflammatory mass, elevated ESR, a Gram stain from the endocervix revealing Gram-negative intracellular diplococci, or a monoclonal smear from the endocervical secretions revealing chlamydia (Sweet & Gibbs, 1985).

Patients may complain of having had numerous episodes of pain associated with fever and may have been given the diagnosis of pelvic inflammatory disease. When these episodes become recurrent, the patient is often considered to have chronic salpingo-oophoritis, although it is not clear that a chronic inflammatory condition exists. Instead, subacute or subclinical disease with recurrent acute infections may be present. An additional possibility is that the patient may not have salpingitis at all. In all these situations, laparoscopy with peritoneal fluid cultures is diagnostic, although an experienced clinician can often make the diagnosis on the basis of clinical criteria. Broad-spectrum antibiotics and anaerobic coverage represent the standard treatment of acute or recurrent salpingo-oophoritis. Only rarely is hysterectomy and salpingo-oophorectomy required.

OVARIAN REMNANT SYNDROME

The ovarian remnant syndrome may cause chronic pelvic pain in a patient who has had a hysterectomy and bilateral salpingo-oophorectomy for severe endometriosis or pelvic inflammatory disease. Ovarian remnant syndrome results from residual ovarian cortical tissue that is left *in situ* after

a difficult dissection in an attempt to perform an oophorectomy (Steege, 1987). Often the patient has had multiple pelvic operations with the uterus and adnexa removed sequentially.

The diagnosis is suspected on the basis of history and physical examination (Price et al., 1990). The patient usually complains of pelvic pain that is often cyclic and may be accompanied by peritoneal signs. The patient may have a history of flank pain and frequent urinary tract infections, and there is on occasion intermittent, partial bowel obstruction. The painful symptoms usually arise 2 to 5 years after surgery. Pelvic exam may reveal a tender mass in the lateral region of the pelvis, and ultrasound following ovarian stimulation with 50 mg of clomiphene daily for 5 days usually confirms a mass with the sonographic characteristics of ovarian tissue. In a patient who has had bilateral salpingo-oophorectomy and is not on hormonal replacement, estradiol and follicle-stimulating hormone (FSH) assays reveal a characteristic premenopausal picture, although on occasion the remaining ovarian tissue may not be active enough to suppress FSH levels. Laparotomy and removal of residual ovarian tissue is necessary for treatment (Pettit & Lee, 1988). Importantly, it has been shown that those who have achieved pain relief with GnRH-agonist hormonal therapy prior to surgery are usually those who also receive relief with surgical removal of the remnant (Carey & Slack, 1996).

CYCLIC PELVIC PAIN

Cyclic pelvic pain consists of primary and secondary dysmenorrhea but also includes atypical cyclic pain, such as pain beginning 1 week prior to menses and lasting for up to 1 week following the cessation of menstrual flow with occasional mid-cycle pain as well. Atypical cyclic pain is a variant of secondary dysmenorrhea. The diagnosis of cyclic pain often depends on the review of a daily pain diary that patients should be asked to maintain. With the availability of NSAIDs and compounds that alter the female sex steroids, cyclic pelvic pain has become significantly more manageable.

Dysmenorrhea or "difficult monthly flow" is a common gynecologic disorder affecting up to 50% of menstruating women (American College of Obstetricians and Gynecologists [ACOG], 1983). Primary dysmenorrhea refers to pain with menses when there is no pelvic pathology, whereas secondary dysmenorrhea is painful menses with underlying pelvic pathology. Primary dysmenorrhea usually appears within 1 to 2 years after menarche, with the establishment of ovulatory cycles. The disorder primarily affects younger women with ovulatory cycles, especially teens, but may persist into the 40s. The pain of primary dysmenorrhea begins a few hours prior to or just after the onset of menstrual flow and usually lasts for 48 to 72 hours. The pain is labor-like with suprapubic cramping that may be accompanied by lumbosacral backache, pain radiating down the anterior thighs, nausea, vomiting, and diarrhea.

Secondary dysmenorrhea, on the other hand, usually, although not always, occurs years after menarche and may occur with anovulatory cycles (ACOG, 1983). The most common cause of secondary dysmenorrhea is endometriosis. Other common causes, listed in Table 30.2, include vaginal, cervical, uterine, fallopian tube, adnexal, and peritoneal pathology. The differential diagnosis of secondary dysmenorrhea includes primary dysmenorrhea and noncyclic pelvic pain and entails ruling out primary dysmenorrhea and confirming the cyclic nature of the pain. The etiology of primary dysmenorrhea has been established due to increased uterine prostaglandin production (Anon., 1979). Prostaglandin synthetase inhibitors are effective for the treatment of primary dysmenorrhea in 70 to 80% of the cases (Anon., 1979). For the patient with primary dysmenorrhea who has no contraindications to oral contraceptive agents and desires contraception, the birth control pill, cyclically or continuously without a menstrual period (newer alternatives include the patch and the vaginal ring or even the levonorgestrel-releasing intrauterine device), is the agent of choice (Chan & Dawood, 1980). More than 90% of women with primary dysmenorrhea have relief with birth control pills.

If the patient does not respond to prostaglandin synthetase inhibitors and does not desire oral contraceptive pills or other forms of contraception, or if either is contraindicated, narcotic analgesics should be administered for 2 to 3 days per month. Prior to the addition of narcotic medication, psychological factors and other organic pathology should be ruled out. Other modes of hormonal menstrual suppression include high-dose progestins (oral or depo intramuscular injection), continuous oral contraceptive pill administration, or GnRH agonists with or without continuous low-dose hormone (menopausal dosage) add-back. Breakthrough bleeding and associated pain are potential problems with these regimens.

A patient with dysmenorrhea who does not respond to prostaglandin synthetase inhibitors and/or estrogen progestin contraceptive formulations and in whom organic disease has been ruled out may also respond to the pain management approach and, in particular, acupuncture or transcutaneous electrical nerve stimulation (Kaplan et al., 1994; Mannheimer & Whaler, 1985). In one study, Kaplan et al. (1994) reported a 30% marked pain relief, 60% moderate pain relief, and 10% no pain relief in women with primary dysmenorrhea undergoing transcutaneous electrical nerve stimulations (TENS). To more fully evaluate the evidence for treating primary dysmenorrhea with TENS or acupuncture, a forthcoming study by the Cochrane Library aims to analyze all prospective randomized controlled trials comparing those modalities with medical treatment or placebo (Wilson et al., 2000).

The distinction between primary and secondary dysmenorrhea requires a thorough history as to the nature and onset of the pain, the duration of pain or symptoms, and a pain diary (if on first query the pain does not appear to be cyclic). A complete physical and pelvic examination is important, with focus on the evaluation of the size, shape, and mobility of the uterus and adnexal structures and for nodularity and fibrosis of the uterosacral ligaments and rectovaginal septum. Genital cultures for gonorrhea and chlamydia and a complete blood count (CBC) with ESR are usually warranted. If no abnormalities are found, a tentative diagnosis of primary dysmenorrhea may be made and the patient started on oral contraceptive pills and/or prostaglandin synthetase inhibitors. Having made a diagnosis of primary dysmenorrhea, a 4- to 6-month trial of combined estrogen/progesterone contraceptives and/or prostaglandin synthetase inhibitors is warranted before laparoscopy is performed to rule out secondary dysmenorrhea and, in particular, endometriosis. A strong family history of endometriosis and any clinical signs of endometriosis on exam may suggest that laparoscopy be performed sooner.

Surgical approaches to dysmenorrhea include laparoscopic uterine nerve ablation, presacral neurectomy, and in selected cases of secondary dysmenorrhea, hysterectomy (Malinak, 1980). The uterosacral ligaments carry the main afferent supply from the uterus, and if complete, the uterosacral ablation should be as effective as the presacral neurectomy, although Doyle (1995) described a 70% success rate. Long-term and controlled studies of the neurectomy procedures are described elsewhere in this chapter. The management of secondary dysmenorrhea involves treatment of the underlying pathology.

GASTROENTEROLOGIC CAUSES OF CHRONIC PELVIC PAIN

Many of the patients referred to gynecologists with chronic pelvic pain actually have GI pathology (Rapkin & Mayer, 1993; Reiter, 1990a). Because the cervix, uterus, adnexa, lower ileum, sigmoid colon, and rectum share the same visceral innervation, with pain signals traveling via the sympathetic nerves to spinal cord segments T10 to L1, it is often difficult to determine whether lower abdominal pain is of gynecologic or enterocoelic origin (Hightower & Roberts, 1981). In addition, as is true with other types of visceral pain, pain sensation from the GI tract is often diffuse and poorly localized. Skillful medical history and examination are usually necessary to make the diagnosis.

Irritable bowel syndrome (IBS) is one of the more common causes of lower abdominal pain and may account for as many as 7 to 60% of referrals to a gynecologist for chronic pelvic pain (Reiter, 1990a). About 70% of patients with IBS are women; 48 to 79% of patients with chronic pelvic pain, dyspareunia, dysmenorrhea, or a history of numerous abdominal surgeries also have IBS (Smith, 2001). Women who have had a hysterectomy for chronic pelvic pain are twice as likely to have IBS (Longstreth, 1997). The predominant symptom of irritable bowel syndrome is abdominal pain (Ritchie, 1979). Other symptoms include excessive flatulence and alternating diarrhea and constipation. The pain is usually intermittent cramp-like and predominantly left lower quadrant in location, but occasionally the pain is constant. Pain is often improved after a bowel movement. The pain may last for only a few minutes, but 50% of patients may have pain for hours to days, and 20% of patients may complain of pain for weeks or longer. Symptoms are usually worse during periods of stress, tension, anxiety, and depression, and with the premenstrual and menstrual phases of the cycle (Ritchie, 1979). Depending on the main symptomatology, a patient with IBS can usually be placed into one of three subgroups including constipation-predominant IBS, diarrhea-predominant IBS, and IBS with alternating bowel habits (or "pain-predominant") (Whitehead, 1999).

Many attempts have been made to determine definite criteria for IBS that do not exclude patients who truly have the disease but are not too sweeping and may mistakenly include individuals with other disorders that may be treated differently. Manning attempted to define criteria in 1978 but these six criteria, although occasionally still used, have been mostly disregarded as not being sensitive enough to differentiate between IBS and other diagnoses such as non-ulcer dyspepsia and other organic GI disease (Talley et al., 1990). The Manning criteria were modified and took the form of Rome I and now Rome II criteria. The Rome II criteria state that the patient must have had at least 12 weeks, which need not be consecutive, in the preceding 12 months of abdominal discomfort or pain that included two of three features: (1) relief with defecation; (2) onset associated with a change in frequency of stool; and/or (3) onset associated with a change in form (appearance) of stool (Thompson et al., 1989, 1999). Using the Rome II criteria, IBS has been found to have around a 3 to 5% prevalence rate in the United States (Boyce et al., 2000; Mearin et al., 2003).

Before a final diagnosis of the IBS is made, other more serious conditions must be excluded especially if the patient complains of any "alarm symptoms" such as weight loss, GI bleeding, anemia, fever, or frequent nocturnal symptoms (Holten et al., 2000). These patients need a CBC, stool occult blood test, thyroid-stimulating hormone level, erythrocyte sedimentation rate, and electrolyte levels along with a gastroenterology referral (Holten et al., 2000). Patients 50 years or older should also be fully evaluated. Sigmoidoscopy, colonoscopy, and barium enema are often necessary and are routinely negative although there may be mucosal hyperemia on sigmoido-

scopy and increased haustral contractions or loss of haustration on barium enema (Hightower & Roberts, 1981). IBS is a waxing and waning disorder and treatment consists of reassurance, education, stress reduction, and symptomatic treatment. Diet changes should include eliminating foods containing lactose, sorbitol, alcohol, fat, and fructose. Products that contain caffeine can also cause abdominal bloating, cramping, and more frequent bowel movements. After a trial of diet change and fiber supplementation, if the patient still continues to be symptomatic, a short-term trial of an antispasmodic such as dicyclomine or hyoscyamine should be initiated (Howard, 2003b; Viera et al., 2002). Tegaserod, a $5-HT_4$ agonist is a newer agent approved by the FDA for women with IBS. It has visceral antinociceptive effects and is beneficial as a short-term treatment (Viera et al., 2002). Please see the chapter on irritable bowel syndrome for further details.

Irritable bowel syndrome, as with chronic pelvic pain, has been associated with underlying psychological factors (either predisposing the patient to disordered sensory perception or as a result of a chronic illness). Patients who have IBS by Rome II criteria are likely to have pan-enteric dysmotility with frequent dyspepsia, associated with psychological morbidity and greatly impaired quality of life (Portincasa et al., 2003); therefore, psychological therapy may improve these patients' outcomes and include cognitive-behavior therapy, dynamic psychotherapy, and hypnosis (Guthrie et al., 1993; Viera et al., 2002). Patients with chronic diarrhea must be evaluated carefully, often with a gastroenterologist in consultation. Although symptoms may have become chronic, it is possible that the patient may have contracted infectious diarrhea due to any one of a number of bacteria or parasites including *Shigella, Escherichia coli, Salmonella, Camphylobacter,* or *Amoeba* (Hightower & Roberts, 1981).

Although appendicitis is a common cause of abdominal pain, the abdominal pain of appendicitis is severe enough that the patient presents to the physician within 12 to 48 hours after the onset of the symptoms. The practitioner treating a patient for chronic pelvic pain should be cautious when the patient suddenly has an increase in abdominal pain, especially if it is accompanied by localized right lower quadrant pain, as well as anorexia, nausea, vomiting, and peritoneal signs on exam. It is not uncommon that a patient under treatment for chronic pelvic pain develops acute appendicitis or other acute pelvic condition while in the process of evaluation for the chronic pain problem. Chronic appendicitis is a controversial entity (Lee et al., 1985).

Another cause of chronic enterocoelic pain is diverticulitis of the colon (Young et al., 1976). Of the adult population over age 40, 5% have been noted to have diverticulae (Painter, 1975). This percentage increases to 40% in individuals over the age of 70 although most patients never develop diverticulitis. Although diverticulosis is usually asymptomatic, diverticulitis results in severe pain. Diverticulitis results from perforation of one or more of the diverticula and usually leads to the formation of a pericolonic abscess. The principal symptom of diverticulitis is left lower quadrant abdominal pain. A tender mass may be palpable on exam. Fever and leukocytosis are usually present. Sigmoidoscopy is diagnostic. These symptoms and signs, however, are usually those of an acute pathological pain process bringing the patient to a physician early in the course of pain.

Inflammatory bowel disease such as ulcerative colitis or granulomatous disease (Crohn's disease) similarly do not usually present as chronic pelvic pain because their presentation is usually more acute with diarrhea, fever, vomiting, and anorexia (Hightower & Roberts, 1981). A sigmoidoscopy or barium enema is diagnostic.

Tumors of the GI tract can cause chronic lower abdominal pain in women (McSherry et al., 1969). The most frequent and early symptoms of bowel carcinomas are change in bowel habits (74% of patients) and abdominal pain (65% of patients). Rectal bleeding and weight loss may be signs of advanced disease (McSherry et al., 1969). Most rectal tumors can be palpated on rectal examination. Sigmoidoscopy and biopsy as well as barium enema are diagnostic.

Included in the differential diagnosis of lower abdominal pain is hernia although there is a relatively low incidence of hernia in females (Hightower and Roberts, 1981). Anterior and posterior perineal hernias, usually limited to cystocele, rectocele, or enterocele, may cause lower abdominal/perineal pain in women although the pain is usually not severe. This type of pain usually responds to a pessary though the management is surgical.

UROLOGIC CAUSES OF CHRONIC PELVIC PAIN

Chronic pelvic pain of urologic origin may be related to recurrent cystoureteritis, urethral syndrome, interstitial cystitis (IC), infiltrating bladder tumors, ectopic pelvic kidney, or various ureteral causes such as ureteral obstructions or endometriosis (Summit, 1993; Vereecken, 1981).

The patient with acute infective cystitis presents with complaints of suprapubic pain, dysuria, frequency, and urgency; has pyuria on urinalysis; and has a positive urine culture (Vereecken, 1981). The symptoms usually respond to adequate antibiotic therapy. Relapses and reinfection can be diagnosed with the aid of history, urinalysis, and culture. The antibiotic and duration of therapy may have to be adjusted and on occasion, if the patient has recurrent cystoureteritis, antibiotics may have to be administered postcoitally for a prolonged period of time (Vereecken, 1981).

The urethral syndrome, more commonly known as urgency frequency syndrome, is a common condition in women and may present as chronic pelvic pain (Bodner, 1988). Symptoms of dysuria, urinary frequency, suprapubic pain, and dyspareunia are prominent and the diagnosis is one of exclusion. Negative urine analysis, urine culture, cervical culture (for gonorrhea and chlamydia), and urethral cultures, as well as negative evaluation for vulvovaginitis, increase the suspicion for the diagnosis of urethral syndrome; however, IC is the usual culprit. Treatment consists of a trial of antibiotics, preferably tetracycline for 2 to 3 weeks, and if without success (although this is controversial), urethral dilatation in reproductive-age women and vaginal estrogen for peri- and postmenopausal women (Bergman et al., 1989). Attention should be paid to psychological factors as well.

When a patient complains of symptoms of urinary frequency, urgency, nocturia, and suprapubic pain but laboratory studies are negative, the patient may actually have IC, an idiopathic chronic inflammatory condition (Karram, 1993; Messing & Stamey, 1978; Wesselmann, 2002). The prevalence of IC in the United States ranges from 10 to 67/100,000 (Held et al., 1990; Speizer et al., 1999).

The evaluation of patients with the preceding symptoms should include urinalysis and culture; urethral culture for chlamydia, mycoplasma, and gonorrhea; and cystoscopy with hydrodistension and possible biopsy. There are no true consensus criteria for the diagnosis of IC, and it is usually a diagnosis of exclusion. Signs and symptoms can consist of pain or bladder filling relieved by emptying, urinary urgency and frequency; nocturia, pressure and pain in suprapubic, pelvic, urethral, vaginal, or perineal region; glomerulations; Hunner's ulcers or patches (these are the only defining pathology); fibrosis on endoscopy, or decreased compliance on cystometrogram (Karram, 1993; Wesselmann, 2002). A validated questionnaire developed by O'Leary et al. called the Interstitial Cystitis Symptom Index and Problem Index measures lower urinary tract symptoms (Clemons et al., 2002; O'Leary et al., 1997). A positive score (≥ 6) on either the symptom or problem index had 90% sensitivity and 95% specificity for diagnosing ICs. Clemons et al. (2002) evaluated the questionnaire as a screening tool and found that a score of 5 or more had 94% sensitivity and 93% negative predictive value in diagnosing IC and, therefore, concluded that it was a useful screening test. The use of a pelvic pain and urgency frequency symptom scale and a provocative bladder potassium intravesical test suggests that many women with pelvic pain or urgency/frequency alone may have early IC (Parsons et al., 2002). Some authors have advocated that during the initial evaluation of chronic pelvic pain, cystoscopy and exploratory laparoscopy should be performed concurrently. Chung found that of 58 patients with cystoscopy-confirmed IC, 54 had a concurrent diagnosis of active or inactive endometriosis (Chung et al., 2002). Of the 54 patients, 47 had biopsy-confirmed active endometriosis.

This very common association is important because of its impact on effective treatment.

Therapy for IC ranges depending on the severity of the patients' symptoms. Change in diet, stress reduction, and behavioral changes such as recording a voiding diary and pelvic floor muscle training can be attempted initially (Wesselmann, 2002). In addition, therapy consisting of intravesical distension with dimethylsulfoxide or lidocaine, intravesical instillation of analogues of glycosaminoglycan, TENS and biofeedback including pelvic floor muscle biofeedback training have all reduced pain in uncontrolled studies of patients with IC. Hydrodistension of the bladder performed under anesthesia at the time of diagnostic cystoscopy has been the most commonly used urological therapy for more than 50 years (Messing, 1989). Because treatment of the condition remains empiric and less than optimal, oral drugs such as anticholinergics, antihistamines, membrane-stabilizing agents, antispasmodics, NSAIDs, tricyclic antidepressants, narcotics, and pentosan polysulfate sodium, which is Food and Drug Administration approved for IC treatment, have all been used with some success (Sant, 1998). Sacral nerve modulation using a permanent InterStim implant or neurolytic surgery using laser destruction of the vesicoureteric plexus has been found to be successful at treating refractory IC (Gillespie, 1994; Peters et al., 2003).

Very severe chronic suprapubic pain may be caused by infiltrating carcinomas of the bladder, cervix, uterus, or rectum (Vereecken, 1981). These conditions should be apparent after performing the history, pelvic examination, urine analysis, and cystoscopy, although intravenous pyelogram or CT urogram may be necessary.

NERVE ENTRAPMENT OR INJURY

Abdominal cutaneous nerve entrapment or injury should always be considered in the differential diagnosis of chronic lower abdominal pain, especially if no visceral etiology is apparent. The syndrome most commonly occurs months to years after Pfannenstiel skin or other lower abdominal and even laparoscopic incisions but can also follow trauma or exercise (Sippo et al., 1987). Commonly involved nerves include ilioinguinal (T12 and L1), iliohypogastric (T12 and L1), and genitofemoral (L1 and L2). In addition to incisional injury, three common ways neurologic injury may occur at the time of gynecological surgery are (1) improper placement or positioning of retractors, especially retractors with deep lateral retractor blades; (2) improper positioning of patients in lithotomy position preoperatively; and (3) radical surgical dissection and subsequent autonomic nerve disruption (Irvin et al., 2004). Abdominal hysterectomy is the number one most common surgical procedure at fault for causing iatrogenic femoral nerve injury (Fardin et al., 1980).

Symptoms of nerve entrapment include pain that is typically elicited by movement and exercise (Sippo et al., 1987). The pain is described as stabbing, colicky, and sudden, and is usually judged as coming from the abdomen and not from the skin. The pain is located along the line of the lateral edge of the rectus margin and may be associated with a burning pain radiating horizontally or diagonally toward the linea alba and back to the flank or sacroiliac region if there is ilioinguinal or iliohypogastric nerve damage. Ilioinguinal and iliohypogastric nerve injury is more likely to occur if a Pfannenstiel incision is extended beyond the lateral border of the rectus abdominus muscle into the muscle of the internal oblique muscle (Irvin et al., 2004). The pathognomonic symptoms include (1) sharp, burning pain arising from the incision site and radiating to the suprapubic, labial, or thigh areas; (2) paresthesia over the corresponding nerve distribution; and (3) pain relief after infiltration with local anesthetic (Stulz & Pfieffer, 1982). Femoral nerve injury results usually after deep lateral retractor blades compress the nerve between the blade and the lateral pelvic sidewall and results in weakness or an inability to flex at the hip joint or to extend at the knee. Paresthesia can occur over the anterior and medial thigh (Irvin et al., 2004; Vosburg & Finn, 1961). Pudendal neuropathy can cause chronic pelvic, vulvar, and perineal pain. Pain due to nerve injury may be exacerbated by constipation, bloating, menstruation, and full bladder (Sippo et al., 1987).

On exam, the pain can usually be localized with the fingertip (McDonald, 1993). The maximal point of tenderness is the neuromuscular foramen at the rectus margin medial and inferior to the anterior iliac spine or, in the case of spontaneous nerve entrapment, at the site of exit from the aponeurosis of the other thoracic/abdominal cutaneous nerves. A maneuver that helps to make the diagnosis is Carnett's test and involves asking the patient to tense the abdominal wall by raising shoulders or raising and extending the lower limbs in a straight leg raising maneuver. The pain is exacerbated if abdominal wall pain is present. With the abdominal wall relaxed, the pain is relieved and becomes more diffuse. The tentative diagnosis is confirmed with a diagnostic nerve block consisting of injection of 2 to 4 ml of 1% lidocaine or 0.25% bupivacaine. Patients usually report immediate relief with symptoms after injection and many patients require no further intervention, although some patients require 3 to 5 weekly injections (McDonald, 1993; Srinivasan & Greenbaum, 2002). Only as a last resort should patients be considered for surgical removal of the involved nerves if no other psychological factors predominate and if visceral pathology can be ruled out. Complete relief of pain after nerve resection occurs in more than 70% of patients (Hahn, 1989; Lee & Dellon, 2000; Nahabedian & Dellon, 1997). On the other hand, deafferentation pain is a probable sequel to surgery. Medications such as low-dose tricyclic antidepressants and anticonvulsants are also useful for pain control. Physical therapy may be necessary to educate the patient concerning strengthening other muscles to prevent reinjury.

MUSCULOSKELETAL CAUSES OF CHRONIC PELVIC PAIN

Women complaining of lower back pain without complaints of pelvic pain rarely have gynecologic pathology as the cause of their pain; however, low back pain may accompany pelvic pathology. Back pain may be caused by gynecologic, vascular, neurological, psychogenic, or spondylogenic (related to the axial skeleton and its structures) pathology (Morscher, 1981). Musculoskeletal abnormalities commonly contribute to the symptoms of chronic pelvic pain (Baker, 1993).

MYOFASCIAL PAIN

"Myofascial pain syndromes constitute a large group of muscle disorders characterized by the presence of hypersensitive points, called trigger points (TPs), within one or more muscles, the investing connective tissue, or both, together with a syndrome of pain, muscle spasm, tenderness, stiffness, limitation of motion, weakness, and occasionally autonomic dysfunction. The symptoms are usually referred to any area distant from the TPs, although local pain may also be present" (Sola & Bonica, 2001, p. 530). Reports of the prevalence of the syndrome vary, but only two papers assessing chronic pelvic pain patients for trigger points have been published. Reiter and Gambone found myofascial syndrome in 15% of their patients with somatic pathology. Patients with somatic pathology represented 47% of all patients referred to their pelvic pain clinic (Reiter, 1990a). Slocumb noted trigger points in most women presenting to the pain clinic with chronic pelvic pain irrespective of underlying pelvic pathology (Slocumb, 1984). Clinically, myofascial pain is exacerbated by activity within the muscle or muscle group and, in the case of abdominal wall trigger points and pelvic floor muscle, is exacerbated by activity in deeper visceral structures (bladder or rectal fullness, menses, and cervical motion and intercourse), which share the same dermatomal innervation (Slocumb, 1984, 1990; Travell, 1976). On digital exam of dermatomas of abdomen, back, or vagina, pressure on the trigger point evokes local and referred pain. Pain is exacerbated by the straight-leg raising maneuver (Carnett's test) described earlier. Treatment of myofascial trigger points includes injecting the trigger points with local anesthetic, as well as treating any physical and psychological factors such as depression, anxiety, learned behavior patterns, and postural elements that may accompany and exacerbate the condition (Slocumb, 1984;

Travell, 1976). Medications such as tricyclic antidepressants and anticonvulsants (medication intended for neuropathic pain) and physical therapy are also be useful.

CENTRAL (BRAIN) FACTORS IN CHRONIC PELVIC PAIN

Descending pain-modulating mechanisms, including those originating in the brain or spinal cord, probably involve various chemicals such as classical neurotransmitter, endogenous endorphin and nonendorphin analgesic systems, and excitatory amino acids. Anxiety, depression, and other psychological states may serve as facilitators or inhibitors of neurological transmission. Wall (1988) has suggested that it is important to consider the lability of central transmission pathways as well as seeking peripheral pathology in all painful conditions. From a psychological perspective, there are various factors that may promote the chronicity of pain. Described as a "diathesis-stress" model of pain, a woman is more susceptible in certain social contexts to develop chronic pain based on her preexisting vulnerabilities including those related to cognitive, affective, biological, and behavioral functioning (Jacob, 1997).

Studies on women with chronic pelvic pain have documented a high level of psychological disturbance. The Minnesota Multiphasic Personality Inventory (MMPI) conversion "V" profile (elevated scores on the hypochondriasis, hysteria, and depression scales) was described by Castelnuova-Tedesco and Krout (1970). In a survey of 40 women with pelvic pain. Gross et al. (1980) reported high levels of psychopathology in women with pelvic pain, as well as a past exposure to childhood sexual abuse in 90% of their sample. Studies using the MMPI have failed to find a correspondence between psychological and physiological findings. Renaer (1979) compared MMPI profiles of women having chronic pain without obvious pathology with those of women having pain arising from endometriosis and a control group. He found the two pain groups differed from controls but not from each other. Interestingly, treatment resulting in subjective improvement in pain severity and increased activity level produces a significant improvement in personality profile (Duleba et al., 1998).

Other studies have focused on the specific diagnosis of depression and pelvic pain. Magni (Richter et al., 1998) examined the role of depression and found higher depression scores for women with chronic pelvic pain without pathology compared with women found to have chronic pelvic pain and pathology as established by laparoscopy. Theses studies have also found a higher likelihood of depressive disorders in the family histories of women whose pain could not be attributed to organic pathology. A comparison of women with pelvic pain of unknown etiology and a pain-free control group revealed the pain group to have a significantly higher prevalence of episodes of major depression (Richter et al., 1998). Most studies find no difference in the psychological profile in women with or without pathology on laparoscopic surgery (Walker et al., 1988). It has been suggested that pain may be augmented by depression, in view of the common neurotransmitter pathways mediating both pain and mood.

Studies have also examined the role of sexual abuse as a specific risk factor for chronic pelvic pain. Gross and associates (1980) reported a high prevalence (90%) of sexual abuse in their sample. A sample of 25 women with chronic pelvic pain of mixed etiology showed no differences in psychological functioning when divided according to presence or absence of organic findings (Harrop-Griffiths et al., 1988). However, when compared with a control group of gynecologic patients without pain, there was a higher prevalence of prior substance abuse, functional dyspareunia, inhibited sexual desire, higher scores on the SCL-90, and greater prevalence of sexual abuse—both as youths prior to age 14 and as adults. The authors identified a history of sexual abuse as a child, along with a past history of depression, as strongly related to the subsequent persistence of pelvic pain.

Rapkin et al. (1990) designed a study to assess whether prior abuse is more likely in patients with pelvic pain than in women with chronic pain in other sites or a painful control group, and whether the abuse was specifically sexual or extended to physical abuse as well. The prevalence of childhood sexual abuse did not differ significantly among the three groups: 19% of pelvic pain, 16% of other pain patients, and 12% of controls. There was a significant difference in the prevalence of physical abuse: highest for the pelvic pain patients (39%), compared with 18 and 9% in the other two groups. This study suggested abuse of any kind is linked to chronic pain (Rapkin et al., 1990). Walling and colleagues (1994) compared women having chronic pelvic pain with women having nonpelvic chronic pain (headache) and pain-free women, finding that women suffering pelvic pain reported a higher lifetime prevalence of major sexual abuse (56%) and physical abuse (50%). A more recent study by Lampe et al. (2003) looked at chronic pain syndromes in general. Of the patients, 40 had chronic low back pain, 43 had chronic pelvic pain, and 22 women made up the control group. The outcomes were assessed by interviews determining childhood sexual and physical abuse and using the Beck Depression Inventory. They found that childhood physical abuse, stressful life events, and depression had a significant affect on the occurrence of chronic pain in general and childhood sexual abuse was correlated with chronic pelvic pain exclusively. In yet another study, the same author determined that there was a significant association between sexual abuse before age 15 and the subsequent development of chronic pelvic pain (Lampe et al., 2000).

Abuse and post-traumatic stress disorders may predispose to chronicity of pain because they increase the vulnerability to depression, and the chronicity is likely fostered by alterations in neural circuitry as a result of early trauma (Grossman et al., 2002). Individuals who have suffered childhood abuse, physical and sexual, may possibly have impaired coping abilities and, as a result, may perceive life events as more stressful (Lampe et al., 2003). There is also evidence for the logical conclusion that chronic pain itself over time reduces physical and mental health, vitality, and social function, so that it leaves the researcher with a "chicken and egg, which came first?" phenomenon (Haggerty et al., 2003). For the above reasons the examining physician should not forget the importance of obtaining sexual and physical abuse histories and including at least a resource for psychological therapy in patients with chronic pelvic pain (Toomey et al., 1993).

Renaer (1980) has suggested that the diagnosis chronic pelvic pain without obvious pathology refers to patients who lack somatic pathology. Often, these patients have been considered to have psychogenic pain. As noted in the previous discussion, the majority of patients with chronic pain have abnormal psychogenic profiles, but those patients without pathology do not appear to be psychologically different from those with visible organic disease (Harrop-Griffiths et al., 1988; Renaer et al., 1979; Richter et al., 1998). Furthermore, the potential role of neurophysiological mechanisms in the brain and spinal cord in the maintenance of chronic pain (neuroplasticity) is well established. Abdominal wall, lower back, and pelvic floor muscle trigger points; nerve entrapment in surgical scars; IBS; and IC represent the most common sources of nonreproductive system chronic pelvic pain (Reiter, 1990b), all of which probably entail alterations of central processing. Interestingly, these patients also have a high incidence of comorbidity with panic disorder, somatization, or depression (Reiter, 1990b; Wood et al., 1990). It is reasonable, therefore, to suggest that chronic pelvic pain regardless of "pathology" is likely to involve all levels of the neuro-axis, and it is necessary to direct management approaches accordingly.

DIAGNOSIS AND MANAGEMENT OF CHRONIC PELVIC PAIN

Successful diagnosis and management of patients with chronic pelvic pain require a meticulous yet compassionate, multidisciplinary approach. As with the investigation of any other physical symptom, a thorough history should be obtained, and often must be acquired in stages. An intake questionnaire form ensures a thorough and in-depth research as to the nature of the patient's pain. In addition, it assists in accurate charting and recollection of the patient's complaints. A commonly used form is the questionnaire compiled by the International Pelvic Pain Society available on line (www.pelvicpain.org). Important on intake is a description of the nature of the pain, severity, location and radiation, aggravating and alleviating factors, timing, relationship to menses, and worsening or improving with exercise, work, stress, intercourse, and orgasm. A pain map can be used that reconstructs the general outline of the female body and is coded for the patient to mark types of pain to their locations (Howard, 2003b). These maps demonstrate that women frequently have multiple pain areas other than pelvic. Up to 60% of women with chronic pelvic pain also have headaches and up to 90% also have backaches (Howard, 2003b). If a patient marks both ventral and dorsal sources of pain, this is more suggestive of intrapelvic source rather than dorsally, which may be due to a musculoskeletal origin. It is important to determine how long the pain lasts and how much it affects the patient's daily life and activities. A visual analogue scale listing numbers 0 through 10 and stating "no pain and worst possible pain" can assess severity.

The context in which the pain arose should be ascertained. Did the pain begin postpartum, postabortal, or after physical or sexual trauma? Pregnancy risk factors include severe lumbar lordosis, delivery of a large infant, muscle weakness and poor physical conditioning, a difficult delivery, vacuum or forceps delivery, and use of gynecological stirrups for delivery (Howard, 2003b). There are additional questions: Have there been previous episodes of pain or inability to perform one's occupation? Is there pending litigation or workers' compensation? Are there other somatic symptoms that should be noted: genital tract (abnormal vaginal bleeding, discharge, Mittelschmerz, dysmenorrhea, dyspareunia, infertility); enterocoelic tract (constipation, diarrhea, flatulence, tenesmus, blood, changes in color or caliber of stool); musculoskeletal system (predominant low back distribution, radiation down posterior thigh, association with injury, fatigue, postural changes); and urologic tract (dysuria, urgency, frequency, suprapelvic pain)? Historical questions specific to all the peripheral pathologies noted in Table 30.2 should be asked.

Past history including medical, surgical, gynecologic, obstetric, medication intake, and prior evaluations for the pain should be documented. Operative and pathology reports are important if the patient has had surgery. It is important to note whether the pain is postoperative and involves the incision site or appears to be from nerve damage due to retractor misplacement.

Current and past psychological history — including psychosocial factors; history of past (or current) physical, sexual, and/or emotional abuse; history of hospitalization; suicide attempts; and chemical dependency — should be asked. The attitude of the patient and her family toward the pain, resultant behavior of the patient's family with respect to the pain, and current upheavals in the patient's life should be discussed. The part of the history addressing sensitive issues may have to be re-obtained after establishing rapport with the patient. Depression is an important predictor of pain severity and responsiveness to treatment in women with chronic pelvic pain, and it is important to use a screening tool such as the Zung or Beck depression inventories. In the multidisciplinary approach the team of clinicians would include a psychologist or social worker who would assist in completing this part of the history.

Symptoms of an acute process such as fever, anorexia, nausea, emesis, significant diarrhea or constipation, hematochezia, abdominal distension, abnormal uterine bleeding, pregnancy, or recent abortion should alert one to the possibility of an acute condition requiring immediate medical or surgical intervention. This is especially called for if accompanied by orthostasis, peritoneal signs, pelvic or abdominal mass, abnormal CBC, positive genital or urinary tract cultures, or positive pregnancy test.

One should perform a complete physical examination, with particular attention to the abdominal, back, vulva, perineum, vaginal, bimanual, and rectovaginal examinations. The goal of the exam is to reproduce the pain by palpation or positioning (Howard, 2003b). The supine part of the exam should include evaluation of the abdomen, looking for distention, abdominal ascites or masses, organomegaly, guarding, rebound, or rigidity suggesting an acute abdomen or peritonitis exists. The Carnett test is done with the abdominal muscles tensed (head raised off the table or with straight leg raising) to differentiate abdominal wall from visceral sources of pain. Abdominal wall pain is augmented and visceral pain is diminished with the preceding maneuvers. The patient should point to the area of pain and the amount of pressure needed to replicate pain, and the point of maximal pain (trigger point or area of nerve injury/entrapment) should be found. Abdominal wall pain or myofascial pain can be due to fibromyalgia, trauma, muscular strain, nerve entrapment, viral myositis, or an abdominal wall hernia. Active leg flexion, knee to chest, can ascertain if there is lower back dysfunction and abdominal weakness (Howard, 2003b). It is important to rule out hernias as a cause of abdominal/pelvic pain. Spigelian hernias are lateral to the lateral margin of the rectus sheath and protrude through the transversus abdominis aponeurosis resulting in severe pain. Surgical scar hernias should also be sought out. Palpation of the pubic symphysis is necessary for a thorough exam to rule out pelvic girdle relaxation, osteomyelitis, osteitis pubis, rectus muscle inflammation, or injury at its fascial insertion (Howard, 2003b).

Very important to the delineation of pelvic pain is the pelvic exam. External genitalia should be inspected for any abnormal findings such as discharge, redness, excoriation, fissures, ulcerations, condylomata, atrophy, abscesses, or trauma. The vulva and introitus should then be examined for hyperalgesia and allodynia. This should be done with cotton tip localization of tender areas. After examination of the external genitalia, a speculum exam should be performed with close attention to not only the cervix but also the vaginal walls. The character of the discharge, lesions, erythema, whitened areas, or areas with atypical vascular patterns should be noted and cultured or biopsied accordingly. At this time cystocele, rectocele, and enterocele can be identified.

A bimanual examination should be performed beginning with a single digit exam noting introital spasm or vaginismus suggestive symptoms. Then the examiner can gently enter the vagina, palpating the levator ani muscles (including the puborectalis, pubococcygeus, and iliococcygeus), and inspecting the pelvic girdle for spasms and tenderness in addition to ruling out abnormal findings such as nodules or masses. The examiner should assess the course of the pudendal nerve for evidence of pudendal neuropathy. It is helpful to have a physical therapist who specializes in chronic pelvic pain to evaluate the patient as part of the multidisciplinary approach. If a muscular etiology is found, these individuals are trained in rehabilitation and are excellent at teaching patients relaxation techniques. The caudal anterior vaginal surface should be examined for tenderness representing a bladder or urethral origin of pain. In addition, any discharge or thickening should be noted and may mean that chronic urethritis, urethral syndrome, urethral diverticulum, a vaginal wall cyst, trigonitis, or interstitial pathology may exist (Howard, 2003b). Deeper vaginal palpation and examination of the uterus is then necessary. Pressing the uterus against the sacrum or between the examiner's abdominal and vaginal hand may illicit tenderness. Posterior uterine pressure that causes tenderness is suggestive of pelvic congestion, adenomyosis, pelvic congestion syndrome, or pelvic infection (Howard, 2003b). Rectovaginal exam should always be performed, not only to adequately evaluate ovaries, but also to check for posterior cul-de-sac pathology (severe endometriosis can result in dense adhesions, a retroflexed uterus, and nodules on the uterosacral ligaments and rectovaginal septum) and stool for occult blood. On rectovaginal exam coccydynia may be diagnosed if an attempt to move the coccyx about 30° results in pain.

Laboratory studies to be obtained the first visit include CBC, ESR, urine analysis and culture, cervical and urethral cultures (gonorrhea and chlamydia), wet mount of vaginal secretions, pap smear, stool guaiac, and—if diarrhea is present—stool culture including *Clostridium difficile* and ova and parasites. If the pelvic or abdominal exam is inadequate due to pain, guarding, or increased abdominal wall thickness or suggestive of a mass, ultrasound evaluation is indicated. If symptoms and signs are suggestive of other system involvement, fiberoptic or other appropriate imaging studies of other organ systems should be considered (e.g., upper and lower gastrointestinal studies, colonoscopy or computerized axial tomography [CAT] scan, CT urogram, and MRI of the spine).

The patient should be given a pain diary in which to note the onset and intensity of pain on a daily basis. Medication intake, menses, and aggravating and alleviating factors should be noted daily in the diary. A simple diary utilizes a visual analogue scale from 1 (no pain) to 10 (most severe pain ever). The diary should be maintained for at least 2 months. Previous medical records, surgical and pathological reports or scans, should be requested at the time of, or prior to, this first visit.

During the second visit, one should again pursue the psychosocial and sexual history. The pain diary, laboratory results, and previous records should be reviewed with the patient. Subacute conditions should be treated (e.g., cervicitis, salpingo-oophoritis, urethritis, cystitis), and the abdominal, back, and pelvic exam should be repeated with thorough evaluation for abdominal, lumbosacral, and vaginal trigger points if not performed on the first exam. A description of the evaluation and treatment of trigger points is provided by Slocumb (1984).

At the time of the second visit a psychologist familiar with the evaluation and management of chronic pain should evaluate the patient. The psychologist should preferably be located within the same office or clinic suite.

Psychological referral accomplishes evaluation, as well as opens the possibility for introducing cognitive behavioral pain management. The assessment should be designed to evaluate the pain complaint, its impact on life circumstances, and the controlling factors and coping mechanisms. Assessment in a chronic context involves a broader range of measures, reflecting social and psychological influences and sequelae, than may apply in the acute setting.

Assessment must evaluate the impact of the pain on the woman's lifestyle. Pelvic pain is likely to affect sexual functioning, which may have additional repercussions in terms of the quality of the patient's relationship and self-esteem. As with mood, a careful history is needed to establish whether the sexual problems existed before the pain or developed subsequently. Previous sexual abuse or trauma should be evaluated, as well as the impact of the pain on day-to-day functioning. Standardized psychological testing is helpful to determine if affective disturbance is present, as well as to establish a baseline against which to measure treatment response and guide treatment approaches.

If peripheral pathology is suspected or confirmed, workup and management should proceed as per treatment of the specific condition. Consultation with a urologist, gastroenterologist, orthopedist, or neurologist should be requested if indicated.

The third visit should include another review of the pain diary. Patients with cyclic or atypical cyclic pain should be evaluated for primary or secondary dysmenorrhea. Evaluation of pelvic pain, especially cyclic pain, may require elimination of the menstrual cycle using continuous estrogen/progesterone combinations, high-dose progesterone alone, or a GnRH analogue with or without add-back hormonal therapy. Pelvic ultrasound or transuterine venography may be helpful if pelvic congestion is suspected, but treatment can proceed on the basis of clinical suspicion. If trigger points or entrapped nerve sites were injected and the pain has persisted, but the initial reduction in pain outlasts the duration of the local anesthetic, injection should be repeated weekly or biweekly up to five injections. In addition, consideration should be given to a physical therapy consultation, especially if activity increases the pain or if low back pain is prominent.

A follow-up appointment (fourth visit) should be scheduled. Before the third and fourth visits, the "pain manager," the gynecologist (if not the pain manager), and the psychologist should consult. If pain persists, the patient should initiate cognitive behavioral pain management and various centrally acting pharmaceutical agents should be tried. Tricyclic antidepressants and membrane-stabilizing agents/anticonvulsants have been used successfully in patients with pelvic pain. To date, only one randomized controlled trial assessed the effect of selective serotonin reuptake inhibitors on pelvic pain, and the short 14-week trial of 23 women failed to show significant difference in measures of pain and functional disability (Engel et al., 1998; for review, see Stones & Mountfield, 2003). The patient should continue to have scheduled visits with the gynecologist on a regular basis.

SURGICAL MANAGEMENT OF CHRONIC PELVIC PAIN

DIAGNOSTIC LAPAROSCOPY

Diagnostic laparoscopy has become a standard procedure in the evaluation of patients with chronic pelvic pain. It has been reported that 40% of gynecologic diagnostic laparoscopies are done for chronic pelvic pain (Howard, 2003a). Between 14 and 77% of patients have no obvious pathology and two thirds of patients have findings of adhesions (85% of all laparoscopic diagnoses) that may or may not play a role in their pain. Furthermore, nonsurgical management of chronic pelvic pain (multidisciplinary pain clinics or trigger point injections) is successful in 65 to 90% of patients regardless of the presence of minimal pathology (Hornstein et al., 1997b; Reiter et al., 1991; Slocumb, 1990). Laparoscopy should probably be reserved for patients in whom other pathology has been ruled out, and for those with signs and/or symptoms of endometriosis, cyclic pelvic pain not responsive to hormonal therapy, or infertility. Some retrospective and prospective evidence suggests that laparoscopy provides patients with pelvic pain a positive psychological impact (Elcome et al., 1997); however, it is costly and not without surgical and anesthetic risks.

A newer approach to diagnostic laparoscopy, called "conscious laparoscopic pain mapping," is performed under local anesthesia, with or without conscious sedation, and is intended to be used as a tool in which the patient can directly report sources of pain upon stimulation (Palter & Olive, 1996). A recently published study on the benefit of conscious pain mapping in 50 patients as compared with 65 others who did not undergo conscious pain mapping showed no improvement in outcome after laparoscopic treatment (Howard et al., 2000).

LYSIS OF ADHESIONS

The role of pelvic adhesions in the genesis of pain is unclear. Lysis of adhesions at laparotomy is frequently undermined by a high incidence of adhesion reformation. Laparoscopic lysis of adhesions may be less likely to result in significant reformation of adhesions; however, adhesions reform or form *de nouveau* after an adhesiolysis procedure. It is not unreasonable, therefore, to lyse adhesions at the time of diagnostic laparoscopy, but controlled studies have yet to be definitive. (See previous section on adhesions for further details.)

HYSTERECTOMY

Hysterectomy has long been performed to cure pelvic pain. In fact, up to 19% of hysterectomies are performed for the sole indication of chronic pelvic pain (Reiter, 1990b). However, 30% of patients presenting to pelvic pain clinics have already undergone hysterectomy without experiencing relief of pain (Chamberlain & La Ferla, 1987). Reiter and associates (1991) note a decline in the incidence of hysterectomy for the indication of chronic pelvic pain from 16.3 to 5.8% after the initiation of a multidisciplinary approach to the diagnosis and treatment of chronic pelvic pain. A prospective cohort study, the Maine Women's Health Study, evaluated the results of hysterectomy on symptom relief, quality of life, and the onset of new medical problems. Of the 418 women, the diagnoses leading to hysterectomy included uterine leiomyomas (35%), chronic pelvic pain (18%), abnormal bleeding (22%), and other (25%). One year later at post-surgical follow-up, pain was reported to have improved in 95% of the women who had pelvic pain before surgery. There were also improvements in scores indicating mental health, general health, and quality of life. New problems that developed after having had a hysterectomy included hot flashes, weight gain, depression, and decreased libido. Finally, before hysterectomy, 63% of the women reported pelvic pain and at the 2 year follow-up visit only 10% of the women reported pelvic pain (Carlson et al., 1994). Hillis et al. (1995) studied a prospective cohort of 308 women who underwent hysterectomy for chronic pelvic pain, thought to be of uterine origin. The outcome revealed a 74% response rate, with observed persistent pain associated with multiparity, prior history of pelvic inflammatory disease, lack of pathology, and Medicaid payer status (Hillis et al., 1995). Hysterectomy remains an option for appropriately selected patients with pain of uterine origin. In recognition of the fact that hysterectomy treats, at best, only some women, the American College of Obstetricians and Gynecologists (1998) established criteria to be met prior to performing such invasive surgery for pelvic pain. The criteria include that no remediable pathology is found on laparoscopic examination and that a 6-month presence of pain occurs with negative effect on the patient's quality of life.

PRESACRAL NEURECTOMY AND UTERINE NERVE ABLATION

Presacral neurectomy or sympathectomy (PSN) was first described by Cotte (1937) for the indication of dysmenorrhea. As is apparent from the discussion of the neuroanatomy of the pelvic organs, the presacral nerve, which is actually the superior hypogastric plexus, receives the major afferent supply from the cervix, uterus, and proximal fallopian tubes. Afferents traveling with the sympathetic nerve supply from the bladder and rectum also pass through the superior hypogastric plexus. Normal micturition and defecation are dependent on an intact sacral autonomic nerve supply and are relatively unaffected by resection of the superior hypogastric plexus. The nerve supply to the adnexal structures bypasses the hypogastric plexus, as the afferents from the ovary travel with sympathetic fibers accompanying the ovarian artery to the superior mesenteric plexus to enter the spinal cord at T9 and T10. These autonomic relationships constitute the rationale for Cotte's (1937) emphasis on differentiating dysmenorrhea with the maximum intensity of the pain localized to the uterus with radiation to the sacrum from lateralizing pain radiating to the lumbar region.

PSN has been studied in the management of central pelvic pain in the setting of both cyclic and noncyclic pain (Ingersoll & Meigs, 1948; Lee et al., 1986; Polan & DeCherney, 1980). Although most studies of PSN are uncontrolled, Polan and DeCherney's (1980) study did include a control group of patients who had had infertility surgery without PSN. In the latter group, only 26% experienced relief of pain as compared with 75% of patients who also underwent PSN. In another randomized controlled study by Tjaden et al. (1992), the study was prematurely terminated due to the overwhelming response to PSN compared with resection of moderate to severe endometriosis (Tjaden et al., 1992). However, when Candiani et al. (1992) studied PSN versus resection of moderate or severe endometriosis, initial central pain was reduced although 6-month follow-up revealed no significant difference in pain. More recently, a randomized controlled study compared laparoscopic surgery with presacral neurectomy versus conservative laparoscopic surgery alone in 140 patients with severe dysmenorrhea (Zullo et al., 2003). The authors found that 87.3% of the patients who had sacral neurectomy performed versus 60.3% of the patients who had conservative laparoscopy alone were pain free at 6 months and 85.7% versus 57.1%, respectively, were pain free in 12 months (Zullo et al., 2003). The value of PSN remains controversial.

An alternative nerve ablation technique, initially tried in order to prevent pelvic pain, yet has fewer complications such as constipation, uterine prolapse, painless labor in subsequent pregnancies, and bladder dysfunction, which has been reported in some studies, is laprascopic uterosacral nerve ablation (LUNA). A randomized trial of women with endometriosis who received therapeutic laparoscopic surgery with LUNA as compared with no treatment showed that 62% of the women in the former group had improved or had complete resolution of their pain at 6 months postoperatively (Dwarakanath et al., 2002; Sutton et al., 1994). This same author found that at 1 year follow-up of the 62% of responsive patients, 90% were still pain free (Sutton et al., 1994). The weakness that exists in studies of this form is the inability to determine whether the therapeutic laparoscopic surgery alone resulted in diminishing the pain or if it was an effect of the LUNA itself. A large multicenter, prospective, randomized trial is being performed using questionnaires at baseline and postoperatively at 3, 6, 12, 24, and 36 months (Birmingham Clinical Trials Unit, 2000).

A Cochrane Database meta-analysis concluded that after review of the literature there was evidence that uterine nerve ablation was more effective for primary dysmenorrhea as compared with no treatment (Proctor et al., 2003). When comparing LUNA with PSN, there was no pain relief difference in the short term; however, PSN was better at relieving pain greater than 6 months or more postoperatively. (Chen et al., 1996; Proctor et al., 2003 They also found that LUNA combined with surgical treatment of endometrial implants as compared with surgical treatment without LUNA did not result in further pain relief (Proctor et al., 2003). The same results were true for PSN but there was a significant difference in relief of midline abdominal pain (Proctor et al., 2003).

IMPLANTABLE STIMULATOR/NEUROMODULATION

An alternative to actual ablation of nerve fibers is neuromodulation. Neuromodulation techniques include sacral nerve stimulation, retrograde nerve root stimulation, and selective stimulation of the S2, S3, and S4 nerve roots. Retrograde stimulation involves implanting four quadripolar leads by a trained specialist with adequate experience because complications can include wet taps and intrathecal electrode implantations (Feler et al., 2003). Another option that has been considered is superior hypogastric nerve block using neurolytic agents such as 10% phenol or 50% ethanol under fluoroscopic guidance. A small uncontrolled study of 10 patients using Transforaminal sacral nerve stimulation with an implantable neuroprosthetic device showed that 9 of 10 patients with the implant had a decrease in the pain severity of the worst pain compared with baseline at a median follow-up of 19 months (Siegel et al., 2001). There was an average decrease in the rate of pain from 9.7 at baseline to 4.4 on a scale of 10 = always to 0 = never having pain (Siegel et al., 2001).

MULTIDISCIPLINARY PAIN MANAGEMENT

MULTIDISCIPLINARY MEDICINE

Multidisciplinary pain management is important in the approach to chronic pelvic pain. Peripheral pathology is managed by the pain manager (gynecologist, anesthesiologist, internist, family practitioner). Spinal cord and central factors related to possible abnormalities of modulation of pain impulses are addressed with trigger point injections, nerve blocks, neuropathic pain medications, acupuncture, or TENS (Helms, 1987; Mannheimer & Whaler, 1985; Rapkin & Kames, 1987; Slocumb, 1984). Cognitive behavioral and other psychological psychosexual factors are addressed by the psychologist.

One program was successful in reducing pain by at least 50% in 85% of the subjects (Rapkin & Kames, 1987). Other studies have suggested that similar results may be obtained with a multidisciplinary team (Milburn et al., 1993; Pearce et al., 1982; Peters et al., 1991; Reiter et al., 1991; Wood et al., 1990;). In a prospective randomized study, the multidisciplinary approach was found to be more effective than traditional gynecologic (medical and surgical) management (Peters et al., 1991).

ALTERNATIVE MANAGEMENT OF CHRONIC PELVIC PAIN

With advances in media and the Internet, the practitioner will find that in general, patients are now more informed than ever before. Many patients not only desire more information about the disease process, but also very often value a practitioner's ability (especially in retractile chronic pelvic pain patients) to present alternative medical management options. Acupuncture is one of the most commonly used alternative forms of therapy. It is a crucial part of the traditional Chinese system of medicine and the oldest form of standardized neuromodulatory therapies. A recent study of men with chronic prostatitis/chronic pelvic pain syndrome assessed 12 men who had undergone at least 6 weeks of acupuncture treatment using a National Institutes of Health (NIH) Chronic Prostatitis Symptom

Index. The investigators showed that at the initial follow-up visit, 10 patients had significant improvement (greater than 50% positive symptomatology decrease) and at an average of 33 weeks post-treatment 8 patients had sustained improvement (Chen & Nickel, 2003). Although this study was in males, it is highly likely that this benefit would translate to women with chronic pelvic pain syndromes. A review by White (2003) of controlled trials of acupuncture and acupressure as self-treatment for infertility and dysmenorrhea concluded that there were only a small number of trials and these varied in quality. However, the techniques of acupuncture and acupressure as determined using these studies seem promising as a treatment for dysmenorrhea and infertility (White, 2003). As of yet, there are no studies using a sham or placebo arm to evaluate these techniques.

Another alternative method that has been proposed by chiropractors is spinal manipulation therapy. This method uses the concept that parasympathetic and sympathetic pelvic nerve pathways are closely associated with the spinal vertebrae, and therefore, mechanical dysfunction in these vertebrae results in disruption of the sympathetic nerve supply to the blood vessels supplying the pelvic viscera. This disruption causes dysmenorrhea due to vasospasm and constriction. With spinal manipulation spinal mobility is improved, the autonomic nerve function improves, and the resultant blood supply improves (Proctor et al., 2003). Alternatively, the theory behind how spinal manipulation therapy works has been explained by assuming dysmenorrhea is referred pain that originally arises from the musculoskeletal structures that share the same pelvic nerve pathways (Proctor et al., 2003). A review of recently published studies concluded that there is no evidence this technique is any more effective than sham manipulation, but it may be more effective than no treatment (Proctor et al., 2003).

Some final techniques are magnetic field therapy and photographic reinforcement during postoperative counseling after diagnostic laparoscopy. A randomized, double-blind placebo-controlled study out of the University of Tennessee Health Sciences Center and Mount Sinai School of Medicine, looked at 51 patients with chronic pelvic pain who had completed 2 to 4 weeks of treatment with either active (500 G) or placebo magnets applied to abdominal trigger points for 24 hours a day (Brown et al., 2002). The study used the McGill Pain Questionnaire, Pain Disability Index, and Clinical Global Impressions Scale as outcome measures. The authors concluded that there was a significant improvement in disability and pain after 4 weeks of continuous use. A randomized trial of photographic reinforcement evaluated 233 women who were randomly assigned to either see or not see a Polaroid print taken of the pelvis during diagnostic laparoscopy concluded that there were no significant differences in pain improvement between these two groups (Onwude et al., 2004). In addition, the authors stated that the patients and the doctors did not feel that the photograph benefited communication regarding intraoperative findings as compared to controls.

The reader can access ACOG for its chronic pelvic pain definitions and guidelines (Williams et al., 2004).

REFERENCES

Adams, J. et al. (1990). Uterine size and endometrial thickness and the significance of cystic ovaries in women with pelvic pain due to congestion. *British Journal of Obstetrics and Gynecology, 97,* 583.

Almeida, O. D., & Val-Gallas, J. M. (1997). Conscious pain mapping. *Journal of American Association of Gynecologic Laparoscopists, 4,* 587.

American College of Obstetricians and Gynecologists. (1983). Dysmenorrhea. *American College of Obstetricians and Gynecologists, 68,* 1.

American College of Obstetricians and Gynecologists criteria set. (1998). Hysterectomy, abdominal or vaginal, for chronic pelvic pain: Number 29, November 27. Committee on Quality Assessment. American College of Obstetricians and Gynecologists, *International Journal of Gynaecology and Obstetrics, 60,* 316.

Anon. (1979). Drugs for dysmenorrhea, *The Medical Letter on Drugs and Therapeutics, 21,* 81.

Bajaj, P. et al. (2003). Endometriosis is associated with central sensitization: A psychophysical controlled study. *The Journal of Pain, 4*(7), 372

Baker, P. K. (1993). Musculoskeletal origins of chronic pelvic pain. In F. W. Ling (Ed.). *Obstetrics and gynecology clinics of North America: Contemporary management of chronic pain* (p. 719). Philadelphia: W. B. Saunders.

Balasch, J. et al. (1997). Pentoxifylline versus placebo in the treatment of infertility associated with minimal or mild endometriosis: A pilot randomized clinical trial. *Human Reproduction, 12,* 2046.

Beard, R. W., Highman, Pearce, & Reginald. (1984). Diagnosis of pelvic varicosities in women with chronic pelvic pain. *Lancet, 2,* 946.

Bergman, A., Karram, M., & Bhatia, N.N. (1989). Urethral syndrome: A comparison of different treatment modalities. *Journal of Reproductive Medicine, 34,* 157.

Berkley, K. J. (1994). Communications from the uterus (and other tissues). In J. M. Besson (Ed.), *Pharmacological aspects of peripheral neurons involved in nociception, pain research and clinical management* (p. 39). Amsterdam: Elsevier.

Berkley, K. J. and Hubscher, C. H. (1995). Visceral and somatic sensory tracks through the neuroaxis and their relation to pain: Lessons from the rat female reproductive system. In G. F. Gebhart (Ed.), *Visceral pain: Progress in pain research and management* (vol. 5, p. 195). Seattle: IASP Press, Seattle.

Bianchi, S. et al. (1999). Effects of 3-month therapy with danazol after laparoscopic surgery for stage III/IV endometriosis: a randomized study. *Human Reproduction, 14,* 1335.

Birmingham Clinical Trials Unit. (2000). *The LUNA Trial.* URL: http://www.cancer.bham.ac.uk/research/luna/luna main.htm Accessed September 10.

Bodner, D. R. (1988). The urethral syndrome. *Office Urology, 15,* 699.

Boyce, P. M., Koloski, N. A, & Talley, N.J. (2000). Irritable bowel syndrome according to varying diagnostic criteria: Are the new Rome II criteria unnecessarily restrictive for research and practice? *American Journal of Gastroenterology, 95,* 3176.

Brosens, J. et al. (2003). Noninvasive diagnosis of endometriosis: The role of imaging and markers. *Obstetrics and Gynecology Clinics, 30*(1), 95.

Brown, C. S. et al. (2002). Efficacy of static magnetic field therapy in chronic pelvic pain: A double-blind pilot study. *American Journal of Obstetrics and Gynecology, 187* (6), 1581.

Bulun, S. E. (1999). Aromatase in aging women. *Seminars in Reproductive Endocrinology, 17,* 349.

Busacca, M. et al. (2001). Post-operative GnRH analogue treatment after conservative surgery for symptomatic endometriosis stage III-IV: A randomized controlled trial. *Human Reproduction, 16,* 2399.

Candiani, G.B., Fedele, Vercellini, Bianchi, & DiNola. (1992). Presacral neurectomy for the treatment of pelvic pain associated with endometriosis: A controlled study. *American Journal of Obstetrics and Gynecology, 167,* 100.

Capasso, P. et al. (1997). Treatment of symptomatic pelvic varices by ovarian vein embolization. *Cardiovascular Interventional Radiology, 20,* 107.

Carey, M. P., & Slack, M. C. (1996). GnRH analogue in assessing chronic pelvic pain in women with residual ovaries. *British Journal of Obstetrics and Gynecology, 103,* 150.

Carlson, K. J., Miller, B. A., & Fowler, F. J., Jr. (1994). The Maine Women's Health Study: I. Outcomes of hysterectomy. *Obstetrics and Gynecology, 83,* 557.

Castelnuova-Tedesco, P., & Krout, B. M. (1970). Psychosomatic aspects of chronic pelvic pain. *Psychiatry in Medicine, 1,* 109.

Cervero, F. (1994). Sensory innervation of the viscera: Peripheral basis of visceral pain. *Physiological Reviews, 74,* 95.

Cervero, F., Tattersall, J. E. H. (1986). Somatic and visceral sensory integration in the thoracic spinal cord. In F. Cervero & J. Morrison (Eds.), *Visceral sensation* (p. 189). New York: Elsevier Science Publications.

Chamberlain, A., & La Ferla, J., (1987). The gynecologist's approach to chronic pelvic pain. In J. D. Burroughs et al. (Eds.), *Handbook of Chronic Pain Management* (vol. 33, p. 371). Amersterdam: Elsevier.

Chan, W. Y., & Dawood, M. Y. (1980). Prostaglandin levels in menstrual fluid of non-dysmenorrheic and of dysmenorrheic subjects with and without oral contraceptive or ibuprofen therapy. *Advances in Prostaglandin and Thromboxane Research, 8,* 1443.

Chapron, C. et al. (1999). Gastrointestinal injuries during gynaecological laparoscopy. *Human Reproduction, 14,* 333.

Chatman, D. L., & Ward, A. B. (1982). Endometriosis in adolescents. *Obstetrics and Gynecology, 27,* 186.

Chen, F. P. et al. (1996). Comparison of laparoscopic presacral neurectomy and laparoscopic uterine nerve ablation for primary dysmenorrheal. *Journal of Reproductive Medicine and Obstetrics and Gynecology, 41* (7), 463.

Chen, R., & Nickel, J. C. (2003). Acupuncture ameliorates symptoms in men with chronic prostatitis/chronic pelvic pain syndrome. *Urology, 61,* 1156.

Chung, M. H., & Huh, C. Y. (2003). Comparison of treatments for pelvic congestion syndrome. *Tohoku Journal of Experimental Medicine, 201*(3), 131.

Chung, M.K. et al. (2002).The evil twins of chronic pelvic pain syndrome: Endometriosis and interstitial cystitis. *Journal of the Society of Laparoendoscopic Surgeons, 6*(4), 311.

Clemons, J. L., Arya, L. A., & Myers, D. L. (2002). Diagnosing interstitial cystitis in women with chronic pelvic pain. *Obstetrics and Gynecology, 100,* 337.

Cornillie, F. J. et al. (1990). Deeply infiltrating pelvic endometriosis: Histology and clinical significance *Fertility and Sterility, 53,* 978.

Cotte, G. (1937). Resection of the presacral nerves in the treatment of obstinate dysmenorrhea. *American Journal of Obstetrics and Gynecology, 33,* 1034.

De Groat, W. C. (1994). Neurophysiology of the pelvic organs. In D. N. Rushton (Ed.), *Handbook of neuro-urology* (p. 55). New York: Marcel Dekker.

Dheenadayalu, K. et al. (2002). Aromatase P450 messenger RNA expression in eutopic endometrium is not a specific marker for pelvic endometriosis. *Fertility and Sterility, 78*(4), 825.

D'Hooghe, T. M. (2003). Immunomodulators and aromatase inhibitors: are they the next generation of treatment for endometriosis? *Current Opinion in Obstetrics and Gynecology, 15*(3), 243.

Doggweiler-Wiygul, R. (2001). Chronic pelvic pain. *World Journal of Urology, 19,* 155.

Doyle, I. B. (1955). Paracervical uterine denervation by transection of the cervical plexus for the relief of dysmenorrhea. *American Journal of Obstetrics and Gynecology, 70,* 1.

Duleba, A J. et al. (1998). Changes in personality profile associated with laparoscopic surgery for chronic pelvic pain. *Journal of American Association of Gynecologic Laparoscopists, 5,* 389.

Dwarakanath, L. S. et al. (2002). Laparoscopic uterosacral nerve ablation (LUNA). *Reviews in Gynaecological Practice, 2,* 69.

Elcombe, S., Gath, D., & Day, A. (1997). The psychological effects of laparoscopy on women with chronic pelvic pain. *Psychological Medicine, 27,* 1041.

Engel, C. C., Jr. et al. (1998). A randomized, double-blind crossover trial of sertraline in women with chronic pelvic pain. *Journal of Psychosomatic Research, 44,* 203.

Fang, Z. et al. (2002). Genetic or enzymatic disruption of aromatase inhibits the growth of ectopic uterine tissue. *Journal of Clinical Endocrinology and Metabolism, 87*(7), 3460.

Fardin, F., Benettello, P., & Negrin, P. (1980). Iatrogenic femoral neuropathy: Considerations on its prognosis. *Electromyography and Clinical Neurophysiology, 20,* 153.

Farquhar, C. et al. (2003). Barrier agents for preventing adhesions after surgery for subfertility. *The Cochrane Library* (issue 4). Chichester: John Wiley & Sons, Ltd.

Farquhar, C. M. et al. (1989). A randomized controlled trial of medroxyprogesterone acetate and psychotherapy for the treatment of pelvic congestion. *British Journal of Obstetrics and Gynaecology, 96,* 1153.

Fedele, L. et al. (1989). Comparison of cyproterone acetate and danazol in the treatment of pelvic pain associated with endometriosis, *Obstetrics and Gynecology, 73,* 1000, 1989.

Feler, C. A., Whitworth, L. A., & Fernandez, J. (2003). Sacral neuromodulation for chronic pain conditions. *Anesthesiology Clinics of North America, 21* (4), 785.

Fields, H. (1987). *Pain* (p. 41). New York: McGraw-Hill.

Foong, L. C. et al. (2002). Microvascular changes in the peripheral microcirculation of women with chronic pelvic pain due to congestion. *British Journal of Obstetrics and Gynecology: An International Journal of Obstetrics and Gynecology, 109,* 867.

Fukaya, T., Hoshiai, H., & Yajima, A. (1993). Is pelvic endometriosis always associated with chronic pain? A retrospective study of 618 cases diagnosed by laparoscopy. *American Journal of Obstetrics and Gynecology, 169,* 719.

Gambone, J. C. et al. (2002). Consensus statement for the management of chronic pelvic pain and endometriosis: Proceedings of an expert-panel consensus process. *Fertility and Sterility, 78*(5), 961.

Gillespie, L. (1994). Destruction of the vesicoureteric plexus for the treatment of hypersensitive bladder disorders. *British Journal of Urology, 74,* 40.

Gross, R. J. et al. (1980). Borderline syndrome and incest in chronic pelvic pain patients. *International Journal of Psychiatry and Medicine, 10,* 79.

Grossman, R., Buchsbaum, M.S., & Yehuda, R. (2002). Neuroimaging studies in post-traumatic stress disorder. *Psychiatry Clinics of North America, 25* (2), 317.

Gupta, A., & McCarthy, S. (1994). Pelvic varices as a cause for pelvic pain: MRI appearance. *Magnetic Resonance Imaging, 12,* 679.

Guthrie, E. et al. (1993), A randomized controlled trial of psychotherapy in patients with refractory irritable bowel syndrome. *British Journal of Psychiatry, 163,* 315.

Haggerty, C. L. Schulz, R., & Ness, R. B. (2003). Lower quality of life among women with chronic pelvic pain after pelvic inflammatory disease. *Obstetrics and Gynecology, 102,* 934.

Hahn, L. (1989). Clinical findings and results of operative treatment in ilioinguinal nerve entrapment syndrome. *British Journal of Obstetrics and Gynecology, 96,* 1080.

Harrop-Griffiths, J. et al. (1988).The association between chronic pelvic pain, psychiatric diagnoses and childhood sexual abuse. *Obstetrics and Gynecology, 71,* 589.

Held, P., Hanno, P., & Wein, A. J. (1990). Epidemiology of interstitial cystitis: 2. In P. M. Hanno et al. (Eds.), *Interstitial Cystitis* (p. 29). New York: Springer-Verlag.

Helms, J. M. (1987). Acupuncture for the management of primary dysmenorrhea. *Obstetrics and Gynecology, 69,* 51.

Hightower, N. C., & Roberts, J. W. (1981). Acute and chronic lower abdominal pain of enterologic origin in chronic pelvic pain. In M. R. Renaer (Ed.), *Chronic pelvic pain in women* (p. 110). New York: Springer-Verlag.

Hillis, S. D., Marchbanks, P. A., & Peterson, H. B. (1995). The effectiveness of hysterectomy for chronic pelvic pain. *Obstetrics and Gynecology, 86,* 941.

Hobbs, J. T. (1976). The pelvic congestion syndrome. *Practitioner, 216,* 529.

Holten, K. B., Wetherington, A., & Bankston, L. (2000). Diagnosing the patient with abdominal pain and altered bowel habits: Is it irritable bowel syndrome? *American Family Physician, 67*(10), 2157.

Hornstein, M. D. et al. (1997a). Retreatment with nafarelin for recurrent endometriosis symptoms: Efficacy, safety, and bone mineral density, *Fertility and Sterility. 67,* 1013.

Hornstein, M. D. et al. (1997b). Use of nafarelin versus placebo after reductive laparoscopic surgery for endometriosis. *Fertility and Sterility, 68,* 860.

Hornstein, M. D. et al. (1998). Leuprolide acetate depot and hormonal add-back in endometriosis: A 12-month study, Lupron add-back study group. *Obstetrics and Gynecology, 91,* 16 and 702.

Howard, F. M. (2003a). The role of laparoscopy in the chronic pelvic pain patient, *Clinical Obstetrics and Gynecology, 46*(4), 749.

Howard, F. M. (2003b). Chronic pelvic pain. *Obstetrics and Gynecology, 101,* 594.

Howard, F. M. et al. (2000). Conscious pain mapping by laparoscopy in women with chronic pelvic pain. *Obstetrics and Gynecology, 96,* 934.

Hurd, W. W. (1998). Criteria that indicate endometriosis is the cause of chronic pelvic pain. *Obstetrics and Gynecology Clinical Commentary, 92*(6), 1029.

Ingersoll, F. M., & Meigs, J. V. (1948). Presacral neurectomy for dysmenorrhea. *New England Journal of Medicine, 823,* 357.

Irvin, W. et al. (2004). Minimizing the risk of neurologic injury in gynecologic surgery. *Obstetrics and Gynecology, 103,* 374.

Jacob, M. C. (1997). Pain intensity, psychiatric diagnosis, and psychosocial factors. In J. Steege, D. Metzger, & B. Levy (Eds.), *Chronic pelvic pain: An integrated approach* (p. 67). Philadelphia: Saunders.

Jacobson, T. Z. et al. (2003). Laparoscopic surgery for pelvic pain associated with endometriosis (Cochrane Review), *The Cochrane library* (issue 4). Chichester: John Wiley and Sons, Ltd.

Janig, W., Haupt-Schade, P., & Kohler, W. (1993). Afferent innervation of the colon: The neurophysiological basis for visceral sensation and pain. In E. A. Mayer & H. E. Raybould (Eds.), *Basic and clinical aspects of chronic abdominal pain* (p. 71). Amsterdam: Elsevier.

Jones, K. D., & Sutton, C. (2003). Patient satisfaction and changes in pain scores after ablative laparoscopic surgery for stage III–IV endometriosis and endometriotic cysts. *Fertility and Sterility, 79*(5), 1086.

Kaplan, B. et al. (1994). Transcutaneous electrical nerve stimulation (TENS) as a relief for dysmenorrhea. *Clinical Experiments in Obstetrics and Gynecology, 21,* 87.

Karram, M. M. (1993). Frequency, urgency, and painful bladder syndrome. In M. D. Walters & M. M. Karram (Eds.), *Clinical Urogynecology* (p. 285). St. Louis: Mosby.

Katz, N. (2002). Coxibs: Evolving role in pain management. *Seminar in Arthritis and Rheumatology, 32*(3 Suppl. 1), 15.

Kauppila, A. et al. (1988). Placebo-controlled study on serum concentrations of CA-125 before and after treatment of endometriosis with danazol or high-dose medroxy-progesterone acetate alone or after surgery. *Fertility and Sterility, 49,* 37.

Keltz, M. D. et al. (1995). Large bowel-to-pelvic sidewall adhesions associated with chronic pelvic pain. *Journal of the American Association Gynecologic Laparoscopists, 3,* 55.

Kettel, L. M. et al. (1996). Treatment of endometriosis with the antiprogesterone mifepristone (RU486). *Fertility and Sterility, 65,* 23.

Kitawaki, J. et al. (1997). Expression of aromatase cytochrome P450 protein and messenger ribonucleic acid in human endometriotic and adenomyotic tissues but not in normal endometrium. *Biology Reproduction, 57,* 514.

Kitawaki, J. et al. (1999). Detection of aromatase cytochrome P450 in endometrial biopsy specimens as a diagnostic test for endometriosis. *Fertility and Sterility, 72,* 1100.

Kitchen, J. D. (1985). Endometriosis. In J. Sciarra (Ed.), *Gynecology and Obstetrics* (p. 1). New York: Harper and Row.

Kresch, A. J. et al. (1984). Laparoscopy in 100 women with chronic pelvic pain. *Obstetrics and Gynecology, 64,* 672.

Kumazawa, T. (1986). Sensory innervation of reproductive organs. In F. Cervero & J. Morrison (Eds.), *Visceral sensation* (p. 115). New York: Elsevier Science Publications.

Kupker, W. et al. (2002). The use of GnRH antagonists in the treatment of endometriosis. *Reproductive Biomedical Online: Molecular Cancer Therapeutics, 5*(1), 12.

Lampe, A. et al. (2000). Chronic pelvic pain and previous sexual abuse. *Obstetrics and Gynecology, 96,* 929.

Lampe, A. et al. (2003). Chronic pain syndromes and their relation to childhood abuse and stressful life events. *Journal of Psychosomatic Research, 54,* 361.

Lee, A.W. et al. (1985). Recurrent appendiceal colic. *Surgical Gynecology and Obstetrics, 161,* 21.

Lee, C. H., & Dellon, A. L. (2000). Surgical management of groin pain of neural origin. *Journal of American College of Surgeons, 191,* 137.

Lee, R. B. et al. (1986). Presacral neurectomy for chronic pelvic pain. *Obstetrics and Gynecology, 68,* 517.

Ling, F., & Pelvic Pain Study Group (1999). Randomized controlled trial of depot leuprolide in patients with chronic pelvic pain and clinically suspected endometriosis. *Obstetrics and Gynecology, 93,* 51.

Liston, W. A. et al. (1972). Laparoscopy in a general gynecologic unit. *American Journal of Obstetrics and Gynecology, 113,* 672.

Longstreth, G. F. (1997). Irritable bowel syndrome: Diagnosis in the managed care era. *Digestive Diseases and Sciences, 42,* 1105.

Lundberg, W. I., Wall, J. E., & Mathers, J. E. (1973). Laparoscopy in the evaluation of pelvic pain. *Obstetrics and Gynecology, 42,* 872.

Malinak, L. R. (1980). Operative management of pelvic pain. *Clinical Obstetrics and Gynecology, 23,* 191.

Mannheimer, J. S., & Whaler, E. C. (1985). The efficacy of transcutaneous electrical nerve stimulation in dysmenorrhea. *Clinical Journal of Pain, 1,* 75.

Manning, A. P., Thompson, W. G., & Heaton, K. W. et al. (1978). Towards a positive diagnosis of irritable bowel syndrome. *British Medical Journal, 2,* 653–654.

Mathias, S. D. et al. (1996). Chronic pelvic pain: Prevalence, health-related quality of life, and economic correlates. *Obstetrics and Gynecology, 87,* 321.

McDonald, J. S. (1993). Management of chronic pain. In F. W. Ling (Ed.), *Obstetrics and gynecology clinics of North America: Contemporary management of chronic pain* (p. 817). Philadelphia: W. B. Saunders.

McDonald, J. S., & Rapkin, A. J. (2001). General considerations. In J. D. Loeser (Ed.), *Bonica's Management of Pain, 3rd ed.* (Chap. 70). Philadelphia: Lippincott Williams & Wilkins.

McSherry, C. K., Cornell, G. N., & Glenn, F. (1969). Carcinoma of the colon and rectum. *Annals of Surgery, 169,* 502.

Mearin, F. et al. (2003). Splitting irritable bowel syndrome: from original Rome to Rome II criteria. *American Journal of Gastroenterology, 10,* 1046.

Messing, E. M. (1989). The diagnosis of interstitial cystitis. *Urology, 29* (Suppl.), 4–21.

Messing, E. M., & Stamey, T. A. (1978). Interstitial cystitis: Early diagnosis, pathology, and treatment. *Urology, 12,* 381.

Milburn, A., Reiter, R. C., & Rhomberg, A. T. (1993). Multidisciplinary approach to chronic pelvic pain. In F. W. Ling (Ed.), *Obstetrics and gynecology clinics of North America: Contemporary management of chronic pain* (p. 643). Philadelphia: W. B. Saunders.

Morgante, G. (1999). Low-dose danazol after combined surgical and medical therapy reduces the incidence of pelvic pain in women with moderate and severe endometriosis. *Human Reproduction, 14*(9), 2371.

Morrison, B. W. et al. (1999). Rofecoxib, a specific cyclooxygenase-2 inhibitor, in primary dysmenorrhea: A randomized controlled trial. *Obstetrics and Gynecology, 94,* 504.

Morscher, E. (1981). Low back pain in women. In M.R. Renaer (Ed.), *Chronic pelvic pain in women* (p. 137). New York: Springer-Verlag.

Nahabedian, M. Y., & Dellon, L. (1997). Outcome of the operative management of nerve injuries in the ilioinguinal region. *Journal of American College of Surgeons, 184,* 265.

Noble, L. S. et al. (1996). Aromatase expression in endometriosis. *Journal of Clinical Endocrinology and Metabolism, 81,* 174.

Nothnick, W. B., Curry, T. E., & Vernon, M. W. (1994). Immunomodulation of rat endometriotic implant growth and protein production. *American Journal of Reproductive Immunology, 31,* 151.

O'Leary M. P. et al. (1997). The interstitial cystitis symptom index and problem index. *Urology, 49,* 58.

Onwude, J. L. et al. (2004). A randomised trial of photographic reinforcement during postoperative counseling after diagnostic laparoscopy for pelvic pain. *European Journal of Obstetrics and Gynecology and Reproductive Biology, 112,* 89.

Ormrod, D., Wellington, K., & Wagstaff, A. J. (2002). Valdecoxib. *Drugs, 62*(14), 2059.

Painter, N. S. (1975). Diverticular disease of the colon, a 20th century problem. *Clinical Gastroenterology, 1,* 3.

Palter, S. F. (1999). Microlaparoscopy under local anesthesia and conscious pain mapping for the diagnosis and management of pelvic pain. *Current Opinion on Obstetrics and Gynecology, 11,* 387.

Palter, S. F., & Olive, D. L. (1996). Office microlaparoscopy under local anesthesia for chronic pelvic pain. *Journal of American Association of Gynecological Laparoscopy, 3,* 359.

Parazzini F. et al. (1994). Postsurgical medical treatment of advanced endometriosis: Results of a randomized clinical trial. *American Journal of Obstetrics and Gynecology, 171,* 1205.

Parsons, C. L. et al. (2002). Increased prevalence of interstitial cystitis: Previously unrecognized urologic and gynecologic cases identified using a new symptom questionnaire and intravesical potassium sensitivity. *Urology, 60* (4), 573.

Pearce, S., Knight, C., & Beard, R. W. (1982). Pelvic pain — A common gynaecological problem. *Journal of Psychosomatic Obstetrics and Gynaecology, 1* (1), 12.

Perry, C. P. (2001). Current concepts of pelvic congestion and chronic pelvic pain. *Journal of the Society of Laparoendoscopic Surgeons, 5*(2), 105.

Peters, A. A. et al. (1991). A randomized clinical trial to compare two different approaches in women with chronic pelvic pain. *Obstetrics and Gynecology, 77,* 740.

Peters, K. M., Carey, J. M., & Konstandt, D. B.(2003). Sacral neuromodulation for the treatment of refractory interstitial cystitis: Outcomes based on technique. *International Urogynecology Journal of Pelvic Floor Dysfunction, 14* (4), 223.

Pettit, P. D., & Lee, R. A. (1988). Ovarian remnant syndrome: Diagnostic dilemma and surgical challenge. *Obstetrics and Gynecology, 71,* 580.

Pieri, S. et al. (2003). Percutaneous treatment of pelvic congestion syndrome. *Radiologia Medica, 105*(1–2), 76.

Polan, M. L., & DeCherney, A. (1980). Presacral neurectomy for pelvic pain in infertility. *Fertility and Sterility, 34,* 557.

Portincasa, P. et al. (2003). Pan-enteric dysmotility, impaired quality of life and alexithymia in a large group of patients meeting Rome II criteria for irritable bowel syndrome. *World Journal of Gastroenterology, 9*(10), 2293.

Prentice, A., Deary, A. J., & Bland, E. (2003). Progestagens and anti-progestagens for pain associated with endometriosis (Cochrane Review). *The Cochrane library* (issue 4). Chichester: John Wiley and Sons, Ltd.

Price, F. V., Edwards, R., and Buchsbaum, H. J. (1990). Ovarian remnant syndrome: Difficulties in diagnosis and management. *Obstetrics and Gynecology Surgery, 45,* 151.

Probst, A. M., & Laufer, M. R. (1999). Endometriosis in adolescents. Incidence, diagnosis and treatment. *Journal of Reproductive Medicine, 44,* 751.

Procacci, P., Zoppi, M., & Maresen, M. (1986). Clinical approach to visceral sensation. In F. Cervero & J. Morrison (Eds.), *Visceral sensation* (p. 21). New York: Elsevier.

Proctor, M. L. et al. (2003). Surgical interruption of pelvic nerve pathways for primary and secondary dysmenorrhea (Cochrane Review), *The Cochrane Library* (issue 4). Chichester: John Wiley and Sons, Ltd.

Proctor, M. L., Johnson, H. W., & Murphy, P.A. (2003). Spinal manipulation for primary and secondary dysmenorrhea (Cochrane Review), *The Cochrane Library* (issue 4), Chichester: John Wiley and Sons, Ltd.

Rapkin, A. J. (1986). Adhesions and pelvic pain: A retrospective study. *Obstetrics and Gynecology, 68,* 13.

Rapkin, A. J., & Kames, L. D. (1987). The pain management approach to chronic pelvic pain. *Journal of Reproductive Medicine, 32,* 323.

Rapkin, A. J., & Mayer, E. A. (1993). Gastroenterologic causes of chronic pelvic pain. *Obstetrics and Gynecology Clinics of North America: Contemporary management of chronic pain* (p. 663). In F.W. Ling (Ed.), Philadelphia: W. B. Saunders.

Rapkin, A. J., Kames, L. D., & Darke, L. L. (1990). History of physical and sexual abuse in women with chronic pelvic pain. *Obstetrics and Gynecology, 76,* 90.

Reiter, R. C. (1990a) Occult somatic pathology in women with chronic pelvic pain. *Clinical Obstetrics and Gynecology, 33,* 154.

Reiter, R .C. (1990b). A profile of women with chronic pelvic pain, *Clinical Obstetrics and Gynecology, 33,* 130.

Reiter, R. C., Gambone, J. C., & Johnson, S.R. (1991). Availability of a multidisciplinary pelvic pain clinic and frequency of hysterectomy for pelvic pain. *Journal of Psychosomatic Obstetrics and Gynaecology, 12* (Suppl.), 109.

Renaer, M. (1980). Chronic pelvic pain without obvious pathology in women: Personal observation and a review of the problem. *European Journal of Obstetrics and Gynecology, 10,* 415.

Renaer, M. (1981). *Chronic pelvic pain in women.* New York: Springer-Verlag.

Renaer, M. et al. (1979). Psychosocial aspects of chronic pelvic pain in women. *American Journal of Obstetrics and Gynecology, 134,* 75.

Rice, V. M. (2002). Conventional medical therapies for endometriosis. *Annals of the New York Academy of Sciences, 955,* 343.

Richter, H. E. et al. (1998). Laparoscopic and psychologic evaluation of women with chronic pelvic pain. *International Journal of Psychiatry in Medicine, 28* (2), 243.

Ritchie, J. (1979). Pain in IBS. *Practical Gastroenterology, 3,* 17.

Rouff, G., & Lema, M. (2003). Strategies in Pain Management: new and potential indications for COX-2 specific inhibitors. *Journal of Pain and Symptom Management, 25*(2S), S21.

Sant, G. R. (1998). Interstitial cystitis – A urogynecologic perspective. *Contemporary Ob/Gyn, 43* (6), 119–130.

Scott, L. J., & Lamb, H. M. (1999). Rofecoxib. *Drugs, 58,* 499, 1999.

Sichlau, M. J., Yao, J.S.T., & Vogelzang, R.L. (1994). Transcatheter embolotherapy for the treatment of pelvic congestion syndrome. *Obstetrics and Gynecology, 83,* 892.

Sidell, N., Han, S. W., & Parthasarathy, S. (2003). Regulation and modulation of abnormal immune responses in endometriosis. *Annals of the New York Academy of Sciences, 955,* 159.

Siegel, S. et al. (2001). Sacral nerve stimulation in patients with chronic intractable pelvic pain. *Journal of Urology, 166* (5), 1742.

Sippo, W. C., Burghardt, A., & Gomez, A.C. (1987). Nerve entrapment after Pfannensteil incision. *American Journal of Obstetrics and Gynecology, 157,* 420.

Slocumb, J. C. (1984). Neurological factors in chronic pelvic pain: Trigger points and the abdominal pelvic pain syndrome. *American Journal of Obstetrics and Gynecology, 149,* 536.

Slocumb, J. C. (1990). Chronic somatic myofascial and neurogenic abdominal pelvic pain. In R. P. Porreco & R. C. Reiter (Eds), *Clinical Obstetrics and Gynecology* (p. 145). Philadelphia: J. B. Lippincott & Co.

Smith, R. P. (2001). Lower gastrointestinal disease in women. *Obstetrics and Gynecology Clinics of North America, 28*(VIII), 351.

Sola, A. E., & Bonica, J. J. (2001). Myofascial pain syndrome. In J. D. Loeser (Ed.), *Bonica's management of pain,* 3rd ed. Philadelphia: Williams & Wilkins.

Somigliana, E. (2002). Use of serum-soluble intercellular adhesion molecule-1 as a new marker of endometriosis. *Fertility and Sterility, 77*(5), 1028.

Somigliana, E. et al. (2003). The therapy of endometriosis. *Minerva Ginecologica, 55*(1), 15.

Soysal, M. E. et al. (2001). A randomized controlled trial of goserelin and medroxyprogesterone acetate in the treatment of pelvic congestion. *Human Reproduction, 16*(5), 931.

Speizer, F. E. et al. (1999). Epidemiology of interstitial cystitis: A population based study. *Journal of Urology, 161,* 549.

Srinivasan, R., & Greenbaum, D. S. (2002). Chronic abdominal wall pain: a frequently overlooked problem. Practical approach to diagnosis and management. *American Journal of Gastroenterology, 97* (12), 3207.

Steege, J. F. (1987). Ovarian remnant syndrome, *Obstetrics and Gynecology, 70,* 64.

Steege, J. F., & Scott, A. L. (1991). Resolution of chronic pelvic pain after laparoscopic lysis of adhesions. *American Journal of Obstetrics and Gynecology, 165,* 278.

Steinleitner, A. et al. (1991). Immunomodulation in the treatment of endometriosis-associated subfertility: Use of pentoxifylline to reverse the inhibition of fertilization by surgically induced endometriosis in a rodent model. *Fertility and Sterility, 56,* 975.

Stones, R. W. et al. (1990). Pelvic congestion in women: Evaluation with transvaginal ultrasound and observation of venous pharmacology. *British Journal of Radiology, 63,* 710.

Stones, R. W., & Mountfield, J. (2003). Interventions for treating chronic pelvic pain in women (Cochrane Review). *The Cochrane Library, 4 ,* Chichester: John Wiley and Sons, Ltd.

Stones, R.W., & Mountfield, J. (2004). Interventions for treating chronic pelvic pain in women (Cochrane Review). In *The Cochrane Library* (issue 1). Chichester: John Wiley & Sons, Ltd.

Stulz, P., & Pfieffer, K. M. (1982). Peripheral nerve injuries resulting from common surgical procedures in the lower abdomen. *Archives of Surgery, 117,* 324.

Summit, R. L. (1993). Urogynecologic causes of chronic pelvic pain. In F. W. Ling (Ed.), *Obstetrics and gynecology clinics of North America: Contemporary management of chronic pain* (p. 685). Philadelphia: W. B. Saunders.

Surrey, E., & Judd, H. (1992). Reduction in vasomotor symptoms and bone mineral density loss with combined norethindrone and long-acting gonadotropin-releasing hormone agonist therapy of symptomatic endometriosis: A prospective randomized trial. *Journal of Clinical Endocrinology and Metabolism, 75,* 558.

Sutton, C. J. et al. (1997). Follow-up report on randomized controlled trial of laser laparoscopy in the treatment of pelvic pain associated with minimal to moderate endometriosis. *Fertility and Sterility, 68,* 1070.

Sutton, C. J. G. et al. (1994). Prospective, randomised, double blind controlled trial of laser laparoscopy in the treatment of pelvic pain associated with minimal, mild and moderate endometriosis. *Fertility and Sterility, 62,* 696.

Swank, D. J. et al. (2002). Complications and feasibility of laparoscopic adhesiolysis in patients with chronic abdominal pain. *Surgical Endoscopy, 16,* 1468.

Swank, D. J et al. (2003). A prospective analysis of predictive factors on the results of laparoscopic adhesiolysis in patients with chronic abdominal pain. *Surgical Laparoscopy, Endoscopy, and Percutaneous Technology, 13*(2), 88.

Sweet, R. L., & Gibbs, R. S. (1985). Pelvic inflammatory disease. In R. L. Sweet & R. S. Gibbs (Eds.). *Infectious diseases of the female genital tract* (part 1, p. 53). Baltimore: Williams & Wilkins.

Takahashi, K. et al. (1996). Studies on the detection of small endometrial implants by magnetic resonance imaging using a fat saturation technique. *Gynecology and Obstetrics Investigations, 41,* 203.

Takayama, K. et al. (1998). Treatment of severe postmenopausal endometriosis with an aromatase inhibitor. *Fertility and Sterility, 69,* 709.

Talley, N. J. et al. (1990). Diagnostic value of the Manning criteria in irritable bowel syndrome. *Gut, 31*(1), 77.

Tarazov, P. G., Prozorovskij, K. V., & Ryzhkov, V. K. (1997). Pelvic pain caused by ovarian varices. Treatment by transcatheter embolization. *Acta Radiologica, 38,* 1023.

Taylor, H. C., Jr. (1954). Pelvic pain based on a vascular and autonomic nervous system disorder. *American Journal of Obstetrics and Gynecology, 67,* 1177.

Telimaa, S. et al. (1987). Placebo-controlled comparison of danazol and medroxyprogesterone acetate in the treatment of endometriosis. *Gynecologic Endocrinology, 1,* 13.

Telimaa, S. et al. (1990). Placebo-controlled comparison of hormonal and biochemical effects of danazol and high-dose medroxyprogesterone acetate. *European Journal of Obstetrics and Gynaecology and Reproductive Biology, 36,* 97.

Telimaa, S., Ronnberg, L., & Kauppila, A. (1987). Placebo-controlled comparison of danazol and high-dose medroxyprogesterone acetate in the treatment of endometriosis after conservative surgery. *Gynecologic Endocrinology, 1,* 363.

Thompson, W. G. et al. (1989) Irritable bowel syndrome: Guidelines for the diagnosis. *Gastroenterology International, 2,* 92.

Thompson, W. G. et al. (1999). Functional bowel disorders and functional abdominal pain. *Gut, 45* (Suppl. 2), I143.

Tjaden, B., Schlaff, Kimball, & Rock. (1992). The efficacy of presacral neurectomy for the relief of midline dysmenorrhea. *Obstetrics and Gynecology, 167,* 100.

Toomey, T. C. et al. (1993). Relationship of sexual and physical abuse to pain and psychological assessment variables in chronic pelvic pain patients. *Pain, 53* (1), 105.

Travell, J. (1976). Myofascial trigger points: Clinical view. *Advances in Pain Research and Therapy, 1* (919) 1976.

Venbrux, A. C., & Lambert, D. L. (1999). Embolization of the ovarian veins as a treatment for patients with chronic pelvic pain caused by pelvic venous incompetence (pelvic congestion syndrome). *Current Opinion in Obstetrics and Gynecology, 11,* 395.

Vercellini, P. et al. (1991). Reliability of the visual diagnosis of ovarian endometriosis. *Fertility and Sterility, 56,* 1198.

Vercellini, P. et al. (1993). A gonadotropin releasing hormone agonist vs. low dose oral contraceptive for pelvic pain associated with endometriosis. *Fertility and Sterility, 60,* 75.

Vercellini, P. et al. (1996). Endometriosis and pelvic pain: Relation to disease stage and localization. *Fertility and Sterility, 65,* 299.

Vercellini, P. et al. (1999). A gonadotrophin-releasing hormone agonist compared with expectant management after conservative surgery for symptomatic endometriosis. *British Journal of Obstetrics and Gynecology, 106,* 672.

Vereecken, R. L. (1981). Chronic pelvic pain of urologic origin. In M. R. Renaer (Ed.), *Chronic Pelvic Pain in Women* (p. 155). New York: Springer-Verlag.

Viera, A. J., Hoag, S., & Shaughnessy, J.(2002). Management of irritable bowel syndrome. *American Family Physician, 66*(10), 1867.

Vigano, P. et al. (2002). Serum leptin concentrations in endometriosis. *Journal of Clinical Endocrinology and Metabolism, 87*(3), 1085.

Vigano, P. et al. (2003). Use of estrogen antagonists and aromatase inhibitors in endometriosis. *Current Opinion in Investigational Drugs, 4*(10), 1209.

Vosburg, L., & Finn, W. (1961). Femoral nerve impairment subsequent to hysterectomy. *American Journal of Obstetrics and Gynecology, 82,* 931.

Walker, E., Katon, W., & Harrop-Griffiths, J. (1988). Relationship of chronic pelvic pain of psychiatric diagnoses and childhood sexual abuse. *American Journal of Psychiatry, 145*, 75.

Wall, P. D. (1988). The John J. Bonica distinguished lecture. Stability and instability of central pain mechanisms. In R. Dubner (Ed.), *Proceedings of the Fifth World Congress on Pain* (p. 13). Amsterdam: Elsevier Science Publishers BV.

Walling, M. K. et al. (1994). Abuse history and chronic pain in women: I. Prevalence of sexual abuse and physical abuse. *Obstetrics and Gynecology, 84*, 193.

Walton, S. M., & Batra, H. K. (1992). The use of medroxyprogesterone acetate 50 mg in the treatment of painful pelvic conditions: Preliminary results from a multicenter trial. *Journal of Obstetrics and Gynecology, 12*(Suppl. 2), S50.

Weaver, A. L. (2001). Rofecoxib: Clinical pharmacology and clinical experience. *Clinical Therapeutics, 23*, 1323.

Wesselmann, U. (2001). Neurogenic inflammation and chronic pelvic pain. *World Journal of Urology, 19*, 180.

Wesselmann, U. (2002). Interstitial cystitis and vulvodynia. *National Vulvodynia Association News, 8* (1), 1.

White, A. R. (2003). A review of controlled trials of acupuncture for women's reproductive health care. *Journal of Family Planning and Reproductive Health Care, 29* (4), 233.

Whitehead, W. E. (1999). Patient subgroups in irritable bowel syndrome that can be defined by symptom evaluation and physical examination. *American Journal of Medicine, 107*, 33S.

Williams, R. E. et al. (2004). Documenting the current definitions of chronic pelvic pain: Implications for research. *Obstetrics and Gynecology, 103* (4), 686.

Wilson, M. et al. (2000). Trans-cutaneous electrical nerve stimulation and acupuncture for primary dysmenorrhea [Protocol]. *The Cochrane library*, Software Update, Oxford.

Winkel, C. A. (1999). Combined medical and surgical treatment of women with endometriosis. *Clinical Obstetrics and Gynecology, 42*, 645.

Wood, D. P., Weisner, M. G., & Reiter, R.C. (1990). Psychogenic chronic pelvic pain. *Clinical Obstetrics and Gynecology, 33*, 179.

Young, S. J. et al. (1976). Psychiatric illness and the irritable bowel syndrome: Practical implications for the primary physician. *Gastroenterology, 70*, 162.

Zullo, F. et al. (2003). Effectiveness of presacral neurectomy in women with severe dysmenorrhea caused by endometriosis who were treated with laparoscopic conservative surgery: A 1-year prospective randomized double-blind controlled trial. *American Journal of Obstetrics and Gynecology, 189* (1), 5.

31

Urologic Pain

Hossein Sadeghi-Nejad, MD, Carin V. Hopps, MD, and Allen D. Seftel, MD

UPPER URINARY TRACT PAIN (RENAL COLIC)

Renal colic is a severe paroxysmal pain that occurs from obstruction of the ureter at any point along its course. The most common cause of ureteral obstruction is a kidney stone that formed within the calyceal system of the kidney, became dislodged, and has been passed along the path of urine flow. In attempting to do so, however, the stone becomes wedged within the ureter somewhere along its course between the point at which the ureter joins the collecting system of the kidney (ureteropelvic junction) and the point at which the ureter enters the bladder (ureterovesical junction). It is estimated that approximately 12% of the population is expected to have urinary stone disease at some time in their lives (Sierakowski, Finlayson, Landes, Finlayson, & Sierakowski, 1978). In 55.4% of these individuals, it has been found that at least one first-degree relative had experienced renal stones, demonstrating that a hereditary component plays a significant role in urolithiasis (Ljunghall et al., 1985). The natural cumulative recurrence rate of calcium oxalate renal stones is approximately 14% within 1 year, 35% within 5 years, and 52% within 10 years (Uribarri, Oh, & Carroll, 1989). The gravity of this pathophysiological process is reflected in the cost incurred to the U.S. economy in 1993 that totaled $1.7 billion, including indirect costs from loss of productivity (Menon & Resnick, 2002). Although discussion of all causes of ureteral obstruction is beyond the scope of this chapter, the etiologies are multiple and diverse: they may be intrinsic or extrinsic, including, for example, congenital anomalies such as ureteral stricture and ureterocele; neoplastic processes such as primary or metastatic carcinomas of the ureter; inflammatory processes such as tuberculosis, schistosomiasis, or endometriosis; and other pathologic processes such as retroperitoneal fibrosis and pelvic lipomatosis.

Obstruction of the upper urinary tract may occur acutely or chronically and it may be complete or partial. Acute obstruction is typically accompanied by sudden onset, severe, colicky pain in the flank that radiates to the groin or to the ipsilateral thigh, occurring usually at night or in the early morning hours while at rest. Following acute obstruction, the kidney continues to produce urine, which in turn leads to distention of the renal pelvis (hydronephrosis) and ureter (hydroureter) proximal to the site of obstruction. Stretching of the renal capsule, which contains splanchnic innervation, with hydronephrosis, may cause nausea, vomiting, and chills (Teichman, 2004). For this reason, acute renal colic may be confused with an acute abdominal process such as appendicitis or gastroenteritis, or a pelvic process such as salpingitis. As the stone descends down the ureter, the location of the pain may course laterally and anteriorly along the individual's abdomen with radiation into the groin and testicle in the male and the labia majora and round ligament in the female. Visceral pain is transmitted by the autonomic nervous system, making localization of the source difficult (Menon & Resnick, 2002). Further descent of a stone toward the ureterovesical junction is associated with irritative voiding symptoms such as frequency, urgency, and dysuria. Patients with renal colic typically cannot position themselves comfortably and, if riding in a car, complain of severe exacerbation of pain with each bump in the road. On physical examination, the individual with acute ureteral obstruction will have severe costovertebral angle (CVA) tenderness such that pressing on the CVA is barely tolerated.

While the symptoms of acute complete obstruction are severe, the symptoms of partial unilateral obstruction may be subtle. For example, partial obstruction may only become symptomatic when the patient consumes a large fluid volume followed by a diuresis, which causes temporary exacerbation of upper tract distention and subsequent pain until diuresis subsides.

Following acute obstruction, the diameter and length of the ureter increase as pressure within the renal pelvis and ureter increases (Biancani, Zabinski, & Weiss, 1976). This is accompanied by pyelolymphatic and pyelovenous urine backflow wherein urine extravasates into lymphatic and small venous channels associated with the kidney (Stenberg et al., 1988). Despite this physiologic pop-off valve, however, the pressure may continue to rise acutely until rupture of the upper tract occurs at the fornix (the location at which the papillae of the kidney converge with the calyx of the collecting system). Rupture of the upper tract may cause a rapid diminution and possibly even complete resolution of pain, as urine may freely drain into the retroperitoneal space and pressure within the upper tract rapidly decreases.

MANAGEMENT OF RENAL COLIC

Fewer than 10% of patients with a newly diagnosed ureteral stone require hospitalization for pain management and treatment (Menon & Resnick, 2002). The majority of ureteral stones smaller than 4 to 5 mm pass spontaneously. Patients without evidence of severe obstruction, renal deterioration, or infection proximal to the site of obstruction may be treated conservatively as outpatients if they do not have nausea and if the renal colic responds to oral medication. Parenteral administration of pain medication may be necessary in the nauseated patient with refractory pain. Both narcotics and nonsteroidal anti-inflammatory drugs (NSAIDs) can be used in the treatment of renal colic. The benefits of narcotics include low cost, titratability, and potency, and the disadvantages include nausea and sedation. In addition, liberal use of narcotics in patients with renal colic may foster drug dependency and possible drug-seeking behavior. NSAIDs are non-narcotic analgesics that have a direct effect on the mechanism of pain through inhibition of cyclooxygenase, which results in decreased eicosanoid production subsequently reducing sensitization of pain receptors. NSAIDs are, however, not titratable and are associated with gastrointestinal bleeding and renal failure. Inhibition of cyclooxygenase also limits vasodilatation, thereby lowering renal blood flow and lessening diuresis, and decreases ureteral smooth-muscle stimulation. Limiting diuresis with an obstructive calculus will limit the extent to which the collecting system becomes distended and therefore the extent to which the patient experiences pain. Ketorolac tromethamine, an NSAID, was found to significantly decrease ureteral pressure and renal blood flow within 15 minutes of administration in a canine model of unilateral ureteral obstruction, which in addition to the analgesic effect of ketorolac synergistically contributed to lessened pain (Perlmutter et al., 1993). However, the rapid decrease in blood flow to an obstructed kidney may adversely affect renal function, and therefore NSAIDs should be used with caution in this patient population.

The first study to compare an NSAID with morphine administered by intravenous (IV) titration evaluated rectally administered indomethacin with IV morphine for analgesia of renal colic in a randomized, double-blind, double-dummy, two-period crossover study and showed that IV morphine produced more rapid analgesia than rectally administered indomethacin, although at 20 and 30 minutes, no significant difference existed between the two groups (Cordell, Larson et al., 1994). A prospective, controlled, randomized, double-blind trial conducted in an academic emergency department comparing the efficacy of intramuscular ketorolac and meperidine (opioid) demonstrated that ketorolac was significantly more effective than meperidine in reducing renal colic at 40, 60, and 90 minutes, and patients who were treated with ketorolac left the hospital significantly earlier than those treated with meperidine, concluding that intramuscular ketorolac as a single agent for renal colic is more effective than meperidine and promotes earlier discharge of renal colic patients from the emergency department (Larkin, Peacock, Pearl, Blair, & D'Amico, 1999). When the analgesic efficacy and safety of IV ketorolac was compared with IV meperidine and with a combination of the two agents for renal colic in a double-blind, randomized, multicenter clinical trial, by 30 minutes, 75% of the ketorolac group and 74% of the combination group had a 50% reduction in pain scores, compared with 23% of the meperidine group, indicating that IV ketorolac, alone or in combination with meperidine, was superior to IV meperidine alone in moderate and severe renal colic, suggesting that clinicians may choose to initiate treatment with a ketorolac–meperidine combination (Cordell, Wright et al., 1996).

To determine the relative efficacy, benefits, and disadvantages of NSAIDs and opioids for the management of acute renal colic, Holdgate and Pollock (2004) performed a rigorous analysis of 20 randomized controlled trials that compared any opioid with any NSAID. The authors found that while both NSAIDs and opioids can provide effective analgesia in acute renal colic, opioids are associated with a higher incidence of adverse events (particularly vomiting observed especially with pethidine), prompting the recommendation that if an opioid is to be used it should not be pethidine. The new generation of NSAIDs, cycolooxygenase-2 (COX-2) inhibitors, does not inhibit cycooxygenase-1, which is located within gastrointestinal mucosa and is responsible for prostaglandin production that maintains gastrointestinal (GI) mucosal integrity. Thus, the use of

TABLE 31.1
Medications Commonly Used to Treat Renal Colic

Class and Name of Drug	Adult Dose
NSAIDs	
Ketorolac	30–60 mg IV or IM loading dose, then 15 mg IV or IM every 6 hours
	Oral continuation dose: 10 mg PO every 4–6 hours (maximum 40 mg/day), not to exceed 5 days
Diclofenac	50 mg PO 2 or 3 times/day
Cyclooxygenase-2 Inhibitors	
Rofecoxib	50 mg PO once/day
Narcotics	
Meperidine	1 mg/kg of bodyweight IM every 3–4 hours
Morphine sulfate	0.1 mg/kg IM or IV every 4 hours
Narcotic Combinations	
Acetaminophen with codeine	300 mg acetaminophen with 30 mg codeine, 2 tablets PO every 4–6 hours

Note: IM = Intramuscular; IV = Intravenous; PO = Orally. Appended from "Clinical Practice. Acute Renal Colic From Ureteral Calculus," by J. M. Teichman, 2004, *New England Journal of Medicine, 350*(7), pp. 684–693.

COX-2 inhibitors for the treatment of renal colic may provide clinical efficacy as has been observed with other NSAIDs while providing a reduced risk of GI toxicity. Teichman (2004) has made suggestions for different medications commonly used to treat renal colic which are detailed in Table 31.1 along with their dosages.

Alternatively, a prospective randomized study performed to compare the effect of acupuncture and an intramuscular narcotic analgesic analogue for the treatment of renal colic showed that acupuncture was as effective in relieving renal colic as the narcotic and had a more rapid analgesic onset in the absence of side effects, whereas 43.8% of the patients in the narcotic group had side effects including paralytic ileus, suggesting that acupuncture can be an excellent alternative for the treatment of renal colic (Atala, Amin, Harty, Liu, & Keeling, 1992). α-Adrenergic and β-adrenergic receptors have been identified in the human ureter, where α-adrenergic receptors are quantitatively predominant (Malin, Deane, & Boyarski, 1970). The efficacy of the α1-adrenergic antagonist tamsulosin in patients with renal colic secondary to a ureterovesical stone was compared with floroglucine-trimetossibenzene (a spasmolytic agent) in a nonblinded randomized trial (Dellabella, Milanese, & Muzzonigro, 2003). Although the mean stone size in this study was statistically larger in the tamsulosin group, the stone expulsion rate was significantly greater and the mean hours to expulsion, the mean number of diclofenac (NSAID) injections, the rate

of hospitalization, and the need for endoscopic stone removal were all lower in the tamsulosin group, suggesting that tamsulosin is effective in hastening the passage of juxtavesical ureteral stones and in decreasing both the severity and duration of renal colic.

BLADDER PAIN

INTERSTITIAL CYSTITIS

Interstitial cystitis (IC) is one of the most enigmatic disease entities in the field of urology. The earliest documented description of this disorder was made in 1808 by Philip Syng Physick, who described an inflammatory condition of the bladder comparable to an ulcer that produced lower urinary tract symptoms similar to a bladder stone (Parsons, 2004). He later expanded his description to include a chronic frequency, urgency, and pain syndrome in the absence of demonstrable etiology which was called tic douloureux of the bladder (Parsons, 2004). Although the disease entity has been recognized for nearly 200 years, the etiology and pathology of the disease remain elusive. IC is characterized by urinary frequency, urgency, and pain in the absence of identifiable inciting factors such as infection, malignancy, radiation, or medication. Pain may be present in the suprapubic area, lower abdomen, lower back, medial thighs, inguinal area, urethra, vagina or vulva in women, or scrotum or testis in men (Parsons, Zupkas, & Parsons, 2001). It is important to remember that the symptoms of IC exist on a spectrum from tolerable to severe, and patients find themselves anywhere between the two ends of the spectrum with alternating exacerbations and remissions.

Recent reports have demonstrated that the prevalence of IC is much greater than was previously thought. The prevalence of IC was calculated to be 8 to 16 per 100,000 female patients in the Netherlands in a study based on a questionnaire administered to urologists (Bade, Rijcken, & Mensink, 1995). The prevalence of IC in 184,583 female participants in the patient questionnaire-based U.S. Nurses' Health Study was between 52 and 67 per 100,000 women (Curhan, Speizer, Hunter, Curhan, & Stampfer, 1999). The disparity observed between these two studies may reflect different diagnostic criteria, detection rates, and study design. While the majority of individuals diagnosed with IC are women, chronic pelvic pain syndrome (CPPS) in men, formerly classified as prostatodynia and nonbacterial prostatitis (see below), shares features similar to IC, and the diagnosis of IC should be considered in patients with CPPS (Dunn, Miller et al., 1995). Early studies report that men make up only 10% of patients with IC (Cristol, Greene, & Thompson, 1944), although contemporary studies suggest that IC in men is underdiagnosed and is commonly misdiagnosed as prostatitis (Forrest & Vo, 2001).

Diagnosis of Interstitial Cystitis

In 1987, the National Institute of Diabetes and Digestive and Kidney Diseases (NIDDK) first developed consensus criteria for the diagnosis of IC, which have subsequently undergone revision. These criteria, detailed in Table 31.2, were not intended to define IC, but rather to standardize criteria for the purpose of patient inclusion in clinical trials (Gillenwater & Wein, 1988). Glomerulations (small, punctate, red lesions) seen within the bladder mucosa at the time of cystoscopic hydrodistention under general anesthesia (technique described below) are essential for the

---

TABLE 31.2
Consensus Criteria for Diagnosis of Interstitial Cystitis from the National Institute of Arthritis, Diabetes, and Digestive and Kidney Diseases Workshop on Interstitial Cystitis

Automatic Exclusion:

Age <18 years
Benign or malignant bladder tumors
Radiation cystitis
Tuberculous cystitis
Cyclophosphamide cystitis or any other chemical cystitis
Vaginitis
Urethral diverticulum
Uterine, cervical, vaginal, or urethral carcinoma
Active genital herpes infection
Diagnosis of bacterial cystitis or prostatitis within a 3-month period
Bladder or ureteral calculi
Waking frequency <8 times per day
Absence of nocturia
Symptoms relieved by antimicrobials, urinary antiseptics,
  anticholinergics, or antispasmodics
Duration of symptoms <9 months
Bladder capacity >350 cc on cystometry
Absence of an intense urge to void with bladder filled to 150 cc of H_2O
  during cystometry, using fill rate of 30–100 cc/min
Involuntary bladder contractions demonstrated on cystometry

Automatic Inclusion:

Hunner's ulcer

Positive Factors:

Pain on bladder filling relieved by emptying
Pain (suprapubic, pelvic, urethral, vaginal, or perineal)
Glomerulations on cystoscopy
Decreased bladder compliance on cystometrogram

Note: Adapted from "Summary of the National Institute of Arthritis, Diabetes, Digestive and Kidney Diseases Workshop on Interstitial Cystitis, National Institutes of Health, Bethesda, Maryland, August 28–29," by J. Y. Gillenwater, & A. J. Wein, 1988, *Journal of Urology, 140*(1), pp. 203-206; and "Interstitial Cystitis: An Introduction to the Problem," by A. J. Wein, P. M. Hanno et al., in *Interstitial Cystitis* (pp. 13–15), edited by P. M. Hanno, D. R. Staskin, R. J. Krane, & A. J. Wein, 1990, London: Springer-Verlag.

---

diagnosis of interstitial cystitis. However, examination with cystoscopy and bladder hydrodistention of 20 asymptomatic women undergoing tubal ligation demonstrated bladder mucosal lesions that are characteristically observed in patients diagnosed with interstitial cystitis (Waxman, Sulak, & Kuehl, 1998). Conversely, not all patients with IC develop glomerulations with hydrodistention (Awad, MacDiarmid, Gajewski, & Gupta, 1992). Given these findings, the diagnosis of IC is commonly one of exclusion. In 1915, Hunner (1915) described red, bleeding areas within the bladders of patients with IC, and while these were at one time thought to be pathognomonic for IC, they are actually very rare, observed in fewer than 5% of patients (Hanno, 2002).

While the exact etiology of IC has not been determined, multiple factors are thought to play a role in the pathogenesis of disease. Changes in urothelial permeability, increased mast cell activity, neuroimmune abnormalities, neuroplasticity of the nervous system, and infectious etiologies have all been implicated (Butrick, 2003). The bladder mucosa is lined by a mucus layer containing glycosaminoglycans (GAGs). This layer forms a physical barrier that prevents small molecules from diffusing through the urothelium into the submucosal tissue containing muscle and nerves (Lilly & Parsons, 1990). Potassium is present in high concentration in urine and normally does not penetrate healthy urothelium. However, individuals with IC, who have defects in the GAG layer, may be subject to potassium diffusion through the urothelium causing depolarization of sensory nerves (C-fibers) in the bladder muscle effecting the symptoms of IC (Parsons, 2004). The intravesical Potassium Sensitivity Test (PST) was developed to detect disruption of urothelial integrity. The PST was found to be positive in 78% of patients with clinical IC and in 0% of controls, suggesting that a positive PST correlates with the presence of an abnormal bladder epithelium (Parsons et al., 2001).

To perform the PST, 40 ml of sterile water is first instilled into the bladder over 2 to 3 minutes followed 3 to 5 minutes later by patient assessment of pain and urgency using a numerical scale from 0 to 5 (0 = none; 5 = severe; Parsons, 1996). The patient voids and 100 ml of a KCl solution (400 mEq/L) is instilled into the bladder over 2 to 3 minutes followed 3 to 5 minutes later by patient assessment of pain and urgency using the numerical scale. The patient voids and the bladder is thoroughly rinsed with water. If the patient experiences severe symptoms, 10,000 to 20,000 units of heparin in 20 cc of 1% lidocaine may be instilled into the bladder until the patient needs to void. Analgesics may be necessary as well. If the patient experiences no pain with instillation of water but scores ≥2 on assessment of pain or urgency, then the test indicates aberrant epithelial permeability.

Parsons et al. (2002) designed a self-administered, eight-item pelvic pain and urgency/frequency (PUF) symptom scale that gives balanced attention to urinary urgency/frequency, pelvic pain, and symptoms associated with sexual intercourse. Answers to the eight-item questionnaire result in a score from 0 to 35; a high score is associated with a high likelihood of having IC. When validated by the PST, high PUF scores correlated with a high likelihood of a positive PST in urologic patients suspected of having IC and in gynecologic patients with pelvic pain, suggesting that the PUF is a valid tool for detecting IC (Parsons et al., 2002). The PUF is also useful in assessing symptoms that the patient is having but does not recognize as abnormal. The symptom complex of an individual with IC usually begins with frequency followed by the development of urgency and finally pain, ultimately prompting the patient to see a physician (Parsons, 2004). IC is associated with significant inter- and intraindividual variation in symptoms, resulting in common misdiagnosis of recurrent urinary tract infection and delay in the correct diagnosis for up to 4 to 7 years before being correctly diagnosed (Butrick, 2003). It is a progressive disease that can result in severe, unremitting pain with time in the absence of treatment to the extent that an end-stage bladder develops, requiring cystectomy with urinary diversion. Prompt identification of IC and timely treatment can lead to improved therapeutic success.

Pathophysiology of Interstitial Cystitis

The symptoms of IC are likely caused by persistent toxic insult on a molecular level that results in tissue injury. The bladder is the most densely innervated organ in the pelvis and has particularly rich innervation by silent afferent fibers (C-fibers) that transmit pain when activated by repeated abnormal noxious stimuli (Cervero, 1994). These fibers transmit a signal to the dorsal horn, which when persistent and repetitive causes activation of N-methyl-D-aspartate (NMDA) receptors in the spinal cord (Bennett, 1999). Subsequently, cells within the dorsal horn undergo neuroplastic changes, causing exaggerated and prolonged pain. The stimulus necessary to induce severe pain is thus significantly reduced; this augmented sensory processing is referred to as non-nociceptive pain, which is characterized by four features (Markenson, 1996):

1. The description of pain seems inappropriate in comparison with the degree of tissue pathology, or no tissue pathology is discernable.
2. Noxious stimuli result in a pain experience that is greater and more unpleasant than would normally be expected (hyperalgesia).
3. Normally non-noxious stimuli may result in pain (allodynia).
4. The extent of the pain boundary is greater than would be expected on the basis of the site of the original tissue pathology.

Neurogenic inflammation may occur as a result of activation of sensory nerves through release of neuropeptides such as substance P, neurokinin A, and calcitonin gene-related protein (Brookoff, 2000). These substances contribute to vascular permeability and mast cell degranulation with release of histamine and other mediators of inflammation causing injury and increased permeability of epithelial surfaces (Elbadawi & Light, 1996).

Increased concentrations of mast cells have been detected in patients with IC. Mast cells have been predominantly located within the detrusor muscle in these individuals and also within the lamina propria, the bladder epithelium, and bladder washings, whereas in control subjects mast cells have been found both in the lamina propria and detrusor muscle, but not in the epithelium nor in bladder washings, suggesting that the mucosal mast cell-IgE system is not only involved in the pathogenesis of IC but also that mast cells in patients with IC migrate across the epithelium (Aldenborg, Fall, & Enerback, 1986, 1989). Bladder washings from patients with ulcerative IC contained well-preserved mast cells and histamine, while only occasional mast cells and traces of histamine were found in washings from patients with non-ulcerative IC (Aldenborg et al., 1989). Mast cells secrete proinflammatory mediators in response to activation by IgE+antigen, acetylcholine, anaphylotoxins, substance P, chemicals, contrast agents, cytokines, opioids, antihistamines, exercise, hormones, viruses, and bacterial toxins (Hanno, 1994; Lagunoff, Martin, & Read, 1983).

Substances that cause mast cell secretion may be released by neurons that innervate the bladder. Investigation of the nerve population within the bladder wall using immunohistochemical stains demonstrated a significantly greater concentration of nerve fibers within the suburothelial and detrusor muscle layers in chronic IC when compared with controls and individuals with chronic bacterial cystitis and systemic lupus erythematosus cystitis, suggesting a specific association between nerve fiber proliferation and IC (Christmas, Rode, Chapple, Milroy & Turner-Warwick, 1990).

Mast cells and neurogenic inflammation may together promote defects in urothelial permeability, all of which contribute together to a cycle of persistent noxious stimulus to the bladder. Tight junctions between urothelial cells provide a barrier between the lumen of the bladder and submucosal tissue. It is suggested that GAGs line the bladder mucosa, providing a continuous physical barrier that prevents small molecules from reaching the underlying tight junctions and cell membranes and, hence, make up a major permeability barrier (Lilly & Parsons, 1990). Different types of GAGs include hyaluronic acid, heparin sulfate, heparin, chondroitin 4-sulfate and chondroitin 6-sulfate, dermatan sulfate, and keratan sulfate. Not only does the GAG layer provide a barrier to permeability but it also provides an antiadherence mechanism. The increased bacterial adsorption that occurs when the bladder is denuded of the GAG layer was prevented by the instillation of heparin (Hanno, Fritz, Wein, & Mulholland, 1978). Parsons et al. (Parsons, Housley, Schmidt, & Lebow, 1994) demonstrated in a rabbit model that the ability of the bladder GAG layer to impair movement of both charged and uncharged small molecules is inhibited by protamine sulfate (heparin antagonist). This protamine effect can be reversed by a treatment with exogenous GAG (heparin), thus demonstrating that the GAG layer plays an important role as a bladder permeability barrier in modulating ion movement (Lilly & Parsons, 1990). Patients with IC were shown to have a leaky epithelium by placing a solution of concentrated urea into the bladder and measuring absorption (Parsons, Lilly, & Stein, 1991). In this study the control subjects absorbed 4.3% in 45 minutes, while the patients with IC absorbed 25%, a difference that was highly significant. Chronic self-administered intravesical heparin was studied to determine if replacement of GAG into the bladder would control the symptoms of IC, and in more than half of patients studied, intravesical heparin controlled the symptoms of IC with continued improvement even after 1 year of therapy (Parsons, Housley, Schmidt, & Lebow, 1994).

While the theory of aberrant epithelial permeability is attractive, not all studies support this mechanism in the etiology of IC. Patients with IC do appear to have a defect in epithelial permeability, but whether this is a primary defect or a result of a separate phenomenon such as mast cell degranulation or neurogenic inflammation is unclear. Likely, the pathogenesis is based on a cycle of events that escalates and in its persistence contributes to chronicity of the disease.

Treatment of Interstitial Cystitis

Hydrodistention

One of the first therapeutic approaches described for the treatment of IC was hydrodistention of the bladder with the patient under anesthesia. In addition to providing therapeutic benefit, hydrodistention also provides information that may facilitate diagnosis as described above. The literature has detailed variable techniques for hydrodistention in terms of pressure and duration of distention. In an early study of 25 patients with IC, treatment by bladder distention was performed at a pressure that was similar to systolic blood pressure for a period of up to 3 hours (Dunn, Ramsden, Roberts, Smith, & Smith, 1977). While 16 patients were symptom-free at a mean follow-up of 14 months, bladder rupture occurred in 2 individuals. Although this study suggested that prolonged bladder distention had a role for the treatment of IC, it also demonstrated that care must be taken to avoid morbidity. Hanno (2002) recommends initial cystoscopy, bladder washings for cytology, and distention of the bladder for 1 to 2 minutes at a pressure of 80 cm H_2O, followed by emptying of the bladder and refilling to assess for the presence of glomerulations or ulceration. A therapeutic distention is then performed for 8 minutes, and if a biopsy is necessary, it is performed following therapeutic distention. In patients with bladder capacity less than 600 ml, therapeutic response was excellent in 26% and fair in 29%, while in patients with larger bladder capacities, response was excellent in 12% and fair in 43% (Hanno & Wein, 1991). Overall, responses were brief, but those patients with a therapeutic benefit lasting 6 months are excellent candidates for repeat hydrodistention. It is thought that therapeutic benefit is secondary to damage of mucosal afferent nerve endings (Dunn, Ramsden et al., 1977).

Conservative Measures

Patients with IC may experience a spectrum of symptoms with alternating exacerbations and remissions. Some may have relatively mild symptoms with nocturia twice per night and a daytime urinary frequency of 2 to 3 hours. These patients may wish to defer medical treatment and instead utilize conservative measures while possible. It is thought that reduction from the diet of acidic foods such as caffeine, alcohol, and juices that acidify the urine may diminish severity of symptoms, although this theory has not been substantiated in clinical trials. Calcium glycerophosphate is a nutraceutical that is marketed for the treatment of IC to neutralize dietary acid, although clinical evidence demonstrating therapeutic benefit of the supplement and supporting its use is lacking. Similarly, the use of potassium citrate as a urinary alkalinizing agent has not been supported by clinical trials. The Interstitial Cystitis Association (www.ichelp.org) is a nonprofit health organization dedicated exclusively to providing a full range of programs, support services, and research funding necessary to help those who suffer with IC. Organizations such as this can be invaluable to individuals with IC in terms of education, which itself can eliminate a great deal of anxiety about the disease process. Awareness regarding the disease history and different types of treatment options as well as a connection not only to other patients with IC, but also to experts in the field may provide some degree of emotional relief.

Oral Medications

Oral medications used in the treatment of IC include tricyclic antidepressants, antihistamines, and pentosan polysulfate sodium (PPS; Elmiron™; Ortho-McNiel Pharmaceuticals, Rantan, NJ).

Tricyclic antidepressants. The most common oral agent used in the treatment of IC is amitriptyline, which may regulate neurological activation. Tricyclic antidepressants have several inherent properties that may benefit patients with IC:

- Anticholinergic actions decrease urinary frequency.
- Reuptake inhibition of serotonin and norepinephrine provide both analgesia and alleviation of potential depression associated with a chronic disease.
- Sedative effects (perhaps mediated by blocking H1-histaminergic receptors) improve sleep.

A clinical trial of amitriptyline for treatment of IC demonstrated that in 28 of 43 (65%) patients who could tolerate the medication for 3 weeks at a dosage of 25 mg that was titrated up to 75 mg over 2 weeks, 18 (64%) had complete remission of symptoms with a mean follow-up of 14.4 months (Hanno, 1994). The most common side effect limiting tolerability of the medication was sedation. Imipramine, a tricyclic antidepressant with general pharmacological properties similar to those of amitriptyline may also be used for the treatment of IC. A starting dose of 25 mg/day of amitriptyline or imipramine at bedtime is recommended (Parsons, 2004). The daily dose is increased to 50 mg/day after 1 to 2 months.

Antihistamines. As described above, mast cell degranulation is thought to be an etiologic factor in IC. Hydroxyzine, a piperazine H1-receptor antagonist, has been shown to inhibit neurogenic stimulus-induced bladder mast cell activation (Minogiannis, El-Mansoury, Betances, Sant, & Theoharides, 1998). An open-label, nonconsecutive case series of patients treated by their local physicians with oral hydroxyzine found that 90 of 140 patients that returned case-report forms reported a 40% reduction in symptom scores, while this rose to 55% in patients with a history of allergies, demonstrating that hydroxyzine is a useful drug for the symptomatic treatment of IC, especially in patients with documented allergies and/or evidence of bladder mast cell activation (Theoharides & Sant, 1997). It is recommended that patients with IC with a history of allergies stay on a continuous regimen of hydroxyzine, beginning with 25 mg/day at bedtime and increasing to 50 to 100 mg/day during allergy seasons (Parsons, 2004).

Pentosan polysulfate sodium. PPS was the first oral drug to receive regulatory agency approval for use in the treatment of IC in the United States in 1996. It is a synthetic sulfated polysaccharide sodium pentosanpolysulfate, a heparin analogue. Heparin sulfate is the predominant GAG located on the bladder surface. The mechanism of action is based on oral administration of a GAG that is then excreted in the urine, with subsequent repair of the GAG layer of the bladder, thereby eliminating the symptoms of IC. To determine the efficacy of 100 mg PPS three times per day in patients with IC, a randomized, prospective, double-blind, placebo-controlled study was conducted at seven clinical centers on 148 patients (Parsons et al., 1993). Of the patients on drug therapy, 32% showed

significant improvement compared with 16% of those on placebo, and more drug patients showed a mean increase of greater than 20 ml in voided volume than did placebo patients. Long-term efficacy and safety of PPS in relieving recurring symptoms of IC were investigated in a long-term, open-label physician's usage study, which demonstrated overall improvement in symptoms in 62% of patients who received therapy for 6 to 35 months (Hanno, 1997). Most patients continued to show improvement over 1 to 2 years, demonstrating that the rate of response to PPS increases with duration of treatment. Adverse events were reported by fewer than 4% of subjects, most commonly reversible alopecia, diarrhea, nausea, headache, and rash. The recommended dosage of PPS is 100 mg given three times per day. In general a trial of PPS lasting up to 6 months is necessary to observe symptom improvement.

Intravesical Treatment

DMSO. Treatment of IC with intravesical agents has the potential benefit of rapid improvement in symptoms when compared with oral agents, as agents instilled into the bladder may locally affect the bladder mucosa directly, thereby effecting a rapid response. Dimethylsulfoxide (DMSO), a derivative of lignin, received regulatory agency approval for treatment of IC in the United States in 1978 (Abber, Lue, Luo, Juenemann, & Tanagho, 1987). DMSO has multiple pharmacological actions including anti-inflammation, analgesia, muscle relaxation, collagen dissolution, and enhancement of drug penetration (Bornman, Franz, Jacobs, & Pretorius, 1986). For treatment, 50 ml of a 50% DMSO solution is instilled into the bladder through a urethral catheter and is retained in the bladder for 15 minutes after which the patient voids to empty the bladder (Parkin, Shea, & Sant, 1997). For patients with difficulty voiding, the catheter may be kept in place and clamped for 15 minutes followed by drainage of the bladder and removal of the catheter. Typically, one instillation is performed once per week for up to 8 weeks, and maintenance therapy may then be instituted once every 2 weeks. Instillation should not be performed sooner than 2 to 3 weeks following a bladder biopsy and urine culture should be proved negative prior to treatment. A review of intravesical DMSO for treatment of IC demonstrated that with this regimen, the overall response rate is 50 to 90% in patients with non-ulcerative disease and 50 to 70% in patients with ulcerated, small-capacity bladders (Parkin et al., 1997). In addition, an overall relapse rate of 35 to 40% with a 4 to 8 week course of DMSO treatment occurred, although 50 to 60% of these patients responded to additional treatment with intravesical DMSO. The most common side effects included chemical cystitis (10%), initial worsening of symptoms (10 to 15%), and transient garlic breath (20 to 40%). Belladonna and opium suppositories, oral anticholinergics, and/or analgesics may be beneficial for patients who develop cystitis following DMSO instillation.

Heparin. Intravesically administered heparin, an exogenous GAG, has been shown to provide an epithelial permeability barrier in bladders injured with protamine, a heparin antagonist (Nickel, Downey, Morales, Emerson, & Clark, 1998). Intravesical heparin is given at a dose of 10,000 to 40,000 IU/day in 10 ml of water held within the bladder for 30 to 60 minutes for chronic therapy, or for maintenance this dose can be given three times/week (Parsons, 2004). To determine the effectiveness of intravesical heparin in treatment of IC, 48 patients underwent intravesical heparin therapy (10,000 units in 10 ml sterile water, three times per week for 3 months), and at 3 months 27 of 48 patients (56%) attained good clinical remissions (Parsons et al., 1994). In this study, the majority of responders that continued with treatment for up to 1 year observed continued improvement.

Pentosan polysulfate sodium. PPS, a semisynthetic GAG, may be dissolved and administered intravesically. To evaluate the therapeutic efficacy of intravesical PPS, a small, double-blind, placebo-controlled study was performed in which 10 patients received intravesical PPS (300 mg in 50 ml of 0.9% sodium chloride) instilled twice per week for 3 months and 10 patients received placebo (Bade, Laseur, Nieuwenburg, van der Weele, & Mensink, 1997). Four patients in the PPS group gained significant symptomatic relief compared with only two receiving placebo, while at 18 months from the start of the study, symptoms were relieved in eight patients still receiving PPS instillations and in four without treatment, suggesting that intravesical PPS provides some benefit in the treatment of IC.

Hyaluronic acid. Hyaluronic acid is a GAG marketed as Cystistat™ (Bioniche Live Sciences, Belleville, Ontario, Canada) in Canada and in Europe that is used intravesically as well. For treatment, 40 mg of hyaluronic acid dissolved in 40 ml of normal saline is instilled weekly for 4 to 8 weeks and monthly thereafter. A 3-year follow-up study of an initial open, nonrandomized trial of Cystistat demonstrated that 58% of patients observed significant long-term improvement in pain and urinary frequency, while approximately 20% of patients recovered to the extent that further treatment was unnecessary (Nordling, Jorgensen, & Kallestrup, 2001). Placebo-controlled, double-blinded investigation of hyaluronic acid for the treatment of IC is in progress.

Lidocaine hydrochloride. Lidocaine is a local anesthetic that belongs to the amide group and is associated with rapid onset of pharmacologic activity. Lidocaine has an anti-inflammatory effect including blockage of mast cell degranulation and inhibition of histamine release, which may contribute to improvement in symptoms of the patient with IC. Because intravesical lidocaine alone is not sufficiently absorbed by human bladders to achieve significant serum levels, it must be administered with sodium bicarbonate to promote absorption (Henry et al., 2001). Henry et al. demonstrated a significant decrease in acute pain scores in a group of patients with IC treated with 5 mg/kg of 5% lidocaine mixed with 8.4% sodium bicarbonate daily for 3 days, indicating that a concentration of local anesthetic within the bladder wall was achieved that was sufficient to block the sensory neurons within the submucosal plexus. For patients with severe IC, Parsons (2004) recommends supplementation of oral pentosan polysulfate with intravesical heparin and lidocaine instillations performed once or twice per day (heparin 40,000 IU in 10 cc 1% lidocaine, or 16 cc 2% lidocaine if 1% is ineffective, and 3 ml of 8.4% sodium bicarbonate). Bupivacaine, an amide group local anesthetic with a longer half-life than lidocaine may have a role in intravesical treatment of IC as well.

Neurotoxins. Capsaicin is a pungent crystalline alkaloid found in chili peppers that acts as a neurotoxin by desensitization of C-fiber afferent neurons. A pilot study of intravesical capsaicin therapy performed on five female patients diagnosed with IC was performed to study the safety and efficacy of this agent (Fagerli et al., 1999). Topical anesthesia (30 ml of 0.5% bupivacaine) was instilled intravesically for 30 minutes prior to each weekly treatment with capsaicin in increasing concentrations of 10, 50, 100, and 250 μM solutions in 1% ethanol given as tolerated by the patient. Four of the five patients experienced subjective improvement in both symptom and pain score with no complications, suggesting that intravesical capsaicin is a safe and promising treatment for IC, potentially functioning through desensitization of bladder C-fiber afferents, which presumably initiate painful sensations in patients with IC. Resiniferatoxin, an ultrapotent analogue of capsaicin, was evaluated for the treatment of IC in a pilot study in which five female patients received a prolonged infusion of a saline solution containing 10 nM of resiniferatoxin at a flow rate of 25 μl/hour through an infusion pump connected to a 5 Fr suprapubic catheter for 10 days (Lazzeri et al., 2004). Patients were evaluated 30 days and >3 months from the end of infusion and showed a significant decrease in frequency, nocturia, and pain score without side effects, demonstrating that the prolonged intravesical instillation of resiniferatoxin by an *in situ* drug delivery system shows promise in the treatment of patients with IC. Clearly, additional investigation is necessary to determine the benefit of neurotoxins in this patient population.

Multimodal Treatment

As no single agent is curative for all patients with IC, a multimodal approach may be necessary. Therapy is directed at the different etiologic mechanisms that have been proposed in IC. Parsons (2004) has made several recommendations for multimodal therapy. Function of the lower urinary tract epithelium may be improved with administration of pentosan polysulfate in a dose of 100 mg given three times per day, or in very difficult to treat patients, the dose may be doubled, although a dose greater than 300 mg per day represents an off-label use of the drug. Intravesical heparin may also help to restore urothelial function, given as frequently as once or twice daily instilled into the empty bladder at a dose of 40,000 IU in 10 cc 1% lidocaine with 3 ml of 8.4% sodium bicarbonate held within the bladder for 30 minutes. If the 1% formulation of lidocaine is ineffective, then 16 cc of 2% lidocaine can be substituted. Alternatively, heparin can be replaced by pentosan polysulfate in this formulation. The PPS capsules can be opened and the contents (100 to 200 mg) dissolved in 10 cc buffered normal saline (Parsons, 2004). Parsons and Davis (2003) report that 85% of patients who used the above intravesical solution three to seven times per week for 2 weeks or longer observed sustained pain relief. Parsons (2004) notes that patients with severe IC may realize improvement with these measures only after long-term treatment (up to 2 years) and therefore treatment with these GAGs should not be discontinued prior to this time period.

To diminish or, ideally, to reverse neural activation, amitriptyline may be added to the treatment regimen at a dosage of 25 mg per day at bedtime. This dosage can be increased to 50 mg after a period of 1 to 2 months as tolerated.

Control of the proposed allergic component of IC can be attempted with administration of hydroxyzine at a starting dose of 25 mg per day at bedtime, increased to 50 to 100 mg as needed and as tolerated. A broad approach to the multiple pathological mechanisms thought to be causative in the development of IC may best benefit the patient when a solitary treatment approach fails.

Nerve Stimulation

Up to 10% of patients with IC are unresponsive to oral or intravesical therapy (Webster & Galloway, 1987), and may benefit from neuromodulation with percutaneous sacral nerve stimulation (PNS). While previously surgical intervention has been considered for patients with refractory IC, PNS may offer a line of therapy prior to implementation of radical surgery. This technique employs electrical nerve stimulation to the third sacral nerve root with a wire electrode that is inserted into the foramen and is connected to an external pulse generator on a temporary basis to assess efficacy, followed by implantation of a permanent device if the trial is successful. The efficacy of PNS in treatment of patients with IC refractory to oral and intravesical treatments who would otherwise have been candidates for surgical intervention was assessed in a multicenter study that included 30 patients wherein statistically significant improvements were seen in frequency, pain, average voided volume (from baseline of 92 ± 73 ml to test average 134 ± 106 ml), maximum voided volume, and in symptom scores, suggesting that PNS is effective in reducing symptom severity and increasing voided volumes in patients with IC previously unresponsive to standard

therapy (Whitmore, Payne, Diokno, & Lukban, 2003). Implementation of sacral neuromodulation for treatment of severe IC provides a reversible option that holds significant promise in this patient population for which the only remaining alternative may be major surgery.

Surgical Therapy

The last resort for end-stage IC remains surgical therapy, although success rates with this approach are variable. While radical surgery is an option, it must be decided on only after prolonged consideration especially because IC is a nonmalignant process with the possibility of temporary remission and does not cause mortality (Hanno, 2002). Transurethral resection of Hunner's ulcers, which are observed in the minority of patients with IC, has been attempted. Complete transurethral resection of visible lesions in 30 patients resulted in initial disappearance of pain in all and a decrease in urinary frequency in 21; 10 patients experienced a relapse in pain at a mean of 10.2 months postoperatively (Fall, 1985).

Laser ablation of Hunner's ulcers may be performed as well. A prospective series of 24 patients who underwent ablative therapy of Hunner's ulcers using a neodymium (Nd):YAG laser showed that all patients had a significant decrease in pain scores, mean urgency score, and nocturia, and a significant increase in mean voiding interval was observed over a mean follow-up of 23 months, though relapse in 11 patients required one to four additional treatments (Rofeim, Hom, Freid, & Moldwin, 2001). This study demonstrated that Nd:YAG laser ablation of Hunner's ulcers represents a minimally invasive method of treating IC that offers patients an opportunity to achieve symptomatic improvement for an extended period and may be repeated as necessary. However, this procedure must be approached with caution, as laser scatter through the thin bladder wall may result in bowel injury.

Supratrigonal cystectomy, in which the majority of the diseased bladder is removed and the remaining bladder is augmented with a large patch of bowel, has been attempted for treatment of IC, and multiple studies investigating the success of this technique are reported in the literature with disparate success rates. Of 13 patients with refractory IC who underwent supratrigonal cystectomy and ileocystoplasty (augmentation of the bladder with ileum), all 10 patients with ulcerative IC experienced relief of symptoms, while 3 patients with non-ulcerative IC had persistent pain (Peeker, Aldenborg, & Fall, 1998). In these latter patients, trigonal resection and urinary diversion with a Koch pouch was performed with resolution of symptoms, suggesting that supratrigonal cystectomy with ileocystoplasty is unsuitable for non-ulcerative disease. Conversely, of 23 patients with IC refractory to conservative therapy treated with subtotal cystectomy and orthotopic bladder substitution with an ileocecal pouch, 20 patients were completely symptom-free at a mean follow-up of 31.5 months, demonstrating that this technique offers significant benefit to the patient with refractory IC (Linn et al., 1998). Review of a series of 100 intestinocystoplasties revealed that 57 had postoperative complications, and of those, 27 patients required either early or late surgical intervention, while 30 were managed non-operatively (Khoury, Timmons, Corbel, & Webster, 1992). The high complication rate of partial cystectomy with bladder reconstruction using bowel must be weighed against the potential benefit.

Alternatively, urinary diversion with or without cystourethrectomy may be performed. If urine is diverted with an ileal loop conduit and the bladder remains *in situ*, complications such as pyocystis, hemorrhage, and pain or spasm may occur potentially requiring eventual cystectomy, and for this reason, cystectomy is recommended at the time of urinary diversion (Adeyoju et al., 1996). In conjunction with cystectomy, continent diversion of the urine (with a catheterizable, continent reservoir created with bowel) or total bladder replacement with creation of a neobladder has been described in the literature for treatment of refractory IC, as well with disparate results. Although the surgical procedure may be technically successful, 40 to 50% of patients can develop "pouch" pain (pain within the urinary diversion) or phantom pain within the pelvis, despite removal of the bladder (Broderick, Gordon, Hypolite, & Levin, 1994; Parsons, 2000). While surgical intervention for the patient with IC for whom all other treatment options have failed may be successful in relieving the patient of debilitating symptoms, surgical complications are not uncommon and no guarantee can be issued that an individual's symptoms will be cured. Surgical intervention for IC must therefore be approached with reservation.

BLADDER CANCER

A study performed by the American Cancer Society estimated that in the year 2000, 53,200 new cases of bladder cancer would be diagnosed in the United States and that, of those, 72% would be detected in men (Greenlee, Murray, Bolden, & Wingo, 2000). For perspective, according to the U.S. Census Bureau, the population of the United States on April 1, 2000, was 281,421,906. In men, bladder cancer is the fourth most commonly diagnosed cancer after prostate, lung, and colorectal carcinomas, representing 6.2% of all newly diagnosed cancers, while in women, bladder cancer is the eighth most commonly diagnosed cancer after breast, lung, colorectal, uterine, ovarian, non-Hodgkins lymphoma, and melanoma, representing 2.5% of newly diagnosed cancers (Greenlee et al., 2000).

While bladder cancer can occur at any age, it is usually detected in middle age or later; the median age at diagnosis for women is 71 years and for men 69 years of age (Lynch & Cohen, 1995). The most common symptom with which

a patient with bladder cancer presents is painless hematuria (macroscopic or microscopic blood in the urine), which occurs in up to 80% of patients with bladder cancer (Schoenberg, 2002). The second most common symptom is one or more of a complex of irritative voiding symptoms including dysuria (pain with urination), frequency, and urgency (Schoenberg, 2002). This type of presentation may be observed with carcinoma *in situ* or invasive bladder cancer. It is unusual for patients with bladder cancer who present with this symptom complex not to have hematuria, although if irritative voiding symptoms are present in the absence of hematuria and in the absence of infection, full evaluation for bladder cancer must be performed. The urinary tract is typically assessed with renal ultrasound to evaluate the renal parenchyma and with intravenous pyelogram and cystoscopy or retrograde pyelogram and cystoscopy to assess the entirety of the urothelium from collecting system within the kidney to the bladder.

Superficial bladder cancer is treated with transurethral resection of the tumor and possible intravesical chemotherapy, while muscle invasive bladder cancer is treated with cystectomy. Although the majority of bladder cancers are painless, large tumors infiltrating the pelvic viscera such as the prostatic stroma, rectum, uterus, or vagina (Stage T4a) or the pelvic sidewalls or abdominal wall (Stage T4b) may cause severe pelvic pain. While rarely curative, locally invasive tumors can be treated with radiation or chemotherapy for palliation, although if refractory to these measures, cystectomy and/or tumor debulking may remain the only alternative for pain relief. Bladder tumors may also have a mass effect on the ureter or extend directly into the ureter resulting in ureteral obstruction. If ureteral obstruction occurs gradually, the patient may not experience renal colic and with chronic obstruction a painless loss of renal function can occur.

PROSTATITIS AND PELVIC PAIN SYNDROMES

EPIDEMIOLOGY AND PATHOPHYSIOLOGY

Adult men of all ages may be affected by prostatitis, a condition that results in more physician visits in the United States than benign prostatic hypertrophy (BPH) or prostate cancer. (Lobel & Rodriguez, 2003; Roberts, Lieber, Bostwick, & Jacobsen, 1997). A national survey of physician visits in the 1990s revealed that more than 2 million office visits per year were attributed to the diagnosis of prostatitis (Collins, O'Leary, & Barry, 1998). In a letter addressed to the editor of the *Journal of Urology* in 1978, Drach, Fair, Meares et al. outlined a scientific and systematic approach to the management of patients with symptoms of prostatitis. In 1995, a National Institute of Diabetes, Digestive, and Kidney Diseases (NIDDK) workshop on prostatitis classified the prostatitis syndromes: (I) acute bacterial prostatitis, (II) chronic bacterial prostatitis, (III) chronic prostatitis/chronic pelvic pain syndrome (CPPS), and (IV) asymptomatic inflammatory prostatitis (Schaeffer et al., 2002). More recently, Krieger et al. (Krieger, Nyberg, & Nickel, 1999) outlined new recommendations for patient evaluation and classification based on the U.S. National Institutes of Health consensus recommendations. The authors recommended patient classification and evaluation based on the segmented urinary specimens (including the seminal fluid) and evaluation of symptoms. The new recommendations expanded the concept of nonbacterial prostatitis by including the seminal fluid in the evaluation and permitted inclusion of seminal inflammation or other urogenital organ abnormalities as potential factors in the etiology of the patients' symptoms (Krieger et al., 1999). In a study of the demographic and clinical characteristics of the chronic prostatitis cohort, Schaeffer et al. (2002) reported that the majority of patients with chronic prostatitis are white, affluent, and well educated. The same investigators noted that lower socioeconomic status, younger age, and lower education were correlated to more chronic pelvic pain symptoms. Furthermore, it is unknown whether decreased income and disability are *caused* by CPPS or whether those who have disability and lower incomes are more prone to developing CPPS (Schaeffer et al., 2002).

The exact pathophysiology of prostatitis has not been clearly elucidated. The presence in prostatic calculi of constituents found only in urine and not in prostatic secretions led Kirby to suggest that inflammatory prostatitis may arise secondary to intraprostatic ductal reflux (Kirby, Lowe, Bultitude et al., 1982). Nickel has nicely summarized the hypotheses based on the concept of intraprostatic ductal urine reflux as follows: Intraductal reflux of urine causes an immunologically mediated inflammatory response in the prostate. Presence of pathogenic bacteria in various segments of the urethra will send the bacteria and the refluxing urine into the prostate, an event that is followed by a quick antibody response resulting in acute bacterial prostatitis *if* the bacterial antigens have not been previously introduced into the prostate (Nickel, 1995). This scenario typically yields to proper antimicrobial therapy and resolution of the acute febrile illness. In a different scenario, recognition of the pathogen by the prostate will result in a slower and milder inflammatory process (chronic bacterial prostatitis). Recurrence of infection occurs because the bacterial microfilm adherent to the ductal epithelium protects these bacteria from host defenses and antibiotics. Given the presence of intraductal reflux, even complete elimination of the bacteria leaves the system open to reinfection with different bacterial strains in the future (Nickel, 1995).

Acute Bacterial Prostatitis

From a purely clinical standpoint, it is important to consider that only a minority of the patients seen in clini-

cians' offices with complaints of pelvic pain have demonstrable "bacterial prostatitis" in the acute or chronic form. Acute bacterial prostatitis is a sudden-onset, febrile illness that results from acute infection of the prostate by aerobic Gram-negative rods, predominantly *Escherichia coli* and *Pseudomonas* spp., that are also commonly encountered in urinary tract infections (UTIs). The latter species, as well as other resistant organisms such as *Enterococcus faecalis* and *Staphylococcus aureus*, are typical causative organisms in bacterial prostatitis that is caused in hospitalized patients whereas nonhospitalized prostatitis is typically caused by coliforms (Meares, 1991). The role of other than enterococci has been questioned in prostatitis. Most Gram-positive organisms (with the exception of enterococcus and possibly *S. aureus*) cannot be reproducibly localized to the prostate in men with prostatitis and do not cause recurrent UTI in untreated patients (Meares, 1991).

Chronic Bacterial Prostatitis

The clinical hallmark of this condition is recurrent UTIs caused by identical bacterial strains due to persistence of the pathogen within the prostate. The recurrence of infections with the same pathogen has been attributed to poor penetrability of most antimicrobials into the prostate and hence reemergence of the unaltered pathogen after cessation of antibiotic therapy. Improved prostate penetration of newer-generation antibiotics such as the fluoroquinolones may result in a gradual decline in the prevalence of chronic bacterial prostatitis in the future. Prostate stones are commonly found in adult men and may be infected. It has been suggested that unrecognized infected prostate stones may account for some cases of persistent chronic bacterial prostatitis despite prolonged antimicrobial therapy (Meares, 1991).

Chronic Prostatitis/Chronic Pelvic Pain Syndrome (Category III)

This syndrome is a broad group that composes the largest segment of symptomatic patients and may be inflammatory (subcategory A) or non-inflammatory (subcategory B). Men in a variety of demographic subgroups may be affected and the disorder has a serious negative impact on the quality of life. Chronic prostatitis/CPPS has a poorly understood etiology that is refractory to most medical therapies and is further characterized by low correspondence of symptoms and objective findings, and association with psychosocial dysfunction, shared features among many chronic pain syndromes (Turner et al., 2002). The primary objective feature of this condition is genitourinary pain of at least 3 months duration in the absence of documented uropathogenic bacteria using standard microbiological procedures. The inflammatory subcategory of this condition is distinguished by the presence of leukocytes in the expressed prostatic secretions (EPS), semen, or prostatic massage urine whereas no bacteria are detected in the non-inflammatory subcategory (Lobel & Rodriguez, 2003). Some investigators are skeptical of the accuracy or clinical significance of this newer National Institutes of Health (NIH) classification and cite lack of a cutoff point for the degree of leukocytosis and the possible pooling in the current system of patients with an autoimmune mechanism responsible for chronic pelvic pain as some of the potential pitfalls of this newest classification (Maake & John, 2003).

The role of cytokines, immunological causes, prostate tissue pressure, and bladder neck morphologic or functional alterations are among the more recent areas of focus. It has been suggested that alterations of the bladder neck may be observed in patients with CPPS. A recent study by Hruz et al. (Hruz, Danuser, Studer, & Hochreiter, 2003) from Germany found that among 48 patients who fulfilled the criteria for NIH classification of non-inflammatory chronic pelvic pain syndrome (III-B), 60% had bladder neck hypertrophy documented in endoscopic studies. The same authors speculated that in those patients with this diagnosis in whom bladder neck hypertrophy may not be visually documented, a functional obstruction in the form of detrusor/internal sphincter dyssynergy may be responsible for the symptoms. An active inflammatory process in the genital tract has been inferred from a number of publications that have shown elevated levels of cytokines — interferon-gamma (IFNγ), interleukin-2 (IL-2), IL-10, tumor necrosis factor-alpha (TNF-α), IL-6, IL-8 — in the seminal plasma or prostatic secretions of men with CPPS (Miller, Fischer, Goralnick et al., 2002; Orhan, Onur, Ilhan, & Ardicoglu, 2001). An adaptive immune response directed against a genital tract antigen(s) (autoimmunity) has been proposed as a possible mediator of this inflammatory reaction. (Batstone, Doble, & Batstone, 2003) Another mediator of an autoimmune process may be a bacterial inflammatory event. This view is supported by demonstration of increased levels of bacterial 16S ribosomal DNA in the prostates of men with chronic prostatitis compared with controls (Krieger & Riley, 2002). The role of increased intraprostatic pressure in the pathophysiology of CPPS has been evaluated by Mehik et al. (Mehik, Alas, Nickel, Sarpola, & Helstrom, 2003) who demonstrated statistically significant elevations of intraprostatic pressure in patients with both the inflammatory and non-inflammatory subtypes of CPPS. The association of rheumatological conditions with CPPS in as many as 21% of patients with prostatitis is suggestive of an immunological process, and the presence of rheumatological disorders in patients with prostatitis is associated with worse quality-of-life scores (but not with more severe symptoms) in questionnaires (Schaeffer et al., 2002). Another support for an autoimmune cause for CPPS comes from Batstone et al. (Batstone, Doble, & Gaston, 2002), who show that the patient's peripheral T cells proliferate to the seminal plasma and propose a T-cell-mediated response to a seminal plasma antigen as the root cause of CPPS.

Asymptomatic Inflammatory Prostatitis

This category is characterized by lack of subjective symptoms in patients in whom white blood cells are found in prostatic tissue or in prostate secretions during evaluation or treatment of other disorders (Schaeffer et al., 2002).

Parsons (2003) has suggested that prostatitis, IC, chronic pelvic pain, and urethral syndrome share a common pathophysiology in lower urinary dysfunctional epithelium and potassium recycling. His group has devised the PST to test for bladder epithelial dysfunction and to test for the hypothesis that potassium cycling is responsible for generating symptoms. He reports that the rate of positive PSTs in men with category IIIA-IIIB CPPS is 84%, similar to the rate found in patients with IC and female patients with pelvic pain (Parsons, 2003).

DIAGNOSIS OF PROSTATITIS

Acute bacterial prostatitis (category I) presents with an acute bacterial urinary tract infection that may manifest with a variety of localized or systemic symptoms. The typical patient will give a history of sudden chills, fever, and low back and/or perineal pain as well as possible irritative or obstructive voiding dysfunction (Meares, 1991). Other reported symptoms include evolving arthralgias, myalgias, and general weakness. In this condition, the prostate is typically swollen, warm, and tender to palpation on digital rectal examination. Evaluation of the prostatic secretions reveals heavy growth of the bacterial pathogen. Numerous white blood cells (WBCs) as well as macrophages that are packed with fat droplets may be demonstrated on microscopic evaluation. Prostate massage is not recommended during the acute phase of the infection because the examination is universally uncomfortable and the responsible uropathogen is readily cultured from the voided urine without the need for prostate massage (Meares, 1991).

Most patients with *chronic bacterial prostatitis (category II)* will complain of nonspecific perineal or lower abdominal pain without systemic signs and symptoms. Prostate examination findings are variable and range from completely normal to indurated or boggy. Diagnosis depends on a culture of a standard uropathogen in the postprostatic massage-voided bladder specimen or in the expressed prostatic secretions that is at least 1 log greater in colony-forming units than the preprostate massage urine specimens as per the Stamey–Meares localization procedure guidelines (Batstone et al., 2003; Meares & Stamey, 1968).

Chronic pelvic pain syndrome/chronic nonbacterial prostatitis: The diagnosis of CPPS relies heavily on the patient's history. Patients frequently complain of prostatic tenderness and pain between the rectum and testes, highlighting the likely role of the prostate in CPPS pathophysiology; however, various socioeconomic influences in the prevalence of this disorder in different groups as well as family histories and IC-like overactive bladder symptoms in a number of these patients suggests the possibility of other organ system (e.g., bladder) involvement (Schaeffer et al., 2002). Because a "gold standard" diagnostic test for chronic prostatitis/CPPS does not exist, CPPS is in some ways a diagnosis of exclusion and all other pathology must be excluded first (Batstone et al., 2003. Perineal and suprapubic pain are the major complaints of patients with chronic prostatitis/CPPS, and it is the presence of pain, particularly post-ejaculatory pain, that differentiates lower urinary tract symptoms (LUTS)/BPH from prostatitis (Nickel, 2003). For accurate follow-up and establishing a reproducible measure of the patient's progress, it is recommended that the Chronic Prostatitis Symptom Index, developed in 1999, be used (Potts, 2003). Potts (2003) and others have suggested that because of the overlapping nature of symptoms in CPPS and many other illnesses, it is critical to complete a thorough review of systems and include potential psychological factors among the possible etiologies for this disorder. Similarly, formal psychological/psychiatric counseling and stress reduction measures should be among the armamentarium of interventions considered in this group. A study of 357 men with CPPS revealed that only 36% were presenting with their first episode of pelvic pain and highlighted the persistent and recurrent nature of this disease as well as the possible beneficial role of cognitive-behavioral and self-management interventions as long-term strategies for symptom control (Turner et al., 2002). Objective differentiation of categories IIIA (inflammatory) and IIIB (non-inflammatory) is made by finding inflammatory cells in the semen, voided bladder specimen (postprostate massage), or the EPS (Batstone et al., 2003. A group of patients with CPPS may have tenderness of the pelvic floor muscles, which may be secondary to inflammation, prostatic infection, or muscle spasm; these patients may benefit from pelvic muscle physiotherapy (Schaeffer et al., 2002).

TREATMENT OF PROSTATITIS

Acute Bacterial Prostatitis

As in most infectious processes, the mainstay of therapy in acute bacterial prostatitis is the administration of antimicrobials. This is a serious bacterial infection that may be potentially fatal and requires immediate attention and antibiotic therapy. Hospitalization for general supportive measures including bed rest, intravenous fluid adminis-

tration, antipyretics, and pain management may be required for the very ill and those who cannot tolerate oral fluids/medications. The severe inflammatory nature of this disease allows excellent accumulation of antibiotics at therapeutic levels in the prostatic secretory system, stroma, and interstitium with usually prompt clinical response (Meares, 1991). Outpatient management may be started with fluoroquinolones (pending final culture and sensitivity results) for those who can tolerate fluids and are not critically ill. The clinician should be aware of the possibility of prostatic abscess formation in cases refractory to antibiotic therapy. Transperineal or transurethral drainage of the abscess may be employed after sonographic or CT scan documentation, but transurethral instrumentation is not recommended during the acute, febrile phase of the disease (Gurunadha Rao Tunuguntla, & Evans, 2002). For the systemically ill patient, hospitalization and initial treatment with intravenous ampicillin and an aminoglycoside, quinolone, or third-generation cephalosporin may be employed and later followed with an appropriate oral agent for a minimum of 4 weeks once the culture and sensitivity results are obtained (Nickel, 1995). Alpha blocker therapy may decrease the chance of urinary retention, and the patient may benefit from alpha blocker combination with a NSAID to subside the inflammatory process in the prostate/bladder neck area. In case of urinary retention, a punch suprapubic cystostomy is recommended to avoid possible epididymitis or prolongation of the infection as a result of urethral catheterization (Gurunadha Rao Tunuguntla & Evans, 2002).

Chronic Bacterial Prostatitis

An extended period of antibiotic therapy forms the backbone of treatment for chronic bacterial prostatitis. Chronic prostatitis due to coliforms is more responsive to therapy than *Pseudomonas aeruginosa* or enterococcal CBP (Lobel & Rodriguez, 2003). In general, antibiotics with lipid solubility and a high pKa such as quinolones, sulfas, macrolides, tetracyclines, and aminoglycosides have the best prostate permeability. However, bacteriologic "cure" may not translate into symptom relief in chronic bacterial prostatitis and, in one study of antibiotics in chronic prostatitis, Nickel et al. (Nickel, Downey, Johnston et al., 2001) demonstrated the least symptom benefit among those patients who had positive cultures (Shoskes, 2003). Furthermore, the particular anatomic and morphological processes affecting the prostate in chronic bacterial prostatitis (i.e., microabscess formation, stasis and obstruction in prostatic ducts and ascini, prostatic calculi, and biofilm-enclosed bacterial colonies) prevent optimal efficacy of even those antibiotics such as fluoroquinolones and trimethoprim-sulfamethoxazole (TMP-SMX) that have been demonstrated to have superior prostate permeability (Nickel, 1995). Consequently, a characteristic of chronic bacterial prostatitis is frequent relapses with the same organism and low-dose. Chronic suppressive antibiotic therapy with nitrofurantoin or TMP-SMX to control the symptoms and prevent bacteriuria is indicated, although even prolonged therapy often does not eradicate the bacteria and symptoms will recur after cessation of therapy (Meares, 1991). Despite a paucity of data pertaining to long-term recurrence and symptom eradication rates, the results of therapy with quinolones appear to be superior to TMP-SMX (Lobel & Rodriguez, 2003). A trial of alpha-blockers or repetitive prostatic massage may be appropriate in patients who fail to respond to antibiotics alone (Barbalias, Nikiforidis, & Liatsikos, 1998; Nickel, Alexander, Anderson et al., 1999; Shoskes, 2003). For those experiencing reflux of a new pathogen into the prostate after eradication of the original bacteria, low-dose prophylactic antibiotic therapy is recommended (Nickel, 1995). Meares (1986) reported success in curing refractory chronic bacterial prostatitis by means of antibiotic therapy combined with "radical" transurethral prostatectomy, but this approach is a "last ditch" effort that is not widely used.

Chronic Pelvic Pain Syndrome/Chronic Nonbacterial Prostatitis

A wide variety of treatment regimens have been proposed for this most common and controversial category of prostatitis. General supportive measures offered by most clinicians caring for the CPPS patients include sitz baths, avoidance of spicy foods, and increased or decreased sexual activity/ejaculation as the last has been shown to alleviate *or* exacerbate symptoms in various groups of patients (Shoskes, 2003; Yavaskaoglu, Oktay, Simsek, & Ozyurt, 1999). Anti-inflammatory medications are also commonly prescribed as more publications have pointed to an autoimmune and inflammatory etiology of CPPS (Batstone et al., 2003; Maake & John, 2003; Orhan et al., 2001).

Therapy directed at relief of pain and spasm of the pelvic floor muscles has been reported through the use of biofeedback and bladder retraining as well as amitriptyline and gabapentin alone or in combination (Shoskes, 2003; Ye et al., 2003).

Despite lack of strong scientific evidence and the fact that complete bacterial localization studies are rarely performed, most clinicians will treat chronic prostatitis/CPPS with an initial trial of antibiotics and use the rationale that cultures may be inconclusive due to "difficult-to-culture bacteria" such as chlamydia, ureaplasma, and mycoplasma and that empiric therapy is easier than performing extensive and inconclusive cultures (Shoskes, 2003). Furthermore, Nickel et al. (2001) have shown that up to 57% of patients with chronic prostatitis/CPPS will respond to empiric antibiotic therapy and that the response to antibiotics is independent of culture results, white blood cell count, or antibacterial antibody status.

In 1981, Osborn et al. (Osborn, George & Rao, 1981) demonstrated the beneficial effects of the nonselective alpha blocker, phenoxybenzamine, in the treatment of the symptoms of prostatodynia. Since then, a number of publications have addressed the possible benefits of different alpha blockers in the management of prostatitis and concomitant relief of voiding symptoms. Mehik et al. (2003) reported on the use of alfuzosin in prostatitis and found that 6 months of alfuzosin therapy for chronic prostatitis/CPPS is safe and well tolerated. Compared with placebo and standard/traditional treatments listed above, the NIH-Chronic Prostatitis Symptom Index (CPSI) showed a modest improvement, particularly in the pain domain, after alfuzosin therapy. The authors further reported that the beneficial effect is not seen until after several months of treatment and disappears when treatment is discontinued. In a nonrandomized study, resolution of symptoms was seen in 76% of patients with prostatodynia after 1 month of alpha-blocker therapy with terazosin and 58% remained asymptomatic 3 months later (Neal & Moon, 1994). Overall, there are four small, placebo-controlled trials addressing the use of alpha blockers in chronic prostatitis/CPPS and this therapy has become increasingly popular among urologists, but there is no consensus regarding the mechanism of action of the alpha blockers' beneficial effects in prostatitis (Nickel, 2003).

The role of prostate massage alone or in combination with antibiotics and other remedies has received renewed attention in a number of publications. Patients who are most likely to benefit are those who have symptom relief with the first massage and have large volume EPS (Nickel et al., 1999; Shoskes, 2003).

Possible anti-inflammatory or 5-alpha reductase inhibitory properties have led to the use of the pollen extract, Cernilton, for treatment of chronic prostatitis/CPPS. An open trial with Cernilton in a group of patients with chronic prostatitis and prostatodynia demonstrated either complete and lasting relief of symptoms or a marked improvement in 13 of 15 patients (Buck, Rees, & Ebeling, 1989). Similarly, Rugendorff et al. (Rugendorff, Weidner, Eberling, & Buck, 1993) reported the results of a prospective study with Cernilton N in 90 patients and found a 78% response rate (36% cure; 42% significant improvement) in those without complicating factors (i.e., urethral strictures, prostatic calculi, bladder neck sclerosis). The same authors reported an overall excellent tolerability (97%) as well as a very poor response in those with the above-mentioned complicating factors. However, rigorous evaluation of these compounds is lacking and they are not widely recommended as standard therapy for chronic prostatitis/CPPS.

A number of investigators have published their findings pertaining to the use of transurethral microwave thermotherapy (TUMT) and prostatic temperature elevation for the treatment of chronic prostatitis/CPPS (Choi, Soh, Yoon & Song, 1994; Gurunadha Rao Tunuguntla & Evans, 2002; Montorsi et al., 1993; Nickel & Sorensen, 1994. Nickel (Nickel & Sorensen, 1996) has demonstrated the beneficial effect of TUMT with lasting results (up to 21 months) compared with sham therapy in a randomized, double blind study using validated questionnaires. Although this mode of therapy, now increasingly popular for treatment of LUTS due to BPH, appears to be potentially effective and safe, its real efficacy and durability of the response have yet to be confirmed with further randomized double-blind, sham-controlled trials before it is routinely adopted.

Based on his ideas pertaining to lower urinary tract dysfunctional epithelium (LUDE), Parsons (2003) advocates the addition of therapies such as hydroxyzine (Atarax™) aimed at suppressing mast cell activity and histamine release, as well as heparinoid therapy with intravesical heparin, intravesical PPS, or oral PPS (Elmiron) to the usual regimen of therapies for prostatitis. The positive effect of Elmiron may also be related to its anti-inflammatory properties (Shoskes, 2003). It should be mentioned that while this approach to therapy is more widely accepted in the treatment of IC, most urologists have not adopted this strategy in the management of prostatitis syndromes.

Among the newer experimental developments, the use of a high-frequency electrostimulation device that can be self-administered is noteworthy. John et al. (2003) reported on a prospective study of urethro-anal high-frequency electrostimulation in 88 patients with non-inflammatory chronic pelvic pain syndrome (Cat IIIB CPPS) and found excellent tolerability, no urethral or anal complications, and improvement of the pain syndrome in 83%.

Finally, Chen and Nickel (2003) reported on the use of acupuncture in 12 men diagnosed with chronic prostatitis/CPPS pain syndrome (NIH criteria) who were refractory to standard therapy (antibiotics, alpha-blockers, anti-inflammatories, phytotherapy) with an average follow-up of 33 weeks. The authors reported that 83% had a sustained greater than 50% decrease in NIH-CPSI at final visit without any adverse events.

PRIAPISM

Epidemiology and Pathophysiology of Priapism

Priapism is defined as a pathological prolonged engorgement or erection of the penis or clitoris that is unrelated to sexual arousal. The word *priapism* is derived from Priapus, a minor god of fertility and luck, and the deity of gardens and fields in Greek mythology (Papadopoulos & Kelami, 1988). Hinman (1914) classified priapism as either mechanical or nervous in etiology in the early 20th

century and suggested corporal vein thrombosis as the cause of "mechanical" priapism. The condition is more common in men and typically involves the paired corpora cavernosa, although rare exceptions with involvement of the corpus spongiosum and sparing of the cavernosal spaces have been reported (Taylor, 1980).

Priapism is generally classified as low flow (ischemic) or high flow (arterial and non-ischemic). Low-flow priapism and the associated severe decrease in venous drainage from the corpora cavernosa is a potential medical emergency and may lead to irreversible ischemic tissue changes. High-flow priapism is less commonly encountered and involves unregulated inflow that is typically secondary to some form of arterial trauma. Unlike the ischemic subtype, arterial priapism is not considered an emergency: spontaneous resolution is the likely outcome in more than half the cases and the patient does not have pain. Therefore, the majority of the discussion in this segment is dedicated to the ischemic, low-flow variant of priapism. Hauri and co-workers (Bruhlmann, Pouliadis, Hauri, & Zollikofer, 1983) were some of the first investigators to suggest that the prognosis of the veno-occlusive (low-flow) priapism is far less favorable than arterial priapism.

The overall incidence rate of priapism in the general population has been estimated to be 1.5 per 100,000 person-years (2.9 per 100,000 person-years in men 40 years old and older; Eland, van der Lei, Stricker, & Sturkenboom, 2001). Because not all patients with priapism will seek medical care, the reported data may underestimate the actual rate in the general population. The incidence of priapism in special "at risk" subpopulations such as those with a history of cocaine drug use or advanced pelvic or hematologic malignancy, and those on antipsychotic medications is much higher (Altman, Seftel, Brown, & Hampel, 1999; Compton & Miller, 2001; Steinhardt & Steinhardt, 1981; Suri et al., 1980). A study of 230 single case reports in the literature revealed the following priapism etiologies: idiopathic causes composed one third of the cases while 21% were attributed to alcohol abuse or medications, 12% to perineal trauma, and 11% to sickle cell anemia (SCA) (Pohl, Pott, & Kleinhans, 1986).

Another "at risk" group of patients are those with erectile dysfunction (ED) who are on intracorporal injection therapy. The incidence range of priapism episodes in this population ranges from 1% for those on prostaglandin E_1 (PGE$_1$) to 17% for patients who receive intracorporal injections of papaverine (Linet & Ogrinc, 1996). Avoidance of overdosage by gradual upward titration of the dose will help decrease this adverse event.

Most cases of priapism associated with sickle cell disease are classically described as ischemic, although rare exceptions (unknown etiology) of high-flow priapism in association with SCA have been reported (Ramos, Park, Ritchey, & Benson, 1995). SCA-related priapism is unusual before puberty with a reported 6% prevalence

(Fowler, Koshy, Strub, & Chinn, 1991; Tarry, Duckett, & Snyder, 1987). However, the probability of experiencing priapism in patients with homozygous SCA (Hb SS) and sickle cell beta(0)-thalassemia (Hb S-beta(0)) by age 20 is as high as 89% (Mantadakis, Cavender, Rogers, Ewalt, & Buchanan, 1999).

A variety of medications, most commonly related to the antihypertensive drugs guanethidine, prazosin, and hydralazine as well as psychotropic medications, have been implicated as etiologic factors in priapism (Rubin, 1968). Among psychotropic medications, trazodone (Desyrel™), thioridazine, and chlorpromazine have been associated with priapism (Ankem et al., 2002). This effect has been attributed to the alpha-adrenergic antagonist properties of these medications (Abber et al., 1987). Antipsychotics that have been reported to cause priapism on rare occasions. The exact pathophysiology has not been elucidated, but is likely multifactorial and may be related to the ratio of alpha-adrenergic blockade to anticholinergic activity. Atypical antipsychotics that have been reported to cause priapism on rare occasions include risperidone, olanzapine, and clozapine (Compton & Miller, 2001).

The recreational drug ecstasy has been associated with episodes of priapism (Dubin & Razack, 2000). More importantly, because trazodone is commonly employed as a hypnotic and is often chosen for polysubstance abusers due to its low abuse potential, it is important to consider that trazodone and cocaine may have synergistic effects in promoting priapism (Myrick, Markowitz, & Henderson, 1998). Cocaine-induced priapism has been reported in association with topical application to enhance sexual performance, as well as intranasal and intracavernous injections (Fiorelli, Manfrey, Belkoff, & Finkelstein, 1990; Mireku-Boateng & Tasie, 2001; Rodriguez-Blaquez, Cardona, & Rivera-Herrera, 1990).

Priapism in patients with degenerative stenosis of the lumbar canal, the cauda equina syndrome (following degenerative stenosis of the lumbar canal and lumbar arachnoiditis), herniated disc, or blockage of the central inhibitory influences such as that seen during general or regional anesthesia are examples of neurologically induced priapism.

Priapism has been reported in patients on high concentration (i.e., 20% rather than 10%) fat emulsion total parenteral nutrition and in a variety of systemic illnesses such as amyloidosis, glucose phosphate isomerase deficiency, and Fabry's disease (glycosphingolipid lipidosis) presenting with a combination of renal insufficiency and priapism (Bschleipfer et al., 2001; Goulding, 1976; Hebuterne, Frere, Bayle, & Rampal, 1992; Lapan, Graham, Bangert, Boyer, & Conner, 1980; Wilson, Klionsky, & Rhamy, 1973; Zimbelman et al., 2000). Table 31.3 lists the important etiologic factors in ischemic (low-flow) priapism.

TABLE 31.3
Etiologic Factors in Low-Flow Priapism

Total parenteral nutrition (high fat content)
Thrombophilia states (lupus, protein C)
Vasculitis
Hematologic
Warfarin/heparin-induced
Fabry's disease
Dialysis
Hemoglobinopathies and sickle cell disease
Malignancies including bladder/prostate cancer and metastatic (e.g., renal) tumors
Psychotropics and antidepressants (chlorpromazine, trazodone, risperidol)
Antihypertensives (guanethidine, hydralazine, prazosin)
Erectogenic agents (intracavernosal vasoactives; sildenafil; intraurethral PGE_1)
Spinal cord stenosis
Amyloidosis
Glucose phosphate isomerase deficiency
Alcohol
Androgens/testosterone

PATHOPHYSIOLOGY

Priapism may be regarded as a failure of erectile regulatory control causing an imbalance between arterial inflow and outflow (Burnett, 2003). Dysregulation of the veno-occlusive mechanism, arterial inflow, or neurogenic processes that can affect inflow or outflow, or malfunction of the normal contractile activities of cavernosal smooth muscle cells may be implicated as causative factors in priapism. The low-flow, ischemic variant of priapism that is the focus of this section is considered a medical emergency. This most common form of priapism is characterized by a painful rigid erection, absent cavernosal blood flow, and severely acidotic corpora. Immediate attention to the problem and decompression of the "compartment syndrome" minimize the chances of long-term adverse events such as penile fibrosis and ED. Trabecular interstitial edema and ultrastructural changes in trabecular smooth muscle cells including functional transformation to fibroblast-like cells may result from the combination of venous outflow obstruction, high pressure chambers, and poor-to-absent inflow. Severe cellular damage and widespread necrosis may occur in cases lasting more than 24 hours (Spycher & Hauri, 1986). Irreversible ED may be caused in cases lasting beyond 48 hours where destruction of the endothelial lining, formation of blood clots within the corpora, and widespread transformation of the smooth muscle cells to fibroblast-like cells or necrosis may be observed (Spycher & Hauri, 1986). These irreversible "late" changes underscore the importance of early intervention and patient education in high-risk groups.

Broderick et al. (1994) have demonstrated that anoxia can eliminate spontaneous and drug-induced contractile activity in an animal model, suggesting a likely explanation for the failure of penile injection of alpha-adrenergic agonists to reverse prolonged ischemic priapism when the penis is in its maximal rigid state. Failed alpha-adrenergic neurotransmission, endothelin deficit, or inactivation of intracellular cofactors of smooth muscle contraction due to hypoxia and/or hypercarbia have been suggested as factors affecting the absence of proper detumescence in low-flow priapism (Broderick et al., 1994). Seftel et al. (Seftel, Haas, Brown et al., 1998) have reported on two cases of veno-occlusive priapism refractory to conventional therapy who later developed high-flow priapism. The high-flow state observed after treatment of veno-occlusive priapism may represent a variant of nonischemic priapism or, alternatively, may represent the pathophysiology of recurrent idiopathic priapism.

Inheritance of one or two genes coding for an abnormal S hemoglobin may result in sickle cell hemoglobinopathy, which is manifested in 0.15% of black Americans in the form of sickle cell disease (homozygous for hemoglobin S) and in 8% as sickle cell trait (heterozygous for hemoglobin S). Inheritance of a combination of a hemoglobin S gene and a second gene coding for an abnormal hemoglobin (e.g., B$^+$ thalassemia or C hemoglobin) is possible and, as in the homozygous type, may result in ischemic complications (Fowler et al., 1991). SCA-induced priapism likely results from decreased oxygen tension and pH developing in stagnant blood within the corporal sinusoids, which in turn leads to a cycle of erythrocyte sickling and sludging followed by even more hypoxemia and acidosis (Siegel, Rich, & Brock, 1993).

DIAGNOSIS

A thorough history and physical examination are prerequisites to diagnostic accuracy.

Many patients with priapism experience significant anxiety and fear in addition to severe penile pain and discomfort. During the initial encounter, often in the emergency room setting, the clinician should make a genuine effort to alleviate the patient's apprehension. The sexual and medical history should especially focus on medications, trauma, and predisposing comorbidities. Presence or absence of pain is a fairly reliable predictor of low-flow versus high-flow priapism, respectively. A history of penile or perineal trauma further suggests high-flow priapism. Absence of pain in arterial priapism frequently results in less patient anxiety and discomfort as compared with veno-occlusive priapism. Consequently, those with arterial priapism may present days or even weeks after the original injury. The fundamental aim of the initial phase of assessment is to distinguish arterial from ischemic priapism. The American Foundation for Urologic Disease (AFUD) panel recommendations for the management of priapism are illustrated in Figure 31.1 and follow a step care model that has been modified and refined over the years (Berger et al., 2001; Jacob & Herschler, 1986; Sadeghi-Nejad, Dogra, Seftel, & Mohamed, 2004).

Physical examination of the penis is critical and will typically reveal firm corpora cavernosa and a soft glans, indicating sparing of the corpus spongiosum in low-flow priapism. Findings in high-flow states usually reveal a partial to full erection and sparing of the corpus spongiosum in most cases (as in low-flow states). Urine toxicology screening for psychoactive drugs and metabolites of cocaine are recommended among the general laboratory diagnostic tests and are especially helpful if the diagnosis is unclear (Altman et al., 1999; Berger et al., 2001). A reticulocyte count, urinalysis, CBC, platelets and differential WBC as well as urologic consultation should be obtained. Men with SCA will typically have an elevated reticulocyte count, but it should be emphasized that hemoglobinopathies are not restricted to African-American men. Other groups, especially those of Mediterranean descent, may be affected (i.e., thalassemia or sickle-thalassemia). The sickledex test and examination of the peripheral smear are less time-consuming than hemoglobin electrophoresis and may be more appropriate for the emergency room setting (Montague et al., 2003).

The corporal blood flow status should be assessed to differentiate low-flow from high-flow priapism. This may be done with a corporal aspirate and visual inspection by color and consistency *or* corporal blood gas including pH, PO_2, and PCO_2 *or* penile duplex Doppler ultrasound (Berger et al., 2001). Low oxygen, high carbon dioxide, and low pH in the blood gas analysis of the aspirate are typical findings in low-flow priapism, whereas a high-flow state is suspected based on the bright red appearance or high oxygen content in the blood gas analysis of the corporal aspirate. In these cases, duplex Doppler sonography may identify a dilated cavernosal artery or pseudocapsule formation at the site of arterial sinusoidal fistula and will be helpful if superselective arterial embolization is performed (Pautler & Brock, 2001). Unlike veno-occlusive priapism, penile aspiration has mainly a diagnostic role in the management of arterial priapism, and nonischemic priapism resolution after aspiration or irrigation is only rarely observed (Berger et al., 2001; Koga, Shiraishi, & Saito, 1990; Montague et al., 2003; Rudick, 2002).

If conventional corporal irrigation and intracavernosal sympathomimetics (i.e., phenylephrine) fail to resolve the initial veno-occlusive priapism, sonography should be considered to identify those patients presenting with refractory low-flow priapism who later convert to a high-flow state. Although this is a very small group of patients with priapism, the distinction is important

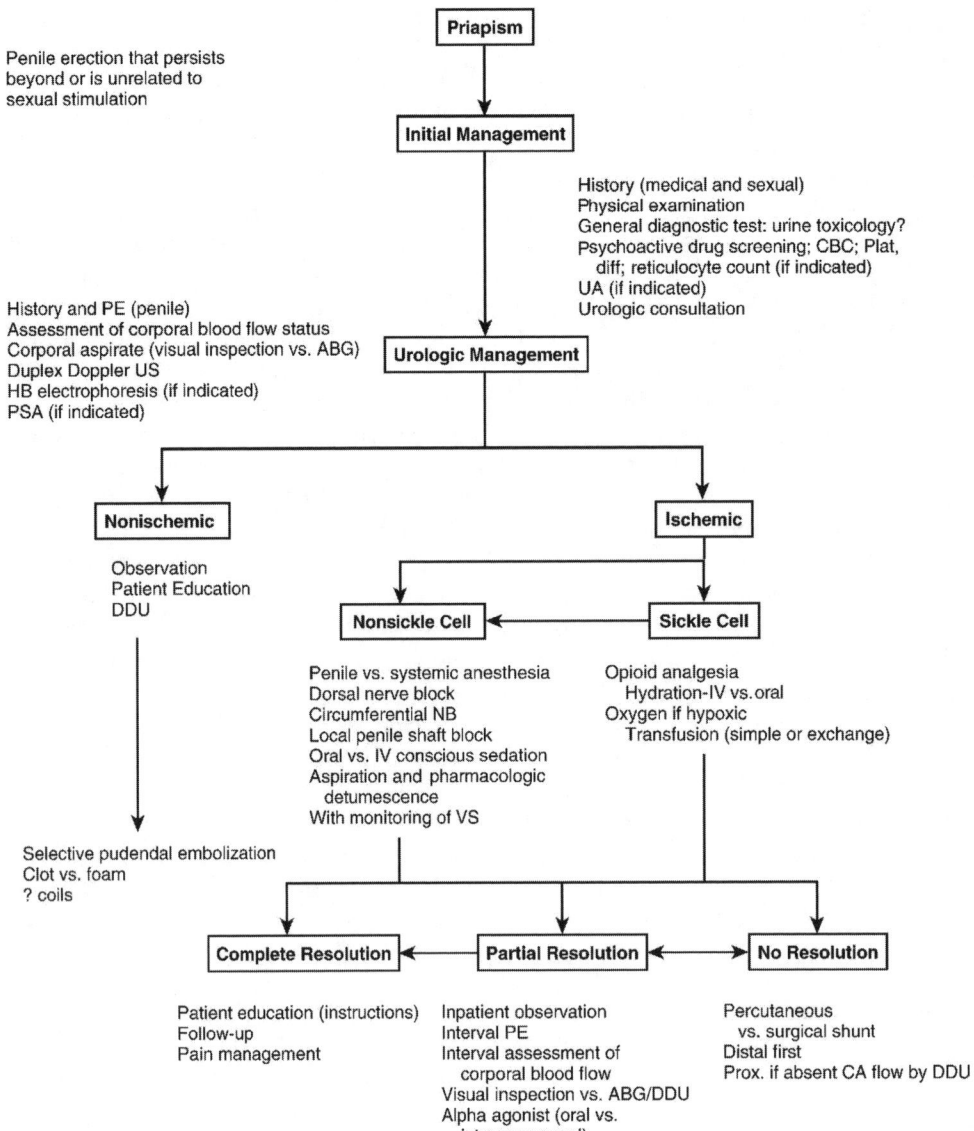

FIGURE 31.1 The American Foundation for Urologic Disease (AFUD) panel recommendations for the management of priapism. ABG = arterial blood gas; CA = cavernosal artery; CBC = complete blood count; DDU = duplex Doppler ultrasound; HB = hemoglobin; IV = intravenous; NB = nerve block; PE = physical examination; PSA = prostate specific antigen; UA = urinalysis; US = ultrasound; VS = vital signs.

because the management of the low-flow and high-flow states is radically different and the high-flow group is usually managed conservatively (Sadeghi-Nejad et al., 2004; Seftel, Haas, Brown et al., 1998.

TREATMENT

Most cases of veno-occlusive priapism treated without excessive delay (<12 hours) will respond to alpha agonist therapy. Failure of resolution after 20 minutes of injection (0.1 ml/min of a 500 μg/ml phenylephrine solution for a total infused dose of 1 mg) is an indication for alternative strategies for management as these patients are unlikely to respond to further injection therapy (Paut-

ler & Brock, 2001). Aspiration and irrigation of the corpora are performed as first-line treatments even in low-flow priapism of more than 4 hours duration; however, these therapies have not shown a benefit in preserving potency when priapism has persisted beyond 72 hours (Berger et al., 2001). Failure of resolution after conservative measures as described will move the "step care" process to the surgical level. A number of different surgical shunts for diversion of blood away from the corpus cavernosum have been described. The consensus among authorities is that, in general, distal corporospongiosal shunts should be undertaken before proximal shunts; however, there is no consensus regarding the choice of percutaneous versus open surgical shunts. We prefer to start with a transglandular Winter shunt (corporoglandular) using a biopsy gun device to create multiple channels between the corpus spongiosum and the corpora (Nelson & Winter, 1977). If this technique is not successful, a larger communication between the corpora cavernosal and the corpus spongiosum may be created by a modified Al-Ghorab shunt in which the distal tunica albuginea of the corpora cavernosa is removed through a transglandular incision. Proximal shunts are rarely performed and are recommended if distal shunts fail and absent cavernosal artery flow is assessed by Doppler sonography (Berger et al., 2001; Sacher, Sayegh, Frensilli, Crum, & Akers, 1972). A few authors have advocated early use of penile prostheses in cases of refractory or recurrent priapism associated with corporal fibrosis and ED (Sundaram, Fernandes, Ercole, & Billups, 1997).

In patients with SCA, initial efforts are directed at relief of pain and anxiety, as well as hydration with hypotonic fluids at 1.5 times maintenance. Intravenous hydration and parenteral narcotic analgesia are started while preparing for aspiration and irrigation, supplemental oxygen, and possible exchange transfusion (Berger et al., 2001). The utility of red cell transfusion in this group of patients has been questioned by Powars and Johnson (1996) who hypothesize that in the static, hypoxic, and acidotic corporal environment, it is unlikely that red cells can reach the target area. Because there is an increased risk of cerebrovascular accident, coma, and intracranial hemorrhage, the blood volume and viscosity must be closely monitored in patients undergoing exchange transfusion or rapid single unit transfusion. Lack of priapism resolution after conservative measures calls for more invasive measures following an algorithm that is very similar to that described for non-SCA priapism. Rutchik et al. (Rutchik, Sorbera, Rayford, & Sullivan, 2001) have reported on a single case of refractory veno-occlusive priapism (failure of response to intracavernosal alpha adrenergic injection/irrigation and recurrence after an Al-Ghorab surgical shunt) that responded to intracavernosal injection of 15-mg tissue plasminogen activator. The authors resorted to this therapy due to severe penile congestion and risk of penile necrosis with further shunting. However, it must be emphasized that experience with this approach is very limited. Methylene blue, a guanylate cyclase inhibitor, has been used as a novel approach for treatment of priapism in a small group of patients. De Holl et al. (de Holl, Shin, Angle, & Steers, 1998) describe the use of methylene blue in 11 patients with priapism and report immediate detumescence in 67%. A possible explanation for the success of this therapy is blockage of cyclic GMP-induced muscle relaxation following the initial aspiration attempts. Recently, successful treatment of recurrent idiopathic priapism with oral baclofen has been reported in two patients (Rourke & Jordan, 2002).

PENILE FRACTURE

Fracture of the penis, *faux pas du coit*, was first reported by Abul Kasem in Cordoba more than 1,000 years ago and follows trauma to the erect penis during coitus or penile manipulation/masturbation (Eke, 2002). This acute condition is a medical emergency that presents with a sudden cracking sound (due to the rupture of the corpora cavernosa) that is accompanied by localized penile pain and immediate detumescence. Many patients present hours (or even days) after the actual injury due to embarrassment. Penile swelling due to hematoma formation at the site of rupture may result in voiding difficulties including possible urinary retention, as well as penile swelling, bruising, and deviation that is often described as an "eggplant" deformity (Cumming & Jenkins, 1991). Some reports have indicated that the condition may be as uncommon as 1 in 175,000 hospital admissions in the United States, but this is likely to be a low estimate due to the stigma associated with penile injury sustained during sexual activity (Farah, Stiles, & Cerny, 1978). Eke (2002) have reviewed a total of 183 publications pertaining to penile fracture from various countries and reported a total of 1,642 cases, but the condition is undoubtedly highly underreported and is commonly seen in most emergency rooms at least a few times per year.

Pathophysiology

Penile fracture occurs as a result of trauma to the erect penis and has been reported in association with intercourse and penile manipulation including forced bending of the phallus to achieve detumescence (Zargooshi, 2000). The acute bending of the penis has been described in association with a variety of situations including reverse coitus with the woman-on-top position or abrupt female rotation during intercourse, as well as accidental injury due to rollover during nocturnal tumescence (Mohapatra & Kumar, 1990; Pruthi, Petrus, Nidess, & Venable, 2000; Seftel, Haas, Vafa, & Brown, 1998; Zargooshi, 2000).

Diagnosis and Treatment

The diagnosis is based on history and physical examination; radiological studies such as MRI or ultrasound, and more invasive measures such as cavernosography are rarely, if ever, required to confirm the diagnosis. A history of acute penile pain after penile trauma and a description of the classic popping sound followed by detumescence is characteristic. The site of injury is often palpable as a distinct defect in the tunica albuginea of the corpus cavernosum, but may be difficult to appreciate if it is covered by a large hematoma. In severe cases, the rupture may involve the corpus spongiosum and urethra with resultant gross hematuria and a possible butterfly-shaped perineal hematoma (Lee et al., 2000).

Treatment of penile fracture consists of surgical repair with evacuation of the hematoma and closure of the cavernosal tunical defect. In comparison with conservative management, immediate repair is associated with faster recovery and lower morbidity (Kalash & Young, 1984; Zargooshi, 2000). Depending on the location of the tunical defect, a circumcising, an inguino-scrotal, or transverse scrotal (with "eversion" of penis) incision may be used to access the site of injury for repair. Both absorbable as well as non-absorbable sutures may be used for tunical closure, but the latter may be associated with long-term discomfort, as the patients can often feel the knots below the skin (Asgari, Hosseini, Safarinejad, Samadzadeh, & Bardideh, 1996; Zargooshi, 2000). Although most authorities recommend aggressive surgical management of penile fracture (especially in the acute setting), those presenting late or refusing therapy will find comfort in knowing that conservative management may also be associated with good long-term outcomes in select cases. Mydlo et al. (Mydlo, Gershbein, & Machia, 2001) reported a series of five patients suspected of having penile fracture who had refused aggressive surgical therapy and who suffered no serious complications (12-month follow-up) as a result of conservative management (Mydlo et al., 2001).

SCROTAL PAIN

In its acute form, scrotal pain is a medical emergency that requires prompt attention to rule out testicular torsion. A full history including the patient's age, sexual history, duration, severity, and onset (gradual vs. sudden) of pain are necessary to focus the clinician's attention on the correct diagnostic path. Contrary to traditional teaching, a few recent reports have shown that the incidence of epididymo-orchitis (EO) is equal to that of testicular torsion and has a peak incidence in infants (McAndrew, Pemberton, Kikiros, & Gollow, 2002). Depending on the study, torsion of the testicular appendages has been reported to peak in 7- to 13-year-old children, whereas testicular torsion is most common in neonates and boys aged 15 years (Marcozzi & Suner, 2001; Van Glabeke, Khairouni, Larroquet, Audry, & Gruner, 1999). The physical examination should be complete and must include a careful evaluation of the abdomen and the inguinal region to assess possible herniation. This section focuses on the acute and non-acute urological causes of scrotal pain.

The physician should be aware of the nonurologic causes of acute scrotal pain (peritonitis, incarcerated hernia, ruptured abdominal aortic aneurysm) as well as referred scrotal pain. Because sensory fibers from both the upper ureter and testis go through the spinal cord segments T11 and T12, upper ureteral distension (e.g., due to a ureteral stone) may cause referred pain to the testis and

lower ureteral distension may result in ipsilateral scrotal pain (Hayden, 1993). The differential diagnosis of scrotal pain also includes Henoch-Schonlein purpura (HSP), a systemic vasculitis that typically affects patients younger than 20 years of age and has a peak incidence at 4 or 5 years of age. This entity may involve the scrotum in 2 to 38% of cases and be misdiagnosed as diseases that require surgical intervention such as testicular torsion or an incarcerated inguinal hernia (Ben-Sira, 2000). HSP has distinct sonographic features (marked edema of the scrotal skin and contents with intact vascular flow in the testicles, epididymal enlargement, and a hydrocele) that allow distinction from testicular torsion in many cases and prevent unnecessary surgical exploration (Ben-Sira, 2000; Laor, Atala, & Teele, 1992). Testicular tumors most often present as a painless scrotal mass, and the teaching that "a painless scrotal mass is testicular cancer until proven otherwise" still holds. However, the astute clinician must be aware that a rapidly growing testicular mass may present with scrotal pain.

When all other causes of chronic scrotal pain described below have been ruled out, low back strain and the resultant radiculitis due to sensory nerve root irritation at the T10 to L1 level may be the source of the discomfort. Holland et al. (Holland, Feldman, & Gilbert, 1994) have proposed that idiopathic orchalgia or "phantom orchalgia" follows an abnormal neural processing where referred scrotal pain is caused by a noxious stimulus. In these cases, the authors recommend correction of bad posture, avoidance of heavy strain or lifting, and use of a scrotal support for 6 weeks. Other recommendations include spermatic cord anesthetic infiltration at the pubic tubercle with lidocaine 1% and bupivacaine 0.5%, physiatrist referral for neuromuscular evaluation, and a possible trial of transcutaneous electrical nerve stimulation unit. Selective ilio-inguinal/genitofemoral blocks or paravertebral nerve root blocks at T10 to L1 may also be attempted in refractory cases (Holland et al., 1994).

Testicular torsion may be intravaginal or extravaginal (typically neonatal and prior to complete testicular descent and scrotal wall fusion) and follows rotation of the spermatic cord with resultant ischemia. The degree of testicular rotation strongly affects the possibility of salvage after torsion and the time until necrosis occurs. *Torsion of the testicular appendages* may present very similarly to testicular torsion, accounts for 24 to 46% of acute scrotal presentations, and is often present in 7- to 13-year-old children (Knight & Vassy, 1984; Marcozzi & Suner, 2001).

DIAGNOSIS

The patient suffering from testicular torsion will typically present with acute-onset, unilateral scrotal pain. As in prostatitis and other parenchymal inflammatory processes, the edema and resultant capsular stretching increase the intensity of the pain (Gerber & Brendler, 2002). Previous episodes of scrotal pain may be related to prior ischemic episodes with spontaneous resolution, and the patient may also complain of systemic symptoms such as nausea and vomiting. A "high riding" testis due to shortening of the cord is often a hallmark of testicular torsion, and the testis may also have an abnormal (e.g., transverse) position in the scrotum (Marcozzi & Suner, 2001). In the pediatric population, the absence of the cremasteric reflex is also characteristic of torsion (Rabinowitz, 1984). The normal reflex is elicited by extra gentle stroking of the inner thigh whereupon elevation of the ipsilateral testis and contraction of the cremasteric muscle is observed; this finding is very rarely seen in a patient with testicular torsion. As in all other causes of painful scrotum, a urinalysis and scrotal ultrasound are helpful in confirming the diagnosis. The presence of hematuria or leukocytosis is more typical of EO as the cause of the acute scrotum. Absence of testicular blood flow on color Doppler ultrasonography is a helpful clinical tool. However, this modality is highly operator dependent and may be subject to false interpretation in young children or neonates with small testicular vessels (Herbener, 1996). Although torsion usually occurs around puberty, whereas epididymitis typically affects sexually active men after age 20, the age distribution may be clinically misleading and should not be relied upon for a definitive diagnosis.

Patients with appendicular torsion (appendix testis or appendix epididymis) rarely have systemic complaints and typically describe a gradual-onset, unilateral scrotal pain that is lesser in intensity compared with testicular torsion and that is localized to the superior pole of the testis (Burgher, 1998). Careful examination of the scrotal skin early in the course of presentation may reveal the "blue dot sign" due to the nonviable appendage.

TREATMENT

When torsion is suspected, immediate surgical intervention with scrotal exploration, detorsion, and orchidopexy is required. In a review of 543 surgical explorations for acute scrotal pain in boys, Van Glabeke et al. (1999) found a 16.6% incidence of testicular torsion and a 46% incidence of appendage torsion. The authors recommend surgical intervention in all male children complaining of acute scrotal pain. When immediate operative intervention is not possible, manual detorsion in the emergency room setting after adequate analgesia may be attempted. It is helpful to recall that torsion typically occurs in a medial direction, and detorsion should therefore be initially tried in a clockwise direction on the left and counterclockwise on the patient's right side (Marcozzi & Suner, 2001). Although surgical exploration is not strictly required for appendicular torsion, the distinction from testicular torsion is not always possible unless unequivocal testicular

blood flow is demonstrated on color Doppler sonography, in which case surgical intervention may be necessary.

EPIDIDYMITIS

Epididymitis is another common cause of the acute scrotum that must be differentiated from torsion of the testis or testicular appendages. This clinical condition is a painful, parenchymal inflammatory process that results in epididymal swelling and may also affect the testicles (epididymo-orchitis). Epididymitis typically results from the spread of microorganisms from the urethra, prostate, or seminal vesicles, but may occur due to hematogenous spread in conditions such as tuberculosis. *Chlamydia trachomatis* and *Neisseria gonorrhea* are the most common causative agents in sexually active men younger than 35 years, whereas Gram-negative enteric epididymitis associated with urinary tract infections is usually seen in older patients, those who have undergone recent genitourinary tract surgery, and those with anatomical abnormalities (Marcozzi & Suner, 2001; Morbity and Mortality Weekly Report [MMWR], 1998). Rarely, fungal agents such as candida have been reported to cause epididymitis (Hori & Tsutsumi, 1995). It has been suggested that the association of infantile epididymitis with other urogenital abnormalities mandates further diagnostic evaluation (Hamdan, 1991). However, Anderson et al. (Anderson, Giacomantonio, & Schwarz, 1989) assessed 48 boys for acutely painful scrota and noted that two of three boys with bacteriuric epididymitis had known predisposing genitourinary anomalies, but boys with sterile urine and epididymitis did not have anatomic abnormalities noted on renal and pelvic ultrasonography or voiding cystourethrography and therefore did not require additional studies. The use of the antiarrhythmic agent amiodarone has been associated with sterile epididymitis in up to 11% of adult patients and, rarely, in children. The pathophysiology of amiodarone-induced epididymitis is unknown, but may be related to high concentration in testicular tissue (Hutcheson, Peters, & Diamond, 1998).

DIAGNOSIS

Unlike the acute nature of the pain experienced by most patients with testicular torsion, epididymitis usually presents as a gradually increasing, dull, unilateral scrotal pain. Possible involvement of the vasa may result in exquisite pain that affects not only the entire hemiscrotum, but the spermatic cord as well. However, milder cases with localized involvement of the epididymis may also be observed. Attempts to distinguish epididymitis from torsion may be frustrated due to this variable presentation, although a history of prior genitourinary tract procedure, sexual activity, and a normal cremasteric reflex on examination are more suggestive of epididymitis. Physical examination reveals a tender and swollen epididymis. A urinalysis and urine culture as well as urethral cultures (for identification of *C. trachomatis* or *N. gonorrhea*) must be performed. When positive, these tests or an elevated white blood cell count favor a diagnosis of epididymitis, but do not exclude torsion. The inflammatory nature of epididymitis causes increased blood flow to the scrotum and its contents. This feature is very helpful in differentiating epididymitis from torsion when interpreting color Doppler ultrasound or nuclear scintigraphy findings. Tuberculous epididymitis has gradually declined in incidence in the western hemisphere. When present, it manifests between the ages of 20 and 50 years in the sexually active years, and more than two thirds of the patients give a history of previous tuberculosis. Scrotal swelling, pain, discharge from draining scrotal sinuses in combination with sterile pyuria are common presenting symptoms (Heaton, Hogan, Michell, Thompson, & Yates-Bell, 1989). Tuberculous orchitis is considered to be a rare entity that may follow tuberculous epididymitis and represents a more severe end of this clinical spectrum.

TREATMENT

When the constellation of clinical findings points to epididymitis, empiric antibiotic therapy until the final culture results are available is recommended. In the younger (less than 35 years old) population in whom a sexually transmitted condition is the more likely etiology of epididymitis, empiric therapy should be started with ceftriaxone and doxycycline or oflaxacin, whereas in the older population, oral fluoroquinolones are recommended (Marcozzi & Suner, 2001). Symptomatic pain relief is achieved with bed rest, scrotal elevation, analgesics, and NSAIDs. A cord block may be used when the pain is severe.

Recognition of amiodarone-induced epididymitis in children and a reduction in dosage or temporary cessation of the drug may result in rapid resolution of the epididymitis and avoidance of unnecessary surgical intervention in a high risk population (Hutcheson et al., 1998).

The patient should be advised that, although the pain and edema usually subside in 7 to 10 days, the epididymal induration may be present for a few weeks despite good response to antimicrobials. An early follow-up (3 days) is advised when the symptoms do not improve within 3 days. Similarly, more unusual organisms (tuberculous or fungal) should be suspected in symptomatic cases that persist 6 to 8 weeks after completion of antimicrobial therapy (Marcozzi & Suner, 2001).

POST-VASECTOMY PAIN

EPIDEMIOLOGY AND PATHOPHYSIOLOGY

A questionnaire-based outcome study of non-oncological post-vasectomy complications revealed that pain after vasectomy is the most common adverse event affecting the patients' quality of life after this operation (Choe & Kirkemo, 1996). Chronic scrotal discomfort is seen in up to one third of men after vasectomy and half of these men consider the pain bothersome and may seek further therapy for relief (McMahon et al., 1992; West, Leung, & Powell, 2000. In one study of 13 patients with post-vasectomy pain, mean time to pain onset after vasectomy was 2 years and the presenting symptoms included testicular pain in 9 cases, epididymal pain in 2, pain at ejaculation in 4, and pain during intercourse in 8 (Nangia, Myles, & Thomas, 2000). The same authors reported the physical examination findings in the same cohort and noted tender epididymides in 6 men, full epididymides in 6, a tender vasectomy site in 4, and a palpable nodule in 4.

The pathophysiology of this condition is not entirely known, but tender sperm granuloma, nerve entrapment, or nerve proliferation at the site of vasectomy, perineural fibrosis, and mechanical duct obstruction with epididymal congestion have been suggested as possible causes (Nangia et al., 2000; Sweeney, Tan, Butler, McDermott, Grainger, & Thornhill, 1998). Epididymal engorgement, complex cystic disease, and chronic epididymitis are the main histological findings in post-vasectomy patients with scrotal pain (West et al., 2000). Other investigators, however, have observed no differences in vasectomy site histological features in patients with the post-vasectomy pain syndrome and matched controls, and no difference in histological findings in patients with the post-vasectomy pain syndrome who did and did not become pain-free postoperatively (after microsurgical vasectomy reversal) (Nangia et al., 2000).

TREATMENT

Some investigators have reported that the incidence of post-vasectomy pain may be significantly reduced by the injection of 1 ml of 0.5% bipuvicaine into the vasal lumen at the time of vasectomy (Paxton, Huss, Loughlin, & Mirakhur, 1995). Inhibition of excitability at the dorsal horn of the spinal cord caused by nociceptive impulses from the injured tissue has been suggested as a possible explanation for the benefits of preemptive bupivacaine anesthesia (Woolf & Chong, 1993).

Conservative measures such as NSAIDs, scrotal elevation, and various analgesics are typically used as first-line therapy. When ineffective, a cord block may be tried, but this requires multiple and possible lifelong therapies and may not be a practical option. A few authors have suggested epididymectomy when surgical intervention is contemplated (Sweeney et al., 1998; West et al., 2000). West et al. (2000) report initial improvement in 14 of 16 patients and lasting symptom relief in 9 of 10 patients who were interviewed 3 to 8 years after epididymectomy. Furthermore, they cite atypical symptoms such as testicular or groin pain, erectile dysfunction, and normal sono-graphic appearance of the epididymis as poor prognostic indicators (West et al., 2000). Although this option precludes ipsilateral vasectomy reversal in the future, the availability of high-level assisted reproductive techniques in combination with testicular sperm retrieval provide the potential for future fatherhood. Finally, a number of studies have reported on microsurgical vasectomy reversal for the treatment of post-vasectomy pain syndrome (Bruning, 1997; Edwards, 1997; Myers, Mershon, & Fuchs, 1997; Nangia et al., 2000). In one of these publications, Bruning (1997) reported relief of post-vasectomy pain in 24 of 32 men who underwent a single microsurgical vasectomy reversal and in 3 of 6 with recurrent pain who had undergone a second procedure.

VARICOCELE

EPIDEMIOLOGY AND PATHOPHYSIOLOGY

Varicocele, an abnormal dilation of the spermatic veins, is a common anatomical abnormality that has an incidence of 10 to 20% in the United States (Meacham, Townsend, Rademacher, & Drose, 1994; Saypol, 1981). In the absence of (or malfunction of) vein valves, retrograde flow of blood from the internal spermatic and cremasteric veins into the veins of the pampiniform plexus in the spermatic cord and scrotum causes varicoceles. Absence of the valve at the left renal–internal spermatic vein and absent/incomplete valves along the internal spermatic vein have been demonstrated by a number of investigators (Ahlberg, Barley, Chidekel, & Fritjofsson, 1966; Comhaire, Kunnen, & Nahoum, 1981; Coolsaet, 1980; Kohler, 1967). Varicoceles can affect various seminal parameters and most authors agree that surgical therapy of varicoceles is an accepted intervention in the treatment of male factor infertility. The varicocele pain is typically reported as a dull, aching, and throbbing sensation in the scrotum without sharp or radiating components (Peterson, Lance, & Ruiz, 1998). Long periods of standing and the resultant increased hydrostatic pressure in the valveless veins of the pampiniform plexus may exacerbate the dull ache. The diagnosis is made by a careful physical examination of the scrotum and spermatic cord after the patient has been standing in a warm room (to allow cremasteric relaxation) for a few minutes. Varicoceles are traditionally classified as grade I (palpable during a Valsalva maneuver), grade II (visible in the standing position during a Valsalva maneuver), or grade III (visible in the standing position through the scrotal skin without increased intra-abdominal pressure). Decreased diameter of the spermatic cord in the recumbent position in comparison with the standing position suggests the presence of varicoceles. Sonographic diagnosis of a clinical varicocele is made when a minimal diameter of 3.5 mm

is demonstrated in the veins of the pampiniform plexus (Meacham et al., 1994).

TREATMENT

It has been estimated that 2 to 10% of men with varicoceles have pain secondary to varicoceles, but surgical intervention for relief of pain is controversial (Peterson et al., 1998). A number of recent studies have published the results of varicocelectomy performed for relief of pain. A large study from Turkey evaluated 119 men who underwent subinguinal microsurgical varicocele ligation for painful varicocele diagnosed based on the findings of both physical examination and color Doppler ultrasound (Yaman, Ozdiler, Anafarta, & Gogus, 2000). Of the 82 patients who were evaluable at the end of this study, 72 (88%) reported complete resolution of pain, 4 patients (5%) partial resolution, 5 patients (6%) no change, and 1 patient (1%) epididymal discomfort that resolved with conservative measures. Similarly, Peterson et al. (1998) (60%) reviewed records from 58 patients who underwent varicocele ligation to establish success of surgical ligation of the painful varicocele and obtained follow-up on 35 of the 58 (60%) patients with painful varicocele in whom initial conservative measures had failed. The authors report resolution of pain postoperatively in 86% and partial resolution in 1 patient, while 4 patients (11%) had persistent or worse symptoms. The excellent results in the two aforementioned studies are corroborated by at least two other recent studies that report 82.8 and 84.5% complete resolution of pain, but are in contrast to the 48% improvement reported by Biggers and Soderdahl in 1981. It should be noted that the diagnostic modalities and follow-up methods are not identical in these reports.

REFERENCES

Abber, J. C., Lue, T. F., Luo, J. A., Juenemann, K. P., & Tanagho, E. A. (1987). Priapism induced by chlorpromazine and trazodone: mechanism of action. *Journal of Urology, 137*(5), 1039–1042.

Adeyoju, A. B., Thornhill, J., Lynch, T., Grainger, R., McDermott, T., & Butler, M. R. (1996). The fate of the defunctioned bladder following supravesical urinary diversion. *British Journal of Urology, 78*(1), 80–83.

Ahlberg, N. E., Bartley, O., Chidekel, N., & Fritjofsson, A. (1966). Phlebography in varicocele scroti. *Acta Radiologia. Series One. Diagnosis (Stockholm), 4*(5), 517–528.

Aldenborg, F., Fall, M., & Enerback, L. (1986). Proliferation and transepithelial migration of mucosal mast cells in interstitial cystitis. *Immunology, 58*(3), 411–416.

Aldenborg, F., Fall, M., & Enerback, L. (1989). Mast cells in interstitial cystitis. *Annales d' Urologie (Paris), 23*(2), 165–166.

Altman, A. L., Seftel, A. D., Brown, S. L., & Hampel, N. (1999). Cocaine associated priapism. *Journal of Urology, 161*(6), 1817–1818.

Anderson, P. A., Giacomantonio, J. M., & Schwarz, R. D. (1989). Acute scrotal pain in children: Prospective study of diagnosis and management. *Canadian Journal of Surgery, 32*(1), 29–32.

Ankem, M. K., Ferlise, V. J., Han, K. R., Gazi, M. A., Koppisch, A. R., & Weiss, R. E. (2002). Risperidone-induced priapism. *Scandinavian Journal of Urology and Nephrology, 36*(1), 91–92.

Asgari, M. A., Hosseini, S. Y., Safarinejad, M. R., Samadzadeh, B., & Bardideh, A. R. (1996). Penile fractures: Evaluation, therapeutic approaches and long-term results. *Journal of Urology, 155*, 148–149.

Atala, A., Amin, M., Harty, J. I., Liu, Y. K., & Keeling, M. M. (1992). Priapism associated with asplenic state. *Urology, 40*(4), 371–373.

Awad, S. A., MacDiarmid, S., Gajewski, J. B., & Gupta, R. (1992). Idiopathic reduced bladder storage versus interstitial cystitis. *Journal of Urology, 148*(5), 1409–1412.

Bade, J. J., Laseur, M., Nieuwenburg, A., van der Weele, L. T., & Mensink, H. J. (1997). A placebo-controlled study of intravesical pentosanpolysulphate for the treatment of interstitial cystitis. *British Journal of Urology, 79*(2), 168–171.

Bade, J. J., Rijcken, B., & Mensink, H. J. (1995). Interstitial cystitis in The Netherlands: Prevalence, diagnostic criteria and therapeutic preferences. *Journal of Urology, 154*(6), 2035-2037; discussion 2037–2038.

Barbalias, G. A., Nikiforidis, G., & Liatsikos, E. N. (1998). Alpha-blockers for the treatment of chronic prostatitis in combination with antibiotics. *Journal of Urology, 159*(3), 883–887.

Batstone, G. R., Doble, A., & Batstone, D. (2003). Chronic prostatitis. *Current Opinion in Urology, 13*(1), 23–29.

Batstone, D., Doble, A., & Gaston, J. (2002). Autoimmune T cell responses to seminal plasma in chronic pelvic pain syndrome (CPPS). *Clinical and Experimental Immunology, 128*, 302–307.

Ben-Sira, L., & Laor, T. (2000). Severe scrotal pain in boys with Henoch-Schonlein Purpura: Incidence and sonography. *Pediatric Radiology, 30*, 125–128.

Bennett, R. M. (1999). Emerging concepts in the neurobiology of chronic pain: Evidence of abnormal sensory processing in fibromyalgia. *Mayo Clinic. Proceedings, 74*(4), 385–398.

Berger, R., Billups, K., Brock, G., Broderick, G. A., Dhabuwala, C. B., Goldstein I. et al. (2001). Report of the American Foundation for Urologic Disease (AFUD) Thought Leader Panel for evaluation and treatment of priapism. *International Journal of Impotence Research, 13*(Suppl 5), S39–S43.

Biancani, P., Zabinski, M. P., & Weiss, R. M. (1976). Time course of ureteral changes with obstruction. *American Journal of Physiology, 231*(2), 393–398.

Biggers, R. D., & Soderdahl, D. W. (1981). The painful varicocele. *Military Medicine, 146*, 440–442.

Bornman, M. S., Franz, R. C., Jacobs, D. J., & Pretorius, H. (1986). Causal relationships between drug-induced hypercoagulability and priapism. *Archives of Andrology, 17*(3), 231–232.

Broderick, G. A., Gordon, D., Hypolite, J., & Levin, R. M. (1994). Anoxia and corporal smooth muscle dysfunction: a model for ischemic priapism. *Journal of Urology, 151*(1), 259–262.

Brookoff, D. (2000). Chronic pain: 1. A new disease? *Hospital Practice. Office Edition, 35*(7), 45–52, 59.

Bruhlmann, W., Pouliadis, G., Hauri, D., & Zollikofer, C. (1983). A new concept of priapism based on the results of arteriography and cavernosography. *Urology and Radiology, 5*(1), 31–36.

Bruning, C. O., 3rd. (1997). Re: Vasectomy reversal for treatment of the post-vasectomy pain syndrome. *Journal of Urology, 158*(4), 1528.

Bschleipfer, T. H., Hauck, E. W., Diemer, T. H., Bitzer, M., Kirkpatrick, Ch. J., Pust, R. A. et al. (2001). Heparin-induced priapism. *International Journal of Impotence Research, 13*(6), 357–359.

Buck, A. C., Rees, R. W., & Ebeling, L. (1989). Treatment of chronic prostatitis and prostatodynia with pollen extract. *British Journal of Urology, 64*(5), 496–499.

Burgher, L. C. D. R. (1998). Acute scrotal pain. *Emergency Medicine Clinics of North America, 16*, 781–809.

Burnett, A. L. (2003). Pathophysiology of priapism: dysregulatory erection physiology thesis. *Journal of Urology, 170*(1), 26–34.

Butrick, C. W. (2003). Interstitial cystitis and chronic pelvic pain: New insights in neuropathology, diagnosis, and treatment. *Clinical Obstetrics and Gynecology, 46*(4), 811–823.

Cervero, F. (1994). Sensory innervation of the viscera: Peripheral basis of visceral pain. *Physiological Reviews, 74*(1), 95–138.

Chen, R., & Nickel, J. C. (2003). Acupuncture ameliorates symptoms in men with chronic prostatitis/chronic pelvic pain syndrome. *Urology, 61*(6), 1156–1159; discussion 1159.

Choe, J. M., & Kirkemo, A. K. (1996). Questionnaire based outcomes study of nononcological post-vasectomy complications. *Journal of Urology, 155*, 1284–1286.

Choi, N. G., Soh, S. H., Yoon, T. H., & Song, M. H. (1994). Clinical experience with transurethral microwave thermotherapy for chronic nonbacterial prostatitis and prostatodynia. *Journal of Endourology, 8*(1), 61–64.

Christmas, T. J, Rode, J., Chapple, C. R., Milroy, E. J., & Turner-Warwick, R. T. (1990). Nerve fibre proliferation in interstitial cystitis. *Virchows Archiv. A. Pathological Anatomy and Histopathology, 416*(5), 447–451.

Collins, M. M., O'Leary, M. P., & Barry, M. J. (1998). Prevalence of bothersome genitourinary symptoms and diagnoses in younger men on routine primary care visits. *Urology, 52*(3), 422–427.

Comhaire, F., Kunnen, M., & Nahoum, C. (1981). Radiological anatomy of the internal spermatic vein(s) in 200 retrograde venograms. *International Journal of Andrology, 4*(3), 379–387.

Compton, M. T., & Miller, A. H. (2001). Priapism associated with conventional and atypical antipsychotic medications: a review. *Journal of Clinical Psychiatry, 62*(5), 362–366.

Coolsaet, B. L. (1980). The varicocele syndrome: Venography determining the optimal level for surgical management. *Journal of Urology, 124*(6), 833–839.

Cordell, W. H., Larson, T. A., Lingeman, J. E., Nelson, D. R., Woods, J. R., Burns, L. B. et al. (1994). Indomethacin suppositories versus intravenously titrated morphine for the treatment of ureteral colic. *Annals of Emergency Medicine, 23*(2), 262–269.

Cordell, W. H., Wright, S. W., Wolfson, A. B., Timerding, B. L., Maneatis, T. J., Lewis, R. H. et al. (1996). Comparison of intravenous ketorolac, meperidine, and both (balanced analgesia) for renal colic. *Annals of Emergency Medicine, 28*(2), 151–158.

Cristol, D. S., Greene, L. F., & Thompson, G. J. (1944). Interstitial cystitis of men: a review of 78 cases. *Journal of the American Medical Association, 126*, 825–828.

Cumming, J., & Jenkins, J.D. (1991). Fracture of the corpora cavernosa and urethral rupture during sexual intercourse. *British Journal of Urology, 67*, 327.

Curhan, G. C., Speizer, F. E., Hunter, D. J., Curhan, S. G., & Stampfer, M. J. (1999). Epidemiology of interstitial cystitis: A population based study. *Journal of Urology, 161*(2), 549–552.

de Holl, J. D., Shin, P. A., Angle, J. F., & Steers, W. D. (1998). Alternative approaches to the management of priapism. *International Journal of Impotence Research, 10*(1), 11–14.

Dellabella, M., Milanese, G., & Muzzonigro, G. (2003). Efficacy of tamsulosin in the medical management of juxtavesical ureteral stones. *Journal of Urology, 70*(6 Pt. 1), 2202–2205.

Drach, G. W., Fair, W. R., Meares, E. M. et al. (1978). Classification of benign diseases associated with prostatic pain: Prostatitis or prostatodynia? *Journal of Urology, 120*, 266.

Dubin, N. N., & Razack, A. H. (2000). Priapism: Ecstasy related? *Urology, 56*(6), 1057.

Dunn, E. K., Miller, S. T., Macchia, R. J., Glassberg, K. I., Gillette, P. N., Sarkar, S. D. et al. (1995). Penile scintigraphy for priapism in sickle cell disease. *Journal of Nuclear Medicine, 36*(8), 1404–1407.

Dunn, M., Ramsden, P. D., Roberts, J. B., Smith, J. C., & Smith, P. J. (1977). Interstitial cystitis, treated by prolonged bladder distension. *British Journal of Urology, 49*(7), 641-645.

Edwards, I. S. (1997). Vasectomy reversal for treatment of the post-vasectomy pain syndrome. *Journal of Urology, 158*(6), 2252.

Eke, N. (2002). Fracture of the penis. *British Journal of Surgery, 89*(5), 555–565.

Eland, I. A, van der Lei, J., Stricker, B. H., & Sturkenboom, M. J. (2001). Incidence of priapism in the general population. *Urology, 57*(5), 970–972.

Elbadawi, A. E., & Light, J. K. (1996). Distinctive ultrastructural pathology of nonulcerative interstitial cystitis: New observations and their potential significance in pathogenesis. *Urologia Internationalis, 56*(3), 137–162.

Fagerli, J., Fraser, M. O., deGroat, W. C., Chancellor, M. B., Flood, H. D., Smith, D. et al. (1999). Intravesical capsaicin for the treatment of interstitial cystitis: A pilot study. *Canadian Journal of Urology, 6*(2), 737–744.

Fall, M. (1985). Conservative management of chronic interstitial cystitis: Transcutaneous electrical nerve stimulation and transurethral resection. *Journal of Urology, 133*(5), 774–778.

Farah, R. N., Stiles, R., & Cerny, J. C. (1978). Surgical treatment of deformity and coital difficulty in healed traumatic rupture of the corpora cavernosa. *Journal of Urology, 120*, 118–120.

Fiorelli, R. L., Manfrey, S. J., Belkoff, L. H., & Finkelstein, L. H. (1990). Priapism associated with intranasal cocaine abuse. *Journal of Urology, 143*(3), 584–585.

Forrest, J. B., & Vo, Q. (2001). Observations on the presentation, diagnosis, and treatment of interstitial cystitis in men. *Urology, 57*(6 Suppl. 1), 26–29.

Fowler, J. E., Jr., Koshy, M., Strub, M., & Chinn, S. K. (1991). Priapism associated with the sickle cell hemoglobinopathies: prevalence, natural history and sequelae. *Journal of Urology, 145*(1), 65–68.

Gerber, G. S., & Brendler, C. B. (2002). Evaluation of the urologic patient: history, physical examination, and urinalysis. In M. F. Campbell, P. C. Walsh, & A. B. Retik (Eds.), *Campbell's urology* (8th ed., pp. 83–110). Philadelphia: Saunders.,

Gillenwater, J. Y., & Wein, A. J. (1988). Summary of the National Institute of Arthritis, Diabetes, Digestive and Kidney Diseases Workshop on Interstitial Cystitis, National Institutes of Health, Bethesda, Maryland, August 28–29, 1987. *Journal of Urology, 140*(1), 203–206.

Goulding, F. J. (1976). Priapism caused by glucose phosphate isomerase deficiency. *Journal of Urology, 116*(6), 819–820.

Greenlee, R. T., Murray, T., Bolden, S., & Wingo, P. A. (2000). Cancer statistics, 2000. *CA: A Cancer Journal for Clinicians, 50*(1), 7–33.

Gurunadha Rao Tunuguntla H. S., & Evans, C. P. (2002). Management of prostatitis. *Prostate Cancer and Prostatic Disease, 5*(3), 172–179.

Hamdan, M. (1991). Epididymitis in infants. Apropos of a case and review of the literature. *Journal d'Urologie (Paris), 97*(4–5), 228–229.

Hanno, P. M. (1994). Amitriptyline in the treatment of interstitial cystitis. *Urologic Clinics of North America, 21*(1), 89–91.

Hanno, P. M. (1997). Analysis of long-term Elmiron therapy for interstitial cystitis. *Urology, 49*(5A Suppl.), 93–99.

Hanno, P. M. (2002). Interstitial cystitis and related disorders. In M. F. Campbell, P. C. Walsh, & A. B. Retik (Eds.), *Campbell's urology* (pp. 631–670). Philadelphia: Saunders.

Hanno, P. M., & Wein, A. J. (1991). Conservative therapy of interstitial cystitis. *Seminars in Urology, 9*(2), 143–147.

Hanno, P. M., Fritz, R., Wein, A. J., & Mulholland, S. G. (1978). Heparin as antibacterial agent in rabbit bladder. *Urology, 12*(4), 411–415.

Hayden, L. J. (1993). Chronic testicular pain. *Australian Family Physician, 22*(8), 1357–1359, 1362, 1365.

Heaton, N. D., Hogan, B., Michell, M., Thompson, P., & Yates-Bell, A. J. (1989). Tuberculous epididymo-orchitis: Clinical and ultrasound observations. *British Journal of Urology, 64*(3), 305–309.

Hebuterne, X., Frere, A. M., Bayle, J., & Rampal, P. (1992). Priapism in a patient treated with total parenteral nutrition. *Journal of Parenteral and Enteral Nutrition, 16*(2), 171–174.

Henry, R., Patterson, L., Avery, N., Tanzola, R., Tod, D., Hunter, D. et al. (2001). Absorption of alkalized intravesical lidocaine in normal and inflamed bladders: A simple method for improving bladder anesthesia. *Journal of Urology, 165*(6 Pt 1), 1900–1903.

Herbener, T. E. (1996). Ultrasound in the assessment of the acute scrotum. *Journal of Clinical Ultrasound, 24*, 405–421.

Hinman, F. (1914). Priapism: report of cases in a clinical study of the literature with reference to its pathogenesis and surgical treatments. *Annals of Surgery, 60*, 689.

Holdgate, A., & Pollock, T. (2004). Nonsteroidal anti-inflammatory drugs (NSAIDs) versus opioids for acute renal colic. *Cochrane Database Systems Review*, (1), CD004137.

Holland, J. M., Feldman, J. L., & Gilbert, H. C. (1994). Phantom orchalgia. *Journal of Urology, 152*, 2291–2293.

Hori, S., & Tsutsumi, Y. (1995). Histological differentiation between chlamydial and bacterial epididymitis: Nondestructive and proliferative versus destructive and abscess forming—Immunohistochemical and clinicopathological findings. *Human Pathology, 26*(4), 402–407.

Hruz, P., Danuser, H., Studer, U. E., & Hochreiter, W. W. (2003). Non-inflammatory chronic pelvic pain syndrome can be caused by bladder neck hypertrophy. *European Urology, 44*(1), 106–110; discussion 110.

Hunner, G. L. (1915). A rare type of bladder ulcer in women: Report of cases. *Boston Medical and Surgical Journal, 172*, 660.

Hutcheson, J., Peters, C. A., & Diamond, D. A. (1998). Amiodarone induced epididymitis in children. *Journal of Urology, 160*(2), 515–517.

Jacob, S. W., & Herschler, R. (1986). Pharmacology of DMSO. *Cryobiology, 23*(1), 14–27.

John, H., Ruedi, C., Kotting, S., Schmid, D. M., Fatzer, M., & Hauri, D. (2003). A new high frequency electrostimulation device to treat chronic prostatitis. *Journal of Urology, 170*(4 Pt. 1), 1275–1277.

Kalash, S. S., & Young, J. D. J. (1984). Fracture of penis: Controversy of surgical versus conservative treatment. *Urology, 24*, 21–24.

Khoury, J. M., Timmons, S. L., Corbel, L., & Webster, G. D. (1992). Complications of enterocystoplasty. *Urology, 40*(1), 9–14.

Kirby, R. S., Lowe, D., Bultitude, M. I. et al. (1982). Intraprostatic urinary reflux: an etiological factor in abacterial prostatitis. *British Journal of Urology, 121*, 729.

Knight, P., & Vassy, L. (1984). The diagnosis and treatment of the acute scrotum in children and adolescents. *Annals of Surgery, 200*, 664–673.

Koga, S., Shiraishi, K., & Saito, Y. (1990). Post-traumatic priapism treated with metaraminol bitartrate: Case report. *Journal of Trauma 30*(12), 1591–1593.

Kohler, F. P. (1967). On the etiology of varicocele. *Journal of Urology, 97*(4), 741–742.

Krieger, J. N., & Riley, D. E. (2002). Bacteria in the chronic prostatitis chronic pelvic pain syndrome: Molecular approaches to critical research questions. *Journal of Urology, 167*, 2574–2583.

Krieger, J. N., Nyberg, L., Jr., & Nickel, J. C. (1999). NIH consensus definition and classification of prostatitis. *Journal of the American Medical Association, 282*, 236–237.

Lagunoff, D., Martin, T. W., & Read, G. (1983). Agents that release histamine from mast cells. *Annual Review of Pharmacology and Toxicology, 23*, 331–351.

Laor, T., Atala, A., & Teele, R. L. (1992). Scrotal ultrasonography in Henoch-Schonlein purpura. *Pediatric Radiology, 22*(7), 505–506.

Lapan, D. I., Graham A. R., Bangert, J. L., Boyer, J. T., & Conner, W. T. (1980). Amyloidosis presenting as priapism. *Urology, 15*(2), 167–170.

Larkin, G. L., Peacock IV, W. F., Pearl, S. M., Blair, G. A., & D'Amico, F. (1999). Efficacy of ketorolac tromethamine versus meperidine in the ED treatment of acute renal colic. *American Journal of Emergency Medicine, 17*(1), 6–10.

Lazzeri, M., Spinelli, M., Beneforti, P., Malaguti, S., Giardiello, G., & Turini, D. (2004). Intravesical infusion of resiniferatoxin by a temporary in situ drug delivery system to treat interstitial cystitis: A pilot study. *European Urology, 45*(1), 98–102.

Lee, J., Singh, B., Kravets, F. G., Trocchia, A., Waltzer, W. C., & Khan, S. A. (2000). Sexually acquired vascular injuries of the penis: A review. *Journal of Trauma, 49*, 599–601.

Lilly, J. D., & Parsons, C. L. (1990). Bladder surface glycosaminoglycans is a human epithelial permeability barrier. *Surgery, Gynecology, and Obstetrics, 171*(6), 493–496.

Linet, O. I., & Ogrinc, F. G. (1996). Efficacy and safety of intracavernosal alprostadil in men with erectile dysfunction. The Alprostadil Study Group. *New England Journal of Medicine, 334*(14), 873–877.

Linn, J. F., Hohenfellner, M., Roth, S., Dahms, S. E., Stein, R., Hertle, L. et al. (1998). Treatment of interstitial cystitis: comparison of subtrigonal and supratrigonal cystectomy combined with orthotopic bladder substitution. *Journal of Urology, 159*(3), 774–778.

Ljunghall, S., Danielson, B. G., Fellstrom, B., Holmgren, K., Johansson, G., & Wikstrom, B. (1985). Family history of renal stones in recurrent stone patients. *British Journal of Urology, 57*(4), 370–374.

Lobel, B., & Rodriguez, A. (2003). Chronic prostatitis: What we know, what we do not know, and what we should do! *World Journal of Urology, 21*(2), 57–63.

Lynch, C. F., & Cohen, M. B. (1995). Urinary system. *Cancer, 75*(1 Suppl), 316–329.

Maake, C., & John, H. (2003). Prostatitis versus pelvic pain syndrome: Immunologic studies. *Current Urology Reports, 4*(4), 327–334.

Malin, J. M., Jr., Deane, R. F., & Boyarsky, S. (1970). Characterisation of adrenergic receptors in human ureter. *British Journal of Urology, 42*(2), 171–174.

Mantadakis, E., Cavender, J. D., Rogers, Z. R., Ewalt, D. H., & Buchanan, G. R. (1999). Prevalence of priapism in children and adolescents with sickle cell anemia. *Journal of Pediatric Hematology and Oncology, 21*(6), 518–522.

Marcozzi, D., & Suner, S. (2001). The nontraumatic, acute scrotum. *Emergency Medicine Clinics of North America, 19*(3), 547–568.

Markenson, J. A. (1996). Mechanisms of chronic pain. *American Journal of Medicine, 101*(1A), 6S–18S.

McAndrew, H. F., Pemberton, R., Kikiros, C. S., & Gollow, I. (2002). The incidence and investigation of acute scrotal problems in children. *Pediatric Surgery International, 18*(5–6), 435–437.

McMahon, A. J., Buckley, J., Taylor, A., Lloyd, S. N., Deane, R. F., & Kirk, D. (1992). Chronic testicular pain following vasectomy. *British Journal of Urology, 69*, 188–191.

Meacham, R. B., Townsend, R. R, Rademacher, D., & Drose, J. A. (1994). The incidence of varicoceles in the general population when evaluated by physical examination, gray scale sonographic and color Doppler sonography. *Journal of Urology, 151*, 1535.

Meares, E. M. (1986). Chronic bacterial prostatitis: Role of transurethral prostatectomy (TURP) in therapy. In W. Weidener, H. Brunner, W. Krause et al. (Eds.), *Therapy of prostatitis* (pp. 193–197). Munich: W. Zuckschwerdt Verlag.

Meares, E. M., & Stamey, T. A. (1968). Bacteriologic localization patterns in bacterial prostatitis and urethritis. *Investigative Urology, 5*, 492–518.

Meares, E. M., Jr. (1991). Prostatitis. *Medical Clinics of North America, 75*(2), 405–424.

Mehik, A., Alas, P., Nickel, J. C., Sarpola, A., & Helstrom, P. J. (2003). Alfuzosin treatment for chronic prostatitis/chronic pelvic pain syndrome: A prospective, randomized, double-blind, placebo-controlled, pilot study. *Urology, 62*(3), 425–429.

Menon, M., & Resnick, M. I. (2002). *Urinary lithiasis: Etiology, diagnosis, and medical management.* In M. F. Campbell, P. C. Walsh, & A. B. Retik (Eds.), *Campbell's urology,* (8th ed., pp. 3229–3305). Philadelphia: Saunders.

Miller, J. L., Fischer, K. A., Goralnick, S. J. et al. (2002). Interleukin-10 levels in the seminal plasma: Implications for chronic prostatitis-chronic pelvic pain syndrome. *Journal of Urology, 167*, 753–756.

Minogiannis, P., El-Mansoury, M., Betances, J. A., Sant, G. R. & Theoharides, T. C. (1998). Hydroxyzine inhibits neurogenic bladder mast cell activation. *International Journal of Immunopharmacology, 20*(10), 553–563.

Mireku-Boateng, A. O., & Tasie, B. (2001). Priapism associated with intracavernosal injection of cocaine. *Urologia Internationalis, 67*(1), 109–110.

Mohapatra, T. P., & Kumar, S. (1990). Reverse coitus: mechanism of injury in the male partner. *Journal of Urology, 144*, 1467–1468.

Montague, D. K., Jarow, J., Broderick, G. A., Dmochowski, R. R., Heaton, J. P., Lue, T. F. et al. (2003). American Urological Association guideline on the management of priapism. *Journal of Urology, 170*(4 Pt. 1), 1318–1324.

Montorsi, F., Guazzoni, G., Bergamaschi, F., Galli, L., Consonni, P., Matozzo, V. et al. (1993). Is there a role for transrectal microwave hyperthermia of the prostate in the treatment of abacterial prostatitis and prostatodynia? *Prostate, 22*(2), 139–146.

Morbidity and Mortality Weekly Report. (1998). *Guidelines for treatment of sexually transmitted diseases.* Centers for Disease Control and Prevention. Report No. 23:47(RR-1).

Mydlo, J. H., Gershbein, A. B., & Machia, R. J. (2001). Nonoperative treatment of patients with presumed penile fracture. *Journal of Urology, 165*, 424–425.

Myers, S. A., Mershon, C. E., & Fuchs, E. F. (1997). Vasectomy reversal for treatment of the post-vasectomy pain syndrome. *Journal of Urology, 157*(2), 518–520.

Myrick, H., Markowitz, J. S., & Henderson, S. (1998). Priapism following trazodone overdose with cocaine use. *Annals of Clinical Psychiatry 10*(2), 81–83.

Nangia, A. K., Myles, J. L., & Thomas, A. J. (2000). Vasectomy reversal for the post-vasectomy pain syndrome: a clinical and histological evaluation. *Journal of Urology, 164*(6), 1939–1942.

Neal, D. E., Jr., & Moon, T. D. (1994). Use of terazosin in prostatodynia and validation of a symptom score questionnaire. *Urology, 43*(4), 460–465.

Nelson, J. H., 3rd, & Winter, C. C. (1977). Priapism: Evolution of management in 48 patients in a 22-year series. *Journal of Urology, 117*(4), 455–458.

Nickel, J. C. (1995). Practical approach to the management of prostatitis. *Techniques in Urology, 1*(3), 162–167.

Nickel, J. C. (2003). The use of alpha1-adrenoceptor antagonists in lower urinary tract symptoms: Beyond benign prostatic hyperplasia. *Urology, 62*(3 Suppl. 1), 34–41.

Nickel, J. C., & Sorenson, R. (1994). Transurethral microwave thermotherapy of nonbacterial prostatitis and prostatodynia: initial experience. *Urology, 44*(3), 458–460.

Nickel, J. C., & Sorensen, R. (1996). Transurethral microwave thermotherapy for nonbacterial prostatitis: A randomized, double-blind sham controlled study using new prostatitis specific assessment questionnaires. *Journal of Urology, 155*, 1950–1954.

Nickel, J. C., Alexander, R., Anderson, R. et al. (1999). Prostatitis unplugged: prostatic massage revisited. *Techniques in Urology, 5*, 1–7.

Nickel, J. C., Downey, J., Johnston, B. et al. (2001). Predictors of patient response to antibiotic therapy for the chronic prostatitis/chronic pelvic pain syndrome: a prospective multicenter clinical trial. *Journal of Urology, 165*, 1539–1544.

Nickel, J. C., Downey, J., Morales, A., Emerson, L., & Clark, J. (1998). Relative efficacy of various exogenous glycosaminoglycans in providing a bladder surface permeability barrier. *Journal of Urology, 160*(2), 612–614.

Nordling, J., Jorgensen, S., & Kallestrup, E. (2001). Cystistat for the treatment of interstitial cystitis: A 3-year follow-up study. *Urology, 57*(6 Suppl. 1), 123.

Orhan, I., Onur, R., Ilhan, N., & Ardicoglu, A. (2001). Seminal plasma cytokine levels in the diagnosis of chronic pelvic pain syndrome. *International Journal of Urology, 8*, 495–499.

Osborn, D. E., George, N. J. R., & Rao, P. N. (1981). Prostatodynia—Physical characteristics and rational management with muscle relaxants. *British Journal of Urology, 53*, 621–623.

Papadopoulos, I., & Kelami, A. (1988). Priapus and priapism. From mythology to medicine. *Urology, 32*(4), 385–386.

Parkin, J., Shea, C., & Sant, G. R. (1997). Intravesical dimethyl sulfoxide (DMSO) for interstitial cystitis—A practical approach. *Urology, 49*(5A Suppl), 105-107.

Parsons, C. L. (1996). Potassium sensitivity test. *Techniques in Urology, 2*(3), 171–173.

Parsons, C. L. (2000). Interstitial cystitis: New concepts in pathogenesis, diagnosis, and management. *AUA News, 5*, 20–31.

Parsons, C. L. (2003). Prostatitis, interstitial cystitis, chronic pelvic pain, and urethral syndrome share a common pathophysiology: Lower urinary dysfunctional epithelium and potassium recycling. *Urology, 62*(6), 976–82.

Parsons, C. L. (2004). Current strategies for managing interstitial cystitis. *Expert Opinion on Pharmacotherapy, 5*(2), 287–293.

Parsons, C. L., & Davis, E. L. (2003, September). Pentosan polysulfate sodium intravesical instillation—End-organ therapy. *Practice Building Today*, 18–22.

Parsons, C. L., Benson, G., Childs, S. J., Hanno, P., Sant, G. R., & Webster, G. (1993). A quantitatively controlled method to study prospectively interstitial cystitis and demonstrate the efficacy of pentosanpolysulfate. *Journal of Urology, 150*(3), 845–848.

Parsons, C. L, Dell, J., Stanford, E. J., Bullen, M., Kahn, B. S., Waxell, T. et al. (2002). Increased prevalence of interstitial cystitis: Previously unrecognized urologic and gynecologic cases identified using a new symptom questionnaire and intravesical potassium sensitivity. *Urology, 60*(4), 573–578.

Parsons, C. L., Housley, T., Schmidt, J. D., & Lebow, D. (1994). Treatment of interstitial cystitis with intravesical heparin. *British Journal of Urology, 73*(5), 504–507.

Parsons, C. L., Lilly, J. D., & Stein, P. (1991). Epithelial dysfunction in nonbacterial cystitis (interstitial cystitis). *Journal of Urology, 145*(4), 732–735.

Parsons, C. L., Zupkas, P., & Parsons, J. K. (2001). Intravesical potassium sensitivity in patients with interstitial cystitis and urethral syndrome. *Urology, 57*(3), 428–432; discussion 432–433.

Pautler, S. E., & Brock, G. B. (2001). Priapism. From priapus to the present time. *Urologic Clinics of North America, 28*(2), 391–403.

Paxton, L. D., Huss, B. K., Loughlin, V., & Mirakhur, R. K. (1995). Intra-vas deferens bupivacaine for prevention of acute pain and chronic discomfort after vasectomy. *British Journal of Anaesthesia, 74*(5), 612–613.

Peeker, R., Aldenborg, F., & Fall, M. (1998). The treatment of interstitial cystitis with supratrigonal cystectomy and ileocystoplasty: Difference in outcome between classic and nonulcer disease. *Journal of Urology, 159*(5), 1479–1482.

Perlmutter, A., Miller, L., Trimble, L. A., Marion, D. N., Vaughan, E. D., Jr., & Felsen, D. (1993). Toradol, an NSAID used for renal colic, decreases renal perfusion and ureteral pressure in a canine model of unilateral ureteral obstruction. *Journal of Urolology, 149*(4), 926–930.

Peterson, A. C., Lance, R. S., & Ruiz, H. E. (1998). Outcomes of varicocele ligation done for pain. *Journal of Urology, 159*(5), 1565–1567.

Pohl, J., Pott, B., & Kleinhans, G. (1986). Priapism: A three-phase concept of management according to aetiology and prognosis. *British Journal of Urology, 58*(2), 113–118.

Potts, J. M. (2003). Chronic pelvic pain syndrome: diagnosis and management. *Current Urology Reports, 4*(4), 316–319.

Powars, D. R., & Johnson, C. S. (1996). Priapism. *Hematology/Oncology Clinics of North America, 10*(6), 1363–1372.

Pruthi, R. S., Petrus, C. D., Nidess, R., & Venable, D. D. (2000). Penile fracture of the proximal corporal body. *Journal of Urology, 164*, 447–448.

Rabinowitz, R. (1984). The importance of the cremasteric reflex in acute scrotal swelling in children. *Journal of Urology, 132*, 89–90.

Ramos, C. E., Park, J. S., Ritchey, M. L., & Benson, G. S. (1995). High flow priapism associated with sickle cell disease. *Journal of Urology, 153*(5), 1619–1621.

Roberts, R. O., Lieber, M. M., Bostwick, D. G., & Jacobsen, S. J. (1997). A review of clinical and pathological prostatitis syndromes. *Urology, 49*(6), 809–821.

Rodriguez-Blaquez, H. M., Cardona, P. E., & Rivera-Herrera, J. L. (1990). Priapism associated with the use of topical cocaine. *Journal of Urology, 143*(2), 358.

Rofeim, O., Hom, D., Freid, R. M., & Moldwin, R. M. (2001). Use of the neodymium: YAG laser for interstitial cystitis: a prospective study. *Journal of Urology, 166*(1), 134–136.

Rourke, K. F., Fischler, A. H., & Jordan, G. H. (2002). Treatment of recurrent idiopathic priapism with oral Baclofen. Journal of *Urology, 168*(6), 2552–2553.

Rubin, S. O. (1968). Priapism as a probable sequel to medication. *Scandinavian Journal of Urology and Nephrology, 2*(2), 81–85.

Rudick, D. H. (2002). Successful treatment of arterial priapism with alpha-agonist irrigation: a rural experience. *Journal of Urology, 167*(5), 2132.

Rugendorff, E. W., Weidner, W., Ebeling, L., & Buck, A. C. (1993). Results of treatment with pollen extract (Cernilton N) in chronic prostatitis and prostatodynia. *British Journal of Urology, 71*(4), 433–438.

Rutchik, S., Sorbera, T., Rayford, R. W., & Sullivan, J. (2001). Successful treatment of recalcitrant priapism using intercorporeal injection of tissue plasminogen activator. *Journal of Urology, 166*(2), 628.

Sacher, E. C., Sayegh, E., Frensilli, F., Crum, P., & Akers, R. (1972). Cavernospongiosum shunt in the treatment of priapism. *Journal of Urology, 108*(1), 97–100.

Sadeghi-Nejad, H., Dogra, V., Seftel, A. D., & Mohamed, M. A. (2004). Priapism. *Radiology Clinics of North America, 42*(2), 427–443.

Saypol, D. C. (1981). The varicocele. *Journal of Andrology, 2* 61.

Schaeffer, A. J., Landis, J. R., Knauss, J. S., Propert, K. J., Alexander, R. B., Litwin, M. S. et al. (2002). Demographic and clinical characteristics of men with chronic prostatitis: The National Institutes of Health chronic prostatitis cohort study. *Journal of Urology, 168*(2), 593–598.

Schoenberg, M. (2002). Management of invasive and metastatic bladder cancer. In M. F. Campbell, P. C. Walsh, & A. B. Retik (Eds.), *Campbell's urology* (8th ed., pp., 2803–2817). Philadelphia: Saunders.

Seftel, A. D., Haas, C. A., Brown, S. L., Herbener, T. E., Sands, M., & Lipuma, J. (1998). High flow priapism complicating veno-occlusive priapism: Pathophysiology of recurrent idiopathic priapism? *Journal of Urology, 159*(4), 1300–1301.

Seftel, A. D., Haas, C. A., Vafa, A., & Brown, S. L. (1998). Inguinal scrotal incision for penile fracture. *Journal of Urology, 159*, 182–184.

Shoskes, D. A. (2003). Treatment response to conventional and novel therapies in chronic prostatitis. *Current Urology Reports, 4*(4), 311–315.

Siegel, J. F., Rich, M. A., & Brock, W. A. (1993). Association of sickle cell disease, priapism, exchange transfusion and neurological events: ASPEN syndrome. *Journal of Urology, 150*(5 Pt.1), 1480–1482.

Sierakowski, R., Finlayson, B., Landes, R. R., Finlayson, C. D., & Sierakowski, N. (1978). The frequency of urolithiasis in hospital discharge diagnoses in the United States. *Investigative Urology, 15*(6), 438–441.

Spycher, M. A, & Hauri, D. (1986). The ultrastructure of the erectile tissue in priapism. *Journal of Urology, 135*(1), 142–147.

Steinhardt, G. F., & Steinhardt, E. (1981). Priapism in children with leukemia. *Urology, 18*(6), 604–606.

Stenberg, A., Bohman, S. O., Morsing, P., Muller-Suur, C., Olsen, L., & Persson A. E. (1988). Back-leak of pelvic urine to the bloodstream. *Acta Physiologica Scandinavica, 134*(2), 223–234.

Sundaram, C. P., Fernandes, E. T., Ercole, C., & Billups, K. L. (1997). Management of refractory priapism with penile prostheses. *British Journal of Urology, 79*(4), 659.

Suri, R., Goldman, J. M., Catovsky, D., Johnson, S. A., Wiltshaw, E., & Galton, D. A. (1980). Priapism complicating chronic granulocytic leukemia. *American Journal of Hematology, 9*(3), 295–299.

Sweeney, P., Tan, J., Butler, M. R., McDermott, T. E., Grainger, R., & Thornhill, J. A. (1998). Epididymectomy in the treatment of intrascrotal disease. *Journal of Urology, 81*, 753–755.

Tarry, W. F., Duckett, J. W., Jr., & Snyder, H. M., 3rd. (1987). Urological complications of sickle cell disease in a pediatric population. *Journal of Urology, 138*(3), 592–594.

Taylor, W. N. (1980). Priapism of the corpus spongiosum and glans penis. *Journal of Urology, 123*(6), 961–962.

Teichman, J. M. (2004). Clinical practice. Acute renal colic from ureteral calculus. *New England Journal of Medicine, 350*(7), 684–693.

Theoharides, T. C., & Sant, G. R. (1997). Hydroxyzine therapy for interstitial cystitis. *Urology, 49*(5A Suppl.), 108–110.

Turner, J. A., Hauge, S., Von Korff, M., Saunders, K., Lowe, M., & Berger, R. (2002). Primary care and urology patients with the male pelvic pain syndrome: symptoms and quality of life. *Journal of Urology, 167* (4), 1768–1773.

Uribarri, J., Oh, M. S., & Carroll, H.J. (1989). The first kidney stone. *Annals of Internal Medicine, 111*(12), 1006–1009.

Van Glabeke, E., Khairouni, A., Larroquet, M., Audry, G., & Gruner, M. (1999). Acute scrotal pain in children: results of 543 surgical explorations. *Pediatric Surgery International, 15*(5–6), 353–357.

Waxman, J. A., Sulak, P. J., & Kuehl, T. J. (1998). Cystoscopic findings consistent with interstitial cystitis in normal women undergoing tubal ligation. *Journal of Urology, 160*(5), 1663–1667.

Webster, G. D. &, Galloway, N. (1987). Surgical treatment of interstitial cystitis. Indications, techniques, and results. *Urology, 29*(4 Suppl), 34–39.

Wein, A. J., & Hanno, P. M. (1990). Interstitial cystitis: An introduction to the problem. In P. M. Hanno, D.R. Staskin, R.J. Krane, & A. J. Wein (Eds.), *Interstitial cystitis* (pp. 13–15). London: Springer-Verlag.

West, A. F., Leung, H. Y., & Powell, P. H. (2000). Epididymectomy is an effective treatment for scrotal pain after vasectomy. *British Journal of Urology International, 85*(9), 1097–1099.

Whitmore, K. E., Payne, C. K., Diokno, A. C., & Lukban, J. C. (2003). Sacral neuromodulation in patients with interstitial cystitis: A multicenter clinical trial. *International Urogynecology Journal and Pelvic Floor Dysfunction, 14* (5), 305–308; discussion 308–309.

Wilson, S. K., Klionsky, B. L., & Rhamy, R. K. (1973). A new etiology of priapism: Fabry's disease. *Journal of Urology, 109*(4), 646–648.

Woolf, C. J., & Chong, M. S. (1993). Preemptive analgesia. *Anesthesia and Analgesia, 77*, 362–379.

Yaman, O., Ozdiler, E., Anafarta, K., & Gogus, O. (2000). Effect of microsurgical subinguinal varicocele ligation to treat pain. *Urology, 55*(1), 107–108.

Yavaskaoglu, I., Oktay, B., Simsek, U., & Ozyurt, M. (1999). Role of ejaculation in the treatment of chronic nonbacterial prostatitis. *International Journal of Urology, 6*, 130–134.

Ye, Z. Q., Cai, D., Lan, R. Z., Du, G. H., Yuan, X. Y., Chen, Z. et al. (2003). Biofeedback therapy for chronic pelvic pain syndrome. *Asian Journal of Urology, 5*(2), 155–158.

Zargooshi, J. (2000). Penile fracture in Kermanshah: Report of 172 cases. *Journal of Urology, 164*, 364–366.

Zimbelman, J., Lefkowitz, J., Schaeffer, C., Hays, T., Manco-Johnson, M., Manhalter, C. et al. (2000). Unusual complications of warfarin therapy: Skin necrosis and priapism. *Journal of Pediatrics, 137*(2), 266–268.

32

Rheumatologic Pain

Thomas Romano, MD, PhD

INTRODUCTION

Pain can be defined as an unpleasant sensation that is thought to originate from a particular body part and that is usually associated with processes capable of causing damage to body tissue. Pain can be acute, such as one might experience in the case of a fractured bone. If pain persists beyond the customary time it takes the affected part to heal or recuperate, the pain is termed " chronic." Acute pain typically occurs when a noxious stimulus activates sensitive peripheral endings of primary afferent nociceptors. The noxious stimulus is then turned into a form of electrochemical energy by a process called *transduction*, whereupon the message is then transmitted via peripheral nerves to the spinal cord and then on to the brain, where the inputs are modulated and pain is consciously perceived (Fields, 1987). It is clear that pain is more than just a sensation. It has two components: (1) sensory and (2) affective. Regardless of the cause of the pain, both of these components must be considered.

No greater interplay between the sensory and affective aspects of pain can be found than in the rheumatic diseases. Not only is the central nervous system of a patient suffering from arthritis bombarded by afferent signals from inflamed swollen tissue, but the conscious (or unconscious) interpretation of the significance of the painful stimuli (perhaps the harbinger of crippling, loss of independence, etc.) may influence pain perception, as can other factors such as the development of a secondary fibromyalgia syndrome (FS) or psychiatric/psychological problems that may complicate the course of a patient with chronic (i.e., incurable and probably progressive) disease.

Rheumatologists are concerned with many problems and/or potential problems that affect the clinical course of the patients under their care. Patients need to be kept ambulatory, or at least their ability to care for themselves has to be maximized to prevent progressive joint and spine deformity. Physicians want to minimize or eliminate the chance that the patient's underlying disease, such as systemic lupus erythematosus (SLE) and rheumatoid arthritis (RA), will affect the internal organs, for example, nephritis in SLE and Felty's syndrome (splenomegaly and neutropenia) in RA, and optimize the length and quality of the patient's life.

When the vast majority of patients first present for consultation and treatment, it is the complaint of pain, above all other symptoms, that dominates the initial patient–physician encounter. Certainly, the fear of having a potentially crippling disease or of not being able to perform certain tasks because of weakness, stiffness, or loss of dexterity comes to the fore after the impact of the illness is explored. However, it is the worsening of pain or the fear of increased pain that has brought the patient to see the rheumatologist at that particular time although other symptoms may have been present for months or even years.

To better appreciate how the rheumatologist approaches the problem of pain and to gain an understanding of the role of pain control in the rheumatic diseases, one must first understand the training of a rheumatologist and what concerns the rheumatologist when confronted with a patient who is in pain, and who often has other symptoms/problems. Frequently, the rheumatologist's patient is confused regarding the diagnosis and prognosis, often having seen numerous other health professionals before consulting the rheumatologist.

A rheumatologist typically treats many types of musculoskeletal diseases. The spectrum of rheumatologic disease is vast, and classifications are constantly being updated. The most recent classification can be found in the latest *Primer on Rheumatic Disease* (Schumacher, 1997). The rheumatologist typically encounters patients with inflammatory conditions, such as RA, SLE, and the like, or degenerative joint disease such as osteoarthritis, or other conditions such as myofascial pain syndromes and fibromyalgia. These latter two conditions are very common problems and each is the subject of a separate chapter in this text.

The rheumatologist is also confronted with musculoskeletal problems that arise out of or complicate other diseases. Infectious disease (e.g., AIDS, tuberculosis, and rheumatic fever), endocrine abnormalities (e.g., diabetes mellitus, thyroid disease, and hyperparathyroidism), malignancy, and other pathologic conditions may first manifest themselves as painful neuromuscular or musculoskeletal problems. Therefore, the rheumatologist must use his or her acumen as an internist to understand and treat patients thus afflicted.

It would be easier to understand the treatment of rheumatologic diseases by establishing general categories and analyzing them separately. For purposes of clarity and trying to follow general pathophysiologic guidelines, this author proposes dividing rheumatologic disorders into four main groups: (1) degenerative conditions, (2) inflammatory diseases, (3) soft tissue problems (e.g., myofascial pain syndrome, fibromyalgia syndrome), and (4) other cause of rheumatologic pain (e.g., infectious, neoplastic, endocrine, congenital).

Naturally, there may be considerable overlap, and any one patient may have several of the above conditions, but these distinctions should prove useful in systematically analyzing and treating patients with either simple or complex problems. Conspicuous in its absence in the above format is the impact of psychological forces that may play a part in the suffering of patients with rheumatologic diseases. Although rheumatologists do not primarily treat psychological disease, its presence is recognized in some patients. Therefore, problems such as depression and anxiety are discussed in terms of their impact on specific diseases, as opposed to creating a separate category.

DEGENERATIVE DISEASES

The category of degenerative diseases contains, but is not limited to, degenerative joint disease; degradation of joint, bone, and other connective tissue by repeated trauma or inflammation; and low back pain that usually arises from a combination of factors.

Degenerative arthritis or osteoarthritis (OA) (also referred to as osteoarthrosis) is probably the most common rheumatic disease affecting bones and joints (Creamer & Hochbery, 1997). It may be primary (idiopathic) or secondary to other diseases (Table 32.1). It is characterized by the narrowing of joint space by progressive loss of

---

TABLE 32.1
Possible Causes of Seconday Osteoarthritis

Joint damage due to:
    Infectious (septic arthritis)
    Hemophilia
    Neuropathy (Charcot joint)
    Gout and other crystal-induced arthritis
    Rheumatoid or other inflammatory arthritis
Multiple epiphyseal dysplasia
Congenital dislocation of the hip
    Slipped capital epiphysis
Inherited metabolic disorders
    Wilson's disease
    Hemochromatosis
    Alkaptonuria
    Morquio's disease
Paget's disease of bone
Acromegaly
Other processes that damage articular cartilage

---

articular cartilage, usually accompanied by reactive changes at the joint margins and underlying subchondral bones. Many patients describe a " bone-on-bone" sensation in weight-bearing joints, such as the knees and/or hips, especially during exercise or simply upon ambulation. It must be remembered that OA is a disease of the joints and has no systemic component (Bergstrom, 1985; Forman, Malamet, & Kaplan, 1983).

The prevalence of OA increases with age and some form of OA is present in almost all patients 65 or older. Many times, the patient experiences transient and/or mild to moderate discomfort and does not see a pain practitioner. Often, over-the-counter analgesics combined with resting of the affected area tend to provide sufficient relief. However, acetaminophen alone may not be effective in providing adequate pain relief in OA (Case et al., 2003). Many patients have more prolonged symptoms or have more severe pain than they can control themselves, so they initially seek relief from their family doctor. Many such patients obtain relief with the chronic use of nonsteroidal anti-inflammatory drugs (NSAIDs). Many NSAIDs in comparatively low doses are available over the counter. These include ibuprofen, naproxen, and ketoprofen. More potent preparations such as indomethacin (Indocin®, Indocin SR®), diclofenac (Voltaren®), and piroxicam (Feldene®) are available by prescription. These have been amply reviewed (Fowler & Arnold, 1983; Fries, Williams, & Boch, 1991) and their effectiveness has been established. A word of caution: if a patient with OA on an NSAID obtains objective improvement (e.g., decreased swelling, redness, warmth) but still complains of pain, a secondary myofascial pain or fibromyalgia syndrome should be considered. Many patients with OA also suffer from regional (e.g., anserine bursitis) or generalized (e.g., fibromyalgia) soft tissue pain syndromes. Unless these are addressed separately and treatment initiated, the patient will continue to complain of pain, which is the main reason he or she sought medical attention in the first place, despite a good response to OA treatment. These are the types of patients the rheumatologist is apt to see. The OA sufferers who do well with NSAID or other therapy prescribed by their family doctor have no reason to visit a rheumatologist's office. While NSAIDs are excellent medications, their use in a cavalier fashion should be discouraged due to potentially severe and even life-threatening side effects. The potential gastrointestinal toxicity of these medications is very well known (Huskisson et al., 1976) as are the effects of these drugs on renal plasma flow (Brezin et al., 1979) and platelet aggregation (Roth & Majerus, 1975). These effects are the result of prostaglandin inhibition and seem to affect patients in direct proportion to their age and the presence of another disease such as peptic ulcer disease, liver disease, and kidney disease.

One way to prevent the untoward effects of prostaglandin inhibitors is the use of anti-inflammatory medications that are selective prostaglandin inhibitors such as nonacetylated salicylate (e.g., salsalate or choline magnesium trisalicylate). Misoprostol (Cytotec®) was introduced to prevent NSAID gastropathy (Graham, Agranval, & Roth, 1988) because it is a synthetic prostaglandin E analogue that allows the stomach to proceed with its endogenous cytoprotective mechanisms even in the presence of NSAID-induced prostaglandin inhibition. It is generally prescribed to patients who are elderly or who have had upper gastrointestinal problems in the past. Patients using nonacetylated salicylates do not need to use misoprostol. Recently, a new class of NSAIDs has been approved for use for arthritis sufferers (Osiri & Moreland, 1999). Celecoxib (Celebrex®) (Simon et al., 1999) and rofecoxib (Vioxx®) (Langman et al., 1999) selectively inhibits cyclooxygenase-2 (COX-2), thus minimizing potential adverse effects on the gastrointestinal tract. The most recently introduced coxib, valdecoxib (Bextra®), has good anti-inflammatory activity and is reported to be relatively safe (Chavez & DeKorte, 2003). Care must be taken when prescribing celecoxib or valdecoxib for patients who are allergic to sulfonamide preparations as such patients may also experience allergic reactions if they are treated with either medication.

Merck, the manufacturer of Vioxx™ (rofecoxib) voluntarily withdrew medication worldwide on September 30, 2004 because of possible adverse reactions. Committees of the FDA met from February 16, 2005 to February 18, 2005. The panel voted unanimously to advise the FDA that all three COX-2 inhibitors could cause heart problems, but the majority of the panel advised against taking them off the market, provided that adequate safety warnings be published.

As adjunct therapies, topical capsaicin (McCarthy & McCarty, 1992) and topical preparations of NSAIDs (Ginsburg & Famaey, 1991; Russell, 1991) have been shown to be effective in relieving symptoms in patients with OA. Often, the combination of such topical therapies and oral NSAIDs is not enough to relieve the pain in a particular joint. In such cases, the use of intra-articular injections of a local anesthetic–corticosteroid mixture can provide prompt, dramatic relief (Hollander, 1972). While the relief is usually temporary, lasting from weeks to months, it can aid the patient in taking advantage of exercise or physical therapy, which previously may have been difficult to endure. The long-term safety and efficacy of intra-articular steroid injections have been recently described (Raynauld et al., 2003). An alternative to intra-articular steroid therapy is the injection of viscous/elastic intra-articular preparations composed of mixtures of hyaluronic acid and saline such as sodium hyaluronate (Hyalgan®; Altman & Moskowitz, 1998) or Synvisc®. These have been employed to treat painful knee OA. While these viscosupplementation medications are superior to oral NSAID treatment alone (Kahan, Lleu, & Salin, 2003), their role in the long-term management of OA has still to be determined, especially because these preparations may be no better than intra-articular corticosteroids (Leopold et al., 2003). Other regimens to help reduce pain and relieve mechanical stress on affected (especially weight-bearing) joints are weight loss, muscle strengthening, use of orthotic (e.g., cane, walker, crutches), and local heat/massage.

A word of warning: NSAIDs should be given with great caution in patients taking oral anticoagulants, sulfonylurea antidiabetes medication, or other highly protein-bound drugs because NSAIDs compete with such medication for plasma protein-binding sites and often displace a sufficient amount of the drug in question to cause untoward effects (e.g., a further prolongation of the prothrombin time or an exaggerated hypoglycemic response). In addition, NSAIDs can interfere with diuretic therapy, and adjustments in type or dosage of these medications may need to be made (Day et al., 1984).

When the pain or deformity of OA becomes overwhelming, consideration should be given to orthopedic consultation, especially if the patient has symptoms involving a weight-bearing joint such as the hip or knee. The technology for the replacement of these joints is superior to that for other joints, and orthopedists generally have more experience with this type of replacement. Significant improvement in pain, function, and quality of life has been documented after total knee (Hawker et al., 1998) or hip (Chang et al., 1996) arthroplasty. Surgery needs to be timely as delays in performing necessary surgery can result in a worse outcome (Fortin et al., 1999).

However, not every patient with recalcitrant knee OA needs total knee replacement. High tibial osteotomy and other corrective procedures may be more appropriate in selected patients.

Often, patients with OA develop associated painful conditions, such as carpal tunnel syndrome, fibromyalgia, or a local myofascial pain syndrome, all of which need to be identified and treated (Romano, 1996).

Joints under increased mechanical stress would seem to be likely candidates for the development of OA, although the medical literature is far from clear on this issue, as illustrated in recent papers regarding runners (Lane et al., 1986; Panush et al., 1986).

Some studies have found that there is a relationship between prolonged stress and OA, for example, spine OA in coal miners (Schlomka, Schroter, & Ocherwal, 1955) and shoulder OA in bus drivers (Lawrence, 1969), while other studies have not found this to be the case (Burkle, Fear, & Wright, 1977; Puranen, et al., 1975).

Each patient's problem must be evaluated individually, and aggravating factors minimized or removed if and when they are identified. This is particularly true for patients with back problems.

Back pain may come from a single problem or a combination of pathologic processes. Spinal OA is a disease of the apophyseal joints. It is frequently associated with disc disease often described by the terms *degenerative disc and joint disease*, or *spondylosis*. While anatomic changes may be well defined by an x-ray or computed tomography (CT) scan showing osteophytic lipping and sclerosis, often these correlate poorly with the clinical picture. The development of spondylosis is probably inevitable in most patients with microtrauma where everyday activities contribute to the symptoms. However, preventive measures, such as the maintenance of ideal weight, good posture, moderate exercise, and proper methods of lifting and carrying, can do much to ease symptoms. The use of NSAIDs as well as adequate rest and the use of heat or cold applications to the affected areas may be helpful. In some patients, traction and/or bracing may be needed (Lee et al., 1989). If the cervical spine is involved, the use of a cervical pillow (preferably a four-in-one cervical pillow or Wal-Pil-O, Los Angeles, CA), which prevents neck flexion and hyperextension, is helpful in relieving night pain. Using a chair with a headrest and avoidance of reading or watching television while recumbent can also help. Posterior neck muscles can be strengthened by using isometric exercises (Thiske, 1969). The patient tightens the muscles in the back of the neck and makes a double chin (military posture) to the count of five; this is repeated 10 times. Patients are encouraged to do this exercise four or five times per day.

As far as the lumbar area is concerned, pain in the buttocks, thighs, and legs can be caused by a combination of entrapment of nerve roots by discs, apophyseal joints, and adjacent soft tissue, which may contribute to foraminal stenosis. There is often a long-standing history of recurrent low back pain related to a congenital narrowing of the neural canal. Aging and degenerative changes bring on further narrowing and the clinical syndrome of spinal stenosis.

Spinal stenosis, especially of the lumbar spine, most commonly occurs in elderly patients with spondylosis with encroachment of osteophytes into the spinal canal or neural foramina. This may manifest as a phenomenon known as *neurogenic claudication* in which the patient experiences calf and/or thigh/buttock pain while walking. Relief typically occurs when the patient sits down, which helps to differentiate the problem from vascular claudication. The symptoms of vascular claudication are often alleviated when ambulation ceases, but sitting down is not usually necessary for relief. The presence of the above history in an elderly patient (or one who suffers from Paget's disease) with strong distal pulses, should make the clinician very suspicious. A CT or magnetic resonance imaging (MRI) scan of the spine should be taken and, if stenosis is present, orthopedic or neurosurgical consultation should be obtained. Corrective surgery often gives dramatic relief. Age alone should not be a deterrent in cases of spinal stenosis, especially because medical management of this condition is far from ideal and the quality of life can be greatly enhanced by a relatively safe and effective procedure.

For those patients who are not surgical candidates and/or have such severe pain that the above remedies are simply inadequate, the use of opioids is, indeed, appropriate. The pain can be so severe that sleep may be adversely affected (Drewes, 1999). Several long-acting preparations such as extended release morphine (Avinza®; Caldwell et al., 2002), controlled-release oxycodone (OxyContin™; Lacouture et al., 1996) and transdermal fentanyl (Duragesic patch™; Milligan et al., 2001) are FDA-approved for moderate to severe pain. While used extensively in the treatment of terminally ill patients with pain related to underlying malignancy, they can be used with success in patients with moderate to severe pain of musculoskeletal origin such as osteoarthritis (Schug et al., 1991). The dose of such medications should be determined by the unique needs of each individual patient (Galer et al., 1992).

The use of short-acting opioids such as oxycodone/acetaminophen (Percocet®) or hydrocodone/acetaminophen (Vicodin®) combinations can be used when pain increases due to weather changes, increased physical activity, or other causes. A word of caution: because of the abuse potential of opioid preparations and regulatory scrutiny, it is prudent for those pain practitioners who prescribe such medications to enter into a formal pain management agreement with each patient receiving such prescriptions. The agreement should clearly specify that the patient must be seen at regular intervals (usually monthly), obtain opioid prescriptions from only one practitioner, and act in a responsible manner. The agreement may call for urine drug screening or other methods, such as random pill counts to test compliance. If the patient fails to abide by the terms of the agreement, no further opioid prescriptions should be written for that patient. The agreement makes it clear that the prescribing and use of opioids can be done only under specified conditions to which both parties (i.e., patient and practitioner) must adhere. This leaves little room for confusion or disagreement. Not intended to be a hardship, this agreement is an aid in the treatment of patients with recalcitrant severe pain.

INFLAMMATORY CONDITIONS

Unlike degenerative diseases such as OA, inflammatory conditions — such as SLE, RA, and vasculitis (e.g., polyarteritis nodosa, giant cell arteritis, or cryoglobulinemia) — are not only painful conditions, but also can be life-threatening. The musculoskeletal manifestations of these systemic diseases can be quite severe and can affect the nervous system directly through the deposition and activation of immune complexes.

RA is a chronic inflammatory connective tissue disease that can be potentially crippling and even life-threatening (Harris, 1990). It typically affects diarthrodial joints, but can also cause such extra-articular manifestations as scleritis, pericarditis, lymphadenopathy, arteritis, nodulosis, splenomegaly, neutropenia, anemia, and pleural effusions/pleuritis. The systemic nature of RA is reflected by the presence of an increased erythrocyte sedimentation rate, the presence of rheumatoid factor, antinuclear antibody, other autoantibodies, anemia (usually anemia of chronic disease, but iron deficiency anemia may also be present), or low plasma albumin in some, but not necessarily all, patients.

RA is found worldwide and is extremely common (approximately 1% of the U.S. population is believed to be affected) with the female to male ratio of 3:1. Peak incidence is between the ages of 40 and 60. Mild cases are usually treated symptomatically by patients using over-the-counter preparations, while more seriously afflicted individuals seek the services of their primary care doctor. The direct and indirect costs of RA are staggering (Clarke et al., 1997; Yelin & Wanke, 1999). Rheumatologists usually see more severe cases, especially when disease-modifying antirheumatic drugs (DMARDs) or remittive agents are needed in addition to NSAIDs and/or oral glucocorticosteroids. DMARDs are slow-acting agents whose function is to prevent RA from crippling, and they are also helpful in controlling systemic problems (Furst, 1990). Gold salts (injectable or oral), *d*-penicillamine, sulfasalazine, and hydroxychlorogorine were used over a decade ago with some success, but more recently immunosuppressive agents, such as methotrexate, azathioprine, and cyclosporin, have been used with greater success in halting the ravages of RA. However, even the immuno-

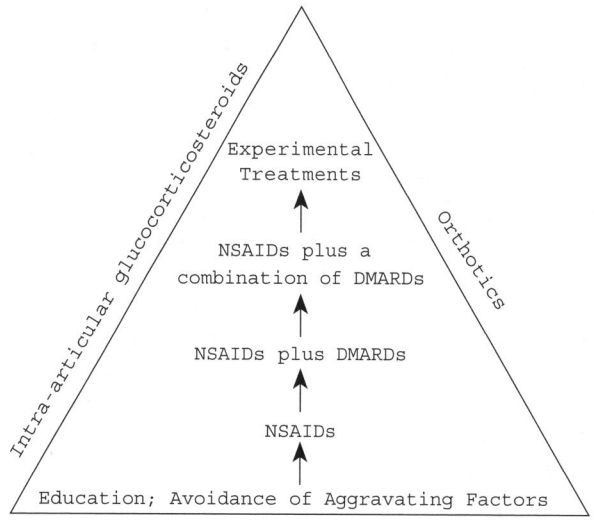

FIGURE 32.1 Treatment pyramid for RA.

suppressive agents were less than ideal due to either unacceptable side effects (e.g., bone marrow failure, hepatotoxicity, nephrotoxicity) or lack of efficacy. Within the past 5 years, leflunomide (Arava®), etanercept (Enbrel®), infliximab (Remicade®), and anakinra (Kineret®) have been introduced. In contrast to the first agent, which is a pharmaceutical, the last three are biological preparations. Each has been shown to be effective in treating many patients with RA already on methotrexate (Maini, Breedveld, & Kalden, 1998; Smolen et al., 1999; Weinblatt, Kremer, & Bankhurst, 1999). Leflunomide inhibits pyrimidine synthesis while etanercept blocks the action of tumor necrosis factor alpha (TNF-alpha), a substance necessary for the autoimmune inflammatory synovitis in RA. Infliximab, a monoclonal antibody, also neutralizes the activity of TNF-alpha, thus reducing disease activity (Lipsky, VanderHeijde, & St. Clair, 2000). Anakinra, on the other hand, inhibits interleukin-1 (IL-1), another cytokine that is produced in excess in patients with RA and contributes to its pathogenesis (Jiang et al., 2000).

For patients with particularly severe RA that is unresponsive to various combinations of one NSAID and a single DMARD, combinations of DMARDs have been used with success (McCarty et al., 1995a). The treatment pyramid for RA is shown in Figure 32.1.

Lately, many rheumatologists have chosen to deal with RA much more aggressively, initiating treatment with NSAIDs plus DMARDs earlier rather than later (Wiske & Healey, 1990). Suffice it to say, the rationale regarding RA therapy has undergone some changes recently (Mikuls & O'Dell, 2000). Many rheumatologists have abandoned the pyramid in patients with severe RA because delays in aggressive therapy can lead to irreversible joint damage and possibly severe systemic pathology. Each patient is unique, and given the variety of medications and techniques now at our disposal, it is more likely than ever that a safe, individualized treatment can be designed to fit each patient.

A word of caution: DMARDs with NSAIDs tend to have potentially more serious side effects than NSAIDs used alone. Alopecia, lowering of blood count (red blood count and/or white blood count and/or platelet count), hepatotoxicity, gastrointestinal upset, and oral ulceration are common to all DMARDs. Gold salts can cause renal problems and rashes, as can *d*-penicillamine, which can also cause such bizarre problems as polymyositis, a myasthenia gravis-type syndrome, and obliterative bronchiolitis. For this reasons, *d*-penicillamine is rarely used these days. Cyclosporin use can cause renal failure. It also is rarely used in the treatment of RA.

Leflonamide can cause hepatotoxicity and other side effects such as rash, diarrhea, and reversible alopecia. Etanercept must not be given to patients at risk for serious infection as it is immunosuppressive and may exacerbate infectious processes. One disadvantage in using etanercept is that it needs to be injected subcutaneously (25 mg.) twice a week. Another is cost — wholesale price for 6 month's treatment would be $6,000 to $7,000. For severe refractory RA, intravenous infliximab has been given in multiple administrations. The cost of three doses for a 70-kg patient would easily be several thousand dollars. This cost must be weighed against the potential benefit and, of course, potential life-threatening side effects.

The other biologic agent, anakinra (Kineret), must also be given subcutaneously (every 2 weeks) and can have the same drawbacks as etanercept and infliximab (Jiang et al., 2000). However, their efficacy has been demonstrated and these preparations have been a godsend for many RA sufferers.

Like OA, RA can involve weight-bearing joints in addition to its capacity to involve the small joints of the hands, wrists, feet, ankles, and elbows in a symmetrical manner. Often when knees are involved, large effusions result in aspiration and injection that can be dramatically effective (McCarty et al., 1995a). Analysis of synovial fluid generally shows an elevated white cell count (usually 10,000 to 50,000/μl) with a predominance of polymorphonuclear leukocytes. Complement levels in RA synovial fluid are generally low and rheumatoid factors are often found; however, this testing tends to be of only limited benefit as it usually does not affect the course of treatment. A more dramatic, convenient, and inexpensive test is the observation that RA synovial fluid is watery compared with the more viscous fluid found in joint fluid from patients wit OA and normal controls. This is because the hyaluronic acid and other macromolecular synovial fluid components have been degraded by the inflammatory mediators, such as superoxides, enzymes, lymphokines present in the affected joint.

If an inflamed RA knee develops a large effusion that becomes chronic, a popliteal or Baker's cyst may develop. Most of the time, the communication between the joint space and the cyst is one-way and this valve effect can cause high pressures in the popliteal space. Because fluid is incompressible, a rupture of the cyst can occur. The release of a large volume of fluid that contains inflammatory mediators posteriorly between the medial head of the gastrocnemius muscle and the tendinous insertion of the biceps femoris muscle can cause the affected calf to become swollen, red, and intensely painful. The patient thus involved can present to the physician with a problem that resembles acute thrombophlebitis. The Homen's sign is frequently positive, thus causing some confusion. A positive arthrogram (with or without a negative venogram, depending on the circumstances) can establish the presence or absence of a Baker's cyst. Treatment with intra-articular steroids, rest, elevation, and attention to the underlying rheumatological conditions should be effective in the vast majority of cases. Surgical synovectomy may occasionally be necessary. A word of caution: treating a patient with a Baker's cyst using an intravenous anticoagulant, like heparin (the preferred treatment for acute thrombophlebitis), is not only ineffective, but may be counterproductive, causing painful ecchymoses in the calf tissues that have become hyperemic from the inflammation.

Although many reports of improved and "unorthodox" treatments for RA are sprinkled throughout the lay press and touted by some health care professionals, it is important to remember that testimonials and endorsements are not a substitute for sound scientific research. However, one must keep an open mind regarding new RA therapies. Three recent studies offer examples of the utility of treatments not ordinarily thought of as antirheumatic that have been shown to be effective in treating RA: fish oil (Kremer et al., 1995) and an antibiotic, minocycline (Kloppenburg et al., 1994; Tilley et al., 1995). The clinician must weigh what he or she feels is the potential benefit versus the possible risks/toxicities of each therapeutic intervention and prescribe accordingly. RA may be unpredictable and often periodic reassessments of the patients' conditions need to be made with attendant adjustments in therapeutic regimen changes in therapy.

Other painful problems that can occur in RA are the development of fibromyalgia, severe metatarsalgia (often helped by wearing 3/8-inch metatarsal bars on the soles of the shoes), carpal tunnel syndrome (median nerve compression neuropathy), chest pain due to either pleuritis or pericarditis, and Sjogren's syndrome (a chronic autoimmune/inflammatory disorder that results in keratoconjunctivitis/sicca and xerostomia). The dry eyes associated with the last condition are painful and annoying, and other mucous membranes can also become affected. The lack of vaginal secretions can make sexual intercourse painful. If food is not chewed well and eaten with frequent sips of water, it may become lodged in the throat. The paucity of saliva (with its attendant antibacterial activity) can lead to painful dental caries and frequently loss of teeth. Other complications of RA are legion but their enumeration and description fall outside the scope of this chapter.

SLE is a potentially very dangerous autoimmune disease that can call attention to itself by pain in various structures. When inflammation affects the pleura (pleuritis), severe chest pain occurs. Joint involvement can cause arthritis. Unlike RA, the arthritis associated with SLE tends not to cause erosion and destruction of bone and cartilage. Other painful manifestations of SLE include myositis, pericarditis, pancreatitis, thrombophlebitis, and mesenteric vasculitis. The pain the patient with SLE experiences may herald a life-threatening situation or be due to concomitant fibromyalgia (Romano, 1992). The clinician must be alert to this disease process affecting virtually any organ or organ system.

SLE tends to occur primarily in young women with a prevalence of about 1 in 2000 individuals (although prevalence and prognosis may vary; Ward, Pyun, & Studenski, 1995). Some medications can cause SLE. The most common offenders are hydralazine, procaineamide, phentoin, and phenothiazines. (Yung & Richardson, 1994). Diagnosis can be made by applying standard criteria (Tan, Cohen, & Fries, 1982). The presence of antinuclear antibody (ANA) is a hallmark of SLE (Tan, 1989) but ANA is nonspecific. Antibodies to double-stranded DNA, low levels of serum complement, and Smith antigen are more specific indicators of SLE and SLE-like processes (Davis, Cumming, & Verrier-Jones, 1977; Schur, 1975). Treatment is aimed at quickly suppressing the overactive immune system and often includes the use of oral corticosteroids such as prednisone or prednisolone. Many patients with SLE require antimalarial drugs such as hydroxy chloroquine; immunosuppressive agents such as cyclophosphamide, azathioprine, and cyclosporin A; or folic acid antagonists such as methotrexate. These agents need to be prescribed with great care due to many potentially serious side effects (Bacon, Treuhaft, & Goodman, 1981; Murtis & Horsman, 1979; Spalton, Verdon Roe, & Hughes, 1993). The use of such dangerous agents is justified because untreated SLE can lead to severe morbidity affecting virtually any organ system (Gladman, 1995) and can be potentially life-threatening.

Hormonal therapy, specifically with male hormones such as dehydroepiandrosterone (DHEA) and danazol, has been shown to favorably affect outcomes in SLE (van Vollenhoven, Engleman, & McGuire, 1995; West et al., 1988). The goal of treatment is not only the alleviation of symptoms such as pain and shortness of breath, but also the protection of organs at risk for serious damage. Often the treatment of drug-induced SLE consists of removing the offending medication and providing symptomatic relief.

However, as with most illnesses and injuries, the patient who is well informed can better collaborate with the health care professional to attain optimal results. An example of an informative booklet written for patients with SLE is *The Lupus Book* (Wallace, 1995). The Arthritis Foundation (Atlanta, GA) publishes pamphlets, each of which provides patients with information regarding many rheumatologic problems including SLE. Because the clinical manifestations of SLE are indeed protean and the potential for serious morbidity so great, the patient with SLE should be armed with adequate information to fully participate in his or her care.

MISCELLANEOUS CONDITIONS

Perhaps in no other area is the skill of the rheumatologist (vis-à-vis internist) put to more of a test than in the realm of such miscellaneous conditions as endocrine, metabolic, infectious, or neoplastic diseases that present with musculoskeletal signs and symptoms. The patient with a disease that fits into one of the above categories has more than a muscle, joint, bone, or soft tissue problem, but this may not be obvious early in the course of the disease, less so if the condition behaves in an atypical manner. One must remember, however, that FS can coexist with any of these disorders (Hudson, Goldenberg, Pope et al., 1992). In fact, FS has even been described in patients infected with human immunodeficiency virus (Simms, Zerbini, Ferrante et al., 1992).

The musculoskeletal problems attendant to certain endocrine diseases may be the first clue that an endocrinopathy is present. The rheumatological signs and symptoms are often eminently treatable and even curable if the underlying endocrine abnormality is rectified (Bland et al., 1979). If the patient presents with myofascial pain (especially fibromyalgia), carpal tunnel syndrome, shoulder capsulitis (periarthritis), crystal deposition disease (e.g., pseudogout due to calcium pyrophosphate deposition disease), proximal myopathy, or osteopenia (osteoporosis and/or osteomalacia), the presence of an underlying endocrine disorder should be strongly considered. Endocrine problems including, but not limited to, parathyroid disease (both hypo- and hyperparathyroidism), adrenal disorders, and diabetes mellitus can be causative or contributing to the development of the above rheumatologic problems.

The patient suffering from hyperparathyroidism often presents with back pain and even vertebral fractures that mimic osteoporosis senilis (Dauphine, Riggs, & Schlotz, 1975). Generalized muscular aching and stiffness, joint laxity and accompanying arthralgia from hypermobility, erosive OA (Resnick, 1974), spontaneous tender avulsion/rupture, and neuromyopathy (Patten et al., 1974) can also raise the suspicion of the presence of hyperparathyroidism, especially if serum calcium determinations are elevated. Some 35% of patients with hyperparathyroidism have chondracalcinosis (Pritchard & Jessop, 1977). Acute arthritis in the setting of an acute myocardial infarction or postoperatively may be due to gout or pseudogout. A synovial fluid analysis that includes a crystal examination helps establish this diagnosis.

At the opposite end of the spectrum, the patient with hypoparathyroidism may present with signs and symptoms (typically back pain) of ankylosing spondylitis (Chaykin, Frame, & Sigler, 1969), carpopedal spasm with tingling due to the low serum calcium, as well as muscle cramps.

Musculoskeletal complaints seem to be associated with adrenal overactivity and adrenal underactivity, the latter condition (Addison's disease) frequently manifesting itself as severe muscle cramping. Cortisol excess (Cushing's syndrome) can be idiopathic or due to treatment with glucocorticosteroids, and severe osteoporosis may ensue with compression fractures of the spine and ribs, proximal muscle wasting, and possible aseptic necrosis of bone (especially the femoral head). When exogenous corticosteroids are withdrawn, pseudorheumatism (diffuse muscle, joint, and bony aching) may occur. It is imperative to be aware of this, as such a problem can have the same symptoms as a flare of certain types of arthritis for which the medication may have been prescribed in the first place. When and if such symptoms occur, their interpretation in light of the patient's clinical course is crucial for optimal management because pseudorheumatism usually abates gradually with a slowing down of the steroid tapering schedule and the administration of mild non-narcotic analgesics. However, a flare of RA, for example, could demand a much more thorough reassessment and revision of the treatment plan.

Thyroid disease often affects the musculoskeletal system and its manifestations are protean. Hypothyroidism often presents with a myopathy, with profound muscle weakness and elevated serum muscle enzymes. It can be confused with inflammatory disorders of muscles, such as polymyositis or dermatomyositis. The peripheral joints of hypothyroid patients with myxedema may be swollen in a symmetrical fashion much like the joints in rheumatoid arthritis (Dorwart & Schumacher, 1975).

In contrast to the joint fluid from patients with RA, the synovial fluid aspirated from the joints of hypothyroid patients is definitely not inflammatory. It is thick and highly viscous, with white cell counts of 1,000 cells/mm³ or less. Thyroid replacement often results in dramatic resolution of the above rheumatic problems.

If a patient has an overactive thyroid, rheumatic problems often manifest. Diffusely swollen and painful hands and feet associated with periostis (thyroid acropachy) can be seen in Graves' disease as can thyrotoxic myopathy, bone pain caused by osteopenia, shoulder periarthritis, and shoulder-hand syndrome complicating adhesive capsulitis (Wohlgethan, 1987). Musculoskeletal pain may also occur

with Hashimoto's thyroiditis. This disorder has been seen with increased frequency in association with RA and possibly other connective tissue disease (Gordon et al., 1981; Smiley, Husain, & Indenbaum, 1980). Ironically, one of the treatments of hyperthyroidism, the administration of propylthiouracil, has been reported to cause such rheumatic diseases as SLE (Amrheim, Kenney, & Ross, 1970) and vasculitis (Houston et al., 1979).

Diabetes mellitus, probably the most common endocrine disease, also has numerous rheumatologic manifestations (Gray & Gottlieb, 1976). Painful neuropathy may first bring the patient with diabetes to the attention of the pain specialist. Other problems, such as Charcot joints are often not completely painless and confused with osteomyelitis (Sinha, Munichoodappa, & Kozak, 1972). Other conditions to which patients with diabetes are susceptible, shoulder periarthritis (Bridgman, 1972), carpal tunnel syndrome and palmar flexor tendinitis (Jung et al., 1971), and a scleroderma-like digital sclerosis (Seibold, 1982), can plague the patient with diabetes. The rheumatologist often encounters patients with both adult and juvenile onset diabetes who have painless contractures of the proximal and distal interphalangeal joints. Recognition of these conditions is important because such microvascular complications as nephropathy and retinopathy may parallel the development and progression of these contractures (Fitzcharles et al., 1984).

Excess pituitary secretion of growth hormone, which causes acromegaly, can result in a characteristic arthropathy that mirrors the enhanced action of this hormone on bone, cartilage, and periarticular soft tissue. With regard to the diarthrodral joints, early cartilage hypertrophy causes the joint space to be abnormally wide, as seen on radiograph. This cartilage tends to break down more easily than normal cartilage, and such patients develop OA at a relatively early age. Carpal tunnel syndrome is also common. Spinal pain and polyarthritis have been reported to respond dramatically when the underlying pituitary disorder is treated successfully (Lachs & Jacobs, 1986). The importance of the identification and treatment of the underlying endocrine problem is crucial to alleviating the pain and suffering of patients with endocrine disease in whom musculoskeletal manifestations may be severe.

It should be noted that FS often coexists with endocrine problems (Crofford, 1996; Griep, Buersmat, & deKloet, 1993) necessitating even more vigilance and circumspection on the part of the clinician. Clearly, the most common metabolic disease that causes musculoskeletal pain in the general population is osteopenia. The scope of this problem is enormous and the differential diagnosis lengthy (Table 32.2). Acute bone fracture can result from osteopenia, and thousands of patients suffer from hip fractures annually, making it a major public health problem with high morbidity and mortality. Metabolic bone disease can also cause muscular pain and weakness, symptoms of which are often

TABLE 32.2
Differential Diagnosis of Generalized Osteopenia in Adults

Osteoporosis	Parallel loss of mineral and matrix
	Predisposing factors including aging, menopause, female sex, white or Asian race, immobilization, low physical activity, inadequate dietary calcium, smoking, alcohol, corticosteroid therapy, family history
Osteomalacia	Inadequate mineralization of bones, matrix
	Differential diagnosis includes:
	Vitamin D deficiency: Inadequate intake, low sunlight exposure, drug-induced catabolism of vitamin D, intestinal malabsorption
	Phosphate-wasting syndrome; Acquired renal tubular defects, with isolated phosphate loss, combined tubular defects (Fanconi's syndrome, renal tubular acidosis, antacid abuse
Osteitis fibrosa	PTH-induced increase in mineral and matrix reabsorption
	Differential diagnosis includes:
	Primary hyperparathyroidism
	Secondary hyperparathyroidism: Vitamin D deficiency states, primary decrease in intestinal calcium absorption with age, reduced renal mass (chronic renal insufficiency)
Glucocorticoid-induced osteopenia	Differential diagnosis includes:
	Iatrogenic
	Adrenal corticosteroid overproduction: Indiopathi (Cushing's syndrome)
Other disorders	Hyperparathyroidism
	Diffuse osteolytic malignancies (e.g., multiple myeloma)
	Congenital disorders: Osteogenesis imperfecta tarda, vitamin D–resistant rickets

confused with other musculoskeletal conditions. Osteopenia can also occur in patients who have other rheumatic diseases, especially those necessitating long-term glucocorticosteroid treatment (Hahn & Hahn, 1976).

The scope of the problem is so vast that a chapter devoted to it could not even begin to outline the problem and discuss therapy. However, some major factors need to be considered. The patient with osteopenia usually has osteoporosis (loss of bone mineral and matrix in parallel), osteomalacia (accumulation of unmineralized matrix after loss of bone mineral), hyperparathyroidism with osteitis fibrosa (replacement of bone by fibrous tissue), or cortisteroid-induced osteopenia. The last problem often is unavoidable due to the patients' need for such medication, but the ability of steroids to interfere with calcium absorption from the intestine may be partially overcome by the

administration of calcium and vitamin D supplementation (Hahn et al., 1979). The use of these medications is recommended for patients with osteoporosis senilis, as is estrogen, fluoride, calcitonin, biphosphonates, or a combination of these agents based on the individual patient's needs. Gastrointestinal distress may accompany the use of diphosphanates (aldetronate, Fosama®; risedtronate, Actonel®). This side effect has been minimized by the introduction of preparations that can be taken once weekly. The best method of treating osteoporosis is prevention, if feasible. Patients at risk, typically sedentary, small-framed women approaching menopause who smoke and drink alcohol and who have low calcium and vitamin D intake, should use preventative measures such as regular exercise, adequate intake of calcium and vitamin D (Matkovic et al., 1979; NIH Consensus Conference, 1984), and consultation with a physician who may feel that other measures, such as estrogen therapy, are necessary.

The most common causes of osteomalacia in adults are decreased absorption of vitamin D due to intestinal or biliary tract disease, accelerated catabolism of vitamin D due to drug-induced increases in hepatic oxidase activity, and acquired renal tubular defects with phosphate wasting. Correcting the cause of the metabolic problem is necessary for reversal of the osteomalacia.

While not as common as osteopenia, Paget's disease of bone is a frequent cause of bony pain and is estimated to affect 1 to 3% of people over the age of 45 in the United States. It is usually polyostotic, and men tend to predominate. While the cause of Paget's disease (osteitis deformans) is unknown, late manifestation of viral infection has been suggested. It is characterized by excessive bone resorption followed by excessive bone formation, culminating in a bizarre mosaic pattern of lamellar bone associated with increased local vascularity and increased fibrous tissue in adjacent marrow (Smiger et al., 1977). The disease is a focal disorder, as normal bone exists even in patients severely affected. The sites most commonly involved are the pelvis, skull, femur, tibia, and spine. In addition to pain, gross deformity, compression of neural structures, fracture of involved bone, and alteration of joint structure/function often result. Increased serum alkaline phosphatase and urinary hydroxproline reflect the increased bone turnover in this disease. An infrequent (<1%) but dreaded complication of Paget's disease is osteosarcoma. Other associated neoplasms include non-neoplastic granulomas and giant cell tumors.

Paget's disease can be asymptomatic with little clinical disability and, therefore, no therapy may be necessary (Altman & Singer, 1980). However, specific therapy is available for patients who are suffering. While NSAIDs help control pain, they do not affect the biochemical abnormalities. Disodium etidronate, a diphophonate compound (Krane, 1982), decreases bone resorption, but this oral agent should be given for no longer than 6 months at a time. Bone pain usually responds to this medication, but a temporary paradoxical increase in bone pain may occur in some patients. Subcutaneous injections of synthetic salmon calcitonin are also used to provide pain relief and help prevent deformity. Clinical improvement usually occurs within a month or two. Some patients may become refractory to this medication if they produce neutralizing antibodies to this salmon protein.

Joint pain can be caused by a variety of pathophysiological mechanisms. While disorders such as RA, OA, and SLE are chronic and incurable causes of arthritis and arthralgia, infectious agents can cause an acute arthritis, which with early detection and proper management can be cured with little or no permanent sequelae.

While any infectious agent can cause septic arthritis, pyogenic bacterial arthritis causes the most rapidly destructive form of infectious arthritis. Bacterial arthritis is usually divided into two groups, that caused by *Neisseria gonorrhea* and that caused by other bacteria (e.g., staphylococci, enteric organisms). Most cases of bacterial arthritis are the result of hematogenous spread to the affected joint(s). Other causes include direct infection from a puncture wound or skin infection. Once inside the joint space, the infectious agent multiplies rapidly, and the inflammatory response can become very severe, causing so much joint swelling and intense pain that the patient can neither actively extend nor flex the affected joint. Usually, such patients are febrile with high peripheral white blood cell counts. If untreated, the infection can cause destruction of cartilage and bone, as a result of a direct toxic effect of the bacteria and enzymatic destruction from purulent inflammatory exudates (Goldenberg & Reed, 1985). *Staphylococcus aureus* and Gram-negative bacilli often destroy joints rapidly, whereas other organisms, such as *Streptococcus pneumoniae* and *N. gonorrhea*, cause damage much more slowly.

To make a correct diagnosis, an aspiration of the affected joint needs to be performed under aseptic conditions and the fluid sent for cell count, differential, and culture. A septic joint typically has a white cell count in excess of 50,000 cells/mm^3 with predominance (often 90%) of polymorphonuclear leukocytes. It may take several days for the offending organism to grow in culture, and therapy should not be delayed. The prompt initiation of intravenous antibiotics, the exact nature of which depends on the likelihood of having a particular organism under certain clinical conditions, may be critical. Periodic joint aspiration and reassessment need to be performed while the patient is hospitalized. Depending on the organism, intravenous antibiotics need to be administered from 2 to 6 weeks. Some patients can be managed with home intravenous therapy at the discretion of the physician.

Patients at risk for the development of septic arthritis include patients taking systemic or locally injected corticosteroids, immunocompromised patients, and patients

TABLE 32.3
Types of Tumors of Joint, Tendon Sheaths, and Bursae

Benign

Neoplasms and tumoral conditions
    Pigmented villonodular synovitis
    Synovial chondromatosis (osteochondromatosis)
    Other benign tumors: lipoma including lipoma arborescens,
      chondroma, hemangioma, fibroma
Tumor-like lesions
    Ganglion bursitis, synovial cyst, parameniscal cyst, nodules

Malignant

Primary
    Synovial sarcoma (malignant synovioma); biphasic and monophasic
    Clear cell sarcoma
    Epithelioid sarcoma
    Synovial chondrosarcoma
Secondary
    Metastatic carcinomatous arthritis
    Joint invasion by leukemia, lymphoma, myeloma
    Continuous spread of malignant bone tumors

with hemarthroses. Among otherwise young, healthy patients, disseminated gonococcal infection is the most common cause of septic arthritis in the urban population. Increasing in prevalence (Veasy et al., 1987), although still considered uncommon, is acute rheumatic fever, which is an inflammatory disease induced by an antecedent group A beta-hemolytic streptococcal pharyngitis. The most common features are carditis and polyarthritis. The Jones criteria enable the physician to establish the diagnosis (Stollerman et al., 1965) and act as a guide in the evaluation of patients with polyarthritis of unknown etiology.

Patients with neoplastic diseases often are seen by a rheumatologist for musculoskeletal symptoms. Primary neoplasms of bursae, joints, and tendon sheaths are uncommon (Jaffe, 1958). Most arise from the synovium and are benign. Tumor-like swelling in and around a joint most likely is the result of inflammatory and traumatic lesions and, hence, should not be considered true neoplasms. However, tumors can occur (see Table 32.3). More often, secondary neoplastic involvement of joints occurs as a complication of contiguous spread of primary bone sarcomas, invasion by hematologic malignancies such as leukemia, lymphoma, myeloma, or carcinomatous metastases (Schajowica, 1982).

Most subtle involvement of the musculoskeletal system with malignancy manifests itself as the group of disorders and is termed paraneoplastic syndromes. True paraneoplastic syndromes include myopathies, arthropathies, and other conditions such as hypertrophic pulmonary osteoarthropathy, amyloidosis, and secondary gout. Polyarthritis resembling RA may be the presenting sign of malignancy (Calabro, 1967). The cause is unknown, but the action of circulating immune complexes and alterations in cellular immunity have been offered as explanations (Awerbuch & Brooks, 1981; Robins & Baldwin, 1978). In addition, a syndrome similar to SLE has been reported in association with underlying malignancies (Pierce et al., 1979; Wallack, 1977). Unfortunately, other rheumatic conditions, such as polymyalgia rheumatica, scleroderma, necrotizing vasculitis, cryoglobulimenia with Raynaud's phenomenon (seen most commonly with metastatic malignancy), and reflex sympathetic dystrophy have been associated with various malignancies. This confusing picture often requires much in the way of energy and expertise to understand and properly treat the specific condition(s).

ROLE OF THE RHEUMATOLOGIST IN THE MULTIDISCIPLINARY APPROACH TO THE TREATMENT OF THE PATIENT WITH PAIN: THE RHEUMATOLOGIST AS A "TEAM PLAYER"

To paraphrase the eminent poet John Donne, no physician is an island, especially when it comes to the treatment of the patient with pain. Often the physician needs to coordinate the efforts of several health care professionals (e.g., orthopedists, neurologists, anesthesiologists, counselors, psychologists, physical therapists) and educate his or her colleagues regarding the special requirements of such patients. Physical therapy, for example, is an extremely useful adjunct in the treatment of many patients who require specialty care. However, the approach of the physical therapist needs to be individualized to each and every patient he or she sees. Most physical therapists see patients with such varied disorders as strokes, arthritis, postsurgical states, sports injuries, and myofascial pain syndromes. The stroke victim has different pathology and hence different needs than the patient with RA or adhesive capsulitis of the shoulder. While general principles of physical therapy usually are the same for all patients, the practical application of these principles can vary greatly from patient to patient depending on the problem. The patient with arthritis of the knees, for example, who requires quadriceps muscle strengthening therapy to combat atrophy of the thigh muscles due to disuse requires different management if a concomitant myofascial pain syndrome (MPS) is also present. The same is true for work-hardening programs. If the deconditioned patient with a regional MPS enrolls in a standard program, he or she will be unable to tolerate the strengthening exercises as they will exacerbate the condition (Travell, 1990, personal communication). It is only when the rheumatologist or other pain specialist treats the MPS successfully, that work-hardening can proceed.

The physical therapist can play a pivotal role in treating MPS with spray-and-stretch techniques, massage, acupressure, local heat, or ultrasound. In fact, the therapist

often can alert the referring physician to the possibility that the patient may have a concomitant regional MPS if the patient in question has a paradoxical response to correctly applied physical therapy modalities. As mentioned above, if work-hardening causes increased pain, one should suspect a regional MPS. The same principle holds true for cervical traction, a very useful treatment for chronic cervical radiculopathies. If, in addition, the patient has a regional MPS in the vicinity of the occiput or cervical musculature or trapezius/rhomboid areas, the force of the correctly applied traction applied to taut muscles usually results in more pain rather than less. Such a scenario should alert the therapist to the possibility of a regional MPS and this information should be shared with the referring physician. If the MPS persists, rheumatologic or physiatric consultation should be obtained.

Often, patients with FS, RA, or SLE with bothersome neuritic symptoms need the expertise of a neurologist to help determine if peripheral neuropathy, nerve entrapment, or another neurological problem exists. Tests such as electromyograms (EMGs), nerve conduction studies, somatosensory evoked potentials (SEPs), and radiographic studies (e.g., CT scans, MRI scans) may need to be done to complement the neurological examination and more precisely define (or rule out) a particular problem. FS sufferers tend to have an exacerbation of their symptoms after EMGs, probably due to their abnormal perception of pain and aberrant central processing. In fact, the first clue that a patient may have FS is often the observation that the patient in question, who is being treated or evaluated by a neurologist for numbness, tingling, or lancinating pain, behaves quite differently from other patients with similar symptoms. The patient may report that the EMG was very painful and may, in fact, terminate his or her participation in the study before it is completed due to unbearable pain. The neurologist can be of great help to the patient referred for neuritic symptoms but for whom no definable neurological abnormality can be found. As mentioned earlier gabapentin may be helpful in the management of neuropathic pain. These patients may be suffering from FS or a polyneuropathy/mononeuritis multiplex and should be referred to a rheumatologist or physiatrist for further evaluation.

The orthopedist is frequently called upon to help the rheumatologist when medical management of rheumatologic conditions fails. As mentioned earlier, patients with end-stage osteoarthritic or rheumatoid arthritic changes in knee or hip joints often require total joint replacement. It is up to the rheumatologist to help select suitable candidates for such procedures. The ideal surgical candidate not only has failed conservative measures but is not overweight (the heavier the patient, the more likely the prosthesis may loosen or dislodge), is motivated and intelligent so as not to take undue risks after the procedure is performed (i.e., avoid activities that put increased mechanical stress on the prosthetic joint), and is sufficiently advanced in years so, statistically speaking, the life span of the prosthesis should exceed that of the patient. Conversely, many practicing orthopedists evaluate patients with joint pain who, inspired by media-hype, self-refer themselves for total joint replacement. Some need the procedure, but many others do not. Their arthritis can be managed quite well with a program of anti-inflammatory drug therapy, weight reduction, physical therapy, and orthotic use such as a cane, if necessary. Conservative medical management of this type can often help patients avoid premature and possible unnecessary surgery while adequately controlling their pain.

The rheumatologist is most likely to call upon the services of his or her colleagues in anesthesiology when a patient requires a nerve block for such diverse conditions as occipital neuralgia (as the cause of some chronic headache conditions) and reflex sympathetic dystrophy (which can often complicate arthritic conditions). Many "failed back" patients benefit from lumbar nerve root blocks, which often give effective, albeit temporary, relief from severe pain. Other modalities (outlined elsewhere in this text) can be extremely effective, especially if timely referrals are made.

Frequently, the orthodontist and the rheumatologist need to work together in the treatment of FS patients with temporomandibular joint (TMJ) disorders, as these two entities frequently coexist in the same patient and one can exacerbate the symptoms of the other (TMJ and related disorders are discussed elsewhere in this text).

A valuable ally in treating patients in pain is the psychologist or counselor. Often, patients with chronic painful states such as RA, fibromyalgia, or OA are anxious or depressed or lack coping skills necessary to deal with their pain. Cognitive behavioral approaches to pain such as pain imaging, for example, may be very useful tools in helping patients take an active role in controlling their pain level not just becoming a victim of their disorder. Biofeedback training may help some patients, especially those afflicted with myofascial pain states. Families whose members have painful diseases often are under a great deal of stress and become dysfunctional. Family counseling and/or marital counseling can go a long way in aiding the patient and those around him or her in coping with chronic illness. The patient suffering from chronic pain must avoid the feelings of helplessness and despair that can occur, especially when the patient feels that he or she is a victim and has no control over his or her pain. Overcoming such obstacles is essential for optimal care of the patient with chronic painful states. Insight into how certain aspects of a patient's lifestyle can aggravate the underlying painful condition can also be attained through counseling, thus further benefiting patients and conceivably lessening their need for analgesics and other medications.

While multidisciplinary pain clinics have been a great boon in the treatment and further understanding of the pain patient, they are beyond the reach of many, and probably most, patients. However, that does not mean that such an approach to patients in pain cannot be attempted at the community level. Such an endeavor requires that the professionals caring for the patient strive to cooperate and communicate with each other in order to provide the most conducive atmosphere for encouragement and eventual improvement.

CONCLUSIONS

For the patient who comes to the rheumatologist with a complaint of pain, it is not sufficient for the physician to offer only symptomatic relief. As an internist, as well as a specialist in the rheumatic diseases, the rheumatologist needs to accurately pinpoint the cause of the pain and take appropriate measures to minimize associated morbidity. Investigations necessary for the accurate and prompt identification of the scope of the patient's illness may be costly in terms of time and money, but the advantages of an accurate, early diagnosis and prompt effective treatment far outweigh these other considerations. Patients trust their physicians to care for them when they are suffering. That trust must never be betrayed; patients deserve no less than the very best we have to offer.

REFERENCES

Altman, R. D., & Singer, F. (Eds.). (1980). Proceedings of the Kroc Foundation Conference on Paget's Disease of Bone. *Arthritis and Rheumatism, 23,* 1073–1240.

Altman, R. D., & Moskowitz, R. (1998). Intra-articular sodium hyaluronate (Hyalgan[R]) in the treatment of patients with osteoarthritis of the knee; A randomized clinical trial. *Journal of Rheumatology, 25,* 2203–2211.

Amrheim, J. A., Kenney, F. M., & Ross, D. (1970). Granulocytopenia, lupus-like syndrome, and other complications of propylthiouracil therapy. *Journal of Pediatrics, 74,* 54–63.

Awerbuch, M. S., & Brooks, P. M. (1981). Role of immune complexes in hypertrophic osteoarthropathy and non-metastatic polyarthritis. *Annals of Rheumatic Disease, 40,* 470–472.

Bacon, B. R., Treuhaft, W. H., & Goodman, A. M. (1981). Azathroprone-induced pancytopenia. Occurrence in two patients with connective tissue disease. *Archives of Internal Medicine, 141,* 223–235.

Bergstrom, G. (1985). Joint impairment and disorders at ages 70, 74 and 79. Thesis, University of Gothenburg, Sweden.

Bland, J. H. et al. (1979). Rheumatic syndromes in endocrine disease. *Seminars in Arthritis & Rheumatism, 9,* 23–65.

Brezin, J. H. et al. (1979). Reversible renal failure and nephrotic syndrome associated with non-steroidal anti-inflammatory drugs. *New England Journal of Medicine, 301*, 1271–1273.

Bridgman, J. F. (1972). Periarthritis of the shoulder and diabetes mellitus. *Annals of Rheumatic Disease, 31*, 9–71.

Burkle, M. J., Fear, E. C., & Wright, V. (1977). Bone and joint changes in pneumatic drillers. *Annals of Rheumatic Disease, 36*, 276–279.

Calabro, J. J. (1967). Cancer and arthritis. *Rheumatism, 10*, 553–567.

Caldwell, J. R., et al. (2002). Efficacy and safety of a once-daily morphine formulation in chronic, moderate to severe osteoarthritis pain. *Journal of Pain and Symptom Management, 23*, 278–291.

Case, J. P. et al. (2003). Lack of efficacy of acetaminophen in treating symptomatic knee osteoarthritis. *Archives of Internal Medicine, 163*, 169–178.

Chang, R. W. et al. (1996). A cost-effectiveness analysis of total hip arthroplasty for osteoarthritis of the hip. *Journal of the American Medical Association, 275*, 858–865.

Chavez, M. L., & DeKorte, C. J. (2003). Valdecoxib: A review. *Clinical Therapeutics, 25*, 817–851.

Chaykin, L. B., Frame, B., & Sigler, J. W. (1969). Spondylitis: A clue to hypoparathyroidism. *Annals of Internal Medicine, 70*, 995–1000.

Clarke, A. et al. (1997). Direct and indirect medical costs incurred by Canadian patients with rheumatoid arthritis: A twelve year study. *Journal of Rheumatology, 24*, 1051–1060.

Creamer, P., & Hochbery, M. C. (1997). Osteoarthritis. *Lancet, 350*, 503–509.

Crofford, L. (1996). Stress-response systems in fibromyalgia. *Lyon Mediterranee Medical Tome, 32*, 2138–2142.

Dauphine, R. T., Riggs, B. L., & Schloltz, D. A. (1975). Back pain and vertebral crush fractures: An unemphasized mode of presentation for primary hyperparathyroidism. *Annals of Internal Medicine, 83*, 365–367.

Davis, P., Cumming, R. H., & Verrier-Jones, J. (1977). Relationship between anti-DNA antibodies, complement consumption, and circulating immune complexes in systemic lupus erythematosus. *Clinical and Experimental Immunology, 28(2)*, 226–234.

Day, R. O. et al. (1984). Anti-rheumatic drug interactions. *Clinics of Rheumatic Disease, 10*, 251–275.

Dorwart, B. B., & Schumacher, H. R. (1975). Joint effusion, chondrocalcinosis, and other rheumatic manifestations in hypothyroidism. *American Journal of Medicine, 59*, 780–790.

Drewes, A. M. (1999). Pain and sleep disturbance with special reference to fibromyalgia and rheumatoid arthritis. *Rheumatology, 38*, 1005–1044.

Fields, H. L. (1987). *Pain*. New York: McGraw Hill.

Fitzcharles, M. A. et al. (1984). Limitation of joint mobility (chiroarthropathy) in adult noninsulin-dependent diabetic patients. *Annals of Rheumatic Disease, 43*, 251–257.

Forman, M. D., Malamet, R., & Kaplan, D. (1983). A survey of osteoarthritis of the knee in the elderly. *Journal of Rheumatology, 10*, 282–287.

Fortin, P. R. et al. (1999). Outcomes of total hip and knee replacement: Preoperative functional status predicts outcomes at six months after surgery. *Arthritis and Rheumatism, 42*, 1722–1728.

Fowler, R. W., & Arnold, K. G. (1983). Non-steroidal analgesic and anti-inflammatory agents. *British Medical Journal, 287*, 835.

Fries, J. F., Williams, C. A., & Bloch, D. A. (1991). The relative toxicity of nonsteroidal anti-inflammatory drugs. *Arthritis and Rheumatism, 34*, 1353–1360.

Furst, D. E. (1990). Rational use of disease-modifying anti-rheumatic drugs. *Drugs, 39*, 19–37.

Galer, B. S. et al. (1992). Individual variability in response to different opioids. *Pain, 49*, 87–91.

Ginsburg, F., & Famaey, J. P. (1991). Double-blind, randomized cross over study of the percutaneous efficacy and tolerability of a topical indomethacin spray versus placebo in the treatment of tendinitis. *Journal of International Medical Research, 19*, 131–136.

Gladman, D. D. (1995). Prognosis and treatment of systemic lupus erythematosus. *Current Opinion in Rheumatology, 7*, 402–408.

Goldenberg, D. L., & Reed, J. I. (1985). Bacterial arthritis. *New England Journal of Medicine, 312*, 764–771.

Gordon, M. B. et al. (1981). Thyroid disease in progressive systemic sclerosis: Increased frequency of glandular fibroids and hypothyroidism. *Annals of Internal Medicine, 95*, 431–435.

Graham, D. J., Agranval, N. M., & Roth, S. H. (1988). Prevention of NSAID-induced gastric ulcer with misoprostol: Multicentre, double-blind, placebo-controlled trial. *Lancet, 2*, 1277–1280.

Gray, R. B. & Gottlieb, N. L. (1976). Rheumatic disorders associated with diabetes mellitus: Literature review. *Seminars in Arthritis & Rheumatism, 6*, 19–34.

Griep, E. N., Boersma, J. W., & DeKloet, E. R. (1993). Altered reactivity of the hypothalamic–pituitary–adrenal axis in the primary fibromyalgia syndrome. *Journal of Rheumatology, 20*, 469–474.

Hahn, T. J. & Hahn, B. H. (1976). Osteopenia in patients with rheumatic disease: Principles of diagnosis therapy. *Seminars in Arthritis & Rheumatism, 6*, 165–188.

Hahn, T. J. et al. (1979). Altered mineral metabolism in glucocorticoid-induced osteopenia: Effect of 25-hydroxyvitamin D administration. *Journal of Clinical Investigation, 64*, 655–665.

Harris, E. D. (1990). Mechanisms of disease: Rheumatoid arthritis. Pathophysiology and implications for therapy. *New England Journal of Medicine, 322*, 1277–1289.

Hawker, G. et al. (1998). Health-related quality of life after knee replacement. *Journal of Bone and Joint Surgery (American Volume), 80*, 163–173.

Hollander, J. L. (1972). Intrasynovial corticosteroid therapy in arthritis. *Maryland Medical Journal, 19*, 62–66.

Houston, B. D. et al. (1979). Apparent vasculitis associated with propylthiouracil use. *Arthritis and Rheumatism, 22*, 925–928.

Hudson, J. I., Goldenberg, D. L., Pope, H. G., Keck, P. E., & Schlesinger, L. (1992). Comorbidity of fibromyalgia with medical and psychiatric disorders. *American Journal of Medicine, 92,* 363–367.

Huskisson, E. C., et al. (1976). Four new anti-inflammatory drugs: Responses and variations. *British Medical Journal, 1*(6017), 1048–1049.

Jaffe, H. L. (1958). *Tumors and tumorous conditions of the bone and joints.* Philadelphia: Lea & Febiger.

Jiang, Y., et al. (2000). A multicenter, double-blind, dose-ranging, randomized, placebo-controlled study of recombinant human interleukin-1 receptor antagonist in patients with rheumatoid arthritis. *Arthritis and Rheumatism, 43,* 1001–1009.

Jung, Y. et al. (1971). Diabetic hand syndrome. *Metabolism, 20,* 1008–1015.

Kahan, A., Lleu, P. L., & Salin, L. (2003). Prospective randomized study comparing the medicoeconomic benefits of hylan GF-20 vs. conventional treatment in knee osteoarthritis. *Journal of Bone and Spine (France), 70,* 276-281.

Kloppenburg, M. et al. (1994). Minocycline in active rheumatoid arthritis. A double-blind, placebo-controlled trial. *Arthritis and Rheumatism, 37(5),* 629–636.

Krane, S. M. (1982). Etidronate disodium in the treatment of Paget's disease of bone. *Annals of Internal Medicine, 96,* 619–625.

Kremer, J.M. et al. (1995). Effects of high-dose fish oil on rheumatoid arthritis after stopping nonsteroidal antiinflammatory drugs. *Arthritis and Rheumatism, 38(8),* 1107–1114.

Lachs, S., & Jacobs, R. P. (1986). Acromeglic arthropathy: A reversible rheumatic disease. *Journal of Rheumatology, 13,* 634–636.

Lacouture, P., Roth, S., Burch, F., Fleishmann, R., Iwan, T., & Kaiko, R. (1996). A short-term trial, placebo-controlled, repeated dose, dose-response evaluation of controlled release (CR) oxycodone in patients with osteoarthritis [Abstr. P1–2]. *Clinical Pharmacology and Therapeutics, 59,* 129.

Lane, N. E. et al. (1986). Long-distance running, bone density, and osteoarthritis. *Journal of the American Medical Association, 255,* 1147–1151.

Langman, M. J. et al. (1999). Adverse upper gastrointestinal effects of Rofecoxib compared with NSAIDs. *Journal of the American Medical Association, 282,* 1929–2933.

Lawrence, J. S. (1969). Generalized osteoarthritis in a population sample. *American Journal of Epidemiology, 90,* 381–389.

Lee, M. H. M., Itoh, M., Yang, G. W., & Eason, A. L. (1989). Physical therapy and rehabilitation medicine. In J. J. Bonica (Ed.), *The management of pain* (2nd ed., pp. 1769–1788). Philadelphia, PA: Lee & Febiger.

Leopold, S. S., et al. (2003). Corticosteroid compared with hyaluronic acid injections for the treatment of osteoarthritis of the knee. A prospective randomized trial. *Journal of Bone and Joint Surgery (American Volune), 85,* 1197–1203.

Lipsky, P. E., VanderHeijde, D., & St. Clair, E. W. (2000). Infliximab and methotrexate in the treatment of rheumatoid arthritis. *New England Journal of Medicine, 343,* 1594–1602.

Maini, R. N., Breedveld, & Kalden, (1998). Therapeutic efficacy of multiple intravenous infusions of anti-tumor necrosis factor-alpha monoclonal antibody combined with low dose weekly methotrexate in rheumatoid arthritis. *Arthritis and Rheumatism, 41,* 1552–1563.

Matkovic, V. et al. (1979). Bone status and fracture rates in two regions in Yugoslavia. *American Journal of Clinical Nutrition, 32,* 540–549.

Mense, S.D. (1994). Referral of muscle pain. New aspects. *American Pain Society Journal, 3,* 1–9.

McCarthy, G. M., & McCarty, D. J. (1992). Effect of topical capsaicin in the therapy of painful osteoarthritis of the hands. *Journal of Rheumatology, 19,* 604–607.

McCarty, D. J., et al. (1995a). Treatment of rheumatoid joint inflammation with intrasynovial triamcinolone hexacetanide. *Journal of Rheumatology, 22,* 1631–1635.

McCarty, D. J. et al. (1995b). Combination drug therapy of seropositive rheumatoid arthritis. *Journal of Rheumatology, 22,* 1636–1645.

Mikuls, T. T., & O'Dell, J. (2000). The changing face of rheumatoid arthritis therapy: Results of serial surveys. *Arthritis and Rheumatism, 43,* 464–465.

Milligan, K. et al. (2001). Evaluation of long-term efficacy and safety of transdermal fentanyl in the treatment of chronic noncancer pain. *The Journal of Pain, 2,* 197–204.

Murtis, L., & Horsman, L. R. (1979). Acute hypersensitivity reaction to cyclophosphamide. *Journal of Pediatrics, 94,* 844–847.

NIH Consensus Conference. (1984). Osteoporosis. *Journal of the American Medical Association, 252,* 799–802.

Osiri, M., & Moreland, L. W., (1999). Specific cyclooxygenase alpha inhibitors: A new choice of nonsteroidal anti-inflammatory drug therapy. *Arthritis Care and Research, 12,* 351–362.

Panush, R. S. et al. (1986). Is running associated with degenerative joint disease? *Journal of the American Medical Association, 255,* 1152–1154.

Patten, B. M. et al. (1974). Neuromuscular disease in primary hyperparathyroidism. *Annals of Internal Medicine, 80,* 172–183.

Pierce, D. A. et al. (1979). Immunoblastic sarcoma with features of Sjogren's syndrome and systemic lupus erythematosus in a patient with immunoblastic lymphadenopathy. *Arthritis and Rheumatism, 22,* 911–916.

Pritchard, M. H., & Jessop, J. D. (1977). Chondrocalcinosis in primary hyperparathyroidism. *Annals of Rheumatic Disease, 36,* 146–151.

Puranen, J. et al. (1975). Running and primary osteoarthritis of the hip. *British Medical Journal, 2,* 424–425.

Raynauld, J. P. et al. (2003). Safety and efficacy of long-term intraarticular steroid injections in osteoarthritis of the knee. *Arthritis & Rheumatism, 48,* 370–377.

Resnick, D. L. (1974). Erosive osteoarthritis of the hand and wrist in hyperparathyroidism. *Radiology, 110,* 263–269.

Robins, R. A., & Baldwin, R. W. (1978). Immune complexes in cancer. *Cancer Immunologic Immunotherapy, 4,* 1–3.

Romano, T. J. (1992). Coexistence of the fibromyalgia syndrome and systemic lupus erythematosus. *American Journal of Pain Management, 2*(4), 211–214.

Romano, T. J. (1996). Fibromyalgia syndrome in other rheumatic conditions. *Lyon Meditaranee Medical Mecidine Sudest, Tome XXXII N 5/6,* 2143-2146.

Roth, G. J., & Majerus, P. W. (1975). The mechanism of the effect of aspirin on human platelets. *Journal of Clinical Investigations, 56,* 624–632.

Russell, A. L. (1991). Piroxicam 0.5% topical gel compared to placebo in the treatment of acute soft tissue injuries: A double-blind study comparing efficacy and safety. *Clinical and Investigative Medicine, 14,* 35–43.

Schajowica, F. (1982). *Tumors and tumor-like lesions of bones and joints.* New York: Springer-Verlag.

Schlomka, G., Schroter, G., & Ocherwal, A. (1955). Uber der Bedentung der bernflischer Belastung far die entsehring der degenerativen. *Gelenkleiden Zeitung Gesamte Internal Medicine, 447*(10), 993.

Schug, S. et al. (1991). Treatment principles for the use of opioids in pain of non-malignant origins. *Drugs, 42,* 228–239.

Schumacher, H. R. (1997). *Primer on rheumatic disease* (11th ed.). Atlanta, GA: Arthritis Foundation.

Schur, P. (1975). Complement in lupus. *Clinics in Rheumatic Disease, 1,* 519–524.

Seibold, J. R. (1982). Digital sclerosis in children with insulin-dependent diabetes mellitus. *Arthritis and Rheumatism, 25,* 1357–1361.

Simms, R. W., Zerbini, C. A. F., Ferrante, N., Anothony, J., Felson, D. T., Craven, D. E., and Boston City Hospital Clinical AIDS Team. (1992). Fibromyalgia syndrome in patients infected with human immunodeficiency virus. *American Journal of Medicine, 92,* 368–374.

Simon, L. D. et al. (1999). Anti-inflammatory and upper gastrointestinal effects of Celecoxib in rheumatoid arthritis. *Journal of the American Medical Association, 282,* 1921–1928.

Sinha, S., Munichoodappa, C. S., & Kozak, G. P. (1972). Neuropathy (charcot joints) in diabetes mellitus. *Medicine, 51,* 191–210.

Smiger, F. R. et al. (1977). Paget's disease of bone. In L. V. Avioli & S. M. Kane (Eds.), *Metabolic Bone Disease* (pp. 490–575). New York: Academic Press.

Smiley, A. M., Husain, M., & Indenbaum, S. (1980). Eosinophilic faciitis in association with thyroid disease: A report of three cases. *Journal of Rheumatology, 7,* 871–876.

Smolen, J. S., et al. (1999). Efficacy and safety of leflunomide compared with placebo and sulphasalazine in active rheumatoid arthritis; a double-blind, randomised, multicentre trial. *Lancet, 353,* 259–266.

Spalton, D. J., Verdon Roe, G. M., & Hughes, G. R. V. (1993). Hydroxychlorozine, dosage parameters and retinopathy. *Lupus, 2,* 355-358.

Stollerman, G. H. et al. (1965). Jones criteria (revised) for guidance in the diagnosis of rheumatic fever. *Circulation, 32,* 664–668.

Tan, E. M., Cohen, A. S., & Fries, J. F. (1982). The 1982 revised criteria for the classification of systemic lupus erythematosus. *Arthritis and Rheumatism, 25,* 1271–1277.

Tan, E. M. (1989). Antinuclear antibodies: Diagnostic markers for autoimmune diseases and probes for cell biology. *Advances in Immunology, 44,* 93–151.

Thiske, M. G. (1969). Neck and shoulder pain: Evaluation and conservative management. *Medical Clinics of North America, 53,* 511–524.

Tilley, B. C. et al. (1995). Minocycline in rheumatoid arthritis. *Annals of Internal Medicine, 122,* 81–89.

van Vollenhoven, R. F., Engleman, E. G., & McGuire, J. L. (1995). Dehydroepiandrosterone in systemic lupus erythematosus: Results of a double-blinded placebo-controlled, randomized clinical trial. *Arthritis and Rheumatism, 38,* 1826–1831.

Veasy, L. G. et al. (1987). Resurgence of acute rheumatic fever in the intermountain area of the United States. *New England Journal of Medicine, 316,* 421–427.

Wallace, D. J. (1995). *The lupus book: A guide for patients and their families.* New York: Oxford University Press.

Wallack, H. W. (1977). Lupus-like syndrome associated with carcinoma of the breast. *Archives of Internal Medicine, 137,* 532–535.

Ward, M. M., Pyun, E., & Studenski, S. (1995). Long-term survival in systemic lupus erythematosus. Patient characteristics associated with poorer outcome. *Arthritis and Rheumatism, 38,* 274, 283.

Weinblatt, M. E., Kremer, J. M., & Bankhurst, A. D. (1999). A trial of etanercept, a recombinant tumor necrosis factor receptor: Fc fusion protein in patients with rheumatoid arthritis receiving methotrexate. *New England Journal of Medicine, 340,* 253–259.

West, S. G., & Johns, S. C. (1988). Danazol for the treatment of refractory autoimmune thrombocytopenia in systemic lupus erythematosus. *Annals of Internal Medicine, 108,* 703-706.

Wiske, K. R., & Healey, L. A. (1990). Challenging the therapeutic pyramid; a new look at treatment strategies for rheumatoid arthritis. *Journal of Rheumatology, 17*(25), S4–S7.

Wohlgethan, J. R. (1987). Frozen shoulder in hyperthyroidism. *Arthritis and Rheumatism, 30,* 936–939.

Yelin, E., & Wanke, L. A. (1999). An assessment of the annual and long-term direct costs of rheumatoid arthritis; the impact of poor function and functional decline. *Arthritis and Rheumatism, 42,* 1209–1218.

Yung, R. L., & Richardson, B. C. (1994). Drug induced lupus. *Rheumatic Disease Clinics of North America, 20,* 61–86.

33

Orthopaedic Pain

Gerald Q. Greenfield, Jr., MD, FACS, FICS

INTRODUCTION

Orthopaedics is typically concerned with the treatment of arthritis, fractures, sprains/strains, infection, cancer/metastasis, spinal care/surgery, nerve injury, and osteoporosis/vertebral compression fractures, all of which are likely to result in a manifestation of pain. Pain is defined as an unpleasant sensory and emotional experience associated with actual or potential tissue damage or described in terms of such damage (Mersky & Trimble, 1979). Pain is not a primary sensation such as smell, taste, touch, or vision, but rather it is an emotional state like sorrow or love. The International Association for the Study of Pain defines neuropathic pain as "pain initiated or caused by a primary lesion or dysfunction of the nervous system" (Mersky & Trimble, 1994). Neuropathic pain is characterized by lesions or dysfunction of the systems that under normal conditions, transmit noxious information to the central nervous system. This definition has been called vague, and the inclusion of "dysfunction" allows it to be assigned to disorders such as chronic regional pain syndrome.

Orthopaedics in the United States is a surgical specialty. However, in many areas of the world orthopaedics is a nonsurgical specialty, which may even be described as orthopaedic medicine. Indeed, the initial approach to many orthopaedic pain problems is nonsurgical. Surgery should be reserved for those situations in which an alteration in anatomy offers the possibility of pain relief or functional improvement. Nevertheless, orthopaedics is concerned with the treatment of complaints of the bones, joints, spine, and peripheral nerves. Pain is the presenting symptom in almost all patients with orthopaedic problems.

The practice of orthopaedics encompasses the treatment of fractures, sprains, strains, arthritis, spinal care, nerve compression, infection, primary cancer and metastatic disease, and osteoporosis. The variety of pain complaints is limited only by the patients' ability to describe the sensation. The first steps are to define whether the pain is local or referred, due to compression or disruption of structures, and mechanical or neurological in origin. Next a differential diagnosis should be made and appropriate laboratory and radiological studies obtained. Interpretation of these studies in conjunction with the patient's history and physical examination will lead to a diagnosis, for which a treatment plan can be formulated.

Most orthopaedic pain is neuropathic (Table 33.1). Clinically, neuropathic pain responds to certain pharmacological, mechanical, or surgical treatments. Also included in the realm of orthopaedic pain is pain that is the result of inflammation, such as an abscess, infection, or an inflammatory process (arthritis, tendonitis, and bursitis). The presence of neuropathic pain does not exclude the possibility of the presence of other types of pain. It has even been suggested that there is a continuum of pain with varying degrees of neuropathic and inflammatory components (Barkonja, 2003). Most importantly, all pain must be regarded as real. The terms that patients use to describe pain may be difficult to understand. Therefore, a high level of competence is needed to translate the patient's subjective description into something objective and useful. This variety of orthopaedic pain etiologies requires both an open mind as well as acceptance of a multidisciplinary approach to the treatment of pain.

TABLE 33.1
Types of Orthopaedic Pain

Fractures	Sprains/strains
Inflammation from overuse	Inflammation from metabolic disease
Arthritis (rheumatoid arthritis, osteoarthritis)	Infection
Postsurgical	Neoplasm/metastasis
Compressive neuropathy (upper extremity, lower extremity)	Spine pathology
Phantom limb pain	Complex regional pain syndrome I and II
Myofascial pain syndrome and fibromyalgia syndrome	

SOURCES OF PAIN FIBER IRRITATION

Pain is *mediated* by impulses carried in specific nerve fibers, but *modulated* by a number of other processes. Pain perception is the result of a combination of the effects of impulses carried by nerves and the physical and psychological factors in the patient's environment. The nerves that carry the impulses (A-delta and C) remain constant in their response to applied stimuli. However, the same noxious stimulus delivered to the same patient can produce different results or be perceived differently depending on environmental, physical, and mental factors. Even in specialized pain research settings, it is sometimes difficult to identify specific neuropathic pain mechanisms. Peripheral sensitization occurs when there is a constant state of hyperexcitability in response to a peripheral nerve injury. Central sensitization occurs as a result of changes in nociceptors resulting in a state of hyperexcitability. If these states do not decay once the stimulus or its effects are removed, the alteration in afferent function may persist and become resistant to treatment. In peripheral sensitization, C-nociceptors and fibers show pathologic adrenergic sensitivity (Baron, 2000; Fields, Rowbotham, & Baron, 1998). These effects can be reversed by the application or injection of local anesthetics. The increased activity in peripheral C-fibers is transmitted centrally by large myelinated A-beta fibers. Through these fibers, stimuli, which would under normal circumstances be innocuous, are transmitted to dorsal horn nuclei and then centrally. Thus, the activity of A-beta fibers is necessary for impulses to reach the central nervous system and incite allodynia. All of these factors may come into play in the evaluation and treatment of orthopaedic pain and its sequelae.

TYPES OF ORTHOPAEDIC PAIN

Fracture treatment is the mainstay of orthopaedic surgery. All fractures cause pain in neurologically intact persons although the character and intensity of the pain may vary from person to person. The pain that results from a fracture may come from a variety of sources. The periostium is richly supplied with free nerve endings. Likewise surrounding tendons and ligaments are innervated with free nerve endings as well as pressure and stretch receptors. Because this pain is acute, it responds to routinely used analgesics given by mouth, by intramuscular injection, or intravenously. The transdermal use of analgesics is not recommended for acute pain management.

Ligament sprains or muscle or tendon strains are also among a number of acute pain problems that are treated by orthopaedic practitioners. Usually the result of low-energy trauma, these injuries may affect a variety of areas. The basis of treatment is signified by the pneumonic R-I-C-E, which stands for rest, ice, compression, and elevation. Analgesic use is typically nonsteroidal anti-inflammatory drugs (NSAIDs). In some severe cases narcotic analgesics may be necessary. Physiotherapy or other rehabilitation methods are also useful. The weekend athlete is usually treated nonsurgically for an acute stretch to ligament, tendon, or muscle. However, for those involved in more organized contests where the degree of injury is greater, surgery may be a consideration. These patients have ligament tears or ruptures (grade III sprain) or muscle/tendon tears.

Inflammation as a source of orthopaedic pain encompasses a wide variety of injuries and disease processes. These include both rheumatoid and osteoarthritis, bursitis, tendonitis, gout and other deposition-type diseases, overuse syndromes, and repetitive motion injuries. The widespread use of computers and occurrence of associated injury has provided a new diagnostic category, which has political and financial overtones for employers and insurance carriers. Although the exact pathophysiology differs, the common process is inflammation with the presence of mast and other cells and the release of lysosyme and other inflammatory agents. Although pain may be the presenting symptom, the underlying process is inflammation; treatment should thus be aimed at relief of that process. Methods of pain relief include ice or heat, bandages, braces or supports, modalities such as ultrasound or trigger point therapy, drugs to limit the body's absorption of certain materials, and simply resting the area. It is not usually necessary to use narcotics, injections, or surgery in the early phases. Because of the potential for disability as the result of deformity in the later stages, some inflammatory processes require surgical intervention or joint replacement.

Infection in the form of a generalized process or an abscess can be a source of pain. The pain may be the result of inflammation associated with the presence of bacteria and their by-products or the result of an expanding lesion such as an abscess. Once thought to be a problem of the past due to the introduction of antibiotics, infection is again a major medical problem. Treatment is aimed at pain relief through the elimination of the infection. While antibiotics alone may be appropriate in some instances, in others, surgical evacuation of the abscess or removal of diseased tissue is necessary. Narcotic or other analgesic agents may be necessary until the infection is resolved.

Postsurgical pain, typically acute, can be treated in a variety of ways. These range from NSAIDs to narcotics, with more complex cases requiring regional anesthetic blocks, to a combination of multiple interventions. Patient-controlled analgesia using a variety of drugs via an intravenous route or transdermal analgesic patches are popular with both patients and nursing staff. Recent studies have shown that local anesthetics injected into the surgical area prior to incision significantly reduce the need for postoperative narcotics. When preoperative NSAIDs are added, there is a further reduction. Finally, the additional use of regional anesthetic techniques (nerve blocks or epidural anesthesia) reduces the blood pressure elevations seen in surgical procedures and decreases the pain and the amount of narcotic required to keep patients comfortable postoperatively. Through the skillful use of NSAIDs and regional anesthetics, the need for narcotics can actually be eliminated in all but a few cases. These and other combination analgesic therapies offer promise for the future.

The pain of cancer or metastatic disease to bone may be referred to the orthopaedic surgeon. In addition to their pain management these patients often have significant psychological problems. Treatment of the latter problem does not fall within the skills of most surgeons and is usually best referred to another professional. Pain treatment or management, however, may be left to the surgeon. A variety of oral agents are now available including tablets as well as pain cocktails. Orthopaedics is mainly concerned with the pain that accompanies expanding or destructive metastatic lesions. Restoration of mechanical stability through surgical stabilization of fractures (current or impending) allows functional recovery as long as there is adequate pain control. Central or peripheral nerve stimulation or lesioning offers another option for pain control. Advances in oncology often mean that patients are already on long-acting analgesics from their oncologist and orthopaedics need only control postoperative pain.

COMPRESSIVE NEUROPATHIES

Compressive neuropathies account for a number of pain syndromes involving the upper and lower extremities. Upper extremity neuropathies (Table 33.2) include thoracic outlet syndrome, radial, ulnar, and median nerve compression, and brachial plexus lesions. Nerve compression in the upper extremity can be a debilitating problem. Lower extremity compression can affect the lateral femoral cutaneous, ilioinguinal, genitofemoral, posterior femoral cutaneous, or several lesser nerves. Gait and ambu-

TABLE 33.2
Compressive Neuropathies (Upper Extremity)

Thoracic outlet	Cubital tunnel
Carpal tunnel	Radial nerve (pronator)
Ulna nerve (Guyon)	Long thoracic nerve
Suprascapular nerve	Axillary nerve
Musculocutaneous nerve	Pancoast tumor
Secretan's disease	

lation are affected by these disorders. They are also not as well understood as those affecting the upper extremity.

The median nerve can be compressed or entrapped at one of four locations in the upper extremity: under the ligament of Struthers (Werrtsch & Melvin, 1982), under the lacertus fibrosis (Laha, Lunsford, & Dujovny, 1978), at the pronator teres (Bell & Goldner, 1956), and at the proximal fibrous arcade of the flexor digitorum superficialis (FDS) (Hill, Niven, & Knussen, 1996). At times vascular leashes around or across the nerve may cause compression. The nerve can also be compressed at the wrist as it passes through the carpal tunnel beneath the transverse carpal ligament. Three named syndromes define compression of the median nerve: carpal tunnel syndrome, pronator teres syndrome, and anterior interosseous syndrome. Sir James Paget first described median nerve entrapment at the carpal tunnel in 1854 (Paget, 1854). It was not until the 1950s when carpal tunnel syndrome (CTS) was formally described (Phalen, Gardner, & Lalonde, 1950). The causes of CTS include inflammation, displaced fractures, gout, acromegaly, amyloidosis, myeloma, and anamolous muscles. Many cases have no identifiable cause. Hand numbness and weakness are the most common symptoms. Treatment includes the use of splints in a neutral or dorsiflexed position, anti inflammatory drugs, and steroid injection into the carpal tunnel. The success of nonsurgical treatment decreases with the presence of risk factors (age > 50 years, positive Phalen's test, symptoms > 10 months, constant paresthesias, and associated trigger finger) (Kaplan, Glickel, & Eaton, 1990). When the above techniques fail surgical intervention is the next option.

Pronator teres syndrome was first described by Seyffarth (1959). The symptoms of anterior forearm pain and paresthesias in the median nerve distribution can be confused with carpal tunnel syndrome. There is pain and tenderness at the point of compression. Nonsurgical treatment involves splinting in slight elbow and wrist flexion with forearm pronation, avoidance of repetitive elbow flexion and pronation/supination, and anti-inflammatory drugs. In most cases these options are successful. Surgery involves wide exposure of the median nerve in the forearm, identification of the median nerve, and release of all potentially compressive structures.

Anterior interosseous nerve syndrome (Kiloh & Nevin, 1952) may be due to amyotrophy, fracture, laceration, or compression. The only sign or symptom is weakness of the flexor pollicus longus (FPL) and flexor digitorum profundus (FDP) of the index finger. There are no sensory findings. Nonsurgical treatment includes avoidance of aggravating activities, NSAIDs, and splinting. If these fail, surgical intervention is a consideration; however, spontaneous recovery has been reported after as long as 18 months. Recovery is faster in surgically treated patients if conservative treatment was not successful after a three-month trial (Howard, 1986).

The ulnar nerve may be entrapped at two sites along its course. The cubital tunnel at the elbow is the most common site by a factor of 10. The other site is Guyon's canal at the wrist (Panas, 1878). After carpal tunnel, cubital tunnel syndrome is the most frequent compressive neuropathy in the upper extremity. Nonsurgical treatment includes splints, activity modification, and NSAIDs. Steroid injection is to be avoided due to the superficial location of the nerve. Surgical treatment in the form of decompression, medial epicondylectomy, or anterior transposition is generally successful in 85 to 90% of cases (Osterman & Davis, 1996). Entrapment of the ulnar nerve at Guyon's canal is often referred to as ulnar tunnel syndrome. It is usually due to repetitive trauma or fracture of the hamate or pisiform bones; other causes are mass lesions, fascial bands, or thrombosis. Conservative treatment depends on the cause and includes splints, activity modification, and NSAIDs. When these fail surgical decompression is considered.

Radial nerve compression syndromes can affect either the superficial or the deep portion. The superficial portion is purely sensory and is rarely affected. The deep or posterior branch provides motor innervation to the extensor muscles of the forearm and sensation to the dorsum of the hand distal to the wrist. Agnew (1963) first described posterior interosseous nerve syndrome. This is also referred to as radial tunnel syndrome. In some cases it may be confused with tennis elbow or lateral epicondylitis. The most common source of compression is an anatomic variant, usually at the arcade of Frohse. Other causes include the vascular leash of Henry, fibrous bands from the supinator, radiocapitellar joint, or extensor carpi radialis brevis (ECRB); mass lesions such as synovitis or bursitis are also implicated. Radial tunnel syndrome can produce pain without muscle weakness as first described by Michele and Kreuger (1956). There are three described signs that differentiate radial tunnel syndrome from tennis elbow: (1) tenderness to palpation distal to the radial head not at the lateral epicondyle, (2) increased pain with forearm supination due to posterior radial nerve compression by the arcade of Frohse, and (3) increased pain with extension of the middle finger against resistance when the wrist and elbow are in extension (middle finger test). Elec-

tromyography can be helpful in distinguishing radial tunnel syndrome from cervical radiculopathy. Conservative trials of splints for elbow flexion with wrist extension, activity modification, NSAIDs, and local injection should be attempted before surgical decompression.

The long thoracic nerve (of Bell) is a pure motor nerve and as such lesions do not present with pain. Injury to the nerve presents as scapular winging, which is accentuated by having the patient push against a wall with the arm flexed. There are three major causes for isolated long thoracic nerve injury: neuralgic amyotrophy, trauma, and stretch or traction on the nerve (Gregg, Labosky, & Harty, 1979). In the military, rucksack palsy is a frequent cause of long thoracic nerve palsy (Hirasawa & Sakakida, 1983; Holzgraefe, Kuwowski, & Eggert, 1994). Because most injuries are due to carrying or stretch and are incomplete, prognosis for spontaneous functional recovery is good. Physical therapy and orthotic devices may be helpful while waiting. Recovery should occur by 2 years postinjury. If there is no recovery, muscle transposition (pectoralis major/minor, rhomboids, teres major) or scapulothoracic fusion are possible treatment options.

Entrapment of the suprascapular nerve at the suprascapular notch or spinoglenoid notch presents as shoulder pain and weakness. This injury is more frequently noted due to the increasing use of backpacks in our society, especially in children. Direct blows to the area may also be a factor. There is deep pain and throbbing along the superior border of the scapula and shoulder joint, with radiation down the arm. Weakness of the supraspinatus and infraspinatus muscles is manifested by decreased shoulder abduction and external rotation strength. The pain is exacerbated by reaching across the body with the involved shoulder while rotating the head away from the affected side. It must be differentiated from inflammatory conditions of the shoulder, cervical radiculopathy, neuralgic amyotrophy, and axillary neuropathy. Electromyography (EMG) may be helpful in these cases. This will also allow exclusion of Parsonage–Turner syndrome, which is idiopathic brachial neuritis. Other causes include ganglion cyst at the spinoglenoid notch, rotator cuff tear, or superior glenoid labrum lesions, shoulder trauma, or repetitive motion injury. Plain radiographs help rule out occult bony pathology and apical lung tumors. Magnetic resonance imaging (MRI) allows evaluation of the shoulder joint and surrounding tissues. Non-operative therapy in the form of physical therapy is often successful. However, if there is a clearly defined pathologic lesion, surgery for release of the transverse scapular ligament or excision of a ganglion cyst is a reasonable option.

Axillary neuropathy presents as a patch of decreased sensation in the deltoid region or atrophy or weakness of the muscle. The most common cause is trauma, especially shoulder dislocation (Toolanen, Hildingsson, & Hedlund, 1993) or humeral fracture. Because partial injuries usually recover fully, physical therapy is important in order to maintain range of motion during the recovery period. Brachial plexus injuries in association with axillary injuries have a less favorable prognosis (Berry & Bril, 1982). Any nerve grafting should be performed by 6 months after injury (Petrucci, Morelli, & Riamondi, 1982).

The musculocutaneous nerve is a mixed motor and sensory nerve. Injury to this nerve presents as weakness in elbow flexion and forearm numbness. Pain in the cubital fossa occurs with more distal injuries. The differential diagnosis includes biceps tendon rupture, cervical radiculopathy, median nerve compression, and lateral epicondylitis. Nerve injury is most often due to trauma to the shoulder or upper arm, especially proximal humeral fractures. Shoulder surgery in which the coracoid is transposed has been shown to injure the nerve (Chaung, Yeh, & Wei, 1992). In the event nonsurgical therapy is ineffective, surgical decompression at the elbow would be indicated (Bassett & Nunley, 1982). Nerve grafting before six months (Chaung et al., 1992; Nagano, Ochiai, & Okinaga, 1992) or free muscle transfer (Alasaka, Hara, & Takahashi, 1990) are options for those patients with electromyography/nerve conduction velocity (EMG/NCV) proven lesions that fail to improve. Isolated stretch lesions of the musculocutaneous have a good prognosis when treated conservatively, while grafting procedures have a variable outcome.

Tumors at the apex of the lung may grow and directly affect the brachial plexus. In Pancoast tumor syndrome this can cause arm pain and in some patients Horner's syndrome. There may also be destruction of the first and second ribs. The pain is neuritic in nature and may develop a deep ache or boring quality. Because the great majority of the patients have no antecedent trauma history, there is often a delay in diagnosis. The diagnosis should be high on the list of any patients who are smokers and present with atypical arm or neck pain. Treatment is directed at the tumor itself and pain management is palliative. Direct surgical treatment of brachial plexus lesions is usually disappointing from both a functional and pain relief perspective. Even direct irradiation of the tumor may cause residual neuropathic pain.

Secretan's disease or post-traumatic edema syndrome, while not due to nerve entrapment, is an enigmatic syndrome of pain and swelling over the dorsum of the hand. The pattern of pain may be mistaken for a radial sensory nerve injury. It is usually associated with minimal trauma. Most often it is seen after minor traumatic events such as bumping the hand against objects. It may not be reported for days and then only because of persistent pain. Wounds or abrasions are seldom noted. There is diffuse swelling over the dorsum of the hand with accompanying restriction of finger motion, especially flexion of the metacarpophalangeal (MCP) joints, due to peritendinous fibrosis. It must be differentiated from reflex sympathetic dystrophy, which presents with accompanying sudomotor or

TABLE 33.3
Compressive Neuropathies (Lower Extremity)

Lateral femoral cutaneous nerve (LFC)	Ilioinguinal nerve
Genitofemoral nerve	Piriformis syndrome
Posterior femoral cutaneous nerve (PFC)	Tarsal tunnel
Morton's neuroma	

vasomotor signs. Treatment is symptomatic including compression, elevation to control swelling, and cast or splint application for support and protection against further trauma. Physical therapy for restoration of range of motion must be gentle in order to avoid exacerbation of painful symptoms. The use of NSAIDs may be helpful. Injection of local anesthetic and steroid into the peritendinous fibrosis is an alternative in recalcitrant cases.

Lower extremity compressive neuropathies (Table 33.3) are sometimes more confusing as the neuroanatomy is generally less familiar to most clinicians. The anatomy of the lumbar plexus is less studied in anatomy class than that of the brachial plexus. These factors make their diagnosis much more challenging. Lower extremity symptoms are usually not reported as quickly as are those in the upper extremity. Meralgia parestetica presents as numbness, tingling, or pain in the anterior and lateral thigh region. The lateral femoral cutaneous nerve is compressed by the inguinal ligament, tight clothing, or belts or due to contusion over the iliac crest and resultant hematoma. In some cases the signs follow iliac crest graft harvest for bone grafting in anterior cervical spinal fusion cases. Because the nerve is purely sensory, no motor deficits are noted. Treatment is nonsurgical using analgesics, NSAIDs, or sometimes physical therapy modalities. Some cases resolve spontaneously.

Ilioinguinal and genitofemoral neuralgia are common causes of lower abdominal and pelvic pain complaints (Starling & Haarms, 1989). Injury to the nerves can occur anywhere along their course. Sources include compression, direct trauma, or damage during pelvic or inguinal procedures. Rarely neuralgia may occur spontaneously. Pain, paresthesias, or numbness occur over the lower abdomen and inner thigh and may radiate to the labia majora or scrotum. Because stretching the nerve by lumbar extension exacerbates symptoms, patients often bend forward at the waist. The diagnosis is best made by clinical examination with the pattern of pain rather than muscle testing. Intra-abdominal tumor or other process needs to be ruled out as well as lumbar plexus lesions or inguinal hernia or infection. Aside from treatment of the primary lesion, management is usually by specific or selective nerve block. Care in examination will prevent mistaking one syndrome for the other.

Piriformis syndrome is an entrapment neuropathy characterized by pain, paresthesias, and sometimes weakness in the distribution of the sciatic nerve. The piriformis muscle compresses the nerve as it passes through the sciatic notch. Patients may develop an altered gait that may precipitate the development of sacroiliac, back, and hip pain. The clinical picture is sometimes so confusing that symptoms are attributed to lumbar disc herniation. In rare cases, patients have even undergone laminectomy and disc excision. Physical findings include sciatic notch tenderness, a positive straight leg raise on the affected side, and pain radiating down the leg into the calf or ankle. If present for a prolonged time or left untreated, weakness of the gluteal muscles and lower extremity may result. In addition to lumbar disc herniation, hip pathology must be excluded. This is best accomplished by careful physical examination, appropriate radiographs, and MRI scans of the spine or hip. Treatment begins with analgesics and NSAIDs along with physical therapy. Local application of modalities such as heat or cold may be of benefit. Steroid combined with local anesthetic is successful in the great majority of cases such that the need for surgical release of the entrapment is rare. Other lower extremity entrapments include the posterior femoral cutaneous nerve, the obturator nerve, the femoral nerve, and saphenous neuropathy. All present as pain in a specific distribution and accompanying motor weakness. Direct trauma from contusion or surgical procedures in the area is the most frequent etiology.

Nerves in the ankle and foot are also injured by compression. The tarsal tunnel is classically located posterior to the medial malleolus. The posterior tibial nerve passes through this osteo-ligamentous tunnel along with the tendons of the posterior tibial and flexor hallicus longus muscles, and the posterior tibial artery. Symptoms of nerve compression include pain and paresthesias on the sole of the foot, weakness of the foot intrinsic muscles, and nighttime pain similar to carpal tunnel syndrome. Tenderness over the tarsal tunnel may also be present. While most cases respond to nonsurgical therapy including NSAIDs, splint or cast application, activity modification, and injection, release of the ligament enclosing the tunnel may be necessary in some cases. The deep peroneal nerve may be compressed as it passes beneath the superficial fascia of the anterior ankle. This has been called anterior tarsal tunnel syndrome. Pain and paresthesias in the nerve distribution are the result. Active plantar flexion of the foot or hyper-dorsiflexion, as in squatting, may exacerbate symptoms. Treatment is again nonsurgical except in recalcitrant cases.

Morton's neuroma occurs when the common digital nerve is compressed between the toes, usually the third and fourth. Presenting symptoms are pain or paresthesias in the toes, pain with prolonged standing or walking, and pain when wearing tight shoes or boots. Physical examination reveals pain with local compression in the interspace or from compression or squeezing the metatarsals

together. Women may complain of pain exacerbated from wearing high heels. Nonsurgical therapy includes metatarsal pads or bars, NSAIDs, or injection of steroid into the area. When this fails, section of the common digital nerve may be necessary.

LOW BACK PAIN

Low back pain is the bane of humankind's upright posture. It is present in all societies from the most technologically advanced to the most primitive. As developed societies have become more technologically and less labor based, fitness of the society has decreased and with this has come an increase in the incidence of low back pain. In most cases the origin of low back pain is not known. The spine is a complex structure consisting of bones and joints, ligaments, muscles, discs, peripheral nerves and nerve roots, and the spinal cord. An appreciation of the anatomy, biomechanics, biochemistry, and pathophysiology of the spine is needed to understand low back pain. Structures that contain unmyelinated nerves or substance P or related peptide are capable of causing pain. There are free nerve endings in the outer one third of the disc annulus, the facet joint and joint capsule, the periosteum, and the paraspinous muscles and ligaments. These various nerve endings are sensitive to stretch, direct trauma, pressure, vibration, and chemical irritation as from inflammation or anaerobic metabolism and can be pain generators. While the nociceptive response is normally a gradual one dependent on the amount of stimulus applied to the tissue, this may not be the case in chronic pain situations. Nerve endings that have been previously sensitized may have a more rapid and sustained response to repeat application of a noxious stimulus. The spinal cord modulates nociceptive stimuli through a number of processes (Melzack & Wall, 1965). Theories include the gate-control (Melzack & Wall, 1965) and the convergence–perception (Hirsch, Ingelmar, & Miller, 1963). There is also evidence that descending seratonogenic pathways and endorphins allow individuals to modify or even turn off their pain responses (Haldeman, 1992). Thus, the pathophysiology of low back pain is extremely complex with multiple points at which it may be modified or modulated, including the dorsal root, the spinal cord, and centrally in the brain and brainstem. Treatments for low back pain are as varied as are the causes. Objective reviews have failed to show efficacy of any single treatment modality over another (Nachemson, 2000). Even in cases of frank disc herniation, surgery may provide only short-term improvement, with no long-term benefit over nonsurgical care. Recent treatment of "discogenic" pain has had at best only marginal success.

Spondylolisthesis is derived from the Greek *spondy*-meaning spine, and -*olisthesis* meaning slip. The anatomic finding in patients with spondylolisthesis is an alteration in the alignment of the spine, usually in the lumbar region.

The condition occurs four to six times more frequently in women than men, and usually after age 50 (Cauchoix, Benoist, & Chassaing, 1976; Newman, 1976). The L4–L5 level is most frequently affected. Displacement of one vertebra on another is slowed and eventually stops due to the onset of degenerative changes in the disc and facet joints (Matsunaga, Sakou, & Morizondo, 1990). The forward slippage of one vertebra on the other causes a decrease in the cross-sectional area of the spinal canal and may result in spinal stenosis and compression of the lumbar nerve roots. Rarely does cauda equine syndrome or myelopathy develop. Patients with spondylolisthesis complain of a deep, dull backache exacerbated by motion of the lumbar spine. Changing from a sitting to a standing position will often produce symptoms. More than one dermatome may be affected, and bowel and bladder function is spared until very late in the process. Likewise, motor function is affected only late in the course. In cases of bowel, bladder, and motor dysfunction, emergent surgical consultation is needed. Careful physical examination will help to identify the level and to rule out a disc herniation. Plain radiographs will usually identify the affected level. Myelography, computerized tomographic scan, or MRI may be necessary to identify nerve root compression. Treatment is multifaceted, including medication, physical therapy, and possibly application of braces. The use of caudal or lumbar epidural blocks with local anesthetic and steroid is also an effective alternative. Surgical intervention is needed for those with severe nerve compression or those who fail nonsurgical treatment. Prior to surgical intervention lytic defects in the pars interarticularis from spondylolysis must be considered. These may be a source of pain and may contribute to segmental instability.

Spinal stenosis was first described in the Netherlands (Verbiest, 1954). It is generally a disease of the aging spine, whether as the result of years or of years of use. It is the result of a combination of factors including disc collapse, "wrinkling" of the ligamentum flavum, facet joint hypertrophy, and the resultant nerve root compression. The hallmark is neurogenic claudication with calf pain and cramping. It must be differentiated from vascular claudication through the use of history, examination, radiographic and laboratory studies, and response to noninvasive treatment trials. Spinal stenosis may respond to epidural injection, but in advanced cases decompressive spinal surgery is usually necessary.

The aging population combined with diets low in calcium has led to a dramatic increase in the incidence of osteoporosis, especially among women (Riggs, 1995). A consequence of this increase is a corresponding increase in vertebral compression fractures. This painful condition affects about 8 million women annually in the United States, according to the National Osteoporosis Foundation. Men are also affected accounting for 20% of all cases of osteoporosis (Licata, 2003). There are roughly 700,000 vertebral compression fractures annually of which more than 80% are due to osteoporosis. While pain is the major presenting symptom, associated conditions include spinal deformity, chest and abdominal compression, decreased lung capacity, sleep disorders, loss of independence, and depression (Gold, 2003; Lyles, Gold, and Shipp, 1993; Silverman 1992). Most vertebral compression fractures heal spontaneously and without residual pain. However, recently a more aggressive approach has been adopted in the treatment of these patients. Injection of bone cement or other bone-space filler is often recommended to treat both the pain and in many cases the deformity associated with the fracture (Gaughen, Jensen, & Schweickert, 2002; Ryu, 2002). While this form of treatment is not applicable to all such fractures it does offer an option where none previously existed.

Coccydynia affects women more frequently than men. Characterized by pain localized to the tailbone region, it is due to direct trauma from a fall or as the result of a difficult vaginal delivery. The pain is due to sprain of the sacrococcygeal ligament, fracture of the coccyx, or a combination of both. Patients present with point pain and tenderness over the coccyx that is exacerbated by movement or pressure as with sitting. Primary pathology of the anus or rectum such as primary or metastatic tumors must be differentiated. Peri-rectal abscess is a frequent mimic as are sacral insufficiency fractures. Treatment is usually symptomatic with use of a pillow or donut for sitting and analgesics or NSAIDs for pain. If radiographic evaluation demonstrates coccyx displacement, especially in acute situations, digital rectal examination and reduction of the displaced fragment can provide sudden and dramatic relief of symptoms. Surgery should be avoided to prevent producing incompetence of the pelvic floor by disruption of supporting muscles and ligaments.

OTHER PAIN SYNDROMES

Ambrose Pare first described phantom limb or post amputation pain in military amputees in the 16th century. While most often described for loss of an extremity, phantom pains of a digit, eye, nose, teeth, breast, bladder, anus, and genital organs have been reported (Davis, 1993; Jensen & Rasmussen, 1989; Loeser, 1990; Marbach, 1993). Nonpainful phantom sensations are divided into three types: kinetic, kinesthetic, and exteroceptive. Kinetic sensations involve the perception of movement and may be perceived as spontaneous or volitional. Kinesthetic perceptions involve the size, shape, and position of the body part. This perception may be either normal or distorted. Exteroceptive perceptions are usually more intense on the involved area and include touch, pressure, temperature, or vibration. Visceral organs may have phantoms related to function of the organ such as the urge to urinate or defecate. Phantom pains are differentiated from annoying sensations and are often described as more intense versions of normal sensations. Stump pain is persistent wound pain that is usually due to a pathologic process such as delayed healing, infection, tumor recurrence, neuromas, or a poorly fitting prosthesis. These pains may even occur as paroxysms or spasms. Patients, however, are able to differentiate annoying or nonpainful sensations from what they classify as pain. More than 80% of amputees experience significant phantom pain (Stein & Warfield, 1982). The intensity is variable (Jensen, Krebs, & Nielsen, 1985) as is the duration (Sherman & Sherman, 1983). The intensity varies from 3 to 7.5 and the duration from seconds (38%) to hours (37%) to continuous (12%). The phantoms can change in character and location over time. The limb may even be perceived as telescoping or shortening (Sherman, Katz, & Marbach, 1997). Some studies imply a pain memory where phantoms replicate preamputation pain (Hill, Niven, & Knussen, 1996). Treatment of phantom pain is as varied as are the descriptions. Included are medications, nerve stimulation, nerve ablation procedures, physical therapy, psychological and behavioral therapy, and complementary or alternative therapies. In several reviews of therapeutic interventions, none was uniformly successful (Davis, 1993; Jensen & Rasmussen, 1989; Loeser, 1990; Sherman, Sherman, & Gall, 1980). Limb amputees report that prosthetic wear may act to either exacerbate or diminish phantom pains. Current research includes brain imaging and mapping, modified surgical techniques, and altered postoperative regimens.

Complex regional pain syndrome I or II (CRPS I or II) is the name now applied to the disorder formerly called reflex sympathetic dystrophy or causalgia. Because traumatic neuropathic pain and neuralgias probably represent more than one specific disease entity, the term *syndrome* is applied to these disorders. According to the new definitions CRPS I is equated with reflex sympathetic dystrophy in which minor lesions of the limb precede the onset of symptoms. CRPS II or causalgia develops after injury to a major peripheral nerve. In CRPS I there is a preceding minor traumatic event (e.g., sprain, fracture, surgery, or other injury) resulting in symptoms whose severity is out of proportion to the severity of the trauma and with a tendency to spread in the affected limb. There is no nerve injury identifiable on EMG testing. Symptoms in CRPS I occur regardless of the type of inciting injury (Evans, 1946) or the site of the injury (Pak, Martin, & Magness, 1970); neither determines symptom location. Mitchell (1865) first described CRPS II as causalgia in soldiers wounded in the Civil War. He noted burning pain; smooth, cold, and sweaty mottled skin; and hypersensitivity of the skin to light touch. In nearly all cases the limb was involved. Partial nerve laceration was the inciting factor. By definition the difference in CRPS I and II is the presence of a partial nerve injury to a major nerve. Patients with CRPS usually experience more that one type of pain

(burning, throbbing, shooting) that is out of proportion to the injury. Temperature differences of as much as 3.5°C occur, comparing side to side. Sweating, edema, and swelling of the affected limb are also noted. Pathogenesis may be inflammatory based on recent investigations (Christiansen, Jensen, & Noer, 1982; Oyen, Arntz, & Claessens, 1993). Although patients are noted to be anxious or depressed, these psychological symptoms are the result not the cause of CRPS (Lynch, 1992). There are no diagnostic tests that are specific for the diagnosis of CRPS; clinical criteria alone must be used. The basic treatment of CRPS relies on pain and symptom relief and rehabilitation of involved limbs. Pharmacologic agents include antidepressants, opioids, local anesthetics, GABA agonists, and oral steroids. Nerve stimulation in the form of transcutaneous electrical stimulation, peripheral or spinal cord stimulation (Hassenbusch, Stanton-Hicks, & Schoppa, 1996), or even deep brain stimulation have been reported to be helpful in CRPS treatment. Physical therapy and rehabilitation are maximally important in functional recovery. Only through regaining the use and strength in the involved limb can there be any confidence in avoiding a relapse.

Fibromyalgia and myofascial pain represent a varied presentation of the same symptoms. Fibromyalgia or fibromyalgia syndrome (FMS) is characterized by widespread muscular aching, pain, and stiffness with tenderness to palpation at multiple sites called tender points (Goldenberg, 1987). *Primary fibromyalgia* is the term used when there is no significant underlying or concomitant condition identified that contributes to the pain (Bengtsson, Henriksson, & Jorfeldt, 1986). However, when there is another condition that may contribute to the pain, such as rheumatoid arthritis or osteoarthritis, the term *concomitant fibromyalgia* is applied. The clinical characteristics of the two are identical (Wolfe, Smyth, & Yunus, 1990). Myofascial pain syndrome (MPS), on the other hand, is defined as regional rather than widespread soft tissue pain. There is evidence that the MPS and FMS overlap clinically (Inanici, Yunus, & Aldag, 1999) and that the former leads to the latter in 40% of cases (Inanici, Yunus, Castillo, & Aldag, 1998). Described as muscular rheumatism in the 17th century, the first controlled study of the clinical characteristics of fibromyalgia was not published until 1981(Yunus, Masi, & Calabro, 1981). In this study the presence of a group of symptoms, including pain, fatigue, sleep disturbance, soft tissue swelling, and tender points, was noted to be more common in patients with fibromyalgia than a group of matched normal controls. This was the first attempt to recognize fibromyalgia as a syndrome. It occurs mostly in White women in the 40- to 60-year-old age group. Symptoms are often present for 6 to 7 years prior to diagnosis (Yunus, 2000). The most common symptoms are generalized pain, stiffness, fatigue, and sleep disturbance. The onset of symptoms usually follows an infection, trauma, or mental stress (Greenfield, Fitzharles, & Esdaile, 1992). Thus far, there are no laboratory studies that are specific for the diagnosis of fibromyalgia, which may be readily diagnosed by its characteristic symptoms and multiple tender points (Wolfe et al., 1990).

Central sensitization is defined as an exaggerated response of the central nervous system to peripheral stimulus that is normally painful (Coderre, Katz, Vaccarino, & Melzack, 1993). Pain is perceived as prolonged or persistent. These same mechanisms may be present in FMS patients (Yunus, 2000). A number of other factors including genetics, psychology, endocrine, and social are involved in fibromyalgia and its treatment. Principles involved in the management of FMS involve a multidisciplinary approach using pharmacologic and nonpharmacologic methods. These principles include positive attitude in the physician, well-established diagnosis, management of comorbid conditions, improved sleep pattern, gradual increase in physical activity, appropriate medications, and psychological therapy. Even with this approach the prognosis in FMS is one of chronic pain and disability (Kennedy & Felson, 1996; Wolfe, Anderson, & Harkness, 1997). Prognosis can be improved by several factors including early diagnosis, younger age (Felson & Goldenberg, 1986), higher education level (Hench, Cohen, & Mitler, 1989), and longer periods of time spent exercising (Granges, Zilko, & Littlejohn, 1994).

TREATMENT TECHNIQUES

First and foremost, there is no silver bullet for the treatment of orthopaedic or neuropathic pain. Any treatment technique must be a component of a comprehensive program that incorporates pharmacology, physical therapy, psychological, anesthesia, and surgical options. While not all will be necessary in all cases, the availability of multiple disciplines assures the greatest possibility for improvement in function, if not pain relief. In addition to treatment, all patients must be involved in an education program about their disorder and pain treatment in general.

Nonsurgical treatment is the appropriate initial effort for many types of orthopaedic pain (Table 33.4). Topical agents from analgesic balms to local anesthetics to transdermal narcotics are also useful. Frequently application of cold (ice) or heat (heating pad) to a painful area will

---

TABLE 33.4
Treatment Techniques (Nonsurgical)

Topical and physiotherapy
Oral agents and medications
Injections and acupuncture
Regional anesthetic/nerve blocks

---

provide some temporary relief and can be a valuable adjunct to any treatment program. This provides a safe and easily available method of pain control that has few if any side effects. Other liniments and salves, including homemade remedies, have been shown to be efficacious in pain management.

Often the first-line treatment selected for any painful situation is an oral medication, either over the counter or prescription. Patients themselves will attempt to treat pain with a variety of medications including acetaminophen, aspirin, or NSAIDs. Other oral agents include opioid analgesics, tricyclic antidepressants, sedative hypnotics, anticonvulsants, tramadol, and gabapentin. Dosages and frequency vary from patient to patient and practitioner to practitioner. There are, however, recommended dosage ranges. In the hands of a skilled practitioner these medications either alone or in combination are a powerful adjunct in the management of orthopaedic pain. Although they may not eliminate the pain completely they allow for enough reduction to restore function and a return to a functional lifestyle.

When topical and oral medications fail to give significant pain relief physical therapy and other manual medicine techniques offer another option. Whether through a formal physical therapy program, chiropractic or osteopathic manipulation, acupressure applied at acupuncture points, yoga or other therapeutic exercise, or massage therapy, the "laying on of hands" itself has proven value in healing. Often in the modern technical medical world practitioners may come to rely on and utilize tests and investigations more than patient inquiry and contact. The establishment of a therapeutic relationship with manual medicine practitioners often results in a more frequent and lengthy meeting than with physicians. This also has therapeutic value. During these more extended contact periods, there is time to ask more questions, explore other options, and sometimes receive more guidance in the recovery process.

When the initial non-invasive options fail to provide symptom relief, more aggressive and invasive methods may be necessary. Injections of materials such as NSAIDs, narcotics, local anesthetics; radiofrequency blocks; and regional anesthetic blocks are treatment options. Local injections in the area of a wound or trigger point are frequently used to either treat the pain or to break the pain–spasm cycle. Injection of local anesthetic agents prior to surgical incision reduces intraoperative anesthetic requirements and also reduces the level of postoperative pain and thus analgesic requirements. The use of NSAIDs has in some cases eliminated the need for any analgesics at all in some minor surgery cases. Injection of local anesthetic either alone or in combination with steroid is a mainstay in the treatment of trigger points. This same technique is sometimes useful in the treatment of muscle spasm or torticollis in adult and pediatric patients. Facet syndrome and other low back pain problems may be treated by injection of local anesthetic or other agents or the application of a radiofrequency generator in the area of the nerves to the facet joint. Because the nerve is not divided, it may regenerate and require repeat application for continued pain relief. Injection of phenol or other neurolytic agents is useful in the treatment of Morton's neuroma, intercostal nerve pain, or other persistent pain syndromes. Acupuncture has been and is currently used in a variety of pain treatment programs. In the hands of a licensed practitioner it is a powerful addition to the range of treatment options.

Regional nerve block or anesthesia is useful in the diagnosis, treatment, and prevention of orthopaedic pain. Based on the location of the pain, anatomy, and patient needs, regional anesthetic blocks can be used to prevent pain as in surgery, block the perception of pain to allow diagnosis, or treat a pain problem to allow return to normal function. The proper selection or agents, location of the block, and timing for length of the block allow the technique to be tailored to particular patients and clinical situations. As an extension of regional techniques nerve or even spinal cord stimulators can be used to modify or eliminate the patient's pain. These offer the possibilities of the generator being turned on or off based on patient needs and of adjusting the degree of nerve stimulation order to achieve the desired effect. Percutaneuos placement or the use of temporary devices adds to the flexibility of the technique. Similar to stimulators in terms of indication is the use of pain pumps or reservoirs that dispense a measured amount of analgesic to a local area or to the spinal cord or cerebral spinal fluid. When narcotics are used, the dose required is lower than parenteral so there is less tolerance. There is also minimal if any central effect so there is neither interference with judgment nor the development of euphoria.

Surgical options are the treatment of choice in many orthopaedic situations or when initial attempts with nonsurgical methods fail to provide pain relief (Table 33.5). Because of the nature of this chapter, surgical techniques are not be described in detail. These techniques can be classified as falling into several categories: (1) decompression/neurolysis, (2) transposition, (3) sectioning/ablative procedures, and (4) nerve grafting. The majority of compressive neuropathies can be treated by relief of the pressure on the nerve through decompression if there is an external source. The use of neurolysis may be necessary when there is residual deformity of the nerve due to scarring of the sheath. Both external and internal neurolysis may be needed to restore anatomy and function to the nerve. Transposition of a nerve may be necessary to relieve excess tension on the nerve as a result of alteration in the course due to injury, abnormal motion or stress, or developmental changes such as growth or muscular development. The procedure, however, carries with it a risk of postsurgical scarring and later compressive problems. Nerve sectioning or ablative procedures are rare and gen-

---

TABLE 33.5
Treatment Techniques (Surgical)

Implants — stimulators, pumps
Surgery — decompression, transposition, stabilization, ablation
    kyphoplasty/vertebroplasty

---

erally irreversible. Thus, great care must be exercised in the evaluation and nonsurgical treatment of these pain conditions. This technique is frequently applied to the treatment of Morton's neuroma, but may also be applied to painful spinal cord or metastatic syndromes.

Kyphoplasty and vertebroplasty are two relatively new procedures aimed at the treatment of painful vertebral compression fractures. Currently, both techniques involve the injection of bone cement into the vertebral body to provide additional strength. While kyphoplasty has as a part of the procedure the restoration of normal anatomy in deformed bodies, its goal is restoration of strength lost as a result of osteoporosis and fracture. Vertebroplasty has as a goal only the restoration of strength. The use of bone cement may in the future be supplanted by "bone filler." There are currently several under investigation. The increasing age of the population indicates that procedures such as these will be more frequent in the future. As a technique for pain relief, they are minimally invasive and can be performed on an outpatient basis using general or even conscious sedation anesthesia. Pain relief is also nearly immediate. If other levels are affected at a later date, the procedure can be repeated at those levels.

SUMMARY

The goal of this chapter has been to present an overview of factors and disorders to consider in the evaluation of patients with pain from an orthopaedic source. Just as the specialty of orthopaedic surgery is broad, the areas to consider as sources of pain are equally broad. Patient evaluation is aided by a thorough history and physical examination, knowledge of musculoskeletal and neurological anatomy and physiology, and use of appropriate laboratory, radiology, and other studies. Only through the application of these principles can a rational approach be developed and a firm diagnosis reached. Once the diagnosis is verified, a treatment plan can be proposed and instituted. The perception of pain is both physical and psychological so a purely physical approach to treatment is not likely to be completely successful.

REFERENCES

Agnew, D. H. (1963). Bursal tumor producing loss of power in the forearm. *American Journal of Science, 46,* 404–405.

Alasaka, Y., Hara, T., & Takahashi, M. (1990). Restoration of elbow flexion and wrist extension in brachial plexus paralysis by means of free muscle transplantation by innervated nerve. *Annals of Hand Surgery, 9,* 341–350.

Barkonja, M. (2003). Defining neuropathic pain. *Anesthesia and Analgesia, 97,* 785–790.

Baron, R. (2000). Peripheral neuropathic pain: From mechanisms to symptoms. *Clinical Journal of Pain, 16,* s12–s20.

Bassett, F. H., & Nunley, J. A. (1982). Compression of the musculotaneous nerve at the elbow. *Journal of Bone and Joint Surgery, 64A*(7), 1050–1052.

Bell, G. E. Jr., & Goldner, J. L. (1956). Compression neuropathy of the median nerve. *Southern Medical Journal, 49,* 966–972.

Bengtsson, A., Henriksson, K. G., & Jorfeldt, L. (1986). Primary fibromyalgia: A clinical and laboratory study of 55 patients. *Scandinavian Journal of Rheumatology, 15,* 340–347.

Berry, H., & Bril, V. (1982). Axillary nerve palsy following blunt trauma to the shoulder region: A clinical and electrophysiological review. *Journal of Neurology, Neurosurgery, and Psychiatry, 45,* 1027–1032.

Cauchoix, J., Benoist, M., & Chassaing, V. (1976). Degenerative spondylolisthesis. *Clinical Orthopaedics, 115,* 122–129.

Christiansen, K., Jensen, E. M., & Noer, I. (1982). The reflex dystrophy syndrome response to treatment with corticosteroids. *Acta Chirugica Scandinavica, 148,* 653–655.

Chaung, D. C. C., Yeh, M. C., & Wei, F. C. (1992). Intercostal nerve transfer of the musculocutaneous nerve in avulsed brachial plexus injuries: Evaluation of 66 patients. *Journal of Hand Surgery, 17A,* 822–828.

Coderre, T. J., Katz, J., Vaccarino, A. L., & Melzack, R. (1993). Contribution of central neuroplasticity to pathological pain: Review of clinical and experimental evidence. *Pain, 52,* 259–285.

Davis, R. W. (1993). Phantom sensation, phantom pain, and stump pain. *Archives of Physical Medicine and Rehabilitation, 74,* 79–91.

Evans, J. A. (1946). Reflex sympathetic dystrophy. *Surgical Clinics of North America, 26,* 435–448.

Felson, D. T., & Goldenberg, D. L. (1986). The natural history of fibromyalgia. *Arthritis and Rheumatism, 29*(12), 1522–1526.

Fields, H. L., Rowbotham, M., & Baron, R. (1998). Postherpetic neuralgia: Irritable nociceptors and deafferentation. *Neurobiology of Diseases, 5,* 209–227.

Gaughen, J. R., Jensen, M. E., & Schweickert P. A. (2002). The therapeutic benefit of repeat vertebroplasty at previously treated vertebral levels. *American Journal of Neuroradiology, 23,* 1657–1661.

Gold, D. T. (2003). The downward spiral of vertebral osteoporosis. A monograph. National Osteoporosis Foundation.

Goldenberg, D. L. (1987). Fibromyalgia syndrome: An emerging but controversial condition. *Journal of the American Medical Association, 257,* 2782–2787.

Granges, G., Zilko, P., & Littlejohn, G. O. (1994). Fibromyalgia syndrome: Assessment of the severity of the condition two years after diagnosis. *Journal of Rheumatology, 21*(3), 523–529.

Greenfield, S., Fitzharles, M. A., & Esdaile, J. M. (1992). Reactive fibromyalgia syndrome. *Arthritis and Rheumatism, 35,* 678–681.

Gregg, J. R., Labosky, D., & Harty, M. (1979). Serratus anterior paralysis in the young athlete. *Journal of Bone and Joint Surgery, 61A,* 825–832.

Haldeman, S. (1992). The neurophysiology of spinal pain. In S. Haldeman (Ed.), Principles and practice of chiropractic (pp. 165–184). East Norwalk, CT: Appleton and Lange.

Hassenbusch, S. J., Stanton-Hicks, M., & Schoppa, D. (1996). Long term results of peripheral nerve stimulation for reflex sympathetic dystrophy. *Journal of Neurosurgery, 84,* 415-423.

Hench, P. K., Cohen, R., & Mitler, M. M. (1989). Fibromyalgia: Effects of amitriptyline, tamazepam and placebo on pain and sleep. *Arthritis and Rheumatism, 32* (Suppl.), S47.

Hill, A., Niven, C. A., & Knussen, C. (1996). Pain memories in phantom limbs: A case study. *Pain, 66,* 381–384.

Hirasawa, Y., & Sakakida, K. (1983). Sports and peripheral nerve injury. *American Journal of Sports Medicine, 11,* 420–426.

Hirsch, C., Ingelmar, K. U. E., & Miller, N. (1963). The anatomic basis for low back pain: Studies on the presence of sensory endings in ligamentous capsular and intervertebral disc structures in the human spine. *Acta Orthopaedica Scandinavica, 33,* 1–15.

Holzgraefe, M., Kuwowski, B., & Eggert, S. (1994). Prevalence of latent and manifest suprascapular neuropathy in high-performance volleyball players. *British Journal of Sports Medicine, 28,* 177–179.

Howard, F. M. (1986). Compression neuropathies in the anterior forearm. *Hand Clinics, 2,* 737–745.

Inanici, F., Yunus, M. B., & Aldag, J. C. (1999). Clinical features and psychologic factors in regional soft tissue pain: Comparison with fibromyalgia syndrome. *Journal of Musculoskeletal Pain, 7*(1/2), 293–301.

Inanici, F., Yunus, M. B., Castillo, L. D., & Aldag, J. C. (1998). Prognosis of regional fibromyalgia: Comparison with fibromyalgia syndrome. *Journal of Musculoskeletal Pain, 6*(Suppl. 2), 97–107.

Jensen, T. S., Krebs, B., & Nielsen, J. (1985). Immediate and long-term phantom limb pain in amputees. Incidence, clinical characteristics and relationship to pre-amputation limb pain. *Pain, 21,* 267–278.

Jensen, T. S., & Rasmussen, P. (1989). Phantom pain and related phenomena after amputation. In P. D. Wall, & R. Melzack (Eds.), *Textbook of pain* (2nd ed., pp. 508–519). New York: Churchill Livingston.

Kaplan, S. J., Glickel, S. Z., & Eaton, R. G. (1990). Predictive factors in the non-surgical treatment of carpal tunnel syndrome. *American Journal of Hand Surgery, 15B,* 106–108.

Kennedy, M., & Felson, D. T. (1996). A prospective long-term study of fibromyalgia syndrome. *Arthritis and Rheumatism, 39*(4), 682–685.

Kiloh, L. G., & Nevin, S. (1952). Isolated neuritis of the anterior interosseous nerve. *British Medical Journal, 1,* 850–851.

Laha, R. K., Lunsford, L. D., & Dujovny, M. (1978). Lacertus fibrosis compression of the median nerve. *Journal of Neurosurgery, 48,* 838–841.

Licata, A. (2003). Osteoporosis in men: Suspect secondary disease first. *Cleveland Clinic Journal of Medicine, 70,* 247–254.

Loeser, J. (1990). Pain after amputation: phantom limb and stump pain. In J. Bonica (Ed.), *The management of pain* (2nd ed., pp. 244–256). Philadelphia: Lea & Febiger.

Lyles, K. W., Gold, D. T., & Shipp, K. M. (1993). Association of osteoporotic vertebral compression fractures with impaired functional status. *American Journal of Medicine, 92*(6), 595–601.

Lynch, M. E. (1992). Psychological aspects of reflex sympathetic dystrophy: A review of the adult and pediatric literature. *Pain, 49,* 337–347.

Marbach, J. J. (1993). Is phantom tooth pain a deafferentation (neuropathic) syndrome? *Oral Surgery, Oral Medicine, Oral Pathology, Oral Radiology and Endodontics, 75,* 95–105.

Matsunaga, S., Sakou, T., & Morizondo, Y. (1990). Natural history of degenerative spondylolisthesis. Pathogenesis and clinical course of the slippage. *Spine, 15,* 1204–1210.

Melzack, R., & Wall, P. D. (1965). Pain mechanisms: A new theory. *Science, 150,* 971–979.

Mersky, H., & Trimble, M. (1979). Personality, sexual adjustment, and brain lesions in patients with conversion symptoms. *American Journal of Psychiatry, 136,* 179–182.

Michele, A. A., & Kreuger, F. J. (1956). Lateral epicondylitis of the elbow treated by fasciotomy. *Surgery, 39,* 277–284.

Mitchell, S. W. (1865). *Injuries to the nerves and their consequences.* New York: Dover.

Nachemson, A. L. (2000). Introduction. In A. L. Nachemson & E. Jonsson (Eds.), *Neck and back pain: The scientific evidence of causes, diagnosis, and treatment* (pp. 1–12). Philadelphia: Lippincott, Williams and Wilkins.

Nagano, A., Ochiai, N., & Okinaga, S. (1992). Restoration of elbow flexion in root lesions of brachial plexus injuries. *Journal of Hand Surgery, 17A,* 815–821.

Newman, P. H. (1976). Stenosis of the lumbar spine in spondylolisthesis. *Clinical Orthopaedics, 115,* 116–121.

Osterman, A. L., & Davis, C. A. (1996). Subcutaneous transposition of the ulnar nerve for the treatment of cubital tunnel syndrome. *Hand Clinics, 12,* 421–433.

Oyen, W. J., Arntz, I. E., & Claessens, R. M. (1993). Reflex sympathetic dystrophy of the hand: An excessive inflammatory response? *Pain, 55,* 151–157.

Paget, J. (1854). *Lectures on surgical pathology* (1st ed.). Philadelphia: Lindsey and Blakiston.

Pak, T. J., Martin, G. M., & Magness, J. L. (1970). Reflex sympathetic dystrophy. Review of 140 cases. *Minnesota Medicine, 53,* 507–512.

Panas, J. (1878). Sur une cause peu comme de paralysie de nerf Cubital. *Archives Generales Chirurgie Medicine, 2,* 5–22.

Petrucci, P. S., Morelli, A., & Riamondi, P. L. (1982). Axillary nerve injuries-21 cases treated by nerve graft and neurolysis. *Journal of Hand Surgery, 7A,* 271–278.

Phalen, G., Gardner, W., & Lalonde, A. (1950). Neuropathy of the median nerve due to compression beneath the transverse carpal ligament. *Journal of Bone and Joint Surgery, 32A,* 109.

Riggs, B. L., & Melton, 3rd, L. J. (1995). The worldwide problem of osteoporosis: Insights afforded by epidemiology. *Bone, 17*(5S), 505S–511S.

Ryu, K. S., Park, C. K., Kim, M. C., & Kang, J. K. (2002). Dose-dependent epidural leakage of polymethylmerthacrylate after percutaneous vertebroplasty in patients with osteoporotic vertebral compression fractures. *Journal of Neurosurgery, 96,* 56–61.

Seyffarth, H. (1959). Primary myoses of the m. pronator teres as cause of compression of the n, medianus (the pronator syndrome). *Acta Psychiatrica Scandinavica, 74*(Suppl.), 251–254.

Sherman, R. A, & Sherman, C. J. (1983). Prevalence and characteristics of chronic phantom limb pain among American veterans: Results of a trial survey. *American Journal of Physical Medicine and Rehabilitation, 62,* 227–238.

Sherman, R., Katz, J., & Marbach, J. (1997). Locations, characteristics and descriptions. In R. A. Sherman, M. Devor, & D. E. Jones (Eds.), *Phantom pain* (pp. 1–32). New York: Plenum Press.

Sherman, R. A., Sherman, C. J., & Gall, N. G. (1980). A survey of current phantom limb treatment in the United States. *Pain, 8,* 85–99.

Silverman, S. L. (1992). The clinical consequences of vertebral compression fracture. *Bone, 13*(Suppl. 2), S27–S31.

Starling, J. R., & Haarms, B. A. (1989). Diagnosis and treatment of genitofemoral and ilioinguinal neuralgia. *World Journal of Surgery, 13,* 586–591.

Stein, J., & Warfield, C. (1982). Phantom limb pain. *Hospital Practices, 17,* 166–167.

Toolanen, G., Hildingsson, C., & Hedlund, T. (1993). Early complications after anterior dislocation of the shoulder in patients over 40 years. *Acta Orthopaedics Scandinavica, 64,* 549–555.

Verbiest, H. (1954). Radicular syndromes from developmental narrowing of the lumbar spinal canal. *Journal of Bone and Joint Surgery, 36B,* 230–237.

Werrtsch, J. J., & Melvin, J. (1982). Median nerve anatomy and entrapment syndrome: A review. *Archives of Physical Medicine and Rehabilitation, 63,* 623–627.

Wolfe, F., Smyth, H. A., & Yunus, M. B. (1990). The American College of Rheumatology 1990 Criteria for the Classification of Fibromyalgia. Report of the Multicenter Criteria Committee. *Arthritis and Rheumatism, 33,* 160–172.

Wolfe, F., Anderson, J., & Harkness, D. (1997). Work and disability status of persons with fibromyalgia. *Journal of Rheumatology, 24,* 1171–1178.

Yunus, M. B. (2000). Central sensitivity syndromes: A unified concept for fibromyalgia and other similar maladies. *Journal of the Indian Rheumatism Association, 8,* 27–33.

Yunus, M. B., Masi, A. T., & Calabro, J. J. (1981). Primary fibromyalgia (fibrositis): Clinical study of 50 patients with matched normal controls. *Seminars in Arthritis and Rheumatism, 11,* 151–171.

34

Treatment of Myofascial Pain Syndromes

Robert D. Gerwin, MD, and Jan Dommerholt, PT, MPS

INTRODUCTION

The treatment of persons with myofascial pain syndrome (MPS) follows the general principles that apply to all medical disorders. The nature of the pain problem first must be understood through developing an appropriate differential diagnosis and evaluating the contributions of coexisting disorders, until a single working diagnosis emerges. Following the initial assessment and formulation of diagnostic hypotheses, new data are collected. A regular review at each encounter and modification of the hypotheses facilitate a more efficient and effective management of patients with MPS and dictate the actual program components (Higgs & Jones, 1995; Jones, 1994). After addressing the issue of diagnosis, the practitioner must determine the structural or biomechanical functioning of the patient and the contribution that any dysfunction may have to the individual's pain. Medical and psychological disorders that may alter the presentation of MPS or that may predispose to its becoming chronic are assessed. Treatment of persons with MPS addresses each of these issues specifically (Figure 34.1). There must be relief of pain by the direct inactivation of the myofascial trigger point (MTrP) itself. The mechanical and structural factors that affect or overload the muscle and aggravate the pain must be resolved or alleviated. The medical and psychological problems that affect muscle function, including those that alter and impair intracellular metabolism, must be identified and corrected where possible. Inactivation of the MTrP may occur with direct intervention at the MTrP itself, through correction of the mechanical factors that produced it or through improvement in the underlying medical disorders that predispose to the development or maintenance of the MTrP.

DIAGNOSIS

The diagnosis of MPS should be suspected when there is a non-neuropathic pain complaint almost anywhere in the body, including headache. At first glance, such a statement may seem to be so nonspecific as to be meaningless, but it emphasizes the need to be aware of the role of soft tissue or muscle in all types of pain. Indeed, MPS has been reported as the most common diagnosis responsible for chronic pain and disability (Fricton, 1990; Masi, 1993; Rosomoff et al., 1989; Skootsky, Jaeger, & Oye, 1989). MPS is often thought of as a regional pain syndrome in contrast to fibromyalgia as a widespread syndrome; however, as many as 45% of patients with chronic MPS have generalized pain in three or four quadrants (Gerwin, 1995b). Thus, regional pain syndromes should certainly raise a suspicion of MPS (Cummings, 2003; Gerwin, 2001), but patients with widespread musculoskeletal pain can also have MPS. Patients with widespread MTrPs should be diagnosed with MPS and not with fibromyalgia, even though the classification criteria for fibromyalgia suggest making the diagnosis of fibromyalgia "irrespective of other diagnoses" (Wolfe et al., 1990, p. 169). In clinical practice the diagnosis of fibromyalgia should not be made without considering all differential diagnoses (Dommerholt, 2001; Dommerholt & Issa, 2003; Gerwin, 1999). A survey of members of the American Pain Society showed general agreement with the concept that MPS exists as an entity distinct from fibromyalgia (Harden et al., 2000).

Muscle pain tends to be dull, poorly localized, and deep, in contrast to the precise location of cutaneous pain. The diagnosis of MPS is confirmed when the MTrP is identified by palpation. Systematic palpation differentiates

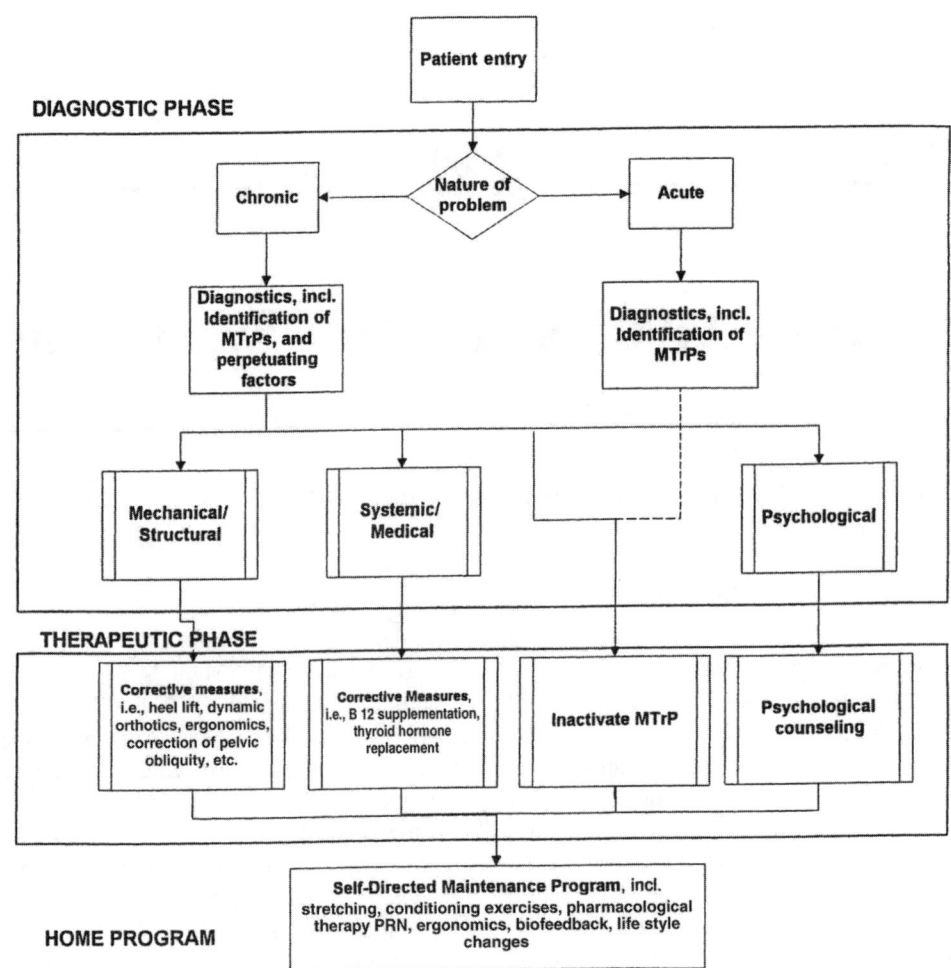

FIGURE 34.1 Treatment program example.

between myofascial taut bands and general muscle spasms (Janda, 1991). An active MTrP is defined as a focus of hyperirritability in a muscle or its fascia that causes the patient pain (Simons & Travell, 1984). The key features of the trigger point have been established by Simons, Travell, and Simons (1999) and are listed in Table 34.1. The interrater reliability of the clinical examination has been established by Gerwin et al. (1997) for the five major

TABLE 34.1
Myofascial Trigger Point Characteristics

1. Focal exquisite tenderness in a taut band of muscle
2. Referral of pain to a distant site upon activation of the trigger point
3. Contraction of the taut band (local twitch response) upon mechanical activation of the trigger point
4. Reproduction of the pain by mechanical activation of trigger point
5. Restriction of range of motion
6. Weakness without muscle atrophy
7. Autonomic phenomenon such as piloerection or changes in local circulation (regional blood flow and limb temperature) in response to trigger point activation

features of the trigger point. Individual features of the trigger point are differentially represented in different muscles. For example, the local twitch response is easier to obtain and therefore more commonly found in the extensor digitorum communis than in the infraspinatus muscle. One should not expect to find each feature of the trigger point in every muscle by physical examination. Reliability of the clinical examination for MTrPs has been confirmed in a study by Sciotti et al. (2001). This study is significant in that is demonstrates that identification of the precise localization of trigger points within a muscle has a high correlation among four examiners. The minimum criteria that must be satisfied in order to distinguish an MTrP from any other tender area in muscle are a taut band and a tender point in that taut band. The presence of a local twitch response, referred pain, or reproduction of the person's symptomatic pain increases the certainty and specificity of the diagnosis.

Making a diagnosis of MPS may itself be therapeutic and may constitute the first step in treatment, as many patients may not have been given a correct diagnosis previously. Patients are often depressed, confused, or frustrated, as they may not have been given an appropriate explanation of their pain in previous evaluations. They often appear relieved when the practitioner can literally put the finger on the source of the pain, which usually results in instant rapport between patient and clinician.

The introduction of pressure algometers has improved the assessment of sensitivity significantly (Fischer, 1986c; Keele, 1954); however, only recently have pressure algometers been applied to the assessment of MTrPs (Fischer, 1984, 1986a, 1986b). Several studies have confirmed the reliability of pressure measurement for the assessment of pain sensitivity (Jensen et al., 1986; Merskey & Spear, 1964), for pressure sensitivity of MTrPs, and for the detection of their location (Delaney & McKee, 1993; Jaeger & Reeves, 1986; Ohrbach & Gale, 1989; Reeves, Jaeger, & Graff-Radford, 1986). Tenderness and the presence of a taut band in muscle may be quantified by pain pressure algometry and tissue compliance measurements (Fischer, 1986a, 1986c, 1993). Fischer (1997) discusses the role of algometry and tissue compliance testing in the diagnosis of MPSs. He incorporates the two main criteria for the diagnosis of MTrPs, local point tenderness (as quantified by algometry) and recognition of patient's symptoms, into his concept of segmental sensitization, radiculopathy, and paraspinal spasm.

Hubbard and Berkoff (1993) identified a characteristic electrical discharge emanating from the trigger point and unique to it. Simons, Hong, and Simons (1995) have further studied this activity, whereas Chu (1995) has reported finding it in the trigger points of persons with lumbosacral radiculopathy. The phenomenon of spontaneous electromyographic activity typical of end plate noise occurring in myofascial trigger points has been further confirmed in a study of young subjects with chronic shoulder and arm pain (Couppé et al., 2001). Studies by Simons, Hong, and Simons (2003) have shown that end plate noise without spikes was found at trigger point sites to a significantly greater degree than at end plate zones outside of trigger points, and not at all in taut band sites outside of an end plate zone. They concluded that end plate noise is characteristic of, but not restricted to, the region of a myofascial trigger point. Phentolamine infusion reduced the average integrated signal of the spontaneous electrical activity by about one third in the experimental animal model. This result shows that there is a modulating effect of the sympathetic nervous system on the motor activity of the trigger point (Chen et al., 1998). Thus, an objective electromyographic (EMG) signature of the trigger point is now available for diagnostic and research purposes.

PRINCIPLES OF TREATMENT

The ultimate goal of treatment of persons with MPS is restoration of function through inactivation of the trigger point, restoration of normal tissue mobility, and elimina-

tion of pain (Dommerholt, 2001; Miller, 1994). The patient and the clinician need to identify appropriate goals and develop the means to implement them through therapy. Inactivation of the trigger point is a means to achieve relief of pain, to improve biomechanical function, and thus to improve the ability of the patient to better perform whatever desired tasks have been selected as goals. Relief of pain or increased range of motion, both of which can be the result of trigger point inactivation, are not in themselves the final goals of treatment. For some individuals, an initial goal may be simply to sleep through the night. For another patient, it may be eating out of bed at a table, or fastening a bra behind the back. For yet another, it may be regaining sexual ability or returning to work or to a recreational activity. Reasonable goals that can be achieved and measured as being reached or not are more important to focus on than simply the inactivation of a tender point or an increase in the range of a particular movement (Gerwin, 2000).

Inactivation of the MTrP can be achieved manually, by correcting structural mechanical stressors, by direct injection of a local anesthetic into the muscle, or by dry needle intramuscular stimulation of the MTrP. Treatment of the patient with MPS can be very effective when used in the context of a comprehensive diagnostic and treatment spectrum (Yue, 1995). After establishing an accurate medical diagnosis with identification of systemic, mechanical, and psychological perpetuating factors, the patient with chronic MPS is best treated through an interdisciplinary team approach (Turk & Okifuji, 1999). The term *interdisciplinary* is preferred to multidisciplinary because it reflects the coordinated working relationship between members of the treatment team (Melvin, 1980; Turk & Rudy, 1994). Essential members of the interdisciplinary team include the patient, physicians, psychologists, clinical social workers, occupational therapists, physical therapists, ergonomists, massage therapists, and others actively involved in patient care (Ghia, 1992; Khalil et al., 1993). Not every patient with MPS necessarily requires such an extensive collaboration. For example, patients with acute MPS may only require treatment by physicians and physical therapists. The treatment plan can be divided into a pain control phase and a training or conditioning phase (Saal & Saal, 1991). During the pain control phase, the most essential components are manual therapy, trigger point injection, dry needling, and elimination of mechanical perpetuating factors. Throughout the treatment process, much attention should be paid to educating the patient concerning the etiology, perpetuating factors, and self-management. Patients must learn to modify their behaviors and avoid overloading the muscles without resorting to total inactivity (Simons & Simons, 1994). Following the pain control phase, patients should be introduced to therapeutic exercises, movement reeducation, and overall conditioning. Too often, patients with chronic myofascial pain dysfunction are introduced too soon to isotonic training and conditioning, causing further aggravation of active trigger points and an increase of pain and dysfunction. Likewise, work hardening programs should never be conducted during this phase of treatment. This can lead to further discouragement and depression, as well as an increase in pain. On the other hand, the pain control phase must be time limited, and patients must understand that progressing to the conditioning phase is imperative. If they do not move beyond the pain control phase, patients can be restricted in their functional abilities and be at greater risk of reinjury (Saal & Saal, 1991). In daily practice, the various aspects of the rehabilitation process are addressed simultaneously and not treated as separate entities.

MANUAL THERAPY

Manual therapy is one of the basic treatment options for MPS. In conjunction with manual therapy approaches, Simons et al. (1999) advocate the stretch-and-spray technique, which combines use of a vapocoolant spray with passive stretching of the muscle. Application of vapocoolant spray stimulates thermal and tactile A-beta skin receptors, thereby inhibiting C-fiber and A-delta fiber afferent nociceptive pathways and muscle spasms, MTrPs, and pain when stretching. Prior to applying the stretch-and-spray method, the patient is positioned comfortably. The muscle involved is sprayed with a few sweeps of a vapocoolant spray, after which the muscle is stretched passively. With the muscle in the stretched position, the spray is applied again over the skin overlying the entire muscle, starting at the trigger zone and proceeding in the direction of, and including, the referred pain zone. Following the stretch and spray, the area is heated with a moist heat pack for 5 to 10 min. The patient is encouraged to move the body part several times through the full range of motion. The stretch-and-spray technique can be used in physical therapy as a separate modality or following MTrP injections.

Lewit (1991) suggests using the stretch technique for short or taut muscles and fascia while promoting postisometric relaxation for treatment of trigger points. Postisometric relaxation is also known as muscle energy technique (Mitchell, 1993) or hold–relax technique (Knott & Voss, 1968) and can easily be combined with stretch-and-spray techniques either in the clinic or as part of the patient's home program. The muscle is gently lengthened, taking up the slack until a barrier is reached. The patient is then asked to contract the muscle isometrically against resistance for about 10 s at approximately 10% of maximal effort. Because it is difficult for patients to gauge a level of effort, the clinician presents a force against which the patient pushes. The patient is instructed, "Meet my force, but do not exceed it." Thus, the clinician is in complete control of the effort exerted by the patient, and an appropriately slight contraction of muscle is achieved. Then the patient relaxes the muscle. Once total relaxation is achieved, the slack is taken up again and the process is repeated three to five times (Lewit, 1991; Lewit & Simons, 1984; Simons & Simons, 1994). Respiratory facilitation of muscle relaxation utilizes the contraction of nonrespiratory muscles that occurs with inspiration and the relaxation of the same muscles during expiration. During the relaxation phase, the patient is asked to exhale and look down to facilitate muscular relaxation (Lewit, 1988). A variation on Lewit's approach combines isometric contractions, reciprocal inhibition, and stretch (Fischer, 1995).

Soft tissue mobilization is an essential component of the treatment. Soft tissue biomechanics including stress–strain patterns; the normal inflammatory, repair, and remodeling stages following soft tissue injury (Carlstedt & Nordin, 1989; Nolan & Nordhoff, 1996; Soderberg, 1992); the reactivity of the tissues; and tolerance level and comfort of the patient are considered (Ellis & Johnson, 1996). The intratissue (muscle tone) and intertissue mobility (muscle play) of the structures involved and of the adjacent muscles, fascia, and joints must be evaluated and treated as well. Myofascial adhesions may develop with secondary or "satellite" trigger points in nearby muscles. MTrPs appearing in muscles that are part of a functional unit must be treated together. Muscles that work together as agonists, or that work in opposition to each other as antagonists, constitute a functional muscle unit. The same muscles can be related to each other both as agonists and antagonists, depending on the action being performed. For example, the muscles that move or stabilize the shoulder form a functional unit. The trapezius and levator scapula muscles display this relationship well. These two muscles work together as agonists in elevation of the shoulder, but are antagonists in rotation of the scapula, the trapezius rotating the glenoid fossa upward and the levator scapula rotating it downward. When one of these two muscles contracts to rotate the scapula, the other must relax. If these or some other shoulder muscles become dysfunctional because of the presence of MTrPs that weaken or shorten them and restrict their range of motion, excessive loading on other muscles in the shoulder functional unit may occur. Trigger points in the levator scapula limit upward rotation of the lateral border of the scapula, thereby placing a greater load on the trapezius, which is unable to accomplish the movement with usual effort, or perhaps is not able to accomplish the movement at all, causing a compensatory lifting of the entire shoulder to raise the arm.

The functional relationships of muscles may differ at each end of the muscle because the agonists and antagonists for each muscle may be different at the proximal and distal ends of the muscle. MTrPs may spread from one region to another because of these relationships.

Bilateral axial muscles such as the trapezius, sterno-cleidomastoid, quadratus lumborum, and iliopsoas act as both agonists and antagonists to each other, facilitating the spread of MTrPs across the midline. Muscles that bridge regions, such as the latissimus dorsi, and those that influence posture, such as the effect of the iliopsoas or quadratus lumborum muscles on scoliosis, also facilitate the spread of MTrPs. Thus, MPS can involve a single region of the body or it can spread to involve all four quadrants of the body. Effective treatment should address all the affected areas. Otherwise, remaining dysfunctional muscle units may lead to the recurrence of active or spontaneously painful MTrPs.

Myofascial release techniques and gentle, sustained pressure may soften or elongate shortened or hardened muscles. The principle of the least possible force is applied, instead of applying high stress to the muscle. Effective myofascial release techniques include strumming, perpendicular and oscillating mobilizations, tissue rolling, and connective tissue massage, among others (Cantu & Grodin, 2001; Ellis & Johnson, 1996). Deep muscle massage consisting of effleurage (stroking massage technique) and pétrissage (kneading massage technique) is also recommended (Lehn, 1990; Vis, Raats, & Van der Voort, 1987). After the introductory superficial approach over the entire muscle and adjacent muscles, massage therapy can be applied directly to the taut band and trigger points. Massage and exercise were found to be effective in reducing the number and intensity of trigger points, but the addition of therapeutic ultrasound did not improve the outcome (Gam et al., 1998).

Soft tissue mobilizations may result in improved local circulation, normalization of muscle tone and muscle play, and reduction of reflex activity and pain (Vis et al., 1987; Wells, 1994). By combining gentle approaches with more aggressive techniques, the Swiss physician and psychologist Dejung (1988a) has developed a seven-step treatment approach to myofascial dysfunction. Dejung's approach combines sustained compression, stretch-and-spray techniques, myofascial release, restoration of muscle play, active and passive movements, and dry needling (Dejung, 1987a, 1988b; Grosjean & Dejung, 1990). As part of Dejung's protocol, the patient actively moves the involved muscle, while the physician or therapist maintains constant pressure over the trigger point (Dejung, 1987b, 1994).

Simons et al. (1999) also describe direct manual compression of the trigger point to inactivate trigger points. Although it previously has been described as ischemic compression, it is now termed trigger point pressure release or trigger point compression. The patient can apply direct compression for self-treatment using a Thera Cane® (Thera Cane Co., Denver, CO) or a similar device. Acupressure may be another form of direct compression of trigger points (Kodratoff & Gaebler, 1993). Following the

Simons et al. (1999) protocol or using acupressure guidelines, compression of trigger points is moderately painful.

Trigger points may also be directly related to underlying articular dysfunction (Ellis & Johnson, 1996). In the treatment of myofascial pain, the practitioner must evaluate and, when indicated, treat both soft tissue and joint dysfunction. Muscular and joint dysfunction are closely related and should be considered as a single functional unit (Janda, 1994). Restrictions in joint capsules inhibit muscle function for those muscles overlying the particular joint. Conversely, muscle dysfunction results in joint capsule restrictions (Dvorák & Dvorák, 1990; Warmerdam, 1992). Zygopophyseal joints may have referred pain patterns similar to MTrPs (Bogduk & Simons, 1993; Dwyer, Aprill, & Bogduk, 1990; McCall, Park, & O'Brien, 1979). In addition, Butler (2000) suggests that impaired mechanics and physiology of the nervous system may be another contributing factor in the overall etiology of various pain problems, including myofascial pain. Somatic dysfunction affecting muscle and joint may result in restricted range of motion and weakness that can be rather quickly reversed by manual therapy.

INVASIVE INACTIVATION OF THE MYOFASCIAL TRIGGER POINT (TRIGGER POINT NEEDLING)

Needling of an MTrP, whether injecting an anesthetic or not, is done for very specific purposes (Table 34.2). It rarely is done to eliminate a trigger point permanently, something that occasionally happens when a localized myofascial pain syndrome is acute (weeks, but not months, old). Facilitation of physical therapy is the most common appropriate use of this technique.

Inactivation of the MTrP by injection appears to be the result of the mechanical action of the needle in the trigger point itself, because it can be successfully accomplished by dry needling without the use of local anesthetics or other materials (Chu, 1995; Gunn, Milbrandt, Little, & Mason, 1980; Hong, 1994b). When using injection needles, the use of a local anesthetic is more comfortable for many patients and results in a longer lasting reduction in trigger point pain (Hong, 1994b; Travell, 1976). However, no credible study exists comparing the two techniques, anesthetic injection versus "dry needling" or needling without anesthetic, in a manner consistent with

---

TABLE 34.2

Indications for Myofascial Trigger Point Needling

1. Therapeutic: Relief of an acute myofascial pain syndrome
2. Diagnostic: To identify a MTrP as the cause of a particular pain
3. Adjunctive: Inactivation of MTrPs to facilitate physical therapy

current standards of medical evidence. The use of solid acupuncture needles versus injection needles has not been examined at this time. Gloves are recommended consistent with the practice of universal precautions. After identifying and manually stabilizing the tender area in the taut band with the fingers, the needle is quickly passed through the skin and then into the trigger zone. A local twitch response or a report of referred pain indicates that the trigger zone has been entered. A small amount, usually 0.1 or 0.2 ml, of local anesthetic may be injected into the trigger zone. The needle is withdrawn to just below the skin, the angle of the needle is changed, and the needle is again passed through the muscle to another trigger zone. A conical volume of muscle can thus be examined for active trigger points without withdrawing the needle through the skin. The trigger zone is explored in this manner until no further local twitch responses are obtained. At this point, the taut band is usually gone, and the spontaneous pain of the trigger point has subsided. Patients who have previously undergone treatment can tell when trigger points remain, and when they have been sufficiently inactivated. A knowledgeable patient urges the clinician to continue in an area until a key trigger point is inactivated, at which time there is a noticeable decrease in pain. The process is repeated until the symptomatic MTrPs are treated throughout the functional muscle unit (Hendler, Fink, & Long, 1983; Hong, 1993, 1994a).

Trigger point injections can be performed without anesthetic, so-called dry needling, or with a local anesthetic (Hong, 1994b). Historically, procaine has been used for this purpose, although lidocaine is used primarily today. Procaine is no longer generally available except in powdered form and has to be reconstituted for use, which for all practical purposes means that it has been replaced by the more readily available lidocaine. Procaine had the advantage of a short half-life, which was pertinent if there was a nerve block. Cummings and White (2001) published a systematic review of needling therapies in myofascial trigger point pain. They concluded that direct needling of myofascial trigger points appears to be an effective treatment, but that there is insufficient evidence that needling therapies have efficacy beyond placebo. Moreover, they found no evidence to suggest that the injection of one material was more effective than another. They found no advantage to adding steroids, ketorolac, or vitamin B_{12} to local anesthetic (Cummings and White, 2001). Steroids have the disadvantage that they are locally myotoxic and that repeated administration can produce all the unwanted side effects associated with steroids. For persons allergic to local anesthetics, saline or dry needling can be used.

Dry needling is the act of inserting a needle into the trigger point without injecting any substance. It can be performed by anyone who is licensed to give injections (physicians, nurses, physician's assistants) and by physical therapists in an increasing number of states in the United States, and in other countries such as Spain and Switzerland, and by acupuncturists. Dry needling elicits a twitch response in the muscle, a response that seems to be related to pain relief. To be most effective, the needle should enter the trigger point itself. A detailed account of dry needling has been published by Dommerholt (2004).

Botulinum toxin has been tried successfully in MTrP inactivation, although it can cause a flu-like myalgia lasting days to a week and occasionally weakness beyond the area of injection (Cheshire, Abashian, & Mann, 1994; Childers et al., 1998; Childers, Wilson, & Simison, 1999; Yue, 1995). It is essentially a long-lasting trigger point injection, capable of about a 3-month inactivation of the trigger point compared with the days to 1 week effect of conventional trigger point injections with local or no anesthetic. Porta (2000) reported in a comparative and randomized, but not double-blinded, study that botulinum toxin type A was as effective in relieving MTrP pain as was steroid injection. There was no placebo control in this study. Lang (2000) proposed injecting botulinum toxin type A into the mid-belly of affected muscles in order to place the toxin where neuromuscular junctions or motor end plates are concentrated. In her uncontrolled, open-label pilot study, 17 to 21% of subjects had an excellent outcome, and an additional 39 to 52% had a good outcome (the range representing different subpopulations of patients).

There is no limit to the number of MTrP that can be needled. Common sense and patient comfort dictate restraint. Nevertheless, when treating a regional MPS, a sufficient number of muscles in the region must be treated to resolve the problem and allow effective post-needling stretching. All the muscles in a functional muscle unit must be released and returned to full length, if possible, either by needling or by trigger point compression and stretching. Inadequate treatment that leaves critical trigger points within a functional muscle unit usually results in the recurrence of trigger points throughout the muscles of the functional unit. From 5 to 10 different MTrP sites can readily be treated per session, and some physicians skilled in MPS management treat considerably more in one session. Repeat injections or dry needling into the same area are best done after an interval of 1 week to allow the muscle to recover. Muscles of the affected functional unit must always be stretched, to their full length if possible, after MTrP needling. Moist heat is applied to the muscle to improve the local circulation and to reduce postinjection soreness. Otherwise, MTrPs recur because of residual significant muscle dysfunction. Local anesthetic patches can be applied to reduce the superficial or cutaneous soreness from needling. Complications of MTrP injections are listed in Table 34.3.

Trigger point injections or dry needling is a highly effective way to reduce the local pain and contraction of the taut band. This does not, however, constitute the whole treatment of MPS. The causes that led to the condition

TABLE 34.3
Complications of Trigger Point Injections

1. Local hemorrhage into muscle
2. Local edema
3. Painful contraction of a taut band from inadequate MTrP inactivation (missing the MTrP)
4. Infection
5. Perforation of a viscous body, most commonly the lung
6. Nerve injury from direct trauma by the needle
7. Transient nerve block
8. Syncope
9. Allergic reaction from the anesthetic

must be corrected, when possible. Mechanical, medical, and psychological perpetuating factors must also be eliminated or alleviated to reduce the chance of recurrence. Inadequate attention to these aspects of treatment leads to failure to relieve the pain (Table 34.4).

Acupuncture is used to treat many different types of pain, including myofascial pain (Baldry, 1993). Acupuncture can be performed by the traditional method of using predetermined acupuncture points along set meridians or by the more recently developed method of placing the needle close to the point of pain (Liao, Lee, & Ng, 1994). Japanese acupuncture (shallow needling) reduced the pain of chronic myofascial neck pain in one study (Birch & Jamison, 1998). Acupuncture, in a randomized, double-blind, sham-controlled study, was found to be superior to sham acupuncture when treating trigger points in chronic neck pain, and was also better than dry needling in improving range of motion (Irnich et al., 2002).

Baldry (1993, 2001) has developed a technique of sub-dermal needling over the trigger point. Edwards and Knowles (2003) reported that patients who received superficial dry needling combined with active stretching improved on the Short Form McGill Pain Questionnaire and improved in their pressure pain thresholds more than controls. Gunn, Milbrandt, Little, and Mason (1980) and Gunn, Sola, Loeser, and Chapman (1990) used a method of dry needling called intramuscular stimulation (IMS). IMS involves the insertion of the needle into the taut band without necessarily considering the actual trigger point. It may be

TABLE 34.4
Causes of Trigger Point Injection Failure

1. Missing the trigger point
2. Injecting the secondary or satellite trigger point and not the primary trigger point
3. Inadequate stretching of the muscle following the injection in the clinic
4. Inadequate stretching of the muscle by the patient at home
5. Failure to correct perpetuating factors

combined with electrical stimulation delivered through the needle (percutaneous electroneural stimulation).

MECHANICAL PERPETUATING FACTORS

Biomechanical perpetuating factors have long been known to cause persistent musculoskeletal pain (Simons et al., 1999; Travell & Simons, 1992). Major mechanical factors to be considered in the management of MPS include anatomic variations, poor posture, and work-related stress (Simons & Simons, 1994).

CORRECTION OF ANATOMIC VARIATIONS

According to Simons et al. (1999), the most common anatomic variations are leg length discrepancy and small hemipelvis, the short upper arm syndrome, and the long second metatarsal syndrome.

The leg length inequality syndrome produces a pelvic tilt that results in a chronic shortening and activation of a chain of muscles in an effort to straighten the head and level the eyes. Any asymmetrical position of the pelvis or spine requires a regulatory adjustment of the neck muscles to maintain equilibrium and an appropriate head position (Janda, 1994). The quadratus lumborum and paraspinal muscles contract to correct the deviation of the spine caused by the pelvic tilt. This correction in turn causes a tilt of the shoulder in the direction opposite to that of the pelvic tilt when a simple C-shaped scoliosis occurs. The shoulder and neck muscles then chronically contract and shorten to correct the subsequent neck tilt. Excessive loading perpetuates MTrPs and may result in low back, head, neck, and shoulder pain (Gerwin, 1995a). Trigger points in these chronically shortened and constantly contracted muscles are not readily inactivated until the muscles are unloaded. The combination of trunk muscles that undergo shortening as they constantly pull the spine toward one side or the other is more complex in an S-shaped scoliosis, but the problem is the same. A similar loading of trunk, shoulder, and neck muscles occurs when one hemipelvis has a diminished height relative to the other or in the presence of pelvic obliquity. According to Grieve (1994), the quadratus lumborum may be less likely to develop trigger points during the teenage years, and typically, unilateral low back pain is located on the side of the shorter leg because of early attenuation of the annulus fibrosis on that side. In adults, it occurs on the side of the longer leg, due to later arthritic and spondylitic changes and shortening of the quadratus lumborum. A true leg length discrepancy is corrected by placing a heel lift on the shorter leg. The asymmetry caused by a small hemipelvis is corrected by placing an ischial or "butt" lift under the ischial tuberosity.

A distinction must be made between a true and an apparent leg length discrepancy. An apparent leg length discrepancy or functional shortening may be caused by a pseudo-scoliosis where the legs are actually of equal or nearly equal length, by hip adductor contractures, by hip capsule tightness, or by posterior innominate rotation, because the acetabulum is anterior to the iliosacral rotation axis (LeVeau, 1994; Mitchell, 1993; Reid, 1992). The cause must be identified and then corrected where possible. If the problem is an ilial rotation, the rotation should be corrected. If it is combined with a sacroiliac joint dysfunction, that should be corrected as well. Quadratus lumborum or iliopsoas muscles shortened by trigger points, a cause of pseudo-scoliosis, must be inactivated by stretching or by other means, such as MTrP injections. Placing a heel lift under an apparent shorter leg may increase the leg length discrepancy. Functional shortening, pseudo-scoliosis, and pelvic obliquity can be corrected via osteopathic mobilizations and muscle energy techniques (Fowler, 1994; Greenman, 1991).

When clinical determination by physical examination is uncertain, a radiographic study of the pelvis and lumbar spine using a plumb line can be helpful (Travell & Simons, 1992). A functional scoliosis can be corrected or reduced by a heel lift, even if it has been present for years. A fixed skeletal cause of scoliosis does not correct with a heel or butt lift. Functional scoliosis must be distinguished from those asymmetries that cannot be corrected before attempting to use a heel or butt lift. Relief of pain in the neck, shoulder, low back, and legs can result from the complete or partial correction of leg length inequality and scoliosis.

Saggini et al. (1996) describe the incomplete resolution of pain in persons with peroneus longus MTrPs and leg length inequality corrected only by a heel lift. The peroneus longus has an increased shear force in the medial-lateral plane when loading, which increases eccentric muscle involvement, leading to muscle injury. Correcting abnormal loading associated with leg length discrepancy with a dynamic insole eliminated both the pain and the trigger points.

Short upper arms result in forward shoulder roll, pectoral muscle shortening, and abnormal loading of neck and trunk muscles as the individual attempts to find a comfortable position when seated. Another cause of biomechanical stress on muscles that can lead to the persistence of MTrPs is a long second metatarsal bone. In this situation, the normal, stable tripod support of the foot created by the first and second metatarsal bones anteriorly and the heel posteriorly may not be present. Instead, in some individuals with this foot configuration, weight is carried on a knife-edge from the second metatarsal head to the heel, overloading the peroneus longus that attaches to the first metatarsal bone. Diagnostic callus formation occurs in these individuals in the areas of abnormal loading, under the second metatarsal head, and on the medial aspect of the foot at the great toe and first metatarsal head.

Correction is accomplished with support under the head of the first metatarsal, restoring the normal tripod support of the foot (Travell & Simons, 1992).

POSTURE CORRECTION

In addition to postural deviations due to anatomic variations, muscle imbalances and altered movement patterns play an extremely important role in the etiology and management of poor posture. The clinician should become familiar with Vladimir Janda's extensive research in posture and muscle dysfunction. Janda distinguished "tonic or postural" muscles from "phasic or dynamic" muscles. Postural and phasic muscles are physiologically different in their oxidative ability and their ability to contract over a specified time period. Tonic muscles are slow-twitch (Type I) muscles. Phasic muscles are fast-twitch (Type II) muscles. MTrPs can develop in both tonic and phasic muscles. Tonic muscles include the hamstrings muscles, rectus femoris, iliopsoas, quadratus lumborum, erector spinae muscles, pectorals, sternocleidomastoids, descending trapezius muscles, and levator scapulae. Phasic muscles include the rectus abdominus, serratus anterior, rhomboids, ascending and transverse trapezius, deep neck flexors, suprahyoid, and mylohyoid (Cantu & Grodin, 2001; Carriere, 1996; Janda, 1983, 1993, 1994). Tonic muscles have a tendency to tighten in response to abnormal stress or dysfunction, whereas phasic muscles have a tendency to become weak. These typical response patterns result in the "upper and lower crossed syndromes" (Janda, 1993, 1994). The upper crossed syndrome or forward head posture is the most common postural deviation in patients with MPS (Fricton et al., 1985; Janda, 1994; Mannheimer, 1994).

In the forward head posture, total body alignment is severely affected. There is posterior cervical rotation with hypomobility of the upper cervical and subcranial motion segments and hypermobility of the mid and lower cervical spine. Muscle imbalances occur between the anterior and posterior cervical muscles and between the anterior and posterior shoulder muscles. The shoulder girdle protracts, and there is an increase in thoracic kyphosis, a loss of lumbar lordosis, and an increase in posterior pelvic rotation. Muscular imbalances may lead to abnormal afferent input and MTrPs (Cantu & Grodin, 2001). There is a statistically significant relation between the degree of forward head posture, posterior cervical rotation, and pain (Haughie, Fiebert, & Roach, 1995). Poor body alignment, forward head posture, and muscle imbalances predispose and perpetuate chronic pain problems including MPS.

Correcting poor body posture and alignment is an important component of treating patients with MPS, even when posture seemingly may not be directly related to the region of musculoskeletal pain. Core (trunk) stabilization as part of a closed kinetic chain rehabilitation allows optimal control of the lumbopelvic complex and improves the recovery of persons with a kinetic chain dysfunction manifest as a postural stress syndrome (Clark, Fater, & Reuteman, 2000). Good posture minimizes stress and improves efficiency in the use of muscles (Sahrmann, 1988). The physical therapist needs to determine on an individual basis whether manual therapy procedures should precede postural corrections or vice versa. In some instances, joint and myofascial restrictions must be removed prior to any postural corrections. Without the mobilizations, shortened muscles may restrict movement so much that treatment to correct postural abnormalities may not succeed. In other cases, patients may be able to alter their posture prior to or even without any manual therapy (Dommerholt & Norris, 1996).

Correction and prevention of abnormal postures require a comprehensive program that includes exercises to restore normal dynamic pelvic and vertebral stabilization and mobility, motor control, muscle balances, strength, endurance, and breathing patterns. Certain activities of daily living may predispose a patient to chronic musculoskeletal overload, increasing the risk of myofascial dysfunction. A dynamically stable trunk in neutral position is essential, as is normal pelvic mobility (Carriere, 1996). Paradoxical breathing should be corrected with functional abdominal breathing. Paradoxical breathing is a common cause of overload of the auxiliary breathing muscles, most notably the scalene muscles (Carriere, 1996; Travell & Simons, 1992). To improve posture, the individual components must be integrated into total motor patterns (Walpin, 1994). Both the Alexander technique (Barlow, 1973; Jones, 1992; Knebelman et al., 1994) and the Feldenkrais method (Feldenkrais, 1977; Rywerant, 1983) aim to restore function to body awareness and movement retraining and can be used in combination with physical therapy (Dommerholt, 2000). It should be noted that postural control and activation of a sequence of muscles when moving or stabilizing a body part can be impaired by MTrPs, which must be inactivated to correct body mechanics. Lucas, Polus, and Rich (2004) have shown that the normal sequential muscle activation pattern in such movements as scapular rotation becomes abnormal when latent MTrPs are present. Treatment of the latent MTrPs to inactivate them restores normal muscle activation sequencing.

Although posture is usually described in terms of relative alignment of body parts, it is important to realize that a person's posture reflects more than just biomechanical principles. Buytendijk (1964) states that "posture is an individual's innermost means of expression." People express their emotions, feelings, and overall well-being through their posture. Therefore, posture must be viewed as a physiological, biomechanical, and psychological phenomenon. Addressing biomechanical issues without consideration of a more phenomenological approach to posture reduces the treatment approach to strict mechanistic intervention.

WORK-RELATED STRESS

Certain jobs and work-related activities are associated with an increased risk of developing cumulative trauma disorders or work-related musculoskeletal disorders (Kuorinka & Forcier, 1995). In certain instances, MPS may be associated with work exposures (Grosshandler & Burney, 1979). In the ergonomics literature, the term *tension neck syndrome* is preferred over MPS (Viikari-Juntura, 1983). Ergonomics is a broad profession and incorporates knowledge from anatomy, physiology, and psychology. More specifically, ergonomics includes anthropometry and biomechanics, work and environmental physiology, and skill and occupational psychology (Singleton, 1972). Thompson (1991) defines *ergonomics* as "the application of the human physical and behavioral sciences together with the engineering sciences in the study of humans working with machines and tools." Ergonomics is based on the so-called human–machine system. In designing the ideal human–machine system, ergonomics recognizes four strategies, namely, stress reduction, machine and task design, match between the job demands and human abilities, and education and training (Ayoub, 1994; Khalil et al., 1993). Pheasant (1991) summarizes the field as "the science of matching the job to the worker and the product to the user."

Awareness of generic risk factors in work-related musculoskeletal disorders is important. They include awkward postures, musculoskeletal loading, task invariability, cognitive demands, and organizational and psychosocial work characteristics (Kuorinka & Forcier, 1995). Prolonged static postures, awkward postures, excessive force, and repetitiveness are the most likely specific risk factors for MPS (Armstrong, 1986a). Several studies have confirmed that occupational groups with repetitive arm movements and constrained work postures have high rates of MPS (Amano et al., 1988; Bjelle, Hagberg, & Michaelsson, 1979; Hünting, Läubli, & Grandjean, 1981). Awkward postures include wrist flexion and extension, ulnar and radial abduction, forearm supination and pronation, extended reaches beyond the shoulder-reach envelope, and pinch grips that are either too wide or too narrow (Armstrong, 1986b; Feuerstein & Hickey, 1992). For example, the intramuscular pressure in the supraspinatus muscle exceeds 30 mmHg at 30° flexion or abduction, resulting in impairment of blood circulation, mechanical overload of the muscle and adjacent muscles, and increased risk for myofascial pain (Järvholm et al., 1988). Particular occupational groups at increased risk include data entry operators, typists (Hünting et al., 1981), musicians (Norris & Dommerholt, 1996), teachers and nurses (Onishi et al.,

1976), and industrial and assembly line workers (Amano et al., 1988; Silverstein, 1985).

Considering work-related aspects of myofascial pain enhances treatment outcomes. Modifying the workplace or the patient's work habits is critical. If a patient continues to be exposed to certain workplace stress factors without modification of the conditions, the potential cause of myofascial dysfunction may not be addressed adequately. Physical therapists and occupational therapists can contribute significantly to integrating basic ergonomic principles into therapeutic practice, although specific training in ergonomics is indicated (Berg Rice, 1995). More complicated ergonomic problems require the assistance of ergonomists (Ayoub, 1994; Khalil et al., 1994).

SYSTEMIC MEDICAL FACTORS

The problem of unresolved or persistent MTrPs can be the result of systemic medical factors that affect muscle metabolism primarily or affect muscle function secondarily. These factors can be categorized broadly as nutritional, hormonal, metabolic, infectious, autoimmune, etc. An important principle that Janet Travell often emphasized in her lectures is that insufficiency states impair the ability of stressed or overloaded muscle to respond adequately to therapy. Levine and Hartzell (1987) have applied this concept to vitamin C insufficiency. They propose that the optimum concentration of an enzyme cofactor (vitamin or mineral) is that which allows each enzymatic reaction to proceed maximally (not rate limited) when required. For example, many vitamin or mineral enzyme cofactors, such as ascorbic acid (vitamin C) or iron, participate in a number of different enzymatic reactions that are not all equally active at any one time. However, if a limited concentration of an enzyme cofactor becomes rate limiting, then the products of the associated reaction may be insufficient, like the underproduction of high-energy organic phosphates for certain iron-dependent enzymes or the underproduction of serotonin or norepinephrine for certain vitamin-C-dependent enzymes. It is postulated that the needs of the body under physical stress are different from those when unstressed and what may be an adequate concentration of enzyme cofactor under normal conditions may be insufficient at times of physical stress. Hence, the concept of nutritional insufficiency states is distinguished from that of disease-producing deficiency states such as scurvy, the disease associated with vitamin C deficiency. Vitamin C taken in the amount of 10 mg/day prevents scurvy, but 250 mg/day is considered the optimum daily intake for good health.

Four nutritional or hormonal factors have repeatedly been found to be low or in the lower quartile of the normal range in persons studied in our clinic who have persistent myofascial pain, namely, insufficiencies of iron, folic acid, vitamin B_{12}, and thyroid hormone. Of women with a chronic sense of coldness and chronic myofascial pain, 65% have a low normal or below normal serum level of ferritin, largely from an iron intake insufficient to replace menstrual iron loss. Other causes of low serum ferritin include blood loss associated with chronic intake of mixed cyclooxygenase-1 and -2 nonsteroidal anti-inflammatory drugs), and gastrointestinal blood loss associated with parasitic disease. Ferritin represents the tissue-bound nonessential iron stores in the body that supply the essential iron for oxygen transport and iron-dependent enzymes. Serum levels of 15 to 20 ng/ml mean that muscle and other storage sites for iron (liver and bone marrow) are depleted of ferritin. Anemia is common at levels of 10 ng/ml or less. The disease of iron deficiency is anemia. Symptoms of iron insufficiency are fatigue, muscle cramps, and coldness. The association between iron insufficiency and chronic myofascial pain suggests that iron-requiring enzymatic reactions such as reduced nicotinamide adenine dinucleotide dehydrogenases and the cytochrome oxidase reaction may be limited in such persons. This may in turn produce an energy crisis in muscle when it is overloaded and thereby produce metabolic stress. MTrPs may not easily resolve in such circumstances. Iron supplementation in persons with chronic MPSs and serum ferritin levels below 30 ng/ml prevents or corrects these symptoms.

Vitamin D deficiency has been shown to be very common in persons with persistent, nonspecific musculoskeletal pain. Measurement of 25-OH vitamin D was very low in 89% of such subjects in one study (Plotnikoff & Quigley, 2003). Persons who are housebound and those whose clothing covers most of their bodies, reducing exposure to sunlight, are at greatest risk.

Vitamin B_{12} and folic acid metabolism are closely related. They function not only in erythropoiesis but also in central and peripheral nerve formation. Studies have shown that in a subset of patients, serum levels of vitamin B_{12} as high as 350 pg/ml may be associated with a metabolic deficiency manifested by elevated serum or urine methylmalonic acid or homocysteine and may be clinically symptomatic (Pruthi & Tefferi, 1994). Preliminary studies show that 16% of patients with chronic MPS either were deficient in vitamin B_{12} or had insufficient levels of vitamin B_{12}, and that 10% had low serum folate levels (Gerwin, 1995b). Replacement of vitamin B_{12} is life-long, either orally, transmucosally, or intramuscularly.

Hypothyroidism is suspected clinically in chronic MPS when there is a complaint of coldness, dry skin or dry hair, constipation, and fatigue. Hypothyroidism occurred in 10% of subjects with chronic MPS in one study (Gerwin, 1995b). The MTrPs tend to be widespread in hypothyroid persons. The thyroid-stimulating hormone level may only be in the upper range of normal but, as shown by thyroid-releasing hormone (TRH) stimulation tests, still be abnormal for a given individual. Thyroid hormone supplementation to restore the thyroid state may resolve many myofascial complaints and allow resolution of the problem by the usual means of physical therapy and trigger point inactivation. Thyroxine (levothyroxine) is generally used to treat hypothyroidism. However, not all tissues are equally able to convert thyroxine to triiodothyronine, the active form of thyroid hormone. The addition of triiodothyronine to thyroxine has been shown to result in an improved sense of well-being, an improvement in cognitive function and mood, and an increase in serum levels of sex-hormone-binding globulins, a sensitive marker of thyroid hormone function (Bunevicius et al., 1999; Toft, 1999).

Other less commonly associated medical problems that are found in patients with chronic MPS and that act as perpetuating factors include recurrent candida yeast infections, particularly in women who have been given courses of antibiotic therapy for recurrent urinary tract infections. Persons with myofascial pain dysfunction syndromes affecting the temporomandibular joint often complain of sore throat or earache and may be given antibiotics, thereby predisposing them to candida overgrowth. Women who present with widespread MTrPs resistant to usual treatment should be investigated for candida infection. If the history is very suggestive, treatment is indicated even if the organism cannot be implicated by hanging drop examination or culture. Men and postmenopausal women who have elevated uric acid levels may also have persistent MTrPs.

Parasitic infections can also be associated with widespread MTrPs, often complicated by fatigue and an often nonspecific sense of discomfort, and occasionally gastrointestinal distress. Amoebiasis is the most common parasite encountered in MPS in the United States, but giardia, trematode, and nematode infection have also been found. Treatment of these infections results in an overall improvement, and often in a diminution of the extent of trigger point involvement of muscle. Lyme disease can cause myalgia, arthralgia, and chronic fatigue. The myalgia may be associated with trigger points. Post-Lyme syndrome in the untreated individual is characterized by high titers of IgG antibody and no elevation of IgM antibodies. The clinical picture is one of diffuse arthralgia, myalgia, and fatigue. The chronic cases show no evidence of borrelial infection by culture or detection of DNA in blood or spinal fluid. Unfortunately, these patients do not improve with antibiotic therapy given for 3 months (Weinstein & Britchkov, 2002).

Persons with osteoarthritis, rheumatoid arthritis, Sjögren's syndrome, carpal tunnel syndrome, or peripheral neuropathy caused by diabetes mellitus are more prone to develop MTrP. The post-laminectomy syndrome is frequently caused by MTrP. Treatment is always directed toward the underlying condition, as well as the trigger point, where possible.

Viscerosomatic pain syndromes include the development of typical myofascial pain, generally in the body wall, but sometimes in a limb. Visceral organs have segmental pain referral patterns derived from their primary sensory innervation (Gerwin, 2002; Hetrick et al., 2003). Hence, interstitial cystitis and irritable bowel syndrome most often display pain referral patterns to the muscles of the pelvic region that can respond to manual or needling therapy of trigger points (Doggweiler-Wiygul & Wiygul, 2002; Weiss, 2001). Ureteral stone commonly refers pain to the flank or abdominal wall muscles (Giamberardino et al., 2003). Treatment of the trigger points referred to the abdominal wall or flank muscles can eliminate local pain and pain that is referred from muscle that mimics the initial visceral pain, such as the pain of renal colic (Iguchi, Katoh, Koike, Hayashi, & Nakamura, 2002). The myofascial representation of a visceral pain syndrome can long outlast the acute visceral pain. A common viscerosomatic pain syndrome is abdominal and pelvic floor pain caused by endometriosis. The pain may be eliminated by treating lower abdominal MTrPs.

Sleep disturbance can be a major factor in the perpetuation of musculoskeletal pain. Pain is magnified in the presence of insomnia, whether the insomnia is caused by pain or by other factors. There is the rare case in which chronic musculoskeletal pain is eliminated by the restoration of normal sleep when caffeine was reduced or eliminated from the diet. More often, however, sleep must be addressed directly, noting that sleep disturbance is increased in persons with chronic pain. Attention is paid to pain control at night, to sleep apnea, and to mood disorders such as depression or anxiety. Management is both pharmacological and nonpharmacological. Pharmacological treatment utilizes drugs that promote normal sleep architecture, induce and maintain sleep through the night, and do not cause daytime sedation. Nonpharmacological treatment emphasizes sleep hygiene, such as using the bed only for sleep and sex, and not for reading, television viewing, and eating (Menefee et al., 2000).

Psychological stress may aggravate MPS and activate MTrP (Lewis et al., 1994; McNulty et al., 1994). Trigger point EMG activity has been shown to increase dramatically in response to mental and emotional stress, whereas adjacent nontrigger point muscle EMG activity remained normal. Thus, the effect of stress on the trigger point can be highly selective, instead of generalized throughout the muscle. MPS may be the major symptomatic expression of psychological distress. In addition, pain-related fear and avoidance can lead to the development of a chronic musculoskeletal pain problem (Vlaeyen & Linton, 2000). Treatment directed toward reducing stress has been shown to diminish MPS symptoms (Banks et al., 1998). The clinician must be sensitive to this possibility and refer the patient for psychological counseling when appropriate.

SUMMARY

In summary, treatment of MPS begins with the identification of the MTrP as a source of the pain or as a contributing factor, and a delineation of the extent of the problem. The problem may be confined to a few muscles or may be more widespread, regional, or generalized. Direct inactivation of the MTrP is accompanied by correction of mechanical and systemic medical factors that contribute to the development of the syndrome. Exercise to restore physical conditioning reduces the chances of recurrence. Persons with chronic MPS who have not responded as expected to appropriate therapy must be evaluated for further mechanical, medical, or psychological problems that have been associated with persistent MPS. Attention to the postural and physical stresses of work and awareness of the effect that psychological stress has on muscle pain identify those areas that need to be addressed. These problems must be corrected or alleviated to effectively treat the MPS. Effective treatment can be provided through the application of a variety of manual techniques, by invasive inactivation of the trigger point, and by carefully identifying and correcting the factors that interfered with recovery.

REFERENCES

Amano, M. et al. (1988). Characteristics of work actions of shoe manufacturing assembly line workers and a cross sectional factor control study on occupational cervicobrachial disorders. *Japanese Journal of Industrial Health, 30*(1), 3–12.

Armstrong, T. J. (1986a). Ergonomics and cumulative trauma disorders: Symposium on occupational injuries. *Hand Clinics of North America, 2*(3), 553–565.

Armstrong, T. J. (1986b). Upper extremity posture: Definition, measurement and control. In N. Corlett, J. Wilson, & I. Manenica (Eds.), *The ergonomics of working postures: Models, methods, and cases.* Proceedings of the First International Occupational Ergonomics Symposium, Zadar, Yugoslavia, 1985. London: Taylor & Francis.

Ayoub, M. A. (1994). Ergonomic considerations in the workplace. In C. D. Tollison, J. R. Satterthwaite, & J. W. Tollison (Eds.), *Handbook of pain management* (pp. 640–666). Baltimore: Williams & Wilkins.

Baldry, P. E. (1993). *Acupuncture, trigger points and musculoskeletal pain.* Edinburgh: Churchill Livingstone.

Baldry, P. E. (2001). *Myofascial pain and fibromyalgia syndromes. A clinical guide to diagnosis and management.* Edinburgh: Churchill Livingstone.

Banks, S. L. et al. (1998). Effects of autogenic relaxation training on electromyographic activity in active myofascial trigger points. *Journal of Musculoskeletal Pain, 6*(4), 23–32.

Barlow, W. (1973). *The Alexander technique.* New York: Alfred A. Knopf.

Berg Rice, V. J. (1995). Ergonomics: An introduction. In K. Jacobs & C. M. Bettencourt (Eds.), *Ergonomics for therapists* (pp. 3–12). Boston: Butterworth-Heinemann.

Birch, S., & Jamison, R. N. (1998). Controlled trial of Japanese acupuncture for chronic myofascial neck pain: Assessment of specific and nonspecific effects of treatment. *Clinical Journal of Pain, 14*, 248–255.

Bjelle, A., Hagberg, M., & Michaelsson, G. (1979). Clinical and ergonomic factors in prolonged shoulder pain among industrial workers. *Scandinavian Journal of Work Environment and Health, 5*, 205–210.

Bogduk, N., & Simons, D. G. (1993). Neck pain: Joint pain or trigger points. In H. Værøy & H. Merskey (Eds.), *Progress in fibromyalgia and myofascial pain* (pp. 267–273). Amsterdam: Elsevier.

Bunevicius, R. et al. (1999). Effects of thyroxine as compared with thyroxine plus triiodothyrinine in patients with hypothyroidism. *New England Journal of Medicine, 340*, 424–429.

Butler, D. S. (2000). *The sensitive nervous system.* Adelaide, Australia: Noigroup Publications.

Buytendijk, F. J. J. (1964). *Algemene theorie der menselijke houding en beweging.* Utrecht, the Netherlands: Het Spectrum.

Cantu, R. I., & Grodin, A. J. (2001). *Myofascial manipulation: Theory and clinical application* (2nd ed.). Gaithersburg, MD: Aspen Publishers.

Carlstedt, C. A., & Nordin, M. (1989). Biomechanics of tendons and ligaments. In M. Nordin & V. H. Frank (Eds.), *Basic biomechanics of the musculoskeletal system* (pp. 59–74). Philadelphia: Lea & Febiger.

Carriere, B. (1996). Therapeutic exercise and self-correction programs. In T. W. Flynn (Ed.), *The thoracic spine and rib cage: Musculoskeletal evaluation and treatment* (pp. 287–307). Boston: Butterworth-Heinemann.

Chen, J.-T. et al. (1998). Phentolamine effect on the spontaneous electrical activity of active loci in a myofascial trigger spot of rabbit skeletal muscle. *Archives of Physical and Medical Rehabilitation, 79*, 790–794.

Cheshire, W. P., Abashian, S. W., & Mann, J. D. (1994). Botulinum toxin in the treatment of myofascial pain syndrome. *Pain, 59*, 65–69.

Childers, M. K. et al. (1998). Treatment of painful muscle syndromes with botulinum toxin: A review. *Journal of Back and Musculoskeletal Rehabilitation, 10*, 89–96.

Childers, M. K., Wilson, D. J. & Simison, D. (1999). *Use of botulinum toxin type A in pain management* (pp. 30–50). Columbia, MO: Academic Information Systems.

Chu, J. (1995). Dry needling (intramuscular stimulation) in myofascial pain related to lumbosacral radiculopathy. *European Journal of Physical and Medical Rehabilitation, 5*(4), 106–121

Clark, M. A., Fater, D., & Reuteman, P. (2000). Core (trunk) stabilization and its importance for closed kinetic chain rehabilitation. *Orthopaedic Physical Therapy Clinics of North America, 9*(2), 119–135.

Couppé, C., Midttun, M., Hilden, J., Jørgensen, U., Oxholm, P., & Fuglsang-Frederiksen, A. (2001). Spontaneous needle electromyographic activity in myofascial trigger points in the infraspinatus muscle: a blinded assessment. *Journal of Musculoskeleten Pain, 9*(3):7–16.

Cummings, M. (2003). Myofascial pain from pectoralis major following trans-axillary surgery. *Acupuncture in Medicine, 21,* 105–107.

Cummings, T. M. & White, A. (2001). Needling therapies in the management of myofascial trigger point pain: A systematic review. *Archives of Physical Medicine and Rehabilitation, 82,* 986–992.

Dejung, B. (1987a). Die Verspannung des M. iliacus als Ursache lumbosacraler Schmerzen. *Manuelle Medizin, 25,* 73–81.

Dejung, B. (1987b). Verspannungen des M. serratus anterior als Ursache interscapularer Schmerzen. *Manuelle Medizin, 25,* 97–102.

Dejung, B. (1988a). Die Behandlung "chronischer Zerrungen." *Schweizerische Zeitschrift fur Sportmedizin, 36,* 16–168.

Dejung, B. (1988b). Triggerpunkt-und Bindegewebebehandlung neue Wege. *Physiotherapie und Rehabilitationsmedizin. Physiotherapeutics, 24*(6), 3–12.

Dejung, B. (1994). Manuelle Triggerpunktbehandlung bei chronischer Lumbosakralgie. *Schweizerische Medizinische Wochenschrift, 124* (Suppl. 62), 82– 87.

Delaney, G. A., & McKee, A. C. (1993). Inter- and intra-rater reliability of the pressure threshold meter in measurement of myofascial trigger point sensitivity. *American Journal of Physical and Medical Rehabilitation, 72,* 136–139.

Doggweiler-Wiygul, R., & Wiygul, J. P. (2002). Interstitial cystitis, pelvic pain, and the relationship of myofascial pain and dysfunction: A report on 4 patients. *World Journal of Urology, 20,* 310–314.

Dommerholt, J. (2000). Posture. In R. Tubiana & P. Amadio (Eds.), *Medical problems of the instrumentalist musician* (pp. 399–419). London: Martin Dunitz.

Dommerholt, J. (2001). Muscle pain syndromes. In R. I. Cantu and A. J. Grodin (Eds.), *Myofascial manipulation* (pp. 93–140). Gaithersburg: Aspen.

Dommerholt, J. & Issa, T. S. (2003). Myofascial pain syndrome. In L. Chaitow (Ed.). *Fibromyalgia: A practitioner's guide to treatment (*2nd ed., pp. 149–177). Edinburgh: Churchill Livingstone.

Dommerholt, J., & Norris, R. N. (1996). Physical therapy management of the injured musician. *Orthopaedic Physical Therapy Clinics of North America, 5,* 185–206.

Dommerholt, J. (2004). Dry needling in orthopedic physical therapy practice. *Orthopedic Practice, 16,* 15–20.

Dvořák, J., & Dvořák, V. (1990). *Manual medicine: Diagnostics.* Stuttgart, Germany: Georg Thieme Verlag.

Dwyer, A., Aprill, C., & Bogduk, N. (1990). Cervical zygapophyseal joint pain patterns. 1. A study in normal volunteers. *Spine, 15*(6), 453–457.

Edwards, J. & Knowles, M. N. (2003). Superficial dry needling and active stretching in the treatment of myofascial pain — A randomized controlled trial. *Acupuncture in Medicine, 21,* 80–86.

Ellis, J. J., & Johnson, G. S. (1996). Myofascial considerations in somatic dysfunction of the thorax. In T. W. Flynn (Ed.), *The thoracic spine and rib cage* (pp. 211–262). Boston: Butterworth-Heinemann.

Feldenkrais, M. (1977). *Awareness through movement.* New York: Harper and Row.

Feuerstein, M., & Hickey, P. F. (1992). Ergonomic approaches in the clinical assessment of occupational musculoskeletal disorders. In D. C. Turk & R. Melzack (Eds.), *Handbook of pain assessment* (pp. 71–99). New York: The Guilford Press.

Fischer, A. A. (1984). Diagnosis and management of chronic pain in physical medicine and rehabilitation. In A. P. Ruskin (Ed.), *Current therapy in psychiatry* (pp. 123–145). Philadelphia: W. B. Saunders.

Fischer, A. A. (1986a). Pressure threshold measurement for diagnosis of myofascial pain and evaluation of treatment results. *Clinical Journal of Pain, 2*(4), 207–214.

Fischer, A. A. (1986b). Pressure threshold meter: Its use for quantification of tender spots. *Archives of Physical and Medical Rehabilitation, 67,* 836–838.

Fischer, A. A. (1986c). Pressure tolerance over muscles and bones in normal subjects. *Archives of Physical and Medical Rehabilitation, 67,* 406–409.

Fischer, A. A. (1993). *Pressure threshold and tolerance meter (manual).* Great Neck, NY: Pain Diagnostics & Thermography.

Fischer, A. A. (1995). Local injections in pain management; trigger point needling with infiltration and somatic blocks. In G. H. Kraft & S. M. Weinstein (Eds.), *Injection techniques: Principles and practice* (pp. 851–870). Philadelphia: W. B. Saunders.

Fischer, A. A. (1997). New developments in diagnosis of myofascial pain and fibromyalgia. *Physical Medicine and Rehabilitation Clinics of North America, 8*(1), 1–21.

Fowler, C. (1994). Muscle energy techniques for pelvic dysfunction. In J. D. Boyling & N. Palastanga (Eds.), *Grieve's modern manual therapy* (pp. 781–791). Edinburgh: Churchill Livingstone.

Fricton, J. R. (1990). Myofascial pain syndrome: Characteristics and epidemiology. *Advances in Pain Research and Therapy, 17,* 107–128.

Fricton, J. R., Kroening, R., Haley, D. et al. (1985). Myofascial pain syndrome of the head and neck: A review of clinical characteristics of 164 patients. *Oral Surgery, Oral Medicine, and Oral Pathology, 60*(10), 615–623.

Gam, A.N. et al. (1998). Treatment of myofascial trigger point with ultrasound combined with massage and exercise in a randomized controlled trial. *Pain, 77,* 73–79.

Gerwin, R. (1995a). Myofascial back and neck pain. In M. A. Young & R. A. Lavin (Eds.), *Physical medicine and rehabilitation state of the art reviews* (Vol. 9, pp. 657–671). Philadelphia: Hanley & Belfus.

Gerwin, R. (1995b). A study of 96 subjects examined both for fibromyalgia and myofascial pain. *Journal of Musculoskeletal Pain, 3*(Suppl 1), 121.

Gerwin R. D. (1999). Differential diagnosis of myofascial pain syndrome and fibromyalgia. *Journal of Musculoskeletal Pain, 7,* 209–215.

Gerwin, R. D. (2000). Management of persons with chronic pain. In M. N. Ozer (Ed), *Management of persons with chronic neurologic illness* (pp. 265–290) Boston: Butterworth-Heinemann.

Gerwin, R. D., (2001). A standing complaint: inability to sit: an unusual presentation of medial hamstring myofascial pain syndrome. *Journal of Musculoskeletan Pain, 9*(4), 81–94.

Gerwin, R. D. (2002). Myofascial and Visceral pain syndromes: visceral somatic pain. *Journal of Musculoskeletan Pain, 10* (1,2), 165–175.

Gerwin, R. D. et al. (1997). Interrater reliability in myofascial trigger point examination. *Pain, 69*, 65–73.

Ghia, J. N. (1992). Development and organization of pain centers. In P. P. Raj (Ed.), *Practical management of pain* (pp. 16–39). St. Louis: Mosby-Year Book.

Giamberardino, M. A., Affaiti, G., Lerze, R., Fano, G., Fuller, S., Belia, S. et al. (2003). Evaluation of skeletal muscle contraction in areas of referred hyperalgesia from an artificial uteric stone in rats. *Neuroscience Letters, 338*, 213–216.

Greenman, P. E. (1991). Osteopathic manipulation of the lumbar spine and pelvis. In A. H. White & R. Anderson (Eds.), *Conservative care of low back pain* (pp. 200–215). Baltimore: Williams & Wilkins.

Grieve, G. P. (1994). The masqueraders. In J. D. Boyling & N. Palastanga (Eds.), *Grieve's modern manual therapy* (pp. 841–856). Edinburgh: Churchill Livingstone.

Grosjean, B., & Dejung, B. (1990). Achillodynie ein unlosbäres Problem? *Schweizerische Zeitschrift für Sportmedizin, 38*, 17–24.

Grosshandler, S., & Burney, R. (1979). The myofascial pain syndrome. *North Carolina Medical Journal, 40*, 562–565.

Gunn, C. C., Milbrandt, W. E., Little, A. S., & Mason, K. E. (1980). Dry needling of muscle motor points for chronic low-back pain. *Spine, 5*, 279–291.

Gunn, C. C., Sola, A. E., Loeser, J. D., & Chapman, C. R. (1990). Dry-needling for chronic musculoskeletal pain syndromes clinical observations. *Acupuncture, 1*, 9–15..

Harden, R.N. et al. (2000). Signs and symptoms of the myofascial pain syndrome: A national survey of pain management providers. *Clinical Journal of Pain, 16*, 64–72.

Haughie, L. J., Fiebert, I. M., & Roach, K. E. (1995). Relationship of forward head posture and cervical backward bending to neck pain. *Journal of Manual and Manipulative Therapy, 3*(3), 91–97.

Hendler, N., Fink, H., & Long, D. (1983). Myofascial syndrome: Response to trigger-point injections. *Psychosomatics, 24*, 990–999.

Hetrick, D. C., Ciol, M. A., Rothman, I., Turner, J. A., Frest, M., & Berger, R. E. (2003). Musculoskeletal dysfunction in men with chronic pelvic pain syndrome type III: A case control study. *Journal of Urology, 170*, 828–831.

Higgs, J., & Jones, M. (1995). Clinical reasoning. In J. Higgs & M. Jones (Eds.), *Clinical reasoning in the health professions* (pp. 3–23). Oxford: Butterworth-Heinemann.

Hong, C.-Z. (1993). Myofascial trigger point injection. *Critical Reviews in Physical Medicine and Rehabilitation, 5*(2) 203–217.

Hong, C.-Z. (1994a). Considerations and recommendations regarding myofascial trigger point injection. *Journal of Musculoskeletal Pain, 2*, 29–59.

Hong, C.-Z. (1994b). Lidocaine injection versus dry needling to myofascial trigger point. *American Journal of Physical and Medical Rehabilitation, 73*, 256–263.

Hubbard, D. R., & Berkoff, G. M. (1993). Myofascial trigger points show spontaneous needle EMG activity. *Spine, 18*, 1803–1807.

Hünting, W., Läubli, T., & Grandjean, E. (1981). Postural and visual loads at VDT workplace. 1. Constrained postures. *Ergonomics, 24*(12), 917–931.

Iguchi, M., Katoh, Y., Koike, H., Hayashi, T., & Nakamura, M. (2002). Randomized trial of trigger point injections for renal colic. *International Journal of Urology, 9*, 475–479.

Irnich, D., Behrens, N., Gleditsch, J. M., Stör, W., Schreiber, M. A., Schöps, P. et al. (2002). Immediate effects of dry needling and acupuncture at distant points in chronic neck pain: Results of a randomized, double-blind, sham-controlled crossover trial. *Pain, 99*, 83–89.

Jaeger, B., & Reeves, J. L. (1986). Quantification of changes in myocardial trigger point sensitivity with the pressure algometer following passive stretch. *Pain, 27*, 203–210.

Janda, V. (1983). *Muscle function testing.* London: Butterworths.

Janda, V. (1991). Muscle spasm: A proposed procedure for differential diagnosis. *Journal of Manual Medicine, 6*, 136–139.

Janda, V. (1993). Muscle strength in relation to muscle length, pain, and muscle imbalance. In K. Harms-Rindahl (Ed.), *Muscle strength* (pp. 83–91). New York: Churchill Livingstone.

Janda, V. (1994). Muscles and motor control in cervicogenic disorders: Assessment and management. In R. Grant (Ed.), *Physical therapy of the cervical and thoracic spine* (pp. 195–216). New York: Churchill Livingstone.

Järvholm, U. et al. (1988). Intramuscular pressure in the supraspinatus muscle. *Journal of Orthopaedic Research, 6*, 230–238.

Jensen, K., et al. (1986). Pressure pain threshold in human temporal pain. Evaluation of a new pressure algometer. *Pain, 25*, 313–323.

Jones, F.P. (1992). Body awareness in action. In M. Murphy (Ed.), *The future of the body.* Los Angeles: Jeremy P. Tarcher.

Jones, M.A. (1994). Clinical reasoning process in manipulative therapy. In J. D. Boyling & N. Palastanga (Eds.), *Grieve's modern manual therapy* (pp. 471–482). Edinburgh: Churchill Livingstone.

Keele, K.D. (1954). Pain-sensitivity tests: Pressure algometers. *Lancet, 1*, 636–639.

Khalil, T.M., et al. (1993). *Ergonomics in back pain.* New York: Van Nostrand Reinhold.

Khalil, T.M., et al. (1994). The role of ergonomics in the prevention and treatment of myofascial pain. In E. S. Rachlin (Ed.), *Myofascial pain and fibromyalgia: Trigger point management* (pp. 487–523). St. Louis: Mosby-Year Book.

Knebelman, S., Ralson Dressler, P., Mathews Brion, M. et al. (1994). The essentials of the Alexander technique. In H. Gelb (Ed.), *New concepts in craniomandibular and chronic pain management* (pp. 177–185). London: Mosby-Wolfe.

Knott, M., & Voss, D.E. (1968). *Proprioceptive neuromuscular facilitation.* New York: Hoeber.

Kodratoff, Y., & Gaebler, T. (1993). *Meridian shiatsu.* Basel: Sphinx Verlag.

Kuorinka, I., & Forcier, L. (1995). *Work related musculoskeletal disorders (WMSDs): A reference book for prevention.* Bristol: Taylor & Francis.

Lang, A. (2000). A pilot study of botulinum toxin type A (Botox®), administered using a novel injection technique, for the treatment of myofascial pain. *American Journal of Pain Management, 10*, 108–112.

Lehn, C. (1990). Massage. In W.E. Prentice (Ed.), *Therapeutic modalities in sports medicine* (pp. 257–285). St. Louis: Times Mirror/Mosby.

LeVeau, B. (1994). Hip. In J. K. Richardson & Z. A. Iglarsh (Eds.), *Clinical orthopaedic physical therapy* (pp. 333–398). Philadelphia: W. B. Saunders.

Levine, M., & Hartzell, W. (1987). Ascorbic acid: The concept of optimum requirements. Third Conference on Vitamin C. *Annals of the New York Academy of Science, 498*, 424–444.

Lewis, C., et al. (1994). Needle trigger point and surface frontal EMG measurements of psychophysiological responses in tension-type headache patients. *Biofeedback and Self-Regulation, 3*, 274–275.

Lewit, K. (1988). Postisometric relaxation in combination with other methods of muscular facilitation and inhibition. *Manuelle Medizin, 2*, 101–104.

Lewit, K. (1991). *Manipulative therapy in rehabilitation of the locomotor system.* Oxford: Butterworth-Heinemann.

Lewit, K., & Simons, D. G. (1984). Myofascial pain: Relief by post-isometric relaxation. *Archives of Physical and Medical Rehabilitation, 65*, 452–456.

Liao, S. J., Lee, M. H. M., & Ng, L. K. Y. (1994). *Principles and practice of contemporary acupuncture.* New York: Marcel Dekker.

Lucas, K. R., Polus, I., & Rich, P. A. (2004). Latent myofascial trigger points: Their effects on muscle activation and movement efficiency. *Journal of Bodywork and Movement Therapies, 8*, 160–166.

Mannheimer, J. S. (1994). Prevention and restoration of abnormal upper quarter posture. In H. Gelb (Ed.), *New concepts in craniomandibular and chronic pain management* (pp. 93–161). London: Mosby-Wolfe.

Masi, A. T. (1993). Review of the epidemiology and criteria of fibromyalgia and myofascial pain syndrome: Concepts of illness in populations as applied to dysfunctional syndromes. In S. Jacobsen, B. Danneskiold-Samsøe, & B. Lund (Eds.), *Musculoskeletal pain, myofascial pain syndrome, and the fibromyalgia syndrome* (pp. 113–136). Binghampton: Haworth Press.

McCall, I. W., Park, W. M., & O'Brien, J. P. (1979). Induced pain referral from posterior lumbar elements in normal subjects. *Spine, 4*, 441–446.

McNulty, W. et al. (1994). Needle electromyographic evaluation of trigger point response to a psychological stressor. *Psychophysiology, 31*, 313–316.

Melvin, J. (1980). Interdisciplinary and multidisciplinary activities and ACRM. *Archives of Physical Medicine, 61*, 379–380.

Menefee, L. A. et al. (2000). Sleep disturbance and nonmalignant chronic pain: A comprehensive review of the literature. *Pain Medicine, 1*, 156–172.

Merskey, H., & Spear, F. G. (1964). The reliability of the pressure algometer. *British Journal of Social and Clinical Psychology, 3*, 130–136.

Miller, B. (1994). Manual therapy treatment of myofascial pain and dysfunction. In E. S. Rachlin (Ed.), *Myofascial pain and fibromyalgia: Trigger point management* (pp. 415–454). St. Louis: Mosby-Year Book.

Mitchell, F.L. (1993). Elements of muscle energy technique. In J. V. Basmajian & R. Nyberg (Eds.), *Rational manual therapies* (pp. 285–321). Baltimore: Williams & Wilkins.

Nolan, R. A., & Nordhoff, L. S. (1996). Basic concepts of soft tissue healing and clinical methods to document recovery. Part 1. Soft tissue injury repair. In L. S. Nordhoff (Ed.), *Motor vehicle collision injuries* (pp. 131–141). Gaithersburg, MD: Aspen Publishers.

Norris, R. N., & Dommerholt, J. (1996). Applied ergonomics: Adaptive equipment and instrument modification for musicians. *Orthopaedic Physical Therapy Clinics of North America, 5*, 159–183.

Ohrbach, R., & Gale, E. N. (1989). Pressure pain thresholds in normal muscles: Reliability, measurement effects, and topographic differences. *Pain, 37*, 257–263.

Onishi, N. et al. (1976). Shoulder muscle tenderness and physical features of female industrial workers. *Journal of Human Ergology, 5*, 87–102.

Plotnikoff, G. A., & Quigley, J. M. (2003). Prevalence of severe hypovitaminosis D in patients with persistent, non-specific musculoskeletal pain. *Mayo Clinic. Proceedings, 78*, 1463–1470.

Porta, M. (2000). A comparative trial of botulinum toxin type A and methylprednisolone for the treatment of myofascial pain syndrome and pain from chronic muscle spasm. *Pain, 85*, 101–105.

Pheasant, S. (1991). *Ergonomics, work and health.* Gaithersburg, MD: Aspen Publishers.

Pruthi, R. K., & Tefferi, A. (1994). Pernicious anemia revisited. *Mayo Clinic. Proceedings, 69*, 144–150.

Reeves, J. L., Jaeger, B., & Graff-Radford, S. B. (1986). Reliability of the pressure algometer as a measure of myofascial trigger point sensitivity. *Pain, 24*, 313–321.

Reid, D. C. (1992). *Sports injury assessment and rehabilitation.* New York: Churchill Livingstone.

Rosomoff, H. L. et al. (1989). Myofascial findings with patients with "chronic intractable benign pain" of the back and neck. *Pain Management, 3*, 114–118.

Rywerant, Y. (1983). *The Feldenkrais method: Teaching by handling.* New Canaan, CT: Keats Publishing.

Saal, J. A., & Saal, J. S. (1991). Rehabilitation of the patient. In A. H. White & R. Anderson (Eds.), *Conservative care of low back pain* (pp. 21–34). Baltimore: Williams & Wilkins.

Saggini, R. et al. (1996). Myofascial pain syndrome of the peroneus longus: Biomechanical approach. *The Clinical Journal of Pain, 12*, 30–37.

Sahrmann, S. A. (1988). Adult posturing. In S. Kraus (Ed.), *TMJ disorders: Management of the craniomandibular complex* (pp. 295–309). New York: Churchill Livingstone.

Sciotti, V. M., Mittak, V. L., DiMarco, L., Ford, L. M., Pleznart, J., Santipadri, E., et al. (2001). Clinical precision of myofascial trigger point location in the trapezius muscle. *Pain, 93*, 259–266.

Silverstein, B. A. (1985). *The prevalence of upper extremity cumulative trauma disorders in industry.* Unpublished Ph.D. thesis, University of Michigan, Ann Arbor.

Simons, D. G., & Simons, L. S. (1994). Chronic myofascial pain syndrome. In C. D. Tollison, J. R. Satterthwaite, & J. W. Tollison (Eds.), *Handbook of pain management* (pp. 556–577). Baltimore: Williams & Wilkins.

Simons, D. G., & Travell, J. G. (1984). Myofascial pain and dysfunction. In P. D. Wall & R. Melzack (Eds.), *Textbook of pain* (pp. 263–276). Edinburgh: Churchill Livingstone.

Simons, D. G., Hong, C. -Z., & Simons, L. (1995). Prevalence of spontaneous electrical activity at trigger spots and control sites in rabbit muscle. *Journal of Musculoskeletal Pain, 3*, 35–48.

Simons, D. G., Hong, C- Z., Simons, L. S. (2003). Endplate potentials are common to midfiber myofascial trigger points. *American Journal of Physical Medicine and Rehabilitation, 81*, 212–222.

Simons, D. G., Travell, J. G., & Simons, L. S. (1999). *Myofascial pain and dysfunction: The trigger point manual,* 2nd ed. (Vol. 1). Baltimore: Williams & Wilkins.

Singleton, W. T. (1972). *Introduction to ergonomics.* Geneva: World Health Organization.

Skootsky, S. A., Jaeger, B., & Oye, R. K. (1989). Prevalence of myofascial pain in general internal medicine practice. *Western Journal of Medicine, 151*, 157–160.

Soderberg, G. L. (1992). Skeletal muscle function. In D. P. Currier & R. M. Nelson (Eds.), *Dynamics of human biologic tissues* (pp. 74–96). Philadelphia: F. A. Davis.

Thompson, D. A. (1991). Ergonomics. In A. H. White & R. Anderson (Eds.), *Conservative care of low back pain.* Baltimore: Williams & Wilkins.

Toft, A. D. (1999). Thyroid hormone replacement — One hormone or two? [Editorial]. *New England Journal of Medicine, 340*, 469–470.

Travell, J. (1976). Myofascial trigger points: Clinical view. In J. J. Bonica, et al. (Eds.), *Advances in pain research and therapy* (pp. 919–926). New York: Raven Press.

Travell, J. G., & Simons, D. G. (1992). *Myofascial pain and dysfunction: The trigger point manual.* Baltimore: Williams & Wilkins.

Turk, D. C., & Okifuji, A. (1999) Assessment of patients' reporting of pain: An integrated perspective. *Lancet, 353*, 1784–1788.

Turk, D. C., & Rudy, T. E. (1994). A cognitive-behavioral perspective on chronic pain: Beyond the scalpel and syringe. In C. D. Tollison, J. R. Satterthwaite, & J. W. Tollison (Eds.), *Handbook of pain management* (pp. 136–151). Baltimore: Williams & Wilkins.

Viikari-Juntura, E. (1983). Neck and upper limb disorders among slaughterhouse workers. *Scandinavian Journal of Work Environment and Health, 9*, 283–290.

Vis, A. J., Raats, G. J., & Van der Voort, E. J. (1987). *Massagetherapie: Een fysiotherapeutische handelen.* Zevenaar, the Netherlands: Van der Voort.

Vlaeyen, J. W. S. & Linton, S. J. (2000). Fear-avoidance and its consequences in chronic musculoskeletal pain: A state of the art. *Pain, 85*, 317–332.

Walpin, L. A. (1994). Posture: The process of body use; principles and determinants. In H. Gelb (Ed.), *New concepts in cranio-mandibular and chronic pain management* (pp. 13–76). London: Mosby-Wolfe.

Warmerdam, A. (1992). *Arthrokinetic therapy: Improving muscle performance through joint manipulation.* Paper presented at the Proceedings of the 5th International Conference of the International Federation of Orthopaedic Manipulative Therapists, Vail, CO.

Weinstein, A. & Britchkov, M. (2002). Lyme arthritis and post-Lyme disease syndrome. *Current Opinion in Rheumatology, 14*, 383–387.

Weiss, J. W. (2001). Pelvic floor myofascial trigger points: Manual therapy for interstitial cystitis and the urgency-frequency syndrome. *Journal of Urology, 166*, 2226–2231.

Wells, P. E. (1994). Manipulative procedures. In P. E. Wells, V. Frampton, & D. Bowsher (Eds.), *Pain management by physical therapy* (pp. 187–212). Oxford: Butterworth-Heinemann.

Wolfe, F. et al. (1990). The American College of Rheumatology 1990 criteria for the classification of fibromyalgia. Report of the Multicenter Criteria Committee. *Arthritis and Rheumatism, 33*,160–172.

Yue, S. K. (1995). Initial experience in the use of botulinum toxin for the treatment of myofascial related muscle dysfunctions. *Journal of Musculoskeletal Pain, 3*(Suppl 1), 22.

35

Fibromyalgia

Richard E. Harris, PhD, and Daniel J. Clauw, MD

INTRODUCTION

Virtually nothing regarding "functional" somatic syndromes is agreed upon in the medical community. There is disagreement about the appropriate semantic terms we should use to describe these conditions, whether these conditions have a primarily "physiologic" or psychologic origin, and in particular, whether these are truly disabling conditions. In this chapter, fibromyalgia, a "prototypical" functional somatic syndrome, is discussed.

Although the terms we now use to describe fibromyalgia are relatively new, the condition is not. For centuries in the medical literature, there have been descriptions of symptom complexes nearly identical to those we now label as fibromyalgia (McKenzie & Straus, 1995). Many terms previously used to describe this condition, such as myofibrositis or fibrositis, were attempts to link the symptom complex to an underlying pathophysiologic process. The more generic terms we now use to describe this illness reflects the recognition that we know what *does not* cause fibromyalgia, not what *does*. We are fairly certain that there is no *-itis* (i.e., inflammation) of the muscles in fibromyalgia and that it is not simply in the minds of those afflicted (Godfrey, 1996; Straus, 1993; Yunus, 1992).

DEFINITION

CLINICAL FEATURES

To fulfill the criteria for fibromyalgia published by an American College of Rheumatology (ACR) committee in 1990, an individual must have both a *history* of chronic widespread pain involving all four quadrants of the body (and the axial skeleton), and the presence of 11 of 18 "tender points" on *physical examination* (Wolfe et al., 1990). These criteria were never intended to be strictly applied to individual patients as diagnostic criteria, and most agree that at least half of the individuals who have the clinical diagnosis of fibromyalgia will not fulfill this definition.

There are problems with the ACR criteria, and especially with the requirement that an individual needs a certain number of tender points to fulfill these criteria. Tender points are predefined anatomic points that are present in various areas of the body, and are considered to be "positive" when an individual complains of pain when 4 kg (approximately 9 pounds) of pressure is applied (approximately the amount of pressure required to blanch the examiner's nail). Although early studies suggested that patients with fibromyalgia experienced tenderness only in these discrete regions, we now know that individuals with fibromyalgia display increased sensitivity to pain throughout the body (Granges & Littlejohn, 1993). Tender points (e.g., the mid-trapezius region, epicondyles) appear to merely represent regions of the body where everyone is tender; thus individuals who are more diffusely tender will generally have a greater number of tender points. Also, tender points measure not only how tender an individual is, but also how "distressed" he or she is (Petzke et al., 2003). Finally, tenderness is influenced by many factors. Female gender, increasing age, poor aerobic fitness, and mood disorders all tend to increase cutaneous pressure sensitivity. Therefore, rigidly adhering to the ACR criteria in clinical practice will skew the diagnosis of fibromyalgia toward older females with poor aerobic fitness, and high levels of distress.

Although both pain and tenderness are defining features of fibromyalgia, the latter is rarely a presenting complaint. The pain of fibromyalgia frequently waxes and wanes, may be quite migratory, and may be accompanied by dysesthesias or paresthesias following a nonderматomal distribution. In some instances, patients will present with "aching all over," whereas in other instances patients experience several areas of chronic regional pain. In this setting, regional musculoskeletal pain typically involves the axial skeleton, or areas of "tender points," and may originally be diagnosed as a local problem (e.g., low back pain, lateral epicondylitis). Regional pain involving nonmusculoskeletal regions is also common, including a higher than expected prevalence of both tension and migraine headaches, temporomandibular joint dysfunction (TMD or TMJ) syndrome, noncardiac chest pain, irritable bowel syndrome, a number of entities characterized by chronic pelvic pain, and plantar or heel pain.

In addition to pain and tenderness, most individuals with this illness also experience a high lifetime and current prevalence of nondefining symptoms (Clauw, 1995). For example, most patients with fibromyalgia experience fatigue, and at least half of individuals who meet ACR criteria for fibromyalgia will also meet criteria for chronic fatigue syndrome (CFS) (Buchwald & Garron, 1994). The fatigue is commonly worse after activities and may be accompanied by memory difficulties. Memory difficulties, especially with attention and short-term memory, may be the most debilitating aspect of their illness (Park et al., 2001). Other constitutional symptoms include fluctuations in weight, heat and cold intolerance, and the subjective sensation of weakness.

Patients with fibromyalgia and related illnesses also display a wide array of "allergic" symptoms, ranging from adverse reactions to drugs and environmental stimuli (as seen in multiple chemical sensitivity), to higher than expected incidences of rhinitis, nasal congestion, and lower respiratory symptoms. Although some of these individuals may truly be atopic, many of these symptoms are due to neural mechanisms (e.g., hypersensitivities, vasomotor rhinitis). Hearing, ocular, and vestibular abnormalities have also been noted, including a high incidence of sicca symptoms, a decreased painful sound threshold, exaggerated nystagmus and ocular dysmotility, and asymptomatic low-frequency sensorineural hearing loss.

Individuals with fibromyalgia likewise suffer from a number of symptoms of "functional" disorders of visceral organs, including a high incidence of recurrent noncardiac chest pain, heartburn, palpitations, and irritable bowel symptoms. However, prospective studies of randomly selected individuals with fibromyalgia have detected a high frequency of *objective* evidence of dysfunction of several visceral organs, including echocardiographic evidence of mitral valve prolapse, esophageal dysmotility, and diminished static inspiratory and expiratory pressures on pulmonary function testing. Neurally mediated hypotension, postural orthostatic tachycardia, and syncope also occur more frequently in these individuals. Similar syndromes characterized by visceral pain and/or smooth muscle dysmotility are also seen in the pelvis, including dysmenorrhea, urinary frequency and urinary urgency, interstitial cystitis, endometriosis, and vulvar vestibulitis or vulvodynia.

ETIOLOGY

There is evidence of familial aggregation for fibromyalgia. First-degree relatives of patients with fibromyalgia display a higher than expected frequency of fibromyalgia, as well as related conditions (Buskila & Neumann, 1997; Hudson et al., 1993). Like many illnesses, the expression of fibromyalgia may occur when a person who is genetically predisposed comes in contact with certain environmental exposures that can trigger the development of symptoms. There are many environmental exposures that are generally accepted triggers of fibromyalgia, all of which can be considered "stressors." Examples of stressors include physical trauma (especially to the axial skeleton), infections (e.g., parvovirus, Hepatitis C), emotional distress (acute or chronic), endocrine disorders (e.g., hypothyroidism), and immune stimulation, as may occur in a variety of autoimmune disorders (Buskila & Neumann, 1997; Hudson et al., 1993). Although studies of *groups* of individuals suggest that there are many "stressors" that can trigger the development of this illness, because of the plethora of potential exposures to which an individual may be exposed, it is sometimes difficult to assess the putative role of a single exposure in an individual.

PATHOGENESIS

Most investigators in this field feel that the primary abnormality that leads to expression of symptoms in fibromyalgia and related conditions is aberrant central nervous system function (Clauw & Chrousos, 1997; Yunus, 1992). Furthermore, there is a general belief that the central components of the "stress response" may be playing a major role in symptom expression. The principal components of the human stress response are the corticotropin-releasing hormone and locus ceruleus-norepinephrine/autonomic (sympathetic/LC-NE) nervous systems. These systems are capable of being activated by a variety of stressors, and disturbances in this system can have effects on sensory processing, autonomic, and neuroendocrine function.

Sensory Processing

The hallmark of fibromyalgia and other central pain syndromes is abnormal sensory processing. Under experimental conditions, individuals display both *hyperalgesia* — an augmentation of pain processing in which a painful stimulus is magnified and perceived with higher intensity than it would be by a normal volunteer — and *allodynia* — perceiving pain even from a nonpainful stimulus such as light touch (Arroyo & Cohen, 1993; Desmeules et al., 2003; Gracely et al., 2002; Mountz et al., 1995). These data are suggestive of a state of heightened pain perception in fibromyalgia (Desmeules et al., 2003; Staud & Smitherman, 2002), which could conceptually result from widespread changes within the target organs (i.e., skin, muscles, etc.), or from alterations in nociceptive processing within the central nervous system, or some combination of both processes.

Some early theories of fibromyalgia pathophysiology posited that peripheral abnormalities (particularly alterations in skeletal muscle) were underlying the pathophysiology of fibromyalgia pain (Olsen & Park, 1998). However, more recent studies have generally failed to confirm the presence of such alterations (Olsen & Park, 1998; Simms, 1998; Simms et al., 1994; Sprott et al., 1998), although it is recognized that changes in the periphery could play a role in instigating or maintaining fibromyalgia (Ernberg et al., 2000; Staud & Smitherman, 2002). On the other hand, several lines of inquiry support the role of altered central pain processing (i.e., "central sensitization") as underlying the pain of fibromyalgia. Several investigators have moved beyond determinations of tender point counts and dolorimeter values in fibromyalgia to more extensively examine the basis for widespread pain and tenderness in this condition. Such studies have demonstrated that patients with fibromyalgia cannot *detect* electrical, pressure, or thermal stimuli at lower levels than normals, but the point at which these stimuli cause pain or unpleasantness is lower (Arroyo & Cohen, 1993; Lautenbacher et al., 1994). Although nearly all of the research on sensory processing in fibromyalgia has focused on the processing of pain, there are some data suggesting a more generalized disturbance in sensory processing. For example, many patients experience sensitivity to loud noises, bright lights, odors, drugs, and chemicals. These data point to a more centralized disturbance in fibromyalgia.

Additional evidence for central nervous system changes in fibromyalgia comes in the form of studies of central neurotransmitters. In particular, four independent studies have demonstrated that levels of substance P (SP) are elevated two- to threefold in the cerebrospinal fluid (CSF) of patients with fibromyalgia versus controls (Bradley et al., 1996; Russell et al., 1994; Vaeroy et al., 1988; Welin et al., 1995), and it appears to act as a neuromodulator, sensitizing (via the neurokinin 1 receptor) neurons to the effects of other excitatory neurotransmitters and thus potentially playing an important role in chronic pain states (Dougherty et al., 1995). However, the meaning of these elevated CSF SP levels is not entirely clear. The SP could theoretically be derived from overactive peripheral nociceptive fibers or from central neurons. An elevated CSF SP is not specific for fibromyalgia because this finding has also been noted in patients with osteoarthritis of the hip and chronic low back pain. It is likely that these findings are related to the presence of pain, because persons with CFS do not display this finding. Russell et al. (1994) have demonstrated that these SP levels in fibromyalgia are stable, or rise, over time, and do not change in response to acute painful stimuli. Also, the same magnitude of elevation of CSF SP is found in patients with fibromyalgia with and without psychiatric co-morbidities.

Finally, functional neuroimaging has been shown to be abnormal in fibromyalgia, another piece of evidence supporting a disorder of central pain processing. Single photon emission computed tomography was the first functional imaging technique used in fibromyalgia, and identified decreased blood flow in several brain regions known to be involved in pain processing (Mountz et al., 1998). More recently, Gracely et al. (2002) used functional nuclear magnetic resonance imaging (fMRI) modality to investigate differences in cortical activation between 16 patients with fibromyalgia and 16 controls while they underwent pressure-pain testing (thumb-nail pressure). Each subject with fibromyalgia had an fMRI performed while subjected to "moderately painful" pressure as defined by the Gracely Scale (Gracely & Kwilosz, 1988). The control subjects were scanned under two conditions: (1) the "stimulus pressure control" condition and (2) the "subjective pain control" condition. The former referred to testing the controls with the same level of mechanical pressure as the patients with fibromyalgia, while the latter involved scanning the controls when they, like the patients with fibromyalgia, reported moderate pain. It was found that the levels of cortical activation between the patients with fibromyalgia and the controls under the "subjective pain control" condition were similar. However, fMRI scans of control subjects under the "stimulus pressure control" condition showed no significant activation. These results are strongly supportive of alterations in the threshold and gain of the nociceptive system in patients with fibromyalgia and are consistent with a model of central sensitization (Gibson et al., 1994; Lorenz, 1998; Lorenz et al., 1996). These findings of augmented pain processing by fMRI have been confirmed by this same group, as well as a different group of investigators using heat instead of pressure stimuli (Cook et al., 2004).

Autonomic and Neuroendocrine Function

Although stress response function is acknowledged to be abnormal in fibromyalgia, the precise nature of the abnormality has been variable among studies (Clauw & Chrousos, 1997; Griep et al., 1993; Pillemer et al., 1997). The most consistent finding in fibromyalgia is hyporesponsiveness of both hypothalamic-pituitary adrenal (HPA) and autonomic function to standardized stressors (Adler et al., 1999; Griep et al., 1993). The baseline HPA activity in fibromyalgia has been shown to be increased or decreased, depending on the clinical setting (i.e., ambulatory determinations or patients in highly controlled environments) and subject selection (patients with and without comorbid chronic fatigue syndrome or depression) (Catley et al., 2000; Crofford & Demitrack, 1996). The precise nature of the defect in HPA function has also yielded somewhat inconsistent findings, but can best be summarized as showing decreased basal cortisol levels, decreased adrenal sensitivity to adrenocorticotropic hormone (ACTH), and exaggerated ACTH response to exogenous or endogenous (e.g., insulin-induced hypoglycemia) corticotropin-releasing hormone (Adler et al., 1999; Crofford & Demitrack, 1996; Riedel et al., 1998). There is also no consensus regarding baseline autonomic function in fibromyalgia, with early reports suggesting hypoactivity, whereas recent better-controlled studies suggest hyperactivity, manifest as abnormal heart rate variability, and sustained hypercatecholaminemia (Martinez-Lavin et al., 1997, 1998; Petzke & Clauw, 2000).

Psychiatric, Psychological, and Behavioral Factors

There has been a long-standing debate over the role of psychiatric, psychological, and behavioral factors in fibromyalgia. Some contend that *all* of these symptoms are "supra-tentorial" in origin or that fibromyalgia represents a state of distress or vulnerability, whereas others counter that the rate of psychiatric comorbidities in these conditions is similar to any chronic disease. Increased levels of psychological distress resulting in psychiatric syndromes are a common accompaniment of many painful chronic illnesses (Katon et al., 2001). Approximately 20 to 30% of patients with fibromyalgia have significant current depression (i.e., meeting DSM IV criteria) and more than 60% of patients with fibromyalgia will have issues with depression over their lifetimes (Epstein et al., 1999). However, some of these differences in the current and lifetime history of mood disorders may be due to health care–seeking behaviors because lower lifetime incidences of affective disorders are typically noted in individuals with fibromyalgia who are identified in the general population.

Other psychosocial factors play a significant role in some individuals with fibromyalgia, as with nearly any chronic medical illness. These include behavioral pathways, such as sick role behavior and maladaptive coping mechanisms, cognitive pathways such as victimization and loss of control, and social pathways, such as interference with role functioning and deterioration of social or other support networks. As pain progresses from the acute phase into chronicity, problems emerge for the individual such as job loss, financial constraints, distancing of friends, etc. If patients' responses to these problems are maladaptive such as avoidance of work, friends, financial responsibilities, and physical activity, the patient may become distressed and overwhelmed by the pain and its negative impact on life. Increased stress, learned helpless-

ness, depression, increased anxiety, anger, distrust, entitlement, and somatization can all emerge and worsen symptoms. All of these factors are important in dictating how individuals report symptoms, how and when they seek health care, and their response to therapy. This may also explain why cognitive-behavioral therapy has generally been effective in the treatment of individuals with fibromyalgia, as well as nearly any other chronic medical condition (NIH, 1996).

Regardless of the precise percentage of individuals with psychiatric comorbidities, at least 60% of individuals with fibromyalgia have no identifiable concurrent psychiatric condition. Furthermore, psychological factors are capable of not only worsening fibromyalgia; in some individuals it appears as though such factors can lead to "resilience" and mitigate against the underlying neurobiological pain amplification processes. The best example of this phenomenon comes from a study that identified three distinct subgroups of individuals with fibromyalgia (Giesecke et al., 2003). In approximately half of the patients with fibromyalgia, there was no evidence of depression or anxiety, nor of cognitive factors associated with a poor prognosis in pain, such as catastrophizing or external locus of control. A second group, which comprised approximately 30% of this sample, had prominent psychological factors that were likely contributing to symptoms. But a third group, which comprised just under 20% of the total subjects in this study, experienced extreme tenderness and had extremely low levels of depressive symptomatology, as well as an absence of catastrophizing, and very strong rating of control over their pain.

ASSESSMENT/DIAGNOSIS

Diffuse pain is a defining symptom of fibromyalgia and also occurs in a number of other settings. The diagnostic evaluation of an individual with diffuse pain varies depending on the duration of symptoms, and the findings in the history and physical examination. Diffuse pain that has been present for years is likely to be due to fibromyalgia, especially if there are accompanying symptoms such as fatigue, memory difficulties, and sleep disturbance, and the individual is tender on examination. In this setting, a minimal workup is necessary.

In contrast, an individual who has diffuse pain for weeks or months needs a more extensive evaluation. In performing the history, particular attention should be focused on the onset and character of the pain, accompanying symptoms, and "exposures" that could be causing the symptoms (especially to both prescription and over-the-counter drugs and supplements). The examination should focus on identifying signs of inflammation (e.g., synovitis) or other findings (e.g., objective weakness) that are not seen in fibromyalgia.

At a minimum, individuals who present with chronic, widespread pain should have a complete blood count, liver and kidney function tests, thyroid stimulating hormone (TSH), and sedimentation rate (or C-reactive protein) performed during the course of their illness. Because fibromyalgia occurs less frequently in males, some have suggested more aggressive diagnostic testing when a male presents with symptoms consistent with fibromyalgia (especially for conditions that are more common in males such as sleep apnea and hepatitis C infection.)

The physical examination is generally unremarkable in fibromyalgia, other than finding tenderness. The tenderness may be virtually anywhere and is not just confined to tender points. The former concept of "control points," previously described as areas of the body that should not be tender, has been abandoned.

Laboratory testing should be used judiciously. Even if the individual has acute or subacute onset of symptoms, ordering serologic assays such as antinuclear antibody (ANA) and rheumatoid factor should generally be avoided unless there is strong evidence for an autoimmune disorder. There are several reasons for this, including the fact that these tests have a low predictive value in the setting of nonspecific symptoms and that the rate of ANA positivity may be higher in persons with illnesses within this spectrum (Bates et al., 1995; Pincus, 1993).

The overlap between fibromyalgia and autoimmune disorders deserves special mention. Many individuals early in the course of autoimmune disorders may present with symptoms reminiscent of fibromyalgia. Symptoms that can be seen in both fibromyalgia and autoimmune disorders include not only arthralgias, myalgias, and fatigue, but also morning stiffness and a history of subjective swelling of the hands and feet. In addition, a Raynaud's-like syndrome (characterized by the *entire hand* turning pale or red instead of just the digits), malar flushing (in contrast to a fixed malar rash), and livedo reticularis are all common in fibromyalgia and can mislead the practitioner to suspect an autoimmune disorder.

Persons with established autoimmune disorders may also suffer from symptoms of fibromyalgia. Studies have suggested that approximately 25% of persons with systemic inflammatory disorders such as systemic lupus erythematosus, rheumatoid arthritis, ankylosing spondylitis will also meet ACR criteria for fibromyalgia. Because both inflammatory and non-inflammatory mechanisms may be causing symptoms in this setting, fibromyalgia should be suspected when an individual with an autoimmune disorder has symptoms despite normal inflammatory indices, or when symptoms are unresponsive to anti-inflammatory regimens. These same symptoms that mimic fibromyalgia may occur when individuals are being tapered from high-dose corticosteroids (this phenomenon previously had been termed "pseudo-rheumatism").

TABLE 35.1
Frequency of Comorbidity in Fibromyalgia

Syndrome	Point Prevalence in Patients with Fibromyalgia	Prevalence in General Population
Chronic low back pain	67%	12–33%
Irritable bowel syndrome	59%	15–20%
Mood disorder	29%	10–15%
Temporomandibular joint disorder	24%	3.7–12%
Chronic tension-type headaches	23%	2–3%
Chronic fatigue syndrome	18%	1%
Multiple chemical sensitivities	18%	Unknown

Both physiologic and psychobehavioral factors are involved in this spectrum of illness. Perhaps when individuals first develop symptoms, physiologic factors may be primarily responsible. However, with the chronicity of illness, some individuals may develop psychological and behavioral cofactors that exacerbate or perpetuate the illness. These factors, in combination with the physiologic factors, are likely to be the biggest determinants of disability in this spectrum of illness. These latter factors are seen much more commonly in individuals who attend tertiary care clinics, and conversely, individuals who are found with these syndromes in the general population, or in primary care, are less likely to have such factors and are likely to respond much better to purely physiologic (e.g., pharmacologic) interventions.

Table 35.1 presents the frequency of comorbidity in fibromyalgia.

TREATMENT

GENERAL CONSIDERATIONS

Patients with fibromyalgia are diagnosed most often in the primary care setting, and almost half of the office visits are to internal medicine and family practice providers (Centers for Disease Control, 2005; Woodwell, 2000). Rheumatologists are the leading specialty group managing patients with fibromyalgia, which make up 16% of their office visits on average. Indeed, fibromyalgia is second only to osteoarthritis as the most common diagnosis in rheumatology offices. Patients with fibromyalgia have been shown to be extremely heavy utilizers of health care, because of both excess diagnostic testing and the costs of treatment (Wolfe et al., 1997a). A wide variety of approaches — both pharmacological and nonpharmacological — have been applied with varying degrees of success in the treatment of fibromyalgia. The management of patients with fibromyalgia involves a complex interplay between pharmacological management of pain and associated symptoms, and the use of nonpharmacological modalities, especially to address functional loss and disability. As the elimination of all fibromyalgia symptoms (i.e., a cure) is not currently possible, the philosophy of management is symptom palliation and functional restoration. The presentation of fibromyalgia symptomatology is highly variable and each patient must have an individualized evaluation before deciding on an initial treatment plan (Bennett, 2002). Regular follow-up and modification of the initial management strategy is usually required, depending upon the response pattern.

It is important to try to understand the complex interplay between symptoms and functional behavior in patients with fibromyalgia. A typical pattern is that as a result of pain and other symptoms of fibromyalgia, individuals begin to function less well in their various roles. They may have difficulties with spouses, children, and work inside or outside the home, which exacerbate symptoms and lead to maladaptive illness behaviors. These include isolation, cessation of pleasurable activities, reductions in activity and exercise, etc. In the worst cases, patients become involved with disability and compensation systems that almost ensure that they will not improve (Hawley & Wolfe, 1991). Many consequences of these symptoms (cessation of exercise, disruption of sleep, distress because of diminished functional status, etc.) are directly capable of worsening pain, fatigue, and other symptoms.

In the above scenario, only the initial symptoms are likely to be responsive to pharmacological therapy. The dysfunction and resultant behaviors will not necessarily improve if the symptoms improve. Thus, a dual approach that addresses symptoms with pharmacological therapy when appropriate, and uses nonpharmacologic therapies to improve function, modify behaviors, etc., may be optimal.

GENERAL APPROACH

Once an individual with this diagnosis is identified, the practitioner first has to consider whether to "label" the individual. For the majority this label will help them understand their symptoms and the most appropriate treatment, but there may be some individuals for whom this is harmful (Hadler, 1997).

The practitioner should schedule a prolonged visit, or series of visits, when this diagnosis is considered. Although there are no data to support this, it is likely that this "upfront" time is extremely useful for both patients and providers, as it helps the physician understand precisely what is bothering the patient and assists the patient in understanding the goals and rationale of treatment. The physician should explore the symptoms that are most bothersome, the impact these symptoms are having on various aspects of the patient's life, the patient's perception about what is causing these symptoms, and the stressors that may be exacerbating the problem.

Some patients who present with symptoms of fibromyalgia want only to be told that this is a benign, nonprogressive condition. These patients generally have milder symptoms that have been present for some time, and they possess adequate strategies for improving symptoms and maintaining function.

But for all patients with fibromyalgia, education about the nature of this disorder is critical. Physicians should describe this condition in terms with which they feel most comfortable, and then refer the patient to reputable sources of information such as the Arthritis Foundation, several national patient support organizations (e.g., American Fibromyalgia Syndrome of America, National Fibromyalgia Research Association, and Fibromyalgia Alliance of America), or up-to-date Web sites (e.g., www.med.umich. edu/painresearch).

PHARMACOLOGIC THERAPIES

As noted above, pharmacologic therapies are very useful for managing the *symptoms* of fibromyalgia. One useful approach is first to introduce pharmacological therapies to improve pain, fatigue, sleep, mood, etc., and then once these symptoms have improved, to aggressively use nonpharmacological therapies (e.g., exercise, cognitive behavioral therapy) to improve function.

Antidepressants

The majority of clinical trials in fibromyalgia have involved antidepressants of one class or another. Trials studying the oldest class of agents, tricyclic antidepressants, are most abundant, although several recent studies have focused on selective serotonin reuptake inhibitors (SSRIs) and "atypical antidepressants" — a class that includes dual reuptake inhibitors and monoamine oxidase inhibitors. Despite the multiplicity of antidepressant classes, practically all of the agents that are currently in clinical use either directly or indirectly increase neurotransmission mediated by the monoamine neurotransmitters, particularly serotonin (5-HT) and/or norepinephrine (NE; also called noradrenaline) (Rao, 2002b). These activities are thought to underlie the antidepressant activity of these compounds, although the exact mechanism by which this occurs is unknown. These pharmacological activities also appear to be an important mechanism by which antidepressant compounds effect centrally mediated analgesia (Rao, 2002b).

Tricyclic Antidepressants

Unfortunately, the anticholinergic and antihistaminergic activities of tricyclic antidepressants (TCAs) contribute to the relatively poor side-effect profile of these agents. This point may be particularly relevant to the fibromyalgia patient population, due to the relatively high prevalence of comorbid chemical intolerance and multiple chemical sensitivity. Despite these tolerability issues, the use of TCAs (particularly amitriptyline) to treat the symptoms of pain, poor sleep, and fatigue associated with fibromyalgia is supported by several randomized, controlled trials (Bennett, 2001; Kranzler et al., 2002). Surprisingly, the story is less clear regarding the mood-elevating effects of these agents in the context of fibromyalgia or other pain states, perhaps as a result of the fact that most trials have evaluated sub-antidepressant doses of TCAs (Bennett, 2001; Kranzler et al., 2002). In most forms of major depressive disorder, however, the efficacy and remission rates of TCAs are equal or superior to those of other classes of agents, an effect that is hypothesized to result from their effects on both the serotonergic and noradrenergic systems (Dwight et al., 1998). TCAs also have an established track record in treating various chronic pain syndromes, including functional somatic syndromes. Double blind, randomized controlled trials also support the use of TCAs in related syndromes such as irritable bowel syndrome (IBS) (Ringel & Drossman, 2002), temperomandibular joint disorder (TMD) (Plesh et al., 2000), and idiopathic chronic low back pain (CLBP) (Salerno et al., 2002).

Selective Serotonin Reuptake Inhibitors

SSRIs have revolutionized the field of psychiatry, providing safe and effective treatment of common psychiatric conditions including major depressive disorder, anxiety, and social phobia. Much of their success is attributable to the fact that SSRIs display improved tolerability compared with TCAs, a result of their much higher degree of pharmacological specificity. As implied by their name, SSRIs primarily inhibit the reuptake of 5-HT, and they typically lack the extra-monoaminergic activities that characterize TCAs. The SSRIs fluoxetine, citalopram, sertraline, and paroxetine have each been evaluated in randomized, placebo-controlled trials in fibromyalgia (Arnold et al., 2002; Capaci & Hepguler, 2002). The results of these trials have been somewhat inconsistent, leaving some debate regarding the relative efficacy of the SSRIs, especially in comparison with TCAs. Two studies have demonstrated positive efficacy for fluoxetine when compared with either placebo or amitriptyline in treating sleep, pain, fatigue, and depression (Arnold et al., 2002; Goldenberg et al., 1996). However, a third study failed to demonstrate any significant improvement in pain, although mild improvements were noted in sleep and depression (Wolfe et al., 1994). Two placebo-controlled trials of citalopram have been performed. The first was convincingly negative, with citalopram failing to demonstrate any improvements in pain, fatigue, sleep, or mood (Norregaard et al., 1995). The second study demonstrated that citalopram significantly improved mood, although other outcome measures did not improve significantly (Anderberg et al., 2000). One study comparing sertraline with amitriptyline demonstrated that the two compounds were equivalent in producing significant improvements in pain, sleep, and fatigue. Finally, a study comparing paroxetine to amitriptyline concluded that while both improve the symptoms of pain, sleep, and depression, amitriptyline had a larger, more robust effect (Capaci & Hepguler, 2002). Further, amitriptyline was beneficial for fatigue, while paroxetine did not improve this symptom. Taken together, SSRIs appear to be effective for treating certain fibromyalgia symptoms, particularly mood. However, overall their effect sizes on pain, sleep, and fatigue appear to be less robust in comparison with amitriptyline and, perhaps, other TCAs. It is possible that SSRIs that are less-selective serotonin inhibitors, and that have noradrenergic effects especially at higher doses (e.g., sertraline, fluoxetine) may be the best drugs in this class to use to treat the cardinal symptoms of fibromyalgia.

Dual Reuptake Inhibitors

Dual reuptake inhibitors (DRIs) are pharmacologically similar to some TCAs in their ability to inhibit the reuptake of both 5-HT and NE, a feature that may improve their analgesic efficacy (Rao, 2002b). Importantly, DRIs differ from TCAs in being generally devoid of significant activity at other receptor systems, and this selectivity results in diminished side effects and enhanced tolerability (Rao, 2002b). Venlafaxine is the only DRI currently available within the United States, and its current labeled indications are depression and anxiety. Data support its use in the management of neuropathic pain (Mattia et al., 2002) and retrospective trial data demonstrate that this compound is effective in the prophylaxis of migraine and tension headaches as well (Adelman et al., 2000). An open-label study suggested venlafaxine is useful in treating multiple symptoms of fibromyalgia (Dwight et al., 1998). However, these results were not replicated by a more recent randomized, placebo-controlled trial (Zijlstra et al., 2002). One significant difference between these two trials was drug dosage: the study by Dwight et al. pushed each patient to the maximally tolerated dose or 375 mg/day (mean 167 mg/day), while the study by Zijlstra et al. had a single drug arm with a dose of 75 mg/day. Like some SSRIs, data suggest that venlafaxine is primarily a 5-HT reuptake inhibitor at lower doses (i.e., <150 mg), with NE effects apparent only at higher doses (Harvey et al., 2000; Roseboom & Kalin, 2000).

Milnacipran is a DRI that is currently available in parts of Europe and in Japan for the treatment of depression. Milnacipran is unique among clinically available DRIs in its preferential blockade of NE reuptake over that of 5-HT; in addition, this compound is a low-affinity N-methyl-D-aspartate (NMDA) antagonist (Rao, 2002a). Milnacipran is now in clinical development for fibromyalgia in the United States, and the results of a Phase II clinical trial were recently announced (Gendreau, 2002). In a double-blind, placebo-controlled, randomized study, treatment with milnacipran resulted in statistically significantly improvements in the pain, sleep, fatigue, and mood of patients with fibromyalgia.

Duloxetine, another dual reuptake inhibitor, has been recently shown to improve multiple symptoms in fibromyalgia (Arnold et al., 2004). In a randomized, double-blind placebo-controlled trial, duloxetine showed significant improvement over placebo for fibromyalgia pain; however, this effect was seen only in the female subjects. The presence of baseline depression did not influence results because participants with and without current major depressive disorder responded well to duloxetine. Duloxetine is a more potent blocker of 5-HT and NE reuptake transporters than venlafaxine.

Antiepileptic Drugs

The majority of the antiepileptic drugs (AEDs) increase the seizure threshold through sodium and/or calcium channel blockade or by increasing inhibitory neurotransmission; this mechanism of action appears to underlie their analgesic activity as well (Kranzler et al., 2002). Indeed, these compounds are widely used in the treatment of various chronic pain conditions, including postherpetic neuralgia and painful diabetic neuropathy (Wiffen et al., 2000). Pregabalin — an AED at present in clinical development — demonstrated efficacy in a Phase II trial against pain, sleep disturbances, and fatigue in patients with fibromyalgia (Crofford et al., 2002). The precise mechanism of action of pregabalin is unknown, although its analgesic activities may result from the agent's ability to block certain calcium channels (Crofford et al., 2002). Neurontin, a compound with similar pharmacology to pregabalin, is specifically indicated for the treatment of postherpetic neuralgia, and studies support its use in the symptomatic treatment of a variety of pain states as well as headache prophylaxis (Redillas & Solomon, 2000; Wiffen et al., 2000).

Nonsteroidal Anti-Inflammatory Drugs

Nonsteroidal anti-inflammatory drugs (NSAIDs; including COX-2-selective agents) and acetaminophen are used by a large number of patients with fibromyalgia (Wolfe et al., 1997b). However, numerous studies have failed to confirm their effectiveness as analgesics in fibromyalgia, although there is limited evidence that patients may experience enhanced analgesia when treated with combinations of NSAIDs and other agents (Lautenschlager, 2000). This phenomenon may be a result of the fact that concurrent "peripheral" pain (i.e., due to damage or inflammation of tissues, e.g., osteoarthritis, rheumatoid arthritis) conditions may be present, or that these comorbid peripheral pain generators might lead to worsening of "central" pain or both.

NONPHARMACOLOGICAL TREATMENT STRATEGIES

Many feel that "multimodal" treatment programs that combine symptom-based pharmacologic therapy with extensive use of nonpharmacologic therapies are the most effective in this illness. The two best-studied nonpharmacological therapies are cognitive behavioral therapy (CBT) and exercise. Both of these therapies have been shown to be efficacious in the treatment of fibromyalgia, as well as a plethora of other medical conditions (Clauw & Chrousos, 1997; Janal, 1996; Keefe et al., 1986; Mannerkorpi et al., 2000; Minor et al., 1989; NIH, 1996; Park et al., 2001; White & Nielson, 1995; Williams et al., 2000).

Extensive excellent reviews of these topics are referenced for specific guidelines (Mannerkorpi & Iversen, 2003; Williams, 2003). Both of these treatments can lead to sustained (i.e., greater than 1 year) improvements and are very effective when an individual complies with therapy. The challenge for new studies examining these treatments is to improve long-term adherence and compliance, and to move toward using modalities (e.g., the Internet, telemedicine) that will allow a larger number of patients access to these therapies. Also new studies need to address the optimal manner to combine pharmacologic and nonpharmacologic therapies.

There are some general recommendations that can be made based on anecdotal experience. When practitioners first encounter a patient with fibromyalgia or a related condition, they should attempt to determine "where" the individual is in this spectrum of illness. At one end of the continuum is an individual with mild or moderate symptoms and no identifiable functional limitation, concurrent distress, etc. This individual may be completely content with an explanation regarding the benign nature of his/her complaints (i.e., this is not a progressive or destructive process) and encouragement to exercise more, sleep better, etc. On the other hand, this individual may instead wish to take a medication to reduce the symptoms, and then the best initial choice would be a low dose of tricyclic compound because of the global effects on pain, sleep, and other symptoms associated with this class of drugs. If the individual fails to respond to a TCA, then any number of other medications described would be reasonable alternatives, using classes of drugs that make the most sense given the cardinal symptoms the patient displays. This less symptomatic and less impaired group may also benefit from a self-directed aerobic exercise program, or "diluted" CBT, as is offered by the Arthritis Foundation self-help courses.

The other end of the continuum is an individual with significant comorbid psychiatric illnesses, significant functional disability, very high levels of distress, etc. Management of these individuals frequently requires a multidisciplinary approach. Again, it may be useful first to attempt to reduce symptoms with pharmacological therapy, but these individuals may require many psychoactive drugs to manage symptoms, depression, anxiety, etc. When exercise and/or CBT is added, it may need to be more intensive, requiring individualized therapists.

COGNITIVE BEHAVIORAL THERAPY

CBT refers to a structured education program that focuses on teaching individuals skills that they can use to improve their illness. CBT has been shown to be effective in improving patient outcomes in nearly every chronic medical illness, including fibromyalgia, and needs to be tailored to the specific condition being treated (Godfrey, 1996). The skills most commonly associated with CBT for pain include relaxation training, activity pacing, pleasant activity scheduling, visual imagery techniques, distraction strategies, focal point and visual distraction, cognitive restructuring, problem solving, and goal setting. A goal of CBT is to allow patients to gain more control of their illness, and to give them the tools to accomplish this.

AEROBIC EXERCISE

Aerobic exercise has likewise been demonstrated to be effective at improving outcomes for a wide range of conditions including fibromyalgia (Minor et al., 1989). The reason for the benefit is likely multifactorial: aerobic exercise has an analgesic as well as antidepressant effect and can enhance the sense of well-being and control.

In designing an aerobic exercise program, it appears that careful planning is required to enhance tolerability and to ensure long-term compliance. Especially in illnesses such as fibromyalgia, patients may experience a worsening of symptoms immediately after exercise and thus fear that any form of exercise will exacerbate their condition. To reduce the pain associated with exercise, low-impact exercises such as aquatic exercise, walking, swimming, or stationary cycling are recommended. Just as with medication, a "start low, go slow" approach appears to be most effective, with a gradual progression in exercise intensity and a focus on adherence to a lifelong program of paramount importance.

COMPLEMENTARY THERAPIES

There are several different types of complementary therapies that are used by physicians and patients to treat fibromyalgia. Some of these are physical modalities such as trigger point injections, myofascial release therapy (or other "hands on" techniques), acupuncture, and chiropractic manipulation, each of which has some data supporting efficacy (for review, see Berman et al., 1999; Harris & Clauw, 2002).

An early randomized clinical trial testing electroacupuncture in fibromyalgia found significant improvement over sham therapy; however, blinding was not assessed (Deluze et al., 1992). Because electroacupuncture can be felt by the patient, blinding may have been compromised in this trial. Two more recent acupuncture trials that were better blinded both failed to show superiority of acupuncture over control conditions (Harris et al., 2003; D. Buchwald, personal communication). However, in both trials, the control interventions produced a significant reduction in pain (approximately one third of participants having a 2 cm or 30% reduction in a pain on a 10 cm visual analogue scale), suggesting that the control treatments were not inert.

Others alternative therapies fall under the general category of "cure *du jour*": nutritional supplements, diets, devices, etc., that are frequently advertised over the Internet, usually accompanied by testimonials to their efficacy. Because there are very few controlled trials to guide the practitioner in how to grapple with these treatment modalities, a general approach is suggested. The practitioner should first evaluate the safety of the proposed treatment and point out to the patient any potential harmful effects. The physician should then consider whether this treatment is reinforcing a maladaptive belief that in the long run will be harmful to the patient (e.g., a treatment program of prolonged bed rest or of isolation). If the treatment is neither harmful nor maladaptive, then the practitioner may suggest that patients conduct the equivalent of a clinical trial on themselves (as is done in "*n* of 1" trials). In this setting, the patient begins a single treatment (keeping all other variables constant) and determines if the treatment is beneficial. If the patient judges the treatment to be helpful, then the treatment should be discontinued to determine if the symptoms worsen. If the treatment withstands this test of efficacy, a placebo effect cannot be excluded, but in clinical practice, especially in an enigmatic condition such as fibromyalgia, it is difficult to argue with success.

CONCLUSION

Fibromyalgia is a complex disease of unknown etiology with multiple symptoms that overlap with other illnesses. In addition the population of patients is heterogeneous, and a single effective treatment for all symptoms does not exist at this time. We suggest a multipronged approach to treatment that takes into consideration where the patient is in the continuum of pain and psychological comorbidity. An effective treatment may include both pharmacologic and nonpharmacologic therapies.

REFERENCES

Adelman, L. C., Adelman, J. U., Von Seggern, R., & Mannix, L. K. (2000). Venlafaxine extended release (XR) for the prophylaxis of migraine and tension-type headache: A retrospective study in a clinical setting. *Headache, 40,* 572–580.

Adler, G. K., Kinsley, B. T., Hurwitz, S., Mossey, C. J., & Goldenberg, D. L. (1999). Reduced hypothalamic-pituitary and sympathoadrenal responses to hypoglycemia in women with fibromyalgia syndrome. *American Journal of Medicine, 106,* 534-543.

Anderberg, U. M., Marteinsdottir, I., & Von Knorring, L. (2000). Citalopram in patients with fibromyalgia — a randomized, double-blind, placebo-controlled study. *European Journal of Pain, 4,* 27–35.

Arnold, L. M., Hess, E. V., Hudson, J. I., Welge, J. A., Berno, S. E., & Keck, P. E., Jr. (2002). A randomized, placebo-controlled, double-blind, flexible-dose study of fluoxetine in the treatment of women with fibromyalgia. *American Journal of Medicine, 112,* 191–197.

Arnold, L. M., Lu, Y., Crofford, L., Wohlreich, M., Detke, M. J., Iyengar, S., & Goldstein, D. J. (2004). A double-blind, multicenter trial comparing duloxetine with placebo in the treatment of fibromyalgia with or without major depressive disorder. *Arthritis & Rheumatism, 50,* 2974–2984.

Arroyo, J. F., & Cohen, M. L. (1993). Abnormal responses to electrocutaneous stimulation in fibromyalgia. *Journal of Rheumatology, 20,* 1925–1931.

Bates, D. W., Buchwald, D., Lee, J., Kith, P., Doolittle, T., Rutherford, C. et al. (1995). Clinical laboratory test findings in patients with chronic fatigue syndrome. *Archives of Internal Medicine, 155,* 97–103.

Bennett, R. M. (2001). Pharmacological treatment of fibromyalgia. *Journal of Functional Syndromes, 1,* 79–92.

Bennett, R. M. (2002). The rational management of fibromyalgia patients. *Rheumatic Disease Clinics of North America., 28,* 181–199.

Berman, B. M., Ezzo, J., Hadhazy, V., & Swyers, J. P. (1999). Is acupuncture effective in the treatment of fibromyalgia? *Journal of Family Practice, 48,* 213–218.

Bradley, L. A., Alberts, K. R., Alarcon, G. S., Alexander, M. T., Mountz, J. M., Wiegent, D. A. et al. (1996). Abnormal brain regional cerebral blood flow and cerebrospinal fluid levels of substance P in patients and non-patients with fibromyalgia. *Arthritis & Rheumatism, 39*[9S], 1109.

Buchwald, D., & Garron, D. C. (1994). Comparison of patients with chronic fatigue syndrome, fibromyalgia, and multiple chemical sensitivities [see comments]. *Archives of Internal Medicine, 154,* 2049–2053.

Buskila, D., & Neumann, L. (1997). Fibromyalgia syndrome (FM) and nonarticular tenderness in relatives of patients with FM. *Journal of Rheumatology, 24,* 941–944.

Buskila, D., Neumann, L., Vaisberg, G., Alkalay, D., & Wolfe, F. (1997). Increased rates of fibromyalgia following cervical spine injury. A controlled study of 161 cases of traumatic injury [see comments]. *Arthritis & Rheumatism, 40,* 446–452.

Capaci, K., & Hepguler, S. (2002). Comparison of the effects of amitriptyline and paroxetine in the treatment of fibromyalgia syndrome. *The Pain Clinic, 14,* 223–228.

Catley, D., Kaell, A. T., Kirschbaum, C., & Stone, A. A. (2000). A naturalistic evaluation of cortisol secretion in persons with fibromyalgia and rheumatoid arthritis. *Arthritis Care Research, 13,* 51–61.

Centers for Disease Control. (2005). www.cdc.gov/nchs/about/major/ahcd/ahcd1.htm.

Clauw, D. J. (1995). Fibromyalgia: More than just a musculoskeletal disease. *American Family Physician, 52,* 843–844.

Clauw, D. J., & Chrousos, G. P. (1997). Chronic pain and fatigue syndromes: Overlapping clinical and neuroendocrine features and potential pathogenic mechanisms. *Neuroimmunomodulation., 4,* 134–153.

Cook, D. B., Lange, G., Ciccone, D. S., Liu, W. C., Steffener, J., & Natelson, B. H. (2004). Functional imaging of pain in patients with primary fibromyalgia. *Journal of Rheumatology, 31,* 364–378.

Crofford, L. J., & Demitrack, M. A. (1996). Evidence that abnormalities of central neurohormonal systems are key to understanding fibromyalgia and chronic fatigue syndrome. *Rheumatic Disease Clinics of North America, 22,* 267–284.

Crofford, L. J. et al. (2002). Pregablin improves pain associated with fibromyalgia syndrome in a multicenter, randomized, placebo-controlled monotherapy trial. *Arthritis & Rheumatism, 46*(9), Suppl. S613.

Deluze, C., Bosia, L., Zirbs, A., Chantraine, A., & Vischer, T. L. (1992). Electroacupuncture in fibromyalgia: Results of a controlled trial. *British Medical Journal, 305,* 1249–1252.

Desmeules, J. A., Cedraschi, C., Rapiti, E., Baumgartner, E., Finckh, A., Cohen, P. et al. (2003). Neurophysiologic evidence for a central sensitization in patients with fibromyalgia. *Arthritis & Rheumatism, 48,* 1420–1429.

Dougherty, P. M., Palecek, J., Paleckova, V., & Willis, W. D. (1995). Infusion of substance P or neurokinin A by microdialysis alters responses of primate spinothalamic tract neurons to cutaneous stimuli and to iontophoretically released excitatory amino acids. *Pain, 61,* 411–425.

Dwight, M. M., Arnold, L. M., O'Brien, H., Metzger, R., Morris-Park, E., & Keck, P. E. J. (1998). An open clinical trial of venlafaxine treatment of fibromyalgia. *Psychosomatics, 39,* 14–17.

Epstein, S. A., Kay, G. G., Clauw, D. J., Heaton, R., Klein, D., Krupp, L. et al. (1999). Psychiatric disorders in patients with fibromyalgia. A multicenter investigation. *Psychosomatics, 40,* 57–63.

Ernberg, M., Voog, U., Alstergren, P., Lundeberg, T., & Kopp, S. (2000). Plasma and serum serotonin levels and their relationship to orofacial pain and anxiety in fibromyalgia. *Journal of Orofacial Pain, 14,* 37–46.

Gendreau, R. M. (2002). Cypress Bioscience Inc.'s Milnacipran Significantly Improves Pain and Fatigue in Fibromyalgia Patients. San Diego, CA: Cypress Bioscience, Inc.

Gibson, S. J., Littlejohn, G. O., Gorman, M. M., Helme, R. D., & Granges, G. (1994). Altered heat pain thresholds and cerebral event-related potentials following painful CO_2 laser stimulation in subjects with fibromyalgia syndrome. *Pain, 58,* 185–193.

Giesecke, T., Williams, D. A., Harris, R. E., Cupps, T. R., Tian, X., Tian, T. X. et al. (2003). Subgrouping of fibromyalgia patients on the basis of pressure-pain thresholds and psychological factors. *Arthritis & Rheumatism, 48,* 2916–2922.

Godfrey, R. G. (1996). A guide to the understanding and use of tricyclic antidepressants in the overall management of fibromyalgia and other chronic pain syndromes. *Archives of Internal Medicine, 156,* 1047–1052.

Goldenberg, D., Mayskiy, M., Mossey, C., Ruthazer, R., & Schmid, C. (1996). A randomized, double-blind cross-over trial of fluoxetine and amitriptyline in the treatment of fibromyalgia. *Arthritis & Rheumatism, 39,* 1852–1859.

Gracely, R. H., & Kwilosz, D. M. (1988). The descriptor differential scale: Applying psychophysical principles to clinical pain assessment. *Pain, 35,* 279–288.

Gracely, R. H., Petzke, F., Wolf, J. M., & Clauw, D. J. (2002). Functional magnetic resonance imaging evidence of augmented pain processing in fibromyalgia. *Arthritis & Rheumatism, 46,* 1333–1343.

Granges, G., & Littlejohn, G. (1993). Pressure pain threshold in pain-free subjects, in patients with chronic regional pain syndromes, and in patients with fibromyalgia syndrome. *Arthritis & Rheumatism, 36,* 642–646.

Griep, E. N., Boersma, J. W., & de Kloet, E. R. (1993). Altered reactivity of the hypothalamic-pituitary-adrenal axis in the primary fibromyalgia syndrome [see comments]. *Journal of Rheumatology, 20,* 469–474.

Hadler, N. M. (1997). Fibromyalgia, chronic fatigue, and other iatrogenic diagnostic algorithms. Do some labels escalate illness in vulnerable patients? [see comments]. *Postgraduate Medicine, 102,* 161–166, 171.

Harris, R. E., & Clauw, D. J. (2002). The use of complementary medical therapies in the management of myofascial pain disorders. *Current Pain and Headache Reports, 6,* 370–374.

Harris, R. E., Tian, X., Cupps, T. R., Groner, K. H., Williams, D. A., Gracely R. H. et al. (2003). The treatment of fibromyalgia with acupuncture: Effects of needle placement, needle stimulation, and dose. *Arthritis & Rheumatism, 48*(9), Suppl. S692.

Harvey, A. T., Rudolph, R. L., & Preskorn, S. H. (2000). Evidence of the dual mechanisms of action of venlafaxine. *Archives of General Psychiatry, 57,* 503–509.

Hawley, D. J., & Wolfe, F. (1991). Pain, disability, and pain/disability relationships in seven rheumatic disorders: A study of 1,522 patients. *Journal of Rheumatology, 18,* 1552–1557.

Hudson, J. I., Goldenberg, D. L., Pope, H. G. J., Keck, P. E. J., & Schlesinger, L. (1993). Comorbidity of fibromyalgia with medical and psychiatric disorders. *American Journal of Medicine, 92,* 363–367.

Janal, M. N. (1996). Pain sensitivity, exercise and stoicism. *Journal of the Royal Society of Medicine, 89,* 376–381.

Katon, W., Sullivan, M., & Walker, E. (2001). Medical symptoms without identified pathology: Relationship to psychiatric disorders, childhood and adult trauma, and personality traits. *Annals of Internal Medicine, 134,* 917–925.

Keefe, F. J., Gil, K. M., & Ross, S. C. (1986). Behavioral approaches in the multidisciplinary management of chronic pain: Programs and issues. *Clinical Psychology Review, 6,* 87–113.

Kranzler, J. D., Gendreau, J. F., & Rao, S. G. (2002). The psychopharmacology of fibromyalgia: A drug development perspective. *Psychopharmacology Bulletin, 36,* 165–213.

Lautenbacher, S., Rollman, G. B., & McCain, G. A. (1994). Multi-method assessment of experimental and clinical pain in patients with fibromyalgia. *Pain, 59,* 45–53.

Lautenschlager, J. (2000). Present state of medication therapy in fibromyalgia syndrome. *Scandinavian Journal of Rheumatology - Supplement, 113,* 32–36.

Lorenz, J. (1998). Hyperalgesia or hypervigilance? An evoked potential approach to the study of fibromyalgia syndrome. *Zeitschrift fur Rheumatologie, 57* (Suppl. 2), 19–22.

Lorenz, J., Grasedyck, K., & Bromm, B. (1996). Middle and long latency somatosensory evoked potentials after painful laser stimulation in patients with fibromyalgia syndrome. *Electroencephalography and Clinical Neurophysiology, 100,* 165–168.

Mannerkorpi, K., & Iversen, M. D. (2003). Physical exercise in fibromyalgia and related syndromes. *Best Practice Research & Clinical Rheumatology, 17,* 629-647.

Mannerkorpi, K., Nyberg, B., Ahlmen, M., & Ekdahl, C. (2000). Pool exercise combined with an education program for patients with fibromyalgia syndrome. A prospective, randomized study. *Journal of Rheumatology, 27,* 2473–2481.

Martinez-Lavin, M., Hermosillo, A. G., Mendoza, C., Ortiz, R., Cajigas, J. C., Pineda, C. et al. (1997). Orthostatic sympathetic derangement in subjects with fibromyalgia. *Journal of Rheumatology, 24,* 714–718.

Martinez-Lavin, M., Hermosillo, A. G., Rosas, M., & Soto, M. E. (1998). Circadian studies of autonomic nervous balance in patients with fibromyalgia: A heart rate variability analysis. *Arthritis & Rheumatism, 41,* 1966–1971.

Mattia, C., Paoletti, F., Coluzzi, F., & Boanelli, A. (2002). New antidepressants in the treatment of neuropathic pain. A review. *Minerva Anestesiologica, 68,* 105–114.

McKenzie, R., & Straus, S. E. (1995). Chronic fatigue syndrome. *Advances in Internal Medicine, 40,* 119–153.

Minor, M. A., Hewett, J. E., Webel, R. R., Anderson, S. K., & Kay, D. R. (1989). Efficacy of physical conditioning exercise in patients with rheumatoid arthritis and osteoarthritis. *Arthritis & Rheumatism, 32,* 1396–1405.

Mountz, J. M., Bradley, L. A., & Alarcon, G. S. (1998). Abnormal functional activity of the central nervous system in fibromyalgia syndrome. *American Journal of Medical Science, 315,* 385–396.

Mountz, J. M., Bradley, L. A., Modell, J. G., Alexander, R. W., Triana-Alexander, M., Aaron, L. A. et al. (1995). Fibromyalgia in women. Abnormalities of regional cerebral blood flow in the thalamus and the caudate nucleus are associated with low pain threshold levels. *Arthritis & Rheumatism, 38,* 926–938.

NIH. (1996). Integration of behavioral and relaxation approaches into the treatment of chronic pain and insomnia. NIH Technology Assessment Panel on Integration of Behavioral and Relaxation Approaches into the Treatment of Chronic Pain and Insomnia. *Journal of the American Medical Association, 276,* 313–318.

Norregaard, J., Volkmann, H., & Danneskiold-Samsoe, B. (1995). A randomized controlled trial of citalopram in the treatment of fibromyalgia. *Pain, 61,* 445–449.

Olsen, N. J., & Park, J. H. (1998). Skeletal muscle abnormalities in patients with fibromyalgia. *American Journal of the Medical Sciences, 315,* 351–358.

Park, D. C., Glass, J. M., Minear, M., & Crofford, L. J. (2001). Cognitive function in fibromyalgia patients. *Arthritis & Rheumatism, 44,* 2125–2133.

Petzke, F. & Clauw, D. J. (2000). Sympathetic nervous system function in fibromyalgia. *Current Rheumatology Reports, 2,* 116–123.

Petzke, F., Gracely, R. H., Park, K. M., Ambrose, K., & Clauw, D. J. (2003). What do tender points measure? Influence of distress on 4 measures of tenderness. *Journal of Rheumatology, 30,* 567–574.

Pillemer, S. R., Bradley, L. A., Crofford, L. J., Moldofsky, H., & Chrousos, G. P. (1997). The neuroscience and endocrinology of fibromyalgia. *Arthritis & Rheumatism, 40,* 1928–1939.

Pincus, T. (1993). A pragmatic approach to cost-effective use of laboratory tests and imaging procedures in patients with musculoskeletal symptoms. *Primary Care, 20,* 795–814.

Plesh, O., Curtis, D., Levine, J., & McCall, W. D., Jr. (2000). Amitriptyline treatment of chronic pain in patients with temporomandibular disorders. *Journal of Oral Rehabilitation, 27,* 834–841.

Rao, S. (2002a). Monoamine reuptake and NMDA antagonist profile of milnacipran: A comparison to duloxetine. Society for Neuroscience, 32nd Annual Meeting, Orlando, FL.

Rao, S. G. (2002b). The neuropharmacology of centrally-acting analgesic medications in fibromyalgia. *Rheumatic Disease Clinics of North America, 28,* 235–259.

Redillas, C., & Solomon, S. (2000). Prophylactic pharmacological treatment of chronic daily headache. *Headache, 40,* 83-102.

Riedel, W., Layka, H., & Neeck, G. (1998). Secretory pattern of GH, TSH, thyroid hormones, ACTH, cortisol, FSH, and LH in patients with fibromyalgia syndrome following systemic injection of the relevant hypothalamic-releasing hormones. *Zeitschrift fur Rheumatologie, 57*(Suppl. 2), 81–87.

Ringel, Y., & Drossman, D. A. (2002). Irritable bowel syndrome: classification and conceptualization. *Journal of Clinical Gastroenterology, 35,* S7–10.

Roseboom, P. H., & Kalin, N. H. (2000). Neuropharmacology of venlafaxine. *Depression and Anxiety, 12*(Suppl. 1), 20–29.

Russell, I. J., Orr, M. D., Littman, B., Vipraio, G. A., Alboukrek, D., Michalek, J. E. et al. (1994). Elevated cerebrospinal fluid levels of substance P in patients with the fibromyalgia syndrome. *Arthritis & Rheumatism, 37,* 1593–1601.

Salerno, S. M., Browning, R., & Jackson, J. L. (2002). The effect of antidepressant treatment on chronic back pain: A meta-analysis. *Archives of Internal Medicine, 162,* 19–24.

Simms, R. W. (1998). Fibromyalgia is not a muscle disorder. *American Journal of Medical Science, 315,* 346–350.

Simms, R. W., Roy, S. H., Hrovat, M., Anderson, J. J., Skrinar, G., LePoole, S. R. et al. (1994). Lack of association between fibromyalgia syndrome and abnormalities in muscle energy metabolism. *Arthritis & Rheumatism, 37,* 794–800.

Sprott, H., Bradley, L. A., Oh, S. J., Wintersberger, W., Alarcon, G. S., Mussell, H. G. et al. (1998). Immunohistochemical and molecular studies of serotonin, substance P, galanin, pituitary adenyl cyclase-activating polypeptide, and secretoneurin in fibromyalgic muscle tissue. *Arthritis & Rheumatism, 41,* 1689–1694.

Staud, R., & Smitherman, M. L. (2002). Peripheral and central sensitization in fibromyalgia: Pathogenetic role. *Current Pain and Headache Reports, 6,* 259–266.

Straus, S. E. (1993). Studies of herpes virus infection in chronic fatigue syndrome. *Ciba Foundation Symposium, 173,* 132–139.

Vaeroy, H., Helle, R., Forre, O., Kass, E., & Terenius, L. (1988). Elevated CSF levels of substance P and high incidence of Raynaud phenomenon in patients with fibromyalgia: New features for diagnosis. *Pain, 32,* 21–26.

Welin, M., Bragee, B., Nyberg, F., & Kristiansson, M. (1995). Elevated substance P levels are contrasted by a decrease in met-enkephalin-arg-phe levels in CSF from fibromyalgia patients. *Journal of Musculoskeletal Pain, 3,* 4.

White, K. P., & Nielson, W. R. (1995). Cognitive behavioral treatment of fibromyalgia syndrome: A followup assessment. *Journal of Rheumatology, 22,* 717–721.

Wiffen, P., Collins, S., McQuay, H., Carroll, D., Jadad, A., & Moore, A. (2000). Anticonvulsant drugs for acute and chronic pain. *Cochrane Database of Systematic Reviews,* CD001133.

Williams, D. A. (2003). Psychological and behavioral therapies in fibromyalgia and related syndromes. *Bailliere's Best Practice and Research. Clinical Rheumatology, 17*(4), 649–665.

Williams, D. A., Cary, M. A., Glazer, L. J., Rodriguez, A. M., & Clauw, D. J. (2000). Randomized controlled trial of CBT to improve functional status in fibromyalgia. *American College of Rheumatology, 43,* S210.

Wolfe, F., Anderson, J., Harkness, D., Bennett, R. M., Caro, X. J., Goldenberg, D. L. et al. (1997a). A prospective, longitudinal, multicenter study of service utilization and costs in fibromyalgia. *Arthritis & Rheumatism, 40,* 1560–1570.

Wolfe, F., Anderson, J., Harkness, D., Bennett, R. M., Caro, X. J., Goldenberg, D. L. et al. (1997b). Health status and disease severity in fibromyalgia: Results of a six- center longitudinal study [see comments]. *Arthritis & Rheumatism, 40,* 1571–1579.

Wolfe, F., Cathey, M. A., & Hawley, D. J. (1994). A double-blind placebo controlled trial of fluoxetine in fibromyalgia. *Scandinavian Journal of Rheumatology, 23,* 255–259.

Wolfe, F., Smythe, H. A., Yunus, M. B., Bennett, R. M., Bombardier, C., Goldenberg, D. L. et al. (1990). The American College of Rheumatology 1990 Criteria for the Classification of Fibromyalgia. Report of the Multicenter Criteria Committee. *Arthritis & Rheumatism, 33,* 160–172.

Woodwell, D. A. (2000). National Ambulatory Medical Care Survey. 1998 Summary. Advance data from vital and health statistics, no. 315. Hyattsville, MD: National Center for Health Statistics.

Yunus, M. B. (1992). Towards a model of pathophysiology of fibromyalgia: Aberrant central pain mechanisms with peripheral modulation. *Journal of Rheumatology, 19,* 846–850.

Zijlstra, T. R., Barendregt, P. J., & van de Laar, M. A. (2002). Venlafaxine in fibromyalgia: Results of a randomized, placebo-controlled, double-blind trial. *Arthritis & Rheumatism, 46*(9), Suppl. S105.

36

Complex Regional Pain Syndrome, Types I and II

Nelson H. Hendler, MD, MS

INTRODUCTION

Complex regional pain syndrome, type I (CRPS I) (formerly known as reflex sympathetic dystrophy, RSD) and complex regional pain syndrome, type II (CRPS II) (formerly known as causalgia) are symptom complexes that evoke a great deal of confusion. Very often, physicians do not recognize that these are separate and distinct entities, and commonly assume that they are disorders of the same etiology, as well as responsive to the same treatment. Clinically, this has not proven accurate. CRPS I is a group of symptoms and clinical signs that usually follows a minor injury to a limb. In contradistinction, CRPS II is usually associated with peripheral nerve injury, classically from a bullet wound or some other partial nerve damage. Throughout this chapter, for the sake of consistency, earlier references that used the terms of RSD are referenced or quoted as CRPS I, despite the original nomenclature. This same approach is used for references using the term causalgia, which are changed, for the sake of continuity, to CRPS II. In a very fine review article, Payne (1986) clearly defined the distinction between CRPS I and CRPS II, although at the time he called them RSD and causalgia, respectively. This has been further expanded by the International Association for the Study of Pain in a supplement edited by Merskey (1986; Table 36.1). A further expansion of this comparison is offered by Baron, Blumberg, and Janig (1996; Table 36.2).

CLINICAL SIGNS AND SYMPTOMS

Clinically, one can make the distinction between the two disorders on the basis of signs and symptoms. This is a more important set of criteria than results of laboratory tests or response to treatment because test results for this disorder are highly variable and the accuracy of diagnosis of this disorder is low. If a disorder is misdiagnosed, then how can a physician rely on the response to treatment as a way of establishing a diagnosis? However, sometimes physicians establish a diagnosis based on a response to treatment. This circular logic predicts that all disorders respond equally well to a given treatment, and those that do not are the fault of the patient. This ego-protective trap is a convenient one into which an unsuspecting physician might easily fall. However, there is valuable information that can be derived from a patient's response to treatment, from both a retrospective and a prospective research position. Obviously, the variables in clinical research are legion and include the variable responses patients have to a single pathological etiology, the similar manifestations patients have to diseases of multiple etiologies, the variability of accurate diagnosis, the variability of the skill of the physician performing a procedure, and the variable response to a single, well-performed procedure. Five variables have already been mentioned, giving rise to a 5-factorial variable, or 120 possible combinations of factors. Therefore, in analyzing the results of clinical research in humans, one has to be very circumspect. As Sir William Osler (Osler

TABLE 36.1
Comparison between CRPS Type I and Type II

<table>
<tr><td colspan="2" align="center">Complex Regional Pain Syndrome, Type II (Causalgia)</td></tr>
<tr><td>Definition</td><td>Burning pain, allodynia, and hyperpathia, usually in the hand or foot, after a partial injury to a nerve or one of its major branches</td></tr>
<tr><td>Site</td><td>In the region of the limb innervated by the damaged nerve, not around the entire limb</td></tr>
<tr><td>Main features</td><td>Onset usually immediately after partial nerve injury or may be delayed for months; CRPS II of the radial nerve very rare; the nerves most commonly involved are the median, the sciatic, and tibial, and the ulnar; spontaneous pain; pain described as constant, burning, exacerbated by light touch, stress, temperature change or movement of involved limb, visual and auditory stimuli (e.g., a sudden sound or bright light, emotional disturbances)</td></tr>
<tr><td>Associated symptoms</td><td>Atrophy of skin appendages, secondary atrophic changes in bones, joints, and muscles
Cool, reddish, clammy skin with excessive sweating; sensory and motor loss in structure innervated by damaged portion of nerve</td></tr>
<tr><td>Signs</td><td>Cool, reddish, clammy, sweaty skin with atrophy of skin appendages and deep structures in painful area</td></tr>
<tr><td>Laboratory findings</td><td>Galvanic skin; responses and plethysmography revealing signs of sympathetic nervous system hyperactivity, roentgenograms possibly showing atrophy of bone</td></tr>
<tr><td>Usual course</td><td>If untreated, the majority of patients having symptoms that persist indefinitely; spontaneous remission occurring</td></tr>
<tr><td>Relief</td><td>In early stages of CRPS II (first few months), sympathetic blockade plus vigorous physical therapy usually providing transient relief; repeated blocks usually leading to long-term relief; when a series of sympathetic blocks not providing long-term relief, sympathectomy indicated; long-term persistence of symptoms reducing the likelihood of successful therapy</td></tr>
<tr><td>Social and physical disabilities</td><td>Disuse atrophy of involved limb; complete disruption of normal daily activities by severe pain; risk of suicide, drug abuse if untreated</td></tr>
<tr><td>Pathology</td><td>Partial injury to major peripheral nerve; actual cause of pain unknown; peripheral central and sympathetic mechanisms involved in an unexplained way</td></tr>
<tr><td>Essential features</td><td>Burning pain and cutaneous hypersensitivity with signs of sympathetic hyperactivity in portion of limb innervated by partially injured nerve</td></tr>
<tr><td colspan="2" align="center">Complex Regional Pain Syndrome, Type I (Reflex Sympathetic Dystrophy)</td></tr>
<tr><td>Definition</td><td>Continuous pain in a portion of an extremity after trauma that may include fracture but does not involve a major nerve, associated with sympathetic hyperactivity</td></tr>
<tr><td>Site</td><td>Usually the distal extremity adjacent to a traumatized area; all around the limb</td></tr>
<tr><td>System</td><td>Peripheral nervous system; possibly the central nervous system</td></tr>
<tr><td>Main features</td><td>The pain follows trauma (usually mild), not associated with significant nerve injury; the pain described as burning, continuous, exacerbated by movement, cutaneous stimulation, or stress; onset usually weeks after injury</td></tr>
<tr><td>Associated symptoms</td><td>Initially vasodilatation with increasing temperature, hyperhidrosis, edema, and reduced sympathetic activity also occurring; atrophy of skin, vasoconstriction, and appendages; cool, red, clammy skin variably present; disuse atrophy of deep structures possibly progressing to Sudeck's atrophy of bone; aggravated by use of body part, relieved by immobilization; sometimes follows a herniated intervertebral disc, spinal anesthesia, poliomyelitis, severe iliofemoral thrombosis, or cardiac infarction; may appear as the shoulder–hand syndrome; later vasospastic symptoms becoming prominent with persistent coldness of the affected extremity, pallor or cyanosis, Raynaud's phenomenon, atrophy of the skin and nails, and loss of hair, atrophy of soft tissues and stiffness of joints; without therapy these symptoms possibly persisting; not necessary for one patient to exhibit all symptoms together; an additional limb or limbs possibly affected as well</td></tr>
<tr><td>Signs</td><td>Variable; may be florid sympathetic hyperactivity</td></tr>
<tr><td>Laboratory findings</td><td>In advanced cases, radiographs possibly showing atrophy of bone, and bone scan changes over time</td></tr>
<tr><td>Usual course</td><td>Persists indefinitely if untreated; small incidence of spontaneous remission</td></tr>
<tr><td>Relief</td><td>Sympathetic block and physical therapy; sympathectomy if long-term results not achieved with repeated blocks; may respond in early phases to high doses of corticosteroids (e.g., prednisone, 50 mg daily)</td></tr>
<tr><td>Complications</td><td>Disuse atrophy of involved limb; risk of suicide and drug abuse if untreated; sometimes spreads to contralateral limb</td></tr>
<tr><td>Social and physical disabilities</td><td>Depression, inability to perform daily activities</td></tr>
</table>

TABLE 36.1 (Continued)
Comparison between CRPS Type I and Type II

	CRPS I	CRPS II
Pathology	Unknown	Partial nerve lesion
Essential features	Burning pain in distal extremity usually after minor injury without nerve damage	Nerve damage
Differential diagnosis	Unrecognized local pathology (fracture, strain, sprain)	Post-traumatic vasospasm, nerve entrapment syndromes radiculopathies, or thrombosis

TABLE 36.2
Criteria for Differential Diagnosis of CRPS Types I and II

	CRPS I	CRPS II
Etiology	Any kind of lesion	Partial nerve lesion
Localization	Distal part of extremity, or entire limb; independent from site of lesion	Any peripheral site of body; mostly confined to territory of affected nerve
Spreading of symptoms	Obligatory	Rare
Spontaneous pain	Common, mostly deep and superficial orthostatic component	Obligatory, predominately superficial, no orthostatic component
Mechanical allodynia	Most of patients with spreading tendency	Obligatory in nerve territory
Autonomic symptoms	Distally generalized with spreading tendency	Related to nerve lesion
Motor symptoms	Distally generalized	Related to nerve lesion
Sensory symptoms	Distally generalized	Related to nerve lesion

Note: From "Classification of Chronic Pain," edited by H. Merskey and the Subcommittee on Taxonomy, 1986, *Pain*, *3*(Suppl), pp. 28–29. Reprinted with permission.

& Churchman, 1907) said about syphilis, "it is almost impossible to describe its clinical symptoms without mentioning almost every symptom of every disease known." The same may be said for CRPS I and CRPS II.

COMPLEX REGIONAL PAIN SYNDROME TYPE I (REFLEX SYMPATHETIC DYSTROPHY)

Following the distinction drawn by Payne (1986), one considers CRPS I as the result of minor trauma; inflammation following surgery, infection, or lacerations resulting in some degree of swelling in the affected limb; infarctions; degenerative joint disease; frostbite; and burns. One should add to this list the possibility of any compression, such as casting or swelling due to injury that may cause prolonged pressure on peripheral nerves. As an example of this, we have seen at least two or three cases per year of CRPS I brought about from arthroscopy. The probable etiology is not injury to the nerve from the use of the arthroscope, but instead from using the tourniquet for a long period of time to create a bloodless operating field. Hendler (2002) has emphasized the need for more refined differential diagnosis between nerve entrapments and CRPS I. This distinction is critical, since proper diagnosis is essential for proper treatment, and is based on the

distribution of the pain, which follows nerve pathways for nerve entrapments, and is circumferential for CRPS I (Hendler, 2002).

According to Schwartzman and McKellan (1987), there seem to be three phases to CRPS I. Importantly, these stages are not temporal in their definition, but rather describe a progression of pathology. Additionally, physicians should recognize that CRPS I is a symptom complex that is a cluster of symptoms and signs, and that patients do not present with all signs and symptoms during the course of their disease. In fact, very often they may have only one or two of the signs and symptoms of the disorder.

As described by Payne (1986) and by Schwartzman and McKellan (1987), the acute stage of CRPS I is characterized by spontaneous pain, usually aching or burning, that follows the distribution of blood vessels or peripheral nerves. The acute stage may manifest as "hyperpathia" (this is described as a painful syndrome of overreaction to a stimulus or after-sensation following a stimulus) and may include hypesthesia or hyperesthesia (described as a decreased or an increased sensation to pain stimulation, respectively), or dysesthesia (described as an unpleasant abnormal sensation). Associated with these tactile sensations are usually warm, dry, red skin or cold, blue, sweaty skin, with some swelling and, surprisingly, increased hair and nail growth. A number of authors have interjected the notion of allodynia, or a painful response to a normally nonpainful stimulus (Chaplan et al., 1994; Kim & Chung, 1995; Lee et al., 1994). Additionally, the patient has dependent redness and reduced motion in the damaged extremity. This summarizes the acute stage of this disorder, which may last several weeks and may begin immediately or several days after the onset of the injury. However, it is possible for CRPS I to remain in this stage, and never progress to stage II or stage III. This is a highly individualized response.

The second stage of CRPS I (which may begin about 3 to 6 months after the injury, or may occur within weeks or may never occur) is called the dystrophic stage by Payne (1986). During this stage, the patient experiences a burning type of pain, which radiates either above or below the site of the injury, and increased hypersensitivity or hyperalgesia (an exquisite sensitivity to touch or temperature — in counterdistinction to allodynia, a painful response to a normally nonpainful stimulus, a most important distinction that is discussed later in the chapter). The patient has changes in the nails on occasion, as well as decreased hair growth. This seems to be a variable finding and certainly is not a *sine qua non* of the diagnosis of CRPS I. Joints may become stiff, with decreased range of motion and possible thickening, associated with some degree of muscle wasting. Edema may be present, as well as bullous skin lesions that are not related to an autoimmune disease (Baron et al., 1996). Osteoporosis may be noted, with proper testing (Payne, 1986). Movement disorders may begin at this stage, with either dystonias or contractures noted (Schwartzman and Kerrigan, 1990; Webster et al., 1991). Symptoms may vary and fluctuate from individual to individual.

The third stage described by Payne is the atrophic stage, which usually occurs 6 months or longer after the injury. According to Payne, the patient experiences pain, decreased skin temperature, trophic changes in the skin associated with a smooth glossy skin, stiff fixed joints associated with contractures, increased or decreased sweating in the affected extremity, and demineralization of the bone associated with wasted muscles and reduced strength (Payne, 1986). Again, the progression to this stage is highly variable and may progress, in a rapidly fulminating case, in less than 2 to 3 months. As always in medicine, there are only guidelines, but no hard and fast rules. (A summary of many of the clinical symptoms is shown in Table 36.3.)

COMPLEX REGIONAL PAIN SYNDROME, TYPE II (CAUSALGIA)

CRPS II is usually associated with peripheral nerve injury and severe pain. According to Payne (1986), pain occurring in CRPS II follows an injury to a nerve trunk, usually a major proximal nerve branch, and is described as a persistent burning pain, but it does not necessarily have to be burning in quality. It is unrelated to associated damage from surrounding tissue and seems to be worsened by emotional or environmental stimuli. Most importantly, the pain seems to persist more than 5 to 6 weeks, which seems to be the length of time needed for surrounding tissue to recover from injury. Typically, the injury is due to damage by a bullet, a knife, sharpened rocks or parts propelled by a machine, or other such objects. When the injury is associated with a high-velocity missile, one must consider not only actual damage to the tissue itself, but also hydrostatic effects caused by shock waves. When one takes into account the fact that the body is made up largely of water, it is easy to see how a high-velocity missile can cause damage not only to the actual tissue that has been penetrated, but also to surrounding tissue as a result of hydrostatically transmitted shock waves. If the reader desires additional information concerning the hydrostatic effects of high-velocity missiles, he or she is referred to a most amazing book entitled *Split Seconds* (Dalton, 1984). Photographs in the book clearly illustrate the hydraulic effect in soft tissue caused by a bullet.

Typically, patients with CRPS II report an onset of pain within several hours to a week after the injury and describe the pain using words such as stinging, aching, burning, or tingling. Patients may experience paroxysms of deep pain (Payne, 1986) superimposed on the regular pain. Long (1982) clearly makes the distinction between CRPS II and CRPS I. CRPS II is secondary to partial injury to major mixed nerves, caused by low- or high-velocity missiles, and manifests as trophic changes in the distribution of the nerve associated with extreme hypersensitivity. The pain is diffuse and burning, and true CRPS II may respond to sympathectomy. However, Payne reports a surgical meta-analysis in which the response to sympathectomy was 12 to 97%. Long suggests performing three or more sympathetic blocks, sometimes every day for up to a week or longer, with the expectation that longer relief should follow each subsequent block. With positive responses to sympathetic blocks, Long would suggest a sympathectomy for CRPS II. On the other hand, CRPS I usually follows a minor injury and does not involve a major nerve root. Frequently, the site of injury for CRPS I is the knee, ankles, or wrist; and the pain seems to get worse with cold but not with emotional upset, unlike CRPS II. Demineralization of the bone occurs more often with CRPS I, with fibrosis of tendons and sheaths and spasm of the muscle. Dysesthesia suggests that there will be less success with sympathectomy.

TABLE 36.3
Clinical Symptoms Associated with CRPS II and CRPS I

Clinical Symptoms	Mechanism	Diagnostic Studies	Treatment
CRPS II			
Burning pain[a,b]	Unmyelinated C-fibers[c]	Rarely have cold hyperalgesia (2/7) or heat hyperalgesia (0/9);[b] do have mechanical hypersensitivity;[b] use a drop of acetone and Von Frey hairs to test	Phenoxybenzamine DREZ[a] sympathectomy 12% to 97% effective, clonazepam,[e] gabapentin[f]
Paroxysms of pain[a]	Nerve stretch and axon disruption[a]	Clinical reports	None
Partial motor paralysis (70%)[d]	Peripheral nerve injury proximal nerve trunk[a,b]	EMG/nerve conduction velocity studies	No relief with sympathetic blocks;[b] no success proximal nerve trunk[a,b] with beta-blockers[d]
Worse with stress[a]	Lots of theory, no proof	Clinical reports	Clonidine
Vasomotor changes, but rare trophic change[d]	Unknown	Clinical observation	Sympathetic blocks
CRPS I			
Hyperalgesia and Allodynia			
Mechanical-hypersensitivity to light touch	Ectopic alpha-adrenergic chemosensitivity;[g] sensitization of WDR neurons in the spinal cord;[i] central nervous system mediated;[k] intact low-threshold mechanoreceptor with A-delta afferents[c]	All patients have mechanical hypersensitivity; use Von Frey hairs to test[b]	Sympathectomy possibly relieving it;[c] sympathectomy not relieving it;[j] low-dose naltrexone possibly working[l] nifedipine?[m] gabapentin?[f]
Thermal-hypersensitivity	No mechanism delineated	Patients having cold either heat or cold,[b,c,k] hyperalgesia (3/4), and/or heat hyperalgesia (4/5); use a drop of acetone to test[b]	6/6 receiving relief with sympathetic blocks or sympathectomy,[b] nifedipine?
Dystrophy Phase			
Osteoporosis[n]	No mechanism delineated	X-ray did not correlate well with clinical symptoms, but bone scan did[r] (abnormal flow images, 83% abnormal static images)[r] (also true for clinical features c. and e.);[a] if clinically had CRPS I, 22/23 had positive delay image bone scan[s]	Maybe calcitonin[n,o,p]
Diffuse or patchy, bony,[n,o,p] demineralization[r]	No mechanism delineated	X-ray and bone scan[s]	Calcitonin[n,o,p,r]
Molted skin[a,b,r]	No mechanism delineated	Themography[t,u]	Prednisone 60 to 80 mg, tapering[r]
Hair loss[b,n]	No mechanism delineated	Clinical observation[r]	Steroids[n,r]
Vasomotor instability[r]	No mechanism delineated	History or longitudinal observation[r]	Sympathetic blocks,[n] steroids[r]
Nail brittleness[a,n]	No mechanism delineated	Clinical observation	Sympathetic blocks,[n] steroids[r]
Muscle spasm[n,v,w]	No mechanism delineated	EMG biofeedback used as test[u]	Trigger point injections[a] baclofen[l]
Contractures[a,n]	May be attributed to disuse, may be central dystonia[x]	Longitudinal observation[n]	Physical therapy,[n] sympathectomy
Contralateral involvement[n,w]	Cross-communication between sympathetic chain in 80% of cadavers[w]	Effective contralateral block[w]	Contralateral sympathectomy[w]
Edema[a,n]	No mechanism delineated[y]	History and clinical observation	Nifedipine,[m] spironolactone, acetazolamide, epidural, spinal cord stimulation[aa]

TABLE 36.3 (Continued)
Clinical Symptoms Associated with CRPS II and CRPS I

Clinical Symptoms	Mechanism	Diagnostic Studies	Treatment
Lower skin temperature[u]	No vasospasm, but may be an afferent and efferent reflex arc[bb]	Thermography[t,u]	Phentolamine;[a,b,t,u] Bier block with reserpine,[bb] guanethidine i.v.,[n] sympathetic blocks[b,n]
Joint stiffness[a,s] and tenderness[r]	No mechanism delineated	Proximal interphalangeal joint 12.9 mm greater (average)[n] affected hand; negative rheumatoid and connective tissue blood studies[r]	Maybe calcitonin[p]
Pathological fractures	May be related to osteoporosis or patchy demineralization	72 hours after a break 95% of bone scans are positive[cc]	Maybe calcitonin,[n,o] maybe Fosamax
Pins and needles[u] and dysesthesias[a]	No mechanism delineated	History	Sympathectomy[u]
Skin lesions[q,y,z,dd]	Disruption of basement membrane and destruction of collagenous anchoring fibrils,[y] circulating immune complexes[q]	Observation and electron microscopy[y]	Prednisone not working,[y] maybe tetracycline[y]
Dystonias,[z] myoclonus[z]	Spinal cord mediated?	Observation	Epidural bupivicaine, epidural baclofen, epidural clonidine, sympathetic blocks[ee]

References: [a] Payne (1986); [b] Raja et al. (1986); [c] Ochoa et al. (1985); [d] Ghostine et al. (1984); [e] Bouckoms & Litman (1985); [f] Mellick & Mellick (1995); [g] Devor (1983); [h] Allen & Morety (1982); [i] Roberts (1986); [j] Hoffert et al. (1984); [k] Meyer et al. (1985); [l] Gillman & Lichtigfeld (1985); [m] Prough et al. (1985); [n] Schott (1986); [o] Gobelet, Waldburger, & Meier (1992); [p] Webster et al. (1993); [q] Van der Laan, Veldman, & Goris (1998); [r] Kozin et al. (1981); [s] Holder & MacKinnon (1984); [t] Uematsu et al. (1981); [u] Hendler et al. (1982); [v] Long (1982); [w] Kleinman (1954); [x] Schwartzman & Kerrigan (1990); [y] Baron et al. (1996); [z] Greipp & Thomas (1994); [aa] Peuschl et al. (1991); [bb] Janoff et al. (1985); [cc] Matin (1979); [dd] Hamamou, Dursun, Ural, & Cakci (1996); [ee] Webster et al. (1991).

SYMPATHETICALLY MAINTAINED PAIN

The term sympathetically maintained pain (SMP) has come into use in an effort to further define diagnostic accuracy, which would then allow better selection of treatment methods and have some predictive value in terms of outcome. Raja and Hendler (1990) report clinical features of sympathetically maintained pain to be (1) spontaneous pain, (2) hyperalgesia to both mechanical and cooling stimuli, (3) soft tissue swelling, (4) vasomotor disturbances, (5) trophic skin changes, (6) diminished motor function, and (7) pain relief after sympathetic blockade. By using these criteria, one can have SMP that could have features of either CRPS I or CRPS II because either of these conditions could have features of SMP.

Hendler (1982) originally described the use of oral phentolamine to treat CRPS I using the rationale that this drug was a postsynaptic alpha-1-blocker. Raja and his coworkers (1991) later described the use of intravenous phentolamine as a diagnostic test to confirm whether the pain a patient had was sympathetic in origin, that is, "sympathetically maintained." There is evidence that the mechanism of SMP is present not only in CRPS I, but also in some cases of CRPS II. However, various authors have reported the benefit of sympathetic blocks and sympathectomies in both disorders (Bosco Vieira Durate et al., 2003a; 2003b; Ghostine et al., 1984; Hannington-Kiff, 1979; Long, 1982). Perhaps the best conceptual framework to use is one that takes into account both neurophysiology (i.e., the presence or absence of major peripheral nerve injury documented by electromyography, EMG; nerve conduction velocities studies, NCV; and the somatosensory-evoked potential, SSEP) and response to pharmacological intervention (i.e., response to I.V. phentolamine testing or sympathetic blocks). A physician might consider six separate types of disorders, as shown in Table 36.4.

USING THE CLINICAL HISTORY AND SENSORY EXAMINATION FOR DIFFERENTIAL DIAGNOSIS

A number of authors have advanced the notion that there are other types of sensory mechanism, other than hyper-

TABLE 36.4
Diagnostic Considerations

Response to I.V.	Positive Response to Phentolamine I.V.	No Response to Phentolamine I.V.	Partial Response to Phentolamine I.V.
EMG/nerve conduction velocity/somatosensory-evoked potential: all negative	CRPS I SMP	Microvascular damage with swelling and mechanical hyperalgesia; sympathetically independent pain (SIP)	Mixed injury
EMG/nerve conduction velocity/somatosensory-evoked potential: at least one positive	CRPS II	Neuroma or nerve entrapment at site of injury; SIP	Mixed injury
Positive response to alcohol drop test	CRPS I, SMP	Too low a dose phentolamine	Too low a dose phentolamine
Positive response nerve to a local nerve block (radial, ulnar, median, peroneal, saphenous, tibial) with 100% relief of all symptoms	Nerve entrapment syndrome with sympathetic component	Nerve entrapment syndrome without any sympathetic component	Nerve entrapment syndrome with sympathetic component
Positive response to sympathetic block, or a warm limb and 100% relief of all symptoms	CRPS I, SMP	Too low a dose of phentolamine; too slow an infusion	Too low a dose of phentolamine; too slow an infusion
Partial relief of pain with local nerve block	Mixed injury	Poor nerve block	Mixed injury

algesia evident in CRPS I and II (Chaplan et al., 1994; Kim and Chung, 1995; Lee et al., 1994; Lee & Yaksh, 1996). Unfortunately, the vast majority of the research reports are in animal models, using animals fairly low on the philogenetic scale. There is always a danger in extrapolating from animal models to clinical work in humans because there are species-specific differences, and some of the sensory values assigned to a rat reveal more about the creativity of the researcher than they do about the sensory experience of the rat. However, bearing these caveats in mind, clinicians should be aware of the research observations that may have significant value for their patients. A sensation called allodynia has been described, which is a painful response to a normally nonpainful stimulus. It is important to make a distinction between this sensation and hyperalgesia, which is a more intense response to a normally painful stimulus. This distinction bears reemphasis, for this is the most commonly confused terminology in the hands of inexperienced clinicians. Clinically, hyperalgesia is seen in the early phases of nerve entrapments and radiculopathies. In counterdistinction, allodynia is seen in CRPS I and II.

Also, it is important to distinguish among cold hyperalgesia, heat hyperalgesia, and mechanical hyperalgesia. Both cold and heat hyperalgesia are rarely seen in CRPS II (Meyer et al., 1985; Raja et al., 1986). Moreover, it is important to make a distinction between cold allodynia and mechanical allodynia. Cold (thermal) allodynia is most often seen in CRPS I and II, whereas mechanical allodynia is seen commonly in CRPS I and

II, nerve entrapment syndromes, and radiculopathies (Hendler & Raja, 1994). This clinical distinction has led to the use of the Hendler alcohol drop and swipe test to make a distinction between CRPS I and II, with cold allodynia (which has a painful response to alcohol dropped on an affected limb); and CRPS I and II, nerve entrapment syndromes, and radiculopathies, with mechanical allodynia, demonstrated by lightly stroking the affected limb with the used alcohol swab (Hendler, 1995). Concisely stated, mechanical allodynia is of less use diagnostically because it may be present in CRPS I and II, nerve entrapment syndromes, and radiculopathies, whereas thermal allodynia is a more useful clinical feature, usually being limited mostly to CRPS I and occasionally to CRPS II (Meyer et al., 1985; Raja et al., 1986). Hendler has also reported a third type of allodynia, chemical allodynia, which is seen with the use of the alcohol swab test. The patient may not respond to the cold produced by evaporation of alcohol, but then 2 to 3 minutes later, the patient reports a burning sensation, as the alcohol presumably diffuses through the skin and reaches the unmyelinated C-fibers associated with producing allodynia in CRPS I.

Additionally, a cool limb is not diagnostic of CRPS I and II, despite many reports in the literature to that effect (Hannington-Kiff, 1979; Prough et al., 1985, Wasner et al., 2002). First and foremost, for a clinician to hold an affected limb in one hand and a normal limb in another, and pronounce that the temperatures are either equal or different is a demonstration of arrogance more than clinical skills. The ability to detect temperature differences varies due to the ambient temperature of the clinical setting and the "physiological zero" of the organism sensing the temperature change, which lowers the "threshold of detection for thermal sensation of the opposite quality" (Geldard, 1962, p. 137). In an extensive report by Uematsu et al. (1981) reviewing 803 cases at Johns Hopkins Hospital, the authors found that (as expected) patients with CRPS I and II had cold limbs most of the time, with ranges of 0.5°C to more than 3.0°C coldness being reported for more than 79% of the cases diagnosed with CRPS I. However, in 89% of the cases in which there were abnormal EMG or NCV studies, the affected limb was also cold, although not to the same severity as the patients with CRPS I. These figures included cases of CRPS II, as well as patients with radiculopathies and nerve entrapment syndromes. Wasner and co-workers (2002) used the response of skin temperature to whole-body cooling and warming in a "thermal suit," measured by infrared thermometry, to compare and contrast 25 patients with CRPS I with 20 healthy controls and 15 patients with "painful limbs of other origins." They found that under normal resting conditions, there were "minor skin temperature asymmetries," with 32% sensitivity, which increased to 76% under artificial changes. However, specificity was 100% at rest and 93% under thermal regulation. Therefore, thermography could be made a more useful diagnostic tool by artificially heating or cooling the torso.

The anatomic distribution of the pain is another important feature to consider. Sympathetic fibers travel with the sensory nerves, so an injured sensory nerve may have a component of sympathetic damage reported, such as coldness or hyperalgesia. However, the actual location of the pain is a critical factor. If the pain is in the distribution of a peripheral nerve, even if all the sensations for CRPS I are present, then the clinical syndrome is really a nerve entrapment, with the sympathetic sensory components of it coming from the sympathetic fibers traveling with the sensory nerve. CRPS I has a circumferential pain distribution (i.e., it is all around the limb, in the pattern of the blood flow, not in a discrete nerve distribution or in a radicular distribution). Failure to recognize this distinction has led to the misdiagnosis of a number of nerve entrapment syndromes, which are mistakenly called CPRS I (Hendler & Kozikowski, 1993; Hendler, Bergson, & Morrison, 1996). Hendler (2002) reported that 71% of the patients sent to Mensana Clinic with the diagnosis of CRPS I had just nerve entrapments, proven by EMG/NCV studies, and total temporary relief to peripheral nerve blocks. Additionally, 10 of 38 (26%) had a combination of CRPS I and nerve entrapments. This means that 37 of all 38 patients in the study actually had unrecognized, and therefore undiagnosed, nerve entrapment syndromes. Only 1 patient of 38 had pure CRPS I.

TREATMENTS

Appropriate treatments for CRPS I and II have been described in the Consensus Report, sponsored by the International Association for the Study of Pain (IASP) (Stanton-Hicks et al., 1998). In this report, the participants emphasized the need for functional restoration and psychological counseling, as well as medical intervention. Not only is there disuse as the result of a painful limb, creating multiple disabilities and atrophy, but there is also evidence that once the disorder of CRPS I spreads, there may be a centrally mediated muscle disorder, resembling dystonia (Schwartzman & Kerrigan, 1990). Therefore, the problem of a painful limb in CRPS I and II is compounded by a real motor disorder.

The psychological problems associated with both CRPS I and II have been well described for patients with chronic pain in general. Hendler (1982, 1984) has long reported that patients with both chronic pain and depression really have become depressed as the result of their chronic pain. The earlier psychiatric "wisdom" of feeling that depression manifests as chronic pain has not been supported by more careful observations (Hendler & Talo, 1989). This is a serious problem to overlook. Fishbain et al. (1991) reported that in patients with chronic pain, white males complete suicide at a rate two times higher than general population, white females three times higher, and white males involved in workers' compensation three times higher. Therefore, the use of group therapy seems to be the most efficient and productive way of providing support for patients with all types of chronic pain problems, and certainly is applicable to patients with CRPS I and II (Hendler et al., 1981). Family counseling and patient education is also of great use, when available.

The pharmacological management of CRPS I and II is complicated (Hendler, 2000). The treatments shown in Table 36.3 are meant to deal with the specific symptoms associated with CRPS I and II. However, there is a role for a more generalized pharmacological approach, especially dealing with the issue of depression and pain relief. Antidepressants, in and of themselves, provide relief of many of the symptoms by (1) reducing depression, (2) reducing anxiety, and (3) promoting natural sleep and actually have some limited pain-relieving properties (Max et al., 1991; Watson et al., 1981; 1991). For symptomatic relief in CRPS I and II, narcotics are problematic. A number of authors have reported reduced efficacy, or variable effects, of narcotics in the palliative treatment of pain in patients with CRPS I and II (Arner & Meyerson, 1988; Lee, Chaplan, & Yaksh, 1995; Portenoy, Foley, & Inturrisi, 1990). The variability and usual lack of efficacy of narcotics for CRPS I and II may be explained by recent elegant research, which shows only a kappa-2 opioid agonist blocks the pain of hyperalgesia and allodynia, seen with peripheral neuritis and neuropathy, by inhibiting the activity of the *N*-methyl-D-aspartate (NMDA) receptor in the spine (Eliav, Herzberg, & Caudle, 1999). Although this research is in animals, with all the attendant problems of translating to human use, this avenue seems to hold a great deal of promise because the formulation of a kappa-2 opioid agonist is a feasible endeavor for major drug companies. However, as of the date of writing this material, there is no practical kappa-2 agonist available for human use; thus, the use of narcotics in CRPS I and II for allodynia and hyperalgesia is of limited usefulness. Opioids may help pain caused by other symptoms of CRPS I and II, such as muscle spasm and pathological fractures. There are even case reports of patients with the associated tremors being treated with carbidopa/levodopa 25/100 mg (Navani et al., 2003). A review of other pharmacological approaches for the management of pain can be found in several chapters by the author (Hendler, 1997, 2000).

Sympathetic blocks have always been the mainstay of diagnosis and treatment. The important feature of these blocks is to be certain of the efficacy of the block before interpreting the result. The clinical criterion that best correlates with an efficacious block is the report of total limb warming. This tells the clinician that the sympathetic block did what it was supposed to do (i.e., blocked the sympathetic input to a limb, thereby producing warming of the limb). At this point, the next question to ask the patient is, "What do you feel?" If the patient has a warm limb and 100% total absolute relief of all pain, then one may consider that the block was (1) effective and (2) appropriate for pain relief. From this, a clinician may conclude that the pain is sympathetic in origin. If, however, the block did not warm the limb, then the clinician must conclude that the block was not effective; and no information of any value can be determined from this type of block, except that another block, at a later date, is needed. If the block produces a warm limb, but only partial relief of the symptoms, then the question is, "Where do you still have pain?" If the remaining pain is reported in a nerve distribution, then the patient has both CRPS I and a nerve entrapment syndrome, which coexist, or a nerve entrapment syndrome with a sympathetic component. If the limb is warm, and the patient has no relief, then the chances are the patient has a pure nerve entrapment syndrome (see Table 36.4).

After a clinician determines a block is effective, then the patient should have a series of 6 to 10 blocks. After this series of blocks, several results are possible: (1) the CRPS I or II may go away; (2) the CRPS I or II may temporarily go away for weeks or months, only to return; or (3) the CRPS I or II may temporarily go away for hours or days following the blocks, only to return. If scenario 1 occurs, the diagnostic blocks have also provided the cure. If scenario 2 or 3 occurs, then the patient is a candidate for sympathectomy. This author favors the surgical sympathectomy because direct visualization of the sympa-

thetic chain and pathology reports on the tissue are more reassuring than blind ablation techniques. Moreover, the author has seen disastrous results in patients, in which phenol was used for a neuroablative procedure. Despite the obvious benefit of direct visualization for sympathectomy, there are still some physicians, mostly anesthesiologists, who continue to use blind chemoablative techniques, with neurolytic agents, such as phenol, or radiofrequency lesions (Stanton-Hicks et al., 1998).

In extreme cases, the use of epidural stimulation has been reported efficacious, although there are only a small number of cases in the literature (Barolat, Schwartzman, & Woo, 1989; Peuschl et al., 1991; Robaina, Dominguez, & Diaz, 1989). The epidural infusion of SNX-111 has been suggested as a possible treatment for CRPS I or II, as has the infusion of baclofen. SNX-111 is a conotoxin that works on specific calcium channels to block the message of pain, whereas baclofen is a gabaminergic muscle relaxer. Epidural opioid infusion has been reported (Broseta, Roldan, & Gonzales-Darder, 1982), but the absence of a kappa-2 agonist may have reduced the potential results (Eliav et al., 1999). Clonidine actually seems more effective than morphine in humans, for deafferentation pain, after spinal cord injury (Hassenbusch, Stanton-Hicks, & Covington, 1995). Other researchers have explained this difference, based on the independence of the opioid and noradrenergic pathways of the spinal cord (Glynn, Dawson, & Sanders, 1988). Opioid receptors exist in only a small group of neurons in the dorsal horn and have various subsets, of which only the kappa-2 subset seems to be effective in reducing the allodynia of CRPS I (Eliav et al., 1999). On the other hand, clonidine has multiple sites of action, such as inhibiting pain transmission in the dorsal horn of the spinal cord and inhibiting norepinephrine release, due to its alpha-2 partial agonist effect, which inhibits the release of norepinephrine.

THEORY

With the clinical descriptions from Table 36.4 in mind, one can make an effort to define the various anatomic, neuroanatomic, and physiological bases for these two disorders. Ghostine and colleagues (1984) have suggested multiple etiologies for CRPS II. Various considerations include ephapse, in which there seems to be an erosion of the insulation between nerve fibers, allowing for short-circuiting between somatic afferent fibers and sympathetic efferent fibers; and experimentally produced neuromas, with resultant ephapses occurring both acutely and chronically between myelinated fibers. Because of the delay in developing the ephapses, which does not correspond to the clinical observations of a relatively rapid onset of CRPS I and II, however, the theory of ephapses as the etiology of CRPS II has fallen from favor. To replace this theory, the concept of nerve sprouts or free nerve endings that are sparsely myelinated seems feasible. Axonal sprouting has been noted to occur early after an injury, with a high frequency and without total axonal disruption. The possibility that causalgia is produced by these sparsely myelinated fibers is supported by evidence that the blood–nerve barrier, which is similar to the blood–brain barrier, has been destroyed in the injured nerve.

Perhaps the most comprehensive review of the neurophysiological basis of CRPS I and II has been advanced by Roberts (1986). In his extensive review article, Roberts deals with the neural mechanisms associated with pain of CRPS II and I. He calls these disorders SMP. His hypothesis concerning SMP is based on two assumptions: "(1) that a high rate of firing in spinal wide dynamic range (WDR) or multireceptive neurons results in painful sensation and (2) that a nociceptor response is associated with trauma which can produce long-term sensitization of the WDR neurons." Furthermore, his theory postulates that SMP is mediated by low-threshold, myelinated mechanoreceptors and that these impulses, which carry messages to the brain, are the result of sympathetic fibers carrying messages from the spine and brain to act on the receptors or to act on the fibers carrying messages to the brain. The most important part of this hypothesis is the fact that Roberts does not postulate the need for nerve injury or for dystrophic tissue. Before one can more fully appreciate Roberts's theories, however, one has to explore the basic anatomy of the sympathetic chains.

Bennett (1991) at the National Institutes of Health has advanced a brilliant theory that integrates clinical observations with basic neurophysiology. Bennett synthesizes three theories that show that damaged nerves, when they regenerate, have sprouts that are sensitive to norepinephrine; they will discharge on exposure to norepinephrine; there is enough norepinephrine produced by sympathetic fibers to trigger firing of damaged nerves; damaged nerves actually produce norepinephrine receptors at the damaged end; and nociceptors (pain receptors) in intact nerves fire more in response to norepinephrine. "All of these mechanisms may be operating in the case of patient nerve damage due to physical trauma," he says, and "these events are likely to sensitize surviving afferent terminals, perhaps to the point of inducing an ongoing discharge." Bennett further differentiates between the types of injury: constriction or entrapment versus partial destruction of a major peripheral nerve. The former injury (constriction) does not seem to respond to sympathetic blocks 1 to 2 weeks after the injury, and this is attributed to the loss of noradrenergic vasomotor innervation, which takes several weeks to develop. The latter injury (partial nerve destruction) becomes painful within hours of the injury, remains painful for months, and responds to sympathetic blocks even months after the injury.

Other researchers have expanded on a purely neuron-mediated mechanism and have suggested that autoimmune factors may be involved. The Schwartzman group at Thomas Jefferson University School of Medicine in Philadelphia found inflammatory skin lesions in the late stages of CRPS I, and attribute these lesions to a deposition of immune complexes in the skin. They believe the skin lesion supports the concept that cytokines and lymphokines such as interleukin-2 (IL-2) are produced as the result of the activation of complement; this in turn is excited by the progression of events beginning with local injury causing nerve growth factor release, thus activating sympathetic neurons and causing recruitment of neutrophils and monocytes, which in turn activate complement (Webster et al., 1991). Interestingly, IL-2 has been found to selectively stimulate sympathetic neurons, whereas nerve growth factor (NGF) is produced in high concentrations after injury, which stimulates inflammation and in turn activates complement. Knobler (1996) has expanded on this and advances the notion of aberrant immunologic mechanism as a cause for CRPS I. He traces trauma as the cause for the release of NGF, which then stimulates inflammation and activates the complement components of the immune response, "promoting the expansion of antibody-producing B cells of the immune system." He reports that substance P and the lymphokine IL-2 are released in response to NGF, with both of these factors acting on the sympathetic nerve to activate it. As research progresses, the various factors described earlier need to be explored with rigorous controls for (1) the type of lesion (crush vs. cut), (2) the stage of the disease correlating with anatomic and neurohumoral changes over time, and (3) the attempt to correlate the clinical symptoms with response to various treatments.

In a discovery that led to her Nobel prize, Rita Levi-Montalcini describes the effect of NGF on sympathetic nerve (Levi-Montalcini et al., 1996). In response to an injury or lack of innervation, the end organ, i.e., the sensory receptor, releases NGF, which chemotaxically stimulates a nerve to grow toward the newly denervated receptor. This chemotaxic agent was found to be NGF. Clearly, sympathetic ganglions grow profusely in response to the addition of NGF to their growth medium. This is not limited to just sympathetic nerves. Skin and sensory nerves also have sprouted after injury (Inball et al., 1987).

A study by Ro et al. (1999) shows that this process can be reversed in rats by the administration of anti-NGF antibodies. Previous work shows that anti-NGF antibodies prevented collateral sprouting of dorsal root ganglion in rats (Mearow & Kril, 1995). Ro and others (1999) studied the specific sensory response to anti-NGF, which showed that in a dosage- and time-dependent fashion, heat and cold hyperalgesia, as well as collateral sprouting, can be reduced.

Finally, one of the most seminal concepts to emerge from animals studies is the idea of plasticity of the central nervous system (i.e., its ability to change in response to stimuli). Nowhere is this more important than for the understanding of CRPS I and II. In response to a chronically painful stimulus, the cells of the dorsal horn of the spinal cord actually alter their cytoarchitecture (the structure of the chemistry of the cell). Hyperalgesia and allodynia are largely created by the enhancement of NMDA receptor activity in the spinal cord and treated by blocking the NMDA receptor (Ren & Dubner, 1993). The central role of NMDA receptor activity in the creation of allodynia must be emphasized. Unfortunately, there is not a practical way to modify the NMDA receptor in humans, so the treatment of hyperalgesia and allodynia remains elusive. Therefore, mechanisms other than NMDA inhibition need to be explored.

To briefly summarize the material presented earlier, three sensations are associated with CRPS I and II: (1) pain, which is a sensation usually experienced when tissue damage occurs; (2) hyperalgesia, which is an increased response to a normally painful stimulus; and (3) allodynia, which is a painful response to a normally nonpainful stimulus. This stimulus can be hot, cold, mechanical, or even chemical. The message of pain is initiated at two receptor sites: (1) a nosioceptor, which is usually a free nerve ending, or unmyelinated C-fiber, which detects tissue damage such as temperature or chemical changes and (2) a mechanoreceptor, such as a Pachinian corpusle, which is sensitive to pressure. When tissue is damaged, it produces a primary hyperalgesia, which is a sensitivity to pain, at the site of the pain, and a secondary hyperalgesia surrounding the zone of primary hyperalgesia, in the absence of tissue damage. A sensitized nosioceptor has a lower threshold to pain and produces hyperalgesia, whereas a sensitized mechanoreceptor transmits a message of pain to a normally nonpainful stimulus (i.e., allodynia).

Both hyperalgesia, and allodynia are the result of spinal dorsal horn body sensitization. The afferent fibers carry the sensory message to the brain, and the efferent fibers modify the sensory input from the brain back to the periphery. They have their origins in the brainstem, medulla, and periaquaductal gray and are called descending afferent pathways. These pathways modify sensation. At the spinal cord level, increased sensory input from the peripheral nosioceptor actually changes cell functioning in the spinal cord by altering chemical mediators and receptor activity. The persistent sensory stimuli activate NMDA at certain cells of the dorsal horn of the spinal cord, called WDR neurons or nociceptive specific (NS). Phosphorylation of the NMDA receptor is the result of constant sensory input, which then activates the NMDA receptor, and this creates central sensitization of the receptor ion channel. Mg^{2+} is removed, so Ca^{2+} enters the channel, which causes cell sensitization. This spinal cord change produces allodynia in the peripheral nerves. Therefore, tissue damage produces damage to the nocioceptor in the periphery, causing sensitization or hyperalgesia; and

the result of this chronic increase in activity at the spinal cord level produces central sensitization. Likewise, damage to the nerve causes growth hormone to produce nerve sprouts; these are very sensitive, which cause continued input the spinal cord, producing central sensitization. This increased sensory input, which produces central sensitization, actually changes the cells in the dorsal horn of the spinal cord, which results in allodynia. The damaged nerve produces sprouts, as the result of NGF stimulation. These sprouts have alpha-2 adreno-receptors on them, which are sensitive to norepinephrine circulating in the bloodstream.

GROSS ANATOMY

The most startling finding, and one that flies in the face of commonly held beliefs, is a report by Kleinman (1954) in which sympathetic chains were found to have communication between them, in up to 80% of cases. This was an important finding because this anatomic consideration is rarely, if ever, discussed in surgical textbooks or clinical papers. This finding also explains why some cases of CRPS I do not respond to sympathetic denervation, and why, paradoxical as it may seem, some cases do respond to contralateral blocks (i.e., if a patient has pain in the left leg, blocking the right lumbar sympathetic chain may produce relief).

Additional anatomy has been described by Allen and Morety (1982). When one traces the pathway of the sympathetic nerves, cell bodies are located in the lateral columns of the cervical, thoracic, and lumbar spinal cord. Cell bodies then give off axons, which form the preganglionic fibers of the sympathetic nervous system. From C7 to L2, these fibers are associated with the anterior spinal nerve roots and leave the spinal cord in this pathway. They then separate from the nerve root and become the white rami communicantes, which then continue on to the paravertebral ganglia, forming a chain running from the skull to the coccyx. From the ganglia themselves postganglionic fibers run back to nerve roots, or become separate nerves supplying various organs.

It is important to note that some ganglion cells are found in the anterior roots, as well as the white and gray rami. By the same token, some pre- and post-ganglionic fibers do not pass through sympathetic trunks, which again indicates that there is residual sympathetic innervation due to either normal variants or aberrant fibers that bypass the sympathetic trunk. This anatomic finding explains the failure of some ganglionectomies and suggests that one might need to do anterior nerve root sections and preganglionic rami sectioning (Smithwick procedure) in patients in whom ganglionectomy has failed.

Cervical outflow, coming from the upper portion of the cervical chain, sends fibers to the pupils and the eyelids. These fibers radiate from the upper stellate ganglion, which also supplies various fibers in the head and face. The upper thoracic sympathetic chain receives preganglionic input from upper thoracic roots and supplies the upper extremity through postganglionic fibers that pass through the brachial plexus. The lower extremities receive input from the T11 to L3 nerve roots, forming ganglia, and from the lower two lumbar and upper sacral nerve roots, with gray rami (postganglionic) to the lumbosacral plexus.

MICROANATOMY

As described earlier in the gross anatomy portion, there are various sites along the sympathetic chain where damage can occur to a nerve. Additionally, there are several sites where chemical intervention is possible, notably at the synapses that occur along the sympathetic pathways. Additionally, the various fibers that carry sympathetic messages are important. It has been widely held that C-fibers, which are small unmyelinated fibers carrying sensory messages, are responsible for the transmission of pain. Some theories consider that SMP is mediated by activity in A fibers, however, because C-fiber blockade fails to eliminate pain in patients with SMP (Roberts, 1986). Therefore, one must start at the very beginning of the onset of pain (i.e., the receptor itself) to fully understand SMP and CRPS I and II. Originally, it was thought that nociceptor afferents (nerves that carry the message of pain from the periphery to the cord and the brain) were responsible for the continuous pain of SMP, CRPS I, and CRPS II (Bonica, 1970; Devor & Janig, 1981; Roberts, 1986). In Roberts's (1986) article, however, he adheres to a theory first advanced by Loh and Nathan (1978) that indicates low-threshold mechanoreceptors are responsible for SMP. Roberts takes this position because nociceptor afferents, which are typically considered unmyelinated C-fibers, do not have appropriate responses to sympathetic activity; therefore, both practically and conceptually they cannot be included as the receptors that mediate SMP. Roberts (1986) reports that mechanoreceptors do respond appropriately to both touch and sympathetic activity, however. For CRPS II, others have proposed a neuroma formation as the cause of pain. Roberts believes that the sympathetic action of a neuroma is not capable of explaining why treatments that occur distal to the injury (in the form of either a nerve block or guanethidine infusion) are able to ameliorate CRPS II. Even so, Roberts (1986) uses the summation theory, or convergence theory, to say that both the peripheral receptors (in this case, mechanoreceptors) that arise in the neuroma and those that arise in the skin itself are transmitting painful messages to the cord and that distal blocks eliminate only the mechanoreceptors from the skin, which is not enough to trigger responses in the WDR neurons in the spinal cord. Additionally, the concept of a neuroma causing prolongation of CRPS

II–type pain does not fit the clinical observation that SMP may occur even in cases in which the nerve is not injured.

Ochoa et al. (1985) advances the theory that mechanical A-delta nociceptor endings become sensitized to multiple sensory inputs. This gives rise to the thermal hyperalgesia that is seen in CRPS I. On the other hand, Ochoa believes that there are abnormalities in distal nociceptor fibers that seem to have a low threshold. These low-threshold mechanoreceptors reside within large myelinated fibers and are nonsympathetic dependent because they transfer their information to nociceptor pathways proximal to the site of injury. These fibers may account for the mechanical hyperalgesia, manifesting as sensitivity to light touch. The previously mentioned receptors, which are the source of the hyperalgesia seen in CRPS I, are different from the burning pain receptors seen in CRPS II. Ochoa and colleagues (1985) believe that the burning pain of CRPS II is mediated by unmyelinated C-fibers, whereas Payne (1986) believes that this pain is due to nerve stretch and axon disruptions. Another consideration is the fact that such pain may be mediated by nerve fascicles where all three types of C-fibers exit (Ochoa et al., 1985). Therefore, in summary, the current thinking seems to suggest that sparsely myelinated C-fibers carry the message of burning pain found in CRPS II, whereas sparsely myelinated afferent fibers or the A-delta nociceptors may be responsible for pain in CRPS I.

SYNAPSES

Both synaptic considerations and axonal considerations have been raised as possible factors controlling both CRPS I and CRPS II. Ephapses, or artificial synapses, have been demonstrated in normal peripheral nerves. The concept of synaptic factors in CRPS I and II pain was first advanced by Granitt, Leksell, and Skoglund (1944) when they found that stimulating the motor root of a damaged mixed motor sensory nerve also produced recordable electrical events in the sensory root. According to the review by Payne (1986), the formation of ephapses after nerve injury may allow a short-circuiting or shunting of current from sympathetic fibers coming from the cord to the peripheral nerve into somatic fibers arising at the site of injury, carrying the message of pain back to the cord. Unfortunately, these cross-connections between fibers coming from the cord to the periphery, and conversely coming from the periphery to the cord, have been demonstrated in animal models, but not in humans (Payne 1986). Another consideration is the possibility of an ectopic impulse resulting from alterations in calcium, sodium, and potassium channels (Payne, 1986). In effect, the damaged nerve becomes "epileptic," and the spontaneous discharges from the sensory nerve may give rise to the episodic pain noted in some individuals. This could be due to lowered threshold or heightened mechanical sensitivity.

Neurosynaptic mediation of CRPS II and I holds great promise for the future. When reviewing the synapses that are present within the sympathetic chain, it is apparent that these provide a potential site of mediation for sensory input. To understand synaptic mediation, one must review the anatomy of a synapse per se. By borrowing heavily from Roberts (1986), one can define the functional neuroanatomy and delineate the location of various synapses. First, the trauma occurs, with receptors in the skin detecting various components of the trauma. Initially, the C-fiber nociceptors carry the message to the dorsal root ganglion and then back to the spinal cord neuron, where they synapse. After synapsing with the neuron in the spinal cord, these multiple neurons transmit information to the WDR neurons, which then send messages, via their axons, to the central nervous system or higher levels of the spinal cord. With use of Roberts' model, additional light touch activates the mechanoreceptors, which travel in the A-fibers instead of the C-fibers. Because the WDR neurons are already sensitized by the C-fiber nociceptors, they respond to what is usually subthreshold stimuli to the A-fiber mechanoreceptors. These mechanoreceptors travel in the A-fiber, reaching a neuron within the spinal cord, which again impinges on the WDR neuron; this, in turn, again sends messages up the spinal cord to the brain.

Sympathetic fibers exist within the lateral portions of the thoracic cord, sending efferent messages to the sensory receptor. These efferent messages (i.e., messages traveling from the cord to the periphery, mainly to the sensory receptors) may occur in the absence of cutaneous stimulation. According to Roberts' theory, however, the sympathetic efferent activity requires no cutaneous stimulation and is the cause of the SMP. In response to this efferent activity, the WDR neurons fire, again sending messages to the spinal cord and brain. The key to Roberts' theory is that the WDR neurons in the spinal cord remain sensitized, and they give a vigorous response to mechanical stimulation of A-fiber mechanoreceptors even after healing has occurred. In this schema, multiple synapses occur within the spinal cord, at the WDR neuron, and in the sympathetic ganglion. Therefore, synaptic regulation can occur at the spinal cord level or at the sympathetic ganglion level. When reviewing the actual synapse, one must conceptualize a presynaptic area wherein various chemicals are formulated, becoming neurosynaptic transmitters. The two synaptic transmitters that are of most interest to the study of CRPS I and II are the indolamines, of which serotonin is an example, and the catecholamines, of which norepinephrine, epinephrine, dopa, and dopamine are examples. In the presynaptic area of the nerve, precursor substances are manufactured into neurosynaptic transmitters, which confer a degree of specificity on nerve transmission. L-Tryptophan becomes 5-hydroxytryptophan, which becomes 5-hydroxytryptamine (serotonin); dopa becomes dopamine, which can be converted to norepinephrine and epinephrine.

The specific type of the neurosynaptic transmitter determines whether it will occupy a specific postsynaptic receptor site. Biogenic amines, such as the indolamines and catecholamines, are constantly being formulated and broken down by monoamine oxidase (MAO). Thus, chemically, the presynaptic area may be described as an area of high flux, with formulation and degradation of the same chemical occurring in the relatively steady state. As electrical impulses travel down the axon, pore diameter changes, altering the permeability of the membrane and causing the release of neurosynaptic transmitters. These synaptic transmitters flow across a minute gap between nerves and occupy postsynaptic receptor sites. The gap, of course, is called the synapse. The postsynaptic receptor sites determine the strength and duration of the electrical impulse that the synapse propagates. This is done by the degree of specificity that the neurosynaptic transmitters have for a particular receptor site. It also depends on the affinity that a specific neurosynaptic transmitter has for a particular receptor site and whether it is easily displaced or forms a tight bond. Almost all neurosynaptic transmitters have their activity ended by presynaptic reuptake; that is, the chemical that occupies the postsynaptic receptor site is taken back into the presynaptic area. Acetylcholine is an exception, being degraded on the postsynaptic receptor site by acetylcholinesterase. Additionally, some small amount of degradation of biogenic amines occurs in the synapse itself by catechol-O-methyltransferase (COMT). It is thought that less than 5% of the chemical degradation of synaptic transmitters occurs in the synapse by COMT, and 95% of the degradation occurs presynaptically by MAO. Of course, there is constant rebuilding of the neurosynaptic transmitter presynaptically, creating the steady state mentioned earlier.

Obviously, there are multiple ways to modify the synapse. One can inhibit MAO, thereby enhancing the buildup of a monoamine neurosynaptic transmitter, such as the indolamines or the catecholamines. In fact, a class of drugs called MAO inhibitors does exactly that. By the same token, certain drugs can function as MAO exciters, which facilitate the degradation of biogenic amine neurosynaptic transmitters, such as the indolamines (serotonin) and the catecholamines (epinephrine, norepinephrine, dopamine, and dopa). Because the majority of the neurosynaptic transmitters have their activity ended by presynaptic reuptake, one can enhance the synaptic transmission by blocking presynaptic reuptake. This is how tricyclic antidepressants work. Conversely, one can diminish synaptic transmission by facilitation of presynaptic reuptake. Finally, one can work at the receptor end by using drugs that mimic the action of the presynaptic transmitters and occupy receptor sites, thereby triggering them as if the actual chemical had been released. By the same token, other drugs can be used that occupy the receptor sites but have no pharmacological activity other than to inhibit the presynaptic transmitter from occupying the receptor site. For example, curare effects a total blockade of the acetylcholine receptor. In this sense, these drugs become inhibitors of neurosynaptic transmission. Receptor sites are found not only postsynaptically but also presynaptically, very often for the same presynaptic neurosynaptic transmitter. As the number and sensitivity of these receptors change, so does the response to the neurosynaptic transmitter itself.

DIAGNOSIS OF COMPLEX REGIONAL PAIN SYNDROME, TYPE II

With the foregoing theoretical information, the clinical components of CRPS I and II should be more readily differentiated by appropriate diagnostic studies. According to both Raja et al. (1986) and Payne (1986), CRPS II manifests as a burning pain, which is not a consistent finding of CRPS I. Additionally, patients with CRPS II may experience paroxysms of pain, especially after stress, whether it be emotional or environmental. In an elegant study, Raja et al. (1986) found that patients with CRPS II rarely have cold hyperalgesia (two of nine), and they do not have heat hyperalgesia (none of nine). Additionally, these patients obtain no relief from sympathetic blocks. Raja et al. (1986) differentiated various types of hyperalgesia using sensory testing with either Von Frey hairs for touch, a drop of acetone for cold, or laser thermal stimulation for heat. Ochoa et al. (1985) believe that CRPS II is not always sympathetically mediated, but instead is mediated by unmyelinated C-fibers. Stretch injuries to the nerve or axon disruption of a major nerve branch is one explanation favored by Payne (1986). Usually, the patient with CRPS II has a history of a nerve injury to a peripheral nerve or surgery that has damaged the proximal portion of the nerve trunk (Payne, 1986; Raja et al., 1986). CRPS II may be related to damage of nerve fascicles where all three types of C-fibers exist (Ochoa et al., 1985).

TREATMENT OF COMPLEX REGIONAL PAIN SYNDROME, TYPE II

Various authors have reported that sympathetic blocks are or are not effective, with efficacy for sympathectomy reported to be between 12 and 97% (Payne, 1986). However, Raja et al. (1986, 1991) reported no relief with sympathetic blocks. Payne has suggested that a dorsal root entry zone (DREZ) procedure may prove effective. Ghostine et al. (1984) have suggested the use of phenoxybenzamine. They reported 40 consecutive cases of CRPS II, all of which involved nerve injuries from bullet or shrapnel wounds. The hydraulic effect of high-speed bullet injuries is well demonstrated by photographs taken of a bullet striking an object. The Ghostine group noted partial motor

paralysis in the distribution of the damaged nerve in 70% of the cases. Over time, these deficits resolved in many of the cases, however. They also noted vasomotor changes, usually severe vasodilatation and sweating and less often vasoconstriction (Ghostine et al., 1984). Rarely were trophic changes noted. The majority of the cases involved the sciatic nerve, median nerve, brachial plexus, cauda equina, and occipital nerve, in descending order. The treatment that Ghostine et al. (1984) used was phenoxybenzamine, which is a postsynaptic alpha-1-blocker and a presynaptic alpha-2-blocker. As mentioned earlier under the etiology of CRPS II, nerve sprouts, which are one of the theoretical origins of this disorder, seem to be highly excitable on the administration of norepinephrine; the excitability can be reversed with alpha-blocking agents such as phentolamine, but are unaffected by beta-blocking agents. The dosage of the drug used by Ghostine et al. initially was 10 mg three times a day, although this varied from patient to patient. Eventually maximum dosages of 40 to 120 mg/day were reached, with treatment lasting 6 to 8 weeks. Common side effects were orthostatic hypotension in about 45% of the patients and reduced ejaculatory ability in about 8% of the patients. In some instances, treatment lasted as long as 16 weeks. It is important to note that the patients were all treated within 2 to 70 days after the onset of their injury.

For this treatment to be effective, it is most important that rapid diagnosis and institution of treatment occur. Another possibility for the pharmacological treatment of CRPS II would be the use of clonazepam, which has been reported by Bouckoms and Litman (1985) to be effective for "burning" pains.

Surgical sympathectomy has been recommended as a treatment for CRPS II, after repetitive sympathetic blocks. Additionally, guanethidine, which is a ganglionic blocking agent, has proved effective in treating some forms of CRPS II. Guanethidine must be used with caution, however, because it causes the release of norepinephrine prior to occupying the receptor sites and the time course of the cessation of activity is variable. The fact that one may occlude an affected limb below the site of the CRPS II and still achieve effective blocks with guanethidine suggests that its activity is not at the ganglion but instead on the peripheral sensory nerves, which produces its effect on CRPS II (Hannington-Kiff, 1979). Surgical intervention, in the form of surgical sympathectomy, has been used to treat CRPS II with variable cure rates, ranging from 12 to 97%. The variability may be ascribed to lack of precision and diagnosis, with an overlap of CRPS I with CRPS II, or CRPS I mistakenly diagnosed as CRPS II; varying skills in performing blocks; collateral reinnervation of postganglionic sympathetic fibers; and delay in performing a sympathectomy (Payne, 1986). For CRPS II that is not responding to sympathectomy, the possibility of a contralateral sympathectomy has been raised (Kleinman, 1954).

DIAGNOSIS OF COMPLEX REGIONAL PAIN SYNDROME, TYPE I

The clinical diagnosis of CRPS I is more complicated than that of CRPS II. Some authors believe that there is a very definite set of criteria to establish the diagnosis, whereas other authors think that only several symptoms from a whole list of symptom complexes need be present to establish the diagnosis of CRPS I. Kozin et al. (1981) have established the criteria for CRPS I as a patient presenting with pain and tenderness in an extremity associated with vasomotor instability (particular temperature or color changes) and generalized swelling in the same extremity. The second group of patients they consider are those with pain and tenderness associated with a vasomotor instability or swelling in an extremity; they call this group "probable CRPS I." This system lacks precision, however, because it does not take into account the particular type of pain that patients with CRPS I experience.

Raja et al. (1986) define patients as having CRPS I if they have pain associated with signs of sympathetic hyperactivity (e.g., lower skin temperature, skin discoloration, increased sweating, and some trophic changes) and symptomatic relief after sympathetic blocks; they found that those with CRPS I also had thermal hyperalgesia either to cold or to heat. In contrast, their patients with CRPS II did not experience thermal hyperalgesia to heat, and only two of seven experienced hyperalgesia to cold. Both patients with CRPS II and with CRPS I experienced hyperalgesia to mechanical stimulation (Raja et al., 1986). On the other hand, Ochoa et al. (1985) found mechanical hyperalgesia, which they called allodynia, in their patients with CRPS I. Additionally, hypersensitivity to temperature was also found in patients with CRPS I, whether it be to heat or to cold (Meyer et al., 1985; Ochoa et al., 1985; Raja et al., 1986).

One proposed mechanism for mechanical hypersensitivity is ectopic alpha-adrenergic chemosensitivity (Devor, 1983). Another consideration is a secondary abnormality in distal nociceptor fibers that escaped injury, or intact low-threshold mechanoreceptors with large myelinated fibers that are not sympathetic dependent because of transfer of information to nociceptor pathways proximal to the site of injury (Ochoa et al., 1985). Additionally, Ochoa et al. advanced the concept of alpha-receptor sensitization, whereas others believe that the hypersensitivity of the mechanoreceptors could possibly be a central nervous system event (Meyer et al., 1985).

TREATMENT OF COMPLEX REGIONAL PAIN SYNDROME, TYPE I

Treatments for the mechanical hypersensitivity or hyperalgesia of CRPS I have been advanced by several authors, without clear-cut definition. One group of authors believes that sympathectomy may relieve mechanical hyperalgesia (Meyer et al., 1985), whereas another group of authors reports that sympathectomy does not. Another group has advanced the notion that nifedipine, a calcium channel-blocking agent, may prove effective (Prough et al., 1985). Finally, a group from South Africa suggested that low-dose naloxone, and possibly longer acting naltrexone, may prove effective for reducing mechanical hyperalgesia, because of the existence of a hypergesic kappa system of opiate receptors (Gillman & Lichtigfeld, 1985). Again, the area of mechanical hyperalgesia is quite muddy, because all the patients with either CRPS II or CRPS I had mechanical hypersensitivity (Raja et al., 1986).

Thermal hypersensitivity to either heat or cold (hyperalgesia) has been reported by several groups (Meyer et al., 1985; Ochoa et al., 1985; Raja et al., 1986). The mechanism behind the thermal hypersensitivity is not well elucidated, but one can clinically differentiate mechanical from thermal hypersensitivity by the use of a drop of acetone. Patients with CRPS I in the series studied by Raja et al. (1986) had hyperalgesia to cold (three of four, as tested by acetone drop) or to heat (four of five, as tested using a laser thermal stimulator). Some patients had hypersensitivity and hyperalgesia to both heat and cold; however, these patients did not have CRPS II, but instead CRPS I. Of the group of patients with hyperalgesia to temperature change, six of six got relief with sympathetic blocks or sympathectomy (Raja et al., 1986). Other authors have reported that nifedipine is effective for treating hyperalgesia (Prough et al., 1985). Specifically, in 13 patients with pain having a burning character, dysesthesia, and cold intolerance, nifedipine beginning at 10 mg three times a day, and increasing to 30 mg three times a day, proved effective in 7 of 13 patients. Nifedipine is a calcium channel-blocking agent, and as such may work by dilating blood vessels and antagonizing the effects of norepinephrine on arterial and venous muscle (Payne, 1986). Also, nifedipine may interfere with ectopic impulse formation that occurs in regenerating nerves by blocking calcium channel protein.

The dystrophic component of CRPS I is more difficult to delineate. Some authors have reported a diffuse or patchy bony demineralization (Kozin et al., 1981), whereas others have reported frank osteoporosis late in the disorder (Schott, 1986). A number of authors have reported molted skin, again late in the disorder (Kozin et al., 1981; Payne, 1986; Raja et al., 1986). Some authors have reported hair loss, yet again late in the disorder (Raja et al., 1986; Schott, 1986). Vague terms such as vasomotor instability have also been reported, as well as trophic skin changes (Kozin et al., 1981). The etiology for these components is not well defined, but the consensus seems to be reduced blood flow to the various involved organs.

A more precise diagnostic assessment was advanced by Holder and MacKinnon (1984). They evaluated patients with CRPS I, which they defined as diffuse hand pain, diminished hand function, joint stiffness, and skin and soft tissue trophic changes with or without vasomotor instability. They also used three other control groups, including patients with diffuse pain, focal pain, or vascular disease. Holder and MacKinnon (1984) found that 22 of the 23 patients who met their criteria for diagnosing CRPS I had positive delayed image bone scans, 12 of the 23 patients had positive blood pool images, and 10 of the 23 patients had positive radionucleotide angiograms. Approximately half the patients with CRPS I had positive early phase bone scans, whereas almost all patients with CRPS I had positive delayed image bone scans.

This study compared favorably with work done by Kozin et al. (1981), who found that radiography is not a useful tool for diagnosing CRPS I. Kozin et al. (1981) did find that 83% of the patients with CRPS I had positive static (delayed) bone scans, however, whereas 69% of the patients had positive flow studies. Therefore, it is apparent that between 50 and 60% of patients with CRPS I will have positive early phase bone scans, but between 83 and 96% of patients will have positive delayed image bone scans (Holder & Mackinnon, 1984; Kozin et al., 1981). Treatment for this component of CRPS I is difficult to assess. Kozin et al. (1981) reported that 90% of patients with positive bone scans had good to excellent steroid response, beginning with steroids at the level of 60 to 80 mg/day and tapering the dosages.

Schott (1986) has reported a variety of therapeutic modalities, including steroids, nonsteroidal anti-inflammatory drugs, alpha- and beta-blocking agents, griseofulvin, calcitonin, transcutaneous electrical nerve stimulation, physical therapy, sympathetic blocks, and intravenous guanethidine. None of these treatments has been studied in a systematized fashion, however.

Nail brittleness has been reported by Schott (1986) and Payne (1986) late in the disorder. The etiology of this is not clear and there is no clear-cut treatment. Muscle spasm has been reported by a number of authors (Kleinman, 1954; Long, 1982; Schott, 1986), again without a clear-cut mechanism describing the etiology (Payne, 1986). Interestingly, EMG nerve conduction velocity studies seem to be relatively negative in CRPS I (Uematsu et al., 1981). The treatments that seemed most effective for muscle spasm were trigger point injections (Payne, 1986) and the use of baclofen. Baclofen is a gamma aminobutyric acid (GABA)-minergic drug that centrally reduces muscle spasm. The inhibition of substance P may be implicated as part of its mechanism for reducing spasm and the pain associated with spasm (Gillman & Lichtigfeld, 1985). Soma and quinine have also been tried, with only limited success (Hendler, unpublished observations). Contractures, usually in the hand, have also been reported (Payne, 1986; Schott, 1986). The etiology of this is unclear but is probably related to disuse. Again, there is an absence of positive EMG-NCV studies (Uematsu et al., 1981), and

the only treatment seems to be preventative, by the use of passive range-of-motion exercises and physical therapy.

Contralateral involvement has been reported by several authors (Kleinman, 1954; Schott, 1986). The etiology for this may be quite direct. In approximately 80% of examined cadavers there is cross-communication between the sympathetic fibers and the sympathetic chains (Kleinman, 1954). Countralateral blocks and denervation have been recommended (Kleinman, 1954). Edema of the affected limb (Payne, 1986; Schott, 1986), as well as swelling of a specific joint (Kozin et al., 1981), has been reported. Again, the etiology is unclear. The diagnosis is established by measuring the proximal interphalangeal joint, which averages 12.9 mm larger in the affected hand than in the control hand (Kozin et al., 1981). No treatment has been advanced for this, although nifedipine is suggested to be effective (Prough et al., 1985). At the Mensana Clinic in Stevenson, MD, we have observed some benefit from the use of spironolactone or carbonic anhydrase inhibitors, but not on a consistent basis.

Lower skin temperature has been reported by a variety of authors (Hendler et al., 1982; Payne, 1986; Raja et al., 1986), but it does not seem to be due to vasospasm (Janoff et al., 1985). Reflex contraction due to altered activity within the afferent and efferent nerves is proposed as the etiology (Janoff et al., 1985). Thermography is an excellent diagnostic tool to document the reduced skin temperature (Hendler et al., 1982; Uematsu et al., 1981). In fact, very often patients with CRPS I are diagnosed as having psychosomatic disorders, and thermography can be a most convincing diagnostic tool to confirm the otherwise subjective complaint (Hendler et al., 1982). However, nerve entrapments and radiculopathies can also lower limb temperature (Uematsu et al., 1981).

Treatment for lower skin temperature associated with pain is best effected using regional sympathetic blocks employing reserpine. It is important to note that these reserpine blocks, or Bier blocks, are not effective for vasospasm, but specifically seem to function best for treating CRPS I. Therefore, vasospasm does not seem to be the etiologic mechanism for the coldness noted in the limb in CRPS I (Janoff et al., 1985). Stiffness (Holder & MacKinnon, 1984; Payne, 1986) and tenderness (Kozin et al., 1981) of the joints have been reported; again, the etiology is not clear (Payne, 1986). Very often, the involvement of the joint leads to misdiagnosis and confusion with other diseases that can affect the joint, notably infective arthritis, rheumatoid arthritis, Reiter's syndrome, systemic lupus erythematosus, and arthritides (Kozin et al., 1981). In one series, 71% of the patients with joint tenderness and stiffness had poor responses to stellate ganglion blocks. Steroids, notably prednisone (60 to 80 mg) for 2 to 4 days, then 40 to 60 mg for 2 to 4 days, and then 30 to 40 mg for 2 to 4 days, in four equally divided doses, were the initial therapy. Subsequently, the dose was rapidly tapered using a single morning dose of 40 mg, then 30 mg, 20 mg, 10 mg, and 5 mg over 2 or 3 days at each dose. By using this regimen, 82% of the patients with joint stiffness and tenderness obtained good or excellent relief.

An unusual complication of CRPS I is the appearance of pathological fractures subsequent to minor trauma. In patients complaining of persistent pain in the limb that seems to be bony in origin, instead of part of the CRPS I, it would be imperative to obtain bone scanning to confirm the presence or absence of an undetected break. In our experience, one patient with long-standing CRPS I received a minor trauma (i.e., bumping her ankle while walking in a train) that resulted in a chronic intense worsening of pain in the heel. Radiographs of this area were within normal limits, but the pain persisted for several days after the event, and a bone scan was obtained. Only on bone scan did the break in the calcaneus appear, which had been totally missed by routine radiograph. Of any breaks present, 95% will have a positive bone scan after 72 h (Matin, 1979). Interestingly, after the fracture is healed, 90% of the bone scans returned to normal 2 years from the date of the injury. Therefore, in patients with CRPS I who have minor injuries and complain of bony pain, it would be prudent to obtain a bone scan and not rely on radiographs.

Payne (1986) has enumerated many attempted treatments for CRPS I. Unfortunately, there seems to be a lack of systematic investigation for these treatments, and most are based on clinical reports instead of systematized trials. Reported pharmacological interventions that may work for CRPS II are the use of propranolol, a beta-blocking agent; prazosin, an alpha-1-adrenergic-blocking agent; phenoxybenzamine, both an alpha-1- and an alpha-2-blocker; and guanethidine, a drug that produces a chemical "sympathectomy." Physical therapy has been advanced for the treatment of CRPS I, specifically to minimize muscle contractures and joint stiffness. It is never a definitive treatment, however, and should not be considered such. Electrical stimulation of the central nervous system, using either electrodes centrally implanted into the periaqueductal or periventricular gray or epidural stimulators, may prove effective, as might transcutaneous electrical nerve stimulation. Tricyclic antidepressants, nonsteroidal anti-inflammatory drugs, narcotics, and anticonvulsants have all been reported as treating some components of CRPS, type I, with varying degrees of success.

Surgical intervention is a treatment that is reserved until all other modalities of treatment have been attempted. In all cases, the criterion for surgical intervention would be repetitive successes with repeat sympathetic blocks. The most commonly employed surgical interventions are resection of the lower third of the stellate ganglion and resection of the upper two thoracic ganglia; however, some surgeons resect the second through fifth thoracic ganglia in an attempt to treat upper-extremity difficulties. There are four surgical approaches to upper extremity sympathectomies (Allen & Morety, 1982):

1. Above the clavicle (anterior cervical approach)
2. Posterior resection of the transverse processes of ribs 2 and 3, and proximal section of ribs 2 and 3
3. Anterior transpleural entry through the pectoralis muscle to the third intercostal space, pressing the lung, to reach the operative area
4. The axillary approach, which is through a transaxillary incision over the second intercostal space

Also, a lumbar approach can be made through the external and internal obliques, and then the transversalis muscle, below the twelfth rib, behind the kidney; others have suggested a thoracolumbar presacral neurectomy. Side effects of surgical approaches are postsympathectomy neuralgia, beginning 7 to 10 days after surgery, and postsympathectomy dysesthesia that may last 2 to 14 weeks and is described as continuous, severe, and worse at night. Anticonvulsants, such as diphenylhydantoin or carbamazepine, may be used to treat this (Allen & Morety, 1982). Medication, such as valproic acid and gabapentin may be useful (Mellick & Mellick, 1995). Dorsal root entry zone procedures, which produce lesions in the dorsal root interrupting the nociceptive pathways in the tract of Lissauer and in laminae I-V of the dorsal horn of the spinal cord, may prove to be an effective modality for treating CRPS II for stretch injuries (Payne, 1986). A treatment guideline is shown in Table 36.5.

CONCLUSIONS

In summary, it is quite apparent that a great deal of confusion has arisen concerning the diagnosis of CRPS I and CRPS II. This is evidenced by the lack of uniformity in clinical criteria for establishing the diagnosis. Because of this lack of uniformity, assessment of various articles detailing treatment of CRPS I and/or CRPS II is difficult. What some clinicians take as symptoms of CRPS I are not always present in their entirety. Unfortunately, if one adheres rigorously to these criteria, proper diagnosis, and more importantly proper treatment, may be withheld. The various clinical symptoms that have been reported as associated with CRPS I and CRPS II are shown in Table 36.3. A patient should be considered to have CRPS I if he or she has both types of allodynia (mechanical and thermal), altered skin temperature, and pain in a circumferential distribution. At a minimum, diagnostic studies that would facilitate the diagnosis of CRPS I would be sympathetic blocks, phentolamine testing, and a bone scan. Clinical diagnostic studies that would prove important would be testing with the Hendler alcohol drop and swipe test, for

TABLE 36.5
Recommended Treatment Flow Sheet

Treatment	Dosage	Time Course	If Ineffective, Next Step
1. Prednisone	80 mg to start and taper by 10 mg q.d.	8 days	Go to 2
2. Physical therapy	3 times a week	2 weeks	Go to 3
3. Transcutaneous electrical stimulation	Wear constantly	1 week	Go to 4
4. Sympathetic blocks	3 times a week	2 weeks	If lasting relief, stop; if 100% pain relief but temporary, go to 5
5. Sympathectomy	—	1-week recovery	If lasting relief, stop; if no relief, go to 6
6. Contralateral blocks	3 times a week	2 weeks	If lasting relief, stop; if 100% pain relief but temporary, go to 7; if no relief, go to 8
7. Contralateral sympathectomy	—	1-week recovery	If relief, stop; if no relief, go to 8
8. Epidural spinal cord stimulator	—	1-week recovery	If relief, stop; if no relief, go to 9
9. Epidural pump	Start with clonidine (Rauck et al., 1993)	1-week recovery	If relief, stop; if no relief, try other meds in combination or alone, go to 10
10. Psychotherapy (supportive)	Use antidepressants	6 months to 2 years	Maintenance

thermal and mechanical allodynia. EMG and NCV studies, SSEP, and neurometer studies should be conducted to detect whether there is an associated nerve entrapment. All patients suspected of having CRPS I should have at least three sympathetic blocks. After that, one should use various diagnostic and treatment techniques, including pharmacological intervention, depending on the patient's type of complaints. If there is residual pain in a peripheral nerve distribution while the limb is warm from the sympathetic block, concomitant nerve blocks should be performed.

To make the diagnosis of CRPS II, one certainly should establish that the symptoms of burning pain are constantly present, in association with a partial peripheral nerve injury. EMG and NCV studies, SSEP, and neurometer studies should be conducted to detect whether there is an associated nerve injury. Certainly, patients should receive a peripheral nerve block, sympathetic blocks, and a trial with phenoxybenzamine, valproic acid, and gabapentin.

Regardless of whether a patient has CRPS I or CRPS II, one must be aware of the need to distinguish between the two diagnoses because the treatments vary. More importantly, if the patient has even a single symptom of CRPS I, a diagnostic assessment involving the previously recommended modalities would be warranted, and further diagnostic studies should be pursued if the diagnosis of CRPS I is not confirmed. Kozin et al. (1981) clearly defines a number of overlapping conditions that may originally be misdiagnosed as CRPS I. Of the patients who were found not to have CRPS I, 25 to 71% had peripheral neuropathy or trapped peripheral nerves, and half the patients misdiagnosed as having CRPS I had inflammatory arthritis (Hendler 2002; Kozin et al., 1981). Therefore, laboratory studies, including erythrocyte sedi-

mentation rate, antinuclear antibody, rheumatoid factor, Lyme disease, HIV, and the like, should be conducted in patients thought to have CRPS I but in whom the diagnosis is not complete. In any event, CRPS II and I require clinical acumen to establish the diagnosis, and persistence to effect appropriate treatment. Aggressively pursuing all the diagnostic studies available, as well as relying on clinical judgment, provides better care for these patients.

REFERENCES

Allen, M. B., Jr., & Morety, W. H. (1982). Sympathectomy. In J. Youmans (Ed.), *Neurological surgery* (vol. 6, 2nd ed., (pp. 3717–3726). Philadelphia: W. B. Saunders.

Arner, S., & Meyerson, B. A. (1988). Lack of analgesic effect of opioids on neuropathic and idiopathic forms of pain. *Pain, 33*, 11–23.

Barolat, G., Schwartzman, R. J., & Woo, R. (1989). Epidural spinal cord stimulation in the management of reflex sympathetic dystrophy. *Stereotactic and Functional Neurosurgery, 53*, 29–39.

Baron, R., Blumberg, H., & Janig, W. (1996). Clinical characteristics of patients with complex regional pain syndrome in Germany, with special emphasis on vasomotor function, in reflex sympathetic dystrophy: A reappraisal. In W. Janig & M. Stanton-Hicks (Eds.). *Progress in pain research and management* (vol. 6, pp. 25–48). Seattle: IASP Press.

Bennett, G. J. (1991). The role of the sympathetic nervous system in painful peripheral neuropathy. *Pain, 45*, 221–223.

Bonica, J. J. (1970). Causalgia and other reflex sympathetic dystrophies. In J. J. Bonica (Ed.), *Advances in pain research and therapy* (vol. 3, pp. 141–166). New York: Raven Press.

Bosco Vieira Durate, J., Kux, P., Magalhaes, & Duarte, D. F., (2003a, December), Endoscopic thoracic sympathicotomy for the treatment of complex regional pain syndrome. *Clinical Autonomic Research, 13*(Suppl 1), 158–162.

Bosco Vieira Durate, J., Kux P., Castro, C. H., Cruvinel, M. G., & Costa, J. R., (2003b), Fast-track endoscopic thoracic sympathectomy, *Clinical Autonomic Research, Dec. (13,* Suppl 1), 163–165.

Bouckoms, A. L., & Litman R. E. (1985). Clonazepam in the treatment of neuralgic pain syndrome. *Psychosomatics, 26,* 933–936.

Broseta, J., Roldan, P., & Gonzales-Darder, J. (1982). Chronic epidural dorsal column stimulation in the treatment of causalgic pain. *Applications in Neurophysiology, 45,* 190–194.

Chaplan, S. R., Bach, F. W., Pogrel, J. W., Chung, J. M., & Yaksh, T. L. (1994). Quantitative assessment of tactile allodynia in the rat paw. *Journal of Neuroscience Methods, 53,* 55–63.

Dalton, S. (1984). *Split seconds — The world of high speed photography* (pp. 21, 28, 30, 31, 32, 34, 36). Salem, NH: Salem House.

Devor, M. (1983). Nerve pathophysiology and mechanisms of pain in causalgia. *Journal of the Autonomic Nervous System, 7,* 371–384.

Devor, M., & Janig, W. (1981). Activation of myelinated afferents ending in a neuroma by stimulation of the sympathetic supply in a rat. *Neuroscience Letters, 24,* 43–47.

Eliav, E., Herzberg, U., & Caudle, R. M. (1999). The kappa opioid agonist GR89 696 blocks hyperalgesia and allodynia in rat models of peripheral neuritis and neuropathy. *Pain, 79,* 255–264.

Fishbain, D. A., Goldberg, M., Rosomoff, R. S., & Rosomoff, H. (1991) Completed suicide in chronic pain, *Clinical Journal of Pain, 7*(1), 29–36.

Geldard, F. A. (1962). *Fundamentals of psychology.* New York: John Wiley and Sons.

Ghostine, S. Y., Comair, Y. G., Turner, D. M. et al. (1984). Phenoxybenzamine in the treatment of causalgia (report of 40 cases). *Journal of Neurosurgery, 6,* 1263–1268.

Gillman, M. A., & Lichtigfeld, R. J. (1985). A pharmacological overview of opioid mechanisms mediating analgesia and hyperalgesia. *Neural Research, 7,* 106–119.

Glynn, C. J., Dawson, D., & Sanders, R. (1988). A double-blind comparison between epidural morphine and epidural clonidine in patients with chronic non-cancer pain. *Pain, 34,* 123–128.

Gobelet, C., Waldburger, M., & Meier, J. L. (1992). The effect of adding calcitonin to physical treatment on reflex sympathetic dystrophy. *Pain, 48,* 171–175.

Granit,t R., Leksell, L., & Skoglund, C. R. (1944). Fiber interaction in injured or compressed region of the nerve. *Brain, 67,* 125–140.

Greipp, M. E., & Thomas, A. F. (1994). Skin lesions occurring in clients with reflex sympathetic dystrophy syndrome. *Journal of Neuroscience Nursing, 26*(6), 342–346.

Hamamou, N., Dursun, E., Ural, C., & Cakci, A. (1996). Calcitonin treatment in reflex sympathetic dystrophy. A preliminary study. *British Journal of Clinical Practice, 50*(7), 373–375.

Hannington-Kiff, J. G. (1979). Relief of causalgia in limbs by regional intravenous guanethedine. *British Medical Journal, 12,* 367–368.

Hassenbusch, S., Stanton-Hicks, M., & Covington, E. C. (1995). Long term intraspinal infusion of opioids in the treatment of neuropathic pain. *Journal of Pain and Symptom Management, 10,* 527–543.

Hendler, N. (2002). Differential diagnosis of complex regional pain syndrome, Type I (RSD), *Pan Arab Journal of Neurosurgery, 6*(2), 1–9.

Hendler, N. (1982). The four stages of pain. In N. Hendler, D. Long, & T. Wise (Eds.), *Diagnosis and treatment of chronic pain* (pp. 1–8). Boston: John Wright-PSG.

Hendler, N. (1984). Depression caused by chronic pain. *Journal of Clinical Psychiatry, 45*(3, Sec. 2), 30–36.

Hendler, N. (1995). Reflex sympathetic dystrophy: Clearing up the misconceptions. *Journal of Workers Compensation, 5*(1), 9–20.

Hendler, N. (1997). Pharmacology of chronic pain. In R. North and R. Levy (Eds.), *Neurosurgical management of pain* (pp. 117–129). Amsterdam: Springer-Verlag.

Hendler, N. (2000). Pharmacotherapy of chronic pain. In P. P. Raj (Ed.), *Practical management of pain* (3rd ed., pp. 145–155). Philadelphia: C.V. Mosby.

Hendler, N., Bergson, C., & Morrison, C. (1996). Overlooked physical diagnoses in chronic pain patients involved in litigation: Part 2. *Psychosomatics, 37*(6), 509–517.

Hendler, N., & Kozikowski, J. (1993). Overlooked physical diagnoses in chronic pain patients involved in litigation. *Psychosomatics, 34*(6), 494–501.

Hendler, N., & Raja, S. (1994). Reflex sympathetic dystrophy and causalgia. In C. D. Tollison (Ed), *Handbook of pain management* (2nd ed., pp. 484–496). Baltimore: Williams and Wilkins.

Hendler, N., & Talo, S. (1989). Chronic pain patients versus the malingering patient. In K. Foley and R. Payne (Eds.), *Current therapy of pain* (pp. 14–22). Philadelphia: B.C. Decker.

Hendler, N., Uematsu, S., & Long, D. (1982). Thermographic validating of physical complaints in "psychogenic pain" patients. *Psychosomatics, 23,* 282–287.

Hendler, N., Vierstein, M., Shallenberger, C., & Long, D. (1981). Group therapy with chronic pain patients. *Psychosomatics, 22*(4), 333–340.

Hoffert, M. I., Greenburg, P. P., Wolskee, P. J. et al. (1984). Abnormal and collateral innervation of sympathetic and peripheral sensory fields associated with a case of causalgia. *Pain, 20,* 1–12.

Holder, L. E., & MacKinnon, S. E. (1984). Reflex sympathetic dystrophy in the hands: Clinical and scintigraphic criteria. *Radiology, 152,* 517–522.

Inball, R., Rousso, N., Ashur, H., Wall, P. D., & Devor, M. (1987). Collateral sprouting in skin and sensory recovery after nerve injury in man. *Pain, 39,* 141–154.

Janoff, K. H., Phinney, E. S., & Porter, I. M. (1985). Lumbar sympathectomy for lower extremity vasospasm. *American Journal of Surgery, 150*, 147–152.

Kim, S. H., & Chung, J. M. (1995). Sympathectomy alleviates mechanical allodynia in an experimental animal model for neuropathy in the rat. *Neuroscience Letters, 134*, 131–134.

Kleinman, A. (1954). Causalgia: Evidence of the existence of crossed sensory sympathetic fibers. *American Journal of Surgery, 87*, 839–841.

Knobler, R. (1996). The pathogenesis of reflex sympathetic dystrophy: Immune and viral mechanisms. *American Journal of Pain Management, 6*(3), 83–85.

Kozin, F., Ryan, L. M., Carerra, G. E. et al. (1981). The reflex sympathetic dystrophy (RSDS). *American Journal of Medicine, 70*, 23–30.

Lee, Y. W., Chaplan, S. R., & Yaksh, T. L. (1995). Systemic and supraspinal, but not spinal opiates suppress allodynia in a rat neuropathic pain model. *Neuroscience Letters, 199*, 111–114.

Lee, Y. W., Kayer, V., Desmeules, J., & Guilbaud, G. (1994). Differential action of morphine and various opioid agonist on thermal allodynia and hyperalgesia in mononeuropathic rats. *Pain, 57*, 233–240.

Lee, Y. W., & Yaksh, T. L. (1996). Pharmacology of the spinal adenosine receptor which mediates the anti-allodynic action of intra-thecal adenosine agonists. *Journal of Pharmacology and Experimental Therapeutics, 277*, 1642–1648

Levi-Montalcini, R., Skaper, S. D., Toso, R. D., Petrelli, L., & Leon, A. (1996). Nerve growth factor: From neurotrophin to neurokine. *Trends in Neuroscience, 19*, 514–520.

Loh, I., & Nathan P. W. (1978). Painful peripheral states and sympathetic blocks. *Journal of Neurology, Neurosurgery, and Psychiatry, 41*, 664–671.

Long, D. M. (1982). Pain of peripheral nerve injury. In J. Youmans (Ed.), *Neurological surgery* (2nd ed., Vol. 6, pp. 3634–3643). Philadelphia: W. B. Saunders.

Matin, P. (1979). The appearance of bone scans following fractures, including immediate and long-term studies. *Journal of Nuclear Medicine, 20*, 1227–1231.

Max, M. B., Kishmore-Kumar, R., Schafer, S. C. et al.(1991). Efficacy of desipramine in diabetic peripheral neuropathy: A placebo controlled trial. *Pain, 45*, 69–73.

Mearow, K. M., & Kril, Y. (1995). Anti-NGF treatment blocks the upregulation of NGF receptor mRNA expression associated with collateral sprouting of rat dorsal ganglion neurons. *Neuroscience Letters, 184*, 55–58.

Mellick, G. A., & Mellick, L. B. (1995). Gabapentin in the management of reflex sympathetic dystrophy. *Journal of Pain Symptoms and Management, 10*, 265–266.

Merskey, H. (Ed.) and the Subcommittee on Taxonomy. (1986). Classification of chronic pain. *Pain, 3*(Suppl.), 28–29.

Meyer, R. A., Campbell, J. N., & Raja, S. N. (1985). Peripheral neural mechanism of cutaneous hyperalgesia. In H. L. Fields, R. Dubner, & F. Cevero (Eds.), *Advances in pain research and therapy* (vol. 9, pp. 53–71). New York: Raven Press.

Navani, A., Rusy, L. M., Jacobson, R. D., & Weisman, S. J. (2003). Treatment of tremors in complex regional pain syndrome, *Journal of Pain Symptom Management, 25*(4), 386–390.

Ochoa, J., Torebjorte, E., Marchetti, H. et al. (1985). Mechanisms of neuropathic pain: Cumulative observations, new experiments and further speculation. In H. L. Fields, R. Dubner, & F. Cevero (Eds.), *Advances in pain research and therapy* (vol. 9, pp. 431–450). New York: Raven Press.

Osler, W., & Churchman, J. W., (1907). *Modern medicine: Its theory and practice* (vol. 3). Philadelphia, Lea Bros.

Payne, R. (1986). Neuropathic pain syndromes, with special reference to causalgia and reflex sympathetic dystrophy. *Clinical Journal of Pain, 2*, 59–73.

Peuschl, G., Blumber, H., & Lucking, C.H. (1991). Tremor in reflex sympathetic dystrophy. *Archives of Neurology, 48*, 1247–1252.

Portenoy, R. K., Foley, K. M., & Inturrisi, C. E. (1990). The nature of opioid responsiveness and its implications for neuropathic pain: A new hypothesis derived from the study of opioid infusions. *Pain, 43*, 273–286.

Prough, D. S., McLeskey, C. H., Poehling, G. G. et al. (1985). Efficacy of oral nifedipine in the treatment of reflex sympathetic dystrophy. *Anesthesiology, 2*, 796–799.

Raja, S. N., Campbell, J. N., Meyer R. A. et al. (1986, November 6–9). *Sensory testing in patients with causalgia or reflex sympathetic dystrophy.* Abstract presented at 6th Annual Meeting of American Pain Society, Washington, D.C.

Raja, S. N., & Hendler N. (1990). Sympathetically maintained pain. In M. Rogers (Ed.), *Current practices in anesthesiology* (pp. 421–425). New York: C. V. Mosby Year Book.

Raja, S. N., Treede R. D., Davis R. D. et al. (1991). Systemic alpha-adrenergic blockade with phentolamine: A diagnostic test for sympathetically maintained pain. *Anesthesiology, 74*, 691–698.

Rauck, R.I., Eisenach, J. C., & Jackson, K. (1993). Epidural clonidine treatment for refractory reflex sympathetic dystrophy. *Anesthesiology, 79*, 1163–1169.

Ren, K., & Dubner, R. (1993). NMDA receptor antagonists attenuate mechanical hyperalgesia in rats with unilateral inflammation of the hindpaw. *Neuroscience Letters, 163*, 22–26.

Ro, L. S., Chen, S. -T., Tang, L. -M., & Jacobs, J. M. (1999). Effect of NGF and anti-NGF on neuropathic pain in rats following chronic constriction injury of the sciatic nerve. *Pain, 79*, 265–274.

Robaina, F., Dominguez, M., & Diaz, M. (1989). Spinal cord stimulation for relief of chronic pain in vasospastic disorders of the upper limbs. *Neurosurgery, 24*, 63–67.

Roberts, M. A. (1986). Hypothesis on the physiological basis for causalgia and related pain. *Pain, 24*, 297–311.

Schott, G. D. (1986). Neurologic manifestation of bone and joint disease. In A. K. Ashbury, G. M. McKham, W. C. McDonald et al. (Eds.), *Diseases of the nervous system* (pp. 1523–1537). Philadelphia: W. B. Saunders.

Schwartzman, R. J., & Kerrigan, J. (1990). The movement disorder of reflex sympathetic dystrophy. *Neurology, 40*, 57–61.

Schwartzman, R. J., & McKellan, T. L. (1987). Reflex sympathetic dystrophy: A review. *Archives of Neurology, 44,* 555–561.

Stanton-Hicks, M., Baron, R., Boas, R., Gordh, T., Harden, N., Hendler, N. et al. (1998). Complex regional pain syndrome: Guidelines for therapy. *The Clinical Journal of Pain, 14*(2), 155–166.

Uematsu, S., Hendler, N., Hugerford, D., Ono, S., & Long, D. M. (1981). Thermography and electromyography in the differential diagnosis of chronic pain syndromes and reflex sympathetic dystrophy. *Electromyography and Clinical Neurophysiology, 21,* 165–182.

Van der Laan, L., Veldman, P. H. J. M., & Goris, R. J. A. (1998). Severe complications of reflex sympathetic dystrophy: Infection, ulcers, chronic edema, dystonia, and myoclonus. *Archives of Physical Medicine and Rehabilitation, 79,* 424–429.

Wasner, G., Schattschneider, J., & Baron, R., (2002), Skin temperature side differences — A diagnostic tool for CRPS? *Pain, 98*(1–2), 19–26.

Watson, C.P., Chipman, M., Reed, K. et. al. (1991). Amitriptyline vs. maprotiline in post herpetic neuralgia: A randomized, double blind, cross-over trial. *Pain, 48,* 29–36.

Watson, C. P., Evans, R. J., Reed, K. et. al. (1981). Amitriptyline vs. placebo in post herpetic neuralgia. *Neurology, 32,* 671–673.

Webster, G. F., Iozzo, R. V., Schwartzman, R. J., Tahmoush, A. J., Knobler, R. L., & Jacoby, R. A. (1993). Reflex sympathetic dystrophy: Occurrence of chronic edema and nonimmune bulious skin lesions. *Journal of the American Academy of Dermatology, 28*(1), 29–32.

Webster, G. F., Schwartzman, R. J., Jacoby, R. A., Knobler, R. L., & Uitto, J. J. (1991). Reflex sympathetic dystrophy: Occurrence of inflammatory skin lesions in patients with stages II and III disease. *Archives of Dermatology, 127,* 1541–1544.

37

HIV and AIDS Pain

Maurice Policar, MD, and Vasanthi Arumugam, MD

INTRODUCTION

The acquired immune deficiency syndrome (AIDS) pandemic has by no means begun to abate. There are more than 38 million cases worldwide. In the United States, there are an estimated 1 million individuals infected with human immunodeficiency virus (HIV) and about 40,000 new infections occur each year. Some evidence suggests that current behavior may result in an increase in these numbers.

The AIDS era can be divided into two major stages: before and after highly active antiretroviral therapy (HAART). The availability of effective medications in 1996, along with the use of triple drug therapy as a treatment strategy (HAART), has had a major impact on those infected, resulting in dramatic decreases in the rates of death, hospitalization, and opportunistic infections. Persons being treated for HIV are now healthier and, in most cases, live otherwise normal lives.

Much is written about treating AIDS-related pain with the same approach used in treating cancer-related pain. This was a reasonable approach in the past when a large proportion of patients with AIDS in care were debilitated and considered to be terminal. Many people with AIDS are still being diagnosed at a late stage of disease, and some harbor virus that has become resistant to all current antiretroviral agents. However, the aspect of pain management in HIV must also be focused on the healthy individuals with active daily lives in whom adequate pain management could dramatically improve quality of life. In a national study of more than 2000 patients infected with HIV from 52 sites, patients surveyed as late as 1998 continued to list various pains as associated with worse perceived health and worse perceived quality of life (Lorenz et al., 2001).

Physician underestimation of pain in HIV-infected individuals has been well described. Providers are often concerned about drug dependence, especially in patients with current or prior substance use. Several reports have demonstrated the underutilization of analgesics in patients with HIV (Breitbart et al., 1996; Larue, Fontaine, & Colleau, 1997). This seems to be more pronounced with opioid analgesia. Poorly controlled pain has been reported as one of the reasons chronically ill patients have asked for physician-assisted suicide (Abrams, 1997).

In discussing the topic of pain in those with HIV infection, it is important to differentiate between pain that is a result of HIV infection or its complications, and pain that is a complication of therapy. In addition, pain syndromes that are unrelated to HIV or its treatment can occur in those infected with HIV.

It is also important for the practitioner to recognize pain syndromes in patients with undiagnosed HIV infection. Painful neuropathy in a patient not known to have a condition that may be associated with pain (i.e., diabetes) is one example. In such situations, it is incumbent on the practitioner to recommend HIV testing to the patient. In the United States today, it is estimated that one of three HIV-infected patients is unaware of his or her diagnosis, and many are first diagnosed when they are afflicted with their first opportunistic infection. Earlier diagnosis of HIV can have a dramatic impact on outcome.

HEADACHE

Headache is one the most common neurologic complaints in patients with HIV infection and may occur at any time from seroconversion to advanced disease (Graham & Wippold, 2001). The causes of headache in persons with HIV infection vary widely. The published incidence of primary headaches versus those caused by an infection or malignancy varied according to the population surveyed.

The evaluation of headache in a patient with HIV infection may include imaging of the head and a lumbar puncture, in addition to history and physical examination. The order and pace of testing should be directed by the acuity and severity of the headache, the accompanying features, and the level of immunosuppression, i.e., the CD4+ lymphocyte count (CD4). Evaluations of HIV-positive patients with headaches suggested little value in computerized tomography (CT) scanning for patients with a CD4 > 200, unless they had focal neurologic signs, altered mental status, or seizures (Gifford & Hecht, 2001; Graham et al., 2000). Complaints of "worst headache of life" should always prompt evaluation for subarachnoid hemorrhage. When accompanied by fever or focal neurologic changes, headache in an HIV-infected individual should prompt a rapid evaluation for infection. Outpatients should probably be referred to a hospital setting where imaging, lab evaluation, and medical treatment are more readily available.

CHRONIC HEADACHE

Chronic headache in patients with HIV is a common complaint. In general, headache is most likely due to a benign, non-infectious cause when it occurs early in the course of HIV infection, before the onset of significant immunologic impairment (Masci, 2001). Causes include muscle tension, vascular headache, depression, or occasionally, chronic sinusitis. Headache may be caused by antiretroviral medications (most commonly zidovidine) and chronic opioid use.

A reasonable approach to the treatment of chronic headache is to begin with acetaminophen or nonsteroidal anti-inflammatory drugs (NSAIDs). Tricyclic antidepressants (TCAs) are used with variable results, but their use is limited at times by their side effects. Gabapentin may be initiated at low doses (i.e., 100 mg tid) and increased gradually to allow for tolerance to side effects. Doses up to 1200 mg tid have been used. Carbamazepine is also sometimes useful, and beta-blockers and calcium channel blockers may be helpful in the prevention of vascular headaches. Opioids may be used for chronic headaches, but chronic use may lead to tolerance and decrease in efficacy.

MENINGITIS

In addition to headache, fever, meningismus, and photophobia, with or without altered mental status, are not unusual in patients with meningitis. In some cases, cranial nerve palsies or seizures may also occur. A lumbar puncture is the study of choice to diagnose meningitis and its etiology. A retinal evaluation to rule out papilledema should always be done prior to a lumbar puncture, in order to avoid herniation in those with increased intracranial pressure. Some advocate an imaging study of the brain in all patients with HIV infection to prevent this complication.

The most common cause of meningitis in AIDS is the fungus *Cryptococcus neoformans*. Most infections occur in patients with CD4 counts below 200. While headache and fever are common, meningismus may be absent. Cerebrospinal fluid (CSF) cell counts and chemistries can vary and may occasionally be normal. A cryptococcal antigen should be positive in the CSF and is usually found in the serum as well. An India ink preparation of the CSF may be positive in more than 50% of cases, showing encapsulated yeast forms, at times with budding.

Other causes of meningitis in the HIV-infected patient include the usual causes of bacterial meningitis such as *Streptococcus pneumoniae*, *Haemophilus influenzae,* and *Neisseria meningitidis*. Among patients infected with HIV, risk for infection is significantly higher with *S. pneumoniae* and marginally increased with *Listeria monocytogenes* (risk is also higher in cirrhosis and pregnancy).

Aseptic or nonbacterial meningitis is usually caused by a self-limited enteroviral infection, but may also be related to HIV itself. With reactivation and skin lesions, Herpes simplex virus (HSV) or Varicella zoster virus (VZV) infection may be related to aseptic meningitis. The presence of genital or skin lesions should suggest these diagnoses. Tuberculous meningitis should be suspected in patients from endemic areas. The course tends to be more chronic than that of bacterial or viral meningitis. The CSF typically reveals a lymphocytic pleocytosis and low glucose, and may have extremely elevated protein levels. Spinal fluid staining and culture for acid-fast bacilli are usually negative; CSF polymerase chain reaction (PCR) for *Mycobacterium tuberculosis* may be helpful, but is frequently nondiagnostic. CT scan may show meningeal enhancement, and about half of patients have findings suggestive of tuberculosis on chest x-ray. Treatment is usually empiric, based on the clinical findings. Occasionally, lymphoma may spread from a primary site to the central nervous system (CNS), causing lymphomatous meningitis. CSF cytology, and/or Epstein–Barr virus (EBV) PCR may be diagnostic.

BRAIN LESIONS

Patients who present with headache and focal neurologic abnormalities or seizures should be evaluated for space occupying lesions (SOL) of the brain. At times, patients with an SOL can present with only headache or mental status changes. The most common diagnosis in this group is toxoplasmosis, a reactivation disease in persons with past exposure to *Toxoplasma gondii*. Less commonly diagnosed are primary lymphoma of the brain and tuberculoma of the brain. In patients with CNS toxoplasmosis, the characteristic finding on CT scan or magnetic resonance imaging (MRI) is multiple ring-enhancing lesions, with a predilection for involvement of the basal ganglia. With appropriate treatment, rapid clinical and/or radiographic improvement is the rule. Rapid improvement with treatment is considered diagnostic, obviating the need for a biopsy. Primary lymphoma of the brain is most commonly seen as a well-defined focal lesion that enhances with contrast. On single positron emission computed tomography imaging, lymphoma shows a greater thallium uptake than infection (Lorberboym et al., 1998). When a lumbar puncture can be safely done, detection of EBV DNA by PCR is diagnostic of lymphoma. EBV infection has been associated with certain lymphomas, especially in the immunocompromised host. Tuberculosis is an uncommon cause of brain lesions in the United States. Tuberculomas or cerebral abscesses may be solitary or multiple, nodular or ring enhancing, and they have a clear predominance in the supratentorial compartment. They are more likely to occur in intravenous drug users and individuals from tuberculosis endemic areas. This form of CNS tuberculosis is less common than meningitis and usually occurs when the CD4 drops below 200. Radiographs of the chest show evidence of tuberculous infection in about half the patients (Lesprit et al., 1997). A host of other organisms can cause abscesses of the brain in patients with HIV, and these may be diagnosed by an aspiration or biopsy of the lesions.

OTHER CONDITIONS

Sinusitis is more common in HIV-infected individuals than in those without HIV. The presentation can be subtle, and headache may be the only symptom. In addition to the usual bacterial and viral pathogens, fungi have been found to be a fairly common cause of sinusitis in HIV, at times becoming invasive into surrounding bone and soft tissue (Hunt et al., 2000). Radiographic evaluation of the sinuses is important to help establish the diagnosis, eliminate other diagnoses, and evaluate for tissue invasion, a rare condition requiring surgical intervention.

Syphilis can cause various manifestations in the HIV-infected patient. Syphilitic meningitis can be seen at any stage of infection with syphilis. Meningovascular syphilis or gummas of the brain are manifestations of tertiary syphilis. Serum testing for syphilis is usually diagnostic, but nontreponemal screening tests may be falsely negative. A treponemal test for syphilis, the VDRL (Venereal Disease Research Laboratory) is usually positive in syphilitic meningitis.

With advanced HIV, headache may be one of several manifestations of infection with "JC virus," the cause of progressive multifocal leukoencephalopathy. JC virus PCR in the CSF is diagnostic. CT scanning reveals white matter lesions.

In patients who have headaches as a result of lumbar puncture, so-called postdural puncture headaches, an autologous epidural blood patch may be helpful in alleviating the symptoms (Tom et al., 1992).

OROPHARYNGEAL PAIN

Patients with HIV/AIDS have frequent oropharyngeal and esophageal conditions that cause pain as one of their manifestations. Significant discomfort can interfere with adequate nutrition and may contribute to weight loss.

ORAL CANDIDA INFECTIONS

Oral candidiasis may be an early manifestation of HIV infection and may have variable presentations: pseudomembranous, erythematous, and angular cheilitis. The most common presentation, pseudomembranous candidiasis or thrush, appears as white or cream-colored patches that are easily scraped off mucosal surfaces. The erythematous form is more subtle and easily overlooked. Patients may complain of pain, burning, or soreness, along with dysguesia. Angular cheilitis results in cracks or fissures at the angles of the mouth. Pain on opening the mouth is a common manifestation. Each of these forms of oral candidiasis can be treated with topical antifungal therapy in the form of solutions or troches (Darouich, 1998). Systemic antifungal agents are also effective. A condition known as hairy leukoplakia can resemble thrush, but is painless, cannot be removed by scraping, and does not respond to antifungal therapy.

GINGIVITIS AND PERIODONTITIS

Gingivitis is common in patients infected with HIV, who most often present with oral pain, inflammation, and receding of gum lines, and at times, progression to bone loss (periodontitis). Spontaneous bleeding can occur. A topical antimicrobial rinse such as chlorhexidine is used as treatment. A form of gingivitis specifically related to HIV has been termed "linear gingival erythema." It presents as a brightly inflamed band of marginal gingiva. The treatment consists of debridement plus antibiotic administration (Obernesser, 2004).

ORAL ULCERS

Oral ulcers are a common finding in HIV-infected patients, and may result from viral infections (HSV, CMV), bacteria (oral fusospirochetosis), fungi (histoplasmosis), or neoplasm or they may be idiopathic (aphthous ulcers). HSV is one of the more common causes of oral ulcerations in patients with HIV. Ulcers due to HSV are usually painful and may be recurrent. In advanced disease, they may be chronic, resolving only after antiviral therapy. Diagnosis is usually by viral culture. Acyclovir 400 mg tid, valacyclovir 500 mg bid, or famciclovir 500 mg bid can be used until the lesions resolve, usually a few days.

Aphthous ulcers are more common in individuals with HIV/AIDS than in those without HIV. These ulcers may be single or multiple, may persist for weeks or longer, and can be extremely painful (Greenspan & Greenspan, 1999). Diagnosis is clinical, and treatment consists of topical steroids such as triamcinolone mixed with orabase and applied topically to the lesions two to three times per day. In patients with multiple ulcers, or those located in the posterior oropharynx, rinsing with dexamethasone elixir (0.5 mg/5 ml), 5 ml tid, may be helpful. Patients should be instructed to expectorate the solution after rinsing. Thalidomide has also been found to be helpful in the treatment of aphthous ulcers in HIV (Jacobson et al., 1997). Topical treatment with 2% viscous lidocaine can help ameliorate pain. At times, narcotic analgesics are required to control pain.

Patients with ulcers that do not respond to empiric treatment with antivirals and topical steroids should probably have a biopsy done to exclude other causes such as *Cytomegalovirus* (CMV), or fungal infection, or malignancy.

NEOPLASMS

Kaposi's sarcoma (KS) and non-Hodgkin's lymphoma (NHL) may present as oral lesions in the patient with HIV infection. The lesions of KS are seen predominantly in men who have sex with men. They usually involve the hard palate, appearing as blue, purple, or red lesions that may be nodular. The oral lesions of KS may be painful because of ulceration and secondary infection (Greenspan & Greenspan, 1999). The diagnosis is made by biopsy, and the treatment may be intralesional or systemic chemotherapy, or radiation therapy. Pain can usually be controlled with oral narcotics. NHL can occur anywhere in the mouth and can present as diffuse swellings, nodules, or ulcers (Greenspan & Greenspan, 1999). Biopsy is required for diagnosis, and treatment is with systemic chemotherapy. Narcotic analgesics in various forms may be required for control of pain.

ESOPHAGEAL CONDITIONS

Chest pain, dysphasia, and odynophagia are all manifestations of esophageal disease in HIV. Esophageal candidiasis is the most common cause of these symptoms. Although common, oral candida may be absent in these patients. Esophageal candidiasis is an AIDS-defining opportunistic infection and is indicative of late-stage disease (CD4 < 200). Patients usually present with dysphasia and/or odynophagia, usually localizing their pain to the substernal area. These symptoms should prompt empiric treatment with a systemic antifungal agent. If there is no response to therapy in 3 to 4 days, endoscopy with biopsy should be done (Darouich, 1998). Other than candidal infections, the most common findings are esophageal ulcers, which may be due to HSV, CMV, or idiopathic aphthous disease. The diagnosis is made by biopsy. Idiopathic ulcers usually respond to systemic steroids. Resolution of pain occurs with treatment of the causative agent. With esophageal ulcers, analgesics may be necessary as pain may respond slowly to specific therapy.

CHEST PAIN

The manifestation of chest pain in the HIV-infected individual is fairly common. When the pain is pleuritic in nature, one should consider bacterial pneumonia, but pleural tuberculosis may be a cause in patients who have been exposed to tuberculosis. In patients with AIDS, spontaneous pneumothorax may occur, usually in relation to *Pneumocystis carinii* pneumonia (PCP). Chest radiographs may indicate infection or pneumothorax. Infection should be treated with the appropriate antimicrobials, and pleuritic pain usually responds well to NSAIDs. Patients with pneumothorax will likely require narcotic analgesics, especially if a chest tube is inserted.

The use of HAART has been associated with insulin resistance and abnormalities of lipid metabolism. Although definitive evidence of an increased risk of coronary disease in HIV/AIDS is still lacking, there are some studies supporting this notion (Hsue et al., 2004; Vittecoq et al., 2003). Coronary disease should be considered in patients with HIV who present with chest pain.

Esophageal manifestations can also present with chest pain (see above).

BACK PAIN

A longitudinal study was done to evaluate the painful symptoms associated with HIV infection and its treatment. Back pain was listed among the most common painful illnesses reported (Singer et al., 1993). In patients who are infected with HIV, back pain is likely caused by the same musculoskeletal conditions that plague uninfected persons.

In persons who are active injecting drug users, osteomyelitis of the spine with or without a spinal epidural abscess can occur. Back pain, most commonly cervical, is the most frequent manifestation, followed by fever. Radiculopathy, myelopathy, and sensory loss may accompany local pain and tenderness. Plain film radiography, CT scan, MRI, and bone scan are useful for diagnosis (Broner, Garland, & Zigler, 1996). Biopsy is indicated for lesions of the bone, and aspiration for abscesses. In patients with neurologic signs of cord compression, high dose steroids and urgent surgical debridement are indicated. Depending on the extent of involvement, pain may be controlled with mild analgesics or may require opioids. Postoperative pain is best relived with narcotics administered via patient-controlled analgesia (PCA) pumps.

Back pain can be a symptom of renal conditions as well. A side effect of indinavir therapy is the development of nephrolithiasis. At times, no stones are found, but crystalluria may cause the classic syndrome of renal colic (Kopp et al., 1997).

ABDOMINAL PAIN

The list of causes of abdominal pain in the HIV-infected individual is extensive. A host of etiologies are similar to those seen in patients without HIV infection. The focus of this section is to list and define entities either that are unique to the patient with AIDS or that occur with a higher frequency in those with HIV infection. We also discuss manifestations that result from complications of antiretroviral therapy.

In the emergency department (ED), abdominal pain in the HIV-infected patient can be especially challenging. Even in the general population, the cause of abdominal pain is not diagnosed in the ED 25 to 46% of the time (Yoshida & Caruso, 2002). In the patient with HIV infection and abdominal pain, one must consider additional diagnoses related to HIV or its management. The CD4 count may help narrow the differential diagnosis. Patients with a CD4 count above 200 are very unlikely to have a condition related to an opportunistic infection. When CD4 counts are <100, diagnoses such as disseminated *Mycobacterium avium* complex (MAC) infection must be considered, while CMV infection of the gastrointestinal tract occurs almost exclusively in patients with a CD4 count <50.

The incidence of opportunistic conditions related to the gastrointestinal tract seems to be decreasing. Monkemuller et al. (2000) reviewed results of gastrointestinal endoscopies in patients with HIV infection, from April 1995 to March 1998. They document a clearly decreasing incidence of opportunistic diseases (69 to 13%), associated with an increase in the use of HAART (0 to 57%).

Yoshida and Caruso (2002) reported on a series of patients with abdominal pain, seen in an inner-city emergency department. Of 108 patients reviewed, two thirds used drugs and/or alcohol and approximately half were taking antiretroviral medication. The most common diagnoses were the same as those in patients without HIV infection: abdominal pain of unknown etiology, gastroenteritis/diarrhea, and ulcer disease/gastritis/dyspepsia. In comparing two groups at different stages of infection (CD4 < 200 vs. CD4 ≥ 200), they found no statistically significant differences in etiologies, except for the presence of disseminated MAC infection in the advanced

group. Opportunistic conditions made up only 10% of diagnoses in the advanced group. Only 8% required surgical procedures. A portion of the apparent reduction in AIDS opportunistic conditions is attributable to HAART. Of note, four patients had nephrolithiasis due to indinavir therapy. The admission rate for HIV-infected patients was 37%, twice that of patients without HIV infection. Other studies have quoted higher rates of opportunistic conditions and surgery, but the populations consisted of inpatients not ED patients.

Presence or absence of fever may be misleading. Although low-grade fever may not be uncommon with advanced HIV infection, one review found that 40% of patients with AIDS with appendicitis had no fever (Whitney et al., 1992). The peripheral white blood count (WBC) in patients with AIDS tends to be low and may rise to normal in the face of infection. For that reason, a normal WBC should not dissuade the practitioner from considering infections or serious conditions, especially if the patient's baseline WBC is known to be low.

Slaven et al. (2003) organize the causes of abdominal pain into five categories, which include HIV-related, iatrogenic (medication- or procedure-related), immune surveillance–related (malignancies), non-HIV-related, and nonspecific (resolution without specific diagnosis). In the following discussion, we focus on only the first three categories, including malignancies as HIV-related conditions because lymphoma and KS have strong associations with HIV infection.

ENTEROCOLITIS

Enterocolitis is one of the most common gastrointestinal manifestations of HIV and is often associated with pain. This condition may be acute or chronic and may be associated with fever and weight loss. Etiologies include a variety of organisms including bacteria, viruses, mycobacteria, parasites, and fungi. Stool studies are most useful, although frequently negative. Endoscopic biopsies may be necessary for the diagnosis of some viral and parasitic infections. *Clostridium difficile*–associated disease can be diagnosed by a toxin assay of the stool. Antimicrobial treatment is usually indicated although antimotility agents may be helpful with some organisms such as cryptosporidium. Specific antimicrobial treatment, with or without antimotility drugs, usually helps relieve the diarrhea along with the pain.

PANCREATITIS

In patients with AIDS, pancreatitis is 35 to 800 times more common than in those without HIV infection. In addition to alcohol use and gallstones, other pathologies related to pancreatitis in HIV infection include medications such as didanosine, Kaletra, and pentamidine, as well as opportunistic infections including CMV, toxoplasmosis, mycobacteria, and cryptosporidium (Dassopoulos & Ehrenpreis, 1999). Infiltration of the pancreas by lymphoma or KS is rare. The presentation is similar to that seen in immunocompetent hosts, but tends to be more severe. Diagnosis relies primarily on symptoms, an elevated amylase and lipase, and ultrasound or CT evidence of pancreatic inflammation. Stool studies or blood cultures may be helpful for some infections, but CMV requires tissue diagnosis. Associated pain will usually respond to pareneterally administered narcotic analgesics, preferably by PCA pump. When pancreatitis is a result of drug toxicity, the offending agent must be discontinued. Patients with a history of pancreatitis should not receive didanosine, Kaletra, or pentamidine. When an infection is the cause, specific antimicrobial therapy should be administered.

APPENDICITIS

The incidence of appendicitis with HIV infection is likely similar to rates in non-infected individuals. The usual causes (i.e., appendoliths) are frequent in HIV, but opportunistic infections may also play a role. AIDS-related pathology was identified in 30% of cases of acute appendicitis in one series (Whitney et al., 1992). The more commonly identified infections associated with appendicitis in HIV are *Mycobacterium tuberculosis* (tuberculosis), MAC, and CMV (Slaven et al., 2003). KS has also been seen in cases of appendicitis in AIDS. The various etiologies could not be predicted from the clinical presentation. As opposed to the findings in immunocompetent hosts, elevated WBC is unusual, and 40% of patients with AIDS with appendicitis have no fever (Whitney et al., 1992). Although perforation rates have been documented to exceed 40%, delays in surgery have also been documented and were likely related to the increased perforation rate (Slaven et al., 2003). Diagnosis is made by clinical and CT findings, and treatment is appendectomy. When an opportunistic infection is identified, specific antimicrobial therapy should be administered.

CHOLECYSTITIS

Cholecystitis in persons with HIV infection may occur with or without stones. Acalculous cholecystitis is approximately twice as common as cholelithiasis (French et al., 1995). Acalculous cholecystitis has been most commonly associated with infection with *Cryptosporidium paarvum*, *Microsporidium,* and CMV although a host of other pathogens have been described (Slaven et al., 2003; Fantry & Chen-Chih, 2002). These opportunistic infections are usually a complication of severe immunosuppression (Walden, 1999). Presentation may be acute or chronic, with right upper quadrant pain in 90%, and fever, nausea, and vomiting in about half. As in appendicitis in

patients with AIDS, leukocytosis is unusual. Transaminase and bilirubin levels are usually unremarkable. Ultrasound evaluation commonly shows a thickened gallbladder wall and/or a distended gallbladder, with or without stones. Cholecystectomy is the treatment of choice. Specific antimicrobial therapy should be used when an infection is diagnosed.

CHOLANGITIS

In HIV, cholangitis is usually associated with opportunistic infection, malignancy, or immunologic destruction of the biliary epithelium. Manifestations include sclerosing cholangitis and/or papillary stenosis. *Cryptosporidium* and CMV are the most commonly identified associated infections. The clinical presentation is similar to that of cholecystitis. The alkaline phosphatase is usually markedly elevated, with minimally elevated transaminases and bilirubin, and a CD4 count <100. Ultrasound or CT will usually show dilated biliary ducts. Evaluation with endoscopic retrograde cholangiopancreatography (ERCP) is indicated, during which biopsy and bile cultures may be obtained. Stents can be placed to relieve obstruction from strictures, and sphincterotomy may help treat pain in some cases (Slaven et al., 2003). Celiac plexus neurolysis should be considered in patients with refractory pain (Collazos et al., 1996). Antimicrobial therapy is indicated when an infection is identified.

INTESTINAL PERFORATION

Intestinal perforation in patients with HIV infection is uncommon, but most commonly caused by ulceration resulting from CMV infection. Manifestations can be misleading, with minimal tenderness, no fever, and a normal WBC. Other causes include lymphoma, KS, histoplasmosis, peptic ulcer disease, and appendicitis. Treatment is surgery, together with antimicrobials or chemotherapy depending on the etiology.

OTHER CONDITIONS

Pain can be due to enlarged intra-abdominal lymph nodes due to MAC, KS, or tuberculosis. In patients with MAC, the infection is disseminated, and patients may also have fever, diarrhea, hepatosplenomegaly, anemia, and increased alkaline phosphatase and gamma-glutamyl transpeptide (GGT). Intestinal obstruction is an unusual manifestation of KS or lymphoma. Intussesception is rare and may be due to lymphoma, KS, or mycobacterial infection. The presence of skin or oropharyngeal lesions of KS may be a clue to visceral disease. Lymphoma in AIDS is usually NHL and may lack peripheral adenopathy as a presenting manifestation. Lactate dehydrogenase (LDH) is frequently elevated. Toxic megacolon has been described in association with CMV, *Clostridium difficile*, or bacterial infection. Surgical resection of affected area is probably the best approach, but endoscopic decompression has been reported to be effective in a few cases. Mortality remains high. Tuberculosis in persons from endemic areas can reactivate in HIV infection. Enteritis is an unusual manifestation and usually affects the ileo-cecal region and causes right lower quadrant pain. Tuberculous peritonitis can manifest with fever, pain, and ascites. The diagnosis of tuberculosis requires pathologic findings on tissue biopsy and is confirmed by culture. In advanced patients, intra-abdominal abscesses may form from tuberculosis or MAC. Abdominal aortic aneurysms have been described as part of a vasculopathy syndrome related to HIV infection. It is caused by a vasculitis in arterioles of the gastrointestinal tract, resulting in ulceration. Some individuals have been reported to have multiple aneurysms. Surgical repair is likely the best approach, but stenting has been used (Chetty, Batitang, & Nair, 2000).

ANTIRETROVIAL MEDICATION-RELATED MANIFESTATIONS

Lactic Acidosis

Although asymptomatic lactic acidosis is often seen with the use of nucleoside reverse transcriptase inhibitors, the syndrome of severe, potentially fatal, lactic acidosis in AIDS is fortunately very rare. Abdominal pain is usually part of the presentation along with marked weakness and fatigue. At times, this entity will progress to profound lactic acidosis, hepatic steatosis, hepatic failure, and frequently death. The only definitive treatment to date is withholding antiretroviral therapy. Zidovidine and stavudine are the most commonly identified culprits (Smith, 2002).

Pancreatitis

See above.

Nephrolithiasis

Nephrolithiasis has been associated with indinavir use, especially with inadequate hydration (Kopp et al., 1997). A case of cholelithiais due to indinavir has also been reported (Verdon et al., 2002).

RHEUMATOLOGIC/MUSCULOSKELETAL PAIN

ARTHRITIS AND ARTHROPATHIES

HIV infection has been associated with various nonspecific arthralgias, reactive arthritis, and psoriatic arthritis. Reiter's syndrome typically affects young men and may be associated with urethritis and conjunctivitis. Some patients may have keratosis blennorrhagia, stomatitis, or balanitis. The arthritis tends to be severe, most often involving knees and shoulders, and treatment with

NSAIDs and or steroids is usually unsuccessful. Psoriasis and seborrheic dermatitis seem to occur more commonly in patients with HIV infection. Psoriasis-associated arthritis may be severe and deforming. NSAIDs, sulfasalazine, or gold therapy may be effective in the treatment of psoriatic arthritis. A form of seronegative arthritis not associated with Reiter's syndrome or psoriasis has been described in patients with advanced HIV infection. The few cases reported were described as having severe and debilitating arthritis of the lower extremities (Masci, 2001). NSAIDs and intra-articular steroid injections are the treatment of choice (Tehranzadeh, Ter-Oganesyan, & Steinbach, 2004). In the past, treatment of Reiter's syndrome or psoriatic arthritis with methotrexate had resulted in clinical deterioration. It is not clear what effect the use of HAART would have on these conditions.

AVASCULAR NECROSIS

The incidence of avascular necrosis (AVN) in HIV-infected patients has increased over the past few years. The increase in the use of HAART might have contributed to the increase in AVN, although the mechanism remains unclear. The most common symptom is hip pain, but the process may affect other locations such as the knee, shoulder, ankle, and wrist. Weight-bearing and activity-associated pain is seen in most cases, but rest pain can occur in two thirds of patients, especially those with advanced disease. The process is usually progressive, resulting in joint destruction within a few years. Conventional radiographs, CT, MRI, and nuclear studies can all be used to diagnose AVN. With a sensitivity around 90%, MRI can reveal the stage of the disease and the extent of the necrosis (Tehranzadeh et al., 2004). The definitive treatment is hip replacement, but the mainstay management is pain control. NSAIDs may be effective in early disease, although opioids are frequently required to control pain.

POLYMYOSITIS

Polymyositis is the most frequent muscle disorder seen in association with HIV. It typically occurs early in the course of HIV infection. The manifestations include proximal muscle weakness, muscle wasting, and elevated creatine kinase (CK) levels. Electromyography (EMG), MRI, and muscle biopsy are the principal diagnostic techniques (Masci, 2001; Tehranzadeh et al., 2004).

ZIDOVIDINE MYOPATHY

Drugs used in the treatment of HIV, particularly zidovidine, have also been associated with the development of myalgias and myositis. Clinically indistinguishable from polymyositis, it is characterized by myalgia, fatigue, proximal muscle weakness, and elevated CK levels. The mechanism is thought to be mitochondrial toxicity. Discontinuation of the medication leads to resolution of the syndrome within several months (Tehranzadeh et al., 2004).

SKIN

Various skin conditions can result in pain in patients with HIV infection. KS is a neoplastic condition, occurring predominantly in men who have sex with men. When it involves the skin, typical lesions are nodular and violaceous in color. Pain is not a usual manifestation unless the lesion ulcerates or, more commonly, it causes lymphatic obstruction. Lesions may occur in the lower extremities causing edema and pain. Radiation and/or systemic chemotherapy are used to treat KS, and pain is usually treated with opioid analgesics. If lesions respond to therapy, pain may resolve; however, persistent pain due to neuropathy as a result of chemotherapy, radiation, or HIV is common. Non-narcotics are more suitable to treat this type of pain (see section on neuropathic pain).

In debilitated patients, most frequently those with advanced AIDS, decubitus ulcers may be seen due to nutritional deficiencies and poor healing. Pain relief can be addressed with small doses of narcotics, if tolerated. Incontinence of stool and urine can result in frequent soiling of the affected area and may prevent healing (Grothe & Gottlieb, 1999). Topical treatments and dressings along with relief of pressure and improved nutrition may help to heal decubitii and relieve pain. In patients with nonhealing or expanding ulcers, viral cultures should be done to exclude herpes simplex infection, and treatment for infection of the soft tissue or underlying bone should be considered.

HSV infection can cause recurrent genital or rectal lesions. In the immunocompromised individual, these can occur more frequently and at times remain as chronic ulcerations. These are usually painful, and symptoms of pain or tingling can herald the onset of an outbreak. Specific treatment of the infection with an antiviral agent is usually all that is necessary to treat the pain. Acyclovir 400 mg tid, valacyclovir 500 mg bid, or famciclovir 500 mg bid can be used until the lesions resolve. Occasionally resistant HSV requires treatment with intravenous foscarnet. The incidence of resistance to oral agents may be rising (Reyes et al., 2003).

Herpes zoster (HZ) can be painful and may lead to postherpetic neuralgia (PHN) (see below).

PERIPHERAL NEUROPATHY

INTRODUCTION

HIV-associated neuropathies have become the most frequent neurological disorders associated with HIV infection. They may be due to a variety of factors, including antiretroviral medication toxicity, immunological dysreg-

ulation produced by HIV infection, opportunistic infection, or a combination of all of these factors. Neuropathy can also result from other causes, such as heavy alcohol consumption, vitamin deficiency, diabetes, or chemotherapy.

PREVALENCE

Symptomatic neuropathies occur in approximately 15 to 50% of patients with HIV (Martin et al., 2003). The prevalence of pain increases in the advanced stages of illness. The risk of peripheral neuropathy increases with higher plasma HIV viral load, lower CD4 cell counts, and increasing age (Lopez et al., 2004; Simpson et al., 2002).

NEUROPATHIES ASSOCIATED WITH HIV INFECTION

Several types of peripheral neuropathies have been diagnosed in patients with HIV and AIDS (Luciano, Perdo, & McArthur, 2003; Pardo, McArthur, & Griffin, 2001). The following discussion is separated into sections on clinical features, diagnosis, and management. Most can have pain as a component of the condition; however, even those that do not present with pain will be mentioned here for the sake of completeness. They include:

1. Distal symmetrical polyneuropathy (DSP)
2. Antiretroviral toxic neuropathies (ATN)
3. Herpes zoster (HZ) and postherpetic neuralgia (PHN)
4. Mononeuropathy mutiplex (MM)
5. Diffuse infiltrative lymphocytosis syndrome (DILS)
6. Lumbosacral polyradiculopathy (cauda equina syndrome)
7. Mononeuropathies
8. Inflammatory demyelinating polyneuropathies
9. Autonomic neuropathy

Clinical Features and Classification

Distal Symmetrical Polyneuropathy

This condition is one of the most common neuropathies in HIV infection and usually presents in the middle and late stages of HIV infection (Keswani et al., 2002; Luciano et al., 2003). It commonly begins as tingling and numbness in the toes bilaterally, then gradually spreads proximally from the lower extremities, rarely involving the upper extremities. Early painful dysesthesias of the lower extremities are common, but patients may also complain of numbness. Ankle jerks are decreased or absent. Knee jerks are occasionally decreased and may be absent in severe cases. Vibratory, pain, and temperature sensation are usually decreased, but muscle weakness is not a prominent symptom of DSP and generally occurs only in advanced disease.

Antiretroviral Toxic Neuropathies

This type of neuropathy may occur at any stage of HIV infection. ATN can be indistinguishable from DSP, except for the temporal association of symptoms with the initiation of antiretroviral medication. ATN is more likely than DSP to be painful, have an abrupt onset, and progress rapidly (Dieterich, 2003). Nucleoside reverse transcriptase inhibitors (NRTIs) are the class of drugs most frequently associated with peripheral neuropathy, particularly the so called "d" drugs: ddI (didanosine), ddC (zalcitabine), and d4T (stavudine) (Luciano et al., 2003; Keswani et al., 2002). Some evidence suggests mitochondrial toxicity as a mechanism for NRTI-associated neuropathy (Luciano et al., 2003).

Herpes Zoster (Shingles) and Postherpetic Neuralgia

HZ or "shingles" is a localized cutaneous eruption that results from reactivation of VZV infection. HZ can occur in anyone who has had varicella, but is more common with increasing age and in immunocompromised patients. Pain of variable severity occurs in virtually all patients with acute herpes zoster. An erythematous macular rash usually occurs in a dermatomal distribution, but may be delayed by up to 5 days after the onset of pain. The rash progresses to clusters of clear vesicles, evolving to pustules and ulcers, and finally to crusted lesions. Healing occurs in 2 to 4 weeks and frequently results in scarring. Pain that persists for more than 30 days after the onset of the rash is termed PHN. Pain and hyperesthesias can persist for months and occasionally years (Gnann and Whitley, 2002).

Mononeuropathy Mutiplex

A condition called mononeuropathy multiplex can occur either early or late in the course of HIV infection. In early stages of HIV infection, MM is immune mediated, whereas in advanced AIDS it can be caused by infection with CMV, hepatitis B, or hepatitis C, particularly when associated with cryoglobulinemia (Stricker et al., 1992; Verma, 2001). Patients can present with numbness, tingling, abnormal sensation, burning pain, dysesthesia, or paralysis. Symptoms are restricted to the territory of the affected nerve, although multiple nerves may be affected. Presentation may be that of an asymmetric sensorimotor polyneuropathy affecting multiple nerves, often in a stepwise progression.

Diffuse Infiltrative Lymphocytosis Syndrome

An unusual cause of peripheral neuropathy, DILS is characterized by a persistent peripheral blood polyclonal CD8+ lymphocyte (CD8) expansion. Peripheral lymphocytosis is present, with lymphocytic infiltration of parotid glands, lungs, lymph nodes, lacrimal glands, kidneys, muscles, and nerves. The most common manifestation is salivary gland enlargement, mainly bilateral parotid gland enlargement (Kazi et al., 1996). Other manifestations include peripheral sensory neuropathy, as well as diffuse lymphadenopathy, xerostomia, hepatosplenomegaly, interstitial pneumonitis, and profound muscle weakness (Berger & Simpson, 1998; Kazi et al, 1996; Nopachai, Garwacki, & Moll, 2004).

Lumbosacral Polyradiculopathy

Lumbosacral polyradiculopathy is usually associated with CMV infection, but may rarely be associated with HSV infection, tuberculosis, syphilis, or cryptococcal infection (Hernandez-Albujar et al., 2000; Kolson & Gonzalez-Scarano, 2001). A rapidly progressing cauda equina syndrome can occur in patients with AIDS, but has not been reported in patients with asymptomatic HIV infection. The clinical picture is one of severe back and leg pain associated with lower extremity weakness. Numbness and tingling can begin in the feet or in the saddle region. Symptoms can be asymmetric, especially early in the course of this condition. Progression occurs rapidly, resulting in a flaccid paraplegia with bowel and bladder incontinence. Most untreated patients die within a few weeks.

Mononeuropathies

Mononeuropathies associated with HIV infection include cranial neuropathies and others such as median neuropathies at the wrist, ulnar neuropathies at the elbow, peroneal neuropathies at the fibular neck, and phrenic neuropathy at the diaphragm (Piliero, Estanislao, & Simpson, 2004). Symptoms and signs depend on the location of the nerve involved and include numbness, decreased sensation, tingling, burning pain, weakness, and paralysis. Other symptoms include impairment of taste and hyperacusis.

Inflammatory Demyelinating Polyradiculoneuropathy

Two major forms of demyelinating polyradiculopathy have been reported in HIV-infected patients: acute inflammatory demyelinating polyneuropathy (AIDP) and chronic inflammatory demyelinating polyneuropathy (CIDP). AIDP, also known as Guillain–Barre syndrome (GBS), has been reported in HIV-infected patients, usually occurring at the time of seroconversion or in asymptomatic individuals with CD4 cell counts > 500.

The AIDP (GBS) clinical course evolves fairly rapidly, over days to weeks. Although AIDP and CIDP share many clinical features, CIDP usually occurs in the advanced stages of illness and evolves over weeks to months. In both disorders, the motor deficit predominates but mild sensory symptoms may be present (Verma, 2001). Patients typically have absent or reduced reflexes as well as patchy numbness and weakness. Cranial palsies, respiratory muscle involvement, and autonomic dysfunction can occur in GBS but are uncommon in CIDP.

Autonomic Neuropathy

Autonomic dysfunction appears to be common in HIV-infected individuals, with as many as 76 to 84% having at least one abnormality on a battery of autonomic tests. The manifestations of autonomic dysfunction in patients infected with HIV appear to be similar to those in non-HIV-infected patients. The severity of autonomic dysfunction generally correlates with the progression of HIV disease. Common symptoms include nausea, vomiting, orthostatic hypotension, heat intolerance, diarrhea, constipation, urinary incontinence, bladder dysfunction, impotence, anhidrosis, or hyperhydrosis (Rogstad et al., 1999).

Diagnosis

The diagnosis of the peripheral neuropathy syndrome in patients infected with HIV is based on the clinical picture supported by electrophysiological studies. Blood tests are frequently obtained to exclude other causes of neuropathy such as vitamin B_{12} or folate deficiencies, thyroid disease, or syphilis. Lumbar puncture is indicated only if neuropathy is associated with encephalopathy or with a presentation suggestive of lymphoma or CMV infection.

Distal Symmetrical Polyneuropathy and Antiretroviral Toxic Neuropathies

1. Laboratory evaluation in DSP/ATN is relatively unrevealing, but it should exclude other causes of this type of neuropathy. Testing should include
   - Vitamin B_{12} and folate levels
   - Thyroid-stimulating hormone assay
   - Fasting blood sugar
   - Liver function tests
   - Blood urea nitrogen and creatinine
   - Serum protein electrophoresis and immuno-electrophoresis
   - Screening test for syphilis (RPR or VDRL)
2. Spinal fluid is mostly acellular and protein levels may be slightly increased.
3. EMG and nerve conduction velocity studies show predominantly axonal sensory-motor polyneuropathy.
4. Nerve biopsy shows axonal degeneration of long axons in distal regions. The density of both small and large myelinated fibers is reduced, and in particular, the density of unmyelinated fibers is reduced.

Herpes Zoster (Shingles) and Postherpetic Neuralgia

Diagnosis is usually based on the distinctive clinical appearance of the rash. However, the appearance may be atypical, especially in the immunocompromised host. A direct immunofluorescent assay is a sensitive and rapid confirmatory test. Viral culture is possible, but VZV is difficult to recover (Gnann & Whitley, 2002).

Mononeuritis Mutiplex

Lab tests are ordered to identify and screen for other causes of MM. These include complete blood count with differential, lyme antibody titer, hepatitis screen, cryoglobulins,

and erythrocyte sedimentation rate (ESR). Diagnosis is made mostly by EMG and nerve conduction studies (electrophysiological studies). Electrophysiological studies show an asymmetric, sensorimotor, axonal polyneurpathy. Patients infected with HIV with mononeuropathy multiplex and CD4 counts less than 200 cells should be evaluated for CMV infection. CNS infection can be diagnosed by identification of CMV by viral culture or PCR of the spinal fluid. CMV can also be diagnosed in other commonly infected organs such as the eye, by characteristic retinal findings on slit lamp exam, and in the gastrointestinal tract by tissue biopsy (Keswani et al., 2002).

Diffuse Infiltrative Lymphocytosis Syndrome

Laboratory testing reveals CD8 lymphocytosis, with peripheral CD8 counts greater than 1,000/µl and CD8 lymphocytes representing more than 60% of peripheral lymphocytes. CD4 counts are variable, ranging from 44 to 847 cells/µl in one review. Antinuclear antibodies and anti-Ro and anti-La antibodies are absent. HLA DR5, DR6, or DR7 is positive in more than 50% of patients with DILS and DR2 present in more than 36% of patients. Nerve biopsy shows focal loss of myelin fiber and intense cellular infiltrate.

Lumbosacral Polyradiculopathy

Suspicion of this diagnosis should prompt immediate treatment. Lumbar puncture reveals a high white blood cell count consisting largely of polymorphonuclear leukocytes, an elevated protein content, and a glucose level that may be normal or significantly reduced. CMV can be cultured from the CSF in approximately 50% of the cases, but testing for CMV DNA PCR in the CSF can provide a more rapid diagnosis. EMG and nerve conduction studies reveal primary evidence of axonal loss in lumbosacral roots with later denervation potentials in leg muscle, sometimes with asymmetric involvement.

Mononeuropathies

Diagnosis is based on the clinical presentation and confirmed by EMG, nerve conduction studies, and nerve biopsy.

Inflammatory Demyelinating Polyradiculoneuropathy

Lumbar puncture should be performed in the evaluation of possible GBS or CIDP. CSF shows elevated protein and lymphocytic pleocytosis of 10 to 50 cells/mm^3, with a normal glucose. EMG may be helpful in the diagnosis of GBS and CIDP. Nerve conduction studies demonstrate slow conduction, delayed latencies and conduction blocks, and reduced sensory and motor amplitudes.

Autonomic Neuropathy

In patients infected with HIV with symptoms of dysautonomia, autonomic function can be assessed by measurement of pulse rate variability on standing, resting, and deep breathing, Valsalva manuever, isometric exercise, cold face test, and mental stress. Blood pressure is measured during standing, lying down face up, resting, and on Valsalva maneuver.

Treatment

Distal Symmetrical Polyneuropathy

Treatment options for HIV-related and drug-induced distal symmetrical polyneuropathy are limited. Management of polyneuropathy is largely symptomatic and usually aimed at ameliorating dysesthesias. NSAIDs, tramadol, narcotics, and transdermal lidocaine are all used empirically. A pilot study of high-dose capsaicin patch has shown benefit in both DSP and ATN Simpson et al., 2004). Although TCAs are used for the treatment of painful diabetic neuropathies, they were ineffective in treating HIV-associated painful neuropathies in one study (Kieburtz et al., 1998). Despite this finding, TCAs are still used by many practitioners, alone or in combination with other agents. Anticonvulsants including gabapentin, carbamazepine, phenytoin, topiramate, and lamotrigine are widely used based on their efficacy with other types of neuropathic pain (Bennett & Simpson, 2004; La Spina et al., 2001).

The use of gabapentin for the treatment of painful HIV-related neuropathy was found to reduce pain in a small group of patients (La Spina et al., 2001). Efficacy with gabapentin has also been demonstrated for the treatment of painful diabetic neuropathy and postherpetic neuralgia. Beneficial effects began with doses greater than 1800 mg/day (Misha-Misroslav, 2002). In our practice, gabapentin is frequently used for the treatment of painful HIV-related neuropathies. The usual starting dose is 100 mg tid, but doses can be increased to 1200 mg tid. There should be a delay of several days between dose adjustments to allow for maximum effect at a given dosage. Slow escalation of doses can also allow for tolerance to side effects such as somnolence and dizziness. In patients requiring higher dosages, the addition of a second agent (antidepressant, anticonvulsant) may help to achieve a more rapid desired effect. In refractory cases, patients may respond to opioid analgesics.

Antiretroviral Toxic Neuropathies

Treatment should include the discontinuation of drugs that cause peripheral neuropathy. About two thirds of patients will eventually respond to NRTI discontinuation, but there may be a "coasting phenomenon," where the neuropathy worsens for 1 to 6 weeks. This is followed by gradual improvement, with recovery in 3 to 19 weeks (Nardin & Freeman, 2004). Remaining symptoms may be due to irreversible toxicity or concomitant DSP. In a small randomized, double-blind, placebo-controlled study, lamotrigine use was associated with a substantial decrease in pain compared with placebo in the treatment of HIV neu-

ropathy. A larger and more recent study demonstrated that the beneficial effect of lamotrigine was seen in patients with ATN rather than DSP. The starting dose was 25 mg given either daily or every other day. Dose escalation occurred over 7 weeks, to reach a maximum of 400 to 600 mg per day in two divided doses. Higher doses were used in patients who were taking drugs known to induce the metabolism of lamotrigine (Simpson et al., 2000, 2003). Recent studies have also shown that nerve growth factor is associated with major improvement of pain compared with placebo. However, there was no improvement in the secondary measures of nerve growth regeneration, and the drug is not commercially available. Amitriptyline, mexiletine, topical capsaicin, acupuncture, 5% lidocaine, and gabapentin may also be useful for treating ATN.

Herpes Zoster (Shingles) and Postherpetic Neuralgia

HZ may be treated with acyclovir, valacyclovir, or famciclovir. In the immunocompetent host, treatment with antivirals may accelerate the rate of healing and reduce the severity of acute pain. Variable benefit has been reported with respect to a reduction in the frequency and duration of postherpetic neuralgia. The addition of corticosteroids may shorten the course of the acute illness, but has no effect on the incidence or duration of postherpetic neuralgia. For acute pain associated with HZ, short-acting narcotic analgesics should be prescribed. For persistent pain, long-acting opioids are preferred, by either oral or transdermal routes. Sympathetic nerve blockade can provide rapid, temporary relief of severe pain (Kotani et al., 2000).

Treatment of PHN may be complex. The value of aspirin is limited, and ibuprofen is ineffective. Topical formulations of aspirin, ibuprofen, lidocaine, and prilocaine have all been reported to be useful. Capsaicin cream may offer modest benefits, but one third of patients may suffer intolerable burning during application (Kost & Strauss, 1996). In various studies, opioids, tricyclic antidepressants, and gabapentin have been shown to reduce the severity and duration of PHN, either as a single agent or in combination (Gnann & Whitley, 2002). A reasonable approach is to use escalating doses of gabapentin, with the addition of TCAs and possibly opioids if necessary. In patients with intractable pain, intrathecal methylprednisolone once weekly for 4 weeks has shown promising results (Kotani et al., 2000).

Mononeuritis Mutiplex

Treatment of mononeuritis mutliplex depends on the underlying cause. For early-stage patients with CD4 counts > 200 cells/µl, only supportive care is recommended as patients may improve spontaneously. If cryoglobulins are found, plasma exchange is the treatment of choice. If CMV is documented in the CSF, in other organs, or by finding typical CMV inclusions on nerve biopsy, treatment with an antiviral agent should be initiated. Ganciclovir is the treatment of choice, but those who are intolerant of this drug can be treated with foscarnet or cidofovir. If a nerve biopsy demonstrates vasculitis, treatment options include intravenous immunoglobulin, plasma exchange, and prednisone (Nardin & Freeman, 2004).

Diffuse Infiltrative Lymphocytosis Syndrome

DILS is treated primarily with antiretroviral drugs, mainly protease inhibitor–containing regimens, with or without corticosteroids. Although DILS often improves with treatment, spontaneous improvement has also been reported.

Lumbosacral Polyradiculopathy

CMV-induced cauda equina syndrome is a medical emergency, and treatment should be started based on clinical suspicion. Ganciclovir intravenously is the treatment of choice. Foscarnet is recommended as an alternative therapy for patients with suspected ganciclovir resistance or ganciclovir-induced leucopenia (Corral et al., 1997).

Mononeuropathies

No clear treatment has been defined. For facial nerve palsy, which may occur during seroconversion, acyclovir with or without prednisone may be considered as this is the treatment for non-HIV-associated Bell's palsy. For other mononeuroathies, a nerve biopsy may provide an etiology, and specific treatment can be administered — immunosuppression for vasculitis or antimicrobials for infection (Nardin & Freeman, 2004).

Inflammatory Demyelinating Polyradiculopathy

The treatment of choice for AIDP (GBS) is plasmapheresis or high-dose intravenous immunoglobulin (IVIG), while that for CIDP is oral corticosteroids. Acute exacerbations of CIDP may require plasmapheresis or IVIG. For patients with advanced disease (CD4 < 100) and evidence of CMV end-organ disease, consideration should be given to treatment with ganciclovir, foscarnet, or cidofovir. In AIDP (GBS), patients may develop significant respiratory muscle weakness, requiring ventilatory support.

Autonomic Neuropathy

Treatment for autonomic neuropathy is supportive. The use of elastic stockings and sleeping with the head elevated may reduce the symptoms of postural hypotension, but some patients may require treatment with Fludrocortisone. Reduced gastric motility can be treated with reglan, small frequent meals, and sleeping with the head elevated. Bladder dysfunction is treated with intermittent catheterization or medication such as bethanechol.

SUMMARY

In dealing with the symptom of pain in the patient infected with HIV, one should be aware of the possible etiologies of the pain, with special attention to the possibility of infection or malignancy. In many cases, diagnosing and treating the underlying condition will be crucial to amelioration of pain. The degree of immunosuppression should direct the pace and extent of medical evaluation. Much of the existing literature regarding treatment of pain in the HIV-infected patient predates the availability of effective treatment for HIV and may not be relevant to patients currently receiving effective antiretroviral medication.

It is likely that inadequate treatment of pain by physicians continues to exist among providers of HIV care. It is important that evaluation and treatment of pain be systematic, with assessment of the impact on daily activities. The aspect of pain management in HIV must also be focused on healthy individuals with active daily lives in whom adequate pain management could dramatically improve quality of life.

REFERENCES

Abrams, D. I. (1997). Physician-assisted suicide and patients with human immunodeficiency virus disease. *New England Journal of Medicine, 336,* 417.

Bennett, M. I. & Simpson, K. H. (2004). Gabapentin in the treatment of neuropathic pain. *Palliative Medicine, 18,* 5.

Berger, J. R., & Simpson, D. M. (1998). The pathogenesis of diffuse infiltrative lymphocytosis syndrome: An AIDS-related peripheral neuropathy. *Neurology, 50,* 855.

Breitbart, W. et al. (1996). The undertreatment of pain in ambulatory AIDS patients. *Pain, 65,* 239.

Broner, F. A., Garland, D. E., & Zigler, J. E. (1996). Spinal infections in the immunocompromised host. *Orthopedic Clinics of North America, 27,* 37.

Chetty, R., Batitang, S., & Nair, R. (2000). Large artery vasculopathy in HIV-positive patients: Another vasculitic enigma. *Human Pathology, 31,* 374.

Collazos, J. et al. (1996). Celiac plexus block as a treatment for refractory pain related to sclerosing cholangitis in AIDS patients. *Journal of Clinical Gastroenterology, 23,* 47.

Corral, I. et al. (1997). Acute polyradiculopathies in HIV-infected patients. *Journal of Neurology, 244,* 499.

Darouich, R. O. (1998). Oropharyngeal and esophageal candidiasis in immunocompromised patients: Treatment issues. *Clinical Infectious Diseases, 26,* 259.

Dassopoulos, T., & Ehrenpreis, D. (1999). Acute pancreatitis in human immunodeficiency virus-infected patients: A review. *Amercan Journal of Medicine, 107,* 78.

Dieterich, D. T. (2003). Long-term complications of nucleoside reverse transcriptase inhibitor therapy. *AIDS Reader, 13,* 176.

Fantry, L. E., & Chen-Chih, J. S. (2002). *Mycobacterium avium* complex-associated cholecystitis in an HIV-infected woman. *AIDS Patient Care STDS, 16,* 201.

French, A. L. et al. (1995). Cholecystectomy in patients with AIDS: Clinicopathologic correlation in 107 cases. *Clinical Infectious Diseases, 21,* 852.

Gifford, A. L., & Hecht, F. M. (2001). Evaluating HIV-infected patients with headache: Who needs computed tomography? *Headache, 41,* 441.

Gnann, J. W., Jr., & Whitley, R. J. (2002). Herpes zoster. *New England Journal of Medicine, 347,* 340.

Graham, C. B., III et al. (2000). Screening CT of the brain determined by CD4 count in HIV-positive patients presenting with headache. *American Journal of Neuroradiology, 21,* 451.

Graham, C. B., III, & Wippold, F. J. II (2001). Headache in the HIV patient: A review with special attention to the role of imaging, *Cephalagia, I,* 169.

Greenspan, J. S., & Greenspan, D. (1999). Oral manifestations of HIV infection and AIDS. In T. C. Merigan, Jr., J. G. Bartlett, & D. Bolognesi (Eds.), *Textbook of AIDS medicine* (2nd ed.). Baltimore: Williams & Wilkins.

Grothe, T., & Gottlieb, M. (1999). Hospice care and symptom management. In T. C. Merigan, Jr., J. G. Bartlett, J.G., & D. Bolognesi (Eds.), *Textbook of AIDS medicine* (2nd ed.). Baltimore: Williams & Wilkins.

Hernandez-Albujar, S. et al. (2000). Tuberculous radiculomyelitis complicating tuberculous meningitis. *Clinical Infectious Diseases, 30,* 915.

Hsue, P. Y. et al. (2004). Progression of atherosclerosis as assessed by carotid intima-media thickness in patients with HIV infection. *Circulation, 109,* 1603.

Hunt, S. M. et al. (2000). Invasive fungal sinusitis in the acquired immunodeficiency syndrome. *Otolaryngologic Clinics of North America, 33,* 335.

Jacobson, J. M. et al. (1997). Thalidomide for the treatment of oral aphthous ulcers in patients with human immunodeficiency virus infection. National Institute of Allergy and Infectious Diseases AIDS Clinical Trials Group, *New England Journal of Medicine, 336,* 1487.

Kazi, S. et al. (1996). The diffuse infiltrative lymphocytosis syndrome: Clinical and immunogenetic features in 35 patients. *AIDS, 10,* 385.

Keswani, S. C. et al. (2002). HIV-associated sensory neuropathies. *AIDS, 16,* 2105.

Kieburtz, K. et al. (1998). A randomized trial of amitriptyline and mexiletine for painful neuropathy in HIV infection. AIDS Clinical Trial Group 242 Protocol Team. *Neurology, 51,* 1682.

Kolson, D. L., & Gonzalez-Scarano, F. (2001). HIV-associated neuropathies: Role of HIV-1, CMV, and other viruses. *Journal of the Peripheral Nervous System, 6,* 2.

Kopp, J. B. et al. (1997). Crystalluria and urinary tract abnormalities associated with indinvir. *Annals of Internal Medicine, 127,* 119.

Kost, R. G., & Strauss, S. E. (1996). Postherpetic neuralgia — pathogenesis, treatment, and prevention. *New England Journal of Medicine, 335,* 32.

Kotani, N. et al. (2000). Intrathecal methylprednisolone for intractable postherpetic neuralgia. *New England Journal of Medicine, 343,* 1514.

La Spina, D. et al. (2001). Gabapentin in painful HIV-related neuropathy: A report of 19 patients, preliminary observations. *European Journal of Neurology, 8,* 71.

Larue, F., Fontaine, A., & Colleau, S. (1997). Underestimation and undertreatment of pain in HIV disease: Multicentre study. *British Medical Journal, 314,* 23.

Lesprit, P. et al. (1997). Cerebral tuberculosis in patients with the acquired immunodeficiency syndrome (AIDS), *Medicine, 76,* 423.

Lopez, L. et al. (2004). Risk modifiers for peripheral sensory neuropathy in HIV infection/AIDS. *European Journal of Neurology, 11,* 97.

Lorberboym, M. et al. (1998). Thallium-201 retention in focal intracranial lesions for differential diagnosis of primary lymphoma and nonmalignant lesions in AIDS patients. *Journal of Nuclear Medicine, 39,* 1366.

Lorenz, K. A. et al. (2001). Associations of symptoms and health-care related quality of life: Findings from a national study of persons with HIV infection. *Annals of Internal Medicine, 134,* 854.

Luciano C. A., Perdo C. A., & McArthur J. C. (2003). Recent developments in the HIV neuropathies. *Current Opinion in Neurology, 16,* 403.

Martin, C. et al. (2003). Painful and non-painful neuropathy in HIV-infected patients: An analysis of somatosensory nerve function. *European Journal of Pain, 7,* 23.

Masci, J. R. (2001). *Outpatient management of HIV infection* (3rd ed.). Boca Raton: CRC Press.

Misha-Misroslav, B. (2002). Use of anticonvulsants for treatment of neuropathic pain. *Neurology, 59,* s14.

Monkemuller, K. E. et al. (2000). Declining prevalence of opportunistic gastrointestinal disease in the era of combination antiretroviral therapy. *American Journal of Gastroenterology, 95,* 457.

Nardin, R. A., & Freeman, R. (2004). Diagnosis, treatment and prognosis of peripheral neuropathy in HIV-infected patients. In B. D. Rose (Ed.), *UpToDate,* version 12.2. Wellesley, MA: UpToDate.

Nopachai, A., Garwacki, C. P., & Moll, S. (2004). Diffuse infiltrative lymphocytosis syndrome. *American Journal of Hematology, 75,* 173.

Obernesser, M. S. (2004). Gingivitis and periodontitis syndromes in adults. In B. D. Rose (Ed.). *UpToDate,* version 12.2, Wellesley, MA: UpToDate.

Pardo, C. A., McArthur, J. C., & Griffin, J. W. (2001). HIV neuropathy: Insights in the pathology of HIV peripheral nerve disease. *Journal of Peripheral Nervous Systems, 6*(1), 21–27.

Piliero, P. J., Estanislao, L., & Simpson, D. (2004). Diaphragmatic paralysis due to isolated phrenic neuropathy in an HIV-infected man. *Neurology, 62,* 54.

Reyes, M. et al. (2003). Acyclovir-resistant genital herpes among persons attending sexually transmitted disease and human immunodeficiency virus clinics. *Archives of Internal Medicine, 163,* 76.

Rogstad, K. E. et al. (1999). Cardiovascular autonomic neuropathy in HIV infected patients. *Sexually Transmitted Infections, 75*(4), 264–267.

Simpson, D. et al. (2004). Novel high concentration capsaicin patch for the treatment of painful HIV-associated distal symmetrical polyneuropathy: Results of an open label trial. Program and abstracts of the 11th Conference on Retroviruses and opportunistic infection, San Francisco, Feb 8–11, Abstract 490.

Simpson, D. M. et al. (2000). A placebo-controlled trial of lamotrigine for painful HIV-associated neuropathy. *Neurology*, *54*, 2115.

Simpson, D. M. et al. (2002). Severity of HIV-associated neuropathy is associated with plasma HIV-1 RNA levels. *AIDS*, *16*, 407.

Simpson, D. M. et al. (2003). Lamotrigine for HIV-associated painful sensory neuropathies: A placebo-controlled trial, *Neurology*. *60*, 1508.

Singer, E. J. et al. (1993). Painful symptoms reported by ambulatory HIV-infected men in a longitudinal study. *Pain*, *54*, 15.

Slaven, E. M. et al. (2003). The AIDS patient with abdominal pain: A new challenge for the emergency physician. *Emergency Medicine Clinics of North America*, *12*, 987.

Smith, K. Y. (2002). Selected metabolic and morphologic complications associated with highly active antiretroviral therapy. *Journal of Infectious Diseases*, *185*, 123.

Stricker, R. B. et al. (1992). Mononeuritis multiplex associated with cryoglobulinemia in HIV infection. *Neurology*, *42*, 2103.

Tehranzadeh, J., Ter-Oganesyan, R.R., & Steinbach, L.S. (2004). Musculoskeletal disorders associated with HIV infection and AIDS. Part II: Non-infectious musculoskeletal conditions. *Skeletal Radiology*, *33*, 311.

Tom, D. J. et al. (1992). Epidural blood patch in the HIV-positive patient. Review of clinical experience. San Diego HIV Neurobehavioral Research Center. *Anesthesiology*, *76*, 94.

Verdon, R. et al. (2002). Indinavir induced cholelithiasis in a patient infected with human immunodeficiency virus. *Clinical Infectious Diseases*, *35*, 57.

Verma, A. (2001). Epidemiology and clinical features of HIV-1 associated neuropathies. *Journal of Peripheral Nervous Systems*, *6*, 8.

Vittecoq, D. et al. (2003). Coronary heart disease in HIV-infected patients in the highly active antiretroviral treatment era. *AIDS*, *17*, S70.

Walden, D. T. (1999). Biliary problems in people with HIV disease, *Current Treament Options in Gastroenterology,l.*, *2*, 147–153.

Whitney, T. M. et al. (1992). Appendicitis in acquired immunodeficiency syndrome. *American Journal of Surgery*, *164*, 467.

Yoshida, D., & Caruso, J. M. (2002). Abdominal pain in the HIV-infected patient. *Journal of Emergency Medicine*, *23*, 111.

38

Injuries from Motor Vehicle Accidents

Christopher R. Brown, DDS, MPS

INTRODUCTION

In the last 30 years, there have been more than 10 million "moderate to severe" injuries and over 1.5 million deaths in the United States from motor vehicle accidents (MVAs). The National Safety Council reported in 1996 that 11.2 million traffic collisions occurred. Of those, 9.6 million were a combination of property damage only and/or non-disabling injury collisions. The economic cost to the United States was estimated to be $176.1 billion, a staggering amount of money.

In terms of the dollar costs involved, Evans in *Traffic Safety and the Driver* indicates property damage to top the list at 37%, with medical costs in fifth place at 6% of the total (1991). Data from the National Highway Traffic Safety Administration (1987) referencing the total cost are presented in Table 38.1 (Evans, 1991).

As presented by the Association for the Advancement of Automobile Medicine in 2003, work-related motor vehicle crash injuries cost employers $41.5 billion in 2000 and required them to pay $18.4 billion in wage–risk premiums. Employer health care spending on MVAs was $7.7 billion in 2003 with another $8.6 billion spent on sick leave and life and disability insurance for crash victims. New York and New Jersey employers carry the highest per cost per employee in the United States at $630 and $540, respectively (Miller, 2003).

Understanding what happens to humans in MVAs takes more than statistics, graphs, and charts. It requires a combination of learning tools, investigative procedures, and a thorough understanding of human anatomy and physiology. There is often an educational gap between clinicians who treat MVA victims and engineers who observe the vehicles involved. As automobiles become relatively "more safe" in terms of death rates, resulting soft tissue injuries probably will increase. People who used to die in car wrecks are now living thanks to improved car safety, an efficient emergency medical (EMS) system, and specialized trauma training, the result of which presents diagnostic, therapeutic, and economic challenges. The more clinicians know about the biomechanics and occupant kinematics (human motion), the more efficient and accurate the care that can be delivered and the more informed the rendering of opinions regarding causation.

From an engineering perspective, certain factors about the automobile such as its weight, speed, and vector (direction of motion) can play a part in the resulting occupant trauma. Other factors that may affect occupants need to be understood as well to fully appreciate and estimate the resulting forces that may contribute to human injury potential.

BIOMECHANICS

Biomechanics is a very inexact science when it comes to human beings and their injuries. Although mathematical predictions are accurate and easily obtainable, human reactions under different stresses are not. How can one explain when a person's parachute fails to open, and he or she beats the odds and survives a multithousand foot fall while another person will trip coming down some stairs, fall several feet, and die? Examples of human response to energy input quickly lead one to the conclusion that the predictability of individual response is based strictly on the individual's response to energy input at a given body location as a function of time; nothing more, nothing less. It is important, however, to understand generalities so that a practicing clinician can approach human injury with logical sense.

543

TABLE 38.1
National Highway Traffic Administration $
Estimate (1987) of U.S. Traffic Crashes

	Dollars Lost/Spent	Percent of Total Expenses
Property	27.0	37.0
Insurance	21.0	28.0
Productivity	16.0	22.0
Legal and court	4.0	6.0
Medical	4.0	6.0
Emergency (transportation, diagnosis, and support)	0.7	0.9
Miscellaneous	0.45	0.6

There are four basis response modes for a body subjected to external forces:

1. Elasticity: Elasticity is defined as deformation induced during forced application, which is completely recovered when the load is recovered. An example of this is the perfect spring. This type of reaction is rarely found in the human body.

2. Plasticity: Plasticity results from deformation of the initial geometry when the load is released. In other words, the loading and unloading paths are different. The absorbed energy is the product of force × motion in the direction of motion. Plastic deformation in essence equals the permanently stored (absorbed) energy. A good example of plastic deformation is the human earlobe's response to weighted earrings or inserts. When pressure is applied over time, the soft tissue of the ear will bend and be permanently changed.

3. Viscoelasticity: Viscoelasticity is body deformation under a load such that it recovers its geometry upon load release, but it does so by following a different loading path. The initial geometry is recovered but the body absorbs some of the applied energy. In a mechanical sense, shock absorbers and tires are good examples. Human soft tissue responds in a viscoelastic manner unless force is applied to the point of actual tissue rupture.

4. Brittleness: A brittle body ruptures with negligent plastic flow. Up to the point of rupture, however, response is purely elastic. The best example of this is glass.

Although each part of the human body under various conditions can exhibit some of these properties, in the true sense of the word, the human soft tissues respond in a viscoelastic manner.

REAR-END MOTOR VEHICLE ACCIDENTS

In reality, actual numbers regarding rear-end motor vehicle accidents (REMVAs) are impossible to track (fatal vs. nonfatal). While statistics on fatalities are easy to track, the statistics on injuries are not. This especially holds true when it comes to REMVAs. Take, for instance, the port of statistical entry for comparing the two. With a fatality, police are involved, certificates are signed. A definite path, which societies have determined as necessary is followed.

With injuries, however, this is not the case. Take into consideration the possible portals of entry into the medical system of the United States. A victim of an MVA may very well start out at the emergency room with a description of minor injuries, which may not need immediate attention. At that point, there may or may not be any type of follow through. The victim may be referred back to a family physician if he or she has one, or the victim may be left to find his or her own way. The choices people have for treatment of pain are varied. For instance, for the treatment of headaches following a REMVA, the person may choose to visit a physician, a chiropractor, a dentist, a massage therapist, an acupuncturist, an optometrist, an ophthalmologist, and so on.

Statistics, as a result, are not accurate and there is no predetermined course of action as in fatalities. In fact, even the accepted terminology varies, depending upon the source, as to how to even describe injuries as a result of REMVAs. They may be described as STI (soft tissue injuries), MIST (minimal impact soft tissue) injuries, or CAD (cervical acceleration/deceleration) injuries. All these descriptions are used to describe a pattern or type of injury as a result of "whiplash." Even with the difficulty of tracking these types of injuries, it has been estimated that 1 million to 2 million CAD injuries occur per year from REMVAs (Evans, 1992). The 2 million per year estimates occur at rates roughly 5,480/day, 1,827/8 hours, 228/hour, 114/half hour, and 4/minute. Not only are REMVA injuries substantial in number, they also can produce long-term residual effects. In fact, the rate of recovery in whiplash injuries is often reported as poor. Literature suggests 20 to 40% of whiplash injuries have debilitating symptoms that persist for years (Carette, 1994).

Most clinicians assume all REMVA vehicular motion and occupant kinematics are predictable and identical. This is far from accurate. There is no such thing as a typical REMVA. Most REMVAs are in actuality offset collisions producing nearly simultaneous torsion, tension, compression, and shear forces to the human body when viewed diagrammatically as a whole, especially when viewing individual anatomical units.

LOW SPEED VERSUS HIGH SPEED

For practical purposes, the working definition of a low-speed impact is a collision in which the change in velocity of the vehicles (usually the one that contains an occupant claiming an injury) is less than 10 mph. It must be emphasized that this definition of low speed is subjective. Clearly, no general consensus among experts exists. This definition is used to delineate automobile speeds not predict occupant injury. In other words a "low speed" collision does not imply the lack of injuries just as "high speed" does not imply more severe injuries. In fact nearly one third of all injuries occur at below 20 miles per hour impact (Watts, Atkinson, & Hennessy, 1996). Essentially, the speed of the impact may not correlate with the severity of injury.

Although it is commonly accepted to describe impact severity and injury potential as functions of change in velocity, caution should be used when considering impacts of grossly dissimilar durations. Comparison of impacts based solely on their respective changes in velocity inherently assumes the impacts occurred over a similar duration, typically 90 to 140 ms for low-speed impacts. For the majority of accidents, this is a reasonable assumption. However, in some collisions, such as underride or sideswipe collisions, the impact duration may be in excess of 300 ms. Given an equal change in velocity, a vehicle that undergoes a longer-duration impact will be exposed to lower peak forces. For this reason, underride and override collisions, although sometimes involving very high dollar amounts of property damage, can be less severe in the resulting occupant injury than a "no damage" collision. There is no correlation between the amount of vehicle damage and occupant injury.

To provide an example, one must first understand the measurement of forces involved. The rate of acceleration, independent of mass, of an object falling to the Earth's surface represents a value due to gravity, referred to as g. The value of g (near the Earth's surface) is a constant measured as 32.2 ft/s^2 (or 9.81 m/s^2). Under normal conditions, this is the acceleration we are accustomed to experiencing in our daily lives, so it is often referred to as 1G. To exemplify the effects of impact duration, consider skidding a vehicle to a stop. In theory, decelerating a vehicle from 30 mph to a stop by applying the brakes involves an impact between the tires and the roadway with a change in velocity of 30 mph, but with impact duration of approximately 2.0 s. The skidding vehicle is decelerated at approximately 0.7 g. Although braking a vehicle to a stop involves a 30-mph change in velocity, this is a quite different event from a 30-mph front-to-barrier impact. The barrier impact occurs over a much shorter duration and typically involves decelerations of 30 to 50 g.

A factor to consider in low-speed rear-end motor vehicle accidents (LSREMVAs) is impact forces, which are concentrated over very small areas. As an everyday event, this may occur while backing into a small-diameter pole in a parking lot or contacting a corner or small area of a bumper. Vehicle structures typically deform in proportion to the amount of force applied. In impacts with narrow objects or to the corners of vehicles, the contact forces are distributed over a very small area producing large local stresses (force per unit area). These large local stresses can damage bumper and vehicle components at changes in velocity below the strength of that area. Testing by the Insurance Institute for Highway Safety indicates that the amount of damage and costs of repair will vary dramatically from car to car and will even vary greatly for the same vehicle depending on the type and angle of low speed collision (Kauffman et al., 1993). These factors have to be taken into consideration to determine forces transferred to the occupants.

In reality, however, the definition changes situationally according to needs; professions that deal with MVAs and human injury may erroneously assume that "one size fits all." In other words, there is a mechanism of injury that either happens or does not happen: people get hurt or they don't. From the perspective of the dental profession it had been assumed that for temporomandibular joints (TMJs) to become injured in an REMVA, the mandible had to go through a full range of motion and in essence hyperextend. Video recordings of LSREMVAs clearly indicate that in low-speed collisions this is often not the mechanism of injury. A few authors, therefore, erroneously assume that because this particular mechanism of injury is not present, the TMJs or other joints cannot be injured. That, of course, is false logic. All parts of the body, no matter where the location, receive injuries from many sources. The mechanisms of soft tissue injury are similar and subject to physiological response. Clinicians need to be aware of these mechanisms to clearly understand, diagnose, and treat the injuries they see. Understanding leads to a more definitive diagnosis and more effective treatment.

Statistics themselves are not applicable when trying to predict individual occurrences. Statistics may be used as an academic yardstick but cannot be used to predict how an individual or small group of occupants will respond in any given situation. Predicting or judging any injury based on a population smaller than what is statistically significant in the measured population is erroneous. There are countless examples of people who "beat the odds" in tremendously potentially destructive situations and escape unscathed. On the other hand, there are also many examples of people in seemingly less traumatic circumstances who are severely injured, even die. To this end, every patient should be evaluated independently. Patients destined to recover will do so in the first 3 to 4 months after initial injury (Barnsley et al., 1994). The consequences are both long term and far reaching, resulting in extended sick leave and increases in disability (Per-

Olof et al., 1998). Beyond that time period, the probability of permanency increases.

While statistics vary greatly, it is safely assumed that up to 50% of all REMVAs will result in some type of neck injury. The risk of occupant disability is approximately 3 to 6%, a staggering amount when one considers the number of motor vehicle accidents per year (Ono et al., 1993). As previously mentioned, future studies might indicate these numbers will increase as the deaths decrease. There is no truth to the assumption that injured people get better after some type of settlement or what is known as "green back poultice."

COLLISION DYNAMICS

There are three different types of collisions in every REMVA:

1. Automobile to automobile
2. Occupant to automobile interior
3. Occupant body part to body part

AUTOMOBILE TO AUTOMOBILE

The easiest type of collision to understand is automobile to automobile. The motion is commonly divided into four different phases:

1. Contact
2. Vehicle at the peak of acceleration
3. Vehicle starting to slow down
4. Vehicle slowing to a stop

All such factors as bumper height, weight of the vehicle, angle of impact, and environment may change the function of time and velocity resulting in an overlap of each phase.

OCCUPANT TO AUTOMOBILE

The second collision, occupant to automobile interior, can also be generalized into four separate phases:

1. 0 to 100 ms. The initial phase occurs at zero to 100 ms. When the vehicle moves forward out under the test subject, initial forward and vertical motion of the hips and low back occurs. Simultaneously, the upper part of the seat begins to flex rearward under the load of the torso, which remains stationary during this time period.
2. 100 to 200 ms. After the first 100 ms, the seatback reaches maximum rearward movement. The subject moves upward and forward resulting in neck compression, cervical spine straightening, and movement upward and rearward. The head is in a chin-up type of position and begins to rotate rearward. By 160 ms, the vertical motion of the torso begins to pull the neck forward as the head continues rearward.
3. 200 to 300 ms. At 200 ms, maximum vertical motion has taken place. At 250 ms, the head starts a forward motion. The seatback returns to its original position while the torso extends back down the seatback.
4. 300 to 400 ms. At 300 ms, the descent of the torso is now complete and is moving at the same velocity as the vehicle. At 400 ms, active deceleration of the neck occurs, all impact-related motions are virtually completed, and the human body is moving at the vehicle's velocity.

The total time for human movement in REMVAs is 0.1 to 0.2 s. Whether the impact results from low or high velocity, the time of energy exchanged is virtually the same. This is due to the biomechanical properties of the elements involved and may vary only by a few fractions of a second.

OCCUPANT BODY PART TO BODY PART

Human injury comes not from the first collision, but from the second and third collisions. Obviously, contact from the human being to parts of the automobile can produce great amounts of soft tissue injury. These can come from movement of the body into the seat, the headrest, a seatbelt, steering wheel, dashboard, automobile pillars, windshield, etc. All are potential injury mechanisms for human beings. However, the third collision (body part to body part) has a great effect, especially in low-impact situations. As the automobile goes through the motions, keeping in mind Newton's laws of motion, the occupants remain stationary relative to the automobile but seem to move toward the impact. The occupant lags behind the car, the torso lags behind the hips, the neck lags behind the torso, the head lags behind the neck, the vertebrae lag behind one another, the mandible lags behind the cranium, etc. As a result, the motion of the human during this time period is a nonphysiological motion resulting in points of injury, which will almost always be at the connective tissue junctions between hard and soft tissues (as commonly seen in the TMJs and cervical vertebrae). The result is injuries to muscles, ligaments, and tendons. In "offset" collisions, which are the most common, a great amount of rotational forces will be placed on the body. The occupants will experience compression and shear forces, which can result in great injury to the soft tissue. The differences in load variations to the human body during cycles of motion result in multiple stress and strain points. One must remember that each REMVA is unique and is not likely to involve pure forward and backward motion. Biomechanical forces applied in REMVAs are always multidimensional. As a result, there is no v (change in velocity as a vector over time) or closing speed under which a person cannot get hurt. For that matter, nor is there a v, or closing speed, over which all people will sustain injury. The injuries are a result of individual response at a moment in time. These principles and conditions apply to soft tissue injuries and all body parts. The rate of acceleration of any given body part is of utmost importance (Newton's second law). The forces increase dramatically with an increase in acceleration. Soft tissue properties differ when applied with time variables.

Crushing of soft tissues can occur in blunt impact when body surface deforms and soft tissues become compressed between impact site and other hard tissues. Examples of these follow:

1. Tissues at the nuchal line and headrest (skull and headrest)
2. Tissues between spinal column and seatback
3. Tissues between vertebrae during ramping and submarining
4. Tissues between the condyles and skull (TMJ injuries)
5. Attachments of muscles (i.e., trapezius) during ramping and contact with friction of the seat, headrest, and body supports built into seats

Because a moving body has inertia, when it collides a force is immediately produced on the impacted surface that starts to slow the body as a whole. The result is a net force that produces differential deceleration between body segments. The resulting biomechanical stresses (shear, compression, torque, etc.) acting simultaneously, and in opposite directions, often yield soft tissue damage. Data studied with high-speed video indicate that facet shearing forces appear to be the most sensitive to increased acceleration. The spinal differentials are magnified by the phenomena of two distinct cervical motions. As the head and cervical spine extend into the head restraint, the greatest intersegmental rotation and posterior shear displacements occur along with peak neuroforaminal pressures. How the head contacts the head restraint is of vital importance when viewing the cervical deformations, which cause soft tissue "pinching" between vertebrae (Tencer, Huber, & Mirza, 2003).

DIRECT VS. INDIRECT TRAUMA

What is the difference between direct and indirect trauma? Can you separate the two when it comes to MVAs? Can you tell the difference clinically and with diagnostic testing? Actually, under the examination by magnetic resonance imaging (MRI) or clinician's diagnostic exam, tissue reaction and dysfunction are the same.

Examples of direct trauma

1. Penetrating — puncture
2. Penetrating — laceration
3. Crush mechanisms (Yes and No)

Examples of indirect trauma

1. Coup–contra-coup brain injury
2. Concussion (e.g., football helmet blow, boxer sustaining blow to the mandible)
3. Fracturing a bone
4. Spraining a knee, elbow, wrist by abnormal/repetitive movement (e.g., tennis elbow)
5. Repetitive strain syndromes of all types (e.g., carpal tunnel)
6. TMJ injuries

As previously mentioned injuries commonly occur at the interfaces between unlike tissues as a result of the following contributing factors:

1. Differential of speed of body parts (lagging behind)
2. Differential of tissue makeup yielding variance of wave transfer
3. Differential of hydraulic pressure
4. Hard tissue rebounding
5. Crush mechanism of hard tissues approximating each other
6. Cellular damage

Each connective tissue junction has potential for suffering stress/strain. These types of mechanisms rarely, if ever, occur by themselves. Biomechanical forces in the real world occur in multiple directions and conflicting degrees simultaneously. The delineation between direct and indirect trauma is not one of physiological origin but rather medicolegal only. Human tissues are limited in their ability to respond and are governed by the same laws of physics as the rest of the universe. To say that, for instance, the soft tissues of the TMJs or their supporting structures cannot be injured unless the mandible is directly struck indicates a lack of understanding, education, truthfulness, or all three. In fact, most injuries to the human body except at the exact point of impact are indirect in nature.

COMMON SOFT TISSUE ACCELERATION/DECELERATION (STAD) MIST INJURIES OF THE HEAD AND NECK RESULTING FROM LSREMVAs

1. Cervical strain/sprain
2. Cervical facet joint inflammation
3. Cervical strain
4. Cervical nerve root damage/compression
5. Occipital neuralgia
6. Myospasm/myalgia
7. Myofascial trigger points
8. Temporal tendonitis
9. Stylomandibular ligament insertion tendinosis (Ernest's syndrome)
10. Injuries to the TMJs
    - Lateral capsulitis
    - Posterior capsulitis
    - Hemarthrosis
    - Disc displacement
        Reducing
        Nonreducing
    - Adhesions in the superior and inferior joint spaces

TESTING METHODS FOR PREDICTING HUMAN INJURY

Testing methods used to determine the kinds and types of injuries received in MVAs fall into five categories:

1. Humans (live)
2. Animals
3. Cadavers
4. Computer modeling
5. Anthropomorphic test dummies

The only totally accurate way to predict human response in REMVAs is to actually use living, breathing humans. Obviously, some restrictions apply for these types of situations.

First of all, humans get injured. A review of studies using live, human testing reveals that humans are brought to the bare minimum level of injuries and then no more. Test situations have very specific parameters, and small variables can result in a great change in human response to input forces. Variables such as occupant seating, anticipation of impact, the weight of apparatus strapped to the patient, helmet versus no helmet greatly modify the parameters of human response, making each individual crash in truth anecdotal. Therefore, the threshold of human injury is not totally statistically accurate and varies greatly based on an almost inexhaustible amount of uncontrolled variables in a real-world situation.

It also should be noted that crash tests are not designed to hurt human beings. They are designed to note human motion and/or response to energy input. All other testing sources, while providing great statistical information, provide no actual correlation to human injury. If one carefully reads published reports through the Society of Automobile Engineers (SAE), it will be obvious with a few biased exceptions that human motion studies do not predict injuries or lack thereof, but carefully note that they are individually dependent.

All other types of testing including cadavers are not accurate for the human response in low-impact REMVAs. In high-speed crashes as the v increases, the correlation between live human response and other factors increases. This is because all other testing measures purely mechanical response but no material response. Pain and dysfunction often result from the material response of viscoelastic human tissue. In other words, the quicker the impact, the higher the forces received, the more mechanical a human will respond and, therefore, mechanical/cadaver/computer modeling becomes more relevant. In low-impact REMVAs, a few good studies with humans exist but virtually none with surrogates that correlate with human motion. As a result, while all crash test studies among living, nonliving, and nonhuman subjects yield good statistics for study and provide cost-effective ways to measure mechanical output, at best they provide unconfirmed approximate vague guidelines for human injury. In a comparison between Hybrid III crash test dummy biofidelity and cadaver variability, Kent and Benson concluded: "Any dummy measurement is relatively unimportant in an injury risk model that includes several experimental and cadaver characteristics as predictors." They also further conclude, "The functional relationship between any Hybrid III injury measure and actual injury risk is highly sensitive to experimental factors such as test speed, restraint condition, and seating position" (Kent & Benson, 2003, pp. 68–69).

Crash and test studies fall short in providing subjective and objective information relating to pain, central nervous system (CNS) information, biological information, physiologic information, kinetic dysfunction following impacts, and latent reaction.

All information gathered from crash test studies is statistical in nature and can never be applied to an individual in a given clinical situation.

PRINCIPLES AFFECTING SOFT TISSUE INJURIES (HOW PEOPLE GET HURT): THRESHOLDS FOR SOFT TISSUE INJURIES- — INDIVIDUAL TOLERANCES AND RISK OF INJURY

In the real world, there are no set thresholds for injuries to soft or hard tissues. Biomechanical trauma is unpredictable and anecdotal with tissue strengths and tolerance varying under different conditions. Body parts accelerate and move at rates different from the car and from one another. To this end, there are several principles affecting soft tissue injuries.

INSTANTANEOUS CENTER OF ROTATION

The instantaneous center of rotation (ICR) of a joint is the mathematical determination of a theoretical point on which all motions rotate. The concept of ICR in a kinematic and biomechanical sense is an important one. It can be considered under healthy conditions to be the physiological center upon which human motions of a given joint will move. Various ICRs have been measured and determined for different body parts. However, in an REMVA, the ICR may change within microseconds, causing a great change in load distribution of the human body. In a landmark study by Kaneoka et al. (1999), the ICR of the spinal column was measured and found to change in as little as a sub-4-mph v resulting in a pathological motion.

The term ICR has been misapplied and misunderstood in some instances of human motion. This is especially true in the TMJs. First of all, the motions of TMJs are not purely rotational and do not move around the fixed axis of rotation. The axis rotation of TMJs will vary in anatomical planes. When subsequent motion of the head and neck apparatus or compressed tissue in the retro-discal area exists, the TMJs translate from the first moment. In this instance, virtually no pure rotation occurs. Under normal circumstances, the initial axis of rotation and resulting translation can very well be different from one TMJ to another within one person, resulting in axes of rotations that are not coupled symmetrically with one another.

The surface of the TMJs can be nongeometric for many reasons, including degenerative joint disease, remodeling, growth, angles of eminentiae, scar tissue, etc. The condition and surface of the articulating surfaces and supporting structures and the resulting musculature function determine the potential motions of the TMJs resulting in a very complex motion system.

For the ICR of the TMJs to be accurately determined, they would have to be rotating cylinders that remain stationary throughout the motion, which of course they do not. The mandible changes its position as it moves throughout the range of motion. The result is not just a change of the head of the mandible, but the mandible itself. As it translates, rotates, and moves in a three-dimensional position, the ICR changes as well. Studies also indicate that the trajectory of the condylar heads along the surfaces can be affected by velocity (distance/time) and is a multiplane vector that can be affected by muscle soreness, speed of forced opening, rotational forces, compressive forces, and shear forces. The ICR of the TMJ will change dramatically in a very slight, fractional opening. When the ICRs of the TMJs are not perfectly matched,

the articulating surfaces of the joints can be either distracted or compressed, depending on which moment in time is measured. Rapid acceleration, such as that experienced in an REMVA, can affect the standardization of motion of the TMJs, creating nonhabitual moment arms resulting in excessive forces not physiologically compatible with the human anatomy involved. These changing patterns from moment to moment will result in gross motor dysfunction, which will produce differing articular motions. The result is that the ICR of the TMJs is a mathematical theory only and not an accurate representation of reality. TMJs and their supporting structures can become excessively damaged from indirect trauma such as that received from whiplash. The following is a list of potential TMJ injury mechanisms.

Wave Motion

Stress waves travel at the speed of sound (square root of the ratio of the Young's modulus to the material density). For the description of the elastic properties of linear objects such as wires, rods, and columns, which are either stretched or compressed, a convenient parameter is the ratio of the stress to the strain, a parameter called the Young's modulus of the material. Young's modulus can be used to predict the elongation or compression of an object as long as the stress is less than the yield strength of the material. These stress waves travel through the body, and are portions to local stresses and forces, resulting in both localized compressions and tensions. Wave speeds for car material are approximately 9,843 to 16,404 ft/s (10 times the speed of sound). Time of energy transfer is 0.1 to 0.2 s, which means the energy travels the length of the car (15 ft) in 1.5 ms. Elastic waves travel 67 times the car length (approximately 33 reverberations) in the energy transfer time of 0.1 to 0.2 s.

Although viscoelastic for the most part at low forces, human soft tissue responds in an elastic manner. At high forces and as a function of time in which the force is applied, soft tissue may respond in a plastic manner resulting in permanent injury. Plastic waves travel much more slowly (slightly faster than the collapsing of impact surfaces) in automobiles and in human tissue as well. In MVAs, both waves are present due to crushed and uncrushed vehicle components. As a result, not surprisingly, injuries often occur at locations remote from the impact site. The velocity (Newton's second law) of deformation is the predominant factor in determining the magnitude of wave created.

High Velocity

Stress waves from impact site travel at the speed of sound in the surrounding tissues. Injuries occur at interfaces of unlike tissues (e.g., meninges, TMJs, muscle to bone attachments, facial lining), as well as tissue/air interfaces (e.g., intestinal wall/gas, sinus cavities/lining). A differentiation of tissue movement is contributed by the following mechanisms of injury: compression and expansion of the stressed tissues, production of pressure differential across a boundary, and "Spalling" energy release as an energy wave attempts to go from a dense to less dense medium (the wave is tensile; most human soft tissues can withstand more compression than tension).

Low Velocity (Most Commonly Experienced in MVAs)

Stress waves travel at less than 15 m/s. Transverse waves of lower velocity and long duration (shear waves) are produced by displacements of body surfaces. The results are differentials created at sites of attachments and sites of body part collisions. These forces will vary more when considering not only a difference in tissue viscosity but structural/architectural differences as well on both micro- and macrolevels.

Hydraulic Pressures

Tremendous amounts of pressure exerted within closed fluid systems cause tearing at micro- and macrolevels. Fluid systems (i.e., shock absorbers) exhibit various mechanical characteristics under different rates of loading. Different types react in a dissimilar manner. The "containers" burst and/or strain when loaded quickly. A study by Tencer et al. (2003) indicates that specimens show greatly increased pressure around the nerve roots during cadaver acceleration tests after the chest has accelerated but before peak head acceleration. In other words, tissue reaction is time sensitive. The forces generated will be released through the path of least resistance. In humans, this path is often the point of connection between soft and hard tissues.

Energy Input and Force $\times$ Compression: $F_{max} \times C_{max}$

This formula relates to how much energy is placed on a subject (or body part) during impact and how much is "lost" during the transfer. Tissues and organs can disrupt and dissipate energy transference. The larger the $F_{max} \times C_{max}$, the more energy loss will be experienced in the soft tissues, and therefore, the greater the potential for destruction.

This relates to Newton's first law (an object at rest tends to stay at rest and an object in motion tends to stay in motion with the same speed and in the same direction unless acted upon by an unbalanced force). How much energy it takes to move tissues will determine injury potential. Tissues that slide over each other and do not resist will not absorb as much energy as those that cannot move as fast as others. The lag time between body part

motion due to differences in location, density, and reaction to forces plays a part in this phenomenon.

Occupant Position at the Time of Impact

Occupant position at the time of impact, one of the most important variables, is commonly overlooked and assumed in REMVAs. Occupant position will greatly reduce the v required to surpass the soft tissue injury threshold. The Biomechanical Assessment Profile (BAP), a position assessment questionnaire developed by the author, allows the clinician and the occupant to help estimate the occupant position at the time of impact. The slightest occupant position variation will greatly affect injury potential resulting in large increases of impact forces (SAE #930211; SAE #700361).

A normal position, such as that assumed by a crash test dummy, is not a normal position for most occupants (SAE #912914). Being out of position is actually more normal for occupants than being in position, if normal is defined by the posture of crash test dummies at the time of impact. Positioning varies by occupants' driving habits, anatomy, seat comfort, and anticipation of a collision.

There are three common actions of bullet vehicle drivers prior to impact; braking, swerving, and spinning/yawing. These motions will have an effect on the impact angle of vehicles, closing speed, and vehicle contact and could potentially negate built-in safety systems as well as directly affect vehicle damage.

These factors also greatly affect the passenger position at the time of impact. Virtually all rear impact testing with dummy and cadaver subjects has been conducted with properly positioned occupants (erect, backs firmly placed against the seat back; Whitman et al., 2003). Being out of position can dramatically change the occupants' reactions to forces and resulting kinematics. Humans react quite differently from crash test dummies especially in low-speed accidents. Variations in occupant positioning may contribute little to injury potential in high-speed crashes but can greatly increase or decrease injury potential in low-speed collisions. Whitman et al. (2003) report that as lateral vehicle motion increased in an REMVA the potential for head contact with vehicle interior surfaces increased. An "offset" REMVA therefore can greatly alter the dynamics of the occupant's kinematics (Pamjabi et al., 1998).

Preexisting Conditions

"Preexisting" is a term that is often misunderstood and abused. Susceptibility to injury does not negate the fact that damage can occur. A preexisting condition can radically lower the amount of energy required to cause soft tissue damage. While there may be evidence of a condition radiographically, such as in localized bone breakdown of the cervical spine or the condylar head of the TMJs, the person may have been asymptomatic and remained so throughout his or her life if not for the large amount of energy transferred in such a short period of time as in an MVA.

In fact, preexisting conditions can make a person more susceptible to injury when the person forced to move faster or more than is habitually required. Conditions that may contribute include, but are not limited to, arthritis, cervical disc disease, fibromyalgia, TMD of many varieties, myofascial disorders, emotional disorders, chronic subluxation, poor spinal alignment, and cranial lesions. The curvature of the spine may also be altered due to tissue conditions or even seating posture at the time of impact.

Muscle Splinting (Pre-Tensed)

The effects of pre-tensing of the muscles can have a varying effect on injury in LSREMVAs. The potential for injury can be increased or decreased, or even not be affected. They may sound contradictory, yet any or all of these can apply to each individual on any occasion or all at once and can apply to various body parts. Examples of pre-tensing of muscles include tightening of the neck, locking the knees, pushing on the brake, and bracing with arms on the steering wheel. Any number of human responses can affect injury potential. The principles of movement are all the same.

All of the above can also relate directly or indirectly to cellular damage. Cell injury can occur when mechanical trauma damages the cell membrane, impairing its ability to act as a barrier to extra cellular calcium. Too much intracellular free calcium can overwhelm the mechanisms that normally maintain a relatively constant calcium concentration. The cell's inability to dispel the calcium can lead to an increase in osmotic pressure causing swelling, cell membrane damage, metabolic depletion, and cell death. This can occur in skeletal muscles, smooth muscles (blood vessel muscle lining), and nerve tissues. Mechanical cellular damage (from stretching) also can alter nerve tissue conduction. This cellular damage can result in muscle spasm, alteration of localized blood flow, hyperirritability, dysfunction, breakdown, and pain. All the aforementioned principles can apply to soft tissue injury on all levels simultaneously. These phenomena can occur from nonphysiologic vertebral intersegmental rotations (Deng et al., 2000), facet capsule tearing (Cusick, Pinitar, & Yoganandan, 2001), facet pinching (Tencer et al., 2003), facet translations which exceed normal limits (SAE #670919), and increased hydraulic pressure around the cervical nerve roots.

Reaction Time

The time span of energy input is rapid; total time is 0.1 to 0.2 s. In contrast, human response time is slow. Even healthy individuals' muscular reactions do not begin until 0.08 to 0.14 s. Total personal response time has been estimated at 2.5 s, but will vary according to each individual and the circumstance at the time of impact.

INDIVIDUAL HUMAN FACTORS AFFECTING INJURY

A preexisting condition will most likely increase the risk of injury. Simply understanding that an acute problem can be superimposed over a chronic condition is significant. As this would tend to lead to a predisposition to injury, it should be taken into consideration when arriving at a differential diagnosis. It is crucial that the clinician has a thorough understanding of the patient's condition. A thorough health history is essential and may include contacting previous treating clinicians.

With regard to gender, women have approximately two times more minor soft tissue injuries than men, in addition to smaller neck diameters and longer necks. As a population, they tend to demonstrate higher frequency of spinal stenosis. According to the National Safety Council, women are involved in a greater number of collisions per million miles driven and tend to have a higher frequency of injury claims with more severe injuries, requiring more extensive and costly treatment. Recovery tends to be slower, with greater disability and poorer prognosis.

Age is another important consideration, as older drivers are likely to be more prone to injury, complicated by a decreased capacity for recovery. The size of the occupant is also important. The larger the occupant's mass, the less likely an injury will occur. Taller occupants have been shown to be at risk for higher neck injury (tall and thin vs. short and fat). Size may correlate with age (children vs. adults; adults vs. elderly people). Size of body parts can also influence injury potential.

AUTOMOBILE COMPONENTS THAT CONTRIBUTE TO HUMAN INJURY POTENTIAL

HEADRESTS

Next to the position of the occupants at the precise time of impact, headrests are the most commonly overlooked contributors to head/neck injuries in REMVAs. They are often the silent contributors to occupant cervical injury. Federal law (Federal Motor Vehicle Safety Standards) requires that "head restraints must be at least 27.5 in. above the seating reference point in the highest position and not deflect more than 4 in. under a 120-lb load." Or, they must not allow the relative angle of the head and torso of a 95th percentile dummy to exceed 45° when exposed to an acceleration of 8 g.

Vans and light trucks from 1991 have had to comply with standards. Studies show an 85-cm seatback height necessary to account for 95% of male occupants and 100% of female occupants. However, the generalization of head-rest design does not allow for individual height differences and resulting cervical strain. The distance an occupant's head has to travel before impacting the headrest in a rear-end collision can greatly increase the forces applied to the head and neck (SAE #670919). This distance can vary not only from structural design but also because of the occupant's build and seating preference. American consumers as a rule prefer adjustable headrests, but rarely have them adjusted to achieve maximum effectiveness. They are often set too low to protect the head/neck complex.

Transfer of energy (0.1 to 0.2 s) and the slowness of human cervical muscles to respond (0.08 to 0.14 s) result in almost no one being able to avoid direct contact with the headrest. Therefore, in almost every case involving a rear-end motor vehicle collision direct impact to the head, neck, and torso of the target vehicle occupants by the seatbacks/headrests occurs, which can result in soft tissue injury.

Factors that affect headrest protection of occupants are positioning; ramping of the body, flexion of the seat-back, head riding above and below, distance the occupant's head travels to make initial contact (longer = more force), occupant positioning, occupant's awareness of impact (bracing), and length of neck, arms, torso. Headrest design and position may contribute greatly to potential cervical/head injury. As a result of occupant motion or pre-impact positioning, the headrest may even increase occupant injury. The contact of the head and cervical spine producing posterior shear translation of the vertebrae can greatly alter injury potential.

SEAT CONSTRUCTION

Federal Standard FMVSS 207 advocates strength require-ments of 20 times the weight of the seatback. Most seats weigh about 40 lb. The resulting strength would be 800 lb, which may not be enough in a significant impact. In fact, impacts may produce forces beyond the seat's designed ability to rebound, resulting in seatback collapse that greatly affects the amount and direction of force to the occupant (SAE #930211). Seat construction is not uniform from one car to the next. It varies in angle, stiff-ness, elasticity, materials, and coefficient of friction. The seat design helps determine relative impact of each body part. It can lead to large differential between head, spine, shoulders, pelvis, and supporting soft tissues. Seat design can directly influence angle of force vectors, compression of the spine in association with bending forces of the rotating pelvis, as well as help determine relative flexibil-ity of the spine. The seat can greatly affect shear and rotational forces on the occupant and influence occupant rebound motion after the input of energy. The seatback's rebound velocity is up to 150% of the initial velocity. If the torso rebounds before the head has reached its rear-most position, the relative velocity between the head and torso will produce unequal rebound speeds (SAE #960665). In LSREMVAs, the rebound of the occupants in the front seat may be due more to the elasticity of the seat back than to vehicle deceleration. Lack of seat uni-formity makes LSREMVA cervical studies difficult to standardize. As previously stated, any given study cannot be used to generalize or apply to a given individual.

RAMPING

The angle of the seat produces forces that may direct the occupant up the seatback. The target vehicle's rear may be deflected upward or downward depending on the rela-tive center of gravity between the target and bullet vehi-cles, resulting in the occupant traveling up the seat in a rearward position (relative to the car but stationary to the Earth). The extent of ramping depends on the angle of seatback deflection. Occupant ramping increases as seat-back angle increases. In addition, the slack of the lap portion of the seatbelt is also crucial. Rearward deflection of the seat causes slack in the seatbelt. Use of a belt or no belt may affect occupant motion.

There are four important factors of body motion lead-ing to occupant injury related to seat construction: head displacement, translation, rotation; differential motion of head, neck, torso; occupant ramping up seatback; and occupant rebound.

No fully instrumented rear impact tests are required by law for seat design. In high impacts, seatbacks cushion the occupants from great accelerations. In low impacts, the same qualities account for greater occupant accelera-tion in the rebound phase. The seatback design and result-ing ramping may increase injury potential to the struck automobile occupants during low-speed collisions. There is a design trade-off between comfort and function/occu-pant protection.

AIR BAGS

More than 103 million (50.3%) of the more than 206 million cars and light trucks on U.S. roads have driver air bags. More than 77 million (37.5%) of these also have passenger air bags. Another 1 million new vehicles with air bags are sold each month.

Through September 2000, driver air bags have inflated in more than 3.3 million vehicles in crashes. More than 560,000 passenger air bags inflated when a passenger was occupying the right front seat.

The National Highway Traffic Safety Administration (Evans, 1991) estimates that more than 5,899 people are alive today because of air bags. Of the 62 drivers killed by air bags (48 females, 14 males), 40 are believed to have been unbelted, 21 are believed to have been using lap/shoulder belts (5 of these may have misused their belts; 2 of these were unconscious and slumped over their steering wheels so they were on top of their air bags; 2 used the shoulder belt only; 1 used the lap belt only). Belt use is unknown for the remaining driver. By 1995, 100% of passenger cars had driver systems. A total of 85% of trucks have driver systems, and 23% have passenger systems (SAE #922523).

The purpose of air bags is to save lives. Overall, air bags have decreased belted fatalities by 12 and 27% of deaths in frontal crashes. It is estimated that 70% of frontal crash fatalities could be prevented by properly wearing safety belts and air bags (SAE #960658). Air bags save lives and decrease severity of major injuries in exchange for increasing the number of minor injuries. There is an increase in abrasions, contusions, and lacerations. The body regions most frequently injured are the head and neck, upper extremities, trunk, and lower extremities. Of injuries received, 90% are Abbreviated Injury Scale I (AIS I; SAE #960658). Air bags actually increase the total number of injuries from vehicle collisions, especially in the Δv of 16 to 32 km/h (10 to 20 mph) (Evans, 1992). There are also certain groups for which air bag deployment may pose a greater risk. These include the unrestrained, elderly people, people of small stature, disabled individuals, children, those with improper seating position, and occupants with compromised health.

There are other significant factors that may influence injuries in MVAs upon inflation: severity of crash; interior compartment intrusion; age of restrained occupant; health status including medications, drug, and alcohol use; occupant height, weight, and proportions; occupant position at time of impact/inflation; safety belt wearing including proper positioning; other occupants in the vehicle affecting the restrained driver; loose objects in the vehicle; pre-crash factors including pre-crash cardiac arrest, drowning, fire, and suicide.

AIR BAG SYSTEMS

Air bag inflation is an explosion (200 mph) capable of killing a person, in which the force is stopped in time by a nylon bag. It comprises four elements: crash sensors and controls, inflator, the air bag itself, and diagnostic circuitry. The sensor comprises a ball in a tube or spring mass sensors, which are mounted in the front of the vehicle. It is designed to activate air bag deployment when a sudden deceleration of approximately 16 to 19 km/h (9 to 11 mph) occurs in the vehicle's forward motion. Deployment starts 15 to 20 ms after initial impact. The inflator is made of a pyrotechnic device that inflates a gas generant (sodium azide) in 18 to 23 ms; 21 to 27 ms after impact. The burning sodium azide produces nitrogen gas that expands the nylon air bag. The actual inflation takes 20 to 40 ms. The force exits and inflates the air bag at approx-

imately 200 mph. The nylon air bag provides a high strength/weight ratio and is abrasion resistant with good elongation properties allowing for uniform stress distribution along seams with equally distributed forces. The driver's side air bag is smaller and circularly shaped. It has less time and distance in which to inflate due to the steering wheel. Passenger side air bags are rectangular and three to five times larger than those on the driver's side.

Air bag tethers limit intrusion of the air bag into the driver's space and allow for more lateral expansion (untethered bags extend 250 to 300 mm toward the driver and untethered bags extend 380 to 510 mm). Air bags deflate in about 80 to 100 ms through vent holes in the back of the bag. The diagnostic circuitry has three main functions: evaluating the entire system every time the vehicle is turned on, continuous monitoring, and operating a backup power source for inflation should there be system power failure.

Soft tissue injuries resulting from air bag inflation are common. Air bag injuries result from both direct and indirect trauma. They include abrasions and contusions to the head neck and chest, as well as abrasions and burns to the hands. Transient/permanent paresthesia of the chin is common as are injuries to the TMJ and supporting structures such as teeth fractures and avulsions. Cervical injuries including sprain/strain and more especially cervical facet inflammation, occipital neuralgia, myospasms, myofascial trigger points, compression neuropathies, paresthesias local to the impact site, and sphenopalatine ganglion neuralgia seem to be commonplace, as is closed head trauma.

"Smart" air bags that adjust their performance characteristics based on the environment present at the time of the collision are being used in many newer vehicles and are likely to be refined even further. They are designed to "sense" the occupant's seat position, the size of occupant (including whether the occupant is a child or infant), and adjust the deployment according to the severity of crash (closing speed). There is a tremendous need for clinical case studies of injuries resulting from air bag deployment. Observations need to be documented and published by treating clinicians so engineers can have accurate information from the field.

SAFETY BELTS

Seatbelts are not perfect but nevertheless are among the most effective and simplest devices that help save lives. Although 49 states have seatbelt laws, it is estimated that only 69% of U.S. citizens use seatbelts even when mandated. Seatbelts are designed to comfortably fit 80% of the U.S. population. Seatbelts are designed to protect the occupants by controlling the ramp up of the seat back, reduce the velocity of the occupant relative to the vehicle interior, and thus reduce injuries resulting from occupant contacts.

The regular use may minimize the potential of occupants to be out of position at the time of impact and allow the driver to be in position to remain in control of the vehicle after an impact. They may be effective in controlling forward rebound of the occupant while keeping the occupant within the vehicle. In frontal impacts, they tend to extend the time of "ride down," thus effectively reducing the force on the occupant. This is accomplished by both structural design and stretching of the fabric. Overall they tend to reduce the frequency and severity of occupant impact with the vehicle's interior (second collision), although occupants can still strike the vehicle's interior including dashboard, steering wheel, and windshield.

Most injuries from lap belts fall into the category of AIS I but can still cause permanent injury or death. The occurrence of certain injuries has increased since the appearance of mandatory seatbelt laws. Such injuries include sternum fractures, neck sprains, thoracolumbar spine injuries, as well as serious cervical spine injuries (SAE #912913). The occurrence of certain injuries appears to be directly related to the type of seatbelt. A lap belt can cause internal injuries upon frontal crashes or rebound from REMVA if the belt is positioned superior to the superior iliac crest of the pelvis. At the very least, severe strain on the lower back due to external forces is likely and may result in "flailing" injuries of the lower extremities. The use of lap belts alone will not stop occupants from striking the dashboard, steering wheel, or windshield with their heads. One of the most important considerations is that use of a lap belt can increase acceleration of the head/neck upon rebound in a REMVA, thus result in greater injury to the head and neck.

A three-point shoulder harness, which is said to be essential for air bag safety, can also cause increased forces to the neck in a MVA even if properly positioned. It will tend to add rotational forces to the head/neck upon rebound as the occupant rotates toward the door. Although it may actually increase likelihood of cervical injury in low-speed collisions, regular use appears to reduce the incidence of serious injury by >57% (Watts, 2003). Shoulder belts, while very effective in saving lives, can directly affect injury patterns and, in fact, cause injuries in low-speed accidents. Some common injuries include bruising and abrasions of shoulder, chest, neck, and abdomen. It is important to note that even with seatbelts, occupants can still directly contact the car's interior with their heads. This can vary according to the severity of the impact, location of the impact, and occupant body proportions.

BUMPERS

Bumpers were first applied to railroad cars to protect cargo rather than the car. However, bumpers were added to automobiles to protect the vehicle rather than to protect the passenger (Watts, 2003). Bumper design in modern automobiles is intended to lessen structural damage in a collision, to keep repair costs down. Most cars have what is known as 5 mph bumpers. This means that a collision 5 mph or less into a rigid barrier will not cause any permanent body damage (Watts, 2003).

There are two types of bumpers commonly used in cars. One is designed of rigid metal and is attached to the frame with pistons (isolators). These oil and gas filled cylinders absorb the forces, collapsing in the process. Another type is made of high-density polyurethane in a honeycombed or foam design with a plastic outer shell cover. The polyurethane has a viscoelastic and plastic response when energy is added in a collision, acting similarly to a spring. As the bumper collapses and expands back, energy is released in the form of motion and heat. Many times plastic bumpers can completely compress without showing any obvious signs of damage (Watts, 2003).

Trucks, vans, and SUVs often do not have the same bumper systems as cars. In fact there are no government regulations on minimal impact or height with which manufacturers have to comply in these vehicles. With so many of these vehicle types on the road, collisions with cars are inevitable. Often in low-speed collisions involving a truck and car, there is more damage to the car than the truck. There can be several reasons for this. The bumpers of the truck are often welded directly to the frame without any shock-absorbing material such as pistons or plastic foam. When contact is made in a truck/SUV–car low-impact collision, the energy absorbed and/or transmitted is different between vehicles because trucks and SUVs have much stiffer frames, making them in essence stronger than the cars. The bumper height is often higher than those in cars, yielding differences in striking heights and force vectors. When an SUV bumper collides with an automobile bumper, more forces can be transmitted to the automobile occupants producing greater occupant injury potential than if the bumper hits the soft bodywork, which is designed to collapse and absorb collision energy (Watts, 2003). The difference in costs of repair would be much greater if the automobile body was struck at the same low speed by the SUV bumper as compared with a bumper-to-bumper contact at the same speed. This scenario supports the fact that the cost of automobile repair, automobile damage, or lack thereof does not correlate with injury potential and energy transfer to the occupants. In fact according to Watts: "Even with the typical low-quality SUV bumper, the heavier and stronger vehicle usually wins when it collides with a typical car, and the SUV occupants rarely suffer injuries in low-speed impacts" (Watts, 2003, p. 126). It is important to note that it is not possible to look at bumper damage and determine if an occupant has been injured, nor is bumper damage a predictor of injuries in a given collision.

TABLE 38.2
Abbreviated Injury Scale (AIS)

0   No injury
1   Minor (may not require professional treatment)
2   Moderate (nearly always requires professional treatment, but is not ordinarily life threatening or permanently disabling)
3   Serious (potential for major hospitalization and long-term disability, but normally not life threatening)
4   Severe (life-threatening and often permanently disabling, but survival is probable)
5   Critical (usually requires intensive medical care, survival uncertain)
6   Maximum (untreatable, virtually unsurvivable)

ABBREVIATED INJURY SCALE

The AIS was developed in 1971 by the Association for the Advancement of Automobile Medicine and the Society of Automobile Engineers to statistically track injury categories. Injuries for each body region area are placed into seven levels (0 to 6). The AIS level (Table 38.2) is based on the level of injury revealed by an examination shortly after the crash by doctors trained in its application (Gennarelli et al., 1998).

As the AIS increases, the cost of medical support greatly increases. However, the purpose of the AIS is for statistics only. No level is supposed to be used as a predictor of final outcome or to estimate the cost of treatment. It is possible for injuries at any AIS level to subsequently prove fatal, although the threat to life potential of the injury increases steeply with increasing AIS level (Evans, 1992).

ADDITIONAL FACTS ABOUT MVAS AND THE RESULTING BIOMECHANICS AND KINEMATICS

1. *Biomechanics is an unpredictable science.* Mathematically, scenarios can be predicted via computer modeling, etc. and information can be gathered following an accident by extensively monitored crash test dummies or other surrogates, but one little change in an almost endless supply of variables can result in dramatically different resulting forces and injury potential. In fact, measurements may differ between individual test subjects in the same carefully monitored crash test, rendering predictions of outcome totally inaccurate. Not everyone is hurt in a low-speed REMVA. Conversely, not everyone escapes uninjured either. Applying the measured outcomes from crash test studies to predict an individual's chance of physical harm in a completely different accident is impossible. In fact, valid scientific papers are quick to point out that the gathered data cannot and should not be used in this manner (SAE #930211).

2. *There is no correlation between the costs of repair of an automobile as a predictor of occupant injury.* If there is truly a cost/injury ratio, then the higher the cost of repair, the more extensive the injuries to the occupants. In fact, often the opposite is true. Whenever a nonbumper impact to a vehicle occurs, large amounts of upper body damage occur to the vehicles involved. Vehicular panels are meant to crush, dispersing energy transfer over a longer period of time, and thus reducing the forces applied to the occupants. In today's vehicles with computerized components, the cost of repair can be quite high with very little energy transfer to the vehicle itself. In fact, a recent crash test demonstrated the cost of repair to the same vehicle at the same impact speed varied by more than $1,000, depending on the angle of impact. In bumper impacts a great amount of force can be transferred to the occupants with little or no vehicular damage. As has been previously discussed, bumpers are not designed to reduce impact to the occupants; they are meant to reduce the costs of repair in a collision (Kauffman et al., 1993).

3. *In no instances does the amount of energy transfer and resulting injury involving humans directly correlate with the cost of repair to plastic, metal, and other materials composing the vehicle.* Each individual vehicle has what is called a critical speed. This term means a speed at which permanent damage occurs. All makes of cars are different and respond differently when comparing types of collisions. Vehicles that respond well (with little cost of repair) in rear-end collisions may not do well in side or frontal impacts. There is not a material, component, or vehicle that responds equally under every circumstance or force vector. People have their own "critical speed" at which they become injured. This "speed" will vary and can only be determined after the fact, not mathematically in advance. People are not made of plastic and metal. Their tissue responses are not the same nor can they be compared. This is easily demonstrated by watching a football game. When a player is hit in the head, do the managers look at the helmet and determine if an injury has truly occurred based on the amount of damage to the plastic helmet? On the other hand, when a person has an internal injury from a fall, is it correct to examine the floor upon which he or she landed and determine if an injury has occurred by the amount of damage to the floor? Of course not, yet this is attempted routinely in injuries resulting from MVAs. The only plea for this correlation is emotional and usually in an effort to deny a claim of bodily harm. There is no scientific basis to back this up.

4. *Each accident must be analyzed as its own separate entity.* When attempts are made to understand injuries that result from motor vehicle accidents, many factors have to be included. The more the treating clinician understands about the forces involved, the more accurately treatment can be rendered. The cost of repair to the vehicles involved, however, is one factor that may be of interest

for academic and epidemiological reasons but cannot be used as a yardstick for measuring the extent of injuries or the length of treatment time, or estimating the cost of service provided.

SUMMARY

Understanding the biomechanics and occupant kinematics in MVAs is essential for the clinician who treats soft tissue injuries. New car safety has dramatically decreased car accident fatalities in the United States. The result, however, is a new challenge to our health care system. People who would have died in the past are now living, but often with extensive injuries. Soft tissue injuries are often dismissed as an annoyance or something that you have to learn to live with. The truth is that they often can be debilitating and greatly affect the quality of life of victims and their families. Learning to live with it is not the answer. The answer lies in partnerships among victims, their families, treating clinicians, and third-party payers based on education and understanding. Too often a battleground is formed with experts representing vested interests lining up on each side. The result is a "double victim": one who is a victim of trauma from the automobile accident and also of the trauma of enduring medicolegal confrontations.

Treating clinicians can also become victims of sorts. It is commonly reported that carefully and thoroughly treating MVA victims may be looked upon with distrust by third-party payers. Suggestions are being made that the practitioner cannot solely govern the formulation of a treatment plan (Farnham, 2001). Treating clinicians can become discouraged by the constant conflict of trying to help the patient heal and being castigated for trying to do so at the same time. As automobiles become more efficient in reducing deaths, the complexity of the injuries of the survivors will increase. Clinicians must strive continually to increase their diagnostic and treatment skills, keeping the best interests of the patient first and foremost.

> "It is one of the most beautiful compensations in life that no person can sincerely try to help another without helping themselves."
>
> **— Ralph Waldo Emerson**

REFERENCES

Barnsley, L. et al. (1994). Clinical review: Whiplash. *Pain*, 283–307.

Carette, S. (1994). Whiplash injury and chronic neck pain. *New England Journal of Medicine, 330*, 1083–1084.

Cusick, J., Pinitar, F.A., & Yoganandan, N. (2001). Whiplash syndrome kinematic factors influencing pain patterns. *Spine, 26*, 1252–1258.

Deng, B. et al. (2000). Kinematics of human cadaver cervical spine during low speed rear-end impacts. *STAPP Car Crash Journal, 44*, 171–188.

Evans, L. (1991). *Traffic safety and the driver*. New York: Van Nostrand Reinhold.

Evans, R. W. (1992). Some observations on whiplash injuries. *Neurology Clinics, 10*, 975–979.

Farnham, E. (2001, April). Workers' Comp abuse: Can we ever tip the scales? *Claims*, p. 53.

Gennarelli, T. et al. (1998). *The abbreviated injury scale*. Des Plaines, IL: Association for the Advancement of Automobile Medicine.

Kaneoka, K. et al. (1999). Motion analysis of cervical vertebrae during whiplash loading. *Spine, 24*(8), 763–770.

Kauffman, M. et al. (1993). *Status report* (Vol. 3, pp. 2–7). Arlington, VA: Insurance Institute for Highway Safety.

Kent, R., & Benson, N. (2003). The Hybrid III dummy as a discriminator of injurious and non-injurious restraint loading. *47th Annual Proceedings, Association for the Advancement of Automobile Medicine*, pp. 68–69. September 22-24.

Miller, T. (2003). What do US traffic crashes cost employers? *47th Annual Proceedings of the Association for the Advancement of Automobile Medicine*, Sept. 22–24.

Ono, K. et al. (1993). *Influence of the physical parameters on the risk to neck injuries in low impact rear-end collisions*. Presented at the International Conference on the Biomechanics of Impacts, Eindhoven, The Netherlands, Sept. 8–10.

Panjabi, M. M. et al. (1998). Whiplash trauma: A biomechanical viewpoint. In *Whiplash injuries: Current concepts in prevention, diagnosis, and treatment of the cervical whiplash syndrome*. Philadelphia: Lippincott-Raven.

Per-Olof, B. et al. (1998). Sick leave and disability pension among passenger car occupants injured in urban traffic. *Spine, 23*, 1023, 1028.

SAE # 670919, Society Automobile Engineers, 400 Commonwealth Drive, Warrendale, PA 15096. Tel. 724-772-7144.

SAE # 700361, Society Automobile Engineers, 400 Commonwealth Drive, Warrendale, PA 15096. Tel. 724-772-7144.

SAE # 912913, Society Automobile Engineers, 400 Commonwealth Drive, Warrendale, PA 15096. Tel. 724-772-7144.

SAE # 912914, Society Automobile Engineers, 400 Commonwealth Drive, Warrendale, PA 15096. Tel. 724-772-7144.

SAE # 922523, Society Automobile Engineers, 400 Commonwealth Drive, Warrendale, PA 15096. Tel. 724-772-7144.

SAE # 930211, Society Automobile Engineers, 400 Commonwealth Drive, Warrendale, PA 15096. Tel. 724-772-7144.

SAE # 960658, Society Automobile Engineers, 400 Commonwealth Drive, Warrendale, PA 15096. Tel. 724-772-7144.

SAE # 960665, Society Automobile Engineers, 400 Commonwealth Drive, Warrendale, PA 15096. Tel. 724-772-7144.

Tencer, A. F., Huber, P., & Mirza, S. K. (2003). A comparison of biomechanical mechanisms of whiplash injury from rear impacts. *47ᵗʰ Annual Proceedings, Association for the Advancement of Automobile Medicine,* pp. 383–398. Sept. 22–24.

Watts, A. (2003). *Low-speed automobile accidents: Accident reconstruction and occupant kinematics, dynamics and biomechanics* (p. 121). Tucson, AZ: Lawyers and Judges Publishing Company.

Watts, A., Atkinson, D., & Hennessy, C. (1996). *Low speed automobile accidents: Accident reconstruction and occupant kinematics, dynamics and biomechanics.* Tucson, AZ: Lawyers and Judges Publishing Co.

Whitman, E. et al. (2003). Human kinematics during non-collinear low velocity rear end collisions. *47th Annual Proceedings, Association for the Advancement of Automobile Medicine,* p. 440, Sept. 22–24.

39

Diagnosis and Management of Electrical Injury

Raphael C. Lee, MD, ScD, PhD, FACS, Elena N. Bodnar, MD,
and Katherine E. Rojahn, MD

INTRODUCTION

Electrical forces can inflict injury in various ways that include both thermal and nonthermal mechanisms. Non-thermal mechanisms include membrane electroporation and electroconformational denaturation of membrane proteins. Nonthermal injury mechanisms produce destructive changes on the timescale of milliseconds or less. Thermal burn mechanisms require field exposure on the scale of seconds or more. Nerve and muscle are prime targets for nonthermal mechanisms of injury. Pain and disability are frequent manifestations expressed by survivors. The injury resulting from the combination of thermal and electric effects depends on several variables, including the tissue field strength, duration of exposure, frequency, and current path. This chapter reviews the destructive changes to cellular structure resulting from exposure to commercial electrical power sources and the resulting manifestations at the organ system level. Several important new therapeutic approaches to treat and possibly reverse the molecular alterations of electrical shock are discussed.

Injury caused by contact with electrical power sources started to become a significant public health problem at the beginning of the 20th century, corresponding to the commercialization of electrical power. It became clear that commercial frequency (i.e., 50 to 60 Hz) electric force was capable of producing very severe and complex injury. Most major electrical injuries occur in the workplace (Hunt, 1992; Lee, Burke, & Cravalho, 1992; Rouge & Dimick, 1978). There are approximately 1000 annual admissions to U.S. burn centers that have been a result of electrical shock (Hunt, 1992). The death rate for individuals that require hospital admission following accidental electrical injury ranges from 3 to 15% (Rouge & Dimick, 1978) and most of the fatalities are due to high-voltage (> 1000 V) electrical shock (Hunt, 1992). Typically, low-voltage accidents requiring hospitalization involve use of electric panels, power hand tools, or industrial machines that use 220 to 440 V (Lee et al., 1992).

Electrical injury involves multiple biophysical mechanisms. To understand the pathophysiology of electrical injury one must consider the effects of Joule heating (Lee & Kolodney, 1987a), electroporation of cell membranes, and electroconformational protein denaturation (Chen & Lee, 1994; Chen et al., 1998; Gaylor, Prakah-Asante, & Lee, 1988; Lee & Kolodney, 1987b; Lee et al., 1988). Injury is also a function of the anatomical distribution of the electric field. If the electrical contact is arc-mediated (no direct mechanical contact), then acoustic blast forces may also add to the magnitude of the injury (Capelli-Schellpfeffer et al., 1998). Injury manifestation is also influenced by the relative susceptibility of tissue to injury. Tissues that communicate by electrical signals, specifically nerve and muscle tissues, are more susceptible to injury. Neuromuscular problems dominate the clinical problems of survivors, with pain being a nearly universal complaint (Pliskin et al., 1998).

This chapter is a review of the pathophysiology and clinical manifestations of injury by electric fields in the extralow frequency (ELF) range (0 to 1 kHz). Current approaches to management of pain are discussed, as well as new methods. This will introduce several of the emerging and potentially effective strategies for the treatment and therapy of electrical trauma that may correct the complex pathophysiological interactions that accompany electrical shock (Lee et al., 1992).

ELECTRIC FIELD TISSUE INTERACTIONS

CURRENT FLOW IN THE BODY

Direct mechanical contact is usually required for electrical contact when the voltage is less than 1,000 V. Arcing usually initiates the electrical contact for high voltages (>1,000 V). Mobile salt ions are the primary charge carriers within the body and the passage of current at the interface is mediated by electrochemical reactions. Heat and toxic chemical by-products are generated by these reactions, which contribute to local tissue injury. The human body is practically a resistive load when in contact with a 50 to 60 Hz power source (Poppendieck et al., 1966).

The epidermis is the outer layer of skin that serves as a transport barrier purpose and is the largest resistive barrier to current flow through the body. However, as voltage applied across the skin increases, skin insulation is at first partially and then ultimately completely destroyed (Freiberger, 1933). The electrical resistance on the epidermis begins to decrease at voltages as small as 20 V. The skin of the palms and soles is able to withstand voltages up to approximately 100 V. It is reported that the magnitude of the voltage applied across the body has negligible effects on internal body resistance until heat denaturation, electrical breakdown of cells, or dehydration occurs. When exposed to an electrical field above the skin breakdown voltage, the body impedance from one hand to one foot is about 1,000 Ω. The internal body impedance between two hands or between two feet is about 500 Ω.

Within tissues, ionic current passes around the cells. As a result of the extracellular water content of the body being 40% of the total body weight and the electrolyte concentrations being highly regulated, the current distribution between the tissues is reflective of the relative volume of the tissues. This is demonstrated by how in the extremities the bulk of the current passes through the skeletal muscles. Because cell membranes are highly resistive, most of the ELF current is shielded from the intracellular fluid. This does not hold true for strong electrical fields that disrupt the cell membranes or for longer cells, which leak current into the cytoplasm.

ELECTRICAL STIMULATION OF MUSCLE AND NERVE

Biological cells utilize transmembrane ion current as a control signal for intracellular and intercellular communication. This is particularly true for muscle and nerve cells

TABLE 39.1
Reported Thresholds for Nerve, Muscle, and Injury Responses to Passage of 60 Hz Electric Current Through the Body

Electrophysiological Response	Threshold Current[a]
Sensation of pain (fingertip)	1.0 mA (M)[b]
	0.5 mA (F)
"No-let-go": involuntary contraction of forearm muscles	16 mA (M)
	11 mA (F)
Cardiac: Arrhythmia	60 mA
Ventricular fibrillation	100 mA
Electroporation of forearm muscle (hand contact)	1,500 mA

Note: Electroporation injury threshold pertains to forearm skeletal muscle and nerve tissue exposed to current passing from an electrical contact point in the hand.

[a] Assumes current path in the upper extremity.

[b] (M) = males; (F) = females.

and a strong example is brain–muscle communication and control. Skeletal muscle contraction is normally triggered by electrical depolarization of the membrane by nerve-mediated signals. Artificially imposed electric fields can also stimulate muscle contraction, as well as alter brain and peripheral nerve function. The magnitude of these effects is dependent on field strength and frequency.

Several distinct effect thresholds may be observed as ELF sinusoidal current passing through tissues is increased. These are listed in Table 39.1. The threshold for human (male) sensitivity to current passed into the finger is approximately 1.0 mA. If the current traveling through the forearm is raised to 16 mA, skeletal musculature of the forearm is stimulated to contract causing involuntary muscle spasm (Dalziel, 1943). During current passage, the hand cannot be voluntarily opened to "let-go" of an object in the palm. This has been called the "let-go" threshold. Because the forearm flexor muscles are more powerful than the extensor muscles, the hand becomes rigidly closed in a fist position.

If electrical current passes through the chest along the path from extremity to extremity (e.g., the hand-to-hand path), a much larger current is required to interfere with breathing and heart function because the current is spread over a wider area in the chest. Therefore, the current density and corresponding electric field strength are much smaller than in the extremity (Figure 39.1). The area available in the thorax for current conduction is greater than in the extremities, and thus the current density will be less. For victims subjected to total currents of approximately 60 mA hand-to-hand, 50% will experience cardiac rhythm disturbances within approximately 30 s (Dalziel, 1960).

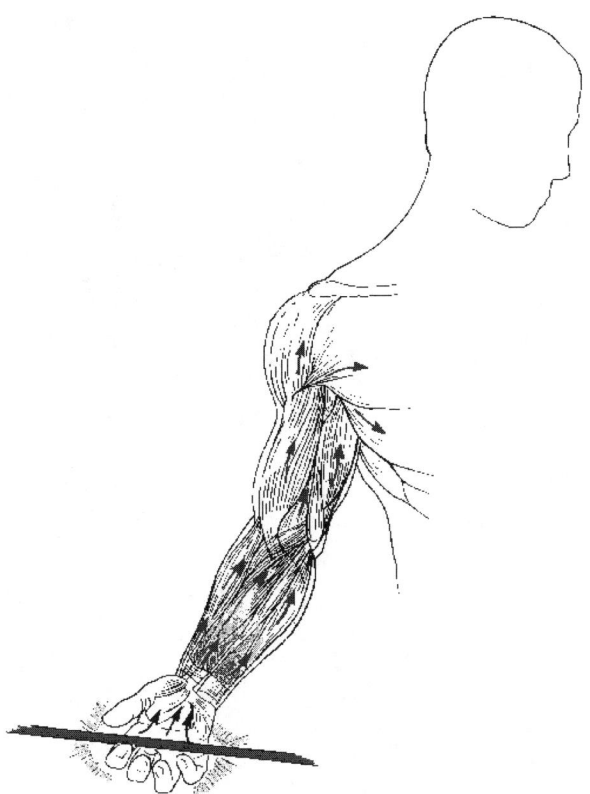

FIGURE 39.1 For a fixed amount of current passing across the body, the current density is quite variable because of variations in anatomical dimensions and, to a much lesser extent, tissue electrical properties.

Electrical current can start and stop cardiac arrhythmias. Ventricular fibrillation is the most life-threatening cardiac arrhythmia. It has been established that ventricular fibrillation can be induced by electric fields of sufficient magnitude during certain phases of the cardiac cycle. It is believed that if the excitable areas of heart muscle are stimulated to contract again before other areas have fully recovered from the previous heartbeat, then the contraction will propagate through the excitable areas and into the other areas of the myocardium that are regaining excitability in time. This leads to an abnormal conduction path and an extremely ineffective discordant muscle contraction. The window for ventricular fibrillation is in the end stage of ventricular contraction systole, which coincides with the most rapid reacquisition of membrane excitability. Electrical shocks to the heart that are strong enough to completely reset the timing of all cardiac cells can result in defibrillation (Wiggers & Wégria, 1939).

THERMAL INJURY

Thermal burning is a well-recognized mode of tissue damage that occurs in electrical shock victims and, until recently, was considered the only mechanism of tissue injury in these patients. Exposure of tissue to supraphys-

iological temperatures in excess of 43°C leads to tissue injury at a temperature-dependent rate (Diller, 1994; Pennes, 1948; Tropea & Lee, 1992). The cell membrane appears to be the cellular component that is the most vulnerable to heat injury.

Tropea and Lee (1992) developed a three-dimensional model of the human arm to address the issue of the relative significance of thermal to nonthermal mechanisms of damage during electrical shock. This preserved basic anatomical details for simulating the thermal response to electrical trauma under worst-case conditions. This worst-case electrical shock scenario assumed perfect mechanical contact with the power source and all current passage was hand-to-hand. The simulation indicated that the rate of heating during contact with 1 to 10 kV was many times faster than circulatory cooling (Pennes, 1948). Blood-flow (tissue perfusion) was observed to be the most important mechanism for transporting thermal energy from Joule-heated tissues (Lee & Kolodney, 1987a; Pennes, 1948). The extent of heat-mediated tissue damage was calculated on the basis of these predicted tissue temperature histories over a range of contact voltages (Pliskin et al., 1998). These Joule heating simulations have also been supported by predictions using a one-dimensional tissue model (Diller, 1994).

Tropea and Lee (1992) also included probability of thermal injury in the model by convolving calculated tissue heating history with damage accumulation rates. Several authors have published damage accumulation rates as a function of high-temperature exposure. Despite the complexity of the process, experimentally measured thermal injury accumulation kinetics seems to obey a first-order chemical reaction process. Therefore, experimental data are reasonably described by the Arrhenius equation. Tropea and Lee (1992) used this approach to arrive at a lethal electrical contact time (LT) in which most of the tissue was lethally heat damaged. Their LT parameter was a function of contact voltage and the location within the extremity. Using the authors' rate constants, contact with a power distribution line (~10-kV contact) requires approximately 0.4 s to cause 50% muscle damage in the distal forearm tissue, 0.9 s in the mid-forearm, and 1.7 s in the mid-arm.

ELECTROPORATION INJURY

Cell membranes are designed to support transmembrane electrical potential differences in the range of 0 to 150 mV, corresponding to normal physiological operating conditions. Cell membranes do not support transmembrane potential magnitudes that are greater than 200 to 300 mV. Once the voltage drop exceeds this magnitude, the membrane becomes hydrated and the transport barrier mechanism of the membrane is lost. This membrane disruption process is called "electroporation" (Lee & Astumanian, 1996), and it is an important mechanism of tissue injury (Block et al.,

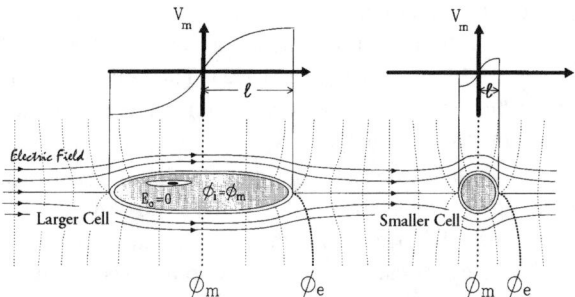

FIGURE 39.2 The cell membrane serves as a transport barrier. This means that the electrical current passes more readily around the cell. The consequence is that most of the voltage drop across the cell is imposed across the cell membrane unless the cell is so large that the resistance of the cytoplasm is equivalent to the membranes.

1995). Electroporation can be transient or permanent, depending on many variables including the magnitude of the field-induced transmembrane potential and the duration of the imposed field (Lee, Canaday, & Hammer, 1993).

To understand the physics of electroporation, the interaction between the electric field and the cells has to be considered. The distribution of current in tissues is governed by the electrical properties of the tissue and the electric field distribution. Cellular membranes are the most resistive of tissues in the body. Cell membrane conductivity is characteristically 10^6- to 10^8-fold less than the intracellular fluid under normal operating conditions. A cell essentially comprises an insulating shell with a highly conductive interior. Electrical current established in the extracellular space by low-frequency fields is to a variable degree shielded from the cytoplasm by the electrically insulating cell membrane. The voltage dropped across the cell by the surrounding current occurs mostly across the cell membrane (Figure 39.2). This induced transmembrane potential is sensitive to several factors including the geometry of the cell and its orientation in the field. For a nonspherical cell, the maximum induced transmembrane potential is dependent on the cell's orientation with respect to the electric field.

The long axes of most skeletal muscle cells and nerve axons in the extremities are oriented approximately parallel to the direction of the field lines (Figure 39.3). These cells have significantly larger transmembrane potentials induced on the membranes than those experienced by skeletal muscle cells in any other orientation or experienced by smaller cell types such as blood cells or tissue fibroblasts. A more precise quantitative appreciation for the magnitude of the induced transmembrane potentials suffered by cells in the current path can be gained by examining the predictions of the basic linear electrical cable model (Gaylor et al., 1988).

The cable model describes both the spatial distribution and kinetics of induced changes in the transmembrane

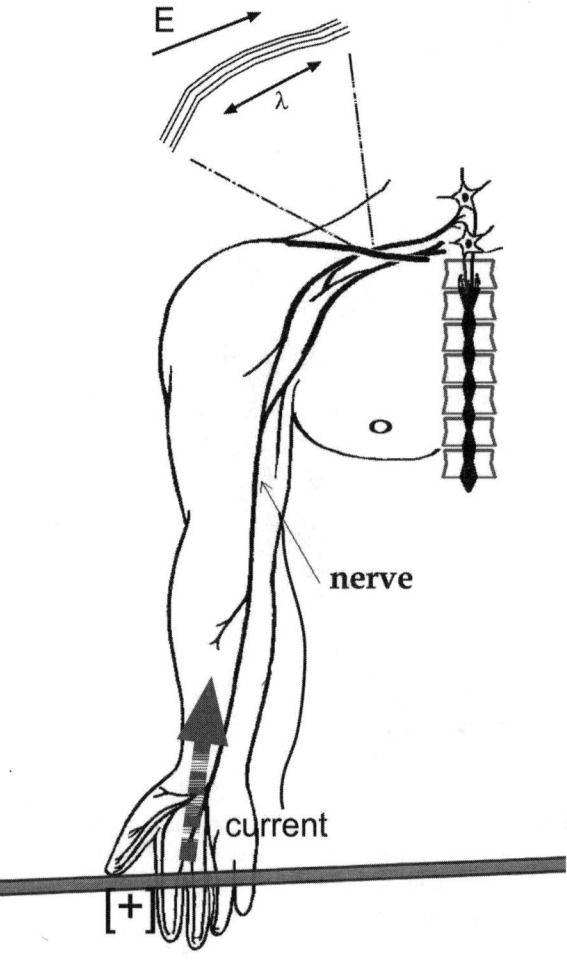

FIGURE 39.3 The physical projection of peripheral nerves and skeletal muscle in direction of current flow is much larger than the electrical space constant of these cells. As a consequence, the voltage imposed across the cell is more dependent on nerve diameter, degree of myelination, and electrical properties of its membrane.

potential. From this basic model two deterministic parameters emerge: the electrical space constant λ and the charging time τ. Dimensionally, λ is in units of distance and τ is in units of time (Figure 39.3). These parameters are very important in understanding the electroporation of skeletal muscle and peripheral nerve cells because the physical dimensions of these cells in the direction of the imposed electric field is much larger than their respective λ. This means that the maximum imposed transmembrane potential of nerve and skeletal muscle while acted upon by an imposed electric field will not exceed the product of the field strength and λ. It also means that the time required for the applied electric field to redistribute the charges across the cell membrane to reach that maximum potential is characterized by τ. For large skeletal muscle cells and large myelinated nerve fibers, the electrical space constant may reach several centimeters. These parameters are only useful in predicting the probability of electroporation injury. Both λ and τ are dependent on the resistance and capacitance of the cell membrane as well as on the physical size of the cell. If the imposed membrane potential reaches values sufficient to electroporate the cells, then both λ and τ change.

It should be noted that the several different types of peripheral nerves differ in diameter and degree of myelination. Thus, they have different space constants and charging times. Small unmyelinated fibers are less susceptible to injury than large heavily myelinated fibers because the large myelinated fibers have larger space constants and shorter charging times. Larger space constants and shorter charging times suggest a higher induced transmembrane potential and increased rate of electroporation.

ELECTROCONFORMATIONAL DENATURATION OF PROTEINS

In addition to disruption of the lipid bilayer component of cell membranes by strong field pulses, the conformation of membrane proteins can also be altered by imposed fields. More than 30% of mammalian cell membranes is composed of proteins. These proteins are composed of amino acids with acidic and basic side groups that can be acted upon directly by an intense intramembrane electric field (Chen & Lee, 1994; Chen et al., 1998; Tsong & Astumian, 1987, 1988). In addition, amino acids of these proteins are electrical dipoles that can align along the length of the transmembrane protein to create a large electric dipole, which can also be acted upon by the field. Many small peptide dipoles in the structure of protein are aligned to effectively form a larger dipole. Generally, a molecule under a strong electric field will tend to shift to having a greater dipole moment in the direction of the field. Hence, membrane proteins will change their conformation in the presence of a strong electric field in a direction to make the effective dipole strength larger.

Effects of this can be observed in several ways, including induced dissociation of ionizable side groups, reorientation of permanent dipoles on the protein within the direction of the field, and other mechanisms. Because voltage-gated ion channels are designed to be sensitive to transmembrane voltage differences, they are the most likely target for this effect. Chen et al. measured the consequences of electrical shock on muscle ion channels (Chen & Lee, 1994; Chen et al., 1998) and found potassium channels to be more susceptible to electroconformational damage than sodium channels (Chen & Lee, 1995). The consequences of this effect may underlie the transient nerve and muscle dysfunction post-shock.

SHOCK WAVE INJURY

If the electrical contact involves high voltages in excess of several thousand volts, the current is likely to be arc-mediated. The arc is a hot ionized plasma reaching tem-peratures of 10^4°C or greater instantaneously (Capelli-Schellpfeffer et al., 1998). The resulting pressure pulse results in an acoustic shock wave that can produce serious injury, particularly to someone in a closed space environment. In addition, the shock wave transmits hot plasma directly to the victim resulting in thermal injury as well.

FACTORS INFLUENCING INJURY PATTERN

Factors that determine the anatomic pattern, extent of tissue injury, and relative contribution of heat versus direct electrical damage include the amount of current, anatomic location, contact duration, physical environment of the contact if an arc blast occurs, and health history of the victim. The type of clothing, use of protective gear, and the power capability of the electrical source also contribute to the wide range of clinical manifestations observed in electrical shock victims. In a small enclosed space, a very high-energy electrical arc can produce a strong thermoacoustic blast force leading to significant barotraumas (Capelli-Schellpfeffer et al., 1998). Associated falls and skin burns are frequent, exacerbating the injury. Cataracts characteristically occur following rapid and brief exposure of the eyes to heat and arc-mediated electrical current (Lee et al., 1992).

Electroporation of extremity skeletal muscle and nerve cell membranes should be expected when more that 0.5 to 1 A is passed through the extremity (Lee & Kolodney, 1987b). Electroporation damage accumulates in the timescale of milliseconds. With more prolonged contacts on the range of seconds, thermal damage in the subcutaneous tissues becomes substantial. Because the vulnerability to supraphysiologic temperature exposure is similar regardless of tissue type, when pathological levels of heating occur, all tissues in the current path are burned. Extensive disruption of cell membranes leads to release of myoglobin and hemoglobin, which enter into the circulation. Acute renal failure can result from intrarenal deposition of these iron-containing molecules.

When heat damage predominates, the injury is not only limited to the cell membrane, but other intracellular membranes also are involved, so the damage is likely to be irreversible. These parameters also determine the pattern of injury. Damage by Joule heating is not known to be dependent on cell size, whereas larger cells are more vulnerable to membrane breakdown by electroporation. Cells do survive transient plasma membrane rupture under appropriate circumstances (Block et al., 1995; Lee & Astumian, 1996; Lee et al., 1993). If electroporation is the primary mechanism of damage, then injured tissue may be salvageable and the challenge for the future is to identify a technique to promptly reseal the damaged membranes.

If the electrical contact time is brief relative to the LT parameter defined earlier, cell damage is more likely to be electroporation related. If the contact time is longer than the LT time, both Joule heating and electroporation would be important. Significant membrane permeabilization can be expected to occur in average-sized human skeletal muscle cells exposed to 60 Hz sinusoidal fields with peak amplitudes greater than 25 V cm⁻¹ for any contact time more than 20 to 40 ms. However, the extent of the Joule heating mediated damage depends on the duration of the contact. The Tropea-Lee model (1992) predicts that if the field strength is less than 25 V cm⁻¹, the Joule-heating rate is insufficient to produce a significant tissue temperature rise.

PAIN IN ELECTRICAL INJURY SURVIVORS

PERIPHERAL NERVE PAIN

Pain is a very common symptom and a complex problem in electrical injury survivors (Mankani et al., 1994; Pliskin et al., 1998; Solem, Fischer, & Strate, 1977; Wilbourn, 1995). Headaches, paresthesias, and dysesthesias within the distribution of peripheral nerves included in the current path are typical. In addition to these problems, many electrical injury survivors experience nerve compression symptoms. This may simply correlate to their occupation. But in our experience, most of the patients do not recall having carpal tunnel or other compression neuropathies before the injury. Complex pain syndromes and causalgia are occasionally reported as well.

Most victims of electrical shock experience transient numbness and weakness, followed by pain. The pain usually subsides over time, particularly with adequate medical help. However, some patients have persistent symptoms. The factors that determine whether the pain resolves remain to be determined. As mentioned previously, heavily myelinated fibers are more susceptible to electroporation than unmyelinated fibers, whereas there should be no difference in their relative susceptibility to heat injury. Figure 39.4 shows a plot of the second action potential as a function of the time interval between the second stimulus and the left (top) and right (bottom) ulnar nerves of an electrical injury survivor. The survivor experienced the shock in the right upper extremity. Note that the faster myelinated fibers are not functioning in the electrically injured extremity. This pattern of abnormality is quite common (Abramov et al., 1996).

In our experience (unpublished), we have often found that the peripheral pain experienced by electrical injury survivors seems to respond to a combination of anti-inflammatory cyclooxygenase inhibitors and vitamin antioxidants (ascorbate and tacopherol). We are currently preparing a clinical trial for further verification.

EMOTIONAL AND COGNITIVE CONSEQUENCES

Electrical injury is associated with a high rate of psychiatric morbidity including major depressive disorders, anx-

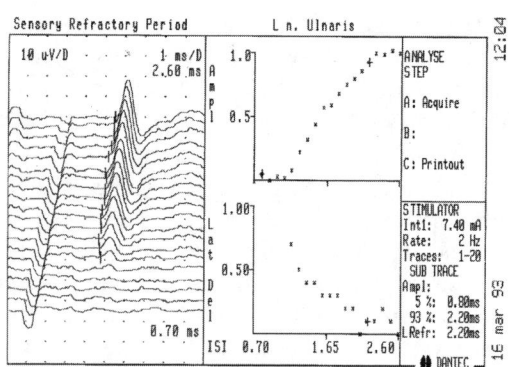

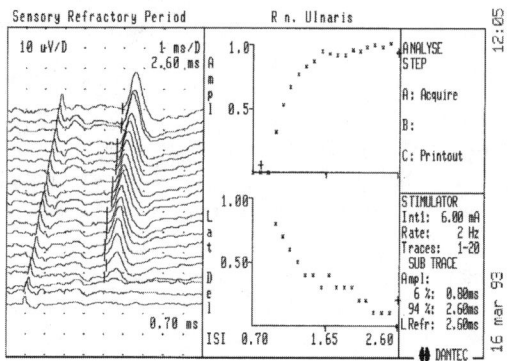

FIGURE 39.4 Refractory period spectral analysis of electrician who received an electrical shock with a current path of left arm to back and legs. Note the loss of fast conducting sensory nerve fibers in the left ulnar nerve.

iety disorders, and post-traumatic stress disorder (Kelley et al., 1999). These problems are commonplace regardless of whether there is direct brain exposure to the electrical shock current. Anxiety and depression certainly have a significant role in pain perception. These psychiatric issues must be managed simultaneously with establishing various approaches to pain management. This requires considerable coordination of effort. A team approach is recommended so that a scheduled dialogue between treating physicians occurs. The treating physician is unlikely to be successful in managing pain related problems without successfully managing the psychiatric problems.

SCAR INFLAMMATION AND PAIN

Lingering effects of wound scar pain is also common in electrical injury survivors (Pliskin et al., 1998). Survivors of major electrical injury heal with scars, which are stiff and often entrap nerves. In addition, burn scars often remain inflamed for a prolonged period leading to painful, pruritic, and hypertrophic scars. The mainstay of clinical management is to reduce inflammation and mechanical tension (Quinby et al., 1978; Roseborough, Grevious, &

Lee, 2004). Topical nonsteriodal agents with an occlusive barrier to increase scar moisture and temperature seem to be effective (Bier et al., 1999). Reconstructive surgery may be necessary to resurface a stiff, scarred, and painful skin surface.

SUMMARY AND CONCLUSIONS

The pathogenesis of electrical injury is now understood to be more complex than the traditional diagnosis of exterior thermal burns (Lee & Astumian, 1996). Treatment and recovery require full comprehension of the mechanism of electrical injury. Injury results by the actions of direct electric force on tissue components and the indirect effect of Joule heating. The kinetics of these injury processes differs so that the clinical presentation depends on the duration of field exposure (Bier et al., 1999). Electrical shock continues to be an important cause of human injury in the workplace. Many victims die immediately from cardiac manifestations, and survivors experience the effects of burn wounds and extensive muscle and nerve damage. Because of increased life support effectiveness, more victims are surviving but with disabling conditions. New diagnostic (Hannig et al., 1999; Hash et al., 1988; Karczmar et al., 1994; Tuch & Lee, 1998) and therapeutic (Basakaran et al., 2001; Lee, 2002; Lee, Capelli-Schellpfeffer & Kelley, 1994) strategies to reduce the tissue loss have been reported by multiple labs. Effective utilization of these strategies will rely on improved diagnostic imaging and on reversing the fundamental problem of cell membrane damage. If successful, these efforts should greatly improve the prognosis of surviving victims following electrical trauma.

ACKNOWLEDGMENTS

The research presented here has been partly supported by the National Institutes of Health Grants R01 GM61101 and R01 GM64757, and The Electric Power Research Institute.

REFERENCES

Abramov, G. et al. (1996). Alteration in sensory nerve function following electrical shock. *Burns, 22*(8), 602.

Basakaran, H. et al. (2001). Poloxamer-188 improves capillary blood flow and tissue viability in a cutaneous burn wound. *Journal of Surgical Research, 101*, 56.

Bier, M. et al. (1999). Kinetics of sealing for transient electropores in isolated mammalian skeletal muscle cells. *Bioelectromagnetics, 20*, 94.

Block, T. A. et al. (1995). Non-thermally mediated muscle injury and necrosis in electrical trauma. *Journal of Burn Care and Rehabilitation, 16*, 581.

Capelli-Schellpfeffer, M. et al. (1998). Correlation between electrical accident parameters and injury. *IEEE. Transactions on Industry Applications, 4*, 25.

Chen, W. et al. (1998). Electric field-induced functional reductions in the K+ channels mainly resulted from supramembrane potential-mediated electroconformational changes. *Biophysical Journal, 75*, 196.

Chen, W., & Lee, R. C. (1994). Altered ion channel conductance and ionic selectivity induced by large imposed membrane potential pulse. *Biophysical Journal, 67*, 603.

Chen, W., & Lee, R. C. (1995). High-intensity electric field-induced reduction of K-channel currents may result from electroconformational changes in channel's voltage sensors: Gating current reduction. *Biophysical Journal, 68*, 354.

Dalziel, C. F. (1943). Effect of frequency on let-go currents. *Transactions. American Institute of Electrical Engineers, 62*, 745.

Dalziel, C. F. (1960). Threshold 60-cycle fibrillating currents. *Transactions. American Institute of Electrical Engineers. III Power Apparatus and Systems, 79*, 667.

Diller, K. R. (1994). The mechanisms and kinetics of heat injury accumulation. Electrical injury: A multidisciplinary approach to therapy, prevention and rehabilitation. *Annals of the New York Academy of Sciences, 720*, 38.

Freiberger, H. (1933). The electrical resistance of the human body to DC and AC currents. (Der elektrische widerstand des menschlichen Korpers gegen technischen gleich und wechselstrom.). *Berlin: Elertrizitatswirtschaft, 32* (17), 373; *32* (2), 442.

Gaylor, D. C., Prakah-Asante, K., & Lee, R. C. (1988). Significance of cell size and tissue structure in electrical trauma. *Journal of Theoretic Biology, 133*, 223.

Hash, M. et al. (1988). Correlation between magnetic resonance imaging and histopathology of an amputated forearm after an electrical injury. *Burns, 24*, 362.

Hannig, J. et al. (1999). Contrast enhanced MRI of electroporation injury. *Journal of Burn Care and Rehabilitation, 20*(1).

Hunt, J. L. (1992). Soft tissue patterns in electric burns. In R. C. Lee, J. F. Burke, & E. G. Cravalho (Eds.), *Electrical trauma: The pathophysiology, manifestations, and clinical management*, New York: Cambridge University Press.

Karczmar, G. S. et al. (1994). Prospects for assessment of the effects of electrical injury by magnetic resonance. Electrical injury: A multidisciplinary approach to therapy, prevention and rehabilitation. *Annals of the New York Academy of Science, 720*, 176.

Kelley, K. M. et al. (1999). Life after electrical injury: Psychiatric and psychosocial sequelae. *Annals of the New York Academy of Science, 888*, 356.

Lee, R. C. (1997). Injury by electrical forces: Pathophysiology, manifestations and therapy. *Current Problems in Surgery, 34*, 677.

Lee, R. C. (2002). Cytoprotection by stabilization of cell membranes. *Annals of the New York Acadamy of Science, 961*, 271.

Lee, R. C. et al. (1988). Role of cell membrane rupture in the pathogenesis of electrical trauma. *Journal of Surgical Research, 44*, 709.

Lee, R. C. et al. (1992). Surfactant-induced sealing of electropermeabilized skeletal muscle membranes *in vivo*. *Proceedings of the National Academy of Sciences*, *89*, 4524.

Lee, R. C., & Kolodney, M. S. (1987a). Electrical injury mechanisms: Dynamics of the thermal response. *Plastic and Reconstructive Surgery, 80*, 663

Lee, R. C., & Kolodney, M. S. (1987b). Electrical injury mechanisms: Electrical breakdown of cell membranes. *Plastic and Reconstructive Surgery, 80*, 672.

Lee, R. C., Burke, J. F., & Cravalho, E.G. (1992). *Electrical trauma: The pathophysiology, manifestations, and clinical management*. New York: Cambridge University Press.

Lee, R. C., Canaday, D. J., & Hammer, S. M. (1993). Transient and stable ionic permeabilization of isolated skeletal muscle cells after electric shock. *Journal of Burn Care and Rehabilitation*, *14*, 528.

Lee, R. C., Capelli-Schellpfeffer, M., & Kelley, K. M. (Eds.). (1994). Electrical injury: A multidisciplinary approach to prevention, therapy and rehabilitation. New York: *Annals of the New York Academy of Science, 720.*

Lee, R.C., & Astumian, R. D. (1996). The physicochemical basis for thermal and non-thermal burn injury. *Burns, 22*, 509.

Mankani, M. et al. (1994). Detection of peripheral nerve injury in electrical shock patients. *Annals of the New York Academy of Sciences, 720*, 206.

Pennes, H. H. (1948). Analysis of tissue and arterial blood temperatures in the resting human forearm. *Journal of Applied Physics, 1*, 93.

Pliskin, N. H. et al. (1998). Neuropsychological symptom presentation following electrical injury. *Journal of Trauma, 44*, 709.

Poppendieck, H. F. et al. (1966). Thermal and electrical conductivities of biological fluids and tissues. Reports under Contract No. ONR 4095(00) specifically: DDC No. Ad 630 712. Solana Beach, CA: Geoscience Ltd.

Quinby, W. C., Jr. et al. (1978). The use of microscopy as a guide to primary excision of high-tension electrical burns. *Journal of Trauma, 18*, 423.

Roseborough, I. E., Grevious, M. A., & Lee, R. C. (2004). Prevention and treatment of excessive dermal scarring. *Journal of the National Medical Association, 96*(1), 108.

Rouge, R. G., & Dimick, A. R. (1978). The treatment of electrical injury compared to burn injury: A review of pathophysiology and comparison of patient management protocols. *Journal of Trauma, 18*, 43.

Solem, L., Fischer, R. P., & Strate, R.G. (1977). The natural history of electrical injury. *Journal of Trauma, 17*, 847.

Tropea, B. I., & Lee, R. C. (1992). Thermal injury kinetics in electrical trauma. *Journal of Biomechical Engineering, 114*(2), 241.

Tsong, T. Y., & Astumian, R. D. (1987). Electroconformational coupling and membrane protein function. *Progress in Biophysics and Molecular Biology, 50*, 1.

Tsong, T. Y., & Astumian, R. D. (1988). Electroconformational coupling: How membrane-bound ATPase transduces energy from dynamic electric fields. *Annual Review of Physiology, 50*, 273.

Tuch D. S., & Lee, R.C. (1998). Three-dimensional wound surface area calculations with a CAD surface element model. *IEEE. Transaction on Biomedical Engineering, 45*, 1397.

Wiggers, C. J. & Wégria, R. (1939). Ventricular fibrillation due to single, localized induction and condenser shocks applied during the vulnerable phase of ventricular systole. *American Journal of Physiology, 128*, 500.

Wilbourn, A. J. (1995). Peripheral nerve disorders in electrical and lightning injuries. *Seminars in Neurology, 15*, 241.

Section IV

Diagnostic Tests and Evaluations

A. Elizabeth Ansel, RN, Section Editor

40

Psychological Assessment Tools in Clinical Pain Management

Kathleen U. Farmer-Cady, PsyD

INTRODUCTION

Assessment tools for the psychologist are as vital as the stethoscope and blood pressure cuff are to the physician. Patients' scores on these tools provide a backdrop for understanding them and setting hypotheses to help them unlock maladaptive behaviors. Individuals with chronic pain are doing the best they can. When they seek treatment in a pain management program, they most likely have failed self-management efforts and are subjugating themselves to the rigors of a pain management program out of a sense of desperation. They do not know what else to do, and they fear that pain will continue to force them into a sub-optimal life in which relief is questionable and being able to function normally, out of reach.

The most effective way to intervene is to see the dilemma through the eyes of the patient. If patients are depressed and at the end of their ropes, the psychologist needs to help them find a stake in life, someone or something that will motivate them to change their perceptions and let go of self-defeating habits. They see themselves as failures and hunger for therapists to say something positive about them. They yearn for hope that this walk through the valley of the shadow of death is nearly over and there is bright sunshine around the next bend. Psychological assessment provides these cues into the inner workings of the patient.

The goal of a psychological evaluation is to learn the best approach for the patient to ameliorate the pain syndrome. It is an investigation of the milestones in that person's life that helps the psychologist hone in on an area that may be especially sensitive to the patient: a married,

menopausal woman who is childless; a 23-year-old female, abandoned by her mother at birth and raised by her maternal grandmother; a police officer who retired after his home was burned and his family assaulted by criminals seeking revenge. These are the barriers to healing that assessment tools uncover, setting the stage for interdisciplinary treatment.

These tools are primarily diagnostic. They are sensitive to disorders that would make active participation in an interdisciplinary program unlikely. These tools include

1. Intelligence: Average intelligence is necessary; a person with an IQ of 89 or below thinks in concrete terms. Abstract ideas, goal setting, and visualizing a brighter future are often incomprehensible to such an intellect.

2. Cognitive functioning: The individual who has suffered a head injury, even whiplash, should be administered neuropsychological testing to identify possible cognitive impairment. Typically, these individuals will attempt to cover-up their inability to make change, follow directions, or read highway signs. Even though they know they are confused, they are ashamed that they cannot function at the level they were pre-injury. Cognitive retraining may be necessary for the person to gain compensatory skills before enrolling in a pain program.

3. Thought disorder: A basic goal of pain management is to change the individual's perception of the discomfort that is interfering with daily

569

functioning. However, when that person has grossly distorted perception (hallucinations) or believes physical problems have occurred through a convoluted thinking process (delusions), there exists no common ground on which to begin the process of therapy and healing. In these cases, the patient needs to be stabilized on a neuroleptic medication before being accepted into a pain program.

4. Personality disorder: The central feature of people with personality disorders is that they accept no responsibility for their behaviors and project blame onto those around them. Within an interdisciplinary pain program, they greatly admire whoever they are with but criticize other members of the staff. In other words, they split the staff. When disagreements arise about a patient at a team meeting, that patient most likely has a personality disorder. To identify such a person ahead of time allows the staff to prepare to treat this individual with firm boundaries and limits and resist requests for special treatment. The diagnosis relies on evaluating the individual's long-term patterns of functioning that are inflexible and maladaptive but stable and cause significant functional impairment. They seek attention (negative as well as positive) to boost self-esteem and they display inconsistency between words and behaviors. They often do not follow through with treatment plans or medication contracts. They also tend to procrastinate and be noncooperative when confronted with a condition or rule of the program. They may be oppositional and self-righteous. Psychological tests designed specifically to identify personality disorders usually yield too many false positives. On the Minnesota Multiphasic Personality Inventory-2 (MMPI-2), an elevated Scale 6, 7, or 8 with a conversion V (Scales 1 and 3 at T-score of 65 or above) is often predictive of a personality disorder.

5. Analgesic rebound headache: An individual who has headaches 15 or more days per month and takes medicine on these days to treat these headaches probably has analgesic rebound headache. That means the medication taken for the headaches is actually perpetuating them. The dilemma is that no other medication will help the headaches until the offending medication is stopped. If the person is taking an opioid or butalbital combination, a tapered withdrawal is indicated; other classes of medication can be stopped abruptly. The patient should not be admitted into the pain program until withdrawal symptoms have subsided, which may take several weeks. A preventative medication (such as an antiepileptic drug) and a clonidine patch are often prescribed to assist the patient through this difficult time of detoxification.

STRUCTURED CLINICAL INTERVIEW

The interviewer has a list of questions to ask the individual directly. However, at the same time, there are questions to be answered covertly through behaviors displayed during the interview and through elaboration of the answers. The following is a list of covert questions in the back of the psychologist's mind during the interview and while interpreting the assessment measures.

COVERT QUESTIONS

1. Is the pain real? Does the patient show obvious or exaggerated signs of being uncomfortable? Does the patient appear well-groomed, smiling during descriptions of excruciating pain, and seemingly unscathed by the reported discomfort?

2. Does the patient have hope or resources for the process of recovery? Does the patient indicate a desire for a new direction or a broader horizon? When hopelessness is reframed as an opportunity, what is the person's reaction? Anger? Ridicule? Excitement?

3. What does pain mean to the patient? Often the person has never considered this question. During the interview, summarize the answers into a formula that may become the focus of treatment.

Meaning of Pain	Focus of Treatment
Punishment/atonement	Self-forgiveness
Strength/taking on others' pain	Set protective boundaries
Victimization	Affirmations: independence
Focus of life	Create other interests
Destruction of quality of life	Define new life path
Numbing to life/emotion	Get in touch with body
Physical pain disguises emotional pain	Identify/release pain memories

4. What are the patient's strengths/resources?
   Supportive relationship with spouse/family
   Employed/desire to return to work
   Impaired but not incapacitated
   Sense of humor
   Religious conviction/faith
   Willing to try new approach
   Able to participate in therapy
   Positive outlook

5. Can the patient give up pain or must residual pain remain?

6. The number of years that pain has been part of the patient's life has taken a toll. Regardless of the years that the current pain has existed, often there is a history of earlier bouts with pain, which were overcome or healed, indicating a positive prognosis. However, the longer that the patient has attempted to cope with chronic pain, the more likely that psychological maladaptations have developed. These include fear that nothing can help, anger at the medical system for being unable to help/fix patient, outrage that God has forgotten him or her, despair over ever functioning "normally" again.

7. Things will get worse before they get better. A breakthrough psychologically will increase pain level temporarily.

STRUCTURED PAIN INTERVIEW

1. When and how did the pain start: injury, illness, assault, spontaneously?
2. What else was going on at that time?
3. How have you coped since then?
4. What medications and treatments have you taken? What worked and what didn't?
5. Education/employment
6. Hobbies
7. Religion
8. Describe typical day

TRENDS THAT DIRECT TREATMENT

During the structured clinical interview, the psychologist listens for themes that direct further investigation and may become the focus of the treatment plan. There are five dominant themes among pain patients from a psychological perspective:

1. *Theme*: Cold hands, cold feet, cannot relax, no power over pain
   Intervention: Temperature biofeedback

Finger temperature is an indicator of the level of stress the individual is carrying within the body. Those with a chronic condition usually have a finger temperature in the 70s, compared with the average finger temperature of 85°F. Biofeedback is the process of training the body to regulate an automatic physiological function. Under the assault of pain, the body responds automatically with the fight-or-flight sympathetic reaction. By warming the finger to 96°F, the emergency response is replaced by the relaxation response. By incorporating biofeedback into daily living, the parasympathetic system balances the sympathetic response to pain and maintains physiological homeostasis. In this way, the process of thermal biofeedback lowers the overall rating of pain and provides the individual with at least a brief reprieve from chronic pain. Biofeedback is a tool that gives the person a level of control over pain. (Finger thermometers or "Plain Stress Meters ST60" can be ordered from www.cliving.org; Conscious Living Foundation, P.O. Box 9, Drain, OR 97435; 800-578-7377.)

2. *Theme*: Negative self-talk. Puts self down. history of abuse. difficult childhood
   Intervention: Cognitive behavioral, using positive affirmations

Negative self-talk is an automatic private conversation that goes on inside a person's mind in response to an occurrence in the environment which degrades or berates the individual. Often these negative evaluations of oneself are unconscious. Under guidance from a psychologist, the individual identifies and records in a diary the downgrading messages that occur. The patient composes positive affirmations to replace the negative self-talk and repeats these affirmations frequently enough to delete the negative self-talk. With patients with pain, the first affirmation is often, "I forgive myself for being imperfect."

3. *Theme*: People pleasers who measure self-worth in terms of acceptance by others
   Intervention: Learn to say no

These individuals believe that by saying "no" or standing up for themselves, they will be rejected, abandoned, or confronted. They actually fear aggression, both from themselves and others, and confuse assertiveness with aggression. They believe the only way to avoid aggression is to be passive and compliant, often to the detriment of their health. They require assertiveness training. The first step is to identify those behaviors that are asked of them but they do not want to do, which is usually signaled by feelings of guilt, anxiety, ignorance, or dread. They are given the assignment to say "no" in unimportant situations, such as to the cashier in a supermarket. The third step is to say "no" to those who will understand, such as a friend. And finally, to successfully achieve assertiveness, they need to say "no" to the person who demands behaviors that they do not want to do.

4. *Theme*: Feels only pain
   Intervention: Get in touch with body; go beneath pain to feel other feelings and sensations

After the onslaught of pain, the body may shut down to other feelings. What's left is a sense of numbness. To begin re-sensitizing the body, the patient needs to attain a state of relaxation, both of the body and the mind. Biofeedback, meditation, yoga, or other mind-clearing exercise helps the body and mind reach a state of detachment. The patient is led through the process of imagining where the body carries various feelings, such as joy, envy, love, jealousy, and anger. One feeling at a time is identified and located. As other feelings surface, the overall level of pain is usually reduced.

5. *Theme*: World is upside down: Existential crisis
   Intervention: Answers to following questions: Who am I? What am I doing here? Where am I going?

Pain forces us to recognize our vulnerability and our lack of control over our lives. It reshuffles our beliefs and pushes us to reevaluate our worth. Often a patient has to give up a profession or a way of life that has served him or her well. There is a sense of being adrift without direction and being drawn into a downward spiraling whirlwind. Can the person regain a stable foundation? A knowledge that better things are ahead?

The three major questions of existence — Who am I? What am I doing here? Where am I going? — are asked of the patient, one at a time. The task is to write "Who am I?" on the top of a sheet of paper and list everything that comes to mind without editing, without censoring. This process takes at least 1 day, sometimes as much as 1 week. The insights and lessons are discussed with the psychotherapist who challenges the patient to greater depth into searching the self for answers.

ASSESSMENT TOOLS

The standard procedure of many interdisciplinary pain programs is to mail background and demographic questionnaires to the patient before the first visit. The patient returns the completed forms to the clinic by mail or at the first visit. The process allows for clinicians to review the data and structure their time with the patient. It is also educational for patients to have them prioritize complaints, summarize previous treatments and their effects, and consider the association among stress, psychological issues, and lifestyle habits on pain. Of the following psychological assessment measures, half of them are administered by a psychologist in the clinic; the other half are sent with the information packet for the patient to answer at home. These are Zung Depression Inventory, Visual Analog Scale, HIT-6 and MIDAS if headaches are part of the pain problem, diary to be filled out until the first visit, and the Symptom Check List.

1. Intelligence test (Wechsler Abbreviated Scale of Intelligence, WASI; Wechsler, 1999) when the patient is having obvious difficulties reading, interacting, comprehending, retaining information. The WASI is similar in format and highly correlated with the Wechsler Adult Intelligence Scales (Goebel & Satz, 1975; Tulsky & Zhu, 2000). This short form provides a valid and reliable measure of intelligence and includes four subtests, two verbal and two performance indicators. These are Vocabulary, Similarities, Block Design, and Matrix Reasoning. Vocabulary measures verbal knowledge and fund of information. It is the single best predictor of general intelligence. Similarities measures verbal concept formation, abstract reasoning, and general intellectual ability. Block Design measures nonverbal concept formation, visual-motor coordination, and perceptual organization by requiring the person to put together geometric designs using two-color cubes to match a picture of the design. Matrix Reasoning measures nonverbal fluid reasoning by requesting the individual to complete a missing portion of an abstract, gridded pattern.

2. Mental Efficiency Workload Test (MEWT), programmed on a Palm 130, is a neuropsychological measure of cognitive efficiency. The score is reported as throughput, which is the number of correct responses over milliseconds. Two tasks, Simple Reaction Time (SRT), which measures the speed of the hardwiring of the nervous system, and Continuous Performance Test (CPT), which measures short-term memory, focus, attention, concentration, were derived from the Automated Neuropsychological Assessment Metrics (ANAM), Version 1.0 (Reeves, Kane, Winter, Raynsford, & Pancella (1994). Developed by the military, the ANAM consists of 30 computerized neuropsychological tests, from which SRT and CPT were chosen specifically to measure the cognitive efficiency of individuals suffering from disabling headaches but have been shown to measure the effects of any type of pain on cognition. However, all 30 tests are highly sensitive to central nervous system integrity and are designed for the repeated-measures paradigm. Through repeated measures, each trial is rated against the baseline performance of the individual. A drop in performance indicates a drop of cognitive efficiency due to a compromised nervous system.

   The MEWT takes only 5 minutes to complete and is especially effective for measuring the impact of different modalities, especially biofeedback and opioids, on patients' performances. Often, even though they may believe they can function better using opioids, they discover that their reaction time is so slow, they cannot tap the button on the Palm 130 to indicate they saw a stimulus on the screen. This is an objective indication that their cognitive performances are being negatively affected by medication. Likewise, biofeedback has the potential to enhance cognitive efficiency, which motivates patients to practice biofeedback every day. Using the Palm, mental efficiency can be tracked daily.

3. Zung Depression Inventory (Zung, 1965, 1973) is a self-rating depression scale for quantifying symptoms of depression. Depression is defined operationally as a syndrome comprising coexisting signs and symptoms that signify the presence of pathological changes in the areas of mood (sad, tearful) and physiological (sleep, libido, appetite, fatigue), psychomotor (agitation, slow moving), and psychological functioning (suicidal, confusion, emptiness). The response to each of the 20 statements of the Zung may be "None or little of the time;" "Some of the time;" "Good part of the time;" or "Most or all of the time." Patients are asked to respond according to how well the statement describes their perceptions during the past week. Half of the statements are worded symptomatically positive and half are presented negatively to interfere with the patient's ability to discern a trend in answers.

The raw scores are converted into an index. An index below 50 indicates no psychopathology; 50 through 59, minimal to mild depression; 60 through 69, moderate to marked depression; and 70 and over, severe to extreme depression. Validation studies compared the scores of depressed versus nondepressed patients as well as depressed patients versus normal subjects ages 20 to 64. The majority of patients with chronic daily headache scored between 60 and 70.

4. Halstead-Reitan Trails A and B are a quick neuropsychological measure of the overall level of functioning of the brain in terms of problem solving. The tasks require an ability to scan the environment quickly and put the stimuli in proper sequence. Trail A consists of 25 circles, each containing a number (1 to 25), printed on a sheet of white 8×11 in. paper. The person is asked to connect the circles in numerical order without lifting the pencil. If there is a mistake, the examiner immediately asks the individual to correct the error. Trail A is the "warm up" test to Trail B, which also consists of 25 circles but half contain numbers 1 through 13 and the other half are lettered A through L. The task is to connect the circles, alternating from numbers to letters, i.e., A, 1, B, 2, etc. The scores for Trails A and B represent the number of seconds required to complete the tests. A normal score for Trail B is 85 seconds or less; 86 to 120 seconds means mildly impaired; more than 120 seconds, seriously impaired (Reitan & Wolfson, 1985).

5. Visual Analog Scale (VAS) of pain severity is presented graphically with a 10-cm line and end point adjective descriptors ("The Worst Imaginable Pain" on one end and "No Pain" on the other). The patient is asked to place a mark along the line to indicate the current pain level. A difference of 13 mm between consecutive ratings of pain is the minimum change in a pain rating that is clinically significant (Gallagher, Liebman, & Bijur, 2001).

6. Verbal Numeric Analog Scale: On a scale of 0 to 10, with 0 being no pain and 10 being the worst pain imaginable, what would the patient rate his/her current pain? This measure is asked and recorded in the patient's chart before and after each treatment modality in the pain program.

7. Many patients with pain complain of headaches. Because there are migraine-specific medications other than analgesics that can treat headaches effectively, it is important to differentiate the impact of headaches from other somatic symptoms on the overall rating of disability associated with pain. The Headache Impact Test (HIT-6™) (Kosinski, Bayliss, Bjorner, Ware et al., 2003) lists six questions by which to measure the impact that headaches have had on the person's life over the past 4 weeks. Scores range from less than 50, little or no impact, to 60 or more, very severe impact. The HIT-6 score has been correlated with the number of hours of lost workplace productivity over the previous 4 weeks; those with no or mild impact lost 2 hours of workplace productivity; some impact, 3 hours; substantial impact, 8 hours; and those with very severe impact (score 60 or more) lost 18 hours of workplace productivity over the previous 4 weeks. In this way, disabling headaches affect not only the individual but also colleagues, employer, family, and others depending on the individual to function at a certain level. The U.S. population mean for recent headache sufferers is 50 with a standard deviation of 10. A score difference as little as 3 points is noteworthy; 5 points is highly significant. The Migraine Disability Assessment (MIDAS) Questionnaire (Stewart,

Lipton, Kolodner, Liberman, & Sawyer, 1999) measures headache-related disability based on five disability questions from three domains of activity: employment (job or school), household work, and family, social, and leisure activities. The score is obtained by summing the number of days of missed activities and reduced productivity over 3 months. Scores range from Grade I (0 to 5), minimal or infrequent disability; Grade II (6 to 10), mild disability; Grade III (11 to 20), moderate disability; and finally Grade IV (21+), severe disability. The drawback of the MIDAS is that headache sufferers often fail to remember or admit that they missed as much of work or other activities as they did.

8. Diary or calendar: Daily log of pain rating, medication taken, and ability to function scale. (See the Headache Care Center Diary in Appendix 40.A at the end of this chapter.)

9. Symptom Check List is essentially a review of systems developed by Headache Care Center personnel for patients to report somatic complaints (see end of this chapter). There is evidence that the more areas of the body with pain, the lower the prognosis for rehabilitation (Freedenfeld, Bailey, Bruns et al., 2002).

10. Minnesota Multiphasic Personality Inventory-2 (MMPI-2) (Butcher, Dahlstrom, Graham, Tellegen, & Kaemmer, 1989; Piotrowski & Lubin, 1990) provides an objective, reliable appraisal of an individual's behavioral adaptation to the current life situation. It consists of 567 true-or-false statements, which usually takes a patient 1 1/2 to 2 hours to complete. The biggest challenge for the psychologist is to motivate the patient to answer all the questions. It is preferable for the patient to complete the inventory in one sitting while at the clinic under supervision. However, patients with pain may require several time periods before completion. The test may be administered by computer or using an answer sheet and pencil. The results can be either scanned or entered by hand into a computer. A computerized report is then produced. A computer printout objectifies the results, making an interpretation of the results to the patient more palatable. The response graphs are explained to the patients as how they scored in relation to the normative sample; that is, they were either high or low on each scale. By expanding the test results into potential goals of the treatment program, the patients are steered toward changes that they may never have previously considered.

MMPI

The MMPI (Graham, 1987; Hathaway & McKinley, 1943) is the most studied objective behavioral assessment tool in the history of psychological testing. The interpretative data available on the MMPI have spanned countless research projects over more than 50 years of clinical use. The MMPI has been the clinical assessment tool most frequently administered in the United States (Lubin, Larsen, & Matarazzo, 1984) and some 12,000 books and articles on the inventory have been published. In addition, the MMPI has been translated into more than 115 languages and is used in 45 countries (Butcher, 1985).

In 1989, the MMPI was revised; 14% of the original items were rewritten and 154 new items were included to measure additional personality dimensions and problems. The MMPI-2 normative data were based on 2,600 subjects randomly solicited from several regions of the United States (Butcher, 1990).

Even though, initially, the MMPI results were categorized into 4 validity scales and 10 basic clinical scales, the MMPI-2 has additional scales and indices that delve deeper into the finer aspects of the person's motivation, much like peeling the proverbial onion. When patients are limited in or lack insight into their maladaptive ways of adjusting to their pain syndrome, the divergence between the results of the MMPI-2 and the patients' histories and backgrounds can become the focus of intervention. Often, these individuals have the "fix me" mentality, where they expect to invest little of themselves yet free themselves from pain. At other times, the MMPI-2 may categorize patients' responses as falling "within normal limits" (no standard validity or clinical scale T-score equaling 65 or higher). This means that their pain syndrome is neither distressing nor upsetting to them, which points to a poor prognosis for intervention.

A computerized interpretation of the MMPI-2 (Greene, Brown, & Kovan, 1998) has a database of 295 code types and corresponding interpretations to which a specific MMPI-2 profile can be matched. Interpretations are possible for 55 spike and two-point codetypes, and 238 three-point codetypes that occurred at least 20 times in the research data set ($N = 32,716$). Data from the MMPI-2 are admissible as evidence in a court of law.

Because patients with pain often score a conversion-V (codetype 1-3/3-1) on the MMPI-2, it is interesting to note that this is the third most popular configuration within the MMPI-2 database, making up 65% of the sample. However, the interpretation of this profile is much different for the pain patient than for the psychiatric patient. The assumption of the 1-3/3-1 codetype is that the individual has somatic complaints that have no basis in reality. These include headaches, chest pain, back pain, and numbness or tremors of the extremities. Eating disorders are common as are complaints of weakness, fatigue, dizziness, and sleep disturbance. These individuals express emotional distress through physical symptoms and generally feel minimal levels of anxiety and depression. They show little concern about their physical problems.

By contrast, the answers by patients with pain that produce a conversion-V accurately portray their experiences. Scale 3 has 60 items that cover two general areas: physical problems and social facility, for example "My sleep is fitful and disturbed" [T]; "I feel weak all over much of the time" [T]; "I am bothered by an upset stomach several times a week" [T]; "It is safer to trust nobody" [F]; "At times I feel like swearing" [F]. For these reasons, after scoring a conversion-V on the MMPI-2, verification of the patient's history is paramount before assuming that the patient's problems are not real.

In terms of pain management, elevated validity scales (lie, L, 15 items; infrequency, F, 60 items; and subtle defensiveness, K, 30 items), paranoia (Scale 4, 40 items), negative work attitudes (WRK, 33 items), and negative treatment indicators (TRT, 26 items) are especially important. The validity scales indicate attitudes that invalidate the test scores and suggest that the person is attempting to present himself or herself in a false manner. The truthfulness of the individual is questioned. Scale 4 measures the patient's trust in interpersonal relationships and the belief that he or she is a target for bad events. These misinterpretations are very difficult to undo during a pain management program because they are based on a lifetime of experiences. This extreme defensive posture is in fact an effort to control and protect the individual. Those with a negative work attitude would not want return to work as a goal. Those with a high negative treatment indicator may not fit into an interdisciplinary treatment program.

The possibility of a personality disorder needs to be further investigated.

CONCLUSIONS

Psychological assessment tools involve more than tests. Central to the process is active listening to the patient, incorporating verbal and nonverbal communication, covert and direct messages, and using the patient's language to reinforce what the psychologist heard. Interpretation of test data is more than reporting scores (Rapaport, Gill, & Schafer, 1986). It is integrating the findings into an understandable, accurate picture of the patient. It also involves sharing the findings with the patient in a therapeutic manner, which helps the patient accept self-attributes or issues that were previously unknown, such as a behavior pattern of ignoring emotional stressors. For this person, the goal of identifying and facing emotional stressors would be an important part of the treatment plan. While scores reflect a slice of a person's response repertoire at the present moment, these are taken from a much richer background of the individual. There are also formal aspects, such as answering all the questions or writing in responses instead of answering True or False. In addition, verbalizations during the testing period should be recorded as well as behaviors, such as affect and expressive style.

Pain is an assault on the individual and as such it produces physical, mental, and spiritual repercussions. Pain invariably changes the person's life, perception, and belief system. The purpose of an interdisciplinary pain program is to reframe these changes into an opportunity for growth and positive redirection. Assessment helps navigate these attempts into channels within the patient that have previously been blocked or are misguided.

APPENDIX A: SYMPTOM CHECK LIST

PLESE CHECK <u>YES</u> OR <u>NO</u>

	YES		NO
	Now	In the past	

GENERAL
Decrease or increase in appetite
Fever / night sweats
Hypoglycemia: shakiness/weakness
Recent weight change _____ pounds ⇑⇓
Skin disorder
Snoring
Weakness / fatigue

HEAD AND NECK
Cataracts / blindness
Change in vision
Injury to eye/ ear
Ear infections
Hearing loss
Ringing in ears
Frequent colds or sinusitis
Nasal / sinus congestion
Frequent nosebleeds

BLOOD
Anemia
Blood transfusion(s): date_____
Easy bruising / bleeding
Swollen glands / mononucleosis

BONES AND JOINTS
Back pain / injury
Gout
Joint pain
Morning joint stiffness
Nightly leg cramps or jerking
Swollen, red, or warm joints

LUNGS
Blood in sputum
Daily cough
Exposure to TB / Positive TB skintest
Falling asleep while working or driving
Lung disease / emphysema
Pleurisy
Shortness of breath
Wheezing / asthma

	YES		NO
	Now	In the past	

KIDNEY AND BLADDER
Blood in urine
Difficulty starting stream
Discomfort with urination
Frequent daytime urination
Hernia in groin area
History of kidney stones
History of urinary tract infections
History of venereal disease
Loss of bladder control
Loss of sexual interest
Nighttime urination:_____ times per night
Practice birth control: Method _____
Sexually active

HEART AND CIRCULATION
Ankle or foot swelling / leg swelling
Chest discomfort / tightness / pain
Heart attack
Heart murmur / rheumatic fever
High blood pressure
Irregular heart beat / palpitations
Leg pain when walking
Mitral valve prolapse
Shortness of breath when lying down
Varicose veins / phlebitis

NERVOUS SYSTEM
Difficulty speaking
Difficulty walking
Difficulty with memory
Difficulty writing
Dizziness / vertigo
Double vision
History of head injury
Loss of consciousness / blacking out
Meningitis
Numbness / tingling
Paralysis / stroke
Sciatica
Seizures / convulsions
Severe headaches
Tremors / shakes

Name: _____   Date: _____   MR#:_____

PLEASE CHECK **YES OR NO**

YES		NO
Now	In the past	

STOMACH AND BOWELS

			Abdominal pain /discomfort
			Black or bloody stools
			Change in bowel habits
			Colon problems
			Constipation
			Crohn's disease / ulcerative colitis
			Diarrhea / frequent loose stools
			Difficulty with swallowing
			Diverticulosis
			Gallbladder disease
			Heartburn / indigestion
			Hemorrhoids
			Jaundice / hepatitis
			Nausea orvomiting
			Pancreatitis
			Poor eating habits
			Ulcers / vomiting blood
			Use antacids: How often?_____

WOMEN

MENSTRUAL HISTORY

Age of onset_____ Last period_____

Last pap smear_____Normal / Abnormal

Number of pregnancies _____

Number of miscarriages _____

Number of abortions _____

			Heavy menstrual flow / clotting
			Hot flashes
			Irregular periods
			Menopause
			Painful intercourse
			Severe menstrual cramps
			Vaginal itching
			Vaginal spotting

BREASTS

			Had mammogram: date of last exam_____
			Lump in breast
			Nipple discharge
			Perform monthly self-exam

MEN

			Hernia / rupture
			Impotence
			Penile sores or discharge
			Prostate infection
			Testicular pain or lumps

YES		NO
Now	In the past	

OTHER SYMPTOMS

			A wish to be dead and away
			Alcohol overuse
			Crying spells
			Depression / frequent unhappiness
			Difficulty falling asleep or staying asleep
			Drug overuse
			Panic attacks
			Severe exhaustion / fatigue
			Stress
			Trouble concentrating
			Trouble sleeping
			Use diet pills

Name: _____   Date: _____   MR#:_____

MY DISCOMFORT REPORT CARD

Directions:

1) Evaluate level of discomfort that you treat.
2) Record results of treatment:
    Y= I obtained the goals outlined.
    N= I did not obtain my goals.
3) Record all medicines used on your calendar.
4) Bring this calendar with you to your next doctor's visit.

Goals:

1) Be able to function.
2) Use medicines as prescribed.

Monday	Tuesday	Wednesday	Thursday	Friday	Saturday	Sunday	Was I able to function? Y or N

Treatment Plan:

1) Treat all discomfort as soon as you know it is likely to interfere with your function.
2) Treat discomfort before the pain is moderate to severe.
3) Rest for 30 minutes after taking meds.
4) Other_____

Tips for Success

1) Keep your discomfort medicines with you.
2) Do not skip meals.
3) Establish consistent wake & sleep schedules.
4) Do something for yourself everyday, ex. go for a walk, relaxation.
5) Analyze each "No" response on the diary and make notes about why your goal was not achieved.

REFERENCES

Butcher, J. N. (1985). Current developments in MMPI use: An international perspective. In J. N. Butcher & C. D. Spielberger (Eds.), *Advances in personality assessment.* Hillsdale, NJ: Lawrence Erlbaum Press.

Butcher, J. N. (1990). *MMPI-2 in psychological treatment.* New York: Oxford University Press.

Butcher, J. N., Dahlstrom, W. G., Graham, J. R., Tellegen, A. M., & Kaemmer, B. (1989). *MMPI-2: Manual for administration and scoring.* Minneapolis: University of Minnesota Press.

Freedenfeld, R., Bailey, B. E., Bruns, D. et al. (2002, August). The ability of the Battery for Health Improvement to predict treatment outcome and barriers to rehabilitation. Poster session presented at International Association for the Study of Pain.

Gallagher, E. J., Liebman, M., & Bijur, P. E. (2001). Prospective validation of clinically important changes in pain severity measured on a visual analog scale. *Annals of Emergency Medicine, 38,* 633.

Goebel, R. A., & Satz, P. (1975). Profile analysis and the Abbreviated Wechsler Adult Intelligence Scale: A multivariate approach. *Journal of Consulting and Clinical Psychology, 43,* 780–785.

Graham, J. R. (1987). *The MMPI, a practical guide* (2nd ed.). New York: Oxford University Press.

Greene, R. L., Brown, R. C., & Kovan, R. E. (1998). *MMPI-2 adult interpretive system.* Lutz, FL: Psych Assessment Resources.

Hathaway, S. R., & McKinley, J. C. (1943). *The Minnesota multiphasic personality schedule.* Minneapolis: University of Minnesota Press.

Kosinski, M., Bayliss, M. S., Bjorner, J. B., & Ware, J. E. et al. (2003). A six-item short-form survey for measuring headache impact: The HIT-6. *Quality of Life Research, 12*(8), 963–974.

Lubin, B., Larsen, R. M., & Matarazzo, J. (1984). Patterns of psychological test usage in the United States. *American Psychologist, 39,* 451.

Piotrowski, C., & Lubin, B. (1990). Assessment practices of health psychologists: Survey of APA Division 38 clinicians. *Professional Psychology: Research & Practice, 21,* 99.

Rapaport, D., Gill, M. M., & Schafer, R. (1986). *Diagnostic psychological testing.* Madison, CT: International Universities Press.

Reeves, D., Kane, R., Winter, K., Raynsford, K., & Pancella, T. (1994). *Automated Neuropsychological Assessment Metrics (ANAM): Test administrators guide version 1.0.* San Diego: National Cognition Recovery Foundation.

Reitan, R. M., & Wolfson, D. (1985). *The Halstead–Reitan neuropsychological test battery.* Tucson, AZ: Neuropsychology Press.

Stewart, W. F., Lipton, R. B., Kolodner, K., Liberman, J., & Sawyer, J. (1999). Reliability of the migraine disability assessment scores in a population-based sample of headache sufferers. *Cephalalgia, 19,* 107–114.

Tulsky, D. S., & Zhu, J. (2000). Could test length or order affect scores on Letter Number Sequencing of the WAIS-III and WMS-III? Ruling out effects of fatigue. *Clinical Neuropsychology, 14,* 474–478.

Wechsler, D. (1999). *Wechsler abbreviated scale of intelligence (WASI).* San Antonio, TX: Psychological Corp.

Zung, W. K. (1965). A self-rating depression scale. *Archives of General Psychiatry, 12,* 63.

Zung, W. W. K. (1973). From art to science: the diagnosis and treatment of depression. *Archives of General Psychiatry, 29,* 328.

41

Laboratory Testing in Pain Disorders

W. John Diamond, MD

INTRODUCTION

Our most primitive indicator of tissue injury, or of a threatening noxious stimulus, is the sensation of pain. Pain is a very subjective symptom employed by our biology to bring attention to a harmful stimulus in our inner or outer environment. As a protective mechanism of homeostasis, pain is defined by the individual patient as to its presence, significance, acuteness, quality, or intensity. Because pain is so personal and nonlinear in its presentation, therefore, does the laboratory have a role in the measurement of pain, or can the laboratory even help in the assessment and management of pain? Young (1979) listed the reasons for ordering laboratory tests in the course of patient care:

- To diagnose disease
- To screen for disease
- To determine the severity of disease
- To determine the appropriate management of the patient
- To monitor progress of the disease and to monitor therapy
- To monitor drug toxicity
- To predict response to treatment

ROLE OF THE LABORATORY IN PAIN MANAGEMENT

Certainly, we cannot diagnose or screen for pain in the clinical laboratory. But we can make underlying diagnoses, that are not normally encountered in everyday practice and that, by their pathophysiology, produce atypical pain, such as the abdominal pain of porphyria or sickle cell anemia. The laboratory can determine the severity of disease or response to treatment, such as monitoring the urine for the quantity of *N*-telopeptide cross-links as an indicator of the rate of osteoporosis or assessment of antiresorptive therapy. Drug screening and therapeutic drug levels of narcotics and anti-inflammatory drugs are now commonplace.

LABORATORY ASSESSMENT OF PAIN SYNDROMES

Margoles (1990) routinely orders the following screening tests for all patients with pain problems and possible underlying perpetuating factors:

- Comprehensive metabolic panel
- Lipid panel
- Complete blood count, platelets, and white cell differential count
- Erythrocyte sedimentation rate
- Urinalysis
- TSH, T_4, and Free T_3

These tests are probably the least one should order and will probably cover the majority of general diseases associated with, or aggravating, a pain syndrome.

The laboratory tests to diagnose or exclude not often encountered specific pain syndromes are listed in an anatomical order below.

1. *Headache*
   - Erythrocyte sedimentation rate (temporal arteritis)

- 24-hour urinary metanephrines (phaeochromocytoma)
2. *Chest pain*
   - Coxsackie B virus (1-6) Antibody (epidemic myalgia and pleurodynia, myocarditis and pericarditis)
3. *Abdominal pain*
   - Lipase and amylase (pancreatitis)
   - Sickle cell hemoglobin (sickle cell anemia)
   - Porphobilinogen and quantitative porphyrins in urine (porphyria)
   - Serum beta hCG (ruptured ectopic pregnancy, hydatidiform mole)
4. *Back pain*
   - Bence-Jones protein in urine (myeloma)
   - Serum electrophoresis, cryoglobulins (malignant gammopathy, Waldenstrom's macroglobulinemia)
   - HLA-B27 (ankylosing spondylitis)
5. *Joint pain*
   - Lyme disease antibodies
   - Uric acid or calcium pyrophosphate dihydrate crystals in synovial fluid (gout and pseudogout)
   - Serum iron and ferritin (hemochromatosis)
6. *Muscle pain*
   - Creatine phosphokinase, lactate dehydrogenase, urinary myoglobin (myopathy, storage disease)
7. *Bone pain*
   - Serum calcium, phosphorus and alkaline phosphatase (Paget's, sarcoidosis, primary, secondary, tertiary hyperparathyroidism, osteoporosis)

HOLISTIC LABORATORY ASSESSMENT IN PAIN SYNDROMES

The clinical laboratory, however, may be much more useful in a more holistic sense by assessing what other global functional disturbances of the entire body affect pain and make its experience all the more distressing or chronic. The body operates as a whole and any disturbance or imbalance in one part of the body will affect the whole body, including the appreciation and perception of pain.

LABORATORY EVALUATION OF PERPETUATING FACTORS

Any time there is an increase in perceived pain or a suboptimal response to adequate treatment in a patient with a pain syndrome, one of the perpetuating factors should be looked for and corrected (Travell & Simons, 1983). These factors include the following.

NUTRITIONAL DEFICIENCIES

- **Vitamins** — Less than optimum levels of the soluble B vitamins: B_1 thiamine, B_2 riboflavin, B_3 niacin, B_5 pantothenate, B_6 pyridoxine, folic acid, B_{12} cobalamin; vitamin C ascorbic acid; and vitamin D cholecalciferol. Travell and Simons (1983) make the point that more than half of patients with chronic myofascial pain syndrome have vitamin deficiencies that require resolution for lasting pain relief. An excess of vitamin A is possible with an excessive vitamin A supplementation.
- **Minerals** — Less than optimum levels of potassium (for rapid membrane repolarization), calcium (for the excitation–contraction mechanism of actin and myosin filaments), magnesium (for the contractile mechanism of the myofilaments), iron, and ferritin (oxygen transport as hemoglobin and myoglobin).

METABOLIC DISTURBANCES

- **Hyperuricemia** — Myofascial trigger points and muscular rheumatism are aggravated by absolute or relative hyperuricemia (Travell & Simons, 1983). Dr. Paul St. Amand (1993) has advocated the use of guaifenesin treatment as a uricosuric in the treatment of fibromyalgia.
- **Low-Grade or Frank Anemia** — Reduced oxygen tension in blood supplied to muscles, fascia, or soft tissue make trigger points more irritable.
- **Hypoglycemia** — Myofascial trigger point activity is aggravated and response to therapy is shortened or reduced by hypoglycemia.
- **Acidosis** — Lactic or metabolic acidosis will cause less efficient muscle contraction, stiffness, and pain.

HORMONAL DISTURBANCES

- **Hypothyroidism** — Absolute low or relative low thyroid levels cause irritable myofascial trigger points and low ATP levels and decrease the concentration of intracellular potassium. Laboratory levels of TSH, free T_3, and free T_4 should all be obtained. In many patients the TSH and T_4 will be normal, while the T_3 will be low. These patients have difficulty in converting T_4 to T_3 and should be supplemented with mixtures of T_4 and T_3 (Armour®, Westhroid®) or supplemented with T_3 (Cytomel®) as well as T_4 (Levoxyl®). In fact, many patients require large supratherapeutic doses of T_3 in order for their intracellular thyroid receptors to respond (Lowe, 2000).

- **Menopausal Syndrome** — The most common pain symptoms attributed to menopause in women are dyspareunia, formications (crawling sensations), mastalgia, paresthesia, myalgia, headache, and arthralgia. These manifestations are relieved by the judicious supplementation of either estradiol and/or micronized progesterone. These symptoms are best explained in a Traditional Chinese Medicine paradigm, where the Liver Blood and Qi become stagnant or deficient and cause an energetic blockage in the organs and structures that Liver controls — the breasts, uterus, muscles, tendons, and joints.

INFECTIONS

All occult or chronic infections will produce a slew of inflammatory proteins and mediators that will ensure ongoing systemic irritation and aggravated myofascial trigger points. The most important *bacterial infection* sites include the tonsils, sinuses, teeth and jaws, and urinary tract. Laboratory measurement of C-reactive protein, sedimentation rate, a urinalysis, and a complete blood count with differential will usually point to these problems. Infected teeth and jaws will often produce clinical pain at an anatomical site distant from the head and neck depending on the energy meridian line being affected by the infected tooth.

Viral infections often worsen underlying chronic pain syndromes such as arthritis and fibromyalgia. Although all viruses can produce these exacerbations, herpes virus type I and coxsackie B virus are the worst culprits. Coxsackie B is often implicated in stressed males with atypical chest pain and unremarkable EKGs. The recent finding of "post polio syndromes" brings into sharp focus many clinical happenings long since forgotten including tertiary syphilis and the sequelae of imprudently administered hepatitis B vaccine and influenza A shots.

Infestations are uncommon, but the increased Western habit of consuming sushi has led to an increase in the incidence of the fish tape worm. *Diphyllobothrium latum,* a worm located in the jejunum, may consume 80 to 100% of all ingested B_{12} and deprive its host of the vitamin.

ALLERGIES

Environmental allergies are not commonly associated with pain syndromes, but Travell and Simons (1983) mention allergic rhinitis as a cause of nonresponsiveness to trigger point therapy due to the release of histamine. Much more common is the effect of food allergies on painful inflammatory conditions such as arthritis. The nightshade family of potatoes, tomatoes, and peppers is implicated in worsening arthritis and should be avoided. Allergies to wheat, gluten, corn, soy, milk, citrus, and eggs are common food intolerances or hypersensitivities that cause a generalized inflammatory diathesis and exacerbate inflammatory pain syndromes. Individual patients will exhibit idiosyncratic reactions to specific foods or food groups and should be screened by an IgG enzyme-linked immunosorbent assay (ELISA) test for those food groups that seem to cause problems. A 4-day rotational diet, or adherence to a caveman diet, will often confirm a clinical impression of food sensitivity. Patients with chemical sensitivity, especially to petrochemicals, will often experience headaches after exposure to smoke and perfumes.

FUNCTIONAL LABORATORY TESTING OF NUTRIENTS, TOXICANTS, AND CELL REGULATORS

INTRODUCTION

Laboratory testing has moved from static one-time snapshot levels of serum or urinary analytes, to dynamic functional testing and screens of associated metabolic pathways and bodily constituents. These new tests enable clinicians to have an overview of the metabolic deficiencies and excesses in a patient and to logically correct them using dietary information, supplements, and phytonutrients.

VITAMIN STATUS

There are many ways of assessing a patient's vitamin status. Vitamin concentrations can be measured in serum and blood cells, or the excretory products formed from vitamins may be measured in the urine. Changes in enzyme activity in response to added vitamins may be measured in leukocytes in cell culture. Measurement of vitamin-dependent, specific metabolic intermediates in the urine may demonstrate the functional adequacy of a particular vitamin. Liquid chromatography and gas chromatography of serum or urine can give very accurate readings of vitamin levels in the body. Vitamins A, D, E, and K are all fat soluble and may build up to toxic levels, as they are not excreted in the urine to any extent but are dissolved into the fat deposits of the body. Vitamin C and all B group vitamins are water soluble and do not usually present a toxic buildup, as any excess vitamin is excreted in the urine.

MINERAL AND TOXIC METAL STATUS

Laboratory testing has the ability to reveal mineral deficiencies and metal toxicities in the human body. The health risks linked to inadequate intakes of nutritionally essential minerals and to increased exposure to toxic elements in industrialized societies are well documented in the scientific literature (Bralley, 2001).

Low concentrations of 13 trace elements are known to be essential for human health. These are iron, copper, zinc, iodine, selenium, boron, cobalt, chromium, molybdenum, manganese, vanadium, silicon, and nickel. The more important minerals present in very large concentrations are calcium, magnesium, and phosphorus. Sodium, potassium, and chloride are classified as electrolytes.

The most important toxic metals, for which exposure is a possibility, are aluminum, lead, mercury, cadmium, and arsenic.

Most mineral action is characterized by a bell-shaped dose–response curve. Low intake results in a deficiency state while over dosage results in a toxic state. The optimal amount of trace element intake is in the middle of the curve where function is maximized and toxicity is minimized.

Selection of what sample to use to assess a mineral's level depends on the clinical situation and the question to be answered. Tissue distribution of most elements is determined by the existence of specific protein factors that bind, transport, and store each element under hormonal or other type of homeostatic control. An ideal sampling tissue for mineral status measurement is one whose mineral stores are exchangeable with other major body pools, with a rate of exchange sufficient to provide the best sensitivity with respect to changes in dietary mineral intake.

The most popular specimens for assessing therapeutic elements are serum and plasma. Whole blood is used in emergency situations to establish acute, toxic heavy metal poisoning. Red blood cell mineral levels tend to follow the individual's general mineral levels and have proved to be popular and useful. Hair is the most popular sample for testing toxic metals in the body.

Chelation challenge or provocation tests are used to mobilize toxic elements from the tissue into the general circulation which are then measured in the urine. EDTA (ethylenediamine tetraacetic acid) in an intravenous drip, or oral DMSA (meso-2,3-dimercaptosuccinic acid) may be used in these provocation tests to reveal sequestered heavy metals in the tissue.

Amino Acid Status

Nine amino acids are considered to be the essential amino acids that must be supplied by our diet. These amino acids are arginine, isoleucine, leucine, lysine, methionine, phenylalanine, threonine, tryptophan, and valine.

Advances in amino acid measurements now enable more than 40+ analytes to be measured, providing information on a wide spectrum of metabolic and nutritional disorders, including protein inadequacy, gastrointestinal insufficiencies, inflammatory responses, vitamin and mineral dysfunctions, detoxification impairments, cardiovas-

cular disease, ammonia toxicity, neurological dysfunction, and inborn errors of metabolism.

Amino acids are measured by high-performance liquid chromatography. The measured analytes are grouped into functional categories, including the nutritionally essential and semi-essential amino acids, dietary peptide-related analytes, the non-essential protein amino acids, and the intermediary metabolites, providing information on nutrient cofactor status and disorders relating to their imbalances.

Lipids and Essential Fatty Acids

A constant supply of fatty acids from the diet or hepatic synthesis is needed for the demands of energy production, cell membrane function, hormones, and eicosanoid synthesis. Changes in the modern diet are largely responsible for the increasing incidence of essential fatty acid (EFA) imbalances and deficiencies. The ratio of omega-6 to omega-3 fats has changed dramatically due to the widespread use of vegetable oils (mostly n-6 fats) in cooking and to the processing of oils to alter omega-3 fats to improve shelf life and eliminate their stronger taste (just think of the distinctive tastes of cod liver or flax oil). In fact, historical estimates place the ratio of n-6 to n-3 oils at nearly 1:1 for prehistoric humans, but by the turn of the 20th century, the ratio had increased to about 4:1.

Current estimates for Americans place the ratio in the range of 20:1 to 25:1! The sharp rise is due to increased vegetable oil consumption: from 2 lb per year in 1909 to 25 lb per year in 1985! The ideal dietary ratio should probably be in the range of 3:1 to 5:1, with a minimum of 1% of our daily calories coming from omega-3 oils. A recent study looked at eight essential fatty acid metabolites in 847 consecutive patients, aged 50 to 70. Of those tested, 322 had at least one EFA outside the normal range, and of those 322 patients, 57% had at least two abnormal values and 7% had five to seven fatty acid deviations (Shamberger, 1997). General trends observed included an increase in abnormal values with age and increased abnormalities in patients with heart disease and cancer.

Many of the chronic inflammatory conditions that accompany an EFA imbalance are currently treated with symptom-specific pharmaceutical drugs such as steroids, prednisone, aspirin, and other nonsteroidal anti-inflammatory drugs (NSAIDs), sulfasalazine, and colchicine. The problem with such drug therapies is that they prevent the formation of "good" anti-inflammatory eicosanoids as well as the "bad" proinflammatory eicosanoids, or they shift production of one type of eicosanoid to another. For effective, long-term management, eicosanoid production should be modified through dietary changes (balancing dietary intake of specific fats, as indicated by testing) and by controlling insulin levels in the circulation.

Maintaining a proper balance between the various families of dietary fats (omega-3, omega-6, omega-9, saturated, and cholesterol) may be one of the most important preventative measures a person can take to reduce the likelihood of developing one of the chronic diseases of modern civilization, such as diabetes, heart disease, obesity, irritable bowel syndrome, and autoimmune disease. And for patients who may already have one of these diseases, EFA testing and therapy has been demonstrated to reduce both morbidity and mortality associated with these diseases.

ORGANIC ACID STATUS

Organic acids are formed in various tissues or by intestinal microbes as metabolic intermediates and end products. Accumulations of organic acids in urine can indicate metabolic dysfunction, hormonal stimulation, or even microbial overgrowth. Abnormal levels of organic acids can be traced to inherited enzyme deficiencies, buildup of toxicants, specific nutrient deficiencies, or drug effects. Every cell is affected when a metabolic pathway is interrupted. Clinical expression is unique to each patient, determined by genomic characteristics, medical history, and recent toxin exposures. Organic acid testing allows one to view the impact of all these factors.

Organic acids in the urine can demonstrate problems in fatty acid oxidation, carbohydrate metabolism, the citric acid cycle, B-complex vitamin activity, detoxification markers, neurotransmitter metabolism, and dysbiosis markers.

TOXIN AND DETOXIFICATION STATUS

One of the body's primary self-defense mechanisms is the conversion and neutralization of metabolic products and toxins into soluble and safe by-products that can then be eliminated. Many challenges to this system — a leaky gut, repeated exposure to food-borne toxic chemicals, environmental pollutants, bacterial endotoxins, and other substances — can increase the detoxification burden. This overload can lead to greater production of free radicals and damage to many body systems. Assessing multiple pathways with challenge substances provides clinical information about individuals with imbalanced detoxification.

All ingested and microbiologically produced toxins are presented to the first-pass clearance system. First-pass clearance involves the biotransformation and clearance of a chemical from the body before it reaches the systemic circulation. This clearance may take place in several organ tissues including the intestinal mucosal wall and the liver.

The liver is the body's primary detoxifying organ. Here, detoxification is carried out in two related processes known as Phase I and Phase II. Phase I serves to biotransform substances through oxidation, reduction, or hydrolysis, using the cytochrome P450 mixed-function oxidase enzymes. This process increases the solubility of molecules and prepares them for Phase II reactions, which will further increase their solubility.

The Phase I reactions are necessary for detoxification, but the resulting production of reactive oxygen species can at times be very damaging. Thus, the liver needs to be able to generate oxidation capacity when needed, yet at the same time generate no more than what is needed. Perhaps this is why Phase I systems are inducible by different compounds.

In Phase II, conjugation reactions add a polar hydrophilic molecule to the metabolite or toxin, converting lipophilic substances to water-soluble forms for excretion and elimination. Phase II reactions may follow Phase I for some molecules or act directly on the toxin or metabolite. Major Phase II pathways include glutathione, sulfate, glycine, and glucuronide conjugations. Individual xenobiotics and metabolites usually follow one or two distinct pathways. While the modification of Phase I and II enzyme activities has its basis in the research setting, there is growing appreciation of the clinical applications of such strategies.

In Phase I, the family of P450 enzyme systems is quite diverse, with specific enzyme systems being inducible by particular drugs or metabolites. Caffeine is a substance capable of testing a number of P450 systems simultaneously.

Measurement of salivary caffeine clearance provides a noninvasive procedure for quantifying hepatic microsomal function, as caffeine is almost completely absorbed by the intestine and is metabolized in the liver by P450 enzymes. Levels are affected only slightly by the presence of liver disease, although they are substantially reduced in patients with cirrhosis. P450 activity and caffeine clearance is reported to be upregulated by smoking. A variety of drugs and xenobiotics are oxidized by the P450 system. Thus, this system plays a crucial role in the detoxification and removal of many potentially toxic substances.

In Phase II pathways, a 650-mg dose of acetaminophen taken in the evening is converted to various conjugation products overnight, and the levels in the urine reflect the respective activities of pathways utilizing glutathione, glucuronic acid, or sulfate as conjugating agents. A 650-mg dose of salicylic acid (aspirin) if taken in the evening can be used as a marker of oxidative damage protection.

OXIDANT STRESS STATUS

Oxidation is a chemical process that allows life for aerobic organisms. It enables the conversion of glucose to carbon dioxide and water with the formation of energy. This action is not harmful to the rest of the cell. In other reactions of oxidation, compounds can enter into unregulated non-enzymatic chemical bond formation, which damages the cell. These oxidation reactions are caused by reactive oxygen species or free radicals. These include the superoxide radical, hydrogen peroxide, and the hydroxyl radical. These reactive species are the responsible for most of the degenerative and chronic diseases in the body. The oxidant stress status of the body can be measured by the following:

Markers of Oxidant Damage
- *Lipid Peroxidation* — Lipid peroxides in serum and urine, serum isoprostanes, HNE (4-hydroxy-2-nonenal), oxidized low-density lipoproteins in plasma: all high.
- *Protein Oxidation* — 3-Nitrotyrosinein plasma and methionine sulfoxide in serum: all high.
- *Nucleotide Oxidation* — 8-Oxoguinasine in serum and white cell DNA strand breakage: all high.

Antioxidant Nutrient Testing
- *Glutathione* — Urinary sulfate (low) and pyroglutamate (high)
- *Fat-Soluble Vitamins* — Vitamins A, E, beta carotene, and serum coenzyme Q_{10} (all low)
- *Antioxidant Minerals* — Selenium, zinc, copper in red blood cells, hair, and urine (all low)

Note: The above information, details, and rationale of testing can be found in the literature, books (especially *Laboratory Evaluations in Molecular Medicine*, by Bralley and Lord), notes, lectures, and Web sites of the following two excellent laboratories:

Great Smokies Diagnostic Laboratory/Genovations™
63 Zillicoa Street, Ashville, NC 28801
Toll Free 1-800-522-4762; Fax 1-828-252-9303
Web site: www.gsdl.com

Metametrix Clinical Laboratory
4855 Peachtree Industrial Blvd., Suite 201, Norcross, GA 30092
Toll Free 1-800-221-4640; Fax 1-770-441-2237
Web site: www.metametrix.com

THERAPEUTIC DRUG MONITORING IN PAIN MANAGEMENT

The application of therapeutic drug monitoring to optimize drug therapy in individual patients should be considered as an adjunct to the physician's clinical judgment in assessing the course and effectiveness of treatment. Always remember that each patient is an individual and no one size fits all. If the serum drug concentration does not fit the clinical picture, it may be that the effects of disease and age, or drug interactions, are responsible for alterations in the pharmacokinetic disposition of the drug.

Therapeutic drug monitoring is inappropriate for acute drug usage and in clinical situations where the clinical end point is easily followed, e.g., blood pressure measurements. For drugs with poor dose–response relationships and with a narrow therapeutic range and a low therapeutic index, and for which toxicity is a problem at upper therapeutic levels, therapeutic drug monitoring is very advantageous to patient safety and clinical drug effectiveness.

PHARMACOKINETIC ISSUES

The time course following administration of a drug is characterized by individualized patterns of absorption, distribution, metabolism, and elimination.

- *Absorption* is the crossing of drugs from the skin, muscle, or gut into the general circulation. Most orally administered drugs have rapid absorption across the gastrointestinal mucosa and reach peak concentrations in 1 to 2 hours. Drugs with limited solubility, or that bind to foods or other drugs, may exhibit poor absorption characteristics.
- *Distribution Phase* is dependent on the degree of plasma protein binding of the drug and the amount of free drug available to stimulate its appropriate receptor. Alterations in the degree of protein binding have been reviewed by Longa and Cross (1984).
- *Metabolism and Elimination* determine the duration of the drug's pharmacological activity and are the result of biotransformations that take place primarily in the liver and are followed by excretion in the bile or by the kidneys. Drugs may undergo activation by the liver or undergo transformation and detoxification into a more soluble substance for renal clearance. Clearance of a drug by glomerular filtration is reduced in patients with reduced renal function, especially in elderly individuals, and this will affect the elimination of the drug and its biological half-life. Appropriate modification of drug dosage in these patients will avoid toxic reactions to increased plasma levels of the drug.
- *Steady-State Concentrations* of the drug provide the best correlation between serum drug concentrations and clinical status. At steady state the amount of drug being eliminated from the body is equal to the amount administered. The steady-state drug concentration is usually achieved after three to five half-lives of a given

drug. Loading doses circumvent the necessity of waiting three to five half-lives to achieve a maximum therapeutic effect.

TIMING OF SPECIMEN COLLECTIONS

In an ideal world, the therapeutic drug specimen should be collected after a steady state has been achieved. For drugs with short half-lives, both a steady-state peak and a trough level should be obtained. Each drug has a different peak collection time, but all trough levels should be taken just prior to the next dose of the drug. A toxic drug evaluation level may be collected at any time.

ALTERED PHARMACOKINETICS

The *in vivo* disposition of drugs varies with age and disease and with drug–drug interactions. These factors are responsible for the intra- and interindividual variations encountered in clinical practice.

- *Age* — There are age-related pharmacokinetic differences among the neonate, infant, child, pubescent child, adult, and geriatric adult, which can be attributed to changing metabolic functions, body composition, and protein-binding characteristics. As a general rule, children metabolize drugs twice as fast as adults. In elderly patients, drugs are cleared at a slower rate than in adults due to a combination of reduced metabolic activity and reduced renal function. As people age, total-body water decreases, lean body mass is reduced, and the percentage of body fat increases. Lipid-soluble drugs will tend to build up and saturate the fat stores and temporarily decrease the serum level of the drug. As the fat compartment becomes saturated with the drug, the serum level will suddenly rise and therapeutic monitoring will alert one to the situation.
- *Disease Processes* — Renal glomerular disease reduces the clearance of drugs and drug metabolites and increases biological half-lives. Diseases that alter the albumen concentration will cause the active drug fraction to alter dramatically. Reduced liver or cardiac functional capacity will cause increased serum levels of administered drugs.
- *Drug–Drug Interactions* — The practice of polypharmacy to treat multiple disease processes, especially in elderly patients, creates the potential of drug–drug interactions with difficulties in interpreting drug levels and adjusting dosages.

THERAPEUTICALLY MEASURED PAIN-ASSOCIATED DRUGS

- *Acetaminophen (Tylenol®)* — Peak plasma concentrations in 30 to 60 minutes; steady state in 10 to 20 hours; therapeutic levels 10 to 20 μg/ml, toxic levels >200 μg/ml. For toxicity, take first sample 6 hours postingestion and a second sample 3 to 4 hours later. Normal half-life is 1 to 3 hours; > 4 hours indicates possible hepatic necrosis.
- *Amitriptyline (Elavil®)* — Peak plasma concentrations at 2 to 6 hours after oral dose; steady state in 3 to 8 days; therapeutic level depends on use. Elavil has significant drug–drug interactions. Elderly patients are prone to postural hypotension, urinary retention, and sedation.
- *Carisoprodol (Soma®)* — Therapeutic levels 6 to 12 μg/ml.
- *Gabapentin (Neurontin®)* — Only 3% bound to plasma proteins and not appreciably metabolized; is cleared by the kidneys and has a half-life of 5 to 7 hours; steady state at 1 to 2 days; for therapeutic monitoring draw trough levels; very little drug–drug interactions.
- *Meperidine (Demerol®)* — Maximum analgesic effect in 30 to 50 minutes after intramuscular injection; duration of action 2 to 4 hours; therapeutic level 50 to 500 ng/ml; 95% efficacy at 700 ng/ml; potentially toxic at levels >1000 ng/ml.

DRUG TOXICOLOGY PROFILES

Every laboratory offers drug toxicology profiles for medical, medicolegal, and preemployment use. Each laboratory has a slightly different menu for blood, urine, and gastric contents. The most important issue is to be in compliance with company, state, or local guidelines or collective bargaining agreements when ordering and collecting samples. Chain-of-custody issues and confirmation of presumptive positive specimens by gas chromatography/mass spectroscopy should be automatic (LabCorp, Directory of Services 2004; Quest Diagnostics, Directory of Services, 2003).

REFERENCES

Bralley, J. A. (2001). *Laboratory evaluations in molecular medicine* (pp. 35–73). Norcross, GA: The Institute for Advances in Molecular Medicine.

Harkness, R., & Bratman, S. (2003). *Handbook of drug–herb and drug–supplement interactions* (pp. v–vi). St. Louis: MO: Mosby.

Laboratory Corporation of America. (2004). *Directory of services and interpretive guide*. Burlington, NC: Laboratory Corporation of America.

Longa, G. J., & Cross, R. E. (1984). Laboratory monitoring of drug rherapy. Part II: Variable protein binding and free drug concentration. *Bulletin of Laboratory Medicine, 80*, 1–6.

Lowe, J. C. (2000). *The metabolic treatment of fibromyalgia*. Lafayette, CO: McDowell Publishing Co.

Margoles, M. (1990). Myofascial pain syndrome. In R. S. Weiner (Ed.), *Innovations in pain management* (pp. 15–24). Orlando, FL: Paul M. Deutsch Press, Inc.

Quest Diagnostics (2003). *Directory of services*. Las Vegas, NV: Quest Diagnostics.

Shamberger, R. J. (1997). Erythrocyte fatty acid studies in patients. *Journal of Advancement in Medicine, 10*(3), 195–205.

St. Amand, R. P. (1993). *What your doctor may not tell you about fibromyalgia*. New York: Time Warner.

Travell, J. G., & Simons, D. G. (1983). *Myofascial pain and dysfunction: The trigger point manual* (pp. 103–163). Baltimore, MD: Williams & Wilkins.

Young, D. S. (1979). Why there is a laboratory. In D. S. Young, H. Nipper, D. Uddin et al. (Eds.), *Clinician and chemistry: The relationship of the laboratory to the physician* (pp. 3–22). Washington, DC: American Association for Clinical Chemistry, Inc.

42

Functional Capacity Evaluations

Barbara L. Kornblau, JD, OT/L, FAOTA, DAAPM, CCM, CDMS,
Max Ito, PhD, OTR/L, and Pam Kasyan-Itzkowitz, MS, OTR/L, CHT

INTRODUCTION

This chapter looks at current practices in functional capacity evaluations as part of the return-to-work process for patients/clients with pain. After describing current practice, the authors provide a discussion of the literature with respect to evidence regarding concerns for the effectiveness, validity, reliability, and limitations of the use of functional capacity assessments.

CASE PRESENTATION

Bill, a 49-year-old airline pilot, was struck by lightning while helping passengers deplane from a corporate jet. The lightning hit the umbrella he was holding, entered his body through his right hand, and exited through his belt buckle. Bill passed out on the tarmac hitting his head and lower back on equipment accidentally left out by one of the airline catering contractors.

Following his acute medical recovery, Bill continued to complain of chronic pain in his lower back and numerous muscles, as well as general fatigue, weakness, and swelling in his right arm. He is not sure what he can and cannot do since he has been out of work for a few months. Although very motivated to return to the workplace, eventually doctors diagnosed Bill with fibromyalgia. He is assigned a case manager by his workers' compensation carrier, and his attorney is pursuing a third-party claim against the catering contractor, who it turns out violated the airport's policies by leaving the equipment on the tarmac. His physician expects Bill to reach Maximum Medical Improvement (MMI) shortly. Once he reaches MMI, his attorney expects to settle his workers' compen-

sation case and Bill is anxious to settle his third-party claim against the caterer.

Bill's situation raises many questions. Will he be able to return to his job safely? Can he work in spite of his pain? How do we know what he is capable of doing? Does he need accommodations in the workplace in order to return to work? Can he benefit from a work conditioning program? Does Bill need a work conditioning program? If so, what kind?

FUNCTIONAL CAPACITY EVALUATION

Functional capacity evaluations attempt to answer these questions by providing specific information about how Bill is functioning in relationship to his work's demands in spite of the pain he experiences. Functional capacity evaluations (FCEs) measure physical abilities or functional capacities through a systematic process of assessment, using a standard protocol (Kornblau, Dahl, Armstrong, Ellexson, & Larson, 1998; Matheson, 1996). Readers will find several related terms for FCE, which are sometimes used interchangeably. These include *work capacity evaluation* (Matheson, 1989), *functional (or physical) capacity assessments* (FCA) (Key, 2004), and *physical capacity evaluation* (Harrand & Hoffman, 1980).

FCEs may contribute valuable information to help in determining job placement, job accommodation, return-to-work assignments after injury, and extent of impairment. Employers, insurance adjusters, rehabilitation specialists, and others have looked to FCEs to help them determine if work restrictions, job modifications, or reasonable accommodations could assist in returning an indi-

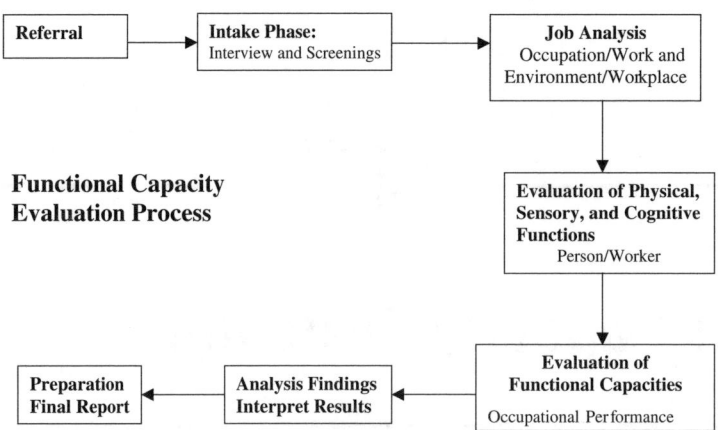

FIGURE 42.1 Functional capacity evaluation process.

vidual to the workplace or help prevent further injury (Kornblau et al., 1998). FCEs have also been used to predict potential ability to perform work tasks following work conditioning or work hardening programs (Kornblau et al., 1998).

FCE tools have long been used to examine the relationship between the individual's abilities and specific job demands through a formal process that involves lengthy and intensive one-on-one contact with the evaluator/clinician. Comprehensive FCEs may take a few hours to a few days to complete, and the time commitment can place a high demand on resources in terms of staffing, training and expertise, equipment, and facility. These factors can lead to high costs of conducting FCEs (Gross, 2004; Matheson, 1996).

FCEs are provided by clinicians or trained evaluators skilled to perform work-related evaluations in free-standing clinics, at job sites, in outpatient and hospital-based rehabilitation programs, and in private practices (Kornblau et al., 1998). Readers may find FCEs performed by multidisciplinary teams of therapists, exercise physiologists, vocational evaluators, rehabilitation professionals, individual occupational therapists or physical therapists, and others. The evaluator/tester or team must possess the necessary skills to assess the physiological, psychophysical, cognitive, and biomechanical functioning of the individual. Clinicians performing FCEs must possess the observational skills, training, and experience necessary to perform complex job and task analysis and assess environmental factors that may affect work performance (Kornblau et al., 1998).

The results of an FCE evaluation may contain objective information that can be used to assist in determining disability status, disability benefits, and whether maximum benefit from rehabilitation and medical interventions has been reached. FCEs may be used as a baseline and final evaluation for work rehabilitation, to determine appropriate job placement, and to confirm an injured worker's self-report of work limitation. Appropriate job placement

reduces the risk of reinjury, which makes the FCE an important component of an injury prevention program.

FUNCTIONAL CAPACITY EVALUATION PROCESS

The FCE involves a seven-step process that allows the evaluator to take a comprehensive look at the fit among the person, the environment, and the everyday occupations that contribute to his or her participation as a worker (Stewart et al., 2003). In other words, the functional capacity assessment looks at the worker, the workplace, and the work tasks and seeks to make a match between them to facilitate safe work performance (Kornblau & Ellexson, 1992).

The FCE process for our airline pilot, Bill, will begin with a referral for the evaluation (Figure 42.1).

REFERRAL

A referral for a functional capacity assessment makes sense for Bill for several reasons. He is approaching MMI shortly, he is motivated to return to work, and he is not sure what he can and cannot do at this point. He wants to settle both his workers' compensation and third-party claims as soon as he can.

Clients are generally referred for FCEs to determine a baseline of what they can do or to compare what they can do with what a given job requires (Kornblau et al., 1998). A client might be referred for an FCE because he or she has reached MMI but continues to have work-related issues interfering with reentry into the workplace (Kornblau et al., 1998). An FCE can provide data needed to initiate settlement in a workers' compensation case or provide evidence of a social security claimant's residual capacity to help determine his or her ability to work. An FCE can provide an individual with information to quantify his or her functional status to facilitate an enlightened, realistic job search (Kornblau et al., 1998). All of these situations may apply to Bill, our hypothetical airline pilot.

Referrals can come from several sources. A rehabilitation professional, such as a rehabilitation counselor or, in Bill's case, a case manager, may refer a client for an FCE. This is the first step in the return-to-work process following discharge from the medical phase of rehabilitation following an accident or injury. Baseline information about one's level of functioning or information comparing the level of function to the job's demands give rehabilitation professionals invaluable information for the return-to-work or job search process. Rehabilitation professionals and/or employers (human resource personnel or risk mangers) may initiate a referral to obtain information about reasonable accommodations the client may need in the workplace to facilitate return-to-work.

Representatives from workers' compensation insurance or disability insurance carriers may refer a client for an FCE to gather information to facilitate claim settlement or to investigate whether the client's claim is legitimate. Referrals from insurance representatives also serve to expedite the return-to-work process.

A physician may refer a patient for an FCE because a case manager, rehabilitation counselor, or attorney desires specific information about how the patient is functioning with the goal of trying to settle a workers' compensation or disability claim. The information from the FCE can provide the physician with the specific details he or she needs to assign the client an impairment rating (American Medical Association [AMA], 1993).

Clients are often referred for functional capacities assessments by physicians who receive a form from the rehabilitation nurse, case manager, or insurance adjuster that asks for information similar in nature to Figure 42.2.

Knowledgeable physicians, physician assistants, and nurse practitioners understand that they can report only on information for which they have knowledge from observation, examinations, or consultations from other practitioners. "Guessing" at the answers to specific questions regarding a patient's physical restrictions and limitations will not sufficiently support their decisions should an attorney question them in detail during a deposition. Finding oneself at a deposition or in court defending a restrictions and limitations form is not unusual considering many clients referred for FCEs are involved in litigation or administrative claims. Readers will find individual state workers' compensation forms potentially more complicated and very specific in the questions they ask (examples: Florida Division of Workers' Compensation form DWC-25, available online at www.fldfs.com/wc/pdf/DWC-25.pdf, and the Texas Rehabilitation Commission form TRC106, available online at http://www.rehab.state.tx.us/forms/trc106.dot).

Attorneys, both plaintiff/claimant and defense/employer, may seek FCEs to obtain information to support their cases in court or in administrative proceedings. These may include workers' compensation claims, social security disability determinations, disability retirement controversies, disability insurance claims, and others. Bill's attorney could certainly benefit from the FCE results in settlement discussions.

Once a referral is made, the clinician will want to confirm that the referral is appropriate for the client, medically and vocationally, and that the client has medical clearance to participate in the FCE. Safety is a feasibility concern, and clients referred for an FCE must not be subjected to an unacceptable risk of injury or an adverse event from testing. Additional safety guidelines should be established and strictly complied with when administering an FCE on clients with medical conditions. Pretest orientation, safety briefing, test procedure training, and warm-up physical exercises may assist in reducing the risk of adverse incidents.

The clinician will review all available records, medical, vocational, and legal; gather pertinent information about the client; evaluate the purpose for the referral; and determine the expected outcome. The clinician should obtain a copy of the client's current or intended job description. What kind of information does the referral source want from the FCE? Is there a job waiting for the client at the end of the process? Does the client have a desire to return to work? Does the client have a realistic vocational goal he or she wishes to work toward? In addition to the answers to these questions, the clinician will also want to know the reimbursement source for the FCE.

Workers' compensation and disability insurance carriers as well as self-insured plans will often pay for FCEs because the information acquired through the assessment helps determine future direction of the claim. In some instances, health insurances may exclude what it considers vocationally related services and may need to be convinced that the functional capacity assessment is a medically necessary intervention, before it will agree to pay for the FCE (Kornblau et al., 1998).

State departments of vocational rehabilitation and other state or local agencies may also reimburse for functional capacities assessments of their clients. Any or all of these reimbursement sources may subject their reimbursement to a set fee schedule. Individuals may also choose to pay privately for an FCE (Kornblau et al., 1998).

INTAKE PHASE

During the intake phase, the clinician will gather information from the client regarding specific past medical history and past vocational and work history through a structured and standardized interview process. Using the job description as an initial focal point for discussion, specific job-related information is collected through inter-

Restriction & Limitations
_____
Fantastic Rehabilitation Company of America
123 Main Street
Anytown, USA
_____

Date: ___October 19, 2023.___

Claimant: Ms. Weary Worker
Carrier: Best Employer Insurance Company

Dear Doctor:

Please answer the following questions and return this form in the enclosed self-stamped addressed envelope:

• How long can the claimant:	Occasionally 0-33%% of the workday	Frequently 34-66% of the workday	Constantly 67-100% of the workday
Walk?	_____	_____	_____
Stand?	_____	_____	_____
Sit?	_____	_____	_____
Stoop?	_____	_____	_____
Climb?	_____	_____	_____
Balance?	_____	_____	_____
Stoop?	_____	_____	_____
Kneel?	_____	_____	_____
Crouch?	_____	_____	_____
Crawl?	_____	_____	_____
Reach?	_____	_____	_____
Handle?	_____	_____	_____
Finger?	_____	_____	_____
Feel?	_____	_____	_____
• How many pounds can the claimant lift?		_____	_____
Floor to table?	_____	_____	_____
Table to shoulder?	_____	_____	_____
Overhead?	_____	_____	_____

• MMI: ☐ No ☐ Yes - If Yes indicate date: _____	Permanent Impairment Rating (PIR) % Body as a whole: _____
May return to work without functional limitations: ☐	May return to work according to the limitations outlined above ☐
May not return to any work at this time: ☐	May return to work with the following reasonable accommodations: ☐ _____ _____ _____ _____

Physician's Signature _____ Date: _____

FIGURE 42.2 Restriction and limitations.

view and/or checklists to acquire a sense of what tasks the client must perform in his or her job as precursor to a preferred onsite job analysis.

The clinician also asks the client about performance of activities of daily living and participation in everyday, non-work-related occupations (*Williams v. Toyota Motor Mfg.,* 534 U.S. 184 [2002]). As part of this phase, the clinician might use forms and checklists, which will help establish how the client perceives his or her own limitations. The format of the intake interview may depend on the specific FCE protocol used.

This step in the process gives the clinician an opportunity to administer psychological tests, pain questionnaires, personality inventories, educational or literacy screenings, and other assessments thought to screen for maximal or submaximal effort. This step in the process

also allows the clinician to discover the client's goals for his or her future and establish mutual goals for the FCE. The clinician can begin to observe pain behaviors and establish a rapport with the client.

Many individuals come to the FCE via a work-related injury or non-work-related accident. Because of the source of the injuries, clinicians may find that many individuals who present themselves for FCEs are often involved in administrative claims or civil litigation. Clients may perceive secondary gains in the form of higher settlements or other non-injury-related benefits should their performance on the FCE show greater than actual limitations. Clinicians have expressed concerns about whether participants are putting forth their true effort. This inquiry has become an integral part of most FCE protocols in one form or another and usually begins during this phase of the process (King, Tuckwell, & Barrett, 1998; Lemstra, Olszynski, & Enright, 2004).

In performing FCEs, test administrators attempt to determine whether the individual tested is putting forth maximal effort or is exaggerating or magnifying his or her symptoms in an effort to "throw" the test in his or her favor. Commercial or proprietary FCE protocols and the therapists who perform FCEs often include a variety of assessments they believe will look at the client's effort and cooperation with the test in an effort to determine the reliability of the client's performance. These may include, among others, the Ransford Pain Drawing and other similar pain drawing scales (Hildebrandt et al., 1988; Ransford, Cairns, & Mooney, 1976), the McGill Pain Questionnaire (Melzack. 1975), Waddell's signs or distraction tests (Waddell, McCulloch, Kummel, & Venner, 1980), visual analog pain scales (Carlson, 1983; Salo et al., 2003), Somatic Amplification Scale (Korbon, DeGood, Schroeder, Schwartz, & Shutty, 1987), EPIC Hand Function Sort (Matheson, Kaskutas, & Mada, 2001), and the Beck Depression Inventory (Beck & Steer, 1984).

Some clinicians have used the rapid grip strength exchange test or other grip or pinch strength tests to try to detect submaximal effort of FCE subjects. They have used them with a variety of diagnoses such as lower back pain but these tests are often performed during the evaluation of physical, sensory, and cognitive functions stage in the FCE process (Mathiowetz, Nelson, Sadoff, & Sadoff, 1984; Smith, 1989).

JOB ANALYSIS (OCCUPATION/WORK AND ENVIRONMENT/WORKPLACE)

The job analysis phase in the process focuses on occupation and the environment or, in other words, the work and the workplace. Job analysis plays a key role in the FCE process. The intended outcome of the return-to-work process, which often begins with an FCE, is a match of some sort between the individual's abilities and work. The work may include the person's preaccident or preinjury job, a different job with the same employer, or a different job with another employer. One must compare the demands of the job with the abilities of the person to accomplish the outcome.

An important aspect of FCE is that the measurement of work capacity is specific to the job demands. This requires a job analysis, an evaluation of specific job tasks. A job analysis then becomes a key part of the overall assessment (Pransky & Dempsey, 2004; Trombly & Radonski, 2002). Work requirements specify components of work along with the requisite skills and abilities to successfully perform work tasks.

The job analysis looks at the skills and abilities the job demands or requires (Kornblau, 1996). Kornblau and Ellexson (1992) describe a job analysis designed to give the evaluator a wealth of information about the job while abiding by requirements of the Americans With Disabilities Act 29 CFR §1630.2(n).

This job analysis incorporates the *Dictionary of Occupational Titles* (DOT) *Physical Demands,* and it also takes a much more comprehensive approach. It goes farther than merely physical demands and looks at cognitive, environmental, and psychosocial demands of work (Ellexson, 2000; Kornblau & Ellexson, 1992).

While the DOT and its intended successor O*NET provide extensive information about jobs and their requirement, these sources do not provide comprehensive information about the work in the specific environment in which the work is performed (O*NET, 2004). Using the methodology described in Figure 42.3, the authors believe one must conduct an onsite job analysis before performing the FCE to truly analyze the job and the environment in which the worker must perform the job. For example, one of the authors performed a job analysis on Jose at a warehouse. Prior to the onsite job analysis, the injured worker was interviewed extensively about the job to look at how injuries could be prevented in the future. Jose reported that one of his job tasks was to open boxcars on the loading dock. He explained that he used his arms to reach the wheel-like mechanism to twist the boxcars open. This did not explain his low back injury. It was only when the occupational therapist went to the worksite did the therapist discover that in order for Jose to reach the boxcars to open the doors, he had to straddle a 28-in. gap between the loading dock and the boxcar. Neither O*NET and the DOT nor the interview with the worker prepared the therapist for the actual, onsite, boxcar scenario. Only with the specific worksite information in hand can clinicians begin to make a close comparison and a match for the person, task, and environment or worker, work, and workplace and proceed to do so with the FCE.

A close match to the specific job demands plays a key role in compliance with the Americans with Disabilities Act (ADA) Title I, 29 C.F.R. §1630.1 *et.seq.* Congress passed the ADA of 1990 to reduce discrimination against individuals with disabilities and promote their inclusion into the workforce and independent life (29 C.F.R. §1630.1 *et.seq*). Employment-related medical testing is one of the areas in which Congress sought to discourage discrimination against individuals with disabilities. The ADA sets specific requirements for tests such as FCEs that may tend to screen out individuals with disabilities. To prevent unnecessary disqualification of an individual with disabilities from employment consideration based on a test such as the FCE, the ADA requires three things: (1) the test be job related, (2) the test must be consistent with business necessity, and (3) the person performing the test on the employer's behalf must provide the subject with reasonable accommodations during the testing process, or

Step	Job Analysis Task
1.	Determine essential functions of the job.
2.	Determine the marginal functions of the job.
3.	Break down each essential function into sequential steps describing the work the worker will perform (task analysis)
4.	Observe and record the physical requirements necessary for the worker to perform the essential function. This includes: • Documenting specific motions, e.g., walking, standing, reaching, climbing, handling, talking, etc. (DOT Physical Demands) (U.S. Department of Labor, 1986) • Measuring the distance, force, and repetition required to perform the physical activities.
5.	Measure the weight, dimensions, pressure required for operation, temperature, and vibration of specific tools, equipment and material used at the worksite.
6.	Record the frequency with which workers perform individual activities.
7.	Document the number of employees available to perform each task.
8.	Document the percent of time spent performing each essential function.
9.	Document the degree of skill or specialization required.
10.	Document psychological considerations
11.	Document physiological considerations.
12.	Record environmental considerations.
13.	Describe cognitive considerations in detail.
14.	Document workplace accommodations or modifications employers can readily make.

FIGURE 42.3 Fourteen point job analysis.

the employer must be able to show that performance of the essential functions of the job cannot be achieved with the provision of a reasonable accommodation (29 C.F.R. §1630.14 (a); EEOC, 2000). By assuring the closest match between the job tasks obtained from the comprehensive onsite job analysis and the FCE tasks, the evaluator/clinician strengthens evidence of the compliance of the FCE with the "job-related" requirements for testing under the ADA.

EVALUATION OF PHYSICAL, SENSORY, AND COGNITIVE FUNCTIONS (PERSON/WORKER)

The evaluation of physical, sensory, and cognitive functions focuses on the person/worker. This part of the evaluation together with the screenings previously mentioned during the intake process focuses the clinician/evaluator on the whole person rather than the impairment or physical limitations.

During this phase, the clinician/evaluator performs a musculoskeletal exam, looking at, among other things, strength, range of motion, flexibility, cardiovascular fitness, and posture. The range of motion evaluation plays an essential role in providing the physician with information he or she will need to assign the patient a permanent impairment rating (AMA, 1993). The comprehensive strength testing provides the clinician/evaluator with significant information regarding weakness following an illness or injury. Weakness can serve as a major contributor to loss of work capacity (Matheson, 1996).

The clinician may use some of the tests for submaximal effort as part of the strength assessment (Mathiowetz

et al., 1984; Smith, Cunningham, & Weinberg, 1989). During this phase, the clinician/evaluator will look at endurance, also called sustained activity tolerance, that combines aerobic, metabolic, and strength capacities (Matheson, 1996).

Pain often plays a major role in interfering with one's ability to return to work. During this stage and throughout the entire FCE process, the therapist/clinician will continue to observe and record the patient's pain behaviors, psychosocial behaviors, and use of body mechanics. Specific methodologies for any or all areas for assessment mentioned herein may be prescribed by the particular FCE protocol in use, proprietary or otherwise.

During this phase, the clinician/evaluator will also look at gait, coordination, balance, sensory abilities, and hand use and dexterity. Some clinicians use coordination tests during this phase such as the Adult 9-hole Peg Test or the Jebsen-Taylor Test of Hand Function (Jebsen, Taylor, Triescsmann, Trotter, & Howard, 1969; Mathiowetz, Weber, Kashman, & Volland, 1985). Other individual tests may be prescribed by the standardized protocol used by the clinician. Clinicians may find the need to do further investigation of activities of daily living during this stage based on results obtained during the intake interviews, written questionnaires, or inventories and the sensory and hand dexterity testing.

One cannot stress enough the need to look at the whole person and those everyday activities of significance to everyday life including those outside work, such as activities of daily living. The U.S. Supreme Court brought this issue to light in the ADA case, *Williams v. Toyota Motor Mfg.* 534 U.S. 184 (2002).

When the ADA originally became law, Title I provided broad protection to individuals with a substantial limitation in their major life activities from discrimination in the employment context, 29 C.F.R. §1630.1 *et.seq.* As the courts interpreted the ADA, judges have narrowed the scope of its coverage to a more limited population of individuals with more involved disabilities.

The Supreme Court set forth the current standard in *Williams v. Toyota Motor Mfg.,* 534 U.S. 184 (2002). Mrs. Williams had cumulative trauma syndrome and tendonitis. She claimed she was limited in the major life activity of performing manual tasks, which interfered with her ability to perform her job.

In examining the facts and applying the law, the Supreme Court explained the broad scope of manual tasks and the importance of looking at how limitations in the performance of manual tasks affect one's participation in everyday activities. The Court said "[m]anual tasks to any particular job are not necessarily important parts of most people's lives. As a result, *occupation specific tasks may have only limited relevance to the manual task inquiry" Williams v. Toyota Motor Mfg,* 534 U.S. at 693. "When addressing the major life activity of performing manual tasks, the central inquiry must be *whether the claimant is unable to perform the variety of tasks central to most people's daily lives,* not whether the claimant is unable to perform the tasks associated with her specific job" (emphasis added).

By putting forth this standard, the Supreme Court reminds those guiding clients through the FCE process that one must look at the "variety of tasks central to most people's daily lives" as part of a comprehensive assessment. Translated into the FCE terminology domain that means participation in one's activities of daily living.

Finally, this phase of the FCE process will give the evaluator a picture of the subject's impairments and limitations. It will also provide an indication of the client's physical safety to proceed to the next level, the evaluation of functional capacities.

EVALUATION OF FUNCTIONAL CAPACITIES (OCCUPATIONAL PERFORMANCE)

There are two types of FCEs, the Baseline FCE and the Job Specific FCE (Kornblau et al., 1998). The Baseline FCE, upon which most of the proprietary products rely, looks to develop a baseline of how the individual functions in relation to the physical demands of work, usually based upon the DOT descriptions (Kornblau et al., 1998).

The Job Specific FCE evaluates the individual worker's ability to function within the specific task demands of his or her job or specific proposed job (Kornblau et al., 1998). This assessment is based on the essential functions of the job identified in the job analysis (Kornblau et al., 1998).

Evaluating functional capacities with the Job Specific FCE involves looking at occupational performance, the interplay among the work, the worker, and the workplace, and often using simulated work tasks in a simulated work environment. The evaluator looks at the subject's occupational performance by analyzing the client's functional capacities within the context of simulated work activities.

Baseline FCEs may involve commercially available or proprietary FCE protocols or the "home grown" variety, a standard protocol developed by the clinician, practice, academic institution, or facility (Gibson & Strong, 2002). Some examples of commercially available or proprietary FCEs include, among others, Blankenship Functional Capacity Evaluation (Blankenship, 1994), EPIC (Matheson, Mooney, Grant, Leggett, & Kenny, 1996), ERGOS Work Simulator (Dusik, Menard, Cooke, Fairburn, & Beach, 1993), Isernhagen Functional Capacity Evaluation (Isernhagen, 1995), Key Method Functional Capacity Evaluation Assessment (Key, 2004), and Ergoscience Physical Work Performance Evaluation (Lechner, Jackson, Roth, & Straaton, 1994).

Although the U.S. Department of Labor intended to replace the DOT with O*NET, an online database of occupational information, the Physical Demands from the DOT still remain a part of the Social Security Federal Regulations, job analysts tools, vocational counselor's repertoire, and many Baseline FCE and some Job Specific protocols that rely on it (King et al., 1998; O*NET, 2004; 20 C.F.R. §404.1567). Most of the commercially available functional capacity systems as well as those "home grown" varieties draw from the physical demands enumerated in the DOT for the functional capacities portion of the process (Fishbain et al., 1994; Jones & Kumar, 2003; King et al., 1998). See Figure 42.4.

Clinicians may evaluate the physical demands using different methods depending on the protocol they employ for their FCE. However, all of the FCEs involve evaluating a variation of the DOT Physical Demands (King et al., 1998; U.S. Department of Labor, 1991). The DOT classifies work into five categories of strength factors, based on lifting, carrying, pushing, and pulling, which the Social Security Administration and some workers' compensation systems use to assist with determining a client's status and future work classification or ability. See Figure 42.5 and Figure 42.6.

During this part of the process, the clinician can make the determination regarding the client's strength factor category to help quantify return-to-work choices available to him or her.

Virtually all FCEs have a lift capacity component in their protocols (King et al., 1998; Matheson, 1996). Many commercially available FCEs and Baseline FCEs include lifting assessment components that seek to determine a

Standing	Stooping
Walking	Kneeling
Sitting	Crouching
Lifting	Crawling
Carrying	Reaching
Pushing	Handling
Pulling	Fingering
Controlling (hand/arm)	Feeling
Controlling (foot/leg)	Talking
Climbing	Seeing (including acuity & visual field)
Balancing	Depth Perception

FIGURE 42.4 *Dictionary of Occupational Titles:* Physical Demands.

Sedentary Work — S

Exerting up to 10 pounds of force occasionally and/or a negligible amount of force frequently to lift, carry, push, pull, or otherwise move objects, like ledgers and small tools and including the human body. Although a sedentary job is defined as one which involves sitting, a certain amount of walking and standing is often necessary in carrying out job duties. Jobs are sedentary if walking and standing are required only occasionally and all other sedentary criteria are met.

Light Work — L

Exerting up to 20 pounds of force occasionally, and/or up to 10 pounds of force frequently, and/or a negligible amount of force constantly to move objects. Physical demand requirements are in excess of those for Sedentary Work. Even though the weight lifted may be only a negligible amount, a job should be rated Light Work: (1) when it requires walking or standing to a significant degree; or (2) when it requires sitting most of the time but entails pushing and/or pulling of arm or leg controls; and/or (3) when the job requires working at a production rate pace entailing the constant pushing and/or pulling of materials even though the weight of those materials is negligible. NOTE: The constant stress and strain of maintaining a production rate pace, especially in an industrial setting, can be and is physically demanding of a worker even though the amount of force exerted is negligible.

Medium Work — M

Exerting 20 to 50 pounds of force occasionally, and/or 10 to 25 pounds of force frequently, and/or greater than negligible up to 10 pounds of force constantly to move objects. Physical Demand requirements are in excess of those for Light Work.

Heavy Work — H

Exerting 50 to 100 pounds of force occasionally, and/or 25 to 50 pounds of force frequently, and/or 10 to 20 pounds of force constantly to move objects. Physical Demand requirements are in excess of those for Medium Work.

Very Heavy Work — V

Exerting in excess of 100 pounds of force occasionally, and/or in excess of 50 pounds of force frequently, and/or in excess of 20 pounds of force constantly to move objects. Physical Demand requirements are in excess of those for Heavy Work.

FIGURE 42.5 *Dictionary of Occupational Titles:* Strength Factor and Social Security Administration physical exertion requirements.

DOT/SSA Term		Definition
Occasionally	O	0–33% of the work day
Frequently	F	34–66% of the work day
Constantly	C	67–100% of the work day
Exerting Force		Lifting, carrying, pushing, and/or pulling

FIGURE 42.6 Key to strength factor and physical exertion terminology.

subject's maximum lift while monitoring heart rate changes and/or biomechanical changes during the test, which can also include the subject's report of pain or discomfort during the test. The tests usually involve lifting a standardized item with light weights and progressing to heavier weights (Matheson et al., 1988; Mayer, Barnes, Kishino, Nichols, Gatchel, Mayer et al., 1988). These assessments often include the use of the NIOSH standards or the National Institute for Occupational Safety and Health (NIOSH) equation for the design and evaluation of manual lifting tasks as an element of their lifting assessment (Waters, Putz-Anderson, Garg, & Fine, 1993).

Evaluators who take a Job Specific FCE approach use tools and materials from the worksite for the lift and other areas of the evaluation. With tools and materials from the actual work performed, evaluators can look at whether the individual can lift the items he or she needs to lift to perform his or her job task, or if the lifting can be eliminated as a reasonable accommodation if necessary.

The Job Specific FCE derives the tasks evaluated, such as lifting, from the job tasks gathered from the job analysis. The subject participates in simulated job tasks with the frequency, weights, measures, and repetitions of the tasks taken directly from the real-life job demands. It is inherently "job-related" within the meaning of the ADA and gives subjects an idea of whether they can perform their own jobs (29 C.F.R. §1630.14 (a); EEOC, 2000).

With both FCE approaches, the clinician must select the task for evaluation based on protocol, job analysis, the subject's physical and psychosocial condition, and professional judgment. The clinician must also use that professional judgment to prevent any further problems from occurring that might injure the test subject and stop the test should the subject experience physical, cardiac, or other problems.

ANALYZE FINDINGS

During this phase, the clinician analyzes and integrates the results of the functional capacity assessment and job analysis with the medical impairment and limitations to determine recommendations for job limitation, safety considerations, job placement, or disability determination. The baseline physical capacities, if performed, must be documented along with recommended work restrictions and/ or reasonable accommodations.

Bill, our airline pilot, may have reached maximum medical improvement, but still experiences lower back pain, general discomfort, fatigue, and right arm weakness. It is determined that he is physically unfit to fly commercially, and no reasonable accommodation is available under the guidelines for commercial pilots. The clinician must determine from documented assessment findings and medical reports Bill's specific medical impairment, functional abilities and limitations, physical capacities or abilities, and job-specific limitations. This information will be used by his case manager and attorney in determining his claims against workers' compensation and his pending litigation against the catering contractor. The information will further assist in Bill's decisions and plans for work conditioning programs, future job placement, or a career change.

PREPARE FINAL REPORT

Professionals who administer FCEs should make sure they write their reports in plain English, understandable to all potential readers. Clinicians should use clear, concise sentences that do not use jargon, medical terminol-

ogy, and other terms of art unfamiliar to those outside. Use of technical language and jargon should include definitions of the terms so the reader can understand them. For example, suppose one reported that Bill could abduct his right shoulder to 90° and externally rotate his right shoulder to 25°. The writer should follow this up with an example to illustrate what this means. One might say, for example, that because of this limitation, Bill could not comb his hair and could not pull down the lever on the presser machine.

Reports should tell a story and paint a picture that readers can understand and explain to others if necessary. Individuals reading these reports, such as attorneys, judges, administrative hearing officers, human resource personnel, and insurance adjusters, do not necessarily have a background in the subject matters and, therefore, use of jargon, minutiae, and technical terminology has the potential to frustrate the reader. Similarly, overly long, computer-generated reports, filled with charts and graphs meaningful only to the writer, may not contribute useful information to those concerned with the client.

The reports should summarize the important information on the first page in plain English. The summary should stress the client's strength and weaknesses as well as the evaluator's recommendations. Clinicians should keep in mind that realistically, in many situations, the summary may be the only part of the report that anyone actually reads and decisions may be based on this summary.

Clinicians should report the sources of their information (i.e., test results, reports by the patient/client, etc.). Objective data should play a significant role in the summary as well as in the body of the report to the extent the writer can abide by the "plain English" rule. Report writers should use well-labeled headings in the body of the report to provide ready access to information.

Clinicians should relate test results directly to recommendations. To whatever extent possible, inclusion in the report of any evidence-based literature references regarding the assessment may assist fact finders (judges or administrative hearing officers) should the FCE subject find himself or herself involved with social security, workers' compensation, insurance disability personal injury, and/or other claims. See, e.g., *Daubert v. Merrell Dow Pharmaceuticals,* 509 US 579 (1993).

FACTORS TO CONSIDER IN SELECTING OR DEVELOPING FCES

Ideally, when selecting an FCE to use or when developing one's own, referral sources and clinicians should consider six basic factors: safety to the test subject, reliability, validity in predicting safe future job performance, content validity, practicality of test administration, and the ability to predict future risk of injury (King et al., 1998). However, while one can consider these six factors, according to the current literature, it is difficult to find or create an FCE that meets all of these criteria.

SCIENTIFIC AND PRACTICAL LIMITATIONS OF FCES

There are scientific and practical limitations to FCEs. Human behavior and performance are not always predictable and accurately measurable, especially when the complex phenomena of motivation, response and tolerance to pain, external environmental, and other internal psychosocial factors may influence task performance. An instrument that measures functional capacity for return-to-work determination should be reliable and valid with the sensitivity and specificity to measure job specific capacities (Innes & Straker, 1999a, 1999b). Most FCEs do not achieve these scientific standards; however, they do have value in documenting progress and performance limitations in relation to a job and in identifying factors influencing abilities (Pransky & Demsey, 2004). FCE results may contribute to job status or disability determination, but one should view these results as part of a broader assessment program that evaluates injury prevention and return-to-work issues. Other limitations identified by Matheson (1996) include the lack of formal or adequate training by clinicians and evaluators in evaluation procedures and test methodologies, availability of standardized test equipment, and reactivity to testing or testing effect.

The nature of FCEs makes them a difficult subject to study. Many of the FCE protocols are proprietary or commercial in nature and, thus, have not appeared in the peer-reviewed literature (Jones & Kumar, 2003). Most studies in the literature review "parts" of a battery of assessments included in an overall FCE, such as lifting or grip strength. This makes it difficult to craft a general statement about a given FCE and virtually impossible to craft statements comparing one FCE with another (Innes & Straker, 1999a). Because protocols vary from FCE to FCE (or FCA or physical capacity assessments [PCA]), and the literature fails to adequately reveal the contents of the evaluations, looking for overall generalizations about "FCEs" is also difficult.

PREDICTING RETURN TO WORK

FCEs may contribute valuable information to help determine job placement, job accommodation, return-to-work assignments after injury, and extent of impairment. FCE tools have long been used to determine the level of work an individual can safely perform. However, while functional capacity theory has long promoted FCEs as an aid to help predict work performance following postinjury rehabilitation (Kornblau et al., 1998; Matheson, 1996;

Smith, Cunningham, & Weinberg, 1986), recent research raises questions about the validity of the FCE's ability to identify those individuals who are "safe" to return to work. One retrospective study (Gross & Battie, 2004) that looked at the prognostic value of sustained recovery in individuals with low back pain showed that better performance on the FCE was associated with a *higher* risk of recurrence and thus not necessarily predictive of those "safe" to return to work.

While the literature indicates the predictive value of the FCE needs more research in terms of return to work as an outcome, the literature does support the ability of the FCE to provide the tools and procedures necessary to quantify present functional capacities (King et al., 1998). In other words, although the FCE might not be able to predict the airline pilot's long-term safe return to work, the FCE would provide quantifiable and qualitative information about his present functional capacities, including the impact of pain on his performance.

VALIDITY AND RELIABILITY

Subjective self-reporting of functional limitations serves as an important element of the evaluation process, but the information provided lacks validity and reliability. FCEs provide a process that may confirm or refute a claim of a functional limitation. The recipients of FCE outcome data (referral sources, insurance companies, workers' compensation case managers, and the injured worker) need some degree of confidence in order to rely on the FCE results. Decision makers need to base return-to-work and disability determinations on accurate and dependable objective measures. These issues point to concerns of validity and reliability of FCE measures and protocols.

Although the literature continues to report additional studies, most commercial FCEs lack adequate documentation of validity (Innes & Straker, 1999a). Validity concerns may stem from inadequately or too broadly defined job demands or inaccurate measures of actual performance capabilities. Further, FCEs based on job simulation test only the physical components of a job and may not include extraneous but significant factors such as the work environment and psychological components (Pransky, 2004). Predictive and concurrent validity are judged the most relevant for FCEs. Currently, the scientific literature does not support predicting return-to-work exclusively on FCE results (Gross, 2004).

Reliability of FCEs also raises concerns in the literature. Reliability threats include motivation, pain, fear, evaluator and equipment, and protocol application. Inconsistent use of practice or training sessions, intra-testing, and interrater testing are also concerns related to FCE reliability (Matheson et al., 1996). Innes and Straker (1999a) conducted an extensive literature review of the existing evidence of the reliability of 28 work-related assessments that included components of FCE batteries. They conclude that older tests that lack sufficient reliability data remain in use simply "because they are there" (Innes & Straker, 1999a). However, the developers of the newer FCE batteries place more emphasis on conducting and reporting reliability studies. Finally, Innes and Straker conclude that a limited number of work-related assessments have an adequate amount of evidence from which to draw conclusions, and they show a moderate to good degree of reliability, with only a few work-related assessments demonstrating reliability sufficient for clinical use. This study points to the need to improve reliability of existing work-related tests and for further reliability studies for other available tests, which need more evidence to prove their worth (Innes & Straker, 1999a).

IDENTIFYING SUBMAXIMAL EFFORT

Those who refer clients for FCEs often seek evidence of whether the client is putting forth full effort in cooperating with the evaluation. The literature suggests significant shortcomings in the effectiveness of the current menu of tests available that are thought to evaluate whether a client is putting forth submaximal or insincere effort. For example, some of literature suggests several shortcomings in the exchange grip strength test and other grip measures used as a means of testing submaximal effort in FCEs. First, no generally accepted standard protocol exists for submaximal effort testing based on grip strength tests (Taylor & Shechtman, 2000), and their reliability is questionable. Westbrook, Tredgett, Davis, and Oni (2002) findings suggest that the exchange grip strength test could not reliably detect submaximal effort. Shechtman and Taylor (2000) found that the rapid grip exchange test may not be sensitive or specific enough to detect insincere effort. The authors warn readers of the likelihood and consequences of mistakenly labeling subjects as putting forth less than a sincere effort, based solely on the rapid exchange grip test (Shechtman & Taylor, 2000).

Gutierrez and Shechtman (2003) found that grip strength testing with a Jamar dynamometer was strength dependent and potentially biased against those with weak hands who were presented with this method to assess sincerity of their effort. They found the Jamar five rung test less effective with women than with men, another potential bias. In light of all of their findings, Gutierrez and Shechtman (2003) recommend against using the five-rung test to assess sincerity of effort.

Lemstra, Olszynski, and Enright (2004) evaluated the effectiveness of 17 tests commonly used to detect maximal effort during FCEs. They found that only 5 of 17 commonly used tests of maximal effort could individually differentiate between subjects' maximal effort and submaximal effort. The five effective tests included 3 of the 6 commonly used hand grip measurement tests presented

to the subjects (Lemstra et al., 2004). In reporting their findings, the authors remind readers of the complexities of determining maximal effort and the medicolegal and ethical implications in labeling a test subject as exerting maximal, or less than maximal, effort and that caution should be taken in relationship to asserting these labels (Lemstra et al., 2004). This study also suggests the need for more effective assessment tools for evaluating maximal effort during FCEs.

LEGAL AND ETHICAL ISSUES

FCEs raise many legal and ethical issues for those who practice in this area. Because the clients referred for FCEs are often already involved in litigation and administrative claims, clinician/evaluators should make sure they maintain comprehensive malpractice insurance. They should put policies in place that promote prevention of client injuries. Documentation plays a key role in protecting one's professional self should something happen during the course of the FCE that puts clients at risk.

With FCE validity and reliability an issue, some question whether courts will accept the results of functional capacity assessments as evidence in court proceedings. One of the reasons for this concern is the case of *Daubert v. Merrell Dow Pharmaceuticals*, 509 U.S. 579 (1993). *Daubert* limits expert witness testimony to theories or techniques the court considers scientific knowledge that will assist the trier of fact or judge.

In *Daubert*, the U.S. Supreme Court articulated four factors for judges to consider in deciding whether to admit scientific expert witness testimony under the Federal Rules of Evidence, *Fed. Rule Evid.* § 104(a).

1. Has the theory or technique been tested?
2. Has the theory or technique been subjected to peer review and publication?
3. In the case of a particular scientific technique, is there a known or potential rate of error, and standards controlling the technique's operation
4. Is the underlying technique generally accepted in the scientific community?

Should the expert not pass muster according to these guidelines set forth in *Daubert*, his or her reports would be considered non-evidence and inadmissible and the FCE professional would not be allowed to testify. Although many pieces of FCEs have appeared in reliability and validity studies in the literature (see, e.g., Brouwer et al., 2003), the literature is certainly not conclusive by any means (Innes & Straker, 1999a, 1999b). However, FCEs have been mentioned in the occupational therapy literature as a part of the return-to-work process since World War I (Crane, 1927; Cranfield, 1947; Office of the Surgeon General, 1968; Reuss, Rawe, & Sundquist, 1958). FCEs have been studied for more than 50 years and are accepted as an integral part of the return-to-work process. The information gathered through FCEs provides fact-finders with objective, quantifiable data.

Federal and state courts have accepted expert witness testimony regarding FCEs and have allowed other experts to give testimony based on results of FCEs that these witnesses relied upon in forming their opinions. (See *Thigpen v. Retirement Board of Firemen's Annuity & Benefit Fund*, 317 Ill.App.3d 1010, 251 Ill.Dec. 682, 741 N.E.2d 276 (2000); *Brennan v. Reinhart Institutional Foods*, 211 F.3d 449, 54 Fed. R. Evid. Serv. 535 (8th Cir., 2000). Clinicians should prepare themselves for court by gathering publications that reference FCEs positively and prepare themselves to defend against those that are not so favorable.

Another significant issue involves the question, "Who is the client?" A typical FCE referral scenario involves a third party — the insurance carrier, defense or claimant's attorney, or case manager — referring our pilot Bill for the FCE and in some cases another party — his employer, for example, paying for the services. In providing occupational therapy interventions in work practice, the professional standards support the concept of client-centered care or intervention. In this situation, one must decide whether the "client" is Bill, our test subject, or the workers' compensation defense attorney representing Bill's employers' workers' compensation insurance carrier — the one who made the referral — or Bill's employer who is ultimately paying the bill. What if the evaluator perceives that Bill is underestimating his subjective complaints and trying too hard because he is so motivated to return to work? With his safety questionable under the circumstances, should the evaluator disclose this information if Bill feels disclosure of the information is not in his best interest? On the other hand, does the evaluator owe a duty to the referral source or the employer to report this information about Bill's risk of safety should he return to work?

One might look at this scenario and think, "Does it really matter?" Doesn't the clinician/evaluator owe a duty to all three parties? However, this situation presents an ethical dilemma to the clinician/evaluator because the three parties may have different interests and one cannot readily determine to whom the tester owes a duty beyond the actual test subject (Kornblau & Starling, 2000).

SUMMARY

Functional capacity evaluations are systematic assessments that measure physical abilities and functional capacity related to work demands. FCEs provide objective information from a trained evaluator to the injured worker/claimant, clinicians, case managers, insurance adjusters, employers, and other payers of compensation or benefit systems. The evaluation findings can verify or refute a worker's subjective report of work limitations resulting from an injury or illness. FCE results provide useful information to assist in determining job placement, recommendations for accommodations, and other return-to-work options. When used together with an injury prevention program, FCEs may be to determine safety guidelines and limits. FCEs serve as a baseline for function and a final evaluation for work rehabilitation programs; they also contribute information to help determine when one has reached maximum medical improvement.

Two types of FCEs have been described: the Baseline and the Job Specific FCEs. The Baseline FCE looks more generally at the baseline of individual function in relation to the physical demands of work. The Job Specific FCE evaluates the worker's abilities within the specific demands of the job. With either type of FCE, a job analysis is seen as an important if not crucial element of the evaluation process. An evaluation with a job analysis better matches the worker to the demands of his or her job or a possible alternative job. An onsite job analysis will, of course, provide more specific job demand information than looking at job descriptions or databases such as the DOT or O*NET.

Clinicians/evaluators use different methodologies depending on the FCE protocol used, but most FCEs assess physical abilities or function, as well as sensory and cognitive functions. The authors stress that clinicians and evaluators look at the whole person and the effect the impairment may have on other aspects of the worker's life in addition to the worker role.

The FCE, as it currently exists, remains the only tool that can provide quantitative and qualitative data about how the individual functions in relationship to work performance and the work environment. The literature paints the FCEs as a necessary but less than perfect system of determining the level of work-related abilities and limitations that result from injury, accident, or illness. The interest in objective measures of functional capacity related to work is expected to continue to rise as more parties demand accurate and reliable information to help with decision making in workers' compensation or other benefit claims, disability determination, work placement, reasonable accommodations, and litigation issues. Ongoing FCE development work and research will continue to improve the reliability and validity of FCE systems and methodologies. The injured worker evaluation process will continue to evolve to better integrate functional assessments from the perspective of the injured individual as a whole, rather than fragmented working parts.

REFERENCES

29 C.F.R. §1630.1 *et.seq.* Americans with Disabilities Act, Title I Regulations.

29 C.F.R. §1630.2(n) Essential functions.

20 C.F.R. §404.1567 Vocational consideration — Physical exertion requirements.

American Medical Association. (1993). *Guides to the evaluation of permanent impairment* (4th ed.). Chicago: AMA.

Beck, A. T., & Steer, R. A. (1984). Internal consistencies of the original and revised Beck Depression Inventory. *Journal of Clinical Psychology, 40*(6), 1365–1367.

Blankenship, K. L. (1994). *The Blankenship system functional capacity evaluation: The procedure manual* (2nd ed.). Macon, GA: The Blankenship Corporation.

Brennan v. Reinhart Institutional Foods, 211 F.3d 449, 54 Fed. R. Evid. Serv. 535, (8th Cir. 2000).

Brouwer, S., Reneman, M. F., Dijkstra, P. U., Groothoff, J. W., Schellekens, J. M., & Goeken, L. N. (2003) Test–retest reliability of the Isernhagen Work Systems functional capacity evaluation in patients with chronic low back pain. *Journal of Occupational Rehabilitation, 13*(4). 207–218.

Carlson, A. (1983). Assessment of chronic pain: I. Aspects of the reliability and validity of the visual analog scale. *Pain, 16,* 87–101.

Crane, A. G. (1927). Medical Department of the Army in the World War, Part 1. Washington, DC: Government Printing Office.

Cranfield, H.V. (1947). Assessment of the working capacity of the physically disabled person. *American Journal of Occupational Therapy, 26,* 128.

Daubert v. Merrell Dow Pharmaceuticals. 509 US 579 (1993).

Dusik, L. A., Menard, M. R., Cooke, C., Fairburn, S. M., & Beach, G. N. (1993). Concurrent validity of the ERGOS work simulator versus conventional functional capacity evaluation techniques in a workers' compensation population. *Journal of Occupational Medicine, 35*(8), 759–767.

Ellexson, M. (2000). Job analysis. In B. L. Kornblau & K. Jacobs (Eds.), *Work: Principles and practice, a self-paced clinical course* (Lesson 5). Bethesda. MD: The American Occupational Therapy Association.

Equal Employment Opportunity Commission (EEOC). (2000). *Enforcement guidance on disability-related inquiries and medical examinations of employees under the Americans with Disabilities Act (ADA).* Retrieved from http://www.eeoc.gov/ada/adadocs.html.

Federal Rule of Evidence. §104(a).

Fishbain, D. A., Abdel-Moty, E., Cutler, R., Khalil, T. M., Sadek, S., Rosomoff, R. S., & Rosomoff, H. L. (1994). Measuring residual functional capacity in chronic low back pain patients based on the *Dictionary of Occupational Titles. Spine, 19,* 872–880.

Gibson, L., & Strong, J. (2002). Expert review of an approach to functional capacity evaluation. *Work, 19,* 231–242.

Gross, D. P. (2004). Measurement properties of performance-based assessment of functional capacity. *Journal of Occupational Rehabilitation, 14*(3), 165–174.

Gross, D. P., & Battie, M. C. (2004). The prognostic value of functional capacity evaluation in patients with chronic low back pain: Part 2: Sustained recovery. *Spine, 29*(8), 920–924.

Gutierrez, Z., & Shechtman, O. (2003). Effectiveness of the five-handle position grip strength test in detecting sincerity of effort in men and women. *American Journal of Physical Medicine and Rehabilitation, 82*(11), 847–855.

Harrand G. M., & Hoffman, P. R. (1980). The physical capacity evaluation in vocational evaluation. *National Reporter,* Stout Vocational Rehabilitation Institute, Spring/Summer. Menomonie, WI: University of Wisconsin-Stout.

Hildebrandt, J., Franz, C. E., Choroba-Mehnen, B., & Temme, M. (1988). The use of pain drawings in screening for psychological involvement in complaints of low back pain. *Spine, 13*(6), 681–685.

Innes, E., & Straker, L. (1999a) Reliability of work-related assessments. *Work, 13,* 107–124.

Innes, E., & Straker, L. (1999b) Validity of work-related assessments. *Work, 13,* 125–152.

Isernhagen, S. J. (1995). Contemporary issues in functional capacity evaluation. In S. J. Isernhagen (Ed.), *The comprehensive guide to work injury management* (pp. 410–429). Gaithersburg, MD: Aspen.

Jebsen, R. H., Taylor, N., Triescsmann, R. B., Trotter, M. J., & Howard, L. A. (1969). An objective and standardized of hand function. *Archives of Physical Medicine and Rehabilitation, 50,* 311–319.

Jones, T., & Kumar, S. (2003). Functional capacity evaluation of manual materials handlers: A review. *Disability and Rehabilitation, 25*(4–5), 179–191.

Key, G. (2004) KEY Method's FCA: The functional capacity assessment. Retrieved June 26, 2004 from http://www.keymethod.com/products/fca.htm.

King, P. M., Tuckwell, N., & Barrett, T. E. (1998). A critical review of functional capacity evaluations. *Physical Therapy, 78*(8), 852–866.

Kornblau, B. L. (1996). The occupational therapist and vocational evaluation. *Work Programs,* Special Interest Section Newsletter, *10*(1), 1–4.

Kornblau, B.L., & Ellexson. M. (1992). *What every rehab professional in the U.S.A. should know about the ADA.* Miami, FL; ADA Consultants.

Kornblau, B. L., & Starling, S. (2000). *Ethics in rehabilitation — A clinical perspective.* Thorofare, NJ: Slack, Inc.

Kornblau, B. L., Dahl, R., Armstrong, F., Ellexson, M., & Larson, B. (1998). *Functional capacity evaluation.* Bethesda, MD: The American Occupational Therapy Association. Retrieved from http://www.aota.org/featured/area6/links/link02o.asp.

Korbon, G. A., DeGood, D. E., Schroeder, M. E., Schwartz, D. P., & Shutty, Jr., M. S. (1987). The development of a somatic amplification rating scale for low-back pain. *Spine, 12*(8), 787–791.

Lechner, D. E., Jackson, J. R., Roth, D. L., & Straaton, K. V. (1994). Reliability and validity of a newly developed test of physical work performance. *Journal of Occupational Medicine, 36*(9), 997–1004.

Lemstra, M., Olszynski, W. P., & Enright, W. (2004). The sensitivity and specificity of functional capacity evaluations in determining maximal effort: A randomized trial. *Spine, 29*(9), 953–959.

Matheson, L. (1989). Work capacity evaluation. In D. C. Tollison & M. L. Kriegel (Eds.), *Interdisciplinary rehabilitation of low back pain* (pp. 232–342). Baltimore, MD: Williams & Wilkins.

Matheson, L. N. (1996). Standardized evaluation of work capacity. In G. B. J. Anderson, S. L. Demeter, & G. H. Smith (Eds.). *Disability evaluation* (pp. 249–264). Chicago: Mosby Yearbook.

Matheson, L. N., Kaskutas, V., & Mada, D. (2001). Development and construct validation of the hand function sort. *Journal of Occupational Rehabilitation, 11*(2), 75–86.

Matheson, L. N., Mooney, V., Grant, J., Leggett, S., & Kenny, K. (1996). Standardization evaluation of work capacity. *Journal of Back and Musculoskeletal Rehabilitation, 6*, 249–264.

Matheson, L. N., Mooney, V., Holmes, D., Grant, J. E., Affleck, M., Hall, H. et al. (1988). A test to measure lift capacity of physically impaired adults: Part 2. Reactivity in a patient sample. *Spine, 20*, 2130–2134.

Mathiowetz, V., Weber, K., Volland, G., & Kashman, N. (1984). Reliability and validity of grip and pinch strength evaluations. *Journal of Hand Surgery, 9*, 222–226.

Mathiowetz, V., Weber, K., Kashman, N., & Volland, G. (1985). Adult norms for the nine hole peg test for finger dexterity. *Occupational Therapy Journal of Research, 5*(1), 25–37.

Mayer, T. G., Barnes, D., Kishino, N. D., Nichols, G., Gatchel, R. J., Mayer, H., & Mooney, V. (1988). Progressive isoinertial lifting evaluation: 1. A standardized protocol and normative database. *Spine, 13*, 993–997.

Melzack, R. (1975). The McGill Pain Questionnaire: Major properties and scoring methods. *Pain, 1*(3), 277–299.

Office of the Surgeon General. (1968). Army Specialist Corps. Washington, DC: Government Printing Office.

O*NET. (2004). Occupational Information Network Consortium (O*NET). Retrieved June 25, 2004 from www.onet-center.org.

Pransky, G. S., & Dempsey, P. G. (2004). Practical aspects of functional capacity evaluations. *Journal of Occupational Rehabilitation, 14*(3), 218–219.

Ransford, A. O., Cairns, D., & Mooney, V. (1976). The pain drawing as an aid to the psychological evaluation of patients with low back pain. *Spine, 1*, 127–123.

Reuss, E. E., Rawe, D. E., & Sundquist, A. E. (1958). Development of a physical capacities evaluation. *American Journal of Occupational Therapy, 12*(1), 1–8.

Salo, D., Eget, D., Lavery, R. F, Garner, L., Bernstein, S., & Tandon, K. (2003). Can patients accurately read a visual analog pain scale? *American Journal of Emergency Medicine, 21*(7), 515–519.

Shechtman, O., & Taylor, C. (2000). The use of the rapid exchange grip test in detecting sincerity of effort, Part II: Validity of the test. *Journal of Hand Therapy, 13*(3), 203–210.

Smith, G. A., Nelson, R. C., Sadoff, S. J., & Sadoff, A. M. (1989). Assessing sincerity of effort in maximal grip strength tests. *American Journal of Physical Medicine and Rehabilitation, 68*, 73–80.

Smith, S. L., Cunningham, S., & Weinberg, R. (1986). The predictive validity of functional capacities evaluation. *American Journal of Occupational Therapy, 40*, 563–567.

Stewart, S., Letts, L., Law, L., Cooper, B. A., Strong, S., and Rigby, P. J. (2003). The person-environment-occupation model. In E. B. Crepearu, E. S. Cohn, & B. A. Shell (Eds.), *Willard & Spackman's occupational therapy* (pp. 227–231). Philadelphia: Lippincott/Williams & Wilkins.

Taylor, C., & Shechtman, O. (2000). The use of the rapid exchange grip test in detecting sincerity of effort, Part I: Administration of the test. *Journal of Hand Therapy, 13*(3), 195–202.

Thigpen v. Retirement Board of Firemen's Annuity and Benefit Fund of Chicago. 317 Ill.App.3d 1010, 741 N.E.2d 276, 251 Ill.Dec. 682 (Ill.App. 1 Dist. Nov 28, 2000) *appeal denied,* Ill.2d 583, 747 N.E.2d 358, 254 Ill.Dec. 318 (Ill. Apr 04, 2001) (TABLE, NO. 90720).

Trombly, C. A., & Radomski, M.V. (Eds.). (2002). *Occupational therapy for physical dysfunction* (5th ed., pp. 720–725). Philadelphia: Lippincott/Williams & Wilkins.

U.S. Department of Labor. (1986). *Dictionary of occupational titles* (fourth edition supplement). Washington, DC: U.S. Government Printing Office.

U.S. Department of Labor. (1991). *The revised handbook for analyzing jobs.* Washington, DC: U.S. Government Printing Office.

Waddell, G., McCulloch, J. A., Kummel, E., & Venner, R. M. (1980). Nonorganic physical signs in low-back pain. *Spine, 5*, 117–125.

Waters, T. R., Putz-Anderson, V., Garg, A., & Fine, L. J. (1993). Revised NIOSH equation for the design and evaluation of manual lifting tasks. *Ergonomics, 36*, 749–776.

Westbrook, A. P., Tredgett, M. W., Davis, T. R., & Oni, J. A. (2002). The rapid exchange grip strength test and the detection of submaximal grip effort. *Journal of Hand Surgery, 27*(2), 329–333.

Williams v. Toyota Motor Mfg., 534 U.S. 184 (2002)

—43—

Diagnostic Musculoskeletal Ultrasound

Kelly Black, MD, and David Chapman, MD, MS

INTRODUCTION

Ultrasound shows musculoskeletal anatomy from a new and unique perspective (Van Holsbeeck & Introcaso, 2001). Musculoskeletal sonography is an advanced application of an established technology to evaluate the acute or chronic painful condition. Diagnostic musculoskeletal ultrasound has been used since the 1970s throughout the world, in the Olympics, and with professional and collegiate athletes, and is recently becoming accepted in the United States (Chapman & Black, 2003). The capability of ultrasound to demonstrate fluid with great sensitivity and specificity proves extremely useful in the diagnosis of osteoarticular diseases (Van Holsbeeck & Introcaso, 2001).

This is a brief introduction to musculoskeletal ultrasound; it is not our intent to make this an exhaustive review of musculoskeletal ultrasound but to point out its uses and benefits. We cover some of the most common uses along with some rare clinical entities.

SONOGRAPHY VERSUS OTHER MODALITIES

The availability, ease of examination, and low cost of sonography in contrast to magnetic resonance imaging (MRI) make follow-up of healing lesions practical. Sonography can provide all the information available with MRI and more with regard to muscle pathology. Its spatial resolution and definition of muscle structure are usually superior to those provided by MRI (Van Holsbeeck & Introcaso, 2001). The basic problem with MRI is that only subtle contrast differences of nerves and surrounding tissues are demonstrated; further, the resolution of MRI is still far below that of sonography. Another reason for the low impact of MRI for diagnosis of peripheral nerve disease is the oblique course of nerves in the extremities — while it is easy to follow a nerve with a longitudinal sonographic scan, this is barely accomplished at all with MRI (Peer, 2003). The interaction with the patient during a sonographic examination helps determine possible pathology and allows for a focused investigation. The examination is easily tailored to the exact location of a patient's pain sensations, or areas of possible coexisting trauma. It is quick and lacks the discomfort caused by pricking with needles during electrodiagnostic studies or by positioning in MRI (Peer, 2003).

Serial ultrasound can be useful in following healing processes, and it provides essential feedback to the athlete and clinician. Real-time ultrasound offers the best dynamic study currently available and allows for prompt image-guided procedures such as aspiration of fluid collections. Bilateral examinations can be performed expeditiously. There is no risk to patients with pacemakers or cochlear implants, and artifacts due to ferromagnetic implants do not occur. Use of Doppler further allows depiction of tissue inflammation and vascularity (Torriani & Kattapuram, 2003). Besides being inexpensive and commonly available, sonography spares the patient from ionizing radiation and is an interactive and nondiscomforting method, which makes it the first choice from a patient's viewpoint (Peer, 2003). Although electrodiagnosis is able to definitely confirm and in many cases localize a nerve lesion, to define the nature of the underlying pathology is often beyond its reach (Torriani & Kattapuram, 2003). The information from the ultrasound examination has a major impact on decision making in competitive athletics, disability, medicolegal cases, and sports injuries in the authors' practice.

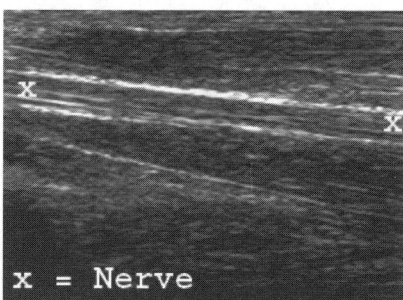

FIGURE 43.1 A normal median nerve (between the x's) in the forearm.

NORMAL NERVES

For inspection of the peripheral nerve, sonography may be regarded as the number one imaging modality. Peripheral nerves are in most cases superficially lying structures easily accessible with sonography, they show a typical and quite distinct sonographic texture, and recent studies have revealed characteristic findings in various disease entities. In comparison with MRI, which is the only competing imaging modality for the workup of nerve compression syndromes, sonography is low cost and generally available. At the same time sonography is nondiscomforting, quickly performed, and easily adjusted to a patient's complaints in static as well as dynamic examinations. The latter are an important adjunct to the standard evaluation of peripheral nerve diseases, and especially valuable for the diagnosis of functional disorders such as the snapping triceps syndrome with ulnar nerve dislocation. This functional evaluation is beyond the abilities of the MRI. A huge advantage of sonography in comparison with MRI is its ability to image longer nerve segments in a single study and its superior resolution. One of the major advantages of sonography compared with other imaging modalities, such as MRI, for example, is its ability to acquire images in virtually every orientation along the course of a peripheral nerve (Peer, 2003).

Figure 43.1 is a longitudinal view of a normal nerve. Nerves have a characteristic appearance on ultrasound. The examination of a peripheral nerve should include transverse and longitudinal scanning (Peer, 2003). At dynamic examination with active or passive movements, the mobility (or immobility) of the nerve in relation to the surrounding musculotendinous structures is assessed. Normal nerves appear as markedly echogenic tubular structures with parallel internal linear echoes on longitudinally oriented scans and as an oval or round echogenic section on transverse scans, occasionally with internal punctate echoes (Fornage, 1988).

NORMAL MUSCLE

Real-time examination available only with ultrasound elucidates some types of muscle lesions that are occult on

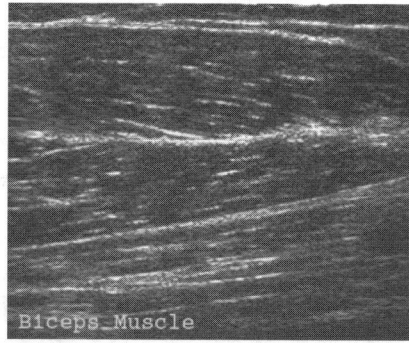

FIGURE 43.2 The bipennate structure of the normal biceps muscle.

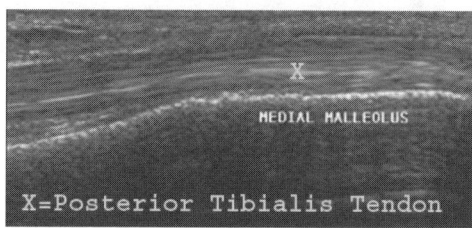

FIGURE 43.3 A normal posterior tibialis tendon.

static examinations. Serial sonographic examinations can accurately evaluate the rate and stage of healing, significantly decreasing the likelihood of reinjury (Van Holsbeeck & Introcaso, 2001).

Figure 43.2 is of normal muscle on a longitudinal view. The typical normal architecture of muscle as seen on longitudinal sections is generally evident; i.e., there is a "herringbone" pattern of hypoechoic skeletal muscle bundles separated by longitudinally aligned echogenic connective tissue (epimysium). In the transverse section the epimysium is seen end-on and therefore appears as an echogenic "dot" (Bohndorf & Kilcoyne, 2002).

NORMAL TENDON

Figure 43.3 shows the appearance of a normal tendon. Tightly packed, longitudinally arranged collagen bundles result in a brightly echogenic structure with a fine internal fibrillar pattern (Gibbon, 1996).

NORMAL JOINT

Figure 43.4 is a longitudinal view of a finger joint. Ultrasound is dramatically changing our approach to the evaluation of joint disease. In Europe, ultrasound has already established its place as the primary means of evaluating periarticular disease of synovial joints. The principal advantage of ultrasound over arthroscopy and MRI is its ability to examine the periarticular soft tissues with a more useful structural and anatomical detail. Many pain syndromes do not originate in bone or articular cartilage.

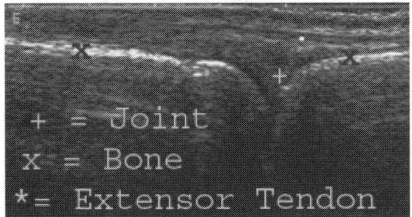

FIGURE 43.4 A normal metacarpal-phalangeal joint.

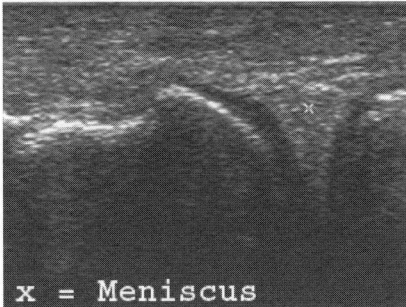

FIGURE 43.5 A normal medial meniscus of the knee.

Until now, these were presumptive clinical diagnoses. Sonography can be used to diagnose disease of the periarticular tissues with great sensitivity and specificity. The densely packed fibers of fibrocartilage result in a relatively homogeneous structure, although occasionally a subtle fibrillar pattern may be identified along the axis of the annularly arranged fibers (Gibbon, 1996). Figure 43.5 is a longitudinal view of the medial meniscus, which is composed of fibrocartilage.

Although hyaline cartilage, subchondral lamellar bone, and trabecular bone can be considered separately, they are now seen increasingly as a functional unit (Bohndorf & Kilcoyne, 2002). Hyaline articular cartilage is anechoic in young adults but its echogenicity slowly increases with age especially if there is chondrocalcinosis. Figure 43.6 is a

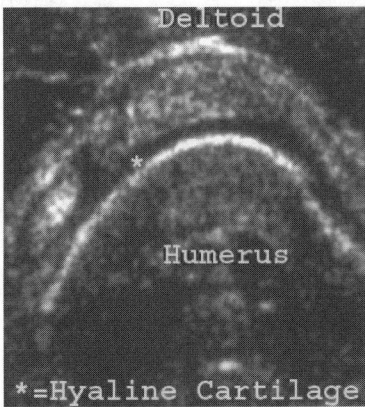

FIGURE 43.6 The normal hyaline cartilage in the shoulder joint, also note the circular hyperechoic biceps tendon on the left-hand side of the image.

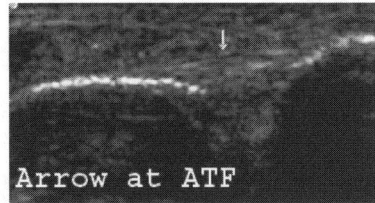

FIGURE 43.7 An intact anterior talofibular ligament bridging the talus and the fibula.

transverse view of the shoulder joint. In bone, the surface is usually brightly echogenic with profound posterior acoustic shadowing.

NORMAL LIGAMENTS

The advantages of ultrasound over MRI are the short examination time, the ability to provide a dynamic examination, reasonable cost, and availability. Computed tomography (CT) lacks sufficient contrast resolution to define ligamentous structures.

Figure 43.7 is a longitudinal view of the anterior talofibular ligament. Ligaments are composed of dense, regular connective tissue similar to that of tendons. Their structure differs from that of tendons in that more interweaving of collagen fibers is observed in ligaments, giving them a less regular histological and sonographic appearance (Van Holsbeeck & Introcaso, 2001).

NORMAL CLINICAL SONOGRAPHIC ANATOMY

In the soft tissues of the neck, many of the diagnostic problems that present to the clinician can be managed with maximal efficiency using ultrasound. The detail that can be seen in lymph nodes is superior to and more clinically useful than that obtained by either CT or MRI. In many cases one is able to make a confident diagnosis before fine needle aspiration cytology or histology, but in those cases where this is still indicated, ultrasound is the imaging technique of choice in guiding the needle to its best target. When one considers that the majority of structures and associated pathology in the neck lie only between 1 and 5 cm below the skin surface, and given the superior resolution that high-resolution ultrasound can attain, it is not surprising that ultrasound is gaining in popularity in the field of head and neck imaging. Ultrasound lends itself to biopsy techniques in the neck, being far superior to MRI and CT in this respect (Ahuja, Cozens, & Berman, 2000). Figure 43.8 shows a transverse view of the neck.

Several pain syndromes can be imaged and guided with ultrasound to help with proper diagnosis and to decrease risks with interventional procedures. Eagle's syndrome is caused by pressure on the internal carotid artery

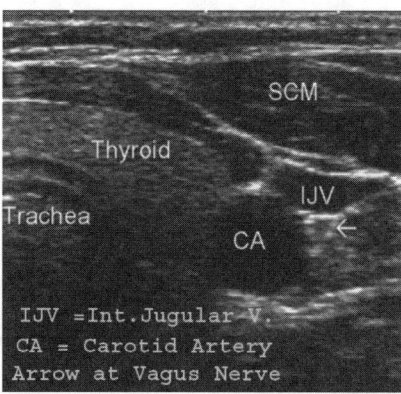

FIGURE 43.8 An example of normal structures in the neck.

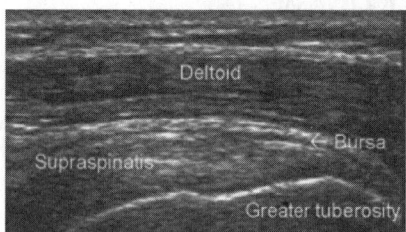

FIGURE 43.9 A normal supraspinatus tendon.

and glossopharyngeal nerve, by an abnormally elongated styloid process and/or a calcified stylohyoid ligament. Injection of the attachment of the stylohyoid ligament to the styloid with local anesthetic and steroid will serve as a therapeutic maneuver (Waldman, 2003). In our practice, we use dynamic ultrasound to evaluate the temporomandibular joint, surrounding musculature, and nerves. We also evaluate the vasculature with Doppler ultrasound. Ernest's syndrome is an insertional tendonosis of the stylomandibular ligament.

The subacromial-subdeltoid bursa lies superficial to the supraspinatis tendon and deep to the deltoid muscle. A thin layer of peribursal fat surrounds the bursa forming an echogenic (white) line between the deltoid and the supraspinatis (Chhem & Cardinal, 1999). The supraspinatus tendon has an outline that has been likened to that of a parrot's beak (Van Holsbeeck & Introcase, 2001). Figure 43.9 is a longitudinal view of a normal supraspinatis tendon.

Figure 43.10 shows a normal humeral epiphysis. Ultrasound has been used to diagnose Salter–Harris fractures in pediatric patients. Hubner et al. (2000) suggest the use of ultrasound in particular cases such as suspected bulge fractures or mildly displaced, simple fractures of the long bones of the forearm, humerus, femur, lower leg, and clavicle (Hubner et al., 2000).

Figure 43.11 shows that the fibrocartilaginous glenoid labrum can be visualized at ultrasound as a triangular, homogeneously hyperechoic structure that caps the bony rim of the glenoid (Sofka & Adler, 2002).

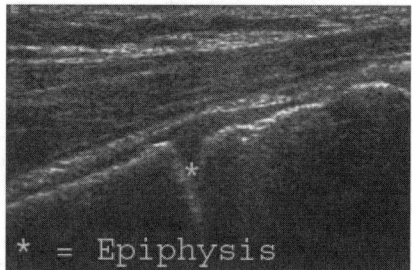

FIGURE 43.10 A normal growth plate in a 12-year-old female.

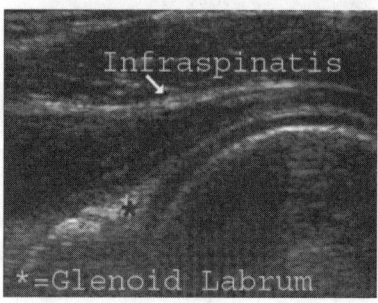

FIGURE 43.11 An example of the posterior aspect of the shoulder joint.

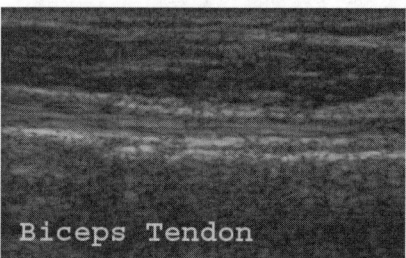

FIGURE 43.12 A normal biceps tendon overlying the proximal humerus.

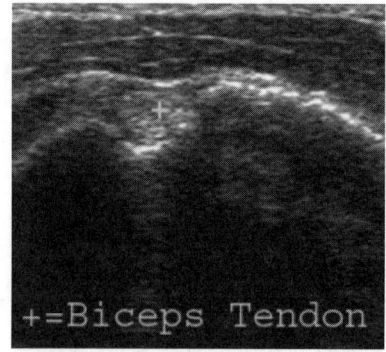

FIGURE 43.13 Transverse view of a normal biceps tendon.

Figure 43.12 shows a longitudinal image of the normal biceps tendon. The tendon will appear as hyperechoic parallel lines (Mack & Matsen, 1995).

Figure 43.13 is a transverse image of a normal biceps tendon. When viewed transversely, the bicipital groove, which contains the tendon of the long head of the biceps

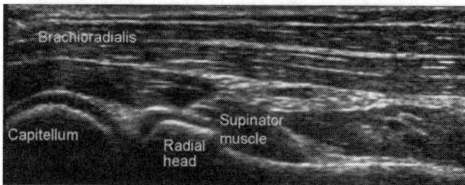

FIGURE 43.14 Normal extended view of the elbow. This type of view makes anatomic recognition more familiar to the clinician.

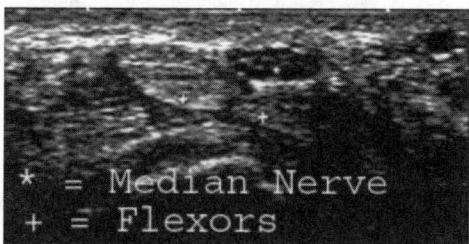

FIGURE 43.15 This view traces the perimeter of the median nerve to determine the cross-sectional area

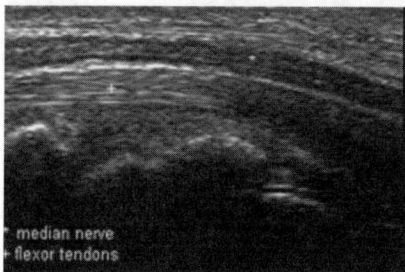

FIGURE 43.16 Visualization of the normal or abnormal glide of the median nerve and its interaction with the surrounding anatomical structures on dynamic examination.

brachii muscle, appears as a concavity in the bony surface of the humerus (Mack & Matsen, 1995).

Figure 43.14 is a panoramic view of a normal elbow. Sonography allows complete evaluation of the elbow and surrounding musculature. At all ages, a frank breach in the cortex is detectable with ultrasound. Children with suspected dislocations at the elbow may benefit in particular from sonography because the unossified cartilage is visible (Barr, 1995).

Figure 43.15 is of a normal carpal tunnel transverse view. Figure 43.16 is a longitudinal view of a normal carpal tunnel. Sonographic guided injection could improve the clinical efficacy of the intralesional treatment of carpal tunnel syndrome by allowing corticosteroid injection into the most appropriate target area. High power resolution plays a key role in ensuring the "step by step" control of needle placement in the target area (Grassi et al., 2002).

De Quervain's syndrome is a stenosing tenosynovitis that causes entrapment of the tendons of the muscles that abduct and extend the thumb. High-resolution ultrasound shows thickening of the tendon sheath of the abductor

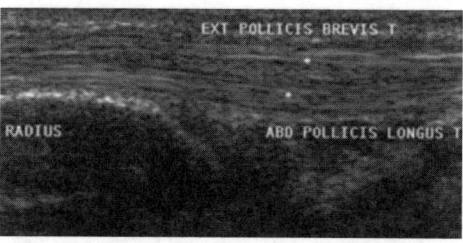

FIGURE 43.17 This view allows determining if each tendon shares a sheath or has a separate sheath, so that accurate injection of medication can be performed.

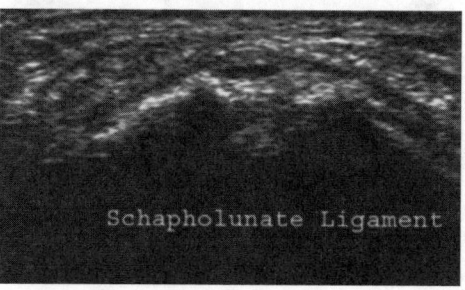

FIGURE 43.18 Scapholunate ligament connecting the scaphoid and lunate bones.

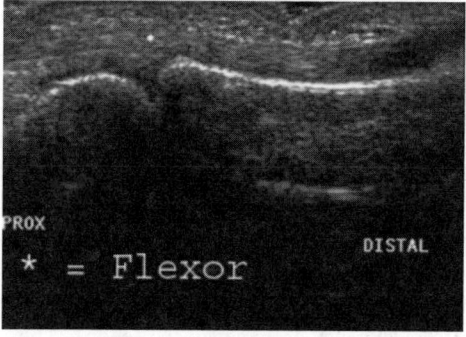

FIGURE 43.19 Dynamic imaging of this finger joint can reveal pulley tears or small tendon tears.

pollicis longus tendon and the extensor pollicis brevis tendon and color Doppler shows hypervascularity of those tendon sheaths (Lin et al., 2000). Figure 43.17 represents a longitudinal view of normal tendons mentioned above.

The scapholunate ligament is one of the important stabilizers of the wrist; abnormalities of this ligament may cause scapholunate dissociation, and rotary subluxation of the scaphoid bone (Totterman & Miller, 2000). The dorsal aspect of the ligament is seen in Figure 43.18.

Figure 43.19 is a longitudinal view of a finger flexor. Dynamic ultrasound with the fingers extended and with the fist clenched enabled excellent visualization of extensor tendon subluxation and dislocation at the metacarpal-phalangeal joint (Lopez-Ben, Lee, & Nicolodi, 2003). Ultrasound is a feasible imaging modality for measurement of the response of rheumatoid small-joint synovitis to therapy (Ribbens et al., 2003).

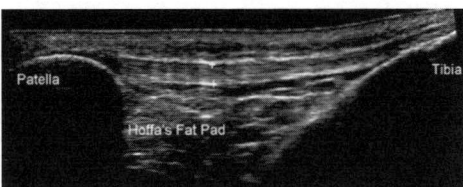

FIGURE 43.20 The extended view aids the clinician in observing a large segment of the infrapatellar region and then concentrating on the injured area.

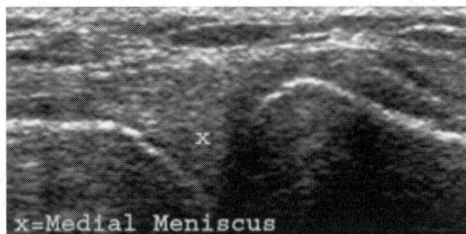

FIGURE 43.21 The peripheral portion of the medial meniscus is readily visualized.

Figure 43.20 represents a panoramic view of a normal infrapatellar ligament. The patellar tendon appears as a cylindrical structure on sonography passing from the inferior pole of the patella to the tibial tuberosity. The normal tendon measures 4 to 5 mm in anteroposterior thickness and broadens at both insertions (Carr et al., 2001).

The meniscus appears as a homogeneous hyperechoic triangle interposed between hypoechoic layers of articular cartilage (Strome, Bouffard, & Van Holsbeek, 1995). Figure 43.21 is a longitudinal view of the knee joint.

The Achilles tendon is the common tendon of soleus and gastrocnemius muscles. The anterior and posterior margins of the tendon should be parallel to each other without fusiform expansion or gap in the tendon. The normal tendon has a uniform fibrillar appearance (Thain et al., 2001). Figure 43.22 is a longitudinal panoramic view of the Achilles tendon.

The normal plantar fascia has a fibrillar echotexture and measures about 3 to 4 mm in thickness (Cardinal et al., 1996). Ultrasound diagnosis of plantar fasciitis includes thickening of the plantar fascia and fat pad edema (Sofka & Adler, 2002). Figure 43.23 is a longitudinal view of the plantar fascia.

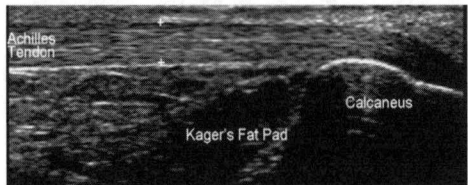

FIGURE 43.22 Panoramic view of the Achilles' tendon, the cursors depict the width of the tendon.

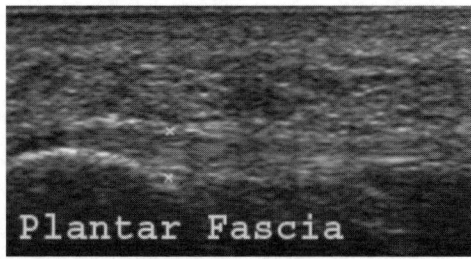

FIGURE 43.23 The x's show the width of the plantar fascia.

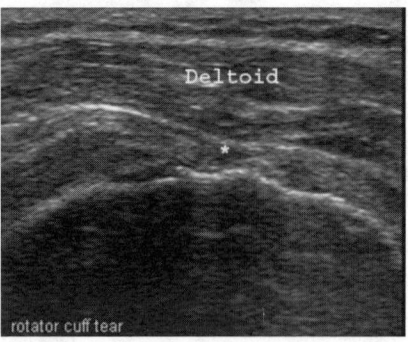

FIGURE 43.24 Full thickness tear of the supraspinatus tendon.

PATHOLOGIC SONOGRAPHY

Musculoskeletal ultrasound is particularly useful in the evaluation of tendons following surgical repair, assessment of soft tissues adjacent to orthopedic hardware, assessment of joint effusion, guidance of procedures and joint aspirations, evaluation of neoplasms, and sonographic assessment of osseous healing as well as focused investigation in stump pain in the amputed limb. Ultrasound offers a fast, effective, and relatively radiation-free method of assessment of postoperative musculoskeletal complications, free of some artifacts encountered on other modalities, including CT and MRI (Jacobson & Lax, 2002).

A full thickness tear is diagnosed when the disruption extends from the articular to the bursal surface of the tendon (Lin et al., 2000). In Figure 43.24, a full thickness tear of the supraspinatis tendon with peribursal fat and deltoid muscle herniation is noted. Also, note the cortical irregularity of the humerus that may accompany a full thickness tear. Sonographic findings of a partial thickness tear include a focal hypoechoic defect reaching either the bursal or articular surface, but not both (Lin et al., 2000). In Figure 43.25 note how the tear does not bridge the bursal and articular surfaces.

Figure 43.26 is a cyst located in the spinoglenoid notch. Suprascapular nerve follows a Z-shaped pattern with two fixed points: the first situated at the suprascapular notch and the second at the spinoglenoid notch. When nerve entrapment occurs at the suprascapular notch, both the infraspinatis and supraspinatis muscles are denervated. When compressed at the base of the scapular spine,

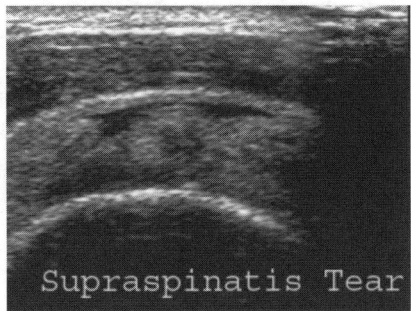

FIGURE 43.25 Partial thickness tear of the supraspinatus tendon.

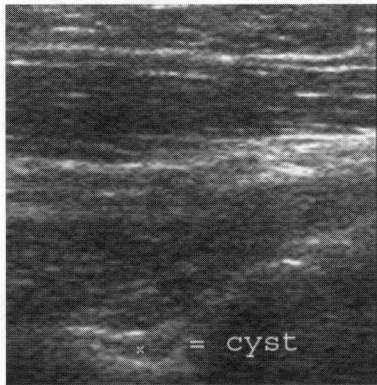

FIGURE 43.26 Spinoglenoid cysts can be drained and injected under ultrasound guidance.

infraspinatis denervation occurs while the supraspinatis remains intact (Ludwig et al., 2001) Ultrasound can detect muscle atrophy and fatty infiltration of the affected muscle. Also, a labral cyst can be detected and aspirated by ultrasound guidance.

Figure 43.27 depicts shoulder impingement test, which is best visualized on dynamic scanning. Stretching of small nerve fibers within the thickened bursal tissues results in pain upon motion and provides less space for the rotator cuff during movement because of the thickened, inflamed tissues (Van Holsbeeck & Introcaso, 2001).

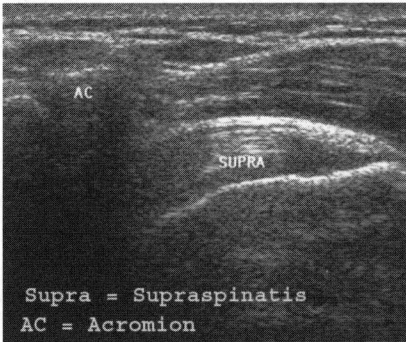

FIGURE 43.27 Dynamic imaging can reveal impingement of the supraspinatus tendon or peribursal fat as it attempts to go under the acromion.

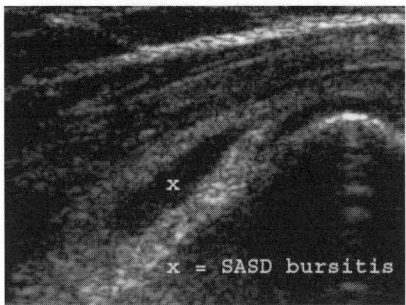

FIGURE 43.28 Large amount of fluid in the subacromial-subdeltoid bursa. In addition to bursitis, this can be a finding in rotator cuff tears.

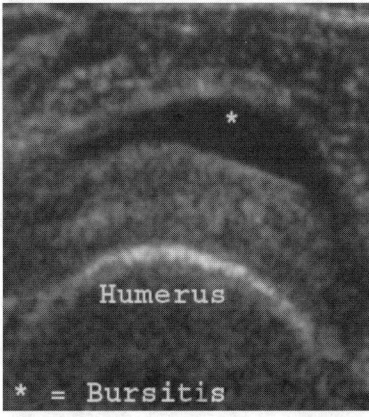

FIGURE 43.29 Curser on a large subacromial-subdeltoid bursitis. Ultrasound-guided aspiration revealed a traumatic hemorrhagic bursitis.

Bursal thickness should be no greater than 2 mm (Van Holsbeeck & Introcaso, 2001). The bursal space may be a potential space or may be seen as a thin hypoechoic (dark) band (due to a small amount of fluid) in normal individuals (Winter et al., 2001). Figure 43.28 shows a longitudinal ultrasound image of fluid in the bursa just inferior to the greater tuberosity and distal to the insertion of the supraspinatis tendon. Figure 43.29 is a transverse view of bursitis.

Figure 43.30 is an epidermal cyst. This cyst is the most common type found in the head and neck. It is surrounded by a fibrous capsule and has an epithelial lining (Ahuja et al., 2000). Ultrasound can help visualize and guide aspiration of loculations of the cyst and help prevent injury to nerves and blood vessels adjacent to the cyst.

Ulnar nerve dislocation represents an abnormal movement of the ulnar nerve out of the cubital tunnel and anterior to the medial epicondyle during flexion of the elbow, which is caused by an absence of the cubital tunnel retinaculum. Neuropathy is induced by abnormal friction and tear to the nerve during recurrent dislocation (Childress, 1975). Snapping triceps syndrome is medial dislocation of the medial head of the triceps muscle

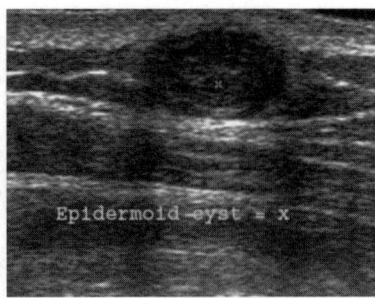

FIGURE 43.30 An epidermoid cyst with no loculations or significant vasculature near the cyst.

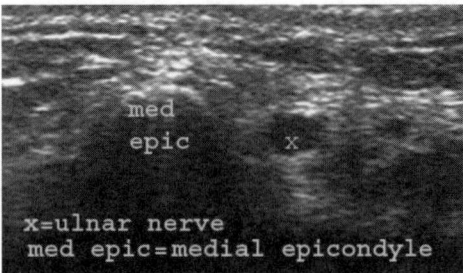

FIGURE 43.31 Ulnar nerve.

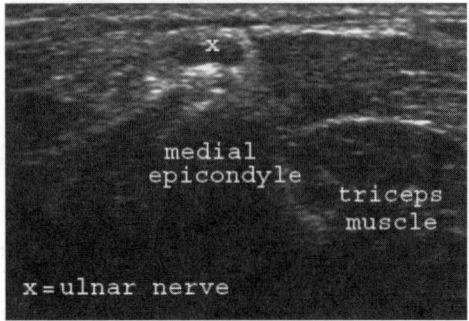

FIGURE 43.32 Ulnar nerve subluxation.

(Spinner & Goldner, 1998). Dynamic ultrasound allows direct visualization of the ulnar nerve and/or triceps dislocation during active flexion of the elbow (Jacobson et al., 2001). Figure 43.31 is of the ulnar nerve at the medial epicondyle in extension. Figure 43.32 is of the ulnar nerve dislocated anterior to the medial epicondyle with the medial head of the triceps muscle in flexion. This is an example of ulnar nerve dislocation with snapping triceps syndrome.

Figure 43.33 shows a tear and severe tendonosis of the flexor tendon origin of the elbow. Dynamic ultrasound also provides a rapid means for evaluating the anterior band of the ulnar collateral ligament in professional baseball pitchers (Nazerian et al., 2003).

Figure 43.34 demonstrates a horizontal tear of the medial meniscus. Sonography reliably demonstrates posterior and peripheral meniscal tears, which are not well demonstrated with arthroscopy (Casser, Sohn,

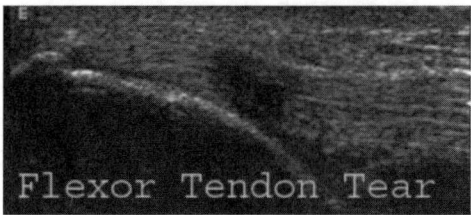

FIGURE 43.33 Flexor tendon tear of the elbow.

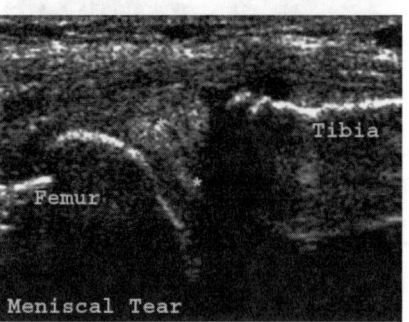

FIGURE 43.34 The black line above the asterisk is a tear.

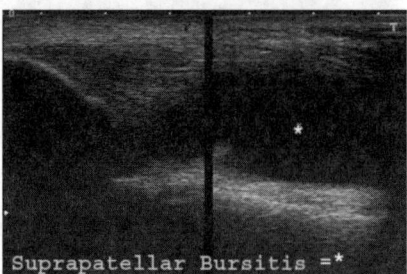

FIGURE 43.35 Ultrasound-guided aspiration and injection simplify procedures.

Kieckenback, 1990). Sonography is also able to identify injuries of the collateral ligaments or periarticular bursae that may mimic meniscal lesions clinically (Casser et al., 1990).

Figure 43.35 shows a suprapatellar bursitis. The suprapatellar bursa acts as a window to intra-articular knee pathology. Inflammatory and noninflammatory arthritis, infections, rheumatoid arthritis, osteoarthritis, gout, spondiloarthropathies, crystalline arthropathies, and trauma all manifest in some way in the suprapatellar bursa (Grobbelaar & Bouffard, 2000).

Figure 43.36 depicts an infrapatellar bursitis. Ultrasound is very sensitive for detecting joint and bursal fluid. An effusion may consist of clear fluid, pus, or blood (Ptasznik, 1999).

Figure 43.37 shows tendonosis of the infrapatellar tendon. Note the increased Doppler signal signifying neovascularization. It may be impossible to distinguish between small intratendon tears and increased gelatinous substance deposition within the tendon because of mucoid degeneration (Grobbelaar & Bouffard, 2000).

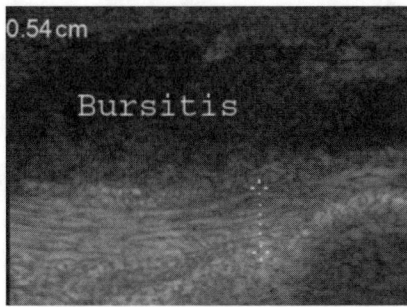

FIGURE 43.36 Cursors on distal infrapatellar tendon.

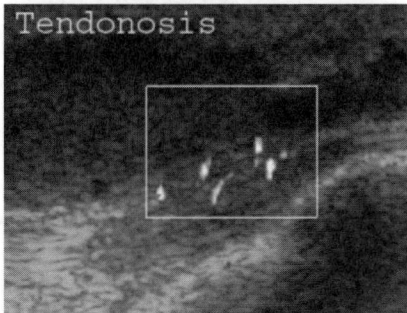

FIGURE 43.37 Doppler activity representing neovascularization.

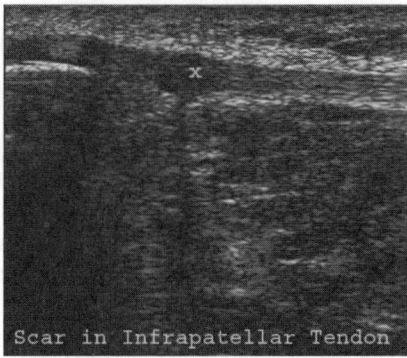

FIGURE 43.38 A 2-year-old trocar scar from arthroscopy.

Hoffa's infrapatellar fat pad can become inflamed with irritation or injury or after arthroscopic surgery. The fat pad may swell, and it may become hyperechoic (Thain et al., 2001). A normal fat pad contains two small vertical arteries with two or three horizontal arteries connecting them (Jacobson et al., 1997). On power Doppler images, a higher number of vessels represents inflammation of the fat pad (Thain et al., 2001). Figure 43.38 shows scar tissue filling in the path of a trocar through the infrapatellar tendon and Hoffa's fat pad from an arthroscopic procedure.

Figure 43.39 shows a Baker's cyst, which is the most commonly described cyst in the knee. The cyst is a pathologic distension of the semimembranosus-gastrocnemius bursa. The most important feature for identifying a Baker's cyst with ultrasound is visualization of the stem of the cyst, which originates in the medial aspect of the popliteal fossa,

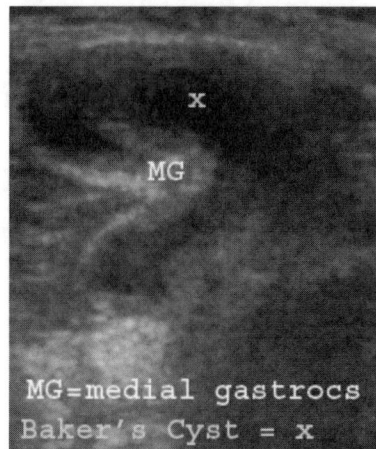

FIGURE 43.39 Fetus-like image of a Baker's cyst.

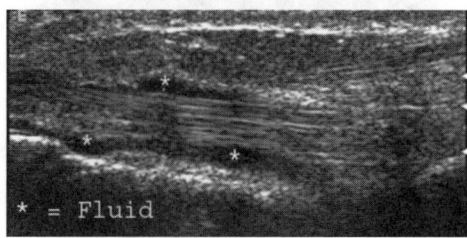

FIGURE 43.40 Peroneal tenosynovitis.

between the semimembranosus tendon and the medial gastrocnemius head (Grobbelaar & Bouffard, 2000).

Peroneal tenosynovitis is a common cause of periarticular pain at the ankle joint (Wang et al., 1999). In Figure 43.40, note the fluid distending the peroneal tendon sheath.

Morton's neuroma is a benign mass of perineural fibrosis affecting the plantar digital nerve (Rawool & Nazarian, 2000). The most common location is the third web space of the foot. On ultrasound, Morton's neuroma appears as a hypoechoic mass with an average size of 5 to 7 mm. Its relationship to the digital nerve can be established with ultrasound (Pollak et al., 1992). Figure 43.41 is a longitudinal view of the digital nerve going into a large hypoechoic mass. Figure 43.42 is a transverse view of a Morton's neuroma.

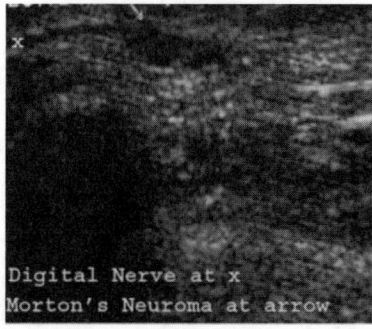

FIGURE 43.41 Morton's neuroma.

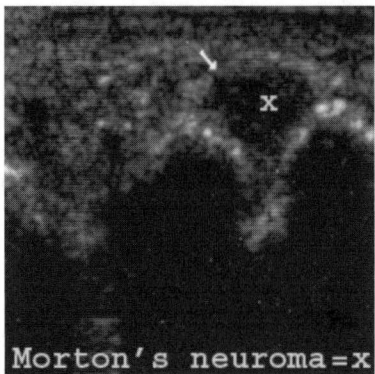

FIGURE 43.42 Morton's neuroma.

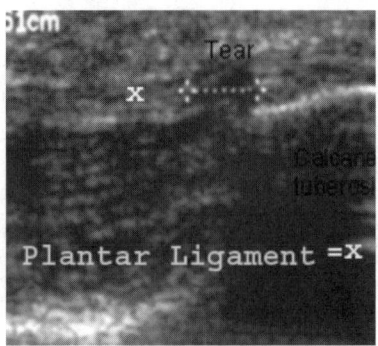

FIGURE 43.43 Plantar fascial ligament tear.

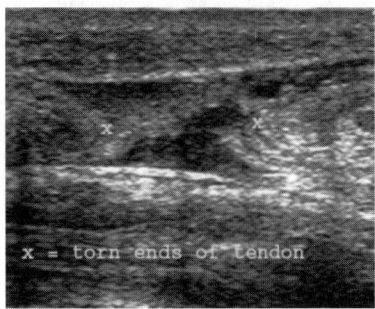

FIGURE 43.44 Achilles' tendon tear.

In Figure 43.43, note the hypoechoic gap in the plantar ligament representing a tear. In plantar fasciitis, ultrasound-guided injection allows accurate placement of medication and improved recovery.

Figure 43.44 is an acute complete rupture of an Achilles tendon. Achilles tendon tear or rupture is frequently caused by sports-related activities, but may also occur with systemic diseases that include inflammatory arthritis, autoimmune disease, diabetes, and gout (Fessell & van Holsbeek, 1999). Rupture most often involves a zone of relative avascularity located 2 to 6 cm proximal to the insertion of the tendon on the calcaneus (Winter et al., 2001). With an acute tear, a hematoma fills the gap

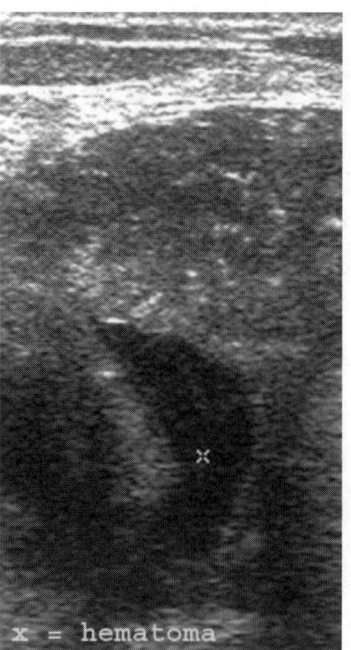

FIGURE 43.45 Pectoralis major muscle tear.

between the torn ends. The mechanism that causes pain in chronic Achilles tendonosis is not known (Astrom, 1997). However, high-resolution color Doppler ultrasound has shown that neovascularization may be involved. Ohberg et al. (2002) have found that sclerosing neovessels appears to be an effective treatment for painful chronic Achilles tendonosis.

Figure 43.45 is a muscle tear with hematoma filling the gap between the torn muscle ends. Ultrasound is also used for guided injection of myofascial trigger points as it can provide accurate placement of the needle and medication into the target tissue. Botulinum toxin can also be injected more accurately with ultrasound assistance with fewer adverse effects.

CONCLUSION

Diagnostic musculoskeletal ultrasound is used by physicians as an extension of the physical examination. Diagnostic musculoskeletal ultrasound can aid the physician in accurate diagnosis, treatment, and monitoring effects of therapy. It is our hope that ultrasound-guided interventions that are videotaped may decrease malpractice premiums for physicians performing office-based procedures. As advances in technology, such as three-dimensional and panoramic musculoskeletal ultrasound, improve we will have an even better and more user-friendly tool in our hands to evaluate patients with pain syndromes. We have given a very brief introduction of the many uses of musculoskeletal ultrasound in pain management.

REFERENCES

Ahuja, A. T., Cozens, N.J., & Berman L. (2000). Lumps and bumps in the head and neck and fine needle aspiration or core biopsy? In A. Ahuja & R. Evans (Eds.), *Practical head and neck ultrasound* (Chap. 5 & 8). London: Greenwich Medical Media.

Astrom, M. (1997). *On the Nature and Etiology of Chronic Achilles Tendonopathy*, Unpublished dissertation. Lund, Sweden: University of Lund.

Barr, L. (1995). Elbow. In B. Fornage (Ed.), *Musculoskeletal ultrasound* (Chap. 10). Philadelphia: Churchill Livingston.

Bohndorf, K., & Kilcoyne, R. F. (2002). Traumatic injuries: Imaging of peripheral musculoskeletal injuries. *European Radiology, 12*, 1605–1616.

Cardinal, E. et al. (1996). Plantar fasciitis: Sonographic evaluation. *Radiology, 201*, 257–259.

Carr, J. et al. (2001). Sonography of the patellar tendon and adjacent structures in pediatric and adult patients. *American Journal of Roentgenology, 176*(6), 1535–1539.

Casser, H. R., Sohn, C., & Kieckenback A. (1990). Current evaluation of sonography of the meniscus. Results of a comparative study of sonographic and arthroscopic findings. *Archives of Orthopaedic and Trauma Surgery, 109*, 150–154.

Chapman, D., & Black, K. (2003). Diagnostic musculoskeletal ultrasound for emergency physicians. *Emergency Medicine News, 25*(10), 60.

Chhem, R. & Cardinal, E. (1999). *Gamuts and guidelines in musculoskeletal ultrasound* (Chap. 2). New York: Wiley–Liss.

Childress, H. M. *(1975).* Recurrent ulnar nerve dislocation at the elbow. *Clinical Orthopaedics, 108*, 168–173.

Fessell, D. P. & Van Holsbeek, M. T. (1999). Foot and ankle sonography. *Radiology Clinics of North America, 37*, 831–858.

Fornage, D. (1988). Peripheral nerves of the extremities: Imaging with US. *Radiology, 167*(1), 179–182.

Gibbon, W. (1996). *Musculoskeletal ultrasound: The essentials,* London: Greenwich Medical Media.

Giovagnorio, F. (1997). Ultrasonographic evaluation of de Quervain disease. *Journal of Ultrasound Medicine, 16*, 685–689.

Grassi, W. et al. (2002). Intralesional therapy in carpal tunnel syndrome: A sonographic-guided approach. *Clinical and Experimental Rheumatology, 20*, 73–76.

Grobbelaar, N. & Bouffard, J.A. (2000). Sonography of the knee, a pictorial atlas. *Seminars in Ultrasound, CT, and MRI, 21*(3), 231–274.

Hubner, V. et al. (2000). Ultrasound in the diagnosis of fractures in children. *Journal of Bone and Joint Surgery* (Britain), *82*, 1170–1173.

Jacobson, J. A., & Lax, M.D. (2002). Musculoskeletal sonography of the postoperative orthopedic patient. *Seminars in Musculoskeletal Radiology, 6*(1), 67–77.

Jacobson, J. A. et al. (1997). MR imaging of the infrapatellar fat pad of Hoffa. *Radiographics, 17*, 675–691.

Jacobson, J. A. et al. (2001). Ulnar nerve dislocation and snapping triceps syndrome: Diagnosis with dynamic sonography — report of three cases. *Radiology, 220*, 601–605.

Lin, J. et al. (2000). An illustrated tutorial of musculoskeletal sonography: Part 2, upper extremity. *American Journal of Roentgenology, 175*(4), 1071–1079.

Lopez-Ben, R., Lee, D. H., & Nicolodi, D. J. (2003). Boxer knuckle (injury of the extensor hood with extensor tendon subluxation): Diagnosis with dynamic US — Report of three cases. *Radiology, 228*(3), 642–646.

Ludwig, T. et al. (2001). MR imaging evaluation of suprascapular nerve entrapment. *European Radiology, 11*(11), 2161–2169.

Mack, L. & Matsen, F. (1995). Rotator cuff. In B. Fornage (Ed.), *Musculoskeletal ultrasound* (Chap. 9). Philadelphia: Churchill Livingstone.

Nazerian, L. N. et al. (2003). Dynamic US of the anterior band of the ulnar collateral ligament of the elbow in asymptomatic major league baseball pitchers. *Radiology, 227*(1), 149–154.

Ohberg, L. et al. (2002). Ultrasound guided sclerosis of neovessels in painful chronic Achilles tendonosis: Pilot study of a new treatment. *British Journal of Sports Medicine, 36*, 1–2.

Peer, S. (2003). High resolution sonography of the peripheral nervous system: General considerations and technical concepts. In S. Peer & G. Bodner (Eds.), *High-resolution sonography of the peripheral nervous system* (Chap. 1, 2, 3). Berlin: Springer-Verlag.

Pollak, R.A. et al. (1992). Sonographic analysis of Morton's neuroma. *Journal of Foot Surgery, 31*, 534–537.

Ptasznik, R. (1999). Ultrasound in acute and chronic knee injury. *Radiology Clinics of North America, 37*(4), 797–817.

Rawool, N., & Nazarian, L. (2000). Ultrasound of the ankle and foot. *Seminars in Ultrasound, CT, and MRI, 21*(3), 275–284.

Ribbens, C. et al. (2003). Rheumatoid hand joint synovitis: Grayscale and power Doppler US quantifications following anti-tumor necrosis factor-alpha treatment: Pilot study. *Radiology, 229*, 562–569.

Schydlowsky, P. et al. (1998). Ultrasonographic examination of the glenoid labrum of healthy volunteers. *European Journal of Ultrasound, 8*, 85–89.

Sofka, C. M., & Adler, R. S. (2002). Ultrasound-guided interventions in the foot and ankle. *Seminars in Musculoskeletal Radiology, 6*(2), 163–168.

Spinner, R. J., & Goldner, R. O. (1998). Snapping of the medial head of the triceps and recurrent dislocation of the ulnar nerve. *Journal of Bone and Joint Surgery* (America), *80*, 239–246.

Strome, G., Bouffard, J. A., & Van Holsbeek, M. (1995). *Musculoskeletal ultrasound,* Philadelphia: Churchill Livingstone, chap. 18.

Thain, L. et al. (2001). Ultrasonography of lower leg: Technique, anatomy and pathologic conditions. *Canadian Association of Radiologists Journal, 52*(5), 325–336.

Torriani, M., & Kattapuram, S. V. (2003). Musculoskeletal ultrasound: An alternative imaging modality for sports-related injuries. *Topics in MRI, 14*(1), 103–110.

Totterman, S. M., & Miller, R. J. (2000). Scapholunate ligament: Normal MR appearance on three-dimensional gradient-recalled-echo images. *Radiology, 200,* 237–241.

Van Holsbeeck, M. T., & Introcaso, J. H. (2001). *Musculoskeletal ultrasound* (2nd ed.). St. Louis: Mosby.

Waldman, S. D. (2003). *Atlas of uncommon pain syndromes,* Philadelphia: Saunders.

Wang, S.-C. et al. (1999). Joint sonography. *Radiology Clinics of North America, 37*(4), 653–668.

Winter, T. C. et al. (2001). Musculoskeletal ultrasound. *Radiology Clinics of North America, 39*(3), 465–483.

44

Electrodiagnosis

Ross E. Lipton, MD, and David M. Glick, DC

INTRODUCTION

The experience of pain is unique to each individual. In spite of the immense strides that have been made in objectively defining the causes and pain perception, there is still much to learn of its pathways and mechanisms. The recording of brief bioelectrical potentials evoked after application of noxious stimuli in humans has aided in the effort to elucidate nociceptive pathways and mechanisms, and simultaneously augmented the clinical and radiological assessment of patients in acute pain. It is not atypical to distinguish acute from chronic pain by its more easily identifiable mechanism (generator). In contrast, chronic pain is far more challenging to characterize, as its localization and pathology tend to be more elusive. Despite these differences, electrodiagnostic assessment is valuable in characterizing both subtypes of pain.

Careful history and physical examination remain the most important tools used to evaluate the patient who complains of pain. The clinician then relies on his or her knowledge and experience to narrow the differential diagnosis and consider the possible underlying causes. It has become routine to consider other forms of assessment to assist in determining a more definitive diagnosis. Laboratory, imaging, and electrodiagnostic studies, whether considered as a group or individually as circumstances may dictate, are relied upon to identify, characterize, and quantify the presence of pathology and the likely cause of pain. In routine clinical practice, imaging studies, such as x-ray and magnetic resonance imaging (MRI) are often considered as the first adjunctive study for evaluating the patient with pain. These provide valuable structural data. While structure and function may overlap, imaging studies alone may not definitively reflect whether a pathology or abnormality is clinically relevant.

All pain has a neurological component. As the technology of physiologic assessment evolves, a means to assess each component of the pain pathway will likely develop. In the mean time, most electrodiagnostic procedures assess general nerve function and play an important role in characterizing neuropathogy. It is the goal of this chapter to provide discussion of those studies, which are considered routine, as well as those that are efficacious, but often overlooked. This chapter is not intended to serve as a comprehensive reference for electrodiagnostic procedures. Rather, it is meant to provide a basic introduction to the clinical utility, method of recording, and understanding the clinical significance of various electrodiagnostic studies.

INSTRUMENTATION

The central issue concerning instrumentation is safety. Vigilance and attention to detail, with respect to grounding, wiring, shielding, and patient-related issues (implantable electronic devices, etc.), goes a long way to ensure a safe laboratory. Once lab safety is secured, the examiner can concentrate on technical excellence and accuracy. To this end, the examiner must understand the capabilities and limitations of each electrodiagnostic testing device. For all of this, a basic conceptual understanding of electricity is key.

We take advantage of the unique characteristics of resistors and capacitors to configure electronic circuits that strategically either permit or block electronic signals. This configuration takes advantage of the difference between high-frequency and low-frequency bioelectric alternating current (AC) signals from the human body, as well as direct current (DC) signals (not biological). Ultimately, the filtering system permits one to manipulate the recorded bioelectrical signal by configuring the electrodiagnostic device to accept or reject specific potentials, based on signal characteristics, such as frequency and amplitude. When it works, the result is a computer screen (oscilloscope) devoid of extraneous noise, leaving a smooth baseline and an accurately assessed bioelectrical signal.

A variety of surface or needle electrodes act to interface between the machine and the patient. The electrode picks up the biological signal (alternating voltage current). Each electrode has inherent impedance (resistance to alternating current). "Good" system impedance is considered to lie in a range between 1,000 and 5,000 ohms. This will confer good signal conduction from the body to the machine. Lower impedance is better. However, if the impedance is too low, one should be suspicious of an unwanted pathway between electrodes on the skin's surface — essentially a "short circuit." This may be caused by imperfect electrode wiring, excessive patient perspiration, or excessive conduction paste (salt bridge). If impedance is too high, it adversely affects conduction, especially of the smaller potentials, such as somatosensory evoked potentials (SEPs). Mismatched impedances can result in a buildup of charge resulting in a battery effect or permit 60 Hz noise (from the power supply) to pollute the signal, masking the electrical potential.

To acquire a bioelectric signal, the active electrode is placed near the expected current source of the action potential (near field) — e.g., the motor point during motor nerve stimulation. When the reference electrode is placed close to the active electrode (i.e., close to the action potential), a bipolar montage is created. This montage is useful for accurate signal localization. Electrodes in a bipolar montage send "like" data to the amplifier. When filtered, like data are subtracted during the processing — leaving the actual signal of interest. The bipolar potential is relatively small, e.g., a sensory nerve action potential (SNAP).

A referential montage is created when the reference electrode is placed a relatively significant distance from the active electrode. Compared with the bipolar system, the referential montage generates a comparatively large potential, as the signal is registered from a relatively larger current field, with little in common between electrodes. This montage is useful for elucidating hard-to-find signals. An example of this montage is seen in electroencephalography (EEG), configured to reference each side of the brain to the ipsilateral ear to propagate the signal.

In either type of setup, the bioelectric potentials of interest remain small in size, necessitating amplification. A signal is amplified when it passes through a system that multiplies it by a fixed factor (gain) that is characteristic of the equipment. Once the signal is amplified, extraneous signal (noise) is removed (filtered). In most machines, the signal is ultimately converted from its original analog characteristic to digital characteristic. The digital representation of the analog signal is then displayed on the cathode ray tube or computer screen.

PHYSIOLOGIC BASIS OF ELECTRODIAGNOSTIC STUDIES

Volume conduction is key to understanding electrophysiology and is defined simply as the propagation of electrical currents from external sources within the body. The human body is a very good volume conductor. As electrical current is conducted along excitable tissue (e.g., nerve), its characteristics can be recorded. The actual individual electrical impulse that is associated with a corresponding phenomenon (e.g., sensation or muscle twitch) may be too small or too far from an electrode to be recorded. But, because of volume conduction, electrical phenomena can be assessed and quantified. Volume conduction occurs because of the characteristics of the excitable tissue (nerve or muscle) and the surrounding ion-rich fluid (Dumitru, 1991a).

In a typical nerve, the lipid-rich semipermeable membrane acts as a barrier to compartmentalize the cell. This membrane is rich in channels and pumps, conferring selectivity to that which can and cannot pass through it. This selectivity of passage is based on ion charge and molecular size. In a typical nerve axon, large negatively charged anions are trapped inside the cell, creating a constant negative intracellular charge. Potassium, a major positively charged ion involved in tissue excitability, moves freely in and out of the cell through the membrane, its direction of flow depending on the relative concentration of the ion on either side of the membrane, as well as the charge difference between the inside and the outside of the cell at any given moment. Sodium, unlike potassium, does not move freely across the membrane. This property permits momentary variations in voltage (charge differences) across the membrane. When the resting state of ion separation is perturbed by the action potential, a complex array of ion flux occurs locally as the action potential (depolarization) and is then reset (repolarization) — on the basis of charge and molecular equilibrium, as well as the specific characteristics of the membrane channels and the ambient charge. These characterize the basis of local charge generation. The action potential is the critical adjacent voltage large enough to stimulate the necessary changes in membrane pumps and channels (Kandal, Schwartz, & Jessell, 2000).

The existence of a transient charge difference between the interior and exterior of the membrane (transient voltage difference) is the key to the generation of a local capacitive current dipole, residing on the extracellular surface. The channels downstream from the local dipole respond to that dipole by generating another series of ion flux, a bit farther "down the membrane."

The dipole represents a local "capacitive current" on the outer surface of the cell membrane. As the dipole effects a contiguous segment of nerve, causing another series of ion fluctuations, further dipoles are generated, and so on. This phenomenon travels incrementally along the nerve (or muscle), giving birth to transmission (Kandal et al., 2000).

Benjamin Franklin postulated that current flowed from positive to negative. This is opposite of what actually occurs, with electrons flowing from the negative to the positive pole. By convention, and based on the polarity of recording electrodes, flow that occurs in the direction of the current is designated as positive, and is represented by a downward deflection of the waveform. Signals propagated along excitable tissue in the human volume conductor have distinct electrical characteristics that translate into the signal that is seen on the computer (oscilloscope). As the biological signal (moving along nerve or muscle) approaches the recording needle, the needle "sees" the approaching edge of the signal. As the signal continues to pass under the needle, the needle records the middle of the signal, followed by the trailing edge, which is moving away. Each component of the biological signal, recorded by the electrode as it passes, is translated into a corresponding component of the waveform seen on the computer screen (oscilloscope). The approaching and trailing signals generate phasic components. Transition zones are associated with wave inflection points. Direction of waveform phase depends on the position of the electrode. By convention, upward (above baseline) is negative and downward (below baseline) is positive (Dumitru, 1991a, b).

In myelinated nerve, an action potential leads to uninterrupted signal transmission of capacitive current along a significant stretch of the insulated axon, without needing any further action potentials until the signal wanes at the next unmyelinated spot (node of Ranvier). This so-called salutatory conduction acts like a slingshot, making transmission along a myelinated axon much faster than that noted along an unmyelinated axon. The classic pain sensory fibers are small and lightly myelinated or unmyelinated. Therefore, transmission along pain fibers is relatively slow.

The speed of pain fibers is exemplified by the situation in which one places a hand on a hot stove. The expectation of pain is realized before the actual pain is felt (Kandal et al., 2000).

Conventional electrodiagnostic studies (e.g., nerve conduction velocity studies) assess the larger, faster myelinated nerves, whereas assessment of smaller fibers that are lightly myelinated or unmyelinated is exacted by indirect means. Painful conditions are often diagnosed by electrodiagnostic studies that reflect the state of large nerve fibers despite the fact that it is small fibers that classically transmit pain signals. It is less common to find small nerve fiber pathology in isolation (Kandal et al., 2000).

ELECTROENCEPHALOGRAPHY

EEG signal reflects activity at the level of the cerebral cortex. Deeper generators of cerebral signal, such as the thalamus and brainstem, are indirectly reflected by these signals (Wyllie, 1997). The EEG signal is of relatively low amplitude because the recorded bioelectrical signal must first pass through dense intervening tissue, to include the scalp. In addition, the cortical convolutions are associated with specific regional geometries, which may be associated with phase cancellation effects, causing a spurious reduction in net regional amplitude. The ability to assess this low-amplitude signal is enhanced by strategic placement of electrodes in geometrically advantaged fields that optimize the capturing of this activity. During acquisition of data, the position of the evenly spaced recording electrodes remains unchanged. Machine-generated variations in polarity and reference points correlate with specific sets of dipoles that characterize each montage. Each montage, in turn, corresponds to a different plane of assessment, each with its own distinct advantage in characterizing different types of regional signal. For example, a transverse montage will more clearly demonstrate stage II sleep activity when compared with that seen in the referential montage (Andriola & Epstein, 1983). Typically, multiple two-dimensional montages are assessed in a single study, to approximate a three-dimensional assessment.

EEG has been used in pain research to map the cerebral topographical perception and modulation of pain, to characterize the processing of nociceptive signal in the central nervous system. EEG augmented with spectral analysis has demonstrated that signal obtained from muscle is processed differently from signal obtained from skin, with both within similar neural matrices of the brain (Chang et al., 2004). As well, brain maps generated by EEG/EMG are used in tandem with PET/fMRI (positron emission tomography/functional MRI), significantly adding to the diagnostic yield. Clinically, EEG is mostly used in the setting of headache (Niedermeyer, 1999).

EMG

The abbreviation EMG has more than one meaning. EMG literally stands for electromyogram, a study that features insertion of a needle into muscle to assess activity during rest, as well as during voluntary contraction. In a broader sense, EMG is the combined study that includes needle EMG when performed in conjunction with nerve conduction velocity (NCV) studies. To help distinguish between the two definitions of EMG, the phrase "needle EMG" is used to describe the specific testing of muscle, whereas "EMG" is used to refer to the entire study.

Surface EMG

Diametrically opposed to needle EMG, the electrode interface of surface EMG (sEMG) does not penetrate the skin, rendering this test unable to directly measure spontaneous activity, insertional activity, motor unit morphology, and motor unit recruitment. Despite its limitations, sEMG plays a role in the diagnosis of muscle impairment syndromes such as fibromyalgia, myofascial pain, muscle injury, and muscle spasms (Cassisi et al., 2000; Pullman, 2000; Nederhand et al., 2003; Wimalaratna et al., 2002). Experimental kinesiology has also proved to be a valuable application of sEMGs (Mannion et al., 1997). A detailed discussion of sEMG can be found elsewhere in this text.

Needle Electromyography

The needle EMG study is complemented by NCV. For example, the abnormal motor NCV in polyneuropathy may be further qualified by severe axonal changes, found on needle EMG. EMG can also help distinguish between neuropathy and radiculopathy or may confirm their coexistence. The information derived from the needle EMG examination also aids in localization of the spinal level(s) of radiculopathy. Irritability of muscle, as exemplified by fibrillations, sharp waves, or myotonia can be demonstrated by needle EMG in a variety of painful muscle disorders. Needle EMG examination also reveals the current state of nerve or nerve root healing after injury and helps approximate the precise date of injury. The latter is particularly valuable in cases where prior injury or pathology is concurrent with new clinical abnormalities.

Needle EMG assessment features both sight and sound. A variety of potentials generate characteristic sounds as well as characteristic waveforms. Audiometric assessment augments visualization. Routine needle EMG is performed using either a monopolar or a concentric needle. The monopolar needle needs a separate ground. Because it is smaller in caliber, the monopolar needle causes relatively less discomfort than does the concentric needle. The concentric needle, which comes in various sizes and is larger than the monopolar needle, contains its own ground (Walker et al., 2001).

Bioelectrical signals obtained during needle EMG are categorized by activity noted at rest versus active muscle contraction. Resting muscle EMG reveals two subtypes of activity: spontaneous activity (that activity noted while the needle is resting in muscle after cessation of insertion) and insertional activity (that activity noted during crisp short insertions). Needle insertion causes a burst of short-lived relatively high frequency activity. Silence immediately follows in normal muscle. Both the examiner and

the subject must hold still after each insertion, to avoid movement artifact. This artifact is sometimes responsible for misdiagnosis of abnormal insertional activity by a less-experienced examiner. Normal insertional activity should last no longer than 0.5 ms. Activity lasting beyond 0.5 s suggests irritability. This may be the earliest evidence of increased insertional activity, especially if coupled with a sharp wave or fibrillation potential (Bromberg, 1993). Needle insertion into the neuromuscular junction begets normal "end plate" activity, exemplified by the miniature end plate potential (MEPP), a tiny sharp monophasic negative wave (less than 10 microvolts, less than 3 ms duration) that occurs randomly and is difficult to isolate, due to coalescence with end plate noise. End plate noise appears as many end plate spikes with an irregular baseline. This activity produces the characteristic "seashell" murmur. Miniature end plate potentials are random, monophasic, upward-deflecting (negative) waves, occurring spontaneously with irregular rhythm representing presynaptic calcium release, leading to subthreshold levels of acetylcholine. Therefore, no action potential is generated (Dumitru, 1991a, b).

Another spontaneously generated potential from muscle is the end plate spike, a potential that is a bit more substantial than the MEPP. It occurs in distinct intervals, approximately every 50 ms. Unlike the miniature end plate potential, the end plate spike results from a suprathreshold action potential, propagating an irregularly fired biphasic waveform: negative–positive. End plate spikes generate a characteristic sound, reminiscent of "sputtering fat in a frying pan." That needle assessment of the neuromuscular junction is particularly painful acts, which is a distinct diagnostic feature.

Abnormal spontaneous and insertional activities are represented by the fibrillation potential and positive sharp wave. The fibrillation potential is a spontaneously generated action potential that is sharp in morphology, owing to its relatively short duration. The potential is characterized by a positive downward deflection followed by a low-amplitude negative upward deflection. It may be triphasic. The potential is about 20 microvolts or higher in amplitude and is 1 to 5 ms in duration. The fibrillation occurs as a result of spontaneous depolarization, a periodic rhythmical twitch excitation of a single sensitized muscle fiber potential (Denny-Brown & Pennymaker, 1938). This activity reflects a muscle fiber that has lost its nerve supply, causing so-called irritability.

Resting muscle membrane of denervated muscle is unstable and irritable, acting as an oscillator that spontaneously depolarizes. The fibrillation may be morphologically similar to an end plate spike, but is classically rhythmic and lower in frequency. Rarely, an end plate spike may demonstrate features of a fibrillation potential, causing confusion for the novice electrodiagnostician. Irritable muscle is seen in many conditions, to include certain myopathies (e.g., necrotizing type), neuropathies with large fiber axonal involvement, and radiculopathy. Needle EMG of paraspinal muscle will confer the best yield for fibrillations and positive sharp waves found in painful irritable myopathies because most myopathic processes preferentially affect the proximal and truncal muscles (Katirji, 1998).

A positive sharp wave carries the same clinical significance as the fibrillation potential (reflecting denervation). The positive sharp wave, like the fibrillation potential, is generated spontaneously. Its significance is thought to equal that of the fibrillation potential, differing only in its point of origin, with its biphasic appearance reflecting electrode position (Dumitru, 1991a, b).

Distinguishing end spikes from fibrillations hinges on rhythm and morphology, the former of relatively high frequency, the latter of lower frequency and regular in rhythm. As well, the deflection of the fibrillation potential is positive, whereas that of end plate spike is negative. Although previously thought to be a rule without exception, characterization by deflection direction is not without potential error (Herbison, 1991).

Other examples of spontaneous needle EMG activity include the complex repetitive discharge (CRD) and the myotonic discharge. Both discharges are prolonged, at times for many seconds. A complex repetitive discharge is generated spontaneously as a result of a nonsynaptic (ephaptic) muscle fiber pacemaker. This is essentially a short circuit of normal synaptic transmission, occurring between groups of adjacent injured nerve fibers, causing repetitive spontaneous firing of the same exact muscle groups, resulting in the production of a complex polyphasic potential, each repetition being identical in morphology. This usually very high frequency rhythmic firing does not waiver in frequency or amplitude. The CRD reflects chronic denervation (Katirji, 1998).

Myotonic discharges are sometimes found in myotonic disorders, but are not exclusive to those disorders, e.g., painful conditions such as myotonia congenita (Sunohara et al., 1996); proximal myotonic myopathy, also called PROMM (Kress et al., 2000); and myotonic dystrophy. The pain experienced as a result of these disorders is mostly due to cramp generation, with cramp discharges a separate issue. Although the CRD is rhythmic, the myotonic discharge waxes and wanes in both amplitude and frequency, generating the characteristic "dive bomber" sound with needle insertion (Bromberg, 1993). Spontaneous activity notwithstanding, myotonic activity obtained during insertion tends to be morphologically sharp. True myotonic discharges last for more than 0.5 s (Daube, 1996).

A fasciculation represents spontaneous activity obtained from an entire motor unit action potential (MUAP), to include the motor neuron and the muscle that it innervates. Fasciculations are noted both in normal sub-jects and in states of diseased motor neuron. Physiological accentuation of fasciculations can be seen secondary to benign exogenous (caffeine) or endogenous (stress) alterations. Fasciculations are usually associated with amyotrophic lateral sclerosis, a classically painless disease. Myokymic discharges are spontaneous, rhythmic to semirhythmic discharges seen with muscle rippling. Myokymia is found in radiation-induced brachial plexopathy, as well as multiple sclerosis (MS), Guillain-Barre syndrome (GBS), pontine tumor, and timber rattlesnake poisoning (Gutmann, 1991).

The neuromyotonic discharge is quite complex, producing bizarre sounds mimicking soldiers marching with sirens ringing. These high-frequency discharges can be sustained or can occur in bursts. They are associated with sustained muscle activity and are unaffected by voluntary movement. This activity is considered to be quite painful, as seen in Isaac's syndrome, anticholinesterase poisoning, achondroplastic dwarfism, tetany, and spinal muscular atrophy (Daube, 1996).

MOTOR UNIT ASSESSMENT

Unlike the aforementioned spontaneous and insertional activity, assessment of the motor unit is performed during voluntary contraction. The motor unit consists of a motor neuron and all of the muscle fibers that it innervates generated by active contraction of skeletal muscle. Assessment of the motor unit aids in the diagnosis of many neuromuscular disorders that are associated with pain, including radiculopathy, plexopathy, and mononeuropathy and characterizing morphology and recruitment pattern. The interference pattern is generated with increasing muscle contraction toward maximal. A full interference pattern is a gross reflection of normal muscle activity but not a sensitive parameter for less obvious motor dysfunction.

Our nervous system responds to gradually increasing muscle contraction by generating a motor unit and increasing its firing frequency. The normal motor unit starts out firing at about 2 to 3 Hz. With further contraction, the first motor unit appears at a higher frequency, toward 10 Hz. Before or at 10 Hz, normal muscle produces a second motor unit. That is to say, once the critical firing frequency is reached, the muscle should produce a second unit that starts at about 2 to 3 Hz, seen concurrently with the first faster unit. This pattern of motor unit recruitment continues with further muscle contraction. By the third or fourth unit, the screen may be filled with so many potentials that it is difficult to identify each individual motor unit (Daube, 1996). The presence of multiple waveforms can create the erroneous impression that some potentials are high in amplitude, by virtue of phase addition. Reduced motor unit recruitment is the earliest electrodiagnostic finding of neurogenic weakness, which is seen concurrently in many painful states, such as plexopathy, radiculopathy, and compressive mononeuropathy. Assessment of motor unit recruitment depends on the ability to isolate a single motor unit, which depends on the cooperation of an alert subject's ability to maintain required muscle tension. Reduced recruitment is synonymous with neurogenic recruitment. In this pattern of recruitment, the initial motor unit fires at an abnormally higher frequency before the next unit is recruited. In severe cases, the second unit may never show and the single unit fires at a very high rate. The most severe recruitment abnormality is characterized when no motor units are obtained, with severe weakness. A lack of fibrillations in the setting of severely reduced recruitment suggests conduction block from a demyelinating lesion, rather than axonal motor nerve damage. However, if the needle EMG study is performed less than 2 to 3 weeks after axonal injury, then fibrillations that are due to develop may not have done so that early, necessitating a follow-up study in about a month.

Myopathies are associated with pain. The electrodiagnostic features of myopathic muscle tend to be inconsistent. Diametrically opposed to neurogenic change, motor unit potentials in myopathic muscle are said to be shorter in duration (thinner) due to fiber loss within the motor unit. They also tend to be polyphasic, due to desynchronization of firing within the unit. Reduced amplitude, a "classic" and most debated myopathic characteristic, is the least reliable feature of myopathy. Myopathic recruitment is marked by many early appearing (fast-onset) muscle fibers of low amplitude (fatigued), in the 50 microvolt range. Recruitment pattern varies, but is usually normal in less severe cases. Increased (early) recruitment is thought due to both weakness and effort, as though the muscle contracts enough to generate potentials, but it does so using several motor units jumping into the fray together, appearing as several suboptimal motor units occurring simultaneously some of which are too "early." Early recruitment is the most common electrodiagnostic finding in myopathy. Neurogenic recruitment is seen in severe late stage muscle disease. Irritable myopathies demonstrate fibrillations and/or sharp waves. This category of myopathy can be due to inflammation, acid maltase deficiency, myotonic dystrophy, myotonia congenita, and many other causes (Katirji, 1998). Pain is a major characteristic of many muscle diseases within this subclass.

Factors that can influence recruitment must be considered to avoid spurious diagnosis. These include pain (inhibition of motor unit activation), co-contraction of antagonist muscle (yielding false assessment of muscle contraction force), electrode movement during muscle contraction (loss of motor unit "focus"), and poor subject cooperation (Petajan, 1991). To accurately assess the motor unit, one must be assured that it is not a distant unit, but the one closest to the needle electrode. The closest units will have the shortest duration and rise time (pointy morphology) and will be of greater amplitude than more distant units (Figure 44.1).

NERVE CONDUCTION VELOCITY STUDY

The motor nerve action potential is more aptly named the compound muscle action potential (CMAP) because it reflects activity from muscle after stimulation by nerve — a combination of both. After motor nerve stimulation, there is a synapse at the neuromuscular junction, where muscle fibers are activated by a calcium-dependent action potential. In a sense, this represents amplification of the motor nerve signal. This also explains why the amplitude of the CMAP (measured in millivolts) is typically 1,000 times larger than that of the SNAP, which is typically measured in microvolts. SNAP morphology is usually "thinner and sharper," marked by a short rise and fall time. The compound muscle action potential is usually biphasic. CMAP amplitude is lost faster than SNAP amplitude after injury.

A stimulated motor nerve has a distal latency and a proximal conduction velocity. The distal latency cannot be referred to as the distal conduction velocity because it involves muscle as well as nerve. The distal motor latency is accounted for by nerve, neuromuscular junction, and muscle conduction combined.

The amplitude of the average adult MUAP ranges from a few hundred microvolts to about 2 millivolts. High amplitude polyphasic motor units suggest reinnervation of muscle after injury. This combination of findings is most consistent with chronic neurogenic change. Denervation caused by an irritable myopathy can be distinguished from that caused by a neurogenic process by distinct morphological and recruitment features. Amplitudes of neurogenic muscle tend to be normal or higher in amplitude, particularly after the healing period. These units may be of longer duration and may also be polyphasic, indicating the healing of motor nerve. The extra phases reflect the sprouting nerve fascicles that have reinnervated new muscle fibers (Bromberg, 1993; Katirji, 1998).

Because of its relatively diminutive size, the normal SNAP is more susceptible to obliteration by artifact, which may be due to improper grounding technique, movement caused by muscle tension, or overstimulation. When a nerve is overstimulated, a component of the CMAP may be incorporated into the SNAP, wiping out that portion of the SNAP or the entire SNAP. In a subject with substantial girth, action potentials may be difficult to obtain, especially the SNAP, leading to higher stimulation current/voltage, which can cause obliteration of the SNAP by the CMAP.

The SNAP is obtained by stimulating the sensory nerve and recording information from that nerve in either the *orthodromic* direction (the same direction in which the nerve naturally propagates its signal) or in the *antidromic*

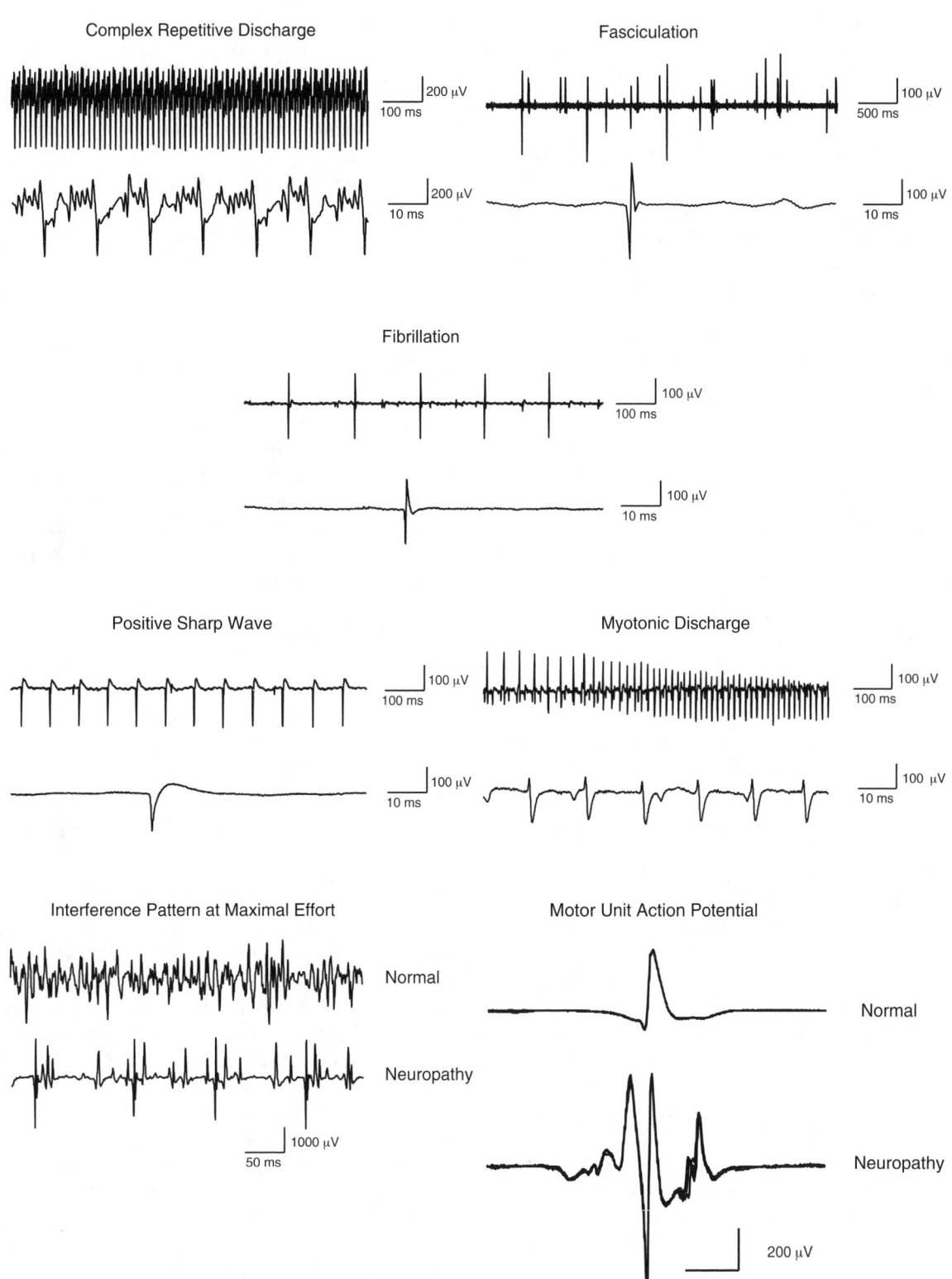

FIGURE 44.1 Sample EMG waveforms demonstrating common normal and abnormal patterns. (Courtesy of Oxford Instruments.)

direction (normal). Therefore, one may stimulate the sensory nerve from either a distal-to-proximal or proximal-to-distal direction. The potential should essentially be the same, unless motor nerve artifact is obtained with stimulation at one end but not at the other end. With respect to the CMAP, only the orthodromic-derived CMAP is considered. With stimulation in the distal-to-proximal (antidromic) direction, one will obtain a large amplitude *M-wave* (CMAP) that is generated by the signal traveling backward. However, a volley also travels proximally, hitting a dead end in the cell body of the motor neuron (in the spinal cord), ultimately being propagated back down the limb to the active electrode. This potential, known as an *F-wave,* is considered a late potential because it arrives many milliseconds after the M-wave is recorded. The F-wave represents conduction through the full course of the motor nerve, up and back (Oh, 1993).

The proximal extent of the F-wave response permits localization of disorders in those regions, e.g., the brachial plexus. Under normal conditions, a series of "rastered" F-wave responses produces a clustered group of late potentials, each differing slightly from one another in both morphology and latency. The variability in latency and morphology is explained on the basis of the signal being propagated along a different component nerve fascicle each time the nerve is stimulated as well as the fact that the local stimulation artifact affects a refractory period for some of the returning F-wave responses during their descent back down the limb.

The *H-wave* (Hoffman reflex) is another type of late response. Stimulation of the tested nerve, usually the tibial nerve at the popliteal fossa, is directed proximally toward the hip girdle, with a descending response expected. Unlike the F-wave response, which spans its entire length in motor nerve, the H-wave signal travels up the afferent sensory component, synapses in the spinal cord, and descends in an efferent motor component, ultimately generating a CMAP at a muscle belly, usually at the medial calf. In most circumstances, the amount of current/voltage used to generate an H-wave is low, whereas the stimulation time is relatively long, usually set at 1 ms. The tibial H-wave reflex recapitulates the clinical muscle stretch tendon reflex (ankle jerk/S1 root). It is performed with the patient lying in the prone position. The H-wave should be triphasic in morphology and should demonstrate little side-to-side latency variation. Unlike the F-wave, the H-wave is nearly invariant in its morphology and latency. Whereas the F-wave is clinically useful in the study of many accessible nerves, the utility of the H-wave in adults is restricted to the tibial nerve, used primarily to aid in diagnosis of an S1 radiculopathy. The median nerve H-wave reflex may be useful in children (Oh, 1993).

Whereas the SNAP is obtainable when the sensory component of a mixed nerve is stimulated in isolation (e.g., median digital branches), the SNAP is obliterated when the sensory and motor components are close to each other. As well, the machine settings (e.g., band-pass filter) and the electrode set up (e.g., ring electrodes on digits that contain no motor nerve component) are modified to "capture" waveforms of various latency and amplitude. Sensory and motor nerve potentials are both affected by the state of the axon, as well as the state of myelination. With a reduction in the quantity of motor fibers, the amplitude of the potential will be reduced proportionally to quantity of fiber loss. When enough fibers are lost, that number will include a percentage of the faster-conducting fiber population. Therefore, with axonal loss, not only does one lose amplitude (expected), but one also loses velocity (Triggs, 1997).

Conduction velocity of demyelinated nerve is slowed due to myelin loss. However, distal stimulation of a demyelinated motor nerve will also show reduced compound muscle action amplitude, not due to axonal injury, but due to temporal dispersion and phase cancellation. When a nerve loses its myelin insulation, it does so unevenly. As a result, different parts of the nerve will conduct signal at different velocities. Dispersed signal loses its synchrony by definition, where fewer fibers to fire at the same time. Phase addition is reduced, and phase cancellation occurs more frequently, both acting to diminish the signal (Daube, 1996). Isolated temporal dispersion (without conduction block) has not been established as a cause of motor or sensory deficits (Olney et al., 1999).

Nerve disorders are either predominantly axonal in nature or predominantly demyelinating in nature. In the setting of so-called conduction block, this distinction has significant prognostic ramifications, as a focal nonpathological demyelinating lesion tends to have a better outcome when compared to conditions of axonal loss. Conduction block of an intact nerve may be axonal in nature, demyelinating, or both (Katirji, 1998). Conduction block is associated with a variety of sensorimotor symptoms. One may also experience pain in a clinical scenario that includes conduction block (e.g., severe carpal tunnel syndrome). Complete conduction block may cause severe weakness along with pain, as exemplified by traumatic injury. Criteria for defining partial conduction block hinge on latency and amplitude. More than one set of accepted criteria to define partial conduction block exists in the literature, revealing the difficult nature of this chore (Olney et al., 1999). Pain is a common symptom experienced by patients with conduction block who suffer acute inflammatory demyelinating polyradiculneuropathy (AIDP) and mixed axonal and demyelinating polyneuropathy, such as that seen in renal disease and diabetes mellitus. Classically, a hereditary predisposition to pressure palsy is not painful, although both nerve compression and secondary nociceptive pain may both play a role in some cases. The finding of conduction block aids in the accurate identification of a primary demyelinating disorder, which is more than an academic exercise, as debilitating disorders such as AIDP and diabetic radiculoplexopathy may be ameliorated with immunotherapeutic intervention, via intravenous immune globulin or plasmaphoresis. Cerebrospinal fluid assessment may be obtained to augment the electrodiagnostic and clinical information in this type of case.

EVOKED POTENTIALS

An evoked potential (EP) is generally defined as an electrical manifestation of the central and peripheral neural pathways in response to an external stimulus. In simple terms, when an electrical, mechanical, visual, auditory, or other stimulus is applied, the body responds in a predictable manner, propagating electrical impulses. These impulses can be recorded and assessed for speed and volume of conduction, as well as aberrance. For the most part, these studies evaluate sensory pathways, including both peripheral and central components, with the exception of motor evoked potentials (MEPs). The three most common EPs in daily clinical practice are (1) somatosensory evoked potentials (SEPs), (2) brainstem auditory evoked potentials (BAEPs), and (3) pattern-shift visual evoked potentials (VEPs). Each of the studies provides an objective measurement of function relating to their respective sensory systems. Although each study is best suited for specific clinical purposes, the clinical benefits of all EPs lie within the ability to demonstrate aberrant function within the sensory systems when clinical examination is equivocal, define the anatomic distribution of a neural pathology, and even monitor the affected pathways over time.

The ability to record EPs is not new. Chiappa (1983) is generally credited with compiling much of the early literature relating to EPs. Although there had been references dating back to the early 1900s with the first EP recorded by Richard Caton in England, it is Dawson (1947) who is responsible for the techniques in use today. Dawson is credited with having made the first systematic recordings of EPs from the human sensory cortex using surface electrodes over the scalp. The initial work was done superimposing photographs of faint traces. He then devised the first mechanical–electric averaging device (Dawson, 1954). Nowadays, signal response averaging and the recording of EPs are taken for granted thanks to electronic and computer technology. For the purposes of this chapter, the detailed discussion of SEPs is felt to be of greater value based on the ability to assist in the differential diagnosis of musculoskeletal pain disorders. Conversely, BAEPs and VEPs are of greater value in assessing loss of function, not necessarily associated with pain, with the exception of intracranial mass, where headache is likely a symptom.

SOMATOSENSORY EVOKED POTENTIALS

SEPs are obtained through direct stimulation of structures in the peripheral nervous system, primarily in the upper and lower limbs, as well as the torso. The acronym SSEP is common to literature, and refers to the term "short-latency" SEPs, in which responses largely occur within 50 ms for nerves stimulated in the upper extremities and 100 ms for the lower. The major clinical application of SEPs is in the detection of physiologic impairment of the sensory pathways including the peripheral nerve, plexus, nerve roots, spinal cord, brainstem, and cerebrum. As one would imagine, these studies are particularly valuable in evaluating conditions that are primarily sensory in nature. For example, in the case of a preganglionic sensory radiculopathy, an SEP is more likely to identify the lesion than the more routine EMG.

An SEP, as are EPs in general, is best understood as a mere continuity check, in this case involving the sensory afferent pathways from the extremities to the sensory cortex. A concise series of waveforms is generated that reflects sequential activation of neural structures along the way. These waveforms can be recorded at specific intervals, most commonly the peripheral nerve, spine, and cortex. If the signal arrives at the cortex at the correct time, with adequate intensity, the study is felt to be normal, reflecting unhindered continuity. If, on the other hand, the signal is late arriving at the cortex, or is attenuated with respect to the volume or strength, the study is abnormal. Localization of the lesion is possible by reviewing the potentials generated along the way, noting where the block or delay first occurred.

Although the term SEP is generally used to describe all types of peripheral nerve stimulation, current literature makes a distinction between the classic stimulation of mixed nerves, such as the median, ulnar, tibial, and peroneal, and other more specialized studies. One of the principal limitations of SEPs that likely contributed to the primary use of EMG for the diagnosis of radiculopathy was the innervation of multiple roots that innervate mixed nerves. To address this problem, several authors described the use of dermatomal SEPs (DSEPs or DEPs) as a means of increasing the sensitivity and specificity of SEPs primarily for radiculopathy (Aminoff & Goodin, 1988; Aminoff et al., 1985a, b; Dvonch et al., 1984; Katifi & Sedgwick, 1987; Liguori, Taher, & Trojaborg, 1991; Machida et al., 1986; Scarff et al., 1981). As the name implies, DEPs are obtained following stimulation of a cutaneous nerve having innervation of a particular nerve root. Credit is largely given though to Slimp et al. (1992) for a paper delineating normative data for dermatomal stimulation from C4 to S1, as the others were primarily limited to distributions such as L5 and S1. There were isolated studies representing the dermatomes of the hand (La Joie & Melvin, 1983). Today the volume of references reporting directly on the clinical utility of SEPs or that rely on SEPs for access to the outcomes or effectiveness of therapeutic interventions or instrumentation is quite extensive.

Before elaborating further on clinical utility of SEPs, there is another term that the literature commonly neglects to differentiate: segmental SEPs (Eisen, Hoirch, & Moll, 1983). Segmental SEPs have factors that are common to both mixed nerve and dermatomal stimulation. Segmental studies involve the direct stimulation of peripheral nerves that have a primary innervation of one nerve root. The most classic of these nerves are the superficial peroneal and the sural, representing the L5 and S1 distributions, respectively. The techniques involving the evaluation of segmental nerves address the limitations regarding sensitivity and specificity related to mixed nerve stimulation, as well as the perceived difficulty in recording the smaller potentials generated with DSEPs, not to mention the overlapping of adjacent dermatomes (Glick, 2001).

The clinical utility of SEPs is highly dependent on the criteria set for abnormality. The classic criteria are well described by the most recent edition of Chaippa's text (1997). The limits of normal are typically portrayed from a statistical standpoint as 2.5 to 3.0 standard deviations (SD) from the mean, as determined from a laboratory set of normal studies by each laboratory. *Latency* is defined as being the time it takes for the potential to travel from the stimulation to the recording side. In practical terms, most clinicians have grown to accept the fact that it takes approximately 19.0 ms for the volley of electrical impulses to reach the cortex following stimulation of the median nerve at the wrist. Coincidentally, 1 SD typically equals 1.02. The normative range assuming 3.0 SD from the mean latency of 19.0 ms would yield a range of 16.0 to 22.0 ms. It should be said that many clinicians rely on the upper limit of 2 SD as clinically significant. To this end, if the left to right side-to-side difference is greater than 2.0 ms, an abnormality is suspected. Localizing this abnormity would be dependent on assessing interpeak latencies, those obtained at the other recording site along the pathway, typically over a peripheral site and the spine. This would be best described by comparison with a road rally, in which the first determination of a problem is reflected by the arrival at the final checkpoint. In this situation, the entire pathway would have to be intact as there are defined limits to the propagation of an electrical impulse along a nerve or neural pathway, and each will function normally. If the potentials recorded over the final destination, i.e., the cerebral cortex, were delayed or late, it is possible to examine the intermediary recording sites or checkpoints to determine the origin of the problem, essentially localizing the pathology.

When it comes to determination of abnormality, most authors concur that latency is clinically diagnostic. There is a notable difference of opinion in the literature regarding the reliability of amplitude measurement. All potentials

that are generated and subsequently recorded are manifested as a waveform. The occurrence of a peak in the waveform is recorded as the latency. In simple terms the height of the waveform is defined as the *amplitude*. The difficulty in relying on amplitude measurements is inherent in factors associated with the recording parameters of the instrumentation, as well as the impedance (reflecting the connection between the patient and the recording instrument) and location of the recording electrodes. As amplitude is a measure of volume conduction, the intensity of the electrical stimulation is also important. From the analytical standpoint, common sense would dictate that by maintaining consistency in recording parameters, and ensuring adequate stimulation of nerves, including when assessing dermatomes, much of the variability is addressed and amplitude variations could be considered more reliable. This would be especially true when comparing nerves evaluated on the ipsilateral side, such as the left median to the left ulnar.

When Slimp et al. (1992) proposed normative data for dermatomes, especially in the thoracic level, they relied on a Z-score concordance analysis to help compare responses from one level to another, as it seemed apparent that comparing a response cephalad and caudal with the level in question could assist in identifying pathology. Their observation was that the response at one level could essentially predict the value of another. This is a very important concept when structuring a study or defining abnormity.

The last consideration in discussing the reliability of SEPs is portrayed in the literature associated with intraoperative monitoring and the predictability of a successful surgical decompression. Early mention of SEPs intraoperatively (Brown, 1983; McCallan & Bennet, 1975) seemed more than promising. That led to further studies such as one by Herron et al. (1987) that acknowledged the ability of DSEPs to determine the adequacy of decompression. The ability of the DSEPs to be sensitive to various surgical events was reported by Toleikis et al. (1993). Other authors presented data that increased the level of confidence in the DSEPs intraoperatively by reporting that the test results at closing could predict the adequacy of decompression (Cohen, Major, & Huizenga, 1991). Studies such as this served well to also demonstrate the clinical significance of small changes in latency as clinically significant by comparing baseline presurgical, intraoperative, and postsurgical studies. Among the early advocates for DSEPs was a study that reported DSEPs as clinically diagnostic of lumbosacral root entrapment in 92% of 300 patients evaluated for the study, suggesting greater diagnostic sensitivity than myelography, without false positives (Scarff, 1981).

No introduction to SEPs would be complete without acknowledging the controversy associated with the studies: the criteria relied on to determine which abnormality is at the forefront, including whether to rely on amplitude measurements. Oddly enough, those that are most critical seem to conclude that SEP and DSEP techniques do not yield clinical information greater than other forms of clinical assessment. Because the studies are efficacious, safe, and cost-effective, logic dictates their use, especially when other methods of examination have not proved effective to identify and treat neuropathic pain.

RECORDING SEPs

The actual performance of SEPs requires a skilled, experienced clinician. To best understand the role of SEPs in the assessment of a patient with pain, it is best to have a basic familiarity as to how SEPs are elicited and recorded. The SEP is first elicited by direct electrical stimulation of a peripheral nerve. The initial volley of electrical impulses is felt to be large-diameter myelinated fibers. In mixed nerve and certain segmental studies they are largely afferents (Ia) from muscle spindles. In dermatomal studies and most segmental studies, cutaneous afferents (IIa) are activated. The electrical volley travels proximally along the nerve entering the cord, then ascends through the dorsal columns. At the cervicomedullary junction, the nucleus gracilis receives signals from the upper extremities, while those from the lower are received by the nucleus cuneatus, more medially. The signals are then carried by the second-order neuron to the opposite side through the medical lemniscus to the ventroposterolateral nucleus of the thalamus. Third-order neurons then project the impulse to the primary sensory cortex, corresponding to the area receiving signals from the stimulation site.

The most important recording site is the final checkpoint over the primary sensory cortex. At least one recording should be made over the proximal portion of the peripheral fibers to help identify or exclude peripheral pathology, as well as to better localize pathology to the plexus or nerve roots. Routine clinical studies seem to show a preference for Erb's point (over the supraclavicular fossa) and the cervical spine for upper extremity studies. Lower extremity studies usually record over the spine at the lower thoracic or upper lumbar.

Although this task might sound trivial, the problem is that these electrical potentials are comparatively small, and are essentially buried with background electrical noise. Endogenous noise (from within the body) comprises electrical potentials associated with muscles, including the heart, as well as the brain, as recorded with EEG. The largest source of exogenous noise can be from the power supply. To this end, there are two considerations that are important to enable the isolation of the comparatively small evoked potentials from the background noise. Improving the signal-to-noise ratio is first and foremost. This is done by ensuring the best possible connection between the recording electrodes and the patient. Adequate stimulation of the nerve is also essential. All too often the clinician does not adequately stimulate the nerve as a result of the discomfort expressed by the patient. It should be noted here that the inverse square law applies. Essentially to make the waveform look twice as good, one would have to stimulate four times as long. This leads to the discussion of signal averaging cited earlier. Modern computers fill the role of sampling EP through the averaging process in a manner very similar to that first accomplished by Dawson (1954). During this process, the nerve is stimulated a constant rate, triggering the computer to record at the same rate. Any electrical potentials that are synchronized to that rate are superimposed or averaged, while all other electrical noise or artifact logarithmically approaches zero. The greater the amount of noise, the longer the averaging necessary for an adequate study. Similarly, the better the signal-to-noise ratio, the shorter the period required to generate and record a potential. Stimulation frequencies are carefully chosen not to coincide with other time synchronized events, such as the 60 cycle sine wave of electrical current. Repetitive stimulation through the averaging process is then replicated to ensure reliability of the test results (Table 44.1).

BASICS OF SEP INTERPRETATION

Although the interpretation of SEPs may require proper experience and training in both recording techniques as well as the pathophysiology of conditions affecting the sensory nervous system, there are fundamental basics that most any clinician can rely on to understand SEP test results. As previously stated, the most important part of the test result is the generation of the cortical potentials. The resultant waveforms from evaluation of nerves in the upper extremities have a pattern that has the appearance of a "mountain-valley" with the peak of the mountain the cortical potentials. By convention, as determined through standardized placement and polarity of recording electrodes, upward deflections are reflected as negative reflection, labeled "N," while deflections downward are positive, labeled "P." For median nerve stimulation, the classic period for the signal to travel from the point of stimulation at the wrist to the cortex is 19.0 ms. On a linear scale measured in milliseconds, the peak of the mountain would appear at approximately 19.0 is the therefore labeled "N19" for the cortical latency.

In looking at test results, even a patient often recognizes the waveform and likens it to a bell curve. That is an appropriate analogy, as the generated waveform represents that sum total of averaged stimulations over time and the average of individual nerve fibers firing synchronously. From the physiologic standpoint, a decrease in the number of individual neurons firing would result in a lower-intensity signal and therefore decreased amplitude. From the technical standpoint, the same effect could occur with poor or inadequate stimulation or with one of the

TABLE 44.1
Sample Evoked Potential Waveforms

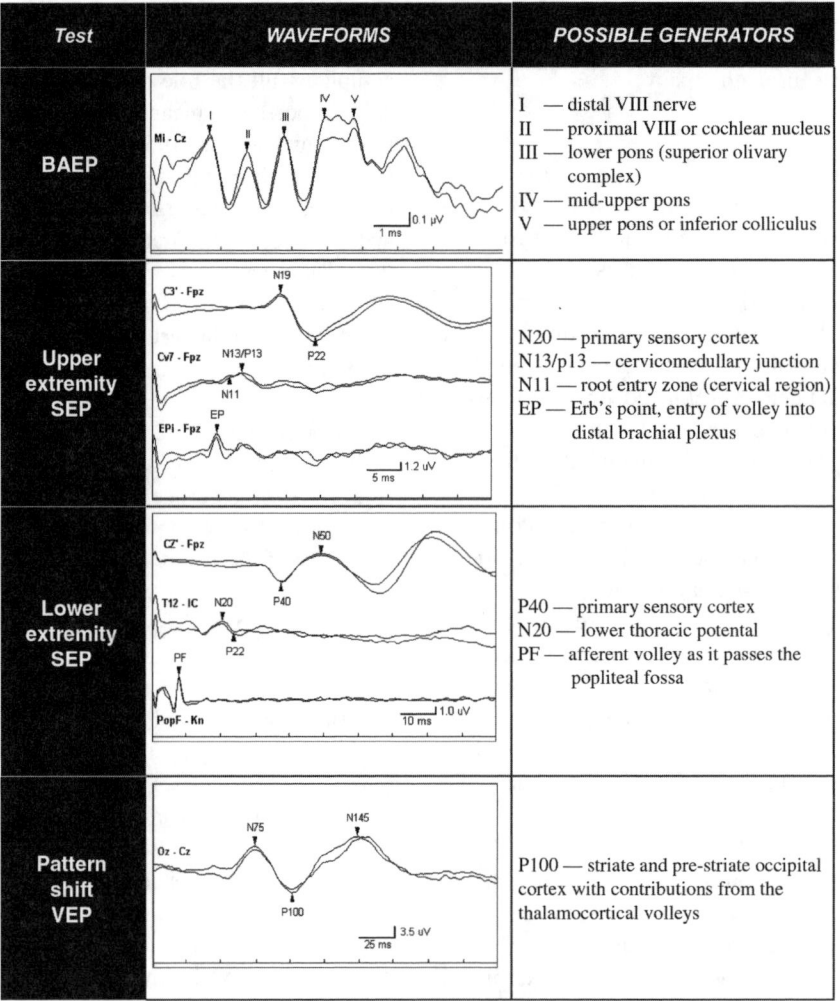

Test	WAVEFORMS	POSSIBLE GENERATORS
BAEP		I — distal VIII nerve II — proximal VIII or cochlear nucleus III — lower pons (superior olivary complex) IV — mid-upper pons V — upper pons or inferior colliculus
Upper extremity SEP		N20 — primary sensory cortex N13/p13 — cervicomedullary junction N11 — root entry zone (cervical region) EP — Erb's point, entry of volley into distal brachial plexus
Lower extremity SEP		P40 — primary sensory cortex N20 — lower thoracic potential PF — afferent volley as it passes the popliteal fossa
Pattern shift VEP		P100 — striate and pre-striate occipital cortex with contributions from the thalamocortical volleys

Note: Courtesy of Cadwell Laboratories, Inc., 2004.

various factors that adversely affect the signal-to-noise ratio. Once again, here lies the controversy in relying on amplitude measurements as a diagnostic criterion. In the hands of a skilled clinician with a properly structured study, amplitude deficiencies may be clinically diagnostic and highly informative in quantifying a neuropathy. Nerve compression is among the most common causes of diminished or attenuated amplitudes. Given this fact, one could argue it would be neglectful to ignore the diagnostic value of such measurements.

Similar to the waveforms generated with upper extremity nerve stimulation, those generated during stimulation of the lower extremities have a pattern that appears as a "W." The first downward deflection of the "W" is the cortical potential. For the tibial nerve this typically occurs at 40.0 ms, as such it is referred to as "P40."

Simply knowing the values for median and tibial nerve evaluation in a normal individual, along with the concept that nerves stimulated more proximal will have a shorter latency and those more distal will have a greater latency, the normative values for any other nerves evaluated can be estimated. It is also important to have a familiarity with nonpathological factors that influence the propagation of SEPs. Among them is patient height. A taller individual with a longer extremity length will require a greater amount of time for the signal to travel, although at approximately 60 m/s the time difference is measured in milliseconds. Gender, temperature, and age represent other factors when considering the test results in the context of a population normal. These variables are less important when considering a patient normal by comparing the results of one nerve with another on the ipsilateral as well as contralateral side of the same patient as described by Slimp et al. (1992). The most basic example of an ipsilateral comparison can be demonstrated by observing median and ulnar SEP in a normal individual, with stimulation sites equidistant from the cortex. If the medial cortical latency is 19.0 ms, the ulnar will approximate 19.0 ms as well. If the ulnar latency measures 21.0 ms, within the limits of normal when relying on population normal, minor pathology affecting the distribution of the ulnar nerve may be overlooked. Clinical correlation should be the deciding factor when considering the significance. An example where such a finding might be clinically important would be in the differential diagnosis of complex regional pain syndrome (Hendler, 2002).

Before leaving the subject of SEPs, although the assessment of typical nerves is commonly discussed, most any nerve accessible to peripheral electrical stimulation can elicit a response. Trigeminal (Soustiel, Feinsod, & Hafner, 1991), facial (McMenomey et al., 1994), glossopharyngeal (Fujii et al., 1994), and pudendal nerve (Haldeman et al., 1982) and even the distal esophagus (Aziz et al., 1995) stimulation are common to literature. Uncommon studies can play an important role in evaluating a patient with an unusual or atypical presentation. In these cases normal values may be gleaned from an unaffected side or ipsilateral adjacent nerves.

BRAINSTEM AUDITORY EVOKED POTENTIALS

Brainstem auditory evoked potentials (BAEPs) are generated by the auditory nerve (CN VIII) and brainstem in response to an external stimulus, in this case a "click." As with SEPs, a waveform is generated. In the case of the BAEP, also commonly referred to as BEAR or BSEAR (brainstem auditory evoked response), the potentials occur within a period of 7 ms from the onset of stimulus. The most common clinical applications are for the evaluation of acoustic neuromas, brainstem tumors, hearing disorders, coma, brain death, strokes, and demyelinating disease (Chiappa, 1983; Donohoe, 1988). There is also much literature regarding the assessment of hearing in children and patients that are unable to provide voluntary response to traditional hearing tests. The resultant waveform comprises five primary components, labeled I through V. The generators responsible for each component of the waveform are the action potential of CN VIII, the cochlear nucleus, the ipsilateral superior olivary nucleus, the nucleus or axons of the lateral lemniscus, and the inferior colliculus, respectively. Determination of the anatomic site of pathology is based on which components of the waveforms are absent or delayed. For the most part, this includes interpeak latencies of I–III, III–V, and I–V and interside comparisons as are amplitudes ratios of I/V or I/IV–V. Absolute latency measurements of III and V are considered when there is difficulty in measuring interpeak latencies (Chiappa, 1983; Hood & Berlin, 1986). Although there seem to be many BAEPs ordered for the assessment of headaches, especially following motor vehicle accidents involving closed head trauma, abnormal studies are rarely found. Recent literature describes changes in BAEPs during acute attacks of migraine reflective of physiologic change, yet the changes were found to be reversible (Kochar et al., 2002). Given the varying findings cited in the literature and described throughout texts such as Chiappa and Hill, BAEPs seem to fill more of a supporting role in the diagnosis of many conditions where brainstem involvement is suspect.

VISUAL EVOKED POTENTIALS

As the name implies, VEPs primarily assist in the investigation of visual pathways from the retina to the occipital cortex. As one would assume, the method of stimulus is visual and the primary clinical application is in the evaluation of optic nerve function. The preferred method in clinical practice is the pattern reversal method accomplished through an alternating reversal of a checkerboard pattern or pattern shift without change in luminance. Other techniques include pattern offset (also called pattern shift) and flash (also called strobe). The most common use of flash stimulation involves the assessment of patients experiencing compromise to the visual pathway from the retina to the visual cortex or with an uncooperative patient. As with SEPs, repetitive stimulation results in a waveform that can be obtained by recording over the cortex. The same basic principles outlined for SEPs apply to VEPs. The test results comprise a waveform that has a characteristic pattern with the first downward deflection typically occurring at 100 ms. As such, it is referred to as "P100." Recording from several sites on the cortex, in certain cases, can better assist in the assessment of visual disturbances. Many early studies report intraocular latency differences largely seen in MS and other nervous system disorders, as well as tumors, infarctions, and migraines, in addition to abnormalities of the visual field (Chiappa, 1983). Clinical applications involving tumors and migraines are among the most prevalent. Rather than yielding a definitive diagnosis, authors investigating transient changes in VEPs during acute migraine attacks (Afra et al., 1998; Drake et al., 1990; Kochar et al., 2002) or comparing differences in patient with and without aura (Bockowski et al., 2003) are leading to a better understanding of the involved pathophysiology.

MOTOR EVOKED POTENTIALS

While EMG and motor NCVs are commonly relied on to assess the motor system, they are primarily useful in identifying lesions in the peripheral nervous system. With the exception of indirect evidence of pathology reflected by abnormal motor unit firing, routine electrodiagnosis was limited in the ability to identify pathology in the central motor pathways. The development of MEPs likely dates to Penfield and Boldrey (1937). They observed that by directly stimulating the human brain with small electrical current in conscious patients undergoing surgery, mapping of the cortex was possible. This work led to the familiar caricature, the homunculus.

During the next 40 years several other authors reported on stimulation of the exposed motor cortex in both human and animal studies. For obvious reasons, such techniques are not useful in routine clinical practice. In 1982 Merton and Morton designed a high-voltage transcranial electrical stimulator that excited the motor cortex using cutaneous electrodes directly over the scalp rather than on an exposed brain (Merton, Hill, Morton, & Marsden, 1982). This was the first report of non-invasive stimulation of the motor cortex to quantitatively assess central motor conduction. A notable disadvantage was the significant discomfort created by the stimulus. The ability to more readily rely on MEPs for routine clinical assessment is largely credited to Barker et al. (1985) for the devolvement of a transcranial magnetic stimulator (TMS). Thus far, the techniques have proved safe and painless.

An MEP may be generated by magnetic or electrical transcranial stimulation. The stimulus activates the cortical motor neuron pathway, which in turn excites spinal motor neuron and generates a CMAP. The CMAP is easily recordable with a surface electrode in a manner similar to a routine nerve conduction study. As the muscle response is a comparatively strong signal, averaging required with other EPs is not necessary to record and measure the potential. The global motor conduction can be measured, and represents the time it takes for the signal to travel from the cortex to the muscle. It is presented as having two distinct components representing central conduction time (CCT) and peripheral conduction times (PCT). The CCT is typically determined by calculating the motor conduction time less the PCT, determined through stimulation at the spine.

The recording of MEPs is accomplished by recording over target muscles with surface electrodes. Needle electrodes are also occasionally used, especially in a research setting. As with other EPs, at least two recordings are obtained to ensure reliability. There is a proper orientation for the current traveling through the coil during magnetic stimulation of the cortex: clockwise when stimulating over the right hemisphere, counterclockwise for the left. Magnetic stimulation directly over the cervical and lumber spine is also possible. Coil current is also important in this application, clockwise for the right, counterclockwise for the left. It is worth mentioning that amplitudes and latencies of MEPs tend to vary over time during repetitive stimulation of relaxed target muscles. It is presumed that this occurrence is indicative of an element of the nervous system that guarantees the consistency of excitatory input to the neural elements, which is theorized to be fluctuations of resting threshold (Keirs et al., 1993). Amplitude and latency measurements of MEPs generated with intensity of the stimulation being constant also vary with the degree of contraction or relaxation by the muscle. With tonic contraction of the target muscle, the latency shortens and amplitude is increased. This process is referred to as facilitation of MEPs. Among the explanations offered was the tendency of a subliminally excited motor neuron to fire more readily when the phasic excitation elicited by the TMS reaches the motor neuron (Hess et al., 1987).

As with other EPs, MEPs are considered essentially safe, although there has been anecdotal mention regarding the risk of seizure. This seems to be limited to a small fraction of the already negligible incidence of seizure following strobe stimulation in EEGs (Pascual-Leone et al., 1993). Conversely, several authors such as Tergau et al. (1999) found that low-frequency transcranial stimulation may actually offer therapeutic benefit in treating epilepsy.

LASER EVOKED POTENTIALS

Among emergent technology is the ability to perform laser evoked potentials (LEPs). SEPs have generally been limited to the evaluation of tactile and proprioceptive pathways. Although SEPs are a sensitive measurement of the somatosensory pathways, many lesions in the sensory system were not detectable. Many recent clinical studies are suggesting that LEPs will permit the assessment of pathways that fall under historical limitations of SEPs (Kakigi, Wananabe, & Yamasaki, 2000; Lefaucheur et al., 2002; Treede, 2003; Treede, Lorenz, & Baumgartner, 2003). Stimulation of receptors associated with temperature and pain perception is accomplished using a pulsed laser. In this case the signal travels along small fibers in the peripheral nerve and the anterolateral spinothalamic tract in the spinal cord and brainstem. The most obvious clinical application will be to assist in differentiating between large and small fiber neuropathies (Kakigi et al., 2000; Treede et al., 2003). While early literature leaned toward the evaluation of peripheral neuropathies and central pain syndromes (Casey et al., 1996; Kakigi et al., 1992), other applications are quickly being reported, such as in the evaluation of painful temporomandibular disorders (Romaniello et al., 2003). LEPs may offer insight into spinal and peripheral sensitization in fibromyalgia (Lorenz, Grasedyck, & Bromm, 1996). Recent literature described the role LEPs may play in the assessment of patients with dorsal root pathologies (Quante et al., 2003). As with other EPs, the study is completely objective. LEPs overcome the subjective component of other tests that have been used to evaluate the small fiber system in the past. For this reason, it is likely LEPs will play a significant role in helping to assess the patient with pain as the technology develops.

ADJUNCTIVE TESTING

There are several other electrodiagnostic studies that are not necessarily considered mainstream for routine clinical assessment. However, there is adequate mention in the literature to warrant discussion in this chapter. It is important to understand that these studies may still aid in the assessment of certain painful conditions, despite inconsistent data concerning their role as diagnostic tools.

QUANTITATIVE SENSORY TESTING

Quantitative sensory testing (QST) comprises a heterogeneous group of tests employed to assess sensory nerve fiber function, although QST is used mainly to assess sensory nerve function of small-caliber sensory nerve fibers. The subgroup of lightly myelinated and unmyelinated small-caliber nerve fiber types includes those which transmit pain signals from the peripheral nervous system to the central nervous system, making QST particularly useful in the realm of pain assessment.

Thermal thresholds are commonly used in quantitative sensory tests. A thermal threshold represents either the lowest perceptible warm temperature or the highest perceptible cool temperature. Assessment is accomplished by comparing age-matched normal values and side-to-side differences. Incremental changes in temperature are called *just noticeable differences* (Siao & Cros, 2003).

The major limitations of QST include its psychophysical subjective nature and the inability to distinguish central and peripheral lesions. Poor performance may be willful or attentional, or may represent a misinterpretation of the instructions (Mendell, Kissel, & Cornblath, 2001). The American Academy of Neurology's 2003 report, *Quantitative Sensory Testing: Report of the Therapeutics and Technology Assessment Subcommittee of the American Academy of Neurology*, corroborated the utility and shortcomings of the test, while noting that QST is more valuable when used to augment the validity of another test, and is less useful when used as the sole electrodiagnostic modality. The report clearly noted that QST could not be used in the medicolegal arena (Shy et al., 2003). Despite these limitations, QST has been a valuable tool in the electrodiagnostic assessment of peripheral nerve disease. Abnormalities must be interpreted in the context of a thorough neurological examination and other appropriate testing such as the EMG, nerve biopsy, skin biopsy, or appropriate imaging studies.

QUANTITATIVE SUDOMOTOR AXON REFLEX TEST

Certain painful neuropathies, such as hereditary sensory and autonomic neuropathies (HSAN) and those associated with porphyria, have a prominent autonomic component. The quantitative sudomotor axon reflex test (QSART) assesses autonomic (small) fiber dysfunction via the sweat response and is considered to be a reliable test with good reproducibility. Acetylcholine (ACH) is the key to QSART. It is used as an exogenous stimulator of the sweat response as well as the endogenous mediator of that response. Iontophoresed (exogenous) ACH activates antidromic axonal transmission, which eventually becomes orthodromic after turning at a branch, ultimately stimulating release of synaptic (endogenous) ACH. The released synaptic ACH that binds to the M3 muscarinic receptor on the sweat gland is quantified by a "sudometer" reading of the multicompartment sweat capsule that collected the released ACH (Jaradeh & Prieto, 2003). In neuropathy, multiple sites are tested. Small fiber nerve damage may be reflected by a reduced or absent sweat response. As well, a small fiber neuropathy may be characterized by an excessive or a persistent sweat response. The sweat response also has a latency, which is measured from commencement of iontophoresis to the moment of sweat secretion. Prolonged latency suggests small fiber dysfunction. Conversely, relatively shortened sweat response latency, less than 1 minute, is consistent with sympathetic overactivity.

THE NEUROMETER®

The Neurometer is a portable constant-current sine wave stimulator, used to quantify peripheral nerve dysfunction by measuring thresholds of constant current stimulation. Stimuli are applied through surface electrodes at three frequencies, with the so-called forced-choice method (as seen in some QST testing) used to determine the minimum detected current amplitude. An investigation by Masson and Boulton (1991) compared neurometric results to those results obtained using more conventional nerve tests, including thermal and vibration detection thresholds in the case of diabetic neuropathy. Their observations suggested that this technology may be useful as a screening instrument, providing a fairly comprehensive assessment of the functional integrity of different nerve fiber populations. A full exam is comparatively short, encompassing 10 to 15 minutes. Although most electrodiagnostic clinicians do not commonly rely on the Neurometer, it may be helpful in the assessment of small fiber pathology. An abundance of clinical research is planned.

BLINK REFLEXES

Terminologically, the clinical blink reflex is distinguished from the electrodiagnostic blink reflex. The clinical blink reflex is carefully elicited by the examiner by lightly touching the cornea of one eye. The electrodiagnostic blink reflex is performed by electrical stimulation of the supraorbital nerve on one side of the face while recording the obicularis oculi muscle response on both sides. Unilateral sensory information is carried from one side of the face, via the supraorbital nerve branch of the V1 segment of the trigeminal nerve. This afferent signal reaches the principal trigeminal nucleus in the pons (Meckel's cave). After pontine nuclear synapse, the efferent limb of the reflex is mediated by the facial nerve (VII) on both sides of the face, resulting in bilateral obicularis oculi muscle contraction.

The so-called ipsilateral R1 response correlates with early efferent signal transmission, occurring after brainstem synapse. The clinical significance of the R1 response remains unclear. The bilateral R2 response correlates with the bilateral blinking of eyes. The normal R1 latency is about 13 ms and is found on the same side of the stimulus. The normal bilateral R2 latency is about 40 ms on each side with potentials noted on each side. The ipsilateral R2 response occurs approximately 3 ms sooner than the contralateral R2 response (Daube, 1996).

The blink reflex test is performed in a variety of suspected disorders that cause pain, such as AIDP (cranial neuropathy) and cerebellopontine angle lesions (e.g., schwannoma or neurofibroma) (Tanaka, Takaki, & Maruta, 1987). Trigeminal neuralgia (TN) is a debilitating syndrome of lancinating pain, which is associated with abnormal blink reflex results. In some cases, TN is associated with a vascular loop that presses the nerve near its nucleus at the skull base (Jannetta, 1980). TN may be caused by connective tissue diseases, such as scleroderma (Serratrice, Pouget, & Saint-Jean, 1986). Blink reflexes are oftentimes abnormal in MS (Novatschkova-Spassova, 1983), with TN the presenting symptom of MS in a minority of cases. Many cases of TN remain idiopathic. The blink reflex may be normal in TN, but when abnormal, the affected component is usually the afferent portion.

NERVE ROOT STIMULATION

The nerve root stimulation (NRS) procedure involves discrete stimulation of a single nerve root using relatively low levels of current/voltage passed through a needle electrode, to assure that only the nerve root of interest is stimulated. This procedure is mostly used to precisely localize the abnormal spinal myotome. NRS is often performed in conjunction with SEP assessment, especially in the context of intraoperative monitoring. NRS is also used to assess atypical neuromuscular disorders, such as bladder abnormalities due to detrusor muscle dysfunction (Markland et al., 1972). NRS is a safe procedure, albeit more invasive than routine EMG. In 2002, Zileli et al. reported the utility of nerve root stimulation to be similar to that of dual diagnostic assessment with needle EMG and NCVs suggesting that the role of NRS will remain limited.

APPROACH TO THE PATIENT

Before performing an electrodiagnostic study on the patient with pain, one must define a diagnostic goal for the investigation. The hypothesis drives the choice of study. Electrodiagnostic findings may, at times, alter the course of the study in midstream if an alternative diagnosis is suggested by those findings. For this reason the examiner must be both prepared and flexible. In some cases, it is vital to know the temporal details of the patient's history. For example, a needle EMG performed 10 days after an apparent axonal injury may show reduced recruitment and be otherwise normal. In this case a repeat study must be performed a few weeks later to assess for delayed onset of axonal injury, as abnormal insertional and spontaneous activity are not apparent until about day 15 after injury.

Before one endeavors the performance of an electrodiagnostic study, normal values and anthropomorphic data should be known, or at least available for reference. Temperature effects must be taken into account during NCV studies. The normal upper limb skin temperature should range from 34 to 36°C, although 32°C is acceptable. The lower limb skin temperature should range from 32 to 34°C, although 30°C is acceptable. Temperature is most important for sensory nerves and in the assessment of symmetrical processes. If a warming apparatus is not available, correction factors may be used, but their use tends to have less accuracy than warming, especially with pathological nerve (Rutkove, 2001). An electrodiagnostic laboratory is considered incomplete if it lacks a temperature probe. Cool limbs can be warmed with direct moist heat. However, in this chapter's first author's opinion, heat from an infrared light is clearly superior. With direct moist heat, the surface is warmed better than deeper tissue, its effects relatively short lasting. Cooling of normal excitable tissue has several effects. It tends to increase amplitude, prolong latency, and slow conduction velocity of nerve responses. Fibrillations are diminished in numbers. Fasciculation amplitude increases, whereas its frequency diminishes. Cooling also reduces compound muscle potential amplitude and initially increases myotonic discharges in paramyotonia (myotonic discharges abate with further cooling). Effects of warming include worsening of conduction block as well as worsening of neuromuscular junction decrement in myasthenia gravis. In PROMM (proximal myotonic myopathy), myotonic activity increases with warming. The effect of temperature on other potentials is not well defined (Rutkove, 2001).

Laboratory safety issues include screening the patient for a history of electronic device implantation, such as a cardiac pacemaker. The American Association of Electrodiagnostic Medicine guidelines for performing studies in patients with implantable electronic devices confirm that NCV, needle EMG, and EP studies are relatively safe, as long as attention to grounding detail is meticulous. Proximal limb studies (e.g., brachial plexus stimulation) may increase the risk of an untoward cardiac event with cardiac pacemaker present. Performance of NCV studies in patients with external cardiac pacemaker is not recommended. Repetitive stimulation can be problematic in the case of sensed-rate triggered implantable defibrillators. Intra-arterial catheters present a significant current-related risk, increasing with current leaks. The patient should be screened for anticoagulant use and for history of coagulopathy, platelet disorder, visceral disease, or proclivity to bruise easily. Universal precautions and protocols are in play at all times. Needle EMG of the chest and abdominal wall musculature carries puncture risks, which should be discussed with the patient and consented to before examination. Electrical safety in the laboratory depends on the proper grounding of the machinery. A low-resistance pathway from the machine to the ground is usually provided through the electrical line in the wall plug. One must never directly ground the patient or permit the patient to make contact with grounded objects while connected to any biomedical equipment. This includes avoiding a scenario in which the patient is hooked up to two different machines simultaneously, as in the case of electrocardiography (EKG) with EEG. Extra care must be taken with electrically sensitive patients who are critically ill (Daube, 1996).

COMMON PAINFUL CONDITIONS

HEADACHE

Hurdles to define the EEG features of migraine include variability in defining migraine as a nosological entity. Inconsistent normal criteria, concurrency of nonmigrainous headache, inclusion of criteria associated with neurologically significant symptoms (e.g., hemiplegia with migraine), age-related differences, and variability in EEG interpretation all contribute to this variability. The interictal EEG is usually normal in migraine, although focal slowing, sharp wave transients, pronounced posthyperventilation delta activity, and hypersynchronous bursts are noted as well. Alpha depression may be noted in the initial (ophthalmic) phase of migraine with aura. Lateralized alpha asymmetry has strongly correlated in common migraine without aura. For the most part, the EEG of patients with migraine does not differ significantly from the EEG of normal individuals (Niedermeyer, 1999).

In the experience of these authors and others, the migraineur demonstrates an occipital driving response at higher flash frequencies (at or above 20 flashes/s) during application of intermittent photic stimulation. This phenomenon is fairly specific for migraine (Golla & Winter, 1959; Slater, 1968; Smythe & Winter, 1964). This premise has been further established by spectral analysis (Simon et al., 1982).

Basilar migraine, common in children and young adults, has a variety of associated EEG findings, depending on the study. Loss of consciousness in basilar migraine is associated with either diffuse or lateralized slowing on EEG. Status migrainosus is not highly corre-

lated with any one particular finding on EEG. Acute migraine is commonly associated with a normal tracing. Predictably, lateralized slowing in the delta and theta frequency range has been noted over the involved hemisphere in cases of hemiplegia that accompanies migraine. Distinguished from adult migraine, childhood migraine is commonly associated with abdominal symptoms and obtundation, either of which may occur without headache. The abdominal component has been shown to be associated with so-called 14 and 6 positive spikes (Niedermyer, 1999).

Intracranial lesions are associated with headache, as well as with seizure. Adults and children with intracranial lesions suffer from headaches. Identified lesions, such as stroke, tumor, and herpes encephalitis are associated with periodic lateralized epileptiform discharges on a fairly consistent basis (Lipton, Chaudry, & Andriola, 1998).

Rolandic spikes have been noted in childhood migraine. Rolandic epilepsy and migraine are relatively common entities, begging the question of linked pathophysiology versus coincidence in this set of patients. An assessment based on extensive data collection was unable to support the theory of a shared genetic susceptibility between migraine and epilepsy (Lipton & Ottoman, 1996). An entity noted as migraine-triggered epilepsy has been described (Niedermeyer, 1999). In this clinical entity, the interictal EEG is mostly normal. Conversely, an epilepsy-triggered migraine has been postulated (Jacobs, Goadsby, & Duncan, 1996).

MONONEUROPATHY

Electrodiagnostic findings in suspected mononeuropathy include prolonged sensory and/or motor nerve latency, reduced SNAP, and reduced CMAP. Significant axonal involvement begets neurogenic changes found on needle EMG. Certain anatomical regions confer a higher susceptibility to compression. The flexor retinaculum at the volar wrist may be the most infamous of those regions (carpal tunnel syndrome, CTS). Entire texts are dedicated to entrapment. Peroneal mononeuropathy may be caused by compression in the thigh (sciatic peroneal), at the fibular head, or at the ankle. Needle EMG study of the biceps femoris short head muscle (the only peroneal-innervated muscle above the knee) helps localize the site of peroneal nerve compression to either above or below the fibular head. An SEP may also be effective in identifying a peroneal nerve entrapment at the piriformis muscle. Axonal changes are common in peroneal mononeuropathy at the fibular head (Katirji & Wilbourn, 1988, 1994; Wilbourn, 1986).

Susceptibility to nerve compression may be conferred by metabolic dysfunction associated with diabetes, likely by microvasculopathic mechanisms involving the vaso nervorum (Dellon, Mackinnon, & Seiler, 1988). Diabetic susceptibility is commonly manifested in median mononeuropathy at the wrist (CTS). Genetic mutation of Connexin-32 causes a hereditary susceptibility to pressure palsy (HNPP). Whereas most other forms of compressive neuropathy are usually painful, HNPP is not (Chance & Lupski, 1994). Vasculitis is a common cause of painful mononeuropathy associated with systemic disease (David, Peine, Schlesinger, & Smith, 1996).

Compressive peripheral neuropathies may coexist with either radiculopathy or plexopathy (double-crush). Limitations in routine electrodiagnostic testing necessitate specialized techniques to identify atypical compressive neuropathies, as in the case of digital mononeuropathy secondary to repetitive finger trauma, as seen in bowlers, hence the term "bowler's thumb" (Nasr & Kaufman, 2001).

The use of SEP studies in the evaluation of peripheral entrapment or injuries is not new (Eisen, 1982; Peterson & Will, 1988; Trainer et al., 1992). SEPs are particularly helpful in the setting of a suspected mononeuropathy that occurs in a region that is difficult or impossible to assess using routine NCV studies. Cordato et al. (2004) demonstrated the reliability of SEPs in identification of lateral femoral cutaneous nerve entrapment in meralgia paresthetica. SEP testing predicts the outcome of surgery that is performed to correct such conditions (Siu & Chandran, 2004).

Carpal Tunnel Syndrome

CTS is the most common peripheral mononeuropathy. In the Western world, CTS is infamously due to repetitive use. Hypothyroidism, rheumatoid arthritis, acromegaly, Lupus, hyperparathyroidism, and diabetes mellitus are felt to account for secondary causes. Brachial plexopathy and cervical radiculopathy may affect a downstream loss of median nerve integrity, increasing susceptibility to compression. This so-called double-crush phenomenon is also seen with involvement of the proximal median nerve (Osterman, 1988; Upton & McComas, 1973). Bilateral CTS is more common than not and, in older males, may be due to amyloid protein deposition, which commonly occurs with multiple myeloma.

Normal electrodiagnostic findings in what appears to be a clinically apparent case of CTS may suggest subclinical CTS or, possibly, another clinical diagnosis, such as de Quervain's tenosynovitis, posterior interosseous (radial sensory) neuropathy, neurogenic thoracic outlet syndrome, cervical radiculopathy, or arthritic changes in the limb. Proximal median nerve lesions are less common (e.g., pronator syndrome). A routine electrodiagnostic assessment includes finger ring electrode stimulation, recording at the volar forearm. One may choose any of the four median-innervated digits to stimulate. The index finger is commonly used. Some experts in the field prefer

the middle digit, likely because this digit is autonomously innervated by the median nerve, with no gross contribution from the radial or ulnar nerves.

Routine laboratory assessment of the median nerve includes the sensory nerve, the motor nerve at the wrist and elbow (some prefer to also stimulate the nerve at the axilla), and the F-wave response. Assessment of the ipsilateral ulnar sensory and motor nerves studies, an ipsilateral radial (posterior interosseous) sensory nerve study, and testing of the contralateral median sensory and motor nerves round out the NCV study. Needle EMG assessment is performed to rule out concurrent cervical radiculopathy and to define, when applicable, the extent of an axonal median nerve lesion. The high incidence of bilateral CTS begs assessment of the median nerve contralateral to the symptomatic side. Prolonged median sensory nerve latency with no other abnormal findings constitutes mild CTS. Involvement of the median motor nerve is consistent with moderate CTS. Although not common, median motor involvement may be seen without concurrent sensory dysfunction. Abnormal needle EMG study suggests severe CTS, usually associated with some level of abductor pollicis brevis (APB) muscle weakness and thenar eminence atrophy. Subtle or focal lesions of the median nerve may not be detected with conventional electrodiagnostic methods, necessitating supplemental techniques of higher precision, including comparison of the median and ulnar mixed nerve latencies (Kaufman, 1996), palmar short segment assessment (Katirji, 1998), and the antidromic inching technique (Kimura, 2001). SEPs are also used to assist in the diagnosis of CTS, or the lack thereof (Glick, 1992; Kawasaki, Saito, & Ogawa, 1995).

Other Mononeuropathies

Radial nerve compression at the humerus (Saturday night palsy) is the usual cause of wrist drop, which is mostly a motor phenomenon, although it may cause pain. The ulnar nerve is classically compressed at the elbow (cubital tunnel syndrome). This is diagnosed when ulnar motor nerve slowing is found with stimulation above the elbow. Ulnar nerve lesions at the wrist are usually noted at Guyon's canal in the wrist or at the pisohamate hiatus in the hand. SEPs can be helpful in confirming an ulnar neuropathy, as well as in ruling out a more proximal medial cord plexopathy or preganglionic C8/T1 radiculopathy.

Although commonly discussed in the electrodiagnostic literature, tarsal tunnel syndrome, as a clinical entity, remains controversial (Dumitru, 1991a). The tarsal tunnel is the site where the descending tibial nerve divides into the calcaneal sensory branch, the medial plantar mixed nerve, and the lateral plantar mixed nerve. Inconsistent ability to obtain mixed and motor plantar nerve potentials necessitates stimulation in both lower limbs for comparison (Katirji, 1998). A routine tibial motor nerve response at the ankle, as well as needle EMG assessment of the adductor hallucis and abductor digit quinti pedis muscles, will improve the diagnostic yield of plantar neuropathy. Plantar neuropathy is also evaluated using SEPs (Dumitru, Kalantri, & Dierschke, 1991).

In suspected piriformis syndrome, the sciatic nerve is thought to be compressed by the piriformis muscle. The literature reveals that compressive denervation of the sciatic nerve is usually due to aberrant myofascial bands, rather than piriformis muscle. NCV studies are rarely corroborative in this setting. A notable percentage of the population demonstrates an anatomical anomaly in which the peroneal division of the sciatic nerve passes either superior to the piriformis muscle or directly through the muscle, piercing it as it goes, increasing the risk of nerve compression (Brazis, Masdeau, & Biller, 1996). In this situation, SEPs can provide a unique means of quantification and confirmatory diagnosis, and are commonly used introperatively to avoid malpositioning injury (Glick, 2001).

Weight loss, crossing of the legs, and trauma are major causes of peroneal mononeuropathy at the fibular head, which may be associated with pain (20% of cases), paresthesias, numbness, and motor findings (e.g., foot drop). The tibialis anterior muscle is the major foot dorsiflexor, conferring functional prognostic value in its assessment. As well, the more distal extensor digitorum brevis (EDB) muscle is commonly atrophic due to "wear and tear," rather than due to pathology, limiting its diagnostic value. Tight footwear may cause denervation (Katirji, 1998). The tibialis anterior muscle is innervated by the L4 and L5 spinal nerve roots and is the only L4-innervated muscle below the knee.

PLEXOPATHY

There are several plexi in the human body. The lumbar plexus is clearly important in the clinical settings of diabetes mellitus, surgical trauma, and pelvic tumors. However, the brachial plexus is the touchstone for electrodiagnostic assessment. Disorders of the brachial plexus include those involving birth trauma (Erb's palsy and Klumpke's palsy), radiation plexopathy seen in breast cancer, Parsonage-Turner syndrome (idiopathic disease of the brachial plexus), a variety of traumas (e.g., avulsion), and neurogenic thoracic outlet syndrome (NTOS). NTOS is due to an abnormality of the lower plexus trunk, associated with local anatomical variations, such as cervical rib and scalene anticus syndrome (Brazis et al., 1996). Plexus lesions tend to be extraordinarily painful. Volume conduction-related error is common with stimulation of Erb's point, causing one to interpret these results with a grain of salt (Herbison, 1996).

Because of its complex anatomy, successful electrodiagnostic assessment of the brachial plexus necessitates solid knowledge of its regional anatomy. Plexus lesions are classified according to lesion level: root, ramus, division, trunk, cord, or terminal nerve branch. Upper plexus lesions (C5, C6, upper trunk) tend to be demyelinating in nature, with or without conduction block, and are more likely. Upper plexus lesions are more likely extraforaminal, i.e., more amenable to surgical repair. Lower plexus lesions tend to be preganglionic and axonal in nature, demonstrating denervation. Neurogenic changes in the lower plexus tend to affect muscles that are distant from the lesion. This feature confers a generally poorer prognosis for lower plexus lesions (Ferrante & Wilbourn, 2002). NTOS affects the lower trunk. However, dysfunction of ramified nerve roots (C8 and T1) and multiple peripheral nerves (median and ulnar) should be considered. Clinically, NTOS features thenar atrophy, hypoesthesia in an ulnar distribution, paresis of the intrinsic muscles of the hand, and pain in the affected limb. Electrodiagnostic findings include low or absent ulnar sensory nerve SNAP, low median CMAP, borderline low ulnar CMAP, and normal median SNAP. Needle EMG will show neurogenic changes in the distal upper limb muscles, more compelling in those innervated by the median nerve (Katirji, 1998). Routine electromyographic plexus evaluation is augmented by SEP studies. The literature demonstrates that SEPs are superior to routine EMG in both localizing plexus injury and assessing the extent of that injury (Brudon et al., 1989; Date, Rappaport, & Ortega, 1991; Stohr, Riffel, & Buettner, 1981; Sugioka, 1984; Synek, 1987a, b; Yilmaz et al., 2003).

RADICULOPATHY

Nerve root pathology (radiculopathy) is considered in the setting of spine- and limb-related pain, as noted with protrusion of disc material, degenerative vertebral changes, arthritis, and fractures of the boney elements. Pathological fractures may occur in the setting of cancer, infection, and rheumatoid arthritis. Muscle, ligament, and tendinous dysfunction often occur with or without deeper spine pathology. The scope of painful root pathology extends to systemic disease, such as that seen in zoster-related root disease and AIDP.

The term *nerve root* refers to a neural bundle contiguous with the spinal cord. The sensory bundle is the *dorsal nerve root*. This extends laterally from the dorsal portion of the spinal cord. The motor bundle is the *ventral nerve root,* which extends laterally from the ventral portion of the spinal cord. The dorsal and the ventral roots meet at a point lateral from the spinal cord, in the vicinity of the neural foramen, where they eventually form the *mixed spinal nerve,* which contains both motor and sensory tissue, as well as autonomic tissue that enters the mixed spinal nerve beyond the neural foramen. As it emerges from the neural foramen, the ramified mixed spinal nerve branches into the primary rami.

The *dorsal primary ramus* extends posteriorly to innervate the axial muscles and the skin of the posterior trunk, whereas the *ventral primary ramus* extends anteriorly to supply the limbs, appendicular skeletal muscles, and the skin of the lateral and anterior trunk and neck. By virtue of the relative volume of innervated structures, the ventral primary ramus is more substantial in size than is the dorsal primary ramus. The dorsal and ventral *roots* are distinguished by functional tissue type — sensory versus motor. The rami are distinguished by their anatomical distribution, i.e., dorsal or ventral structures (Brazis et al., 1996). The dorsal root ganglion lies just proximal to the junction of the sensory root and the mixed nerve. A chemical synapse at the ganglion separates sensory information transmitted from the periphery to the ganglion from the sensory information transmitted from the preganglionic region to the brain. A lesion, therefore, proximal to the dorsal root ganglion, will not affect the sensory nerve distal to it. This relationship reveals an extremely important clinical pearl that describes a clinical scenario in which a painful dorsal root lesion is associated with a completely normal sensory nerve conduction velocity study. As well, if the dorsal root is affected in isolation, without ventral root involvement, the needle EMG and motor F-wave evaluations will be normal.

In this special circumstance of an isolated preganglionic lesion, only the SEP can diagnose this lesion, as the SEP is the only study that assesses the sensory system in continuity and is superior to EMG (Aminoff et al., 1985a; Dvonch et al., 1984; Pape, Eldevik, & Vandvik, 2002; Rodriquez et al., 1987; Slimp et al., 1992; Snowden et al., 1992; Talavera-Carbajal et al., 2003). Therefore, SEPs should be considered when more routine electromyography is equivocal and when a preganglionic radiculopathy is suggested.

One study assessing EMG in radiculopathy revealed that a six-muscle limb screen confers "good" yield for neurogenic activity, limiting the need for a more extensive muscle study (Hong, Lee, & Lum, 1986). Although each muscle is innervated by different nerve roots, each muscle is considered to have one predominant level of innervation. An upper limb nerve root screen should include needle EMG assessment of at least one representative muscle from each nerve root level. For example, C5 is represented by the deltoid muscle. As well, the proximal-to-distal gradient should be appropriately assessed by testing two anatomically separate muscles that represent the same predominant nerve root, e.g., triceps (proximal) and the extensor digitorum communis (distal) muscles, both predominantly innervated by C7.

To help localize cervical spinal nerve root pathology, one should understand that the C1 nerve exits the spine above the C1 vertebra. This pattern of the nerve exiting above the vertebral level of the same number continues until the T1 vertebral level, at which point the C8 nerve root exits on top and the T1 root exits below. From this point, as one descends the spine, the root exits below the corresponding numbered vertebra. The anatomical consistency of this pattern breaks down at the L1 vertebra, where the distance between the spinal cord levels shortens, but the intervertebral distance does not. Thus, proximal bunching of lumbar nerve root egress is noted; the result is the cauda equina. The longer the distance a motor neuron nucleus lies from its synapse with muscle, the more time it takes to generate neurogenic activity after injury. As well, it takes that much longer for that nerve to heal after injury. In addition, proper healing is less likely with increased nerve length. Therefore, by virtue of its midline axial location, the paraspinal muscles are more apt to demonstrate normal EMG activity after a monophasic injury than are limb muscles. Evidence of radiculopathy may be masked by the overlapping of paraspinal nerve root levels. Paraspinal neurogenic activity manifests by about day 7, but may be gone, if mild, by the time that activity shows in the limb. The tibial nerve H-wave reflex examination may augment needle EMG in the setting of an S1 radiculopathy, especially if it is unilateral. In the setting of polyneuropathy, the H-reflex is typically prolonged symmetrically, assuming no other focal lesion (Johnson & Pease, 1997).

SPINAL STENOSIS

Clinically speaking, spinal stenosis represents tightening of the spinal and foraminal spaces due to congenitally small size and/or abnormal changes in spinal tissue. Spinal stenosis can produce pain and reduced mobility and may also cause neurological dysfunction (Benini, 1992). Clinically, spinal stenosis is recognized as a generic entity of heterogeneous pathology, but is entertained as a singular electrodiagnostic construct. Recent literature suggests that compared with MRI, paraspinal needle EMG is a superior study in the diagnostic assessment of symptomatic spinal stenosis (Haig et al., 2001). In the asymptomatic elderly patient with spinal stenosis, the sural sensory nerve action potentials and tibial nerve H-wave reflexes tend to be absent, causing potential false electrodiagnostic positives for polyneuropathy. The most common EMG finding associated with lumbar stenosis is bilateral symmetrical L5, S1, and S2 radiculopathies. The literature shows that SEPs augment electrodiagnostic assessment of spinal stenosis, especially in the setting of surgical decompression for this clinical entity (Herron et al., 1987; Kraft, 2003; Norcross-Nechay, Mathew, Simmons, & Hadjipavlou, 1999; Seyal et al., 1992; Snowden et al., 1992).

POLYNEUROPATHY

Entire texts are dedicated to the classification and categorization of this diverse group of disorders, with a plethora of subtypes. Many polyneuropathies cause pain, either due to small fiber involvement or secondary to other causes that are characteristic of a particular pathological process (e.g., inflammation or susceptibility to compression). The length-dependent polyneuropathy is common and is exemplary of the bunch. The length-dependent polyneuropathy affects the most distal portion of the limbs first, that is, the toes. In diabetic neuropathy, it is thought that both metabolic and microvascular pathology play a role. The process progresses with a gross symmetry characterized by abnormal sensation slowly ascending the lower limbs. If motor fibers are involved, the most distal foot muscles are affected first, i.e., toe extensors, explaining why "hammertoes" develop in polyneuropathy (unopposed flexion). Early nerve conduction velocity study findings include slowing of sensory nerve conduction velocity, along with reduced SNAP and CMAP amplitudes. Significant motor dysfunction begets neurogenic changes on needle EMG. Atrophy of the extensor digitorum brevis muscle is a classic motor sign of polyneuropathy. Besides pain, small fiber manifestations may include autonomic changes such as postural syncope, as well as an array of dermatological changes (Periquet, Mendell, & Kissel, 1999).

The most common cause of symmetrical painful polyneuropathy in the Western world is diabetes mellitus. Alcohol polyneuropathy is second, associated with the direct toxic effect or nutritional deficiency or both. Genetic factors play a role in predisposition to alcoholic neuropathy (Kucera et al., 2002). Other painful neuropathies include those secondary to B vitamin deficiency, hypothyroidism, renal insufficiency, paraneoplastic (variety), HIV, treatment for HIV (didanosine, zalcitabine), Lyme disease, sarcoidosis, amyloidosis (familial or acquired), dysprotenemia (e.g., multiple myeloma), INH (isoniazid without B_6), vincristine, cisplatin, paclitaxel, D4T, porphyria, vasculitis, cryoglobulinemia, Fabry's disease, Tangier's disease, multiple myeloma, Sjögren's syndrome, cancer, macroglobulinemia, lapromatous compression, perhexiline poisoning, hereditary sensory and autonomic (HSAN), idiopathic, and cryptogenic causes, just to name a few (Mendell et al., 2001). Early detection of diabetes mellitus is correlated with improved outcome, but it must be looked for. A simple sensory examination followed by electrodiagnostic assessment may lead not only to the discovery of diabetes, but also to the recognition of other serious illnesses associated with neuropathy, such as multiple myeloma, lung cancer, and connective tissue disease.

Painful Hereditary Neuropathies

HSAN is a group of congenital neuropathies associated with abnormalities of neurotrophin. There are five major types, many of which cause burning and lancination pain. Subtypes vary clinically and electrodiagnostically, with respect to motor, large fiber sensory, and small fiber sensory changes on EMG. Amyloid neuropathies may be congenital or acquired, such as those that occur with multiple myeloma. Genetic testing and nerve biopsy are usually not needed for family members who are already classified. Electrodiagnostic findings include large fiber axonal changes. The small fiber electrodiagnostic studies (QSART, QST) may corroborate the painful and autonomic symptoms, respectively.

The spectrum of Charcot-Marie-Tooth disease (CMT) exemplifies an inherited large fiber polyneuropathy, originally referred to as peroneal muscular atrophy by Dyck and Lambert (1968). Experience reveals that abnormal sensory symptoms associated with inherited polyneuropathy are associated with pain that is both nociceptive (e.g., cramps, hammertoes) and neuropathic, although CMT is not classically considered a painful neuropathy. In a prospective study of 52 patients with CMT, positive sensory symptoms were reported by 28 of those patients (54%), including neuropathic pain in 6 of those patients. Pain, either neuropathic or nociceptive, was present in 29 patients (56%) and in 15 patients as a main symptom (Gemignani et al., 2004).

Sensory Ganglionopathy (Neuronopathy)

Sensory neuronopathies represent impaired function of the unipolar sensory neurons that reside in the spinal dorsal root ganglia or trigeminal ganglia of the pons. The large fiber component is well documented, but the painful component is less obvious. Sensory ataxia is typically profound, as is the gravity of etiologies, such as cancer (e.g., paraneoplastic from lung cancer) and autoimmune disease (e.g., Sjögren's syndrome). Treatment tends to be more academic than efficacious (Bryer & Chad, 1999).

Myopathy and Neuromyopathy

Muscle pain secondary to myopathy has many causes. Myopathies can be myotonic, inflammatory, metabolic, and storage disorder categories. Recruitment patterns of myopathic muscle may vary and are usually abnormal in more severe cases. Because myopathic processes preferentially affect the proximal and trunk muscles (Katirji, 1998), needle EMG of paraspinal muscle confers the best yield of abnormal activity manifested through denervation potentials found in irritable myopathies (fibrillations and positive sharp waves).

Rhabdomyolysis is an acute, painful, and life-threatening myopathy, associated with a disturbance of thermoregulation. Fibrillation potentials abound; high CPK levels cause concern for renal failure. The three classic inflammatory myopathies (polymyositis, inclusion body myositis, and dermatomyositis) have their own distinct pathologies. Dermatomyositis features classic skin lesions, to include periorbital edema with an upper eyelid heliotrope, Grotten's dorsal hand nodules, and fiery erythema of the chest, representing telangectasias (Fitzpatrick et al., 1992). Needle EMG findings reflect denervation due to inflammation. Specific EMG features of dermatomyositis include fibrillations, pseudomyotonic discharges, and positive sharp waves. In this particular disease, evidence of denervation portends occult tumor. Myopathy, whether acquired (e.g., HIV, alcohol) or congenital (e.g., Duchenne's muscular dystrophy, McCardle's disease), irritable or non-irritable, and with or without myotonic or dystrophic components, comprises a vast heterogeneous group of entities, many causing pain and amenable to electrodiagnostic assessment.

Muscle disease associated with alcohol abuse is more common than previously realized. The acute painful variety is associated with swelling, hyperalgesia, cramps, and weakness. This typically occurs after a binge and may be difficult to differentiate clinically from deep vein thrombosis. Ethanol and its metabolite acetaldehyde exact direct pathologic effects on skeletal muscle (Ford, Cadwell, & Kilgo, 1984).

SYRINGOMYELIA AND MYOPATHIOSIS

A syrinx refers to a pathological expansion of the central spinal cord canal (syringomyelia), which may extend to the brainstem (syringobulbia), associated with Chiari malformation. Burning pain is typically localized to the trunk and limbs. Myelopathic signs and symptoms, such as urinary incontinence and lower limb paresis, may be noted. The complaint of burning trunk and/or limb pain is not uncommon. Traumatic syringomyelia is common, although most cases are associated with tumor or are noted as congenital variants.

A study of 48 subjects with syringomyelia revealed that 70% suffered from pain, many of them localizing that pain to the neck and upper extremities. In 68.7% of these subjects, an associated cervical *myopathiosis* was found to be the principal cause of the manifestations. This phenomenon was noted in subjects with no evidence of cervical osteochondrosis. The myopathiosis was electromyographically characterized by a persistent mixture of shortened and prolonged motor unit potentials noted during cervical spinal needle EMG assessment. Regional upper extremity circulatory changes correlated with the intensity of muscle pain. Segmental massage was found to be effective in helping reduce and eliminate local myopathiosis (Ivanichev, Khasanova, & Aleeva, 1982). SEP may be useful in the electrodiagnosis of syringomyelia (Wagner et al., 1995).

PSEUDOMYOPATHY (HYPOPHOSPHATEMIA)

Painful proximal muscle weakness that clinically simulates polymyositis can be found in cases of hypophos-phatemia, which may result from antacid overuse. CPK (creatine phosphokinase) and muscle enzymes are normal. This metabolic "pseudomyopathy" exemplifies the myriad of rheumatic diseases that may be mimicked by hypophosphatemia (Searles et al., 1977).

CRAMPS

Cramps can be profoundly painful, especially if they are sustained. Cramps are benign in subjects with no known pathology. They may be idiopathic or associated with stress, as well as exogenous substances, such as theophylline. They are also seen in a litany of systemic disorders. Individual potentials resemble motor unit potentials. They fire rapidly at 40 to 60 Hz, usually with abrupt onset and cessation. These potentials may fire irregularly, in a sputtering fashion, especially just before termination. Typically, increasing numbers of potentials that fire at similar rates are recruited as the cramp develops. Those potentials, then, drop out as the clinical cramp subsides (Daube, 1996).

LANDRY–GUILLAIN–BARRE–STORHL SYNDROME

Landry–Guillain–Barre–Storhl syndrome, commonly known as GBS, is an umbrella term for the array of idiopathic inflammatory disorders that subacutely affect the nerves and nerve roots. The flagship disorders under this group are AIDP and chronic inflammatory demyelinating polyradiculoneuropathy (CIDP). Both of these disorders are associated with pain, which can be debilitating. AIDP is considered a monophasic illness, marked by the clinical hallmark of ascending weakness. Its onset, clinical nadir, and recovery phase occur over a span of weeks. Despite its motor flavor, the pathological process affects both large and small nerve fiber types, affecting a variety of sensory symptoms, with pain prominent. Classic presentations of AIDP may feature low back pain as the presenting symptom. Dysautonomia may have grave consequences, including cardiovascular instability. Intensive care admissions are not uncommon. Electrodiagnostic confirmation of AIDP expedites immunotherapy. Early recognition leads to early treatment. Mitigation of the autoimmune process improves long-term motor prognosis as well as potentially preserving life.

The usual targets of the inflammatory attack against mixed fiber populations in AIDP are characterized electrodiagnostically, being clustered at the anatomical extremes of the peripheral nervous system. That is, the foci of pathology tend to cluster proximally, at the nerve root, as well as at the distal extents of the peripheral nerve. Involvement of the nerve root sleeve confers a high cerebrospinal fluid protein level, noted without a rise in cerebrospinal fluid white count (the so-called cytoalbuminemic dissociation). Criteria for diagnosis include EMG evidence of primary demyelination (including significant slowing of conduction and/or conduction block), with clinical findings such as lower limb areflexia and ascending paresis. Axonal involvement, as reflected by low CMAP amplitude at clinical plateau, portends a poorer prognosis for recovery of motor function. Other electrodiagnostic characteristics of AIDP include absent H-waves, prolonged or absent F-waves, reduced SNAP amplitude, and temporal dispersion (which causes lower amplitude but does not affect volume under the curve). An electrodiagnostic pearl for AIDP is the finding of a reduced median nerve SNAP accompanied by a normal sural nerve SNAP. Specific electrodiagnostic criteria differ among authors (Katirji, 1998).

PORPHYRIA

Porphyria refers to a set of disorders caused by a defect in heme metabolism. Clinical symptoms mimic those of AIDP. Paroxysmal attacks of debilitating pain, as well as specific urine findings, aid in distinguishing between the two disorders. The paroxysmal attacks of hepatic porphyria, due to neuropathy, are precipitated by stress, drugs, dietary indiscretion, and endocrinological factors. Porphyric neuropathy affects the small, lightly myelinated or unmyelinated nerve fibers, mediating visceral autonomic dysfunction along with regional pain. Besides distinct patterns of pain, proximal limb weakness and the persistence of the muscle stretch tendon reflexes help distinguish this disorder from AIDP (Mendell et al., 2001). A study of 115 patients with acute intermittent porphyria, seen during a 20-year period, revealed that 11 of them suffered an acute episode of quadriparesis. Nerve conduction studies performed on 8 of these 11 patients demonstrated low-amplitude compound action potentials with normal velocity measurements. Needle EMG demonstrated prominent fibrillation potentials, especially in proximal muscles. The changes in these findings with time confirm that this disorder, at least a major component of this disorder, is an acute axonal neuropathy with proximal predilection (Albers, Robertson, & Daube, 1978).

POST-POLIO SYNDROME

Post-polio syndrome tends to cause pain. Electrodiagnostic findings of polio include giant motor units and tiny fibrillations. The large-amplitude motor unit represents the large population of muscle fibers that are reinnervated by the motor neurons that survived the viral infection. Years after motor function has stabilized, a later-life motor decompensation becomes manifest as weakness, fatigue, and myalgias. Tiny fibrillation potentials suggest ongoing denervation and reinnervation. This post-polio phenomenon may be secondary to the collateral sprouting of motor neurons that do not actually fully stabilize. Denervation becomes more prominent with time. A post-infectious autoimmune syndrome is suggested in late-onset destabilization of motor dysfunction (Younger, 1999).

DIABETES MELLITUS

Neurological manifestations of diabetes mellitus are diffuse and well defined. From cerebral stroke to muscle hemorrhage, the entire neuraxis is fair game for the assault by metabolic and vascular pathology. Lesions associated with pain are usually those that are involved with polyneuropathy (which secondarily predisposes to painful mononeuropathy), plexopathy, and radiculopathy. Serum glucose control, weight loss, and blood pressure control contribute to a favorable outcome. Several types of neuropathy are seen in diabetes, and more than one type may manifest in the same patient. The length-dependent, so-called "dying-back" polyneuropathy is one of the more common types and may involve multiple fiber types. Polyneuropathy in diabetes may be primarily axonal, but may also be mixed demyelinating/axonal. Isolated painful small fiber polyneuropathy cannot be diagnosed using conventional EMG/NCV studies. Thermal threshold QST, QSART, and skin biopsy are appropriate studies in the diagnostic assessment of isolated small fiber painful polyneuropathy. Length-dependent neuropathy correlates with a stocking-glove sensory loss, as well as weak distal lower limb muscles. Hammertoes are formed when the most distal foot muscles, the extensor muscles, become affected before the toe flexors, which contract unopposed. Sensory nerve studies are more sensitive than motor nerve studies for diagnosing polyneuropathy. Needle EMG changes may precede nerve conduction study changes. The comparison of central and conduction times recorded by SEP in a group of diabetic patients revealed what had been an unapparent lesion of the spinal cord in addition to peripheral nerve involvement (Varsik et al., 2001).

Other painful neuropathies such as CTS and meralgia paresthetica (entrapment of the lateral femoral nerve at the anterior hip) are common in patients with diabetes. The later causes pain and numbness in the anterolateral proximal lower limb. Obesity further increases the risk of this phenomenon, as it does the risk for diabetes. Femoral neuropathy, distinguished from lateral femoral cutaneous nerve, tends to occur as part of diabetic lumbosacral radiculoplexopathy (Mendell et al., 2001). Diabetic truncal neuropathy can be very painful and may present as symptoms of a myocardial infarction, an ironic assertion, due to the proclivity of patients with diabetes to suffer from painless infarction of heart muscle. Diabetic amyotrophy (Brun-Garland syndrome) is a distinctly proximal lower limb phenomenon in which electrodiagnostic studies tend to reveal concurrent large fiber polyneuropathy. Fibrillations in proximal and distal lower limb muscles are seen. Cranial neuropathies are also seen in diabetes mellitus. Oculomotor neuropathy, which can be painful, is diagnosed on clinical grounds. In this so-called diabetic third nerve, it is key to differentiate between a vaso nervorum stroke and a compressive third nerve aneurysm. Painful hemorrhagic muscle infarction can also be seen in diabetes mellitus. MRI assessment supports the characterization of this entity as a primary infarct, associated with secondary hemorrhage (Sharma et al., 2000). Literature also suggests as association with immune defects (Ali et al., 2003).

LYME DISEASE

Neurological abnormalities in Lyme disease result from the direct effect of *Borrelia burgdorferi* as well as from the effect of the host's immune response. Lyme vasculitis has been implicated in painful peripheral Lyme neuropathy. Electrodiagnostic tests suggest peripheral nerve demyelination in Lyme neuropathy. An autoimmune etiology is implicated. Subarachnoid inflammation is implicated in both spinal radiculitis and cranial neuritis (e.g., trigeminal neuralgia) caused by Lyme disease. In Lyme radiculopathy, EMG usually reveals axonal involvement in both nerves and nerve roots, in a pattern reminiscent of AIDP. Peripheral nerve findings include slowing of conduction velocity and prolongation of distal latency. Sensory and motor nerve potentials may be reduced in amplitude. F-waves are prolonged in as many as 50% of patients. Lyme radiculoneuritis tends to improve spontaneously within a few months of onset. Painful muscle disease due to Lyme disease is associated with stiffness, cramps, swelling, and myalgias. The symptoms begin between 1 to 6 months after tick bite. Significant weakness is rare. EMG findings in Lyme myositis include short-duration, low-amplitude polyphasic potentials (myopathic potentials), positive sharp waves, and fibrillation potentials. Early manifestations of neurological Lyme disease also include syringomelia, cauda equine syndrome, mononeuropathy multiplex, isolated painful radiculitis, and ulnar nerve entrapment. Late neurological sequelae of Lyme disease include "late" polyneuropathy, CTS, and radiculopathy (Coyle, 1993). Radiculoplexitis and focal nodular myositis round out an array of painful late onset neurological syndromes of Lyme disease (Coyle, 1993).

COMPLEX REGIONAL PAIN SYNDROME

Complex regional pain syndrome (CRPS) is an extraordinarily painful condition, which varies in its presentation, etiology, and progression. Definitive pathophysiology and nosology of CRPS are yet to be accepted by the scientific community. EMG may rule out CRPS by virtue of diagnosing an ulterior entity, such as an occult plexopathy. QSART can help verify an autonomic component, although is not specific for the sympathetic nervous system. SEP can confirm a preganglionic radiculopathy that mimics CRPS. CRPS is discussed in greater detail elsewhere in this text.

CONCLUSION

The information contained within this chapter addresses merely the tip of the iceberg. Electrodiagnostic studies augment the clinical analysis by reflecting neuronal function while concurrently providing information regarding anatomical localization. A well-crafted, well-performed study is invaluable. Although these studies confirm and characterize the clinical hypothesis, they may also divulge important prognostic information. The reader should have obtained a framework for understanding the basic electrophysiological underpinnings of electrodiagnostic tests, particularly those crafted for patients in pain. A grasp of the major clinical entities that cause pain is key to choosing the appropriate electrodiagnostic study or studies to provide a differential diagnosis and localize pathology. Ultimately, the reader should develop a flavor for the utilization pattern for these tests.

REFERENCES

Afra, J., Cecchini, A. P., De Pasqua, V., Albert A., & Schoenen J. (1998). Visual evoked potentials during long periods of pattern-reversal stimulation in migraine. *Brain, 121,* 233–241.

Albers, D. J., Robertson, W., & Daube, J. (1978). Electrodiagnostic findings in acute porphyric neuropathy. *Muscle & Nerve, 1*(4), 292–296.

Ali, A., Conti, M., Massucco, P., & Trovati, M. (2003). Diabetic muscle infarction associated with multiple autoimmune disorders, IgA deficiency and a catastrophically poor glycaemic control: A case report. *Diabetes Nutrition & Metabolism, 16*(2), 134–137.

Aminoff, M. J., & Goodin, D. S. (1988). Dermatomal somatosensory evoked potentials in lumbosacral root compression. *Journal of Neurology, Neurosurgery, and Psychiatry, 51,* 740–741.

Aminoff, M. J., Goodin, D. S., Barbaro, N. M., Weinstein, P. R., & Rosenblum, M. L. (1985a). Dermatomal somatosensory evoked potentials in unilateral lumbosacral radiculopathy. *Annals of Neurology, 17,* 171–176.

Aminoff, M. J., Goodin, D. S., Parry, G. J., Barbaro, N. M., Weinstein, P. R., & Rosenblum M. L. (1985b). Electrophysiological evaluation of lumbosacral radiculopathies: Electromyography, late responses, and somatosensory evoked potentials. *Neurology, 35,* 1514–1518.

Andriola, M., & Epstein, C. (1983). *Introduction to EEG and evoked potentials.* Philadelphia, PA: J. B. Lippincott Company.

Aziz, Q., Furlong, P. L., Barlow, J., Hobson, A., Alani, S., Bancewicz, J. et al. (1995). Topographic mapping of cortical potentials evoked by distension of the human proximal and distal esophagus. *Electroencephalography and Clinical Neurophysiology, 96(3),* 219–228.

Barker, A. T., Freeston, I. L., & Jalinous, R. (1985). Noninvasive magnetic stimulation of human motor cortex. *Lancet, 2,* 1106–1107.

Benini, A. (1992). Clinical aspects, pathophysiology and surgical treatment of lumbar spinal stenosis. *Schweizerische Rundschau fur Medizin Praxis* (Switzerland), *81*(13), 395–404.

Bockowski, L., Spbaniec, W., Smigielska-Kuzia, J., Kulak, W., & Solowiej, E. (2003). The pattern-reversal visual evoked potentials in children with migraine with aura and without aura. *Roczniki Akademii Medycznej in Juliana Marchlewskiego w Bialmstoku, 48,* 154–157.

Brazis, P., Masdeau, J., & Biller, J. (1996). *Localization in neurology* (3rd ed.). New York, NY: Little, Brown, & Company.

Bromberg, M. (1993). Electromyographic (EMG) findings in denervation. *Critical Reviews in Physical and Rehabilitation Medicine, 5(1),* 83–127.

Brown, M. D. (1983). *Intraoperative somatosensory evoked potentials in compressive lumbar root lesions.* Presented at the International Society for the Study of the Lumbar Spine, Cambridge, England.

Brudon, J. R., Brudon, F., Bady, B., & Descotes, J. (1989). Value of somatosensory evoked potentials in thoraco-brachial outlet syndrome. *Journal des Maladies Vasculaires, 14*(4), 303–306.

Bryer, M. A., & Chad, D. A. (1999). Sensory neuronopathies. *Massachusetts Neurologist, 5*(2), 90–100.

Casey, K. L., Baydoun, A., Boivie, J., Sjolund, B., Holmgren, H., Leijon, G., & Morrow, T. J. (1996). Laser-evoked cerebral potentials and sensory function in patients with central pain. *Pain, 64*(3), 485–491.

Cassisi, J. E., Levin, J. B., et al. (2000). The incremental validity of lumbar surface EMG, behavioral observation, and a symptom checklist in the assessment of patients with chronic low-back pain. *Applied Psychophysiological Biofeedback, 25*(2), 67–78.

Chance, P. F., & Lupski, J. R. (1994). Inherited neuropathies: Charcot-Marie-Tooth disease and related disorders. *Baillieres Clinical Neurology* (England), *3*(2), 373–85.

Chang, P. F., Arendt-Nielsen, L., Graven-Nielsen, T., Svensson, P., & Chen, A. C. (2004). Comparative EEG activation to skin pain and muscle pain induced by capsaicin injection. *International Journal of Psychophysiology, 51*(2), 117–126.

Chiappa, K. H. (1983). *Evoked potentials in clinical medicine.* New York: Raven Press.

Chiappa, K. H. (1997). Short latency somatosensory evoked potentials: Interpretation. In K. H. Chiappa (Ed.), *Evoked potentials in clinical medicine* (3rd ed., pp. 341–400). Philadelphia, PA: Lippincott-Raven.

Cohen, B. A., Major, M. R., & Huizenga, B. A. (1991). Predictability of adequacy of spinal root decompression using evoked potentials. *Spine, 16*(8), S379–S384.

Cordato, D. J., Yiannikas, C., Stroud, J., Halpern, J. P., Schwartz, R. S., Akbunar, M., & Cook, M. (2004). Evoked potentials elicited by the stimulation of the lateral and anterior femoral cutaneous nerves in meralgia paresthetica. *Muscle & Nerve, 29*(1), 139–142.

Coyle, P. K. (1993). *Lyme disease* (pp. 101–112). St. Louis, MO: Mosby.

Date, E. S., Rappaport, M., & Ortega, H. R. (1991). Dermatomal somatosensory evoked potentials in brachial plexus injuries. *Clinical Electroencephalography, 22*(4), 236–249.

Daube, J. (1996). *Clinical neurophysiology.* Philadelphia, PA: F.A. Davis.

David, W. S., Peine, C., Schlesinger, P., & Smith, S. A. (1996). Nonsystemic vasculitic mononeuropathy multiplex, cryoglobulinemia, and hepatitis C. *Muscle & Nerve, 19*(12), 1596–1602.

Dawson, G. D. (1947). Cerebral responses to electrical stimulation of peripheral nerve in man. *Journal of Neurology, Neurosurgery, and Psychiatry, 10,* 134–140.

Dawson, G. D. (1954). A summation technique for the detection of small evoked potentials. *Electroencephalography and Clinical Neurophysiology, 6,* 65–84.

Dellon, A. L., Mackinnon, S. E., & Seiler, W. A. (1988). Susceptibility of the diabetic nerve to chronic compression. *Annals of Plastic Surgery, 20*(2), 117–119.

Denny-Brown, D., & Pennymaker, J. F. (1938). Fibrillation and fasciculation in voluntary muscle. *Brain, 61,* 311.

Donohoe, C. (1988). *Clinical atlas of auditory evoked potential.* New York: Grune & Stratton.

Drake, M. E., Pakalnis, A., Hietter, S. A., & Padamadan, H. (1990). Visual and auditory evoked potentials in migraine. *Electromyography and Clinical Neurophysiology, 30(2),* 77–81.

Dumitru, D. (1991a). Volume conduction & instrumentation. *Video CME Seminar.* University of Texas Health Science Center at San Antonio, TX.

Dumitru, D. (1991b). Instrumentation in clinical electrophysiology & volume conduction. *Video CME Seminar.* University of Texas Health Science Center at San Antonio, TX.

Dumitru, D., Kalantri, A., & Dierschke, B. (1991). Somatosensory evoked potentials of the medial and lateral plantar and calcaneal nerves. *Muscle & Nerve, 14*(7), 665–671.

Dvonch, V., Scarff, T., Bunch, W. H., Smith, D., Boscardin, J., Lebarge, H., & Ibrahim, K. (1984). Dermatomal somatosensory evoked potentials: Their use in lumbar radiculopathy. *Spine, 9*(3), 291–293.

Dyck, P. J., & Lambert, E. H. (1968). Lower motor and primary sensory neuron diseases with peroneal muscular atrophy. I & II. Neurologic, genetic, and electrophysiologic findings in various neuronal degenerations. *Archives of Neurology, 18*(6), 603–618, 619–625.

Eisen, A. A. (1982). The somatosensory evoked potential. *Canadian Journal of Neurological Sciences, 9*(2), 65–77.

Eisen A., Hoirch M., & Moll, A. (1983). Evaluation of radiculopathies by segmental stimulation and somatosensory evoked potentials. *Canadian Journal of Neurological Sciences, 10,* 178–182.

Ferrante, R., & Wilbourn, A. (2002). *Brachial plexus assessment.* Presented at the American Academy of Neurology 52nd Annual Meeting, San Diego, CA.

Fitzpatrick, T., Johnson, R., Polano, R., Suurmond, D., & Wolff, K. (1992). *Color atlas and synopsis of clinical dermatology: Common and serious diseases* (2nd ed.). New York: McGraw-Hill.

Ford, C. S., Caldwell, S. H., & Kilgo, G. R. (1984). Acute alcoholic myopathy. *American Family Physician, 29*(5), 249–252.

Fujii, M., Toleikis, J. R., Logemann, J. A., & Larson, C. R. (1994). Glossopharyngeal evoked potentials in normal subjects following mechanical stimulation of the anterior faucial pillar. *Electromyography and Clinical Neurophysiology, 92*(3), 183–195.

Gemignani, F., Melli, G., Alfieri, S., Inglese, C., & Marbini, A. J. (2004). Sensory manifestations in Charcot-Marie-Tooth disease. *Peripheral Nervous System, 9*(1), 7–14.

Glick, D. M. (1992). *The use of a new somatosensory evoked potential protocol in the diagnosis of carpal tunnel syndrome.* Presented at the Foundation for Chiropractic Education and Research International Conference on Spinal Manipulation, Chicago, IL.

Glick, D. M. (2001). *Somatosensory evoked potential for the diagnosis of low back pain.* Presented at the American Academy of Pain Management Clinical Meeting, Arlington, VA.

Golla, F., & Winter, A. (1959). Analysis of cerebral responses to flicker in patients complaining of episodic headache. *Electromyography and Clinical Neurophysiology, 11,* 539–549.

Gutmann, L. (1991). AAEM Minimonograph #37: Facial & limb myokymia. *Muscle & Nerve, 14*(11), 1043–1049.

Haig, A. J., Levine, J. W., Ruan, C., & Yamakawa, K. (2001). Describing paraspinal EMG findings: Inadequacy of the single 0-4+ score. *American Journal of Physical Medicine and Rehabilitation, 80*(5), 400–401.

Haldeman, S., Bradley, W. E., Bhatia, N. N., & Johnson, B. K. (1982). Pudendal evoked responses. *Archives of Neurology, 39,* 280–282.

Hendler, N. (2002). Differential diagnosis of complex regional pain syndrome, Type I (RSD). *Pan Arab Journal of Neurosurgery, 6*(2), 1–9.

Herbison, G. (1991). Volume conduction. *Video CME Seminar.* University of Texas Health Science Center at San Antonio, TX.

Herbison, G. (1996). Uselessness of proximal conduction; electrodiagnostic medicine: Pitfalls and analysis. *Syllabus of the American Academy of Electrodiagnostic Medicine 19th Annual Meeting*, Minneapolis, MN.

Herron, L. D., Trippi, A. C., & Gonyeau, M. (1987). Intraoperative use of dermatomal somatosensory evoked potentials in lumbar stenosis surgery. *Spine, 12*(4), 379–383.

Hess, C. W., Mills, K. R., & Murray, N. M. F. (1987). Responses in small hand muscles from magnetic stimulation of the human brain. *Journal of Physiology, 388,* 397–420.

Hong, C. Z., Lee, S., & Lum, P. (1986). Cervical radiculopathy. Clinical, radiographic and EMG findings. *Orthopedic Review, 15*(7), 433–439.

Hood, L. J., Berlin, C. I. (1986). *Auditory evoked potentials, pro-ed studies in communicative disorders.* Austin, TX: Pro-Ed.

Ivanichev, G. A., Khasanova, R. B., & Aleeva, L. L. (1982). Role of the muscle factor in the pathogenesis of painful forms of syringomyelia. *Zhurnal Nevropatologii I Psikhiatrii imemo S S Korsakova, 82*(4), 49–52.

Jacobs, J., Goadsby, P., & Duncan, J. (1996). Use of sumatriptan in postictal migraine headache. *Neurology, 47,* 1104.

Jannetta, P. (1980). Neurovascular compression in cranial nerve and systemic disease. *Annals of Surgery, 192*(4), 518–525.

Jaradeh, S., & Prieto, T. (2003). Evaluation of the autonomic nervous system. *Physical Medicine and Rehabilitation Clinics of North America, 14,* 287–292.

Johnson, E., & Pease, W. (1997). *Practical Electromyography* (3rd ed.). Baltimore, MD: Lippincott, Williams, & Wilkins.

Kakigi, R., Shibasaki, H., Ikeda, T., Neshige, R., Endo, C., & Kuroda, Y. (1992). Pain related somatosensory evoked potentials following CO2 laser stimulation in peripheral neuropathies. *Acta Neurologica Scandinavica, 85*(5), 347–352.

Kakigi, R., Watanabe, S., & Yamasaki, H. (2000). Pain-related somatosensory evoked potentials. *Journal of Clinical Neurophysiology. 17*(3), 295–308.

Kandel, E., Schwartz, J., & Jessell, T. (2000). *Principles of Neural Science* (4th ed.). New York: McGraw-Hill Professional Publishing.

Katifi, H. A., & Sedgwick E. M. (1987). Evaluation of the dermatomal somatosensory evoked potential in the diagnosis of lumbosacral root compression. *Journal of Neurology, Neurosurgery, and Psychiatry, 50,* 1204–1210.

Katirji, B. (1998). *Electromyography in clinical practice.* Philadelphia, PA: Mosby.

Katirji, B., & Wilbourn, A. J. (1988). Common peroneal mononeuropathy: A clinical and electrophysiologic study of 116 lesions. *Neurology, 38(11),* 1723–1728.

Katirji, B., & Wilbourn, A. J. (1994). High sciatic lesion mimicking peroneal neuropathy at the fibular head. *Journal of the Neurological Sciences* (Netherlands), *121*(2), 172–175.

Kaufman, M. A. (1996). Differential diagnosis and pitfalls in electrodiagnostic studies and special tests for diagnosing compressive neuropathies. *Orthopedic Clinics of North America, 27*(2), 245–252.

Kawasaki, M., Saito, T., & Ogawa, R. (1995). Somatosensory evoked potentials for the diagnosis of carpal tunnel syndrome. *Nippon Seikeigeka Gakkai Zasshi, 69*(10), 891–898.

Keirs, L., Cros, D., Chiappa, K. H., & Fang, J. (1993). Variability of motor potentials evoked by transcranial magnetic stimulation. *Electromyography and Clinical Neurophysiology, 89,* 415–423.

Kimura, J. (2001). *Electrodiagnosis in diseases of nerve & muscle: Principles & practice* (3rd ed.). New York: Oxford University Press.

Kochar, K., Sirvastava, T., Maurya, R. K., Jain, R., & Aggarwal, P. (2002). Visual evoked potentials & brainstem auditory evoked potentials in acute attack and after attack of migraine. *Electromyography and Clinical Neurophysiology, 42*(3), 175–179.

Kraft, G. H. (2003). Dermatomal somatosensory-evoked potentials in the evaluation of lumbosacral spinal stenosis. *Physical Medicine and Rehabilitation Clinics of North America* [Review], *14*(1), 71–75.

Kress, W., Mueller-Myhsok, B., Ricker, K., et al. (2000). Proof of genetic heterogeneity in the proximal myotonic myopathy syndrome (PROMM) and its relationship to myotonic dystrophy type 2 (DM2). *Neuromuscular Disorders, 10*(7), 478–480.

Kucera, P., Balaz, M., Varsik, P., & Kurca, E. (2002). Pathogenesis of alcoholic neuropathy. *Bratislavske Lekarske Listy* (Slovakia)*, 103*(1), 26–29.

La Joie, W. J., & Melvin, J. L. (1983). Somatosensory evoked potentials elicited from individual cervical dermatomes represented by different fingers. *Electromyography and Clinical Neurophysiology, 23,* 403–411.

Lefaucheur, J. P., Brusa, A., Creange, A., Drouot, X., & Jarry, G. (2002). Clinical application of laser evoked potentials using the Nd:YAG laser. *Neurophysiologie Clinique, 32*(2), 91–98.

Liguori, R., Taher, G., & Trojaborg, W. (1991). Somatosensory evoked potentials from cervical and lumbosacral dermatomes. *Acta Neurologica Scandinavica, 84,* 161–166.

Lipton, R. B., & Ottoman, R. (1996). Is the comorbidity of epilepsy and migraine due to shared genetic susceptibility? *Neurology, 47,* 918–924.

Lipton, R. E., Chaudhry, F., & Andriola, M. (1998). Clinical assessment of patients with periodic lateralized epileptiform discharges on electroencephalography. *Epilepsia, 39*(6), S110–S111.

Lorenz, J., Grasedyck, K., & Bromm, B. (1996). Middle and long latency somatosensory evoked potentials after painful laser stimulation in patients with fibromyalgia syndrome. *Electromyography and Clinical Neurophysiology, 100*(2), 165–168.

Machida, M., Asai, T., Sato, K., Toriyama, S., & Yamada, T. (1986). New approach for diagnosis in herniated lumbosacral disc. *Spine, 11*(4), 380–384.

Mannion, A. F., Connolly, B., Wood, K., & Dolan P. (1997). The use of surface EMG power spectral analysis in the evaluation of back muscle function. *Journal of Rehabilitation Research and Development. 34* (4), 427–439.

Markland, C., Merrill, D., Chou, S., & Bradley, W. (1972). Sacral nerve root stimulation: A clinical test of detrussor innervation. *Journal of Urology, 107*(5), 772–776.

Masson, E. A., & Boulton, A. J. (1991). The Neurometer: Validation and comparison with conventional tests for diabetic neuropathy. *Diabetic Medicine, 8,* S63–66.

McCallan, J. E., & Bennet, M. H. (1975). Electrophysiologic monitoring of spinal cord function during intraspinal surgery. *Surgical Forum, 26,* 469.

McMenomey, S. O., Glasscock, M. E., 3rd, Minor, L. B., Jackson, C. G., & Strasnick, B. (1994). Facial nerve neuromas presenting as acoustic tumors. *American Journal of Otology, 15*(3), 307–312.

Mendell, J., Kissel, J., Cornblath, D. (2001). *Diagnosis and management of peripheral nerve disorders.* New York: Oxford University Press.

Merton, P. A., Hill, D. K., Morton, H. B., & Marsden, C. D. (1982). Scope of a technique for electrical stimulation of human brain, spinal cord, and muscle. *Lancet, 2*(8298), 597–600.

Nasr, J. T., & Kaufman, M. A. (2001). Electrophysiologic findings in two patients with digital neuropathy of the thumb. *Electromyography and Clinical Neurophysiology, 41*(6), 353–356.

Nederhand, M., Hermens, H., Ijzerman, M., Turk, D., & Zilvold, G. (2003). Chronic neck pain and disability due to acute whiplash injury. *Pain, 102*(1–2), 63–71.

Niedermeyer, E. (1999). EEG in patients with migraine and other forms of headache. In E. Niedermeyer, F. L. DaSilva (Eds.), *Electroencephalography: Basic principles, clinical applications, related fields* (4th ed., pp. 595–602). Baltimore, MD: Lippincott/Williams, & Wilkins.

Norcross-Nechay, K., Matthew, T., Simmons, J. W., & Hadjipavlou, A. (1999). Intraoperative somatosensory evoked potential findings in acute and chronic spinal canal compromise. *Spine, 24*(10), 1029–1033.

Novatschkova-Spassova, S. (1983). [Electromyographic studies of the blink reflex in patients with multiple sclerosis]. *Psychiatrie, Neurologie, und Medizinische Psychologie* (Leipz)*, 35*(2), 79–84.

Oh, Shin. (1993). *Clinical electromyography/nerve conduction studies* (3rd ed.). Baltimore, MD: Williams & Wilkins.

Olney, R., et al. (1999). Guidelines in electrodiagnostic medicine: Consensus criteria for the diagnosis of partial conduction Block. *Muscle & Nerve, 22*(8), S225–229.

Osterman, A. L. (1988). The double crush syndrome. *Orthopedic Clinics of North America, 19*(1), 147–155.

Pape, E., Eldevik, P., & Vandvik, B. (2002). Diagnostic validity of somatosensory evoked potentials in subgroups of patients with sciatica. *European Spine Journal, 11*(1), 38–46.

Pascual-Leone, A., Houser, C. M., Reese, K., Shotland, L. I., Grafman, J., Sato, S. et al. (1993). Safety of rapid-rate transcranial magnetic stimulation in normal volunteers. *Electromyography and Clinical Neurophysiology, 89,* 120–130.

Penfield, W. G., & Boldrey, E. (1937). Somatic motor and sensory representation in the cerebral cortex of man as studied by electrical stimulation. *Brain, 60,* 389–443.

Periquet, M., Mendell, J., & Kissel, J. (1999). Painful sensory neuropathy: Prospective evaluation using skin biopsy. *Neurology, 53,* 1641–1164.

Periquet, M. I., Novak, V., Collins, M. P., Nagaraja, H. N., Erdem, S., Nash, S. M. et al. (1999). Painful sensory neuropathy: Prospective evaluation using skin biopsy. *Neurology, 53*(8), 1641–1647.

Petajan, J. (1991). Motor unit recruitment. *Muscle & Nerve, 14,* 489–502.

Peterson, G. W., & Will, A. D. (1988). Newer electrodiagnostic techniques in peripheral nerve injuries. *Orthopedic Clinics of North America, 19*(1), 13–25.

Pridmore, S., & Oberoi, G. (2000). Transcranial magnetic stimulation: Applications and potential use in chronic pain: Studies in waiting. *Journal of Neurological Sciences, 182*(1), 1–4.

Pullman, S., Goodin, D., Marquinez, A., Tabbal, S., & Rubin, M. (2000). Clinical utility of surface EMG: Report of the Therapeutics and Technology Assessment Subcommittee of the American Academy of Neurology. *American Academy of Neurology Guidelines.*

Quante, M., Lampe, F., Hauck, M., Bromm, B., Hille, E., & Lorenz, J. (2003). Laser-evoked potentials: Diagnostic approach to the dorsal root. *Orthopade, 32*(10), 852–858.

Rodriquez, A. A., Kanis, L., Rodriquez, A. A., & Lane, D. (1987). Somatosensory evoked potentials from dermatomal stimulation as an indicator of L5 and S1 radiculopathy. *Archives of Physical Medicine & Rehabilitation, 68,* 366–368.

Romaniello, A., Cruccu, G., Frisardi, G., Arendt-Nielsen, L., Svensson, P., Iannetti, G. D., & Truini, A. (2003). Assessment of nociceptive trigeminal pathways by laser-evoked potentials and laser silent periods in patients with painful temporomandibular disorders. *Pain, 103*(1–2), 31–39.

Rutkove, S. (2001). AAEM Minimonograph #14: The effects of temperature in neuromuscular electrophysiology. *Muscle & Nerve, 24*(7), 867–882.

Scarff, T. (1981). Dermatomal somatosensory evoked potentials in the diagnosis of lumbar root entrapment. *Surgical Forum, 32,* 489–491.

Searles, R.P., Bankhurst, A. D., Ahlin, T. D., & Messner, R. P. (1977). Antacid-induced hypophosphatemia: An unusual cause of "pseudo-myopathy." *Journal of Rheumatology, 4*(2), 176–178.

Serratrice, G., Pouget, J., & Saint-Jean, J. C. (1986). [Sensory trigeminal neuropathy in systemic diseases: 4 cases with study of the trigeminal reflex.] *Revue Neurologique* (Paris), *142*(5), 535–540.

Seyal, M., Sandhu, L. S., & Mack, Y. P. (1992). Spinal segmental somatosensory evoked potentials in the diagnosis of lumbosacral spinal stenosis: Comparison with imaging studies. *Muscle & Nerve, 15,* 1036–1044.

Sharma, P., Mangwana, S., Kapoor, R. K., & Sara, K. (2000). Diabetic muscle infarction: atypical MR appearance. *Skeletal Radiology, 29*(8), 477–480.

Shy, M.E., Frohman, E. M., So, Y. T., Arezzo, J. C., Cornblath, D. R., Giuliani, M. J. et al. (2003). Quantitative sensory testing: Report of the Therapeutics and Technology Assessment Subcommittee of the American Academy of Neurology. *Neurology, 60*(6), 898–904.

Siao, P., & Cros, D. (2003). Quantitative sensory testing. *Physical Medicine and Rehabilitation Clinics of North America, 14,* 261–286.

Simon, R., Zimmerman, A., Tasman, A., & Hale, M. (1982). Spectral analysis of photic stimulation in migraine. *Electromyography and Clinical Neurophysiology, 53,* 270–276.

Siu, T. L., & Chandran, K. N. (2004). Somatosensory evoked potentials predict neurolysis outcome in meralgia paresthetica. *ANZ Journal of Surgery, 74*(1–2), 27–30.

Slater, K. (1968). Some clinical and EEG findings in migraine. *Brain, 91,* 85–98.

Slimp, J. C., Rubner, D. E., Snowden, M. L., & Stolov, W. C. (1992). Dermatomal somatosensory evoked potentials: Cervical, thoracic, and lumbosacral levels. *Electromyography and Clinical Neurophysiology, 94*(1), 55–70.

Smythe, V., Winter, A. (1964). The EEG in migraine. *Electromyography and Clinical Neurophysiology, 16,* 194–202.

Snowden, M. L., Haselkorn, J. K., Kraft, G. H., Bronstein, A. D., Bigos, S. J., Slimp, J. C. et al. (1992). Dermatomal somatosensory evoked potentials in the diagnosis of lumbosacral spinal stenosis: Comparison with imaging studies. *Muscle & Nerve, 15*(9), 1036–1044.

Soustiel, J. F., Feinsod, M., & Hafner, H. (1991). Short latency trigeminal evoked potentials: Normative data and clinical correlations. *Electromyography and Clinical Neurophysiology, 80*(2), 119–125.

Stohr, M., Riffel, B., & Buettner, U. W. (1981). Diagnostic value of somatosensory evoked potentials (SEP) in lesions of the brachial plexus (author's transl.). *EEG EMG Zeitschrift fur Elektronenzephalogrphie Elektromyographie und Verwandte Gebiete, 12*(4), 195–197.

Sugioka, H. (1984). Evoked potentials in the investigation of traumatic lesions of the peripheral nerve and the brachial plexus. *Clinical Orthopedics, 184,* 85–92.

Sunohara, N., Tomi, H., Nakamura, A., et al. (1996). Myotonia congenita with painful muscle cramps. *Internal Medicine* (Japan), *35*(6), 507–511.

Synek, V. M. (1987a). Short latency somatosensory evoked potentials in patients with painful dysaesthesias in peripheral nerve lesions. *Pain, 29*(1), 49–58.

Synek, V. M. (1987b). Role of somatosensory evoked potentials in the diagnosis of peripheral nerve lesions: Recent advances. *Journal of Clinic Neurophysiology, 4*(1), 55–73.

Talavera-Carbajal, M. R., Estanol-Vidal, B., Lopez-Lomeli, M. M., Garcia-Ramos, G., & Corona, V. (2003). Monitoring dermatomal somatosensory evoked potentials at the ERB point, the cervical spinal cord and the cerebral cortex in the diagnosis of cervical radiculopathy. *Revue Neurologique, 36*(10), 917–924.

Tanaka, A., Takaki, T., & Maruta, Y. (1987). Neurinoma of the trigeminal root presenting as atypical trigeminal neuralgia: diagnostic values of orbicularis oculi reflex and magnetic resonance imaging; a case report. *Neurosurgery, 21*(5), 733–736.

Tergau, F., Naumann, U., Paulus, W., & Steinhoff, B. J. (1999). Low-frequency transcranial magnetic stimulation improves intractable epilepsy. *Lancet, 353*(9171), 2209.

Toleikis, J. R., Carlvin, A. O., Shapiro, D. E., & Schafer, M. F. (1993). The use of dermatomal evoked responses during surgical procedures that use intrapedicular fixation of the lumbosacral spine. *Spine, 18*(16), 2401–2407.

Trainer, S., Durey, A., Chevallier, B., & Liot, F. (1992). Value of somatosensory evoked potentials in saphenous entrapment neuropathy. *Journal of Neurology, Neurosurgery, and Psychiatry, 55*(6), 461–465.

Treede, R. D. (2003). Neurophysiological studies of pain pathways in peripheral and central nervous system disorders. *Journal of Neurology, 250*(10), 1152–1161.

Treede, R. D., Lorenz, J., & Baumgartner, U. (2003). Clinical usefulness of laser-evoked potentials. *Neurophysiologie Clinique, 33*(6), 303–314.

Triggs, W. (1997). The neurophysiology of demyelination. *Electromyography and clinical neurophysiology: Practical approach to physiological assessment of nerve and muscle disease.* Boston, MA: Harvard Medical School Department of Continuing Medical Education.

Upton, A. R., & McComas, A. J. (1973). The double crush in nerve entrapment syndromes. *Lancet, 2*(7825), 359–362.

Varsik, P., Kucera, P., Buranova, D., & Balaz, M. (2001). Is the spinal cord lesion rare in diabetes mellitus? Somatosensory evoked potentials and central conduction time in diabetes mellitus. *Medical Science Monitor, 7*(4), 712–715.

Wagner, W., Peghini-Halbig, L., Maurer, J. C., Huwel, N. M., & Perneczky, A. (1995). Median nerve somatosensory evoked potentials in cervical syringomyelia: correlation of preoperative versus postoperative findings with upper limp clinical somatosensory function. *Neurosurgery, 36*(2), 336–345.

Walker, W., Keyser-Marcus, L., Johns, J., & Seel, R. (2001). Relation of electromyography-induced pain to type of recording electrodes. *Muscle & Nerve, 24*(3), 417–420.

Wilbourn, A. (1986). AAEE Case Report #12: Common peroneal mononeuropathy at the fibular head. *Muscle & Nerve* (United States), *9*(9), 825–836.

Wimalaratna, H. S., Tooley, M. A., Churchill, E., Preece, A. W., & Morgan, H. M. (2002). Quantitative surface EMG in the diagnosis of neuromuscular disorders. *Electromyography and Clinical Neurophysiology, 42*(3), 167–174.

Wyllie, E. (1997). *The treatment of epilepsy: Principles and practice* (2nd ed.). Baltimore, MD: Williams & Wilkins.

Yilmaz, C., Kayahan, I. K., Avci, S., Milcan, A., & Eskandari, M. M. (2003). The reliability of somatosensory evoked potentials in the diagnosis of thoracic outlet syndrome. *Acta Orthopaedic et Traumatologica Turcica, 37*(2), 150–153.

Zileli, B., Ertekin, C., Zileli, M., & Yunten, N. (2002). Diagnostic value of electrical stimulation of lumbosacral roots in lumbar spinal stenosis. *Acta Neurologica Scandinavica, 105*(3), 221–227.

Younger, D. (1999). *Motor disorders*. Philadelphia, PA: Lippincott, Williams, & Wilkins.

——45——

SEMG: Objective Methodology in Muscular Dysfunction Investigation and Rehabilitation

Gabriel E. Sella, MD, MPH, MSc, PhD (HC)

INTRODUCTION

Surface electromyography (SEMG) is a methodology discovered in the 1930s and used more and more in the clinical field since the 1950s. The advent of the computer allowed for an exponential development of its use since the 1980s. John Basmajian and collaborators were major early contributors to the field (Basmajian, 1974). The Association of Applied Psychobiology and Biofeedback (and its predecessor) was the leading research society, which disseminated the research results of the researchers across the past 30 to 40 years in the field of SEMG. The medical field needed further development of the clinical applications of SEMG beyond the original contributions (Fernando & Basmajian, 1978). Development of clinical dynamic protocols and their standardization was an awaited event. The author has contributed to the field since the early 1990s and continues to perform clinical and applied research and dissemination thereof.

THE INVESTIGATIVE ARM OF SEMG

SEMG aims to assess the muscular electric tonus during rest or during activity (Sella, 2000b).

Muscle functions in two modes, the resting and the active modes. During the resting mode, it does not move a joint or body region through any segment of motion. The muscle is actively reenergizing while using action potentials only to maintain the body part against gravity in the resting position and to maintain the "alertness state" tonus required by the sympathetic nervous system at any given moment in time. The energy consumption is generally minimal compared with that needed for any motion.

During the active mode, the muscle works together with the other muscles in its primary myotatic unit and vector to move a joint or a body region in space, with or against gravity. The body musculature as a whole works on a "saving mode" system in which multiple muscles are active at the least level of force or electrical potential effort such that no muscle is particularly prone to fatigue (and, by extension, pain) for a determined action.

THE RESTING TONUS

The muscular tonus at rest comprises the alpha-motor neuron component and the sympathetic system input component. The muscle has to sustain the body part it pertains to against gravity. It must also maintain the turgor of the particular body part, such that the vascular and neural components or visceral components should not be compressed and damaged. In addition, even when the body does not move, such as when supine at rest, all the muscles of the trunk are still participating, even if minimally, in the act of breathing and in the slow movement of the abdominal visceral components.

The electrical potentials used during rest are generally 2 to 3 μV rms, except in the case of the muscles of expression. More likely than not, the sympathetic tone contributes to maintain a more elevated resting potential level (>2 and <6 μV rms). The resting tonus electric potential can be modulated by the individual who has learned basic relaxation techniques. As such, it can be decreased to levels <1 μV rms in any given muscle.

THE ACTIVITY TONUS

The electrical potentials used by an active muscle vary with the intensity of the activity. SEMG measures mainly the amount of effort that any active muscle contributes to the overall motion or motions in space, with or against gravity. The muscles that move a given joint or region work together in a well-orchestrated fashion to promote, modulate, and effectuate the motion in such a way that each one provides the least amount of effort. The activity amplitude level is a number of times the multiple of the action potentials needed to maintain the resting tonus. The ballistic muscles, i.e., the limb muscles, have an *A/R* (activity/rest) ratio >10:1 on the average while the postural muscles have an *A/R* ratio on the average of <5:1 (Sella, 2000a, 2000d). The ratio increases with the amount of energy expended both in the postural and in the ballistic muscles. The resting tonus remains rather constant, provided that the muscle returns to rest for an appropriate amount of time (i.e., >3 seconds). Dysfunctional muscles activity disrupts the natural modulation. If the resting tonus increases while the activity tonus stays rather stationary, the *A/R* ratio will decrease. If both the resting and the activity tonus increase proportionally, the *A/R* ratio may not change.

Pain occurs usually following the advent of muscular fatigue (De Luca, 1985). It also occurs in conditions of muscular spasm and hypertonus or in conditions associated with repeated co-contractions or co-activation (Donaldson et al., 2001a, 2001b). This subject is developed later in this chapter.

The activity tonus is normally an electric potential multiple of the resting tonus. The *A/R* ratio is usually 2 to 3 in the components of the axial skeleton and between 5 and 18 in the components of the appendicular skeleton. This fact corroborates the principle that the axial muscles function mainly as "postural" muscles while the appendicular muscles function mainly as "ballistic" muscles.

Muscles may be hypoactive or hyperactive, according to the level of control imparted by a number of physiological or pathological conditions, as well as the result of dysfunctional learning. This subject will be developed further later in this chapter.

STATIC SEMG PROTOCOLS

A number of protocols have been developed to enable the assessment of axial muscles electric potentials in a given static position against gravity (Sella, 2002b). While the intent was commendable, such protocols suffer, at present, principally from a technical limitation: only a pair of homologous contralateral muscles can be assessed simultaneously. The subsequent pair, usually tested from a cephalad-to-caudad direction, is tested a number of seconds later. Thus, the idea of static testing suffers from the fact that the body may change posture, in a physiological or pathological sense, over time.

Nonetheless, after having considered this limitation, one can test repeatedly the paraspinal musculature and observe if the same electric potential static pattern occurs over time, and one can gather the statistics of the average potentials at each paraspinal level and compare contralateral potentials over a number of trials in a number of ways.

DYNAMIC SEMG PROTOCOLS

A number of dynamic protocols have been written and standardized (Sella, 2002b, 2003b; Sella & Donaldson, 1996; Sella & Finn, 2001). All dynamic protocols involve testing a number of homologous contralateral muscles through a given number of segments of motion, within a well-defined clinical and neuroanatomic context.

According to the standard protocols, muscles may be tested simultaneously bilaterally or in a sequence of one side at rest while the other is moving through well-defined segments of motion in space.

Although the number of potential dynamic protocols is quite large, the following protocols have been written and standardized by the author.

ROM PROTOCOLS

This is a series of protocols following the standard range of motion (ROM) of the joints and regions of the body. The dynamic protocols follow closely the inclinometry derived degrees of motion from a standardized text (Gerhardt & Sella, 2002).

The joints tested with SEMG dynamic protocols are the following:

1. Shoulder (6 to 7 segments of motion)
2. Elbow (4 segments of motion)
3. Wrist (4 segments of motion)
4. Hand/fingers (7 segments of motion)
5. Hip (6 segments of motion)
6. Knee (2 segments of motion)
7. Ankle (4 segments of motion)
8. Foot (4 segments of motion)

The regions tested are the following:

1. Cervical (6 segments of motion)
2. Trunk (6 segments of motion)
3. Pelvis (2 segments of motion)

Each dynamic protocol follows an identical pattern:

1. Screen 1 involves initial rest, pretesting rest in the neutral position for 30 seconds

2. Screen 2-n represents the number of screens following the number of segments of motion. Thus, the elbow SEMG dynamic protocol requires testing through elbow flexion, extension, pronation, and supination. Each screen is performed identically: Starting with the particular activity for 7 seconds of sustained motion and 2 seconds of returning to the original resting position, with 9 seconds of resting in the neutral position following the activity. The sequence of activity and rest is repeated five times or more, if necessary. Thus, any screen of activity and rest will take 90 seconds or longer.

3. Final rest or post-exercise resting of 30 seconds in the neutral position.

Statistics are compiled from the quantitative data accumulated from the test through activity and rest. Those statistics involve gathering data for the average activity (x) (μV rms) of any muscle tested through any segment of motion five times. This will involve calculating the standard deviation (SD) of the average described above, the coefficient of variation (CV) derived from the SD/x ratio, and other statistics, as necessary (Sella, 2001d). Such statistics may involve contralateral comparisons, regression analysis, etc. The most valuable statistic of the resting tonus is that of the minimal resting tonus, derived from the average of the central 3-second period of the 9-second resting interval. The first 3 seconds of the resting period are "biased" by the returning to rest momentum and the last 3 seconds are "biased" by the tendency to start the motion again, i.e., anticipatory movement.

The overall purpose of the ROM dynamic protocols is to identify the muscular response through any given segment of motion. The particular myotatic unit tested or any muscular component of it may respond with "normal" amplitudes of electrical potentials through a given segment of motion and "abnormal" amplitude through other segments of motion. Thus, performing only one segment of motion of a given joint or region may not reflect the true picture of functional or dysfunctional muscular behavior. The performance of several segments of motion allows also for the identification of any degree of dysfunction of any given muscle through the test, as performed bilaterally. Furthermore, it allows for the identification of unilateral dysfunction with the muscles at rest while the contralateral muscles are performing any given segment of motion, i.e., ruling out the presence of co-contractions or co-activation.

The SEMG dynamic protocols allow also for the identification of improvement of amplitude electric potentials at rest or through motion during the period of neuromuscular rehabilitation following the diagnostic testing. Figure 45.1 exemplifies the process of testing with SEMG

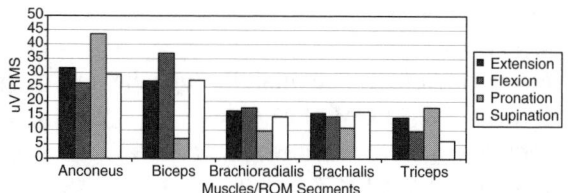

FIGURE 45.1 Average SEMG amplitude potentials of the five muscles tested with SEMG through elbow region ROM segments. From Sella, G. E., 2004. Presentation given at the 8th Annual BFE (Biofeedback Foundation of Europe) Meeting & Workshops. Winterthur, Switzerland. February 24–28. Reprinted with permission.)

through a given joint classic ROM segments of motion (Sella, 2003a).

NEUROMUSCULAR PROTOCOLS

The neuromuscular protocols follow in format the ROM protocols described above in terms of the type of screens and statistics. The aim of these protocols is to rule out any neurological abnormality that may affect a muscle or a muscle group, ranging from central to peripheral neuropathy (Sella, 2003b). The following examples aim to clarify the general protocols.

The musculocutaneous nerve (C5–C6–C7) innervates the following muscles: coracobrachialis, biceps brachii, and brachialis. The first muscle is anatomically located too deep for SEMG testing at the present time. The testing is performed on the biceps and brachialis, in the appropriate segments of motion, i.e., the segment of motion with the highest and lowest activity found from the database for each muscle. If only one muscle is affected, the diagnosis will lead to mononeuropathy, whereas if both muscles are affected, the diagnosis will lead to musculocutaneous neuropathy as a whole. Because the nerve has a three-root innervation, one may need to proceed with differential diagnosis of radiculopathy. In this case, the deltoid muscle may be tested for C5 radiculopathy, the brachioradialis may be tested to rule out C6 radiculopathy, and the triceps may be tested to rule out C7 radiculopathy. In each case, testing for each muscle needs to be done in the clinically chosen segments of motion, most often those found in the database to produce the highest and lowest amplitude potentials. Thus, neuromuscular testing can serve to rule out mononeuropathy or radiculopathy with no invasiveness, in an effective and efficient manner, with quantitative analysis. The procedure can be quite useful in the overall diagnostic process, as well as in the process of neuromuscular rehabilitation.

The neuromuscular protocols follow the anatomic outline of 29 nerves and include also the differential diagnosis for all the roots. The only limitation is the ability to test muscles that are too deeply located anatomically for the SEMG testing at the present time. SEMG neuro-

TABLE 45.1

Electrical Activity Potentials through the Primary Joint ROM of Muscles Innervated by the *Suprascapular Nerve* (µV rms), C5–C6–C7

Shoulder ROM	Supraspinatus	Infraspinatus
Abduction	25.2	26.4
Anterior flexion	15.8	27.8
Lateral flexion	29.6	22.1
Posterior flexion	17.8	23.9
External rotation	24.3	26.8
Internal rotation	18.7	16.4
Total activity	131.4	143.4

Note: Based on Gerhardt & Sella, 2002; Sella, 2003a.

TABLE 45.2

Electrical Activity Potentials through the Shoulder Joint ROM of Muscles Innervated by the *Axillary Nerve* (µV rms), Representative of Root C5

Ranking	Anterior Deltoid		Middle Deltoid		Posterior Deltoid		Teres Minor	
Highest	Abduction	54.1	Lat. flex.	61.2	Post. flex.	38	Ext. rot.	10
Lowest	Post. flex.	20.5	Post. flex.	17.7	Ant. flex.	12.2	Int. rot.	6.2

Note: From *Surface Electromyography: A Neurological Clinical Approach*, by G. E. Sella, 2003. Martins Ferry, OH: GENMED Publishing. Reprinted with permission.

muscular testing allows for the finding of pathological signs such as fasciculations. Thus, the testing can help to distinguish central from peripheral or mixed neuropathy without invasiveness (Sella, 2003b). Table 45.1 shows the process of differential diagnosis used with SEMG neuromuscular protocols.

The examiner can use the knowledge from the database and Table 45.2 through Table 45.4 to assess the normalcy of the electric potentials amplitude through the segments of motion representative of the expected highest and lowest activity for each muscle described. In general, the confidence interval (CI) of 95% is within 20% of the averages of µV rms cited above. Therefore, results, which would be above those values, would be indicative of loss of strength, more commonly resulting from peripheral neuropathy, including radiculopathy. The testing needs to be done bilaterally following the general outline described in the dynamic SEMG joint ROM protocols section. Because most neuropathy is unilateral, that should provide a good frame of reference in the sense that the expectation would be that the asymptomatic side values would fall within the reference values frame of reference. Thus, SEMG is an objective electrophysiological modality that can be applied in a noninvasive fashion in the differential diagnosis needed for neurologic workup.

MYOFASCIAL PROTOCOLS

Myofascial pain syndrome (MPS) is a common clinical occurrence in the muscular pain field (Sella & Finn, 2001). The authors have devised at least 75 SEMG dynamic protocols to be used in the diagnostic and rehabilitation process of the MPS. The SEMG dynamic testing or biofeedback can be used simultaneously with physical testing or myofascial trigger points massage treatment or trigger point injections.

The testing procedure is similar to that described for the ROM testing. In terms of the diagnostic findings and the rehabilitation process, the ranking sequence of amplitude potentials through the classic or functional ROM is of relevance in MPS or other such conditions (e.g., fibromyalgia). This involves comparing the patient's results with those in the database. Figure 45.2 exemplifies this point. As Figure 45.2 indicates, there is a "ranking" of all

TABLE 45.3

Electrical Activity Potentials through the Elbow Joint ROM of Muscles Innervated by the *Musculocutaneous Nerve* (µV rms), Representative of Root C6

Ranking	Biceps Brachii		Brachialis	
Highest	Ext.	27.6	Ext.	16.4
Lowest	Flex.	4.8	Supin.	10.9

Note: From Sella, G. E., 2003. *Surface Electromyography: A Neurological Clinical Approach*, Martins Ferry, OH: GENMED Publishing. Reprinted with permission.

TABLE 45.4

Electrical Activity Potentials through the Elbow Joint ROM of Muscles Innervated by the *Radial Nerve* (µV rms), Representative of Root C7

Ranking	Extensor Carpi Radialis		Brachioradialis		Triceps		Anconeus	
Highest	Ext.	11.7	Flex.	18	Pron.	17.9	Pron.	43.6
Lowest	Flex.	8.8	Pron.	9.7	Supin.	6.3	Flex.	26.3

Note: From Sella, G. E., 2003. *Surface Electromyography: A Neurological Clinical Approach*, Martins Ferry, OH: GENMED Publishing. Reprinted with permission.

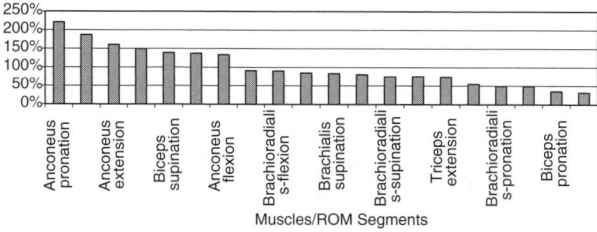

FIGURE 45.2 Normalized activity potentials of the elbow muscles through the elbow region ROM (%). (From Sella, G. E., 2003. *The Journal of Neurological and Orthopaedic Medicine and Surgery*, *21*(3). Reprinted with permission.)

the segments of motion of the muscles tested through the elbow joint ROM. The clinician will note that the highest amplitude of motion (normalized to the average of the group) is that of the anconeus muscle in pronation and the lowest amplitude is that of the triceps in supination. It stands to reason that the rehabilitation sequence of the elbow joint myotatic unit should be performed "from easy to hard," i.e., from motions that require the least amount of energy to those requiring the highest amount of energy. Thus, the clinician will choose the triceps muscle and work with that muscle first in supination to enable the person to regain appropriate proprioception and muscular control of energy expenditure. This will avoid fatigue and unnecessary pain. As the patient progresses through the different muscles/segments of motion from "low to high," the elbow region is more exercised and enabled to proceed with higher and higher energy requirements for motion. By this token, the pronation of the anconeus muscle will be last in the rehabilitation sequence. This is the general situation obtained from the database of 373 muscles tested through the elbow joint ROM (Sella, 2001a).

Any particular patient whose elbow myotatic unit muscles are tested through the elbow joint ROM may show a different ranking pattern of amplitude potentials. The clinician is enabled to compare that pattern with the expected pattern from the database.

FORENSIC PROTOCOLS

SEMG dynamic testing can be used in the field of forensic sciences or legal medicine (Sella & Donaldson, 1996). The testing results can help to rule out objectively a number of features of muscular behavior of relevance in the forensic field (Sella, 1997a, 2001c, 2002d). The principle of internal consistency of muscular behavior through given joint classic segments of motion can help rule out symptom magnification, functional overlay, or malingering (Sella, 2000c) The author uses protocols of bilateral simultaneous testing of four homologous contralateral muscles through the classic joint/region ROM. In the forensic arena, one may have to add any number of functional motions relevant to the target case. It is expected

that if a person performs the testing consistently, i.e., without a secondary agenda to show "pain" or any other symptom, the coefficient of variation for any given segment of motion of the eight muscles tested should be ≤10% (CV ≤ 0.10).

The literature shows that this is the case in >93% of the tests done on more than 2,800 muscles (Sella, 2000a). Furthermore, it may be expected that if one muscle is dysfunctional, it will be the only muscle that may show a CV > 10% through any given motion or at rest. The author has shown that persons who intend consciously or unconsciously to magnify their symptoms will show aberrant types of muscle motions and electrical potentials thereof with high coefficients of variation.

The presence of a number of asymptomatic muscles acting in an aberrant fashion through any given segment of motion is indicative of functional overlay or symptom magnification (Figure 45.3). In the case of malingering, by definition, the claimant should not have any muscular symptom or sign because there was no involvement in any actual injury. The pattern described above shows that muscular behavior is subject to voluntary control aimed at deceiving the examiner and will show a generalized pattern of CV > 10% for any given muscle and segment of motion.

Forensic testing with SEMG may also be useful to rule out muscle weakness. In general, muscles that suffer from loss of strength show a high-amplitude electrical potential pattern through any given segment of motion (Sella, 2003d). This is the result of the need to recruit a higher number of myofibrils to produce that given motion. Thus, it may be expected that if the right biceps is weak, it may show an amplitude potential at least 20% superior to the expected 36.9 μV rms in elbow flexion (CI < 95%, >95% 29.9 to 43.9 μV rms). If the asymptomatic left biceps of the claimant shows an amplitude potential within 29.9 to 43.9 μV rms, while the right symptomatic muscle shows a value above 43.9 μV rms, the symptom of weakness may be credible. On the other hand, the credibility factor is decreased if the flexion value is within the expected range for asymptomatic biceps in flexion. If there is any question, the credibility may be enhanced if the weakness can be demonstrated on all the classic segments of motion and also on a functional motion such as ball throwing. Thus, SEMG testing and the ability to compare

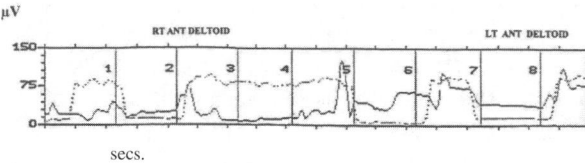

FIGURE 45.3 Symptom magnification: there is no pattern of activity to either muscle through five identical repetitions of motion and rest. Based on Sella, 1997b; Sella, 1999.

amplitude potential values of a given claimant with those of the asymptomatic population can help in the diagnosis process of symptom magnification.

The forensic testing may have to rely also on the presence or absence of a number of electric dysfunctions of symptomatic muscles. Those dysfunctions may involve spasm, hypertonus, loss of mirror image, fasciculations, co-contractions or co-activations, the presence of myokimia, etc. Those electric dysfunctions are defined and discussed later in the chapter.

To summarize, normal findings rule out against the presence of muscular symptoms. Internal inconsistency shown by CV > 10% rules in favor of symptom magnification, functional overlay, or malingering. Findings of weakness rule against unfounded complaints. Findings of abnormal electric potential patterns in the target muscles preclude the performance of adequate statistics and rule in the favor of the plaintiff.

ERGONOMIC PROTOCOLS

Those protocols may follow the outline of the joint/region ROM protocols, the neuromuscular protocols or the myotatic protocols. The performance procedure during the investigation is similar to that described for the SEMG dynamic ROM protocols (Sella, 2002d, 2002e). The ergonomic requirements of motion are usually above and beyond those of the classic ROM segments of motion. The procedure will usually require the performance of the classic joint/region ROM tests to allow the clinician or ergonomist to compare the electric potential amplitude results derived from the client to those from the database (Sella, 2001b, c, d). The overall aim of ergonomic SEMG testing, including athletic utilization is to assess the fitness of any given muscle and myotatic unit to prepare them through SEMG/biofeedback reeducation to give optimal function.

The SEMG meaning of optimal function is that of utilization of the least amount of action potentials for the active myofibrils in the most efficient and effective manner, in unison within the myotatic unit and primary and secondary vectors in order to achieve the best rendition for the longest period of time without fatigue. This can be achieved by training each individual muscle involved and then the entire primary myotatic unit and vectors above to act within the lowest possible amplitude of activity and greatest control and possible effort and strength.

The muscles of a given myotatic unit are assessed at first and then ranked according to a "high to low" ranking fashion. The examiner has to compare the values of any given client to those of the existing database (Sella, 2001a). Then, the muscles are trained from "low to high" at the minimal effort level of activity. Finally, they are trained at the level of activity that is necessary for the objective target work function or athletic endeavor.

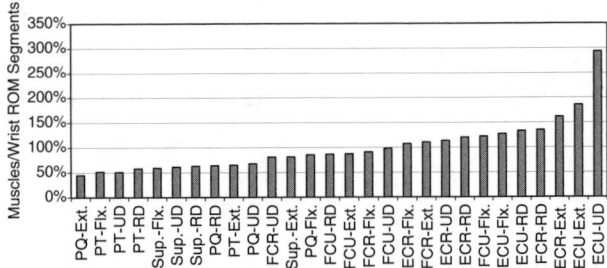

FIGURE 45.4 Wrist joint ROM: sequential activity potential tonus of the muscles and motions tested. The normalization (%) is performed as a ratio of each muscle/motion by the average of the whole group (19.7 μV rms). (From Sella, G. E., 2004. Presentation given at the International Symposium of Cerebral Palsy. Munich, Germany, March 17–20. Reprinted with permission.)

Figure 45.4 and Table 45.5 illustrate the point of ergonomic/athletic SEMG testing and neuromuscular reeducation procedure. The examiner will modify the ranking of the muscular retraining per muscle and motion after training the client to proceed in harmony with the muscle segmental motions at the least amount of effort. The new or modified engram of the participant will help in the ergonomic retraining procedure. Thus, different ergonomic or athletic needs will determine different patterns of muscular utilization either for the classic wrist segmental motions described above or for any functional motions such as needed for the purpose of the training. The final aim is to utilize the least amount of energy to provide the best rendition with the least fatigue. The database allows the ergonomic/athletic trainer to modify different ergonomic protocols within a solid framework, which would avoid fatigue, pain, or injury.

THE THERAPEUTIC ARM OF SEMG/BIOFEEDBACK

The SEMG modality can be used not only for investigative or diagnostic purposes but also for neuromuscular retraining or reeducation (Basmajian, 1981; Schwartz et al., 1995). With the diagnostic framework in mind, the clinician can proceed to establish a rehabilitation program (Sella, 2000b). The first step is to compare the results of any given muscular activity with those of the database. The next step needs to be to establish a program that, in most cases, will involve a plurality of therapeutic methods and SEMG/biofeedback.

The main aim of the addition of the SEMG/biofeedback is to modify and improve the existing neuromotor engram (Donaldson et al., 2001c; Sella, 2002e). It is taken for granted in most cases, except for very small children, that the individual has learned a movement pattern involving a given number of muscles or myotatic units through life. Because of the injury or other causes, this engram

TABLE 45.5
Wrist Joint ROM: Primary Myotatic Unit Muscles and Classic Segments of Motion (μV rms)

Muscle	Wrist joint ROM segments				
	Ulnar Deviation	Extension	Radial Deviation	Flexion	Avg.
Extensor carpi ulnaris	57.9	36.6	26.3	25.1	36.5
Extensor carpi radialis	22.4	31.8	23.7	21.2	24.8
Flexor carpi radialis	15.9	21.8	26.6	17.9	20.6
Flexor carpi ulnaris	19.3	17.2	17.03	24.1	19.4
Supinator	12.02	16	12.4	11.6	13.0
Pronator quadratus	13.3	8.8	12.6	16.8	12.9
Pronator teres	10	12.8	10.7	10.13	10.9
Average	21.5	20.7	18.5	18.1	19.7

Note: From "SEMG/Biofeedback: General Methodology & Utilization in Central Paresis," by G. E. Sella, 2004. Presentation given at the International Symposium of Cerebral Palsy. Munich, Germany, March 17–20. Reprinted with permission.

will have been disrupted or disturbed. Consequently, the pattern of movement of the target myotatic unit has been disrupted and the individual had lost some proprioception and ability to control the muscular movements in the most effective fashion.

SEMG/biofeedback can retrain the proprioceptive ability (Sella, 2004b). Although the nerve endings responsible for proprioception reside uniquely or mainly in the capsular apparatus rather than in muscles, muscular movement or controlled resting helps to reestablish the normal proprioception regarding a joint via new learning involving a complexity of visuocorticomotor or audiocorticomotor pathways. The body–brain–SEMG equipment connection needs to be performed by applying the surface electrodes to the skin overlying the target muscles in the vectorial direction of the muscle action's main vectorial direction. The electrode wires, the SEMG equipment, the computer, and the computer screen serve to connect the muscular message with the brain motor terminals. This is usually accomplished via a visual message found on the computer screen. Occasionally, the message may be of auditory or vibratory origin. The final muscle–SMG equipment message is transmitted to the subject's sensory-cortical (and subcortical) brain terminals and is relayed to the homunculus motorius and, via complex pathways, to the corticospinal motor tracts leading peripherally to the target muscles (Sella, 2000c).

The original engram will be modified or actually partially replaced by the new SEMG/biofeedback learning in time, through a number of clinical sessions. The end result will be a better proprioception involving the particular joint or region as well as an improved level of control of the muscles targeted with the learning for either activity or rest. If the new engram is exercised properly, in time

it will remain as the actual functional engram. If it is not exercised properly and the individual returns to old habits and dysfunctional pathways, it will be of little use.

Research done in the past 40 years has shown that the brain is not a "black box" but a vibrant organ able to undergo neuromodulation (Changeux, 1985). This ability enables the individual with dysfunctional muscular activity from neurologic, traumatic, or other etiology to learn anew to utilize the target muscles in the most effective manner. SEMG/biofeedback and other forms of biofeedback are main tools that can be used in the realm of helping the brain in the act of neuromodulation (Donaldson et al., 2001c). This is done, in terms of SEMG/biofeedback, by involving either the ancient motor pathways not used since early infancy or by involving new neuronal associations, which permit adequate muscular behavior through the new learning pattern (Donaldson et al., 2001a, 2001b, 2001c).

Rehabilitation of the resting tonus, the activity tonus, is the main task of the SEMG/biofeedback neuromuscular reeducation program.

The resting tonus has been assessed for more than 180 muscles. The total number of muscles tested is around 7,000 (Sella, 2000d). As described above, the resting tonus as investigated by the author represents the minimal resting value obtained in the central range of the resting period of 9 seconds between any two repeated movements of any given muscle. Overall, the resting tonus of the untrained muscles ranges between 2 and 3 μV rms. The resting tonus of the muscles of expression is usually higher in untrained persons. It may be reduced to below 2 μV rms in any muscle in trained individuals. The resting tonus depends largely on the input of the α-motor neurons and the sympathetic nervous system (SNS) input. The general outline of the clinical assessment of the magnitude of the SNS component is that it would affect all muscles tested, not only the target, symptomatic muscle. Other factors showing a high sympathetic input of different systems would be ruled out by the demonstration of elevated heart rate, breathing rate, sweat, etc. The α-motor neuron input may be different in the target muscle than in its homologous contralateral, depending on a number of factors. Pain may increase the overall SNS input and the α-motor neuron input. On the other hand, some individuals learn to adapt to pain by reducing the overall muscular tonus.

A normal individual may learn through SEMG/biofeedback to reduce the resting tonus of any given muscle within a matter of minutes and retain the new learning (Sella, 2000b). The lower the resting tonus, the less the energy expenditure required to maintain the target muscle in any given tonic state. It would stand to reason that a higher tonus would be tantamount to a decreased arteriolar and capillary blood and oxygen intake and a decreased appropriate emptying of catabolic substances through the lymphatic and venous channels. The accumulated catabolic products and local edema would be detrimental to the normal metabolism of the muscular tissue (Travell & Simons, 1983). In time, the individual concerned would perceive symptoms, such as pain, muscle sluggishness, and early fatigue. In terms of ergonomic and/or athletic endeavor, it is most appropriate to maintain the muscular tonus at its optimal resting level, usually within 0.5 to 1 μV rms.

In the biofeedback world, there is some confusion between the expression "baseline" and the expression "resting tonus." Baseline is a general, nonspecific expression that has no power of structural definition of the muscle at rest nor of any pathological or functional significance. Resting tonus refers to the dynamic muscular electrical activity of a given muscle that is not moving a joint and is not moved concentrically, eccentrically, or in a rotatory fashion at any given moment of time. The dynamics of the resting tonus depend on the nervous factors above as well as other factors such as temperature and vascular system.

A lot of work has been done in the past in the area of muscle relaxation for a variety of emotional, psychological, or other etiologies (Basmajian, 1981; Schwartz et al., 1995). In general, well-documented therapy has proved successful in relaxing muscles and reducing the resting tonus. A note of caution needs to be added at this point. Some clinicians chose to place electrodes *across* muscles rather than *on* the same muscle. They found that, in time, the amplitude potentials "quieted down" and deduced therefore that the muscles or the region had "globally" relaxed. These hypotheses and conclusions were clinically and electrophysiologically unfounded, as *electromyography* requires specific electrode placements in the main vectorial direction of a particular muscle. They used the volume conduction parameter applicable to SEMG as a

substitute for actual *myographic* properties and derived the wrong conclusions, which are simply not applicable clinically. As an example, electrode placements at 2 cm interelectrode distance on the main vectorial direction of a given muscle, e.g., biceps brachii, may result in an electric potential difference of approximately 2 μV rms while the muscle is at rest, compatible with the definition of the resting tonus. If electrodes are placed one on the right biceps and one on the left biceps (with the ground electrode placed elsewhere), and if the resulting amplitude potential is 2 μV rms, that can only happen if the electric potential difference between the two electrodes across the chest volume and the upper limbs volume is 2 μV rms. In other words, if the voltage potential on the right side is 30 μV rms and on the left it is 28 μV rms, the difference would be 2 μV rms, thus not a value compatible with resting tonus. Yet, those clinicians mistakenly believed that the volumetric conduction difference equated that of relaxed resting potential.

It is important for any clinician to understand that SEMG refers to specific muscular measurement and rehabilitation. Volumetric work is not to be equated or confused with SEMG.

ACTIVITY TONUS

The electric tonus of any given muscle during any given activity is a multiple of that of the resting tonus. Table 45.6 illustrates the average activity/rest ratio for different joints and regions through the classic ROM.

Table 45.6 summarizes important data from many studies. The average value represents the average amplitude potential for the number of motions and the number of muscles tested through the ROM segments for each joint or region. The average resting tonus values represent the average minimal resting values during the resting periods as defined above.

It is easy to notice that the limb joint overall activity and the *A/R* ratio are quite larger than those of the axial regions. The hip joint seems to be an exception, save for the fact that the joint motions were tested in the supine position (except for extension). The testing was done at all times at the minimal effort level of muscular contraction. The actual degrees of motion for any given muscular movement followed the pattern described in the standardized text (Gerhardt & Sella, 2002).

The activity tonus required for any movement that needs more effort than to move the muscle/joint/region against gravity is greater than the activity levels described above or in the database (Sella, 2000d, 2001d). Two things need to be stressed again at this point: (1) if a muscle is weak it will require more active myofibrils, thus resulting on SEMG amplitude potentials that are generally at least 20% higher than the amplitude potentials seen at the upper 95% CI of the general sample tested in the database (Sella,

TABLE 45.6
SEMG Testing of the Activity and Resting Tonus in 11 Joints and Body Regions

Joint/Region	No. of Muscles	No. of Segments of Motion	Overall Avg. Muscle/Seg. (µV rms)	Avg. Min. Resting Tonus (µV rms)	A/R
Head — TMJ and facial expressions	7	6	13.4	2.9	4.6
Neck	4	4	14.6	5	2.9
Trunk	9	4	6.5	2.4	2.8
Shoulder	19	6	19.4	2.3	8.4
Elbow	5	4	19.7	1.6	12.3
Wrist	7	4	19.7	1.7	11.6
Hand	15	7	31.9	1.8	17.7
Hip	8	6	8.5	1.9	4.5
Knee	13	2	11.4	2.2	5.2
Ankle	5	4	14.9	1.0	14.3
Foot	4	4	15.5	1.2	12.9

Note: Adapted from Gerhardt & Sella, 2002; Sella, 2001a, 2000d.

2000d); (2) the amount of conditioning or deconditioning of the tested individual will either decrease the amplitude potential levels of the muscles tested or increase it.

Ergonomic reeducation aims at producing overall activity potentials that are no larger than those found within the upper and lower 95% CI of the asymptomatic persons tested and described in the database. Rehabilitation patients need to be trained to produce activity potentials that reflect the same pattern.

MUSCULAR DYSFUNCTION

MUSCLE SHORTENING

Skeletal muscle gives its best rendition at a length that is at least equal to that of the well-conditioned muscle at rest. All athletes and ballet dancers start with a period of stretching exercises before any given performance. Those exercises actually "warm-up" the viscoelastic elements; improve the arteriolar, capillary, venous, and lymphatic circulation; and prime the muscle fibers for the activity to follow.

Deconditioned muscles, such as related to a number of factors, e.g., joint ROM limitations, lose the optimal length and can actually shorten structurally. Any fascial scar or muscular scar from previous injuries can contribute to the tendency to stretch less and give less of an effort when required to move the joint.

Acute muscular splinting and ensuing protective guarding can promote the muscular shortening. The target engram of the person suffering from such symptoms and signs will undergo changes whereby the muscle tends to use fewer and fewer myofibrils and action potentials. The

joint in question will rely, in time, more and more on other structural elements for motion and the overall effort of motion will decrease accordingly, e.g., in whiplash injuries, a few months after the injury, in untreated cases.

Figure 45.5 shows that the SEMG amplitude potentials of shortened muscles will decrease compared with the expected range found in the database. Simple clinical observation of the individual in motion will note an ongoing fear of motion and tendency toward protective guarding. Shortened muscles fatigue more easily from any level of effort that normal muscles would not. If the muscles are subjected to greater levels of effort, fatigue may be transformed into pain.

Shortening of muscles is a problem that cannot be solved too quickly. A program of exercises aimed at gradual joint/region ROM increase may be given jointly with an SEMG/biofeedback program aimed at increasing the muscular amplitude potentials to reach the range of the asymptomatic muscles described in the database. The process of improvement in the ROM and in the amplitude potentials may take several sessions.

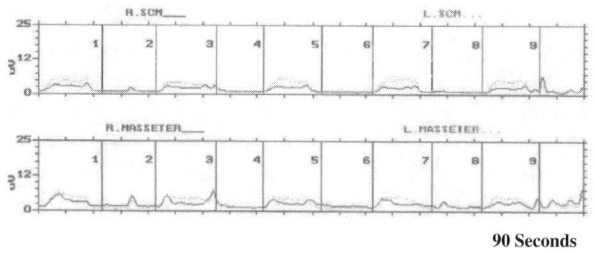

FIGURE 45.5 Muscular shortening: presentation of symptomatic (whiplash) subject.

Loss of Joint ROM

The joint is a complex structure. Whatever etiology may be responsible for joint lost ROM (LROM), muscular, tendinal, capsular, etc., the end result is muscular suffering. The muscle may respond to poor ROM or partial ankylosis with loss of optimal functional strength, deconditioning, early fatigue, or pain. The response is not immediate but can be found very frequently in subacute or chronic joint LROM. The SEMG amplitude is usually higher in a muscle that is subject to joint LROM as compared with its homologous contralateral. This may be expected because the muscular disuse may beget loss of strength (LOS). Such loss of strength may be responsible for the muscle's needing to recruit more contractile elements to effectuate any contraction, concentric or eccentric, of the target joint.

Loss of Strength

This subject has been alluded to in the previous sections. Loss of strength could be defined clinically as a loss of >10% of tensile strength from a given group of muscles compared with the homologous contralaterals. Normally, for example, in the hand grip, there is a difference of ≤6% between the two hands when gripping a Jamar dynamometer. Published studies have shown that the dominant hand is within 6% stronger than the nondominant hand 53% of the time, weaker than the nondominant hand 36% of the time, and equal in strength to the nondominant hand 11% of the time (Gerhardt & Sella, 2002; Sella, 2001a, 2001b, 2002a).

There are no methodologies currently that can rule out loss of strength of one single muscle in a particular group. SEMG is the only methodology that comes close to it. Several studies have shown consistently that a weaker muscle has a higher amplitude potential curve for any given motion performed at the minimal level of effort. This has been theoretically explained by the fact that the weaker the muscle, the higher the recruitment of more myofibrils and the higher the number of action potentials required for the performance of the given activity (Sella, 2000a, 2000b, 2000d). Thus, SEMG can be used in the diagnostic workup to rule out muscular weakness in terms of its characteristic of more elevated amplitude potential curves on the weaker side. By the same token, therapeutic success can be documented with SEMG by showing that the previously weaker muscle performs better in time through the rehabilitation period as it shows a decreasing pattern of amplitude potential curves for given motions and finally the amplitude and pattern fall within the expected range of the database (Sella, 2000b, 2001d).

Muscle Fatigue

Fatigue is a complex phenomenon, partly of physical origin and partly of emotional or even motivational ori-gin. Muscular fatigue has been shown on the SEMG spectral analysis to correspond most closely with the median frequency (Anderson et al., 1978; Arendt-Nielsen & Mills, 1988; Bigland-Ritchie, 1981; Christensen, 1986; De Luca, 1985). The author has noticed empirically that the median frequency curve tends to lower far earlier than the change in amplitude potentials curves in persons complaining of early fatigue. Spectral analysis is the domain of choice at the present time in terms of investigation and also of therapeutic documentation of rehabilitation success.

Muscle Pain

A number of factors can contribute directly or indirectly to muscular pain. The sensation can be primary or secondary such as in referred pain (Travell & Simons, 1983). Pain may be referred from visceral tissue as well such as in anginal pain referred to either upper limb. The sensation is actually perceived in the muscular tissue. Muscular pain may be direct and acute such as in traumatic etiology. It may coincide with splinting of a joint and/or protective guarding of the same joint. It may be of myofascial origin or of diffuse central nervous system origin such as in fibromyalgia. Muscular pain may be the result of vascular, metabolic, endocrine disease, or more rarely, intrinsic muscular diseases.

Because a person would tend to "protect" a muscle or a group of muscles in pain, the descriptions given above under the sections of "Muscular Fatigue," "Loss of Joint ROM," and "Loss of Strength" do apply fully within the present context. In general, a muscle in pain has a decreased pattern in the median frequency amplitude. It is able to contract concentrically or eccentrically in a consistent manner (Sella, 2000d). It may show a higher amplitude potential through a given ROM than its homologous contralateral (Sella, 2000b, 2000d). It may act in a "protective guarding" mode by performing at a lower amplitude of contraction such as the case in whiplash. When the symptom of pain is reduced via different therapeutic means, the amplitude potentials of contraction tend to normalize (Simons & Mense, 2001). Muscular pain may change from the acute state to the chronic state although the characteristics of intensity or frequency may not change. Generally, the person affected with muscular pain feels more comfort at rest than with motion and that tends to create overall deconditioning.

Muscular pain may also be a characteristic of hyperalgesia and allodynia, such as in fibromyalgia or related disorders. SEMG/biofeedback may be a useful modality not only in terms of investigation and ruling out the presence of electrical dysfunctions compatible with pain (see below), but also in terms of engram modification and neuroplasticity during the rehabilitation program.

TABLE 45.7
Laterality: Right and Left Muscle Pair Percentage (%) Differences

Joint/region	N	Normal Rest	Abnormal Rest	Normal Activity	Abnormal Activity	Weighted Normal Rest	Weighted Abnormal Rest	Weighted Normal Activity	Weighted Abnormal Activity
Head	16	24	64	25	35	5	14	6	8
Neck	137	25	39	28	36	48	75	54	69
Trunk	191	20	37	20	24	53	99	53	64
Shoulder	127	30	47	25	46	53	83	44	82
Elbow	23	31	38	33	36	10	12	11	12
Wrist/hand	18	21	103	49	66	6	31	13	19
Hip and knee	33	31	36	28	33	14	17	13	15
Ankle	27	18	38	40	40	7	14	15	15
Total	572	25	50.25	31	39.5	25	43	26	35

Note: From *Surface Electromyography: A Neurological Clinical Approach* (table II, p. 43), by G. E. Sella, 2003. Martins Ferry, OH: GENMED Publishing. Adapted with permission.

TABLE 45.8
Summary: Laterality Percentage (%) Differences for 10 Joints/Regions (572 muscles)

Right and Left % Difference	Normal Rest %	Abnormal Rest %	Normal Activity %	Abnormal Activity %
Min.–max. difference range	7–53	14–99	6–54	8–82
Average difference	25	43	26	35
Median difference	12	24	14	17

Note: From *Surface Electromyography: A Neurological Clinical Approach* (table I, p. 42), by G. E. Sella, 2003. Martins Ferry, OH: GENMED Publishing. Adapted with permission.

MUSCULAR DYSEQUILIBRIUM (LOSS OF NORMAL LATERALITY)

Appropriate posture and gait require equilibrium on both sides of the body. Homologous contralateral muscles function most effectively when they are required to use the least amount of energy for the effort of contraction and when they function in equilibrium, i.e., generally within 25% difference of electric potential activity during motion and rest (Sella, 2000d). This empirical observation applies for the appendicular muscles and for the axial muscles, as well.

Table 45.7 shows that there are striking percentage differences in laterality of amplitude potentials between normal and abnormal values, as compared with the database. The data in the table have been weighed and the results are presented as such. Table 45.8 is a summary of Table 45.7. Of interest is the fact that there are several overlaps in the percentage differences between the normal and abnormal resting and activity amplitude potential values. The median difference and the average differences are quite different between the two groups. At all times, the differences are larger either for the resting tonus or the activity tonus during motion than during rest.

The clinician may interpret the data from Tables 45.7 and 45.8 in terms of assessing myotatic units of the appendicular skeleton or of the axial skeleton.

Table 45.9 shows that the average resting range muscular differences between the right and left side of the body in the normal (asymptomatic) muscles and the abnormal (symptomatic) were generally less, with no overlap between the two groups. The same did not hold true for the similar ranges of the muscles during activity. In general, the differences were less in the asymptomatic groups of the axial and appendicular muscles than in the symptomatic groups. There was significant overlap between the symptomatic/asymptomatic group differences.

SEMG-DEFINED PARAMETERS OF MUSCULAR DYSFUNCTION

SPASM

From a clinical perspective, it is difficult to define the presence of spasm. A very taut muscle or group of muscles could be called "in spasm" during palpation if the person complains of pain at the time of the visit. On the other

TABLE 45.9
Laterality: Right and Left Muscle Pair Percentage (%) Differences in the Appendicular and Axial Skeleton

Joint/region	N	Normal Rest	Abnormal Rest	Normal Activity	Abnormal Activity	Weighted Normal Rest	Weighted Abnormal Rest	Weighted Normal Activity	Weighted Abnormal Activity
Axial skeleton*	344	69	140	73	95	106	188	113	141
Average difference		23	47	24	32	35	63	38	47
Range		20–25	37–64	20–28	24–36	5–53	14–99	6–54	8–69
Appendicular skeleton**	228	131	262	175	221	90	157	96	143
Average difference		26	52	35	44	18	31	19	29
Range		18–31	36–103	25–49	33–66	6–53	12–83	11–44	12–82

* Sum total of the average differences in the head, neck, and trunk muscles tested.

** Sum total of the average differences in the shoulder, elbow, wrist, hand, hip, knee, and ankle muscles tested.

Note: From Sella, G. E., 2003b. *Surface Electromyography: A Neurological Clinical Approach.* Martins Ferry, OH: GENMED Publishing. Reprinted with permission.

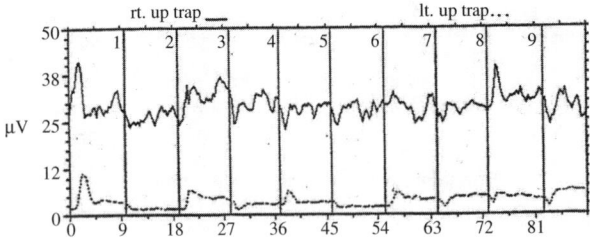

FIGURE 45.6 Spasm.

hand, the same palpation in an individual who has no complaints would not be called "spasm." Therefore, the tautness of a muscle or a group of muscles cannot be defined as "spasm" without further documentary proof.

The complaint of pain alone may not be sufficient, especially in the forensic environment. SEMG is the only electrophysiological modality that can throw light onto this problem (Sella, 2000d). Muscles that are simply taut, without the presence of any symptom, will show a normal resting tonus and an activity tonus. Muscles that are indeed in pain show no visible differences in the amplitude potentials during any ROM activity. Figure 45.6 illustrates this point and the SEMG derived definition of spasm.

Figure 45.6, deriving from a whiplash case, illustrates that the right upper trapezius is in spasm from the SEMG perspective. One can see no tendency to increase or decrease the amplitude potential through the five repetitions of neck flexion. The left upper trapezius (shown at the bottom of the graph) has an overall amplitude that is far less than that of the right side of the same muscle. Its activity is likewise mildly abnormal, but there is a tendency to return to normal resting tonus in the first three repetitions of the motion.

HYPERTONUS

From a clinical perspective, it is difficult to define the presence of hypertonus. Many a clinician will define

loosely a very taut muscle or group of muscles as being "hypertonic." This is a very nonspecific term, as it is dependent on the ability of palpation of the clinician involved. If the person complains of pain at the time of the visit, then the taut muscle or group of muscles could be considered symptomatic and the "proof" of it is the tautness. On the other hand, the same palpation in an individual who has no complaints would not be called "hypertonus."

The complaint of pain alone may not be sufficient to consider the tautness of the muscle or muscle group as dysfunctional or pathologic, especially in the forensic environment. SEMG is the only electrophysiological modality that can throw light onto this problem. Muscles that are simply taut, without the presence of any symptom, will show a normal resting tonus and an activity tonus.

The SEMG-derived definition of hypertonus is that of a muscle that performs activity with an increased amplitude, commonly above that of the database range, while in the same time the resting tonus does not return to real resting values (Sella, 2000d). The tendency is commonly there in terms of the return to rest; however, that does not quite happen.

There are three versions of hypertonus: (1) the resting tonus is elevated but rather constant among the five repetitions of a given segment of motion; (2) the resting tonus tends to increase in amplitude within the space of the 90 seconds and the five repetitions of motion, i.e., "scale-up hypertonus"; and (3) the resting tonus tends to decrease in amplitude within the space of the 90 seconds and the five repetitions of motion, i.e., "scale-down hypertonus." Occasionally, it could be seen that scale-up hypertonus may become spasm and spasm may become scale-down hypertonus. Figure 45.7a illustrates the SEMG-derived definition of hypertonus. This figure illustrates at the same time two versions of hypertonus. The left supraspinatus shows a scale up of the hypertonus. The right and left pectoralis major illustrates the "constant" elevated resting

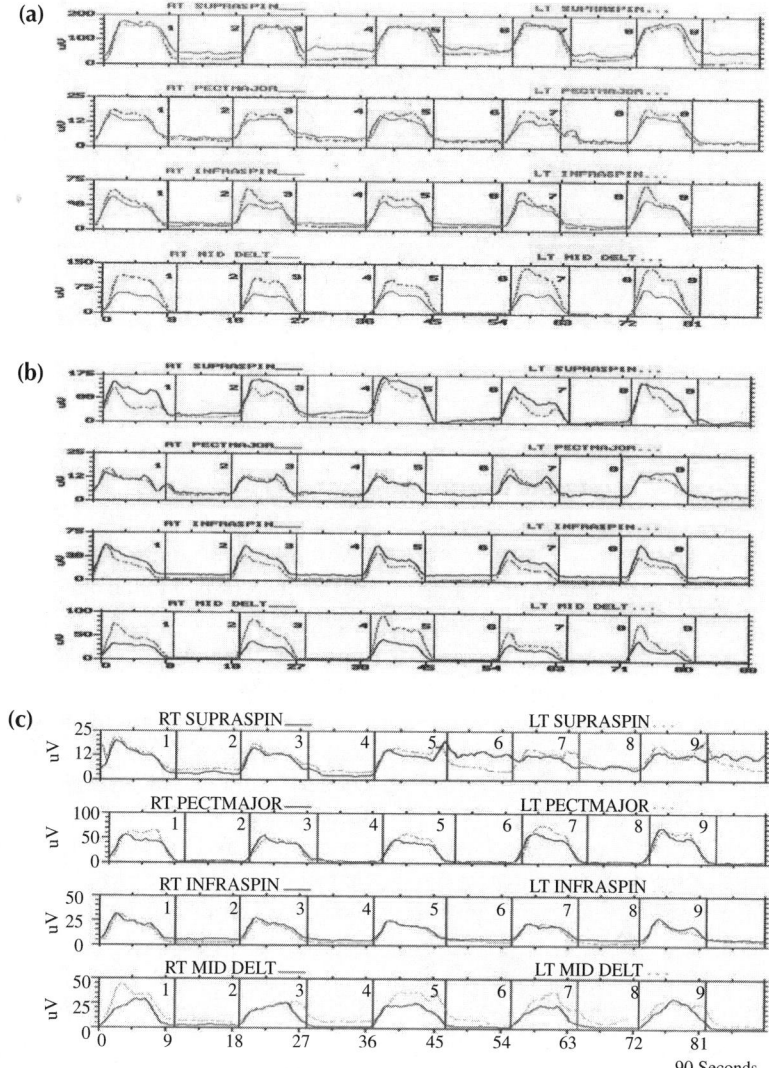

FIGURE 45.7 (a) Hypertonus: constant and scale-up versions; (b) hypertonus: scale-down version; (c) hypertonus and spasm transformation.

tonus through the motions (compare with middle deltoid) on the lower side of the figure. Figure 45.7b illustrates the scale-down version of hypertonus. The right supraspinatus shows a scale down of the hypertonus phenomenon and the five repetitions end with a normal resting tonus.

Hypertonus and spasm are thus phenomena on the same continuum. It is possible that warming up of the muscles through repeated motion improves the symptoms and the muscles tend to act more normally such as in the case of scale-down hypertonus. It is possible that repeated motions irritate the peripheral nerves and/or the muscles, which then act in a more abnormal fashion such as in scale-up hypertonus or spasm. It has been shown that either phenomenon is bound to be more particular in a given segment of motion and may change its aspect in a different segment of motion to follow. Thus, both hypertonus and spasm are functional electric dysfunctions.

Figure 45.7c illustrates the continuum between hypertonus and spasm. One may note on the supraspinatus muscle the change of the resting tonus to that compatible with spasm and then a tendency to normalize via change to hypertonus.

HYPOTONUS

From a clinical perspective, it is difficult to define the presence of hypotonus. Many a clinician will define loosely a "soft feeling" muscle or group of muscles as "hypotonic." This is a very nonspecific term as it is dependent on the ability of palpation of the clinician involved. If the person complains of pain at the time of the visit, then the "soft" muscle or group of muscles could be considered symptomatic and the "proof" of it is the softness. On the other hand, the same palpation in an individual

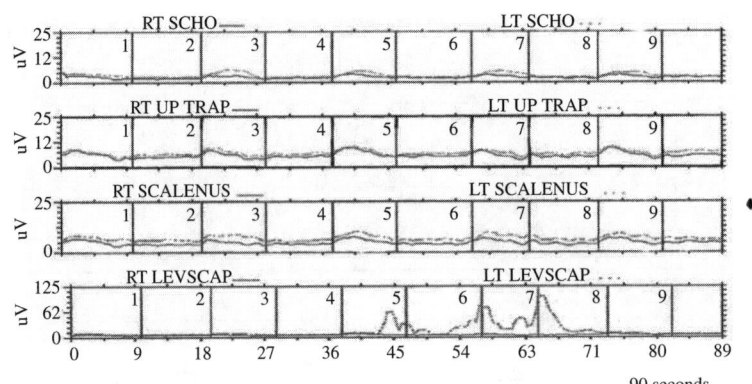

FIGURE 45.8 Fasciculations.

who has no complaints would not be called "hypotonus." At most, the clinician will consider the muscle or group of muscles as "deconditioned."

The complaint of pain alone may not be sufficient to consider the lack of tautness of the muscle or muscle group as dysfunctional or pathologic, especially in the forensic environment. SEMG is the only electrophysiological modality that can throw light on this problem. Muscles that are simply "soft," without the presence of any symptom, will show a normal resting tonus and an activity tonus. The SEMG-derived definition of hypotonus is that of a muscle that performs activity with a decreased amplitude, commonly below that of the database range, while in the same time the resting tonus does not return to real resting values (Sella, 2000d).

The tendency is commonly there in terms of the return to rest; however, that does not quite happen. Just as in the case of hypertonus, there are three versions of hypotonus: (1) the resting tonus is elevated but rather constant among the five repetitions of a given segment of motion; (2) the resting tonus tends to increase in amplitude within the space of the 90 seconds and the five repetitions of motion, i.e., scale-up hypotonus; (3) the resting tonus tends to decrease in amplitude within the space of the 90 seconds and the five repetitions of motion, i.e., scale-down hyportonus. Occasionally, it could be seen that scale-up hypotonus may become spasm and spasm may become scale-down hypotonus. The author has observed empirically the "transformation" of hypotonus into spasm and spasm into hypotonus, but not that of hypotonus into hypertonus, or vice versa.

FASCICULATIONS

Fasciculations are unconscious paroxystic muscular contractions, usually part of lower motor neuron pathology, but occasionally, an asymptomatic normal variant (Dumitru, 1996). Usually, only one muscle in a group shows fasciculations. Occasionally, they can recur with a certain constancy and the twitch may be visible at the surface level if the amplitude is high enough. SEMG can demonstrate fasciculations with no interference with the neuromotor plate, such as may be the case with needle EMG testing. The fasciculations seen on SEMG may be recorded according to the clinical need of the investigator. Figure 45.8 illustrates repeated fasciculations of the left levator scapulae. Fasciculations may be found more commonly in conditions of muscular irritation and pain.

Myokimia is a form of spasm. The individual cannot control the muscular tremor voluntarily. It occurs more commonly on muscles of expression innervated by the facial nerve, such as orbicularis oris (Dumitru, 1996). The myokimia may last for several minutes or even longer. It may be recorded on SEMG with no fear that the methodology may have induced it. It is more common in lower motor-neuron disease.

CO-CONTRACTIONS/CO-ACTIVATION

It has been observed clinically that when one joint (joint A) moves and the other is at rest, occasionally one muscle becomes active in the contralateral joint (joint B) at rest. The other muscles from the same myotatic unit do not show any change in amplitude from the resting tonus, thus documenting that there is no conscious or unconscious attempt at moving that joint. The contracting muscle that should be resting along with the rest of the myotatic unit is *co-contracting* (Sella, 2003b). It can be shown that most of the time when the previously resting joint (joint B) is moving through any segment of the primary ROM, no muscle on the previously moving joint (joint A). Occasionally, there is likewise a co-contracting homologous contralateral to the muscle initially noted to be co-contracting.

The usual history is that joint B has suffered from central or peripheral neuropathy, e.g., stroke or plexopathy, or a history of diffuse allodynia and hyperalgesia such as found in fibromyalgia. The hypothesis of the author is that the co-contraction takes place as a result of new internuncial associations.

Co-contraction by definition refers to a muscle contracting minimally while supposedly at rest and surrounded

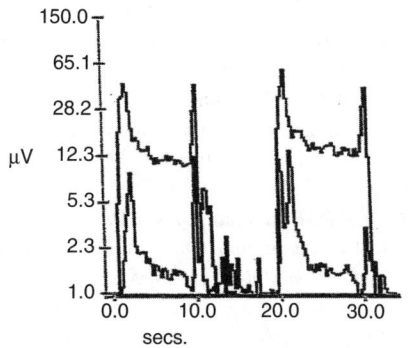

FIGURE 45.9 Co-contraction of right biceps.

by other muscles from the same myotatic unit, while those other muscles show no tendency to contract. It is a situation occurring only when the homologous contralateral joint is going through the primary segmental ROM.

Figure 45.9 shows a co-contracting right biceps while the right upper limb is at rest in the neutral position and the left elbow is moving through flexion. The right upper limb or elbow exhibits no actual movement, but the right biceps shows obvious electric activity, both during elbow flexion of the left side and during rest. This is a situation found in an individual with right brachial plexopathy.

Co-activation is a situation where a contralateral muscle from a different joint (joint C) is active while supposedly at rest when the contralateral different joint (joint D) is moving. This has been observed in situations such as fibromyalgia while the patient was sitting on a chair with a back support and moving one shoulder at a time. There was no co-contraction on the homologous contralateral muscles but there was co-contraction on the contralateral hip.

This could only be explained via a hypothesis whereby the condition, i.e., fibromyalgia, associated with allodynia and hyperalgesia produced a generalized spinal disinhibition of the primitive motor associations, which allowed the co-contraction (Donaldson et al., 2001a, 2001b). The authors' hypothesis relates to the fact that the disinhibition resulted in the activation of primitive impulses of movement of the quadruped type motion, which would have required concomitant motion of one shoulder and the contralateral hip.

Figure 45.10 illustrates the point of the co-contraction. Figure 45.10a shows that when a normal, asymptomatic subject moves the shoulder (upper area of the graph) there is no co-contraction or co-activation of any other muscle. Figure 45.10b shows that in a fibromyalgia sufferer there are multiple co-activation sites, active during a shoulder contraction (Donaldson et al., 2001b).

Loss of Mirror Image

SEMG dynamic testing of the axial skeleton allows for the observation of mirror image of the muscles tested in the segments of lateral flexion or rotation. Logic would say that for the same degrees of motion, the target muscles

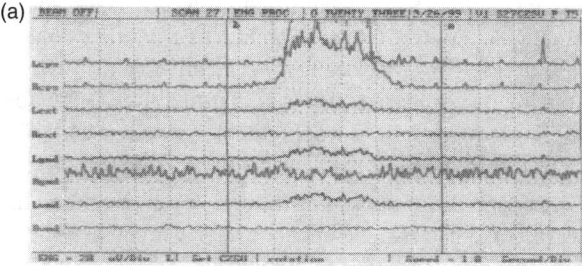

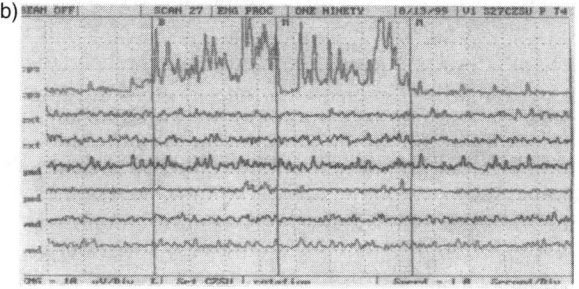

FIGURE 45.10 (a) Co-activation: presentation of asymptomatic subject; (b) co-activation: presentation of fibromyalgia subject. (From Donaldson, C. C. S., MacInnis, A. L., Snelling, L. S., Sella, G. E., & Mueller, H. H., 2001. *Neuro Rehabilitation*, *17*. Reprinted with permission.)

should express similar activity in the target motions (Sella, 2000d). For example, the right sterno-cleido-mastoid (SCM) should express an activity of 14.7 to 17.4 μV rms (95% upper and lower CI) in left rotation while the left SCM should express similar activity in right rotation, for the same degree of motion. That would be normal mirror image. If, on the other hand, for the same movement pattern and degree of motion, the activity range is >25% or <25% the upper or lower CI limits described above, that would define loss of mirror image. This may be important within the clinical rehabilitation context and would be even more important in the ergonomic or athletic competition context.

Contracture

By clinical definition, a muscle that loses the trophic nervous factor, such as in poliomyelitis, atrophies in time to become just a fibrous band (McAnelly & Faulkner, 1996). The SEMG aspect of such a contractured muscle would show an amplitude level ≤1 μV rms. This would be the situation both at rest and during any given passive or active activity level of the primary myotatic unit. Of course, in this situation, the clinician needs to rule out the possibility of a technical artifact before coming to the conclusion of "contracture."

SUMMARY

The soft tissue injury and pain field suffered for a long time from lack of credible, objective methodologies of documentation. Such documentation is necessary within the clinical context where palpation or any other clinical observation could be deemed "subjective" and different from one examiner to the next. Furthermore, very few investigative modalities would be able to focus specifically on one muscle rather than a whole region.

SEMG dynamic testing allows for a much higher degree of objective documentation of various aspects of muscular dysfunction or pathology. It allows for a superior differential diagnosis of upper versus mixed or lower neuron disease, muscle tension derived from sympathetic nervous system hyperactivity, engram changes related to protective guarding or emotional shock, etc. Furthermore, SEMG dynamic studies allow for a much more objective identification of pain and pain-related parameters in soft tissue injury or disease. Moreover, the rehabilitation arm of this methodology allows for a better engram repair or reeducation and consequent improved control on muscles and movements.

REFERENCES

Anderson, J. A. D. et al. (1978) An electromyographic investigation of postural fatigue in low back pain — A preliminary study. *Electromyography and Clinical Neurophysiology, 18,* 191–198.

Arendt-Nielsen, L., & Mills, R. K. (1988). Muscle fibre conduction velocity, mean power frequency, mean EMG voltage and force during sub-maximal fatiguing contractions of human quadriceps. *European Journal of Applied Physiology, 58,* 20–25.

Basmajian, J. V. (1974). *Muscles alive* (3rd ed.). Baltimore, MD: Williams & Wilkins.

Basmajian, J. V. (1981). Biofeedback in rehabilitation: A review of principles and practices. *Archives of Physical Medicine and Rehabilitation, 62,* 469–475.

Bigland-Ritchie, B. (1981). EMG/force relations and fatigue of human voluntary contractions. *Exercise Sports Science, 9,* 75–117.

Changeux, J. (1985). *Neuronal man: The biology of the mind.* (L. Garey, Trans.). New York: Pantheon Books.

Christensen, H. (1986). Muscle activity and fatigue in shoulder muscles of assembly plant employees. *Scandinavian Journal of Work, Environmental Health, 12,* 582–587.

De Luca, C. J. (1985). Myoelectric manifestation of localized muscular fatigue in humans. *CRC Critical Reviews in Biomedical Engineering, 11,* 251–279.

Donaldson, C. C. S., MacInnis, A. L., Snelling, L. S., Sella, G. E., & Mueller, H. H. (2001a). Diffuse muscular co-activation (DMC) as a potential source of pain in fibromyalgia – Part 1. *NeuroRehabilitation, 17,* 33–39.

Donaldson, C. C. S., MacInnis, A. L., Snelling, L. S., Sella, G. E., & Mueller, H. H. (2001b). Diffuse muscular co-activation (DMC) as a potential source of pain in fibromyalgia – Part 2. *NeuroRehabilitation, 17,* 41–48.

Donaldson, C. C. S., Sella, G. E., & Mueller, H. H. (2001c). The neural plasticity model of fibromyalgia. *Practical Pain Management, 6,* 25–29.

Dumitru, D. (1996). Electrodiagnostic medicine. I: Basic aspects. In R. L. Braddom et al. (Eds.), *Physical medicine & rehabilitation* (pp. 104–131). Philadelphia: W.B. Saunders.

Fernando, C. K., & Basmajian, J. V. (1978). Biofeedback in physical medicine and rehabilitation. *Biofeedback and Self-Regulation, 39*(4), 435–455.

Gerhardt, J. J., & Sella, G. E. (2002). *Inclinometry, SEMG & hand dynamometry in clinical & disability medicine.* Martins Ferry, OH: GENMED Publishing.

McAnelly, R.D., & Faulkner, V. W. (1996). Lower limb prostheses. In R. L. Braddom et al. (Eds.), *Physical medicine & rehabilitation* (pp. 289–320). Philadelphia: W.B. Saunders Company.

Schwartz, M. et al. (1995). *Biofeedback. A practitioner's guide.* (2nd ed.). New York: The Guilford Press

Sella, G. E. (1997a). SEMG utilization in the evaluation of soft tissue injury. *Forensic Examiner: The Official Journal of the American College of Forensic Examiners, 6*(5 & 6), 36–37.

Sella, G. E. (1997b, November 13–15). Surface EMG utilization in ruling out soft tissue injury symptom magnification or malingering. Presentation given at the 11th Annual Scientific Session & Business Meeting of AADEP. Nashville, TN.

Sella, G. E. (1999). *Neuro-muscular testing with surface EMG.* Martins Ferry, OH: GENMED Publishing.

Sella, G. E. (2000a, March). Internal consistency, reproducibility & reliability of SEMG testing. *Europa Medico Physica, 36*(1), 31–38.

Sella, G. E. (2000b). *Guidelines for neuro-muscular re-education with SEMG/biofeedback.* Martins Ferry, OH: GENMED Publishing.

Sella, G. E. (2000c). Internal consistency, reproducibility & reliability of SEMG testing. *Europa Medico Physica, 36*(1), 31–38.

Sella, G. E. (2000d). *Muscular dynamics: Electromyography assessment of energy and motion.* Martins Ferry, OH: GENMED Publishing.

Sella, G. E. (2001a). The hand grip: A differential factor in the evaluation of symptom magnification. *Disability: The International Journal of the American Academy of Disability Evaluating Physicians, 10*(1), 33–50.

Sella, G. E. (2001b). The hand grip: Gender, dominance and age considerations. *Europa Medico Physica, 37*(3), 161–170.

Sella, G. E. (2001c). SEMG: Clinical research and utilization in neuromuscular rehabilitation. *Europa Medico Physica, 37*(3), 629–636.

Sella, G. E. (2001d). *SEMG muscular assessment reference manual.* Martins Ferry, OH: GENMED Publishing.

Sella, G. E. (2002a). Forensic applications of hand dynamometry. *Forensic Examiner, 11*(5 & 6), 29–34.

Sella, G. E. (2002b). *Muscles in motion: Surface EMG analysis of the human body range of motion* (3rd ed., revised, Vols. I & II). Martins Ferry, OH: GENMED Publishing.

Sella, G. E. (2002c). Neuro-orthopedic impairment rating. In R. S. Weiner (Edi.), *Pain management: A practical guide for clinicians* (6th ed., pp. 549–562). Boca Raton, FL: CRC Press.

Sella, G. E. (2002d). Objective assessment of soft tissue injury. In N. D. Zasler & M. F. Martelli (Eds.), *Functional disorders: Physical medicine & rehabilitation, State of the art reviews* (pp. 77–94). Philadelphia, PA: Hanley & Belfus, Inc.

Sella, G. E. (2002e). Objective evaluation & treatment outcome measurements in soft tissue injury. In R. S. Weiner (Ed.), *Pain management: A practical guide for clinicians* (6th ed., pp. 1039–1056). Boca Raton, FL: CRC Press.

Sella, G. E. (2003a). Elbow muscular relationships: An SEMG view of muscular agonism & antagonism. *The Journal of Neurological and Orthopaedic Medicine and Surgery, 21*(3).

Sella, G. E. (2003b). *Surface electromyography: A neurological clinical approach.* Martins Ferry, OH: GENMED Publishing.

Sella, G. E. (2004a). Muscular harmony through motion as view by SEMG investigation & biofeedback. Presentation given at the 8th Annual BFE (Biofeedback Foundation of Europe) Meeting & Workshops. Winterthur, Switzerland. February 24–28, 2004.

Sella, G. E. (2004b). SEMG/biofeedback: General methodology & utilization in central paresis. Presentation given at the International Symposium of Cerebral Palsy. Munich, Germany. March 17–20, 2004.

Sella, G. E. & Donaldson, C. C. S. (1996). *Soft tissue injury evaluation: Forensic criteria: A practical manual.* Martins Ferry, OH: GENMED Publishing & Myosymmetries.

Sella, G. E. & Finn, R. E. (2001). *Myofascial pain syndrome: Manual trigger point & SEMG biofeedback therapy methods.* Martins Ferry, OH: GENMED Publishing.

Simons, D. G., & Mense, S. (2001). *Muscle pain. Understanding its nature, diagnosis & treatment.* Baltimore, MD: Lippincott/Williams & Wilkins.

Travell, J. G., & Simons, D. G. (1983). *Myofascial pain & dysfunction: The trigger point manual.* Baltimore, MD: Williams & Wilkins.

46

Impairment and Disability Determination

Gabriel E. Sella, MD, MPH, MSc, PhD (HC)

DEFINITIONS

The field of disability medicine or forensic evaluation has a number of rules of procedure and definitions, which are functional within the field. Those definitions may differ somewhat from the dictionary definitions of certain words or principles (Garner, 1999).

By definition, *physical* or *mental impairment* refers to the following: (1) a permanent situation whereby an individual is not expected to change substantially in the physical or mental status in the targeted respect within the foreseeable 24 months without the advent of major, unexpected medical discoveries; (2) the impairment refers to the inability to perform one or more activities of daily living commonly necessary for maintaining a normal lifestyle; (3) the impairment may also refer to the inability to perform certain occupational functions, although this part of the definition does not always hold true (World Health Organization, 1980).

The definition of *disability* includes parts 1 and 2 above and will also include part 3 in administrative, legal, insurance, or occupational terms. One example illustrates the differences between impairment and disability. A right-handed surgeon may have the right index finger amputated for a traumatic reason. An amputation is by definition a permanent impairment. The impairment may not be sufficient to impede the performance of most or all activities of daily living around the house. However, the surgeon may not be able to perform any more surgeries because the function of the index finger is essential for such performance. Therefore, that surgeon may be considered permanently disabled in terms of the essential duties of his surgical profession. It is clear that he or she may teach medicine or surgery or perform office kind of

duties. However, that will not change the status of the permanent disability in terms of performance of surgery. The same impairment may be of less consequence to a medical practitioner who does not perform surgery. There is no question that the surgeon may perform quite well most activities of daily living. On the other hand, there are situations where the performance of activities of daily living are impaired and the performance of a working function may not be impaired. Therefore, it is important to consider all the factors within the perspective of any individual requesting an impairment evaluation.

Specialized physicians may perform the duties of impairment evaluation. The complexity of this performance is described summarily below for the remainder of this chapter. The final goal of the performance of an impairment evaluation is to produce a complete report, which would include the conclusions about whether the person has indeed a permanent impairment. If the person has such impairment, then, according to the legal and administrative rules of the evaluation, the specialist may have to give a quantitative assessment of the impairment.

This can be done by following the guidelines of the *Guides to the Evaluation of Permanent Impairment* of the American Medical Association or similar texts (American Medical Association, 1993; Minnesota Medical Association, 1989). This assessment is referred to as the "permanent percentage of impairment" and it is a percentage ranging between 1 and 100%. The administrative, insurance, or legal authorities use that percentage number in their calculation of the disability relative to the governing laws and regulations. Therefore, the physician participates in the process of establishing the range or limits of the *disability* by performing the *impairment* evaluation. The rest is performed by the accredited administrative, legal, or insurance specialists.

It is common to talk about "disability"; however, in reality, the physician performs only the impairment component of the disability evaluation process.

It may be relevant at this point to describe the activities of daily living commonly evaluated by the impairment-evaluating physician in a historical perspective (LaPlante, 1991). They are as follows:

1. *Communication* — This refers to the ability of the individual to communicate with other persons. The ability to hear or speak is evaluated in a functional way. The ability to write, read, or use a computer or other keyboard may be evaluated by giving the individual a questionnaire to complete.
2. *Sensory functions* — The evaluee is examined for hearing, seeing, and speaking; indirectly or directly, the evaluee is also examined for the touch or, if necessary, for the smell or taste perception.
3. *Hand functions* — The evaluee is examined for the hand grip. As necessary, an individual is also evaluated for the ability to dress and undress or to discriminate between two points, stereognosis, etc.
4. *Physical activities* — The evaluee may have traveled independently to the examiner's office and be able to sit, stand, walk, lift a light weight, and carry the same. Or the evaluee may have traveled in a wheelchair and be unable to perform any of the above ambulation and lift/carry activities. The evaluee may be evaluated for the abilities to push, pull, climb, or perform light exercises.
5. *Travel* — The evaluee is asked about the way he or she traveled to the examiner's office, i.e., driving, being driven, etc. If necessary, one inquires about the abilities to travel by other means such as bicycling, boating, or using an airplane.
6. *Personal hygiene* — As necessary, from the personal appearance, the examiner finds out about bathing, grooming, or dressing habits. As necessary, one can inquire about the ability to perform the acts related to hygiene or dressing. The examiner takes the vital signs including the weight of the person. The eating habits are inquired about. Routinely, there are questions about incontinence or constipation/diarrhea problems.
7. *Sleep* — The evaluee is asked routinely if there are any problems with sleeping or changes in the sleeping pattern. The examiner finds out if the evaluee has to take any sleeping medications.
8. *Sexual functions* — The examiner asks routinely if there are any problems with the usual sexual functions related to age, gender, or social status. Furthermore, the examiner may ask questions about sexual habits or need for medication such as Viagra or oral contraception.
9. *Social/recreational activities* — The examiner inquires if there are any changes related to the impairment under question in terms of the accomplishment of personal and family social and recreational activities.

ELEMENTS OF IMPAIRMENT EVALUATION

THE CLAIM

The claim depends on the legal context involved. For example, a claim for similar symptoms may be valid under one type of legislation, e.g., workers' compensation, and not fall within the legal criteria of another legislation, e.g., social security disability. Therefore, at all times the word *claim* should be understood within the exact administrative or legal context to which it pertains.

In general, a claim will refer to some type of body or mental impairment whereby the individual requests a monetary compensation related to that impairment.

THE CAUSALITY

In some legal perspectives, the claim does not necessarily have to fulfill the clause of *causality*. For example, in terms of social security disability claims, it is irrelevant why a claimant has a condition such as neck pain related to whiplash from a car accident. What matters is the presence of the neck pain and related symptoms and signs, with regard to the diagnostic criteria under the social security disability law. In another context, such as in accident insurance context, the issue of the whiplash and the motor vehicle accident may be quite relevant. For example, at issue may be the question of *fault*. The targeted insurance company may recognize a whiplash claim if the motor vehicle accident could be demonstrated to be caused by its insured but not if the accident was caused by the person who got the whiplash. Therefore, the validity of the claim may be the first issue under consideration. Once the claim is demonstrated to be valid, the next question is that of *causality* (Sella, 1997a). For example, in this case, the issue is the type of impact that may have caused the type of whiplash.

A back-to-front vehicular impact may be compatible with a flexion–extension whiplash but not with a lateral bending or rotation whiplash. Therefore, if the claimant presents with symptoms of lateral bending whiplash in a back-to-front (or front-to-back) collision, then causality may not be established and the claim may not be recognized. Clearly, physical or other type of causality must coincide with the symptoms and signs it produced. One issue that needs to be addressed as early as possible is that of malingering.

The definition of *malingering* within this context is that of a physical or mental symptomatology presentation of an injury or other valid etiology, when it could be shown that the claimant was not actually present in the location and at the time of the injury (Sella, 1997b). One variant of malingering could be demonstrated to be within the context of a somatoform disorder. There are a number of psychiatric conditions that may present with symptoms of injuries that never occurred as stated. Therefore, it is important to demonstrate for the purpose of the claim that the injured or impaired party was actually present at the time and location of the injury. That is done commonly by presenting physical witnesses who saw the events of the injury and the claimant at that time. Other such "witnessing" could be offered by police officers, tape recordings, or video recordings of the injury events. Within the context of somatoform disorders, such witnessing may be provided by the clinical authorities in favor or in the disfavor of the causality presented in the claim.

There are several types of causality and the interested reader is referred to standard legal texts (Garner, 1999). While they are important to know, they are not necessarily relevant within the context of this chapter. Suffice it to say that the impairment evaluator may need to know those definitions within the working context and also within the potential expert witness context.

CHRONOLOGY OF INJURY — DESCRIPTION OF THE INJURY EVENT

A verbal report is nice; however, in legal terms it may serve only as "hearsay" because the examiner may be cross-examined in court or in deposition to prove that the series of events of the injury happened the way that he or she described in the written report (Sella, 1996c). Taking for granted that the issue of the validity of the claim has been established and that the causality has been determined, the evaluee needs to render a written statement in which the injury event is as fully described as possible. The author advises every impairment evaluator to obtain a written statement from the claimant in terms of the actual description of the events of the injury. Such a statement could be attached to the examiner's report or paraphrased. It can be used in court as documentation of the examiner in the course of one's medical/legal work. If the description is demonstrated not to be truthful or accurate, then the problem cannot be imputed to the examiner but to the claimant. Clearly, in such a case, the claimant would have broken the trust relationship and willfully misled the examiner (unless it can be documented that this occurred within the context of a somatoform disorder).

Usually, the symptomatology presented at the time of the evaluation should fit well the expected development of symptoms/signs resulting from the injury under the claim in the course of time. At times, the situation is rendered more complex and yet it could follow a direct causality pattern. Such is the case where an injury requires surgery, e.g., lumbosacral disk herniation surgery, and the scar resulting from the surgery produces further damage, chronic pain, lumbosacral radiculopathy, etc. Such a series of events may be considered legally acceptable in terms of the final impairment evaluation. However, in other cases, the symptomatic presentation cannot be fairly associated with the original injury or subsequent treatment.

The issues of symptom magnification and malingering need to be touched on again at this point. If there was an injury, one may expect a number of symptoms and signs to exist as a result of that injury. Within the reasonable knowledge and experience of medical practitioners, the intensity (and frequency) of such symptoms will have been known from the experience gathered from other patients with similar conditions. Therefore, if a claimant presents with exaggerated symptoms in spite of lack of physical signs that may corroborate such symptoms, the examiner should be alerted to the possibility of symptom magnification. The same would apply for the possibility of malingering or for that of somatoform disorders. Only a clear review of objective data, including prior medical and other documentation, may help to rule out those possibilities.

CHRONOLOGY OF THE HEALTH CARE TREATMENT RELATED TO THE INJURY UNDER THE CLAIM

By the technical nature of things, an impairment evaluator usually sees an evaluee for a final evaluation at least 6 months after the injury under the claim. This is the general rule because most symptoms following injuries would either disappear or tend to become permanent in at least that period of time. The only major exceptions would be amputations. Therefore, the evaluee has to have a chronology of diagnoses and treatment leading to the time of the impairment evaluation. Most typically, an injured person would be seen immediately after the injury in an emergency department or by the plant physician, family physician, or other such health care provider. That would be followed by a period of investigation of a few days. After the general diagnosis or diagnoses are posed, there follows a period of treatment or rehabilitation. Such a period lasts a number of weeks or even months.

Because most injuries result in soft tissue pathology or dysfunction, the physical/occupational therapy period lasts usually within a range of 3 months. After that, most persons affected by an injury will have returned to work either in their previous line of duty or in modified duties, if there are any remnants of symptoms. A rather small percentage of persons affected by injury develop chronic pain and related symptoms. These form the bulk of cases seen by impairment evaluators.

The impairment evaluator has to review the documentation available and perform a rather comprehensive physical examination on the claimant (Sella, 1996c). The impairment evaluator does not treat the claimant and does not give medical advice, but may have to report such treatment suggestions or follow-up suggestions in the final written report.

A number of issues merit individual consideration:

1. Was the original diagnosis appropriate for the injury under claim? Were there any additional factors involved that may have affected the presence of the diagnosis? Such factors may include, for example, high habitual alcohol intake and the presence of an injury from a fall from a ladder. The question is, in this case, whether the claimant had a high alcohol level at the time of the injury which may have contributed to the actual fall. The converse would be, of course, that the injury would not have occurred if it were not for the alcohol factor.

2. Were the diagnostic investigations appropriate for the clinical presentation and were they done in a timely manner? One recurrent example, at this point, is the ever presence of the emergency room diagnosis of "sprain/strain" in cases of acute myofascial pain syndrome, in the presence of clear symptoms of trigger points, etc. The lack of appropriate diagnosis more often than not may lead to very expensive and unnecessary diagnostic procedures such as MRIs (magnetic resonance imagings) and unnecessary consults to neurosurgery and even to the practice of neurosurgery in questionable cases. The appropriate diagnosis is very important in itself and in the timeliness of it. The second point is the costly and ineffective radiologic procedures in the presence of documentation, which shows that such procedures do not usually result in useful information for the case under consideration. A case in point is that at least 30% of lumbosacral MRIs of asymptomatic adults are "positive," which represents a very large "false-positive" factor when it comes to interpreting the MRI of an injured person who presents with back pain. Many people with symptoms and such positive MRI results end up with neurosurgery only to be followed by either no change in the original symptoms or complications in time related to the presence of

scar. Many a time, an impairment evaluator has to review or even grant a percentage of permanent impairment in such cases, where no surgery was appropriate to begin with. Practically speaking, such impairment results in an addition of at least 10% more than would have been necessary for the same symptoms in the absence of surgery.

3. The next issue refers to the duration, frequency, and intensity of the treatment. Medical experience shows that most common rehabilitation treatments last 3 to 6 months, start with a frequency of three times a week, and taper off as necessary to once a week, once every 2 weeks, and then once a month for the duration. The intensity may refer to the number of treatment modalities and to the ratio of active to passive modalities. At the same time, the evaluator needs to know if an overall program of reconditioning, mainly a home program with review in the physical therapy department, was part of the overall treatment. The examiner needs to know if the factors of duration, frequency, and intensity applied as well in a proper manner to programs in alternative medicine, as these programs become more frequent in our society. In either case, appropriate objective notes from the treatment providers are very important in terms of the examination of the results of the treatment. Many times, the impairment evaluator is asked to provide an opinion about the appropriateness of the treatment program for the injury under the claim. Such objective notes are paramount for the formation of that opinion. Therefore, the clinicians involved in the treatment program would be well advised to do a quantitative analysis of their treatment results because, in many cases, they may be denied payment unless they can document the effectiveness and efficiency of their program.

4. Factitious treatment must be ruled out. An experienced examiner should know what treatment generally works for a particular injury and resulting symptoms and what treatment could be continued for a very long period of time without any documentation of improvement. It is very important to assess the effectiveness and efficiency of any given program, and alternative medicine programs cannot be an exception to this. At times, the examiner finds evidence of completely unproven treatments, alternative or not, and, of course, no positive results. The examiner needs to report such treatments and the fact that the claimant has been treated with a factitious type of treatment. The question may

arise then whether the symptoms would still be present at the time of the impairment evaluation if the injured person had been treated appropriately. Therefore, the examiner may conclude and opine for a change of venue in the treatment pattern for a given period of time, such as 2 to 3 months, with a treatment modality or combination thereof that is known to work.

5. The principle of maximal medical improvement (MMI) must be considered. According to the governing rules, the impairment evaluator has to decide whether one can grant, at a given time, a permanent percentage of impairment for a given claimant. That granting is dependent on the "MMI factor" (Sella, 1996a). In other words, permanent situations such as amputations result automatically in the MMI simply because there is no further expectation of change, for better or worse. On the other hand, a surgical treatment such as lumbosacral surgery does not result in immediate MMI. A period of rehabilitation usually follows such surgery. It is only after an adequate period of physical rehabilitation, including perhaps work reconditioning, that one could learn if the claimant is at the "plateau" point of rehabilitation where no further improvement may be expected. By definition, if no further improvement in the physical or mental status may be expected within a 24-month time from the date of the evaluation, a person may be declared to have reached the status of MMI. The only condition that the examiner may add to the reporting of the MMI is that of "barring" unexpected medical discoveries or treatments.

6. Determining the principle of permanent impairment. Once the examiner has decided that a person has not attained the status of MMI, no granting of any percentage of permanent impairment can be given. The examiner has to write in the report that the evaluee may have to return for further examination within the number of months when the MMI would have been expected to occur. On the other hand, once the examiner has decided that MMI has occurred, he or she can grant the status of "permanent impairment." Because the MMI was conditional on no change from a "plateau" state within the foreseeable 24 months from the date of the evaluation, the same applies to the granting of the percentage of permanent impairment (% PPI). At that time, the report must contain either no actual percentage of impairment if the governing law requires no such percentage (e.g., civil law) or it must contain a given numerical per-

centage if the governing law (e.g., workers' compensation) requires such a percentage (Sella, 1996b). In the latter case, the examiner has to obtain and calculate the given percentage from authoritative texts, which give such numerical percentages, such as the AMA *Guides to the Evaluation of Permanent Impairment*. Impairment evaluators are specialized physicians who know how to find and interpret, as well as calculate, the figures necessary for the final percentage of permanent impairment. It is clear that the impairment evaluator needs to support the data of the percentage of permanent impairment either on the report or in deposition, including that of court testimony. A whole case may falter if the impairment evaluator does not give an appropriate percentage or does not support such a percentage (Stamp et al., 1996).

CONSIDERATIONS OF TEMPORARY PARTIAL IMPAIRMENT

In a number of administrative or legal conditions, a person may be granted a "temporary partial impairment." Such conditions usually refer to workers' compensation cases, as part of the continuum leading to the final rendering of the "permanent partial impairment."

A temporary partial impairment may be granted under certain governing laws without the status of MMI and without a percentage of permanent impairment. Under such circumstances, the claimant may have some benefits in the financial sense and may not have to work until declared either free of symptoms and fit for duty or suffering from symptoms related to the injury and such symptoms would have achieved the status of MMI, would be permanent, and may be granted a percentage of permanent impairment. Usually, the temporary partial impairment lasts a number of months, and the impairment evaluator reviews each case at the end of the "temporary period."

CONSIDERATIONS OF TEMPORARY TOTAL IMPAIRMENT

The difference between "partial" and "total" impairment is that of a degree of physical and/or mental dysfunction related to a claim. The actual percentage numbers, which distinguish "total" from "partial," are relative and may vary among different legislations. Suffice it to say that, if an evaluator considers that a person may be granted 75 to 80% PPI or more if the temporary period were to become permanent, that would be compatible with the definition of the word "total." Any percentage below that of the legally accepted definition of "total" would be considered "partial."

A clear example would be a person with an occupational respiratory impairment of Class II (10 to 25%) versus one affected by a Class IV (50 to 100%), calculated to have impaired pulmonary function tests in the range of >80% (AMA, 1993). If, in either case, the pulmonary condition should resolve, the person affected would not be given any particular percentage of impairment in terms of its permanency. Clinically, it would be quite unlikely that this would be the case in the situation of a person with a Class IV impairment and, although the examiner would grant a "temporary" status for a determined period of rehabilitation, e.g., 6 months until the final evaluation, it would be expected that a certain percentage of permanent impairment would be granted at the end of that period.

CONSIDERATIONS OF PERMANENT PARTIAL IMPAIRMENT

Most injured persons who reach MMI can be considered for the purpose of granting a permanent partial (%PPI) or total (%PTI) impairment percentage. In most cases, the injured party may be granted a permanent partial percentage of impairment. This percentage represents what is legally acceptable to grant based on authoritative texts such as the AMA *Guides to the Evaluation of Permanent Impairment*. One must stress at this point that the expression "Guides" refers exactly to what it states.

The textbook is a major compendium based on consensus of opinion and agreement of several medical societies and authorities. It is mostly based on consensus and minimally based on scientific studies of the highest credibility. However, it is the best that the medicolegal and forensic community has at the present time. The fact that the text has undergone five editions and the sixth is on its way shows that the AMA committees are working hard at ever improving the way that one can grant such a percentage of permanent impairment.

The AMA *Guides* is not the only authoritative text on the subject; several states or legal authorities use other texts of a rather similar nature. In general, most U.S. state legislations have adopted the AMA *Guides* to be the basis for granting percentages of partial or total permanent impairment as if the "guides" have become "written in stone." At times, the impairment evaluator has the opportunity to explain, during a deposition or court testimony, that the AMA *Guides* or such other authoritative text means to provide guidelines only, not precise numbers that have to be utilized at all times. Even though that is the case, the legislatures took the concept of "guidelines" and transformed it into a legal obligation (Sella, 1998).

What is the procedure of granting the percentage of partial permanent impairment? As described above, the impairment evaluator has to decide first of all the actual merit of a case. If the decision is positive, then the evaluator

has to decide whether the case has reached the state of MMI. Only when that status has been reached, could one grant a percentage according to the rules in the case. If the person has an injury that could be granted a %PPI deriving from only one source of data from the AMA *Guides* or such other text, then the evaluator has to cite that in the report. To give a simple example, if the person suffered from a lumbosacral impairment compatible with the description of "DRE lumbo-sacral category II: Minor impairment," then the evaluator could grant 5% PPI and state that this was based on the AMA *Guides to the Evaluation of Permanent Impairment*, 4th edition, Chapter 3, Paragraph 3.3g, p. 102. If, on the other hand, the decision is that the %PPI to be granted is to be based on more than one source of impairment data, then the total would be composed either from the addition of the two percentages of PPI if the sum total would be ≤14% PPI or from the combination of such numbers resulting in a PPI ≤ 15% PPI, according to the AMA *Guides*. An example in point would be as follows: A person who had disk surgery at C6 followed by loss of cervical range of motion (ROM), and documented pain and rigidity could be granted 9% PPI according to Table 75, p. 113 of the *Guides* as well as 4% for loss of motion in right rotation and 4% for loss of motion for left rotation. In this case, the first two percentages are added up, i.e., 9% + 4% = 13%. Then 13% is combined with 4%, according to the rules of the Combined Values Chart on p. 322 of the AMA *Guides*, and the resulting combination is 16%. How can that be explained when in reality, the addition of 13% + 4% = 17%? The explanation is quite simple and clear. The person already has 13% whole-body permanent percentage impairment before the last addition or combination. Therefore, the addition/combination of the last 4% is really to the body, which is only at 87% whole capacity. That, combined with the last 4%, comes out to 16% rather than 17%. If a new permanent percentage is to be "added," the combination would take into consideration the fact the body is now at only 84% of the original whole-body full capacity.

For a better and clearer understanding of the issue, an abstract example would be a first permanent impairment percentage of 10%. Therefore, if a second permanent impairment of 10% should occur at a later time, the second impairment would come from 100% − 10% = 90% and would actually count as 10% of 90%, i.e., 9%. The same would apply to any later percentage. Otherwise, if this type of calculation were not done, a successive number of impairments could total more than 100%, which would be impossible.

CONSIDERATIONS OF PERMANENT TOTAL IMPAIRMENT

In theory, a person would be granted "total permanent" impairment only upon a condition such as permanent coma or complete paralysis. In reality, this is rarely the case. Most workers' compensation legislatures and other such legal bodies define total impairment as 80 ± 5% permanent impairment. That percentage is reached by calculating the pertaining figures in the same way as was described above for the calculation of partial permanent impairment. If the target is attained for the pertinent legislature definition of permanent total impairment, then that can be granted as such. It should be clear that a person receiving a *total permanent impairment percentage* cannot do any kind of activity of daily living, and certainly not any kind of occupational activity. This applies to a number of major organs damage such as advanced chronic obstructive pulmonary disease (COPD), most severe CHF, major paresis, Meniere's disease, etc.

While it is technically possible to review a case granted a permanent partial percentage of impairment after a number of years and be enabled to increase or decrease the original percentage, this is rarely the case with persons who have been granted a total percentage of permanent impairment. The only difference that may apply is that if the percentage of permanent impairment is, say, 80% in one state legislature and the person moves to another state where the definition for total permanent impairment is 85%, that would induce the legal issue regarding which definition should apply to the case. In either situation, however, the impairment evaluator would still find basically the same total percentage.

THE "PAIN" FACTOR IN INJURY

The first principle to be applied in this context is that the pain should be of a chronic and permanent nature under the applicable definition (AMA, 1993). The impairment evaluator will need to take into consideration the injury, its causality, and the presence of pain within the overall symptoms and signs of the issue under claim. The evaluator will also need to consider the chronology of the treatment, especially focusing on specific treatment to alleviate pain and the appropriateness and results of such treatment. It is relevant to document whether the pain factor increased or decreased within the context of the history of the injury and whether the pain has increased in terms of becoming part of a secondary set of symptoms within the context of "chronic pain syndrome." If the latter is the case, then the presence and intensity/frequency of the pain needs to be interpreted within the context of the overall psychiatric evaluation and treatment for the depression component of the chronic pain syndrome. Of course, depending on the legal context, the evolution and presence of the chronic pain syndrome may have to be accepted within the legal framework of the claim. If it is not, although that does not exclude its presence, the evaluator needs to note it as such.

If pain is to be considered in terms of granting a PPI, a number of considerations apply. The first involves a holistic approach. The examiner needs to define the pain of the individual within a number of biological and psychosocial parameters (Sella & Donaldson, 1996). These parameters include the physical context of the injury, the social context involving the claimant and his or her family, the economic context, including factors such as the economic contribution to the family of the claimant before the injury and at them time of the evaluation, the mental status prior to the injury and at the time of the evaluation; and eventually, the spiritual context of the individual with pain within the family and within the community.

If pain is present within the framework of "chronic pain syndrome," then the eight defining factors of this syndrome need to be considered in terms of presence, intensity, and frequency. Those factors refer to the substance dependence and/or abuse, psychological dependence of the claimant on the health care system, the presence of depression/anxiety, the number of contextual diagnoses, the duration of the injury period, and the aspect of dramatization of the pain symptom, as well as factors such as physical deconditioning and physical and mental dysfunction (AMA, 1993).

Should pain be granted its own percentage? That is a question referred to time and again by impairment evaluators when the pain appears more as an autonomous factor rather than a clear and focused component of a particular symptom. The AMA *Guides* 5th edition tries to relate to this question from a slightly different perspective than that of previous guides. In fact, every edition of the text has considered this subject slightly differently. This shows that the complexity of this matter has not been resolved to date.

The author opines in favor of granting specific permanent percentage of impairment for the presence of pain, where such impairment cannot be fit directly and properly within the context of any particular permanent symptom/sign that is considered for granting a particular percentage of permanent impairment. In the author's opinion, the pain percentage would be granted after due consideration of the grid of the usual activities of daily living (ADL), in the format shown in Table 46.1. This format contains two components: (1) the manner in which any ADL component is impeded by the presence of pain and (2) the manner in which the performance of any ADL component affects the intensity/frequency of the pain.

Any item would be considered within 100% for each category of ADL. The total percentage for the involvement of the pain factor in terms of intensity/frequency would be 30% partial permanent impairment. The actual calculations are described in an earlier text (Sella, 1999).

As such, when the presence of pain is relevant as a chronic and permanent factor, not expected to change in

TABLE 46.1

Total Percentage of Permanent Impairment Related to the Presence of Chronic Pain and Its Association with the Accomplishment of Activities of Daily Living

ADL	Pain Affecting ADL (%)	ADL Affecting Pain (%)	Total %
Communication			
Hand functions			
Physical activity			
Self-care (hygiene)			
Sensory function			
Sexual function			
Sleep			
Social/recreational activities			
Travel			
Total			

frequency or intensity within the foreseeable 24 months, it should be granted its own percentage rather than trying to fit it as a "square peg in a round hole."

This would fit quite well in cases of malignant pain such as in cancer or in failed back syndrome. Society as a whole and the legal/insurance/administrative authorities have to change their mentality and accept in some cases, where they are well-defined, the presence of permanent chronic pain in a given claim. Of course, the intensity/frequency of the pain and its involvement in the ADL such as shown in Table 46.1 may change in time and should be reevaluated at appropriate intervals within the context of reevaluation of any given claim.

REFERENCES

American Medical Association. (1993). *Guides to the Evaluation of Permanent Impairment*, 4th Edition. Chicago: AMA.

Garner, B. A. (Ed.). (1999). *Black's Law Dictionary.* Eagan, MN: West Group.

LaPlante, M.P. (1991). *Disability in basic life activities across the life span.* Washington, DC: National Institute on Disability and Rehabilitation Research, U.S. Department of Education.

Minnesota Medical Association (1989). *Revised temporary disability duration guide.* Minneapolis, MN: MMA.

Sella, G. E. (1996c). File review. *Forensic Examiner, The Official Journal of the American College of Forensic Examiners,* 5(7 & 8).

Sella, G. E. (1996a). The cornerstone of the maximum medical improvement in impairment evaluations. *Forensic Examiner, The Official Journal of the American College of Forensic Examiners,* 5(5 & 6).

Sella, G. E. (1996b). Disability evaluations: The percentage of permanent impairment. *Forensic Examiner, The Official Journal of the American College of Forensic Examiners,* 5(3 & 4).

Sella, G. E. (1997a). Causation. *Forensic Examiner, The Official Journal of the American College of Forensic Examiners,* 6(3 & 4).

Sella, G. E. (1997b). Consideration on symptom magnification and malingering. *Forensic Examiner, The Official Journal of the American College of Forensic Examiners,* 6(1 & 2).

Sella, G. E. (1998). Common sense shall prevail. *Forensic Examiner, The Official Journal of the American College of Forensic Examiners,* 7(1 & 2), 40–41.

Sella, G. E. (1999). Chronic pain: Permanent evaluation, objective techniques. Presentation given at the American Academy of Pain Management's 10th Annual Clinical Meeting. Las Vegas, NV. September 23–26, 1999.

Sella, G. E. & Donaldson, C. C. S. (1996). *Soft tissue injury evaluation: Forensic criteria: A practical manual.* Calgary, Canada & Martins Ferry, OH: Myosymmetries & GENMED Publishing.

Stamp, F., Fitzsimmons, R., Hess, T., & Sella, G. E. (1996). What do the legal authorities expect from the independent medical evaluator? *Disability: The International Journal of the America Academy of Disability Evaluating Physicians.*

World Health Organization (1980). *International classification of impairments, disabilities and handicaps.* Geneva, Switzerland: WHO.

Section V

Behavioral Approaches

Nelson H. Hendler, MD, MS, Section Editor

47

The Biopsychosocial Perspective: Psychiatric Disorders and Related Issues in Pain Management

Raphael J. Leo, MD, FAPM

INTRODUCTION: THE BIOPSYCHOSOCIAL PERSPECTIVE

For psychiatrists and mental health practitioners, the contemporary view of pain adopts a biopsychosocial perspective. In this model, the experience of pain and the patient's presentation and response to treatment are determined by the interaction of biological, psychological, and social/environmental derivatives. There is no dichotomizing between physical versus psychological origins. Rather, the experience of pain and the response to treatment can be influenced by the patient's psychological makeup, the presence of psychological comorbidities, and the extent of social support and extenuating environmental circumstances (Leo, 2003). The array of variables exerting an impact on the patient with pain can exceed the capabilities of sole pain practitioner. Hence, a multidisciplinary treatment approach is advocated (Gallagher, 1999).

Patients with chronic, enduring, frequently recurring, or unremitting pain can report a number of psychological experiences. For many, there is the experience of emotional roller coasters, with hopes for relief dashed by unsuccessful treatment endeavors or only transient relief. They may experience significant losses, e.g., loss of work with resultant loss of income and health insurance. There may be a greater dependency on others and a loss of a sense of self-efficacy, and perhaps even a loss of their customary level of autonomy. There may be a reduction in capacity to maintain their level of activity. Patients may have less physical energy and emotional reserve to invest in others, and their ability to pursue and maintain relationships may diminish. Other relationships, e.g., those within the home, may require modification as a result of the limitations imposed on the life of the patient with pain. This may lead to increased levels of stress within the home and contribute to strained relationships. Patients may experience guilt for their inability to overcome or master their pain.

While any of the aforementioned psychological and social factors may seem plausible and even intuitive, the pain practitioner must also bear in mind that there are several psychiatric comorbidities that can accompany pain. If present, it is prudent to enlist the support of psychiatric and other mental health practitioners into the comprehensive treatment of the patient with pain.

PSYCHIATRIC COMORBIDITIES

A comorbidity refers to a coexisting disorder that can accompany an index disease or illness (Feinstein, 1970). Common psychiatric comorbidities arising among patients with chronic pain (Fishbain, 1999a; Katon, Egan, & Miller, 1985; Koenig & Clark, 1996) include those listed in Table 47.1. Such psychiatric disorders are likely to contribute to the experience of pain, influencing prognosis and long-term outcome. It is important to remember that the presence of a comorbid psychiatric

TABLE 47.1
Common Psychiatry Comorbidities Accompanying Pain

Disorder	Percent (%) of Occurrence in Various Series
Depression	30–54[a]
Substance abuse/dependence	2–34[b]
Somatoform disorders	16–53[c]
Anxiety disorders	1–62.5[d]

[a] Banks & Kerns, 1996.
[b] Fishbain, 1999; Fishbain et al., 1992.
[c] Dworkin & Caligor, 1988.
[d] Fishbain et al., 1986.

disorder does not render a patient's pain complaints less credible. Identification of psychiatric comorbidities can influence the selection of, and response to, treatment for the index condition. The rates of psychiatric disorders vary among various studies due to the diversity in patients with chronic pain examined; estimates vary depending upon whether one examines patients in clinic or community samples (Chapman, 1986; Crook, 1986; Crook, Weir, & Tunks, 1989; King & Strain, 1989). The psychiatric diagnostic criteria employed may also vary across the studies. In addition, diagnostic techniques employed in the studies were diverse; e.g., some employed diagnostic interviews, while others employed pencil-and-paper assessments.

MOOD DISORDERS

Most healthy individuals experience a wide range of emotional states and feel as though they have a repertoire of skills to deal with life situations and moods. Disturbances of mood, e.g., depression or anxiety, refer to clinical entities that by virtue of their duration and intensity, are sufficiently severe to adversely influence one's functioning. The mood is so overwhelming that one often feels no control over it. The prevailing mood colors one's existence, limiting the individual's capacity for pursuing interests, pleasure, relationships, work, or other achievements, or maintaining self-care.

The experience of pain is associated with a number of distressing life consequences that are likely to precipitate and exacerbate emotional distress. Patients with chronic pain are often plagued with distress, experiencing unpleasant changes in lifestyle and loss of rewarding activities and interpersonal reinforcement. It would be a fallacy to ascribe the depression and/or anxiety to such circumstances. The potential pitfall is that clinicians might assume the depression and/or anxiety is expected given the pain, overlooking potentially treatable disorders.

Emerging evidence suggests that mood disorders and pain share common physiological substrates. First, mood disturbances (i.e., depression and anxiety) and pain modulation involve common central nervous system (CNS) neurotransmitter systems (Blier & Abbott, 2001; Cross, 1994; Fields & Basbaum, 1999; Nelson, 1999), i.e., norepinephrine (NE) and serotonin (5-HT). The relationship between pain and mood disturbances might simultaneously involve disruptions in the NE and 5-HT neurotransmission.

Second, substance P, a neurotransmitter essential to pain processing and transmission from the periphery (Doyle & Hunt, 1999), has likewise been implicated to have a role in depression and anxiety. Recent evidence has suggested that substance P is abundantly present in limbic system structures, i.e., the repository of emotions within the CNS (Santarelli & Saxe, 2003). Increased activity of substance P centrally may contribute to the experience and expression of emotional distress, e.g., depression and fear. Current efforts are being directed at treating depression and anxiety through the development of centrally acting substance P antagonists (Rupniak & Kramer, 1999).

Third, the opioid system is intimately linked with the development of emotions. Measures of μ opioid receptor binding within the limbic system, as measured in positron emission tomography, revealed that dynamic changes occur in the activity of the μ opioid receptor system during various emotional states. Deactivation of μ opioid neurotransmission has been observed to occur during periods of sadness, presumably reflecting generalized states of dysphoria (Zubieta et al., 2003).

While further clarification is required, the physiological factors that subserve both pain and mood disorders may account for the high co-occurrence rates between them. It is necessary, therefore, to inquire into, accurately diagnose, and treat comorbid mood disorders occurring in the context of pain.

DEPRESSION

Among patients with chronic pain, depression prevalence rates are much higher than in the general population (Banks & Kerns, 1996; Gamsa, 1990). Patients with medical illnesses of sustained duration, e.g., chronic back pain and migraine, were twice as likely to develop major depression than individuals without long-term medical illnesses (Patten, 2001; Sullivan et al., 1992). Therefore, one should keep a high index of suspicion of the possibility of concurrent depression among patients with chronic pain (Ohayon & Schatzberg, 2001). The causal relationships between depression and pain are unclear. Depression may develop as a consequence of pain (Gamsa, 1990) or medical treatment (Massie & Holland, 1990), e.g., from medication use such as opiate use, baclofen use, and treatment with other medications (Browning, 1996; Sommer & Petrides, 1992). Alternatively, depression may precede the pain and may be related to the maintenance of pain. The biopsychosocial approach recognizes that the relationship between pain and emotional disturbances, e.g., depression, is likely to be reciprocal. Depressed patients tend to focus on several somatic complaints and concerns. Almost 60% of patients with depression report pain symptoms (Magni, Schifano, & DeLeo, 1985; Von Knorring et al., 1983). A number of studies demonstrate that the severity of depressive symptoms predicted the number and severity of pain complaints (Dworkin, von Korff, & LeResche, 1990; Faucett, 1994; Hotopf et al., 1998), but these improve once the depression is successfully treated. Conversely, patients with pain with comorbid depression tend to rate their pain severity higher than those without comorbid depression, a phenomenon referred to as pain scale augmentation (Gamsa, 1990).

Clinical depression is a pervasive sense of sadness, tearfulness, or dysphoria that colors one's existence, with a restricted range in the affective states of the individual. Major depressive disorder is associated with significant dysphoria or sadness, for a minimum of 2 weeks in duration, but often longer. The tearfulness and sadness influences all aspects of life, incapacitating patients from engaging in usual role responsibilities, interfering with academic and occupational functioning. Patients are incapable of taking in any comfort or relief. There may be a commensurate reduction in their ability to take in pleasure, notable as a decline in their pursuit of interests, hobbies, and normally rewarding relationships. Patients may experience a number of symptoms, including sleep disturbances (either too much or insomnia) and appetite changes (either too much leading to significant weight gain or too little intake leading to significant weight loss). The individual may experience energy changes with commensurate fatigue, a sense of restlessness or conversely retardation of activity, and indecisiveness and poor concentration. This can manifest as an inability of the patient to attend to and adhere to prescribed and proscribed treatment measures to treat the pain. Afflicted individuals may report preoccupations with guilt, or an intense focus on their worthlessness, and preoccupations with death and dying, or suicidal ideation (American Psychiatric Association [APA], 2000).

The presence of a depressive disorder can influence one's view of life circumstances, health, and long-term prognosis. Expectations can be jaded by the presence of a depressive disorder, leading individuals to "expect the worst" and view the outlook as bleak, and predisposing them to hopelessness. The depressed patient might conclude that participation in any rehabilitative efforts is futile. The patient might, therefore, be prone to helplessness and passivity, self-blaming, and other self-defeating tendencies, along with a tendency to abdicate responsibility for self-care, rehabilitation, and recovery. It is essential, therefore, that we consider the depression a serious medical condition that warrants treatment (Leo, 2003).

ANXIETY

Anxiety is also commonly associated with acute and chronic pain states, encompassing a number of distressing symptoms. Anxious people are likely to report apprehension and worry, chest palpitations, chest tightness, dyspnea, chest discomfort or throat closing off, feeling faint, tremulousness, restlessness, muscle tension, a sense of impending doom, a sense that they will not survive or will die, a sense of separation from their body, paresthesias, hot flashes, and cold chills. Such symptoms can be quite distressing, and without a particular means of alleviating these symptoms, patients might be inclined to seek out medical attention, fearing that there is something seriously wrong (Dworkin & Caligor, 1988).

When confronting stressful situations (e.g., taking an exam, encountering an unfamiliar barking dog, racing to avoid being late for an important meeting), it is appropriate for one to experience a heightened sense of arousal. The activity of the autonomic nervous system stimulates one's inclinations for fight-or-flight, serving to mobilize one's defenses to face challenges, forestall danger, and alleviate distress.

On the other hand, pathological anxiety can take on a life of its own, whereby one not only experiences bouts of severe anxiety and distress but becomes apprehensive about the possibility of recurrences. Patients may experience new worries and new reasons to experience fear. Pathological anxiety can become so incapacitating that it interferes with their ability to think, reason, concentrate, and accurately perceive the significance of events.

Anxiety, similar to depression, is associated with an increased incidence of somatic symptoms and may augment pain perception (Beidel, Christ, & Long, 1991). Preoperative anxiety can predict postoperative pain ratings and severity (Thomas et al., 1998), and anxiety may be a powerful predictor of pain ratings among patients with various forms of arthritis (Smith & Zautra, 2003). Anxiety may be related to fears of engaging in activities that precipitate pain. As a result, the patient may be inclined to avoid activity, physical therapy, and even basic self-care activities. This may have the net effect of leading to muscle wasting, deconditioning, and physical weakness with reduced physical endurance, compromising rehabilitative measures (Leo, 2003).

There are a number of anxiety disorders that can accompany chronic pain. Among these, the clinician is apt to encounter:

- Post-Traumatic Stress Disorder — Persistent anxiety associated with intrusive recollections and reexperiencing of a traumatic event, e.g., motor vehicle accidents, work-related accidents, etc. Often, the experience of anxiety can be precipitated by reminders of the traumatic event, may result in a generalized state of heightened arousal and irritability, with poor sleep and concentration difficulties (McFarlane, 1986).

- Generalized Anxiety Disorder — Relentless apprehension regarding the potential outcomes of events, life circumstances, and the future (often about matters that do not warrant that degree of worry), associated with experience muscle tension, fatigue, sleep disturbances, and irritability. Patients may appear restless, tense, vigilant, and scanning (a watchful feeling and hyperarousal). Patients have difficulty controlling the worry, will often even recognize that it is excessive, but feel an inability to distract themselves from it (Banks & Kerns, 1996).
- Existential Anxiety — Patients with painful terminal disorders may experience anxiety related to end-of-life issues, unachieved aspirations, and failure to leave a legacy. They may come to question the meaning of their life and then question whether their life has been productive and worthwhile (Leo, 2003).

TREATMENT OF MOOD DISORDERS ACCOMPANYING PAIN

The clinical symptoms of depression and/or anxiety require recognition, accurate diagnosis, and expedient treatment. Psychiatric consultation may be helpful when there is doubt about the patient's clinical presentation and when there are uncertainties about treatment approaches.

There is an array of options from which to select treatment for comorbid anxiety and/or depression. A number of antidepressants have efficacy in treating both anxiety and depression. Selection of an anxiolytic and/or antidepressant agent can be based on a number of factors, including response of the individual (or a member of the individual's family) to prior antidepressant therapy, the tolerability of side effects, concerns related to potential interactions with concurrently administered medications, and medication cost.

In addition, a number of antidepressants can be effective in treating pain. To simplify the medication regimen, it may be prudent to select from among those agents that can treat both pain and the underlying mood disorder. Some antidepressants are thought to have a pain-mitigating effect due to their influence on NE and 5-HT neurotransmission of the supraspinal modulatory systems influencing dorsal horn pain transmission. It is possible that antidepressants that influence both neurotransmitters may have an advantage over those antidepressants exerting influences over a single neurotransmitter system (Max et

al., 1992; Sindrup & Jensen, 1999). Thus, tricyclic antidepressants such as amitriptyline and imipramine, venlafaxine, and a new agent, duloxetine, may hold particular promise in this regard while antidepressants with predominantly NE effects such as despiramine or those with predominantly 5-HT effects such as fluoxetine, citalopram, or sertraline may have less efficacy in pain mitigation (Leo, 2003; Max et al., 1992; Sussman, 2003).

Other ways in which antidepressants can influence pain is by influencing opiate activity (Schreiber, Bleich, & Pick, 2002) and by potentiation of opioid analgesia (Ventafridda et al., 1990). Venlafaxine and mirtazapine have been found to influence μ and κ opioid receptors, in addition to their influences on monamine neurotransmission essential for treatment of depression (Schreiber et al., 2002).

Sometimes the side effects associated with some of these agents can be particularly difficult for patients to tolerate, e.g., anticholinergic side effects associated with some of the tricyclic antidepressants. As such, consideration of alternative agents might need to be explored based on the monitoring of the tolerability of the agents employed. On the other hand, selection of an antidepressant might be based on certain of the side effects, e.g., for patients with insomnia selection of a sedating antidepressant might help to eradicate the dysphoria as well as facilitate sleep.

The influence on mood of antidepressants might not be appreciated for as long as 4 to 6 weeks after initiation and dose optimization. However, the effect on pain can occur much more rapidly. Failure to achieve antidepressant and/or anxiolytic efficacy might warrant psychiatric consultation and evaluation.

Psychotherapeutic approaches might be simultaneously invoked to help patients achieve an understanding of the illness, development of more effective coping strategies, mobilization of their social support network, and modifications in their cognitive appraisals and life view that may have become distorted and disturbed by the prevailing depression. Psychotherapeutic endeavors may exceed the purview and skills available to the pain management clinician. As such, referrals to a mental health specialist, e.g., psychiatrist, psychologist, or social worker, with skills in psychotherapy may be helpful in mitigating some of the sequelae of depressive disorders.

SOMATOFORM DISORDERS

Somatic concerns, including a variety of pain states, bowel disturbances, dizziness, palpitations, fatigue, and respiratory symptoms, account for approximately half of outpatient physician visits. Most of these remit spontaneously or respond to simple treatment interventions; however, as many as one fourth of these symptoms remain chronic.

TABLE 47.2
Common Pain Complaints

Source of Pain Complaint	Estimated No. of Outpatient Medical Visits Annually (in Millions)
Back	19.8
Knee	9.8
Abdominal	12.3
Headache	9.6
Chest	8.4
Neck	8.1
Nonspecific	3.2

Note: Adapted from Schappert, 1992.

As many as one third of symptoms remain medically unexplained (Kroenke, 2003; Kroenke & Mangelsdorff, 1989; Kroenke & Price, 1993; Marple et al., 1997). Pain complaints of a variety of sorts are likely to be the basis for patient presentations to ambulatory medical settings (Schappert, 1992; see Table 47.2).

Clinicians may be apt to question the veracity of the patient's pain when the complaints appear disproportionate to the nature of the pathology of a given disease or the complaints of most others with comparable disease states. Psychological factors are often invoked when complaints persist beyond the expected course of the illness or despite customarily reasonable treatment endeavors. Such complaints are often deemed to be psychogenic or "all in one's head." The reality is, there can be quite a range of diversity in the pattern and experience of pain and distress in response to medical conditions.

A number of psychiatric disorders have long been recognized in which physical complaints, including pain, are the predominant focus, which cannot be reasonably accounted for by a medical condition or disease. Such disorders, broadly categorized under the rubric of somatoform disorders (APA, 2000), can include the following:

- Hypochondriasis is characterized by preoccupations with fears of having a dreaded medical condition, based on the misinterpretation of bodily sensations. The disturbance is a cognitive one, whereby individuals misconstrue the significance of a common, perhaps normal, sensation, e.g., a momentary twinge in the shoulder is believed to signal myocardial disease. Such individuals are characterized by a conviction that they are ill and will seek out medical consultation and diagnostic tests to confirm the suspicion that they are, indeed, ill. Medical reassurances are not well received; the patient is likely to become persistent, perhaps seeking out other medical evaluations and consultation with specialists, to affirm the suspected disease.

- Somatization disorder involves distortions in physical sensations. Patients seek out medical attention for multiple unexplained symptoms, several of which are pain symptoms, gastrointestinal symptoms, genitourinary symptoms, and even pseudo-neurological symptoms.

- Pain disorder is characterized as a condition in which psychological factors are thought to contribute to the patient's subjective experience of pain by exacerbating the level of pain, maintaining the pain, precipitating bouts of pain, and aggravating it. Currently, there is no stipulation that the pain cannot be accounted for by a general medical condition. However, it is accepted that even pain conditions may not be fully accounted for by our current knowledge of physical conditions.

Generally speaking, patients with somatoform disorders present with bodily preoccupations and concerns, often with vague, sweeping, and confusing features. They frequently and persistently seek out physician evaluations, laboratory, and other diagnostic investigations, and frequently perceive themselves as chronically ill (Barsky, 1996). However, despite the seeming similarity between alleged symptoms and medical symptoms, there is little or no evidence to support a medical diagnosis. It should be borne in mind that any of these conditions can co-occur with medical conditions and chronic pain disorders.

There are controversies about the utility of the psychiatric diagnostic criteria of somatoform disorders (Mayou, Levenson, & Sharpe, 2003). The biggest of these is the contention that the classification of somatoform disorders perpetuates the outmoded dualistic definitions of disease couched in physical versus psychological origins. Another criticism is that the taxonomy outlined by the *Diagnostic and Statistical Manual of Mental Disorders-IV* (DSM-IV; APA, 2000) really is only understood and employed by psychiatrists, i.e., is not widely understood or acceptable. Primary care clinicians may address the same sorts of symptoms and disturbances by employing medical taxonomies, e.g., labeling a constellation of symptoms or syndromes as fibromyalgia, irritable bowel syndrome, multiple chemical sensitivities, or chronic fatigue syndrome.

Even within psychiatry, there are alternative viewpoints of how to conceptualize somatic preoccupations (DeGucht & Fischler, 2002). For example, a broad concept of somatizing is sometimes referred to in the literature, whereby patients with mood disturbances present with preoccupations about physical symptoms. In such conceptualizations, there is less emphasis placed on characterization of the number and type of symptoms as defined in the DSM-IV, but rather an emphasis on the "function" that the somatic preoccupations serve. For some patients, there may be a vested interest in presenting the worst of their plight. In this way, they may be apt to convince the clinician of the seriousness of the complaints and the legitimacy of their disorder. For some patients, there is much to be gained by focusing on somatic complaints, e.g., to avoid unpleasant tasks, to achieve secondary gains (e.g., compensation, disability payments), to avoid family conflicts (e.g., by diverting attention away from more pressing issues), to communicate displeasure with others in their life (Ford, 1986).

Nonetheless, patients with somatoform disorders and/or manifesting functional somatization can become quite focused on their ailments, to the point of compromising most aspects of their lives, their relationships, and adaptive functioning. Regardless of whether one construes such conditions as predominantly psychological or an as yet unexplained physical phenomenon, psychological treatment may be warranted. Otherwise, the physician may erroneously be caught up in the endless and futile attempts to provide patients with relief from their symptoms, rather than attempting to address adaptation to the physical concerns and the psychological factors underlying the somatic concerns (Barsky, Geringer, & Wood, 1988). Psychological interventions may be particularly helpful in assisting patients to develop strategies with which to take control of many aspects of their lives that had been subterfuged to the focus on somatic concerns, fears, and preoccupations with disability. Psychiatric treatment would attempt to assess and address the impact of the somatic complaints on patients' ability to sustain work, experience pleasure, and improve the quality of interpersonal relationships.

SUBSTANCE ABUSE AND DEPENDENCE

Many clinicians still have a tendency to underutilize opiate analgesics for their patients with pain. For many, this is driven by concerns related to the federal regulation of opiate analgesics and concomitant fears of prescribing agents that will be abused, misappropriated, or diverted (Potter et al., 2001).

Such apprehensions have been fueled by media attention and legal pursuits. In recent years, a great deal of attention has been directed to the abuse and diversion of opiate analgesics, e.g., OxyContin SR abuse (Baumrucker, 2001; Tough, 2001). When crushed, so that its analgesic and euphoric effects become immediate, OxyContin SR has been ingested intranasally or injected intravenously to produce euphoria. As a result, acquisition and illegal distribution of OxyContin SR has become an epidemic in some parts of the country. Clinicians have also been implicated in legal suits related to the emergence of

drug dependence from the prescription of analgesic agents (Albert, 2002).

While opiates have been a focus of media attention, there are several other agents used in the armamentarium of pain treatment that are likewise prone to abuse and dependence. These can include the muscle relaxant carisoprodol (Soma®), which, when metabolized, is converted to methocarbamol, a barbiturate-like substance with sedative qualities; ketamine; ergot alkaloids and barbiturates employed in migraine treatment; and benzodiazepines, employed in patients with pain to address insomnia and muscle tension.

Consequently, clinicians may be reluctant to employ optimal analgesia in their patients with pain, especially for patients with chronic, nonmalignant pain. While there are anecdotal experiences with patients abusing the doctor–patient relationship to acquire analgesics for purposes of abuse, the literature has been lacking with regard to accurate estimates of the degree to which such patterns of behavior occur. Estimates of substance abuse and dependence among patients with chronic pain have varied in the literature (see Table 47.1). The difficulty in interpreting such varied results is related to how dependence/addiction was defined; i.e., varying rates of addiction were reported depending on the criteria employed to classify abuse and addictive behaviors (Fishbain, Rosomoff, & Rosomoff, 1992).

According to the DSM-IV, substance dependence has been defined by physiological and psychological symptoms. Physiological symptoms of dependence include tolerance (higher amounts of a substance are required to produce the same effects that previously lower amounts had achieved) and withdrawal (symptoms emerge with abrupt cessation of use) (APA, 2000). Some clinicians erroneously rely on such physiological parameters to define addiction. However, the presence of tolerance and dependence alone does not constitute addiction. For example, any patient with chronic pain who has received an opiate analgesic for an extended period of time is likely to experience a diminution of the analgesic effect over time, requiring higher doses of the analgesic (i.e., tolerance) and can experience withdrawal symptoms upon abrupt cessation of the use of the analgesic. Such physiological reactions to long-standing analgesic use do not necessarily constitute addiction.

Instead, for patients with pain, the presence of psychological symptoms of dependence, suggesting a lack of control over the use of the substance, may be better indicators of dependence (APA, 2000; Miotto et al., 1996; Portenoy, 1996). Dependence is suggested when the individual's use of the substance not only has become excessive, but has taken on a life of its own. The individual may experience craving of the substance and the person's activities become centered on acquiring more of the substance, using it (oftentimes to feel "normal"), and recovering from misuse. The individual may resort to extreme measures to acquire the substance, even though such activities can incur significant legal and health consequences (e.g., prescription drug forgery, prostitution, drug trafficking). The addicted individual may persist in his or her use of the substance despite deleterious effects. For example, the person's capabilities at functioning socially, taking interest in normally pleasurable activities and interpersonal exchanges might suffer as a result of the attempt to acquire and use substances. Similarly, the person's basic self-care, as well as pursuit of adaptive academic and occupational endeavors may suffer as a result.

In such cases, patients may require formal detoxification from the agents to which they are addicted. Inpatient treatment may be required in those situations in which safe detoxification on an outpatient basis may be too uncomfortable or unsafe, e.g., in situations in which severe physical sequelae can arise from too abrupt a discontinuation of the substance, as would be the case for opiates, benzodiazepines, and barbiturates.

The patient with pain who simultaneously has ongoing alcohol or illicit substance abuse (or a prior history) can pose significant treatment challenges. Addiction to such agents can compromise functioning and full participation in the rehabilitation process. While effective pain management should never be withheld because of an abuse/addiction history, effective treatment may require use of an array of pain-reducing approaches, e.g., use of adjunctive agents, agents with low abuse potential, physical and psychological therapies, as well as participation in concurrent substance abuse treatment programs (Leo, 2003).

Inpatient detoxification may be indicated for alcohol and selected illicit substance dependence, especially those with significant withdrawal symptoms upon cessation of use. Outpatient treatment is likely to be required to facilitate maintaining health, reducing health risk behaviors, and maintaining abstinence from illicit substances. Psychological interventions, along with prudent psychopharmacologic interventions may be warranted especially when patients abuse substances as a means of controlling psychological distress, e.g., cannabis and/or benzodiazepine abuse to alleviate anxiety.

PAIN AND SUICIDE

The impact of painful conditions and psychiatric comorbidities can be so compromising that patients may despair. Suicide risk is increased among persons with medical illnesses (Druss & Pincus, 2000) and, therefore, warrants clinical attention and intervention. Medical disorders associated with increased risk of suicide include terminal illnesses (e.g., cancer and AIDS), heart disease, renal failure (especially for those on dialysis), CNS disorders, and chronic inflammatory conditions (Work Group, 2003).

Furthermore, the risk of suicide is increased among those persons with medical illnesses in which there is distress over disfigurement (Work Group, 2003), pain (Chochinov et al., 1995; Fishbain, 1999b; Fishbain et al., 1991), comorbid mood disorders (Work Group, 2003), substance abuse (Borges, Walters, & Kessler, 2000), severe functional impairments (Waern et al., 2002), and increased perceived levels of disability. Hopelessness on the part of the patient can be an additional significant predictor of suicide risk as well as the individual views his or her plight as unremitting and may believe that there is nothing to look forward to (Chochinov et al., 1998).

The medical clinician can be the first to expect, anticipate, and intervene for the suicidal patient. The clinician caring for the patient with pain should be attentive to the prospect that despair has seeped into the patient's existence. Clinicians may be reluctant to inquire into the possibility that their patients may be entertaining thoughts of suicide, fearing incorrectly that making such inquiries may be offensive to patients or may "plant" such thoughts into their head (Henderson & Ord, 1997). Inquiries should be framed in a matter-of-fact, nonjudgmental, concerned, and empathic manner. It is probably best to inquire frankly whether the patient is experiencing distress and harboring thoughts of suicide. Patients may actually find that such frank inquiry is relieving. If the patient is given an opportunity to verbalize their concerns, thoughts, feelings, and despair, the physician–patient relationship may be strengthened, particularly if the clinician is concerned and not particularly shocked by the admission of despair. Admission of thoughts of suicide should be taken seriously and never minimized or dismissed as manipulative ploys.

The clinician should, in turn, appropriately direct the patient to psychiatric treatment. It is incumbent upon the clinician to arrange for psychiatric referral or transfer to an emergency psychiatric facility to be certain that a comprehensive lethality assessment is conducted and to ensure that all reasonable measures are undertaken to maintain the patient's safety. Psychiatric hospitalization may be required in cases in which there is significant psychiatric comorbidity, imminent lethality risk, suicidal intent/plans, and when the patient's cooperation in mobilizing available resources to ensure their safety is not forthcoming (Work Group, 2003).

PSYCHOLOGICAL VARIABLES AFFECTING THE EXPERIENCE OF PAIN

Psychological variables, separate from psychiatric comorbidities, can have a profound impact on the experience of pain. Patients' beliefs and expectations regarding the pain experience and its ramifications can have a profound impact on their functioning and well-being.

The individual who believes that even if the pain is not totally eradicated, he or she may have the capacity to develop ways of dealing with it may be more inclined to develop a proactive approach to the treatment process. By contrast, patients with pain may harbor unreasonable expectations and beliefs about pain and its treatment. So often, such patients expect that their pain will be unremitting and that there is no hope for relief over the horizon. Hence, patients who harbor belief that regardless of what they do, "the pain seems to get worse" will be less inclined to be active participants in prescribed treatment and rehabilitation endeavors. Similarly, one cannot be expected to be optimistic or anticipate much in the way of pleasure in life if the person appraises that his or her life "is hardly worth living." Patients will be less inclined to engage in collaborative endeavors with treating sources if they believe that the "doctors don't take my pain seriously enough." It becomes extremely difficult to manage the pain of patients who harbor maladaptive beliefs and expectations. Indeed, maladaptive cognitions may lie at the very center of the pain problem.

The experience of chronic pain can be associated with a number of stressors (see Table 47.3). Patients' ability to cope with a stressor is contingent on their appraisal of the significance and severity of the stressors, their appraisal of their intrinsic repertoire of coping strategies (and the

---

TABLE 47.3
Biopsychosocial Factors Encountered in Chronic Pain

Physical
    Pain
    Physical deconditioning
    Complications arising from treatment interventions,
      diagnostic tests, and medication use
Marital/Family
    Role responsibility modifications
    Communication difficulties
    Reduced emotional reserve to invest in other family members
    Sexual dysfunction
Vocational
    Loss of work
    Job restrictions
Financial
    Loss of income
    Costs of medical care
    Concerns over health insurance and medical coverage
Social
    Depletion of social support networks
    Strained relationships
    Little emotional reserve to pursue customary interests
    Decline in recreational interests
Legal
    Litigation regarding disability
    Workers' Compensation issues

---

utility of those measures), the availability of social supports and their ability to make use of those supports. Distress may result if patients believe they lack the requisite abilities to deal with such stressors effectively, or when the severity of the stressors is overly magnified. The distress, in turn, can aggravate and exacerbate the experience of pain.

In reality, individuals often cannot control or avoid distressing life events. However, the patient can almost always exert some control over how much distress and life disruption those events produce. A number of psychotherapy approaches can be helpful in assisting the patient's ability to cope with the disorder and the ramifications of having a chronic disorder (Leo, 2003).

Psychological and psychiatric endeavors might well be invoked to address concurrent stressors, and beliefs can be instrumental in optimizing the patient's response to treatment. Psychotherapeutic measures would attempt to foster patient empowerment by addressing maladaptive and ineffective beliefs and by developing effective coping strategies and mobilizing social supports in such a way as to assist individuals assert control over their reactions to pain and its ramifications. These interventions might be beyond the scope of the sole pain practitioner, and referral for psychiatric and psychological consultation might prove to be a necessary adjunct to manage the patient's condition.

Psychotherapy can be quite individualized, contoured to the needs of the patient. Thus, for patients whose pain appears to be exacerbated by perceived stress, patient instruction on the use of a variety of relaxation techniques and hypnosis might prove helpful (Turner & Chapman, 1982a,b]. For those experiencing marked difficulties with conceptualizing their pain and ineffective coping, a variety of psychotherapeutic approaches, e.g., cognitive-behavioral therapy, might be of use (Turner & Chapman, 1982b). Other therapy approaches, e.g., interpersonal psychotherapy, might address the way in which patients relate to other social supports in their life. Individuals sustaining marked marital and family stress might benefit from couples/marital and family therapies. For those facing intense distress over loss of work and concomitant loss of self-efficacy, vocational rehabilitation may be essential to improve adaptive functioning (Leo, 2003).

PSYCHOLOGICAL ASSESSMENT

Consistent with comprehensive pain management approaches, it is useful to organize how we think about our patients with chronic pain in terms of biopsychosocial variables. While clinical interview is probably most useful, it can sometimes be helpful to employ standardized scales and assessment instruments to conceptualize patients in terms of psychological characteristics, personality traits, and social supports. Useful assessment instruments might include those listed in the Table 47.4. Consultation with

---

TABLE 47.4

Psychometric Scales Used in Assessing Chronic Pain

Coping Strategies Questionnaire — Assesses coping strategies in one's repertoire to deal with chronic pain. May predict the level of activity, physical impairment, and psychological functioning associated with pain (Rosenstiel & Keefe, 1983).

Fear Avoidance Beliefs Questionnaire — Assesses beliefs characterized by danger, threat, or harm associated with pain. The degree to which patients assign threat to activities may limit their participation in, and lead to avoidance of, activities related to work (Waddell et al., 1993).

McGill Pain Questionnaire — Assesses the features of pain severity and intensity. Allows patients to qualify pain in emotional, cognitive/evaluative, and sensory terms (Melzack, 1975, 1987).

Minnesota Multiphasic Personality Inventory — Provides personality profiles and pathological assessment of patients with chronic pain (Hathaway et al., 1989).

Quality of Life Indices — Assess the impact of chronic pain states on various aspects of one's life, activity, recreation and leisure time activities, social interactions, work, and adaptive self-care (Ferrell, Wisdom, & Wenzl, 1989).

West Haven-Yale Multidimensional Pain Inventory — Assesses one's appraisals of pain, its impact on functioning, and perceived responses of others in response to pain (Kerns, Turk, & Rudy, 1985).

Note: From Leo, R. J. *Concise Guide to Pain Management for Psychiatrists* (p. 50), Washington, DC: American Psychiatric Publishing. Reprinted with permission.

---

psychologists skilled in the administration, scoring, and interpretation of such instruments is warranted.

CONCLUSIONS

As clinical practice within the realm of pain management has evolved, it has become increasingly apparent that the effective treatment of patients with pain requires recognition of prevailing psychiatric issues. In addition to the physical discomfort associated with pain, patients likewise experience marked emotional and psychosocial distress. A number of biological, psychological, and social factors can have an impact on the experiences and life of the patient with chronic pain. Emotional factors, e.g., depression and anxiety, not only emerge as a consequence of pain but can, in addition, contribute to pain, exacerbating and maintaining it. Psychological factors can likewise interfere with treatment adherence and efficacy. The frustration caused by ongoing pain, the effects on functioning, and the impact on families and other relationships can contribute significantly to psychiatric morbidity. The comprehensive approach to the patients with pain requires assessment of each of these dimensions. Barriers may be ascertained which pose impediments to the recovery of the patient. A number of psychiatric disorders can coexist

with chronic pain disorders. The presence of such psychiatric comorbidities can add to the complexities of the presentation of the patient with pain, and warrant treatment as part of the comprehensive rehabilitation program offered to the patient.

A multidisciplinary approach to the management of patients with pain is advocated. Treatment of coexistent psychiatric disorders would require the cooperation and assistance of psychiatrists and other mental health professionals who can lend their knowledge and skills to such endeavors. In addition, a multimodal approach to the patient, involving somatic treatments and psychological interventions, would be required to manage the complexities encountered among the patients suffering from chronic pain disorders.

REFERENCES

Albert, T. (2002). Florida physician guilty of manslaughter. *American Medical News, 45*(10), 1, 4.

American Psychiatric Association. (2000). *Diagnostic and statistical manual of mental disorders – TR* (4th ed.). Washington, DC: American Psychiatric Association.

Banks, S. M., & Kerns, R. D. (1996). Explaining high rates of depression in chronic pain: A diathesis-stress framework. *Psychological Bulletin, 119*, 95–110.

Barsky, A. J. (1996). Hypochondriasis — Medical management and psychiatric treatment. *Psychosomatics, 37*(1), 48–56.

Barsky, A. J., Geringer, E., & Wood, C. A. (1988). A cognitive-educational treatment for hypochodriasis. *General Hospital Psychiatry, 10*, 322–327.

Baumrucker, S. J. (2001). Oxycontin, the media, and law enforcement. *American Journal of Hospice and Palliative Care, 18* (3), 154–156.

Beidel, D. C., Christ, M. A. G., & Long, P. J. (1991). Somatic complaints in anxious children. *Journal of Abnormal Child Psychology, 19*, 659–670.

Blier, P., & Abbott, F. V. (2001). Putative mechanisms of action of antidepressant drugs in affective and anxiety disorders and pain. *Journal of Psychiatry and Neuroscience, 26*, 37–43.

Borges, G., Walters, E. E., & Kessler, R. C. (2000). Association of substance use, abuse and dependence with subsequent suicidal behavior. *American Journal of Epidemiology, 151*, 781–789.

Browning, C. H. (1996). Nonsteroidal anti-inflammatory drugs and severe psychiatric side effects. *International Journal of Psychiatry in Medicine, 26*(1), 25–34.

Chapman, C. R. (1986). Illness behavior and depression in pain center and private pain practice patients. *Pain, 27*, 1–43.

Chochinov, H. M. et al. (1995). Desire for death in the terminally ill. *American Journal of Psychiatry, 152*, 1185–1191.

Chochinov, H. M. et al. (1998). Depression, hopelessness, and suicidal ideation in the terminally ill. *Psychosomatics, 39*, 366–370.

Crook, J. (1986). Epidemiologic comparison of persistent pain sufferers in a specialty pain clinic and in the community. *Archives of Physical Medicine and Rehabilitation*, 67, 451–455.

Crook, J., Weir, R., & Tunks, E. (1989). An epidemiological follow-up survey of persistent pain sufferers in a group family practice and specialty pain clinic. *Pain*, 36, 49–61.

Cross, S. A. (1994). Pathophysiology of pain. *Mayo Clinic Proceeding*, 69, 375–383.

DeGucht, V., & Fischler, B. (2002). Somatization: A critical review of conceptual and methodological issues. *Psychosomatics*, 43(1), 1–9.

Doyle, C. A., & Hunt, S. P. (1999). Substance P receptor (neurokinin-1)-expressing neurons in lamina I of the spinal cord encode for the intensity of noxious stimulation: A c-fos study in rat. *Neuroscience*, 89(1), 17–28.

Druss, B., & Pincus, H. (2000). Suicidal ideation and suicide attempts in general medical illnesses. *Archives of Internal Medicine*, 160, 1522–1526.

Dworkin, R. H. & Caligor, E. (1988) Psychiatric diagnosis and chronic pain: DSM-III-R and beyond. *Journal of Pain and Symptom Management*, 3, 87–98.

Dworkin, S. F., von Korff, M., & LeResche, L. (1990). Multiple pains and psychiatric disturbance — An epidemiologic investigation. *Archives of General Psychiatry*, 47, 239–244.

Faucett, J. A. (1994). Depression in painful chronic disorders: the role of pain and conflict about pain. *Journal of Pain and Symptom Management*, 9, 520–526.

Feinstein, A. (1970). The pre-therapeutic classification of comorbidity in chronic disease. *Journal of Chronic Disease*, 23, 455–468.

Ferrell, B. R., Wisdom, C., & Wenzl, C. (1989). Quality of life as an outcome variable in the management of cancer pain. *Cancer*, 63, 2321–2327.

Fields, H. L. & Basbaum, A..I. (1999). Central nervous system mechanisms of pain modulation. In P. D. Wall & R. Melzack (Eds.), *Textbook of pain* (4th ed., pp. 309–329). Endinburgh: Churchill Livingstone.

Fishbain, D. A. (1999a). Approaches to treatment decisions for psychiatric comorbidity in the management of the chronic pain patient. *Medical Clinics of North America*, 83(3), 737–760.

Fishbain, D. A. (1999b). The association of chronic pain and suicide. *Seminars in Clinical Neuropsychiatry*, 4(3), 221–227.

Fishbain, D. A., Rosomoff, H. L., & Rosomoff, R. S. (1992). Drug abuse, dependence, and addiction in chronic pain patients. *Clinical Journal of Pain*, 8(2), 77–85.

Fishbain, D. A. et al. (1986). Male and female chronic pain patients categorized by DSM-III psychiatric diagnostic criteria. *Pain*, 26(2), 181–197.

Fishbain, D. A. et al. (1991). Completed suicide in chronic pain. *Clinical Journal of Pain*, 7, 29–36.

Ford, C. U. (1986). Somatizing disorders. *Psychosomatics*, 27(5), 327–337.

Gallagher, R. M. (1999). Treatment planning in pain medicine. Integrating medical, physical and behavioral therapies. *Medical Clinics of North America*, 83(3), 823–849.

Gamsa, A. (1990). Is emotional disturbance a precipitator or a consequence of chronic pain? *Pain*, 42, 183–195.

Hathaway, S. R. et al. (1989). *Minnesota Multiphasic Personality Inventory–2: Manual for administration*. Minneapolis, MN: University of Minnesota Press.

Henderson, J. M. & Ord, R. A. (1997). Suicide in head and neck cancer patients. *Journal of Oral and Maxillofacial Surgery*, 55, 1217–1221.

Hotopf, M. et al. (1998). Temporal relationships between physical symptoms and psychiatric disorder: Results from a national birth cohort. *British Journal of Psychiatry*, 173, 255–261.

Katon, W., Egan, K., & Miller, D. (1985). Chronic pain: Lifetime diagnoses and family history. *American Journal of Psychiatry*, 142, 1156–1160.

Kerns, R. D., Turk, D. C., & Rudy, T. E. (1985). The West Haven-Yale Multidimensional Pain Inventory (WHYMPI). *Pain*, 23, 345–356.

King, S. A., & Strain, J. J. (1989). The problem of psychiatric diagnosis for the pain patient in the general hospital, *Clinical Journal of Pain*, 5, 329–335.

Koenig, T. W., & Clark, M. R. (1996). Advances in comprehensive pain management. *Psychiatric Clinics of North America*, 19(3), 589–611.

Kroenke, K. (2003). The interface between physical and psychological symptoms. *Primary Care Companion Journal of Clinical Psychiatry*, 5(Suppl. 7), 11–18.

Kroenke, K., & Mangelsdorff, A.D. (1989). Common symptoms in ambulatory care: Incidence, evaluation, therapy, and outcome. *American Journal of Medicine*, 86, 262–266.

Kroenke, K., & Price, R. K. (1993). Symptoms in the community: Prevalence, classification, and psychiatric comorbidity. *Archives of Internal Medicine*, 153, 2474–2480.

Leo, R. J. (2003). *Concise guide to pain management for psychiatrists*. Washington, DC: American Psychiatric Publishing, Inc.

Magni, G., Schifano, F., & DeLeo, D. (1985). Pain as a symptom in elderly depressed patients: Relationship to diagnostic subgroups. *European Archives of Psychiatry and Neurological Sciences*, 235, 143–145.

Marple, R. L. et al. (1997). Concerns and expectations in patients presenting with physical complaints: Frequency, physician perceptions and actions, and 2-week outcome. *Archives of Internal Medicine*, 157, 1482–1488.

Massie, M. J., & Holland, J. C. (1990). Depression and the cancer patient. *Journal of Clinical Psychiatry*, 51(Suppl. 7), 12–17.

Max, M.B. et al. (1992). Effects of desipramine, amitriptyline, and fluoxetine on pain in diabetic neuropathy. *New England Journal of Medicine*, 326, 1250–1256.

Mayou, R., Levenson, J., & Sharpe, M. (2003). Somatoform disorders in DSM-V. *Psychosomatics*, 44(6), 449–451.

McFarlane, A. C. (1986). Posttraumatic morbidity of a disaster: a study of cases presenting for psychiatric treatment. *Journal of Nervous and Mental Disease*, 174, 4–14.

Melzack, R. (1975). The McGill Pain Questionnaire: Major properties and scoring methods. *Pain*, 1, 277–299.

Melzack, R. (1987). The short-form McGill Pain Questionnaire. *Pain*, 30, 191–197.

Miotto, K. et al. (1996). Diagnosing addictive disease in chronic pain patients. *Psychosomatics*, *37*(3), 223–235.

Nelson, J. (1999). A review of the efficacy of serotonergic and noradrenergic reuptake inhibitors for treatment of major depression. *Biological Psychiatry*, *46*, 1301–1308.

Ohayon, M. M., & Schatzberg, A.F. (2003). Using chronic pain to predict depressive morbidity in the general population. *Archives of General Psychiatry*, *60*, 39–47.

Patten, S. B. (2001). Long-term medical conditions and major depression in a Canadian population at waves 1 and 2. *Journal of Affective Disorders*, *63*, 35–41.

Portenoy, R.K. (1996). Opioid therapy for chronic nonmalignant pain: A review of the critical issues. *Journal of Pain and Symptom Management*, *11*(4), 203–217.

Potter, M. et al. (2001). Opioids for chronic nonmalignant pain. Attitudes and practices of primary care physicians in the UCSF/Stanford collaborative research network. *Journal of Family Practice*, *50*(2), 145–151.

Rosenstiel, A. K. & Keefe, F. J. (1983). The use of coping strategies in chronic low back pain patients: Relationship to patient characteristics and current adjustment. *Pain*, *17*, 33–44.

Rupniak, N. M. J., & Kramer, M. S. (1999). Discovery of the antidepressant and anti-emetic efficacy of substance P receptor (NK1) antagonists. *Trends in Pharmacological Sciences*, *20*(12), 485–490.

Santarelli, L., & Saxe, M. D. (2003). Substance P antagonists: Meet the new drugs, same as the old drugs? Insights from transgenic animal models. *CNS Spectrums*, *8*(8), 589–596.

Schappert, S. M. (1992). National Ambulatory Medical Care Survey: 1989 summary. National Center for Health Statistics, *Vital Health Statistics*, *13*(110), 1–80.

Schreiber, S., Bleich, A., & Pick, C. G. (2002). Venlafaxine and mirtazapine: different mechanisms of antidepressant action, common opioid-mediated antinociceptive effects: A possible opioid involvement in severe depression? *Journal of Molecular Neuroscience*, *18*, 143–150.

Sindrup, S. H., & Jensen, T. S. (1999). Efficacy of pharmacologic treatments of neuropathic pain: An update and effect related to mechanism of drug action. *Pain*, *83*, 389–400.

Smith, R., & Zautra, A. (2003). Anxiety and depression as predictors of pain in older women with arthritis. Abstract presented at 156th Annual Meeting of the American Psychiatric Association, San Francisco, California (Abstract No. NR 368).

Sommer, B. R., & Petrides, G. (1992). A case of baclofen-induced psychotic depression. *Journal of Clinical Psychiatry*, *53*(6), 211–212.

Sullivan, M. J. et al. (1992). The treatment of depression in chronic low back pain: Review and recommendations. *Pain*, *50*(1), 5–13.

Sussman, N. (2003). SNRI's versus SSRI's: Mechanisms of action in treating depression and painful physical symptoms. *Primary Care Companion Journal of Clinical Psychiatry*, *5*(Suppl. 7), 19–26.

Thomas, T. et al. (1998). Prediction and assessment of the severity of post-operative pain and of satisfaction with management. *Pain*, *75*, 177–185.

Tough, P. (2001, July 29). The oxycontin underground. *New York Times*.

Turner, J. A. & Chapman, C. R. (1982a). Psychological interventions for chronic pain: A critical review. I. Relaxation training and biofeedback. *Pain*, *12*, 1–21.

Turner, J. A. & Chapman, C. R. (1982b). Psychological interventions for chronic pain: A critical review. II. Operant conditioning, hypnosis, and cognitive-behavioral therapy. *Pain*, *12*, 23–46.

Ventafridda, V. et al. (1990). Studies on the effects of antidepressant drugs on the antinociceptive action of morphine and on plasma morphine in rat and man. *Pain*, *43*, 155–162.

Von Knorring, L. et al. (1983). Pain as a symptom in depressive disorders II. Relationship to personality traits as assessed by means of KSP. *Pain*, *17*(4), 377–384.

Waddell, G. et al. (1993). A fear-avoidance beliefs questionnaire (FABQ) and the role of fear-avoidance beliefs in chronic low back pain and disability. *Pain*, *52*, 157–168.

Waern, M. et al. (2002). Burden of illness and suicide in elderly people: Case-control study. *British Medical Journal*, *324*, 1355–1357.

Work Group on Suicidal Behaviors. (2003). Practice guidelines for the assessment and treatment of patients with suicidal behaviors. *American Journal of Psychiatry*, *160*(Suppl. 11), 1–60.

Zubieta, J. K. et al. (2003). Regulation of human affective responses by anterior cingulate and limbic μ-opioid neurotransmission. *Archives of General Psychiatry*, *60*, 1145–1153.

48

Psychotherapeutic Approaches in Pain Management

Kathleen Sitley Brown, PhD, and Lorie T. DeCarvalho, PhD

HISTORICAL VIEWS OF PAIN

It has been said that "pain upsets and destroys the nature of the person who feels it" (Aristotle, *Nicomachean Ethics*). Centuries have come and gone, and the message behind this statement still rings true for individuals who suffer from persistent pain. Philosophers, physicians, and psychologists alike have struggled with the issue of how to best deal with and treat people suffering from pain. Historically, one argument was given by Descartes (1596–1650), who ushered in a new paradigm of viewing the human experience with his argument that the mind or "soul" was separate from the physical body, and that the mind was a passive, dependent entity, incapable of directly affecting either physical or somatic processes (Gatchel, 1999). Damasio (1994) claimed that Descartes's ideas of such a separation between the mind and body "have shaped the peculiar way in which Western medicine approaches the study and treatment of diseases" (p. 251). Even in today's health care system, psychologically based problems or contributing factors are often disregarded, while the diseased body part is examined solely as the cause of pain and illness.

Kossman and Bullrich (1997) brought to light a new theory, initially proposed by von Bertalanffy in the 1960s, which stated that the study of general systems necessitated an understanding of the "whole" rather than the sum of parts. This gestalt-like theory led to a shift from former biomedical reductionism as science began to look at human functions in terms of the whole. And by the late 1980s, pain researchers realized that both organic pain *and* psychogenic pain resulted in an experience of pain. This led to the *Biopsychosocial Model* of pain, which proposed that the assessment, diagnosis, and treatment of organically caused pain should incorporate both the physiological and psychological factors that contribute to patients' experiences with pain (Gatchel, 1999).

THE CHALLENGE OF PAIN

Chronic pain has been defined by the International Association for the Study of Pain as "an unpleasant sensory and emotional experience associated with actual or potential tissue damage" (Merskey & Bogduk, 1994). Indeed, individuals who suffer from chronic pain not only experience physical pain but they may also become disabled as a result of their condition(s). For example, chronic low back pain is the leading cause of physical disability in persons under the age of 45 in the United States, and after the age of 45, it is the third leading cause of disability (Mayer & Gatchel, 1998). Along with the physical manifestations of chronic pain and disability, these individuals also tend to experience the psychological effects of fear, anxiety, and depression. Of course, no two individuals respond the same way to a similar injury. Consequently, "one individual may view pain as disabling, whereas the other continues to function in spite of his or her pain and returns to a productive lifestyle" (Koestler & Doleys, 2002). But as practitioners treating these individuals, it is vital that we are mindful of their experience in its entirety, to incorporate the biopsychosocial perspective.

Cognitive, affective, and behavioral factors have all been shown to play essential roles in the perception and behavioral responses to chronic pain. Given this complex perceptual experience of chronic pain, treatment must address the reciprocal interactions between the physical consequences and psychological factors, as well as the social sequelae of chronic pain. Chronic pain also affects family functioning as their support of the person with pain often results in role changes, financial difficulties, changes in lifestyle, and emotional distress in family members (Turk, Flor, & Rudy, 1987). Therefore, treatment must address the psychophysiological processes, as well as the inter- and intrapersonal challenges posed by chronic pain.

In the perception of pain, cognitive appraisals of nociceptive stimuli based on prior learning history, the meaning of the context in which this stimuli is perceived, and the evaluation of resources for controlling pain all directly affect an individual's emotional state. Furthermore, emotional factors influence physiological functioning, appraisal processes, and behavioral responses. And, environmental reinforcement contingencies subsequently influence thoughts, feelings, and behavior.

In this chapter, we first review psychotherapeutic issues related to chronic pain that should be addressed (i.e., depression, suicidality, and post-traumatic stress disorder, or PTSD) and integrated into a comprehensive pain management treatment plan. This incorporates use of a model for PTSD and chronic pain (DeCarvalho, 2004), with specific application to clinical treatment of patients with chronic pain. We then discuss issues related to chronic pain and grief work, which we follow with a discussion of psychotherapeutic approaches for effective pain management. This includes sections on cognitive-behavioral therapy, behavior therapy/operant conditioning, stress inoculation therapy, self-directed treatments, adjunctive treatments, and relapse prevention for patients with chronic pain. Finally, we address barriers encountered in the practice of pain management and how to overcome them. As a note, biofeedback and hypnosis, which can be used as stand alone treatment approaches or integrated as adjuncts to psychotherapy, are discussed in other chapters and thus are not included in this chapter.

PSYCHOTHERAPEUTIC ISSUES RELATED TO CHRONIC PAIN

CHRONIC PAIN, DEPRESSION, AND SUICIDALITY

According to the *Diagnostic and Statistical Manual of Mental Disorders* (APA, 2000; DSM-IV-TR), symptoms of depression incorporate marked changes in mood, diminished interest or pleasure, and vegetative changes (e.g., weight loss or gain, insomnia or hypersomnia, fatigue, psychomotor agitation or retardation). Additionally, individuals who experience depression may have

feelings of worthlessness, difficulty concentrating, and suicidal ideation, thoughts, or impulses (APA, 2000).

A large body of literature acknowledges that there is a high incidence of depressive symptoms in persons with chronic pain (Lindal, 1990; Trief, Carnricke, & Drudge, 1995; Turk, 1994). For example, Schuster and Smith (1994) assessed 101 patients with chronic pain and found that 47% of the patients exhibited significant depressive symptoms. They found that nearly 90% of the patients' depression was explained by symptoms of hopelessness, decreased interest, and sadness. Other researchers have indicated that within the United States, depression is the single most common psychiatric diagnosis in patients with chronic pain in general (Fishbain, 1986) and chronic low back pain specifically (Magni, 1987). Prevalence rates for depression as a comorbid disorder with some chronic pain conditions have been found to range from 10 to 100% (Romano & Turner, 1985). Most studies report prevalence rates between 30 and 60% (Magni, 1987). Although it is frequently assumed that patients with pain have a premorbid history of depression, Hendler (1989) found that although the incidence of depression in patients with chronic pain admitted to his clinic was 77%, 89% did not have a pre-morbid history of depression prior to the onset of pain.

It is well-known that patients with chronic pain who are depressed secondary to their conditions are more likely to physically function more poorly and demonstrate more significant levels of physical disability (Fields, 1987). Further, there is some research evidence that patients with chronic pain who scored higher on depressive symptomatology reported greater intensity of perceived pain, more pain behaviors, and pain tending to interfere with daily living more so than in patients experiencing fewer depressive symptoms (Haythornthwaite, Sieber, & Kerns, 1991). It is important to note that the generalizability of this study is questionable due to the sample demographics. Despite the methodological problems in the Haythornthwaite et al. (1991) study, their findings were remarkably similar to those of a more recent study by Burns et al. (1998), who found that feelings of helplessness decreased as pain severity decreased. This study demonstrated that depression significantly relates to levels of perceived pain.

Similarly, there is a clear relationship among personal control, learned helplessness, anxiety, and chronic pain disability (Abramson, Garber, & Seligman, 1980; DelVecchio-Good, Brodwin, Good, & Kleinman, 1992). For example, Lackner, Carosella, and Feurstein (1996) concluded that chronic pain disability and perceived levels of severity of pain correlated negatively with functional self-efficacy, or patients' confidence in their abilities to cope with their pain. Burns et al. (1998) found that pre- to post-treatment decreases in pain helplessness were related to improvement in pain severity, activity, and downtime. Thus, patients who experience greater disability and have reduced functional self-efficacy are likely to experience greater psychological distress, which can be evidenced in the form of secondary depressive symptoms.

Overall, patients with chronic pain who use positive, active coping strategies tend to have lower levels of self-reported pain severity, depression, and functional disability while the opposite is true of those patients who use passive coping strategies (Brown & Nicassio, 1987; Brown, Nicassio, & Wallston, 1989; Keefe & Williams, 1992; Kores, Murphy, Rosenthal et al., 1990). As such, it may be said that patients' beliefs in themselves that they are able to take a proactive approach in the healing process, or self-efficacy, is key in helping patients with chronic pain to manage their condition. Those who perceive that they are unable to control their physical pain may use passive-avoidant coping strategies and tend to rely upon wishful thinking and avoidance to cope with their pain (Weickgenant, Slater, Patterson, Atkinson, Grant, & Garfin, 1993).

Of paramount importance is the acknowledgment that those suffering from uninterrupted, extreme pain and disability are highly vulnerable to suicidal ideation (Fuerst, 1993; Heller, Flohr, & Zegans, 1989; Ivey, Ivey, & Simek-Morgan, 1993; Jourard, 1971). These individuals may feel guilty and humiliated because they have suicidal ideation (Herman, 1992). Fishbain, Goldberg, Rosomoff, and Rosomoff (1991) found that males with chronic pain complete suicide at a rate two times higher than the general population, while those involved in workers' compensation litigation completed suicide at a rate three times higher than the general population. Females with chronic pain were found to complete suicide at a rate three times higher than the general population. A limitation of this study was that the ethnic composition of the sample was limited only to Caucasians. Further research is needed to determine whether such suicide rates are similar in other ethnic groups with chronic pain.

As clinicians, screening individuals for depression, as well as assessing for suicidal ideation and risk of danger to self or others, should be incorporated as a fundamental part of the treatment process for any person suffering from chronic pain. This is particularly true if the individual has a history of psychiatric illness, or if this is true of his or her family, as well as if the individual lacks adequate social support that can buffer the stress entailed in coping with ongoing, persistent severe pain and/or disability.

CHRONIC PAIN AND POST-TRAUMATIC STRESS DISORDER

Although PTSD has been recognized as "shell shock" and related to wars, especially World War II (Kizer, 1996), it may occur with *any* serious trauma that involves helplessness and potential loss of physical or mental integrity. In fact, the experience of chronic pain is a traumatic event involving serious injury and/or threat to one's physical integrity of self, and the person's response involves fear and helplessness. PTSD is categorically defined in the DSM-IV-TR (APA, 2000) as a disorder wherein both of the following are present:

1. The person experienced, witnessed, or was confronted with an event or events that involved actual or threatened death or serious injury, or threat to the physical integrity of self or others, and
2. The person's response involved intense fear, helplessness, and horror.

According to the DSM-IV, the individual persistently reexperiences the trauma. This may take on different forms: intrusive images, thoughts, or perceptions; nightmares or night terrors; behaviors or feelings related to the event; psychological and/or physiological reactivity to internal or external cues resembling aspects of the traumatic event. As a response to the reexperiencing of the trauma, the individual reacts with (1) persistent avoidance (e.g., of thoughts, feelings, conversations, activities concerning the trauma) and (2) arousal (e.g., sleep difficulties, irritability or difficulty controlling anger, difficulties with concentration, hypervigilance, exaggerated startle response). Individuals experience clinically significant distress or impairment for at least 1 month. With delayed-onset PTSD, the presentation of symptoms is at least 6 months after the traumatic event took place (APA, 2000). To appreciate the relationship to and impact of PTSD on patients with chronic pain, we first examine the relationship for individuals in the general population.

In the general population, PTSD has been found to be one of the most common anxiety disorders, having a lifetime prevalence of 5 to 10% in the general population (Ballenger et al., 2000). The long-term prognosis or outcome of persons with PTSD can vary, depending on factors such as the individual's social support network; however, it has been determined that approximately 40% of persons do *not* experience a resolution of symptoms in the long term (McFarlane, 2000). The U.S. National Comorbidity Survey determined that the median duration of PTSD is approximately 3 years if the individual obtains treatment; yet this estimate neglects the fact that many individuals do *not* get treatment and could potentially experience more than one traumatic event in their lifetime (Kessler, Sonnega, Bromet, et al., 1995).

More recent studies indicate that the average duration of a PTSD episode is more than 7 years (Ballenger et al., 2000). Shalev (1996) concluded that there might be a progressive instability of the underlying neurobiological systems, which may lead to a continuation of the disorder. Ballenger et al. (2000) concluded that PTSD, along with depression, heads the list in terms of disability resulting in the individual, as well as in terms of the financial costs to society. Persons with PTSD tend to have difficulties sustaining stable employment, have more relationship strife, and have more troubles with the law when compared with nonsufferers of PTSD (Shalev, 2000). PTSD has been associated with misuse of psychotropic medications, illicit drugs, and alcohol; and persons with PTSD also tend to engage in risky behaviors more frequently than nonsufferers (Hearst, Newman, & Hulley, 1986).

Yet another serious ramification of PTSD is its correlation with suicidality. More specifically, PTSD is more strongly associated with suicidal behaviors when compared with other anxiety disorders (Kessler, Borges, & Walters, 1999). In fact, it has been found that the rate of attempted suicide in persons with PTSD is approximately 19% (Hendin & Haas, 1991), which is comparable with the suicide attempt rate for persons experiencing major depressive disorder (Buda & Tsuang, 1981).

Consequently, the prevalence of PTSD has been found to be substantially elevated in patients with chronic pain when compared with the general population (15 to 35% vs. 2%, respectively) (Asmundson, Bonin, Frombach, & Norton, 2000). For example, diagnoses of PTSD in patients with chronic pain following motor vehicle accidents have been found in numerous studies (Blanchard et al., 1995; Chibnall & Duckro, 1994; Kuch, Swinson, & Kirby, 1985; Muse, 1986). Hickling and Blanchard (1992), in a study of patients being treated for chronic headache pain and pain resulting from motor vehicle accidents, found that 50% of the patients met criteria for PTSD. A more recent study showed that approximately 51% of patients with chronic low back pain assessed evidenced clinically significant levels of PTSD symptoms (DeCarvalho, 2004). Furthermore, another 24% of the patients evidenced a mild PTSD symptom severity level, reporting at least one to eight symptoms of PTSD (DeCarvalho, 2004). The findings resembled those of other investigators (DeCarvalho, 2001; Hickling & Blanchard, 1992). DeCarvalho (2004) also found that 77% of those patients with chronic low back pain who experienced a combination of trauma (back-related and non-back-related) reported clinically significant levels of PTSD symptoms. A very significant finding, however, was that pain alone appears to be a sufficient trauma to trigger clinically significant levels of PTSD symptoms for some patients (DeCarvalho, 2004), which supports the conclusions of Schreiber and Galai-Gat (1993); Buckley, Blanchard, and Hickling (1996); and Geisser, Roth, Bachman, and Eckert (1996).

As is true with depression, not every individual who suffers from chronic pain will develop PTSD. As such, it is important to attempt to determine certain possible predictive factors. By doing so, clinicians can better treat these individuals. DeCarvalho (2001, 2004) proposed a model for the predictors of PTSD in patients with chronic low back pain. While the model has not yet been researched with individuals with different forms of chronic pain, it is believed that this model may tentatively serve as a means of improving the assessment and treatment of persons with chronic pain. Essentially, DeCarvalho (2004) found that (1) the characteristics of the person, (2) history of antecedent trauma(s), (3) complicated physical involvement, (4) proactive measures, and (5) perceptions of pain are intricately woven together to predict PTSD symptom severity level. Because patients with chronic pain tend to be more difficult to treat, not only because of slow-going clinical improvements, but also because of the emotional component, it is strongly recommended that a very thorough history be taken for each patient. These aforementioned areas inherent in the model (DeCarvalho, 2004) may be used as a guide for assessing each patient's needs. The relevance of each of these areas to the treatment of chronic pain is now discussed.

PERSONAL CHARACTERISTICS

Pre-Trauma Vulnerability

The characteristics of the person would include such things as an individual's sex, age, family history of psychiatric or other illness, and personal history of psychiatric illness. This would also include personality style or traits, including tendencies to be neurotic, or to the other extreme, it would incorporate axis II or long-term personality disorders of some kind. Individuals who possess negative histories or personality makeups are essentially predisposed to other psychiatric or psychological problems in the future. Thus, pre-trauma vulnerability means that those individuals who have these person characteristics, as well as a history of trauma, are already psychologically more fragile and vulnerable should another traumatic event occur in the future. Pre-trauma vulnerability can ensue from several possible factors, including genetics, family history of mental illness, personality traits such as neuroticism, and previous traumatic experiences (McFarlane & Yehuda, 1996; Shalev, 1996). As clinicians, this means that we must address more than the individual's physical pain in treatment. We must inquire about personal history, particularly a history of trauma, as this will significantly affect treatment outcomes.

Age, Chronic Pain, and PTSD

Other personal characteristics that significantly predict PTSD symptom level are age and what has been labeled as perceived uncontrollability (DeCarvalho, 2004) over pain. We know that exposure to trauma appears to decrease with age, including certain traumatic events (i.e., physical and sexual assaults; Norris, 1992). However, it is known that aging tends to increase the prevalence of acute and chronic diseases, as well as disabilities (Kemp, 1985). In fact, disability has been commonly accepted as a normal and prevalent characteristic of older age (Ben-Sira, 1991). Because elderly persons are likely to view disease and disability as a normal part of the aging process, they may actually dismiss warning signals (e.g., pain) (Kart, 1981). Further, it is possible that many elderly persons internalize societal expectations for degeneration and deactivation, which could lead to many elderly persons assuming that pain and disability are normal aging processes (Ben-Sira, 1991; Kovar, 1980).

In working with elderly patients who suffer from chronic pain, it is important to be aware that, because of societal expectations and individual perceptions about ageism, they may cope with their pain in one of two ways. Some older persons who have an *internal locus* of control tend to use less escape-avoidance, hostility, and self-blame as coping mechanisms when compared with younger persons (Blanchard-Fields & Irion, 1988). Conversely, older individuals who have an *external locus* of control in coping with their conditions tend to catastrophize more, thereby having a more difficult time in reducing their pain (Gibson & Helme, 2000). Those who perceive they have less control over their pain are more likely to report greater levels of pain and disability, and to develop PTSD (DeCarvalho, 2004). Thus, treatment goals should include helping patients to feel more in control and empowering them to own responsibility for their treatment.

ANTECEDENT TRAUMA

As discussed earlier, pre-trauma vulnerability strongly predicts individuals developing PTSD symptoms a second time; this is essentially because persons who have experienced trauma before must heal from it, and if another trauma occurs prior to "resolution" of this, it is more likely that these individuals feel more out of control and anxious. This means they experience a compounding effect of trauma upon trauma, and it predisposes them to PTSD. Patients who have a history of antecedent trauma(s) are more likely to manifest these experiences in the form of chronic pain.

Childhood trauma (physical, sexual, or psychological abuse) is one form of antecedent trauma that has been linked to somatic and behavioral manifestations in adulthood. Moreover, adult survivors of childhood trauma are predisposed to predictable physical and behavioral problems (Scaer, 2001). Examples of physical syndromes include pelvic, lower back, orofacial, and chronic bladder pain, as well as fibromyalgia, interstitial cystitis, nonremitting whiplash syndromes, and eating disorders. Scaer (2001) added that infants and young children who experienced abuse will have permanent neuronal patterns or procedural memories imprinted in their brains, which may result in long-term personality traits, behaviors, and coping styles for dealing with traumas (Grigsby & Hartlaub, 1994; Perry, Pollard, Blakely, Baker, & Vigilante, 1995). Similarly, Damasio

(1994) proposed that memories of emotions and sensations comprise somatic markers, which contribute to future behaviors when faced with trauma. Thus, in clinical practice, integrating psychodynamic, gestalt, interpersonal, and cognitive-behavioral therapies is invaluable in helping such patients heal from their traumatic experiences, as well as to reduce symptoms of pain. Neglecting to address antecedent trauma and focusing solely on the pain condition will hamper therapeutic gains, particularly as tension-related problems have both somatic and emotional underpinnings.

COMPLICATED PHYSICAL INVOLVEMENT

Patients who have more complicated presentations of chronic pain are generally harder to treat. As a form of chronic pain, chronic low back pain secondary to a herniated or ruptured disk(s) usually involves pain at the site of the injury, as well as referred pain, which involves the sciatic nerve root (Rosomoff & Rosomoff, 1991). Thus, patients experience a "double dose" of severe pain, which when combined with a longer duration, results in disability. Such disability may include (but is not limited to) difficulty ambulating or poor gait; paralysis; frequent urination or, in cases of extreme nerve impingement, incontinence; loss of reflex(s); sensory or proprioceptive losses; bilateral foot-drop; rigid and tight muscles; and loss of functional activity (Deyo, 1988). Patients with ruptured disk(s) are also more likely to undergo more back surgery(s).

The experience of surgery incurs fears of death, injury, postoperative pain, and helplessness. Studies with patients who have undergone breast cancer surgery have indicated that even 1 year after surgery, one third of the patients continued to have insomnia because of intrusive thoughts or images of their illness; one fifth of the patients had nightmares; 12% continued to meet criteria for PTSD; and over 50% had dissociative symptoms (Tjemsland, Soreide, & Malt, 1998). Therefore, Tjemsland et al.'s (1998) study reinforced the importance of addressing fears and experiences associated with surgeries and invasive procedures, as patients generally tend to have long-term symptoms of dissociation, nightmares, flashbacks, panic, and fear.

Previous studies in both the general population and with patients with chronic pain have indicated that perception of life threat and significant physical impairment were major predictors of the development of PTSD (Blanchard et al., 1995; Butler, Moffic, & Turkal, 1999; Helzer, Robins, & McEnvoi, 1987; Kilpatrick et al., 1989; Martini, Ryan, Nakayama, & Ramenofsky, 1990; Pitman, Orr, Forgue, De Jong, & Claiborn, 1989), as is the physical experience of severe, unrelenting pain (Geisser et al., 1996). Furthermore, nagging physical injuries may be constant reminders of the trauma, which would maintain or exacerbate PTSD (Buckley et al., 1996). In clinical practice, therefore, reducing patients' sense of helplessness and lack of control is crucial. Using guided imagery and relaxation exercises such as diaphragmatic breathing and visualization are simple and quick, yet effective techniques that can help patients with chronic pain feel less threatened. In the long run, this may prevent them from developing anxiety disorders such as PTSD.

PROACTIVE MEASURES

It is important to find out what types of treatments patients are trying and using for their chronic pain condition, as well as how frequently they are engaging in these treatments. This will provide you, as the clinician, with an indication of how compliant the patient is and will be in treatment with you, as well as how proactive the patient is in taking necessary measures to feel better. The converse of this is that patients who try numerous treatments and are hopeful they will help may experience disappointment when the treatments do not work. Such disappointment tends to result in frustration, anger, and even depression as the individual begins to feel more and more helpless and out of control of the situation. In general, the more treatments a patient tries that fail, the greater the anxiety he or she will experience, which strongly contributes to greater levels of PTSD. By the same token, such patients who tend to be very proactive and who have more self-efficacy are more likely to try other treatments that are offered to them, provided they believe there is a glimmer of hope and that possibility that the treatment can help.

PAIN PERCEPTIONS

The physical experience of severe, unrelenting pain as a result of trauma relates to the development of PTSD symptoms (e.g., Geisser et al., 1996). Geisser et al. (1996) also found that PTSD symptoms were positively related to increased affective distress, self-report of pain, and functional disability among patients with chronic pain. In another significant study, Schreiber and Galai-Gat (1993) presented a case study of a patient with chronic pain stemming from the loss of an eye. Their case study suggested that uncontrolled and prolonged chronic pain may be a strong enough stressor to lead to the onset of PTSD. This valuable study also supported that accidents or traumatic injuries are not necessary prerequisites for the development of PTSD in patients with chronic pain. Of course, as a case study based on only one participant, results are not generalizable.

Another study found that nagging physical injuries in patients with chronic pain may be constant reminders of the trauma, which would maintain or exacerbate PTSD (Buckley et al., 1996). The authors made an important contribution to an understanding of the relationship between chronic pain and PTSD. Their findings suggest that the presence of an injury could, in itself, maintain or exacerbate PTSD.

Perceived loss of control is a central facet in the experience of trauma. Patients suffering from chronic pain who utilize an internal locus of control tend to believe that their actions and efforts contribute to reduced pain (Crisson & Keefe, 1988). Therefore, individuals with an *internal locus*, or a decreased sense of perceived uncontrollability, are more likely to be proactive in their efforts to minimize or reduce pain. On the other hand, patients with chronic pain who utilize an *external locus* of control tend to believe that their own personal efforts will not reduce their pain. They tend to rely on the efforts of powerful others (e.g., physicians, health care providers, friends, family), or luck to bring relief from their pain (Crisson & Keefe, 1988). Patients who have an external locus of control (chance locus) tend to catastrophize and divert their attention, and they typically report being in more pain (Gibson & Helme, 2000; Toomey, Mann, Abashian, & Thompson-Pope, 1991). These individuals tend to experience greater helplessness and are less able to effectively cope with their chronic pain conditions (Crisson & Keefe, 1988; Skevington, 1983).

We have discussed each of these areas of the model (DeCarvalho, 2004). The most important thing to understand is that each of these areas plays a role in how patients individually perceive and cope with their chronic pain conditions. Of course, individuals may have different chronic pain conditions. The most common type, as discussed throughout this chapter, is chronic low back pain. As one example, in its most severe forms, chronic low back pain may cause paralysis and numbness, loss of gross motor control, loss of bowel and bladder control, loss of reflexes in lower limbs, spasticity, and degeneration of nerves. Chronic pain in general most often results in disability, and with chronic pain disability comes a cognitive reevaluation and reintegration of one's belief systems, values, emotions, and feelings of self-worth (Miller, 1990).

Coping with a chronic pain condition and being told that one will need to "live with it" and "manage the pain" for the rest of one's life is certainly more easily said than done. Being faced with the news of impending health problems, ongoing severe pain, and disability is extremely difficult. Learning to live with chronic pain presumes that the patient accepts that the diagnosis and prognosis are accurate. However, research demonstrates that misdiagnosis of patients with chronic pain occurs 40 to 60% of the time (Hendler & Kozikowski, 1993; Hendler, Bergson & Morrison, 1996). Hendler and Kozikowski (1993) reexamined 60 patients consecutively admitted to their chronic pain clinic and found that approximately 66% were referred with diagnoses that were considered incomplete as they did not reflect the complexity of the underlying pathology. Of this group, half of these patients were found to have surgically correctable lesions. Considering the large number of missed and treatable diagnoses, the formulation of differential diagnoses must be based on patient complaints, history, and physical examination rather than negative test results.

The process of acceptance of living with chronic pain is very much like that designated by Elizabeth Kubler-Ross (1969) for death and dying, wherein the person experiences feelings of shock/denial, anger, bargaining, depression, and acceptance. Such people have lost a part of themselves. They have lost their physical abilities, and they have lost the assurance that they can fully control whatever is going on in their lives. This process of grief work is now discussed.

CHRONIC PAIN, DISABILITY, AND GRIEF WORK

In being told that they will be living with chronic, painful, and potentially disabling conditions, individuals will initially experience shock or denial. They may attempt to deny that they are having such an experience; for example, patients who face dangerous and invasive surgical procedures may experience shock and deny that they are subject to the risks involved. And, as patients become more anxious from severe chronic pain, there may also be other factors that contribute to the disruption in their lives. Wheeler (1995) stated that fear of reinjury and panic may reinforce patients' anxieties, and complicate recovery. Patients with chronic pain and disability may experience deep uncertainty about the meaning of the events and circumstances that have occurred and how they are to deal with life from the present onward (Mishel & Braden, 1988). All these factors may result in a person either feeling numb inside or expressing to clinicians or others that they are really doing okay and will be getting better soon. This is an attempt to maintain control over the situation.

As the situation becomes worse and the pain and disability worsen, the individuals may attempt to try more treatments to relieve the pain. However, when their pain is not relieved, and their condition worsens, they are likely to start to feel anger (Miller, 1990). Because anger is strongly related to fear, some patients will express this in the form of anxiety (McCracken, 1993), deep-seated frustration, and/or decreased self-efficacy (Altmaier, 1993). These individuals may feel powerless and have a sense of uncontrollability in their situation (Carpenito, 1989). The more powerless an individual feels, the more likely he or she is to be angry.

Patients may express anger at themselves for getting injured in the first place, toward their loved ones for not being more helpful or supportive, against agencies such as the government or workers' compensation departments for not financially compensating them, and at their providers for not taking away the pain like they believe they should be able to. At this point, it is important to understand that when patients become angry and frustrated, it is a normal human response to pain. Being empathetic and gently confronting the patients may mean reminding the patients that you want to help them, but that they need to own a share of the work too. Generally, this is the most difficult point in the psychotherapy process, as it tends to involve the most resistance, and it can trigger a great deal of frustration and anxiety in the therapist. Coming to an understanding that this is a normal process that each patient, as a person, must go through to be able to make sense of his or her condition, can facilitate a smoother therapy process as well as a stronger therapeutic alliance with the patient.

As the anger turns more into fear, patients may begin bargaining in their healing process. While this process varies from person to person, this may involve blame and judgment. For example, some patients with chronic pain may reach a point where they attribute their pain to their behaviors or personal life decisions; for example, some individuals will blame their self-judged "bad behavior" for their pain, which they view as a punishment from God. Other chronic pain sufferers feel that their pain provides for their moral and spiritual atonement (Hawthorn & Redmond, 1998). When their pain gets to a point of unbearability, many patients with such beliefs will bargain with God or their Higher Power for respite, and in return, they promise to "be good" in the future (Kubler-Ross, 1969). By doing so, these individuals are, again, attempting to restore their sense of control over their condition. Referring the individual to a chaplain, pastor, or minister can be very therapeutic and should be done when possible if you are not trained to deal with such issues.

As they realize their efforts have failed, the individuals experience depression. Again, it is crucial to assess for any suicidal ideation, as persons with chronic pain are far more likely to attempt suicide than the general population. Kubler-Ross (1969) indicated that, eventually, patients who face severe illness, pain, and/or loss reach a point of acceptance. One common concern that pain practitioners have is that labeling a person as having a specific diagnosis of a chronic nature will strongly relate to the individual coping in maladaptive ways, which may lead to a state of chronicity (e.g., Abenhaim, Rossignol, & Gobeille, 1995). This phenomenon is commonly referred to as the "labeling effect." However, Fishbain (2003) disputes this position and states, "The patient with intractable pain needs to stop looking for a cure and thus stop doctor shopping. The patient needs to understand that they have a chronic condition which has no cure in most situations, but which can be managed" (p. 68).

Understandably, individuals who perceive that they cannot attain their goals in finding relief from their pain and who are unable to be flexible in accommodating negative stressors tend to have poorer psychological functioning (Brandtstadter & Renner, 1992). Thus, such individuals are also more likely to be depressed and to report greater levels of pain intensity and disability (Schmitz, Saile, & Nilges, 1996). Acceptance takes time, and this may mean that the patients come to accept a particular aspect of their condition, but not others at that time. Acceptance can be an ongoing process for many individuals with chronic pain. As professionals working with these patients, the key to their healing lies in the acknowledgment that the process is different for everyone.

Any psychotherapeutic interventions on our part will be futile if we ignore the bigger picture, which is that each individual has a unique history and present experience. We need to respect, honor, and accommodate treatments that fit each individual based on where the individual is in life. In addition, it is fundamental that we are cognizant of the fact that chronic pain and disability tend to alter one's self-image and body image. By nature, human beings are considered to be fundamentally meaning-making creatures (Baumeister, 1991). As the implications of the pain condition unfold, individuals will begin to consider the meaning of the losses associated with their pain in the broader context of their ongoing lives. The subjective meanings associated with interpersonal loss are evident on a continuum, which extends from relatively mundane appraisals, to concrete evaluations of specific problems caused by the loss, to deeper and more encompassing questions about emotional well-being and identity, to the most profound existential concerns about the meaning of life (Bonanno & Kaltman, 1999). In respecting that each individual copes with chronic pain differently, we will now address specific psychotherapeutic approaches in the practice of pain management.

PSYCHOTHERAPEUTIC INTERVENTIONS IN PAIN MANAGEMENT

COGNITIVE BEHAVIORAL THERAPY

Overview of Cognitive Behavioral Therapy in Pain Management

Cognitive behavioral therapy (CBT) for pain management is based on a cognitive-behavioral model of pain (Turk, Meichenbaum, & Genest, 1983) and has become the common standard of psychosocial intervention for pain (Morley, Eccleston, & Williams, 1999). Pain is defined in this model as a complex experience that is influenced not only by its underlying psychophysiology, but also by the individual's cognitions, affect, and behavior (Keefe & Gil, 1986). CBT is designed to reduce emotional distress and covert self-statements concerning pain. By altering negative self-talk, which directly reduces anxiety and/or depression, indirect modification of pain perception and tolerance will occur and allow the patient to increase activity levels and decrease medication use.

Several cognitive-behavioral models have been developed in which fear and avoidance variables were postulated as critical mechanisms by which acute pain develops into

chronic pain (Letham, Slade, Troup, & Bentley, 1983; Phillips, 1987; Waddell, Newton, Henderson, & Somerville, 1993). For example, Vlaeyen, Haazen, Schuerman, Kole-Snijders, and van Eek (1995a, 1995b) developed a cognitively oriented model in which pain catastrophizing and pain-related fear are central in the development of chronic pain. Pain catastrophizing promotes avoidance behavior and hypervigilance to bodily sensations, followed by disuse, depression, and disability. These factors then maintain the pain experience and reinforce fear reactions and avoidant behaviors (Asmundson, Norton, & Norton, 1999; Vlaeyan & Linton, 2000). Thorn, Boothby, and Sullivan (2002) developed a group treatment program specifically to reduce catastrophizing and promote adaptive coping. This program incorporates principles from stress management training (Meichenbaum, 1986), cognitive therapy for depression (Beck, 1995), communal coping methods (Coyne & Smith, 1991), and assertiveness training (Turk et al., 1983). By reducing catastrophizing and increasing adaptive coping, the patient's attention is diverted away from his or her pain and onto mastery of activities and achievement of tasks.

Application of CBT to Pain Management

In using CBT for pain management, there are three basic components involved in the treatment process. First, there must be a treatment rationale that helps patients understand that cognitions and behaviors can affect the pain experience (Holzman, Turk, & Kerns, 1986). This rationale must emphasize the role that patients can play in controlling their own pain. Psychoeducation is used to teach patients about the relationship between their thoughts, feelings, behaviors, and chronic pain. It is also the point at which a therapeutic alliance begins to build, and we explain the importance of a collaborative relationship with the patients. Thus, we emphasize to the patients that we will guide and support them, but that they will need to do the work in order to get better and find some relief from their pain. This part of the treatment also involves being very honest with patients and letting them know that while the treatment is very effective for most people, we are not trying to set up false hopes for them. It is at this point in treatment where we work with patients to derive attainable short- and long-term goals for management of their pain.

The second part of treatment involves coping-skills training to help patients manage their chronic pain. For instance, progressive relaxation and cue-controlled brief relaxation exercises are used to decrease tension, reduce emotional distress, and divert attention from pain. Pacing of activities and scheduling of pleasant events are used to help patients increase the levels and range of their activities. Training in distraction techniques such as pleasant imagery, counting methods, and use of a focal point can help patients learn to divert attention away from severe pain episodes. Cognitive restructuring is used to help patients identify and challenge overly negative pain-related thoughts and to replace these thoughts with more adaptive, coping thoughts. Cognitive restructuring emphasizes alteration of the patient's irrational beliefs through Socratic dialogue and rational self-examination of cognitive responses. Thus, an individual learns to discriminate irrational self-defeating thoughts from rational alternatives. Through this process, patients begin to generate more rational cognitive responses surrounding their pain experience and their capacity to manage it more effectively. Cognitive strategies may also address past illness experiences, learned patterns, and schemas related to personal and family developmental issues (Looper & Kirmayer, 2002).

Finally, the third component involves the application and maintenance of learned coping skills. During this phase of treatment, we encourage patients to apply their coping skills to a progressively wider range of daily situations. Patients learn to use behavioral techniques in place of illness behaviors such as help seeking, avoidance, and disability (Looper & Kirmayer, 2002). Strategies may include the following: graduated increases in activity to promote a return to prior functioning levels, desensitization and exposure techniques to treat avoidance, and response prevention to diminish maladaptive responses to distressing thoughts and situations. Problem-solving methods enable individuals with pain to analyze and develop plans for dealing with pain flares and other challenging situations. Teaching patients to self-monitor and hold to behavioral contracts can prompt and reinforce patients in frequently practicing these various coping skills and strategies.

CBT for pain management is typically carried out in small group (four to eight patients) sessions that are held weekly for 8 to 10 weeks. Numerous studies have shown that CBT generally decreases pain, improves functioning, and decreases physical and psychosocial disability among patients with chronic pain (Bradley et al., 1987; James, Thorn, & Williams, 1993; Keefe et al, 1990; Kole-Snijders et al., 1999; Syrjala, Donaldson, Davis, Kipps, & Carr, 1995; Thorn & Williams, 1993; Turner & Clancy, 1986, 1988; Vlaeyan, Haazen, Schuerman, Kole-Snijders, & van Eek, 1995). Thus, evidence suggests that CBT is effective in treating both chronic pain conditions, such as back pain, and persistent disease-related pain conditions, such as arthritis and cancer. However, as it does not benefit everyone, individual differences play a role in treatment success or failure (Thorn et al., 2002).

BEHAVIOR MODIFICATION/OPERANT CONDITIONING

Overview of Behavior Modification in Pain Management

The learning theory model of chronic pain emphasizes the role and importance of environmental factors in chronic

pain states (Fordyce, 1976). The most widely used definition of chronic pain looks at pain in terms of behavior, that is, how the person behaves and communicates his or her pain to others. In some patients, pain behaviors occur as a result of environmental contingencies rather than from antecedent stimuli, such as tissue damage. Behaviors originally respondent in nature can become operant through learning. This is a result of pain behaviors receiving direct positive reinforcement, or being negatively reinforced because they lead to avoidance of aversive situations, as well as non-reinforcement of activity related to "well behavior." The operant conditioning approach to chronic pain management demonstrates that all voluntary behaviors are influenced by their contingent consequences and the surrounding environment in which they occur (Sanders, 2003).

Anxiety has been identified as a part of the motivational-affective dimension of pain as discussed by Melzack and Torgerson (1971) in their three-component model of pain. The motivational-affective component compels an organism in pain to act in a way that relieves the aversive stimulation. Physical withdrawal, rest, and immobility are innate survival skills in acute pain, but are maladaptive in chronic pain. Often individuals in pain anticipate future increases in pain intensity and thus avoid physical activities that have previously been associated with increased pain. Another effect is the tendency to be "on guard" by tensing certain skeletal muscles or using protective movements and postures (Hanson & Gerber, 1990). Consistent guarding and decreases in physical movements and activities usually result in a physical deactivation syndrome, which is associated with increased levels of chronic pain and disability.

The goal of this operant approach to pain management is not to directly modify or "cure" pain, but to modify the maladaptive pain behaviors by extinction and to reinforce "well behavior" by teaching patients to be more functional in their environment despite their pain experience. The patient's experience of pain decreases significantly as a result of change in pain behavior and/or reduced levels of muscle tension. In Sanders' (2003) review of 30 studies during the past 25 years using operant and other behaviorally based therapies with patients with pain, clinically significant improvement was shown in physical functioning, activity, reduced analgesics, and subjective pain intensity ratings in the application of operant conditioning therapy for patients with low back pain. However, he noted a lack of research on the efficacy of operant approaches in other chronic pain states; other developmental age groups, such as pediatric and geriatric patients; and other cultural populations.

Application of Operant Conditioning to Pain Management

In essence, in using behavior therapy in the form of operant conditioning, we use "reinforcement" (both a procedure and a behavioral effect) to diminish ineffective coping strategies and to increase positive coping. The basic procedure is to follow a well-defined behavior with a consequence, which in turn leads to an increase in the frequency, strength, and duration of the behavior. For example, we can use positive reinforcement with patients by providing social attention with praise following active participation in physical therapy; this is likely to increase the probability of active participation in the next session. The reverse of reinforcement, extinction, may be used to reduce the frequency of an unwanted behavior.

In using extinction, we do a behavioral assessment to identify naturally occurring reinforcers that can be removed. We then remove those reinforcers to decrease the negative behaviors that patients are engaging in to "cope" with their chronic pain. For example, if pain behavior, as evidenced by grimacing or limping, co-occurs upon the solicitous attention of a partner, the partner is instructed to ignore and not attend to the person in pain when displaying such behaviors but to provide this attention only during socially appropriate, nonpain-related behavior. Over time, this will extinguish reinforcement of pain behavior as a means of communication in the relationship.

The implementation of rehearsal in behavioral treatment emphasizes the importance of practicing and consolidating those skills learned in sessions. Rehearsal techniques can include mental practice, role-playing, and role reversal (Holtzman & Turk, 1986). For example, individuals with chronic pain may role-play an employment interview with their therapist to answer questions about missed periods of work or a conversation with their spouse to negotiate changing household roles. To increase the likelihood of successful behavior change, we can assign homework to patients so that they can practice skills learned during treatment sessions (Turk et al., 1983). Homework assignments could use various modalities, such as written exercises, behavioral skills to practice in specific situations or with certain people, or mental practice of affirmative self-statements or images.

STRESS INOCULATION TRAINING

Overview of Stress Inoculation Training in Pain Management

Within the coping literature, the term *stress* has been defined by the transactional view of stress and coping conceived by Lazarus and Folkman (1984). This viewpoint addressed the efforts people make, regardless of whether those efforts are successful. Losses, threats, and other stressful demands, such as the pain itself, are appraised cognitively along with available coping resources. Based on this appraisal process, specific coping responses are used to focus either on the perceived problem or on the resulting emotional reactions. Because of the importance placed on appraisal processes, cognitive therapy to address maladaptive thinking patterns influencing the perception of pain is part of the standard of care.

More recently, the psychophysiological interconnection between the mind and body have been referred to as *allostatic load* rather than the historical term *stress* (Ray, 2004). Allostasis refers to the psychophysiological system of communication between the brain, endocrine system, and the immune system (McEwen, 2002). Allostatic load, or stress, occurs when there is an inadequate match between an individual's coping skills and the environmental demands that the individual believes these skills must confront. Patients with pain must learn the cyclical relationship in which stress increases pain and increased pain, in turn, is a stressor. Pain is just one stressor among many, and only one source of their suffering. Training on coping skills focuses on helping patients to separate pain from other sources of stress and that which they are unable to control.

Application of Stress Inoculation Training to Pain Management

Stress inoculation training (SIT) helps clients cope with stress by teaching them coping skills and then having them practice the skills while they are exposed to stress-evoking events (Meichenbaum & Turk, 1976). Stress inoculation therapy is commonly used for treating anxiety, anger, and pain. The treatment consists of three phases: conceptualization, coping skills acquisition, and application. Stress inoculation is a behavioral analogue of biological immunization. Thus, the coping skills clients learn can be considered "psychological antibodies," which increase resistance to potentially stress-evoking events.

In using SIT with patients, we teach them to view coping as a four-part process. We have summarized these as 4 Cs, and they are listed below.

1. *Consideration* of preparing for a pain episode
2. *Confronting* and handling the pain
3. *Coping* with feelings at critical moments
4. *Consistently* practicing reinforcement to increase effective pain management

SELF-DIRECTED TREATMENT

Overview of Self-Directed Treatment in Pain Management

Self-directed treatment broadens pain management to permit individual responsibility for as much of the treatment of pain and maintenance of health as is possible. Self-management training primarily focuses on changing thoughts (cognitions) and actions (behaviors), which in turn changes negative emotions and pain sensations. Goals of self-management include the following: (1) improving the ability to divert attention away from pain sensations through activities and mental techniques, (2) improving overall physical conditioning, (3) improving pacing of daily activities, and (4) learning how to manage depression, anger, pain flares, and interpersonal conflict more effectively (Hanson & Gerber, 1990; Turk et al., 1983). The advantage to using a self-directed treatment approach lies in the greater specificity of therapy procedures, which enhances the uniformity of training and evaluation, client-centered control, and the probability of maintaining therapeutic effects after contact with the provider has ended.

Application of Self-Directed Treatment to Pain Management

Self-directed treatment goals are typically framed in the context of life-long learning as individuals learn healthy patterns of responding and continue to adjust their goals as interpersonal and environmental changes occur in their lives. This approach involves the following components:

1. *Physical*: Exercise regimen, use of proper body mechanics, appropriate rest, and use of analgesics when warranted, decreasing pain behaviors such as guarding and bracing
2. *Emotional*: Using positive self-statements, enhancing self-efficacy
3. *Cognitive-Behavioral*: Relaxation training, distraction techniques for pain flare-ups, reduction of maladaptive self-statements (i.e., catastrophizing, wishful thinking)

Note. Goals adapted and modified from Jensen et al. (1994), Loeser and Turk (2001), and Jensen, Nielson, and Kerns (2003).

Self-instructional training can be used in pain management. This approach focuses primarily on covert responses rather than hypothesized belief systems and thought processes (Meichenbaum, 1986). The patient gradually learns to use self-instructions and replace maladaptive self-statements with adaptive coping self-statements. In self-instructional training, individuals learn to instruct themselves to cope effectively with difficult situations. Self-instructions serve to prepare individuals to focus attention, guide behavior, provide encouragement, evaluate performance, and reduce anxiety. The five steps of self-instructional training are (1) cognitive modeling, (2) cognitive participant modeling, (3) overt self-instructions, (4) fading of overt self-instructions, and (5) covert self-instructions.

TREATMENTS FOR INSOMNIA RELATED TO CHRONIC PAIN

Overview of Treatments for Insomnia in Pain Management

Sleep disturbance has been associated with chronic pain across a variety of diagnostic groups, such as headaches, fibromyalgia, and Sjögren's syndrome (Burckhardt et al., 1997; Perlis et al., 1997; Tishler, Barak, Paran, & Yaron, 1997); rheumatoid arthritis (Stone, Broderick, Porter, & Kaell, 1997); osteoarthritis and back pain (Hyyppa & Kronholm, 1995; Ingernarsson, Sivik, & Nordholm, 1996). However, despite this association, the causal relationship between sleep disturbances and pain remains unknown. Multiple types of sleep disturbance have been identified across chronic pain populations and may include difficulty falling asleep, difficulty staying asleep, early awakening, and interrupted sleep. Lack of sleep has long been associated with daytime fatigue (Dinges et al., 1997). Depression may potentiate pain and sleep disturbances, although that relationship is neither consistent nor linear. Depression has been associated with frequent awakenings and decreased quality of sleep (Burckhardt et al., 1997).

A review of the merits of behavioral interventions in improving outcomes in the treatment of pain and insomnia demonstrated the efficacy of multiple behavioral treatments (National Institutes of Health, 1990). The degree of functional impairments and associated economic costs of the suffering and distress associated with these disorders led the panel to conclude, "Conventional medical and surgical approaches have failed — at considerable expense — to adequately address these problems" (p. 3).

Application of Treatments for Insomnia to Pain Management

Relaxation and behavioral approaches for the treatment of insomnia in patients with chronic pain include sleep hygiene (Turner, 1986), stimulus control therapy (Bootzin & Nicassio, 1978), and sleep restriction therapy (Spielman, Saskin, & Thorpy, 1987). When administered by experienced clinicians as part of a complete treatment program, behavioral interventions can produce reductions in sleep-related symptoms for up to 73% of patients with insomnia referred for treatment (Chambers & Alexander, 1991). Behavioral techniques primarily provide improvements in sleep latency and time awake after sleep onset.

Sleep restriction, stimulus control, and multimodal treatment were the three most effective treatments in reducing insomnia. In using the technique of stimulus control, we use cueing strategies to gradually reduce and eliminate stimuli that are likely to elicit undesirable behaviors; conversely, we increase stimuli that are likely to elicit desirable behaviors. For example, we may instruct the patient to fall asleep at specified times and places, while excluding other activities, such as watching television, reading, or worrying. Inconsistencies in the assessment measures of insomnia and the lack of established criteria for what constitutes a therapeutic outcome reveal the need for the use of valid objective measures of insomnia, more meaningful outcome criteria relevant to a patient's quality of life, and empirically established guidelines for the selection of treatment techniques (Chambers, 1992).

ADJUNCTIVE TREATMENTS

Behavioral medicine focuses on altering behavior or physiology to enhance medical treatment. Relaxation training and biofeedback specifically address changing the physiological response of the sympathetic nervous system in response to pain stimuli.

An integrated adjunctive treatment approach may include use of biofeedback and various forms of relaxation training, which can incorporate the three major sources of data — physiological, self-report, and behavioral observations. Application of these treatments are not discussed, because it is discussed in a separate chapter of this book.

RELAPSE PREVENTION FOR CHRONIC PAIN

Overview of Relapse Prevention in Pain Management

Turk, Holzman, and Kerns (1987) modified the relapse prevention approach applied to addictive behaviors for use with chronic pain to help individuals learn to identify and successfully cope with factors that might trigger pain flares. Such an approach allows the patient to anticipate and plan for future events. It also provides the individual with the expectation that although minor setbacks may in fact occur, they do not signal complete failure. Setbacks are considered as means of implementing coping skills previously learned in a more effective manner. As the patient generalizes the use of learned coping skills across problem situations that arise in his or her experience with chronic pain, greater perceived self-efficacy will occur. Ultimately, this will directly affect the expectation that changes will be maintained.

Application of Treatments for Relapse Prevention to Pain Management

Maintaining and generalizing learned skills requires practice and graduated, stepwise increases in behavior across different situations. Similar to the treatment for phobias, based on exposure to fear-arousing stimuli, alternative coping behaviors must be substituted for the maladaptive avoidant tendencies typically used in patients experiencing pain.

Exposure and relapse prevention strategies for chronic pain include six steps, which we have summarized as the 3Es/3Rs method. Thus, patients with pain

can reduce the risk of relapse by applying the following to their everyday lives:

1. *Eliminating* habit-forming central nervous system medications
2. *Exposing* themselves gradually to previously avoided physical activities
3. *Exercising* to physically recondition and reduce postural guarding
4. *Relaxing* by using techniques such as diaphragmatic breathing, progressive muscle relaxation, visualization, guided imagery, meditation, yoga, and body self-awareness to decrease muscle tension
5. *Reinforcing* themselves in a positive manner for successful behaviors and interactions with others
6. *Rethinking* things by using cognitive-behavioral strategies during increased pain flares

Note. List adapted and modified from Hanson & Gerber (1990).

BARRIERS TO EFFECTIVE PAIN MANAGEMENT

ADHERENCE AND COMPLIANCE ISSUES

Poor adherence to treatment has historically been a major and costly problem. An estimated 50 to 55% of patients with chronic medical conditions fail to adequately adhere to their treatment regimens (Rapoff, 1999). Turk and Rudy (1991) note the negative effects of non-adherence in the chronic pain population include a greater number of medical emergencies, increased number and strength of prescriptions, worsening of disability and prognosis, increased likelihood of secondary complications, and suboptimal recovery following injury.

There is speculation, but little available documentation, that a substantial proportion of present-day health care costs could be significantly reduced by improving patient compliance. Clinicians and researchers may erroneously conclude that therapeutic trials are ineffective when they fail to recognize, identify, and control for compliance. Reviews of the literature have revealed no clear or consistent patterns in the association of demographic variables with adherence (Kaplan & Simon, 1990; Meichenbaum & Turk, 1987). Clay and Hopps (2003), in their review of the literature, found no studies that addressed the factors governing treatment refusals, premature terminations, or receipt of fewer treatment sessions than prescribed, even though these circumstances occur with regularity in pain management. They advocate for the treatment of choice, and its delivery must be customized to the lifestyle and personality of the patient.

When speaking of noncompliance, the focus is often on the individual and his or her characteristics. When talking of adherence, the focus is on what people do. This shift of perspective led researchers away from the study of attributes or character to studies of behavioral cues, triggers, and consequences (Gatchel, 1999). The treatment of chronic pain is often perceived by health care professionals as complex, demanding, and challenging. Problematic family and work relationships, conflicts with health care providers, and ongoing battles with the disability compensation system are common co-occurrences. There has been extensive research to no avail to identify predictors of personality and psychosocial factors that predispose individuals to problems with chronic pain (Gatchel & Weisberg, 2000). In fact, these efforts have been challenged extensively (Gatchel, 1991; Turk & Salovey, 1984) given the lack of empirical support.

Hendler (1984) initially described a four-stage response to chronic pain that paralleled the stages of dying described by Kubler-Ross (1969). In the acute state (0 to 2 months), the individual expects to get well and is without psychological changes. During the second pain stage (2 to 6 months), the person begins to get anxious as a transient response to continued pain. When chronic pain persists beyond 6 months, depression ensues with the realization that the pain may be permanent. In the acceptance stage, which could take from 3 to 12 years from onset of pain, the individual becomes reconciled to the need to make accommodations for coping with chronic pain.

Gatchel (1991, 1999; Gatchel & Weisberg, 2000) later proposed a three-stage model of developmental changes that occur in an individual in response to pain. As pain or hurt is associated with harm, Stage 1 is associated with the emotional reactions as a consequence of the perception of pain, such as fear, anxiety, and worry. If the pain persists beyond a 2 to 4 month course, the time period when acute pain typically resolves, the individual progresses to Stage 2 in which a wider array of behavioral and psychological reactions occur. These reactions, such as depression or anger, depend on the preexisting psychological characteristics of the individual, as well as the environmental conditions, such as social or economic supports. The model presumes a general nonspecificity in terms of the relationship between personality, psychological problems, and pain rather than an inherent personality type associated with the development of chronic pain. The persistence of psychological and behavioral problems then leads to Stage 3, which results in the acceptance of the "sick role." This assumption of the "sick role" serves as a powerful reinforcer for disability. If compensation issues are present, these serve as further disincentives for becoming well. Compensation has been found to be a critical factor in the persistence of disabilities (Beals, 1984). Mayer and Gatchel (1988) also found that physical deconditioning, in which disuse and subsequent atrophy of the injured area result in physical incapacity, serves as an interaction variable to reduce psychological well-being and self-esteem and thus maintain the pain cycle.

The prevalence of personality disorders is higher in patients with chronic pain (Gatchel, Garofolo, Ellis, & Holt, 1996; Livengood & Johnson, 1998; Weisberg & Keefe, 1997) than in the general population, although it is similar to rates found within the outpatient psychiatric population (Weisberg, Vittengl, Clark, Gatchel, & Gorin, 2000).

The diasthesis-stress model (Weisberg & Keefe, 1997) was postulated as an explanation for the emergence of personality disorders activated by the stress of chronic pain when no such disorder was found to be present on examinations of patients' premorbid functioning. The model has been applied to various chronic pain populations (Banks & Kerns, 1996; Dworkin & Banks, 1999; Flor & Turk, 1994; Turk & Flor, 1984; Weisberg & Keefe, 1997). The diasthesis is the underlying personality predisposition that is activated by the extreme stress of pain and its physical, psychological, and social consequences. Turk and Salovey (1984) suggest that low back pain develops when stress and sympathetic arousal become activated in an individual who has a predisposition to develop hyperactive back muscles, has inadequate coping resources, and experiences recurrent problems, such as family or work stressors. As the pain cycle begins, with pain as an additive factor to these already existing issues, muscle tension increases and the cycle is maintained. The relevance of this model to multidisciplinary treatment in general, and psychotherapy in particular, is the importance of shifting the focus from the personality deficit of the individual to the situational context in which the behaviors are being expressed and maintained (Weisberg et al., 2000).

Research indicates that it is futile to attempt to define a noncompliant personality; thus, the task remains to identify those individuals who are the least likely to adhere and focus on intervention efforts to improve their adherence rates. Physicians and health care providers tend to poorly predict which of their patients will comply, although they often assume that they can identify potentially noncompliant patients by their patient's educational level, income, gender, or personality. One survey indicated that 76% of physicians attributed non-adherence to one or more of these characteristics, but in fact the accuracy of predictions based on these variables is no better than chance (Meichenbaum & Turk, 1987). In general, there are no characteristics that consistently identify noncompliant patients, with one exception: Across all studies and all diseases, individuals who are experiencing depression or psychological distress tend to be less compliant with treatment (Chesney, 1997).

One of the most consistent findings of research on compliance is that there is a direct association between poor compliance and the extent to which an assigned regimen interferes with daily life, the complexity of drug regimens, the number of specific medications that are prescribed, and poor communication between patient and provider (Dunbar-Jacob, Burke, & Puczynski, 1995). Clinicians can promote compliance by providing patients with tools that will help them achieve and maintain a high level of compliance, by devising dosing schedules that can be integrated into their patients' daily routines, and by encouraging compliance in every encounter with every patient (Chesney, 1997).

Rapoff (1999) has proposed a model of treatment adherence that specifically addressed the importance of treatment characteristics, such as the face validity, duration, and complexity of the treatment regimen; the deviation required from normal routine; adverse side effects of medication; technical skills required; and the self-awareness needed to implement treatment. Clay and Hopps (2003) focused on treatment accommodations for rehabilitation patients, which refers to the extent to which a specific treatment is adaptable to better fit into the unique and complex lifestyles and limitations of patients. Providers must focus on the values and desired outcome of the patient and the content of the treatment.

The purpose and goals of treatment must reflect the values and desired outcomes of the patient and family (Clay & Hopps, 2003). Pain rehabilitation providers generally establish treatment goals that include optimal medical outcomes (i.e., decreased pain intensity, and maximization of physical functioning and functional capacity). Our aim as clinician should be to encourage patients to make the goals as achievable as possible while still demanding some change.

TREATMENT GOAL SETTING TO IMPROVE COMPLIANCE/ADHERENCE

It cannot be stressed enough how important goal setting is in the treatment process, particularly with patients with chronic pain. As stated earlier, building strong rapport with the patient and establishing a collaborative therapeutic alliance will serve not only to build trust in the patient, but also to increase the patient's motivation and sense of self-efficacy and mastery. Therefore, we recommend the following suggestions that may help increase adherence and compliance, and ultimately help the patients heal and manage their chronic pain more effectively.

Goals should therefore be

Specific: Well-defined goals must be written in terms of what clients will be doing rather than what they will not be doing or thinking. Goals should be broken down into the short and long terms and should be as specific and detailed as possible.
Personal: Goals should be written so that patients know they are in control of fulfilling and meeting those goals, irrespective of other people.

Additionally, goals should be described in the patient's language to ensure that we are working toward a goal that the patient wants, not what we want or what we think the patient should want.
Present-focused: Goals should be anchored in the here-and-now so that the patient can start the solution immediately.

Along with monitoring goal progress throughout treatment, it is also important to assess and monitor the patient's motivation for pain management, or readiness to change, as patients must engage in an active role to manage their pain. Readiness to change was first proposed by Prochaska, DiClemente, and Norcross (1992) who developed the transtheoretical model of behavior change to integrate existing models of psychotherapy into a single model of positive change. Five stages of change were delineated: precontemplation, contemplation, preparation, action, and maintenance. Individuals who change their behavior use different behavior change strategies to progress from one stage to the next.

Motivational interviewing (MI) is a therapeutic approach, based on Prochaska's transtheoretical model, to help clients address and resolve feelings of ambivalence about initiating positive behavioral changes. According to Miller and Rollnick (2002), there are three critical components of motivation: importance (value or incentives), confidence (self-efficacy), and readiness. Change is more likely to occur in a collaborative relationship in which each of these components is elicited from the patient. Despite its efficacy having been demonstrated in other patient populations, no study to date has yet directly tested the efficacy of MI-based treatments for enhancing the efficacy of chronic pain treatment.

Individuals living with chronic pain vary in their degree of readiness to adopt a self-management approach to their chronic pain. Kerns and Rosenberg (2000) have proposed that understanding a patient's stage of change might predict both engagement in self-management strategies and outcomes of these interventions. The measurement of pain stages of change has lent support to the relevance of the model in understanding the processes of engagement, adherence, and change during self-management treatments for chronic pain (Biller, Arnstein, Caudill, Federman, & Guberman, 2000; Dijkstra et al., 2001; Jensen, Nielson, & Kerns, 2003; Jensen, Nielson, Romano, Hill, & Turner, 2000; Keefe, Lefebvre, Kerns, Rosenberg, Beaupre, Prochaska et al., 2000; Nielson, Jensen & Kerns, 2003).

Jensen et al. (2003) developed a preliminary model of understanding motivation for chronic pain self-directed treatment and the implications for enhancing adherence to chronic pain treatment. They define motivation as the readiness to change pain, and postulate that patients will engage in specific pain self-management strategies as a function of their readiness to use these strategies. Readiness is influenced by the individuals' beliefs both about the importance of and about their ability to engage in pain self-management behaviors. Nielson et al. (2003) have demonstrated that readiness to adopt a self-management approach to pain might be multidimensional in nature. Other researchers believe that the commitment to the learning and application of skills more accurately reflects a continuum of change rather than a stepwise movement through discrete changes (Bandura, 1997; Little & Girvin, 2002).

Interventions for compliance and health behavior change have included strong educational components and behavioral strategies for change and maintenance. For health behavior interventions, specific interventions for pain management, such as pacing activities and relaxation training, can benefit from the basic research and intervention developments within these respective content areas (Dubbert, 2002). Research based on an understanding of the factors involved in the persuasion, social influence, and social control must be directed at educational strategies to alter patients' values, expectations, and belief systems.

SUMMARY

Psychotherapeutic interventions in the management of chronic pain typically involve a cognitive-behavioral approach. The cognitive-behavioral model of chronic pain integrates the physical, psychological, and behavioral aspects of the chronic pain experience. Assessment should be an ongoing process throughout treatment. Interventions are oriented toward the assumption of patients' responsibility for self-management of pain and maintenance of their health. A comprehensive multimodal approach, as reviewed in Turk and Rudy (1994), should include education, skills acquisition, cognitive and behavioral rehearsal, homework, and generalization and maintenance. As clinicians, our primary objective is to assist patients in learning self-regulation and self-control skills, while shaping the patient to owning greater personal responsibility for lifestyle habit changes.

It is crucial that we, as clinicians, understand that treatment of chronic pain cannot operate in a vacuum. By integrating psychotherapeutic interventions with a multidisciplinary approach, not only will we help our patients to better manage their chronic pain, but in addition we will help facilitate their healing from other problems or painful life experiences that have resulted in emotional pain and turmoil. This, as a whole, is effective pain management.

REFERENCES

Abenhaim, L., Rossignol, M., & Gobeille, D. (1995). The prognostic consequences in the making of the initial medical diagnosis of work-related injuries. *Spine, 20*, 791–795.

Abramson, L.Y., Garber, J., & Seligman, M. E. (1980). Learned helplessness in humans: An attributional analysis. In J. Garber & M. E. Seligman (Eds.), *Human helplessness: Theory and application*. New York: Academic Press.

Altmaier, E. M. (1993). Role of self-efficacy in rehabilitation outcome among chronic low back pain patients. *Journal of Clinical Psychology, 40*, 335–339.

American Psychiatric Association. (2000). *Diagnostic and statistical manual of mental disorders*. (4th ed, Text Revision). Washington D.C.: Author.

Asmundson, G. J., Bonin, M. F., Frombach, I. K., & Norton, G. R. (2000). Evidence of a disposition toward fearfulness and vulnerability to posttraumatic stress in dysfunctional pain patients. *Behaviour Research and Therapy, 38*, 801–812.

Asmundson, G. J. G., Norton, P. J. & Norton, G. R. (1999). Beyond pain: The role of fear and avoidance in chronicity. *Clinical Psychology Review, 19*, 97–119.

Ballenger, J. C., Davidson, J. R., Lecrubier, Y., Nutt, D. J., Foa, E. B., Kessler, R. C., et al.(2000). Consensus statement on posttraumatic stress disorder from the international consensus group on depression and anxiety. *Journal of Clinical Psychiatry, 61*(Suppl. 5), 60–66.

Bandura, A. (1997). The anatomy of stages of change. *American Journal of Health Promotion, 12,* 8–10.

Banks, S. M., & Kerns, R. D. (1996). Explaining the high rates of depression in chronic pain: A diathesis-stress framework. *Psychological Bulletin, 119*(1), 95–110.

Baumeister, R. F. (1991). *Meanings of life*. New York: Guilford Press.

Beals, R. (1984). Compensation and recovery from injury. *Western Journal of Medicine, 140*, 233–237.

Beck, J. S. (1995). *Cognitive therapy: Basics and beyond*. New York: Guilford Press.

Ben-Sira, Z. (1991). *Regression, stress, and readjustment in aging: A structured biopsychosocial perspective on coping and professional support*. New York: Praeger Publishers.

Biller, N., Arnstein, P., Caudill, M., Federman, C., & Guberman, C. (2000). Predicting completion of a cognitive-behavioral pain management program by initial measures of a chronic pain patient's readiness for change. *Clinical Journal of Pain, 16*, 352–359.

Blanchard, E. B., Hickling, E. J., Mitnick, N., Taylor, A. E., Loos, W. R., & Buckley, T. C. (1995). The impact of severity of physical injury and perception of life threat in the development of post-traumatic stress disorder in motor vehicle accident victims. *Behavior Research and Therapy, 33*, 529–534.

Blanchard-Fields, F., & Irion, J. C. (1988). The relation between locus of control and coping in two contexts: Age as a moderator variable. *Psychology of Aging, 3* (2), 197–203.

Bonanno, G. A., & Kaltman, S. (1999). Toward an integrative perspective on bereavement. *Psychological Bulletin, 125*(6), 760–776.

Bootzin, R. R., & Nicassio, P. M. (1978). Behavioral treatments for insomnia. In M. Herson, R. M. Eisler, & P. M. Miller (Eds.), *Progress in behavior modification* (Vol. 6, pp. 1–45). New York: Academic Press.

Bradley, L. A., Young, L. D., Andeerson, J. O., Turner, R. A., Agudelo, C. A., McDaniel, L. K. et al. (1987). Effects of psychological therapy on pain behavior of rheumatoid arthritis patients: Treatment outcome and six-month follow-up. *Arthritis & Rheumatism, 30*, 1105–1114.

Brandtstadter, J., & Renner, G. (1992). Coping with discrepancies between aspirations and achievements in adult development: A dual-process model. In L. Montada, S. H. Filipp, & M. J. Lerner (Eds.), *Crises and experiences of loss in adulthood*. Hilsdale, NJ: Erlbaum.

Brown, G. K., & Nicassio, P. M. (1987). The development of a questionnaire for the assessment of active and passive coping strategies in chronic pain patients. *Pain, 31*, 53–65.

Brown, G. K., Nicassio, P. M., & Wallston, K. A. (1989). Pain coping strategies and depression in rheumatoid arthritis. *Journal of Consulting and Clinical Psychology, 57*(5), 652–7.

Buckley, T. C., Blanchard, E. B., & Hickling, E. J. (1996). A prospective examination of delayed onset PTSD secondary to motor vehicle accidents. *Journal of Abnormal Psychology, 105*(4), 617–625.

Buda, M., & Tsuang, M. T. (1981). The epidemiology of suicide: Implications for clinical practice. In S. Blumenthal & D. J. Kupfer (Eds), *Suicide over the life cycle: Risk factors, assessments, and treatments of suicide patients*. Washington, DC: American Psychiatric Press.

Burckhardt, C. S., Clark, S. R., O'Reilly, C. A., & Bennen, R. M. (1997). Pain coping strategies of women with fibromyalgia: Relationship to pain, sleep and quality of life. *Journal of Musculoskeletal Pain, 5*(3), 5–20.

Burns, J. W., Johnson, B. J., Mahoney, N., Devine, J., & Pawl, R. (1998). Cognitive and physical capacity process variables predict long-term outcome after treatment of chronic pain. *Journal of Consulting and Clinical Psychology, 66*, 434–439.

Butler, D. J., Moffic, H. S., & Turkal, N. W. (1999, August). Posttraumatic stress reactions following motor vehicle accidents. *American Family Physician* (online edition).

Carpenito, L. (1989). *Handbook of nursing diagnoses* (3rd ed). Philadelphia: Lippincott.

Chambers, M. J. (1992). Therapeutic issues in the treatment of insomnia. *Professional Psychology: Research and Practice, 23* (2), 131–138.

Chambers, M. J., & Alexander, S. (1991). Insomnia treatment outcome: Factor analysis of a follow-up questionnaire. *Sleep Research, 20*, 222.

Chesney, M. (1997, June). Compliance: How physicians can help. *HIV Newsline*.

Chibnall, J. T., & Duckro, P. N. (1994). Posttraumatic stress disorder in chronic posttraumatic headache patients. *Headache, 34*, 357 –361.

Clay, D. L. & Hopps, J.A. (2003). Treatment adherence in rehabilitation: The role of treatment accommodation. *Rehabilitation Psychology, 48* (3), 215–219.

Coyne, J. C., & Smith, D. A. (1991). Couples coping with myocardial infarction: A contextual perspective on wives' distress. *Journal of Personality and Social Psychology, 61*, 404–412.

Crisson, J. E., & Keefe, F. J. (1988). The relationship of locus of control to pain coping strategies and psychological distress in chronic pain patients. *Pain, 35*, 147–154.

Damasio, A. R. (1994). A passion for reasoning. *Descartes' error: Emotion, reason, and the human brain*. New York: Avon Books.

DeCarvalho, L. T. (2001). *The nature of the traumatic event as a predictor of posttraumatic stress disorder in chronic low back pain patients*. Loma Linda, CA: Loma Linda University.

DeCarvalho, L. T. (2004, Feb.). Predictors of posttraumatic stress disorder symptom severity level in chronic low back pain patients. *Dissertation Abstracts International, B 64/08, p. 4030*.

DeCarvalho, L. T. (submitted). Perceived pain severity as a predictor of PTSD in chronic low back pain patients. *Journal of Traumatic Stress*.

DelVecchio-Good, M., Brodwin, P. E., Good, B. J., & Kleinman, A. (Eds.). (1992). *Pain as human experience: An anthropological perspective*. Berkeley, CA: University of California Press.

Deyo, R. A. (1988). Measuring the functional status of patients with low back pain. *Archives of Physical Medicine and Rehabilitation, 69*, 1044–1053.

Dijkstra, A., Vlaeyan, J., Rijnen, H., & Nielson, W. (2001). Readiness to adopt the self-management approach to cope with chronic pain in fibromyalgia patients. *Pain, 90*, 37–45.

Dinges, D. F. (1995). An overview of sleepiness and accidents. *Journal of Sleep Research, 4* (S2), 4–14.

Dubbert, P. (2002). Exercise. *Journal of Consulting and Clinical Psychology, 70*, 526–536.

Dunbar-Jacob J., Burke L. E., & Puczynski S. (1995). Clinical assessment and management of adherence to medical regimens. In P. M. Nicassio and T. W. Smith (Eds.), *Managing chronic illness* (pp. 313–350). Washington, D.C.: American Psychological Association.

Dworkin, R., & Banks, S. (1999). A vulnerability-diathesis-stress model of chronic pain: Herpes zoster and the development of postherpetic neuralgia. In R. J. Gatchel & D. C. Turk (Eds.), *Psychosocial factors in pain* (pp. 247–269). New York: Guilford Press.

Fields, H. (1987). *Pain*. New York: McGraw-Hill.

Fishbain, D. A. (1986). Suicide pacts and homicide. *American Journal of Psychiatry, 143*, 1319–1320.

Fishbain, D. A. (2003). Aspects of the chronic pain history and its application to treatment decisions. In T. S. Jensen, P. R. Wilson, & A. S. Rice (Eds.). *Clinical pain management: Chronic pain* (pp. 63–88). New York: Oxford University Press, Inc.

Fishbain, D. A., Goldberg, M., Meagher, B. R., & Rosomoff, H. (1986). Male and female chronic pain patients categorized by DSM-III psychiatric diagnostic criteria. *Pain, 26*, 181–97.

Fishbain, D. A., Goldberg, M., Rosomoff, R. S., & Rosomoff, H. (1991). Completed suicide in chronic pain. *Clinical Journal of Pain, 7* (1), 29–36.

Flor, H. & Turk, D. C. (1984). Etiological theories and treatments for chronic pain. I. Somatic models and interventions. *Pain, 19*, 105–121.

Fordyce, W. E. (1976). Behavioral methods for chronic pain and illness. Mosby: St. Louis.

Fuerst, M. L. (1993). Doctors and suicide. *American Health, 12* (3), 25.

Gatchel, R. J. (1991). Early development of physical and mental deconditioning in painful spinal disorders. In T. G. Mayer, V. Mooney & R. J. Gatchel (Eds.), *Contemporary conservative care for painful spinal disorders* (pp. 278–289). Philadelphia: Lea & Febiger.

Gatchel, R. J. (1999). Perspectives on pain: A historical overview. In R. J. Gatchel & D. C. Turk (Eds.), *Psychosocial factors in pain: Critical perspectives* (pp. 3–17). New York: Guilford Press.

Gatchel, R. J. & Weisberg, J. N. (Eds.). (2000). *Personality characteristics of patients with pain*. Washington, D.C.: American Psychological Association.

Gatchel, R. J., Garofolo, J. P., Ellis, E., & Holt, C. (1996). Major psychological disorders in acute and chronic TMD: An initial examination. *Journal of the American Dental Association, 127*, 1365–1374.

Geisser, M. E., Roth, R. S., Bachman, J. E., & Eckert, T. A. (1996). The relationship between symptoms of post-traumatic stress disorder and pain, affective disturbance and disability among patients with accident and non-accident related pain. *Pain, 66*, 207–214.

Gibson, S. J., & Helme, R. D. (2000). Cognitive factors and the experience of pain and suffering in older persons. *Pain, 85*, 375–383.

Grigsby, J., & Hartlaub, G. (1994). Procedural learning and the development and stability of character. *Perceptual and Motor Skills, 79*, 355–370.

Hanson, R. W. & Gerber, K. E. (1990). *Coping with chronic pain: A guide to patient self-management*. New York: Guilford Press.

Hawthorn, J., & Redmond, K. (1998). *Pain: Causes and management*. Malden, MA: Blackwell Science.

Haythornthwaite, J. A., Sieber, W. J., & Kerns, R. D. (1991). Depression and the chronic pain experience. *Pain, 46*, 177–184.

Hearst, N., Newman, T. B., & Hulley, S. B. (1986). Delayed effects of the military draft on mortality: A randomized natural experiment. *New England Journal of Medicine, 314*, 620–624.

Heller, B. W., Flohr, L. M., & Zegans, L. S. (Eds). (1989). *Psychosocial interventions with physically disabled persons*. Piscataway, NJ: Rutgers University Press.

Helzer, J. E., Robins, L. N., & McEnvoi, L. (1987). Post-traumatic stress disorder in the general population. *New England Journal of Medicine, 317*, 1630–1634.

Hendin, H., & Haas, A. P. (1991). Suicide and guilt as manifestations of PTSD in Vietnam combat veterans. *American Journal of Psychiatry, 148*, 586–591.

Hendler, N. H. (1984). Depression caused by chronic pain. *Journal of Clinical Psychiatry, 45*, 30–36.

Hendler, N. (1989). Validating and treating the complaint of chronic back pain: The Mensana Clinic approach. In P. Black (Ed.), *Clinical Neurosurgery* (pp. 385–397). Baltimore: Williams and Wilkins.

Hendler, N., & Kozikowski, J. (1993). Overlooked physical diagnoses in chronic pain patients involved in litigation. *Psychosomatics, 34* (6), 494–501

Hendler, N., Bergson, C. and Morrison, C. (1996). Overlooked physical diagnoses in chronic pain patients involved in litigation, part 2. *Psychosomatics, 37* (6), 509–517.

Herman, J. L. (1992). Complex PTSD: A syndrome in survivors of prolonged and repeated trauma. *Journal of Traumatic Stress, 5* (3), 377–391.

Hickling, E. J., & Blanchard, E. B. (1992). Post-traumatic stress disorder and motor vehicle accidents. *Journal of Anxiety Disorders, 6*, 285–291.

Holtzman, A. D. & Turk, D. C. (1986). *Pain management: A handbook of psychological treatment approaches*. Elmsford, NY: Pergamon Press.

Holzman, A. D., Turk, D. C., & Kerns, R. D. (1986). The cognitive-behavioral approach to the management of chronic pain. In A. D. Holzman & D. C. Turk (Eds.), *Pain management: A handbook of psychological treatment approaches*. New York: Pergamon Press.

Hyyppa, M. T., & Kronholm, E. (1995). Poor sleep among rehabilitation patients. *International Journal of Rehabilitation and Health, 1* (4), 237–245.

Ingemarsson, A. H., Sivik, T., & Nordholm, L. (1996). Sick leave among patients with lumbar and cervical pain: Relationship to sick leave, education, nationality, sleep disturbance and experience of pain. *Physiotherapy Theory and Practice, 12*, 143–149.

Ivey, A. E., Ivey, M. B., & Simek-Morgan, L. (1993). *Counseling and psychotherapy: A multicuultural perspective*. (3rd ed.). Boston: Allyn & Bacon.

James, L. D., Thorn, B. E., & Williams, D. A. (1993). Goal specification in cognitive behavioral therapy for chronic headache pain. *Behavior Therapy, 24*, 305–320.

Jensen, M. P., Nielson, W. R., & Kerns, R. D. (2003). Toward the development of a motivational model of pain self-management. *Journal of Pain, 4* (9), 477–492.

Jensen, M. P., Nielson, W. R., Romano, J., Hill, M., & Turner, J. (2000). Further evidence of the Pain Stages of Change Questionnaire: Is the transtheoretical model of change useful for patients with chronic pain? *Pain, 86*, 255–264,

Jensen, M. P., Turner, J. A., Romano, J. M. & Lawler, B. K. (1994). Relationship of pain-specific belief to chronic pain adjustment. *Pain, 57*, 301–309.

Jourard, S. (1971). *The transparent self: Self-disclosure and well-being*. (Rev. ed.). New York: Van Nostrand Reinhold.

Kaplan, R. M., & Simon, H. J. (1990). Compliance in medical care: Reconsideration of self predictions. *Annals of Behavioral Medicine, 12*, 66–71.

Kart, C. (1981). Experiencing symptoms: Attribution and misattribution of illness among the aged. In M. R. Huang (Ed.). *Elderly patients and their doctors*. New York: Springer.

Keefe, F. J. (1996). Cognitive behavioral therapy for managing pain. *The Clinical Psychologist, 49*(3), 4–5.

Keefe, F. J. & Gil, K.M. (1986). Behavioral concepts in the analysis of the chronic pain syndromes. *Journal of Consulting and Clinical Psychology, 54*, 776–783.

Keefe, F. J., & Williams, D. A. (1992). Pain behavior assessment. In D. C. Turk & R. Melzack (Eds.), *Handbook of pain assessment* (pp. 277–292). New York: Guilford.

Keefe, F. J., Caldwell, D. S., Williams, D. A., Gil, K. M., Mitchell, D., Robertson, D., et al. (1990). Pain coping skills training in the management of osteoarthritis knee pain: A comparative study. *Behavior Therapy, 21*, 49–62.

Keefe, F. J., Lefebvre, J., Kerns, R., Rosenberg, R., Beaupre, P., Prochaska, J. et al. (2000). Understanding the adoption of arthritis self-management: Stages of change profiles among arthritis patients. *Pain, 87*, 303–313.

Kemp, B. (1985). Rehabilitation and the older adult. In J. E. Birren & K. W. Schaie (Eds.), *Handbook of the psychology of aging.* (2nd ed). New York: Van Nostrand Reinhold.

Kerns, R., & Rosenberg, R. (2000). Predicting responses to self-management treatments for chronic pain: Application of the pain stages of change model. *Pain, 84*, 49–55.

Kessler, R. C., Sonnega, A., Bromet, E. et al., (1995). Posttraumatic stress disorder in the National Comorbidity Survey. *Archives of General Psychiatry, 52*, 1048–1060.

Kessler, R. C., Borges, G., & Walters, E. E. (1999). Prevalence of and risk factors for lifetime suicide attempts in the National Comorbidity Survey. *Archives of General Psychiatry. 56*, 617–626.

Kilpatrick, D. G., Saunders, B. E., Amick-McMullan, A., Best, C. L., Veronen, L. J., & Resnick, H. S. (1989). Victim and crime factors associated with the development of crime-related posttraumatic stress disorder. *Behavior Therapy, 20*, 199–214.

Kizer, K. (1996). Progress on posttraumatic stress disorder. *Journal of the American Medical Association, 275* (15), 1149.

Koestler, A., & Doleys, D. M. (2002). The psychology of pain. In C. D. Tollison, J. R. Satterthwaite, & J. W. Tollison (Eds.), *Practical pain management* (3rd ed., pp. 26–39). Philadelphia, PA: Lippincott Williams & Wilkins.

Kole-Snijders, A. M. J, Vlaieyen, J. W. S., Goossens, M. E. J. B., Rutten-van Molken, M. P. M. H., Heuts, Ph. H. T. G., vanBreukelin, G. et al. (1999). Chronic low-back pain: What does cognitive coping skills training add to operant behavioral treatment? Results of a randomized clinical trial. *Journal of Consulting and Clinical Psychology, 67*, 931–944.

Kores, R. C., Murphy, W. D., Rosenthal, T. L., Elias, D. B., & North, W. C. (1990). Predicting outcome of chronic pain treatment via a modified self-efficacy scale. *Behaviour Research and Therapy, 28*, 165–169.

Kossman, M. R., & Bullrich, S. (1997). Systematic chaos: Self-organizing systems and the process of change. In F. Masterpasqua & P. A. Perna (Eds.), *The psychological meaning of chaos: Translating theory into practice.* Washington, DC: American Psychological Association Press.

Kovar, M. G. (1980). Morbidity and health care utilization. In S. G. Haynes & M. Feinlib (Eds.), *Second conference on the epidemiology of aging.* Bethesda, MD: NIH.

Kubler-Ross, E. (1969). *On death and dying.* New York: Collier Books.

Kuch, K., Swinson, R. P., & Kirby, M. (1985). Posttraumatic stress disorder after car accidents. *Canadian Journal of Psychiatry, 30*, 426–427.

Lackner, J. M., Carosella, A. M., & Feurstein, M. (1996). Pain expectancies, pain, and functional self-efficacy expectancies as determinants of disability in patients with chronic low back disorders. *Journal of Consulting and Clinical Psychology, 64* (1), 212–220.

Lazarus, R. S., & Folkman, S. (1984). *Stress, appraisal and coping.* New York: Springer.

Letham, J., Slade, P. D., Troup, J. D., & Bentley, G. (1983). Outline of a fear-avoidance model of exaggerated pain perception: I. *Behaviour Research and Therapy, 21*, 401–408.

Lindal, E. (1990). Interaction between constant levels of low back pain and other psychological parameters. *Psychological Reports, 67*, 1223–1234.

Little, J., & Girvin, H. (2002). Stages of change: A critique. *Behavior Modification, 26*, 223–273.

Livengood, J., & Johnson, B. (1998). Personality disorders in chronic pain patients. *Pain Digest, 8*, 292–296.

Loeser, J. & Turk, D. C (2001). Multidisciplinary pain management. In J. Loeser, S. Batler, C. Chapman, & D. C. Turk (Eds.), *Bonica's management of pain* (pp. 2069–2079). Philadelphia, PA: Lippincott Williams & Wilkins.

Looper, K. J. & Kirmayer, L. J. (2002). Behavioral medicine approaches to somatoform disorders. *Journal of Consulting and Clinical Psychology, 70*(5), 810–827.

Magni, G. (1987). On the relationship between chronic pain and depression where there is no organic lesion. *Pain, 51*, 1–21.

Martini, D. R., Ryan, C., Nakayama, D., & Ramenofsky, M. (1990). Psychiatric sequalae after traumatic injury: The Pittsburgh Regatta accident. *Journal of American Academic Child Adolescent Psychiatry, 29*, 181–184.

Mayer, T. G., & Gatchel, R. J. (1988). *Functional restoration for spinal disorders: The sports medicine approach.* Philadelphia, PA: Lea & Febiger.

McCracken, L. M. (1993). Prediction of pain in patients with chronic low back pain: Effects of inaccurate prediction and pain-related anxiety. *Behavior Research and Therapy, 31*, 647–652.

McEwen, B. S. (2002). *The end of stress as we know it.* Washington, DC. Joseph Henry Press.

McFarlane, A. C. (2000). Posttraumatic stress disorder: A model of the longitudinal course and the role of risk factors. *Journal of Clinical Psychiatry, 61*(Suppl. 5), 15–20.

McFarlane, A.C., & Yehuda, R. (1996). Resilience, vulnerability, and the course of posttraumatic reactions. In B. A. van der Kolk, A.C. McFarlane, & L. Weisaeth (Eds.), *Traumatic stress: The effects of overwhelming experience on mind, body, and society.* (pp. 102–114). New York: Guilford Press.

Meichenbaum, D. (1986). Cognitive behavioral modification. In F. H. Knfer & A. P. Goldstein (Eds.), *Helping people change: A textbook of methods* (pp. 346–380). New York: Pergamon.

Meichenbaum, D. H., & Turk, D. C. (1976). The cognitive-behavioral management of anxiety, anger and pain. In P. O. Davidson (Ed.), *The behavioral management of anxiety, depression and pain.* New York: Bruner/Mazel.

Meichenbaum, D. & Turk, D. C. (1987). *Facilitating treatment adherence: A practitioner's guidebook.* New York: Plenum Press.

Melzack, R. & Torgerson, W. S. (1971). On the language of pain. *Anesthesiology, 34*(1), 50–59.

Merskey, H., & Bogduk, N. (1994). *Classification of chronic pain.* Seattle: IASP Press.

Miller, T. W. (Ed.). (1990). *Chronic pain.* (Vol. 1–2). Guilford, CT: International Universities Press, Inc.

Miller, W. R. & Rollnick, S. (2002). *Motivational interviewing, Second edition: Preparing people for change.* New York: Guilford Press.

Mishel, M. H., & Braden, C. J. (1988). Finding meaning: Antecedents of uncertainty in illness. *Nursing and Research, 37* (2), 98–127.

Morley, S., Eccleston, C., & Williams, A. (1999). Systematic review and meta-analysis of randomized controlled trials of cognitive behaviour therapy and behaviour therapy for chronic pain in adults, excluding headache. *Pain, 80* (1–2), 1–13.

Muse, M. (1986). Stress-related posttraumatic chronic pain syndrome: A behavioral treatment approach. *Pain, 25,* 389–394.

National Institutes of Health Assessment Panel. (1996). Integration of behavioral and relaxation approaches into the treatment of chronic pain and insomnia. *Journal of the American Medical Association, 176*(4), 313–318..

Nielson, W., Jensen, M., & Kerns, R. (2003). Initial development and validation of a Multidimensional Pain Readiness to Change Questionnaire (MPRCQ). *Journal of Pain, 4,* 148–158.

Norris, F. H. (1992). Epidemiology of trauma: Frequency and impact of different potentially traumatic events on different demographic groups. *Journal of Consulting and Clinical Psychology, 60,* 409–418.

Perlis, M. L., Giles, D. E., Bootzin, R. R., Dikman, Z. V., Fleming, G. M., Drummond, S. P. A. et al. (1997). Alpha sleep and information processing, perception of sleep, pain and arousability in fibromyalgia. *International Journal of Neuroscience, 89,* 265–280.

Perry, B., Pollard, R., Blakely, T., Baker, W., & Vigilante, D. (1995). Childhood trauma, the neurobiology of adaptation, and "use-dependent" development of the brain: How "states" become "traits." *Infant Mental Health Journal, 16* (4), 271–291.

Phillips, H. C. (1987). Avoidance behaviour and its role in sustaining chronic pain. *Behaviour Research and Therapy, 25,* 273–279.

Pitman, R. K., Orr, S. P., Forgue, D. F., De Jong, J. B., & Claiborn, J. M. (1989). Prevalence of post-traumatic stress disorder in wounded Vietnam veterans. *American Journal of Psychiatry, 146,* 667–669.

Prochaska, J. O., DiClemente, C. C., & Norcross, J. C. (1992). In search of how people change: Applications to addictive behaviors. *American Psychologist, 47,* 1102–1114.

Rapoff, M. A. (1999). *Adherence to pediatric medical regimens.* New York: Kluwer Academic/Plenum Publishers.

Ray, O. (2004). How the mind hurts and heals the body. *American Psychologist, 59* (1), 29–40.

Romano, J. M, & Turner, J. A. (1985). Chronic pain and depression: Does the evidence support a relationship. *Psychological Bulletin, 97,* 18–34.

Rosomoff, H. L., & Rosomoff, R. S. (1991). Comprehensive multidisciplinary pain center approach to the treatment of low back pain. *Neurosurgery Clinics of North America, 2*(4), 877–890.

Sanders, S. H. (2003). Operant therapy with pain patients: Evidence for its effectiveness. In A. H. Lebovits (Ed.), *Seminars in pain medicine, 1* (pp. 90–98). Philadelphia: W.B. Saunders.

Scaer, R. C. (2001). *The body bears the burden: Trauma, dissociation, and disease.* New York: Haworth Medical Press.

Schmitz, U., Saile, H., & Nilges, P. (1996). Coping with chronic pain: Flexible goal adjustment as an interactive buffer against pain-related distress. *Pain, 67,* 41–51.

Schreiber, S., & Galai-Gat, T. (1993). Uncontrolled pain following physical injury as the core-trauma in post-traumatic stress disorder. *Pain, 54,* 107–110.

Schuster, J. M., & Smith, S. S. (1994). Brief assessment of depression in chronic pain patients. *American Journal of Pain Management, 4* (3), 115–117.

Shalev, A. Y. (1996). Stress versus traumatic stress: From acute homeostatic reactions to chronic psychopathology. In B. A. van der Kolk, A. C. McFarlane, & L. Weisaeth (Eds.), *Traumatic stress: The effects of overwhelming experience on mind, body, and society* (pp. 77–101). New York: Guilford Press.

Shalev, A. Y. (2000). Measuring outcome in posttraumatic stress disorder. *Journal of Clinical Psychiatry, 61*(Suppl. 5), 33–39.

Skevington, S. M. (1983). Chronic pain and depression: Universal of personal helplessness. *Pain, 15,* 309–317.

Spielman, A. J., Saskin, P., & Thorpy, M. J. (1987). Treatment of chronic insomnia by restriction of time in bed. *Sleep, 10,* 45–56.

Stone, A. A., Broderick, J. E., Porter, L. S., & Kaell, A. T. (1997). The experience of rheumatoid arthritis pain and fatigue: Examining momentary reports and correlates over one week. *Arthritis Care and Research, 10* (3), 185–193.

Syrjala, K. L., Donaldson, G. W., Davis, M. W., Kippes, M. E., & Carr, J. E. (1995). Relaxation and imagery and cognitive-behavioral training reduce pain during cancer treatment: A controlled clinical trial. *Pain, 63,* 189–198.

Thorn, B. E. & Williams, D. A. (1993.) Cognitive-behavioral management of chronic pain. In L. VandeCreek & T. Jackson (Eds.), *Innovations in clinical practice: A sourcebook* (pp. 169–191). Sarasota, FL: Professional Resource Exchange.

Thorn, B. E., Boothby, J. L., & Sullivan, M. J. L. (2002). Targeted treatment of catastrophizing for the management of chronic pain. *Cognitive and Behavioral Practice, 9,* 127–138.

Tishler, M., Barak, Y., Paran, D., & Yaron, M. (1997). Sleep disturbances, fibromyalgia and primary Sjogren's syndrome. *Clinical and Experimental Rheumatology, 15,* 71–74.

Tjemsland, L., Soreide, J., & Malt, U. (1998). Traumatic distress symptoms in early breast cancer III: Breast cancer research and treatment. *Psychology and Oncology, 47,* 141–151.

Toomey, T. C., Mann, J. D., Abashian, S., and Thompson-Pope, S. (1991). Relationship between perceived self-control of pain, pain description, and functioning. *Pain, 45,* 129–133.

Trief, P. M., Carnricke, C. L., & Drudge, O. (1995). Chronic pain and depression: Is social support relevant? *Psychological Reports, 76,* 227–236.

Turk, D. C. (1994). Detecting depression in chronic pain patients: Adequacy of self-reports. *Behavior Research and Therapy, 32,* 9–16.

Turk, D. C., & Rudy, T. E. (1988). Toward an empirically derived taxonomy of chronic pain patients: Integration of psychological assessment data. *Journal of Consulting & Clinical Psychology, 56,* 233–238.

Turk, D. C., & Rudy, T. E. (1991). Neglected topics in the treatments of chronic pain patients: relapse, noncompliance and adherence enhancement. *Pain, 44,* 5–28.

Turk, D. C., & Rudy, T. E. (1994). Methods for evaluating treatment outcomes. Ways to overcome potential obstacles. *Spine, 19* (15),1759–1763.

Turk, D. C., & Salovey, P. (1984). Chronic pain as a variant of depressive disease: A critical reappraisal. *Journal of Nervous and Mental Disease, 172,* 398–404.

Turk, D. C., Flor, H., & Rudy, T. E. (1987). Pain and families: Role in etiology, maintenance, and psychosocial impact. *Pain, 30,* 3–28.

Turk, D. C., Holzman, A. D., & Kerns, R. D. (1987). Chronic pain: Emphasis on self-management. In K. A. Holroyd & T. Creer (Eds.), *Self-management in health psychology and behavioral medicine.* New York: Academic Press.

Turk, D. C., Meichenbaum, D., & Genest, M. (1983). *Pain and behavioral medicine: A cognitive-behavioral perspective.* New York: Guilford Press.

Turner, J. A., & Clancy, S. (1986). Strategies for coping with chronic low back pain: Relationship to pain and disability. *Pain, 24,* 355–364.

Turner, J. A., & Clancy, S. (1988). Comparison of operant-behavioral and cognitive-behavioral group treatment for chronic low back pain. *Journal of Consulting and Clinical Psychology, 58,* 573–579.

Turner, R. M. (1986). Behavioral self-control procedures for disorders of initiating and maintaining sleep (DIMS). *Clinical Psychology Review, 6,* 27–38.

Vlaeyen, J. W. S., & Linton, S. J. (2000). Fear-avoidance and its consequences in chronic musculoskeletal pain: A state of the art. *Pain, 85,* 317–332.

Vlaeyen, J. W. S., Haazen, I. W. C. J., Schuerman, J. A., Kole-Snijders, A. M. J., & van Eek, H. (1995). Behavioral rehabilitation of chronic low back pain: Comparison of an operant treatment and operant-cognitive treatment and an operant-respondent treatment. *British Journal of Clinical Psychology, 34,* 95–118.

Vlaeyen, J. W. S., Kole-Snijders, A. M. J., Boeren, R. G. B., & van Eek, H. (1995a). Fear of movement/(re)injury in chronic low back pain and its relation to behavioral performance. *Pain, 62,* 363–372.

Vlaeyen, J. W. S., Kole-Snijders, A. M. J., Rotteveel, A. M., & Ruesink, R. (1995b). The role of fear of movement/(re)injury in pain disability. *Journal of Occupational Rehabilitation, 5,* 235–252.

Waddell, G., Newton, M., Henderson, I., & Somerville, D. (1993). A Fear-Avoidance Beliefs Questionnaire (FABQ) and the role of fear-avoidance in chronic low back pain and disability. *Pain, 52,* 157–168.

Weickgenant, A. L., Slater, M. A., Patterson, T. L., Atkinson, J. H., Grant, I., & Garfin, S. R. (1993). Coping activities in chronic low back pain: Relationship with depression. *Pain, 53,* 95–103.

Weisberg, J. N. & Keefe, F. J. (1997). Personality disorders in the chronic pain population: Basic concepts, empirical findings and clinical implications. *Pain Forum, 6* (1), 1–9.

Weisberg, J. N., Vittengl, J. R., Clark, L. A., Gatchel, R. J., & Gorin, A. A. (2000). Personality and pain: Summary and future perspectives. In J. N. Weisberg & R. J. Gatchel (Eds.), *Personality characteristics of patients with pain.* Washington, DC: American Psychological Association.

Wheeler, A. H. (1995). Evolutionary mechanisms in chronic low back pain and rationale for treatment. *American Journal of Pain* Management, *5* (2), 62–66.

49

Relaxation and Biofeedback Self-Management for Pain

Frank Andrasik, PhD

INTRODUCTION

Pain is a complex experience that typically requires a multifaceted, multidimensional, multidisciplinary approach. Relaxation and biofeedback are often components of treatment and, although this chapter focuses on these treatments as isolated techniques, rarely are they applied in this fashion. More typically they are combined with one another, various aspects of cognitive-behavior therapy (Gatchel, Robinson, Pulliam, & Maddrey, 2003; Thorn, 2004; Waters, Campbell, Keefe, & Carson, 2004), and ongoing medical care. Consequently, they are one of many options that patients and therapists consider and find of value.

Relaxation, biofeedback, and related self-management treatments (such as hypnotherapy; see Chapter 51 this volume by Burte) share common features that distinguish them from standard medical care. Self-management treatments place less emphasis on physical procedures applied by others; place more emphasis on patient involvement and personal responsibility; expand the scope of treatment to include emotional, mental, behavioral, and social factors that impact pain; and seek to enable patients to cope more effectively with pain and associated symptoms. Active involvement of patients can lead to an increased confidence in their ability to prevent and manage pain and promote new and different ways of dealing with pain, which can lead to less pain-related disability (French, Holroyd, Pinell, Malinoski, O'Donnell, & Hill, 2000). Additionally, patients who attribute therapy improvements to their own efforts demonstrate better long-term outcome than patients who attribute improvement to the interventions of health care providers (Spinhoven et al., 1992).

This chapter begins with a detailed look at varied generalized relaxation techniques, including biofeedback-assisted relaxation approaches. Next follows discussion of more focused or specific approaches to biofeedback and then various procedural matters. The chapter concludes with a brief review of the evidence base for the approaches discussed in this chapter.

RELAXATION THERAPIES

Several rationales justify the use of relaxation with patients experiencing pain. First, a reduction in general arousal leads to reduced central processing of peripheral sensory inputs. Another assumption derives from the pain–negative affect cycle (Fernandez, 2002). Pain often produces negative affective states (depression, anxiety, and fear), which in turn decrease pain tolerance and increase reports and complaints of pain. Achieving a more relaxed state can help to reverse these trends. A final consideration is based on the association of stress and pain, which Melzack (1999) has discussed in detail. Prolonged activation of the stress system increases cortisol levels, which is related to a number of physiological changes that can give rise to pain. Stress is also directly linked to the negative affective triad. Based on these considerations, a case can be made that most patients with pain could benefit from some form of general relaxation.

A number of procedures have been used to promote generalized relaxation. Chief among these are guided imagery, relaxed breathing, autogenic training, and progressive muscle relaxation training. Recent research with functional magnetic resonance imaging (MRI) has shown that distraction, a common component of relaxation, leads to significant activation within the periaqueductal gray region, a site recognized for higher cortical control of pain (Tracey et al., 2002). Thus, these treatments may be exerting an impact on central mechanisms as well.

GUIDED IMAGERY

The first and simplest approach involves teaching a patient how to create a mental image ("picture in your mind's eyes") of a pleasant or relaxing scene, such as lying on a blanket at the beach while listening to the waves roll in and back out or walking through a pleasant meadow on a warm, sunny day. Patients are advised to avoid images that involve sexual content or vigorous physical activity (as these activities can increase rather than decrease arousal) and to include as many sensory modalities (auditory, olfactory, tactile, and even gustatory) and details as possible (Arena & Blanchard, 2002), as these are believed to deepen the experience. It is recommended that patients practice employing several different relaxing images, so that they can switch to another image if the selected one is not working at a given time. With practice, images can be recalled quickly and vividly and can be used effectively to provide mental escape when situations become seemingly overwhelming. A more detailed discussion of this topic may be found in Bresler (Chapter 52 in this volume).

RELAXED BREATHING

Regulating breathing is a particularly useful procedure because breathing can be readily brought under voluntary control, and it is an activity that is vital to survival. The notion of relaxed breathing is deceptively simple, so most patients need detailed instructions for correct use. Improper application can lead to blood gas imbalance and hyper- or hypoventilation. Also, patients whose initial respiration rate is high (greater than 30 breaths per minute) may feel quite strange as their breathing rate approaches the relaxed range. Such patients are instructed to pay no particular attention to this and are informed that these peculiar feelings will pass with time.

Diaphragmatic breathing is commonly used. It involves teaching the patient to draw air more deeply into the lungs by moving the diaphragm downward toward the umbilicus, thus causing a notable expansion of the abdomen upon inspiration. Gevirtz and Schwartz (2003) provide an excellent discussion of this topic, which includes a brief review of the physiology of breathing and provides instructions on how to teach patients to breathe slowly (to a target range of five to eight breaths per minute), deeply (to full lung capacity), and evenly (to facilitate approximately the same rate for exhaling and for inhaling), while concentrating on the associated physiological sensations.

Having the patient subvocalize a word associated with relaxation on each exhalation can help "cue" subsequent relaxation, just by recalling the word.

Three methods can be used to illustrate this technique. Patients can practice breathing while: (1) holding their arms straight overhead (which minimizes chest movement); (2) lying on a firm surface, placing a medium-weight book on the abdomen, and raising and lowering the text with each breath cycle; and (3) placing one hand on the chest and the other just below the rib cage, breathing in a manner that limits movement of the hand on the chest and maximizes movement of the hand on the abdomen.

When breathing is the sole or main focus, certain instruments may be useful to quantify and shape proper breathing. These include nasal airflow temperature gauge, strain gauge, electromyography (EMG) from accessory breathing muscles, capnometer and oximeter methods, spirometry, arterial blood oxyhemoglobin saturation, and the like. Gevirtz and Schwartz (2003) discuss other approaches for promoting more relaxed breathing as well, including paced respiration, breath meditation, breath mindfulness, rebreathing, pursed-lip breathing, and instrument-based approaches. These very portable procedures can be easily combined (and often are) with other relaxation techniques.

AUTOGENIC TRAINING

A third form of relaxation borrows from the well-developed body of literature on autogenic training, a meditation-type of relaxation that is made up of six components. Autogenic training has an extensive history and involves having patients passively concentrate on key words and phrases selected for their ability to promote desired somatic responses (Schultz & Luthe, 1969). Clinicians typically use two of autogenic training's six components. Patients are instructed to focus on feelings or sensations of *warmth* and *heaviness* in the extremities, as this is believed to facilitate increased blood flow to the extremities, which accounts for peripheral warming and a reduction in sympathetic nervous arousal. It is recommended that patients develop their own phrasing and subvocalize these phrases numerous times (50 to 100) during practice to maximize effects (Arena & Blanchard, 1996). Autogenic training is commonly added to thermal biofeedback (to be discussed later), leading to a technique termed "autogenic feedback" (Sargent, Green, & Walters, 1972)

PROGRESSIVE MUSCLE RELAXATION TRAINING

This form of relaxation involves active tensing and relaxing of groups of muscles as a way to facilitate overall relaxation. The following points are stressed when introducing this form of relaxation training: (1) relaxation training consists of systematic tensing and relaxing of

TABLE 49.1
Outline of Progressive Muscle Relaxation Training Program

Week	Session	Introduction and Treatment Rationale	No. of Muscle Groups	Deepening Exercises	Breathing Exercises	Relaxing Imagery	Muscle Discrimination Training	Relaxation by Recall	Cue-controlled Relaxation
1	1	x	14	x	x				
	2		14	x	x	x			
2	3		14	x	x	x	x		
	4		14	x	x	x	x		
3	5		8	x	x	x	x		
	6		8	x	x	x	x	x	
4	7		4	x	x	x	x	x	
5	8		4	x	x	x	x	x	x
6	9		4	x	x	x	x	x	x
7	None								
8	10		4	x	x	x	x	x	x

Note: From Andrasik, F. & Walch, S. 2003. In *Handbook of Psychology* (Vol. 9), A. M. Nezu, C. M. Nezu, & P. A. Geller (Eds.). New York: Wiley. Reprinted with permission.

major muscle groups; (2) tensing muscles even for a brief period results in their reflexively achieving a subsequent lower level of tension; (3) experiencing a broad range of muscle tension levels enables patients to better discriminate when muscle tension is building; (4) with improved discrimination abilities and newly acquired skills for rapidly relaxing muscles, this technique can be used to counteract tension buildup as it occurs throughout the day (termed "applied relaxation"); (5) achieving a deep state of relaxation is a learned skill and requires regular practice; and (6) the focus is initially on all major muscle groups, but groups are subsequently combined over time to permit rapid deployment.

The procedure described here is based on Andrasik (1986) and is summarized in Table 49.1. It begins by having the patient sequentially tense and relax 14 separate muscle groupings in the 18 steps indicated in Table 49.2. Prior to formal instruction, the patient is observed when completing a few practice tension–release cycles, to ensure that the tension generated is proper (neither incomplete nor overly zealous) and is confined to the target group (as this is important to developing discrimination skills). Muscles that are very painful or that have been strained or injured are omitted so as not to cause further problems. Target muscle groups are tensed for 5 to 7 seconds and then relaxed for 20 to 30 seconds, which constitutes a complete cycle. The patient is instructed to attend to the sensations associated with tension and relaxation during each cycle. If a patient prefers a different muscle sequence, it is acceptable to modify the sequence. Once modified, it is important that the patient adhere to the same order, as consistency and routine facilitate training effects. Patients may be periodically instructed to mentally scan select muscle groups that have been targeted

previously in order to identify any residual tension. If detected, another tension–release cycle may be completed. Various procedures, all involving therapist suggestions, may also be used to promote a deepened sense of relaxation (such as having the therapist count out loud backwards from 5 to 1 and instructing the patient that a deeper level of relaxation will be experienced with each successive count, picture oneself descending a staircase and becoming more relaxed as each floor is passed). These deepening strategies are similar to hypnotic techniques, but they are not typically labeled as such. Relaxed breathing and imagery are added early on, in the manner discussed previously. Once the patient has made adequate progress at tensing and relaxing the 14 major muscle groups, the therapist begins to combine various muscle groups in order to abbreviate the procedure first to eight total muscle groupings, and then to four groupings (see Table 49.3).

More specific training for muscle discrimination can be added for areas of difficulty. To demonstrate this aspect, a patient is asked to engage in a complete tension–release cycle involving the hand and arm, then to tense these muscles by only half as much. This is followed by a tension cycle involving only a quarter as much force and so on. Once the concept of differential tension is understood, the patient is instructed to apply differential muscle tensing to the muscles most associated with pain (another procedure for enhancing muscle discrimination abilities is presented later). Final techniques concern relaxation by recall and cue-controlled relaxation. To implement relaxation by recall, the patient is instructed first to recall the sensations associated with relaxation and then to attempt to reproduce these sensations without the aide of tension and release cycles. Actual tension–release

TABLE 49.2
The 14 Initial Muscle Groups and Procedures for Tensing in 18 Steps

1. Right hand and lower arm (have client make fist, simultaneously tense lower arm)
2. Left hand and lower arm
3. Both hands and lower arms
4. Right upper arm (have client bring his or her hand to the shoulder and tense biceps)
5. Left upper arm
6. Both upper arms
7. Right lower leg and foot (have client point his or her toe while tensing the calf muscles)
8. Left lower leg and foot
9. Both lower legs and feet
10. Both thighs (have client press his or her knees and thighs tightly together)
11. Abdomen (have client draw abdominal muscles in tightly, as if bracing to receive a punch)
12. Chest (have client take a deep breath and hold it)
13. Shoulders and lower neck (have client "hunch" his or her shoulders or draw his or her shoulders up toward the ears)
14. Back of the neck (have the client press head backwards against headrest or chair)
15. Lips/mouth (have client press lips together tightly, but not so tight as to clench teeth; or have client place the tip of the tongue on the roof of the mouth behind upper front teeth)
16. Eyes (have client close the eyes tightly)
17. Lower forehead (have client frown and draw the eyebrows together)
18. Upper forehead (have client wrinkle the forehead area or raise the eyebrows)

Note: From "Headaches," by F. Andrasik & S. Walch, 2003. In *Handbook of Psychology* (Vol. 9), edited by A. M. Nezu, C. M. Nezu, & P. A. Geller, New York: Wiley. Reprinted with permission.

TABLE 49.3
Abbreviated Muscle Groups

8 Muscle Groups

1. Both hands and lower arms
2. Both legs and thighs
3. Abdomen
4. Chest
5. Shoulders
6. Back of neck
7. Eyes
8. Forehead

4 Muscle Groups

1. Arms
2. Chest
3. Neck
4. Face (with a particular focus on the eyes and forehead)

Note: From "Headaches," by F. Andrasik & S. Walch, 2003. In *Handbook of Psychology* (Vol. 9), edited by A. M. Nezu, C. M. Nezu, & P. A. Geller, New York: Wiley. Reprinted with permission.

cycles are used only as needed to promote the desired somatic state. Practice outside of the office is necessary to maximize effects and patients are typically instructed to practice techniques taught them once or twice per day, and then on an as-needed basis for everyday coping. Pairing relaxing words or cues with the feelings of relaxation can help to evoke relaxation later on (cue-controlled relaxation). Audiotapes prepared commercially or by the therapist during an actual session with the patient facilitate home practice. See Andrasik (1986), Arena and Blanchard (1996), Bernstein and Borkovec (1973), Lichstein (1988), and Smith (1990) for further information about relaxation in general.

BIOFEEDBACK-ASSISTED RELAXATION

BIOFEEDBACK DEFINED

"Feedback" is a process in which the factors that produce a result are themselves modified, corrected, or strength-

ened by the result. "Bio" is commonly referred to as pertaining to self. Hence, biofeedback is a technique in which information about the self is used to modify, correct, or strengthen processes within the self. More specifically, biofeedback is a therapeutic or research technique that involves monitoring an individual's physiological processes or responses, such as muscular contraction or heart rate, and providing information about that physiological process back to the individual in a meaningful way so that he or she can modify the physiological process (Blanchard & Epstein, 1978). In therapeutic settings the goal is to help individuals alter their physiology to a healthier standard. We all use biofeedback every day. Looking into a mirror to guide how makeup is applied or how our hair is combed are examples of elementary uses of biofeedback.

Feedback is most often presented in auditory or visual modalities, in either binary or continuous proportional fashion. Binary feedback uses a signal that comes on or goes off at a specified value and is used when the therapist is having the patient strive for a specific target level (a shaping procedure). Many applications involve obtaining the lowest possible level of arousal, and these use continuous feedback to produce ever-increasing degrees of relaxation (e.g., a tone is provided that decreases in pitch or volume as relaxation occurs). On occasion, combinations of both are used. The information that is presented to the individual has reinforcing or rewarding qualities when the desired response is produced. Typically the information is presented to the individual in real time, so that the individual can immediately see the results of his or her actions. The individual will eventually cultivate a greater awareness of his or her physiological processes that are ordinarily beyond conscious control and will eventually develop greater voluntary control over the processes. Voluntary control is developed initially through trial and error, then by successively getting closer and closer to the desired training goal and repeated practice (Andrasik & Lords, 2004).

When recording physiology, care must be taken to ensure that areas for sensor placements are prepared adequately and that the sensors are placed on the proper locations. Electrode sites may need to be cleaned and lightly abraded (although advances in instrumentation are making this less necessary), and a conductive gel applied to facilitate conductance and reduce measurement artifact in certain instances. More detailed discussion of physiology, electrical theory, and bases of the primary responses used in biofeedback may be found in Peek (2003) and various chapters within Andreassi (2000); Cacioppo, Tassinary, and Bernston (2000); and Stern, Ray, and Quigley (2001). Various theories have been used to account for biofeedback, ranging from operant learning to cognitive and expectancy models (Schwartz & Schwartz, 2003).

The goal of biofeedback, in its most common application, is quite complementary to relaxation and other self-management approaches. The distinguishing characteristic is that biofeedback uses instruments that record information about a person's body as a way of gauging targets for treatment and evaluating progress. Biofeedback can give concrete evidence that relaxation is actually occurring. Think of it as *instrument-aided* relaxation. Feedback is a critical link and an additional distinguishing feature of this approach. Imagine how difficult it would be to learn to play tennis if you were blindfolded and were not told when a ball would be served your way. If you should happen to hit the ball, you would have little idea where it went. Removing the blindfold establishes a feedback loop that allows learning to take place more quickly (Andrasik & Lords, 2004).

THREE BASIC APPROACHES

Any response modality indicative of heightened arousal theoretically can serve as a target for promoting relaxation, although three are used most commonly — muscle tension (EMG), skin conductance (or sweat gland activity), and peripheral temperature. These modalities, termed the "workhorses" of the biofeedback general practitioner (Andrasik, 2000, 2004), are easily collected, quantified, and interpreted and are discussed below. Other responses, such as heart rate, respiration, blood volume, and electroencephalogram, can be useful, but these will not be addressed further (see Andrasik, 2000; Andrasik & Lords, 2004; Cacioppo et al., 2000; Flor, 2001; Stern et al., 2001; and Othmer & Othmer, Chapter 50 of this volume, for discussion).

EMG-Assisted Relaxation

The rationale for employing muscle tension (and skin conductance, too; see next section) feedback to facilitate relaxation is straightforward. The basis of the EMG signal is the small electrochemical changes that occur when a muscle contracts. By placing a series of electrodes along the muscle fibers, the muscle action potentials associated with the ion exchange across the membrane of the muscles can be detected and processed (when single motor units are the focus of treatment, as in the case of muscle rehabilitation, fine wire electrodes that penetrate the skin surface are used). EMG monitoring from surface sites is accomplished by the use of two active electrodes, separated by one ground electrode, to set up two separate circuits to detect electrical activity that leaks up to the skin surface. With this arrangement, the resultant signal is the difference between the two circuits (with the amount subtracted out considered to be noise).

When EMG is used for generalized relaxation, sensors are typically placed on the forehead region (one active sensor about 1 inch above the pupil of each eye, with the ground or reference sensor placed above the bridge of the nose), or along the neck or trapezius (shoulder) muscles. The frontal placement, which employs large-diameter sensors, is sensitive to muscle tension from adjacent areas, possibly down to the upper rib cage (Basmajian, 1976). Reducing forehead muscle tension can affect other adjacent untrained muscles, promoting a state of "cultivated low arousal." This does not automatically occur (Surwit & Keefe, 1978), so clinicians may need to train patients from several sites in the course of general relaxation treatment (or combine biofeedback with other approaches).

Surface EMG has a power spectrum ranging from 20 to 10,000 Hz. Some of the commercially available biofeedback machines sample a very limited amount of this range. For example, some machines filter out EMG occurring below 100 Hz and/or above a certain value (sometimes as low as 200 Hz). This misses much of the EMG power spectrum and results in lower readings overall. Clinicians need to be aware of the "band pass" of their equipment and to realize that readings obtained from one machine may not be comparable with those obtained on another machine where different settings may be employed. Some of the other factors affecting measurement quantity include sensor type and size, sensor placement on the muscle, distance between sensors, and patient adiposity (as fat acts as an insulator and dampens the electrical signal).

EMG activity can be summarized and presented in various ways. The EMG signal is an alternating response with a very high frequency. These characteristics make it difficult or nearly impossible for subjects to discriminate the small changes in EMG activity that must be detected for learning to occur. Consequently the raw signal is hardly ever used. EMG signals are rectified, smoothed, and averaged over time periods to provide useful feedback, with the values expressed as microvolts. The microvolt information is provided back to the person via some type of computer presentation that is pleasing and understandable to the patient.

Skin Conductance-Assisted Relaxation

Electrical activity of the skin or sweating has long been assumed to be a good measure of arousal. In fact, in the late 1800s Romain Virouroux included measures of skin resistance to facilitate understanding when working with cases of hysterical anesthesias. Electrodermal activity became popular and was thought of as a way to read the mind when used by Carl Jung in the early 1900s in word-association experiments (Neumann & Blanton, 1970; Peek, 2003).

Two separate portions of the central nervous system are believed to be responsible for control of electrodermal activity (Boucsein, 1992). Sensors are typically placed on body surface areas that are most densely populated with "eccrine" sweat glands (such as the palm of the hand or the fingers), as these respond primarily to psychological stimulation and are innervated by the sympathetic branch of the autonomic nervous system (Stern et al., 2001). Sweat contains electrically conductive salts, and sweaty skin is more conductive to electricity than dry skin. A skin conductance biofeedback device applies a very small electrical voltage to the skin (so small it is undetectable to the person). Conductance measures (the reciprocal of resistance; measured in microomhs or microsiemens), as opposed to resistance measures, are preferred in clinical application because the former measures have a linear relationship to the number of sweat glands that are activated. This permits a straightforward explanation to patients (as arousal increases, so does skin conductance; focusing on decreasing skin conductance helps to lower arousal and to achieve a state of relaxation).

Skin-Temperature-Assisted Relaxation

It is less obvious why skin temperature has been targeted for general relaxation. This is because the first clinical application resulted from a serendipitous finding by clinical researchers at the Menninger Clinic. During a standard laboratory evaluation it was noticed that spontaneous termination of a migraine was accompanied by flushing in the hands and a rapid, sizable rise in surface hand temperature (Sargent et al., 1972). This led Sargent et al. to pilot-test as a treatment a procedure wherein migraineurs were given feedback to raise their hand temperatures as a way to regulate stress and headache activity. Treatment was augmented by components of autogenic training (Schultz & Luthe, 1969), leading to a procedure

they termed "autogenic feedback." Noting that constriction of peripheral blood flow is under control of the sympathetic branch of the nervous system, these researchers reasoned that decreases in sympathetic outflow lead to increased vasodilation, blood flow, and a resultant rise in peripheral temperature (due to the warmth of the blood). Thus, temperature feedback may best be thought of at the moment as yet another way to affect the sympathetic nervous system and facilitate general relaxation.

Temperature is monitored by highly sensitive probes, called thermistors, whose resistance changes in a lawful, linear manner as a function of temperature change. They are typically composed of a semiconductor, although thermocouples, composed of two different metals in juxtaposition, are used occasionally. It is important to note that the laboratory, clinic, and outdoor temperature and humidity influence heat buildup if sensors are not attached properly, and wind/air conditioning currents within the room can influence the accuracy of skin-temperature measurements.

SPECIFIC BIOFEEDBACK APPROACHES

"Specific" approaches begin by identifying precisely the physiological dysfunction or response system underlying the pain condition, using a psychophysiological assessment (or "psychophysiological stress profile") (Andrasik & Flor, 2003; Arena & Schwartz, 2003; Flor, 2001), before launching into a course of biofeedback. Psychophysiological assessment is designed to identify the physiological dysfunction or response modalities assumed to be relevant to the pain condition and to do so under varied stimulus conditions, psychological and physical, that mimic work and rest (reclining, bending, stooping, lifting, working a keyboard, simulated stressors, etc.) in order to guide treatment efforts and gauge progress (Andrasik, Thorn, & Flor, in press). This assessment may or may not precede biofeedback-assisted relaxation approaches.

Flor (2001) points out the various functions, utility, and advantages of psychophysiological data collection: (1) providing evidence for the role of psychological factors in maladaptive physiological functioning; (2) justifying pursuit of biofeedback therapy; (3) facilitating tailoring treatments to patients; (4) making it possible to document efficacy, generalization, and transfer of treatment; (5) helping to identify predictors of treatment response; and (6) serving as a source of motivation (e.g., as patients realize they are able to influence bodily processes by their own thoughts, emotions, and actions, their feelings of helplessness decrease and they become more open to psychological approaches).

This data collection involves the following phases or periods:

Adaptation allows patients to become familiar with the therapist, setting, and recording procedure; minimizes pre-session effects (rushing to the appointment, temperature and humidity differences between the office or laboratory and outdoors); and permits habituation of the orienting response and response stability to occur. Meeting the therapist for the first time, coming into a novel environment, and being attached to unfamiliar equipment may result in temporary increases in arousal for the patient. Without a proper adaptation, the therapist or experimenter may mistake a habituation effect for a training effect. Adaptation refers to the client becoming comfortable and returning to a "normal" level of functioning. Patients are instructed merely to sit quietly during this period.

Although the importance of having an adequate adaptation period is widely acknowledged, little research has been conducted to help identify key parameters of adaptation, the amount of time needed to achieve stability, or how best to define *stability*. Most but not all individuals will adapt within 15 minutes (some may not adapt for the entire appointment; Lichstein, Sallis, Hill, & Young, 1981; Taub, 1977; Taub & Emurian, 1976; Taub & School, 1978). Practitioners may not always be able to wait until stability is observed for key responses of interest (defined as minimal to no fluctuation within a specified period of time). They need to remain mindful of how initial levels may affect subsequent training.

Baseline serves as the basis of comparison for subsequent assessment phases and as the basis for gauging progress within and across future treatment sessions. In clinical practice, a baseline of from 1 to 5 minutes will provide a reasonable representation of the patient's current physiological state.

When the goal of biofeedback is generalized relaxation, therapists may collect a **second baseline** during which the patient is instructed something like the following: "I would now like to see what happens when you try to relax as deeply as you can. Use whatever means you believe will be helpful. Please let me know when you are as relaxed as possible." This serves as a test of preexisting abilities to relax and can be used as a comparison for judging future training effects.

It once was thought that elevated resting levels of muscle tension might be a unique characteristic of patients experiencing chronic pain. A review of 60 psychophysiological investigations including patients with headache, back, and temporomandibular joint disorder (TMD) found minimal support for this (Flor & Turk, 1989).

Reactivity assesses responses to simulated stressors that are personally relevant or conditions that approximate real-world events that are associated with pain onset or exacerbation. There are no standard empirically validated approaches. Some examples of commonly used stimulus conditions are (1) negative imagery, wherein a patient concentrates on a personally relevant unpleasant situation (the details of which are obtained during an intake interview); (2) cold exposure (e.g., for Raynaud's) or cold pressor test (as a general physical stressor); (3) movement, such as sitting, rising, bending, stooping, or walking; (4) load bearing, such as lifting or carrying an object; and (5) operation of a keyboard or other work device. Although baseline differences for EMG have not been found to reliably characterize pain disorders, symptom-specific responses to stimuli have been found for certain pain conditions on a more consistent basis (see Flor, 2001, for a review).

In assessing reactivity in muscles, some researchers have turned their attention to the psychophysiological model of Travell and Simons (1983) who postulate that a large percentage of chronic muscle pain results from trigger points. Hubbard (1996) has expanded upon their view using the following line of reasoning: (1) muscle tension and pain are sympathetically mediated hyperactivity of the muscle stretch receptors, or the muscle spindles; (2) muscle spindles, which are scattered throughout the muscle belly (hundreds within the trapezius muscle), are encapsulated organs that contain their own muscle fibers; (3) although traditionally viewed as a stretch sensor, the muscle spindle is recognized now to be a pain and pressure sensor and an organ that can be activated by sympathetic stimulation; and (4) thus, the pain associated with trigger points arises in the spindle capsule.

Support for this model comes from studies where careful needle (indwelling) electrode placements have detected high levels of EMG activity in the trigger point itself, but data collected from adjacent nontender sites just 1 cm away are relatively silent (Hubbard & Berkoff, 1993). Further, when exposed to a stressful stimulus, EMG activity increases at the trigger point but not at the adjacent site (McNulty, Gevirtz, Hubbard, & Berkoff, 1994). This work provides further evidence of the link between behavioral and emotional factors and mechanisms of muscle pain. As a result of this basic research, Gevirtz, Hubbard, and Harpin (1996) have developed a comprehensive treatment program that uses EMG biofeedback to facilitate muscle tension awareness in sessions and in daily life activities, to identify stressors triggering increased EMG activity, and to assist patients in finding improved ways to cope with tension producing situations.

Recovery from stress assesses how and when a patient's physiology returns to a value close to that observed prior to stimulus presentation (often responses do not fully return to their starting values).

Figure 49.1 (from Flor, 2001) provides a sample psychophysiological profile. EMG was recorded bilaterally from three sites (masseter, frontal, and trapezius muscles), during baseline, imaginal neutral, stress, and pain situations, and during extended mathematical problems (another mental stressor) and extended movement. Heart rate and skin conductance were also monitored. The following was gained from this evaluation. EMG resting values were markedly elevated and asymmetrical. EMG

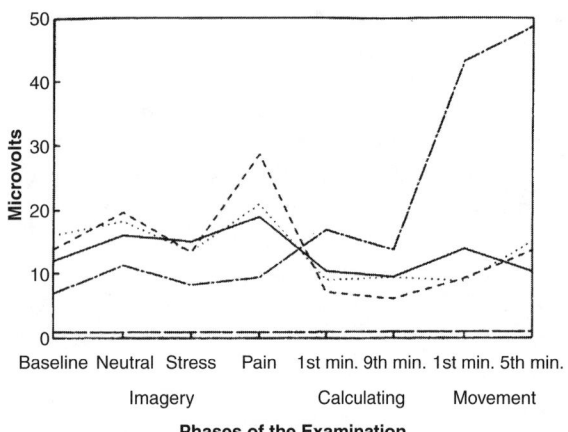

FIGURE 49.1 EMG profile of Mr. F. (From Flor, H. 2001.) *Handbook of Pain Assessment* (2nd ed., pp. 76–96). D. C. Turk & R. Melzack (Eds.). New York: Guilford. Reprinted with permission.)

values increased in response to imagery, particularly so for the pain episodes, and they were markedly exacerbated by movement. Heart rate and skin conductance were found to be unresponsive. Treatment focused on tension reduction in relevant muscles and alteration of responding during simulations of aversive situations (e.g., therapist displayed "aggressive verbalization" toward the patient).

The above components constitute the basic approach to psychophysiological assessment. One additional component can be very useful.

Muscle discrimination assesses a person's ability to perceive bodily states accurately. Flor and colleagues (Flor, Fürst, & Birbaumer, 1999; Flor, Schugens, & Birbaumer, 1992) have shown that patients with chronic pain are unable to perceive muscle tension levels accurately both in the affected and nonaffected muscles and that, when exposed to tasks requiring production of muscle tension, these patients overestimate physical symptoms, rate the task as more aversive, and report greater pain. These findings point to a heightened sensitivity.

Muscle discrimination abilities can easily be assessed in a clinical setting (Flor, 2001). This involves (1) presenting the patient with a bar of varying height on a monitor, (2) instructing the patient to tense a muscle to the level reflected in the height of the bar, which is varied from low to high, (3) correlating the obtained EMG readings with the actual heights of the bars, and (4) defining as "good" discrimination abilities correlation coefficients ≥0.80 and "bad" or poor discrimination abilities as correlation coefficients ≤ 0.50.

SELECT EXAMPLES OF SPECIFIC APPLICATIONS AND SPECIFIC SENSOR PLACEMENTS

Arena (cited within Arena & Blanchard, 2002) describes a somewhat straightforward approach to a more individ-

ualized biofeedback treatment for chronic low back pain. Treatment begins with EMG biofeedback-assisted relaxation, initially from the frontal or forehead area, which is then followed by feedback of the trapezius muscles, all performed with the patient sitting in a comfortable chair or recliner. Once the basic strategies are acquired, positions are changed to facilitate generalization of training effects. The patient practices in a comfortable office chair (with arms supported), then moves to an office chair without arm support, and then to a standing position. This phase of training continues for 12 to 16 sessions.

If improvement is insufficient and the patient has not had a prior course of general relaxation training, then this may be pursued. If this is unwarranted or has been unsuccessful, then an abbreviated psychophysiological assessment, based on the logic of biomechanical theory, is conducted to analyze the problem further. EMG sensors are placed bilaterally on the paraspinals (L4–L5) and the biceps femoris (back of the thigh). Recordings are made in at least two positions: sitting with back supported in a recliner and standing with arms by the side. These sites were selected because they provided greater information than other sites (such as quadriceps femoris or gastrocnemius) in prior examinations. References for these, and other EMG placement sites, may be found in Basmajian and DeLuca (1985) and Lippold (1967).

The resulting data reveal one of three patterns of abnormality: (1) unusually low muscle tension levels (which Arena states most typically occurs when nerve damage and muscle atrophy are present), (2) unusually high muscle tension levels (which Arena states is the most common finding), and (3) left–right asymmetry, wherein one side has normal muscle and the other side is either abnormally high or low. Treatment centers on returning EMG values to normal levels. Arena notes that much can be learned by examining gait and posture and correcting faulty positions as well. Sella (2003a, 2003b, and elsewhere in this volume) has commented on these postural aspects as well.

The approach that Arena describes is appealing because of its simplicity. The difficulty is in determining normal versus abnormal values. Experience with a considerable number of patients is necessary for this. Some researchers are approaching this problem in a more systematic manner and developing normative data banks for multiple muscle sites to help identify aberrant values, as these may be suggestive of bracing or favoring of a position or posture and, thus, targets for EMG treatment (Cram, 1990, and Sella, Chapter 45 this volume).

In this approach, multiple bilateral recordings need to be made in fairly rapid succession. To make this feasible, Cram uses two hand-held "post" electrodes to obtain brief (around 2 seconds per site) sequential bilateral recordings while the patient is sitting and standing (rather than having to apply multiple leads or apply and reapply the same set of leads). Although seemingly straightforward, this approach is actually complex because a number of factors can influence the results (angle and force of sensor application; amount of adipose tissue present, as fat acts as an insulator and dampens the signal; and the exactness of sensor placement).

Studies used to support claims for efficacy of EMG biofeedback for recurrent headache (and summarized in the concluding section) have monitored muscle activity almost exclusively from the forehead area, despite patients reporting other sites as central to their pain (such as occipital, temporal, neck, and shoulders). Support exists for feedback from the upper trapezius muscles (Arena, Bruno, Hannah, & Meador, 1995), and an interesting and creative novel approach, termed the Frontal-Posterior Neck placement, is presented by Nevins and Schwartz (1985). This placement seeks to provide an indirect measure of activity in the occipitalis and temporalis areas, as they are frequent sites of headache activity for certain tension-type patients but sites that are not easily accessed (covered with hair). This is accomplished by placing one active electrode on the frontal area and the remaining active electrode on the posterior neck on the same side. The summated electrical activity between these sites closely approximates that which occurs in the occipital and temporalis areas (when direct comparisons have been made). This approach has been found useful for discriminating patients with headache from patients without headache and headache from headache-free periods in patients with headache (Hudzynski & Lawrence, 1988, 1990). For TMD, in addition to frontal sites, biofeedback is provided from masseter and temporalis muscles (Crider & Glaros, 1999; Glass, Glaros, & McGlynn, 1993; Glaros & Lausten, 2003).

Finally, work undertaken by Sherman and colleagues (Sherman, 1997) has helped to identify the most appropriate biofeedback treatment for patients experiencing phantom limb pain. Pain described as burning, throbbing, and tingling was associated with decreased temperature in the stump, while pain described as cramping was preceded by and associated with EMG changes. Targeting biofeedback accordingly leads to the greatest outcome.

SELECT TREATMENT CONSIDERATIONS

Individuals presenting for biofeedback and relaxation are often confused about the nature of their disorder and are anxious, fearful, depressed, discouraged, and uncertain about their chances for improvement. Brief instruction about factors underlying the condition, pointing out variables that potentially may be controlled by the patient, is often helpful in counteracting the patient's initial feelings of helplessness and in mobilizing interest in treatment. This is followed by a description of treatment and what will be required (frequency and number of sessions, home practice, etc.), and any ancillary treatment that may be

used. The explanation of biofeedback is best understood when accompanied by a live demonstration, which points out the steps involved in measurement and provision of feedback. Education remains an integral part of treatment, as patients continue to discover more about causes and newfound ways to react.

Self-management involves learning skills and this requires regular practice and eventually incorporating learned skills into day-to-day activities. In biofeedback, some patients become successful simply by concentrating on the feedback stimulus and becoming aware of corresponding sensations. Others engage in various mental games or attempt to empty their minds completely and think of nothing (Arena & Blanchard, 2002). In early sessions, patients are encouraged to experiment with various techniques, but to remain with a given technique long enough to give it an ample trial period.

The biofeedback therapist is best viewed as a "coach," someone who has special skills the patient does not yet have, but who can impart these skills by properly timed guidance. This involves (1) sharing observations for discussion ("I noticed that your EMG signal suddenly increased. It seemed you might have been clenching your teeth then. How about dropping your lower jaw and moving it just a bit forward? I wonder if anything particular might have been on your mind then?"); (2) determining when breaks and encouragement might be needed (early attempts to lower EMG or skin conductance or to raise hand temperature often are met with the opposite effect and this situation is paradoxically worsened as patients try harder and harder; these occurrences can be of great therapeutic value as they help to demonstrate the relationship between thoughts and physiological functioning and illustrate to the patient how present means of coping are actually "backfiring"; explaining how and why this is happening helps to counteract frustration and get the patient back on track); (3) helping patients to articulate and consolidate learning; and (4) augmenting biofeedback with other self-management procedures as appropriate. With experience, the therapist learns when the patient needs uninterrupted time to practice biofeedback and when support and assistance would be valuable (and refrains from being overly active and intrusive; Borgeat, Hade, Larouche, & Bedwani, 1980).

A typical biofeedback treatment session involves the following components: (1) sensor attachment and time for adaptation, (2) initial progress review, (3) resting baseline, (4) "self-control" baseline (defined as the patient's ability to regulate the target response in the desired direction once training has begun but in the absence of feedback [Blanchard & Epstein, 1978], which provides an index of the ability to perform the biofeedback skills outside of the treatment setting), (5) 20 to 30 minutes of actual feedback (continuous or interrupted by breaks), (6) final resting or self-control baseline (to assess extent of learning within the session), and (7) final progress review, homework assignment, etc.

Each session should end by reviewing the strategies explored and appraising their effectiveness. Once the patient has shown some abilities to regulate target physiological levels in the clinic, practice outside of the office is encouraged. Initially this practice is performed in a setting maximally conducive to achieving a relaxed state or concentrating on the task at hand. Subsequently, patients are instructed to practice during everyday, but low stress/low pain activities (when driving, shopping, standing in line, during a coffee break, etc.). The final goal is to employ learned self-management skills to counteract the buildup of stress and physiological arousal. Skills have to be highly developed to be successful at this step.

Thus, the goals of self-management are for the patient to be able to discriminate when the target response is in need of control, effect the necessary change in the absence of feedback, apply the learned skills in the real world, and continue use of these skills over the long term. Therapists need, then, to be concerned with generalization and maintenance of learned skills. Lynn and Freedman (1979) have identified a number of procedures for helping to make biofeedback training effects more durable, for example, overlearning the response; incorporating booster treatments; fading or gradually removing feedback during treatment; training under stimulating or stressful conditions, such as during noise and distractions, while engaged in a physical or mental task; employing multiple therapists, which is possible in group practices; varying the physical setting; providing patients portable biofeedback for use in real-life situations; and augmenting biofeedback with other physiological interventions and with cognitive and behavioral procedures (see Bresler, Chapter 52, and Burte, Chapter 51, this volume; Thorn, 2004; Waters et al., 2004).

There are no firm criteria for deciding when to terminate biofeedback. In research investigations of biofeedback as a general relaxation technique, patients are commonly provided a set number of treatments, typically ranging from 8 to 12. Research conducted with patients with headache has shown that a much-abbreviated form of treatment can be effective, when accompanied by detailed manuals and relaxation tapes that patients study and use at home (Haddock et al., 1997). In practice, the number of sessions is determined according to clinical response, as gauged by degree of symptom relief and/or adequacy of control of the target response. Skilled therapists come to sense when treatment has reached the point of diminishing returns or marginal utility (i.e., response reaches a plateau and further effort does not alter matters much). Some have argued for using a physiological training criterion as a deciding factor; e.g., ability to reduce and keep EMG levels below a certain value for a specified time, ability to raise hand temperature above a certain

value within a specified time period. This intuitive notion has great clinical appeal, but we are not yet at a point where it is possible to advocate for a specific approach.

Although relaxation and biofeedback treatments most commonly lead to positive outcomes, a small number of patients can experience initial negative outcomes (muscle cramps, disturbing sensory, cognitive or emotional reactions) and/or other problems that affect adherence and practice. A small portion of clients may experience what has been termed "relaxation-induced anxiety," defined as a sudden increase in anxiety during deep relaxation that can range from mild to moderate intensity and that can approach the level of a minor panic attack (Heide & Borkovec, 1983). It is important for the therapist to remain calm, reassure the patient that the episode will pass, and when possible, have the patient sit up for a few minutes or even walk about the office when this happens. With patients who are believed to be at risk for relaxation-induced anxiety, it may be helpful to instruct them to focus more on the somatic aspects as opposed to the cognitive aspects of training (Arena & Blanchard, 2002). Schwartz, Schwartz, and Monastra (2003) provide detailed discussions of these potential problems, as well as solutions for addressing them.

BIOFEEDBACK AS AN "INDIRECT" APPROACH

Belar and Kibrick (1986) point out how biofeedback can be considered as an "indirect" approach for certain patients. Their use of this term is based more on clinical than empirical reasons. Here the approach is used as a means for facilitating psychosomatic therapy. Consider the example of the patient with pain who steadfastly holds to a purely somatic view and refuses to accept the notion that other factors (emotional, behavioral, and environmental) may be precipitating, perpetuating, or exacerbating pain and somatic symptoms. With this type of patient, a referral for biofeedback is likely to be less threatening (it is construed as a "physical" treatment for a "physical" problem) and to at least open the door for help. As "physiological insight" is acquired, such patients may begin to see the broader picture, i.e., the interplay of physical and psychological factors. In fact, it is not all that uncommon for a patient with pain, who denies psychological factors upon entry to therapy, to make a request like the following after just a few sessions of biofeedback: "Doc, how about turning off the biofeedback equipment today. I want to talk about a few things." From this point on, session time is divided between biofeedback and psychotherapy.

BIOFEEDBACK: THERAPISTS, CREDENTIALING, AND RESOURCES

The increasing popularity of biofeedback has led to a significant increase in the number of professionals providing this service to the public. Biofeedback clinicians can be found in a variety of settings: mental health centers, universities, medical schools, hospitals, rehabilitation clinics, and private practice. These clinicians hold degrees in psychology, social work, mental health, medicine, physical therapy, occupational therapy, nursing, and related disciplines. Their training may have been formal, such as at one of the few professional training programs in the country, or as informal as a self-directed literature review. As the issue of reimbursement for biofeedback services becomes increasingly important, professionals are moving toward more formal training and credentialing in the area. Insurance companies and other reimbursement agencies are beginning to require credentialing in biofeedback, in line with their expectation for other modes of treatment. Although credentials are not always required to deliver biofeedback, the extended training and knowledge that is acquired through the credentialing process can only add to a practitioner's competence.

Because anyone can purchase biofeedback equipment and provide treatment, it is important that biofeedback providers be properly trained and credentialed. The applications of biofeedback are diverse and there are many types of training programs. The Biofeedback Certification Institute of America (BCIA) provides accreditation of educational programs that are not based at universities, and this institute also provides certification for basic or general biofeedback and for one specialized use, that concerning EEG biofeedback (or neurotherapy). Both certifications require professional training and an internship period where the applicant works under the supervision of a certified member. Following the internship period, the applicant must then take a written examination and a practical examination. If the applicant is successful, he or she must then participate in ongoing continuing certification to maintain certified status (which is renewed every 4 years).

The Association for Applied Psychophysiology Biofeedback (www.aapb.org), the Society for Neuronal Regulation (www.snr-jnt.org), and the Biofeedback Foundation of Europe (BFE; www.bfe.org) sponsor various training programs at their annual conferences and at other times as well. The BFE has available on its Web site treatment protocols for various conditions developed by experienced clinicians/researchers.

When selecting a biofeedback therapist, consider the following: Is the provider credentialed? Has the provider received extended training (attendance at workshops or professional training in biofeedback)? Does the provider engage in academic pursuits involving biofeedback (present or teach courses on the topic)? Is the person licensed or certified in his or her specific field? Is the provider familiar with the diagnosis you are seeking to have treated? A list of certified providers may be found at the BCIA Web site (www.bcia.org).

EVIDENCE BASE

The aforementioned procedures have been extensively researched in the literature, with this literature evaluated both by efficacy or task force panels conducting evidence-based reviews and by scientists conducting quantitative or meta-analytic reviews. The chapter closes by providing a brief summary of the extant literature.

The most extensive empirical support for relaxation and biofeedback pertains to treatment of headache. Evidence-based reviews have been performed by various task forces within the Association for Applied Psychophysiology and Biofeedback (Andrasik & Blanchard, 1987; Blanchard & Andrasik, 1987; Yucha & Gilbert, 2004), the Task Force on Promotion and Dissemination of Psychological Procedures (1995), the U.S. Headache Consortium (composed of the American Academy of Family Physicians, American Academy of Neurology, American Headache Society, American College of Emergency Physicians, American College of Physicians–American Society of Internal Medicine, American Osteopathic Association, and National Headache Foundation; Campbell, Penzien, & Wall, 2000), the NIH Technology Assessment Panel on Integration of Behavioral and Relaxation Approaches into the Treatment of Chronic Pain and Insomnia (1996), among others for adult patients. Similar reviews have been conducted for children and adolescents (Holden et al., 1999). Further, meta-analytic reviews have been performed for both adults (Blanchard & Andrasik, 1987; Blanchard et al., 1980; Bogaards & ter Kuile, 1994; Haddock et al., 1997; Holroyd & Penzien, 1986; Goslin et al., 1999; McCrory et al., 2001) and children (Eccleston et al., 2002, 2004; Hermann & Blanchard, 2002; Hermann et al., 1995; Sarafino & Goehring, 2000). All show strong support for relaxation, biofeedback, and related approaches (cognitive behavior therapy). Some research suggests that biofeedback may offer an advantage over relaxation with certain patients (Blanchard et al., 1982). Finally, a meta-analytic comparison revealed similar outcomes for relaxation and biofeedback when compared with various standard prophylactic medications (Holroyd & Penzien, 1990).

Biofeedback-based treatments for TMD have also been the subject of a meta-analysis (Crider & Glaros, 1999). This work primarily involves EMG biofeedback from the following sites: masseter, temporalis, frontal, or intraoral locations. This analysis revealed a mean improvement rate of 68.6% for biofeedback treatments compared with 34.7% for various control conditions. Effect size scores for pain measures were 1.04 and 0.47 and for actual examination results were 1.33 and 0.26 for biofeedback and controls, respectively. Effects noted at the end of treatment were either maintained or improved during follow-up evaluations, some of which extended over 2 years.

Finally, biofeedback and related procedures do have value in isolation when treating patients with chronic pain (Arena & Blanchard, 2001; Flor & Birbaumer, 1994), but effects are maximized when combined with other inventions, as is the practice in most comprehensive treatment centers (Flor et al., 1992; Gatchel et al., 2003; Morley et al., 1999).

REFERENCES

Andrasik, F. (1986). Relaxation and biofeedback for chronic headaches. In A. D. Holzman & D. C. Turk (Eds.), *Pain management: A handbook of psychological treatment approaches* (pp. 213–329). New York: Pergamon.

Andrasik, F. (2000). Biofeedback. In D. I. Mostofsky & D. H. Barlow (Eds.), *The management of stress and anxiety disorders in medical disorders* (pp. 66–83). Boston: Allyn & Bacon.

Andrasik, F. (2004). The essence of biofeedback, relaxation, and hypnosis. In R. H. Dworkin & W. S. Breitbart (Eds.), *Psychosocial aspects of pain: A handbook for health care providers, progress in pain research and management* (vol. 27, pp. 285–305). Seattle: IASP Press.

Andrasik, F., & Blanchard, E. B. (1987). The biofeedback treatment of tension headache. In J. P. Hatch, J. G. Fisher, & J. D. Rugh (Eds.), *Biofeedback: Studies in clinical efficacy* (pp. 281–321). New York: Plenum.

Andrasik, F., & Flor, F. (2003). Biofeedback. In H. Breivik, W. Campbell, & C. Eccleston (Eds.), *Clinical pain management: Practical applications and procedures* (pp. 121–133). London: Arnold Publishers.

Andrasik, F., & Lords, A. O. (2004). Biofeedback. In L. Freedman (Ed.), *Mosby's complementary & alternative medicine: A research-based approach* (2nd ed., pp. 207–235). Philadelphia: Elsevier Science.

Andrasik, F., & Walch, S. E. (2003). Headaches. In A. M. Nezu, C. M. Nezu, & P. A. Geller (Eds.), *Handbook of psychology: Health Psychology* (pp. 245–266). New York: Wiley.

Andrasik, F., Thorn, B. E., & Flor, F. (in press). Psychophysiological assessment of pain. In R. F. Schmidt & W. D. (Eds.), *Encyclopedic reference of pain*. Heidelberg, Germany, Springer-Verlag.

Andreassi, J. L. (2000). *Psychophysiology: Human behavior & physiological response* (4th ed.). Mahwah, NJ: Lawrence Erlbaum Associates.

Arena, J. G., & Blanchard, E. B. (1996). Biofeedback and relaxation therapy for chronic pain disorders. In R. J. Gatchel & D. C. Turk (Eds.), *Psychological approaches to pain management: A practitioner's handbook* (pp. 179–230). New York: Guilford Press.

Arena, J. G. & Blanchard, E. B. (2001). Biofeedback therapy for chronic pain disorders. In J. D. Loeser, S. D. Butler, C. R. Chapman, & D. C. Turk, (Eds.), *Bonica's management of pain* (3rd ed., pp. 1755–1763). Baltimore, MD: Williams & Wilkins.

Arena, J. G., & Blanchard, E. B. (2002). Biofeedback training for chronic pain disorders: A primer. In R. J. Gatchel & D. C. Turk (Eds.), *Psychological approaches to pain management: A practitioner's handbook*, 2nd edition (pp. 159–187). New York, NY: Guilford Press.

Arena, J. G., & Schwartz, M. S. (2003). Psychophysiological assessment and biofeedback baselines: A primer. In M. S. Schwartz & F. Andrasik (Eds.), *Biofeedback: a practitioner's guide* (3rd ed., pp. 128–158). New York: Guilford Press.

Arena, J. G., Bruno, G. M., Hannah, S. L., & Meador, K. J. (1995). A comparison of frontal electromyographic biofeedback training, trapezius electromyographic biofeedback training, and progressive muscle relaxation therapy in the treatment of tension headache. *Headache, 35,* 411–419.

Basmajian, J. V. (1976). Facts versus myths in EMG biofeedback. *Biofeedback and Self-Regulation, 1,* 369–371.

Basmajian, J. V., & DeLuca, C. J. (1985). *Muscles alive: Their functions revealed by electromyography.* Baltimore: Williams & Wilkins.

Belar, C. D., & Kibrick, S. A. (1986). Biofeedback in the treatment of chronic back pain. In A. D. Holzman & D. C. Turk (Eds.), *Pain management: A handbook of psychological treatment approaches* (pp. 131–150). New York: Pergamon Press.

Bernstein, D. A., & Borkovec, T. D. (1973). *Progressive relaxation training.* Champaign, IL: Research Press.

Blanchard, E. B., & Andrasik, F. (1987). Biofeedback treatment of vascular headache. In J. P. Hatch, J. G. Fisher, & J. D. Rugh (Eds.), *Biofeedback: Studies in clinical efficacy* (pp. 1–79). New York: Plenum.

Blanchard, E. B., Andrasik, F., Ahles, T. A., Teders, S. J., Jurish, S. E., & O'Keefe, D. (1980). Migraine and tension headache: A meta-analytic review. *Behavior Therapy, 14,* 613–631.

Blanchard, E. B., & Epstein, L. H. (1978). *A biofeedback primer,* Reading, MA: Addison-Wesley Publishing.

Blanchard, E. B., Andrasik, F., Neff, D. F., Teders, S. J., Pallmeyer, T. P., Arena, J. G. et al. (1982). Sequential comparisons of relaxation training and biofeedback in the treatment of three kinds of chronic headache or, the machines may be necessary some of the time. *Behaviour Research and Therapy, 20,* 469–481.

Bogaards, M. C., & ter Kuile, M. M. (1994). Treatment of recurrent tension headache: A meta-analytic review. *Clinical Journal of Pain, 10,* 174–190.

Borgeat, F., Hade, B., Larouche, L. M., & Bedwani, C. N. (1980). Effect of therapist's active presence on EMG biofeedback training of headache patients. *Biofeedback and Self-Regulation, 5,* 275–282.

Boucsein, W. (1992). *Electrodermal activity.* New York: Plenum.

Cacioppo, J. T., Tassinary, L. G., & Bernston, G. G. (Eds.) (2000). *Handbook of psychophysiology.* Cambridge, U.K.: Cambridge University Press.

Campbell, J. K., Penzien, D. B., & Wall, E. M. (2000). *Evidence-based guidelines for migraine headaches: Behavioral and physical treatments.* Available at: http://www.aan.com/public/practiceguidelines/headache_g1.htm.

Cram, J. R. (1990). EMG muscle scanning and diagnostic manual for surface recordings In J. R. Cram et al. (Eds.), *Clinical EMG for surface recordings* (Vol. 2). Nevada City, CA: Clinical Resources.

Crider A. B., & Glaros, A. G. (1999). A meta-analysis of EMG biofeedback treatment of temporomandibular disorders. *Journal of Orofacial Pain, 13,* 29–37.

Eccleston, C., Morley, S., Williams, A., Yorke, L., & Mastroyannopoulou, K. (2002). Systematic review of randomised controlled trials of psychological therapy for chronic pain in children and adolescents, with a subset meta-analysis of pain relief. *Pain, 99,* 157–165.

Eccleston, C., Yorke, L., Morley, S., Williams, A. C., & Mastroyannopoulou, K. (2004). Psychological therapies for the management of chronic and recurrent pain in children and adolescents. *The Cochrane Library, Issue 1.*

Fernandez, E. (2002). *Anxiety, depression, and anger in pain.* Dallas: Advanced Psychological Resources.

Flor, H. (2001). Psychophysiological assessment of the patient with chronic pain. In D. C. Turk & R. Melzack (Eds.), *Handbook of pain assessment* (2nd ed., pp. 76–96). New York: Guilford.

Flor, H., & Birbaumer, N. (1994). Psychophysiological methods in the assessment and treatment of chronic musculoskeletal pain. In J. G. Carlson, R. R. Seifert, & N. Birbaumer (Eds.), *Clinical applied psychophysiology* (pp. 171–184). New York: Plenum.

Flor, H., & Turk, D. C. (1989). Psychophysiology of chronic pain: Do chronic pain patients exhibit symptom-specific psychophysiological responses? *Psychological Bulletin, 105,* 219–259.

Flor, H., Fürst, M., & Birbaumer, N. (1999). Deficient discrimination of EMG levels and overestimation of perceived tension in chronic pain patients. *Applied Psychophysiology and Biofeedback, 24,* 55–66.

Flor, H., Fydrich, T., & Turk, D. C. (1992). Efficacy of multidisciplinary pain treatment centers: A meta-analytic review. *Pain, 49,* 221–230.

Flor, H., Schugens, M. M., & Birbaumer, N. (1992). Discrimination of muscle tension in chronic pain patients and healthy controls. *Biofeedback and Self-Regulation, 17,* 165–177.

French, D. J., Holroyd, K. A., Pinell, C., Malinoski. P. T., O'Donnell, F., & Hill, K. R. (2000). Perceived self-efficacy and headache-related disability. *Headache, 40,* 647–656.

Gatchel, R. J., Robinson, R. C., Pulliam, C., & Maddrey, A. M. (2003). Biofeedback with pain patients: Evidence for its effectiveness. *Seminars in Pain Medicine, 1,* 55–66.

Gevirtz, R. N., & Schwartz, M. S. (2003). The respiratory system in applied psychophysiology. In M. S. Schwartz & F. Andrasik, (Eds.), *Biofeedback: A practitioner's guide,* 3rd. ed., pp. 212–244). New York: Guilford Press.

Gevirtz, R. N., Hubbard, D. R., & Harpin, R. E. (1996). Psychophysiologic treatment of chronic lower back pain. *Professional Psychology: Research and Practice, 27,* 561–566.

Glaros, A. G., & Lausten, L. (2003). Temporomandibular disorders. In M. S. Schwartz & F. Andrasik (Eds.), *Biofeedback: A practitioner's guide,* 3rd. ed., pp. 349–368). New York: Guilford Press.

Glass, E. G., Glaros, A. G., & McGlynn, F. D. (1993). Myofascial pain dysfunction: Treatments used by ADA members. *Journal of Craniomandibular Practice, 11,* 25–29.

Goslin, R. E., Gray, R. N., McCrory, D. C., Penzien, D. B., Rains, J. C., & Hasselblad, V. (1999, February). *Behavioral physical treatments for migraine headache. Technical review 2.2.* (Prepared for the Agency for Health Care Policy and Research under Contract No. 290-94-2025. Available from the National Technical Information Service; NTIS Accession No. 127946).

Haddock, C. K., Rowan, A. B., Andrasik, F., Wilson, P. G., Talcott, G. W., & Stein, R. J. (1997). Home-based behavioral treatments for chronic benign headache: A meta-analysis of controlled trials. *Cephalalgia, 17,* 113–118.

Heide, F. J., & Borkovec, T. D. (1983). Relaxation-induced anxiety: Paradoxical anxiety enhancement due to relaxation training. *Journal of Consulting and Clinical Psychology, 51,* 171–182.

Hermann, C., & Blanchard, E. B. (2002). Biofeedback in the treatment of headache and other childhood pain. *Applied Psychophysiology and Biofeedback, 27,* 143–162.

Hermann, C., Kim, M., & Blanchard, E. B. (1995). Behavioral and prophylactic pharmacological intervention studies of pediatric migraine: An exploratory meta-analysis. *Pain, 60,* 239–256.

Holden, E. W., Deichmann, M. M., & Levy, J. D. (1999). Empirically supported treatments in pediatric psychology: Recurrent pediatric headache. *Journal of Pediatric Psychology, 24,* 91–109.

Holroyd, K. A., & Penzien, D. (1986). Client variables and the behavioral treatment of recurrent tension headache: A meta-analytic review. *Journal of Behavioral Medicine, 9,* 515–536.

Holroyd, K. A., & Penzien, D. (1990). Pharmacological versus non-pharmacological prophylaxis of recurrent migraine headache: A meta-analytic review of clinical trials. *Pain, 42,* 1–13.

Hubbard, D. (1996). Chronic and recurrent muscle pain: Pathophysiology and treatment, and review of pharmacologic studies. *Journal of Musculoskeletal Pain, 4,* 123–143.

Hubbard, D., & Berkoff, G. (1993). Myofascial trigger points show spontaneous EMG activity. *Spine, 18,* 1803–1807.

Hudzynski, L. G., & Lawrence, G. S. (1988). Significance of EMG surface electrode placement models and headache findings. *Headache, 28,* 30–35.

Hudzynski, L. G., & Lawrence, G. S. (1990). EMG surface electrode normative data for muscle contraction headache and biofeedback therapy. *Headache Quarterly, 1,* 224–229.

Lichstein, K. L. (1988). *Clinical relaxation strategies.* New York: Wiley & Sons.

Lichstein, K. L., Sallis, J. F., Hill, D., & Young, M. C. (1981). Psychophysiological adaptation: An investigation of multiple parameters. *Journal of Behavior Assessment, 3,* 111–121.

Lippold, D. C. J. (1967). Electromyography. In P. H. Venables & I. Martin (Eds.), *Manual of psychophysiological methods* (pp. 245–297). New York: Wiley.

Lynn, S. J., & Freedman, R. R. (1979). Transfer and evaluation of biofeedback treatment. In A. P. Goldstein & F. Kanfer (Eds.), *Maximizing treatment gains: Transfer enhancement in psychotherapy* (pp. 445–484). New York: Academic Press.

McCrory, D. C., Penzien, D. B., Hasselblad, V., & Gray, R. N. (2001). *Evidence report: Behavioral and physical treatments for tension-type and cervicogenic headache.* Des Moines, IA: Foundation for Chiropractic Education and Research (Product No. 2085).

McNulty, E., Gevirtz, R., Hubbard, D., & Berkoff, G. (1994). Needle electromyographic evaluation of trigger point response to a psychological stressor. *Psychophysiology, 31,* 313–316.

Melzack, R. (1999). Pain and stress: A new perspective. In R. J. Gatchel & D. C. Turk (Eds.), *Psychosocial factors and pain: Critical perspectives* (pp. 89–106). New York: Guilford Press.

Morley, S., Eccleston, C., & Williams, A. (1999). Systematic review and meta-analysis of randomized controlled trials of cognitive behaviour therapy and behaviour therapy for chronic pain in adults, excluding headache. *Pain, 80,* 1–13.

Neumann, E., & Blanton, R. (1970). The early history of electrodermal research. *Psychophysiology, 6,* 453–475.

Nevins, B. G., & Schwartz, M. S. (1985). An alternative placement for EMG electrodes in the study and treatment of tension headaches. Paper presented at the 16th annual meeting of the Biofeedback Society of America, New Orleans, LA.

NIH Technology Assessment Panel on Integration of Behavioral and Relaxation Approaches into the Treatment of Chronic Pain and Insomnia. (1996). Integration of behavioral and relaxation approaches into the treatment of chronic pain and insomnia. *Journal of the American Medical Association, 276,* 313–318.

Peek, C. J. (2003). A primer of biofeedback instrumentation. In M. S. Schwartz & F. Andrasik (Eds.), *Biofeedback: A practitioner's guide* (3rd ed., pp. 43–87). New York: Guilford Press.

Sarafino, E. P., & Goehring, P. (2000). Age comparisons in acquiring biofeedback control and success in reducing headache pain. *Annals of Behavioral Medicine, 22,* 10–16.

Sargent, J. D., Green, E. E., & Walters, E. D. (1972). The use of autogenic training in a pilot study of migraine and tension headaches. *Headache, 12,* 120–124.

Schultz, J. H., & Luthe, W. (1969). *Autogenic training* (Vol. 1). New York: Grune & Stratton.

Schwartz, N. M., & Schwartz, M. S. (2003). Definitions of biofeedback and applied psychophysiology. In M. S. Schwartz & F. Andrasik (Eds.), *Biofeedback: a practitioner's guide,* 3rd ed., pp. 27–39). New York: Guilford Press.

Schwartz, M. S., Schwartz, N. M., & Monastra, V. J. (2003). Problems with relaxation and biofeedback-assisted relaxation, and guidelines for management. In M. S. Schwartz & F. Andrasik (Eds.), *Biofeedback: A practitioner's guide,* 3rd ed., 251–264). New York: Guilford Press.

Sella, G. E. (2003a). Back pain: Musculoskeletal pain syndrome. In D. Moss, A. McGrady, T. C. Davies, & I. Wickramasekera (Eds.), *Handbook of mind-body medicine for primary care* (pp. 259–273). Thousand Oaks, CA: Sage Publications.

Sella, G. E. (2003b). Neuropathology considerations: Clinical and sEMG /biofeedback applications. *Applied Psychophysiology and Biofeedback, 28,* 93–105.

Sherman, R. (1997). *Phantom pain.* New York: Plenum Press.

Smith, J. C. (1990). *Cognitive-behavioral relaxation training: A new system of strategies for treatment and assessment.* New York: Springer.

Spinhoven, P., Lenssen, A. C., Van Dyck, R., & Zitman, F. G. (1992). Autogenic training and self-hypnosis in the control of tension headache. *General Hospital Psychiatry, 14,* 408–415.

Stern, R. M., Ray, W. J., & Quigley, K.S. (2001). *Psychophysiological recording* (2nd ed.). Oxford, U.K: Oxford University.

Surwit, R. S. & Keefe, F. J. (1978). Frontalis EMG-feedback training: An electronic panacea? *Behavior Therapy, 9,* 779–772.

Task Force on Promotion and Dissemination of Psychological Procedures. (1995). Training in and dissemination of empirically-validated psychological treatments: Report and recommendations. *The Clinical Psychologist, 48,* 3–23.

Taub, E. (1977). Self-regulation of human tissue temperature. In G. E. Schwartz & J. Beatty (Eds.), *Biofeedback theory and research* (pp. 265–300). New York: Academic Press.

Taub, E., & Emurian, C. S. (1976). Feedback-aided self-regulation of skin temperature with a single feedback locus. *Biofeedback and Self Regulation, 1,* 147–168.

Taub, E., & School, P. J. (1978). Some methodological considerations in thermal biofeedback training. *Behavior Research Methods & Instrumentation, 10,* 617–622.

Thorn, B. E. (2004). *Cognitive therapy for chronic pain: A step-by-step guide.* New York: Guilford.

Tracey, I., Proghaus, A., Gati, J. S., Clare, S., Smith, S., Menon, R. S. et al. (2002). Imaging attentional modulation of pain in the periaqueductal gray in humans. *Journal of Neuroscience, 22,* 2748–2752.

Travell, J., & Simons, D. (1983). *Myofascial pain and dysfunction: The trigger point manual.* New York: Williams & Wilkins.

Waters, S. J., Campbell, L. C., Keefe, F. J., & Carson, J. W. (2004). The essence of cognitive-behavioral pain management. In R. H. Dworkin & W. S. Breitbart (Eds.), *Psychosocial aspects of pain: A handbook for health care providers, progress in pain research and management* (Vol. 27; pp. 261–283). Seattle, WA: IASP Press.

Yucha, C., & Gilbert, C. (2004). *Evidence-based practice in biofeedback and neurofeedback.* Wheat Ridge, CO: Association for Applied Psychophysiology and Biofeedback.

50

Efficacy of Neurofeedback for Pain Management

Siegfried Othmer, PhD, and Susan Othmer, BA, BCIAC

INTRODUCTION

It has been known for some time that self-regulation strategies can alter the perception of pain. The evidence for this is strongest in certain very specific areas such as application to migraines (see Andrasik, Chapter 49 of this volume), tension headaches (Middaugh & Pawlick, 2002), and myofascial pain (Meyers, White, & Heft, 2002). Other applications of traditional autonomic biofeedback have been to arthritis pain, fibromyalgia, temporomandibular disorders, tinnitus, vulvodynia, complex regional pain syndrome, and other kinds of chronic pain (Yucha & Gilbert, 2004). In recent years, we have seen the reemergence of electroencephalography (EEG)-based biofeedback in application to a variety of psychopathologies and neurological disorders. In the context of this work, clinical benefit for certain pain syndromes was also observed. In some instances, this is simply corroborative of what had already been established with peripheral biofeedback. In others, it represents new departures.

The evidentiary basis in the literature for these new findings is still sparse. This is for many of the obvious reasons. Pain syndromes do not present clean targets for research. They are heterogeneous in clinical presentation and often obscure in terms of etiology. They are rarely seen in isolation from other clinical syndromes and/or psychiatric involvement. Self-regulation strategies, in turn, are almost never used as a stand-alone treatment. Chronic pain is rarely addressed with a single clinical approach, particularly in the complex cases where neurofeedback might be most helpful. This fact, plus the strong emotional involvement with pain, renders the demonstration of specific efficacy of neurofeedback problematic. Moreover, self-regulation strategies have traditionally been regarded as part of the discipline of psychology and, hence, have been published largely in psychology journals, most specifically biofeedback journals, with little cross-pollination occurring with medical disciplines (Masterpasqua & Healey, 2003). Further, behavioral interventions have not been favored in the current funding environment. They also present many methodological challenges to placebo-controlled evaluations that are typically mandated in the modern era. Sham training has even been ruled unethical by institutional review boards (IRBs). Finally, there is little motivation for neurofeedback research in the private sector, because nothing patentable is likely to be forthcoming. The process is straightforward and already solidly established within the public domain.

On the other hand, clinicians who have employed self-regulation techniques for pain management have been amply rewarded. Because the utilization of peripheral biofeedback for pain management is already well established, peripheral measures have remained the default choice. Efficacy of neurofeedback for pain control was therefore only discovered fortuitously, reported anecdotally, and studied nonsystematically over the years. In line with increasing interest in brain function and growth in the neurosciences, neurofeedback has recently eclipsed conventional biofeedback in terms of clinical interest, but with respect to cumulative published research, neurofeedback remains far behind. A sober appraisal finds much commonality between the disciplines as well as areas of unique strengths. We can only hope to bring order to this untidy state of affairs by means of an overarching model.

For present purposes, we intend to construct our argument that neurofeedback represents an alternative mechanization of an overall strategy for improved self-regulation. For purposes of such argument, traditional biofeedback and neurofeedback can be seen as making fundamentally the same case, and the evidence for each is mutually supportive of a single proposition, namely, the responsiveness of pain syndromes to a general self-regulation strategy. Choice between various feedback modalities would then be a matter of relative efficiency rather than of relative efficacy. For other applications, such as neuropathic pain, episodic pain such as migraine, and chronic pain, neurofeedback appears to offer some unique clinical opportunities. Something very specific is being accomplished, and that cannot be understood entirely based on the more comprehensive models.

In sum, then, we build on the surprisingly robust body of research in peripheral biofeedback for headache, plus the strands of evidence that have been forthcoming on neurofeedback specifically, to make the case for a key role of self-regulation in comprehensive pain management strategies. From that vantage point, the case can be made for the specific and perhaps unique role that can be played by neurofeedback for such conditions as neuropathic pain, migraines, and chronic pain in general.

The case for self-regulation-based remedies is compatible with modern conceptions of pain as a homeostatically regulated and emotionally modulated sensory system (Craig, 2002). These centrally mediated, homeostatic mechanisms can become disregulated, and pain itself over time can contribute to further dysregulation through positive feedback. It is easiest to think of self-regulation strategies as targeting dysregulation itself, rather than the pain response directly, in the general case. This makes it reasonable to invoke self-regulatory strategies that on the surface have no obvious direct involvement with pain pathways. Similarly, strategies may be invoked that target emotional regulation rather than pain, with a favorable consequence for pain then being a second-order effect of improved emotional stability.

The principal utility of peripheral biofeedback in pain management has been the calming of high arousal and of hyperexcitability, with beneficial fallout for reactivity to pain and for excessive focusing on the pain experience. With neurofeedback, a more comprehensive approach to arousal dysregulation appears to be possible, so that in addition to the vulnerabilities of high-arousal states one is also able to address the consequences of depressive tendencies and low-arousal conditions. These include lowered pain threshold and adverse impacts on sleep that militate against recovery. Hence, neurofeedback appears to confer improved bilateral control of arousal, both on the high-arousal and low-arousal domains. It should there-fore be seen as enhancing the regulation of arousal generally (Othmer, Othmer, & Kaiser, 1999).

As central arousal regulation is trained through neurofeedback, it is found that autonomic arousal is better managed as well. In this respect, neurofeedback and biofeedback strongly overlap. In addition, however, nervous system stability is enhanced, which has beneficial fallout for episodic pain syndromes such as migraines. The kindling of a migraine becomes progressively less likely as training proceeds. Benefits are also observed for fibromyalgia pain and for episodic pain events such as trigeminal neuralgia. It is in the stabilization of brain function that particular advantage may exist for neurofeedback, with favorable implications for a number of pain syndromes.

In its role for pain management, neurofeedback must be regarded at the systems level as impinging on primary regulatory functions such as arousal regulation, in which capacity it has varied, diffuse, and multiple effects. Because it impinges at such a basic level on brain function, neurofeedback can be thought of as targeting neuroregulation itself, with the arousal dimension primary. Additionally, however, one aspect of neuroregulation is active management of sensitivity to pain. Here the pain response is considered as a regulatory system in its own right, with its own internal feedback pathways. There are indications that neurofeedback can have a specific effect on the regulatory set points of nociception as well as more general effects on modulatory influences on that system. Hence, neurofeedback can be expected to help not only with centrally mediated pain, but also with nociceptive pain and neuropathic pain.

Finally, neurofeedback offers help for chronic pain that is not fully recoverable because organic injury to the pathways of nociception has already occurred. In these cases, neurofeedback can still favorably affect the pain experience. In this application, one is addressing (in addition to central modulatory mechanisms) the psychological and subjective dimension of the pain response with a technique that is experiential rather than directly ameliorative. The rationale for this approach is the observation that there is an intimate connection between the chronic pain experience and a history of prior psychological or physical trauma. The correspondence is so high that one would not be far wrong to start therapy with the working hypothesis that any case of chronic pain most likely involves trauma as a priming event, irrespective of whether the individual is aware of a specific trauma history.

A particular kind of neurofeedback can be used as an induction technique into regressed, low-arousal states that facilitate the recall and benign processing of traumatic material. Once such processing has occurred, the individual may be in a position to acquire mastery over his or her pain that would not have been possible otherwise. Whereas the primary driver for this aspect of neurofeedback is the experiential, psychological realm, there is also an EEG training aspect involved. The experience of deep states supports and fortifies the individual's gradual movement out of hyperexcitable states. The training helps to abolish excessive fear responses and, on the positive side, promotes a more secure and stable sense of self. Of most immediate interest is that this training allows the patient to shed victim status with respect to pain, which is quite possibly a signal factor in the successful treatment of chronic pain.

In summary, then, neurofeedback can impinge favorably on the pain experience indirectly through arousal regulation, as well as through enhanced central nervous system and autonomic nervous system stability and improved homeostatic control. These can affect reactivity to pain and reduce vulnerability to episodic pain events. Neurofeedback may also be able to affect pain regulation directly by influencing the pain threshold. Moreover, it can prepare the individual to relieve the psychological factors that sustain the chronic pain experience in an unremitting state. This addresses the degree of suffering experienced because of unremediated pain.

In the following discussion, we focus on a number of pain syndromes and attempt to document the impact that neurofeedback can have even at its current state of novelty and relative immaturity. Brevity compels us to ignore a great deal of clinical detail that has been diligently amassed in this field. We apologize in advance, in that we are single-mindedly focused on the particular contribution that might be made by self-regulation approaches, based on a dysregulation model that establishes connections above the level of such clinical details (Othmer, Othmer, & Kaiser, 1999). It is implicitly understood that self-regulation strategies must find their place alongside a variety of other interventions and work synergistically. It is not the purpose of this chapter to establish that proper balance, nor even to illuminate all of the issues involved, and certainly not to seek an exalted or unique role for the proposed methods.

WHAT IS NEUROFEEDBACK?

Neurofeedback is biofeedback with the EEG used as the physiological variable being measured. Typically, it is some aspect of the amplitude and frequency distribution of the EEG that is placed in feedback configuration with an external feedback loop that involves auditory, visual, or tactile cues to the individual sourcing the EEG. Historically it has been the most prominent features of the EEG spectral distribution that have received the most attention. In the human, waking EEG is the alpha rhythm, which for present purposes can be considered the resting rhythm of the visual system. Also subject to training has been the sensorimotor rhythm, observable most prominently as the sleep spindle in Stage II sleep, which can be considered the idling rhythm of the motor system. Sterman has

recently reviewed this work in application to the control of seizures (Sterman, 2000).

Training an individual to enhance either of these amplitudes typically takes that person toward a lower state of arousal for the duration of the experience. More significantly, however, extended training improves the person's autonomous capacity to regulate arousal appropriately, if that capacity had been in any way deficient. It has become apparent that the EEG reflects the state of central arousal in both the frequency and amplitude properties of the EEG generally (Othmer et al., 1999). Empirically it has been found that the brain responds in terms of arousal regulation in both a general and a specific fashion when reinforcement occurs at any of a variety of EEG frequencies and cortical sites. The response can be thought of in terms of the activation or deactivation of specific brain networks. Thus, arousal dysregulation can now be targeted with a delineated strategy of reinforcements that take into account what is known about localization of function, hemispheric laterality of functional organization, and the particular dysregulation that the patient brings to the task. The entire EEG spectral range has become a target of training in neuro-regulation; similarly, the entire cortex has been targeted by one or another strategy of functional re-normalization.

The EEG also reveals aspects of dysregulation that are of clinical interest. In recognition of the inherent complexity of EEG morphology, an operational solution has emerged in which the EEG is treated self-referentially, and any excursions far beyond "typical" behavior for an individual are deemed to reflect states of dysregulation. Given our still limited understanding of the myriad underlying proximal mechanisms that connect these electro-chemical patterns with overt behavior and function, extreme deviation from norms is equated with deviance, i.e., dysregulation. When such excursions are used in a negative feedback configuration over an extended period, a more stable distribution of brain states can be brought about. Clinical phenomenology associated with such dysregulations will then be observed to drop away.

Three main strategies of remediation have emerged in the field. The first targets known physiological mechanisms such as the alpha and sensorimotor rhythm. This was historically the first approach and is referred to as mechanisms-based training. It still dominates the field, and benefits from the most robust literature support. The second strategy attempts to normalize steady-state EEG deviations as discerned by comparison with normative databases. This is referred to as QEEG-based training. As it is very strongly data-driven, this approach has flourished particularly in the medical applications such as traumatic brain injury, stroke, dementia, and seizure disorder. Finally, an approach based on brain function as a nonlinear dynamical system has emerged, in which the targets are dynamically established through a multivariate assessment of the quality of self-regulation manifested in the EEG at any moment. This is referred to as NLD-based training. There has now been considerable cross-fertilization between these disparate approaches, and the distinctions among them will be obscured in what follows. We refer the reader to other resources for more detailed discussion. The entire issue of *Clinical Encephalography*, 31(1), January 2000, is devoted to neurofeedback and serves as a comprehensive reference (see also Othmer, 2002a, b).

In its most common implementations, EEG neurofeedback has emerged as a dual strategy in which there is both a narrow targeting of specific frequency activity and a broad targeting of what has come to be called dysregulation. The narrow range of target frequencies is reinforced in amplitude, in the hope of establishing the individual in a particular state, namely, one of calm focus. Once that state is achieved, the person is reinforced for maintaining that state. Hence, the exercise may be seen as training the individual in the maintenance of continuity of states. The second aspect of the training involves a comprehensive appraisal of the EEG throughout the frequency domain to discern, and then to discourage through negative reinforcement, excursions into disregulated states.

The two aspects of EEG neurofeedback are generally referred to as reward-based training and inhibit-based training, respectively. By means of reward, the person effectively exercises certain brain rhythms that are important in the regulation of state. These rhythms are always observable and can always be appealed to, irrespective of any dysfunction. Through the feedback pathway, the brain is gently led out of its prevailing state (of arousal, vigilance, attention, emotional set point, etc.). Because the brain actively manages its own states, it will react to this perturbation by way of countering it and restoring the state that it had intended for itself. A kind of push–pull situation is set up in which the brain is provoked to change state through the feedback mechanism, and the brain both yields to this intervention in first instance and then resists it. The brain will not allow its state to be changed arbitrarily. The continuing exercise of this push–pull operation eventuates in improved regulatory control of arousal, and commonly also in the gradual movement toward more functional states.

The information density involved in this feedback process is very high because the EEG is so highly dynamic. When the EEG is surveyed with a narrow-band filter to focus on the part of the spectrum of immediate clinical interest, we tend to observe wavelets of some 300 ms in duration. Evidently, the neuronal ensembles under observation organize themselves transiently to subserve some aspect of brain function, and then that organization dissipates, followed by the formation of another ensemble. Hence, there is a very prominent ebb and flow of EEG amplitudes in any subband even on the 1-s timescale. This makes for potentially highly dynamic, information-rich feedback to the brain, which is then coached to enhance these amplitudes in the moment. The feedback signal to the brain is updated at normal computer monitor frame rates of 30 to 90/s. Discrete rewards for meeting goals may be given as rapidly as two times per second. Hence, the reinforcement schedule amounts to many thousands of cues in the analog domain, along with a thousand or more discrete (binary) cues in a typical half-hour session. Additionally, the information may be presented simultaneously through visual, auditory, and tactile cues for a still more reinforcing ambience.

This kind of work was originally conceptualized in terms of conventional operant conditioning. However, conventional operant conditioning typically refers to discrete rewards for discrete behavioral contingencies, and in its current implementation, we have moved essentially to a continuous data stream and more toward analog representations. Although discrete reinforcements still play a significant role, they do not index discrete events in most cases but rather signal a state in which all goals of training are being simultaneously met. Because such goals are generously set in order to motivate the client, the nearly continuous stream of discrete rewards becomes the expectation. The disappearance of the reward becomes the uncommon event that draws attention. An analogy can be drawn here to the oddball paradigm in continuous performance tests. In view of such changes, the classical operant conditioning model no doubt needs to be modified or augmented to accommodate these new methods.

An example of a highly disregulated EEG is shown in Figure 50.1. The full-bandwidth EEG shown in the top trace (with 0.5 to 30 Hz bandwidth), and clinically relevant limited-bandwidth traces derived from the raw signal are shown in the remaining three traces. The wavelets referred to above can be readily seen in the band-limited traces.

Insofar as its organization of synaptic information processing is concerned, the human brain is clearly organized exquisitely toward pattern recognition. When such explicit information is provided to the brain about its own function, the brain appears to be able to readily "recognize itself" in the information being presented. We have come to understand the reward-based training based on such pattern recognition. The brain can often respond rather quickly (i.e., within a timeframe of seconds to minutes) in a frequency-specific and cortically localized manner to the proffered signal. The initial consequence is a shift in state of arousal. This shift can then be appraised by the clinician as to its appropriateness to the clinical objective. Is the person moving toward a calmer, more alert state? Is pain subsiding? Is drowsiness increasing or decreasing? Is agitation and anxiety subsiding? Over the longer term, improved self-regulation of arousal and other state variables ensues. Because the patient is often highly labile, the clinician must assure that the training takes place within the envelope of stability of the patient's nervous

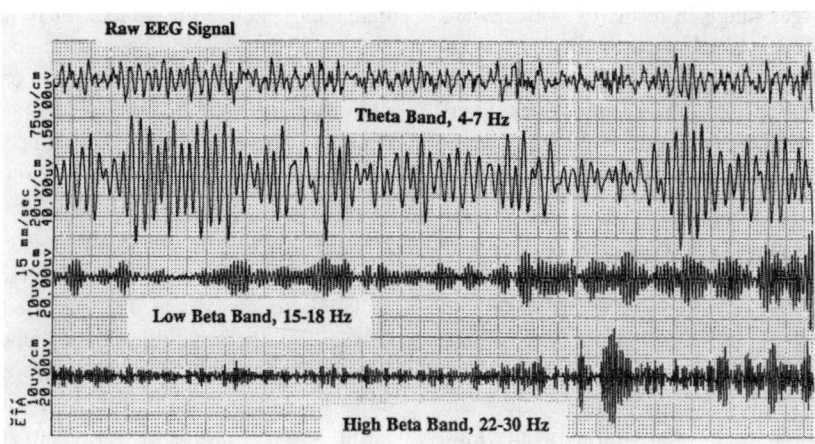

FIGURE 50.1 Raw and filtered EEG signals as utilized in EEG neurofeedback. The exemplar shows a highly disregulated EEG. The raw waveform is elevated in amplitude, itself a signature of dysregulation. It also shows epochs of rhythmic EEG dominated by frequencies falling into the theta band. This is a key signature of dysregulation, and it shows up prominently in the second trace, the theta band filtered signal. The reward band (15 to 18 Hz) shown in the third trace reveals the characteristic brief wavelets mentioned in the text. Note the change in average amplitude over the 14-s timescale of the plot, a signature of instability. The same is even more evident in the high-frequency filtered data, where the change in average amplitude is even more abrupt. Note also the sharp, high-amplitude burst in the high-frequency plot, which is also a signature of instability. All of these features are incorporated into multidimensional feedback to cue the brain toward better regulation.

system at that moment, and the magnitude of the challenge has to be adjusted to suit the capacities of the patient.

The inhibit-based training, by contrast, is opportunistic in character. One detects the brain in a trajectory toward dysregulation, and then inhibits any reward as long as this state of dysregulation persists. This repetitive, gentle negative reinforcement eventually moves the brain toward better internal regulation. In contrast to the reward-based training, which is very specific and directive in nature, the inhibits are nonspecific with regard to remedy. The brain simply has to figure out how to respond to the challenge. An advantage of the inhibit-based training is that it can be performed with almost no clinical discernment involved with respect to the nexus of EEG extrema and specific clinical phenomenology. Inhibit-based training is the embodiment of the principle that dysregulation itself is the target of the training. However, refinements are possible here in terms of the subtlety with which incipient dysregulation may be detected. At worst, even normal excursions in the EEG are called out for inhibition (that is, if the threshold for inhibition were to be set inappropriately). For that reason, the training is carried out under baseline conditions of no overt challenge to the patient, whose only duty is to witness the feedback and to rejoice in his or her success in achieving the rewards that the instrument metes out. Under such baseline conditions, episodic excursions in the EEG should be more unambiguously indicative of dysfunction than would be the case under challenge conditions.

In the final application of neurofeedback, namely, to the remediation of psychological trauma, the feedback technique is deployed in a manner that gently encourages movement toward states dominated by low-frequency activity, in the range of 12 Hz or less. The individual is thus moved toward states of low arousal, and toward internal engagement, shutting off the outside world. Under such benign circumstances, traumatic material has increased likelihood of reaching consciousness, where the material becomes available for resolution or for subsequent processing in a therapeutic setting.

The first utilization of neurofeedback can be considered as primarily impinging on physiological mechanisms: the improved regulation of central and autonomic arousal. The second utilization is intended predominantly to facilitate psychodynamic interventions. Indeed, it appears important to address both physiological and psychological aspects of pain (Singer et al., 2004; Wager et al., 2004) with an aim of reducing it. In practice, a combination of the conventional neurofeedback and the low-frequency inductions are deployed in cases of treatment-resistant chronic pain. The first, or conventional, approach is commonly referred to as SMR/beta training, because of the historical circumstance that the primary training initially took place at the sensorimotor strip, and targeted the sensorimotor rhythm (hence SMR). The sensorimotor rhythm is the 12 to 15 Hz subset of the broader beta band that extends from the top of the alpha band out to gamma (nominally 35 Hz). The second of these techniques is commonly referred to as alpha–theta training because the alpha and theta bands are jointly or alternately reinforced in that procedure. The alpha band is nominally 8 to 12 Hz, and the theta band typically 4 to 7 Hz (although in our mechanization we have adopted the variation of 5 to 8 Hz).

In view of the larger range in terms of both reward frequencies and electrode placement that now characterizes the "SMR/beta" training, the term has become anachronistic, and we now prefer to call this simply "eyes-open" training. For parallelism, then, the lower-frequency training may be referred to as eyes-closed training.

HOW IS NEUROFEEDBACK DONE?

A variety of strategies has emerged in the clinical world to effect both kinds of neurofeedback training. These approaches, or protocols, differ primarily in the relative emphasis given to the single-frequency enhancement and the broadband inhibition strategy, as well as in the kind of decision making that enters into placement of electrodes and targeting strategy. The robustness of the technique becomes apparent when it is considered that a variety of different techniques can all yield positive clinical outcomes. The fact that there is no uniqueness to the remedy also speaks to the issue that what is sought is improved regulation, not a specific set point of function. The term *homeostasis* has been gradually eased out of common usage in the field of biofeedback, as we are recognizing that we do not so much seek a particular brain state as much as we seek the capacity for improved regulation. The focus has shifted from static set points to the dynamics of brain function. Homeostasis is not a point in state space, but rather a trajectory, and a very dynamic one at that.

In the most common implementation of neurofeedback, including our own, the primary emphasis remains on the reward signal. The particular reward frequency that leaves the patient or client in a calm and focused state turns out to be highly individual. It is determined by iterative trial and frequent communication with the patient as to mental, physical, and emotional state. In sensitive individuals, discernment of change in state of arousal can often be achieved within just a few minutes. Patients with pain, however, may be so involved with their pain that they cannot report well on subtle changes. They may have lost some degree of discrimination. In that event, we work session to session to optimize the reward frequency for best outcome. To this end, we inquire as to quality of sleep and other factors. (Peripheral physiology can be helpful in this appraisal as well. Autonomic measures such as finger temperature and galvanic skin response are sensitive to state shifts that are beneath the level of awareness of the untutored patient.) In this application, however, the autonomic measures are made available to the clinician rather than to the patient, as they would be in conventional biofeedback (Schwartz & Andrasik, 2003).

In our reinforcement of the target frequency, there need be no concern about whether we are targeting a particular deficit in the EEG. It is best to think of this in terms of an exercise of the mechanisms by which the brain manages its activation–relaxation dynamics. Such an exercise could presumably be conducted at a number of EEG frequencies. However, it is also necessary to maintain the individual in a good state of functioning throughout the exercise. This constraint makes it necessary to assure precise targeting of the reward frequency. This is most particularly true in patients who are highly reactive, patients with pain foremost among them.

The inhibit strategy can either target the whole range of EEG frequencies at once, as we commonly do, or it can selectively target those bands where the dysregulation is most likely to manifest. The difference in training strategies falls out in terms of relative training efficiency, but not in terms of basic efficacy. Dysregulation simply needs to be systematically detected, and that can be done in a variety of ways using any number of variables by which the EEG may be characterized. One now increasingly takes the perspective of nonlinear dynamical systems theory to argue that normal EEG behavior is of bounded variation. Any extreme excursions in any EEG variable are deemed signatures of dysregulation, particularly in the benign baseline state in which the training takes place. The particulars need not even be understood in order for this strategy to be successful, although our understanding of the EEG is advancing rapidly.

Sessions are conducted with nominally 30 min on the instrument. Reinforcement schedules are set to maximize motivation of the client throughout the process — not too difficult to prevent frustration, and not too easy to forestall boredom. Hence, reinforcement thresholds are set according to psychological criteria more than psychophysiological or neurological ones. A discrete criterion is needed, but the specific choice involves some arbitrariness. Sessions can be conducted at rates from 1 to 10 per week, essentially up to the tolerance of the individual. Learning rates appear to scale with session time over that entire range.

Assessment to guide neurofeedback training is done comprehensively. This follows from the fact that the immediate objective of the training is improved self-regulation of central states and the autonomic nervous system. Pain is just one index of such function. The quality of sleep must be assessed, as well as daytime functioning in terms of arousal level, affect, energy level, and executive function. Other factors that may be brought to bear are cognitive function (e.g., Egner & Gruzelier, 2001; Vernon et al. 2003) and the variation in any other symptoms that the patient may have reported or to which the patient is known to be vulnerable.

PAIN FROM THE PERSPECTIVE OF THE SELF-REGULATION TECHNOLOGIES

In the following, various pain syndromes are discussed in terms of the general categories that have been identified:

(1) pain that is significantly connected to arousal level and to nervous system hyperexcitability, (2) episodic pain associated with central nervous system instability, (3) pain that is exacerbated by prior traumatic experience, and (4) specific pain categories such as neuropathic pain. This is admittedly an unusual partitioning, but it fits with the remedy that is being brought to bear. From the standpoint of neurofeedback, the genetic endowment and any organic factors exacerbating the pain response are simply givens that are oblique to our concerns. What matters is how regulation of physiological state can be recruited to diminish or even abolish the ongoing pain experience, to diminish severity of episodic pain and reduce incidence of events, and to remediate the trauma response and the general emotional vulnerability that sustains and infuses the pain experience.

The case of migraines is discussed first because of the foundation of evidentiary support available from research in traditional biofeedback. Migraines are most representative of the class of episodic pain phenomena grounded in central nervous system instabilities. The case of migraines illustrates what is perhaps the greatest contribution of neurofeedback, namely, a general strategy for the stabilization of cortical/subcortical regulatory networks. This example is also featured first because it represents one of the few categories of debilitating pain in which essentially complete resolution is a prospect for the large majority of cases.

APPLICATION TO MIGRAINE HEADACHE: CEREBRAL INSTABILITY

The diagnostic category that has benefited from the most solid research support in biofeedback is migraine and what has been called tension headache. This application area is covered in another part of this volume with respect to autonomic or peripheral biofeedback and, therefore, is not treated here. The collective import of numerous studies on migraine is that peripheral biofeedback matches medication efficacy in the short term and exceeds it in the long-term. Moreover, the two modalities can have additive benefits. The solidity of the evidence notwithstanding, there has not been a groundswell toward the adoption of biofeedback for migraines over the years.

This might be primarily because neither the culture of medicine nor the constraints of the reimbursement environment favor the adoption of a time-consuming training strategy. However, there are at least three additional reasons relating to the shortcomings of traditional biofeedback. First, biofeedback is not generally relied upon to abort ongoing migraines. If despite biofeedback training a migraine eventuates, little can be done in terms of traditional biofeedback to help in the moment. Therefore, biofeedback is not an emergency treatment. (However,

biofeedback countermeasures taken during the prodrome may be helpful prophylactically.) Second, biofeedback approaches tend not to be successful with hormonally mediated migraines, a large subset because migraines tend to afflict females predominantly and to occur preferentially either at ovulation or in the late luteal phase. Finally, there appears to be quite commonly the need for ongoing physiological self-regulation practice. Few chronic migraineurs "graduate" from biofeedback with any finality.

These three critical shortcomings of traditional biofeedback appear to be largely resolved with new developments in neurofeedback. First, with emerging EEG training strategies there is now a high likelihood of aborting an ongoing migraine or at least of setting it upon a largely irreversible course toward resolution some time after the session is completed. With current practice, some 50% of migraines can be aborted within a 30-min session, and 80% of the remainder will be redirected from their normal trajectory toward resolution over the succeeding few hours. Second, there appears to be no residual distinction in terms of efficacy between hormonally mediated and other migraines. Third, migraines may resolve so completely, even in long-term case histories of medically intractable migraines, that no further intervention is required, at least over typical periods of post-treatment follow-up care.

These findings are now merely observational, but they have gained empirical confirmation over more than a decade of clinical work. Jointly they appear to make the case that EEG neurofeedback offers something unique in migraine management that happens to address all of the principal shortcomings of the standard autonomic self-regulation approach. On the other hand, there have been complementary developments in conventional thermal biofeedback as well, which bear on this question.

Carmen (2004) reports startling results for a technique of thermal reinforcement of cortical activity prefrontally. This finding emerged fortuitously out of an attempt to recover from the terminal stage of migraines by use of thermal down training of cortical vascular activity. Migraines are commonly attended, after all, by elevations in thermal emissions from the scalp surface. It was found that thermal down training was relatively ineffective in the intended role of aborting migraines, but not, however, thermal up training. With a simple scheme of rewarding the person for increasing output in the thermal band of 12 to 14 μm using an infrared sensor, recovery from an ongoing migraine could be routinely achieved. Similarly, the long-term outcomes of such training were more satisfactory. In addition, there was no longer any talk of hormonally mediated migraines being refractory to treatment.

Thus, it appears that a "conventional" biofeedback technique was, in fact, capable of matching the results of neurofeedback in nearly every respect. While both of these techniques are unambiguously superior in outcome to the standard biofeedback that has been the subject of so much published research, the relative advantage of the two emerging techniques can be established only by formal comparative studies. In the meantime, claims of exceptionalism for neurofeedback with respect to migraine have to be set aside as well.

Interestingly, Carmen makes the case that this kind of thermal training should be considered a neurofeedback technique, rather than fitting within traditional thermal biofeedback. The reasoning goes as follows: Traditional temperature training of hands or feet finds its rationale in the normalization of autonomic — in particular, sympathetic — arousal. This is clearly not the case with thermal training of cortical activity. It is well known by now that neuronal activity (including glial cell activity) is the source of heat in the brain, and that the vasculature is the thermal sink on which we critically depend. An increase in thermal emissions from cortex could arise either from greater cortical neuronal activation or from reduction in heat removal. Given the traditional preoccupation with vascular phenomena in migraines as well as the direct tie-in with heat removal, Carmen calls his technique hemoencephalography (HEG), and by virtue of detection of infrared cortical emissions, more specifically pIR HEG (for passive infrared). His paper reporting on 100 cases of migraine has been recently published (Carmen, 2004).

The startling finding was that if one counted only those subjects who came for at least six sessions of training, men in the study were successful in 100% of the cases in significantly reducing their migraines. Women were successful at a 92% level. The overall success rate was 95%. One may conjecture that in women there tend to be more severe comorbidities and, in particular, more trauma histories that may not have been disclosed to the (male) practitioner. Carmen also reports that migraine-like (i.e., episodic) phenomena may continue to be observed after the completion of training, but these events may not involve pain at all.

We are confronted with the emerging reality that unprecedented results can be achieved in migraine management using two techniques that have essentially nothing in common methodologically. Moreover, when one delves into the details with respect to both techniques, the results appear to depend on very particular circumstances. For example, the most favorable outcomes in pIR HEG seem to require training at Fpz vis-à-vis Fp1 or Fp2 (in the Standard International 10–20 System), for example. The EEG training proceeds most efficiently, on the other hand, by training at temporal sites, T3–T4 in bipolar placement (vs. C3–C4, F3–F4, T5–T6, or P3–P4, for example). Even if a migraineur requires training at Fp1–Fp2 for one issue or another, when it is a matter of obtaining migraine relief it appears preferable to repair back to T3–T4. Carmen is developing a rationale that involves frontal lobe

training to underpin this technique. That same model could not serve to explain the neurofeedback results.

It is possible, of course, that the particularity follows from the unique features of each kind of training, rather than from any properties of the migraine mechanism itself. In that event, one may argue that both techniques simply cue the brain toward restoration of the normal state of self-regulation. The fact that neither T3–T4 EEG training nor pIR HEG is targeting a known deficit supports this more general view. The great disparity in techniques, combined with high similarity in clinical outcome, further supports the case for the general self-regulation model. In this view, any physiological variable that either manifests the dysregulation directly or simply ties into the disregulated networks could serve equally well in principle. However, the training of any such variable may also have other effects that are not strictly related to the migraine mechanism, yet need to be taken into account. The training not only serves to stabilize the brain over the long term, but as an immediate consequence also profoundly alters the person's state. In migraineurs who are very sensitive to such changes in state, the training parameters end up being very circumscribed. Thus, training with pIR HEG at Fp1 or Fp2 could, in principle, be equally efficacious from the standpoint of migraines, but also have implications for anxiety, depression, and affective regulation that may be an issue in the same subject. Indeed, this appears to be the case. Moreover, with regard to neurofeedback at T3–T4, a small shift in reinforcement frequency can serve to induce a migraine, or exacerbate migraine pain, as effectively as the "correct" frequency is able to expunge it.

At this point in our understanding, and in cognizance of the Zeitgeist respecting the emergence of integrative medicine, we would be inclined to promulgate the more inclusive view that both EEG and HEG neurofeedback cue the brain toward a more regulated state, each in its own way. The details are important clinically and tactically but are of lesser import in the basic mechanism sense. Both lines of evidence then give independent and complementary support to the same proposition, namely, that migraine susceptibility yields systematically and consistently to a targeted self-regulation strategy.

At the current state of maturity of EEG training procedures, the expectation is that migraine pain should significantly subside or abate entirely within a 30-min training session in the vast majority of cases. In-session changes in levels of pain are also found to be a reliable guide to the optimum training frequency. For obvious reasons, it is preferable to conduct the training when the person is not thus afflicted. However, if the person is able, then there is no reason not to attempt training even with a migraine. Visual hypersensitivity under those circumstances may require resorting to auditory training under eyes-closed conditions or to tactile means of reinforcement.

If migraines occur very frequently, a reduction in both incidence and severity should typically be observable within six sessions, whether these occur via pIR HEG or EEG neurofeedback. Migraine incidence should be eliminated in the vast majority of cases within 20 to 40 sessions. If migraines recur over time, some additional booster sessions may be scheduled. If migraines are observed as comorbidity to other conditions such as fibromyalgia, complex regional pain syndrome, or irritable bowel disease, more extended training is commonly necessary. That is discussed further below.

Efficacy of neurofeedback and biofeedback for migraines needs to be understood. However, the technique itself does not give us much of a handle because it engages with the cerebrum at such a high level. A presumptive deficit in self-organization must exist that renders the brains of migraineurs susceptible to occasional excursions into migraine. The neurofeedback apparently rebalances the excitatory/inhibitory network relations to the point where such an excursion becomes much less likely. The observation that ongoing migraines can also be systematically disrupted by the same technique is intriguing, and most satisfying, but it is not required to support the first claim and may quite possibly require additional explanation.

The complexity of cortical networks is such that the brain satisfies the condition of a nonlinear dynamical system (Llinas, Ribary, Jeanmonod, Kronberg, & Mitra, 1999) and, as such, has to satisfy a variety of stability criteria. If for the sake of argument we refrain from drawing on other hypotheses for insights into the migraine generator, i.e., we confine the discussion to the realm of control theory, then it is possible to say that the problem is one of marginal function with respect to requisite stability criteria. The problem is instability itself. The problem of instability, moreover, now has an operational remedy. The brain can be trained toward greater stability of function, even in the absence of any other intervention. The target of the intervention is the identified instability. Such instability in this case is the property of distributed networks. It cannot simply be assigned to the presumptive migraine generator.

The hypothesis finds support in the extraordinary success rate of this intervention. The essentially equivalent clinical success achieved with pIR HEG supports the hypothesis as well. It is a secondary issue of whether we target the bioelectrical activity of the brain or the thermodynamic measures because the target in each case is the source of the instability in the dysregulation of cortical/subcortical networks. Any variable that reveals such dysregulation to us is a potential target for a strategy of functional renormalization.

One other argument that can be made for the instability model of migraine is that the arousal model does not fit. Migraine susceptibility does not map into high arousal states, for example, as the phenomenon of rebound migraines attests. On the other hand, rapid change in arousal level can trigger the instability, and this includes, in particular, rapid decrease in arousal level. By virtue of their clinical preoccupation with high-arousal states, biofeedback therapists have historically been misled into thinking that parasympathetic dominance was inherently a zone of stability. This has delayed coming to terms with instabilities in the parasympathetic subsystem such as migraine and asthma attacks. Instability can be found anywhere on the arousal curve and anywhere on the sympathetic/parasympathetic continuum.

Another argument is that seizures respond to the same protocol that has been found optimal for migraine. So does bipolar disorder. These three conditions have little in common. They cover a wide variety of possible triggers of unstable state shifts. Yet they all respond to the same intervention. This is not unprecedented, as all three conditions are treated with anticonvulsants. These pharmacological agents target neuronal (i.e., cell membrane) hyperexcitability generally. By analogy, one may think of neurofeedback as changing network excitability through bioelectrical rather than neurochemical means. Just as anticonvulsants do not specifically and differentially target the seizure focus or the migraine generator, but rather the stability of neuronal networks, so does neurofeedback.

There is, in fact, one published study on neurofeedback for migraines that is relevant to the issue of the instability model. In this technique, slow cortical potentials in the EEG are trained transiently in order to shift neuronal populations at that location toward hyperpolarization, i.e., toward reduced excitability, under voluntary control. Evidently, there is a residual effect from this exercise that leaves cortical networks less excitable. This technique has also had a long research history and is known primarily for its use in brain-based communication for locked-in syndrome, as well as for the control of medically refractory seizures. With this technique, a 50% reduction in migraine incidence could be achieved (Kropp, Siniatchkin, & Gerber, 2002). This evidence can serve as independent validation of the efficacy of the neurofeedback intervention. In addition, its use for both seizure control and migraine supports the more inclusive instability model. In terms of clinically significant results, however, this technique has clearly been eclipsed by the new techniques devised with frequency-based training.

FIBROMYALGIA AND REFLEX SYMPATHETIC DYSTROPHY: HYPEREXCITABILITY

It was pointed out above that outcomes are not nearly so straightforward when migraines are seen in the context of other pain syndromes such as fibromyalgia and reflex sympathetic dystrophy (RSD). This is closer to the clinical reality when dealing with chronic pain, in that we rarely have the luxury of addressing one symptom per patient. The essential difference here is that in these comorbidities one encounters a high degree of cortical hyperexcitability across the board. This feature may be seen in the context of over-arousal, but it is not to be identified with it. It is not a unitary phenomenon. There are various ways in which such hyperexcitability can be expressed. Just as with the instability model above, this particular formulation is chosen because neurofeedback appears to moderate hyperexcitability in the general case. One can think of arousal as a more global variable, whereas hyperexcitability can arise from inadequate inhibition at the level of a particular neuronal network and, thus, can characterize specific systems such as visual or auditory processing.

Hyperexcitability is an issue in migraines as well, for example, visual hypersensitivity. Moreover, instability in turn is an issue in fibromyalgia and RSD. It is a question of which model has the greater explanatory power in each case. Hyperexcitability can be developmental in origin, but more likely is the result of specific physical injury and/or psychological trauma. A deficit in inhibitory control develops that allows neuronal pools to be too responsive to weak inputs, to respond too broadly to inputs (e.g., enlarged sensory receptive fields), and to respond too strongly to inputs that should be handled benignly. These circuits could even activate in the absence of any provocation whatsoever, or they can recruit other cortical regions into what we call a dysregulation cascade.

The essential nonlinearity of the organization of synaptic activity comes to the fore particularly when the system goes into dysregulation. A bowling analogy comes to mind, which leads us to the concept of a dysregulation cascade. On the short timescale of minutes, hours, to days, one can often observe patients slip into states of more profound dysregulation, and one can observe the same on long time scales of months to years. The dysregulation of one system gradually disregulates another. The nonlinearity of this process explains the paradox that whenever one intervenes successfully with one aspect of such dysregulation, the entire physiology appears to benefit. Thus, one may target sleep dysregulation, depression, or the pain response itself, and obtain a certain amount of relief for pain. In addition, once we move the person into the right direction physiologically, the nonlinearity is our ally. Symptom improvement should be greater than the change we produce in constituent variables, or in a particular subsystem. Put simply, even a little progress can do much good.

We have found it necessary to accept a certain lack of tidiness when it comes to chronic pain and to realize that however re-regulation is brought about, we are having an impact on dysregulation itself and, in particular, on the dysregulation cascade, its nonlinearities, and mutual couplings. The consequences do not fall out narrowly for one symptom or another but rather to the whole bouquet of symptomatology, including, in addition to pain, the quality of sleep, the anxiety/depression domain, energy level, perceived level of cognitive function, as well as emotional tone and equilibrium.

FIBROMYALGIA

There have been two published studies that bear on the application of neurofeedback to fibromyalgia. The first of these, by Donaldson and colleagues (Donaldson, Sella, & Mueller, 1998) employs a mix of techniques that includes both peripheral biofeedback and EEG biofeedback modalities. Even with regard to the neurofeedback component, the study deviates from convention. It employs a relatively novel technique in which extremely small electromagnetic fields, modulated at EEG frequencies, are delivered to the scalp to alter the EEG. First, such stimulation can be used to disrupt the brain's residence in pathological states. Second, the brain apparently detects even such low-level disturbance and attempts to compensate for it to maintain its desired function. Such a reaction exercises the regulatory circuits, with the longer-term consequence of improved regulatory function.

The second study, by Xavier Caro, evaluates one of the standard neurofeedback protocols for fibromyalgia when used in conjunction with a comprehensive medical treatment (Caro & Winter, 2001). Amazingly, Caro finds that patients maintain the intensive training schedule with surprising regularity. Such unusual compliance with a time-intensive regimen is itself an argument for the neurofeedback contribution to recovery. In a comparison study of 15 patients with long-term fibromyalgia who received at least 40 sessions of neurofeedback (average of 58 sessions; range of 40 to 98) and a group of 63 patients who had been involved in long-term follow-up, Caro found significant improvement in physician-assessed tenderness, self-reported pain, and fatigue ($p < 0.006$). Visual attention measures also improved (although not auditory ones), as indexed by a continuous performance test ($p < 0.008$).

Somatic symptoms had not changed significantly in the historical controls over a median of 6.4 years of longitudinal observation. Quantitative EEG measurements were also used in his clinic to document progress with the training. The experimental group of 15 was drawn from 42 subjects who had entered into the study. Of these, 19 received at least 40 sessions of EEG training. Of these, 4 were excluded from the analysis because of conflicting medical or psychological problems. Forty sessions were thought to be a reasonable cutoff to judge the effect of the training, but it turns out that a number of patients did not reach the 40-session milestone because their symptoms remediated sooner. Others dropped out for lack of insurance company support.

Caro's work involved the use of one of the standard neurofeedback protocols that was commonplace at the time and had much literature support in application to attention-deficit hyperactivity disorder (ADHD). The technique involved reinforcement of the SMR band (12 to 15 Hz) with simultaneous inhibition of excessive amplitudes in the 4 to 7 Hz and 22 to 30 Hz bands, with placement at Cz, the vertex of the International 10/20 System (Jasper, 1958). This particular protocol had been devised for working with ADHD (Nash, 2000). Could this same technique help with the attentional and cognitive deficits of fibromyalgia? Also, "In our experience many FMS symptoms correlate with one another, i.e., when one symptom worsens or improves, other symptoms tend to worsen or improve simultaneously" (Caro & Winter, 2001). This empirical finding supports the dysregulation model for fibromyalgia. Indeed, a correlation was observed between the improvement in attentional measures and the pain assessments.

Over time, with the growth of the field of neurofeedback, there has also been an increased diversity of protocols. In our own work, the evolution has taken us to the point where a variety of techniques are used to address different aspects of the clinical presentation. Substantial reduction or even elimination of fibromyalgia pain is now possible in the vast majority of cases within 20 to 40 sessions of neurofeedback. Improvement in the quality of sleep is likely to be reported. There should be improvements in energy level when fatigue is an issue. Moreover, improved cognitive function is often reported anecdotally, even if that cannot always be documented.

Although assessments are necessarily subjective when it comes to pain and self-perceived energy level, it should be possible to quantify the improvement in cognitive function. Paradoxically it has not often been possible to verify the cognitive deficits of which patients complain. One possible explanation is that we are dealing with patients who have historically been high performers, and who are suddenly reduced to performance that still lies within the normal range of function, but is experienced as a deficit. Another explanation may lie in the fact that typical assessment tools tend to cover the range of more profound cognitive deficits, and suffer from ceiling effects when applied to those who are more functional. It is also possible that these patients can briefly rally to meet a cognitive challenge in a testing environment, without necessarily being in a position to sustain such a level of mental efficacy.

Over time, it may be necessary to undergo an occasional neurofeedback session in order to maintain gains. The vulnerability to symptoms manifestly persists, and the vicissitudes of life often plunge the patient with fibromyalgia back into symptoms. This is in contrast to migraines, where training may reach a definable end point. It may be considered paradoxical that instability conditions such as migraine can respond more completely and more comprehensively to neurofeedback than conditions grounded in hyperexcitability. This may be understood in

the following way. The brain of a migraineur may be considered quasi-stable against migraine formation. It may not take much in terms of brain training to confer sufficient stability to the brain so that migraine formation does not propagate from the presumptive migraine generator. Hyperexcitability, on the other hand, may be a more fundamental, general, or intrinsic property of a particular brain, whether by virtue of developmental history, learned behavior, or organically acquired dysfunction. It may take longer to normalize.

In fibromyalgia cases, we may find certain characteristic EEG anomalies that constrain our operational space. Often, for example, excess alpha amplitudes are observed in the waking EEG, and alpha intrusion in sleep is sometimes observed. In consequence of this, a lack of restorative sleep is often reported. EEG training can serve to normalize the EEG in such cases, and sleep behavior may normalize as well. The underlying vulnerability may remain, however. If one later initiates alpha–theta training in order to access prior traumas, the alpha signature of dysregulation may resurface. As with other conditions of chronic pain, a high likelihood prevails of a trauma history among those with severe and intractable cases of fibromyalgia. If these cannot be accessed via alpha–theta training, then other techniques, such as eye movement desensitization and reprocessing or hypnotherapy, may need to be brought to bear.

REFLEX SYMPATHETIC DYSTROPHY

Reflex sympathetic dystrophy or complex regional pain syndrome is one of the most challenging conditions confronted in the neurofeedback practice. We are not aware of any published report, and the following is simply a reflection on our clinical work with this condition. The extent of symptom relief that can be achieved appears correlated with the length of time that the person has been symptomatic. What may start out as a largely functional deficit may progressively become a more intractable organic condition. In application to RSD, we expect neurofeedback to be only moderately ameliorative in severe cases. Patients report improvement in sleep, in energy level, in the ability to undertake life tasks, and perhaps in the level of pain. However, sleep improvements may be transient, in some cases lasting only one to three nights after a neurofeedback session. In these cases, it is advantageous for the person to conduct training sessions at home between visits to the clinic.

In RSD, we may be engaged through neurofeedback in an ongoing campaign of symptom suppression. A variety of techniques may be used in that effort, including, in particular, peripheral biofeedback and possibly cortical electrical stimulation (CES). No matter what array of techniques is employed, the patient will usually identify some unique benefit with the neurofeedback, even if that benefit

TABLE 50.1
Self-Reported Symptom Severity before and after Neurofeedback in RSD

Pre–Post Comparison Variable	n-Value	p-Value
Average pain level for five sites	19	0.001
Headaches	17	0.000
Muscle tension	12	0.000
Muscle spasms	13	0.046
Anxiety–agitation	13	0.002
Feeling more rested	7	0.007
Falling asleep	7	0.021
Staying asleep	7	0.033
Depression	15	0.017
Mental clarity	12	0.000
Ability to cope with the pain	15	0.000
Perceived energy level	12	0.018
Feeling of well-being	16	0.001

is only transient in nature. For cases such as this, we may find it beneficial to move to "always on" neurofeedback using ambulatory monitoring of the EEG and auditory feedback, in order that the patient may continuously optimize his or her state, and in order to be able to take advantage of the most propitious times to train the brain.

The objective first is to reduce the high arousal level in which the person is living. Second is to help normalize autonomic arousal. Third, the objective is to improve sleep architecture. Fourth is to address the anxiety–depression continuum. Specific training is undertaken to bring about a sense of body calmness. In each of these aspects of training, the level of pain is used as one index of progress. Training generally has to be maintained over the long term, and for that purpose transition to home training, with continual clinical supervision, is facilitated.

Although no published data on neurofeedback for RSD are available, we have been furnished preliminary statistical data on a clinical study being undertaken with standard protocols (Tracy-Smith, personal communication). Areas of concern where significant improvement was observed with the neurofeedback are listed in Table 50.1. Some additional variables where the improvement was not significant included the following: swelling at RSD sites, discoloration at RSD sites, utilization of spinal cord stimulator, tics, cold or burning skin, light sensitivity, sound sensitivity, memory function, language skills, feeling centered, and relaxation. All assessments were by self-appraisal using a 10-point scale.

It is noteworthy that there were significant improvements in the depression category, in mental clarity, in sleep criteria, in muscle tension, and in the feeling of well-being. Improvements in these disparate variables tend to support the dysregulation model. Finally, it may be seen as ironic that the nonlisted category of "relaxation"

showed no significant change. Actually, this highlights that the objective of relaxation training is not relaxation in the colloquial sense, but rather control. Success in that enterprise may not necessarily be accompanied by the subjective feeling of relaxation.

TRIGEMINAL NEURALGIA

Only a single published report is available on the use of neurofeedback for trigeminal neuralgia, and in this case a combination of neurofeedback and peripheral biofeedback was used (Sime, 2004). The response to the biofeedback was often immediate, however, which supported the clinician's view that each of the features of the protocol contributed to the ultimate resolution of the symptoms. The case concerned a person who was poorly regulated on medical management, and the next planned intervention was the severing of the trigeminal nerve. Some 10 sessions of electromyography (EMG) biofeedback were conducted over a period of 9 months, plus 29 sessions of neurofeedback. Left-hemisphere training appeared best for sleep issues, and interhemispheric training at T3–T4, identical to what is used with migraines, was best for the pain episodes.

The patient experienced a substantial reduction in pain and bruxism as well as improved sleep quality. Symptom reduction varied with the specifics of the protocols used in neurofeedback and later, in follow-up symptom reduction, fluctuated with life stresses. Counseling on stress management was provided in addition to the biofeedback. The success of the treatment was such that surgery could be avoided, and even medication could be discontinued, except for an occasional resort to Ultram. There was some continuing need for self-regulation practice, and the patient returned once for maintenance neurofeedback over the subsequent year.

A number of cases have been seen in clinical settings over the years. Generally, it has emerged that the same techniques are useful for this condition as have been evolved for the remediation of migraines and seizures. Hence, an enhancement of cortical stability appears to serve also to thwart painful episodes of tic douloureux.

MYOFASCIAL PAIN

Insofar as the self-regulation technologies are concerned, myofascial pain has been firmly in the domain of peripheral biofeedback. It was presumed that elevated muscle tension was implicated in the pain mechanism, and EMG training was brought to bear in consequence. For many years, this was considered the standard biofeedback treatment of the condition. More recently, it has been established that the presumptive excess of muscle tension could not be universally identified in this condition.

Rather, it was found that the problem could be traced to an inappropriate set point of the muscle spindles. These set points are sympathetically mediated, so any biofeedback impinging on sympathetic nervous system regulation should have beneficial fallout for myofascial pain, not only EMG training.

At the same time, it was found that a different biofeedback modality, namely, heart rate variability training, gave superior relief clinically (Lehrer, 2003). In this modality, paced breathing is used to drive blood pressure regulation and heart rate over a wider dynamic range. In a well-regulated system, heart rate varies in approximate synchronization with the breath, a phenomenon known as respiratory sinus arrhythmia. The baroreflex system that modulates blood pressure fluctuates at the same frequency, but at a different phase. At a sufficiently slow breathing rate, nominally 6/min, the system achieves resonance, with the forcing function of the breath "pumping" the baroreflex system and the oscillations in heart rate to larger cyclical excursions. This process can be thought of as exercising the relevant autonomic regulatory loops. These are enervated both sympathetically and parasympathetically, so that both arms of the autonomic nervous system are trained in a dance of mutual regulation.

It is important to observe that the target here is pure self-regulation. There is no bias in favor of a particular set point of function. There is no direct nexus to myofascial pain. Yet this is observed to be the strongest available remedy in the arsenal of self-regulation technologies. There is a comforting similarity in the language now being applied to heart rate variability training and to neurofeedback by its respective practitioners. Both are challenging regulatory systems somewhat nonprescriptively, simply allowing them to renormalize or reequilibrate. Given this new understanding of the mechanism of relief of myofascial pain, it should be equally appropriate to apply neurofeedback to the task.

Only one publication is available that speaks to the point. Ibric (1996) reports on the response of nine patients diagnosed with myofascial pain. The data are compromised by the fact that each of the patients had at least one additional diagnosis among the following: depression, sleep disorder, anxiety, diabetes, and attention-deficit disorder. The EEG biofeedback training was also provided in the context of other therapies, including other biofeedback. Significant pain reduction could usually be achieved within a neurofeedback session, to the accompaniment of measurable EEG change. Results on one patient are reproduced in Figure 50.2, with pain levels going from 10/10 (maximal rating) at the outset to 1 to 2/10 (minimal rating) by the end of the session, accompanied by substantial (albeit transient) normalization of the EEG. In this particular patient, there was transient recovery from ptosis during the session as well. The patient reported that she had not experienced equivalent relief from relaxation training or any other therapy. No data were provided on long-term outcome.

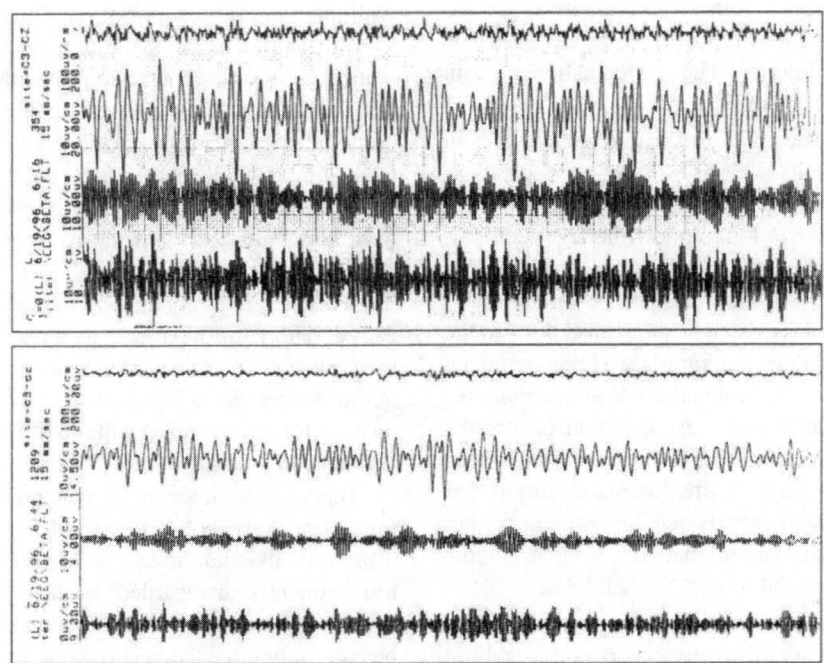

FIGURE 50.2 Comparison of two EEG plots in the same patient, one taken at the beginning of a neurofeedback session, and one taken near the end. Observe the profound change in EEG amplitudes produced within the session. The change correlates with reported symptom improvement. The initial amplitudes are elevated with respect to norms, so that a reduction in amplitude is to be expected. Significantly, all the bands are elevated in amplitude in the first plot, a feature often seen in severe patterns of dysregulation. As in Figure 50.1, the raw waveform is depicted at the top within each panel, with 4–7 Hz, 15–18 Hz, and 22–30 Hz bands, respectively, below.

TRAUMATIC BRAIN INJURY

There are certain similarities in the history of the medical treatment of minor traumatic brain injury to that of pain. Many of the sequelae involve subjective judgments. Many lack an identifiable organic foundation for which objective evidence can be adduced. There is often very poor prognosis for the most severe cases. Largely, one relies on whatever resources for self-recovery may exist. One defaults to the tincture of time. It took a long time for pain to become recognized as a disease process in its own right. Similarly, it has taken the emergence of functional imaging to reveal the full dimensions of the disease process in minor traumatic brain injury. Meanwhile, a tradition of denial carried the day in the medical management of pain, and accusations of malingering became commonplace in traumatic brain injury. Physician perceptions of malingering in patients with chronic pain, for example, ranged up to 75% (Fishbain et al., 1999).

Both of these find their resolution in the recognition that we must look to the domain of functional illness — of dysregulation — for explanations of the panoply of typical symptoms reported in traumatic brain injury. Such dysregulations need leave no trace in standard tests of structural injury. They may be observable in functional imagery. Prominent in head injury symptoms are various pain syndromes, in particular head pain. Dysregulation of arousal, of sleep, of vigilance, of cognitive function, of emotional stability, of attention and other aspects of executive function, of appetite — these go a long way toward explaining the dysfunctions reported as the consequence of even minor head injuries. The dysregulation of pain mechanisms fits this pattern.

Given the relative dearth of medical remedies for even apparently minor insults such as whiplash and postconcussion syndrome, victims have sought recourse to legal redress. It is instructive to look at how the legal community, largely in service to the insurance industry, has responded. A defense is usually mounted by finding evidence that the symptoms existed at some level prior to the traumatic event. This does not surprise. Minor traumatic brain injury is best seen as a signal event in a cumulative dysregulation cascade, in this case one that covers the entire lifespan of the victim. There may well have been priming events in the person's life that placed him or her at the threshold of significant dysregulation upon further physical insults to the central nervous system. In the extreme, these are referred to as "eggshell" cases.

What interests us at this moment is that this entire trajectory into dysfunction is to be understood largely in the domain of functional illness — of the disordering of central regulatory networks. Pain in traumatic brain injury fits this model as well. Thus, it makes little sense to discuss pain in traumatic brain injury as a distinct entity. Rather, traumatic brain injury presents perhaps the most cogent demonstration of the dysregulation model of functional illness: the sudden appearance of a wide variety of disparate symptoms as the result of a singular event. Once that model is understood, then pain fits readily within its framework as an exemplar.

It is in application to traumatic brain injury that neurofeedback distinguishes itself even from peripheral biofeedback and other general psychophysiological remedies. Unfortunately, very little of this promising work has reached the literature. In one study recently published, Walker reported on the recovery through neurofeedback of some 17 people who had been totally disabled by their traumatic experience. All were more than 2 years posttrauma, by which time self-recovery processes have reached a plateau. The average recovery with neurofeedback was >80% by self-report. Pain was the most prominent symptom and recovered substantially, but the pain data were not broken out. Significantly, more than 60% of the subjects were back at work within months of beginning neurofeedback (those who had been employed prior to their injury), whereas the expectation when they initiated neurofeedback was that none of these people was capable of further recovery (Walker, Gilbert, & Weber, 2002).

Walker had previously made available to us data on a prior cohort of traumatic brain injury subjects that had been treated with a single protocol, one that has historically been used for seizure management. The data were virtually identical in terms of self-report of progress and average number of sessions (just over 30) to that obtained with the more refined protocols. This tends to support the view that most of the symptoms refer to general dysregulation accessible to generic protocols.

The import of the above for pain management in general is that traumatic brain injury of sufficient magnitude to be clinically relevant is often entirely overlooked. Emergency room treatments are not oriented toward the long-term consequences, with the result that patients are discharged under the impression that all is well, when in fact the worst is yet to come. It is in practice very difficult to extract reports from patients with respect to such events in their personal histories. In our intake interview, we ask the question about head injury in six different ways before we take no for an answer. Additionally, birth trauma is often shrouded in ambiguity, particularly with adopted children.

Based on such scrupulous attention to traumatic brain injury, we have come to regard it as a kind of stealth disease — like pain itself — commonplace among us but too frequently disregarded. Both play a role in the dysregulation cascade, with the likelihood that attention will be paid only after the best opportunity for remediation is already past. Pain treatment specialists may want to inquire more diligently into traumatizing events in the patient's history, or else simply to test the hypothesis that pain may be remediable with neurofeedback by recommending a trial.

EMOTIONAL TRAUMA

The intimate association of emotional trauma with chronic pain syndromes has been known for some time. This association was statistically robust even when the focus was almost entirely on what may be called event-related trauma, or post-traumatic stress disorder. By analogy to physical injury, such event-related trauma exposes in clearest relief the sudden thrust into dysregulation. Emotional trauma is therefore to be seen as another singular event in the dysregulation cascade. Because this cuts so close to the "self," it is perhaps no surprise that emotional trauma can have consequences that are just as significant as those of physical trauma. In fact, there is a surprising overlap in symptoms attributable to both kinds of trauma: the dysregulation of arousal, of sleep, of attentional and memory capacities, of emotional stability, of executive function, etc. On the one hand, this unitary quality helps to make the case for the general dysregulation model. On the other, it can be argued that emotional trauma must be part of physical trauma as well. The sudden loss of function and of mental capacities is a blow to self-hood, to the basis of one's self-regard, and a threat to all of one's social ties. In addition, at the level of brain function, it can be argued that just as physical trauma can disregulate attentional networks, emotional trauma can disturb the networks that govern emotional stability.

Ross has put the case for general dysregulation in trauma victims most succinctly (Ross, 2000). If we were to adopt the assumptions of the *Diagnostic and Statistical Manual of Mental Disorders* (DSM) and regard all of the diagnostic categories of mental disorders as representing discrete, independent entities, then it is trivial to calculate the joint probability of finding, say, 10 such diagnostic categories to be represented in one individual. If each of these categories had a population incidence of 10%, we would still expect fewer than one person on Earth to satisfy criteria for 10 conditions. Yet such findings are plentiful among those with a trauma history. Quite clearly, the different classifications cannot be seen as independent.

Among mental disorders, diagnostic entities are manifestly coupled. There is likely, then, to be a fundamental explanatory principle that underlies many of them, or at least a much smaller set of basic mechanisms than the more than 400 disorders represented within the DSM. Moreover, trauma can be seen as inducing dysregulation generally. If the trauma occurs to a vulnerable individual, e.g., one that has had a history of traumatically priming events, then the particular trauma at issue may be the signal event that catastrophically initiates the dysregulation cascade, leading to a gradual and cumulative progression of symptomatology. Pain dysregulation simply fits this pattern and, with respect to central mechanisms of pain modulation, may not be understandable apart from this more inclusive model. For example, Fishbain reports

that the likelihood of more than one Axis I diagnosis in chronic pain is 60% (Fishbain, Goldberg, Meagher, Steele, & Rosomoff, 1986). Add to that the 35% of patients with chronic pain exhibiting one such diagnosis, and it is apparent that chronic pain is highly correlated with psychiatric disorders, and that they cannot be understood independently of each other.

To this point, the focus has been on event-related trauma because it makes the most persuasive case for the dysregulation model in general and for the dysregulation cascade in particular. In recent years, growing insights into child development have revealed that other trauma mechanisms can possibly contribute to the same syndromes. It is now known that mere neglect can be as damaging to the mental health of a growing infant as overt abuse (Schore, 1999). There is also the trauma of grief and the trauma of shame. Even life with one's disabled child can predispose a parent to the kindling of the dysregulation cascade.

We are mindful of the hazard of trivializing the concept of trauma by invoking it so broadly. That would be counterproductive to our intentions. We seek simply to put forward a new organizing principle for our conceptualizations: traumatizing events or steady-state conditions with traumatizing potential have as their primary physiological consequence the disruption of key regulatory modalities. We should not fall once again into the trap of asking whether the particular provocation — the ostensibly traumatic event — could really have been sufficient to explain the clinical phenomenology that now confronts us. A traumatic event is one to which the patient responded with a classical trauma response, quite irrespective of the magnitude of the triggering event. Depending on where this event falls in a person's particular status with respect to the dysregulation cascade, an even minor trauma can be one's undoing. This is the same dilemma that we confronted with apparently minor cases of whiplash, and with apparently minor provocations in chronic pain cases, not to mention cases with no identified antecedent.

If dysregulation is the primary consequence of trauma, then the clinical target should be the state or condition of dysregulation itself, rather than any particular symptom. Putting this kind of construction on these clinical presentations would not be very meaningful if we did not also have a remedy at hand in the form of neurofeedback, peripheral biofeedback, and related psychophysiological techniques. This remedy constitutes the final argument in support of the dysregulation model. In the first instance, it is remarkable that most of the clinical objectives can be met with a very small number of protocols. This speaks to parsimony of underlying mechanisms. Second, there appears to be no obvious or consistent target of the neurofeedback, no universal EEG deviation that characterizes the disorders. It appears that neurofeedback targets dysregulation itself. The mere exercise of the regulatory loops effects improved regulation.

The neurofeedback approach to trauma consists of two parts. The first consists of challenge training under eyes-open conditions in which the brain is active and engaged. The intent here is to enhance stability of state and to move homeostatic set points to more appropriate levels with regard to central arousal, autonomic arousal, vigilance, attention, and pain. The second consists of reinforcement of low-frequency states under eyes-closed conditions. This phase places the individual in a state more conducive to the psychological resolution of trauma. It is important to make clear at this point just what it means to "resolve" psychological trauma. After all, the reference is presumably to a historical event. Neurofeedback does not produce amnesia.

The clinical pattern issues from the fact that the traumatic experience is registered in memory in its totality, including the entire set of physiological responses. Subsequent spontaneous recall therefore recruits the physiological responding as well. Whereas this process of association can clearly happen in single-shot learning, cumulative traumas reinforce this "whole-body" memory. Early traumas (i.e., threats to the integrity and viability of the self) establish a kind of template or scaffolding with respect to which subsequent traumas are processed and recorded. Each trauma, then, reawakens and reinforces what went before. The body memory is simply carried forward essentially intact, and is reinforced by events that call to mind the original traumas. We postulate that the traumatic experience serves as a kind of wick that perpetually nourishes the state of dysregulation of the patient. It is as if the person in some sense remains in a trauma status. The state of living with unprocessed trauma allies pain to suffering in a mutually reinforcing, progressive descent into abject misery.

The clinical objective is therefore to separate the event memory from the pattern of adverse physiological responding and thus to allow the event to take its appropriate place in historical or declarative memory. Historically this has been done through sequences of reexperiencing the event in the attempt to gradually desensitize the individual. The hazard is further traumatization. Neurofeedback represents a fresh alternative that avoids these hazards first by working at low arousal, where a sudden excursion into hyperreactivity, hypervigilance, and hyperarousal is less likely. Second, the process is self-pacing. Third, the process is nonverbal. Finally, any abreaction that may nevertheless occur tends to abort the process.

Physiologically the neurofeedback takes the person toward states of more whole-brain EEG synchrony. Such states of synchrony prevail when the brain is least challenged and least engaged. Hence they promote states of calmness and internal stillness, states that the traumatized person is unable to reach unaided. Additionally, these states replicate conditions that may have prevailed during early life stages, when the EEG was less mature. Such low-frequency EEGs facilitate recall of traumatic material,

and they may particularly favor the recall of traumatic material that was laid down during such EEG states, i.e., during the early years of life, and even preverbally.

The promotion of both alpha-band activity and theta-band activity in this eyes-closed training may facilitate not only the recall but also the visual processing of the traumatic material even while the person is in the regressed and protected state. It may also be significant that this involves no verbal processing of the material. Deep trauma seems to be encoded preferentially in the right hemisphere, whose "language" is through visualization and through feeling states (Baker & Kim, 2004). It is apparent that there is some difference in the quality of consciousness during alpha-dominant and theta-dominant states. The visualization is more dreamlike and linearly progressive in alpha-dominated states, whereas it is more hypnagogic, episodic, and disjointed in theta-dominant states. It may well be that traumatic material is accessed in the theta state and then processed in the alpha-dominant state. In any event, excursion into high arousal, hypervigilance, or other visceral responding is disfacilitated in this state, and any reexposure to the traumatic material is experienced as benign.

Once the traumas have been rendered innocuous, the person can gradually achieve improved autonomic regulation and progress toward the normalization of the pain response. Whereas the low-frequency training is an important if not essential step, the actual symptom relief comes with the higher-frequency eyes-open training. The eyes-open training is also required to stabilize the brain at the outset to the point where the low-frequency work can even be undertaken. Moreover, in some cases of seizure disorder or of traumatic brain injury the low-frequency work may be contraindicated. The trauma work may instead have to be done with hypnotherapy, which does not involve reinforcement of states of high synchrony at low EEG frequencies.

The whole sequence of steps suggested to address the problem of intractable chronic pain has not yet been subjected to formal study. Rather, the above understandings emerge from clinical work. The first claim, that chronic pain is ineluctably bound up with prior traumatic experience, can be challenged on the contemporary theory that traumatic memories can be introduced into the therapeutic setting by an overly zealous therapist. This hazard does not exist in the neurofeedback setting, however, where the process is largely nonverbal. Nor is the therapist likely to make things worse, because no sooner is the traumatic memory recovered than it is already on the pathway to resolution.

A further objection is that traumatic memories are not reliable. This objection is also not relevant in the present context. We are not in a court of law where this might matter. The only relevant question is whether the particular memory is still "radioactive" for the patient now. Rightly or wrongly, the trauma is the patient's reality, and the only question of clinical import is whether recall recruits inappropriate physiological responding. It does not have to have historical truth on its side. In fact, the therapeutic approach is based on the knowledge that memory is alterable. The objective is to alter the memory of the event that resides in the body–mind. Remedy lies in a benign re-experiencing and re-scripting process that is largely under the direction of the patient.

Then there is the question of whether trauma desensitization can in fact be achieved with the low-frequency training. In support of this proposition, we draw upon a controlled study by Peniston, working with post-traumatic stress disorder in Vietnam veterans with this approach (Peniston & Kulkosky, 1989, 1991). After neurofeedback, done in conjunction with conventional treatment for alcoholism in the VA (Veterans' Administration), these individuals no longer met diagnostic criteria for post-traumatic stress disorder, whereas all the controls (who received only the conventional treatment) stayed true to pattern.

The proposed low-frequency training also bears a similarity to the technique called eye movement desensitization and reprocessing (EMDR). This technique also involves inducing low-frequency modulation of states. It is used to aid in the processing of traumas. Whereas in EMDR the therapist directs the action and determines both the reinforcement frequency and the pacing of the process, neurofeedback merely invites participation in the process. This absence of external forcing and constraint may be one of the key virtues accounting for its clinical efficacy on the one hand, and for the absence of significant abreactive experiences on the other.

A REPRESENTATIVE CASE HISTORY

The following is a clinical case history from the practice of Richard Soutar, one that illustrates the issues that have been raised in this chapter.

The client was a 45-year-old male who had been diagnosed first with multiple sclerosis (MS) by a neurologist and later with fibromyalgia by a rheumatologist. The tender points tended to be in his lower rather than upper body. The client had been on Paxil for 10 years, as well as Zoloft for sleep. He had also been taking hydrocodone for some time for pain. He reported that he had been to "every pain specialist in the area," and that he had consulted many alternative health practitioners as well.

At the time of his brain map at intake, he was moderately depressed but still functioned effectively at his work in spite of the severe episodes of pain. The pain was usually severe in the morning and dissipated as the day progressed. It was accompanied by numbness, tingling, weakness, and fatigue. Sometimes he required a cane to walk. His symptoms were aggravated by sudden changes in weather.

The most outstanding feature on his brain map was significantly elevated 12 to 14 Hz amplitudes as well as mildly elevated 23 and 24 Hz amplitudes in the posterior

region. There was also significant global beta hypercoherence between key regions of the anterior (F7, F8) and posterior region (O1, O2). We often see elevations of 12 to 14 Hz in the posterior regions with somatic symptoms. The beta hypercoherence and elevated posterior beta are commonly present in anxiety conditions.

We began by training 12 to 14 Hz amplitudes down at Pz as indicated by his map. The patient had difficulty gaining control over beta suppression and showed few symptom changes. At the fifth session, the target of training was moved to the location between O1 and O2 (Oz) and two trials of alpha (8 to 10 Hz) up training were introduced into each session. The patient demonstrated better control of alpha, and the beta came down during this training. The client began to experience relief from pain for 2 days after each session. By the 12th session, he had experienced a week without pain. By the 16th session, it was more than 2 weeks without pain. By the 19th session, he was reporting unusual levels of energy, reduced irritability, and improved mood. By the 29th session, he was pain-free and remained so until his brain map on session 40. At this point, he was on a very low dose of Paxil and would be off it completely by the 45th session. By the 50th session, he was off his Zoloft and we began to wean him off the neurofeedback treatments. He comes in periodically for a booster session.

Pre–post subjective rating scales indicate clear relief globally from both mental and physical suffering. The comparison of self-rating at sessions 5 and 29 are shown in Figure 50.3. The upper tier shows categories where the rating is expected to increase with successful intervention, and the lower tier shows categories where the score is expected to decrease.

Pre–post maps show almost complete normalization of the hypercoherence as well as reduction of beta amplitudes below significance levels in all posterior areas except P3 and P4. The coherence data are shown in Figure 50.4a and b.

First, the improvements across the board tend to support the dysregulation model. Second, it is observed that the most significant quantitative electroencephalography (QEEG) deviations, and the most numerous, consisted of coherence anomalies. This indicates deficits in cortical–cortical communication relationships. Finally, it is observed that the successful training did not directly target the observed deviations. In particular, when suppression of the excess 13-Hz amplitude was first tried, it was found to be relatively ineffectual. Yet a different challenge at a slightly different frequency was found to resolve nearly all of the anomalies. Perhaps surprisingly, single-site training was even effective in normalizing the two-site coherence anomalies. This again supports the dysregulation model. An appropriate challenge, empirically derived, effects broad and nonspecific functional renormalization that will be generally reflected in a tendency toward normalization of EEG parameters.

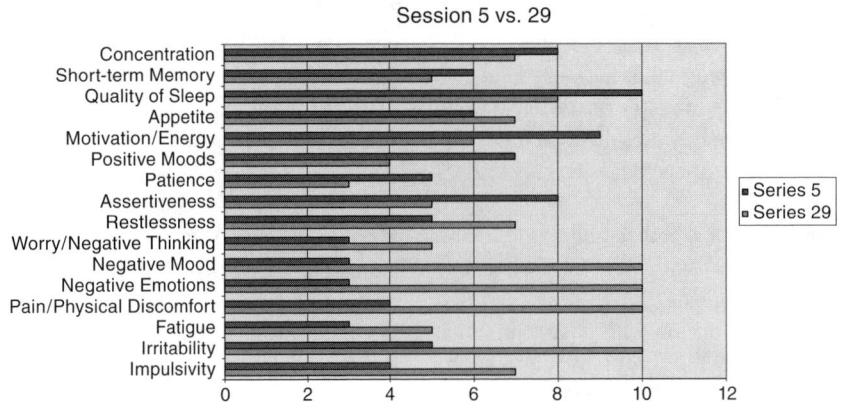

FIGURE 50.3 Progress from session 5 to 29 by self-assessment. Data are shown in two blocks, with the upper tier referring to categories where an increase in score is expected, and the lower tier referring to adverse criteria where a decrease in score is expected.

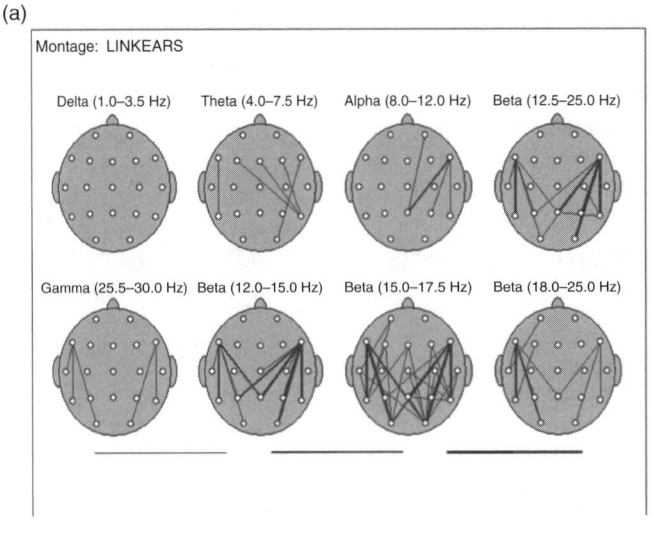

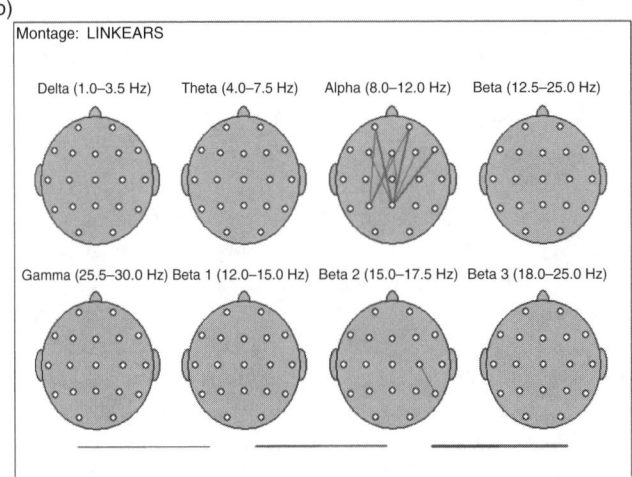

FIGURE 50.4 (a) Initial coherence data, expressed in Z-scores (units of a standard deviation). Only deviations greater than a nominal $Z = 2$ are shown. (b) Coherence data after 29 sessions of neurofeedback. Observe that most coherence anomalies have resolved.

EEG CHARACTERISTICS OF DYSREGULATION

The above case was distinctive in that it was characterized by numerous coherence anomalies in the absence of many other deviations. More typically, deviations will be found across the board: in terms of spectral amplitudes or spectral power measures, in relative power, in amplitude asymmetries across the hemispheric fissure, as well as in coherence and/or spectral comodulation. All these measures refer to the stationary properties of the EEG. The most significant feature of dysregulation may in fact be the transient behavior, in the observation of elevated variability. Such transients are typically quite apparent on visual inspection of clinical EEGs, but they may also be sufficiently sparse as to leave no obvious impression on the stationary measures. The latter should therefore not be taken as an index to the severity of the dysregulation independent of other assessments, in particular of the EEG waveform morphology. For a realistic appraisal, it may even be necessary to evaluate the EEG dynamics under challenge, much as neurologists evaluate the EEG under conditions of hyperventilation or sleep deprivation. Even at this late date in the evolution of our tools for EEG quantitative analysis, there is still no substitute for looking at the EEG.

Some pain conditions have been shown to be correlated with specific deviations in the EEG. Thus, fibromyalgia is often characterized by intrusion of alpha dominance in non-REM sleep (Roizenblatt, Moldofsky et al., 2001). Both tonic and phasic alpha activity have been identified in fibromyalgia, with the phasic type (seen in half of all such patients) showing the greatest correlation with symptoms. Some 30% of patients with fibromyalgia do not show these alpha elevations, however, and some normal individuals show alpha elevations in absence of symptoms. Therefore, this particular EEG feature has limited predictive power diagnostically. (It is, however, a consideration with respect to how the patient is trained.) The existence of a single, obvious EEG feature may actually distract from what may be more meaningful ultimately, namely, the more general state of dysregulation manifested in the EEG upon more comprehensive quantitative analysis and inspection of EEG morphology.

Roizenblatt may have already hinted at a greater complexity of EEG morphology by pointing out that the phasic alpha activity in fibromyalgia occurs simultaneously with delta activity. This may be the more significant observation, as we see in the following.

A PHYSIOLOGICAL MODEL

Given the emergence of a general pattern of dysregulation in the EEG in chronic pain conditions, there is a need for equally general physiological models. In this we are handicapped by the belated recognition in the neurosciences of the frequency basis of organization of neuronal assemblies (Buzsaki & Draguhn, 2004). The core principles in a possible model are intimated in the following. Synaptic transport is contingent on the organization of simultaneity of action potentials over large regions of cortex on a timescale of milliseconds, and the persistence of states imposes the condition of periodicity on such processes. Synaptic transport further serves as a nexus of explicit processing of information and implicit modulation by homeostatic mechanisms. By such processes, the brain achieves a transient "binding" of neuronal assemblies into functional entities. The defining signature of such binding is temporal simultaneity of action potentials, i.e., time does binding. The Hebbian principle that "what fires together wires together" may extend also to the ensemble level, under the rubric that "what fires together functions together" (Gray, Koenig, Engel, & Singer, 1989).

The resulting ensembles must be bounded in frequency and space. That is to say, the binding problem brings together the boundary problem and the extinction problem — in effect the unbinding problem. How is the ensemble managed so that it does not recruit larger resources than necessary (amplitude deviations, spatial spread), couple too tightly or too poorly to other cortical regions (hemispheric asymmetries, coherence and phase anomalies), couple inappropriately the high and low EEG frequencies (dysrhythmias), or fail to extinguish upon completion of the task at hand (amplitude and/or coherence deviations)?

One may ground functional dysregulation, as referred to in this chapter, to an inadequacy in the organization of ensemble dynamics as suggested above. To understand this further, the architecture by which brain timing is organized at the ensemble level must be taken into account. It is most economical to propose that timing is the result of distributed network relations, i.e., that every element in the neuronal network in fact contributes to the overall unfolding of temporal relationships. Nevertheless, a hierarchy of control can be identified, and evolutionary arguments brought to bear on the proposition that commitments made early in our evolutionary history have been largely conserved.

One must therefore look to the earliest structures, the brainstem and the diencephalon, for the top of the hierarchy. Among these, only the thalamus has the topographical complexity to permit full description of the phenomenology of interest. Hence, it may be no surprise that the first candidate to emerge for a comprehensive neurological model for psychopathologies arises out of the study of thalamocortical networks over the past several decades. The model has been termed "thalamocortical dysrhythmia," and it is based on the observation of a profound distinction in bispectral couplings in the EEG between psychiatric patients and normal subjects. In the first presentation of this model, Rodolfo Llinas (Llinas et al.,

1999) found identical patterns of dysrhythmia in a patient with chronic pain as in a patient suffering from Parkinson's disease, one suffering major depression, and one suffering tinnitus. Only because the data were so dramatic in their contrast between pathology and normalcy would one have the courage to draw such generalized conclusions from such a meager database of only four disparate cases representing four different diagnostic categories.

It now seems obvious in retrospect that in addition to organizing spatial relationships between different cortical sites at any given EEG frequency, the brain must also organize the coupling or interaction of different frequencies at any one cortical site. Crudely speaking, the higher-frequency activity is more associated with processing "text," and the lower frequencies are involved more in organizing "context." Their interrelationship is crucial. Such frequency-to-frequency coupling has not surfaced much previously because bispectral analysis is not commonplace in clinical practice. For present purposes, the model of thalamocortical dysrhythmia is not yet being proposed as a definitive explanation applicable to all the chronic pain conditions discussed in this chapter. It is simply recruited as an exemplar of a generalized model in which EEG phenomenology is a point of departure to understand much of psychopathology in terms of disorders of dysregulation. Other such comprehensive models are needed for a full understanding of dysregulation in the bioelectrical domain: spatial correlations need to be modeled, and there needs to be an understanding of brain function under challenge. Only after "normal" brain function is successfully modeled can we hope to understand what happens under the constraint of organic injury or of acquired dysfunction.

Fortunately, the deficiencies in our fundamental understanding of bioelectrical mechanisms need not stand in the way of the clinical exploitation of the technique of neurofeedback, which can be accomplished through empirically derived and clinically validated techniques of functional renormalization. The history of medical science is full of examples in which the practice preceded our understanding.

SUMMARY

Self-regulation approaches in general, and neurofeedback in particular, should play a key role in the management of chronic pain. A model is suggested in which pain is recognized as a homeostatically regulated, affectively modulated sensory system, and that the excursion into chronic pain should be regarded from the perspective of a more inclusive dysregulation model. Such dysregulation manifests in the bioelectrical organization of neuronal networks and is observable in both the dynamic and stationary properties of the EEG. Neurofeedback is a self-regulation strategy that broadly targets the dysregulation of

central states through reinforcement of certain favored EEG behavior and the discouragement of disfavored activity. Pain relief is then obtained as a secondary consequence of improved self-regulation status. The key role of the emotions in pain perception is recognized. Chronic pain cannot be considered independently of the psychodynamic milieu in general and of trauma status in particular.

A neurofeedback strategy has been devised to address affect regulation in general and the trauma response specifically, to prepare the ground for resolution of pain syndromes with conventional neurofeedback techniques. Research data have been brought to bear on this discussion to the extent that such published data exist. However, the evidentiary support for the model presented is still fragmentary, and embarrassingly out of scale with the considerable promise of neurofeedback. Clinical data are good enough, however, to establish both EEG neurofeedback and pIR HEG neurofeedback as a categorical remedy for migraine pain. This observation alone is sufficient to commend neurofeedback to the attention of the pain community.

ACKNOWLEDGMENTS

The authors are grateful to Victoria Ibric, Richard Soutar, Veronica Tracy-Smith, and Caroline Grierson for making their unpublished data available to us.

REFERENCES

American Psychiatric Association. (1994). *Diagnostic and statistical manual of mental disorders* (4th ed., Text Revised). Washington, DC: American Psychiatric Press.

Baker, K. B., & Kim, J. J. (2004). Amygdalar lateralization in fear conditioning: Evidence for greater involvement of the right amygdala. *Behavioral Neuroscience, 118*(1), 15–23.

Buzsaki, G., & Draguhn, A. (2004). Neuronal oscillations in cortical networks. *Science, 304*, 1926–1929.

Carmen, J. A. (2004). Passive infrared hemoencephalography, four years and 100 migraines later. *Journal of Neurotherapy, 8*(3), 23–51.

Caro, X. J., & Winter, E. F. (2001). Attention measures improve in fibromyalgia patients receiving EEG biofeedback training: A pilot study. *Arthritis & Rheumatism, 44*(9S), S71.

Craig, A. D. (2002). How do you feel? Interoception: The sense of the physiological condition of the body. *Nature Reviews Neuroscience, 3*(8), 655–666.

Donaldson, C., Sella, G., & Mueller, H. (1998). Fibromyalgia: A retrospective study of 252 consecutive referrals. *Canadian Journal of Clinical Medicine, 5*(6), 116–127.

Egner, T., & Gruzelier, J. (2001). Learned self-regulation of EEG frequency components affects attention and event-related brain potentials in humans. *Neuroreport, 12*(18), 4155–4159.

Fishbain, D. A., Cutler, R., Rosomoff, H. L., & Rosomoff, R. S. (1999). Chronic pain disability exaggeration/malingering and submaximal effort research. *Clinical Journal of Pain, 15*(4), 244–274.

Fishbain, D. A., Goldberg, M., Meagher, B. R., Steele, R., & Rosomoff, H. (1986). Male and female chronic pain patients categorized by DSM-III psychiatric diagnostic criteria. *Pain, 26*(2), 181–197.

Gray, C. M., Koenig, P., Engel, A. K., & Singer, W. (1989). Oscillatory responses in cat visual cortex exhibit intercolumnar synchronization which reflects global stimulus properties. *Nature, 338*, 334.

Ibric, V. L. (1996). Components in long-term, comprehensive care of patients with myofascial pain syndrome: Part II — The usefulness of biofeedback. contemporary management of myofascial pain syndrome (pp. 29–39). Beverly Hills, CA: Discovery International Symposium, Oct 19th.

Jasper, H. (1958). The ten–twenty electrode system of the International Federation. *Electroencephalography and Clinical Neurophysiology, 10*, 371–375.

Kropp, P., Siniatchkin, M., & Gerber, W. D. (2002). On the pathophysiology of migraine — Links for "empirically based treatment" with neurofeedback. *Journal of Applied Psychophysiology and Biofeedback, 27*(3), 203.

Lehrer, P. M. (2003). For a Treatment of Heart Rate Variability Training (in application to asthma). Presentation at California Biofeedback Society Annual Conference. See also Lehrer, P. M., Vaschillo, E., Vaschillo, B., Lu, S. E., Scardella, A., Siddique, M. et al. (2004), Biofeedback treatment for asthma, *Chest, 126*, 352–361.

Llinas, R. Ribary, U., Jeanmonod, D., Kronberg, E., & Mitra, P. (1999). Thalamocortical dysrhythmia. A neurological and neuropsychiatric syndrome characterized by magnetoelectroencephalography. *Proceedings of the National Academy of Sciences, 96*(26), 15222–15227.

Masterpasqua, F., & Healey, K. (2003). Neurofeedback in psychological practice. *Professional Psychology: Research and Practice, 34*(6), 652–656.

Meyers, C., White, B., & Heft, M. (2002). A review of complementary and alternative medicine use for treating chronic facial pain. *Journal of the American Dental Association, 133*(9), 1189–1196.

Middaugh, S., & Pawlick, K. (2002). Biofeedback and behavioral treatment of persistent pain in the older adult: A review and a study. *Applied Psychophysiology and Biofeedback, 27*(3), 185–202.

Nash, J. K. (2000). Treatment of attention deficit hyperactivity disorder with neurotherapy. *Clinical Electroencephalography, 31*(1), 30–37.

Othmer, S. (2002a). Emerging trends in neurofeedback: I. On the status and future of mechanisms-based training. *Biofeedback, 30*(2), p.21.

Othmer, S. (2002b). Emerging trends in neurofeedback: II. The challenge of QEEG-based and NLD-based neurofeedback protocols. *Biofeedback, 30*(3 / 4), p.43.

Othmer, S., Othmer, S. F., & Kaiser, D. (1999). EEG biofeedback: An emerging model for its global efficacy. In J. R. Evans & A. Abarbanel (Eds.), *Introduction to quantitative EEG and neurofeedback* (pp. 243–310). San Diego, CA: Academic Press.

Peniston, E. G., & Kulkosky, P. J. (1989). Alpha-theta brainwave training and beta-endorphin levels in alcoholics. *Alcohol — Clinical and Experimental Research, 13*(2), 271–279.

Peniston, E. G., & Kulkosky, P. J. (1991). Alpha-theta brain wave neurofeedback for Vietnam veterans with combat related posttraumatic stress disorder, *Medicine and Psychotherapy, 4*, 1–14.

Roizenblatt, S., Moldofsky, H., Benedito-Silva, A. A., & Tufik, S. (2001). Alpha sleep characteristics in fibromyalgia. *Arthritis & Rheumatism, 44*(1), 222–230.

Ross, C. A. (2000). *The trauma model: A solution to the problem of comorbidity in Psychiatry.* Richardson, TX: Manitou Communications.

Schore, A. N. (1999). *Affect regulation and the development of the self: The neurobiology of emotional development.* Hillsdale, NJ: Lawrence Erlbaum Associates.

Schwartz, M. S., & Andrasik, F. (Eds.). (2003). *Biofeedback, third edition: A practitioner's guide.* New York: The Guilford Press.

Sime, A. (2004). Case study of trigeminal neuralgia using neurofeedback and peripheral biofeedback. *Journal of Neurotherapy, 8*(1), 59–70.

Singer, T., Seymour, B., O'Doherty, J., Kaube, H., Dolan, R., & Frith, C. (2004). Empathy for pain involves the affective but not sensory components of pain. *Science, 303*, 1157–1163.

Sterman, B. (2000). Basic concepts and clinical findings in the treatment of seizure disorders with EEG operant conditioning. *Clinical Electroencephalography, 31*(1), 45–55.

Vernon, D., Egner, T., Cooper, N., Compton, T., Neilands, C., Sheri, A. et al. (2003). The effect of training distinct neurofeedback protocols on aspects of cognitive performance. *International Journal of Psychophysiology, 47*, 75–85.

Wager, T., Rilling, J., Smith, E., Sokolik, A., Casey, K., Davidson, R. et al. (2004). Placebo-induced changes in fMRI in the anticipation and experience of pain. *Science, 303*, 1162–1166.

Walker, J. E., Gilbert, C., Weber, R. C. (2002). Impact of qEEG-guided coherence training for patients with a mild closed head injury. *Journal of Neurotherapy, 6*(3), 31–43.

Yucha, C., & Gilbert, C. (2004). *Evidence-based practice in biofeedback and neurofeedback.* Wheat Ridge, CO: AAPB Monograph.

——————— 51 ———————

Hypnotherapeutic Advances in Pain Management

Jan M. Burte, PhD, MS Psychopharm, DAAPM

Hypnosis as a form of pain management has shown increasing favor within the past decade. This may be attributable to numerous factors including the increase of solid research demonstrating its efficaciousness with various forms of pain and the experiences of practitioners and patients utilizing it.

In situations where pharmacotherapy is limited by other factors and in situations of intractable pain, it has been shown to be an excellent adjunct to standard care. Research has helped to define its limitations (i.e., high vs. low susceptible subjects), its biophysiological and neurophysiological basis, and its interaction with the sensory and emotional pain receptor sites in the brain. The diversity of conditions to which it is currently being applied continues to expand with varied degrees of clinical success. In this brief chapter, I hope to provide an overview of hypnotic application based on recent peer-reviewed research and textual materials.

HISTORY

There is little doubt that the induction of hypnoidal states utilizing chanting and breathing exercises dates back to earliest history. Meditation and hypnosis have been frequently compared regarding their impact on concentration, altered states, and suggestibility (Holroyd, 2003). The earliest clinical records of hypnosis are attributed to John Elliotson (1792–1869), an English surgeon, who used hypnosis for pain management in his practice and James A. Esdaile (1808–1859), who performed more than 300 operations using hypnosis as analgesia while practic-

ing in India (Bassman & Wester, 1992). One such operation reportedly entailed the removal of a 103-lb tumor (Jackson, 1999). Although hypnosis and trance represent an age-old treatment for a variety of conditions including pain, hypnosis has been embraced as a legitimate therapy consequent to continuing research only over the past 50 years (Hrezo, 1998).

Hypnosis as a form of pain management fell in and out of favor from the early 1940s until the 1960s when Milton H. Erickson demonstrated its utility with acute and chronic pain control (Erickson, 1966, 1986). The application of hypnosis within the medical and pain setting has continued to develop from the work of Hilgard and Hilgard (1975), Hilgard and LeBaron (1982), Barber and Adrian (1982), and Melzack and Wall (1965, 1983).

Zohaurek (1985) points out two historical misconceptions of pain that have affected the role of hypnosis in treating pain.

Pain was considered to be only a symptom of an underlying disease or trauma. Therefore, research and treatment focused on the etiological cause and ignored the pain, assuming it would disappear when the cause was addressed. Historically, pain reporting was by necessity heavily relied upon as part of the initial diagnostic procedure, where severity, location, and nature of the pain often assisted in proper diagnosis. Although pain reporting maintains a significant role in diagnosis, the advent of additional diagnostic procedures (i.e., computerized axial tomography [CAT] and magnetic resonance imaging [MRI] scans), goes beyond pain reports and reduces their unique significance. The reliance on pain reports was especially true in certain acute pain situations although not as much in chronic pain situations where a diagnosis had been reached (Bonica, 1990). It was postulated that hypnosis could mask the symptoms of pain and might interfere with obtaining a proper diagnosis and treatment (i.e., using hypnosis to mask pain associated with appendicitis could result in delaying care until the appendix has ruptured).

Fordyce (1976) and Sternbach (1978) point out that historically pain was seen as evolving from either a physical or a psychological origin rather than from both. Pain was perceived to have either a "real/organic" basis or a "functional/imaginary" basis. Current thinking might view the impact of pain as an etiological factor. As a result of its bidirectional psychoneuroimmunological role (on the psychological, endocrinological, and immunological systems), pain may contribute to the maintenance of illness or enhance the progression or metastasis of certain illnesses (Paige & Ben-Eliyahu, 1997).

Since 1958, hypnosis has been recognized by the American Medical Association as a legitimate form of medical treatment when administered by an appropriately trained practitioner (Simon & James, 1999). Fortunately, with the resurgence of integrative, mind/body, psychoneuroimmunological approaches, current thought and research have begun to view hypnosis as a potentially significant modality in the treatment of pain and illness.

CURRENT CONCEPTIONS OF PAIN

In this chapter, I focus on the hypnotherapeutic advances in pain management and discuss the applicability of hypnosis in the treatment of specific illnesses. Due in part to its historical misportrayal in the popular media, patients referred for hypnosis often ask, "But does it really work?" Contemporary popular media portray hypnosis as an effective means of pain control (Foderaro, 1996). Currently, sufficient experimental and clinical research exists to allow clinicians to respond affirmatively to the question. However, certain caveats, discussed later, still exist. An extensive review analysis of recent published research by Hawkins (2001) concludes that there is sufficient evidence of good quality in favor of views that hypnosis is an effective modality in the treatment of pain.

What then is medical or clinical hypnosis and what are the contemporary views of both practitioners and the public, especially within the realm of pain management? One recent survey indicates, "most people have a positive view of the therapeutic benefits with a vast majority of respondents believing that it reduces the time that is usually required to uncover causes of a person's problems, and that hypnotized persons can undergo dental and medical procedures without pain" (Johnson & Hauck, 1999).

Retrospectively, it is important to recognize that "pain," until the 20th century, was considered an untreat-able consequence of illness or injury. Indeed, Chaves and Dworkin (1997) astutely point out that hypnoanalgesia did not fully emerge until the 19th century, due largely in part to the societal belief that pain relief and reduced suffering were not a primary goal in treatment. Prior to effective clinical techniques for pain management, pain was an accepted aspect of life. One might wonder whether the introduction of pharmacological forms of pain relief such as analgesia and anesthesia altered patients' perceptions of the importance of pain relief and ultimately their thresholds for pain.

If pain can act as a mediator in trance production with patients experiencing pain, then did our progenitors and do perhaps third world cultures that had/have limited access to various forms of pain relief intuitively rely on hypnosis and self-hypnosis to alter their pain thresholds? For these individuals, pain, whether from childbirth, dental procedures, illness, or injury, was anticipated.

Today, the application of hypnotic analgesia in acute and chronic pain treatment has grown substantially. Both patients and clinicians are demonstrating increased knowledge and experience with hypnosis. In many cases, patients bring clinical experiences with hypnosis for related or unrelated issues to the treating physician (Lynch, 1999), thereby opening a door to increased complementary approaches to standard interventions. Where this may be significantly prevalent is in the non-pharmacological strategies employed in managing cancer pain. As Zaza, Sellick, Willan, Reyno, and Browman (1999) point out, while pharmacological treatments are appropriately the central component of cancer pain management, the under-utilization of effective non-pharmacological strategies may contribute to the problems of pain and suffering among cancer patients. In a study of 214 health professions, Zaza et al. (1999) found that the healthcare professionals recommended "imagery" exercises 54% of the time and meditation 43% of the time. They expressed interest in learning more about hypnosis and other non-pharmacological strategies, suggesting its under-utilization as a complementary or adjunctive treatment to standard care. In a critical review of the literature, Sellick and Zaza (1998) found that in randomized controlled studies of hypnosis in managing cancer pain, substantial evidence exists for its effectiveness when non-pharmacoligcal pain management approaches are being sought. Given the side effects frequently seen with many pain medications including sedations, gastrointestinal problems, and tolerance issues, it is not surprising to find patients seeking adjunctive means to reduce their reliance on analgesic.

BASIC CONSTRUCTS OF HYPNOSIS

This concept, then, of unifying both the confidence of the practitioner and the trust and belief of the patient, may represent the components necessary to obtain efficacious pain relief. Barber (1998) aptly delineates a two-component model explaining why hypnosis may work for pain management. He suggests that in the first component the "clinician communicates specific ideas that strengthen the patient's ability to derive therapeutic support and to develop a sense of openness to the unexplored possibilities of pain relief within the security of a nurturing therapeutic relationship." In so doing, the patient is led to relax in the clinician's confidence in hypnosis. In the second component, "the clinician employs posthypnotic suggestions that capitalize on the patient's particular pain experiences which simultaneously ameliorate the pain experience and which, in small repetitive increments, tend to maintain persistent pain relief over increasing periods of time." This second component offers the patient a sense of voluntary learned control over his or her pain, thereby reducing anxiety and learned helplessness.

A somewhat more constructionistic view is offered by Chapman and Nakamura (1998), who suggest that hypnosis alters the learned pain experience (pain schemata) by interacting with feedback processes that prime the associations and memories tied to the pain, thereby shaping the formation of pain expectations and processes and ultimately reducing the experience of pain.

Holroyd (2003) notes that for highly suggestible subjects it may be that hypnosis alters the experience of suffering and not as much the experience of sensory pain. He contrasts the effects of hypnosis to meditation, pointing out the added effects of hypnosis and the different neurocognitive components of each. Of primary importance is that it is the superior attentional abilities of these areas of the brain, which are found only in highly susceptible individuals, that enables them to experience significant hypnoanalgesic effects.

NEUROCOGNITIVE COMPONENTS

As mentioned previously, hypnosis has fallen in and out of favor over the years due in part to arguments concerning the lack of hard scientific data to support its efficacy or pathophysiology. With increasing frequency, studies are demonstrating the impact of hypnosis on pain from the perspective of changes occurring in the brain itself. Rainville et al. (1997) demonstrated that positron emission tomography (PET) revealed significant changes in pain-evoked activity within the anterior cingulate cortex consistent with the encoding of perceived unpleasantness, thereby linking frontal lobe limbic activity with pain susceptible to hypnotic suggestion.

In an examination of exposure to noxious stimuli presented to subjects, Faymonville et al. (2000) found that hypnosis could reduce the intensity and unpleasantness of the exposure. By examining cerebral blood flow of subjects both with and without hypnotic intervention, they concluded that hypnotic modulation of pain appears to be mediated by the anterior cingulate cortex.

Rainville and colleagues (1999a) in their examination of cerebral blood flow using PET scans found that the hypnotic experience may result in increased occipital regional cerebral blood flow (RCBF) and delta activity as measured by electroencephalography (EEG) by altering the consciousness associated with decreased arousal via facilitation of visual imagery. Frontal increases in RCBF may be associated with verbal mediation of suggestions, working memory, and top-down processes involved in reinterpreting the perceptual experience of the noxious stimuli. They concluded that specific patterns of cerebral activation appear to be associated with the hypnotic state.

Other researchers have demonstrated the effectiveness of hypnotic analgesia on raising pain thresholds by examining the nociceptive flexion reflex and EEG patterns (Danziger et al., 1998). The actual mechanism on a neurophysiological basis has become an area of more recent research. Crawford et al. (1998) suggest that hypnotic analgesia is a function of the activity of the supervisory, attention control system involving the anterior frontal cortex, which then works with the cortical and subcortical processes in the allocation of thalamocortical activities. In addition, the anticipation of pain causes different adaptive behaviors, emotional states, attentional focus, and perceptual changes that affect the activity of the brain in the areas of the rostral anterior cingulated cortex, posterior cerebellum, ventromedial prefrontal cortex, mid cingulated cortex, and hippocampus (Ploghaus et al., 2003).

Crawford et al. (1998a) report that recent research "supports the proposal that hypnotic analgesia is an active inhibitory process involving several brain systems mediating attentional and nociceptive processes" (p. 22). More specifically, it appears that it is the anterior frontal (prefrontal) cortex that responds to pain. Pain has two components. The first is the physical sensory experience and the other, the emotional distress component. Through a process of "active disattention" individuals learned to disregard incoming pain/sensory signals during hypnoanalgesia (Crawford et al., 1998a).

Gruzelier (1998) notes that the significant role of the anterior cingulate cortex in managing sensory input in conjunction with the frontolimbic inhibitory processes allowing patients to suspend reality testing and critical evaluation. From the perspective of the emotional context of pain, research suggests that hypnosis resulted in inhibition of the amygdala and activation of the hippocampus. In addition, hypnosis appears to have an electrophysiological profile of its own, which shares electrophysiological features with lowered vigilance but other features with increased attention (Lehman, Faber, Isotani, & Wohlgemuth, 2001).

For the individual seeking an in-depth understanding of the interrelationship of hypnoanalgesia and brain activity the recent work of Crawford and coauthors (1998a, b) provides an excellent overview of the subject. For the role of social, environmental, and situational variable in pain interpretation and integration through neural activation of the cortical and subcortical systems, Chudler and Dong (1995) offer a discussion on the topic.

Raz and Shapiro (2002) notes that hypnotic analgesia is regarded as an active process requiring inhibitory effort. In contrast, Wagstaff (2000) in responding to the work of Gruzelier (2002) and others suggest it may be relevant to focus on the "various psychological activities and physiological processes involved in responding to a varied range of suggestions, hypnotic and otherwise, rather than attempting to identify an atypical brain state that we can specifically associate with hypnosis" (p. 161).

For those in the pain field this is especially relevant in being able to better treat the broadest range of patients available (low to high susceptible). Research continues to better delineate and specify the neurophysiological basis of sensory pain perception and emotional context. Hypnosis appears to trigger activation, "active disattention" to pain signals, and congruent emotional content at sites within the brain that are associated with pain perception. Hypnosis consequently may play a role in reducing both pain and suffering as well as function as a research instrument in defining how the brain neurophysiologically and cognitively processes the emotional and sensory pain experiences. Of interest is that with hypnosis pain reception centers in the brain can be activated with no external peripheral sensory input.

PAIN CONTROL

However, the real question for clinicians is: Can learning to develop hypnoanalgesia to noxious stimuli in a laboratory (an acute short-term artificial environment) be generalized to a patient's ability to control real nocioceptive acute or chronic pain? Crawford et al. (1998) found that patients with chronic back pain could be trained to use hypnotic analgesia on a noxious stimulus and then generalize the hypnotic analgesia to their back pain. They suggest that hypnotic analgesia is an active process that requires an inhibitory effort dissociated from conscious awareness where the anterior frontal cortex participates in a topographically specific inhibitory feedback circuit that cooperates in the allocation of the thalamocortical activities. They further point out that the subjects could successfully transfer the experimental pain reduction to reduction of their own chronic pain and, in so doing, experience increased well-being and increased sleep quality.

Using a modulated form of pain management, patients can learn the hypnotic skill of pain control or the raising of their pain thresholds. They can then be taught to generalize this skill to pain situations that are more a function of their illness or injuries.

Hypnotic analgesia has also been shown to reduce subjective pain perceptions and the nociceptive flexion reflex in highly hypnotizable subjects (Sandrini et al., 2000). This raises yet another question. If pain can be unlearned via hypnoanalgesia, does it imply that at least to some degree it is a psychoneurologically learned behavior? The concept of the existence of a "neural signature of pain" that acts as a progenitor of subsequent pain experiences is offered by Melzack & Wall (1983). If this is so, we should teach patients how to communicate more positively when in acute pain stages before they develop chronic pain. Meta-analyses of 18 studies revealed a moderate-to-large hypnoanalgesia effect supporting the efficacy of hypnotic technique for pain management in both clinical and experimental pain settings (Montgomery et al., 2000).

HYPNOTIC SUSCEPTIBILITY

When we speak of patients with pain and hypnosis, another important question is raised. Does hypnosis work equally well for all patients? The literature seems to suggest that numerous variables must be considered in drawing any conclusions. Issues of patients' hypnotic susceptibility, chronic vs. acute pain, and the origin and etiology of the pain are relevant factors. The term *hypnosis* as it is described in the pain literature represents a broad concept ranging from indirect suggestion to direct suggestion, Ericksonian, traditional, New Hypnosis, self-hypnosis, and hypnosis via face to face interactions versus audio and videotaped teaching modules (Araoz, 2001; Laidlaw & Willet, 2002). However, one common denominator, which appears prevalent within the literature, is that the type of hypnosis used is less important than the hypnotizability of the subject. The variance observed in determining the efficacy of hypnosis may be partially washed out by a lack of proper selection of subjects. As such, just as in pharmacotherapy where one medication may not fit all, hypnosis may prove to be more effective for some individuals than for others.

In the realm of hypnosis, the question of the importance of hypnotic susceptibility and trance depth has long been debated (Frankel et al., 1979; Hilgard & Hilgard, 1979; Perry et al., 1979), especially with regard to pain (Hilgard & LeBaron, 1982). Recent studies that have examined the importance of hypnotic susceptibility of patients experiencing pain (as opposed to patients not experiencing pain) appear to indicate that when dealing with acute pain issues, hypnotic susceptibility is very important. Sandrini et al. (2000) examined subjects rated as both high or low susceptibles on the Harvard Group Scale of Hypnotic Susceptibility (Shor & Orne, 1963) and the Stanford Hypnotic Susceptibility Scale (Weitzenhoffer & Hilgard, 1959). Using a noxious stimulus, they concluded, "the susceptibility of the subject is critical in hypnotically induced analgesia." Similarly, high hypnotic but not low hypnotic subjects demonstrated significant reductions in pain intensity and reduced nociceptive receptive reflexes during hypnotic analgesia (Holroyd, 2003; Zachariae et al., 1998).

Increased hypnotizability was also found to positively affect sensory and pain thresholds during dissociated imagery and focused analgesia as measured by skin conductance responses, somatosensory event-related potentials, and pain perceptions (De Pascalis et al., 1999). The ability to modulate pain was greater when subjects demonstrated higher hypnotic suggestibility (Rainville et al., 1999b). Controlled associative ability (Agagun et al., 1998) and the ability to use internal (guided imagery) and external distractors (word memory and pursuit of motor tasks) were found to be effective only in high susceptibility subjects fulfilling analgesic suggestions (Farthing et al., 1997).

Is the low suggestibility patient subjugated to not being able to use hypnosis or is suggestibility trainable? In a brief training experience, Milling et al. (1999), using the Carlton Skill Training Program, found that training failed to increase overall suggestibility scores or to enhance the effects of a suggestion for pain reduction. However, pain reduction was more highly correlated with post-traumatic levels of suggestibility than with pretreatment suggestibility.

Many authors have thought that hypnotizability is a skill that is enhanced with practice but occurring at a rate set by the patient. It has been further suggested that "hypnosis may be best conceived as a set of skills to be deployed by the individual rather than as a state" (Alden & Heap, 1998). Others have suggested that hypnotic susceptibility may not be a factor in treatment. In a study of hypnotic susceptibility and the treatment of irritable bowel syndrome, hypnotic susceptibility to suggestion was not a factor in the positive effect found for hypnosis (Galovski & Blanchard, 1998). Utilizing the Hypnotic Induction Profile as part of the hypnotic experience, clinicians can within 5 to 10 minutes assess a patient's hypnotic response capabilities and provide the patient with an initial firsthand experience (skill acquisition trial) of what hypnosis is like (Spiegel & Spiegel, 1987). Any patient, but especially patients with pain, may spontaneously shift to an altered state of awareness increasing their suggestibility merely as a function of their motivation to develop rapid rapport and trust in the clinician in an effort to escape the pain (Araoz, 1985).

A simple but effective means of incorporating the patient's willingness to accept suggestion is presented by Eimer (2000) who, at the end of an induction concludes, "As you go deeper and deeper into relaxation and hypnosis, the door way to your unconscious opens and, with your permission, I have the opportunity to talk directly to

your unconscious and give it the information it needs to help you make the changes you want to make" (p. 20).

CLINICAL APPLICATIONS

BURNS

A review of the literature points to an increasingly broadening range of applications of hypnosis in treating medical conditions with associated pain. One area where hypnosis has been used for both acute pain and healing is with burn victims. Hypnosis has been shown to reduce pain even in situations where opioids fail to bring relief (Ohrbach et al., 1998). Treatment and dressing changes can be an extremely painful part of burn care. Wright and Drummond (2000) found that rapid induction analgesia was effective in reducing pain and anxiety associated with dressing changes, and Ewin (1986) found that hypnosis positively reduced pain in adults during debridement. Similar indications were also found with pediatric patients (Foertsch et al., 1998). Indeed, burn victims may demonstrate enhanced receptivity to hypnotic suggestion secondary to issues of motivation, dissociation, and regression (Patterson et al., 1997), especially within the subset of burn patients who report high levels of baseline pain (Patterson & Ptacek, 1997).

SURGERY

Another area where hypnosis has been extensively utilized is in the arena of surgical intervention. Hypnoanesthesia, the use of hypnotic suggestion rather than general anesthesia to mediate pain during surgical intervention, has been successfully employed for endocrine cervical surgery (Defochereux et al., 1999; Meurisse et al., 1999b). Hypnosedation (hypnosis in combination with conscious intravenous sedation and local anesthesia) has been employed as an alternative to traditional anesthetic techniques (Faymonville et al., 1999; Meurisse et al., 1999).

Hypnosis has also been shown to provide proprioceptive pain and anxiety relief, reduced Alfenta and Midazolam requirements, and increased patient satisfaction and surgical conditions when compared with other surgical stress strategies in patients receiving conscious sedation (Faymonville et al., 1997).

Audiotaped hypnotic instructions produced reduced anxiety (Ghoneim et al., 2000) while preoperative hypnosis resulted in a reduction of consumption of analgesics (Engvist & Fischer, 1997) in third molar surgeries.

Self-hypnosis has been employed as an anesthesia for liposuction surgery (Botta, 1999) and for postoperative levels of pain control and relaxation in coronary artery bypass surgery (Ashton et al., 1997) and arteriotomies (Austan et al., 1997). It is attributed to reduced reported pain and anxiety and improved hemodynamic stability during invasive medical interventions such as percutaneous vascular and renal procedures (Lang et al., 2000). In particular, hand surgery that requires painful rapid remobilization of the hand is especially benefited by hypnosis. Hypnosis reduces perceived pain intensity allowing patients to be more compliant and able to withstand physical rehabilitative interventions (Mauer et al., 1999), as well as increased rates of anatomical and functional healing (Ginandes & Rosenthal, 1999).

Hypnosis has demonstrated its utility in the surgical setting resulting in decreased anesthetic utilization, more hemodynamic stability, and decreased recovery time (Lang et al., 2000). Using numerous outcome measures it was observed that postsurgical wound healing was significantly greater in patients who had received eight adjunctive hypnosis sessions targeting wound healing versus adjunctive supportive attention session or usual care. At 1- and 7-week follow-up the hypnosis group was significantly more healed than the usual care group. The hypnosis group also reported lower levels of postsurgical pain and higher scores on quality of life measures (Ginandes et al., 2003).

Hypnosis also has demonstrated its efficacy with children dealing with the pain and anxiety associated with invasive medical procedures (Hilgard & LeBaron, 1984), including bone marrow aspiration (Liossi & Hatira, 1999), resulting in lower levels of reported pain, reduced anxiety, and shorter hospital stays (Lambert, 1996; Smith & Barabasz, 1996). Distraction and imagery techniques have been shown to be highly effective in reducing pain in painful procedures (Broome et al., 1992). Scripts and metaphors for children with painful conditions are readily available to the pediatric pain practitioner (Mills & Crowley, 1986; Wester & O'Grady, 1991).

CANCER

Another significant area where hypnosis has continued to demonstrate its utility is cancer intervention. Numerous books and articles on the use of imagery and healing (Gaynor, 1994; Siegel, 1998) have discussed the psychoneuroimmunological benefits of hypnosis.

Pain, illness, injury, trauma, and loss are significant precipitants of a stress response, which may lead to a reduction in the efficacy of the functioning of the immune system. Hypnosis has been frequently demonstrated to reduce the psychological and physiological impact of stress on these systems. Hypnosis has demonstrated its utility in reducing physical and emotional stress reactions and in improving the functioning of these individuals and improving the quality of their lives (Shea, 2003).

Furthering this concept to examine the effects of unconscious motivations and metaphors, Araoz (2001) suggests that patients with pain should explore via hypnosis the somatopsychic connections that contribute to the maintenance of their pain, suffering, and negativistic experience of life.

Williamson (2002) reports that a single hypnosis session, which released suppressed anger and a revivification of a previous successful experience with acupuncture, resulted in a significant reduction in reported intractable pain. John Sarno (1998) recently continued his concept of repressed rage and intolerable emotional conflicts as contributing to reduced blood flow and autonomic system imbalance as significant factors in most back pain. Self-hypnosis has been shown to be effective in reducing the effects of stress on the immune system resulting in reduced expression of disorders associated with immunosuppression (e.g., virulent genital herpes recurrences significantly reduced, with increased cytotoxicity of natural killer cells for the virus; Gruzelier, 2002).

Chronic pain often results in lowered self-esteem, hopelessness, and despondency and decreased sense of control over pain and may be benefited by hypnosis (Turk & Holzman, 1986). Hunter (1996) furthers the concept through a metaphor of a dance that patients with chronic pain must develop "a relationship with their pain." In so doing, she emphasized that pain can be better tolerated and self-confidence improved via techniques such as hypnosis and stress management.

Liossi and White (2001) evaluated terminally ill patients with chronic pain. Using the Rotterdam Symptom Check List (DeHaes et al., 1996), a quality of life measure, she concluded that a 4-week hypnosis intervention resulted in reported enhancement of quality of life for patients with far advanced cancer. Reduced suffering was attributed to diminished pain and cognitive changes in the levels of anxiety and depression. Patients who wished to be active participants in their pain management are especially well suited for hypnosis as a means of pain control (Loitman, 2000).

Laidlaw and Willet (2002) note that terminal illness often results in strong feelings of sadness and anxiety, which can lower self-esteem, impair relationships, and lead to feelings of helplessness and despair and may result in a poor response to treatment. In what they refer to as a pilot study using a brief 10-minute audiotape intervention, they report a trend toward positive changes in patient functioning and reduced anxiety in patients with cancer.

For many years hypnosis has also been shown to provide specific pain relief and reduced suffering for patients with cancer (Hilgard & Hilgard, 1975; Hilgard & LeBaron, 1984; Sacerdote, 1966), and more recently, by employing physical relaxation coupled with imagery that provides a substitute focus of attention for painful situations (Spiegel & Moore, 1997). Patients demonstrate an increased awareness of the willingness to employ hypnosis adjunctively to their standard medical care, resulting in new programs that incorporate hypnosis into their treatment protocols (Lynch, 1999). As recently as 1996, the

NIH Technology Assessment Panel presented its conclusion in the *Journal of the American Medical Association* that strong evidence exists for the use of hypnosis in alleviating pain associated with cancer.

Irritable Bowel Syndrome

The use of hypnosis has been shown in controlled trial cases to be highly effective (Whorwell et al., 1984) and may well be the treatment of choice for refractory patients with irritable bowel syndrome (IBS) (Zimmerman, 2003). Zimmerman presents a hypnotic metaphor of a river that is used to evoke both a smooth coordinated flow through the normal digestive tract and a normal flow in the management of the patient's emotions.

Using hypnotic suggestion for an induced emotional state, Houghton et al. (2002) brought an awareness of the role of emotions in the motility of the gastrointestinal tract and IBS. With seven biweekly sessions and audiotapes for practice at home, Palsson et al. (2002) demonstrated the effectiveness of hypnosis. The authors concluded that hypnosis improves IBS symptoms through reductions in psychological distress and somatization.

Vidavic-Vukic (1999) notes that IBS is a frequently observed painful disorder, but its etiology and pathogenesis are still unknown. However, it is clear that individual perceptions may play an important role in its pathogenesis. Vidavic-Vukic points out that in recent years hypnotherapy has been shown to be successful in the treatment of IBS, resulting in either reduction or complete disappearance of pain and flatulence or a normalization of bowel habits. Similar results with a hypnotic treatment where the focus of intervention was "gut directed" and "symptom driven" found that abdominal pain, constipation, and flatulence improved while anxiety scores decreased (Galovski & Blanchard, 1998).

McGrath (1998), based on the studies of P. J. Whorwell and those of O. S. Palsson, presents hypnosis as a significant component in the treatment of IBS with success rates approaching 80% reported in the literature. The focus of hypnosis for IBS should be on the gut-directed and associated symptomology. In a review article, Camilleri (1999) points out that in addition to various medicinal interventions and fiber intake, hypnosis may play an important role in relief of pain in patients with IBS. Notwithstanding recent medical and pharmacological advances, the treatment of IBS can be adjunctively enhanced with the addition of hypnosis.

ACUTE PAIN

Hypnosis also has been shown to be effective in acute pain care settings such as emergency room settings with burn pain, pediatric procedures, psychiatric presentations, and obstetric situations (Peebles-Klieger, 2000; Zahourek,

1985). Iserson (1999) describes a simple method of hypnosis used in pediatric fracture reduction on four cases of angulated forearm fractures employing distraction techniques when no other form of analgesia was available. Interestingly, fracture healing also may be enhanced using hypnosis. Faster edge healing, improved ankle mobility, greater function mobility to descend stairs, lower use of analgesic, and trends toward lower self-reported pain were found in patients who received hypnotic intervention in addition to standard orthopedic emergency room care (Ginandes & Rosenthal, 1999).

Hypnotically induced glove anesthesia with transference to the pain site for acute pain relief is a commonly used technique. This is accomplished by using suggestions of creating a numbing sensation in the hand. Patients may be asked to imagine their hands in a bucket of anesthetic gel or a glove or other such images. This numbing or pleasant sensation is then transferred to the pain site with a pleasant increase in numbness. An excellent example of this technique is offered by Basserman and Wester (1984). Other techniques include distraction techniques and dissociative techniques (Burte, 1999; Eastwood et al., 1998). In all cases, a trusting rapport with the clinician appears to be a critical factor in achieving the desired goals. In addition, as has been noted earlier, pain may act as a mediator toward an altered state of increased suggestibility to pain alleviation.

Patients with acute pain may willingly and rapidly transfer their pain to the hypnotherapist or anyone willing to accept the pain. Patients should be reassured that proper medical care is forthcoming and they can let go of their pain. As Schafer (1996) points out, perhaps as many as half the patients in an emergency room may be in spontaneous trance. An alternative approach is to focus on the imagery the patient spontaneously reports associated with the pain. Psychosemantics and somatopsychic queues are observed when utilizing the patient's perceptions, internal representations, and understandings of the pain to alter the cognitive, emotional, and sensory experience (Burte & Araoz, 1994).

Using the New Hypnosis Model developed by Daniel Araoz (1985), patients are helped to achieve an altered state of internally directed experiencing of their symptomology. By focusing on the way they interpret and communicate their pain through any or all of their five senses, patients are led to a reinterpretation and understanding of their ability to modulate their pain. How patients integrate pain sensations will affect their pain thresholds. Positive suggestions to pain altered the amount of time that patients could keep their hands immersed in ice water (Staats et al., 1998).

For example, in the case of a man with recently fractured ribs, he may be asked to experience or visualize the ribs as they appear to him. He is then asked to visualize ways to soothe, protect, or heal the ribs (e.g., an anesthetic band wrapped around the chest, relaxing, protecting, and healing the area of injury), while communicating calming, relaxing, and possibly "in control of the situation" thoughts. At times, visualizing being in a safe or pleasant situation helps induce a hypnoidal form of relaxation or mild dissociation. Although creating relaxation has often been seen as an important element in inducing trance for the patient experiencing pain, it may be a secondary goal with the imaging or individualized experience of the pain as the primary pathway to the hypnotic state. In this regard hypnosis can be viewed as a state of focused internally directed learning experiences (FIDLE).

Acute pediatric pain represents a somewhat different issue in that children often lack clinical insight regarding their condition, an understanding of the etiology, potential longevity, or plausible interventions available for ameliorating their pain, concepts that help adults cope with acute pain more effectively. Patients provided appropriate preoperative information demonstrate less acute pain (Stevensen, 1995). Hypnosis may represent a complementary treatment in conjunction with other forms of intervention such as pharmacological pain management (Rusy & Weisman, 2000). By providing cognitive and behavioral schemata via modalities easily accessed by children (e.g., imagery, fantasy), the pediatric patient with acute pain can be empowered similarly to the way adults use reason to empower coping ability with pain. Pediatric pain management has been augmented by the utilization of hypnotic intervention in a broad array of conditions. Whereas there are numerous scales available to help young and preverbal children rate their pain (Wong & Baker, 1988), they may have drawbacks, which reduce their accuracy (Lehmann et al., 1990).

An area where hypnosis has proved helpful with children is in reducing acute procedural pain (Howard, 2003). Hart & Hart (1998) notes that hypnosis is the most frequently used intervention for acute procedure pain and distress in pediatric patients with cancer. The utilization of hypnosis in pediatric pain control is well presented in Hilgard and LeBaron's (1982) work and is now found throughout the pediatric pain literature. Chronic pediatric pain was suggested to result in long-term emotional distress and may contribute to physical and emotional disability in later life (Campo et al., 2001; Hotopf et al., 1998; Howard, 2003).

Neuropathic pain appears to benefit from the adjunctive application of hypnosis to standard pharmacological and physical treatment. Often cognitive and hypnotherapeutic interventions can help children better understand and create a sense of mastery over their pain. In so doing, an increased sense of control can lead to reduced anxiety and potentially improved immunological functioning. Gastrointestinal disorders such as IBS may show an equal benefit from hypnotherapy in both pediatric and adult populations. A combined acupuncture/hypnosis interven-

tion was successfully employed in treating chronic pediatric pain. Improvement was found in both pain levels and emotional well-being (Zeltzer et al., 2002).

From a biophysical perspective, it may be relevant to recognize that much of the adult literature concerning hypnotic procedures for treating acute pain may apply equally for adults and children. As we develop greater understanding of the central nervous system and physiological mechanisms of hypnotic analgesia, its applicability should be relevantly generalizable to the pediatric population. Hypnosis has demonstrated a reliable and significant impact on both acute procedural pain and chronic pain conditions (Patterson & Jensen, 2003).

A procedure common to many pediatric patients with acute and chronic pain as well as patients without pain is the painful experience of venipuncture and intravenous insertion. Fear, anxiety, and conditional responding to procedures associated with venipuncture and intravenous insertions often result in elevated levels of pain and anticipatory pain. Hypnosis and distraction techniques can help children to reinterpret painful experiences and reduce negative associations with pain (Carlson et al., 2000).

In a recent article on the use of imagination and hypnosis in the treatment of children with pain and anxiety, LeBaron (2003) presents a strong case for the effectiveness of hypnosis utilizing vignettes illustrating its implementation. He points out that through hypnosis, fantasies and wishes and desires can be vivified and that in so doing, it may "create enough renewed excitement and interest that the child experiences an increase in energy and motivation and a new connection with their family."

Anbar (2001) found that children with recurrent abdominal pain in the absence of an identifiable physiological cause respond following a single hypnotic session. One cannot discuss pediatric pain without referring to where it all begins. Hypnosis and self-hypnosis have proved effective in reducing pain and fear associated with induced pain in labor during childbirth (albeit we are talking about the mother's pain and not the child's) (Jackson, 2003; Ketterhagen et al., 2002; Mongan, 1998).

Hypnosis may be a means of reducing both pain and pain-related distress (Chen et al., 2000). For example, Adam, a young patient with cancer was treated using hypnosis for pain. First, he was taught glove anesthesia, which he applied to areas where he was to have finger sticks, Broviac changes, and later bone marrow aspirations. He was taught to visualize himself as a cartoon superhero named He-Man. He was taught how to enter a trance state. A signal was then used to initiate rapid induction. By lifting his crutch and later his finger into the air and reciting the words, "By the power of Grey Skull, I am He-Man," Adam was magically (hypnotically) transformed into He-Man, the strongest man in the universe. At such times, he could withstand increased levels of pain and invasive procedures.

Recurrent pediatric headaches appear to show a positive response to hypnotic intervention when relaxation and/or thermal feedback techniques are employed (Holden et al., 1999). The use of autogenic training (hand warming) with imagery has also been useful in reducing or eliminating pediatric migraines when done early in the migraine episode at the first signs of visual aura or muscular discomfort.

GERIATRICS

Lamberg (1998) reported on the new guidelines on managing chronic pain in older persons. At the other end of the lifespan within the over-65-year-old population and geriatric population, pain is reported in 45 to 80% of individuals. The most common treatment for pain in older persons is analgesic drugs. She states that the American geriatric panel included hypnosis among these coping skills. "Non pharmacological interventions used in combination with appropriate drug regimes often improve overall pain management."

CHRONIC PAIN

Crawford et al. (1998), in drawing attention to the transition of the patient with acute pain to the patient with chronic pain, note that by utilizing hypnosis, patients could alter acute pain experiences. They further suggest that learned hypnotic analgesia resulted in reported chronic pain reductions, increased psychological well-being, and increased sleep quality. The "neuro signature of pain" can influence subsequent pain experiences (Melzack & Wall, 1983). Specific pain-reduction hypnotic skills may indeed be essential in developing lasting pain relief, especially in situations where chronic pain based on medical conditions (e.g., cancer tumors, herniated discs) is anticipated. In this context, hypnotic pain control may be conceived as a set of skills rather than a state (Alden & Heap, 1998).

Patients with chronic pain clearly represent a population different from patients with acute pain. The most common form of chronic pain, other than from illness, is chronic low back pain, accounting for $50 billion to $100 billion a year in lost wages and medical care (Burte et al., 1994). Unlike acute pain, chronic pain may result in significant changes in individuals, personalities, and clinical presentations as evidenced by performance on Minnesota Multiphasic Personality Inventory (MMPI) profiles (Strassberg et al., 1992), as well as on specific pain measures such as the Posttraumatic Personality Profile (P3) and the behavioral assessment of pain (BAP).

Clinically, we commonly find that patients with chronic pain demonstrate elevated levels of feelings of hopelessness, helplessness, and despair. They often report ongoing struggles with depression, somatic preoccupations, and obsessive concerns with fatal illness. When chronic pain becomes a central issue in the individual's life, it may function as a coping mechanism altering the patient's capacities, both psychopathophysiologically and etiologically (Kuhn, 1984).

In addition to its direct impact on pain alleviation, hypnosis can play a key role with the depression and hopelessness the patient with chronic pain experiences. Metaphors and hypnotic scripts can address both the pain and psychological distress (Havens & Walters, 1989). Margaret Jack (1999) cites the case of a patient with chronic pain syndrome (CPS) for whom hypnosis played a critical role in her emotional recovery with some additional pain relief. Individuals who are diagnosed with CPS are often overwhelmed by the impact of their pain. For patients with CPS, the pain often takes on an all-encompassing life of its own, dictating the patient's quality of life both psychologically and physically. Issues of learned behaviors, conditioned avoidances, and conscious and unconscious secondary gains often complicate the alleviation of the pain patients with CPS experience.

Hypnotherapy represents a complementary component in a multidisciplinary approach that should first acknowledge that the patient with CPS is not primarily a psychiatric patient but rather a composite of both psychological and physical distress. Melzack (1990) points out the advantages of a multidisciplinary approach, inclusive of narcotics, for rescuing people in chronic pain. As Hitchcock (1998) points out, there are significant myths and misconceptions about the patient with chronic pain that the pain practitioner must address in formulating a treatment plan. She further points out that in many ways the patient is a valuable contributor to the understanding of his or her own condition. As such, hypnosis may assist patients in that understanding via uncovering techniques and experiential insights into various aspects of their pain.

In addition to low back pain, many other conditions can result in CPS. Patients experiencing temporomandibular disorders who underwent hypnotic intervention demonstrated significant decreases in pain severity and frequency, which were maintained for at least 6 months after treatment (Simon & Lewis, 2000). Ray and Page (2002) demonstrated how even a single session of hypnotherapy brought about reductions in subjectively reported pain in patients with chronic pain.

Hypnosis has helped adolescent teens and adults with cystic fibrosis (CF) develop improved attitudes about health and a sense of independence and decreased anxiety (Belsky & Kahanna, 1994; Olness & Kohen, 1996). Using a technique introduced by Bressler (1990), Anbar (2000) taught patients with CF to seek an inner advisor while in self-hypnosis to uncover information pertaining to their physical or psychological symptoms. In so doing, they achieved greater levels of physical comfort and reduced anxiety levels.

Hypnotic intervention resulted in improvement in symptoms resulting from multiple sclerosis (Sutcher, 1997); fibromyalgia syndrome, especially when used as part of a multidisciplinary treatment (Berman & Swyers, 1999); procedures associated with dermatological disorders (Shenefelt, 2003); and phantom limb pain (Muraoka et al., 1996; Sthalekar, 1993). Using a hypnotically induced "virtual mirror" to allow patients to create hypnotic movement in imagery, Oakley and Halligan (2002) were able to modify long-standing intractable phantom limb pain. Tinnitus has been described as what pain would sound like if it made a sound (McSpaden, 1993). The cognitive distress that often overwhelms these patients has been treated hypnotically with some success (Burte, 1993; Harosymczuk, 2002). The list of illnesses, disease conditions, and injury-induced pain conditions for which hypnosis has historically been utilized and for which its application may apply is beyond the scope of one chapter. A review of the literature suggests that its clinical application is continually expanding.

PSYCHOGENIC AND PSYCHOSOMATIC PAIN

Another arena in which hypnosis may play a significant role in pain management and suffering is with patients experiencing psychogenic and psychosomatic pain. Using the affect bridge initially described by Watkins (1971) and listening to the patient's somatopsychic language (Araoz, 1985; Burte et al., 1994), patients can gain insight into the range and variety of symptoms they are experiencing. The psychosemantics the patient uses in describing his or her life situations or pain offers insight into the non-organic etiology of the conditions. Cues and stimuli associated with past trauma may maintain the patient's symptoms, whereas reassociating those symptoms to positive images may result in symptom reduction or alleviation (Burte, 1993).

With the psychosomatic patient with no known organic etiological basis for the pain, the exploration of the negative self-hypnotic (NSH) statements associated with the condition will lend insight into the symptom output. Patients' expectations of pain may result in the need for the therapist to "dehypnotize" patients out of their expectation of pain (i.e., painful childbirth). In a study by Whalley and Oakley (2003), psychogenic pain was hypnotically induced in highly hypnotic subjects, reinforcing the cognitive element in pain perception. This is especially relevant with patients experiencing sexual dysfunction associated with pain (Araoz, 1998; Burte & Araoz, 1994).

Techniques and case histories are presented in the above-noted works, but the essence of the hypnotherapy is to have the patient, by experiencing these NSH statements in trance, identify the bridges between his or her

psychic conflicts (semantic input) and the pain or dysfunctional symptoms (somatic output).

DENTAL PAIN

As stated earlier, learned emotional responses and anticipation of pain (anxiety) are very common. One area where this is seen is with dental patients. Whether the result of childhood trauma associated with painful procedures or the result of painful procedures in adulthood or issues of loss of control, many individuals demonstrate anxiety and fear reactions to dental care resulting in avoidance of proper or timely treatment. Hypnosis can prove to be an effective intervention in reducing anticipatory anxiety.

In addition, hypnosis can reduce anxiety during procedures and be used hypnoanalgesically within the dental setting. Dyas (2001) compared 40 subjects (20 per group), who received intravenous drug administration of Midazolam and Fentanyl for mandibular third molar surgical removal either with or without hypnosis. He found that heart rate (an indicator of stress and anxiety), electrocardiographic, and pulse oximeter recordings were better for patients who received hypnosedation. Further, the hypnosedative group required less intravenous sedation, their heart rate increase was significantly lower, and their recovery time was significantly shorter.

Hypnosis effectively allowed for reduced intravenous doses in dental treatments (Lu & Lu, 1996). Hypnosis in general dentistry has been shown to be an effective intervention for pain management, increasing rate of healing, reducing analgesic medication, and reducing anxiety and phobia (Hammond, 1990).

CONCLUSION

In conclusion, the field of hypnosis for pain management is diverse. Its range encompasses hypnoanalgesia, treatment of acute and chronic pain, pre- and postsurgical intervention, distress and suffering, neurophysiological intervention, and psychosomatic pain, to mention but a few areas. It continues to grow as an accepted modality in pain management and has been endorsed as an effective adjunctive treatment by many professional societies and organizations for intervention with all age populations from pediatric to geriatric. It has shown its utility with intractable conditions such as cancer pain and has been used for pain with terminal illness. Hypnosis has been suggested to be effective in enhancing immune functioning via stress reduction and increased cognitive coping.

For the health care provider seeking a broader range of knowledge about hypnosis, there is a plethora of information available. Works such as the *Handbook of Hypnotic Suggestions and Metaphors* (Hammond, 1990) offer an overview of hypnotic intervention, whereas for the pain practitioner, the work of Elmer and Freeman (1998) focuses on hypnotic interventions more relevant to the cognitive and sensory aspects of pain (Munafo, 1998). Rossi (1993) presents a good introduction into the field of psychobiology of mind, body connectedness, and healing. Fredericks (2002) provides an excellent text on surgery and anesthesia, an overview of which is presented by Rogerson (2002). For practitioners seeking applications to clinical cases, Frank and Mooney's (2002) work on hypnosis and counseling in the treatment of chronic illness is an excellent resource.

As cited earlier, hypnosis with pharmacotherapy has been shown to be more effective than either alone and should not be overlooked by professionals seeking to help manage patients' pain.

REFERENCES

Alden, P., & Heap, M. (1998). Hypnotic pain control: Some theoretical and practical issues. *International Journal of Clinical and Experimental Hypnosis, 46*(1), 62–67.

Anbar, R. D. (2000). Hypnosis, Theodore Roosevelt and the patient with cystic fibrosis. *Pediatrics, 106*(2), 339–346.

Araoz, D. L. (1985). *The new hypnosis.* New York: Brunner/Mazel.

Araoz, D. L. (1998). *The new hypnosis in sex therapy.* Northvale, NJ: Jason Aronson Inc.

Araoz, D. L. (2001). The unconscious in Ericksonian hypnotherapy. *Australian Journal of Clinical Hypnotherapy and Hypnosis, 22* (2) 78–90.

Arargun, M. Y., Tegeoglu, I., Kara, H., Adak, B., & Ercan, M. (1998). Hypnotizability, pain threshold and dissociative experiences. *Biological Psychiatry, 44*(1), 69–71.

Ashton, Jr., C., Whitworth, G. C., Seldonridge, J. A., Shapiro, P. A., Weinberg, A. D., Michler, R. E. et al.(1997). Self-hypnosis reduces anxiety following coronary artery bypass surgery. A prospective randomized trial. *Journal of Cardiovascular Surgery* (Torino), 38(1), 69–75.

Austan, F., Polise, M., & Schultz, T. R. (1997). The use of verbal expectancy in reducing pain associated with arteriotomies. *American Journal of Clinical Hypnosis, 39*(3), 182–186.

Barber, J. (1998). The mysterious persistence of hypnotic analgesia. *International Journal of Clinical and Experimental Hypnosis, 46*(1), 28–43.

Barber, J. & Adrian, C. (1982). *Psychological approaches to the management of pain.* New York: Brunner/Mazel, Inc.

Basserman, S. W., & Wester, W. C. (1984). In W. C. Wester & A. H. Smith, Jr. (Eds.), *Hypnosis and pain control in clinical hypnosis: A multidisciplinary approach.* Philadelphia: Lippincott.

Bassman, S. W., & Wester, II, W. C. (1992). *Hypnosis, headache and pain control, an integrated approach.* Columbus, OH: Psychology Publications Inc.

Belsky, J., & Kahanna, P. (1994). The effects of self-hypnosis for children with cystic fibrosis: A pilot study. *American Journal of Clinical Hypnosis, 36,* 282–292.

Berman, B. M., & Swyers, J. P. (1999). Complementary medicine treatments for fibromyalgia syndrome. *Bailliere's Best Practice and Research in Clinical Rheumatology, 13*(93), 487–492.

Bonica, J. J. (1990). *The management of pain* (Vol. 1, 2nd ed.). Philadelphia: Lea & Febiger.

Botta, S. A. (1999). Self-hypnosis as anesthesia for liposuction surgery. *American Journal of Clinical Hypnosis, 41*(4), 299–331.

Bressler, D. E. (1990). Meeting an inner advisor. In D.C. Hammond (Ed.), *Handbook of hypnotic suggestion and metaphors.* New York: W.W. Norton.

Broome, M. E., Lillis, P. P., McGahee, T. W., & Bates, T. (1992). The use of distraction and imagery with children during painful procedures. *Oncology Nursing Forum, 19,* 499–502.

Burte, J. M. (1993). The role of hypnosis in the treatment of tinnitus. *Australian Journal of Clinical Hypnotherapy and Hypnosis, 14*(2), 41–52.

Burte, J. M. (1999). Introduction for creating a dissociative state. In S. Rosenberg, (Ed.), *Course workbook.* New York: New York Society of Clinical Hypnosis.

Burte, J. M. (2002). Psychoneuroimmunology. In R. Weiner (Ed.), *Pain management: A practical guide for clinicians* (6th ed.). Boca Raton, FL: CRC Press.

Burte, J. M. & Araoz, D. L. (1994). Cognitive hypnotherapy with sexual disorders. *Journal of Cognitive Psychotherapy, 8*(4), 299–312.

Burte, J. M., Burte, W., & Araoz, D. L. (1994). Hypnosis in the treatment of back pain. *Australian Journal of Clinical Hypnotherapy and Hypnosis, 15*(2), 93–115.

Camilleri, M. (1999). Review article: Clinical evidence to support current therapies of irritable bowel syndrome. *Alimentary Pharmacology and Therapeutics, 13*(Suppl. 2), 48–53.

Campo, J. V., Di, L. C., Chiappetta, L. et. al. (2001). Adult outcomes of pediatric recurrent abdominal pain. Do they just grow out of it? *Pediatrics, 108,* El.

Carlson, K. L, Broom, M., & Vessey, J. A. (2000) Using distraction to reduce reported pain, fear and behavioral distress in children and adolescents. A multi-site study. *Journal of the Society of Pediatric Nurses 5*(2), 75–91.

Chapman, C. R., & Nakamura, Y. (1998). Hypnotic analgesia: A constructivist framework. *International Journal of Clinical and Experimental Hypnosis, 6*(1), 6–27.

Chaves, J. F., & Dworkin, S. F. (1997). Hypnotic control of pain: historical perspectives and future prospects. *International Journal of Clinical and Experimental Hypnosis, 45*(4), 356–376.

Chen, E., Joseph, M. H., & Zeltzer, L. K. (2000). Behavioral and cognitive interventions in the treatment of pain in children. *Pediatric Clinics of North America, 47*(3), 513–525.

Chudler, E. H., & Dong, W. K. (1995). The role of the basal ganglia in nociception and pain. *Pain, 60,* 3–38.

Crawford, M. J., Knebel, T., Kaplan, L., Vendemia, J. M., Xie, M., Jamison, S. et al. (1998). Hypnotic analgesia: 1. Somatosensory event related potential changes to noxious stimuli and 2. Transfer learning to reduce chronic low back pain. *International Journal of Clinical and Experimental Hypnosis, 46*(1), 92–132.

Crawford, H., Knebel, T., & Vendemia, J. M. C. (1998). The nature of hypnotic analgesia: Neurophysiological foundation and evidence. *Contemporary Hypnosis, 15*(1), 22–34.

Danziger, N., Fournier, E., Bouhassira, D., Michaud, D., DeBroucher, T., Santarcangelo, E., Carli, G., Chertock, L., & Willer, J.C. (1998). Different strategies of modulation can be operative during hypnotic analgesia, a neuro-physiological study. *Pain, 75*(1), 85–92.

Defochereux, T., Meurisse, M., Hamoir, E., Gollogly, L., Joris, J., & Faymonville, M. E. (1999). Hypnoanesthesia for endocrine cervical surgery: a statement of practice. *Journal of American Complementary Medicine, 5*(6), 509–520.

DeHaes, J., Olschewski, M., Fayers, P., Visser, M., Culla, A., Hopwood P. et al. (1996). *The Rotterdam symptom checklist.* The Netherlands: Northern Centre for Health Care Research, University of Groningen.

DePascalis, V., Maguarano, M. R., & Bellusci, A. (1999). Pain perception, somatosensory event related potentials and skin conductance responses to painful stimuli in high, mid, and low hypnotizable subjects: Effects of differential pain reduction strategies. *Pain, 83*(3), 499–508.

Dinges, D. F., Whitehouse, W. G., Onre, E. C., Bloom, P. B., Carlin, M. M., Bauer, N. K., et al. (1997). Self-hypnosis training as an adjunct treatment in the management of pain associated with sickle cell disease. *International Journal of Clinical and Experimental Hypnosis, 45*(4), 417–432.

Dyas, R. (2001). Augmenting intravenous sedation with hypnosis, a controlled retrospective study. *Contemporary Hypnosis, 18*(3), 128–134.

Eastwood, J. D., Gaskowski, P., & Bowers, K. S. (1998). The folly of effort: Ironic effects in the mental control of pain. *International Journal of Clinical and Experimental Hypnosis, 46*(1), 77–91.

Eimer, B. N. (2000). Clinical applications of hypnosis for brief and efficient pain management psychotherapy, *American Journal of Hypnosis, 43*(1), 17–40.

Elmer, B. N., & Freeman, A. (1998). *Pain management psychotherapy: A practical guide.* New York: John Wiley and Sons.

Engvist, B., & Fischer, K. (1997). Preoperative hypnotic techniques reduce consumption of analgesics after surgical removal of third mandibular molars: A brief communication. *International Journal of Clinical and Experimental Hypnosis, 45*(2), 102–108.

Erickson, M. H. (1966). The interspersal hypnotic technique for symptoms correction and pain control. *American Journal of Clinical Hypnosis, 8*, 198–209.

Erickson, M. H. (1986). Mind-body communication in hypnosis. In E. Rossi & M. Ryan (Eds.), *The seminars, workshops and lectures of Milton H. Erickson* (Vol. III). New York: Irvington Publishers Inc.

Ewin, D. M. (1986). The effect of hypnosis and mental sets on major surgery and burns. *Psychiatric Annals, 16*(2) 115–118.

Farthing, G. W., Vonturino, M., Brown, S. W., & Lazar, J. D. (1997). Internal and external distraction in the control of cold pressor pain as a function of hypnotizability. *International Journal of Clinical and Experimental Hypnosis, 45*(4), 433–446.

Faymonville, M. E., Mambourg, P. H., Joris, J., Vrijens, B., Fissette, J., Albert, A. et al. (1997). Psychological approaches during conscious sedation. Hypnosis versus stress reducing strategies: A prospective randomized study. *Pain, 73*(3), 361–367.

Faymonville, M. E., Meurisse, M., & Fissette, J. (1999). Hypnosedation: A valuable alternative to traditional anaesthetic techniques. *Acta Chirurgica Belgica, 99*(4), 141–146.

Faymonville, M. E., Laureys, S., Degueldre, C., DelFiore, G., Luxen, A., Franck, G., et al. (2000). Neural mechanisms of antinociceptive effects of hypnosis. *Anesthesiology, 92*(5), 1257–1267.

Foderaro, L. W. (1996, February 24). Hypnosis gains credence as influence on the body. *New York Times.* p. 23.

Foertsch, C. E., O'Hara, M. W., Stoddard, F. J., & Kealey, G. P. (1998). Treatment resistant pain and distress during pediatric burn dressing changes. *Journal of Burn Care and Rehabilitation, 19*(3), 219–224.

Fordyce, W. E. (1976). *Behavioral methods from chronic pain and illness.* St. Louis: C.V. Mosby.

Frank, D., & Mooney, B. (2002). *Hypnosis and counseling in the treatment of chronic illness.* Wales, U. K.: Crown House Publishing.

Frankel, F. H., Apfel, R. J., Kelly, S. F., et al. (1979). The use of hypnotizability scales in the clinic: A review after six years. *International Journal of Clinical and Experimental Hypnosis, 27*, 63–67.

Fredericks, L. (2002). *The use of hypnosis in surgery and anesthesiology: Psychological preparation of the surgical patient.* Springfield, IL: Charles C Thomas.

Galovski, T. E., & Blanchard, E. B. (1998) The treatment of irritable bowel syndrome with hypnotherapy. *Applied Psychophysiological Biofeedback, 23*(4), 219–232.

Gaynor, M. (1994). *Healing E.S.S.E.N.C.E.: A cancer doctor's practical program for hope and recovery.* New York: Kodansha International.

Ghoneim, M. M., Block, R. I., Sarasin, D. S., Davis, C. S., & Marchman, J. N. (2000). Tape recorded hypnosis instructions as adjuvant in the care of patients scheduled for third molar surgery. *Anesthesia & Analgesia, 90*(1), 64–68.

Ginandes, C. S., & Rosenthal, D. I. (1999). Using hypnosis to accelerate the healing of bone fractures: A randomized controlled pilot study. *Alternative Therapies Health and Medicine, 5*(2), 67–75.

Ginandes, C., Brooks, P., Sando, W., Jones, C., & Aker, J. (2003). Can medical hypnosis accelerate post-surgical wound healing? Results of a clinical trial. *American Journal of Clinical Hypnosis 45*(4), 333–350.

Gruzelier, J. (1998). A working model of neurophysiology of hypnosis: A review of evidence. *Contemporary Hypnosis, 15*(1), 3–19.

Gruzelier, J. (2002). Self-hypnosis and immune function, health, well being, and personality. *Hypnosis, 29*(4), 186–191.

Hammond, D. C. (1990). *Handbook of hypnotic suggestions and metaphors.* New York: Norton and Co.

Harosymczuk, M. (2002). Hypnosis as an adjunct to tinnitus retaining therapy in the treatment of persistent tinnitus – A case. *Hypnosis, 29*(4), 192–195.

Hart, C., & Hart, B., (1998). Discussion commentary: Hypnosis in the alleviation of procedure related pain and distress in pediatric oncology patients. *Contemporary Hypnosis, 15*(4), 208–211.

Havens, R. A., & Walters, C. (1989). *Hypnotherapy scripts: A neo-Ericksonian approach to persuasive healing.* New York: Brunner/Mazel.

Hawkins, R. M. F. (2001). A systematic meta-review of hypnosis as an empirically supported treatment for pain. *Pain Reviews, 8*, 47–73.

Hilgard, E. R., & Hilgard, J. R. (1975). *Hypnosis in the relief of pain.* Los Altos, CA: William Kaufman.

Hilgard, J. R., & Hilgard, E. R. (1979). Assessing hypnotic responsiveness in a clinical setting: A multi-item clinical scale and the advantages over single item scales. *International Journal of Clinical and Experimental Hypnosis, 27*, 134–150.

Hilgard, J. R., & LeBaron, S. (1982). Relief of anxiety and pain in children and adolescents with cancer: Quantitative measures and clinical observations. *International Journal of Clinical and Experimental Hypnosis, 30*, 417–442.

Hilgard, J. R., & LeBaron, S. (1984). *Hypnotherapy of pain in children with cancer.* Los Altos, CA. William Kaufman.

Hitchcock, L. (1998). Myths and misconceptions about chronic pain. In R. Weiner (Ed.), *Pain management: A practical guide* (5th ed.). Boca Raton, FL: CRC Press.

Holden, E. W., Deichman, M. M., & Levy, J. D. (1999). Empirically supported treatments in pediatric psychology: Recurrent pediatric headache. *Journal of Pediatric Psychology, 24*(2), 91–109.

Holroyd, J. (2003). The science of meditation and the state of hypnosis. *American Journal of Clinical Hypnosis, 46*(2), 109–128.

Hotopf, M., Carr, S., Mayou, R., Wadsworth, M., & Wossely, S. (1998). Why do children have chronic abdominal pain and what happens to them when they grow up? Population based cohost study. *British Medical Journal, 316*, 1196–1200.

Houghton, L. A., Calvert, E. L., Jackson, N. A., Cooper, P., & Whorwell, P. J. (2002). Visceral sensation and emotion: A study using hypnosis. *Gut, 51*(5), 701–704.

Howard, R. F. (2003). Current status of pain management in children. *Journal of the American Medical Association, 290*(18), 2464–2469.

Hrezo, R. J. (1998). Hypnosis, an alternative in pain management for nurse practitioners. *Nurse Practical Forum, 9*(4), 217–226.

Hunter, M. E. (1996). *Making peace with chronic pain: A whole-life strategy.* New York: Brunner/Mazel.

Iserson, K. V. (1999). Hypnosis for pediatric fracture reduction. *Journal of Emergency Medicine, 17*(1), 53–56.

Iserson, K. V. (1999). Hypnosis for pediatric fracture reduction. *Journal of Emergency Medicine, 17*(1), 53–56.

Jack, M. A. (1999). Clinical reports: The use of hypnosis for a patient with chronic pain. *Contemporary Hypnosis, 16*(4), 231–236.

Jackson, D. D. (1999). You will feel no pain. *Smithsonian, 29*(12), 126–137.

Jackson, P. (2003). Hypnosis for birthing – A natural option: Part 2. *Australian Journal of Clinical Hypotherapy and Hypnosis, 24*(2) 112–122.

Johnson, M. E., & Hauck, C. (1999). Beliefs and opinions about hypnosis held by the general public: A systematic evaluation. *American Journal of Clinical Hypnosis, 42*(1), 10–20.

Ketterhagen, D., Vande Vusse, L., & Berner, M. A. (2002). Self-hypnosis: Alternative anesthesia for childbirth. *American Journal of Maternity and Child Nursing, 27*(6) 335–340.

Kuhn, W. (1984). Chronic pain. *Southern Medical Journal, 77*, 1103–1106.

Laidlaw, T. M., & Willet, M. J. (2002). Self-hypnosis tapes for anxious cancer patients: An evaluation using personalized emotional index (PEI). Diary Data. *Contemporary Hypnosis, 19*(1), 25–35.

Lamberg, L. (1998). New guidelines on managing chronic pain in older persons. *Journal of the American Medical Association, 280*(4), 311.

Lambert, S. A. (1996). The effects of hypnosis/guided imagery on the postoperative course of children. *Journal of Developmental and Behavioral Pediatrics, 17*(5), 307–310.

Lang, E. V., Benotsch, E. G., Fick, L. J., Lutgendorf, S., Berbaum, M. L., Berbaum, K. S. et al. (2000). Adjunctive non-pharmacological analgesia for invasive medical procedures: A randomized trial. *Lancet, 29*, 355(9214), 1486–1490.

LeBaron, S. (2003). The use of imagination in the treatment of children with pain and anxiety. *Australian Journal of Clinical Hypnotherapy and Hypnosis, 24*(1), 1–13.

Lehmann, H. P., Bendebba, M., & DeAngelis, C. (1990). The consistency of young children's assessment of remembered painful events. *Journal of Developmental and Behavioral Pediatrics, 11*, 128–134.

Lehman, D., Faber, P., Isotani, T., & Wohlgemuth, P., (2001). Source locations of EEG frequency bands during hypnotic arm levitation. A pilot study. *Contemporary Hypnosis, 18*(3), 120–128.

Levitan, A. A. (1992) Hypnosis – The hypnotic brain: Hypnotherapy and social communication (book review). *Journal of the American Medical Association, 267*(24), 3357.

Lioss, C., & White, P. (2001). Efficacy of clinical hypnosis in the enhancement of quality of life of terminally ill cancer patients. *Contemporary Hypnosis, 18*(3), 145(Book Review)161.

Liossi, C., & Hatira, P. (1999). Clinical hypnosis versus cognitive behavioral training for pain management with pediatric cancer patients undergoing bone marrow aspirations. *International Journal of Clinical and Experimental Hypnosis, 47*(2), 104–116.

Loitman, J. E. (2000). Pain management: Beyond pharmacology to acupuncture and hypnosis. *Journal of the American Medical Association, 283*(1) 118–119.

Lu, D. P., & Lu, G. P. (1996). Hypnosis and pharmacological sedation for medically compromised patients. *Compendium of Continuing Education in Dentistry, 17*, 34–36.

Lynch, D. F. Jr. (1999). Empowering the patient: Hypnosis in the management of cancer, surgical disease and chronic pain. *American Journal of Clinical Hypnosis, 42*(2), 122–130.

Mauer, M. H., Burnett, K. F., Ouelette, E. A., Ironson, G. H., & Dandes, H. M. (1999). Medical hypnosis and orthopaedic hand surgery: Pain perception, post-operative recovery and therapeutic comfort. *International Journal of Clinical and Experimental Hypnosis, 47*(2), 144–161.

McGrath, M. (1998). Gimme a break! *Prevention, 50*(6), 98–103.

McSpaden, J. B. (1993). Tinnitus aurium. *Tinnitus Today, 18*(2), 15–17.

Medd, D. Y. (2001) Fear of injections: The value of hypnosis in facilitating clinical treatment. *Contemporary Hypnosis, 18*(2), 100–107.

Melzack, R. (1990). The tragedy of needless pain. *Scientific American, 262*(2), 27–33.

Melzack, R., & Wall, P. D. (1965). Pain mechanisms: A new theory. *Science, 150*, 971–979.

Melzack, R., & Wall, P. D. (1983). *The challenge of pain.* New York: Basic Books.

Meurisse, M., Defechereux, T., Homoir, E., Maweja, S., Marchettini, P., Gollogly, L. et al. (1999), Hypnosis with conscious sedation instead of general anesthesia? Applications in cervical endocrine surgery. *Acta Chirurgica Belgica, 99*(4), 151–158.

Meurisse, M., Hamoir, E., Defechereux, T., Gollogly, L., Derry, O., Postal, O. et al. (1999). Bilateral neck exploration under hypnosedation: A new standard of care in primary hyperparathyroidism. *Annals of Surgery, 229*(3), 401–408.

Milling, L. S., Kirsch, I., & Burgess, C. A. (1999). Brief modification of suggestibility and hypnotic analgesia: Too good to be true? *International Journal of Clinical and Experimental Hypnosis, 46*(1), 62–67.

Mills, J. C., & Crowley, R. J. (1986). *Therapeutic metaphors for children and the child within.* New York: Bruner/Mazel.

Mongan, M. (1998). Hypnobirthing: A celebration of life. River Tree Publishing, N.H.

Montgomery, G. H., DuHamel, K. N., & Redd, W. H. (2000). A meta-analysis of hypnotically induced analgesia: How effective is hypnosis? *International Journal of Clinical and Experimental Hypnosis, 48*(2), 138–153.

Munafo, M. R. (1998). Pain management psychotherapy: A practical guide. (book review). *Psychology, Health and Medicine, 3*(4), 443.

Muraoka, M., Komiyama, H., Hosoi, M., Mine, K., & Kubo, C. (1996). Psychosomatic treatment of phantom limb pain with post traumatic stress disorder: A case report. *Pain, 66*(2–3), 385–388.

NIH Technology Assessment Panel on Integration of Behavioral and Relaxation Approaches into the Treatment of Chronic Pain and Insomnia. (1996). Integration of behavioral and relaxation approaches into the treatment of chronic pain and insomnia. *Journal of the American Medical Association, 276*(4), 313–318.

NIH Technology Assessment Panel on Integration of Behavioral and Relaxation Approaches into the Treatment of Chronic Pain and Insomnia. (1996). Integration of behavioral and relaxation approaches into the treatment of chronic pain and insomnia. *Journal American Medical Association, 276*(4), 313–318.

Oakley, D. A., & Halligan, P. W. (2002). Hypnotic mirrors and phantom pain. A single case study. *Contemporary Hypnosis, 19*(2), 75–84.

Ohrbach, R., Patterson, D. R., Carroughen, G., & Gibram, N. (1998). Hypnosis after an adverse response to opioids in an ICU burn patient. *Clinical Journal of Pain, 14*(2), 167–175.

Olness, K., & Kohen, D. P. (1996). *Hypnosis and hypnotherapy with children.* (3rd ed.). New York: Guilford Press.

Paige, G. G., & Ben-Eliyahu, S. (1997). The immune-suppressive nature of pain. *Seminars in Oncology Nursing, 13*(1), 10–15.

Palsson, O. S., Turner, M. I., Johnson, D. A., Burnett, C. K., & Whitehead, W. E. (2002). Hypnosis treatment for severe irritable bowel syndrome: Investigation of mechanism and effect on symptoms. *Digestive Diseases and Sciences, 47*(11), 2605–2614.

Patterson, D. R., & Ptacek, J. T. (1997). Baseline pain as a moderator of headache hypnotic analgesia for burn injury treatment. *Journal of Consulting and Clinical Psychology, 65*(1), 60–67.

Patterson, D. R., Adcock, R. J., & Bobardier, C. H. (1997). Factors predicting hypnotic analgesia in clinical burn pain. *International Journal of Clinical and Experimental Hypnosis, 45*(4), 377–395.

Patterson, D. R., & Jensen, M. P. (2003). Hypnosis and clinical pain. *Psychological Bulletin, 129*(4), 495–521.

Peebles-Klieger, M. J. (2000). The use of hypnosis in emergency medicine. *Emergency Medicine Clinics of North America, 18*(2), 327–338.

Perry, C., Gelfand, R., & Marcovitch, P. (1979). The relevance of hypnotic susceptibility in the clinical context. *Journal of Abnormal Psychology, 88*, 592–603.

Ploghaus, A., Becerra, L., Borros, C., & Borsook, D. (2003). Neural circuitry underlying pain modulation, expectation hypnosis, placebo. *Trends in Cognitive Science, 7*(5) 197–200.

Rainville, P., Duncan, G. H., Price, D. D., Carrier, B., & Bushnell, M. C. (1997). Pain affect encoded in human anterior cingulate but not somatosensory cortex. *Science, 277*(5328), 968–971.

Rainville, P., Hofbauer, R. K., Paus, T., Duncan, G. H., Bushnell, M. C., & Price, D. D. (1999a). Cerebral mechanisms of hypnotic inductions and suggestions. *Journal of Cognitive Neuroscience, 11*(1), 110–125.

Rainville, P., Carrier, B., Hobauer, R. K., Bushnell, M. C., & Duncan, G. H. (1999b). Dissociation of sensory and affective dimensions of pain using hypnotic modulation. *Pain, 82*(2), 159–171.

Ray, P., & Page, A. C. (2002). A single session of hypnosis and eye movement desensitization and reprocessing (EMDR) in the treatment of chronic pain. *Australian Journal of Clinical and Experimental Hypnosis, 30*(2), 170–178.

Raz, A., & Shapiro, T., (2002) Hypnosis and neuroscience: A cross talk between clinical and cognitive research. *Archives of General Psychiatry, 59*(1), 85–97.

Rogerson, D. (2002) The use of hypnosis in surgery and anesthesiology: Psychological preparation of the surgical patient. (Book Review). *Contemporary Hypnosis, 19*(1), 44..

Rossi, E. L. (1993). *The psychology of minds – Body healing. New concepts of therapeutic hypnosis.* New York: W.W. Norton and Co.

Rowe, P. M. (1995). Better ways of treating chronic pain and insomnia. *Lancet, 346*(8984), 1220.

Rusy, L. M. & Weisman, S. J. (2000). Complementary therapies for acute pediatric pain management. *Pediatric Clinics of North America, 47*(3), 589–599.

Sacerdote, P. (1966). The uses of hypnosis in cancer patients. *Annals of the New York Academy of Science, 125,* 1011–1019.

Sandrini, G., Mianov, I., Malaguti, S., Nigrelli, M. P., Moglia, A., & Nappi, G. (2000). Effects of hypnosis on diffuse noxious inhibitory controls. *Physiological Behavior, 69*(3), 295–300.

Sarno, J. E. (1998). *The mind–body prescription: Healing the body, Healing the pain.* New York: Warner Books.

Schafer, D. W. (1996). *Relieving pain: A basic hypnotherapeutic approach.* Northvale, NJ: Jason Aronson Inc.

Sellick, S. M., & Zaza, C. (1998). Critical review of five non-pharmacologic strategies for managing cancer pain. *Cancer Prevention and Control, 2*(1), 7–14.

Shea, J. D. (2003). Hypnosis with cancer patients. *Australian Journal of Clinical Hypnotherapy and Hypnosis, 24*(2), 98–111.

Shenefelt, P. D., (2003). Hypnosis – Facilitated relaxation using self-guided imagery during dermatologic procedures. *American Journal of Clinical Hypnosis, 45*(3), 225–233.

Shor, R. E., & Orne, E.C. (1963). Norms on the Harvard group scale of hypnotic susceptibility, Form A. *International Journal of Clinical Hypnosis, 11,* 47–49.

Siegel, B. (1998). *Love medicine and miracles.* New York: Harper & Row.

Simon, E. P., & James, L. C. (1999). Clinical applications of hypnotherapy in a medical setting. *Hawaii Medical Journal, 58*(12), 344–347.

Simon, E. P., & Lewis, D. M. (2000). Medical hypnosis for temporomandibular disorders: Treatment efficacy and medical utilization outcome. *Oral Surgery, Oral Medicine, Oral Pathology, Oral Radiology, and Endodontics, 90*(1), 54–63.

Smith, J., & Barabasz, A. (1996). Comparison of hypnosis and distraction in severely ill children. *Journal of Counseling Psychology, 43*(2), 187–193.

Spiegel, D., & Moore, R. (1997). Imagery and hypnosis in the treatment of cancer patients. *Oncology* (Huntington), *11*(8), 1179–1189, 1189–1195.

Spiegel, H., & Spiegel, D. (1987). *Trance and treatment: Clinical uses of hypnosis.* Washington, D.C.: American Psychiatric Press, Inc.

Staats, P., Hekmat, H., & Staats, A. (1998). Suggestion/placebo effects on pain: Negative as well as positive. *Journal of Pain and Symptom Management, 15*(4), 235–243.

Sternbach, R. A. (1978). Clinical aspects of pain. In R. A. Steinbach (Ed.), *The psychology of pain.* New York: Raven Press.

Stevensen, C. (1995). Non-pharmacological aspects of acute pain management. *Complementary Therapy in Nursing and Midwifery, 1*(3), 77–84.

Sthalekar, H. (1993). Hypnosis for relief of chronic phantom pain in a paralyzed limb. *The Australian Journal of Clinical Hypnotherapy and Hypnosis, 14*(2), 75–80.

Strassberg, D. S., Tilley, D., Bristone, S., & Oei, T. P. S. (1992). The MMPI and chronic pain: A cross-cultural view. *Psychiatric Assessment, 4*(4), 493–497.

Sutcher, H. (1997). Hypnosis as adjunctive therapy for multiple sclerosis: A progress report. *American Journal of Clinical Hypnosis, 39*(4), 283–290.

Turk, D.C., & Holzman, A.D. (1986). Chronic pain: Interfaces among physical, psychological and social parameters. In A. D. Holzman & D. C. Turk (Eds.), *Pain management. A handbook of psychological approaches* (pp. 59). New York: Pergamon.

Turk, D. C., & Kerns, R. D. (1986). Chronic pain. In K. A. Holroyd & T. L. Creer (Eds.), *Self-management of chronic disease: Handbook of Clinical interventions and research* (pp. 441–472). Orlando, Fl: Academic Press.

Vidavic-Vukic, M. (1999). Hypnotherapy in the treatment of irritable bowel syndrome: Methods and results in Amsterdam. *Scandinavian Journal of Gastroenterology Supplement, 203,* 49–51.

Walker, L. G., Heys, S. D., Walker, M. B., Ogston, K., Miller, I. D., Hucheon, A. W. et al. (1999). Psychological factors can predict response to primary chemotherapy in patients with locally advanced breast cancer. *European Journal of Cancer, 35,* 1783–1788.

Wagstaff, G. F. (2000). On the physiological redefinition of hyponisis: A reply to Gruzlier. *Contemporary Hypnosis, 17*(4), 154–161.

Watkins, J. G. (1971). The affect bridge: A hypnoanalytic technique. *International Journal of Clinical and Experimental Hypnosis, 19,* 21–27.

Weitzenhoffer, M. M., & Hilgard, E. R. (1959). *Stanford hypnotic susceptibility scale: Forms A and B.* Palo Alto, CA: Consulting Psychologist Press.

Wester, W. C., & O'Grady, D. J. (1991). *Clinical hypnosis with children.* New York: Brunner/Mazel.

Wester, W. C., & O'Grady, D. J. (1991). *Clinical hypnosis with children.* New York: Brunner/Mazel.

Whalley, M. G., & Oakley, D. A. (2003). Psychogenic pain: A study using multi-dimensional scaling. *Contemporary Hypnosis, 20*(1), 16–24.

Whorwell, P. J., Houghton, L. A., Taylor, E. E., & Maxton, D. G. (1992). Physiological effects of emotion assessment via hypnosis. *Lancet, 340*(8811), 69–72.

Whorwell, P. J., Prior, A., & Favaghor, E. B. (1984). Controlled trial of hypnotherapy in the treatment of severe refractory bowel syndrome. *Lancet, 2,* 1232–1234.

Williamson, A. (2002). Chronic psychosomatic pain alleviated by brief therapy. *Contemporary Hypnosis, 19*(3), 118–124.

Wong, D. L., & Baker, C. M. (1988). Pain in children: Comparison of assessment scales. *Pediatric Nursing, 14,* 9–17.

Wright, B. R., & Drummond, P. D. (2000). Rapid induction analgesia for the alleviation of procedural pain during burn care. *Burns, 26*(3), 275–282.

Zachariae, R., Andersen, O. K., Bjerring, P., Jorgensen, M. M., & Arendt-Nielsen, L. (1998). Effects of opioid antagonist on pain intensity and withdrawal reflexes during induction of hypnotic analgesia in high and low hypnotizable volunteers. *European Journal of Pain*, *2*(1), 25–34.

Zaza, C., Sellick, S. M., Willan, A., Reyno, L., & Browman, G. P. (1999). Health care professionals' familiarity with non-pharmacological strategies for managing cancer pain. *Psychooncology*, *8*(2), 99–111.

Zeltzer, L. K., Tsao, J. C., Stelling, C., Powers, M., Levy, S., & Waterhouse, M. (2002). A phase I study on the feasibility and acceptability of an acupuncture/hypnosis intervention for chronic pain. *Journal of Pain Symptom Management, 24*(4), 437–446.

Zimmerman, J. (2003). Cleaning up the river: A metaphor for functional digestive disorders. *American Journal of Clinical Hypnosis, 45*(4), 353–359.

Zohourek, R. (1985). *Clinical hypnosis and therapeutic suggestion in nursing.* New York: Grune & Stratten.

52

Clinical Applications of Interactive Guided Imagery℠ for Diagnosing and Treating Chronic Pain

David E. Bresler, PhD, LAc

INTRODUCTION

Chronic pain has become the Western world's most expensive, disabling, and common disorder. An estimated 45 million Americans suffer from some form of chronic headache, which costs the U.S. economy $50 billion directly and indirectly (National Headache Foundation, 2003). Arthritis afflicts nearly 50 million Americans and accounts for 36 million outpatient visits and 750,000 hospitalizations annually (Centers for Disease Control, 2004).

Back pain generates nearly 12.5 million office visits per year and has disabled 7 million Americans (Cherry & Woodwell, 2002). Add facial and dental pain, neuralgia, cancer pain, chronic neck and shoulder pain, fibromyalgia, and other common pain syndromes, and it's easy to understand why pain is estimated to cost the nation's economy $100 billion per year (American Pain Society, 2000; Marcus, 1996). The cost in human suffering is incalculable.

The focus of this chapter is on the uses of a particular form of mental imagery, called Interactive Guided Imagery℠, to diagnose and treat chronic pain, increase pain tolerance, and reduce amplification and the emotional toll of pain, and its ability, in short, to alleviate suffering.

Of all the modalities and techniques studied and developed during the past 30 years of treating patients with chronic pain and other chronic illnesses, I have found Interactive Guided Imagery℠ to be highly effective in increasing compliance, relieving symptoms, enhancing tolerance, reducing feelings of hopelessness and help-lessness, promoting healing, and increasing functional abilities in our patients, while carrying few, if any, significant risks.

WHAT IS INTERACTIVE GUIDED IMAGERY℠?

Mental images, formed long before we learn to understand and use words, lie at the core of who we think we are, what we believe we can do, what we think the world is like, what we feel we deserve, and even how motivated we are to take care of ourselves. They also strongly influence our beliefs and attitudes about how and why we fall ill, what will help us get better, and whether any medical and/or psychological interventions will be effective.

Images also have profound physiological consequences that powerfully influence the healing systems of the body, including the immune, endocrine, and nervous systems. Images can affect the cardiovascular, respiratory, and gastrointestinal systems, and probably all other bodily systems, as well. For example, does not a vivid scary (or erotic) thought cause powerful changes to occur in many of these systems?

Positive images can stimulate and support the healing systems of the body, and the remarkable healings that have been documented following religious or faith-based healing ceremonies, while often difficult to explain, may be related to the positive healing images that they evoke. Scientists have coined a term that they use to describe the impact of positive expectant faith on health and healing — it is called the "placebo effect."

Research on the omnipresent placebo effect, the standard to which we compare all other modalities and interventions (and find relatively few more powerful), has provided some of the strongest evidence for the power of the imagination and positive expectant faith in healing. It is well documented that from 30 to 55% of all patients given inactive placebos respond as well or better than those given active treatments or agents (Frank, 1974).

Although we do not completely understand the mechanisms involved, *it is clear that people can derive not only symptomatic relief, but actual physiologic healing in response to treatments that work primarily through beliefs and attitudes about an imagined reality.*

Thus, learning how to better mobilize and amplify this "mind/body" phenomenon in a purposeful, conscious way is an important, if not critical, area of investigation for modern medicine and psychology. Marty Rossman, cofounder of the Academy for Guided Imagery, often remarks that there should be a new discipline in medicine called "placebology" to train health care professionals how to mobilize and enhance the placebo effect in the service of healing.

In addition to its potential for stimulating and accelerating physical healing, imagery provides a powerful window of insight into unconscious processes, rapidly and graphically revealing underlying unconscious psychological dynamics that may support either health or illness. To the trained imagery clinician, this "window" is an invaluable tool for quickly identifying unique opportunities for positive change, subtle manifestations of resistance to change, and ways to work effectively with both.

Guided imagery is a term used to describe a wide range of techniques from simple visualization and direct imagery-based suggestion, through metaphor and storytelling, to unscripted free association and fantasizing. Guided imagery is most commonly used to help teach psychophysiologic relaxation, to relieve symptoms, to stimulate healing responses in the body, and to enhance tolerance to procedures and treatments.

Most people do imagery all the time, primarily by worrying, for what we worry about usually is not going on anywhere except in our imagination. We regret the past, recalling moments when we should have acted differently, and then we drag them into our imagination in the present time to be "ruminated," analyzed, reviewed, re-scripted, and/or grieved.

Alternatively, we fear the future as we think about all the possible negative things that could happen, but all those things are happening only in our imagination. In a sense, we poison the present by attending to (and growing) our past worries and future fears. Remember, all images can have profound physiological consequences. It has

been said, "Yesterday is history. Tomorrow is a mystery. Today is a gift. That's why it's called the present."

Fortunately, more and more people are realizing that they can use this same mind/body connection to facilitate healing and to self-treat a variety of chronic pain problems, including back pain, headaches, arthralgia, neuralgia, myalgia, and even secondary pain-related problems, such as anxiety, depression, insomnia, and relationship issues.

According to a nationwide survey by the National Center for Complementary and Alternative Medicine (NCCAM), up to 25% of Americans use mind/body techniques for health (including deep breathing, relaxation, meditation, hypnosis, and guided imagery). If you add prayer, it is up to 68% (Centers for Disease Control and Prevention, 2002).

Interactive Guided Imagery[sm] (IGI) is a service-marked term used by the Academy for Guided Imagery to represent its highly interactive, nonjudgmental, content-free style of guiding imagery, which is particularly effective for enhancing patient self-management and self-care, and for evoking greater patient autonomy.

This autonomy is often critical to achieving long-term success, for people living with chronic pain can become highly dependent on health care providers, family members, and others. Unfortunately, this can reinforce the sense of helplessness, hopelessness, and worthlessness (i.e., depression), which is already problematic.

Rather than processing patients through a standardized program or protocol that may or may not be appropriate to meet their unique needs, IGI helps people in pain to draw upon their own inner resources to explore the meaning of their pain symptoms, to relieve symptoms and support healing, to choose the most appropriate interventions, to identify and deal with their resistance to change and issues that sabotage compliance, and to find creative solutions to challenges that they previously thought were insoluble.

IGI is particularly useful in our current health care climate, where briefer yet more effective, efficient, and empowering mind/body approaches to health care are becoming highly valued by patients, providers, and insurers alike. Before explaining the principles and practices of IGI, let us briefly examine some of the unique aspects of chronic pain that illuminate the unique value of using mind/body approaches such as IGI to achieve long-term success.

CHRONIC PAIN DEMANDS TREATMENT DIFFERENT FROM ACUTE PAIN

Modern technology has created a huge variety of pharmaceutical products and interventional techniques for acute or self-limiting pain. These agents are usually highly effective and patients who undergo operative or other acute invasive procedures are generally spared all but the slightest degree of pre- or postsurgical discomfort. Likewise, for patients with acute sprains, strains, menstrual cramps, or headaches, a variety of effective medications are available over the counter.

Yet, the approaches that have proved to be so successful in the management of acute pain are often ineffective or even counterintentional for controlling *chronic* or long-term pain. Although acute pain usually gets better by itself, and pain medications can provide greater comfort as the body heals, *chronic pain typically becomes worse with time*. Its victims are referred endlessly from doctor to doctor, for even if temporary relief can be obtained, the pain inevitably returns for most people with chronic pain diagnoses.

For example, when opiate-based analgesic medications are used over a prolonged period of time, pharmacologic tolerance can develop and effectiveness becomes progressively reduced. As tolerance develops, patients often increase their dosages with the idea that "if a little is good, a lot will be even better." Unfortunately, higher dosages only produce greater side effects, and tolerance continues to develop. In addition, many of the most effective analgesic agents also carry a high risk of dependency.

As a result, it is common to find patients with chronic pain taking large amounts of medications that they say are not really helping to ease their pain. These medications may also be producing significant side effects, some of which could be contributing to the pain experience. When patients or their doctors attempt to reduce these medications, withdrawal symptoms can make pain even less tolerable, and the patients return in desperation to their former regimens, feeling as though they have been total failures and are doomed to be hopeless victims of pain and suffering.

When medications or other medical interventions fail, patients are often told, "Nothing more can be done. You'll have to learn to live with it." This statement has two iatrogenic implications. First, it destroys one of the most significant healing assets that chronic pain (or other chronic illness) sufferers possess — namely, hope or positive expectant faith. Second, it conveys the subtle message that if you "have to learn to live with it," the only time you *won't* have it is when you are no longer alive. This may add to the significant suicidal ideation experienced by many people already severely depressed from being in chronic pain.

The way we communicate with patients in pain and the images that our communications evoke can have an important, if not critical, influence on the outcome of any interventions we recommend or provide. As I discuss below, negative communications may actually retard the body's intrinsic healing abilities, while more positive, imagery-based suggestions may enable patients to unlock the door to the most potent and varied pharmacy yet discovered — the one in our own brain.

WHAT IS PAIN?

As I have discussed in detail elsewhere (Bresler & Trubo, 2002), one of the greatest challenges in researching and treating chronic pain is to resolve the inherent ambiguity in the terms and concepts we use to describe it. For example, I find it helpful to distinguish between a painful *sensation* (mental awareness of an unpleasant physical stimulus) and the pain *experience* (the total subjective, cognitive, and emotional experience of pain). Furthermore, it is important to recognize that *there is not necessarily any direct relationship between the sensation and experience of pain*.

This is seen in several studies that reported that soldiers seriously wounded in battle complained of only mild discomfort compared with civilians with similar injuries, for they were elated to learn that the war was over for them and that they were to be sent home. In contrast, patients with phantom limb pain often report agonizing discomfort even though the entire stump has been anesthetized.

In our language, we often talk about pain as if it were a tangible, *invasive thing*, much like a splinter is an *invasive thing* — that is, an object or substance from outside that infiltrates or penetrates the body. Thus, if you accidentally strike your thumb with a hammer, you might say you that you "feel pain in the thumb which is radiating to your hand."

Such a notion is very inaccurate, for there is no pain "in" your thumb, any more than there is pleasure "in" your mouth when you eat something that tastes good. You probably would not say, "Umm. My mouth is full of pleasure which is radiating to my stomach."

When you injure your thumb, you stimulate local neural receptors that send a barrage of electrochemical messages up through the nerves in your hand and arm to your spinal cord and brain. *Whether or not we become aware of a potentially painful stimulus depends upon the way the stimulus information is interpreted by the nervous system.*

If the nervous system decides that the messages from the thumb are urgent and require immediate action, it creates an experience of pain that is identified with the thumb so that you will give it proper attention. If it decides that the messages are unimportant, the messages may be ignored altogether until they become important (e.g., when your thumb swells).

For example, as you read this, your shoes may be stimulating neural receptors in your toes and feet, and if so, these are generating electrical and neurochemical messages that ascend the neuraxis to your brain. There, probably in the thalamic nuclei, your brain interprets those messages as being unimportant, and thus, information about your shoes is usually not communicated to higher centers. You may have had no awareness whatsoever that your shoes were pressing against your toes and feet unless your attention was called to them, as I just did.

The same is true if you are wearing a watch, jewelry, or any tight clothing. If your brain can choose to ignore unimportant information generated from neural receptors in your feet, can it not choose to ignore information from a neuralgia or pain-related injury if it interprets that information as being no longer important? What if your brain could interpret a painful stimulus as being pleasurable? For example, if you have ever scratched an itch hard, you know that it is often difficult to determine if it hurts or really feels good. All of this reminds us that the main pain receptor is between our ears, and that is where pain usually resides.

Like many *perceptions*, pain is well known to be influenced by learning and early developmental predispositions. For example, animals raised in a pain-free environment showed insensitivity to noxious stimuli in later life. Social, cultural, and ethnic differences in the experience of pain also are well documented. Vivid examples are the horrific initiation rituals of many primitive tribes. These would be considered nothing short of torture if practiced by members of Western cultures.

Aristotle was the first to suggest "pain is an *emotion*," as pervasive as anger, terror, or joy. The emotional component of pain is inexorably bound to other aspects of the pain experience, for anxiety and agitation are the natural consequence of a painful sensation that tells higher cognitive centers "something is wrong." If the "something" can be clearly identified and appropriate corrective action can be taken, the (acute) pain experience is usually terminated as the body heals.

However, for most patients with chronic pain, the "something" is vague, unknown, or untreatable, and fear of continued pain for an indefinite future produces even greater stress and anxiety. On a physiologic level, this anxiety causes sympathetic hyperactivity, as manifested by increased heart rate, blood pressure, respiration, palmar sweating, and muscle tension.

In patients with musculoskeletal pain, this increased muscle tension often augments the sensation of pain, which further increases stress and anxiety, which, in turn, produces even greater muscular tension and more pain. The amplifying relationship among stress and anxiety, muscle tension, and pain is well known to clinicians, for treatment of one frequently provides relief of the others as well. This relationship is also one of the reasons that chronic pain symptoms can be temporarily alleviated by providing stress management training or antianxiety agents, physical therapy or muscle relaxants, or pain medications.

However, over time, exhaustion of sympathetic hyperactivity is inevitable, and more vegetative signs and symptoms soon emerge, such as feelings of helplessness, hopelessness, worthlessness, and despair, sleep and appetite disturbances, irritability, decreased interests, low libido, erosion of personal relationships with family and friends, as well as increased somatization of complaints.

Thus, acute pain and anxiety become chronic pain and depression.

It is well known that the most notable emotional change in patients with chronic pain is the development of depression, the "crash" that occurs after a long period of unrelenting stress. This depression may be overt or masked to both patient and health practitioner alike. In a sense, depression can be thought of as "emotional pain," and when its symptoms are effectively treated, the chronic pain experience is often relieved, as well. This is why antidepressant agents can be helpful in the management of chronic pain.

It is important to emphasize the psychophysiological basis of chronic pain, for it is a complex subjective experience that involves physical, perceptual, cognitive, emotional, and spiritual factors. When a patient with low back pain complains that "my back hurts," his or her pain experience also may involve anxiety or depression (producing insomnia, loss of appetite, and decreased sexual desire); drug dependence or addiction; separation from work, family and friends; loss of avocational interests and hobbies; numerous secondary gains; and a host of other problems. These may remain indelibly associated with the experience of back pain, even after the entire spine has been chemically anesthetized.

Thus, it is easy to see why no simple pill or shot is the cure-all for chronic pain. The most common error made by clinicians is to primarily evaluate and treat the physical symptoms associated with the problem, for they assume that the objective of therapy is to *treat pain in people*.

To me, however, the objective of therapy is to treat *people in pain*, which takes a much broader perspective. From this point of view, it is unnecessary to wonder if a patient has "real" versus "unreal" pain, "organic" versus "psychologic" pain, or "legitimate" versus "hysterical" pain. Pain is an intensely subjective and personal experience, and even if no physical explanation for it can be found, *all pain is real*. According to the scientific method, the absence of data does not disprove a hypothesis, and simply because we cannot find the source of pain does not mean that it is not real.

PAIN VERSUS SUFFERING

In our Western culture, pain is usually considered an enemy to be fought and overcome, and as a result, our first approach is usually to search for a "pain killer." This overlooks and ignores the survival value of pain, which can be a warning signal, a protector, a potential teacher, a guide, a motivator, or even an incentive for change.

While some believe that chronic pain is a symptom that has lost its meaning and become "an illness in itself," I believe that this is the result of our health care system's tendency to medicalize and externalize symptoms rather than to examine their meaning in a more holistic context, as discussed below.

Whatever the cause, if an individual cannot tolerate or cope effectively with pain, he or she *suffers*, which is manifested as an inability to sleep, eat, work, function, or fully enjoy life. Life, in the most personal, meaningful sense, stops. As we discuss below, I believe that suffering is primarily an epiphenomenon of one's attitude and beliefs, and that it is *possible to have pain, and yet not suffer,* depending on how we relate to the pain we experience.

In the more traditional psychological literature, a distinction is often made between pain sensitivity and pain tolerance. To illustrate the clinical importance of pain tolerance, when teaching fellows and residents at UCLA, I found it helpful to compare x-ray films of two patients, both of who complained of knee pain.

The first patient was a professional football player who had undergone six prior knee surgeries. While reviewing his films, I wondered how this individual could walk, much less continue to play football. However, he reported only minor pain or discomfort, took no pain medications (because they made him "feel less ferocious"), and only desired treatment that would increase the strength, stability, and range of motion in his knees.

The second patient was injured on-the-job and had filed extensive workers' compensation litigation. Although his knee x-rays appeared to be completely normal, he suffered greatly and was unable to climb stairs, drive a car, or sleep for more than 2 to 3 hours at a time. He was totally disabled, despondent and depressed, and completely dependent on his family, four medical doctors, and seven different pain medications.

The first patient had significant pathology but high tolerance and barely complained of pain. The second had minimal, if any, pathology, but little tolerance to the pain he experienced and lots of suffering.

In the clinical situation, we often confront limitations in our ability to reverse severe physical pathology (e.g., degeneration of cartilage in a joint). However, our ability to help patients reduce their suffering by enhancing their tolerance of pain appears to have no upper limit. Thus, practitioners who help patients embrace a more positive belief or attitude about pain can often successfully help reduce their suffering and enhance tolerance, even when "nothing more (medically) can be done."

There is evidence that positive imagery and the placebo effect can stimulate the production of endorphins, naturally occurring pain-relieving substances in the central nervous system. I have long believed that endorphins have nothing to do with pain, and everything to do with suffering. For example, when a patient is given an injection of morphine (which mimics the effects of endorphins), he or she will often state that "it still hurts, but it doesn't bother me." This represents enhanced pain tolerance, not a reduced pain sensation, which is why morphine is considered to be an analgesic (that enhances pain tolerance), not an anesthetic (that blocks all sensation)

The extent to which a patient's suffering can be reduced through psychophysiological approaches such as IGI depends on many complex variables including the patient's belief systems and attitudes, early life experiences, the degree of physical pathology, and perhaps most importantly, the *meaning* of pain in the context of the patient's life.

THE MEANING OF PAIN

Since the dawn of creation, pain has provided critically important information concerning our relationship to our inner and outer environments. Pain strongly conveys the message that "something is wrong," and it encourages the body to take action to prevent further injury. From an evolutionary point of view, it is one of the most powerful ways to ensure the survival of an organism in a dangerous world.

While most authorities acknowledge these positive aspects of acute pain, many believe that chronic pain is a "biological mistake" or "obsolete symptom" that serves "no useful purpose." To correct this "mistake," they recommend strong medications or surgical interventions in an attempt to obliterate the sensation of pain.

It is interesting to note that the exact technique utilized will depend more on the type of specialist consulted than on the patient's unique needs. For example, an internist may prescribe medication; an orthopedist, physical therapy or surgery; a psychologist, family psychotherapy; an acupuncturist, needles or herbs; a chiropractor, manipulation; and so forth. Abraham Maslow used to say, "When you are holding a hammer, you tend to look for nails."

In my opinion, the best long-term interests of the patient usually are not well served when the major goal of therapy is to mask or suppress the symptoms of pain without first attempting to understand its underlying meaning. To do so is like responding to a ringing fire alarm by cutting its wires to stop the annoying clamor, rather than by leaving the burning building.

I invite patients to consider the notion that like the oil light in a car, their nervous system may be generating the experience of chronic pain *for a reason.* I invite them to explore the possibility that their chronic pain is not a disease or "mistake" but a symptom generated through the wisdom of the body.

I then teach them about the extraordinary healing, regeneration, repair, and regulatory systems that are at work in their body, and remind them that *symptoms are the way that the body tries to heal itself or prevent further injury.* Like the oil light and the fire alarm, once the message is heard and appropriate action is taken, symptoms usually will decrease and ultimately disappear, for they are no longer needed or important.

Western medical practitioners consider a fever to be a pathologic symptom that is best treated by prescribing antipyretic medications that will reduce it. Oriental practitioners do not treat a fever at all, unless it becomes so high as to be imminently dangerous. They consider a fever to be a healthy symptom that represents the body's attempt to raise its core temperature to destroy an invading microorganism.

Unfortunately, much of contemporary Western medicine is focused on reducing or suppressing symptoms. For example, if a patient has high blood pressure, antihypertensives are prescribed to reduce it. If a patient is unable to sleep, medications are given for sedation at night. If a patient has excessive anxiety, antianxiety agents are often utilized. However, should not a health care practitioner first determine *why* that particular patient has hypertension, sleep disorders, or anxiety neurosis? What is the message that these symptoms are trying to convey? Exploring the meaning of symptoms in a nonjudgmental way can be the key to finding answers to many intractable health challenges, including chronic pain.

Pain is a message that alerts us to danger. Through the primitive, survival-oriented wisdom of the nervous system, it motivates us to correct the situation by changing and adapting to the shifting demands of the world in which we live. Through pain, we are warned about *all* of the dangers we face, and if we continue to ignore them, our nervous system will often increase the intensity of pain in an attempt to get our attention and/or to elicit some change.

Perhaps this is why many patients with chronic pain receive only temporary relief after symptomatic treatment. Although symptoms can be suppressed for a short period by drugs or surgical interventions, if their meaning remains unacknowledged and the nervous system believes that something important is still not being attended to, it will cause pain to increase, break through, and continue to return until the message is heard and appropriate corrective action is taken.

PRINCIPLES OF INTERACTIVE GUIDED IMAGERYᔆᴹ

GIVE ATTENTION TO WHAT YOU WANT TO GROW

Although no one really knows what "consciousness" is, I believe that it is critically related to the process of *attention*, for we only experience what we personally attend to. There is an old saying "whatever you give your attention to grows," whether it be your garden, your children, your worries and fears, or your pain.

Over the years, most of us learn to give our attention to the conscious, verbal part of our mind that narrates a linear, logical, rational, analytic monologue describing its perspective of the world, and how we *think* about it. It is the "little voice inside your head" that talks all the time,

the "person" who most of us think we are. Because we have given it so much attention and reinforcement (e.g., reading, writing, and arithmetic are highly rewarded in our culture), it is a very strong presence in our lives.

However, who we really are is much more than simply what we "think." We are also the richness of our intuitions, emotions, feelings, memories, drives, fantasies, goals, appetites, aspirations, expectations, ambitions, values, passions, beliefs, perceptions, and sensations. Any or all of these aspects of self may require and even demand attention, finding ways to compete by intruding on everyday consciousness through physical, cognitive, emotional, or even behavioral symptoms, if need be.

Rather than suffer the results from neglecting these parts of ourselves, we can focus attention on them in a relaxed state of mind and invite images that seek attention to "come to mind." By properly dialoguing interactively with these images, we can reconnect with important and powerful inner resources that are deeply dedicated to protecting us, healing us, and improving the quality of our lives.

IMAGERY IS THE PRIMARY ENCODING LANGUAGE OF THE BODY'S HEALING SYSTEMS

Imagery can be thought of as one of the brain's higher-order information processing and encoding systems or "languages." The language we are most familiar with is the verbal one spoken by the "little voice in our head." It uses *sequential information processing* that provides a linear, analytic, and conscious verbal perspective of the world. It makes linear associations and connections, and most health professionals are highly educated and rewarded for their abilities in using this mode of information processing, e.g., associating specific symptoms with specific illnesses.

Images, on the other hand, are the language of the emotions, which use *simultaneous information processing*. This provides an instantaneous, holistic, synthetic perspective that includes vital input and information from the unconscious mind. As is said, "a picture is worth a thousand words," and imagery can reveal to us how seemingly disparate areas of our lives are intimately related. A brief clinical example can help to bring the importance of this relational quality to life.

> A 52-year-old cardiologist named John was suffering from excruciating low back pain following treatment for rectal cancer. Although surgery and radiation therapy apparently had eradicated the cancer, he described the pain that remained as unbearable. Because the area had been so heavily irradiated, neither repeated nerve blocks nor further surgery could be used to help relieve his terrible discomfort, and he had long ago developed tolerance to his pain medications.

When John first came in, he already had narrowed down his personal alternatives to three: (1) successful treatment, (2) voluntary commitment to a mental institution, or (3) suicide. John was convinced that under no circumstances could he continue to live with pain and, at the same time, maintain his sanity.

In reviewing his medical records, I noticed that during a psychiatric workup, John had described his pain as "a dog chewing on my spine." This image was so vivid that I suggested we make contact with the dog, using guided imagery. With his training in traditional medicine, he thought the idea was silly, but he was willing to give it a try.

In John's case, our initial goal was to encourage the dog to stop chewing on his spine. Over the next few sessions, the dog began to reveal critically important information. According to the dog (named Skippy), John never had wanted to be a physician — his own career choice was architecture — but he had been pressured into medical school by his mother. Consequently, he felt resentment not only toward his mother, but also toward his patients and colleagues. Skippy suggested that this hostility had in turn contributed to the development of his cancer and to the subsequent pain problem as well.

During one session, Skippy told John, "You're a damn good doctor. It may not be the career you wanted, but it is time you recognized how good you are at what you do. When you stop being so resentful and start accepting yourself, I'll stop chewing on your spine." These insights were accompanied by an immediate alleviation of the pain, and in only a few weeks' time, John became a new person, and his pain progressively subsided.

This type of experience demonstrates how powerfully the imagery process can reveal meaning in a supposedly "meaningless" symptom, and illuminate the path to healing. While IGI does not always lead so dramatically to relief, it usually leads to better self-understanding and enhanced coping skills for dealing with a chronic illness or condition.

IMAGERY HAS POWERFUL PHYSIOLOGICAL CONSEQUENCES

As mentioned previously, numerous research studies have shown that imagery can affect almost all major physiologic control systems of the body, including respiration, heart rate, blood pressure, metabolic rates in cells, gastrointestinal mobility and secretion, sexual function, and even immune responsiveness (Sheikh & Kunzendorf, 1984).

Imagery is essentially a way of thinking that uses sensory attributes, and in the absence of competing sensory cues, the body tends to respond to imagery as it would to a genuine external experience. For example, take a moment to imagine that you have a big, fresh, juicy, yellow lemon in your hand. Experience what it might feel like to hold it. Imagine it in your mind's eye until you sense its heaviness and fresh tartness. Now, imagine taking a knife and slicing into the lemon. Carefully cut out a thick, juicy section. Now, if you're willing, imagine taking a deep bite of the lemon slice, feeling how sour the lemon juice tastes, saturating every taste bud of your tongue so fully that your lips pucker, and your tongue begins to curl.

If you are able to imagine this vividly in your mind's eye, the image probably caused some salivation, for the autonomic nervous system easily understands the language of imagery and responds as if it is real. While the image of the lemon may be imaginary, the salivation is real.

Here is the crux of the matter: *If imagining a lemon makes you salivate, what happens if you imagine that you are a hopeless, helpless victim of chronic pain?* Does it not tell your nervous system to give up? Is it not likely to create neural and biochemical signals that indicate you are getting worse rather than actively healing? From another perspective, if you believed you were able to resolve various life problems, improve communications and relationships, and learn how to modulate pain, would this not create a healthier and more functional physiology in the body?

IMAGERY IS THE LANGUAGE OF THE EMOTIONS

Imagery is a powerful tool in the healing arts also because of its close relationship to the emotions. Imagery is the expressive language of the arts — poetry, drama, painting, sculpture, music, and dance — and it reflects various aspects of the emotional self. Emotions reveal what is personally important to us, and they can be either potent motivators that promote healing or barriers to changing dangerous lifestyle habits.

Emotions motivate us to action and they produce characteristic physiologic changes in the body, including varying patterns of muscle tension, blood flow, respiration, metabolism, and neurologically and immunologically reactive peptide secretions. Modern research in psychoneuroimmunology points to the emotions as the key modulators of neuroactive peptides secreted by the brain, gut, and immune systems (Pert & Chopra, 1997).

Our emotions represent communications about basic survival that originate from our primitive, reptilian-like limbic system. There are four primary emotions: sad, mad, glad, and frightened. In short, fear is about *flight*. Frightening feelings let you know that the object you fear may be dangerous or stronger than you, and this motivates you to get away from it so you don't lose something of value (e.g., your possessions, your health, or even your life).

Anger, on the other hand, is about *fight*. It is a message implying that something has been taken from you (e.g., your possessions, safety, pride, self-esteem), and it motivates you to fight to get it back so you do not lose even more.

Grief motivates us to detach and move away. It lets us know that the object of our grief has been lost and that we most likely will not get it back. Joy, on the other hand, is about *attachment*, and it motivates us to move closer to the things that make us feel good.

PATIENT AUTONOMY IS MOST EFFECTIVELY SUPPORTED BY USING A TWO-WAY INTERACTIVE GUIDING STYLE

One key to the extraordinary clinical effectiveness of Interactive Guided Imagery^{sm} is the unique interactive communications component that it incorporates. By working interactively instead of simply reading an imagery script, the Interactive Imagery Guide^{sm} ensures that the experience has personal meaning for the client, and that it proceeds at a pace determined by the client's actual needs and abilities rather than the guide's "best guess estimate."

For example, an Interactive Imagery Guide might ask, "Of all the different problems, symptoms, and challenges now going on in your life, allow an image to form that represents the single most important and critical issue for us to work on now, and then describe it to me." The guide can then facilitate a dialogue between the client and the image to find out what the image wants, needs, and has to offer.

Because the content, direction, and pace of the imagery experience are set by the client, not by the guide, it is the client who actually (unconsciously) guides the process to the resources most needed to support healing, change, and positive therapeutic results.

PATIENT AUTONOMY IS MOST ENCOURAGED BY USING CONTENT-FREE LANGUAGE AND NONJUDGMENTAL GUIDING

Whenever possible, the Interactive Imagery Guide uses nonjudgmental, content-free language that encourages clients to tap their own inner resources to find solutions for solving their own problems. I often like to say, "while the guide provides the setting, it's the client that provides the jewel."

At a time when there is so much concern about "false memory syndrome" (Pope, 1996), this type of content-free guiding also ensures that the client's experience is not unduly contaminated or influenced by the suggestions of the guide.

PATIENT AUTONOMY IS MOST ENCOURAGED BY SPECIFIC QUALITIES AND SKILLS UTILIZED BY THE GUIDE

There are important personal qualities that the well-trained Interactive Imagery Guide brings to the therapeutic experience, including a nonjudgmental attitude, patience, and trust in clients' own abilities to identify healing resources and to find solutions to their problems. The guides provide

vital support as clients explore their inner world and inner issues, and emphasize the notion that clients have within them more healing resources than they had previously imagined. This approach leads to minimal transference, greater client self-confidence, increased opportunities for effective self-care, an enhanced sense of self-efficacy, and the rapid development of greater patient autonomy.

PROVIDER–PATIENT/CLIENT INTERACTIONS

DIAGNOSTIC AND ASSESSMENT PROCEDURES AND TECHNIQUES

The Interactive Imagery Guide must first decide whether there are any contraindications to introducing imagery to the patient, such as a medical or surgical condition requiring emergency treatment, or a mental illness precluding its use. Having decided that imagery may offer some benefit, a history is taken regarding the client's prior experience with imagery, visualization, hypnosis, relaxation, meditation, biofeedback, or related approaches. This allows the guide to utilize prior positive experiences or to address relevant issues in the case of negative experiences.

If the client has no prior experience with relaxation or imagery, the guide usually begins with a brief relaxation technique. The client is invited to imagine being in a beautiful, safe, and peaceful place and, then, to describe what he or she sees, hears, smells, feels, or experiences there. The guide may ask, "What's the weather like there?" or "What time of day is it there?" Such questions encourage the client to more vividly imagery the "Personal Place" in order to answer them.

The guide may suggest that the client choose a personal place with specific qualities that could be uniquely helpful. For example, fearful clients might be encouraged to imagine themselves protected in a "sanctuary," a "powerful place," or a "place where you are completely safe and free from any harm." A client who feels too exhausted to deal with a situation might be encouraged to imagine a place of "great energy and vitality" or "a place of rest, renewal, and nourishment."

Imagining a visit to a quiet, safe personal place is one of the quickest ways to teach people in pain how to relax, and it powerfully illustrates the profound effects a simple imagery experience can have. Occasionally, clients have difficulty imagining such a place or become more anxious as they close their eyes and begin to relax. If their anxiety does not respond to reassurance that they are completely in control, and to gentle encouragement that it might be helpful to see what comes next, this can simply reflect inexperienced clients' insecurity that they won't do it correctly, or it may be a signal that relaxing their vigil may be psychologically dangerous to them.

Such relaxation-induced anxiety can be a marker for early trauma, as is the experience of having an imaginary safe place suddenly turn dangerous or foreboding. When early trauma is identified and found to be producing strong resistance to inner exploration, it is essential that the guide be appropriately trained to handle such situations in order to prevent the occurrence of traumatic insight or regression panic.

Once relaxation is introduced and a personal place is established, clients may be guided in one of several directions, depending upon their unique needs, as determined by the guide. Clients might be invited to turn their attention to specific symptoms, then to allow images to form for them, and then to invite healing imagery to come to mind. The client may be invited to dialogue with an image representing a specific symptom in order to find out why it is there, what it wants, needs, has to offer, and importantly, under what circumstances it is willing to leave.

Clients may also be invited to meet with an imaginary, kind, wise "Inner Advisor" who can provide previously inaccessible information about their issues or illness, as well as loving support and encouragement.

In this relaxed state, clients can invite images to form for almost anything they want to know more about, and by dialoguing with these images, they can expand their awareness of previously unknown connections and identify new options that can promote greater healing.

Typically, clients are initially seen one to three times to explore their history, status, and the potential benefits of working with guided imagery. The guide must consider whether the client will be able to use imagery most effectively as part of an individual counseling or therapy relationship, in a group or class, or as a self-care technique. Self-help books, CDs, and tapes are an inexpensive option for many clients who are capable of using imagery techniques on their own.

In practice, most well-trained guides recommend the imagery methods and techniques that suit a given client's situation and needs the best, considering the unique nature of the issue, the client's innate coping responses and worldview, and the amount of time, energy, and funds the client is willing or able to invest in the process.

In the course of only a few imagery sessions, most clients will have solved their problem, found a successful way to work it out by themselves, identified issues that require additional work, or found that the method or practitioner is not suitable for them or their situation.

DESCRIPTION OF COMMONLY USED TREATMENT TECHNIQUES

The list of techniques used in IGI is quite extensive, and this approach has been applied to problems ranging from severe depression, chronic pain, post-traumatic stress, and relationship conflicts, to enhanced creativity and the search for meaning and life purpose. However, some of the most basic techniques include the following.

1. Conditioned Relaxation

This powerful relaxation technique is based on Pavlovian classical conditioning techniques and utilizes imagery-linked breathing and body awareness techniques that train the client to relax automatically by taking a special "signal breath." Instead of tensing when pain starts to flare, patients become conditioned to relax and imagine gently moving any painful symptoms out of their body.

2. Symptom Suppression Techniques

Symptomatic imagery techniques reduce the physical symptoms of pain without concern for their cause. They are a useful alternative to analgesic or anesthetic medications, and they are particularly helpful when discomfort is so intense that the patient cannot concentrate enough to use other guided-imagery approaches.

Symptom suppression techniques include a wide variety of methods, such as "glove anesthesia," a two-step imagery exercise in which patients are first taught to imagine developing feelings of numbness in the hand, as if it were being placed into an imaginary anesthetic glove. Next, they learn to transfer these feelings of numbness to any part of the body that hurts, simply by placing the "anesthetized" hand upon it.

Glove anesthesia often helps to "take the edge off" the pain sensation, thus permitting patients to explore other aspects of the pain experience more fully. In addition, glove anesthesia provides a dramatic illustration of the power of self-control. When patients realize that they can produce feelings of numbness in their hands at will, they recognize that they may be able to control their discomfort, too. This is profoundly therapeutic for pain sufferers who previously felt totally helpless and unable to affect their discomfort in any way.

3. Symptom Substitution Techniques

Symptom substitution techniques invite the nervous system to move the discomfort to a new area of the body where it will be less disruptive. For example, patients can learn to experience their headaches in their little finger instead of their head. This technique does not require the nervous system to suppress or stop the experience of pain, or to cover up the message it is trying to communicate. Rather, it moves the symptom to a less traumatized area so that patients can work more effectively to identify what the pain message is really trying to communicate.

4. Interactive Imagery Dialogue

This interactive technique can be used with an image that represents anything the client or therapist wants to know more about, and in many ways, it is the ultimate insight-oriented technique. It can be used to explore an image of a symptom (whether physical, emotional, or behavioral); an image that represents resistance that arises anywhere in the process; an image for an inner resource that can help the client deal with the current problem; or an image of the solution.

When using Interactive Imagery, the point is not to analyze the images, but to communicate with them as if they are alive, which of course, they are. This is not to say that they have an existence apart from the client, but rather that the images represent living complexes of thoughts, beliefs, attitudes, expectations, memories, feelings, body sensations, and values that at different times can function as distinct and relatively autonomous aspects of the personality. These constellations have been referred to as "subpersonalities" by Assagioli (1971), or "ego states" by Watkins and Watkins (1979).

Conflicts are often generated by subpersonalities that appear to have completely opposite beliefs, attitudes, and motivations. This is seen most clearly in issues related to habit control such a smoking, where people are of "two minds" about it. One part of them desperately wants to quit, while another part is determined to maintain the habit. The same is usually true when dealing with drug dependence, eating disorders, and other habits.

IGI is uniquely suited to mediate this conflict and to bring the parts closer together. By dialoguing with each of the parts, and finding out what they are willing to give up in order to get what they really want, unique solutions often arise. It is like conducting marriage counseling inside the skin.

5. The Inner Advisor

After learning to relax in their personal place, clients are frequently invited to dialogue with an imaginary figure that is designed to be both wise and loving, or as characterized in analytic terms, an "Ego Ideal." This figure is called an "Inner Advisor," and it is sometimes referred to as an "Inner Guide," "Inner Healer," "Inner Wisdom," "Inner Helper," "Inner Physician," "Higher Self," or any other term that is meaningful and comfortable for the client.

By dialoguing with their Inner Advisor, clients often receive creative and imaginative suggestions for how to alleviate their primary and secondary pain symptoms. Even more significantly, they can also often find answers to puzzling questions related to the etiology of their pain, as well as ideas for raising their pain tolerance.

6. Evocative Imagery

This state-dependent technique helps clients to shift moods and affective states at will, thus making new behaviors and insights more accessible to consciousness. Through the structured use of memory, fantasy, and sensory recruitment, clients are encouraged to identify a per-

sonal quality or qualities that would serve them especially well in their current situation. For instance, clients may feel they need "calmness" or "peace of mind" in order to deal more effectively with pain.

The guide then invites the client to relax and recall a time when peace of mind was actually experienced. Using sensory recruitment and present tense recall, clients are encouraged to imagine they are there again now, feeling that peace of mind. Once this peaceful feeling state has been well established and amplified, patients are invited to let the past images go, and to return to the present, bringing back with them the feelings of peace of mind. As they become aware of their pain problem while strongly in touch with this feeling, they are usually able to tolerate it far more effectively.

Evocative imagery was researched by Dr. Sheldon Cohen (personal communication) at Carnegie-Mellon University and found to be highly effective in shifting affective states. Research aimed at assessing the effects of those altered affective states on subsequent behavior, problem solving, and self-efficacy remains to be done, and this approach offers a fertile field for future psychological and behavioral research.

7. Grounding: Moving From Insight to Action

Grounding is the process by which the insights evoked using imagery are turned into actions, and where the increased awareness and motivation that result are focused into a specific plan for attitudinal, emotional, and/or behavioral change.

This process of adding the will to the imagination involves clarification of insights, brainstorming, choosing the best option, affirmations, action planning, imagery rehearsal, and constant reformulation of the plan until it actually succeeds. It is often the "missing link" in insight-oriented therapies, for it connects the new awareness to a specific action plan. It is where the "rubber meets the road," and imagery can be used to enhance this process by providing creative options for action and by using imagery rehearsal to troubleshoot and anticipate obstacles to success.

TREATMENT EVALUATION

The time spent preparing the client before entering into a formal guided imagery exploration is called the "foresight" part of the process. Along with evaluating the appropriateness of using imagery with the client, the guide works with the client to establish the desired goals and objectives for their work together.

As with any medical or psychological situation, goals can be defined in physical, emotional, or behavioral terms, and a reasonable trial period for exploration is agreed upon. Typically, patients are asked to participate in three exploratory sessions and then to decide whether this approach seems useful to them; whether they can best employ it as self-care in a brief, time-limited period of work (10 to 15 sessions); or whether it looks as if longer-term work will be needed.

At the end of each formal imagery experience (called "insight'), the goals of the work are reviewed and progress assessed (this phase is called "hindsight"). After this evaluation, an agreement is made to continue for another period of time, to define a period of time in which the client will do "ownwork" and then return to report progress, to terminate treatment, and/or to refer to another practitioner.

CONTRAINDICATIONS AND PRECAUTIONS

1. Do not substitute imagery for necessary medical or surgical interventions.

The primary danger in using imagery to augment healing in medical situations is when it is used in lieu of appropriate medical diagnosis and/or treatment. I have emphasized the necessity of an accurate diagnosis prior to using any psychophysiologic approach, so that the client is also aware of the medical options for treatment.

At times, patients may decide that they do not like the risks associated with the accepted medical treatments available and will then choose to use guided imagery or other mind/body approaches as their first-line treatment alternative. Although there are some situations in which this may make sense, each situation must be evaluated individually to ascertain patients' abilities to judge wisely for themselves and to make such important choices on their own.

2. Do not use imagery inappropriately with patients with unstable or poorly managed psychopathology.

There are several diagnostic categories of mental illness where the practitioner must use extreme care when utilizing exploratory imagery techniques. In particular, patients who are psychotic or who are on the verge of psychotic breaks, patients with dissociative identity disorders, and patients with borderline personality disorders must be treated with extreme caution, and only by well-trained and experienced imagery guides.

While these diagnoses do not represent absolute contraindications for imagery work, they require treating health professionals to have appropriate training and expertise in these areas. While many clients with these diagnoses may benefit from certain types of imagery (usually directed imagery focusing on centering, calmness, self-control, safety, etc.), great caution should be taken when using potentially disorganizing exploratory imagery techniques.

In proper therapeutic hands, guided imagery techniques may be one of the most effective ways available to work with clients who are survivors of traumatic abuse and who tend to experience pathological dissociation. However, such treating practitioners must be extremely well trained and experienced both in working with survivors of abuse and in working with exploratory IGI approaches.

3. Do not confuse responsibility with blame.

The fact that an illness can be helped through mental means does not necessarily mean it was caused by mental means. When using exploratory techniques such as the Imagery Dialogue with Symptoms or Working with an Inner Advisor, there is a tendency to confuse the ability to learn from illness with blame for causing the illness. What I usually tell clients is, "We may never know to what extent you or your unconscious is responsible for this pain problem, and that's really not the most important question. While it may not be clear to what extent you are responsible for your problem, it's absolutely clear that you are responsible for how you *deal* with your pain problem, and that's what we need to address."

This issue needs to be handled with skill and sensitivity, and while the practitioner may not be able to prevent certain clients from self-blaming (this may be an important issue to address with them), they can remind clients that using positive images to stimulate healing does not necessarily mean that it was their negative images that *caused* their problem in the first place.

4. Do not underestimate the power of the client's inner resources.

Imagery is a potent form of communication and suggestion. Whenever possible, we advocate using the patient's own imagery and an interactive guiding style with the conviction that clients have within them a great deal of information, experience, knowledge, and problem-solving resources that they are not yet using most effectively.

While there are certainly places and situations where an imagery guide may need to provide suggestions or even starting images, these are relatively rare when using IGI, and they risk robbing clients of the opportunity to learn an important way to help themselves. This can also create or sustain a sense of dependency on the expertise of the guide, rather than attention to the inner abilities that have always been available to help them to help themselves.

SCOPE OF PRACTICE FOR INTERACTIVE GUIDED IMAGERY^sm

This has been an important and problematic area for the Academy for Guided Imagery. When initially considering the criteria for formal certification in IGI, certification eligibility was restricted to professionals licensed to provide counseling services in their states of residence.

However, it was quickly determined that many states have no such licensing for therapists, and people with highly varying levels of training and experience were providing counseling, psychotherapy, hypnosis, and guided imagery. As a result, the academy evaluates each candidate on an individual basis, assessing the candidates for both competence and ethical standards as they are observed in clinical supervision as part of their IGI certification training.

Health professionals must ethically practice within the scope of their licensure, education, experience, and competence. Within these guidelines, certification in IGI can significantly help health professionals to become more effective at what they already do. Using guided imagery or IGI does not turn a physician into a psychotherapist, or a psychotherapist into a physician. Instead, it gives each a greater range of skillfulness in working with issues that involve both mind and body, and with issues involving emotions and behavioral change.

Certified IGI practitioners must discriminate between psychotherapy and psychoeducation, and between enhancing healing responses and practicing medicine. To maintain their certification status, they must also ethically practice within their scope of licensure, training, experience, and competence.

TRAINING, CERTIFICATION, AND ISSUES OF COMPETENCE

Many health professionals already utilize guided imagery in their work, although they may have learned how to guide someone only by reading a non-interactive script. The quality of training and competence of practitioners using this approach is highly variable. Because there is always the potential for doing harm when these techniques are used inappropriately or without adequate skills, standards of practice and quality control is an issue of critical importance.

The Academy for Guided Imagery has established specific standards of competence and ethical behavior that must be met before certification in Interactive Guided Imagery^{sm} is awarded. Quality assurance is based largely on direct observation of clinical work in small group and individual supervision sessions during the training program. During 52 hours of direct supervision, several different faculty members carefully observe the candidates and provide specific feedback to help them enhance their guiding skills.

Except for the academy's Professional Certification Training Program, there are no other such standards of quality assurance established for imagery practitioners.

REIMBURSEMENT STATUS

Imagery practitioners usually bill and are reimbursed for their guided imagery work in the same way they are for other professional services they render. Sessions are usually billed as psychotherapy, counseling, stress reduction training, or medical hypnosis. When applied for medical purposes, medical practitioners may ethically bill for medical services, although insurance companies may challenge this if services are lengthy and repetitive. There are currently no separate billing codes for guided imagery or IGI.

PROSPECTS FOR THE FUTURE

When you look closely at nearly every form of human therapeutic interaction and communication, imagery is usually centrally involved, primarily because it is a fundamental language of the body's healing systems. As this is better recognized, we are hopeful that health professionals will learn more about the best ways to utilize this potent form of thinking to support optimal health and healing.

Feedback from the thousands of health professionals who have taken the academy's training program in IGI confirms that it is a rapid route to insight, growth, and change. One constant piece of feedback received is that learning to use imagery interactively has improved the listening, communicating, and therapeutic skills of the academy's graduates, whether they are mental health professionals, physicians, or nurses.

Competence in effectively yet respectfully guiding the imagery process should be a fundamental part of every health professional's education and training, and the Academy for Guided Imagery is working toward that goal by co-sponsoring many of its professional training programs with well-established schools of medicine, nursing, and psychology, and with other professional medical and psychological associations.

In addition to professional training and certification in Interactive Guided Imagery^{sm}, the academy's Imagery Store is a valuable resource for self-help books, CDs, tapes, and reliable information on imagery (Academy for Guided Imagery, www.interactiveimagery.com). The academy is also participating in research studies exploring the uses of imagery in pain control, surgical preparation and recovery, and cancer chemotherapy, and it recently established the nonprofit Imagination Foundation to support further research in these and other areas. The Imagination Foundation (www.imaginationfoundation.org) is currently soliciting both funds and research proposals investigating various applications of imagery in healing.

Humans have always used their imagination to solve problems that threatened their survival. These times demand more than ever that we now learn to use this powerful information processing and problem-solving mechanism to help heal ourselves, our families, our communities, and our planet. A sustainable future depends in part on our ability to imagine it in both personal and global terms, and we are committed to supporting the healing potential of this much underutilized resource — the human imagination.

ACKNOWLEDGMENTS

The author gratefully acknowledges the assistance of Marty Rossman, who co-authored a previous version of this chapter, and to Diane Sternbach, who provided invaluable research assistance.

RESOURCES

PROFESSIONAL TRAINING

The Academy for Guided Imagery
Professional Certification Training in Interactive
    Guided Imagery^sm
30765 Pacific Coast Hwy #369
Malibu, CA 90265
800-726-2070
Fax 800-727-2070
www.interactiveimagery.com

TAPES, CDS, VIDEOS, BOOKS, AND RELATED MATERIALS

The Imagery Store (Academy for Guided Imagery)
30765 Pacific Coast Hwy #369
Malibu, CA 90265
www.imagerystore.com
800-726-2070

Health Journeys (BelleRuth Naparstek, Ph.D.)
891 Moe Drive, Suite C
Akron, OH 44310
800-800-8661

Source Cassettes (Emmett Miller, M.D.)
P.O. Box W
Stanford, CA 94309
800-528-2737

REFERENCES

American Pain Society. (2000). *Chronic pain in America: Roadblocks to relief.* New York: Roper Starch Worldwide.

Assagioli, R. (1971). *Psychosynthesis.* New York: Penguin.

Bresler, D. E., & Trubo, R. (2002). *Free yourself from pain.* Malibu, CA: Alphabooks.

Centers for Disease Control and Prevention. (2002). *2002 National Health Interview Survey (NHIS).* Atlanta: CDC.

Centers for Disease Control and Prevention. (2004). Targeting arthritis: The nation's leading cause of disability. Retrieved from http://www.cdc.gov/nccdphp/aag/aag_arthrit.htm.

Frank, J. (1974). *Persuasion and healing,* New York: Schocken Books.

Marcus, N. J. (1996). Loss of productivity due to pain. New York: New York Pain Treatment Program, Lenox Hill Hospital. Retrieved from http://www.medscape.com/viewarticle/405853_print.

National Headache Foundation. (2003). HNHF Headache Facts 2003. Retrieved from http://www.headaches.org.consumer/generalinfo/factsheet.html.

Pert, C. B., & Chopra, D. (1997). *Molecules of emotion: Why you feel the way you feel,* New York: Scribner.

Pope, K. S. (1996, September). Memory, abuse, and science, *American Psychologist,* 957–974.

Sheikh, A., & Kunzendorf, R. G. (1984). Imagery, physiology and psychosomatic illness. In A. Sheikh (Ed.), *International review of mental imagery* (Vol. 1, pp. 95–138). New York: Human Sciences Press.

Vargiu, J. (1974). *Subpersonalities, synthesis 1.* Redwood City, CA: Synthesis Press.

Watkins, J. G., & Watkins, H. H. (1979). The theory and practice of ego-state therapy. In H. Grayson (Ed.), *Short-term approaches to psychotherapy.* New York: Human Sciences Press.

Section VI

Pharmacotherapy

Robert B. Supernaw, PharmD, Section Editor

53

Nonsteroidal Anti-Inflammatory Drugs

Grace M. Kuo, PharmD

INTRODUCTION

Nonsteroidal anti-inflammatory drugs (NSAIDs) are used frequently to treat mild to moderate pain and have been shown to be most effective in treating pain related to muscle ache, headache, dysmenorrhea, toothache, osteoarthritis, and rheumatoid arthritis. Natural products, such as willow bark, that contain salicylates have been used for pain relief for more than 3,500 years (Vane, 2000; Warner & Mitchell, 2002). Many NSAIDs used today (e.g., aspirin, ibuprofen, naproxen) are available as over-the-counter products. An estimated 100 million prescriptions for NSAIDs are written by clinicians in the United States each year, and the use of over-the-counter NSAIDs may be as much as seven times higher (Jouzeau et al., 1997). Currently, more than 30 million Americans use prescription or over-the-counter NSAIDs regularly (Singh, 2000).

MECHANISMS OF ACTION: PAIN RELIEF FROM NSAIDS

The pain associated with inflammation results from the production of prostanoids in the inflamed body tissues that sensitize nerve endings and lead to the sensation of pain (Gordon et al., 2002). Pain reduction is achieved through the inhibition of prostaglandin synthesis, specifically, of cyclooxygenase (COX). COX is the key enzyme for the conversion of arachidonic acid into prostaglandins. Two main isoforms of the COX enzyme have been discovered — COX-1 and COX-2 — which are structurally similar and produce the same prostaglandins. COX-1 is a constitutive isoenzyme that has a protective function and is continuously produced in tissues throughout the body (e.g., gastric mucosa, platelets, kidneys) (Vane & Botting,

1997). COX-2 is predominantly an inducible isoenzyme that is produced by stimuli such as inflammation, although it also has a constitutive property in the brain, kidneys, synovium, and female reproductive tract (Hawkey, 1999). A third isoform, COX-3, is expressed constitutively, particularly in the cerebral cortex and the heart (Bazan & Flower, 2002).

NSAIDs inhibit COX by interfering with the conversion of arachidonic acid into prostaglandins (Vane & Botting, 1997). Traditional NSAIDs are a mixture of COX-1 and COX-2 inhibitors, such as salicylates (e.g., aspirin) and nonsalicylate anti-inflammatory agents (e.g., acetaminophen, etodolac, ibuprofen, naproxen, sulindac). Although salicylates have been used to treat pain for millennia, their mechanism of action was not known until 1971, when Nobel laureate John Vane discovered the mechanism by which aspirin and other traditional NSAIDs exert their therapeutic effects (Vane & Botting, 2003). Aspirin undergoes acetylation, a process that leads to the inhibition of COX, which, in turn, prevents the formation of prostaglandins. Traditional NSAIDs are nonselective in their mechanism of action, have different inhibitory effects on the COX-1 and COX-2 isoenzymes, and cause different complications (e.g., gastrointestinal and renal) (Cryer & Feldman, 1998). For example, etodolac and meloxicam inhibit COX-2 strongly and COX-1 weakly. This difference in inhibition explains why etodolac and meloxicam have fewer gastrointestinal side effects while exerting potent anti-inflammatory effects (Bazan & Flower, 2002).

In the late 1980s, Dan Simmons discovered a second, distinct COX gene from which the newer NSAIDs have been derived (Vane & Botting, 2003). These newer NSAIDs (e.g., celecoxib, rofecoxib, valdecoxib) are primarily COX-2 inhibitors (Dionne, 2003). Although COX-

2 inhibitors (e.g., celecoxib) do not affect platelet aggregation as much as nonselective NSAIDs, they can produce renal complications that are similar to those encountered with traditional NSAIDs. Both celecoxib and rofecoxib were approved by the U.S. Food and Drug Administration (FDA) in 1999; however, rofecoxib was withdrawn from the market by its manufacturer in 2004 because of concerns about an increased incidence in adverse cardiovascular effects. Celecoxib is currently approved by the FDA for the treatment of osteoarthritis, adult rheumatoid arthritis, familial adenomatous colorectal polyps, acute pain, and primary dysmenorrhea. Second-generation COX-2 inhibitors (e.g., valdecoxib, parecoxib, etoricoxib, lumiracoxib) that have different selectivity for COX-1 and COX-2 and different pharmacokinetic properties are currently being developed (Capone et al., 2003; Stichtenoth & Frolich, 2003). Valdecoxib has greater biochemical selectivity for COX-1 *in vitro* than does celecoxib and may be clinically important for improving gastrointestinal safety; valdecoxib was approved by the FDA in 2001 for the treatment of the signs and symptoms of osteoarthritis and adult rheumatoid arthritis and for the treatment of primary dysmenorrhea. In April 2005, the Food and Drug Administration requested sales of valdecoxib be suspended in the United States due to concerns related to cardiovascular risk and rare serious skin reactions. Parecoxib is a prodrug of valdecoxib and is the only injectable COX-2 inhibitor that is available; however, the FDA disapproved its manufacturer's new drug application in 2001 because of concerns related to its adverse effect profile. Etoricoxib has a slightly greater selectivity of COX-2 *in vitro* than does refecoxib and may also clinically improve gastrointestinal safety. As it is the only acidic COX-2 inhibitor, lumiracoxib is the most selective COX-2 inhibitor *in vitro*. The Food and Drug Administration has not yet approved the use of etoricoxib and lumiracoxib.

Acetaminophen is a weak inhibitor of COX-1 and COX-2, lacking strong anti-inflammatory effects. The mechanism of its analgesic effect was a mystery until the recent discovery of the COX-3 enzyme (Simmons et al., 1999). COX-3 is derived from the COX-1 gene with alternative splicing of the COX-1 messenger RNA (Bazan & Flower, 2002). It is suggested that acetaminophen selectively inhibits COX-3 (Chandrasekharan et al., 2002; Swierkosz et al., 2002), thereby exerting its analgesic effect by dulling the pain sensory system. In addition to the COX-3 enzyme, Simmons et al. (1999) identified two partial COX-1 (PCOX-1) proteins derived from the COX-1 gene. Although the PCOX-1 proteins are abundant in the brain, their mechanism of action and functions are not clearly known at this time (Simmons et al., 1999). The discovery of COX-3 and the PCOX-1 proteins is significant because it will contribute to the continual search for potential drugs that can target these isoenzymes.

THERAPEUTIC USES

NSAIDs are commonly used to relieve mild to moderate pain (e.g., myalgia, dysmenorrhea, dental pain, arthritis). Evidence-based therapeutic uses of NSAIDs for commonly encountered pain are summarized below, with the focus on COX-2 inhibitors.

LOW BACK PAIN

The prevalence of low back pain varies from 7.6 to 37% in different U.S. populations (Borenstein, 1997). Back pain is the most common reason for claiming workers' compensation. The prevalence of back pain among industrial workers is 4.6%, projecting to an estimated 101.8 million lost workdays per year (Guo et al., 1999). The rationale for using NSAIDs to treat low back pain is based on their analgesic property, as well as their anti-inflammatory action. In a Cochrane meta-analysis, van Tulder et al. (2000) concluded from the data of 51 clinical trials ($N = 6,057$) that NSAIDs were effective for short-term relief of pain in patients with acute low back pain. The pooled relative risk for global improvement was 1.24 (95% CI 1.10, 1.41). Additional qualitative analysis showed conflicting evidence that NSAIDs were more effective than acetaminophen, and the evidence for various types of NSAIDs being equally effective for acute low back pain was strong (van Tulder et al., 2000).

DYSMENORRHEA

Dysmenorrhea is a common complaint that affects as many as 50% of women; 10% of affected women report being incapacitated for up to 3 days during each menstrual cycle (Dawood, 1999). Women who have dysmenorrhea have higher levels of prostaglandin than women who do not have it (Pickles, 1979). For this reason, NSAIDs are thought to bring pain relief to women with menstrual cramps. In a Cochrane meta-analysis, Marjoribanks, Proctor, & Farquhar (2003) compared the effectiveness and safety of traditional NSAIDs with placebo and paracetamol and of different NSAIDs in relieving pain related to primary dysmenorrhea. The review included 63 randomized controlled trials ($N = 4,066$); 19 of the studies had a parallel design and 44 had a crossover design. Overall, NSAIDs were found to be significantly more effective than placebo (OR 7.91, 95% CI 5.65, 11.09) in relieving menstrual pain, but they were also found to be significantly more likely to be associated with adverse effects—combined gastrointestinal adverse effects (e.g., nausea, vomiting) and neurological adverse effects (e.g., headaches, fatigue). There was little evidence showing any significant difference between traditional NSAIDs and paracetamol or among the various NSAIDs.

Selective COX-2 inhibitors (e.g., celecoxib and valdecoxib) have been shown to be as effective as traditional

NSAIDs (e.g., naproxen) in the management of dysmenorrhea (Chavez & DeKorte, 2003; Fenton, Keating, & Wagstaff, 2004; Malmstrom et al., 2003; Ruoff & Lema, 2003).

ACUTE PAIN

The analgesic effects and safety profiles of the various NSAIDs used to treat acute pain (e.g., postoperative pain) have been evaluated by Cochrane reviewers. In 72 randomized single-dose trials that together included 3,253 patients in an aspirin group and 3,297 patients in a placebo group, aspirin was shown to be significantly more beneficial than placebo in its relief of acute pain (Edwards et al., 2000). The numbers needed to treat (NNTs) to achieve at least 50% relief of pain were found to be 4.4 (95% CI 4.0, 4.9) with the 600/650-mg dose, 4.0 (95% CI 3.2, 5.4) with the 1,000-mg dose, and 2.4 (95% CI 1.9, 3.2) with the 1,200-mg dose (Edwards et al., 2000). In addition, the side effects of drowsiness and gastric irritation were also shown to be significantly greater in the aspirin group than in the placebo group (Edwards et al., 2000). In 47 clinical studies that together included 2,561 patients in an acetaminophen group and 1,625 patients in a placebo group, the NNTs for at least 50% relief of pain over 4 to 6 hours were found to be 3.8 (95% CI 2.2, 13.1) with the 325-mg dose, 3.5 (95% CI 2.7, 4.8) with the 500-mg dose, 4.6 (95% CI 3.9, 5.5) with the 600/650-mg dose, 3.8 (95% CI 3.4, 4.4) with the 975/1,000-mg dose, and 3.7 (95% CI 2.3, 9.5) with the 1,500-mg dose (Barden et al., 2004b). Adverse effects were generally mild and transient, and the reported adverse effects between the 975/1,000-mg dose and placebo were not statistically significant (Barden et al., 2004).

In 32 trials comparing ibuprofen and placebo (3,591 total patients), the NNTs for at least 50% relief of acute pain were 3.3 (95% CI 2.8, 4.0) with the 200-mg dose, 2.7 (95% CI 2.5, 3.0) with the 400-mg dose, and 2.4 (95% CI 1.9, 3.3) with the 600-mg dose (Collins et al., 2000). In seven trials that included 581 patients treated with diclofenac and 364 patients treated with placebo, the NNTs for at least 50% relief of acute pain were 2.8 (95% CI 2.1, 4.3) with the 25-mg dose, 2.3 (95% CI 2.0, 2.7) with the 50-mg dose, and 1.9 (95% CI 1.6, 2.2) with the 100-mg dose (Barden et al., 2004a). The side-effect profiles of the 50-mg diclofenac and placebo groups were not statistically different (Barden et al., 2004).

In two trials that compared 200-mg celecoxib with placebo (418 total subjects), the NNT for at least 50% relief of acute pain was found to be 4.5 (95% CI 3.3, 7.2) with the 200-mg dose (Barden et al., 2003a). Celecoxib has also been shown to display efficacy comparable with naproxen in relieving pain associated with acute shoulder tendonitis/bursitis and acute ankle sprain (Petrella et al., 2004; Petri et al., 2004). Preliminary findings from two trials have demonstrated that 40-mg valdecoxib has a quicker onset of action and has a longer time-to-rescue than does 50-mg rofecoxib (Christensen & Cawkwell, 2004; Fenton et al., 2004). In a quantitative systematic review conducted by Barden et al. (2003b), the NNTs for at least 50% relief of acute postoperative pain were found to be 1.7 (95% CI 1,4, 2.0) with the 20-mg dose of valdecoxib, 1.6 (95% CI 1.4, 1.8) with the 40-mg dose of valdecoxib, 3.0 (95% CI 2.3, 4.1) with the 20-mg dose of parecoxib, and 2.3 (95% CI 2.0, 2.6) with the 40-mg dose of parecoxib.

OSTEOARTHRITIS

More than 20 million Americans have osteoarthritis (National Institute of Arthritis and Musculoskeletal and Skin Diseases, 2004). NSAIDs do not prevent or slow the progression of the disease; they are used only to help relieve pain associated with osteoarthritis. The efficacy of NSAIDs in the treatment of osteoarthritis has been widely studied. A search for NSAIDs and osteoarthritis using the Cochrane Database (EBM [evidence-based medicine] Reviews) yielded 36 meta-analyses and systematic reviews. In a meta-analysis, Towheed et al. (2003) evaluated the effects of NSAIDs on pain reduction, patient global assessments, and improvements in functional status. The objectives of the review were to assess the efficacy and safety of (1) acetaminophen versus placebo and (2) acetaminophen versus other NSAIDs (including ibuprofen, arthrotec, celecoxib, naproxen, and rofecoxib) in the treatment of patients with osteoarthritis. Six randomized controlled trials ($N = 1,689$) were included in the review; one trial compared acetaminophen with placebo and five trials compared acetaminophen with other NSAIDs. In the trial comparing acetaminophen with placebo ($n = 25$), acetaminophen was found to be more significant in reducing pain while at rest (RR 8.0, 95% CI 2.08, 30.73) and while in motion (RR 3.75, 95% CI 1.48, 9.52) and in improving patient global assessment (RR 18.0, 95% CI 2.66, 121.64). Differences in the safety profiles of these two groups were not statistically significant. In the trials comparing acetaminophen and various other NSAIDs, the other NSAIDs were found to be more effective than acetaminophen in reducing pain while at rest (effect sizes were 0.32, 95% CI 0.08, 0.56 and 0.34, 95% CI 0.10, 0.58), but all of them were similar in improving functional status and in the safety profile. Patients taking NSAIDs were more likely to experience a gastrointestinal adverse event (RR 2.24, 95% CI 1.23, 4.08).

A second search of the English-language medical literature in PubMed on NSAIDs using the search terms "osteoarthritis and celecoxib efficacy," "osteoarthritis and rofecoxib efficacy," and "osteoarthritis and valdecoxib efficacy" and limiting the search to reports on human adults (≥19 years) enrolled in clinical trials yielded 12, 17, and 4 journal articles, respectively, for each set of

TABLE 53.1
Selected Clinical Trials Using NSAIDs for Osteoarthritis (OA) Treatment (sorted by recent publication year)

Study	Year	Study Design[a]	N	OA	Treatment	Duration (Months)	Outcome Measures[b]	Results
Gibofsky et al.	2003	R, DB, PC, MC	475	Knee	Celecoxib 200 mg/day; rofecoxib 25 mg/day; placebo	1.5	1. VAS 2. Total domain score on WOMAC	1. Similar efficacy between celecoxib and rofecoxib 2. Celecoxib and rofecoxib were superior to the placebo ($p < 0.02$)
Geba et al.	2002	R, P, DB	382	Knee	Rofecoxib 12.5 or 25 mg/day; celecoxib 200 mg/day; acetaminophen 4,000 mg/day	1.5	1. Pain on VAS by WOMAC 2. Global response to therapy	1. Patients in the acetaminophen group discontinued treatment early due to lack of efficacy (31% vs. 18% to 19% of patients in other treatment groups) 2. Efficacy showed greatest response to rofecoxib 25 mg/day, followed by rofecoxib 12.5 mg/day, celecoxib, and acetaminophen
Kivitz et al.	2002	R, DB, PC, MC	1,016	Knee	Valdecoxib 5, 10, or 20 mg once daily; naproxen 500 mg BID; placebo	3.0	1. PaGAA, PhGAA, VAS, WOMAC 2. Upper GI ulceration from endoscopy	1. Valdecoxib 10 mg and 20 mg once daily (but not 5 mg once daily) were similar to naproxen; all three dosages were superior to placebo for the PaGAA, PhGAA, VAS, and WOMAC osteoarthritis indices ($p < 0.05$) 2. The incidence of ulcers was significantly higher in the naproxen group than in the 5- and 10-mg valdecoxib groups, but not in the 20-mg valdecoxib group; all three valdecoxib doses were comparable with placebo
Makarowski et al.	2002	R, DB, MC	467	Hip	Valdecoxib 5, 10 mg once daily; naproxen 500 mg BID; placebo	3.0	1. PaGAA, PhGAA, WOMAC 2. Incidence of adverse events	1. Valdecoxib was clinically and statistically superior to placebo for PaGAA, PhGAA, WOMAC ($p \leq 0.05$) 2. Valdecoxib 10 mg was similar to naproxen in terms of efficacy and superior to valdecoxib 5 mg 3. Valdecoxib 5 and 10 mg were similar in tolerability when compared with placebo and had a lower incidence of GI-related adverse effects when compared with naproxen
Tindall et al.	2002	OL, MC	2,327	Knee Hip	Celecoxib 200 mg/day to 400 mg/day	12.0	1. Radiographs in subsets of patients	1. Significant hip joint-space narrowing ($p = 0.029$); the observed increase in narrowing was small, was observed prior to celecoxib exposure, and was not dose related
Kivitz et al.	2001	R, PC, MC	1,061	Hip	Celecoxib 100, 200 or 400 mg/day; naproxen 1,000 mg/day; placebo	3.0	1. Standard measures of efficacy	1. Celecoxib (all doses) and naproxen were superior to the placebo 2. Celecoxib 200 mg/day, 400 mg/day, and naproxen were similar in pain relief and improvement in functional capacity
McKenna et al.	2001	DB, PC, MC	600	Knee	Celecoxib 100 mg BID; diclofenac 50 mg TID; placebo	1.5	1. Index joint pain by VAS, WOMAC index 2. Tolerability and safety profile	1. VAS and WOMAC index showed superior efficacy for both celecoxib and diclofenac but not for the placebo 2. No differences in efficacy between celecoxib and diclofenac 3. More diclofenac patients reported GI side effects, elevations in mean hepatic transaminases and serum creatinine, and reductions in hemoglobin concentration

Truitt et al.	2001	R, PC	341	OA	Rofecoxib 12.5 or 25 mg/day; nabumetone 1,500 mg/day; placebo	1.5	PaGAA WOMAC IGADS	1. Rofecoxib and nabumetone were superior to the placebo ($p < 0.001$) 2. Renal safety was similar for rofecoxib and nabumetone; no GI ulcers occurred
Williams et al.	2001	DB, PC, P, MC	718	Knee	Celecoxib 100 mg BID or 200 mg once daily; placebo	1.5	1. PaGAA, PhGAA, VAS 2. Lequesne Osteoarthritis Severity Index	1. Both celecoxib groups were superior to the placebo group in all measures of efficacy ($p < 0.05$) 2. No significant differences in efficacy or adverse events were shown between the celecoxib groups
Cannon et al.	2000	R, DB, C	784	Knee Hip	Rofecoxib 12.5 or 25 mg once daily; diclofenac 50 mg TID; placebo	12.0	1. VAS, WOMAC 2. PaGAA 3. PhGAA	1. Clinical efficacy of rofecoxib and diclofenac was similar 2. All treatments were well tolerated.
Day et al.	2000	R, DB	809	Knee Hip	Rofecoxib 12.5 or 25 mg once daily; ibuprofen 800 mg TID; placebo	1.5	1. WOMAC 2. PaGAA, IGADS	1. Both rofecoxib and ibuprofen were superior to the placebo ($p < 0.001$) 2. All treatments were well tolerated
Saag et al.	2000	R, DB, P, PC	736 693	Knee Hip	Rofecoxib 12.5 or 25 mg once daily; ibuprofen 800 mg TID; placebo Rofecoxib 12.5 or 25 mg once daily; diclofenac 50 mg TID; placebo	1.5 12.0	1. VAS, WOMAC 2. PaGAA, IGADS, PhGAA 3. Study joint tenderness	1. Rofecoxib and ibuprofen were similar in clinical efficacy 2. Both rofecoxib and ibuprofen were superior to the placebo at 6 weeks 3. Both rofecoxib and diclofenac showed similar efficacy over 1 year 4. All treatments were well tolerated
Bensen et al.	1999	R, DB, PC, MC	1,003	Knee	Celecoxib 50, 100, or 200 mg BID; naproxen 500 mg BID; placebo	3.0	1. Standard measures of efficacy	1. All celecoxib doses were efficacious when compared with the placebo, although the celecoxib 50 mg BID dose had only minimal efficacy 2. Celecoxib 100 mg and 200 mg BID were similarly efficacious, and the efficacy was comparable with naproxen 500 mg BID 3. All doses of celecoxib and naproxen were well tolerated
Ehrich et al.	1999	DB, P, R, MC	219	Knee	Rofecoxib 25 or 125 mg once daily; placebo	1.5	1. WOMAC	1. Clinical improvement was similar in the rofecoxib 25-mg and 125-mg groups
Zhao et al.	1999	R, DB, P	1,004	Knee	Celecoxib 50, 100, or 200 mg BID; naproxen 500 mg BID; placebo	3.0	1. Functional status by WOMAC index 2. Pain scores	1. Celecoxib and naproxen were superior to the placebo 2. The celecoxib 100 mg BID group had significantly better improvement in pain scores than did the placebo and naproxen groups

[a] C, controlled; DB, double-blind; MC, multicenter; OL, open-label; P, parallel; PC, placebo control; R, randomized.

[b] IGADS, The Investigator's Global Assessment of Disease Status; PaGAA, The Patient's Global Assessment of Arthritis; PhGAA The Physician's Global Assessment of Arthritis; VAS, visual analog scale; WOMAC, Western Ontario and McMaster Universities Osteoarthritis Index.

search terms. The clinical efficacy of COX-2 inhibitors is superior to the placebo and is similar to traditional NSAIDs in the treatment of osteoarthritis. Table 53.1 summarizes information from selected articles pertaining to the efficacy of COX-2 inhibitors in the management of osteoarthritic pain (Bensen et al., 1999; Cannon et al., 2000; Day et al., 2000; Ehrich et al., 1999; Geba et al., 2002; Gibofsky et al., 2003; Kivitz et al., 2001, 2002; Makarowski et al., 2002; McKenna et al., 2001; Saag et al., 2000; Tindall et al., 2002; Truitt et al., 2001; Williams et al., 2001; Zhao et al., 1999).

RHEUMATOID ARTHRITIS

Rheumatoid arthritis affects 2.1 million Americans and costs the U.S. economy nearly $125 billion per year in medical care and indirect costs. It is a disease that causes inflammation of the membranous lining of the joints, producing symptoms of pain, stiffness, and swelling (Arthritis Foundation, 2004). NSAIDs are frequently used to decrease inflammation, as well as to control associated symptoms.

In a systematic review, Wienecke and Gltzsche (2004) found that the comparison between NSAIDs and acetaminophen in the treatment of rheumatoid arthritis was inconclusive because of insufficient information with regard to study methods, blinding methods, and collection of data on adverse effects. Nevertheless, NSAIDs were preferred as the treatment of choice by patients and study investigators.

In a systematic review that included five randomized controlled trials ($N = 4,465$), Garner et al. (2002a) found that celecoxib was as efficacious as other NSAIDs, such as naproxen, diclofenac, and ibuprofen, in treating pain related to rheumatoid arthritis. In the same review, celecoxib was also found to be superior to the placebo (51% celecoxib 200 mg twice daily and 52% celecoxib 400 mg twice daily vs. 29% placebo) in achieving the 20 improvement criteria of the American College of Rheumatology (ACR).

In a second systematic review that included two clinical trials, Garner et al. (2002b). found the efficacy of 25-mg and 50-mg rofecoxib to be similar and both forms of rofecoxib to be more efficacious than placebo in reducing pain associated with rheumatoid arthritis, as measured by the number of ACR improvement criteria achieved. Although the safety profiles of rofecoxib and placebo were similar, the difference in the efficaciousness of rofecoxib and placebo was statistically significant (RR 1.39, 95% CI 1.07, 1.80 with rofecoxib 25 mg and RR 1.55 CI: 1.20, 1.99 with rofecoxib 50 mg). In the same review, Garner et al. (2002b) also found that the efficacy of rofecoxib at a dose of 50 mg/day was similar to that of naproxen at a dose of 500 mg twice daily. Rofecoxib produced fewer gastrointestinal adverse events than naproxen did (RR 0.46, 95% CI 0.34, 0.63) but was associated with a higher rate of cardiovascular adverse events (RR 2.36, 95% CI

1.38, 4.02 with any cardiovascular event and RR 4.48, 95% CI 1.52, 13.23 with nonfatal myocardial infarction).

UNLABELED USES

NSAIDs have several unlabeled uses, including the treatment of Alzheimer's disease and various types of cancer. Epidemiological studies found that patients taking NSAIDs had a 50% lower risk of developing Alzheimer's disease than those who were not (Turini & DuBois, 2002). NSAIDs may delay the onset and slow the progression of Alzeimer's disease by suppressing the inflammatory processes in the brain and by decreasing the production of beta-amyloid peptides (Blasko & Grubeck-Loebenstein, 2003; Giovannini et al., 2003; McGeer & McGeer, 2002; Michaelis, 2003; Pasinetti, 2002; Turini & DuBois, 2002; Zandi, Breitner, & Anthony, 2002). Several epidemiological studies found that NSAID users had a 40 to 50% decrease in the relative risk of having colon cancer (Turini & DuBois, 2002), possibly due to the role of NSAIDs in regulating COX-2 expression in tumorigenesis (Chan, 2003; Ferrandez, Prescott, & Burt, 2003; Kawai, Tsujii, & Tsuji, 2002; Ricchi et al., 2003; Yamamoto & Viale, 2003). Overexpression of COX has also been found in other epithelial tumors, such as those of the breast (Howe & Dannenberg, 2003; Singh-Ranger & Mokbel, 2002) lung (Natale, 2003; Saha, Pyo, & Choy, 2003), and cervix (Dannenberg & Howe, 2003).

USUAL DOSES

Table 53.2 lists the therapeutic uses of common NSAIDs, including acetylsalicylic acid, acetaminophen, celecoxib, diclofenac, etodolac, ibuprofen, indomethacin, ketoprofen, ketorolac, nabumetone, naproxen, sulindac, and valdecoxib, for pain management. Specifically, the indications approved by the FDA are listed with the corresponding doses. The cytochrome P450 enzymes are listed as a reference source for assessing potential interactions with drugs that are substrates, inhibitors, or inducers of these enzymes. Therapeutic monitoring related to hepatic and renal dosage adjustment recommendations are included, as well as the pregnancy categories recommended by the FDA.

CONTRAINDICATIONS

NSAIDs are generally contraindicated in persons who have hypersensitivities to NSAIDs and to salicylates. Celecoxib and valdecoxib have sulfonamide groups that confer selectivity and, consequently, are contraindicated in persons who are allergic to sulfonamide-related compounds.

PHARMACOKINETICS

In general, COX-1 inhibitors bind with isoenzymes competitively and reversibly, whereas COX-2 inhibitors bind

TABLE 53.2
Therapeutic Uses of Selective NSAIDs for Pain Management

Generic Name	Brand Name	FDA-Approved Indications	Common Doses[a]	Mechanism of Action	Drug Interaction	Therapeutic Monitoring
Acetaminophen	Tylenol	Mild pain, dysmenorrhea, OA	*Adults and children ≥ 12 years:* 325–650 mg PO/PR q 4–6 h, PRN; do not exceed 1 g/dose or 4 g/day *Children < 12 years and infants:* 10–15 mg/kg PO/PR q 4–6 h; do not exceed 5 doses in 24 hours *Neonates:* 10–15 mg/kg PO/PR q 6–8 h PRN; do not exceed 75 mg/kg/day	COX-3	Substrate (minor) of CYP1A2, 2A6, 2C8/9, 2D6, 2E1, 3A4 Inhibits CYP3A4 (weak) Interactions: ↑hepatotoxicity with CYP2E1 and CYP1A2 inducers (e.g., carbamazepine, rifampin, barbiturate, isoniazid)	*Hepatic:* use with extreme caution *Renal:* analgesic of choice for episodic pain in patients with underlying renal disease, but chronic use should be discouraged. Cl$_{cr}$ 10–50 ml/min: administer q 6 h; Cl$_{cr}$<10 ml/min: administer q 8 h; moderately dialyzable (20% to 50%) Pregnancy category C[b]
Acetylsalicylic acid	Bayer aspirin; Ecotrin	Mild to moderate pain, dysmenorrhea, OA, RA	*Adults and Adolescents:* 325–650 mg PO/PR q 4 h, PRN; do not exceed 4 g/day *Pediatrics:* 10–15 mg/kg PO/PR q 4–6 h, PRN; do not exceed 4 g/day	COX-1 and COX-2	Substrate of CYP2C8/9 (minor) Interactions: ↑ bleeding ↑ nephrotoxicity	Salicylate toxicity when the total salicylate level is usually >300–350 μg/ml *Hepatic:* at increased risk of salicylate-related adverse reaction *Renal:* avoid in patients with severe renal dysfunction, CrCl < 10 ml/min; dialyzable (50 to 100%) Pregnancy category C[b]
Celecoxib	Celebrex	Moderate to severe acute pain, dysmenorrhea, OA, RA	*Pain and dysmenorrhea:* 200 mg PO BID PRN OA: 100 mg PO BID or 200 mg PO QD RA: 100–200 mg PO BID; do not exceed 800 mg/day (adults) or 400 mg/day (elderly adults); lower doses for patients weighing < 50 kg	COX-2	Substrate of CYP P450 2C9 Inhibits CYP P450 2D6 (weak) Interactions: ↑ bleeding in the elderly	*Hepatic:* reduce dose by 50% and not recommended in patients with severe hepatic impairment *Renal:* no adjustment recommendation *Contraindications:* sensitivities to sulfonamide Pregnancy category C[b]
Diclofenac	Voltaren	Mild to moderate pain, dysmenorrhea, OA, RA	50 mg PO TID; do not exceed 150 mg/day	COX-1 and COX-2	Substrate (minor) of CYP1A2, 2B6, 2C8/9, 2C19, 2D6, 3A4 Inhibits CYP1A2 (moderate), 2C8/9 (weak), 2E1 (weak), 3A4 (strong) Interactions: ↑ bleeding	*Hepatic:* no adjustment recommendation *Renal:* close monitoring *Contraindications:* hematological disease or bone marrow suppression Pregnancy category B[b]
Etodolac	Lodine	Mild to moderate pain, OA, RA	*Pain:* 200–400 mg PO q 6–8 h, up to 1,000 mg/day as needed; do not exceed 1,200 mg/day *OA and RA:* 300 mg PO BID–TID, or 400–500 mg PO BID	COX-1 and COX-2	Interactions: ↑ bleeding	*Hepatic:* dosage adjustment in cases of severe liver disease or failure *Renal:* no adjustment needed Pregnancy category C[b]

TABLE 53.2 (Continued)
Therapeutic Uses of Selective NSAIDs for Pain Management

Generic Name	Brand Name	FDA-Approved Indications	Common Doses[a]	Mechanism of Action	Drug Interaction	Therapeutic Monitoring
Ibuprofen	Advil, Motrin	Mild to moderate pain, dysmenorrhea, OA, RA	Pain and dysmenorrheal: Adults and adolescents: 400 mg PO q 4–6h PRN; self-treatment: 200 mg q 4–6 h PRN; do not exceed 1,200 mg/day and/or 10 days OA and RA: 400–800 mg PO TID–QID; do not exceed 3,200 mg/day	COX-1 and COX-2	Substrate of CYP P450 CYP2C8/9, 2C19 Inhibits CYP2C8/9 (strong) Interactions: ↑ bleeding	*Hepatic:* avoid use in severe liver disease or failure *Renal:* no adjustment recommendation Pregnancy category B[b]
Indomethacin	Indocin	Moderate to severe pain, OA, RA	*Pain:* 75 mg (sustained-release)/day PO QD–BID; usually 7 to 14 days *OA and RA:* 25 mg PO BID–TID; may increase dose by 25 mg/day PO every 7 days up to 150–200 mg/day; reduce dosage by 25% in the elderly	COX-1 and COX-2	Substrate of CYP2C8/9, 2C19 Inhibits CYP P450 2C8/9 (strong), 2C19 (weak) Interactions: ↑ bleeding	*Hepatic:* dosage adjustment in hepatic dysfunction *Renal:* no adjustment recommendation Pregnancy category B[b]
Ketoprofen	Orudis	Mild to moderate pain, dysmenorrhea, OA, RA	*Pain:* 25–50 mg PO 6–8 h PRN; self-treatment: 12.5 mg PO q4–6h PRN, do not exceed 75 mg/day *OA and RA:* 50 mg PO TID to 75 mg PO QID	COX-1 and COX-2	Inhibits CYP2C8/9 (weak) Interactions: ↑ bleeding ↑ nephrotoxicity	*Hepatic:* dosage adjustment in liver dysfunction or when albumin < 3.5 g/dl; daily dose not to exceed 100 mg *Renal:* dosage adjustments according to renal function CrCl < 25 ml/min: 25–50 mg PO BID CrCl ≥ 25 and < 90 ml/min: 25–50 mg PO TID Pregnancy category B[b]
Ketorolac	Toradol	Moderate pain	60 mg IM or 30 mg IV × 1; then 30 mg IM/IV q 6 h.; do not exceed 5 consecutive days *Oral dose:* 20 mg PO × 1 after IV/IM dose, then 10 mg PO q 4–6 h; do not exceed 5 consecutive days	COX-1 and COX-2	Interactions: ↑ bleeding ↑ nephrotoxicity	*Renal:* use with caution *Renal:* reduce dose by 50% if CrCl < 30 ml/min; avoid use in patients with severe renal impairment *Contraindications:* breast-feeding, bleeding disorders, dehydration, renal failure, epidural or intrathecal administration, prophylactic use before or during surgery, labor Pregnancy category C[b]
Nabumetone	Relafen	OA, RA	Initially, 1,000 mg PO once daily or 500 mg PO BID; adjust dose according to patient response; do not exceed 2,000 mg/day	COX-1 and COX-2	Interactions: ↑ bleeding ↑ nephrotoxicity	*Hepatic:* dosage reduction may be needed *Renal:* discontinue if renal function worsens (CrCl < 30 ml/min) Pregnancy category C[b]

Drug	Brand/Status	Indication	Dosage	COX selectivity	Metabolism/Interactions	Hepatic/Renal/Pregnancy
Naproxen	Aleve, Naprosyn	Mild to moderate pain, OA, RA	*Pain:* 250 mg PO q 6–8 h PRN (do not exceed 1,000 mg/day); self-treatment: 220 mg PO q 8–12 h (do not exceed 660 mg/day PO or 440 mg in any 8–12 hour period) *OA and RA:* 250–500 mg PO twice daily	COX-1 and COX-2	Substrate (minor) of CYP1A2, 2C8/9 Interactions: ↑ bleeding ↑ nephrotoxicity	*Hepatic:* 50% dosage reduction in hepatic impairment *Renal:* dosage reduction may be needed if CrCl < 20 ml/min Pregnancy category B[b]
Rofecoxib	Vioxx	Voluntarily withdrawn by Merck & Co. on September 30, 2004	N/A	COX-2	Substrate of CYP2C8/9 (minor) Inhibits CYP1A2 (strong) Induces CYP3A4 (weak) Interactions: ↑ bleeding	*Hepatic:* not recommended in hepatic insufficiency *Renal:* avoid use in severe renal impairment Pregnancy category C[b]
Sulindac	Clinoril	OA, RA	150 mg PO twice daily; do not exceed 400 mg/day	COX-1 and COX-2	Substrate of CYP2C8/9 (minor) Interactions: ↑ bleeding ↑ nephrotoxicity	*Hepatic:* dosage reduction needed in hepatic impairment *Renal:* dosage reduction may be needed Pregnancy category B[b]
Valdecoxib	Bextra	Dysmenorrhea, OA, RA	*Dysmenorrhea:* 20 mg PO BID PRN *OA, RA:* 10 mg PO once daily	COX-2	Substrate (minor) of CYP2C8/9, 3A4 Inhibits CYP2C8/9, 2C19 (weak) Interactions: ↑ nephrotoxicity	*Hepatic:* avoid in severe hepatic impairment *Renal:* avoid in severe renal impairment Pregnancy category C[b]

Note: CYP = cytochrome isoenzymes; OA = osteoarthritis; RA = rheumatoid arthritis. Based on Harrison's online database. Retrieved March 25, 2004 from http://harrisons.accessmedicine.com/cgi-bin/search_drugDb.cgi. U.S. Food and Drug Administration database. Retrieved March 25, 2004 from http://www.accessdata.fda.gov/scripts/cder/drugsatfda/. Lexi-Comp's Clinical Reference Library Online. Available from the American Pharmacist Association (member's) Website: http://www.pharmacist.com/drug_information.cfm.

[a] Common doses are dosages based on the adult population (< 65 years old and ≥ 50 kg) unless otherwise indicated.

[b] FDA Pregnancy Categories (regardless of the designated pregnancy category or presumed safety, no drug should be administered during pregnancy unless it is clearly needed and potential benefits outweigh potential hazards to the fetus). A = Adequate studies in pregnant women have not demonstrated a risk to the fetus in the first trimester of pregnancy and there is no evidence of risk in later trimesters. B = Animal studies have not demonstrated a risk to the fetus but there are no adequate studies in pregnant women, or animal studies have shown an adverse effect, but adequate studies in pregnant women have not demonstrated a risk to the fetus during the first trimester of pregnancy and there is no evidence of risk in later trimesters. C = Animal studies have shown an adverse effect on the fetus but there are no adequate studies in humans; the benefits from the use of the drug in pregnant women may be acceptable despite its potential risks, or there are no animal reproduction studies and no adequate studies in humans. D = There is evidence of human fetal risk, but the potential benefits from the use of the drug in pregnant women may be acceptable despite its potential risks. X = Studies in animals or humans demonstrate fetal abnormalities or adverse reaction reports indicate evidence of fetal risk. The risk of use in a pregnant woman clearly outweighs any possible benefit.

with isoenzymes tightly, dissociate slowly, and form irreversible binding that is time dependent (Hawkey, 1999). Traditional NSAIDs, such as salicylates, are acidic; newer COX-2 agents, such as celecoxib and rofecoxib, are nonacidic (Brune & Neubert, 2001). Celecoxib binds tightly to plasma proteins and has an elimination half-life of 11 hours; changes in the pharmacokinetics of celecoxib have been reported in elderly individuals and differences in the disposition of the drug have been found among various racial groups (Davies et al., 2000). The pharmacokinetic profile of rofecoxib is complex and nonlinear, with an elimination half-life that ranges from 9 to 17.5 hours after multiple dosing (Depre et al., 2000). Rofecoxib binds tightly to plasma protein and is eliminated predominantly by the liver; its termination half-life is about 17 hours at a steady state (Ahuja, Singh, & Singh, 2003). Valdecoxib also binds tightly (98%) to plasma protein; its steady-state plasma concentrations can be achieved on the fourth day, and its oral bioavailability is 83% with rapid absorption and maximal plasma concentrations in 3 hours (Alsalameh et al., 2003). Valdecoxib is metabolized extensively in the liver and has an elimination half-life of approximately 8 to 11 hours (Alsalameh et al., 2003).

The COX-2 inhibitors differ from each other in biochemical selectivity. *In vitro,* valdecoxib (COX-1/COX-2 ratio: 60) has greater biochemical selectivity than does celecoxib (COX-1/COX-2 ratio: 30) and may lead to improved gastrointestinal safety. Etoricoxib (COX-1/COX-2 ratio: 344) exhibits slightly greater biochemical selectivity than does rofecoxib (COX-1/COX-2 ratio: 272) and may have a gastrointestinal safety profile similar to that of valdecoxib. Lumiracoxib is the most biochemically selective COX-2 inhibitor *in vitro* (COX-1/COX-2 ratio: 400); as it is the only acidic COX-2 inhibitor, a high concentration of the drug may be found in inflamed body tissues (Capone et al., 2003).

ADVERSE EFFECTS

More than 100,000 hospitalizations, at an estimated cost of $20,000 per event, are associated with NSAID use each year. Some 16,000 deaths are attributed to NSAID use yearly among NSAID users who have osteoarthritis or rheumatoid arthritis (Singh, 2000; Wolfe, Lichtenstein, & Singh, 1999). Some common adverse effects are listed below.

Gastrointestinal Effects

NSAIDs that inhibit both COX-1 and thromboxane synthetase increase the risk of bleeding. Aspirin, in particular, acetylates platelets irreversibly and interferes with coagulation. NSAID-induced gastritis is common, with an estimated 30 to 40% of NSAID users having gastrointestinal side effects (Garcia Rodriguez, 1997). In one study, the

relative risk of gastrointestinal complications in 4,164 patients seen at eight Arthritis, Rheumatism, and Aging Medical Information System centers was three to four times greater with NSAID use (Singh, 2000). Aspirin can cause severe gastric irritation and erosion of the gastric mucosa. Unlike nonselective NSAIDs, COX-2 inhibitors do not inhibit COX-1-dependent platelet aggregation and, therefore, are associated with a lower risk of bleeding.

In the Celecoxib Long-term Arthritis Safety Study (CLASS), Silverstein at al. (2000) found that fewer patients treated with celecoxib than patients treated with NSAIDs experienced chronic gastrointestinal blood loss and gastrointestinal intolerance. The Vioxx® GI Outcomes Research (VIGOR) Trial also found a gastrointestinal protective effect from rofecoxib compared with traditional NSAIDs (Bombardier et al., 2000). In general, COX-2 inhibitors are associated with a significant reduction in gastric irritation; they have been shown to be more cost-effective than NSAIDs in reducing gastrointestinal side effects while continuing to be efficacious in relieving pain (Lee et al., 2003).

Cardiovascular Effects

Through inhibition of prostaglandin synthesis, NSAIDs may have a deleterious cardiovascular effect (FitzGerald, 2002). Heerdink et al. (1998) followed a cohort of 10,519 patients older than 55 years and found an overall increased risk of hospitalization for congestive heart failure in those taking diuretics and NSAIDs in combination than in those taking diuretics only (crude relative risk 2.2, 95% CI 1.7, 2.9). In patients with established cardiovascular disease, NSAIDs may interfere with the cardioprotective effects of aspirin (MacDonald & Wei, 2003). In the 6-month CLASS trial, the incidence of cardiovascular events associated with celecoxib and NSAIDs, irrespective of aspirin use, was similar (Silverstein et al., 2000). In the SUCCESS VI Study, Whelton et al. (2001) found that celecoxib was associated with less edema and fewer changes in blood pressure than was rofecoxib. In the VIGOR study, the incidence of myocardial infarction (MI) was lower in the naproxen group (0.1% in the naproxen group vs. 0.4% in the rofecoxib group; relative risk 0.2, 95% CI 0.1, 0.7) (Bombardier et al., 2000). Even though the overall mortality rate in both groups was similar, the incidence of MI in the rofecoxib group increased by a factor of five when compared with the naproxen group (Fitzgerald, 2004). Likewise, the Adenomatous Polyp Prevention on Vioxx (APPROVe) trial that enrolled 2600 patients also showed a significant increase by a factor of 3.9 (45 of the 3,041 patients in the rofecoxib group vs. 25 of the 3,315 patients in the placebo group; relative risk 2.0, 95% CI 1.2, 3.2) in the incidence of thromboembolic adverse events (MI and stroke) associated with long-term (>18 months) use of rofecoxib. Based on the finding of an excess risk of MI and strokes in the APPROVe trial, Merck & Co., Inc., announced voluntary worldwide withdrawal of rofecoxib (Vioxx) on September 30, 2004 (Topol, 2004).

It is possible that the entire class of COX-2 inhibitors has the potential to produce adverse cardiovascular effects (Fitzgerald, 2004). For example, in the Therapeutic Arthritis Research and Gastrointestinal Event Trial (TARGET), more cardiovascular events (nonfatal and silent MI, stroke, or cardiovascular death) were found to have occurred in the lumiracoxib group than in the naproxen/ibuprofen group (0.65% vs. 0.55%; hazard ratio 1.14, 95% CI 0.78, 1.66) after 1 year; however, the difference was not statistically significant (Farkouh et al., 2004). COX-2 is believed to affect the cardiovascular system by (1) selectively inhibiting prostaglandin I_2 over thromboxane A_2 in the eisocanoid pathway, which disrupts the normal homeostatic balance and promotes thrombosis, and (2) by inhibiting prostaglandins E_2 and I_2 in the kidney, thus causing blood pressure elevation and sodium and water retention (Krum et al., 2004; Mukherjee & Topol, 2003). Both the European Medicines Agency and the U.S. FDA are conducting safety reviews of COX-2 inhibitors to assess whether all drugs in this class adversely effect the cardiovascular system. Meanwhile, it is suggested that patients who have cardiovascular disease or who are at risk for it should avoid taking COX-2 inhibitors (Fitzgerald, 2004).

HEPATIC EFFECTS

Traditional NSAIDs are metabolized predominantly in the liver. In a review of 14 controlled clinical trials, Maddrey and colleagues (2000) found that the overall incidence of hepatic adverse events related to celecoxib use was similar to that related to placebo use and was significantly lower than that related to the use of a combination of celecoxib and other NSAIDs. Nevertheless, the steady-state area under the plasma-concentration time curve (AUC) of celecoxib is increased in patients with mild to moderate hepatic impairment (Davies et al., 2000); for this reason, a dosage reduction of 50% is recommended for patients who have hepatic dysfunction. Furthermore, celecoxib and valdecoxib are not recommended for patients who have severe hepatic impairment.

RENAL EFFECTS

NSAIDs reduce renal function and increase both sodium and water retention because they block the production of renal prostaglandins by regulating renal blood flow, glomerular filtration, and the release of rennin (Palacioz, 2001). A post hoc analysis of the safety of celecoxib with data from more than 50 clinical trials ($N > 13,000$) showed that the overall incidence of renal adverse events related to celecoxib use was similar to that related to the use of other NSAIDs but was higher than that related to placebo use

(Whelton, 2000). The adverse drug reactions report issued by the World Health Organization/Uppsala Monitoring Center showed that rofecoxib use resulted in more renal complications than occurred with the use of celecoxib or nonselective NSAIDs (Zhao et al., 2001). Pooled safety data from the etoricoxib clinical development program showed that the renal effects of etoricoxib were similar to those of naproxen and ibuprofen (Curtis et al., 2004).

EFFECTS ON PREGNANCY

Because NSAIDs inhibit prostaglandin synthesis, NSAID use during pregnancy may prolong gestation and labor and increase anemia and peripartum blood loss (Shaver, 2001). Use of NSAIDs during pregnancy may be associated with an increased risk of miscarriage. In a population-based cohort study of 1,055 pregnant women, Li, Liu, & Odouli (2003) found that NSAID users had an 80% greater risk of miscarriage (adjusted hazard ratio 1.8, 95% CI 1.0, 3.2); the association was stronger if they used NSAIDs around conception (35%) and if they used NSAIDs for longer than a week (52%). This trend was similar for aspirin users but not for acetaminophen users. Women attempting to become pregnant should be advised not to use NSAIDs because animal studies have shown that these drugs could block embryo implantation (Shaver, 2001).

NSAID use by pregnant women poses potential adverse effects on the fetus, including premature closure of the ductus arteriosus, kidney dysfunction, pulmonary hypertension, and increased risk of intracranial hemorrhage. The adverse effects are thought to be less common if NSAID use is discontinued at least 6 to 9 weeks before delivery (Shaver, 2001). NSAIDs usually meet the criteria in the FDA Pregnancy Category C, but most NSAIDs meet the criteria in Pregnancy Category D during the third trimester.

DRUG INTERACTIONS

The adverse effects most commonly associated with the use of NSAIDs include an increased risk for bleeding with concomitant use of anticoagulants, corticosteroids, or ginkgo biloba and an increased risk of nephrotoxicity with concomitant use of aminoglycosides or cyclosporin. NSAIDs impair the metabolic effects of anti-hypertensive medications. Celecoxib does not appear to interact with angiotensin-converting enzyme inhibitors, beta-blockers, calcium channel blockers, diuretics, ketoconazole, methotrexate, or warfarin (Davies et al., 2000; Karim et al., 1999, 2000; Whelton et al., 2000); however, clinically significant interactions of celecoxib with fluconazole and lithium have been reported (Davies et al., 2000). Because celecoxib is a substrate of CYP2C9, it may potentially interact with either CYP2C9 inhibitors (e.g., fluvastatin, fluconozole) or inducers (e.g., rifampin). Valdecoxib is predominantly metabolized by the hepatic cytochrome P450 isoenzymes 3A4 and 2C9; the plasma concentration of valdecoxib has been shown to increase by 38% when coadministered with the CYP3A4 inhibitor ketoconazole and by 62% when coadministered with the CYP2C9/3A4 inhibitor fluconazole (Alsalameh et al., 2003). Coadministration of valdecoxib with warfarin was found to produce a small but statistically significant increase in the International Normalized Ratio (Alsalameh et al., 2003).

CLINICAL GUIDELINES AND EDUCATIONAL CAMPAIGN

Clinical guidelines for pain management have been endorsed by several medical organizations. Guidelines for the management of osteoarthritis and rheumatoid arthritis from the American College of Rheumatology (ACR) are available via http://www.rheumatology.org. For the management of osteoarthritis, the ACR recommends that NSAID users exploit nonpharmacologic adjunctive treatments (e.g., patient education, physical therapy, muscle-strengthening exercise) for more effective pain relief. For mild to moderate joint pain, the ACR states that acetaminophen and COX-2 inhibitors are as efficacious as traditional NSAIDs. The ACR also recommends that NSAIDs be used with caution in patients with risk factors for upper gastrointestinal adverse events — patients who are older than 65 years, with comorbid medical conditions or with smoking and alcohol consumption, who are taking oral glucocorticoids or anticoagulants, or who have a history of peptic ulcer disease or upper gastrointestinal bleeding. For the management of rheumatoid arthritis, the ACR recommends that salicylates, nonsalicylate NSAIDs, or COX-2 inhibitors be used in combination with disease-modifying antirheumatic drugs. NSAIDs are used to reduce joint pain and swelling but do not alter the progression of rheumatoid arthritis or prevent joint destruction. In terms of clinical efficacy, the ACR states that COX-2 inhibitors are no more effective than traditional NSAIDs, although COX-2 inhibitors have a significantly lower risk of serious gastrointestinal side-effects. The ACR does not recommend the routine use of H_2 blockers to prevent NSAID-induced gastropathy. However, the ACR does recommend concomitant use of low-dose aspirin with highly selective COX-2 inhibitors because there is evidence that COX-2 inhibitors are associated with a higher rate of thrombotic events and myocardial infarctions than are traditional NSAIDs.

To prevent NSAID-induced ulcers, the American College of Gastroenterology (ACG) recommends that patients at high risk for bleeding be considered for prophylaxis with misoprostol (e.g., 100 to 200 µg by mouth four times a day with meals) or proton pump inhibitors; to treat patients with NSAID-induced ulcers, the ACG recommends discontinuation of NSAIDs and treatment with any approved therapy for ulcer disease (Lanza, 1998).

In their guidelines for the management of persistent pain in older persons, the American Geriatrics Society (http://www.americangeriatrics.org) recommends that COX-2 inhibitors or nonacetylated salicylates be used to treat patients who require long-term daily analgesia. Both the American Chronic Pain Association (http://www.theacpa.org) and the American Pain Foundation (http://www.painfoundation.org/) provide good educational resources for health care professionals and consumers. In addition, the Department of Defense Veterans Health Administration has useful clinical practice guidelines for the management of low back pain or sciatica in the primary care setting (http://www.oqp.med.va.gov/ cpg/LBP/LBP_Base.htm). The Agency for Healthcare Research and Quality has compiled clinical guidelines on acute low back problems in adults and has indicated that acetaminophen is the safest effective therapy and that muscle relaxants are no more effective than NSAIDs (Agency of Healthcare Research and Quality, 2004).

Two educational campaigns have been launched recently to educate health care professionals and consumers about the adverse effects of NSAIDs (e.g., gastrointestinal bleeding). The first is the Risk Education to Decrease Ulcer Complications and Their Effects from NSAIDs (REDUCE) Campaign developed collaboratively by the American Gastroenterological Association and the American Pharmacists Association to educate physicians, pharmacists, and consumers about the risks caused by prescription and over-the-counter NSAIDs. The Roper Starch Worldwide Survey revealed that nearly 75% of the estimated 30 million Americans who regularly use NSAIDs were unaware or unconcerned about serious adverse effects (e.g., gastrointestinal bleeding) that may be associated with the use of these medications. The educational programs of the REDUCE Campaign include public service announcements and other educational materials. Additional information can be found at www.2REDUCE.org.

On January 22, 2004, the FDA launched a national education campaign to provide advice on the safe use of over-the-counter pain relief products. Concerns the FDA raised about the prolonged used of over-the-counter pain relief products include the potential hepatoxicity associated with acetaminophen and the gastrointestinal bleeding and renal toxicity associated with other NSAIDs. Through this campaign, the FDA aims to increase the public's awareness and to minimize potential risks associated with NSAIDs. Additional information can be found via the MedWatch Web-link http://www.fda.gov/medwatch/SAFETY/2004/safety04.htm#otc or http://www.fda.gov/cder/drug/analgesics/default.htm.

THERAPEUTIC MONITORING

Monitoring of NSAID-related toxicities includes assessments at baseline and during therapy and continual follow-up. Before NSAID therapy is initiated, patients should have a complete blood cell count and kidney and liver function tests. During therapy, the following signs and symptoms of NSAID-related complications should be monitored: dark stool, dyspepsia, nausea and vomiting, abdominal pain, edema, and shortness of breath. Continual follow-up should include an annual complete blood cell count and kidney and liver functions tests (American College of Rheumatology, 2002).

REFERENCES

Agency of Healthcare Research and Quality. (2004). Clinical practice guideline 14: Acute lower back problems in adults. Retrieved March 29, 2004 from: http://hstat.nlm.nih.gov.

Ahuja, N., Singh, A., & Singh, B. (2003). Rofecoxib: An update on physicochemical, pharmaceutical, pharmacodynamic and pharmacokinetic aspects, *Journal of Pharmacy and Pharmacology, 55,* 859.

Alsalameh, S. et al. (2003). Review article: The pharmacological properties and clinical use of valdecoxib, a new cyclooxygenase-2-selective inhibitor. *Alimentary Pharmacology and Therapeutics, 17,* 489.

American College of Rheumatology Subcomittee on Rheumatoid Arthritis Guidelines. Guidelines for the management of rheumatoid arthritis: 2002 Update. *Arthritis & Rheumatism, 46,* 328.

Arthritis Foundation. (2004). Rheumatoid arthritis. Retrieved March 29 from http://www.arthritis.org/conditions/DiseaseCenter/ra.asp.

Barden, J. et al. (2003a). Oral valdecoxib and injected parecoxib for acute postoperative pain: A quantitative systematic review. *BMC Anesthesiology, 3,* 1.

Barden, J. et al. (2003b). Single dose oral celecoxib for postoperative pain. *Cochrane Database Systems Review,* CD004233.

Barden, J. et al. (2004a). Single dose oral diclofenac for postoperative pain. *Cochrane Database Systems Review,* CD004768.

Barden, J. et al. (2004b). Single dose oral paracetamol (acetaminophen) for postoperative pain. *Cochrane Database Systems Review,* CD004602.

Bazan, N. G., & Flower, R. J. (2002). Medicine: Lipid signals in pain control. *Nature, 420,* 135.

Bensen, W. G. et al. (1999). Treatment of osteoarthritis with celecoxib, a cyclooxygenase-2 inhibitor: A randomized controlled trial. *Mayo Clinic Proceedings, 74,* 1095.

Blasko, I., & Grubeck-Loebenstein, B. (2003). Role of the immune system in the pathogenesis, prevention and treatment of Alzheimer's disease. *Drugs & Aging, 20,* 101.

Bombardier, C. et al. (2000). Comparison of upper gastrointestinal toxicity of rofecoxib and naproxen in patients with rheumatoid arthritis. VIGOR Study Group. *New England Journal of Medicine, 343,* 1520.

Borenstein, D. G. (1997). Epidemiology, etiology, diagnostic evaluation, and treatment of low back pain. *Current Opinion in Rheumatology, 9,* 144.

Brune, K., & Neubert, A. (2001). Pharmacokinetic and pharmacodynamic aspects of the ideal COX-2 inhibitor: A pharmacologist's perspective. *Clinical and Experimental Rheumatology, 19,* S51.

Cannon, G. W. et al. (2000). Rofecoxib, a specific inhibitor of cyclooxygenase 2, with clinical efficacy comparable with that of diclofenac sodium: Results of a one-year, randomized, clinical trial in patients with osteoarthritis of the knee and hip. Rofecoxib Phase III Protocol 035 Study Group. *Arthritis & Rheumatism, 43,* 978.

Capone, M. L. et al. (2003). Clinical pharmacology of selective COX-2 inhibitors. *International Journal of Immunopathology and Pharmacology, 16,* 49.

Chan, T. A. (2003). Cyclooxygenase inhibition and mechanisms of colorectal cancer prevention. *Current Cancer Drug Targets, 3,* 455.

Chandrasekharan, N. V. et al. (2002). COX-3, a cyclooxygenase-1 variant inhibited by acetaminophen and other analgesic/antipyretic drugs: cloning, structure, and expression. *Proceedings of the National Academy of Sciences of the United States of America, 99,* 13926.

Chavez, M. L., & DeKorte, C. J. (2003). Valdecoxib: A review. *Clinical Therapeutics, 25,* 817.

Christensen, K. S., & Cawkwell, G. D. (2004). Valdecoxib versus rofecoxib in acute postsurgical pain: Results of a randomized controlled trial. *Journal of Pain and Symptom Management, 27,* 460.

Collins, S. L. et al. (2000). Single dose oral ibuprofen and diclofenac for postoperative pain. *Cochrane Database Systems Review,* CD001548.

Cryer, B., & Feldman, M. (1998). Cyclooxygenase-1 and cyclooxygenase-2 selectivity of widely used nonsteroidal anti-inflammatory drugs. *American Journal of Medicine, 104,* 413.

Curtis, S. P. et al. (2004). Renal effects of etoricoxib and comparator nonsteroidal anti-inflammatory drugs in controlled clinical trials. *Clinical Therapeutics, 26,* 70.

Dannenberg, A. J., & Howe, L. R. (2003). The role of COX-2 in breast and cervical cancer. *Progress in Experimental Tumor Research, 37,* 90.

Davies, N. M. et al. (2000). Clinical pharmacokinetics and pharmacodynamics of celecoxib: A selective cyclo-oxygenase-2 inhibitor. *Clinical Pharmacokinetics, 38,* 225.

Dawood, M. Y. (1999). Efficacy and safety of piroxicam-B-cyclodextrin (PBCD, Brexidol). Comparison studies with ibuprofen, naproxen sodium and placebo in the relief of moderate to severe abdominal pain associated with primary dysmenorrhoea. The Brexidol Study Group. *Today's Therapeutic Trends, 17,* 273.

Day, R. et al. (2000). A randomized trial of the efficacy and tolerability of the COX-2 inhibitor rofecoxib vs ibuprofen in patients with osteoarthritis. Rofecoxib/Ibuprofen Comparator Study Group. *Archives of Internal Medicine, 160,* 1781.

Depre, M. et al. (2000). Pharmacokinetics, COX-2 specificity, and tolerability of supratherapeutic doses of rofecoxib in humans. *European Journal of Clinical Pharmacology, 56,* 167.

Dionne, R. (2003). Relative efficacy of selective COX-2 inhibitors compared with over-the-counter ibuprofen. *International Journal of Clinical Practice* (Suppl.), 18.

Edwards, J. E. et al. (2000). Single dose oral aspirin for acute pain. *Cochrane Database Systems Review,* CD002067.

Ehrich, E. W. et al. (1999). Effect of specific COX-2 inhibition in osteoarthritis of the knee: A 6-week double-blind, placebo-controlled pilot study of rofecoxib. Rofecoxib Osteoarthritis Pilot Study Group. *Journal of Rheumatology, 26,* 2438.

Farkouh, M. E. et al. (2004). Comparison of lumiracoxib with naproxen and ibuprofen in the Therapeutic Arthritis Research and Gastrointestinal Event Trial (TARGET), cardiovascular outcomes: Randomised controlled trial. *Lancet, 364,* 675.

Fenton, C., Keating, G. M. & Wagstaff, A. J. (2004). Valdecoxib: A review of its use in the management of osteoarthritis, rheumatoid arthritis, dysmenorrhoea and acute pain. *Drugs, 64,* 1231.

Ferrandez, A., Prescott, S., & Burt, R. W. (2003). COX-2 and colorectal cancer. *Current Pharmaceutical Design, 9,* 2229.

FitzGerald, G. A. (2002). Cardiovascular pharmacology of nonselective nonsteroidal anti-inflammatory drugs and coxibs: Clinical considerations. *American Journal of Cardiology, 89,* 26D.

Fitzgerald, G. A. (2004). Coxibs and cardiovascular disease. *New England Journal of Medicine, 351,* 1709.

Garcia Rodriguez, L. A. (1997). Nonsteroidal antiinflammatory drugs, ulcers and risk: A collaborative meta-analysis. *Seminars in Arthritis and Rheumatism, 26,* 16.

Garner, S. et al. (2002a). Celecoxib for rheumatoid arthritis. *Cochrane Database Systems Review,* CD003831.

Garner, S. et al. (2002b). Rofecoxib for the treatment of rheumatoid arthritis. *Cochrane Database Systems Review,* CD003685.

Geba, G. P. et al. (2002). Efficacy of rofecoxib, celecoxib, and acetaminophen in osteoarthritis of the knee: A randomized trial. *Journal of the American Medical Association, 287,* 64.

Gibofsky, A. et al. (2003). Comparing the efficacy of cyclooxygenase 2-specific inhibitors in treating osteoarthritis: Appropriate trial design considerations and results of a randomized, placebo-controlled trial. *Arthritis & Rheumatism, 48,* 3102.

Giovannini, M. G. et al. (2003). Experimental brain inflammation and neurodegeneration as model of Alzheimer's disease: Protective effects of selective COX-2 inhibitors. *International Journal of Immunopathology and Pharmacology, 16,* 31.

Gordon, S. M. et al. (2002). Peripheral prostanoid levels and nonsteroidal anti-inflammatory drug analgesia: replicate clinical trials in a tissue injury model. *Clinical Pharmacology and Therapeutics, 72,* 175.

Guo, H.R. et al. (1999). Back pain prevalence in US industry and estimates of lost workdays. *American Journal of Public Health, 89,* 1029.

Hawkey, C. J. (1999). COX-2 inhibitors. *Lancet, 353,* 307.

Heerdink, E. R. et al. (1998). NSAIDs associated with increased risk of congestive heart failure in elderly patients taking diuretics. *Archives of Internal Medicine, 158,* 1108.

Howe, L. R., & Dannenberg, A. J. (2003). COX-2 inhibitors for the prevention of breast cancer. *Journal of Mammary Gland Biology Neoplasia, 8,* 31.

Jouzeau, J. Y. et al. (1997). Cyclo-oxygenase isoenzymes. How recent findings affect thinking about nonsteroidal anti-inflammatory drugs. *Drugs, 53,* 563.

Karim, A. et al. (1999). Celecoxib, a specific COX-2 inhibitor, has no significant effect on methotrexate pharmacokinetics in patients with rheumatoid arthritis. *Journal of Rheumatology, 26,* 2539.

Karim, A. et al. (2000). Celecoxib does not significantly alter the pharmacokinetics or hypoprothrombinemic effect of warfarin in healthy subjects. *Journal of Clinical Pharmacology, 40,* 655.

Kawai, N., Tsujii, M., & Tsuji, S. (2002). Cyclooxygenases and colon cancer. *Prostaglandins & Other Lipid Mediators, 187,* 68–69.

Kivitz, A. et al. (2002). Randomized placebo-controlled trial comparing efficacy and safety of valdecoxib with naproxen in patients with osteoarthritis. *Journal of Family Practice, 51,* 530.

Kivitz, A. J. et al. (2001). Comparative efficacy and safety of celecoxib and naproxen in the treatment of osteoarthritis of the hip. *Journal of International Medical Research, 29,* 467.

Krum, H. et al. (2004). Cardiovascular effects of selective cyclooxygenase-2 inhibitors. *Expert Reviews of Cardiovascular Therapy, 2,* 265.

Lanza, F. L. (1998). A guideline for the treatment and prevention of NSAID-induced ulcers. Members of the Ad Hoc Committee on Practice Parameters of the American College of Gastroenterology. *American Journal of Gastroenterology, 93,* 2037.

Lee, K. K. et al. (2003). Economic analysis of celecoxib versus diclofenac plus omeprazole for the treatment of arthritis in patients at risk of ulcer disease. *Alimentary Pharmacology and Therapeutics, 18,* 217.

Li, D. K., Liu, L., & Odouli, R. (2003). Exposure to non-steroidal anti-inflammatory drugs during pregnancy and risk of miscarriage: Population based cohort study. *British Medical Journal, 327,* 368.

MacDonald, T. M., & Wei, L. (2003). Effect of ibuprofen on cardioprotective effect of aspirin. *Lancet, 361,* 573.

Maddrey, W. C. et al. (2000). The hepatic safety and tolerability of the novel cyclooxygenase-2 inhibitor celecoxib. *American Journal of Therapeutics, 7,* 153.

Makarowski, W. et al. (2002). Efficacy and safety of the COX-2 specific inhibitor valdecoxib in the management of osteoarthritis of the hip: A randomized, double-blind, placebo-controlled comparison with naproxen. *Osteoarthritis Cartilage, 10,* 290.

Malmstrom, K. et al. (2003). Analgesic efficacy of etoricoxib in primary dysmenorrhea: results of a randomized, controlled trial. *Gynecologic and Obstetric Investigation, 56,* 65.

Marjoribanks, J., Proctor, M. L., & Farquhar, C. (2003). Nonsteroidal anti-inflammatory drugs for primary dysmenorrhoea. *Cochrane Database Systems Review,* CD001751.

McGeer, P. L., & McGeer, E. G. (2002). Local neuroinflammation and the progression of Alzheimer's disease. *Journal of Neurovirology, 8,* 529.

McKenna, F. et al. (2001). Celecoxib versus diclofenac in the management of osteoarthritis of the knee. *Scandinavian Journal of Rheumatology, 30,* 11.

Michaelis, M. L. (2003). Drugs targeting Alzheimer's disease: some things old and some things new. *Journal of Pharmacology and Experimental Therapeutics, 304,* 897.

Mukherjee, D., & Topol, E. J. (2003). Cox-2: Where are we in 2003? Cardiovascular risk and Cox-2 inhibitors. *Arthritis Research and Therapy, 5,* 8.

Natale, R. B. (2003). Irinotecan, cisplatin/carboplatin, and COX-2 inhibition in small-cell lung cancer. *Oncology (Huntingt), 17,* 22.

National Institute of Arthritis and Musculoskeletal and Skin Diseases. (2004). Handout on Health: Osteoarthritis. Retrieved March 29, 2004 from: http://www.niams.nih.gov/hi/topics/arthritis/oahandout.htm.

Palacioz, K. (2001). COX-2 inhibitors and cardiorenal effects, *Pharmacist's Letter, 17,* 170602.

Pasinetti, G. M. (2002). Cyclooxygenase as a target for the antiamyloidogenic activities of nonsteroidal anti-inflammatory drugs in Alzheimer's disease. *Neurosignals, 11,* 293.

Petrella, R. et al. (2004). Efficacy of celecoxib, a COX-2-specific inhibitor, and naproxen in the management of acute ankle sprain: Results of a double-blind, randomized controlled trial. *Clinical Journal of Sports Medicine, 14,* 225.

Petri, M. et al. (2004). Celecoxib effectively treats patients with acute shoulder tendinitis/bursitis. *Journal of Rheumatology, 31,* 1614.

Pickles, V. R. (1979). Prostaglandins and dysmenorrhea. Historical survey. *Acta Obstetrica et Gynecologica Scandinavica. Supplement, 87,* 7.

Ricchi, P. et al. (2003). Nonsteroidal anti-inflammatory drugs in colorectal cancer: From prevention to therapy. *British Journal of Cancer, 88,* 803.

Ruoff, G., & Lema, M. (2003). Strategies in pain management: New and potential indications for COX-2 specific inhibitors. *Journal of Pain and Symptom Management, 25,* S21.

Saag, K. et al. (2000). Rofecoxib, a new cyclooxygenase 2 inhibitor, shows sustained efficacy, comparable with other nonsteroidal anti-inflammatory drugs: A 6-week and a 1-year trial in patients with osteoarthritis. Osteoarthritis Studies Group. *Archives of Family Medicine, 9,* 1124.

Saha, D., Pyo, H., & Choy, H. (2003). COX-2 inhibitor as a radiation enhancer: New strategies for the treatment of lung cancer. *American Journal of Clinic Oncology, 26,* S70.

Shaver, K. (2001). The use of NSAIDs during pregnancy. *Pharmacist's Letter, 17,* 170305.

Silverstein, F. E. et al. (2000). Gastrointestinal toxicity with celecoxib vs nonsteroidal anti-inflammatory drugs for osteoarthritis and rheumatoid arthritis: The CLASS study: A randomized controlled trial. Celecoxib Longterm Arthritis Safety Study. *Journal of the American Medical Association, 284,* 1247.

Simmons, D. L. et al. (1999). Induction of an acetaminophensensitive cyclooxygenase with reduced sensitivity to nonsteroid antiinflammatory drugs. *Proceedings of the National Academy of Sciences of the United States of America, 96,* 3275.

Singh, G. (2000). Gastrointestinal complications of prescription and over-the-counter nonsteroidal anti-inflammatory drugs: A view from the ARAMIS database. Arthritis, Rheumatism, and Aging Medical Information System. *American Journal of Therapeutics, 7,* 115.

Singh-Ranger, G., & Mokbel, K. (2002). The role of cyclooxygenase-2 (COX-2) in breast cancer, and implications of COX-2 inhibition. *European Journal of Surgical Oncology, 28,* 729.

Stichtenoth, D. O., & Frolich, J. C. (2003). The second generation of COX-2 inhibitors: What advantages do the newest offer? *Drugs, 63,* 33.

Swierkosz, T. A. et al. (2002). Actions of paracetamol on cyclooxygenases in tissue and cell homogenates of mouse and rabbit. *Medical Science Monitor, 8,* BR496.

Tindall, E. A. et al. (2002). A 12-month, multicenter, prospective, open-label trial of radiographic analysis of disease progression in osteoarthritis of the knee or hip in patients receiving celecoxib. *Clinical Therapeutics, 24,* 2051.

Topol, E. J. (2004). Failing the public health — Rofecoxib, Merck, and the FDA. *New England Journal of Medicine, 351,* 1707.

Towheed, T. E. et al. Acetaminophen for osteoarthritis. *Cochrane Database Systems Review,* CD004257.

Truitt, K. E. et al. (2001). A multicenter, randomized, controlled trial to evaluate the safety profile, tolerability, and efficacy of rofecoxib in advanced elderly patients with osteoarthritis. *Aging* (Milano), *13,* 112.

Turini, M. E., & DuBois, R. N. (2002). Cyclooxygenase-2: A therapeutic target. *Annual Review of Medicine, 53,* 35.

van Tulder, M. W. et al. (2000). Non-steroidal anti-inflammatory drugs for low back pain. *Cochrane Database of Systems Reviews,,* CD000396.

Vane, J. R. (2000). The fight against rheumatism: From willow bark to COX-1 sparing drugs. *Journal of Physiology and Pharmacology, 51,* 573.

Vane, J. R., & Botting, R. M. (1997). Mechanism of action of aspirin-like drugs. *Seminars in Arthritis and Rheumatism, 26*, 2.

Vane, J. R., & Botting, R. M. (2003). The mechanism of action of aspirin. *Thrombosis Research, 110*, 255.

Warner, T. D., & Mitchell, J. A. (2002). Cyclooxygenase-3 (COX-3): Filling in the gaps toward a COX continuum? *Proceedings of the National Academy of Sciences of the United States of America, 99*, 13371.

Whelton, A. (2000). COX-1 sparing and COX-2 inhibitory drugs: the renal and hepatic safety and tolerability profiles of celecoxib. *American Journal of Therapeutics, 7*, 151.

Whelton, A. et al. (2000). Renal safety and tolerability of celecoxib, a novel cyclooxygenase-2 inhibitor. *American Journal of Therapeutics, 7*, 159.

Whelton, A. et al. (2001). Cyclooxygenase-2--specific inhibitors and cardiorenal function: A randomized, controlled trial of celecoxib and rofecoxib in older hypertensive osteoarthritis patients. *American Journal of Therapeutics, 8*, 85.

Wienecke, T., & Gotzsche, P. (2004). Paracetamol versus nonsteroidal anti-inflammatory drugs for rheumatoid arthritis. *Cochrane Database Systems Review, 1*, CD003789.

Williams, G. W. et al. (2001). Comparison of once-daily and twice-daily administration of celecoxib for the treatment of osteoarthritis of the knee. *Clinical Therapeutics, 23*, 213.

Wolfe, M. M., Lichtenstein, D. R., & Singh, G. (1999). Gastrointestinal toxicity of nonsteroidal antiinflammatory drugs. *New England Journal of Medicine, 340*, 1888.

Yamamoto, D. S., & Viale, P. H. (2003). Cyclooxygenase-2: From arthritis treatment to new indications for the prevention and treatment of cancer. *Clinical Journal on Oncological Nursing, 7*, 21.

Zandi, P. P., Breitner, J. C., & Anthony, J. C. (2002). Is pharmacological prevention of Alzheimer's a realistic goal? *Expert Opinion on Pharmacotherapt, 3*, 365.

Zhao, S. Z. et al. (1999). Evaluation of the functional status aspects of health-related quality of life of patients with osteoarthritis treated with celecoxib. *Pharmacotherapy, 19*, 1269.

Zhao, S. Z. et al. (2001). A comparison of renal-related adverse drug reactions between rofecoxib and celecoxib, based on the World Health Organization/Uppsala Monitoring Centre safety database. *Clinical Therapeutics, 23*, 1478.

54

Opioids Used in Primary Care for the Management of Pain: A Pharmacologic, Pharmacotherapeutic, and Pharmacodynamic Overview

Robert L. Barkin, MBA, PharmD, FCP, DAAPM, Arcangelo M. Iusco, MD, and Stacie J. Barkin, MEd, MA, PsyD

INTRODUCTION

Opioid analgesics are drugs that bind to opioid receptors and share properties of the naturally occurring endogenous opioids. The term *narcotic* is derived from the Greek word narkotikos, meaning to numb or deaden (narcotic can refer to non-opioids as well as opioids and is not a pharmacologic term, but does appear in legislative, judicial, and government documents). This chapter provides an overview of the pharmacology, pharmacokinetics, and pharmacodynamics of this diverse group of analgesics (American Academy of Pain Medicine and American Pain Society, 1997; Ashburn & Ready, 2001; Ashburn & Staats, 1999; Ballantyne et al., 1993; Barkin & Barkin, 2001; Barkin, Barkin, & Barkin, 2005; Barkin, Fawcett, & Barkin, 2002; Bartleson, 2002; Carr & Goudas, 1999; Carr et al., 2002; de Leo-Casasola & Lema, 1996; DeRuiter, 2000; Edwards & Breed, 1990; Foley, 2003; Resnik et al., 2001; Zenz, Strumpf, & Tryba, 1992).

MECHANISMS OF ACTION

Opioids are primarily employed for their ability to reduce the perception of pain. Their analgesic activity is mediated by opioid receptors in the central nervous system (CNS).

Opioids act as agonists at stereospecific endogenous opioid receptors, which are found at both presynaptic and postsynaptic central and peripheral nervous system sites. Four major categories of opioid receptors are known; three provide analgesia mu (μ), kappa (κ), delta (δ). The sigma (σ) receptor has biologic effects, but is no longer considered to be an opioid receptor. Opioid drugs bind to the same receptors as endogenous opioid peptides (enkephalins, endorphins, and dynorphins). These three families of opioid peptides differ in their protein precursors, anatomic distributions, and receptor affinities. Both the endogenous agonists and opioid analgesics alter the central release of neurotransmitters. The actions of the opioid analgesics now available can be defined by their activity at three specific opiate receptor types: mu, kappa, and delta. Some opioids also have mechanism as partial agonists and mixed agonist antagonist (Barkin et al., 2005) (Table 54.1 and Table 54.2).

OPIOID RECEPTORS

Opioids are classified as agonists, partial agonists, mixed agonist–antagonists, and antagonists (naloxone) (Table 54.1). Only drugs with agonist effects provide analgesia.

Mu receptors (Barkin et al., 2002; Zenz et al., 1992) mediate analgesia, euphoria, respiratory and physical

TABLE 54.1
Overview of Opioid Receptors

Receptor	Proposed Location	Proposed Events
Mu$_1$ (μ_1)	Supraspinal, peripheral analgesia, spinal cord, nucleus raphe magnus, locus ceruleus, cerebral cortex (lamina IV), thalamus, periaqueductal gray, periventricular gray, substantial gelatinosa	Analgesia
Mu$_2$ (μ_2)	Spinal analgesia, spinal trigeminal nucleus, gastrointestinal tract, Limbic area, reticular activating system (RAS), striatum medulla, medullar raphe nuclei	Sedation, vomiting, urinary retention, respiratory depression, euphoria, miosis, physical dependence, delayed gastrointestinal motility
Kappa (κ)	K$_1$ spinal cord K$_3$ supraspinal	Spinal analgesia, dyspnea, psychomimetic effects, respiratory depression, miosis, diuresis, sedation, physical dependence, euphoria, dysphoria

Delta (δ)	δ_1 spinal
	    supraspinal
	δ_2 frontal cortex
	    limbic area
	    olfactory tubercle
	    spinal
		Analgesia, spinal analgesia

TABLE 54.2
Chemical Classification of Opioid Medications

Chemical Class for Opioid Agonists	Opioid Agonist	Opioid Agonist–Antagonist and Partial Agonist
Phenanthrenes	Codeine	Buprenorphine (partial agonist)
	Hydrocodone	Butorphanol (agonist/antagonist/mixed)
	Hydromorphone	Nalbuphine (mixed agonist/antagonist)
	Levorphanol	Pentazocine (mixed agonist/antagonist)
	Morphine	
	Oxycodone	
	Oxymorphone	
Phenylpiperidines	Alfentanil	
	Fentanyl	
	Meperidine	
	Sufentanil	
Diphenylheptanes	Levomethadyl	
	Methadone	
	Propoxyphene	
Anilidopiperidines	Remifentanil	

depression, miosis, and reduced gastrointestinal (GI) motility. These receptors have been further subtyped as mu-1 and mu-2 receptors, and there may be affinity and pharmacologic differences between two. For example, mu-1 receptors may mediate high-affinity supraspinal analgesia, whereas mu-2 receptors have been implicated in opioid side effects, such as respiratory depression, euphoria, and GI motility (see Table 54.1). Enkephalins are the endogenous ligands for these receptors and morphine is the prototypic exogenous ligand.

Delta receptors (δ) mediate spinal and supraspinal analgesia and potentiate the action of μ agonists. These receptors have been subtyped delta 1 and delta 2 and are implicated in terms of analgesia, location, function.

Kappa receptors (κ) mediate spinal analgesia, sedation, miosis, and dysphoria. Dynorphins are endogenous ligands at these receptors and morphine functions as the exogenous ligand. These receptors have been further subtyped as kappa 1, which mediates supraspinal analgesia, and kappa 2 whose function is not known (see Table 54.1).

Sigma receptors (σ), which are not considered opioid receptors (although opioid agonists may bind to sigma receptors), have been implicated in psychotomimetic and dysphoric side effects. They possibly cause dilation of the pupils (American Academy, 1997; Barkin & Fawcett, 2000; Barkin et al., 1998, 2002, 2005; Bartleson, 2002; Bonica, 1990; DeRuiter, 2000).

Opioid-receptor activation inhibits the presynaptic release and postsynaptic response to excitatory neurotransmitters (e.g., substance P) from nociceptive neurons. The cellular mechanism for this neuromodulation may involve alterations in potassium and calcium ion conductance leading to an influx of potassium and resultant hyperpolarization, which limits calcium intracellular entry. Furthermore, coupling of opioid receptors to G proteins results in decreased formation of intracellular cyclic adenosine monophosphate (cAMP), leading to a decrease in calcium channel phosphorylation and consequent diminished calcium entry. Opioid action on G proteins, which is independent of cAMP formation, directly diminishes calcium channel opening and enhances the opening of potassium channels. This sequence of events blocks substance P release, resulting in blockade of nociceptive transmission. Transmission of pain impulses can be interrupted at the level of the dorsal horn of the spinal cord with intrathecal or epidural administration of opioids. Modulation of a descending inhibitory pathway from the periaqueductal gray through the nucleus raphe magnus to the dorsal horn of the spinal cord may also play a role in opioid analgesia. These CNS areas are involved with pain perception, impulse integration, and pain response. Although opioids exert their greatest effect within the central nervous system, opioid receptors have also been isolated from somatic and sympathetic peripheral nerves. Effects on organ systems are listed in Table 54.1 (Barkin et al., 1998, 2002; Ellenhorn, 1997; McEvoy, 2004; Reves, 2002; Sabbe & Yaksh, 1990; Wickersham, 2003). Drug formulations of various opioid analgesics are arranged by chemical class in Table 54.2.

EFFECTS OF OPIOIDS ON SPECIFIC ORGAN SYSTEMS

CARDIOVASCULAR

Generally, opioids do not seriously affect cardiovascular (CV) function. However, high doses of certain opioids are associated with a vagus-mediated bradycardia. With the exception of meperidine, opioids do not depress contractility. However, blood pressure often falls as a result of bradycardia and decreased sympathetic activity. Also, opioids may evoke histamine release that can lead to decreases in arterial blood pressure and systemic vascular resistance. Areas in the brainstem that integrate CV responses and homeostasis include nucleus solitaris, dor-

sal vagal nucleus, nucleus ambiguous, and parabrachial nucleus (Barkin et al., 1998, 2005; Bonica, 1990; Cherny et al., 2001; Ellenhorn, 1997; McEvoy, 2004; Ready et al., 1995; Reisine & Pasternak, 1996; Reves, 2002; Rogers, 1991; Wickersham, 2003).

CENTRAL NERVOUS SYSTEM

In general, following a dose–response relationship, opioids decrease cerebral oxygen consumption cerebral blood flow and intracranial pressure. Stimulation of the medullary area postrema chemoreceptor trigger zone is responsible for the high incidence of nausea and vomiting. Physical dependence is a significant problem associated with chronic administration. Opioids do not reliably produce amnesia. Other effects on the CNS include euphoria, drowsiness, apathy, mental confusion, and mood alterations (Barkin & Barkin, 2001;. Barkin et al., 1998, 2005; Bonica, 1990; Cherny et al., 2001; Ellenhorn, 1997; McEvoy, 2004; Reisine & Pasternak, 1996; Reves, 2002; Wickersham, 2003).

RESPIRATORY

Opioids, by a dose–response relationship depress ventilation through brainstem respiratory centers, particularly respiratory rate and depth of respiration (minute ventilation) in patients at risk, especially with comorbidity. $PaCO_2$ (arterial partial pressure of carbon monoxide) increases and the response to a CO_2 challenge is blunted. This results in a shift of the CO_2 response curve down and to the right. These effects are mediated in the brainstem at the respiratory center. The hypoxic drive is decreased, and the apneic threshold (highest $PaCO_2$ at which a patient remains apneic) is increased. These effects are not usually clinically significant at typical therapeutic doses in otherwise healthy patients. Opioids, such as morphine, may induce histamine release causing bronchospasm in susceptible patients. Also, opioids cause a depression of the cough reflex center in the medulla creating antitussive activity (Barkin & Barkin, 2001; Barkin et al., 2005; Bonica, 1990; Cherny et al., 2001; McEvoy, 2004; Reisine & Pasternak, 1996; Reves, 2002; Sabbe & Yaksh, 1990; Wickersham, 2003).

GASTROINTESTINAL

Opioids slow gastric emptying time by decreasing peristalsis. The effect may be mediated by CNS mechanisms, as well as local organ effects. This may lead to constipation and esophageal reflux (lowers esophageal sphincter activity producing sphincter relaxation). In the biliary tract, the sphincter of Oddi constricts, leading to epigastric distress or biliary colic and increased biliary duct pressure and increased sphincter of Oddi tone in a dose-dependent manner (Barkin et al., 2002, 2005; Ellenhorn, 1997; McEvoy, 2004; Reisine & Pasternak, 1996; Wickersham, 2003; Zenz et al., 1992).

PHARMACOKINETICS AND PHARMACODYNAMICS

Patients exhibit interpatient/intrapatient variation in dose responses to opioids (see CV, CNS, respiration, GI discussion). A single opioid may not be appropriate for every patient; which to use is a multifactoral decision that includes considering the types of pain (eudynia or maldynia), pharmacokinetics, pharmacogenetics, and pharmacodynamics in a specific patient. The cytochrome P450 (CYP450) system is partially responsible for the metabolism of opioids, especially CYP450 2D6 and 3A4. An overview of this material is presented with each specific opioid and is reviewed in several references (Barkin & Barkin, 2001; Barkin et al., 2002, 2005; Barkin, Schwer, & Barkin, 1999; Cepeda et al., 2001; Davis & Walsh, 2001; DeRuiter, 2000; Gear et al., 1999; Hansten & Horn, 2004; McCarberg & Barkin, 2001; Raffa et al., 1992; Rogers, Nafziger, & Bertino, 2002; Tatro, 2004). See abbreviations list for an explanation of the abbreviations used in the specific opioid listings.

ABBREVIATIONS

2D6 cytochrome 2D6
3A cytochrome 3A
3A4 cytochrome 3A4
5-HT serotonin
AAG α_1 acid glycoprotein
ADR adverse drug reaction
APAP acetaminophen
ARF acute renal failure
AUC area under the curve
BBB blood–brain barrier
BP blood pressure
BZ benzodiazepine
C/I contraindications
Cl clearance
Cl$_{cr}$ creatine clearance
C$_{max}$ maximum concentration
C$_{min}$ minimum concentration
CNS central nervous system
CO cardiac output
CR controlled release
CRI chronic renal insufficiency
C$_{ss}$ steady-state concentration
CV cardiovascular
CYP cytochrome P450
D distribution

D/C discontinue
DPH diphenhydramine
epi epinephrine
EPS extrapyramidal side effects
ER extended release
F bioavailability
GI gastrointestinal
GIT gastrointestinal tract
H$_1$, H$_2$ histamine receptors
HA headache
HCl hydrochloride
HD hemodialysis
HR heart rate
HTN hypertension
IM intramuscular
IR immediate release
IV intravenous
LE lower extremity
M metabolism
M-3-G morphine-3-glucoride
M-6-G morphine-6-glucoride
M-1 O-desmethyltramadol
MAOI monoamine oxidase inhibitor
ml milliliter
MOA mechanism of action
N nausea
NE norepinephrine
NMDA *N*-methyl-D-aspartate
NS nasal spray
OH hydroxy
PCP phencyclidine
PCTA patient-controlled transdermal analgesia
PG pregnancy category
P-kin pharmacokinetics
PO oral route
PPB plasma protein binding
PR per rectum
RR respiratory rate
RUB reuptake blockers
S/E side effect
SC subcutaneous
SR sustained release
Sz seizure
τ dosing interval
T 1/2 β plasma elimination half-life
T$_{max}$ time to maximum concentration
V vomiting
Vd volume of distribution

CODEINE (PHENANTHRENE)

Weak analgesic mu (μ) and to a much lesser extent K$_1$, K$_3$, by its active metabolite morphine responsible for codeine analgesic effect; alone very weak mu affinity.

Duration of action: 4 to 6 h

Absorption: Rapid, and adequate oral

PPB%: 7% (plasma protein binding)

T 1/2 β: 3 h (codeine, 1.5 h; but increased up to 18.7 h with hemodialysis)

Metabolism: Prodrug: 10% to morphine by CYP2D6 and 3A3/4 dependent: followed by conjugation, 1% hydrocodone

Vd: 3.5 L/kg

Time to peak plasma level: 30 to 60 min all routes

Subject to genetic polymorphism (unable to metabolize) CYP 2D6 is absent in >10% of population

Onset: SC 15 to 30 min, duration analgesia 4 to 6 h, Peak analgesia 1 to 1.5 h

Onset analgesia PO: 30 to 60 min (peak PO analgesia 1 to 1.5 h)

Elimination: Unchanged, norcodeine, morphine, conjugated morphine, hydrocodone

Cl$_{cr}$ 10 to 50 ml/min: Administer ≤75% of dose utilized

Cl$_{cr}$ ≤ 10 ml/min: Administer ≤50% of dose utilized

Hepatic insufficiency: Dose adjustment

Renal dysfunction: Narcosis sedation may occur

Caution: Sulfite content

PG: C (D if chronic use or high doses at term), crosses placenta, in breast milk

References: Abramowitz, 2000; American Pain Society, 2003; Barkin & Barkin, 2001; Barkin et al., 2002, 2005; Carr et al., 1995; deGroot & Conemans, 1986; DeRuiter, 2000; Ellenhorn, 1997; Hansten & Horn, 2004; Kaiko et al., 1982; Lubenow, Ivankovich, & Barkin, 2005; McEvoy, 2004; Mokhlesi et al., 2003; Reisine & Pasternak, 1996; Tatro, 2003; Wickersham, 2004

DIHYDROCODEINE (PHENANTHRENE)

Mu and kappa agonist

Onset: ≤30 min

Duration: 4 to 6 h

Bioavailability (F): (21% range 12 to 34%) due to first pass

T 1/2 β: 3.3 to 4.5 h (similar in normal and renally impaired patients)

Similar to codeine in most respects pharmacokinetically, pharmacologically, and pharmacotherapeutically; a CYP450 2D6 substrate

Time to peak plasma levels: 1.6 to 1.8 h (greater in renally impaired)

AUC: Greater in renally impaired (area under the curve – plasma concentration time curve)

Prodrug: Morphine

PG: B: (D if chronic use or high doses at term) no information on lactation available

Metabolite: morphine salt

Renal dysfunction/impairment: Narcosis sedation may occur

Renal failure: Reduced systemic clearance or increased bioavailability

References: American Pain Society, 2003; Carr et al., 1995; Ellenhorn, 1997; Hansten & Horn, 2004; Kaiko et al., 1982; Lubenow et al., 2005; McEvoy, 2004; Mokhlesi et al., 2003; Reisine & Pasternak, 1996; Tatro, 2003; Wickersham, 2004

PENTAZOCINE

Partial agonist–antagonist

Mixed kappa 1 and kappa 3, sigma agonist, partial mu agonist/antagonist (supra spinal level); partial mu antagonist may precipitate abstinence in opiate dependence

F: About 20%, ↑ 60 to 70% in cirrhosis

PPB%: 60 to 70%

T 1/2 β: 2 to 3 h, ↑ with ↓ hepatic function

Metabolism: First pass hepatic metabolism 80%, Phase I/II pathways; CYP450 2D6 substrate

Side effects/ADRs: Euphoria, psych. (see below), weakness, miosis

C/I: Myocardial ischemia

Note: ↓ analgesic ceiling due to partial K agonist

CNS psychomimetic effects: Disorientation, confusion, dysphoria, hallucinations, delusions, seizure, CNS depression

Onset: PO, IM, SC: ≤15 to 30 min, IV ≤2 to 3 min

Parenteral dosage form may contain sulfites

Note: Smokers may require a 40 to 50% greater dose due to hepatic induction, another reason to avoid this opioid

Duration: PO: 4 to 5 h; parenteral: 2 to 3 h

Vd: 4.4 to 7.8 L/kg

Cl$_{cr}$ 10 to 50 ml/min: ≤75% of dose

Cl$_{cr}$ ≤ 10 ml/min: ≤50% of dose

Note: Infrequent use is recommended

PG: B (D if used chronically or high dose at term) crosses placenta

References: Abramowitz, 2000; Alexander & Spence, 1974; American Pain Society, 2003; Barkin & Barkin, 2001; Barkin et al., 2002; Carr et al., 1995; Challoner, McCaroon, & Newton, 1990; De Bard & Jagger, 1982; DeRuiter, 2000; Ellenhorn, 1997; Hansten & Horn, 2004; Hanunen et al., 1993; Kaiko et al., 1982; Lubenow et al., 2005; McEvoy, 2004; Mokhlesi et al., 2003; Reed & Schnoll, 1994; Reisine & Pasternak, 1996; Tatro, 2003; Wickersham, 2003

FENTANYL (PHENYLPIPERIDINE)

Mu agonist, lesser kappa agonist

Peak plasma level: ≤30 min IM

PPB%: 84 (range 80 to 86), basic drug binds to α_1 AGP (acid glycoprotein)

Peak analgesia: 3 to 5 min

IV analgesia: Onset ≤ 3 to 5 min

Analgesia duration: 30 to 60 min

T 1/2 β: 1.5 to 6 h (average: 2 to 4 h) transmucosal T 1/2 β 5 to 15 h (average 6.6 h)

F: Transmucosal ≈ 50% (range 36 to 71%); transdermal = 92%

Metabolism: Rapid hepatic n-dealkylation via CYP450–3A4 enzyme and hydroxylation, ≤10% unchanged

Elimination: Up to 85% in urine ≈ 3 to 4 days; 6 to 10% unchanged; metabolites

ADRs: Respiratory depression (especially with doses > 200 μg, rigidity (skeletal muscle and thoracic) — some irritation and pruritus (perinasal)

Onset: Transdermal 8 to 12 up to 24 h, duration 72 h (duragesic dose form only)

Transmucosal: Onset: 5 to 15 min; peak: 20 to 30 min; absorption: rapid 25% buccal, 75% if swallowed, and slowly from GI tract; cancer pain indication

BBB alterations change active transport in and out of brain tissue

Transdermal semipermeable membrane system: 25 μg/10 cm² increments (duragesic dose form only); avoid silicone base matrix forms, interchange or substitute not recommended

Distribution Vd: 4 L/kg; highly lipophilic, redistributes into the muscle and fat up to 75% of an initial dose undergoes first pass pulmonary uptake

Note: Almost no H_2 release, $T \geq 104$ ↑ fentanyl transdermal absorption

If Cl_{cr} is 10 to 50, use 75% of the normal dose, and if the Cl_{cr} is lower, use 50% or less of the normal dose

Patient-controlled transdermal fentanyl delivery system for acute postoperative pain management (PTCA, a needle-less credit card–sized system using the E-trans® (IONSYS®) system, is a self-contained, on-demand preprogrammed system utilizing iontophoresis for transdermal delivery of 40 μg per demand dose and operates for up to 24 h with no more than 80 doses, whichever comes first)

PG: B (D if chronic use or high dose at term), crosses placenta

References: Abramowitz, 2004; American Pain Society, 2003; Barkin & Barkin, 2001; Barkin et al., 2002; Bennett & Adams, 1983; Carr et al., 1995; DeRuiter, 2000;Ellenhorn, 1997; Fine, 1997; Hansten & Horn, 2004; Jeal & Benfield, 1997; Kaiko et al., 1982; Lubenow et al., 2005; McCarberg & Barkin, 2001; McEvoy, 2004; Mokhlesi et al., 2003; Reisine & Pasternak, 1996; Schechter et al., 1995; Scholz, Steinfath, & Schulz, 1996; Simpson et al., 1997; Stoukides & Stegman, 1992; Tatro, 2004; Wickersham, 2004

MORPHINE (PHENANTHRENE)

Mu agonist, less kappa, agonist (K_1 K_2) generally in the midbrain, medulla, and spinal cord and more specifically in periaqueductal and periventricular gray matter, the ventromedial medulla, and the dorsal horn on the spinal cord. CNS tissues involved in pain perception, integration responses: frontal cortex, limbic system (amygdala, hypothalamus, thalamus), area postrema chemoreceptor trigger zone (CRTZ), nucleus solitary tract cough center. Peripheral tissues: substantia gelatinosa dorsal horn spinal cord.

Duration: 4 to 5 h (IR)

F (oral): ≤40% (20 to 40% range)

Absorption: Oral route interindividual variable, rapid and incomplete 2.5 to 7 h due to variable extensive presystemic metabolism (bioavailability increased in hepatic dysfunction)

PPB%: 20 to 35% primarily to plasma albumins (M-6-G) α_1 acid glycoprotein (stress, surgery, inflammation, chronic pain, and carcinoma)

T 1/2 β: 3 h (M) range 2 to 4 h; 15 for 48 h blood levels

Vd: 1 to 6 L/kg; average 3 to 4 L/kg (lower in elderly patients)

Distribution: Following absorption: skeletal muscle, renal tissue, hepatic tissue, GI tract, spleen, and the CNS

Cl: Hepatic for morphine, renal for M-6-G

P-kin: Linear

C_{ss}: Several days

Hydrophilic (small amounts cross the BBB)

M-6-G analgesia ≥ than parent (T 1/2 β: 1.75 h)

M-3-G T 1/2 β: 2.75 h

Peak plasma level: ≤1 h SC/IM route

Metabolism: A CYP450-2D6 substrate followed by Phase II pathway. Hepatic: M-3-G (major metabolite) M-6-G (minor metabolite) causes seizures and some respiratory depression, nausea, and sedation under special circumstances; extrahepatic gut metabolism (gastric, small intestine) and enterohepatic recycling

PO plasma levels: 1/5 to 1/3 of parenteral route

Elimination: Bile 7 to 10%

S/E: Hypotension, dizziness, histamine release, pruritus (more common with epidural and intrathecal administration), peripheral vasodilation, sinus bradycardia, constipation

Onset: Analgesia PO (IR): 15 to 60 min, duration 4 to 6 h

Onset: Analgesia PO (SR): 2 to 4 h duration 8/12 to 17 h or more (24 h) (Kadian)

Onset: Analgesia parenteral route SC 30 to 50 min, IM 30 to 60 min

Peak analgesia, IV: 20 min

Duration of analgesia by IM or IV route: 4 to 5 h

Elimination: Excreted unchanged in the urine 8.5 to 12%, and 7 to 10% as glucuronidation in the feces

Constipation: Enhancing the tone in the long segments of the longitudinal muscle and inhibiting propulsive contraction of both circular and longitudinal muscle (prophylactic bowel management)

Cl_{cr} 10 to 50 ml/min: Utilize 75% of normal dose

Cl_{cr} ≤ 10 ml/min: Utilize 50% or less of normal dose

PG: B (D if chronic use or high dose at term)

References: Abramowitz, 2000; American Pain Society, 2003; Barkin, 1988; Barkin & Barkin, 2001; Barkin et al., 2002; Braunwald et al., 2003; Brunk & Delle, 1974; Caldwell et al., 2002; Dampler et al., 1995; Carr et al., 1995; DeRuiter, 2000; Duthie & Nimmo, 1987; Ellenhorn, 1997; Hansten & Horn, 2004; Henry & Volans, 1985; Holdsworth et al., 1995; Jacobi et al., 2003; Jadad et al., 1992; Kaiko, 1980; Kaiko et al., 1982; Lorenz, Beck, & Bromm, 1997; Lubenow et al., 2005; Maier et al., 2002; McCarberg & Barkin, 2001; McEvoy, 2004; McRorie et al., 1982; Mokhlesi et al., 2003; Reisine & Pasternak, 1996; Richtsmeier, Barnes, & Barkin, 1997; Schug, Zech, & Grond, 1992; Tatro, 2003; Wickersham, 2004

MEPERIDINE (PETHIDINE)

Phenylpiperidine

Mu_1 Mu_2 agonist supraspinally and reuptake blockade monoamines spinally

Peak plasma level PO or IM: 1 to 2 h

F: 50 to 60%, ↑ liver disease

Duration: 2 h to 5 h, onset 10 to 45 min, peak: 0.5 to 1 h

PPB%: 55 to 75 (α_1 acid glycoprotein, an acute phase reactant) basic drug

T 1/2 β meperidine: 2.5 to 4 h (3 to 4 by IV route); liver disease: 7 to 11 h

T 1/2 β (normeperidine): Nonopioid, 15 to 30 h renal function dependent, accumulates with high doses and/or renal function compromised

Metabolism: CYP450-2D6 substrate n-demethylation → normeperidine → Phase II → de-esterified to normeperidinic acid; reduced metabolism in hepatitis; repeat doses accumulate

Lipophilic

Higher dose: Normeperidine produces anxiety, hyperactivity, dysphoria, tremors, myoclonus, seizures, and hyperflexia upon accumulation and/or repeated dosing not naloxone reversible; atropinic

Now falling into disuse, avoid administration during renal or hepatic dysfunctions

Normeperidine: CNS excitation producing neurotoxicity

Elimination: 50% as unchanged

Note: Sulfites; some preparations; may produce serotonin syndrome with SSRIs; anticholinergic, local anesthetic, orthostatic hypotension, fatality

C/I: MAOI agents (delirium, hypertensive crisis, serotonin syndrome)

PG: B (D if used chronically or at high doses at term), appears in breast milk

References: Abramowitz, 2000; American Pain Society, 2003; Armstrong & Bersten, 1986; Barkin & Barkin, 2001; Barkin & Stein, 1989; Barkin et al., 2002; Carr et al., 1995; DeRuiter, 2000; Ellenhorn, 1997; Hansten & Horn, 2004; Kaiko et al., 1982; Latta, Ginsberg, & Barkin, 2002; Leikin et al., 1990; Lubenow et al., 2005; McCarberg & Barkin, 2001; McEvoy, 2004; Mokhlesi et al., 2003; Reisine & Pasternak, 1996; Tatro, 2003; Wickersham, 2004

METHADONE

A racemic mixture (diphenylheptane)

Mu agonist, non-opioid NMDA antagonism (d-isomer) blocks Ca^{2+} channel, lesser kappa agonist, possibly strong delta receptor activity; chronic exposure desensitizes mu and delta receptors-l-isomer, 5-HT/NE RUB (reuptake blockers)-d-isomer

Duration: 4 to 6 h (up to 8 h following chronic dosing) for analgesia, analgesic onset 30 to 60 min, analgesic peak 0.5 to 1 h; following repeat dosing, the drug accumulated with repeated dosing, necessitating frequent monitoring and dosage reductions, particularly during the first several days after starting the medication

PPB%: 80 to 89%

F: 92%

T 1/2 β: 15 to 25 h/single dose, range 13 to 47 h, 48 to 72 h (average 24 to 36 h) with multiple dosing, prolonged with alkaline pH

Vd: 3.8 L/kg — wide tissue distribution

S/E: LE, edema, (antidiuretic effect) sedation, dizziness, hypotension, bradycardia, peripheral vasodilation, palpitations, histamine release, (less euphoria), libido decrements, dysphoria

Metabolism: CYP 1A2, 2D6, 3A4, substrate N-demethylation; metabolite: active N-demethylated methadone, which is 2-ethyldene-1,5-dimethyl-3,3-diphenylpyrrolidene (EDDP) accumulation: due to long T 1/2

Elimination: 52% urine (10% unchanged)

Note: Avoid use in hepatic disease; may cause dose-related interpatient variation (torsades de pointes, which is dose related, particularly at high doses)

Absorption: PO rapid, incomplete

$Cl_{cr} \leq 10$ ml/min: tilize 50 to 75% or less of the dose

PG: C, crosses placenta

References: Abramowitz, 2000; American Pain Society, 2003; Barkin & Barkin, 2001; Barkin et al., 2002; Bartolome & Kuhn, 1983; Carr et al., 1995; DeRuiter, 2000; Ellenhorn, 1997; Fishman et al., 2002; Gardner-Nix, 1996; Garrido & Troconiz, 1999; Hansten & Horn, 2004; Kaiko et al., 1982; Krantz et al., 2002; Lubenow et al., 2005; McCarberg & Barkin, 2001; McEvoy, 2004; Mokhlesi et al., 2003; Morley et al., 1993; Olkkola, Hamunen, & Maunuksela, 1995; Reisine & Pasternak, 1996; Tatro, 2003; Wasserman & Yahr, 1980; Weschules et al., 2003; Wheeler & Dickerson, 2000; Wickersham, 2004

LEVORPHANOL (PHENANTHRENE, MORPHINAN DERIVATIVE)

Mu agonist, K_3 agonist, NMDA receptor antagonist

Peak plasma level: 1.5 to 2 h PO; 0.5 to 1.0 h IM

T 1/2 β: 12 to 16 h

C_{ss}: 2 to 4 days

Metabolism: Phase II, adipose tissue accumulates

S/E: Less nausea, vomiting, and constipation than morphine; fatigue, drowsiness, bradycardia, CNS depression, pruritus, peripheral vasodilation, palpitations, hypotension

Onset: Analgesia 10 to 30 min

Peak: Analgesia 0.5 to 1 h

Duration: Analgesia 6 to 8 h

Accumulates within 2 to 3 days of continuous administration

Elimination: 60% in the urine within 4 days, 7% unchanged, feces: 37% in approximately 4 days

PG: B (D if chronic use or high dose at term)

References: Abramowitz, 2000; American Pain Society, 2003; Barkin & Barkin, 2001; Barkin et al., 2002; Carr et al., 1995; DeRuiter, 2000; Ellenhorn, 1997; Hansten & Horn, 2004; Kaiko et al., 1982; Lubenow et al., 2005; McCarberg & Barkin, 2001; McEvoy, 2004; Mokhlesi et al., 2003; Reisine & Pasternak, 1996; Tatro, 2003; Wickersham, 2003

BUPRENORPHINE

Semisynthetic lipophilic thebaine derived opioid

Mu_1, partial agonist, centrally acting, some kappa opioid receptor antagonist activity seen at higher doses

Onset: Analgesia IM 10 to 30 min (mean 15 min), peak analgesia 1 h (IV: shorter onset and peak)

Duration: 6 to 8 h or longer

F: 90 to 100% IM

Peak plasma level: 4 to 5 min IV, 30 to 60 min following the IM

PPB%: 96 (α and β globulin)

Absorption: 90 to 100% parenterally, sublingually 31%

T 1/2 β: 2 to 3.5 (mean 3.7 h)

Vd: 97 to 187 L

Elimination: 70% in feces by bile, 30% in urine unchanged, up to 11 days post D/C of the drug

Metabolism: n-Dealkylation, CYP450-3A4; a weak analgesic; 3-G buprenorphine

Compared to placebo no significant differences in BP, HR, RR

Very slow disassociation from mu_1 receptor

Mixed agonist (mu_1) antagonist (K) (detox, opiate dependent) due in part to low physical dependence

Renal failure: Both norbuprenorphine and 3-G buprenorphine are increased

PG: C

Note: Established safety and effectiveness in children 2 to 12 years; SL dosage form alone and in combination with N haloxone is available for chemical dependency treatment

References: Abramowitz, 2000; American Pain Society, 2003; Barkin & Barkin, 2001; Barkin et al., 2002; Carr et al., 1995; DeRuiter, 2000; Ellenhorn, 1997; Gal, 1989; Hansten & Horn, 2004; Harcus, Ward, & Smith, 1980; Kaiko et al., 1982; Lubenow et al., 2005; Mac Evilly & O'Carroll, 1989; McCarberg & Barkin, 2001; McEvoy, 2004; Mokhlesi et al., 2003; Reisine & Pasternak, 1996; Rolandi et al., 1983; Tatro, 2003

NALBUPHINE

Kappa, sigma agonist, mu antagonism

F: 6 to 20% PO absorbed

Peak plasma level: 30 min IM

Onset: Analgesia IV 12 to 30 min, 10 to 15 min SC/IM

Peak: (IM) 60 min, IV 30 min

Duration: Analgesia 3 to 6 h

Elimination: Renal

T 1/2 β: 5 h, 2 to 3 h (elderly)

Vd: 3 to 14 L/kg

Metabolism: *n*-Dealkylation: first pass; Phase II, excreted in the stool via the bile; and excreted in the urine about 7%; no active metabolites

S/E: Limited ceiling effects, opiate abstinence, dysphoria, psychomimetic effects (less than pentazocine), HA, histamine release

May precipitate abstinence in some opiate-dependent patients

Some products contain sulfites

PG: B (D if used chronically at high doses at term)

References: Abramowitz, 2000; American Pain Society, 2003; Barkin & Barkin, 2001; Barkin et al., 2002; Carr et al., 1995; DeRuiter, 2000; Ellenhorn, 1997; Errick & Heel, 1983; Gear et al., 1999; Hansten & Horn, 2004; Hoskin & Hanks, 1991; Jallion et al., 1989; Kaiko et al., 1982; Leikin et al., 1990; Lubenow et al., 2005; McCarberg & Barkin, 2001; McEvoy, 2004; Mokhlesi et al., 2003; Reisine & Pasternak, 1996; Tatro, 2003; Wickersham, 2004; Yoo et al., 1995

HYDROMORPHONE (PHENANTHRENE)

Dihydromorphone

Chemistry: 4,5 α-Epoxy-3-hydroxy-17-methylmorphinan-6-one HC1

$Mu_{1,2}$ (μ_1 μ_2) agonist, (δ) lesser K agonist and delta

Metabolism: To three major metabolites — hydromorphone-3-glucuronide (H-3-G) and 3-glucoside and dihydroisomorphine-6-glucuranide — and three other but minor metabolites, inhibitor (mild) of $CYP1A^2$, 2A6, 2C8, 2D6, 3A4; hydrophilic

Vd: 4 L/kg oral, 295 L (IV route)

C_{max}: 3 ng/ml (maximum exposure)

T_{max}: Poorly defined IR-AUC (0 to 24) ng.h/ml

Mean minimum plasma concentration ng/ml.7 ng/ml

C_{min}: 0.7 ng/ml

Cl: 1.66 L/h for IV

F: 51 to 62% (immediate release)

Accumulates in renal impairment (neurotoxicity, H-3-G metabolism, also seizures, myoclonus, allodynia)

Distribution: Skeletal muscle, liver, GIT, lungs, spleen, brain, plasma, urine

S/E: Myoclonus (clonazepam responsive), feelings of relaxation, euphoria, restlessness, palpitations, histamine release, (pruritus, flushing, red eye, diaphoresis, orthostatic, hypotension), peripheral vasodilation, $\uparrow$ transaminases, elevated asthenia, respirator decrements, headache, constipation, nausea, emesis, somnolence

Onset: Analgesia (IR) 30 to 60 min, duration analgesia 4 to 6 h, 5 min parenterally (peak $\leq$ 20 min)

Onset: Analgesia (CR) 2 to 4 h; duration analgesia 8 to 24 h

T 1/2 β: 2 to 3 h, 18.6 h (CR)

Elimination: 6% renally unchanged in $\leq$24 h; and elimination: $\uparrow$ concentration in bile of both parent and metabolite, found in feces

PG: B (D if used chronically or at term) crosses placenta; C, for CR form

Renal impairment: Modify doses

Metabolites found in plasma, urine, hepatocytes; two CR (24-h) dosage forms; currently one has a 10% bolus dose release action

References: Abramowitz, 2000; American Pain Society, 2003; Barkin & Barkin, 2001; Barkin et al., 2002; Carr et al., 1995; DeRuiter, 2000; Ellenhorn, 1997; Hansten & Horn, 2004; Honigberg & Stewart, 1980; Kaiko et al., 1982; Lubenow et al., 2005; McCarberg & Barkin, 2001; McEvoy, 2004; Mokhlesi et al., 2003; Moulin et al., 1991; Nasraway, 2001; Reisine & Pasternak, 1996; Tatro, 2003; Wickersham, 2004

HYDROCODONE (PHENANTHRENE)

Differs from codeine by a single bond between C-7 and C-8 and a ketone rather than OH group at C-6

Dihydrocodeinone

Absorption: Well absorbed

Elimination: Urine (26% in 72 h, 12% as unchanged)

Metabolism: Liver to hydromorphone via CYP (2D6), nor-codeine, and 12% unchanged drug by *O*-demethylation

Onset: Analgesia 30 to 60 min

Duration: Analgesia 3 to 8 h

T 1/2 β: 3.8 to 4.5 h; peak serum level: 1 h

Peak: Analgesia 2 h

PG: C

Renal: $\downarrow$ dose in ARF or CRI

Note: Association with abuse noted (euphoria), similar to oxycodone

ADRs: Anxiety; euphoria at the therapeutic doses 5 to 10 mg; addiction potential exceeds codeine and may rival oxycodone abuse

References: Abramowitz, 2000; American Pain Society, 2003; Barkin & Barkin, 2001; Barkin et al., 2002; Carr et al., 1995; DeRuiter, 2000; Ellenhorn, 1997; Hansten & Horn, 2004; Kaiko et al., 1982; Lubenow et al., 2005; McCarberg & Barkin, 2001; McEvoy, 2004; Mokhlesi et al., 2003; Reisine & Pasternak, 1996; Tatro, 2003; Wickersham, 2004

OXYCODONE (PHENANTHRENE)

Morphinan-6-one, 4,5 epoxy-14-hydroxy-3-methoxy-17-methyl hydrochloride (5α)(7,8-dihydro-14-hydroxycodeinone; or 4,5α-epoxy-14-hydroxy-3-methoxy-17-methylmorhpinan-6-one-HCl) receptors: mu_1, mu_2 agonist via its metabolite, kappa agonist (strong)

F: 60 to 80% (due to lower presystemic or first-pass metabolism); increased by 15% in elderly and 50% in renal dysfunction

T 1/2 β: 3.5 to 4 h (single dose)

Onset: Analgesia (IR): 15 to 60 min; duration analgesia: 4 to 6 h

Onset: Analgesia (CR): ≤ 1 (rapid absorption bolus dose release phase); duration analgesia 6 to 12 h, bolus release $\approx 37\%$ release ≤ 2 h post-ingestion

C_{max}: 13 to 19 ng/ml

AUC: 72 to 84 ng × h/ml (multiple dosing)

Peak analgesia: ≤ 60 min

Vd: 2.6 L/kg

T_{max}: 1 to 1.6 h

PPB: 45%

C_{ss}: 24 to 36 h (CR form) with 12-h dosing

Vd at steady state: 2.39 L/kg

Distribution: Highly perfused tissues: muscle (skeletal), intestinal tract, pulmonary, spleen, CNS (brain), hepatic

ADRs: Euphoria, feeling of relaxation, constipation (decreased gastrointestinal motility), ataxia, sedation, diaphoresis, histamine release, confusion, anorexia, memory deficits, hypotension, fatigue, drowsiness, nervousness, HA, restlessness, malaise, miosis, endocrine changes, autonomic nervous system changes, respiratory depression

Metabolism: Oxymorphone (1/10 plasma concentration of oxycodone), noroxycodone by *N*-demethylated to noroxycodone and *O*-demethylation (for oxycodone to oxymorphone) to glu-

curonides — a pharmacologically active weaker analgesic

CYP450: 2D6 substrate to oxymorphone

Cl systemic: 16.7 ml/kg/min

Elimination: Excretion in urine: 33 to 61% in 24 h, 13 to 19% free (unchanged conjugated $\leq 50\%$ and noroxycodone conjugated oxymorphone $\leq 14\%$ not quantified free or conjugated)

Renal failure (anesthetized patient): T 1/2 β = 3.9 h

End stage renal disease: Prolonged T 1/2 β due to $\uparrow$ Vd and $\downarrow$ Cl, if $Cl_{cr} \leq 60$ ml/min then $\downarrow Cl_{cr}$ and $\uparrow$ AUC

Hepatic impairment: If occurs $\uparrow$ AUC

AUC = Extent of absorption

PG: B (D if used chronically or in high doses found in breast milk)

Gender: Opiate-naïve females have 25% higher plasma concentration than males

Note: Opiate dependence, prominent, addiction liability, CR dosage form provides a bolus dose of $\approx 38\%$ within 1 to 2 h of ingestion

References: Abramowitz, 2000; American Pain Society, 2003; Barkin & Barkin, 2001; Barkin et al., 2002; Bruera et al., 1998; Carr et al., 1995; DeRuiter, 2000; Ellenhorn, 1997; Hansten & Horn, 2004; Kaiko et al., 1982; Kalso & Vainio, 1990; Lubenow et al., 2005; McCarberg & Barkin, 2001; McEvoy, 2004; Mokhlesi et al., 2003; Reisine & Pasternak, 1996; Roth et al., 2000; Tatro, 2003; Turturro & O'Toole, 1991; Wickersham, 2004

PROPOXYPHENE

Weak mu binding for analgesia is 1/2 that of codeine and possible kappa subtype affinity, noncompetitive NMDA antagonist

Structurally similar to methadone

F: 30 to 70% due to significant hepatic first pass

Absorption: Complete

Metabolism: First pass to norpropoxyphene (a non opioid) arrhythmogenic agent and local anesthetic effect, also associated with pulmonary edema and seizures

PPB: 78%

T 1/2 β: 6 to 12 h up to 15 h parent (37 h in elderly); norpropoxyphene: 30 to 36 h (up to 42 h in elderly patients)

Onset: Analgesia 30 to 60 min; Duration 4 to 6 h; peak plasma concentration in 2 to 2.5 h

S/E: Euphoria, false sense of well-being, hypotension, dizziness, lightheadedness, nausea, vomiting, sedation, malaise, paradoxical excitation, nightmares, insomnia, fatigue, drowsiness, auditory hallucinations, weakness, histamine release, depression, pulmonary edema, PQRS prolongation, arrhythmias, trembling, tinnitus, subacute painful myopathy, seizures

Elimination: 20 to 25% excreted in urine

Nor-propoxyphene not reversible by naloxone and leads to cardiac arrhythmias and pulmonary edema, and accumulates

An agent falling into significant disuse; discourage use in elderly patients

A CYP450 system inhibitor at 3A 3/4

Poor analgesia but prominent euphoria, avoid use in elderly patients (metabolism reduced)

PG: C (D if chronic use); possible human teratogen, cranial/facial abnormalities, limbs absent

References: Abramowitz, 2000; American Pain Society, 2003; Barkin & Barkin, 2001; Barkin et al., 2002; Carr et al., 1995; DeRuiter, 2000; Ellenhorn, 1997; Finkle, 1984; Hansten & Horn, 2004; Kaiko et al., 1982; Lawson & Northridge, 1987; Lubenow et al., 2005; McCarberg & Barkin, 2001; McEvoy, 2004; Mokhlesi et al., 2003; Proudfoot, 1984; Reisine & Pasternak, 1996; Stork et al., 1995; Tatro, 2003; Tennant, 1973; Wetli & Bednarczyk, 1980; Wickersham, 2004

BUTORPHANOL

Kappa$_1$ agonist and antagonist effects (methadone, propoxyphene)

Peak: IM ≤ 30 to 60 min, NS and IV ≤ 4 to 5 min

Absorption: Rapid and well

S/E: Psychomimetic anxiety, confusion, dysphoria, euphoria, somnolence, hallucinations, S, D, N, V, insomnia, peripheral edema, dizziness, vasodilation palpitations, nausea, emesis

PPB: 83%

Metabolism: Extensive first pass in the liver: hydroxylation, N-demethylation

T 1/2 β: 2.5 to 4 h

Elimination: 11 to 15% excreted in bile, 72% in urine within 96 h

Cl$_{cr}$: When ≤60, consider decreasing dose by 50 to 75%

Onset of analgesia: IM within 10 min

PG: B (D with chronic use or high dose at term) crosses placenta, distributes to breast milk

References: Abramowitz, 2000; American Pain Society, 2003; Barkin, 1996a; Barkin & Barkin, 2001; Barkin et al., 2002; Bennie et al., 1998; Carr et al., 1995; DeRuiter, 2000; Ellenhorn, 1997; Gaver et al., 1980; Hansten & Horn, 2004; Kaiko et al., 1982; Lubenow et al., 2005; McCarberg & Barkin, 2001; McEvoy, 2004; Melanson et al., 1997; Mokhlesi et al., 2003;

Pachter & Evens, 1985; Ramsey et al., 1986; Reisine & Pasternak, 1996; Shyu, Morgenthien, & Barbhaiya, 1996; Tatro, 2003; Vachharajani et al., 1996, 1997; Wickersham, 2004

TRAMADOL

Cyclohexanol

Mu$_1$, opioid receptor effects supraspinally

5-HT, NE, reuptake blockade spinally

CYP450 substrate: 2D6 → M1 metabolite, 3A4 for MI metabolite

Analgesia ≥ codeine, hydrocodone, oxycodone, meperidine, propoxyphene

T 1/2 β: With APAP: 325 mg/tramadol/37.5 mg dosage form: 7 to 9 h (preferred dosage form)

T 1/2 β: Tramadol alone: 6 h, M1: metabolite 7 h

Maximum dosage: 8 tablets per day

Elimination: Renal: ≤10% removed by HD (hemodialysis)

F: 75%

Onset analgesia: ≤1 h, Peak analgesia 2 to 4 h, duration analgesia 6 h

Relative lack of opiate dependence

PPB: 20%

Metabolism: Demethylation, glucuronidation, sulfation

Metabolite: M1 (N-demethylation by CYP 2D6; M1 (deomethyltramadol) is six times more potent an analgesic with 200 more times affinity for mu$_1$ receptor

PG: C; placenta crossing

References: Abramowitz, 2000; American Pain Society, 2003; Barkin, 1995a, b, 1996b; Barkin & Barkin, 2001; Barkin et al., 2002; Carr et al., 1995; Collins et al., 1997; Dayer, Collart, & Desmeules, 1994; DeRuiter, 2000; Ellenhorn, 1997; Gaver et al., 1980; Gaynes & Barkin, 1999; Hansten & Horn, 2004; Lewis & Han, 1997; Kaiko et al., 1982; Lubenow et al., 2005; McCarberg & Barkin, 2001; McCarberg et al., 2003; McEvoy, 2004; Mehlisch, Brown, Lefner et al., 1993; Mokhlesi et al., 2003; Rauck, Ruoff, & McGillen, 1994; Reisine & Pasternak, 1996; Ruoff, 1999; Tatro, 2003; Wickersham, 2004

KETAMINE

MOA: NMDA (N-methyl-D-aspartate) antagonist, chiral compound, administered as racemic mixture, S(+) isomer 2× analgesic; some opiate agonist effects (PCP similarity)

P-kin: Bi- or tri-exponential elimination pattern; potency of mixture; S(+) is 3× potency of R(−) isomer

Analgesia duration: 30 to 40 min

Unconsciousness duration: 10 to 15 min

Amnesia duration: up to 1-2 hours

Vd: 3 to 5 L/kg

PPB: 30%; basic to α_1 AAG

Metabolism: Hepatic (hydroxylation, N-demethylation; nor-ketamine (π activity of parent), dihyronorketamine

T 1/2 β: 1 to 3 h; α: 10 to 15 min anesthetic phase, redistribution to the peripheral tissues (from the CNS) followed by hepatic metabolism T 1/2 β: 2.5 h

Elimination: Renal, with renal impairment increased plasma concentration of metabolites (norketamine; glucuronides)

ADRs:

CV: catecholamine (NE/epi) released/elevated → sympathomimetic effects: tachycardia, ↑ CO, HTN

GI: N, V

CNS: Visual hallucinations, vivid unpleasant dreams, confusion, irrational behaviors, ↑intracranial pressure

Neuromuscular: Tonic-clonic, myoclonic movements, tremors

Miscellaneous: Emergence reaction (dysphoria/euphoria), vocalization (avoid in psychosis prone patients); residual psychomotor impairment upon awakening (hangover)

BZs useful for delirium, dysphoria, hallucinations, Sz

BZs and DPH: Useful for EPS (benzodiazepine, diphenhydramine)

BZs, α_2 agonist (clonidine), beta-blockers, calcium channel blockers

(verapamil) useful for ↓ cardiac stimulation

Atropine for hypersalivation

PG: D (crosses placenta)

References: Abramowitz, 2000; American Pain Society, 2003; Barkin & Barkin, 2001; Barkin et al., 2002; Carr et al., 1995; Clements & Nimmo, 1981; DeRuiter, 2000; Ellenhorn, 1997; Felser & Orban, 1982; Hansten & Horn, 2004; Hartvig et al., 1995; Kaiko et al., 1982; Lubenow et al., 2005; McCarberg & Barkin, 2001; McEvoy, 2004; Mokhlesi et al., 2003; Reisine & Pasternak, 1996; Tatro, 2003; Wickersham, 2004

OXYMORPHONE (PHENANTHRENE)

Chemistry: 4,5α-Epoxy-3-14-dihydroxy-17-methyl morphinan-6-one HCI (similar chemistry to hydromorphone)

Mu_1 agonist specifically

Linear pharmacokinetics

Absorption: PO: rapid IR: T_{max} = 0.5 h; ER: T_{max} = 2.5 to 4 h

Onset: Parenteral: 5 to 10 min

PR: 15 to 30 min

Duration: PR/parenteral 3 to 4 h

Metabolism: (1) Phase II hepatic glucuronidation; extensive first pass (PO); (2) reduction to 6-OH; 6-OH analgesic potency similar to parent, about 70% of AUC; (3) very minor Phase I metabolism; CYP450 1A2, 2D6, 3A4; (4) not sufficiently metabolized CYP450

Metabolites: 0-3-G (plasma, urine), 33 to 38% 0-3-G; 6-OH 0.25 to 0.62%

Excretion: Enterohepatic recycling bilary — parent and metabolite, urine (≤1% unchanged, parent)

PPB: Not extensive (10 to 12%)

C_{max} (μg/ml):1.16 (0.17)

T 1/2 β: 13.46 (3.38) h

C_{ss}: 3 days

Solubility: Lipophilic (access to neurovascular membrane–BBB–spinal cord)

Remains in CNS aqueous phase without redistribution; slow dissociation from CNS receptor sites

Linear dose–response curve

ADRs:

CV: Hypotension

CNS: Fatigue, drowsiness, dizziness

Skeletal/neuromuscular: Weakness

Miscellaneous: Histamine release, ureteral spasm, diminished micturation

CNS: Nervousness, cephalgia, restlessness, malaise, confusion

GI: anorexia, abdominal cramps and xerostomia, biliary spasms

Local: Injection site pain

PG: B/D, prolonged use or high dose at term; excreted in breast milk

Sulfites: Some preparations (parenteral) contain

Forms: Oral (IR, ER as 12 h), these two new dosage forms to be released shortly; CR: low fluctuations; parenteral rectal

References: Abramowitz, 2000; Adams & Ahdieh, 2004; American Pain Society, 2003; Barkin & Barkin, 2001; Barkin et al., 2002; Carr et al., 1995; DeRuiter, 2000; Eddy & Lee, 1959; Ellenhorn, 1997; Hansten & Horn, 2004; Kaiko et al., 1982; Lubenow et al., 2005; McCarberg & Barkin, 2001; McEvoy, 2004; Mokhlesi et

al., 2003; Reisine & Pasternak, 1996; Sinatra
& Harrison, 1989; Sinatra, Hyde, & Harrison,
1988; Tatro, 2003; Wickersham, 2004

REFERENCES

Abramowitz, M. (Ed.). (2004). Drugs for pain. *Medical Letter on Drugs and Therapeutics, 42*, 73.

Adams, H., & Ahdieh, H. (2004). Single- and multiple-dose pharmacokinetics and dose-proportionality study of oxymorphone immediate-release tablets, *Pharmacotherapy, 24*(4), 468–476.

Alexander, J. L., & Spence, A. A. (1974). Central nervous effects of pentazocine. *British Medical Journal, 2*, 224.

American Academy of Pain Medicine and American Pain Society. (1997). *The use of opioids for the treatment of chronic pain.* Glenview, IL: Author.

American Pain Society. (2003). *Principles of analgesic use in the treatment of acute pain and chronic cancer pain* (5th ed.), Glenview, IL: Author.

Armstrong, P. J., & Bersten, A. (1986). Normeperidine toxicity. *Anesthesia and Analgesia, 65*, 536.

Ashburn, M., & Ready, L. (2001). Postoperative pain. In J. Loeser, S. Butler, C. Chapman, & D. Turk (Eds.), *Bonica's management of pain* (Chap. 41). Philadelphia, PA: Lippincott Williams & Wilkins.

Ashburn, M. A., & Staats, P. S. (1999). Management of chronic pain. *Lancet, 353*(9167), 1865–1869.

Ballantyne, J. C, et al. (1993). Postoperative patient-controlled analgesia: Meta-analyses of initial randomized control trials. *Journal of Clinical Anesthesia, 5*, 182.

Barkin, R. L. (1988). Pain management update: IV morphine infusions in children. *Resident and Staff Physician, 34*(8), 11.

Barkin, R. L. (1995a). Focus on tramadol: A centrally acting analgesic for moderate to moderately severe pain. *Formulary, 30*, 321.

Barkin, R. L. (1995b). Alternative dosing for tramadol aids effectiveness. *Formulary, 30*, 542.

Barkin, R. L. (1996a). Withdrawal syndrome is not precipitated when butorphanol is added to opiate or opioid therapy: A comment on intranasal butorphanol-induced apraxia (Reversed by Naloxone). *Pharmacotherapy, 16*(5), 969.

Barkin, R. L. (1996b). Focus on tramadol: A centrally acting analgesic for moderate to moderately severe pain. *Analgesic Digest, 1*, 11–12.

Barkin, R. L., & Barkin, D. S. (2001). Pharmacologic management of acute and chronic pain. *Southern Medical Journal, 94*(8), 798.

Barkin, R. L., & Fawcett, J. (2000, November). The management challenges of chronic pain: The role of antidepressants. *Pharmacologic Management of Chronic Pain.* San Diego, CA: U.S. Psychiatric & Mental Health Congress. Session 425.

Barkin, R. L., & Stein, Z. L. G. (1989). Drugs with anticholinergic side effects. *Southern Medical Journal, 82*(12), 1547.

Barkin, R. L., Barkin, S. J., & Barkin, D. S. (2005). Perception, assessment, treatment, and management of pain in the elderly. *Clinics in Geriatric Medicine, 21*(3), 465–490.

Barkin, R. L., Fawcett, J., & Barkin, S. J. (2002). Chronic pain management with a focus on the role of newer antidepressants and centrally acting agents. In R. S. Weiner (Ed.), *Pain management. A practical guide for clinicians* (6th ed., Chap. 35). Boca Raton, FL: CRC Press.

Barkin, R. L., Schwer, W. A., & Barkin, S. J. (1999). Recognition and management of depression in primary care: A focus on the elderly. A pharmacotherapeutic overview of the selection process among the traditional and new antidepressants. *American Journal of Therapeutics, 7*, 205.

Barkin, R. L. et al. (1998). Opiate, opioids, and centrally acting analgesics and drug interactions: The emerging role of the psychiatrist. *Medical Update for Psychiatrists, 3*(6), 172.

Bartleson, J. D. (2002). Evidence for and against the use of opioid analgesics for chronic nonmalignant low back pain: A review. *Pain Medicine, 3*, 260.

Bartolome, M. B., & Kuhn, C. M. (1983). Endocrine effects of methadone in rats: acute effects in adults. *European Journal of Pharmacology, 95*, 231.

Bennett, M. R., & Adams, A. P. (1983). Postoperative respiratory complications of opiates. *Clinical Anesthesiology, 1*, 41.

Bennie, R. E. et al. (1998). Transnasal butorphanol is effective for postoperative pain relief in children undergoing myringotomy, *Anesthesiology, 89*, 385.

Bonica, J. J. (1990). Anatomic and physiologic basis of nociception and pain. In J. J. Bonica (Ed.), *The management of pain* (2nd ed., pp. 28–94). Philadelphia, PA: Lea and Febiger.

Braunwald, E. et al. (2003). ACC/AHA 2002 guideline update for the management of patients with unstable angina and non-ST-segment elevation myocardial infarction – Summary article: A report of the American College of Cardiology/American Heart Association Task Force on Practice Guidelines (Committee on the Management of Patients with Unstable Angina). *Journal. American College of Cardiology, 40*(7), 1366.

Bruera, E. et al. (1998). Randomized, double-blind, cross-over trial comparing safety and efficacy of oral controlled-release oxycodone with controlled-release morphine in patients with cancer pain. *Journal of Clinical Oncology, 16*, 3222.

Brunk, S. F., & Delle, M. (1974). Morphine metabolism in man. *Clinical Pharmacology and Therapeutics, 16*, 51.

Caldwell, J. R. et al. (2002). Efficacy and safety of a once-daily morphine formulation in chronic, moderate-to-severe osteoarthritis pain: Results from a randomized, placebo-controlled, double-blind trial and an open-label extension trial. *Journal of Pain Symptom Management, 23*, 278.

Carr, D. B. et al. (1995). *Acute Pain Management: Guideline Technical Report No. 1* (AHCPR Publication No. 95-0034). Rockville, MD: U.S. Dept. of Health and Human Services, Public Health Service Agency for Health Care Policy and Research.

Carr, D. B. et al. (2002). *Management of cancer symptoms: Pain, depression, and fatigue* (AHRQ Publication No. 02-E032). Rockville, MD: Agency for Healthcare Research and Quality.

Carr, D. B., & Goudas, L. (1999). Acute pain. *Lancet, 353,* 2051.

Cepeda, M. S. et al. (2001). Ethnicity influences morphine pharmacokinetics and pharmacodynamics. *Clinical Pharmacology and Therpeutics, 70,* 351.

Challoner, K. R., McCaroon, M. M., & Newton, E. J. (1990). Pentazocine (Talwin®) intoxication: Report of 57 cases, *Journal of Emergency Medicine, 8,* 67.

Cherny, N. et al. (2001). Strategies to manage the adverse effects of oral morphine: An evidence-based report. *Journal of Clinical Oncology, 19,* 2542.

Clements, J. A., & Nimmo, W. A. (1981). Pharmacokinetics and analgesic effect of ketamine in man. *British Journal of Anaesthesia, 53,* 27.

Collins, M. et al. (1997). The effect of tramadol on dento-alveolar surgical pain. *British Journal of Oral and Maxillofacial Surgery, 35,* 54.

Dampler, D. C. et al. (1995). Intravenous morphine pharmacokinetics in pediatric patients with sickle cell disease. *Journal of Pediatrics, 126,* 461.

Davis, M. P., & Walsh, D. (2001). Methadone for relief of cancer pain: A review of pharmacokinetics, pharmacodynamics, drugs interactions and protocols of administration,. *Supportive Care in Cancer, 9,* 73.

Dayer, P., Collart, L., & Desmeules, J. (1994). The pharmacology of tramadol. *Drugs, 47*(1), 3.

De Bard, M. L., & Jagger, J. A. (1982). Ts and Bs. Midwestern heroin substance. *Clinical Toxicology, 18,* 1117.

de Groot, A. C., & Conemans, J. (1986). Allergic urticarial rash from oral codeine. *Contact Dermatitis, 14,* 209.

de Leo-Casasola, O. A., & Lema, M. J. (1996). Postoperative epidural opioid analgesia: What are the choices? *Anesthia and Analgesia, 83,* 867.

DeRuiter, J. (2000, Fall). *Principles of drug action, 2.*

Duthie, D. J., & Nimmo, W. S. (1987). Adverse effects of opioid analgesic drugs. *British Journal of Anaesthesia, 59,* 61.

Eddy, N. B., & Lee, L. E. J. (1959). The analgesic equivalence to morphine and relative side action liability of oxymorphone (4-hydroxydihydromorphinone). *Journal in Pharmacology and Experimental Therapeutics, 125,* 116.

Edwards, W., & Breed, R. (1990). Treatment of postoperative pain in the post anesthesia care unit. *Anesthesiology Clinics of North Amererica, 8,* 235.

Ellenhorn, M. J. (1997). *Ellenhorn's medical toxicology, diagnosis and treatment of human poisoning* (2nd ed.). Baltimore, MD: Williams & Wilkins.

Errick, J. K., & Heel, R. C. (1983). Nalbuphine: A preliminary review of its pharmacological properties and therapeutic efficacy. *Drugs, 26,* 191.

Felser, J. M., & Orban, D. J. (1982). Dystonic reaction after ketamine abuse. *Emergency Medicine, 11,* 673.

Fine, P. G. (1997). Fentanyl in the treatment of cancer pain. *Seminars in Oncology, 24*(5), S16.

Finkle, B. S. (1984). Self-poisoning with dextropropoxyphene and dextropropoxyphene compounds: The USA experience. *Human Toxicology, 3,* 115S.

Fishman, S. M. et al. (2002). Methadone reincarnated: Novel clinical applications with related concerns. *Pain Med, 3*(4), 1.

Foley, K. M. (2003). Opioids and chronic neuropathic pain [Editorial]. *New England Journal of Medicine, 348*(13), 1279.

Gal, T. J. (1989). Naloxone reversal of buprenorphine-induced respiratory depression. *Clinical Pharmacology and Therapeutics, 45,* 66.

Gardner-Nix, J. S. (1996). Oral methadone for managing chronic nonmalignant pain. *Journal of Pain Symptom Management, 11,* 321.

Garrido, M. J., & Troconiz, I. F. (1999). Methadone: A review of its pharmacokinetic/pharmacodynamic properties. *Journal of Pharmacology and Toxicology Methods, 42*(2), 61.

Gaver, R. C. et al. (1980). Disposition of parenteral butorphanol in man. *Drug Metabolism and Disposition, 8,* 230.

Gaynes, B. L., & Barkin, R. L. (1999). Analgesics in ophthalmic practice: A review of the oral non-narcotic agent tramadol, optometry and vision science. *Optometry and Vision Science, 76*(7), 455.

Gear, R. W. et al. (1999). The kappa opioid nalbuphine produces gender- and dose-dependent analgesia and antianalgesia in patients with postoperative pain. *Pain, 83,* 339.

Hansten, P. D., & Horn, J. P. (2004). *The top 100 drug interactions.* Edmonds, WA: Hanah Publication.

Hanunen, K. et al. (1993). Pharmacokinetics and pharmacodynamics of pentazocine in children. *Pharmacology and Toxicology, 73,* 120.

Harcus, A. H., Ward, A. E., & Smith, D. W. (1980). Buprenorphine: Experiences in an elderly population of 975 patients during a year's monitored release. *British Journal of Clinical Practice, 34,* 144.

Hartvig, P. et al. (1995). Central nervous system effects of subdissociative emission of tomography in healthy volunteers. *Clinical Pharmacology and Therapeutics, 58,* 165.

Henry, J., & Volans, G. (1985). *ABCs of poisoning.* London: BMJ Publishing Group.

Holdsworth, M. T. et al. (1995). Continuous midazolam infusion for the management of morphine-induced myoclocus. *Annals of Pharmacotherapeutics, 29,* 25.

Honigberg, I. L., & Stewart, J. T. (1980). Radioimmunoassay of hydromorphone and hydrocodone in human plasma. *Journal of Pharmaceutical Sciences, 69,* 1171.

Hoskin, P. J., & Hanks, G. W. (1991). Opioid agonist-antagonist drugs in acute and chronic pain states. *Drugs, 41,* 326.

Jacobi, J. et al. (2003). Clinical practice guidelines for the sustained use of sedatives and analgesics in the critically ill adult. *Critical Care Medicine, 30*(1), 119.

Jadad, A. R. et al. (1992). Morphine responsiveness of chronic pain double-blind randomized crossover study with patient-controlled analgesia. *Lancet, 339,* 1367.

Jallion, P. et al. (1989). Pharmacokinetics of nalbuphine in infants, young healthy volunteers and elderly patients. *Clinical Pharmacology and Therapeutics, 46,* 226.

Jeal, W., & Benfield, P. (1997). Transdermal fentanyl: A review of its pharmacological properties and therapeutic efficacy in pain control. *Drugs, 53,* 109.

Kaiko, R. F. (1980). Age and morphine analgesia in cancer patients with postoperative pain. *Clinical Pharmacology and Therapeutics, 28*, 823.

Kaiko, R. F. et al. (1982). Narcotics in the elderly. *Medical Clinics of North America, 66*, 1079.

Kalso, E., & Vainio, A. (1990). Morphine and oxycodone hydrochloride in the management of cancer pain. *Clinical Pharmacology and Therapeutics, 47*, 639.

Krantz, M. J. et al. (2002). Torsade de pointes associated with very-high-dose methadone. *Annals of Internal Medicine, 137*, 501.

Latta, K. S., Ginsberg, B., & Barkin, R. L. (2002). Meperidine: A critical review. *American Journal of Therapeutics, 9*, 53.

Lawson, A. A., & Northridge, D. B. (1987). Dextropropoxyphene overdose. Epidemiology, clinical presentation and management. *Medical Toxicology and Adverse Drug Experience, 2*, 430.

Leikin, J. B. et al. (1990). Nalbuphine vs. meperidine in sickle cell anemia: DICP. *Annals of Pharmacotherapy, 24*, 781.

Lewis, K. S., & Han, N. H. (1997). Tramadol: A new centrally acting analgesic, *American Journal of Health-System Pharmacy, 54*, 643.

Lorenz, J., Beck, H., & Bromm, B. (1997). Cognitive performance, mood and experienced pain before and during morphine-induced analgesics in patients with chronic non-malignant pain. *Pain, 73*, 369.

Lubenow, T. R., Ivankovich, A. D., & Barkin, R. L. (2005). Management of acute postoperative pain. In P. G. Barash, B. F. Cullen, & R. Stoelting, *Clinical anesthesia* (3rd ed.). Philadelphia: J. R. Lippincott Co.

Mac Evilly, M., & O'Carroll, C. (1989). Hallucinations after epidural buprenorphine. *British Medical Journal, 298*, 928.

Maier, C. et al. (2002). Morphine responsiveness, efficacy and tolerability in patients with chronic non-tumor associated pain – Results of double blind placebo-controlled trial (MONTAS). *Pain, 97*, 223.

McCarberg, B., & Barkin, R. L. (2001). Long-acting opioids for chronic pain: Pharmacotherapeutic opportunities to enhance compliance, quality of life, and analgesia. *American Journal of Therapeutics, 8*, 151.

McCarberg, B. et al. (2003). Tender points as predictors of distress and the pharmacologic management of fibromyalgia syndrome, *American Journal of Therapeutics, 10*, 176.

McEvoy, G. K. (Ed.). (2004). *AHFS drug information*. Bethesda, MD: American Society of Health-System Pharmacists.

McRorie, T. I. et al. (1982). Narcotics in the elderly. *Medical Clinics of North America, 66*, 1079.

Mehlisch, D. R., Brown, P., Lefner, A. et al. (1993). Tramadol hydrochloride: Short term efficacy in pain following dental surgery. *Clinical Pharmacology and Therapeutics, 53*, 223.

Melanson, S. W. et al. (1997). Transnasal butorphanol in the emergency department: Management of migraine headache. *American Journal of Emergency Medicine, 15*, 57.

Mokhlesi, B. et al. (2003). Adult toxicology in critical care: Part II: Specific poisonings. *Chest, 123*, 897.

Morley, J. S. et al. (1993). Methadone in pain uncontrolled by morphine. *Lancet, 342*, 1243.

Moulin, D. E. et al. (1991). Comparison of continuous subcutaneous and intravenous hydromorphone infusions for management of cancer pain. *Lancet, 337*, 465.

Nasraway, S. A. (2001). Use of sedative medications in the intensive care unit. *Sem. Resp. Crit. Care Med, 22*, 165.

Olkkola, K. T., Hamunen, K., & Maunuksela, E. L. (1995).. *Clinical Pharmacokinetics, 28*, 385.

McEvoy, G. K. (Ed.) (2004). Opiate Agonists General Statement. *AHFS drug information*. Bethesda, MD: American Society of Health-System Pharmacists.

Pachter, I. J., & Evens, R. P. (1985). Butorphanol. *Drug and Alcohol Dependence, 14*, 325.

Proudfoot, A. T. (1984). Clinical features and management of Distalgesic overdose. *Human Toxicology, 3*, 85S.

Raffa, R. et al. (1992). Opioid and nonopioid components independently contribute to the mechanism of action of tramadol, an atypical opioid analgesic. *Journal of Pharmacology and Experimental Therapeutics, 260*, 275.

Ramsey, R. et al. (1986). Influence of age on the pharmacokinetics of butorphanol. *Acute Care, 12*(1), 8.

Rauck, R. L., Ruoff, G. E., & McGillen, J. I. (1994). Comparison of tramadol and acetaminophen with codeine for long-term pain management in elderly patients. *Current Therapeutics Research, 55*, 1417.

Ready, L. et al. (1995). Practice guidelines for acute pain management in the perioperative setting. A report of the American Society of Anesthesiologists Task Force on Pain Management (Acute Pain Section). *Anesthesiology, 82*, 1071.

Reed, D. A., & Schnoll, S. H. (1994). Abuse of pentazocine as analgesic in pediatric cases. *Journal. Indian Medical Association, 92*, 77.

Reisine, T., & Pasternak, G. (1996). Opioid analgesics and antagonists. In J. G. Hardman & L. E. Limbird (Eds.), *Goodman & Gilman's the pharmacological basis of therapeutics* (9th ed., Chap. 23). New York: McGraw-Hill.

Resnik, D. B. et al. (2001). The undertreatment of pain: Scientific, clinical, cultural, and philosophical factors. *Med. Health Care Philos., 4*, 277.

Reves, J. G. (2002). Profiles in anesthetic practice: Rational administration of intravenous anesthesia. In G. E. Morgan, Jr., M. S. Makhail, & M. J. Murray (Eds.), *Clinical anesthesiology* (3rd ed., Chap. 8). New York: McGraw-Hill..

Richtsmeier, A., Barnes, S. D., & Barkin, R. L. (1997). Ventilatory arrest with morphine patient-controlled analgesia in a child with renal failure. *American Journal of Therapeutics, 4*, 255.

Rogers, A. G. (1991). Considering histamine release in prescribing opioid analgesics. *Journal of Pain Symptom Management, 6*, 44.

Rogers, J. F., Nafziger, A. N., & Bertino, J. S., Jr. (2002). Pharmacogenetics affects dosing, efficacy, and toxicity of cytochrome P450-metabolized drugs. *American Journal of Medicine, 113*, 746.

Rolandi, E. et al. (1983). Changes in pituitary secretion induced by an agonist-antagonist opioid drug, buprenorphine, *Acta Endocrinologica* (Copenhagen), *104*, 257.

Roth, S. H. et al. (2000). Around-the-clock, controlled-release oxycodone therapy for osteoarthritis-related pain placebo-controlled trial and long-term evaluation. *Archives of Internal Medicine, 160*, 853.

Ruoff, G. E. (1999). Slowing the initial titration rate of tramadol improves tolerability. *Pharmacotherapy, 19*, 88.

Sabbe, M. B., & Yaksh, T.L. (1990). Pharmacology of spinal opioids. *Journal of Pain Symptom Management, 5*, 191.

Schechter, N. L. et al. (1995). The use of oral transmucosal fentanyl citrate for painful procedures in children. *Pediatrics, 95*, 335.

Scholz J., Steinfath M., & Schulz, M. (1996). Clinical pharmacokinetics of alfentanil, fentanyl, and sufentanil. An update. *Clinical Pharmacokinetics, 31*, 275.

Schug, S. A., Zech, D., & Grond, S. (1992). Adverse effects of systemic opioid analgesics. *Drug Safety, 7*, 200.

Shyu, W. C., Morgenthien, E. A., & Barbhaiya, R. H. (1996). Pharmacokinetics of butorphanol nasal spray in patients with renal impairment. *British Journal of Clinical Pharmacology, 41*, 397.

Simpson, Jr., R. K. et al. (1997). Transdermal fentanyl for chronic low back pain. *Journal of Pain Symptom Management, 14*, 218.

Sinatra, R. S., & Harrison, D. M. (1989). Oxymorphone in patient-controlled analgesia. *Clinical Pharmacy, 8*(8), 541.

Sinatra, R. S., Hyde, N. H., & Harrison, D. M. (1988). Oxymorphone revisited. *Seminars in Anesthesia, 7*, 209.

Stork, C. M. et al. (1995). Propoxyphene-induced wide WRS complex dysrhythmia responsive to sodium bicarbonate — A case report. *Journal of Toxicology, Clinical Toxicology, 33*, 179.

Stoukides, C. A., & Stegman, M. (1992). Diffuse rash associated with transdermal fentanyl. *Clinical Pharmacy, 11*, 222.

Tatro, D. S. (Ed.). (2003). *Drug interactions. Drug Facts and Comparisons* (8th ed).

Tennant, F. S., Jr. (1973). Complications of propoxyphene abuse. *Archives of Internal Medicine, 132*, 191.

Turturro, M. A., & O'Toole, K. S. (1991). Oxycodone-induced pulmonary edema. *American Journal of Emergency Medicine, 9*, 201.

Vachharajani, N. N. et al. (1996). The absolute bioavailability and pharmacokinetics of butorphanol nasal spray in patients with hepatic impairment. *Clinical Pharmacology and Therapeutics, 60*, 283.

Vachharajani, N. N. et al. (1997). The pharmacokinetics of butorphanol and its metabolites at steady state following nasal administration in humans. *Biopharmaceutics and Drug Disposition, 18*, 191.

Wasserman, S., & Yahr, M. D. (1980). Choreic movements induced by the use of methadone. *Archives of Neurology, 37*, 727.

Weschules, D. J. et al. (2003). Methadone and the hospice patient: Prescribing trends in the home care setting. *Pain Medicine, 4*(3), 269.

Wetli, C. V., & Bednarczyk, L. R. (1980). Deaths related to propoxyphene overdose: A ten year assessment. *Southern Medical Journal, 73*, 1205.

Wheeler, W. L., & Dickerson, E. D. (2000). Clinical applications of methadone. *American Journal of Hospital Palliative Care, 17*(3), 196.

Wickersham, R. M. (Ed.). (2004). *Drug facts & comparison*. St. Louis, MO: Walters Klewer Health Inc.

Yoo, Y. C. et al. (1995). Determination of nalbuphine in drug abusers' urine. *Journal of Analytical Toxicology, 19*, 120.

Zenz, M., Strumpf, M., & Tryba, M. (1992). Long-term oral opioid therapy in patients with chronic nonmalignant pain. *Journal of Pain and Symptom Management, 7*, 69.

55

Natural Supplements in Pain Management: A Primer and Evidence-Based Review

Robert A. Bonakdar, MD

INTRODUCTION

Herbal and dietary supplements account for more than $15 billion in yearly sales, with pain management as one of the most common reasons for utilization. The use of dietary supplements, which is often done without the input or monitoring of a clinician, introduces many important issues of which the health care provider should be aware. These primarily include understanding the regulation, marketing, and efficacy of supplements as well as sensitivity to the demographics and ideology of those using supplements in order to improve discussion and management. Dietary supplements commonly used for pain management and evaluated in clinical trials are reviewed.

The typical journey of the patient with pain (and similarly patients with a chronic condition) involves consultations and information gathering regarding potential treatment options. At some point during this investigation, the possibility of using dietary supplements will inevitably be introduced. Compared with the general population, patients experiencing pain as a whole, as well as those fitting certain demographics, will be more likely to consider, use, and continue with dietary supplementation as a treatment option. This scenario inspires several important questions for the practitioner:

- How many of my patients are using supplements?
- Are my patients discussing their supplement use with me?
- Why did the patient start using supplements?

- Are the supplements safe and well-regulated?
- Are the supplements effective?
- Where did my patients learn about and obtain their supplements?
- How do I effectively counsel and manage patients on supplements?
- How do I find evidence-based resources and information on supplements?

The answers to these questions can be quite surprising and contrast sharply with respect to the properties of prescription medications. An overview of dietary supplements, including definition, prevalence, rationale, and regulation is offered in the first section of the chapter as a primer for the clinician. The second section discusses efficacy and utilization issues related to common pain management supplements evaluated in clinical trials.

DIETARY SUPPLEMENTS OVERVIEW

DEFINITION

Dietary supplements have various definitions and are typically thought of as commonly used herbal products — *Echinacea,* feverfew — or nonherbal products — glucosamine, *S*-adenosyl methionine (SAMe). However, the definition as listed in the Dietary Supplement Health and Education Act (DSHEA) of 1994 is more encompassing and includes any single or combination ingredient products containing the following (with examples in parentheses):

- A vitamin (riboflavin)
- A mineral (magnesium)
- An herb or other botanical (feverfew)
- An amino acid (L-tryptophan)
- A dietary substance for use by humans to supplement the diet by increasing the total dietary intake (proteolytic enzymes from pineapple)
- A concentrate, metabolite, constituent or extract (white willow bark extract) (Food and Drug Administration, 2002)

The definition effectively incorporates most substances used by consumers or patients outside the realm of prescription or over-the counter (OTC) medications. Because of the broad definition, clinician should be clear in asking about all categories of dietary supplements potentially used.

PREVALENCE AND RATIONALE

Dietary supplement sales have grown steadily, at times dramatically, since the early 1990s with an approximate 400% increase since that time (Eisenberg et al., 1993, 1998). Since the late 1990s supplements have demonstrated a variable picture where certain markets (Internet, catalogs, and health food stores) have increased while others have slowed. Additionally, individual supplements demonstrate stronger (glucosamine) or weaker (Kava) sales based on recent studies, advertising, or government warnings. Overall, the supplement industry continues to demonstrate impressive numbers with greater than $15 billion in total sales by the most recent estimates (*Nutrition Business Journal,* 2001).

Currently, 50% or more of Americans use a vitamin/mineral formula and 18% an herbal formula on a regular basis (Gugliona, 2000; Harris Interactive Health Care News, 2002). The use of dietary supplements is predicted by several demographic characteristics. The typical user of dietary supplement tends to be a female with higher education and income, with potentially more severe and long-standing medical issues than a nonuser (Astin, 1998; Begbie et al., 1996; Gray et al., 2002; Leung et al., 2001). The rationale for supplement use is additionally correlated with a number of factors including the type of medical diagnoses as well as patient belief systems. A diagnosis of pain is one of the top conditions prompting supplement use (Astin, 1998; Consumer Health Products Association, 2001; Leung et al., 2001). Surveys have demonstrated that those in chronic pain have greater than 40% use of at least one complementary and alternative medicine (CAM) modality. The most common modalities vary by condition but typically including dietary supplements, acupuncture, massage, and manipulation (Bruneli et al., 2004; Nayak et al., 2001). Certain pain conditions (such as osteoarthritis and fibromyalgia) tend to attract greater

CAM and supplement use due to several factors including the psychosocial factors associated with the condition as well as availability of effective conventional treatments. For example, in patients with osteoarthritis awaiting joint replacement, 40% used some type of dietary supplement with usage correlated with higher levels of pain (Zochling et al., 2004). One of the highest levels of dietary supplement usage is seen with patients with fibromyalgia who had a 91% CAM utilization rate versus 63% in a matched rheumatology population (Pioro-Boisset et al., 1996).

The health beliefs and values of the person considering supplements are also quite important and often misinterpreted. Those who are involved in "active coping behaviors," such as greater physical activity, tend to view supplement use in a similar manner. Also, several surveys demonstrate that those with a more "holistic outlook" wish to utilize complementary methods including dietary supplements, which may take this viewpoint into consideration. Although there has been speculation regarding the use of CAM and dietary supplements as secondary to dissatisfaction with conventional care, the more prevalent theme is that of CAM utilization for optimization of care. In fact, dissatisfaction with conventional care did not predict use of CAM in a previous national survey and less than 5% of CAM users did so in isolation from conventional care. Most CAM users state their motivations for CAM incorporation encompass more global control over their health care with up to 80% reporting substantial benefit from its use (Astin, 1998). In their pursuit of CAM, users have actually been found to have more frequent relationships with a primary care physician, regular physician follow-up, and compliance with recommended preventative health behaviors such as regular mammography (Astin et al., 2000).

KNOWLEDGE BASE

The knowledge base of the average clinician and consumer regarding dietary supplements has been shown to be suboptimal. Physician surveys have found that physicians in training may have a low general understanding of commonly used supplements as well as their safety, interaction, and regulation profiles. Similarly, consumers and patients tend to receive their information regarding supplements from nonclinical sources including magazines, friends, and family, with clinician consultation occurring rarely. As pointed out by a recent Harris Poll, the outcome of inaccurate or biased supplement information may be overestimation of the regulatory and evidence basis of dietary supplements. The poll demonstrated that 55% of consumers believed that the government does not allow claims of safety without supporting evidence, 59% believed that products must be preapproved by the FDA before sale, and 68% believed the government required labels to have warnings about potential side effects (Harris Interactive, 2002).

DISCUSSION

One of the other key deficiencies in the dietary supplement scenario is the level of clinician–patient discussion. Initial survey found that in approximately 70% of encounters, there was no discussion of CAM use, including dietary supplements (Eisenberg et al., 1993). More recently the percentage appears to be lower and closer to 50%, which still leaves many encounters in which neither the patient nor clinician introduces the topic. More disconcerting is the fact that if a patient is hospitalized by a specialist, CAM use is not identified up to 88% of the time (Azaz-Livshits et al., 2002). The importance of identifying, discussing, and charting CAM and supplement use cannot be understated. The immediate motivation for discussing dietary supplements involves identification of any potential interactions or adverse effects of which the patient may not be aware. More importantly, full discussion enables a better understanding of patient rationale for consideration and utilization of supplements. As mentioned previously, supplement users share health behaviors which, when identified by clinicians, enable improved coordination and guidance of conventional and complementary treatment options.

To help improve discussion, it is important to better understand why patients do not disclose supplement (or other CAM) use. Surveys indicate that factors including anticipation of negative or disinterested clinician response, as well as belief that the clinician will not provide useful information, motivated nondisclosure (Adler et al., 1999). However, most important may be clinician inquiry, with patients demonstrating willingness to disclose supplements use, but only if asked by a clinician directly (Hansrud et al., 1999). Unfortunately, a recent survey of physicians found that few of those surveyed felt comfortable discussing CAM with their patients. One of the major reasons for the lack of comfort was related to a need to improve their knowledge base regarding CAM (84% of responders). It is hypothesized that with improved education about CAM, physicians may be more willing to discuss CAM and counsel patients (Corbin-Winslow et al., 2002).

There are a number of resources available to clinicians interested in better understanding dietary supplements as a means of increasing and improving patient communication. These resources are listed in Table 55.1 and include print and online information on evidence-based use of supplements as well as continuing medical education courses available to clinicians. In addition, the H-E-R-B-A-L mnemonic is offered in Table 55.2 as an additional practice tool for alerting clinicians to the most important steps involved in managing dietary supplement use.

REGULATION

The general regulation of dietary supplements in the United States is in evolution, but is currently based on the DSHEA of 1994. The key components of this act are important for all practitioners to review to better understand how regulation differs from prescription medications. First, unlike prescription medications that need to proceed through multiphase trials to gain premarketing approval from the FDA, supplements (with established ingredients) are not required to have safety, efficacy, or bioavailability data prior to marketing. Ensuring these important qualities, along with having a clear and truthful label, is solely the responsibility of the manufacturer. Second, because supplements are not required to go through premarketing clearance, they also fall into a different labeling scheme than prescription products. In short, supplements may have only "structure or function" claims that cannot imply prevention, treatment, or cure of a condition. The line can at times be difficult to distinguish with a number of manufacturers being cited for going beyond allowed standards (Federal Trade Commission [FTC] for the Consumer Newsletter, 2003).

The key role of the FDA (and in the case of advertising, the FTC) begins after the supplement is marketed and involves monitoring safety, label claims, and product advertising. Thus, the typical premarketing steps needed for prescription medication approval are replaced with postmarketing surveillance. In this scenario, the FDA must utilize adverse drug reports and product analysis to prove a supplement poses significant health risks. Two recent examples of this are the banning of ephedra secondary to adverse reactions and "PCSPES" (a dietary supplement marketed to patients with prostate cancer) because of product adulteration (FDA Press Release, 2002, 2003).

As it currently stands, the supplement regulatory system contrasts greatly to that for prescription medication and will likely see additional scrutiny and amendments in the near future. Although many manufacturers utilize proper standards, the publicity of an adulterated or unsafe supplement tarnishes the standing of well-regulated supplements as well as decreases the confidence of practitioners and consumers wishing to incorporate evidence-based supplements. The incorporation of new good manufacturing practice (GMP) standards as published in 2003 will be helpful in standardizing the manufacturing process. Also greater organizational support for monitoring claims, advertising, and adverse events should improve the enforcement of existing statutes.

EXTERNAL REGULATION

Several independent agencies now offer testing and monitoring services, allowing manufacturers the opportunity to demonstrate their adherence to regulatory standards.

TABLE 55.1
Selected Dietary Supplement and CAM Resources

Internet

CAM on PubMed (www.nlm.nih.gov/medlineplus/alternativemedicine.html) Focused search on PubMed for articles with a focus on alternative and complementary medicine

Cochrane Library (www.cochrane.org) Collection of systematic reviews with a complementary medicine field

European Scientific Cooperative on Phytotherapy (ESCOP) (www.escop.com) International perspective on herbal supplements and adverse effects

FDA Division of Dietary Supplement (http://vm:cfsan.fda.gov/~dms/supplmnt/html) Discussion of dietary supplement regulation including list of recalls and warnings

HerbMed (www.HerbMed.org) Botanical information collections including background, clinical, and adverse effect profiles of select herbal supplements; organized by the Alternative Medicine Foundation

International Bibliographic Information on Dietary Supplements (IBIDS) (http://ods.od.nih.gov/showpage.aspx?pageid=48) Collaborative database of available abstract on dietary supplements

Longwood Herbal Taskforce (www.mcp.edu/herbal) Collection of clinically oriented monographs and reviewed Internet links

Natural Medicines Comprehensive Database (www.naturaldatabase.com) An extensive collection of supplement information including uses, indication, efficacy, and adverse effects with a drug interactions checker

Natural Products Alert (NAPRALERT) (www.ag.uiuc.edu/~ff/napra.html) Review of foundation topics relevant to supplements including chemistry, pharmacology, and ethnomedicinal considerations

Office of Dietary Supplements (http://ods.od.nih.gov/index.aspx) NIH division with information and background on dietary supplements

Books

Blumenthal, M. (2000). *The ABC guide to herbs.* Austin, TX: American Botanical Council.

Blumenthal, M. et al. (2000). *Herbal medicine: Expanded German E monographs.* Newton, MA: Integrative Medicine Communications.

Brinker, F. (2001). *Herb contraindications and drug interactions* (3rd ed.). Sandy, OR: Eclectic Medicine Publications.

Duke, J. A. (1977). *The green pharmacy.* Emmaus, PA: Rodale/St. Martin's Press.

Huan, K. C. (1999). *The pharmacology of Chinese herbs* (2nd ed.). Boca Raton, FL: CRC Press.

Kapoor, L. D. (1990). *CRC handbook of Ayurvedic medicinal plants.* Boca Raton, FL: CRC Press.

Journals

Alternative Medicine Alert (www.ahcpub.com) Concise summary of available evidence on pertinent alternative medicine topics including dietary supplements

HerbalGram (www.herbalgram.org) Article and summary of research in the field of herbal medicine, produced by the American Botanical Council.

Planta Medica (www.thieme.de/plantamedica/fr_inhalt.html) Review of natural products and medicinal plant research

Continuing Medical Education

Botanical Medicine in Modern Clinical Practice. Organized by Columbia University Medical Center. Date: yearly in June

Natural Supplements in Practice: An evidence-based update. Organized by the Scripps Center for Integrative Medicine and University of California, San Diego. Date: yearly in January

Peered-Reviewed Information for Patients

MedlinePlus (www.nlm.nih.gov/medlineplus/alternativemedicine.html) Patient-oriented summary of Medline published research and international health news

Healthfinder (www.healthfinder.gov) A portal for peer-reviewed Internet health sites including subheadings on CAM and herbal medicine

National Center for Complementary and Alternative Medicine (NCCAM) (www.nccam.nih.gov) NIH clearinghouse of government-funded initiatives in CAM including research, fellowships, grants, and patient education materials

Manufacturers may voluntarily submit their product for review, which can take various forms including ingredient verification, manufacturing site monitoring, and random off-the-shelf testing. Those that pass inspection may carry an independent "Seal-of-Approval" on their label and advertising. Several of the government agencies as well as independent agencies currently involved in testing are listed in Table 55.3. Although there is no absolute standard for external regulation, nor is external regulation a replacement for continued vigilance by the consumer or federal regulators, it may help to improve and establish stronger manufacturing standards.

SAFETY AND ADVERSE EFFECTS

The rate and severity of adverse effects associated with dietary supplements are difficult to estimate. This is due to minimal if any premarketing safety data as well as a suboptimal system of capturing and verifying postmarketing events. One of the proposed DSHEA regulatory changes is establishment of a mandatory adverse events reporting system by manufacturers. Currently, because of the lack of initial communication and subsequent discussion regarding dietary supplements, the involvement of the clinician in detecting and reporting adverse effects and potential inter-

TABLE 55.2
The H-E-R-B-A-L Mnemonic©

Hear the Patient out with Respect

More patients will disclose supplement use when asked openly and directly

Most patients desire discussion but do not initiate it on their own

Ask in a nonjudgmental, inclusive manner: "Some of my other patients are using herbs and supplements for various conditions. Have you tried any of these?"

Remember that there may be a fear of ridicule or indifference with disclosure

Understand that the patient may have important personal reasons for choosing supplements which may include:

- Previous positive experience
- More time to discuss health issues with alternative health practitioner or health food salespersons
- Anecdotal evidence, "It worked for my friend"
- Issues with current conventional care

Thank them for taking an active role in their health care. Discuss other ways they can do this that you can agree upon: diet, exercise, stress management, etc.

Educate the Patient

Supplements are potentially powerful agents that can have benefit as well as serious side effects and interactions, just like prescription medication

Your job is not to be an expert, but simply to dispel the myths and balance the picture

Give the patient resources that are objective and reliable (www.healthfinder.gov, http://NCCAM.NIH.GOV, www.naturaldatabase.com)

Record

Treat supplements like other medications: chart all supplement use in the progress note and medication section for your benefit as well as for other practitioners viewing the chart

Try to record an evaluation date to discuss if the supplement has shown any benefit for treatment. If no benefit is seen discuss options including changing dosage or brand, stopping or switching supplements.

Beware

If the patient develops new or worsening side effects or abnormal laboratory values (especially prothrombin time/international normalized ratio [PT-INR]) and the usual suspects have been ruled out — **Think Supplements**

Monitor patients with polypharmacy, especially those on anticoagulants

Agreement to Discuss

Forge an agreement that all new supplements will be discussed before commencement, which gives you and your staff a chance to balance the mostly anecdotal/testimonial information the patient hears through the media, mailings, and the Internet

Learn about New Supplements

Try to keep up with what the patient is hearing about and considering using

A wide variety of peer-reviewed resources are available to help decipher the increasing amount of information on supplements (see Table 55.1)

---

action is hindered. Additionally, patient reporting of adverse effects to dietary supplements appears to occur less often than with prescription medication. A 1998 study that interviewed dietary supplement users found that they would act differently based on the type of product that caused the adverse effect. Surprisingly, 26% would consult their primary care provider for serious adverse effects of a conventional OTC medication, but not for a similar adverse effect of an herbal remedy (Barnes et al., 1998).

The discrepancy in how patients view supplements, their safety, and the need for reporting is especially important in certain populations who may have relative or absolute contraindications to supplement use. These populations include pregnant or breastfeeding women, young children, or patients with certain conditions (such as dialysis or transplant patients) who may be on a narrow therapeutic regimen or medications with high interaction

potential. These advisories are unfortunately currently more theoretical than actual and largely based on mechanistic studies, varying quality case studies, and rare prospective trials. An example of this model would be a pregnant patient considering supplements for headache management. She may not know the difference in safety between feverfew, which has been correlated with uterine activity, and magnesium, which is generally considered safe in typical doses. Thus, in many cases, the pregnant patient, as a model of the vulnerable patient, should have a higher level of clinician counseling regarding the safety issues of any supplement she may be considering.

The reported adverse effects in clinical trials of dietary supplement for pain management appear to be low. As detailed in several of the trials in the next section, the most common side effects tend to be minor gastrointestinal (GI) reactions. These may include bloating, nausea, or changes

TABLE 55.3
Governmental and Independent Regulatory Agencies

Agency	Web Site
Governmental	
Food and Drug Administration (FDA) Medwatch Program for collecting adverse reactions to prescription and OTC medications as well as dietary supplements	www.fda.gov/medwatch
Federal Trade Commission (FTC) site for submitting complaints on false or misleading advertising	www.ftc.gov/ftc/complaint.htm
American Association of Poison Control Centers for reporting and management of adverse effects	www.poison.org or (800)222-1222
Independent Labs Providing Supplement Testing	
The Consumerlab Product Review	www.Consumerlab.com
Dietary Supplement Verification Program (DSVP) through the United States Pharmacopeia (USP)	www.uspverified.org
National Sanitation Foundation (NSF)	www.NSF.ORG/consumer/dietary_supplements
National Nutritional Foods Association Good Manufacturing Practices (NNFA GMP)	www.nnfa.org/services/science/gmp.htm

in gastric motility, typically because of GI active ingredients such as tannins. Other side effects tend to occur rarely and are not more common than placebo, other than when reported below. Of particular comparison are GI side effects including symptomatic ulceration and bleeding, which are increased fourfold with chronic nonsteroidal anti-inflammatory drug (NSAID) use (Garcia-Rodriguez et al., 2004; Hernandez-Diaz et al., 2000). According to Arthritis, Rheumatism, and Aging Medical Information System prospective data, of every 1,000 patients on chronic NSAIDs, 7.3 patients with osteoarthritis and 13 patients with rheumatoid arthritis will develop serious GI complications (Singh et al., 1999). Although reporting and monitoring need to improve, these serious GI adverse events have thus far not been associated with dietary supplements and may be one particularly attractive feature for patients needing alternative therapeutic options for chronic pain management.

Data on the occurrence or potential for herb–drug interactions (HDIs) also are quite preliminary. Broad estimates indicate that from approximately 20 to 43% of patients take dietary supplements along with prescription medications (Eisenberg et al., 1998; Peng et al., 2004). In most cases this use may pose little actual danger as determined by a recent survey that found a 3 to 6% occurrence of concomitant use of a medication with a potentially interacting supplement. However, certain scenarios should prompt further discussion, monitoring, or supplement/medication alteration to avoid the potential for negative interactions. The most common scenario for the pain clinician is that of a patient on dietary supplements with a bleeding potential. When the supplement is concomitantly used with prescription agents with similar properties or in the setting of surgery, increased caution is advised. In

recent surveys, up to 22% of presurgical patients routinely used herbs (8% reported multiple herbs) and 51% routinely used vitamins. Of the products reviewed 27% of patients used herbs that could potentially interfere with blood clotting (Norred, Zamudio, & Palmer, 2000; Tsen et al., 2000). A list of dietary supplements with such a potential is given in Table 55.4. Although extremely rare, this combination has been implicated in cases of hemorrhage (Norred et al., 2000). Overall, the field of HDI identification, monitoring, and management is quite preliminary and likely overstating its true impact. However, until more is known on the subject, it behooves the clinician to have continued vigilance in discussing and monitoring patients in certain clinical scenarios to minimize patient risk.

Last, the topic of interactions would not be complete without a brief discussion of the potentially beneficial GI interactions of several supplements. This type of interaction can be described as an antagonistic pharmacodynamic interaction in nature in which one agent counteracts the actions of another agent at a specific site. In this case, supplements may counteract the depletion of mucosal integrity potentiated by pain medications (NSAIDs and corticosteroids) by mechanisms including promotion of mucin production. Several animal and human studies of capsicum (*Capsicum* spp.), licorice (*Glycyrrhiza glabra*), turmeric (*Curcuma longa),* ginger (*Zingiber officinale*), and cat's claw (*Uncaria tomentosa*) have demonstrated a decrease in various models of GI toxicity (Al-Yahya et al., 1989; Goso et al., 1996; Rafatullah et al., 1990; Yeoh et al., 1995). Additionally, many of the potentially GI protective supplements also possess pain-modulatory properties. This has translated into drug (NSAID)-sparing effects in some trials that may portend a decreased adverse effects incidence.

TABLE 55.4
Herbs Associated with Antiplatelet/Blood Thinning Potential

Herb	Botanical Name	Herb	Botanical Name
Agrimony	*Agrimonia eupatoria*	Horse chestnut	*Aesculus hippocastanum*
Alfalfa	*Medicago sativa*	Horseradish	*Armoracia rusticana*
Angelica	*Angelica archangelica*	Licorice	*Glycyrrhiza glabra*
Anise	*Pimpinella anisum*	Northern prickly ash	*Zanthoxylum americanum*
Asafoetida	*Ferula assa-foetida*	Onion	*Allium cepa*
Aspen	*Populi cortex*	Papain	*Carica papaya*
Bladderwrack	*Fucus vesiculosis*	Passionflower	*Passiflora incarnata*
Black cohosh	*Cimicifuga racemosa*	Pau d'arco	*Tabebuia impetiginosa*
Bogbean	*Menyanthes trifoliate*	Plantain	*Plantago major*
Dong quai	*Angelica sinensis*	Poplar	*Populus tacamahacca*
Boldo	*Peumus boldus*	Quassia	*Quassia amara*
Borage seed oil	*Borago officinalis*	Red clover	*Trifolium pratense*
Bromelain	*Ananas comosus*	Roman chamomile	*Chamaemelum nobile*
Capsicum	*Capsicum frutescen*	Safflower	*Carthamus tinctorius*
Celery	*Apium graveolens*	Southern prickly ash	*Zanthoxylum clava-herculis*
Clove	*Syzygium aromaticum*	Stinging nettle	*Urtica dioica*
Danshen	*Salvia miltiorrhiza*	Sweet clover	*Melilotus officinalis*
European mistletoe	*Viscum album*	Sweet vernal grass	*Anthoxanthum odoratum*
Fenugreek	*Trigonella foenum-graecum*	Tonka bean	*Dipterux odorata*
Feverfew	*Tanacetum parthenium*	Turmeric	*Curcuma longa*
Garlic	*Allium sativum*	Wild carrot	*Daucus carota*
Ginkgo	*Ginkgo biloba*	Wild lettuce	*Lactuca virosa*
Ginseng, Panax	*Asian ginseng*	Yarrow	*Achillea millefolium*
Goldenseal	*Hydrastis canadensis*		

Source: This listing compiled from various sources including www.NaturalDatabase.com.

NATURAL SUPPLEMENTS IN PAIN MANAGEMENT: AN EVIDENCE-BASED REVIEW

This summary focuses on natural supplements commonly utilized for pain management with special focus on those evaluated in clinical trials. Categorization is performed on a clinical basis (phyto-anti-inflammatories, joint pain, and headaches) as opposed to supplement type (vitamin, herb, mineral). Several supplements can be placed in more than one heading, but are placed in categories based on their mechanism or more common indication. White willow bark (WWB) is discussed in detail because of its prototypic role as a phyto-anti-inflammatory. It has benchmark data related to its use and research, including history of traditional use, evidence for biomarkers/bioactivity, efficacy data against placebo and prescription medications, and statistics on safety and cost efficacy. A listing of pain management supplements as evaluated in clinical trials appears in Table 55.5. Listings of additional pain management supplements, which are beyond the scope of this review, are found in Table 55.6. These additional supplements deserve mention because they possess various levels of use in the traditional, clinical, or research setting and

may be recommended or sold for pain management in the United States. The reader looking for more comprehensive or detailed dietary supplement information is again referred to Table 55.1 for additional resources.

Phyto-Anti-Inflammatories

Willow Bark (*Salix* spp.)

WWB has a long history of use in medicine with records describing Hippocrates recommending its use for pain relief. Rev. Edmond Stone formally described WWB in 1763 as helpful in the treatment of inflammatory and febrile conditions with the active component salicylic acid being isolated in 1860. Shortly thereafter in 1898, aspirin (acetylsalicylic acid) was discovered and became a leading pain-relieving agent. Although WWB led the way to aspirin's discovery, these two compounds are not simply natural and synthetic counterparts; WWB has many additional constituents that deserve attention.

As an example, a clinically therapeutic WWB dose in healthy subjects resulted in a blood salicylate level of 1.4 µg/ml, which is subtherapeutic compared with the 35 to 50 µg/ml level obtained from a 500-mg dose of aspirin (Schmid, Kotter, & Heide, 2001). Therefore,

TABLE 55.5
Pain Management Supplements Reviewed in Clinical Trials

Name	Source/Botanical Name	Dosage in Trials
Anti-Inflammatory		
White willow bark	*Salix* spp.	Dose varies, typically standardized to 240 mg salicin/day
Essential oils	Marine animal fat and vegetable oils: various sources: fish oils, GLA, borage and flax seed oil, etc.	1–3 g/day starting dose
Phytodolor	*Populus tremula, Fraxinus excelsior, Solidago virguarea* standardized to 1 mg salicin/ml, 0.07 mg/ml flavanoids, and 0.14 mg/ml isofraxidine	30 drops (ml) of standardized extract, three times daily
Devil's claw	*Harpa gophytum procumbens*	50–100 mg harpagosides/iridoid content of 1.5–3%
Stinging nettle	*Utica dioica*	Varies based on formulation
Ginger	*Zingiber officinale*	Typical 500–1,500 mg/day
Joint Health		
Glucosamine	Marine exoskeletons	1,500 mg/day
Chondroitin	Bovine cartilage	1,200 mg/day
SAMe	Methionine by-product	200–600 mg/day with titration to 1,600 mg/day
Avocado–soybean unsaponifiables (ASU)	Vegetable oil derivative	300–600 mg/day
Headache		
Feverfew[+]	*Tanacetum parthenium*	50–100 mg/day
Magnesium[+]	Magnesium salts	300 mg/day or higher
Riboflavin[+]	Vitamin B$_2$	400 mg/day
Butterbur*	*Petasites hybridus*	100 mg/day 2–10 mg/day
Capsicum	*Capsicum* spp.	Intranasal spray
Coenzyme Q-10	Proprietary fermentation process with beets, sugar cane, and yeast	150–300 mg/day

[+] Available as Migralief, a proprietary combination of feverfew, magnesium, and riboflavin.

* Available as Petadolax, a proprietary butterbur product.

the clinical efficacy of WWB as described below cannot be explained by its salicin content alone and may be attributed to WWB's other active ingredients including glycosides, phenolic glucosides, flavanoids, polyphenols, procyanidins, and tannins. *In vitro*, WWB has demonstrated cyclooxygenase-2 (COX-2), prostaglandin E$_2$ (PGE-2), and leukotriene (LT) inhibitory activity. The inflammatory cascade is pictured in Figure 55.1 to illustrate how WWB and other supplements mentioned below can block or shift inflammatory mediators. Another departure from aspirin comes in the GI tolerability and platelet activity of WWB. One of the main constituents of WWB, salicin, is relatively inactive until traveling past the stomach and appears to have minimal GI ulceration and platelet deactivation potential. Although GI and bleeding potential warnings typically used with aspirin are paralleled for WWB, these may

become less pertinent as more research draws definitive distinction between these two compounds.

Clinically, WWB has been tested for efficacy in several conditions including low back pain and arthritis. A randomized, double-blind, placebo-controlled (RDBPC) study of 78 patients with hip or knee osteoarthritis treated with placebo or WWB containing 240 mg of salicin over a 2-week period demonstrated a statistically significant improvement in WOMAC (Western Ontario and McMaster Universities Osteoarthritis Index) pain scores in the WWB group (Schmid et al., 1998). Similar results were exhibited in a smaller randomized, double-blind, placebo-controlled trial (RDBPCT) of 21 subjects taking WWB containing 240 mg of salicin over a 2-week period for knee and hip osteoarthritis. Results of the study demonstrated a decrease in WOMAC scores of 40% in the WWB group vs. 18% in the placebo group (Schaffner, 1997).

TABLE 55.6
Listing of Dietary Supplements Utilized for Pain Management

Herbal Supplements

Ashwaganda (*Withania somnifera*)
Ash bark (*Fraxinus spp.*)
Barberry (*Berberis vulgaris*)
Birch bark (*Betula alba*)
Boswellia (*Boswellia serrata*)
California poppy (*Eschscholzia californica*)
Cat's claw (*Uncaria tomentosa*)
Holy basil (*Ocimum sanctum*)
Garlic (*Allium sativum*)
Jamaica dogwood (*Piscidia piscipula*)
Motherwort (*Leonurus cardiaca*)
Passion flower (*Passiflora incarnata*)
Poplar (aspen) bark (*Populus tremula*)
Rue (*Ruta graveolens*)
Skullcap (*Scutellaria laterfilora*)
St. John's wort (*Hypericum perforatum*)
Tea (*Camellia sinensis*)
Thunder god vine (*Tripterygium wilfordii*)
Turmeric (*Curcuma longa*)
Wild lettuce (*Lactuca virosa*)

Nonherbal Supplements

5-HTP
Adenosine
Boron
Calcium
Dietary enzymes
L-Arginine
L-Tryptophan
Manganese
Methylsulfonylmethane

Topical Agents Including Essential or Volatile Oils

Aloe (*Aloe* spp.)
Arnica (*Arnica montana*)
Calendula (*Calendula officinalis*)
Camphor (*Cinnamomum camphora*)
Capsicum (*Capsicum* spp.)
Lemongrass (*Cymbopogon citrates*)
Peppermint (*Mentha piperita*)
Spearmint (*Mentha spicata*)
Wintergreen (*Gaultheria procumbens*)

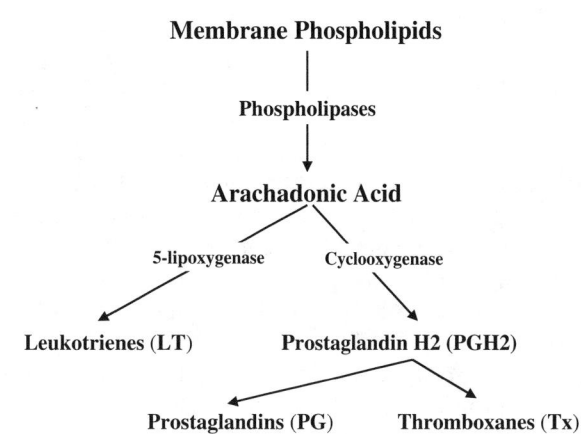

FIGURE 55.1 The inflammatory cascade. (From Crosby, V., Wilcock, A., & Corcoran R. (2000). *Journal of Pain and Symptom Management,* 19, 35–39.)

within 1 week of initiating treatment. Additionally, one patient suffered an allergic reaction attributed to WWB (Chrubasik et al., 2000). In addition to dose responsivity, WWB is one of the few natural products with comparative data against a prescription analgesic (see also devil's claw and SAMe). A randomized, open-label study of standardized WWB (Assalix) containing 240 mg salicin versus 12.5 mg of rofecoxib (Vioxx®) in 228 patients with acute exacerbation of low back pain was carried out for 4 weeks. When compared by visual analogue scale (VAS), Total Pain Index, and need for additional medication, no significant difference in efficacy was noted between groups. Additionally, treatment with WWB was noted to be approximately 40% less expensive than that with rofecoxib (Chrubasik et al., 2001).

The safety profile of WWB appears to demonstrate better GI tolerability and decreased platelet interaction than typically seen with NSAIDs. However, because of its salicylate content, WWB has been implicated in rare allergic reactions, including as a probable source of anaphylaxis in a patient with a history of aspirin allergy (Boullata et al., 2003). Patients should continue to be asked about their medications and allergies, as well as GI and bleeding disorders and receive appropriate counsel regarding the risks and benefits of WWB use. Currently, WWB, standardized to 240 mg of salicin, appears to be a relatively safe, effective, and cost-effective option, especially in the setting of acute exacerbation of low back pain.

Essential Oils

The use of essential oils for the treatment of pain is a broad and difficult-to-summarize topic. The variation in research results stems from factors including the source (e.g., fish oil, borage oil, evening primrose oil). the constituent concentration (i.e., eicosapentaenoic acid or EPA, docosahexaenoic acid or DHA), as well as background dietary pro- and anti-inflammatory intake, which can

WWB appears to be a therapeutic option as well as demonstrating a dose–response range in the difficult scenario of acute exacerbation of low back pain. In one study, 119 subjects with acute exacerbation of low back pain were randomized to WWB standardized to 120 or 240 mg of salicin vs. placebo over 4 weeks. The study demonstrated complete relief of pain in 39% in the high-dose WWB group, 21% in the low-dose WWB group, and 6% in the placebo group (*P* < 0.001). Of note, the pain relief in the high-dose group was not immediate, but typically occurred strongly influence results. In general, polyunsaturated fats are sources for both omega-3 fatty acids and omega-6 fatty acids with the latter producing gamma linoleic acid (GLA) as a by-product. Omega-3s have *in vitro* anti-inflammatory effects, shifting both the cyclo- and lipo-oxygenase pathways by decreasing PGE-1 and PGE-2, increasing PG-3 with eventual decease in proinflammatory markers including interleukins (IL-1, IL-6) and tumor necrosis factor-alpha (TNFα). GLA appears to have anti-inflammatory effects through inhibition of leukotriene B 5 and 12 with subsequent decrease of PGE-2 and prostaglandin I (MacLean et al., 2004). See Figure 55.1 for further details of the inflammatory cascade.

Several trials have attempted to ascertain the dietary and supplement intake necessary for clinical efficacy. In one, 51 patients with rheumatoid arthritis were randomized to 3.6 mg of omega-3 fish oils versus capsules containing standard dietary fats. After 12 weeks, those on fish oil were noted to have small but significant improvement in morning stiffness, joint tenderness, and C-reactive protein values while not showing any benefit in other category measures. There were also no serious side effects noted versus the placebo group (Faarvang et al., 1994). A previous multicenter study utilizing the same protocol found similar findings in morning stiffness and joint tenderness (Nielsen et al., 1992). Similar modest, but clinically significant improvements were demonstrated in a DBPCT of 56 patients with rheumatoid arthritis with use of 2.8 g/day of GLA (Zurier et al., 1996). A recent survey of the literature concluded that in patients with rheumatoid arthritis, doses of 2 to 8 g of GLA/day are required for 12 weeks in order to exhibit an anti-inflammatory effect that compared to therapy with NSAIDs.

The effect of background diet on the potential benefit of essential oil supplementation was shown to be additive to an anti-inflammatory diet. In one study, 68 patients with rheumatoid arthritis were randomized for 3 months with a 2-month washout to a typical Western diet (WD) or an anti-inflammatory diet (AID) in which arachidonic acid intake was less than 90 mg/day. Patients in both groups were additionally randomized to receive placebo or fish oil supplements at 30 mg/kg. With placebo supplementation, the AID decreased swollen joints by 14% as compared with WD. With addition of fish oil, a significant difference in tender (28% vs. 11%) and swollen (34% vs. 22%) joints was noted ($P < 0.01$). Serological studies also demonstrated that the AID, especially with the combination of fish oils, has significant decreases in LT B(4), 11-dehydro-thromboxane B(2), and PG metabolites. The authors concluded that an anti-inflammatory diet improves symptoms of rheumatoid arthritis and can augment the beneficial effects of fish oil supplements Adam et al., 2003).

Essential oils have also been studied in nonrheumatologic pain conditions, including sickle cell disease, with benefit possibly secondary to modulation of vascular

inflammation. One study examined the ability of dietary n-3FA (omega-3 fatty acid) to alter pain episodes in 10 patients with sickle cell disease. Over the course of a year, n-3FA decreased yearly hospital pain episodes from 7.8 to 3.8 ($p < 0.01$) with no significant change noted in the placebo group. n-3FA dietary modification was also associated with decrease in serum markers of thrombosis including D-dimer and plasmin-antiplasmin complex (Tomer et al., 2001).

Although essential fatty acids have clearly documented positive changes in *in vitro* and *in vivo* markers controlling inflammation, there are a number of important notes regarding its use. First, not all clinical trials have demonstrated benefits. There have been a number of non-significant trials with use of essential fatty acid including the use of alpha-linoleic acid from flax seeds as a precursor of EPA and DHA to treat rheumatoid arthritis (Nordstrom et al., 1995). Side effects with use of essential oils are typically dose dependent and include GI symptoms of belching, bloating, increased peristalsis, and diarrhea. The potential for symptoms or drug-sparing benefit appears to be strongly related to the type and dose of the treatment as well as the disease state and background diet of those studied. At this point the strongest evidence appears in the literature for those consuming a 2 g or greater amount of GLA or fish oil supplement while limiting their proinflammatory intake of arachadonic acid (<90 mg/day) or (n-6) fatty acid intake (<10 g/day) (Volker et al., 2000). The latter dietary factor deserves greater attention when developing future trials or when considering recommendation of essential fatty acids in practice.

Phytodolor

Phytodolor is a patented supplement from Germany that contains *Populus tremula, Fraxinus excelsior, Solidago virguarea* standardized to 1 mg salicin/ml, 0.07 mg/ml flavanoids, and 0.14 mg/ml isofraxidine. The active constituents are diverse and including the previously discussed anti-inflammatory actions of salicin (as discussed under WWB), as well as other potential activity including the antispasmodic actions of *Solidago* (von Kruedener et al., 1995). A number of trials have examined Phytodolor in various conditions including osteoarthritis, rheumatoid arthritis, low back pain, and epicondylitis. The studies include a randomized controlled trial (RCT) of 108 inpatients with rheumatic pain randomized to 30 drops three times a day of Phytodolor, placebo, or piroxicam 20 mg/day for up to 4 weeks. There were significant benefits in reducing pain at 2 and 4 weeks for both active groups over placebo without significant differences noted between active groups. Additionally, a DBPCT of 40 subjects with mixed rheumatologic diagnosis already on medication management demonstrated a significant reduction in conventional medication dosing required at 3 weeks when using 30 drops of Phytodolor three times daily. At least four other small trials demonstrate Phytodolor's efficacy in reducing pain or medication requirement with no serious side effects noted (Ernst & Chrubasik, 2000).

Ginger (*Zingiber officinale*)

Ginger (*Zingiber officinale*) has been used for longer than 2,500 years in traditional Chinese, Ayurvedic (Indian), and Tibetan medicine for rheumatological, GI, and oncological conditions. More recently, a number of active ingredients have been isolated from the ginger plant. These include the gingeroles, which exert direct anti-inflammatory activity, as well as galanolactones that have serotonin receptor activity and likely modulate GI actions as well as indirectly affect pain inhibitory activities. Additionally, animal studies have demonstrated that some ginger subspecies have documented COX-2 and PGE-2 inhibitory activities (Garcia-Rodriguez et al., 2004; Hernandez-Diaz & Rodriguez, 2000; Murakami, 1992; Thomson, 2002).

In clinical pain trials, ginger has been utilized mostly for osteoarthritis of the knee. In a 6-week RDBPCT of 261 subjects with knee osteoarthritis, a specialized ginger species containing *Z. officinale* and *Alpinia glanga* (EV.EXT 77) was evaluated in an intent-to-treat analysis. There was moderate improvement noted in knee pain on standing ($P = 0.048$) and pain on walking ($P = 0.016$). There were mild GI side effects in the ginger group that were statistically greater than in the control group (Altman et al., 2001). In a more recent small trial, an extract of *Zingiberis Rhizoma* (Zintona EC) was tested versus placebo in 29 patients with knee osteoarthritis. Patients were randomized to 1,000 mg/day or to placebo with crossover taking place at 3 months. The results demonstrated significant improvement over placebo starting only at the 6-month mark (Wigler et al., 2003). At this point, ginger is known to have a number of pain modulatory constituents with future research requiring a focus on the type of ginger used, dosage titration, proper blinding, and long-term treatment in order to measure clinical significance.

Devil's Claw (*Harpagophytum procumbens*)

Devil's claw is a traditional South African plant used for arthritis and myalgia, and as an external ointment for burns and sores. Its efficacy has been attributed to a number of active ingredients, most notably harpagosides, which have demonstrated *in vitro* activity against the lipo- and cyclooxygenase-mediated inflammatory pathways as well as inhibiting PGE-2 and TNFα synthesis (Fiebich et al., 2001; Jang et al., 2003; Loew et al., 2001). Clinically it has been used most commonly in the setting of osteoarthritis and low back pain. Four RCTs (two examining osteoarthritis, two low back pain) with 50 to 197 treated with 50 to 100 mg harpagosides for up to 8 weeks demonstrated a positive trend (statistically significant in three of four trials) for pain reduction and/or joint mobility with mild and infrequent GI symptoms reported in the active group (Nielsen et al., 1992).

Devil's claw, similar to WWB, has been tested against rofecoxib (Vioxx) for treatment of acute exacerbations of low back pain. In an RDBPCT, 88 patients were randomized to a standardized devil's claw extract (Doloteffin) containing 60 mg of harpagoside daily or 12.5 mg/day of rofecoxib for 6 weeks. Clinical response was measured with the Arhus Index, with the mean pain component decreasing by 23 in devil's claw and 26 in the NSAID group. Additionally, 18 devil's claw and 12 rofecoxib subjects had greater than 50% reduction in weekly averages of their pain scores between the start and end of the trial. Side-effect profiles were similar, although rofecoxib had more dropouts secondary to GI symptoms. Overall, there were no significant differences between groups with the authors noting that larger trials are required before definitive efficacy and safety differentiations can be made Chrubasik et al., 2003).

Stinging Nettle (*Utica dioica*)

Stinging nettle, whose active ingredients include caffeic malic acid and caffeoylmalic acid, has been shown, mostly *in vitro*, to alter numerous aspects of the inflammatory cascade including IL-1B, IL-2, interferon-gamma, NF-κB, lipopolysaccharide-induced release of the cytokine TNFα, and cyclo- and lipooxygenase by-products (Klinghoefer et al., 1999; Riehemann et al., 1999). Clinically, stinging nettle containing 20 mg of caffeoylmalic acid was administered for 2 weeks in a controlled trial to 26 patients with acute arthritis. The subjects were also on a subtherapeutic dose of diclofenac at 50 mg (therapeutic dosing is typically 150 mg/day). The combination of 50 mg diclofenac and stinging nettle was comparable in pain relief with 200 mg of diclofenac administered to 19 control patients (Chrubasik et al., 1997). Adverse effects were minor in this stinging nettle group.

Bromelain Extract (*Ananus comosus*)

Bromelain is an extract of the pineapple plant containing a number of enzymatic complexes including glycoproteins, glucosidases, peroxidases, and phosphates. Bromelains *in vitro* activity centers on decreases in kinnins and bradykinnins, as well as more traditional decreases in PGE-2 and thromboxane B2. In an RDBPCT of 73 patients with osteoarthritis of the knee, a mixture of bromelain, trypsin, and rutin was compared with diclofenac. The trials demonstrated similar improvement in pain and joint mobility (Klein et al., 2000).

NATURAL SUPPLEMENT FOR JOINT PAIN

Glucosamine and Chondroitin

Glucosamine and chondroitin are discussed here jointly because of their general similarity in structural joint function as well as their combination use in commonly used preparations. Both ingredients have been implicated in reducing the progressive degradation of articular cartilage as well as helping to stimulate proteoglycan synthesis in *in vitro* trials (Bassleer et al., 1998; Uelbelhart et al., 1998). In clinical trials, glucosamine and chondroitin have been evaluated for their ability to improve pain and functional ability, typically of the knee and hip. Additionally, isolated glucosamine has some data demonstrating joint space narrowing. The Cochrane Review of glucosamine summarizes that 15 of 16 trials versus placebo were positive, and in 4 trials vs. an NSAID, 2 were equivalent and 2 demonstrated superiority over medication in long-term pain relief (Towheed et al., 2001). Two additional meta-analyses, one by McAlindon et al. and more recently Richy et al. have examined glucosamine and chondroitin in the treatment of osteoarthritis. These trials examined approximately 15 RDBPC trials with greater than 1,500 patients. The later analysis found that glucosamine at 1,500 mg/day was associated with decrease in progression of joint space narrowing. Additionally, glucosamine at this dose, as well as chondroitin at varying doses (200 to 1,200 mg/day), was associated with statistically significant pain relief and improvement in joint mobility at 4 weeks. The number needed to treat (NNT) was 5 with no significant adverse effects as compared with placebo (McAlindon et al., 2000; Richy et al., 2003).

Several important clinical notes exist regarding these formulations. First, the Cochrane Review points out in its conclusions that the majority of studies were performed on the Dona Glucosamine brand and that results may be difficult to extrapolate to other brands (Towheed et al., 2001). Additionally, studies have demonstrated wide variations in glucosamine formulations. Last, the Richy et al. (2003) meta-analysis deemed the chondroitin trials to be of overall low quality with the combination of the two products not being evaluated. Products with glucosamine and chondroitin typically state that the two combined work better than either alone. Unfortunately, this has not yet been established nor has the question of who may benefit more from one therapy over the other. In clinical practice, when combination therapy does not have a clear advantage, it is prudent to start with a single ingredient to assess clinical response before changing or adding therapy. The results of the ongoing National Institutes of Health Glucosamine/Chondroitin Arthritis Intervention Trial (2004) should be helpful in determining the answers to important questions regarding combination dosing.

SAMe

S-Adenosyl methionine is a sulfur-containing dietary supplement synthesized from reactions between adenosine triphosphate (ATP) and methionine and promoted for treatment of a number of conditions including depression, liver, and joint disease. Its role in these conditions is derived from possible intrinsic anti-inflammatory, serotonergic, and proteoglycan stimulatory mechanisms (Harmand et al., 1987; Parcell, 2002; Stramentinoli et al., 1987). A number of earlier clinical trials demonstrated the treatment potential of SAMe in open trials. A recent meta-analysis of RCTs found 11 trials demonstrating improvement in functional ability and pain levels when compared with placebo or NSAIDs (Soeken et al., 2002). Also there were significantly fewer complaints of side effects when compared with NSAID therapy and similar complaints to placebo.

A more recent RDBPCT compared SAMe (1,200 mg) with celecoxib (200 mg) in 61 subjects with knee osterarthritis over 16 weeks (Najm et al., 2004). After 1 month of intervention, celecoxib demonstrated greater pain reduction over SAMe ($p = 0.024$). However, from the second month onward, there was no significant difference between groups, with both interventions demonstrating improvement in pain scores and functional joint ability. The authors concluded that SAMe had a slower onset of action but similar efficacy as celecoxib. Those considering SAMe should be monitored for concomitant use of serotonergic medication because of synergistic potential. One significant drawback to this supplement is its current cost that makes it one of the more expensive supplements on the market. Typical initial dosing is 600 mg/day usually divided into three daily doses with titration up to 1,200 mg/day. Doses up to 1,600 mg/day have been used in selected settings with monitoring.

Avocado–Soybean Unsaponifiables (ASU)

Although not yet readily available in the United States, this combination product does deserve mention because of it promising results in osterarthritis. The unsaponifiable portion of vegetables oils has been regarded for its potential bioactivity due to its sterol, tocopherol, and squalene levels (Rosenblat et al., 1995). A specific mixture derived from the unsaponifiables of avocado and soybean, typically in a ratio of 2:1, has been examined since the 1970s for use in several conditions including scleroderma and periodontal and degenerative diseases (Reginster et al., 2000). Recent *in vitro* chrondrocyte research has demonstrated the ability of ASU to decrease several key agents implicated in joint degradation and inflammation including IL-1-beta-induced collagenase release, stromelysin, IL-6 and IL-8, and PGE-2 (Henrotin et al., 2003). In addition, there is *in vitro* evidence regarding its supportive role in maintaining the joint matrix including upregulation of transforming growth factor-beta and aggrecan synthesis (Boumediene et al., 1999; Reginster et al., 2000.)

Clinically, ASUs have been utilized mainly in the symptomatic treatment of knee and hip osterarthritis. In one multicenter RCT, 300 or 600 mg/day of ASU was compared with placebo in patients with knee osterarthritis. At 3 months the number of patients decreasing NSAID or analgesic intake by more than 50% in the either ASU dosage group was 71% versus 36% in the placebo group. There were also clinical improvements noted ($P < 0.01$) in a number of parameters included Lequesne's index, which decreased by 3.2 and 2.9 points (with the 600 and 300 mg dosing, respectively) versus 1.6 points in the placebo group (Appelbloom et al., 2001). A second trial demonstrated treatment benefit up to 8 months, including a 2-month follow-up while not on the supplement (Maheu et al., 1998).

A more recent systematic review of RCTs meeting high methodological criteria found that three of four trials demonstrated efficacy with use of ASUs (Ernst, 2003). The negative trial was one with the longest length of follow-up. Joint space narrowing has also been discussed with use of ASUs, but only seen in research populations with the worst levels of joint deterioration. Of note, there were no significant differences between 300 and 600 mg dosage efficacy, and side effects have been shown to be similar to placebo and typically GI in nature. At this point the use of ASUs is promising with long-term efficacy trials needed to confirm their clinical and potential structural benefit in practice.

NATURAL SUPPLEMENTS FOR HEADACHE

Feverfew (*Tanacetum parthenium*)

Feverfew is a member of the chrysanthemum family originally recognized by first century A.D. Greek physicians for its analgesic and antipyretic properties. It was typically used in a number of clinical scenarios including treatment of fever and dysmenorrhea. Feverfew has exhibited a number of active constituents including the sesquiterpene lactone parthenolide (typically used for standardization), tanetin, and many other bioflavanoids. Unfortunately, previous examination of feverfew samples has identified certain products that in contrast to label claims, contained little or no actual parthenolide, thus emphasizing the importance of finding well-regulated supplements (Nelson, Cobb, & Shelton, 2002). Feverfew has also demonstrated a number of activities related to inflammation and headache activation including inhibition of PG synthetase, 5-lipoxygenase, cyclooxygenase, platelet phospholipase, and serotonin secretion in platelets (Heptinstall et al, 1985; Makheja & Bailey, 1982; Pugh & Sambo, 1988; Sumner et al., 1992).

Clinically, four DBPCTs have been performed with three trials demonstrating a reduction in the severity, duration, and frequency (of approximately 24%) of migraine headaches using a dried powder preparation. The fourth trial using an alcohol extract had nonsignificant results (De Weerdt, Bootsma, & Hendriks, 1996; Johnson et al., 1985; Murphy, Heptinstall, & Mitchell, 1988; Palevitch, Earon, & Carasso, 1997). A meta-analysis of these trials states that further long-term trials with focus on the type of preparation utilized are needed to better establish feverfew's efficacy (Pittler, Vogler, & Ernst, 2000). Feverfew extracts utilized should be standardized to a minimum of 0.2% parthenolide content and those using the herb should be told that 1 to 2 months of use may be needed before any appreciable improvement is noted. Allergies are rarely reported in subjects with sensitivity to the chrysanthemum family. Side effects are also rare and typically reported as GI upset or withdrawal headache with rapid discontinuation. Because of feverfew's platelet inhibitory activity, caution should be taken in patients on other blood thinners or with history of platelet dysfunction.

Magnesium

Magnesium (Mg) is a ubiquitous mineral necessary for >300 enzymatic reactions including nerve conduction, skeletal and cardiac muscle contraction, protein synthesis, and energy reactions involving ATP. Magnesium is also involved in functions that may be especially influential on headaches including platelet aggregation, vasospasm, and calcium channel antagonism. Subjects with poor neurovascular tone demonstrate low cerebrospinal fluid Mg levels, and low Mg with high calcium/Mg ratios also appear to modulate cerebral serotonin receptors (Altura, 1985; Ramadan et al., 1989).

Clinical studies on magnesium demonstrate that intravenous Mg has a variable effect on acute treatment of migraine that may depend on magnesium levels. In one trial using intravenous Mg, 85% of responders had low ionized Mg levels <0.54 mmol/L with 85% of nonresponders having normal ionized Mg levels with no correlation noted with levels of serum Mg. Studies of oral Mg as a prophylactic agent have noted two short-term positive DBPCTs in adults with an approximate 25% decrease in headache frequency and one DBPCT in children demonstrating improvement in headache frequency ($P = 0.0037$) and severity ($P = 0.0029$) relative to the placebo group (Faccinetti et al., 1991; Peikert, Wilimzig, & Kohne-Volland, 1996; Wang et al., 2003). A negative study involving Mg aspartate was discontinued early secondary to drop out mainly from GI symptoms (Pfaffenrath et al., 1996). The dosage and Mg formulation may be critical in potential benefit and tolerability of Mg. Various formulations, including those that are chelated, in addition to consideration of intracellular testing to monitor titration, may be needed to improve compliance and subgroup efficacy variations. The typical dose used for prophylaxis is Mg at 300 mg/day or higher with dose titration based on GI tolerance.

Riboflavin (Vitamin B₂)

Riboflavin is an important vitamin in its actions as a precursor of flavin adenine dinucleotide and flavin mononucleotide. Dysfunction of these coenzymes has been linked to electron transport chain abnormalities and poor cerebrovascular tone, both of which have a potential role in migraine pathogenesis (Welch & Ramadan, 1995). An intention-to-treat analysis of 55 patients using 400 mg/day over 3 months demonstrated decreased headache days by 59% versus 15% for placebo. In this study the NNT to reach significance was 2.3. As with other supplements, an extended use of supplement for several months was necessary before clinical improvement was noted. Side effects are rare and typically GI in nature.

Of note, a patented formulation of feverfew (50 mg), Mg (300 mg), and riboflavin (400 mg) is available under the brand name Migralief. This formulation is currently undergoing an RDBPCT to demonstrate clinical efficacy beyond that seen with the isolated ingredients.

Butterbur (*Petasites hybridus*)

Butterbur is an herbal supplement with a history of benefits in a number of conditions including asthma, hypertension, and migraine. The active ingredients include the sesquiterpene petasines, which have demonstrated activity including LT inhibition and calcium channel antagonism. Clinically, butterbur is available most commonly as Petadolax®, which is an unsaturated pyrrolizidine alkaloids-free formulation standardized to 7.5 mg of the constituents petasin and isopetasin. One trial of Petadolax randomized 60 patients to 100 mg/day or placebo. Results at 3 months demonstrated a significant improvement in headache frequency and headache responder rate (improvement of migraine frequency ≥ 50%) of 45% versus 15% in the placebo group (Diener, Rahlfs, & Danesch, 2004). A more recent three-arm, parallel group, randomized trial compared 50 and 75 mg of Petadolax (p = 0.0012 vs. placebo), 36% at 50 mg bid (p = 0.127 vs. placebo), and 26% with the placebo. Side effects were minimal and included GI upset.

Butterbur's safety has been demonstrated in animal and human trials with the most likely adverse effect seen at a typical daily dosage of 100 mg/day, GI intolerance, occurring rarely (Danesch & Rittinghausen, 2003). There has been some concern regarding pyrrolizidine alkaloid levels in some butterbur preparations, which have been linked to rare cases of cholestatic hepatitis with incidence by one estimate of 1:175,000 (Kalin, 2003). Newer methods for extraction make this possibility less likely, with monitoring still prudent in patients on long-term therapy.

Other Supplements for Headache (Melatonin, Capsicum, and Coenzyme Q10)

A number of additional supplements have preliminary data for the treatment of headache. Melatonin has demonstrated variable results in treatment of cluster headache in several small trials. The trend may have to do with circadian influences as well as dosing, with the nonsignificant trial dosing at 2 mg/day and the two positive trials utilizing 9 to 10 mg/day (May & Leone, 2003). Topical intranasal capsicum has one RCT demonstrating efficacy in cluster headaches (Marks et al., 1993). An open-label trial of coenzyme Q10 at 150 mg/daily in 32 patients with migraine demonstrated a reduction in migraine frequency of 13% at 1 month and 53% at 3 months (Rozen et al., 2002). A more recent randomized controlled trial evaluated CoQ10 taken 100 mg TID versus placebo in 42 migraine patients. In the third treatment month, CoQ10's 50% responder rate for attack frequency was 47.6% versus 14.4% for placebo. This response demonstrates a low number-needed-to-treat of 3. Additionally, CoQ10 was well tolerated and demonstrated superiority versus placebo for headache-days and days-with-nausea by the third treatment month. The potential benefit of CoQ10, once confirmed in further studies, may be attributed to regulation of the electron transport chain, similar in many respects to the actions of riboflavin.

MISCELLANEOUS SUPPLEMENTS IN PAIN MANAGEMENT

A number of supplements, including several of those reviewed above, have been used in additional pain-related clinical trials. Minerals with preliminary benefits include intravenous Mg for short-term relief of cancer-associated neuropathic and posthysterectomy pain and oral calcium at 1,200 mg/day for premenstrual syndrome-associated pain (Crosby, Wilcock, & Corcoran, 2000).

Topical agents such as camphor and capsicum are found in OTC approved preparations for temporary pain relief, with positive results, especially for the latter in rheumatoid arthritis, osterarthritis, and diabetic- or shingles-associated neuropathy. Ginkgo biloba and L-arginine have also been associated with a decrease in vascularly mediated pain in claudication and angina pectoris, respectively (Blum et al., 1999; Pittler & Ernst, 2000).

CONCLUSIONS

Although the type and avenue for purchase of dietary supplements will change over time, they will continue to be an increasingly present aspect of patient care. This phenomenon appears even more prevalent for pain practitioners whose patients often turn to dietary supplement as a treatment option. The first section of this chapter served as a primer offering key points regarding the regulation, utilization, and management of dietary supplements in the United States. With dietary supplement use expanding, it is imperative for clinicians to be aware of key regulatory distinctions as well as to be able to discuss them openly with patients.

The second section reviewed commonly used supplements that have been evaluated in preclinical and clinical trials in order to demonstrate their safety and efficacy. Several of these supplements have pain modulatory properties that should prompt careful considerations regarding their incorporation in patient care. Additionally, the review provides many areas of opportunity for research to explore and expand what is known regarding supplements. Ultimately, the field of natural supplements is dynamic and requires increased patient–clinician discussion and collaboration in order to best guide care. The following key points are offered regarding natural supplements in pain management:

- Discussion is key. Pain patients have a high rate of supplement use, which influences their conventional care and deserves education and guidance.
- Patients are mostly using supplements in conjunction with conventional care. In this setting clinicians should be cognizant of the potential drug-sparing effects of supplements.
- The background diet of patients may influence the efficacy of certain supplements. This needs to be discussed to optimize the potential benefit of supplements.
- All supplements are not created or researched equally. Regulation is variable and vigilance is needed by clinicians and patients to find the best-researched and regulated supplements.
- Supplements, especially botanical products, have diverse bioactivity that cannot typically be explained by one isolated constituent. This may be beneficial in treating multiple conditions (e.g., magnesium: headache and hypertension; butterbur: headache and allergic rhinitis) or problematic, especially when other medication are involved (St. John's Wort and indinivar).
- Supplements may often have a slower onset of action than conventional prescription agents. Warn patients to expect this so that expectations are reasonable and compliance is optimized.
- Supplements often combat more than inflammatory mediated pain. In addition to inflammation, vascular, thrombotic, neurogenic, psychogenic, hormonal, and environmental factors my cause or contribute to pain. Supplements may influence one or more of these factors through their individual or synergistic mechanisms of action.

REFERENCES

Adam, O. et al. (2003). Anti-inflammatory effects of a low arachidonic acid diet and fish oil in patients with rheumatoid arthritis. *Rheumatology International, 23*(1), 27–36.

Adler, S. R. et al. (1999). Disclosing complementary and alternative medicine use in the medical encounter: A qualitative study in women with breast cancer. *Journal of Family Practice, 48*(6), 453–458.

Al-Yahya, M. A. et al. (1989). Gastroprotective activity of ginger, *Zingiber offinale Res*, in albino rats. *American Journal of Chinese Medicine, 17*(1–2), 51–56.

Altman, R. D. et al. (2001). Effects of a ginger extract on knee pain in patients with osteoarthritis. *Arthritis and Rheumatism, 44*(11), 2531–2538.

Altura, B. M. (1985). Calcium antagonist properties of magnesium: Implications for antimigraine actions. *Magnesium, 4*(4), 169–175.

Appelbloom, T. et al. (2001). (2001). Symptoms modifying effect of avocado–soybean unsaponifiables (ASU) in knee osteoarthritis. A double blind, prospective, placebo-controlled study. *Scandinavian Journal of Rheumatology, 30*(4), 242–247.

Astin, J. A. (1998). Why patients use alternative medicine: Results of a national study. *Journal of the American Medical Association, 279*(19), 1548–1553.

Astin, J. A. et al. (2000). Complementary and alternative medicine use among elderly persons: One-year analysis of a Blue Shield Medicare supplement. *Journals of Gerontology. Series A. Biological Sciences and Medical Sciences, 55*(1), M4–9.

Azaz-Livshits, T. et al. (2002). Use of complementary alternative medicine in patients admitted to internal medicine wards. *International Journal of Clinical Pharmacology and Therapeutics, 40*(12), 539–547.

Barnes, J. et al. (1998). Different standards for reporting ADRs to herbal remedies and conventional OTC medicines: Face-to-face interviews with 515 users of herbal remedies. *British Journal of Clinical Pharmacology, 45,* 495–500.

Bassleer, C. et al. (1998). Stimulation of proteoglycan production by glucosamine sulfate in chondrocytes isolated from human osteoarthritic articular cartilage *in vitro*. *Osteoarthritis Cartilage, 6,* 427–434.

Begbie, S. D. et al. (1996). Patterns of alternative medicine use by cancer patients. *Medical Journal of Australia, 165,* 545–548.

Blum, A. et al. (1999). Clinical and inflammatory effects of dietary L-arginine in patients with intractable angina pectoris. *American Journal of Cardiology, 15,* 1488–1490.

Boullata, J. I. et al. (2003). Anaphylactic reaction to a dietary supplement containing willow bark. *Annals of Pharmacotherapy, 37*(6), 832–835.

Boumediene, K. et al. (1999). Avocado–soya unsaponifiables enhance the expression of transforming growth factor beta1 and beta2 in cultured articular chondrocytes. *Arthritis and Rheumatism, 42,* 148–156.

Bruneli, B. et al. (2004). The use of complementary and alternative medicine by patients with peripheral neuropathy. *Journal of the Neurological Sciences, 218*(1–2), 59–66.

Chrubasik, S. et al. (1997). Evidence for antirheumatic effectiveness of *Herba Urticae Dioicae* in acute arthritis: A pilot study. *Phytomedicine, 4*(2), 105–108.

Chrubasik, S. et al. (2000). Treatment of low back pain exacerbations with willow bark extract: A randomized double-blind study. *American Journal of Medicine, 109*(1), 9–14.

Chrubasik, S. et al. (2001). Treatment of low back pain with a herbal or synthetic anti-rheumatic: A randomized controlled study. Willow bark extract for low back pain. *Rheumatology* (Oxford), *40*(12), 1388–1393.

Chrubasik, S. et al. (2003). A randomized double-blind pilot study comparing Doloteffin and Vioxx in the treatment of low back pain. *Rheumatology* (Oxford), *42*(1), 141–148.

Consumer Health Products Association. (2001, May 22). Self care in the new millennium: American attitudes toward maintaining personal health and treatment.

Consumer Health Products Association Report released 5/22/2001. Retrieved April 27, 2004 from http://www. chpa-info.org/web/press_room/statistics/pdfs/chpa_final_ report_revised_03_20.pdf.

Corbin-Winslow, L. et al. (2002). Physicians want education about CAM to enhance communication with their patients. *Archives of Internal Medicine, 162*(10), 1176–1181.

Crosby, V., Wilcock, A., & Corcoran R. (2000). The safety and efficacy of a single dose (500 mg or 1 g) of intravenous magnesium sulfate in neuropathic pain poorly responsive to strong opioid analgesics in patients with cancer. *Journal of Pain and Symptom Management, 19*, 35–39.

Danesch, U., & Rittinghausen, R. (2003). Safety of a patented special butterbur root extract for migraine prevention. *Headache, 43*(1), 76–78.

De Weerdt, C. J., Bootsma, H. P. R., & Hendriks, H. (1996). Herbal medicines in migraine prevention. *Phytomedicine, 3*, 225–230.

Diener, H. C., Rahlfs, V. W., & Danesch, U. (2004). The first placebo-controlled trial of a special butterbur root extract for the prevention of migraine: Reanalysis of efficacy criteria. *European Neurology, 51*(2), 89–97.

Eisenberg, D. M. et al. (1993). Unconventional medicine in the United States. Prevalence, costs, and patterns of use. *New England Journal of Medicine, 32*(4), 246-252.

Eisenberg, D. M. et al. (1998). Trends in alternative medicine use in the United States, 1990–1997: Results of a follow-up national survey. *Journal of the American Medical Association, 280*, 1569–1575.

Ernst, E. (2003). Avocado–soybean unsaponifiables (ASU) for osteoarthritis — A systematic review. *Clinical Rheumatology, 22*(4–5), 285–288.

Ernst, E., & Chrubasik, S. (2000). Phyto-anti-inflammatories. A systematic review of randomized, placebo-controlled, double-blind trials. *Rheumatic Disease Clinics of North America, 26*(1), 13–27.

Faarvang, K. L. et al. (1994). Fish oils and rheumatoid arthritis. A randomized and double-blind study. *Ugeskrift for Laeger, 156*(23), 3495–3498.

Faccinetti, F. et al. (1991). Magnesium prophylaxis of menstrual migraine: Effects on intra-cellular magnesium. *Headache, 31*, 298–304.

Federal Drug Administration Medwatch Press Release. (2002, June 5). 2002 Safety Alert — SPES, PC SPES. Retrieved May 1, 2004 from http://www.fda.gov/medwatch/SAFETY/2002/spes_press2.htm.

Federal Drug Administration Press Release. (2003, December 30). FDA announces plans to prohibit sales of dietary supplements containing Ephedra. Retrieved from http://www.fda.gov/oc/initiatives/ephedra/december2003/.

Federal Trade Commission for the Consumer Newsletter. (2003, June 10). FTC and FDA take new actions in fight against deceptive marketing. Retrieved May 1, 2004 from http://www.ftc.gov/opa/2003/06/trudeau.htm.

Fiebich, B. L. et al. (2001). Inhibition of TNFa synthesis in LPS-stimulated primary human monocytes by Harpagophytum extract SteiHap 69. *Phytomedicine, 8*, 28–30.

Food and Drug Administration. (2001, March 17). "Overview." Retrieved April 7, 2004 from http://www.cfsan.fda.gov/~dms/supplmnt.html.

Garcia-Rodriguez, L. A. et al. (2004). Risk of uncomplicated peptic ulcer among users of aspirin and nonaspirin nonsteroidal anti-inflammatory drugs. *American Journal of Epidemiology, 159*(1), 23–31.

Glucosamine/Chondroitin Arthritis Intervention Trial (GAIT) begins patient recruitment. Retrieved September 20, 2004 from http://nccam.nih.gov/news/19972000/121100.

Goso, Y. et al. (1996). Effects of traditional herbal medicine on gastric mucin against ethanol-induced gastric injury in rats. *Comparative Biochemistry and Physiology, 113C*(1), 7–21.

Gray, C. et al. (2002). Complementary and alternative medicine use among health plan members. A cross-sectional survey. *Effective Clinical Practice, 5*(1), 17–22.

Gugliona, G. (2000, March 19). Health concerns grow over herbal aids: As industry booms, analysis suggests rising toll in illness and death. *Washington Post.*

Hansrud, D. D. et al. (1999). Underreporting the use of dietary supplements and nonprescription medication among patients undergoing a periodic health examination. *Mayo Clinic. Proceedings, 74*, 443–447.

Harmand, M. F. et al. (1987). Effects of S-adenosylmethionine on human articular chondrocyte differentiation. An *in vitro* study. *American Journal of Medicine, 83*(5A), 48--54.

Harris Interactive Health Care News. (2002). Widespread ignorance of regulation and labeling of vitamins. *Minerals and Food Supplements, 2*(23).

Henrotin, Y. E. et al. (2003). Avocado/soybean unsaponifiables increase aggrecan synthesis and reduce catabolic and proinflammatory mediator production by human osteoarthritic chondrocytes. *Journal of Rheumatology, 30*(8), 1825-34.

Heptinstall, S. et al. (1985). Extracts of feverfew inhibit granule secretion in blood platelets and polymorphonuclear leukocytes. *Lancet, 1*, 1071–1074.

Hernandez-Diaz, S., & Rodriguez, L. A. (2000). Association between nonsteroidal anti-inflammatory drugs and upper gastrointestinal tract bleeding/perforation: An overview of epidemiologic studies published in the 1990s. *Archives of Internal Medicine, 160*(14), 2093–2099.

Jang, M. H. et al. (2003). *Harpagophytum procumbens* suppresses lipopolysaccharide-stimulated expressions of cyclooxygenase-2 and inducible nitric oxide synthase in fibroblast cell line L929. *Journal of Pharmacological Science, 93*(3), 367–371.

Johnson, E. S. et al. (1985). Efficacy of feverfew as prophylactic treatment of migraine. *British Medical Journal, 291,* 569–573.

Kalin, P. (2003). Försh Komplementarmed Klass. *Naturheikd 10*(Suppl. 1), 41–44.

Klein, G. et al. (2000). Short-term treatment of painful osteoarthritis of the knee with oral enzymes. *Clinical Drug Investigation, 19*(1), 15–-23.

Klinghoefer, S. et al. (1999). Antirheumatic effect of IDS 23, a stinging nettle leaf extract, on *in vitro* expression of T helper cytokines. *Journal of Rheumatology, 26,* 2517–2522.

Leung, J. M. et al.(2001). The prevalence and predictors of the use of alternative medicine in presurgical patients in five California hospitals. *Anesthesia and Analgesia, 93,* 1062–1068.

Lipton, R. B., Gobel, H., Einhaupl, K. M., Wilks, K., & Mauskop, A. (2004). *Petasites hybridus* root (butterbur) is an effective preventive treatment for migraine. *Neurology, 63*(12), 2240–2244.

Loew, D. et al. (2001). Investigations on the pharmacokinetic properties of Harpagophytum extracts and their effects on eicosanoid biosynthesis *in vitro* and *ex vivo*. *Clinical Pharmacology and Therapeutics, 69,* 356–364.

MacLean, C. H. et al. (2004). Effects of omega-3 fatty acids on lipids and glycemic control in type II diabetes and the metabolic syndrome and on inflammatory bowel disease, rheumatoid arthritis, renal disease, systemic lupus erythematosus, and osteoporosis. Summary, Evidence Report/Technology Assessment No. 89. (Prepared by the Southern California/RAND Evidence-based Practice Center, Los Angeles, CA.) AHRQ Publication No. 04-E012-1. Rockville, MD: Agency for Healthcare Research and Quality. March.

Maheu, E. et al. (1998). Symptomatic efficacy of avocado–soybean unsaponifiables in the treatment of osteoarthritis of the knee: A prospective, randomized, double-blind, placebo-controlled, multicenter trial with a six-month treatment period and a two-month follow up demonstrating a persistent effect. *Arthritis and Rheumatism, 41*(1), 81–91.

Makheja, A. N., & Bailey, J. M. (1982). A platelet phospholipase inhibitor from the medicinal herb feverfew (*Tanacetum parthenium*). *Prostaglandins, Leukotrienes, and Medicine, 8,* 653–660.

Marks, D. R. et al. (1993). A double-blind placebo-controlled trial of intranasal capsaicin for cluster headache. *Cephalalgia, 13* (2), 114–116.

May, A., & Leone, M. (2003). Update on cluster headache. *Current Opinion in Neurology, 16*(3), 333–340.

McAlindon, T. et al. (2000). Glucosamine and chondroitin for the treatment of osteoarthritis. *Journal of the American Medical Association, 283,* 1469–1475.

Murakami, A. (1992). Zerumbone, a southeast Asian ginger sesquiterpene, markedly suppresses free radical generation, proinflammatory protein production, and cancer cell proliferation accompanied by apoptosis: The alpha, beta-unsaturated carbonyl group is a prerequisite. *Carcinogenesis, 23*(5), 795–802.

Murphy, J. J., Heptinstall, S., & Mitchell, J. R. A. (1988). Randomised double-blind placebo-controlled trial of feverfew in migraine prevention. *Lancet, 2,* 189–192.

Najm, W. I. et al. (2004). S-adenosyl methionine (SAMe) versus celecoxib for the treatment of osteoarthritis symptoms: A double-blind cross-over trial. *BioMed Central Musculoskeletal Disorders, 5*(1), 6.

Nayak, S. et al. (2001). The use of complementary and alternative therapies for chronic pain following spinal cord injury: A pilot study. *Journal of Spinal Cord Medicine, 24*(1), 54–62.

Nelson, M. H., Cobb, S. E., & Shelton, J. (2002). Variations in parthenolide content and daily dose of feverfew products. *American Journal of Health-System Pharmacy, 59*(16), 1527–1531.

Nielsen, G. L. et al. (1992). The effects of dietary supplementation with n-3 polyunsaturated fatty acids in patients with rheumatoid arthritis: A randomized, double blind trial. *European Journal of Clinical Investigation, 22*(10), 687–691.

Nordstrom, D. C. et al. (1995). Alpha-linolenic acid in the treatment of rheumatoid arthritis. A double-blind, placebo-controlled and randomized study: Flaxseed vs. safflower seed. *Rheumatology International, 14*(6), 231–234.

Norred, C. L. et al. (2000). Hemorrhage after the preoperative use of complementary and alternative medicines. *American Association of Nurse Anesthetists Journal, 68*(3), 217–220.

Norred, C. L., Zamudio, S., & Palmer, S.K. (2000). Use of complementary and alternative medicines by surgical patients. *American Association of Nurse Anesthetists Journal, 68*(1), 13–18.

Nutrition Business Journal. (2001), *6,* 1–3.

Palevitch, D., Earon, G., & Carasso, R. (1997). Feverfew (*Tanacetum parthenium*) as a prophylactic treatment for migraine: A double-blind placebo-controlled study. *Phytotherapy Research, 11,* 508–511.

Parcell, S. (2002). Sulfur in human nutrition and applications in medicine. *Alternative Medicine Review, 7*(1), 22–44.

Peikert, A., Wilimzig, C., & Kohne-Volland, R. (1996). Prophylaxis of migraine with oral magnesium: Results from a prospective, multicenter, placebo-controlled and double-blind randomized study. *Cephalalgia, 16,* 257–263.

Peng, C. et al. (2004). Incidence and severity of potential drug-dietary supplement interactions in primary care patients. *Archives of Internal Medicine, 164,* 630–636.

Pfaffenrath, V. et al. (1996). Magnesium in the prophylaxis of migraine — A double-blind, placebo-controlled study. *Cephalalgia, 16,* 436–440.

Pioro-Boisset, M. et al. (1996). Alternative medicine use in fibromyalgia syndrome. *Arthritis Care Research, 9*(1), 13–17.

Pittler, M. H., & Ernst, E. (2000). Ginkgo biloba extract for the treatment of intermittent claudication: A meta-analysis of randomized trials. *American Journal of Medicine, 108,* 276–281.

Pittler, M. H., Vogler, B. K., & Ernst, E. (2000). Feverfew for preventing migraine. *Cochrane Database Systems Review*, (3), CD002286.

Pugh, W. J., & Sambo, K. (1988). Prostaglandin synthetase inhibitors in feverfew. *Journal of Pharmacy and Pharmacology, 40*, 743–745.

Rafatullah, S. et al. (1990). Evaluation of turmeric (*Curcuma longa*) for gastric and duodenal antiulcer activity in rats. *Journal of Ethnopharmacology, 29*, 25–34.

Ramadan, N. M. et al. (1989). Low brain magnesium in migraine. *Headache, 29*(7), 416–419.

Reginster, J. Y. et al. (2000). Evidence of nutraceutical effectiveness in the treatment of osteoarthritis. *Current Rheumatology Reports. 2*, 472–477.

Richy, F. et al. (2003). Structural and symptomatic efficacy of glucosamine and chondroitin in knee osteoarthritis. *Archives of Internal Medicine, 163*, 1514–1522.

Riehemann, K. et al. (1999). Plant extracts from stinging nettle (*Urticae Dioicae*), an antirheumatic remedy, inhibit the proinflammatory transcription factor nF-KB. *Federation of European Biochemical Societies Letters, 442*, 89–94.

Rosenblat, G. et al. (1995). Chemical characteristics of lysyl oxidase inhibitor from avocado seed oil. *Journal of the American Oil Chemists' Society, 72*(2), 225–229.

Rozen, T. D. et al. (2002). Open label trial of coenzyme Q10 as a migraine preventive. *Cephalalgia, 22*(2), 137–141.

Sandor, P. S. et al. (2005). Efficacy of coenzyme Q10 in migraine prophylaxis: A randomized control trial. *Neurology, 64*(4), 713–715.

Schaffner, W. (1997). Eidenrinde-Ein Antiarrheumatikum der modernen Phytotherapie. In S. Chrubasik & M. Wink (Eds.), *Rheumatherapie mit Phytopharmaka* (pp. 125–127). Stuttgart: Hippokrates Verlag.

Schmid, B. et al. (1998). Analgesic effects of willow bark extract in osteoarthritis: Results of a clinical double-blind trial. FACT: Focus. *Alternative and Complementary Therapeutics, 3*, 86.

Schmid, B., Kotter, I., & Heide, L. (2001). Pharmacokinetics of salicin after oral administration of a standardized willow bark extract. *European Journal of Clinical Pharmacology, 57*(5), 387–391.

Singh, G. et al. (1999). Epidemiology of NSAID-induced GI complications. *Journal of Rheumatology, 26*(Suppl.), 18–24.

Soeken, K. et al. (2002). Safety and efficacy of S-adenosylmethionine (SAMe) for osteoarthritis. *The Journal of Family Practice, 51*(5), 425–430.

Stramentinoli, G. et al. (1987). Pharmacologic aspects of S-adenosylmethionine. *American Journal of Medicine, 83* (Suppl. 5A), 35–42.

Sumner, H. et al. (1992). Inhibition of 5-lipoxygenase and cyclo-oxygenase in leukocytes by feverfew. *Biochemical Pharmacology, 43*, 2313–2320.

Thomson, M. (2002). The use of ginger (*Zingiber officinale Rosc.*) as a potential anti-inflammatory and antithrombotic agent. *Prostaglandins Leukotrienes and Essential Fatty Acids, 67*(6), 475–478.

Tomer, A. et al. (2001). Reduction of pain episodes and prothrombotic activity in sickle cell disease by dietary n-3 fatty acids. *Thrombosis and Haemostasis, 85*(6), 966–974.

Towheed, T. E. et al. (2001). Glucosamine therapy for treating osteoarthritis. *Cochrane Database Systems Review,* CD002946.

Tsen, L. C. et al. (2000). Survey of residency training in preoperative evaluation. *Anesthesiology, 93* (4), 1134–1137.

Uelbelhart, D. et al. (1998). Protective effect of exogenous chondroitin 4,6-sulfate in the acute degradation of articular cartilage in the rabbit. *Osteoarthritis Cartilage, 6*(Suppl. A), 6–13.

Volker, D. et al. (2000). Efficacy of fish oil concentrate in the treatment of rheumatoid arthritis. *Journal of Rheumatology, 27*(10), 234–236.

von Kruedener, S. et al. (1995). A combination of *Populus tremula, Solidago virguarea,* and *Fraxinus excelsior* as an anti-inflammatory and antirheumatic drug. A short review. *Arzneimittelforschung, 45*(2), 169–171.

Wang, F. et al. (2003). Oral magnesium oxide prophylaxis of frequent migrainous headache in children: A randomized, double-blind, placebo-controlled trial. *Headache, 43*(6), 601–610.

Welch, K. M., & Ramadan, N. M. (1995). Mitochondria, magnesium and migraine, *Journal of the Neurological Sciences, 134*, 9–14.

Wigler, I. et al. (2003). The effects of Zintona EC (a ginger extract) on symptomatic gonarthritis. *Osteoarthritis Cartilage, 11*(11), 783–789.

Yeoh, K. G. et al. (1995). Chili protects against aspirin-induced gastroduodenal mucosal injury in humans. *Digestive Diseases and Sciences, 40*(3), 580–583.

Zochling, J. et al. (2004). Use of complementary medicines for osteoarthritis — A prospective study. *Annals of the Rheumatic Diseases, 63*(5), 549–554.

Zurier, R. B. et al. (1996). Gamma-linolenic acid treatment of rheumatoid arthritis. A randomized, placebo-controlled trial. *Arthritis and Rheumatism, 39*(11), 1808–1817.

56

The Role of Cannabis and Cannabinoids in Pain Management

Ethan Russo, MD

INTRODUCTION

The herb cannabis is derived from the Old World species *Cannabis sativa* L. It is generally conceived that cannabis is a monotypic species (Merzouki, 2001), but *C. afghanica* may also merit species status (Clarke, 1998). Cannabis has a history as an analgesic agent that spans at least 4,000 years, including a century of usage in mainstream Western medicine. Quality control issues and, ultimately, political fiat eliminated this agent from the modern pharmacopoeia, but it is now resurgent. The reasons lie in the remarkable pharmacological properties of the herb, and new scientific research that reveals the inextricable link that cannabinoids possess with our own internal biochemistry. In essence, the cannabinoids form a system in parallel with that of the endogenous opioids (endorphins/enkephalins) in modulating pain. More importantly, cannabis, and its endogenous and synthetic counterparts, may be uniquely effective in pain syndromes such as neuropathic pain and migraine where opiates and other analgesics fail.

Despite hundreds of supportive journal articles over the last 15 years, the news about cannabis and cannabinoids has only slowly filtered into public and even professional acknowledgment. The attendant politics remain contentious, with certain states and countries acknowledging a role for cannabis in medicine, while other governmental bodies languish in inactivity or outright opposition.

Before the previous edition of this book (E. B. Russo, 2002a), no major medical text on pain had covered this topic to the author's awareness. This chapter may then represent a point of departure in what the author believes will be a major renaissance of interest in this plant, its healing attributes, and what it may tell us about our own internal mechanisms of analgesia. A unique set of clinical tools may be added to an armamentarium in pain management that never seems wholly adequate to the task at hand.

We examine the use of cannabis and cannabinoids historically, scientifically, and anecdotally in relation to a variety of pain syndromes. The author has previously addressed this topic with respect to migraine (E. Russo, 1998; E. B. Russo, 2001a, 2001b), chronic musculoskeletal pain (E. B. Russo et al., 2002a), obstetrics and gynecology (E. Russo, 2002b), and fibromyalgia and idiopathic bowel syndrome (E. B. Russo, 2004a). Additional history of medicinal cannabis usage is also available (E. B. Russo, 2001, 2004b).

CANNABIS AND PAIN TREATMENT: A HISTORICAL SURVEY

CHINA

Traditional knowledge of cannabis in China may span 5,000 years, dating to the legendary emperor and "Divine Plowman," Shên-Nung. Julien (1849) wrote of the physician Hoa-tho in the early second century and his use of a cannabis extract in surgical anesthesia (p. 197):

> He gave to the sick person a preparation of hemp (Mayo), and, in a few moments, he became so insensible that it were as if he was plunged into rapture of loss of

life. Then, following this instance, he practiced some overtures, incisions, amputations, and removed the cause of the malady; then he repaired the tissues with suture points, and applied liniments. [translation EBR]

INDIA

The *Atharvaveda* of India dates to between 1400 and 2000 B.C.E. and mentions a sacred grass, *bhang,* which remains a modern term of usage for cannabis. Medical references to cannabis date to Susruta in the sixth to seventh centuries B.C.E. (Chopra & Chopra, 1957). Dwarakanath (1965) described a series of Ayurvedic and Arabic tradition preparations containing the herb indicated for migraine, neuralgic, and visceral pains. These ancient claims in cannabis therapeutics have almost uniformly been supported by modern experimentation (E. B. Russo, 2005).

EGYPT

Previous scholars had thought cannabis to be absent from Ancient Egypt, but Nunn (1996) cited six supporting experts that it was utilized medicinally. These authors agree with the view of Dawson that the hieroglyphic *shemshemet* represents cannabis. Physical proof includes discoveries of hemp remnants in the tomb of Akhenaten (Amenophis IV) around 1350 B.C.E., and cannabis pollen in the tomb of Rameses II, who died in 1224 B.C.E. (Mannische, 1989). Cannabis has remained in the Egyptian pharmacopoeia since pharaonic times, administered orally, rectally, vaginally, on the skin, in the eyes, and by fumigation.

Mannische cites the following from Papyrus Ramesseum III, 1700 B.C.E. (Mannische, 1989, p. 82): "A treatment for the eyes: celery; hemp; is ground and left in the dew overnight. Both eyes of the patient are to be washed with it early in the morning." This suggests a parallel to modern use of cannabis in glaucoma treatment (Jarvinen, Pate, & Laine, 2002).

Another passage (Ebers Papyrus 821) is reminiscent of 19th century use of cannabis as an aid to childbirth (Ghalioungui, 1987, p. 209): "Another: *smsm-t* [shemshemet]; ground in honey; introduced into her vagina *(iwf)*. This is a contraction." The passage E618 refers to treatment of a toenail with a bandage containing hemp resin (Ghalioungui, 1987).

SUMER/AKKAD/ASSYRIA

Thompson (1924, 1949) documented 29 citations of use of cannabis in Assyrian medical documents, and attested to its analgesic and psychogenic effects by various methods including fumigation. The bulk of the references date to the second millennium B.C.E. and pertain to *A.ZAL.LA* in Sumerian, and *azallû* in Akkadian. Through philological arguments the author concluded (Thompson, 1924, p. 101):

The evidence thus indicates a plant prescribed in AM [Assyrian manuscripts] in very small doses, used in spinning and rope-making, and at the same time a drug used to dispel depression of spirits. Obviously, it is none other than hemp, *Cannabis sativa,* L.

Specifically, according to Thompson (1949), hemp, or *azallû,* was employed to bind the temples (possibly for headache?). Furthermore, the Sumerian texts recommended internal use for depression and staying the menses, and "for 'poison' of all limbs, dry, pound, sift, and fumigate."

ANCIENT ISRAEL/PALESTINE/JUDEA

Physical evidence of medicinal cannabis use in Israel has been discovered (Zias et al., 1993) in a burial tomb in Beit Shemesh where the skeleton of a 14-year-old girl was found along with fourth century bronze coins. Contained in her pelvic area was the skeleton of a term fetus, of sufficient size to render a successful vaginal delivery unlikely. In her abdominal area, gray carbonized material was noted and analyzed, yielding chromatographic and nuclear magnetic resonance spectroscopy evidence of delta-6-tetrahydrocannabinol, a stable metabolite of cannabis. The authors stated (p. 215), "We assume that the ashes found in the tomb were cannabis, burned in a vessel and administered to the young girl as an inhalant to facilitate the birth process." They further remarked that cannabis retained an indication as an aid to parturition into the 19th century.

GREEK AND ROMAN EMPIRES

In the first century of the Common Era, Dioscorides published his *Materia Medica* and described the analgesic role of cannabis (1968, 3.165, p. 390): "Cannabis is a plant of much use in this life for ye twistings of very strong ropes, … but being juiced when it is green is good for the pains of the ears."

Pliny described additional indications for hemp (1951, Book XX, XCVII, p. 153): "The root boiled in water eases cramped joints, gout too and similar violent pains. It is applied raw to burns."

THE ISLAMIC WORLD

In the ninth century, Sabur ibn Sahl in Persia cited use of cannabis several times in his dispensatorium, *Al-Aqrabadhin Al-Saghir* (Kahl, 1994). According to the translation and interpretation of the text by Dr. Indalecio Lozano (personal communication, 2000), ibn Sahl prescribed a compound medicine containing cannabis juice that was used to treat a variety of aching pains and migraine that was instilled into the nostril of the afflicted patient.

Also in the 12th century, Al-Biruni noted (Biruni, Said, & Hamdard National Foundation-Saydanah, 1973, p. 346): "Galen says: 'The leaves of this plant [cannabis] cure flatus — Some people squeeze the fresh (seeds) for use in ear-aches. I believe that it is used in chronic pains.'"

Umar ibn Yusuf ibn Rasul also suggested cannabis for ear and head pains (Lewis, Menage, Pellat, & Schacht, 1971) at the end of the 13th century.

Some time later, an electuary named *bars,* or *barsh,* containing a variety of ingredients, sometimes including cannabis, became popular as an analgesic treatment in the Arab world (Lozano Camara & Arabe, 1990).

At the close of the 17th century in Indonesia, Rumphius studied cannabis use (Rumpf & Beekman, 1981) including treatment of pleuritic chest pains and hernias.

WESTERN MEDICINE

Medicinal use of cannabis also evolved from early times involving hemp strains that in all likelihood contained cannabidiol (CBD), but no Δ^9-tetrahydrocannabinol (THC), unlike the cannabis strains of the East. An early citation derives from the ninth century in the *Old English Herbarium Manuscript V,* translated from Anglo-Saxon (Pollington, 2000, p. 301): "For pain of the innards take the same plant [hemp], give it to drink, it takes away the pain." Such uses persisted in England, as Gerard continued to recommend hemp for colic in 1597 (Gerard & Johnson, 1975). Similarly, in 1640 in the *Theatrum Botanicum, The Theater of Plantes* (Parkinson, Bonham, & L'Obel, 1640), Parkinson indicated (p. 598):

> Hempe is cold and dry ... the *Dutch* as one saith doe make an Emulsion out of the seede, ... for it openeth the obstructions of the gall, and causeth digestion of choller therein: ... the Emulsion or decoction of the seede, stayeth laskes and fluxes that are continuall, easeth the paines of the collicke: and allayeth the troublesome humours in the bowels: ... The decoction, of the roote is sayd to allay inflammations in the head or any other part, the herbe it selfe, or the distilled water thereof performeth the like effect; the same decoction of the rootes, easeth the paines of the goute, the hard tumours, or knots of the joynts, the paines and shrinking of the sinewes, and other the like paines of the hippes: it is good to be used, for any place that hath beene burnt by fire, if the fresh juyce be mixed with a little oyle or butter.

In 1758, Marcandier published his *Traité du chanvre* [Treatise on hemp] (Marcandier, 1758), which was translated into English several years later (Marcandier, 1764, pp. 24, 26):

> The grain and the leaves being squeezed, while they are green, and applied, by way of cataplasm, to painful tumours, are reckoned to have a great power of relaxing and stupefying.... The root of it boiled in water, and

applied in the form of a cataplasm, softens and restores the joints of fingers or toes that are dried and shrunk. It is very good against the gout, and other humours that fall upon the nervous, muscular, and tendinous parts. It abates inflammations, dissolves tumours, and hard swellings upon the joints. Beat and pounded in a mortar, with butter, when it is still fresh, it is applied to burns, which it relieves greatly when it is often renewed.

Linnaeus acknowledged the pain-reducing properties of cannabis in his list of its medical applications in his *Materia Medica* (Linné, 1772, pp. 213–214), "narcotica, phantastica, dementans, anodyna, repellens."

In France, Chomel (1782) noted once more the benefits of hemp seed oil on burn treatment, promoting both pain and healing.

The medical use of cannabis, or what became known as "Indian hemp" was reintroduced to the West by O'Shaughnessy in 1839 (O'Shaughnessy, 1838–1840). His treatise on the subject dealt with the apparent utility of a plant extract administered to patients suffering from rabies, cholera, tetanus, and infantile convulsions, but also a series of painful rheumatological conditions.

Shortly after Indian hemp came to England, Clendinning described his results of treatment of 18 patients (1843): three with headaches, one with abdominal pain secondary to tumor, one with pain secondary to a laceration, two with rheumatic joint pain, and one with gout. In each case, the tincture of Indian hemp provided relief, even in cases of morphine withdrawal symptoms. He observed (p. 209):

> I have no hesitation in affirming that in my hand its exhibition has usually, and with remarkably few substantial exceptions, been followed by manifest effects as a soporific or hypnotic in conciliating sleep; as an anodyne in lulling irritation; as an antispasmodic in checking cough and cramp; and as a nervine stimulant in removing languor and anxiety, and raising the pulse and spirits; and that these effect have been observed in both acute and chronic affections, in young and old, male and female.

In Ireland in 1845, Donovan extensively described his own extensive trials with small doses of cannabis resin, mainly in patients with various types of neuropathic and musculoskeletal pain. Effects were fairly uniformly impressive, with few side effects. He also described the benefits of local application of hemp leaf oil on hemorrhoids and neuralgic pains.

Christison (1851) endorsed benefits of cannabis in treating tetanus, augmenting labor, and treatment of neuralgic and musculoskeletal pain.

Grigor in 1852 examined the role of cannabis in facilitating childbirth. In nine cases, little was noticeable, but in seven, including five primiparous women (p. 125), "the contractions acquire great increase of strength … it is capable of bringing the labour to a happy conclusion considerably within a half of the time that would other have been required." No ontoward effects were observed on mother or child.

Over the next decades, numerous authorities recognized cannabis as helpful for painful conditions. Sir John Russell Reynolds was eventually to become Queen Victoria's personal physician. Popular legend supports that he successfully treated her dysmenorrhea with a cannabis extract throughout her adult life. Reynolds (1868) reported on various successes with Indian hemp, theorizing (p. 160):

> This medicine appears capable of reducing over-activity of the nervous centres without interfering with any one of the functions of organic, or vegetal life. The bane of many opiates and sedatives is this, that the relief of the moment, the hour, or the day, is purchased at the expense of tomorrow's misery. In no one case to which I have administered Indian hemp, have I witnessed any such results.

In 1870, Silver reported five cases in detail of menorrhagia and dysmenorrhea, all relieved nicely with cannabis. He also referred to a colleague, who had never failed in over 100 cases to control pain and discomfort in these disorders within three doses.

In 1874, a popular textbook, *Practical Therapeutics,* stated of cannabis (Waring, 1874, p. 159): "Of a good extract, gr. 1/4 to gr. 1/2, rarely gr. j, in the form of pill, is very effective in some forms of neuralgia."

In the French literature, Michel (1880) extensively reviewed and endorsed the success of cannabis in treating neuralgic afflictions.

In 1883, two letters to the *British Medical Journal* attested to the benefits of extract of *Cannabis indica* in menorrhagia, treating both pain and bleeding successfully with a few doses (Batho, 1883; Brown, 1883).

Rennie reported from India on the therapeutic value of a cannabis tincture in curing acute and chronic dysentery and its attendant pain in some dozen patients (Rennie, 1886).

In 1887, Dr. Hobart Hare published an article that dealt at length with the indications of cannabis (pp. 225–226):

> CANNABIS INDICA has been before the profession for many years as a remedy to be used in combating almost all forms of pain, yet, owing to the variations found to exist as to its activity, it has not received the confidence which I think it now deserves.… I have found the efficient dose of a pure extract of hemp to be as powerful in relieving pain as the corresponding dose of the same preparation of opium.… During the time that this remarkable drug is relieving pain a very curious psychical condition sometimes manifests itself; namely, that the diminution of the pain seems to be due to its fading away in the distance, so that the pain becomes less and less, just as the pain in a delicate ear would grow less and less as a beaten drum was carried farther and farther out of the range of hearing.

Soon after, Farlow penned a treatise on the use of rectal preparations of cannabis (1889, p. 508), "Cannabis has few equals in its power over nervous headaches such as women with pelvic troubles are subject to."

Aulde (1890) lauded the drug as follows (p. 526): "As a remedy for the relief of *supraorbital neuralgia* no article perhaps afford better prospects than cannabis."

In the French literature, Sée submitted a detailed report on use of cannabis in the treatment of various disorders producing gastric and intestinal pain (1890). He found it preferable in efficacy and side effects to other agents of the day, including opiates and bismuth that remain on the modern scene.

In the article "On the Therapeutic Value of Indian Hemp," Suckling (1891) declared (p. 12), "I have met with patients who have been incapacitated for work from the frequency of the attacks [of migraine], and who have been enabled by the use of Indian hemp to resume their employment." This echoes modern claims of clinical cannabis users who partake lightly of the drug and return to work or study.

Mattison was effusive in his praise in 1891 (pp. 270–271):

> Indian hemp is not here lauded as a specific. It will, at times, fail. So do other drugs. But the many cases in which it acts well, entitle it to a large and lasting confidence. My experience warrants this statement: cannabis indica is, often, a safe and successful anodyne and hypnotic.

Mackenzie (1894) described the utility of cannabis in treating neuralgias, headache (including chronic daily headache), tabetic (syphilitic) pain, functional gastrointestinal pain (corresponding to modern idiopathic bowel syndrome), and pruritic disorders.

That year in India, among many other indications, the encyclopedic Indian Hemp Drugs Commission (1894) reported that a small piece of *charas* (hashish) placed in a carious tooth would relieve aching pain.

An 1898 American drug handbook stated the following quaint prose under "Actions and uses" for cannabis (Lilly, 1898, p. 32): "Not poisonous according to best authorities, though formerly so regarded. Antispasmodic, analgesic, anesthetic, narcotic, aphrodisiac. Specially recommended in spasmodic and painful affections."

Dixon (1899), a famed British pharmacologist, studied cannabis extensively and recognized its value "as a useful food accessory," supporting its current indications in the cachexia of cancer chemotherapy and HIV-positive patients in 1899. He also reintroduced the concept of smoking the drug to Western medicine (p. 1356):

In cases where an immediate effect is desired the drug should be smoked, the fumes being drawn through water. In fits of depression, mental fatigue, nervous headache, and exhaustion a few inhalations produce an almost immediate effect, the sense of depression, headache, feeling of fatigue disappear and the subject is enabled to continue his work, feeling refreshed and soothed. I am further convinced that its results are marvelous in giving staying power and altering the feelings of muscular fatigue which follow hard physical labour.

The same year, Shoemaker (1899) reported on a large series of patients with pain conditions, including migraine, dental neuralgia, gastralgia, enteralgia, cerebral tumor, and herpes zoster, all successfully treated with *Cannabis indica*.

As late as 1915, Sir William Osler, the acknowledged father of modern medicine stated of migraine treatment (Osler & McCrae, 1915, p. 1089): "*Cannabis indica* is probably the most satisfactory remedy. Seguin recommends a prolonged course of the drug." This statement provided support of its use for both acute and prophylactic treatment of migraine.

In 1918, *The Dispensatory of the United States of America* stated (Remington et al., 1918, p. 280), "Cannabis is used in medicine to relieve pain, to encourage sleep, and to soothe restlessness.... For its analgesic action it is used especially in pains of neuralgic origin, such as *migraine,* but is occasionally of service in other types."

In 1922, Hare still advocated use of cannabis noting (p. 181), "For the relief of *pain,* particularly that depending on nerve disturbance, hemp is very valuable."

As late as 1930, the ability of cannabis to achieve a labor with pain burden substantially reduced or eliminated, followed by a tranquil sleep, was noted (Anonymous, 1930). It was stated (p. 1165), "As far as is known, a baby born of a mother intoxicated with cannabis will not be abnormal in any way."

In 1941, despite its political disenfranchisement, Morris Fishbein, the editor of the *Journal of the American Medical Association* still advocated oral preparations of cannabis in treatment of menstrual (catamenial) migraine (Fishbein, 1942).

Cannabis remained in the British armamentarium until 1961, and was extolled above opiates and barbiturates in the treatment of the pain of hospitalized patients with duodenal ulcers (Douthwaite, 1947).

MODERN ETHNOBOTANY OF CANNABIS IN ANALGESIA

In Tashkent in the 1930s, cannabis or *nasha* was employed medicinally, despite Soviet prohibition (Benet, 1975; pp. 46–47): "A mixture of lamb's fat with *nasha* is recommended for brides to use on their wedding night to reduce the pain of defloration. The same mixture works well for headache when rubbed into the skin; it may also be eaten spread on bread."

In Southeast Asia, cannabis remains useful (M. A. Martin, 1975, p. 70):

Everywhere it is considered to be of analgesic value, comparable to the opium derivatives. Moreover, it can be added to any relaxant to reinforce its action. Cooked leaves, which have been dried in the sun, are used in quantities of several grams per bowl of water. This decoction helps especially to combat migraines and stiffness.

A very recent study documents the ethnobotanical uses of cannabis by the Hmong minority in the China–Vietnam border region (Gu & Clarke, 1998, p. 6): "Some older Hmong men may rarely smoke cannabis to 'relieve discomfort,' but they are not daily smokers."

In a book about medicinal plants of India (Dastur, 1962), we see the following (p. 67):

Charas is the resinous exudation that collects on the leaves and flowering tops of plants [equivalent to the Arabic *hashish*]; it is the active principle of hemp; it is a valuable narcotic, especially in cases where opium cannot be administered; it is of great value in malarial and periodical headaches, migraine, acute mania, whooping cough, cough of phthisis, asthma, anaemia of brain, nervous vomiting, tetanus, convulsion, insanity, delirium, dysuria, and nervous exhaustion; it is also used as an anaesthetic in dysmenorrhea, as an appetizer and aphrodisiac, as an anodyne in itching of eczema, neuralgia, severe pains of various kinds of corns, etc.

In Colombia the analgesic effects of a cannabis tincture were lauded (Partridge, 1975, p. 161): "the knowledge that cannabis can be used for treatment of pain is widespread." Rubin documented extensive usage of cannabis in Jamaica for a variety of conditions (V. Rubin, 1976; V. Rubin & Comitas, 1972), including headache. In Brazil, Hutchinson noted (1975, p. 180):

Such an infusion [of marijuana leaves] is taken to relieve rheumatism, "female troubles," colic and other common complaints. For toothache, marijuana is frequently packed into and around the aching tooth and left for a period of time, during which it supposedly performs an analgesic function.

MODERN DATA ON CANNABIS AND ANALGESIA

RECENT THEORY AND CLINICAL DATA

A popular treatise on marijuana noted medicinal effects (Margolis & Clorfene, 1969, p. 26):

You'll also discover that grass is an analgesic, and will reduce pain considerably. As a matter of fact, many women use it for dysmenorrhea or menorrhagia when they're out of Pamprin or Midol. So if you have an upset stomach, or suffer from pain of neuritis or neuralgia, smoke grass. If pains persist, smoke more grass.

Solomon Snyder (1971), the discoverer of opiate receptors, examined the pros and cons of cannabis as an analgesic commenting (p. 14):

For there are many conditions, such as migraine headaches or menstrual cramps, where something as mild as aspirin gives insufficient relief and opiates are too powerful, not to mention their potential for addiction. Cannabis might conceivably fulfill a useful role in such conditions.

Subsequent experimental studies by Noyes explored these reported analgesic effects of cannabis. One article examined pain tolerance thresholds (Milstein, MacCannell, Karr, & Clark, 1975). Both naïve (8% increase) and experienced human subjects (16% increase) noted statistically significant increases in pain threshold after smoking cannabis. Noyes (Noyes & Baram, 1974) described case studies of five patients who voluntarily employed it to treat their painful conditions.

Another study pertained to oral THC in patients with cancer (Noyes, Brunk, Baram, & Canter, 1975). Pain relief with escalating doses significant to the $P < 0.001$ level was observed. Peak effects occurred at 3 hours with doses of 10 and 15 mg, but were delayed until 5 hours after the 20-mg oral dose.

Noyes's research group compared the analgesic effect of THC with codeine (Noyes, Brunk, Avery, & Canter, 1975). In short, 10 mg of oral THC reduced subjective pain burdens by similar decrements to 60 mg of codeine, as did 20 mg of THC versus 120 mg of codeine. The 20-mg dose was sedative and not as well tolerated in some elderly, cannabis-naïve subjects.

Hollister (1986) addressed possible cannabis indications including analgesia. He concluded that it seemed that no THC homologue would be an analgesic of choice, but that "It is too early to be sure, however" (p. 15). These were prophetic words in light of upcoming cannabinoid receptor research.

In 1991, a series of case studies on utility of cannabis in treating chronic pain were published (Randall, 1991). One pertained to Lynn Hastings, an Idaho woman with severe juvenile rheumatoid arthritis, whose symptoms of pain, spasm, and depression were resistant to standard medicine, but were effectively treated with cannabis. A state Supreme Court finding of "medical necessity" followed her initial arrest for cultivation of cannabis. Eventually, charges were dropped.

In 1993, the landmark book, *Marihuana, the Forbidden Medicine,* was first published by Grinspoon and Bakalar, and since revised (Grinspoon & Bakalar, 1997). Although criticized in some quarters as anecdotal, the book contains numerous compelling testimonials from patients and their doctors attesting to the clinical efficacy of cannabis where conventional pharmacotherapy failed. Cases of painful conditions responding to cannabis are legion: osteoarthritis, ankylosing spondylitis, pruritus from allergic dermatitis, premenstrual syndrome (PMS), menstrual cramps, labor pains, gingival pain (with local application of cannabis tincture), migraine, phantom limb pain, Crohn's disease, and "functional" gastrointestinal pain. Often these patients improved with cannabis, worsened without it, and improved once more upon its resumption. These accounts fulfill criteria of "*N*-of-1 studies" and have been accepted by epidemiologists as proof of efficacy in rare conditions or ones in which blinded, controlled trials are technically difficult (Guyatt et al., 1990; Larson, 1990).

The *American Journal of Public Health* issued a particularly strong plea for liberalization of laws pertaining to medical cannabis (Anonymous, 1996) in 1996, citing its activity in "decreasing the suffering from chronic pain."

Hollister (2000) reviewed indications for cannabis, "for exploratory purposes, any patient with pain unrelieved by conventional analgesics should have access to smoked marijuana if they so desire" (p. 5).

CANNABINOID AND ENDOCANNABINOID NEUROCHEMISTRY

In recent years, scientists have provided elucidation of the mechanisms of action of cannabis and THC, the primary psychoactive component, with the discovery of an endogenous cannabinoid (endocannabinoid) ligand, arachidonylethanolamide, nicknamed anandamide, from the Sanskrit word *ananda,* or "bliss" (Barinaga, 1992; Devane et al., 1992; Marx, 1990; Matsuda, Lolait, Brownstein, Young, & Bonner, 1990). Anandamide inhibits cyclic AMP mediated through G protein coupling in target cells, which cluster in nociceptive areas of the CNS (Herkenham, 1993). Early testing of its pharmacological action and behavioral activity indicate similarity to THC (Fride & Mechoulam, 1993), although anandamide differs from THC in some respects. Pertwee (1997) has examined the pharmacology of cannabinoid receptors in detail. CB_1 receptors are mainly confined to the CNS, while CB_2 receptors are found in the periphery, often in conjunction with immune mechanisms.

Further research has elucidated analgesic mechanisms of cannabinoids, which will be examined system by system.

Cannabinoids and Serotonergic Systems

Serotonergic mechanisms are implicated in many pain conditions, especially migraine and cluster headaches. THC reduces serotonin release from the platelets of human migraineurs (Volfe, Dvilansky, & Nathan, 1985). Cannabis has been observed to stimulate 5-HT synthesis, its brain content, decrease its synaptosomal uptake, while stimulating its release (Spadone, 1991). Anandamide and other cannabinoid agonists inhibit rat serotonin type 3 (5-HT_3) receptors (Fan, 1995) that mediate emetic and pain responses. The recent advent of alosetron, a 5-HT_3 blocker employed in treatment of irritable bowel syndrome (Letter, 2000), would seem to support claims of the efficacy of cannabis in that disorder on the basis of this mechanism.

Recently, Boger and his group have demonstrated an 89% relative potentiation of the 5-HT_{1A} receptor response, and a 36% inhibition of the 5-HT_{2A} receptor response by anandamide (Boger, Patterson, & Jin, 1998). Similar effects by THC are likely, supporting efficacy for cannabinoids in acute symptomatic migraine treatment due to agonistic activity at 5-HT_{1A} or 5-HT_{1D}, and in prophylactic treatment of chronic headache due to antagonistic activity at 5-HT_{2A} (Peroutka, 1990a, b).

Kimura et al. (Kimura, Ohta, Watanabe, Yoshimura, & Yamamoto, 1998) showed that high concentrations of anandamide decreased serotonin and ketanserin binding (a 5-HT_{2A} antagonist). 11-OH-delta 8-THC and 11-oxo-delta 8-THC metabolites of cannabis were also observed to modify serotonin receptor binding.

Ultimately, this author and colleagues have shown that essential oil components of cannabis demonstrate potent serotonin receptor activity (E. B. Russo, Macarah, Todd, Medora, & Parker, 2000) that supports putative synergism with THC in the modulation of analgesia. Similarly, CBD seems to harbor similar activity that would help to explain prophylactic benefits of cannabis in migraine (Hall et al., 2004).

Dopaminergic Systems

The importance of dopaminergic mechanisms in treatment of migraine and other types of pain has received recent emphasis (Peroutka, 1997). However, existing neuroleptics are significantly sedating. Ferri et al. (Ferri, Cavicchini, Romualdi, Speroni, & Murari, 1986) were able to demonstrate that 6-hydroxydopamine, which causes degeneration of catecholamine terminals, was able to block THC antinociception. In a review article (Mechoulam, Fride, & Di Marzo, 1998, p. 12), a number of studies were reviewed as demonstrating that cannabimimetic drugs cause "inhibition of the dopaminergic nigrostriatal system."

Müller-Vahl and her colleagues cited Mailleux (Mailleux & Vanderhaeghen, 1992) in their discussion of cannabinoid interactions with the dopaminergic system (Müller-Vahl, Kolbe, Schneider, & Emrich, 1998) stating, "Cannabinoid receptors were found to be co-localized both with dopamine D_1 receptors on striatonigral dynorphin/substance-P-containing neurones and with dopamine D_2 receptors on striatopallidal enkephalinergic neurones" (p. 504).

Carta et al. demonstrated that antinociceptive effects of THC are mediated by CB_1 and dopamine D_2 receptors, and that combination of the agents improved analgesic effects in rats (Carta, Gessa, & Nava, 1999).

Inflammatory Mechanisms

Modern authors (S. Burstein, 1992; A. T. Evans, Formukong, & Evans, 1987; Formukong, Evans, & Evans, 1988, 1989) have examined the relationship between cannabinoids and inflammation. McPartland (2001a) provides an excellent summary and analysis of the subject.

Burstein et al. demonstrated that THC and other cannabinoids inhibit prostaglandin E_2 synthesis (S. Burstein, Levin, & Varanelli, 1973). In 1979, experiments showed that smoked cannabis reduced platelet aggregation (Schaefer, Brackett, Gunn, & Dubowski, 1979).

In 1981, cannabichromene was demonstrated to be a more effective anti-inflammatory agent than phenylbutazone in carrageenan-induced rat paw edema and the erythrocyte membrane stabilization method (Turner & ElSohly, 1981). The authors stated, "The activity of cannabichromene through the oral route, its safety and its lack of behavioral-type (psychotomimetic) activity characteristic of THC(I) indicate its therapeutic potential for the treatment of inflammatory diseases" (pp. 288S–289S).

Evans stated (1991, p. S65), "Experiments involving oral administration of THC suggested that THC was 20 times more potent than aspirin and twice as potent as hydrocortisone." Cannabidiol (CBD) functioned as a dual cyclooxygenase and lipoxygenase inhibitor in various assays.

Klein noted that THC had variable effects on tumor necrosis factor (TNF-α) production depending on the cells and culture system selected (Klein, Friedman, & Specter, 1998).

In 1998, Jaggar et al. issued two reports addressing visceral and inflammatory pain in rats (Jaggar, Hasnie, Sellaturay, & Rice, 1998; Jaggar, Sellaturay, & Rice, 1998). The endocannabinoid anandamide, a CB_1 ligand, prevented and reduced viscero-visceral hyperreflexia (VVH) in the inflamed bladder. In contrast, palmitylethanolamide, a presumptive endogenous CB_2 ligand that accumulates in inflamed tissues and reduces edema by downmodulating mast cells, only reversed VVH once previously established. The authors posited the possibility of development of nonsedating analgesic anti-inflammatory drugs based on CB_2 receptor agonism.

In a 1999 review, Fimiani et al. note, "Delta-9-THC blocks the conversion of arachidonic acid into all metabolites derived by cyclooxygenase activity, whereas it stimulates lipoxygenase, resulting in an increase in lipoxygenase products" (p. 27). Clinically, no increased incidence of gastric ulceration was reported in chronic cannabis users (New York [City] Mayor's Committee on Marihuana, Wallace, & Cunningham, 1973; V. D. Rubin & Comitas, 1975; Stefanis, Dornbush, & Fink, 1977). In 1978, cannabis was felt to reduce gastric acidity in humans (Nalin et al., 1978), while another group demonstrated THC to have antiulcer effects in rats (Sofia, Nalepa, Harakal, & Vassar, 1973). In fact, one essential oil sesquiterpene component of cannabis, caryophyllene, has recently been demonstrated to have a gastric cytoprotective effect (Tambe, Tsujiuchi, Honda, Ikeshiro, & Tanaka, 1996).

The above authors (Fimiani et al., 1999) also observed that the morphine-cannabinoid system modulates the eicosanoid cascade and its proinflammatory cytokine activity through induction of nitric oxide synthesis, averting damaging effects on tissues. They state in summary, "Thus, we can surmise cannabinoid-morphine systems are down-regulators of inflammatory processes in an attempt to restore homeostasis" (p. 30).

A recent report has demonstrated the efficacy of oral cannabidiol (CBD), a minimally psychoactive cannabis component, at a dose of 5 mg/kg/day in treating mice against collagen-induced arthritis, a model for human rheumatoid arthritis (Malfait et al., 2000). Benefits were produced through a combination of immunosuppressive effects (diminished CII-specific proliferation and interferon-gamma production) and anti-inflammatory effects (decreased release of tumor necrosis factor by synovial cells).

Cannabis seed also has dietary benefits as an anti-inflammatory agent. It yields linolenic acid, which promotes formation of anti-inflammatory metabolites, and gamma-linolenic acid, which inhibits the formation of proinflammatory products from arachidonate (Conrad, 1997; Haines et al., 2000; Wirtshafter, 1997).

Flavonoid and terpenoid essential oil components of cannabis demonstrate anti-inflammatory effects at physiologically appropriate levels (McPartland & Russo, 2001). Cannflavin A and B inhibited prostaglandin E_2 production in human rheumatoid synovial cells 30 times more potently than aspirin (Barrett, Scutt, & Evans, 1986).

The cannabis flavonoid apigenin has anti-inflammatory actions on interleukin, TNF-α, and carrageenan-induced edema and by inhibition of upregulation of cytokine-induced genes (Gerritsen et al., 1995). Quercetin, another flavonoid in cannabis, serves as an antioxidant, and inhibits hydrogen peroxide–mediated nuclear factor (NF)-kappa B activity (Musonda & Chipman, 1998). Burstein et al. have demonstrated eugenol to be a potent prostaglandin inhibitor (S. Burstein, Varanelli, & Slade,

1975). Subsequently, both the alpha-pinene and caryophyllene components of cannabis have proved to demonstrate anti-inflammatory activity in the rat hindpaw edema model (S. Martin et al., 1993).

Cannabinoid Interactions with Opiates and Endogenous Opioids

THC experimentally increases beta-endorphin levels (Wiegant, Sweep, & Nir, 1987). Depletion of endorphins has been measured in the cerebral spinal fluid of migraineurs during attacks (Fettes, Gawel, Kuzniak, & Edmeads, 1985) and theoretically contributes to migraine effects such as hyperalgesia and photophobia. Early exposure to THC in rat pups boosted adult levels of beta-endorphins in specific brain areas (Kumar et al., 1990).

Mailleux and Vanderhaeghen (1994) have also demonstrated that THC regulates substance P and enkephalin mRNA levels in the basal ganglia. Manzanares et al. (1998) have shown THC is able promote increases in beta-endorphin in rats. Meng and his group demonstrated that THC is involved in an analgesic brainstem circuit in the rostral ventromedial medulla that interacts with opiate pathways (Meng, Manning, Martin, & Fields, 1998).

Cichewicz and her group examined the enhancement of opioid antinociception by oral THC in rodents (Cichewicz, Martin, Smith, & Welch, 1999). THC (20 mg/kg) preceding morphine rendered it significantly more analgesic with an ED_{50} dropping from 28.8 to 13.1 mg/kg. For codeine, the ED_{50} dropped phenomenally from 139.9 to 5.9 mg/kg, with enhancement also noted for oxymorphone, hydromorphone, methadone, diacetylmorphine (heroin), and meperidine. This THC enhancement was decreased by naloxone, but not by other opiate-blockers, suggesting an effect on μ-opioid receptors.

In a subsequent study, Cichewicz, Haller, and Welch (2001) demonstrated that continued low doses of THC and morphine in mice produce no behavioral tolerance to the opioid, and that the combination circumvented the expected downregulation of opioid receptor protein in the mouse midbrain observed in tolerant animals. Extension of this work (Cichewicz & McCarthy, 2003) demonstrated that oral doses of THC with either morphine or codeine produced synergistic increases in analgesia.

Perhaps the most exciting development from this group surrounds the suggestion that THC blocks opiate withdrawal effects and prevents the development of opiate tolerance (Cichewicz & Welch, 2003). Such tolerance in chronic opioid-treated mice was circumvented with nonanalgetic doses of oral THC, while THC also significantly reduced naloxone-precipitated withdrawal effects in such mice. Substantiation is thus provided for 19th century claims of utility of cannabis in treatment of opiate addiction, suggesting a new indication for clinical trials.

Finally, Cichewicz presented findings indicating that late administration of THC will restore opioid analgesic effects after low doses or ones that had previously worn off (Cichewicz, Rubo, & Welch, 2003), thus scientifically verifying the anecdotal reports of cannabis-opiate alternation from the 19th century.

Welch and Eads (1999) note cannabinoid-induced analgesia produced antinociception through spinal dynorphin release with synergistic effects with opiates. They state, however, "THC, in comparison to the morphine derivatives, has a greater therapeutic range" (p. 188).

Many analgesic effects of cannabinoids cannot be reproduced by opiates, however, particularly in cases of neuropathic pain (Hamann & di Vadi, 1999). Nicolodi (1998) examined opiate aggravation of migraine. Manzanares (Manzanares et al., 1999) cited that chronic cannabinoid administration could similarly promote hypothalamic production of beta-endorphin.

Strangman and Walker (1999) demonstrated that a cannabinoid antagonist was able to decrease wind-up in spinal nociceptive neurons producing hyperalgesia and allodynia in chronic pain states. A similar group (Walker et al., 1999) showed that cannabinoids selectively affect nociceptive neurons in the spinal cord and ventroposterolateral nucleus of the thalamus in a manner that promotes antinociception without anesthesia. In all, seven sites in the CNS involved in pain processing produced effects after microinjections of cannabinoids, effecting a circuit that mediates the descending pain suppressing effects of opiates.

Cannabinoids and the Periaqueductal Gray Area

In 1996, researchers demonstrated antinociceptive effects of delta-9-THC and other cannabinoids in the periaqueductal gray (PAG) matter in rats (Lichtman, Cook, & Martin, 1996). The PAG is a putative migraine generator area (Goadsby & Gundlach, 1991; Raskin, 1988) and has received a lengthy analysis (Behbehani, 1995) citing its importance in the processes of ascending and descending pain pathways. A detailed review of effects of the PAG and cannabinoids in migraine is contained in Russo (E. B. Russo, 2001a).

Manzanares (Manzanares et al., 1998) suggested that cannabinoid-mediated antinociception in the PAG is produced by activation of endogenous opioids, supported by the fact that subchronic THC administration elevates proenkephalin gene expression in the area.

Walker, Huang, Strangman, Tsou, and Sanudo-Pena (1999) demonstrated that electrical stimulation of PAG in the rat stimulated anandamide release and CB_1 receptor-mediated analgesia. The system seemed to be tonically active, and cannabinoid antagonists produced hyperalgesia. The authors posited that this cannabinoid-modulated

pain system would support the prospect of approaches with cannabinoids to opiate-resistant syndromes.

NMDA and Glutamate

A trigeminovascular system, which has long been implicated as subserving pain, inflammatory and vascular effects, has again been reviewed (E. B. Russo, 2001a).

In 1996, Shen et al. elucidated basic mechanism of cannabinoids in glutamatergic systems (Shen, Piser, Seybold, & Thayer, 1996). Through G protein coupling, cannabinoid receptors inhibit voltage-gated calcium channels, and activate potassium channels to produce presynaptic inhibition of glutamate release. Subsequently, it has been shown (Shen & Thayer, 1999) that THC is a partial agonist acting presynaptically via CB_1 to modulate glutamatergic transmission through a reduction without blockade.

Hampson and colleagues demonstrated a 30 to 40% reduction in delta-calcium-NMDA responses by THC (Hampson, Bornheim et al., 1998), which was eliminated by a cannabinoid antagonist. THC and CBD components of cannabis act as neuroprotective antioxidants against glutamate neurotoxicity and cell death mediated via NMDA, AMPA, and kainate receptors (Hampson, Grimaldi, Axelrod, & Wink, 1998). Effects are independent of cannabinoid receptors. The natural cannabinoids were more potent in their antioxidant effects than either alphatocopherol or ascorbate.

Italian researchers Nicolodi and Sicuteri have recently elucidated the role of NMDA antagonists in eliminating hyperalgesia in migraine, chronic daily headache, fibromyalgia, and possibly other mechanisms of chronic pain (Nicolodi & Sicuteri, 1995, 1998; Nicolodi, Del Bianco, & Sicuteri, 1997; Nicolodi, Volpe, & Sicuteri, 1998). Gabapentin and ketamine were suggested as tools to block this system and provide amelioration. Given the above observations and relationships, it is logical that prolonged use of THC prophylactically may exert similar benefits, as was espoused in cures of chronic daily headache claimed in the 19th century with regular use of extract of Indian hemp (Mackenzie, 1887).

This concept is bolstered by examination of another series of articles by Richardson and her group. One study examined peripheral mechanisms (Richardson, Kilo, & Hargreaves, 1998), wherein cannabinoids acted on CB_1 to reduce hyperalgesia and inflammation via inhibition of neurosecretion of calcitonin gene-related peptide (CGRP) in capsaicin-activated nerve terminals.

At the spinal level, her group noted an antihyperalgesic effect of cannabinoids (Richardson, Aanonsen, & Hargreaves, 1998a), mediated by the CB_1 receptor. Additionally, experimental cannabinoid receptor blockade induced a glutamate-dependent hyperalgesia, suggesting a tonic activity of cannabinoids in averting such a development. The authors suggested the clinical use of cannabinoids in disorders, "characterized by primary afferent barrage" (p. 152). An increased potency of cannabinoids observed in hyperalgesia "may mean that there are dosages of cannabinoids that would be effective as antihyperalgesic agents but sub-threshold for the untoward psychomimetic effects" (p. 152). This is akin to Dixon's observations of patients able to return to work after having treated their headaches with a few inhalations of cannabis (Dixon, 1899).

Elaborating on these themes, Richardson noted that a decrease in lumbar cannabinoid receptor numbers correlated with hyperalgesia (Richardson, Aanonsen, & Hargreaves, 1998b) and could provide an etiology for certain chronic pain states, especially those unresponsive to opiates.

In another study (Li et al., 1999), the synthetic cannabinoid agonist WIN 55,212-2 was employed to block capsaicin-induced hyperalgesia in rat paws much as has been observed for THC in formalin treatment. Ko and Woods (1999) examined local THC administration and its activity on capsaicin-induced pain in rhesus monkeys. THC effectively reduced pain, which was blocked by a CB_1 antagonist and was effective at a parenteral dose that produced no behavioral change or sedation.

Maneuf, Nash, Crossman, and Brotchie (1996) examined similar issues at higher CNS levels and were able to show a tonic activation of the cannabinoid system serving to reduce GABA uptake in the globus pallidus.

These tonic endocannabinoid systems subserving analgesic pathways are strongly suggestive that certain pain disorders long conceived as at least partially "psychogenic," including migraine, fibromyalgia, idiopathic bowel syndrome, complex regional pain syndromes, and others may be attributable to a "clinical endocannabinoid deficiency" (CECD). This concept is explored elsewhere in depth (E. B. Russo, 2004a).

Synergism and the Entourage Effect

Palmitylethanolamide (PEA) is another endogenous cannabinoid with analgesic effects, released from a phospholipid in conjunction with anandamide (Calignano, La Rana, Giuffrida, & Piomelli, 1998). In ensemble, the two substances effect a 100-fold synergism on CB_1 type peripheral receptors in cutaneous tissues.

Endocannabinoids and their inactive metabolites combine to boost physiological responses (the "entourage effect"; Mechoulam & Ben-Shabat, 1999). Given the likely contributions of cannabis flavonoids and essential oils to therapeutic effects on mood, inflammation, and pain reviewed in McPartland and Russo (2001), one may readily accept Mechoulam's quotation (Mechoulam & Ben-Shabat, 1999, p. 136): "This type of synergism may play a role in the widely held (but not experimentally based) view that in some cases plants are better drugs than the natural products isolated from them."

PRACTICAL APPLICATION OF CANNABINOIDS TO ANALGESIA

Marinol (Dronabinol): Pros and Cons

Marinol,® developed by Unimed Pharmaceuticals, is a synthetically derived THC dissolved in sesame oil. It is available in capsules of 2.5, 5, and 10 mg and is marketed in the United States, Canada, Australia, and some areas in Europe (Grotenhermen, 2001a). Until 1999, Marinol was a Schedule II drug in the United States with close scrutiny to its usage, which was restricted to indications of AIDS-associated anorexia and cancer chemotherapy. After safety studies revealed a low potential for abuse or diversion (Calhoun, Galloway, & Smith, 1998), dronabinol was "down-scheduled" to Schedule III in 1999, allowing refill prescriptions for up to 6 months, and its "off-label" administration for any indication.

Clinicians have used Marinol only to a limited degree. Its bioavailability is only 25 to 30% of an equivalent smoked dose of THC (Association, 1997). Additional problems include the first pass effect of hepatic metabolism, which results in the production of a possibly more psychoactive metabolite 11-hydroxy-THC, and its considerable cost, which may exceed U.S. $600 per month for the lowest dosage of 2.5 mg TID. Considerable anecdotal data supports preference by patients of herbal cannabis over dronabinol (Grinspoon & Bakalar, 1997; E. B. Russo et al., 2002).

Reports of dronabinol use in painful clinical conditions are few, but it has had some variable success in migraine prophylaxis (Mikuriya, 1997; E. Russo, 1998; E. B. Russo, 2001a).

Maurer et al. demonstrated efficacy of analgesia of 5 mg per oris THC to 50 mg codeine in treatment of pain in a young paraplegic patient after removal of a spinal tumor (Maurer, Henn, Dittrich, & Hofmann, 1990). However, THC also limited spasticity whereas codeine and placebo did not.

Holdcroft et al. (1997) were able to demonstrate an analgesic benefit ($p < 0.001$) of THC 50 mg per day in five split doses in a patient with relapsing familial Mediterranean fever in a double-blind, placebo-controlled trial.

Nabilone

Nabilone is a synthetic cannabinoid said to be pharmacologically similar to THC, but more potent, less apt to produce euphoria, and possessing lower "abuse potential" (Association, 1997). It is produced by Eli Lilly Company as Cesamet® and is available in the United Kingdom, Canada, Australia, and certain countries in Europe (Grotenhermen, 2001a) as an agent for nausea in chemotherapy. Some scattered reports have noted benefit on spasticity in multiple sclerosis (MS) and effects on dyskinesias.

Lethal toxicity in dogs has been noted with chronic use (Mechoulam & Feigenbaum, 1987).

A group in the United Kingdom recently assessed analgesic effects of nabilone in patients including some with neuropathic pain (Notcutt, Price, & Chapman, 1997). Side effects of drowsiness and dysphoria were troubling. Several patients claimed improved pain relief and fewer side effects with smoked cannabis and preferred it to this legal alternative. Nabilone's cost was also estimated to be 10 times higher than cannabis even at black market rates.

LEVONANTRADOL

Levonantradol is a synthetic cannabinoid developed by Pfizer. In 1981, levonantradol was studied in double-blind fashion versus placebo with single intramuscular exposures in acute postoperative or trauma pain (Jain, Ryan, McMahon, & Smith, 1981). Various doses were analgesic for up to 6 hours compared with placebo ($P < 0.05$), but no dose–response effect was evident, and side effects were prominent with levonantradol (57 vs. 12.5%), including prominent drowsiness with less degrees of dry mouth, dizziness, "weird dreams," mild hallucinations, and anxiety. These adverse events were labeled "unacceptable" according to the British Medical Association (Association, 1997).

AJULEMIC ACID (CT3)

Ajulemic acid is a synthetic derived from delta-8-THC that does not bind to cannabinoid receptors. CT3 was developed by Atlantic Pharmaceuticals. It has shown analgesic and anti-inflammatory properties in animal models without COX-1 inhibition side effects (S. H. Burstein, 2000, 2001). It has shown strong analgesic and anti-inflammatory properties in animal models of arthritis without COX-1 inhibition side effects such as ulcer production, and is in advanced clinical trials (S. H. Burstein 2000, 2001). Ajulemic acid binds to the peroxisome proliferator-activated receptor gamma, part of the nuclear receptor superfamily involved in inflammatory processes (Liu, Li, Burstein, Zurier, & Chen, 2003), and also suppresses human monocyte interleukin-1beta production *in vitro* (Zurier, Rossetti, Burstein, & Bidinger, 2003). Ajulemic acid may represent a valuable addition to cannabinoid pharmaceuticals used for anti-inflammatory and analgesic effects.

DEXANABINOL (HU-211)

Dexanabinol is a synthetic cannabinoid agent developed at Hebrew University from Δ^8-THC. It is a nonpsychoactive enantiomer of the extremely potent cannabis agonist, HU-210 (Pop, 2000). It has several interesting properties including antioxidant and anti-inflammatory effects, as well as suppression of TNF-α production. Additionally, it reduced damage in experimental focal ischemia, as may be associated with closed head injury (Lavie, Teichner, Shohami, Ovadia, & Leker, 2001). In one human Phase II clinical trial of 67 patients with closed-head injury, dexanabinol reduced intracranial pressure and perfusion significantly with few adverse events (Knoller et al., 2002). Improvements in clinical outcome scales were seen after 3 and 6 months, but were relatively subtle.

Dexanabinol is currently in Phase III clinical trials. Parenteral injection of dexanabinol is required.

HU-308

HU-308 is another agent emerging from the research of Raphael Mechoulam's laboratories in Israel. It is a synthetic and specific CB_2 agonist demonstrating no cannabinoid behavioral effects in laboratory animals (Hanus et al., 1999). Its pharmacological properties include inhibition of forskolin-stimulated cyclic AMP production, blood pressure reduction, inhibition of defecation, and production of peripheral analgesia with anti-inflammatory effects. An important therapeutic role for HU-308 as a peripherally acting agent may eventuate on further testing.

CANNABIS PROPER

Use of cannabis for pain conditions is extensive in the United States and some European nations. A survey of patients attending the Oakland Cannabis Buyers' Club revealed (Gieringer, 2001):

> By far the largest category of patients interviewed by Mikuriya use cannabis for analgesia to treat conditions including: migraines and neuralgias; arthritis and rheumatism; spinal, skeletal and back disorders due to injury, deformity, or degenerative disease; inflammatory gastrointestinal disorders, and a host of miscellaneous diseases.

Analysis of the totals revealed that at least 1,133 of 2,480 patients or 46% sought cannabis for analgesia in treatment of chronic pain conditions.

Cannabis is traditionally employed therapeutically by smoking, ingestion, or vaporization. Each has advantages and disadvantages. Grotenhermen has produced an excellent summary of "Practical Hints" (Grotenhermen, 2001b), as have Brazis and Mathre (1997). Dosing of therapeutic cannabis must be titrated to the patient's need. In general, 5 mg of THC represents a threshold dose for noticeable effects in the average adult. While tolerance to cardiovascular effects (tachycardia) and psychoactive effects ("high") are achieved after some days to weeks of chronic usage, observed clinical and "anecdotal" reports support retention of analgesic efficacy over the long term. Occasionally, upward dose titration is necessary, as is true for any agent.

Allergies to cannabis are rare, although some may experience rhinitis symptoms, particularly when exposed to the smoke of the unrefined product.

More severe psychiatric conditions present a relative contraindication to use of cannabis, while many milder emotional afflictions may benefit from the drug (Grinspoon & Bakalar, 1997; Grinspoon, Bakalar, & Russo, 2005; E. B. Russo, 2001c). Although concerns have been raised about subtle neuropsychological sequelae in children born to mothers employing cannabis in pregnancy, other studies have shown no significant abnormalities (Dreher, 1997). Certainly, no mutagenic or teratogenic potential has been demonstrated in humans (E. Russo, 2002b).

Concerns about our youth employing cannabis are often well intentioned. However, there is some evidence that very young children may be relatively resistant to its psychoactive properties. A research group in Israel examined the antiemetic effects of delta-8-tetrahydrocannabinol (a natural isomer) in a series of children undergoing chemotherapy (Abrahamov & Mechoulam, 1995). Excellent efficacy and tolerance was observed at doses that would be expected to produce significant psychoactivity in adults. People employing cannabis therapeutically must be warned of the usual caveats assigned to any potentially sedative drug: due care with operation of machinery, motor vehicles, etc.

Acute overdosages of cannabis are self-limited, and most frequently consist of panic reactions. These are uniquely sensitive to reassurance ("talking down") and are quite unusual once a patient becomes familiar with the drug. Cannabis has a unique distinction of safety over four millennia of analgesic usage: No credible deaths due to direct toxicity of cannabis have ever been documented in the medical literature. An extremely detailed review of chronic cannabis effects in a medical context is available (E. B. Russo et al., 2002).

Some cannabis–drug interactions are apparent, but are few in number or consequence. Additive sedative effects with other agents, including alcohol, may be observed. Similarly, however, additive or synergistic antiemetic and analgesic benefits may accrue when combining dopamine agonist neuroleptics and cannabis (Carta et al., 1999). Cannabis may accelerate metabolism of theophylline, while slowing that of barbiturates. Anticholinergic-induced tachycardia may be accentuated by cannabis, while this effect is countered by beta-blockers (Grotenhermen, 2001b). Indomethacin seems to reduce slightly the psychoactive and tachycardic effects of cannabis (Perez-Reyes, Burstein, White, McDonald, & Hicks, 1991). As discussed above, synergistic analgesic benefits may accrue with concomitant usage of cannabis and opioids (Cichewicz et al., 1999; Hare, 1887).

Crude cannabis contains most of its THC in the form of delta-9-THC acids that must be decarboxylated by heating to be activated. This occurs automatically when cannabis is smoked, whereas herbal cannabis that is employed orally should be heated to 200 to 210°C for 5 minutes prior to ingestion (Brenneisen, 1984).

Contrary to political opinion in the United States, *average* cannabis potency has varied little over the last three decades (ElSohly et al., 2000; Mikuriya & Aldrich, 1988). It is true that the *maximum* potency has increased through applied genetics, cultivation, and harvesting techniques. This goal is achieved through production of clonal cultivation of the preferred female plants and maximization of the yield of unsterilized flowering tops known as *sinsemilla* (Spanish for "without seed"). In this manner a concentration of stalked trichomes where THC and therapeutic terpenoids are produced is effected. Resultant yields of THC may exceed 20% by weight. This is potentially advantageous, particularly if smoked, because a therapeutic dosage of THC is obtained with fewer inhalations, thereby decreasing lung exposure to tars and potential carcinogens.

A considerable concentration of THC, other cannabinoids, and terpenoids may also be achieved through some simple processing of crude dried cannabis. Techniques for sieving or washing of cannabis to isolate the trichomes to produce hashish are well described (Clarke, 1998; Rosenthal, Gieringer, & Mikuriya, 1997), and may produce potential yields of 40 to 60% THC. Clarke demonstrates a simple method of rolling the resultant powdery material into a joint of pure hashish, termed "smoking the snake" (Clarke, 1998), providing a relatively very pure product for inhalation.

Cultivation techniques are beyond the scope of this review, but are freely available through a variety of guidebooks (Clarke, 1981; Rosenthal et al., 1997), magazines such as *Cannabis Culture* or *High Times,* or via the Internet to those who live in jurisdictions where this endeavor is legal. Outdoor, indoor, or hydroponic techniques are possible. Recent reviews outline good agricultural practice in cultivation of cannabis (Anonymous, 2003), its husbandry for medical usage in an industrial setting (Potter, 2004; E. B. Russo, 2003), and a primer on cannabis genetics (E. P. de Meijer et al., 2003). Emphasis should focus on potent medicinal strains, scrupulous organic cultivation of female plants, clonal selection and augmentation, and appropriate processing, all combined with best available techniques of harm reduction.

Oral Use of Cannabis

A variety of issues attend this mode of cannabis administration. The most important one concerns bioavailability. Oral absorption of cannabinoids is slow and erratic at best, often requiring 30 to 120 minutes. In HIV-positive or chemotherapy patients and in acute migraine, nausea and emesis may preclude oral usage altogether. Additionally, oral THC is subject to the "first pass effect" of hepatic metabolism yielding 11-hydroxy-THC, which may be more psychoactive than THC itself. Thus, some patients clearly become "too high" even on low doses of medicine, such as 2.5 mg of THC as dronabinol.

Advantages of oral usage are its avoidance of lung exposure in those who are immunosuppressed or have impaired pulmonary function, and its prolonged half-life. This may be of advantage for nocturnal complaints where sedation is less of an issue.

Grotenhermen suggests dose titration beginning with 2.5 mg of oral THC bid with increases as needed and tolerated (Grotenhermen, 2001b). For cannabis of 5% THC content, this would represent 50 mg of herb per dose. For 10% THC cannabis, only 25 mg of plant material would be required. Most painful clinical conditions require tid dosing of cannabis.

THC, CBD, and terpenoids are all highly lipophilic. Gastrointestinal absorption is markedly enhanced by inclusion of lipids in the cooked preparations. Traditional Indian cannabis cookery makes good use of *ghee,* or clarified butter. When cannabis tea is employed, added cream will enhance clinical benefits. Therapeutic tincture extraction in alcohol is also possible.

Smoked Cannabis

Techniques of smoking cannabis are legion, and include marijuana cigarettes ("joint," "reefer," etc.), pipes, waterpipes ("hookahs"), bongs etc. Pharmacodynamically, smoking might seem a reasonable administration of clinical cannabis, but for its attendant pulmonary sequelae, lack of standardization, risks of intoxication, and illegality in most jurisdictions (E. B. Russo et al., 2002). Clinical effects are noted within seconds to minutes after smoking. Inhalation avoids the first pass effect that hampers oral use and allows effective dosage titration. Doses as low as 5 mg of THC equivalent may provide relief of clinical symptoms, while anecdotal evidence claims the ability to continue work or study with unimpaired effectiveness. When symptoms return, repeat dosage may be achieved quickly and easily. Overdosage is possibly avoidable.

In chronic usage of smoked cannabis, isolated cases of upper airway carcinogenesis have been noted (Tashkin, 2001). Precancerous cytological changes in the airways of heavy cannabis smokers have been observed via bronchoscopy but do not seem to lead to emphysematous deterioration (Tashkin, Simmons, Sherrill, & Coulson, 1997). There still has never been a documented case of a pulmonary malignancy in a cannabis-only smoker. That not withstanding, smoked cannabis is unlikely to be a vehicle that can achieve FDA approval as a prescription medicine, due to the irritant effects, lack of standardization, quality control, and similar issues herein discussed.

The "amotivational syndrome" has been largely relegated to the dustbin of drug war propaganda (Zimmer & Morgan, 1997). In fact, the interested reader may wish to seek out three rare books of the past generation on chronic usage that are remarkable for their careful documentation of the few distinguishing features between chronic cannabis smokers and age-matched controls (Carter, Coggins, Doughty, University of Florida Center for Latin American Studies, & National Institute on Drug Abuse, 1976; V. D. Rubin & Comitas, 1975; Stefanis et al., 1977). These are hardly ever mentioned in alarmist reviews of the dangers of cannabis.

Some old myths die hard. Traditional smoking techniques in the United States make prolonged holding of a marijuana "toke" *de rigueur.* From a dose–response standpoint, this is unnecessary. Inhaled THC is well absorbed after a very brief interval, and subjective high and serum THC levels do not increase beyond a maximum 10-second inhalation (Azorlosa, Greenwald, & Stitzer, 1995). Furthermore, prolonged breath holding under pressure increases the potential for hypoxia or pneumothorax (Tashkin, 2001).

Contamination of herbal cannabis by pesticides, herbicides, and bacterial or fungal agents is possible and may represent a threat to the smoker, especially immunosuppressed patients (McPartland, 2001b; McPartland & Pruitt, 1997; Tashkin, 2001). Scrupulous cultivation techniques avoid some of these issues. McPartland recommends pasteurization of herbal cannabis by heating in an oven of 150°C for 5 minutes (McPartland, 2001b).

Waterpipes and bongs are popular techniques for cooling smoke. While they may reduce particulate matter as well, THC content and pharmaceutical efficiency also seem to be compromised (Gieringer, 1996a, b). Surprisingly, the unfiltered "joint" seems to represent a relatively efficient means for conventional smoking, although use of hashish in a pipe (without tobacco) was not examined.

Vaporizers for Cannabis Administration

Vaporization of herbal cannabis may allow THC and terpenoid components below the flash point of the leaf, thereby reducing exposure to smoke, tar, and carcinogens. The technology has been hampered in its development by paraphernalia laws. Initial investigations of available second-generation devices were quite disappointing in their results (Gieringer, 1996a, b), but additional studies with the Volcano® vaporizer are more promising (E. B. Russo & Stortz, 2003). In a recent assay of the device, there was reasonable preservation of available THC, and a reduction, *but not elimination,* of potential carcinogens down to 5% of yield (Gieringer, St. Laurent, & Goodrich, 2004). A clinical trial of the Volcano vs. smoked cannabis was approved by the FDA in late 2003.

Rectal Administration

Suppository preparations of cannabis were employed in the 19th century and may be an acceptable alternative route of administration for some conditions. The first pass effect is largely avoided, although the ability for close dose titration is lost. THC suppositories as a hemisuccinate have proved to be twice as bioavailable as oral THC (Brenneisen, Egli, ElSohly, Henn, & Spiess, 1996; Broom, Sufka, ElSohly, & Ross, 2001; ElSohly et al., 1991; Mattes, Engelman, Shaw, & ElSohly, 1994). No studies have examined use of this preparation with respect to analgesia, but one might expect comparison with dronabinol at least with regard to the spectrum of activity. Synergistic combinations of cannabis components may be more valuable. Additionally, suppositories are not a popular method of drug delivery in the United States.

Transdermal Administration

The American Cancer Society has received a large grant to examine the use of a THC skin patch. Limited pharmacokinetic data are currently available to ascertain whether transdermal THC administration is a viable option (Brenneisen, 2001; Challapalli & Stinchcomb, 2002), but results to date have fallen far short of goals. Additionally, the gradient required to drive THC through the skin necessitates a large residual would remain in the patch that could represent a danger of diversion.

Sublingual/Oro-Mucosal Tincture of Cannabis

The oro-mucosal method of administration was first used in the 19th century, wherein Marshall described symptoms of cannabis intoxication after 45 minutes, as opposed to 4 hours after oral ingestion of a cannabis extract (Marshall, 1897). It has been under investigation by GW Pharmaceuticals in the United Kingdom employing combinations of specific strains of cannabis that are rich in THC or CBD. Terpenoids and other minor components that may be important to therapeutic effects of cannabis are retained in this fashion (Whittle & Guy, 2001; Whittle, Guy, & Robson, 2001). Dose-metered sublingual/oromucosal sprays are currently in Phase I to III clinical trials for a variety of indications, and approval as a prescription medicine for Sativex®, a whole cannabis extract with equal proportions of THC and CBD, was confirmed for central neuropathic pain in multiple sclerosis in Canada in 2005, and is expected for other indications in the United Kingdom, European Union, and British Commonwealth nations subsequently.

Further data on the raising of the plant material through application of Mendelian genetics are available (E. de Meijer, 2004; E. P. de Meijer et al., 2003), as is further information on its organic husbandry (Potter, 2003; E. B. Russo, 2003), processing with supercritical carbon dioxide extraction and production of cannabis-based medicine extracts (CBME; E. B. Russo, 2003; Whittle & Guy, 2003; Whittle, Guy, & Robson, 2003).

Phase I pharmacokinetic data on the material are available (Guy & Flint, 2003; Guy & Robson, 2003a, b). Clinical studies support good bioavailability, patient tolerance, and clinical effects. A Phase II clinical study in England with 24 patients with MS and intractable pain was performed as a consecutive series of double-blind, randomized, placebo-controlled single-patient cross-over trials with oro-mucosal CBME (Wade, Robson, House, Makela, & Aram, 2003). Pain scores on visual analogue scales were significantly improved over placebo with both high THC and high CBD CBME. Subjectively, spasm was significantly improved with high THC and THC:CBD fixed ratio extracts. Spasticity was also subjectively improved with the high THC CBME. All three extracts significantly improved objective measures of spasticity, while the high THC and THC:CBD fixed ratio CBME significantly improved objective measures of spasm (all improvements were $P < 0.05$).

In 34 patients with intractable pain in England (Notcutt et al., 2004), 7 experienced substantial improvement over best available conventional treatment with CBME, 13 moderate, and 8 some benefit. Many extended the range of their activities of daily living with acceptable levels of adverse effects.

Preliminary results of four Phase III clinical trials of CBME by GW Pharmaceuticals have revealed highly significant benefits ($P < 0.01$)in neuropathic pain in MS, pain and sleep disturbance in MS and other neurological diseases, multiple symptoms in MS, and neuropathic pain in brachial plexus injury. Most patients attained good symptomatic control with minimal side effects. Results are available online at http://www.gwpharm.com/news_pres_05_nov_02.html.

Aerosol THC Preparations

Cannabis has a long history of use in asthma, even as a smoked preparation. A pure THC aerosol has been attempted numerous times in the past. Physical and delivery issues have been challenging, but more interestingly, pure THC seems to have an irritating and even bronchoconstrictive effect when employed in isolation (Tashkin et al., 1977). This author believes that anti-inflammatory effects of concomitant terpenoid and flavonoid administration are necessary for full effects and tolerance in pursuit of the pulmonary route. Further research is under way by GW Pharmaceuticals, Inhale Therapeutic Systems, and possibly others. Preliminary Phase I data from GW Pharmaceuticals indicate that very rapid effects within seconds to minutes are produced, comparable with those from smoking cannabis (Guy & Flint, 2003). Although this rapid onset is not necessary for most chronic pain condition treatments, it may be of value in paroxysmal disorders such as treatment of trigeminal neuralgia, or for breakthrough pain or spasm.

REFERENCES

Abrahamov, A., & Mechoulam, R. (1995). An efficient new cannabinoid antiemetic in pediatric oncology. *Life Sciences, 56*(23–24), 2097–2102.

Anonymous. (1930). Effects of cannabis and alcohol during labor. *Journal of the American Medical Association, 94*, 1165.

Anonymous. (1996). Access to therapeutic marijuana/cannabis. *American Journal of Public Health, 86*, 441–442.

Anonymous. (2003). Guidelines for cultivating cannabis for medicinal purposes [Voorschriften voor de verbouw van cannabis voor medicinale doeleinden]. *Journal of Cannabis Therapeutics, 3*(2), 51–61.

Association, B. M. (1997). *Therapeutic uses of cannabis.* Amsterdam: Harwood Academic Publishers.

Aulde, J. (1890). Studies in therapeutics: *Cannabis indica. Therapeutic Gazette, 14*, 523–526.

Azorlosa, J. L., Greenwald, M. K., & Stitzer, M. L. (1995). Marijuana smoking: effects of varying puff volume and breathhold duration. *Journal of Pharmacology and Experimental Therapeutics, 272*(2), 560–569.

Barinaga, M. (1992). Pot, heroin unlock new areas for neuroscience. *Science, 258*, 1882–1884.

Barrett, M. L., Scutt, A. M., & Evans, F. J. (1986). Cannflavin A and B, prenylated flavones from *Cannabis sativa* L. *Experientia, 42*(4), 452–453.

Batho, R. (1883, May 26). *Cannabis indica. British Medical Journal*, 1002.

Behbehani, M. M. (1995). Functional characteristics of the midbrain periaqueductal gray. *Progress in Neurobiology, 46*(6), 575–605.

Benet, S. (1975). Early diffusion and folk uses of hemp. In V. Rubin (Ed.), *Cannabis and culture* (pp. 39–49). The Hague: Mouton.

Biruni, M. I. A., Said, H. M., & Hamdard National Foundation-Saydanah. (1973). *al-Biruni's book on pharmacy and materia medica.* Karachi: Hamdard Academy.

Boger, D. L., Patterson, J. E., & Jin, Q. (1998). Structural requirements for 5-HT2A and 5-HT1A serotonin receptor potentiation by the biologically active lipid oleamide. *Proceedings. National Acadamy of Sciences (USA), 95*(8), 4102–4107.

Brazis, M. Z., & Mathre, M. L. (1997). Dosage and administration of cannabis. In M. L. Mathre (Ed.), *Cannabis in medical practice: A legal, historical and pharmacological overview of the therapeutic use of marijuana* (pp. 142–156). Jefferson, NC: McFarland.

Brenneisen, R. (1984). Psychotrope Drogen. II. Bestimmung der Cannabinoide in *Cannabis sativa* L. und in Cannabisprodukten mittels Hochdruckflüssigkeitschromatographie (HPLC). [Psychotropic drugs. II. Determination of cannabinoids in *Cannabis sativa* L. and in cannabis products with high pressure liquid chromatography (HPLC)]. *Pharmeutica Acta Helvetiae, 59*(9–10), 247–259.

Brenneisen, R. (2001). Pharmacokinetics. In F. Grotenhermen & E. Russo (Eds.), *Cannabis and cannabinoids: Pharmacology, toxicity and therapeutic potential.* Binghamton, NY: Haworth Press.

Brenneisen, R., Egli, A., ElSohly, M. A., Henn, V., & Spiess, Y. (1996). The effect of orally and rectally administered delta 9- tetrahydrocannabinol on spasticity: A pilot study with 2 patients. *International Journal of Clinical Pharmacology and Therapeutics, 34*(10), 446–452.

Broom, S. L., Sufka, K. J., ElSohly, M. A., & Ross, R. A. (2001). Analgesic and reinforcing properties of delta9-THC-hemisuccinate in adjuvant-arthritic rats. *Journal of Cannabis Therapeutics, 1*(3–4), 171–182.

Brown, J. (1883, May 26). *Cannabis indica*; A valuable remedy in menorrhagia. *British Medical Journal, 1*, 1002.

Burstein, S. (1992). Eicosanoids as mediators of cannabinoid action. In L. Murphy & A. Bartke (Eds.), *Marijuana/cannabinoids: Neurobiology and neurophysiology of drug abuse* (pp. 73–91). Boca Raton: CRC Press.

Burstein, S., Levin, E., & Varanelli, C. (1973). Prostaglandins and cannabis. II. Inhibition of biosynthesis by the naturally occurring cannabinoids. *Biochemical Pharmacology, 22*(22), 2905–2910.

Burstein, S., Varanelli, C., & Slade, L. T. (1975). Prostaglandins and cannabis-III. Inhibition of biosynthesis by essential oil components of marihuana. *Biochemical Pharmacology, 24*(9), 1053–1054.

Burstein, S. H. (2000). Ajulemic Acid (CT3): A potent analog of the acid metabolites of THC. *Current Pharmaceutical Research, 6*(13), 1339–1345.

Burstein, S. H. (2001). The therapeutic potential of ajulemic acid (CT3). In F. Grotenhermen & E. Russo (Eds.), *Cannabis and cannabinoids: Pharmacology, toxicology and therapeutic potential.* Binghamton, NY: Haworth Press.

Calhoun, S. R., Galloway, G. P., & Smith, D. E. (1998). Abuse potential of dronabinol (Marinol). *Journal of Psychoactive Drugs, 30*(2), 187–196.

Calignano, A., La Rana, G., Giuffrida, A., & Piomelli, D. (1998). Control of pain initiation by endogenous cannabinoids. *Nature, 394*(6690), 277–281.

Carta, G., Gessa, G. L., & Nava, F. (1999). Dopamine D(2) receptor antagonists prevent delta(9)-tetrahydrocannabinol-induced antinociception in rats. *European Journal of Pharmacology, 384*(2–3), 153–156.

Carter, W. E., Coggins, W. J., Doughty, P. L., University of Florida. Center for Latin American Studies, & National Institute on Drug Abuse. (1976). *Chronic cannabis use in Costa Rica: A report by the Center for Latin American Studies of the University of Florida to the National Institute on Drug Abuse.* Gainesville: University of Florida Press.

Challapalli, P. V., & Stinchcomb, A. L. (2002). *In vitro* experiment optimization for measuring tetrahydrocannabinol skin permeation. *International Journal of Pharmacy, 241*(2), 329–339.

Chomel, P. J. B. (1782). *Abrégé de l'histoire des plantes usuelles.* Paris: Libraires Associés.

Chopra, I. C., & Chopra, R. W. (1957). The use of cannabis drugs in India. *Bulletin on Narcotics, 9*, 4–29.

Christison, A. (1851). On the natural history, action, and uses of Indian hemp. *Monthly Journal of Medical Science of Edinburgh, Scotland, 13*, 26–45, 117–121.

Cichewicz, D. L., & McCarthy, E. A. (2003). Antinociceptive synergy between delta(9)-tetrahydrocannabinol and opioids after oral administration. *Journal of Pharmacology and Experimental Therapeutics, 304*(3), 1010–1015.

Cichewicz, D. L., & Welch, S. P. (2003). Modulation of oral morphine antinociceptive tolerance and naloxone-precipitated withdrawal signs by oral Delta 9-tetrahydrocannabinol. *Journal of Pharmacology and Experimental Therapeutics, 305*(3), 812–817.

Cichewicz, D. L., Haller, V. L., & Welch, S. P. (2001). Changes in opioid and cannabinoid receptor protein following short-term combination treatment with delta(9)-tetrahydrocannabinol and morphine. *Journal of Pharmacology and Experimental Therapeutics, 297*(1), 121–127.

Cichewicz, D. L., Martin, Z. L., Smith, F. L., & Welch, S. P. (1999). Enhancement of mu opioid antinociception by oral delta9-tetrahydrocannabinol: Dose-response analysis and receptor identification. *Journal of Pharmacology and Experimental Therapeutics, 289*(2), 859–867.

Cichewicz, D. L., Rubo, A., & Welch, S. P. (2003). *Recovery of morphine- and codeine-induced antinociception by delta-9-tetrahydrocannabinol.* Paper presented at the 2003 Symposium on the Cannabinoids, NAV Centre, Cornwall, ON, Canada.

Clarke, R. C. (1981). *Marijuana botany: An advanced study: The propagation and breeding of distinctive cannabis.* Berkeley, CA: And/Or Press.

Clarke, R. C. (1998). *Hashish!* Los Angeles: Red Eye Press.

Clendinning, J. (1843). Observation on the medicinal properties of *Cannabis sativa* of India. *Medico-Chirurgical Transactions, 26*, 188-210.

Conrad, C. (1997). *Hemp for health: The medicinal and nutritional uses of Cannabis sativa.* Rochester, VT: Healing Arts Press.

Dastur, J. F. (1962). *Medicinal plants of India and Pakistan; A concise work describing plants used for drugs and remedies according to Ayurvedic, Unani and Tibbi systems and mentioned in British and American pharmacopoeias.* Bombay: D.B. Taraporevala Sons.

de Meijer, E. (2003). The breeding of cannabis cultivars for pharmaceutical end uses. In B. A. Whittle, G. W. Guy, & P. Robson (Eds.), *Medicinal uses of cannabis and cannabinoids.* London: Pharmaceutical Press.

de Meijer, E. P., Bagatta, M., Carboni, A., Crucitti, P., Moliterni, V. M., Ranalli, P., et al. (2003). The inheritance of chemical phenotype in *Cannabis sativa* L. *Genetics, 163*(1), 335–346.

Devane, W. A., Hanus, L., Breuer, A., Pertwee, R. G., Stevenson, L. A., Griffin, G., et al. (1992). Isolation and structure of a brain constituent that binds to the cannabinoid receptor. *Science, 258*(5090), 1946–1949.

Dioscorides, P. (1968). *The Greek herbal of Dioscorides* (J. Goodyer & R. W. T. Gunther, Trans.). London New York: Hafner Publishing.

Dixon, W. E. (1899). The pharmacology of *Cannabis indica. British Medical Journal, 2*, 1354–1357.

Donovan, M. (1845). On the physical and medicinal qualities of Indian hemp *(Cannabis indica)*; with observations on the best mode of administration, and cases illustrative of its powers. *Dublin Journal of Medical Science, 26*, 368–402, 459–461.

Douthwaite, A. H. (1947). Choice of drugs in the treatment of duodenal ulcer. *British Medical Journal*, 43–47.

Dreher, M. C. (1997). Cannabis and pregnancy. In M. L. Mathre (Ed.), *Cannabis in medical practice: A legal, historical and pharmacological overview of the therapeutic use of marijuana* (pp. 159-170). Jefferson, NC: McFarland.

Dwarakanath, C. (1965). Use of opium and cannabis in the traditional systems of medicine in India. *Bulletin on Narcotics, 17*, 15–19.

ElSohly, M. A., Little, T. L., Jr., Hikal, A., Harland, E., Stanford, D. F., & Walker, L. (1991). Rectal bioavailability of delta-9-tetrahydrocannabinol from various esters. *Pharmacology, Biochemistry, and Behavior, 40*(3), 497–502.

ElSohly, M. A., Ross, S. A., Mehmedic, Z., Arafat, R., Yi, B., & Banahan, B. F., 3rd. (2000). Potency trends of delta9-THC and other cannabinoids in confiscated marijuana from 1980-1997. *Journal of Forensic Science, 45*(1), 24–30.

Evans, A. T., Formukong, E. A., & Evans, F. J. (1987). Actions of cannabis constituents on enzymes of arachidonate metabolism: anti-inflammatory potential. *Biochemistry and Pharmacology, 36*(12), 2035–2037.

Evans, F. J. (1991). Cannabinoids: The separation of central from peripheral effects on a structural basis. *Planta Medica, 57*(7), S60–S67.

Fan, P. (1995). Cannabinoid agonists inhibit the activation of 5-HT3 receptors in rat nodose ganglion. *Journal of Neurophysiology, 73*, 907–910.

Farlow, J. W. (1889). On the use of belladonna and *Cannabis indica* by the rectum in gynecological practice. *Boston Medical and Surgical Journal, 120*, 507–509.

Ferri, S., Cavicchini, E., Romualdi, P., Speroni, E., & Murari, G. (1986). Possible mediation of catecholaminergic pathways in the antinociceptive effect of an extract of *Cannabis sativa* L. *Psychopharmacology, 89*(2), 244–247.

Fettes, I., Gawel, M., Kuzniak, S., & Edmeads, J. (1985). Endorphin levels in headache syndromes. *Headache, 25*(1), 37–39.

Fimiani, C., Liberty, T., Aquirre, A. J., Amin, I., Ali, N., & Stefano, G. B. (1999). Opiate, cannabinoid, and eicosanoid signaling converges on common intracellular pathways nitric oxide coupling. *Prostaglandins and Other Lipid Mediators, 57*(1), 23–34.

Fishbein, M. (1942). Migraine associated with menstruation. *Journal of the American Medical Association, 237*, 326.

Formukong, E. A., Evans, A. T., & Evans, F. J. (1988). Analgesic and antiinflammatory activity of constituents of *Cannabis sativa* L. *Inflammation, 12*(4), 361–371.

Formukong, E. A., Evans, A. T., & Evans, F. J. (1989). The inhibitory effects of cannabinoids, the active constituents of *Cannabis sativa* L. on human and rabbit platelet aggregation. *Journal of Pharmacy and Pharmacology, 41*(10), 705–709.

Fride, E., & Mechoulam, R. (1993). Pharmacological activity of the cannabinoid receptor agonist, anandamide, a brain constituent. *European Journal of Pharmacology, 231*(2), 313–314.

Gerard, J., & Johnson, T. (1975). *The herbal: or, General history of plants* (The complete 1633 ed.). New York: Dover Publications.

Gerritsen, M. E., Carley, W. W., Ranges, G. E., Shen, C. P., Phan, S. A., Ligon, G. F., et al. (1995). Flavonoids inhibit cytokine-induced endothelial cell adhesion protein gene expression. *American Journal of Pathology, 147*(2), 278–292.

Ghalioungui, P. (1987). *The Ebers papyrus: A new English translation, commentaries and glossaries.* Cairo: Academy of Scientific Research and Technology.

Gieringer, D. (1996a). Waterpipe study. *Bulletin of the Multidisciplinary Association for Psychedelic Studies, 6*, 59–63.

Gieringer, D. (1996b). Why marijuana smoke harm reduction? *Bulletin of the Multidisciplinary Association for Psychedelic Studies, 6*(64–66).

Gieringer, D. (2001). Medical use of cannabis: Experience in California. In F. Grotenhermen & E. Russo (Eds.), *Cannabis and cannabinoids: Pharmacology, toxicology, and therapeutic potential* (pp. 153–170). Binghamton, NY: Haworth Press.

Gieringer, D., St. Laurent, J., & Goodrich, S. (2004). Cannabis vaporizer combines efficient delivery of THC with effective suppression of pyrolytic compounds. *Journal of Cannabis Therapeutics, 4*(1), 7–27.

Goadsby, P. J., & Gundlach, A. L. (1991). Localization of 3H-dihydroergotamine-binding sites in the cat central nervous system: relevance to migraine. *Annals of Neurology, 29*(1), 91–94.

Grigor, J. (1852). Indian hemp as an oxytocic. *Monthly Journal of Medical Sciences, 14*, 124.

Grinspoon, L., & Bakalar, J. B. (1997). *Marihuana, the forbidden medicine* (Rev. and exp. ed.). New Haven: Yale University Press.

Grinspoon, L., Bakalar, J. B., & Russo, E. (2005). Marihuana. In J. H. Lowinson, L. Ruiz, R. B. Millman, & J. G. Langrod (Eds.), *Substance abuse: A comprehensive textbook* (4th ed., pp. 263–276). New York: Lippincott, William & Wilkins.

Grotenhermen, F. (2001a). Definitions and explanations. In F. Grotenhermen & E. Russo (Eds.), *Cannabis and cannabinoids: Pharmacology, toxicology and therapeutic potential.* Binghamton, NY: Haworth Press.

Grotenhermen, F. (2001b). Practical hints. In F. Grotenhermen & E. B. Russo (Eds.), *Cannabis and cannabinoids: Pharmacology, toxicology and therapeutic potential.* Binghamton, NY: Haworth Press.

Gu, W., & Clarke, R. C. (1998). A survey of hemp (*Cannabis sativa* L.) use by the Hmong (Miao) of the China/Vietnam border region. *Journal of the International Hemp Association, 5*(1), 4–9.

Guy, G. W., & Flint, M. E. (2003). A single centre, placebo-controlled, four period, crossover, tolerability study assessing pharmacokinetic effects, pharmacokinetic characteristics and cognitive profiles of as single dose of three formulations of cannabis based medicine extracts (CBMEs)(GWPD9901), plus a two period tolerability study comparing pharmacodynamic effects and pharmacokinetic characteristics of a single dose of a cannabis based medicine extract given via two administration routes (GWPD9901 EXT). *Journal of Cannabis Therapeutics, 3*(3), 35–77.

Guy, G. W., & Robson, P. (2003a). A phase I, double blind, three-way crossover study to assess the pharmacokinetic profile of cannabis based medicine extract (CBME) administered sublingually in variant cannabinoid ratios in normal healthy male volunteers (GWPK02125). *Journal of Cannabis Therapeutics, 3*(4), 121-152.

Guy, G. W., & Robson, P. (2003b). A phase I, open label, four-way crossover study to compare the pharmacokinetic profiles of a single dose of 20 mg of a cannabis based medicine extract (CBME) administered on 3 different areas of the buccal mucosa and to investigate the pharmacokinetics of CBME *per oral* in health male and female volunteers (GWPK0112). *Journal of Cannabis Therapeutics, 3*(4), 79–120.

Guyatt, G. H., Keller, J. L., Jaeschke, R., Rosenbloom, D., Adachi, J. D., & Newhouse, M. T. (1990). The n-of-1 randomized controlled trial: clinical usefulness. Our three-year experience. *Annals of Internal Medicine, 112*(4), 293–299.

Haines, T., Adler, C. D., Farley, T. P., Russo, E. B., Grinspoon, L., & Sweet, R. W. (2000). Living with our drug policy. *Fordham Urban Law Journal, 28*(1), 92–129.

Hall, B., Burnett, A., Christians, A., Halley, C., Parker, L. A., Russo, E., et al. (2004, January 25–29). *Pharmacology of cannabidiol at serotonin receptors.* Paper presented at the Western Pharmacology Society, Honolulu, HI.

Hamann, W., & di Vadi, P. P. (1999). Analgesic effect of the cannabinoid analogue nabilone is not mediated by opioid receptors. *Lancet, 353*(9152), 560.

Hampson, A. J., Bornheim, L. M., Scanziani, M., Yost, C. S., Gray, A. T., Hansen, B. M., et al. (1998). Dual effects of anandamide on NMDA receptor-mediated responses and neurotransmission. *Journal of Neurochemistry, 70*(2), 671–676.

Hampson, A. J., Grimaldi, M., Axelrod, J., & Wink, D. (1998). Cannabidiol and (–)delta9-tetrahydrocannabinol are neuroprotective antioxidants. *Proceedings. National Academy of Sciences (USA), 95*(14), 8268–8273.

Hanus, L., Breuer, A., Tchilibon, S., Shiloah, S., Goldenberg, D., Horowitz, M., et al. (1999). HU-308: A specific agonist for CB(2), a peripheral cannabinoid receptor. *Proceedings. National Academy of Sciences (USA), 96*(25), 14228–14233.

Hare, H. A. (1887). Clinical and physiological notes on the action of *Cannabis indica. Therapeutic Gazette, 2*, 225–228.

Hare, H. A. (1922). *A text-book of practical therapeutics, with especial reference to the application of remedial measures to disease and their employment upon a rational basis* (18th ed.). Philadelphia, New York: Lea & Febiger.

Herkenham, M. A. (1993). Localization of cannabinoid receptors in brain: relationship to motor and reward systems. In S. G. Korman & J. D. Barchas (Eds.), *Biological basis of substance abuse* (pp. 187–200). London: Oxford University.

Holdcroft, A., Smith, M., Jacklin, A., Hodgson, H., Smith, B., Newton, M., et al. (1997). Pain relief with oral cannabinoids in familial Mediterranean fever [see comments]. *Anaesthesia, 52*(5), 483–486.

Hollister, L. E. (1986). Health aspects of cannabis. *Pharmacological Reviews, 38*(1), 1–20.

Hollister, L. E. (2000). An approach to the medical marijuana controversy. *Drug and Alcohol Dependence, 58*(1–2), 3–7.

Hutchinson, H. W. (1975). Patterns of marihuana use in Brazil. In V. Rubin (Ed.), *Cannabis and culture* (pp. 173–183). The Hague: Mouton.

Indian Hemp Drugs Commission. (1894). *Report of the Indian Hemp Drugs Commission, 1893–1894*. Simla: Government Central Print. Office.

Jaggar, S. I., Hasnie, F. S., Sellaturay, S., & Rice, A. S. (1998). The anti-hyperalgesic actions of the cannabinoid anandamide and the putative CB2 receptor agonist palmitoylethanolamide in visceral and somatic inflammatory pain. *Pain, 76*(1–2), 189–199.

Jaggar, S. I., Sellaturay, S., & Rice, A. S. (1998). The endogenous cannabinoid anandamide, but not the CB2 ligand palmitoylethanolamide, prevents the viscero-visceral hyperreflexia associated with inflammation of the rat urinary bladder. *Neuroscience Letters, 253*(2), 123–126.

Jain, A. K., Ryan, J. R., McMahon, F. G., & Smith, G. (1981). Evaluation of intramuscular levonantradol and placebo in acute postoperative pain. *Journal of Clinical Pharmacology, 21*(8–9 Suppl), 320S–326S.

Jarvinen, T., Pate, D., & Laine, K. (2002). Cannabinoids in the treatment of glaucoma. *Pharmacology and Therapeutics, 95*(2), 203–220.

Julien, M. S. (1849). Chirugie chinoise. Substance anesthétique employée en Chine, dans le commencement du III-ième siecle de notre ère, pour paralyser momentanement la sensibilité. *Comptes Rendus Hebdomadaires de l'Académie des Sciences, 28*, 195–198.

Kahl, O. (1994). *Sabur ibn Sahl: Dispensatorium parvum (al-Aqradhin al-Saghir)*. Leiden: E.J. Brill.

Kimura, T., Ohta, T., Watanabe, K., Yoshimura, H., & Yamamoto, I. (1998). Anandamide, an endogenous cannabinoid receptor ligand, also interacts with 5-hydroxytryptamine (5-HT) receptor. *Biological and Pharmaceutical Bulletin, 21*(3), 224–226.

Klein, T. W., Friedman, H., & Specter, S. (1998). Marijuana, immunity and infection. *Journal of Neuroimmunology, 83*(1–2), 102–115.

Knoller, N., Levi, L., Shoshan, I., Reichenthal, E., Razon, N., Rappaport, Z. H., et al. (2002). Dexanabinol (HU-211) in the treatment of severe closed head injury: A randomized, placebo-controlled, phase II clinical trial. *Critical Care Medicine, 30*(3), 548–554.

Ko, M. C., & Woods, J. H. (1999). Local administration of delta9-tetrahydrocannabinol attenuates capsaicin-induced thermal nociception in rhesus monkeys: a peripheral cannabinoid action. *Psychopharmacology* (Berlin), *143*(3), 322–326.

Kumar, A. M., Haney, M., Becker, T., Thompson, M. L., Kream, R. M., & Miczek, K. (1990). Effect of early exposure to delta-9-tetrahydrocannabinol on the levels of opioid peptides, gonadotropin-releasing hormone and substance P in the adult male rat brain. *Brain Research, 525*(1), 78–83.

Larson, E. B. (1990). N-of-1 clinical trials. A technique for improving medical therapeutics [clinical conference] [see comments]. *Western Journal of Medicine, 152*(1), 52-56.

Lavie, G., Teichner, A., Shohami, E., Ovadia, H., & Leker, R. R. (2001). Long term cerebroprotective effects of dexanabinol in a model of focal cerebral ischemia. *Brain Research, 901*(1–2), 195–201.

Letter, M. (2000). Alosetron (Lotronex) for the treatment of irritable bowel syndrome. *Medical Letter, 42*(1081), 53–54.

Lewis, B., Menage, V. L., Pellat, C. H., & Schacht, J. (1971). *The encyclopedia of Islam*. Leiden: E.J. Brill.

Li, J., Daughters, R. S., Bullis, C., Bengiamin, R., Stucky, M. W., Brennan, J., et al. (1999). The cannabinoid receptor agonist WIN 55,212-2 mesylate blocks the development of hyperalgesia produced by capsaicin in rats. *Pain, 81*(1–2), 25–33.

Lichtman, A. H., Cook, S. A., & Martin, B. R. (1996). Investigation of brain sites mediating cannabinoid-induced antinociception in rats: Evidence supporting periaqueductal gray involvement. *Journal of Pharmacology and Experimental Therapeutics, 276*(2), 585–593.

Lilly. (1898). *Lilly's Handbook of Pharmacy and Therapeutics*. Indianapolis: Lilly and Company.

Linné, C. A. (1772). *Materia medica per regna tria naturae*. Lipsiae et Erlangae: Wolfgang Waltherum.

Liu, J., Li, H., Burstein, S. H., Zurier, R. B., & Chen, J. D. (2003). Activation and binding of peroxisome proliferator-activated receptor gamma by synthetic cannabinoid ajulemic acid. *Molecular Pharmacology, 63*(5), 983–992.

Lozano Camara, I., & Arabe, I. (1990). *Tres tratados arabes sobre el Cannabis indica: Textos para la historia del hachis en las sociedades islamicas S. XIII-XVI*. Madrid: Agencia Española de Cooperacion Internacional, Instituto de Cooperación con el Mundo Arabe.

Mackenzie, S. (1887). Remarks on the value of Indian hemp in the treatment of a certain type of headache. *British Medical Journal, 1*, 97–98.

Mackenzie, S. (1894). Thérapeutique médicale: De la valeur thérapeutique spéciale du chanvre indien dans certains états morbides. *Semaine Médicale, 14*, 399-400.

Mailleux, P., & Vanderhaeghen, J. J. (1992). Localization of cannabinoid receptor in the human developing and adult basal ganglia. Higher levels in the striatonigral neurons. *Neuroscience Letters, 148*(1–2), 173–176.

Mailleux, P., & Vanderhaeghen, J. J. (1994). Delta-9-tetrahydro-cannabinol regulates substance P and enkephalin mRNAs levels in the caudate-putamen. *European Journal of Pharmacology, 267* 1), R1–R3.

Malfait, A. M., Gallily, R., Sumariwalla, P. F., Malik, A. S., Andreakos, E., Mechoulam, R., et al. (2000). The non-psychoactive cannabis constituent cannabidiol is an oral anti-arthritic therapeutic in murine collagen-induced arthritis. *Proceedings. National Academy of Science (USA), 97*(17), 9561–9566.

Maneuf, Y. P., Nash, J. E., Crossman, A. R., & Brotchie, J. M. (1996). Activation of the cannabinoid receptor by delta 9-tetrahydrocannabinol reduces gamma-aminobutyric acid uptake in the globus pallidus. *European Journal of Pharmacology, 308*(2), 161–164.

Mannische, L. (1989). *An ancient Egyptian herbal.* Austin: University of Texas.

Manzanares, J., Corchero, J., Romero, J., Fernandez-Ruiz, J. J., Ramos, J. A., & Fuentes, J. A. (1998). Chronic administration of cannabinoids regulates proenkephalin mRNA levels in selected regions of the rat brain. *Brain Research and Molecular Brain Research, 55*(1), 126–132.

Manzanares, J., Corchero, J., Romero, J., Fernandez-Ruiz, J. J., Ramos, J. A., & Fuentes, J. A. (1999). Pharmacological and biochemical interactions between opioids and cannabinoids. *Trends in Pharmacological Sciences, 20*(7), 287–294.

Marcandier, M. (1764). *Treatise on hemp.* London: T. Becket and P.A. de Hondt.

Margolis, J. S., & Clorfene, R. (1969). *A child's garden of grass (The official handbook for marijuana users).* North Hollywood, CA: Contact Books.

Marshall, C. R. (1897). The active principle of Indian hemp: A preliminary communication. *Lancet, 1,* 235–238.

Martin, M. A. (1975). Ethnobotanical aspects of cannabis in Southeast Asia. In V. Rubin (Ed.), *Cannabis and Culture* (pp. 63–75). The Hague, Paris: Mouton Publishers.

Martin, S., Padilla, E., Ocete, M. A., Galvez, J., Jimenez, J., & Zarzuelo, A. (1993). Anti-inflammatory activity of the essential oil of *Bupleurum fruticescens. Planta Medica, 59*(6), 533–536.

Marx, J. (1990). Marijuana receptor gene cloned. *Science, 249*(4969), 624–626.

Matsuda, L. A., Lolait, S. J., Brownstein, M. J., Young, A. C., & Bonner, T. I. (1990). Structure of a cannabinoid receptor and functional expression of the cloned cDNA. *Nature, 346*(6284), 561–564.

Mattes, R. D., Engelman, K., Shaw, L. M., & ElSohly, M. A. (1994). Cannabinoids and appetite stimulation. *Pharmacology, Biochemistry, and Behavior, 49*(1), 187–195.

Mattison, J. B. (1891). *Cannabis indica* as an anodyne and hypnotic. *St. Louis Medical and Surgical Journal, 61,* 265–271.

Maurer, M., Henn, V., Dittrich, A., & Hofmann, A. (1990). Delta-9-tetrahydrocannabinol shows antispastic and analgesic effects in a single case double-blind trial. *European Archives of Psychiatry and Clinical Neuroscience, 240*(1), 1–4.

McPartland, J. M. (2001a). Cannabis and eicosanoids: A review of molecular pharmacology. *Journal of Cannabis Therapeutics, 1*(1), 71–83.

McPartland, J. M. (2001b). Contaminants and adulterants in herbal cannabis. In F. Grotenhermen & E. Russo (Eds.), *Cannabis and cannabinoids: Pharmacology, toxicology, and therapeutic potential.* Binghamton, NY: Haworth Press.

McPartland, J. M., & Pruitt, P. L. (1997). Medical marijuana and its use by the immunocompromised. *Alternative Therapies in Health and Medicine, 3*(3), 39–45.

McPartland, J. M., & Russo, E. B. (2001). Cannabis and cannabis extracts: Greater than the sum of their parts? *Journal of Cannabis Therapeutics, 1*(3–4), 103–132.

Mechoulam, R., & Ben-Shabat, S. (1999). From gan-zi-gun-nu to anandamide and 2-arachidonoylglycerol: The ongoing story of cannabis. *Natural Product Reports, 16*(2), 131–143.

Mechoulam, R., & Feigenbaum, J. J. (1987). Toward cannabinoid drugs. In G. Ellis & G. West (Eds.), *Progress in medicinal chemistry* (Vol. 24, pp. 159–207). Amsterdam: Elsevier Science.

Mechoulam, R., Fride, E., & Di Marzo, V. (1998). Endocannabinoids. *European Journal of Pharmacology, 359,* 1–18.

Meng, I. D., Manning, B. H., Martin, W. J., & Fields, H. L. (1998). An analgesia circuit activated by cannabinoids. *Nature, 395*(6700), 381–383.

Merzouki, A. (2001). *El cultivo del cáñamo (Cannabis sativa L.) en el Rif, Norte de Marruecos, taxonomía, biología y etnobotánica.* Unpublished doctoral dissertation, Universidad de Granada, Granada, Spain.

Michel, L. (1880). Propriétés médicinales de l'Indian hemp ou du *Cannabis indica. Montpellier Medical, 45,* 103–116.

Mikuriya, T. H. (1997). *Chronic migraine headache: Five cases successfully treated with marinol and/or illiciit cannabis.* Retrieved from http://www.druglibrary.org/schaffer/hemp/migrn1.htm

Mikuriya, T. H., & Aldrich, M. R. (1988). Cannabis 1988. Old drug, new dangers. The potency question. *Journal of Psychoactive Drugs, 20*(1), 47–55.

Milstein, S. L., MacCannell, K., Karr, G., & Clark, S. (1975). Marijuana-produced changes in pain tolerance. Experienced and non-experienced subjects. *International Pharmacopsychiatry, 10*(3), 177–182.

Müller-Vahl, K. R., Kolbe, H., Schneider, U., & Emrich, H. M. (1998). Cannabinoids: Possible role in patho-physiology and therapy of Gilles de la Tourette syndrome. *Acta Psychiatrica Scandinavica, 98*(6), 502–506.

Musonda, C. A., & Chipman, J. K. (1998). Quercetin inhibits hydrogen peroxide (H_2O_2)-induced NF-kappa B DNA binding activity and DNA damage in HepG2 cells. *Carcinogenesis, 19*(9), 1583–1589.

Nalin, D. R., Levine, M. M., Rhead, J., Bergquist, E., Rennels, M., Hughes, T., et al. (1978). Cannabis, hypochlorhydria, and cholera. *Lancet, 2*(8095), 859–862.

New York (City). Mayor's Committee on Marihuana, Wallace, G. B., & Cunningham, E. V. (1973). *The marihuana problem in the city of New York.* Metuchen, NJ: Scarecrow Reprint Corp.

Nicolodi, M. (1998). Painful and non-painful effects of low doses of morphine in migraine sufferers partly depend on excitatory amino acids and gamma-aminobutyric acid. *International Journal of Clinical Pharmacology Research, 18*(2), 79–85.

Nicolodi, M., & Sicuteri, F. (1995). Exploration of NMDA receptors in migraine: Therapeutic and theoretic implications. *International Journal of Clinical Pharmacology Research, 15*(5–6), 181–189.

Nicolodi, M., & Sicuteri, F. (1998). Negative modultors [sic] of excitatory amino acids in episodic and chronic migraine: preventing and reverting chronic migraine. Special lecture 7th INWIN Congress. *International Journal of Clinical Pharmacology Research, 18*(2), 93–100.

Nicolodi, M., Del Bianco, P. L., & Sicuteri, F. (1997). Modulation of excitatory amino acids pathway: A possible therapeutic approach to chronic daily headache associated with analgesic drugs abuse. *International Journal of Clinical Pharmacology Research, 17*(2–3), 97–100.

Nicolodi, M., Volpe, A. R., & Sicuteri, F. (1998). Fibromyalgia and headache. Failure of serotonergic analgesia and N-methyl-D-aspartate-mediated neuronal plasticity: Their common clues. *Cephalalgia, 18*(Suppl. 21), 41–44.

Notcutt, W., Price, M., & Chapman, G. (1997). Clinical experience with nabilone for chronic pain. *Pharmaceutical Sciences, 3*, 551–555.

Notcutt, W., Price, M., Miller, R., Newport, S., Phillips, C., Simmonds, S., et al. (2004). Initial experiences with medicinal extracts of cannabis for chronic pain: Results from 34 "N of 1" studies. *Anaesthesia, 59*, 440–452.

Noyes, R., Jr., & Baram, D. A. (1974). Cannabis analgesia. *Comprehensive Psychiatry, 15*(6), 531–535.

Noyes, R., Jr., Brunk, S. F., Avery, D. A. H., & Canter, A. C. (1975). The analgesic properties of delta-9-tetrahydrocannabinol and codeine. *Clinical Pharmacology and Therapeutics, 18*(1), 84–89.

Noyes, R., Jr., Brunk, S. F., Baram, D. A., & Canter, A. (1975). Analgesic effect of delta-9-tetrahydrocannabinol. *Journal of Clinical Pharmacology, 15*(2–3), 139–143.

Nunn, J. F. (1996). *Ancient Egyptian medicine*. Norman: University of Oklahoma Press.

O'Shaughnessy, W. B. (1838–1840). On the preparations of the Indian hemp, or gunjah *(Cannabis indica)*; Their effects on the animal system in health, and their utility in the treatment of tetanus and other convulsive diseases. *Transactions of the Medical and Physical Society of Bengal*, 71–102, 421–461.

Osler, W., & McCrae, T. (1915). *The principles and practice of medicine*. New York, London: Appleton and Company.

Parkinson, J., Bonham, T., & L'Obel, M. (1640). *Theatrum botanicum: The theater of plants; or, An herball of a large extent ... distributed into sundry classes or tribes, for the more easie knowledge of the many herbes of one nature and property, with the chiefe notes of Dr. Lobel, Dr. Bonham, and others inserted therein*. London: Tho. Cotes.

Partridge, W. L. (1975). Cannabis and cultural groups in a Colombian *municipio*. In V. Rubin (Ed.), *Cannabis and culture* (pp. 147–172). The Hague: Mouton.

Perez-Reyes, M., Burstein, S. H., White, W. R., McDonald, S. A., & Hicks, R. E. (1991). Antagonism of marihuana effects by indomethacin in humans. *Life Sciences, 48*(6), 507–515.

Peroutka, S. J. (1990a). Developments in 5-hydroxytryptamine receptor pharmacology in migraine. *Neurologic Clinics, 8*(4), 829–839.

Peroutka, S. J. (1990b). The pharmacology of current antimigraine drugs. *Headache, 30* (Suppl. 1), 5–11; discussion 24–18.

Peroutka, S. J. (1997). Dopamine and migraine [see comments]. *Neurology, 4 9*(3), 650–656.

Pertwee, R. G. (1997). Cannabis and cannabinoids: Pharmacology and rationale for clinical use. *Pharmaceutical Science, 3*, 539–545.

Pliny. (1951). *Pliny: Natural history* (W. H. S. Jones, Trans., Vol. 6). Cambridge, MA: Harvard University.

Pollington, S. (2000). *Leechcraft: Early English charms, plant lore, and healing*. Hockwold-cum-Wilton, Norfolk, UK: Anglo-Saxon Books.

Pop, E. (2000). Dexanabinol pharmos. *Current Opinion on Investigative Drugs, 1*(4), 494-503.

Potter, D. (2004). Growth and morphology of medicinal cannabis. In B. A. Whittle, G. W. Guy, & P. Robson (Eds.), *Medicinal uses of cannabis and cannabinoids*. London: Pharmaceutical Press.

Randall, R. C. (1991). *Muscle spasm, pain & marijuana therapy: Testimony from federal and state court proceedings on marijuana's medical use in the treatment of multiple sclerosis, paralysis, and chronic pain*. Washington, DC: Galen Press.

Raskin, N. H. (1988). *Headache* (2nd ed.). New York: Churchill Livingstone.

Remington, J. P., Wood, H. C., Sadtler, S. P., LaWall, C. H., Kraemer, H., & Anderson, J. F. (1918). *The dispensatory of the United States of America* (20th ed.). Philadelphia; London: J.B. Lippincott.

Rennie, S. J. (1886). On the therapeutic value of *tinctura Cannabis indica* in the treatment of dysentery, more particularly in its sub-acute and chronic forms. *Indian Medical Gazette, 21*, 353–354.

Reynolds, J. R. (1868). On some of the therapeutical uses of Indian hemp. *Archives of Medicine, 2*, 154–160.

Richardson, J. D., Aanonsen, L., & Hargreaves, K. M. (1998a). Antihyperalgesic effects of spinal cannabinoids. *European Journal of Pharmacology, 345*(2), 145–153.

Richardson, J. D., Aanonsen, L., & Hargreaves, K. M. (1998b). Hypoactivity of the spinal cannabinoid system results in NMDA-dependent hyperalgesia. *Journal of Neuroscience, 18*(1), 451–457.

Richardson, J. D., Kilo, S., & Hargreaves, K. M. (1998). Cannabinoids reduce hyperalgesia and inflammation via interaction with peripheral CB1 receptors. *Pain, 75*(1), 111–119.

Rosenthal, E., Gieringer, D., & Mikuriya, T. (1997). *Marijuana medical handbook: A guide to therapeutic use*. Oakland, CA: Quick American Archives.

Rubin, V. (1976). Cross-cultural perspectives on therapeutic uses of cannabis. In S. Cohen & R. C. Stillman (Eds.), *The therapeutic potential of marihuana* (pp. 1–17). New York: Plenum Medical.

Rubin, V., & Comitas, L. (1972). *Effects of chronic smoking of cannabis in Jamaica. Report. Research Institute for the Study of Man.* Washington, DC: National Institute of Mental Health.

Rubin, V. D., & Comitas, L. (1975). *Ganja in Jamaica: A medical anthropological study of chronic marihuana use.* The Hague: Mouton.

Rumpf, G. E., & Beekman, E. M. (1981). *The poison tree: Selected writings of Rumphius on the natural history of the Indies.* Amherst: University of Massachusetts Press.

Russo, E. (1998). Cannabis for migraine treatment: The once and future prescription? An historical and scientific review. *Pain, 76*(1–2), 3–8.

Russo, E. B. (2001a). Hemp for headache: An in-depth historical and scientific review of cannabis in migraine treatment. *Journal of Cannabis Therapeutics, 1*(2), 21–92.

Russo, E. B. (2001b). Migraine: Indications for cannabis and THC. In F. Grotenhermen & E. B. Russo (Eds.), *Cannabis and cannabinoids.* Binghamton, NY: Haworth Press.

Russo, E. B. (2001c). *Handbook of psychotropic herbs: A scientific analysis of herbal remedies for psychiatric conditions.* Binghamton, NY: Haworth Press.

Russo, E. B. (2002a). Role of cannabis and cannabinoids in pain management. In R. S. Weiner (Ed.), *Pain management: A practical guide for clinicians.* (6th ed., pp. 357–375). Boca Raton, FL: CRC Press.

Russo, E. (2002b). Cannabis treatments in obstetrics and gynecology: A historical review. *Journal of Cannabis Therapeutics, 2*(3–4), 5–35.

Russo, E. B. (2003). Cannabis — From pariah to prescription. *Journal of Cannabis Therapeutics, 3*(3–4), 1–29.

Russo, E. B. (2004a). Clinical endocannabinoid deficiency (CECD): Can this concept explain therapeutic benefits of cannabis in migraine, fibromyalgia, irritable bowel syndrome and other treatment-resistant conditions? *Neuroendocrinology Letters, 25*(1–2), 25–39.

Russo, E. B. (2004b). The history of cannabis as medicine. In B. A. Whittle, G. W. Guy & P. Robson (Eds.), *Medicinal uses of cannabis and cannabinoids.* London: Pharmaceutical Press.

Russo, E. B. (2005). Cannabis in India: Ancient lore and modern medicine. In R. Mechoulam (Ed.), *Cannabinoids as therapeutics.* Boston, MA: Birkhäuser.

Russo, E. B., & Stortz, M. (2003). An interview with Markus Storz: June 19, 2002. *Journal of Cannabis Therapeutics, 3*(1), 67–78.

Russo, E. B., Macarah, C. M., Todd, C. L., Medora, R., & Parker, K. (2000, July 22–26). *Pharmacology of the essential oil of hemp at 5HT1A and 5HT2a receptors.* Paper presented at the 41st Annual Meeting of the American Society of Pharmacognosy, Seattle, WA.

Russo, E. B., Mathre, M. L., Byrne, A., Velin, R., Bach, P. J., Sanchez-Ramos, J., et al. (2002). Chronic cannabis use in the Compassionate Investigational New Drug Program: An examination of benefits and adverse effects of legal clinical cannabis. *Journal of Cannabis Therapeutics, 2*(1), 3–57.

Schaefer, C. F., Brackett, D. J., Gunn, C. G., & Dubowski, K. M. (1979). Decreased platelet aggregation following marihuana smoking in man. *Journal of the Oklahoma State Medical Association, 72*(12), 435–436.

Sée, M. G. (1890). Usages du *Cannabis indica* dans le traitement des névroses et dyspepsies gastriques. *Bulletin de l'Academie Nationale de Médecine, 3,* 158–193.

Shen, M., & Thayer, S. A. (1999). Delta-9-tetrahydrocannabinol acts as a partial agonist to modulate glutamatergic synaptic transmission between rat hippocampal neurons in culture. *Molecular Pharmacology, 55*(1), 8–13.

Shen, M., Piser, T. M., Seybold, V. S., & Thayer, S. A. (1996). Cannabinoid receptor agonists inhibit glutamatergic synaptic transmission in rat hippocampal cultures. *Journal of Neuroscience, 16*(14), 4322–4334.

Shoemaker, J. V. (1899). The therapeutic value of *Cannabis indica. Texas Medical News, 8*(10), 477–488.

Silver, A. (1870). On the value of Indian hemp in menorrhagia and dysmenorrhoea. *Medical Times and Gazette, 2,* 59–61.

Snyder, S. H. (1971). *Uses of marijuana.* New York: Oxford University Press.

Sofia, R. D., Nalepa, S. D., Harakal, J. J., & Vassar, H. B. (1973). Anti-edema and analgesic properties of delta9-tetrahydrocannabinol (THC). *Journal of Pharmacology and Experimental Therapeutics, 186*(3), 646–655.

Spadone, C. (1991). Neurophysiologie du cannabis [Neurophysiology of cannabis]. *Encephale, 17*(1), 17–22.

Stefanis, C. N., Dornbush, R. L., & Fink, M. (1977). *Hashish: Studies of long-term use.* New York: Raven Press.

Strangman, N. M., & Walker, J. M. (1999). Cannabinoid WIN 55,212-2 inhibits the activity-dependent facilitation of spinal nociceptive responses. *Journal of Neurophysiology, 82*(1), 472–477.

Suckling, C. (1891). On the therapeutic value of Indian hemp. *British Medical Journal, 2,* 12.

Tambe, Y., Tsujiuchi, H., Honda, G., Ikeshiro, Y., & Tanaka, S. (1996). Gastric cytoprotection of the non-steroidal anti-inflammatory sesquiterpene, beta-caryophyllene. *Planta Medica, 62*(5), 469–470.

Tashkin, D. P. (2001). Respiratory risks from marijuana smoking. In F. Grotenhermen & E. Russo (Eds.), *Cannabis and cannabinoids: Pharmacology, toxicology and therapeutic potential.* Binghamton, NY: Haworth Press.

Tashkin, D. P., Reiss, S., Shapiro, B. J., Calvarese, B., Olsen, J. L., & Lodge, J. W. (1977). Bronchial effects of aerosolized delta 9-tetrahydrocannabinol in healthy and asthmatic subjects. *American Review of Respiratory Diseases, 115*(1), 57–65.

Tashkin, D. P., Simmons, M. S., Sherrill, D. L., & Coulson, A. H. (1997). Heavy habitual marijuana smoking does not cause an accelerated decline in FEV1 with age. *American Journal of Respiratory and Critical Care Medicine, 155*(1), 141–148.

Thompson, R. C. (1924). *The Assyrian herbal.* London: Luzac and Co.

Thompson, R. C. (1949). *A dictionary of Assyrian botany.* London: British Academy.

Turner, C. E., & ElSohly, M. A. (1981). Biological activity of cannabichromene, its homologs and isomers. *Journal of Clinical Pharmacology, 21*, 283S–291S.

Volfe, Z., Dvilansky, A., & Nathan, I. (1985). Cannabinoids block release of serotonin from platelets induced by plasma from migraine patients. *International Journal of Clinical Pharmacology Research, 5*(4), 243–246.

Wade, D. T., Robson, P., House, H., Makela, P., & Aram, J. (2003). A preliminary controlled study to determine whether whole-plant cannabis extracts can improve intractable neurogenic symptoms. *Clinical Rehabilitation, 17*, 18–26.

Walker, J. M., Hohmann, A. G., Martin, W. J., Strangman, N. M., Huang, S. M., & Tsou, K. (1999). The neurobiology of cannabinoid analgesia. *Life Sciences, 65*(6–7), 665–673.

Walker, J. M., Huang, S. M., Strangman, N. M., Tsou, K., & Sanudo-Pena, M. C. (1999). Pain modulation by the release of the endogenous cannabinoid anandamide. *Proceedings of the National Academy of Sciences, 96*(21), 12198–12203.

Waring, E. (1874). *Practical Therapeutics*. Philadelphia: Lindsay and Blackiston.

Welch, S. P., & Eads, M. (1999). Synergistic interactions of endogenous opioids and cannabinoid systems. *Brain Research, 848*(1–2), 183–190.

Whittle, B. A., & Guy, G. W. (2001). Formulations for sublingual delivery. UK.

Whittle, B. A., & Guy, G. W. (2003). Development of cannabis-based medicines; risk, benefit and serendipity. In B. A. Whittle, G. W. Guy & P. Robson (Eds.), *Medicinal uses of cannabis and cannabinoids*. London: Pharmaceutical Press.

Whittle, B. A., Guy, G. W., & Robson, P. (2001). Prospects for new cannabis-based prescription medicines. *Journal of Cannabis Therapeutics, 1*(3–4), 183–205.

Whittle, B. A., Guy, G. W., & Robson, P. (2003). *Cannabis and cannabinoids as medicines*. London: Pharmaceutical Press.

Wiegant, V. M., Sweep, C. G., & Nir, I. (1987). Effect of acute administration of delta 1-tetrahydrocannabinol on beta-endorphin levels in plasma and brain tissue of the rat. *Experientia, 43*(4), 413–415.

Wirtshafter, D. (1997). Nutritional value of hemp seed and hemp seed oil. In M. L. Mathre (Ed.), *Cannabis in medical practice* (pp. 181–191). Jefferson, NC: McFarland and Company.

Zias, J., Stark, H., Sellgman, J., Levy, R., Werker, E., Breuer, A., et al. (1993). Early medical use of cannabis. *Nature, 363*(6426), 215.

Zimmer, L. E., & Morgan, J. P. (1997). *Marijuana myths, marijuana facts: A review of the scientific evidence*. New York: Lindesmith Center.

Zurier, R. B., Rossetti, R. G., Burstein, S. H., & Bidinger, B. (2003). Suppression of human monocyte interleukin-1beta production by ajulemic acid, a nonpsychoactive cannabinoid. *Biochemistry and Pharmacology, 65*(4), 649–655.

Section VII

Procedures and Techniques

Laxmaiah Manchikanti, MD, Section Editor

57

Guidelines for the Practice of Interventional Techniques

Laxmaiah Manchikanti, MD, Vijay Singh, MD, Andrea M. Trescot, MD, Timothy R. Deer, MD, and Mark V. Boswell, MD, PhD

INTRODUCTION

Guidelines for the practice of interventional pain management are statements developed to assist physician and patient decisions about appropriate health care related to chronic pain.[1-4] These recommendations are professionally derived for practices in the diagnosis and treatment of chronic or persistent pain.

These guidelines do not constitute inflexible treatment recommendations. It is recommended that a provider establish a plan of care on a case-by-case basis, taking into account an individual patient's medical condition and the physician's experience. Based on an individual patient's needs, treatment different from that outlined here may be warranted. Each practice should develop their policies considering their needs. This document may be used as a template.

These guidelines have not been approved or endorsed by any agency or organization. Individual carriers including third-party payers, Medicare, and Medicaid operate under their own coverage, utilization, and local medical review policies. Thus, while each practice may have separate guidelines, it is always prudent to check with payors to make certain that guidelines correlate. However, the information from these guidelines may assist in providing an appropriate rationale for appeals, etc.

EVALUATION AND MEDICAL NECESSITY

Appropriate history, physical examination, and medical decision making comprise the initial evaluation of a patient's presenting symptoms. A patient's evaluation should not only meet the required medical criteria but also pertinent regulatory requirements.[5-9] The guidelines of the Centers for Medicare and Medicaid, formerly the Health Care Financing Administration, provide various criteria for five levels of service. The three crucial components of evaluation and management services are history, physical examination, and medical decision making. Other components include counseling, coordination of care, nature of presenting problem, and time.

HISTORY

The history includes

- Chief complaint
- History of present illness
- Review of systems
- Past, family, and/or social history

Chief Complaint

The chief complaint is a concise statement describing the symptom, problem, condition, diagnosis, or other factor that is the reason for the encounter; it is usually stated in the patient's words.

History of Present Illness

The history of present illness is a chronological description of the development of the patient's present illness from the first sign and/or symptom. It includes the following elements:

- Location
- Quality
- Severity
- Duration
- Timing
- Context
- Modifying factors
- Associated signs and symptoms

Review of Systems

The review of systems is an inventory of body systems obtained through a series of questions seeking to identify signs and/or symptoms that the patient may be experiencing or has experienced.

Past, Family, and/or Social History

Past, family, and/or social history consists of a review of the past history of the patient including past experiences, illnesses, operations, injuries, and treatment; family history, including a review of medical events in the patient's family, hereditary diseases, and other factors; and social history, appropriate for age, reflecting past and current activities.

Past history in interventional pain medicine includes history of past pain problems and motor vehicle, occupational, or non-occupational injuries; history of headache, neck pain, upper-extremity pain, pain in the upper or mid back or chest wall, pain in the lower back or lower extremities, and pain in joints; and disorders such as arthritis, fibromyalgia, or systemic lupus erythematosus.

Family history includes history of pain problems in the family, degenerative disorders, familial disorders, drug dependency, alcoholism, or drug abuse; and psychological disorders such as depression, anxiety, schizophrenia, suicidal tendencies, etc. Family history of medical problems is also important.

Social history includes environmental information such as education, marital status, children, habits, hobbies, and occupational history, whenever available.

PHYSICAL EXAMINATION

Physical examination in interventional pain medicine involves general, musculoskeletal, and neurological examination.

Examination of other systems, specifically cardiovascular, lymphatic, skin, eyes, and cranial nerves is recommended, based on the presenting symptomatology.

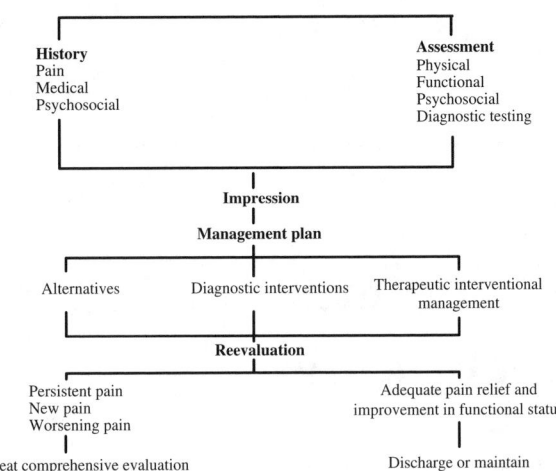

EVALUATION AND MANAGEMENT

FIGURE 57.1 Suggested algorithm for comprehensive evaluation and management of chronic pain. From Evidence-based practice guidelines for interventional techniques in the management of chronic spinal pain, by L. Manchikanti et al. (2003), *Pain Physician, 6,* 3–80. Reproduced with permission of the authors and the American Society of Interventional Pain Physicians (ASIPP).

MEDICAL DECISION MAKING

Medical decision making refers to the complexity of establishing a diagnosis and/or selecting a management option as measured by three components:

1. Diagnosis/management options with a number of possible diagnoses and/or the number of management options
2. Review of records/investigations, with number and/or complexity of medical records, diagnostic tests, and other information that must be obtained, reviewed, and analyzed
3. Risk(s) of significant complications, morbidity, and mortality, as well as comorbidities associated with the patient's presenting problem(s), the diagnostic procedure(s), and/or the possible management options

Psychological evaluation, laboratory evaluation, imaging techniques, electromyography, and nerve conduction and somatosensory evoked potentials are also an extension of the evaluation process. It is beyond the scope of these guidelines to discuss these assessment techniques.

Appropriate history and physical examination with the assistance of other evaluations should direct a physician to formulate a provisional diagnosis. A suggested algorithm for comprehensive evaluation and management of chronic pain is illustrated in Figure 57.1.

MEDICAL NECESSITY DOCUMENTATION

The following criteria should be considered carefully in performing interventional techniques:

1. Complete initial evaluation, including history and physical examination
2. Physiological and functional assessment, as necessary and feasible
3. Definition of indications and medical necessity, as follows:
   - Suspected organic problem
   - Nonresponsiveness to less invasive modalities of treatment except in acute situations such as acute disc herniation, herpes zoster and postherpetic neuralgia, reflex sympathetic dystrophy, and intractable pain secondary to carcinoma
   - Pain and disability of moderate to severe degree
   - No evidence of contraindications such as severe spinal stenosis resulting in intraspinal obstruction, infection, or predominantly psychogenic pain
   - Responsiveness to prior interventions with improvement in physical and functional status for repeat blocks or other interventions
   - Repeating interventions only upon return of pain and deterioration in functional status

INTERVENTIONAL TECHNIQUES

The overall benefit of various types of injection techniques includes pain relief outlasting by days, weeks, or months the relatively short duration of pharmacologic action of the local anesthetics and other agents used.[1–4,10] Clear-cut explanations for these benefits are not currently available. It is believed that neural blockade alters or interrupts nociceptive input, reflex mechanisms of the afferent limb, self-sustaining activity of the neuron pools and neuraxis, and the pattern of central neuronal activities. The explanations are based in part on the pharmacological and physical actions of local anesthetics, corticosteroids, and other agents. It is also believed that local anesthetics interrupt the pain–spasm cycle and reverberating nociceptor transmission, whereas corticosteroids reduce inflammation either by inhibiting the synthesis or release of a number of proinflammatory substances. Various modes of action of corticosteroids include membrane stabilization, inhibition of neural peptide synthesis or action, blockade of phospholipase A_2 activity, prolonged suppression of ongoing neuronal discharge, suppression of sensitization of dorsal horn neurons, and reversible local anesthetic effect. In addition, local anesthetics have been shown to produce prolonged dampening of C-fiber activity.[10]

Physical effects include clearing adhesions or inflammatory exudates from the vicinity of the nerve root sleeve. The scientific basis of some of these concepts, at least in part, is proven for spinal pain management with epidural injections of betamethasone and intravenous methylprednisolone.

DIAGNOSTIC INTERVENTIONAL TECHNIQUES

Diagnostic blockade of a structure with a nerve supply that can generate pain can be performed to test the hypothesis that the target structure is a source of the patient's pain. Testing the hypothesis by provoking pain in any structure is an unreliable criterion except in provocative discography. Although neurodiagnostics of the involved nerve pathways have proven valuable, the relief of pain is the essential criterion in almost all structures, including analgesic discography in the cervical spine, the only deviation being lumbar discs. If the pain is not relieved, the source may be in another structural component of the spine similar to the one tested such as a different facet joint or a different nerve root or some other structure. Thus, precision diagnostic injections directed toward specific spinal pathology are potentially powerful tools for diagnosis of chronic spinal pain, but are often technically challenging.[11,12] Identifying the specific pathology responsible for pain is often difficult, leading to frustrated patients and clinicians. Nevertheless, these injections may be safely performed by properly trained anesthesiologists, physiatrists, neurologists, radiologists, spine surgeons, and physicians from other related specialties who take the time to learn the basis for, and perfect, the application of these techniques.

When the source of pain is more than one structure or multiple levels, it is not expected that all the pain will be relieved. For example, there may be painful facet joints bilaterally at a given segmental level, in which case anesthetizing the left joint should relieve the left side, but not the right side; there may be pain from two consecutive joints on one side, in which case anesthetizing the lower joint alone may relieve only the lower half of the pain; or there may be more than one structure involved, such as pain contributed by discs and facet joints or facet joints and nerves.

True-positive responses are secured by performing controlled blocks. Ideally, this should be in the form of placebo injections of normal saline, but logistical and/or ethical considerations prohibit the use of normal saline in conventional practice.

Rationale

The rationale for diagnostic neural blockade in the management of spinal pain stems from the fact that in the absence of disc herniation and neurological deficit clinical

TABLE 57.1
Profile of Commonly Used Epidural Steroids

Drug	Equivalent Dose	Epidural Dose	Anti-Inflammatory Potency	Sodium Retention Capacity	Duration of Adrenal Suppression		
					IM	Single Epidural	Three Epidurals
Hydrocortisone	20 mg	N/A	1	1	N/A	N/A	N/A
Depo-methylprednisolone (Depo-Medrol®)	4 mg	40–80 mg	5	0.5	1–6 weeks	1–3 weeks	N/A
Triamcinolone diacetate (Aristocort®)	4 mg	25–50 mg	5	0	1–2 weeks	1–5 weeks	N/A
Triamcinolone acetonide (Kenalog®)	4 mg	40–80 mg	5	0	2–6 weeks	N/A	2–3 months
Betamethasone (Celestone Soluspan®)	0.6 mg	6–12 mg	25	0	1–2 weeks	N/A	N/A

Source: From L. Manchikanti, Role of neuraxial steroids in interventional pain management, *Pain Physician, 5,* 182. Reproduced with permission of the author and ASIPP.

features and imaging or neurophysiologic studies do not permit the accurate diagnosis of the causation of spinal pain in the majority of patients. Further rationale is based on the recurring facts showing the overall rate of inaccurate or incomplete diagnosis in patients referred to pain treatment centers as ranging from 40 to 67%, the incidence of psychogenic pain to be only 1 in 3,000 patients, and the presence of organic origin of the pain mistakenly branded as psychosomatic in 98% of cases.[13,14] Finally, chronic low back pain is a diagnostic dilemma in 85% of patients, even in experienced hands with all the available technology.[11,12,15,16] Structural basis of spinal pain has been well established.[17–22] It has been determined that utilizing alternative means of diagnosis, including precision diagnostic blocks in cases where there is a lack of definitive diagnostic radiologic or electrophysiologic criteria, can enable an examiner to identify the source of pain in the majority of patients, thus reducing the proportion of patients who cannot be given a definite diagnosis from 85 to 30% or even as low as 15%.[4,11,12,20,21]

THERAPEUTIC INTERVENTIONAL TECHNIQUES

The rationale for therapeutic interventional techniques in the spine is based on several considerations: the cardinal source of chronic spinal pain, namely, discs and joints, is accessible to neural blockade; removal or correction of structural abnormalities of the spine may fail to cure and may even worsen painful conditions; degenerative processes of the spine and the origin of spinal pain are complex; and the effectiveness of a large variety of therapeutic interventions in managing chronic spinal pain has not been demonstrated conclusively. It has been shown that there is no conclusive evidence supporting the effectiveness of numerous conservative modalities used in managing chronic low back pain, including drug therapy, manipula-

tion, back schools, electromyographic biofeedback therapy, exercise therapy, traction and orthoses, behavioral/cognitive/relaxation therapy, and transcutaneous electrical nerve stimulation. There are a multitude of interventional techniques in the management of chronic pain, including not only neural blockade but also minimally invasive surgical procedures such as peripheral nerve blocks, trigger-point injections, epidural injections, facet joint injections, sympathetic blocks, neuroablation techniques, intradiscal thermal therapy, disc decompression, morphine pump implantation, and spinal cord stimulation.

DELIVERY

There is no consensus among interventional pain management specialists with regards to type, dosage, frequency, total number of injections, or other interventions, yet significant attention in the literature seems to be focused on the complications attributed to the use of epidural steroids in the entire arena of interventional pain management. Thus, various limitations of interventional techniques, specifically neural blockade, have arisen from basically false impressions. Based on the available literature and scientific application, the most commonly used formulations of long-acting steroids (see Table 57.1), which include methylprednisolone (Depo-Medrol®), triamcinolone diacetate (Aristocort®), triamcinolone acetonide (Kenalog®), and betamethasone acetate and phosphate mixture (Celestone Soluspan®), appear to be safe and effective.[10] Based on the present literature, it appears that if repeated within 2 weeks, betamethasone probably would be the best choice in avoiding side effects; whereas if treatment is carried out at 6-week intervals or longer, any one of the four formulations would be safe and effective.

Frequency and total number of injections or interventions are a key issue, although controversial and rarely addressed. Some authors recommend one injection for diagnostic as well as therapeutic purposes; others advocate three injections in a series irrespective of the patient's progress or lack thereof; still others suggest three injections followed by a repeat course of three injections after 3-, 6-, or 12-month intervals; and, finally, there are some who propose an unlimited number of injections with no established goals or parameters. Limitation of 3 mg/kg of body weight of steroid or 210 mg per year in an average person and a lifetime dose of 420 mg of steroid, equivalent to methylprednisolone, also have been advocated. While some investigators recommend one injection and do not repeat if there has been no response to the first, others recommend one or two more injections in the absence of response to the first injection. Some authors have reported good pain relief in previously unresponsive patients after an additional one or two injections. Similarly, some have believed that more than three injections do not result in additional improvement,[23] whereas others have reported the use of 6 to 10 injections if they are of benefit, however, not to exceed 3 if they are not beneficial.[24,25] Such descriptions for other interventional techniques have been extrapolated from the limitations described for epidural steroid injections, even though there is no scientific basis or justification for such an extrapolation, as the techniques and type and dosage drugs are vastly different. It also has been shown in a multitude of publications that relief following multiple injections or interventions demonstrated a staircase-type phenomenon, even though it reached a plateau after three to four interventions.

AN ALGORITHMIC APPROACH

In the changing paradigm of modern medicine, with its major focus on evidence-based medicine, interventional pain physicians are forced to learn and practice evidence-based interventional pain management. The necessary ingredients to provide evidence-based care include the following:

- Precise definition of the problem/diagnosis
- Research of best evidence
- Critical appraisal of the evidence
- Consideration of the evidence and its implications, in the context of the patient's condition, circumstances, and values

Even though a basic understanding of these ingredients may appear not only easy, but simple, developing expertise with the incorporation of evidence, and meticulous application of evidence to a patient's situation, is difficult and time-consuming. Thus, an algorithmic approach, if developed properly, may assist a physician in the clinical practice of interventional pain management.

We have developed an algorithmic approach based on the structural basis of spinal pain, moderate to strong evidence of diagnostic techniques available in arriving at a structural diagnosis of spinal pain (not available by means of radiological evaluation, physical examination, and electrodiagnostic testing), and employing effective interventional techniques available in managing chronic spinal pain. Consensus was used in the absence of evidence. Figure 57.2 and Figure 57.3 describe proposed algorithmic approaches for diagnosis and management of chronic low back pain, whereas Figure 57.4 describes a proposed algorithmic approach for diagnosis of chronic neck pain.

EPIDURAL INJECTIONS[26–53]

DESCRIPTION

Spinal pain generates from multiple structures in the spine with a nerve supply capable of causing pain similar to that seen in clinically normal volunteers, and that are susceptible to diseases or injuries that are known to be painful. Certain conditions may not be detectable using currently available technology or biochemical studies. However, for a structure to be implicated, it should have been shown to be a source of pain in patients, using diagnostic techniques of known reliability and validity. The structures responsible for pain in the spine include the intervertebral discs, spinal cord, nerve roots, facet joints, ligaments, muscles, and sacroiliac joints.

One of the most common structures responsible for pain in the spine is the intervertebral disc. Even though disc herniation is seen only in a small number of patients, degeneration of the disc resulting in primary discogenic pain is seen much more commonly. In contrast to a ruptured disc with pain arising from the nerve root, in discogenic pain a disc with or without internal disruption is implicated rather than the nerve root.

Postlaminectomy syndrome, or pain following operative procedures of the spine, sometimes also known as failed management syndrome, is becoming a common entity in modern medicine. It is estimated that 20 to 30% of spinal surgeries, occasionally up to as high as 60%, may not be successful as a result of the surgery being either inadequate, incorrect, or unnecessary; but also it may result following a well-indicated and well-performed surgical procedure. Even in cases of successful surgery, pain and subsequent disability have returned after variable periods of 6 months to 20 years. However, surgical results are extremely poor in patients after a failed surgical procedure. Other spinal conditions include various degenerative disorders such as spinal stenosis, spondylolysis, spondylolisthesis, degenerative scoliosis, idiopathic vertebrogenic sclerosis, diffuse idiopathic spinal hyperostosis, and segmental instability. Degenerative conditions other

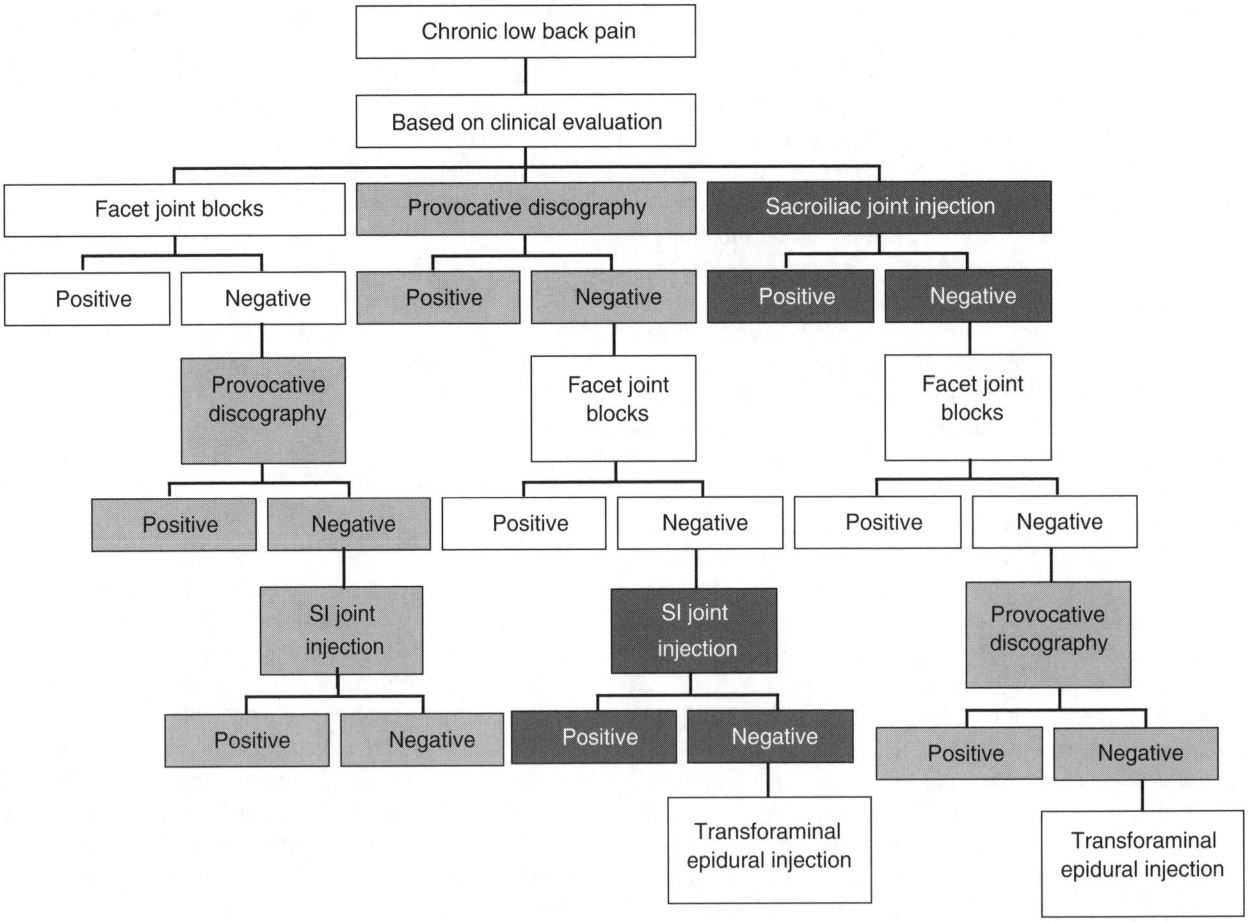

```
                        ┌──────────────────────┐
                        │ Chronic low back pain │
                        └──────────────────────┘
                                   │
                        ┌──────────────────────┐
                        │ Based on clinical evaluation │
                        └──────────────────────┘
```

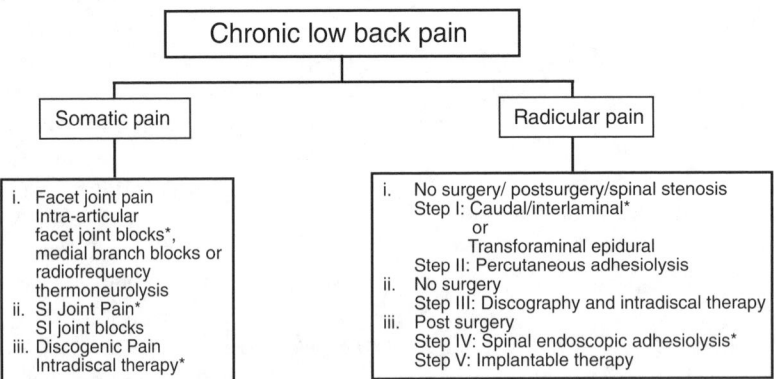

FIGURE 57.2 An algorithmic approach to diagnosis of chronic low back pain without diagnosis of disc herniation. From Evidence-based practice guidelines for interventional techniques in the management of chronic spinal pain, by L. Manchikanti et al. (2003), *Pain Physician, 6,* 3–80. Reproduced with permission from authors and ASIPP.

FIGURE 57.3 A suggested algorithm for application of therapeutic interventional techniques in management of chronic low back pain. * Intra-articular facet joint blocks, interlaminar epidurals, SI joint blocks, and intradiscal therapy are not based on evidence synthesis. From Evidence-based practice guidelines for interventional techniques in the management of chronic spinal pain, by L. Manchikanti et al. (2003), *Pain Physician, 6,* 3–80. Reproduced with permission of authors and ASIPP.

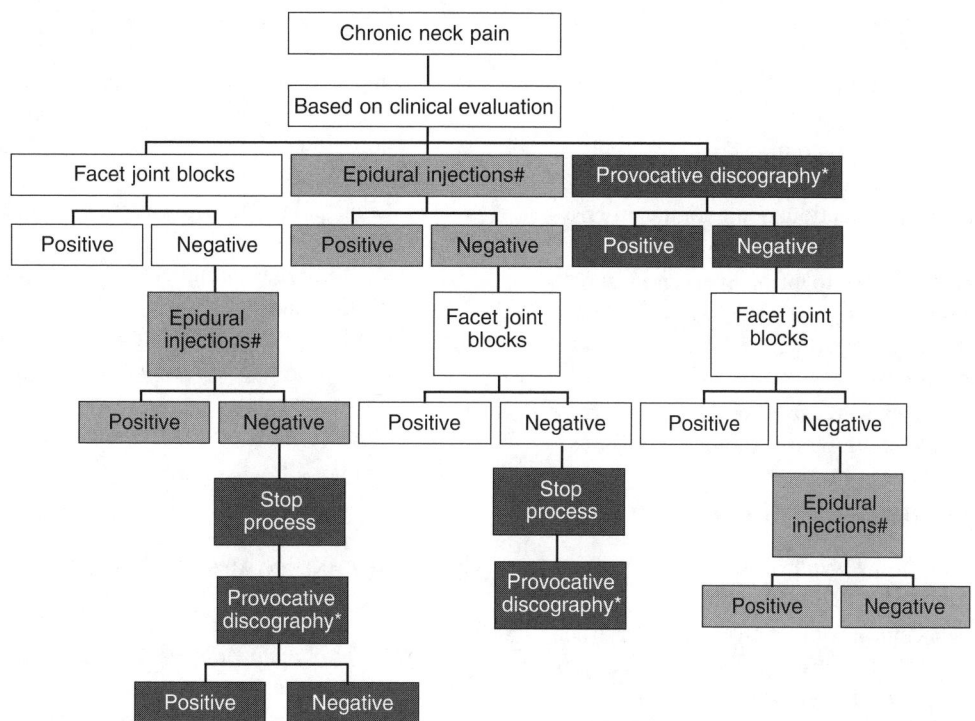

FIGURE 57.4 An algorithmic approach to diagnosis of chronic neck back pain without diagnosis of disc herniation. *Not based on evidence. #Transforaminal epidural injections have been associated with reports of risk. From Evidence-based practice guidelines for interventional techniques in the management of chronic spinal pain, by L. Manchikanti et al. (2003), *Pain Physician, 6*, 3–80. Reproduced with permission by authors and ASIPP.

than disc disruption and facet arthritis may contribute to approximately 5 to 10% of spinal pain.

CURRENT PROCEDURAL TERMINOLOGY (CPT) CODES

- 62310 Injection, single, not including neurolytic substances, with or without contrast of diagnostic or therapeutic substance(s); epidural or subarachnoid; cervical or thoracic
- 62311 Injection, single, not including neurolytic substances, with or without contrast of diagnostic or therapeutic substance(s); epidural or subarachnoid; lumbar, sacral (caudal)
- 62318 Catheter placement, continuous infusion for intermittent bolus; epidural or subarachnoid; cervical or thoracic
- 62319 Catheter placement, continuous infusion for intermittent bolus; epidural, lumbar, sacral (caudal)
- 64479 Cervical/thoracic transforaminal epidural, single level
- 64480 Cervical/thoracic transforaminal epidural, each additional level
- 64483 Transforaminal epidural; lumbar or sacral, single level
- 64484 Transforaminal epidural; lumbar or sacral, each additional level

- 72275 Epidurography, radiological supervision and interpretation
- 76005 Fluoroscopic guidance and localization of needle or catheter tip for spine or paraspinous diagnostic or therapeutic injection procedures (epidural, transforaminal epidural, subarachnoid, paravertebral facet joint, paravertebral facet joint nerve, or sacroiliac joint), including neurolytic agent destruction

INDICATIONS AND MEDICAL NECESSITY

The following criteria should be considered carefully when performing epidural injections:

1. Complete initial evaluation including history and physical examination
2. Physiological and functional assessment, as necessary and feasible
3. Definition of indications and medical necessity, as follows:
   - Suspected organic problem
   - Nonresponsiveness to less invasive modalities of treatments except in acute situations such as acute disc herniation, herpes zoster and postherpetic neuralgia, reflex sympa-

thetic dystrophy, and intractable pain secondary to carcinoma

- Pain and disability of moderate to severe degree
- No evidence of contraindications such as severe spinal stenosis resulting in intraspinal obstruction, infection, or predominantly psychogenic pain
- Responsiveness to prior interventions with improvement in physical and functional status to proceed with repeat blocks or other interventions
- Repeating interventions only upon return of pain and deterioration in functional status

ICD-9[1] CODES THAT SUPPORT MEDICAL NECESSITY

1. Postlaminectomy syndrome: 722.81 cervical, 722.82 thoracic, 722.83, lumbosacral
2. Disc displacement without myelopathy (disc herniation, radiculitis, disc extrusion, disc protrusion, disc prolapse, discogenic syndrome): 722.0 cervical, 722.11 thoracic, 722.10 lumbosacral
3. Disc displacement with myelopathy: 722.71 cervical, 722.72 thoracic, 722.73 lumbosacral
4. Degeneration of intervertebral disc (includes narrowing of disc space): 722.4 cervical, 722.51 thoracic, 722.52 lumbosacral
5. Radiculitis: 723.4 cervical, 724.4 thoracic, 724.4 lumbosacral
6. Spinal stenosis: 723.0 cervical, 724.04 thoracic, 724.02 lumbosacral
7. Spondylosis with myelopathy: 721.1 cervical, 721.41 thoracic, 721.42 lumbosacral
8. Closed fracture of spine: 805.0 cervical, 805.2 thoracic, 805.4 lumbar, 805.6 sacral
9. Congenital spondylolysis: 756.11 cervical, 756.11 thoracic, 756.11 lumbosacral
10. Acquired/degenerative spondylolysis or acquired spondylolisthesis: 738.4 cervical, 738.4 thoracic, 738.4 lumbosacral
11. Congenital spondylolisthesis: 756.12 cervical, 756.12 thoracic, 756.12 lumbosacral
12. Coccygodynia: 724.79
13. Sciatica: 724.3
14. Complex regional pain syndrome (Type I or reflex sympathetic dystrophy): 337.20 reflex sympathetic dystrophy unspecified, 337.21 reflex sympathetic dystrophy upper limb, 337.22 reflex sympathetic dystrophy lower limb, 337.29 reflex sympathetic dystrophy other unspecified site
15. Complex regional pain syndrome (Type II or causalgia): 355.9 causalgia, 354.4 causalgia upper limb, 355.71 causalgia lower limb
16. Peripheral neuropathy: 356.4 idiopathic, 356.0 hereditary, 357.2 diabetic, 357.5 alcoholic, 357.6 due to drug
17. Limb pain: 353.6 phantom limb pain, 997.60 stump pain, 997.61 neuroma of amputation stump, 342.0 hemiplegia–flaccid, 342.1 hemiplegia–spastic
18. Postherpetic neuralgia: 053.10 with unspecified nerve system complication, 053.13 postherpetic polyneuropathy
19. Pain syndromes secondary to neoplasm 141.0–239.9
20. Vascular ischemic pain 440.22

FREQUENCY AND NUMBER OF INJECTIONS OR INTERVENTIONS

- In the diagnostic phase, a patient may receive injections at intervals of no shorter than 1 week or preferably, 2 weeks, except for blockade in cancer pain or when a continuous administration of local anesthetic is employed for reflex sympathetic dystrophy.
- In the therapeutic phase (after the diagnostic phase is completed), the frequency of interventional techniques should be 2 months or longer between each injection, provided that at least ≥50% relief is obtained for 6 to 8 weeks. However, if the neural blockade is applied for different regions, it can be performed at intervals of no sooner than 1 week and preferably 2 weeks for most types of blocks. The therapeutic frequency must remain at least 2 months for each region. It is further suggested that all regions be treated at the same time, provided all procedures are performed safely.
- In the diagnostic phase, the number of injections should be limited to no more than two times except for reflex sympathetic dystrophy, in which case three times is reasonable.
- In the treatment or therapeutic phase, the interventional procedures should be repeated only as necessary judging by the medical necessity criteria, and these should be limited to a maximum of six times.
- Under unusual circumstances with a recurrent injury, carcinoma, or reflex sympathetic dystrophy, blocks may be repeated at intervals of 6 weeks after diagnosis/stabilization in the treatment phase.
- Total number of interventions are applied separately for each region.

---

[1] *International Classification of Diseases,* Ninth Revision.

COMBINATIONS OF BLOCKS/INTERVENTIONS

It may be essential to combine, in certain circumstances, more than one block. This may include an epidural for the cervical region and facet-joint blocks for the lumbar region, or epidural and facet-joint blocks for the same region in the case of identification of pain generators from both sources.

DOCUMENTATION REQUIREMENTS

The patient's medical record must contain documentation that fully supports the medical necessity for epidural injections.

It is preferable to perform interlaminar epidural injections (CPT 62310, 62311) in interventional pain management under fluoroscopy. It is mandatory to perform transforaminals under fluoroscopy. If interlaminar or caudal epidurals are performed without fluoroscopy, response to the first epidural injection must always be documented. If the response to the first injection is inadequate either in quality (level of pain relief ≤ 50%) or quantity (less than 1 week), the next treatment must be performed under fluoroscopy.

Documentation must also support the frequency and the appropriateness of this procedure, as opposed to alternative forms of therapy.

FACET JOINT BLOCKS[11,12–21,54–77]

DESCRIPTION

Spinal pain generates from multiple structures in the spine with a nerve supply capable of causing pain similar to that seen in clinically normal volunteers; these structures are susceptible to diseases or injuries that are known to be painful. Certain conditions may not be detectable using currently available technology or biochemical studies. However, for a structure to be implicated, it should have been shown to be a source of pain in patients, using diagnostic techniques of known reliability and validity. The structures responsible for pain in the spine include the intervertebral discs, spinal cord, nerve roots, facet joints, ligaments, and muscles.

Disc herniation, strained muscles, and torn ligaments have been attributed in the past to be the cause of most spinal pain. However, in the neck and upper extremities, upper and mid back, or low back and lower extremities; disorders of the spinal joints, which include facet joints, have been implicated more commonly than disc herniation, attributing some 50% of spinal pain to these joints. Facet joints were described as a potential source of low back pain as early as 1911, 20 years earlier than ruptured discs. The existence of lumbar facet joint pain is supported by a preponderance of scientific evidence, even though a few detractors have disputed this. The prevalence of facet joint pain in patients with chronic spinal pain has been established as 15 to 45% in low back pain, 42 to 48% in chronic thoracic pain, and 54 to 67% in neck pain, utilizing controlled diagnostic blocks, based on type of setting and population studied.

In managing low back pain, local anesthetic injection into the facet joints or interruption of the nerve supply to the facet joints has been accepted as the standard for diagnosis of facet joint pain. Because a single joint is innervated by at least two medial branches, two adjacent levels should always be blocked.

If the pain is relieved, the joint may be considered to be the source of pain. However, false-positive responses, which may be seen in 27 to 63% in cervical spine, 45 to 58% in thoracic spine, and 17 to 47% in lumbar spine of the patients, must be ruled out.

- All the patient's pain need not be relieved, for it is possible that a patient may have several sources of pain.
- Comparative local anesthetic blocks, should be administered so that the same joint is anesthetized on two separate occasions, but using local anesthetics with different durations of action or placebo blocks.
- A true-positive response confirms that the joint is the source of the pain, with a confidence of 85%.

It is recognized that it may be necessary to provide additional blocks such as selective nerve root or selective epidural blocks and disc injections in conjunction with facet-joint blocks. It is also recognized that multiple levels of facet-joint blocks may be performed in one setting, either in the same region or in multiple regions, more commonly than not.

Multiple blocks are provided only with proper evaluation to determine pain generator(s). Once a structure is proved to be negative, no interventions must be directed at that structure.

Therapeutic facet joint blocks are based on the outcome of a diagnostic facet-joint block, with the patient obtaining sufficient relief for a meaningful period of time; but when pain recurs, a repeat block using a small dose of local anesthetic and steroid provides longer-lasting relief (4 to 8 weeks).

If facet joint pain is present in conjunction with radiculopathy, both ailments should be managed.

CURRENT PROCEDURAL TERMINOLOGY (CPT) CODES

- 64470 Cervical paravertebral facet joint nerve block, single level
- 64472 Injection, cervical facet joint nerve block, each additional level

- 64475 Injection, lumbar facet joint nerve block, single level
- 64476 Injection, lumbar facet joint nerve block, each additional level
- 76005 Fluoroscopic guidance and localization of needle or catheter tip for spine or paraspinous diagnostic or therapeutic injection procedures (epidural, transforaminal epidural, subarachnoid, paravertebral facet joint, paravertebral facet joint nerve, or sacroiliac joint), including neurolytic agent destruction

INDICATIONS AND MEDICAL NECESSITY

The following criteria should be considered carefully when performing facet blocks:

1. Complete initial evaluation, including history and physical examination
2. Physiological and functional assessment, as necessary and feasible
3. Definition of indications and medical necessity:
   - Suspected organic problem
   - Nonresponsiveness to less invasive modalities of treatments except in acute situations such as acute disc herniation, herpes zoster and postherpetic neuralgia, reflex sympathetic dystrophy, and intractable pain secondary to carcinoma
   - Pain and disability of moderate to severe degree
   - No evidence of contraindications such as intraspinal obstruction, infection, or predominantly psychogenic pain
   - Responsiveness to prior interventions with improvement in physical and functional status to proceed with repeat blocks or other interventions
   - Repeating interventions only upon return of pain and deterioration in functional status

ICD-9 CODES THAT SUPPORT MEDICAL NECESSITY

1. Spondylosis without myelopathy, dorsal arthritis, osteoarthritis, and spondyloarthritis (facet-joint arthropathy): 721.0 cervical, 721.2 thoracic, 721.3 lumbar, and 721.7 traumatic spondylopathy
2. Spondylolysis: 756.11 congenital, 738.4 acquired
3. Spondylolisthesis: 756.12 congenital, 738.4 acquired

FREQUENCY AND NUMBER OF INJECTIONS OR INTERVENTIONS

- In the diagnostic phase, a patient may receive injections at intervals of no sooner than 1 week or, preferably, 2 weeks.

- In the therapeutic phase (after the stabilization is completed), the frequency should be 2 months or longer between each injection, provided that at least ≥50% relief is obtained for 6 weeks. However, if the neural blockade is applied for different regions, it can be performed at intervals of no sooner than 1 week or preferably 2 weeks for most types of blocks. The therapeutic frequency must remain at 2 months for each region. It is further suggested that all regions be treated at the same time, provided all procedures are performed safely. AdminaStar Federal of Kentucky and Indiana limits to a total of six blocks per year, per region.
- In the diagnostic or stabilization phase, the number of injections should be limited to no more than four per year.
- In the treatment or therapeutic phase, the interventional procedures should be repeated only as necessary judging by the medical necessity criteria, and these should be limited to a maximum of six times for local anesthetic and steroid blocks for a period of 1 year per region.
- Under unusual circumstances with a recurrent injury or cervicogenic headache, blocks may be repeated at intervals of 6 weeks after stabilization in the treatment phase.

DOCUMENTATION REQUIREMENTS

The patient's medical record must contain documentation that fully supports the medical necessity for facet joint injections as described above.

Documentation must also support the frequency and the appropriateness of this procedure, as opposed to alternative forms of therapy.

Facet joint blocks must always be performed under fluoroscopy.

MEDIAL BRANCH NEUROTOMY[54–86]

DESCRIPTION

Spinal pain generates from multiple structures in the spine with a nerve supply capable of causing pain similar to that seen in clinically normal volunteers; these structures are susceptible to diseases or injuries that are known to be painful. Certain conditions may not be detectable using currently available technology or biochemical studies. However, for a structure to be implicated, it should have been shown to be a source of pain in patients, using diagnostic techniques of known reliability and validity. The structures responsible for pain in the spine include the intervertebral discs, spinal cord, nerve roots, facet joints, ligaments, and muscles.

Even though disc herniation, strained muscles, and torn ligaments have been attributed in the past to be the cause of most spinal pain in the neck and upper extremities, the upper and mid back, or the low back and lower extremities, disorders of the spinal joints, which include facet joints, have been implicated more commonly than disc herniation, attributing some 50% of spinal pain to these joints. Facet joints were described as a potential source of low back pain as early as 1911, 20 years earlier than ruptured discs. The existence of lumbar facet joint pain is supported by a preponderance of scientific evidence, even though a few detractors have disputed this. The prevalence of facet joint pain in patients with chronic spinal pain has been established as 15 to 45% in low back pain, 42 to 48% in chronic thoracic pain, and 54 to 67% in neck pain utilizing controlled diagnostic blocks.

Facet joint denervation is based on the outcome of a diagnostic facet joint block, with the patient obtaining sufficient relief for a meaningful period of time; but, when pain recurs, a repeat block using a small dose of local anesthetic and steroid does not provide longer-lasting relief. This is performed either by injecting neurolytic substance or by denervation utilizing radiofrequency thermoneurolysis or cryoneurolysis.

If facet joint pain is present in conjunction with radiculopathy, both ailments should be managed.

CPT Codes

- 64626 Destruction by neurolytic agent, paravertebral facet joint nerve; cervical or thoracic, single level
- 64627 Destruction by neurolytic agent, paravertebral facet joint nerve; cervical or thoracic, each additional level
- 64622 Destruction by neurolytic agent, paravertebral facet joint nerve; lumbar or sacral, single level
- 64623 Destruction by neurolytic agent, paravertebral facet joint nerve; lumbar or sacral, each additional level
- 76005 Fluoroscopic guidance and localization of needle or catheter tip for spine or paraspinous diagnostic or therapeutic injection procedures (epidural, transforaminal epidural, subarachnoid, paravertebral facet joint, paravertebral facet joint nerve, or sacroiliac joint), including neurolytic agent destruction

Indications and Medical Necessity

The following criteria should be considered carefully in performing facet neurolytic blocks:

1. Complete initial evaluation, including history and physical examination
2. Physiological and functional assessment, as necessary and feasible
3. Definition of indications and medical necessity:
   - Suspected organic problem
   - Nonresponsiveness to less invasive modalities of treatments except in acute situations such as acute disc herniation, herpes zoster and postherpetic neuralgia, reflex sympathetic dystrophy, and intractable pain secondary to carcinoma
   - Pain and disability of moderate to severe degree
   - No evidence of contraindications such as intraspinal obstruction, infection, or predominantly psychogenic pain
   - Responsiveness to prior interventions with improvement in physical and functional status to proceed with repeat blocks or other interventions
   - Repeating interventions only upon return of pain and deterioration in functional status
4. Confirmation of facet joint pain with double diagnostic blocks

ICD-9 Codes That Support Medical Necessity

1. Spondylosis without myelopathy, dorsal arthritis, osteoarthritis, and spondyloarthritis (*facet-joint arthropathy*): 721.0 cervical, 721.2 thoracic, 721.3 lumbar, and 721.7 traumatic spondylopathy
2. Spondylolysis: 756.11 congenital, 738.4 acquired
3. Spondylolisthesis: 756.12 congenital, 738.4 acquired

Frequency and Number of Interventions

- The frequency should be limited to 3 months or longer between each injection, provided that at least ≥50% relief is obtained for 10 weeks. However, if the neurotomy is applied for different regions, it can be performed at intervals of no sooner than 1 month. The therapeutic frequency must remain at 3 months for each region. AdminaStar Federal of Kentucky and Indiana (www.astar-federal.com/anthem/affiliates/adminastar) limits to a total of two neurotomies per year.
- The interventional procedures should be repeated only as necessary judging by the medical necessity criteria.

DOCUMENTATION REQUIREMENTS

The patient's medical record must contain documentation that fully supports the medical necessity for the diagnosis of facet joint pain and neurolytic blocks.

Documentation must also support the frequency and the appropriateness of this procedure, as opposed to alternative forms of therapy.

Medial branch neurotomy must always be performed under fluoroscopy.

PERCUTANEOUS LYSIS OF EPIDURAL ADHESIONS[1,87-96]

DESCRIPTION

Postlaminectomy syndrome or pain following operative procedures of the spine, sometimes known as failed management syndrome, is becoming a common entity in modern medicine. It is estimated that 20 to 30% of spinal surgeries, occasionally up to as high as 40%, may not be successful as a result of the surgery being inadequate, incorrect, or unnecessary, or may result following a well-indicated and well-performed surgical procedure. Even in cases of successful surgery, pain and subsequent disability have returned after variable periods of from 6 months to 20 years. In these cases, scar tissue development, destabilization of the spinal joints, and recurrent or repeat disc herniation may be responsible for continued pain problems. However, surgical results are extremely poor in patients after a failed surgical procedure. Epidural fibrosis may also develop without surgery.

Percutaneous nonendoscopic adhesiolysis and injection of hypertonic saline in the lumbar spine, its utilization, and its studies have been reasonable and acceptable. This modality of treatment appears to be reasonable in the management of refractory low back pain secondary to failed back surgery, disc disruption, and multilevel degenerative arthritis, even though there are a few detractors.

Percutaneous epidural adhesiolysis is also indicated for patients suffering with refractory low back pain secondary to a multitude of causes, including postlumbar laminectomy syndrome, lumbar epidural fibrosis, spinal stenosis and multilevel disc disruption, or multilevel degenerative arthritis. However, this should only be used after the failure of the conservative modalities of treatment, including caudal and transforaminal epidural injections.

CPT CODES

- 62263 Percutaneous lysis of epidural adhesions using solution injection, e.g., hypertonic saline, enzyme, or mechanical means, e.g., catheter, including radiologic localization (includes contrast when administered), multiple adhesiolysis sessions; 2 or more days
- 62264 Percutaneous lysis of epidural adhesions using solution injection, e.g., hypertonic saline, enzyme, or mechanical means, e.g., catheter, including radiologic localization (includes contrast when administered); 1 day

Note: Epidurography (CPT 72275) and fluoroscopic guidance (CPT 76005) are component codes of CPT 62263 and 62264.

INDICATIONS AND MEDICAL NECESSITY

The following criteria should be considered carefully in performing lysis of epidural adhesions:

1. Complete initial evaluation, including history and physical examination
2. Physiological and functional assessment, as necessary and feasible
3. Definition of indications and medical necessity:
   - Suspected organic problem
   - Presence of facet joints has been ruled out by clinical evaluation or diagnostic controlled facet joint blocks
   - Non-responsiveness to less invasive modalities of treatments including fluoroscopically directed caudal, interlaminar, or transforaminal epidural steroid injections
   - Pain and disability of moderate to severe degree
   - No evidence of contraindications such as intraspinal obstruction, infection, or predominantly psychogenic pain
   - Responsiveness to prior interventions with improvement in physical and functional status to proceed with repeat blocks or other interventions
   - Repeating interventions only upon return of pain and deterioration in functional status

ICD-9 CODES THAT SUPPORT MEDICAL NECESSITY

1. Postlaminectomy syndrome: 722.81 cervical, 722.82 thoracic, 722.83 lumbosacral
2. Epidural fibrosis: 349.2
3. Disc displacement with myelopathy: 722.71 cervical, 722.72 thoracic, 722.73 lumbosacral
4. Disc displacement without myelopathy (disc herniation, radiculitis, disc extrusion, disc protrusion, disc prolapse, discogenic syndrome): 722.0 cervical, 722.11 thoracic, 722.10, lumbosacral

5. Degeneration of intervertebral disc (includes narrowing of disc space): 722.4 cervical, 722.51 thoracic, 722.52 lumbosacral

FREQUENCY AND NUMBER OF INTERVENTIONS

- In the diagnostic or stabilization phase, a patient may receive injections at intervals of no sooner than 4 weeks.
- In the treatment or therapeutic phase, the number of procedures should be limited to:
  - With a 3-day protocol, two interventions per year
  - With a 1-day protocol, a maximum of four interventions per year.

DOCUMENTATION REQUIREMENTS

The patient's medical record must contain documentation that fully supports the medical necessity for lysis of epidural adhesions.

Documentation must also support the frequency and the appropriateness of this procedure, as opposed to alternative forms of therapy.

SPINAL ENDOSCOPIC ADHESIOLYSIS[1,97–105]

DESCRIPTION

Spinal endoscopy with epidural adhesiolysis is an invasive but important treatment modality in managing chronic low back pain that is nonresponsive to other modalities of treatment, including percutaneous spring guided adhesiolysis and transforaminal epidural injection(s).

Low back pain is the most common ailment in the modern era, burdening approximately 15 to 39% of the population with serious financial and social consequences, and ranking first among musculoskeletal disorders. Multiple investigators have shown that as many as 79% of patients continue to suffer with chronic or recurrent low back pain 1 year after its onset. Among various causes of low back pain, postlumbar laminectomy syndrome is increasingly recognized as a cause. It is estimated that 5 to 40% of lumbar surgeries result in failed back surgery syndrome, with some statistics showing failure rates reaching as high as 68%. Postlumbar laminectomy syndrome may result from surgery that may have been inadequate, incorrect, or unnecessary, but it may also result following a well-indicated and well-performed surgical intervention or without surgery. Endoscopic adhesiolysis is based on the premise that the three-dimensional visualization of the contents of the epidural space provides the operator with the ability to steer the catheter toward structures of interest, allowing the examination of a specific nerve root and its pathology, lysis of adhesions, and target-specific injection of a drug(s).

The purpose of spinal or epidural endoscopy is to directly visualize the contents of the epidural space, lyse the adhesions, and directly apply drugs, thus assuring delivery of high concentrations of injected drugs to the target areas. Thus, spinal endoscopy with lysis of adhesions incorporates multiple therapeutic goals into one treatment, similar to percutaneous lysis of adhesions with a spring-guided catheter, with added advantages of direct visualization of the epidural space and its contents, a three-dimensional view, and increased steerability of endoscopic equipment with a fiber-optic catheter. Nomenclature used to describe this procedure includes *spinal canal endoscopy, spinal epiduroscopy, myeloscopy, spinal or lumbar epiduroscopy,* and *endoscopic adhesiolysis.*

Percutaneous epidural endoscopic adhesiolysis is also indicated for patients suffering with refractory low back pain secondary to a multitude of causes, including postlumbar laminectomy syndrome, lumbar epidural fibrosis, and multilevel disc disruption, or multilevel degenerative arthritis. However, this should only be used after the failure of conservative modalities of treatments, as well as other interventional procedures, including caudal and transforaminal epidural steroid injections and percutaneous lysis of adhesions.

CPT CODE

1. 0027T Endoscopic lysis of epidural adhesions with direct visualization using mechanical means, e.g., spinal endoscopic catheter system, or solution injection, e.g., normal saline, including radiologic localization and epidurography, which retained its approval even though EBI opposed the code.

Note: Epidurography (CPT 72275) and fluoroscopic guidance (CPT 76005) are component codes of CPT 0027T.

INDICATIONS AND MEDICAL NECESSITY

The following criteria should be considered carefully in performing lysis of epidural adhesions:

1. Complete initial evaluation, including history and physical examination
2. Physiological and functional assessment, as necessary and feasible
3. Definition of indications and medical necessity:
   - Suspected organic problem without facet joint arthropathy
   - Nonresponsiveness to other invasive modalities of treatments including fluoroscopically directed epidurals and percutaneous adhesiolysis

- Pain and disability of moderate to severe degree
- No evidence of contraindications such as severe spinal stenosis resulting in intraspinal obstruction, infection, or predominantly psychogenic pain
- Responsiveness to prior interventions with improvement in physical and functional status to proceed with repeat blocks or other interventions
- Repeating interventions only upon return of pain and deterioration in functional status

ICD-9 CODES THAT SUPPORT MEDICAL NECESSITY

1. Postlaminectomy syndrome: 722.83 lumbosacral
2. Epidural fibrosis: 349.2
3. Disc displacement with myelopathy: 722.73 lumbosacral
4. Disc displacement without myelopathy (disc herniation, radiculitis, disc extrusion, disc protrusion, disc prolapse, discogenic syndrome): 722.10 lumbosacral
5. Degeneration of intervertebral disc (includes narrowing of disc space): 722.52 lumbosacral

FREQUENCY AND NUMBER OF INJECTIONS OR INTERVENTIONS

- Spinal endoscopy with adhesiolysis may not be repeated within 6 months after the procedure.

DOCUMENTATION REQUIREMENTS

The patient's medical record must contain documentation that fully supports the medical necessity for lysis of epidural adhesions.

Documentation must also support the frequency and the appropriateness of this procedure, as opposed to alternative forms of therapy.

PROVOCATIVE DISCOGRAPHY[106–116]

DESCRIPTION

Disc herniation, strained muscles, and torn ligaments have been attributed in the past as the cause of most spinal pain, in the neck and upper extremities, the upper and mid back, or the low back and lower extremities. However, disc herniation is seen only in a small number of patients, whereas degeneration of the disc resulting in primary discogenic pain is seen much more commonly. In contrast to a ruptured disc having pain arising from the nerve root, in discogenic pain a disc with or without internal disruption is implicated rather than the nerve root.

Even though riddled with controversy, disc stimulation is used quite frequently for diagnosis of discogenic syndrome, as well as a precursor to surgical intervention such as fusion. Stringent standards of practice have been established to ensure that the results of discography are not polluted by false-positive responses.

CPT CODES

- 62290 Injection procedure for discography, each level; lumbar
- 62291 Injection procedure for discography, each level; cervical or thoracic
- 72285 Discography, cervical or thoracic, radiological supervision and interpretation
- 72295 Discography, lumbar, radiological supervision and interpretation
- 76003 Fluoroscopic guidance for needle placement

Note: 76003 should not be used with discography interpretation codes CPT 72285 and CPT 72295. CPT 76005 is a component code of discography.

INDICATIONS AND MEDICAL NECESSITY

The following criteria should be considered carefully in performing disc interventions:

1. Complete initial evaluation, including history and physical examination
2. Physiological and functional assessment, as necessary and feasible
3. Definition of indications and medical necessity:
   - Suspected organic problem
   - Pain and disability of moderate to severe degree
   - No evidence of contraindications such as intraspinal obstruction, infection, or predominantly psychogenic pain
4. Indications for discography:
   - Unremitting spinal pain, with or without extremity pain, of greater than 4 months' duration
   - The pain has been unresponsive to all appropriate methods of conservative therapy including fluoroscopically directed epidural steroid injections
   - Before discography, the patient should have undergone investigations with other modalities which have failed to explain the source of pain; such modalities should include, but not be limited to, computed tomography (CT) scanning, magnetic resonance imaging (MRI) scanning, and/or myelography. In

these circumstances, discography may be the only study capable of providing a diagnosis or permitting a precise description of the internal anatomy of the disc.

- To rule out secondary internal disc disruption or recurrent herniation in the postoperative patient
- To determine the number of levels to include in a spine fusion
- To determine the primary symptom-producing level when annular denervation (via thermocoagulation with an intradiscal catheter or a radiofrequency probe) is contemplated

ICD-9 CODES THAT SUPPORT MEDICAL NECESSITY

1. Disc displacement without myelopathy (disc herniation, radiculitis, extrusion, protrusion, prolapse, discogenic syndrome): 722.0 cervical, 722.11 thoracic, 722.10 lumbosacral
2. Degeneration of intervertebral disc including narrowing of disc space: 722.4 cervical, 722.51 thoracic, 722.52 lumbosacral

DOCUMENTATION REQUIREMENTS

The patient's medical record must contain documentation that fully supports the medical necessity for discography.

Documentation must also support the frequency and the appropriateness of this procedure, as opposed to alternative forms of therapy.

SYMPATHETIC BLOCKS[3,4,117–127]

DESCRIPTION

The evolution of the nomenclature, conceptual understanding, and management of complex regional pain syndrome, formerly known as reflex sympathetic dystrophy and causalgia, has been dynamic. *Reflex sympathetic dystrophy, causalgia, sympathetically maintained pain, sympathetically independent pain*, and *complex regional pain syndrome* encompass some of the commonly used nomenclature. As per the International Association for the Study of Pain Committee on Taxonomy, to satisfy the diagnosis of complex regional pain syndrome Type I (reflex sympathetic dystrophy), the clinical findings include regional pain, sensory changes, e.g., allodynia, abnormalities of temperature, abnormal pseudomotor activity, edema, and an abnormal skin color that occurs after a noxious event. Complex regional pain syndrome Type II, or causalgia, includes all of the above-described features, in addition to a peripheral nerve lesion. However, the pathophysiology of these syndromes is poorly understood.

Sympathetically maintained pain, by definition, is eliminated by an anesthetic blockade of the sympathetic efferents that serve the painful area. Similarly, neuropathic pain, which is similar to reflex sympathetic dystrophy, however, represents various heterogeneous conditions, which can be explained neither by one single etiology nor by a particular anatomical lesion.

Visceral pain also may be caused by sympathetic overactivity. Temporary relief of abdominal visceral pain can therefore be obtained by blockade of the celiac plexus or lumbar or thoracic sympathetic chain.

In addition to the above conditions, sympathetic blockade may also be used for treatment of other painful conditions, including vascular ischemic pain, phantom limb pain, herpes zoster, postherpetic neuralgia, facial pain of unknown origin, neuropathic pain, pain secondary to carcinoma, headache, and other painful conditions, which may not be differentiated.

Numerous modalities of treatments include sympathetic ganglion blocks, intravenous regional blocks, physical therapy, administration of a host of pharmacological agents, behavioral interventions, and surgical interventions with either sympathetectomy or radiofrequency neurotomy.

CPT CODES

- 64505 Injection, anesthetic agent; sphenopalatine ganglion block
- 64510 Injection, anesthetic agent; stellate ganglion (cervical sympathetic)
- 64517 Injection, anesthetic agent; superior hypogastric plexus block
- 64520 Injection, anesthetic agent; lumbar or thoracic (paravertebral sympathetic)
- 64530 Injection, anesthetic agent; celiac plexus, with or without radiological monitoring
- 64680 Destruction by neurolytic agent; with or without radiologic monitoring; celiac plexus
- 64681 Destruction by neurolytic agent; with or without radiologic monitoring; superior hypogastric plexus
- 76003 Fluoroscopic guidance for needle placement

Note: A physician may use modifier 22 with sphenopalatine ganglion code, stellate ganglion code, or thoracic or lumbar paravertebral sympathetic code if neurolysis is performed.

INDICATIONS AND MEDICAL NECESSITY

Sympathetic blocks are indicated and are considered appropriate to confirm the diagnosis of sympathetically maintained pain. The following criteria should be considered carefully in performing sympathetic blocks:

1. Complete initial evaluation, including history and physical examination
2. Physiological and functional assessment, as necessary and feasible
3. Definition of indications and medical necessity:
   - Suspected organic problem
   - Pain and disability of moderate to severe degree
   - No evidence of contraindications such as intraspinal obstruction, infection, or predominantly psychogenic pain
   - Responsiveness to prior interventions with improvement in physical and functional status to proceed with repeat blocks or other interventions
   - Repeating interventions only upon return of pain and deterioration in functional status

FREQUENCY AND NUMBER OF INJECTIONS OR INTERVENTIONS

- In the diagnostic or stabilization phase, a patient may receive injections at intervals of no sooner than 1 week or, preferably, 2 weeks except for cancer pain or when a continuous administration of local anesthetic for sympathetic block is employed. However, the total number of injections in the stabilization phase should be limited to four to six per year.
- In the treatment or therapeutic phase, that is, after the stabilization phase, the frequency of sympathetic blocks should be limited to 6 weeks or longer between each injection, provided that at least >50% relief is obtained for 4 to 6 weeks.

ICD-9 CODES THAT SUPPORT MEDICAL NECESSITY

1. Complex regional pain syndrome Type I (reflex sympathetic dystrophy) and Type II (causalgia):
   - 337.20 reflex sympathetic dystrophy unspecified, 337.21 reflex sympathy dystrophy upper limb, 337.22 reflex sympathetic dystrophy lower limb, 337.29 reflex sympathetic dystrophy other unspecified site
   - 355.9 causalgia, 354.4 causalgia upper limb, 355.71 causalgia lower limb
2. Peripheral neuropathy: 356.4 idiopathic, 356.0 hereditary, 357.2 diabetic, 357.5 alcoholic, 357.6 due to drug
3. Limb pain: 353.6 phantom limb pain, 997.60 stump pain, 997.61 neuroma of amputation stump, 342.0 hemiplegia–flaccid, 342.1 hemiplegia–spastic
4. Plexus lesions: 353.0 thoracic outlet syndrome, 353.1 lumbar plexus lesions
5. Postherpetic neuralgia: 053.10 with unspecified nerve system complication, 053.11 geniculate herpes zoster, 053.12 postherpetic trigeminal neuralgia, 053.13 postherpetic polyneuropathy, 053.19 other, 053.12 herpes zoster dermatitis of upper eyelid, 053.21 herpes zoster keratoconjunctivitis, 053.22 herpes zoster iridocyclitis, 053.29 other ophthalmic complications
6. Pain syndromes secondary to neoplasm: 141.0 to 239.9
7. Chronic pancreatitis
8. Abdominal pain
9. Pelvic pain
10. Vascular ischemic pain
11. Headache: 346.01 intractable migraine with aura, 346.11 intractable migraine without aura, 346.21 intractable cluster, 346.20 nonintractable cluster, 346.9 unspecified migraine

DOCUMENTATION REQUIREMENTS

The patient's medical record must contain documentation that fully supports the medical necessity for sympathetic blocks.

Documentation must also support the frequency and the appropriateness of this procedure, as opposed to alternative forms of therapy.

INTERCOSTAL NERVE BLOCKS AND NEUROLYSIS[128]

DESCRIPTION

Intercostal/chest wall pain usually results from irritation or inflammation of the intercostal nerve, which may result from, but is not limited to, trauma, rib fracture, cancer, injury from a thoracotomy incision, osteoarthritis or degenerative arthritis of the thoracic spine, herpes zoster or postherpetic neuralgia, compression fracture of vertebrae, sternal fracture, injury to the nerve trunk, compression of nerves, or nerve-root lesions. This type of pain can be managed with either an intercostal nerve block or neurolysis (via radiofrequency ablation, cryoablation, or injection of a neurolytic agent such as phenol).

CPT CODES

- 64420 Injection, anesthetic agent; intercostal nerve, single
- 64421 Intercostal nerves, multiple, regional block
- 64620 Destruction by neurolytic agent; intercostal nerve

- 76003 Fluoroscopic guidance for needle placement

INDICATIONS AND MEDICAL NECESSITY

The following criteria should be considered carefully when performing either intercostal nerve blocks or intercostal neurolysis:

1. Complete initial evaluation including history and physical examination
2. Physiological and functional assessment, as necessary and feasible
3. Definition of indications and medical necessity as follows:
   - Suspected organic problem
   - Nonresponsiveness to conservative modalities of treatments
   - Pain and disability of moderate to severe degree
   - No evidence of contraindications such as infection or pain of predominantly psychogenic origin
   - Responsiveness to prior interventions, with improvement in physical and functional status for repeat blocks or other interventions
   - Repeating interventions only upon return of pain and deterioration in functional status

ICD-9 CODES THAT SUPPORT MEDICAL NECESSITY

1. Herpes zoster, with unspecified nervous system complication: 053.10
2. Postherpetic polyneuropathy: 053.13
3. Pain syndromes secondary to neuroplasm: 114.02 to 239.9
4. Malignant neoplasm of ribs, sternum, and clavicle: 170.3
5. Secondary malignant neoplasm of other specified sites, bone and bone marrow: 198.5
6. Benign neoplasm of ribs, sternum, and clavicle: 213.3
7. Thoracic root lesions, not elsewhere classified (intercostal neuritis): 353.3
8. Other nerve root and plexus disorders: 353.8
9. Unspecified nerve root and plexus disorder: 353.9
10. Pathologic fracture of other specified site: 733.19
11. Fracture of rib(s) closed: 807.00
12. Of rib(s) open: 807.1
13. Of sternum, closed: 807.2
14. Of sternum, open: 807.3
15. Flail chest: 807.4
16. Injury to other nerve(s) of trunk, excluding shoulder and pelvis girdles, other specified nerve(s) of trunk: 954.8

FREQUENCY AND NUMBER OF INJECTIONS OR INTERVENTIONS

- In the diagnostic or stabilization phase, a patient may receive injections at intervals of no sooner than 1 week or, preferably, 2 weeks.
- In the treatment or therapeutic phase (after the stabilization is completed), the frequency should be 2 months or longer between each injection, provided that at least >50% relief is obtained for 6 weeks. However, if the neural blockade is applied for different regions, it can be performed at intervals of no sooner than 1 week or, preferably, 2 weeks for most types of blocks. The therapeutic frequency must remain at 2 months for each region. It is further suggested that all regions be treated at the same time, provided all procedures are performed safely.
- In the diagnostic or stabilization phase, the number of injections should be limited to no more than four per year.
- In the treatment or therapeutic phase, the interventional procedures should be repeated only as necessary judging by the medical necessity criteria, and these should be limited to a maximum of six times for local anesthetic and steroid blocks, and four times for interventions such as radiofrequency thermoneurolysis, and cryoneurolysis, for a period of 1 year.

CODING GUIDELINES

For multiple levels of neurolytic blocks for additional levels, CPT 64620-51 may be used. For fluoroscopic guidance, CPT 76003 may be used.

DOCUMENTATION REQUIREMENTS

The patient's medical record must contain documentation that fully supports the medical necessity for intercostal nerve blocks and neurolysis.

Documentation must also support the frequency and the appropriateness of this procedure, as opposed to alternative forms of therapy.

SACROILIAC JOINT INJECTIONS

DESCRIPTION

The sacroiliac joint includes a joint capsule, synovial fluid, and hyaline cartilage on the sacral side and fibrocartilage on the iliac side. The sacroiliac joint possesses widespread neural innervation, anatomic variability, and unique biomechanical properties. Now there is evidence that the sacroiliac joint is a source of mechanical low back and lower extremity pain. Provocative injections and arthrography have described sacroiliac joint pain referral patterns in asymptomatic volunteers, predicted symptomatic sacroiliac joints in patients with suspected lumbar discogenic or facet joint pain, described morphologic futures of sacroiliac joint capsule, and defined contrast extravasation patterns on sacroiliac joint arthrography and post-arthrography CT in subjects with low back or groin pain.

Sacroiliac joint block may be diagnostic or therapeutic. In the diagnostic sacroiliac joint block, an anesthetic agent is introduced into the sacroiliac joint under fluoroscopic guidance. At least 75% resolution of the patient's pain over the ipsilateral sacroiliac joint is considered diagnostic of pain emanating from the sacroiliac joint. Incidence of sacroiliac joint pain has been highly variable.

CPT CODES

- 27096 Injection procedure for sacroiliac joint, arthrography, and/or anesthetic/steroid
- 73542 Radiologic examination, sacroiliac joint arthrography, radiological supervision and interpretation
- 76005 Fluoroscopic guidance and localization of needle or catheter tip for spine or paraspinous diagnostic or therapeutic injection procedures (epidural, transforaminal epidural, subarachnoid, paravertebral facet joint, paravertebral facet joint nerve, or sacroiliac joint), including neurolytic agent destruction

INDICATIONS AND MEDICAL NECESSITY

The following criteria should be considered carefully in performing sacroiliac joint blocks:

1. Complete initial evaluation, including history and physical examination
2. Physiological and functional assessment, as necessary and feasible
3. Definition of indications and medical necessity, as follows:
   - Suspected organic problem
   - Nonresponsiveness to conservative modalities of treatments
   - Pain and disability of moderate to severe degree
   - No evidence of contraindications such as infection or predominantly psychogenic pain

- Responsiveness to prior interventions with improvement in physical and functional status for repeat blocks or other interventions
- Repeating interventions only upon return of pain and deterioration in functional status

ICD-9 CODE THAT SUPPORTS MEDICAL NECESSITY

- Sacroiliitis: 720.2

FREQUENCY AND NUMBER OF INTERVENTIONS

- In the diagnostic phase, a patient may receive injections at intervals of no sooner than 1 week or, preferably, 2 weeks.
- In the therapeutic phase (after stabilization is completed), the frequency should be 2 months or longer between each injection, provided that at least ≥50% relief is obtained for 6 weeks. However, if the neural blockade is applied for different regions, it can be performed at intervals of no sooner than 1 week or preferably 2 weeks for most types of blocks. The therapeutic frequency must remain at 2 months for each region.
- In the diagnostic or stabilization phase, the number of injections should be limited to no more than four times per year.
- In the treatment or therapeutic phase, the interventional procedures should be repeated only as necessary judging by the medical necessity criteria, and these should be limited to a maximum of six times for local anesthetic and steroid blocks for a period of 1 year.

DOCUMENTATION REQUIREMENTS

The patient's medical record must contain documentation that fully supports the medical necessity for sacroiliac joint injections.

Documentation must also support the frequency and the appropriateness of this procedure, as opposed to alternative forms of therapy.

TRIGEMINAL NERVE BLOCKS[146–151]

DESCRIPTION

Trigeminal nerve block with local anesthetic and steroid is used in managing pain of trigeminal neuralgia or cancer pain when pharmacological measures fail.

CPT CODES

- 64400 Injection, anesthetic agent; trigeminal nerve, any division or branch

- 64600 Destruction by neurolytic agent, trigeminal nerve; supraorbital, infraorbital, mental, or inferior alveolar branch
- 64605 Destruction by neurolytic agent, trigeminal nerve; second and third branches at foramen ovale
- 64610 Destruction by neurolytic agent, trigeminal nerve; second and third division branches at foramen ovale under radiological monitoring
- 76003 Fluoroscopic guidance for needle placement

FREQUENCY AND NUMBER OF INJECTIONS OR INTERVENTIONS

- In the diagnostic or stabilization phase, a patient may receive injections at intervals of no sooner than 1 week or, preferably, 2 weeks.
- In the treatment or therapeutic phase (after stabilization is completed), the frequency should be 2 months or longer between each injection, provided that at least 50% relief is obtained for 6 to 8 weeks. However, if the neural blockade is applied for different regions, it can be performed at intervals of no sooner than 1 week or, preferably, 2 weeks for most types of blocks. The therapeutic frequency must remain at 2 months for each region. It is further suggested that all regions be treated at the same time, provided all procedures are performed safely.
- In the diagnostic or stabilization phase, the number of injections should be limited to no more than four per year.
- In the treatment or therapeutic phase, the interventional procedures should be repeated only as necessary judging by the medical necessity criteria, and these should be limited to a maximum of six times for local anesthetic and steroid blocks, and four times for interventions such as radiofrequency thermoneurolysis, and cryoneurolysis, for a period of 1 year.

ICD-9 CODES THAT SUPPORT MEDICAL NECESSITY

1. Trigeminal neuralgia: 350.1
2. Atypical facial pain: 350.2
3. Trigeminal neuralgia, specified: 350.8
4. Trigeminal neuralgia, unspecified: 350.9
5. Postherpetic trigeminal neuralgia: 053.12

DOCUMENTATION REQUIREMENTS

The patient's medical record must contain documentation that fully supports the medical necessity for trigeminal nerve blocks and neurolytic procedures.

Documentation must also support the frequency and the appropriateness of this procedure, as opposed to alternative forms of therapy.

SUPRASCAPULAR NERVE BLOCKS[3,152]

DESCRIPTION

Pain secondary to irritation or inflammation of the suprascapular nerve may be caused by multiple variants such as soft tissue trauma, arthritis, cysts, or lesions. The irritation of the suprascapular nerve is manifested with pain in the distribution of the shoulder and shoulder–girdle area. This may be associated with weakness of the supraspinatus and infraspinatus muscles. Weakness of these muscles may be diagnosed by weakness of abduction of the shoulder, as well as lateral rotation.

A suprascapular nerve block, which results in relief of pain, can confirm the diagnosis of suprascapular neuritis. This may be followed by injection of depo-steroids.

CPT CODES

- 64418 Suprascapular nerve block
- 76003 Fluoroscopic guidance for needle placement

INDICATIONS AND MEDICAL NECESSITY

The following criteria should be considered carefully in performing either intercostal nerve blocks or intercostal neurolysis:

1. Complete initial evaluation, including history and physical examination
2. Physiological and functional assessment, as necessary and feasible
3. Definition of indications and medical necessity, as follows:
   - Suspected organic problem
   - Nonresponsiveness to conservative modalities of treatments
   - Pain and disability of moderate to severe degree
   - No evidence of contraindications such as infection or pain of predominantly psychogenic origin
   - Responsiveness to prior interventions, with improvement in physical and functional status for repeat blocks or other interventions
   - Repeating interventions only upon return of pain and deterioration in functional status

ICD-9 CODES THAT SUPPORT MEDICAL NECESSITY

1. Brachial neuritis or radiculitis: 723.4

2. Degeneration of cervical intervertebral disc, including narrowing of disc space: 722.4

3 Cervical disc displacement without myelopathy (disc herniation, radiculitis, disc extrusion, disc protrusion, disc prolapse, discogenic syndrome): 722.0

4. Frozen shoulder: 726.0

FREQUENCY AND NUMBER OF INJECTIONS OR INTERVENTIONS

- In the diagnostic or stabilization phase, a patient may receive injections at intervals of no sooner than 1 week or, preferably, 2 weeks.

- In the treatment or therapeutic phase (after stabilization is completed), the frequency should be 2 months or longer between each injection, provided that at least 50% relief is obtained for 6 weeks. However, if the neural blockade is applied for different regions, it can be performed at intervals of no sooner than 1 week or, preferably, 2 weeks for most types of blocks. The therapeutic frequency must remain at 2 months for each region. It is further suggested that all regions be treated at the same time provided all procedures are performed safely.

- In the diagnostic or stabilization phase, the number of injections should be limited to no more than four times per year.

- In the treatment or therapeutic phase, the interventional procedures should be repeated only as necessary judging by the medical necessity criteria, and these should be limited to a maximum of six times for local anesthetic and steroid blocks and four times for interventions such as radiofrequency thermoneurolysis, and cryoneurolysis for a period of 1 year.

DOCUMENTATION REQUIREMENTS

The patient's medical record must contain documentation that fully supports the medical necessity for suprascapular nerve block.

Documentation must also support the frequency and the appropriateness of this procedure, as opposed to alternative forms of therapy.

GREATER OCCIPITAL NERVE BLOCKS

DESCRIPTION

Cervicogenic headache may result from cervical facet joint syndrome, cervical spinal disease, or occipital neuritis. Cervicogenic headache may be caused by either arthritis of the facet joints or whiplash syndrome causing facet joint mediated pain or irritation of the greater occipital nerve. Rarely, the greater occipital nerve may be entrapped; however, more commonly it is inflamed.

A diagnostic block or greater occipital nerve can confirm the clinical impression of occipital neuralgia. Headaches secondary to occipital neuralgia are either unilateral or bilateral. They may be constant or intermittent. Headaches may be radiating behind the ear or to the face. Therapeutically, injection of local anesthetic with or without steroids along the greater occipital nerve in its course also may provide relief which may be long-lasting in some cases, particularly if chronic muscle spasm is present and in conjunction with other modalities of treatments, including physical therapy and an exercise program.

CPT CODES

- 64405 Greater occipital nerve block
- 76003 Fluoroscopic guidance for needle placement

INDICATIONS AND MEDICAL NECESSITY

The following criteria should be considered carefully in performing either intercostal nerve blocks or intercostal neurolysis:

1. Complete initial evaluation, including history and physical examination

2. Physiological and functional assessment, as necessary and feasible

3. Definition of indications and medical necessity, as follows:

   - Suspected organic problem
   - Nonresponsiveness to conservative modalities of treatments
   - Pain and disability of moderate to severe degree
   - No evidence of contraindications such as infection or pain of predominantly psychogenic origin
   - Responsiveness to prior interventions, with improvement in physical and functional status for repeat blocks or other interventions
   - Repeating interventions only upon return of pain and deterioration in functional status

ICD-9 CODES THAT SUPPORT MEDICAL NECESSITY

1. Occipital neuritis: 729.2
2. Cervical spondylosis or cervical facet joint arthropathy: 721.0
3. Cervical intervertebral disc disease: 722.4

FREQUENCY AND NUMBER OF INJECTIONS OR INTERVENTIONS

- In the diagnostic or stabilization phase, a patient may receive injections at intervals of no sooner than 1 week or, preferably, 2 weeks.
- In the treatment or therapeutic phase (after the stabilization is completed), the frequency should be 2 months or longer between each injection, provided that at least 50% relief is obtained for 6 weeks. However, if the neural blockade is applied for different regions, it can be performed at intervals of no sooner than 1 week or, preferably, 2 weeks for most types of blocks. The therapeutic frequency must remain at 2 months for each region. It is further suggested that all regions be treated at the same time, provided all procedures are performed safely.
- In the diagnostic or stabilization phase, the number of injections should be limited to no more than four per year.
- In the treatment or therapeutic phase, the interventional procedures should be repeated only as necessary judging by the medical necessity criteria and these should be limited to a maximum of six times for local anesthetic and steroid blocks and four times for interventions such as radiofrequency thermoneurolysis, and cryoneurolysis for a period of 1 year.
- Under unusual circumstances with a recurrent injury or cervicogenic headache, blocks may be repeated at intervals of 6 weeks after stabilization in the treatment phase.

DOCUMENTATION REQUIREMENTS

The patient's medical record must contain documentation that fully supports the medical necessity for occipital nerve blocks.

Documentation must also support the frequency and the appropriateness of this procedure, as opposed to alternative forms of therapy.

PERIPHERAL NERVE BLOCKS[2,154]

DESCRIPTION

Peripheral nerve blocks may be performed to manage pain emanating from irritation or inflammation of peripheral nerve(s). If response to a peripheral nerve block with local anesthetic is significant and predictable, a peripheral neurolytic block may be performed, either by injection of neurolytic agent or cryoablation.

CPT CODES

- 64450 Peripheral nerve block
- 64640 Peripheral neurolytic block
- 76003 Fluoroscopic guidance for needle placement

INDICATIONS AND MEDICAL NECESSITY

The following criteria should be considered carefully in performing either intercostal nerve blocks or intercostal neurolysis:

1. Complete initial evaluation, including history and physical examination
2. Physiological and functional assessment, as necessary and feasible
3. Definition of indications and medical necessity, as follows:
   - Suspected organic problem
   - Nonresponsiveness to conservative modalities of treatments
   - Pain and disability of moderate to severe degree
   - No evidence of contraindications such as infection or pain of predominantly psychogenic origin
   - Responsiveness to prior interventions with improvement in physical and functional status for repeat blocks or other interventions
   - Repeating interventions only upon return of pain and deterioration in functional status

ICD-9 CODES THAT SUPPORT MEDICAL NECESSITY

Codes describing peripheral neuritis are considered to support medical necessity.

DOCUMENTATION REQUIREMENTS

The patient's medical record must contain documentation that fully supports the medical necessity for peripheral nerve blocks or neurolysis as it is covered by Medicare as described above.

Documentation must also support the frequency and the appropriateness of this procedure, as opposed to alternative forms of therapy.

FREQUENCY AND NUMBER OF INJECTIONS OR INTERVENTIONS

- In the diagnostic or stabilization phase, a patient may receive injections at intervals of no sooner than 1 week or, preferably, 2 weeks.
- In the treatment or therapeutic phase (after the stabilization is completed), the frequency

should be 2 months or longer between each injection, provided that at least 50% relief is obtained for 6 weeks. However, if the neural blockade is applied for different regions, it can be performed at intervals of no sooner than 1 week or, preferably, 2 weeks for most types of blocks. The therapeutic frequency must remain at 2 months for each region. It is further suggested that all regions be treated at the same time, provided all procedures are performed safely.

- In the diagnostic or stabilization phase, the number of injections should be limited to no more than four per year.
- In the treatment or therapeutic phase, the interventional procedures should be repeated only as necessary judging by the medical necessity criteria, and these should be limited to a maximum of six times for local anesthetic and steroid blocks and four times for neurolytic blocks for a period of 1 year.

TRIGGER POINT INJECTIONS[2,155–164]

DESCRIPTION

Myofascial pain syndrome, which is a regional muscle pain disorder accompanied by trigger points, appears to be a common phenomenon in multiple regions, specifically in the cervical spine. In the head and neck region, it is believed that myofascial pain syndrome can manifest not only with mechanical symptoms in the neck, but also as headache, tinnitus, shoulder pain, temporomandibular joint pain, eye symptoms, and torticollis. However, there is absolutely no epidemiologic data on the prevalence of myofascial pain in the neck. The authors, exploring the role of trigger points and myofascial pain in whiplash injuries, believe that the theory of trigger points lacks demonstrated internal validity. Formal studies also have shown that myofascial experts have difficulty agreeing on the presence of a trigger point, which is the cardinal feature of regional myofascial pain syndrome. In addition to this, it has been shown that, topographically, trigger points of the neck overlie the cervical facet joints, and it has been reported that pain patterns of cervical trigger points are identical to those of referred pain from the facet joints.

Similar to the cervical spine, the most common diagnosis for low back pain is acute or chronic lumbosacral strain or sprain; however, the scientific evidence for low back pain of muscle origin is not overwhelming.

Myofascial trigger points are self-sustaining, hyperirritative foci that may occur in any skeletal muscle in response to strain produced by acute or chronic overload. Classically, these trigger points produce a referred-pain pattern characteristic for that individual muscle. Thus,

each pattern becomes part of a single muscle myofascial pain syndrome. To successfully treat chronic myofascial pain syndrome, each single muscle syndrome needs to be identified, along with every perpetuating factor.

As there is no laboratory or imaging test available for establishing or confirming the diagnosis of trigger points, diagnosis mainly depends on detailed history and specific musculoskeletal examination. Some of the cardinal features of trigger points are as follows:

1. Distribution pattern of the pain consistent with the referral pattern of trigger points that are described in the literature
2. The presence of trigger points with focal tenderness with a specific referral pattern of pain
3. A palpable taut band of muscle in which the trigger point is located
4. Reproduction of referred-pain pattern upon stimulation of the trigger point

CPT CODES

- 20552 Injection, single or multiple trigger point(s), one or two muscle groups
- 20553 Injection, single or multiple trigger point(s), three or more muscle groups

INDICATIONS AND MEDICAL NECESSITY

The following criteria should be considered carefully in performing trigger point injections:

1. Complete initial evaluation, including history and physical examination
2. Physiological and functional assessment, as necessary and feasible
3. Definition of indications and medical necessity, as follows:
   - Suspected organic problem
   - Nonresponsiveness to conservative modalities of treatments
   - Pain and disability of moderate to severe degree
   - No evidence of contraindications such as infection or pain of predominantly psychogenic origin
   - Responsiveness to prior interventions with improvement in physical and functional status for repeat blocks or other interventions
   - Repeating interventions only upon return of pain and deterioration in functional status

ICD-9 CODES THAT SUPPORT MEDICAL NECESSITY

1. Myalgia and myositis, unspecified: 729.1
2. Rheumatism, unspecified, and fibrositis: 729.0

Frequency and Number of Injections or Interventions

- In the diagnostic or stabilization phase, a patient may receive injections at intervals of no sooner than 1 week or, preferably, 2 weeks.
- In the treatment or therapeutic phase (after the stabilization is completed), the frequency should be 2 months or longer between each injection, provided that at least 50% relief is obtained for 6 weeks. However, if the neural blockade and/or injections are applied for different regions, it/they can be performed at intervals of no sooner than 1 week or, preferably, 2 weeks for most types of blocks. The therapeutic frequency must remain at 2 months for each region. It is further suggested that all regions be treated at the same time provided all procedures are performed safely.
- In the diagnostic or stabilization phase, the number of trigger point injections should be limited to no more than four times per year.
- In the treatment or therapeutic phase, the trigger point injections should be repeated only as necessary judging by the medical necessity criteria, and these should be limited to a maximum of six times for local anesthetic and steroid blocks.

Documentation Requirements

The patient's medical record must contain documentation that fully supports the medical necessity for trigger point injections.

Documentation must also support the frequency and the appropriateness of this procedure, as opposed to alternative forms of therapy.

SPINAL CORD STIMULATORS[1-4,165-179]

Description

Spinal cord or epidural stimulation involves an electric field, and a specified waveform, pulse width, and rate, and is reported to diminish pain intensity in select cases of chronic neurogenic pain. In spinal cord stimulation used to treat chronic neurogenic pain, most typically dorsal or sensory fibers of the spinal cord are stimulated. Spinal cord stimulation is indicated for the treatment of a number of conditions that are intractable and nonresponsive to many of the other modalities of treatments. The neurostimulator electrodes used for this purpose are implanted percutaneously in the epidural space through a special needle. Some patients may need an open procedure requiring a laminectomy to place the electrodes.

Prior to placement of the permanent electrodes, trial electrodes are placed and stimulation is carried out with an external stimulator. The trial period may be extended up to 4 weeks if necessary. If, during the trial period, it is determined that the spinal cord stimulation is not effective or is not acceptable to the patient, the electrodes may be removed. However, if the trial has been successful, a spinal neurostimulator and pulse generator are inserted subcutaneously and connected to the electrodes already in place or to new electrodes.

In some cases, neurostimulator electrodes migrate or move from the area that needs to be stimulated, in which case the electrodes require realignment. Additionally, in very few cases, electrodes may need to be removed if the patient cannot tolerate the electrodes, the spinal cord stimulation becomes ineffective after a period of time, or the leads and/or the impulse generator become infected.

CPT Codes

- 63650 Percutaneous implantation of neurostimulator electrode array, epidural
- 63655 Laminectomy for implantation of neurostimulator electrodes, plate/paddle, epidural
- 63660 Revision or removal of spinal neurostimulator electrode percutaneous array(s) or plate/paddle(s)
- 63685 Incision and subcutaneous placement of spinal neurostimulator pulse generator or receiver, direct or inductive coupling
- 63688 Revision or removal of implanted spinal neurostimulator pulse generator or receiver

Indications and Medical Necessity

The following criteria should be considered carefully in performing spinal cord simulation procedures:

1. Complete initial evaluation, including history and physical examination
2. Physiological and functional assessment, as necessary and feasible
3. Psychological evaluation as necessary
4. Definition of indications and medical necessity, as follows:
   - Suspected organic problem
   - Nonresponsiveness to almost all conservative modalities of treatments, including fluoroscopically directed epidural injections
   - Pain and disability of severe degree
   - No evidence of contraindications such as intraspinal obstruction, infection, or predominantly psychogenic pain
5. Implantation of the spinal cord stimulator used only as a choice of last resort and after other

treatment modalities have been tried and did not prove to be satisfactory, or these have been judged to be unsuitable or contraindicated for the given patient

6. In addition to the physical, functional, and psychological assessment, which is basic, careful screening and evaluation by a multidisciplinary team prior to implantation, which should include physical and functional as well as psychological evaluation

7. Prior to implantation of the permanent electrodes, demonstrated relief of pain with a temporarily implanted electrode, without deleterious effects

ICD-9 CODES THAT SUPPORT MEDICAL NECESSITY

1. Postlaminectomy syndrome: 722.81 cervical, 722.82 thoracic, 722.83 lumbosacral

2. Disc displacement without myelopathy (disc herniation, radiculitis, disc extrusion, disc protrusion, disc prolapse, discogenic syndrome): 722.0 cervical, 722.11 thoracic, 722.10 lumbosacral

3. Disc displacement with myelopathy: 722.71 cervical, 722.72 thoracic, 722.73 lumbosacral

4. Epidural fibrosis: 349.2 cervical, 349.2 thoracic, 349.2 lumbosacral

5. Complex regional pain syndrome (Type I or reflex sympathetic dystrophy): 337.20 reflex sympathetic dystrophy unspecified, 337.21 reflex sympathetic dystrophy upper limb, 337.22 reflex sympathetic dystrophy lower limb, 337.29 reflex sympathetic dystrophy other unspecified site

6. Complex regional pain syndrome (Type II or causalgia): 355.9 causalgia, 354.4 causalgia upper limb, 355.71 causalgia lower limb

7. Limb pain: 353.6 phantom limb pain, 997.60 stump pain, 997.61 neuroma of amputation stump, 342.0 hemiplegia–flaccid, 342.1 hemiplegia–spastic

8. Postherpetic neuralgia: 053.10 with unspecified nerve system complication, 053.13 postherpetic polyneuropathy

9. Cauda equina injury: 952.4

10. Chronic arachnoiditis: 322.2

11. Arthrosclerosis of extremities with wrist pain: 440.22

12. Mechanical complications of nervous system device implanted graft: 996.2 (to be used to indicate intolerance of the device by the patient or failure of equipment/loss of effectiveness)

13. Infection and inflammatory reaction due to internal prosthetic device, implant, and graft; due to nervous system device, implant, and graft: 996.63

DOCUMENTATION REQUIREMENTS

The patient's medical record must contain documentation that fully supports the medical necessity for spinal cord stimulators.

Documentation must also support the frequency and the appropriateness of this procedure, as opposed to alternative forms of therapy.

INTRATHECAL INFUSION SYSTEMS[180–191]

DESCRIPTION

Chronic opioid therapy in the treatment of persistent pain of noncancer origin has gained broad acceptance. The multiple routes of administration available to the practitioner are the oral, transdermal, epidural, and intrathecal. This policy addresses intrathecal administration of opioids and other drugs. Opioid agonists produce analgesia at the spinal cord level when administered in the intrathecal or epidural space. This technique may be used for the management of chronic intractable pain when it is not controlled by less invasive techniques, as well as oral narcotics. Intrathecal baclofen is used for the treatment of intractable spasticity of the spine or brain etiology. For intrathecal administration of drugs, a reservoir is inserted subcutaneously; it is attached to the proximal portion of the catheter, which is tunneled beneath the skin.

With the epidural catheterization, preservative-free morphine sulfate, hydromorphone hydrochloride (Dilaudid®, Palladone), Fentanyl, or baclofen can be administered every 8 to 12 hours in the epidural space through an indwelling catheter, which can be placed percutaneously.

CPT CODES

- 62350 Implantation, revision, or repositioning of tunneled intrathecal or epidural catheter, for long-term medication administration via an external pump or implantable reservoir/infusion pump; without laminectomy

- 62351 Implantation, revision, or repositioning of tunneled intrathecal or epidural catheter, for long-term medication administration via an external pump or implantable reservoir/infusion pump; with laminectomy

- 62355 Removal of previously implanted intrathecal or epidural catheter

- 62360 Implantation or replacement of device for intrathecal or epidural drug infusion; subcutaneous reservoir

- 62361 Implantation or replacement of device for intrathecal or epidural drug infusion; non-programmable pump
- 62362 Implantation or replacement of device for intrathecal or epidural drug infusion; programmable pump, including preparation or pump, with or without programming
- 62365 Removal of subcutaneous reservoir or pump, previously implanted for intrathecal or epidural infusion
- 62367 Electronic analysis of programmable, implanted pump for intrathecal or epidural drug infusion (includes evaluation of reservoir status, alarm status, drug prescription status); without reprogramming
- 62368 Electronic analysis of programmable, implanted pump for intrathecal or epidural drug infusion (includes evaluation of reservoir status, alarm status, drug prescription status); with reprogramming
- 62310 Injection, single, epidural or subarachnoid; cervical or thoracic
- 62311 Lumbar, sacral (caudal)
- 62318 Catheter placement, continuous infusion or intermittent bolus; epidural or subarachnoid; cervical or thoracic
- 62319 Lumbar, sacral (caudal)
- 96530 Refilling or maintenance of implantable pump or reservoir for drug delivery, systemic (e.g., intravenous, intra-arterial)

INDICATIONS AND MEDICAL NECESSITY

The following criteria should be considered carefully in performing intrathecal pump placements:

1. Complete initial evaluation, including history and physical examination
2. Physiological and functional assessment, as necessary and feasible
3. Psychological evaluation as necessary
4. Definition of indications and medical necessity, as follows:
   - Suspected organic problem
   - Nonresponsiveness to almost all conservative modalities of treatments, including fluoroscopically directed epidural injections
   - Pain and disability of severe degree
   - No evidence of contraindications such as intraspinal obstruction, infection, or predominantly psychogenic pain
5. Implantation of the morphine pump or epidural catheterization for long-term purposes used only as a choice of last resort and after other treatment modalities have been tried and did

not prove to be satisfactory; or these have been judged to be unsuitable or contraindicated for the given patient
6. In addition to the physical, functional, and psychological assessment, which is basic, careful screening and evaluation by a multidisciplinary team prior to implantation, which should include physical and functional, as well as psychological, evaluation
7. Prior to implantation of the pump, demonstrated relief of pain with subarachnoid or epidural injections of morphine reliably on at least two occasions, without any deleterious effects
8. A patient with the diagnosis of cancer with a likely life expectancy of at least 3 months and unresponsiveness to less invasive medical therapy or that may no longer be the choice of therapy

ICD-9 CODES THAT SUPPORT MEDICAL NECESSITY

For implantation of catheter/pump services:

1. Postherpetic trigeminal neuralgia: 053.12
2. Postherpetic polyneuropathy: 053.13
3. Carcinomas: 141.0 to 239.9
4. Chronic arachnoiditis: 322.2
5. Reflex sympathetic dystrophy: 337.20 to 337.29
6. Unspecified disease of spinal cord: 336.9 (to be used only for the diagnosis of myelopathy)
7. Phantom limb pain: 353.6
8. Causalgia of upper limb: 354.4
9. Causalgia of lower limb: 355.71
10. Postlaminectomy syndrome, cervical region: 722.81
11. Postlaminectomy syndrome, thoracic region: 722.82
12. Postlaminectomy syndrome, lumbar region: 722.83

For removal/revision of catheter/pump services:

1. Other complications of internal (biological) (synthetic): 996.70 due to unspecified device, implant, and graft

DOCUMENTATION REQUIREMENTS

The patient's medical record must contain documentation that fully supports the medical necessity for pump implantation and administration of drugs.

Documentation must also support the frequency and the appropriateness of this procedure, as opposed to alternative forms of therapy.

REFERENCES

1. Manchikanti, L., Shah, R. V., Everett, C. R. et al. (2005). Evidence-based practice guidelines for interventional techniques in the management of chronic spinal pain. *Pain Physician, 8*, 1–47.
2. Manchikanti, L., Staats, P. S., Singh, V. et al. (2003). Interventional techniques in the management of chronic spinal pain. Evidence-based practice guidelines. *Pain Physician, 6*(1), 3–80.
3. Manchikanti, L., Singh, V., Kloth, D. et al. (2001). Interventional techniques in the management of chronic pain: Part 2.0. *Pain Physician, 4*, 24–96.
4. Manchikanti, L., Singh, V., Bakhit, C. E. et al. (2000). Interventional techniques in the management of chronic pain. Part 1.0. *Pain Physician, 3*, 7–42.
5. Manchikanti, L. (2000). Appropriate documentation, billing and coding of interventional pain procedures. *Pain Physician, 3*, 218–236.
6. Manchikanti, L. (1999). The role of evaluation and management services in pain management. *Pain Physician, 2*, 10–32.
7. Manchikanti, L. (2000). Evaluation and management services in interventional pain practice: Doing it right! *Pain Physician, 3*, 322–341.
8. DeParle, N. A. (2000). Evaluation and management services guidelines. *Journal of the American Medical Association, 283*, 3061.
9. Health Care Financing Administration. *Evaluation and Management Services Guidelines.* (2000). Health Care Financing Administration, Washington, D.C., June 22.
10. Manchikanti, L. (2002). Role of neuraxial steroids in interventional pain management. *Pain Physician, 5*, 182–199.
11. Boswell, M. V., Singh, V., Staats, P. S. et al. (2003). Accuracy of precision diagnostic blocks in the diagnosis of chronic spinal pain of facet or zygapophysial joint origin. *Pain Physician, 6*, 449–456.
12. Bogduk, N. (1997). International Spinal Injection Society guidelines for the performance of spinal injection procedures. Part 1: Zygapophyseal joint blocks. *Clinical Journal of Pain, 13*, 285–302.
13. Hendler, N. H., Bergson, C., & Morrison, C. (1996). Overlooked physical diagnoses in chronic pain patients involved in litigation. Part 2. *Psychosomatics, 37*, 509–517.
14. Hendler, N. H., & Kolodny, A. L. (1992, May 15). Using medication wisely in chronic pain. *Patient Care, 125*.
15. Bogduk, N., & McGuirk, B. (2002). Causes and sources of chronic low back pain. In N. Bogduk & B. McGuirk (Eds.), *Medical management of acute and chronic low back pain. An evidence-based approach. Pain research and clinical management* (Vol. 13, pp. 115–126). Amsterdam: Elsevier Science BV.
16. Bogduk, N. (1997). Low back pain. In *Clinical anatomy of the lumbar spine and sacrum* (3rd ed., pp. 187–214). New York: Churchill Livingstone.
17. Gagliese, L., & Katz, J. (2000). Medically unexplained pain is not caused by psychopathology. *Pain Research & Management, 5*, 251–257.
18. Kuslich, S. D., Ulstrom, C. L., & Michael, C. J. (1991). The tissue origin of low back pain and sciatica: A report of pain response to tissue stimulation during operation on the lumbar spine using local anesthesia. *Orthopedic Clinics of North America, 22*, 181–187.
19. Cavanaugh, J. M., Ozaktay, A. C., Yamashita, T. et al. (1997). Mechanisms of low back pain: A neurophysiologic and neuroanatomic study. *Clinical Orthopedics, 335*, 166–180.
20. Pang, W. W., Mok, M. S., Lin, M. L. et al. (1998). Application of spinal pain mapping in the diagnosis of low back pain — Analysis of 104 cases. *Acta Anaesthesiol Sinica, 36*, 71–74.
21. Manchikanti, L., Fellows, B., Pampati, V. et al. (2001). Evaluation of the relative contributions of various structures in chronic low back pain. *Pain Physician, 4*, 308–316.
22. Manchikanti, L., Singh, V., & Fellows, F. (2002). Structural basis of chronic low back pain. In. L. Manchikanti, C. W. Slipman, & B. Fellows (Eds.), *Interventional pain management: Low back pain — Diagnosis and treatment.* Paducah, KY: ASIPP Publishing.
23. Brown, F. W. (1977). Management of discogenic pain using epidural and intrathecal steroids. *Clinical Orthopedics, 129*, 72–78.
24. Jurmand, S. H. (1972). Cortiotherapie peridurale des lombalgies et des sciatiques d'origine discale. *Concours Medicale, 94*, 5061–5070.
25. Ito, R. (1971). The treatment of low back pain and sciatica with epidural corticosteroids injection and its pathophysiologic basis. *Journal of the Japanese Orthopedic Association, 45*, 769–777.
26. Boswell, M. V., Hansen, H. C., Trescot, A. M. et al. (2003). Epidural steroids in the management of chronic spinal pain and radiculopathy. *Pain Physician, 6*, 319–334.
27. Koes, B. W., Scholten, R., Mens, J. M. A. et al. (1999). Epidural steroid injections for low back pain and sciatica. An updated systematic review of randomized clinical trials. *Pain Digest, 9*, 241–247.
28. Abdi, S., Datta, S., & Lucas, L. F. (2005). Role of epidural steroids in the management of chronic spinal pain: A systematic review of effectiveness and complications. *Pain Physician, 8*, 127–143.
29. Bush, K., & Hillier, S. (1991). A controlled study of caudal epidural injections of triamcinolone plus procaine for the management of intractable sciatica. *Spine, 16*, 572–575.
30. Matthews, J. A., Mills, S. B., Jenkins, V. M. et al. (1987). Back pain and sciatica: Controlled trials of manipulation, traction, sclerosant and epidural injections. *British Journal of Rheumatology, 26*, 416–423.
31. Beliveau, P. (1971). A comparison between epidural anesthesia with and without corticosteroids in the treatment of sciatica. *Rheumatology and Physical Medicine, 11*, 40–43.
32. Helsa, P. E., & Breivik, H. (1979). Epidural analgesia and epidural steroid injection for treatment of chronic low back pain and sciatica. *Tidsskrift fur den Norske Laegeforening, 99*, 936–939.

33. Breivik, H., Hesla, P. E., Molnar, I. et al. (1976). Treatment of chronic low back pain and sciatica. Comparison of caudal epidural injections of bupivacaine and methylprednisolone with bupivacaine followed by saline. In J. J. Bonica & D. Albe-Fesard (Eds.). *Advances in pain research and therapy* (vol. 1, pp. 927–932). New York: Raven Press.

34. Meadeb, J., Rozenberg, S., Duquesnoy, B. et al. (2001). Forceful sacrococcygeal injections in the treatment of postdiscectomy sciatica. A controlled study versus glucocorticoid injections. *Joint Bone Spine, 68,* 43–49.

35. Yates, D. W. (1978). A comparison of the types of epidural injection commonly used in the treatment of low back pain and sciatica. *Rheumatology and Rehabilitation, 17,* 181–186.

36. Manchikanti, L., Singh, V., Rivera, J. et al. (2002). Effectiveness of caudal epidural injections in discogram positive and negative chronic low back pain. *Pain Physician, 5,* 18–29.

37. Hauswirth, R., & Michot, F. (1982). Caudal epidural injection in the treatment of low back pain. *Ischweizerische Medizinische Wochenschrift, 112,* 222–225.

38. Ciocon, J. O., Galindo-Clocon, D., Amarnath, L. et al. (1994). Caudal epidural blocks for elderly patients with lumbar canal stenosis. *Journal of the American Geriatrics Society, 42,* 593–596.

39. Carette, S., Lecaire, R., Marcoux, S. et al. (1997). Epidural corticosteroid injections for sciatica due to herniated nucleus pulposus. *New England Journal of Medicine, 336,* 1634–1640.

40. Snoek, W., Weber, H., & Jorgensen, B. (1977). Double-blind evaluation of extradural methylprednisolone for herniated lumbar disc. *Acta Orthopaedica Scandinavica, 48,* 635–641.

41. Cuckler, J. M., Bernini, P. A., Wiesel, S. W. et al. (1985). The use of epidural steroid in the treatment of radicular pain. *Journal of Bone and Joint Surgery, 67,* 63–66.

42. Dilke, T. F. W., Burry, H. C., & Grahame, R. (1973). Extradural corticosteroid injection in the management of lumbar nerve root compression. *British Medical Journal, 2,* 635–637.

43. Klenerman, L., Greenwood, R., Davenport, H. T. et al. (1984). Lumbar epidural injections in the treatment of sciatica. *British Journal of Rheumatology, 23,* 35–38.

44. Ridley, M. G., Kingsley, G. H., Gibson, T. et al. (1988). Outpatient lumbar epidural corticosteroid injection in the management of sciatica. *British Journal of Rheumatology, 27,* 295–299

45. Rogers, P., Nash, T., Schiller, D. et al. (1992). Epidural steroids for sciatica. *The Pain Clinic, 5,* 67–72.

46. Castagnera, L., Maurette, P., Pointillart, V. et al. (1994). Long-term results of cervical epidural steroid injection with and without morphine in chronic cervical radicular pain. *Pain, 58,* 239–243.

47. Kraemer, J., Ludwig, J., Bickert, U. et al. (1997). Lumbar epidural perineural injection: A new technique. *European Spine Journal, 6,* 357–361.

48. Stav, A., Ovadia, L., Sternberg, A. et al. (1993). Cervical epidural steroid injection for cervicobrachialgia. *Acta Anaesthesiologica Scandinavica, 37,* 562–566.

49. Bush, K., & Hillier, S. (1996). Outcome of cervical radiculopathy treated with periradicular/epidural corticosteroid injections: A prospective study with independent clinical review. *European Spine Journal, 5,* 319–325.

50. Riew, K. D., Yin, Y., Gilula, L. et al. (2000). Can nerve root injections obviate the need for operative treatment of lumbar radicular pain? A prospective, randomized, controlled, double-blind study. *Journal of Bone and Joint Surgery, 82A,* 1589–1593.

51. Karppinen, J., Ohinmaa, A., Malmivaara, A. et al. (2001). Cost effectiveness of periradicular infiltration for sciatica: Subgroup analysis of a randomized controlled trial. *Spine, 26,* 2587–2595.

52. Vad, V., Bhat, A., Lutz, G. et al. (2002). Transforaminal epidural steroid injections in lumbosacral radiculopathy: A prospective randomized study. *Spine, 27,* 11–16.

53. Botwin, K. P, Thomas, S., Gruber, R. D. et al. (2002). Radiation exposure of the spinal interventionalist performing fluoroscopically guided lumbar transforaminal epidural steroid injections. *Archives of Physical Medicine and Rehabilitation, 83,* 697–701.

54. Schwarzer, A. C., Derby, R., Aprill, C. N. et al. (1994). The value of the provocation response in lumbar zygapophysial joint injections. *Clinical Journal of Pain, 10,* 309–313.

55. Schwarzer, A. C., Wang, S., Laurent, R. et al. (1992). The role of the zygapophysial joint in chronic low back pain. *Australia and New Zealand Journal of Medicine, 22,* 185.

56. Schwarzer, A. C., Derby, R., Aprill, C. N. et al. (1994). Pain from the lumbar zygapophysial joints: A test of two models. *Journal of Spinal Disorders, 7,* 331–336.

57. Schwarzer, A. C., Aprill, C. N., Derby, R. et al. (1994). Clinical features of patients with pain stemming from the lumbar zygapophysial joints. Is the lumbar facet syndrome a clinical entity? *Spine, 19,* 1132–1137.

58. Schwarzer, A. C., Wang, S., Bogduk, N. et al. (1995). Prevalence and clinical features of lumbar zygapophysial joint pain: A study in an Australian population with chronic low back pain. *Annals of the Rheumatic Diseases, 54,* 100–106.

59. Manchikanti, L., Pampati, V. S., Fellows, B. et al. (1999). Prevalence of lumbar facet joint pain in chronic low back pain. *Pain Physician, 2,* 59–64.

60. Manchikanti, L., Pampati, V. S., Bakhit, C. E. et al. (2000). The diagnostic validity and therapeutic value of lumbar facet joint nerve blocks with or without adjuvant agents. *Current Review of Pain, 4,* 337–344.

61. Manchikanti, L., Pampati, V., Fellows, B. et al. (2000). The inability of the clinical picture to characterize pain from facet joints. *Pain Physician, 3,* 158–166.

62. Manchikanti, L., Hirsch, J. A., & Pampati, V. (2003). Chronic low back pain of facet (zygaphysial) joint origin: Is there a difference based on involvement of single or multiple spinal regions? *Pain Physician, 6,* 399–405.

63. Manchikanti, L., Boswell, M. V., Singh, V. et al. (2004). Prevalence of facet joint pain in chronic spinal pain of cervical, thoracic, and lumbar regions. *BioMed Central Musculoskeletal Disorders, 5*, 15.

64. Manchikanti, L., Pampati, V. S., Fellows, B. et al. (2001). Influence of psychological factors on the ability to diagnose chronic low back pain of facet joint origin. *Pain Physician, 4*, 349–357.

65. Manchikanti, L., Singh, V., Pampati, V. (2003). Are diagnostic lumbar medial branch blocks valid? Results of 2-year follow up. *Pain Physician, 6*, 147–153.

66. Barnsley, L., Lord, S. M., Wallis, B. J. et al. (1995). The prevalence of chronic cervical zygapophyseal joint pain after whiplash. *Spine, 20*, 20–26.

67. Lord, S. M., Barnsley, L., Wallis, B. J. et al. (1996). Chronic cervical zygapophysial joint pain with whiplash: A placebo-controlled prevalence study. *Spine, 21*, 1737–1745.

68. Manchikanti L., Singh, V., Rivera, J. J. et al. (2002). Prevalence of cervical facet joint pain in chronic neck pain. *Pain Physician, 5*, 243–249.

69. Manchikanti, L., Pampati, V. S., Damron, K. et al. (2004). A randomized, prospective, double-blind, placebo-controlled evaluation of the effect of sedation on diagnostic validity of cervical facet joint pain. *Pain Physician, 7*, 301–309.

70. Manchikanti, L., Singh, V., Pampati, V. et al. (2002). Evaluation of the prevalence of facet joint pain in chronic thoracic pain. *Pain Physician, 5*, 354–359.

71. Manchikanti, L., Boswell, M. V., Singh, V. et al. (2004). Prevalence of facet joint pain in chronic spinal pain of cervical, thoracic, and lumbar regions. *BioMed Central Musculoskeletal Disorders, 5*, 15.

72. Manchikanti, L., Damron, K. S., Rivera, J. et al. (2004). Evaluation of effect of sedation as a confounding factor in the diagnostic validity of lumbar facet joint pain: A prospective, randomized, double-blind, placebo-controlled evaluation. *Pain Physician, 7*, 407.

73. Manchikanti, L., Pampati, V. S., Damron, K. S. et al. (2004). A randomized, prospective, double-blind, placebo-controlled evaluation of the effect of sedation on diagnostic validity of cervical facet joint pain. *Pain Physician, 7*, 301.

74. Carette, S., Marcoux, S., Truchon, R. et al. (1991). A controlled trial of corticosteroid injections into facet joints for chronic low back pain. *New England Journal of Medicine, 325*, 1002–1007.

75. Barnsley, L., Lord, S. M., Wallis, B. J. et al. (1994). Lack of effect of intra-articular corticosteroids for chronic pain in the cervical zygapophyseal joints. *New England Journal of Medicine, 330*, 1047–1050.

76. Manchikanti, L., Pampati, V. S., Bakhit, C. et al. (2001). Effectiveness of lumbar facet joint nerve blocks in chronic low back pain: A randomized clinical trial. *Pain Physician, 4*, 101–117.

77. Manchikanti, L., Manchikanti, K. N., Damron, K. S. et al. (2004). Effectiveness of cervical medial branch blocks in chronic neck pain: A prospective outcome study. *Pain Physician, 7*, 195–202.

78. Manchikanti, L., Singh, V., Vilims, B. et al. (2002). Medial branch neurotomy in management of chronic spinal pain: Systematic review of the evidence. *Pain Physician, 5*, 405–418.

79. Geurts, J. W., van Wijk, R. M., Stolker, R. J. et al. (2001). Efficacy of radiofrequency procedures for the treatment of spinal pain: A systematic review of randomized clinical trials. *Regional Anesthesia and Pain Medicine, 26*, 394–400.

80. Niemistö, L., Kalso, E., Malmivaara, A. et al. (2003). Radiofrequency denervation for neck and back pain: A systematic review within the framework of the Cochrane Collaboration Back Review Group. *Spine, 28*, 1877–1888.

81. Lord, S. M., Barnsley, L., Wallis, B. J. et al. (1996). Percutaneous radio-frequency neurotomy for chronic cervical zygapophyseal-joint pain. *New England Journal of Medicine, 335*, 1721–1726.

82. Van Kleef, M., Liem, L., Lousberg, R. et al. (1996). Radiofrequency lesions adjacent to the dorsal root ganglion for cervicobrachial pain. A prospective double blind randomized study. *Neurosurgery, 38*, 1127–1131.

83. Dreyfuss, P., Halbrook, B., Pauza, K. et al. (2000). Efficacy and validity of radiofrequency neurotomy for chronic lumbar zygapophysial joint pain. *Spine, 25*, 1270–1277.

84. Boswell, M. V., Colson, J. D., & Spillane, W. F. (2005). Therapeutic facet joint interventions: A systematic review of their role in chronic spinal pain management and complications. *Pain Physician, 8*, 101–114.

85. Leclaire, R., Fortin, L., Lambert, R. et al. (2001). Radiofrequency facet joint denervation in the treatment of low back pain: A placebo-controlled clinical trial to assess efficacy. *Spine, 26*, 1411–1417.

86. Sapir, D., Gorup, J.M. (2001). Radiofrequency medial branch neurotomy in litigant and non-litigant patients with cervical whiplash. *Spine, 26*, E268–E273.

87. Manchikanti, L., & Bakhit, C. E. (2000). Percutaneous epidural adhesiolysis. *Pain Physician, 3*, 46–64.

88. Chopra, P., Smith, H. S., Deer, T. R. et al. (2005). Role of adhesiolysis in the management of chronic spinal pain: A systematic review of effectiveness and complications. *Pain Physician, 8*, 87–100.

89. Manchikanti, L., Rivera, J. J., Pampati, V. et al. (2004). One day lumbar epidural adhesiolysis and hypertonic saline neurolysis in treatment of chronic low back pain: A randomized, double-blind trial. *Pain Physician, 7*, 177–186.

90. Manchikanti, L., Pakanati, R. R., Bakhit, C. E. et al. (1999). Role of adhesiolysis and hypertonic saline neurolysis in management of low back pain. Evaluation of modification of Racz protocol. *Pain Digest, 9*, 91–96.

91. Heavner, J. E., Racz, G. B., & Raj, P. (1999). Percutaneous epidural neuroplasty. Prospective evaluation of 0.9% NaCl versus 10% NaCl with or without hyaluronidase. *Regional Anesthesia and Pain Medicine, 24*, 202–207.

92. Manchikanti, L., Pakanati, R. R., Bakhit, C. E. et al. (1999). Non-endoscopic and endoscopic adhesiolysis in post lumbar laminectomy syndrome. A one-year outcome study and cost effectiveness analysis. *Pain Physician, 2*, 52–58.

93. Manchikanti, L., Pampati, V., Fellows, B. et al. (2000). The inability of the clinical picture to characterize pain from facet joints. *Pain Physician, 3*, 158–166.

94. Manchikanti, L., Pampati, V. S., Fellows, B. et al. (2001). Role of one day epidural adhesiolysis in management of chronic low back pain: A randomized clinical trial. *Pain Physician, 4*, 153–166.

95. Manchikanti, L., Pampati, V., Rivera, J. J. et al. (2001). Effectiveness of percutaneous adhesiolysis and hypertonic saline neurolysis in refractory spinal stenosis. *Pain Physician, 4*, 366–373.

96. Hammer, M., Doleys, D., & Chung, O. (2001). Transforaminal ventral epidural adhesiolysis. *Pain Physician, 4*, 273–279.

97. Manchikanti, L., & Singh, V. (2002). Epidural lysis of adhesions and myeloscopy. *Current Pain and Headache Report, 6*, 427–435.

98. Manchikanti, L., Saini, B., & Singh, V. (2001). Spinal endoscopy and lysis of epidural adhesions in the management of chronic low back pain. *Pain Physician, 4*, 240–265.

99. Manchikanti, L. Boswell, M. V., Rivera, J. J. et al. (in press). Evaluation of spinal endoscopic adhesiolysis in chronic refractory low back pain with a randomized, double-blind trial with one year follow-up. *BioMed Central Anesthesiology*.

100. Geurts, J. W., Kallewaard, J. W., Richardson, J. et al. (2002). Targeted methylprednisolone acetate/hyaluronidase/clonidine injection after diagnostic epiduroscopy for chronic sciatica: A prospective, 1-year follow-up study. *Regional Anesthesia and Pain Medicine, 27*, 343–352.

101. Richardson, J., McGurgan, P., Cheema, S. et al. (2001). Spinal endoscopy in chronic low back pain with radiculopathy: A prospective case series. *Anaesthesia, 56*, 454–460.

102. Manchikanti, L., Pampati, V., Bakhit, C. E et al. (1999). Non-endoscopic and endoscopic adhesiolysis in post lumbar laminectomy syndrome: A one-year outcome study and cost effective analysis. *Pain Physician, 2*, 52–58.

103. Manchikanti, L. (2000). The value and safety of epidural endoscopic adhesiolysis. *American Journal of Anesthesiology*, 275–278.

104. Krasuski, P., Poniecka, A. W., Gal, E. et al. (2001). Epiduroscopy: Review of techniques and results. *The Pain Clinic, 13*, 71–76.

105. Igarashi, T., Hirabayashi, Y., Seo, N. et al. (2004). Lysis of adhesions and epidural injections of steroid/local anesthetic during epiduroscopy potentially alleviate low back and leg pain in elderly patients with lumbar spine stenosis. *British Journal of Anaesthesia, 93*, 181–187.

106. Guyer, R. D., & Ohnmeiss, D. D. (2003). NASS. Lumbar discography. *Spine Journal, 3*, 11S–27S.

107. Bogduk, N. (1996). The argument for discography. *Neurosurgery Quarterly, 6*, 152–153.

108. Shah, R. V., Everett, C. R., McKenzie-Brown, A. M. et al. (2005). Discography as a diagnostic test for spinal pain: A systematic and narrative review. *Pain Physician, 8*, 187–209.

109. Fortin, J. D. (2000). Precision diagnostic disc injections. *Pain Physician, 3*, 271–288.

110. Carragee, E. J., Tanner, C. M., Yang, B. et al. (1999). False-positive findings on lumbar discography. *Spine, 24*, 2542–2547.

111. Carragee, E., Tanner, C., Khurana, S. et al. (2000). The rates of false-positive lumbar discography in select patients without low back symptoms. *Spine, 25*, 1373–1381.

112. Walsh, T. R., Weinstein, J. N., Spratt, K. P. et al. (1990). Lumbar discography in normal subjects. *Journal of Bone and Joint Surgery, 72A*, 1081–1088.

113. Schwarzer, A. C., Aprill, C. N., Derby, R. et al. (1995). The prevalence and clinical features of internal disc disruption in patients with chronic low back pain. *Spine, 20*, 1878–1883.

114. Merskey, H., & Bogduk, N. (1994). Classification of chronic pain. In H. Merskey & N. Bogduk (Eds.), *Descriptions of chronic pain syndromes and definition of pain terms* (2nd ed., pp. 180–181). Seattle: IASP Press.

115. Manchikanti, L., Singh, V., Pampati, V. S. et al. (2001). Provocative discography in low back pain patients with or without somatization disorder: A randomized, prospective evaluation. *Pain Physician, 4*, 227–239.

116. Bogduk, N. (1996). The argument for discography. *Neurosurgery Quarterly, 6*, 152–153.

117. Stanton-Hicks, M., Baron, R., Boas, R. et al. (1988). Complex regional pain syndromes: Guidelines for therapy. *Clinical Journal of Pain, 14*, 155–166.

118. International Association for the Study of Pain Subcommittee on Taxonomy. (1986). Classification of chronic pain: Description of chronic pain syndromes and definitions of pain terms. Prepared by the subcommittee on taxonomy. *Pain, (Suppl.), 3*, S29–S30.

119. Raj, P. P. (1998). Complex regional pain syndrome-reflex sympathetic dystrophy and causalgia. *Current Review of Pain, 2*, 242–253.

120. Rocco, A. G. (1995). Radiofrequency lumbar sympatholysis. The evolution of a technique for managing sympathetically maintained pain. *Regional Anesthesia, 20*, 3–12.

121. Elias, M. (2000). Cervical sympathetic and stellate ganglion blocks. *Pain Physician, 3*, 294–304.

122. Manchikanti, L. (2000). The role of radiofrequency in managing complex regional pain syndrome. *Current Review of Pain, 24*, 437–444.

134. Rauck, R. L. (2001). Stellate ganglion block. *Techniques in Regional Anesthesia and Pain Management, 5*, 88–93.

124. Stanton-Hicks, M. (2001). Thoracic sympathetic block: A new approach. *Techniques in Regional Anesthesia and Pain Management, 5*, 94–98.

125. Raj, P. (2001). Celiac plexus/ splanchnic nerve blocks. *Techniques in Regional Anesthesia and Pain Management, 5*, 102–115.

126. Haynsworth, R. F., & Noe, C. E. (1991). Percutaneous lumbar sympathectomy: A comparison of radiofrequency denervation versus phenol neurolysis. *Anesthesiology, 74*, 459–463.

127. Kantha, K. S. (1989). Radiofrequency percutaneous lumbar sympathectomy: Technique and review of indications. In Racz (Ed.), *Techniques of neurolysis* (pp. 71–183). Boston: Academic Publishers, Kluwer.

128. Thompson, G. E. (1996). Intercostal nerve block. In S. D. Waldman & A. Winnie (Eds.), *Interventional pain management* (pp. 311–318). Phildadelphia: WB Sanders Company.

129. Fortin, J. D. (1993). The sacroiliac joint: A new perspective. *Journal of Back Musculoskeletal Rehabilitation, 3*, 31–43.

130. Fortin, J. D, Dwyer A., West, S. et al. (1994). Sacroiliac joint pain referral patterns upon application of a new injection/arthrography technique. Part I: Asymptomatic volunteers. *Spine, 19*, 1475–1482.

131. Fortin, J. D, Dwyer, A., Aprill, C. et al. (1994). Sacroiliac joint pain referral patterns. Part II: Clinical evaluation. *Spine, 19*, 1483–1489.

132. Dreyfuss, P., Dreyer, S., Griffin, J. et al. (1994). Positive sacroiliac screening tests in asymptomatic adults. *Spine, 19*, 1138–1143.

133. Dreyfuss, P., Michaelsen, M., Pauza, K. et al. (1996). The value of medical history and physical examination in diagnosing sacroiliac joint pain. *Spine, 21*, 2594–2602.

134. Maigne, J. Y., Aivaliklis, A., & Pfefer, F. (1996). Results of sacroiliac joint double block and value of sacroiliac pain provocation tests in 54 patients with low back pain. *Spine, 21*, 1889–1892.

135. Vogler, J. B., III, Brown, W. H., Helms, C. A. et al. (1984). The normal sacroiliac joint: A CT study of asymptomatic patients. *Radiology, 151*, 433–437.

136. Norman, G. F., & May, A. (1956). Sacroiliac conditions simulating intervertebral disc syndrome. *Western Journal of Surgery, 64*, 461–462.

137. Slipman, C. W., Plastaras, C. T., Yang, S. T. et al. (1996). Outcomes of therapeutic fluoroscopically guided sacroiliac joint injections for definitive SIJS. *Archives of Physical Medicine and Rehabilitation, 77*, 937.

138. Hansen, H. C. (2003). Is fluoroscopy necessary for sacroiliac joint injections? *Pain Physician, 6*, 155–158.

139. Hansen, H. C, & Helm, S. (2003). Sacroiliac joint pain and dysfunction. *Pain Physician, 6*, 179–190.

140. McKenzie-Brown, A. M., Shah, R. V., Seghal, N. et al. (2005). A systematic review of sacroiliac joint interventions. *Pain Physician, 8*, 115–125.

141. Maugers, Y., Mathis, C., Berthelot, J. M. et al. (1996). Assessment of the efficacy of sacroiliac corticosteroid injections for spondyloarthropathies: A double-blind study. *British Journal of Rheumatology, 35*, 767–770.

142. Hanly, J. G., Mitchell, M., MacMillan, L. et al. (2000). Efficacy of sacroiliac corticosteroid injections in patients in inflammatory spondyloarthropathy. Results of a 5-month controlled study. *Journal of Rheumatology, 27*, 719–722.

143. Ferrante, F. M., King, L. F., Roche, E. A. et al. (2001). Radiofrequency sacroiliac joint denervation: The devil is in the details. *Regional Anesthesia and Pain Medicine, 26*, 137–142.

144. Yin, W., Willard, F., Carreiro, J. et al. (2003). Sensory stimulation-guided sacroiliac joint radiofrequency neurotomy: Technique based on neuroanatomy of the dorsal sacral plexus. *Spine, 28*, 2419–2425.

145. Cohen, S. P., & Abdi, S. (2003). Lateral branch blocks as a treatment for sacroiliac joint pain: A pilot study. *Regional Anesthesia and Pain Medicine, 28*, 113–119.

146. Waldman, S. D. (2001). Blockade of the gasserian ganglion and the distal trigeminal nerve In S. D. Waldman (Ed.), *Interventional pain management*, second edition (pp. 316–320). Philadelphia: WB Sanders Company.

147. Taha, J. M., & Tew, J. M. (1996). Comparison of surgical treatments for trigeminal neuralgia: Reevaluation of radiofrequency rhizotomy. *Neurosurgery, 38*, 865–871.

148. Taha, J. M., & Tew, J. M. (1997). Treatment of trigeminal neuralgia by percutaneous radiofrequency rhizotomy. *Neurosurgery Clinics of North America, 8*, 31–39.

149. Oturai, A. B., Jensen, K., & Eriksen, J. (1996). Neurosurgery for trigeminal neuralgia: Comparison of alcohol block, neurectomy and radiofrequency coagulation. *Clinical Journal of Pain, 12*, 311–315.

150. Taha, J. M., Tew, J. M., & Buncher, C. R. (1995). A prospective 15-year follow up of 154 consecutive patients with trigeminal neuralgia treated by percutaneous stereotactic radiofrequency thermal rhizotomy. *Journal of Neurosurgery, 83*, 989–993.

151. Scrivani, S. J., Keith, D. A., Mathews, E. S. et al. (1999). Percutaneous stereotactic differential radiofrequency thermal rhizotomy for the treatment of trigeminal neuralgia. *Journal of Oral and Maxillofacial Surgery, 57*, 104–111.

152. Waldman, S. D. (2001). Suprascapular nerve block. In S. D. Waldman (Ed.), *Interventional pain management* (2nd ed., pp. 388–389). Philadelphia: WB Saunders Company.

153. Brown, D. L., & Wong, G. Y. (2001). Occipital nerve block. In S. D. Waldman (Ed.), *Interventional pain management* (2nd ed., pp. 312–315). Philadelphia: WB Saunders Company.

154. Raj, P. P., & Anderson S. R. (2001). Peripheral neurolysis in the management of pain. In S. D. Waldman (Ed.), *Interventional pain management* (2nd ed., pp. 541–553). Philadelphia: WB Saunders Company.

155. Manchikanti, L. (1999). Neural blockade in cervical pain syndromes. *Pain Physician, 2*, 65–84.

156. Travell, J. (1976). Myofascial trigger points. Clinical view. In J. J. Bonica & D. Able-Fessardi (Eds.), *Advances in pain research and therapy* (Vol. 1, pp. 919–926). New York: Raven Press.

157. Skootsky, S. A., Jaeger, B., & Oye, R. K. (1989). Prevalence of myofascial pain in general internal medicine practice. *Western Journal of Medicine, 151*, 157–160.

158. Han, S. C., & Harrison, P. (1997). Myofascial pain syndrome and trigger point management. *Regional Anesthesia and Pain Medicine, 22*, 89–101.

159. Barnsley, L., Lord, S., & Bogduk, N. (1994). Whiplash injury. *Pain, 58*, 283–307.

160. Wole, F., Simons, D. G., Fricton, J. et al. (1992). The fibromyalgia and myofascial pain syndromes. A preliminary study of tender point and trigger points in persons with fibromyalgia pain and no disease. *Journal of Rheumatology, 19*, 944–951.

161. Bogduk, N., & Simons, D. G. (1993). Neck pain: Joint pain or trigger points. In H. Vaeroy & J. Merskey (Eds.), *Progress in fibromyalgia and myofascial pain* (pp. 267–273). Amsterdam: Elsevier.

162. Gerwin, R. D. (1999). Myofascial pain syndromes from trigger points. *Pain 3*, 153–159.

163. Rauck, R. L. (1996). Myofascial pain syndrome and fibromyalgia. *Pain, 64,*, 41–53.

164. Harden R. N, Bruehl, S. P., Gass, S. et al. (2000). Signs and symptoms of the myofascial pain syndrome: A national survey of pain management providers. *Clinical Journal of Pain, 16*, 64–72.

165. North, R., Kidd, D., Zahurak, M. et al. (1993). Spinal cord stimulation for chronic intractable pain: Experience over two decades. *Neurosurgery, 32*, 384–394.

166. North, R. B., & Wetzel, F. T. (2002). Spinal cord stimulation for chronic pain of spinal origin. *Spine, 27*, 2584–2591.

167. Turner, J. A., Loeser, J. D., & Bell, K. G. (1995). Spinal cord stimulation for chronic low back pain. A systematic literature synthesis. *Neurosurgery, 37*, 1088–1096.

168. North, R. B., Kidd, D. H., Lee, M. S. et al. (1994). Spinal cord stimulation versus reoperation for the failed back surgery syndrome: A prospective, randomized study design. *Stereotactic and Functional Neurosurgery, 62*, 267–272.

169. Kemler, M. A., Barendse, G. A., van Kleef, M. et al. (2000). Spinal cord stimulation in patients with chronic reflex sympathetic dystrophy. *New England Journal of Medicine, 343*, 618–624.

170. Burchiel, K.J., Anderson, V. C., Brown, F. D. et al. (1996). Prospective: Multicenter study of spinal cord stimulation for relief of chronic back and extremity pain. *Spine, 21*, 2786–2794.

171. Barolat, G., Oakley, J., Law, J. et al. (2001). Epidural spinal cord stimulation with a multiple electrode paddle lead is effective in treating low back pain. *Neuromodulation, 2*, 59–66.

172. Kumar, K., Malik, S., & Demeria, D. (2002). Treatment of chronic pain with spinal cord stimulation versus alternative therapies: Cost-effectiveness analysis. *Neurosurgery, 51*, 106–116.

173. Bell, G., & North, R. (1997). Cost-effectiveness analysis of spinal cord stimulation in treatment of failed back surgery syndrome. *Journal of Pain and Symptom Management, 13*, 285–296.

174. Kemler, M., & Furnee, C. (2002). Economic evaluation of spinal cord stimulation for chronic reflex sympathetic dystrophy. *Neurology, 59*, 1203–1209.

175. May, M. et al. (2002). A retrospective, long term, third-party follow-up of patients considered for spinal cord stimulation. *Neuromodulation, 3*, 137–144.

176. Sarubbi, F., & Vasquez, J. (1997). Spinal epidural abscess associated with the use of temporary epidural catheters: Report of two cases and review. *Clinical Infectious Diseases, 25*, 1155–1158.

177. Oakley, J., & Prager, J. (2002). Spinal cord stimulation: Mechanism of action. *Spine, 22*, 2574.

178. Taylor, R. S., Taylor, R. J., Van Buyten, J. P. et al. (2004). The cost effectiveness of spinal cord stimulation in the treatment of pain: A systematic review of the literature. *Journal of Pain and Symptom Management, 27*, 370.

179. Turner, J., Loeser, J., Deyo, R. et al. (2004). Spinal cord stimulation for patients with failed back surgery syndrome or complex regional pain syndrome: A systemic review of effectiveness and complications. *Pain, 108*, 137.

180. Prager, J. P. (2002). Neuraxial medication delivery. The development and maturity of a concept for treating chronic pain of spinal origin. *Spine, 27*, 2593–2605.

181. Hassenbusch, S. (2000). Current practices in intraspinal therapy – A survey of clinical trends and decision making. *Journal of Pain and Symptom Management, 20*, S4–11.

182. van den Bosch, G. (2001). Driving and intrathecal morphine administration. *European Journal of Pain, 5*, 443–447.

183. Bennett, G. (2000). Clinical guidelines for intraspinal infusion: Report of an expert panel. *Journal of Pain and Symptom Management, 20*, S37–S43.

184. Siddall, P. J. (2000). The efficacy of intrathecal morphine and clonidine in the treatment of pain after spinal cord injury. *Anesthesia & Analgesia, 91*, 1493–1498.

185. van Hilten, B. J., van de Beek, W. J., Hoff, J. I. et al. (2000). Intrathecal baclofen for the treatment of dystonia in patients with reflex sympathetic dystrophy. *New England Journal of Medicine, 343*, 654–656.

186. Smith, T. J., Staats, P. S., Deer, T. et al. (2002). Randomized clinical trial of an implantable drug delivery system compared with comprehensive medical management for refractory cancer pain: Impact on pain, drug-related toxicity, and survival. *Journal of Clinical Oncology, 20*, 4040–4049.

187. Hassenbusch, S. J., & Stanton-Hicks, M. (1995). Long-term intraspinal infusions in the treatment of neuropathic pain. *Journal of Pain and Symptom Management, 10*, 527–543.

188. Angel, I. F., Gould, H. J., Jr., & Carey, M. E. (1998). Intrathecal morphine pump as a treatment option in chronic pain of nonmalignant origin. *Surgical Neurology, 49*, 92–99.

189. Anderson, V. C., & Burchiel, K. J. (1999). A prospective study of long-term intrathecal morphine in the management of chronic nonmalignant pain. *Neurosurgery, 44*, 289–301.

190. Corrado, P., Gottlieb, H., Varga, C. A. et al. (2000). The effect of intrathecal morphine infusion on pain level and disability in pain patients with chronic intractable low back pain. *American Journal of Pain Management, 10*, 160–166.

191. Kumar, K. (2001). Continuous intrathecal morphine treatment for chronic pain of nonmalignant etiology: Long-term benefits and efficacy. *Surgical Neurology, 55*, 79–88.

58

Evidence for the Use of Interventional Techniques for Chronic Spinal Pain

Laxmaiah Manchikanti, MD, Vijay Singh, MD, and Elmer E. Dunbar, MD

STRUCTURAL BASIS OF CHRONIC SPINAL PAIN

Chronic spinal pain continues to be an epidemic and treatment often remains inadequate.[1-16] The devastating nature of chronic pain, which can destroy the quality of life by eroding the will to live, disturbing sleep and appetite, creating fatigue, and impairing recovery from illness or injury, is not well appreciated.[7-10,16] Consequences may be especially difficult for the elderly patient in chronic pain, resulting in vocational, social, and family discord, which may make the difference between a reasonable quality of life and loss of function and comorbidity.[11-13]

Chronic spinal pain is recognized as a multidimensional problem with both sensory and affective components. The biopsychosocial model, which emerged in the 1980s, views chronic spinal pain as a biopsychosocial phenomenon, in which biological, psychological, and social factors dynamically interact with each other. In the 1990s, the biopsychosocial approach dominated chronic spinal pain management, at least among academicians, with efforts to introduce "psychosocial" approaches.

The concept of psychogenic pain has stimulated controversy in the field of pain medicine, not only regarding its prevalence, but indeed, its very existence.[17] Essentially, psychogenic pain is considered within the context that "since there is nothing wrong with your body, there must be something wrong with you." Some state that the term *psychogenic pain* is fundamentally meaningless.[18]

The diagnosis of psychogenic pain not only fails to provide a valid organic diagnosis, but it also fails to pro-

vide validation of patient symptomatology and complaints. Thus, psychogenic pain also implies it is unreal or illusional. The concept of psychogenic pain is weakened by the fact that its diagnostic signs have been challenged. Gagliese and Katz[18] believe that medically unexplained pain is not a symptom of a psychological disorder and that it is time to abandon thinking that separates mind and body. Thus, the challenge remains for proponents to provide empirical evidence to prove that psychopathology causes pain and, in doing so, to specify the mechanisms by which it is generated.

Modern technology, including magnetic resonance imaging (MRI), computed axial tomographic scanning (CT), neurophysiologic testing, and comprehensive physical examination with psychological evaluation, can identify the cause of low back pain in only 15% of patients in the absence of disc herniation and neurological deficit.[1-3,19] In addition, overall inaccurate or incomplete diagnoses in patients referred to pain treatment centers have been described as ranging from 40 to 67%, and the incidence of psychogenic pain has been shown to be present only in 1 of 3,000 patients, with the presence of pain of organic origin mistakenly branded as psychosomatic in 98% of the cases.[20,21] Psychogenic pain should not be confused with factitious illness and malingering, which are distinct psychiatric disorders.

Providing a structural basis of pain will invalidate the theory that maladaptive psychological processes are primarily responsible for causing regional pain syndromes, and therefore, the assumption that psychological or behavioral interventions are the most logical treatment modalities. The majority of painful conditions include various types of pain originating from the spine with pain in the neck, upper back, mid back, low back, and upper or lower extremities.

Bogduk[22] postulated that, for any structure to be deemed a cause of back pain: (1) the structure should have a nerve supply; (2) the structure should be capable of causing pain similar to that seen clinically, ideally demonstrated in normal volunteers; (3) the structure should be susceptible to diseases or injuries that are known to be painful; and (4) the structure should have been shown to be a source of pain in patients, using diagnostic techniques of known reliability and validity. The same philosophy may be applied for cervical and thoracic pain.

PATHOPHYSIOLOGIC BASIS

Kuslich et al.[23] identified intervertebral discs, facet joints, ligaments, fascia, muscles, and nerve root dura as tissues capable of causing pain in the low back. Thus, the structures responsible for pain originating in the spine and afflicting the neck, mid back, upper back and low back, upper extremities, and lower extremities may originate from the vertebrae, intervertebral discs, spinal cord, nerve roots, facet joints, ligaments, muscles, and sacroiliac or atlanto-axial and atlanto-occipital joints. However, vertebrae, muscles, and ligaments have not been proved to be common sources of spinal pain. In contrast, facet joint pain, discogenic pain, and sacroiliac joint pain have been proved to be common causes of pain with proven diagnostic techniques.[1,22,24]

Cavanaugh et al.[25] describe how idiopathic low back pain has confounded health care practitioners for decades and how the cellular and neural mechanisms that lead to facet pain, discogenic pain, and sciatica are not well understood. In a series of neurophysiologic and neuroanatomic studies, they show the evidence in support of facet pain, including an extensive distribution of small nerve fibers and endings in the lumbar facet joint, nerves containing substance P, high threshold mechanoreceptors in the facet joint capsule, and sensitization and excitation of nerves in facet joint and surrounding muscle when the nerves were exposed to inflammatory or algesic chemicals. Evidence for pain of disc origin included an extensive distribution of small nerve fibers and free nerve endings in the superficial anulus of the disc, as well as small fibers and free nerve endings in the adjacent longitudinal ligaments. They also described possible mechanisms of sciatica including vigorous and long-lasting excited discharges when dorsal root ganglia were subjected to moderate pressure, excitation of dorsal root fibers when the ganglia were exposed to autologous nucleus pulposus, and excitation and loss of nerve functions in nerve roots exposed to phospholipase A_2. These findings render support for a structural and chemical basis for low back pain.

Pang et al.[26] by applying spinal pain mapping, which is a sequence of well-organized nerve block procedures, analyzed 104 cases in a pain clinic. They prospectively evaluated consecutive adult patients with intractable low back pain (who had failed conservative therapy) of undetermined etiology after medical history, physical examination, x-ray, CT, MRI, EMG/NCV (electromyography/nerve conduction velocity) evaluation of the lumbar spine. By using pain mapping, the source of pain was facet joint(s) in 24%, combined lumbar nerve root and facet disease in 24%, combined facet(s) and sacroiliac joint(s) in 4%, lumbar nerve root irritation in 20%, internal disc disorder in 7%, sacroiliac joint in 6%, and sympathetic dystrophy in 2% of the patients. Pain mapping failed to demonstrate causes of pain in the remaining 13% of the patients. However, Pang et al.[26] used a single block technique with the potential for false-positive results.[1,2,27]

Manchikanti et al.[27] evaluated the relative contributions of various structures in patients with chronic low back pain who had failed to respond to conservative modalities of treatments including physical therapy, chiropractic, and drug therapy. These patients had lack of radiological evidence to indicate disc protrusion or radiculopathy. Utilizing precision diagnostic injections (controlled comparative double diagnostic blocks), they showed that 40% of the patients suffered from facet joint pain, 26% from discogenic pain, 2% from sacroiliac joint pain, and possibly 13% from segmental dural/nerve root pain with no cause identified in 19% of the patients.

INTERVENTIONAL TECHNIQUES

The overall benefit of various types of injection techniques includes pain relief that outlasts by days, weeks, or months the relatively short duration of pharmacologic action of the local anesthetics and other agents used. Clear-cut explanations for these prolonged improvements are not currently available. It is believed that neural blockade alters or interrupts nociceptive input, reflex mechanisms of the afferent limb, self-sustaining activity of the neuron pools and neuraxis, and the pattern of central neuronal activities.[28] Explanations for improvements are based in part on the pharmacological and physical actions of local anesthetics, corticosteroids, and other agents. It is believed that local anesthetics interrupt the pain–spasm cycle and reverberating nociceptor transmission, whereas corticosteroids reduce inflammation either by inhibiting the synthesis or release of a number of proinflammatory substances or by causing a reversible local anesthetic effect.[29–45]

MECHANISM OF ACTION

Various modes of action of corticosteroids include:

- Membrane stabilization
- Inhibition of neural peptide synthesis or action
- Blockade of phospholipase A_2 activity
- Prolonged suppression of ongoing neuronal discharge
- Suppression of sensitization of dorsal horn neurons.

Local anesthetics have been shown to produce prolonged dampening of C-fiber activity.[46–48] Physical effects include clearing adhesions or inflammatory exudates from the vicinity of the nerve root sleeve. The scientific basis of some of these concepts, at least in part, is proved for spinal pain management with epidural injections of betamethasone and intravenous methylprednisolone.[29,33,35–39]

Various mechanisms of benefits for longer periods of time than the duration of the anesthetics used have been described.[40] This phenomenon has been documented in the literature and is regularly observed by clinicians. The mechanisms by which local anesthetics abolish chronic pain for several days when they are effective for a maximum of 4 hours if used for acute or "physiological" pain are not known.[40] Several theories have been suggested. In an essay on the future of local anesthetics,[41] several theories were listed including the sympathetic nervous system.[42] Others[43–45] have speculated that such blocks cause temporary abolition of spontaneous ectopic discharges, resulting in abolition of dynamically maintained central hyperexcitability, as well as reinforcing endogenous G-protein-couple receptor inhibition of N-type voltage-sensitive calcium channels. In addition, the data on glial activation in pathological pain[45] also may cast doubt on the utility of cognitive behavioral therapy and other psychological interventions, while lending new legitimacy to local anesthetic block procedures. Activation of spinal cord glia has been demonstrated in response to a variety of stimuli including tissue injury and infections.[45] The activated glia produces a number of proinflammatory cytokines associated with central sensitization. This activation spreads from cell to cell across "gap junctions," following no particular neuronal pathways or anatomical boundaries. In an editorial on nerve blocks and cognitive therapy, Merskey and Thompson[40] commented:

> It now seems highly likely that "unexplained" regional pain is the result of organic or neurochemical changes; therefore, they are medically explained. Hence, therapeutic modalities that can, even temporarily, reduce neuronal excitability and sympathetic nervous system malfunction may result in just the sort of benefits from local anesthetic blocks documented.... The time is right for renewed interest in nerve block models for the relief of pain. Those models are the ultimate foundation of the truly multidisciplinary pain clinic, and their results encouraged pioneers such as Bonica and Travell to take chronic pain seriously. A look at their work may help

to renew some well-established approaches that are currently neglected or out of favor (p. 175).

DIAGNOSTIC INTERVENTIONAL TECHNIQUES

It has been postulated that for any structure to be deemed a cause of back pain, the structure should have been shown to be a source of pain in patients, using diagnostic techniques of known reliability and validity.[49] The diagnostic blockade of a structure with a nerve supply with the ability to generate pain can be performed to test the hypothesis that the target structure is a source of the patient's pain. Evidence-based interventional diagnostic techniques include facet joint blocks, discography, and sacroiliac joint injections. Other techniques including transforaminal epidural or selective nerve root blocks and sympathetic blocks also are used. The descriptions in this chapter are limited to evidence-based techniques.

RATIONALE

The popularity of neural blockade as a diagnostic tool in painful conditions is due to several features.[50] Multiple challenging clinical situations include the characteristics of chronic spinal pain, which are purely subjective. Various painful conditions, in most cases, are inexactly defined with uncertain pathophysiology. Precision diagnostic blocks are used to clarify these challenging clinical situations, in order to determine the pathophysiology of clinical pain, the site of nociception, and the pathway of afferent neural signals. Precise anatomical diagnosis in low back pain has been described not only as elusive, but also as often frustrating for both physicians and patients.[51,52] History, physical examination, and imaging provide limited information.[52]

RELIABILITY AND VALIDITY

Clinical studies of precision diagnostic techniques are variable, not only in quality, but also in quantity. Important considerations include entrance criteria, study size, and the use of controlled subjects. The importance of the false-positive rate (how often patients without a condition will nonetheless have a positive test) and false-negative rate (how often a patient with disease will have a negative test) is extremely crucial because they vary inversely with specificity and sensitivity. Specificity is a relative measure of the prevalence of false-positives, whereas sensitivity is the relative prevalence of false-negative results. The general parameters of accuracy are described as the specificity and sensitivity of the diagnostic test. The most sensitive test will be positive for all cases in which the disease is present. The specificity is greatest when there is a positive test result only when the disease is present. Thus, the ideal diagnostic test would have a sensitivity of 100% and a specificity of 100%. Placebo response also needs to be taken into consideration. Because none of the tests available in clinical medicine has these ideal features, there is a degree of uncertainty regarding the accuracy of each and every diagnostic test as applied to an individual clinical case. In addition, for many painful conditions, a credible standard to document the disease for comparison with test results is unavailable.

Hildebrandt[53] published an extensive review on the relevance of nerve blocks in treating and diagnosing low back pain. He described zygapophysial joint blocks, sacroiliac joint blocks, disc stimulation, and nerve root blocks. Hildebrandt[53] concluded that the diagnostic use of neural blockade rests on three premises:

1. The pathology causing pain is located in an exact peripheral location, and impulses from this site travel via unique and consistent neural route.
2. Injection of local anesthetic totally abolishes the sensory function of intended nerves and does not affect other nerves.
3. Relief of pain after local anesthetic block is attributable solely to the block of the target afferent neural pathway.

However, the validity of these assumptions is limited by complexities of anatomy, physiology, and psychology of pain perception, and by the effect of local anesthetics on impulse conduction.

In contrast, others[54,55] have concluded that various studies outside imaging have rarely demonstrated clinical utility in assessment of patients with neck and back pain. It was described that diagnostic and treatment devices lacking in scientific rigor included facet blocks, discography, and diagnostic nerve root infiltration, along with other tests including EMG, stress radiographs and flexion and extension x-rays, bone scintigraphy, thermography, diagnostic ultrasound, and temporary external fixation.[55] It is generally described that the accuracy of a diagnostic test is best determined by comparing it with an appropriate reference standard (gold standard) such as biopsy, surgery, autopsy, or long-term follow-up.[56,57] A reference standard allows accurate comparison of a given diagnostic test's capacity to yield positive results when the clinical condition is present and negative results when the clinical condition is not present. Thus, a gold standard or reference standard facilitates accurate determination of the specificity and sensitivity of a test. Tissue confirmation of the presence or absence of a disease at surgery, with a biopsy, or at autopsy, which has served as the accepted gold standard across multiple medical disciplines, is not applicable to interventional pain management. Thus, most pain provocative or relieving tests used to diagnose painful conditions of the spine are more closely related to a physical examination than to a laboratory test.[58] Stability of the diagnosis over a long period of time with long-term follow-up may also be used as a gold standard.[59] These facts are especially true in the diagnosis of facet joint pain, discogenic pain, and sacroiliac joint pain. Thus, there is no completely reliable gold standard with which to compare the diagnostic test of precision diagnostic injection in conditions where the evaluation is dependent on pain relief or functional improvement as the end point. Consequently, a true calculation of clinical accuracy of these tests may not be possible.

The clinical setting in which the test is performed and the prevalence of the disease in that setting also affect the meaningfulness of the test results. The prevalence refers to the frequency of the disease in the general population and to the population seen in a specific setting where the test is used. When the prevalence is high, there is a higher probability that a positive test result indicates the presence of the disease. Consequently, evaluation of a diagnostic test in a population for which the prevalence is low or absent has either limited meaning or no meaning. Thus, the predictive value of a diagnostic test is a function of the prevalence, sensitivity, and specificity.

Although diagnostic blockade of a structure with a nerve supply that can generate pain can be performed to test the hypothesis that the target structure is the source of the patient's pain,[49,60] testing the hypothesis by provoking pain in any structure is an unreliable criterion except in provocative discography.[61] Thus, relief of pain is the essential criterion in almost all structures. If the pain is not relieved, the source may be in another structural component of the spine similar to the one tested, such as a different facet joint, different nerve root, or some other structure.[49] Ideally, all controlled blocks should include placebo injections of normal saline, but it may be neither logistically feasible nor ethical to use placebo injections of normal saline in conventional practice in each and every patient. In addition, one may be required to perform three blocks of the same structure if a placebo is used. As an alternative, the use of comparative local anesthetic blocks, on two separate occasions, during which the same joint is anesthetized using two local anesthetics with different duration of actions, has been proposed. The use of comparative local anesthetic blocks with facet joint injections has been validated and found to be robust against challenge with placebo.[62, 63]

FACILITIES

The requirements for diagnostic interventional techniques include a sterile operating room or a procedure room, monitoring equipment, radiological equipment, sterile preparation with all the resuscitative equipment, needles, gowns, injectate agents, intravenous fluids, sedative agents, and trained personnel for preparation and monitoring of the patients. Minimum requirements include history and physical examination, informed consent, and appropriate documentation of the procedure.

CONTRAINDICATIONS

Contraindications include bacterial infection, possible pregnancy, bleeding diathesis, and anticoagulant therapy. Precautions are warranted in patients with antiplatelet or anticoagulant therapy, diabetes mellitus, and artificial heart valves.

FACET OR ZYGAPOPHYSIAL JOINT BLOCKS

Blocks of a facet or zygapophysial joint can be performed in order to test the hypothesis that the target joint is the source of the patient's pain.[49,60]

RATIONALE

The rationale for using facet joint blocks for diagnosis is based upon the following:

- **Innervation:** Spinal facet joints are well innervated[2,49,60]
- **Sources of pain:**
  Cervical facet joints have been shown to be capable of being a source of neck pain and referred pain in the head or upper limb girdle.
  Thoracic facet joints have been shown to be capable of being a source of thoracic pain and referred pain over the chest wall.
  Lumbar facet joints have been shown to be capable of being a source of low back pain and referred pain in the lower limbs in normal volunteers.
- **Referral patterns:**
  Various patterns of referred pain described for facet joints in the spine are variable and restricted.[64–75]
  Other structures, such as the disc, in the same segment may produce the same pattern of pain.
- **Physical examination:**
  None of the features of physical examination is diagnostic.
  Most maneuvers used in physical examinations are likely to stress several structures simultaneously, especially the discs, muscles, and facet joints, thus failing to provide any reasonable diagnostic criteria.
  Presented evidence thus far has been controversial.[49,60,76–85]
- **History:**
  Demographic features, pain characteristics, and other signs and symptoms may not be corre-

lated with diagnosis of facet joint pain and are unreliable.[49, 60, 76–85]

- **Imaging:**
  There are no valid and reliable means of identifying symptomatic lesions of the facet joint using currently available imaging technologies.[86–95]
  On retrospective review of radiographs of specimens known to have lesions, radiologists could identify lesions in only a small minority of instances,[95] if at all.[87]
  The results of most studies fail to show a correlation between radiologic imaging, including MRI, CT scanning, dynamic bending films, single photon emission computed tomography (SPECT), and radionuclide bone scanning, and facet joint pain.[76,77,86,88–96]

VALIDITY

Controlled diagnostic blocks with two separate local anesthetics (or placebo controlled) are the only means of confirming diagnosis of facet joint pain. The face validity of medial branch blocks has been established by injecting small volumes of local anesthetic onto the target points for these blocks and by determining the spread of contrast medium in posteroanterior and lateral radiographs.[58–61] Construct validity of facet joint blocks is also extremely important, as the placebo effect is the single greatest confounder of diagnostic blocks. Patients are liable to report relief of pain after a diagnostic block for reasons other than the pharmacologic action of the drug administered.[63] Thus, it is essential to know in every individual case whether the response is a true-positive. The theory that testing a patient first with lidocaine and subsequently with bupivacaine provided a means of identifying placebo response has been tested and proved.[62,63]

The specificity of the effect of cervical and lumbar facet joint blocks was demonstrated in controlled trials.[58–61] Provocation response was shown to be unreliable in one study.[61] The false-negative rate of diagnostic facet joint blocks was shown to be 8% due to unrecognized intravascular injection of local anesthetic.[60] Confounding psychological factors showed lack of influence of psychological factors on the validity of comparative controlled diagnostic local anesthetic blocks of facet joints in the lumbar spine.[59] False-positive rates were evaluated in multiple investigations.[27,80,101–113] Reported false-positive rates varied from 27 to 63% in cervical spine, 55 to 58% in thoracic spine, and 22 to 47% in lumbar spine.

PREVALENCE

Based on multiple evaluations, using controlled diagnostic blocks, facet or zygapophysial joints have been implicated as the source of chronic spinal pain in 15 to 45% of the heterogeneous groups of patients with chronic low back pain,[27,79,80,84,101,102,104,106,107] 42 to 48% of the patients with thoracic pain,[105] and 54 to 67% of the patients with chronic neck pain.[103,104,107,114–16]

Based on a multitude of evaluations, Manchikanti et al.[1] and Boswell et al.[117] conclude that the validity, specificity, and sensitivity of facet joint nerve blocks were strong in the diagnosis of facet joint pain.

SAFETY AND COMPLICATIONS

Safety of facet joint interventions with intra-articular injections and medial branch blocks has been demonstrated. The most common and worrisome complications of facet joint injections or nerve blocks are related to needle placement and drug administration. These complications include dural puncture, spinal cord trauma, infection, intravascular injection, spinal anesthesia, chemical meningitis, neural trauma, pneumothorax, radiation exposure, and hematoma formation.[118–130] Steroid side effects were attributed to the chemistry or to the pharmacology of the steroids.[129,130] Facet capsule rupture also may occur, if large volumes of injectate are used for intra-articular injections.[67]

Vertebral artery damage or entry is a potential risk with cervical facet blockade. Such complications occur more frequently with a lateral intra-articular technique than with blockade of the medial branches because the former technique requires deeper penetration of the needle toward the spinal structures. Local anesthetic leakage out of the joint into spinal canal may cause motor and sensory blockade with its risks and complications. In the cervical spine, third occipital nerve blocks can cause transient ataxia and unsteadiness due to partial blockade of the upper cervical proprioceptive afferents and the righting response.[131] Furthermore, when C3/4, C4/5, or C5/6 facet joint blocks are performed, the phrenic nerve may be compromised, especially if a large volume of local anesthetic is employed.

DISCOGRAPHY

Discography is a diagnostic procedure designed to determine whether a disc is intrinsically painful.

RATIONALE

Formal studies have shown that the discs are innervated and can be a source of pain that has pathomorphologic correlates.[132–151] Biologic basis for lumbar discography has been well established. However, embryologically and morphologically, the cervical discs differ from lumbar discs and do not suffer the same pathology.[152, 153] In addition, there is no evidence that cervical discs suffer

the internal disc disruption widely described in lumbar discs. Thoracic discs with anular tears, intrinsic degeneration, and/or associated vertebral body end plate infractions were painful in approximately 75% of the patients.[154] Cervical discs also have been shown to have prelesions in the anterior anulus, which may be the basis for cervical discogenic pain but they have not been shown to be painful.[155,156]

The rationale is well established for lumbar discography.[152,153,157,158] Discography is helpful in patients with lumbar or leg pain to acquire information about the structure and sensitivity of their lumbar intervertebral discs and to make informed decisions about treatment and modifications of activity. The injected substance in the disc pushes anular fibers aside to form pools of contrast, which indicate the location of fissures.[159] Contrast exiting from the disc indicates tears in the outer wall of the anulus. Extruded contrast may outline fragments of anulus and nucleus outside the disc and adjacent tissues, such as peridural membranes.

Discography was performed in asymptomatic volunteers without spinal pain in cervical spine,[160] thoracic spine,[161] and lumbar spine.[162] It was shown that discographically normal cervical discs were never painful in either symptomatic or asymptomatic groups.[160–162] For many years, disc degeneration was considered as the sole or dominant factor predisposing to spinal pain. However, spinal pain without disc herniation or secondary to involvement of other structures is well known.[22] Even though the mechanism of pain that arises within the disc continues to be poorly understood, it is accepted that damage to the disc can produce pain without consensus on the responsible mechanisms.[22]

VALIDITY

Examination of cadaver discs provided good correlation with which images were compared.[159,163–165] Multiple authors also have investigated the accuracy of discographic and CT/discographic findings based on the ability to demonstrate accurate pathology confirmed at the time of surgery. While many authors[166-171] have demonstrated significant correlation with reliable and accurate diagnosis, some[172,173] have demonstrated poor correlation. In addition, discography was compared with myelography, CT, MRI, and results of surgical and conservative management. CT discography was reported to be more accurate than myelography.[167,168,173–180] On similar grounds, discography was shown to be superior to plain computed tomography.[176,179,181] While comparing the results of discography with MRI, some found discography to be as good as MRI, even though MRI was preferable as it was non-invasive and allowed assessment of more levels with one test with minimal risks of complication and minimal discomfort.[182,183] However, others have identified advantages of discography with pain provocation when MRIs were normal or equivocal.[160,161,184–188] Some have identified its poor sensitivity and specificity.[136–142] Thus, the role of discography in a normal MRI is of questionable value and is not suggested to be performed routinely.

The good correlation between MRI, discography, and high intensity zone (HIZ) related pain have been established by some,[196–200] while others have reported poor correlation and limited value of discography in evaluating the clinical significance of the HIZ and the need for treatment.[201–204] Finally, the relationship of discography to outcomes, including conservative management, minimally invasive surgery, and open procedures also has been controversial.[1,157]

While the accuracy of discography as an imaging test is high, with high specificity and sensitivity for diagnosis of disc degeneration, the question that revolves around discography is whether this test is accurate for the diagnosis of discogenic pain. An integral part of the problem is the lack of an adequate reference or gold standard. Surgical exposure can confirm the presence of disc degeneration or disruption, but it cannot definitely confirm the presence or absence of discogenic pain. However, the results from both surgical and minimally invasive treatment of discogenic pain in patients whose diagnosis was confirmed by discography should provide a reference standard for discogenic pain. Positive results have been provided in multiple publications.

The face validity of discography has been established by injecting small volumes of contrast into the disc and by determining the concordant pain with spread of the contrast medium in posteroanterior and lateral radiographs and/or computed tomography. Construct validity of the discograms is also extremely important, as a false-positive result is the single greatest confounder of diagnostic discography. Patients are liable to report pain after insertion of the needle for reasons other than stimulation of the nociceptors. Thus, it is essential in each and every case for a response to be considered positive, that concordant pain be produced; and for the test to be valid, there must be at least one disc (preferably two) that do not illicit pain upon injection, thereby serving as control discs.[205]

Validity of discography has been established in asymptomatic patients. However, there are no modern normative data that establish that cervical discography is a specific test for cervical discogenic pain.[152] There is also evidence indicating that up to 40% of the positive cervical discograms may be false-positive.[206] Further, it was shown that cervical discography induced neck pain in 50% of the patients with neurological symptoms due to cervical spondylosis but with no neck pain.[207] With thoracic discography, unfamiliar or disconcordant pain was produced in lifelong asymptomatic individuals.[161] Thus, any evidence of value for cervical and thoracic discography is inconclusive at the present time.

In the 1960s, Holt[208, 209] reported a significant number of false-positive (37%) lumbar spine discograms[208] in an asymptomatic prison population;[208] similar findings were reported with cervical spine discograms.[209] Simmons et al.[210] reassessed Holt's data[208] and pointed out that discography as performed by Holt, although appropriate for its time, was quite different from discography as performed in 1988. The necessity for accurate needle tip positioning was proven by Urasaki et al.[211] Walsh et al.,[162] in a carefully controlled series of disc injections in asymptomatic volunteers, showed a 0% false-positive rate refuting the findings of Holt.[208] Studies by Carragee et al.[212–217] have shown a higher rate of false-positives than the study of Walsh et al.[162] However, a multitude of methodological flaws have been pointed out with each of these similarly structured studies.[58,218–221]

Multiple drawbacks described include the technique of disc puncture, interpretation, presence of negative discs, small number of patients, inability to compare pain provocation to clinical or typical pain, post-test and pre-test probability, and accuracy of psychological evaluation. Discography is most accurate and useful when the diagnosis of discogenic pain is highly probable, as determined by the history, physical examination, imaging data analyzed, and inability to isolate another source of pain. Manchikanti et al.[220] evaluated 50 patients with discography, of which 25 patients were without somatization disorder and 25 patients were with documented somatization disorder. They concluded that provocative discography provided similar results in patients with or without somatization, with or without depression, with somatization but with or without depression or with other combinations of the psychological triad of somatization disorder, depression, and generalized anxiety disorder. Saal[58] points out that some of the issues raised by Carragee et al.[212–217] may be resolved on the basis that disc stimulation is related to reflex reaction in the groin and lower abdomen; L5/6 disc was innervated by the L1 or L2 spinal nerves; and the sacroiliac joints are dually innervated, including those arising from L1 to L3. Others also have reported psychological influences, perhaps causing false-positive results.[222,223]

INDICATIONS

Much of the controversy about discography has arisen because the results of discography have been used to help decide whether a certain patient should or should not have surgery, even though patients have usually undergone other diagnostic tests, the results of which were either equivocal or nondiagnostic. Thus, discography should be performed only if the patient has failed to respond to adequate attempts of non-operative care, and if diagnostic tests such as MRI have not provided sufficient diagnostic information. Generally, discography should be viewed as an invasive test to be used to seek abnormalities when results from other tests are equivocal or inconsistent, in a patient with symptoms severe enough to require further evaluation.[157] Thus, specific uses for discography include, but are not limited to,

- Further evaluation of demonstrably abnormal discs to help assess the extent of abnormality or correlation of the abnormality with clinical symptoms (in case of recurrent pain from a previously operated disc or a lateral disc herniation)
- Evaluation of patients with persistent, severe symptoms in whom other diagnostic tests have failed to reveal clear confirmation of a suspected disc as the source of pain
- Assessment of patients who have failed to respond to surgical procedures to determine if there is painful pseudoarthrosis or asymptomatic disc in a posteriorly fused segment, or to evaluate possible recurrent disc herniation
- Assessment of discs before fusion to determine if the discs within the proposed fusion segment are symptomatic and to determine if discs adjacent to this segment are normal
- Assessment of minimally invasive surgical candidates to confirm a contained disc herniation or to investigate contrast distribution pattern before chemonucleolysis or other intradiscal procedures

PREVALENCE

Prevalence of pain due to internal disc disruption was reported as 39% in patients suffering with chronic low back pain.[224] In contrast, primary discogenic pain was reported to be 26% in a sample of 120 patients, but 43% in patients undergoing discography in lumbar spine.[27] However, in another study of patients with intractable low back pain, using spinal pain mapping with nerve blocks, the authors estimated lumbar nerve root involvement in 20% and internal disc disorder in only 7% of the patients.[26]

EVIDENCE

Review of the available evidence regarding discogenic pain[1] shows that the validity for cervical and thoracic discography is limited, whereas the validity for lumbar discography is strong for the diagnosis of discogenic pain.

SAFETY AND COMPLICATIONS

Complications related to discography include infection, neural trauma, intravascular penetration, and spinal cord trauma. Lack of permanent effects secondary to discography has been reported.[225–228] Significant complications

from diagnostic cervical discography procedures occurred in 0.6 to 2.5% of the patients and 0.16 to 1.5% of the cervical disc injections.[229–231] In contrast, in the lumbar spine, overall incidence of discitis has been reported to be 2 to 3%, with an overall complication rate of 13%.[177–181] However, postdiscography discitis represents approximately 30% of all cases of pyogenic discitis and has been reported after almost every type of open and minimally invasive spinal surgical procedure.[236-239] Similar to postoperative vertebral osteomyelitis, postprocedural discitis frequently affects elderly and immunocompromised individuals and is an important cause of postoperative back pain in the patient with a spine disorder. Other reported complications include subdural empyema,[240] pulmonary embolism of nucleus pulposus,[241] herniated cervical disc,[242] quadriplegia,[243] and epidural abscess.[244,245]

Prophylactic intradiscal antibiotic administration may also result in disastrous complications, including death.[246]

SACROILIAC JOINT BLOCKS

The sacroiliac joint is accepted as a potential source of low back and/or buttock pain with or without lower extremity pain. Diagnostic blocks of a sacroiliac joint can be performed in order to test the hypothesis that the sacroiliac joint is the source of the patient's pain. The sacroiliac joint can be anesthetized with intra-articular injection of local anesthetic.

RATIONALE

The rationale for sacroiliac joint blocks for diagnosis is based on the fact that sacroiliac joints have been shown to be capable of being a source of low back pain and referred pain in the lower extremity. There are no definite historical, physical, or radiological features to provide definite diagnosis of sacroiliac joint pain.[247–257] Nevertheless, multiple authors[85,258–260] have advocated a positive predictive value in diagnosing sacroiliac joint pain in patients with positive provocative maneuvers. However, a corroborative history and physical examination may enter into the differential diagnosis of sacroiliac joint pain but cannot make a definitive diagnosis of sacroiliac joint syndrome.[261,262] Many studies have reported on the efficacy of plain films,[263] computed tomography,[255] single photon emission computed tomography,[264] bone scans,[265,266] nuclear imaging,[267–270] and MRI.[271] However, these radiologic studies can only help in assessing anatomic integrity of other possible nociceptive sources that may mimic sacroiliac joint pain, such as the lumbar intervertebral disc. Imaging studies may be helpful in other disorders, which may affect the sacroiliac joint, such as hyperparathyroidism, fracture, Reiter's syndrome, psoriatic arthritis, ankylosing spondylitis, rheumatoid arthritis, and septic sacroiliitis.

VALIDITY

The face validity of sacroiliac joint block has been established by injecting small volumes of local anesthetic with contrast into the target joint and determining the contrast spread in posterior, anterior, and lateral radiographs. Construct validity of sacroiliac joint blocks is also extremely important to avoid the placebo effect. Maigne et al.[248] established that the false-positive rate of single, uncontrolled, sacroiliac joint injections was 20%. False-positive injection may occur with extravasation of anesthetic agent out of the joint secondary to defects in the joint capsule. False-negative results may occur from faulty needle placement, intravascular injection, or inability of the local anesthetic agent to reach the painful portion of the joint due to loculations.

PREVALENCE

Multiple authors have shown sacroiliac joint pain to be 10 to 30% by a single block[26,247] and 10 to 19% by a double-block paradigm.[27,248]

EVIDENCE

The validity of sacroiliac joint diagnostic injections has been established as moderate.[1]

SAFETY AND COMPLICATIONS

Complications of sacroiliac joint injection include infection, trauma to the sciatic nerve, and others related to drug administration. Without fluoroscopy, successful joint injection, as documented with CT, is successful in only 22% of procedures.[272] Notable in the study was epidural spread in 24% of the procedures or foraminal filling in 44% sacroiliac joint injections. Others have demonstrated similar findings.[251,252,273]

THERAPEUTIC INTERVENTIONAL TECHNIQUES

Interventional techniques in the management of chronic spinal pain include neural blockade and minimally invasive surgical procedures ranging from epidural injections, facet joint injections, and neuroablation techniques, to intradiscal thermal therapy, disc decompression, morphine pump implantation, and spinal cord stimulation.

RATIONALE

The rationale for therapeutic interventional techniques in the spine is based on several considerations:

- Cardinal source(s) of chronic spinal pain, namely discs and joints, are accessible to neural blockade

- Removal or correction of structural abnormalities of the spine may fail to cure and may even worsen painful conditions
- Degenerative processes of the spine and the origin of spinal pain are complex
- The effectiveness of a large variety of therapeutic interventions in managing chronic spinal pain has not been demonstrated conclusively

FACILITIES

The requirements for therapeutic interventions include a sterile operating room or procedure room, monitoring equipment, radiological equipment, special equipment based on technique, sterile preparation with all the resuscitative equipment, needles, gowns, injectate agents, intravenous fluids, sedative agents, and trained personnel for preparation and monitoring of the patients. Minimum requirements include history and physical examination, informed consent, appropriate documentation of the procedure.

CONTRAINDICATIONS

Contraindications include bacterial infection, possible pregnancy, bleeding diathesis, and anticoagulant therapy. Precautions are warranted in patients with anticoagulant or antiplatelet therapy, diabetes mellitus, or artificial heart valves.

FACET JOINT INTERVENTIONS

A preponderance of evidence supports the existence of facet joint pain;[1–3,22–27,49,58–81,84–86,88,97–117,274–315] however, there are also a few detractors.[316–318] Facet joint pain may be managed by either intra-articular injections, medical branch blocks, or neurolysis of medial branches. An extensive, evidence-based review[1] considered relief with intra-articular injections or medial branch blocks as short term if it was documented for less than 3 months and long-term if it was documented for longer than 3 months. Relief with medial branch neurotomy was considered short-term if it was less than 6 months and long-term it if was longer than 6 months.

INTRA-ARTICULAR BLOCKS

Therapeutic benefit has been reported with the injection of corticosteroids, local anesthetics, or normal saline into the facet joints. The literature describing the effectiveness of these interventions is abundant. However, no systematic reviews have been performed. Five randomized clinical trials offer data on the use of intra-articular injections in the spine.[274–278] Controlled and uncontrolled clinical studies that evaluated the long-term relief of back and leg pain from intra-articular facet joint injections are abundant.

The well-controlled trials of both Carette et al.[274] and Barnsley et al.[275] were described as negative by the authors. Manchikanti et al.[1] concluded that only one randomized trial by Carette et al.[274] was considered positive in contrast to the second randomized trial by Barnsley et al.,[275] which was negative. Among the nonrandomized trials, positive results were noted for short-term relief in all the studies; however, long-term relief was noted only in three of the five studies.[94,283–286,315]

Manchikanti et al.[1] concluded that the evidence of intra-articular injections of local anesthetics and steroids from randomized trials, complemented with that of nonrandomized trials (prospective and retrospective evaluations), provided moderate evidence of short-term relief and limited evidence of long-term relief of chronic neck and low back pain.

MEDIAL BRANCH BLOCKS

Medial branch blocks have been extensively used for diagnostic and prognostic purposes with limited use for therapeutic purposes. The therapeutic role of medial branch blocks was evaluated in three randomized clinical trials[276,277,291] and five nonrandomized clinical trials.[97,101,319–321]

Based on the review of the current studies, it appears that the evidence of medial branch blocks is strong for short-term relief and moderate for long-term relief of pain of facet joint origin.

MEDIAL BRANCH NEUROTOMY

Percutaneous radiofrequency neurotomy of medial branches is a procedure that offers temporary relief of pain by denaturing the nerves that innervate the painful joint. However, the pain returns when the axons regenerate. This return of pain can be managed by repeating the procedure and reinstating the relief.[297] Radiofrequency neurotomy is a neurolytic technique.

There have been three systematic reviews of medial branch neurotomy.[322–324] Two[322,324] of the three reviews were marred with inappropriate methodology and inaccurate conclusions. Manchikanti et al.[323] also evaluated the medial branch neurotomy in the management of chronic spinal pain. This review used inclusion/exclusion criteria and search strategy, and followed key domains in rating quality of systematic reviews as described by the Agency for Healthcare Research and Quality (AHRQ).[325]

Manchikanti et al.[1,323] concluded that the evidence for radiofrequency neurotomy of medial branches was strong for short-term relief (less than 6 months) and moderate for long-term relief (6 months or longer) of chronic spinal pain of facet joint origin.

SAFETY AND COMPLICATIONS

Potential side effects with radiofrequency denervation include painful cutaneous dysesthesias, increased pain due to neuritis or neurogenic inflammation, anesthesia dolorosa, cutaneous hyperesthesia, pneumothorax, and deafferentation pain.

EPIDURAL INJECTIONS

Epidural injection of corticosteroids is one of the commonly used interventions in managing chronic spinal pain.[1–3,327,328] Several approaches are available to access the lumbar epidural space: caudal, interlaminar, and transforaminal. Epidural administration of corticosteroids is one of the subjects most studied in interventional pain management with the most systematic reviews available.

Numerous systematic reviews of effectiveness of epidural steroid injections have reached contradictory conclusions, mostly negative and a few positive.[1–3,327–338]

Epidural injections may be performed by three approaches. There are substantial differences between the three approaches.[1–3,327,328]

- The interlaminar entry is directed more closely to the assumed site of pathology, requiring less volume than the caudal route.
- The caudal entry is relatively easily achieved, with minimal risk of inadvertent dural puncture.
- The transforaminal approach is target specific with smallest volume in fulfilling the aim of reaching the primary site of pathology, namely, ventrolateral epidural space.

Disadvantages of the caudal approach include[1–3,327,346–367]

- Requirement of substantial volume of fluid
- Dilution of the injectate
- Extra-epidural placement of the needle
- Increased risk for intravascular placement of the needle

Disadvantages of interlaminar approach include[1–3,325,326,346–367]

- Dilution of the injectate
- Extra-epidural placement of the needle
- Intravascular placement of the needle
- Preferential cranial flow of the solution
- Preferential posterior flow of the solution
- Difficult placement (with increased risk) in postsurgical patients
- Difficult placement below L4/5 interspace
- Deviation of needle to nondependent side
- Dural puncture
- Trauma to spinal cord

Disadvantages of the transforaminal approach include[1–3,327,328,368–380]

- Intraneural injection
- Neural trauma
- Technical difficulty in presence of fusion and/or hardware
- Intravascular injection
- Spinal cord trauma

Due to the inherent variations, differences, advantages, and disadvantages applicable to each technique (including the effectiveness and outcomes), caudal epidural injections, interlaminar (cervical, thoracic, and lumbar) epidural injections, and transforaminal (cervical, thoracic, and lumbosacral) epidural injections are considered separate entities within epidural injections and are discussed as such below.

Manchikanti et al.[1] and Boswell et al.,[328] after considering a multitude of systematic reviews, along with randomized, as well as nonrandomized trials for each category, namely, interlaminar, caudal, and transforaminal epidural injections, considered short-term effect as significant relief of less than 3 months and long-term effect as 3 months or longer.

CAUDAL EPIDURAL INJECTIONS

There was only one systematic review[328] and one evidence-based review[1] evaluating caudal epidural injections. There were nine studies either randomized or double blind,[381–389] three prospective trials,[390–392] and many retrospective evaluations[1–3] examining the effectiveness of caudal epidural injections.

Boswell et al.[328] and Manchikanti et al.[1] included eight randomized or double-blind trials, of which five were positive for short-term relief and five were positive for long-term relief with multiple injections.[381,382,386–388] Further, all prospective trials[390–392] and all (four) retrospective trials[1] were positive for short-term and long-term relief with multiple injections.

The combined evidence of caudal epidural steroid injections with randomized trials and nonrandomized trials (prospective and retrospective trials) is strong for short-term relief and moderate for long-term relief.

INTERLAMINAR EPIDURAL INJECTIONS

Multiple systematic reviews provided contradictory and confusing opinions. Further, most of the systematic reviews utilized combined caudal and interlaminar epidural steroid injections, thus, no reasonable conclusions may be drawn from these systematic reviews, and their conclusions may not be applied in clinical practice settings. However, studies in the literature evaluating the effectiveness of interlaminar epidural injections, specifically the lumbar epidural injections, are extensive. Multiple evaluations included 16 randomized or double-blind trials,[393–408]

eight non-randomized prospective trials, and multiple other observational trials.[1,409–417]

Of the 16 randomized trials, 10 included an evaluation, 7 were positive for short-term relief, whereas only 3 were positive for long-term relief. Numerous nonrandomized trials, both prospective and retrospective, reported good results in 18 to 90% of patients receiving cervical or lumbar interlaminar epidural steroid injections.

Among the three prospective trials included for evaluation, one was positive, one was indeterminate, and one was negative. Boswell et al.[328] and Manchikanti et al.[1] concluded that the evidence for the overall effectiveness of interlaminar epidural steroid injections in managing chronic low back pain was moderate for short-term relief and limited for long-term relief. There was no evidence of effectiveness of interlaminar epidural steroids in managing spinal stenosis.[410,411] Further, multiple evaluations[412–414] failed to identify predictive factors in administration of interlaminar epidural steroid injections.

TRANSFORAMINAL EPIDURAL INJECTIONS

Transforaminal epidural injections have emerged recently as a target-specific modality of treatment for management of spinal pain. Review of the literature showed seven randomized trials,[405,417–423] nine prospective evaluations,[409,412–415,424–431] one prospective evaluation of change in disc herniation,[432] and multiple retrospective reports.[1,433–435]

Manchikanti et al.[1] and Boswell et al.[328] synthesized the evidence with inclusion of multiple evaluations, all of them showing positive short-term and long-term effectiveness of transforaminal epidural steroids in managing nerve root pain. Based on all the evidence, transforaminal epidural injections provide strong evidence for short-term relief and moderate evidence for long-term relief. Their effectiveness in postlumbar laminectomy syndrome and disc extrusions was inconclusive.

SAFETY AND COMPLICATIONS

The most common and worrisome complications of caudal, interlaminar, and transforaminal epidural injections are of two types: those related to the needle placement, and those related to drug administration. Complications include dural puncture, spinal cord trauma, infection, hematoma formation, abscess formation, subdural injection, intracranial air injection, epidural lipomatosis, pneumothorax, nerve damage, headache, death, brain damage, increased intracranial pressure, intravascular injection, vascular injury, cerebral vascular or pulmonary embolus, and effects of steroids.[1–3,129,130,368–380,433–486] Spinal cord trauma and spinal cord or epidural hematoma formation are catastrophic complications that are rarely seen following interventional procedures in the cervical spine, thoracic spine, or upper lumbar spine.[357–361] There are growing concerns about the potential risk of unintended intravascular injections that occur during the performance of transforaminal epidural steroid injections. Disastrous, but apparently rare injuries have occurred, which may be due to injection of particulate steroid into spinal arteries that enter the spinal canal adjacent to exiting nerve roots.[369–380] Complications have been reported with cervical and lumbar transforaminal injections.

Side effects related to the administration of steroids are generally attributed either to the chemistry or to the pharmacology of the steroids. The major theoretical complications of corticosteroid administration include suppression of pituitary-adrenal axis, hypercorticism, Cushing's syndrome, osteoporosis, avascular necrosis of bone, steroid myopathy, epidural lipomatosis, weight gain, fluid retention, and hyperglycemia.[1–3,129,474–486] However, evaluation of the effect of neuraxial steroids on weight and bone mass density noted no significant difference in patients undergoing various types of interventional techniques with or without steroids.[130] The most commonly used steroids in neural blockade in the United States, methylprednisolone acetate, triamcinolone acetonide, and betamethasone acetate and phosphate mixture, have all been shown to be safe at epidural therapeutic doses in both clinical and experimental studies.[1–3,129]

ADHESIOLYSIS

The purpose of epidural lysis of adhesions is to eliminate deleterious effects of scar formation, which can physically prevent direct application of drugs to nerves or other tissues to treat chronic back pain. The goal of percutaneous lysis of epidural adhesions is to assure delivery of high concentrations of injected drugs to the target areas. Epidural lysis of adhesions and direct deposition of corticosteroids in the spinal canal are also achieved with a three-dimensional view provided by epiduroscopy or spinal endoscopy.

PERCUTANEOUS ADHESIOLYSIS

Manchikanti et al.[1] in their evaluation, considered duration of relief of less than 3 months as short-term and longer than 3 months as long-term, for percutaneous adhesiolysis. In contrast, for spinal endoscopic adhesiolysis, 6 months of relief was considered short-term and longer than 6 months was considered long-term.

In the evidence synthesis for percutaneous epidural adhesiolysis using a spring-guided catheter with or without hypertonic saline neurolysis to evaluate the clinical effectiveness, three randomized controlled trials[487–489] and multiple nonrandomized evaluations[490–493] were included. Thus, it appears that evidence for effectiveness of percutaneous adhesiolysis is strong for short-term and moderate for long-term relief with repeat interventions.

SPINAL ENDOSCOPIC ADHESIOLYSIS

Evidence synthesis for spinal endoscopy included one randomized, double-blind trial,[494,495] two prospective evaluations,[496,497] and two retrospective evaluations[493,498] showing strong evidence for short-term relief (less than 6 months) and moderate for long-term relief (greater than 6 months).

SAFETY AND COMPLICATIONS

The most common and worrisome complications of adhesiolysis and spinal endoscopy with lysis of adhesions are related to dural puncture, spinal cord compression, catheter shearing, infection, steroids, hypertonic saline, hyaluronidase, instrumentation with endoscope, and administration of high volumes of fluids potentially resulting in excessive epidural hydrostatic pressures. Hypertonic saline injected into the subarachnoid space has been reported to cause cardiac arrhythmias, myelopathy, paralysis, and loss of sphincter control.[499] Aldrete, Zapata, & Ghaly,[500] in a case report, attributed incidences of arachnoiditis following epidural adhesiolysis with hypertonic saline to subarachnoid leakage of hypertonic saline. However, there were multiple variations in the technique and injection of hypertonic saline, (intraoperatively or injecting in spite of subarachnoid blockade), which may be responsible for these complications. While there are multiple reports with experience of hypertonic saline solution, there are no controlled reports of potential adverse effects.[501–505]

Another specific complication of percutaneous epidural adhesiolysis is related to catheter shearing and its retention in the epidural space.[506] Additionally, a troublesome complication is that of excessive intraspinal pressure development with its potential to affect both local and distant profusion, and resulting in visual changes and even blindness. Even though the incidence is rare, it appears that this would be much higher with spinal endoscopic procedures with a combination of high volumes of fluid and generation of high hydrostatic pressures.[507] It is also possible with catheter-based adhesiolysis if excessive amounts of fluids are injected rapidly.

Spinal cord trauma or spinal cord or epidural hematoma formation is a catastrophic complication possible with both catheter-based or endoscopic adhesiolysis, however, more so with endoscopic adhesiolysis. But, there are no such case reports in the literature. Understanding fluoroscopic imaging is crucial to avoid disastrous complications.[508]

INTRADISCAL THERAPIES

Commensurate with our improved ability to identify painful discs and image spinal anatomy are the advances achieved in the treatment of spinal disorders.[509] During the past few decades, numerous authors have reported on percutaneously administered minimally invasive spinal surgery techniques to manage discogenic pain. Procedures investigated have been chymopapain injection to achieve nucleolysis, percutaneous disc decompression with nucleotomy using coblation technology (nucleoplasty), and intradiscal electrothermal therapy (IDET). Manchikanti et al.[1] defined relief of 6 months or less as short-term, whereas long-term was over 6 months.

INTRADISCAL ELECTROTHERMAL THERAPY

IDET intervention is applicable solely for the patient with axial symptoms and is not indicated for radicular pain.[509] IDET is performed by introducing a flexible catheter, containing a resistive coil, into the disc. IDET has been shown to provide precision temperature control.[510–512]

The present evidence for intradiscal electrothermal therapy appears to be controversial with limited evidence for short-term as well as long-term relief.[510,512–516]

Safety and Complications

Infrequent complications were reported, including catheter breakage in 19 of 35,000 catheters used (0.05%) and six nerve root injuries; there were six cases of post-IDET disc herniation at the treated level transpiring 2 to 12 months post-treatment in 1,675 patients.[517] Two separate case reports of cauda equina syndrome have been reported.[518,519]

PERCUTANEOUS DISC DECOMPRESSION

Percutaneous disc decompression (PDD) with nucleoplasty (coblation technology) is performed with radiofrequency energy, used to dissolve nuclear material through molecular dissociation.[520–522] It is believed that this reduced volume of disc material results in reduced intradiscal pressure. Bipolar radiofrequency coagulation further denatures proteoglycans, changing the internal environment of the affected nucleus pulposus, which showed changes in intradiscal pressure following coblation. The present evidence for PDD is limited.

Safety and Complications

Safety and complications are expected to be similar to those for discography and IDET, even though none have been reported thus far.

IMPLANTABLE THERAPIES

Spinal cord stimulation systems and implantable intrathecal devices are frequently used in managing chronic intractable pain.[523,524]

SPINAL CORD STIMULATION

The mechanism of action of spinal cord stimulation is not completely understood. However, recent research has given us insight into effects occurring at the local and supraspinal levels, and through dorsal horn interneuron and neurochemical mechanisms.[525,526]

There have been multiple reviews evaluating the effectiveness of spinal cord stimulation in low back and lower extremity pain,[1,527] along with a few prospective controlled trials.[528–530] Based on this, it appears that the evidence for spinal cord stimulation in properly selected population with neuropathic pain is moderate for long-term relief (longer than 6 months).

Safety and Complications

Complications with spinal cord stimulation range from simple, easily correctable problems, such as lack of appropriate paraesthesia coverage, to devastating complications such as paralysis, nerve injury, and death.[529–533]

IMPLANTABLE INTRATHECAL DRUG ADMINISTRATION SYSTEMS

Spinal administration of opioid and non-opioid medication has been increasingly advocated for those patients who fail to achieve pain relief or experience undue side effects with oral opioid regimens.[534]

With inclusion of multiple trials,[535–542] in the evidence synthesis, there is moderate evidence indicating the long-term effectiveness of intrathecal infusion systems (longer than 6 months).

Safety and Complications

The complication rate appears to average about 20%. The most common immediate problems include postdural puncture headache, infection, nausea, urinary retention, and pruritus. Long-term complications seen post-implant include catheter and pump failure. The high rate of device-related complications identified in the literature is certainly concerning from a patient safety and cost-effectiveness perspective. Catheter complication rates tend to range from 10 to 40% with pump complications somewhat lower. The incidence of granuloma based on reporting to the FDA and device manufacturers appears to be less than 1%.[543] Commonly reported drug-related complications include pedal edema and hormonal changes leading to decreased libido and sexual dysfunction.

REFERENCES

1. Manchikanti, L. et al. (2003). Evidence-based practice guidelines for interventional techniques in the management of chronic spinal pain. *Pain Physician, 6*, 3.

2. Manchikanti, L. et al. (2001). Interventional techniques in the management of chronic pain: Part 2.0. *Pain Physician, 4,* 24.

3. Manchikanti, L. et al. (2000). Interventional techniques in the management of chronic pain. Part 1.0. *Pain Physician, 3,* 7.

4. Practice guidelines for chronic pain management. (1997). Report by the American Society of Anesthesiologists Task Force on Pain Management, Chronic Pain Section. *Anesthesiology, 86,* 995.

5. American Geriatrics Society. (1998). The management of chronic pain in older persons: New guidelines from the American Geriatrics Society. *Journal of the American Geriatrics Society, 46,* 128.

6. Sanders, S. H. et al. (1999). Clinical practice guidelines for chronic non-malignant pain syndrome patients II: An evidence-based approach. *Journal of Back Musculoskeletal Rehabilitation, 13,* 47.

7. Verhaak, P. F. M. et al. (1998). Prevalence of chronic benign pain disorder among adults: A review of the literature. *Pain, 77,* 231.

8. Elliott, A. M. et al. (1999). The epidemiology of chronic pain in the community. *Lancet, 354,* 1248.

9. Blyth, F. M. et al. (2001). Chronic pain in Australia: A prevalence study. *Pain, 89,* 127.

10. Menefee, L. A. et al. (2000). Sleep disturbance and nonmalignant chronic pain: A comprehensive review of the literature. *Pain Medicine, 1,* 156.

11. Bressler, H. B. et al. (1999). The prevalence of low back pain in the elderly. A systemic review of the literature. *Spine, 24,* 1813.

12. Pahor, M., Guralnik, J. M., & Wan J. Y. (1999). Lower body osteoarticular pain and dose of analgesic medications in older disabled women: The women's health and aging study. *American Journal of Public Health, 89,* 930.

13. VanDen Kerkhof, E. G. et al. (2003). The impact of the sampling and measurement on the prevalence of self-reported pain in Canada. *Pain Research and Management, 8,* 157.

14. Asch, S. M. et al. (2000). Measuring underuse of necessary care among elderly Medicare beneficiaries using inpatient and outpatient claims. *Journal of the American Medical Association, 284,* 2325.

15. Hoffmann, D. E. (1998). Pain management and palliative care in the era of managed care: Issue for health insurers. *Journal of Law, Medicine, & Ethics, 26,* 267.

16. Gureje, O. et al. (1998). Persistent pain and well being: A World Health Organization Study in primary care. *Journal of the American Medical Association, 280,* 147.

17. Covington, E. C. (2000). Psychogenic pain – What it means, why it does not exist, and how to diagnose it. *Pain Medicine, 1,* 287.

18. Gagliese, L., & Katz, J. (2000). Medically unexplained pain is not caused by psychopathology. *Pain Research and Management, 5,* 251.

19. Bogduk, N., & McGuirk, B. (2002). Causes and sources of chronic low back pain. In N. Bogduk & B. McGuirk (Eds.), *Medical management of acute and chronic low back pain. An evidence-based approach: Pain research and clinical management* (Vol. 13, pp. 115). Amsterdam: Elsevier Science BV.

20. Hendler, N. H., Bergson, C., & Morrison, C. (1996). Overlooked physical diagnoses in chronic pain patients involved in litigation. Part 2. *Psychosomatics, 37,* 509.

21. Hendler, N. H., & Kolodny, A. L. (1992). Using medication wisely in chronic pain. *Patient Care, 15,* 125.

22. Bogduk, N. (1997). *Clinical anatomy of the lumbar spine and sacrum* (3rd ed.). New York: Churchill Livingstone.

23. Kuslich, S. D., Ulstrom, C. L., & Michael, C. J. (1991). The tissue origin of low back pain and sciatica: A report of pain response to tissue stimulation during operation on the lumbar spine using local anesthesia. *Orthopedic Clinics of North America, 22,* 181.

24. Manchikanti, L., Singh, V., & Fellows B. (2002). Structural basis of chronic low back pain. In L. Manchikanti, C. W. Slipman, & B. Fellows (Eds.), *Interventional pain management: Low back pain – Diagnosis and treatment* (p. 77). Paducah, KY: ASIPP Publishing.

25. Cavanaugh, J. M. et al. (1997). Mechanisms of low back pain: A neurophysiologic and neuroanatomic study. *Clinical Orthopedics, 335,* 166.

26. Pang, W. W. et al. (1998). Application of spinal pain mapping in the diagnosis of low back pain — Analysis of 104 cases. *Acta Anaesthesiologica. Sinica, 36,* 71.

27. Manchikanti, L. et al. (2001). Evaluation of the relative contributions of various structures in chronic low back pain. *Pain Physician, 4,* 308.

28. Fox, E. J., & Melzack, R. (1976). Transcutaneous electrical stimulation to acupuncture. Comparison of treatment of low back pain. *Pain, 2,* 141.

29. Byrod, G. et al. (2000). Methylprednisolone reduces the early vascular permeability increase in spinal nerve roots induced by epidural nucleus pulposus application. *Journal of Orthopedic Research, 18,* 983.

30. Flower, R. J., & Blackwell, G. J. (1979). Anti-inflammatory steroid induced biosynthesis of a phospholipase A2 inhibitor which prevents prostaglandin generation. *Nature, 278,* 456.

31. Devor, M., Govrin-Lippmann, R., & Raber, P. (1985). Corticosteroids suppress ectopic neural discharges originating in experimental neuromas. *Pain, 22,* 127.

32. Johansson, A., Hao, J., & Sjolund, B. (1990). Local corticosteroid application blocks transmission in normal nociceptor C-fibers. *Acta Anaesthesiologica Scandinavica, 34,* 335.

33. Olmarker, K. et al. (1994). Effects of methylprednisolone on nucleus pulposus-induced nerve root injury. *Spine, 19,* 1803.

34. Hua, S. Y., & Chen, Y. Z. (1989). Membrane receptor-mediated electrophysiological effects of glucocorticoid on mammalian neurons. *Endocrinology, 124,* 687.

35. Hayashi, N. et al. (1998). The effect of epidural injection of betamethasone or bupivacaine in a rat model of lumbar radiculopathy. *Spine, 23,* 877.

36. Lee, H. M. et al. (1998). The role of steroids and their effects on phospholipase A2. An animal model of radiculopathy. *Spine, 23,* 1191.

37. Minamide, A. et al. (1998). Effects of steroids and lipopolysaccharide on spontaneous resorption of herniated intervertebral discs. An experience study in the rabbit. *Spine, 23,* 870.

38. Kingery, W. S., Castellote, J. M., & Maze, M. (1999). Methylprednisolone prevents the development of autotomy and neuropathic edema in rats, but has no effect on nociceptive thresholds. *Pain, 80,* 555.

39. Johansson, A., & Bennett, G. J. (1997). Effect of local methylprednisolone on pain in a nerve injury model. A pilot study. *Regional Anesthesia, 22,* 59.

40. Merskey, H., & Thompson, E. N. (2002). Nerve blocks and cognitive therapy: A beneficial failure. *Pain Research and Management, 7,* 175.

41. Wall, P. D. (1998). New horizons. an essay. In M. J. Cousins & P. O. Bridenbaugh (Eds.), *Neural blockade* (3rd ed., p. 1135). Philadelphia: Lippincott-Raven.

42. Kim, S. H. et al. (1993). Effects of sympathetectomy on a rat model of peripheral neuropathy. *Pain, 55,* 85.

43. McCormack, K. (1999). Signal transduction in neuropathic pain, with special emphasis on the analgesic role of opioids – Part I: The basic science of phenotype expression in normal and regenerating nerves. *Pain Review, 6,* 3.

44. McCormack, K. (1999). Signal transduction in neuropathic pain, with special emphasis on the analgesic role of opioids – Part II: Moving basic science towards a new pharmacotherapy. *Pain Review, 6,* 99.

45. Watkins, L., Milligan, E. D., & Maier, S. F. (2001). Spinal glia: New players in pain, *Pain, 93,* 201.

46. Li, Y. M. et al. (1995). Local anesthetics inhibit substance P binding and evoked increases in intracellular Ca2+. *Anesthesiology, 82,* 166.

47. Bonica, J. J., Backup, P. H., & Anderson, C. E. (1957). Peridural block, an analysis of 3,637 cases. A review. *Anesthesiology, 18,* 723.

48. Fink, B. R., & Cairns, A. M. (1987). Differential use-dependent (frequency-dependent) effects in single mammalian axons: Data and clinical considerations. *Anesthesiology, 67,* 477.

49. Bogduk, N. (1997). International Spinal Injection Society guidelines for the performance of spinal injection procedures. Part 1: Zygapophyseal joint blocks. *Clinical Journal of Pain, 13,* 285.

50. Hogan, Q. H., & Abram, S. E. (1997). Neural blockade for diagnosis and prognosis. *Anesthesiology, 86,* 216.

51. Deyo, R. A., & Weinstein, J. N. (2001). Low back pain. *New England Journal of Medicine, 344,* 363.

52. Deyo, R. A., Rainville, J., & Kent, D. L. (1992). What can the history and physical examination tell us about low back pain? *Journal of the American Medical Association, 268,* 760.

53. Hildebrandt, J. (2001). Relevance of nerve blocks in treating and diagnosing low back pain – Is the quality decisive? *Schmerz, 15,* 474.

54. Nachemson, A., & Vingård, E. (2000). Assessment of patients with neck and back pain: A best-evidence synthesis. In A. Nachemson & E. Jonsson (Eds.), *Neck and back pain. The scientific evidence of causes, diagnosis and treatment* (p. 189). Philadelphia: Lippincott Williams & Wilkins.

55. Ramsey, S. D. et al. (1998). The limited state of technology assessment for medical devices: Facing the issues. *American Journal of Managed Care, 4,* 188.

56. Jaeschke, R., Guyatt, G., & Lijmer, J. (2002). Diagnostic tests. In G. Guyatt & D. Rennie (Eds.), *Users' guides to the medical literature – A manual for evidence-based clinical practice* (p. 121). Chicago: AMA Press.

57. Sackett, D. L. et al. (1991). *Clinical epidemiology, a basic science for clinical medicine* (2nd ed., p. 53). Boston: Little, Brown and Company.

58. Saal, J. S. (2002). General principles of diagnostic testing as related to painful lumbar spine disorders. *Spine, 27,* 2538.

59. Manchikanti, L., Singh, V., & Pampati, V. (2003). Are diagnostic lumbar medial branch blocks valid? Results of 2-year follow up. *Pain Physician, 6,* 147.

60. Bogduk, N., & Lord, S. (1998). Cervical zygapophysial joint pain. *Neurosurgery Quarterly, 8,* 107.

61. Schwarzer, A. C. et al. (1994). The value of the provocation response in lumbar zygapophysial joint injections. *Clinical Journal of Pain, 10,* 309.

62. Barnsley, L., Lord, S., & Bogduk, N. (1993). Comparative local anesthetic blocks in the diagnosis of cervical zygapophysial joints pain. *Pain, 55,* 99.

63. Lord, S. M., Barnsley, L., & Bogduk, N. (1995). The utility of comparative local anesthetic blocks versus placebo-controlled blocks for the diagnosis of cervical zygapophysial joint pain. *Clinical Journal of Pain, 11,* 208.

64. Fukui, S. et al. (1996). Referred pain distribution of the cervical zygapophyseal joints and cervical dorsal rami. *Pain, 68,* 79.

65. Dwyer, A., Aprill, C., & Bogduk, N. (1990). Cervical zygapophyseal joint pain patterns: A study in normal volunteers. *Spine, 15,* 453.

66. Aprill, C., Dwyer, A., & Bogduk, N. (1990). The prevalence of cervical zygapophyseal joint pain patterns II: A clinical evaluation. *Spine, 15,* 458.

67. Pawl, R. P. (1977). Headache, cervical spondylosis, and anterior cervical fusion. *Surgery Annals, 9,* 391.

68. Dreyfuss, P., Tibiletti, C., & Dreyer, S. J. (1994). Thoracic zygapophyseal joint pain patterns: A study in normal volunteers. *Spine, 19,* 807.

69. Mooney, V. and Robertson, J. (1976). The facet syndrome. *Clinical Orthopedics, 115,* 149.

70. McCall, I. W., Park, W. M., and O'Brien, J. P. (1979). Induced pain referral from posterior elements in normal subjects. *Spine, 4,* 441.

71. Marks, R. (1989). Distribution of pain provoked from lumbar facet joints and related structures during diagnostic spinal infiltration. *Pain, 39,* 37.

72. Fukui, S. et al. (1997). Distribution of referral pain from the lumbar zygapophyseal joints and dorsal rami. *Clinical Journal of Pain, 13,* 303.

73. Hirsch, C., Ingelmark, B. E., & Miller, M. (1963). The anatomical basis for low back pain. *Acta Orthopaedica Scandinavica, 33*, 1.

74. Windsor, R. E. et al. (2002). Electrical stimulation induced lumbar medial branch referral patterns. *Pain Physician, 5*, 405.

75. Windsor, R. E. et al. (2003). Electrical stimulation induced cervical medial branch referral patterns. *Pain Physician, 6*, 411.

76. Helbig, T., & Lee, C.K. (1988). The lumbar facet syndrome. *Spine, 13*, 61.

77. Revel, M. E. et al. (1992). Facet joint block for low back pain: identifying predictors of a good response. *Archives of Physical Medicine and Rehabilitation., 73*, 824.

78. Revel, M. et al. (1998). Capacity of the clinical picture to characterize low back pain relieved by facet joint anesthesia. Proposed criteria to identify patients with painful facet joints. *Spine, 23*, 1972.

79. Schwarzer, A. C. et al. (1994). Clinical features of patients with pain stemming from the lumbar zygapophysial joints. Is the lumbar facet syndrome a clinical entity? *Spine, 19*, 1132.

80. Manchikanti, L. et al. (2000). The inability of the clinical picture to characterize pain from facet joints. *Pain Physician, 3*, 158.

81. Schwarzer, A. C. et al. (1994). Pain from the lumbar zygapophysial joints: A test of two models. *Journal of Spinal Disorders, 7*, 331.

82. Faye, L. J., & Wiles, M. R. (1992). Manual examination of the spine. In S. Haldeman (Ed.), *Principles and practice of chiropractic* (2nd ed., p. 301). San Mateo, CA: Appleton & Lange.

83. Schafer, R. C., & Faye, L. J. (1990). *Motion palpation and chiropractic technique* (2nd ed.). Huntington Beach, CA: The Motion Palpation Institute.

84. Schwarzer, A. C. et al. (1995). Prevalence and clinical features of lumbar zygapophysial joint pain: A study in an Australian population with chronic low back pain. *American Rheumatic Diseases, 54*, 100.

85. Young, S., Aprill, C., & Laslett, M. (2003). Correlation of clinical examination characteristics with three sources of chronic low back pain. *Spine Journal, 3*, 460.

86. Schwarzer, A. C. et al. (1992). The role of bone scintigraphy in chronic low back pain: A comparison of SPECT and planar images and zygapophysial joint injection. *Australian and New Zealand Journal of Medicine, 22*, 185.

87. Taylor, J. R., & Twomey, L. T. (1993). Acute injuries to cervical joints: An autopsy study of neck sprain. *Spine, 9*, 1115.

88. Schwarzer, A. C. et al. (1995). The ability of computed tomography to identify a painful zygapophysial joint in patients with chronic low back pain. *Spine, 20*, 907.

89. Binet, E. F. et al. (1977). Cervical spine tomography in trauma. *Spine, 2*, 163.

90. Abel, M. S. (1975). Occult traumatic lesions of the cervical vertebrae. *Critical Reviews in Clinical Radiology and Nuclear Medicine, 6*, 469.

91. Woodring, J. H., & Goldstein, S. J. (1982). Fractures of the articular processes of the cervical spine. *American Journal of Roentgenology, 139*, 341.

92. Magora, A. et al. (1994). The significance of medical imaging findings in low back pain. *Pain Clinic, 7*, 99.

93. Wiesel, S. W. et al. (1984). A study of computer assisted tomography I: The incidence of positive CAT scans in an asymptomatic group of patients. *Spine, 9*, 549.

94. Murtagh, F. R. (1988). Computed tomography and fluoroscopy guided anesthesia and steroid injection in facet syndrome. *Spine, 13*, 686.

95. Jonsson, H. et al. (1991). Hidden cervical spine injuries in traffic accident victims with skull fractures. *Journal of Spinal Disease, 4*, 251.

96. Destouet, J. M., & Murphy, W. A. (1985). Lumbar facet blocks: Indications and techniques. *Orthopedic Review, 14*, 57.

97. Barnsley, L., & Bogduk, N. (1993). Medial branch blocks are specific for the diagnosis of cervical zygapophyseal joint pain. *Regional Anesthesia, 18*, 343.

98. Manchikanti, L. et al. (2001). Influence of psychological factors on the ability of diagnose chronic low back pain of facet joint origin. *Pain Physician, 4*, 349.

99. Dreyfuss, P. et al. (1997). Specificity of lumbar medial branch and L5 dorsal ramus blocks. *Spine, 22*, 895.

100. Kaplan, M. et al. (1998). The ability of lumbar medial branch blocks to anesthetize the zygapophysial joint. *Spine, 23*, 1847.

101. Manchikanti, L. et al. (2000). The diagnostic validity and therapeutic value of medial branch blocks with or without adjuvants agents. *Current Review of Pain, 4*, 337.

102. Manchikanti, L. et al. (1999). Prevalence of lumbar facet joint pain in chronic low back pain. *Pain Physician, 2*, 59.

103. Manchikanti, L. et al. (2002). Prevalence of cervical facet joint pain in chronic neck pain. *Pain Physician, 5*, 243.

104. Manchikanti, L et al. (2002). Is there correlation of facet joint pain in lumbar and cervical spine? *Pain Physician, 5*, 365.

105. Manchikanti, L. et al. (2002). Evaluation of the prevalence of facet joint pain in chronic thoracic pain. *Pain Physician, 5*, 354.

106. Manchikanti, L. et al. (2003). Chronic low back pain of facet (zygapophysial) joint origin: Is there a difference based on involvement of single or multiple spinal regions? *Pain Physician, 6*, 399.

107. Manchikanti, L. et al. (2004). Prevalence of facet joint pain in chronic spinal pain of cervical, thoracic, and lumbar regions. *BioMed Central Anesthesiology, 5*, 15.

108. Manchikanti, L. et al. (2001). Contribution of facet joints to chronic low back pain in postlumbar laminectomy syndrome: a controlled comparative prevalence evaluation. *Pain Physician, 4*, 175.

109. Manchikanti, L. et al. (2001). Role of facet joints in chronic low back pain in the elderly: A controlled comparative prevalence study. *Pain Practice, 1*, 332.

110. Manchikanti, L. et al. (2002). Evaluation of influence of gender, occupational injury, and smoking on chronic low back pain of facet joint origin: A subgroup analysis. *Pain Physician, 5*, 30.

111. Barnsley, L. et al. (1993). False-positive rates of cervical zygapophysial joint blocks. *Clinical Journal of Pain, 9*, 124.

112. Schwarzer, A. C. et al. (1994). The false-positive rate of uncontrolled diagnostic blocks of the lumbar zygapophysial joints. *Pain, 58*, 195.

113. Manchikanti, L. et al. (2001). Evaluation of role of facet joints in persistent low back pain in obesity: A controlled, perspective, comparative evaluation. *Pain Physician, 4*, 266.

114. Barnsley, L. et al. (1995). The prevalence of chronic cervical zygapophyseal joint pain after whiplash. *Spine, 20*, 20.

115. Lord, S. M. et al. (1996). Chronic cervical zygapophysial joint pain with whiplash: A placebo-controlled prevalence study. *Spine, 21*, 1737.

116. Speldewinde, G. C., Bashford, G. M., & Davidson, I. R. (2001). Diagnostic cervical zygapophyseal joint blocks for chronic cervical pain. *Medical Journal of Australia, 174*, 174.

117. Boswell, M. V. et al. (2003). Accuracy of precision diagnostic blocks in the diagnosis of chronic spinal pain of facet or zygapophysial joint origin. *Pain Physician, 6*, 449.

118. Thomson, S. J., Lomax, D. M., & Collett, B. J. (1991). Chemical meningism after lumbar facet joint nerve block with local anesthetic and steroids. *Anesthesia, 46*, 563.

119. Gladstone, J. C., & Pennant, J. H. (1987). Spinal anaesthesia following facet joint injection. *Anaesthesia, 42*, 754.

120. Gladstone, J. C., & Pennant, J. H. (1987). Spinal anaesthesia following facet joint injection. *Anaesthesia, 42*, 754.

121. Marks, R., & Semple, A. J. (1988). Spinal anaesthesia after facet joint injection. *Anaesthesia, 43*, 65.

122. Cook, N. J., Hanrahan, P., & Song, S. (1999). Paraspinal abscess following facet joint injection. *Clinical Rheumatology, 18*, 52.

123. Magee, M. et al. (2000). Paraspinal abscess complicating facet joint injection. *Clinical Nuclear Medicine, 25*, 71.

124. Berrigan, T. (1992). Chemical meningism after lumbar facet joint block. *Anesthesia, 47*, 905.

125. Manchikanti, L. et al. (2002). Radiation exposure to the physician in interventional pain management. *Pain Physician, 5*, 385.

126. Windsor, R. E., Storm, S., & Sugar, R. (2003). Prevention and management of complications resulting from common spinal injections. *Pain Physician, 6*, 473.

127. Manchikanti, L. et al. (2003). Effectiveness of protective measures in reducing risk of radiation exposure in interventional pain management: A prospective evaluation. *Pain Physician, 6*, 301.

128. Manchikanti, L. et al. (2003). Risk of whole body radiation exposure and protective measures in fluoroscopically guided interventional techniques: A prospective evaluation. *BioMed Central Anesthesiology, 3*, 2.

129. Manchikanti, L. (2002). Role of neuraxial steroids in interventional pain management. *Pain Physician, 5*, 182.

130. Manchikanti, L. et al. (2000). The effect of neuraxial steroids on weight and bone mass density: A prospective evaluation. *Pain Physician, 3*, 357.

131. Bogduk, N., & Marsland, A. (1986). On the concept of third occipital headache. *Journal of Neurology, Neurosurgery, and Psychiatry, 49*, 775.

132. Bogduk, N., Wilson, A. S., & Tynan, W. (1982). The human lumbar dorsal rami. *Journal of Anatomy, 134*, 383.

133. Inman, V. T., & Saunders, J. B. C. M. (1947). Anatomicophysiological aspects of injuries to the intervertebral disc. *Journal of Bone and Joint Surgery, 29*, 461.

134. Bogduk, N., Windsor, M., & Inglis, A. (1988). The innervation of the cervical intervertebral discs. *Spine, 13*, 2.

135. Mendel, T., Wink, C. S., & Zimny, M. L. (1992). Neural elements in human cervical intervertebral discs. *Spine, 17*, 132.

136. Jackson, H. C., Winkelmann, R. K., & Bickel, W. H. (1966). Nerve endings in the human lumbar spinal column and related structures. *Journal of Bone and Joint Surgery, 48A*, 1272.

137. Roofe, P. G. (1940). Innervation of annulus fibrosis and posterior longitudinal ligament. *Archives of Neurology and Psychiatry, 44*, 100.

138. Malinsky, J. (1959). The ontogenetic development of nerve trigeminations in the intervertebral discs of man. *Acta Anatomica, 38*, 96.

139. Yoshizawa, H. et al. (1980). The neuropathology of intervertebral discs removed for low back pain. *Journal of Pathology, 132*, 95.

140. Bogduk, N., Tynan, W., & Wilson, A. S. (1981). The nerve supply to the human lumbar intervertebral discs. *Journal of Anatomy, 132*, 39.

141. Freemont, A. J. et al. (1997). Nerve ingrowth into diseased intervertebral disc in chronic back pain. *Lancet, 350*, 178.

142. Coppes, M. H. et al. (1990). Innervation of annulus fibrosus in low back pain. *Lancet, 336*, 189.

143. Coppes, M. H. et al. (1997). Innervation of "painful" lumbar discs. *Spine, 22*, 2342.

144. Nakamura, S. et al. (1996). Origin of nerves supplying the posterior portion of lumbar intervertebral discs in rats. *Spine, 21*, 917.

145. Suseki, K. et al. (1998). Sensory nerve fibers from lumbar intervertebral discs pass through rami communicantes. *Journal of Bone and Joint Surgery, 80B*, 737.

146. Morinaga, T. et al. (1996). Sensory innervation to the anterior portion of lumbar intervertebral disc. *Spine, 21*, 1848.

147. Ohtori, S. et al. (1999). Sensory innervation of the dorsal portion of the lumbar intervertebral disc in rats. *Spine, 24*, 2295.

148. Groen, G., Baljet, B., & Drukker, J. (1990). Nerves and nerve plexuses of the human vertebral column. *American Journal of Anatomy, 188*, 282.

149. Edgar, M. A., & Ghadially, J. A. (1976). Innervation of the lumbar spine. *Clinical Orthopedics, 115*, 35.

150. Luschka, H. V. (1850). Die Nerven des menschlichen Wirbelkanales. *H. Laupp. Tubingen: H. Laupp.*

151. Bogduk, N. (1982). The clinical anatomy of the cervical dorsal rami. *Spine, 7*, 319.

152. Bogduk, N. (1994). Diskography. *APS Journal, 3*, 149.

153. Bogduk, N., & Modic, M. (1996). Controversy lumbar discography. *Spine, 21*, 402.

154. Schellhas, K. P., Pollei, S. R., & Dorwart, R. H. (1994). Thoracic discography. A safe and reliable technique. *Spine, 19*, 2103.

155. Davis, S. J. et al. (1994). Cervical spine hyperextension injuries: MRI findings. *Radiology, 180*, 245.

156. Taylor, J. R., & Kakulas, B. A. (1991). Neck injuries. *Lancet, 338*, 1343.

157. Guyer, R. D., & Ohnmeiss, D. D. (2003). Lumbar discography. *Spine Journal, 3*, 11S.

158. Fortin, J. D. (2000). Precision diagnostic disc injections. *Pain Physician, 3*, 271.

159. Adams, M.A., Dolan, P., & Hutton, W. C. (1986). The stages of disc degeneration as revealed by discograms. *Journal of Bone & Joint Surgery* (Britain), *68*, 36.

160. Schellhas, K. P. et al. (1996). Cervical discogenic pain. Prospective correlation of magnetic resonance imaging and discography in asymptomatic subjects and pain sufferers. *Spine, 21*, 300.

161. Wood, K. B. et al. (1999). Thoracic discography in healthy individuals. A controlled prospective study of magnetic resonance imaging and discography in asymptomatic and symptomatic individuals. *Spine, 24*, 1548.

162. Walsh, T. R. et al. (1990). Lumbar discography in normal subjects. *Journal of Bone and Joint Surgery* (America), *72*, 1081.

163. Yasuma, T., Ohno, R., & Yamauchi, Y. (1988). False-negative lumbar discograms: Correlation of discographic and histologic findings in postmortem and surgical specimens. *Journal of Bone and Joint Surgery* (America), *70*, 1279.

164. Yu, S. W. et al. (1989). Comparison of MR and discography in detecting radial tears of the annulus: A postmortem study. *American Journal of Neuroradiology, 10*, 1077.

165. Saternus, K. S., & Bornscheuer, H. H. (1983). Comparative radiologic and pathologic-anatomic studies on the value of discography in the diagnosis of acute intravertebral disk injuries in the cervical spine. *Fortschritte auf dem Gebiete der Rontgenstrahlen und der Nuklearmedizin, 139*, 651.

166. Jackson, R. P. et al. (1989). The neuroradiographic diagnosis of lumbar herniated nucleus pulposus: I. A comparison of computed tomography (CT), myelography, CT-myelography, discography, and CT-discography. *Spine, 14*, 1356.

167. Gresham, J. L., & Miller, R. (1969). Evaluation of the lumbar spine by diskography and its use in election of proper treatment of the herniated disk syndrome. *Clinical Orthopedics, 67*, 29.

168. Brodsky, A. E., & Binder, W. F. (1979). Lumbar discography: Its value in diagnosis and treatment of lumbar disc lesions. *Spine, 4*, 110.

169. Birney, T. J. et al. (1992). Comparison of MRI and discography in the diagnosis of lumbar degenerative disease. *Journal of Spinal Disorders, 5*, 417.

170. Bernard, T. N., Jr. (1993). Repeat lumbar spine surgery: Factors influencing outcome. *Spine, 18*, 2196.

171. Southern, E. P. et al. (2000). Disc degeneration: A human cadaveric study correlation magnetic resonance imaging and quantitative discomanometry. *Spine, 25*, 2171.

172. Simmons, J. W. et al. (1991). Awake discography. A comparison study with magnetic resonance imaging. *Spine, 16*, S216.

173. Simmons, E. H., & Segil, C. M. (1975). An evaluation of discography in the localization of symptomatic levels in discogenic disease of the spine. *Clinical Orthopedics, 108*, 57.

174. Lehmer, S. M., Dawson, M. H., & O'Brien, J. P. (1994). Delayed pain response after lumbar discography. *European Spine Journal, 3*, 28–31.

175. Jackson, R. P., & Glah, J. J. (1987). Foraminal and extraforaminal lumbar disc herniation: Diagnosis and treatment. *Spine, 577*, 12.

176. Ohnmeiss, D. D., Guyer, R. D., & Mason, S. L. (2000). The relation between cervical discographic pain responses and radiographic images. *Clinical Journal of Pain, 16*, 1.

177. Winter, R. B., & Schellhas, K. P. (1996). Painful adult thoracic Scheuermann's disease. Diagnosis by discography and treatment by combined arthrodesis. *American Journal of Orthopedics, 25*, 783.

178. Wiley, J. J., Macnab, I., & Wortzman, G. (1968). Lumbar discography and its clinical applications. *Canadian Journal of Surgery, 11*, 280.

179. Sachs, B. L. et al. (1987). Dallas discogram description: A new classification of CT/discography in low-back disorders. *Spine, 12*, 287.

180. Grubb, S. A., Lipscomb, H. J., & Guilford, W. B. (1987). The relative value of lumbar roentgenograms, metrizamide myelography, and discography in the assessment of patients with chronic low back syndrome. *Spine, 12*, 282.

181. Milette, P. C., Raymond, J., & Fontaine, S. (1990). Comparison of high-resolution computed tomography with discography in the evaluation of lumbar disc herniations. *Spine, 15*, 525.

182. Gibson, M. J. et al. (1986). Magnetic resonance imaging and discography in the diagnosis of disc degeneration: A comparative study of 50 discs. *Journal of Bone and Joint Surgery* (Britain), *68*, 369.

183. Schneiderman, G. et al. (1987). Magnetic resonance imaging in the diagnosis of disc degeneration: Correlation with discography. *Spine, 12*, 276.

184. Whitecloud, T. S., & Seago, R. A. (1987). Cervical discogenic syndrome: results of operative intervention in patients with positive discography. *Spine, 12*, 313.

185. Horton, W. C., & Daftari, T. K. (1992). Which disc as visualized by magnetic resonance imaging is actually a source of pain? A correlation between magnetic resonance imaging and discography. *Spine, 17*, S164.

186. Kornberg, M. (1989). Discography and magnetic resonance imaging in the diagnosis of lumbar disc disruption. *Spine, 14*, 1368.

187. Zucherman, J. et al. (1988). Normal magnetic resonance imaging with abnormal discography. *Spine, 13*, 1355.

188. Parfenchuck, T. A., & Janssen, M. E. (1994). A correlation of cervical magnetic resonance imaging and discography/computed tomographic discograms. *Spine, 19*, 2819.

189. Ito, M. et al. (1988). Predictive signs of discogenic lumbar pain on magnetic resonance imaging with discography correlation. *Spine, 23*, 1252.

190. Osti, O. L., & Fraser, R. D. (1992). MRI and discography of anular tears and intervertebral disc degeneration. A prospective clinical comparison. *Journal of Bone and Joint Surgery* (Britain), *74*, 431.

191. Greenspan, A. et al. (1992). Is there a role of discography in the era of magnetic resonance imaging? Prospective correlation and quantitative analysis of computed tomography-diskography, magnetic resonance imaging, and surgical findings. *Journal of Spinal Disorders, 5*, 26.

192. Buirski, G., & Silberstein, M. (1993). The symptomatic lumbar disc in patients with low-back pain: Magnetic resonance imaging appearances in both a symptomatic and control population. *Spine, 18*, 1808.

193. Gill, K., & Blumenthal, S. L. (1992). Functional results after anterior lumbar fusion at L5/S1 in patients with normal fusion at L5/S1 in patients with normal and abnormal MRI scans. *Spine, 17*, 940.

194. Milette, P. C. et al. (1999). Differentiating lumbar disc protrusions, disc bulges, and discs with normal contour but abnormal signal intensity: Magnetic resonance imaging with discographic correlations. *Spine, 24*, 44.

195. Buirski, G. (1992). Magnetic resonance signal patterns of lumbar discs in patients with low back pain: A prospective study with discographic correlation. *Spine, 17*, 1199.

196. Aprill, C., & Bogduk, N. (1992). High-intensity zone: A diagnostic sign of painful lumbar disc on magnetic resonance imaging. *British Journal of Radiology, 65*, 361.

197. Schellhas, K. P. et al. (1996). Lumbar disc high-intensity zone. Correlation of magnetic resonance imaging and discography. *Spine, 21*, 79.

198. Saifuddin, A. et al. (1998). The value of lumbar spine magnetic resonance imaging in the demonstration of anular tears. *Spine, 23*, 453.

199. Smith, B. M. et al. (1998). Interobserver reliability of detecting lumbar intervertebral disc high-intensity zone on magnetic resonance imaging and association of high-intensity zone with pain and anular disruption. *Spine, 23*, 2074.

200. Lappalainen, A. K. et al. (2002). The diagnostic value of contrast-enhanced magnetic resonance imaging in the detection of experimentally induced anular teras in sheep. *Spine, 27*, 2806.

201. Ricketson, R., Simmons, J. W., & Hauser, B. O. (1996). The prolapsed intervertebral disc. The high-intensity zone with discography correlation. *Spine, 21*, 2758.

202. Schellhas, K. P. (1997). Comment on Ricketson et al. The prolapsed intervertebral disc. The high-intensity zone with discography correlation [Letter]. *Spine, 22*, 1538.

203. Carragee, E.J., Paragiodakis, S. J., & Khurana, S. (2000). Lumbar high-intensity zone and discography in subjects without low back problems. *Spine, 25*, 2987.

204. Lam, K. S., Carlin, D., & Mulholland, R. C. (2000). Lumbar disc high-intensity zone: The value and significance of provocative discography in the determination of the discogenic pain source. *European Spine Journal, 9*, 36.

205. Merskey, H., & Bogduk, N. (1994). *Classification of chronic pain: Descriptions of chronic pain syndromes and definitions of pain terms* (2nd ed.). Seattle: IASP Press.

206. Bogduk, N., & Aprill, C. (1993). On the nature of neck pain, discography, and cervical zygapophyseal joint blocks. *Pain, 54*, 213.

207. Shinomiya, K. et al. (1993). Evaluation of cervical discography in pain origin and provocation. *Journal of Spinal Disease, 6*, 422.

208. Holt, E. P., Jr. (1968). The question of lumbar discography. *Journal of Bone and Joint Surgery* (America), *50*, 720.

209. Holt, E. P., Jr. (1964). Fallacy of cervical discography. Report of 50 cases in normal subjects. *Journal of the American Medical Association, 188*, 799.

210. Simmons, J. W. et al. (1988). A reassessment of Holt's data on: "The question of lumbar discography." *Clinical Orthopedics, 237*, 120.

211. Urasaki, T. et al. (1998). Consistency of lumbar discograms of the same disc obtained twice at a 2-week interval: Influence of needle tip position. *Journal of Orthopedic Science, 3*, 243.

212. Carragee, E. et al. (2000). The rates of false-positive lumbar discography in select patients without low back symptoms. *Spine, 25*, 1373.

213. Carragee, E. J. et al. (2000). Provocative discography in patients after limited lumbar discectomy. *Spine, 25*, 3065.

214. Carragee, E. J. et al. (1999). False-positive findings on lumbar discography: Reliability of subjective findings on lumbar discography. Reliability of subjective concordance assessment during provocative disc injection. *Spine, 24*, 2542.

215. Carragee, E. J. et al. (2002). Provocative discography in volunteer subjects with mild persistent low back pain. *Spine Journal, 2*, 25.

216. Carragee, E. J. (2003). Low pressure positive discography in subjects without significant LBP illness. *Spine Journal, 3*, 68.

217. Carragee, E. J. et al. (2000). The rates of false-positive lumbar discography in select patients without low back symptoms. *Spine, 25,* 1373.

218. Bogduk, N. (2001, Summer). An analysis of the Carragee data on false-positive discography. *International Spine Intervention Society Newsletter, 3.*

219. Tsou, P.M. (2001). Mislabeling the articles, and then injecting strong bias against lumbar provocation discography as a diagnostic tool. *Spine, 26,* 994.

220. Manchikanti, L. et al. (2001). Provocative discography in low back pain patients with or without somatization disorder: A randomized prospective evaluation. *Pain Physician, 4,* 227.

221. Vilims, B. D., Carragee, E. J., & Alamin, T. E. (2002). Letter to the editor. *Spine Journal, 2,* 387.

222. Block, A. R. et al. (1996). Discographic pain report: Influence of psychological factors. *Spine, 21,* 334.

223. Ohnmeiss, D. D., Vanharanta, H., & Guyer, R. D. (1995). The association between pain drawings and computed tomographic/discographic pain responses. *Spine, 20,* 729.

224. Schwarzer, A. C., et al. (1995). The prevalence and clinical features of internal disc disruption in patients with chronic low back pain. *Spine, 20,* 1878.

225. Carragee, E. et al. (2000). Can discography cause long-term back symptoms in previously asymptomatic subjects? *Spine, 25,* 1803.

226. Johnson, R. G. (1989). Does discography injure normal discs? An analysis of repeat discograms. *Spine, 14,* 424.

227. Heggeness, M. H., & Doherty, B. J. (1993). Discography causes end plate deflection. *Spine, 18,* 1050.

228. Reitman, C. A. et al. (2001). Posterior annular strains during discography. *Journal of Spinal Disorders, 14,* 347.

229. Zeidman, S. M., Thompson, K., & Ducker, T. B. (1995). Complications of cervical discography: Analysis of 4400 diagnostic disc injections. *Neurosurgery, 37,* 414.

230. Grubb, S. A., & Kelly, C. K. (2000). Cervical discography: Clinical implications from 12 years of experience. *Spine, 25,* 1382.

231. Guyer, R. D. et al. (1997). Complications of cervical discography: Findings in a large series. *Journal of Spinal Disorders, 10,* 95.

232. Connor, P. M., & Darden, B.V., II. (1993). Cervical discography complications and clinical efficacy. *Spine, 18,* 2035.

233. deSeze, S., & Levernieux, J. (1952). Les accidents de la discographie. *Revue du Rhumatisme et des Maladies Osteo-Articulaires, 19,* 1027.

234. Goldie, I. (1957). Intervertebral disc changes after discography. *Acta Chirurgica Scandinavica, 113,* 438.

235. Fraser, R. D., Osti, O. L., & Vernon-Roberts, B. (1987). Discitis after discography. *Journal of Bone and Joint Surgery* (Britain), *69,* 26.

236. Silber, J. S. et al. (2002). Management of postprocedural discitis. *Spine Journal, 2,* 279.

237. Osti, O. L., Fraser, R. D., & Vernon-Roberts, B. (1990). Discitis after discography. *Journal of Bone and Joint Surgery* (Britain), *72,* 271.

238. Guyer, R. D. et al. (1988). Discitis after discography. *Spine, 13,* 1352.

239. Bajwa, Z. H. et al. (2002). Discitis associated with pregnancy and spinal anesthesia. *Anesthesia & Analgesia, 94,* 415.

240. Lownie, S. P., & Ferguson, G. G. (1989). Spinal subdural empyema complicating cervical discography. *Spine, 14,* 1415.

241. Schreck, R. I. et al. (1995). Nucleus pulposus pulmonary embolism. A case report. *Spine, 20,* 2463.

242. Smith, M. D., & Kim, S. S. (1990). Herniated cervical disc resulting from discography: An unusual complication. *Journal of Spinal Disorders, 3,* 392.

243. Laun, A., Lorenz, R., & Agnoli, N. L. (1981). Complications of cervical discography. *Journal of Neurosurgical Science, 25,* 17.

244. Tsuji, N., Igarashi, S., & Koyama, T. (1987). Spinal epidural abscess. *No Shinkei Geka, 15,* 1079.

245. Junila, J., Niinimäki, T., & Tervonen, O. (1997). Epidural abscess after lumbar discography. *Spine, 22,* 2191.

246. Boswell, M. V. et al. (2004). Intrathecal cefazolin-induced seizures following attempted discography. *Pain Physician, 7,* 103.

247. Schwarzer, A. C., Aprill, C. N., & Bogduk, M. (1995). The sacroiliac joint in chronic low back pain. *Spine, 20,* 31.

248. Maigne, J. Y., Aivakiklis, A., & Pfefer, F. (1996). Results of sacroiliac joint double block and value of sacroiliac pain provocation test in 54 patients with low back pain. *Spine, 21,* 1889.

249. Fortin, J. D. et al. (1994). Sacroiliac joint: Pain referral maps upon applying a new injection/arthrography technique. Part I: Asymptomatic volunteers. *Spine, 19,* 1475.

250. Fortin, J. D. et al. (1994). Sacroiliac joint: Pain referral maps upon applying a new injection/arthrography technique. Part II: Clinical evaluation. *Spine, 19,* 1483.

251. Hansen, H. C. (2003). Is fluoroscopy necessary for sacroiliac joint injections? *Pain Physician, 6,* 155.

252. Hansen, H. C., & Helm S. (2003). Sacroiliac joint pain and dysfunction. *Pain Physician, 6,* 179.

253. Dreyfuss, P. et al. (1996). The value of medical history and physical examination in diagnosing sacroiliac joint pain. *Spine, 21,* 2594.

254. Dreyfuss, P. et al. (1994). Positive sacroiliac screening tests in asymptomatic adults. *Spine, 19,* 1138.

255. Vogler, J. B., III et al. (1984). The normal sacroiliac joint: A CT study of asymptomatic patients. *Radiology, 151,* 433.

256. Tullberg, T. et al. (1998). Manipulation does not alter the position of the sacroiliac joint: A roentgen stereophotogrammatic analysis. *Spine, 23,* 1124.

257. Slipman, C. W. et al. (2000). Sacroiliac joint pain referral zones. *Archives of Physical Medicine and Rehabilitation, 81,* 334.

258. Slipman, C. W. et al. (1998). The predictive value of provocative sacroiliac joint stress maneuvers in the diagnosis of sacroiliac joint syndrome. *Archives of Physical Medicine and Rehabilitation, 79,* 288.

259. Young, S. B. et al. (2000). The sacroiliac joint: Comparing physical examination and diagnostic block arthrography. *Journal of Orthopedic and Sports Physical Therapy, 30*, A34.

260. Broadhurst, N. A., & Bond, M. J. (1998). Pain provocation tests for the assessment of sacroiliac joint dysfunction. *Journal of Spinal Disorders, 11*, 341.

261. Meijne, W. et al. (1999). Intraexaminer and interexaminer reliability of the Gillet test. *Journal of Manipulative Physiological Therapy, 22*, 4.

262. Carmichael, J. P. (1987). Inter- and intra-examiner reliability of palpation for sacroiliac joint dysfunction. *Journal of Manipulative Physiological Therapy, 10*, 164.

263. Ebraheim, N. A. et al. (1997). Radiology of the sacroiliac joint. *Spine, 22*, 869.

264. Resnik, C. S., & Resnick, D. (1985). Radiology of disorders of the sacroiliac joints. *Journal of the American Medical Association, 253*, 2863.

265. Slipman, C. W. et al. (1996). The value of radionuclide imaging in the diagnosis of sacroiliac joint syndrome. *Spine, 21*, 2251.

266. Maigne, J. Y., Boulahdour, H., & Charellier G. (1998). Value of quantitative radionuclide bone scanning in the diagnosis of sacroiliac joint syndrome in 32 patients with low back pain. *European Spine Journal, 7*, 328.

267. Goldberg, R. et al. (1978). Applications and limitations of quantitative sacroiliac joint scintigraphy. *Radiology, 128*, 683.

268. Lantto, T. (1990). The scintigraphy of sacroiliac joints: a comparison of 99-mTc-VPB and 99mTc-MDP. *European Journal of Nuclear Medicine, 16*, 677.

269. Lentle, B. et al. The scintigraphic investigation of sacroiliac disease. *Journal of Nuclear Medicine, 6*, 529.

270. Verlooy, H. et al. (1992). Quantitative scintigraphy of the sacroiliac joints. *Clinical Imaging, 16*, 230.

271. Hanly, J. G. et al. (1994). Early recognition of sacroiliitis by magnetic resonance imaging and single photon emission computed tomography. *Journal of Rheumatology, 21*, 2088.

272. Rosenberg, J. M., Quint, T. J., & de Rosayro, A. M. (2000). Computerized tomographic localization of clinically-guided sacroiliac joint injections. *Clinical Journal of Pain, 16*, 18.

273. Saha A. K. et al. (1999). To do or not to do under fluoroscopy, that is the question: An analysis of sacroiliac joint and caudal epidural injections in a pain center. *American Journal of Anesthesiology, 26*, 269.

274. Carette, S. et al. (1991). A controlled trial of corticosteroid injections into facet joints for chronic low back pain. *New England Journal of Medicine, 325*, 1002.

275. Barnsley, L. et al. (1994). Lack of effect of intra-articular corticosteroids for chronic pain in the cervical zygapophyseal joints. *New England Journal of Medicine, 330*, 1047.

276. Marks, R. C., Houston, T., & Thulbourne, T. (1992). Facet joint injection and facet nerve block. A randomized comparison in 86 patients with chronic low back pain. *Pain, 49*, 325.

277. Nash, T. P. (1990). Facet joints. Intra-articular steroids or nerve blocks? *Pain Clinic, 3*, 77.

278. Lilius, G. et al. (1989). Lumbar facet joint syndrome. A randomized clinical trial. *Journal of Bone and Joint Surgery* (Britain), *71*, 681.

279. Carrera, G. F. (1980). Lumbar facet joint injection in low back pain and sciatica: Preliminary results. *Radiology, 137*, 665.

280. Carrera, G. F., & Williams, A. L. (1984). Current concepts in evaluation of the lumbar facet joints. *CRC Critical Reviews in Diagnostic Imaging, 21*, 85.

281. Lewinnek, G. E., & Warfield C. A. (1986). Facet joint degeneration as a cause of low back pain. *Clinical Orthopedics, 213*, 216.

282. Wedel, D. J., & Wilson, P. R. (1985). Cervical facet arthrography. *Regional Anesthesia, 10*, 7.

283. Destouet, J. M. et al. (1982). Lumbar facet joint injection: Indication, technique, clinical correlation, and preliminary results. *Radiology, 145*, 321.

284. Lippitt, A. B. (1984). The facet joint and its role in spine pain. Management with facet joint injections. *Spine, 9*, 746.

286. Lau, L. S., Littlejohn, G. O., & Miller M. H. (1985). Clinical evaluation of intra-articular injections for lumbar facet joint pain. *Medical Journal of Australia, 143*, 563.

287. Roy, D. F. et al. (1988). Clinical evaluation of cervical facet joint infiltration. *Canadian Association of Radiologists Journal, 39*, 118.

288. Dussault, D. G., & Nicolet, V. M. (1985). Cervical facet joint arthrography. *Canadian Association of Radiologists Journal, 36*, 79.

289. Dory, M. A. (1983). Arthrography of the cervical facet joints. *Radiology, 148*, 379.

290. Hove, B., & Glydensted, C. (2001). Cervical analgesia facet joint arthrography. *Neuroradiology, 32*, 456.

291. Manchikanti, L. et al. (2001). Effectiveness of lumbar facet joint nerve blocks in chronic low back pain: A randomized clinical trial. *Pain Physician, 4*, 101.

292. Lord, S. M., Barnsley, L., & Bogduk, N. (1995). Percutaneous radiofrequency neurotomy in the treatment of cervical zygapophyseal joint pain: A caution. *Neurosurgery, 35*, 732.

293. McDonald, G. J., Lord, S. M., & Bogduk, N. (1999). Long-term follow-up of patients treated with cervical radiofrequency neurotomy for chronic neck pain. *Neurosurgery, 45*, 61.

294. Van Kleef, M. et al. (1999). Randomized trial of radiofrequency lumbar facet denervation for chronic low back pain. *Spine, 24*, 1937.

295. Dreyfuss, P. et al. (2000). Efficacy and validity of radiofrequency neurotomy for chronic lumbar zygapophysial joint pain. *Spine, 25*, 1270.

296. Van Kleef, M. et al. (1996). Radiofrequency lesions adjacent to the dorsal root ganglion for cervicobrachial pain. A prospective double blind randomized study. *Neurosurgery, 38*, 1127.

297. Lord, S. M. et al. (1996). Percutaneous radio-frequency neurotomy for chronic cervical zygapophyseal-joint pain. *New England Journal of Medicine, 335*, 1721.

298. Katz, S. S., & Savitz, M. H. (1986). Percutaneous radiofrequency rhizotomy of the lumbar facets. *Mt. Sinai Journal of Medicine, 7*, 523.

299. Koning, H. M., & Mackie, D. P. (1994). Percutaneous radiofrequency facet denervation in low back pain. *Pain Clinic, 7*, 199.

300. Sluijter, M. E. (1988). The use of radiofrequency lesions for pain relief in failed back patients. *International Disabilities Studies, 10*, 37.

301. Bogduk, N., & Marsland, A. (1988). The cervical zygapophyseal joints as a source of neck pain. *Spine, 13*, 610.

302. Schaerer, J. P. (1988). Treatment of prolonged neck pain by radiofrequency facet rhizotomy. *Journal of Neurological and Orthopedic Medicine and Surgery, 9*, 74.

303. Vervest, A. C. M., & Stolker, R. J. (1991). The treatment of cervical pain syndromes with radiofrequency procedures. *Pain Clinic, 4*, 103.

304. Schaerer, J. P. (1978). Radiofrequency facet rhizotomy in the treatment of chronic neck and low back pain. *International Surgery, 63*, 53.

305. Gallagher, J., Vadi, P. L. P., & Wesley, J. R. (1994). Radiofrequency facet joint denervation in the treatment of low back – A prospective controlled double-blind study to assess efficacy. *Pain Clinic, 7*, 193.

306. Holzer, J., & Holzer, F. (1997). Percutaneous radiofrequency facet denervation: Treatment of chronic low back pain. *Revista Chilena de Neuro-Psiquiatria, 35*, 355.

307. Faclier, G., & Kay, J. (2000). Cervical facet radiofrequency neurotomy. *Techniques in Regional Anesthesia and Pain Management, 4*, 120.

308. Stolker, R. J., Vervest, A. C., & Groen, G. J. (1994). The treatment of chronic thoracic segmental pain by radiofrequency percutaneous partial rhizotomy. *Journal of Neurosurgery, 80*, 986.

309. Sanders, M., & Zuurmond, W. W. A. (1999). Percutaneous intraarticular lumbar facet joint denervation in the treatment of low back pain: A comparison with percutaneous extra-articular lumbar facet denervation. *Pain Clinic, 11*, 329.

310. Leclaire, R. et al. (2001). Radiofrequency facet joint denervation in the treatment of low back pain: A placebo-controlled clinical trial to assess efficacy. *Spine, 26*, 1411.

311. Sapir, D., & Gorup, J. M. (2001). Radiofrequency medial branch neurotomy in litigant and nonlitigant patients with cervical whiplash. *Spine, 26*, E268.

312. Stolker, R. J., Vervest, A. C., & Groen, G. J. (1993). Percutaneous facet denervation in chronic thoracic spinal pain. *Acta Neurochirurgia, 122*, 82.

313. Tzaan, W. C., & Tasker, R. R. (2000). Percutaneous radiofrequency facet rhizotomy – Experience with 118 procedures and reappraisal of its value. *Canadian Journal of Neurological Sciences, 27*, 125.

314. Wallis, B. J. et al. (1997). Resolution of psychological distress of whiplash patients following treatment by radiofrequency neurotomy: A randomized, double-blind, placebo-controlled trial. *Pain, 73*, 15.

315. Lynch, M. C., & Taylor, J. F. (1986). Facet joint injection for low back pain. A clinical study. *Journal of Bone and Joint Surgery* (Britain), *68*, 138.

316. Jackson, R. P., Jacobs, R. R., & Montesano, P. X. (1988). Facet joint injection in low back pain. A prospective statistical study. *Spine, 13*, 966.

317. Jackson, R. P. (1992). The facet syndrome: myth or reality? *Clinical Orthopedics, 279*, 110.

318. Deyo, R. A.(1991). Fads in the treatment of low back pain. *New England Journal of Medicine, 325*, 1039.

319. North, R. B. et al. (1994). Radiofrequency lumbar facet denervation: Analysis of prognostic factors. *Pain, 57*, 77.

320. Manchikanti, L. et al. (2004). Effectiveness of cervical medial branch blocks in chronic neck pain: A prospective, outcome study. *Pain Physician, 7*, 195.

321. Manchikanti, L. et al. (2002). Therapeutic lumbar facet joint nerve blocks. In L. Manchikanti, S. W. Slipman, & B. Fellows (Eds.), *Low back pain: Diagnosis and treatment* (p. 447). Paducah, KY: ASIPP Press.

322. Geurts, J. W. et al. (2001). Efficacy of radiofrequency procedures for the treatment of spinal pain: A systematic review of randomized clinical trials. *Regional Anesthesia and Pain Medicine, 26*, 394.

323. Manchikanti, L. et al. (2002). Medial branch neurotomy in management of chronic spinal pain: Systematic review of the evidence. *Pain Physician, 5*, 405.

324. Niemistö, L. et al. (2003). Radiofrequency denervation for neck and back pain: A systematic review within the framework of the Cochrane Collaboration Back Review Group. *Spine, 28*, 1877.

325. *Systems to rate the strength of scientific evidence.* (2002). Evidence Report/Technology Assessment No. 47. University of North Carolina: Agency for Healthcare Research and Quality, AHRQ Publication No. 02-E016, April.

326. Manchikanti, L. et al. (2003). Methods for evidence synthesis in interventional pain management. *Pain Physician, 6*, 89.

327. Bogduk, N. et al. (1994). *Epidural use of steroids in the management of back pain.* Report of working party on epidural use of steroids in the management of back pain. National Health and Medical Research Council. Canberra, Commonwealth of Australia, 1.

328. Boswell, M. V. (2003). Epidural steroids in the management of chronic spinal pain and radiculopathy. *Pain Physician, 6*, 319.

329. Nelemans, P. J. et al. (2001). Injection therapy for subacute and chronic benign low back pain. *Spine, 26*, 501.

330. van Tulder, M. W. V., Koes, B. W., & Bouter, L. M. (1997). Conservative treatment of acute and chronic nonspecific low back pain. A systematic review of randomized controlled trials of the most common interventions. *Spine, 22*, 2128.

331. Rozenberg, S. et al. (1999). Efficacy of epidural steroids in low back pain and sciatica: A critical appraisal by a French task force of randomized trials. *Revue du Rhumatisme, 66*, 79.

332. Nachemson, A. L., & Jonsson, E. (2000). *Neck and back pain. The scientific evidence of causes, diagnosis, and treatment.* Philadelphia: Lippincott Williams & Wilkins.

333. Kepes, E. R., & Duncalf, D. (1985). Treatment of backache with spinal injections of local anesthetics, spinal and systemic steroids. *Pain, 22,* 33.

334. Benzon, H. T. (1986). Epidural steroid injections for low back pain and lumbosacral radiculography. *Pain, 24,* 277.

335. Koes, B. W. et al. (1999). Epidural steroid injections for low back pain and sciatica. An updated systematic review of randomized clinical trials. *Pain Digest, 9,* 241.

336. Watts, R. W., & Silagy, C. A. (1995). A meta-analysis on the efficacy of epidural corticosteroids in the treatment of sciatica. *Anaesthesia and Intensive Care, 23,* 564.

337. McQuay, H. J., & Moore, R. A. (1998). *Epidural corticosteroids for sciatica. An evidence-based resource for pain relief* (p. 216). Oxford, NY: Oxford University Press.

338. Bernstein, R. M. (2001). Injections and surgical therapy in chronic pain. *Clinical Journal of Pain, 17,* S94.

339. Manchikanti, L., Bakhit, C. E., & Pampati V. (2001). Role of epidurography in caudal neuroplasty. *Pain Digest, 8,* 277.

340. Botwin, K. P. et al. (2001). Complications of fluoroscopically guided caudal epidural injections. *American Journal of Physical Medicine and Rehabilitation, 80,* 416.

341. Renfrew, D. L. et al. (1991). Correct placement of epidural steroid injections: fluoroscopic guidance and contrast administration. *American Journal of Neuroradiology, 12,* 1003.

342. Stewart, H. D., Quinnell, R. C., & Dann, N. (1987). Epidurography in the management of sciatica. *British Journal of Rheumatology, 26,* 424.

343. El-Khoury, G. et al. (1988). Epidural steroid injection: A procedure ideally performed with fluoroscopic control. *Radiology, 168,* 554.

344. Stitz, M. Y., & Sommer, H. M. (1999). Accuracy of blind versus fluoroscopically guided caudal epidural injection. *Spine, 24,* 1371.

345. Manchikanti, L. et al. (2004). Evaluation of fluoroscopically guided caudal epidural injections. *Pain Physician, 7,* 81.

346. Sullivan, W. J. et al. (2000). Incidence of intravascular uptake in lumbar spinal injection procedures. *Spine, 25,* 481.

347. White, A. H., Derby, R., & Wynne, G. (1980). Epidural injections for diagnosis and treatment of low back pain. *Spine, 5,* 78.

348. Saberski, L. R., Kondamuri, S., & Osinubi, O. Y. O. (1997). Identification of the epidural space: Is loss of resistance to air a safe technique? *Regional Anesthesia, 22,* 3.

349. Fredman, B. et al. (1988). Epidural steroids for treating "failed back surgery syndrome": Is fluoroscopy really necessary? *Anesthesia & Analgesia, 88,* 367.

350. Manchikanti, L. et al. (1999). Fluoroscopy is medically necessary for the performance of epidural steroids. *Anesthesia & Analgesia, 89,* 1326.

351. Mehta, M., & Salmon, N. (1985). Extradural block. Confirmation of the injection site by X-ray monitoring. *Anaesthesia, 40,* 1009.

352. Nishimura, N., Khahara, T., & Kusakabe, T. (1959). The spread of lidocaine and 1-131 solution in the epidural space. *Anesthesiology, 20,* 785.

353. Burn, J. M., Guyer, P. B., & Langdon L. (1973). The spread of solutions injected into the epidural space: A study using epidurograms in patients with lumbosciatic syndrome. *British Journal of Anaesthesiology, 45,* 338.

354. Kim, K. M. et al. (2001). Cephalic spreading levels after volumetric caudal epidural injections in chronic low back pain, *Journal of Korean Medical Science, 16,* 193.

355. Liu, S. S. et al. (2001). Prospective experience with a 20-gauge Tuohy needle for lumbar epidural steroid injections: Is confirmation with fluoroscopy necessary? *Regional Anesthesia and Pain Medicine, 26,* 143.

356. Stojanovic, M. P. et al. (2002). The role of fluoroscopy in cervical epidural steroid injections: An analysis of contrast dispersal patterns. *Spine, 27,* 509.

357. Bromage, P. R., & Benumof, J. L. (1998). Paraplegia following intracord injection during attempted epidural anesthesia under general anesthesia. *Regional Anesthesia and Pain Medicine, 23,* 104.

358. Krane, E. J. et al. (1998). The safety of epidurals during general anesthesia. *Regional Anesthesia and Pain Medicine, 23,* 433.

359. Hodges, S. D. et al. (1998). Cervical epidural steroid injection with intrinsic spinal cord damage. Two case reports. *Spine, 23,* 2137.

360. Derby, R. (1998). Cervical epidural steroid injection with intrinsic spinal cord damage. Point of view. *Spine, 23,* 2141.

361. Manchikanti, L. (1999). Cervical epidural steroid injection with intrinsic spinal cord damage. *Spine, 24,* 1170.

362. Andrade, A., & Eckman, E. (1992, January). The distribution of radiologic contrast media by lumbar translaminar and selective neural canals in normal human volunteers. In *Proceedings of the Annual Meeting of the International Spinal Injection Society*, Keystone, CO.

363. Saal, J. S., & Saal, J. A. (1998). Comprehensive cervical and lumbar intra-spinal injection course. Stanford University School of Medicine, Stanford, CA, July 11–12.

364. Botwin, K., Castellanos, R., & Rao, S.(2003). Complications of fluoroscopically guided interlaminar cervical epidural injections. *Archives of Physical Medicine and Rehabilitation, 84,* 627.

365. Kim, Y. C., Lim, Y. J., & Lee, S. C. (1998). Spreading pattern of epidurally administered contrast medium in rabbits. *Acta Anaesthesiologica Scandinavica, 42,* 1092.

366. Kopacz, D., & Allen, H. W.(1995). Comparison of needle deviation during regional anesthetic techniques in a laboratory model. *Anesthesia & Analgesia, 81,* 630.

367. Botwin, K.P., Natalicchio, J., & Hanna, A. (2004). Fluoroscopic guided lumbar interlaminar epidural injections: A prospective evaluation of epidurography contrast patterns and anatomical review of the epidural space. *Pain Physician, 7,* 77.

368. Manchikanti, L. (2000). Transforaminal lumbar epidural steroid injections. *Pain Physician, 3,* 374.

369. McMillan, M. R., & Crumpton, C. (2003). Cortical blindness and neurologic injury complicating cervical transforaminal injection for cervical radiculopathy. *Anesthesiology, 99*, 509.

370. Rozin, L. et al. (2003). Death during transforaminal epidural steroid nerve root block (C7) due to perforation of the left vertebral artery. *American Journal of Forensic Medicine and Pathology, 24*, 351.

371. Furman, M. B. et al. (2000). Incidence of intravascular penetration in transforaminal lumbosacral epidural steroid injections. *Spine, 25*, 2628.

372. Botwin, K. P. et al. (2000). Complications of fluoroscopically guided transforaminal lumbar epidural injections. *Archives of Physical Medicine and Rehabilitation, 81*, 1045.

373. Houten, J. K., & Errico, T. J. (2002). Paraplegia after lumbosacral nerve root block: Report of three cases. *Spine Journal, 2*, 70.

374. Furman, M. B., Giovanniello, M. T., & O'Brien, E. M. (2003). Incidence of intravascular penetration in transforaminal cervical epidural steroid injections. *Spine, 28*, 21.

375. Brouwers, P. J. et al. (2001). A cervical anterior spinal artery syndrome after diagnostic blockade of the right C6-nerve root. *Pain, 91*, 397.

376. Baker, R. et al. (2003). Cervical transforaminal injection of corticosteroids into a radicular artery: A possible mechanism for spinal cord injury. *Pain, 103*, 211.

377. Helm, S., Jasper, J. F., & Racz, G. B. (2004). Complications of transforaminal epidural injections. *Pain Physician, 6*, 389.

378. Schultz, D. M. (2004). Risk of transforaminal epidural injections, *Pain Physician, 7*, 289.

379. Kloth, D. S. (2003). Risk of cervical transforaminal epidural injections by anterior approach. *Pain Physician, 6*, 392.

380. Windsor, R. E. et al. (2003). Cervical transforaminal injection: review of the literature, complications, and a suggested technique. *Pain Physician, 6*, 457.

381. Breivik, H. et al. (1976). Treatment of chronic low back pain and sciatica. Comparison of caudal epidural injections of bupivacaine and methylprednisolone with bupivacaine followed by saline. In J. J. Bonica & D. Albe-Fesard (Eds.), *Advances in pain research and therapy* (Vol. 1, pp. 927–932). New York: Raven Press.

382. Bush, K., & Hillier, S. (1991). A controlled study of caudal epidural injections of triamcinolone plus procaine for the management of intractable sciatica. *Spine, 16*, 572.

383. Matthews, J. A. et al. (1987). Back pain and sciatica: Controlled trials of manipulation, traction, sclerosant and epidural injections. *British Journal of Rheumatology, 26*, 416.

384. Beliveau, P. (1971). A comparison between epidural anesthesia with and without corticosteroids in the treatment of sciatica. *Rheumatology and Physical Medicine, 11*, 40.

385. Czarski, Z. (1965). Leczenie rwy kulszowej wstrzykiwaniem hydrokortyzonu inowokainy do rozworu kryzowego. *Przeglad Kekarski, 21*, 511.

386. Manchikanti, L. et al. (2001). Caudal epidural injections with Sarapin steroids in chronic low back pain. *Pain Physician, 4*, 322.

387. Hesla, P. E., & Breivik, H. (1979). Epidural analgesia and epidural steroid injection for treatment of chronic low back pain and sciatica. *Tidsskrift fur den Norske Laegeforening, 99*, 936.

388. Revel, M. et al. (1996). Forceful epidural injections for the treatment of lumbosciatic pain with post-operative lumbar spinal fibrosis. *Revue du Rhumatisme* (English), *63*, 270.

389. Meadeb, J. et al. (2001). Forceful sacrococcygeal injections in the treatment of postdiscectomy sciatica. A controlled study versus glucocorticoid injections. *Joint, Bone, and Spine, 68*, 43.

390. Manchikanti, L. et al. (2002). Effectiveness of caudal epidural injections in discogram positive and negative chronic low back pain. *Pain Physician, 5*, 18.

391. Yates, D. W. (1978). A comparison of the types of epidural injection commonly used in the treatment of low back pain and sciatica. *Rheumatology and Rehabilitation, 17*, 181.

392. Waldman, S. D. (1998). The caudal epidural administration of steroids in combination with local anesthetics in the palliation of pain secondary to radiographically documented lumbar herniated disc: A prospective outcome study with 6-months follow-up. *Pain Clinic, 11*, 43.

393. Carette, S. et al. (1997). Epidural corticosteroid injections for sciatica due to herniated nucleus pulposus. *New England Journal of Medicine, 336*, 1634.

394. Snoek, W., Weber, H., & Jorgensen, B. (1977). Double-blind evaluation of extradural methylprednisolone for herniated lumbar disc. *Acta Orthopaedica Scandinavica, 48*, 635.

395. Cuckler, J. M. et al. (1985). The use of epidural steroid in the treatment of radicular pain. *Journal of Bone and Joint Surgery* (America), *67*, 63.

396. Dilke, T. F. W., Burry, H. C., & Grahame R. (1973). Extradural corticosteroid injection in the management of lumbar nerve root compression. *British Medical Journal, 2*, 635.

397. Serrao, J. M. et al. (1992). Intrathecal midazolam for the treatment of chronic mechanical low back pain: A controlled comparison with epidural steroid in a pilot study. *Pain, 48*, 5.

398. Klenerman, L. et al. (1984). Lumbar epidural injections in the treatment of sciatica. *British Journal of Rheumatology, 23*, 35.

399. Rocco, A. G. et al. (1989). Epidural steroids, epidural morphine and epidural steroids combined with morphine in the treatment of post-laminectomy syndrome. *Pain, 36*, 297.

400. Ridley, M. G. et al. (1988). Outpatient lumbar epidural corticosteroid injection in the management of sciatica. *British Journal of Rheumatology, 27*, 1003.

401. Rogers, P. et al. (1992). Epidural steroids for sciatica. *Pain Clinic, 5*, 67.

402. Castagnera, L. et al. (1994). Long-term results of cervical epidural steroid injection with and without morphine in chronic cervical radicular pain. *Pain, 58,* 239.

403. Hernandez, R., & Lopez, F. (1999). Assessment of pain intensity in patients with diabetic polyneuropathy treated with peridural 2% lidocaine methylprednisolone acetate vs peridural 2% lidocaine. *Anestesia en Mexico, 11,* 65.

404. Kikuchi, A. et al. (1999). Comparative therapeutic evaluation of intrathecal versus epidural methylprednisolone for long-term analgesia in patients with intractable postherpetic neuralgia. *Regional Anesthesia and Pain Medicine, 24,* 287.

405. Kraemer, J. et al. (1997). Lumbar epidural perineural injection: A new technique. *European Spine Journal, 6,* 357.

406. Helliwell, M., Robertson, J. C., & Ellia, R. M. (1985). Outpatient treatment of low back pain and sciatica by a single extradural corticosteroid injection. *British Journal of Clinical Practice, 39,* 228.

407. Stav, A. et al. (1993). Cervical epidural steroid injection for cervicobrachialgia. *Acta Anaesthesiologica Scandinavica, 37,* 562.

408. Buchner, M. et al. (2000). Epidural corticosteroid injection in the conservative management of sciatica. *Clinical Orthopaedics and Related Research, 375,* 149.

409. Bush, K., & Hillier, S. (1996). Outcome of cervical radiculopathy treated with periradicular/epidural corticosteroid injections: A prospective study with independent clinical review. *European Spine Journal, 5,* 319.

410. Rivest, C. et al. (1998). Effects of epidural steroid injection on pain due to lumbar spinal stenosis or herniated discs: A prospective study. *Arthritis Care Research, 11,* 291.

411. Fukusaki, M. et al. (1998). Symptoms of spinal stenosis do not improve after epidural steroid injection. *Clinical Journal of Pain, 14,* 148.

412. Warfield, C. A., & Crews, D. A. (1987). Epidural steroid injection as a predictor of surgical outcome. *Surgery Gynecology & Obstetrics, 164,* 457.

413. Jamison, R. N., VadeBoncouer, T., & Ferrante F. M. (1991). Low back pain patients unresponsive to an epidural steroid injection: Identifying predictive factors. *Clinical Journal of Pain, 7,* 311.

414. Ferrante, F. M. et al. (1993). Clinical classification as a predictor of therapeutic outcome after cervical epidural steroid injection. *Spine, 18,* 730.

415. Hopwood, M. B., & Abram, S. E. (1993). Factors associated with failure of lumbar epidural steroids. *Regional Anesthesia, 18,* 238.

416. Klein, R. G. et al. (2000). Efficacy of cervical epidural steroids in the treatment of cervical spine disorders. *American Journal of Anesthesiology, 9,* 547.

417. Silva, J. et al. (1999). Management of radicular pain from lumbar herniated disc using betamethasone epidural injection. *Revista Brasileira de Ortopedia, 34,* 165.

418. Riew, K. D. et al. (2000). The effect of nerve-root injections on the need for operative treatment of lumbar radicular pain. *Journal of Bone and Joint Surgery* (America), *82,* 1589.

419. Karppinen, J. et al. (2001). Periradicular infiltration for sciatica. *Spine, 26,* 1059.

420. Karppinen, J. et al. (2001). Cost effectiveness of periradicular infiltration for sciatica. *Spine, 26,* 2587.

421. Vad, V. et al. (2002). Transforaminal epidural steroid injections in lumbosacral radiculopathy: A prospective randomized study. *Spine, 27,* 11.

422. Kolsi, I. et al. (2000). Efficacy of nerve root versus interspinous injections of glucocorticoids in the treatment of disc-related sciatica. A pilot, prospective, randomized, double-blind study. *Joint, Bone, and Spine, 67,* 113.

423. Thomas, E. et al. (2003). Efficacy of transforaminal versus interspinous corticosteroid injection in discal radiculalgia — A prospective, randomised, double-blind study. *Clinical Rheumatology, 22,* 299.

424. Lutz, G. E., Vad, V. B., & Wisneski, R. J. (1998). Fluoroscopic transforaminal lumbar epidural steroids: an outcome study. *Archives of Physical Medicine and Rehabilitation, 79,* 1362.

425. Devulder, J. et al. (1999). Nerve root sleeve injections in patients with failed back surgery syndrome: A comparison of three solutions. *Clinical Journal of Pain, 15,* 132.

426. Berger, O. et al. (1999). Evaluation of the efficacy of foraminal infusions of corticosteroids guided by computed tomography in the treatment of radicular pain by foraminal injection. *Journal of Radiology, 80,* 917.

427. Melzer, A., & Seibel, R. M. (1999). Magnetic resonance (MR)-guided percutaneous pain therapy of degenerative spinal diseases. *Seminars in Interventional Radiology, 16,* 143.

428. Sequeiros, R. B. et al. (2002). MRI-guided periradicular nerve root infiltration therapy in low-field (0.23-T) MRI system using optical instrument tracking. *European Radiology, 12,* 1331.

429. Zennaro, H. et al. (1998). Periganglionic foraminal steroid injections performed under CT control. *American Journal of Neuroradiology, 19,* 349.

430. Groenemeyer, D. H. et al. (2002). CT-guided periradicular injections of corticosteroids in the management of lumbar radiculopathy associated with disk herniation. *Journal of Radiology, 1.*

431. Koning, H. M., & Koning, A. J. (2003). Prolonged pain relief following selective nerve root infiltration. *Pain Clinic, 15,* 225.

432. Buttermann, G. R. (2002). Lumbar disc herniation regression after successful epidural steroid injection. *Journal of Spinal Disorders and Techniques, 15,* 469.

433. Weiner, B. K., & Fraser, R. D. (1997). Foraminal injection for lateral lumbar disc herniation. *Journal of Bone and Joint Surgery, 79B,* 804.

434. Rosenberg, S. K. et al. (2002). Effectiveness of transforaminal epidural steroid injections in low back pain: A one year experience. *Pain Physician, 5,* 266.

435. Wang, J. C. et al. (2002). Epidural injections for the treatment of symptomatic lumbar herniated discs. *Journal of Spinal Disorders Tech., 15,* 269.

436. Nelson, D. A., & Landau, W. M. (2001). Intraspinal steroids: History, efficacy, accidentality, and controversy with review of United States Food and Drug Administration reports. *Journal of Neurology, Neurosurgery, and Psychiatry, 70*, 433.

437. Benzon, H. T., & Molly, R. E. (2000). Outcomes, efficacy, and complications from management of low back pain. In P. P. Raj et al. (Eds.), *Practical management of pain*, 3rd ed. (pp. 891–903). Philadelphia: Mosby.

438. Waldman, S. D. (1989). Complications of cervical epidural nerve blocks with steroids: A prospective study of 790 consecutive blocks. *Regional Anesthesia, 14*, 149.

439. Katz, J. A. et al. (1991). Subdural intracranial air: An unusual cause of headache after epidural steroid injection. *Anesthesiology, 74*, 615.

440. Mateo, E. et al. (1999). Epidural and subarachnoid pneumocephalus after epidural technique. *European Journal of Anesthesiology, 16*, 413.

441. MacLean, C. A., & Bachman, D. T. (2001). Documented arterial gas embolism after spinal epidural injection. *Annals of Emergency Medicine, 38*, 592.

442. Williams, K. N., Jackowski, A., & Evans, P. J. (1990). Epidural hematoma requiring surgical decompression following repeated cervical epidural steroid injections for chronic pain. *Pain, 42*, 197.

443. Reitman, C. A., & Watters, W. (2002). Subdural hematoma after cervical epidural steroid injection. *Spine, 27*, E174.

444. Locke, G. E. et al. (1976). Acute spinal epidural hematoma secondary to aspirin-induced prolonged bleeding. *Surgical Neurology, 5*, 293.

445. Ghaly, R. F. (2001). Recovery after high-dose methylprednisolone and delayed evacuation: A case of spinal epidural hematoma. *Journal of Neurosurgical Anesthesiology, 13*, 323.

446. Mastronardi, L. et al. (1996). Cervical spontaneous epidural hematoma as a complication of non-Hodgkin's lymphoma. *European Spine Journal, 5*, 268.

447. Waldman, S. D. (1991). Cervical epidural abscess after cervical epidural nerve block with steroids [Letter]. *Anesthesia & Analgesia, 72*, 717.

448. Mamourian, A. C. et al. (1993). Spinal epidural abscess: Three cases following spinal epidural injection demonstrated with magnetic resonance imaging. *Anesthesiology, 78*, 204.

449. Knight, J. W., Cordingley, J. J., & Palazzo, M. G. A. (1997). Epidural abscess following epidural steroid and local anesthetic injection. *Anaesthesia, 52*, 576.

450. Yue, W. M., & Tan, S. B. (2003). Distant skip level discitis and vertebral osteomyelitis after caudal epidural injection: A case report of a rare complication of epidural injections. *Spine, 28*, E209.

451. Elias, M. (1994). Cervical epidural abscess following trigger point injection. *Journal of Pain and Symptom Management, 9*, 71.

452. Chan, S. T., & Leung, S. (1989). Spinal epidural abscess following steroid injection for sciatica: Case report. *Spine, 14*, 106.

453. Goucke, C. R., & Graziotti, P. (1990). Extradural abscess following local anaesthetic and steroid injection for chronic low back pain. *British Journal of Anaesthesiology, 65*, 427.

454. Lindner, A. et al. (1997). Iatrogenic spinal epidural abscesses: Early diagnosis essential for good outcome. *European Journal of Medical Research, 2*, 201.

455. O'Brien, D. P., & Rawluk, D. J. (1999). Iatrogenic mycobacterium infection after an epidural injection. *Spine, 24*, 1257.

456. Yamaguchi, M. et al. (1999). Epidural abscess associated with epidural block in a patient with immunosuppressive disease. *Japanese Journal of Anesthesiology, 48*, 506.

457. Sabel, M. et al. (2000). Enlargement of a chronic aseptic lumbar epidural abscess by intraspinal injections — A rare cause of progressive paraparesis. *Zentralblatt fur Neurochirurgie, 61*, 111.

458. Pounder, D., & Elliott, S. (2000). An awake patient may not detect spinal cord puncture. *Anaesthesia, 55*, 194.

459. Dougherty, J. H., & Fraser, R. A. R. (1978). Complications following intraspinal injections of steroids. *Journal of Neurosurgery, 48*, 1023.

460. Lehmann, L. J., & Pallares, V. S. (1995). Subdural injection of a local anesthetic with steroids: Complication of epidural anesthesia. *Southern Medical Journal, 88*, 467.

461. Siegfried, R. N. (1997). Development of complex regional pain syndrome after a cervical epidural steroid injection. *Anesthesiology, 86*, 1394.

462. Rovira, E. et al. (1997). Chronic adhesive arachnoiditis following epidural paramethasone. *Revista de Neurologia, 25*, 2067.

463. Gorski, D. W. et al. (1982). Epidural triamcinolone and adrenal response to hypoglycemic stress in dogs. *Anesthesiology, 57*, 364.

464. Ling, C., Atkinson, P. L., & Munton, C. G. F. (1993). Bilateral retinal hemorrhages following epidural injection. *British Journal of Ophthalmology, 77*, 316.

465. Young, W. F. (2002). Transient blindness after lumbar epidural steroid injection. *Spine, 27*, E476.

466. Clark, C. J., & Whitwell, J. (1961). Intraocular hemorrhage after epidural injection. *British Medical Journal, 2*, 1612.

467. Kushner, F. H., & Olson, J. C. (1995). Retinal hemorrhage as a consequence of epidural steroid injection. *Archives of Ophthalmology, 113*, 309.

468. Purdy, E. P., & Gurjit, S. A. (1998). Vision loss after lumbar epidural steroid injection. *Anesthesia & Analgesia, 86*, 119.

469. Victory, R. A., Hassett, P., & Morrison, G. (1991). Transient blindness following epidural analgesia. *Anaesthesia, 46*, 940.

470. Kao, L. Y. (1998). Bilateral serous retinal detachment resembling central serous chorioretinopathy following epidural steroid injection. *Retina, 18*, 479.

471. Sandberg, D. I., & Lavyne, M. H. (1999). Symptomatic spinal epidural lipomatosis after local epidural corticosteroid injections: case report. *Neurosurgery, 45*, 162.

472. McCullen, G. M., Spurling, G. R., & Webster, J. S. (1999). Epidural lipomatosis complicating lumbar steroid injections. *Journal of Spinal Disorders, 12*, 526.

473. Trattner, A. et al. (1993). Kaposi's sarcoma with visceral involvement after intraarticular and epidural injections of corticosteroids. *Journal of the American Academy of Dermatology, 29*, 890.

474. Knight, C. L., & Burnell, J. C. (1980). Systemic side-effects of extradural steroids. *Anaesthesia, 35*, 593.

475. Jacobs, A. et al. (1983). Adrenal suppression following extradural steroids. *Anaesthesia, 38*, 953.

476. Mikhail, G. R., Sweet, L. C., & Mellinger, R. C. (1973). Parenteral long-acting corticosteroid effect on hypothalamic pituitary adrenal function. *Annals of Allergy, 31*, 337.

477. Mikhail, G. R. et al. (1969). Effect of long-acting parenteral corticosteroids on adrenal function. *Archives of Dermatology, 100*, 263.

478. Melby, J. C. (1974). Drug spotlight program: Systemic corticosteroid therapy; pharmacologic and endocrinologic considerations. *Annals of Internal Medicine, 81*, 505.

479. Boonen, S. et al. (1995). Steroid myopathy induced by epidural triamcinolone injection. *British Journal of Rheumatology, 34*, 385.

480. Ward, A. et al. (2002). Glucocorticoid epidural for sciatica: metabolic and endocrine sequelae. *Rheumatology, 41*, 68.

481. Delaney, T. J. et al. (1980). Epidural steroid effects on nerves and meninges. *Anesthesia & Analgesia, 58*, 610.

482. MacKinnon, S. E. et al. (1982). Peripheral nerve injection injury with steroid agents. *Plastic and Reconstructive Surgery, 69*, 482.

483. Chino, N., Awad, E. A., & Kottke, F. J. (1974). Pathology of propylene glycol administered by perineural and intramuscular injection in rats. *Archives of Physical Medicine and Rehabilitation, 55*, 33.

484. Benzon, H. T. et al. (1987). The effect of polyethylene glycol on mammalian nerve impulses. *Anesthesia & Analgesia, 66*, 553.

485. Abram, S.E., Marsala, M., & Yaksh, T. L. (1994). Analgesic and neurotoxic effects of intrathecal corticosteroids in rats. *Anesthesiology, 81*, 1198.

486. Latham, J. M. et al. (1997). The pathologic effects of intrathecal betamethasone. *Spine, 22*, 1558.

487. Heavner, J. E., Racz, G. B., & Raj, P. (1999). Percutaneous epidural neuroplasty. Prospective evaluation of 0.9% NaCl versus 10% NaCl with or without hyaluronidase. *Regional Anesthesia and Pain Medicine, 24*, 202.

488. Manchikanti, L. et al. (2004). One day lumbar epidural adhesiolysis and hypertonic saline neurolysis in treatment of chronic low back pain: A randomized, double blind trial. *Pain Physician, 7*, 177.

489. Manchikanti, L. et al. (2001). Role of one day epidural adhesiolysis in management of chronic low back pain: A randomized clinical trial. *Pain Physician, 4*, 153.

490. Manchikanti, L. et al. (1999). Role of adhesiolysis and hypertonic saline neurolysis in management of low back pain. Evaluation of modification of Racz protocol. *Pain Digest, 9*, 91.

491. Manchikanti, L. et al. (2001). Effectiveness of percutaneous adhesiolysis and hypertonic saline neurolysis in refractory spinal stenosis. *Pain Physician, 4*, 366.

492. Racz, G. B., & Holubec, J. T. (1989). Lysis of adhesions in the epidural space. In G. B. Racz (Ed.), *Techniques of neurolysis* (p. 57). Boston: Kluwer Academic Press.

493. Manchikanti, L. et al. (1999). Non-endoscopic and endoscopic adhesiolysis in post lumbar laminectomy syndrome. A one-year outcome study and cost effective analysis. *Pain Physician, 2*, 52.

495. Manchikanti, L. et al. (2003). Spinal endoscopic adhesiolysis in the management of chronic low back pain: A preliminary report of a randomized, double-blind trial. *Pain Physician, 6*, 259.

494. Manchikanti, L. et al. (in press). Evaluation of spinal endoscopic adhesiolysis in chronic refractory low back pain with a randomized, double-blind trial with one year follow-up. *Anesthesiology*.

496. Geurts, J. W. et al. (2002). Targeted methylprednisolone acetate/hyaluronidase/clonidine injection after diagnostic epiduroscopy for chronic sciatica: A prospective, 1-year follow-up study. *Regional Anesthesia and Pain Medicine, 27*, 343.

497. Richardson, J. et al. (2001). Spinal endoscopy in chronic low back pain with radiculopathy: A prospective case series. *Anaesthesia, 56*, 454.

498. Manchikanti, L. (2000). The value and safety of epidural endoscopic adhesiolysis. *American Journal of Anesthesiology, 27*, 275.

499. Kim, R.C. et al. (1988). Myelopathy after intrathecal administration of hypertonic saline. *Neurosurgery, 22*, 942.

500. Aldrete, J. A., Zapata, J. C., & Ghaly, R. (1996). Arachnoiditis following epidural adhesiolysis with hypertonic saline report of two cases. *Pain Digest, 6*, 368.

501. Hitchcock, E. R., & Prandini, M. N. (1973). Hypertonic saline in management of intractable pain. *Lancet, 1*, 310.

502. Lucas, J. T., Ducker, T. B., & Perot, P. L. (1975). Adverse reactions to intrathecal saline injections for control of pain. *Journal of Neurosurgery, 42*, 57.

503. Dagi, T. F. (1988). Comments on myelopathy after the intrathecal administration of hypertonic saline. *Neurosurgery, 22*, 944.

504. Lundy, J. S., Essex, H. E., & Kernohan, J. W. (1936). Experiments with anesthetics. IV. Lesions produced in the spinal cord of dogs by a dose of procaine hydrochloride sufficient to cause permanent and fatal paralysis. *Journal of the American Medical Association, 101*, 1546.

505. Gentili, M. E., & Samii, K. (1991). Accidental epidural injection of hypertonic sodium chloride solution. *Annales Francaises d'Anesthesie et le Reanimation, 10*, 401.

506. Manchikanti, L., & Bakhit, C.E. (1997). Removal of torn Racz catheter from lumbar epidural space. *Regional Anesthesia, 22*, 579.

507. Tabandeh, H. (2000). Intraocular hemorrhages associated with endoscopic spinal surgery. *American Journal of Ophthalmology, 129,* 688.

508. Hammer, M. (2002). Safety of spinal endoscopy is contingent on basic image interpretation. *Regional Anesthesia and Pain Medicine, 27,* 621.

509. Singh, V., & Slipman, C. W. (2002). Discogenic pain and intradiscal therapies. In L. Manchikanti, C, W. Slipman, & B. Fellows (Eds.), *Interventional pain management: Low back pain – Diagnosis and treatment* (p. 411). Paducah, KY: ASIPP Publishing.

510. Bogduk, N., & Karasek, M. (2002). Two-year follow-up of a controlled trial of intradiscal electrothermal anuloplasty for chronic low back pain resulting from internal disc disruption. *Spine Journal, 2,* 343.

511. Shah, R. V. et al. (2001). Intradiscal electrothermal therapy: a preliminary histologic study. *Archives of Physical Medicine and Rehabilitation, 82,* 1230.

512. Wetzel, F. T., McNally, T. A., & Phillips, F. M. (2002). Intradiscal electrothermal therapy used to manage chronic discogenic low back pain. *Spine, 27,* 2621.

513. Pauza, K. et al. (2004). A randomized, placebo-controlled trial of intradiscal electrothermal therapy for the treatment of discogenic low back pain. *Spine Journal 4,* 27.

514. Derby, R. et al. (2000). Intradiscal electrothermal annuloplasty (IDET): A novel approach for treating chronic discogenic back pain. *Neuromodulation, 3,* 82.

515. Webster, B. S., Verma, S., & Pransky, G. S. (2004). Outcomes of workers' compensation claimants with low back pain undergoing intradiscal electrothermal therapy. *Spine, 29,* 435.

516. Derby, R. et al. (2004). Comparison of intradiscal restorative injections and intradiscal electrothermal treatment (IDET) in the treatment of low back pain. *Pain Physician, 7,* 63.

517. Saal, J. A. et al. (2001). IDET related complications: A multi-center study of 1,675 treated patients with a review of the FDA MDR data base. In *Proceedings of the North American Spine Society, 16th Annual Meeting,* Seattle, 187.

518. Hsia, A. W., Isaac, K., & Katz, J. S. (2000). Cauda equina syndrome from intradiscal electrothermal therapy. *Neurology, 55,* 320.

519. Ackerman, W. E. (2002). Cauda equina syndrome after intradiscal electrothermal therapy. *Regional Anesthesia and Pain Medicine, 27,* 622.

520. Singh, V. et al. (2002). Percutaneous disc decompression, using coblation (nucleoplasty), in the treatment of discogenic pain. *Pain Physician, 5,* 250.

521. Sharps, L. S., & Isaac, Z. (2002). Percutaneous disc decompression using nucleoplasty. *Pain Physician, 5,* 121.

522. Zhou, Y. et al. (2005). Role of percutaneous disc decompression using coblation in managing chronic discogenic low back pain. *Pain Physician, 8,* 49.

523. Krames, E. (1999). Spinal cord stimulation: Indications, mechanism of action, and efficacy. *Current Review of Pain, 3,* 419.

524. Deer, T. R. (2001). Current and future trends in spinal cord stimulation for chronic pain. *Current Pain and Headache Report, 5,* 503.

525. Oakley, J., & Prager, J. (2002). Spinal cord stimulation: Mechanism of action. *Spine, 22,* 2574.

526. Huber, S., & Vaglienti, R. (2000). Spinal cord stimulation in severe, inoperable, peripheral vascular disease. *Neuromodulation, 3,* 131.

527. Turner, J. A., Loeser, J. D., & Bell, K. G. (1995). Spinal cord stimulation for chronic low back pain. A systematic literature synthesis. *Neurosurgery, 37,* 1088.

528. North, R. B. et al. (1994). Spinal cord stimulation versus reoperation for the failed back surgery syndrome: A prospective, randomized study design. *Stereotactic and Functional Neurosurgery, 62,* 267.

529. Burchiel, K. J. et al. (1996). Prospective: Multicenter study of spinal cord stimulation for relief of chronic back and extremity pain. *Spine, 21,* 2786.

530. Barolat, G. et al. (2001). Epidural spinal cord stimulation with a multiple electrode paddle lead is effective in treating low back pain. *Neuromodulation, 4,* 59.

531. May, M., Banks, C., & Thomson, S. J. (2002). A retrospective, long term, third-party follow-up of patients considered for spinal cord stimulation. *Neuromodulation, 5,* 137.

532. Sarubbi, F., & Vasquez, J. (1997). Spinal epidural abscess associated with the use of temporary epidural catheters: Report of two cases and review. *Clinical Infectious Diseases, 25,* 1155.

533. North, R. B., & Wetzel, F. T. (2002). Spinal cord stimulation for chronic pain of spinal origin. *Spine, 27,* 2584.

534. Prager, J. P. (2002). Neuraxial medication delivery. The development and maturity of a concept for treating chronic pain of spinal origin. *Spine, 27,* 2593.

535. Siddall, P. J. et al. (2000). The efficacy of intrathecal morphine and clonidine in the treatment of pain after spinal cord injury. *Anesthesia & Analgesia, 91,* 1493.

536. van Hilten, B. J. et al. (2000). Intrathecal baclofen for the treatment of dystonia in patients with reflex sympathetic dystrophy. *New England Journal of Medicine, 343,* 654.

537. Smith, T. J. et al. (2002). Randomized clinical trial of an implantable drug delivery system compared with comprehensive medical management for refractory cancer pain: Impact on pain, drug-related toxicity, and survival. *Journal of Clinical Oncology, 20,* 4040.

538. Hassenbusch, S. J., & Stanton-Hicks, M. (1995). Long-term intraspinal infusions in the treatment of neuropathic pain. *Journal of Pain and Symptom Management, 10,* 527.

539. Angel, I. F., Gould, H. J., Jr., & Carey, M. E. (1998). Intrathecal morphine pump as a treatment option in chronic pain of nonmalignant origin. *Surgical Neurology, 49,* 92.

540. Anderson, V. C., & Burchiel, K. J. (1999). A prospective study of long-term intrathecal morphine in the management of chronic nonmalignant pain. *Neurosurgery, 44,* 289.

541. Corrado, P. et al. (2000). The effect of intrathecal morphine infusion on pain level and disability in pain patients with chronic intractable low back pain. *American Journal of Pain Management, 10*, 160.

542. Kumar, K., Kelly, M., & Pirlot, T. (2001). Continuous intrathecal morphine treatment for chronic pain of nonmalignant etiology: Long-term benefits and efficacy. *Surgical Neurology, 55*, 79.

543. Coffey, R., & Burchiel, K. (2002). Inflammatory mass lesions associated with intrathecal infusion catheters: Report and observations on 41 patients. *Neurosurgery, 50*, 78.

59

Psychological Evaluation in Interventional Pain Practice

Jeffrey W. Janata, PhD

INTRODUCTION

Two phenomena currently characterize the field of pain medicine. First is the dramatic rise of interventional pain practice. Invasive, nonsurgical procedures are playing an increasingly prominent role in the treatment of chronic pain.[1] Simultaneously, research points out how psychologically and behaviorally complex are the patients who present to pain physicians. Recent informal studies indicate that an alarming proportion of patients in carefully managed practices are abusing narcotics or other substances and are escaping routine detection.[2] Depression as a consequence of chronic pain is considered normative.[3] Demoralization and passivity typically characterize this population, which increases the implicit demand on physicians to provide cures. Physicians, and particularly their staffs, complain of the high incidence of personality disorders in their practices. The physicians who care for people with chronic pain often find themselves feeling overwhelmed and at a loss regarding how to provide compassionate care while developing and protecting their practices and finding a sense of satisfaction in their work.

This chapter is written with the intention of aiding clinicians in identifying strategies used to elucidate psychological and behavioral factors, which contribute to and are consequent of chronic pain, particularly for patients who may be candidates for interventional pain procedures.

Comprehensive evaluation of people experiencing chronic pain definitionally includes assessment of the behavioral and social factors that contribute to the subjective experience of pain. This is distinct from the assessment of psychiatric pathology, which may constitute a comorbid condition, in the case, for example, of a patient presenting with chronic pain who incidentally carries a diagnosis of schizophrenia, which is otherwise well controlled on antipsychotic medication.

SOURCES OF EVALUATIVE INFORMATION

Psychological and behavioral information can come from a variety of sources each informing clinicians in unique ways.

CLINICAL INTERVIEW AND PATIENT QUESTIONNAIRES

The clinical interview can be a rich source of information and often provides the initial indication that a more comprehensive psychological evaluation is indicated.[4,5] Experienced clinicians follow a general interview outline to ensure obtaining a complete picture but not so rigidly as to get in the way of hearing the patient's story.[6] Table 59.1 provides a suggested outline for the clinical interview, which can be paralleled in a questionnaire given to patients to complete in advance of their initial appointment or in the waiting room.

PAIN

The clinical interview (and questionnaire) should always begin with the complaints that bring the patient to the

TABLE 59.1
Outline of the Clinical Interview and Waiting Room Questionnaire

1. Pain
   a. Pattern and distribution, including pain drawing
   b. Pain rating: best, worst, average levels
   c. Qualitative pain perception: adjectival descriptions of pain
   d. Activities, events, interventions that increase, decrease pain
   e. Coping with pain: the patient's adaptive and maladaptive strategies
2. Pain History
   a. Precipitating event
   b. Duration
   c. Treatment history: Physicians consulted, diagnostic procedures, medications (prescribing physician, dosage, response), interventional procedures (physician, response)
   d. Patient's understanding, beliefs about his/her pain, diagnosis and prognosis
3. General medical history and status
   a. Medical and surgical history
   b. Medications for conditions other than pain
   c. Physical status: height, current weight and weight history, sleep patterns
   d. Sexual function
   e. Nicotine, caffeine use
   f. Substance use: history, any treatment, family history, CAGE* questions
4. Financial and legal history
   a. Pursuit of disability, family history of disability
   b. Pending litigation, family history of litigation
   c. Current sources of financial support
5. Educational and occupational history
   a. Educational history
   b. Occupational history
   c. Perceived future occupational opportunity
6. Psychosocial information
   a. Behavioral observation, how the patient expresses pain verbally and physically, obtained from staff waiting room observation and during interview
   b. Mental status examination
   c. Psychological, psychiatric history: personal and family
   d. Family and marital status and history
   e. Impact of pain on personal functioning, degree of independence, dependence
   f. Impact of pain on family functioning
   g. Daily activity, description of typical day

*1. C: Have you ever felt that you should **Cut down** on your drinking?
 2. A: Have people **Annoyed** you by criticizing your drinking?
 3. G: Have you ever felt bad or **Guilty** about your drinking?
 4. E: Have you ever had a drink first thing in the morning to steady your nerves or get rid of a hangover? (**Eye-opener**)

Interpretation:
Answering yes to two questions is a strong indication for alcoholism. Answering yes to three questions confirms alcoholism.

Source: Adapted from Ewing, J.A., 1984, *Journal of the American Medical Association, 252,* 1905–1907.

office. Patients typically want to be able to provide a narrative of their pain experience and history, which can be full of emotion, attribution, and expectation and "present the thread necessary to weave the facts of the clinician's evaluation into the fabric of pain".[7] Pain drawings can provide valuable information about the patient's experience of pain. Pain ratings often indicate not only perception of the intensity of pain but also provide clues about the patient's cognitive set. For example, it is not uncommon that patients are better able to describe what makes pain worse than what helps to decrease pain. This helps define a negative cognitive set on the part of the person in pain, symptomatic of the situational depression that is so commonly seen in chronic pain presentations[8] and provides the clinician an early opportunity to help the patient recalibrate his or her sense of the topography of pain intensity through the day.

PAIN HISTORY

Pain history provides the patient's perspective on causes of pain and the types of interventions used to date. This again gives the clinician a view of the patient's emotional response to the circumstances surrounding the onset of pain and to prior attempts by physicians to alleviate the pain. A careful examination of pain medications used and the patient's response to those medications helps to begin the process of understanding the patient's expectations of relief provided by medications and the potential evolving dependence on those medications. Behavior indicative of physical tolerance, psychological dependence, and addiction deserves careful attention.[9,10] Addiction is defined by a pervasive preoccupation with obtaining a substance, use or misuse despite negative consequences to the patient, and an increased risk that illegal means will be employed (e.g., prescription forgery or alteration) or illegal substances sought to satisfy the patient's craving. Addiction has been likened to experiencing a "hole in the soul" (T. Parran, personal communication) that only the substance of choice can fill. By contrast, pseudo-addiction is an iatrogenic condition created when a beneficial medication is provided in inadequate doses or with unnecessarily rigid restrictions on the part of the prescribing physician. An example of the latter condition might be the physician who provides prescription refills only every 30 days to the day to a patient whose work requires frequent travel. What appears to be drug-seeking behavior may in fact be reasonable relief-seeking.

GENERAL MEDICAL INFORMATION

Obtaining general medical information helps complete the medical context in which painful conditions reside. It also provides the first opportunity to observe any vegetative signs of depression in chronic pain. Recent history of weight loss or gain may be symptomatic of depression, and sleep disturbance is among the most common complaints of patients experiencing pain. While patients may report that sleep is disturbed by virtue of the difficulty they face in finding comfortable sleeping positions, sleep disturbance may represent another of the vegetative signs of affective disorder. Sexual function is often overlooked in medical history-taking and yet to ignore patients' concerns about the quality of their sex lives is to avoid an important aspect of their experience. Sexual function can be impaired by pain itself and by medications used to manage pain, particularly the selective serotonin reuptake inhibitors (SSRI) class of antidepressants. Decreased sexual drive can be symptomatic of depression, and sexual difficulties can contribute to marital distress. Use of substances represents a critical line of inquiry, particularly given the aforementioned high rate of undetected substance abuse in the chronic pain population. Embedding the CAGE questions[11] in a questionnaire can provide clinicians important clues regarding the risk of misuse of analgesics.

Financial and Legal History

The financial and legal portions of the interview are often overlooked in clinical practice. Clinicians are as likely to experience discomfort when asking about patient finances as when inquiring about sexual function. However, the patient's financial status and concerns about financial security can set the context for anticipatory anxiety, thereby increasing the urgency with which a cure is demanded of the physician. Pursuing legal aspects of the patient's presentation is equally critical. A patient intent on seeking disability has different expectations of medical care than does one who is intent on return to occupational function, yet this intention is often difficult to detect. Inquiry both in questionnaire and interview form may increase the likelihood that clinicians have an accurate sense of the patient's motivation. Finally, asking simply whether a patient has contacted or retained an attorney can open an important line of inquiry.

Educational and Occupational History

Educational and occupational history provides a sense of premorbid functioning and may set the stage for inquiry about the patient's anxiety about the future. A patient employed historically as a laborer presenting with chronic low back pain is entitled to considerably greater anxiety about future employability than one who has a long history of stable white collar employment.

Psychosocial Information

The psychosocial section completes the interview process and indications already obtained of psychological diffi-

culty can be more fully pursued. In addition to asking about previous psychological diagnosis and treatment, obtaining family history of psychopathology is also helpful in determining possible genetic risk. The history can aid, for instance, in establishing that a biological risk of depression exists in addition to a situational depressive response to pain. The degree of patient stability in marital and familial relationships, along with employment stability, can provide initial indications of possible personality disorders, defined by the DSM IV[12] as persistent, maladaptive patterns of behavior affecting cognition, affect, interpersonal function, and/or impulse control. Personality disorders influence how one relates to others and are expressed frequently in the interpersonal relationship that a patient develops with his or her physician and staff. Because personality disorders are developmentally present as early as adolescence, these long-term patterns of dysfunction are likely to be present prior to the onset of pain. However, the distress accompanying pain can amplify the symptoms of personality disorders.[13,14]

Mood evaluation is central to the comprehensive evaluation of pain. In addition to the vegetative signs of affective disorders, chronic pain routinely and predictably precipitates emotional responses such as anger, irritability, and agitation. As pain persists despite ameliorative efforts, patients can become demoralized and experience *learned helplessness* characterized by passivity and increased dependence. *Locus of control* is a psychological construct that describes a continuum from internal to external. Internal locus of control suggests an individual who relies primarily on internal resources to manage life stresses, while external locus of control describes one who relies primarily on resources outside his or her own control. Patients with long histories of pain inevitably have learned from their own failed attempts at managing pain and increasingly depend on external strategies. Eventually, this can create a pattern of overreliance on physicians, procedures, and medications. A pattern of passivity and evidence of external locus of control provides clues to the clinician that intervention strategies should be paired with, or even made conditional upon, evidence of the patient's engaging in self-managed efforts.

The mood assessment should also explore suicidality and impulsivity. Depression is the strongest correlate of suicidal ideation and behavior. Impulsivity, often expressed in a history of substance misuse, helps establish risk for impulsive misuse of medications. Finally, clinicians prescribing narcotics and antidepressants (particularly tricyclics) need to be aware that another correlate of suicidal behavior is access to lethal means.

Observations about a patient's demeanor and personal interactions while in the office may provide insight regarding the patient's cognitive state. However, a mental status examination should be included in the interview to provide more specific information about memory and cognition, particularly if traumatic brain injury is suspected.

Inquiry into a patient's typical day can be revelatory. Evidence of the impact of pain on personal and family function, on physical activity and functional capacity, and on quality of life can be revealed and explored further as indicated.

The interview and waiting room questionnaires can generate a rich, initial source of data, setting the stage for determining whether additional psychological evaluation is indicated. Moreover, these data help to determine what particular consultative questions are being asked of a pain-informed psychologist or psychiatrist. Establishing a comprehensive psychological understanding of the patient in chronic pain often is aided by the process of *convergent validation*, in which history, observations, patterns of behavior and assessment results coalesce to create a more valid and reliable diagnostic and prognostic picture than any of these means alone can provide. The high probability of psychological and behavioral distress in the chronic pain population argues for routine inclusion of psychological opinion in comprehensive, team-based assessment of pain.

PSYCHOLOGICAL ASSESSMENT

Formal psychological assessment employs instruments that have been thoroughly researched and provide established reliability and validity. *Reliability* refers to the capacity of an instrument to provide the same data over time. Scales have established reliability coefficients that quantify this capacity for stable measurement. *Validity* measures indicate the degree to which an instrument measures what it purports to measure.

PERSONALITY

Although the search for the pain-prone personality has been roughly as fruitful as the search for the Holy Grail,[15] personality issues specific to particular individuals can be revelatory. The utility of personality testing per se continues to be debated,[16] yet the potential for describing one's general psychological status, detecting prognostic behavioral information, and the reliance of the medicolegal system on personality testing preserve an important role for personality assessment.

The Minnesota Multiphasic Personality Inventory (MMPI-2)[17] is a widely used and highly validated general measure of personality. Among its strengths is the use of validity scales that provide a profile of test-taking set. The MMPI's capacity to estimate whether an examinee provided a valid self-description, tried to appear healthy, or tried to appear unhealthy can be beneficial to clinicians. The 10 primary clinical scales and a host of subscales and research scales help explain the prominence of the MMPI

in personality testing. Computer scoring provides scale scores and a brief, initial interpretive narrative. The test comprises 576 true–false questions, so the time it takes a patient to complete the test is significant. Clinicians need to weigh the cost in patient time against the possible diagnostic benefits of MMPI administration.

The Symptom Checklist-90 (SCL-90-R)[18] comprises 90 items describing both physical and psychological symptoms. Each item is scored using a five-point scale representing the degree to which a particular symptom was bothersome to the patient in the past week. Nine clinical scales are derived, estimating, for example, obsessive-compulsive tendencies, somatization, depression, and anxiety. Like the MMPI, the SCL-90-R has been widely used in pain populations.

The Millon Behavioral Health Inventory (MBHI)[19] was designed to assess personality function in medical populations. The instrument is a 150-item scale, deriving 20 clinical scales: eight scales assessing styles of relating to providers, six that assess stressors, and six that assess probable response to illness. Advantages of the MBHI include having fewer items than the MMPI, its items having low somatic content, and the instrument having been validated in a medical (rather than psychiatric) population.

MOOD

The relationship between mood and pain has been well established.[20,21] The experience of pain has been associated with vegetative symptoms (e.g., sleep disturbance, weight changes), affective symptoms (e.g., demoralization, irritability, anger), and cognitive symptoms (e.g., concentration, attention). Several instruments have been found to be useful in the assessment of mood.

The Beck Depression Inventory (BDI-2)[22] has been extensively used in pain populations.[23,24] It is brief and well validated, consisting of 21 items each with four possible answers. Easily scored in the office, the BDI provides clinicians with information in cognitive-affective as well as somatic-performance domains. The Beck provides a well-accepted criterion for psychological distress that has been used frequently in studies of chronic pain.[25]

The Center for Epidemiological Studies-Depression Scale (CES-D)[26] was designed as an alternative to the BDI, arising out of a concern that the somatic content on the BDI might artificially inflate estimation of depression in medical populations.[27] One study suggests that the CES-D was somewhat more sensitive to changes in the severity of depression than the BDI,[28] which may reflect its deemphasis of somatic content.

The Profile of Mood States (POMS)[29] provides an assessment of six mood states (tension–anxiety, anger–hostility, depression–dejection, vigor–activity, fatigue–inertia, and confusion–bewilderment). The

POMS is being employed in an increasing number of pain treatment studies.[30,31]

MEASURES OF PHYSICAL FUNCTIONING

Pain-specific, health quality of life measures quantify the degree to which pain interferes with daily functioning. A series of studies has demonstrated that pain and function are only modestly correlated,[32] however, which argues for the inclusion of measures of function in pain assessment.

The SF-36 Health Survey[33] is a widely used general measure of health-related quality of life. The instrument provides an eight-scale profile of functional health scores, along with indices of physical and mental health. Although much used in the surveys of general health, its utility in pain populations has been tempered by concern that it may lack adequate sensitivity to change in pain populations.[28]

The Sickness Impact Profile[34] assesses perception of general health and, as such, is not specific to pain. However, scales derived, such as ambulation, mobility, body care, and social activity, may be useful in some pain subtypes in which a patient's perception of his or her level of disability is in question.

The Multidimensional Pain Inventory (MPI)[35] more specifically assesses pain and function using 56 items scored on a seven-point scale. Nine clinical scales are derived, including particularly interference of pain on physical functioning. Other scales include ratings of pain severity, life control, affective distress, social support, punishing and distracting responses from others, and a measure of activity level. The MPI assigns the probability that a patient falls into one of three profiles: dysfunctional, interpersonally distressed, or active coper.

The Brief Pain Inventory (BPI)[36] measures intensity of pain and interference of pain, including interference with sleep, a clinically significant concern. The inventory is well validated and reliable and has been used in a variety of painful conditions.

Additional instruments of note include the Oswesty Low Back Pain Disability Questionnaire;[37] the Coping Strategies Questionnaire,[38] used to evaluate how patients are coping with pain (e.g., catastrophizing, praying, reinterpreting pain sensations); the Pain Cognitions Questionnaire,[39] which assesses patient beliefs and expectations about pain and its treatment; and the Pain Disability Index,[40] which provides disability evaluation of seven areas of function.

SCREENING FOR USE OF INVASIVE PROCEDURES

Most clinicians are in agreement with the use of psychological exclusion criteria when considering use of interventional procedures, particularly spinal cord stimulators, which can inform clinical thinking when considering the use of narcotics as well. Nelson, Kennington, Novy et al.[41] have proposed the following criteria:

1. Active psychosis. With evidence of delusions, hallucinations, or somatic preoccupation, the validity of pain complaints must be suspect. However, patients who are well controlled on antipsychotic medications, who are not currently or recently psychotic, may be candidates for interventional procedures if carefully psychiatrically monitored.

2. Major depression, untreated or poorly treated. Patients with severe mood disturbance may, as a consequence, experience intensification of pain or be at risk for responding poorly to treatment. Moreover, the relationship between mood and pain is likely bidirectional; failure to isolate and aggressively treat significant mood disturbance puts clinicians at risk for underappreciating that pain report is inflated and maintained by depression. Significant sleep disturbance should also indicate pretreatment prior to considering pain intervention. It should be emphasized that depression is a normal consequence of pain and does not preclude adequate response to treatment; it is the severity of depression that is at issue.

3. Active suicidal ideation or behavior. Suicidal thoughts, preoccupations, intentions, or plans require psychological or psychiatric intervention before pain treatment can be considered. Suicidal patients cannot reliably participate in the process of treatment and are at risk to respond to failed treatment with a fatal solution to pain.

4. Active homicidal thinking or behavior. Patients who are preoccupied with thoughts of violence or who have a history of difficulty controlling violent impulses are considered too unstable to engage in treatment. Rarely are such individuals candidates for spinal cord stimulation at any point, given the difficulty achieving adequate psychological stabilization. This poor prognosis should inform clinical use of other pain interventions as well.

5. Untreated or poorly treated substance abuse or addiction. A patient with drug-seeking behavior cannot be relied on to adhere to a medication or treatment regimen. Moreover, addicts are at risk to pursue medicinal narcotics over street drugs, given relative purity, low cost, and diminished legal risk. Clinicians should refer patients with alcohol or drug addiction for evaluation and treatment and reconsider such patients for inter-

vention only after a minimum of 3 months of appropriate control of substance use.

6. Somatization or somatoform disorder. These diagnoses carry the risk that the patient will be preoccupied with physical complaints that are unsupported by or exceed evidence obtained in diagnostic evaluations. The dilemma here, of course, is that pain mechanisms in many conditions are not well understood. What may appear to be a non-organic complaint may originate with an undetected or undetectable physical cause. Referral to a psychologist or psychiatrist who is familiar with the somatoform disorders can help to clarify this complex issue.

7. Unresolved compensation or litigation issues. Active disability pursuit or involvement in a lawsuit can create a significant disincentive for patients to report positive response to treatment. This should not suggest that every patient on disability or pursuing legal remedy is a poor candidate for interventional pain treatment, only that the influence of these contingencies should be carefully examined.

8. Lack of adequate social support. To be successful, pain treatment and rehabilitative efforts require the daily practical and psychological support of family members or friends. Our experience suggests that social support is an important prognostic indicator.

9. Serious cognitive deficits. When reason, judgment, or memory are significantly impaired, a patient cannot be expected to actively partner with a treating physician or team in participating in treatment or reliably reporting pain symptoms.

10. Inadequate self-efficacy. Self-efficacy,[42] or the perception that a person has in him or her the ability to effect behavior change, predicts response to treatment and may mediate the relationship between pain and disability.[43] As noted earlier, patients who overrely on external strategies to try to control pain are disinclined to actively engage in the behavior change efforts that are the necessary companions to pain interventions.

ASSESSMENT OF OUTCOME

Dworkin, Turk, and colleagues[31] have advocated the standardized use of behavioral measures to assess the outcome of pain treatment. The Initiative on Methods, Measurement and Pain Assessment in Clinical Trials (IMMPACT) convened 35 specialists representing academics, patient advocates, governmental institutions, and the pharmaceutical industry to recommend core outcome measures for pain treatment trials. Included in their recommendations was the routine use of (1) pain intensity ratings (using a 0 to 10 numerical rating); (2) measures of physical functioning, such as the Brief Pain Inventory or the Multidimensional Pain Inventory Interference Scale; (3) measures of emotional function, specifying either the Beck Depression Inventory or the Profile of Mood States; (4) ratings of overall improvement as estimated by the Patient Global Impression of Change scale; (5) comprehensive review of history and symptoms, with particular emphasis on prospective assessment of predictable adverse or stressful events that appear contribute to pain exacerbation; and (6) comprehensive documentation of treatment adherence and reasons for discontinuation of a treatment trial.

Especially in the field of pain, where long-term benefits of particular treatment strategies have not been demonstrated, the kind of standardization that IMMPACT calls for is more than justified. As pain management and interventional strategies evolve and develop, the use of standard sets of outcome measures can aid in the process of developing research protocols, provide comparability across treatment types and settings, and create a basis for determining which treatment outcomes constitute clinically meaningful differences.[44]

REFERENCES

1. Krames, E. S. (1999). Interventional pain management. Appropriate when less invasive therapies fail to provide adequate analgesia. *Medical Clinics North America, 83,* 787–808.

2. Atluri, S. et al. (2003). Guidelines for the use of controlled substances in the management of chronic pain. ASIPP controlled substances guidelines. *Pain Physician, 6,* 233–257.

3. Romano, J. M., & Turner, J. A. (1985). Chronic pain and depression: Does the evidence support a relationship? *Psychological Bulletin, 97,* 18–34.

4. Deyo, R. A., Rainville, J., & Kent, D. L. (1992). What can the history and physical tell us about low back pain? *Journal of the American Medical Association, 268,* 760.

5. Feuerstein, M., & Beattie, P. (1995). Biobehavioral factors affecting pain and disability in low back pain: Mechanisms and assessment. *Physical Therapy, 75,* 267.

6. Morris, D. B. (1997). The plot of suffering [abstract]. *Proceedings of the American Pain Society.* New Orleans: American Pain Society.

7. Doleys, D. M., & Doherty, D. C. (2003). Psychologic Evaluation. In P. P. Raj (Ed.), *Pain Medicine: A comprehensive review.* St. Louis: Mosby.

8. Roy, R., Thomas, M., & Matas, M. (1984). Chronic pain and depression: A review. *Comprehensive Psychiatry, 25*(1), 96–105.

9. Portenoy, R. K. (1996). Opioid therapy for chronic nonmalignant pain: A review of the critical issues. *Journal of Pain and Symptom Management, 11*(4), 203–217.

10. Krames, E. (2002). Implantable devices for pain control: spinal cord stimulation and intrathecal therapies. *Best Practice and Research. Clinical Anesthesiology, 16*(4), 619–649.

11. Ewing, J. A. (1984). Detecting alcoholism: The CAGE questionnaire. *Journal of the American Medical Association, 252*, 1905–1907.

12. American Psychiatric Association. (1994). *Diagnostic and statistical manual of mental disorders* (4th ed.). Washington, DC: Author.

13. Weisberg, J. N. (2000). Personality and personality disorders in chronic pain. *Current Review of Pain, 4*(1), 60–70.

14. Weisberg, J. N., & Villaincourt, P. D. (1999). Personality factors and disorders in chronic pain. *Seminars in Clinical Neuropsychiatry, 4*(3), 155–166.

15. Roy, R. (1982). Pain-prone patient: A revisit. *Psychotherapy and Psychosomatics, 37*, 202–213.

16. Nelson, D. V., Kennington, M., & Novy, D. M. (1996). Psychological selection criteria for implantable spinal cord stimulators. *Pain Forum, 5*(2), 93–103.

17. Butcher, J. N. (1989). *Minnesota multiphasic personality inventory (MMPI-2).* Minneapolis, MN: University of Minneapolis Press.

18. Kinney, R. K., Gatchel, R. J., & Mayer, T. G. (1991). The SCL-90-R evaluated as an alternative to the MMPI for psychological screening in chronic low back pain patients. *Spine, 16*, 940–943.

19. Millon, T., Green, C., & Meagher, R. (1982). *Millon behavioral health inventory* (3rd ed.). Minneapolis, MN: National Computer Systems.

20. Von Korff, M., & Simon, G. (1996). The relationship between pain and depression. *British Journal of Psychiatry – Supplementum, 30*, 101–108.

21. Faucett, J. A. (1994). Depression in painful chronic disorders: the role of pain and conflict about pain. *Journal of Pain and Symptom Management, 9*(8), 520–526.

22. Beck, A. T. (1996). *Beck depression inventory.* New York: Harcourt, Brace.

23. Novy, D. M., Nelson, D. V., Berry, L. A., & Averill, P. M. (1995). What does the Beck depression inventory measure in chronic pain? *Pain, 61*(2), 261–270.

24. Williams, A. C., & Richardson, P. H. (1993). What does the BDI measure in chronic pain? *Pain, 55*(2), 259–266.

25. Kerns, R. D. (2003). Assessment of emotional functioning in pain treatment outcome research. Presented at the second meeting of the Initiative on Moods, Methods and Pain Assessment in Clinical Trials (IMMPACT-II), (www.immpact.org/meetings.html).

26. Roberts, R. E., & Vernon, S. W. (1983). The Center for Epidemiological Studies depression scale: Its use in a community sample. *American Journal of Psychiatry, 140*(1), 41–46.

27. Wesley, A. L., Gatchel, R. A., Polatin, P. B. et al. (1991). Differentiation between somatic and cognitive/affective components in commonly used measures of depression with chronic low back pain. *Spine,* (Suppl. 16), S213–S215.

28. Wittink, H., Turk, D. C., Carr, D. B., Sukiennik, A., & Rogers, W. (2004). Comparison of the redundancy, reliability and responsiveness to change among the SF-36, Oswestry Disability Index and Multidimensional Pain Inventory. *Clinical Journal of Pain, 20*(3), 133–142.

29. McNair, D. M., Lorr, M., & Droppleman, L. F. (1971). *Profile of mood states.* San Diego: Educational and Industrial Testing Service.

30. Dworkin, R. H., Corbin, A. E., Young Jr., J. P. et al. (2003). Pregabalin for the treatment of postherpetic neuralgia: A randomized, placebo-controlled trial. *Neurology, 60*(8), 1274–1283.

31. Dworkin, R. H., Turk, D. C., Farrar, J. T. et al. (2005). Core outcome measures for chronic pain clinical trials: IMMPACT recommendations. *Pain, 113*(1–2), 9–19.

32. Turk, D. C. (2002). Clinical effectiveness and cost effectiveness of treatments for patients with chronic pain. *Clinical Journal of Pain, 18*, 355–365.

33. Ware, J. E., & Sherbourne, C. D. (1992). The MOS 36-item short-form health survey (SF-36). *Medical Care, 30*, 473–483.

34. Bergner, M., Bobbitt, R.A., Carter, W. B. et al (1981). The Sickness Impact Profile: Development and final revision of a health status measure. *Medical Care, 119*, 787–805.

35. Kerns, R. D., Turk, D. C., & Rudy, T. E. (1985). The West Haven-Yale Multidimensional Pain Inventory (WHYMPI). *Pain, 23*, 345–356.

36. Cleeland, C. S., & Ryan, K. M. (1994). Pain assessment: Global use of the Brief Pain Inventory. *Annals of the Academy of Medicine, 23,* 129–138.

37. Fairbank, J. C., Couper, J., Daviess, J. B. et al. (1980). The Oswestry low back pain disability questionnaire. *Physiotherapy, 66*(8), 271–273.

38. Rosenstiel, A. K., & Keefe, F. J. (1983). The use of coping strategies in chronic low back pain patients: Relationship to patient characteristics and current adjustment. *Pain, 17*(1), 33–44.

39. Boston, K., Pearce, S. A., & Richardson, P. H. (1990). The pain cognitions questionnaire. *Journal of Psychosomatic Research, 34*(1), 103–109.

40. Pollard, C. A. (1985). Preliminary validity study of the pain disability index. *Perceptual and Motor Skills, 59*, 974–981.

41. Nelson, D. V., Kennington, M., Novy, D. M. et al. (1996). Psychological selection criteria for implantable spinal cord stimulators. *Pain Forum, 5*(2), 93–103.

42. Bandura, A. (1997). *Self-efficacy: The exercise of control.* New York: WH Freeman.

43. Lumley, M. A., Smith, J. A., & Longo, D. J. (2002). The relationship of alexythymia to pain severity and impairment among patients with chronic myofascial pan: Comparisons with self-efficacy, catastrophizing, and depression. *Journal of Psychosomatic Research, 53*(3), 823–830.

44. Jadad, A. R., & Cepeda, M. S. (2000). Ten challenges at the intersection of clinical research, evidence-based medicine, and pain relief. *Annals of Emergency Medicine, 36*, 247–252.

60

Epidural Steroid Injections

W. David Leak, MD

INTRODUCTION

Epidural injection of corticosteroids is commonly used for managing chronic spinal pain and other painful conditions. Several approaches are available to access the lumbar epidural space: caudal, interlaminar, and transforaminal. The mechanisms of action of epidural injections are not well understood, but it is believed that neural blockade alters or interrupts nociceptive or neuropathic mechanisms. Explanations for improvement are based in part on the pharmacological and physical actions of local anesthetics, corticosteroids, and other agents. Effects may occur at spinal roots, dorsal root ganglia, and the dorsal horn. It is probable that the steroid component of the injection has an anti-inflammatory component, although there may be effects on neural excitability as well.

The placement of chemicals for diagnostic, prognostic, and therapeutic purposes in the epidural space is widely practiced and published. More than 1,817 references were cited in 2004, up from 447 in 2000, in the National Library of Medicine, using the search phrase "epidural injection." The search for the keyword "epidural" yielded 20,471 citations in 2000. The search in 2004 produced 25,607 references.

Approximately 140 citations referenced transforaminal epidural injections. The advent of sensitive and specific electrophysiological diagnostic testing and the standard application of fluoroscopy make precision needle localization the most practical approach for epidural injections for advanced practitioners of interventional pain management. The use of epidural injections, although a useful clinical tool, is underappreciated and thus undervalued relative to associated risk.

Key clinical pearl: Transforaminal epidural injections may be used as a diagnostic, prognostic, or therapeutic tool. Current literature affirms that transforaminal epidural injection is neither experimental nor investigational.

HISTORICAL BACKGROUND

Clinical reports of the earliest use of epidural anesthesia were credited to James Corning. Corning used intraspinal cocaine on a human with "spinal weakness and seminal incontinence." These were classified as neurological illnesses. The results were reported in the fall of 1885 in the *New York Medical Journal*. European urologists Cathelin and Sicard of France documented epidural placement via the sacral route in the early 1900s. Epidural injection to treat sciatica was described by Viner in 1925. Edwards and Hingson reported continuous caudal epidural anesthesia in 1942 (Kafiluddi & Hahn, 2000). Interventional procedures can be partitioned into three major purposes: (1) diagnostic, (2) prognostic, and (3) therapeutic.

Historically, epidural steroid injections were viewed as therapeutic, applied in many cases to treat sciatica. Epidural injection with various agents may be diagnostic. Injection of epidural steroids yielding relief suggests inflammatory disease. Injection of epidural local anesthetics for lower extremity pain relief that lasts well beyond the duration of the local anesthetic suggests neuropathic or autonomic dysfunction. Should pain return after a short duration of relief (hours, days, weeks), the procedure is prognostic for future interventions. If pain relief is prolonged after the diagnostic injection, the procedure is therapeutic.

Key clinical pearl: Epidural injection and infusion are neither new nor investigational.

ANATOMY

The epidural space is confined to the cranial and spinal canal. The most common reference is the space between the walls of the vertebral canal and the dura mater of the spinal cord (Stedman, 1999). It extends from the most cephalad aspect of the cranium surrounding the brain with compartmental interruption at the foramen magnum. In the spinal canal, it extends caudally to the sacrococcygeal junction. Thus, epidural therapies and pathology may occur from the cranium to the caudal canal.

Accessing the epidural space in the spinal column had been traditionally taught as a "blind technique," palpating vertebral spinous processes and advancing the needle using proprioceptive feedback. Numerous terms have been used to describe the sensations one should appreciate during various phases of this "blind procedure." The terms include words such as *give, pop, release,* and *loss of resistance.* When taught by experts, an appreciation of these mystical sensations can be regarded as universal truths that guarantee proper procedural performance. The subcutaneous fascial planes and intervertebral ligaments have give, will pop, release, and lose resistance but may direct a needle far away from the epidural space.

The advent of fluoroscopic guidance for spinal injection procedures has revealed that massive amounts of misinformation existed relative to the anatomy, proprioception, and behavior of infusions into the epidural space. When compared with fluoroscopy, vertebral interspaces (specifically the L3–4) could not be identified using conventional anatomy surface landmarks in patients in the prone position. Clinicians and researchers have published prospective studies demonstrating the essential need for fluoroscopy when performing epidural blocks for painful diseases (Bogduk, Aprill, & Derby, 1995; Manchikanti & Bakhit, 1999). White (White, Derby, & Wynne, 1980) noted a missed target rate of 25% using blind techniques for epidurals. The traditional teachings suggested that the spread of injection solutions in the epidural space could be calculated. Teaching that the volume of an anesthetic solution would cover predictable anatomic areas has been proved erroneous by numerous clinical reports (Bogduk et al., 1995).

A recent review by Boswell et al. (2005) concluded that there is strong evidence for transforaminal epidural steroid injections in managing lumbar nerve root pain. Evidence for caudal epidural steroid injections in managing lumbar radicular pain also was strong. Evidence for other conditions was either limited or inconclusive.

THE WORK-UP

Although mastery of anatomy for execution of the epidural injection is required, the most important components of the procedure are performing it correctly, for the right reasons. Guidelines regarding technical aspects of the procedure and clinical indications are available (Boswell et al., 2003, 2005).

Patient history and physical examination should generate substantial subjective and objective evidence to support the need for the procedure. The impressions and plan should be consistent with the history and physical examination. Avoidance of being the "itinerant surgeon" is of paramount importance. A patient may be referred for a series of epidural injections for back pain or sciatica. The performance of a transient palliative procedure may result in masking or delaying the diagnosis of cancer, exacerbating undiagnosed diabetes, propagation of discitis, worsening of osteomyelitis, all of which are preventable. Thus, a review of records, history, and relevant laboratory and radiographic studies, and physical examination constitute the minimum standard prior to performance of the procedure.

Precise diagnosis is important, as the transforaminal epidural has become the most appropriate injection of choice. An appropriate medical evaluation prior to injection is medically indicated and necessary. The application of electrophysiological studies to evaluate the status of sensory, vasomotor, thermal, and/or sudomotor activity of specific nerve roots may provide additional useful diagnostic information.

The specific components of the medical evaluation should include the following.

HISTORY

1. Chief complaint
2. History of present illness (include other work-ups and treatment for the current problem)
3. Past medical and surgical history (e.g., age is an important factor in the work-up of complaints of low-back pain from a 20-year-old subject)
4. Social history (e.g., work, smoking, substance abuse, and secondary gain factors should be explored)
5. Family history (rheumatoid disease, coagulopathy, cancer, etc.)
6. Allergies and specific reactions and where the events are documented:
   a. Beware of patients who are allergic to "all nonsteroidal anti-inflammatory drugs"
   b. Supplementation of pain relief with scheduled drugs must be based on appropriate medical evaluation

c. When total classes of nondependency producing agents are reported without any health care professional's objective documentation, consider allergy testing

7. Medication history (a copy of pharmacy printouts from the previous 12 months is recommended)

8. Review of systems

Physical Examination

1. Vital signs:
   a. They will change in association with performance of epidurals.
   b. Noxious stimulation associated with traumatic introduction of a trochar into an already hyperalgesic area may produce a clinically significant changes in hemodynamics.
   c. A patient rendered "normotensive" by antihypertensive agents may be volume deficient and suffer physiologic consequences from epidural infusions and associated vasodilation.

2. Cardiovascular exam:
   a. Mortality associated with epidural injections in the face of uncompensated aortic stenosis is a preventable circumstance. The epidural may cause vasodilatation that may not be adequately compensated for in an individual with severe aortic stenosis, resulting in profound hypotension.

3. Neurologic exam:
   a. Sensory, motor, and reflex findings should be documented prior to commencing a procedure with the capacity to cause neurologic damage.

4. Musculoskeletal exam:
   a. Tenderness pre- and postprocedure
   b. Noxious range of motion
   c. Pain-alleviating range of motion
   d. Documentation of range of motion

5. Integument:
   a. Infectious lesions of the skin in the path of the epidural are direct contraindications to performing the procedure.
   b. Psoriatic lesions should not be traversed if in the path of an epidural injection.
   c. Displacing keratinotic and possibly nonsterile tissue into the epidural space may be hazardous.
   d. Bruises may suggest coagulation problems: epidural hematomas are associated with severe morbidity and mortality.

Laboratory

1. Complete blood count (CBC):
   a. Evidence of infection or, more important, absence of infection should be documented.
   b. Leukopenia may identify risk of serious infection.
   c. Anemia may become clinically significant with required volume expansion.
   d. Thrombocytopenia may result in insufficient clotting.

2. Coagulation profile:
   a. Prolonged bleeding times may result in bleeding and anemia.
   b. Prolonged coagulation times may result in paralyzing intraspinal hematomas.

3. Electrolytes and blood tests as clinically indicated:
   a. Glucose may have dangerous fluxes in susceptible individuals, such as those with diabetes, when epidural steroids are administered.

4. Erythrocyte sedimentation rate (ESR) and C-reactive protein (CRP):
   a. Inflammatory processes, both infectious and noninfectious, may yield elevated ESR and CRP. Elevated studies should prompt additional testing.
   b. The CRP can be followed to determine whether the inflammation is progressive, because it responds very quickly to circulating pyrogens and complement complexes.

5. Urinalysis may be helpful:
   a. Urinalysis provides a broad snapshot of endocrine, immune, and metabolic functions.
   b. Infectious processes revealed in the urine are a relative contraindication to epidural injection.

Radiographic Studies

1. Plain radiographs:
   a. The target region must be imaged in the anterior/posterior and lateral views to eliminate the presence of anatomic anomalies that may create complications in an otherwise uncomplicated procedure.
   b. Spina bifida should be known prior to needle introduction.
   c. Hypertrophic spinous processes and facets may impede successful injection.
   d. Calcification of interspinous ligaments may complicate a midline approach.

2. Nuclear medicine scans:
   a. Primary metastatic oncologic disease may be revealed.
   b. Discitis or osteomyelitis may be discovered.
3. Computerized axial tomography (CT):
   a. Depending on the history and physical examination, a CT scan may be indicated.
   b. With a history of cancer, a CT or MRI is necessary to visualize potential metastatic or recrudescent disease.
4. Magnetic resonance imaging (MRI):
   a. Prior to embarking on an invasive therapeutic trial, comprehensive information concerning soft tissue structures of the spine should be known.

ELECTROPHYSIOLOGIC STUDIES

1. Somatosensory evoked potentials (SSEP):
   a. Measures sensory (the pain) aspects of nerve function
2. Nerve conduction velocities and electromyography (NCV/EMG) to evaluate for conduction abnormalities and denervation
3. Selective tissue conductance (STC):
   a. A direct measure of autonomic dysfunction that responds instantly to change
   b. Evaluates changes in sudomotor and vasomotor activity

Note that overlapping abnormalities in three electrophysiological studies direct the clinician to a more focused work-up. Objective data reflect the presence or absence of nociception. The STC, cold pressor, and SSEP studies allow the physician to quantify physiologic improvements brought about through therapeutic intervention.

Invasive and non-invasive modalities are associated with side effects and complications. Interventions are associated with expected benefits as well as risks. The possibilities of bleeding, infection, intravascular injection, adverse reactions, and neurological damage are notable complications. Clinical reports of complications including paralysis and death have been associated with transforaminal epidural injection.

The diagnosis must be specific and match the procedural plan. Transforaminal epidural injections have been used clinically as a localization procedure for chemoneuroloysis. The procedure has been part of the treatment paradigm in predicting the probability of success of spinal cord stimulator implantation. Transforaminal epidural injections appear to be more therapeutic in late inflammatory conditions than diffuse intervertebral epidural injections. Postlaminectomy patients experiencing post lumbar puncture cephalgia can have successful epidural blood patches safely performed via the bilateral transforaminal

approach. Unlike interlaminar epidural injections, there is no expert opinion supporting nonfluoroscopically guided needle placement using the transforaminal approach.

The term "rule out" negates a diagnosis and leads to third-party rejection of the procedural claim. The cancellation of the work-up may be included in the denial as the impression was reduced to "rule out." The Center for Medicare and Medicaid Services (CMS), formerly the Healthcare Finance Administration (HCFA), the administrative and regulatory body for Medicare, requires that the documentation for epidural injection meet their criteria for diagnosis and treatment, prior to issuing reimbursement. Each state has published polices administered by the Medicare contracting administrative company. The policies are known as local Medicare review policies (LMRPs). Appropriate *International Diagnosis of Coding, 9th edition* (ICD-9) and *Current Procedural Terminology* (CPT) codes supporting the performance of epidural injections are provided in Chapter 57 by Manchikanti et al. entitled, "Guidelines for Practice of Interventional Techniques" in this volume.

Giving a disease a name does not necessarily prove that that is what the patient has; thus, objective criteria should be used when possible. The U.S. health care culture may contain numerous third-party administrative encumbrances. The administrative information request for documentation can be overcome with proper radiographs, laboratory, and electrophysiology studies. Objective evidence of motor, sensory, or autonomic function allows the practitioner to practice evidence-based medicine. The known hazards of the procedure mandate the laboratory assessment.

PHARMACOLOGY

Numerous agents are used for epidural injections. Agents include, but are not limited to,

1. Saline
2. Local anesthetics
3. Steroids
4. Alpha-2-adrenergic agonists
5. Neurolytics

Below is a description of the two classes of agents most frequently injected into the epidural space — steroids and local anesthetics.

STEROIDS

Methylprednisolone acetate is an anti-inflammatory steroid with glucocorticoid properties, formulated for intramuscular, intrasynovial, soft tissue, or intralesional injections. It is available in three strengths: 20 mg/ml, 40 mg/ml, and 80 mg/ml.

Preparations of triamcinolone are preferred by some because the formulation may be less prone to clumping when suspended in local anesthetic solution. Clumping is worrisome because of the risk of unintentional intravascular injection and spinal cord injury from embolization of particulate steroid. However, there are few studies supporting the use of one depo-steroid preparation over another.

Prolonged use of corticosteroids may produce posterior subcapsular cataracts or glaucoma with possible damage to the optic nerves and may enhance the establishment of secondary ocular infections due to fungi or viruses. Avascular necrosis has been reported with a wide variety of doses and durations of recurrent exposures to steroids.

The appropriate number of injections is a clinical decision, and guidelines are available to aid the clinician (see Chapter 57 of this volume). In addition, one should follow electrolytes, glucose, weight, CBCs, and manufacturer recommendations for diagnosing and management of toxicity when using these agents. Methylprednisolone is indicated for many inflammatory diseases. However, the indication for intraspinal injections is an off-label use of the steroid preparations. The Food and Drug Administration updated its position on "Off-Label" and "Investigational Use of Marketed Drugs, Biologics, and Medical Devices" in 1998 (see http://www.fda.gov/oc/ohrt/irbs/offlabel.html).

LOCAL ANESTHETICS

Local anesthetics block the conduction of nerve impulses, by increasing the threshold for electrical excitation in the nerve, by slowing the propagation of the nerve impulse, and by reducing the rate of rise of the action potential. Systemic absorption of local anesthetics can produce effects on the cardiovascular and central nervous systems. However, at blood concentrations achieved with usual therapeutic doses, changes in cardiac conduction, excitability, refractoriness, contractility, and peripheral vascular resistance are minimal. On the other hand, toxic blood concentrations can depress cardiac conduction and excitability, which may lead to atrioventricular block, ventricular arrhythmias, and cardiac arrest. Myocardial contractility is depressed and peripheral vasodilation occurs, leading to decreased cardiac output and arterial blood pressure. Incremental dosing is necessary with blind injection. Fluoroscopy with contrast reduces the incidence of adverse reactions associated with injection of local anesthetics.

TECHNICAL CONSIDERATIONS

Interlaminar epidural injections performed with fluoroscopic guidance and injection of non-ionic contrast such as iohexol help ensure proper needle placement and flow of injectate. Fluoroscopy confirms that needle placement is adjacent to the presumed site of nerve root irritation.

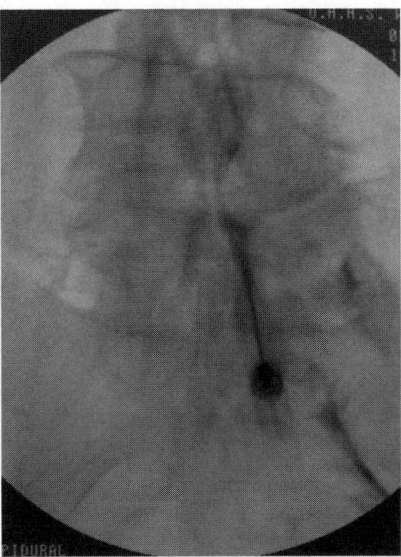

FIGURE 60.1 Interlaminar epidural steroid injection in a patient with spinal stenosis. A right paramedian epidural was performed using the loss of resistance technique. Fluoroscopy was helpful to guide and confirm proper needle placement. Note the hourglass appearance of the non-ionic contrast in the epidural space. The S1 nerve root opacified.

The procedure may involve using the "loss of resistance" technique, in conjunction with visual confirmation of needle position by fluoroscopy. After proper needle position is obtained, confirmation of epidural drug flow is confirmed with injection of contrast agent (Figure 60.1).

The transforaminal epidural steroid injection technique, as described in detail by Derby (Derby, Bogduk, & Kine, 1993), allows more precise placement of the epidural needle, without damaging the target nerve root. Typically, needle placement is at the anterior and superior aspect of the intervertebral foramen, at the 6 o'clock position of the pedicle on anteroposterior view (Figure 60.2). This localizes the tip of the needle above and lateral to the nerve root, adjacent to the dorsal root ganglion. Optimal position should allow flow of injectate to the anterior epidural space, adjacent to the intervertebral disc (Figure 60.3).

Precision diagnostic and therapeutic injections are possible with the transforaminal technique. However, dural puncture or subdural injection, which may traumatize the nerve root or dorsal root ganglion, should be avoided. Intravascular injection must be meticulously avoided, to prevent unintentional intravascular embolization of particulate steroid, which could compromise blood flow to the spinal cord (Figure 60.4 a and b).

COMPLICATIONS

Informed consent is critical as complications do occur. Patients should be asked to make decisions that a reasonable person would make, if placed in a similar circum-

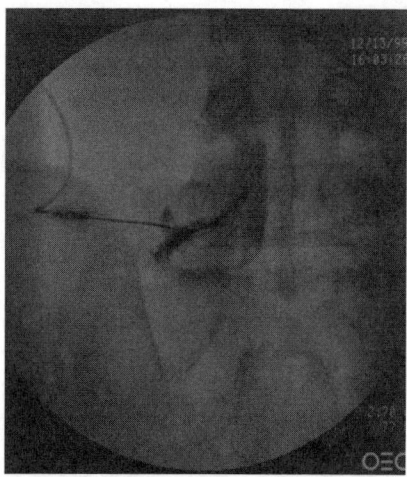

FIGURE 60.2 Transforaminal epidural steroid injection. Needle placement at the L5 intervertebral foramen outlines the nerve root with extension of iohexol contrast to the adjacent intracanal spinal dura. There is no evidence of intrathecal or intravascular uptake.

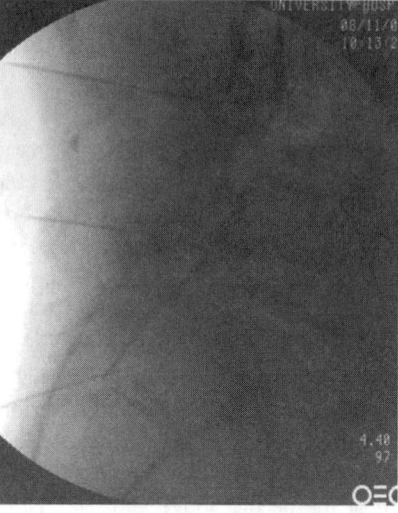

FIGURE 60.3 Transforaminal epidural steroid injection; lateral view. Needles placed at L4, L5, and S1. Iohexol contrast is seen to outline the anterior epidural space.

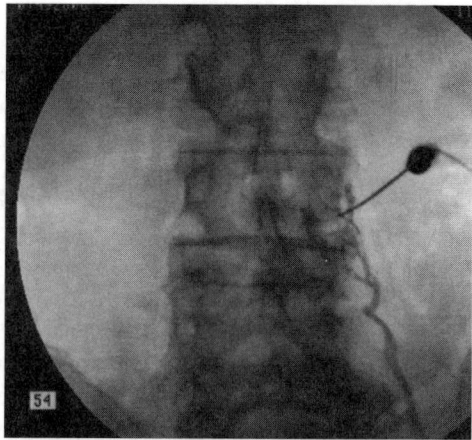

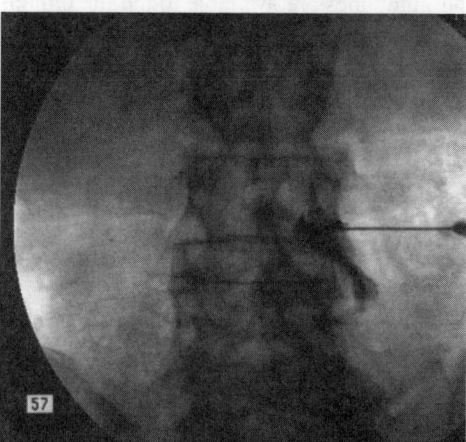

FIGURE 60.4 (a) Intravascular transforaminal injection. The epidural needle is positioned appropriately at the L3 intervertebral foramen. Iohexol injection opacified a blood vessel adjacent to the foramen. Intravascular contrast is seen to enter the spinal canal through the foramen. The needle was repositioned with a subsequent normal epidurogram and the steroid injection was completed without complication. (b) Needle repositioned after intravascular injection. The transforaminal epidural needle was repositioned slightly, and the subsequent injection was satisfactory.

stance as the patient. Guarantees and assurances should not be promised, but failure of expectation constitutes a perceived breach of contract. Do not say, "This will definitely take all your pain away, and there is no risk of anything bad happening to you." The following components should be included in the informed consent and thought process for treating complications:

1. The patient should be aware of the nature (invasive vs. noninvasive) of the procedure.
2. The patient should be aware of the purpose (diagnostic, prognostic, or therapeutic) of the procedure.
3. The patient should be aware of the alternatives to the procedure (e.g., behavioral, pharmacological, physiotherapy, less-invasive procedures).
4. The patient should be aware of the course of the disease without the procedure (e.g., remain the same with unacceptable pain, get worse relative to pain and physiologic dysfunction).
5. The patient should be aware of the risk of the procedure. This is the predominant issue relative to informed consent in liability cases. The consent as a whole is important, but lack of disclosure of salient risks is often an important point of contention. The following is a brief list of possible complications that should be disclosed when seeking consent for epidural procedures:

a. Bleeding (perioperative CBC and vital signs)

b. Infection (perioperative CBC and vital signs)

c. Adverse reactions to drugs (monitoring, perioperative CBC, and vital signs)

d. Allergic reactions to materials used (monitoring, perioperative CBC, and vital signs)

e. Injury to organs/organ systems (monitoring, perioperative CBC, and vital signs)

f. Pain not be relieved (monitoring, pain rating scales, vital signs, SSEPs, and STCs)

g. May need further procedures

h. Paralysis (monitoring with emphasis on neurological function, pain rating scales), e.g., intravascular injections of particulate medications

i. Headache (monitoring, vital signs, CBC, electrolytes, bed rest, fluid, caffeine, adrenocorticotropic hormone, dural repair)

j. Numbness (CBC, monitoring with emphasis on neurological function, pain rating scales, vital signs, SSEPs, and STCs)

k. Weakness (CBC, monitoring with emphasis on neurological function, pain rating scales, vital signs, SSEPs, and STCs)

l. Bladder dysfunction (monitoring with emphasis on urological function, pain rating scales, vital signs, SSEPs, and STCs)

SUMMARY

The clinical benefits of indicated epidural injections in properly selected patients are positive. The agents commonly used are frequently applied in an off-label but widely published and acceptable manner.

Knowledge of radiographic anatomy, pharmacology, physiology, and medical management of perioperative comorbid diseases is critical. Equal importance must be placed on early recognition of complications by appropriate monitoring and patient follow-up.

The procedure can be performed safely by properly trained physicians, but must always be respected for its capacity cause injury. The development of additional agents that may be effective in long-term pain relief makes epidural injection one of the most valuable current and future skills in the physician's repertoire.

REFERENCES

Bogduk, N., Aprill, C., & Derby, R. (1995). Epidural steroid injections. In A. White (Ed.), *Spine care operative treatment* (Vol. 1, pp. 322–343). St. Louis, MO: Mosby Yearbook.

Boswell, M.V. et al. (2003). Epidural steroids in the management of chronic spinal pain and radiculopathy. *Pain Physician, 6*, 319–334.

Derby, R., Bogduk, N., & Kine, G. (1993). Precision percutaneous blocking procedures for localizing spinal pain: Part 2. The lumbar neuraxial compartment. *Pain Digest, 3*, 175–188.

Kafiluddi, R., & Hahn, M. B. (2000). Epidural neural blockade. In P. P. Raj (Ed.), *Practical management of pain* (3rd ed., pp. 637–650). St. Louis, MO: Mosby Yearbook.

Manchikanti, L., & Bakhit, C. E. (1999). Fluoroscopy is medically necessary for the performance of epidural steroids response. *Anesthesia & Analgesia, 89*, 1330.

Manchikanti L. et al. (2003). Evidence-based practice guidelines for interventional techniques in the management of chronic spinal pain. *Pain Physician, 6*, 3–81

Stedman, T. L. (1999). *Stedman's medical dictionary*. Baltimore, MD: Williams & Wilkins.

White, A. H., Derby, R., & Wynne, G. (1980). Epidural injections for the diagnosis and treatment of low-back pain. *Spine, 5*, 78–86.

61

Sympathetic Neural Blockade in the Evaluation and Treatment of Pain

Steven D. Waldman, MD, JD

INTRODUCTION

The role of the sympathetic nervous system as a factor in a variety of painful conditions in humans has been a part of conventional medical wisdom for over 100 years. Early interest in the role of the sympathetic nervous system as part of the pain puzzle was limited primarily to its role as an anatomic pathway to carry the pain impulses to the brain in a manner analogous to the somatic nervous system. The unique anatomic nature of the sympathetic nervous system relative to the better anatomically defined somatic nervous system doomed this line of inquiry to raising more questions than were ultimately answered. It took the landmark work of Melzak and Wall and their gate control theory to move the prosaic thinking of the nerve as simply a wire to carry a pain message from a receptor to the brain to allow early pain clinicians such as Alon Winne to more clearly delineate the role of the sympathetic nervous system as a unique contributor to the evolution and continuation of pain in humans. As our specialty began to understand the unique way that the sympathetic nervous system interacted at both the peripheral and spinal cord levels, many of the things we were observing clinically begin to make sense, and for the first time, the specialty could put forth a rational explanation of how interruption of the sympathetic nervous system could provide prolonged pain relief. The advent of computerized tomography and magnetic resonance imaging further advanced our understanding of the structure and functional anatomy sympathetic nervous system in health and disease, enabling refinement of the techniques described below to allow for improved safety and efficacy. This chapter provides the reader with an overview of the current clinical thinking on the uses and abuses of sympathetic neural blockade in the treatment of pain.

STELLATE GANGLION BLOCK: ANTERIOR APPROACH

INDICATIONS

Stellate ganglion block is indicated in the treatment of acute herpes zoster in the distribution of the trigeminal nerve and cervical and upper thoracic dermatomes as well as frostbite and acute vascular insufficiency of the face and upper extremities. Stellate ganglion block is also indicated in the treatment of reflex sympathetic dystrophy of the face, neck, upper extremity, and upper thorax, and Raynaud's syndrome of the upper extremities, as well as sympathetically mediated pain of malignant origin. There are clinical reports to suggest that stellate ganglion blocks may also be useful in the acute palliation of some atypical vascular headaches.

CLINICALLY RELEVANT ANATOMY

The stellate ganglion is located on the anterior surface of the longus colli muscle. This muscle lies just anterior to the transverse processes of the seventh cervical and first thoracic vertebrae. The stellate ganglion is made up of the fused portion of the seventh cervical and first thoracic sympathetic ganglia. The stellate ganglion lies anterome-

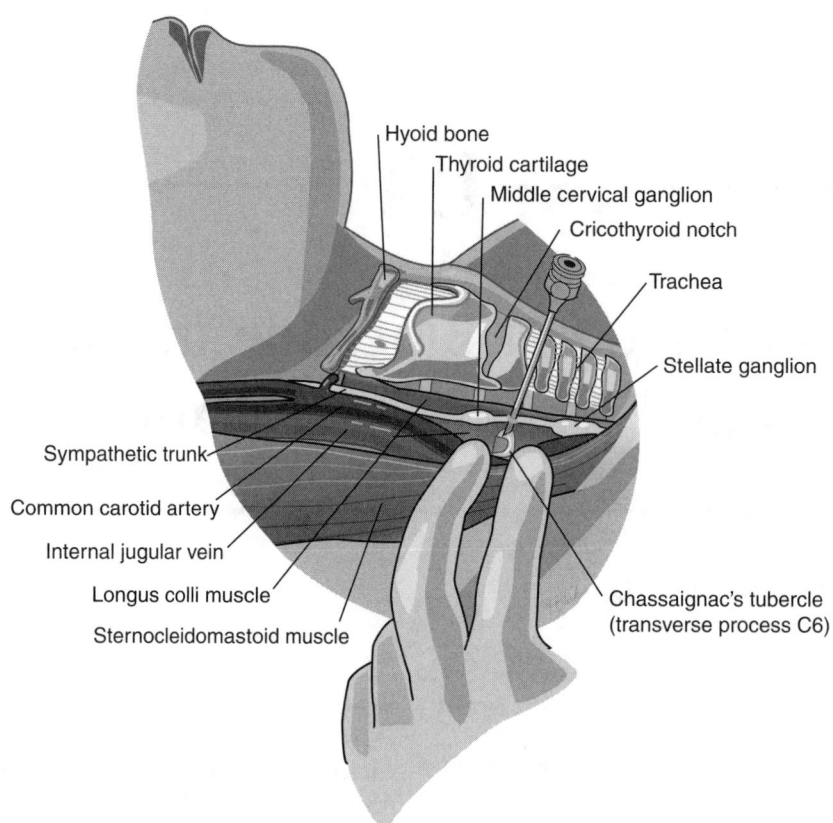

Hyoid bone
Thyroid cartilage
Middle cervical ganglion
Cricothyroid notch
Trachea
Stellate ganglion
Chassaignac's tubercle
(transverse process C6)
Sympathetic trunk
Common carotid artery
Internal jugular vein
Longus colli muscle
Sternocleidomastoid muscle

FIGURE 61.1 Technique for stellate ganglion block.

dial to the vertebral artery and is medial to the common carotid artery and jugular vein. The stellate ganglion is lateral to the trachea and esophagus.

TECHNIQUE

The patient is placed in the supine position with the cervical spine in neutral position, and 7 to 10 mL of local anesthetic without preservative is drawn into a 12-mL sterile syringe. For disease processes that have a component of inflammation, such as acute herpes zoster, or disease processes with associated edema, such as reflex sympathetic dystrophy, 80 mg of methylprednisolone is added for the first block and 40 mg of methylprednisolone is added for subsequent blocks.

The medial edge of the sternocleidomastoid muscle is identified at the level of the cricothyroid notch (C6). The sternocleidomastoid muscle is then displaced laterally with two fingers, and the tissues overlying the transverse process of C6 (Chassaignac's tubercle) are compressed. The pulsations of the carotid artery are then identified under the palpating fingers (Figure 61.1). The skin medial to the carotid pulsation is prepared with antiseptic solution, and a 22-gauge, 1.5-inch needle is advanced until contact is made with the transverse process of C6 (Figure 61.2). If bony contact is not made with needle insertion to a depth of 1 inch, the needle is probably between the

transverse processes of C6 and C7. If this occurs, the needle should be withdrawn and reinserted with a more cephalad trajectory. After bony contact is made, the needle is then withdrawn approximately 2 mm to bring the needle tip out of the body of the longus colli muscle. Careful aspiration is carried out, and 7 to 10 mL of solution is then injected (Figure 61.3).

SIDE EFFECTS AND COMPLICATIONS

This anatomic region is highly vascular, and because of the proximity of major vessels, the pain specialist should carefully observe the patient for signs of local anesthetic toxicity during injection. This vascularity and proximity to major blood vessels also give rise to an increased incidence of post-block ecchymosis and hematoma formation, and the patient should be warned of such. In spite of the vascularity of this anatomic region, this technique can safely be performed in the presence of anticoagulation by using a 25- or 27-gauge needle, albeit at increased risk of hematoma, if the clinical situation dictates a favorable risk-to-benefit ratio. These complications can be decreased if manual pressure is applied to the area of the block immediately after injection. Application of cold packs for 20-minute periods after the block will also decrease the amount of post-procedure pain and bleeding the patient may experience.

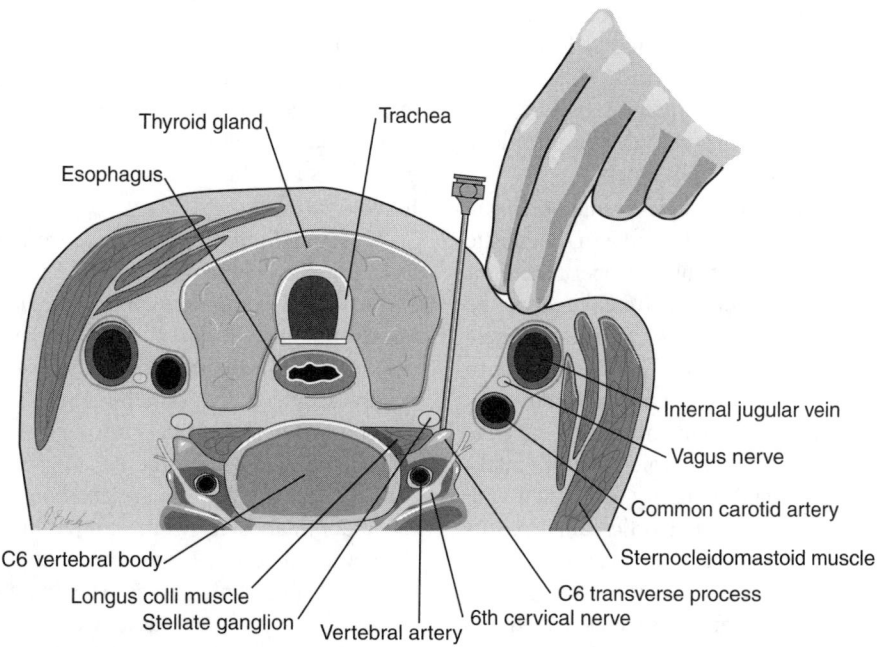

Thyroid gland
Trachea
Esophagus
Internal jugular vein
Vagus nerve
Common carotid artery
Sternocleidomastoid muscle
C6 vertebral body
Longus colli muscle
C6 transverse process
Stellate ganglion
6th cervical nerve
Vertebral artery

FIGURE 61.2 Technique for stellate ganglion block. Cross-sectional view.

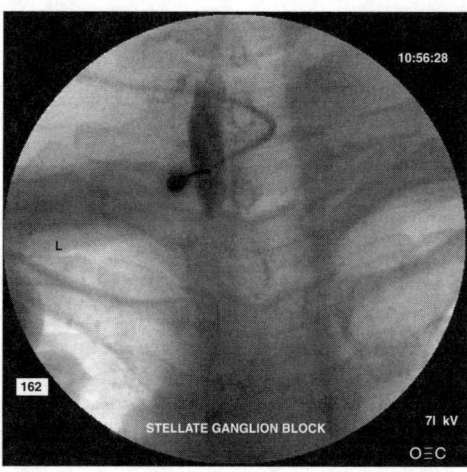

FIGURE 61.3 Stellate ganglion block. Fluoroscopic view.

Because of the proximity to the spinal column and its contents, it is also possible to inadvertently inject the local anesthetic solution into the epidural, subdural, or subarachnoid space. At this level, even small amounts of local anesthetic placed into the subarachnoid space may result in a total spinal anesthetic. If needle placement is too inferior, pneumothorax is possible, because the dome of the lung lies at the level of the C7–T1 interspace.

Additional side effects associated with stellate ganglion block include inadvertent block of the recurrent laryngeal nerve with associated hoarseness and dysphagia and the sensation that there is a lump in the throat when swallowing. Horner's syndrome occurs when the superior cervical sympathetic ganglion is also blocked during stellate ganglion block. The patient should be forewarned of

the possibility of these complications prior to stellate ganglion block.

CLINICAL PEARLS

Properly performed stellate ganglion block is a safe and effective technique for treatment of the previously mentioned pain syndromes. Improperly performed, it can be one of the most dangerous regional anesthetic techniques used in pain management. Almost all the complications associated with stellate ganglion block can be avoided if two simple rules are always followed: (1) the C6 level must always be accurately identified and double-checked by identifying the cricothyroid notch; and (2) the needle tip must always make bony contact with the transverse process of C6 before the injection of any drugs. Always forewarn the patient of the potential side effects associated with this technique, as side effects invariably occur.

CELIAC PLEXUS BLOCK: SINGLE-NEEDLE PERIAORTIC TECHNIQUE

INDICATIONS

Pain management specialists began performing celiac plexus block using a single needle after it was recognized that, when using the two-needle transcrural approach to celiac plexus block under computed tomographic guidance, contrast injected via the left-sided needle would spread around the aorta, obviating the need for injection through the second needle. The use of a single needle decreases needle-related complications as well as the pain associated with the procedure. The single-needle periaortic approach to celiac plexus block has the added advantage over the classic two-needle retrocrural technique in that the single needle is placed in the precrural space, thus avoiding the higher incidence of neurologic complications associated with retrocrural needle placement.

Celiac plexus block using the single-needle periaortic approach with local anesthetic is indicated as a diagnostic maneuver to determine whether flank, retroperitoneal, or upper abdominal pain is sympathetically mediated via the celiac plexus. Daily celiac plexus block with local anesthetic is also useful in the palliation of pain secondary to acute pancreatitis and other acute pain syndromes subserved by the celiac plexus. Early implementation of celiac plexus block with local anesthetic, steroids, or both markedly reduces the morbidity and mortality associated with acute pancreatitis. Single-needle periaortic celiac plexus block is also used to palliate the acute pain of arterial embolization of the liver for cancer therapy as well as to treat the pain of abdominal "angina" associated with visceral arterial insufficiency. Single-needle periaortic celiac plexus block with local anesthetic may also be used prognostically prior to celiac plexus neurolysis.

Neurolysis of the celiac plexus via the single-needle periaortic approach with alcohol or phenol is indicated to treat pain secondary to malignancies of the retroperitoneum and upper abdomen. This approach may also be useful in some chronic benign abdominal pain syndromes, including chronic pancreatitis, in carefully selected patients.

CLINICALLY RELEVANT ANATOMY

The sympathetic innervation of the abdominal viscera originates in the anterolateral horn of the spinal cord. Preganglionic fibers from T5–T12 exit the spinal cord in conjunction with the ventral roots to join the white communicating rami on their way to the sympathetic chain. Rather than synapsing with the sympathetic chain, these preganglionic fibers pass through it to ultimately synapse on the celiac ganglia. The greater, lesser, and least splanchnic nerves provide the major preganglionic contribution to the celiac plexus. The greater splanchnic nerve has its origin from the T5–T10 spinal roots. The nerve travels along the thoracic paravertebral border through the crus of the diaphragm into the abdominal cavity, ending on the celiac ganglion of its respective side. The lesser splanchnic nerve arises from the T10–T11 roots and passes with the greater nerve to end at the celiac ganglion. The least splanchnic nerve arises from the T11–T12 spinal roots and passes through the diaphragm to the celiac ganglion.

Interpatient anatomic variability of the celiac ganglia is significant, but the following generalizations can be drawn from anatomic studies of the celiac ganglia. The number of ganglia vary from one to five and range in diameter from 0.5 to 4.5 cm. The ganglia lie anterior and anterolateral to the aorta. The ganglia located on the left are uniformly more inferior than their right-sided counterparts by as much as a vertebral level, but both groups of ganglia lie below the level of the celiac artery. The ganglia usually lie approximately at the level of the first lumbar vertebra.

Postganglionic fibers radiate from the celiac ganglia to follow the course of the blood vessels to innervate the abdominal viscera. These organs include much of the distal esophagus, stomach, duodenum, small intestine, ascending and proximal transverse colon, adrenal glands, pancreas, spleen, liver, and biliary system. It is these postganglionic fibers, the fibers arising from the preganglionic splanchnic nerves, and the celiac ganglion that make up the celiac plexus. The diaphragm separates the thorax from the abdominal cavity while still permitting the passage of the thoracoabdominal structures, including the aorta, vena cava, and splanchnic nerves. The diaphragmatic crura are bilateral structures that arise from the anterolateral surfaces of the upper two or three lumbar vertebrae and discs. The crura of the diaphragm serve as a barrier to effectively separate the splanchnic nerves from the celiac ganglia and plexus below.

The celiac plexus is anterior to the crus of the diaphragm. The plexus extends in front of and around the aorta, with the greatest concentration of fibers anterior to the aorta. With the single-needle periaortic approach to celiac plexus block, the needle is placed close to this concentration of plexus fibers. The relationship of the celiac plexus to the surrounding structures is as follows. The aorta lies anterior and slightly to the left of the anterior margin of the vertebral body. The inferior vena cava lies to the right, with the kidneys posterolateral to the great vessels. The pancreas lies anterior to the celiac plexus. All of these structures lie within the retroperitoneal space.

TECHNIQUE

Pre-block preparation includes the administration of adequate amounts of oral or intravenous fluids to attenuate the hypotension associated with celiac plexus block. Evaluation of the patient for coagulopathy is indicated if the patient has undergone antiblastic therapy or has a history of significant alcohol abuse. If radiographic contrast is to be used, evaluation of the patient's renal status is also indicated.

The patient is placed in the prone position with a pillow under the abdomen to flex the thoracolumbar spine. For comfort, the patient's head is turned to the side and the arms are permitted to hang freely off each side of the table. The inferior margins of the 12th ribs are identified and traced to the T12 vertebral body. The spinous process of the L1 vertebral body is then identified and marked with a sterile marker. A point approximately 2.5 inches

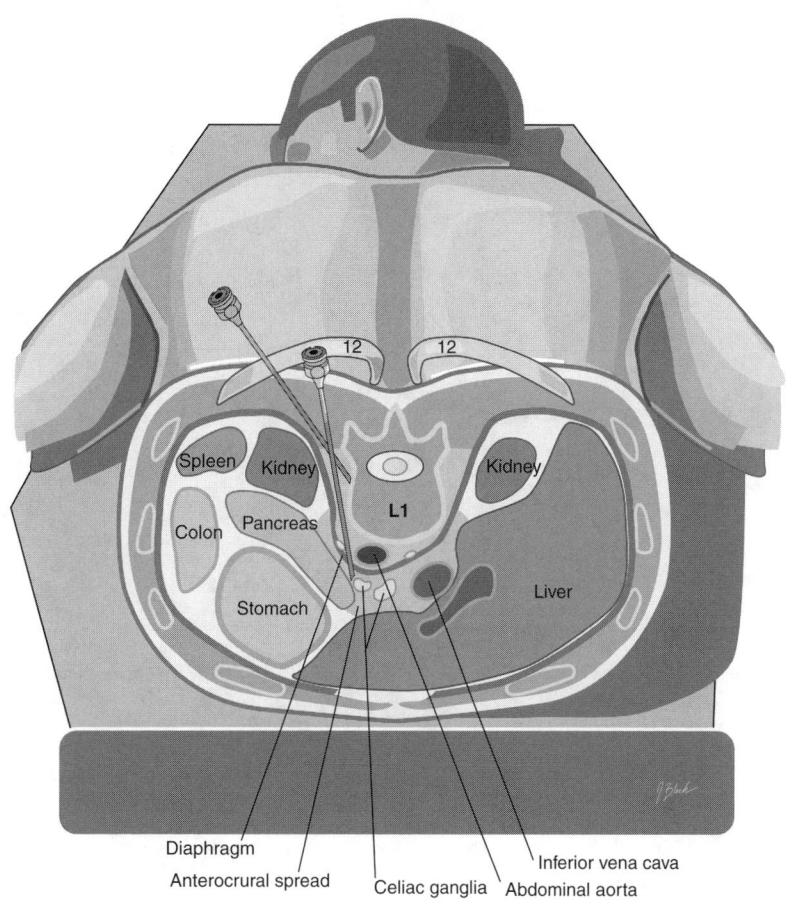

FIGURE 61.4 Celiac plexus block. Cross sectional view.

just inferior and lateral to the left side of the transverse process of L1 is identified. The injection site is then prepared with antiseptic solution.

The skin, subcutaneous tissues, and musculature are infiltrated with 1.0% lidocaine at the point of needle entry. A 20-gauge, 13-cm styletted needle is inserted bilaterally through the previously anesthetized area. The needle is initially oriented 45° toward the midline and about 15° cephalad to ensure contact with the L1 vertebral body. Once bone is contacted and the depth noted, the needle is withdrawn to the level of the subcutaneous tissue and redirected less mesiad (about 65° from the midline) so as to "walk off" the lateral surface of the L1 vertebral body (Figure 61.4). The needle is reinserted to the depth at which the vertebral body was first contacted. At this point, if no bone is contacted, the needle is gradually advanced 3 to 4 cm, or until the pulsation emanating from the aorta and transmitted to the advancing needle is noted. If aortic pulsations are noted, the pain specialist may either convert the block into a transaortic celiac plexus technique or note the depth to which the needle has been placed, withdraw the needle into the subcutaneous tissues, and then redirect the needle less mesiad to slide laterally to the aorta. Ultimately, the tip of the needle should be just lateral and anterior to the side of the aorta (Figure 61.5). This periaortic precrural placement decreases the incidence of inadvertent spread of injected solutions onto the lumbar somatic nerve roots.

The stylet of the needle is removed, and the needle hub is inspected for the presence of blood, cerebrospinal fluid, or urine. If radiographic guidance is being used, a small amount of contrast material is injected through the needle, and its spread is observed radiographically. On the fluoroscopic anteroposterior view, contrast is confined primarily to the left of the midline near the L1 vertebral body. A smooth curvilinear shadow can be observed that corresponds to contrast in the pre-aortic space on the lateral view. Alternatively, if computed tomographic guidance is used, contrast should appear periaortic or, if adenopathy or tumor is present, contrast should be confined to the periaortic space to the left of the aorta. If this limitation of spread of contrast occurs, one should consider redirecting the needle more medially to pass through the aorta to place the needle tip just in front of the aorta. If the contrast is entirely retrocrural, the needle should be advanced to the precrural space to avoid any risk of spread of local anesthetic or neurolytic agent posteriorly to the somatic nerve roots.

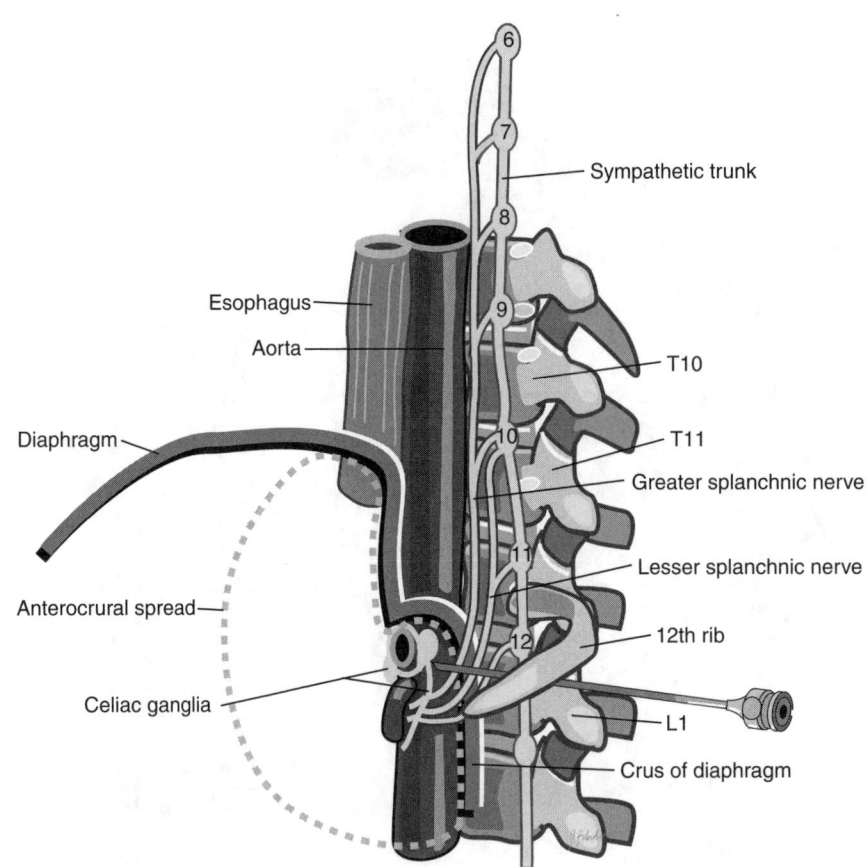

FIGURE 61.5 Celiac plexus block. Oblique view.

If radiographic guidance is not used, a rapid-onset local anesthetic is used in sufficient concentration to produce motor block (such as 1.5% lidocaine or 3.0% 2-chloroprocaine) prior to administration of neurolytic agents. If the patient experiences no motor or sensory block in the lumbar dermatomes after an adequate time, additional drugs injected through the needles will probably not reach the somatic nerve roots if given in like volumes.

For diagnostic and prognostic block via the single-needle periaortic technique, 12 to 15 mL of 1.0% lidocaine or 3.0% 2-chloroprocaine is administered through the needle. For therapeutic block, 10 to 12 mL of 0.5% bupivacaine is administered through the needle. Because of the potential for local anesthetic toxicity, all local anesthetics should be administered in incremental doses. When treating acute pancreatitis or pain of malignant origin, 80 mg of depot methylprednisolone is advocated for the initial celiac plexus block, with a 40-mg dose given for subsequent blocks.

A 10- to 12-mL volume of absolute alcohol or 6.0% aqueous phenol is injected through the needle for neurolytic block. Alternatively, 25 mL of 50% ethyl alcohol can be injected via the needle. After neurolytic solution is injected, the needle should be flushed with sterile saline solution because there have been anecdotal reports of neu-

rolytic solution being tracked posteriorly with the needle as it is withdrawn.

SIDE EFFECTS AND COMPLICATIONS

Because of its proximity to vascular structures, celiac plexus block using the single-needle periaortic approach is contraindicated in patients who are on anticoagulant therapy or suffer from coagulopathy secondary to antiblastic cancer therapies or liver abnormalities associated with ethanol abuse. Intravascular injection of solutions may result in thrombosis of the nutrient vessels to the spinal cord with secondary paraplegia. Local or intra-abdominal infection and sepsis are absolute contraindications to celiac plexus block.

Because blockade of the celiac plexus results in increased bowel motility, this technique should be avoided in patients with bowel obstruction. Post-block diarrhea occurs in approximately 50% of patients. Celiac plexus block should be deferred in patients who suffer from chronic abdominal pain, who are chemically dependent, or who exhibit drug-seeking behavior until these issues have been adequately addressed. Alcohol should not be used as a neurolytic agent in patients on disulfiram therapy for alcohol abuse.

The proximity to the spinal cord, exiting nerve roots, pleura space, and viscera makes it imperative that this procedure be carried out only by those well versed in the regional anatomy and experienced in interventional pain management techniques. Needle placement that is too medial may result in epidural, subdural, or subarachnoid injections or trauma to the spinal cord and exiting nerve roots. Such incorrect needle placement can result in severe neurologic deficits, including paraplegia. Medial needle placement may also result in intradiscal placement and resultant discitis. Because the needle terminus is precrural with the single-needle periaortic approach to celiac plexus block, there is a decreased incidence of neurologic complications, including neurolysis of the lumbar nerve roots with resultant hip flexor weakness and lower extremity numbness, compared with the classic two-needle approach to celiac plexus block.

Given the proximity of the pleural space, pneumothorax after celiac plexus block may occur if the needle is placed too cephalad. Trauma to the thoracic duct with resultant chylothorax may also occur. If the needle is placed too laterally, trauma to the kidneys and ureters is a distinct possibility.

CLINICAL PEARLS

When using the classic two-needle retrocrural approach to celiac plexus block, the needles will almost always be retrocrural in proximity to the splanchnic nerves rather than the celiac ganglia. That is to say that the needles and injected solution will be placed posterior and cephalad to the crura of diaphragm. Computed tomographic and cadaver studies have given rise to the recent suggestion that the classic method of retrocrural block is more likely to produce splanchnic nerve block than blockade of the celiac plexus. This is because this approach does not result in the deposition of injected material around and anterior to the aorta and directly onto the celiac plexus at the level of the L1 vertebral body, as previously thought. Rather, the injectate appears to (1) concentrate posterior to the aorta and in front of and along the side of the L1 vertebral body, where it may anesthetize retroaortic celiac fibers, (2) diffuse cephalad to anesthetize the splanchnic nerve at a site rostral to the origin of the plexus, and (3) only finally encircle the aorta at the site of the celiac plexus when enough drug is injected to transgress the diaphragm by diffusing caudad through the aortic hiatus. Unfortunately, this larger volume of drug is also associated with an increased incidence of blockade of the lumbar somatic nerve roots.

Radiographic guidance, especially computed tomographic guidance, offers the pain specialist an added margin of safety during neurolytic celiac plexus block via the single-needle periaortic approach and hence should be used routinely unless the patient's clinical status requires

that celiac plexus block be performed at the bedside. Given the increased incidence of damage to the lumbar nerve roots due to the retrocrural placement of needles with the classic two-needle technique, the transcrural, single needle periaortic, or transaortic approaches to celiac plexus block should be preferred.

Most pain specialists report a lower success rate when using celiac plexus block to treat chronic benign abdominal pain than when treating abdominal pain of malignant origin. Patients with chronic benign abdominal pain should be tapered off narcotic analgesics prior to consideration of celiac plexus neurolysis. It should be noted that the phrenic nerve also transmits nociceptive information from the upper abdominal viscera. This information is perceived as poorly localized pain referred to the supraclavicular region; this source of pain should be considered in all patients suffering from upper abdominal pain.

LUMBAR SYMPATHETIC GANGLION BLOCK

INDICATIONS

Lumbar sympathetic ganglion block is useful in the evaluation and management of sympathetically mediated pain of the kidneys, ureters, genitalia, and lower extremity. Included in this category are phantom limb pain, reflex sympathetic dystrophy, causalgia, and a variety of peripheral neuropathies. Lumbar sympathetic ganglion block is also useful in the palliation of pain secondary to vascular insufficiency of the lower extremity, including pain secondary to frostbite, atherosclerosis, Buerger's disease, and arteritis secondary to collagen vascular disease, and in maximizing blood flow after vascular procedures on the lower extremities. Lumbar sympathetic ganglion block with local anesthetic can be used as a diagnostic tool when performing differential neural blockade on an anatomic basis in the evaluation of flank, pelvic, and lower extremity pain. If destruction of the lumbar sympathetic chain is being considered, this technique is useful as a prognostic indicator of the degree of pain relief that the patient may experience. Lumbar sympathetic ganglion block with local anesthetic is also useful in the treatment of acute herpes zoster and postherpetic neuralgia involving the lumbar and sacral dermatomes. Destruction of the lumbar sympathetic chain is indicated for the palliation of pain syndromes that have responded to lumbar sympathetic blockade with local anesthetic.

CLINICALLY RELEVANT ANATOMY

The preganglionic fibers of the lumbar sympathetics exit the intervertebral foramina along with the lumbar paravertebral nerves. After exiting the intervertebral foramen, the lumbar paravertebral nerve gives off a recurrent branch that loops back through the foramen to provide innervation to the spinal ligaments, meninges, and its respective vertebra. The upper lumbar paravertebral nerve also interfaces with the lumbar sympathetic chain via the myelinated preganglionic fibers of the white rami communicantes. All five of the lumbar nerves interface with the unmyelinated postganglionic fibers of the gray rami communicantes. At the level of the lumbar sympathetic ganglia, preganglionic and postganglionic fibers synapse. Additionally, some of the postganglionic fibers return to their respective somatic nerves via the gray rami communicantes. Other lumbar sympathetic postganglionic fibers travel to the aortic and hypogastric plexus and course up and down the sympathetic trunk to terminate in distant ganglia.

In many patients, the first and second lumbar ganglia are fused. These ganglia and the remainder of the lumbar chain and ganglia lie at the anterolateral margin of the lumbar vertebral bodies. The peritoneal cavity lies lateral and anterior to the lumbar sympathetic chain. Given the proximity of the lumbar somatic nerves to the lumbar sympathetic chain, the potential exists for both neural pathways to be blocked when performing blockade of the lumbar sympathetic ganglion.

TECHNIQUE

The patient is placed in the prone position with a pillow under the abdomen to gently flex the lumbar spine. The spinous process of the vertebra just above the nerve to be blocked is palpated. At a point just below and 3 inches lateral to the spinous process, the skin is prepared with antiseptic solution. A 22-gauge, 3.5-inch needle is attached to a 12-mL syringe and is advanced at a 35° to 45° angle to the skin, aiming for the lateral aspect of the vertebral body. The needle should impinge on bone after being advanced approximately 2 inches. If the needle comes into contact with bone at a shallower depth, it has probably impinged on the transverse process. If this occurs, the needle should be directed in a slightly more cephalad trajectory to pass above the transverse process to impinge on the lateral aspect of the vertebral body. After bony contact is made with the vertebral body, the needle is withdrawn into the subcutaneous tissues and redirected at a slightly steeper angle and walked off the lateral margin of the vertebral body. As soon as bony contact is lost, the needle is slowly advanced approximately 0.5 inch deeper (Figure 61.6). Given the proximity of the lumbar sympathetic chain to the somatic nerve, a paresthesia in the distribution of the corresponding lumbar paravertebral nerve may be elicited. If this occurs, the needle should be withdrawn and redirected slightly more cephalad. The needle is then again slowly advanced until it passes the lateral border of the vertebral body. The needle should ultimately rest at the anterior lateral margin of the vertebral body (Figure 61.7). If fluoroscopy is used,

a small amount of contrast medium may be added to the local anesthetic (Figure 61.8). The contrast medium should appear just anterior to the vertebral body on the lateral view and just lateral to the vertebral body on the PA view. If computed tomographic guidance is used, the contrast can be seen surrounding the sympathetic chain, anterolateral to the vertebral body. Once the needle is in position and careful aspiration reveals no blood or cerebrospinal fluid, 12 to 15 mL of 1.0% preservative-free lidocaine is injected.

SIDE EFFECTS AND COMPLICATIONS

The proximity to the spinal cord and exiting nerve roots makes it imperative that this procedure be carried out only by those well versed in the regional anatomy and experienced in performing interventional pain management techniques. Given the proximity of the peritoneal cavity, damage to the abdominal viscera during lumbar sympathetic ganglion block is a distinct possibility. The incidence of this complication will be decreased if care is taken to place the needle just beyond the anterolateral margin vertebral body. Needle placement too medial may result in epidural, subdural, or subarachnoid injections or trauma to the intervertebral disc, spinal cord, and exiting nerve roots. Although uncommon, infection remains an ever-present possibility, especially in the immunocompromised patient with cancer. Early detection of infection, including discitis, is crucial to avoid potentially life-threatening sequelae.

CLINICAL PEARLS

Lumbar sympathetic ganglion block is a simple technique that can produce dramatic relief for patients suffering from the previously mentioned pain complaints. Neurolytic block with small quantities of absolute alcohol or phenol in glycerin, or by cryoneurolysis or radiofrequency lesioning, has been shown to provide long-term relief for patients suffering from sympathetically maintained pain that has been relieved with local anesthetic. As mentioned earlier, the proximity of the lumbar sympathetic chain to the neuraxis and pleural space makes careful attention to technique mandatory.

HYPOGASTRIC PLEXUS BLOCK: SINGLE-NEEDLE TECHNIQUE

INDICATIONS

Hypogastric plexus block with the single-needle technique is useful in the evaluation and management of sympathetically mediated pain of the pelvic viscera. Included in this category is pain secondary to malignancy, endometriosis, reflex sympathetic dystrophy, causalgia, proctalgia fugax, and radiation enteritis. Hypogastric plexus block is also

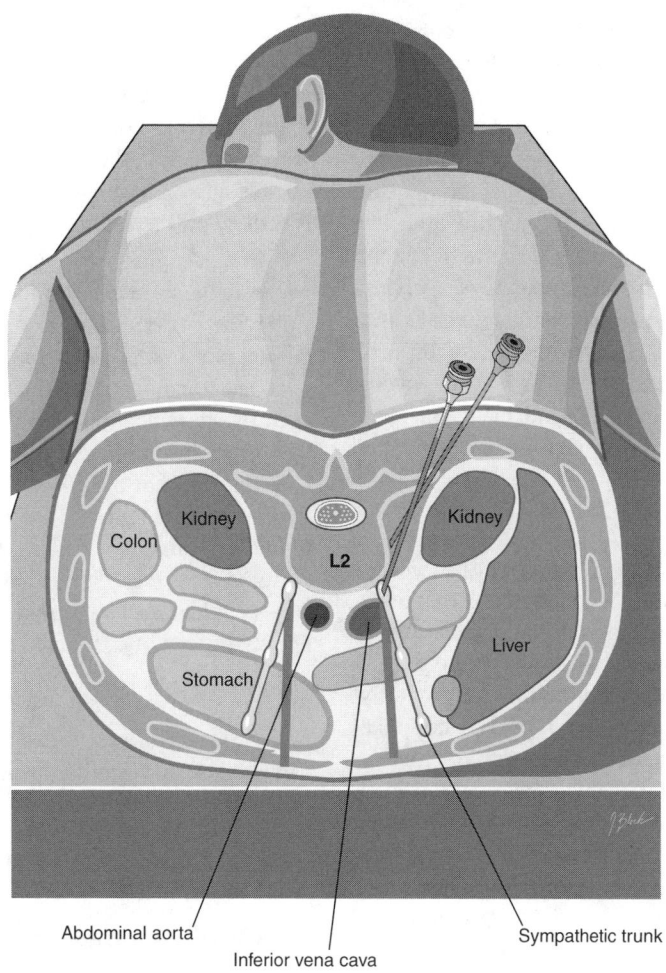

FIGURE 61.6 Diagram for lumbar sympathetic block.

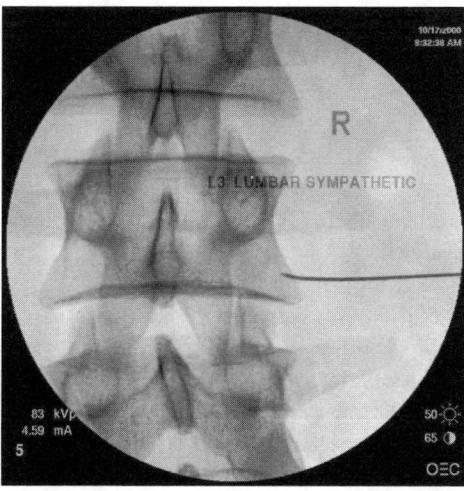

FIGURE 61.7 Needle placement for lumbar sympathetic block. Fluoroscopic view. (Courtesy of Milton Landers, D.O.)

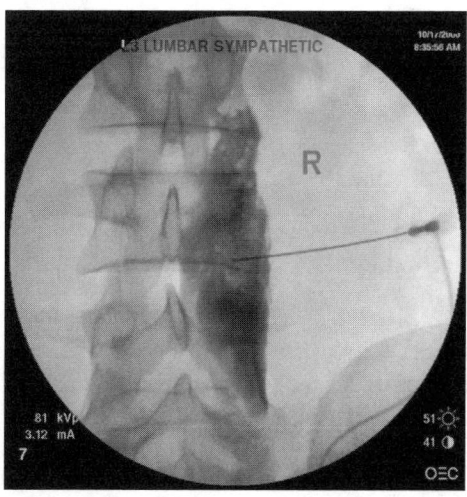

FIGURE 61.8 Needle placement for lumbar sympathetic block. Fluoroscopic view demonstrating proper contrast spread along the vertebral column. (Courtesy of Milton Landers, D.O.)

useful in the palliation of tenesmus secondary to radiation therapy to the rectum. Hypogastric plexus block with local anesthetic can be used as a diagnostic tool when performing differential neural blockade on an anatomic basis in the evaluation of pelvic and rectal pain. If destruction of the hypogastric plexus is being considered, this technique is useful as a prognostic indicator of the degree of pain relief that the patient may experience. Hypogastric plexus block with local anesthetic is also useful in the treatment of acute herpes zoster and postherpetic neuralgia involving the sacral dermatomes. Destruction of the hypogastric plexus is indicated for the palliation of pain syndromes that have temporarily responded to blockade of the hypogastric plexus with local anesthetic and have not been controlled with more conservative measures.

CLINICALLY RELEVANT ANATOMY

In the context of neural blockade, the hypogastric plexus can simply be thought of as a continuation of the lumbar sympathetic chain that can be blocked in a manner analogous to lumbar sympathetic nerve block. The preganglionic fibers of the hypogastric plexus find their origin primarily in the lower thoracic and upper lumbar region of the spinal cord. These preganglionic fibers interface with the lumbar sympathetic chain via the white communicantes. Postganglionic fibers exit the lumbar sympathetic chain and, together with fibers from the parasympathetic sacral ganglion, make up the superior hypogastric plexus. The superior hypogastric plexus lies in front of L4 as a coalescence of fibers. As these fibers descend, at a level of L5, they begin to divide into the hypogastric nerves following in close proximity the iliac vessels. As the hypogastric nerves continue their lateral and inferior course, they are accessible for neural blockade as they pass in front of the L5–S1 interspace. The hypogastric nerves pass downward from this point, following the concave curve of the sacrum and passing on each side of the rectum to form the inferior hypogastric plexus. These nerves continue their downward course along each side of the bladder to provide innervation to the pelvic viscera and vasculature.

TECHNIQUE

Blind Technique

The patient is placed in the prone position with a pillow placed under the lower abdomen to gently flex the lumbar spine and maximize the space between the transverse process of L5 and the sacral alae. The L4–L5 interspace is located by identifying the iliac crests and finding the interspace at that level. The skin at this level is prepared with antiseptic solution. A point 6 cm from the midline at this level is identified, and the skin and subcutaneous tissues are anesthetized with 1.0% lidocaine. A 20-gauge, 13-cm needle is then inserted through the previously anesthetized

area and directed approximately 30° caudad and 30° mesiad toward the anterolateral portion of the L5–S1 interspace. If the transverse process of L5 is encountered, the needle is withdrawn and redirected slightly more caudad. If the vertebral body of L5 is encountered, the needle is withdrawn and redirected slightly more lateral until, in a manner analogous to lumbar sympathetic block, the needle is walked off the anterolateral aspect of the vertebral body.

A 5-mL glass syringe filled with preservative-free saline is then attached to the needle. The needle is then slowly advanced into the prevertebral space while maintaining constant pressure on the plunger of the syringe in a manner analogous to the loss-of-resistance technique used for identification of the epidural space. A "pop" and loss of resistance will be felt as the needle pierces the anterior fascia of the psoas muscle and enters the prevertebral space (Figure 61.9). After careful aspiration for blood, cerebrospinal fluid, and urine, 10 mL of 1.0% preservative-free lidocaine is slowly injected in incremental doses while observing the patient closely for signs of local anesthetic toxicity. If there is believed to be an inflammatory component to the pain, the local anesthetic is combined with 80 mg of methylprednisolone and is injected in incremental doses. Subsequent daily nerve blocks are carried out in a similar manner, substituting 40 mg of methylprednisolone for the initial 80-mg dose. The needle is then removed, and an ice pack is placed on the injection site to decrease post-block bleeding and pain.

Computed Tomographic Guided Technique

The patient is placed in the prone position on the computed tomography gantry with a pillow placed under the lower abdomen to gently flex the lumbar spine and maximize the space between the transverse process of L5 and the sacral alae. A computed tomography scout film of the lumbar spine is taken, and the L4–L5 interspace is identified. The skin overlaying the L4–L5 interspace is prepared with antiseptic solution, and sterile drapes are placed. At a point approximately 6 cm from midline, the skin and subcutaneous tissues are anesthetized with 1% lidocaine using a 25-gauge, 3.8-cm needle. A 20-gauge, 13-cm needle is then inserted through the previously anesthetized area and directed approximately 30° caudad and 30° mesiad toward the anterolateral portion of the L5–S1 interspace. If the transverse process of L5 is encountered, the needle is withdrawn and redirected slightly more caudad. If the vertebral body of L5 is encountered, the needle is withdrawn and redirected slightly more lateral and walked off the anterolateral aspect of the vertebral body in a manner analogous to lumbar sympathetic block. A 5-mL glass syringe filled with preservative-free saline is then attached to the needle. The needle is then slowly advanced into the prevertebral space while maintaining constant pressure on the plunger of the syringe. A "pop"

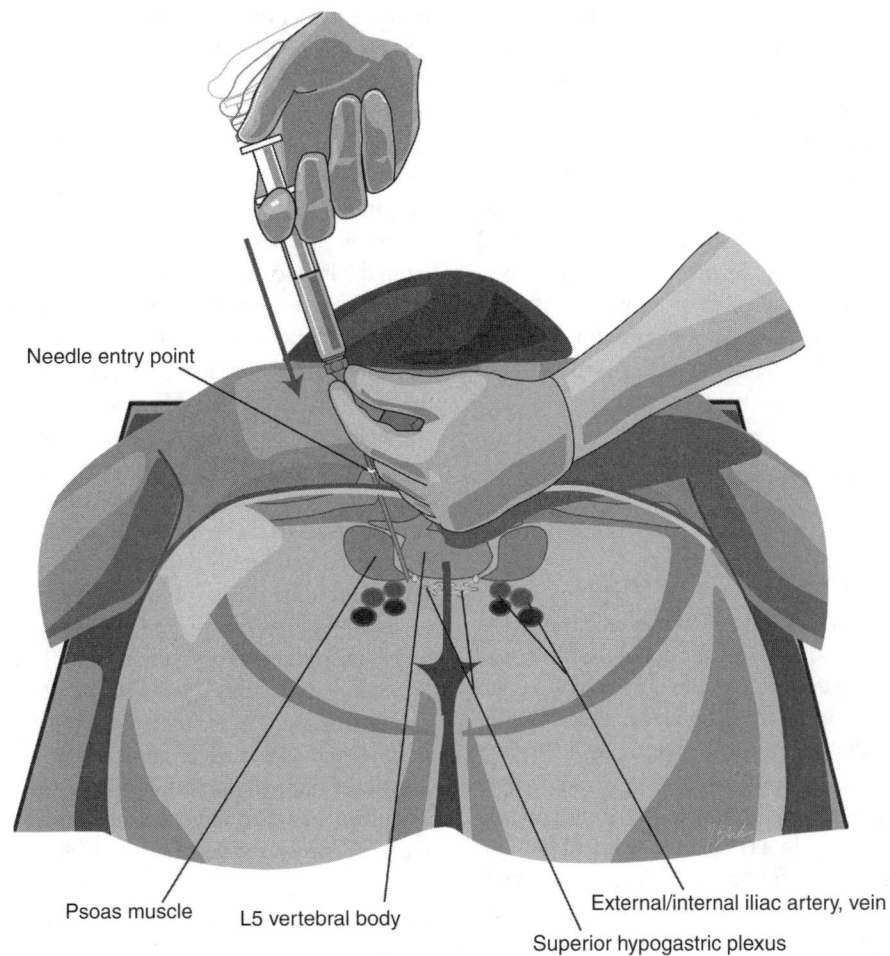

Needle entry point

Psoas muscle   L5 vertebral body   External/internal iliac artery, vein

Superior hypogastric plexus

FIGURE 61.9 Diagram showing superior hypogastric plexus block.

and loss of resistance will be felt as the needle pierces the anterior fascia of the psoas muscle. After careful aspiration, 2 to 3 mL of water-soluble contrast medium is injected through the needle and a computed tomography scan is taken to confirm current retroperitoneal needle placement. Because of contralateral spread of the contrast medium in the prevertebral space, it is often unnecessary to place a second needle as is advocated by some pain specialists. A total volume of 10 mL of 1.0% preservative-free lidocaine is then injected in divided doses after careful aspiration for blood, cerebrospinal fluid, and urine. If adequate pain relief is obtained, incremental doses of absolute alcohol or 6.5% aqueous phenol may be injected in a similar manner after it is ascertained that the patient is experiencing no untoward bowel or bladder effects from blockade of the hypogastric plexus.

SIDE EFFECTS AND COMPLICATIONS

The proximity of the hypogastric nerves to the iliac vessels means that the potential for bleeding or inadvertent intravascular injection remains a distinct possibility. The relationship of the cauda equina and exiting nerve roots makes

it imperative that this procedure be carried out only by those well versed in the regional anatomy and experienced in performing lumbar sympathetic nerve block. Given the proximity of the pelvic cavity, damage to the pelvic viscera including the ureters during hypogastric plexus block is a distinct possibility. The incidence of this complication will be decreased if care is taken to place the needle just beyond the anterolateral margin of the L5–S1 interspace. Needle placement too medial may result in epidural, subdural, or subarachnoid injections or trauma to the intervertebral disc, spinal cord, and exiting nerve roots. Although uncommon, infection remains an ever-present possibility, especially in the immunocompromised patient with cancer. Early detection of infection, including discitis, is crucial to avoid potentially life-threatening sequelae.

CLINICAL PEARLS

Hypogastric plexus block is a simple technique that can produce dramatic relief for patients suffering from the previously mentioned pain complaints. Neurolytic block with small quantities of absolute alcohol or phenol in glycerin or by cryoneurolysis or radiofrequency lesioning has been shown to provide long-term relief for patients suffering from sympathetically maintained pain that has been relieved with local anesthetic. As with the celiac plexus and lumbar sympathetic nerve blocks, the proximity of the sympathetic nerves to vascular structures mandates repeated careful aspiration and vigilance for signs of unrecognized intravascular injection. Computed tomographic guidance allows visualization of the major blood vessels and their relationship to the needle, which is a significant advance over blind or fluoroscopically guided techniques. As mentioned earlier, the proximity of the hypogastric plexus to the neuraxis and pelvic viscera makes careful attention to technique mandatory.

GANGLION OF WALTHER (IMPAR) BLOCK

INDICATIONS

Ganglion of Walther (also known as the ganglion impar) block is useful in the evaluation and management of sympathetically mediated pain of the perineum, rectum, and genitalia. This technique has been used primarily in the treatment of pain secondary to malignancy, although theoretical applications for benign pain syndromes including pain secondary to endometriosis, reflex sympathetic dystrophy, causalgia, proctalgia fugax, and radiation enteritis can be considered if the pain has failed to respond to more conservative therapies. Ganglion of Walther block with local anesthetic can be used as a diagnostic tool when performing differential neural blockade on an anatomic basis in the evaluation of pelvic and rectal pain. If destruction of the ganglion of Walther is being considered, this technique is useful as a prognostic indicator of the degree of pain relief that the patient may experience. Destruction of the ganglion of Walther is indicated for the palliation of pain syndromes that have temporarily responded to blockade of the ganglion with local anesthetic and have not been controlled with more conservative measures.

CLINICALLY RELEVANT ANATOMY

In the context of neural blockade, the ganglion of Walther can simply be thought of as the terminal coalescence of the sympathetic chain. The ganglion of Walther lies in front of the sacrococcygeal junction and is amenable to blockade at this level. The ganglion receives fibers from the lumbar and sacral portions of the sympathetic and parasympathetic nervous system and provides sympathetic innervation to portions of the pelvic viscera and genitalia.

TECHNIQUE

Blind Technique

The patient is placed in the jackknife position to facilitate access to the inferior margin of the gluteal cleft. The midline is identified, and the skin just below the tip of the coccyx that overlies the anococcygeal ligament is prepared with antiseptic solution. The skin and subcutaneous tissues at this point are anesthetized with 1.0% lidocaine. A 3.5-inch spinal needle is then bent at a point 1 inch from its hub to a 30° angle to allow placement of the needle tip in proximity to the anterior aspect of the sacrococcygeal junction. The needle may be bent again at a point 2 inches from the hub to accommodate those patients with an exaggerated coccygeal curve to allow placement of the needle tip to rest against the sacrococcygeal junction.

The bent needle is then placed through the previously anesthetized area and is advanced until the needle tip impinges on the anterior surface of the sacrococcygeal junction (Figure 61.10 and Figure 61.11). However, fluoroscopic visualization is advocated, and contrast injection can be used to confirm proper needle placement (Figure 61.12). After careful aspiration for blood, cerebrospinal fluid, and urine, 3 mL of 1.0% preservative-free lidocaine is slowly injected in incremental doses. If there is believed to be an inflammatory component to the pain, the local anesthetic is combined with 80 mg of methylprednisolone and is injected in incremental doses. Subsequent daily nerve blocks are carried out in a similar manner, substituting 40 mg of methylprednisolone for the initial 80-mg dose. The needle is then removed, and an ice pack is placed on the injection site to decrease post-block bleeding and pain.

Computer Tomographic Guided Technique

The patient is placed in the prone position on the computed tomography gantry with a pillow placed under the pelvis to facilitate access to the inferior gluteal cleft. A computed tomography scout film is taken, and the sacrococcygeal junction and the tip of the coccyx are identified. The midline is also identified, and the skin just below the tip of the coccyx that overlies the anococcygeal ligament is prepared with antiseptic solution. The skin and subcutaneous tissues at this point are anesthetized with 1.0% lidocaine. A 3.5-inch spinal needle is then bent at a point 1 inch from its hub to a 30° angle to allow placement of the needle tip in proximity to the anterior aspect of the sacrococcygeal junction. The needle may be bent again at a point 2 inches from the hub to accommodate patients with an exaggerated coccygeal curve to allow the needle tip to rest against the anterior sacrococcygeal junction.

The needle is then placed through the previously anesthetized area and is advanced until the needle tip impinges on the anterior surface of the sacrococcygeal junction. After careful aspiration for blood, cerebrospinal fluid, and urine, 2 to 3 mL of water-soluble contrast medium is injected through the needle and a computed tomography scan is taken to confirm the spread of contrast medium just anterior to the sacrococcygeal junction. After correct needle placement is confirmed, a total volume of 3 mL of

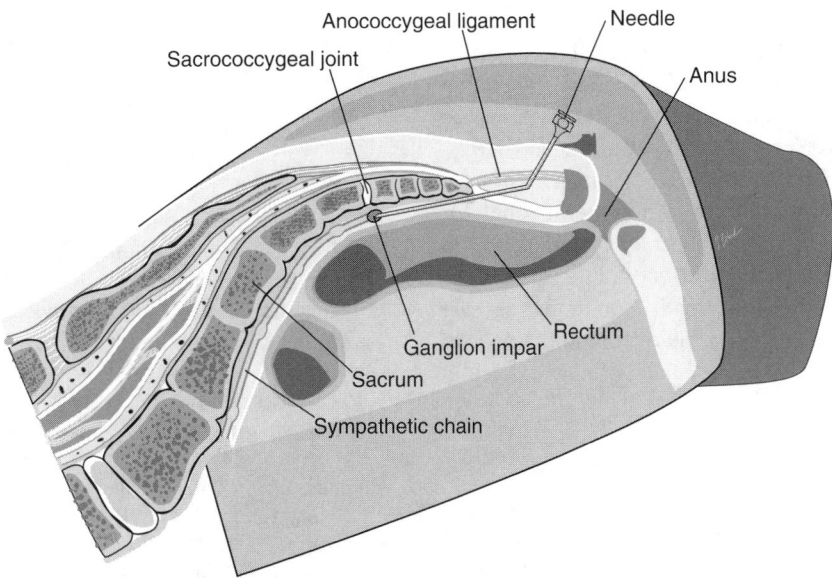

FIGURE 61.10 Diagram showing ganglion impar block. Lateral view.

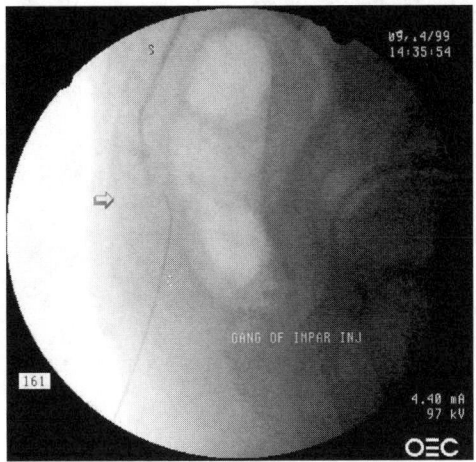

FIGURE 61.11 Needle placement for ganglion impar block. Lateral fluoroscopic view.

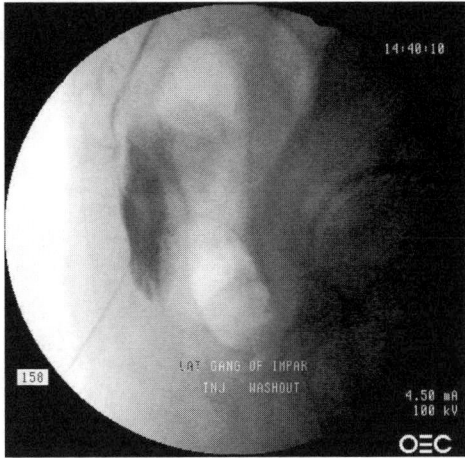

FIGURE 61.12 Needle placement for ganglion impar block. Lateral fluoroscopic view with contrast injection.

1.0% preservative-free lidocaine is injected in divided doses after careful aspiration for blood, cerebrospinal fluid, and urine. If adequate pain relief is obtained, incremental doses of absolute alcohol or 6.5% aqueous phenol may be injected in a similar manner after it is ascertained that the patient is experiencing no untoward bowel or bladder effects from local anesthetic blockade of the ganglion of Walther. The needle is then removed, and an ice pack is placed on the injection site to decrease post-block bleeding and pain.

SIDE EFFECTS AND COMPLICATIONS

The proximity of the ganglion of Walther to the rectum makes perforation and tracking of contaminants back through the needle track during needle removal a distinct possibility. Infection and fistula formation, especially in those patients who are immunocompromised or have received radiation therapy to the perineum, can represent a devastating and potentially life-threatening complication to this block. The relationship of the cauda equina and exiting sacral nerve roots makes it imperative that this procedure be carried out only by those well versed in the regional anatomy and experienced in performing interventional pain management techniques.

CLINICAL PEARLS

Ganglion of Walther block is a straightforward technique that can produce dramatic relief for patients suffering from the previously mentioned pain complaints. Given the localized nature of this neural structure when compared with the superior hypogastric plexus, neurolytic block with small quantities of absolute alcohol or phenol in glycerin or by cryoneurolysis or radiofrequency lesioning may be a reasonable choice over superior hypogastric plexus block, at least insofar as bowel and bladder dysfunction is concerned. Destruction of the ganglion of Walther has been shown to provide long-term relief for patients suffering from sympathetically maintained pain that has been relieved with local anesthetic. Computed tomographic guidance allows visualization of the regional anatomy and the relationship of the rectum to the needle. This is a significant advance over blind or fluoroscopically guided techniques.

ACKNOWLEDGMENTS

The author thanks colleague and friend Milton Landers, D.O., Ph.D., for the use of several radiographs used in the preparation of this chapter.

BIBLIOGRAPHY

Bonica, J. J. (1953). *The management of pain*. Philadelphia: Lea & Febiger.

De Leon-Casasola, O. A., Kent, E., & Lema, M. J. (1993). Neurolytic superior hypogastric plexus block for chronic pelvic pain associated with cancer. *Pain, 54*, 145–151.

Eriksson, E. (1980). *Illustrated handbook of local anaesthesia*. Copenhagen: Munksgaard.

Ischia, S., Luzzani, A., Ischia, A. et al. (1983). A new approach to the neurolytic block of the celiac plexus: The transaortic technique. *Pain, 16*, 34.

Lieberman, R. P., Lieberman, S. L., Cuka, D. J. et al. (1988). Celiac plexus block and splanchnic nerve block: A review. *Seminars in Interventional Radiology, 5*, 213.

Plancarte, R., Amescua, C., Patt, R. et al. (1990). Superior hypogastric plexus block for pelvic cancer pain. *Anesthesiology, 73*, 236.

Stanton-Hicks, M. D. A. (1990). Blocks of the sympathetic nerve system. In M. D. A. Stanton-Hicks (Ed.), *Pain and the sympathetic nervous system* (p. 155). Boston: Kluwer Academic.

Waldman, S. D. (1992). Management of acute pain. *Postgraduate Medicine, 87*, 17, 1992.

Waldman, S. D. (1993). Acute and postoperative pain management. In R. Weiner (Ed.), *Innovations in pain management* (pp. 28–29). Orlando, FL: PMD Press.

Waldman, S. D. (2004). Celiac plexus block. In S. Waldman, *Atlas of interventional pain management* (pp. 277–278). Philadelphia, PA: Saunders.

Waldman, S. D. (2004). Ganglion of Walther block. In S. Waldman, *Atlas of interventional pain management* (pp. 419–420). Philadelphia, PA: Saunders.

Waldman, S. D., & Portenoy, R. K. (1991). Recent advance is the management of cancer pain. Part II. *Pain Management, 4*, 19.

62

Pain Management with Regenerative Injection Therapy

Felix S. Linetsky, MD, Richard Derby, MD, Rafael Miguel, MD,
Lloyd Saberski, MD, and Michael Stanton-Hicks, MD

INTRODUCTION

The purpose of this chapter is to provide pain management clinicians with a review of the pertinent literature and clinical and anatomic considerations in relation to an interventional regenerative treatment for chronic musculoskeletal pain.

Connective tissues are ubiquitous throughout the body. Structurally and biomechanically, they represent a heterogeneous group with variations in collagen orientation cross-linking, shape, cell properties, and presence of synovial lining. They constitute the essence of the musculoskeletal system.

A large variety of functions depend on the proper homeostasis of connective tissue. For example, without the storage and release of energy in connective tissue during locomotion, much higher energy expenditure would be required (Bannister et al., 1995; Dorman, 1992). Conversely, many dysfunctional and painful syndromes may arise from pathologic conditions of the connective tissue.

The injury occurs when the internal or external forces exceed the threshold of failure for the specific connective tissue. This may be in the form of a ruptured or strained ligament, tendon, fascia, or a bone fracture, or a disrupted disc.

Pain arising from connective tissue pathology, such as posttraumatic changes in the intervertebral disc, ligaments, tendons, aponeuroses, fasciae, sacroiliac, and zygapophyseal joint capsular ligaments, is often difficult to differentiate based solely on clinical presentation. Individual variations in innervation further complicate the differential diagnosis. Left untreated, post-traumatic and overuse injuries of ligaments and tendons can linger indefinitely, leading to the progression of degenerative changes, loss of function, deconditioning, and perpetuation of disability and chronic pain (Bogduk et al., 1996a, b; Dreyfuss, 1997; Hackett, 1958, 1991; Merskey & Bogduk, 1994; Shuman, 1958; Steindler et al., 1938).

Interventional regenerative modalities for painful musculoskeletal pathologies have been described for more than two millennia. For example, the technique of collagen thermomodulation, now known as thermocapsulorraphy, was originally described by Hippocrates, who performed thermocoagulation of the anteroinferior capsule for treatment of recurrent shoulder dislocations "with red hot slender irons" (Dorman et al., 1991; Shuman, 1958). It is currently recognized that sufficient thermomodulation of collagen can be achieved with lower temperatures to stimulate a proliferative and regenerative/reparative response. This concept has led to the development of intradiscal electrothermal (IDET) procedures, currently used with the intent to achieve nuclear shrinkage, seal annular fissures, and thermocoagulate nociceptors (Derby et al., 1998; Saal et al., 1998a, b).

The coexistence of physical and chemical methods is well demonstrated in the contemporary practice of dermatology and plastic surgery, where chemical (carbolic acid/phenol) and laser-induced facial peels are used for regeneration and rejuvenation by chemo- and thermomodulation of the skin collagen.

Regenerative injection therapy (RIT), also known as prolotherapy or sclerotherapy, is one of the long-practiced methods of pain management. It was originally described by Celsus for treatment of hydroceles, with injections of saltpeter (Hoch, 1939; Linetsky, 1999a). From inception to date, the general principles of injection techniques and differential diagnosis employed in RIT are those advocated by American Academy of Pain Management, American Society of Interventional Pain Physicians, International Spinal Injection Society, and the International Association for the Study of Pain (Aprill et al., 1990; Bogduk, 1982, 1986, 1988, 1996, 1997; Bogduk et al., 1996b; Bonica, 1990; Derby, 2002; Manchikanti, 2002; Merskey & Bogduk, 1994; Steindler, 1938). The difference is that painful chronic tissue bed pathology is the primary target for differential diagnosis and therapeutic application of RIT. Response to the blocks and nerve supply to the tissue are continuously taken into account during procedure. Differential diagnosis encompasses a wide variety of painful tissue including large synovial joints with their components and extends beyond the spinal segmental innervation (Cyriax, 1969, 1982; Dorman, 1993; Dorman et al., 1991; Hackett et al., 1991; Linetsky et al., 2002a, b, c; Ombregt et al., 1995; Waldman, 1998).

Application of RIT for low back pain has been described in numerous textbooks and articles; comparable, adequate applications for cervical and thoracic pain are lacking. We choose to emphasize cervicothoracic pain problems treated with RIT in this chapter (Cyriax, 1969, 1982; Dorman et al., 1991, 1993; Hackett, 1991; Ombregt et al., 1995).

ETYMOLOGY OF SOME TERMINOLOGY

Biegeleisen (1984) first used the term "sclerotherapy" in 1936. *Sclero* is derived from the word *skleros* (Greek, hard). Hackett (1958) felt that sclerotherapy implied scar formation; therefore, he coined the term "prolotherapy" and defined it as "the rehabilitation of an incompetent structure by the generation of new cellular tissue" (derived from the word *proli,* Latin, offspring). "Proliferate": to produce new cells in rapid succession. Proliferation, however, is an integral attribute of a malignant, unsuppressed growth. Moreover, with advances in basic science and the contemporary understanding of the healing process, contemporary exponents prefer RIT because it is recognized that regeneration extends beyond the proliferative stage. On a cellular level, RIT induces chemomodulation of collagen through repetitive stimulation of the inflammatory and proliferative phases in a sophisticated process of tissue regeneration and repair, mediated by numerous growth factors leading to the restoration of tensile strength, elasticity, increased mass, and load-bearing capacity of the affected connective tissue (Klein et al., 1989; Liu et al., 1983; Maynard et al., 1985; Ongley et al., 1987). These

capabilities make RIT a specific treatment for chronic, degenerative, painful conditions such as enthesopathy, tendinosis, and ligament laxity, in place of commonly used steroid injections and denervation procedures (Klein & Eek, 1997; Reeves, 1995).

LOCAL ANESTHETICS IN DIAGNOSIS OF MUSCULOSKELETAL PATHOLOGY: BRIEF HISTORY

In 1930, Leriche introduced the application of procaine for differential diagnosis and treatment of ligament and tendon injuries of the ankle and other joints at their fibroosseous insertions. In 1934, Soto-Hall and Haldeman reported on the benefits of procaine injections in the diagnosis and treatment of painful shoulders. Subsequently in 1938, they published a study on diagnosis and treatment of painful sacroiliac dysfunctions with procaine injections. After infiltration of the posterior sacroiliac ligaments, interspinous ligaments at L4–5 and L5–S1 levels, and zygapophyseal joint capsules with procaine, they observed a marked relaxation of spastic musculature. They added the routine use of sacroiliac joint manipulations, establishing manipulation of axial joints under local anesthesia (Haldeman et al., 1938).

In 1938, Steindler and Luck made a significant contribution to currently validated approaches in the diagnosis and treatment of low back pain based on procaine injections. The authors pointed out that posterior divisions of the spinal nerves provide the sensory supply to the musculature; tendons; supraspinous, interspinous, iliolumbar, sacroiliac, sacrotuberous, and sacrospinous ligaments; and origins and insertions of aponeurosis of tensor fascia lata, gluteal muscles, and thoracolumbar fascia. They proposed and postulated that five criteria must be met to prove that a causal relationship exists between the structure and pain symptoms (Table 62.1).

Subsequently, in 1948, Hirsch demonstrated relief from sciatica following intradiscal injection of procaine (Hirsch, 1948).

TABLE 62.1
Radiating/Referral Pain Postulates

1. Contact with the needle must aggravate the local pain.
2. Contact with the needle must aggravate or elicit the radiation of pain.
3. Procaine infiltration must suppress local tenderness.
4. Procaine infiltration must suppress radiation of pain.
5. Positive leg signs must disappear.

Note: From "Differential Diagnosis of Pain Low in the Back: Allocation of the Source of Pain by the Procaine Hydrochloride Method," by A. Steindler et al., 1938, *Journal of the American Medical Association, 110,* 106–113. Reproduced with permission.

Local anesthetic diagnostic blocks are currently the most reliable and objective confirmation of the precise tissue source of pain and clinical diagnosis (Bonica, 1990; Cousins et al., 1988; Merskey & Bogduk, 1994; Wilkinson, 1992).

HISTORY AND EVOLUTION OF RIT

The rationale for implementing RIT in chronic painful pathology of ligaments and tendons evolved from clinical and histologic research performed for injection treatment of hernias, hydroceles, and varicose veins. The therapeutic action of the newly formed connective tissue was different in each condition. In hernias, the proliferation and subsequent regenerative/reparative response led to fibrotic closure of the defect (Riddle, 1940; Warren, 1881; Watson, 1938). In hydroceles, hypertrophied subserous connective tissue reinforced the capillary walls of serous membrane and prevented further exudate formation (Hoch, 1939; Linetsky, 1999c). The latter mode of action was employed in the treatment of chronic olecranon and pre-patellar bursitis by Poritt in 1931. He drained the fluid from the sac and injected 5% sodium morrhuate. In cases of persistence, he injected a 5% phenol solution into the bursae (Poritt, 1931).

In 1935, Schultz, while searching for a better way to treat painful subluxations of temporomandibular joints (TMJs), conceived the idea that strengthening of the joint capsule by induced ligament fibrosis would lead to capsular contraction and prevent subluxations. Animal experiments were conducted with several solutions. Among those, Sylnasol provided the best outcomes and therefore was chosen for the clinical trials. (Sylnasol-sodium psyllate was an extract of psyllium seed oil produced by Searle Pharmaceutical and discontinued in 1960s.) A clinical study of 30 human subjects after biweekly injections of 0.25 to 0.5 ml Sylnasol demonstrated "entire patient satisfaction." Schultz (1937) concluded that the principle of induced hypertrophy of the articular capsule by injecting a fibrosing agent might be applied to other joints capable of subluxations or recurrent dislocations. He also concluded that Sylnasol was a dependable agent. Injections restored normal joint function and the method was within the scope of treatment of a general practitioner. Twenty years later, Schultz presented the positive results of Sylnasol injections on several hundred patients, successfully cured of painful hypermobility of TMJ (Schultz, 1956). Also in 1937, Gedney reported some details of collateral ligament injections for painful unstable hypermobile knees and posterior sacroiliac ligaments of unstable painful sacroiliac articulations. Small amounts of sclerosant solutions were injected along the entire affected structures. He extended this treatment 6 months later to recurrent shoulder dislocations, acromioclavicular separations, and sternoclavicular subluxations (Gedney, 1937, 1938).

In 1939, Kellgren injected volunteers with hypertonic saline and implicated interspinous ligaments as a significant source of local and referred pain. He published maps of referred pain from deep somatic structures, including interspinous ligaments (Kellgren, 1939).

In 1940, Riddle included a chapter on "The Injection Treatment of Joints" in his text and described the injection treatment of TMJs and shoulders in great detail, giving Schultz the appropriate credit for initiation of this treatment. Shuman described injection treatment of recurrent shoulder dislocations via strengthening of the inferior capsular ligaments with Sylnasol in 1941. Subsequently, in 1949, he adopted the term "sclerotherapy" for this injection modality, modifying it later that year to "joint sclerotherapy" (Shuman, 1949a, 1949b).

In 1945, Bahme published the first retrospective study of 100 patients who improved after injection of Sylnasol to the sacroiliac ligaments. Patients were under his care for an average of 4 months. The average number of injection treatments was five; 80% reported complete resolution of symptoms. He also found these injections to be very helpful in the treatment of unstable ribs, and reported improvement in 12 patients. He described a significant coexistence of painful hypermobile ribs with hypermobile sacroiliac joints, explaining the phenomenon by concomitant functional scoliosis.

By 1944, Lindblom demonstrated radial annular fissures during cadaveric disc injections and later described nucleographic patterns of 15 discs in 13 patients. Thereafter, in 1948, Hirsch relieved sciatic pain with intradiscal injection of procaine. These two articles prompted Gedney, and subsequently Shuman, to explore therapeutic applications of sclerosants for pain related to intervertebral disc (IVD) pathology.

By 1951, Gedney had extended treatment with sclerosant injections to painful degenerative lumbar disc syndromes and described the detailed technique of Sylnasol injections into the lateral annulus of the lumbar disc without fluoroscopic guidance. He reported L4 disc involvement in 95% of cases and a 50% clinical improvement after treatment of this disc alone (Gedney, 1952b). In the treatment of hypermobile sacroiliac joints, he emphasized that the amount of solution and quantity of treatments were highly individual and depended on the patient's response (Gedney, 1952a). In a retrospective study, Gedney (1954b) emphasized the significant statistical coexistence of sacroiliac pathology with IVD pathology at L3, L4, and L5 levels. By 1954, he had completed a prospective study of 100 patients; 65 were initially treated with the injections into the disc, and 35 were initially treated with injections into the posterior sacroiliac ligaments. The latter group required fewer intradiscal injections. Thus, he concluded that in the presence of sacroiliac pain and hypermobility, adequate stabilization of the sacroiliac joint should be achieved in all cases prior to addressing discogenic pain (Gedney, 1954b). He emphasized the importance of interspinous and iliolumbar ligament injections in the treatment of lumbar spondylolisthesis (Gedney, 1954a).

In 1954, Shuman evaluated the effectiveness of sclerosant injections to the sacroiliac joints, intervertebral discs, spondylolisthesis, zygapophyseal joint capsules, knees, and shoulders in 93 respondents in a retrospective survey. Improvements ranged from 75 to 98%. Only those patients who were able to perform their usual occupations were considered to have positive results. Subsequently, he detailed many aspects of treatment with integration of manipulative techniques, including manipulation under local anesthesia as introduced 20 years earlier by Haldeman and Soto-Hall. Shuman stated that zygapophyseal joint pathology (emphasized by Hackett in 1956) and disc pathology were the more common causes of lower back pain than sacroiliac joint pathology (Shuman, 1958).

Hackett, the inventor of prolotherapy, postulated in 1939 that ligaments were responsible for the majority of back pain (Hackett, 1953). By 1958, he came to the conclusion that tendons at the fibro-osseous junctions were another significant source of chronic pain syndromes (Hackett, 1958). In a retrospective study, he reported on 84 patients with sacroiliac pain treated by sclerosant injections of Sylnasol, five to seven times to each affected area. In this study, 82% reported themselves entirely symptom free for a duration of 6 to 14 years (Hackett & Henderson, 1955). In the initial animal experiments, he demonstrated a 30 to 40% increase in tendon size after injections of Sylnasol (Hackett, 1956; Figure 62.1). Not satisfied with the term "sclerotherapy," because it implied hardening of the tissue and scar formation, Hackett introduced the term "prolotherapy" in 1956. He did this because the results of his experimental study did not support scarring but rather hypertrophy induced by proliferation of connective tissue in a linear fashion (Hackett, 1956). Hackett employed and emphasized the importance of the earlier referenced postulates of Steindler. He confirmed ligament or tendon involvement as pain generators reproducing local and referred pain by "needling" and abolishing the pain by infiltration of local anesthetic prior to injecting the proliferants (Hackett, 1956). He published maps of referred pain from ligaments and tendons, initially of the lumbopelvic region. These were derived from 7,000 injections in more than 1,000 patients treated over 17 years. He subsequently developed maps of the cervicothoracic region (Hackett, 1958; Figure 62.2). Later, he pointed out that loose-jointed individuals have a lesser ability to recuperate from sprains, because of the congenital laxity of their ligaments, and have a predisposition to chronic lingering pain for decades. He emphasized their positive response to prolotherapy (Hackett, 1959a).

In several subsequent publications, Hackett emphasized the common pathogenesis of impaired local circu-

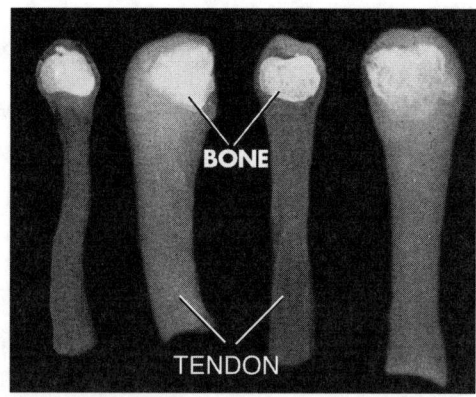

FIGURE 62.1 Paired radiograph of hypertrophied rabbit tendons, fibro-osseous attachment 1 and 3 months after injection of proliferant. Treated tendons are on the right side of each pair, controls on the left. From *Ligament and Tendon Relaxation (Skeletal Disability) — Treated by Prolotherapy (Fibro-Osseous Proliferation)* (3rd ed.), by G. Hackett, 1958, Springfield, IL: Charles C Thomas.

lation in chronic conditions such as neuritis, headaches, whiplash, osteoporosis, bone dystrophy, bronchospasm, and arteriosclerosis. Excess antidromic, sympathetic, and axon reflex stimulation caused local vasodilatation and edema, with a perpetuating vicious cycle of "tendon relaxation," the condition now understood as degenerative changes, enthesopathy, tendinosis, and laxity (Hackett 1959a, 1959b, 1960a, 1960b, 1961, 1966a, 1966b, 1966c, 1967; Hackett et al., 1961, 1962).

Extended subsequent animal experiments with multiple solutions conducted by Hackett revealed that the strongest fibro-osseous proliferations were achieved with Sylnasol, zinc sulfate solutions, and silica oxide suspensions. The strongest acute inflammatory reaction was obtained with Sylnasol and zinc sulfate, followed by silica oxide. Whole blood moderately stimulated fibro-osseous proliferation. Hydrocortisone used alone or in combination with proliferants inhibited proliferation for 3 to 4 weeks. At the fracture sites, proliferants increased callus formation in 3 weeks, whereas when used in combination with steroids, the callus formation was markedly inhibited (Hackett et al., 1961).

Hackett's positive results were initially corroborated by others (Compere et al., 1958; Green, 1956, 1958; Myers, 1961; Neff, 1959). In fact, Myers reported improvement in 82% of patients.

In 1961, Blaschke reported the first prospective study of 42 patients treated with prolotherapy for lower back pain. Of the patients 32 were workers' compensation cases, notoriously the most difficult cases to treat, and 10 were private insurance cases. Complete recovery was achieved in 20 patients observed for 3 years, 13 patients reported no change in their condition, and 9 underwent surgery. The 4 patients with clinical presentation of acute

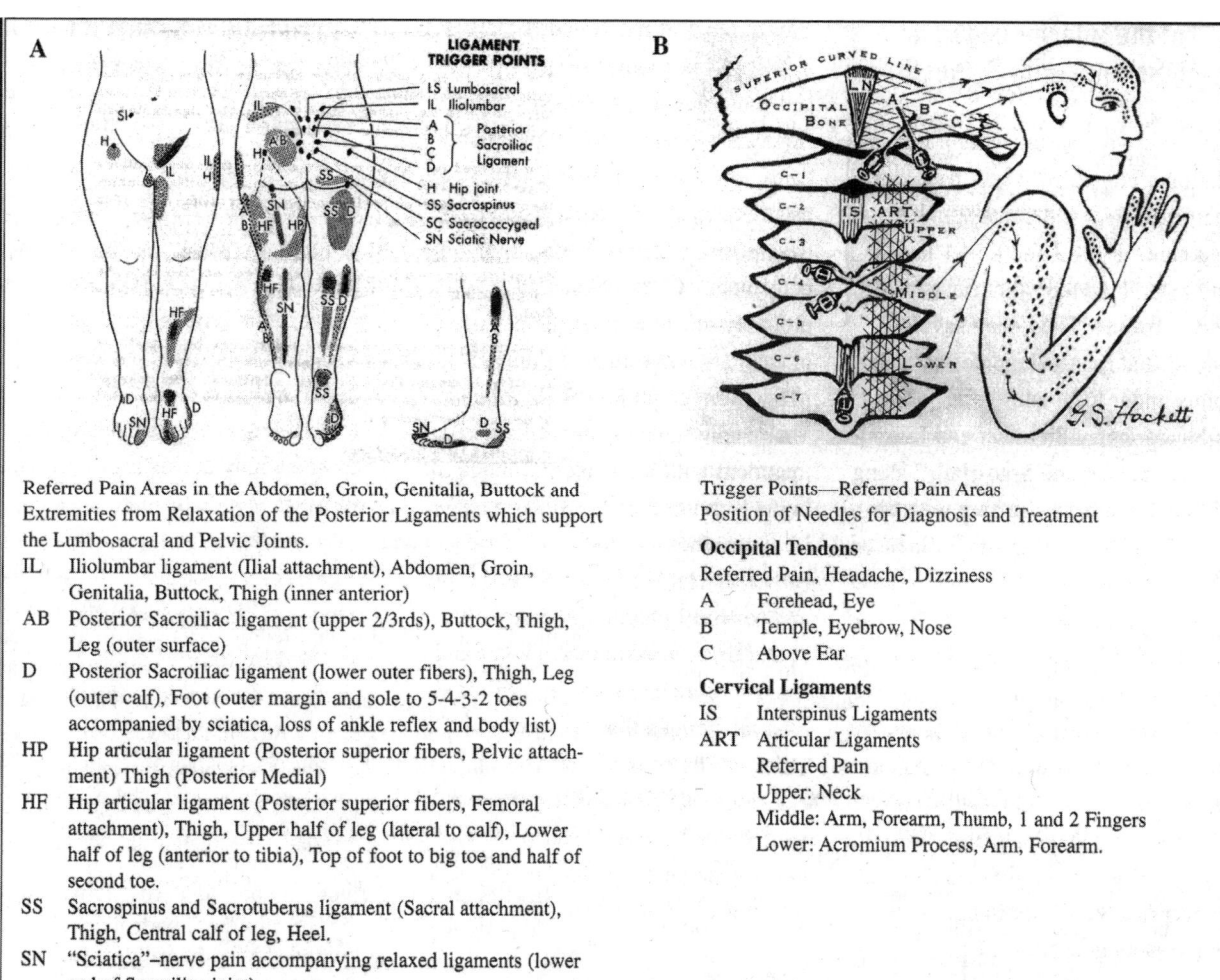

FIGURE 62.2 Hackett's maps of referred pain from ligaments and tendons. (A) The initial maps of the lumbopelvic region derived from 7,000 injections in more than 1,000 patients treated over 17 years. (B) Subsequent maps were of the cervicothoracic region. From *Ligament and Tendon Relaxation (Skeletal Disability) — Treated by Prolotherapy (Fibro-Osseous Proliferation)* (3rd ed.), by G. Hackett, 1958, Springfield, IL: Charles C Thomas. Reproduced with permission.

herniated disc, in whom prolotherapy was used without hope of success, had better results than any other patients in this study. In three instances of surgical intervention, specimens were obtained from the sites of injections and were reported as "normal fibrous tissue."

A multicenter study (Kayfetz et al., 1963b) was published in 1963. Of 264 patients treated by prolotherapy for headaches, 78% had headaches of traumatic origin, 58% had nontraumatic headaches, and 56% had symptoms of Barre–Lieou syndrome. In addition, 86% had symptoms longer than 1 month and 46% had symptoms longer than 1 year. The traumatic group reported satisfactory results in 79%, with excellent results in 60%. The nontraumatic group reported satisfactory results in 47% and excellent results in 29%. Of 264 cases, 60% of patients were followed for over 1 year and 27% were followed for 3 to 5 years. There were no infections or other complications following prolotherapy.

Kayfetz (1963b) also reported a 5-year follow-up study of 189 cases with whiplash injuries treated by prolotherapy. Of these, 149 cases (79%) were due to automobile accidents, 153 (81%) had associated injuries to the thoracic and lumbar areas, 98 (52%) had an associated Barre–Lieou syndrome, and 55% had symptoms longer than 1 month duration and 21% longer than 1-year duration. A majority of patients received 6 to 30 injections in one setting and were treated on 1 to 10 occasions. Duration of treatment was from 1 to 6 months. Excellent results, in terms of pain, were obtained by 113 (60%), good results by 15 (8%), and fair results by 34 (18%). Some 75% of patients considered themselves cured of pain.

In response to adverse effects published after alleged incidental intrathecal injections of zinc sulfate, experiments were conducted with intrathecal injections of this solution in rabbits (Hunt, 1961; Keplinger et al., 1960; Schneider, 1959). Clinical doses (4 to 5 drops) did not produce any noticeable effect. Those animals receiving increased doses that produced spinal anesthesia completely recovered after the anesthetic wore off. "It was necessary to use much greater than clinical dosage to induce paraplegia for a few weeks duration, which also cleared up" (Hackett et al., 1961).

In 1967, Coleman brought medicolegal aspects of prolotherapy to the attention of the medical community. He pointed out that Hackett's technique was accepted as a standard of care. It was declared by a California court that a physician treating a patient had deviated from the method as described by Hackett. Conclusion was made that one did not have to follow the method of treatment followed by the majority of the physicians in the community. A physician is permitted to follow a method or a form of treatment followed by a minority of physicians if they are reputable and in good standing. But if physicians vary from the minority method of treatment they do so in violation, just as if they deviated from the generally accepted method of treatment.

The court concluded: "as a matter of law that prolotherapy as a method of treatment cannot be said to be inappropriate or to be malpractice even though it has not been accepted as a common method of treatment by the medical profession generally" (Coleman, 1968, p. 348).

Abroad, positive results with Hackett's method were obtained by Ongley, Cyriax (1969, 1982), Barbor (1964), and Coplans (1972). Barbor presented a study of 153 patients with back pain for up to 20 years duration. Of 153, 111 (74%) of them reported relief to their satisfaction, 17 (11%) failed to improve; 25 (16%) were lost for follow-up, and 31 (23%) required periodic booster injection for relief. The solution utilized was dextrose, phenol, and glycerin (DPG) mixed in proportions of 2 cc DPG to 3 cc local anesthetic.

Cyriax (1969, 1982, 1993) included detailed descriptions of "sclerosant injections" to interspinous and facet joint capsular ligaments of the cervical, thoracic, and lumbar regions in his texts. Further, he described "a clinical blind study of 'sclerosant therapy' presented by Sanford in 1972. Of 100 patients, only 3 were lost for follow-up." The following three solutions were compared: (1) 2 ml DPG sclerosant mixed with 8 ml saline; (2) 10 ml of 0.5% procaine; and (3) 10 ml normal saline. The diluted sclerosant and procaine solutions were almost equally effective, by relieving pain in more than 50% of cases. Procaine and normal saline were equally ineffective by not helping in 50% of cases. Saline solution helped less than a third of patients. The dilution of DPG sclerosant down to 20% of the original strength significantly impaired its proliferant action.

In 1974, Blumenthal reported two cases of migraine headache and one case of cluster headache successfully cured by prolotherapy and a minor modification of Hackett's technique in the treatment of cervicodorsal pain.

By 1976, Leedy had reported a 70% improvement in the condition of 50 patients with low back pain treated with sclerosant injections and followed for 6 years. He also published several descriptive articles of the method (Leedy et al., 1976).

Also in 1976, Vanderschot compared prolotherapy with acupuncture in the treatment of chronic musculoskeletal pain and concluded that prolotherapy has a faster onset of action and longer-lasting pain relief (Vanderschot, 1976a, 1976b).

In 1978, Chase reported up to 70% or better improvement in long-standing cases of painful head, neck/shoulder, and low back syndromes.

Also in 1978, Koudele reported findings of Haws and Willman on histologic changes in human tissue treated up to five times with sclerosant injections for low back pain. The following changes were observed and documented on slides. DPG solution produced early coagulation necrosis, followed by early collagen formation. By 6 months, a small zone of residual inflammatory cells was documented in an area of very dense collagen. In two other specimens treated with DPG, a dense collagen with fibrosis, occluded blood vessels, and a dense whirl of scar was observed.

After injection of a pumice suspension, an area of dense collagen and fibrosis surrounding a "lake" of pumice was documented without foreign body reaction but with a capsule formation (Koudele, 1978).

In 1982, Hirschberg et al. reported a prospective study of 16 patients with the iliolumbar syndrome. Of the patients, 9 were treated with infiltration of lidocaine at the insertion of the posterior iliolumbar ligament to the iliac crest, and 7 were injected with a mixture containing equal amounts of 50% dextrose and 2% xylocaine (a total of 5 cc). Significant recovery was reported by 10 patients. Of the 7 treated with dextrose/xylocaine, 6 recovered, whereas only 4 of the 9 treated with xylocaine recovered.

Liu et al., in a 1983 double-blind study, injected rabbit medial collateral ligaments (MCLs) and demonstrated that repeated injections of 5% sodium morrhuate at the fibroosseous attachments (enthesis) significantly increased its bone–ligament–bone junction strength by 28%, ligament mass by 44%, and thickness by 27%, when compared with saline controls. Morphometric analysis of electron micrographs demonstrated a highly significant increase in the diameter of collagen fibrils in the experimental ligaments vs. controls. These findings confirmed that sodium morrhuate had a significant regenerative influence on dense connective tissue at the insertion sites.

Maynard and co-workers (1985) reported a decrease in collagen fibrils and hydroxyproline content and an overall increase in the mass of tendons in experimental animals injected with sodium morrhuate. The average tendon circumference increased up to 25%.

Ongley et al. (1987) in a double-blind, randomized study of chronic low back pain in 81 subjects, statistically demonstrated a significant improvement greater than 50% in patients injected with a DPG solution vs. saline. In terms of disability scores, the experimental groups demonstrated a greater improvement than the control group ($p < 0.001$, $p < 0.004$, and $p < 0.001$, respectively; Ongley et al., 1987). Subsequently, Ongley demonstrated a significant statistical improvement in five patients treated for painful instability of the knees with prolotherapy. Ligament stability data was obtained via three-dimensional computerized goniometry, integrated with force measurements (Ongley et al., 1988).

Bourdeau (1988) published a 5-year retrospective survey of patients with low back pain treated with prolotherapy; 17 patients (70%) reported excellent to very good results.

Klein et al. (1989) histologically documented proliferation and regeneration of ligaments in human subjects in response to injections of DPG solution, accompanied by decreased pain and increased range of motion, as documented by computerized inclinometry.

Roosth (1991) described gluteal tendinosis as a distinct clinical entity, and Klein (1991) described the treatment of gluteus medius tendinosis with proliferant injections.

Also in 1991, Schwartz et al. reported a retrospective study of 43 patients with chronic sacroiliac strain who received three series of proliferant injections at biweekly intervals. Improvement was reported by all but 3 patients, and ranged from 95% reported by 20 patients to 66% reported by 4 patients; 10 patients reported recurrence. Schwartz concluded that induced proliferation of collagen and dense connective tissue of the ligament is associated with a reduction of painful subluxations.

Hirschberg et al. (1992) reported positive results in treating iliocostal friction syndrome in elderly individuals with proliferant injections and a soft brace.

Klein et al. (1993) reported a double-blind clinical trial of 79 patients with chronic low back pain who had failed to respond to previous conservative therapy. Subjects were randomly assigned to receive a series of six injections in a double-blind fashion at weekly intervals of either lidocaine/saline or lidocaine/DPG solution into the posterior sacroiliac and interspinous ligaments, fascia, and facet capsules of the low back from L-4 to the sacrum. All patients underwent pretreatment magnetic resonance imaging (MRI) or computed tomography (CT) scans. Patients were evaluated with visual analogue, disability, and pain grid scores, and with objective computerized triaxial tests of lumbar function 6 months following the conclusion of injections. Of the 39 patients randomly assigned to the proliferant group, 30 achieved a 50% or greater decrease in pain or disability scores at 6 months compared with 21 of 40 in the group that received lidocaine/saline ($p = 0.042$). Improvements in visual analogue ($p = 0.056$), disability ($p = 0.068$), and pain grid scores ($p = 0.025$) were greater in the proliferant group.

Massie et al. (1993) reported that it was possible to stimulate fibroplasia in the intervertebral discs with proliferant injections. Also in 1993, Mooney advocated proliferant injections for chronic painful recurrent sacroiliac sprains if the clinician was skilled (Mooney, 1993a, 1993b).

Grayson (1994) reported a case of sterile meningitis after injection of lumbosacral ligaments with proliferating solutions. Matthews (1995) found significant improvement in painful osteoarthritic knees after injection of the ipsilateral sacroiliac ligaments with proliferant solutions. Also in 1995, Reeves pointed out those degenerative changes of enthesopathy may be painful, and prolotherapy with a less aggressive solution such as 12% dextrose with xylocaine is the only type of specific treatment for these pathologic changes of ligaments and tendons.

Eek (1996) reported on the benefit of proliferating injections for intradiscal pain. Klein and Eek have described proliferant injections for low back pain in detail (Klein, 1997).

The clinical anatomy in relation to RIT/prolotherapy for low back pain was reviewed recently. The presence of the connective tissue stocking surrounding various lumbar structures, dictating their function as a single unit in a normal state and the necessity to include multiple segmental and extrasegmental structures in differential diagnosis of low back pain, was emphasized (Linetsky & Willard, 1999; Linetsky et al., 2000).

Subsequently, in March of 2000, Reeves demonstrated in a randomized, double-blind, placebo-controlled study the beneficial effects of 10% dextrose with lidocaine in knee osteoarthritis with anterior cruciate ligament laxity. Goniometric measurements of knee flexion improved by 12.8% ($p = 0.005$) and anterior displacement difference improved by 57% ($p = 0.025$). By 12 months (six injections), the dextrose-treated knees improved in pain (44% decrease), swelling complaints (63% decrease), knee buckling frequency (85% decrease), and flexion range (14° increase). He concluded that proliferant injection with 10% dextrose stimulated growth factors and regeneration and resulted in statistically significant clinical improvements in knee osteoarthritis (Reeves et al., 2000). The history of RIT/prolotherapy from the 1930s through the 1980s was recently reviewed (Linetsky et al., 2000, 2001).

Two recent pilot studies demonstrated significant pain reduction and return to previous levels of activity in patients treated with intradiscal injections of 25% dextrose and combined dextrose-based solutions (Klein et al., 2003; Matthews et al., 2001). Comparison of intradiscal RIT and intradiscal electrothermal therapy (IDET) demonstrated a statistically significant and better results from intradiscal RIT, 47.8% of IDET patients reported improvement while 65.6% of RIT patients reported the same results. Worsening of the conditions was reported by 35.8% of IDET patients and by none of the RIT patients (Derby et al., 2004).

A retrospective study demonstrated a statistically significant improvement in patients treated with phenol-based solution (Wilkinson et al., 2002). An Australian pilot study demonstrated visual analog scale (VAS) scores of back pain improved 60% and VAS scores for leg pain improved 76% after injection of 20% dextrose/xylocaine solution (Yelland et al., 2000). The randomized study by the same senior author comparing 20% dextrose/xylocaine solution and normal saline demonstrated a sustained, statistically significant improvement in a group of patients with chronic low back pain of up to 14 years duration and post-procedural follow-up for 2 years. The role of volume and concentration in the injectate has been brought to light by this study and appears to be much more complex than previously thought; normal saline injected at 3-cc increments (which had never been done by previous investigators) demonstrated significantly positive results (Yelland et al., 2003). Further studies in this direction may provide a better grasp on the indirectly induced stimulation of growth factors in regenerative reparative cascade. Yelland's study also suggests that the volume of injectate may change the concentration of prevailing catabolic interleukin (IL-1) to anabolic interleukin (IL-8). The latter changes have been demonstrated in the injured porcine discs after percutaneous plasma decompression (O'Neill, 2003). A small group of patients improved after intra-articular injection of 25% dextrose or 2.5% phenol into the cervical synovial joints (Linetsky et al., 2004).

To understand the essence of RIT/prolotherapy, it is important to review the basic science related to the healing process, as well as some anatomical and biomechanical properties of connective tissue and clinical anatomy.

INFLAMMATORY-REGENERATIVE/ REPARATIVE RESPONSE AND DEGENERATIVE PATHWAYS

The inflammatory response is intertwined with the regenerative, reparative process. A complex inflammatory reaction induced in vascularized connective tissue by endogenous or exogenous stimuli may lead to two distinct repair pathways. The first is regeneration, which replaces injured cells with the same type of cells; and the second is fibrosis, or the replacement of injured cells with fibrous connective tissue. Often, a combination of both processes contributes to the repair. Initially in both processes a similar pathway takes place with migration of fibroblasts, proliferation, differentiation, and cell–matrix interaction. The last, together with the basement membrane, provides a scaffold for regeneration of preexisting structures (Cotran et al., 1999). Leadbetter (1992) stated, "modulation of these cell matrix responses regardless of the method provides an intriguing challenge" (p. 572). Cell replication is controlled by chemical and growth factors. Chemical factors

may inhibit or stimulate proliferation, whereas growth factors such as cytokines/chemokines, TGF-b1 (transforming growth factor-b1), PDGF (platelet-derived growth factor), FGF (fibroblast growth factor), VEGF (vascular endothelial growth factor), IGF (insulin-like growth factor), CTF (connective tissue growth factor), and NGF (nerve growth factor) stimulate proliferation. The regenerative potential depends on cell type, genetic information, and the size of the defect. In the presence of a large connective tissue defect, fibrotic healing takes place (Cotran et al., 1999; Reeves, 2000).

Under the best circumstances, natural healing restores connective tissue to its preinjury length but only 50 to 75% of its preinjury tensile strength (Leadbetter, 1992; Reeves, 1995). Connective tissues are bradytrophic (their reparative capability is slower than that of muscle or bone). In the presence of repetitive microtrauma, injudicious use of nonsteroidal anti-inflammatory drugs (NSAIDs) and steroid medications, tissue hypoxia, metabolic abnormalities, and other less-defined causes, connective tissue may divert toward a degenerative pathway (Leadbetter, 1992, 1994, 1995; Reeves, 1995, 2000). "A judicious utilization of anti-inflammatory therapy remains useful, albeit adjunctive therapy" (Leadbetter, 1995, p. 402). Biopsies of these tissues demonstrate disorganized collagen, excessive matrix, insufficient elastin, disorganized mesenchymal cells, vascular buds with incomplete lumen, few or absent white blood cells, neovasculogenesis, and neoneurogenesis (Jozsa & Kannus, 1997; Leadbetter, 1994). Degenerative changes in tendons may be hypoxic, mucoid, mixoid, hyaline, calcific, fibrinoid, fatty, fibrocartilaginous and osseous metaplasia, and any combination of the above (Jozsa & Kannus, 1997).

Similar degenerative changes were found in fibromyalgia syndrome with dense foci of rough, frequently hyalinized fibrillar connective tissue. Vascularization occurred at the periphery of these foci, only where thin nervous fibrils and sometimes small paraganglions were seen with severe degenerative changes of the collagen fibers, and marked decrease of fibroblasts. Inflammatory markers were absent (Tuzlukov et al., 1993).

Neoneurogenesis and neovascularization always accompanies the proliferative phase of the healing process and regresses during the contraction phase. Neovascularization has been demonstrated by ultrasound in the injured Achilles tendons (Zanetti et al., 2003). The presence of hyaline cartilage in extruded disc material can suppress neovascularization and subsequent size reduction of herniated mass leading to persistent radiculopathy. Modic types of MRI bone marrow changes are highly suggestive of hyaline cartilage defects at the end plates (Schmid et al., 2004). There is a high correlation between gene defects of COL9A3 and intervertebral disc degeneration, Scheuermann disease, Schmorl's nodules, dorsal annular tears, end plate degeneration, and hyperintense lesions on sagittal T2-weighted lumbar MRIs (Karppinen et al., 2003).

Repeated eccentric contractions diminish muscle function and increase intramuscular pressure. For example, the intramuscular pressure in the supraspinatus and infraspinatus is four to five times higher than that in the deltoid or trapezius at the same relative load (Ranney, 1997). Edema arising in one muscle compartment secondary to overuse does not spread to adjacent compartments. Prolonged static muscular efforts predispose to edema, which leads to a decrease in perfusion pressure and a subsequent reduction of blood flow with granulocyte plugging of the capillaries and further metabolite accumulation and vasodilatation (Jozsa & Kannus, 1997; Leadbetter, 1994; Ranney, 1997).

Further repeated eccentric contractions are notorious for microtraumas with microruptures at the fibro-osseous junctions, in the mid substance of the ligaments and tendons, or at the myotendinous interface. Repetitive microtrauma with insufficient time for recovery leads to an inadequate regenerative process that turns to a degenerative pathway in tendons, muscles, discs, joint ligaments, and cartilage. Improper posture, in combination with eccentric contractions (such as driving with both hands on a steering wheel or typing on a computer with improperly positioned keyboard and monitor), are the most common examples of eccentric contraction (Jozsa, 1997; Leadbetter, 1992, 1994, 1995; Ranney, 1997; Reeves, 2000).

Impaired circulation at the fibromuscular and fibro-osseous interface eventually leads to impaired intraosseous circulation with diminished venous outflow and increased intraosseous pressure. This, in turn, stimulates intraosseous baroreceptors and contributes to nociception transmitted through fine myelinated and nonmyelinated fibers that accompany nutrient vessels into bone and located in perivascular spaces of Haversian canals. Decreased circulation leads to hypoxia, affects calcium metabolism, and contributes to the progression of osteoarthritis (Bannister, 1995; Hackett, 1959b, 1960a, 1960b, 1961, 1966a, 1966c, 1966d, 1967; Hackett et al., 1961, 1962; Shevelev et al., 2000; Sokov et al., 2000; Zoppi et al., 2000).

There is a high coincidence of degenerative changes in syndesmotic, symphyseal (IVD), and uncovertebral joints of the anterior column with degenerative painful changes in synovial and syndesmotic joints of the posterior column. Communications have been reported between the IVD and costovertebral joints (CVJ) through uncovertebral joints. An S-shaped deformity of zygapophyseal joints invariably accompanies disc degeneration with disc height narrowing throughout cervical, thoracic, and lumbar regions (Giles & Singer, 2000, 2001). Degenerative changes in IVD coincide with degenerative changes in tendinous tissue of the posterior spinal syndesmotic joints, i.e., supraspinous, interspinous, and ligamentum flavum representing themselves with disorganization and quantitative decrease of proteoglycan (PG) bonds, chondrifications, and calcifications. Further degenerated spinal ligaments may be a precursor of IVD protrusions (Yahia et al., 1990).

Neoneurogenesis and neovasculogenesis have been documented in chronic connective tissue pathology. The nerve and vascular tissue ingrowth into diseased intervertebral discs, posterior spinal ligaments, hard niduses of fibromyalgia, together with neuropeptides in the facet joint capsules, have been observed (Ashton et al., 1992; El-Bohy et al., 1988; Freemont et al., 1997; Tuzlukov et al., 1993).

Substance P has been recently identified in chronically painful posterior sacroiliac ligaments, joint capsule, and periarticular adipose tissue. There is a strong possibility that it may be present at chronically painful enthesopathy sites throughout the body (Fortin, Vilensky, & Merkel, 2003).

Insertion pathology of the trunk muscles (enthesopathy) at the fibro-osseous junctions most commonly affects the following sites: occiput, scapulas, spinous processes, especially at the cervicodorsal and thoracolumbar regions; sternum, ribs, posterior lateral and anterior surfaces; iliac crest; and symphysis pubis (Figure 62.3 through Figure 62.9). Histopathologically, the following findings were observed: calcium deposits and mineralization of the fibrocartilaginous zone (Jozsa & Kannus, 1997). A large study examined traumatically ruptured tendons from 891 patients in comparison with 445 tendon specimens obtained from similar local sites in similar age and gender groups of "healthy" individuals who died accidentally. Degenerative changes were well documented in 865 ruptured tendons (97%) and only in 149 control tendons (27%). Similar statistical differences were observed comparing tendons of individuals who died 3 years after quadriplegia and those who died accidentally. Irreversible lipoid degenerations at the muscle tendon junctions were documented as early as 3 months after onset of quadriplegia (Jozsa & Kannus, 1997).

There is a high coincidence of degenerative change in syndesmotic and symphyseal joints of the anterior column and uncovertebral arthroses with degenerative painful changes in synovial and syndesmotic joints of the posterior column. Communications have been reported between the IVD and CVJ through uncovertebral joints. An S-shaped deformity of zygapophyseal joints invariably accompanies disc degeneration with disc height narrowing throughout cervical, thoracic, and lumbar regions (Giles & Singer, 2000, 2001). This makes intra-articular needle placement from the posteroinferior pole difficult even with fluoroscopic guidance. Degenerative changes in IVD correspond with degenerative changes in the posterior spinal syndesmotic joints, i.e., supraspinous, interspinous, and ligamentum flavum, where they are represented by disor-

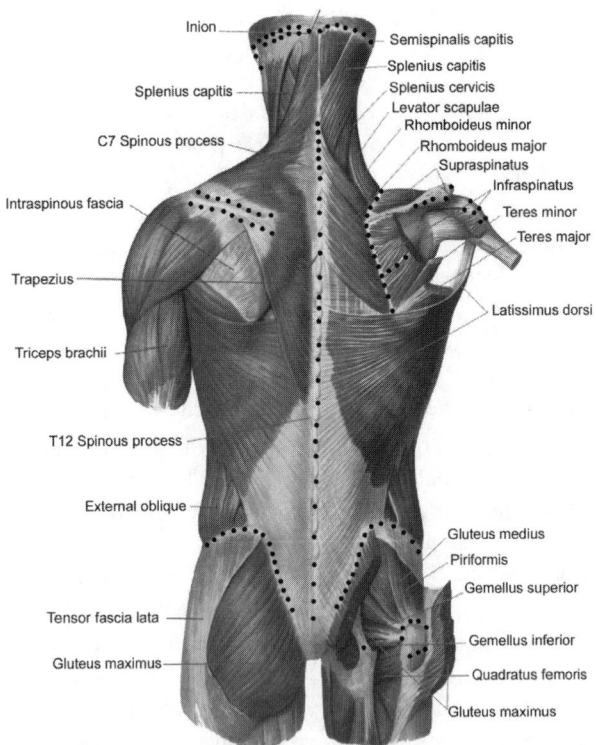

FIGURE 62.3 Dots represent some of the common enthesopathy areas at the fibro-osseous insertions (enthesis), at the occiput, scapulas, humerus, trochanter, iliac crests, and spinous processes. Dots also represent the most common needle locations during RIT infiltrations. (*Note:* Selected locations are treated at each visit.) From *Atlas of Anatomy* (Vol. 1), by R. D. Sinelnikov, 1972, Moscow: Meditsina. Modified for publication by David M. Paul.

ganization and quantitative decrease of proteoglycan bonds and chondrification (Yahia et al., 1990).

The ability of RIT to regenerate and repair connective tissue has been documented by multiple experimental and clinical studies (Klein et al., 1989; Koudele, 1978; McPheeters et al., 1949; Rice, 1936; Riddle, 1940; Warren, 1881; Yeomans et al; 1939).

SOME ANATOMICAL AND BIOMECHANICAL PROPERTIES OF LIGAMENTS AND TENDONS

Ligaments are dull white, dense connective tissue structures that connect adjacent bones. They may be intra-articular, extra-articular, or capsular. Collagen fibers in ligaments may be parallel, oblique, or spiral. These orientations represent adaptation to specific directions in restriction of joint displacements.

Tendons are glistening white collagenous bands interposed between muscle and bone that transmit tensile forces during muscle contraction. There are considerable variations in shape of fibro-osseous attachments from cylindrical, fan shaped to wide, flat, and ribbon shaped.

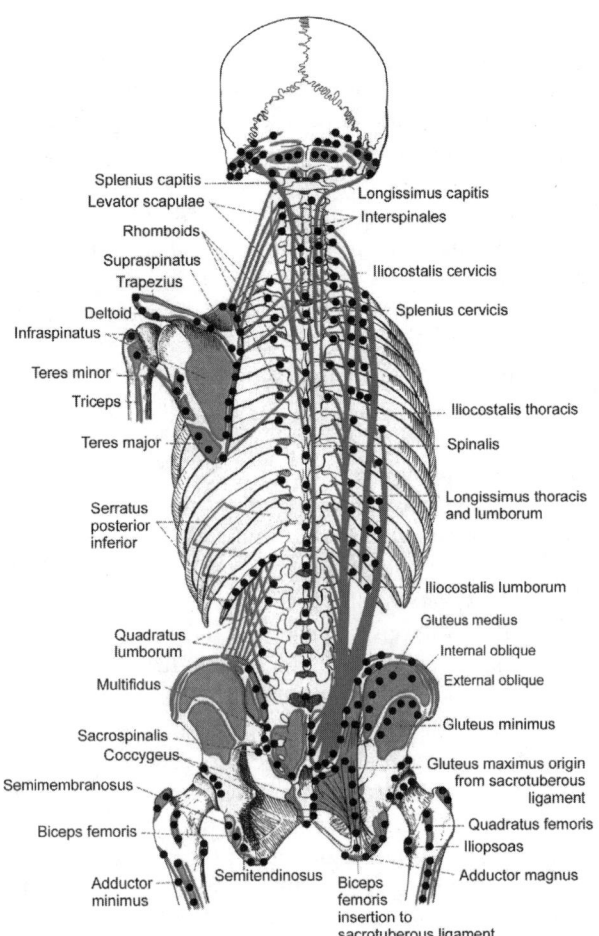

FIGURE 62.4 Schematic drawing demonstrates sites of tendon origins and insertions (enthesis) of the vertebral, paravertebral, and peripheral musculature in the cervical, thoracic, and lumbar regions and part of the upper and lower extremities. Clinically significant painful enthesopathies are common at these locations defined by dots. Dots also represent most common locations of needle insertions and infiltration during RIT. (*Note:* Selected locations are treated at each visit.) From *Atlas of Anatomy* (Vol. 1), by R. D. Sinelnikov, 1972, Moscow: Meditsina. Modified for publication by David M. Paul.

The myotendinous junctions have significant structural variations from end to end, to oblique and singular intermuscular fibers. The collagen content of tendons is approximately 30% wet weight, 70% dry weight (Bannister, 1995; Butler et al., 1978).

Under a light microscope, ligaments and tendons have a crimped, waveform appearance. This crimp is a planar zigzag pattern that unfolds during initial loading of collagen (Bannister, 1995; Butler et al., 1978). Elongated below 4% of original length, ligaments and tendons return to their original crimped wave appearance; beyond 4% elongation, they lose the elasticity and become permanently laxed. However, in degenerative ligaments, subfailure was reported as early as 1.5% elongation. Laxity of ligaments obviously leads to joint hypermobility. Experi-

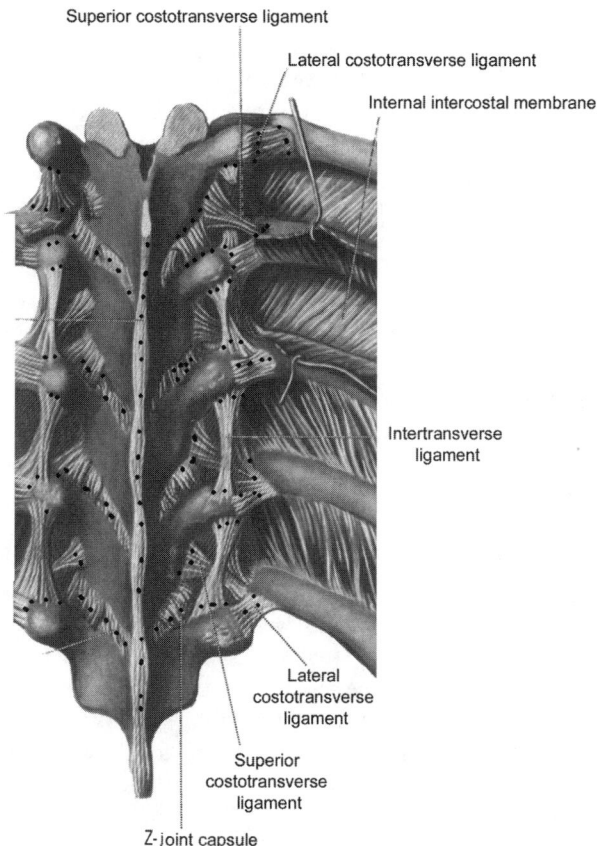

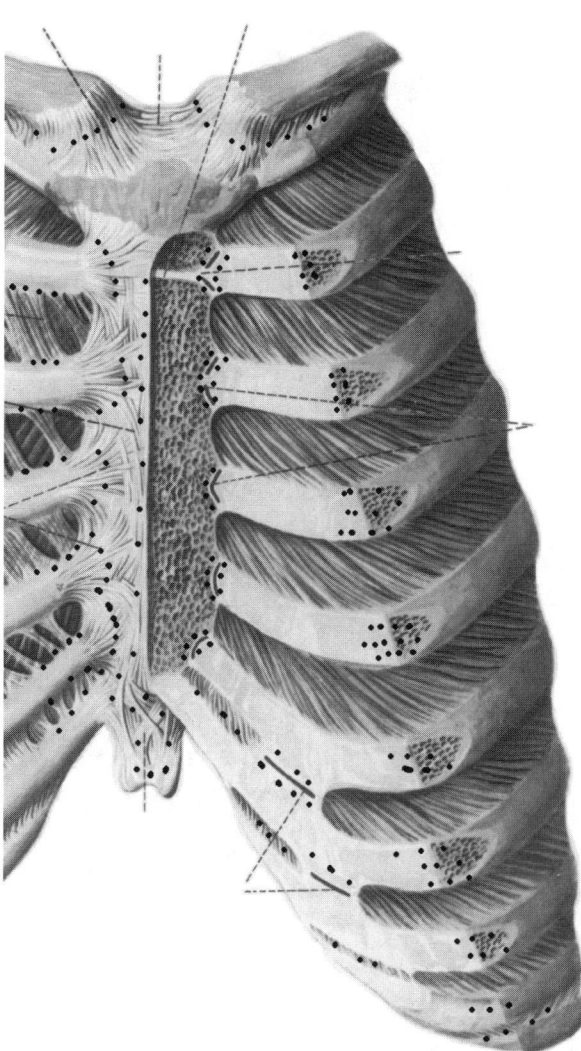

FIGURE 62.5 Sites of common posterior thoracic vertebral and paravertebral arthropathies and enthesopathies. Dots also represent the most common needle locations during RIT infiltrations. (*Note:* Selected locations are treated at each visit.) From *Atlas of Anatomy* (Vol. 1), by R. D. Sinelnikov, 1972, Moscow: Meditsina. Modified for publication by David M. Paul.

FIGURE 62.6 Common sites of painful enthesopathies on the anterior thoracic wall, including sternoclavicular, costosternal, interchondral synovial articulations, various syndesmotic joints, and costochondral synchondroses. (*Note:* Selected locations are treated at each visit.) From *Atlas of Anatomy* (Vol. 1), by R. D. Sinelnikov, 1972, Moscow: Meditsina. Modified for publication by David M. Paul.

mental studies have confirmed that the MCL failed more abruptly than either the capsular ligaments or the anterior cruciate ligament (ACL). This happens because the MCL has more parallel fibers with uniformity in length, and therefore, they fail together. The capsular fibers are less organized than the MCL or ACL, and their lengths and orientations vary. Because these fibers are loaded and fail at different times a large joint displacement is needed before capsular failure is complete.

Three principal failure modes exist. The first and most common is ligament failure. The second is a bone avulsion fracture, and the third, the least common, is a shear or cleavage failure at the fibro-osseous interface.

Collagenous tissues are deleteriously affected by inactivity and are favorably influenced by physical activity of an endurance nature. They are also deleteriously affected by NSAIDs and steroid administrations.

In fact, "Administration of even a single dose of corticosteroids directly into ligaments or tendons can have debilitating effects upon their strength. Intra-articular injections of methyl-prednisolone acetate given either

once or at intervals of several months may be less detrimental to ligament or tendon mechanical properties" (Butler et al., 1978).

Tendons are strongly attached to the bones by decussating and perforating Sharpey's fibers. Current understanding of OTJ (osseo tendinous junction, also called enthesis, fibro-osseous junction) is such that the fibers insert to the bone via four zones: tendon zone, fibrocartilage zone, mineralized fibrocartilage zone, and lamellar bone. However, it does not shed much light on the mechanism of tendon avulsion and overuse-induced pathology, as was emphasized by Hackett et al. (1991) and Jozsa and Kannus (1997). The tensile strength of tendons is similar to that of bone and is about half that of steel. A tendon

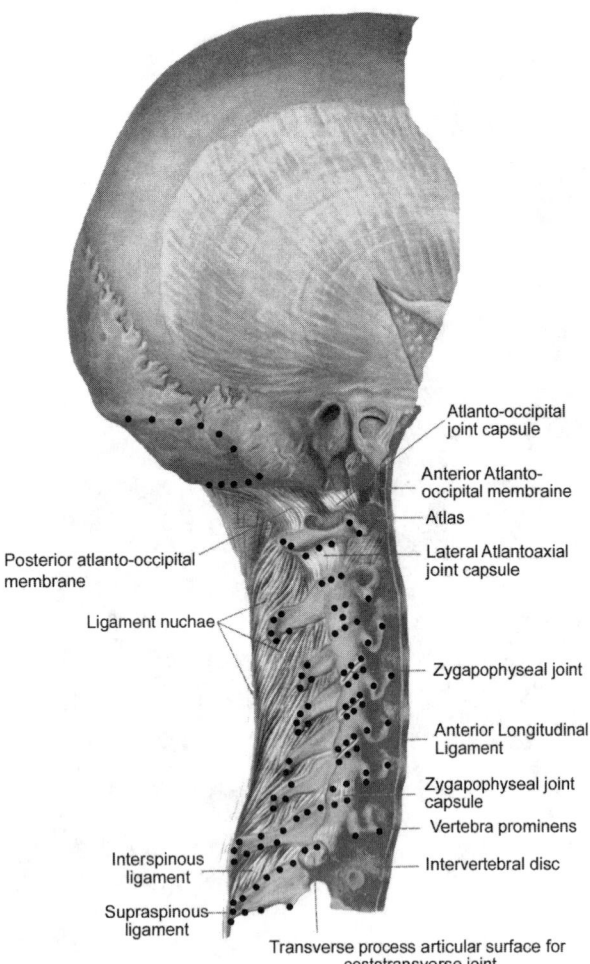

Atlanto-occipital
joint capsule

Anterior Atlanto-
occipital membraine

Atlas

Lateral Atlantoaxial
joint capsule

Posterior atlanto-occipital
membrane

Ligament nuchae

Zygapophyseal joint

Anterior Longitudinal
Ligament

Zygapophyseal joint
capsule

Vertebra prominens

Interspinous
ligament

Intervertebral disc

Supraspinous
ligament

Transverse process articular surface for
costotransverse joint

FIGURE 62.7 Clinically significant painful enthesopathies and arthropathies are common at the locations defined by dots. Dots also represent most common needle locations during RIT infiltrations. (*Note:* Selected locations are treated at each visit.) From *Atlas of Anatomy* (Vol. 1), by R. D. Sinelnikov, 1972, Moscow: Meditsina. Modified for publication by David M. Paul.

with a cross section of 10 mm in diameter can support a load of 600 to 1,000 kg (Bannister, 1995; Butler et al., 1978; Jozsa & Kannus, 1997).

During postnatal development, tendons enlarge by interstitial growth, particularly at the myotendinous junction (also called the fibromuscular interface) where there is a high concentration of fibroblasts. The nerve supplies are largely sensory (Bannister, 1995; Best, 1994; Butler et al., 1978; Jozsa & Kannus, 1997).

GROSS ANATOMY OF CRANIOVERTEBRAL, CERVICAL AND THORACIC REGIONS IN RELATION TO RIT

The shape of a human body and its components is irregularly tubular. This shape is maintained by continuous compartmentalized connective tissue stocking that incor-

porates, interconnects, and supports various ligaments, tendons, fascia, muscles, osseous and neurovascular structures. Collagenous connective tissues, despite slightly different biochemical content, blend at their boundaries and at the osseous structures, functioning as a single unit (Agur, 1991; Bannister, 1995; Linetsky et al., 1999, 2002a, 2002b, 2004; Sinelnikov, 1972; Willard, 2003). This arrangement provides bracing and a hydraulic amplification effect to the muscles, increasing contraction strength in the lumbar region up to 30% (Bogduk, 1997). If only the connective tissues were left in place and all other tissue removed, the shape of a human body would not change.

Movements of the spine and cranium are accomplished through various well-innervated joints, located in the anterior and posterior columns. These joints are syndesmotic, synovial, and symphyseal in nature. Syndesmotic joints of the anterior column are anterior and posterior longitudinal ligaments; anterior and posterior atlanto-occipital membranes; and transverse, apical, and alar ligaments. Symphyseal joints are IVDs and their extensions; unique to the cervical and upper thoracic spine are the so-called uncovertebral joints of Luschka, which are lateral and posteriolateral elevations of the uncinate processes. Synovial joints are atlanto-axial (AA), atlanto-occipital (AO), and CVJ. Syndesmotic joints of the posterior column are posterior atlanto-occipital membrane, supraspinous and interspinous ligaments, ligamentum flavum and nuchae. Synovial joints are costotransverse and zygapophyseal (ZJ). The following joints are indirectly related to the spine: costosternal, interchondral, and sternoclavicular (Agur et al., 1991; Bannister, 1995; Giles & Singer, 2000, 2001; Sinelnikov, 1972).

Segmental innervation of the aforementioned compartments and their contents is provided by the spinal nerves and their respective ventral and dorsal rami (VR, DR). The DRs further divide into medial and lateral branches (MBDR, LBDR) providing innervation to the posterior structures. Anteriorly, spinal segments are innervated by sympathetic fibers (SF); laterally, by gray rami communicantes (GRC); and posteriorly, by the sinuvertebral nerve of Luschka (SN). The extrasegmental communications are widely present on the anterior surface of the spine between the SF, laterally between GRCs and posteriorly between branches of SN (Agur et al., 1991; Bannister, 1995; Bogduk, 1986, 1996; Cramer & Darby 1995; Linetsky et al., 2002a, 2002b, 2004; Willard, 1995).

The first dorsal ramus, also called the sub-occipital nerve, supplies the muscles of the sub-occipital region, rectus capitis posterior minor and major, inferior and superior oblique, and semispinalis capitis. It has an ascending cutaneous branch that connects with the greater and lesser occipital nerves and may contribute to the occipital and sub-occipital headaches (Bannister, 1995; Bogduk, 1982, 1986, 1988). The second cervical dorsal ramus also sup-

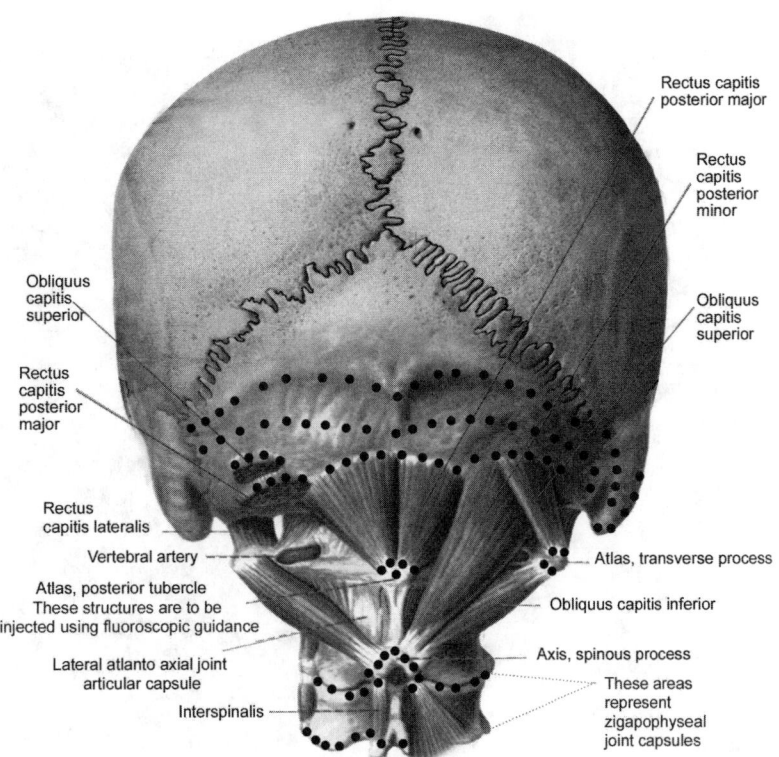

FIGURE 62.8 Sites of tendon origins and insertions (enthesis) of the vertebral and paravertebral musculature in the upper cervical and occipital region. Clinically significant painful enthesopathies are common at locations defined by dots. Dots also represent most common locations of needle insertions and infiltration during RIT. (*Note:* Selected locations are treated at each visit.) From *Atlas of Anatomy* (Vol. 1), by R. D. Sinelnikov, 1972, Moscow: Meditsina. Modified for publication by David M. Paul.

plies the inferior oblique, connects with the first one, and divides into LMBDR. Its medial branch, the greater occipital nerve, pierces the semispinalis capitis and trapezius at their insertion to the occipital bone on its ascending course. Thereafter, it connects with the branches from the third occipital nerve along the course of the occipital artery supplying the skin of the skull up to the vertex (Bannister et al., 1995; Bogduk, 1982, 1986, 1988).

Lateral branches supply the iliocostalis, longissimus cervices, and longissimus capitis. Similar anatomic relationships are observed in the thoracic region where medial branches of the upper six thoracic dorsal rami supply the zygapophyseal joints, semispinalis thoracis, multifidi, piercing trapezius, and rhomboid, and reach the skin most proximal and lateral to the spinous processes (Agur et al., 1991; Bannister et al., 1995; Bogduk, 1982).

Current trends in therapeutic and diagnostic blocks are based on the fact that the anatomy and course of the MBDRs is fairly constant, and that it arises from the intertransverse space and wraps around the waist of the respective articular pillars (Aprill et al., 1990; Bogduk, 1982, 1986, 1988). Recent clinical observations supported by ongoing research and microdissections of Willard (Figure 62.10) concur with the previous investigations (Bogduk, 1982). MBDR furnishes twigs to zygapophyseal joint capsules and continues along the lamina and spinous

process toward its apex, innervating structures inserting or originating at the lamina and the spinous process on its course often terminating in interspinalis muscles (Bogduk, 1982, 1988, 1996; Bogduk et al., 1996; Willard, 2003, see Figure 62.10 and Figure 62.11). For example, the fourth and fifth cervical MBDRs supply the semispinalis cervices and capitis, multifidi, interspinalis, splenius and trapezius, and supraspinous ligaments, and end in the skin. The lowest three MBDRs have a similar course (Figure 62.10).

However, variations in innervation occur, their incidence is unknown. Floating dorsal rami have been described in the cervical and thoracic regions, sometimes descending from the level of C5–6, C6–7, or C7–T1 to the level of T3–4, T4–5, T5–6. The latter "so-called" causes of thoracic pain of cervicogenic origin, which may complicate the differential diagnosis, explain failures after MBDR blocks or radiofrequency procedures, and *make tissue nociceptors specific targets for RIT* (Linetsky et al., 2004; Maigne, 1996; Willard, 2003; Figure 62.11).

Three types of nerve endings in posterior ligamentous structures of the spine were confirmed microscopically. They are free nerve endings and Pacini and Ruffini corpuscles. The free nerve endings were found in superficial layers of all ligaments, including supraspinous and interspinous, with a sharp increase in their quantity at the spinous processes attachments (enthesis). Paciniform corpuscles are

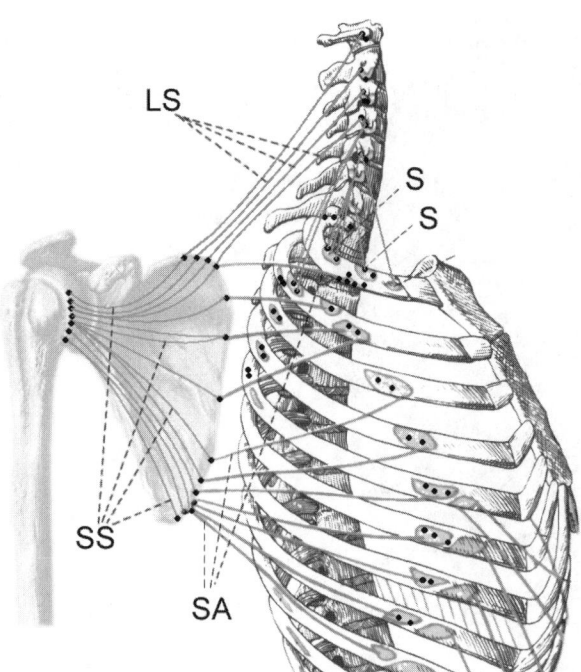

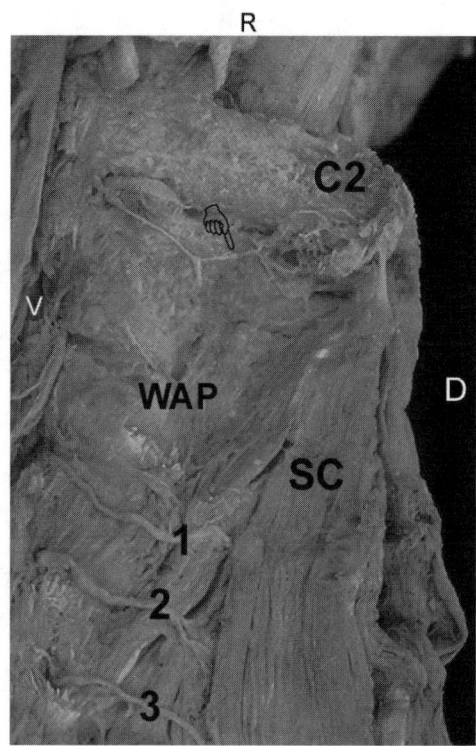

FIGURE 62.9 Commonly overlooked painful enthesopathies of levator scapula (LS), subscapularis (SS), and serratus anterior (SA) especially superior fascicle often mimic upper trapezial pain. Contribution of rhomboid, scalenes (S), omohyoid (inferior belly), splenius services, posterior and anterior column structures including first costotransverse joint should be considered in differential diagnosis. (*Note:* Selected locations are treated at each visit.) From *Atlas of Anatomy* (Vol. 1), by R. D. Sinelnikov, 1972, Moscow: Meditsina. Modified for publication by David M. Paul.

FIGURE 62.10 Left dorsolateral view of the cervical medial branches of the dorsal rami (MBDRs). C–2 = apex of C2 spinous process, SC = semispinalis cervices, WAP = waist of articular pillar with the medial branch displaced anteriolaterally, 1 2 3 = MBDRs wrapping around the waists of articular pillars ramifying into multifidi. One of the two MBDRs that usually arise separately, innervating structures at the apex of C2. Slide and microdissections are courtesy of Professor Frank Willard, Ph.D. Modified for publication by David M. Paul.

located in adipose tissue between supraspinous ligaments and lumbosacral fascia and in the deep layers of supraspinous and interspinous ligaments acting as nociceptors in all locations and as mechanoreceptors with a low threshold, and are stimulated by stretch of the ligaments and muscle actions. Ruffini receptors are located in the interspinous and flaval ligaments; they respond to stretch and control the reflex inhibitory mechanism (Yahia et al., 1989).

Variously shaped, synovium-covered menisci composed of adipose, fibroadipose, collagenous, and cartilaginous tissue extend into cervical synovial joint space and anchor at their periphery to the joint capsule where they receive their blood supply. Their shape and position changes with age and degeneration (Mercer & Bogduk, 1993; Yu et al., 1987). The nerve supply to the inferior synovial folds of lumbar z-joints has also been documented (Giles, 1988; Giles & Taylor, 1987).

CLINICAL ANATOMY OF CRANIOVERTEBRAL, CERVICAL, AND THORACIC REGIONS IN RELATION TO RIT

The subjective nature of pain and especially chronic pain, because of the suffering characteristics, is a major com-

munication problem. Quite often a physician has not had a comparable experience and will have difficulty understanding what the patient is trying to communicate. Physicians, especially those involved in pain management, have to accept patients' "pain and tenderness" at face value without dismissal or allocation to a distant "proven" source. It is the knowledge of clinical anatomy, pain patterns, and pathology that should guide the clinical investigation, versus insurance policies and reimbursement especially in the current mismanaged care environment.

Hilton's law is clear that a nerve passing a joint is also supplying that joint, muscles are moving that joint, and the skin is covering insertions of these muscles (Hilton, 1891). This is in accord with anatomical, histological, experimental, and human studies that followed and are too numerous to count.

Scientifically verified are the following data. Cervical ZJ is responsible for 54% of chronic neck pain after "whiplash" injury. Intra-articular corticosteroid injections are ineffective in relieving chronic cervical ZJ pain (Barnsley et al., 1994, 1995). In cervicogenic headaches after whiplash, more than 50% stem from the C2–3 ZJ

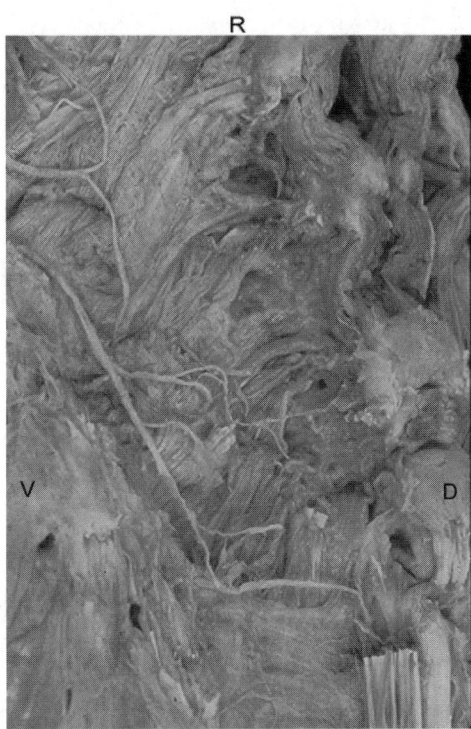

FIGURE 62.11 Left dorsolateral view of cervical micro-dissection. Descending floating cervical MBDR with multiple branches reaching lateral aspects of the spinous processes at the enthesis of multifidi. Slide and micro-dissections are courtesy of Professor Frank Willard, Ph.D. Modified and prepared for publication by David M. Paul.

(Bogduk, 1986, 1996; Bogduk et al., 1996; Lord, 1996). Prevalence of cervical ZJ pain is as high as 67%; thoracic is 48% (Boswell et al., 2003; Lord, 1996; Manchikanti et al., 2002). The preceding statistical data were obtained by a painstaking adherence to precision protocols and strongly suggest a presence of nociceptors other than ZJ and IVD. Lack of statistical data on these "other, hidden, unproven pain generators" could not be misconstrued as their absence. Cervical and thoracic facet syndromes comprise the pathology of capsular ligaments, periarticular tendons with their enthesis, extrapment, and entrapment of menisci, and fractures of the articular pillars, which are not detected by current radiologic modalities. Also S-shaped intra- and periarticular degenerative changes of ZJ predispose intra-articular inclusions and subchondral bone to contusions during trauma (similar to an inadvertent bite on the buccal mucosa). The same changes make intra-articular needle placement from the inferior pole difficult even with fluoroscopic guidance.

Pain patterns resembling those of facet syndromes have been described from structures located distally on the course of MBDRs, lateral branches (LBs), and those receiving extrasegmental innervation. Further, patterns from AO and AA joints overlap with patterns from the lower z-joints (Aprill et al., 1990; Dreyfuss et al., 1994a),

as well as sub-occipital and posterior cervical soft tissues (Feinstein et al., 1954; Hackett 1958, 1960a; Hackett et al., 1962, 1991; Kellgren, 1939; Linetsky et al., 2004; Travell et al., 1983). AO and AA contribution to nociception requires confirmation with intra-articular blocks under fluoroscopic guidance by a practitioner with a significant amount of experience (Dreyfuss et al., 1994a). Usually it is a diagnostic procedures of exclusion and is employed after failure of mid-cervical and C2–3 ZJ interventions to provide a relief. (Bogduk, 1988; Dreyfuss et al., 1994a, 1994b). Conversely RIT injections are capsular ZJ injections that provide relief without fluoroscopic assistance in the cervicothoracic region as high as C2–3 ZJ capsule which is the highest palpable ZJ in the cervical spine, at a comparatively much lower cost (Blumenthal, 1974; Cyriax 1969, 1982, 1993; Hackett, 1958, 1962, 1991; Kayfetz, 1993a, b; Linetsky, 2002b, 2004; Maigne, 1996; Waldman, 1998). Current prevailing trends in diagnostic efforts are variable and are as follows. Cervical facetogenic pain is confirmed by MBDR block but AO, AA, CVJ, and sacroiliac joints are diagnosed by intra-articular blocks. Thoracic ZJ pain is diagnosed by both intra-articular and MBDR block, without consideration for chronic degenerative, painful changes in the tissue bed. Neuralgic spinal pain is diagnosed by translaminar or transforaminal block. Discogenic pain is addressed by needle placement and tissue distention with contrast or what is known as tissue bed block (Aprill et al., 1990; Bogduk, 1982; Linetsky & Willard, 1999; Linetsky et al., 2002a, 2004).

Consequently, therapy is directed toward neuromodulation or neuroablation with radiofrequency generators or corticosteroid injections for neuralgic pain. Surgical interventions and fusions are aimed to correct the mass effects in neurocompressive models or discogenic pain. The rest of pain generators are not included in differential diagnosis because of the spinal uncertainty principle. According to the principle even for a simple example of two motion segments, where disc, facets, and musculotendinous compartments, each considered as one putative nociceptive unit, the total number of clinically indistinguishable combinations rises to 63 possibilities. It is practically impossible to address such a magnitude of possibilities under fluoroscopic guidance (Dickey, 2001).

The tissue bed pathology and pain are the primary targets for RIT taking innervation into account. Therefore, RIT affords evaluation of many putative pain generators from the variety of pain presentations in the craniocervicothoracic region in addition to the posterior column. When correctly implemented, RIT offers an attractive, practical alternative that is accomplished at the same office visit.

The apices of the spinous processes (SP) and their entheses are well innervated and considered a "spinous rotator cuff" especially at C2 and C6–T12.

Standard MBDR blocks interrupt orthodromic and antidromic transmission at the proximal segment of MBDR. Other putative nociceptors located distally on MBDR course are excluded from the differential diagnosis without consideration to individual variation in the locations of terminal filaments of MBDR and LB. For RIT purpose, the blocks are performed beginning from the terminal filaments at SP enthesis, towards origins of innervation located proximally on the course of MBDR or LB (Hackett et al., 1991; Linetsky et al., 2002b, 2004; Steindler et al., 1938).

For example, at the cervicocranial junction, lateral aspects of the apex at the C2 spinous process (specifically enthesis of rectus capitus posterior major, obliquus capitus inferior, semispinalis services) are addressed initially. If pain persists, respective enthesis are addressed at the superior and inferior nuchal lines. If pain persists, the C2–3 posterior z-joint capsule is injected (Linetsky, 2002b, 2004; Figure 62.7, Figure 62.8, Figure 62.10, Figure 62.11). At the mid-cervical segments, central tenderness is rare while facet capsular tenderness is more prevalent, which is the reason the posterior ZJ capsules are blocked initially if this is the only presenting pain. Should this fail, subsequent intra-articular fluoroscopically guided injections are indicated. This approach may fail in the presence of paramedian pain and trapezial pain because it does not take into account extrasegmental innervation to some of the cervical and thoracic structures commonly involved in chronic pain syndromes that receive innervation from the cranial nerves or the ventral rami.

Multilevel C6–T9 midline pain with variable degree of tenderness in the projection of posterior syndesmotic joints and rhomboid-shaped trapezius (TR) aponeurosis is by far one of the most common presenting complaints encountered in pain practice (exact prevalence unknown) (Figure 62.3 through Figure 62.5). This is combined with variations of paramedian, lateral, middle and upper TR pain, and tenderness commonly ascribed to "trigger points" (TPs). Injections of these TPs often do not resolve the pain. What to do next? Search for all other tender sites in the region. This usually reveals exquisite tenderness at the superomedial angle of the scapula where levator scapulae (LS) share the insertion site, enthesis, with serratus anterior (SA) and subscapularis (SS). Innervation of these structures is as follows: TR — by the XIth pair, the accessory nerve; LS — by ventral rami (VR) from (C3–C4) and dorsal scapular nerve (C5); SA — by long thoracic nerve (C5–C7 VR); and SS — by superior and inferior subscapular nerves (C5–C6 VR). To base differential diagnosis and treatment of this condition on diagnostic blocks of all these nerves in one setting is impossible (Dickey, 2001).

Conversely, block of the common enthesis at the superomedial scapular angle addressing both dorsal and ventral surface may provide instant relief including disappearance of TPs. The following case will demonstrate

the necessity to consider all potential nociceptors in a given presentation (Figure 62.9).

For the purpose of RIT, when trapezial pain is accompanied by midline tenderness at C6–T6, those structures are injected initially. If TR pain persists and is accompanied by paramedian pain and tenderness, ZJ capsules are injected. If TR pain persists, the first CVJs are injected if tender. If not, scalene medius enthesis at the first rib is injected if tender. If pain persists, iliocostalicis services, thoraces, and serratus superior enthesis at the respective ribs are injected. If pain persists, LS and SA enthesis at superomedial angle of the scapula are blocked. This site may be blocked initially if it is the sole area of presenting complaint, pain, and tenderness. If pain persists, the above-described sequence may be initiated.

MECHANISM OF ACTION

The exact mechanism of action is unknown. The proposed and postulated RIT mechanisms of action are complex and multifaceted.

- Temporary neurolysis with chemoneuromodulation of peripheral nociceptors is achieved by chemical properties of the injectates and provides stabilization of antidromic, orthodromic, sympathetic and axon reflex transmissions.
- Temporary neurolysis is achieved via mechanical transsections of some small myelinated and unmyelinated C fibers by the needle or hydraulic pressure of the injected volume.
- Mechanical transsections of cells and extracellular matrix by the needle causes cellular damage, stimulates inflammatory cascade and release of growth factors.
- Compression of cells by relatively large extracellular volume as well as cell expansion or constriction due to osmotic properties of injectate stimulates the release of intracellular growth factors.
- Chemomodulation of collagen through inflammatory, proliferative, regenerative/reparative response is induced by the chemical properties of the injectates and mediated by cytokines and multiple growth factors.
- Modulation of local haemodynamics with changes in intra-osseous pressure leads to reduction of pain. Empirical observations suggest that dextrose/lidocaine action is much more prolonged than that of lidocaine alone.
- Temporary repetitive stabilization of the painful hypermobile joints, induced by inflammatory response to the injectates, provides a better environment for regeneration and repair of the affected ligaments and tendons.

- The large volume of injectate disrupts adhesions that were created by the original inflammatory attempts to heal the injury, akin to epidural or intra-abdominal lyses of adhesions.
- A relatively large volume of osmotically inert injectate assumes the role of a space occupying lesion in a tight and slowly equilibrating extracellular compartment of the connective tissue. It initiates inflammatory cascade and also irrigates catabolic interleukins

Putative Pain-Generating Structures Addressed by RIT/Prolotherapy

1. Ligaments: Intra-articular, periarticular, capsular
2. Tendons
3. Fascia
4. Enthesis: The zone of insertion of ligament, tendon, or articular capsule to bone (Anderson, 1988; Jozsa & Kannus, 1997; Klein & Eek, 1997) (also called fibro-osseous junctions of ligaments and tendons). In the orthopedic literature, this is referred to as OTJ (osseo/tendinous junction) (Jozsa & Kannus, 1997; Leadbetter, 1992, 1994, 1995; Linetsky et al., 2002a, b, c, 2004; Reeves, 2000). For the purpose of this chapter, enthesis and fibro-osseous junction are interchangeable.
5. Intervertebral discs

TISSUE PATHOLOGY TREATED WITH RIT/PROLOTHERAPY

1. *Sprain*: Ligamentous injury at the fibro-osseous junction or intersubstance disruption. A sudden or severe twisting of a joint with stretching or tearing of ligaments; also, a sprained condition (Leadbetter, 1994; Reeves, 1995; Simon et al., 1987).
2. *Strain*: Muscle/tendon injury at the fibromuscular or fibro-osseous interface. When concerned with the peripheral muscles and tendons sprains and strains are identified as separate injuries and in three-stage gradations: first-, second-, and third-degree sprain, and similarly for strain. With regard to vertebral and paravertebral ligaments and tendons, no consensus exists among authors and the definitions are quite vague (Anderson, 1985; Leadbetter, 1994).
3. *Enthesopathy*: A painful degenerative pathological process that results in the deposition of poorly organized tissue, degeneration and tendinosis at the fibro-osseous interface, and transition toward loss of function (Jozsa & Kannus, 1997; Klein & Eek, 1997; Leadbetter, 1994; Linetsky, 1999b; Reeves, 1995).

4. *Tendinosis/ligamentosis*: A focal area of degenerative changes due to a failure of cell matrix adaptation to excessive load and tissue hypoxia, with a strong tendency toward chronic recurrent pain and dysfunction (Best, 1994; Jozsa & Kannus, 1997; Klein & Eek, 1997; Leadbetter, 1994; Reeves, 1995; Roosth, 1991).
5. *Pathologic ligament laxity*: A post-traumatic or congenital condition leading to painful hypermobility of the axial and peripheral joints (Anderson, 1985; Dorman et al., 1991; Hackett, 1958; Reeves, 1995, 2000; Reeves et al., 2000; Simon et al., 1987).

INDICATIONS FOR RIT/PROLOTHERAPY

1. Chronic pain from ligaments or tendons secondary to sprains or strains
2. Pain from overuse or occupational conditions known as repetitive motion disorders (i.e., neck and wrist pain in typists and computer operators, "tennis" and "golfer's" elbows, chronic supraspinatus tendinosis)
3. Painful chronic postural neck and cervicodorsal junction problems
4. Painful recurrent somatic dysfunctions secondary to ligament laxity that improve temporarily with manipulation; hypermobility and subluxation at a given peripheral or spinal articulation or mobile segment(s), accompanied by a restricted range of motion at reciprocal segment(s)
5. Thoracic vertebral compression fractures with a wedge deformity that exerts additional stress on the posterior ligamento-tendinous complex
6. Recurrent painful subluxations of ribs at the costotransverse, costovertebral, and/or costosternal articulations
7. Spondylolisis and spondylolisthesis
8. Intolerance to NSAIDs, steroids, or opiates and failure of manipulative treatments or physical therapy
9. RIT is the treatment of choice when corticosteroid injections, RF, and surgery failed or are contraindicated

SYNDROMES AND DIAGNOSTIC ENTITIES CAUSED BY LIGAMENT AND TENDON PATHOLOGY THAT HAVE BEEN SUCCESSFULLY TREATED WITH RIT/PROLOTHERAPY

1. Cervicocranial syndrome (cervicogenic headaches, alar ligaments sprain, atlanto-axial and atlanto-occipital joint sprains)

2. Temporomandibular pain and dysfunction syndrome
3. Barre–Lieou syndrome
4. Spasmodic torticollis
5. Cervical segmental dysfunctions
6. Cervical and cervicothoracic spinal pain of "unknown" origin
7. Cervicobrachial syndrome (shoulder/neck pain)
8. Hyperextension/hyperflexion injury syndromes
9. Cervical, thoracic, and lumbar facet syndromes
10. Cervical, thoracic, and lumbar sprain/strain syndromes
11. Costotransverse joint pain
12. Costovertebral arthrosis/dysfunction
13. Slipping rib syndrome
14. Sternoclavicular arthrosis and repetitive sprain
15. Thoracic segmental dysfunction
16. Tietze's syndrome/costochondritis/chondrosis
17. Costosternal arthrosis
18. Intercostal arthrosis
19. Xiphoidalgia syndrome
20. Acromioclavicular sprain/arthrosis
21. Shoulder–hand syndrome
22. Recurrent shoulder dislocations
23. Scapulothoracic crepitus
24. Myofacial pain syndromes
25. Ehlers–Danlos syndrome
26. Marie–Strumpell disease
27. Failed back surgery syndrome

CONTRAINDICATIONS TO RIT/PROLOTHERAPY

1. Allergy to anesthetic or proliferant solutions or their ingredients, such as dextrose, sodium morrhuate, or phenol
2. Acute nonreduced subluxations or dislocations
3. Acute sprains or strains of axial and peripheral joints
4. Acute arthritis (septic or post-traumatic with hemarthrosis)
5. Acute bursitis or tendinitis
6. Capsular pattern shoulder and hip designating acute arthritis accompanied by tendinitis
7. Acute gout or rheumatoid arthritis
8. Recent onset of a progressive neurologic deficit, including but not limited to severe intractable cephalgia, unilaterally dilated pupil, bladder dysfunction, and bowel incontinence
9. Requests for a large quantity of sedation and/or narcotics before and after treatment
10. Paraspinal neoplastic lesions involving the musculature and osseous structures

11. Severe exacerbation of pain or lack of improvement after local anesthetic blocks
12. Relative contraindications: central spinal canal, lateral recess and neural foraminal stenosis

CLINICAL PRESENTATIONS

Patients may present with a variety of complaints ranging from one area of localized pain and tenderness to any combination of referred pain patterns known with cervical disc, cervicocranial, and cervicobrachial or cervical and thoracic facet syndromes. Headaches accompanied by cervical muscle spasms are a common complaint. Other complaints include (1) exacerbation of pain while standing or sitting in the same position for a given period of time, and increased pain after exertion or physical activity; (2) a feeling of weakness in the neck, back, or extremities and extreme fatigability; (3) pseudoradicular patterns of change in sensation, such as burning, numbness, and tingling; (4) difficulties in maintaining balance, ringing in the ears, and blurred vision; (5) feeling the need for repetitive self-manipulations, or chiropractic or osteopathic manipulations; (6) painful clicking, popping, or locking of axial or peripheral joints; (7) dropping of objects, weakness of the hands, and "heaviness of the head" (Dorman et al., 1991; Hackett et al., 1991; Kayfetz, 1963; Kayfetz et al., 1963; Reeves, 1995, 2000).

Physical Examination

Tenderness is the most common finding over the chronically strained or sprained ligaments or tendons. Provoked tenderness rarely reproduces radiating or referral pain; it is a local phenomenon. However, intensity of such tenderness may be changed or abolished completely after manipulation. Patients are able to point out such pain with their finger in the posterior cervicodorsal region.

Such local tenderness, as well as referred and radiating pain, can often be abolished by infiltration of nociceptors in the involved tissue with local anesthetic. Tenderness is an objective finding, especially when elicited at posterior structures (Borenstein et al., 1996; Broadhurst et al., 1996; Hackett, 1958; Hackett et al., 1991; Linetsky, 1999).

RADIOLOGIC EVALUATION PRIOR TO RIT/PROLOTHERAPY

1. Plain radiographs are of limited diagnostic value in painful pathology of the connective tissue; however, they may detect
   a. Structural or positional osseous abnormalities
   b. Anterior or posterior listhesis on lateral views (flexion, extension)
   c. Degenerative changes in general and deformity of zygapophyseal articulation

(Browner et al., 1998; Harris et al., 1981; Resnick, 1995; Watkins, 1996)

2. Videofluoroscopy has been popularized in the previous edition of this chapter; based on the experience of the last 3 years, our current opinion is that the findings of the interpreting practitioners do not correlate with the findings of clinical evaluation augmented by diagnostic blocks (Fielding, 1957)

3. MRI may detect intervertebral disc pathology, enthesopathy, ligamentous injury, interspinous bursitis, zygapophyseal joint disease and sacro-iliac joint pathology, evaluation of the neural foraminal pathology, bone contusion, and neoplasia infection or fracture, as well as exclude or confirm spinal cord disease and pathology related to intradural, extramedullary, and epidural space (Resnick, 1995; Stark et al., 1999)

4. CT scan may detect small avulsion fractures of the facets, laminar fracture, fracture of vertebral bodies and pedicles, or degenerative changes (Resnick, 1995)

5. Bone scan is useful in the assessment of the entire skeleton, ruling out metabolically active disease processes (Resnick, 1995)

6. Ultrasound has been long practiced in Europe for diagnosis of "soft tissue" pathology (Jozsa & Kannus, 1997). It has been widely used in veterinary medicine in the United States (Herthel, 2003). Current radiologic publications also demonstrate the effectiveness of diagnostic ultrasound in soft tissue pathology (Zanetti et al., 2003; Jacobson et al., 2003). A case has recently been reported of trapezius rupture diagnosed by ultrasound and successfully treated with xylocaine/dextrose injections followed by ultrasound confirming the closure of the defect (Saberski, 2003).

TECHNICAL CONSIDERATIONS AND INJECTION SITES

Painful enthesopathies and arthropathies in the craniocervicothoracic region commonly affect the following sites: apices of spinous processes, occipital bone at inferior and superior nuchal lines, mastoid processes, anterior and posterior tubercles of transverse processes, tubercles, angles and tuberosities of the ribs, proximal and distal portions of the clavicle, superomedial and inferomedial margins and the spine of the scapula, sternum, and xyphoid, capsular ligaments of the cervical and thoracic synovial joints such as AA, AO, z-joints, costovertebral, costotransverse joints, and TMJs. (Figure 62.4 through Figure 62.9).

There is a significant overlap in published pain maps from the structures innervated by the DRs. which have been grouped for practical purposes into the dorsal ramus syndrome (DRS). Consequently, in the craniocervicodorsal area, only structures that receive innervation from DRs are considered potential pain generators. However, there are also many structures receiving extrasegmental innervation that do not fit into DRS. The question is, "How to navigate in this sea of unknown?" The physician continuously follows the main objective of RIT, specifically the painful tissue bed as the primary target of investigation, taking the nerve supply into account. For the purpose of RIT, the following step-by-step approach to differential diagnosis is implemented to investigate all potential nociceptors in the distribution of the medial and lateral branches extending it beyond z-joints.

Initially, pain generators are identified by reproducible tenderness and the areas are marked. Tenderness of the posterior structures is an objective finding, especially in the midline (Broadhurst et al., 1996; Hackett et al., 1991; Kayfetz et al., 1963; Linetsky et al., 2002b, 2002c, 2004; Maigne, 1996; Reeves, 2000; Wilkinson, 1992). Confirmation is obtained by needling and local anesthetic blocks of the tissue at the enthesis, taking the nerve supply into account (Figure 62.3 and Figure 62.4).

The C2 spinous process is the most prominent palpable structure of the upper cervical region, and because of bifurcation, it should be addressed from a lateral approach. C6–T2 are the most prominent structures at the cervicodorsal junction (Figure 62.7, Figure 62.8, and Figure 62.10).

In experienced hands, using palpable landmarks for guidance, the following posterior column elements innervated by the dorsal rami may be safely injected without fluoroscopic guidance: enthesis of ligaments and tendons at the spinous processes, from C2 caudad, lamina, posterior zygapophyseal joint capsule, posterior and anterior tubercles of the cervical transverse processes, and cervicodorsal fascia insertions when palpable. Transverse processes of C1 are rarely palpable and sometimes may be injected without fluoroscopy. It is easier to inject them under fluoroscopic guidance during upper cervical synovial joint injections. Fluoroscopy itself does not prevent intravascular or intraneural needle placement.

Lidocaine is usually used for diagnostic purposes. However, the dextrose/lidocaine solution is also an effective initial diagnostic and therapeutic option for pain arising from posterior column elements when used in increments of 0.2 to 1.0 ml injected at each bone contact, initially blocking the terminal filaments of the MBDRs with the sequence as follows:

1. In the presence of midline pain and tenderness, the superior aspect of the SP is blocked initially in the midline at the enthesis. This is achieved with the caudal direction of the needle.

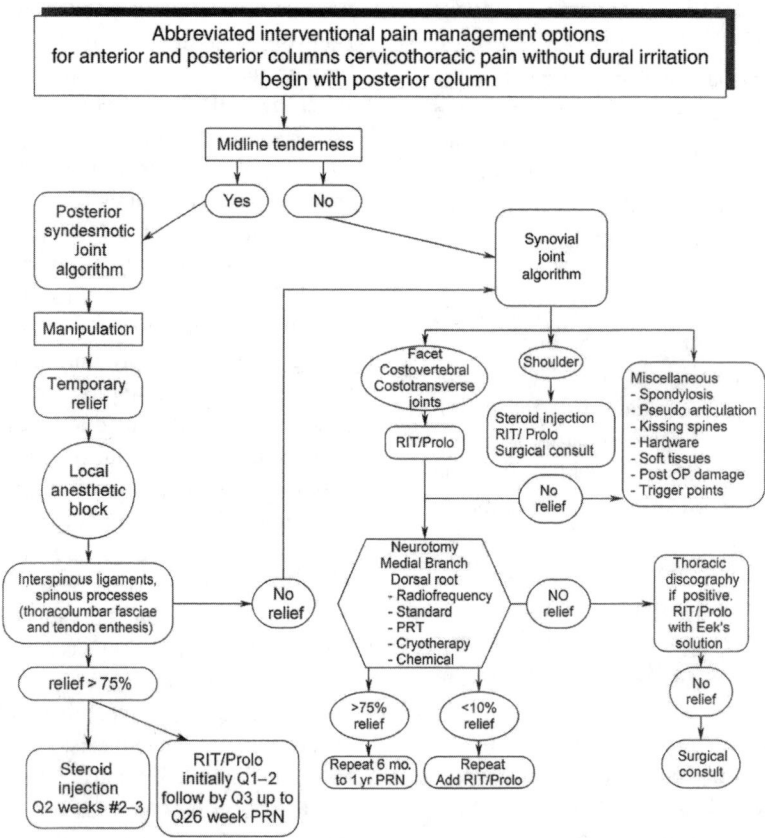

FIGURE 62.12 Modified excerpt from "Percutaneous Management Options for Cervical and Thoracic Spinal Pain" by Richard Derby, February 9–10, 2002, in *ISIS 9th Annual Scientific Meeting Syllabus, ISIS Presents: The Guidelines* (pp. 1476–1485), Orlando, FL.

2. If tenderness remains at the lateral aspects and the apices of the SP, then injections are carried out to the lateral aspects and the apices of the SPs, thus continuing on the course of MBDR. However, it should be noted that all cervical, and some thoracic, SPs are asymmetrically bifurcated at their apices. Therefore, the needle direction is from lateral to medial to prevent inadvertent intrathecal injections.

3. Persistence of paramedial pain dictates blocks of the facet joint capsules, costotransverse joints, or posterior tubercle of the transverse processes in the cervical region at their respective enthesis.

4. Perseverance of lateral tenderness dictates investigation of the structures innervated by the LBDR (i.e., iliocostalis tendon insertions to the ribs or structures receiving extrasegmental innervation such as serratus anterior and trapezius).

In this fashion, all of the potential nociceptors on the course of MBDR are investigated from its periphery to the origin. Using the previously described sequence, a differential diagnosis of pain developing from vertebral and paravertebral structures innervated by MBDRs and LBDR is made (Figure 62.3 through Figure 62.9). Modified percutaneous management options for cervical and thoracic spinal pain are a broad algorithm to follow while more specific algorithms are being developed.

Pain from the upper cervical synovial joints presents a diagnostic and therapeutic challenge. Because pain patterns overlap, it usually is a diagnosis of exclusion (Figure 62.12).

Intra-articular, atlanto-axial, and atlanto-occipital joint injections of 3 to 4% phenol in the final injectate have secured a long-lasting therapeutic effect in selected patients (Stanton-Hicks, 2003). Positive therapeutic effects with intra-articular injections of 25% dextrose to the same joints and mid-cervical synovial joints also were reported to relieve persistent pain after radiofrequency and capsular injection failure (O'Neill, 2003). All of the synovial intra-articular injections of the spine should be performed under fluoroscopic guidance.

To prevent complications, the following cardinal rules should be followed:

1. Injections should be made only after the needle contacts the bone and the pain is reproduced by the needle placement(s).

2. The needle should be slightly withdrawn to prevent subperiosteal placement of the injectate.

3. Should the needle fail to contact the bone at the expected depth, it must be withdrawn to the level of superficial fascia and redirected.

4. If blood or cerebrospinal fluid appears in the syringe, the injection should be aborted.

5. Should the needle contact the nerve (this may present itself with lancinating, lightening pain), the procedure should be aborted. If pain remains intolerable, the area should be infiltrated with corticosteroids and local anesthetic.

SOLUTIONS UTILIZED

The most common solution employed for RIT is dextrose 10%, 12.5%, 16.5%, 20%, and 25%. Dilutions are achieved with local anesthetic in 1:4, 1:3, 1:2, 2:5, and 1:1 proportions (i.e., 1 ml of 50% dextrose mixed with 3 ml of 1% lidocaine will produce a final 12.5% dextrose/lidocaine solution) (Hackett et al., 1991; Linetsky, 2002b, 2002c, 2004; Reeves, 1995, 2000).

For intra-articular knee injections, Hemwall recommended a 25% dextrose solution (Hackett et al., 1991). Reeves et al. (2000) have pointed out that a 10% dextrose solution may be equally effective. If this proves ineffective, gradual progression to sodium morrhuate full strength has been described (Dorman et al., 1991; Hackett et al., 1991).

Sodium morrhuate (5%) is a mixture of sodium salts of saturated and unsaturated fatty acids of cod liver oil and 2% benzyl alcohol, which acts as a local anesthetic and a preservative. Note that benzyl alcohol is chemically very similar to phenol.

Dextrose/phenol/glycerin solution, originally produced in England by Boots Company Ltd. of Nottingham, England, for treatment of varicose veins, was introduced to pain management by Ongley et al. (1988). The solution consists of 25% dextrose, 2.5% phenol, and 25% glycerin and is referred to as DPG (or P2G). Prior to injection it is diluted in concentrations of 1:2; 1:1, or 2:3 with a local anesthetic of the practitioner's choice. Some authors exclusively use this solution in 1:1 dilution (Dorman et al., 1991). Others modify it, reducing the percentage of glycerin to 12.5%.

The 6% phenol in glycerin solution was used by Poritt in 1931 and reintroduced in the late 1950s by Maher (1957) of England for intrathecal injections in the treatment of spasticity. Subsequently, after gaining sufficient experience with intrathecal use of this solution, Wilkinson (1992), a neurosurgeon trained at Massachusetts General Hospital, began injecting it at the donor harvest sites of the iliac crests for neurolytic and proliferative responses.

COMPLICATIONS

As with any interventional procedure, complications do occur with RIT, but statistically they are rare. The most recent statistical data are from a survey of 450 physicians performing prolotherapy. In the study, 120 respondents revealed that 495,000 patients received injections. Of the 29 pneumothoraces reported, two of them required chest tube placement; 24 non-life-threatening allergic reactions were also reported. Thus, the occurrence of pneumothoraces requiring chest tube is 1 per 247,500 patients, self-limited pneumothoraces is 1 per 18,333, and allergic reaction is 1 per 20,625. Assuming that each patient receives at least three visits and during each visit receives at least 10 injections, the numbers are relatively miniscule.

In the late 1950s and early 1960s, five cases of post-injectional arachnoiditis were reported (Keplinger et al., 1960). Two of them were fatal (Schneider, 1959; Hunt, 1961). One was a direct sequence of arachnoiditis; another was a sequence of incompetent shunt and persistent hydrocephalus with increased intracranial pressure (Schneider, 1959). Of the three other cases, the first, with mild paraparesis, recovered after a ventriculo-jugular shunt. The second recovered spontaneously with a mild neurological deficit (Hunt, 1961). The third case remained paraplegic (Keplinger et al., 1960). There have been a few recent cases of intrathecal injections not reported in the literature because of medicolegal issues. Two of them resulted in paraplegia. The first occurred after injection at the thoracic level, the second after lumbar injection. A third case was performed by a naturopath who injected solution containing zinc sulfate at the craniocervical level, which resulted in immediate onset of severe neurologic deficit, quadriplegia, and subsequent hydrocephalus.

One case of self-limiting sterile meningitis after lumbosacral sclerosing injections was reported 10 years ago (Grayson, 1994). A more recent report described a case of adjacent end plate fractures associated with intradiscal dextrose injections (Whitworth, 2002). Post-spinal puncture headaches are common, especially after lumbosacral injections (Yelland et al., 2003). Two such cases have occurred in Dr. Linetsky's practice during the past 14 years. Patients recovered after 1 week with bed rest and fluids without sequelae. Among the overall rare complications, pneumothoraces are the most common, occurring during injections of the costovertebral; costotransverse articulations; insertions of the tendons to the ribs such as iliacostalicis, serratus posterior, superior, and inferior, scalene insertions to the ribs, and levator and rhomboid insertions to the scapula especially in very muscular or significantly overweight patients. Anterior synovial joint injections, such as sternoclavicular, costosternal, and interchondral, may also result in pneumothorax in the same subset of patients.

CONCLUSIONS

As stated recently by Dr. Mooney, this treatment has advanced "from the fringe to the frontier of medical care" (Mooney, 2003).

1. RIT/prolotherapy is a valuable method of treatment for correctly diagnosed, chronic painful conditions of the locomotive systems.
2. Thorough familiarity of the physician with normal, pathologic, cross-sectional, and clinical anatomy, as well as anatomical variations and function is necessary.
3. Current literature supports manipulation under local joint anesthesia.
4. The use of RIT in an ambulatory setting is an acceptable standard of care in the community.
5. The current literature suggests that NSAIDs and steroid preparations have limited utility in chronic painful overuse conditions and in degenerative painful conditions of ligaments and tendons. Microinterventional regenerative techniques and proper rehabilitation up to 6 months or a year, supported with mild opioid analgesics, are more appropriate.

The future is such that, instead of indirect stimulation of growth factors through inflammatory cascade, specific growth factors will become available. The challenge will remain as to what specific growth factors to utilize. Most probably, a combination of several growth factors will be utilized, together with specific genes responsible for production of these growth factors. It appears that the delivery mode will be injections for deep structures; however, superficial structures will probably be addressed through transdermal delivery systems (Cook, 2000; DesRosiers et al., 1996; Kang et al., 1999; Lee et al., 1998; Marui et al., 1997; Nakamura et al., 1998; Reeves, 1995, 2000; Rudkin et al., 1996; Spindler et al., 1996).

Physicians versed in manipulation as well as diagnostic and therapeutic injection techniques as described in this chapter may find ample opportunity to use RIT in their pain management practice.

PRACTICAL SUGGESTIONS

Though Hackett's textbook is used by many as a primary source of information, even the 1991 edition is rudimentary and does not adequately explain the differential diagnosis. Standard anatomical texts are not current regarding innervation; therefore, it behooves physician to familiarize themselves with referral pain patterns and review clinical anatomy from primary sources referenced in this chapter. RIT/prolotherapy is not a panacea but another

powerful tool in the armamentarium of many interventional procedures.

Readers interested in incorporating RIT/prolotherapy in their pain management practice may attend the courses and workshops conducted by The Florida Academy of Pain Medicine (http://fapm.med.new.net) and The American Association of Orthopedic Medicine (www.aaomed.org).

ACKNOWLEDGMENTS

The authors extend special thanks to Carolyn Lower and Dianne Zalewski for their invaluable help in the preparation of this manuscript, and to Tracey Welsh and David M. Paul for preparing the illustrations for publication.

REFERENCES

Agur, A. et al. (1991). *Grant's atlas of anatomy* (9th ed.). Baltimore: Williams & Wilkins.
Anderson, D. M. (Ed.). (1985). *Dorland's illustrated medical dictionary* (26th ed.). Philadelphia: W. B. Saunders.
Aprill, C. et al. (1990). Cervical zygapophyseal joint pain patterns II: A clinical evaluation. *Spine, 15*, 6.
Ashton, I. et al. (1992). Morphological basis for back pain: The demonstration of nerve fibers and neuropeptides in the lumbar facet joint capsule but not in the ligamentum flavum. *Journal of Orthopaedic Research, 10*, 72–78.
Bahme, B. (1945). Observations on the treatment of hypermobile joints by injections. *Journal of the American Osteopathic Association, 45*(3), 101–109.
Bannister, L. H., Berry, M. M., Collins, P., & Dussek, L. E. (Eds.) (1995). *Gray's anatomy* (38th British ed.). New York: Churchill Livingston, Pearson Professional Limited.
Barbor, R. (1964, September 6–11). A treatment for chronic low back pain. *Proceedings from the IV International Congress of Physical Medicine*, Paris, pp. 661–663.
Barnsley, L. et al. (1994). Lack of effect of intra-articular corticosteroids for chronic pain in the cervical zygapophyseal joints. *New England Journal of Medicine, 330*(15), 1047–1050.
Barnsley, L. et al. (1995). The prevalence of chronic cervical zygapophysial joint pain after whiplash. *Spine, 20*, 20–26.
Best, T. (1994). Basic science of soft tissue. In J. C. Delee & D. Drez, Jr. (Eds.), *Orthopedic sports medicine principles and practice* (Vol. 1, pp. 7–35). Philadelphia: W.B. Saunders.
Biegeleisen, H. I. (1984). *Varicose veins, related diseases and sclerotherapy: A guide for practitioners*. Montreal: Eden Press.
Blaschke, J. (1961, September). Conservative management of intervertebral disk injuries. *Journal of the Oklahoma State Medical Association, 54*, 9.
Blumenthal, L. (1974, September). Injury to the cervical spine as a cause of headache. *Postgraduate Medicine, 56*, 3.

Bogduk, N. (1982). The clinical anatomy of the cervical dorsal rami. *Spine, 7*(4), 319–330.

Bogduk, N. (1986). On the concept of third occipital headache. *Journal of Neurology, Neurosurgery, and Psychiatry, 49,* 775–780.

Bogduk, N. (1988). Back pain: Zygapophyseal blocks and epidural steroids. In M. Cousins et al. (Eds.), *Neural blockage in clinical anesthesia and management of pain* (pp. 935–954). Philadelphia: J.B. Lippincott.

Bogduk, N. (1996). Post-traumatic cervical and lumbar spine zygapophyseal joint pain. In R. W. Evans (Ed.), *Neurology and trauma* (pp. 363–375). Philadelphia: W.B. Saunders.

Bogduk, N. (1997). *Clinical anatomy of the lumbar spine and sacrum* (3rd ed.). New York: Churchill Livingstone.

Bogduk, N. et al. (1996). Precision diagnosis of spinal pain. In T. S. Jensen (Ed.), *Pain 1996 — An updated review refresher course syllabus* (pp. 507–525). IASP refresher courses on pain management, held in conjunction with the 8th World Congress on Pain, Vancouver, B.C., August 17–22.

Bonica, J. (with collaboration of Loeser, J. D., Chapman, C. R., & Fordyce, W. E.). (1990). *Management of pain* (Vol. 1, 2nd ed., pp. 7, 136–139). Philadelphia: Lea & Febiger.

Borenstein, D. et al. (1996). Neck pain medical diagnosis and comprehensive management. Philadelphia: W. B. Saunders.

Boswell M. et al. (2003). Accuracy of precision diagnostic blocks in the diagnosis of chronic spinal pain of facet or zygapophysial joint origin: A systematic review. *Pain Physician, 6,* 449–456.

Bourdeau, Y. (1988). Five-year follow-up on sclerotherapy/prolotherapy for low back pain. *Manual Medicine, 3,* 155–157.

Broadhurst, N. et al. (1996). Vertebral mid-line pain: Pain arising from the interspinous spaces. *Journal of Orthopaedic Medicine, 18*(1), 2–4.

Browner, B. et al. (1998). *Skeletal trauma* (Vol. 1, 2nd ed.). Philadelphia: W. B. Saunders.

Butler, D. et al. (1978). Biomechanics of ligaments and tendons. *Exercise and Sport Sciences Reviews, 6,* 125–182.

Chase, R. (1978, December). Basic sclerotherapy. *Osteopathic Annals, 6,* 514–517.

Coleman, A. (1968). Physician electing to treat by prolotherapy alters the method at his peril. *Journal of the National Medical Association, 60*(4), 346–348.

Compere, E. et al. (1958). Persistent backache. *Medical Clinics of North America, 42,* 299–307.

Cook, P. (2000, August/September). Wound repair system assists body in regenerating tissue. *Outpatient Care Technology, 1.*

Coplans, C. (1972). The use of sclerosant injections in ligamentous pain. In A. Heflet, L. Grueble, & M. David (Eds.), *Disorders of the lumbar spine* (pp. 165–169). Philadelphia: Lippincott.

Cotran, R. S. et al. (1999). *Robbins pathologic basis of disease.* Philadelphia: W. B. Saunders.

Cousins, M. et al. (1988). *Neural blockage in clinical anesthesia and management of pain.* Philadelphia: J. B. Lippincott.

Cramer G., & Darby S. (1995). *Basic and clinical anatomy of the spine, spinal cord and ANS.* St. Louis: Mosby-Year Book.

Cyriax, J. (1969). *Textbook of orthopaedic medicine. Vol. 1, Diagnosis of soft tissue lesion* (5th ed.). Baltimore: Williams & Wilkins.

Cyriax, J. (1982). *Textbook of orthopaedic medicine. Volume 1: Diagnosis of soft tissue lesion* (8th ed.). London: Bailliere Tindall.

Cyriax, J. (1993). *Illustrated manual of orthopaedic medicine* (2nd ed.). Oxford: Butterworth-Heinemann.

Derby, R. et al. (1998, May). *Intradiscal electro-thermal annuloplasty.* Presentation at IITS 11th Annual Meeting, San Antonio, TX.

Derby R. (2002, February 9–10). Percutaneous management options for lumbar and thoracic pain. In *ISIS 9th Annual Scientific Meeting Syllabus, ISIS Presents: The Guidelines* (pp. 1476–1485). Orlando, FL.

Derby, R. et al. (2004). Comparison of intradiscal restorative injections and intradiscal electrothermal treatment (IDET) in the treatment of low back pain. *Pain Physician. 7,* 63-66.

DesRosiers, E. et al. (1996). Proliferative and matrix synthesis response of canine anterior cruciate ligament fibroblasts submitted to combine growth factors. *Journal of Orthopaedic Research, 14,* 200–208.

Dickey, S. P. (2001) The spinal uncertainty principle. *The Pain Clinic, 3*(2), 42–47.

Dorland's illustrated medical dictionary, 28th ed. (1988). Philadelphia, PA: W.B. Saunders.

Dorman, T. (1992). Storage and release of elastic energy in the pelvis: Dysfunction, diagnosis and treatment. In A. Vleeming, V. Mooney, C. Snijders, & T. Dorman (Eds.), *Low back pain and its relation to the sacroiliac joint* (pp. 585–600). San Diego, CA: E.C.O.

Dorman, T., (1993). Prolotherapy: A survey. *Journal of Orthopaedic Medicine, 15*(2), 49–50.

Dorman, T. (1995). *Prolotherapy in the lumbar spine and pelvis.* Philadelphia: Hanley & Belfus.

Dorman, T. et al. (1991). *Diagnosis and injection techniques in orthopedic medicine.* Baltimore: Williams & Wilkins.

Dreyfuss, P. (1997, December). Differential diagnosis of thoracic pain and diagnostic/therapeutic injection techniques. *ISIS Newsletter, 2*(6), 10–29.

Dreyfuss, P. et al. (1994a). Atlanto-occipital and lateral atlanto-axial joint pain patterns. *Spine, 19*(10), 1125–1131.

Dreyfuss, P. et al. (1994b). Thoracic zygapophyseal joint pain patterns: A study in normal volunteers. *Spine, 19*(7), 807–811.

Dreyfuss, P. et al. (1995). MUJA: Manipulation under joint anesthesia/analgesia: A treatment approach for recalcitrant low back pain of synovial joint origin. *Journal of Manipulative & Physiological Therapeutics, 18*(8), 537–546.

Dussault, R. et al. (1994, June). Facet joint injection: Diagnosis and therapy. *Applied Radiology, 23,* 35–39.

Dwyer, A. et al. (1990). Cervical zygapophyseal joint pain patterns. I: A study in normal volunteers. *Spine, 15,* 6.

Eek, B. (1996, August 16). New directions in the treatment of disc pain. In *Diagnosis and treatment of discogenic pain*. International Spinal Injection Society 4th annual meeting syllabus (pp. 47–48), Vancouver, BC.

El-Bohy, A. et al. (1988). Localization of substance P and neurofilament immunoreactive fibers in the lumbar facet joint capsule and supraspinous ligament of the rabbit. *Brain Research, 460*, 379–382.

Feinstein, B., Langton, J., Jameson, R. et al. (1954). Experiments on pain referred from deep somatic tissues. *Journal of Bone and Joint Surgery, 36-A*(6), 281–996.

Fielding, J. (1957). Cineroentgenography of the normal cervical spine.. *The Journal of Bone and Joint Surgery, 39A*(6), 1280–1288.

Fortin, J., Vilensky J., & Merkel G. (2003). Can the sacroiliac joint cause sciatica? *Pain Physician, 6*, 269–271.

Freemont, A. et al. (1997). Nerve ingrowth into diseased intervertebral disc in chronic back pain. *Lancet, 22*, 178–181.

Gedney, E. (1937, June). Special technique hypermobile joint: A preliminary report. *The Osteopathic Profession*, 30–31.

Gedney, E. (1938). *The hypermobile joint — Further reports on injection method*. Paper presented at Osteopathic Clinical Society of Pennsylvania, February 13.

Gedney, E. (1951, September). Disc syndrome. *The Osteopathic Profession*, 11–13, 34, 38, 40.

Gedney, E. (1952a, August). Technique for sclerotherapy in the management of hypermobile sacroiliac. *The Osteopathic Profession*, 16–19, 37–38.

Gedney, E. (1952b, April). Use of sclerosing solution may change therapy in vertebral disk problem. *The Osteopathic Profession, 34*, 38 & 39. 11–13.

Gedney, E. (1954a, September). The application of sclerotherapy in spondylolisthesis and spondylolysis. *The Osteopathic Profession*, 66–69, 102–105.

Gedney, E. (1954b, August). Progress report on use of sclerosing solutions in low back syndromes. *The Osteopathic Profession*, 18–21, 40–44.

Giles, L. (1988). Human zygapophysial joint inferior recess synovial folds: A light microscope examination. *Journal of Anatomic Research, 220*, 117–124.

Giles, L., & Singer K. (Eds.). (2000). *Clinical anatomy and management of thoracic spine pain*. I ed. *The clinical anatomy and management of back pain series* (Vol. 2). Oxford, UK: Butterworth-Heinemann.

Giles, L., & Singer K. (Eds.). (2001). *Clinical anatomy and management of cervical spine pain*. II ed. *The clinical anatomy and management of back pain series* (Vol. 3). Oxford, U.K.: Butterworth-Heinemann.

Giles, L., & Taylor J. (1987). Innervation of lumbar zygapophysial joint synovial folds. *Acta Orthopaedica Scandinavica, 58*, 43–46.

Grayson, M. (1994a). Sterile meningitis after lumbosacral ligament sclerosing injections. *Journal of Orthopaedic Medicine, 16*(3), 98–99.

Grayson, M. F. (1994b). Sterile meningitis after lumbosacral ligament sclerosing injections. *Journal of Orthopaedic Medicine, 16* (3).

Green, S. (1956, April). Hypermobility of joints: Causes, treatment and technique of sclerotherapy. *The Osteopathic Profession, 26*–27, 42–47.

Green, S. (1958, January). The study of ligamentous tissue is regarded as key to sclerotherapy. *The Osteopathic Profession, 26*–29.

Hackett, G. (1953). Joint stabilization through induced ligament sclerosis. *Ohio State Medical Journal, 49*, 877–884.

Hackett, G. (1956). *Joint ligament relaxation treated by fibro-osseous proliferation*. Springfield, IL: Charles C Thomas.

Hackett, G. (1958). *Ligament and tendon relaxation (skeletal disability) — Treated by prolotherapy (fibro-osseous proliferation)* (3rd ed.). Springfield, IL: Charles C Thomas.

Hackett, G. (1959a). Ligament relaxation and osteoarthritis, loose jointed vs. closed jointed. *Rheumatism* (London), *15*(2), 28–33.

Hackett, G. (1959b, September). Low back pain. *Industrial Medicine and Surgery, 28*, 416–419.

Hackett, G. (1960a). Prolotherapy in low back pain from ligament relaxation and bone dystrophy. *Clinical Medicine, 7*(12), 2551–2561.

Hackett, G. (1960b). Prolotherapy in whiplash and low back pain. *Postgraduate Medicine, 27*, 214–219

Hackett, G. (1961). Prolotherapy for sciatic from weak pelvic ligament and bone dystrophy. *Clinical Medicine, 8*, 2301–2316.

Hackett, G. (1966a, July). Cause & mechanism of headache, pain and neuritis. *Headache, 6*, 88–92.

Hackett, G. (1966b, August). Uninhibited reversible antidromic vasodilatation in bronchiogenic pathophysiologic diseases. *Lancet, 86*, 398–404.

Hackett, G. (1966c, February). Uninhibited reversible antidromic vasodilation in pathophysiologic diseases: Arteriosclerosis, carcinogenesis, neuritis and osteoporosis. *Angiology, 17*(2), 109–118.

Hackett, G. (1967, September). Prevention of cancer, heart, lung and other diseases. *Clinical Medicine, 74*, 19.

Hackett, G., & Henderson, D. (1955, May). Joint stabilization: An experimental, histologic study with comments on the clinical application in ligament proliferation. *American Journal of Surgery, 89*, 968–973.

Hackett, G. et al. (1961, July). Back pain following trauma and disease prolotherapy. *Military Medicine*, 517–525.

Hackett, G. et al. (1962, April). Prolotherapy for headache: Pain in the head and neck, and neuritis. *Headache, 2*, 20–28.

Hackett, G. et al. (1991). *Ligament and tendon relaxation — Treated by prolotherapy* (5th ed.). Oak Park, IL: Gustav Hemwall, M.D.

Haldeman, K. et al. (1938). The diagnosis and treatment of sacroiliac conditions by the injection of procaine (novocain). *Journal of Bone and Joint Surgery, 20*(3), 675–685.

Harris, J. et al. (1981). *The radiology of emergency medicine* (2nd ed.). Baltimore: Williams & Wilkins.

Herthel, D. (2003). Injections of stem cells from bone marrow aspirate into damaged ligaments and tendons. In *Soft tissue injuries of the spine: New concepts in diagnosis and treatment*. San Francisco.

Hilton J. (1891). *Rest and pain. A course of lectures.* Cincinnati: P.W. Gardfield.

Hirsch, C. (1948). An attempt to diagnose the level of a disc lesion clinically by disc puncture. *Acta Orthopaedia Scandinavica, 18,* 131–140.

Hirschberg, G. et al. (1982). Treatment of the chronic iliolumbar syndrome by infiltration of the iliolumbar ligament. *Western Journal of Medicine, 136,* 372–374.

Hirschberg, G. et al. (1992). Diagnosis and treatment of iliocostal friction syndromes. *Journal of Orthopedic Medicine, 14*(2), 35–39.

Hoch, G. (1939). Injection treatment of hydrocele. In F. Yeoman (Ed.), *Sclerosing therapy, the injection treatment of hernia, hydrocele, varicose veins and hemorrhoids* (pp. 141–156). London: Bailliere, Tindall & Cox.

Hunt, W. (1961). Complications following injections of sclerosing agent to precipitate fibro-osseous proliferation. *Journal of Neurosurgery, 18,* 461–465.

Jacobson J., Propeck T., Jamadar D. et al. (2003). US of the anterior bundle of the ulnar collateral ligament: Findings in five cadaver elbows with MR arthrographic and anatomic comparison – Initial observations. *Radiology, 227*(2), 561–566.

Jozsa, L., & Kannus, P. (1997). *Human tendons, anatomy, physiology and pathology.* Champaign, IL: Human Kinetics.

Kang, H. et al. (1999). Ideal concentration of growth factors in rabbit's flexor tendon culture. *Yonsei Medical Journal, 40*(1), 26–29.

Karppinnen J., Paakko E., Paassilta P. et al. (2003). Radiologic phenotypes in lumbar MRI imaging for a gene defect in the COL9A3 gene of type IX collagen. *Radiology, 227,* 143–148.

Kayfetz, D. (1963a, June). Occipito-cervical (whiplash) injuries treated by prolotherapy. *Medical Trial Technique Quarterly,* 109–112, 147–167.

Kayfetz, D. et al. (1963b). Whiplash injury and other ligamentous headache. Its management with prolotherapy. *Headache, 3*(1), 1–8.

Kellgren, J. H. (1939). On the distribution of pain arising from deep somatic structures with charts of segmental pain areas. *Clinical Science, 4,* 35–46.

Keplinger, J. et al. (1960). Paraplegia from treatment with sclerosing agents — Report of a case. *Journal of the American Medical Association, 73,* 1333–1336.

Klein, R. (1991). Diagnosis and treatment of gluteus medius syndrome. *Journal of Orthopaedic Medicine, 13,* 1373–1376.

Klein, R., & Eek, B. (1997). Prolotherapy: An alternative approach to managing low back pain. *Journal of Musculoskeletal Medicine, 16*(5), 45 –59.

Klein, R. et al. (1989). Proliferation injections for low back pain: Histologic changes of injected ligaments and objective measurements of lumbar spine mobility before and after treatment. *Journal of Neurological and Orthopaedic Medicine and Surgery, 10*(2), 123–126.

Klein, R. et al. (1993). A randomized double-blind trial of dextrose-glycerin-phenol injections for chronic, low back pain. *Journal of Spinal Disorders, 6*(1), 23–33.

Klein, R. et al. (2003). Biochemical injection treatment for discogenic low back pain: A pilot study. *Spine Journal, 3,* 220–226.

Koudele, C. (1978). Treatment of joint pain. *Osteopathic Annals, 6*(12), 42–45.

Leadbetter, W. (1992). Cell-matrix response in tendon injury. *Clinical Sports Medicine, 11,* 533–578.

Leadbetter, W. (1994). *Soft tissue athletic injuries: Sports injuries: Mechanisms, prevention, treatment.* Baltimore: Williams & Wilkins.

Leadbetter, W. (1995). Anti-inflammatory therapy and sport injury: The role of non-steroidal drugs and corticosteroid injections. *Clinical Sports Medicine, 14,* 353–410

Lee, J. et al. (1998). Growth factor expression in healing rabbit medial collateral and anterior cruciate ligaments. *Iowa Orthopaedic Journal, 18,* 19–25.

Leedy, R. et al. (1976). Analysis of 50 low back cases 6 years after treatment by joint ligament sclerotherapy. *Osteopathic Medicine, 6,* 15–22.

Leriche, R. (1930). Effets de l'anesthesia a la novocaine des ligaments et des insertion tenineuses periarticulares dans certanes maladies articulares et dans les vices de positions foncitionnells des articulations. *Gazette des Hopitaux Civils et Militaires, 103,* 1294.

Lindblom, K. (1944). Protrusions of the discs and nerve compression in the lumbar region. *Acta Radiologica Scandinavica, 25,* 192–212.

Linetsky, F.S., & Willard, F. (1999). Regenerative injection therapy for low back pain. *The Pain Clinic, 1*(1), 27–31.

Linetsky, F. S. (1999). History of sclerotherapy in urology. *The Pain Clinic, 5*(2), 30–32.

Linetsky, F. S. et al. (2000). Regenerative injection therapy: History of applications in pain management, Part 1, 1930–1950s. *The Pain Clinic, 2*(2), 8–13.

Linetsky, F. S. et al. (2001). A history of the applications of regenerative injection therapy in pain management, Part II, 1960s–1980s. *The Pain Clinic, 3*(2), 32–36.

Linetsky, F. S. et al. (2002a). Effectiveness and appropriate usage. Positional Paper of the Florida Academy of Pain Medicine on Regenerative Injection Therapy. *The Pain Clinic, 4*(3), 38–45.

Linetsky, F. S. et al. (2002b). Pain management with regenerative injection therapy (RIT). In R. S. Weiner (Ed.), *Pain management: A practical guide for clinicians* (6th) ed., pp. 381–402), Boca Raton, FL: CRC Press.

Linetsky, F. S. et al (2002c). Regenerative injective therapy. In L. Manchikanti, C. Slipman, & B. Fellows (Eds.), *Low back pain: Diagnosis and treatment* (pp. 519–540). Paducah, KY: ASIPP Publishing.

Linetsky, F. S., et al. (2004). Treatment of cervicothoracic pain and cervicogenic headaches with regenerative injection therapy, *Current Pain and Headache Reports, 8*(1), 41–48

Liu, Y. et al. (1983). An *in situ* study of the influence of a sclerosing solution in rabbit medial collateral ligaments and its junction strength. *Connective Tissue Research, 11,* 95–102.

Lord, S. (1996). Chronic cervical zygapophyseal joint pain after whiplash: A placebo-controlled prevalence study. *Spine, 21*(15), 1737–1745.

Maher, R. (1957, January). Neuron selection in relief of pain. Further experiences with intrathecal injections. *Lancet*, 16–19.

Maigne, R. et al. (Eds.). (1996). *Diagnosis and treatment of pain of vertebral origin: A manual medicine approach* (1st ed.) Baltimore: William & Wilkins.

Manchikanti, L. (2002). In L. Manchikanti, C. Slipman, & B. Fellows (Eds.), *Low back pain, diagnosis and treatment* (Vol. 1, p. 651). Paducah: ASIPP Publishing.

Manchikanti, L. et al., (2002). Evaluation of the prevalence of facet joint pain in chronic thoracic pain. *Pain Physician*, 5(4), 354–359.

Marui, T. et al. (1997). Effect of growth factors on matrix synthesis by ligament fibroblasts. *Journal of Orthopaedic Research, 15*, 18–23.

Massie, J. et al. (1993). Is it possible to stimulate fibroplasia within the intervertebral disc? *Journal or Orthopaedic Medicine, 15*(3), 83.

Matthews, J. (1995). A new approach to the treatment of osteoarthritis of the knee: Prolotherapy of the ipsilateral sacroiliac ligaments. *American Journal of Pain Management, 5*(3), 91–93.

Matthews, R. et al. (2001). Treatment of mechanical and chemical lumbar discopathy by dextrose 25%. *Journal of Minimally Invasive Spinal Technique, 1*(1), 57–61.

Maynard, J. et al. (1985). Morphological and biochemical effects of sodium morrhuate on tendons. *Journal or Orthopaedic Research, 3*, 234–248.

McPheeters, H. et al. (1949). *The injection treatment of varicose veins and hemorrhoids* (2nd ed.). Philadelphia, PA: FA Davis Co.

Mercer S., & Bogduk, N. (1993). Intra-articular inclusions of the cervical synovial joints. *British Journal of Rheumatology, 32*, 705–710.

Merskey, H., & Bogduk, N. (1994). *Classification of chronic pain, descriptions of chronic pain syndromes and definitions of pain terms* (2nd ed.). Seattle: IASP Press.

Mooney, V. (1993a, January). Sclerotherapy in back pain? Yes, if clinician is skilled. *Journal of Musculoskeletal Medicine*, 13.

Mooney, V. (1993b, July). Understanding, examining for, and treating sacroiliac pain. *Journal of Musculoskeletal Medicine*, 37–49.

Mooney, V. (2003). Prolotherapy at the fringe of medical care, or is it the frontier? *Spine Journal, 3*, 253–254.

Myers, A. (1961). Prolotherapy treatment of low back pain and sciatica. *Bulletin, Hospital for Joint Diseases, 22*, 48–55.

Nakamura, N. et al. (1998). Early biological effect of *in vivo* gene transfer of platelet-derived growth factor (PDGF)-B into healing patellar ligament. *Gene Therapy, 5*, 1165–1170.

Neff, F. (1959, March). A new approach in the treatment of chronic back disabilities. *Family Physician, 9*, 3.

Neff, F. (1960). Low back pain and disability. *Western Medicine, 1*, 12.

Ombregt, L. et al. (1995). *A system of orthopaedic medicine*. Philadelphia: W. B. Saunders.

O'Neill C. (2003). *Intra-articular dextrose/glucosamine injections for cervical facet syndrome, atlanto-occipital and atlanto-axial joint pain, combined ISIS AAOM approach*. Presentation at the 20th American Association of Orthopedic Medicine Annual conference and scientific seminar; A common sense approach to "hidden" pain generators. Orlando, FL.

O'Neill C., Liu J., Leibenberg E. et al. (2004). Percutaneous plasma decompression alters cytokine expression in injured porcine intervertebral discs. *Spine Journal, 4*, 88–98.

Ongley, M. et al. (1987, July 18). A new approach to the treatment of chronic low back pain. *Lancet*, 143–146.

Ongley, M. et al. (1988). Ligament instability of knees: A new approach to treatment. *Manual Medicine, 3*, 152–154.

Poritt, A. (1931). The injection treatment of hydrocele, varicocele, bursae and nevi. *Proceedings, Royal Society of Medicine, 24*, 81.

Ranney, D. (1997). *Chronic musculoskeletal injuries in the workplace*. Philadelphia: W. B. Saunders.

Reeves, D. (1995). Prolotherapy: Present and future applications in soft-tissue pain and disability. *Physical Medicine and Rehabilitation Clinics of North America, 6*(4), 917–926.

Reeves, D. (2000). Prolotherapy: Basic science clinical studies and technique. In T. A. Lennard (Ed.), *Pain procedures in clinical practice* (pp. 172–189). Philadelphia: Hanley & Belfus.

Reeves, K. et al. (2000). Randomized prospective double-blind placebo-controlled study of dextrose prolotherapy for knee osteoarthritis with or without ACL laxity. *Alternative Therapy, 6*(2), 68–74, 77–80.

Resnick, D. (1995). *Diagnosis of bone and joint disorders* (Vol. 1–6, 3rd ed.). Philadelphia: W. B. Saunders Co.

Rice, C. (1936). Hernia — Its cure by injection of irritating solutions. *Journal of the Iowa Medical Society, 26*, 279–283.

Riddle, P. (1940). *Injection treatment*. Philadelphia: W. B. Saunders.

Roosth, H. (1991, November). Low back and leg pain attributed to gluteal tendinosis. *Orthopedics Today, 10* et seq.

Rudkin, G. et al. (1996). Growth factors in surgery. *Plastic and Reconstructive Surgery, 97*(2), 469–476.

Saal, J. et al. (1998a, April). *A novel approach to painful internal disk derangement: Collagen modulation with a thermal percutaneous navigable intradiscal catheter*. A prospective trial presented at the NASS-APS first joint meeting. Charleston, SC.

Saal, J. et al. (1998b). Percutaneous treatment of painful lumbar disc derangement with a navigable intradiscal thermal catheter: A pilot study presented at the NASS-APS first joint meeting. Charleston, SC, April.

Saberski, L. (2003). Trapezius midsubstance rupture diagnosed by ultrasound and treated with dextrose/xylocaine injections. 20th American Association of Orthopedic Medicine Annual conference and scientific seminar. A common sense approach to "hidden" pain generators. Orlando, FL.

Schmid G., Witteler A., Willburger R. et al. (2004). Lumber disk herniation: Correlation of histologic findings with marrow signal intensity changes in vertebral endplates at MR imaging. *Radiology, 231*(2), 352–358.

Schneider, R. (1959). Fatality after injecting of sclerosing agent to precipitate fibro-osseous proliferation. *Journal of the American Medical Association, 170*, 1768–1772.

Schultz, L. (1937, September). A treatment for subluxation of the temporomandibular joint. *Journal of the American Medical Association,* 256.

Schultz, L. (1956, December). Twenty years' experience in treating hypermobility of the temporomandibular joints. *American Journal of Surgery,* 92.

Schwartz, R. et al. (1991). Prolotherapy: A literature review and retrospective study. *Journal of Neurologic and Orthopaedic Medicine and Surgery, 12,* 220–223.

Shevelev, A. et al. (2000, July 15–21). Interosseous receptor system as the modulator of trigeminal afferent reactions. *Worldwide Pain Conference* [Abstract] p. 34.

Shuman, D. (1941). Luxation recurring in shoulder. *The Osteopathic Profession, 8*(6), 11–13.

Shuman, D. (1949a, March). Sclerotherapy — Injections may be best way to restrengthen ligaments in case of slipped knee cartilage. *The Osteopathic Profession* (preprint).

Shuman, D. (1949b, October). The place of joint sclerotherapy in today's practice. *Bulletin of the New Jersey Association of Osteopathic Physicians and Surgeons* (preprint).

Shuman, D. (1954, July). Sclerotherapy: Statistics on its effectiveness for unstable joint conditions. *The Osteopathic Profession,* 11–15, 37–38.

Shuman, D. (1958). *Low back pain.* Philadelphia: David Shuman.

Simon, R. et al. (1987). *Emergency orthopedics: The extremities* (2nd ed.). Norwalk, CT: Appleton & Lange.

Sinelnikov, R. D. (1972). *Atlas of anatomy* (Vol. 1). Moscow: Meditsina.

Sokov. E. et al. (2000). Are herniated disks the main cause of low back pain? In abstract book of Worldwide Pain Conference, p. 74.

Spindler, K. et al. (1996). Patellar tendon and anterior cruciate ligament have different mitogenic responses to platelet-derived growth factor and transforming growth factor b. *Journal of Orthopaedic Research, 14,* 542–546

Stanton-Hicks, M. (2003). *Cervicocranial syndrome: Treatment of atlanto-occipital and atlanto-axial joint pain with phenol/glycerin injections.* Presented at 20th American Association of Orthopedic Medicine Annual conference and scientific seminar; A common sense approach to "hidden" pain generators. Orlando, FL.

Stark, D. et al. (1999). *Magnetic resonance imaging* (Vol. 1 & 2, 3rd ed.). St. Louis, MO: Mosby.

Steindler, A. et al. (1938). Differential diagnosis of pain low in the back allocation of the source of pain by the procaine hydrochloride method. *Journal of the American Medical Association, 110,* 106–113.

Travell, J. et al. (1983). Myofacial pain and dysfunction-trigger point manual — The upper extremities (Vol. 1). Baltimore: Williams & Wilkins.

Tuzlukov, P. et al. (1993). The morphological characteristics of fibromyalgia syndrome. *Arkhiva Patelogie, 4*(2), 47–50.

Vanderschot, L. (1976a). The American version of acupuncture. Prolotherapy: Coming to an understanding. *American Journal of Acupuncture, 4,* 309–316.

Vanderschot, L. (1976b). Trigger points vs. acupuncture points. *American Journal of Acupuncture, 4,* 233–238.

Vleeming, A. et al. (1997). *Movement, stability and low back pain: The essential role of the pelvis.* New York: Churchill Livingstone.

Waldman, S. (1998). *Atlas of interventional pain management.* Philadelphia: W.B. Saunders Co.

Warren, J. (1881). *Hernia-strangulated and reducible with cure by subcutaneous injection.* Boston: Charles C Thomas.

Watkins, R. (1996). *The spine in sports.* St. Louis: Mosby.

Watson, L. (1938). *Hernia* (2nd ed.). St. Louis: C.V. Mosby.

Whitworth, M. (2002). Endplate fracture associated with intradiscal dextrose injection. *Pain Physician, 5*(4), 379–386.

Wilkinson, H. A. (1992). *The failed back syndrome etiology and therapy* (2nd ed.). Berlin: Springer-Verlag.

Wilkinson, H. A. et al. (2002). Injection therapy of periosteal trigger points with steroids or prolotherapy. *The Pain Clinic. 4*(5), 40–48.

Willard, F. (1995, November 9–11). The lumbosacral connection: The ligamentous structure of the low back and its relation to back pain. In A. Vleeming, U. Mooney, C. Snijders, & T. Dorman (Eds.), *Proceedings of the Second Interdisciplinary World Congress on Low Back Pain, the Integrated Function of the Lumbar Spine and Sacroiliac Joints,* Part I (pp. 29–58), San Diego, CA.

Willard, F. (2003). *Gross anatomy of the cervical and thoracic regions: Understanding connective tissue stockings and their contents.* 20th AAOM Annual Conference and Scientific Seminar. Orlando, FL.

Yahia, H. et al. (1989). A light and electron microscopic study of spinal ligament innervation. *Zeitschrift fuer Mikroskopische-Anatomische, 103,* 664–674.

Yahia, L., Garzon S., Strykowski H. et al. (1990). Ultrastructure of the human interspinous ligament and ligamentum flavum: A preliminary study. *Spine, 15*(4), 262–268.

Yelland, M. J. et al. (2000). Prolotherapy injections for chronic low back pain: Results of a pilot comparative study. *Australian Musculoskeletal Medicine, 5,* 20–23.

Yelland, M. J. et al. (2003) Prolotherapy injection, saline injections, and exercises for chronic low-back pain: A randomized trial. *Spine, 29*(1), 9–16

Yeomans, F. C. et al. (1939). *Sclerosing therapy, the injection treatment of hernia, hydrocele, varicose veins and hemorrhoids.* London: Bailliere, Tindall & Cox.

Yu, S., Sether, L., & Haughton, V. (1987). Facet joint menisci of the cervical spine: Correlative MR imaging and Cryomicrotomy study. *Radiology, 164*(1), 79–82.

Zanetti, M. et al. (2003). Achilles tendons: Clinical relevance of neovascularization diagnosed with power Doppler US. *Radiology, 227*(2), 556–560.

Zoppi, M. et al. (2000). From "intraosseous pain syndrome" to osteoarthritis. *Worldwide Pain Conference* [abstract] p. 412.

63

Cervical Facet Joint Interventions

Laxmaiah Manchikanti, MD, David M. Schultz, MD, and Vijay Singh, MD

INTRODUCTION

Among chronic pain complaints, pain arising in the cervical spine is one of the most common problems. The lifetime prevalence of spinal pain from the cervical spine has been reported as 65 to 80%.[1-14] Further, chronicity of neck pain has been demonstrated with chronic persistent pain resulting in 26 to 44% of the patients after an initial episode of neck pain or whiplash.[12-16] The prevalence of persistent neck pain due to the involvement of cervical facet joints has been described in controlled studies as varying from 54 to 67%.[17-21]

HISTORY

While Goldthwait[22] described lumbar facet joints as potential sources of back pain in 1911, it was not until 1977 that Pawl[23] reported the reproduction of pain in patients with neck pain and headache after injections of hypertonic saline into the cervical facet joints. However, cervical facet joints attracted relatively little attention as possible sources of neck pain and referred pain in the upper extremities in the late 1970s and early 1980s. Bogduk and Marsland[24] studied the role of cervical facet joints in causation of idiopathic neck pain by using diagnostic cervical medial branch blocks and facet joint injections. Dwyer et al.[25] mapped out specific locations of referred neck pain by performing facet joint injections in normal volunteers while Aprill et al.[26] confirmed the accuracy of the pain chart reported by them earlier following anesthesia of the medial branches of the dorsal rami above and below the symptomatic joint. Fukui et al.[27] also studied the referred pain distribution of cervical facet joints and cervical dorsal rami with similar results. Windsor et al.[28] investigated

electrical stimulation–induced cervical medial branch referral patterns. They concluded that electrical stimulation of the third occipital nerve, as well as the medial branch of the C3–C8 posterior primary rami, produced discrete reproducible referral patterns, which differ from those reported from other causes of neck pain.

PREVALENCE

Cervical facet joints have been shown to be capable of being a source of pain in the neck and referred pain in the head and upper extremities.[23-28] Based on responses to controlled diagnostic blocks of cervical facet joints in accordance with the criteria established by the International Association for the Study of Pain,[29] the prevalence of cervical facet joint pain has been shown to be 54 to 67% in patients with chronic neck pain.[17-21]

PATHOPHYSIOLOGY

As with any synovial joint, degeneration, inflammation, and injury of facet joints can lead to pain upon joint motion. Pain leads to restriction of motion, which eventually leads to overall physical deconditioning. Irritation of the facet joint innervation in itself also leads to secondary muscle spasm. It has been assumed that degeneration of the disc would lead to associated facet joint degeneration and subsequent spinal pain. These assumptions were based on the pathogenesis of a degenerative cascade in the context of a three-joint complex that involves the articulation between two vertebrae consisting of the intervertebral disc and adjacent facet joints, as changes within each member of this joint complex will result in changes in others.[30–32] Many of the studies during the past 30 to 40 years have proposed that disc degeneration initiates degenerative changes in the facet joints by altering the mechanical function of the entire motion segment.[33] Further, facet joints have been implicated as responsible for chronic neck pain, headache, and upper extremity pain.

DIAGNOSTIC FACET JOINT BLOCKS

Blocks of a cervical facet or zygapophysial joint can be performed to test the hypothesis that the target joint is the source of the patient's pain.[34–36] Cervical facet joints can be anesthetized either with intra-articular injections of local anesthetic or by anesthetizing the medial branches of the dorsal rami that innervate the target joint. True-positive responses are secured by performing controlled blocks, in the form of either placebo injections of normal saline or comparative local anesthetic blocks, in which on two separate occasions, the same joint is anesthetized but using local anesthetics with different durations of action. However, an injected capsule may leak into the adjacent neural foramen and result in blockade of the dorsal root ganglion and segmental nerves, and produce a false-positive result.

The rationale for using facet joint blocks for diagnosis is based on the fact that cervical facet joints have been shown to be capable of being a source of neck pain and referred pain in the head and upper extremities. Consequently, facet joints are possible sources of pain in patients presenting with neck pain and referred pain. Historical and clinical features may be indicative, but not diagnostic of facet joint pain. However, there is no definitive valid indicator or clinical means to implicate cervical facet joints as the source of neck pain, headache, or upper extremity pain in a given patient. Numerous attempts by investigators to correlate neurophysiologic findings, radiologic findings, physical findings, and other signs and symptoms with the diagnosis of facet joint pain have been unsuccessful.[1] Thus, controlled diagnostic blocks with two separate local anesthetics or placebo-controlled blocks are the only means of confirming the diagnosis of facet joint pain in the neck.

Indications for diagnostic blocks are also based on the strong evidence demonstrating the reliability of cervical facet joint nerve blocks in the diagnosis of neck pain, upper extremity pain, and headaches.[1,34–36] The face validity of intra-articular injections and medial branch blocks is demonstrated under fluoroscopic visualization by determining the spread of contrast medium to confirm proper needle placement, then by injecting a small volume of local anesthetic.[37] Construct validity of facet joint blocks, which is an extremely important aspect to rule out placebo effect, also has been demonstrated.[38] Further, the theory that testing a patient first with lidocaine and subsequently with bupivacaine provided a means of identifying placebo

---

TABLE 63.1

Common Indications for Cervical Diagnostic Facet Joint Blocks

- Somatic or nonradicular neck and/or upper extremity pain
- Cervicogenic headache and/or upper back pain
- Lack of obvious evidence for discogenic pain
- Lack of disc herniation or evidence of radiculitis
- Duration of pain of at least of 3 months
- Failure to respond to more conservative management, including physical therapy modalities with exercises, chiropractic management, and nonsteroidal anti-inflammatory agents
- Average pain levels of greater than 5 on a scale of 1 to 10
- Intermittent or continuous pain causing functional disability
- No contraindications with understanding of consent, nature of the procedure, needle placement, or sedation
- No history of allergy to contrast administration, local anesthetic steroids, Sarapin, or other drugs potentially used
- Contraindications or inability to undergo physical therapy or chiropractic management or inability to tolerate nonsteroidal anti-inflammatory drugs

---

response has been tested and proved.[39–42] The reported false-positive rates of single facet joint blocks in the cervical spine have been demonstrated to be 27 to 63%.[19,20,43,44]

Indications for diagnostic facet joint blocks include neck pain, for which no cause is otherwise evident, and for which pain patterns resemble those evoked in normal volunteers upon stimulation of the facet joints. Table 63.1 illustrates indications for diagnostic cervical facet joint injections, whereas Table 63.2 indicates contraindications.

Contraindications are quite obvious and include bacterial infection, possible pregnancy, and bleeding diathesis. Relative contraindications include allergy to contrast media or local anesthetics and treatment with non-aspirin anti-platelet drugs, which may compromise coagulation. Raj et al.[45] provided a detailed description on the role of anticoagulants in interventional pain management.

TABLE 63.2

Common Contraindications for Cervical Facet Joint Blocks

- Infection
- Arnold Chiari malformation
- Inability of the patient to understand consent, nature of the procedure, needle placement, or sedation
- Allergies to contrast, local anesthetic, steroids, Sarapin, or other drugs
- Needle phobia
- Psychogenic pain
- Suspected discogenic pain or disc herniation
- Pregnancy
- Anticoagulant therapy
- Non-aspirin anti-platelet therapy
- Bleeding diathesis

THERAPEUTIC INTERVENTIONS

A significant role has been described for therapeutic facet joint injections, either intra-articular or by medial branch blocks in addition to medial branch neurotomy.[1] However, the evidence is poor for short-term, as well as long-term relief for intra-articular blocks of cervical spine based on one randomized controlled trial.[46] Manchikanti et al.[1] extensively reviewed the literature in preparing evidence-based guidelines for managing spinal pain. They concluded that except for the one negative randomized trial for intra-articular injections, there were no other non-observational trials qualifying to be included for evidence synthesis.

In addition to the intra-articular blocks, medial branch blocks have been used for therapeutic purposes in the cervical spine. One recent prospective, nonrandomized, observational study[47] showed significant effectiveness of medial branch blocks in managing chronic neck pain.

In addition to intra-articular cervical facet joint blocks and medial branch blocks, medial branch neurotomy has been described with well-controlled trials. The effectiveness of medial branch neurotomy has been described in case reports, observational studies, randomized trials, and systematic reviews, though yielding mixed results.[1,48–54]

ANATOMIC CONSIDERATIONS

The cervical facet joints are paired, diarthrodial, synovial joints located between the superior and inferior articular pillars in the posterior cervical column.[55] While cervical facet joints extend from C2/3 to C7/T1, the atlanto-occipital and atlanto-axial synovial joints are also present in the cervical spine. However, these are not considered facet joints. Cervical facet joints exhibit the features of typical synovial joints. The articular facets are covered by articular cartilage and a synovial membrane bridges the margins of the articular cartilage of the two facets in each joint.[56,57] Further, these joints, along with a meniscus, may contain a variety of intra-articular inclusions, with fibroadipose meniscoids the most common inclusions. The fibrous joint capsule is richly innervated with mechanoreceptors, as well as nociceptors.[58–60] The cervical facet joint surfaces are essentially planar and slope backward and downward. The articular surfaces of facet joints in the cervical spine are generally flat with only minimal concavity and convexity.[61] The obliquity of cervical facet joints averages about 45° but is flatter at C2/3 and steeper at C6/7.[62] The C2/3 joint is more oblique in its orientation than its adjacent counterpart. Thus, the inclination of lower joints is steeper.[63] The average joint volume is less than 1 mL.[25]

Cervical facet joints are well innervated by the medial branches of the dorsal rami.[35,37,64–67] The cervical facet joints below C2/3 are supplied by medial branches of the cervical dorsal rami above and below the joint, which also innervate the deep paramedian muscles. The C2/3 joint is supplied by the third occipital nerve.[37,68] However, innervation of the atlanto-occipital and atlanto-axial joints is derived from the C1 and C2 roots, respectively.[37,68,69] Each C3 to C7 dorsal ramus crosses the same segments transverse process and divides into lateral and medial branches. The medial branch curves around the waist of the articular pillar of the same numbered vertebra. The medial branch nerves are bound by fascia, held against the articular pillar, and covered by the tendinous slips of the origin of the semispinalis capitus.[65]

The vertebral artery ascends through the cervical transverse foramina of C1 to C6, which is located anteriorly. At C2 to C7, it is located anterior to the facet joints from both posterior and lateral injection approaches. However, the vertebral artery passes directly superior in the neck to the level of the transverse process of the axis, where it courses upward and laterally to the transverse foramina of the atlas.[70]

TECHNICAL CONSIDERATIONS

INTRA-ARTICULAR INJECTIONS

Even though they were described later than lumbar facet joint blocks, numerous techniques have been described for the cervical spine. In 1980 Sluijter and Koetsveld-Baart[71] described a technique for blocking the cervical dorsal rami near their origin and a percutaneous radiofrequency technique to coagulate these nerves. In 1988 Bogduk and Marsland[24] described cervical medial branch blocks distal to the target sites used by Sluijter and Koetsveld-Baart[71] in 1988. Okada[72] in 1981 introduced intra-articular cervical facet joint blocks using a lateral approach. Dory[73] described a posterior approach based on a pillar view of the cervical facet joints. Subsequently, others[74–77] have described intra-articular cervical facet joint blocks.

Cervical facet joint injections may be performed using posterior, lateral, or anterior approaches. The posterior approach is the most commonly used method, followed by the lateral approach. Hence, we describe both techniques.

Posterior Intra-Articular Blocks

The posterior approach for cervical intra-articular blocks can be performed with the patient in a prone position, or if required, in a sitting position. It involves introducing a 22- or 25-gauge needle into the target joint from behind, along an oblique trajectory that coincides with the plane of the joint. Commonly, the patient is positioned in the prone position on an operating room table with a cushion under the chest and the neck rotated to the opposite side. Under aseptic conditions, the skin entry is carried out

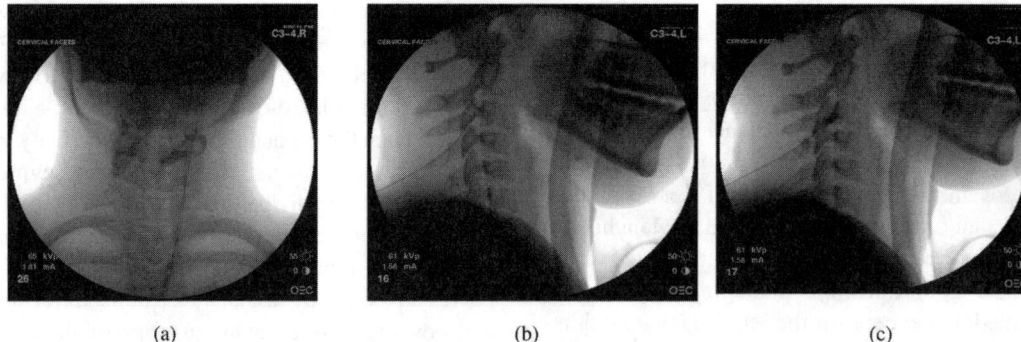

(a)   (b)   (c)

FIGURE 63.1 Intra-articular needle placement with a posterior approach. (a) C3/4 anteroposterior view; (b) C3/4 needle placement lateral view; (c) C3/4 arthrogram lateral view.

approximately two or more segments below the target joint. The skin entry point may be determined either by directing an imaginary line to the skin along the plane of the joint (as determined by a lateral view) or by direct visualization of the joint via a pillar view and making a skin mark along the plane of the X-ray beam into the center of the joint lucency.[78]

The needle is passed with caution through the skin at approximately a 45° angle upward and ventrally through the posterior neck muscles until it makes the contact with the back of the target joint. At this point, the needle may be readjusted until it enters the joint cavity. One should be aware that directing the needle medially toward the interlaminar space or excessively laterally away from the joint will make the injection extremely difficult and dangerous. After satisfactory localization of the needle into the joint, contrast medium is injected to obtain an arthrogram and to verify accurate placement and then to inject local anesthetic and/or corticosteroid is injected. Figure 63.1 illustrates intra-articular needle placement with a posterior approach.

Overall, the posterior approach is considered safer because the needle penetrates only the skin and posterior neck muscles, with the deep cervical artery the only structure at risk of inadvertent puncture. Further, the posterior cervical artery poses minimal risk of morbidity, as it supplies no major structures. However, if the needle is inserted too deeply or too aggressively, it could penetrate the anterior joint capsule. Further, the risk is not only leakage of local anesthetic and steroid over to the dorsal root ganglion, but also the risk of puncture to the vertebral artery or ventral ramus of the spinal nerve lying in front of the joint. In addition, the needle may also enter the epidural space or spinal cord.

Lateral Intra-Articular Blocks

Proponents of the lateral approach argue that it is technically less demanding and may be performed with smaller-gauge needles.[25,72] In addition, it may be more comfortable for the patient because less soft tissue is traversed. Similar

to the posterior approach during insertion, the risk of morbidity is minimal because only the skin and postero-lateral neck muscles are penetrated with no other overlying structures at risk of puncture. However, an aggressive approach or overpenetration may lead the needle into the epidural space or spinal cord.

The lateral approach to the cervical facet joints is performed with the patient lying on his/her side. The target joint is identified on lateral screening of the neck and the needle is introduced through the skin over the midpoint of the joint. It is advanced deeply until it makes contact with the bone of either the superior or inferior articular process. Lateral fluoroscopic imaging identifies the left and right joints simultaneously. The object is to identify the image of the target joint, which lies uppermost in the patient. This may also be confirmed by insertion of the needle after it contacts the bone. Once the correct joint is clearly identified, the needle is advanced until the superior articular process is contacted just above the joint line. The needle is then directed and advanced through the joint capsule. The needle may be felt to pierce the capsule and to enter the joint space. Only minimal penetration is required and the operator may also notice loss of resistance as the needle pierces the capsule. The appropriate position into the joint may be confirmed either by injection of a small dose of contrast medium to obtain an arthrogram or by multiple x-ray views.

The C2/3 joint may be technically more difficult to visualize and more difficult to cannulate, due to anatomic features. The C2/3 joint is more angulated vertically and medially and is not clearly evident on lateral views. In such cases, the approach may be modified by rotating the patient's head to face the table. This will accentuate the cavity of the C2/3 joint into view as it rotates forward of the long axis of the vertebral column. Other modifications with the fluoroscopic unit may also be made. Figure 63.2 illustrates intra-articular placement with a lateral approach.

It is of paramount importance that low volumes be injected into the cervical facet joints. If volumes of

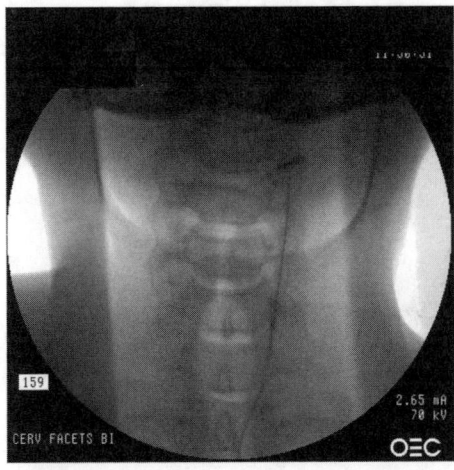

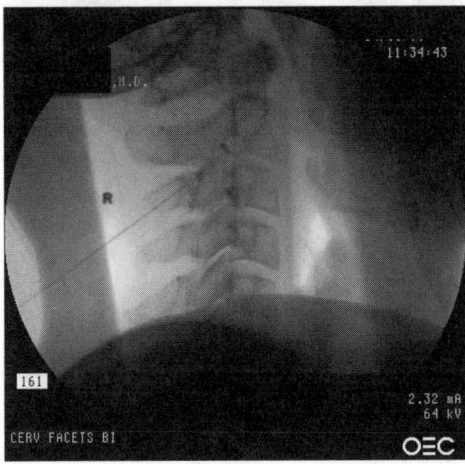

FIGURE 63.2 Intra-articular placement of C2/3 with a lateral approach.

more than 1 mL are injected, or injection is carried out rapidly or forcefully, the joint capsule may rupture and result in spread onto nearby structures. Extra-articular spread is extremely important, specifically when the diagnostic blocks are performed, as this will compromise the specificity.

MEDIAL BRANCH BLOCKS

The cervical facet joints can be anesthetized by blocking the nerves that supply them, namely, medial branches of the cervical dorsal rami. Table 63.3 illustrates the nerves to be blocked for each joint. The target points for these nerves, other than the third occipital nerve, are the crossing points of the waists of the articular pillars — a point proximal to the origin of the articular branches and a point where the nerves have a constant relationship to the bone.[34,78] These points may be reached by needles using a posterior, lateral, or anterior approach. Posterior and lateral approaches are the commonly used techniques.

Posterior Approach

The patient is placed in prone position with a pillow under the chest with the head turned opposite to the procedure site; turn head left for a right side procedure, and right for a left side procedure. Under sterile conditions and fluoroscopic visualization, a posteroanterior view is obtained to identify the posterior aspect of the waists of the articular pillars from C3 to C7. In some patients, the articular pillars of the superior cervical spine (C3 and C4) may be difficult to identify, specifically with the patient's head in neutral position. Turning the head to the opposite side will facilitate this. An additional maneuver may be to ask the patient to open the mouth to remove the mandible from the radiologic field. After identification of the waists of the articular pillars of the levels to be blocked, a 22- or 25-gauge, 2 or 2.5 inch spinal needle is inserted through the skin and posterior neck muscles aiming first for the dorsal aspect of the articular pillar medial to its lateral concavity. Once the needle has made the contact with the bone, it is readjusted laterally to the deepest of this concavity where C3 to C7 medial branches lie. Initially, directing the needle medially to bone ensures that the needle is not placed too deeply. The needle is then directed laterally until the tip reaches the lateral margin of the waist of the articular pillar. The needle should be felt to barely slip off the bone laterally in a ventral direc-

TABLE 63.3
Facet Joint Nerves Required to Be Blocked for Each Facet Joint in Cervical Region

Facet Joint	Facet Joint Nerves to be Blocked	Level of Transverse Process
C2/3	Third occipital nerve or C2 and C3 medial branches	At C2/3 joint
C3/4	C3 and C4 medial branches	At C3 and C4 articular pillars
C4/5	C4 and C5 medial branches	At C4 and C5 articular pillars
C5/6	C5 and C6 medial branches	At C5 and C6 articular pillars
C6/7	C6 and C7 medial branches	At C6 and C7 articular pillars
C7/T1	C7 and C8 medial branches	At C7 articular pillar, and at T1 transverse process for C8

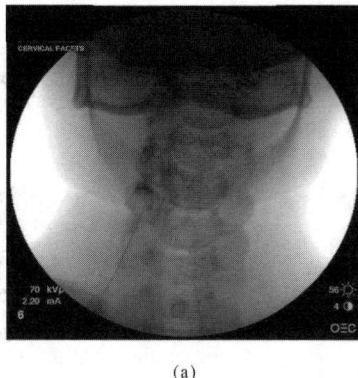
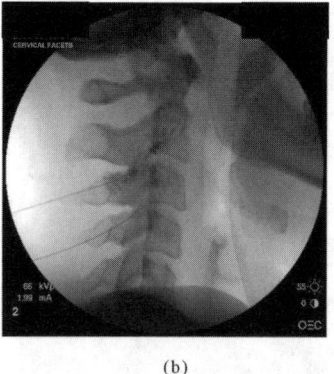

(a)   (b)

FIGURE 63.3 Medial branch blocks with posterior approach. (a) Needle placement posteroanterior (PA) view; (b) needle placement lateral view.

tion at the deepest point of articular pillars concavity (Figure 63.3).[78]

Lateral Approach

For the lateral approach, the patient is positioned on his/her side and the needle is directed through the skin and posterolateral neck muscle toward the centroid of the articular pillar as seen on a true lateral radiograph.[78] If necessary, the uppermost articular pillar can be distinguished from the opposite side either by moving the fluoroscope or by rolling the patient. The needle will be seen to travel with the uppermost articular pillar as the two articular pillars separate on the fluoroscopic image. This approach is well suited for C3 to C6 medial branches.[78] However, the lateral approach for C7 medial branch is somewhat different.

To block the C7 medial branch by lateral approach, the needle is advanced so that it stays within the confines of the C7 superior articular process, which prevents excessive advancement into the C8 foramen and toward the vertebral artery.[78] Once the superior articular process is contacted, anteroposterior imaging should verify that the needle lies against the lateral aspect of the superior articular process. Figure 63.4 illustrates medial branch blocks with a lateral approach.

With posterior and lateral approaches, contrast in doses of 0.1 to 0.2 mL may be injected to confirm appropriate needle placement. However, it is not mandatory. After the confirmation of the needle position, local anesthetic in small doses with or without steroids is injected around the nerve.

Cervical medial branch blocks are extremely safe. Other than general risks associated with cervical injections, including fluoroscopic exposure, infection, needle trauma, etc., no specific complications are reported. The safety lies in the fact that these blocks are performed on the external surface of the vertebral column well away from any vital structures.

Local anesthetic injection for intra-articular injections, as well as medial branch blocks, should be limited

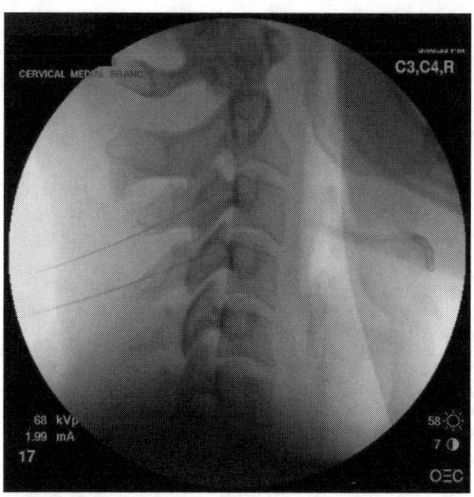

FIGURE 63.4 C3, C4 medial branch blocks with a lateral approach.

to 0.5 mL (0.3 to 0.6 mL) for a diagnostic block and approximately 1 mL for a therapeutic block. Authors[17,18,34] pioneering the concept of comparative local anesthetic blocks recommended potent local anesthetics such as 4% lidocaine and 0.75% bupivacaine to minimize the risk of false-negative medial branch blocks, which can occur at a 10% rate with 2% lidocaine in lumbar spine. Further, for diagnostic as well as therapeutic blocks, the literature has been limited to using local anesthetic agents of different durations of action, namely, lidocaine and bupivacaine. Manchikanti et al.[1,19–21] in multiple investigations used concentrations of lidocaine of 1% and bupivacaine of 0.25%, in contrast to 4% lidocaine and 0.75% bupivacaine as recommended by others, without compromising validity of diagnostic blocks and responsiveness to therapeutic blocks.

MEDIAL BRANCH NEUROTOMY

Radiofrequency lesioning is performed using either a heat lesion or pulsed mode radiofrequency. A thermal radiofrequency neurotomy lesion for facet denervation is performed at 80 to 85°C. A radiofrequency lesion is performed when the temperature exceeds 45°C. Clinically, a higher temperature allows for a larger lesion to be made. The size of the lesion is influenced by the vascularity of the surrounding tissue. The greater the vascularity of the tissue, the smaller the lesion. Top mode equilibrium is achieved in about 60 seconds. The pulsed mode radiofrequency is an application of a strong electric field to the tissue that surrounds the electrode and the temperature of the tissue surrounding the tip of the electrode does not exceed 42°C. Essentially, the radiofrequency current is applied in a pulsed fashion and heat is dissipated during the silent period.[79]

Most commonly, radiofrequency thermoneurolysis of the cervical medial branches is performed in prone position, even though some clinicians use a supine or an oblique approach. Prone position is considered an optimal position providing maximal parallel needle placement to the target nerves with the least complication profile.

In the prone position, exposure to the medial branches is obtained as described earlier. The needles are placed directly down the beam into the target waist of the articular pillar that corresponds to the same numbered target nerve. Some have recommended that two to three lesions be made to account for superior to inferior nerve position variability. With this, the needle is placed at the middle of the articular pillar in a cephalad-to-caudad plane and then additional lesions can occur. One lesion is one radiofrequency needle diameter superior and the other is one radiofrequency needle diameter inferior. As many as six lesions have been performed.

SAFETY AND COMPLICATIONS

Complications from intra-articular injections or medial branch blocks in the cervical spine are exceedingly rare.[1,17–21,23–26,34,42–44,46,64,75–90] However, disastrous complications with cervical facet joint injections may occur. The complications include those related to the technique with placement of the needle and complications related to the administration of various drugs. Proximity to the vertebral artery and spinal cord, along with nerve root ganglion, make these injections highly vulnerable. Complications may include dural puncture, spinal cord trauma, subdural injection, neural trauma, injection into the intervertebral foramen and intervertebral formation; intravascular injection into the veins or, in a worst-case scenario, vertebral artery; infectious complications including epidural abscess and bacterial meningitis; and side effects related to the administration of steroids, local anesthetics, and other drugs. Vertebral artery and ventral ramus damage, along with a risk of embolus resulting in serious neurological sequelae with spinal cord damage and cerebral

infarction, is an exceedingly rare but potential complication with cervical facet joint injections.

Other, minor complications include lightheadedness, flushing, sweating, nausea, hypotension, syncope, pain at the injection site, and headaches. Side effects related to the administration of steroids are generally attributed to the steroid's chemistry or the pharmacology of the steroids.[80] These include separation of pituitary-adrenal access, hypocorticism, Cushing syndrome, osteoporosis, avascular necrosis of the bone, steroid myopathy, epidural lipomatosis, weight gain, fluid retention, and hypoglycemia.

Reported complications of radiofrequency thermoneurolysis include a worsening of the usual pain, burning or dysesthesias, decreased sensation and allodynia in the paravertebral skin or the facets denervated, transient leg pain, persistent leg weakness, and inadvertent lesioning of the spinal nerve or ventral ramus resulting in motor deficits, sensory loss, and possible deafferentation pain.[79] A spinal cord lesion can lead to paraplegia; loss of motor, proprioception, and sensory function; bowel and bladder dysfunction; Brown-Séquard syndrome; and spinal cord infarction.

CONCLUSION

Cervical facet joints are commonly identified as the cause of neck pain, upper extremity pain, and headaches. Cervical facet joint blocks can be performed to test the hypothesis that the target joint is the source of the patient's pain. The rationale for using facet joint blocks for diagnosis, as well as therapy, is based upon the facts that cervical facet joints have been shown to be capable of being a source of neck pain and referred pain in the head and upper extremities; cervical facet joint pain may not be diagnosed based on referral patterns, physical examination, history, neurophysiologic testing, or radiological evaluation; diagnostic cervical facet joint blocks have been shown to be highly valid and specific; degenerative process of the cervical spine and the origin of cervical spine is extremely complex; and the effectiveness of a large variety of therapeutic interventions in managing chronic pain arising from the cervical spine has not been demonstrated conclusively.

The validity of diagnostic facet joint blocks has been demonstrated conclusively. However, the value of therapeutic intra-articular joint injections is limited, the value of medial branch nerve blocks is moderate, and the value radiofrequency neurotomy is strong.

REFERENCES

1. Manchikanti, L. et al. (2003). Evidence-based practice guidelines for interventional techniques in the management of chronic spinal pain. *Pain Physician, 6*, 3.

2. Bovim, G., Schrader, H., & Sand, T. (1994). Neck pain in the general population. *Spine, 19,* 1307.

3. Côté, D. C., Cassidy, J. D., & Carroll, L. (1998). The Saskatchewan Health and Back Pain Survey. The prevalence of neck pain and related disability in Saskatchewan adults. *Spine, 23,* 1689.

4. Côté, D. C., Cassidy, J. D., & Carroll, L. (2000). The factors associated with neck pain and its related disability in the Saskatchewan population. *Spine, 25,* 1109.

5. Lau, E. M. C., Sham, A., & Wong, K. C. (1996). The prevalence of and risk factors for neck pain in Hong Kong Chinese. *Journal of Public Health Medicine. 18,* 396.

6. Johnson, G. (1996). Hyperextension soft tissue injuries of the cervical spine: A review. *Journal of Accident and Emergency Medicine, 13,* 3.

7. Ariëns, G. A., Borghouts, J. A., & Koes, B. W. (1999). Neck pain. In I. K. Crombie et al. (Eds.), *Epidemiology of pain* (p. 235). Seattle: IASP Press.

8. Frederiksson, K. et al. (1999). Risk factors for neck and upper limb disorders: Results from 24 years of follow up. *Occupational and Environmental Medicine, 56,* 59.

9. Leclerc, A. et al. (1999). One-year predictive factors for various aspects of neck disorders. *Spine, 24,* 1455.

10. Marshall, P. D., O'Connor, M., & Hodgkinson, J. P. (1995). The perceived relationship between neck symptoms and precedent injury. *Injury, 26,* 17.

11. Linton, S. J., Hellsing, A. L., & Hallden, K. (1998). A population based study of spinal pain among 35-45-year old individuals. *Spine, 23,* 1457.

12. Miles, K. et al. (1988). The incidence and prognostic significance of radiological abnormalities in soft tissue injuries to the cervical spine. *Skeletal Radiology, 17,* 493.

13. Pennie, B., & Agambar, I. (1991). Patterns of injury and recovery in whiplash. *Injury, 22,* 57.

14. Ylinen, J., & Ruuska, J. (1994). Clinical use of neck isometric strength measurement in rehabilitation. *Archives of Physical and Medical Rehabilitation, 75,* 465.

15. Hallgern, R. C., Greenman, P. E., & Rechtien, J. J. (1994). Atrophy of suboccipital muscles in patients with chronic pain: A pilot study. *Journal of the American Osteopathic Association, 12,* 1032.

16. Hildingsson, C., & Toolanen, G. (1990). Outcome after soft-tissue injury of the cervical spine: A prospective study of 93 car accident victims. *Acta Orthopaedica Scandinavica, 61,* 357.

17. Barnsley, L. et al. (1995). The prevalence of chronic cervical zygapophyseal joint pain after whiplash. *Spine, 20,* 20.

18. Lord, S. M. et al. (1996). Chronic cervical zygapophysial joint pain with whiplash: A placebo-controlled prevalence study. *Spine, 21,* 1737.

19. Manchikanti, L. et al. (2002). Prevalence of cervical facet joint pain in chronic neck pain. *Pain Physician, 5,* 243.

20. Manchikanti, L. et al. (2002). Is there correlation of facet joint pain in lumbar and cervical spine? *Pain Physician, 5,* 365.

21. Manchikanti L., Boswell M. V., Singh V., Pampati V., Damron K. S., & Beyer C. D. (2004). Prevalence of facet joint pain in chronic spinal pain of cervical, thoracic, and lumbar regions. *BioMed Central Musculoskeletal Disorders, 5,* 15.

22. Goldthwait, J. E. (1911). The lumbosacral articulation: an explanation of many cases of lumbago, sciatica, and paraplegia., *Boston Medical and Surgical Journal, 164,* 365.

23. Pawl, R. P. (1977). Headache, cervical spondylosis, and anterior cervical fusion. *Surgery Annual, 9,* 391.

24. Bogduk, N., & Marsland, A. (1988). The cervical zygapophyseal joints as a source of neck pain. *Spine, 13,* 610.

25. Dwyer, A., Aprill, C., & Bogduk, N. (1990). Cervical zygapophyseal joint pain patterns: A study in normal volunteers. *Spine, 6,* 453.

26. Aprill, C., Dwyer, A., & Bogduk, N. (1990). The prevalence of cervical zygapophyseal joint pain patterns II: A clinical evaluation. *Spine, 6,* 458.

27. Fukui, S. et al. (1996). Referred pain distribution of the cervical zygapophyseal joints and cervical dorsal rami. *Pain, 68,* 79.

28. Windsor, R. E. et al. (2003). Electrical stimulation induced cervical medial branch referral patterns. *Pain Physician, 6,* 411.

29. Merskey, H., & Bogduk, N. (1994). *Classification of chronic pain: Descriptions of chronic pain syndromes and definitions of pain terms* (2nd ed., p. 180). Seattle: IASP Press.

30. Handel, J. A., Knap, J., & Poletti, S. (1995). The structural degenerative cascade. The cervical spine. In A. H. White & J. A. Schofferaian (Eds.), *Spine care. Diagnosis and conservative treatment* (p. 16). St. Louis: Mosby.

31. Thompson, R. E., Pearcy, M. J., & Downing, K. J. W. (2000). Disc lesions and the mechanics of the intervertebral joint complex. *Spine, 25,* 3026.

32. Ziv, I. et al. (1993). Human facet cartilage: Swelling and some physicochemical characteristics as a function of age. Part 2: Age changes in some biophysical parameters of human facet joint cartilage. *Spine, 18,* 136.

33. Nachemson, A. L., Schultz, A. B., & Berkson, M. H. (1979). Mechanical properties of human lumbar spine motion segments. Influence of age, sex, disc level and degeneration. *Spine, 4,* 1.

34. Bogduk, N. (1997). International Spinal Injection Society guidelines for the performance of spinal injection procedures. Part 1: Zygapophyseal joint blocks. *Clinical Journal of Pain, 13,* 285.

35. Bogduk, N., & Lord, S. (1998). Cervical zygapophysial joint pain. *Neurosurgery, 8,* 107.

36. Boswell, M. V. et al. (2003). Accuracy of precision diagnostic blocks in the diagnosis of chronic spinal pain of facet or zygapophysial joint origin. *Pain Physician, 6,* 449.

37. Barnsley, L., & Bogduk, N. (1993). Medial branch blocks are specific for the diagnosis of cervical zygapophyseal joint pain. *Regional Anesthesia and Pain Medicine, 18,* 343.

38. Lord, S.M., Barnsley, L., & Bogduk, N. (1995). The utility of comparative local anesthetic blocks versus placebo-controlled blocks for the diagnosis of cervical zygapophysial joint pain. *Clinical Journal of Pain, 11*, 208.

39. Bonica, J. J. (1989). Local anesthesia and regional blocks. In P. D. Wall & R. Melzack (Eds.), *Textbook of pain* (2nd ed., p. 724). Edinburgh: Churchill Livingstone.

40. Bonica, J. J., & Buckley, F. P. (1990). Regional analgesia with local anesthetics. In J. J. Bonica (Ed.), *The management of pain* (p. 1883). Philadelphia: Lea & Febiger.

41. Boas, R. A. (1991). Nerve blocks in the diagnosis of low back pain. *Neurosurgery Clinics of North America, 2*, 806.

42. Barnsley, L., Lord, S., & Bogduk, N. (1993). Comparative local anesthetic blocks in the diagnosis of cervical zygapophysial joints pain. *Pain, 55*, 99.

43. Speldewinde, G. C., Bashford, G. M., & Davidson, I. R. (2001). Diagnostic cervical zygapophyseal joint blocks for chronic cervical pain. *Medical Journal of Australia, 174*, 174.

44. Barnsley, L. et al. (1993). False-positive rates of cervical zygapophysial joint blocks, *Clinical Journal of Pain, 9*, 124.

45. Raj, P. P. et al. (2004). Bleeding risk in interventional pain practice: Assessment, management, and review of the literature. *Pain Physician, 7*, 3.

46. Barnsley, L. et al. (1994). Lack of effect of intra-articular corticosteroids for chronic pain in the cervical zygapophyseal joints. *New England Journal of Medicine, 330*, 1047.

47. Manchikanti, L. et al. (2004). Effectiveness of cervical medial branch blocks in chronic neck pain: A prospective outcome study. *Pain Physician, 7*, 195.

48. Lord, S. M. et al. (1996). Percutaneous radio-frequency neurotomy for chronic cervical zygapophyseal-joint pain. *New England Journal of Medicine, 335*, 1721.

49. Sapir, D., & Gorup, J. M. (2001). Radiofrequency medial branch neurotomy in litigant and nonlitigant patients with cervical whiplash. *Spine, 26*, E268.

50. McDonald, G. J., Lord, S. M., & Bogduk, N. (1999). Long-term follow-up of patients treated with cervical radiofrequency for chronic neck pain. *Neurosurgery, 45*, 1499.

51. Geurts, J. W. et al. (2001). Efficacy of radiofrequency procedures for the treatment of spinal pain: A systematic review of randomized clinical trials. *Regional Anesthesia and Pain Medicine, 26*, 394.

52. Manchikanti, L. et al. (2002). Medial branch neurotomy in management of chronic spinal pain: Systematic review of the evidence. *Pain Physician, 5*, 405.

53. Niemistö, L. et al. (2003). Radiofrequency denervation for neck and back pain: A systematic review within the framework of the Cochrane Collaboration Back Review Group. *Spine, 28*, 1877.

54. Bogduk, N. (2002). In defense of radiofrequency neurotomy [Letter to the editor]. *Regional Anesthesia and Pain Medicine, 27*, 439.

55. Bland, J. H. (Ed.) (1987). Anatomy and biomechanics. In *Disorders of the cervical spine* (p. 9). Philadelphia: W.B. Saunders.

56. Yu, S., Sether, L., & Haughton, V. M. (1987). Facet joint menisci of the cervical spine: Correlative MR imaging and cryomicrotomy study. *Radiology, 164*, 79.

57. Mercer, S., & Bogduk, N. (1993). Intra-articular inclusion of the cervical synovial joints. *British Journal of Rheumatology, 32*, 705.

58. McClain, R. F. (1994). Mechanoreceptor endings in human cervical facet joints. *Spine, 19*, 495.

59. Wyke, B. (1979). Neurology of the cervical spinal joints. *Physiotherapy, 65*, 72.

60. Wyke, B. (1981). Articular neurology: A review. *Physiotherapy, 58*, 563.

61. Grieve, G. P. (Ed.) (1988). Applied anatomy – Regional. In *Common vertebral joint problems* (2nd ed., p. 7). London: Churchill Livingstone.

62. Nowitzke, A., Westaway, M., & Bogduk, N. (1994). Cervical zygapophyseal joints. Geometrical parameters and relationship to cervical kinematics. *Clinical Biomechanics, 9*, 342.

63. Dvorak, J., & Dvorak, V. (1990). *Manual medicine-diagnostics* (2nd ed., p. 1). New York: Thieme.

64. Bogduk, N. (1990). Back pain: Zygapophyseal joint blocks and epidurals. In M. J. Cousins & P. O. Bridenbaugh (Eds.), *Neural blockade in clinical anesthesia and pain management* (2nd ed., p. 935). Philadelphia: J.B. Lippincott.

65. Lord, S. M., Barnsley, L., & Bogduk, N. (1998). Cervical zygapophyseal joint pain in whiplash injuries. *Spine State of the Art Review, 12*, 301.

66. Bogduk, N. (1982). The clinical anatomy of the cervical dorsal rami. *Spine, 7*, 35.

67. Stilwell, D. L. (1956). The nerve supply of the vertebral column and its associated structures in the monkey. *Anatomical Record, 125*, 139.

68. Dreyfuss, P., Michaelsen, M., & Fletcher, D. (1994). Atlanto-occipital and lateral atlanto-axial joint pain patterns. *Spine, 19*, 1125.

69. Bogduk, N., & Marsland, A. (1986). On the concept of third occipital headache. *Journal of Neurology, Neurosurgery, and Psychiatry, 49*, 775.

70. Schultz, D. (2004). Risk of transforaminal epidural injections. *Pain Physician, 7*, 289.

71. Sluijter, M. E., & Koetsveld-Baart, C. C. (1980). Interruption of pain pathways in the treatment of the cervical syndrome. *Anaesthesia, 35*, 302.

72. Okada, K. (1981). Studies on the cervical facet joints using arthrography of the cervical facet joint. *Journal of the Japanese Orthopedic Association, 55*, 563.

73. Dory, M. A. (1983). Arthrography of the cervical facet joints. *Radiology, 148*, 379.

74. Dussault, R. G., & Nicolet, V. M. (1985). Cervical facet joint arthrography. *Journal of the Canadian Association of Radiologists, 36*, 79.

75. Wedel, D. J., & Wilson, P. R. (1985). Cervical facet arthrography. *Regional Anesthesia, 10*, 7.

76. Hove, B., & Glydensted, C. (1990). Cervical analgesic facet joint arthrography. *Neuroradiology, 32*, 456.

77. Roy, D. F. et al. (1988). Clinical evaluation of cervical facet joint infiltration. *Journal of the Canadian Association of Radiologists, 39*, 118.

78. Dreyfuss, P., Kaplan, M., & Dreyer, S. J. (2000). Zygapophyseal joint injection techniques in the spinal axis. In T. A. Lennard (Ed), *Pain procedures in clinical practice* (2nd ed., p. 276). Philadelphia: Hanley & Belfus, Inc.

79. Curran, M. A. (2002). Lumbosacral facet joint radiofrequency. In L. Manchikanti, C. W. Slipman, & B. Fellows (Eds.), *Interventional pain management: Low back pain — Diagnosis and treatment* (p. 463). Padukah, KY: ASIPP Publishing.

80. Manchikanti, L. (2002). Role of neuraxial steroids in interventional pain management. *Pain Physician, 5*, 182.

81. Windsor, R. E., Storm, S., & Sugar, R. (2003). Prevention and management of complications resulting from common spinal injections. *Pain Physician, 6*, 473.

82. Windsor, R. E., Pinzon, E. G., & Gore, H. C. (2000). Complications of common selective spinal injections: Prevention and management. *American Journal of Orthopedics, 29*, 759.

83. Gladstone, J. C., & Pennant, J. H. (1987). Spinal anaesthesia following facet joint injection. *Anaesthesia, 42*, 754.

84. Marks, R., & Semple, A. J. (1988). Spinal anaesthesia after facet joint injection. *Anaesthesia, 43*, 65.

85. Cook, N. J., Hanrahan, P., & Song, S. (1999). Paraspinal abscess following facet joint injection. *Clinical Rheumatology, 18*, 52.

86. Magee, M. et al. (2000). Paraspinal abscess complicating facet joint injection, *Clinical Nuclear Medicine, 25*, 71.

87. Manchikanti, L. et al. (2002). Radiation exposure to the physician in interventional pain management. *Pain Physician, 5*, 385.

88. Orpen, N. M., & Birch, N. C. (2003). Delayed presentation of septic arthritis of a lumbar facet joint after diagnostic facet joint injection. *Journal of Spinal Disorders and Techniques, 16*, 285.

89. Manchikanti, L. et al. (2003). Effectiveness of protective measures in reducing risk of radiation exposure in interventional pain management: A prospective evaluation. *Pain Physician, 6*, 301.

90. Berrigan, T. (1992). Chemical meningism after lumbar facet joint block. *Anesthesia, 7*, 905.

64

Thoracic Facet Joint Interventions

Laxmaiah Manchikanti, MD, David M. Schultz, MD, and Vijay Singh, MD

INTRODUCTION

Thoracic facet joints have been implicated as the source of chronic pain in 45 to 48% of patients with chronic thoracic pain.[1,2] These figures were based on responses to controlled diagnostic blocks of these joints, in accordance with the criteria established by the International Association for the Study of Pain.[3] The role of thoracic facet joints in chronic upper or mid back pain has received very little attention with only a few publications discussing these joints as the source of pain.[1,2,4–11] Even though thoracic spinal pain is less common, it can be as chronic and disabling as neck and low back pain. In the interventional pain management environment, the proportion of patients with thoracic disorders is relatively small, ranging from 3 to 22%.[12,13] Linton et al.[14] estimate the prevalence of all spinal pain in the general population as 66%, with 15% reporting thoracic pain, 44% reporting neck pain, and 56% reporting low back pain.

HISTORY

Diagnosis of thoracic facet joint pain is a relatively recent development. Involvement of lumbar facet joints in low back pain had been described by Goldthwait[15] as early as 1911. In 1927, the Italian surgeon Putti[16] published an article on articular facet degeneration as a cause of pain that supported the findings of Goldthwait. In 1963, Hirsch et al.[17] demonstrated that low back pain could be induced by injecting hypertonic saline in the region of facet joints. Pawl,[18] in 1977, reported the reproduction of neck pain and headache after injection of hypertonic saline into the cervical facet joints. However, thoracic facet syndrome was not described until 1987.[7] Subsequently, further men-

tions were made about thoracic facet joint pain in 1991.[6] In 1994, Dreyfuss et al.[4] described thoracic zygapophysial joint pain patterns in normal volunteers.

ANATOMY

The facet joints are paired diarthrodial articulations between the posterior elements of the adjacent vertebrae.[19,20] The facet joints are formed by the articulation of the inferior articular processes of one vertebra with the superior articular processes of the next vertebra. The joints exhibit the features of typical synovial joints. The articular facets are covered by articular cartilage, and a synovial membrane bridges the margins of the articular cartilage of the two facets in each joint.

In the thoracic region, the articular surface of the joints is inclined 60° from the horizontal to the frontal plane and rotated 20° from the frontal to the sagittal plane in a medial direction. Thus, the lateral aspect of the joint is placed anterior and the medial aspect of the joint posterior.[21,22] The superior articular facet from the inferior vertebrae is almost flat and faces posterior, superior, and slightly lateral. The inferior articular facet is oriented in a reciprocal manner. There is some variation in the inclination of the joints by region with the midthoracic level approximately 60° off the horizontal plane, while the upper segments achieve a more vertical orientation. The lower thoracic segments show some characteristics of the lumbar segments as their angle approaches the sagittal plane.[23]

A tough fibrous capsule composed of several layers of fibrous tissue and a synovial membrane, separated by a layer of loose alveolar tissue, is present on the posterolateral aspect of the facet joint. However, there is no fibrous capsule on the ventral aspect of the joints. Instead, in its place the ligamentum flavum is in direct contact with the synovial membrane. Facet joints appear to be anatomically designed to restrain excessive mobility and distribute axial loading over a broad area.

Thoracic facet joints are innervated from branches of the thoracic dorsal rami arising from the spinal nerves. Chua and Bogduk[24] showed that the medial branches of the thoracic dorsal rami were found to assume a reasonably constant course except at mid-thoracic levels (T5–T8). They showed that the medial branches of the thoracic dorsal rami at mid-thoracic levels do not run on bone. Instead, they are suspended in the intertransverse space. They also reported that thoracic medial branches are not that close to the facet joint, as they swing laterally to circumvent the multifidus. Free nerve endings have been demonstrated in the capsules of the facet joints. In an analogy to the innervation of the cervical and lumbar facet joints, the thoracic facet joints receive a bisegmental innervation from the medial branches of the dorsal ramus of the upper segment and one or more cephalad levels.[24,25]

PATHOPHYSIOLOGY

Degeneration, inflammation, and injury of facet joints can lead to pain upon joint motion, leading to restriction of motion secondary to pain, which eventually leads to overall physical deconditioning and irritation of the facet joint innervation in itself, leading to secondary muscle spasm. It has been assumed that degeneration of the disc would lead to associated facet joint degeneration and subsequent spinal pain. These assumptions are based on the pathogenesis model of a degenerative cascade involving the three joint complex of a spinal motion segment consisting of the intravertebral disc and the two adjacent facet joints that make up the articulation between two vertebrae. Changes within one member of this joint complex will result in changes within the other members. This model should apply to cervical and thoracic as well as lumbar spinal segments.[26] However, this hypothesis was shown to be realistic in post-traumatic neck pain, and opposite conclusions were reached in low back pain.[27,28] Causes such as rheumatoid arthritis and ankylosing spondylitis, small fractures, capsular tears, splits in the articular cartilage, hemorrhage, osteoarthritis, meniscoid entrapment, synovial impingement, joint subluxation, chondromalacia, capsular and synovial inflammation, excessive mechanical injury to the joint capsule, and restriction to normal articular motion from various causes, synovial cysts, and infection have been described as sources of facet joint pain. However, radiographic changes of osteoarthritis have been shown to be equally common in patients with and without low back pain, and degenerative joints seen on computed tomography (CT) are not always painful, even though

some studies report severely degenerated joints are more likely to be symptomatic.

Thoracic facet joint pain is considered relatively uncommon compared with pain from the lumbar and cervical spine. Van Kleef et al.[29] showed that thoracic pain was the presenting symptom in 12% of new patients attending a pain clinic in the Netherlands.

DIAGNOSIS

There is no evidence that thoracic facet joint pain can be diagnosed by clinical examination or by medical imaging.[30] The principles established for facet joint blocks utilizing controlled comparative local anesthetic blocks are the only means available to identify facet joint pain in the thoracic region. These joints can be blocked either by intra-articular injections or by anesthetizing the medial branches of the dorsal rami that innervate the target joint.

The rationale for using thoracic facet joint blocks for diagnosis is based on the fact that the thoracic facet joints have been shown to be capable of being a source of mid or upper back pain and referred pain into the chest wall in normal volunteers. Consequently, thoracic facet joints are possible sources of pain in patients presenting with mid back or upper back pain. There are no historical or clinical features that are pathognomonic for thoracic facet joint pain. Attempts by investigators to correlate demographic features, pain characteristics, physical findings, and other signs and symptoms with the diagnosis of facet joint pain in the cervical and lumbar spine have been proved to be unreliable. In addition, imaging technologies do not provide valid or reliable means of identifying symptomatic lesions. Thus, controlled diagnostic blocks with two separate local anesthetics (standard practice within the United States) or placebo-controlled blocks (standard practice in Australia and certain other countries) are the only means of confirming a diagnosis of facet joint pain. The diagnostic accuracy of controlled local anesthetic facet joint blocks has been reviewed and was determined to be high in the diagnosis of chronic low back pain and neck pain.[30,31]

The face validity of intra-articular injections for medial branch blocks has been established by injecting small volumes of local anesthetic into the joint or onto the target points of the nerve. Construct validity of facet joint blocks is determined by removing the placebo effect with controlled comparative local anesthetic blocks.[30,31] The indications and contraindications[32] for diagnostic facet joint blocks are described in Table 64.1 and Table 64.2.

Contraindications are quite obvious and include bacterial infection, possible pregnancy, and bleeding diathesis. Relative contraindications include allergy to contrast media or local anesthetics and treatment with non-aspirin antiplatelet therapy, which may compromise coagulation.[33,34] Patients on warfarin therapy should be checked

TABLE 64.1
Common Indications for Diagnostic Thoracic Facet Joint Blocks

- Somatic or nonradicular mid or upper back pain
- Lack of obvious evidence for discogenic pain
- Lack of disc herniation or evidence of radiculitis
- Duration of pain of at least of 3 months
- Failure to respond to more conservative management, including physical therapy modalities with exercise, chiropractic management, and nonsteroidal anti-inflammatory agents
- Average pain levels of greater than 5 on a scale of 1 to 10
- Intermittent or continuous pain causing functional disability
- No contraindications with understanding of consent, nature of the procedure, needle placement, or sedation
- No history of allergy to contrast administration, local anesthetic steroids, Sarapin, or other drugs potentially utilized
- Contraindications or inability to undergo physical therapy or chiropractic management or inability to tolerate nonsteroidal anti-inflammatory drugs

TABLE 64.2
Common Contraindications for Thoracic Facet Joint Blocks

- Infection
- Inability of the patient to understand consent, nature of the procedure, needle placement, or sedation
- Allergies to contrast, local anesthetic, steroids, Sarapin, or other drugs
- Needle phobia
- Psychogenic pain
- Suspected discogenic pain or disc herniation
- Pregnancy
- Anticoagulant therapy
- Non-aspirin antiplatelet therapy
- Bleeding diathesis

for prothrombin time (PT), and it should be at acceptable levels. In stopping anticoagulant therapy, one should take into consideration the risk/benefit ratio and also consult with the physician in charge of anticoagulant therapy. In our practice, we advise the patients to contact the physician in charge of anticoagulant therapy and let that physician make the decision of the date to stop, and for how long. Raj et al.[33] provide a detailed description of the role of anticoagulants in interventional pain management.

Stoppage of warfarin for 3 days should be sufficient. Longer intervals may only increase risk of thromboembolism. However, prior to facet joint injections, a PT must be performed. Various other drugs such as low-molecular-weight heparins — for example, enoxaparin (Lovenox®) or ardeparin ([Normiflo®) — or other antithrombotics such as danaparoid (Organ®) should also be discontinued as

they increase the risk of bleeding. Similarly, antiplatelet agents such as ticlopidine (Ticlid®) and clopidogrel (Plavix®) are also relative contraindications.

Patients with diabetes mellitus should be informed about increases in blood sugar if steroids are used. They also should monitor their blood glucose after corticosteroid injection. Precautions should also be taken by patients with artificial heart valves, who may require the use of antibiotics before and after the procedure, as determined by the treating physician. However, use of preprocedural antibiotics for patients with mitral valve prolapse is controversial.

THERAPEUTIC FACET JOINT INTERVENTIONS

Thoracic facet joint pain may be treated with intra-articular injections, medial branch blocks, or radiofrequency thermoneurolysis. However, there is a paucity of literature on the role of therapeutic interventions of thoracic facet joints.

INTRA-ARTICULAR BLOCKS

There are no descriptions in the literature concerning the role of thoracic intra-articular blocks in managing chronic pain.

MEDIAL BRANCH BLOCKS

There is no literature available describing the role of medial branch blocks as a therapeutic measure in managing chronic thoracic pain.

RADIOFREQUENCY NEUROTOMY

In a nonrandomized prospective trial, Stolker et al.[8] evaluated the effectiveness of percutaneous facet denervation in chronic thoracic spinal pain. They evaluated 40 patients with chronic thoracic spinal pain of greater than 12 months' duration, which failed to respond to conservative treatment. All patients were evaluated by specialists, mainly neurologists and orthopedic surgeons. The diagnosis of facet syndrome was made by clinical criteria and a transient positive response to a prognostic blockade of the medial branch of the dorsal ramus of the thoracic spinal nerve. The results showed that 40 patients underwent 51 percutaneous thoracic facet denervations. After 2 months, 19 patients (47.5%) were pain free and 14 patients (35%) had more than 50% pain relief, with a total of 82.5% of the patients reporting greater than 50% relief. With a long-term follow-up average of 31 months in 36 patients, 44% were pain free and 39% had more than 50% pain relief, with a total of 83% of the patients presenting greater than 50% relief.

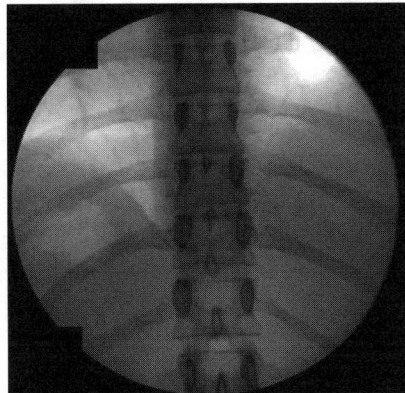

FIGURE 64.1 Thoracic pedicles darkened.

TECHNICAL CONSIDERATIONS

Patients are placed in the prone position for thoracic intra-articular facet injections, medial branch blocks, and radiofrequency neurotomy. Posteroanterior (PA) view of the thoracic spine is essential for all interventions (Figure 64.1). Although thoracic facet joints are not quite evident in a PA view, their location can be estimated from the location of the thoracic pedicles (Figure 64.1).[30]

The joints slide behind the intervertebral foramina, and these foramina lie between the pedicles. The location of the target joint is determined by counting vertebrae and ribs from above.

INTRA-ARTICULAR INJECTIONS

The target joint will not be visible in the posteroanterior views but can be gauged to lie between the two pedicles bearing the same segmental number as the target joint.[30] Thoracic facet joints are difficult to enter directly from behind due to orientation in the coronal plane, and laterally they may carry the risk of pneumothorax.

Thus, the safest entry is from below, which requires an initial insertion of the needle approximately one to two segments below the target joint.

With intermittent fluoroscopic visualization, the needle is inserted through the skin cephalad pointing toward the superior articular process. The needle should remain on an imaginary vertical line connecting the midportion of the targeted facet joint and the one below. If the needle stays in this line without deviation, either medial or lateral, it will be safe. However, the risks with deviation of the needle include entering the epidural space and spinal cord, or pleural space and lung. After the insertion of the needle approximately 4 to 5 cm, or once the needle tip is seen to lie at the mid to inferior aspect of the pedicle, the fluoroscope is rotated away from the side being injected until the outline of the joint is clearly visible (almost a lateral position). Following this, the needle is advanced through the capsule into the inferior aspect of the joint (Figure 64.2).

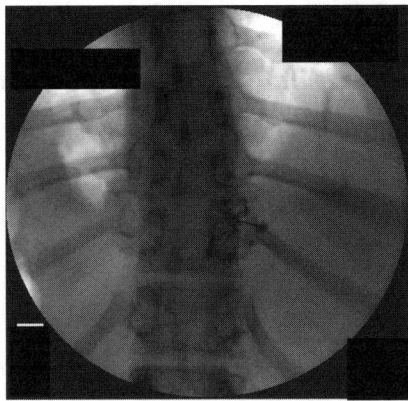

FIGURE 64.2 Needle in thoracic facet.

After the needle is inserted into the inferior aspect of the joint, contrast is injected. After confirmation, local anesthetic and/or steroid may be injected.

The description provided is ideal for the joints below T6/7. However, for superior levels from T1/2–T5/6, a more perpendicular approach to the facet joints is needed. At these levels on PA imaging, skin entry is usually at the midportion of the vertebral body rather than its inferior aspect. Figure 64.2 illustrates intra-articular injection of a thoracic facet joint.

MEDIAL BRANCH BLOCKS

For thoracic medial branch blocks the target points are, in general, the superolateral corners of the thoracic transverse processes (Figure 64.3). The nerves to a particular joint are the ones that cross the transverse process above the joint and the transverse process below the joint. Numerically, if the joint to be blocked is the Tx/y joint, the transverse processes required are the Tx–1 and Tx transverse processes.[30] Respectively, these are crossed by the Tx–2 and Tx–1 medial branches. The numerical rela-

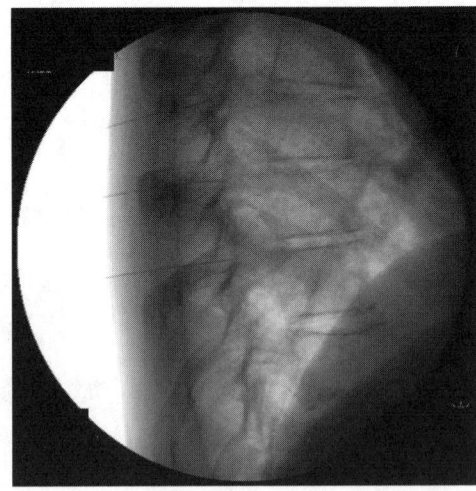

FIGURE 64.3 Thoracic medial branch blocks.

TABLE 64.3
Facet Joint Nerves Required to Be Blocked for Each Facet Joint in Thoracic Region

Facet Joint	Facet Joint Nerves (medial branches) to be Blocked	Level of Transverse Process
T1/2	C8 and T1 medial branches	At T1 transverse process for C8
		At T2 transverse process for T1
T2/3	T1 and T2 medial branches	At T2 transverse process for T1
		At T3 transverse process for T2
T3/4	T2 and T3 medial branches	At T3 transverse process for T2
		At T4 transverse process for T3
T4/5	T3 and T4 medial branches	At T4 transverse process for T3
		At T5 transverse process for T4
T5/6	T4 and T5 medial branches	At T5 transverse process for T4
		At T6 transverse process for T5
T6/7	T5 and T6 medial branches	At T6 transverse process for T5
		At T7 transverse process for T6
T7/8	T6 and T7 medial branches	At T7 transverse process for T6
		At T8 transverse process for T7
T8/9	T7 and T8 medial branches	At T8 transverse process for T7
		At T9 transverse process for T8
T9/10	T8 and T9 medial branches	At T9 transverse process for T8
		At T10 transverse process for T9
T10/11	T9 and T10 medial branches	At T10 transverse process for T9
		At T11 transverse process for T10
T11/12	T10 and T11 medial branches	At T11 transverse process for T10
		At T12 transverse process for T11
T12/L1	T11 and T12 medial branches	At T12 transverse process for T11
		At L1 transverse process for T12

tionships between nerves, transverse processes, and joints are, therefore, like those of the lumbar region. Caution should be taken to accurately interpret and report the level to be blocked, in terms of both the joint anesthetized and the nerves anesthetized.[30]

For medial branch blocks C8 to T10, the target transverse processes should be differentiated from the rib that lies in front and whose upper margin projects slightly above the transverse process.[30]

At the T12 level the medial branches of the thoracic dorsal rami assume a course that is similar to lumbar. The T12 medial branch assumes a course exactly analogous to that of typical lumbar medial branches, lying on the junction of the superior articular process and the transverse process.

Table 64.3 illustrates the nerve supply of thoracic facet joints.

Medial Branch Blocks T1 to T4 and T9 to T10

For the needle placement from T1 to T4 and T9 to T10, the needle is positioned directly overlying the target point of the nerve. The needle must be advanced until the contact is made with the target transverse process, with subsequent adjustment of the needle to rest on the back of the superolateral corner of the transverse process. Injectate may be instilled at this time.

Medial Branch Blocks at T5 to T8

At these levels, a single-needle or two-needle technique may be applied. The aim is to position the needle onto the nerve that is passing dorsally and caudally just above and slightly dorsal to the typical target joint on the superolateral corner of the transverse process. Consequently, the depth of the needle placement is the same as the depth of the transverse process.

With a two-needle technique, the first needle is introduced as for a typical thoracic medial branch block and left in place on the superolateral corner of the transverse process. Following this, a second needle is introduced parallel to the first but aiming at the back of the rib just above the corner of the transverse process. When the second needle touches the rib, it is a sign that it has been introduced more deeply than the first one. At this point, the second needle is withdrawn until its hub is at the same height from the skin as that of the first needle, indicating that its tip lies at the same depth as the back of the transverse process. At this point, local anesthetic injection may be carried out.

Medial Blocks of T11 and T12

Medial branch blocks of T11 and T12 are performed similarly to medial branch blocks of lumbar spine. The target location for the T11 and T12 medial branches is at the junction of the superior articular process and the transverse process that the nerve crosses, midway between the transverse process and the location of the mammillo-accessory notch. On AP imaging, the tip of the needle should be at least in line with the lateral margin of the silhouette of the superior articular process and, if possible, medial to this margin.

RADIOFREQUENCY THERMONEUROLYSIS

Radiofrequency lesioning is performed using either a heat lesion or pulsed mode radiofrequency. A radiofrequency neurotomy lesion for facet denervation is performed at 80 to 85°C. A radiofrequency lesion is performed when the temperature exceeds 45°C. Clinically, a higher temperature allows for a larger lesion to be made. The size of the lesion is influenced by the vascularity of the surrounding tissue. The greater the vascularity of the tissue, the smaller the lesion. Top mode equilibrium is achieved in about 60 seconds. The pulsed mode radiofrequency is an application of a strong electric field to the tissue that surrounds the electrode and the temperature of the tissue surrounding the tip of the electrode, does not exceed 42°C. Essentially, the radiofrequency current is applied in a pulsed fashion and heat is dissipated during the silent period.[35]

The approach and views for radiofrequency thermoneurolysis are the same as described for the medial branch blocks. Once satisfactory needle placement is confirmed via fluoroscopic imaging and contrast injection, the radiofrequency electrode is placed through the needle. Motor testing, injection of local anesthetic, and subsequent lesioning may be performed.

SIDE EFFECTS AND COMPLICATIONS

Complications from facet joint nerve blocks or intra-articular injections in the thoracic spine, though rare, may be serious.[36–50] The most common complications of this technique are twofold. These include complications related to the technique with placement of the needle and complications related to the administration of various drugs. The majority of the problems are short-lived and self-limiting to local swelling and pain at the site of the needle insertion, as well as pain in the upper or mid back. Complications may include pneumothorax, dural puncture, spinal cord trauma, subdural injection, neural trauma, injection into the intervertebral foramen and hematoma formation; infectious complications including epidural abscess and bacterial meningitis; and side effects related to the administration of steroids, local anesthetics, and other drugs.[36–47]

Other minor complications include lightheadedness, flushing, sweating, nausea, hypotension, syncope, pain at the injection site as described earlier, and nonpostural headaches. Side effects related to the administration of steroids are generally attributed to the steroid's chemistry or to the pharmacology of the steroids.[47] The major theoretical complications of corticosteroid administration include suppression of pituitary-adrenal axis, hypocorticism, Cushing syndrome, osteoporosis, avascular necrosis of bone, steroid myopathy, epidural lipomatosis, weight gain, fluid retention, and hypoglycemia. However, Manchikanti et al.[48] in evaluating the effect of neuraxial steroids on weight and bone mass density, showed no significant differences in patients undergoing various types of interventional techniques with or without steroids.

Reported complications of radiofrequency thermoneurolysis include a worsening of the usual pain, burning or dysesthesias, decreased sensation and allodynia in the paravertebral skin or the facets denervated, transient leg pain, persistent leg weakness, and inadvertent lesioning of the spinal nerve or ventral ramus resulting in motor deficits, sensory loss, and possible deafferentation pain.[8–11,35,49,56] A spinal cord lesion can lead to paraplegia, loss of motor, proprioception and sensory function, bowel and bladder dysfunction, Brown-Séquard syndrome, and spinal cord infarction.

CONCLUSION

Thoracic facet joints are identified as the cause of thoracic pain. Thoracic facet joint blocks can be performed in order to test the hypothesis that the target joint is the source of the patient's pain. The rationale for using facet joint blocks for diagnosis, as well as therapy, is based on the facts that thoracic facet joints have been shown to be capable of being a source of thoracic pain and referred pain in the chest; thoracic facet joint pain may not be diagnosed based on referral patterns, physical examination, history, neurophysiologic testing, or radiological evaluation; diagnostic facet joint blocks have been shown to be highly valid and specific; degenerative process of the thoracic spine and the origin of thoracic pain is extremely complex; and the effectiveness of a large variety of therapeutic interventions in managing pain arising from the thoracic spine has not been demonstrated conclusively. Literature evaluating therapeutic facet joint interventions is insufficient at the present time.

REFERENCES

1. Manchikanti, L. et al. (2002). Evaluation of the prevalence of facet joint pain in chronic thoracic pain. *Pain Physician, 5*, 354.

2. Manchikanti, L. et al. (2004). Prevalence of facet joint pain in chronic spinal pain of cervical, thoracic, and lumbar regions. *BioMed Central Musculoskeletal Disorders, 5*, 15.

3. Merskey, H., & Bogduk, N. (1994). *Classification of chronic pain: Descriptions of chronic pain syndromes and definitions of pain terms* (2nd ed.). Seattle: IASP Press.

4. Dreyfuss, P., Tibiletti, C., & Dreyer, S. J. (1994). Thoracic zygapophyseal joint pain patterns: A study in normal volunteers. *Spine, 19*, 807.

5. Dreyfuss, P. et al. (1994). Thoracic zygapophyseal pain: A review and description of an intraarticular block technique. *Pain Digest, 4*, 44.

6. Skubic, J. W., & Kostuik, J. P. (1991). Thoracic pain syndromes and thoracic disc herniation. In J. W. Frymoyer (Ed.), *The adult spine* (p. 1443). New York: Raven Press.

7. Wilson, P. R. (1987). Thoracic facet joint syndrome — A clinical entity? *Pain Supplement, 4*, S87.

8. Stolker, R. J., Vervest, A. C., & Groen, G. J. (1993). Percutaneous facet denervation in chronic thoracic spinal pain. *Acta Neurochirurgia, 122*, 82.

9. Stolker, R. J., Vervest, A. C., & Groen, G. J. (1994). Parameters in electrode positioning in thoracic percutaneous facet denervation: an anatomical study. *Acta Neurochirurgia, 128*, 32.

10. Stolker, R. J., Vervest, A. C., & Groen, G. J. (1994). The treatment of chronic thoracic segmental pain by radiofrequency percutaneous partial rhizotomy. *Journal of Neurosurgery, 80*, 986.

11. Stolker, R. J. et al. (1994). Electrode positioning in thoracic percutaneous partial rhizotomy: An anatomical study. *Pain, 57*, 241.

12. Singer, K. P., & Edmondston, S. J. (2000). Introduction: The enigma of the thoracic spine. In G. F. Giles & K. P. Singer, (Eds.), *Clinical anatomy and management of thoracic spine pain* (p. 3). Boston: Butterworth Heineman.

13. Manchikanti, L., & Pampati, V. (2002). Research designs in interventional pain management: Is randomization superior, desirable or essential? *Pain Physician, 5*, 275.

14. Linton, S. J., Hellsing, A. L., & Hallden, K. (1998). A population based study of spinal pain among 35–45-year old individuals. *Spine, 23*, 1457.

15. Goldthwait, J. E. (1911). The lumbosacral articulation: an explanation of many cases of lumbago, sciatica, and paraplegia. *Boston Medical and Surgical Journal, 164*, 365.

16. Putti, V. (1927). Lady Jones' lecture on new concepts in pathogenesis of sciatic pain. *Lancet, 2*, 53.

17. Hirsch, D., Inglemark, B., & Miller, M. (1963). The anatomical basis for low back pain. *Acta Orthopaedica Scandinavica, 33*, 1.

18. Pawl, R. P. (1977). Headache, cervical spondylosis, and anterior cervical fusion. *Surgery Annual, 9*, 391.

19. Stein, M. et al. (1993). Percutaneous facet joint fusion. Preliminary experiences. *Journal of Vascular and Interventional Radiology, 4*, 69.

20. Maldague, B., Mathurien, P., & Malghern, J. (1981). Facet joint arthrography in lumbar spondylolysis. *Radiology, 140*, 29.

21. Dvorak, J., & Dvorak, V. (1990). *Manual medicine – Diagnostics* (2nd ed.). New York: Thieme Medical Publishers.

22. Schiowitz, S. (1991). Biomechanics of joint motion. In S. DioGiovanna & S. Schiowitz (Eds.), *An osteopathic approach to diagnosis and treatment* (p. 71). Philadelphia: JB Lippincott.

23. Valencia, F. (1988). Biomechanics of the thoracic spine. In R. Grant (Ed.), *Physical therapy of the Cervical and thoracic spine* (p. 27). Edinburgh: Churchill Livingstone.

24. Chua, W. H., & Bogduk, N. (1995). The surgical anatomy of thoracic facet denervation. *Acta Neurochirurgia, 136*, 140.

25. Stolker, R. J et al. (1994). On the innervation of the dorsal compartment of the thoracic spine. In R. J. Stolker, & A. C. Vervest (Eds.), *Pain management by radiofrequency procedures in the cervical and thoracic spine: A clinical and anatomical study* (p. 133). University of Utrecht, Thesis.

26. Kirkaldy-Wills, W. H. et al. (1978). Pathology and pathogenesis of lumbar spondylosis and stenosis. *Spine, 3*, 319.

27. Bogduk, N., & Aprill, C. (1993). On the nature of neck pain, discography, and cervical zygapophyseal joint blocks. *Pain, 54*, 213.

28. Schwarzer, A. C. et al. (1994). The relative contributions of the disc and zygapophyseal joint in chronic low back pain. *Spine, 19*, 801.

29. Van Kleef, M. et al. (1995). Effects of producing a radiofrequency lesion adjacent to the dorsal root ganglion in patients with thoracic segmental pain. *Clinical Journal of Pain, 11*, 325.

30. Bogduk, N. (1997). International Spinal Injection Society guidelines for the performance of spinal injection procedures. Part 1: Zygapophyseal joint blocks. *Clinical Journal of Pain, 13*, 285.

31. Boswell, M. V. et al. (2003). Accuracy of precision diagnostic blocks in the diagnosis of chronic spinal pain of facet or zygapophysial joint origin. *Pain Physician, 6*, 449.

32. Manchikanti, L., & Singh, V. (2002). Diagnostic lumbar facet joint injections. In L. Manchikanti, C. W. Slipman, & B. Fellows (Eds.), *Interventional pain management: Low back pain — Diagnosis and treatment* (p. 239). Padukah, KY: ASIPP Publishing.

33. Raj, P. P. et al. (2004). Bleeding risk in interventional pain practice: assessment, management, and review of the literature. *Pain Physician, 7*, 3.

34. Horlocker, T. T. et al. (2003). Regional anesthesia in the anticoagulated patient: Defining the risks. The second American Society of Regional Anesthesia and Pain Medicine Consensus Conference of Neuraxial Anesthesia and Anticoagulation. *Regional Anesthesia and Pain Medicine, 28*, 163.

35. Curran, M. A. (2002). Lumbosacral facet joint radiofrequency. In L. Manchikanti, C. W. Slipman & B. Fellows (Eds.), *Interventional pain management: Low back pain — Diagnosis and treatment* (p. 463). Paducah, KY: ASIPP Publishing.

36. Dreyfuss, P., Kaplan, M., & Dreyer, S. J. (2000). Zygapophyseal joint injection techniques in the spinal axis. In T. A. Leonard (Ed.), *Pain procedures in clinical practice* (2nd ed., p. 276). Philadelphia: Hanley & Belfus, Inc.

37. Windsor, R. E., Storm, S., & Sugar, R. (2003). Prevention and management of complications resulting from common spinal injections. *Pain Physician, 6,* 473.

38. Windsor, R. E., Pinzon, E. G., & Gore, H. C. (2000). Complications of common selective spinal injections: Prevention and management. *American Journal of Orthopedics, 29,* 759.

39. Gladstone, J. C., & Pennant, J. H. (1987). Spinal anaesthesia following facet joint injection. *Anaesthesia, 42,* 754.

40. Marks, R., & Semple, A. J. (1988). Spinal anaesthesia after facet joint injection. *Anaesthesia, 43,* 65.

41. Cook, N. J., Hanrahan, P., & Song, S. (1999). Paraspinal abscess following facet joint injection. *Clinical Rheumatology, 18,* 52.

42. Magee, M. et al. (2000). Paraspinal abscess complicating facet joint injection. *Clinical Nuclear Medicine, 25,* 71.

43. Manchikanti, L. et al. (2002). Radiation exposure to the physician in interventional pain management. *Pain Physician, 5,* 385.

44. Orpen, N. M., & Birch, N. C. (2003). Delayed presentation of septic arthritis of a lumbar facet joint after diagnostic facet joint injection. *Journal of Spinal Disorders and Techniques, 16,* 285.

45. Manchikanti, L. et al. (2003). Effectiveness of protective measures in reducing risk of radiation exposure in interventional pain management: A prospective evaluation. *Pain Physician, 6,* 301.

46. Berrigan, T. (1992). Chemical meningism after lumbar facet joint block. *Anesthesia, 7,* 905.

47. Manchikanti, L. (2002). Role of neuraxial steroids in interventional pain management. *Pain Physician, 5,* 182.

48. Manchikanti, L. et al. (2000). The effect of neuraxial steroids on weight and bone mass density. A prospective evaluation. *Pain Physician, 3,* 357.

49. Tzaan, W., & Tasker, R. (2000). Percutaneous radiofrequency facet rhizotomy — Experience with 118 procedures and reappraisal of its value. *Canadian Journal of Neurological Sciences, 27,* 125.

50. Hammer, M., & Meneese, W. (1998). Principles and practice of radiofrequency neurolysis. *Current Review of Pain, 2,* 267.

65

Lumbar Facet Joint Interventions

Laxmaiah Manchikanti, MD, David M. Schultz, MD, and Vijay Singh, MD

INTRODUCTION

The prevalence of persistent low back pain due to the involvement of lumbosacral facet joints has been described in controlled studies as varying from 15 to 45% based on types of population and settings studied.[1–17] Even though evidence is lacking for diagnosis of lumbar facet syndrome,[1–21] a preponderance of evidence supports the existence of lumbar facet joint pain.[1–50] However, the existence of facet joint pain has been questioned.[51-57]

As with the epidemiology and clinical significance of facet joint pain, significant controversy surrounds various treatments used in the management of chronic low back pain arising from lumbosacral facet joints. Long-term therapeutic benefit for facet joint pain has been reported with three types of interventions. These include intra-articular injections,[21,25–29,33,38–40] medial branch nerve blocks,[2,30,39–41] and neurolysis of medial branch nerves by means of radiofrequency, chemical neurolysis, or cryo-neurolysis.[41–45,46–50] The long-term therapeutic benefit of intra-articular injections of facet joints is equivocal.[24–29,46] The evidence for long-term benefits of medial branch nerve blocks is preliminary,[2,30,39–41,46] and radiofrequency neurotomy is supported with moderate evidence.[42–49] However, all the treatments have been controversial.

HISTORY

As early as 1911, Goldthwait[58] recognized lumbar facet joints as potential sources of back pain and explained facet joints as a cause of many cases of lumbago, sciatica, and paraplegia. Some 20 years later in 1933, Ghormley[59] coined the term *facet syndrome* and defined it as lumbosacral pain with or without sciatic pain, particularly

occurring suddenly after a twisting or rotatory strain of the lumbosacral region. Further, in 1941, Badgley[60] suggested that facet joints themselves would be a primary source of pain separate from the nerve compression component and made a plea for continuing focus on the facets to explain the large numbers of patients with low back pain whose symptoms were not due to a ruptured disc. Hirsch et al.[61] demonstrated that the low back pain distributed along the sacroiliac and gluteal areas with radiation to the greater trochanter could be induced by injecting hypertonic saline into the region of the facet joints. In subsequent studies, Mooney and Robertson[21] and McCall et al.,[18] using fluoroscopic visualization to confirm the location of intra-articular lumbar facet joint injections in asymptomatic volunteers, demonstrated causation of back and lower extremity pain after injection of hypertonic saline. Marks[22] and Fukui et al.[23] also described the distributions of pain patterns and confirmed the findings of previous researchers. Windsor et al.[62] also confirmed the ability of lumbar facet joints to be a source of pain in the low back. While Mooney and Robertson[21] and McCall et al.[18] showed that the stimulation of the facet joints with injections of hypertonic saline or contrast medium produces back pain and somatic referred pain identical to that commonly seen in patients, Kaplan et al.[36] and Dreyfuss et al.[37] showed that this pain can be relieved by anesthetizing the facet joints responsible for low back pain.

PATHOPHYSIOLOGY

Facet joints have been shown to produce low back pain in normal volunteers. Stimulation of facet joints with injections of hypertonic saline or contrast medium produces back pain and somatic referred pain identical to that commonly seen in patients.[16,18,21–23,62] In addition, this pain can be relieved by anesthetizing the facet joints deemed to be responsible for low back pain.[16,17,21,36,37] Pain originating from facet joints is predominantly present in the low back, buttocks, and thighs; however, it does not follow a reliable segmental pattern.[16–21] Even though radiation of referred pain below the knee as far as the foot has been described,[21] typically pain involves predominantly the proximal parts of the lower extremity. Mooney and Robertson[21] postulated that the distance of radiation of pain is proportional to the intensity of pain in the back.

Even though the prevalence of facet joint pain as a cause of low back pain has been extensively studied, its pathophysiology remains elusive. The lumbar facet joints can be affected by rheumatoid arthritis,[63–65] ankylosing spondylitis,[66] or inferior articular processes epiphyses that are not united.[66–69] It has been repeatedly documented by radiological surveys, as well as by postmortem studies, that the lumbar facet joints are frequently affected by osteoarthritis.[70–74] Further, intraoperative reports excising the facet joints have demonstrated changes similar to that of chondromalacia of the patella.[75] Even though it continues to be stressed that facet joint pain is due to osteoarthritis of facet joints, the evidence from controlled studies has been unable to establish this fact. It also has been shown on plain radiographs that facet joint arthritis appears as commonly in asymptomatic individuals as in patients with back pain.[66–69] Evaluation of facet joint arthritis with computed tomography (CT) scans also revealed the same results; even though CT scans were once hailed as indicative of facet joint pain,[76–78] controlled studies have shown that CT is of no diagnostic value for lumbar facet joint pain.[31] Thus, evidence to date shows that data from radiological evaluation preclude making the diagnosis of pain for facet joint arthropathy on the basis of either plain radiography or CT scanning, and also indicates either that osteoarthritis is not a cause of facet joint pain or that when it is, the pain is due to some factor other than the simple radiological presence of this condition. Further, assertions that facet joint arthritis is usually secondary to disc degeneration or spondylosis[72,79–83] may not be true, as in approximately 20% of the cases facet joint arthritis can be a totally independent disease;[70] correlation between discogenic pain and facet joint pain or a combination of discogenic and facet joint pain has not been established thus far.

Multiple injuries of facet joints have been described in the literature. These include capsular tears, capsular evulsions, subchondral fractures, intra-articular hemorrhage, and fractures of the intra-articular processes in both biomechanical studies and postmortem studies.[67,70,84–95] However, none of these abnormalities was observed on plain radiographs. Even though fractures are visible on CT scans, no such reports exist in the literature with proven painful lumbar facet joint pain.[27] Lesions such as capsular tears cannot be detected by radiography, CT, or magnetic resonance imaging (MRI). Hence, the importance of these lesions, if they are present, is not known. Finally, the theoretical possibility of meniscus entrapment causing low back pain also appears to be only hypothetical, as it is difficult to visualize meniscoids radiologically. However, it may be one of the plausible explanations for some cases of acute low back pain, particularly in those responding to manipulative therapy.[96]

DIAGNOSTIC FACET JOINT BLOCKS

Lumbosacral facet joints can be anesthetized either with intra-articular injections of local anesthetic or by anesthetizing the medial branches of the dorsal rami that innervate the target joint.[16,17] The joint may be considered to be the source of pain if the pain is relieved. However, steps need to be taken to ensure that the observed response is not false-positive. True-positive responses are secured by performing controlled blocks, in the form of either placebo injections of normal saline or comparative local anesthetic blocks, in which the same joint is anesthetized on two separate occasions but using local anesthetics with different duration of action.

The rationale for using lumbosacral facet joint blocks for diagnosis is based on the fact that lumbar facet joints have been shown to be capable of being a source of low back pain and referred pain in the lower limb in normal volunteers. There are no historical or clinical features that are conclusively diagnostic of facet joint pain. There are no reliable clinical means of implicating zygapophysial or facet joints as the source of low back pain in a given patient. Referral patterns described for various joints are not only variable, but also restricted.[16,18,21–23] In addition, many of the other structures in the lumbosacral spine, such as the disc, in the same segment may produce the same pattern of pain. Attempts by multiple investigators to correlate demographic features, pain characteristics, physical findings, and other signs and symptoms with the diagnosis of facet joint pain have been proved to be unreliable.[1–6,16,17,20,31,35,97–99] In addition, imaging technologies provide neither valid nor reliable means of identifying symptomatic lesions.[31,99,100] Thus, in the United States, controlled diagnostic blocks with two separate local anesthetics or placebo-controlled blocks are the only means of confirming diagnosis of facet joint pain. The diagnostic accuracy of controlled local anesthetic facet joint blocks has been reviewed and was determined to be high in the diagnosis of chronic low back pain.[16,17,101]

The face validity of intra-articular injections or medial branch blocks is established by injecting small volumes of local anesthetic into the joint or onto the target points of the nerve.[37] Further, construct validity of facet joint blocks is also extremely important, as placebo effect is the single greatest confounder of diagnostic blocks. The theory that testing a patient first with lidocaine and subsequently with bupivacaine provides a means of identifying placebo response has been tested and proven.[102–106] The specificity of controlled diagnostic blocks has been demonstrated in multiple controlled trials. Provocation response was shown to be unreliable.[98] The false-negative rate of diagnostic facet joint blocks was shown to be around 8% due to unrecognized intravascular injection of local anesthetic.[37] Confounding psychological factors also were shown to have lack of influence on the validity of comparative, controlled diagnostic local anesthetic blocks of facet joints in the lumbar spine.[11] False-positive rates as evaluated in multiple investigations were reported to be 22 to 47% in lumbar spine.[2–17,107]

The indications and contraindications for diagnostic facet joint blocks are listed in Tables 65.1 and 65.2.[108]

TABLE 65.1
Common Indications for Lumbar Diagnostic Facet Joint Blocks

- Somatic or nonradicular low back and/or lower extremity pain
- Lack of evidence, either for discogenic or sacroiliac joint pain
- Lack of disc herniation or evidence of radiculitis
- Duration of pain of at least 3 months
- Failure to respond to more conservative management, including physical therapy modalities with exercises, chiropractic management, and nonsteroidal anti-inflammatory agents
- Average pain levels of greater than 5 on a scale of 1 to 10
- Intermittent or continuous pain causing functional disability
- No contraindications with understanding of consent, nature of the procedure, needle placement, or sedation
- No history of allergy to contrast administration, local anesthetic steroids, Sarapin, or other drugs potentially utilized
- Negative provocative discography and sacroiliac joint blocks
- Contraindications or inability to undergo physical therapy, chiropractic management, or inability to tolerate nonsteroidal anti-inflammatory drugs

---

TABLE 65.2
Common Contraindications for Lumbosacral Facet Joint Blocks

- Infection
- Inability of the patient to understand consent, nature of the procedure, needle placement, or sedation
- Allergies to contrast, local anesthetic, steroids, Sarapin, or other drugs
- Needle phobia
- Psychogenic pain
- Suspected discogenic, sacroiliac joint, or myofascial pain
- Pregnancy
- Anticoagulant therapy
- Non-aspirin antiplatelet therapy
- Bleeding diathesis

Contraindications are quite obvious and include bacterial infection, possible pregnancy, and bleeding diathesis. Relative contraindications include allergy to contrast media or local anesthetics and treatment with non-aspirin antiplatelet drugs, which may compromise coagulation. Raj et al.[109] provides a detailed description on the role of anticoagulants in interventional pain management. Even then, there is no consensus as to the importance of discontinuation of aspirin before lumbar facet joint injection procedures. Patients on warfarin therapy should be checked for prothrombin time (PT), and it should be at acceptable levels.

THERAPEUTIC FACET JOINT INTERVENTIONS

There is a paucity of literature on the role of therapeutic facet joint blocks. However, facet joint pain may be managed by either intra-articular injections or medial branch blocks, in addition to neurolysis of medial branches.

Therapeutic benefit has been reported with the injection of corticosteroids, local anesthetics, or normal saline into the facet joints. The literature describing the effectiveness of these interventions is abundant. Manchikanti et al.,[46] in developing evidence-based practice guidelines for interventional techniques in managing chronic spinal pain, reviewed the available literature which included four randomized clinical trials[24,28,39,40] and multiple nonrandomized and observational reports.[26,27,29,32] Based on the definition of short-term relief as relief of less than 3 months and long-term relief as relief of 3 months or longer, the only randomized trial[24] meeting the inclusion criteria showed positive results at 6 months; however, authors of this study, Carette et al.,[24] described it as negative. Among the nonrandomized trials, positive results were noted for short-term relief in all the studies, whereas long-term relief was noted in only three of the five studies. Thus, Manchikanti et al.[46] conclude that the evidence of intra-articular injections of local anesthetics and steroids from randomized trials, complemented with that of nonrandomized trials (prospective and retrospective evaluations), provided moderate evidence of short-term relief and limited evidence of long-term relief of chronic low back pain.

Medial branch blocks have been extensively used for diagnostic and prognostic purposes with limited use for therapeutic purposes. The therapeutic role of medial branch blocks was evaluated in three randomized clinical trials,[30,39,40] and one nonrandomized clinical trial.[2] Based on the definition (short-term < 3 months and ≥ 3 months long-term) with one randomized trial and one nonrandomized evaluation, evidence for medial branch blocks appears to be strong for short-term relief and moderate for long-term relief of pain of lumbar facet joint origin. Indications and contraindications for therapeutic lumbar facet joint blocks are the same as for diagnostic blocks except that a negative response to diagnostic facet joint blocks is a contraindication for therapeutic facet joint blocks.

Multiple investigators have studied the effectiveness of radiofrequency denervation of medial branches in the lumbar spine. Percutaneous radiofrequency neurotomy is a procedure that offers temporary relief of pain by denaturing the nerves that innervate the painful joint. However, pain may return when the axons regenerate. At this time, the procedure may need to be repeated to reinstate the relief. Radiofrequency neurolysis as a treatment of chronic intractable pain began in the early 1930s. Multiple systematic reviews have been performed recently[30,46–49] with controversial results. While Geurts et al.[47] and Niemistö et al.[49] showed that radiofrequency was not effective, Manchikanti et al.[48] in a systematic review showed that there may be strong evidence that radiofrequency denervation offers short-term relief and moderate evidence of long-term relief of chronic low back pain. These conclusions were based on the studies by Van Kleef et al.[43] and Dreyfuss et al.[42]

ANATOMIC CONSIDERATIONS

The lumbar facet joints are formed by the articulation of the inferior articular processes of one lumbar vertebra with the superior articular processes of the subjacent vertebra. The joints exhibit the features typical of synovial joints. The articular facets are covered by articular cartilage, and a synovial membrane bridges the margins of the articular cartilages of the two facets in each joint.[128] Surrounding the synovial membrane is a joint capsule that attaches to the articular processes a short distance beyond the margin of the articular cartilage.

Histological studies have shown that capsules of the lumbar facet joints are richly innervated with encapsulated, unencapsulated, and free nerve endings.[110–113]

The medial branches are of paramount clinical importance and relevance because of their distribution to the facet joints. The medial branches of the L1–L4 dorsal rami run across the top of their respective transverse processes and pierce the dorsal leaf of the intertransverse ligament at the base of the transverse process.[111] Subsequently, each nerve runs along bone at the junction of the root of the transverse process with the root of the superior articular process hooking medially around the base of the superior articular process, which is covered by the mamillo-accessory ligament. Finally, the nerve crosses the vertebral lamina, where it divides into multiple branches that supply the multifidus muscle, the interspinous muscle and ligament, and two facet joints. Thus, each medial branch supplies the facet joints above and below its course.[36,37,111,112,114,115] Two articular branches in an ascending and a descending branch arise from the nerve, the ascending branch arising from the nerve just beyond the mamillo-accessory ligament where the nerve starts to cross the lamina, in contrast

to the descending articular branch, which arises slightly more distally and courses downward to the joint below. The medial branch of the L5 dorsal ramus has a different course and distribution than those of the L1–L4 dorsal rami in that instead of crossing a transverse process, it crosses the ala of the sacrum. Thus, the medial branch of the L5 dorsal ramus runs in the groove formed by the junction of the ala and the root of the superior articular process of the sacrum before hooking medially around the base of the lumbosacral facet joint.[111] The medial branch of the L5 dorsal ramus sends an articular branch to the facet joint before ramifying in multifidus.

TECHNIQUE

LUMBAR FACET JOINT INTRA-ARTICULAR INJECTIONS

The patient is placed in a prone position on the fluoroscopy table. A towel roll or pillow can be placed under the abdomen to distract the intended facet joint. This may allow for an easier entry into the joint. The target area is then prepped and draped in a sterile manner. The fluoroscopy beam is then rotated to gain an anterior-posterior view of the target facet joint. This view is most commonly used in the upper lumbar facet joints secondary to their sagittal plane alignment. An oblique view may be required for optimal visualization of the lower lumbar segments due to their more frontal plane orientation.[116] The target joint is then visualized under fluoroscopic guidance and the skin entry point is identified.

A skin wheal with 1 mL of 1% lidocaine is then raised at the site of entry. Care is taken not to infiltrate the deep subcutaneous area overlying the target site. Diffusion of this anesthetic could possibly cause a false-positive response to the zygapophysial joint injection. A 22- to 25-gauge, 3.5-in. spinal needle is then inserted through the anesthetized area. The needle is directed down toward the selected joint under direct fluoroscopic visualization. Contact is made with the inferior articular processes. This confirms the depth of the needle. The needle is then withdrawn slightly and redirected to enter the target facet joint. As the needle is felt to penetrate the joint, advancement is stopped to prevent any potential articular cartilage damage. If there is difficulty in obtaining capsular penetration, then one may try to access the articular recesses by redirection of the needle just off the margins of the inferior articular processes. Another method of gaining intracapsular entry is to redirect the needle slightly medially or laterally to the posterior joint line so the needle gains access via its medial placement to the insertion of the capsule on the articular process.[32] Once the needle is in an appropriate position, 0.2 to 0.5 mL of contrast is then injected into the joint to confirm proper placement. An arthrographic image should then be visualized.[117] During contrast injection, lack of vascular flow and no epidural

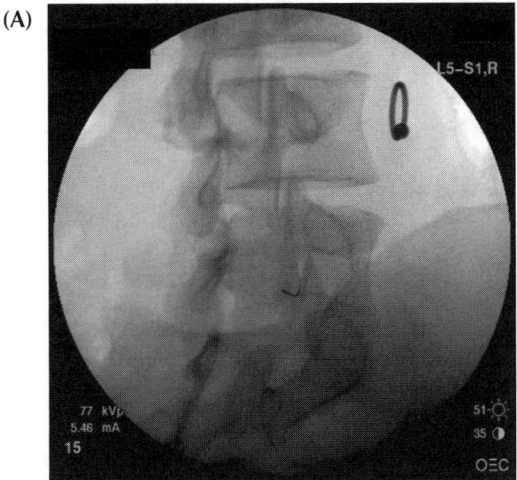

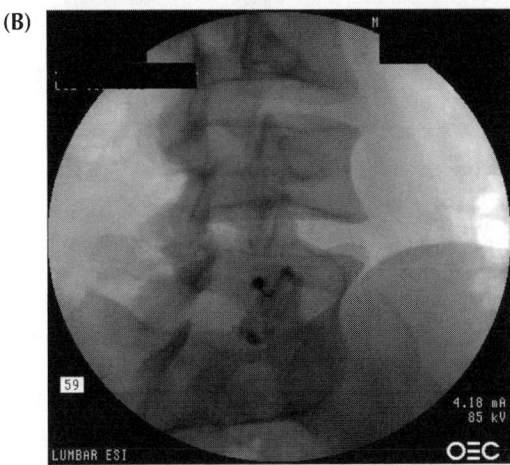

FIGURE 65.1 (A) 25-gauge spinal needle curving into L5–S1 facet joint. (B) L5–S1 arthrogram.

spread should be observed. After confirmation of placement with contrast, the joint is injected with anesthetic agent to complete a diagnostic block or in combination with a steroid agent for a therapeutic zygapophysial joint injection.[32,117] Figure 65.1 illustrates intra-articular placement of needles and injection of contrast.

MEDIAL BRANCH BLOCKS

To block the nerves supplying a lumbar facet joint, two medial branch blocks are necessary due to its dual innervation. Table 65.3 illustrates the nerves to be blocked for each facet joint in the lumbar region. It is extremely simple to remember to block a particular joint. The medial branch at the transverse process at the same level and the level below must be blocked. Thus, to block the L3/4 facet joint, two medial branches need to be blocked, which include the L2 medial branch at the transverse process of L3 and the L3 medial branch at the transverse process of L4. Similarly, to block the L5/S1 facet joint, the L4 medial branch at the L5 transverse process and the L5 dorsal

ramus at the sacral ala must be blocked. For the L5/S1 facet joint, it has been suggested that a communicating branch from the dorsal ramus of the S1 may provide additional supply, which may be blocked just above the exit from the S1 posterior foramina.[117] However, it has been suggested that blockade of the L4 medial branch and the L5 dorsal ramus alone adequately anesthetizes the L5/S1 facet joint from an experimental stimulus without the need for anesthetization of a potential ascending branch from S1.[36]

L1 to L4 Medial Branch Blocks

The nerves should be blocked proximal to the mamillo-accessory ligament and notch for L1–L4 medial branch blocks.[37] Dreyfuss et al.[37] described that the target location for the L1–L4 medial branch is at the junction of the superior articular process and the transverse process that the nerve crosses, midway between the superior border of the transverse process and the location of the mamillo-accessory notch. Dreyfuss et al.[37] believed that this point is not associated with an inadvertent spread of injectate into the intervertebral foramen or epidural space for L1–L4 medial branch blocks. They also described that on oblique views, the target point lies high on the "eye" of the "Scottie dog." Placement more superior at the most superior junction of the superior articular process and transverse process as previously recommended apparently leads to an unacceptable incidence of spread into the foramen. Dreyfuss et al.[37] validated a slight superior-to-inferior and lateral-to-medial needle approach to medial branch blocks. However, if an inferior-to-superior needle approach is used, the injected anesthetic theoretically may spread toward the spinal nerve root or the sinuvertebral nerve, thereby substantially decreasing the specificity of the block. For all medial branch blocks a 22- or 25-gauge spinal needle may be used.

The procedure is performed, generally, with the patient in the prone position. The C-arm must be adjusted either straight anteroposterior or oblique position from the skin entry point laterally using anteroposterior imaging, which is usually just above the tip of the target transverse process. The needle is advanced toward the back of the root of the transverse process to ensure safe needle depth away from the ventral ramus. However, it can also be achieved in an oblique view. Using an oblique view with a "Scottie dog," the needle is advanced "down the beam" toward the target using a slightly superior starting position to the final target. To maximally visualize the landmarks of the "Scottie dog," approximately a 25° to 30° angle is necessary based on the level of the injection from L1–L4 medial block(s). Thus, the needle will be directed anterior, medial, and caudad to reach the target location. However, if this is started in an oblique position, switching to an anteroposterior view is necessary to ensure that the needle

TABLE 65.3
Facet Joint Nerves Required to Be Blocked for Each Facet Joint in Lumbar Region

Facet joint	Facet Joint Nerves to be Blocked (medial branches or L5 dorsal ramus)	Level of Transverse Process or Sacral Ala
L1/2	T12 and L1 medial branches	At L1 transverse process for T12
		At L2 transverse process for L1
L2/3	L1 and L2 medial branches	At L2 transverse process for L1
		At L3 transverse process for L2
L3/4	L2 and L3 medial branches	At L3 transverse process for L2
		At L4 transverse process for L3
L4/5	L3 and L4 medial branches	At L4 transverse process for L3
		At L5 transverse process for L4
L5/S1	L4 medial branch L5 dorsal ramus	At L5 transverse process for L4 medial branch at sacral ala groove for L5 dorsal ramus

is placed medial enough despite contact on the oblique view, and an oblique view is necessary to ensure needle placement on the target if the needle is initially advanced on anteroposterior imaging.

L5 Dorsal Ramus Blocks

The target point for the L5 dorsal ramus is at the junction of the ala of the sacrum with the superior articular process of the sacrum. This target point is recognized as a notch between these two bones with a minor amount of ipsilateral obliquity. The target point lies opposite the middle of the base of the superior articular process and thus slightly below the silhouette at the top of the sacral ala. Higher placement is associated with spread into the L5/S1 epidural space and lower placement with spread to the S1 posterior sacral foramen.

For L5 dorsal ramus block, an approximately 10 to 15° oblique view can be helpful to optimally visualize the junction of the sacral ala and the superior articular process of S1. Further obliquity usually places the medial iliac crest in front of the trajectory to the target position. The needle is advanced directly down the beam to the target position on slight oblique imaging. Anteroposterior imaging is then obtained to verify that the needle is placed at or preferably medial to the lateral silhouette of the S1 superior articular process. After the needle is in the proper location, the bevel opening should be medial. This has been shown to reduce inadvertent spread to the S1 posterior foramen or the L5 vertebral foramen.[36,117] Figure 65.2 illustrates the technique of medial branch blocks under fluoroscopy.

Local anesthetic injection should be limited to 0.4 to 0.6 mL for a diagnostic block and approximately 1 mL for a therapeutic block. Dreyfuss et al.[37,117] recommend potent local anesthetics, e.g., 4% lidocaine and 0.75% bupivacaine, to minimize the risk of false-negative medial branch blocks, which can occur at a 10% rate with 2% lidocaine. Kaplan et al.[36] describes that failure to obtain relief with lumbar medial branch blocks in a case in which venous uptake of contrast is observed, despite needle redirection with avoidance of subsequent venous uptake, carries a 50% risk for false-negative results.

For diagnostic, as well as therapeutic blocks, the literature has been limited to using local anesthetic agents of different durations of action, namely, lidocaine and bupivacaine. However, Manchikanti et al.[1] have shown the validity of diagnostic blocks is maintained with addition of adjuvant agents such as Sarapin and methylprednisolone, along with provision of a therapeutic benefit much longer than the local anesthetic alone. In addition, in multiple investigations, Manchikanti et al.[2,4–15] utilized concentrations of lidocaine of 1% and bupivacaine of 0.25% rather than 4% lidocaine and 0.75% bupivacaine, as recommended by others.

MEDIAL BRANCH NEUROTOMY

Radiofrequency lesioning is performed using either a heat lesion or pulsed mode radiofrequency. A thermal radiofrequency neurotomy lesion for facet denervation is performed at 80 to 85°C. A radiofrequency lesion is performed when the temperature exceeds 45°C. Clinically, a higher temperature allows for a larger lesion to be made. The size of the lesion is influenced by the vascularity of the surrounding tissue. The greater the vascularity of the tissue, the smaller the lesion. Top mode equilibrium is achieved in about 60 seconds. The pulsed mode radiofrequency is an application of a strong electric field to the tissue that surrounds the electrode and the temperature of the tissue surrounding the tip of the electrode does not exceed 42°C. Essentially, the radiofrequency current is applied in a pulsed fashion and heat is dissipated during the silent period.[118]

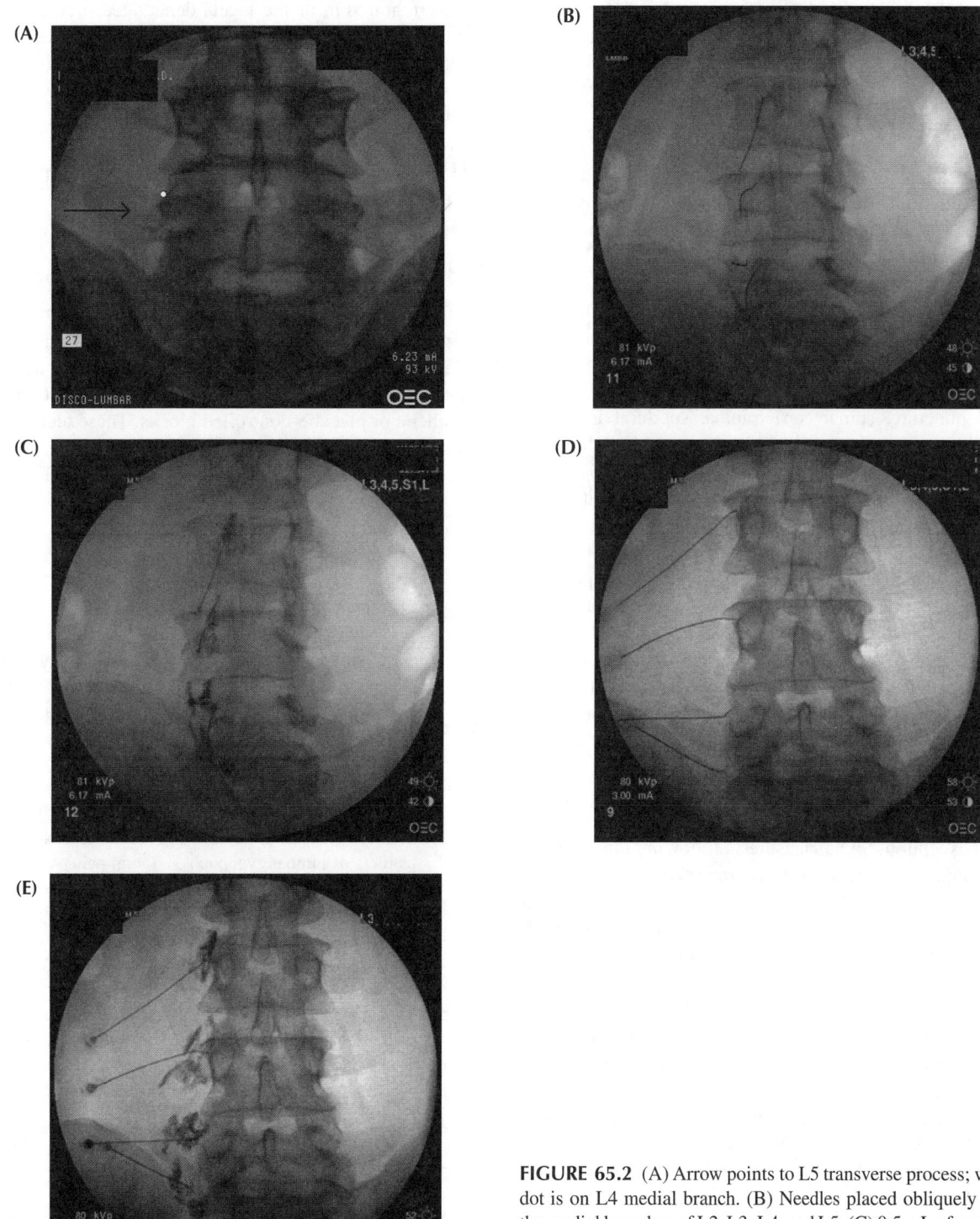

FIGURE 65.2 (A) Arrow points to L5 transverse process; white dot is on L4 medial branch. (B) Needles placed obliquely onto the medial branches of L2, L3, L4, and L5. (C) 0.5 mL of contrast injected, oblique view. (D) Needle placement for medial branch blocks in PA view. (E) 0.5 mL of contrast injected, PA view.

The patient is placed in a prone position. Appropriate preparation is performed. Following this, under fluoroscopic visualization in a posteroanterior (PA) view or oblique view, needles are positioned similarly to the descriptions of the medial branch blocks. For radiofrequency thermoneurolysis, the cannula is placed along the course of the medial branch or at the L5 level on the posterior primary ramus. A larger interruption of the nerve is made if the lesion is made parallel to the nerve, that is, along the course of the nerve, rather than placing the cannula more at a tangent to the nerve.[118] Theoretically, a larger lesion of the nerve allows for a prolonged and improved pain relief. However, for pulsed radiofrequency, the needles may be positioned in a fashion similar to medial branch blocks.

SIDE EFFECTS AND COMPLICATIONS

Complications from facet joint nerve blocks or intra-articular injections in the lumbar spine are exceedingly rare.[42,43,117–127] However, the two most common complications of this technique include complications related to the technique with placement of the needle and complications related to the administration of various drugs. The majority of the problems are short-lived and self-limiting to local swelling and pain at the site of the needle insertion, as well as pain in the low back. Complications may include dural puncture, spinal cord trauma, subdural injection, neural trauma, injection into the intervertebral foramen and hematoma formation; infectious complications including epidural abscess and bacterial meningitis; and side effects related to the administration of steroids, local anesthetics, and other drugs.[119–127] Thompson et al.[126] reported instances of chemical meningism from penetration of the dural cuff leading to subarachnoid entry with two level facet joint injections and a one level medial branch block. However, large volumes of injectate were used and the descriptions of the needle placement and contrast flow under fluoroscopic imaging prior to injection were not discussed. Berrigan[125] also reported chemical meningism. With the use of fluoroscopy alone or fluoroscopy and contrast, damage to a spinal nerve root or needle placement into the epidural or subarachnoid spaces should be an exception. Spinal anesthesia following lumbar facet joint injections also has been reported.[120,121] Infection associated with facet joint injections has been reported.[119,123,125] Facet capsule rupture may occur, with large volumes of injectate, leading to diagnostic and therapeutic uncertainty.

Other minor complications include lightheadedness, flushing, sweating, nausea, hypotension, syncope, pain at the injection site as described earlier, and nonpostural headaches. Side effects related to the administration of steroids are generally attributed to the steroid's chemistry or to the pharmacology of the steroids.[127] The major theoretical complications of corticosteroid administration include suppression of pituitary-adrenal axis, hypocorticism, Cushing syndrome, osteoporosis, avascular necrosis of bone, steroid myopathy, epidural lipomatosis, weight gain, fluid retention, and hypoglycemia. However, Manchikanti et al.,[128] in evaluating the effect of neuraxial steroids on weight and bone mass density, showed no significant differences in patients undergoing various types of interventional techniques with or without steroids.

Reported complications of radiofrequency thermoneurolysis include a worsening of the usual pain, burning or dysesthesias, decreased sensation and allodynia in the paravertebral skin or the facets denervated, transient leg pain, persistent leg weakness, and inadvertent lesioning of the spinal nerve or ventral ramus resulting in motor deficits, sensory loss, and possible deafferentation pain.[42,43,118] A spinal cord lesion can lead to paraplegia, loss of motor, proprioception, and sensory function, bowel and bladder dysfunction, Brown-Séquard syndrome, and spinal cord infarction.

CONCLUSION

Lumbar facet joints are sources of local and referred pain in approximately 40% of patients with low back and lower extremity pain. The definitive diagnosis of facet joint pain relies on properly performed, controlled, diagnostic local anesthetic or placebo-controlled blocks. These techniques maintain an important diagnostic and potentially therapeutic role in the management of low back pain and should not be performed in isolation but rather in the context of other diagnostic and therapeutic methodology.

REFERENCES

1. Schwarzer, A. C. et al. (1994). Clinical features of patients with pain stemming from the lumbar zygapophysial joints. Is the lumbar facet syndrome a clinical entity? *Spine, 19*, 1132.
2. Manchikanti, L. et al. (2000). The diagnostic validity and therapeutic value of medial branch blocks with or without adjuvants. *Current Review of Pain, 4*, 337.
3. Schwarzer, A. C. et al. (1995). Prevalence and clinical features of lumbar zygapophysial joint pain. A study in an Australian population with chronic low back pain. *Annals of the Rheumatic Diseases, 54*, 100.
4. Manchikanti, L. et al. (2000). The inability of the clinical picture to characterize pain from facet joints. *Pain Physician, 3*, 158.
5. Manchikanti, L. et al. (1999). Prevalence of facet joint pain in chronic low back pain. *Pain Physician, 2*, 59.
6. Manchikanti, L. (1999). Facet joint pain and the role of neural blockade in its management. *Current Review of Pain, 3*, 348.
7. Manchikanti, L. et al. (2001). Evaluation of the relative contributions of various structures in chronic low back pain. *Pain Physician, 4*, 308.
8. Manchikanti, L. et al. (2001). Evaluation of the role of facet joints in persistent low back pain in obesity: A controlled, prospective, comparative evaluation. *Pain Physician, 4*, 266.
9. Manchikanti, L. et al. (2001). Contribution of facet joints to chronic low back pain in postlumbar laminectomy syndrome: a controlled comparative prevalence evaluation. *Pain Physician, 4*, 175.
10. Manchikanti, L. et al. (2001). Role of facet joints in chronic low back pain in the elderly: A controlled comparative prevalence study. *Pain Practice, 1*, 332.

11. Manchikanti, L. et al. (2001). Influence of psychological factors on the ability to diagnose chronic low back pain of facet joint origin. *Pain Physician, 4,* 349.

12. Manchikanti, L. et al. (2002). Evaluation of influence of gender, occupational injury and smoking on chronic low back pain of facet joint origin. *Pain Physician, 5,* 30.

13. Manchikanti, L. et al. (2002). Is there correlation of facet joint pain in lumbar and cervical spine? An evaluation of prevalence in combined chronic low back and neck pain. *Pain Physician, 5,* 365.

14. Manchikanti, L., Hirsch, J. A., & Pampati, V. (2003). Chronic low back pain of facet (zygapophysial) joint origin: is there a difference based on involvement of single or multiple spinal regions? *Pain Physician, 6,* 399.

15. Manchikanti, L., Boswell, M. V., Singh, V., Pampati, V., Damron, K. S., & Beyer C. D. (2004). Prevalence of facet joint pain in chronic spinal pain of cervical, thoracic, and lumbar regions. *BioMed Central Musculoskeletal Disorders, 5,* 15.

16. Bogduk, N. (1997). International spinal injection society guidelines for the performance of spinal injection procedures. Part 1. Zygapophysial joint blocks. *Clinical Journal of Pain, 13,* 285.

17. Boswell, M. V. et al. (2003). Accuracy of precision diagnostic blocks in the diagnosis of chronic spinal pain of facet or zygapophysial joint origin. *Pain Physician, 6,* 449.

18. McCall, I. W., Park, W. M., & O'Brien, J. P. (1979). Induced pain referral from posterior elements in normal subjects. *Spine, 4,* 441.

19. Dreyfuss, P. H., & Dreyer, S. J. (2003). Lumbar zygapophysial (facet) joint injections. *Spine Journal, 3,* 50S.

20. Schwarzer, A. C. et al. (1994). Pain from the lumbar zygapophysial joint. A test of two models. *Journal of Spinal Disorders, 7,* 331.

21. Mooney, V., & Robertson, J. (1976). The facet syndrome. *Clinical Orthopedics, 115,* 149.

22. Marks, R. (1989). Distribution of pain provoked from lumbar facet joints and related structures during diagnostic spinal infiltration. *Pain, 39,* 37.

23. Fukui, S. et al. (1997). Distribution of referral pain from the lumbar zygapophyseal joints and dorsal rami. *Clinical Journal of Pain, 13,* 303.

24. Carette, S. et al. (1991). A controlled trial of corticosteroid injections into facet joints for chronic low back pain. *New England Journal of Medicine, 325,* 1002.

25. Murtagh, F. R. (1988). Computed tomography and fluoroscopy guided anesthesia and steroid injection in facet syndrome. *Spine, 13,* 686.

26. Lau, L. S., Littlejohn, G. O., & Miller, M. H. (1985). Clinical evaluation of intra-articular injections for lumbar facet joint pain. *Medical Journal of Australia, 143,* 563.

27. Lippitt, A. B. (1984). The facet joint and its role in spine pain. Management with facet joint injections. *Spine, 9,* 746.

28. Lilius, G. et al. (1989). Lumbar facet joint syndrome. A randomized clinical trial. *Journal of Bone and Joint Surgery* (Britain), *71,* 681.

29. Lynch, M. C., & Taylor, J. F. (1986). Facet joint injection for low back pain. A clinical study. *Journal of Bone and Joint Surgery* (Britain), *68,* 138.

30. Manchikanti, L. et al. (2001). Effectiveness of lumbar facet joint nerve blocks in chronic low back pain: A randomized clinical trial. *Pain Physician, 4,* 101.

31. Schwarzer, A. C. et al. (1995). The ability of computed tomography to identify a painful zygapophysial joint in patients with chronic low back pain. *Spine, 20,* 907.

32. Destouet, J. M., Gilula, L. A., & Murphy, W. A. (1982). Lumbar facet joint injection: indication, technique, clinical correlation and preliminary results. *Radiology, 145,* 321.

33. Helbig, T., & Lee, C. K. (1988). The lumbar facet syndrome. *Spine, 13,* 61.

34. Revel, M. E. et al. (1992). Facet joint block for low back pain. Identifying predictors of a good response. *Archives of Physical and Medical Rehabilitation, 73,* 824.

35. Revel, M. et al. (1998). Capacity of the clinical picture to characterize low back pain relieved by facet joint anesthesia. Proposed criteria to identify patients with painful facet joints. *Spine, 23,* 1972.

36. Kaplan, M. et al. (1998). The ability of lumbar medial branch blocks to anesthetize the zygapophysial joint. *Spine, 23,* 1847.

37. Dreyfuss, P. et al. (1997). Specificity of lumbar medial branch and L5 dorsal ramus blocks: A computed tomography study. *Spine, 22,* 895.

38. Carrera, G. F. (1980). Lumbar facet joint injection in low back pain and sciatica: Preliminary results. *Radiology, 137,* 665.

39. Marks, R. C., Houston, T., & Thulbourne, T. (1992). Facet joint injection and facet nerve block: A randomized comparison in 86 patients with chronic low back pain. *Pain, 49,* 325.

40. Nash, T. P. (1990). Facet joints: Intra-articular steroids or nerve blocks? *Pain Clinic, 3,* 77.

41. North, R. B. et al. (1994). Radiofrequency lumbar facet denervation: analysis of prognostic factors. *Pain, 57,* 77.

42. Dreyfuss, P. et al. (2000). Efficacy and validity of radiofrequency neurotomy for chronic lumbar zygapophysial joint pain. *Spine, 25,* 1270.

43. Van Kleef, M. et al. (1999). Randomized trial of radiofrequency lumbar facet denervation for chronic low back pain. *Spine, 24,* 1937.

44. Gallagher, J., Vadi, P. L. P., & Wesley, J. R. (1994). Radiofrequency facet joint denervation in the treatment of low back pain: a prospective controlled double-blind study to assess efficacy. *Pain Clinic, 7,* 193.

45. Leclare, R. et al. (2001). Radiofrequency facet joint denervation in the treatment of low back pain. *Spine, 26,* 1411.

46. Manchikanti, L. et al. (2003). Evidence-based practice guidelines for interventional techniques in the management of chronic spinal pain. *Pain Physician, 6,* 3.

47. Geurts, J. W. et al. (2001). Efficacy of radiofrequency procedures for the treatment of spinal pain: A systematic review of randomized clinical trials. *Regional Anesthesia and Pain Medicine, 26,* 394.

48. Manchikanti, L. et al. (2002). Medial branch neurotomy in management of chronic spinal pain: Systematic review of the evidence. *Pain Physician, 5*, 405.

49. Niemistö, L. et al. (2003). Radiofrequency denervation for neck and back pain: A systematic review within the framework of the Cochrane Collaboration Back Review Group. *Spine, 28*, 1877.

50. Bogduk, N. (2002). In defense of radiofrequency neurotomy [Letter to the editor]. *Regional Anesthesia and Pain Medicine, 27*, 439.

51. Jackson, R. P., Jacobs, R. R., & Montesano, P. X. (1988). Facet joint injection in low back pain. A prospective study. *Spine, 13*, 966.

52. Deyo, R. A. (1991). Fads in the treatment of low back pain. *New England Journal of Medicine, 325*, 1038.

53. Jackson, R. P. (1992). The facet syndrome. Myth or reality? *Clinical Orthopedics, 279*, 110.

54. Nachemson, A. L. (1992). Newest knowledge of low back pain. A critical look. *Clinical Orthopedics, 279*, 8.

55. Nachemson, A. L., & Vingard, E. (2000). Assessment of patients with neck and back pain: A best-evidence synthesis. In A. L. Nachemson & E. Jonsson (Eds.), *Neck and back pain. The scientific evidence of causes, diagnosis and treatment* (p. 189). New York: Lippincott Williams & Wilkins.

56. Ramsey, S. D. et al. (1998). The limited state of technology assessment for medical devises: Facing the issues. *American Journal of Managed Care, 4*, 188.

57. Nelemans, P. J. et al. (2001). Injection therapy for subacute and chronic benign low back pain. *Spine, 26*, 501.

58. Goldthwait, J. E. (1911). The lumbosacral articulation: An explanation of many cases of lumbago, sciatica, and paraplegia. *Boston Medical and Surgical Journal, 164*, 365.

59. Ghormley, R. K. (1933). Low back pain. With special reference to the articular facets, with presentation of an operative procedure. *Journal of the American Medical Association, 101*, 1773.

60. Badgley, C. E. (1941). The articular facets in relation to low back pain and sciatic radiation. *Journal of Bone and Joint Surgery, 23*, 481.

61. Hirsch, D., Inglemark, B., & Miller, M. (1963). The anatomical basis for low back pain. *Acta Orthopaedica Scandinavica, 33*, 1.

62. Windsor, R. E. et al. (2002). Electrical stimulation induced lumbar medial branch referral patterns. *Pain Physician, 5*, 347.

63. Jayson, M. I. V. (1976). Degenerative disease of the spine and back pain. *Clinical Rheumatic Diseases, 2*, 557.

64. Lawrence, J. S., Sharpe, J., & Ball, J. (1964). Rheumatoid arthritis of the lumbar spine. *Annals of the Rheumatic Diseases, 23*, 205.

65. Sims-Williams, H., Jason, M. I. V., & Baddeley, H. (1977). Rheumatoid involvement of the lumbar spine. *Annals of the Rheumatic Diseases, 36*, 524.

66. Ball, J. (1971). Enthesopathy of rheumatoid and ankylosing spondylitis. *Annals of the Rheumatic Diseases, 30*, 213.

67. Bailey, W. (1937). Anomalies and fractures of the vertebral articular processes, *Journal of the American Medical Association, 108*, 266.

68. Fulton, W. S., & Kalbfleisch, W. K. (1934). Accessory articular processes of the lumbar vertebrae. *Archives of Surgery, 29*, 42.

69. King, A. B. (1955). Back pain due to loose facets of the lower lumbar vertebrae. *Bulletin of Johns Hopkins Hospital, 97*, 271.

70. Lewin, T. (1964). Osteoarthritis in lumbar synovial joints. *Acta Orthopaedica Scandinavica, 73*, 1.

71. Shore, L. R. (1935). On osteo-arthritis in the dorsal intervertebral joints: A study in morbid anatomy. *British Journal of Surgery, 22*, 833.

72. Vernon-Roberts, B., & Pirie, C. J. (1977). Degenerative changes in the intervertebral discs of the lumbar spine and their sequelae. *Rheumatology and Rehabilitation, 16*, 13.

73. Lawrence, J. S., Bremner, J. M., & Bier, F. (1966). Osteoarthrosis: Prevalence in the population and relationship between symptoms and X-ray changes. *Annals of the Rheumatic Diseases, 25*, 1.

74. Magora, A., & Schwartz, A. (1976). Relation between the low back pain syndrome and x-ray findings. 1. Degenerative osteoarthritis. *Scandinavian Journal of Rehabilitation Medicine, 8*, 115.

75. Eisenstein, S. M., & Parry, C. R. (1987). The lumbar facet arthrosis syndrome. *Journal of Bone and Joint Surgery* (Britain), *69B*, 3.

76. Abel, M. S. (1984). The radiology of low back pain associated with posterior element lesions of the lumbar spine. *CRC Critical Reviews in Diagnostic Imaging, 20*, 311.

77. Carrera, G. F., & Williams, A. L. (1984). Current concepts in evaluation of the lumbar facet joints. *CRC Critical Reviews in Diagnostic Imaging, 21*, 85.

78. Hermanus, N. et al. (1983). The use of CT scanning for the study of posterior lumbar intervertebral articulations. *Neuroradiology, 24*, 159.

79. Kirkaldy-Willis, W. H. et al. (1978). Pathology and pathogenesis of lumbar spondylosis and stenosis. *Spine, 3*, 319.

80. Fujiwara, A. et al. (1999). The relationship between facet joint osteoarthritis and disc degeneration of the lumbar spine: An MRI study. *European Spine Journal, 8*, 396.

81. Fujiwara, A., Tamai, K., & An, H. S. (2000). The relationship between disc degeneration, facet joint osteoarthritis, and stability of the degenerative lumbar spine. *Journal of Spinal Disorders, 13*, 444.

82. Thompson, R. E., Pearcy, M. J., & Downing, K. J. W. (2000). Disc lesions and the mechanics of the intervertebral joint complex. *Spine, 25*, 3026.

83. Fujiwara, A. et al. (2000). The effect of disc degeneration and facet joint osteoarthritis on the segmental flexibility of the lumbar spine. *Spine, 25*, 3036.

84. Adams, M. A., & Hutton, W. C. (1981). The relevance of torsion to the mechanical derangement of the lumbar spine. *Spine, 6*, 241.

85. Farfan, H. F. (1973). *Mechanical disorders of the low back*. Philadelphia: Lea & Febiger.

86. Farfan, H. F. (1977). A reorientation in the surgical approach to degenerative lumbar intervertebral joint disease. *Orthopedic Clinics, 8*, 9.

87. Farfan, H. F., & Kirkaldy-Willis, W. H. (1981). The present status of spinal fusion in the treatment of lumbar intervertebral joint disorders. *Clinical Orthopedics, 158*, 198.

88. Farfan, H. F. et al. (1970). The effects of torsion on the lumbar intervertebral joints: The role of torsion in the production of disc degeneration. *Journal of Bone and Joint Surgery (America), 52A*, 468.

89. Lamy, C., Kraus, H., & Farfan, H. F. (1975). The strength of the neural arch and the etiology of spondylosis. *Orthopedic Clinics of North America, 6*, 215.

90. Taylor, J. R., Twomey, L. T., & Corker, M. (1990). Bone and soft tissue injuries in post-mortem lumbar spines. *Paraplegia, 28*, 119.

92. Twomey, L. T., Taylor, J. R., & Taylor, M. M. (1989). Unsuspected damage to lumbar zygapophyseal (facet) joints after motor-vehicle accidents. *Medical Journal of Australia, 151*, 210.

93. Jacoby, R. K. et al. (1976). Radiographic stereoplotting: A new technique and its application to the study of the spine. *Annals of the Rheumatic Diseases, 35*, 168.

94. Mitchell, C. L. (1933). Isolated fractures of the articular processes of the lumbar vertebrae. *Journal of Bone and Joint Surgery, 15*, 608.

95. Sims-Williams, H., Jayson, M. I. V., & Baddeley, H. (1978). Small spinal fractures in back pain patients. *Annals of the Rheumatic Diseases, 37*, 262.

96. Bogduk, N., & Jull, G. (1985). The theoretical pathology of acute locked back: a basis for manipulative therapy. *Manuelle Medizin, 1*, 78.

97. Manchikanti, L., & Singh, V. (2002). Review of chronic low back pain of facet joint origin. *Pain Physician, 5*, 83.

98. Schwarzer, A. C. et al. (1994). The value of the provocation response in lumbar zygapophysial joint injections. *Clinical Journal of Pain, 10*, 309.

99. Schwarzer, A. C. et al. (1992). The role of bone scintigraphy in chronic low back pain: A comparison of SPECT and planar images and zygapophysial joint injection. *Australia and New Zealand Journal of Medicine, 22*, 185.

100. Magora, A. et al. (1994). The significance of medical imaging findings in low back pain. *Pain Clinic, 7*, 99.

101. Manchikanti, L., Singh, V., & Pampati, V. (2003). Are diagnostic lumbar medial branch blocks valid? Results of 2-year follow up. *Pain Physician, 6*, 147.

102. Bonica, J. J. (1989). Local anesthesia and regional blocks. In P. D. Wall & R. Melzack (Eds.), *Textbook of pain* (2nd ed., p. 724). Edinburgh: Churchill Livingstone.

103. Bonica, J. J., & Buckley, F. P. (1990). Regional analgesia with local anesthetics. In J. J. Bonica (Ed.), *The management of pain* (p. 1883). Philadelphia: Lea & Febiger.

104. Boas, R. A. (1991). Nerve blocks in the diagnosis of low back pain. *Neurosurgery Clinics of North America, 2*, 806.

105. Barnsley, L., Lord, S., & Bogduk, N. (1993). Comparative local anesthetic blocks in the diagnosis of cervical zygapophysial joints pain. *Pain, 55*, 99.

106. Lord, S. M., Barnsley, L., & Bogduk, N. (1995). The utility of comparative local anesthetic blocks versus placebo-controlled blocks for the diagnosis of cervical zygapophysial joint pain. *Clinical Journal of Pain, 11*, 208.

107. Schwarzer, A. C. et al. (1994). The false-positive rate of uncontrolled diagnostic blocks of the lumbar zygapophysial joints. *Pain, 58*, 195.

108. Manchikanti, L., & Singh, V. (2002). Diagnostic lumbar facet joint injections. In L. Manchikanti, C. W. Slipman, & B. Fellows (Eds.), *Interventional pain management: Low back pain — Diagnosis and treatment* (p. 239). Paducah, KY: ASIPP Publishing.

109. Raj, P. P. et al. (2004). Bleeding risk in interventional pain practice: assessment, management, and review of the literature. *Pain Physician, 7*, 3.

110. Bogduk, N. (1997). *Clinical anatomy of the lumbar spine and sacrum* (p. 33). New York: Churchill Livingstone.

111. Bogduk, N. (1997). Nerves of the lumbar spine. In *Clinical anatomy of the lumbar spine and sacrum* (p. 127). New York: Churchill Livingstone.

112. Bogduk, N. (1983). The innervation of the lumbar spine. *Spine, 8*, 286.

113. Jackson, H. C., Winkelmann, R. K., & Bickel, W. H. (1966). Nerve endings in the human lumbar spinal column and related structures. *Journal of Bone and Joint Surgery* (America), *48A*, 1272.

114. Bogduk, N., Wilson, A. S., & Tynan, W. (1982). The human lumbar dorsal rami. *Journal of Anatomy, 134*, 383.

115. Pedersen, H. E., Blunck, C. F. J., & Gardner, E. (1956). The anatomy of lumbosacral posterior rami and meningeal branches of spinal nerves (sinu-vertebral nerves): With an experimental study of their function. *Journal of Bone and Joint Surgery (America), 38A*, 377.

116. Derby, R., Bogduk, N., & Schwarzer, A. (1993). Precision percutaneous blocking procedures for localizing spinal pain. Part 1: The posterior lumbar compartment. *Pain Digest, 3*, 89.

117. Dreyfuss, P., Kaplan, M., & Dreyer, S. J. (2000). Zygapophyseal joint injection techniques in the spinal axis. In T. A. Lennard. (Ed.), *Pain procedures in clinical practice* (2nd ed., p. 276). Philadelphia: Hanley & Belfus, Inc

118. Curran, M. A. (2002). Lumbosacral facet joint radiofrequency. In L. Manchikanti, C. W. Slipman, & B. Fellows (Eds.), *Interventional pain management: Low back pain — Diagnosis and treatment* (p. 463). Paducah, KY: ASIPP Publishing.

119. Windsor, R. E., Storm, S., & Sugar, R. (2003). Prevention and management of complications resulting from common spinal injections. *Pain Physician, 6*, 473.

120. Gladstone, J. C., & Pennant, J. H. (1987). Spinal anaesthesia following facet joint injection. *Anaesthesia. 42*, 754.

121. Marks, R., & Semple, A. J. (1988). Spinal anaesthesia after facet joint injection. *Anaesthesia, 43*, 65.

122. Cook, N. J., Hanrahan, P., & Song, S. (1999). Paraspinal abscess following facet joint injection. *Clinical Rheumatology, 18*, 52.

123. Magee, M. et al. (2000). Paraspinal abscess complicating facet joint injection. *Clinical Nuclear Medicine, 25*, 71.

124. Manchikanti, L. et al. (2003). Risk of whole body radiation exposure and protective measures in fluoroscopically guided interventional techniques: A prospective evaluation. *BioMed Central Anesthesiology, 3*, 2.

125. Berrigan, T. (1992). Chemical meningism after lumbar facet joint block. *Anesthesia, 7*, 905.

126. Thomson, S. J., Lomax, D. M., & Collett, B. J. (1991). Chemical meningism after lumbar facet joint block with local anaesthetic and steroids. *Anaesthesia, 46*, 563.

127. Manchikanti, L. (2002). Role of neuraxial steroids in interventional pain management. *Pain Physician, 5*, 182.

128. Manchikanti, L. et al. (2000). The effect of neuraxial steroids on weight and bone mass density: A prospective evaluation. *Pain Physician, 3*, 357.

66

Cervical Discography

Vijay Singh, MD, and Laxmaiah Manchikanti, MD

INTRODUCTION

Neck pain is a common complaint among the general population in the United States.[1,2] Reports show that 35 to 40% of individuals will suffer from neck and arm pain and 30% may develop chronic pain symptoms. Of 100,000 people, there are 83.2 cases per year that demonstrate cervical radiculopathy,[3] and 38.4 cases per 100,000 who display definite radiculopathy proven to be due to disc prolapse.[4] In spite of attempts to use rational selection algorithms to choose the methods to diagnose the source of cervical pain, discussion in the literature continues concerning the selection and value of procedures because no one modality can provide the information required in every case. Complementary procedures are used to acquire the fullest picture of pathology. Techniques such as magnetic resonance imaging (MRI), computed tomography (CT) scanning, and myelography provide detailed resolution of abnormal anatomy. The images, however accurate, do not report a particular lesion as the cause or source of symptoms.[5] Correlation of reported symptoms with information obtained in imaging may not be sufficiently reliable to unequivocally determine the location or degree that symptoms and pathology coincide.[6–9]

This was the position taken by Roth[10] in 1976 when he defined a cervical discogenic (painful disc) syndrome to be uniquely diagnosed by analgesic discography. Over 2 years he found the technique of analgesic discography to be able precisely to locate and identify a pain-producing disc. His study marked the first time analgesic disc injection was advocated for diagnosis in the cervical discogenic pain syndrome. Provocative discography, the practice of reproducing a patient's pain with injection of contrast followed by local anesthetic injection to confirm the presence of a painful disc, has emerged as a useful technique in the evaluation of chronic cervical pain.

HISTORY

Although Lindblom[11] studied the effects of disc puncture in 1948 and coined the term *discography*, Schmorl[12] in 1921 first injected a disc for radiographic visualization. Hirsch[13] in 1948 followed Lindblom's work with the first clinical study of disc injection in 16 patients using saline and procaine to localize lumbar pain. Subsequent surgery showed an absence of signs of disc injury. Early data on intradiscal pressure were obtained by Erlacher[14] in 1952 who pressurized 200 discs removed at autopsy to 300 kPa without any instance of disc rupture. Also in the 1950s, Smith and Nichols,[15] and independently Cloward,[16] in work done to evaluate patients with chronic neck, shoulder, and headache pain, published procedures for the direct injection of cervical discs. Each group published nearly simultaneously, without the knowledge of the other's work. The techniques were similar, with similar indications and clinical findings reported in a series of papers. The authors reported that injection into an abnormal disc could produce pain and that the finding of painful disc correlated well with increasing age. Each considered the pain response upon injection more relevant than the radiographic appearance of the disc. Each also found that normal cervical discs accepted fairly small volumes (0.25 to 0.5 mL) and that injection of normal discs was not painful.

These surgeons developed their techniques for cervical disc excision and bony fusion using an anterior approach. To select the disc level for the surgical procedure, both groups used cervical disc injection as a diagnostic technique to support their choice. As a diagnostic technique, cervical discography in the 1960s was accepted by some and criticized by others. Still a relatively new procedure, basic clinical findings and their relevance were under study and evaluation.

Holt's 1964 study[17] of volunteer, asymptomatic prison subjects is noted for its negative conclusions, that discography was ineffective and useless. Simmons et al.[18] did a careful reexamination of Holt's study and conclusions in 1988 and exposed significant deficiencies and flaws in the study. The selection process of inmate subjects was questioned because bias was not controlled, the contrast agent used was an irritant itself, fluoroscopic guidance was not utilized, monitored anesthesia was not used, and the technique itself was suspect in the Simmons group's opinion. As an example, extravasation of contrast material was noted with every injection; it continued even with reduction in the amount injected. Its significance had not been investigated by Holt. Holt had rejected correlation of pain with any amount of material injected as without value. Control subjects had not been used. Any critical look at this study today is harsh in its appraisal. Briefly, Simmons et al.[18] concluded that the Holt paper should no longer be considered as either scientific or authoritative evidence in any discussion of discography.

Since that time, the basic knowledge of the physiology and pathology of the disc has expanded. The technique of cervical discography has undergone modification and significant advancement. Fluoroscopic guidance is routine, contrast dye media is far less toxic, and with greater numbers of discograms successfully done, experience has been gained so that the practice of cervical discography is safe and well established. Although cervical may be considered controversial by some, most discographers consider discography to be an essential part of a diagnostic evaluation of chronic cervicogenic pain.[19]

ANATOMY

Differences as well as similarities exist between cervical discs and others in the spinal column. Symptoms solely due to disc herniation are less common in the cervical region than in the lumbar region. Herniation posteriorly and laterally is prevented first by cervical facet joints, which form a bony barrier between the disc and the nerve root, and second, by the dense posterior longitudinal ligament that encloses the disc posteriorly. The nucleus also lies much more anteriorly in the cervical disc than in the lumbar disc, and its movement posteriorly is correspondingly much more difficult and unlikely. In adults, the cervical disc is composed of fibrocartilaginous material, which makes up the annulus fibrosus, with very little nucleus pulposus present. The cervical disc annulus does not consist of concentric laminae of collagen fibers as are found in lumbar discs. Rather, a crescent-shaped mass of collagen fibers thicker anteriorly and tapered laterally toward the uncinate process characterizes the annulus fibrosus. It is more like a crescent-shaped anterior interosseous ligament than a ring of circular fibers surrounding a nucleus pulposus.[20,21] For the discographer, this has some practical meaning, as healthy cervical discs accept only small amounts of contrast media, usually on the order of 0.25 to 0.5 mL, due to the very small nucleus and small size of the disc. Injection of greater volumes usually means extravasation of contrast, with little resistance upon injection being appreciated by the discographer.

The volume of nucleus in the adult cervical intervertebral disc has been studied in cadavers in 1983 by Saternus and Bornscheuer.[22] They report that 75% of discs at C2–C3, C3–C4, and C7–T1 accepted less than 0.5 mL and 50% of discs at C4–C5, C5–C6, and C6–C7 accepted less than 0.5 mL. They also found that discs accepting more than 0.5 mL frequently demonstrated leakage from the posterolateral or uncovertebral portions of the annulus.

Kambin et al.[23] in 1980 made intradiscal volumetric determinations during discography at the time of cervical disc surgery and found that normal-appearing discs accepted 0.2 to 0.4 mL of contrast while maintaining sustained intradiscal pressures. Lower pressures were associated with higher volumes and posterior escape of solution. It can be concluded that a normal cervical nucleus will be filled by less than 0.5 mL of solution.

Anatomists usually make a distinction between the posterior or thinner part and the anterior or thicker portion of the cervical disc. A feature of cervical discs is the usual development in the first two decades of life of horizontal clefts or fissures in the annular tissue, thought to be a functional adaptation to maintain rotational ability as the elastic nature of the annulus decreases with age.[3] These are referred to as joints of Luschka by many authors.[20,21,24–26]

The uncovertebral articulations, or the joints of Luschka, warrant consideration. The lateral and posterolateral areas of the disc are relatively thinner than the anterior areas and this thinning of the annulus results in linear clefts that communicate with the nucleus. The clefts have not been reported in any patients except adults.[20,21] Clefts filling with contrast during discography also have been noted only in adults. They vary in size and configuration and may fill asymmetrically with contrast. Dispersal of contrast posterolaterally into clefts or joints of Luschka is not a result of degeneration of the disc but rather reflects maturation of the adult disc.[24] Degeneration in adulthood is common.

The cervical discs may dehydrate earlier than lumbar discs. Deterioration of the nucleus occurs early in the adult, and it may be absent after the age of 35 to 40. Characterization of the pathologic changes in adult intervertebral cervical discs was done by Gen[27] in 1990 in discs obtained at autopsy. He examined discs by plain roentgenography, discography, and CT discography, and histologically with morphologic measurements. His data revealed that the anterior portion of discs became thinner with aging. The nucleus, initially located slightly anterior to the center of the disc, tended to migrate to the posterior with aging, and the anteroposterior diameter showed a gradual decrease with aging.

Cervical nerve roots branch off the spinal cord laterally through the intervertebral foramina. Radicular symptoms result if the posterior cervical disc herniates laterally and impinges on the nerve root. In 1993, Dubuisson et al.[28] reported on a retrospective series of 100 patients with soft cervical disc herniations. All were surgically treated and those with radiculopathy only as the presenting symptom had better outcomes than those with combined radicular and spinal cord involvement. Other than as presenting symptoms, the hernias were not further characterized.

Until the work of Yamazaki et al.,[29] no study had characterized the courses of herniated masses in cervical disc herniations. He found using CT discography that most herniated masses causing myelopathy have median penetration in the deep layer of the longitudinal ligament and oblique courses of herniation are common. He also noted that among herniated masses causing radiculopathy, most masses took an oblique course from the median penetration to the paramedian or lateral section.

Lateral disc herniation was found to be uncommon where the bony barrier of the uncovertebral junction exists on both sides of the disc. If the cervical disc herniates obliquely, it can impinge on the spinal cord, producing myelopathy that may cause upper and lower extremity neurologic signs.

PATHOPHYSIOLOGY

Innervation of the cervical intervertebral discs has been shown to be similar to that found in lumbar discs. Cervical sinuvertebral nerves have an upward course in the vertebral canal and supply the disc at their level of entry as well as the more cranial.[30–32] Both nerve fibers and proprioceptive receptors are found in the outer third of the annulus fibrosus, and these have been postulated by Bogduk to be the substrate for primary disc pain in disease and for the pain response of provocative cervical discography.[30]

Additionally, there have been advances in the past decade in understanding the biologic aspects of intervertebral disc cell function.[33] Disc cellular function produces the extracellular matrix components of the disc, which in turn shape the physiologic and biomechanical function of the disc. Ongoing research points to the cellular basis of disc degeneration and the very complex intradiscal metabolism involved in the interrelated phenomena of end-plate nutrient diffusion, the role of cytokines in modulating the inflammatory and pain responses of the disc, and how mechanical stimuli modify disc cell activity.

Injuries to the disc may evoke pain by the activation of sensory nociceptors. Injury of the annulus can lead to release of significant amounts of inflammatory chemicals that may in turn irritate or sensitize the annulus and adjacent structures in the spinal and intervertebral foramina. Inflammatory and immunological reaction to herniated disc material is well recognized as a pain-generating mechanism.[34] Determination of a particular disc as the pain-producing site is the goal of cervical discography.

An atypical case presentation of cervical disc herniation causing localized ipsilateral popliteal pain was described by Neo et al.,[35] using MRI as a diagnostic modality. An adult woman gave a 4-month history of increasing pain, eventually being unable to stand or walk. Physical examination and conventional radiography could not explain the pain. An MRI examination showed a large disc herniation on the right at C3/4 and narrowing of the spinal canal at C4/5. Following anterior decompression and fusion to prevent impending myelopathy, the popliteal pain resolved immediately and completely. The pain has not recurred in almost 3 years after surgery. This case exemplifies the infrequent but significant findings that cervical herniations can cause. The utility of discography in solving puzzling presentations of atypical pain resulting from cervical lesions was shown most recently in a patient with atypical cervicogenic headache, reported by Singh,[36] in which MRI did not disclose the pain-producing lesion. This particular patient had given a 6-year history of intractable pain and until the pain-producing lesion was identified by discography, no diagnostic modality or treatment had given any benefit.

Cervical discography has been used to establish a diagnosis of cervical angina or pseudoangina, which Wells[37] reported as chest pain resembling true cardiac pain coming from C7 nerve root compression. Guler et al.[38] defined cervical angina as chest pain that resembles true cardiac angina but originates from cervical discopathy with nerve root compression. Cervical discography can establish the diagnosis after coexisting coronary artery disease as been ruled out. Guler reported in his paper the first cases of cervical angina associated with acute electrocardiographic (ECG) changes brought on by neck motion. In a more extensive survey, Jacobs[39] reported his series of 164 patients with cervical angina giving similar presentations.

RATIONALE AND INDICATIONS

Discography is not a screening or initial examination in the investigation cervical pain. That role is met by patient history and physical examination, MRI examinations, CT scans, and myelography. Radiographic anatomy disclosed by these techniques is often precise and descriptive but it may not identify the origin of pain, and there can be discrepancies between the degree of pain and the apparent severity of changes observed in radiographic images.[40]

Parfenchuck and Janssen[41] in a 1994 study suggested that while several patterns seen with MRI correlate well with discography findings, others are equivocal. His opinion was that discography was required to diagnose the discogenic pain syndrome. A study by Schellhas et al.[42] in 1996 compared chronic head and neck pain sufferers undergoing MRI or cervical discography. He concluded that discographically normal discs were never painful, whereas painful discs exhibited annular tears that often escaped MRI detection and that MRI could not reliably discern the source of discogenic pain. Collins[43] noted the useful adjunct role played by cervical discography: it was particularly helpful in determining the level of fusion and the selection of patients with cervical discs that needed to be fused.

Cervical discography is indicated for the following situations:

1. Presence of persistent neck pain for which usual diagnostic modalities have failed to identify a cause
2. Findings using traditional modalities are equivocal for the cause of pain
3. Planning for surgical fusion requiring precise identification of painful levels
4. Persistent pain following fusion requiring levels above and below fusion to be examined as pain generators
5. Differentiation cannot be made of scar tissue from recurrent herniation by usual modalities

Guyer and Ohnmeiss[44] delineated indications for lumbar discography in the position statement of the North American Spine Society (NASS) in 1995. Points stressed in the NASS statement define the appropriate use of discography, with attention given that patients may recognize pain provoked in the procedure as similar or identical to their presenting complaint.

Disc injection has been used for well over two decades to select levels for surgical discectomy and fusion. Riley et al.[45] in 1969 used cervical disc injection at the time of surgery, with discometry and epidural leakage the primary diagnostic factors. Simmons and Segil[46] in 1975 used pain responses from saline injection distention of the disc to select disc levels for surgery. Both groups found high percentage rates of success determining the level for surgery. Different groups, such as Whitecloud and Seago,[47] Siebenrock and Aebi,[48] and Hubach,[49] report similarly high percentage success rates for discectomy and fusion of painful discs at levels diagnosed by discography. When discography *was* not employed preoperatively, success rates were reported only half as high.

Contraindications to cervical discography include known allergies to contrast dye, suspected or confirmed patient sepsis, infection at the site of injection, known coagulopathy, or patient refusal. Symptoms of cord compression or myelopathy are absolute contraindications.

TECHNICAL CONSIDERATIONS

Cervical discography is a technique in which proficiency and expertise are essential. The precise detailed knowledge of the anatomy of the cervical spine and the vital structures in the anterior cervical region is of utmost importance. The discographer must be skilled in airway management and cardiovascular resuscitation.

Pre-procedural preparations include usual preoperative considerations as well as a crucial aspect of cervical discography: the review of prior imaging studies of the cervical spine before beginning discography. The procedure should not be performed at any level where spinal cord compression exists, with or without myelopathy. Any cervical disc level revealing spinal cord deformity should be avoided or studied under extreme care, depending on the individual circumstances.

Prophylactic antibiotics are given within an hour before the procedure begins, usually Cefazolin or a similar antibiotic with known intradiscal diffusion characteristics and activity against staphylococcal and streptococcal skin inhabitants.

The procedure is performed with the patient in supine position and with support under the shoulders, the head and neck slightly hyperextended, and the head rotated away from the side used by the discographer. The disc cannot be entered posteriorly due to the spinal cord or anteriorly because of the trachea. Therefore, entry into the cervical disc is usually done from the right anterolateral approach. Complete aseptic technique is used throughout the procedure. The skin is prepped with Betadine or chlorhexidine solution and the solutions should remain on the skin for at least 2 minutes to kill any *Staphylococcus aureus* or *Streptococcus epidermidis* spp., which are the most common skin bacteria usually implicated in risk of deep tissue infections following skin puncture. An alcohol rinse of the site is done for maximal antibacterial effect.

A right paratracheal approach is used and the C-arm is placed in oblique position and the uncovertebral junction is identified. Unlike lumbar discography, where the disc is punctured on the side opposite the patient's symptoms, a right-sided approach is used by most discographers because of concern of accidental puncture of the esophagus with the left-side approach. The skin is anesthetized with 1% buffered, preservative-free lidocaine. Light intravenous sedation, usually with midazolam, may be used; however, the patient must always remain alert enough to respond to pain sensations and communicate them. The patient is monitored closely for vasovagal signs, which may be caused by compression of the carotid artery during manual displacement with needle entry. The C-arm

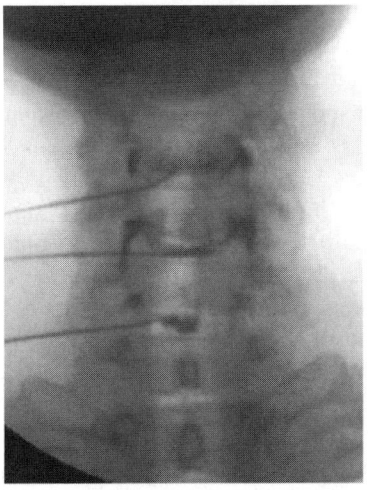

(A) AP view

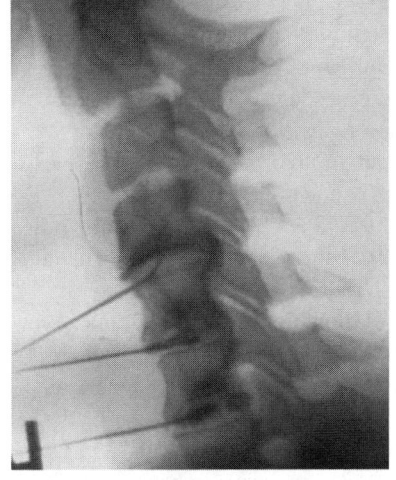

(B) Lateral view

FIGURE 66.1 Illustration of cervical discography at C4/5, C5/6 and C6/7.

is placed in an oblique position with a slight cranial angulation to best visualize the disc space.

Skin puncture is made with an 18-gauge needle, medial to the anterior border of the sternocleidomastoid muscle, between the carotid sheath and trachea. A 22-gauge 3.5-inch styletted spinal needle is inserted through the puncture hole and slowly advanced to the target point just medial to the uncovertebral junction of the lower vertebral body. The carotid pulse is palpated and carotid sheath structures are displaced laterally by digital pressure. Additional local anesthetic is given along the needle tract. Slow, deliberate needle advancement is key to the successful procedure. The needle is advanced either into the disc or against the vertebra adjacent to the disc. The position is confirmed in the anteroposterior and lateral projections with the fluoroscope. Careful adjustment and redirection of the needle as necessary is made into the annulus of the disc.

Two levels, one superior and one inferior, to the level being examined should also be punctured to serve as necessary controls for the patient pain response.

From 0.25 to 0.5 mL of contrast solution is injected into the nucleus at each level and the pain response is noted. The discogram is positive when the patient reports concordant pain that closely resembles symptomatic pain in intensity and location. Injection of local anesthetic into a painful disc is used to further evaluate symptomatic relief and confirm a disc as a pain generator. Leakage of contrast out of the disc space is noted, as well as the overall disc appearance. Figure 66.1 illustrates cervical discography.

Intradiscal antibiotics may be injected at the discretion of the discographer, but with careful attention to leakage of antibiotic solution into the epidural space. Some discographers use antibiotic solution in combination with contrast. It is preferable and safer to not mix antibiotic with contrast and use antibiotic only when the pattern of

dye has been fully visualized and subarachnoid spread has been completely ruled out.

INTERPRETATION

Interpretation of the pain response is the *sine qua non* of the effective use of cervical discography. Pain is a subjective response that individuals report differently. Pain reporting cannot be objectively treated for bias-free analysis. Various methods have been used to rate the patient pain response; most incorporate self-reporting using a visual analogue scale, an independent observer rating pain appearance and behavior, and patient reporting the similarity of injection pain to chronic pain. The alleviation of pain following injection of local anesthetics is recorded to note the analgesic effect in an abnormal disc.

Cervical discography and the pain response are discussed by Klafta and Collis.[50] In their work a very low percentage of discs was judged to be normal, as pain occurred in the majority of injections, and this was taken as an indicator of disc abnormality but not diagnostic of disc protrusion. A subsequent paper addressed this finding; the authors did not consider pain from injection to be of significance and of concern only if a mass lesion in the disc itself was demonstrable.[51] This contrasts with current discographic practice, as exemplified by the report of Ohnmeiss et al.[40] Pain response and radiographic appearance of discs showed good agreement, with clinical pain provoked in 78% of discs appearing abnormal and in only 14% of normal discs.

Beginning with the report of Roth[10] in 1976, with discogenic pain accurately diagnosed prior to surgery by analgesic disc injection, many authors report that the most effective test for the identification and localization of a painful disc is cervical discography. Patients with cervicogenic pain are accurately and consistently diagnosed by cervical discography reproducing their characteristic pain. Other modalities can identify pathology, but only discography can correlate abnormalities with pain.

The purpose of the procedure is to identify a source of pain. The information to be recorded for every procedure includes, but is not limited to, injection volumes; characteristics of all end points of injections reached; pain responses at each level examined on a 0 to 10 scale with 0 meaning no pain and 10 the worst pain possible; whether the pain felt is identical, similar, or not at all the same as the pain that led to the examination; location of pain from the examination; the morphology of the disc revealed by the examination (annular tears, end plate defects, anatomical abnormalities, fissures, or leakage of contrast media); correlation of these findings with MRI or CT imaging studies; and an opinion from the discographer concerning the apparent validity of the examination — patient pain response and cooperation.

Even though the pattern of contrast dispersal is the least important finding in cervical discography, some characteristic patterns of abnormal discs have been described. These include the following: escape of contrast beneath the longitudinal ligament or into the epidural space reveals rupture of the annulus; a deflated balloon appearance filling the disc space indicates degeneration of the nucleus; escape of contrast through the vertebral end plates shows interosseous herniation; leakage of contrast beneath an unfused ring epiphysis shows vertebral edge separation; escape of contrast into a communicating hemangioma related to end plate fracture.

COMPLICATIONS

Although very beneficial as a diagnostic tool, the procedure is not without risks.[52–60] Complications can occur due to incorrect needle placement in which the hypopharynx, esophagus, or even spinal cord could be punctured, with the attendant risks of infection or neurologic damage. Very deliberate and careful needle advancement and good fluoroscopic visualization prevent such occurrences and their sequelae.

Unusual complications are also possible. In one reported case, quadriplegia developed within seconds after injection into the intervertebral space. During the injection the patient reported having severe pain in her arm. Surgical evidence showed sequestered portions of a degenerate disc were pushed into the spinal canal during the examination. Slow recovery of neurologic deficits took place after the operation.[58] A recent study of a large group of patients undergoing cervical discography gave a 1.49% complication rate based on the number of discs injected.[54] There were two cases of discitis, one post-injection hematoma, and one patient developed headache.

The cord compression syndrome due to soft central disc herniation can be a potential complication with exacerbation of herniation causing myelopathy and even quadriplegia in extreme cases.

Another rare but significant potential complication, that of spinal epidural abscess mimicking disc herniation, was reported by Sawada et al.[59] His patient developed fever, sore throat, and nuchalgia with a sudden onset of quadriplegia following partial sigmoidectomy, and MRI showed characteristic findings of a cervical herniation. At discectomy, cervical discitis was discovered with an associated spinal epidural abscess. With antibiotic follow-up, he improved. A high index of suspicion must be accorded any MRI image and associated clinical signs of infection. Discitis, although rare, must remain in the differential diagnosis.

Discitis, one of the most dreaded complications of disc injection, is rarely reported and in reviews of the literature, rates of 0.1 to 0.2% are found. Guyer et al.[60] in their series report a rate of infection of 0.1 to 0.5%.

The author typically uses both intravenous and intradiscal antibiotics for prophylaxis. Although an intravenous bolus before the procedure can produce antibiotic penetration into the disc, timing of the bolus is critical. Studies have found that the minimum inhibitory concentration (MIC) for the most common agent responsible for discitis, *Staphylococcus epidermidis*, was not exceeded using cefazolin except in a well-defined time period of 15 to 80 minutes after an intravenous bolus.[61] Moreover, if the disc has undergone degeneration, it is likely that antibiotic concentrations intradiscally would be further reduced. Thus, intradiscal antibiotics are usually considered.[59–67] Studies support the use of appropriate broad-spectrum intradiscal antibiotics to minimize the risk of discitis; typical skin inhabitants *Staphylococcus aureus* and *Streptococcus epidermidis* are the organisms most likely to be contaminants. Cefazolin has been widely used because of its activity against these organisms and its documented inhibitory levels intradiscally.[61]

The argument has been made for the use of intradiscal antibiotics for prophylaxis of disc infection during discography and that with proper timing and choice of antibiotic, intradiscal placement of antibiotic should obviate the need for systemic administration to avoid the risk of generating antibiotic resistance.[63–66] Several antibiotics meet the requirement to be above the minimum inhibitory concentration of *Staphylococcus aureus* and *Streptococcus epidermidis* among them cefazolin, gentamycin, and clindamycin; ceftriaxone meets this requirement and also has been shown to persist at levels above the MIC for these organisms as long as 5 hours in the intervertebral disc space with administration systemically 1 hour prior to the procedure.[63,67]

There are, then, several classes of antibiotics shown to be efficacious. With proper selection and use, any allergic or sensitivity reaction should be avoided.

A recent case report by Boswell and Wolfe[68] details the first reported post-discography seizures associated with a cephalosporin, cephazolin. Caution would be advised mixing beta-lactam antibiotics or cephalosporins with contrast prior to disc injection. Accidental or inadvertent intrathecal injection with this class of antibiotic may provoke this reaction.

With the exercise of meticulous care at all times, discography can be done with few, if any, complications, when performed in sterile conditions and by those well experienced in the procedure. It is not a procedure to be attempted by the novice because it is very easy to pass a needle through the disc and into the spinal cord.

CONCLUSION

Cervical discography is a specialized procedure requiring the skill of a highly trained and competent interventionalist with expertise in the procedure. Diagnostic disc injection may be indicated in the evaluation of patients with symptomatology without a discernible etiology from other imaging studies. Discography is used to determine the presence of pathology and to reproduce pain felt by the patient, so-called concordant pain. It is not a screening procedure but rather a confirmatory one when cervical disc pathology is suspected and is best utilized with MRI and clinical examination.

There is a very low level of reported complications; patient selection, skilled operation, and maintenance of sterility are essential. Cervical discography has a unique position in the diagnosis and localization of the painful disc syndrome, correlating MRI findings with symptomatology and in determining the levels for successful surgical fusion of the cervical spine.

REFERENCES

1. Bogduk, N. (1984). Neck pain. *Australian Family Physician, 13,* 26.
2. Goodman, B. W., Jr. (1988). Neck pain. *Primary Care, 15,* 689.
3. Bovim, G., Schrader, H., & Sand, T. (1994). Neck pain in the general population. *Spine, 19,* 1307.
4. Radhakrishnan, K. et al. (1994). Epidemiology of cervical radiculopathy. A population-based study from Rochester, Minnesota, 1976 through 1990. *Brain, 117,* 325.
5. Motimaya, A. et al. (2000). Diagnostic value of cervical discography in the management of cervical discogenic pain. *Connecticut Medicine, 64,* 395.
6. Slipman, C. et al. (2002). Provocative cervical discographic symptom mapping. *Spine Journal, 2,* 112.
7. Kaiser, J. A., & Holland, B. A. (1998). Imaging of the cervical spine. *Spine, 23,* 2701.
8. Chevrot, A. et al. (2003). Imaging the painful cervical spine. *Journal of Radiology, 84,* 181.
9. Gelehrter, G. (1975). The addition of nucleography to discography as an extended method of examination. *ROFO Fortschritte auf dem Gebiete der Rontgenstrahlen und Nuklearmedizin, 122,* 517.
10. Roth, D. A. (1976). Cervical analgesic discography. A new test for the definitive diagnosis of the painful disc syndrome. *Journal of the American Medical Association, 235,* 1713.
11. Lindblom, K. (1948). Diagnostic puncture of intervertebral discs in sciatica. *Acta Orthopaedica Scandinavica, 17,* 231.
12. Schmorl, G. (1926). Die pathologie der wirbelsaule. *Deutschen Orthopadischen Gessellschaft, 21,* 3.
13. Hirsch, C. (1948). An attempt to diagnose level of disc lesion clinically by disc puncture. *Acta Orthopaedica Scandinavica, 18,* 132.
14. Erlacher, P. R. (1952). Nucleography. *Journal of Bone and Joint Surgery* (Britain), *34B,* 204.
15. Smith, G. W., & Nichols, P., Jr. (1957). Technic for cervical discography. *Radiology, 68,* 718.
16. Cloward, R. B. (1958). Cervical discography. Technique, indications and use in the diagnosis of ruptured cervical discs. *American Journal of Roentgenology, 79,* 563.
17. Holt, E. P. (1964). Fallacy of cervical discography. *Journal of the American Medical Association, 188,* 799.
18. Simmons, J. W. et al. (1988). A reassessment of Holt's data. *Clinical Orthopedics, 237,* 120.
19. Fortin, J. D. (2000). Precision diagnostic disc injections. *Pain Physician, 3,* 271.
20. Bland, J. H. (1994). Basic anatomy. In J. H. Bland (Ed.), *Disorders of the cervical spine* (2nd ed., p. 41). Philadelphia: W.B. Saunders.
21. Van Roy, P., Barbaix, E., & Clarijs, J. P. (2001). Functional anatomy of the cervical spine. In M. Szpalski & R. Gunzburg (Eds.), *The degenerative cervical spine* (p. 3). Philadelphia: Lippincott Williams & Wilkins.
22. Saternus, K. S., & Bornscheuer, H. H. (1983). Comparative radiologic and pathologic-anatomic studies on the value of discography in the diagnosis of acute intravertebral disc injuries in the cervical spine. *ROFO Fortschritte auf dem Gebiet der Rontgenstrahlen und der Bildgebenden Verfahre, 139,* 651.
23. Kambin, P., Abda, S., & Kurpicki, F. (1981). Intradiscal pressure and volume recording: Evaluation of normal and abnormal cervical discs. *Clinical Orthopedics, 146,* 144.
24. Kumaresan, S. et al. (2000). Morphology of young and old cervical spine intervertebral discs tissues. *Biomedical Sciences Instrumentation, 36,* 141.
25. Mercer, S., & Bogduk, N. (1999). The ligaments and annulus fibrosus of human adult cervical intervertebral discs. *Spine, 7,* 619.
26. Pooni, J. S. et al. (1986). Comparison of the structure of human intervertebral discs in the cervical, thoracic and lumbar regions of the spine. *Surgical and Radiologic Anatomy, 8,* 175.
27. Gen, H. (1990). A clinicopathologic study of cervical intervertebral discs. Part 2: Morphological and roentgenological findings. *Nippon Seikeigeka Gakkai Zasshi, 7,* 572.

28. Dubuisson, A., Lenelle, J., & Stevennaert, A. (1993). Soft cervical disc herniation: a retrospective study of 100 cases. *Acta Neurchirurgia (Wein), 125*, 115.

29. Yamazaki, S. et al. (2003). Courses of cervical disc herniation causing myelopathy or radiculopathy. *Spine, 28*, 1171.

30. Bogduk, N., Windsor, M., & Inglis, A. (1988). The innervation of the cervical intervertebral discs. *Spine, 13*, 2.

31. Bogduk, N., Tynan, W., & Wilson, A. S. (1981). The nerve supply to the human lumbar intervertebral disc. *Journal of Anatomy, 132*, 39.

32. Mendel, T., Wink, C. S., & Zimny, M. L. (1992). Neural elements in human cervical intervertebral discs. *Spine, 17*, 132.

33. Gruber, H. F., & Hanley, E. N., Jr. (2003). Recent advances in disc cell biology. *Spine, 28*, 186.

34. Bibby, S. R. et al. (2001). The pathophysiology of the intervertebral disc. *Joint Bone Spine, 68*, 537.

35. Neo, M. et al. (2002). Cervical disc herniation causing localized ipsilateral popliteal pain. *Journal of Orthopedic Science, 7*, 147.

36. Singh, V. (2004). Percutaneous disc decompression for the treatment of chronic atypical cervical discogenic pain. *Pain Physician, 7*, 115.

37. Wells, P. (1997). Cervical angina. *American Family Physician, 5*, 2262.

38. Guler, N. et al. (2000). Acute ECG changes and chest pain induced by neck motion in patients with cervical hernia — A case report. *Angiology, 51*, 861.

39. Jacobs, B. (1990). Cervical angina. *New York State Journal of Medicine, 90*, 8.

40. Ohnmeiss, D. D., Guyer, R. D., & Maxon, S. L. (2000). The relation between cervical discographic pain responses and radiographic images. *Clinical Journal of Pain, 16*, 1.

41. Parfenchuck, T. A., & Janssen, M. E. (1994). A correlation of cervical magnetic resonance imaging and discography/computed tomographic discograms. *Spine, 18*, 2819.

42. Schellhas, K. P. et al. (1996). Cervical discogenic pain. Prospective correlation of MRI and discography in asymptomatic subjects and pain sufferers. *Spine, 21*, 300.

43. Collins, H. R. (1975). An evaluation of cervical and lumbar. *Clinical Orthopedics, 107*, 133.

44. Guyer, R. D., & Ohnmeiss, D.D. (1995). Position statement from North American Spine Society diagnostic and therapeutic committee. *Spine, 20*, 248.

45. Riley, L. H., Jr. et al. (1969). The results of anterior interbody fusion of the cervical spine. Review of 93 consecutive cases. *Journal of Neurosurgery, 30*, 127.

46. Simmons, E. H., & Segil, C. M. (1975). An evaluation of discography in the localization of symptomatic levels in discogenic disease of the spine. *Clinical Orthopedics, 108*, 57.

47. Whitecloud, T. S., & Seago, R. A. (1987). Cervical discogenic syndrome. Results of operative intervention in patients with positive discography. *Spine, 2*, 313.

48. Siebenrock, K. A., & Aebi, M. (1994). Cervical discography in discogenic pain syndrome and its predictive value for cervical fusion. *Archives of Orthopedic and Trauma Surgery, 113*, 199.

49. Hubach, P. (1994). A prospective study of anterior cervical spondylodesis in intervertebral disc disorder. *European Spine Journal, 3*, 209.

50. Klafta, L. A., Jr., & Collis, J. S., Jr. (1969). An analysis of cervical discography with surgical verification. *Journal of Neurosurgery, 30*, 38.

51. Klafta, L. A., Jr., & Collis, J. S., Jr. (1969). The diagnostic inaccuracy of the pain response in cervical discography. *Cleveland Clinic Quarterly, 36*, 35.

52. Guyer, R. D. et al. (1997). Complications of cervical discography: Findings in a large series. *Journal of Spinal Disorders, 10*, 95.

53. Roosen, K., Bettag, W., & Fiebach, O. (1975). Complications of cervical discography. *ROFO Fortschritte auf dem Gebiete der Rontgenstrahlen und Nuklearmedizin 122*, 520.

54. Grubb, S. A., & Kelly, C. K. (2000). Cervical discography: Clinical implications from 12 years experience. *Spine, 25*, 1382.

55. Zeidman, S. M., Thompson, K., & Ducker, T. B. (1995). Complications of cervical discography: Analysis of 4400 diagnostic disc injections. *Neurosurgery, 37*, 414.

56. Fraser, R. D., Osti, O.L., & Vernon-Roberts, B. (1989). Iatrogenic discitis: The role of intravenous antibiotics in prevention and treatment. An experimental study. *Spine, 14*, 1025.

57. Smith, M. D., & Kim, S. S. (1990). A herniated cervical disc resulting from discography: An unusual complication. *Journal of Spinal Disorders, 3*, 392.

58. Laun, A., Lorenz, R., & Asgnoli, A.L. (1981). Complications of cervical discography. *Journal of Neurosurgery Science, 1*, 17.

59. Sawada, M. et al. (1996). Cervical discitis associated with spinal epidural abscess caused by methicillin-resistant *Staphylococcus aureus. Neurologia. Medico-Chirurgica* (Tokyo), *36*, 40.

60. Guyer, R. D. et al. (1988). Discitis after discography. *Spine, 13*, 1352.

61. Boscardin, J. B., Ringus, J. C., & Feingold, D. J. (1992). Human intradiscal levels with cefazolin. *Spine, 17*, S145.

62. Osti, O. L., Fraser, R. D., & Vernon-Roberts, B. (1990). Discitis after discography. The role of prophylactic antibiotics. *Journal of Bone and Joint Surgery* (Britain), *72*, 271.

63. Lang, R. et al. (1994). Penetration of ceftriaxone into the intervertebral disc. *Journal of Bone and Joint Surgery* (America), *76*, 689.

64. Rhoten, R. L. et al. (1995). Antibiotic penetration into cervical discs. *Neurosurgery, 37*, 418.

65. Riley, L. H., 3rd et al. (1994). Tissue distribution of antibiotics in the intervertebral disc. *Spine, 23*, 2619.

66. Klessig, H. T., Showsh, S. A., & Sekorski, A. (2003). The use of intradiscal antibiotics for discography: An *in vitro* study of gentamycin, cefazolin and clindamycin. *Spine, 28*, 1735.

67. Lang, R. et al. (1995). Sequential levels of ceftriaxone in intervertebral disc removed as part of scoliosis surgery. *Clinical Orthopedics, 315*, 209.

68. Boswell, M. V., & Wolfe, J. R. (2004). Intrathecal cefazolin-induced seizures following attempted discography. *Pain Physician, 7*, 103.

67

Thoracic Discography

Vijay Singh, MD, and Laxmaiah Manchikanti, MD

INTRODUCTION

Discography was first named by Lindblom[1] when he described diagnostic disc puncture. Hirsch[2] used the procedure to identify painful discs in patients with sciatica and lumbar pain. The foundation of the practice of discography was thus begun, and Lindblom did further work using the injection of contrast media to visualize radial tears in the annulus, thus expanding the diagnostic information from intervertebral discs. Pain provocation upon injection served to localize the painful disc, and radiographic appearance with contrast gave information about the internal morphology of the disc.

The clinical use of discography has expanded enormously in the ensuing years.[3–5] Lumbar discography and, to a somewhat lesser extent, cervical discography have been extensively documented and practiced over the past three decades. The technique of thoracic discography is very similar to that of lumbar discography.[6] Although thoracic disc herniation in association with spinal cord compression is documented as a source of back pain, cases of thoracic disc pathology with back pain and an absence of neurological deficits as the major findings are not as well documented in the literature. Imaging studies such as computed tomography (CT) or magnetic resonance imaging (MRI) showing an absence of disc herniation do not exclude the thoracic disc as the source of pain.[7,8] Here, as in lumbar and cervical studies, the well-known attribute of discography and its ability to identify exactly which disc is pain producing, makes it a valuable and unique procedure.

ANATOMY

Thoracic intervertebral discs have a well-defined nucleus pulposus surrounded by a denser fibroelastic aggregation of fibers comprising the outer portion of the disc, the annulus fibrosus. Like other discs, the annular layer is innervated by nociceptor fibers in the outer regions of the annulus, receiving them posteriorly from the sinuvertebral nerves. The anterior portion of the disc receives some fibers from the thoracic sympathetic chain. Dorsal and ventral rami branch from the spinal cord and exit via the intervertebral foramina laterally. Radicular symptoms can result if the disc herniates laterally and impinges on the thoracic nerve root as it leaves the foramen. Myelopathy causing lower extremity or bowel and bladder symptoms can result if the thoracic disc herniates posteromedially. More severe compression of the cord can result in paraparesis.

Neurological occurrences are a result of the spinal cord occupying a fuller extent of the canal. It is a more critical issue neurologically to identify precisely the disc level involved in a suspected disc herniation and the relationship of the herniation to the cord in the thoracic region. The corresponding case is the cauda equina occupying the larger diameter lumbar canal. With a larger diameter canal and a smaller diameter structure filling it, direct neurological insult is less likely.

PATIENT SELECTION AND INDICATIONS

Criteria for performing thoracic discography are not significantly different from those used in cervical or lumbar procedures. The desired result is the same in all three uses of discography — the identification and confirmation of a particular disc as a pain-generator. Thoracic discogenic pain without evidence of a true disc herniation is not a well-known or documented clinical entity. Application of the same principles guiding the use of discography pertain: discography is a useful procedure for patients who have failed to benefit or are refractory to conventional therapies and have unremitting pain, as determination can be made whether a particular disc is a source of thoracic back pain.[9–14] These criteria apply to patients (1) having persistent thoracic radicular or spinal pain, for whom traditional diagnostic modalities have failed to identify the source of pain; (2) for whom traditional methods have identified abnormalities and to make the determination if they are responsible for the pain; (3) planning to undergo spinal fusion, where discography identifies the levels to be fused; (4) having post-fusion pain, to identify whether levels above or below those fused are pain producing; (5) for whom recurrent disc herniation cannot be differentiated from scar tissue using traditional imaging methods.

CONTRAINDICATIONS

These are similar to the contraindications for cervical or lumbar discography, with the added precautions due to the anatomical site and physiologic function: anatomy distorted by disease or deformity may preclude the procedure, and with the attendant risk of inadvertent lung puncture and pneumothorax, pulmonary function should be assessed. Thus, contraindications include thoracic deformity, inadequate pulmonary function, coagulopathy, infection at the puncture site, allergy or sensitivity to medications used, and patient refusal for the procedure.

TECHNICAL CONSIDERATIONS

The technique in thoracic discography is very much like that used for lumbar procedures. Prior imaging studies, ideally including an MRI, are reviewed. The discontinuation of aspirin or other anticoagulants is an important aspect, which needs to be discussed with the primary care provider. Prothrombin time/partial thrombin time (PT/PTT) with a platelet count is done if the medications are continued. Some patients will need anticoagulant therapy. In those patients undertaking an interventional procedure, it poses a high risk, but is not contraindicated.

The consent form is checked with the patient, with particular attention given to the risks and benefits of the procedure and of long-term administration of antibiotics should they be necessary. Specifically, the risk of pneumothorax is fully discussed. Post-procedural transportation is confirmed. ECG, blood pressure, and pulse oximetry monitoring is begun and done during and immediately after the completion of the procedure. Intravenous access is established and prophylactic antibiotics are given within 1 hour of the procedure. When the pre-procedural checklist is complete, the patient is taken to the procedural room.

The patient is positioned prone on the fluoroscopic table. The C-arm is positioned to visualize the pedicle, which projects beneath the superior articulating process

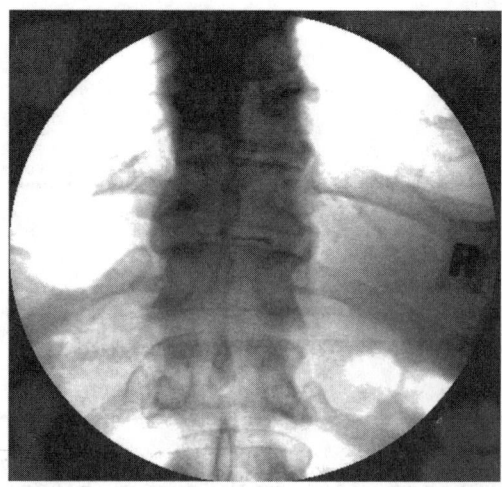

FIGURE 67.1 AP view. Thoracic discograms: T9/10 and T10/11.

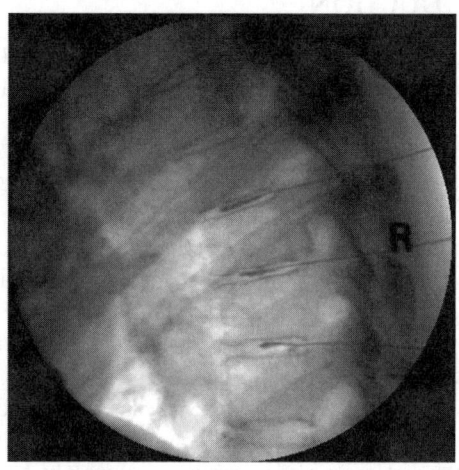

FIGURE 67.2 Lateral view discography: T9/10, T10/11, T11/12.

of the vertebral body of the desired level. A steeper angle of needle insertion is required in the thoracic procedure than in the lumbar. By fluoroscopy, the superior articulating process can be positioned 30 to 40% of the distance across the ipsilateral ventral aspect of the vertebral body. It is important to keep the needle track along the lateral aspect of the superior articulating process and medial to the costotransverse junction to avoid pleural puncture. In lower thoracic levels some discographers have patients hold an expired breath to deflate the lung to reduce the chance of inadvertent pleural puncture, although at the time it is not necessary to make the patient more anxious and hence more motile. (See Figure 67.1 and Figure 67.2.)

Strict aseptic technique is maintained throughout the procedure. The skin at the site is prepped with betadine or chlorhexidine, which is left on the skin for at least 2 minutes followed by an alcohol wipe for maximal antiseptic effect. A fenestrated sterile drape is then applied. If it has

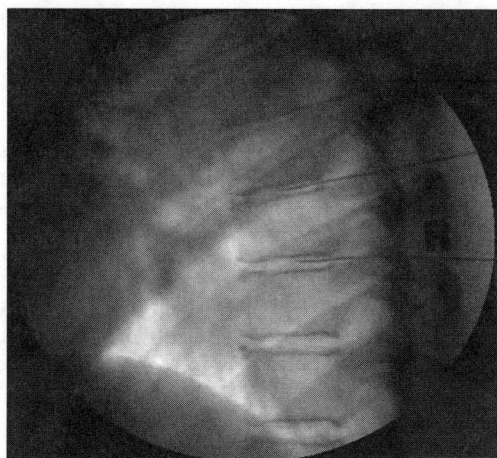

FIGURE 67.3 Lateral view, needle placement, thoracic discography: T9/10, T10/11, T11/12.

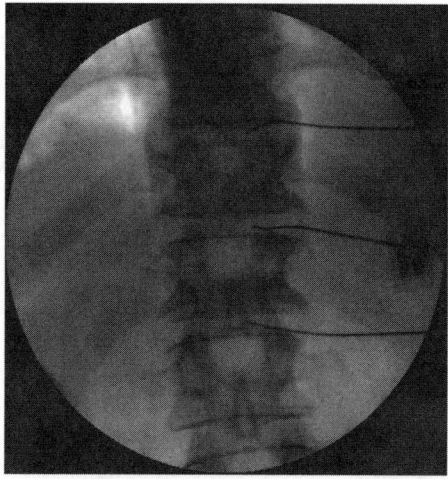

FIGURE 67.4 AP needle placement for discography at T10/11, T11/12, and T12/L1.

been decided to use conscious sedation, usually 1 to 2 mg of Versed and 50 to 100 mg of Fentanyl is sufficient to provide a mild degree of anxiolysis and analgesia. A skin wheal is raised with 0.25 mL 1% lidocaine; deeper tissues are anesthetized with 1% lidocaine or local anesthetic of choice. Before any injection of anesthetic, aspiration should be confirmed to be negative for blood or fluid to prevent accidental intravascular or subarachnoid injection.

Skin puncture may be done with a 22-gauge needle. A 25-gauge styletted needle is introduced through the puncture hole and the needle visualized in both antero-posterior and lateral projections to be in correct position similar to the lumbar procedure. One or two levels adjacent (one superior and one inferior) may be punctured to serve as controls as in the lumbar procedure. Injection of contrast follows with the removal of the needle stylet. Appearance of the contrast should be noted in two projection planes to be certain of injection location in the thoracic disc. For each level injected pain response and volume of injectate is noted. Pain responses are noted to be absent, concordant, or discordant. Intradiscal antibiotic is injected as needed. Needles are removed and skin puncture sites are dressed. (See Figure 67.3 and Figure 67.4.)

Patients are transferred to the recovery area and monitored until ready for discharge. Nonrenewable prescriptions appropriate for pain are given along with printed discharge instructions. Patients are advised that some pain or discomfort can be expected for up to 4 days later. If rare events such as fever, night sweats, chills, malaise, or worsening pain occur within a week, patients are instructed to call immediately as a disc infection could be developing. Patients are carefully monitored for signs of pneumothorax and advised to watch for breathing difficulties or pain. All patients are advised to rest for 24 hours after the procedure, with someone with them for that period in case breathing difficulty or another problem develops. Instruction is given to avoid immersion in water

for the 24 hours after the procedure to minimize the risk of infection. Transport is made to the CT facility as previously arranged. Attempts are made to contact all patients by phone within the next 24 hours to check their status.

As with other discography procedures, reporting of results completes the procedure:

1. Injection volumes and pressures reached, points of injection (end point, absence of end point, voluntary termination of injection) are recorded.
2. Pain response on a 0 to 10 Visual Analogue Scale (0 = none, 10 = worst possible) is recorded.
3. The amount of sedation and effect of sedation on the pain response should not be discounted.
4. Whether the pain was discordant or concordant is recorded for each level.
5. Locations of perceived pain and intensities are recorded.
6. Disc morphology as revealed by the spread of contrast should be recorded, especially annular tears, fissures, leakage of contrast media, and loss of disc height. The spread of contrast can provide very useful information. Annular spread of contrast will vary depending on the amount of degeneration and extent of annular disruption. Radial or concentric tears have different patterns. Although it is not easy for an untrained eye to decipher the pattern of an annular tear, the experienced discographer can certainly study the pattern of contrast spread. Anterior and lateral spread of contrast indicates annular incompetence in the anterior and lateral portion. These findings should be correlated with the MRI findings and the patient's symptoms.
7. Discometry records if pressure measurements were taken — opening pressure (first sign of

contrast media), pressure at which pain was first noted, maximum pressure reached during procedure.

COMPLICATIONS

Pneumothorax has been mentioned as a possible complication. By using meticulous technique and care this can be avoided. The same applies to damaging any retroperitoneal structure. Unintended puncture or damage can be minimized with strict attention to detail.

The most watched-for and serious complication in discography is discitis.[15] Prophylaxis with appropriate antibiotics given at proper times before any procedure can ensure that the disc achieves minimal inhibitory concentrations against the most common skin contaminants, *Staphylococcus aureus* and *Staphylococcus epidermidis*. Several antibiotics are suitable, including cefazolin, gentamycin, ceftriaxone, and clindamycin.[16] With several families of acceptable antibiotics, allergies and sensitivities should not be an issue. The use of intradiscal antibiotics is favored by some authorities, and all the previously mentioned agents have been used successfully.[17]

Note is made of a reported complication using cefazolin. Inadvertent or accidental introduction of cephalosporins to the intrathecal space may lead to the development of seizure activity, even if there is an absence of prior history.[18]

PAIN RESPONSE

As in lumbar and cervical discography, pain response is reason for the procedure. The result is called positive if the injection of contrast causes pain the patient recognizes as the same as pain leading to medical consultation. If the patient recognizes pain as same or very similar to the presenting pain, it is called concordant pain and grading on a sliding scale of 10 (worst) to 0 (none) is commonly done. The disc is considered to be the cause of the symptoms and noted. Although it is not fully elucidated what a finding of painful discordant disc means, it should not be regarded as normal. Some authors believe this finding is a discovery of a disc that is destined to become symptomatic although it may be asymptomatic at present. If the pain is unfamiliar, regardless of grade, it is called discordant and at that particular level is felt not to be implicated. Any equivocal response is usually an indication that the explanation for pain lies elsewhere and not in a thoracic disc, with further evaluation needed.

OUTCOMES

Thoracic discography does diverge from lumbar and cervical discography at the completion of the procedure.

Patients with thoracic disc herniations causing neurologic deficits are very likely to undergo immediate spinal fusion following discography for stabilization; other therapy is not considered.[3]

While lumbar and cervical patients have a range of interventional procedures as well as medical management available to them, thoracic patients usually have options of open discectomy and fusion for severe cases or traditional therapies involving medications and time. Disc herniations in the thoracic spine are reported in the literature as manyfold less likely to cause pain; there is a definite prevalence but apparently many are asymptomatic. Conservative therapy is appropriate.[8]

CONCLUSION

Discography, whether cervical, thoracic, or lumbar, has similar indications. The technique varies with the site of the anatomy. In conjunction with other imaging modalities, it can help provide a complete picture of disc pathology. There are common concerns over complications and risks; they can be accounted for with appropriate preparation and patient selection. The information produced by the procedure is quite similar, dependent on the patient's subjective reporting of concordant/discordant pain. Whether planning surgery, percutaneous procedures, medical management, or physical therapy and rehabilitation, it has proved to be invaluable as a tool to differentiate spinal pain.

REFERENCES

1. Lindblom, K. (1948). Diagnostic puncture of intervertebral discs in sciatica. *Acta Orthopaedica Scandinavica, 17,* 231.
2. Hirsch, C. (1948). An attempt to diagnose level of disc lesion clinically by disc puncture. *Acta Orthopaedica Scandinavica, 18,* 132.
3. Vanichachorn, J. S., & Vaccaro, A. R. (2000). Thoracic disk disease: diagnosis and treatment. *Journal of the American Academy of Orthopedic Surgeons, 8,* 159.
4. Schellhas, K. P., Pollei, S. R., & Dorwart, R.H. (1994). Thoracic discography. A safe and reliable technique. *Spine, 19,* 2103.
5. O'Leary, P. F. et al. (1984). Thoracic disc disease. Clinical manifestations and surgical treatment. *Bulletin of the Hospital for Joint Diseases Orthopaedic Institute, 44,* 27.
6. Wood, K. B. et al. (1999). Thoracic discography in healthy individuals. A controlled prospective study of magnetic resonance imaging and discography in asymptomatic and symptomatic individuals. *Spine, 24,* 1548.
7. Dietze, D. D., Jr., & Fesler, R. G. (1993). Thoracic disc herniations. *Neurosurgery Clinics of North America, 4,* 75.

8. Brown, C. W. et al. (1992). The natural history of thoracic disc herniation. *Spine, 17*, S97.

9. Boriani, S. et al. (1994). Two-level thoracic disc herniation. *Spine, 19*, 2461.

10. Levi, N., & Dons, K. (1998). Two-level thoracic disc herniation. *Mt. Sinai Journal of Medicine, 65*, 404.

11. Morgan, H., & Abood, C. (1998). Disc herniation at T1-2. Report of four cases and literature review. *Journal of Neurosurgery, 88,* 148.

12. Okada, Y. et al. (1997). Multiple thoracic disc herniations: Case report and review of the literature. *Spinal Cord, 35,* 183.

13. Korovessis, P. G. et al. (1997). Three-level thoracic disc herniation: Case report and review of the literature. *European Spine Journal, 6*, 74.

14. Oppenheim, J. S., Rothman, A. S., & Sachdev, V. P. (1993). Thoracic herniated discs: Review of the literature and 12 cases. *Mt. Sinai Journal of Medicine, 60,* 321.

15. Guyer, R. D. et al. (1988). Discitis after discography. *Spine, 13,* 1352.

16. Klessig, H. T., Showsh, S. A., & Sekorski, A. (2003). The use of intradiscal antibiotics for discography: An in vivo study of gentamycin, cefazolin, and clindamycin. *Spine, 28*, 1735.

17. Boscardin, J. B., Ringus, J. C., & Feingold, D. J. (1992). Human intradiscal levels with cefazolin. *Spine, 17,* S145.

18. Boswell, M. V., & Wolfe, J. R. (2004). Intrathecal cefazolin-induced seizures following attempted discography. *Pain Physician, 7*, 103.

68

Lumbar Discography

Vijay Singh, MD, and Laxmaiah Manchikanti, MD

INTRODUCTION

Provocative lumbar discography is an invasive diagnostic procedure in which contrast is injected into the intervertebral disc. It is a procedure that has been practiced for over 50 years and is accepted by many as a valid investigative tool. In the evaluation of spinal pain, it is of critical importance to diagnose accurately precise origins of pain or structural derangement.[1] It is also important to evaluate findings of pathological significance from imaging studies and correlate them with patient symptoms.[2] When a disc problem is suspected by history or physical examination, imaging studies such as magnetic resonance imaging (MRI) can determine disc pathology in many cases, but they do not always identify a particular abnormal finding as coincident with painful symptoms.

Lumbar provocative discography is a complementary examination to confirm if an abnormal disc determined by radiologic imaging and patient complaint is the pain-generating entity.[3] Discography has been shown by formal investigation, when performed by experienced and knowledgeable interventionalists, to improve both surgical and nonsurgical outcomes.[4] Clinical questions such as the following may be answered using discography:

- Is disc pathology observed by imaging studies of clinical significance?
- What therapeutic intervention is indicated?
- Is a satisfactory surgical outcome likely?
- Which spinal segments should be treated?
- What prognosis is likely?

HISTORY

The study of lumbar disc puncture to obtain clinically relevant information was begun by Lindblom in 1948.[5] In the same year Hirsch injected discs with saline and procaine.[6] His hypothesis that pressurization of an injured or degenerative disc would reproduce pain was confirmed. Procaine injection alleviated the pain response following pressurization. The importance of this work was that it showed disc puncture could be used to make a clinical diagnosis of the cause of a patient's back pain.

In the 1950s, Cloward[7] developed techniques for lumbar disc injection and its indications. Erlacher[8] documented the dispersal pattern of dye in cadaveric discs and established radiographic correlation between dispersal patterns and radiographic images. The suggestions that mechanisms other than simple nerve root compression could cause pain were made first by Fernstrom.[9] Discography was relevant for its role in the development of this concept, as painful discs were diagnosed without a nerve compression being present.

Holt's[10,11] papers critical of discography have been challenged and are not considered today other than for their historical significance in the development of techniques for successful discography. His papers have been thoroughly reviewed and several issues raised to question their relevance to current discographic practice, including patient selection, contrast dyes used, techniques employed, and interpretation made of observed findings.

Important developments over the last three decades include the use of water-soluble and less irritating contrast media, fluoroscopic guidance for accurate needle placement, styleted needles to minimize infection, stricter criteria for patient selection, and the use of axial computed tomography (CT) scanning after discography to enable viewing the discs in three planes. Derby et al.[4] developed the practice of manometric measurement of injection pressures during the assessment, adding further information useful to the interpretation of the status of the disc.

Advancements and technological development have made lumbar discography the standard by which painful discs are diagnosed. It is a useful test in the evaluation of candidates for surgery, and for patients undergoing minimally invasive procedures for low back pain.

There is now recognition of the metabolic complexity of the intervertebral disc and the manner in which it responds to injury. The early theory of disc rupture and nerve root compression from the work of Mixter and Barr[12] has been extensively developed and work continues today. Crock[13] put forth the idea of symptomatic disc lesions, from internal disruption to prolapse and protrusion, with different mechanisms causing each particular pathology. The exact mechanism of pain production by an injured or damaged disc is unknown, but active research implicates inflammatory and immunological mediators as well as the interaction of metabolic mechanisms and enzyme activation.[14] Lumbar discography is required to differentiate symptomatic from asymptomatic discs and establish the diagnosis of internal disc disruption.

ANATOMY

The lumbar intervertebral disc is made up of an external layer of concentric rings of fibrocartilage composed of collagen and fibroblastic cells, the annulus fibrosus surrounding the nucleus of the disc, and the nucleus pulposus. The collagenous end plates consist of collagen fibers and chondrocytes, and through this layer all nutrients vital to the maintenance of the disc diffuse. These end plates cover the superior and inferior aspects of the disc, and collagen fibers from the most superficial aspects of the annulus join the end plate fiber and inset directly into the bone of the vertebral body.

The lamellae or layers in the annulus are not continuous; many are found to extend 40 to 50% or less of the circumference of the disc. They are thicker in the center of the disc and in the anterolateral portion, becoming thinner posteriorly.[15] The nucleus is a three-dimensional intricate network of glycoproteins, collagen fibers, and aminoglycans. The water content may be as high as 70%, decreasing with age. This water–glycoprotein–aminoglycan gelatinous combination gives the disc its shock-absorbing capacity and its multiaxial weight-bearing properties during flexion and extension of the spine. Innervation of the disc has been shown histologically with the outer third of the annulus being innervated with fibers

from the sinuvertebral nerve. Both nerve fibers and mechanico-receptors are found in the outer third of the annulus fibrosus. These have been characterized by Bogduk et al.[16] and postulated as the substrate for primary disc pain in disease and for the pain response of provocative lumbar discography.

Activities of daily living, trauma, and age cause changes in the disc found clinically as degeneration. With disc degeneration not only is the internal structure of the disc jeopardized as well as its function, but pain results from a variety of mechanisms.[17] The release of potent mediators of inflammation, direct stimulus of intradiscal nerve fibers, the action of proteolytic enzymes from the nucleus itself, and activation of potent cell cytokines all are documented to be involved in the production of pain from injured lumbar discs.[18–23]

INDICATIONS

Indications for discography follow the position statement per the North American Spinal Society (1995):[24]

1. A primary indication for lumbar discography is the identification of a particular disc as a pain source or the correlation of pain with a disc with a known abnormality.
2. Patients with persistent low back pain in whom an equivocal MRI has not confirmed a disc as a source of pain.
3. Further assessment of patients who have had surgery who continue to have persistent pain. A painful disc in a fused segment or possible recurrent disc herniation can be determined by provocative lumbar discography.
4. Disc assessment prior to surgery to determine if discs in the proposed fusion segment are painful and to find if discs adjacent to this disc are normal and nonpainful.
5. Assessment of patients prior to undergoing minimally invasive procedures to confirm a painful contained disc herniation or to identify the distribution pattern of dye in disc to fully discern disc degeneration.

CONTRAINDICATIONS

Absolute contraindications to the procedure include discitis, local skin infection, cord compression, known coagulopathies, and allergies to contrast media. Relative contraindications are allergies to other medications used, pregnancy, and known disc herniations. Patients with abnormal profiles on psychological screening examinations require careful evaluation and may give variable, difficult-to-interpret pain responses.

TECHNIQUE

Discographers must be experienced in the technique and knowledgeable in anatomy, as well as skilled in the interpretation of results. The techniques specific to the performance of lumbar provocative discography are presented in several texts; it is not a procedure for amateurs. Consultation and close communication with the primary care physician is maintained, especially in matters of discontinuing aspirin or anticoagulants. Consent is checked with the patient with attention given to the risks involved and the potential risk of long-term antibiotic therapy should it be necessary.

PREMEDICATION

For purposes of premedication or intravenous sedation, it is preferable to use only anxiolytics if sedation is deemed necessary. Analgesics such as Fentanyl should be avoided but in rare cases they may become necessary for those patients who have needle phobia or a very low pain threshold. A broad-spectrum antibiotic should be given intravenously 30 minutes before the start of a procedure, as a prophylactic measure to prevent discitis. Cefazolin is commonly used; if there is sensitivity to cephalosporins or penicillins, clindamycin or gentamycin may be substituted.

Needle placement is accomplished under fluoroscopic guidance in the operating room or special diagnostic procedure suite. Meticulous attention to asepsis is of paramount importance.

INJECTION OF CONTRAST

A normal disc can accept 1 to 2 mL of contrast agent without eliciting pain. Injection without resistance or injection exceeding 2 mL of contrast should alert the interventionalist to the likelihood of extravasation of contrast and should be discontinued immediately. Resistance to injection should be noted as well as any pain response. The location and character of any pain are part of the evaluation. Concordant pain is pain produced upon disc injection, which matches the chief complaint pain as perceived by the patient. Pain that is elicited but of a different character intensity or location as perceived by the patient is termed discordant. This may signify an injured or damaged disc but is not considered the disc producing the patient's pain. A disc level that, upon injection, does not elicit pain is termed a control level. The recording of clinical information for later interpretation is detailed below.

Following disc injection, it may be deemed appropriate to inject antibiotic intradiscally. A range of 0.5 to 2.0 mg antibiotic is typically used. (The range of intradiscal antibiotic use varies. Some use much higher doses.) The needles are removed and the puncture site is dressed with antibiotic ointment and a sterile dressing.

INTERPRETATIONS OF DISCOGRAMS

Patterns of dye dispersal consistently show one of five sets of features that can be correlated with distinct stages of disc degeneration. The discogram pattern is created by the distribution of contrast intradiscally. The descriptions of the contrast pattern seen on radiographs and the subsequent correlation of their relationship to actual disc degeneration is derived from the work of Adams et al.[25] in his cadaveric study.

ADAMS CLASSIFICATION OF RADIOGRAPHIC APPEARANCE

1. Cottonball discogram: The contrast medium appears to be contained within the nucleus and is of uniform density. The shape tends to be round or central. Discs giving this pattern of contrast do not show signs of degeneration. No fissures into the annulus are seen. The injection pressure into the nucleus is low; if the needle is moved into the annulus the injection, pressures rise significantly, as the intact annulus does not easily deform to accept fluid.

2. Lobular: The contrast appears to be contained within the nucleus and has more of a lobulated appearance, with greater density toward the end plates and lesser or absent density in the center. A shape suggesting a hamburger is perceived by many observers. These patterns are shown by mature discs with the nucleus beginning to coalesce into fibrous lumps separated by clefts or lines of fracture. The annulus is intact, without obvious fissures extending from the nucleus. Contrast injected may not appear to move freely from one part of the intradiscal space to another. As in the previous case, injection into the annulus was difficult.

3. Irregular: The contrast pattern first begins to show disc degeneration. There is poor differentiation between the nucleus and annulus, with a fibrous-appearing nucleus and multiple small clefts and fissures between the nucleus and inner annulus. Injection pressures are usually low except in the outer margins of the annulus, which appears relatively intact.

4. Fissured: The discogram shows contrast extending to the outer edge of the annulus, even beyond the edge of the vertebral body in some cases. No contrast is observed to escape from the annulus of the disc. One or more radial fissures are seen in the annulus and these extend to the posterior or posterolateral margin of the

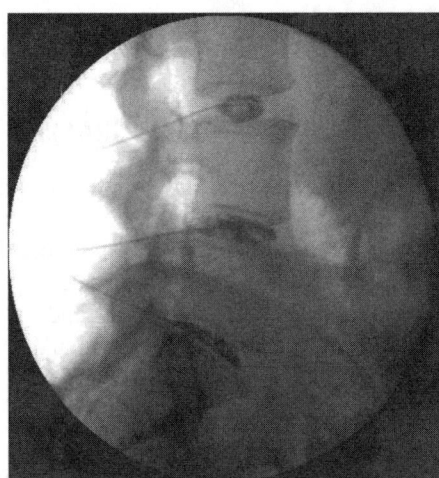

FIGURE 68.1 Lateral view. L3/4: Cotton ball appearance (normal/control disc); L4/5: Degenerated disc with posterior leakage of contrast material into the epidural space; L5/S1: Posterior bulging and degeneration.

annulus. The posterior annulus often bulges and extends well beyond the edge of the vertebral body. Injectate tends to form pools in the nucleus and annulus, filling the fissures but not escaping from the disc itself. Injection is relatively easy into any region.

5. Ruptured: Contrast material is observed extending to the outer margin of the annulus and escaping from the disc. A large quantity of contrast might be seen in the disc; there is no limit on the volume of contrast that can be injected. Almost always a complete fissure is identified, usually in the posterior annulus. The escaping contrast can be readily identified, even if hindered by the posterior longitudinal ligament. (See Figure 68.1 and Figure 68.2.)

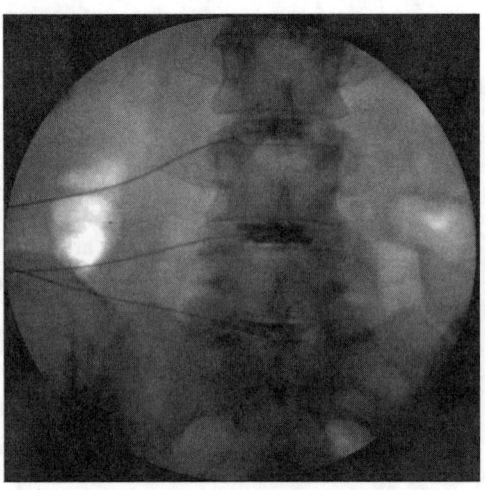

FIGURE 68.2 AP view L3/4, L4/5, L5/S1.

MODIFIED DALLAS DISCOGRAM DESCRIPTION

Sachs et al.[26] developed the Dallas Discogram Description classification system, modified by Schellhas et al.,[27] using five grades (0 to 4) to delineate the appearances of annular tears found in discograms:

Grade 0: Normal discs with an intact annulus
Grade 1: Fissure/tear involving inner one third of annulus
Grade 2: Fissure/tear involving inner two thirds of annulus
Grade 3: Tear extending from the nuclear space either into or through the outer one third of the disc annulus, involving up to 30° of the disc circumference
Grade 4: Tear extending from the nuclear space either into or through the outer one third of the disc annulus, involving greater than 30° of the disc circumference

This modified system of Grade 0 to Grade 4 is straightforward and is commonly used to describe the appearance of tears seen in lumbar discography.

INTERPRETATION OF PAIN RESPONSES

The provocation of pain from injection of an abnormal disc is the *sine qua non* of contemporary discography, along with the confirmation of relief with injection of analgesics. Pain provocation with disc injection is not fully understood. Different hypotheses have been advanced, including pain provocation by raised intradiscal pressure, causing nerve fibers in the annulus to be stretched, pain from biochemical or neurochemical stimulation, or disc injection increases pressure at the vertebral end plates resulting in pain or, similarly, intraosseous pressure increase in the vertebral body itself from pressure transfer across the end plates, resulting in pain.

The topic of pain responses in lumbar discography has generated a voluminous literature. By its subjective and changeable nature, pain itself is difficult to report and record, making statistically valid conclusions or even inferring results for comparison subject to issues of bias, placebo effect, and psychological interpretation. Several authors have made and expounded on this point, and it still enters the literature as a viable topic, when the natural history of lumbar pain is discussed or treatment modalities are compared.[28–30] It will continue to be one point of potential controversy until an objective, quantifiable means of measuring the pain response is found. Close attention should be paid to the interpretation of the pain response during the injection of the disc, that is, reports of whether the pain and the intensity of the pain are similar to or exactly like that for which the patient seeks relief.

Pressure-controlled discography is one measure for the determination of the level of pain response. A disc is determined to be symptomatic or asymptomatic based on the provocation of pain and the pressure at which that pain is produced. The opening pressure at which the patient reports pain, which may be similar or dissimilar to the usual pain experienced by the patient, is used to produce a manometric classification of the intervertebral disc. This classification is based on the work of Derby et al.,[4] which classifies discs as chemically sensitive, mechanically sensitive, or indeterminate according to the pressure giving the onset of pain. In a chemically sensitive disc, pain appears at pressure less than 15 psi greater than opening pressure, mechanically sensitive discs replicate pain with pressures between 15 and 50 psi, and indeterminate discs are those giving a painful response at greater than 50 psi; these findings usually warrant further investigation of a pain source other than the disc. The clinical correlation suggested by Derby is that chemically sensitive discs may be candidates for an IDET (intradiscal electrothermal therapy) procedure (annular pathology), mechanically sensitive discs may be candidates for laser or other discectomy, and indeterminate discs should be reevaluated as the source of pain.

Along with a lack of definitive evidence of the source or mechanism of pain from disc injection, other factors make the assessment of pain difficult — psychological factors are reported to have a profound influence on the accuracy of pain reporting, and a perplexing situation exists whereby some patients report pain upon injection of otherwise normal, nonpathogenic discs. There may exist subtle disc changes with respect to prolapsed annular fibers not contiguous with the disc, or this may be a manifestation of a psychological factor. Nonetheless, patients report pain with radiographically normal-appearing discs. The salient point is that recognition of psychological factors must not be ignored and information given that is pertinent to a patient's prognosis may contribute to the patient's sense of well-being apart from any immediate treatment decision.[29,30]

COMPLICATIONS

The risk of disc infection, discitis, is one of the most respected potential complications. Prophylactic antibiotic use and adherence to strict sterile technique has reduced this risk to very low levels.[31–34] Other complications, which are rare, include meningitis, spinal headache, subdural and epidural abscess, intrathecal hemorrhage, severe reaction to accidental intrathecal injection, disc herniation, retroperitoneal hemorrhage, nausea, convulsions, and increased pain.[35] Poor needle placement may cause damage to the vertebral end plate, leading to vertebral end plate necrosis. Infrequent reports also include the cauda equina syndrome, febrile reactions, and myalgias.[35]

CONCLUSION

Lumbar provocative discography provides information about the structure and pain sensitivity of the disc that cannot be obtained by any other method. Its role is to identify a particular disc as a pain generator and aid in the correlation of abnormal radiographic imaging with that pain. It should be performed by those who are well experienced in the procedure, under strict sterile conditions and with fluoroscopic guidance. There is ample evidence for the use of antibiotics, either intradiscally or intravenously, for prophylaxis against discitis. Correspondingly, maintenance of strict and meticulous sterile technique may accomplish the same end. Information from the procedure should include the volume injected into the disc, the pressure eliciting pain, the patient's pain response with emphasis on the location and similarity to the patient's symptomatic pain, and the observed pattern of contrast distribution. The interpretation and correlation of the pain response is the reason for the examination; increased knowledge of the disc morphology may lead to better treatment planning.

REFERENCES

1. Colhoun, E. et al. (1988). Provocation discography as a guide to planning operations on the spine. *Journal of Bone and Joint Surgery, 70*, 267.
2. Milette, P. C. et al. (1999). Differentiating lumbar disc protrusions, disc bulges, and discs with normal contour but abnormal signal intensity. Magnetic resonance imaging with discographic correlations. *Spine, 24*, 44.
3. Fortin, J. D., Sehgal, N., & Nieves, R. A. (2000). Lumbar and thoracic discography with CT and MRI correlation. In T. A. Lennard (Ed.), *Pain procedures in clinical practice* (p. 241). Philadelphia: Hanley and Belfus, Inc.
4. Derby, R. et al. (1999). The ability of pressure-controlled discography to predict surgical and nonsurgical outcomes. *Spine, 24*, 364.
5. Lindblom, K. (1948). Diagnostic puncture of intervertebral discs in sciatica. *Acta Orthopaedica Scandinavica, 17*, 231.
6. Hirsch, C. (1948). An attempt to diagnose level of disc lesion clinically by disc puncture. *Acta Orthopaedica Scandinavica, 18*, 132.
7. Cloward, R. B. (1958). Cervical discography. Technique, indications and use in the diagnosis of ruptured cervical discs. *American Journal of Roentgenology, 79*, 563.
8. Erlacher, P. R. (1952). Nucleography. *Journal of Bone and Joint Surgery* (Britain), *34B*, 204.
9. Fernstrom, U., & Goldie, I. (1960). Does granulation tissue in the intervertebral disc provoke low back pain? *Acta Orthopaedica Scandinavica, 30*, 202.
10. Holt, E. P. (1964). Fallacy of cervical discography. *Journal of the American Medical Association, 188*, 799.

11. Holt, E. P. (1968). The question of lumbar discography. *Journal of Bone and Joint Surgery, 50*, 720.

12. Mixter, W. J., & Barr, J. S. (1934). Rupture of the intervertebral disc with involvement of the spinal canal. *New England Journal of Medicine, 211*, 210.

13. Crock, H. V. (1970). An appraisal of intervertebral disc lesions. *Medical Journal of Australia, 1*, 983.

14. Guiot, B., & Fessler, R. (2000). Molecular biology of degenerative disc disease. *Neurosurgery, 47*, 1034.

15. Mirza, S. K., & White, A. A. (1995). Anatomy of intervertebral disc and pathophysiology of herniated disc disease. *Journal of Clinical Laser Medicine and Surgery, 13*, 131.

16. Bogduk, N., Tynan, W., & Wilson, A. S. (1981). The nerve supply to the human lumbar intervertebral disc. *Journal of Anatomy, 132*, 39.

17. Schwarzer, A. et al. (1995). The prevalence and clinical features of internal disc disruption in patients with chronic low back pain. *Spine, 20*, 1878.

18. Freemont, A. J. et al. (2002). Current understanding of cellular and molecular events in intervertebral disc degeneration: Implications for therapy. *Journal of Pathology, 196*, 374.

19. Goupille, P. et al. (1998). The role of inflammation in disc herniation-associated radiculopathy, *Seminars in Arthritis and Rheumatism, 28*, 60.

20. Aoki, Y. et al. (2002). Local application of disc-related cytokines on spinal nerve roots. *Spine, 27*, 1614.

21. Rannou, F. et al. (2000). Sensitivity of anulus fibrosus cells to Interleukin 1 beta. Comparison with articular chondrocytes. *Spine, 25*, 17.

22. Doita, M. et al. (2001). Influence of macrophage infiltration of herniated disc tissue on the production of matrix metalloproteinase leading to disc resorption. *Spine, 26*, 1522.

23. Goupille, P. et al. (1998). Matrix metalloproteinases: The clue to intervertebral disc degeneration? *Spine, 23*, 235.

24. Guyer, R. D., & Ohnmeiss, D. D. (1995). Position statement from North American Spine Society diagnostic and therapeutic committee. *Spine, 20*, 248.

25. Adams, M. A., Dolan, P., & Hutton, W. C. (1986). The stages of disc degeneration as revealed by discograms. *Journal of Bone and Joint Surgery* (Britain), *68*, 36.

26. Sachs, B. L. et al. (1987). Dallas discogram description. A new classification of CT/discography in low-back disorders. *Spine, 12*, 287.

27. Schellhas, K. P. et al. (1996). Lumbar disc high-intensity zone: Correlation of MRI and discography. *Spine, 21*, 79.

28. Block, A. R. et al. (1996). Discogenic pain report: Influence of psychological factors. *Spine, 1*, 334.

29. Manchikanti, L. et al. (2001). Provocative discography in low back pain patients with or without somatization disorder: A randomized, prospective evaluation. *Pain Physician, 4*, 227.

30. Manchikanti, L. et al. (2002). Evaluation of the psychological status in chronic low back pain: Comparison with the general population. *Pain Physician, 5*, 149.

31. Schulitz, K. P., Assheuer, J., & Wiesner, L. (1995). Early diagnosis of post-operative discitis. *Zeitschrift fur Orthopadie und Ihre Grenzgebiete, 133*, 148.

32. Osti, O. L., Fraser, R. D., & Vernon-Roberts, B. (1990). Discitis after discography. The role of prophylactic antibiotics. *Journal of Bone and Joint Surgery* (Britain), *72*, 271.

33. Schnoring, M., & Brock, M. (2003). Prophylactic antibiotics in lumbar disc surgery: Analysis of 1030 procedures. *Zentralblatt fur Neurochirurgie, 64*, 24.

34. Boscardin, J. B., Ringus, J. C., & Feingold, D. J. (1992). Human intradiscal levels with cefazolin. *Spine, 17*, S145.

35. Collins, H. R. (1975). An evaluation of cervical and lumbar discography. *Clinical Orthopedics, 107*, 133.

69

Intradiscal Therapies

Vijay Singh, MD, and Laxmaiah Manchikanti, MD

INTRODUCTION

"Intradiscal therapies" is a term commonly used for the minimally invasive, percutaneous techniques applied to the treatment of symptomatic contained disc herniation and discogenic pain due to internal disc disruption or annular fissures.

Historically, intradiscal therapies were directed to the disc nucleus pulposus to remove portions of nuclear material and decompress the disc and reduce pain. Later, methods were introduced to treat fissures or tears in the annulus fibrosus of the disc. The development of intradiscal therapies began with the introduction of chymopapain use in the 1950s. Percutaneous injection of chymopapain was done by Lyman Smith in 1964.[1] This led to a gradual evolution of intradiscal therapies.

Open laminectomies and discectomies have been widely performed and have been established as treatment for disc herniations for many years. Small, contained disc herniations investigated by Carragee and Kim[2] were found less amenable to laminectomy than large herniations. In these subsets of patients with small, contained herniations, percutaneous disc decompressions have been found to be effective with reported success rates of 50 to 70%. Since the introduction of chymopapain injection by Smith, others have done clinical evaluations and patient studies using various techniques of percutaneous disc decompression. Choy[3] produced data for laser discectomy, Onik et al.[4,5] published work done with an automatic technique, automated percutaneous lumbar discectomy (APLD), and more recently several others[6–10] have published data and patient studies with coblation technology, which was introduced in 2000. All of these methods targeted the nucleus pulposus. Derby[11–13] published a review and early clinical data of the technique termed IDET (intradiscal electrothermal therapy), a minimally invasive method targeting the disc annulus for annuloplasty based on the observations that the fibers of the annulus shortened when heat was applied. Saal and Saal[14–16] also published clinical studies of this intradiscal technique in the same year.

The indications for the use of these annuloplasty techniques are similar to those for other intradiscal therapies. Understanding the pathomechanisms of discogenic pain whether from internal disc disruption or from a small contained disc herniation with or without internal disc disruption is vital to a successful outcome.

DISCOGENIC PAIN

Intervertebral discs are innervated by fibers from a branch of the sinuvertebral nerve, but only in the outer third of the annulus in healthy discs. In pathological discs, the nerve endings have been found to extend into the inner portion of the annulus. Mechanical stimulation of these annular fibers results in some cases of discogenic pain, but this is not the only mechanism capable of causing pain. Pain from a degenerated or otherwise damaged disc is now also thought to derive from complex interaction of chemicals released by the disc itself and the interaction of these proinflammatory chemicals with the mediators of the inflammatory cascade beginning with phospholipase A_2 released from damaged cell membranes.[17–19]

Damaged lumbar discs may also herniate portions of nucleus material posterolaterally and increase mechanical pressure on nerve roots, causing radicular pain. Herniation of nuclear material itself may induce the above-mentioned painful inflammatory cascade. Minor trauma, including that resulting from normal activities of daily living and aging, may result in tears or fissures developing in the annulus of the intervertebral disc and, by either direct irritation on nerve endings or activation of the inflammatory cascade, cause pain. Fissures or tears in the annulus may be extensive enough to allow extrusion of disc tissue into the spinal canal and this may also be a pain-producing event. In summary then, the intervertebral disc may undergo insult sufficient to lead to the development of pain, so-called discogenic pain. Regardless of the cause, treating discogenic pain has been a challenge to the medical community for many years and only in the past three decades has real progress been achieved in creating therapies specifically directed to this problem.

There is discussion and ongoing research concerning the exact mechanisms of discogenic pain and the relative importance of each in clinical situations. It is commonly accepted that stretching (mechanical) irritation of the disc by whatever means is not the only method of pain generation. Chemical mediators, enzymes from the disc itself, inflammatory moieties, and proinflammatory intermediates, along with immunological factors and members of the cytokine cascade increase the sensitivity of nociceptors and play a role in the production of discogenic pain.

INTRADISCAL THERAPIES

Open surgical procedures and techniques, which began in the 1930s to relieve radicular pain from a mechanical standpoint, continue to be performed; however, it is increasingly recognized that they may not offer the optimal therapy for some patients with discogenic low back pain. Open surgical intervention to treat spinal pain is indicated for diagnoses of nerve root compression or spinal stenosis with an abnormal neurological examination. Omitting the obvious need for surgery in cases of trauma or mechanical instability, spinal surgery to relieve pain without a confirmed lesion may not be successful if only because of the complex nature of the etiology of spinal pain.

According to the discussion of O'Brien,[20] the diagnosis and treatment of painful degenerative disc disease is one of the more controversial topics in the spine literature today. The points of contention concern the reliability of the diagnosis of the painful site and the reported inadequacies of surgical outcomes combined with the risks and costs of surgery.

Advocates of the surgical approach usually follow guidelines that include failure of previous conservative therapies and confirmation of an involved disc as the source of pain. Even with strict criteria for patient selection many sources report 10 to 30% failure rates in efforts to control pain with open surgery or to achieve the preoperative goals of pain relief and return to normal func-

tioning. This remains an area of controversy and discussion in the literature.[21]

The impetus behind the development of intradiscal therapies was to offer an option to those who were not candidates for surgery. The development of intradiscal therapies has been directed at relieving pain, focusing on either the nucleus or the annulus of the disc and using minimally invasive percutaneous methods. In the last few decades many authors have proposed methods to effect disc decompression by percutaneous routes to relieve pain. One, chymopapain, is no longer available in the United States. Others include manual or automated percutaneous nucleotomy, using a nucleotome, percutaneous laser disc decompression, and percutaneous disc decompression using coblation; another technique (IDET) uses a resistive coil in an attempt to enhance the integrity of the annulus of the disc and control discogenic pain.

CHEMONUCLEOLYSIS

Chemonucleolysis or the injection of enzymes or chemically active agents into the nucleus was introduced in the mid-1960s and developed the concept of removing nuclear material, sparing other intradiscal tissues, which would lead to a reduction in external pressure on an affected nerve root. The enzymes were numerous; including chymopapain, Chymodiactin, and collagenase, among others, and the chemicals included denaturants such as ethanol and others with proteolytic function such as aprotinin. This was the initial attempt to decompress a disc that targeted the disc itself. A wide array of enzymes and enzymatically active chemicals were used to dissolve nuclear material to cause a volumetric decrease in nuclear material and thus a reduction in intradiscal pressure. The difficulty in this method was the control of the chemical activity in the disc and the real potential for spread outside the disc where inflammation and tissue damage could occur and not be monitored or known to the interventionalist. The possibility this could lead to irreversible nerve root damage and rare occurrences of anaphylactic reactions put a damper on its use in the United States. Eventually the manufacturer decided to stop producing chymopapain for the U.S. market, and the method is now available only outside the United States. Research in its use continues in Europe.

Indications: Discogenic pain, contained herniated disc with intact annular margin, failure of other therapy.

Contraindications: Allergy or hypersensitivity to chemical, fissured annulus with communication to the subarachnoid space.

Outcomes: Due to variety of enzymes and chemicals used, and that the amounts and exposure times were different, it is difficult to make valid comparisons.

Complications: Concerns arose because it was found difficult to control where enzymes/chemicals would go and because they could cause anaphylactic reaction outside the discal environs and scar adjacent tissues and nerves irreversibly.

PERCUTANEOUS INTRADISCAL NUCLEOTOMIES

The concept of a minimally invasive approach to treat discs responsible for radicular pain by the volumetric removal of intradiscal tissue to cause a reduction in internal pressure, introduced by chemonucleolysis, was further developed and refined in techniques designed to perform percutaneous discectomies. These were introduced in the 1970s and have been modified in several ways, utilizing endoscopic visualization and an automatic disc shaver technique with aspiration of nuclear material. Reports of efficacy varied with different patient populations and methods used to evaluate outcomes. Nevertheless, most reported series showed reasonably favorable outcomes.

Kambin[22] developed a procedure using an arthroscope for direct visualization in microdiscectomy. He was able to evacuate herniated disc material through a posterolateral approach as well as perform elimination of central disc nuclear mass and effect a decompressive nucleotomy. The method was further enhanced with direct video and fluid management through a single portal approach.

Onik[4,5] introduced an automatic suction shaver to perform an APLD. By drawing and cutting with a reciprocating blade under fluid suction, a percutaneous microdiscectomy could be done. Percutaneous endoscopic lumbar discectomy (PELD) using a rigid endoscope for visualization was described by Mayer and Brock[23] in 1987.

There have been extensive reviews involving many patients. These methods are more technically demanding and patient acceptance is complicated by occasional occurrences of muscles spasm and a sense of post-procedural instability. Reported infection rates in some series have approached 1%, which is higher than that found with other intradiscal methods.

Indications: Discogenic pain, contained herniated disc, failure of other therapies.

Contraindications: Local infection, cord compression, coagulopathies.

Outcomes: Usually reported as successful in 60 to 70%.

Complications: Higher risk of infection often reported; somewhat longer recovery times due to the nature and time of the procedure.

LASER-ASSISTED PERCUTANEOUS DISC DECOMPRESSION

Laser procedures for disc decompression were introduced about 10 years after the emergence of the manual methods. Percutaneous laser disc decompression treated herniated intervertebral discs by using laser energy to vaporize small amounts of intradiscal tissue. The small amount of tissue removed caused a fall in intradiscal pressure with subsequent migration of the herniated portion of the disc away from the affected nerve root.[3] An ongoing concern with this method is the need to control unintentional or inadvertent thermal damage to surrounding tissue. Pulsed lasers gave more of an opportunity to achieve this over the use of continuous lasers, with some types and wavelengths being far more efficacious than others. Success rates were reported in the 70 to 80% range in most series of patients, with relatively few discernible complications. Thermal damage to the vertebral body end plate was reported in several series, and infection rates and other complications remained in the <1% range. Although seemingly an improvement in procedural time and complication rates was found over those of manual methods, the method has some drawbacks.

Indications: Failure of conservative therapy, contained herniated disc with discogenic pain, positive provocative discogram.

Contraindications: Large herniations, local infection, coagulopathies.

Outcomes: Generally reported as favorable in 70% range.

Complications: Inadvertent thermal damage to tissues due to difficulty controlling laser; difficult to control amount of tissue vaporized, thermal damage to vertebral end plates a risk.

PERCUTANEOUS DISC DECOMPRESSION USING COBLATION

Coblation technology uses radiofrequency (RF) energy to effect dissolution of nuclear material and denaturation of intradiscal proteoglycans. By reducing intradiscal volume, intradiscal pressure is reduced, and this is thought to be a factor in the reduction of pain.

Effects on the intradiscal environment may also decrease the inflammatory-cascade mediated stimulus for pain. Animal studies have shown that the application of RF energy results in minimal damage to the surrounding tissue. A lower temperature than other methods is used and results in the absence of necrotic tissue intradiscally. Significant reductions in intradiscal pressure have been reported in human cadaveric specimens, and measurement of intradiscal temperature variations showed an absence of temperature increase 5 mm from the RF source.

Prospective trials have given similarly favorable results. Reduction of pain, reduction in use of medications for pain, and decreases in numeric pain scores all have been significant in patients followed for 6 to 12 months.[8,9] Patient acceptance has been equally high and, with lessened tissue damage, its use for discogenic low back pain provides another option with short recovery times.

> **Indications:** Failure of conservative regimens, discogenic pain, including that from small contained disc herniations, inadequate pain control with medication, positive provocative discogram.
> **Contraindications:** Local infection, sepsis, coagulopathies.
> **Outcomes:** Generally in the 70+% range, excellent patient acceptance.
> **Complications:** None reported to date.

INTRADISCAL ELECTROTHERMAL THERAPY

This method is a minimally invasive one in which the annulus and not the nucleus is the targeted entity. Unlike the other methods, it is not indicated for radicular pain. IDET is a therapy directed toward tears in the annulus; by resistive heating these tears are thought to be coagulated and stabilized, and annular nerve fibers are rendered nonviable.[24] A normal neurological examination without deficits is required, with 6 months of persistent symptoms. Imaging studies are performed to confirm the absence of disc herniation. The procedure uses a resistive coil, inserted percutaneously and positioned to assume a circular configuration within the annulus. This coil is heated to a temperature and for a time sufficient to coagulate annular collagen and destroy annular neural elements. The actual mechanism of action, however, remains unverified. Neither collagen denaturation nor nerve ablation has been confirmed in patients. However, successful outcome percentages have been reported with the method that are comparable to those reported with the nuclear procedures. In a large, randomized, controlled prospective study Pauza et al.[25] examined 64 patients who met eligibility requirements including 6 months discogenic pain, positive discography, and an absence of comorbidity. Improvement in pain scores and disability scales was seen only in the IDET group, but 50% of those treated experienced no benefit. This report supports strict inclusion criteria to provide relief for a small proportion of patients undergoing the IDET procedure.

Restricted activities and back bracing are usually advised for 6 to 8 weeks; many patients wear a brace for 12 months or longer.[26] In many instances pain relief is not apparent until 6 months.

> **Indications:** Failure of aggressive conservative therapy, discogenic pain with confirmed annular lesions, positive provocative discogram.
> **Contraindications:** Presence of herniated disc tissue, stenosis, evidence of neural compression on magnetic resonance imaging (MRI), previous lumbar surgery, presence of significant psychological issues.
> **Outcomes:** Generally favorable over 2-year period in uncontrolled reports; one controlled study found success rates varying from 23 to 60% depending on the criteria used. The percentage of patients on disability is reported as unchanged. Somewhat longer recovery times; bracing and restricted activities for up to 1 year post-procedure.
> **Complications:** Poorer results when patient is obese, presence of pain continuing after the procedure with half of patients reporting dissatisfaction in one retrospective analysis.

CONCLUSION

Intradiscal therapies have emerged as an option for patients who have failed conservative therapies and are not candidates for open surgery. For many, they are an option for treatment of pain and can reduce or eliminate the need for long-term medication, with its well-known costs and risks. There is ample evidence that long-term use of nonsteroidal anti-inflammatory drugs (NSAIDs) is not without risks, even life-threatening risks in some cases due to renal effects of NSAIDs, as well as more well-known gastrointestinal bleeding problems. The long-term use of opioids for pain carries another set of medical and social costs. Frequent monitoring for compliance, risks of tolerance, and potential addiction are common concerns for patients and providers alike.

The impetus for these intradiscal treatments has come out of a need to provide an option to the number of people who would prefer not to take medications long term and who are not considered able to benefit from open surgical intervention. Ideally, treatments would reduce pain and the need for medication, and not impede a return to desired function. Among the most important criteria for the use of these methods is patient selection. Accurate diagnosis and fundamentally sound correlation of symptoms with findings are essential to the success of any of these therapies.

REFERENCES

1. Smith, L. (1964). Enzyme dissolution of the nucleus pulposus in humans. *Journal of the American Medical Association, 187*, 137.

2. Carragee, E. J., & Kim, D. H. (1997). A prospective analysis of magnetic resonance imaging findings in patients with sciatica and lumbar disc herniation. Correlation of outcomes with disc fragment and canal morphology. *Spine, 22,* 1650.

3. Choy, D. S. (1998). Percutaneous laser disc decompression (PLDD): Twelve years' experience with 752 procedures in 518 patients. *Journal of Clinical Laser Medicine and Surgery, 16,* 322.

4. Onik, G. et al. (1988). Automated percutaneous discectomy: Preliminary experience. *Acta Neurochirurgia Supplement* (Wein), *43,* 58.

5. Onik, G. et al. (1985). Percutaneous lumbar discectomy using a new aspiration probe. *American Journal of Neuroradiology, 6,* 290.

6. Yetkinler, D. N., Nau, W. H., & Brandt, L. L. (2002, September 4-7). *Disc temperature measurements during the nucleoplasty and IDET procedures.* Paper presented at 6th International Conference on Spinal Surgery. Ankara Turkey.

7. Chen, Y. C. et al. (2001, September). Nucleoplasty (volumetric tissue ablation and coagulation of the nucleus) for chronic discogenic back pain and/or radiculopathy: A preliminary 6-month follow-up study. In *Proceedings of the International Spinal Injection Society (ISIS) 9th Annual Meeting,* Boston, MA.

8. Sharps, L. S., & Isaac, Z. (2002). Percutaneous disc decompression using nucleoplasty. *Pain Physician, 5,* 120.

9. Singh, V. et al. (2002). Percutaneous disc decompression using coblation (nucleoplasty) in the treatment of discogenic pain. *Pain Physician, 5,* 250.

10. Slipman, C. W. et al. (2002, September). Preliminary outcomes of percutaneous nucleoplasty for treatment of axial low back pain. A comparison of patients with versus without associated central focal protrusion. In *Proceedings of the International Spinal Injection Society (ISIS) 9th Annual Meeting,* Austin, TX.

11. Derby, R. et al. (1999, August). Intradiscal electrothermal therapy by catheter: 12 month follow-up. *Proceedings of the 7th Annual Scientific Meeting of the International Spinal Injection Society,* Las Vegas.

12. Derby, R. et al. (2000). Intradiscal electrothermal annuloplasty (IDET): A novel approach for treating chronic discogenic back pain. *Neuromodulation, 3,* 82.

13. Derby, R. (2003). Intradiscal electrothermal annuloplasty: current concepts. *Pain Physician, 6,* 383.

14. Saal, J. S., & Saal, J. A. (2000). Management of chronic discogenic low back pain with a thermal intradiscal catheter: A preliminary study. *Spine, 25,* 382.

15. Saal, J. A., & Saal, J. S. (1999, October). Intradiscal electrothermal annuloplasty (IDET) treatment for multilevel discogenic pain: Prospective 1 year follow-up outcome study. *Proceedings of the 14th Annual Meeting of the North American Spine Society.* Chicago.

16. Saal, J. S., & Saal, J. A. (1999, October). Intradiscal electrothermal annuloplasty (IDET) for chronic disc disease: Outcome assessment with minimum 1-year follow-up. *Proceedings of the 14th Annual Meeting of the North American Spine Society,* Chicago.

17. Groupille, P. et al. (1998). The role of inflammation in disc herniation-associated radiculopathy. *Seminars in Arthritis and Rheumatism, 28,* 60.

18. Guoit, B., & Fessler, R. (2000). Molecular biology of degenerative disc disease. *Neurosurgery, 47,* 1034.

19. Freemont, A. J. et al. (2002). Current understanding of cellular and molecular events in intervertebral disc degeneration: Implications for therapy. *Journal of Pathology, 196,* 374.

20. O'Brien, J. P. (1996). Lumbar disc disease with discogenic pain: What surgical treatment is most effective? *Spine, 21,* 1836.

21. Zdeblick, T. A. (1996). Lumbar disc disease with discogenic pain: What surgical treatment is most effective? *Spine, 21,* 1836.

22. Kambin, P. (1993). Arthroscopic microdiscectomy of the lumbar spine. *Clinical Sports Medicine, 12,* 143.

23. Mayer, H. M., & Brock, M. (1993). Percutaneous endoscopic lumbar discectomy (PELD). *Neurosurgery Review, 16,* 115.

24. Davis, T. T. et al. (2004). The IDET procedure for chronic low back pain. *Spine, 29,* 752.

25. Pauza, K. J. et al. (2004). A randomized, placebo-controlled trial of intradiscal electrothermal therapy for the treatment of discogenic low back pain. *Spine Journal, 4,* 27.

26. Chen, S. P. et al. (2003). Risk factors for failure and complications of intradiscal electrothermal therapy: A pilot study. *Spine, 28,* 1142.

—— 70 ——

Percutaneous Lysis of Lumbar Epidural Adhesions and Hypertonic Saline Neurolysis

Laxmaiah Manchikanti, MD, and Vijay Singh, MD

INTRODUCTION

Treatment of chronic back pain, specifically for postsurgical patients and patients with epidural fibrosis, continues to be a challenge. The effectiveness of epidural steroid injections in patients with epidural fibrosis has not been studied. Further surgery for peridural scarring has resulted in disappointing results, with success rates as low as 12%.[1–3] One of the techniques described to effectively manage chronic low back pain secondary to epidural fibrosis is adhesiolysis of epidural scar tissue.[4–18] The purposes of percutaneous epidural lysis of adhesions are to eliminate deleterious effects of a scar, which can physically prevent direct application of drugs to nerves or other tissues, and to assure delivery of high concentrations of injected drugs to the target areas. In a 2002 review describing the role of decompressive surgery in managing chronic pain of spinal origin after lumbar surgery, Phillips and Cunningham[19] reported that no form of surgical treatment or adhesion lysis procedure for this diagnosis has proved to be safe and effective.

HISTORY

Epidural injection for chronic low back pain was performed by Sicard[20] in 1901. Eight years later, reports on cures of sciatica with epidural anesthesia were made by Caussade and Queste.[21] The initial epidurography was performed in 1921 by Sicard and Forestier.[22] Hitchcock[23] administered cold hypertonic saline in 1967 for the treatment of chronic pain intrathecally. Ventrafridda and Spreafico[24] reported the use of intrathecal saline to relieve pain in patients with cancer. Hitchock[25] also reported that the determining factor in the therapeutic effect of this solution was its hypertonicity rather than the temperature.

Racz and Holubec[6] reported the first use of epidural hypertonic saline to facilitate lysis of adhesions. In 1989, Racz et al.[26] evaluated dural permeability in dogs, demonstrating slow transdural equilibration of hypertonic saline. Payne and Rupp[27] used hyaluronidase in an attempt to alter the rapidity of onset and extent, intensity, and duration of caudal anesthesia. Moore[28] also described the addition of hyaluronidase to caudal epidural injections to enhance the spread of local anesthetic.

Cyriax's[29] extensive experience with 20,000 patients showing significant improvement with large volumes of caudal epidural anesthetic was reported by Ombregt and Ter Veer.[29] Brown[30] also injected large volumes ranging from 40 to 100 mL of normal saline, which was followed by the injection of 80 mg of methylprednisolone in an attempt to mechanically disrupt and prevent preformation of presumably fibrotic lesions in patients with sciatica. Hyaluronidase was introduced as an alternative agent by Stolker et al.[31] Over the years, multiple investigators[6–18, 26] have studied the effectiveness of adhesiolysis and hypertonic saline neurolysis with or without hyaluronidase.

PURPOSE

Adhesiolysis of epidural scar tissue, followed by the injection of hypertonic saline, described by Racz et al.,[6,7–11,26] involved epidurography, adhesiolysis, and injection of hyaluronidase, bupivacaine, triamcinolone diacetate, and 10% sodium chloride solution on day 1, followed by injections of bupivacaine and hypertonic sodium chloride solution on days 2 and 3. Manchikanti et al.[10,12–17] described and studied a modification of the Racz protocol from a 3-day procedure to a 1-day procedure.

The purpose of percutaneous epidural lysis of adhesions is to eliminate deleterious effects of scar formation, which can physically prevent direct application of drugs to nerves or other tissues to treat chronic back pain with or without radiculopathy. The goal of percutaneous lysis of epidural adhesions is to assure delivery of high concentrations of injected drugs to the target areas.

PATHOPHYSIOLOGY

Kuslich et al.[32] identified intervertebral discs, nerve root dura, facet joints, ligaments, fascia, and muscles as tissues capable of transmitting pain in the low back and lower extremity. The pathophysiology of spinal radicular pain continues to be a subject of ongoing research and controversy. Proposed etiologies include neural compression with dysfunction, vascular compromise, inflammation, and biochemical influences.[33] Multiple causes described for chronic low back and lower extremity pain include not only disc herniation with neural compression and dysfunction, but also vascular compromise, inflammation, biochemical influences, postlumbar laminectomy syndrome, and spinal stenosis. Postlumbar laminectomy syndrome or pain following operative procedures of the lumbar spine is estimated in approximately 5 to 40% of patients after surgical intervention.[11,13,34–37] Although there are multiple etiologies responsible for postlumbar laminectomy pain, descriptions of causes of continued pain after surgical intervention have included epidural fibrosis, facet joint arthritis, spinal stenosis, and other causes.

Among patients with postlumbar laminectomy syndrome, epidural fibrosis is seen as a common phenomenon, which contributes to approximately 60% of the patients with recurring symptoms in conjunction with instability.[37] McCarron[38] reported an inflammatory reaction in the spinal cord sections taken from dogs sacrificed after the initial injection of homogenized nucleus pulposus. Cooper et al.[39] reported periradicular fibrosis and vascular abnormalities occurring with herniated intervertebral disc. Hoyland et al.,[40] in a cadaveric study, found significant pathological changes within and around the nerve root complex, including peri- and intraneural fibrosis, edema of nerve roots, and focal demyelination, proposing that venous obstruction may be an important pathogenic mechanism in the development of perineural and intraneural fibrosis. Epidural adhesions were also demonstrated in cadavers with lumbar disc herniation, with 40% of cadavers showing adhesions at L4/5 level, 36% at L5/S1

level, and 16% at L3/4 level.[41] Further, it was shown that perineural fibrosis, which interferes with cerebrospinal fluid–mediated nutrition, can render nerve roots hyperesthetic and hypersensitive to compression forces.[42,43] Songer et al.[44] showed that postoperative scar tissue renders the nerve susceptible to injury. Even though epidural fibrosis is commonly seen in patients with recurring symptoms in conjunction with instability in postlumbar surgery syndrome,[19,34,35,37,45–50] its role as a causative factor of chronic spinal pain or as a pain generator continues to be questioned.[13,19,35,45,48,49] In a study of the relationship between peridural scar evaluated by magnetic resonance imaging (MRI) and radicular pain after lumbar discectomy, Ross et al.[50] showed that subjects with extensive peridural scarring were three times more likely to experience recurrent radicular pain.

Multiple investigators have stated that epidural adhesions are difficult to diagnose by conventional studies such as myelography, computerized tomography (CT), and MRI, even though modern technology has made significant improvements in this area.[4–18,51,52] Thus, it is believed that epidural adhesions are best diagnosed by performing an epidurogram, which is most commonly performed via the caudal route, followed by the other routes, including the lumbar interlaminar route.[4–18,51–57] Epidural filling defects have been reported in a significant number of patients after surgical intervention, but also in patients with no history of prior surgery.[51]

It is accepted that while peridural scarring in itself is not painful, it can produce pain by "trapping" spinal nerves so that movement places tension on the nerves, thus eliciting pain in an inflamed nerve.[8,9,32,44] Kuslich et al.[32] reported that back pain was produced by stimulation of several lumbar tissues, even though the outer layer of the annulus fibrosis and posterior longitudinal ligament innervated by sinuvertebral nerves was the most common source of pain.

RATIONALE

The rationale for adhesiolysis and hypertonic saline neurolysis in the management of spinal pain stems from the concept that epidural adhesions are a common source of chronic low back pain. The epidural space restricted by adhesions is safely accessible using a special catheter. Removal or correction of structural abnormalities of the lumbar spine may fail to cure and may even worsen painful conditions; degenerative processes of the lumbar spine and the origin of spinal pain are complex; the effectiveness of a large variety of therapeutic interventions in managing low back pain has not been demonstrated conclusively; and the reasonable effectiveness of adhesiolysis and hypertonic saline neurolysis has been demonstrated.[4,6–19]

It was rationalized by Racz et al.[7–9,53] that in patients requiring adhesiolysis, the following may be present:

TABLE 70.1

Results of Published Reports of Percutaneous Adhesiolysis and Hypertonic Saline Neurolysis for One to Three Procedures

Ref.	Study Characteristics	No. of Patients	No. of Days of Procedure	3 Months	6 Months	12 Months
Manchikanti et al.[17]	P, C, RA, DB	Group I = 25*	1	0%	0%	0%
		Group II = 25**		60%	60%	60%
		Group III = 25***		72%	72%	72%
Heavner et al.[9]	P, C, RA, DB	59	3	49%	43%	49%
Manchikanti et al.[16]	P, RA, C	45	1	97%	93%	47%
Racz and Holubec[6]	R, RA	72	3	43%	13%	N/A
Manchikanti et al.[14]	R, RA	103	2	70%	28%	15%
Manchikanti et al.[14]	R, RA	129	1	68%	36%	13%
Manchikanti et al.[12]	R	18	1	89%	61%	17%

Note: R = retrospective; C = controlled; RA = randomized; DB = double blind; P = prospective.

* Control.

** Adhesiolysis only.

*** Adhesiolysis with hypertonic saline neurolysis.

inflammation, edema, fibrosis, and venous congestion; mechanical pressure on posterior longitudinal ligaments, annulus fibrosus, and spinal nerve; reduced or absent nutrient delivery to the spinal nerve or nerve root; and central sensitization. Hence, it was postulated that it is reasonable to treat back pain with or without radiculopathy with local application of anti-inflammatory medication (e.g., corticosteroids), agents aimed at reducing edema (e.g., hypertonic sodium chloride solution), corticosteroids, local anesthetics, and hyaluronidase to promote lysis. Thus, percutaneous lysis of adhesions is indicated in patients with appropriate diagnostic evaluation and after failure or ineffectiveness of conservative modalities of treatment has been proved.

While most commonly used methods involve entry into the epidural space through the sacral hiatus, medication placed in the posterior or posterolateral epidural space may not reach pathology in an intravertebral foramen or in the anterior epidural space.[4,5,18,58–71] The rationale for transforaminal approach is based on lesion-specific adhesiolysis and delivery of medication to fulfill the aim of reaching the primary site of pathology, thus improving the ultimate outcome. In fact, present evidence evaluating the effectiveness of transforaminal steroids is encouraging compared with that for interlaminar and caudal epidural steroid injections.

CLINICAL EFFECTIVENESS

Clinical effectiveness of percutaneous adhesiolysis was evaluated in three randomized, controlled trials[9,16,17] and five retrospective evaluations,[6,12,14,15] and is summarized in Table 70.1.

Manchikanti et al.[17] in a randomized, double-blind trial evaluated the effectiveness of 1-day lumbar epidural adhesiolysis and hypertonic saline neurolysis in the treatment of chronic low back pain. In this study, they evaluated the effectiveness of not only adhesiolysis, but also hypertonic saline neurolysis. The results showed significant improvement in patients undergoing adhesiolysis with hypertonic saline neurolysis and in patients with adhesiolysis and hypertonic saline neurolysis at 3 months, 6 months, and 12 months, compared with baseline measurements, as well as compared with control group without adhesiolysis, for numerous parameters measured. In the study, 72% of patients with adhesiolysis and hypertonic saline neurolysis (Group III), 60% of patients with adhesiolysis only without hypertonic saline neurolysis (Group II), compared with 0% in control group (Group I), showed significant improvement at 12-month follow-up. Figure 70.1 through Figure 70.3 and Table 70.2 illustrate improvement in multiple outcome parameters.

Heavner et al.[9] studied percutaneous epidural adhesiolysis, with a prospective evaluation of 0.9% sodium chloride solution versus 10% sodium chloride solution with steroids, with prospective 1-year follow-up. They concluded that percutaneous epidural neuroplasty, as part of an overall pain management strategy, reduces pain in 25% or more of patients with radiculopathy plus low back pain refractory to conventional therapies. They also noted that the use of hypertonic saline and hyaluronidase may reduce the number of patients that require additional treatments. However, adhesiolysis was effective, even in the patients receiving normal saline. They also showed that the percent of patients requiring additional treatments during 1-year follow-up was approximately 70%, at, on average, around

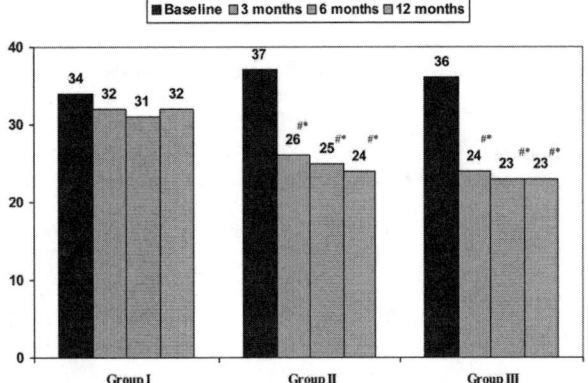

# Indicates significant difference within the group compared to baseline (p < 0.001).
* Indicates significant difference with group I, at the time of evaluation (p < 0.001).

FIGURE 70.1 The outcome measurements based on Oswestry Disability Index 2.0. (From L. Manchikanti et al., 2004, *Pain Physician*, 7, 177. Reproduced with permission from authors and ASIPP.)

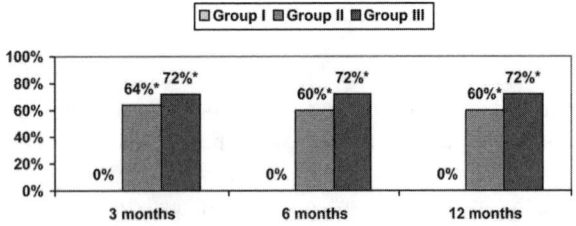

* Indicates significant difference with Group I, at the time of evaluation (p < 0.001).

FIGURE 70.2 Proportion of patients with significant relief (≥50%) at 3 months, 6 months, and 12 months. (From L. Manchikanti et al., 2004, *Pain Physician*, 7, 177. Reproduced with permission from authors and ASIPP.)

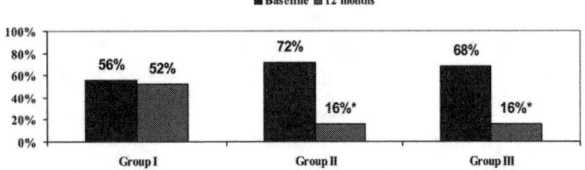

* Indicates significant difference with baseline values within the group (p < 0.001).

FIGURE 70.3 Change in proportion of patients with significant opioid intake. (From L. Manchikanti et al., 2004, *Pain Physician*, 7, 177. Reproduced with permission from authors and ASIPP.)

70 days. This figure was approximately 60% in patients receiving hypertonic saline, and 80% in patients receiving normal saline. Finally, Heavner et al.[9] concluded that the most significant finding of the study was that at 1-year follow-up, 49% of the patients had pain relief in the body area targeted for the lesion-specific therapy.

Manchikanti et al.[6] evaluated the role of 1-day epidural adhesiolysis in the management of chronic low back pain in a randomized clinical trial involving 45 patients. In the study, 15 patients were randomly assigned to the

control group and treated with conservative modalities including medication, physical therapy, and an exercise program; and 30 patients in group II were treated with percutaneous epidural adhesiolysis and hypertonic saline neurolysis. The patients were evaluated over a period of 1.5 to 3 years. The study showed that overall health status improved significantly in the treatment group in all parameters, including average pain, physical health, mental health, functional status, psychological status, and narcotic intake.

The effectiveness of percutaneous adhesiolysis with hypertonic saline neurolysis was also evaluated in refractory spinal stenosis. Manchikanti et al.[12] studied patients failing to respond to multiple modalities of treatment, including fluoroscopically directed epidural steroid injections with spinal stenosis. This retrospective evaluation included 18 patients derived from a total sample of 239 patients undergoing adhesiolysis and hypertonic saline neurolysis over a period of 3 years. The results showed significant improvement with reduction in pain and improvement of physical health, mental health, and functional status. They also reported improvements in psychological status and decrease in narcotic intake. The results showed that with one to three injections, cumulative relief with greater than 50% relief was seen in 89% of the patients at 1 month and 3 months, declining to 61% of the patients at 6 months. They also evaluated cumulative relief (greater than 50%) with 1 to 10 injections and reported 89% of patients achieving greater than 50% relief at 3 months, 72% at 6 months, 17% at 1 year, and 11% at 2 years.

In contrast to the above reports, Devulder et al.[57] concluded that epidurography might confirm epidural filling defects, but a better contrast spread, assuming scar lysis does not guarantee sustained pain relief, as filling defects were confirmed in 88% of the patients with epidurography; but significant pain relief was seen in only 33% of the patients at 1 month, 13% at 3 months, and 0% at 12 months. However, the problem with this study was that lysis of adhesions was not lesion specific. Consequently, the delivery of drugs was also nonspecific.

The quality of evidence presented in clinical effectiveness studies reviewed for this report includes two randomized clinical trials[9,17] that are of high quality, one randomized trial[16] of moderate quality, followed by five retrospective reports, two of which were randomized. The type and strength of efficacy evidence are strong for short-term and long-term relief.

INDICATIONS

Percutaneous epidural adhesiolysis and hypertonic saline neurolysis are indicated in patients with chronic low back pain who have failed to respond to conservative modalities of treatments, including epidural injections administered

TABLE 70.2
Analysis of Psychological Outcome Measurements

		Baseline			12 Months		
		I	II	III	I	II	III
		25	25	25	25	25	25
Depression	Diagnosis	15 (60%)	18 (72%)	16 (64%)	13 (52%)	6*# (24%)	6*# (24%)
	Score	57 ± 8.7	59 ± 11.3	58 ± 13.0	55 ± 8.6	49*# ± 7.6	47*# ± 11.9
	Mean ± SD						
Anxiety	Diagnosis	14 (56%)	16 (64%)	13 (52%)	12 (48%)	4*# (16%)	5*# (20%)
	Score	56 ± 10.6	58 ± 10.5	55 ± 11.4	54 ± 9.2	47*# ± 8.5	46* ± 10.3
	Mean ± SD						
Somatization	Diagnosis	14 (56%)	19 (76%)	16 (64%)	12 (48%)	4*# (16%)	5*# (20%)
	Score	55 ± 8.0	59 ± 8.5	57 ± 8.3	54 ± 7.8	48*# ± 7.5	46*# ± 9.3
	Mean ± SD						

* Indicates significant difference with Group I, at the time of evaluation.

# Indicates significant difference with baseline values within the group various pints of evaluation.

Note: From "One Day Lumbar Epidural Adhesiolysis and Hypertonic Saline Neurolysis in Treatment of Chronic Low Back Pain: A Randomized Controlled Trial," by L. Manchikanti et al., 2004, *Pain Physician*, 7, 177. Reproduced with permission from authors and ASIPP.

TABLE 70.3
Indications for Lysis of Epidural Adhesions

- Postlaminectomy syndrome
- Epidural fibrosis
- Spinal stenosis
- Radiculopathy
- Small herniated discs
- Fractures of the vertebral bodies
- Vertebral metastases
- Degenerative diseases
- Disc disruption

Note: Adapted from Racz et al.[6–9,11]

under fluoroscopic guidance and other well-documented therapeutic modalities. Racz et al.[6–9,11] described various conditions in which epidural lysis of adhesions is indicated, including postlaminectomy syndrome, epidural adhesions, disc disruption, traumatic or pathologic vertebral body compression fracture, spinal stenosis, and resistant multilevel degenerative arthritis (Table 70.3).

COMPLICATIONS

The most common and worrisome complications of adhesiolysis in the lumbar spine are related to dural puncture, spinal cord compression, catheter shearing, infection, steroids, hypertonic saline, and hyaluronidase.[4,5,29,72–94] Unintended subarachnoid or subdural puncture with injection of local anesthetic or hypertonic saline is one of the major complications of the procedure. Hypertonic saline injected into the subarachnoid space has been reported to cause cardiac arrhythmias, myelopathy, paralysis, and loss of sphincter control.[76] In fact, Aldrete et al.[74] attributed incidences of arachnoiditis following epidural adhesiolysis with hypertonic saline to subarachnoid leakage of hypertonic saline. A case of myelopathy has been reported after intrathecal administration of hypertonic saline of 15%, 10 mL, diluted with cerebrospinal fluid to a volume of 12 mL, preceded by an injection of 1 mL of an aqueous solution of morphine sulfate without preservative, 10 mg/mL, diluted with cerebrospinal fluid to a volume of 10 mL, and 1 mL of which was slowly administered intrathecally.[76] Autopsy findings of this patient, who died 16 months after intrathecal administration of hypertonic saline, showed peripheral accentuated loss of myelinated fibers within the spinal cord from T12 downward, as well as dense collagenous thickening of the dorsal leptomeninges from T9 to T11. This case report was a devastating complication.[76] However, in a large study of 108 patients suffering from intractable pain and treated with intrathecal hypertonic saline, it was reported that sphincter disorders occurred in 8% of the patients, with 2.7% experiencing cauda equina syndromes with paraplegia.[76] They also reported rapid recovery in one patient, but quite slow and incomplete recovery in the others, attributing the cauda equina syndromes to preexisting arachnoiditis in one patient and two arteriovascular diseases in the others. In a survey of 648 neurosurgeons, it was reported that 31.2% had used intrathecal hypertonic saline to treat pain in 1,943 patients with adverse reactions in 11.2% of the patients compared with 7.6% of those treated with normal or diluted saline injections.[78]

Further, 22 patients, or 1%, suffered significant morbidity with paraplegia or tetraplegia in 16, or 0.76% of the patients, and monoparesis in 1 patient (0.05%).[78] Other reports of spinal cord lesions by subdural injection of neurolytic agents and local anesthetics included descriptions of exuberant pachymeningitis reaction in dogs.[80] However, the other postmortem examinations in humans after saline injections were more sobering.[78]

The second specific complication of percutaneous epidural adhesiolysis is related to catheter shearing and its retention in the epidural space. Even though the RK™ needle (Epimed International, Inc.) and Racz™ catheter (Epimed International, Inc.) have been specifically designed for this procedure, catheter shearing has been reported. This problem was reported as occurring in five such cases by Racz and others.[10] Manchikanti and Bakhit[75] also reported a torn Racz catheter in the lumbar epidural space, which was successfully removed.

Spinal cord compression following rapid injections into the epidural space, which may cause large increases in intraspinal pressure with a risk of cerebral hemorrhage, visual disturbance, headache, and compromise of spinal cord blood flow, has been mentioned. However, the only complication reported following epidural injection has been vision loss, but no such complications have been reported following adhesiolysis and hypertonic saline neurolysis.

Epidural infection following this procedure is a distinct possibility due to the procedure itself, as well as potential immunosuppression secondary to steroid injection. Racz et al.[6-9,11] have reported no instances of epidural abscess in their patient population. Manchikanti et al.[12-17] reported serious infection in one patient with the development of an abscess; however, no involvement of the spinal canal was noted. They also reported a suspicion of infection in 2% of the cases. In a 1-year study of the incidence of spinal epidural abscess, nine cases of epidural abscess formation from a total of 17,372 epidural catheters were noted.[88] Others described epidural abscess formation as an uncommon but devastating complication that has been associated with continuous epidural analgesia, as well as single-shot epidural injections.[90] They also noted that epidural abscess most often arises in association with systemic infection, but it rarely occurs following epidural analgesia.[90]

Direct trauma to the spinal cord following lumbar epidural injections has been rarely reported, but it can result in disastrous complications.[89] None of the case reports has involved percutaneous lysis of epidural adhesions. The potential for spinal cord trauma is more likely with percutaneous adhesiolysis with hypertonic saline injection than with other epidural procedures, as the injection of adjuvant agents with preservatives may be unforgiving. Additional issues with transforaminal epidural adhesiolysis include intravascular penetration and neural trauma that may be higher than with the caudal or intralaminar approaches. The incidence of vascular epidural injections documented by contrast-enhanced fluoroscopic imaging and negative blood aspiration has varied from 5 to 11%.[95,96]

Neural trauma is a potential complication, even though there are no such case reports with either caudal or transforaminal epidural adhesiolysis.[97,98] Once again, this emphasizes the risks associated with all types of neural blockade, specifically epidural adhesiolysis, with either the caudal or transforaminal routes, even when performed with precautions; following the protocol and diligence are extremely crucial. Thus, no injection should be performed without confirming the location of the needle under fluoroscopic visualization with contrast injection.

Occasional sensitivity (3%) to hyaluronidase has been reported in a series of 1,520 epidural administrations of hyaluronidase.[28] However, Racz et al.[6-9] reported no such incidences of hyaluronidase sensitivity and postulated that the steroid leaves the space more slowly than hyaluronidase, which may help protect against allergic reaction, as the steroid is placed exactly at the site where the hyaluronidase is also deposited.

Other side effects are related to the administration of steroids and are generally attributed to the chemistry or pharmacology of the steroids. The safety of steroids and preservatives at epidural therapeutic doses has been demonstrated in both clinical and experimental studies.[99-109] The major theoretical complications of corticosteroid administration include arachnoiditis, suppression of the pituitary-adrenal axis, hypocorticism, Cushing syndrome, osteoporosis, avascular necrosis of bone, steroid myopathy, weight gain, fluid retention, and hyperglycemia.[107-117] Other potential complications include hypertension, hypokalemia, epidural lipomatosis, retinal hemorrhage, increased intraocular pressure, subcapsular cataract formation, insomnia, mood swings, psychosis, facial flushing, headache, gastrointestinal disturbances, and menstrual disturbances. Although the use of corticosteroids repeatedly for days or even a few weeks does not lead to adrenal insufficiency upon cessation of treatment, prolonged therapy with corticosteroids occasionally may result in the suppression of pituitary–adrenal function that can be slow in returning to normal. Rare hypothalamic–pituitary–adrenal suppression during corticosteroid administration with epidural injections and after its withdrawal has been reported. However, no such reports have implicated percutaneous adhesiolysis and hypertonic saline neurolysis. Table 70.4 illustrates the comparative pharmacology of commonly used steroids in neural blockade in general and adhesiolysis and hypertonic saline neurolysis in particular.

TABLE 70.4

Pharmacologic Profile of Commonly Used Steroids

Name of Drug	Equivalent Dose	Epidural Dose	Anti-Inflammatory Potency	Sodium Retention Capacity	Duration of Adrenal Suppression		
					IM	Single Epidural	Three Epidurals
Triamcinolone acetonide (Kenalog®)	4 mg	40–80 mg	5	0	2–6 weeks	N/A	2–3 months
Betamethasone (Celestone Soluspan®)	0.6 mg	6–12 mg	25	0	1–2 weeks	N/A	N/A
Triamcinolone diacetate (Aristocort®)	4 mg	40–80 mg	5	0	1–2 weeks	1–5 weeks	N/A
Methylprednisolone acetate (Depo-Medrol®)	4 mg	40–80 mg	5	0.5	1–6 weeks	1–3 weeks	N/A

Note: IM = Intramuscular. Adapted from Manchikanti et al.[5]

TECHNICAL CONSIDERATIONS

The technique of adhesiolysis involves accessing the lumbar epidural space by utilizing a caudal, an interlaminar, or a transforaminal approach. Entry is performed with a 16-gauge RK needle (Epimed), followed by advancement of a Racz catheter into the epidural space, with appropriate lysis of adhesions under radiographic control using nonionic contrast medium. Subsequently, a combination of local anesthetic and steroid is injected into the epidural space through the catheter, following which hypertonic saline neurolysis is carried out by slow and intermittent injection of hypertonic saline, either by infusion or in incremental doses. In the classic Racz technique, the procedure is repeated without steroids on day 2 and day 3; whereas, with other modifications, the catheter is removed after the initial procedure is performed. Racz and his followers also recommend hyaluronidase with these injections.

RACZ TECHNIQUE

The technique employed by Racz and colleagues[6–9,11] is described as percutaneous epidural neuroplasty and outlined in Table 70.5.

General Principles

- The consent form should include all possible complications related to the procedure.
- Intravenous access is recommended. It may be necessary to sedate the patient with midazolam and fentanyl. Injection of solutions into the epidural space of a patient with adhesions is usually quite painful because of distention of affected nerve roots. The patient typically experiences pain in the dermatomal distribution of the nerve roots being stretched. Although sedation is given, it is important that the patient be awake and responsive during the procedure to

TABLE 70.5

Percutaneous Epidural Neuroplasty Technique as per Racz and Colleagues

In the operating room:

Place epidural needle.

Inject iohexol (Omnipaque-240) and visualize spread of contrast medium (epidurogram).

If filling defect corresponding to area of pain is present, thread Racz Tun-L-Kath® (Epimed) catheter into filling defect (scar), while injected normal saline through the catheter; observe fluoroscopically to visualize washout of contrast and opening of scar.

Inject additional iohexol to ascertain opening of scar and spread of injectate within the epidural space.

Inject preservative-free saline with or without hyaluronidase (Wydase).

Inject 0.25% bupivacaine and triamcinolone.

Tape catheter in place.

In the postoperative care unit:

Inject 10% saline 30 minutes after steroid/local anesthetic injection.

In clinic area:

Once on each of the following 2 days, inject 0.25% bupivacaine; 30 minutes later, inject 10% saline.

After the last treatment, remove the epidural catheter

Note: Adapted from Heavner et al.[9]

ensure that the spinal cord is not compressed during the injection.

- Fluoroscopy is mandatory for lysis of adhesions.
- A water-soluble, nonionic contrast medium is used because of the possibility of unintended subarachnoid injection. Even in the most careful of hands, scar tissue may dissect during injection of contrast and enter the subarachnoid space. Nonwater-soluble ionic contrast medium in the subarachnoid space can cause spinal cord irritation, spinal cord injury, seizures or clonus, arachnoiditis, and paralysis.
- The steroid that is currently used for this procedure by Racz et al.[6–9] is triamcinolone acetate.

Methylprednisolone is discouraged due to clumping when mixed with local anesthetics or normal saline.

- Hypertonic saline is used to prolong pain relief because of its local anesthetic effect.

The Caudal Approach

- The patient is placed prone with a pillow under the abdomen to straighten the lumbar spine. Monitors are applied, including electrocardiography sensors, a pulse oximeter, and a blood pressure cuff. The sacral area is then prepared with sterile technique and draped from the top of the iliac crest to the bottom of the buttocks. Abduction of the legs and inversion of the feet ("pigeon toe") facilitate entry into the sacral hiatus.

- The sacral cornua and the sacral hiatus are palpated with the index finger of the operator's nondominant hand. The entry point through the skin, approximately 1 to 2 cm lateral and 2 cm inferior to the sacral hiatus, is in the gluteal fold opposite the affected side. This allows the needle and the catheter to be directed toward the affected side. Lateral needle placement also tends to avoid penetration of the dural sac or subdural area with either the needle or the catheter. The entry point is infiltrated with a local anesthetic such as lidocaine. A 16-gauge epidural needle (preferably an RK needle) is passed through the described entry point and into the sacral hiatus, using the sacral cornua as landmarks to locate the hiatus. The needle is advanced to a point below the S3 foramen to prevent S3 nerve root damage. To verify that the needle is within the bony canal, placement is confirmed by a lateral fluoroscopic view before any injections. This is important because anatomic variations of the sacrum could lead to incorrect needle placement that nevertheless "feels" correct. Next, an anteroposterior view should verify that the needle tip points toward the affected side.

- After aspiration is negative for blood and cerebrospinal fluid, 10 mL of iohexol (Omnipaque®-240) or metrizamide (Amipaque®) is injected under fluoroscopy. As the medium is injected into the epidural space, a Christmastree shape develops as the dye spreads into the perineural structures inside the bony canal and along the nerves as they exit the vertebral column. Epidural adhesions prevent dye spread so dye does not outline the involved nerve roots. A lateral view likewise shows no dye outlining the scarred nerve roots. If cerebrospinal fluid is aspirated, it is best to abort the procedure and repeat it another day. If blood is aspirated, the needle is first retracted caudad in the sacral canal until no blood can be aspirated. If this is unsuccessful, an attempt can be made to proceed with catheter placement into the proper site. Aspiration through this catheter should be negative for blood, and lack of venous runoff should be confirmed with injection of contrast medium.

- The ideal epidural catheter is a stainless steel, fluoropolymer-coated, spiral-tipped Racz Tun-L-Kath-XL (Epimed International, Inc.). The bevel of the needle should face the ventrolateral aspect of the caudal canal on the affected side. This facilitates passage of the catheter to the desired side and decreases the chance of shearing the catheter. Because scar formation is usually uneven, multiple passes may be necessary to place the catheter into the scarred area. For this reason, it is best to use a 16-gauge RK epidural needle, which has been specially designed to allow multiple passes of the catheter. To facilitate steering of the catheter into the desired location, a 15° bend is placed at its distal end. After final placement of the catheter and negative aspiration, another 5 to 10 mL of contrast medium is injected through the catheter. This additional dye should spread into the area of previous filling defect and outline the targeted nerve root. Then 1,500 units of hyaluronidase (Wydase®) in 10 mL of preservative-free saline is injected rapidly. Afterward and after negative aspiration, 10 mL of 0.2% ropivacaine and 40 mg of triamcinolone are injected through the catheter in divided doses. This additional volume promotes further lysis of adhesions, because the catheter tip is in the scar tissue. The area of scarring and subsequent scar dissection should be noted and recorded. Because steroids cannot be injected through the 0.2-m bacteriostatic filter, the steroid must be injected before the in-line filter is installed.

- When the procedure is completed, the catheter should be secured to the skin with 2-0 nylon on a cutting needle. The puncture site where the catheter exits is covered by a large clump of a triple-antibiotic ointment such as polymyxin, and two 2 × 2-inch split venous gauze dressings are used to cover the antibiotic ointment and prevent its spread outside the area of the gauze. The surrounding skin is sprayed or covered with tincture of benzoin, and with a single curve of the catheter toward the midline, all of the above are covered with a 4 × 6-inch Tegaderm

(OpSite®) dressing. The catheter is connected to an adapter and the bacteriostatic filter, which is not removed until three daily injections have been completed. The filter is capped, and the catheter is taped to the flank of the patient. During the hospitalization, the patient is given intravenous antibiotics in the form of cephalosporin (Rocephin®), 1 g/day, to prevent bacterial colonization that is especially hazardous because of the epidurally administered steroid.

- Once the patient is taken to the recovery room and vital signs are checked, 9 mL of 10% hypertonic saline is infused over 20 to 30 minutes. Occasionally, the patient may complain of severe, burning pain during the infusion. The cause is usually the introduction of hypertonic saline into unanesthetized epidural tissue. Should this occur, the infusion must be stopped; and another 3- to 5-mL bolus of local anesthetic is given. After 5 minutes, the hypertonic saline infusion can be restarted without incident. After completion of the hypertonic saline infusion, 1.5 mL of preservative-free normal saline is used to flush the catheter. Once this task is completed, the cap is replaced on the filter.

- The catheter is left in place for 3 days. On the second and third days, it is injected once a day with 10 mL of 0.2% ropivacaine after negative aspiration from the catheter. Then, 15 minutes later, 10 mL of 10% saline is infused over 20 minutes for patient comfort. As in any hypertonic saline infusion series, the catheter must be flushed with 1.5 mL of preservative-free normal saline. On the third day, the catheter is removed 10 minutes after the last injection. A triple antibiotic ointment is placed on the wound, which is covered with a bandage or another appropriate dressing.

Interlaminar Lumbar Approach

The technique for lysis of epidural adhesions in these areas of the spinal cord must be modified to ensure that initially the needle is positioned in the epidural space and that spinal cord compression by subsequent injections is avoided.

- The patient is placed in the left lateral position on the fluoroscopy table. With the fluoroscopy C-arm in the vertical position, which actually provides a lateral view of the spine, the bases of the spinous processes are visualized. Sterile preparation and draping are carried out.

- A 16-gauge epidural needle (preferably an RK needle) is advanced with the stylet in place to the ligamentum flavum. Skin entry should be 1.5 to 2 levels below the desired epidural entry to facilitate catheter placement. After local anesthetic is used on the skin, an 18-gauge needle is inserted through the same puncture site to form an entry wound. Through the puncture site, a 16-gauge epidural needle is first advanced under fluoroscopic guidance (anteroposterior view) to determine the *direction* of the needle. Next, in the lateral view, the needle is advanced to the point just before the "straight line" formed by the fluoroscopic image of the anterior border of the spinous process in the lateral view (the insertion site of the ligamentum flavum). The lateral view under fluoroscopy demonstrates the *depth* of needle placement. Last, an anteroposterior view is checked again to confirm the *direction* of the needle. When the direction is satisfactory, the loss-of-resistance technique with a Pulsator (Concord Labs) syringe filled halfway with normal (0.9%) saline and halfway with air is used to advance the needle into the epidural space.

- A Racz Tun-L-Kath or Racz Tun-L-Kath-XL epidural catheter is passed in an anterocephalad direction toward the filling defect outlined by the dye, until the catheter tip enters the scarred area. The catheter adapter is attached to the external end of the catheter for injection. After negative aspiration, 1 to 3 mL of nonionic dye is injected while observing the fluoroscope screen for spread within the adhesions. Once an outflow or runoff tract is seen, i.e., either opening of the neuroforamina or caudal spread, 3 to 5 mL of 0.9% preservative-free saline with 1,500 units of hyaluronidase is injected. Last, 0.2% ropivacaine (4 mL) and 40 mg (1 mL) triamcinolone diacetate are injected after negative aspiration, while attention is directed to watch for displacement of the contrast. For safety purposes, the local anesthetic is given in divided doses to first rule out intrathecal subdural (1 to 2 mL) or intravascular injection. After 5 minutes, the remaining volume of the local anesthetic and steroid is injected.

- The procedure may also be performed in the prone position similar to the caudal approach, but with interlaminar entry.

- The volume of ropivacaine injected depends on the level where the tip of the catheter lies, with 10 mL injected in the lumbar and caudal area. The catheter is then secured as described for the caudal approach. After 30 minutes, 10% saline is injected after negative aspiration, in small increments or by slow infusion over 20

TABLE 70.6
Percutaneous Epidural Neuroplasty Technique, as per Manchikanti et al.

In the operating room:
> Place epidural needle.
> Inject Omnipaque 240 and visualize spread of contrast medium with caudal or lumbar epidurogram.
> After identification of the filling defect corresponding to the area of the pain, thread a Racz catheter into filling defect.
> Inject additional Omnipaque 240 to ascertain opening of the scar and spread of injectate within the epidural space and nerve roots.
> Inject preservative-free saline 10 to 20 mL.
> Inject 2% Xylocaine 5 mL.
> Tape the catheter in place in a sterile fashion.

In the recovery room:
> After ascertaining for motor blockade, inject 6 mL of 10% saline in two divided doses of 3 mL each, 15 to 30 minutes after injection of local anesthetic.
> Inject 6 to 12 mg of Celestone Soluspan, or 40 to 80 mg of alcohol-free Depo Medrol, or 40 to 80 mg of triamcinolone.
> Inject 0.5 to 1 mL of normal saline and remove the catheter.

Note: Adapted from Manchekanti et al.[16]

minutes. Again, the volume used is dependent on the location of the tip of the catheter, with 9 mL used in the lumbar area.

MODIFIED TECHNIQUE

Multiple modifications have been applied to the above-described technique. Some modifications were developed by Racz et al.[6–9,11] themselves; others were introduced by others. The technique utilized by Manchikanti et al.[16] as outlined in Table 70.6, is as follows.

Procedure Environment

The procedure is performed in a sterile operating room under appropriate sterile precautions using fluoroscopy and a specially designed RK needle, as well as a spring-wire Racz catheter (Epimed International).

Preparation

After the initial evaluation, the patient is transferred to the holding area, where appropriate preparation is carried out, including preoperative evaluation, with intravenous access, and administration of antibiotic, based on protocol and patient condition.

Consent

An appropriate detailed consent is obtained from the patient.

Operating Room

Following this, the patient is taken to the operating room or a sterile procedure room where preparation is carried out with iodophor solution skin preparation. Draping is carried out to cover the patient, extending into the midthoracic or cervical region, even if the procedure is performed in the lumbosacral region. Appropriate monitoring is carried out, with monitoring of blood pressure and pulse and pulse oximetry. Sedation is slowly administered.

The fluoroscope is adjusted over the lumbosacral region for anteroposterior and lateral views. A physician, scrubbed and in sterile gown and gloves, infiltrates the area for needle insertion with local anesthetic. Following this, an RK needle is introduced into the epidural space under fluoroscopic guidance. Once the needle placement is confirmed to be in the epidural space, a lumbar epidurogram is carried out using approximately 2 to 5 mL of contrast. Finding the filling defects by examining the contrast flow into the nerve roots is the purpose of the epidurogram. Intravascular or subarachnoid placement of the needle or contrast is avoided; if such malpositioning occurs, the needle is repositioned.

After appropriate determination of epidurography, a Racz catheter, which is a spring-guided, reinforced catheter, is slowly passed through the RK needle to the area of the filling defect or the site of pathology determined by MRI, CT, or patient symptoms. Following the positioning of the catheter into the appropriate area by mechanical means, adhesiolysis is carried out.

After completion of the adhesiolysis, a repeat epidurogram is carried out by additional injection of contrast. If appropriate adhesiolysis is completed, nerve root filling as well as epidural filling will be noted. Figure 70.4 through Figure 70.8 illustrate examples of the procedure.

At this time, variable doses of local anesthetic are injected. Commonly injected are 5 to 10 mL of 2% lidocaine hydrochloride or 5 to 10 mL of 0.25% bupivacaine.

Following completion of the injection, the catheter is taped using bio-occlusive dressing; the patient is turned to the supine position and transferred to the recovery room.

Recovery Room

The patient is very closely monitored for any potential complications or side effects. If no complications are observed and the patient reports good pain relief without any motor weakness, hypertonic saline neurolysis is carried out at this time by injection of variable doses of 10% sodium chloride solution. This may be carried out by an infusion pump or repeat injections in doses of 2 to 3 mL, ranging from 6 to 10 mL total, followed by injection of steroid (Celestone 6 to 12 mg or Depo-Medrol 40 to 80 mg).

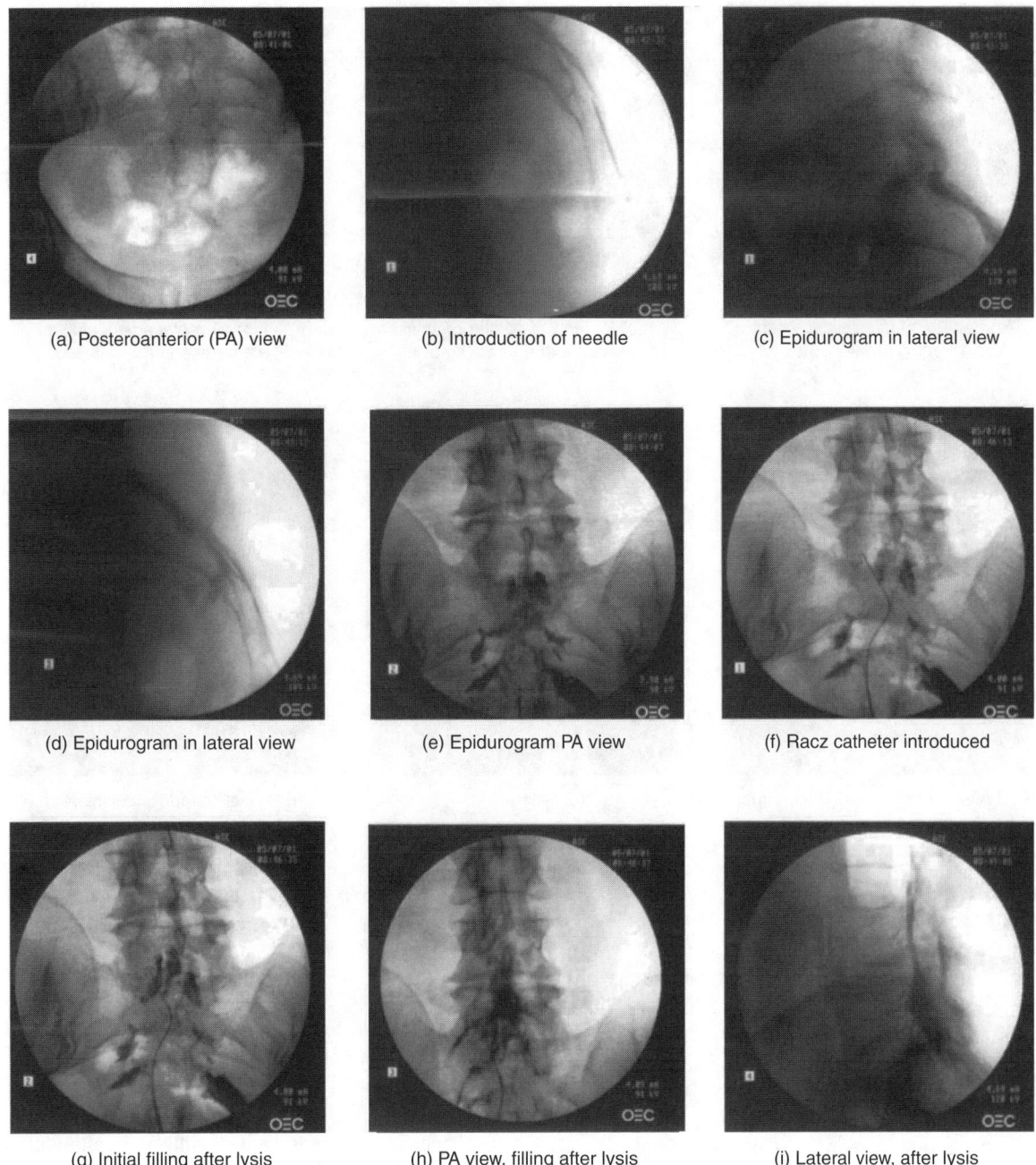

(a) Posteroanterior (PA) view   (b) Introduction of needle   (c) Epidurogram in lateral view

(d) Epidurogram in lateral view   (e) Epidurogram PA view   (f) Racz catheter introduced

(g) Initial filling after lysis   (h) PA view, filling after lysis   (i) Lateral view, after lysis

FIGURE 70.4 Illustration transforaminal adhesiolysis. From L. Manchikanti, C. W. Slipman, & B. Fellows, Eds., *Interventional Pain Management: Low Back Pain — Diagnosis and Treatment* (p. 373), Paducah, KY: ASIPP Publishing. Reproduced with permission of the authors *Pain Physician,* and the American Society of Interventional Pain Physicians.

The catheter is flushed with normal saline and removed and checked for intactness. The wound is also checked at this time. The patient is ambulated if all parameters are satisfactory, intravenous access is removed, and the patient is discharged home with appropriate instructions.

TRANSFORAMINAL ADHESIOLYSIS

Transforaminal adhesiolysis is described by Hammer et al.[18]

Procedure

To reach the anterior portion of the nerve, a needle is placed obliquely through the intervertebral foramen. Double rotation, fluoroscopic images are required. After squaring off the vertebral endplates, the fluoroscope is directed in a 35° to 40° oblique angle to visualize the opening of the intervertebral foramen. A 17-guage Tuohy or blunt trocar is advanced using tunnel vision under the pedicle. Once bone contact has been confirmed, the fluoroscopic beam is

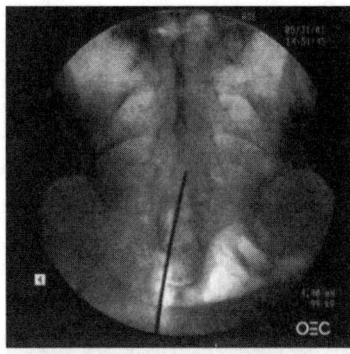

(a) PA view of needle placement
directed toward right

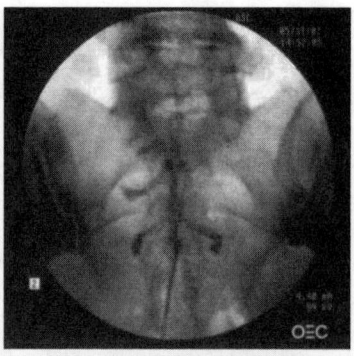

(b) PA view of epidurogram in
patient with right S1 fibrosis

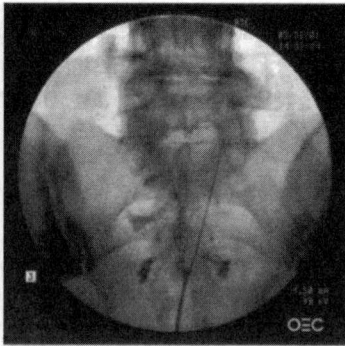

(c) PA view placement of Racz
catheter and adhesiolysis

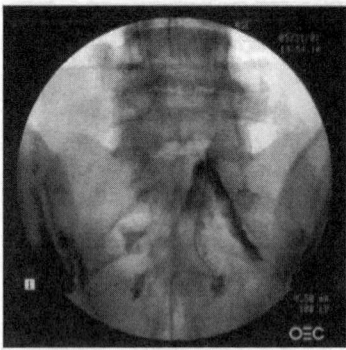

(d) PA view of filling of S1 nerve root

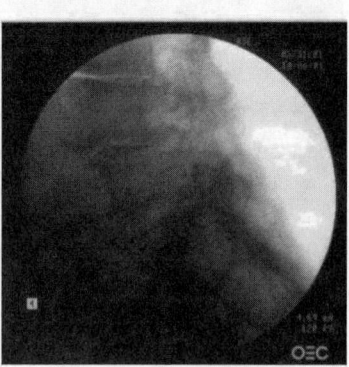

(e) Lateral view

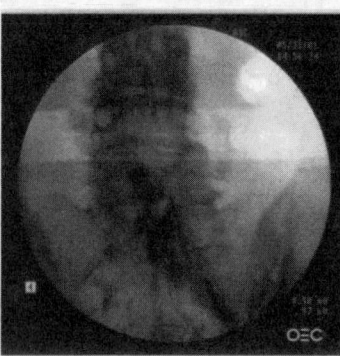

(f) PA view of additional injection of
contrast

FIGURE 70.5 Illustration of the technique of adhesiolysis involving right S1 nerve root. From L. Manchikanti, C. W. Slipman, & B. Fellows, Eds., *Interventional Pain Management: Low Back Pain — Diagnosis and Treatment* (p. 374), Paducah, KY: ASIPP Publishing. Reproduced with permission of the authors *Pain Physician,* and the American Society of Interventional Pain Physicians.

directed posteroanteriorly to demonstrate proximity of the needle trocar tip to the lateral foraminal zone. The fluoroscope is then redirected to a cross-table (lateral) view to prepare for final positioning. The needle/trocar is then slowly advanced from the posterior (dorsal) border of the neuroforamina to the retrovertebral space parallel to and "hugging" the inferior border of the pedicle. Paresthesia should not be elicited, or very minimally so, while advancing to the posterior vertebral body. After contact, a posteroanterior image should reveal the tip to be in the mid foraminal or subarticular zone. With the needle bevel facing posteriorly a BreviKath (Epimed International, Inc.) catheter is gently advanced under the exiting nerve root and into the ventral epidural space. The bevel may be rotated cephalad to steer the catheter appropriately if needed.

Having achieved a confirmation of ventrolateral epiradicular contrast spread, initial injection of 3.5 cc of 0.5% bupivacaine with or without 100 mg of fentanyl followed by hyaluronidase 1,500 units (1 mL) and slow infusion of 10% sodium chloride (hypertonic saline) and injection of triamcinolone acetate 40 mg (1 to 3 mL) are carried out.

CAUTION

Whatever the technique and whatever the route applied, it is of paramount importance that a physician pay attention to subarachnoid spread of the contrast and local anesthetic blockade following the injection. Injection of local anesthetic prior to lysis of adhesions, although practiced widely in the past, is no longer recommended. In addition, hypertonic saline should never be injected directly into the epidural space through the needle; rather it should be injected through the catheter in incremental doses after waiting at least 15 minutes following short-acting local anesthetics and 30 minutes following long-acting local anesthetics. Deviation from these descriptions may include:

- Injection of steroid at the end after the injection of hypertonic saline; however, the deviation should never occur with regard to injection of local anesthetic, specifically a long-acting local anesthetic, prior to the lysis and confirmation

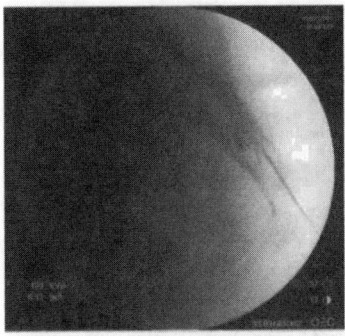

(a) Lateral view, caudal epidurogram

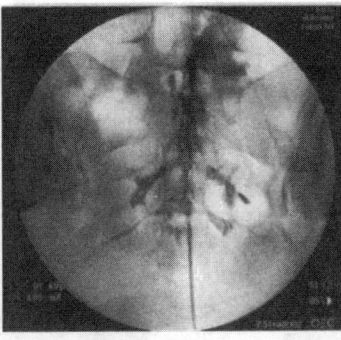

(b) PA view, caudal epidurogram

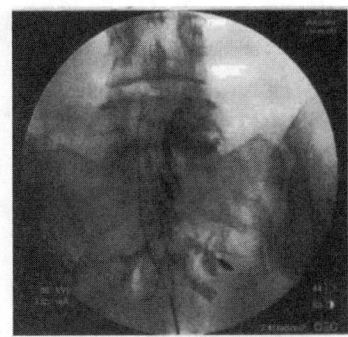

(c) PA view, placement of Racz catheter on left side

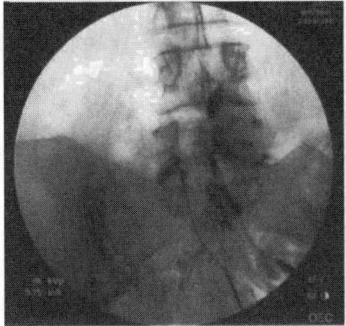

(d) PA view, early filling L5 nerve on left side

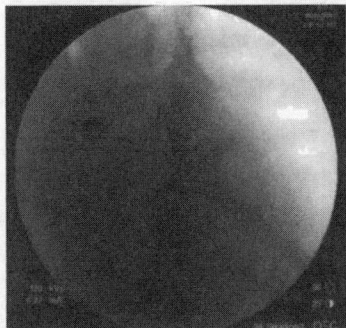

(e) Lateral view showing epidural and L5 nerve root filling

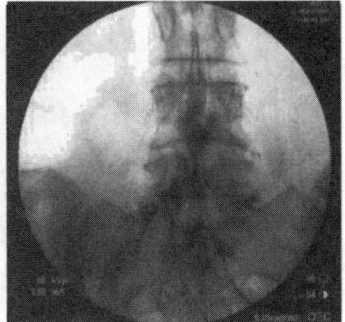

(f) PA view, final view after adhesiolysis of left L5 nerve root

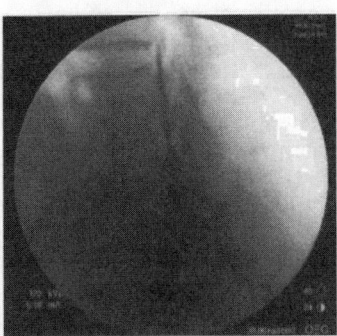

(g) Lateral view; final view after adhesiolysis

FIGURE 70.6 Illustration of left L5 epidural adhesiolysis. From L. Manchikanti, C. W. Slipman, & B. Fellows, Eds., *Interventional Pain Management: Low Back Pain — Diagnosis and Treatment* (p. 374), Paducah, KY: ASIPP Publishing. Reproduced with permission of the authors *Pain Physician,* and the American Society of Interventional Pain Physicians.

of the position of the catheter and lack of subarachnoid spread

- Injection of hypertonic saline through the needle
- Injection of hypertonic saline, without appropriate waiting time, through the catheter

The injection procedures with such deviations as described above may result in disastrous complications, including arachnoiditis, which may be attributed to the injection, even though there is no substantial proof at the present time to indicate that 10% sodium chloride solution in fact causes arachnoiditis.

CONCLUSION

Chronic low back pain is a major health care and social problem. Much of the confusion surrounding epidural adhesiolysis in managing refractory low back pain results

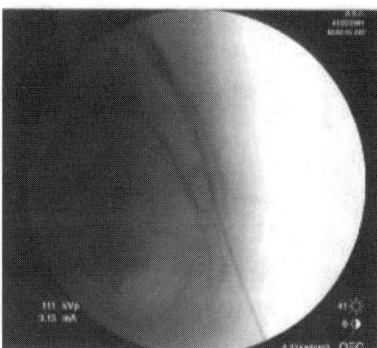

(a) Lateral view with needle placement
and contrast injection

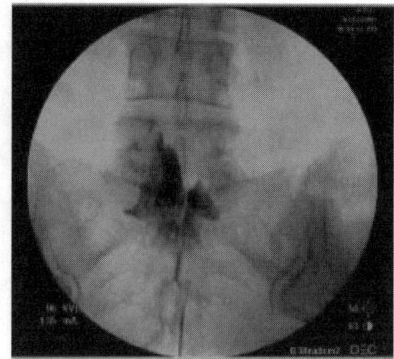

(b) PA view of lumbar epidurogram with filling
defect on right side

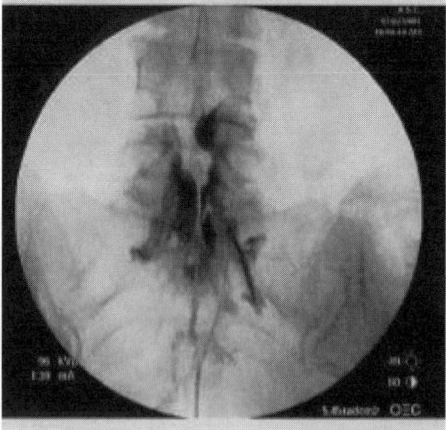

(c) PA view contrast injection with
right S1 nerve root filling

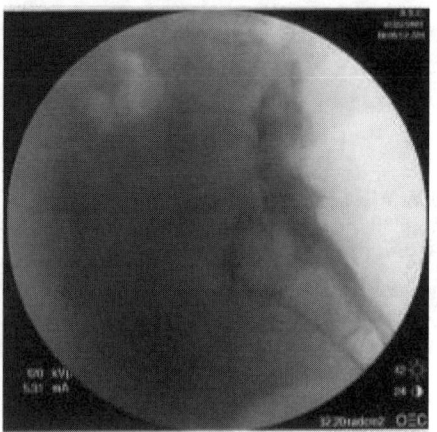

(d) Lateral view of (c)

FIGURE 70.7 An example of caudal epidural adhesiolysis with right S1 radiculitis. From L. Manchikanti, C. W. Slipman, & B. Fellows, Eds., *Interventional Pain Management: Low Back Pain — Diagnosis and Treatment* (p. 375), Paducah, KY: ASIPP Publishing. Reproduced with permission of the authors *Pain Physician,* and the American Society of Interventional Pain Physicians.

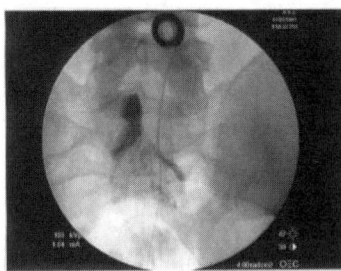

(a) PA view showing defect on
right with Racz catheter in place

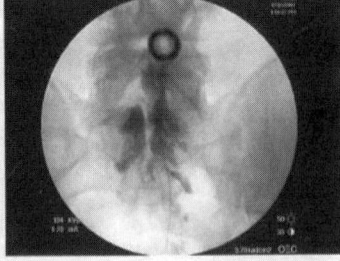

(b) PA view following appropriate
adhesiolysis

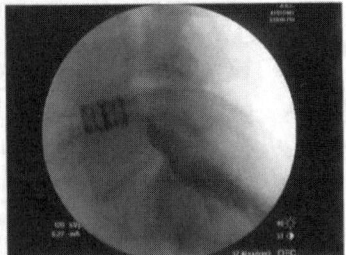

(c) Lateral view of (b)

FIGURE 70.8 Right-sided epidural fibrosis with symptomatic S1 nerve root following disc prosthesis, with adhesiolysis. From L. Manchikanti, C. W. Slipman, & B. Fellows, Eds., *Interventional Pain Management: Low Back Pain — Diagnosis and Treatment* (p. 376), Paducah, KY: ASIPP Publishing. Reproduced with permission of the authors *Pain Physician,* and the American Society of Interventional Pain Physicians.

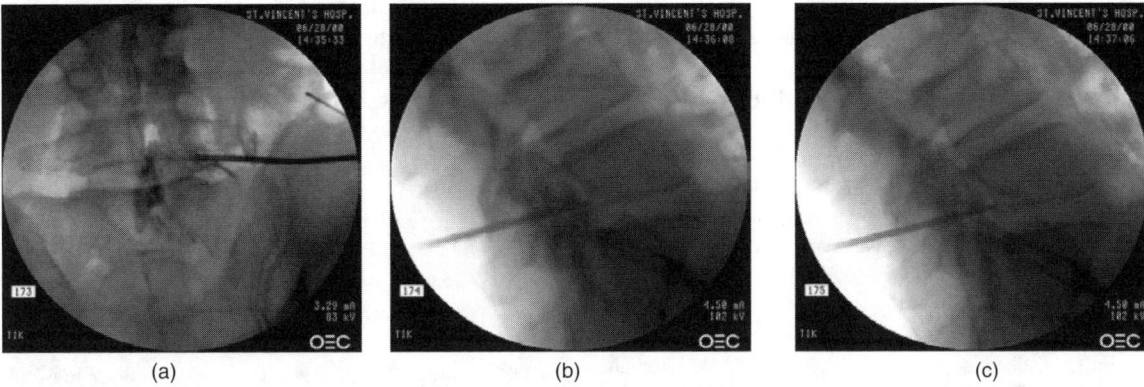

(a)

(b)

(c)

Needle placement in the lateral recess of the L5 neral foramen. Contrast study shows a filling defect.

Lateral view demonstrates a similiar filling defect as in (a). Note that the needle is flush against the vertebral body under the L5 pedicle (retrovertebral contact).

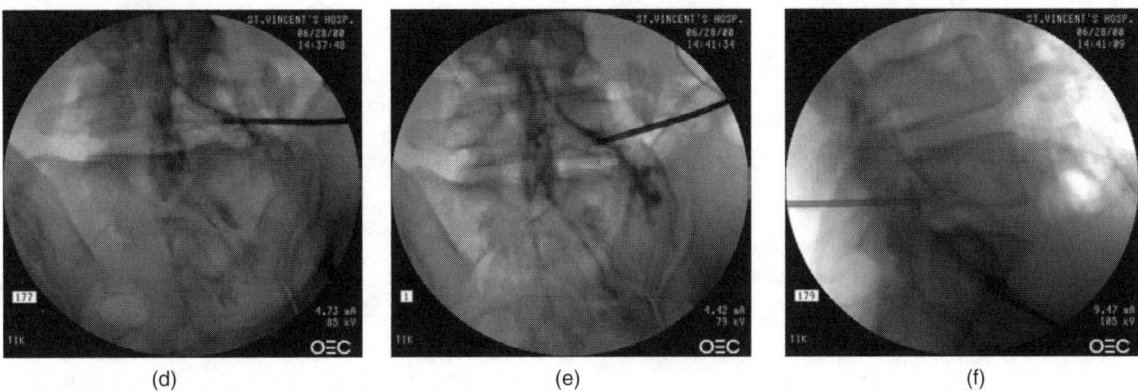

(d)

(e)

(f)

After hydromechanical dissection/irrigation with 20 cc of sterile saline, a repeat contrast study clearly demonstrates free flow of contrast along the epidural space, exiting nerve root, dorsal root ganglion, and exiting ventral ramus.

Final confirmation of 360° circumferential PA adhesiolysis by a lateral view demonstrating an unobstructed L5 nerve root.

FIGURE 70.9 Illustration of transforaminal adhesiolysis. From L. Manchikanti, C. W. Slipman, & B. Fellows, Eds., *Interventional Pain Management: Low Back Pain — Diagnosis and Treatment* (p. 377), Paducah, KY: ASIPP Publishing. Reproduced with permission of the authors *Pain Physician,* and the American Society of Interventional Pain Physicians.

from overemphasis on biopsychosocial problems and inappropriate selection of patients for this treatment modality. Considering the cumulative evidence available in the literature on epidural adhesiolysis, the efficacy of this procedure is similar, if not superior, to various other modalities of treatment available in managing chronic low back pain, including surgical intervention.

While this is a very effective technique in managing chronic low back pain, caution must be exercised, as there are significant risks of complications. While a pain practitioner needs to individualize the choice of treatment to each patient and personal experience, we recommend epidural adhesiolysis. This has proved to be a valuable, safe, and cost-effective technique for relieving chronic intractable pain in a patient nonresponsive to other conservative treatment modalities. Epidural adhesiolysis can also be performed in an out-patient setting, with reasonable and customary charges for the facility and physician services.

REFERENCES

1. Wilkinson, H. A. (1992). *The failed back syndrome. Etiology and therapy* (2nd ed., p. 1). New York: Springer-Verlag.

2. Waddell, G. et al. (1979). Failed lumbar disc surgery and repeat surgery following industrial injury. *Journal of Bone and Joint Surgery* (America), *61*, 201.

3. North, R. B. et al. (1991). Failed back surgery syndrome: 5 year follow-up in 102 patients undergoing repeated operation. *Neurosurgery, 28*, 685.

4. Manchikanti, L. et al. (2003). Evidence-based practice guidelines for interventional techniques in the management of chronic spinal pain. *Pain Physician, 6*, 3.

5. Manchikanti, L. et al. (2001). Interventional techniques in the management of chronic pain: Part 2.0. *Pain Physician, 4*, 24.

6. Racz, G. B., & Holubec, J. T. (1989). Lysis of adhesions in the epidural space. In G. B. Racz (Ed.), *Techniques of neurolysis* (p. 57). Boston: Kluwer Academic Publishers.

7. Racz, G. B., Haynsworth, R. F., & Lipton, S. (1986). Experiences with an improved epidural catheter. *Pain Clinic, 1,* 21.

8. Racz, G. B., Heavner, J. E., & Raj, P. P. (1999). Percutaneous epidural neuroplasty. Prospective one-year follow up. *Pain Digest, 9,* 97.

9. Heavner, J. E., Racz, G. B., & Raj, P. P. (1999). Percutaneous epidural neuroplasty. Prospective evaluation of 0.9% NaCl versus 10% NaCl with or without hyaluronidase. *Regional Anesthesia and Pain Medicine, 24,* 202.

10. Manchikanti, L., Saini, B., & Singh, V. (2002). Lumbar epidural adhesiolysis. In L. Manchikanti, C. W. Slipman, & B. Fellows (Eds.), *Interventional pain management: Low back pain – Diagnosis and treatment* (p. 353). Paducah, KY: ASIPP Publishing.

11. Anderson, S. R., Racz, G., & Heavner, J. (2000). Evolution of epidural lysis of adhesions. *Pain Physician, 3,* 262.

12. Manchikanti, L. et al. (2001). Effectiveness of percutaneous adhesiolysis and hypertonic saline neurolysis in refractory spinal stenosis. *Pain Physician, 4,* 366.

13. Manchikanti, L., & Bakhit, C. E. (2000). Percutaneous lysis of epidural adhesions. *Pain Physician, 3,* 46.

14. Manchikanti, L. et al. (1999). Role of adhesiolysis and hypertonic saline neurolysis in management of low back pain. Evaluation of modification of Racz protocol. *Pain Digest, 9,* 91.

15. Manchikanti, L. et al. (1999). Non-endoscopic and endoscopic adhesiolysis in post lumbar laminectomy syndrome. A one-year outcome study and cost effective analysis. *Pain Physician, 2,* 52.

16. Manchikanti, L. et al. (2001). Role of one day epidural adhesiolysis in management of chronic low back pain: A randomized, double blind trial. *Pain Physician, 4,* 153.

17. Manchikanti, L. et al. (2004). One day lumbar epidural adhesiolysis and hypertonic saline neurolysis in treatment of chronic low back pain: A randomized controlled trial. *Pain Physician, 7,* 177.

18. Hammer, M., Doleys, D., & Chung, O. (2001). Transforaminal ventral epidural adhesiolysis. *Pain Physician, 4,* 273.

19. Phillips, F. M., & Cunningham, B. (2002). Managing chronic pain of spinal origin after lumbar surgery. *Spine, 27,* 2547.

20. Sicard, M. A. (1901). Les injections medicamenteuse extraduraqles per voie saracoccygiene. *Comptes Rendus des Senances de la Societe de Biolgie et de ses Filliales, 53,* 396.

21. Caussade, G., & Queste, P. (1909). Traitement de al neuralgia sciatique par la mèthode de Sicard. Résultats favorables même dans les cas chroniues par la cocaïne à doses élevées et répétées à intervalles raproches. *Bulletin de la Societe Medicales Hospitales, 28,* 865.

22. Sicard, J. A., & Forestier, J. (1921). Méthode radiographique d'exploration de la cavité épidurale par le Lipiodol. *Revue Neuroligique, 28,* 1264.

23. Hitchcock, E. (1967). Hypothermic subarachnoid irrigation for intractable pain. *Lancet, i,* 1133.

24. Ventrafridda, V., & Spreafico, R. (1974). Subarachnoid saline perfusion. In J. J. Bonica (Ed.), *Advances in neurology (*Vol. 4, p. 477). New York: Raven Press.

25. Hitchcock, E. (1969). Osmolytic neurolysis for intractable facial pain. *Lancet, i,* 434.

26. Racz, G. B. et al. (1989). Hypertonic saline and corticosteroid injected epidurally for pain control. In P. Raj (Ed.), *Techniques of neurolysis* (p. 73). Boston: Kluwer Academic Publishers.

27. Payne, J. N., & Rupp, N. H. (1951). The use of hyaluronidase in caudal block anesthesia. *Anesthesiology, 2,* 164.

28. Moore, D. C. (1951). The use of hyaluronidase in local and nerve block analgesia other than spinal block. 1520 cases. *Anesthesiology, 12,* 611.

29. Ombregt, L., & Ter Veer, H. J. (1995). Treatment of the lumbar spine. In L. Omebregt et al. (Eds.), *A system of orthopaedic medicine* (p. 633). London: WB Saunders.

30. Brown, J. H. (1960). Pressure caudal anesthesia and back manipulation. *Northwest Medicine, 59,* 905.

31. Stolker, R. J., Vervest, A. C. M., & Gerbrand, J. G. (1994). The management of chronic spinal pain by blockades. A review. *Pain, 58,* 1.

32. Kuslich, S. D., Ulstrom, C. L., & Michael, C. J. (1991). The tissue origin of low back pain and sciatica: A report of pain response to tissue stimulation during operation on the lumbar spine using local anesthesia. *Orthopedic Clinics of North America, 22,* 181.

33. Wheeler, A. H., & Murrey, D. B. (2002). Chronic lumbar spine and radicular pain: Pathophysiology and treatment. *Current Pain and Headache Report, 6,* 97.

34. Nachemson, A. L. (1999). Failed back surgery syndrome is syndrome of failed back surgeons. *Pain Clinic, 11,* 271.

35. Anderson, S. R. (2000). A rationale for the treatment algorithm of failed back surgery syndrome. *Current Review of Pain, 4,* 395.

36. Slosar, P. J. (2002). Indications and outcomes of reconstructive surgery in chronic pain of spinal origin. *Spine, 27,* 2555.

37. Fritsch, E. W., Heisel, J., & Rupp, S. (1996). The failed back surgery syndrome. Reasons, intraoperative findings, and long-term results: A report of 182 operative treatments. *Spine, 21,* 626.

38. McCarron, R. F. (1989). Epidural fibrosis: Experimental model and therapeutic alternatives. In G. B. Racz (Ed.), *Techniques of neurolysis* (p. 87). Boston: Kluwer Academic Publishers.

39. Cooper, R. G. et al. (1995). Herniated intervertebral disc-associated periradicular fibrosis and vascular abnormalities occur without inflammatory cell infiltration. *Spine, 20,* 591.

40. Hoyland, J. A., Freemont, A. J., & Jayson, M.I . (1989). Intervertebral foramen venous obstruction. A cause of periradicular fibrosis? *Spine, 14,* 558.

41. Parke, W. W., & Watanabe, R. (1990). Adhesions of the ventral lumbar dura. Adjunct source of discogenic pain? *Spine, 15,* 300.

42. Rydevik, B. L. (1992). The effects of compression on the physiology of nerve roots. *Journal of Manipulative Physiological Therapy, 1*, 62.

43. Olmarker, K., & Rydevik, B. (1999). Pathophysiology of spinal nerve roots as related to sciatica and disc herniation. In H. N. Herkowitz et al. (Eds.), *Rothman-Simeone studies, the spine* (p. 159). Philadelphia: WB Saunders.

44. Songer, M., Ghosh, L., & Spencer, D. (1990). Effects of sodium hyaluronate on peridural fibrosis after lumbar laminectomy and discectomy. *Spine, 15*, 550.

45. Pawl, R. P. (1998). Arachnoiditis and epidural fibrosis: The relationship to chronic pain. *Current Review of Pain, 2*, 93.

46. Van Goethem, J. W. et al. (1996). MRI after successful lumbar discectomy. *Neuroradiology, 38*, S90.

47. Grane, P. et al. (1996). Postoperative lumbar magnetic resonance imaging with contrast enhancement: Compression between symptomatic and asymptomatic patients. *Acta Radiologica, 37*, 366.

48. Annertz, M. et al. (1995). No relationship between epidural fibrosis and sciatica in the lumbar postdiscectomy syndrome: A study with contrast-enhancement magnetic resonance imagery in symptomatic and asymptomatic patients. *Spine, 20*, 449.

49. Cervellini, P. et al. (1988). Computed tomography of epidural fibrosis after discectomy. A comparison between symptomatic and asymptomatic patients. *Neurosurgery, 6*, 710.

50. Ross, J. S. et al. (1996). Association between peridural scar and recurrent radicular pain after lumbar discectomy: Magnetic resonance evaluation. *Neurosurgery, 38*, 855.

51. Manchikanti, L., Bakhit, C. E., & Pampati, V. (1998). Role of epidurography in caudal neuroplasty. *Pain Digest, 8*, 277.

52. Manchikanti, L. et al. (2004). Evaluation of fluoroscopically guided caudal epidural injections. *Pain Physician, 7*, 81.

53. Racz, G. B., Noe, C., & Heavner, J. E. (1999). Selective spinal injections for lower back pain. *Current Review of Pain, 3*, 333.

54. Hatten, H. P., Jr. (1980). Lumbar epidurography with metrizamide. *Radiology, 137*, 129.

55. Robertson, G. H., Hatten, H. P., Jr., & Hesselink, J. H. (1979). Epidurography. Selective catheter technique and review of 53 cases. *American Journal of Radiology, 132*, 787.

56. Stewart, H. D., Quinnell, R. C., & Dann, N. E. (1987). Pidurography in the management of sciatica. *British Journal of Rheumatology, 26*, 424.

57. Devulder, J. et al. (1995). Relevance of epidurography and epidural adhesiolysis in chronic failed back surgery patients. *Clinical Journal of Pain, 11*, 147.

58. Manchikanti, L. (2000). Transforaminal lumbar epidural steroid injections. *Pain Physician, 3*, 374.

59. Andrade, S., & Eckman, E. (1992, October 6–8). Distribution of radiographic contrast media in the epidural space of normal volunteers using a midline transligamentum flavum vs. a selective epidural nerve canal injection technique. *International Spinal Intervention Society Newsletter.*

60. Bogduk, N. et al. (1994). Epidural use of steroids in the management of back pain. Report of working party on epidural use of steroids in the management of back pain (p. 1). National Health and Medical Research Council, Canberra, Commonwealth of Australia.

61. Bogduk, N. (1999). Epidural steroids for low back pain and sciatica. *Pain Digest, 9*, 226.

62. Manchikanti, L., Pakanati, R. R., & Pampati, V. (1999). Comparison of three routes of epidural steroid injections in low back pain. *Pain Digest, 9*, 277.

63. Lutz, G. E., Vad, V. B., & Wisneski, R. J. (1998). Fluoroscopic transforaminal lumbar epidural steroids. An outcome study. *Archives of Physical and Medical Rehabilitation, 79*, 1362.

64. Riew, D. K. et al. (2000). The effect of nerve-root injections on the need for operative treatment of lumbar radicular pain: A prospective, randomized, controlled, double blind study. *Journal of Bone and Joint Surgery* (America), *82*, 1589.

65. Vad, V. D. et al. (2002). Transforaminal epidural steroid injections in lumbosacral radiculopathy: A prospective randomized study. *Spine, 27*, 11.

66. Boswell, M. V. et al. (2003). Epidural steroids in the management of chronic spinal pain and radiculopathy. *Pain Physician, 6*, 319.

67. Botwin, K. P. et al. (2000). Complications of fluoroscopically guided transforaminal lumbar epidural injections. *Archives of Physical and Medical Rehabilitation, 81*, 1045.

68. Thomas, E. et al. (2003). Efficacy of transforaminal versus interspinous corticosteroid injection in discal radic. algia – A prospective, randomised, double-blind study. *Clinical Rheumatology, 22*, 299.

69. Botwin, K. P., Natalicchio, J., & Hanna, A. (2004). Fluoroscopic guided lumbar interlaminar epidural injections: A prospective evaluation of epidurography contrast patterns and anatomical review of the epidural space. *Pain Physician, 7*, 77.

70. Windsor, R. E. et al. (2003). Cervical transforaminal injection: Review of the literature, complications, and a suggested technique. *Pain Physician, 6*, 457.

71. Manchikanti, L. et al. (2004). Evaluation of lumbar transforaminal epidural injections with needle placement and contrast flow patterns: A prospective descriptive report. *Pain Physician, 7*, 217.

72. Racz, G. B., & Heavner, J. E. (1991). Aristocort and Depo-Medrol passage through a 0.2-micron filter [Abstract]. *Regional Anesthesia, 15*, 25.

73. Lewandowski, E. M. (1997). The efficacy of solutions used in caudal neuroplasty. *Pain Digest, 7*, 323.

74. Aldrete, J. A., Zapata, J. C., & Ghaly, R. (1996). Arachnoiditis following epidural adhesiolysis with hypertonic saline report of two cases. *Pain Digest, 6*, 368.

75. Manchikanti, L., & Bakhit, C. E. (1997). Removal of torn Racz catheter from lumbar epidural space. *Regional Anesthesia, 22,* 579.

76. Kim, R. C. et al. (1988). Myelopathy after intrathecal administration of hypertonic saline. *Neurosurgery, 22,* 942.

77. Hitchcock, E. R., & Prandini, M. N. (1973). Hypertonic saline in management of intractable pain. *Lancet, 1,* 310.

78. Lucas, J. S., Ducker, T. B., & Perot, P. L. (1975). Adverse reactions to intrathecal saline injections for control of pain. *Journal of Neurosurgery, 42,* 57.

79. Dagi, T. F. (1988). Comments on myelopathy after the intrathecal administration of hypertonic saline. *Neurosurgery, 22,* 944.

80. Lundy, J. S., Essex, H. E., & Kernohan, J. W. (1936). Experiments with anesthetics. IV. Lesions produced in the spinal cord of dogs by a dose of procaine hydrochloride sufficient to cause permanent and fatal paralysis. *Journal of the American Medical Association, 101,* 1546.

81. Rojiani, A. M., Prineas, J. W., & Cho, E. S. (1994). Electrolyte-induced demyelination in rats. Ultrastructural evolution. *Acta Neuropathologica* (Berlin), *88,* 293.

82. Rojiani, A. M., Prineas, J. W., & Cho, E. S. (1987). Protective effect of steroids in electrolyte-induced demyelination. *Journal of Neuropathology and Experimental Neurology, 46,* 495.

83. Lake, D. A., & Barnes, C. D. (1980). Effects of changes in osmolality on spinal cord activity. *Experimental Neurology, 68,* 555.

84. Abram, S. E., & O'Connor, T. C. (1996). Complications associated with epidural steroid injections. *Regional Anesthesia, 212,* 149.

85. Nelson, D. A. (1993). Intraspinal therapy using methylprednisolone acetate. *Spine, 18,* 278.

86. Kushner, F. H., & Olson, J. C. (1995). Retinal hemorrhage as a consequence of epidural steroid injection. *Archives of Ophthalmology, 113,* 309.

87. Clark, C. J., & Whitwell, J. (1961). Intraocular hemorrhage after epidural injection. *British Medical Journal, 2,* 1612.

88. Wang, L. P., Haverberg, J., & Schmidt, J. F. (1999). Incidence of spinal epidural abscess after epidural analgesia. *Anesthesiology, 91,* 1928.

89. Bromage, P. R., & Benumof, J. L. (1998). Paraplegia following intracord injection during attempted epidural anesthesia under general anesthesia. *Regional Anesthesia and Pain Medicine, 23,* 104.

90. Rathmell, J. P., Garahan, M. B., & Alsofrom, G. F. (2000). Epidural abscess following epidural analgesia. *Regional Anesthesia and Pain Medicine, 25,* 79.

91. Hlavin, M. L. et al. (1990). Spinal epidural abscess: a ten year perspective. *Neurosurgery, 27,* 177.

92. Darouiche, R. O. et al. (1992). Bacterial spinal epidural abscess. Review of 43 cases and literature survey. *Medicine, 71,* 369.

93. Mackenzie, A. R. et al. (1998). Spinal epidural abscess: The importance of early diagnosis and treatment. *Journal of Neurology, Neurosurgery, and Psychiatry, 65,* 209.

94. Yuste, M. et al. (1997). An epidural abscess due to resistant *Staphylococcus aureus* following epidural catheterization. *Anaesthesia, 52,* 150.

95. Sullivan, W. J. et al. (2000). Incidence of intravascular uptake in lumbar spinal injection procedures. *Spine, 25,* 481.

96. Furman, M. B., O'Brien, E. M., & Zgleszewski, T. M. (2000). Incidence of intravascular penetration in transforaminal lumbosacral epidural steroid injections. *Spine, 25,* 2628.

97. Houten, J. K., & Errico, T. J. (2002). Paraplegia after lumbosacral nerve root block: Report of three cases. *Spine Journal, 2,* 70.

98. Cousins, M. J. (2000). An additional dimension to the efficacy of epidural steroids. *Anesthesiology, 93,* 565.

99. Delaney, T. J. et al. (1980). Epidural steroid effects on nerves and meninges. *Anesthesia & Analgesia, 58,* 610.

100. Cicala, R. S. et al. (1990). Methylprednisolone acetate does not cause inflammatory changes in the epidural space. *Anesthesiology, 72,* 556.

101. MacKinnon, S. E. et al. (1982). Peripheral nerve injection injury with steroid agents. *Plastic and Reconstructive Surgery, 69,* 482.

102. Chino, N., Awad, E. A., & Kottke, F. J. (1974). Pathology of propylene glycol administered by perineural and intramuscular injection in rats. *Archives of Physical and Medical Rehabilitation, 55,* 33.

103. Benzon, H. T. et al. (1987). The effect of polyethylene glycol on mammalian nerve impulses. *Anesthesia & Analgesia, 66,* 553.

104. Abram, S. E., Marsala, M., & Yaksh, T. L. (1994). Analgesic and neurotoxic effects of intrathecal corticosteroids in rats. *Anesthesiology, 81,* 1198.

105. Latham, J. M. et al. (1997). The pathologic effects of intrathecal betamethasone. *Spine, 22,* 1558.

106. Slucky, A. V. et al. (1999). Effects of epidural steroids on lumbar dura material properties. *Journal of Spinal Disorders, 12,* 331.

107. Manchikanti, L. (2000). The value and safety of steroids in neural blockade. Part I. *American Journal of Pain Management, 10,* 69.

108. Manchikanti, L. (2000). The value and safety of steroids in neural blockade. Part II. *American Journal of Pain Management, 10,* 122.

109. Manchikanti, L. et al. (2000). The effect of neuraxial steroids on weight and bone mass density: A prospective evaluation. *Pain Physician, 3,* 357.

110. Knight, C. L., & Burnell, J. C. (1980). Systemic side-effects of extradural steroids. *Anesthesia, 35,* 593.

111. Edmonds, L. C., Vance, M. L., & Hughes, J. M. (1991). Morbidity from paraspinal depo corticosteroid injections for analgesia. Cushing's syndrome and adrenal suppression. *Anesthesia & Analgesia, 72,* 820.

112. Jacobs, A. et al. (1983). Adrenal suppression following extradural steroids. *Anesthesia, 38,* 953.

113. Mikhail, G. R., Sweet, L. C., & Mellinger, R. C. (1973). Parenteral long-acting corticosteroid effect on hypothalamic pituitary adrenal function. *Annals of Allergy, 31*, 337.

114. Mikhail, G. R. et al. (1969). Effect of long-acting parenteral corticosteroids on adrenal function. *Archives of Dermatology, 100*, 263.

115. AHFS. (2003). *AHFS 2003 Drug Information*. Bethesda, MD: American Society of Health-System Pharmacists.

116. Roonen, S. et al. (1995). Steroid myopathy induced by epidural triamcinolone injection. *British Journal of Rheumatology, 34*, 385.

117. Roy-Camille, R. et al. (1991). Symptomatic spinal epidural lipomatosis induced by a long-term steroid treatment. *Spine, 16*, 1365.

71

Endoscopic Lysis of Lumbar Epidural Adhesions

Laxmaiah Manchikanti, MD, and Vijay Singh, MD

INTRODUCTION

Spinal endoscopic lysis of epidural adhesions is an interventional pain management technique that emerged during the 1990s.[1-11] It is an invasive, but important, treatment modality in managing chronic refractory low back pain that is resistant to fluoroscopically directed epidural steroid injections and percutaneous adhesiolysis. Endoscopic adhesiolysis is based on the premise that the three-dimensional visualization of the contents of the epidural space provides the operator with the ability to steer the catheter toward structures of interest, allowing the examination of a specific nerve root and its pathology, lysis of adhesions, and target-specific injection of a drug(s).

HISTORICAL CONSIDERATIONS

Epidural injections for chronic low back pain were performed independently by Sicard,[12] Cathelin,[13] and Pasquier and Leri[14] to treat low back pain, sciatica, relief of pain due to inoperable carcinoma of the rectum, and to provide anesthesia for surgical procedures. The initial epidurography was performed by Sicard and Forestier.[15] Over the years, various authors[1-11,16-20] have studied the effectiveness of epidural steroid injections and percutaneous adhesiolysis facilitated by a spring-guided catheter. Development of endoscopic adhesiolysis added a third dimension to epidural delivery of drugs.

Medical literature has described various types of endoscopes for 60 years.[21] Integration of fiber-optic technology with computer-enhanced imaging provided a new medium for viewing the central nervous system.[21] Burman[22] first described the possibility of direct visualization of the spinal canal and its contents in 1931. However, direct visualization of spinal contents could not be achieved until the advent of flexible fiber-optic light sources and optics.[23] Burman[22] concluded that myeloscopy was limited by the available technology, but with higher quality instrumentation, he felt that the ability to visualize the contents of the spinal canal might be especially important in establishing a diagnosis of tumor or inflammation. Stern,[24] in 1936, described a spinascope, which was specifically designed for the *in vivo* examination of the spinal canal contents during spinal anesthesia.

Pool[25] in 1937, attempted to improve the preoperative diagnostic assessment of lumbar-sciatic syndrome by examining an anesthetized patient. However, only a fleeting glimpse of the lumbosacral nerve roots was possible due to hemorrhage, which obscured the field of vision. In subsequent evaluations[26,27] of the cauda equina and blood vessels in seven volunteers, blood flow through epidural vessels was visualized. Pool[26,27] subsequently summarized his experience with 400 patients with endoscopic evaluation.

In the late 1960s and 1970s, Ooi et al.[28-31] developed a miniature endoscope for intradural and extradural examinations. Ooi et al.[32,33] and Satoh et al.[34] performed 208 myeloscopies using various types of equipment from 1967 to 1977. With publication of their technique of myeloscopy and cauda equina blood flow changes during Lasègue's test in 1981, Ooi et al.[35] also reported that abdominal straining, coughing, and sneezing did not alter the blood flow and caused only mild movements of the cauda equina in the lateral position.

Blomberg[36] studied the anatomical variations of the epidural space and the appropriate delivery of epidural anesthetics, under epiduroscopy or spinaloscopy. Blomberg[36] reported that epidural adhesions between the dura mater and the ligamentum flavum restricted the opening of the epidural space. Blomberg and Olsson[37] reported experience with 10 epiduroscopies of patients scheduled for partial laminectomies for herniated lumbar discs. Following the experience of endoscopy in live patients, Blomberg[38] concluded that the opinions drawn from previous autopsy work were not applicable to the clinical setting. He also confirmed the presence of a dorsomedian connective tissue band that divided the epidural space into compartments.[38]

Modern era evaluations of several fiber-optic systems for use in clinical epiduroscopy in 1991 were started by Saberski and Brull.[21] Heavner et al.[39,40] in the early 1990s reported endoscopic evaluation of the epidural and subarachnoid spaces in rabbits, dogs, and human cadavers, with the aid of a flexible endoscope. Since then, multiple publications[5–11,41–45] have described various aspects of spinal endoscopy, including clinical basis, safety, and cost effectiveness.

PURPOSE AND GOALS

Since the introduction of epidural corticosteroids, it has always been the objective of pain specialists to deliver them close to the site of pathology, presumably onto an inflamed nerve root. For many reasons, this objective has been hindered in caudal as well as interlaminar delivery of epidural corticosteroids. Consequently, the reports of effectiveness of epidural corticosteroids have shown a wide disparity, ranging from 18 to 90%.[3]

The purpose of spinal or epidural endoscopy is to directly visualize the contents of the epidural space, lyse the adhesions, and directly apply drugs, thus assuring delivery of high concentrations of injected drugs to the target areas. Thus, spinal endoscopy with lysis of adhesions incorporates multiple therapeutic goals into one treatment, similar to percutaneous lysis of adhesions with a spring-guided catheter, with added advantages of direct visualization of the epidural space and its contents, a three-dimensional view, and increased steerability of endoscopic equipment with a fiber-optic catheter. Nomenclature used to describe this procedure includes spinal canal endoscopy, spinal epiduroscopy, myeloscopy, spinal or lumbar epiduroscopy, and endoscopic adhesiolysis.

PATHOPHYSIOLOGY

Epidural fibrosis is described as an inflammatory reaction of the arachnoid, a fine nonvascular and elastic tissue enveloping the CNS. Anular tear, hematoma, infection, surgical trauma, and injection of intrathecal contrast media are considered potential etiologies of epidural fibrosis. The invasion of fibrous connective tissue into the postoperative hematoma resulting in epidural fibrosis was demonstrated by LaRocca and MacNab.[46] The irritative effect of material from the nucleus pulposus upon the dural sac, adjacent nerve roots, and nerve root sleeves independent of the influence of direct compression upon these structures was investigated by McCarron et al.[47,48] They also further reported an inflammatory reaction in the spinal cord sections taken from dogs after an initial injection of homogenized nucleus pulposus, while the spinal cord remained grossly normal after an injection of normal saline.

Epidural fibrosis, recurrent disc herniation, new disc herniation at a different level, local arachnoiditis, facet joint arthritis, spinal stenosis, instability, and spondylitis or spondylodiscitis are common causes of continued or recurrent low back and/or lower extremity pain following surgical interventions. Epidural fibrosis is considered a major cause of continued or recurrent pain following surgical intervention, if not surgical failure, in almost 60% of cases in conjunction with instability in postlumbar surgery syndrome. The role of epidural fibrosis as a causative factor of chronic pain or a pain generator, however, has been questioned.[48–53] In spite of the debate on whether epidural fibrosis causes pain, it is widely accepted that postoperative scar tissue renders the nerve susceptible to injury.[54]

Ross et al.[55] showed that subjects with extensive peridural scarring were 3.2 times more likely to experience recurrent radicular pain. Parke and Watanabe[56] in cadavers with lumbar disc herniation showed significant evidence of adhesions in 40% at L4/5 levels, in 36% at L5/S1 levels, and in 16% at L3/4 levels. Berger and Davis[57] diagnosed epidural fibrosis preoperatively in 0.67% and postoperatively in 11%. Further, in a study of 400 patients with multiple operations, they confirmed that, at the time of the second operation, the incidence of periradicular fibrosis had risen to 47%. Epidural adhesions have also been seen without surgery. Leakage of the irritants of the nucleus pulposus into the epidural space has been documented to cause an inflammatory response, resulting in an increase in fibrocytic deposition, resulting in epidural fibrosis.[16–20,47,48,56–60]

Mooney[61] postulated that persistent low back pain without segmental instability or another structural cause may result form poor healing of annular injuries due to inadequate blood supply. Wheeler and Murrey[62] described pathophysiology of chronic lumbar spine and radicular pain. In experimental studies, trauma to canine discs resulted in elevated concentrations of multiple neuropeptides, including substance P, calcitonin gene-related peptide, and vasoactive intestinal peptide in the dorsal root ganglion.[63,64] The noxious inflammatory and neurochemical influences on spinal tissues may explain induction of lumbar and radicular pain. Proposed etiologies of radicular pain include neural compression with dysfunction, inflammation, vascular compromise, and biochemical influences. Perineural fibrosis can render nerve roots hyperesthetic with heightened sensitivity to compressive forces.[61,62,65,66] It was also shown that compensatory nutrition from cerebrospinal fluid (CSF) diffusion during low-pressure radicular compression in the face of epidural inflammation or fibrosis is probably inadequate.[55,56] Thus, present evidence suggests that the etiology of radiculitis is multifactorial beyond neural dysfunction due to impingement. Numerous authors[62–66] have identified the likely role of chemical irritation of the nerve root by the nucleus pulposus. Soon after Mixter and Barr's[67] landmark description of mechanical compression in 1934, it was noticed that the removal of the disc did not always result in pain relief.[68] Barr[69] reported that a patient may have persistent low back pain, sciatica, or both, in spite of surgical intervention. Mixter and Ayers,[70] soon after their own discovery of neurocompressive lesion, reported that low back and leg pain may occur without disc herniation and with normal appearance of a disc. It has been long recognized that mechanical factors are not the only causative factors of radicular pain. Histological injury may occur without compression, resulting in persistence of radicular symptoms. Nerve roots may be exposed to chemical irritant substances from degenerated intervertebral discs or facet joints, which can generate pain.[17] Structures in the ventral epidural space may become highly sensitized by chemical irritation, resulting in axial pain. These structures include ventral dura, posterior longitudinal ligament, vertebral periosteum, dural attachments, and epiradicular components.[71]

Innervation to the ventral epidural space is extensive and, thus, may become highly sensitized, resulting in chronic low back pain. Histopathological studies have demonstrated sinuvertebral nerve and sympathetic innervation pain.[17] Thus, evolved the concept of noncompressive lesion and irritation of the nerve root, as well as the definition of failed back surgery syndrome or postlumbar laminectomy syndrome with persistent or recurring low back pain, with or without radiculitis following one or more lumbar operations, which followed the theories of neurocompressive lesion and its decompression.

Prior to 1935, the condition of chronic adhesional arachnoiditis was generally described as chronic spinal meningitis.[49] Thus, epidural fibrosis or arachnoiditis was a relatively rare entity prior to the introduction of lumbar spine surgery for degenerative conditions. The speculation of the association of recurrent symptomatology with perineural scarring originated from multiple authors reporting epidural fibrosis at repeat surgery.[49,72] The prevalence of recurrent disc herniation and facet joint pain in postlumbar laminectomy syndrome was shown to be 5 to 11%[73] and 32%.[74] The prevalence of epidural

scarring, arachnoiditis, and mechanical instability is not accurately known.

Kuslich et al.[75] postulated that the presence of scar tissue compounded pain associated with the nerve root by fixing it in one position and thus increasing the susceptibility of the nerve root to tension or compression. They also concluded that sciatica can only be reproduced by direct pressure or stretch on the inflammatory, stretched, or compressive nerve root. Further, compromised delivery of nutrition has also been described.[61,66]

Epidural fibrosis is found in the three compartments of the epidural space: dorsal, ventral, and lateral. Dorsal epidural scar tissue is formed by resorption of surgical hematoma and may be involved in pain generation.[76] Ventral epidural scar tissue, often dense, is formed by ventral defects in the disc, which may persist despite surgical treatment and continue to produce either chronic low back or lower extremity pain after the surgical healing phase.[47] The lateral epidural space includes epiradicular structures out of the root canals or sleeves, containing the exiting nerve root and dorsal root ganglia, susceptible to lateral disc defects, facet overgrowth, neuroforaminal stenosis, etc.[77] Thus, it is postulated that various changes producing low back pain and lower extremity pain include inflammation, edema, fibrosis, venous congestion, mechanical pressure on the posterior longitudinal ligament, reduced or absent nutrient delivery to the spinal nerve or nerve root, and central sensitization.

Epidural fibrosis with or without symptoms of back pain is not readily diagnosed by conventional studies such as myelography, computerized tomography (CT), and magnetic resonance imaging (MRI), in spite of modern technology and its significant improvements. Epidural fibrosis is best diagnosed by performing an epidurogram. The presence of epidural filling defects has been demonstrated in a significant number of patients with no history of prior surgery.[60]

RATIONALE

Although Phillips and Cunningham[78] reported that surgical decompression or surgical lysis of adhesions was not effective for postlumbar laminectomy syndrome, the rationale for spinal endoscopy and adhesiolysis in the management of chronic, resistant spinal pain stems from the concept that epidural adhesions are a common source of chronic low back pain. Indeed, the effectiveness of percutaneous adhesiolysis with a spring-guided catheter has been demonstrated.[3]

The epidural space that is restricted by adhesions is safely accessible to a fiber-optic endoscope, and spinal endoscopy and therapeutic application of drugs in selected cases have been shown to be clinically effective and safe.[1] Additional aspects of the rationale include the mechanical and hydrostatic effect of the procedure with high-volume

TABLE 71.1
Results of Published Reports of Spinal Endoscopy

Ref.	Study Characteristic(s)	No. of Patients	Relief 3 Months	Relief 6 Months	Relief 1 Year
Manchikanti et al.[11]	P, RA, DB	C = 33	0%	0%	0%
		T = 50	80%	56%	48%
Geurts et al.[8]	P	20	40%	35%	35%
Richardson et al.[7]	P	34	Sig	Sig	Sig
Manchikanti et al.[5]	R	60	75%	40%	22%
Manchikanti[6]	R	85	77%	52%	21%

Note: P = prospective; RA = randomized; DB = double-blind; R = retrospective, Sig = significant number of patients; C = control; T = treatment.

fluid administration and direct access to the target site, removing or diluting the chemical irritants.

CLINICAL EFFECTIVENESS

Clinical effectiveness of endoscopic adhesiolysis with direct visualization was evaluated in one randomized, double-blind trial,[11] two prospective case series,[7,8] four retrospective trials,[5,6,9,44] and some case reports.[41,43] The results of those trials eligible are summarized in Table 71.1.

In a prospective, randomized, double-blind trial with a 1-year follow-up of spinal endoscopic adhesiolysis in patients with chronic low back pain, refractory to multiple other modalities of treatments, including percutaneous adhesiolysis, Manchikanti et al.[11] showed that significant improvement was seen without any adverse events in 80% of the patients at 3 months, 56% at 6 months, and 48% at 12 months. They considered that short-term relief was noted in 80% and long-term relief was noted in 56% based on the definition of short-term improvement as less than 6 months and long-term improvement as greater than 6 months.

Geurts et al.[8] in a prospective case series reported results of spinal endoscopic adhesiolysis in 20 patients with greater than 50% reduction in pain in 40% of the patients at 3 months, 35% at 6, 9, and 12 months.

Richardson et al.[7] evaluated the role of spinal endoscopy in a prospective case series of 34 patients suffering with chronic, severe low back pain, with 50% of the patients having failed back surgery syndrome. They reported the presence of epidural adhesions in 100% of the patients, with 41% having dense adhesions. A follow-up over a 1-year period showed significant reductions in pain scores and disability.

Manchikanti et al.[5] in a study evaluating the effectiveness of endoscopic adhesiolysis in postlumbar laminectomy syndrome in 60 patients, showed that 100% of the patients reported significant pain relief at 1 month, whereas 75% reported significant relief at 3 months, 40%

reported significant relief at 6 months, and 22% reported significant relief at 12 months.

Manchikanti et al.[6] in a retrospective evaluation of 85 consecutive patients undergoing 112 epidural endoscopic procedures reported significant pain relief in 100% of the patients initially. However, this relief decreased to 94% at 1 to 2 months, to 77% at 2 to 3 months, to 52% at 3 to 6 months, to 21% at 6 to 12 months, and to 7% after 12 months.

Krasuski et al.[9] reviewed 22 cases. They reported initial improvement in 64% of the patients. The relief declined to 50% of the patients after 1 month and 32% after 3 months. Medication decrease was noted in 32% of the patients.

INDICATIONS

Endoscopic epidural adhesiolysis is indicated in patients with chronic low back pain who have failed to respond to conservative modalities of treatment, including epidural injections administered under fluoroscopic guidance, percutaneous lysis of adhesions with a spring-guided catheter, and other well-documented therapeutic modalities. Various conditions in which spinal endoscopy is indicated include postlumbar laminectomy syndrome, epidural adhesions, and disc disruption resulting in chronic, intractable pain nonresponsive to other modalities of treatment. Probable indications include low back pain nonresponsive to other modalities of treatments and chemical irritation.

COMPLICATIONS

The most common and worrisome complications of spinal endoscopy with lysis of adhesions are related to instrumentation and administration of high volumes of fluids, resulting in excessive epidural hydrostatic pressures, which may cause spinal cord compression, excessive intraspinal and intracranial pressures, epidural hematoma, bleeding, infection, increased intraocular pressures with resultant visual deficiencies, and even blindness and dural puncture.[79–125] Even though dural puncture was noted in 8 of 112 procedures[6] and 7 of 77 procedures,[5] subarachnoid blockade was seen in only 30 to 40% of patients, without any other complications. However, excessive pressure development has the potential to affect both local and distant perfusion, possibly resulting in visual changes and even blindness. Even though the incidence is rare, it appears that it would be much higher with spinal endoscopic procedures with a combination of high volumes of fluid and generation of high hydrostatic pressures.[79] This also has been reported with routine epidural injections, presumably resulting from transmission of spinal canal pressures cephalad into the brain by the CSF, affecting retinal perfusion or causing macular hemorrhage.

Kushner and Olson[80] evaluated patients who complained of visual-field defects or blurred vision after receiving epidural steroid injections and conclude that retinal hemorrhage is uncommon but significant and a previously unemphasized complication of epidural steroid injections in general. Retinal hemorrhages mainly have been attributed to rapid epidural injections of high volumes, causing a sudden increase in intracranial pressure, resulting in the increase of retinal venous pressure.[80–86] Hence, there may be a causal relationship between these complications and spinal endoscopy and adhesiolysis with administration of high volumes of saline, and other agents, specifically with rapid injections.

Epidural infection following this procedure is a distinct possibility due to the procedure itself, as well as potential immunosuppression secondary to steroid injection.[80–114] Manchikanti et al.[6] reported a serious infection in one patient requiring prolonged antibiotic therapy and skin grafting. In this report, infection occurred following 2 of 112 procedures, was suspected in 6 others, which were managed by prophylactic antibiotics.[6] Manchikanti et al.[5] in another study also report suspicion of infection following 8 of 77 procedures, with no major complications. Sampath and Rigamonti,[87] in a review of epidemiology, diagnosis, and treatment of spinal epidural abscess, note that spinal nerve block was responsible for 7% of the patients, whereas a multitude of other predisposing factors included intravenous (IV) drug use, diabetes neuritis, multiple medical illnesses, trauma, prior spinal surgery, morbid obesity, HIV disease, and end-stage renal disease in a descending order of frequency. Wang et al.,[88] in a 1-year study of the incidence of spinal epidural abscess after epidural analgesia, report nine cases of epidural abscess formation from a total of 17,372 epidural catheters.

Direct trauma to the spinal cord following spinal endoscopy in the lumbar spine is only a theoretical possibility. Neural trauma is a potential complication, even though there are no such case reports. Subdural injection, neural trauma, injury to the spinal cord, and hematoma formation have been described with epidural injections,

even though there are no specific descriptions relating to spinal endoscopy.[115–120] Spinal cord trauma or spinal cord or epidural hematoma formation is a catastrophic complication possible with spinal endoscopic adhesiolysis, although there are no case reports in the literature.

Potential complications include increased or continued pain, transient dysesthesias, paresis, paralysis, local surgical site bleeding, allergic reactions, and side effects related to the administration of steroids. While paresis, paralysis, and intractable pain may be related to needle trauma, epidural hematoma, elevated hydrostatic pressures, ischemia, or nerve injury, severe headache, dysesthesia, and intractable acute back pain may indicate epidural hematoma, cord ischemia, and elevated hydrostatic pressure. However, the safety of steroids and preservatives at epidural therapeutic doses has been demonstrated in both clinical and experimental studies.[121–131] The major theoretical complications of corticosteroid administration include arachnoiditis, suppression of the pituitary-adrenal axis, hypocorticism, Cushing syndrome, osteoporosis, avascular necrosis of bone, steroid myopathy, weight gain, fluid retention, and hyperglycemia.[130,131]

Additional complications include hypertension, hypokalemia, epidural lipomatosis, retinal hemorrhage, subcapsular cataract formation, insomnia, mood swings, psychosis, facial flushing, headache, gastrointestinal disturbances, and menstrual disturbances. The use of corticosteroids repeatedly for days or even a few weeks does not lead to adrenal insufficiency upon cessation of treatment, but prolonged therapy with corticosteroids occasionally may result in the suppression of pituitary-adrenal function that can be slow in returning to normal. Rare hypothalamic-pituitary-adrenal suppression during corticosteroid administration with epidural injections and after its withdrawal has been reported.[130,131] However, no such reports have implicated spinal endoscopy and administration of steroids. Manchikanti et al.[132] evaluated the effect of neuraxial steroids on weight and bone mass density (BMD) prospectively. The results of serial determination of weight and BMD showed no significant change at any interval or at the end of 1 year in any of 123 patients with or without steroid administration.

Houten and Errico[123] report three cases of paraplegia after lumbosacral nerve root block in post laminectomy patients. They report that in each case, performed at three different facilities, in the hands of two different physicians, the needle placement was verified with injection of contrast in conjunction with CT or biplanar fluoroscopy. In each patient, paraplegia was reported suddenly after injection of steroid solution, and in each instance, postprocedure MRI revealed spinal cord edema in the low thoracic region. The authors postulate that in these patients the spinal needle penetrated or caused injury to an abnormally low dominant radiculomedullary artery, a recognized anatomical variant. This vessel, also known as the artery of Adamkiewicz, in 85% of individuals arises between T9 and L2, usually from the left, but in a minority of people, it may arise from the lower lumbar spine and rarely even from as low as S1.[123] This artery travels with the nerve root through the neural foramen, supplying the anterior spinal artery. Injury of the artery or injection of particulate steroid may result in infarction of the lower thoracic spinal cord.

Cousins[124] also reports similar complication as above.[123] He reports a potential complication of particulate depo-corticosteroids related to inadvertent intravascular administration, producing occlusion of small end arteries, which resulted in visual defects in one case and hearing loss in another case, involving suboccipital nerve block. It is felt that prednisolone acetate tends to form aggregates of the steroid material when mixed with local anesthetic and may pose more of a risk for this problem than other depo-steroids.

TECHNICAL ASPECTS

Spinal endoscopy is best performed by a caudal approach based on anatomy, equipment, and experience with epidural adhesiolysis with spring-guided catheter. The straight entry into the epidural space through the caudal approach is much easier and more practical than entry into the lumbar epidural space through a paramedian approach, even with a steep angle. This facilitates not only the easy passage of the fiber-optic endoscope but also reduces damage to the device.

ANATOMY

The spinal canal extends from the foramen magnum to the sacrum, which is bounded posteriorly by the ligamentum flavum and periosteum and anteriorly by the posterior longitudinal ligament that lies over the dorsal aspects of the vertebral bodies and discs. The spinal cord ends at L1, and the dural sac continues to the level of S2.

The dural sac rests on the floor of the vertebral canal.[133] The anterior relations of the dural sac, therefore, are the backs of the vertebral bodies and the intervertebral discs, and covering these structures is the posterior longitudinal ligament.[133] Thus, anterior spinal arteries and sinuvertebral nerves run across the floor of the vertebral canal and are located anterior to the dural sac. The dural sac posteriorly is related to the roof of the vertebral canal, the laminae, and ligamentum flava.

The epidural space is a potential space intervening between the dural sac and the osseo-ligamentous boundaries of the vertebral canal. The epidural membrane is a thin layer of areolar connective tissue, which varies from diaphanous to pseudomembranous in structure.[134,135] The membrane surrounds the dural sac and lines the deep surface of the laminae and pedicles.[133] Ventrally, opposite the vertebral bodies, the membrane lines the back of the vertebral body and then passes medially deep to the posterior longitudinal ligament, where it detaches from the anterior surface of the deep portion of the ligament.[134] However, the membrane does not cover the back of the anulus fibrosus and is prevented from doing so by the posterior longitudinal ligament as it expands laterally over the back of the disc. The size of the posterior epidural space averages 4 to 6 mm at the lumbar level.

TECHNIQUE

Prior to undergoing spinal endoscopy, all the patients must be assessed with a comprehensive physical and psychological evaluation. All less invasive and conservative modalities of treatment, including fluoroscopically directed epidural steroid injections and spring-guided catheter lysis of adhesions, should be exhausted. In addition, appropriate laboratory studies should be considered to rule out bleeding disorders. Nonsteroidal anti-inflammatory drugs, aspirin, and anticoagulants should be discontinued prior to spinal canal endoscopy to avoid unusual bleeding.

An antibacterial scrub with a shower the night before should be considered. In addition, the patient should have an empty stomach. No general anesthesia should be contemplated. The patient should understand all the implications of the procedure and sign an informed consent.

After the initial evaluation, the patient is transferred to the holding area, where appropriate preparation is carried out with preoperative evaluation, checking of vital signs, and establishment of IV access, as well as antibiotic administration.

Following this, the patient is taken to the operating room or a sterile procedure room where preparation is carried out with iodophor solution. Draping is carried out to cover the entire patient, extending into the cervical region. At this time, under appropriate monitoring with blood pressure and pulse oximetry, sedation is administered and continuous monitoring is performed.

The procedure is performed in a sterile operating room under appropriate sterile precautions using fluoroscopy. The fluoroscope is adjusted over the lumbosacral region to perform the procedure in the lumbosacral region for a lumbar or caudal procedure, both anteroposterior and lateral views.

After appropriate positioning of fluoroscopy, a physician scrubbed and with sterile gown and gloves infiltrates the area for needle insertion with local anesthetic. Following this, an epidural needle is introduced into the epidural space using fluoroscopic visualization. Once the needle placement is confirmed to be in the epidural space, a lumbar epidurogram is carried out using approximately 2 to 5 ml of non-ionic contrast. Finding the filling defects by examining the contrast flow into the nerve roots is the purpose of the epidurogram. Intravascular or subarachnoid placement of the needle or contrast is avoided; if such malpositioning occurs, the needle is repositioned.

A 0.9-mm guide wire is inserted through the needle, which is advanced under fluoroscopic guidance to the level of suspected pathology, followed by advancement of a 2-mm × 17.8-cm dilator with catheter (sheath) over the guide wire. Once the catheter is advanced to the tip of the guide wire, the wire is removed. At this time, a 0.8-mm fiber-optic spinal endoscopy is introduced into the catheter through the valve and is advanced until the tip is positioned at the distal end of the catheter, as determined by video and fluoroscopic images. In conjunction with gentle irrigation using normal saline, the catheter and fiber-optic myeloscope are manipulated and rotated in multiple directions, with visualization of the nerve roots at various levels. Gentle irrigation may also be carried out by slow, controlled infusion. Adhesiolysis and decompression are carried out by distension of the epidural space with normal saline and by mechanical means using the fiber-optic endoscope. Figure 71.1 through Figure 71.3 illustrate the procedural considerations.

Confirmation is accomplished with injection of nonionic contrast material. An epidurogram is performed on at least two occasions. Following completion of the procedure, generally, lidocaine 1%, preservative free, mixed with 6 to 12 mg of betamethasone acetate and phosphate mixture or methylprednisolone or triamcinolone is injected in each case after assuring that there is no evidence of subarachnoid leakage of contrast. If there is a question of subarachnoid leakage of the contrast, a Racz catheter may be passed into the epidural space, and a mixture of local anesthetic injected very slowly in incremental doses, followed by injection of the steroid.

Following completion of the procedure, if necessary, self-absorbed sutures are applied, followed by sterile Bioclusive dressing. Subsequently, the patient is turned to the supine position and transferred to the recovery room. In the recovery room, the patient is very closely monitored for any potential complications or side effects. If a patient has a catheter and no complications are observed and good pain relief is reported without any motor weakness, steroid is injected.

CONCLUSION

Chronic low back pain is a major health care and social problem. Much of the confusion surrounding spinal endoscopy and adhesiolysis in managing refractory low back pain results from overemphasis on biopsychosocial problems and inappropriate selection of patients for this treatment modality. Considering the cumulative evidence available, the efficacy of this procedure is similar, if not superior, to multiple other modalities of treatments available in managing chronic low back pain, including surgical intervention.

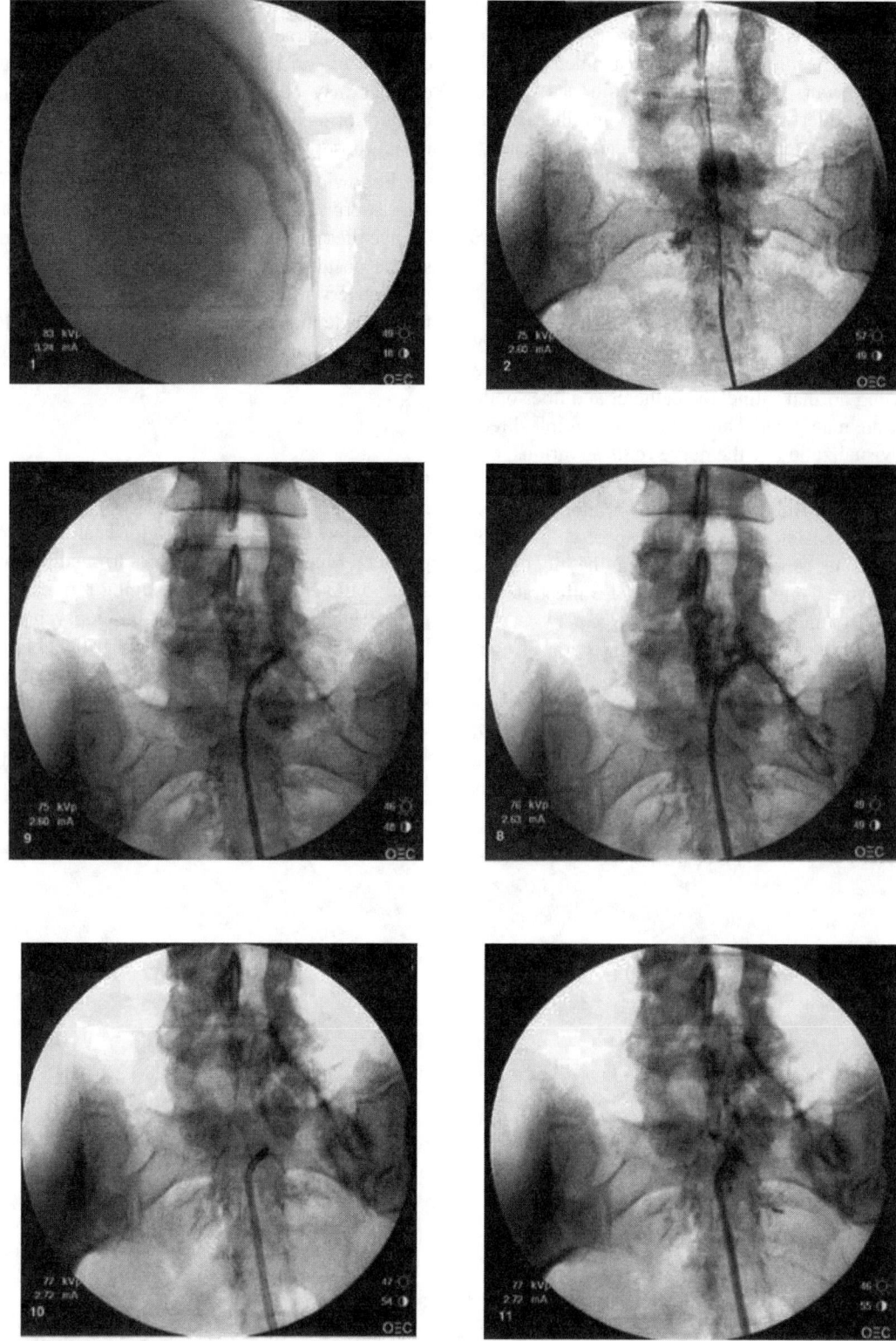

FIGURE 71.1 Fluoroscopic illustration of placement of needle, contrast injection, videocatheter placement, and adhesiolysis.

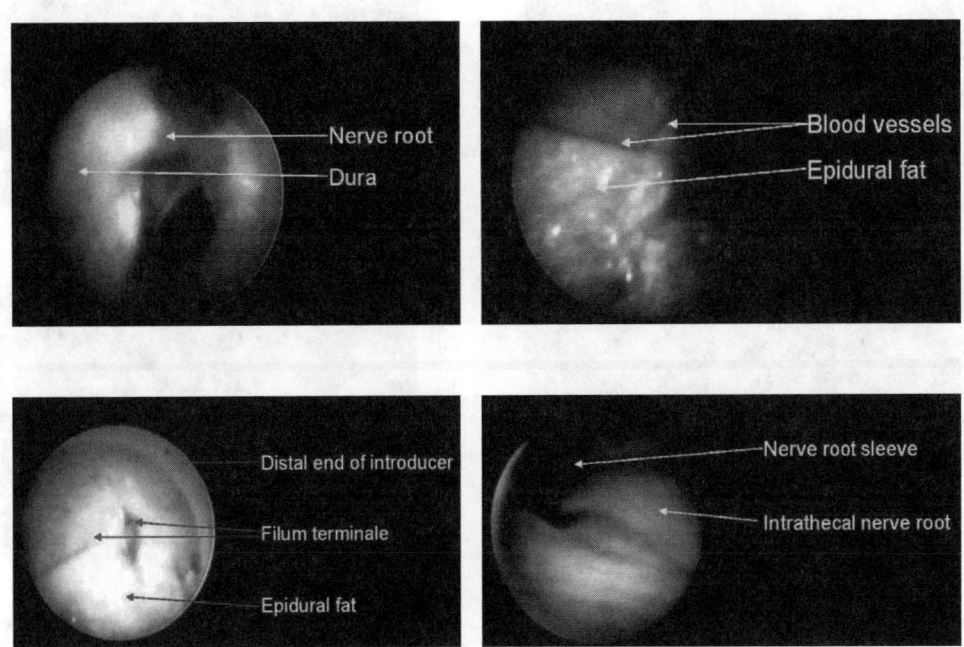

FIGURE 71.2 Normal endoscopic anatomy of lumbar epidural space. (Courtesy of Visionary Biomedical [Myelotec], Inc.)

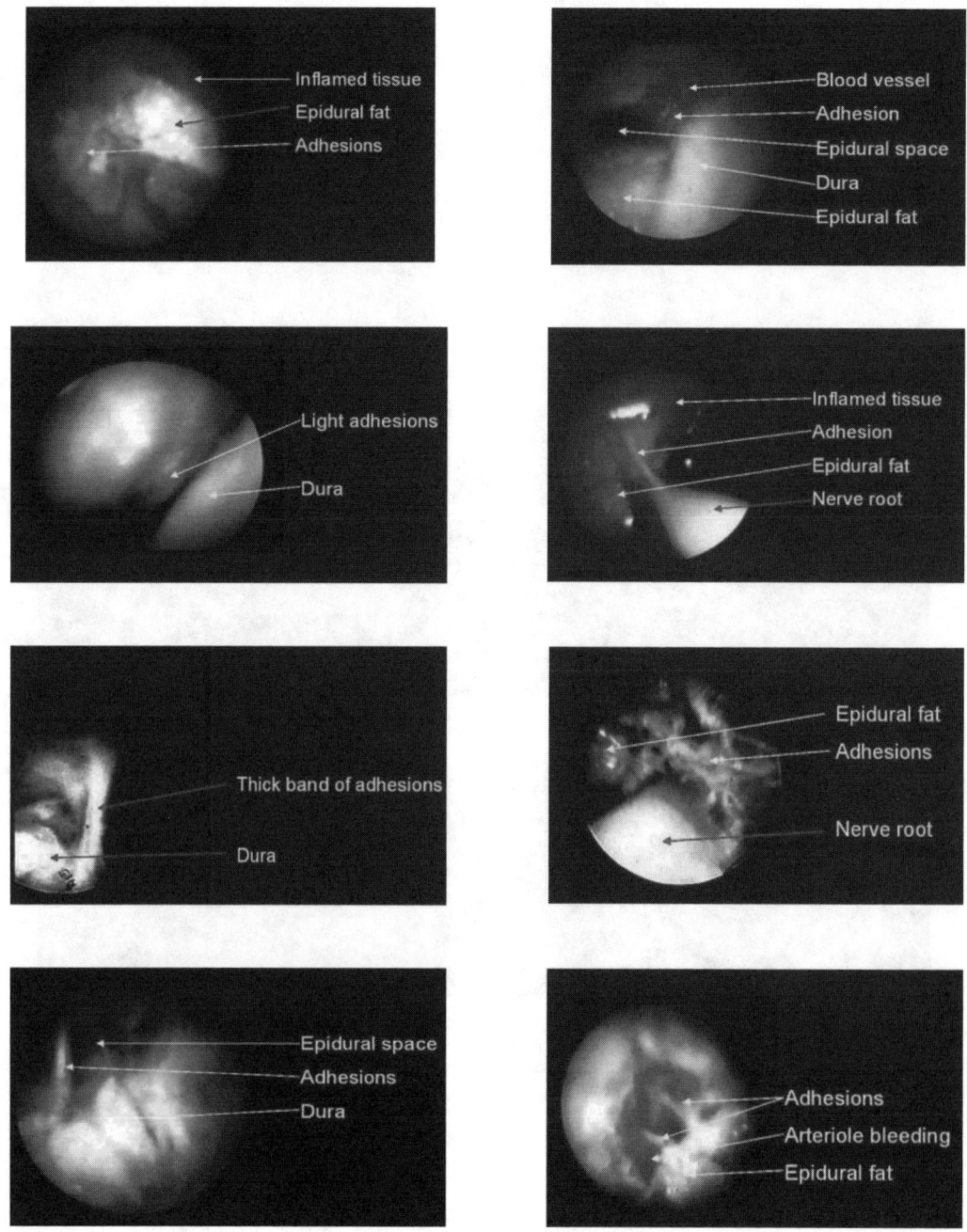

FIGURE 71.3 Typical findings of endoscopic anatomy and adhesiolysis of lumbar epidural space. (Courtesy of Visionary Biomedical [Myelotec], Inc.)

REFERENCES

1. Manchikanti, L., & Singh, V. (2002). Epidural lysis of adhesions and myeloscopy. *Current Pain and Headache Report, 6,* 427.

2. Manchikanti, L., Saini, B., & Singh, V. (2001). Spinal endoscopy and lysis of epidural adhesions in the management of chronic low back pain. *Pain Physician, 4,* 240.

3. Manchikanti, L. et al. (2003). Evidence-based practice guidelines for interventional techniques in the management of chronic spinal pain. *Pain Physician, 6,* 3.

4. Manchikanti, L., & Singh, V. (2002). Lumbar endoscopic adhesiolysis. In L. Manichikanti, C. W. Slipman, & B. Fellows (Eds.), *Interventional pain management: Low back pain — Diagnosis and treatment* (pp. 391–410). Paducah, KY: ASIPP Publishing.

5. Manchikanti, L. et al. (1999). Non-endoscopic and endoscopic adhesiolysis in post lumbar laminectomy syndrome: A one-year outcome study and cost effective analysis. *Pain Physician, 2,* 52.

6. Manchikanti, L. et al. (2000). The value and safety of epidural endoscopic adhesiolysis. *American Journal of Anesthesiology, 27,* 275.

7. Richardson, J. et al. (2001). Spinal endoscopy in chronic low back pain with radiculopathy: A prospective case series. *Anaesthesia, 56,* 454.

8. Geurts, J. W. et al. (2002). Targeted methylprednisolone acetate/hyaluronidase/clonidine injection after diagnostic epiduroscopy for chronic sciatica: A prospective, 1-year follow-up study. *Regional Anesthesia and Pain Medicine, 27,* 343.

9. Krasuski, P. et al. (2001). Epiduroscopy: Review of techniques and results. *Pain Clinic, 13,* 71.

10. Shutse, G. et al. (1996). Endoscopic method for the diagnosis and treatment of spinal pain syndromes. *Anaesthesiologie und Reanimation, 4,* 62.

11. Manchikanti, L. et al. (in press). Evaluation of spinal endoscopic adhesiolysis in chronic refractory low back pain with a randomized, double-blind trial with one year follow-up. *BioMed Central Anesthesiology.*

12. Sicard, M. A. (1901). Les injections medicamenteuse extraduraqles per voir saracoccygiene. *Comptes Rendus des Senances de la Societe de Biolgie et de SES Filliales, 53,* 396.

13. Cathelin, F. (1901). Mode d'action de a cocaine injete daus l'escapte epidural par le procede canal sacre. *Comptes Rendus des Senances de la Societe de Biologic et de SES Filliales, 53,* 452.

14. Pasquier, N. M., & Leri, D. (1901). Injection-intra-et extraudrales de cocaine a dose minime daus le traitment de la sciatique. *Bulletin General de Therapeutique, 142,* 196.

15. Sicard, J. A., & Forestier, J. (1921). Méthode radiographique d'exploration de la cavité épidurale par le Lipiodol. *Revue Neurologique, 28,* 1264.

16. Racz, G. B. et al. (1982). Intractable pain therapy using a new epidural catheter. *Journal of the American Medical Association, 248,* 579.

17. Heavner, J. E., Racz, G. B., & Raj, P. (1999). Percutaneous epidural neuroplasty. Prospective evaluation of 0.9% NaCl versus 10% NaCl with or without hyaluronidase. *Regional Anesthesia and Pain Medicine, 24,* 202.

18. Manchikanti, L. et al. (1999). Role of adhesiolysis and hypertonic saline neurolysis in management of low back pain. Evaluation of modification of Racz protocol. *Pain Digest, 9,* 91.

19. Manchikanti, L. et al. (2001). Role of one-day epidural adhesiolysis in management of chronic low back pain: A randomized clinical trial. *Pain Physician, 4,* 153.

20. Manchikanti, L. (2004). One day lumbar epidural adhesiolysis and hypertonic saline neurolysis in treatment of chronic low back pain: A randomized, double blind trial. *Pain Physician, 7,* 177.

21. Saberski, L., & Brull, S. (1995). Spinal and epidural endoscopy: A historical review. *Yale Journal of Biology and Medicine, 68,* 7.

22. Burman, M. S. (1931). Myeloscopy or the direct visualization of the spinal cord. *Journal of Bone and Joint Surgery, 13,* 695.

23. Shimoji, K. et al. (1991). Observation of spinal canal and cisternae with the newly developed small-diameter, flexible fiberscopes. *Anesthesiology, 75,* 341.

24. Stern, E. L. (1936). The spinascope: A new instrument for visualizing the spinal canal and its contents. *Medical Record* (NY), *143,* 31.

25. Pool, J. L. (1938). Direct visualization of dorsal nerve roots of the cauda equina by means of a myeloscope. *Archives of Neurology, 39,* 1308.

26. Pool, J. L. (1938). Myeloscopy: Diagnostic inspection of the cauda equina by means of an endoscope. *Bulletin Neurological Institute of New York, 7,* 178.

27. Pool, J. L. (1942). Myeloscopy: Intraspinal endoscopy. *Surgery, 11,* 169.

28. Ooi, Y., & Morisaki, N. (1969). Intrathecal lumbar endoscope. *Clinical Orthopedic Surgery* (Japan), *4,* 295.

29. Ooi, Y., Satoh, Y., & Morisaki, N. (1973). Myeloscopy. *Clinical Orthopedic Surgery* (Japan), *24,* 181.

30. Ooi, Y., Satoh, Y., & Morisaki, N. (1973). Myeloscopy: Possibility of observing lumbar intrathecal space by use of an endoscope. *Endoscopy, 5,* 91.

31. Ooi, Y., Satoh, Y., & Morisaki, N. (1973). Myeloscopy: A preliminary report. *Journal of the Japanese Orthopedic Association, 47,* 619.

32. Ooi, Y., Satoh, Y., & Morisaki, N. (1977). Myeloscopy. *International Orthopaedics, 1,* 107.

33. Ooi, Y. et al. (1978). Myeloscopy. *Acta Orthopaedica Belgica, 44,* 881.

34. Satoh, Y. et al. (1978, July 2–9). Myeloscopy in the diagnosis of low back pain syndrome. In *Proceedings of Third Congress of International Rehabilitation Medicine Assoc.*, Basel, Switzerland: Raven Press.

35. Ooi, Y. et al. (1981). Myeloscopy with special reference to blood flow changes in the cauda equina during Lasegue's test. *International Orthopaedics, 4,* 307.

36. Blomberg, R. G. (1985). A method of epiduroscopy and spinaloscopy: Presentation of preliminary results. *Acta Anaesthesiologica Scandinavica, 29,* 113.

37. Blomberg, R. G., & Olsson, S. S. (1989). The lumbar epidural space in patients examined with epiduroscopy. *Anesthesia & Analgesia, 68,* 157.

38. Blomberg, R. G. (1988). Technical advantages of the paramedian approach for lumbar epidural puncture and catheter introduction. A study using epiduroscopy in autopsy subjects. *Anaesthesia, 43,* 837.

39. Heavner, J. E., Cholkhavatia, S., & Kizelshteyn, G. (1991). Percutaneous evaluation of the epidural and subarachnoid space with the flexible fiberscope. *Regional Anesthesia, 15S,* 85.

40. Heavner, J. et al. (1993, August). Diagnostic and therapeutic maneuvers in the epidural space via a flexible endoscope [Abstract 1534]. In *Abstracts of the Seventh World Congress on Pain,* Paris: Raven Press.

41. Saberski, L., & Kitahata, L. (1995). Direct visualization of the lumbosacral epidural space through the sacral hiatus. *Anesthesia & Analgesia, 80,* 839.

42. Saberski, L., & Kitahata, L. (1996). Review of the clinical basis and protocol for epidural endoscopy. *Connecticut Medicine, 60,* 71.

43. Saberski, L., & Kitahata, L. (1996). Persistent radiculopathy diagnosed and treated with epidural endoscopy. *Journal of Anesthesia, 10,* 292.

44. Saberski, L. (2000). A retrospective analysis of spinal canal endoscopy and laminectomy outcomes data. *Pain Physician, 3,* 193.

45. Witte, H. et al. (1997). Epiduroscopy with access via the sacral canal. Some constructional equipment requirements from the anatomic and biomechanical viewpoint. *Biomedizinische Technik, 42,* 24.

46. LaRocca, H., & MacNab, I. (1974). The laminectomy membrane: studies in its evolution, characteristics, effects and prophylaxis in dogs. *Journal of Bone and Joint Surgery, 56,* 545.

47. McCarron, R. F. et al. (1987). The inflammatory effect of the nucleus pulposus. A possible element in the pathogenesis of low back pain. *Spine, 12,* 760.

48. McCarron, R. F. (1989). Epidural fibrosis: Experimental model and therapeutic alternatives. In G. B. Racz (Ed.), *Techniques of neurolysis* (p. 87). Boston: Kluwer Academic Publishers.

49. Pawl, R. P. (1998). Arachnoiditis and epidural fibrosis: The relationship to chronic pain. *Current Review of Pain, 2,* 93.

50. Van Goethem, J. W. et al. (1996). MRI after successful lumbar discectomy. *Neuroradiology, 38,* S90.

51. Grave, P. et al. (1996). Postoperative lumbar magnetic resonance imaging with contrast enhancement: Compression between symptomatic and asymptomatic patients. *Acta Radiologica, 37,* 366.

52. Annertz, M. et al. (1995). No relationship between epidural fibrosis and sciatica in the lumbar postdiscectomy syndrome: A study with contrast-enhancement magnetic resonance imagery in symptomatic and asymptomatic patients. *Spine, 20,* 449.

53. Cervellini, P. et al. (1988). Computed tomography of epidural fibrosis after discectomy. A comparison between symptomatic and asymptomatic patients. *Neurosurgery, 6,* 710.

54. Songer, M., Ghosh, L., & Spencer, D. (1990). Effects of sodium hyaluronate on peridural fibrosis after lumbar laminectomy and discectomy. *Spine, 15,* 550.

55. Ross, J. S. et al. (1996). Association between peridural scar and recurrent radicular pain after lumbar discectomy: Magnetic resonance evaluation. *Neurosurgery, 38,* 855.

56. Parke, W. W., & Watanabe, R. (1990). Adhesions of the ventral lumbar dura. Adjunct source of discogenic pain? *Spine, 15,* 300.

57. Berger, E., & Davis, J. M. B. (1999, August). Chronic pain following lumbar spinal surgery in 1000 patients. In *Proceedings of 9th World Congress on Pain* (p. 181). Basel, Switzerland: Raven Press.

58. Quiles, M., Marchisello, P. J., & Tsairis, P. (1978). Lumbar adhesive arachnoiditis: Etiological and pathological aspects. *Spine, 3,* 45.

59. Cooper, R. et al. (1995). Herniated intervertebral disc-associated periradicular fibrosis and vascular abnormalities occur without inflammatory cell infiltration. *Spine, 20,* 591.

60. Manchikanti, L., Bakhit, C. E., & Pampati, V. (1998). Role of epidurography in caudal neuroplasty. *Pain Digest, 8,* 277.

61. Mooney, V. (1987). Where is the pain coming from? *Spine, 12,* 754.

62. Wheeler, A. H., & Murrey, D. B. (2002). Chronic lumbar spine and radicular pain: Pathophysiology and treatment. *Current Pain Headache Report, 6,* 97.

63. Kawakami, M., Chatenia, K., & Weinstein, J. N. (1995). Anatomy, biochemistry, and physiology of low back pain. In A. G. White & J. A. Schofferman (Eds.), *Spine care: Diagnosis and conservative treatment* (p. 84). St. Louis: Mosby Press.

64. Weinstein, J. N., Claverie, W., & Gibson, S. (1988). The pain of discography. *Spine, 13,* 1344.

65. Rydevik, B. L. (1992). The effects of compression on the physiology of nerve roots. *Journal of Manipulative Physiological Therapy, 1,* 62.

66. Olmarker, K., & Rydevik, B. (1999). Pathophysiology of spinal nerve roots as related to sciatica and disc herniation. In H. N. Herkowitz et al. (Eds.), *Rothman-Simeone studies, the spine* (p. 159). Philadelphia: WB Saunders.

67. Mixter, W. J., & Barr, J. S. (1934). Rupture of the intervertebral disc with involvement of the spinal cord. *New England Journal of Medicine, 211,* 210.

68. Ford, L. T., & Lam, R. L. (1952). The psychiatric aspects of low back pain. *Journal of Bone and Joint Surgery, 38,* 931.

69. Barr, J. S. (1951). Low back pain and sciatic pain. *Journal of Bone and Joint Surgery, 33,* 633.

70. Mixter, W. J., & Ayers, J. B. (1935). Herniation or rupture of the intervertebral disc into the spinal canal. *New England Journal of Medicine, 213,* 385.

71. Cautico, W. et al. (1988). An anatomical and clinical investigation of spinal meningeal nerves. *Acta Neurochirurgie* (Wien), *90,* 139.

72. Barsa, J. E., & Charlton, J. E. (1984). Diagnosis of epidural scarring and its possible contribution to chronic low back pain syndrome. *Pain, S4*, 376.

73. Suk, K. S. et al. (2001). Recurrent lumbar disc herniation. Results of operative management. *Spine, 26*, 672.

74. Manchikanti, L. et al. (2001). Contribution of facet joints to chronic low back pain in postlumbar laminectomy syndrome: A controlled comparative prevalence evaluation. *Pain Physician, 4*, 175.

75. Kuslich, S. D., Ulstrom, C. L., & Michael, C. J. (1991). The tissue origin of low back pain and sciatica. *Orthopedic Clinics of North America, 22*, 181.

76. Key, J. A., & Ford, L. T. (1948). Experimental intervertebral disc lesions. *Journal of Bone and Joint Surgery, 30*, 621.

77. Imai, S., Hukuda, S., & Maeda, T. (1995). Dually innervating nociceptive networks in the rat lumbar posterior longitudinal ligaments. *Spine, 19*, 2086.

78. Phillips, F. M., & Cunningham, B. (2002). Managing chronic pain of spinal origin after lumbar surgery. *Spine, 27*, 2547.

79. Tabandeh, H. (2000). Intraocular hemorrhages associated with endoscopic spinal surgery. *American Journal of Ophthalmology, 129*, 688.

80. Kushner, F. H., & Olson, J. C. (1995). Retinal hemorrhage as a consequence of epidural steroid injection. *Archives of Ophthalmology, 113*, 309.

81. Ling, C., Atkinson, P. L., & Munton, C. G. (1993). Bilateral retinal hemorrhages following epidural injection. *British Journal of Ophthalmology, 77*, 316.

82. Purdy, E. P., & Ajimal, G. S. (1998). Vision loss after lumbar epidural steroid injection. *Anesthesia & Analgesia, 86*, 119.

83. Victory, R. A., Hassett, P., & Morrison, G. (1991). Transient blindness following epidural analgesia. *Anesthesia, 46*, 940.

84. Amirikia, A. et al. (2000). Acute bilateral visual loss associated with retinal hemorrhages following epiduroscopy. *Archives of Ophthalmology, 118*, 287.

85. Usubiaga, J. E., Wikinski, J. A., & Usubiaga, L. E. (1967). Epidural pressure and its relation to spread of anesthetic solution in epidural space. *Anesthesia & Analgesia, 46*, 440.

86. Morris, D. A., & Henkind, P. (1967). Relationship of intracranial, optic-nerve sheath, and retinal hemorrhage. *American Journal of Ophthalmology, 64*, 853.

87. Sampath, P., & Rigamonti, D. (1999). Spinal epidural abscess: A review of epidemiology, diagnosis, and treatment. *Journal of Spinal Disorders, 12*, 89.

88. Wang, L. P., Haverberg, J., & Schmidt, J. F. (1999). Incidence of spinal epidural abscess after epidural analgesia. *Anesthesiology, 91*, 1928.

89. Rathmell, J. P., Garahan, M. B., & Alsofrom, G. F. (2000). Epidural abscess following epidural analgesia. *Regional Anesthesia and Pain Medicine, 25*, 79.

90. Martin, R. J., & Yuan, H. A. (1996). Neurosurgical care of spinal epidural, subdural, and intramedullary abscesses and arachnoiditis. *Orthopedic Clinics of North America, 27*, 125.

91. Kuker, W. et al. (1997). Epidural spinal infection: Variability of clinical and magnetic resonance imaging findings. *Spine, 22*, 544.

92. Baker, A. S. et al. (1975). Spinal epidural abscess. *New England Journal of Medicine, 293*, 463.

93. Knight, J. W., Cordingley, J. J., & Palazzo, M. G. A. (1997). Epidural abscess following epidural steroid and local anesthetic injection. *Anesthesia, 52*, 576.

94. Sharif, H. S. (1992). Role of imaging in the management of spinal infections. *American Journal of Roentgenology, 158*, 1333.

95. DuPen, S. L. et al. (1990). Infection during chronic epidural catheterization: Diagnosis and treatment. *Anesthesiology, 73*, 905.

96. Brookman, C. A., & Rutledge, M. L. C. (2000). Epidural abscess: Case report and literature review. *Regional Anesthesia and Pain Medicine, 25*, 428.

97. Hlavin, M. L. et al. (1990). Spinal epidural abscess: A ten year perspective. *Neurosurgery, 27*, 177.

98. Darouiche, R. O. et al. (1992). Bacterial spinal epidural abscess. Review of 43 cases and literature survey. *Medicine, 71*, 369.

99. Mackenzie, A. R. et al. (1998). Spinal epidural abscess: The importance of early diagnosis and treatment. *Journal of Neurology, Neurosurgery and Psychiatry, 65*, 209.

100. Nussbaum, E. S. et al. (1992). Spinal epidural abscess: A report of 40 cases and review. *Surgical Neurology, 38*, 225.

101. Sarubbi, F. A., & Vasquez, J. E. (1997). Spinal epidural abscess associated with the use of temporary epidural catheters: Report of two cases and review. *Clinical Infectious Diseases, 25*, 1155.

102. Yuste, M. et al. (1997). An epidural abscess due to resistant *Staphylococcus aureus* following epidural catheterization. *Anesthesia, 52*, 150.

103. Mamourian, A. C. et al. (1993). Spinal epidural abscess: Three cases following spinal epidural injection demonstrated with magnetic resonance imaging. *Anesthesiology, 78*, 204.

104. Strong, W. E. (1991). Epidural abscess associated with epidural catheterization: A rare event? Report of two cases with markedly delayed presentation. *Anesthesiology, 74*, 943.

105. Bromage, P. R. (1993). Spinal extradural abscess: Pursuit of vigilance. *British Journal of Anaesthesiology, 70*, 471.

106. Kaul, S. et al. (2000). Spinal extradural abscess following local steroid injection. *Neurology India, 48*, 181.

107. Chan, S. T., & Leung, S. (1989). Spinal epidural abscess following steroid injection for sciatica: Case report. *Spine, 14*, 106.

108. Goucke, C. R., & Graziotti, P. (1990). Extradural abscess following local anesthetic and steroid injection for chronic low back pain. *British Journal of Anaesthesiology, 65*, 427.

109. Scott, D. B., & Hibbard, B. M. (1990). Serious non-fatal complications associated with extradural block in obstetric practice. *British Journal of Anaesthesiology, 64*, 537.

110. Pegues, D. A., Carr, D. B., & Hopkins, C. C. (1994). Infectious complications associated with temporary epidural catheters. *Clinical Infectious Diseases, 19*, 970.

111. Darchy, B. et al. (1996). Clinical and bacteriologic survey of epidural analgesia in patients in the intensive care unit. *Anesthesiology, 85*, 988.

112. Carson, D., & Wildsmith, J. A, W. (1995). The risk of extradural abscess [Editorial]. *British Journal of Anaesthesiology, 75*, 520.

113. Del Curling, O., Gower, D. J., & McWhorter, J. M. (1990). Changing concepts in spinal epidural abscess: A report of 29 cases. *Neurosurgery, 27*, 185.

114. Yue, W. M., & Tan, S. B. (2003). Distant skip level discitis and vertebral osteomyelitis after caudal epidural injection: A case report of a rare complication of epidural injections. *Spine, 28*, E209.

115. Bromage, P. R. (1978). Complications and contraindications. In P. R. Bromage (Ed.), *Epidural analgesia* (p. 469). Philadelphia: WB Saunders.

116. Bromage, P. R., & Benumof, J. L. (1998). Paraplegia following intracord injection during attempted epidural anesthesia under general anesthesia. *Regional Anesthesia and Pain Medicine, 23*, 104.

117. Horlocker, T. T., & Wedel, D. J. (2000). Neurologic complications of spinal and epidural anesthesia. *Regional Anesthesia and Pain Medicine, 25*, 83.

118. Raj, P. P. et al. (2004). Bleeding risk in interventional pain practice: Assessment, management, and review of the literature. *Pain Physician, 7*, 3.

119. Sandhu, H., Morley-Fost, P., & Spadafora, S. (2000). Epidural hematoma following epidural analgesia in a patient receiving unfractionated heparin for thromboprophylaxis. *Regional Anesthesia and Pain Medicine, 25*, 72.

120. Osmani, O., Afeiche, N., & Lakkis, S. (2000). Paraplegia after epidural anesthesia in a patient with peripheral vascular disease: Case report and review of the literature with a description of an original technique for hematoma evacuation. *Journal of Spinal Disorders, 13*, 85.

121. Furman, M. B. et al. (2000). Incidence of intravascular penetration in transforaminal lumbosacral epidural steroid injections. *Spine, 25*, 2628.

122. Botwin, K. P. et al. (2000). Complications of fluoroscopically guided transforaminal lumbar epidural injections. *Archives of Physical and Medical Rehabilitation, 81*, 1045.

123. Houten, J. K., & Errico, T. J. (2002). Paraplegia after lumbosacral nerve root block: Report of three cases. *Spine Journal, 2*, 70.

124. Cousins, M. J. (2000). An additional dimension to the efficacy of epidural steroids. *Anesthesiology, 93*, 565.

125. Schultz, D. M. (2003). Risk of transforaminal epidural injections. *Pain Physician, 6*, 390.

126. Delaney, T. J. et al. (1980). Epidural steroid effects on nerves and meninges. *Anesthesia & Analgesia, 58*, 610.

127. Cicala, R. S. et al. (1990). Methylprednisolone acetate does not cause inflammatory changes in the epidural space. *Anesthesiology, 72*, 556.

128. Abram, S. E., Marsala, M., & Yaksh, T. L. (1994). Analgesic and neurotoxic effects of intrathecal corticosteroids in rats. *Anesthesiology, 81*, 1198.

129. Latham, J. M. et al. (1997). The pathologic effects of intrathecal betamethasone. *Spine, 22*, 1558.

130. Manchikanti, L. (2000). The value and safety of steroids in neural blockade. Part I. *American Journal of Pain Management, 10*, 69.

131. Manchikanti, L. (2000). The value and safety of steroids in neural blockade. Part II. *American Journal of Pain Management, 10*, 122.

132. Manchikanti, L. et al. (2000). The effect of neuraxial steroids on weight and bone mass density: A prospective evaluation. *Pain Physician, 3*, 357.

133. Bogduk, N. (1997). *Clinical anatomy of the lumbar spine and sacrum* (p. 127). New York: Churchill Livingstone.

134. Parkin, I. G., & Harrison, G. R. (1985). The topographical anatomy of lumbar epidural space. *Journal of Anatomy, 141*, 211.

135. Wiltse, L. L. et al. (1993). Relationship of the dura, Hoffman's ligaments, Batson's plexus, and a fibrovascular membrane lying of the posterior surface of the vertebral bodies and attaching to the deep layer of the posterior longitudinal ligament: An anatomical, radiological, and clinical study. *Spine, 18*, 1030.

72

Cryoneurolysis: Principles and Practice

Andrea M. Trescot, MD

DEFINITION

Cryoanalgesia, cryoneuroablation, or cryoneurolysis is a specialized technique for providing long-term pain relief when pain has been shown to be caused by sensory nerves.

HISTORY

Humans have known about the use of cold for analgesia for thousands of years. Hippocrates (460–377 B.C.) left us the first written records of the use of ice for pain relief, describing how snow was brought down from the mountains in ancient Greece and applied to wounds for pain relief.[1] The ancient Egyptians documented the use of low temperature for analgesia.[2] Avicenna of Persia (A.D. 982–1070), an early physician, described the use of cold for preoperative analgesia.[3] Baron Dominique Jean Larre, Napoleon's Surgeon General, noted in 1812 that half-frozen soldiers in the Moscow battle were able to tolerate limb amputation with little or no pain.[4] In addition, Hunter noted in 1777 that when rooster comb tissues were killed by cold, the base of the comb healed without scarring.[5] In 1851, Arnott[6] avidly promoted the application of cold to relive certain types of cancer and nerve pain, using mixtures of ice and salt at –20°C. He also noted the hemostatic and anesthetic effects of cold. Richardson[7] introduced ether spray in 1866 for topical anesthesia, which was followed by ethyl chloride spray in 1891; thus "to freeze" became synonymous with "to numb." Trendelenberg[8] demonstrated that freezing tissues caused severe nerve damage and loss of function, but noted that the nerves regenerated without neuroma formation.

Modern cryoanalgesia traces its roots to Cooper et al.[9] who developed in 1961 a device that used liquid nitrogen in a hollow tube that was insulated at the tip and achieved a temperature of –190°C. Amoils,[10] an ophthalmic surgeon, developed a simpler handheld device in 1967, which used carbon dioxide or nitrous oxide and could achieve temperatures of –70°C. Lloyd and his co-workers[11] coined the term *cryoanalgesia* for its use in pain management. They proposed that this technique was superior to other methods of peripheral nerve destruction, e.g., alcohol, phenol, or surgical lesions, because it is not followed by neuritis or neuralgia.[12]

Current probes range in size from 1.4 to 2 mm in size and have as well a built-in nerve stimulator for localization of the nerve and a thermistor to identify temperature at the tip. Barnard and Lloyd,[13] Evans,[5] and Glynn and Carrie[14] popularized cryoneuroablation in the early 1980s, but relatively little has been written on the technique since then. This chapter is an attempt to describe the contemporary role of cryoneuroablation.

PHYSICS AND EQUIPMENT

The cryoprobe consists of a hollow tube with a smaller inner tube. Pressurized gas (usually N_2O or CO_2) at 600 to 800 psi travels down the inner tube and is released into the larger outer tube, which is at a low pressure of 10 to 15 psi through a very fine aperture (0.002 mm), allowing the gas to rapidly expand (Figure 72.1) into the distal tip. This extracts heat from the tip of the probe, dropping the temperature to as cold as –89°C at the tip itself (Joule-Thompson effect). This forms an ice ball, creating temperatures in the range of –70°C.[15] The gas is then vented back to the machine itself through the outer tube, and is scavenged through a ventilated outlet. The "closed system" construc-

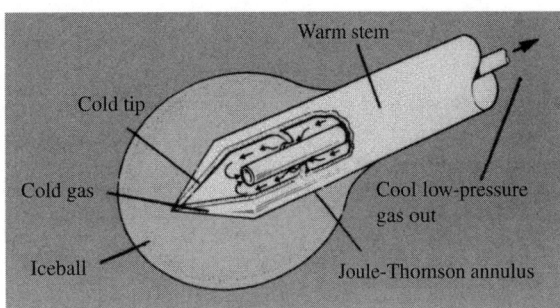

FIGURE 72.1 Probe.

tion of the probe and machine assures that no gas escapes into the patient's tissues. The 2.0-mm probe forms a 5.5-mm ice ball while the 1.4-mm probe forms a 3.5-mm ice ball. Precise gas flows are necessary for safe and effective cryoneuroablation; inadequate gas flows will not produce an ice ball while excessive flows can cause freezing proximally up the probe, which may increase the risk of skin burns. The probe also includes a nerve stimulator, with sensory and motor capabilities, which allow precise localization of the target nerve.

The application of cold to tissues creates a conduction block, similar to the effect of local anesthetics. At 10°C, larger myelinated fibers stop conducting, but all nerve fibers stop conducting at –20°C. The extent and duration of the analgesic effect, therefore, is a function of the degree of cold obtained and the length of exposure.[16] Long-term pain relief from nerve freezing occurs because ice crystals create vascular damage to the vasa nervorum, which produces severe endoneural edema. Endoneural fluid pressure increases about 20 mm within 90 minutes of the cryolesioning. Changes in the elastic properties of the perineurium cause a decrease in extracellular fluid pressure within 24 hours, which increases again and then reaches a plateau about 6 days post-lesion, disrupting the nerve structure and creating Wallerian degeneration but leaving the myelin sheath and endoneurium intact.[17] The Schwann cell basal lamina is spared and ultimately provides the structure for regeneration. Although demyelination and degeneration of the axon occurs, Sunderland[18] demonstrated that when the endoneurium remains intact, neuroma formation does not occur, and the nerve is typically able to regenerate at a rate of 1 to 1.5 mm/week. He described five categories of nerve injury based on histology and prognosis:

- First degree (neurapraxia) — An injury with minimal histologic changes with neurons failing to conduct impulses for several days to months.
- Second degree (axonotmesis) — An injury with loss of axonal continuity without breaching the endoneurium. This is the goal of cryoneuroablation, and occurs when a short section of a peripheral nerve is frozen to –20°C.

- Third, fourth, and fifth degree (neurotmesis) are associated with neural and stromal destruction.

Autoimmune phenomena are also implicated in the long-term effects of cryoneuroablation, with a release of sequestered proteins that may trigger an autoimmune response to the targeted lesioned tissues, which might explain the prolonged analgesic effect.[19–21]

The extent of the freezing (and subsequent nerve damage) is a function of the following:

1. The proximity of the probe to the nerve
2. The size of the cryoprobe
3. The size of the ice ball formed
4. The completeness of the freezing (rate and duration)
5. The temperature of the tissues in proximity to the probe, which is affected by local heat sinks (such as cerebrospinal fluid/blood flow)

The intensity and duration of analgesia is dependent on the degree of nerve damage from the ice ball.[22] For example, exposure of the fingers or toes to winter cold can lead to numbness (which is reversible) up to frostbite (which may result in permanent changes). The use of the nerve stimulator, meticulous localization of the nerve, the use of the largest probe appropriate, and the use of appropriate freeze and defrost cycles will increase the degree of nerve disruption and therefore the success rate. Repeat cycles decrease the temperature at sites farther from the probe, increasing the size of the ice ball formed and increasing the length of nerve incorporated into the ice ball. The use of saline with epinephrine injected in proximity to the target structure may decrease the "heat sink" of the nearby warm blood flow and at the same time potentially decrease bruising from the placement of the probe, which would be expected to decrease post-procedure soreness. The cryoprobe should typically be withdrawn only after the ice ball has thawed, as trying to withdraw the probe with the ice ball present could tear the attached tissues and avulse a nerve segment.

Current probes range from 1.4 to 2 mm in size. Most have a built-in nerve stimulator for localization of the nerve and a thermistor to identify temperature at the tip. The nerve stimulator allows a frequency choice for sensory (100 Hz) or motor (2 Hz) responses. Use of an introducer is recommended because the introducer can be used to infiltrate local anesthetic, isolate the electrical current stimulation to the tip of the probe (should the Teflon coating fail over time), and afford skin protection from the ice ball during treatment of superficial structures. The most commonly used introducer is a large-gauge intravenous (IV) catheter. The sharp tip pierces the tissues more easily than the probe itself, and the stylet can be removed to allow introduction of the probe. A 12-gauge catheter is used for the 2.0-mm probe and a 14- or 16-gauge catheter is used for the 1.4-mm probe.

CLINICAL ASPECTS

"You cannot treat what you cannot diagnose," is the tenet of the effective interventional pain management specialist. The cryoneurolysis technique is only as good as the diagnostic technique that precedes it. It is critical that a precise diagnosis be made prior to an attempt to freeze any nerve. In fact, the first step is to confirm that pathology is primarily isolated to sensory nerves. Performing a meticulous diagnostic block, using small volumes of local anesthetic no greater than the volume of the freeze that would be created (0.2 to 0.8 cc), does this. Use of a nerve stimulator as well as fluoroscopic guidance, direct exposure, or absolute anatomic location of the structure is critical. Because the nerve is *expected* to regrow, it is critical that the period of pain relief after the cryoneuroablation be used to restore as normal environment as possible so that, as the nerve regenerates, the original pathology (entrapment) does not recur. Cryoneuroablation may address the issue of "wind up" (the continued stimulation of a nerve causes increased sympathetic outflow and thus more stimulation), resulting in a period of reduced sympathetic stimulation that may allow aggressive rehabilitation. There is no evidence of permanent neurologic damage as a result of multiple cryoneuroablation procedures.[23] Success of cryoanalgesia is directly related to patient selection, accurate probe placement, and the post-procedure rehabilitation process.

PATIENT PREPARATION

Informed consent is as important for this technique as it is for any other interventional procedure. Risk, potential complications, and specific contraindications should be discussed and that discussion documented. The machine and gas supply should be checked, and the cryoprobe purged of the room air gases. The patient is placed in the appropriate position, and the nerve location confirmed by palpation and, when appropriate, by fluoroscopic localization. Minimal, if any, sedation should be used, as it is critical that the patient be awake enough to respond to the stimulation.

TECHNIQUE

The technique requires precise localization of the target nerve. Depending on the anatomy and ease of locating landmarks, cryoneuroablation can be done with or without fluoroscopy. After a sterile prep and drape, a small amount of local anesthetic is infiltrated subcutaneously. A 27-gauge, 1.5-inch needle is then advanced into the subcutaneous tissues, and 1 cc of saline with freshly added epinephrine 1:200,000 is then infiltrated for hemostasis. A small incision is made in the skin, and an IV introducer is then advanced to the target area. Small doses of additional local anesthetic can be injected through the introducer, as it is advanced, taking care not to anesthetize the actual target area.

When the introducer comes in contact with the target area, the stylet is removed and the cryoprobe is then advanced through the catheter and the tip of the probe is then exposed by withdrawing the catheter into the subcutaneous tissues. (Most of the techniques described it this chapter use bone as the "backstop," allowing the nerve to be "pinned" against the bone to facilitate maximal nerve contact with the probe.) Not all catheters are created equally. It is important, especially when changing brands, to confirm that the probe will fit through the catheter prior to introducing the catheter through the skin. There is little worse than getting the catheter placed perfectly, only to be unable to advance the probe through the catheter.

Accurate and meticulous sensory stimulation is critical for success. As the probe moves across the periosteum, sensory stimulation (100 Hz), first at 2 volts and then as low as 0.5 volts, is used to identify the nerve. Particular care must be used in the movement of the probe, because the movement itself may cause a paresthesia that is not an actual sensory stimulation but rather a "piezoelectric" or traction effect. As soon as the patient perceives stimulation in, or paresthesia to, the target nerve, the stimulation should be immediately turned to zero to avoid overstimulation of the nerve. Turning the stimulator back on its previous setting should again provide stimulation without movement of the probe, confirming the actual electrical and not mechanical stimulation of the nerve. The procedure is repeated with progressively decreasing voltages, until stimulation can be reliably obtained at 0.5 volts. At this time motor stimulation (2 Hz) is used at its highest voltage to confirm that the probe is not too close to nearby motor nerves. Gas flows are then turned up to 10 to 12 liters/minute (for the 2.0-mm probe) or 8 to 10 liters per minute (for the 1.4-mm probe) and a series of 2- to 3-minute freezes with 30 seconds defrosting between each cycle is performed. There is usually a burning pain on initiation of the first freeze cycle, which often replicates the pain and should resolved within approximately 30 seconds. The rest of the procedure should be completely painless.

Freeze cycles of 2 to 3 minutes result in optimal density of the ice ball. It is clear that freeze cycles longer than 3 minutes do not result in any additional benefit because the ice acts as its own insulation. Adequate thawing (more than 20 seconds but less than 40 seconds) allows subsequent freezes to increase the size of the freeze zone. After the last defrost cycle, the probe is withdrawn from the catheter and 1 cc of 0.5% bupivacaine is used to infiltrate the tissues as the catheter is withdrawn. This provides post-procedure analgesia.

It is critical that minimal sedation be used for the procedure, allowing the patient to interact fully with the determination of sensory stimulation. Done with a gentle technique, this should not be a painful procedure, and it is commonly done with no sedation at all. Small doses of a short acting opioid (50 to 100 µg of fentanyl) should be more than adequate for analgesia.

ALTERNATIVES

There are few options other than cryoneuroablation for the ablation of large sensory nerves. Surgical resection has been used, but is all too often associated with postoperative neuroma formation. One of the clinical uses for cryoneuroablation is the treatment of those postoperative neuromas. Alcohol and phenol will destroy the nerve but are also associated with neuroma formation. Opioids do not treat nerve pain, rather they only "mask" the pain. Anticonvulsants should be used before attempting cryoablation. Pulse radiofrequency lesioning has recently been used. The theoretic advantage would be the use of smaller (22-gauge) probes; however, long-term results are not available, and the mechanism is not yet well elucidated.

CONTRAINDICATIONS

General contraindications to percutaneous cryoneurolysis are quite basic: bleeding diathesis, infection (local or systemic), and an uninformed patient. The bleeding contraindication is relative and is important primarily in those situations where bleeding could go unnoticed, such as an intercostal cryoneurolysis with bleeding into the thorax or an obturator nerve cryoneurolysis where there could be hidden bleeding into the pelvis. Placing the probe through infected tissue could seed the infection into deeper tissues. Patients must be warned of the risks of depigmentation or hyperpigmentation at the cryolesion site. In addition, a diagnostic block should be used to let the patient "preview" the effect, stressing that the lesion creates numbness and not just pain relief. Some patients have actually felt distressed by the numbing effect, for instance, complaining about numbness when brushing their hair after an occipital cryolesion. Alopecia may also occur at the cryo site, especially at the eyebrow when performing a supraorbital cryolesion. There is only one reported case of neuritis after cryoneuroablation.[24] With a well-informed patient, outcomes will be improved and patients' expectations are more likely to be met.

CLINICAL USES

CRANIOFACIAL PAIN

Supraorbital Nerve

The supraorbital nerve is the termination of the first division of the trigeminal nerve. Irritation of the nerve occurs primarily at the supraorbital notch. A small ligament completes the inferior border of a foramen through which the nerve passes prior to passage through the orbicularis oculi. Commonly confused with migraine headaches and frontal sinusitis, the pain of supraorbital neuralgia most typically manifests as frontal headache, often associated with blurred vision, nausea, and photophobia. Vulnerable to blunt trauma, this nerve can be injured by trauma caused by being hit on the forehead by an automobile windshield or an abuser's fist. This neuralgia tends to worsen with time following the trauma as the injured tissue slowly develops a cicatrix, which eventually envelopes the nerve. Contraction of the orbicularis oculi (such as frowning or squinting) exacerbates the entrapment. This etiology is supported by the efficacy of botulism toxin in the forehead region in the treatment of "migraines." However, the relief from botulism is expected to last only 2 to 3 months, whereas cryoneuroablation relief can be for up to a year. Less commonly, the nerve can be injured as the result of acute herpetic infection (e.g., shingles), Paget's disease, and neoplasm. Patients will often experience an increase in headache intensity and frequency with menstruation (associated with fluid retention), salt intake, stress, and bright light (which causes squinting).

Technique: Cryoneuroablation of the supraorbital nerve can be accomplished via an "open" operative technique involving dissection under local anesthesia. The nerve can then be frozen under direct vision. The "closed" technique involves using the 1.4-mm probe, passed via a 14-gauge intravenous catheter introducer. Two or three 2-minute cycles are usually sufficient. The supratrochlear nerve, located at the medial aspect of the orbit, may also be involved and is lesioned in a similar manner. In this cosmetically important area, particular care must be used to avoid thermal damage to the sensitive skin around the eye. Entry of the catheter and probe should be below or above the eyebrow line. This avoids damage to the brow follicles, which could cause subsequent alopecia. Changes in skin color can be expected, but generally resolve in a matter of months; however, the patient must be counseled appropriately.

Infraorbital Nerve

The infraorbital nerve is the termination of the second division of the trigeminal nerve. Irritative peripheral neuropathy occurs principally at the infraorbital foramen. Also vulnerable to blunt trauma, this nerve is often injured by pugilistic blows. This neuralgia tends to worsen with time following the trauma as the injured tissues slowly develop a cicatrix, which entraps the nerve. This nerve can also be injured as the result of fracture of the zygoma, with entrapment of the nerve from the formation of bony callus. Commonly confused with maxillary sinusitis, the pain of infraorbital neuralgia typically presents as maxillary pain worsened by smiling and laughter (which put tension on the zygomaticus musculatures). Because of referred pain to the teeth, patients often undergo futile dental procedures prior to presentation. As with the aforementioned entrapments, these patients will often experience an increase in headache intensity and frequency with menstruation, salt intake, stress, and bright light.

Technique: Cryoneuroablation of the infraorbital nerve can be accomplished via an open operative technique involving dissection under local anesthesia, and the nerve can be thereby frozen under direct vision. This is usually performed submucosally. The closed technique involves using the 1.4-mm probe, passed via a 14-gauge introducer, as close as possible to the foremen. This can be accomplished by a direct percutaneous approach, but this area is also cosmetically important; so to minimize cosmetic damage, the intraoral approach can be employed. The same or a larger introducer and probe are inserted through the superior buccal-labial fold. The probe is then advanced until it lies over the infraorbital foramen. Two or three 2-minute cycles seem to be sufficient.

Mandibular Nerve

The mandibular nerve derives from the third division of the trigeminal nerve. This nerve can be injured or irritated at many locations along its path. It is most commonly injured as the result of muscular hypertrophy of the pterygoids, which in turn results from chronic bruxism. It may also be injured as the result of loss of vertical dimension of the oral cavity, i.e., loss of posterior dentition resulting in dysfunctional dental occlusion and subsequent pressure on the mandibular nerve as it passes through the pterygoid fossa.

Technique: Cryoneuroablation of the mandibular nerve can be accomplished using an open or closed technique. In the closed extraoral approach, the patient is placed in the semirecumbent position and the jaw is opened 3 to 5 mm, allowing the coronoid process of the mandible to rotate rostrally. An inverted equilateral triangle can be imagined with the base of this triangle being formed by the zygoma, one segment of the triangle being formed by the neck of the mandible, and the last segment of the triangle being formed by the coronoid process of the mandible. After injecting a small amount of local anesthetic into the skin and subcutaneous tissues, a 27-gauge needle is passed to the center of this triangle until a second "pop" is felt as the needle enters the fascial plane between the temporalis and the lateral pterygoid muscles. Saline containing epinephrine 1:200,000 is injected in the area to minimize bruising. Notation is made as to the depth of the needle, and the needle is withdrawn. A 14-gauge intravenous catheter is then placed to this depth, and a 1.4-mm cryoprobe is advanced using a peripheral nerve stimulator. After location of the nerve, two or three 2-

minute freeze cycles are generally sufficient. Patients need to be warned about potential tongue anesthesia because this technique would affect the lingular branch of the mandibular nerve. A similar approach to the maxillary nerve can be used, angling the probe anteriorly and using the sensory nerve stimulator. Because of cosmetic considerations, an intraoral approach to the mandibular nerve can be used, locating the inferior alveolar branch of the mandibular nerve at the medial superior border of the lingular mandible. Because the lingular branch takes off prior to this, tongue sensation is usually preserved.

Mental Nerve

The mental nerve is the termination of the third division of the trigeminal nerve. Irritative peripheral neuropathy occurs principally at the mental foramen. Less vulnerable to blunt trauma, this nerve is most often injured as the result of bony impingement following changes in mandibular bone architecture. Occurring chiefly in elderly edentulous patients, the pain of mental neuralgia most typically manifests as pain in the chin, lower lip, and gum line; however, trauma from tooth extractions or telephone receivers can also irritate this nerve.

Technique: The closed cryoneuroablative technique for the mental nerve involves using the 1.4-mm probe, passed via a 14-gauge introducer, percutaneously or intraorally. Two or three 2-minute cycles seem to be sufficient. Insofar as this area is also cosmetically important, the considerations mentioned above should be entertained for this area as well.

Auriculotemporal Nerve

The auriculotemporal nerve derives from the third division of the trigeminal nerve. Irritative peripheral neuropathy occurs principally at two sites along the course of this nerve. The most common site of entrapment is immediately proximal to the parietal ridge at the attachment of the temporalis musculature. Less commonly, the nerve can be injured posterior to the ramus of the mandible. This is often triggered by clenching or bruxism. Clinical presentation of the auriculotemporal pathology consists of temporal pain associated with retroorbital pain. Referred pain to the teeth is often seen. The patient often awakens at night or in the early morning with temporal headache (especially at 3 or 4 A.M.). The pain is described as throbbing, aching, and pounding, and the pain can be unilateral or bilateral. Because it is associated with blurry vision, nausea, and emesis, this headache is mistaken for vascular "migraine." Most commonly associated with cross bite, bruxism, and functional abnormality of the temporomandibular joint, this syndrome is also associated with malformation or dysmorphia of the mandible or maxilla, as well as trauma (including dental work). Patients will often experience an increase in headache intensity and frequency with menstruation, salt intake, or stress.

Technique: To locate the auriculotemporal nerve distally, the base of an equilateral triangle is imagined between the corner of the eye and the anterior tragus. The apex of the triangle locates the parietal attachment of the temporalis musculature and the distal site of entrapment of the auriculotemporal nerve. A 12-gauge intravenous catheter is used as the introducer for the 2.0-mm cryoprobe. Three 2-minute cycles are used. The proximal entrapment occurs just in front of the temporomandibular joint as the nerve curves in front of the joint. Particular care must be taken to avoid the facial nerve, which exits at this level. The smaller 14-gauge catheter is used with the 1.4-mm probe to limit possible trauma to the facial nerve.

It is not usually necessary to destroy the trigeminal nerve itself because pathology is mostly confined to individual branches; however, occasionally, the entire nerve needs neuroablation. Tic douloureux pain that does not have a distal trigger zone may respond to lesioning of the nerve, as it leaves the cranium.

Technique: Using fluoroscopy with the patient supine and neck extended, the foramen ovale is identified, and a 27-gauge needle is used to infiltrate the region with saline containing epinephrine 1:200,000 to minimize bruising. The 1.4-mm probe is advanced through a 14-gauge intravenous catheter, which has been positioned under fluoroscopy, and using sensory stimulation, the area of maximal stimulation identified. With care, the ophthalmic portion of the trigeminal nerve can sometimes be avoided, but clearly the patient needs to be warned regarding the risks of hypoesthesia of the eye with this technique, which obviously limits this approach.

Posterior Auricular Neuralgia

Posterior auricular neuralgia is often seen weeks to years after blunt injury to the mastoid area. Seen commonly in physically abused women, the left side is most often involved, due to the preponderance of right-handed spouse abusers. The clinical presentation consists of pain in the ear, along with a feeling of "fullness" and tenderness. This syndrome is often misdiagnosed as a chronic ear infection, and again is often worse with menstruation and salt intake. The nerve may also be entrapped by the sternocleidomastoid (SCM) muscle. Klein et al.[25] described the diagnosis and treatment of "cryptogenic earache" with posterior auricular nerve blocks. Trigger point treatment of the SCM may be adequate for most patients; but, some will need more aggressive treatment such as cryoablation.

Technique: The posterior auricular nerve runs along the posterior border of the sternocleidomastoid musculature, superficially and immediately posterior to the mastoid. A 12-gauge intravenous catheter is used as the introducer for the 2.0-mm cryoprobe, employing three 2-minute cryocycles. The skin is quite thin here, and special care must be taken to avoid freezing the skin. Approaching the nerve from inferiorly, as far down on the cranium as possible, gives one more skin depth with which to work.

Glossopharyngeal Neuralgia

The glossopharyngeal nerve exits the skull, with the vagus and spinal accessory nerves, through the jugular foramen. It descends anteriorly to the carotid artery and passes deep to the styloid. Then it turns to the tongue, where it passes through the tonsillar fossa. Both a motor and sensory nerve, it provides sensation to the middle ear, the posterior third of the tongue, the palatine tonsils, and the pharynx. There is a paroxysmal glossopharyngeal neuralgia that presents with lacinating pain similar to trigeminal neuralgia; but, it is with pain in the throat instead of the face. Although the glossopharyngeal nerve block is primarily used as an anesthesia block for intubations, cryoneuroablation may be appropriate for postoperative pain relief for tonsillectomies as well as for cancer-related throat and neck pain or to break the reflex cycle of intractable hiccups.

Technique: Cryoneuroablation at the styloid process is not recommended, as the carotid artery is directly behind the target, and a 12-gauge hole in the carotid artery from the introducer would be difficult to manage. In addition, the vagus and spinal accessory nerve also pass through this area, and it would be difficult to avoid lysis of these nerves as well. As a result, the usual site for cryoneuroablation is at the tonsillar fossa. The patient is placed supine and the tongue retracted medially. The nerve is located at the inferior portion of the tonsillar pillar. The mucosa is anesthetized with a topical spray or pledget, and 1 cc of saline with epinephrine 1:200,000 is infiltrated for homeostasis. Intravascular epinephrine from an unrecognized blood vessel injection may cause a rapid increase in heart rate, and should caution the practitioner regarding needle placement. The 12-gauge introducer is then advanced subcutaneously, and the 2-mm probe advanced through the catheter. Sensory stimulation should refer to the ear and throat, and there may be a throat motor stimulation. Care must be used to avoid the palatine artery. This may be done most easily at surgical tonsillectomy when the nerve is exposed.

Clinical Effectiveness

Intractable face pain from a variety of causes may be treatable with cryoneuroablation. Bernard et al.[26] reported on 21 patients with intractable face pain, unresponsive to medical and surgical management. They diagnosed pain secondary to entrapments of several nerves, including supraorbital, infraorbital, mental, and lingual. All the nerves were treated with open (or exposed) cryoneuroablation. Barnard et al.[27] reported on 54 patients with chronic facial pain. Patients were selected for cryoneuroablation after they had a temporary response to local anesthetic injections. The mean duration of sensory loss was 60 (5 to 117) days. The success of the blockade appeared to be an "all or nothing" effect; i.e., the patients with only 5-day duration of pain relief reflected the failure to adequately freeze the nerve. They emphasized the difference between nerve "killing" and simple nerve "cooling." Diagnoses included nonherpetic neuralgia, tic douloureux, postsurgical neuralgia, atypical facial neuralgia, and postherpetic neuralgia (PHN). Of the patients other than the those with PHN, 30 to 40% had relief for more than 6 months. No patients with PHN had relief for greater than 1 year; however, the other groups had more than a year's relief in 17 to 20% of the cases.

Trigeminal neuralgia or tic douloureux has caused debilitating pain in a group of very unfortunate patients. The advances in anticonvulsant therapy have helped, but the lancinating pain that may occur spontaneously or with the lightest touch of a "trigger zone" can be extremely debilitating. Nally and Zakrzewski[28] looked at 112 patients with paroxysmal trigeminal neuralgia. Intraoral or periorbital dissections of the peripheral branches of the trigeminal were performed. These included the supraorbital, supratrochlear, infraorbital, mental, posterior and middle superior dental, greater palatine, lingular, and long buccal nerves. An average of 2.2 procedures per patient over a 5-year period was reported. As an example, 68% of the 78 mental nerves treated remained pain free over 52 months. Similar results were seen with the other nerves, and patients noted that if and when the pain returned, it was at a lower level. Several patients noted that when the pain returned it was to a different site, but freezing the new site also provided relief. Nally[29] looked at 211 patients over a 22-year period and concluded that cryotherapy offered significant long-term relief.

In 1988, Zakrzewska and Nally[30] initially reported a 6-year experience with cryoanalgesia in the treatment of paroxysmal trigeminal neuralgia. Then in 1991, Zakrzewska[30a] further reviewed 475 patients with trigeminal neuralgia followed over a 10-year period. Of those patients, 145 underwent cryotherapy, 265 underwent radiofrequency thermocoagulation, and 65 underwent microvascular decompression. Mean follow-up was 45 months in each group. Morbidity after cryotherapy was low, whereas radiofrequency thermocoagulation resulted in more prolonged sensory loss (88%), anesthesia dolorosa (8%), and eye problems (15%). Microvascular decompression was associated with eighth cranial nerve problems in 11% of the patients and a 1% mortality rate. None of the cryoneuroablation patients developed anesthesia dolorosa. Of the patients treated with radiofrequency, 75% continued to have sensory loss. In the cryoablation patients, the area of sensory loss was small but in the radiofrequency patients it sometimes extended

across all three divisions of the trigeminal nerve, and 62% of these patients felt the sensory loss affected their lives.

One of the most commonly preformed surgical procedures is a tonsillectomy, and pain management has been a significant problem. Postoperative tonsillectomy pain is thought to be due to a combination of nerve irritation, inflammation, and pharyngeal muscle spasms. In a prospective, randomized, double-blinded study of 59 patients, Robinson and Purdie[31] reported that bilateral tonsillectomies were performed and the patients randomized to cryoneuroablation of the glossopharyngeal nerve or a control group. The cryoprobe was inserted superficially into the tonsillar fossa at surgery. Treatment resulted in a reduction of pain for 10 days and a faster return to work or school compared with controls.

Occipital Nerve

The occipital nerve is one of the most discussed nerves for cryoneuroablation. When diagnostic injections have given excellent but only temporary relief, cryoneuroablation may be an excellent option.

Clinical Presentation: Occipital neuralgia is a frequent cause of occipital and retro-orbital headaches. The greater occipital nerve is made up of the dorsal rami of C2 and C3 and causes occipital pain. However, because the ganglion of this nerve interconnects with the trigeminal nerve ganglion in the brainstem, pain may be referred to any branch of the trigeminal nerve. The occipital nerve pierces the nuchal fascia at the base of the skull and is prone to trauma from flexion/extension injuries and well as entrapment by spasm of the trapezius muscle. The lesser occipital nerve comes from the cervical plexus and is located slightly more laterally. The third occipital nerve consists of the posterior ramus of C3. Standard anesthesia texts describe occipital nerve blocks as injections of large volumes (10 cc) at the nuchal ridge in a "fan" fashion; however, this type of injection is not diagnostic and will not predict a response to cryoneuroablation. The technique recommended by Trescot et al.[32] identify the injection site (in this case describing the right side) by placing the thumb of the right hand at the foramen magnum (which identifies midline and avoids the cisternal injection); the index finger is placed at the conjoined tendon attachment, and the second finger identifies the injection site at the base of the skull. Small volumes (less than 2 cc) of local and steroid are thereby injected underneath the tendon where the nerve pierces the tendon. Cryoneuroablation is done at the same site.

Technique: The technique requires precise localization of the target nerve. With the patient positioned prone or seated with head flexed and resting on the patient's hands, the tenderness at the base of the skull is identified by palpation. After local anesthetic infiltration subcutaneously, 1 cc of saline with epinephrine 1:200,000 is infil-

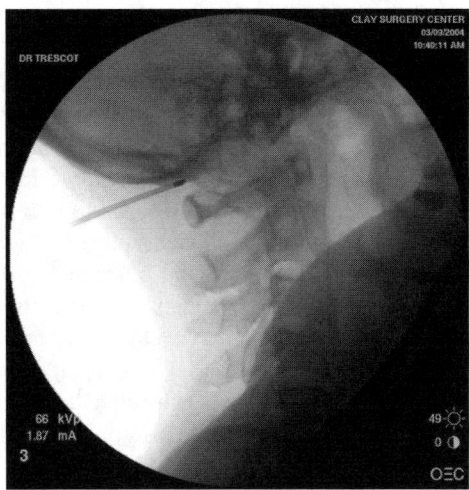

FIGURE 72.2 Occipital.

trated to the periosteum, using the 27-gauge needle as a "seeker needle" to find the periosteum. The 12-gauge IV catheter is then advanced to the periosteum. When the introducer comes in contact with the target bone, the stylet is removed and the 2.0-mm probe is then advanced through the catheter and the tip of the probe exposed by withdrawing the catheter into the subcutaneous tissues (Figure 72.2). The "gritty" feeling of the periosteum should be appreciated; if not, replace the stylet and advance the catheter farther. Accurate and meticulous sensory stimulation is critical for success. As the probe moves across the periosteum in a medial to lateral direction, sensory stimulation (100 Hz), first at 2 volts, and then as low as 0.5 volts, is used to identify the median branch nerve. Particular care must be used in the movement of the probe, as the movement itself may cause a parasthesia that is not an actual sensory stimulation but rather a "piezoelectric" or traction effect. The procedure is repeated with progressively decreasing voltage, until stimulation can be reliably obtained at 0.5 volts. Three 2-minute freeze cycles are usually adequate.

Clinical Effectiveness: Kappes[33] described cryoablation of the occipital nerve in 72 patients with intractable headaches: 62% of the total patients had 75% or greater improvement in symptoms, 90% enjoyed a reduction of 50% or more, 47% were symptom free for 6 weeks to 1 year.

UPPER EXTREMITY PAIN

Suprascapular Nerve

The suprascapular nerve arises from the upper trunk of the brachial plexus and travels downward and laterally to pass through the suprascapular notch to provide innervation to the supraspinatus, infraspinatus, and shoulder joint. Clinically, the patient complains of a poorly localized upper shoulder pain, usually triggered by a lifting injury

with the arm internally rotated. Tenderness is elicited by palpation of the suprascapular notch (the "Vulcan death grip"). Diagnostic blocks should be performed using a peripheral nerve stimulator. The classic approach to the suprascapular notch is to advance the needle perpendicular to the scapular spine from above, and then "walk it off" anteriorly until the needle drops into the suprascapular notch. This technique, however, has a high risk of pneumothorax. I recommend instead that the needle (with a peripheral nerve stimulator) be directed perpendicular to the scapula itself, using the scapular wall as a "backstop," and then directed medially or laterally to find the nerve. This technique works for both the diagnostic nerve block and the cryoneuroablation.

Technique: The patient is positioned prone with the chest supported on pillows, letting the arm hang anteriorly. Alternatively, the patient can be positioned seated with the affected arm hanging by the patient's side. The 12-gauge catheter is advanced into the supraspinatus notch parallel to the direction of the nerve. Consider using fluoroscopic guidance to locate the superior border of the scapula if the scapula is not easily palpated. The 2.0-mm probe is then advanced through the catheter and the suprascapular nerve is identified using sensory or motor stimulation; this is one of the few mostly motor nerves amenable to cryoneuroablation. Three 2-minute freeze cycles are usually sufficient.

Superficial Radial Nerve

The superficial radial nerve runs under cover of the brachioradialis into the forearm and onto the posterior surface of the wrist to supply the skin along the radial portion of the wrist and fingers including portions of the dorsum of the hand. This is the nerve injured when the hand is bumped on a table, the classic "trivial injury" resulting in sympathetic overstimulation and CRPS (chronic regional pain syndrome). This nerve is also injured after chronic wrist movements and Colles fractures. Cryoanalgesia may address the "wind up" phenomenon seen with these injuries.

Technique: The area of maximal tenderness is identified, usually between the brachioradialis and extensor carpi radialis muscles. If possible, the 12-gauge intravenous catheter is used, advanced distally parallel to the nerve (similar to starting an IV). The 2.0-mm probe is then placed through the catheter. Sometimes the tissues in this area are too tight to accept the larger probe, and the 14-gauge catheter and 1.4-mm probe must be used. The skin may be quite thin in this region, and extra caution regarding skin burns must be observed.

Palmar Branch of the Median Nerve

The palmar median branch of the median nerve travels over the carpal ligament at the wrist and thus bypasses possible median nerve entrapment from carpal tunnel syndrome (CTS). Unfortunately, it is therefore vulnerable to trauma to the palmar structures, such as seen with falls onto an outstretched hand, or the chronic repetitive trauma of pounding a stapler with the palm. It may be misdiagnosed as CTS, and neuromas of this nerve may also occur as a result of CTS surgery. Diagnosis is made by small local anesthetic injections proximal to the carpal crease, and cryoneuroablation is done via the smallest probe available.

Clinical Effectiveness

Wang[34] performed percutaneous cryoneurolysis on various peripheral nerves (ulnar, median, sural, occipital, palmar branch of the median, and digital) in 12 patients with 6 patients reporting relief of 1 to 12 months' duration.

CHEST WALL PAIN

Intercostal Nerve

Of all the postoperative indications for cryoneurolysis, lesioning of the intercostal nerve intraoperatively has been the most extensively studied. The nerve is very easily identified at thoracotomy, and intraoperative cryoneuroablation can provide significant and long-lasting postoperative analgesia. It has been somewhat more difficult to address post-thoracotomy neuromas, persistent pain after rib fractures, or thoracic post herpetic neuralgia, but a percutaneous technique can provide excellent analgesia.

Technique: In the open technique, after the thoracotomy is complete, the cryoprobe is placed directly on the nerve at the posterior rib angle. The nerve is easily visualized beneath the parietal pleura. Meticulous use of diagnostic nerve blocks is critical for accurate nerve localization. Because each rib has an innervation contribution from the rib below and the rib above, it is advisable to lesion the intercostal nerves above and below the incision line as well. Because the nerves are exposed, one or two 1-minute freeze cycles should be adequate.

With the percutaneous approach, the technique has to take into consideration the underlying lung and the intercostal artery, which acts as a heat sink. Physicians are traditionally taught to perform intercostal nerve blocks by advancing the needle perpendicular to the inferior edge of rib and then "walking it off the edge of the bone," dropping to just before the parietal pleura. However, the nerve is actually up under the curve of the rib. In addition, the intercostal artery acts as a huge "heat sink," limiting the size of the ice ball and therefore the effectiveness of the cryolesion. By introducing the probe perpendicular to the nerve, the area of freezing is limited, which also limits the effectiveness of the cryolesion. In addition, the temptation is to use a smaller probe because of the concern regarding advancing a 12-gauge needle into the pleural

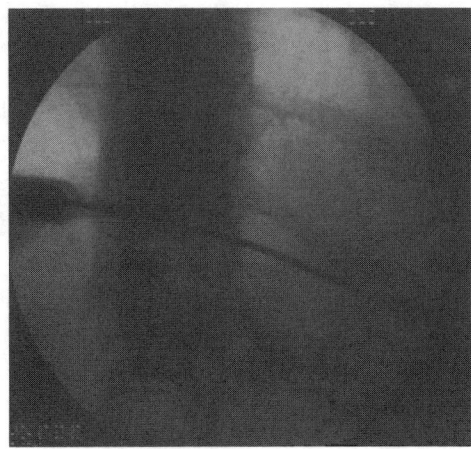

FIGURE 72.3 Rib picture.

space, causing a pneumothorax. The technique I recommend somewhat different. I recommend approaching the rib edge tangentially from posterior to anterior (medial to lateral), then pushing the tip up under the edge of the rib (Figure 72.3). This accomplishes several things. It dramatically reduces the risk of pneumothorax, and it increases the length of contact of the probe on the nerve, which increases the effectiveness of the cryolesion. It is important to use the largest probe possible to overcome the arterial heat sink.

Clinical Effectiveness

Nelson et al.[35] first described intraoperative intercostal cryoneurolysis. The technique is most effective in relieving incisional pain and provides relatively little relief of visceral pleuritic pain or the pain of ligamentous or muscle pains. It provides no relief for chest tube pain. The multiple pain generators involved in post-thoracotomy pain make cryoneuroablation difficult to use as a sole treatment. Despite these limitations, studies have shown that patients have less postoperative pain and less opioid requirement, both in the immediate postoperative period and in the weeks following the procedure. Orr et al.[36] studied 45 patients randomized into three groups: a control group that received intramuscular morphine postoperatively, a cryoanalgesia group, and a morphine infusion group. All patients underwent a general anesthetic, and while the chest was open, the control and infusion groups had rib blocks performed with 0.5% bupivacaine while the cryoanalgesia group underwent a sharp dissection of the nerves followed by a 45-second freeze cycle under direct vision. The number of requests for analgesics was less for the cryoanalgesia group than for the controls, and the morphine infusion and control groups used the same total dose of morphine. The authors noted that the cryoneuroablation added about 10 minutes to the procedure but gave better postoperative pain relief. This same group did a further study comparing the original patients with an additional group of patients that included 23 patients who received the cryoneuroablation as well as a continuous infusion of morphine.[37] Pain relief was best in the cryo-plus-infusion group, and at 8 days postoperatively the cryoanalgesia patients had the best pain relief at rest (although there was no significant difference in pain with movement). Although a morphine infusion gave good relief and required very little special equipment or expertise, the authors felt that cryoneuroablation of the intercostals nerves at the time of surgery gave enough extra relief to be worth the extra 10 minutes of surgical time.

It must be noted that cryoanalgesia of the third and fourth intercostals can cause ipsilateral nipple anesthesia. Riopelle et al.[38] suggested using a lower incision and not freezing nerves above the fifth intercostal nerve. Denervation of the intercostal nerves appear to have no consequence, but loss of tone from the external and internal oblique muscles can cause a subtle but definite subcostal bulge that resolves with the return of sensation.[39] There has been one case report of a neuroma formation after the use of cryoneuroablation for post-thoracotomy pain,[24] and several patients have noted sensory deficits for up to 6 months. Comparative studies suggest superior relief with epidural analgesia,[40] and the time necessary to perform lesions at multiple levels limits the usefulness of the technique. However, with the elimination of reimbursement for preoperative epidurals, the need for continuous monitoring during the epidural infusion, and the weeks of postoperative relief available with cryoneuroablation, thoracic surgeons may be interested in resurrecting the technique.

It is the experience with post-thoracotomy pain and cryoneuroablation that leads to its use in other chronic chest wall pains. The postoperative neuroma, costochondritis, postherpetic neuralgia, and rib fractures have all been treated with cryoneuroablation. Two large series suggest improved pain relief and few complications. Green et al.[41] studied the effectiveness of cryoanalgesia on 43 patients with postherpetic neuralgia or intercostal neuralgia: 50% of the patients noted significant relief of 3 month's duration, no patients developed neuritis, and the pain relief outlasted the return of sensory function. Another study of 70 patients with chest wall pain of a variety of etiologies resulted in pain relief from 1 week to 12 months, with the patients with postherpetic neuralgia uniformly noting a poorer response.[42]

ABDOMINAL AND PELVIC PAIN

Ilioinguinal, Iliohypogastric, Genitofemoral, Subcostal Neuralgia

Arising from the anterior primary ramus of the first lumbar nerve root via the lumbar plexus, the ilioinguinal nerve pierces the internal oblique muscle mediocaudally to the anterior superior iliac spine and then passes through the inguinal canal and accompanies the spermatic cord through the superficial inguinal ring to supply the thigh and scrotum or labia. This nerve is often injured at the lateral border of the rectus sheath, approximately 5 cm from midline and 10 cm inferior to the umbilicus, where it perforates the superior crus of the superficial inguinal ring. The ilioinguinal nerve may be injured during inguinal herniorrhaphy, and as the result of compression from the bladder retractor during abdominal surgery, particularly when the Pfannenstiel incision is employed. Even midline incisions may be associated with entrapment of the nerves, often months or years later as the scar cicatrix contracts. Occasionally, this nerve is injured by tight-fitting garments, e.g., belts and weapon holsters. The iliohypogastric nerve pathology will present in a similar manner but this nerve entrapment occurs about two fingerbreadths higher. There may be a communication between these two nerves, and their sizes are often inversely related. Both can be traumatized by the expanding abdomen of late pregnancy or ascites. Both can mimic appendicitis (on the right) or diverticulitis (on the left). The fluid retention associated with the perimenstrual timeframe can also result in entrapment of the nerves and subsequent "endometriosis" pain.

The genitofemoral nerve (GFN) rises from the first and second lumbar nerves. The genital branch of the nerve passes under the inguinal ligament and over the symphysis pubis immediately lateral to the pubic tubercle. This sensory nerve then travels to the labia or scrotum. Vulnerable to trauma as it passes over the ramus of the pubis, the genitofemoral nerve can be injured as the result of blunt surgical trauma, and the pain tends to worsen with time. Pfannenstiel incisions for hysterectomy or cesarean section, and inguinal herniorrhaphy (especially with mesh because of the "bite" taken on Poupart's ligament) can result in chronic, intractable pain. A slowly developing cicatrix can entrap this nerve, and the pain generally develops months to years following the surgery. Less commonly, this nerve can be injured as the result of compression of the nerve during late pregnancy. A similar syndrome results from entrapment of the subcostal nerve, which arises from the T10 to T12 nerve roots and passes around the ribs anteriorly to the rectus sheath. This neuropathy results in an upper quadrant pain that may mimic cholecystitis or pancreatitis or may be caused by the surgical treatment of upper abdominal pathology.

Clinical presentation of genitofemoral, ilioinguinal, or iliohypogastric pathology consists of dull, aching pain in the lower lateral abdomen. This pain is worse with Valsalva's maneuver, cough, bowel movement, and lifting. Patients will often experience increase in pain intensity and frequency with menstruation, salt intake, and sexual intercourse. Irritation of either nerve can result in referred pain to the testicle or vulva, interior thigh, or upper lumbar region. A localized tenderness and pain with digital pressure worsened during Valsalva's maneuver is observed.

Occasionally the ilioinguinal nerve is trapped more laterally at the attachment of the external oblique onto the iliac crest. A "double crush" situation may result from pathology at both places, requiring the more proximal treatment for complete relief. The genitofemoral nerve entrapment is usually found at the pubic tubercle. Unfortunately, in the case of surgical scar entrapment, it may be difficult to address the pathology more proximally, as the nerve becomes intra-abdominal at that point.

Technique: After superficial infiltration with local anesthetic and deep infiltration with saline containing epinephrine 1:200,000, a 12-gauge intravenous catheter is used as the introducer for the 2.0-mm cryoprobe. After precise confirmation of probe placement employing the peripheral nerve stimulator, three 2-minute cryocycles seem to be sufficient. Fluoroscopic localization may be useful for the identification of the nerves at the pubic tubercle or iliac crest in the obese patient. Occasionally, especially in the face of surgical scarring from multiple surgeries, the abdominal and pelvic nerves must be addressed more proximally. Paravertebral nerve blocks under fluoroscopy, with a peripheral nerve stimulator at T12 or L1 (depending on the nerve target) will predict response to cryoneuroablation. If the diagnostic injections give temporary relief, cryoablation of the nerve root can give good relief distally into the groin or lower abdomen. The transverse process of the target nerve root is identified by fluoroscopy. After local anesthetic subcutaneous injection and saline with epinephrine infiltration, the 12-gauge catheter is advanced tangentially to the foramen, taking care not to advance into the foramen itself. The 2.0-mm probe is then advanced through the catheter, and using the sensory stimulation mode, stimulation into the groin is obtained. Special care must be taken not to have motor stimulation down the leg, although motor stimulator into the groin is acceptable. Proximal treatment of the GFN nerve is more problematic. The GFN runs most of its course along the surface of the psoas muscle. At laparotomy, the nerve can be easily visualized, and lesioned under direct vision. Recent descriptions of pelvic pain mapping under sedation and minimal insufflation laparoscopy have confirmed the GFN as a common cause of chronic pelvic pain, and it may be amenable to transabdominal lesioning under laparoscopic visualization.[43]

Sacral Neuralgia

Perineal pain and coccydynia can be due to pathology of the sacral nerve roots. If the patient has failed nonsteroidal anti-inflammatory drugs (NSAIDs) and caudal epidurals, then coccygeal nerve blocks done bilaterally as the S5 nerve roots leave the sacral foramen may be an option. The diagnostic blocks assist in confirming the lack of rectal dysfunction and predict the success. The nerve is identified under fluoroscopy at the medial border of the sacral cornu, and sensory stimulation at 50 Hz aids in localization of the nerve. In the same way, cryoneuroablation of the dorsal S4 nerve roots can provide pain relief of the scrotum, vagina, perineum, and anus without affecting bowel or bladder function. The probe is either placed through the sacral hiatus up to the level of the fourth sacral foramen or passed through each foramen laterally to medially. Diagnostic transforaminal nerve blocks (I use a peripheral nerve stimulator and contrast to confirm location) will give a temporary block, which allows the patient to "preview" the pain relief.

Clinical Effectiveness: Intraoperative lesioning of the ilioinguinal nerve at the time of inguinal hernia surgery adds only a minute to the procedure but can provide significant pain relief. After repair of the inguinal ring and the posterior wall, the ilioinguinal nerve is isolated and elevated onto a retractor. The cryoprobe is placed directly on the nerve and the freeze cycle initiated. A visible ice ball forms, and a 1-minute freeze (with perhaps a second freeze cycle, taking care not to pull on the ice ball which can tear the nerve) should be adequate. Wood et al.[44] first described cryoanalgesia after herniorrhaphy in 1979. Open cryoneurolysis of the ilioinguinal nerve decreased the analgesic requirements postoperatively. The follow-up study[45] looked at three groups of patients after hernia repair: those who received cryoneurolysis, paravertebral nerve blocks, or as needed oral narcotics. Not only did the cryoneurolysis patients have less postoperative pain, but they used fewer narcotics, ate a regular diet earlier, and returned to work sooner. In contrast, Khiroya et al.[46] found no significant difference in pain scores, pulmonary function, or analgesic use in a randomized, double-blinded study of 36 patients. Callesen et al.[47] studied cryoneuroablation of the ilioinguinal and iliohypogastric nerves compared with sham cryoneuroablation and found no statistical difference. The authors postulated that the post-herniorrhaphy pain might originate from deep muscle layers innervated by nerves other than the ilioinguinal and iliohypogastric nerves (such as the subcostal and genitofemoral nerves). Abdominal pain relief, when diagnostic blocks have given excellent but only temporary relief, may be provided by cryoneuroablation. In one study, 15 patients with chronic abdominal pain underwent cryoneuroablation of the ilioinguinal and iliohypogastric nerves. Of the 15, 7 (47%) noted good to excellent relief; 3 of the 7 had permanent relief, while the other 4 had relief lasting between 4 and 30 months.[48] Raj[23] describes the use of cryoneuroablation of the ilioinguinal nerve to treat the abdominal pain of late pregnancy, which results in severe traction on the ilioinguinal nerve, especially if the nerve is tethered by scar tissue from prior surgery. Glynn and Carrie[14] reported on the use of cryoanalgesia to treat pelvic pain at the symphysis pubis during pregnancy (most likely treating the genitofemoral nerve at that level).

Evans and colleagues[49] performed cryoneurolysis of the lower three sacral nerve roots in 40 patients with intractable perineal pain; 78% of the patients received at least 30 days of relief. At the Hospital of the University of Pennsylvania, Loev et al.[50] described a novel cryolesion approach to the ganglion impar in a patient with rectal pain, which provided more than 6 months of relief. Jain et al.[51] described a case report of a 38-year-old multiparous woman complaining of severe sacrococcygeal pain of 6 years' duration. The pain began after the birth of her second child and was not relieved by oxycodone. Diagnostic blocks with 1% lidocaine on several occasions gave temporary relief. A cryoprobe was inserted into the sacral extradural canal under fluoroscopy, two 60-second freeze cycles were performed, and the patient was noted to be pain free at follow-up 1.5 years later.

Pudendal Neuralgia

The pudendal nerve can be a cause of intractable perineal, vaginal, penile, scrotal, and rectal pain. Providing almost sole enervation of the perineum, the pudendal nerve arises from the second, third, and fourth sacral nerves in the pelvis, passes through the sciatic notch medial and inferior to the sciatic nerve, and then crosses the ischial spine to enter the perineal region. Familiar to obstetricians, the pudendal nerve is often traumatized during vaginal deliveries. However, it can be a cause of pain in both males and females and may be triggered by trauma from bicycle seats, surgery, radiation, or perirectal infections. The pain is often hard for the patient to localize, and a meticulous physical exam, including rectal and pelvic exam, may be necessary to identify the nerve entrapment.

Technique: The nerve can be approached vaginally or percutaneously. The vaginal approach is a simple modification of the obstetrician's pudendal nerve block done during delivery to anesthetize the perineum. Using a modified Iowa trumpet with the patient in the lithotomy position, first the 12-gauge introducer and then the 2.0-mm probe are advanced through the trumpet to the ischial spine. Cryoneurolysis at this site will lead to profound hypoesthesia, including the possibility of loss of clitoral sensation. The percutaneous approach can be much more selective in the isolation of specific branches of the pudendal nerve. If the pain is primarily vaginal or penile, I will place the patient in a modified lithotomy position with the feet on the table instead of in stirrups. The 12-gauge catheter is directed toward the sacrospinous ligament instead of the ischial spine itself, and the 2.0-mm probe sensory stimulation is used to select the stimulation field needed. In the same way, if the pain is primarily rectal, I position the patient prone in a jackknife position, placing the 12-gauge catheter and then the 2.0-mm probe more inferiorly, using stimulation to direct the probe toward the rectal branches.

SPINAL PAIN

Facet Joint Pain

The most common use for cryoanalgesia for low back pain is the long-term treatment of lumbar facet pathology. When diagnostic lumbar facet blocks (either intra-articular or median branch blocks) have given good but only temporary relief, one option for further treatment is cryoneuroablation of the median dorsal rami.

Clinical Presentation: The clinical presentation, anatomy, and innervation of the lumbar facet disease and pain syndrome have been described in many texts. Facet pain is often considered a "biomechanical "pain, typically made worse on movement, particularly with hyperextension. There may be significant myofascial spasms in the paravertebral region as the muscles try to "splint" the injured joint. Patients will often fail a physical therapy program because therapy will aggravate the pain. There are usually no neurologic signs despite the referred pain down the leg ("pseudosciatica"). Cervical pain as well as thoracic or abdominal pain can also be due to facet pathology. Radiographs may or may not show facet sclerosis, and there may be a history of trauma such as "whiplash" in the cervical region or twisting injuries in the lumbar region. Pain is transmitted to the spinal cord via the articular facet nerves, the nerves of Luschka, the dorsal median nerve, the meningeal nerves, the anterior communicating ramus, and other branches of the posterior ramus. Palpation reveals exquisite tenderness along the paravertebral muscles. Other biomechanical problems are also often seen, including leg discrepancy (functional vs. anatomy), sacroiliac (SI) joint dysfunction, and scoliosis. Median branch blocks may give a better predictive indication of potential success from cryoneuroablation than do intra-articular injections. In the neck or thorax, facet pathology can refer down the arm, between the shoulders, or around to the anterior chest. These are commonly seen after "whiplash" injuries, because of the mobility of the neck and upper thorax. Because the pain relief is expected to be temporary, it is critical to use the pain-free period to facilitate a rehabilitation program. The success of the cryolesion is a direct function of the patient selection, accurate probe placement, and the rehabilitation.

Technique: The technique requires precise localization of the target nerve. The inferior border of the transverse process at the level of the inferior articular process is identified by fluoroscopy. When the introducer comes in contact with the target bone, the stylet is removed, the 2.0-mm probe is advanced through the catheter, and the tip of the probe exposed by withdrawing the catheter into the subcutaneous tissues. Accurate and meticulous sensory stimulation is critical for success. As the probe moves across the periosteum in a medial to lateral direction, sensory stimulation (100 Hz), first at 2 volts, and then as

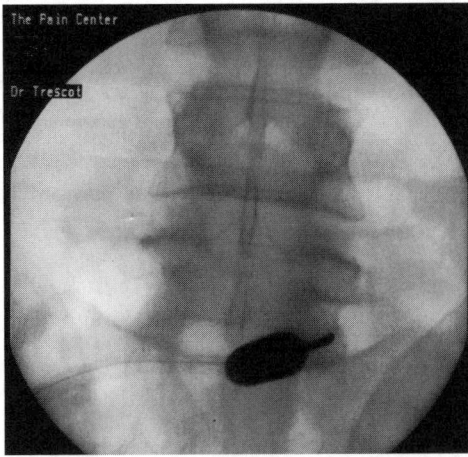

FIGURE 72.4 Lumbar facet.

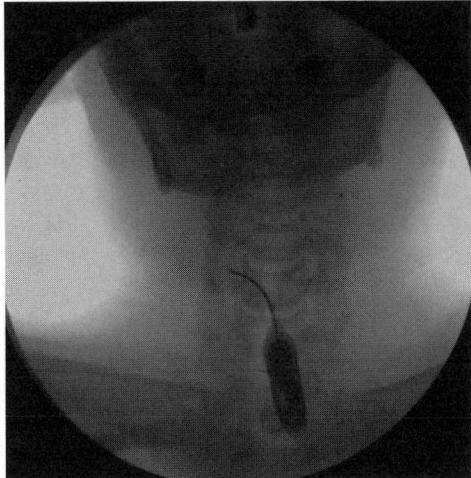

FIGURE 72.5 Cervical facet.

low as 0.5 volts, is used to identify the median branch nerve. Particular care must be used in the movement of the probe, as the movement itself may cause a paresthesia that is not an actual sensory stimulation but rather a "piezoelectric" or traction effect. The procedure is repeated with progressively decreasing voltage, until stimulation can be reliably obtained at 0.5 volts. This position is usually at the "neck of the Scottie dog," consistent with the position of a "collar" or at the junction of the transverse process and pedicle — the Scottie dog's eye (Figure 72.4). Similar techniques are used for the neck and thorax (Figure 72.5). At this time motor stimulation (2 Hz) is used at its highest voltage to confirm that the probe is not too close to the spinal nerve root. Three 2-minute freeze cycles are usually adequate.

Clinical Effectiveness: Brechner[52] studied the effects of percutaneous cryoneuroablation of the lumbar facet in patients with neck and low back pain. There was 70% pain relief after 1 hour and relief lasted 1 week. Pain relief decreased to 50% at 3 weeks and, by 3 months, had

returned to baseline. Schuster[53] studied 52 patients followed for a 13-month period: 47 patients had significant relief of low back pain after cryoneuroablation, and only 1 patient had a repeat cryoneuroablation when the pain recurred after a 9-month pain-free period. Ross[54] described 23 patients with complete but only short-term relief from lumbar facet blocks, who were treated with cryoneurolysis of the dorsal median nerve: 21 had complete relief for a follow up of 6 months to 2 years; 2 patients had return of pain 6 to 8 months later and underwent subsequent cryoneurolysis with complete relief. These studies are limited by a lack of certainty that the facet was the sole pain generator. Prognostic blocks, if performed, did not utilize currently recommended techniques.

Prognostic blocks should be performed one level at a time, one side at a time, and repeated to assure validity. All too often, pain generators are assumed based on a single trial of anesthetic (remember the placebo effect) with multiple levels injected and volumes of anesthetic far in excess of that needed to anesthetize the median dorsal ramus, a nerve a fraction of a millimeter in diameter. Small volumes, less than 0.2 cc, are more than sufficient for adequate precision prognostic blocks. Volumes larger than that only serve to spread throughout the area and to confuse the issue.

As described above, it is well known that there is dual innervation of the facet joint. Median branch block diagnostic injections are commonly done both above and below the level of pathology. However, complete denervation of the joint does not appear to be necessary for adequate pain relief. There are theoretic advantages to avoidance of a Charcot joint. In at least one case, an experienced pain physician treated another pain physician with a neurolytic facet block, resulting in a Charcot joint situation with resultant paraparesis when a listhesis developed at the treated segment.[55] Fortunately, recovery ensued, but the concern about multiple neurolytic facet blocks is very real.

In addition, in "virgin backs" the goal is to provide a period of "analgesia" to allow appropriate rehabilitation; this does not necessarily require complete "anesthesia." My practice is usually to freeze only the most symptomatic level, with a goal of "good" rather than "complete" analgesia. Sensation to the joint is expected to return in 2 to 6 months as the nerve regenerates, but this timeframe usually provides ample rehabilitation time, and most patients who have not undergone prior surgery will note long-term relief. In patients with operated backs, however, the formation of postoperative neuromas from the surgery itself, coupled with the surgical destabilizing of the posterior muscle and ligamentous structures, sets the stage for continued instability and pathology. Although these patients will also get relief with a cryoneuroablation, the effect is shorter-lived due to the multiple pain generators. However, the procedure can be repeated, and it has not been uncommon in my practice to have post-laminectomy patients returning every 6 to 8 months to have the facet nerves refrozen, noting significant relief in the interim.

Pseudosciatica

Since Mixter and Barr[56] described herniations of the nucleus pulposus as a cause of pain going down the leg, the term *sciatica* has become synonymous with herniated discs. The definition of *sciatica* from *Taber's Cyclopedic Medical Dictionary* is "compression or trauma of the sciatic nerve or its roots, especially that resulting from ruptured intervertebral disc."[57] However, both physicians and patients use the term to describe pain going down the leg, despite the fact that there are several clinical entities that will cause similar or identical pain going down the leg, which are not related to disc disease. These I have termed "pseudosciaticas," and several are quite amenable to treatment with cryoneuroablation. While facet pathology could also be considered a pseudosciatica, this section discusses interspinous ligament pathology, superior gluteal neuralgia, sacroiliac joint, and cluneal neuralgia.

Intraspinous Ligament

The intraspinous segment of the dorsal ramus (ISDR) is the termination of the medial branch of the dorsal ramus of the spinal nerve. Injury to the soft tissues of the axial skeleton occur as the result of hyperextension or hyperflexion of the spine with injury to the ligamentous structures between the spinous processes, segmental muscle spasm, and bursitis. The ISDR is responsible, in large part, for sensory innervation of these structures. Irritation of this nerve will refer pain down the leg (one or both sides) in a dermatomal pattern consistent with the level involved.[58,59] This pathology is seen commonly after spinal surgery, and patients will present with well-localized midline tenderness with localized swelling over the intervertebral space and may benefit from injection of small volumes of local anesthetic and steroid solutions. When this provides only temporary relief, cryoneuroablation may be indicated.

Technique: With the patient in the prone position, a large pillow is placed under the abdomen, and the patient is thereby flexed forward. Local anesthetic is infiltrated 2 cm lateral to the targeted interspace. Infiltration with local anesthetic containing epinephrine 1:200,000 is performed deeply until contact is made with the lamina. The 2.0-mm probe is passed via a 12-gauge introducer aimed at the junction of the lamina and the spinous process. A nerve stimulator is used to ensure that the probe is away from the spinal nerve itself. Three 2-minute cycles seem to be sufficient. This procedure is performed bilaterally at each desired level, and

can be performed with fluoroscopic guidance, or can be done using bony landmarks.

Clinical Effectiveness: Klein and Trescot[60] reported in a poster presentation on the clinical effectiveness of the cryoneurolysis technique, describing 10 patients with low back pain treated effectively with dorsal median nerve cryoneuroablation.

Superior Gluteal Neuralgia

Superior gluteal nerve (SGN) entrapment may also be a source of pseudosciatica. The superior gluteal nerve, formed from the posterior branches of L4, L5, and S1, passes from the pelvis above the piriformis muscle. Deep to the gluteus maximus and medius muscles, the nerve accompanies the superior gluteal artery and vein over the surface of the gluteus minimus muscle. It supplies the gluteus medius and gluteus minimus muscles and innervates the tensor fascia lata muscle by a branch, which accompanies the lower branch of the deep division of the superior gluteal artery.

Clinical Presentation: Neuralgia due to irritation of the SGN is commonly seen after a lifting injury involving the lower back and hip. After exiting the sciatic notch, the SGN passes caudal to the inferior border of the gluteus minimus and penetrates the gluteus medius. Vulnerable as it passes in the fascial plane between the gluteus medius and gluteus minimus musculature, the SGN is injured as a result of shearing between the gluteal musculature with forced external rotation of the leg, and with extension of the hip under mechanical load. Occasionally, this nerve is injured with forced extension of the hip, as might occur in a head-on automobile collision where the foot is pressed against the automobile floorboards with the knee in extension, as the patient anticipates impact. The clinical presentation consists of sharp pain in the lower back, dull pain in the buttock, and vague pain to the popliteal fossa and occasionally down to the foot. Patients generally experience pain with prolonged sitting, leaning forward, or twisting to the contralateral side. Often, patients will describe a "giving away" of the leg. Patients will sit with the weight on the contralateral buttock or cross their legs in such a manner as to minimize pressure on the involved side.[61] Clinically, the presentation can be similar to SI pathology, but examination will show the SI tenderness medial to the posterior iliac crest while the SGN is lateral. Diagnostic blocks under fluoroscopy, with nerve stimulation, are critical for accurate diagnosis, as it is easy to confuse this nerve with a piriformis entrapment syndrome or the myofascial pain of the gluteus medius muscle itself.

Technique: With the patient in the prone position, the medial border of the ilium is palpated. The nerve is located about 5 cm lateral and inferior to the attachment of the gluteus medius (Figure 72.6). Infiltration with local anesthetic is followed by a saline solution with epinephrine 1:200,000. A 12-gauge intravenous catheter is again used

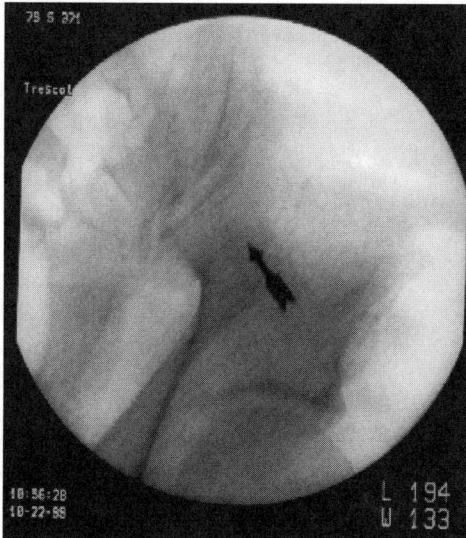

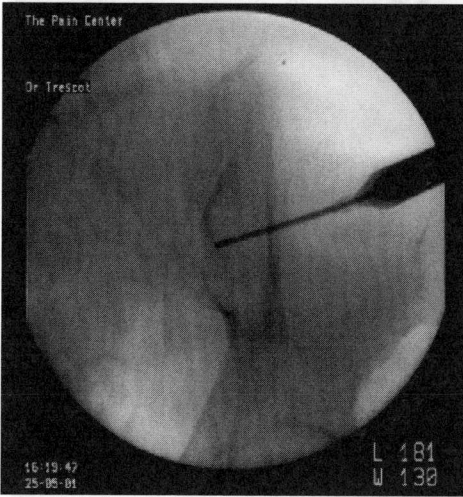

FIGURE 72.6 Superior gluteal nerve (marker and cryo).

as the introducer for the 2.0-mm cryoprobe. The nerve is approached from superior-laterally and the probe is directed inferior-medially. The nerve stimulator is employed to ensure the avoidance of motor nerves (e.g., sciatic nerve). Three 2-minute freeze cycles seem sufficient.

Prospective data regarding clinical and/or cost-effectiveness have not yet been reported.

Sacroiliac Joint

Prior to 1934, the SI joint was considered the most common cause of idiopathic low back pain;[62] however, that was the year Mixter and Barr described the herniated nucleus pulposus. The sacroiliac joint then was ignored for many years. The difficulty of imaging this joint also contributed to its obscurity. New appreciation of the SI joint as a cause of lumbosacral and leg pain has been triggered by new diagnostic physical exam techniques, injection approaches, and treatment options. It is estimated that 22% of low back pain (and 33% of low back

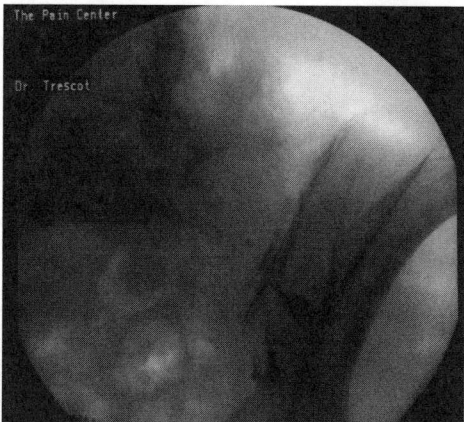

FIGURE 72.7 SI joint injection.

pain in elementary and high school students) is from SI pathology.[63]

Clinical Presentation: The SI joint is not fused, as is often taught, but rather is a joint with a fibrous lateral surface and a cartilaginous medial surface. The joint is designed to lock while in stance position and unlock as part of the stride. It is therefore vulnerable to "dislocation" and "jamming." Slamming on brakes during motor vehicle collisions or falling on the buttocks or a sudden twisting injury can cause pain in the buttocks radiating down the leg. Physical exam shows tenderness at the medial aspect of the posterior iliac crest — the "Fortin finger test"[64] — and diagnosis is confirmed by fluoroscopic injection of local anesthetic and contrast into the joint with subsequent resolution of pain (Figure 72.7). The innervation of the sacroiliac joint is primarily by way of the dorsal rami of S1 through S3.[62] Because these nerves enter the spinal column at the level of the leg nerves, pathology of the sacroiliac joint will refer pain down the leg in a radicular pattern. The most common major innervation in my experience is usually S2. The exiting dorsal ramus leaves the foramen usually at the 4 o'clock position on the right and the 8 o'clock position on the left. A diagnostic block using a peripheral nerve stimulator can aid in the determination of the most significant level of nerve innervation, and a small dose of contrast will outline the nerve root, giving a good "roadmap" for the subsequent cryoneuroablation procedure (Figure 72.8). The subcutaneous structures overlying the joint are innervated by branches of the L5–S1 facet nerves and medial cluneal.

Technique: For the cryoneuroablation procedure, the patient is positioned prone and the target sacral foramina identified by fluoroscopy. After prep, a small dose of local anesthetic is infiltrated subcutaneously, and deeper infiltration is performed with the saline/epinephrine solution, again about 1 cc. After a small skin nick is made, the 12-gauge introducer is advanced to the inferior border of the foramen laterally (as described above, at 4 o'clock on the right and 8 o'clock on the left). The stylus is then removed

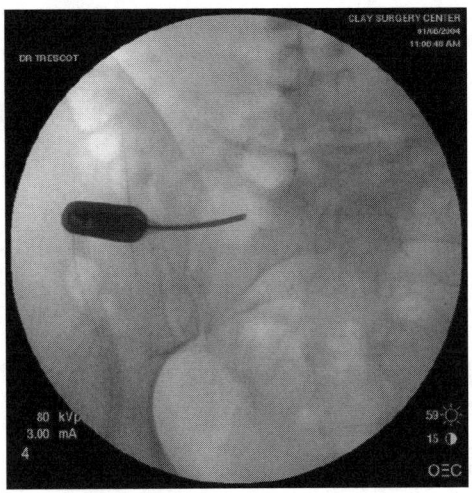

FIGURE 72.8 S2 nerve root.

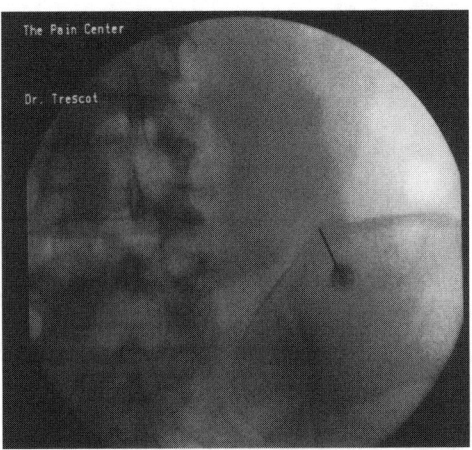

FIGURE 72.9 Cluneal injection.

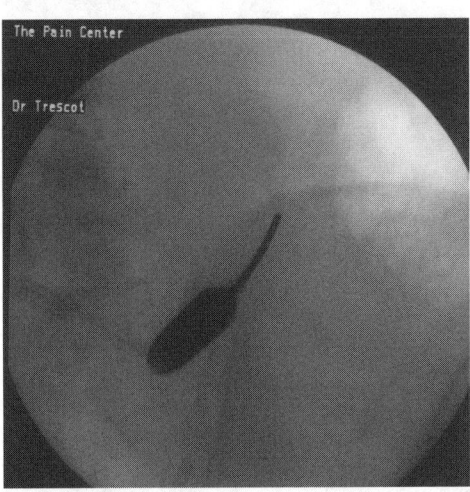

FIGURE 72.10 Cluneal cryo.

and the 2.0-mm probe advanced through the catheter. Using the stimulation pattern described for facets, the area of maximal stimulation is identified. Care must be taken to avoid actually cannulating the foramen, as this could potentially affect the nerves to the bowel and bladder.

Clinical Effectiveness: Lloyd et al.[11] and Evans et al.[5] used cryoanalgesia to treat the sacral nerve roots in patients with intractable "sciatica" and perineal pain. Prospective data regarding clinical and/or cost-effectiveness have not yet been reported.

Cluneal Neuralgia

The superior cluneal nerves are an under recognized source of hip, back, and leg pain. These nerves are the lateral cutaneus branches of the dorsal rami of the upper three lumbar nerves. They pierce the quadratus lumborum fascia at the lateral border of the erector spinae muscle, cross the iliac crest a short distance in advance of the posterior iliac spine, and distribute to the skin of the gluteal region as far as the greater trochanter. Pain can refer to the posterior thigh, calf, and foot.

Clinical Presentation: Two recognized nerve pathologies will cause pain in this region. One pathology is of the cluneal nerve itself, either after surgical iliac crest graft harvesting or, much more commonly, secondary to entrapment of the nerve as it pierces the quadratus lumborum fascia. Thus, the muscle spasm of a "pulled muscle" would entrap the cluneal nerve, causing a referred pain down the leg, potentially all the way to the foot. This "pseudosciatica" would clinically mimic a radiculopathy. Diagnosis is made by physical exam because palpation of the iliac crest will be markedly tender and will usually replicate the leg pain. At fluoroscopy, the maximal tenderness is usually seen at the medial iliac crest (Figure 72.9), and a traction spur of the attachment of the quadratus lumborum is often seen just medial to the area of maximal tenderness. Injection of 1 cc of local anesthetic using a peripheral

nerve stimulator is diagnostic and depo-steroids at this spot are often very effective in completely relieving the pain. If the relief is complete but only temporary, placement of the cryoprobe (Figure 72.10) at that same spot (confirmed by sensory stimulation and lack of motor stimulation), using the technique previously discussed, can give dramatic and long-term relief. Maigne's syndrome is a T12–L1 facet pathology referring pain to the iliac crest via the cluneal nerves. There is tenderness of the skin over the iliac crest, and the diagnosis is made by the use of a thoracolumbar (T12–L1) facet block. Treatment would then include cryoneuroablation of the median branch at that level, identical to that described above for lumbar facets.

Technique: The initial steps are as described above, and as noted, accurate and meticulous sensory stimulation is critical for success. As the probe moves across the periosteum, sensory stimulation at first at 2 volts, then 1 volt, and then 0.5 volts is used to identify the cluneal nerve. Small movements of the probe are used as described above. The position of the probe is where the quadratus lumborum attaches to the periosteum. At this time motor stimulation is used at its highest voltage to confirm that the probe is not too close to the L5 nerve root. Gas flows are then turned up to 10 to 12 liters per minute and a series of three 2-minute freezes with 30 seconds defrosting between each cycle is performed as for the facet cryoneuroablation. There is usually a burning pain on initiation of the first freeze cycle, which often replicates the pain and should resolve within approximately 30 seconds.

Clinical Effectiveness: Saberski et al.[65] described a syndrome of "painful iliac crest donor site" in a patient who had undergone iliac crest bone harvesting for a lumbar fusion. This patient experienced 1 year of complete relief after cryoneuroablation of the region of the iliac crest. Although this was not identified as the cluneal nerve, the clinical description appears to be consistent with a cluneal nerve pathology. Long-term (in excess of 5 years) relief has been obtained with open cryoneurolysis of cluneal nerves injures during bone graft harvesting. Noback[66] presented a technique of exposure of the graft site by reopening the surgical incision with dissection to the iliac crest. Cluneal neuromata are often found where the chiseled nerve has retracted to the upper anterior (abdominal) portion of the graft site. After exposure and stimulation during the procedure performed with local anesthetic, the severed nerve is cryoablated just proximal to its severed end with the 2 mm probe according to previously described techniques.

LOWER EXTREMITY PAIN

Obturator Nerve

The obturator nerve is rarely a pain problem except in cases of spasticity. It has, however, also been observed after surgical manipulation and in association with retroperitoneal hemorrhage. The obturator nerve has both sensory and motor components, and provides sensation to the medial distal thigh and knee. Diagnostic blocks may be useful in the evaluation of hip pain, as the articular branch of the obturator nerve is involved with sensation to the hip. The obturator is formed from branches of the second and third sacral nerve roots and passes anteriorly into the pelvis and then out onto the thigh via the obturator canal.

Technique: The patient is placed supine, with the affected limb abducted slightly. Fluoroscopy may be useful in the obese or severely spastic patient. The pubic tubercle is the palpated, and local anesthetic is infiltrated subcutaneously approximately one fingerbreadth laterally and inferiorly to the tubercle. After saline with epinephrine infiltration, the 12-gauge catheter is carefully and gently advanced to the inferior border of the ramus. If done blindly, hitting the edge of the ramus will confirm depth. If done under fluoroscopy, the catheter can be directed to

just below the inferior border of the ramus. To treat spasticity, this is one of the few times that motor stimulation for localization is appropriate. Adduction of the thigh at low voltages (0.5 to 1 mV) will confirm position. Spastic muscles should relax quickly, usually during the first freeze cycle. For pain, on the other hand, localization with the sensory mode is more effective, and an effort is made to avoid strong motor simulation, repositioning the probe if needed.

Clinical Effectiveness: Kim and Ferrante[67] reported cryoneuroablation of the obturator nerve for the treatment of adductor spasticity and obturator neuropathy. However, with the increased use of botulium toxin, this technique may be less useful.

Infrapatellar Saphenous Nerve

Neuralgia due to irritation of the infrapatellar branch of the saphenous nerve is seen weeks to years after blunt injury to the tibial plateau, or following knee replacement. The nerve is vulnerable as it passes superficially to tibial collateral ligament, piercing the sartorius tendon and fascia lata, inferior to the medial tibial condyle. The clinical presentation consists of dull pain in the knee joint, and achiness below the knee. Patients have trouble localizing the pain and tend to ambulate in such a manner as to minimize flexion of the knee joint. Physical exam shows tenderness to palpation just inferior to the medial tibial plateau. Pain with digital pressure is diagnostic, and most patients respond extremely well to a small volume local anesthetic and depo-steroid injection. Cryoneuroablation can be very useful for those patients in whom the injection gives only temporary relief.

Technique: A 12-gauge intravenous catheter is used as the introducer for the 2.0-mm cryoprobe, employing three 2-minute cryocycles. Special care must be taken to prevent frostbite injury to the skin. Approaching the nerve from a caudad to cephalad direction and keeping the probe positioned at an acute angle will help keep the ice ball below skin level and thereby decrease the frostbite risk.

Superficial Peroneal and Saphenous Nerves

Neuralgia due to irritation of the superficial peroneal and saphenous nerves can be seen weeks to years after injury to the foot and ankle. These superficial sensory nerves pass through strong ligamentous structures and are vulnerable to stretch injury with inversion of the ankle, compression injury due to edema, and sharp trauma due to bone fragmentation.

The superficial peroneal nerve runs superficial and medial to the lateral malleolus and continues superficial to the inferior extensor retinaculum, terminating in the fourth and fifth toes. Particularly vulnerable to injury following sprains of the lateral ankle, the clinical presentation consists of dull ankle pain, worse with passive inversion of the ankle. Signs and symptoms consistent with reflex sympathetic dystrophy or CRPS (a disproportionate swelling, vasomotor instability, and allodynia) are remarkably common. Patients tend to ambulate in such a manner as to minimize weight bearing on the lateral aspect of the foot. Pain with digital pressure in the area between the lateral malleolus and extensor retinaculum is diagnostic. Sometimes the patients are so diffusely tender that it is hard to determine where the worst tenderness is. The history can be very helpful here because the mechanism of injury is consistent enough that almost all of these injuries result in superficial peroneal neuralgia. Small-volume diagnostic injections with local anesthetic and depo-steroid can give rapid and dramatic relief, sometimes decreasing the swelling "right before your eyes." The saphenous nerve at the ankle passes anterior to the medial malleolus, and is injured by eversion ankle trauma. The pain, swelling, and hyperesthesia from this entrapment can result in a chronic regional pain syndrome (CRPS). Pain will radiate up the medial shin and down to the great toe, but the patient may have difficult identifying the exact location. It is important, therefore, to explore the mechanism of injury to predict the likely pathology.

Technique: A 12-gauge intravenous catheter is used as the introducer for the 2.0-mm cryoprobe, employing three 2-minute cryocycles. Special care must be taken to prevent frostbite injury to the skin. Approaching the nerve from a caudad to cephalad direction and keeping the probe positioned at an acute angle will help keep the ice ball below skin level and thereby decrease the frostbite risk.

Deep Peroneal Neuralgia

The deep peroneal nerve runs beneath the tendon of the extensor hallucis brevis, superficial to the dorsal interosseous muscle, between the first and second metatarsal heads, terminating in the first and second toes. Individuals with diabetes and women seem to be most vulnerable to this compression injury, which results from tightly fitting shoes. Seen less commonly following blunt injury to the dorsum of the foot, the clinical presentation consists of dull pain in the great toe, often worse after prolonged standing. There may also be pain at ball of the foot, poorly localized and occasionally burning in nature. Patients tend to ambulate in such a manner as to minimize weight bearing on the anterior foot. Pain with digital pressure in the area between first and second metatarsal heads (especially with concomitant pressure on the metatarsal heads) is diagnostic. Morton's neuromas (digital neuromas, intermetatarsal space neuromas) will present similarly but are located between the second and third metatarsal space or between the third and fourth (Figure 72.11). Neuromas that have not been surgically treated

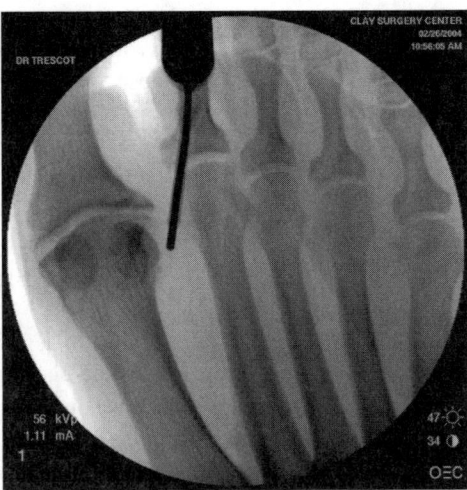

FIGURE 72.11 Digital neuroma.

are easier to treat because there is room for the large (2.0-mm) probe, which increases the success rate. Unfortunately, many patients are sent for evaluation only after the surgical treatment has failed. The cryoprobe must be placed proximal to the surgical trauma to be effective, and there is not much room in the proximal portion of the metatarsal triangle apex, necessitating the use of the smaller (1.4-mm) probe.

Technique: The appropriate introducer (12 gauge for "virgin" nerves and the 1.4 gauge for postoperative neuromas) is introduced through the skin perpendicular to the nerve and directed toward the apex of the metatarsal bones. Care must be used with the saline and epinephrine because of the risk of digital ischemia. Placing the non-introducing hand at the plantar surface will detect if the probe is too close to the skin of the sole of the foot. Stimulation should replicate the patient's usual pattern of pain. Nonsurgically treated neuromas and the deep peroneal nerve can use the 12-gauge catheter and the 2.0-mm probe.

Clinical Effectiveness: Cryoneurolysis of an intermetatarsal space neuroma has been reported to provide at least 6 months of relief.[68] Wang[34] performed percutaneous cryoneurolysis on various peripheral nerves (ulnar, median, sural, occipital, palmar branch of the median, and digital) in 12 patients with 6 patients reporting relief of 1 to 12 months' duration.

Medial and Lateral Calcaneal Nerves

Heel pain, especially on the plantar surface, is often diagnosed as plantar fasciitis. However, occasionally the heel pain is caused, instead, by entrapment of the medial and less commonly the lateral calcaneal nerves. The medial calcaneal nerve is a terminal branch of the posterior tibial nerve and passes under the flexor retinaculum at the bony attachment of the abductor hallucis. The small overhang of bone is the site of entrapment and the target for the cryolesion. A similar anatomy exists laterally, although the bony outcropping is less distinct and therefore a harder landmark to find.

Technique: A 14-gauge intravenous catheter is used as the introducer for the 1.4-mm cryoprobe, employing three 2-minute cryocycles. Care must be used to avoid frostbite, and the technique seems to work best when the probe is directed cephalad to caudad along the groove in the bone.

Peripheral Neuropathy

Patients who have been diagnosed as having peripheral neuropathies may actually have distal nerve entrapments. The digital, superficial peroneal, and saphenous nerves described above have been implicated in all or a vast majority of the foot pain attributed to peripheral neuropathy. The patient is questioned regarding the area of initial pain onset, and a diagnostic block in that area is performed. If this results in good but only temporary relief, cryoneuroablation of that nerve is attempted.

Clinical Effectiveness: Milleret[69] described the use of cryoanalgesia in elderly patients with distal arteritis. Dellon[70] described surgical decompression of peripheral nerves for the symptoms of diabetic peripheral neuropathy. However, he noted up to 1 year for wound healing. Cryoneuroablation, which is much less invasive and results in minimal tissue trauma, would be expected to be at least as effective.

PHANTOM LIMB PAIN

Brief Review of Phantom Limb Pain

Phantom-limb pain is a common sequela of amputation, occurring in up to 80% of people who undergo the procedure.[71] It must be differentiated from nonpainful phantom phenomena, residual-limb pain, and nonpainful residual-limb phenomena. The term *phantom-limb pain* was coined for this sensation by Mitchell.[72] Phantom-limb pain is commonly classified as neuropathic, and it is assumed to be related to damage of central neurons. However, it was Ambroise Paré in 1552 who postulated that peripheral factors as well as a central pain memory might be causing phantom-limb pain, and he was actually the first to describe the phenomenon.[73] Searching for peripheral triggers for phantom pain symptoms can be guided by the nerve pattern of the phantom pain, tracing the known path of the nerve proximally, and examining for proximal tender regions. Diagnostic injections will confirm the site, and cryoanalgesia can give long-term relief.

CONCLUSION

In conclusion, cryoneuroablation is an effective interventional pain management technique, providing significant analgesia in an outpatient or office setting. The effect is routinely reversible, relatively painless, and not associated with neuroma formation. An accurate diagnosis with specific diagnostic injections of small volumes of local anesthetic and meticulous localization of the nerve is critical for successful outcome. Remember, "*You cannot treat what you cannot diagnose.*"

REFERENCES

1. Hippocrates. (1931). Aphorisms. In *Heracleitus on the universe* (Vol. 4, trans. by W. H. S. Jones). London: Heinemann, 5:165; 7:201.
2. Breasted, J. G. (1930). *Ancient records of Egypt — Historical documents from the earliest times to the Persian conquest* (Vol. III, p. 217). Chicago: University of Chicago Press.
3. Gruner, O. C. (1930). *A treatise on the canon of medicine of Avicenna.* London: Luzac.
4. Larre, D. (1832). *Surgical memoirs of the campaigns of Russia, Germany and France* (trans. by J. C. Mercer). Philadelphia: Carey & Lea.
5. Evans, P. J., Lloyd, J. W., & Jack, T. M. (1981). Cryoanalgesia for intractable perineal pain. *Journal of the Royal Society of Medicine, 74,* 804.
6. Arnott, J. (1851). *On the treatment of cancer by the regulated application of an anesthetic temperature.* London: J. Churchill.
7. Richardson, B. W. (1866). *Medical Times and Gazette, 1,* 115.
8. Trendelenberg, W. (1917). Uber Landauende Nerveausschaltung mit siche Regenerationsfahigkeit. *Zeitschrift fur die Gesamte Experimentelle Medizin, 5,* 371.
9. Cooper, I. S. Grissman, F. & Johnson, R. (1962). *Saint Barnabas Hospital Medical Bulletin, 11.*
10. Amoils, S. P. (1967). The Joules Thompson cryoprobe. *Archives of Ophthalmology, 78,* 201.
11. Lloyd, J. W., Barnard, J. D. W., & Glynn, C. J. (1976). Cryoanalgesia, a new approach to pain relief. *Lancet, 2,* 932–934.
12. Warfield, C. A. (1987). Cryoanalgesia: Freezing of peripheral nerves. *Hospital Practice,* 71.
13. Barnard, J. D. W. and Lloyd, J. W. (1977). Cryoanalgesia. *Nursing Times, 73,* 897.
14. Glynn, C. J., & Carrie, L. E. (1985). Cryoanalgesia to relieve pain in diastasis of the symphysis pubis during pregnancy. *British Medical Journal, 290,* 1946.
15. Garamy, G. (1968). Engineering aspects of cryosurgery. In R. W. Rand, A. Rinfret, & H. von Leden (Eds.), *Cryosurgery* (pp. 92–132). Springfield, IL: Charles C Thomas.
16. Evans, P. (1981). Cryoanalgesia. The application of low temperatures to nerves to produce anesthesia or analgesia. *Anaesthesia, 36,* 1003.
17. Myers, R. R. et al. (1981). Biophysical and pathological effects of cryogenic nerve lesion. *Annals of Neurology, 10,* 478.

18. Sunderland, S. (1968). *Nerves and nerve injuries* (p. 180). Edinburgh: Livingstone.

19. Holden, H. (1973). Cryosurgery: Its scientific basis and clinical application. *Practitioner, 210,* 543.

20. Gander, M., Soanes, W. A., & Smith, V. (1967). Experimental prostate surgery. *Investigations in Urology, 1,* 610.

21. Soanes, W. A., Ablin, R. J., & Gander, M. J. (1970). Remission of metastatic lesions following cryosurgery in prostate cancer: Immunologic considerations. *Journal of Urology, 104,* 154.

22. Myers, R. R., Heckman, H. M., & Powell, H. C. (1996). Axonal viability and the persistence of thermal hyperalgesia after partial freeze lesions of nerve. *Journal of Neurological Sciences, 139,* 28.

23. Raj, P. (1986). Cryoanalgesia. In *Practical management of pain* (p. 779). Chicago: Year Book Medical Publishers.

24. Johannesen, N., Madsen, G., & Ahlburg, P. (1990). Neurological sequelae after cryoanalgesia for thoracotomy pain relief. *Ann. Chir. Gynaecol., 79,* 108–109.

25. Klein, D. S., Edwards, L. W., & Klein, P. W. (1992). Treatment of cryptogenic earache with posterior auricular nerve block. Poster. American Academy of Pain Management.

26. Bernard, J., Lloyd, J., & Glynn C. (1998–1999). Cryosurgery in the management of intractable facial pain. *British Journal of Oral Surgery, 16,* 135.

27. Barnard, D., Lloyd, J., & Evans, J. (1981). Cryoanalgesia in the management of chronic facial pain. *Journal of Maxillofacial Surgery, 9,* 101.

28. Nally, F. F. and Zakrezewska, J. (1984). Cryotherapy for trigeminal neuralgia. *Lancet, 8384*(1), 1021.

29. Nally, F. F. (1984). A 22-year study of paroxysmal trigeminal neuralgia in 211 patients with a 3-year appraisal of the role of cryotherapy. *Oral Surgery, Oral Medicine, Oral Pathology, 58,* 17.

30. Zakrzewska, J. M., & Nally, F. F. (1988). The role of cryotherapy (cryoanalgesia) in the management of paroxysmal trigeminal neuralgia: A six year experience. *British Journal of Oral & Maxillofacial Surgery, 26,* 18.

30a. Zakrzewska, J. M. (1991). Cryotherapy for trigeminal neuralgia: A ten-year audit. *British Journal of Oral Maxillofacial Surgery, 29,* 1–4.

31. Robinson, S. R., & Purdie, G. L. (2000). Reducing post-tonsillectomy pain with cryoanalgesia: A randomized controlled trial. *Laryngoscope, 110,* 1128.

32. Trescot, A. M., Saberski, L., & Klein, D. S. (2001). Interventional pain management: Applications of cryoablative procedures. *Pain Clinic, 3,* 11.

33. Kappes, T. J. (2003). Cryoablation of the occipital nerves for prolonged relief of cervicogenic headache. *American Journal of Pain Management, 13,* 118.

34. Wang, J. K. (1985). Cryoanalgesia for painful peripheral nerve lesions. *Pain, 22,* 191.

35. Nelson, K., Vincent, R.. & Bourke, R. (1974). Intraoperative intercostal nerve freezing to prevent postthoracotomy pain. *Annals of Thoracic Surgery, 18,* 280.

36. Orr, I., Keenan, D., & Dundee, J. (1981). Improved pain relief after thoracotomy: use of cryoprobe and morphine infusion. *British Medical Journal, 283,* 945.

37. Orr, I. A. et al. (1983). Post-thoracotomy pain relief: Combined use of cryoprobe and morphine infusion. *Annals of the Royal College of Surgeons of England, 65,* 366.

38. Riopelle, J. M. et al. (1985). Cryoanalgesia: Present day status. *Seminars in Anesthesia, 4,* 305.

39. Maiwand, O., & Makey, A. (1981). Cryoanalgesia for the relief of pain after thoracotomy. *British Medical Journal, 282,* 1749.

40. Brichon, P. Y. et al. (1994). Comparison of epidural analgesia and cryoanalgesia in thoracic surgery. *European Journal of Cardiothoracic Surgery, 8,* 482.

41. Green, C. R. et al. (1993). Long term followup of cryoanalgesia for chronic thoracic pain. *Regional Anesthesia, 18,* 46.

42. Jones, M., & Muffin, K. R. (1987). Intercostal block with cryotherapy. *Annals of the Royal College of Surgeons of England, 69,* 261.

43. Rosser, J. C. et al. (2001). The use of mini-laparoscopy for conscious pain mapping. *Regional Anesthesia and Pain Management, 5.*

44. Wood, G. et al. (1979). Cryoanalgesia and day case herniorrhaphy. *Lancet, 2,* 479.

45. Wood, G. et al. (1981). Postoperative analgesia for day case herniorrhaphy patients. A comparison of cryoanalgesia, paravertebral blockade and oral analgesia. *Anesthesia, 36,* 603.

46. Khiroya, R. C., Davenport, H. T., & Jones, J. G. (1986). Cryoanalgesia for pain after herniorrhaphy. *Anaesthesia, 41,* 73.

47. Callesen, T. et al. (1998). Cryoanalgesia: Effect on post-herniorrhaphy pain. *Anesthesia & Analgesia, 87,* 896.

48. Racz, G., & Angstrom, D. (1992). Iliohypogastric and ilioinguinal nerve entrapment: Diagnosis and treatment. *Pain Digest, 2,* 43.

49. Evans, P. J., Lloyd, J. W., & Green, C. J. (1981). Cryoanalgesia: The response to alterations in freeze cycle and temperature. *British Journal of Anaesthesia, 53,* 1121.

50. Loev, M. A. et al. (1998). Cryoablation: A novel approach to neurolysis of the ganglion impar, *Anesthesiology, 88,* 1391.

51. Jain, S., Rooney, S. M. and Goldiner, P. L. (1983). Managing the cancer patient's pain. *The Female Patient, 8,* 1.

52. Brechner, T. (1981). Percutaneous cryogenic neurolysis of the articular nerve of Luschka. *Regional Anesthesia, 6,* 18.

53. Schuster, G. D. (1982). The use of cryoanalgesia in the painful facet syndrome. *Journal of Neurological and Orthopaedic Surgery, 4,* 271.

54. Ross, E. L. (1991, April 6). *Cryoneurolysis of lumbar facet joints for the treatment of chronic lower back pain.* Presented at the American Society of Regional Anesthesia.

55. Sassano, J. Personal communication.

56. Mixter, W. J., & Barr, J. S. (1934). Rupture of the intervertebral disc with involvement of the spinal canal. *New England Journal of Medicine, 211,* 210.

57. Taber, C. W. (1993). *Taber's Cyclopedic Medical Dictionary* (17th ed.). Philadelphia: FA Davis Company.

58. Feinstein, R. et al. (1954). Experiments on pain referred from deep somatic tissues. *Journal of Bone and Joint Surgery* (America), *36A*, 981.

59. Kellgren, J. H. (1939). On the distribution of pain arising from deep somatic structures with charts of segmental pain areas. *Clinical Science, 4*, 35.

60. Klein, D. S., & Trescot, A. M. (1994). Dorsal median nerve cryoanalgesia. Poster presented at American Pain Society, New Orleans, Oct. 23–26.

61. Trescot, A. M., Klein, D. S., & Edwards, L. W. (1995, November). Proximal auriculotemporal neuralgia. *APS Abstracts*.

62. Fortin, J. D., & Falco, F. J. E. (1997). The Fortin finger test: An indicator of sacroiliac pain. *American Journal of Orthopedics, 26*(7), 477.

63. Bernard, P. N., & Cassidy, J. D. (1991). Sacroiliac joint syndrome: Pathophysiology, diagnosis and management. In J. Frymoyer (Ed.), *The adult spine: Principles and practice* (pp. 2107–2131). New York: Raven Press.

64. Fortin, J. D., Kissling, R. O., O'Connor, B. L. et al. (1999). Sacroiliac joint innervation and pain. *American Journal of Orthopedics, 28*(12), 687–690.

65. Saberski, L. R. et al. (2000). Identification of a new therapeutic approach for prolonged pain relief in chronic iliac crest donor site pain: A case report. *Pain Clinic, 2*, 37.

66. Noback, C. R. (1999, June). *Interventional pain management techniques and technologies*. Lecture. Bethesda, MD.

67. Kim, P. S., & Ferrante, F. M. (1998). Cryoanalgesia: A novel treatment for hip adductor spasticity and obturator neuralgia. *Anesthesiology, 89*, 534.

68. Hodor, L., Barkal, K., & Hatch-Fox, L. D. (1997). Cryogenic denervation of the intermetatarsal space neuroma. *Journal of Foot and Ankle Surgery, 36*, 311.

69. Milleret, R. (1983). Cryoanalgesia of the nerves of the feet in distal arteritis in the elderly. *Journal des Maladies Vasculaires, 8*(4), 307.

70. Dellon, A. L. (2001). Decompression of peripheral nerves for symptoms of diabetic neuropathy: Pain management considerations. *Pain Clinic, 3*, 11.

71. Jensen, T. S., & Nikolajsen, L. (1999). Phantom pain and other phenomena after amputation. In P. D. Wall & R. A. Melzack (Eds.), *Textbook of pain* (pp. 799–814). Edinburgh: Churchill Livingstone.

72. Mitchell, S. W. (1872). *Injuries of nerves and their consequences*. Philadelphia: Lippincott.

73. Keil, G. (1990). So-called initial description of phantom pain by Ambroise Paré. "Chose digne d'admiration et quasi incredible": The "douleur es parties mortes et amputees." *Fortschritte der Medizin, 108*, 62.

73

Endoscopic Surgery and Minimally Invasive Techniques

Anthony T. Yeung, MD, and Christopher Alan Yeung, MD

INTRODUCTION

EVOLUTION OF ENDOSCOPIC SPINE SURGERY

Spinal endoscopy is poised to parallel the development and evolution of knee, shoulder, and ankle arthroscopy.[1] Without endoscopy, spine surgeons must depend heavily on imaging systems that while extremely sensitive in identifying pathologic conditions, do not always correlate that condition with the patient's pain. Endoscopic disc surgery is evolving rapidly due to the introduction of improvements in endoscope design and instrumentation (Figure 73.1).[2] The introduction of various cannula configurations combined with excellent optics gives the endoscopic spine surgeon the ability to probe spinal anatomy in a conscious patient while protecting sensitive spinal nerves, allowing the surgeon to evaluate the pathologic process causing the patient's pain. When spinal endoscopy can be performed, conditions previously not even considered for surgery may be evaluated and managed.[3]

ENDOSCOPIC SURGERY COMPLEMENTING INTERVENTIONAL PAIN MANAGEMENT

Patients who find temporary relief with interventional pain management injections directed toward a pain generator may find more lasting and definitive relief with surgical correction or modification of the pathoanatomy. Our understanding of discogenic back pain is enhanced by diagnostic and surgical endoscopy of the lumbar spine, as endoscopic visualization of pathologic lesions not previously seen with traditional techniques is increasing our understanding of the pain generators in the lumbar spine.

The pain pattern does not always match the anatomic dermatome, which confuses many surgeons dependent on identifying a mechanical condition compressing sensitive spinal nerves and on correcting the spinal condition. With endoscopy, aided by discography, epidurography, and therapeutic injections, it is possible to evaluate, diagnose, and treat spinal conditions not usually considered for the more invasive open surgical techniques.[4] The technique first depends on directing a needle to the pain generator, desensitizing or anesthetizing it, dilating a path that will allow a tubular retractor to be inserted, followed by an operating endoscope. With this capability, we will gain a better understanding of the biology of back pain and sciatica, and also will be able to study the pathoanatomy and pathophysiology of pain in specific individuals. It is also well known that although a spinal structure is capable of pain, spinal pathology on imaging studies does not always correlate with the debilitating pain. What may be very painful in one person may be well tolerated or painless in another. Evocative discography™ is helpful in identifying the disc as a pain generator in axial back pain and sciatica.[5] Spinal endoscopy and probing in a sedated, awake patient can identify painful and nonpainful structures and help correlate the patient's pain to imaging studies. This increased knowledge of back pain can eventually lead to more targeted and alternative treatment options.

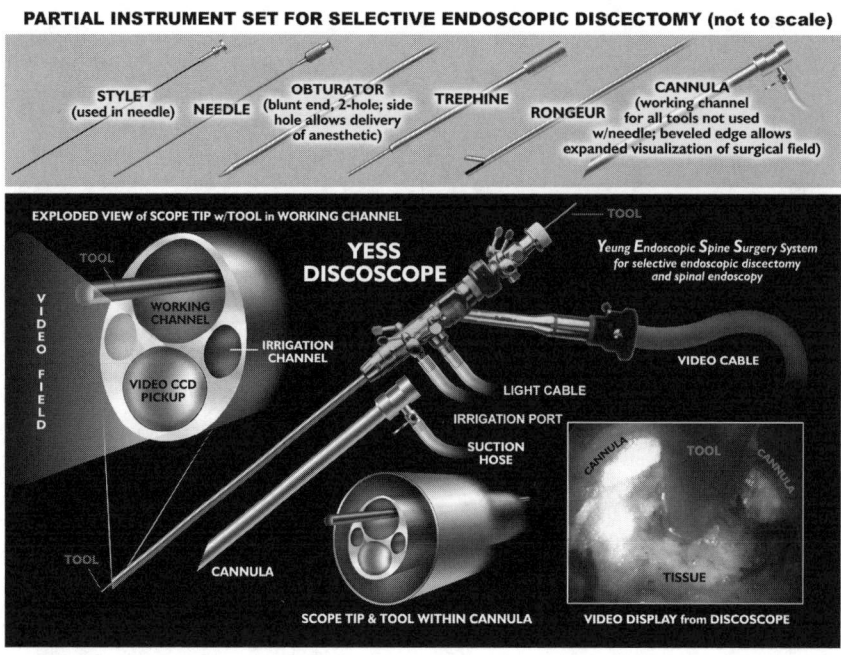

FIGURE 73.1 The YESS discoscope and partial instrument set. The spinal endoscope is designed with multichannel irrigation and a cannula system that allows access to targeted areas while protecting sensitive nerves.

INDICATIONS

Any pathologic lesion accessible, visible, treatable, or requiring endoscopic confirmation through the foramen may ultimately become an indication for diagnostic and therapeutic endoscopy.[6] Patient selection for pain and radiculopathy from disc herniation is similar to selection criteria for traditional spine procedures, but endoscopic surgical indications may be dictated by the limitations of the endoscopic procedure itself with respect to the patient's anatomy or the surgeon's skill and experience with endoscopic spinal surgery.[7] At L5–S1, anatomic restrictions may cause the surgeon to opt for the posterior transcanal approach (Figure 73.2a). For herniations from T-10 to L5, the foraminal approach provides excellent access to the disc and epidural space (Figure 73.2b). As the surgeon's experience increases, previous contraindications become relative, dependent partly on the surgeon's ability to endoscopically visualize, probe, and access the pathologic lesion. Restrictions are dictated only by anatomic considerations in accessing the patient's spinal pathology and the rationale of the endoscopic procedure itself.[8] Anatomic structures within reach of the spine endoscope transforaminally are illustrated in Figure 73.3.

INCLUSION CRITERIA

Discogenic pain as determined by evocative discography may implicate the disc as a pain generator. Symptomatic disc herniation is the obvious indication, with surgical decompression limited only by the accessibility of endoscopic instruments to the herniated fragment.[9,10] Because of the posterolateral foraminal approach, the ideal lesion for endoscopic discectomy is a far lateral, extraforaminal disc herniation. Traditional approaches to far-lateral, extraforaminal disc herniations are more difficult, requiring a paramedian incision through the vascular intertransverse ligament. This surgical area is often called the "hidden zone" for traditional surgeons. Although a traditional spinal surgeon can access the lateral zone of the disc with a paramedian incision, it is easier to access the extraforaminal zone endoscopically via the posterolateral portal. A typical foraminal view of nucleus pulposus extruded past the posterior annulus is shown in Figure 73.4. With this approach to the disc, relatively easy access is possible from T-10 to L5 (Figure 73.2b). This is also the preferred approach for disc herniations in the upper lumbar and lower thoracic spine because the transcanal approach will require more extensive laminectomy that may destabilize the spinal segment if the herniation is above L3–L4.

Recurrent herniations after posterior discectomies are another good indication. The posterior scar usually limits any migration of the herniated disc, and the postero-lateral endoscopic approach avoids going through the scar tissue. Endoscopic excisional biopsy and disc space debridement are ideal for surgically treating infectious discitis (Figure 73.5).[11] Currently treated with immobilization and parenteral antibiotics, discitis is much more effectively treated when augmented by endoscopic debridement. Unlike the open posterior approach, no dead space is

(a)

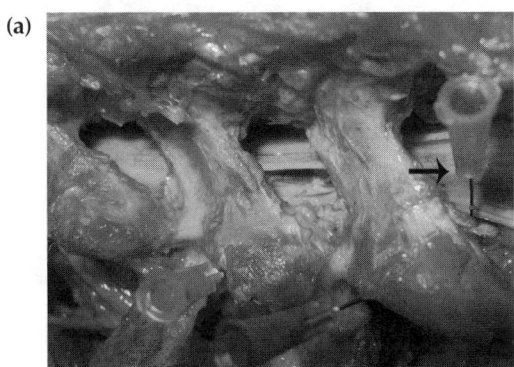

(b)

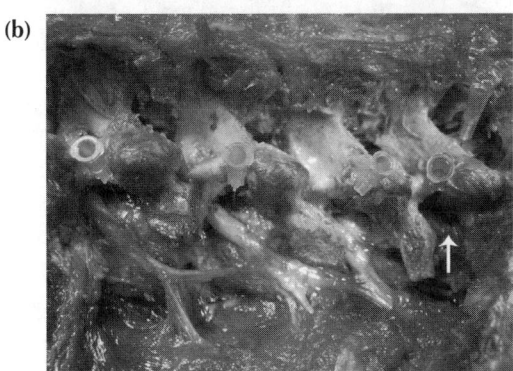

FIGURE 73.2 (a) The anatomy of the posterior portal provides easier access to the posterior disc and spinal canal at L5–S1, but with planning, most contained disc herniations can be removed posterolaterally. (b) Anatomy of the posterolateral foraminal portal from L2 to S1. Only at the L5–S1 disc space is access to the spinal canal restricted due to the pelvis and the relatively wide facet. High lumbar disc herniations from L1 to L3 are easier to reach endoscopically through the posterolateral foraminal portal. L4–5 provides ample room for either approach. Note the furcal nerve branches entering the psoas muscle.

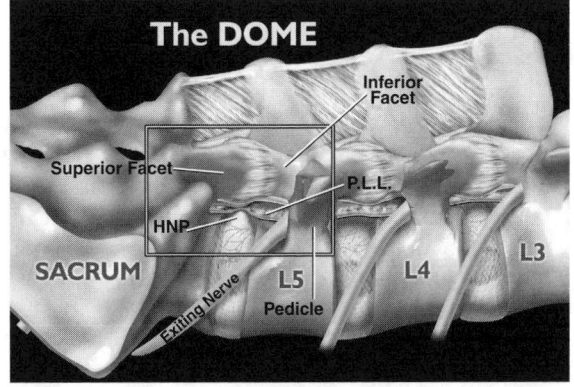

FIGURE 73.3 The dome. Spinal structures in the foramen accessible to visualization and surgical intervention and probing via the posterolateral approach.

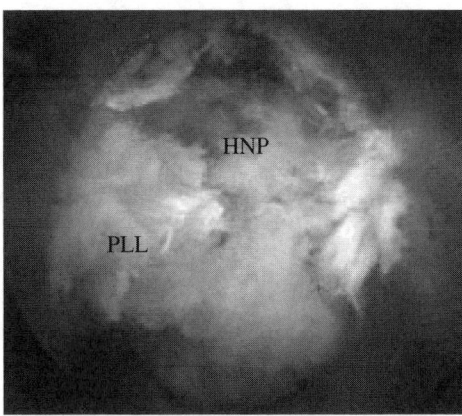

FIGURE 73.4 Foraminal view of an extruded disc herniation through the posterior annulus. The vital dye stains the disc for easier identification and extraction. Here, the herniation has clearly extruded through the posterior annulus.

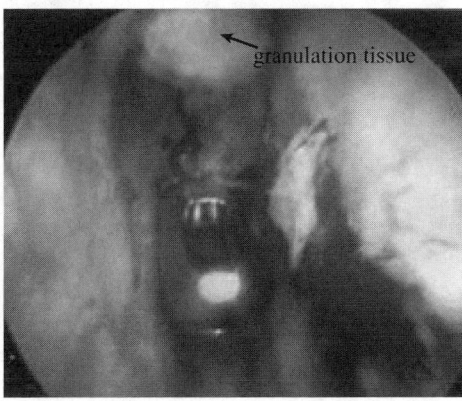

FIGURE 73.5 Intradiscal view of discitis post-debridement. Usual findings of inflammatory disc material and loose end plate cartilage are readily removed from the disc space. Pain relief is immediate, and abundant tissue is available for laboratory analysis. The micropituitary forceps is visualized through a biportal fenestration of the disc.

created. Thus, the surgeon will not have to worry about spreading the infection. The clinical results are dramatic, and tissue biopsy is more accurate than needle aspiration in identifying the cause of discitis. Even sterile discitis will benefit from intradiscal debridement and irrigation.

Endoscopic foraminoplasty by endoscopic techniques is also possible for experienced endoscopic surgeons.[3,7,12] Although trephines, rasps, and burrs can be used, the Ho:Yag laser has enhanced the procedure technically as the laser is a very precise cutting tool for visually controlled soft tissue and bone ablation. Endoscopic laser foraminoplasty is further validated by research studies by Osman and Panjabi[13] demonstrating that decompression through the foramen can be as effective as posterior decompression, but will not produce further instability (Figure 73.6). The foramen can be enlarged up to 45.5% versus the 34.2% attainable with the standard posterior

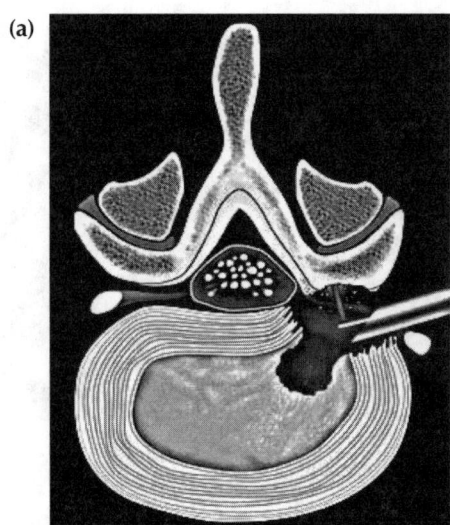

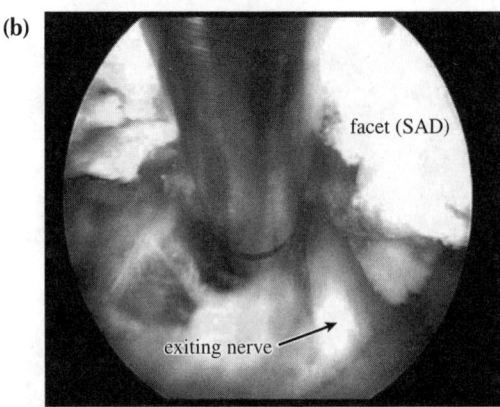

FIGURE 73.6 (a) The technique of endoscopic foraminal decompression. The annulus can be decompressed and even resected, while the capsule, ligamentum flavum, and inferior facet surface can be ablated with a side-firing laser to enlarge the foramen and free the traversing as well as the exiting nerve. (b) Side firing laser ablating bone under the superior articular process. Intraoperative view of foraminoplasty at L5–S1. Note exiting nerve at 5 o'clock.

technique of removing only the medial third of the facet. Posterior decompression of the lamina with removal of the medial third of the facet will produce increased extension and axial rotation postoperatively.[13] Endoscopic foraminal plasty has not been shown to cause increased instability even in spondylolisthesis.[3] The technique is most useful for lateral recess stenosis, a condition that is responsible for atypical leg pain rather than true intermittent claudication of central spinal stenosis. In central spinal stenosis, when there is concomitant posterior disc protrusion, decompression of the spinal canal can be effectively accomplished by resecting the bulging annulus in a collapsed disc, thus lowering the floor of the foramen. In isthmic and degenerative spondylolisthesis, when there is more leg than back pain, this is usually due to impingement on the exiting nerve by the pars pseudoarthrosis

defect or the undersurface of the superior articular facet. The goal is then to decompress the compromised exiting nerve by elevating the dome formed by the superior facet and lamina without further destabilizing the spinal column segment.

EXCLUSION CRITERIA

Except perhaps for pregnancy, there are no absolute exclusion criteria but only relative contraindications dependent on the surgeon's skills and experience. Spinal endoscopy and spinal probing can be used for diagnostic purposes in a very difficult or confusing clinical problem. Therefore, if endoscopy is helpful for diagnostic purposes, exclusion criteria may depend mainly on the accessibility of the spinal pathology and the endoscopic skills of the surgeon. A high narrow pelvis may make it difficult to access the posterior aspect of the L5–S1 disc and extract the herniation. If the herniation is sequestered and a free fragment, then a posterior microdiscectomy may be a better option for herniation removal. The risks and benefits of the procedure must be weighed against the need to use this fluoroscopically guided procedure under local anesthesia or sedation.

FUTURE CONSIDERATIONS

It is not inconceivable that the spine scope will eventually be used for all conditions where visual inspection is desired. The senior author (A.T.Y.) has utilized spinal endoscopy to inspect a spinal nerve suspected to be irritated by orthopedic hardware adjacent to the pedicle, to remove suspected recurrent or residual disc herniations that do not show up on imaging studies, to decompress the lateral recess by foraminoplasty, to remove osteophytes and facet cysts that cause unrelenting sciatica, and to locate painful lateral annular tears or small disc herniations not evident on physical examination or on magnetic resonance imaging (MRI). Some of these correctable lesions are responsible for failed back surgery syndrome. The lateral "hidden" zone is rarely visualized by surgeons. It has been reported that most tears that do not heal are too extensive or are caused by interpositional disc material keeping the tear open. Simply removing the interpositional disc tissue will then allow the tear to heal, and the pain to resolve. It has been demonstrated that with endoscopy, it is possible to perform isolated disc and annulus surgery using a visualized thermal modulation procedure (Figure 73.7), challenging the old concept that disc surgery is merely nerve decompressive surgery. For example, discogenic pain from annular tears is currently being evaluated and correlated with the pathoanatomic conditions visualized.[14–25] Some minimally invasive spinal surgeons use an endoscope, but only through the traditional transcanal approach. Because most surgeons are more com-

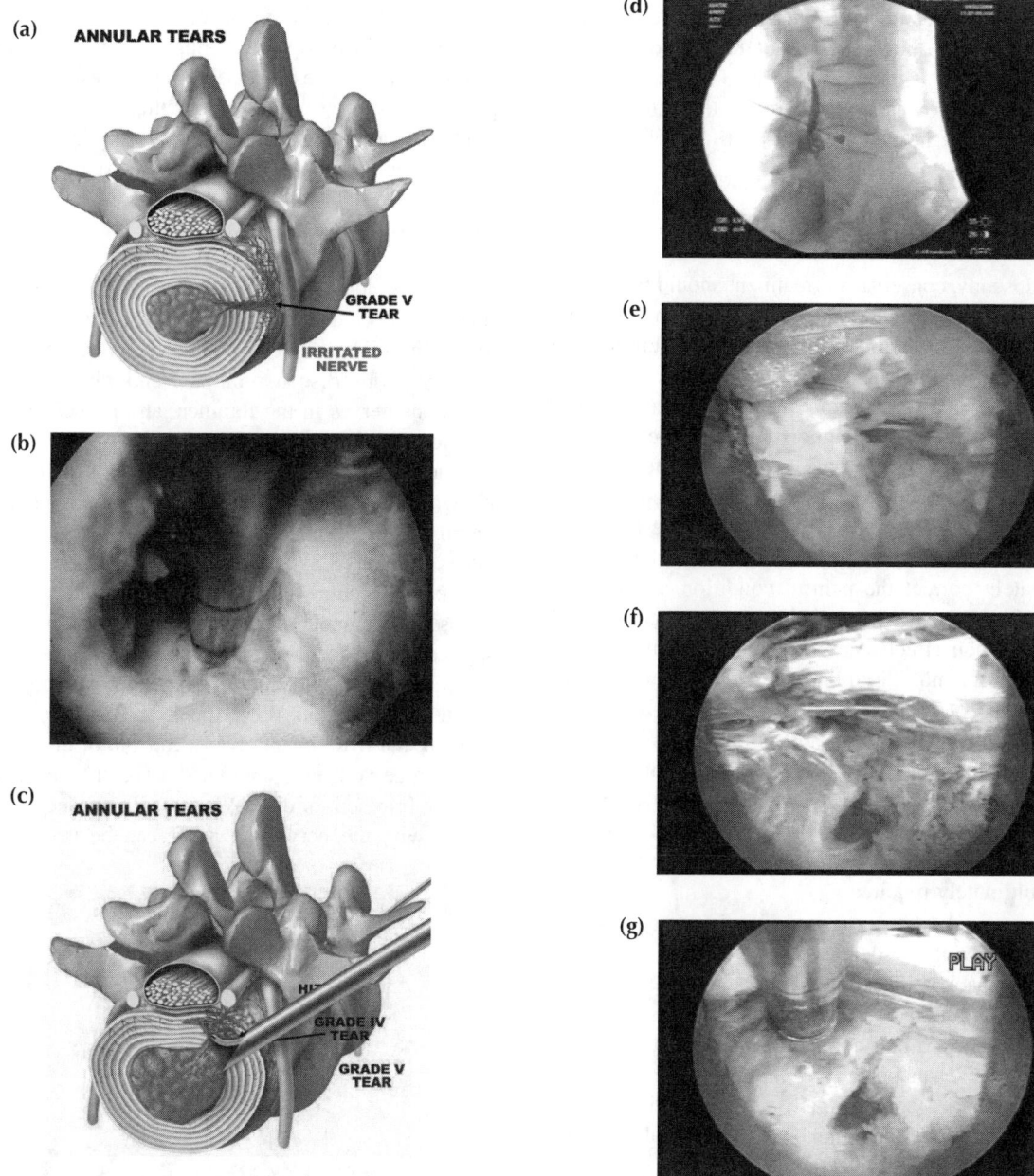

FIGURE 73.7 (a) Annular tears. Grade V annular tears open into the epidural space or psoas muscle, allowing the ingrowth of nerves and capillaries that create an inflammatory response that, if next to a spinal nerve or the dorsal root ganglion, can cause pain out of proportion to what may be anticipated from traditional imaging studies. If patients with annular tears get relief from foraminal epidural blocks, more lasting relief of 1 or 2 years is possible with selective endoscopic discectomy (SED™) and thermal annuloplasty. (b) Far-lateral annular tear. This far-lateral annular tear is thermally modulated by a side-firing Ho:Yag laser ablating the interpositional disc tissue that kept the tear open and prevented healing. The laser probe was inserted on the side opposite the tear. (c) Illustration of the Ellman bipolar trigger-flex probe treating a grade IV annular tear. Interpositional disc material embedded in the annular layers is the usual cause of annular tears not healing. Nucleus pulposus should be removed from the annular layers to treat the annular tear effectively. (d) Intraoperative evocative chromo-discography identifies a large grade V annular tear. (e) Nucleus pulposus found in annulus, demonstrating a small herniated foraminal disc fragment unrecognized on MRI. (f) Annular tear exposed after removal of herniation. Vascularization of the tear is demonstrated. (g) Thermomodulation of the annular tear with a bipolar radiofrequency probe helps close the defect.

fortable with the anatomy encountered in a traditional approach, this is a good way to begin the transition to other endoscopic techniques. Once they feel comfortable with the endoscope, however, it is not difficult to transition to the posterolateral portal. Those who take the time to learn other approaches, including the posterolateral approach, will be in the best position to do what is best for their patients.

Non-Operative Treatment

With endoscopy, conservative treatment should be labeled non-operative treatment. Physicians specializing in spinal medicine, rehabilitation, and pain management are becoming more sophisticated in their ability to identify the tissue source of back pain. Once the source is identified, physical therapy and diagnostic and therapeutic injection methods are used for pain relief. These techniques, such as foraminal epidural blocks and selective nerve blocks, may be labeled "conservative," but are therapeutically beneficial. They may also be limited in their ability to ultimately correct the painful condition. Endoscopic spine surgeons are still needed to address correctable lesions, but their effectiveness is enhanced by incorporating the help of a multidisciplinary team. The senior author has devised a new technique for performing foraminal epidurography and therapeutic injections that is done with a far-lateral trajectory into the foramen, mimicking the surgical approach.[4] Familiarity with foraminal injections will enhance the endoscopic surgeon's surgical skills and provide the surgeon with a "trial run" if endoscopic surgery is ultimately required.

The world literature on conservative treatment has presented strong evidence that a multidisciplinary approach to back pain, coupled with behavioral modification and exercise therapy, gives the best results. With spinal endoscopy, a new concept for treatment should be non-operative versus operative treatment, as the ability to more specifically diagnose a painful condition in the lumbar spine with endoscopy makes early surgical intervention the more "conservative" approach.

PLANNING

Patients with chronic back pain and atypical sciatica are the most difficult to treat. Traditional methods of nonsurgical treatment are often not effective or relief is very transient, and the patient is often labeled drug seeking or psychologically unstable. In this situation it is extremely helpful to utilize a multidisciplinary team approach. Psychologic profiling, behavioral modification, active exercise, and manual therapy help the patients overcome their pain and focus on becoming functional. The team approach with psychologists, physiatrists, addictionologists, and pain management specialists who are working with each

other and agree on the overall treatment plan has helped rescue many chronic pain sufferers from total disability and reliance on salvage procedures. Around the disc, foraminal epiduroscopy and foraminal epidural blocks will help determine the ease of reaching the disc and epidural space. A temporary response to the foraminal epidural injection is a good indicator for a foraminal approach to the pathologic lesion to be addressed surgically.

Current Imaging Methods

In the senior author's experience, imaging studies are only about 70% accurate and specific for predicting pain.[3,6,26–29] Conditions such as lateral annular tears, rim tears, small subligamentous disc herniations, end plate separations, anomalous nerves in the foramen, and miscellaneous discogenic conditions are cumulatively missed about 30% of the time. These conditions are diagnosable and often treatable with spinal endoscopy. Tears that are in the lateral and ventral aspect of the disc are routinely missed by MRI studies (Figure 73.8). Very small disc herniations that protrude past the outer fibers of the annulus are also missed because the fragment may be flattened against the posterior longitudinal ligament or nerve, appearing on the MRI as a thickened or bulged annulus, but really containing a subligamentous herniation. When the nerve root is "swollen" or enlarged, the MRI is not always capable of distinguishing a swollen nerve from a conjoined nerve or a nerve with an adherent fragment of disc. When the disc tissue is in direct contact with the nerve, the nerve can be irritated and a

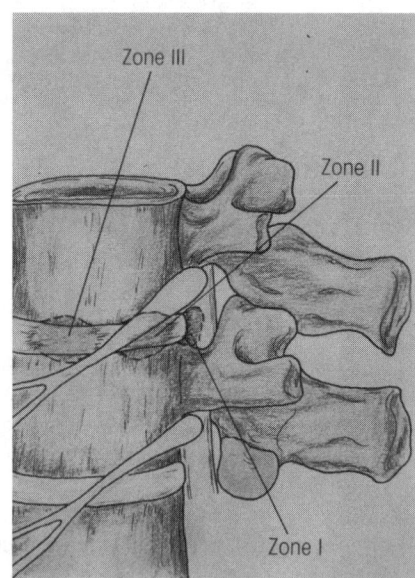

FIGURE 73.8 The three zones of disc herniation and annular tears. Zone III is usually missed on routine imaging studies, often produces nondermatomal symptoms, and is often only identified by evocative discography. Zone III annular tears can cause groin pain at L5–S1, and small extraforaminal disc herniations are difficult to diagnose by physical examination.

painful inflammatory membrane forms. Even an epidural venous plexus that is inflamed can contribute to back pain and sciatica. Anomalous nerve branches known as furcal nerves are never seen on MRI but can be visualized with spinal endoscopy of the foramen.[22,30]

When an inflammatory membrane is present, the patient's pain pattern can be confusing. Diagnostic spinal endoscopy has confirmed "nondermatomal" pain in scores of patients with proximal thigh, buttock, and groin pain at levels distal to the root origin of the anatomic area. Removal of the source of irritation will resolve or improve the patient's pain.

EVOCATIVE DISCOGRAMS

The senior author uses evocative chromo-discography™ as an integral part of spinal endoscopy.[5] The literature on discography is currently considered controversial because of the high interobserver variability by discographers in reporting the patient's subjective pain as well as the ailing patient's ability to give a clear response, especially if the pain response is altered by the use of analgesics or sedation during the procedure. Surgeons who are accomplished in endoscopic spine surgery prefer to do the discography themselves to decrease the interobserver variability interpreting the patient's response. When the surgeon compares his own assessment of the patient's pain response with another discographer's report, there can be some variability in diagnosis and interpretation. This variability may result in unpredictable treatment outcomes. False-positive discography, however, can be significantly decreased in an experienced endoscopic surgeon's hands. The surgeon learns to correlate the patient's response to the discogram pattern of the painful disc the surgeon is treating. There is good correlation of discograms with different types of annular tears and disc herniations. The surgical result can then be predicted on the basis of the visualized condition. For example, the discogram can be used to predict the presence of a collagenized disc fragment versus a soft herniation, the extrusion of a disc fragment as a noncontained herniation, or the presence of the type, grade, and location of a painful versus nonpainful annular tear.

TECHNIQUE

ENDOSCOPIC SPINE SURGERY: THE POSTEROLATERAL APPROACH

The current technique used by the senior author has evolved over a 13-year period beginning in 1991 after learning arthroscopic discectomy from Parviz Kambin. Previously the author had experience in the use of chymopapain, automated percutaneous discectomy, laser discectomy, and discography. The current technique combines the best features of each endoscopic procedure into a visu-

alized method that is described as selective endoscopic discectomy (SED™) and thermal discoplasty and annuloplasty. It continues by incorporating endoscopic foraminoplasty techniques for degenerative conditions of the lumbar spine. The foraminal approach is refined further by a standardized surgical protocol that helps decrease the learning curve. A prospective, Institutional Review Board-approved study of 56 patients undergoing SED and thermal discoplasty by the senior author for conditions ranging from discogenic pain to spondylolisthesis, targeting the pain generator, revealed a satisfactory outcome of 89% by modified MacNab criteria and 91% by patient questionnaire.[8] Surgical results continue to improve, consistent with the refinement of indications and techniques for specific conditions treatable by this endsocopic method.

Accessing the foramen is simplified and standardized by drawing coordinates on the patient's skin to determine the optimal skin window and annular window for positioning the surgical instruments to the center of the disc (Figure 73.9). Reference points are the anatomic center of the disc, the superior facet of the inferior vertebra, and the skin window. The needle trajectory must also be in a line of inclination between the end plates of the adjacent vertebrae. Adjustments in the trajectory will be made to accommodate individual anatomic considerations and the pathology to be accessed. Once the optimal trajectory is established, the cannulas are inserted to allow for endoscopic surgery under direct visualization.

The spinal structures accessible with this technique are the facet joints, the pedicles of the superior and inferior vertebra, the traversing and exiting nerve roots, and the disc annulus. The epidural space is accessible with flexible instruments and special cannulas (Figure 73.3). The posterolateral approach can avoid the spinal canal if desired and does not require the stripping of muscle or ligament to access the disc. A third-generation system, the Yeung Endoscopic Spine System (YESS), features a cannula set with configured openings that allow instruments to exit the cannula for surgical work, while a protruding tongue protects and retracts adjacent structures. The beveled cannula allows visualization of the disc and epidural space at the same time, facilitating the removal of subligamentous, extruded, and sequestered disc fragments. Its configuration also allows for dilation of the disc space for intradiscal surgery. The foramen can be enlarged by foraminoplasty to decompress foramenal and lateral recess stenosis. Adjuvant tools and therapies such as radiofrequency, chymopapain, steroids, intradiscal injections, and laser can be employed for tissue modulation or ablation when the visualized spinal pathology dictates its use.

POSTOPERATIVE CARE

Postoperative management may differ from the typical postoperative program used for disc herniations with

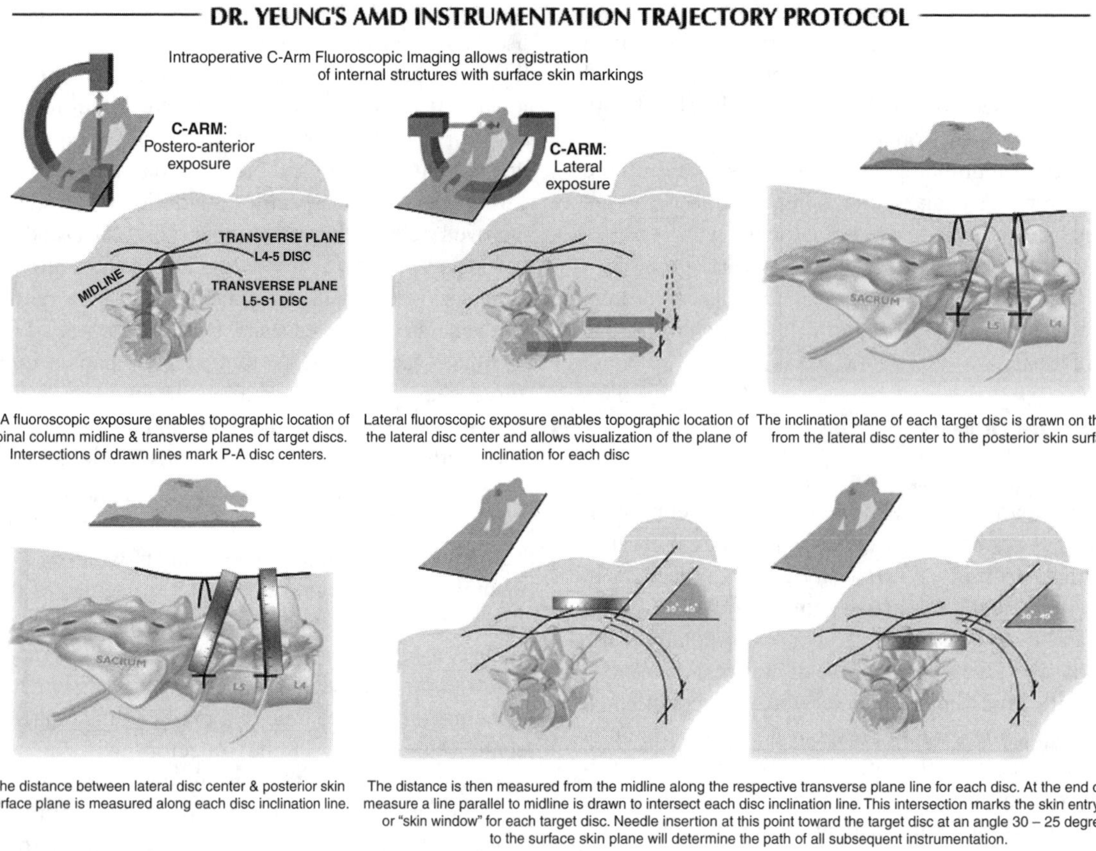

DR. YEUNG'S AMD INSTRUMENTATION TRAJECTORY PROTOCOL

Intraoperative C-Arm Fluoroscopic Imaging allows registration
of internal structures with surface skin markings

C-ARM:
Postero-anterior
exposure

C-ARM:
Lateral
exposure

TRANSVERSE PLANE
L4-5 DISC

MIDLINE

TRANSVERSE PLANE
L5-S1 DISC

SACRUM

LS L4

P-A fluoroscopic exposure enables topographic location of spinal column midline & transverse planes of target discs. Intersections of drawn lines mark P-A disc centers.

Lateral fluoroscopic exposure enables topographic location of the lateral disc center and allows visualization of the plane of inclination for each disc

The inclination plane of each target disc is drawn on the skin from the lateral disc center to the posterior skin surface.

SACRUM

LS L4

30 - 45

30 - 45

The distance between lateral disc center & posterior skin surface plane is measured along each disc inclination line.

The distance is then measured from the midline along the respective transverse plane line for each disc. At the end of this measure a line parallel to midline is drawn to intersect each disc inclination line. This intersection marks the skin entry point or "skin window" for each target disc. Needle insertion at this point toward the target disc at an angle 30 – 25 degrees to the surface skin plane will determine the path of all subsequent instrumentation.

FIGURE 73.9 Determination of optimal instrument path.

radiculopathy. Endoscopic treatment for discogenic back pain often involves multiple levels, and disc segments with extensive circumferential annular tears that involve the entire 360° circumference. This differs from a disc herniation that involves only one quadrant of the annulus that after disc extraction, has a better chance of healing when the disc extrusion no longer acts as a barrier to healing. With an extensive annular delamination and tear, the annulus of the spinal segment must be protected while the collagen of the annulus heals, and only light non-axial loading movement is allowed. After 6 to 8 weeks, gauged by the patient's response to decompression and thermal modulation, a therapeutic exercise program is initiated consisting of lumbar stabilization exercises and MacKenzie extension maneuvers. Ultimately, the goal of mobilization and aerobic conditioning is functional recovery.

PROBLEMS AND COMPLICATIONS

As with arthroscopic knee surgery, the risks of serious complications or nerve injury are low — about 1 to 3% in the senior author's experience.[31] The usual risks of infection, nerve injury, dural tears, bleeding, and scar tissue formation are always present as with any spine surgery. Fenestration past the anterior annulus is a potential hazard creating a bowel or vascular injury. Although this

is a rare complication because the thickness of the anterior annulus will usually prevent fenestration, it must be recognized as a potential risk if the annulus is weakened or fenestrated by an anterior disc herniation. This risk is also present with the posterior approach. One limitation of the endoscopic technique is the need to use some instruments in a "blind" fashion. That is, shavers, pituitary rongeurs, and basket forceps are too large to fit in the working channel of the endoscope, and must be monitored with fluoroscopy. The surgeon must be cognizant of the depth of the instruments and develop a feel for the working instruments while in the disc. The cannulas are designed to protect vital structures by utilizing windows as surgical portals. Spinal nerves may be adherent to the disc and annulus, and can be extracted along with the disc or annulus by shavers or cutting instruments. In addition, the author has identified anomalous autonomic and peripheral nerves in the foramen (furcal nerves), buried in the annular fat, that connect with the sacral plexus or the traversing nerve. These nerves are described in the medical literature and can be symptomatic (Figure 73.10a). The inflammatory membrane may contain tiny nerves and blood vessels that contribute to severe discogenic pain (Figure 73.10b).

Dysesthesia, the most common postoperative complaint, occurs about 5 to 15% of the time but is almost always transient. Its cause is still incompletely understood

(a)

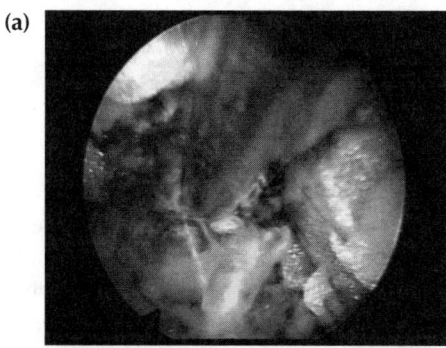

(b)

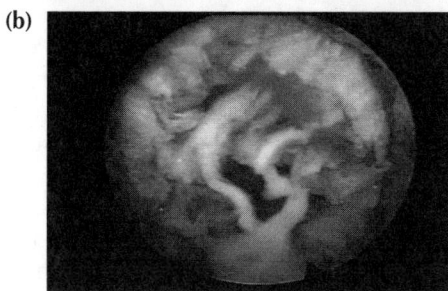

FIGURE 73.10 Anomalous nerves. (a) Anomalous nerve identified in the annular fat in the foramen. When found in the foramen, it is considered an anomalous branch, but furcal nerves are common branches from the exiting nerve entering the psoas muscle. These communicating branches are described as furcal nerves in the anatomy and literature. Small sympathetic nerves are occasionally seen. (b) Neo-angiogenesis and neo-neurogenesis are commonly present in the inflammatory membrane adjacent to annular tears in patients who have severe discogenic pain and sciatica, but a rather benign MRI.

and may be related to nerve recovery, as it can occur days or weeks after surgery, or it may be due to irritation of the dorsal root ganglion. This condition cannot be completely avoided, as neuromonitoring with dermatomal somatosensory evoked potentials (SEP) and continuous electromyography, the most sensitive means of monitoring, has not identified the cause of dysesthesia.[32] The symptoms can be similar to complex regional pain syndrome (CRPS), but less severe, and usually without the skin changes that accompany CRPS. Stimulation of the doral root ganglion of the exiting spinal nerve can also result in dysesthesia when foraminoplasty is performed, even with the exiting nerve clearly identified and protected.

Endoscopic spine surgery has a high learning curve, but is within the grasp of every endoscopic surgeon with proper training. As with any new procedure, the complication rate is higher during the learning curve and may vary with each surgeon's skills and experience. The endoscopic technique, because of its approach, may incur additional risk for iatrogenic injury, but it is possibly safer than traditional surgery for the patient as the patient is awake and able to provide immediate input to the surgeon when pain is generated. The surgeon's ability to perform the surgery without causing the patient undue pain will self-select for surgeons who can master the technique to the extent that the surgeon prefers endsocopic to traditional surgery for the same condition. For most disc herniations and discogenic pain, experienced endoscopic spine surgeons will opt for the endoscopic approach as the treatment of choice for their patients. New neuromonitoring techniques and equipment help warn the surgeon of nerve irritation even when there is no direct contact of surgical instruments with the nerve proper. About 66% of the time, there is EMG activity recorded that warns the surgeon that there is nerve irritation. Neuromonitoring may make the procedure safer, but it has not been demonstrated to be safer than the use of dilute local anesthetic. It is imperative for the surgeon to insist that the anesthesiologist not use general or spinal anesthesia. The senior author requires anesthesiologists to not use propofol or any anesthetic that has the potential for the patient not to feel pain, as the patient's ability to feel pain becomes the surgeon's main safety net. The author also uses only a dilute solution of local anesthetic such as 0.5% lidocaine or its equivalent. The patient's ability to report pain during the procedure will also help the surgeon recognize the pain generators in the spine when the surgeon correlates the production of pain with the anatomy the surgeon is probing.

Frequently observed improvement in nerve conduction latencies and abnormal preoperative EMGs immediately postoperation may help predict the surgical efficacy of each procedure.[32]

ALTERNATIVES TO FUSION FOR THE TREATMENT OF BACK PAIN

Fusion has traditionally been reserved for spinal instability and deformity. More recently, the utilization of spinal instrumentation and intervertebral fusion cages has extended the indications to discogenic pain from internal disc disruption and degenerative disc disease, but, overall, the results remain disappointing; adjacent-level disease remains a problem. Discogenic pain has been discovered to arise primarily from the annulus, but can also involve the end plates (intranuclear herniations), the inflammatory membrane surrounding the annulus, and sensitized tissue surrounding the annulus. Patients with debilitating back pain are currently offered surgical fusion as a treatment option to stabilize the motion segment. However, patients with recurrent, relatively annoying or debilitating pain from annular tears in the lumbar disc may be also be helped by electrothermal treatment. Type III and IV pain nociceptors in the annulus are deformed by heat at 42 to 45°C. When the heat is increased to 65°C, the annulus contracts and thickens. This novel approach, touted in the literature as intradiscal electrothermal therapy (IDET), is limited because of the lack of endoscopic visualization. Patient selection is critical, but even if initially successful in the immediate postoperative period, follow-up studies have reported significant deterioration of results months to years later. A visualized endoscopic variation of the technique, SED and thermal annuloplasty, overcomes some of the pitfalls of the blind technique. The tear is detected by evocative discography. Indigo carmine dye, mixed with a non-ionic contrast material, Isovue 300, stains the degenerative disc and annular tear a light blue. The degenerative disc is removed from the posterior disc quadrant, exposing the annular tear for thermal annuloplasty. When imaging studies identify these lesions as a high intensity zone, there is a high incidence of concordant pain by evocative discography and endoscopic confirmation of a focus of ingrown granulation tissue. This tissue can then be ablated under direct visualization. The senior author's endoscopic version of IDET has converted 80% of IDET failures to satisfactory results.[33] Spinal endoscopy has enabled surgeons to identify interpositional disc tissue as the single most common finding preventing annular tears from healing. Other novel approaches are currently being studied to help the tears heal, as annular modulation may incorporate injection of therapeutic solutions utilizing hypertonic dextrose, glucosamine sulfate, and chondroitin sulfate. These novel approaches deserve study and may provide a viable alternative to fusion as a first line of surgical treatment for debilitating discogenic back pain from annular tears and internal disc disruption. Ultimately, techniques to enhance disc healing, regeneration, or arthroplasty may replace fusion as treatments of choice.

OUTCOMES

The results of percutaneous spine surgery in the literature focus on blind techniques such as laser disc decompression and automated percutaneous lumbar discectomy. The visualized technique, however, as described by Kambin, ranges from 85 to 93% good/excellent in studies with a minimum 2-year follow-up. In a prospective manner, Kambin has also validated the visualized technique as a valuable tool in the armamentarium of a spinal surgeon. When performed in an experienced endoscopic surgeon's hands, Kambin found results equal to a traditional microdisectomy, but with less morbidity and an earlier return to work.[35–37] The high learning curve has curtailed its universal acceptance at this time, but those surgeons willing to invest the time in learning this technique will soon earn the loyalty and acceptance of their patients and referring physicians.

The evolution of endoscopic surgery is enhanced when physicians document their findings by video-imaging and then study the tapes postoperatively. By studying the video of their surgeries in the early part of the learning curve, surgeons will soon learn to associate visualized conditions with their ability to affect those conditions. This will help surgeons evolve their diagnostic and surgical skills faster.

THE AUTHOR'S EXPERIENCE WITH ENDOSCOPIC SPINE SURGERY

Since 1991, the senior author has used a rod–lens system for endoscopic disc excision through a posterolateral approach as described by Parviz Kambin. Kambin coined the term *arthroscopic microdiscectomy* to describe his method of disc removal from the dorsal half of the intervertebral disc using uniportal and biportal techniques. In 1997, a newly designed spinal endoscope (YESS) featured a working channel and multiple inflow and outflow ports. This allowed consistent clear visualization through fluid volume and pressure control, to provide consistent hemostasis. The ability of the surgeon to visualize structures clearly and the concomitant development of flexible instruments to be used with slotted cannulas opened the door for true endoscopic spine surgery and spinal probing in a sedated, but awake patient. From 1991 to 2004, the senior author treated more than 2,400 patients with discogenic pain, degenerative conditions of the lumbar spine, and the whole spectrum of disc herniations including extruded and sequestered fragments. The success rate in the first 500 patients was 432/500 (86%) good/excellent using modified MacNab criteria.[26] A subsequent retrospective study of 219 consecutive patients with radiculopathy secondary to large intracanal noncontained lumbar disc herniations revealed a satisfactory outcome in 204 (93.1%) by modified MacNab criteria, but even higher (94.8%) when patients were asked to respond to a study patient-based outcome questionnaire.[9] The evolving methodology in the treatment of discogenic back pain by SED is reviewed in a prospective study that validates SED as an alternative for a variety of spinal conditions treated by traditional methods (Yeung & Gore, 2001). *The Practice of Minimally Invasive Spinal Technique* is a recent book edited by Martin Savitz, John Chiu, and Anthony Yeung. A journal by the same name has been endorsed by multiple spine specialty societies to bring endoscopic spine surgery into the next millennium.

NEW HORIZONS — THE FUTURE OF ENDOSCOPIC SPINE SURGERY

The learning curve in endoscopic spine surgery is steep compared with knee surgery because surgical misadventures are unforgiving in the spine. Intensive surgical instruction with preceptorship programs has produced small numbers of spinal endoscopists worldwide. It is strongly recommended, however, for further advancement of endoscopic spinal surgery, that a preceptorship be completed before attempting endoscopic spine surgery. Eventually, for further advancement, endoscopic spine surgery may have to be a subspecialization for most surgeons. If young surgeons could obtain their training in their fellowship or post-fellowship program, endoscopic spine surgery would advance faster. For now, the small number of surgeons should hone their endoscopic skills by limiting their indications to contained small, soft disc herniations. With the development of artificial nucleus disc replacements, interest in posterolateral spinal endoscopy is expected to surge, as this represents the best surgical approach for nucleus replacements.

CONCLUSION

The future of endoscopic spine surgery is extremely bright. There will soon be an explosion of new imaging systems, endoscopes, and endoscopic instruments. Refined techniques and image-guided systems may help shorten the learning curve. Coupled with advancements in tissue regeneration and enhancement of tissue healing, and the trend toward tissue healing instead of removal, regeneration over healing, and arthroplasty instead of fusion, the spinal surgeon may no longer have to consider spine surgery as paradoxical. As a treatment modality, it will no longer be considered a last resort in a desperate patient. There will be a paradigm shift in the way we view and approach patients with back pain, especially when endoscopic spinal surgery is further validated with outcome studies and becomes routinely available.

KEY POINTS

1. The endoscopic foraminal posterolateral surgical approach to the lumbar disc offers the least trauma to normal anatomy.
2. Spinal endoscopy offers expanded diagnostic as well as therapeutic benefits not possible with traditional surgery.
3. Spinal endoscopy is a complement to interventional pain management, and techniques are beginning to merge.
4. New terminology and concepts, evocative discography, evocative chromo-discography, selective endoscopic discectomy, and thermal annuloplasty, are introduced and explained in the text.
5. The learning curve is steep, but once mastered, this approach will revolutionize surgical treatment of the lumbar disc, and provide the delivery system for emerging technology in tissue repair and regeneration.

REFERENCES

1. Yeung, A. T. (2001a). Endoscopic spinal surgery: What future role? *Journal of Musculoskeletal Medicine, 18*(11), 518–528.
2. Yeung, A. T. (2000, June). Minimally invasive disc surgery with the Yeung endoscopic spine system (YESS). *Surgical Technology International, 8,* 267–277.
3. Yeung, A. T., & Yeung, C. A. (2003). Advances in endoscopic disc and spine surgery: Foraminal approach. *Surgical Technology International, 11,* 253–261.
4. Yeung, A. T. (2004, January 20–30). Discography, foraminal epidurography and therapeutic foraminal injections: Its role in endoscopic spine surgery. *International 22nd Course for Percutaneous Endoscopic Spinal Surgery and Complementary Techniques.* Zurich, Switzerland.
5. Yeung, A. T. (2000). The role of provocative discography in endoscopic disc surgery. In M. H. Savitz, J. Chiu, & A. T. Yeung (Eds.), *The practice of minimally invasive spinal technique* (pp. 231–236). Richmond, VA: AAMISMS Education.
6. Yeung, A. T., & Porter, J. (2002). Minimally invasive endoscopic surgery for the treatment of lumbar discogenic pain. In R. Weiner (Ed.), *Pain management: A practical guide for clinicians* (5th ed., pp. 1073–1078). Boca Raton, FL: CRC Press.
7. Yeung, A. T. (2003, October 21–25). Endoscopic decompressive approaches to the disc. North American Spine Society Annual Meeting Symposium: Minimally Invasive Surgical Treatments of Spinal Pathologies: A Rational Approach. San Diego, CA.
8. Yeung, A. T., & Gore, S. A. (2001). Evolving methodology in treating discogenic back pain by selective endoscopic discectomy (SED). *Journal of Minimally Invasive Spinal Technique, 1,* 8–16.
9. Tsou, P. M., & Yeung, A. T. (2002). Transforaminal endoscopic decompression for radiculopathy secondary to intracanal noncontained lumbar disc herniations: Outcome and technique. *Spine Journal, 2*(1), 41–48.
10. Yeung, A. T., & Tsou, P. M. (2002). Posterolateral endoscopic excision for lumbar disc herniation: Surgical technique, outcome, and complications in 307 consecutive cases. *Spine, 27*(7), 722–731.
11. Savitz, S. I., Savitz, M. H., & Yeung, A. T. (2001). Antibiotic prophylaxis for percutaneous discectomy. *Journal of Minimally Invasive Spinal Technique, 1,* 49–51.
12. Yeung, A. T. (2001, January 25–26). Endoscopic access for degenerative disorders of the lumbar spine. International Society for Minimal Intervention in Spinal Surgery – 19th Course for Percutaneous Spinal Surgery and Complementary Techniques. Zurich, Switzerland.
13. Osman, S. G. et al. (1997). Transforaminal and posterior decompressions of the lumbar spine. A comparative study of stability and intervertebral foramen area. *Spine, 22*(15), 1690–1695.
14. Tsou, P. M., Yeung, A. T., & Yeung, C. A. (2004). Posterolateral transforaminal selective endoscopic discectomy and thermal annuloplasty for chronic lumbar discogenic pain. *Spine Journal, 4*(5), 564–573.

15. Yeung, A. T. (1998). Arthroscopic electro-thermal surgery for discogenic low back pain: A preliminary report. International Intradiscal Therapy Society Annual Meeting. San Antonio, Texas.

16. Yeung, A. T. (1998, December 12). Classification and electro-thermal treatment of annular tears. American Back Society Annual Meeting. Las Vegas, NV.

17. Yeung, A. T. (1999, August 1–5). Annular tears: Correlating discogram and endoscopic findings with electro-thermal response. International Intradiscal Therapy Society and International Society for Minimally Invasive Spine Surgery Annual Meeting. Cambridge, England.

18. Yeung, A. T. (1999, July 8–10). Endoscopic thermal modulation as an alternative to fusion for discogenic pain. International Meeting for Advanced Spine Technologies. Vancouver, British Columbia, Canada.

19. Yeung, A. T. (1999, November 5–8). Patho-anatomy of discogenic pain. In *Minimally Invasive Spine Update.* 1999. Disney Magic Cruise.

20. Yeung, A. T. (2000, December 7–10). Thermal modulation of disc pathology. 1st World Congress American Academy of Minimally Invasive Spinal Medicine and Surgery. Las Vegas, NV.

21. Yeung, A. T. (2000, December 7–10). Thermal modulation: SED versus IDET. 1st World Congress American Academy of Minimally Invasive Spinal Medicine and Surgery. Las Vegas, NV.

22. Yeung, A. T. (2003, April 2–5). Macro- and micro-anatomy of degenerative conditions of the lumbar spine (Best Paper Presentation Award). International Intradiscal Therapy Society 16th Annual Meeting. Chicago, IL.

23. Yeung, A. T. et al. (2000). Intradiscal thermal therapy for discogenic low back pain. In M. H. Savitz, J. Chiu, & A. T. Yeung (Eds.), *The practice of minimally invasive spinal technique.* Richmond, VA: AAMISMS Education.

24. Yeung, A. T., & Savitz, M. H. (2002). Treatment of multi-level lumbar disc disease by selective endoscopic discectomy and thermal annuloplasty: Case report. *Journal of Minimally Invasive Spinal Technique, 2*(Spring), 36–38.

25. Yeung, A. T., & Yeung, C. A. (in press). Microtherapy in low back pain. In M. Mayer (Ed.), *Minimally invasive spine surgery.* Berlin: Springer Verlag.

26. Yeung, A. T. (2000). The evolution of percutaneous spinal endoscopy and discectomy: State of the art. *Mt. Sinai Journal of Medicine, 67*(4), 327–332.

27. Yeung, A. T. (2000). Selective discectomy with the Yeung endoscopic spine system. In M. H. Savitz, J. Chiu & A. T. Yeung (Eds.), *The practice of minimally invasive spinal technique* (pp. 115–122). Richmond, VA: AAMISMS Education.

28. Yeung, A. T. (2002). Minimal invasive techniques in the lumbar spine: Evolving methodology since 1991 (Magistral speaker). International 20th Jubilee Course for Percutaneous Endoscopic Spinal Surgery and Complementary Techniques. Zurich, Switzerland.

29. Yeung, A.T. (2002). Transforaminal endoscopic selective nuclectomy and annuloplasty for chronic lumbar discogenic pain: An alternative to fusion. Spine Arthroplasty II Spine Arthroplasty Society. Montpellier, France, May 5–8.

30. Yeung, A. T. (2003, July 27–31). Rauschning's anatomy for minimally invasive spine surgery. *Spine Across the Sea* Conference.

31. Yeung, A. T., & Savitz, M. H. (2004). Complications of percutaneous spinal surgery. In A. Vacarro (Ed.), *Complications in adult and pediatric spine surgery.*

32. Yeung, A. T., Porter, J., & Merican, C. (2001, December). SEP as a sensory integrity check in selective endoscopic discectomy using the Yeung endoscopic spine system. 2nd World Congress American Academy of Minimally Invasive Spinal Medicine and Surgery. Las Vegas, NV.

33. Yeung, A. T. (2001). Factors affecting IDET Outcome: An edoscopic analysis of IDET. Western Orthopedic Association Annual Meeting. 2001. San Francisco, CA.

34. Hermantin, F. U., Peters, T., Quararo, L., & Kambin, P. (1999). A prospective, randomized study comparing the results of open discectomy with those of video-assisted arthroscopic microdiscectomy. *Journal of Bone and Joint Surgery* (America), *81*(7), 958–965.

35. Kambin, P. (1991). Posterolateral percutaneous lumbar discectomy and decompression: Arthroscopic microdiscectomy. In P. Kambin (Ed.), *Arthroscopic microdiscectomy: Minimal intervention in spinal surgery* (pp. 67–100). Baltimore: Urban & Schwarzenberg.

36. Kambin, P., Gennarelli, T., & Hermantin. F. (1998). Minimally invasive techniques in spinal surgery: Current practice. *Neurosurgery Focus, 4,* 1.

37. Kambin, P., O'Brien, E., Zhou, L. et al. (1998). Arthroscopic microdiscectomy and selective fragmentectomy. *Clinical Orthopaedics and Related Research, 347,* 150–167.

RECOMMENDED READING

Aprill, C., & Boduk, N. (1992). High intensity zone: A diagnostic sign of painful lumbar disc on magnetic resonance imaging. *British Journal of Radiology, 65,* 361–369.

Freemont, A. J. (1997). Nerve ingrowth into diseased intervertebral disc in chronic back pain. *Lancet, 350,* 178–181.

Javid, M. J., Nordby, E. J., Ford, L. T. et al. (1983). Safety and efficacy of chymopapain in herniated nucleus pulposus with sciatica. *Journal of the American Medical Association, 249,* 2489–2494.

Jensen, M. C. et al. (1994). Magnetic resonance imaging of the lumbar spine in people without back pain. *New England Journal of Medicine, 331,* 69–73.

Kuslich, S. D. (1990). Microsurgical lumbar nerve root decompression utilizing progressive local anesthesia. In W. Williams, J. McCullouch, & P. Young (Eds.), *Microsurgery of the lumbar spine.* Rockville, MD: Aspen.

Matthews, H. H., & Long, B. H. (2003). Posterior minimally invasive techniques. In *Principles and practice of spine surgery* (pp. 288–294). Philadelphia: Mosby.

Osti, O. L., Vernon-Roberts, B., Moore, R., & Fraser, R. D. (1992). Annular tears and disc degeneration in the lumbar spine. A post mortem. *Journal of Bone and Joint Surgery* (Britain), *74*(5), 678–682.

Saal, J. A., & Saal, J. S. (2000). Intradiscal eletrothermal treatment for chronic discogenic low back pain: A prospective outcome study with minimum 1-year follow-up. *Spine, 25*(20), 2622–2627.

Sachs, B,, Vanharanta, H., Spivey, M. A. et al. (1987). Dallas discogram description: A new classification of CT/discography in low back pain disorders. *Spine, 12*(3), 287–94.

Savitz, M. H., Chiu, J. C., & Yeung, A. T. (2000). *The practice of minimally invasive spinal technique.* Richmond, VA: AAMISMS Education.

Schaffer, J., & Kambin, P. (1991). Percutaneous posterolateral lumbar discectomy and compression with 6.9 millimeter cannula: Analysis of operative failures and complications. *Journal of Bone and Joint Surgery, 73*, 882

Schellhas, K. P. et al. (1996). Lumbar disc high intensity zone: Correlation of magnetic resonance imaging and discography. *Spine, 21*, 79–86.

Yeung, A. T. (1999, June). Minimally invasive disc surgery with the Yeung endoscopic spine system (YESS). Surgical Technology International, *8*, 267–277.

74

Spinal Cord Stimulation

Milan P. Stojanovic, MD, and Salahadin Abdi, MD, PhD

INTRODUCTION

Spinal cord stimulation (SCS), also known as "dorsal column stimulation," is a common mode of neuromodulation technique used for the treatment of a variety of pain syndromes — e.g., failed back surgery syndrome (FBSS), complex regional pain syndrome, postherpetic neuralgia, peripheral vascular disease, and diabetic neuropathy. The SCS implantation involves placement of the stimulating electrodes in the epidural space. The SCS lead is connected to the subcutaneously internalized pulse generator (IPG) and the internal or external power source. Generally, an SCS screening trial is performed before permanent SCS implantation.

SCS has recently gained in popularity for treatment of chronic low back pain. SCS is minimally invasive and is reversible as opposed to nerve ablation. The recent improvements in hardware design have made implantation techniques simpler and prolonged equipment longevity. Stimulation trials become less invasive, allowing patients to test its effects before final implantation. The scientific evidence has shown better outcomes of SCS in comparison with other modalities for treatment of some forms of low back pain.

Up until 10 years ago, the SCS was considered as the last treatment option, "only when everything else failed." However, the current practice of many clinicians is to utilize this mode of treatment earlier in the course of the above-mentioned pain syndromes. In fact, SCS can arguably be the best treatment option in some forms of chronic low back pain, such as FBSS, considering the relative low cost of the trials, low risk/benefit ratio, and positive outcome studies.

One can argue that the SCS trial and possible permanent implant may have better long-term risk/benefit ratio than the trial of chronic opioid therapy. Although many studies support opioid therapy for nonmalignant pain, no long-term studies on iatrogenic addiction rate with chronic opioid treatments have been published.

HISTORY

Humans opened an era of SCS, by utilizing the electrical power of torpedo fish, in 600 B.C. The first attempts of brain electrical stimulation were reported in 1874. However, the first implantation of brain electrodes was performed in 1948 for treatment of psychiatric disorder. Many attempts to use electrical central nervous system (CNS) stimulation for treatment of pain emerged in 1950s and 1960s. Based on the gate theory of pain proposed by Melzack and Wall,[1] Shealy et al.[2] introduced SCS in 1967. Initial SCS procedures involved open intrathecal implantation of electrodes via laminotomy. The lack of adequate hardware and the paucity of clinical outcome studies significantly slowed the development of neurostimulation in the 1970s.

Recently, the hardware technology has substantially improved. The development of minimally invasive percutaneous stimulation trials enabled a variety of patients with low back pain to test SCS. Electrodes have become smaller and easier to navigate through the epidural space. Internal pulse generators have new programming capabilities and longer battery lifespan.

ANATOMY AND HARDWARE

For chronic low back pain treatment, the SCS electrode leads are placed in thoracic epidural space, with a lead tip location at the T8–T10 level. An electrical field from the SCS lead acts on the dorsal columns of the spinal cord and modulates its pain transmission. The anatomical position of the SCS lead can influence the pain relief and SCS "coverage." Holsheimer et al.[3] measured the thickness of cerebrospinal fluid (CSF) layers in thoracic areas corresponding to SCS electrodes placement and correlated results with paresthesia perception from SCS coverage. They concluded that the thickness of the dorsal CSF layer is the main factor determining the perception threshold and paresthesia coverage in spinal cord stimulation: an increasing CSF layer thickness raises the threshold and reduces the coverage, and vice versa. In the same study, the effects of an asymmetrical electrode position with respect to the spinal cord midline were also analyzed by computer modeling. It is concluded that a lateral asymmetry of less than 1 mm gives a significant reduction of perception threshold and may result in unilateral SCS coverage.

The same group of investigators using magnetic resonance imaging (MRI) found that spinal cord midline and vertebral midline are apart by at least 1 to 2 mm in all levels investigated in 40% of patients. Adequate symmetrical SCS coverage of low back and lower extremity is in many cases difficult to achieve. Barolat et al.[4] found that only 27% of paresthesia was felt symmetrically when the stimulating contacts were perfectly located at the radiological midline.

The permanent SCS hardware consists of SCS lead, an extension cable, a power source, and a pulse generator. Many leads contain a removable stylet, which eases lead steering during implantation. The lead design varies in the number of electrodes from four (Medtronic and Advanced Neuromodulation Systems, ANS) to eight (ANS). The distance between the electrodes and the length of the leads also can differ. It is not clear if an increased number of electrodes provides better coverage, but it might be beneficial in case of lead migration. The leads with minimal space between electrodes (such as Medtronic Quad compact lead) might be better suited for isolated axial low back pain without radiating component to the lower extremity.

There are two types of pulse generators: (1) the completely implantable pulse generator (IPG) containing a battery and (2) IPG supplied by external power through a radiofrequency antenna applied to the skin. The implanted pulse generator is more convenient to use and can be easily adjusted by the patient using a small telemetry device. Patients can turn the stimulator on and off and control the stimulation amplitude, frequency, and pulse width. A separate external programmer allows for more complex IPG reprogramming by the physician. In case of inadequate stimulation, the physician can change polarity and number of functioning electrodes in order to provide better stimulation coverage. The batteries have to be changed every 3 to 6 years, which requires a brief visit to the operating room. The battery life depends on how many hours a day the system is used and the intensity of the stimulation. The externally powered IPG has an advantage over the implanted one in patients requiring higher amplitudes of stimulation, which would deplete the implanted batteries in a short period of time.

The permanent SCS implant can be achieved by placing the percutaneous lead via epidural needle or "paddle" lead via open laminotomy. The configuration of SCS electrodes varies in these two techniques. Percutaneous electrodes are the same configuration as the ones used for stimulation trial. Paddle electrodes are larger, and can be anchored directly to the dura, potentially minimizing migration.

PATHOPHYSIOLOGY AND MECHANISM OF ACTION

The basic foundation for initial SCS trials was Melzak and Wall's gate control theory.[1] Their theory proposed that stimulation of Aβ-fibers modulates the dorsal horn "gate" and thus reduces the nociceptive input from periphery. Indeed, several studies demonstrated that dorsal horn neuronal activity caused by peripheral noxious stimuli could be inhibited by concomitant stimulation of the dorsal columns.[5] However, it seems that other mechanisms may play a more significant role in the mechanisms of action of SCS.[6,7]

Many animal studies have shown a suppressive effect of SCS on tactile allodynia, which is mediated via Aβ-fibers[8] and represents a state of central hyperexcitability.[9] Allodynic animals have lower extracellular levels of γ-aminobutyric acid (GABA), and that GABA antagonists abolish the allodynia suppressive effect of SCS indicates that one of the proposed mechanisms of actions of SCS is augmenting the dorsal horn inhibitory action of the GABAergic system.[9–11] Furthermore, intrathecal administration of $GABA_B$ agonist, baclofen, enhances the antinociceptive action of SCS in an animal model of neuropathic pain.[12] In humans, the intrathecal baclofen infusion produces significant augmentation of SCS effects.[13] Future studies must clarify if concomitant use of SCS and intrathecal $GABA_B$ agonists may have a synergistic effect in treating certain forms of neuropathic pain.

Apart from that, several other putative mechanisms may be responsible for the pain relief induced by SCS. Recent animal and human studies revealed a potential role of adenosine in mechanisms of action of SCS. Intrathecal administration of adenosine$_A$ receptor agonist was found to have potentiating effect with SCS and also synergistic effect with baclofen.[6] The disinhibition of descending analgesia pathways originating in periaqueductal gray and the release of serotonin and substance P can be other explanations for the mechanism of actions of SCS.[14,15]

SCS may abolish peripheral ischemic pain by rebalancing the oxygen demand and supply and preventing ischemia.[7] At low levels of stimulation, SCS may act by suppressing the sympathetic activity via α-adrenoreceptors. However, at increased levels of stimulation, the nitric oxide–dependent release of calcitonin gene-related peptide (CGRP) may be more responsible for the vasodilatation effect.[16] Better survival of skin flaps during SCS seems to be due to the CGRP-mediated mechanism.[17] However, recent studies utilizing Doppler imaging did not reveal any changes in peripheral blood flow despite good SCS effects.[18]

Patients with end-stage myocardial ischemia respond well to SCS. Many possible explanations exist for SCS mechanism of action in myocardial ischemia. The most likely mechanism for pain relief consists of redistribution of the coronary blood flow from regions with normal perfusion in favor of regions with impaired myocardial perfusion.[19] The anti-ischemic effect of SCS was shown by coronary blood flow measurements and positron emission tomography. Other lines of evidence show that modulation of the intrinsic cardiac nervous system might contribute to the therapeutic effects of SCS in patients with angina pectoris.[20] In this proposed mechanism, SCS may suppress the excitatory effects of myocardial ischemia on intrinsic cardiac neurons.

The effects of SCS on human brain activity were studied using functional magnetic resonance imaging. The SCS produced increased activity in human somatosensory cortex (SI and SII areas), contralateral to the side of pain and cingulate gyri. The somatosensory cortex activation becomes more pronounced with increased SCS activity.[21] These brain areas activated by SCS correspond to CNS pain pathways involved in processing of somatosensory (SI, SII) and affective components (cingulate gyri) of pain. Further research may better define the role of higher CNS structures during SCS.

RATIONALE

SCS is not a neurodestructive procedure, as opposed to neuroablation. Thus, its effects are easily reversible. The relative low invasiveness of SCS trial (similar invasiveness as an epidural catheter placement) makes SCS the treatment of choice for certain forms of low back pain. In the long term, this treatment modality can be more cost-effective than conservative treatment options. Many studies have confirmed good outcomes of SCS for low back pain and highlighted its advantages over repeat back surgery.

INDICATIONS

FAILED BACK SURGERY SYNDROME

FBSS is the most common indication for SCS placement in the United States.[22] It is defined as persistent pain after attempted surgical treatment for low back pain. FBSS occurs in 20 to 40% of more than 200,000 American patients who undergo lumbar spine surgery each year.[23] In patients who have failed medical management, physical therapy, and nerve blocks, SCS may be the best treatment choice. Many studies support the role of SCS in these patients, emphasizing its advantages over reoperation.[24]

LOW BACK PAIN AND LUMBAR RADICULOPATHY

Surgically naive patients who are poor candidates for surgery may respond well to SCS. The chronic radicular pain in these patients is often of neuropathic origin. However, it is important to rule out other sources of pathology (e.g., facet disease, internal disc disruption, piriformis syndrome, myofascial pain) before choosing SCS.

AXIAL VERSUS RADICULAR PAIN

Traditionally, patients with a radiating pattern of pain to the leg seem to respond better to SCS than patients with isolated axial low back pain.[23,25,26] Further, axial low back pain in combination with bilateral leg pain responds well to SCS.[27–29]

COMPLEX REGIONAL PAIN SYNDROME

Complex regional pain syndrome (CRPS), previously known as reflex sympathetic dystrophy and causalgia, was first described by Mitchell in 1864.[30] CRPS I and II respond well to SCS with reported effectiveness ranging from 50 to 91%.[31–33] Typically, patients with upper or lower extremity pain are the best candidates. In a randomized trial by Kemler et al.[33] patients with CRPS who received SCS treatment and physical therapy had better improvement (56% success rate) than patients who received physical therapy alone. A 2-year follow-up in the same study confirmed the long-term benefits.[34]

It seems that a subgroup of patients with neuropathic pain (sympathetically dependent/maintained pain) respond better to SCS than patients with sympathetically independent pain. Recent study by Hord et al.[35] reports that patients with good response to sympathetic block before SCS are more likely to have a positive response during their SCS trial and long-term pain relief after placement of a permanent SCS device.[35] Therefore, the SCS is an excellent treatment option in carefully selected patients with CRPS. However, SCS should be combined with other treatment modalities in a multidisciplinary setting.

DIABETIC NEUROPATHY

SCS is effective treatment for certain cases of diabetic neuropathy. It can provide pain relief and possibly help in salvaging the affected limb. Because of a higher infection risk, special precautions in patients with diabetic neuropathy should be used when SCS implantation is anticipated.[36] The patients with an increase in transcutaneous oxygen tension (TcpO$_2$) during SCS trial seem to respond better to SCS.[37]

POSTHERPETIC NEURALGIA

Although the scientific evidence on the efficacy of SCS for postherpetic neuralgia is scarce, a recent European study shows excellent outcomes with this modality.[38] To date, SCS treatment of postherpetic neuralgia is considered investigational in United States. Further randomized studies are needed to better establish a role for SCS in postherpetic neuralgia.

OTHER NEUROPATHIC PAIN STATES

Other neuropathic pain pathologies such as deafferentation pain (e.g., phantom-limb pain) and spinal cord injury do not seem to respond well to SCS, most likely due to a cortical reorganization in these painful conditions.

PERIPHERAL VASCULAR DISEASE

Peripheral vascular disease in nonsurgical candidates is currently one of the most common indications for SCS implantation in Europe. Several studies reported excellent pain relief with SCS in these patients, ranging from 60 to 100%. Besides providing pain relief, SCS may increase the peripheral blood flow, promote ulcer healing, and potentially contribute to limb salvage. Studies have shown that an increase in TcpO$_2$ during the first 2 weeks post-implantation predicts future limb salvage. Additionally, ischemic ulcers of less than 3 cm^2 are likely to heal with SCS treatment.[39–42]

CORONARY ARTERY DISEASE

Coronary artery disease with anginal pain responds well to SCS.[43] The best indication for SCS trial is angina refractory to pharmacologic and surgical treatments. Patients with ischemic heart disease treated with SCS demonstrated an increase in exercise capacity, reduction in anginal complaints, decreased use of short-acting nitrates, and improved quality of life. In 60% of the patients, SCS was effective 5 years after implantation and more than 80% patients benefited from SCS for at least 1 year.[44]

In a randomized trial setting, SCS proved advantageous to coronary artery bypass surgery in certain patients with severe angina pectoris.[45] More studies are needed to support this treatment modality for the use in anginal pain in United States.

The fear of potentially masking myocardial ischemia does not seem to be justified, as SCS does not completely abolish anginal pain, but only raises the anginal threshold. It is also important to point out that it does not seem

to affect left ventricular ejection fraction or cardiac arrhythmias.[46]

CONTRAINDICATIONS

Severe psychiatric diseases present major contraindications for SCS implantation. Before SCS implantation, a psychological evaluation of the patient is recommended. One should use caution in SCS placement in patients with cervical and thoracic spinal canal stenosis. This applies in particular to dual-lead systems. Infection, drug abuse, and coagulopathies are also contraindications for SCS placement.

TECHNIQUE

STIMULATION TRIAL

A stimulation trial is warranted before proceeding with permanent SCS implantation. The percutaneous SCS trial is a minimally invasive procedure and can positively predict a long-term outcome in 50 to 70% of cases. The trial allows patients to evaluate the SCS analgesic activity in their everyday surroundings. The criteria for a successful trial include at least a 50% reduction in pain intensity, a decrease in analgesic intake, and significant functional improvement.

There is no consensus on technical approach and the length of an SCS trial. Minimal trial time should be 24 hours, although many centers perform 3- to 5-day trials. The initial inpatient trial allows for proper SCS adjustment after which the patient is discharged home for several days of "home" trial. In cases of equivocal results, the trial time can be extended.

There are two technical approaches for SCS trials. In the first approach, the SCS lead is placed percutaneously. Once the trial is completed, the lead is removed. At a later date, a new lead and internal pulse generator (IPG) are placed. The other approach is to tunnel and anchor the trial lead via surgical incision and to later internalize it for permanent SCS placement. This approach simplifies the final procedure and assures that stimulation coverage remains the same during both the trial period and permanent implantation. Its major disadvantage is the need for a second visit to the operating room for lead removal, in case of an unsuccessful trial. The advantage of a percutaneous trial is its minimal invasiveness, with similar low risk of complications as in routine epidural catheter placement.

The percutaneous trial followed by lead placement via laminectomy is another, less frequently used approach for SCS. In this case a lead with wider electrodes is placed via laminotomy during permanent implantation. Wider electrodes might provide better coverage in certain

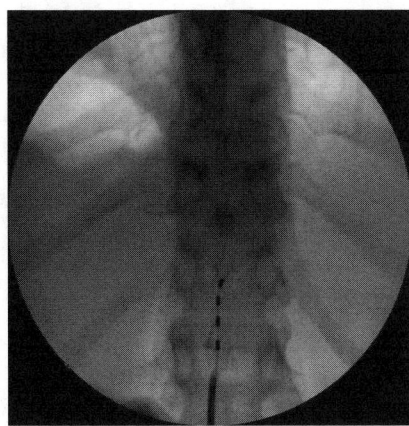

FIGURE 74.1 Anteroposterior fluoroscopic view of the position of percutaneously placed SCS lead. The lead electrodes are positioned at T12–L1 level.

patients and are less prone to migration in comparison with standard SCS leads.[47]

IMPLANTATION TECHNIQUES

The patient is placed in prone position, with a pillow under the abdomen, to facilitate approach to the epidural space. Both trial and permanent implantation are performed under local anesthesia with light intravenous sedation. The most common entry sites for the lumbar area are the T12–L1 or L1–L2 spinal interspaces.

For the cervical area, the entry sites at T1–T2 or spinal levels in close proximity are recommended. Alternatively, the entry site can be in lumbar (T12–L1) area and a long SCS lead can be treaded up to the cervical levels.

True anteroposterior (AP) fluoroscopic images are obtained, making sure that the spinous processes are placed midline to the pedicles. The needle entry site is just lateral to the spinous process. The epidural space is identified by loss of resistance technique. It is recommended that the lateral fluoroscopic views be checked during needle insertion, in order to assess the needle depth. The SCS lead is inserted into the epidural space under continuous fluoroscopic guidance. The curved lead tip can facilitate desired lead positioning and treading (Figure 74.1). The goal is to position the lead midline to the spinous process or to its lateral margin if unilateral coverage is intended. This is verified with fluoroscopic image

in the AP view. A too-lateral position of SCS lead can cause SCS lead dislodgement to the lateral or even anterior epidural space and, consequently, inadequate coverage. It is noteworthy to mention that some cases of lumbar radiculopathy may require SCS lead placement directly through the neural foramina (retrograde lead placement).[48]

Once adequate lead position is obtained (Table 74.1), the trial stimulation is performed. It is important that stimulation paresthesias provide at least 70 to 80% overlap with the patient's pain location. At the end of the procedure, it is recommended that the lateral views be saved to assure epidural placement (Figure 74.2 and Figure 74.3).

The permanent stimulator placement technique is similar to the trial. While the trial is usually done in the pain clinic setting, permanent SCS placement is reserved for the operating room. Under local anesthesia and intravenous sedation, skin incision is made along the lumbar insertion site where the stimulator lead is placed and anchored to the skin. A separate subcutaneous pocket is made for a pulse generator in the gluteal or abdominal area. The SCS lead is then connected with the IPG through an extension cable tunneled through the skin. The skin and subcutaneous tissues are closed in layers.

Patients should avoid any extreme activity for the first 6 to 8 weeks following permanent SCS implantation to prevent lead migration and to allow for epidural scar tissue formation.

During trial and permanent lead implantation, care should be taken to obtain the best possible pain coverage ("sweet spot placement"). The SCS topographic coverage depends on the spinal level where the SCS lead tip is positioned. For low back pain and lower extremity pain the T8–10 levels are recommended; however, there is a high intersubject variation in these guidelines.

CLINICAL EFFECTIVENESS

There is substantial scientific evidence on the efficacy of SCS for treatment of low back and lower extremity pain of neuropathic nature. Clinical studies have revealed from 50 to 70% success rates with certain methods of SCS.[23,49–51] Those studies have shown decreased pain intensity scores, functional improvement, and decreased medication use with SCS treatment. The main drawback

TABLE 74.1
Recommended Anatomical SCS Lead Placement

Pain Location	Upper Extremity	Lower Extremity	Foot	Low Back	Chest	Pelvic Pain
Recommended SCS lead tip placement	C2–C5	T9–T10	T11–L1	T8–T10	T1–T3	S2–S4

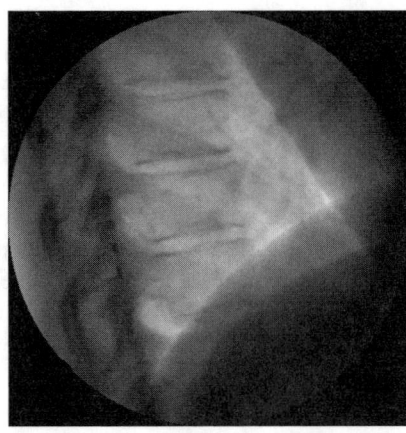

FIGURE 74.2 Lateral fluoroscopic view of properly positioned SCS lead in thoracic area.

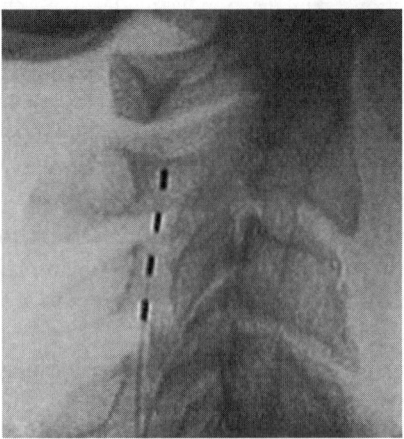

FIGURE 74.3 Cervical SCS lead in lateral fluoroscopic view.

of neurostimulation is a decrease in its effectiveness over time, as seen in 20 to 40% of patients. It seems that this "tolerance" to treatment is due to reorganization of CNS (CNS plasticity) that takes place in neuropathic pain states. Anecdotal evidence suggests that not using the SCS continuously (e.g., shutting it off overnight) may decrease the development of tolerance.

North et al.[24] reported that patients with FBSS respond better to SCS than to reoperation. According to the literature, the success rate of treating FBSS using SCS varies from 12 to 88%, with higher efficacy reported in recent studies.[27,52,53] A systematic review of literature by Turner et al.[54] revealed that an average of 59% of patients with FBSS treated with SCS had ≥50% pain relief. The average complication rate in the same study was 42% and was related to mainly minor complications. Besides pain relief, the SCS improves functional status in a significant number of patients, with a 25% return-to-work rate[27] and up to 61% improvement in activities of daily living.[55] Moreover, the reduced consumption of analgesics with SCS treatment varies from 40 to 84% in published reports.[50,56] It is critical to utilize an appropriate psychological screening

test to appropriately select patients who might benefit from the procedure. Certain psychological tests have been shown to correlate with outcomes to SCS.[57]

Although SCS is an excellent treatment choice for patients with FBSS,[28,58] more studies are needed to further narrow the patient selection criteria and improve long-term success rates.

COST-EFFECTIVENESS AND OUTCOMES

If compared with the more conservative treatments, such as medical regimens and physical therapy, SCS may appear costly. However, the overall cost of SCS can actually be lower than conservative management costs, provided a good outcome is achieved. If taken together, the cost of medications, emergency room visits, multiple physician visits, radiological workups, and absence from work can easily surpass the cost of an SCS implant. Bell et al.[59] have shown that for those patients for whom SCS is clinically efficacious, the SCS pays for itself within 2.1 years.

COMPLICATIONS AND TROUBLESHOOTING

SCS complications can be divided into surgical complications and hardware complication. The most common surgical complication is infection. Wound hematoma and seroma are the other commonly encountered surgical complications. Turner et al.[54] performed a meta-analysis of SCS for FBSS publications and found the incidence of infection and other surgical complications to be 5 and 9%, respectively. The authors further report that hardware complications — lead migration, lead failure, and pulse generator failure — to be 7, 2, and 24%, respectively. As Turner et al.'s study analyzed publications that used old hardware systems, we speculate this incidence to be much lower with the current hardware system. Nevertheless, we see much lower complication rates with SCS in our institution.

SURGICAL COMPLICATIONS

Bleeding at the IPG site (subcutaneous hematoma) is usually self-limiting and gradually reabsorbs in a few weeks. Frequent observation of the hematoma is important because hematoma can lead to infection.

Antibiotic prophylaxis regimens for SCS vary. The minimal prophylaxis should consist of preoperative antibiotic coverage (Cefazolin 1 g intravenously). However, at many institutions prophylactic antibiotics are given up to 10 days post-implantation. Obtaining a complete blood count with differential and sedimentation rate is important to rule out infection. Although not proven advantageous, some centers obtain a urine specimen for culture 3 to 10 days before anticipated implantation.

Other clinical signs of infection are increased temperature and tenderness at incision site. Redness, swelling, and discharge at insertion site can also occur. If infection occurs at the IPG insertion site, one should make sure to first aspirate the site for cultures before initiating antibiotic coverage and removing the hardware.

INADEQUATE COVERAGE OR SCS MALFUNCTION

In case of SCS malfunction, one should obtain AP and lateral fluoroscopic images of the SCS lead tip, IPG, and all connections to rule out lead migration, breakage, or disconnection. If the cause is not found by fluoroscopy, one should analyze the IPG using the programmer. The battery status and impedance of each electrode in relation to the IPG should be checked. Exactly the same impedance of two electrodes raises a possibility of a short circuit between the two electrodes, most commonly located at the connector or IPG site. Some mechanical failures might require surgical revision and replacement of affected SCS components.

DECREASE IN STIMULATION AMPLITUDE

The decreased stimulation threshold can be caused by intrathecal migration of the SCS lead. If migration stays unnoticed, it can lead to serious complications such as spinal cord injury. This complication seems to be most common in patients with significant spinal canal stenosis. If intrathecal migration is suspected, an MRI of the targeted spinal level should be obtained before anticipated SCS replacement.

PACEMAKERS AND SCS

The interference and inhibition of the cardiac pacemaker can be caused by SCS. However, SCS can be used in a patient with a preexisting pacemaker if certain precautions are taken: (1) both devices should be programmed in bipolar mode; (2) the SCS frequency should be set at 20 Hz; (3) SCS programming should be performed using continuous electrocardiographic monitoring; and (4) the manufacturer's recommendations should be strictly followed and the input of a cardiologist is recommended.

CONTROVERSIES

SINGLE- VERSUS DUAL-LEAD SYSTEM

Adequate relief of axial low back pain using SCS remains a challenge. It is not clear if SCS is indicated for isolated axial low back pain or only for axial low back pain combined with lower extremity pain. If the goal of SCS is to cover low back pain and bilateral lower extremity pain, single- or dual-lead systems can be considered. Using a dual-lead system can potentially provide "deeper" electrical field penetration in the dorsal column and therefore provide better axial low back pain coverage.[29,60] North et

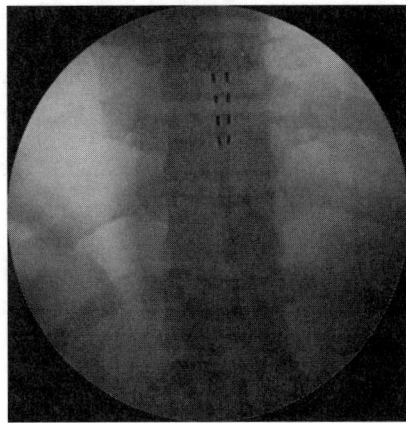

FIGURE 74.4 AP fluoroscopic view of dual lead system in thoracic area.

al.[28,61] have shown that there is no advantage to using the dual over single lead for axial low back pain and that a failure rate is higher in dual electrodes. However, the dual system is justified when it is expected that separate programming of two leads is necessary (Figure 74.4).

FOUR VERSUS EIGHT ELECTRODE SYSTEM

Both four and eight electrodes were shown to be effective in treatment of low back and lower extremity pain with no apparent advantages of one system over the other. Eight electrodes may have the potential advantage in case of the lead migration but this has not been shown in clinical trials. Putatively, the increased number of electrodes may offer more combinations for stimulation coverage but its clinical significance is not clear.

INTERNAL VERSUS EXTERNAL POWER SOURCE

An internalized, fully implanted power source offers apparent advantages. It is more convenient for the patient to use, it is aesthetically more appealing, and it does not require frequent external battery changes.

However, in certain situations, the external power source can be indicated. This applies to all the cases where high amplitudes of stimulation are needed during the trial phase. In particular, the required stimulation amplitude should be monitored when dual-lead systems are used. Dual-lead systems tend to empty batteries faster than a single-lead system even at modest stimulation amplitudes. In case an internal power source is used, these patients may require frequent battery replacements.

PERCUTANEOUS VERSUS LAMINECTOMY APPROACH

Although both approaches can be used, percutaneous placement of the SCS lead is a less invasive procedure, minimizing immediate complications and requiring less operating room time. Because percutaneous electrodes are placed under monitored anesthesia care, adequate SCS coverage can be confirmed during permanent implantation. This has advantage over the laminectomy approach, which is generally done under regional or general anesthesia, which makes it difficult if not impossible to confirm appropriate stimulation coverage.

Nevertheless, the laminectomy electrodes provide several advantages over percutaneously placed one[47]: (1) they are anchored to the dura and thus have minimal chance of migration[62–64] and (2) they are in closer contact with the dura, and thus they do not cause unnecessary posterior epidural space stimulation.

CONCLUSION

The SCS is an excellent treatment modality for carefully selected patients with low back and lower extremity pain. It may be a treatment of choice for patients with FBSS. The main advantages of SCS are its minimal invasiveness, reversibility, and excellent studies supporting its use. In carefully selected patients, SCS is cost-effective in comparison with the medical approaches. However, further studies are needed to better identify patient selection criteria for SCS.

REFERENCES

1. Melzack, R., & Wall, P. (1965). Pain mechanism: A new theory. *Science, 150,* 951.

2. Shealy, C., Mortimer, J., & Reswick, J. (1967). Electrical inhibition of pain by stimulation of the dorsal columns: Preliminary report. *Anesthesia & Analgesia, 46,* 489.

3. Holsheimer, J. et al. (1995). Significance of the spinal cord position in spinal cord stimulation. *Acta Neurochirurgia Supplement, 64,* 119.

4. Barolat, G., Zeme, S., & Ketcik, B. (1991). Multifactorial analysis of epidural spinal cord stimulation. *Stereotactic and Functional Neurosurgery, 56,* 77.

5. Dubuisson, D. (1989). Effect of dorsal-column stimulation on gelatinosa and marginal neurons of cat spinal cord. *Journal of Neurosurgery, 70,* 257.

6. Meyerson, B., & Linderoth, B. (2000). Mechanisms of spinal cord stimulation in neuropathic pain. *Neurological Research, 22,* 285.

7. Linderoth, B., & Foreman, R. (1999). Physiology of spinal cord stimulation: Review and update. *Neuromodulation, 2,* 150.

8. Yakhnitsa, V., Linderoth, B., & Meyerson, B. A. (1999). Spinal cord stimulation attenuates dorsal horn neuronal hyperexcitability in a rat model of mononeuropathy. *Pain, 79,* 223.

9. Bennett, G. (1993). An animal model of neuropathic pain: A review. *Muscle & Nerve, 16,* 1040.

10. Stiller, C. O. et al. (1996). Release of GABA in the dorsal horn and suppression of tactile allodynia by spinal cord stimulation in mononeuropathic rats. *Neurosurgery, 39,* 367.

11. Cui, J. G. et al. (1997). Spinal cord stimulation attenuates dorsal horn release of excitatory amino acids in mononeuropathy via a GABAergic mechanism. *Pain, 73,* 87.

12. Cui, J. G., Linderoth, B., & Meyerson, B. A. (1996). Effects of spinal cord stimulation on touch evoked allodynia involve GABAergic mechanisms: An experimental study in mononeuropathic rat. *Pain, 66,* 287.

13. Meyerson, B. A. et al. (1997). Modulation of spinal pain mechanisms by spinal cord stimulation and the potential role of adjuvant pharmacotherapy. *Stereotactic and Functional Neurosurgery, 68,* 129.

14. Stiller, C. O. et al. (1995). Repeated spinal cord stimulation decreases the extracellular level of gamma-aminobutyric acid in periaqueductal grey matter of freely moving rats. *Brain Research, 699,* 231.

15. Linderoth, B. et al. (1992). Dorsal column stimulation induces release of serotonin and substance P in the cat dorsal horn. *Neurosurgery, 31,* 289.

16. Croom. J. E. et al. (1997). Cutaneous vasodilatation during dorsal column stimulation is mediated by dorsal roots and CGRP. *American Journal of Physiology, 272,* H950.

17. Gheradini, G. et al. (1999). Spinal cord stimulation improves survival in ischemic skin flaps: An experimental study of the possible mediation by calcitonin gene-related peptide. *Plastic and Reconstructive Surgery, 103,* 1221.

18. Kemler, M. A. et al. (2000). Pain relief in complex regional pain syndrome due to spinal cord stimulation does not depend on vasodilation. *Anesthesiology, 92,* 1653.

19. Hautvast, R. W. et al. (1996). Spinal cord stimulation causes redistribution in myocardial perfusion during dipyridamole stress testing in patients with refractory angina pectoris as assessed by 13 NH3-positron emission tomography. *American Journal of Cardiology, 77,* 462.

20. Foreman, R. D. et al. (2000). Modulation of intrinsic cardiac neurons by spinal cord stimulation: Implications for its therapeutic use in angina pectoris. *Cardiovascular Research, 47,* 367.

21. Kiriakopoulos, E. T. et al. (1997). Functional magnetic resonance imaging: A potential tool for the evaluation of spinal cord stimulation: technical case report. *Neurosurgery, 41,* 501.

22. North, R. B. et al. (1992). Automated "pain drawing" analysis by computer-controlled, patient-interactive neurological stimulation system. *Pain, 50,* 51.

23. Kumar, K., Nath, R., & Wyant, G. M. (1991). Treatment of chronic pain by epidural spinal cord stimulation: A 10 year experience. *Journal of Neurosurgery, 75,* 402.

24. North, R. B. et al. (1994). Spinal cord stimulation versus reoperation for the failed back surgery syndrome: A prospective randomized study design. *Stereotactic and Functional Neurosurgery, 62,* 267.

25. Sweet, W., & Wepsic, J. (1974). Stimulation of the posterior columns of the spinal cord for pain control, *Clinical Neurosurgery, 21*, 278.

26. Meilman, P. W., Leibrock, L. G., & Leong, F. T. L. (1989). Outcome of implanted spinal cord stimulation in the treatment of chronic pain: Arachnoiditis versus single nerve root injury and mononeuropathy. *Clinical Journal of Pain, 5*, 189.

27. North, R. B., Ewend, M. G., & Lawton, M. T. (1991). Failed back surgery syndrome: Five year follow up after spinal cord stimulator implantation. A prospective, randomized study design. *Neurosurgery, 28*, 692.

28. North, R. B. et al. (1993). Spinal cord stimulation for chronic intractable pain: Two decades' experience. *Neurosurgery, 32*, 384.

29. Law, J. D. (1992). Spinal cord stimulation in the "failed back surgery syndrome." Comparison of technical criteria for palliating pain in the leg vs. in the low back. *Acta Neurochirurgia, 117*, 95.

30. Mitchell, S. W., Morehouse, G., & Keen, W. W. (1864). *Gunshot wounds and other injuries to the nerves.* Philadelphia: J.B. Lippincott.

31. Stanton-Hicks, M. (1999). Spinal cord stimulation for the management of complex regional pain syndromes. *Neurostimulation, 2*, 193.

32. Kumar, K., Toth, C., & Nath, R. K. (1997). Spinal cord stimulation is effective in reflex sympathetic dystrophy. *Neurosurgery, 40*, 503.

33. Kemler, M. A. et al. (2000). Spinal cord stimulation in patients with chronic reflex sympathetic dystrophy. *New England Journal of Medicine, 343*, 618.

34. Kemler, M. A. et al. (2004). The effect of spinal cord stimulation in patients with chronic reflex sympathetic dystrophy: Two years' follow-up of the randomized controlled trial. *Annals of Neurology, 55*, 13.

35. Hord, E. D. et al. (2003). The predictive value of sympathetic block for the success of spinal cord stimulation. *Neurosurgery, 53*, 626.

36. Torrens, J. K. et al. (1997). Risk of infection with electrical spinal-cord stimulation [Letter, comment]. *Lancet, 349*, 729.

37. Petrakis, I. E., & Sciacca, V. (2000). Spinal cord stimulation in diabetic lower limb critical ischaemia: Transcutaneous oxygen measurement as predictor for treatment success. *European Journal and Vascular and Endovascular Surgery, 19*, 587.

38. Harke, H. et al. (2002). Spinal cord stimulation in postherpetic neuralgia and in acute herpes zoster pain. *Anesthesia and Analgesia, 94*(3), 694.

39. Claeys, L. Spinal cord stimulation for peripheral vascular disease: A critical review-European studies. *Pain Digest, 9*, 337.

40. Kumar, K. et al. (1997). Improvement of limb circulation in peripheral vascular disease using epidural spinal cord stimulation: A prospective study. *Journal of Neurosurgery, 86*, 662.

41. Huber, S. et al. (1996). Enhanced limb salvage for peripheral vascular disease with the use of spinal cord stimulation. *West Virginia Medical Journal, 92*, 89.

42. Petrakis, E., & Sciacca, V. (2000). Prospective study of transcutaneous oxygen tension (TcPO2) measurement in the testing period of spinal cord stimulation in diabetic patients with critical lower limb ischaemia. *International Angiology, 19*, 18.

43. DeJongste, M. J. (2000). Spinal cord stimulation for ischemic heart disease. *Neurology Research, 22*, 293.

44. Hautvast, R. W. et al., Spinal cord stimulation in chronic intractable angina pectoris: A randomized, controlled efficacy study. *American Heart Journal, 136*, 1114.

45. Mannheimer, C. et al. (1998). Electrical stimulation versus coronary artery bypass surgery in severe angina pectoris: The ESBY study. *Circulation, 97*, 1157.

46. Jessurun, G. A. et al. (1997). Sequelae of spinal cord stimulation for refractory angina pectoris. Reliability and safety profile of long-term clinical application. *Coronary Artery Diseases, 8*, 33.

47. Villavicencio, A. T. et al. (2000). Laminectomy versus percutaneous electrode placement for spinal cord stimulation. *Neurosurgery, 46*, 399.

48. Alo, K. M. et al. (1999). Lumbar and sacral nerve root stimulation (NRS) in the treatment of chronic pain. A novel anatomic approach and neuro stimulation technique. *Neuromodulation, 2*, 19.

49. Krames, E. (1999). Spinal cord stimulation: Indications, mechanism of action, and efficacy. *Current Review of Pain, 3*, 419.

50. LeDoux, M. S., & Langford, K.H. (1993). Spinal cord stimulation for the failed back syndrome. *Spine, 18*, 191.

51. Meglio, M. et. al. (1994). Spinal cord stimulation in low back and leg pain. *Stereotactic and Functional Neurosurgery, 62*, 263.

52. Burchiel, K. J. et al. (1996). Prospective multicenter study of spinal cord stimulation for relief of chronic back and extremity pain. *Spine, 21*, 2786.

53. Kolin, M. T., & Winkelmuller, W. (1990). Chronic pain after multiple lumbar diskectomies. Significance of intermittent spinal cord stimulation. *Pain, 5*, S241.

54. Turner, J. A., Loeser, J. D., & Bell, K. G. (1995). Spinal cord stimulation for chronic low back pain: A systematic literature synthesis. *Neurosurgery, 37*, 1088.

55. De Laporte, C., & Van de Kelft, E. (1993). Spinal cord stimulation in failed back surgery syndrome. *Pain, 52*, 55.

56. Ohnmeiss, D. D., Rashbaum, R. F., & Bogdanffy, G. M. (1996). Prospective outcome evaluation of spinal cord stimulation in patients with intractable leg pain. *Spine, 21*, 1344.

57. Dumoulin, K. et. al. (1996). A psychoanalytic investigation to improve the success rate of spinal cord stimulation as a treatment for chronic failed back surgery syndrome. *Clinical Journal of Pain, 12*(1), 43.

58. North, R. B., & Guarino, A. (1999). Spinal cord stimulation for failed back surgery syndrome: Technical advances, patient selection and outcome. *Neuromodulation, 2*(1), 171.

59. Bell, G. K., Kidd, D., & North, R. B. (1997). Cost-effectiveness analysis of spinal cord stimulation in treatment of failed back surgery syndrome. *Journal of Pain and Symptom Management, 13*, 286.

60. Bartolat, G. (1999). A prospective multicenter study to assess the efficacy of spinal cord stimulation utilizing multi-channel radio-frequency system for the treatment of intractable low back pain and lower extremity pain. Initial considerations and methodology. *Neuromodulation, 2*, 179.

61. North, R. B. (1998). Spinal cord stimulation for axial low back pain: Single versus dual percutaneous electrodes [Abstract]. *International Neuromodulation Society Abstracts* (Lucerne, Switzerland), 212.

62. Hassenbusch, S. J., Stanton-Hicks, M., & Covington, E. C. (1995). Spinal cord stimulation versus spinal infusion for low back and leg pain. *Acta Neurochirurgia, 64*, 109.

63. Law, J. (1983, November 11–13). Results of treatment for pain by percutaneous multicontact stimulation of the spinal cord. Presented at the Annual Meeting of the American Pain Society, Chicago.

64. Law, J. D., & Miller, L. V. (1982). Importance and documentation of an epidural stimulating position. *Applied Neurophysiology, 45*, 461.

75

Intrathecal Pumps

Timothy R. Deer, MD

INTRODUCTION

Pain persisting after the expected time for healing is defined as chronic pain. More than 40 million people in the United States suffer from chronic musculoskeletal pain. Chronic low back pain is a major public health problem in the United States, serving as the second most common cause of hospital admissions. Each year, approximately $25 billion is spent on direct medical costs for low back pain. When indirect costs, such as lost productivity and economic hardship, are included, the figure exceeds $100 billion annually.[1] After an initial presentation of spine-related pain, 80 to 90% of patients resolve within 6 weeks with conservative treatment. Unfortunately, a number of these patients will have relapses while others will never recover fully. This can lead to a prevalence of low back pain of 40% at 1 year after initial presentation. Chronic pain after cervical injury, or whiplash, occurs in up to 45% of patients 1 year after initial presentation.

This epidemic of chronic spine-related pain syndromes leads to more than 600,000 spine surgeries and over 2 million interventional pain procedures per year. The costs of caring for these patients exceed those of coronary disease, cancer, and AIDS.[2] In another large group of patients, osteoporosis leads to long-term sequelae, with as many as 700,000 patients per year suffering from debilitating compression fractures. Unfortunately, despite the growing number of surgeries, injections, and alternative modes of treatment, a number of patients fail in both noncancer and cancer disease states. The increasing prevalence of chronic pain is due to those with noncancer pain, along with as many as 75% of patients suffering with cancer pain. This has led to an increase in the use of oral opioids.

The increased use of opioids has resulted in a consensus statement from the American Pain Society and the American Academy of Pain Medicine regarding the appropriate use of oral and transdermal medications.[3] Unfortunately, even when using these guidelines, a large number of patients fail with opioids over time. The most common causes of failure are unacceptable side effects or lack of efficacy. This has led to a growing number of patients becoming candidates for intrathecal drug delivery. In the past decade, there has been a growing problem of drug diversion and opioid abuse. The spreading epidemic of opioid abuse has also led many physicians to offer intrathecal therapies earlier in the course of therapy to avoid escalating opioid doses. Despite continued debate, these factors have helped chronic intrathecal therapy for the treatment of persistent pain of noncancer origin to gain acceptance. The use of these systems in cancer pain has become the standard of care in patients with severe pain who do not do well with conventional medical therapy.

HISTORY AND GENERAL PRINCIPLES

The use of intrathecal drug delivery systems (IDDS) to administer morphine intrathecally for the treatment of chronic pain was introduced in the early 1980s.[4] An IDDS consists of two implantable components: an infusion pump and an intraspinal catheter. The pump is usually placed abdominally in a subcutaneous pocket, while the catheter is inserted into the intrathecal space of the spine, tunneled under the skin, and connected to the pump. The pump reservoir is filled with medication by inserting a needle through a septum in the pump. Medication is delivered through the catheter to the intrathecal space.

The development of chronically infusing drug delivery systems has been a point of controversy in the medical community for three decades. In the early 1980s pioneers such as Penn and Coombs initiated this therapy for the treatment of intractable spasticity related to cerebral palsy and spinal cord injuries. This therapy then evolved to use in unrelenting cancer pain. Several years ago, the Food and Drug Administration (FDA) approved the use of preservative-free baclofen and preservative-free morphine in intrathecal solution for the treatment of moderate to severe spasticity and moderate to severe pain, respectively. Krames and Lanning[5] noted that morphine alone was unacceptable in many patients because of side effects, allergies, and lack of clinical success. In the last 20 years, research has been performed on several other drugs including intrathecal bupivacaine, hydromorphone, clonidine, and fentanyl. This led others to search for new agents, some of which have been very helpful, and some of which have led to toxicity and bad outcomes. Since the initiation of such therapies, we have learned about neurotoxicity and adverse outcomes that have changed the practice of interventional pain medicine. The last few decades have also been significant for the advancement of technology for both pumps and catheters. Since the work of the pioneers, many papers have been written on the acceptable drugs and techniques for the use of intrathecal therapies. This chapter reviews the critical points that may result in optimal outcomes with this therapy.

PHYSIOLOGY

The theory behind intrathecal drug delivery is that by directly depositing drugs into the cerebral spinal fluid (CSF), we can avoid the first pass effect. For example, it has been estimated that intrathecal morphine is 300 times as effective as oral morphine for equipotent pain treatment.[6] By direct drug action, the number of central nervous system (CNS)–derived side effects can be reduced. The effect of spinal opioid administration may be more complex than simply the delivery route. Eisenach et al.[7] recently concluded that spinal opioids caused the release of adenosine in humans. This effect appears to be caused by local opioid receptor activation of an opioid-adenosine mechanism. Further research is needed into this area as to the action of adenosine in the spinal cord.

The mechanism of action of intrathecal-administered opioids appears to be at the spinal cord level as well as at receptors in the supraspinal region. The supraspinal effect may lead to side effects despite the relatively low dose of medication delivered as compared with other routes.[8]

DISEASE STATES

The use of intrathecal catheters attached to totally implantable pumps first came to clinical utilization for the treatment of spasticity. Implantation for pain soon followed. The initial pain-related disease state in which this therapy was used involved cancer-related syndromes. In a recent study, Smith et al.[9] showed a major improvement using intrathecal devices in cancer pain when compared with comprehensive medical management in the areas of fatigue, level of consciousness, and survival. Despite this evidence of efficacy, the use of intrathecal pumps for cancer pain has shown no recent increases in requests from oncologists. This lack of increase in use in patients with cancer has resulted in cancer becoming a secondary use of this device.

Other disease states have been found to respond well to this therapy. Spinal disorders result in chronic disabling pain in many patients. Spinal stenosis, radiculitis, compression fractures, spondylosis, spondylolisthesis, foraminal stenosis, arachnoiditis, syrinx, and ankylosing spondylitis are only a few of the debilitating conditions that can result in severe pain in the cervical, thoracic, or lumbar spine. Intrathecal drug delivery has been used in each of these disease states. In more severe syndromes such as spinal cord trauma, spinal infarction, paraplegia, and cauda equina syndrome, the use of intrathecal therapy may involve treatment of both pain and spasticity.

In addition to spinal disease, other conditions may be appropriate for this treatment. Peripheral neuropathy, phantom-limb pain, rheumatoid arthritis, radiation neuritis, postherpetic neuralgia, post-thoracotomy syndrome, interstitial cystitis, and chronic pain of the abdomen and pelvis have successfully been treated by intrathecal drug treatment.[10] The development of new drugs will expand the efficacy of the therapy and also expand the number of diseases that may be amenable to the therapy.

PATIENT SELECTION

Proper selection of patients for this therapy is more important than technique, trialing, or management. The presence of an intrathecal pump in a patient who is not a good candidate for the therapy is doomed to fail, even if all parameters of clinical practice are at the highest level. In choosing the proper patient for intrathecal drug delivery several essential questions must be answered:

- Does the patient have an acceptable physiological explanation for the pain syndrome? Does the diagnosis warrant aggressive pain treatment?
- Has the patient failed less invasive therapies? What were those therapies? Are they documented in the record? Does this include physical therapy and oral medications?
- Are less invasive therapies unacceptable, not desired, or contraindicated?

- Does the patient have a life expectancy of 3 months or longer? This criterion is required for both patients with cancer and patients without cancer.
- Do the symptoms of pain affect the ability to function?
- Has the patient been reasonably compliant with past treatment recommendations?
- Does the patient have a contraindication to pump placement? Examples may include untreated coagulopathy, bacteremia, or localized infection.
- Is the patient psychologically stable?
- Has the patient had a successful neuroaxial trial? The physician should document acceptable symptom relief, side effects, and overall patient acceptance.
- Does the patient have reasonable expectations?
- Does the patient accept the risks of the procedure and future drug therapies?

In general the patient should meet some or all of the noted criteria. In the event that a patient does not meet these criteria, but other therapies have been exhausted, a pump may be placed at the discretion of the physician. In these rare cases the physician should consider other options, the risk-to-benefit ratio, and the possibility of obtaining a second opinion prior to proceeding. As noted, if the patient meets the appropriate criteria, a trial should be performed prior to placing a permanent pump.[11]

PSYCHOLOGICAL ASSESSMENT

Prior to pump placement many physicians treating non-cancer pain obtain a consultation with a psychologist to help finalize the selection process. Psychologists use interviewing, MMPI testing, Beck inventories, IQ testing, EQ testing, and other measurement tools to form an opinion of the patient's mental status and stability. Outcomes have been shown to worsen with the presence of untreated depression, untreated anxiety disorders, and suicidal or homicidal ideation. Outcomes have also been seen to be negatively influenced by the presence of untreated drug addiction. The presence of these factors is not seen as an absolute contraindication, but the problems should be treated and stabilized prior to going to a permanent implant. The presence of a personality disorder diagnosed as borderline, antisocial, or multiple should be viewed with extreme caution, and only implanted with a intrathecal pump in rare cases.[12] Psychological clearance is not needed in the patient with cancer pain; however, many of these patients may benefit from counseling to better cope with the disease process.

PUMP TRIAL

A patient trial for potential pump placement can be performed in several different clinical settings. The clinician must decide on the method of a single bolus or continuous infusion. Other decisions include anatomical position of the trial. Options include intrathecal or epidural trialing. Other considerations include length of trial, site of service, and medication selection for trialing. Recently, an expert panel met to discuss recommendations for trialing for pump placement. The panel included 19 experienced implanters, with a broad diversity of geographic locations, practice type, and specialties. The expert panel agreed that there is strong theoretical justification for a trial that mimics the conditions that will be achieved by the implanted system as closely as possible. Relevant parameters include (1) delivery site (intrathecal vs. epidural; spinal level); (2) delivery modality (infusion vs. bolus); (3) rate of infusion; and (4) dose/concentration range.[13]

A recent multicenter prospective analysis compared trialing methods in patients selected for an intrathecal drug delivery system. Deer and colleagues[14] analyzed the results of patient outcomes based on initial trialing success and outcomes at 1 year based on functional analysis, pain scores, quality of life ratings, and patient satisfaction. In each center the physician used the trialing method of choice based on patient profiles, usual clinical practice specific to the trialing physician, and primary pain type. To estimate primary pain type, the physicians were asked to classify the pain as nociceptive, neuropathic, or mixed. Trialing methods were grouped into single-shot intrathecal, continuous intrathecal, or continuous epidural. In the final analysis at 12 months post-implant it was determined that there was no statistical difference in trialing method in outcomes with nociceptive pain. In trialing for neuropathic syndromes, the initial success of trialing was significantly better if a continuous method was used. There was no difference in outcome between trialing via the epidural route as compared with the intrathecal route. It was interesting to note that the primary difference in patients with successful trials in neuropathic and mixed pain syndromes was the use of more than one agent to improve the success of the trial.

Continuous catheter trialing may be performed by placement of an epidural or intrathecal catheter. The FDA has approved morphine for continuous intrathecal infusion. Because of the regulatory approval, morphine is often the initial drug of choice for patient trialing. For patients with burning or lancinating extremity pain, some physicians will add a local anesthetic or alpha receptor-acting drug to improve the chances of trial success. With patients who have side effects from morphine or fail to achieve relief at reasonable doses, the drug infusate may be rotated to an alternative opioid.

Trialing success should include three significant outcomes:

1. The patient should have significant pain relief.
2. The patient should have controllable side effects.
3. In noncancer pain the patient should achieve some objective functional improvement.

TECHNIQUES

Once a patient has been selected for intrathecal therapy and an acceptable trial has been performed, a permanent placement is scheduled. Prior to going to the operating suite, the patient should have appropriate preoperative assessment. Preoperative laboratory assessment should be consistent with the American Society of Anesthesiologists Criteria for the selected anesthetic based on the patient's age and health status. In relation to the proposed procedure, an evaluation of the white blood cell count and differential, hemoglobin, platelet count, and metabolic profile should be obtained. In patients with diabetes, the patient should be encouraged to maintain appropriate control of serum glucose in the weeks preceding the implant. A hemoglobin A1C may be helpful in assessing compliance. If any high risks of infection exist such as a history of poorly controlled diabetes, AIDS, cancer, Addison's disease, prolonged oral steroid use, or infectious skin conditions, an infectious disease consult should be considered in the preoperative period.[15]

Several decisions and steps that are critical for a successful pump implant program are discussed below.

ANTIBIOTIC PROPHYLAXIS

In the past the use of prophylactic antibiotics has been controversial. Over time the use of prophylactic antibiotics has become the standard of care in most cases. Practices vary in the antibiotic choice with the most common a third-generation cephalosporin or vancomycin. Oral antibiotics are given during the course of the trial in most cases, and for 7 to 10 days after permanent implant. Acceptable choices include cephalosporins, penicillin derivatives, and quinolones. Intraoperatively, it may be helpful to irrigate the wound with antibiotic solution. The most common choices are bacitracin, a polypeptide, or an aminoglycoside such as kanamycin. Modifications to antibiotic choices should be made based on common pathogens seen in the institution and community.[16]

PREPPING, DRAPING, AND POSITIONING

Patients should undergo a vigorous prep that is outside of the margins of the planned surgical field. It is also helpful to use an adhesive drape to prevent migration of the sterile

field with patient movement. Common prepping solutions include chlorhexidine, alcohol, and iodophor solutions. Positioning should include vigilance to pressure points and peripheral nerves. The patient may be positioned in the prone position for catheter placement, but this requires repositioning for pocket creation. In the majority of cases the patient is placed in the lateral decubitus position, with the hips flexed, and the knees bent.

CATHETER PLACEMENT

Once the patient is prepared the fluoroscopic image is used to properly identify anatomy and pathology of the spine. In most cases the point of entry will be below the level of L2. In rare cases the entry point will be at the level of the cord. In the event that the entry point is above L2, the patient should be conversant, and the angle should be as shallow as possible. If the patient experiences paraesthesias, the needle should be removed and repositioned. Prior to starting the case the physician should have a planned level for the catheter placement. Once the catheter is in place, a purse-string suture should be placed to help secure the tissue around the catheter, and a silastic anchor should be used to secure the catheter. Two theories are common regarding the appropriate level of catheter placement. Some clinicians choose to place the catheter tip as close to the primary pain generator as possible. This type of placement allows for the delivery of a lipophilic drug in an effective manner. Others suggest that the benefit of direct catheter placement is outweighed by the recently described problem of inflammatory catheter mass. Currently, no studies give a clear answer to this debate, and the decision remains a matter of physician judgment and preferred practice.[17]

POCKET PLACEMENT

The most common location for pump placement is the lateral anterior abdominal wall at the level of the umbilicus. In deciding the appropriate place for incision, one should consider the location of the anterior superior iliac spine, the rib, and the patient's preferred belt line. Anatomical considerations such as the presence of an osteotomy should be considered in the planning. The pump should be anchored with either suture loops or a Dacron pouch to avoid flipping. Prior to placing the pump in the pocket, it should be prepared based on the manufacturer's recommendations, and filled with the appropriate drug based on the trial response.

HEMOSTASIS AND SKIN CLOSURE

Prior to wound closure, great care should be taken to assure that hemostasis has been achieved. After extensive antibiotic irrigation of the newly created pump pocket, the wound should be retracted to allow good visualization.

This will allow the recognition of small venous and arterial vessel bleeders. If bleeders are identified, an appropriate technique should be used to control bleeding; options include the following:

1. Simple pressure may alleviate bleeding.
2. Sponges soaked in hydrogen peroxide 3% solution may be packed into the wound for 3 to 5 minutes. This may be helpful with very small vessels.
3. Electrocautery can be used to control more aggressive bleeding. Care should be taken in the application of cautery to limit its use to the specific vessel. Overheating of tissue can create skin trauma or seroma formation. This can lead to delayed healing, dehiscence, or infection of the wound.
4. Suturing a vessel is still the "gold standard." Once the vessel has been clamped with a hemostat, a simple suture or "figure of eight" type suture using 00 or 000 absorbable material on a noncutting needle can be used to stay the bleeding. If space allows, a simple tie may be used. Another method for hemostasis would the use of metal ligature clips. Just prior to insertion of the pump, the wound should be irrigated again and reinspected for hemostasis. Once the pump has been inserted the subcutaneous tissue and skin must be closed over the pump. The pump should fit snugly in the pocket but still allow the skin edges to be brought together without tension. If this cannot be achieved, further tissue undermining may be required. The subcutaneous tissue should be brought together using a 00 or 000 monofilament absorbable suture. When closing the wound, care should be taken to obliterate any "dead space." This can be done with careful suture placement using an interrupted or running suture. The skin edges should be touching slightly, everted, and then closed with a monofilament non-absorbable material or metal skin clips (Figure 75.1).

A bulky sterile pressure dressing should be applied over the wound. An abdominal binder could be used for compression and support, which may reduce the risk of seroma and bleeding. The use of antibiotic ointment may be of some help in preventing infection. Dressing changes may be performed daily, or only if dressings are saturated. This is a physician judgment issue.

POSTOPERATIVE CARE

The patient is generally seen 7 to 10 days postoperatively. At this time stitches or staples can be removed and adhe-

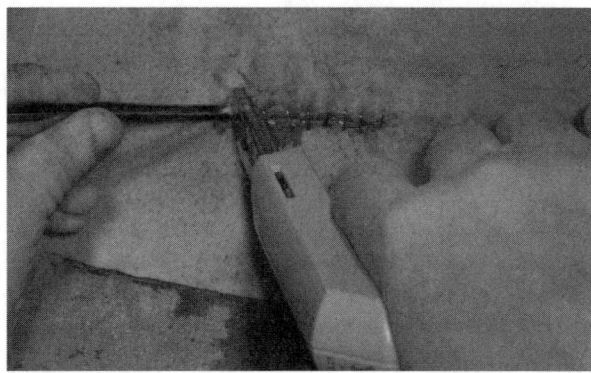

FIGURE 75.1 Pocket closure

sive strips applied to support the wound. The time may be extended in those patients who are immunocompromised or have a nutritionally poor status. Any signs of wound breakdown or infection should be approached aggressively.

SURGICAL COMPLICATIONS AND MANAGEMENT

The most important aspect in the management of complications is early recognition of the problem and quick action to remediate the problem. Bleeding at the wound site will be fairly self-evident, manifested by swelling, discoloration, and erythema. Treatment may include ice and compression, but may require surgical exploration. Infection may be a minor, limited, superficial problem, or may lead to a loss of the device and significant sequelae. Infection may present as elevated body temperature, purulent wound drainage, erythema, or frank pus. Urgent action is required to incise and drain the wound, identify the pathogen, and initiate antibiotics (Figure 75.2, Figure 75.3). The decision to excise the pump is based on the presence of necrotic tissue, the overall condition of the wound, and the condition of the patient. The collection of non-infectious fluid is called a seroma. Treatment may be limited to pressure dressings and time for reabsorption. If conservative treatment fails, a sterile aspiration of fluid may be required (Figure 75.4, Figure 75.5). Another cause of fluid collection is a hygroma. This represents a collection of CSF. The most common cause of hygroma is fluid seepage around the catheter entry point to the pocket. The

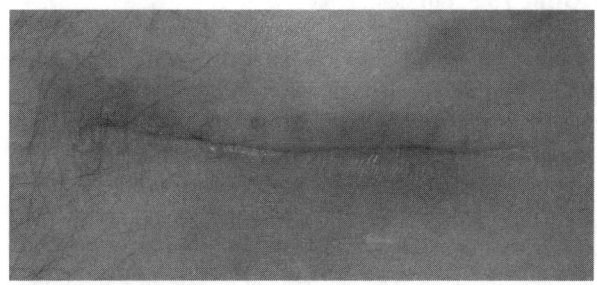

FIGURE 75.2 Early wound.

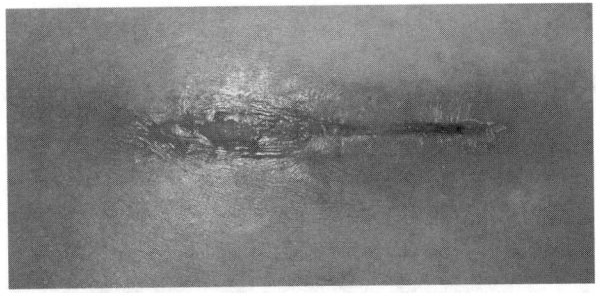

FIGURE 75.3 Wound infected with cellulites.

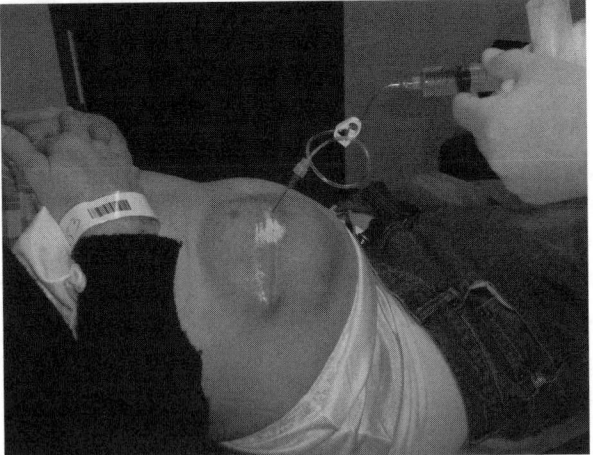

FIGURE 75.4 Aspiration.

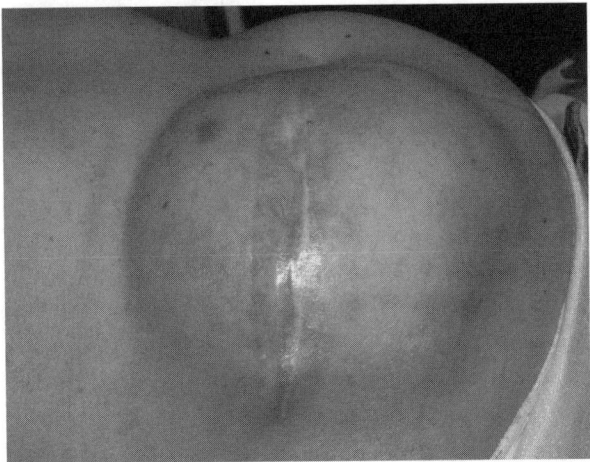

FIGURE 75.5 Effusion 2.

problem can be treated by abdominal pressure, increased fluids, and caffeine. In addition to the complications noted, two disastrous problems must be identified if present. These include epidural hematoma, which may result in paralysis. Any change in the neurological exam postoperatively should be viewed as an emergency and an MRI should be obtained as soon as possible to rule out spinal cord compression. The presence of an intrathecal pump is not a contraindication to MRI, and should not delay the

use of this imaging modality. The second serious complication is the presence of neuroaxial infection. This may include meningitis or epidural abscess. Both of these diagnoses must be made in an expedient fashion to allow initiation of the appropriate treatment.

MEDICATION SELECTION

The FDA has approved morphine as the drug of choice for chronic intrathecal infusion in the United States. A survey in 1999 involving physicians from North America, Europe, and Australia showed that physicians use many other drugs in patients with chronic cancer and noncancer pain.[18] Based on available world literature and the information obtained from the survey, a consensus panel of experts created an algorithm for intrathecal use. This algorithm suggested using morphine as a first-line drug, followed by hydromorphone in patients with side effects from morphine. In patients with no side effects, but lack of analgesia with morphine, a combination of morphine with bupivacaine or morphine with clonidine was suggested as second-line treatment. In patients failing those combinations, a third-line therapy involved the use of hydromorphone with bupivacaine or clonidine, the use of morphine with clonidine and bupivacaine, or the use of more potent lipophilic opioids such as fentanyl or sufentanil.[19] In an update of the consensus algorithm in 2003, the panel elevated hydromorphone to first-line therapy along with morphine. This decision was based on recent studies in laboratory models showing safety that may be better than morphine. In a study of chronic infusion in a sheep model, hydromorphone was not associated with inflammatory mass formation. This may suggest this drug is safer in humans, although more extensive research is needed.[19]

Local anesthetics are often added to opioids in patients experiencing burning or lancinating pain. The drug with the most experience in clinical use is bupivacaine. Clinical experience shows the drug is safe and shows efficacy when compared with opioid alone. The drug is most commonly used at doses of 1 to 20 mg per day (Deer et al., 2002).[20] Work in the laboratory shows that bupivacaine is stable, compatible, and safe when administered via an implantable delivery system.[21] Tetracaine has shown signs of neurotoxicity and has been discouraged for clinical use. Ropivacaine has now been used clinically, but data on this drug are limited and its use should be approached cautiously.[22]

In a landmark study, Staats and colleagues[23] found that ziconotide provided clinically and statistically significant analgesia in patients with pain from cancer and AIDS. Ziconotide, formerly called SNX-111, works by selectively blocking N-type voltage sensitive calcium channels. In theory, this drug may provide relief in patients who have failed or do not tolerate opioids. This drug, which is formed by modification of a snail toxin, shows the possibilities of future non-opioid drug development. Presley and colleagues[24] conducted a double-blind, placebo-controlled trial that comprised 257 patients with noncancer pain, 78% of whom had neuropathic pain. Pain relief was assessed for 5 or 6 days in a blinded fashion, followed by an additional 5- to 6-day maintenance period. Significantly lower Visual Analog Scale of Pain Intensity (VASPI) scores (mean percent change in VASPI score from baseline to titration phase; $P = 0.0002$) were reported by 31% of the ziconotide-treated patients, compared with 6% of the placebo-treated patients. Moderate to complete pain relief was achieved in 43% of patients in the ziconotide arm versus 18% placebo ($P = 0.001$). Patients who received ziconotide reported improved mood, sleep, and enjoyment of life, and were able to decrease their use of opioid compared with patients receiving placebo (mean of >300 mg/day morphine equivalents by +24.3% vs. –5.3%).

Opioid research has been limited in chronic noncancer pain. In a retrospective analysis of 29 patients who received intraspinal drug therapy for pain, 8 patients received fentanyl 10.5 to 115 µg/day for a mean duration of 31 months. These patients experienced an average of 68.4% improvement in pain and an average overall satisfaction of 3.25 on a scale of 1 (poor) to 4 (excellent).[25] Another retrospective study ($n = 122$) reviewed the complications associated with implantable drug delivery systems, including two patients with the combination of fentanyl and bupivacaine combination. In this study the group was seen to have minimal complications with this combination. The efficacy was 74% in the group compared with fentanyl alone.[26] Three studies, two prospective ($n = 24$ and $n = 70$) and one retrospective ($n = 47$), were performed to evaluate the use of methadone in neuroaxial infusion. The surveys involved both patients with cancer and patients without cancer; methadone was administered at total daily doses of 5 to 60 mg, and duration of treatment ranged from 3 days to 37 months. Overall effectiveness, based on greater than 50% reduction in pain only or pain reduction combined with improved quality of life survey scores ranged from 37.5 to 80%. Transient blurred vision was noted as an adverse event in one patient.[27–29]

Deer et al.[30] recently reviewed the use of intrathecal bupivacaine with and without opioids. They note that stability, bacteriologic studies, toxicology data, and clinical reports of infrequent complications support the safety of this regimen. Intrathecal bupivacaine, a clinically effective combination partner, was also noted to be more efficacious than epidural administration. The authors conclude that intrathecal bupivacaine is a safe and efficacious treatment for malignant/nonmalignant pain. They suggest that the data warranted further studies of compatibility with combination partners, and outcome analyses based on the source and mechanism of pain.

Hassenbusch et al.[31] report a 20-month prospective Phase I/II cohort study of 31 patients (6 with cancer pain, 25 with nonmalignant pain) who received intrathecal clonidine at a total daily dose of 144 to 1,200 µg/day (mean 872 µg/day). In the study, 22 patients (achieving >50% pain/symptom reduction without intolerable side-effects) who progressed through the dose escalation stage were evaluated. At 6 months, 77.3% (17/22) of this cohort achieved continued good pain relief, and 59% of the cohort (42% of the accrued study population) were considered long-term successes (mean follow-up 16.7 months). Consistently, clonidine dose did not change significantly over time in this group. Moreover, there was no change in patients' Karnofsky performance status. Inability to achieve long-term pain relief was related to inadequate pain relief ($n = 4$) and intolerable side effects (hypotension, $n = 2$; impotence, lethargy, and malaise, 1 each).[31]

A retrospective survey observed that only 2 of the 10 patients treated with clonidine alone (75 to 950 µg/day) had good pain relief after 7 to 11 months of intrathecal therapy. The addition of clonidine (75 to 950 µg/day) to either morphine 0.15 to 15 mg/day (5 patients) or hydromorphone 200 to 800 µg/day (10 patients) similarly yielded very limited effect; only 3 of these patients achieved long-term pain relief (7 to 11 months). Adverse events reported by Ackerman et al. include hypotension (5 patients), catheter complications (1 patient), sedation (3 patients), confusion (1 patient), constipation (1 patient), nausea (2 patients), pruritus (2 patients), and catheter-tip granuloma (1 patient). It is unclear whether the adverse events in this and other prospective studies were related to clonidine or opioid administration.[32]

In a prospective cohort study, Uhle et al.[33] report data from 10 patients with neuropathic pain syndromes (2 of whom had cancer pain) who received clonidine (average, 44 µg/day) in combination with morphine sulfate or buprenorphine. These patients realized a 70 to 100% reduction in pain. Four of eight patients with non-neuropathic pain also appeared to benefit from the addition of clonidine. The frequency of adverse events was hypotension (10 patients), fatigue (4 patients), dry mouth (3 patients), and impaired bowel (1 patient). Studies have shown that clonidine is stable in combination with morphine and when infused in intrathecal pumps over 90 days. Clonidine has also been shown to be stable at 90 days with bupivacaine and morphine. In animal studies there has been no evidence of neurotoxicity in preservative free midazolam. Continuous infusions in sheep and pigs have shown no changes in mental status or toxicity. In the sheep studies, the pain thresholds were improved and the overall ability to tolerate painful stimulus was improved.[34]

CLINICAL MANAGEMENT

The chronic successful management of intrathecal delivery systems requires a group of professionals working as a team with a compliant, motivated patient. The team

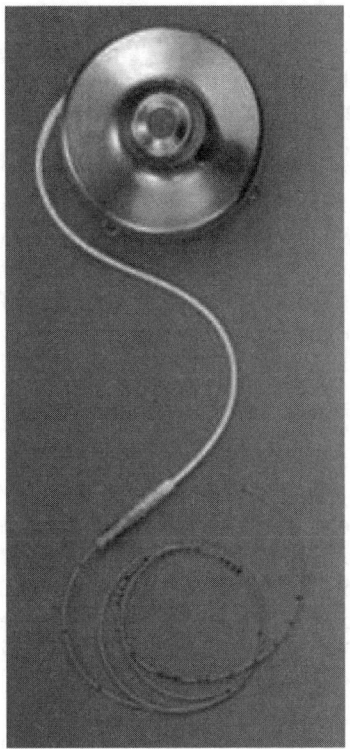

FIGURE 75.6 Continuous flow pump.

should include a physician leader who prescribes the therapy and makes clinical decisions based on patient response and side effects. Other members of the team should include nursing personnel, well educated in patient assessment and pump management; a pharmacist who is familiar with appropriate drug preparation and dosing; and support staff who assure proper materials are present for the refill. Refills should be performed by the physician or team member with appropriate training in refilling and, when appropriate, reprogramming the pump.

PUMP AND CATHETER TYPE

Pumps are of two basic types. In the constant-flow pump a pressurized, hydraulic mechanism drives the flow of drug into the catheter (Figure 75.6). In this type of pump there is no internal battery. The downside of a constant-flow pump is the inability to program the pump for bolus dosing and daily infusion variable doses, and the inability to obtain a history of infusion or reservoir volume.

In the programmable pump, an internal battery is used to drive a rotor to deliver drug to the catheter (Figure 75.7). In this type of pump the battery must be replaced over time. The advantage of this type of pump is the ability to rapidly change dose and boluses, and to track reservoir volume.

The catheter type selected is important in reducing the complications rate of the catheter. Catheters vary on the number of exit points at the end of the catheter. Catheters

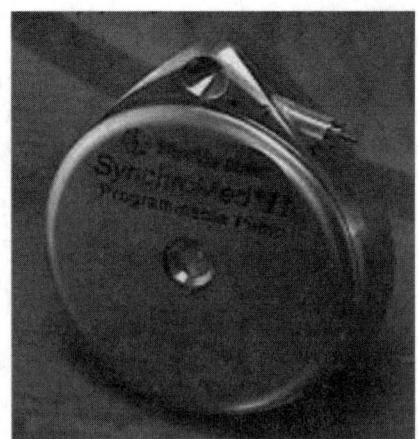

FIGURE 75.7 Programmable pump.

also vary in the internal structure. Options include silastic materials or wire-reinforced catheters. The wire reinforcement theoretically limits the complications of catheter fracture and kinking.[35]

COMPLICATIONS

A large retrospective study involving 429 patients showed a high complication rate. In this report by Paice and colleagues,[36] 21.6% of patients show system malfunction. The most common reason for this problem was catheter related, including catheter kinking and fracture (Figure 75.8 and Figure 75.9). In a limited study of cancer patients Commbs and colleagues[37] report no complications, such as infection, catheter problems, or respiratory depression, in a very early study of a limited number of patients

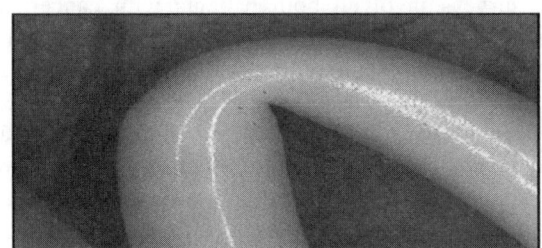

FIGURE 75.8 Catheter kinking.

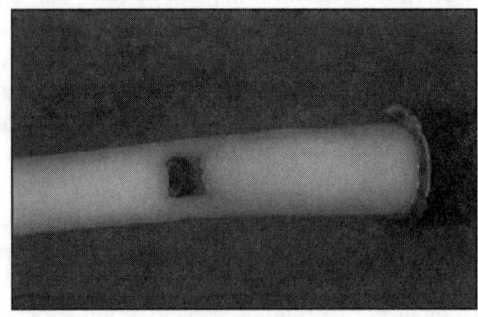

FIGURE 75.9 Catheter fracture.

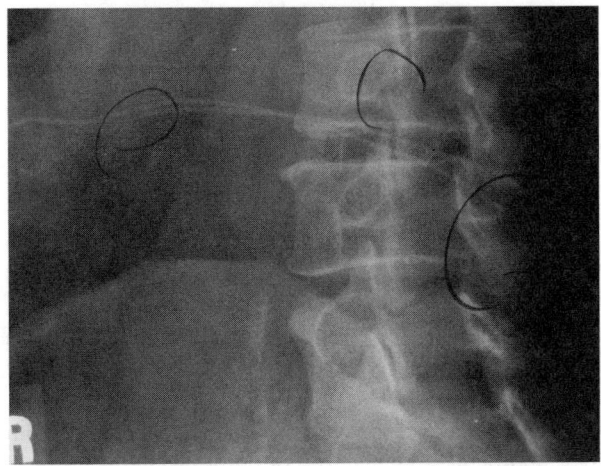

FIGURE 75.10 Lateral of Fx.

receiving intrathecal therapies for cancer pain. There have been reports of migration of a catheter into the subdural space causing drug withdrawal. This diagnosis should be considered with cases of acute catheter failure. The diagnosis is made by catheter injection with post-injection computed tomography (CT) scanning.[38] As noted, the number of complications with catheters with wire reinforcement has been reported to be less than 1% over the life of the implant. This design avoids the risk of kinking and is more resistant to fracture (Figure 75.10).

Hormonal changes have been reported with long-term opioid use regardless of the route of delivery. Naturally occurring opioids diminish testosterone levels at both the central and end organ locations. The use of long-term sustained-release oral opioids has been shown to contribute to subnormal sex hormone levels.[39] Willis and Doleys[40] studied several patients receiving long-term opioids by intrathecal infusion for at least 1-year duration. In this group several patients experienced hypogonadism and fatigue related to clinically proven decreased testosterone. Many have hypothesized that there may be an effect on other hormonal systems as well, and more studies are needed to determine the extent of this problem.

Recently, another complication issue has led to a great deal of discussion in the pain management community: inflammatory mass or granuloma (Figure 75.11, Figure 75.12). This complication results from buildup of inflammatory material at the tip of the catheter. This condition leads to a compressive disorder that causes complications ranging from asymptomatic patients to catastrophic neurological sequelae. Coffey and Burchiel[41] analyzed 41 cases of inflammatory mass lesions in intrathecal drug infusion catheters. Their conclusions were that those requiring high-dose intraspinal opioids should be monitored closely for signs of this problem. They also concluded that early recognition may lead to prevention of neurological damage. Both physi-

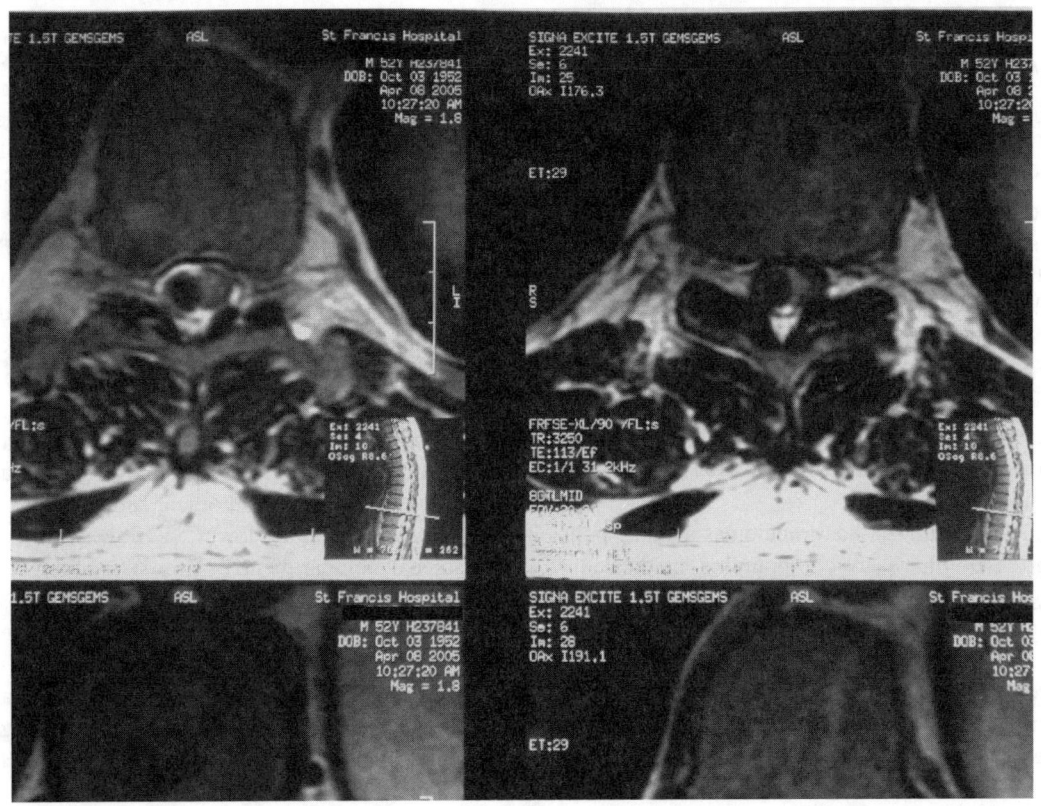

FIGURE 75.11 Large thoracic.

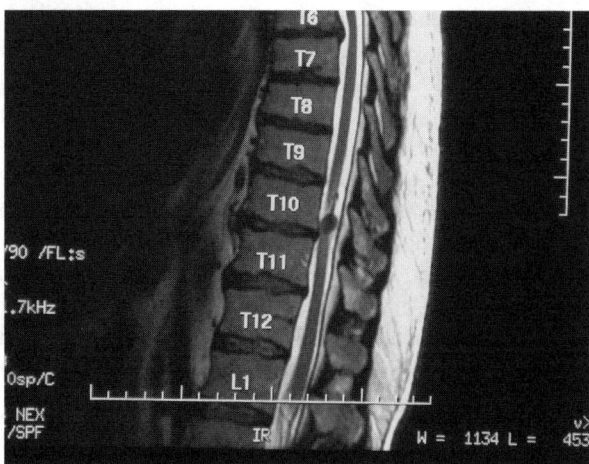

FIGURE 75.12 Lateral of granuloma.

cians served on a consensus panel that made recommendations on the cause, prevention, diagnosis, and management of inflammatory mass.[17]

The true incidence of inflammatory mass in clinical practice is unknown. Coffey and Burchiel mention clusters of reports in their analysis. McMillan and colleagues[42] report a significant percentage in their practice. They report three of seven patients with confirmed inflammatory masses on diagnostic imaging. In one of these patients, left lower-extremity paralysis developed. The other two patients were treated conservatively with no complications. Deer[43] recently reported a much lower incidence in his group with only 3% of patients having inflammatory mass by diagnostic imaging. In this study, 208 consecutive patients underwent MRI or CT myelogram. In the cases that were recognized, no patients had any long-term sequelae.

The etiology of granuloma has been reviewed extensively. Based on work by Yaksh et al.,[44,45] the appearance of granulomas suggests an inflammatory reaction to an opioid. The mechanism may be related to a mitogen-activated protein kinase cascade that causes increased lymphocyte activity. This inflammatory reaction appears to dissipate once the offending opioid is removed. Some have suggested an allergy to silicone, but the absence of these lesions in patients receiving baclofen for spasticity argues against that thought.

It has been postulated that granulomas are a response to impurities in pharmacy-compounded medications; however, granulomas have been seen just as frequently in commercially purchased preparations.[41] Granulomas have been reported most commonly with morphine. Other drugs have also been implicated in causing this complication including hydromorphone, fentanyl, and ziconotide.[41,43] Clonidine has been theorized to have a protective effect in humans, although this has not been shown in any clinical study to date. Walker et al.,[46] who routinely combine clonidine with opioid, have reported no

granulomas in Australia. Yaksh et al.[45] has shown a protective effect of clonidine in the dog model. More data are needed on the prophylactic effect of clonidine.

Admixtures of opioid with clonidine and/or bupivacaine have led to dose reduction in the opioid. Dosage reduction allows for lower concentrations of drug (because higher doses must be concentrated to allow for a reasonable period of time between refills). Indeed, not only is the drug that is infused thought to be important in the formation of granuloma, but also the concentration of drug. With morphine, the majority of cases have been described in patients receiving concentrations of 40 mg/cc or greater.

The same concentration-effect has been reported with hydromorphone; the majority of described cases received concentrations of 10 mg/cc or greater. Despite this increased incidence in patients with higher concentrations of drug, there are reported cases at markedly lower concentrations of morphine and hydromorphone. These granulomas, seen at low concentrations, suggest the need for vigilance in all patients.[47]

It is often noted that granuloma formation is more common in catheters with a single exit site. Catheters with single orifices allow for a high concentration of drug to settle at one point in the CSF. The theory suggests that the concentration gradient leads to an inflammatory reaction. New catheters with multiple drug exit sites may be safer. However, the issue has not yet been addressed in a randomized study. Indeed, because time is required for granulomas to become clinically significant, the possibility exists that the majority of granulomas have been noted with single-orifice catheters because these catheters have been in use the longest. If this is true, problems may become evident with multiple exit catheters in the future.[48]

The most controversial area in the etiology of granulomas involves the issue of catheter placement. The majority of granulomas have been reported in the area of the thoracic spine. This has led many to conclude that catheters should be placed in the lumbar or cervical region avoiding the site of most granuloma formation. The science behind this thought process involves the fact that CSF volume and flow in the region of the thoracic cord are relatively reduced, compared with other parts of the spinal cord. The ventral thoracic subarachnoid space has the longest region of low CSF flow within the entire intrathecal compartment.[49] This stagnation of flow has been postulated to cause higher concentrations of drug. The confounding issue in the catheter placement debate is the number of catheters placed in that region compared with the lumbar and cervical spine. For technical reasons, the number of current indwelling catheters is higher in the thoracic spine as compared with other regions. Therefore, it is difficult to be sure whether concentration effects explain the high number of granulomas seen in the thoracic spine.[17]

The possibility that granulomas result from a low-grade infection has also been considered. In animal studies, analysis of cytology and cultures shows no evidence of infection. The same can be said of tissue samples and catheter analysis in postoperative patients with granulomas. Many cultures have been performed in these patients and have been negative. Based on this information, it appears that infection does not play a role in the formation of granuloma.[17]

A retrospective cohort analysis of 23 patients with leg edema associated with long-term (greater than 24 months) administration of intrathecal morphine found an association between edema during neuroaxial infusion and the presence of leg edema and venous stasis prior to pump implantation; a dose–effect relationship for leg edema was suggested by these observations. The etiology of this leg edema has been theorized to arise from an effect on the pituitary. Opioids may have an effect on antidiuretic hormone, causing edema. Further research is needed to examine this issue.[50]

OUTCOMES

Outcomes in patients suffering from severe pain secondary to cancer have been very positive by physician report. Most studies have been retrospective or based on case reports. Smith and colleagues[9] report a multicenter, international, randomized, prospective study comparing intrathecal drug delivery versus comprehensive medical management. In this study the patients were randomized to the intent-to-treat group and then underwent a trial for intrathecal pump placement. The trials were performed based on the physician's normal technique. At 4 weeks after the enrollment of the patient, the data were analyzed based on the initial enrollment group. The results showed a clinically significant advantage of intrathecal pumps in overall toxicity (based on national cancer toxicity criteria), pain relief, fatigue, and level of consciousness. Perhaps the most impressive finding was a trend toward improved survival in the pump group ($P = 0.06$). This study suggests more patients with moderate to severe cancer pain should be considered for intrathecal drug delivery. In a large retrospective study involving both cancer (32.7%), and noncancer (67.3%) pain, a mean pain reduction of 61% was seen in both groups. In those patients with neuropathic pain, improved efficacy was reported when using drugs such as clonidine or bupivacaine. Minimal long-term adverse drug events occurred in this group.[36] One of the earliest outcome studies presented a negative impression of intrathecal infusions in patients with cancer. In this study, Commbs and colleagues[37] found in a small group of 14 patients that there was no difference in patients receiving intrathecal morphine when compared with other routes of delivery.

De Lissovoy and colleagues[51] found a positive outcome in cost-effectiveness. An analytic study with computer simulation was used to project outcomes in a group of patients with failed back surgery syndrome. In this model, a patient receiving intrathecal therapy would be cost-effective to society at 12 to 22 months when compared with alternative methods of treatment. It should be noted that in a more care-intensive patient such as an end-of-life cancer patient, Bedder et al.[52] have shown cost-effectiveness at 3 months when compared with epidural home infusion. Kumar et al.[53] published their analysis comparing conventional pain therapy with intrathecal drug delivery. In this 5-year study, the data were collected regarding function, hardware costs, professional fees, diagnostic imaging, nursing visits, hospitalization costs, and alternative medicines. The conclusion of this study was a cost-effectiveness of intrathecal therapies at 28 months. This is even more impressive when considering that the intrathecal therapy patients had improved function when compared with conventional treatment using the Oswestry Disability Index. The National Outcomes Registry for Low Back Pain has collected prospective data on outcomes for 136 patients with chronic low back pain who received neuroaxial infusion via implanted devices (morphine in 81% of patients). Patients were entered into the registry by a group of participating clinicians. Pain and function ratings were measured by the visual analogue scale and Oswestry Low Back Pain Disability Scale, respectively. Impressively, at the 12-month follow-up period both indices improved by more than 47% for patients with back pain and by more than 31% for those with leg pain.[14]

Willis and Doleys[40] in a retrospective evaluation of 29 consecutive patients with a follow-up duration of 31 months report an average 63% improvement in pain, 46% improvement in activity level, and 54% improvement in ease of performing activities. Paice et al.[36] also showed 61% relief in a large, retrospective, multicenter survey. In other studies, Tutak and Doleys[54] report a good or excellent outcome in 78% of the patients, and Krames and Lanning[5] report good or excellent outcome in 81% of patients. Other drugs also have been used for pain treatment in implantable systems. Van Hilten et al.[55] studied intrathecal baclofen for the treatment of painful dystonia in patients with reflex sympathetic dystrophy. They performed a double-blind, randomized, controlled, crossover of bolus intrathecal injections of 25, 50, and 75 mg of baclofen as well as placebo. The results showed that in six women, bolus injections of 50 and 75 mg of baclofen resulted in complete or partial resolution of focal dystonia of the hands but little improvement in dystonia of the legs. In chronic infusions, two of the patients with lower extremity dystonia improved. The conclusions made were that painful dystonia can be improved by intrathecal baclofen. This study, a double-blind, placebo-controlled study, is limited based on the low number of patients enrolled for analysis.

Unfortunately, despite numerous studies of existing and novel drugs, outcome data pertaining to long-term neuroaxial infusion are limited. An algorithmic process to choose drugs based on clinical and animal studies must be a critical part of patient decision making. As new drugs are developed for intrathecal use, the medical community must continue to take a critical look at safety, efficacy, and indications.

COMPOUNDING

Infumorph® (preservative-free morphine sulfate sterile solution/Elkins-Sinn) is the only drug currently approved by the U.S. FDA for the intrathecal treatment of pain. In up to 65% of patients, morphine alone will fail to provide appropriate relief because of side effects, dose escalation, and failure of safe concentrated drugs to provide a reasonable length of time between device refills. This has led clinicians to use off-label drugs to treat patient's long term. Unfortunately, most commercially available drugs labeled for other uses are not acceptable for human use. The drugs are unacceptable because of the presence of preservatives, excipients, or unacceptable solubility at body temperature. It is important to note that drugs labeled as "preservative-free" may still be neurotoxic because of excipients or pH buffers. Another issue is the compatibility of drugs with intrathecal devices. Several drugs including dopamine, mitomycin C, cyclosporin A, apomorphine, meperidine, octreotide pH 4.11, interleukin II with 25 mg human serum albumin (HAS)/ml, and diamorphine have been reported to be incompatible with, and cause malfunction of, the SynchroMed Infusion System (Medtronic Neurological, Minneapolis, MN).

In an era in which the cost of drug development is high and the use of intrathecal drug infusions is challenged because of financial restraints, many pharmaceutical companies are unwilling to spend large amounts of revenue on this patient group. Because of the lack of acceptable drugs, drug compounding has become common practice in patients requiring polyanalgesia.

Drug compounding is defined as the mixing of ingredients to prepare a medication for patient use. Compounding is a complicated practice that requires vigilance with sterile technique and attention to drug solubility and drug compatibility. Incorrectly prepared products can lead to nerve injury, paralysis, and death when administered into the CNS.

The U.S. Pharmacopoeia and the American Society of Health-System Pharmacists have issued guidelines on compounded sterile products that have practical and legal significance. These guidelines apply to the compounding of solutions for neuroaxial drug delivery.[44,56,57] When a compounding pharmacy is chosen, it is important for patient safety that it comply with these guidelines.

FUTURE ADVANCES

Advances in intrathecal drug delivery will occur on many fronts. Developments in new drugs, devices, and catheters must occur for this therapy to gain wider acceptance. For new drugs to be considered they must be put through stringent evaluations. Recommendations include drug formulation, chemical stability/compatibility, pharmacokinetics, and toxicology during the development and approval phase.[58]

Current research on new drugs is promising. Tizanidine and gabapentin are two drugs of interest. In a dog model by Kroin et al.,[59] a comparison of tizanidine and clonidine at doses of 3.0 to 18.0 mg/day yielded equivalent analgesia on a thermal withdrawal test but greater toxicity hypotension, bradycardia, and bradyarrhythmias from the clonidine. An additional tizanidine toxicity study with 3 to 6 mg/day in dogs found no significant side effects (neurotoxicity, body weight, temperature, respiratory rate, heart rate, sedation, or motor coordination) or histopathologic effects (spinal cord gray and white matter).

The analgesic efficacy of intrathecal gabapentin has been evaluated in rodent models. Administered by bolus intrathecal injection (100 to 1000 µg), gabapentin reduced mechanical allodynia, neuropathic pain, and hyperalgesia in rats and chronic allodynia in mice. Gabapentin had no effect on acute nociceptive pain as assessed using the Phase I formalin test in rats or the hot-plate test in mice. In these rodent studies, the potency of gabapentin was markedly higher (greater than 10-fold) when the drug was administered intrathecally as compared with other routes of administration. Intrathecal administration yielded no effect on hemodynamics, but produced mild neurological toxicity at doses greater than 300 µg.[60–62]

The work on gabapentin is exciting when viewed in terms of a single agent; however, new data suggest it may act synergistically when administered with clonidine and agents acting at the NMDA receptor. In rat models, using a ligature model of neuropathic pain, the use of the drugs concomitantly was significantly better than either drug alone, or the additive effect of the drugs independently.[63]

Other exciting work is ongoing with hormonal therapies. Deer et al.[64] recently completed a double-blind, randomized study of intrathecal octreotide for the treatment of chronic pain. In the final analysis, the overall improvement versus placebo was not statistically significant. However, when the subset of patients with neuropathic pain was analyzed separately, a statistically significant improvement was seen. Other drugs that are currently undergoing clinical studies include aspirin, neostigmine, adenosine, methadone, Demerol, and NMDA antagonist.

CONCLUSIONS

The decision for a physician or practice to add intrathecal therapies should be approached with a great deal of thought. Once that decision has been made, a commitment must be made by the entire team. This includes physicians, nurses, support staff, and pharmacists. With proper use of intrathecal therapies, many patients who have no hope for improvement may receive treatment that significantly enhances quality of life. It is imperative that advances continue with intrathecal drugs, devices, and outcome measures.

REFERENCES

1. Bigos, S. et al. (1994, December). *Acute low back problems in adults.* Clinical practice guideline no. 14. AHCPR Publication No. 95-0642, Rockville, MD: Agency for Health Care Policy and Research, Public Health Service, U.S. Department of Health and Human Services.

2. Lenrow, N. et al. (1990). *The 50 most frequent diagnosis-related groups, diagnoses, and procedures: Statistics by hospital size and location.* Rockville, MD: Public Health Service, DHHS publication 90-3465.

3. The American Academy of Pain Medicine and The American Pain Society. (2005). The use of opioids for the treatment of chronic pain: A consensus statement. Available at www.ampainsoc.org/advocacy/opioids.htm.

4. Coombs, D. W. et al. (1983). Relief of continuous chronic pain by intraspinal narcotics infusion via an implanted reservoir. *Journal of the American Medical Association, 250,* 2336.

5. Krames, E. S., & Lanning, R. M. (1993). Intrathecal infusional analgesia for nonmalignant pain: Analgesic efficacy of intrathecal opioid with or without bupivacaine. *Journal of Pain and Symptom Management, 8,* 539.

6. Onofrio, B. M. (1983). Treatment of chronic pain of malignant origin with intrathecal opiates. *Clinical Neurosurgery, 31,* 304.

7. Eisenach, J. et al. (2004). Intrathecal but not intravenous opioids release adenosine from the spinal cord. *Pain, 5,* 64.

8. Goodchild, C., Nadeson, R., & Cohen, E. (2004). Supraspinal and spinal cord opioid receptors are responsible for antinociception following intrathecal morphine injections. *European Journal of Anaesthesiology, 21,* 179.

9. Smith, T. et al. (2002). Randomized clinical trial of an implantable drug delivery system compared with comprehensive medical management for refractory cancer pain: Impact on pain, drug-related toxicity, and survival. *Journal of Clinical Oncology, 20,* 4040.

10. Manchikanti, L. et al. (2003). Evidence-based practice guidelines for the interventional techniques in the management of chronic spinal pain. *Pain Physician, 6,* 3.

11. Shetter, A. G., Hadley, M. N., & Wilkinson, E. (1986). Administration of intraspinal morphine sulfate for the treatment of intractable pain. *Journal of Neurosurgery, 18,* 740.

12. Brown, J. et al. (1999). Disease-specific and generic health outcomes: A model for the evaluation of long-term intrathecal opioid therapy in noncancer low back pain patients. *Clinical Journal of Pain, 15,* 122.

13. Katz, K. (2002). The impact of pain management on quality of life. *Journal of Pain and Symptom Management, 24,* S38.

14. Deer, T. et al. (2004). Intrathecal drug delivery for treatment of chronic low back pain: Report from the National Outcomes Registry for Low Back Pain. *Pain Medicine, 5,* 6.

15. Nguyen, H., Garber, J. E., & Hassenbusch, S. J. (2003). Spinal analgesics. *Anesthesiology Clinics of North America, 21,* 805.

16. Simpson, R. K., Jr. (2003). Mechanisms of action of intrathecal medications. *Neurosurgery Clinics of North America, 14,* 353.

17. Hassenbusch, S. et al. (2002). Management of intrathecal catheter-tip inflammatory masses: A consensus statement. *Pain Medicine, 3,* 313.

18. Hassenbusch, S. J., & Portenoy, R. K. (2000). Current practices in intraspinal therapy — A survey of clinical trends and decision-making. *Journal of Pain and Symptom Management, 20,* S4.

19. Bennet, G. et al. (2000). Clinical guidelines for intraspinal infusion: report of an expert panel. PolyAnalgesic Consensus Conference 2000. *Journal of Pain and Symptom Management, 20,* S37.

20. Deer, T. et al. (2002). Clinical experience with intrathecal bupivacaine in combination with opioid for the treatment of chronic pain related to failed back surgery syndrome and metastatic cancer pain of the spine. *Spine Journal, 2,* 274.

21. Hildebrand, K., Elsberry, D., & Deer, T. (2001). Stability, compatibility, and safety of intrathecal bupivacaine administered chronically via an implantable delivery system. *Clinical Journal of Pain, 17,* 239.

22. Dahm, P. et al. (2000). Comparison of 0.5% intrathecal bupivacaine with 0.5% intrathecal ropivacaine in the treatment of refractory cancer and noncancer pain conditions: Results from a prospective, crossover, double-blind, randomized study. *Regional Anesthesia and Pain Medicine, 25,* 480.

23. Staats, P. et al. (2004). Intrathecal ziconotide in the treatment of refractory pain in patients with cancer or AIDS: A randomized controlled trial. *Journal of the American Medical Association, 291,* 63.

24. Presley, R. W. et al. (submitted). Intrathecal ziconotide in the treatment of opioid-refractory neuropathic and nonmalignant pain: A controlled clinical trial. *Anesthesia & Analgesia,* submitted.

25. Roberts, L. J. et al. (2001). Outcome of intrathecal opioids in chronic non-cancer pain. *European Journal of Pain, 5,* 353.

26. Mironer, Y. E., & Grumman, S. (1999). Experience with alternative solutions in intrathecal treatment of chronic nonmalignant pain. *Pain Digest, 9,* 299.

27. Mironer, Y. E., & Tollison, C. D. (2001). Methadone in the intrathecal treatment of chronic nonmalignant pain resistant to other neuroaxial agents: The first experience. *International Neuromodulation Society, 4,* 25.

28. Mironer, Y. E. et al. (1999). Successful use of methadone in neuropathic pain: A multicenter study by the National Forum of Independent Pain Clinicians. *Pain Digest, 9,* 191.

29. Shir, Y. et al. (1991). Continuous epidural methadone treatment for cancer pain. *Clinical Journal of Pain, 7,* 339.

30. Deer, T. R. et al. (2002). Intrathecal bupivacaine for chronic pain: A review of current knowledge, *Neuromodulation, 5,* 196.

31. Hassenbusch, S. J. et al. (2002). Intrathecal clonidine in the treatment of intractable pain: A phase I/II study. *Pain Medicine, 3,* 85.

32. Ackerman, L. L., Follett, K. A. and Rosenquist, R. W. (2003). Long-term outcomes during treatment of chronic pain with intrathecal clonidine or clonidine/opioid combinations. *Journal of Pain and Symptom Management, 26,* 668.

33. Uhle, E. I. et al. (2000). Continuous intrathecal clonidine administration for the treatment of neuropathic pain. *Stereotactic and Functional Neurosurgery, 75,* 167.

34. Johansen, M. J. et al. (2002). Toxicity and efficacy of continuous intrathecal midazolam infusion in the sheep model. *Pain Medicine, 3,* 188.

35. Codman Interventional Pain. (2003). Data on file. Boston, MA: Author.

36. Paice, J., Penn, R., & Shott, S. (1996). Intraspinal morphine for chronic pain: A retrospective, multicenter study. *Journal of Pain and Symptom Management, 11,* 71.

37. Commbs, D., Maurer, L., & Saunders, R. (1984). Outcomes and complications of continuous intraspinal narcotic analgesia for cancer pain control. *Journal of Clinical Oncology, 2,* 1414.

38. Pasquier, Y., Cahana, A., & Schnider, A. (2003). Subdural catheter migration may lead to baclofen pump dysfunction. *Spinal Cord, 41,* 700.

39. Daniell, H. (2002). Hypogonadism in men consuming sustained-action oral opioids. *Journal of Pain, 3,* 377.

40. Willis, K. D., & Doleys, D. M. (1999). The effects of long-term intraspinal infusion therapy with noncancer pain patients: Evaluation of patient, significant-other, and clinic staff appraisals. *Neuromodulation, 2,* 241.

41. Coffey, R., & Burchiel, K. (2002). Inflammatory mass lesions associated with intrathecal drug infusion catheters: Report and observations on 41 patients. *Neurosurgery, 50,* 78.

42. McMillan, M., Doud, T., & Nugent, W. (2003). Catheter-associated masses in patients receiving intrathecal analgesic therapy. *Anesthesia & Analgesia, 96,* 186.

43. Deer, T. (2004). A prospective analysis of intrathecal granuloma in chronic pain patients: A review of the literature and report of a surveillance study. *Pain Physician, 7,* 225.

44. Yaksh, T. L. et al. (2002). Inflammatory masses associated with intrathecal drug infusion: A review of preclinical evidence and human data. *Pain Medicine, 3,* 300.

45. Yaksh, T. L. et al. (2003). Chronically infused intrathecal morphine in dogs. *Anesthesiology, 99,* 174.

46. Walker, S. M., Cousins, M. J. and Carr, D. B. (2002). Combination spinal analgesic chemotherapy: A systematic review. *Anesthesia & Analgesia, 95,* 674.

47. Gradert, T. L. et al. (2003). Safety of chronic intrathecal morphine infusion in a sheep model. *Anesthesiology, 99,* 188.

48. Baledent, O. et al. (2004). Relationship between cerebrospinal fluid and blood dynamics in healthy volunteers and patients with communicating hydrocephalus. *Investigational Radiology, 39,* 45.

49. Follett, K. A., & Naumann, C. P. (2000). A prospective study of catheter-related complications of intrathecal drug delivery systems. *Journal of Pain and Symptom Management, 19,* 209.

50. Aldrete, J. A., & Couto da Silva, J. M. (1997). Leg edema from intrathecal opiate infusions. *European Journal of Pain, 4,* 361.

51. de Lissovoy, G. et al. (1997). Cost-effectiveness of long-term intrathecal morphine therapy for pain associated with failed back surgery syndrome. *Clinical Therapeutics, 19,* 96.

52. Bedder, M., Soifer, B., & Mulhall, J. (1991). A comparison of patient-controlled analgesia and bolus PRN intravenous morphine in the intensive care environment. *Clinical Journal of Pain, 7,* 205.

53. Kumar, K., Hunter, G., & Demeria, D. (2002). Treatment of chronic pain by using intrathecal drug therapy compared with conventional pain therapies: A cost-effectiveness analysis. *Journal of Neurosurgery, 97,* 803.

54. Tutak, U., & Doleys, D. M. (1996). Intrathecal infusion systems for treatment of chronic low back and leg pain of noncancer origin. *Southern Medical Journal, 89,* 295.

55. van Hilten, B. J. et al. (2000). Intrathecal baclofen for the treatment of dystonia in patients with reflex sympathetic dystrophy. *New England Journal of Medicine, 343,* 625.

56. Grouls, R. J. E., Korsten, E. H. M., & Yaksh, T. L. (1999). General considerations for the formulation of drugs for spinal delivery. In T. L. Yaksh (Ed.), *Spinal drug delivery* (p. 371). Amsterdam: Elsevier Science B.V.

57. Yaksh, T. L., Rathbun, M. L., & Provencher, J. C. (1999). Preclinical safety evaluation for spinal drugs. In T. L. Yaksh (Ed.), *Spinal drug delivery* (p. 417). Amsterdam: Elsevier Science B.V.

58. Bennett, G. et al. (2000). Future directions in the management of pain by intraspinal drug delivery. *Journal of Pain and Symptom Management, 20,* S44.

59. Kroin, J. S., McCarthy, R. J., & Penn, R. D. (2003). Continuous intrathecal clonidine and tizanidine in conscious dogs: Analgesic and hemodynamic effects. *Anesthesia & Analgesia, 96*, 776.

60. Yoon, M. H., & Yaksh, T. L. (1999). The effect of intrathecal gabapentin on pain behavior and hemodynamics on the formalin test in rats. *Anesthesia & Analgesia, 89*, 434.

61. Wallin, J. et al. (2002). Gabapentin and pregabalin suppress tactile allodynia and potentiate spinal cord stimulation in a model of neuropathy. *European Journal of Pain, 6*, 261.

62. Lu, C., & Westlund, K. (1999). Gabapentin attenuates nociceptive behaviors in an acute arthritis model in rats. *Journal of Pharmacology and Experimental Therapeutics, 290*, 214.

63. Cheng, J. K., Pan, H. L., & Eisenach, J. C. (2000). Antiallodynic effect of intrathecal gabapentin and its interaction with clonidine in a rat model of postoperative pain. *Anesthesiology, 92*, 1126.

64. Deer, T. et al. (submitted). Intrathecal octreotide in the treatment of chronic noncancer pain, *Neuromodulation,* Submitted.

Section VIII

Integrative and Complementary Approaches

Robert A. Bonakdar, MD, Section Editor

76

Acupuncture and Traditional Chinese Medicine

James E. Williams, OMD, LAc, AP, FAAIM

INTRODUCTION

Chronic pain is one of the fastest growing health problems in the United States with an estimated one third of Americans suffering from pain at an annual cost of $80 billion to $100 billion (Eshkevari, 2003). It is also one of the most challenging conditions clinicians face and the most common reason patients seek alternative care. Acupuncture, of all alternative therapies, has considerable potential in the treatment and management of chronic pain. Much of the evidence on acupuncture is relevant and convincing, and suggests that in some cases it may be useful on its own while in others it may be part of an integrative approach to pain management. The integrative model may offer the most potential benefit to the patient. This chapter reviews and summarizes the scientific basis and clinical evidence for acupuncture and related traditional Chinese medicine modalities in the treatment and management of chronic and acute pain. It also discusses safety and the most common therapeutic course for conditions treatable by these therapies.

ACUPUNCTURE

Acupuncture and traditional Chinese medicine (TCM), the use of Chinese herbal medicines to treat disease and promote health, are collectively referred to as Oriental medicine (OM) and sometimes as East Asian medicine. With a history of several thousand years, OM is still widely practiced in Asia and has gained acceptance in Western countries. In fact, since the 1950s acupuncture has evolved rapidly as a modern therapy. First in China and Japan, followed by other Asian countries, Europe, and lately North America, acupuncture is gaining the respect of both the public and medical sectors. Interest in TCM followed in the mid-1980s, stimulating a surge of basic research in antiviral compounds, immunomodulating compounds for cancer, and adaptogenic compounds for neuroendocrine regulation, as well as anti-inflammatory and analgesic compounds for pain.

In the United States, acupuncture caught the public imagination in 1971 when James Reston, a reporter for the _New York Times_, published an article about his experience in China. In 1973, the U.S. Food and Drug Administration (FDA) classified acupuncture needles as experimental medical devices. Acupuncture needles were reclassified as "safe and effective" in 1995. In 1997, the National Institutes of Health published a consensus statement, the _NIH Consensus Development Conference on Acupuncture_, reporting favorable findings for the use of acupuncture in a select number of conditions. With such achievements, it is understandable that between 1992 and 1998 the demand for acupuncturists nearly doubled, climbing from 5,525 to 10,512.

At present in the United States, roughly 3,500 physicians and 12,000 licensed acupuncturists use this medical specialty for the treatment of a wide range of illnesses including chronic pain. Currently, 50 acupuncture and OM schools train nonphysicians, and about 500 to 600 physicians train yearly to American Acupuncture Medical Association standards (Erickson, 2003). Costs for acupuncture treatments vary according to locale, specialization, and experience of practitioners with an average range from $40 to $75 per visit. Workers' compensation and insurance fee schedules vary from state to state, but apply for those covered. However, most patients pay for acupuncture out-of-pocket.

Although now practiced worldwide, acupuncture has its roots in Chinese cosmology and philosophy. In this model, the universe is an orderly series of ever-changing cycles and events. Human biology is looked on as a reflection of the natural environment. For example, blood vessels are like rivers and fever or inflammation is likened to fire. Animating both the human and natural worlds is the non-Western concept of *qi*, an invisible but palpable energy pervading the body that flows in specialized networks or meridian systems and that is concentrated at specific sites along the course of those meridians — the acupuncture points (acupoints). Although *qi* and the meridians have defied scientific proof of their existence, they remain the central paradigm by which acupuncture is understood and practiced.

For now, most researchers leave the question of whether *qi* is real to philosophers and newly founded specialized fields such as human bioenergy, turning their attention to investigating the underlying neurophysiology of how acupuncture works. Practitioners are equally affected by a similar quandary as researchers: are *qi* and traditional theory necessary to achieve clinical success or can acupuncture be just as effective when performed as a medical technique based on neurophysiology or other Western methodology? Some acupuncturists base their practice on traditional Chinese medical philosophy; others combine points based on protocols matched to specific diseases; and some practitioners have suggested models integrating both Eastern and Western medical paradigms. Such modernized systems only utilize traditional acupuncture theory to the extent of selection of optimal therapeutic sites for the placement of needles, electrical stimulating devices, point injections, laser, or microcurrent stimulation.

NEEDLE MECHANICS

Traditionally, needle insertion is thought to stimulate and regulate the quality and flow of *qi*, described specifically in the acupuncture literature as *de qi* or needle sensation resulting in a particular numbing response that is associated with greater therapeutic effect. Because of the extreme thinness of acupuncture needles, specialized manual skill is required to insert it without bending. In some cases, an insertion tube made of stainless or plastic is used to keep the needle from flexing during initial insertion.

Once inserted, each needle is manually manipulated or electrically stimulated to maximize the needle sensation. Concurrent with needle insertion and manipulation, patients frequently report sensations in other areas of their body distant from the needle insertion site, which are known to correspond to meridians.

Scientific studies, on the other hand, contend that needle insertion has a wide range of neurochemical, immunological, and neurobiological effects. For example, inserting an acupuncture needle into normal tissue causes cellular disruption and corresponding immunological reactions. The multiple "mini-wounds" caused by needle insertion stimulate the release of growth factors such as platelet-derived growth factor, which induces DNA response and in turn promotes cell and tissue repair through increased protein synthesis (Filshie & White, 1998).

In the United States, acupuncturists favor pre-sterilized disposal needles in gauges between 0.12 and 0.30 mm in lengths from 15.0 to 60.0 mm. Depending on the area of the body treated and the technique employed, insertion depths range from 1 to 2 mm up to several centimeters, with an average depth of 14 mm. The number of needles used per treatment varies ranging from 2 to 12 on average.

SCIENTIFIC BASIS

Of all complementary and alternative therapies, acupuncture is the most researched, particularly for its use for pain management. Since 1976 numerous scientific studies have investigated the effects and possible mechanisms of acupuncture analgesia (AA) with a critical mass of acupuncture research accumulated between 1976 and 1988. By 2004, PubMed listings for acupuncture research included 8,916 papers of which 2,292 were related to pain. Bruce Pomeranz, a leader in acupuncture research, published more than 100 papers on AA. Other prominent researchers include Lixing Lao, Richard Hammerschlag, Jeanette Ezzo, Adrian White, Edzard Ernst, and Zang Hee Cho. In addition, research centers in China, Japan, South Korea, Hong Kong, Taiwan, and Singapore continue to contribute substantial information, as do centers in Germany and other European countries. Unfortunately, most of the results of this research is unavailable in English.

BASIC MECHANISMS

Chronic pain is thought to be the outcome of one or more causes: (1) ongoing nociception as from an unhealed fracture, a torn ligament, or chronic inflammation; (2) psychogenic factors without a known physiological basis; (3) stress-induced abnormal regulation of the hypothalamic-pituitary-adrenal axis; and (4) functional disturbances in the nervous system causing hypersensitivity without nociception as with sympathetically mediated pain. Acupuncture and related modalities, particularly electrostimulation, have the ability to regulate all four of these causes.

Acupuncture needling and electrical stimulation to acupuncture points have been shown to affect nociceptive, proprioceptive, and autonomic nerve pathways. Both needle acupuncture and electroacupuncture (EA) increase enkephalin and dynorphin in the spine and mid-brain, and raise endorphins in the pituitary–hypothalamus complex. The flow of enkephalins in mid-brain stimulates the release of monoamines, serotonin, and norepinephrine in the spine. It is theorized that these substances are responsible for the inhibition of pain. As early as 1979, Han et al. found that serotonin turnover is increased with acupuncture, and conversely, when serotonin is depleted, the acupuncture analgesic effect is reduced (Han, Chou, Lu, Lu, Yang, & Jen, 1979). According to this hypothesis, needle stimulus acts to restore neurotransmitter chemical balance and thereby neutralizes pain initiated by a painful stimulus (Pomeranz, 2001).

Inflammatory mediators may also be involved in AA. Endorphins inhibit substance P, a short-chain polypeptide that functions as a neurotransmitter involved in pain and inflammation. Neuropeptides, such as substance P, are involved in the production of cytokines such as tumor necrosis factor-alpha, interleukin 1-beta, interleukin 2, and interleukin 6. These cytokines along with substance P are involved in the inflammatory cascade and influence the rate of wound healing (Delgado, McManus, & Chambers, 2003). The anti-inflammatory actions of acupuncture are linked to the complex interactions between substance P and beta-endorphin, which may influence the balance between proinflammatory and anti-inflammatory activity (Zijlstra, van den Berg-de Lange, Huygen, & Klein, 2003). EA has been shown to influence substance P in the dorsal vagal complex in rat models (Liu et al., 2004).

NEWER MODELS: GENE EXPRESSION

Part of the long-term effect of acupuncture beyond opioid changes may lie in gene expression. Several studies demonstrate that levels of c-Fos, a gene that produces a protein, which functions in the control of the transcription of DNA to mRNA, increase in affected brain areas following acupuncture. Usually the amount of c-Fos in cells is low until the cell is stimulated by a stressor. c-Fos is useful as a marker for increased cellular activity and has been studied in the expression of GABAergic and serotonergic activity in the brainstem and spinal cord (Maloney, Mainville, & Jones, 2000). In animal studies, acupuncture has shown to increase c-Fos expression in the hypothalamus (Medeiros, Canteras, Suchecki, & Mello, 2003), hippocampus (Kang et al., 2003), spinal cord (Kim et al., 2003), and pituitary gland (Pan, Castro-Lopes, & Coimbra, 1996). However, in a paper by Jiang et al., EA was found to inhibit c-Fos expression during brain injury (Jiang, Zhao, Shui, & Xia, 2004). As with many research models of acupuncture, it is possible that a regulatory effect may eventually be found in which acupuncture acts as both an agonist and antagonist for c-Fos expression.

NEUROENDOCRINE MODULATION

Neuromodulators and functional changes in the neuroendocrine system may also be involved in the acupuncture response and its ability to mediate pain. In one study, researchers demonstrated that melatonin combined with EA suggested a relationship between AA with an increase in pro-opimelanocortin (POMC) mRNA (Zhou, Yu, & Wang, 2001). POMC is a single precursor molecule for peptides such as melanocortin that effect energy homeostasis (Schwartz, Woods, Porte, Seeley, & Baskin, 2000). In another study, electrostimulation to auricular points increased plasma levels of growth hormone (Debreceni, 1991). Less is known on how the pituitary–hypothalamic complex functions than neural response; however, it is thought that acupuncture modulates hypothalamic release of β-endorphin and adrenocorticotrophic stimulating hormone by the pituitary (Masala et al., 1983). Studies suggest that both peptides continue to increase up to 80 minutes after acupuncture (Zhou et al., 2001). Dopamine may also play a role in chronic widespread pain (Wood, 2004) and may be increased by acupuncture (Han, Yoon, Cho, Kim, & Min, 1999). Neuronal circuits that influence hormone regulation in the hypothalamus, such as POMC expression, suggest at the complexity of neuroendocrine activity in the body. These and other studies suggest how acupuncture might play a neuroendocrine regulatory role in the management of pain.

IMAGING AND BRAIN SCANNING

Historically, acupuncture research seems to have taken on the technology of the times. After endorphins, a group of 10 neurotransmitters that activate opiate receptors, were discovered by Hughes and Kosterlitz in 1975 (Kosterlitz & Hughes, 1977), for more than a decade acupuncture researchers favored opioid models. In the early 1980s, neuroendocrine models were investigated. In the early 1990s, models of gene expression were explored. As computerized scanning technology became available in the late 1990s, researchers such as Alavi and La Riccia demonstrated by single photon emission computed tomography (SPECT) scan abnormal blood flow in some brain areas of patients with chronic pain, which normalized with acupuncture (Alavi & La Riccia, 1997). In a study of five patients with chronic pain, SPECT scanning employed before and after acupuncture treatment revealed thalamic asymmetrical blood flow, which was normalized after treatment coinciding with reported pain relief from the test subjects (Alavi, La Riccia, Sadek, & Lattanand, 1996).

More recently, using functional magnetic resonance imaging, Cho investigated models for acupuncture research using neuroimaging based on molecular science and pharmacokinetics. Although far from a unifying theory of how acupuncture works, such research provides objective and quantitative analyses in an "East meets West" approach toward understanding the mechanisms of acupuncture.

In groundbreaking work, Cho examined needling response to acupoints LI4 and ST36, both commonly used sites for amelioration of pain in the upper and lower body, respectively, in normal subjects (Cho et al., 1998; Cho, Oleson, Alimi, & Niemtzow, 2002). Significant brain activity was noted in the brainstem, midbrain, and cerebral cortex. In further studies, Cho expanded acupoints to include UB67 on the foot, GB 37 on the lower lateral leg, and GB 43 on the lateral distal foot. Armed with promising results from his imaging studies, Cho formulated an acupuncture pain relief hypothesis involving higher cortical areas (Cho, 2001). In this model, the effects of acupuncture are mediated through the central nervous system affecting corresponding areas of the cerebral cortex where communication takes place, theorized principally in the hypothalamus, where further neural communication occurs resulting in pain modulation. This may also help to explain the healing effects of acupuncture on a wide range of diseases.

CLINICAL EVIDENCE

Although an overwhelming body of observational information in nonpeer-reviewed journals and books describes the effects of acupuncture and Chinese medicine, and the body of scientific research into the mechanisms of acupuncture is extensive and growing, the overall number of clinical studies remains small. The reason for this is twofold. First, initial efforts in acupuncture research have focused on amassing a sizable body of evidence evaluating the mechanisms of AA and establishing safety before conducting human trials. At the time, no one knew how acupuncture worked; therefore, animals were ethically acceptable models for investigation. Second, there are several inherent difficulties in acupuncture clinical research. These include whether single- or double-blinded studies are best, how to establish a true control group since sham acupuncture itself may have greater effect than placebo; and if placebo in fact is the standard against which acupuncture should measured (Hammerschlag, 2003).

Blinded, placebo-controlled trials may be the gold standard for studying drugs, but obviously acupuncture is not a drug and, if anything, is more like a surgical procedure. Perhaps the only reason clinical studies for acupuncture have been compared against placebo is because of the early stance of the American Medical Association that acupuncture was no more effective than placebo or that it was similar to hypnosis. It seems strange that this debate is still going on when the first NIH grant for acupuncture headed by Ulett delivered convincing evidence in 1983 that acupuncture successfully modulated experimental pain and was not hypnosis (Ulett, 1983, 1996).

In addition, assessing the adequacy of acupuncture trials emphasizes study design but, in the West, rarely addresses whether the method used was in fact sufficiently adequate to achieve effective results (White & Ernst, 1998). The problem of effectiveness arises because of the many different techniques and styles of acupuncture used by practitioners; some methods are more effective for certain conditions than others and some practitioners are more effective than others. Compounding this is that there are no definitive studies comparing one form of acupuncture with another, such as Chinese versus Japanese acupuncture, for the treatment of a specific condition.

Systematic reviews of existing acupuncture studies also suffer from a variety of problems. These include reviewers' bias, limited number of well-designed studies, and lack of clustering of similarly designed studies. In addition, until recently there was no method of assessing the adequacy of acupuncture treatments used in the studies. To address this concern, White and Ernst devised a checklist of data required in studies using acupuncture treatments, including specifics of patient posture, number of needles used, needle size, use of international standards for acupuncture point names and locations, and depth of insertion (White & Ernst, 2003). Defining universal standards for acupuncture studies is a significant step toward establishing evidence.

In contrast to these limitations, the Cochrane Collaboration rigorously reviews methodology and outcomes and is considered the leading method for summarizing evidence (Ezzo, 2003). To date, seven Cochrane Reviews have been completed on acupuncture for rheumatoid arthritis, asthma, headache, induction of labor, lateral elbow pain, low back pain, and smoking cessation, with reviews in progress on stroke, postoperative nausea and vomiting, Bell's palsy, chronic constipation, depression, opioid dependence, and osteoarthritis. The interest in evidence-based information on acupuncture is shown by the number of reviews conducted or in progress. However, due to lack of well-designed, placebo-controlled, and randomized studies available in English, results of these reviews are equivocal.

Several important areas of study in pain management with acupuncture remain to be investigated. Because acupuncture needle therapy is time and labor intensive, it is important to learn if electrical stimulation provides equal benefit (Ceccherelli, Gagliardi, Seda, Corradin, & Giron, 1999). If so, which type is more effective? Is auricular acupuncture, in practice much easier to administer to a patient, equal or better than whole-body needle acupuncture (Lein, Clelland, Knowles, & Jackson, 1989)? Does electrostimulation of auricular acupuncture points work better than manual auricular acupuncture? In one study comparing auricular acupuncture with electrical stimulation for the treatment of chronic cervical pain, continuous electrical stimulation of auricular acupuncture points sig-

TABLE 76.1
Selected WHO-Listed Pain Conditions

System	Condition
Dental	Toothache, post-extraction pain
Neurological	Headache, migraine, trigeminal neuralgia, peripheral neuropathies, intercostals neuralgia
Musculoskeletal	Cervicobrachial syndrome, "frozen" shoulder, "tennis elbow," sciatica, low back pain, osteoarthritis

TABLE 76.2
NIH Consensus Statement on Acupuncture Listed Conditions

Conditions with Substantial Evidence	Acceptable Conditions for Treatment
Postoperative pain	Addiction
Chemotherapy-induced and pregnancy-associated nausea and vomiting	Asthma
Postoperative dental pain	Carpal tunnel syndrome
	Fibromyalgia
	Headache
	Low back pain
	Menstrual cramps
	Myofascial pain
	Osteoarthritis
	Stroke
	Tennis elbow

nificantly decreased pain, improved psychological well-being, and improved sleep (Sator-Katzenschlager et al., 2003). The challenge for researchers has been in finding a fair and objective way to evaluate the clinical evidence of acupuncture so that the foundational studies necessary are rigorously conducted (Sherman & Cherkin, 2003).

EVIDENCE BASE FOR SPECIFIC CONDITIONS

Acupuncture is used for a broad range of health conditions. Chinese acupuncture textbooks list anesthesia during surgery, infectious diseases such as the common cold and malaria, respiratory conditions such as asthma and bronchitis, cardiovascular conditions such as congestive heart failure, diabetes, hyperthyroidism, facial paralysis, headache, mastitis, and many other conditions (Bensky, 1981). However, it was not until 1979 when the World Health Organization (WHO) upon review of traditional claims for acupuncture listed more than 40 conditions that are suitable for treatment by acupuncture (Table 76.1). However, these conditions were selected without strong evidence for their efficacy. They include conditions of the upper and lower respiratory tract; eye, ear, and dental problems, gastrointestinal disorders, neurological, and musculoskeletal pain.

In 1998, almost two decades after the WHO list, the NIH Consensus Statement on Acupuncture (NIH, 1998) concluded that there was substantial evidence for the efficacy of acupuncture for postoperative, chemotherapy-induced, and pregnancy-associated nausea and vomiting, and for postoperative dental pain (Table 76.2). In addition, the panel concluded that a number of conditions are acceptably treated with acupuncture although further research is necessary. These include addiction, stroke, headache, menstrual cramps, tennis elbow, fibromyalgia, myofascial pain, osteoarthritis, low back pain, carpal tunnel syndrome, and asthma.

Recent acupuncture literature suggests that many other pain conditions respond to acupuncture and related modalities including musculoskeletal pain, sciatica, urogenital pain, labor pains, neuropathy, facial pain, neck pain, and pain associated with malignancy (Filshie & White, 1998).

In a study of 73 patients with symptomatic osteoarthritis of the knee, acupuncture proved effective as long as 4 weeks after treatment (Singh, Berman, Hadhazy, Bareta, Lao, Zarow et al., 2001). In another study on knee osteoarthritis, psychosocial factors were measured in patients to study possible placebo effects of acupuncture. As in other arthritis studies, response to acupuncture was favorable, while no evidence of a link between psychosocial variables was found (Creamer, Singh, Hochberg, & Berman, 1999).

Acupuncture and EA have been found to ameliorate symptoms in men with chronic prostatitis and pelvic pain (Antolak, 2004) and renal colic (Antolak, 2004), dysmenorrhea (Thomas, Lundeberg, Bjork, Lundstrom-Lindstedt et al., 1995), and pelvic pain in women (Slocomb, 1984).

Chronic low back pain (cLBP) is a commonly seen condition in the pain clinic. Several studies show that acupuncture is useful in all age groups. In a 2003 randomized, controlled trial on subjects older than 60 years, Meng et al. (2003) found that acupuncture was effective and safe in older patients. In blinded, randomized, controlled studies comparing electrical stimulation with manual acupuncture, both therapies have been shown to be effective in managing cLBP (Kerr, Walsh, & Baxter, 2003). Policy setting studies are currently under way in Europe for the treatment of cLBP and osteoarthritis. To date, the largest study on cLBP is the German Acupuncture Trial for Chronic Low Back Pain study. In a multicenter, randomized, partially blinded trial 102 patients were treated. In another study 300 patients were studied for osteoarthritis under protocols developed by Acupuncture Randomized Trials, and another 300 subjects for cLBP (Brinkhaus et al., 2003). Results from these studies were due for release in 2004 but have not been published in time for inclusion here.

Studies comparing different treatments and combining modalities have also been performed. As orthopedists refer patients for physical therapy, most acupuncturists

TABLE 76.3
Comprehensive List of Pain Conditions Responsive to Acupuncture

Conditions with Substantial Evidence	Conditions with Reasonable Evidence or Consensus	Conditions Potentially Responsive to Acupuncture Based on Observational Studies
Postoperative dental pain	Carpal tunnel syndrome	Malignancy-associated pain
Headache	Fibromyalgia	Neck pain
Low back pain	Intercostal neuralgia	Neurofibromatosis
Osteoarthritis	Menstrual cramps	Neuralgia
	Migraine	Post-arthroscopic pain
	Myofascial pain	Reflex sympathetic dystrophy
	Peripheral neuropathies	Rheumatoid arthritis
	Tennis elbow	Sciatica
	Trigeminal neuralgias	

prescribe back exercises in addition to providing treatment. In one study combining EA and back exercises, 52 patients were treated with results indicating that the combination was effective in managing pain and reducing disability associated with cLBP (Yeung, Leung, & Chow, 2003). In a randomized trial with 115 patients comparing medication, spinal manipulation, and acupuncture for spinal pain, results suggest that manipulation may be better for short-term pain relief and increased mobility, but it does not provide the longer-term anti-inflammatory relief as does acupuncture or steroid medications (Giles & Muller, 2003). In a randomized, controlled trial on chronic neck pain, laser acupuncture was more effective than conventional massage therapy (Konig et al., 2003). Acupuncture is useful following musculoskeletal surgery as found in a controlled study on arthroscopic acromioplasty. Findings with 35 patients indicated lower postsurgical pain levels, less use of analgesics, increased range of motion, and a high rate of patient satisfaction (Gilbertson, Wenner, & Russell, 2003).

Malignancy-associated pain causes considerable suffering among cancer patients. In France, auricular acupuncture has been used to alleviate cancer pain for more than 30 years. In a randomized, blinded, controlled trial of 90 patients, statistically significant evidence was found for the reduction of pain intensity (Alimi, Rubino, Leandri, & Brule, 2000; Alimi et al., 2003).

Other conditions for which acupuncture has been shown to be effective include neurofibromatosis, low back pain of pregnancy, soft tissue disorders of the shoulder, rheumatoid arthritis, neuropathic pain following spinal cord injury, reflex sympathetic dystrophy, sciatica, and fibromyalgia (Table 76.3).

MERIDIAN SYSTEM AND ACUPUNCTURE POINT RESEARCH

The problem of solving or disproving the existence of *qi*, acupoints, and the meridians has been of little interest to Western researchers. However, because these concepts are the basis of acupuncture theory and practice, and derive from Chinese culture, Asian researchers have taken the challenge more seriously. *Qi* research is largely carried on in China and Japan, where it is culturally acceptable, with international conferences annually where results of studies are presented, little of which has been taken seriously by Western scientists. Detection of acupoints has focused on electrical conductivity or resistance, with researchers theorizing that acupoints should manifest at the dermal surface as sites of lowered resistance and increased conduction.

Since the 1950s, Chinese, Japanese, French, German, and Austrian researchers have developed devices that confirm this suggesting that acupoints are anatomically real but instead are part of a non-neurological system in communication with the nervous, endocrine, and immune systems: in a sense, a homeostatic system regulating the internal physiological milieu with the outer environment.

A number of electrical point detection devices are used by acupuncturists and researchers including Electro-Acupuncture According to Voll originally developed in Germany by Reinhold Voll in 1953. This system measures galvanic skin resistance at distal acupuncture points on the fingers and toes using a 1 volt, 6 to 12 microampere current. Ryodoraku, first researched in Japan by Yoshio Nakatani in 1951 and followed by Odo and Hyodo of the pain clinic at Osaka Medical College (Hyodo, 1980), is based on autonomic nervous system function and uses a 12 volt, 200-microampere current to measure points.

Validating the existence of acupuncture meridians is equally challenging. Based on animal models, Ma et al. hypothesize that a perivascular space around blood vessels independent of lymphatic vessels constitutes an interstitial space within loose tissue through which acupuncture-induced signals are transmitted (Ma et al., 2003). Motoyama's Apparatus for Meridian Identification device is under investigation for its diagnostic capabilities in establishing meridian and organ system disturbances and as means of monitoring effectiveness of acupuncture intervention (Borg, 2003).

SAFETY

Acupuncture safety falls into several categories: transmission of infectious diseases, infection from unsanitary needles or improper clean needle technique, direct injury to tissue or organs from needle insertion, allergic reactions, and needle breakage within the tissue. Lao, Hamilton, Fu, and Berman (2003), in a systematic review of 98 published papers between 1965 and 1999, identified 202 cases of complications associated with acupuncture. The most common complication found between 1974 and 1988 was hepatitis B with 94 cases reported. There have been no epidemiological reports of transmission of hepatitis C virus or HIV through acupuncture.

Common side effects of acupuncture include pain from needling, anxiety, and syncope. First-time patients are most susceptible; therefore, to prevent syncope the supine position is recommended over the seated position. Hematoma is another possible side effect, as are light-headedness, tiredness, drowsiness, and induction of sleep during treatment. Transient, localized skin irritation including erythema is not uncommon in patients with allergic dispositions. All of these side effects can be significantly minimized by an experienced practitioner who explains each step of treatment to new patients, and applies localized massage to acupuncture points after treatment, applies pressure when a hematoma is observed, and makes sure patients are positioned in a comfortable manner on the treatment table. Bruising may also occur in patient with a tendency for easy bruising and in elderly individuals with aged and fragile skin. Because of their blood-thinning properties, precaution should be taken with patients taking drugs such as coumadin and aspirin (Peuker, White, Ernst, Pera, & Filler, 1999).

Some patients do not react favorably to acupuncture. These nonresponders may be deficient, genetically or otherwise, in opiate receptors (Peets & Pomeranz, 1978). Nonresponder results may be improved by the addition of DL-phenylalanine, an essential amino acid, at 750 to 1,000 mg daily to potentiate endorphin release (Hendler, 2001). Other factors influencing acupuncture efficacy are under investigation. In animal models, Lee et al. (2003) demonstrated that the analgesic effect of acupuncture is closely related to the amount of genetic expression of cholecystokinin-A receptors. Cholecystokinin is a peptide prehormone secreted from mucosal epithelial cells in the small intestine and produced by neurons in the enteric nervous system. It is widely distributed in the brain and may be the most abundant neuropeptide in the central nervous system.

Considering an estimated 5.4 million acupuncture visits in 1997 alone, the risks of acupuncture are small and the incidence of side effects minimal and uncommon. According to the 2002 National Health Interview Survey, the largest and most comprehensive survey of complementary and alternative medicine use by American adults, an estimated 8.2 million U.S. adults have used acupuncture safely (Barnes et al., 2004).

ACUPUNCTURE THERAPY

Acupuncture is both a practice and a technique. The practice of acupuncture rests upon several thousand years of empirical experience and an ancient, comprehensive theory of health and disease. The technique of acupuncture consists of inserting specialized stainless steel needles into specific sites on the body, manipulating these needles manually or with electrostimulation, and then removing them. Point selection is based on the condition, location, and symptoms, and is guided by the theory of practice. The procedure is repeated at subsequent visits for a course of treatment, which on average consists of between 5 and 10 visits.

In China, it is common to perform acupuncture in a series of 10 to 30 daily treatments for two to four courses, with a rest of several days to a few weeks between each course. In the West and particularly in the HMO environment, we cannot emulate this economically, which brings up the question of cost-to-benefit ratio. But what is the most effective number of treatments for specific conditions? It is well known that repeated treatment with acupuncture or low-frequency, high-intensity electrical stimulation as with transcutaneous electric nerve stimulation (TENS) produce cumulative benefit for the patient (Pomeranz & Warma, 1988). Due to this cumulative effect, Western practitioners find that 10 to 15 treatments provided two to three times weekly produce sufficient pain-modulating effects.

Needle insertion combined with electrical stimulation, heat from moxibustion, and massage to acupoints before or after insertion are common additions to traditional acupuncture. In fact, in China acupuncture is traditionally called *zhen jiu* meaning needle and moxibustion, which is the burning of a prepared form of *Artemesia vulagaris*, a mugwort species, indirectly to an acupoint or directly to a needle inserted into a point. Other modalities include injection therapy, adaptation of microcurrent stimulation to acupoints using small probes or pads, EA without needles, retention of magnets or interdermal needles, and laser therapy.

Acupoint injection therapy uses small dosages of vitamin B_{12}, herbal extracts, homeopathic medications, biological substances such as Botox, as well as anti-inflammatory pharmaceutical agents such as cortisone and analgesics for the treatment of pain. Often referred to as "wet" acupuncture (vs. "dry" when needle only is employed), this method has a long history in Germany but is only in the early stages of use in the United States.

Microcurrent has been shown to reduce symptoms of muscle damage following competitive sports (Lambert, Marcus, Burgess, & Noakes, 2002), neck and shoulder pain (Kim, 2001), and other pain conditions (Wieder, 1991). Devices have been adapted specifically for the acupuncture clinic using handheld probes to identify and treat problem areas such as the temporomandibular joint and other small joints.

EA devices that do not use needles but that simulate results of acupuncture are attractive for use in the pain clinic. TENS has a long history of use in the pain clinic. Grant, Bishop-Miller, Winchester, Anderson et al. (1999) demonstrated statistically significant improvement with both TENS and acupuncture, with acupuncture offering additional benefits over TENS. Home use of TENS units can complement acupuncture treatments, especially when patients can come for treatment only once or twice weekly.

Correlations among acupuncture, auricular acupuncture, EA, and vagal response have long been speculated with research conducted on heart rate (Shi, 1997; White & Ernst, 1999) and gastric secretion (Noguchi & Hayashi, 1996), as well as in the treatment of pain. In particular, auricular acupuncture according to Nogier of France has received wide acceptance (Oleson, 2002). In a study of 90 patients with cancer pain, Alimi, Rubino, Leandri, and Brule (2003) demonstrated clear benefit using auricular acupuncture over placebo.

Magnets and interdermal needles retained subcutaneously have wide use in Asia; however, there is scanty evidence in the literature for their use. Interest in using magnets applied to acupoints is increasing in the United States and may play an adjunctive role by applying magnets to affected areas in patients with pain between treatments as with TENS. In one double-blind study, Hinman, Ford, and Heye (2002) found that patients with chronic knee pain had statistically significantly less pain than the control group. In another study on osteoarthritis of the knee, Wolsko, Eisenberg, Simon, Davis et al. (2004) demonstrated statistically significant efficacy of magnetic therapy as compared with placebo after 4 hours.

Low-power lasers (LPL) have been employed in Europe since the 1970s for the treatment of pain and the promotion of tissue healing. The most frequently used types are visible red light helium–neon gas lasers, infrared gallium–aluminum–arsenide lasers, and gallium–arsenide lasers. Irradiated tissue is not heated as with surgical lasers. Trials involved LPL for pain have been conducted for trigeminal neuralgia (Walker & Akhanjee, 1985), postherpetic neuralgia (Moore, Hira, Kumar et al., 1988), rheumatoid disease (Oyamada & Izu, 1985), and myofascial pain. LPL therapy has been adapted for stimulation of acupoints as "needleless" acupuncture. Although the mechanisms behind laser efficacy remains poorly under-

stood, there is wide acceptance among acupuncture professionals for tissue-healing, reduction in soft tissue inflammation, and in some cases, reduction of pain.

TRADITIONAL CHINESE MEDICINE

Traditionally, Chinese herbal medicine has been used in Asia for a wide range of acute and chronic pain conditions such as osteoarthritis, rheumatoid arthritis, cervicalgia, low back pain, headache, fibrositis and myositis, neuritis, and other pain conditions. Herbal drugs have been shown to exert antioxidant activity, modulate cytokines and chemokines, effect gene expression, and regulate the inflammatory cascade. Modern Chinese herbal preparations include concentrated extracts, standardized dry extracts, and injectable medications. Numerous traditional Chinese herbal medicines have been shown to have analgesic and anti-inflammatory activity in the laboratory and in animal models. These include *Panax ginseng radix*, *Scutellaria radix*, *Aconiti radix*, *Stephaniae tetrandrae radix*, and others.

Ginsenosides Rb1, Rb2, Rd, Rf, Rg1, and Rg3 have antinociceptive effects on substance P–induced pain models (Choi, Han, Han, Lee, & Suh, 2003). In a study involving *Aconiti* and *Stephaniae*, analgesia was demonstrated in a rat model (Li, Zhang, & Qin, 2000). In another animal model, the flavanoid wogonin derived from *Scutellaria* inhibited inflammatory-associated enzymes much as cyclooxygenases (Chi, Lim, Park, & Kim, 2003).

However, few randomized, controlled clinical studies on large numbers of subjects have been performed. Because safety and drug–herb interactions are a controversial topic, until further investigation provides sufficient data on efficacy and safety, the practice of using Chinese herbal compounds in the integrative pain clinic should be avoided.

CONCLUSIONS

Both medical and traditional acupuncture are effective and safe methods for the treatment and management of chronic pain. Although a unifying model of the scientific mechanisms of acupuncture reconciled with TCM theory and modern human bioenergy hypotheses remains illusive, researchers continue to investigate the evidence underlying acupuncture. Further investigation is required for use of Chinese herbal preparations before they are integrated into common use in the pain clinic. It may be that bringing Western and Chinese medical paradigms into concert with each other, both in the research and clinical setting, will provide the necessary relevance needed to learn how they can benefit patients and fully integrate acupuncture and related traditional Chinese medicine therapies into the pain clinic.

REFERENCES

Alavi, A., & La Riccia, P. (1997). Neuroimaging of acupuncture in patients with chronic pain. *Journal of Alternative and Complementary Medicine, 3*(1), S47–S53.

Alavi, A., La Riccia, P., Sadek, H., & Lattanand, G. (1996). Objective assessment of the effects of pain and acupuncture on regional brain function with Tc99 mm HMPAO SPECT imaging. *Journal of Nuclear Medicine, 37*(Suppl. 5), 278.

Alimi, D., Rubino, C., Leandri, E. P., & Brule, S. F. (2000). Analgesic effects of auricular acupuncture for cancer pain. *Journal of Pain and Symptom Management, 19*(2), 81–82.

Alimi, D., Rubino, C., Pichard-Leandri, E., Fermand-Brule, S. et al. (2003). Analgesic effect of auricular acupuncture for cancer pain: A randomized, blinded, controlled trial. *Journal of Clinical Oncology, 21*(22), 4120–4126.

Alimi, D., Rubino, C., Pichard-Leandri, E., Fermand-Brule, S., Dubreuil-Lemaire, M. L., & Hill, C. (2003). Analgesic effect of auricular acupuncture for cancer pain: A randomized, blinded, controlled trial. *Journal of Clinical Oncology, 21*(22), 4120–4126.

Antolak, S. J., Jr. (2004). Acupuncture ameliorates symptoms in men with chronic prostatitis/chronic pelvic pain syndrome. *Urology, 63*(1), 212.

Barnes, P. M., Powell-Griner, E., McFann, K., & Nahin, R. L. (2004). Complementary and alternative medicine use among adults: United States, 2002. *CDC Advance Data Report, 343.*

Bensky, D. (Ed.). (1981). *Acupuncture, A comprehensive text.* Chicago: Eastland Press.

Borg, H. (2003). Alternative method of gifted identification using the AMI: An apparatus for measuring internal meridians and their corresponding organs. *Journal of Alternative and Complementary Medicine, 9*(6), 861–867.

Brinkhaus, B., Becker-Witt, C., Jena, S., Linde, K., Streng, A., Wagenpfeil, S. et al. (2003). Acupuncture randomized trials (ART) in patients with chronic low back pain and osteoarthritis of the knee — design and protocols. *Research in Complementary and Classical Natural Medicine, 10*(4), 185–191.

Ceccherelli, F., Gagliardi, G., Seda, R., Corradin, M., & Giron, G. (1999). Different analgesic effects of manual and electrical acupuncture stimulation of real and sham auricular points: A blind controlled study with rats. *Acupuncture & Electro-Therapeutics Research, 24*(3–4), 169–179.

Chi, Y., Lim, H., Park, H. J., & Kim, H. (2003). Effects of woganin, a plant flavone from *Scutellaria radix* on skin inflammation: *In vivo* regulation of inflammation-associated gene expression. *Biochemical Pharmacology, 66*(7), 1271–1278.

Cho, Z. H. (2001). Functional magnetic resonance imaging of the brain in the investigation of acupuncture. In G. Strux & R. Hammerschlag (Eds.), *Clinical Acupuncture: Scientific Basis* (pp. 83–95). Berlin: Springer Verlag.

Cho, Z. H., Chung, S. C., Jones, J. P., Park, J. B., Park, H. J., Lee, H. J. et al. (1998). New findings of the correlation between acupoints and corresponding brain cortices using functional MRI. *Proceedings of the National Academy of Sciences of the United States of America, 95*(5), 2670–2673.

Cho, Z. H., Oleson, T. D., Alimi, D., & Niemtzow, R. C. (2002). Acupuncture: The search for biologic evidence with functional magnetic resonance imaging and positron emission tomography techniques. *Journal of Alternative and Complementary Medicine, 8*(4), 399–401.

Choi, S. S., Han, E. J., Han, K. J., Lee, H. K., & Suh, H. W. (2003). Antinociceptive effects of ginsenosides injected intracerebroventricularly or intrathecally in substance P-induced pain model. *Planta Medica, 69*(11), 1001–1004.

Creamer, P., Singh, B. B., Hochberg, M. C., & Berman, B. M. (1999). Are psychosocial factors related to response to acupuncture among patients with knee osteoarthritis? *Alternative Therapies in Health and Medicine, 5*(4), 72–76.

Debreceni, L. (1991). The effect of electrical stimulation of the ear points on the plasma ACTH and GH level in humans. *Acupuncture & Electro-Therapeutics Research, 16*(1–2), 45–51.

Delgado, A. V., McManus, A. T., & Chambers, J. P. (2003). Production of tumor necrosis factor-alpha, interleukin 1-beta, interleukin 2, and interleukin 6 by rat leukocyte subpopulations after exposure to substance P. *Neuropeptides, 37*(6), 355–361.

Erickson, R. J. (2003). *Guide for physicians seeking hospital and HMO privileges.* American Academy of Medical Acupuncture. Available at http://www.medicalacupuncture.org/acu_info/priv.html.

Eshkevari, L. (2003). Acupuncture and pain: A review of the literature. *American Association of Nurse Anesthetists Journal, 71*(5), 361–370.

Ezzo, J. (2003). From the five blind men to Cochrane Complementary Medicine Systematic Reviews. *Journal of Alternative and Complementary Medicine, 9*(6), 969–972.

Filshie, J., & White, A. (Eds.). (1998). *Medical acupuncture, a western scientific approach.* London: Churchill Livingston.

Gilbertson, B., Wenner, K., & Russell, L. C. (2003). Acupuncture and arthroscopic acromioplasty. *Journal of Orthopedic Research, 21*(4), 752–758.

Giles, L. G., & Muller, R. (2003). Chronic spinal pain: A randomized clinical trial comparing medication, acupuncture, and spinal manipulation. *Spine, 28*(14), 1490–1502; discussion 1502–1493.

Grant, D., Bishop-Miller, J., Winchester, D., Anderson, L. et al. (1999). A randomized comparative trial of acupuncture versus transcutaneous electrical nerve stimulation for chronic back pain in the elderly. *Pain, 82*(1), 9–13.

Hammerschlag, R. (2003). Acupuncture: On what should its evidence base be based? *Alternative Therapies in Health and Medicine, 9*(3), 34–35.

Han, C., Chou, P., Lu, C., Lu, L., Yang, T. H., & Jen, M. E. (1979). The role of central 5-hydroxytrptamine in acupuncture analgesia. *Scientia Sinica, 22,* 91–104.

Han, S.-H., Yoon, S.-H., Cho, Y.-W., Kim, C.-J., & Min, B.-I. (1999). Inhibitory effects of electroacupuncture on stress responses evoked by tooth-pulp stimulation in rats. *Physiology and Behavior, 66*(2), 217–222.

Hendler, S. (Ed.). (2001). *PDR for nutritional supplements.* Montvale, NJ: Medical Economics, Thomson Healthcare.

Hinman, M.R., Ford, J., & Heyl, H., (2002). Effects of static magnets on chronic knee pain and physical function: A double-blind study. *Alternative Therapies in Health and Medicine, 8*(4), 50–55.

Hyodo, M. (1980). *Recent advances on acupuncture treatment.* Osaka, Japan: Pain Clinic, Department of Anesthesiology, Osaka Medical College.

Jiang, K., Zhao, Z., Shui, Q., & Xia, Z. (2004). Electro-acupuncture preconditioning abrogates the elevation of *c-Fos* and *c-Jun* expression in neonatal hypoxic-ischemic rat brains induced by glibenclamide, an ATP-sensitive potassium channel blocker. *Brain Research, 998*(1), 13–19.

Kang, J. E., Lee, H. J., Lim, S., Kim, E. H., Lee, T. H., Jang, M. H. et al. (2003). Acupuncture modulates expressions of nitric oxide synthase and c-Fos in hippocampus after transient global ischemia in gerbils. *American Journal of Chinese Medicine, 31*(4), 581–590.

Kerr, D. P., Walsh, D. M., & Baxter, D. (2003). Acupuncture in the management of chronic low back pain: A blinded randomized controlled trial. *Clinical Journal of Pain, 19*(6), 364–370.

Kim K. H. (2001). Atlanto-axial subluxation syndrome and management of intractable headache, neck pain and shoulder pain with auricular stimulation: A clinical case report. *Acupuncture & Electro-Therapeutics Research, 26*(4), 263–275.

Kim, H. W., Kwon, Y. B., Ham, T. W., Roh, D. H., Yoon, S. Y., Lee, H. J. et al. (2003). Acupoint stimulation using bee venom attenuates formalin-induced pain behavior and spinal cord fos expression in rats. *Journal of Veterinary Medical Science, 65*(3), 349–355.

Konig, A., Radke, S., Molzen, H., Haase, M., Muller, C., Drexler, D. et al. (2003). Randomised trial of acupuncture compared with conventional massage and "Sham" laser acupuncture for treatment of chronic neck pain range of motion analysis. *Zeitschrift fur Orthopadie und Ihre Grenzgebiete, 141*(4), 395–400.

Kosterlitz, H., & Hughes, J. (1977). Peptides with morphine-like action in the brain. *British Journal of Psychiatry, 130,* 298–304.

Lambert, M. I., Marcus, P., Burgess, T., & Noakes, T. D. (2002). Electro-membrane microcurrent therapy reduces signs and symptoms of muscle damage. *Medicine and Science in Sports and Exercise, 34*(4), 602–607.

Lao, L., Hamilton, G. R., Fu, J., & Berman, B. M. (2003). Is acupuncture safe? A systematic review of case reports. *Alternative Therapies in Health and Medicine, 9*(1), 72–83.

Lee, G. S., Han, J. B., Shin, M. K., Hong, M. C., Kim, S. W., Min, B. I. et al. (2003). Enhancement of electroacupuncture-induced analgesic effect in cholecystokinin-A receptor deficient rats. *Brain Research Bulletin, 62*(2), 161–164.

Lein, D. H., Jr., Clelland, J. A., Knowles, C. J., & Jackson, J. R. (1989). Comparison of effects of transcutaneous electrical nerve stimulation of auricular, somatic, and the combination of auricular and somatic acupuncture points on experimental pain threshold. *Physical Therapy, 69*(8), 671–678.

Li, X., Zhang, S., & Qin, L. (2000). Experimental study of analgesic effect of combined Radix Aconiti and Radix Stephaniae Tetrandrae. *Zhongguo Zhong Xi Yi Jie He Za Zhi, 20*(3), 202–204.

Liu, J. H., Yan, J., Yi, S. X., Chang, X. R., Lin, Y. P., & Hu, J. M. (2004). Effects of electroacupuncture on gastric myoelectric activity and substance P in the dorsal vagal complex of rats. *Neuroscience Letters, 356*(2), 99–102.

Ma, W., Tong, H., Xu, W., Hu, J., Liu, N., Li, H. et al. (2003). Perivascular space: Possible anatomical substrate for the meridian. *Journal of Alternative and Complementary Medicine, 9*(6), 851–859.

Maloney, K. J., Mainville, L., & Jones, B. E. (2000). c-Fos expression in GABAergic, serotonergic, and other neurons of the pontomedullary reticular formation and raphe after paradoxical sleep deprivation and recovery. *Journal of Neuroscience, 20*(12), 4669–4679.

Masala, A., Satta, G., Alagna, S., Zolo, T. A., Rovasio, P. P., & Rassu, S. (1983). Suppression of electroacupuncture (EA)-induced beta-endorphins and ACTH release by hydrocortisone in man. Absence of effects on EA-induced anaesthesia. *Acta Endocrinologica, 103*(4), 469–472.

Medeiros, M. A., Canteras, N. S., Suchecki, D., & Mello, L. E. (2003). c-Fos expression induced by electroacupuncture at the Zusanli point in rats submitted to repeated immobilization. *Brazilian Journal of Medical and Biological Research, 36*(12), 1673–1684.

Meng, C. F., Wang, D., Ngeow, J., Lao, L., Peterson, M., & Paget, S. (2003). Acupuncture for chronic low back pain in older patients: A randomized, controlled trial. *Rheumatology* (Oxford), *42*(12), 1508–1517.

Moore, K., Hira, N., Kumar, P. et al. (1988). A double-blind crossover trial of low-level laser therapy in the treatment of post herpetic neuralgia. *Laser Therapy, 1*(1), 7–9.

National Institute of Health. (1998). NIH Consensus Development Panel on Acupuncture. *Journal of the American Medical Association, 280*(17), 1518–1524.

Noguchi, E., & Hayashi, H. (1996). Increases in gastric acidity in response to electroacupuncture stimulation of the hindlimb of anesthetized rats. *Japanese Journal of Physiology, 46*(1), 53–58.

Oleson, T. D. (2002). Auriculotherapy stimulation for neuro-rehabilitation. *NeuroRehabilitation, 17*(1), 49–62.

Oyamada, Y., & Izu, S. (1985). *Application of low energy laser in chronic rheumatoid arthritis and related rheumatoid diseases.* Paper presented at the 6th Congress of the International Society for Laser Surgery and Medicine.

Pan, B., Castro-Lopes, J. M., & Coimbra, A. (1996). Activation of anterior lobe corticotrophs by electroacupuncture or noxious stimulation in the anaesthetized rat, as shown by colocalization of Fos protein with ACTH and beta-endorphin and increased hormone release. *Brain Research Bulletin, 40*(3), 175–182.

Peets, J. M., & Pomeranz, B. (1978). CXBK mice deficient in opiate receptors show poor electroacupuncture analgesia. *Nature, 273*(5664), 675–676.

Peuker, E. T., White, A., Ernst, E., Pera, F., & Filler, T. J. (1999). Traumatic complications of acupuncture. Therapists need to know human anatomy. *Archives of Family Medicine, 8*(6), 553–558.

Pomeranz, B. (2001). Acupuncture analgesia — Basic research. In G. Strux & R. Hammerschlag (Eds.), *Clinical acupuncture: Scientific basis* (pp. 1–28). Berlin: Springer-Verlag.

Pomeranz, B., & Warma, N. (1988). Electroacupuncture suppression of a nociceptive reflex is potentiated by two repeated electroacupuncture treatments: The first opioid effect potentiates a second non-opioid effect. *Brain Research, 452*(1–2), 232–236.

Sator-Katzenschlager, S. M., Szeles, J. C., Scharbert, G., Michalek-Sauberer, A., Kober, A., Heinze, G. et al. (2003). Electrical stimulation of auricular acupuncture points is more effective than conventional manual auricular acupuncture in chronic cervical pain: A pilot study. *Anesthesia & Analgesia, 97*(5), 1469–1473.

Schwartz, M. W., Woods, S. C., Porte, D., Jr., Seeley, R. J., & Baskin, D. G. (2000). Central nervous system control of food intake. *Nature, 404*(6778), 661–671.

Sherman, K. J., & Cherkin, D. C. (2003). Developing methods for acupuncture research: Rationale for and design of a pilot study evaluating the efficacy of acupuncture for chronic low back pain. *Alternative Therapies in Health and Medicine, 9*(5), 54–60.

Shi, X. N. (1997). Relative specificity of acupoint as observed from influence of acupuncture on heart rate variability. *International Journal of Clinical Acupuncture, 8*(3), 237–240.

Singh, B. B., Berman, B. M., Hadhazy, V., Bareta, J., Lao, L., Zarow, F. M. et al. (2001). Clinical decisions in the use of acupuncture as an adjunctive therapy for osteoarthritis of the knee. *Alternative Therapies in Health and Medicine, 7*(4), 58–65.

Slocomb, J. (1984). Neurologic factors in chronic pelvic pain: Trigger points and the abdominal pelvic pain syndrome. *American Journal of Obstetrics and Gynecology, 149*, 536–543.

Takeshige, C. (2001). Mechanisms of acupuncture analgesia produced by low frequency electrical stimulation of acupuncture points. In G. Strux & R. Hammerschlag (Eds.), *Clinical acupuncture* (pp. 29–50). Berlin: Springer-Verlag.

Thomas, M., Lundeberg, T., Bjork, G., Lundstrom-Lindstedt, V. et al. (1995). Pain and discomfort in primary dysmenorrhea is reduced by preemptive acupuncture or low frequency TENS. *European Journal of Physical and Medical Rehabilitation, 5*, 71–76.

Ulett, G. (1983). Acupuncture is not hypnosis: Physiologic studies. *American Journal of Acupuncture, 11*(1), 5–13.

Ulett, G. (1996). Conditioned healing with electroacupuncture. *Alternative Therapies in Health and Medicine, 2*(5), 56–60.

Walker, J., & Akhanjee, L. (1985). Laser therapy for pain of trigeminal neuralgia. *Clinical Journal of Pain, 3*(4), 183–187.

White, A. R., & Ernst, E. (1998). A trial method for assessing the adequacy of acupuncture treatments. *Alternative Therapies in Health and Medicine, 4*(6), 66–71.

White, A., & Ernst, E. (1999). The effect of auricular acupuncture on the pulse rate: An exploratory randomized controlled trial. *Acupuncture in Medicine, 17*(2), 86–88.

White, A., & Ernst, E. (2003). Pitfalls in conducting systematic reviews of acupuncture. *Rheumatology* (Oxford), *42*(10), 1271–1272; author reply, 1272–1273.

Wieder, D. (1991). Microcurrent therapy: Wave of the future? *Rehabilitation Management, 4*(2), 34–35.

Wolsko, P., Eisenberg, D., Simon, L., Davis, R. et al. (2004). Double-blind placebo-controlled trial of static magnets for the treatment of osteoarthritis of the knee results of a pilot study. *Alternative Therapies in Health and Medicine, 10*(2), 36–43.

Wood, P. B. (2004). Stress and dopamine: Implications for the pathophysiology of chronic widespread pain. *Medical Hypotheses, 62*(3), 420–424.

Yeung, C. K., Leung, M. C., & Chow, D. H. (2003). The use of electro-acupuncture in conjunction with exercise for the treatment of chronic low-back pain. *Journal of Alternative and Complementary Medicine, 9*(4), 479–490.

Zhou, M. M., Yu, C. X., & Wang, M. Z. (2001). Changes of cerebral beta-endorphin in rats treated with combination therapy of melatonin and electroacupuncture. *Zhongguo Zhong Xi Yi Jie He Za Zhi, 21*(2), 115–118.

Zijlstra, F. J., van den Berg-de Lange, I., Huygen, F. J., & Klein, J. (2003). Anti-inflammatory actions of acupuncture. *Mediators of Inflammation, 12*(2), 59–69.

77

Aromatherapy for Pain Relief

Alan R. Hirsch, MD

INTRODUCTION

In explaining the persuasive attraction of alternative medicine, Kaptchuk and Eisenberg (1998) note, "The fundamental premises are an advocacy of nature, vitalism, science, and spirituality." Use of aromatherapy has burgeoned along with the other forms of complementary and alternative medicine. As of 1997, out-of-pocket money spent for alternative medicine products and services was $27 billion and equaled that for all out-of-pocket U.S. physician services (Yager, Siegfried, & DiMatteo, 1999). There has been a growth of 900% in the use of aromatherapy from the 1980s and 1990s (Kessler, Davis, Foster et al., 2001). Pain, including headache, is one of the most common reasons for seeking complementary alternative medicine treatment (Eisenberg, David, Ettner et al., 1998), and in particular aromatherapy because it is suggested that, "almost all essential oils have some analgesic properties" (Gatefoss, as quoted in Buckle, 1999b).

DEFINITIONS

One of the difficulties in understanding aromatherapy is that it means different things to different people. One part of its definition that is agreed upon is that aromatherapy uses odorous compounds to promote health and healing (Kaptchuk & Eisenberg, 1998). Beyond this, opinions differ. Aromachologists speak of using odors not to treat disease, but to promote wellness. Aromatologists believe in ingestion of the substance being used as well as its inhalation (Price & Price, 1995). Many aromatherapists believe in using massage and topical application coinci-

dent with inhalation (Tisserand, 1977, Wood, 2003). In this chapter, aromatherapy for pain relief is defined as the use of odorants as inhalants. This definition excludes any effects of ingestion or percutaneous absorption, although this may be significant depending on the method of application (Weyers & Brodbeck, 1989). This definition is consistent with the literature indicating that real aromatherapy involves the uptake of fragrant compounds only through inhalation, not by other methods (Buchbauer, 1993). As defined, aromatherapy is also independent of any coincident, noninhalational therapies, such as massage, interpersonal interaction, or bathing.

Many in the aromatherapy community believe that natural or essential oils are effective and that artificial synthesized compounds are not. However, in the treatment of neurologic and psychiatric diseases, the literature does not substantiate this dichotomy (King, 1994). No distinction will be made herein between the use of synthetic as opposed to naturally occurring oils.

BACKGROUND

Why is the concept of aromatherapy under consideration today? One reason is its history. Throughout the ages, odorants have been used to treat various diseases. More than 5,000 years ago the Egyptians treated disease using odors (Lindsay, Pitcaithly, & Geelen, 1997), and 3,500 years ago the Babylonians used odors to exorcise demons of disease (Roebuck, 1988). The ancient Aztecs also used odors to treat disease. Aromatherapy has known no cultural or geographic boundaries. Virtually all cultures have fumigated the sick (Buchbauer, 1993).

ANATOMY OF OLFACTION

Neuroscience provides insight into the mechanisms by which odors may influence behavior and neurologic functioning.

There is an anatomic basis for the belief that odors can affect the brain and behavior (Brodal, 1969). Once an odor passes through the olfactory epithelium, it stimulates the olfactory nerve, which consists of unmyelinated olfactory filia. The olfactory nerve has the slowest conduction rate of any nerve in the body. The olfactory filia pass through the cribiform plate of the ethmoid bone and enter the olfactory bulb. During trauma, damage often occurs in this bulb (Hirsch & Wyse, 1993). Different odors localize in different areas of the olfactory bulb.

Inside the olfactory bulb is a conglomeration of neuropil called the glomeruli. Approximately 2,000 glomeruli reside in the olfactory bulb. Four different cell types make up the glomeruli: processes of receptor cell axons, mitral cells, tufted cells, and second-order neurons that give off collaterals to the granule cells and to cells in the periglomerular and external plexiform layers. The mitral and tufted cells form the lateral olfactory tract and establish a reverberating circuit with the granule cells. The mitral cells stimulate firing of the granule cells, which, in turn, inhibit firing of the mitral cells. A reciprocal inhibition exists between the mitral and tufted cells. This results in a sharpening of olfactory acuity.

The olfactory bulb receives several afferent projections, including the primary olfactory fibers, the contralateral olfactory bulb and the anterior nucleus, the prepiriform cortex (inhibitory), the diagonal band of Broca (with neurotransmitters acetylcholine and gamma amino butyric acid [GABA]), the locus coeruleus, the dorsal raphe, and the tuberomamillary nucleus of the hypothalamus.

The olfactory bulb's efferent fibers project into the olfactory tract, which divides at the olfactory trigona into the medial and lateral olfactory stria. These project to the anterior olfactory nucleus, the olfactory tubercle, the amygdaloid nucleus (which, in turn, projects to the ventral medial nucleus of the hypothalamus, a feeding center), the cortex of the piriform lobe, the septal nuclei, and the hypothalamus, in particular the anterolateral regions of the hypothalamus, which are involved in reproduction. The neurotransmitters by which the olfactory bulb conducts its information include glutamate, aspartate, *N*-acetyl-aspartylglutamate, cholecystokinin, and GABA.

The anterior olfactory nucleus receives afferent fibers from the olfactory tract and projects efferent fibers, which decussate in the anterior commissure and synapse in the contralateral olfactory bulb. Some of the efferent projections from the anterior olfactory nucleus remain ipsilateral and synapse on internal granular cells of the ipsilateral olfactory bulb.

The olfactory tubercle receives afferent fibers from the olfactory bulb and the anterior olfactory nucleus. Efferent fibers from the olfactory tubercle project to the nucleus accumbens as well as the striatum. Neurotransmitters of the olfactory tubercle include acetylcholine and dopamine.

The area on the cortex where olfaction is localized, that is, the primary olfactory cortex, includes the prepiriform area, the periamygdaloid area, and the entorhinal area. Afferent projections to the primary olfactory cortex include the mitral cells, which enter the lateral olfactory tract and synapse in the prepiriform cortex (lateral olfactory gyrus) and the corticomedial part of the amygdala. Efferent projections from the primary olfactory cortex extend to the entorhinal cortex (area 28), the basal and lateral amygdaloid nuclei, the lateral preoptic area of the hypothalamus, the nucleus of the diagonal band of Broca, the medial forebrain bundle, the dorsal medial nucleus and submedial nucleus of the thalamus, and the nucleus accumbens.

It should be noted that the entorhinal cortex is both a primary and a secondary olfactory cortical area. Efferent fibers, from the cortex, project via the uncinate fasciculus to the hippocampus, the frontal cortex, and the anterior insular cortex (next to the gustatory cortical area). This may explain why temporal lobe epilepsy that involves the uncinate often produces parageusias of burning rubber, known as uncinate fits (Acharya, Acharya, & Luders, 1996).

Some of the efferent projections of the mitral and tufted cells decussate in the anterior commissure and form the medial olfactory tract. They then synapse in the contralateral parolfactory area and contralateral subcallosal gyrus. The exact function of the medial olfactory stria and tract is not clear. The accessory olfactory bulb receives afferent fibers from the bed nucleus of the accessory olfactory tract and the medial and posterior corticoamygdaloid nuclei. Efferent fibers from the accessory olfactory bulb project through the accessory olfactory tract to the same afferent areas, for example, the bed nucleus of the accessory olfactory tract and the medial posterior corticoamygdaloid nuclei. It should be noted that the medial and posterior corticoamygdaloid nuclei project secondary fibers to the anterior and medial hypothalamus, the areas associated with reproduction. Therefore, the accessory olfactory bulb in humans may be the mediator for human pheromones (Hirsch, 1998b).

Some unique aspects of the anatomy of the olfactory system are worth mentioning. Smell is the only sensation to reach the cortex before reaching the thalamus. The only sensory system that is primary ipsilateral in its projection, olfaction does not depend upon the cortex, as has been demonstrated in decorticate cats (Dusser de Barenne, 1933).

Neurotransmitters of the olfactory cortex are multiple, including glutamate, aspartate cholcystekinin, luteinizing hormone releasing factor, and somatastatin. Furthermore, perception of odors causes modulation of olfactory neurotransmitters within the olfactory bulb and the limbic system. Virtually all known neurotransmitters are present in the olfactory bulb. Thus, odorant modulation of neurotransmitter levels in the olfactory bulb, tract, and limbic system intended for transmission of sensory information may have unintended secondary effects on a variety of different behaviors and disease states that are regulated by the same neurotransmitters. For example, odorant modulation of dopamine in the olfactory bulb/limbic system may effect manifestations of Parkinson's disease. Non-olfactory mesolimbic override to many of the components of Parkinson's disease have been well documented, for example, motoric activation associated with emotional distress and fear of injury in a fire (Adams, Victor, & Roper, 1997).

EMOTIONAL AND BEHAVIORAL EFFECTS OF ODORS

Odors can affect behavior by acting as alternative sensory stimuli. The phenomena of visual system modification of the movements of Parkinsonian gait through the visual stimulation of lines placed on the floor (Dietz, Goetz, & Steddings, 1990) are an example of alternative stimuli. Other sensory input, including pain, has been shown to inhibit the Jacksonian march in epilepsy (Gowers, 1881, cited in Efron, 1957). Similarly, odors may act as competing sensory stimuli during an uncinate seizure (Efron, 1957). It seems possible that other sensory input, including odors, could modify Parkinson's disease as well as other neurologic conditions, including pain, by acting as competing sensory stimuli.

Using another mechanism of action, odors can affect behavior and mood by producing a primary effect on the emotions of the individual (Ersser, 1990). This is different from a direct neurophysiologic effect on the limbic system. Rather, the odor can change the mood of the individual, which then has secondary neurologic effects. For example, mood or level of alertness can affect the perceptual threshold of a stimulus, including the perception of pain (Loring & Meador, 2001). A soldier who is severely wounded in battle may continue to fight and not feel pain until the battle is over. Studies also suggest that persons in a positive state of mind are less bothered by pain (Fields, 1967). Thus, aromatherapy's analgesic effect may be due to its ability to induce happiness.

Substantial evidence exists that odors can affect mood (Broughan, 2002). As early as 1908, Freud stressed the importance of olfaction on emotion in his description of a patient with an obsessional neurosis.

By his own account, when a child, he recognized everyone by their smell, like a dog, and even when he was grown up he was more susceptible to sensations of smell than other people ... and I have come to recognize that a tendency towards osphresiolagnia which has become

extinct since childhood may play a part in the genesis of neuroses.

In a general way I should like to raise the question whether the inevitable shunting of the sense of smell as a result of man's turning away from the earth and the organic repression of smell pleasure produced by it does not largely share in his predisposition to nervous diseases. It would thus furnish an explanation for the fact that with the advance of civilization it is precisely the sexual life which must become the victim of repression. For we have long known what an intimate relation exists in the animal organization between the sexual impulse and the function of the olfactory organs.

Of all the sensations, olfaction is the one most intertwined with limbic system functioning (MacLean, 1973). The profuse anatomic and physiologic interconnections through the olfactory bulb, stria, and nuclei to the olfactory tubercle, and from there to the prepiriform cortex, the amygdala, and numerous other limbic system structures elucidated earlier support this (Brodal, 1969).

Smells are described differently from other sensory modalities, adding credence to their connection to emotion. Other sensory modalities are first described cognitively; a picture, for example, is identified as being of a ship, a woman, or a house and only secondarily is it described affectively: "I like," or "I dislike it" (Ehrlichman & Halpern, 1988). But odors are first and foremost described affectively: "I like," or "I dislike" it.

The olfactory/limbic/hippocampal connections help to explain olfactory-evoked nostalgia, the phenomenon whereby an odor induces a vivid recall of a scene from the distant past (Hirsch, 1992). In 86% of 989 subjects queried, certain odors triggered vivid associations analogous to a flashbulb memory. Classically, an event must induce strong emotions for deposition of such memories to occur (Brown & Kulik, 1977; Squire, 1987). By directly stimulating the limbic system, odors also can act as the inducing agent. This phenomenon was vividly described by Proust (1934), who wrote that the aroma of madeleine dipped in tea evoked a flood of memories and nostalgic feelings. Olfactory-evoked recall is usually a positive experience, but it can be negative, as in the olfactory flashbacks of post-traumatic stress disorder (Kline & Rausch, 1985). Hence, it seems possible that olfactory-evoked nostalgia may affect pain because approximately 90% of these memories are associated with strong affective tones (Laird, 1988).

Odorants' effect on mood may be mediated through more short-term influence — through a Pavlovian conditioned response. In this mechanism, a recent exposure to an odor is linked to a mood or behavioral state, and when the odor is reintroduced, this same emotional tone also returns (Broughan, 1998; Engen, 1991). This suggests that for each person the same odor will have a different effect because the emotions paired with the odor will be unique, dependent on each individual's past experiences and memories (Van Toller & Dodd, 1988). Superimposed on individual preferences are cultural mores, trends, and prohibitions, which also act to guide members of each culture for use of specific odors for group occasions, like incense in a church or cotton candy at a carnival (Classen, Howes, & Synnott, 1994). In these situations, specific odors are more likely to be associated with specific emotions common to their respective cultural groups — i.e., happiness with cotton candy and contrition with incense (Broughan, 1998). Thus, not only will there be cultural differences from odor to odor in terms of preference and use, but even within the culture, there will be individual variability (Davis & Panboro, 1982).

The above brings to the forefront the question of how odors exert an impact on behavior or mood. The answer can be represented by either of two constructs: the lock and key theory or the general affective theory of odors.

THE LOCK AND KEY THEORY OF ODORS

The lock and key theory of odors (also called the systemic effect theory) (Buchbauer, 1993) suggests that odor acts very much like a specific neurotransmitter, a drug, or an enzyme. In this paradigm, an odorant has a specific effect on behavior or emotion — one odor for one emotion or one odor for, at most, a few emotions. Thus, an odor could be viewed like a medication in the pharmacopoeia. For example, in the world of neurology, propranolol is used for modulation of essential tremor, migraine headache, and anxiety. However, one would not use propranolol as a treatment for insomnia, dementia, or multiple sclerosis. The lock and key theory suggests that specific odors have specific effects. This theory has been proposed in virtually every book about aromatherapy in which specific odors are recommended for specific health effects (Cunningham, 1995; Damian & Damian, 1995; Feller, 1997; Keville & Green, 1995; Price, 1991; Price & Price, 1995; Schnaubelt, 1995).

An argument supporting the lock and key theory is that odorants exert central nervous system (CNS) effects outside a subject's conscious awareness. In test animals, the more lipophilic an odor is, the greater its sedative effect. In addition, steric differences in odors create different effects despite similarities in perceived odor and volatility (Buchbauer, 1993; Buchbauer et al., 1993). In humans, conscious detection is not necessarily required for an odorant to have its effects. For example, subliminal aromas of vanilla enhances mood (Lorig, 1994) and the subliminal aromas of mixed flowers increase both the perceived value and the desire to buy inanimate objects (Nike shoes) (Hirsch & Gay, 1991).

According to the lock and key theory, odors act as a drug (Buchbauer, 1993) with a potentially pharmacologic mechanism of action. The odorants are integrated in the membrane of the cells causing an increase in membrane volume due to disruption of the membrane lipids. This leads to electrical stabilization of the membrane, thus blocking the inflow of calcium ions and suppressing permeability for sodium ions. As a result, action potential production is inhibited, which induces narcosis or local anesthesia. At higher concentrations of odorant, the conductivity of potassium ions is reduced. It also is possible that the odorants act on protein kinase C, which could affect the spontaneous rhythm of nerve cells (Buchbauer, 1993).

This mechanism of action is further supported by established pharmacology for the action of the target organ, in this case, a drug on the brain. If the odorant did not directly infiltrate the olfactory neurons and then spread transaxonally to specific neural nuclei as has been postulated (Buckle, 1993, 1999a), inhalation of an odorant would have to produce measurable levels in the blood, sufficient to pass through the blood–brain barrier. Parts per billion levels in blood have been seen after minimum inhalation of oils of rosemary (Kovar, Gropper, Friess et al., 1987), sandalwood (Jirovetz, 1992), and lavender (Buchbauer, Jirovetz, Jäger, Dietrich et al., 1991; Jellinek, 1998/1999). Stimpfl et al. (1995) demonstrated that this does occur in humans. One subject inhaled 1,8-cineol for 20 minutes, which produced a linear increase of 1,8-cineol in the blood, up to 275 ng/ml, a level high enough to allow penetration of the blood–brain barrier (Stimpfl et al., 1995).

Battaglia (1997) postulates that part of the efficacy of aromatherapy for analgesia lies in its pharmacologic effects: anti-inflammatory and prostaglandin-inhibiting properties. Göbel, Schmidt, and Soyka (1994) suggests that antinociceptive influences of aromas are derived either through afferent segmental inhibition at the posterior horn or through central efferent inhibition, or through a combination of these.

THE GENERAL AFFECTIVE THEORY OF ODORS

An alternative theory, the general affective theory of odors, also called the reflectorial effect theory (Buchbauer, 1993), holds that an odor experienced as hedonically positive induces a positive, happy mood, and when in a happy mood, an individual does almost everything better, and pain is less bothersome. For example, when a person feels happy, it is easier to learn and to sleep, and headaches are less frequent. According to the general affective theory, a single odor could have a multitude of diverse effects, thus affecting virtually all behaviors.

The major premise that hedonically positive odors induce happier moods was demonstrated by Alaoui-Ismaili et al. (1997); 44 subjects inhaled five odorants, namely, vanillin, menthol, eugenol, methyl methacrylate, and propionic acid. Six autonomic nervous system parameters were recorded: skin potential, skin resistance, skin temperature, skin blood flow, instantaneous respiratory frequency, and instantaneous heart rate. Evaluation of these parameters demonstrated a pattern consistent with known emotional states. Hedonically pleasant odors evoked mainly happiness and surprise, and unpleasant ones induced mainly disgust and anger (Alaoui-Ismaili et al., 1997).

Miltner et al. (1994) also showed that exposure to odors could change emotions in the same direction as the hedonic valence of the odor. Using the startle reflex amplitude as a physiologic indicator of emotional valence, he found that the odor of hydrogen sulfide increased the startle reflex amplitude and the odor of vanillin reduced it.

Aromatherapists recognize the affective impact of odors as the mechanism of action. Buchbauer notes, "A pleasant odor has always been, and still is, an important factor for people to feel good, and feeling well is synonymous with good health. Therefore, we can conclude that all substances which are able to create a certain amount of well-being and well-feeling possess therapeutic properties and, therefore, can be called therapeutic agents" (Buchbauer, 1990). The general affective theory of odors might be extended to include non-odorants in the pharmacologic arena, such as Valium. Valium may be useful for virtually all medical conditions because reducing anxiety makes conditions such as chronic pain, movement disorders, or insomnia less bothersome. Hence, an entire branch of medicine could be built around Valium: "Valiotherapy." If one ascribes aromatherapeutic results to the general affective theory as the mechanism of action, it follows that any odor that one likes induces a happier state and, hence, would have a positive effect on any disease. Again, the concept could be expanded beyond odors to any environmental stimuli, for example, a bird singing or a pretty landscape. A *Star Wars* movie might induce happiness in some observers and could be seen as inducing a positive mood state. The positive mood might lead to a reduction in pain, anxiety, and negative feelings. One could then categorize this as a form of alternative therapy: "Lucastherapy!" Thus, reliance on the general affective theory of odors implies that virtually any sensory stimulus could be used as a therapeutic tool. This largely trivializes the definition of therapy.

Another problem with the general affective theory of odors is that the same odor, in different contexts, may induce opposite emotional tones (Sugawara, Hino, & Kawasaki, 1999). In "The Invalid's Story," Mark Twain compares the disgust at the odor of a rotting corpse to the delight at the smell of cheese (Clemens, 1882). The odors were the same but perceived to be from different sources. This suggests that an odor that is contextually appropriate in one situation might be considered totally inappropriate in another. Smelled in a positive context, it would be appreciated as hedonically positive and would enhance a positive affective state; smelled in a negative context, it would be perceived as hedonically negative and would, thus, induce a negative affective state. Therefore, the same odor could produce opposite mood states and opposite effects. This suggests that it is the perception of the odor rather than the odor itself that is essential in the mechanism of aromatherapy (Broughan, 1998). This was demonstrated for neroli, which had either an activating or an opposite, deactivating response, depending upon whether the subject believed it was a floral or a citrus-based aroma (Torii, 1996).

A variant of the general affective theory is that odors may induce a mood more congruent with the demands of the external environment. For example, if the external environment requires that the individual be alert, the odor induces awareness of this; therefore, the individual responds by becoming more alert. Alternatively, if the external environment is such that it is more appropriate to be relaxed, the odor induces that awareness and the individual responds by becoming more relaxed. Evidence for the validity of this variant comes from studies of muguet odor. Where the external demand is for a greater degree of relaxation, individuals do become more relaxed, and in an environment where they are required to be more alert and vigilant, they become more alert. Warm, Dember, and Parasuraman (1991) demonstrated this effect of odorant-induced recognition of affective demands. A total of 40 subjects underwent vigilance tasks for 40 minutes during which they received periodic 30-second whiffs of air or one of two hedonically positive fragrances: muguet (independently judged as relaxing) or peppermint (independently judged as alerting). Those who received either the relaxing or alerting fragrance detected more signals during the vigilance task than the unscented air controls ($p = 0.05$).

This odorant-induced congruence of mood may also be applied to the pharmacologic agent diazepam or Valium. Valium can induce opposite mood states in the same individual at different times. It can reduce anxiety to enhance concentration on a test, or it can reduce concentration to act as a soporific when the same individual is suffering with insomnia.

A corollary to the general affective theory is that hedonically negative odors or malodors have a negative effect on mood (Baron & Thomley, 1994). If this were true, the simple elimination or masking of malodors with neutral or hedonically positive odors would induce positive effects; in this paradigm, in the hospital setting, the true aromatherapist is actually the hospital janitor!

Literature supports the deleterious and cephalogenic effects of hedonically unpleasant odors. Miner (1980) described some health effects of exposure to the odor of livestock waste. They included annoyance, depression, nausea, vomiting, headache, shallow breathing, coughing, insomnia, and impaired appetite.

One of the malodorous pollutants that has been studied, trichloroethylene, a universally present air pollutant, can cause cephalgia (Hirsch & Rankin, 1993). Acute exposure to nitrogen tetroxide can cause cephalgia (Hirsch, 1995a) and chronic neurotoxicity (Hirsch, 1995d). Acute exposure to chlorine gas can cause neurotoxicity (Hirsch, 1995c). In 1991, Neutra et al. reported that people living near hazardous waste sites suffer more physical symptoms during times when they can detect malodors than when they are unaware of them. Shusterman (1992) demonstrated that even at levels considered nontoxic, chemical effluviums can cause physical symptoms.

Health effects of malodors can be divided into six categories: respiratory, chemosensory, cardiovascular, immune, neurologic, and psychologic.

Respiratory. Individuals with asthma are especially affected by malodors. Any strong odor may induce an attack in persons with unstable asthma, and even in people without asthma, malodors have been demonstrated to affect the cardiorespiratory system. Increased ambient oxidant levels correlate with slower cross-country running times in high school students (Wayne, Wehrle, & Carroll, 1967).

Chemosensory. Chronic exposure to malodors from pulp mills can cause permanent olfactory loss (Maruniak, 1995).

Cardiovascular. Certain malodors can induce an adrenocortical and adrenomedullary response leading to elevated blood pressure and a subsequent increase in stroke and heart disease (Evans, 1994).

Immune. Immune function may be compromised either directly, as a result of olfactory/neural projections to lymphoid tissue (Evans, 1994), or indirectly, as a result of malodor-induced depression or other negative mood states (Weisse, 1992).

Neurologic. Chronic exposure to intermittent malodors from a U.S. Navy dump site in Port Orchard, Washington, induced cortical and subcortical dysfunction, which was manifested by encephalopathy: limbic encephalopathy and cephalgia (Hirsch, 1995b). Both ambient NO_2 and SO_2 impair visual adaptation to darkness and sensitivity to brightness, and increase alpha wave desynchronization on electroencephalogram (EEG) (Izmerov, 1971).

Psychologic. Recognized for centuries and noted by Freud and others, psychologic effects of odors vary widely among individuals. Persons under major stress are particularly vulnerable to the psychologic effects of ambient malodors (Evans, 1994). Persons with a distorted or impaired olfactory sense may be annoyed by odors that other persons usually consider pleasant (Evans, 1994).

Certain bad odors irritate nasal passages. Resultant trigeminal stimulation releases adrenaline, leading to a tense and angry state. Thus, bad odors can trigger aggression that may then be covertly expressed. For example, in one experiment college men were instructed to apply electric shocks of varying intensity to their colleagues, supposedly for the purpose of training them. When bad odors were present, the subjects chose to inflict greater degrees of pain upon their colleagues (Rotton et al., 1979). Another example involves air pollution. On days when malodorous air pollution is high, the number of motor vehicle accidents increases, indicating that people drive more aggressively in a polluted environment (Ury, Perkins, & Goldsmith, 1972).

Various studies show how mood and well-being suffer in the presence of malodors. Residents exposed to the effluvium from nearby commercial swine operations reported that they suffered increased tension, fatigue, confusion, depression, and anger, and that their vigor decreased (Schiffman et al., 1995). According to one study (Rotton et al., 1978) ambient pollutants decreased personal attraction. In a German urban area, the moods of young adults fluctuated in synchrony with the daily fluctuations in quality of environmental air, a pattern especially marked among more emotionally unstable individuals (Brandstatter, Fuhrwirth, & Kitchler, 1988). Further, daily diary entries of women in Bavaria showed that variations in their psychologic well-being coincided with variations in ambient air quality. The correlation was particularly marked among women suffering from chronic diseases such as diabetes (Bullinger, 1989a, 1989b). In Israel, negative health effects were significantly associated with levels of urban pollution (Zeidner & Schecter, 1988).

The number of family disturbances and the number of 911 emergency psychiatric calls also were linked to malodors in the environment, as determined by ozone levels (Rotton & Frey, 1985). In several cities, the number of psychiatric admissions paralleled the quality of environmental air (Briere, Downes, & Spensley, 1983).

In a study of the malodorous emanations from a mulching site southeast of Chicago, it was found that on days when the miasma wafted from the site to the school across the street, children at the school demonstrated increased behavioral problems (Hirsch, 1998a).

Malodorous ambient SO_2 levels correlate with psychiatric admissions, child psychiatric emergencies (Valentine et al., 1975), and behavioral difficulties with decreased cooperation (Cunningham, 1979). Ambient NO_2 levels covary with psychiatric emergency room visits (Strahilevitz, Strahilevitz, & Miller, 1979). In nonsmokers, the odor of cigarette smoke has been demonstrated to exacerbate aggressive behavior (Jones & Bogat, 1978).

The fatigue and annoyance caused by ambient malodors undoubtedly reduce individuals' capacities to function normally. Their abilities to tolerate frustration and pain, to learn, and to cope with other stressors are impaired. In one laboratory study, subjects exposed to unpleasant odors experienced increased feelings of helplessness (Rotton, 1983).

CONTRADICTORY THEORIES

If the general affective theory of odors is true, a single odor can induce a positive mood in one person and a negative mood in another. This negates the lock and key theory in which odors' effects are produced outside of conscious awareness. Robin et al. (1999) demonstrated this using eugenol. Eugenol, which is often associated with the smell of dental cement, was rated pleasant by nonfearful dental subjects and unpleasant by fearful subjects ($p = 0.036$). Changes in subjects' autonomic nervous system measurements were consistent with their emotional states; 19 subjects were exposed to eugenol while recording six autonomic nervous system parameters, including two electrodermal, two thermovascular, and two cardiorespiratory. The results of 7 subjects with high dental fear were compared with those of 12 without such fear. Those with dental fear had a stronger electrodermal response ($p = 0.006$), suggesting that eugenol triggered different emotional responses depending on the unpleasantness of the subject's past dental experiences. Thus, the same odor can have different effects depending on the past experience of the individual (Robin et al., 1998).

On the other hand, if the lock and key theory is true, and an odor's behavioral effects are produced independent of affective reaction, this negates the general affective theory of odors. Ludvigson and Rottman do just that, demonstrating that the scent of lavender enhances mood state while impairing arithmetic reasoning ($p = 0.01$) (Ludvigson & Rottman, 1989).

Given the previous information, several factors must be taken into account in reviewing the literature regarding efficacy of aromatherapy in the treatment of pain. Can odors elevate mood as the general affective theory maintains or do they act in a lock and key fashion? Were the odors tested considered hedonically positive by each subject? This question is essential because what is hedonically positive for one person can be hedonically negative for another, and an odor that is hedonically positive at one concentration may be hedonically negative at another (Distel et al., 1999). Was an associated change in mood independent of the desired effect? Was there a placebo control group (Miller et al., 2004)? Was it a single-blind or double-blind procedure? Was the subject size sufficient to obviate falsely positive test results? Did the subjects of the experiment have a normal or near-normal sense of smell?

Could suggestion have an effect? This is particularly relevant because various studies suggest that as in traditional pharmacologic intervention (Flaten, Simonsen, & Olsen, 1999), odors have both placebo and nocebo effects as demonstrated by Knasko, Gilbert, and Sabini, (1990). Knasko and co-workers subjected 90 people to water vapor sprayed in a room; 30 subjects were told that the water vapor odor was pleasant, 30 that it was unpleasant, and 30 that it was neutral. Those who had been told that the odorant was pleasant reported being in a better mood than did the other two groups ($p = 0.05$). Subjects who had been told the odor was unpleasant reported having more health symptoms ($p < 0.0003$). The strong effect of belief over actuality in the perception of odor pleasantness (Martin, 1996) begs the question, if a scent is even needed at all for the aromatherapy's effects to occur or is it enough just to have the belief that an effective aroma is present (Buckle, 1999b). Martin posits, "If an odour is not required, simply the manipulation of belief, the use of odour in aromatherapy becomes redundant."

Were the experiments controlled not only for the effect of suggestion, but also for the effect of expectation of outcome? It seems possible that persons with a positive view of aromatherapy, and who believe that odors can have a positive effect, will be more predisposed to experience a positive effect from odors because of their bias independent of any true effect of the aroma (Broughan, 1998/1999). The effect of expectation has been demonstrated neurophysiologically by Lorig and Roberts (1990) who measured the contingent negative variation (CNV) of the EEG in 18 subjects presented with a mixed odor of lavender, jasmine, and galbanium. They found CNV amplitude for the mixed odors varied depending on what the subjects were told about the odorant ($p = 0.05$).

One way of eliminating expectancy effects is by using subjects with no preconceived notions of efficacy of aromatherapy for pain relief. One such group is infants and young children. A variety of studies of aromatherapy for pain relief have been performed on this population.

In one study, 20 HIV-infected hospitalized children aged 3 months and older were provided Roman chamomile and *Lavandula angustifolia* for pain relief and comfort (Styles, 1987). While it was reported that all the children responded well to these blends with a reduction of need for analgesic drugs and relief of chest pain, muscle spasm, and peripheral neuropathy associated pain, the exact amount and responses were not described and no statistical analysis was provided.

The effect of aromas to reduce pain has also been evaluated in even younger children. Full-term newborns displayed *no* reduction in pain expression in response to a painful heelstick when presented the aroma of maternal milk (Mellier et al., 1997; Rattaz et al., 2001), unfamiliar milk, or lavender (Kawakami et al., 1997).

In another study 51 preterm infants (average 32-weeks gestational age) assessed at 1 week postnatal age had no reduction in crying in response to heelstick pain during exposure to the pre-familiarized odor of vanillin or the novel, unfamiliar odor of vanillin as compared with a no odor control (Goubet, Rattaz, Pierrat, Bullinger, & Lequien, 2003). In response to a less severe painful stimuli (venipuncture), those exposed to the familiar odor of vanillin had a reduction in perceived pain as displayed by no increase in crying as compared with baseline. Thus, the familiar odor of vanillin prevented preterm infants from crying during mild pain, but had no effect on more intense pain, whereas the same aroma, if unfamiliar, had no effect on either painful situation. This implies that vanillin's analgesic effect was based not on the inherent properties of the vanillin, but rather, on the perception of the odor as familiar. Familiar odors may reduce pain because there is a preference for familiarity early in life, or from odor-induced affective memory and an associated happy (non-painful) mood state.

Did the experimenter consider the effect of social desirability whereby subjects try to please the examiner by biasing their answers (Visser, 1999)?

Were the subjects' individual personality factors, which could influence their response to odors, taken into account (Warrenburg & Schwartz, 1990)? For example, those with field dependence tend to be more susceptible to the effects of external cues like ambient aromas on affect and mood state, than field independent personalities, who are more influenced by their own internal milieu and more resistant to impact of ambient aroma (Ehrlichman & Bastone, 1992; Goodenough, 1978; Jellinek, 1998/1999).

In an analysis of all randomized controlled clinical trials of aromatherapy referenced in Medline, Embase, British Nursing Index, CIS-CO, and AMED from June 1999 back to the origin of each database, no studies that had independent replication for the treatment of pain were found in *any* language (Cooke & Ernst, 2000). The authors suggest that use of aromatherapy for anxiety is best considered "a pleasant diversion," and for pain or any other indication, "is not supported by the findings of vigorous clinical trials."

In light of the above, one must be circumspect regarding articles touting aromatherapeutic efficacy in the treatment of pain. Because the basic physiologic mechanism of aromatherapy's antinociceptive effect has not been fully established, skepticism seems all the more appropriate.

As a general rule, pain can be positively influenced by improving the patient's mood or allaying anxiety. Virtually all pain is made worse with depression and/or high anxiety. If these moods can be ameliorated by aromatherapy, it would suggest that aromatherapy could have a positive role in treating pain (Ching, 1999). Aromatherapy's analgesic effects may be secondary to its anxiolytic effect because relaxation or anxiolysis reduces perception

of pain (Buckle, 2001). Thus, aromas may act like diazepam, which activates GABA-mediated inhibitor neurons in the amygdala (LeDoux, 1996). True lavender may induce anxiolysis through a similar mechanism (Tisserand, 1993).

But, do aromas have efficacy as anxiolytics or antidepressants? Aromatherapists recommend numerous odors as anxiolytics, including chamomile, cypress, orange blossom, lavender, marjoram, rose, sandalwood, clary sage (Tisserand, 1977), basil, bergamot, cedarwood, geranium, jasmine, juniper, neroli, petitgrain, ylang-ylang (Damian & Damian, 1995), melissa (Feller, 1997), benzoin, camphor, cardamom, fennel, frankincense, nutmeg, parchouly, peppermint, pine, rosemary, rosewood (Keville & Green, 1995), mandarin, lemon verbena (Schnaubelt, 1995), neroli, and juniper berry (Price, 1991).

Studies of the effects of odorants on anxiety have relied primarily on individuals' self-appraisals of their feeling state. In one instance, apple/nutmeg odor associated with the task of performing certain mathematical calculations led to an attenuated increase in anxiety as determined by subjects' self-reports and blood pressure measurements (Warren & Warrenburg, 1993).

In a nonrandomized, uncontrolled study of eight female day hospital psychiatric patients with anxiety with depression, psychotic depression, or schizophrenia, unnamed oils reduced self-reports of anxiety and depression, although no statistical analysis was performed to demonstrate this (Edge, 2003).

Aromatherapy induced a self-reported relaxed state in five patients with stroke and one patient with spinal injury in a nonrandomized uncontrolled study (Papadopoulos, Wright, & Ensor, 1999). Again, no statistical analysis of efficacy was provided. These results should also be viewed skeptically as olfactory ability was not determined in these subjects and olfactory ability is frequently impaired after a stroke (Murphy et al., 2003) and after spinal cord injury (Hirsch & Cleveland, 1998).

Similarly, the odor of green apple eased the anxiety of being in a space-deprivation booth for six normosmic subjects as demonstrated in a double-blind, controlled, randomized experiment (Hirsch & Gruss, 1998).

Not all studies of the impact of aromatherapy on anxiety have shown positive results, even when outcome parameters were based only on self-appraisals. Among 66 women awaiting surgical abortion, 10 minutes of inhalation of a mixture of the essential oils of vertivert, bergamot, and geranium was no more effective at reducing pre-procedure anxiety than inhalation of the placebo hair conditioner, based on self-reports on a verbal anxiety scale (Wiebe, 2000).

Physiologic evidence is even less conclusive regarding the potential of odorants as anxiolytics. Lavender odor was found to reduce the CNV among perfumers, and the lavender correlated with a more relaxed state (Torii, 1988).

This change on the CNV, however, may also indicate a distracting effect of the odorant (Warren & Warrenburg, 1993). The physiologic manifestations of the anxiolytic effects of the odors of nutmeg–apple, mace, valerian, neroli (orange flowers), and lavender have been demonstrated (Brodal, 1969; Roebuck, 1988). EEG studies support observations that lavender increases alpha waves posteriorly, which is associated with relaxation (Acharya et al., 1996).

Mild reduction in systolic blood pressure, an indicator of anxiolysis (Langewitz, Ruddel, & VonEiff, 1987), with inhaled odors was assessed in a double-blind, controlled, randomized fashion in normosmic and anosmic, awake and anesthetized adults (Allen, 1929). No significant effect was noted with inhalation of hedonically positive odors, but inhalation of an irritant (ammonia) caused an increase in blood pressure.

Studies have also addressed the anxiolytic effects of aromatherapy in the clinical setting with, at best, ambiguous results. In a case-controlled study of 36 men with public speaking anxiety, jasmine and apple spice were no more effective than the odorless control condition in reducing speech anxiety (Spector et al., 1993).

Likewise, no clear efficacy has been demonstrated for aromatherapy for anxiety reduction in patients confined to the hospital. Aromas of marjoram, lavender, rose, eucalyptus, geranium, chamomile, and neroli were used in combination with massage and music therapy to treat 69 terminally ill patients (Evans, 1995). An 80% rate of success, defined as "deriving benefit in some way," was found, but this must be viewed critically for the following reasons: statistical significant was not determined; treatments ancillary to the aromatherapy included talking, massage, or music may have been the true agents; concomitant medical treatment, for example, pharmacologic agents used to decrease pain, may have been the agent of beneficial effects which were misattributed to aromatherapy; different odors were used for each subject; and no consideration was given to hedonics, olfactory ability, a control group, randomization, expectation bias, or examiner bias.

In 122 patients in intensive care, aromatherapy with massage was no more effective than either massage alone or no treatment (the control subgroup) in either subjective perception of aromas ($p > 0.05$) or physiologic parameters of anxiety (systolic blood pressure, respiratory rate, and heart rate) (Dunn, 1992; Dunn, Sleep, & Collett, 1995).

Similarly, a randomized, double-blind trial of aromatherapy with two different species of lavender and massage was performed on 24 postoperative intensive care cardiac patients. No statistically significant self-perceived anxiolytic effect for either species of lavender was found ($p = 0.09$) (Buckle, 1993).

The same results were documented with inhaled neroli aroma combined with massage in 100 1-day post-operative intensive care cardiac patients (Stevensen, 1994). In this randomized, controlled study, again, no statistical significance was found in physiologic parameters of anxiety (heart rate, systolic blood pressure) or subjects' self-perceptions of anxiety as reported in a modified Spielberger State Trait Anxiety Inventory (STAI) self-evaluation questionnaire.

Wilkinson (1995) also used the STAI and the psychologic scale of the Rotterdam Symptom Checklist (RSCL) to assess anxiolytic effects of aromatherapy. In the study, 51 patients with cancer receiving palliative care were randomly assigned to receive three sessions of either full-body massage with carrier oil only or full-body massage with carrier oil and 1% Roman Chamomile essential oil. Upon completion of the sessions, there was no statistically significant effect ($p = 0.08$) of aromatherapy with massage as opposed to massage alone on the psychologic scale of the RSCL or the STAI. Definitive evidence validating aromatherapy in anxiolysis remains to be seen.

Depressed mood is associated with exacerbation of states of pain, and with reduction of depression with elevation of mood, there is a reduction of perception of pain. Thus, if aromatherapy can reduce depression, associated pain would also be expected to be reduced.

A variety of odorants, including basil, bergamot, chamomile, frankincense, geranium, jasmine, lavender, neroli, patchouli, peppermint, rose, sandalwood, ylang-ylang (DeGroot, 1996), clary sage, grapefruit, lemon, mandarin orange (Damian & Damian, 1995), camphor, hyssop, melissa, petitgrain, pine, thyme (Feller, 1997), coriander, helichrysum, rosewood, vetivert (Keville & Green, 1995), marjoram, and thyme (Walji, 1996), have been advocated for the treatment of depression (Tisserand, 1977).

However, scientific studies of aromatherapy for elevation of mood have yielded disappointing results. A mixed citrus odor (a combination of lemon oil, orange oil, bergamot oil, and cis-4-hexenol) was applied to the ambient air for 4 to 11 weeks in the rooms where 12 men were hospitalized for DSM-III-R major depression (Komori et al., 1995). During this time, antidepressant medications were reduced or eliminated for 11 of the 12 men and kept constant for another 8 control patients whose rooms were not perfumed. The criteria for medication tapering were not informal, but rather, on a clinical basis. Comparing effects of odorant and antidepressant treatment versus antidepressant treatment alone, the odorant had no statistically significant effect on objective measures of depression including the Hamilton Rating Scale for Depression, a self-rating depression scale, and the number of days of hospital treatment. Despite this, the results of the study are difficult to interpret because levels of antidepressants were not kept constant. Furthermore, olfactory ability was never assessed and because many antidepressants impair olfactory ability, this is particularly important (Estrem &

Renner, 1987). Also, depression itself is associated with olfactory impairment (Hirsch & Trannel, 1996).

Kite, Maher, Anderson et al. (1998) suggested that aromatherapy significantly improved depression as determined by the Hospital Anxiety Depression Scale ($p < 0.001$) and reduced parameters consistent with adjustment disorders and major depressive disorders. These results must be viewed critically for the following reasons: (1) Of 89 entrants, only 58 (65%) completed the study, an indication that the dropouts may have been treatment failures. (2) The majority of subjects (74%) had breast cancer and were receiving oncologic therapy including radiation therapy or surgery. Olfactory ability was not assessed, yet chemotherapy, radiation therapy, and simply having breast cancer (estrogen receptor positive type; Lehrer, Levine, & Bloomer, 1985) are associated with olfactory impairment (Hirsch & Bailey, 2004). Thus, any positive results could be spurious and unrelated to the aromatherapy. The experimental design supports that this may have been the case. (3) No control group was provided; therefore, mood improvement could have been due to the coincident improvement of the underlying disease state. (4) Aromatherapy was not provided alone, but along with massage and empathic therapeutic sessions, either of which might have been effective. (5) One third of the patients concomitantly received counseling and some were on antidepressants, both of which could improve depression. (6) In all, 20 different essential oils were used, alone or in various combinations. The odors were different for each subject and changed during the course of treatment in more than one third of the cases. Thus, even though relief of depression was reported, the effects of the odorants are indeterminate. Thus, primary anxiolytic or antidepressant influence as a mechanism of aromatherapy antinociceptive effects is, at best, tenuous.

However, a dissociation between analgesic and antidepressant/anxiolytic effects of aromas have been seen, suggesting aromas antinociceptive action may be mediated through nonlimbic mechanisms. Stevensen demonstrated this dissociation in a study of 50 post-cardiac surgery intensive care patients, half of whom underwent 20 minutes of foot massage with plain vegetable oil, while the other half had foot massage with neroli essential oil (Stevenson, 1992). While the aromatherapy group had a marked reduction in anxiety, a significant reduction of pain was not observed.

This same analgesic–anxiolytic dissociation was demonstrated in a study of 40 healthy (8 to 25 years old) volunteers (Marchand and Arsenault, 2002). In this experiment, thermal nociception was induced through immersion of the hand for 3 minutes in a hot (46 to 48°C) circulating bath, 10 different times per subject. During each epoch, in a randomized fashion, a different essence was presented for inhalation: massage oil, orange water, aftershave, distilled water, baby oil, vanilla extract, white vinegar, perm product (hair care), and zonalin (a dentistry product). For the 20 men, there was no significant effect of aromas on pain perception. For the women, however, pain perception was significantly reduced in the presence of pleasant aromas. In both men and women, no correlation was found between mood and pain perception, suggesting analgesic effects of aromas are through other mechanisms such as distraction or even more specific action: both pleasant touch and odors activate the same region in the orbitofrontal cortex, and thus, odors may act to stimulate cortically mediated pain-inhibiting pathways (Francis, Rolls, Bowtell et al., 1999).

Possibly, aromas act to reduce pain through distraction — by focusing attention away from the pain, central supraspinal inhibition occurs and perceived pain is less (Adams, 1998; Buckle, 1999b). Distraction has been suggested as the mechanism whereby lavender suppresses contingent negative variation magnitude (Torii et al., 1988). If this is aromatherapy's antinociceptive mechanism of action, almost all aromas should be effective and those of higher intensity or with greater trigeminal component should be even more effective because they have greater distracting qualities. However, use of essential oils as trigeminal stimulants for pain relief has not been heretofore evaluated.

Another posited mechanism of action of aromatherapy is through potentiation of the analgesic effect of orthodox pain medication (Buckle, 1999b). To date, no studies have been published that substantiate this claim.

AROMATHERAPY FOR VARIOUS PAIN CONDITIONS

Given the above, let us review the literature discussing the antinociceptive effects of aromatherapy in specific complaints and diseases.

HEADACHE

Nontraditional therapies, such as acupuncture, massage, and biofeedback, are frequently used in the management of headache (Matteliano, 2003).

Historically, odors have been recognized to have analgesic effects. When Roman soldiers returned from battle, they placed bay leaves in their baths to reduce their pains (Genders, 1972). In ancient Greece, the Corinthian physician Philonides recommended pressing cool, scented flowers against the temples to relieve headaches (Genders, 1972).

In contemporary lay literature, a multitude of unsupported claims are made for headache and pain reduction using specific odorants. These claims do not indicate whether the mechanism of action is primarily analgesic, soporific, or anxiolytic. Suggested odorants include benzoin, chamomile, lavender, and rosemary for pain (Mantle,

1996); cloves for dental pain (Price & Price, 1995); wintergreen for muscle pain (Göbel et al., 1995; Price & Price, 1995); menthol, ginger, lemongrass, rosewood, clary sage (Damian & Damian, 1995), cajeput, tea tree, juniper, pepper, and rose (Walji, 1996) for headaches (Price & Price, 1995); lavender (Passant, 1990; Waldman et al., 1993), *Lavandula angustifolia, Chamaemelum mobile, Ocimum basilicum, Origanum majorana, Rosmarinus officinalis* (Price & Price, 1995), eucalyptus (Damian & Damian, 1995), and true melissa (Price, 1991; Keville, 1999) for migraine; sweet marjoram for catamenial migraine (Lim, 1997); mentha × piperita for "headache caused by digestive disorder" (Price & Price, 1995); Roman chamomile, lemon, lavender, and peppermint for migraine related to digestion (Lim, 1997); peppermint and eucalyptus for tension headache (Saller, Hellstein, & Hellenbrecht, 1988; Waldman, 1993); basil, cardamom, and eucalyptus radiata for sinus headaches (Worwood, 1995); helichrysum, chamomile, marjoram, and lavender for neuralgia (Keville & Green, 1995).

Experimental studies of odors for pain management are few. Hirsch and Kang (1998) studied 50 chronic sufferers whose headaches met International Headache Society (IHS) criteria. Upon olfactory testing, only 31 demonstrated normal olfactory ability. Green apple odor was given in an aromatherapy inhaler. Only 15 subjects found the odor hedonically pleasant. In this open-label, non-blinded study, subjects served as their own controls. The control condition consisted of resting in a dark, quiet room, and the experimental condition involved inhaling the green apple odor while resting in the same dark, quiet room. Results indicated that green apple odor produced no statistically significant improvement over simple resting in a dark, quiet room. However, in the subgroup of 15 subjects who liked the odor, there was a statistically significant reduction in the severity of the headache ($p < 0.03$). Therefore, the efficacy of the green apple odor was hedonically dependent. Subjects who liked the smell experienced a statistically significant reduction in the severity of the headaches, but patients who disliked the smell experienced no significant improvement.

The mechanism of the odor's action in reducing headaches in these 15 patients is subject to speculation. The odor may have induced a variety of psychologic effects. The therapeutic result may have been mediated through Pavlovian conditioning. For example, the respondents may have consciously or unconsciously associated (Kirk-Smith, Van Toller, & Dodd, 1983) the green apple odor with past anxiolytic or pain-alleviating experiences so that the association reproduced this same effect during the headache episodes. The odor also might have worked through olfactory-evoked recall, because olfactory-evoked recall is usually pleasant and associated with a positive mood state. The green apple scent, by inducing a positive mood state in the 15 patients, could thus have reduced

perception of pain (Fields, 1967). This corresponds with the general affective theory of odors described previously.

The lack of response in those who found the green apple scent unpleasant indicates that hedonics was more important than the particular odor used. This does not preclude the possibility of a neurophysiologic effect of the odor, including a change in serotonin, dopamine, acetylcholine, norepinephrine, GABA, gastrin, beta endorphin, or substance P, all of which are known to be modulators of headache, including migraine (Willis & Westlund, 1997). Because these neurotransmitters exist within the olfactory bulb, they could, theoretically, be influenced by odors (Anselmi et al., 1980; Appenzeller, Atkinson, & Standefer, 1981; Foote, Bloom, & Aston-Jones, 1983; Gall et al., 1987; Haberly & Price, 1978; Halasz & Shepherd, 1983; Hardebo et al., 1985; Igarashi et al., 1987; Leston et al., 1987; Macrides & Davis, 1983; Mair & Harrison, 1991; Moskowitz, 1984; Nattero et al., 1985; Shipley, Halloran, & Torre, 1985; Sjaastad, 1986; Zaborsky et al., 1985). Alternatively, aromatherapy's analgesic effect may be mediated in the nucleus accumbens by way of dopamine, serotonin, and norepinephrine (Buckle, 2001).

Despite its hedonic dependence, green apple odor may have worked somewhat like pharmacologic agents used in the treatment of headache, for example, amitriptyline or propranolol, by modifying the neurotransmitters in the pain pathway. In patients who disliked the odor, a strong negative mood state may have been induced that overwhelmed the odor's neurophysiologic effect. Therefore, the pain was not alleviated.

Göbel also studied the effects of odors on headaches (Göbel et al., 1994, 1995). In that study, 32 healthy subjects underwent a double-blind, placebo-controlled, randomized crossover study of the effects of peppermint oil, eucalyptus, and ethanol. The odors were used in different combinations on various measures of headache pain, including the relaxation of pericranial muscles and contingent negative variation. In this study, three applications of odorant were placed on the skin of the forehead and temples at 15-minute intervals using a small sponge. After 45 minutes, parameters were assessed. To avoid factors of circadian rhythm, all testing took place between 3 and 6 P.M. To prevent subjects from recognizing the presence or the absence of odors and thereby breaking the double-blind nature of the study, "traces" of peppermint oil and eucalyptus oil were added to all applications. Eucalyptus had no effect. Peppermint combined with eucalyptus and ethanol relaxed pericranial muscles ($p < 0.05$) as did a combination of peppermint and ethanol. The most reduction of pain sensitivity as measured by algesimetry was from a combination of peppermint oil and ethanol. Regulation of pericranial muscles was a postulated mechanism of action of the peppermint.

This study has several potential problems. Because the traces of peppermint and eucalyptus were sufficient to cause olfactory response, they also may have been sufficient to produce an effect, although they were described as inert. Hence, the authors may not have tested the particular odors they thought they were testing. Furthermore, no parameter was measured to determine whether the effect was based on hedonics, to eliminate any influence of the general affective theory of odors. No assessment was made of subjects' olfactory abilities, nor was the preconceived notion or the expectancy effect addressed.

The author postulated that the odors, through a peripheral mechanism in the gate control theory of pain, acted by segmental inhibition of the posterior horn (Göbel et al., 1995). However, this same pathway could have been activated totally independently of the odors. The experimental procedure of applying the odors by rubbing cold oils on the skin may, in and of itself, have influenced the pain pathway. The cold stimuli could have induced firing of A-delta fibers, which would have increased blood flow in the skin and created a counterstimulus to reduce the headache pain. Alternatively, the inhalation of odors may have affected central serotonergic systems leading to a change in mood state and, thus, a reduction in pain (general affective theory of odors).

In another study, Göbel and colleagues found aromatherapy with peppermint oil was effective in treating tension headaches meeting IHS classification (Göbel et al., 1996). Peppermint oil was applied locally in a randomized, placebo-controlled, double-blind, crossover fashion; 10 g of peppermint oil and 90% ethanol were used. The placebo was 90% ethanol solution to which traces of peppermint oil were added for blinding purposes. During their headache attacks, peppermint oil was applied across the foreheads and temples of 41 patients. The application was repeated after 15 and 30 minutes. Compared with the placebo, peppermint oil significantly reduced headache intensity after 15 minutes ($p < 0.01$). The analgesic effect equaled that of 1,000 mg of acetaminophen. Very few studies that claim to have demonstrated efficacy of aromatherapy have been as carefully performed (Woolfson & Hewitt, 1992).

Another possible mechanism by which peppermint may relieve headache is by noncompetitive inhibition of serotonin and substance P (Saller et al., 1988). Odors may inhibit headaches by acting as calcium channel blockers. *Romarinus officinalis*, for example, has been demonstrated to relax tracheal smooth muscle by way of its calcium antagonistic property (Aqel, 1991).

OTHER PAIN CONDITIONS

Aromatherapy has been suggested as a treatment option for a variety of nonheadache acute and chronic pain conditions. Foremost among these is the pain association with labor and delivery (Jardine, 2002; Reid, 2001).

Among 635 postpartum women with acute perineal pain (Dale & Cornwell, 1994), use of lavender in the daily bath was compared with an aromatic placebo consisting of 2-methyl-3-isobutyl tyrosine diluted in distilled water. Of the women, 217 received lavender, 213 synthetic, and 205 control. This study demonstrated no statistically significant effect of using lavender in treating perineal pain.

In a retrospective, nonrandomized, nonblinded, non-placebo-controlled study, the analgesic effect of aromas was assessed in 534 women in labor and delivery pain (Burns & Blamey, 1994). Essential oils assessed included, individually or in combinations of up to four: lavender, clary sage, peppermint, eucalyptus, chamomile, frankincense, jasmine, rose, lemon, and mandarin. They were either administered through inhalation or directly placed on the skin, with or without massage. Expectation effect was encouraged: only those who wanted aromatherapy were chosen and the subjects themselves chose the aroma combination and the method of application. Despite this bias, this study did not support any antinociceptive properties of aromatherapy; there were 225 uses of analgesia before use of essential oils, compared with 624 uses after essential oil application.

In another study, Burns (Burns, Blamey, Ersser et al., 2000) assessed the effect of the same 10 aromas on labor pain among 564 women as compared with a nonaromatherapy control group. Aromatherapy was administered through inhalation, massage, footbath, cutaneous application, or perineal lavage and spray; 54% of those who used lavender and 64% of those who used frankincense reported efficacy in pain reduction, and fewer women required epidural analgesic when aromatherapy was used to reduce anxiety and pain. These results remain suspect because no statistical analysis, randomization, blinding, or control for expectation bias was performed, nor was olfactory ability assessed. Furthermore, their data revealed internal inconsistencies. They report that 7% of 8,058 mothers or 564, used aromatherapy to relieve pain, but later state that *only* 537 administrations of essential oil for pain were provided!

In an attempt to determine efficacy of complementary and alternative therapy for pain management during labor, assessment of aromatherapy was performed through an analysis of all published and unpublished randomized controlled trials that appeared in the Cochrane Pregnancy and Childbirth Group Trials Register (*The Cochrane Library*, Issue 2, 2002), Medline (1966 to July 2002), Embase (1980 to July 2002), and Cinahl (1980 to July 2002) (Smith, Collins, Cyna, & Crowther, 2003). Only one trial of aromatherapy was found that met these criteria (Calvert, as referenced in Smith, 2003). This was a double-blinded, randomized study involving 22 multiparous women with a singleton pregnancy, who, for pain relief, received either the essential oil of ginger, the essential oil of lemongrass, or both. These were applied by bath. There was no statistically significant effect of any of the aromas as measured by the McGill pain visual analogue scales or in the use of pharmacological pain relief. This study suggested the absence of efficacy of aromatherapy for labor pain.

An open-label, non-placebo-controlled study of *Vitex agnus-castus*, applied dermally (presumably at a level high enough for an inhalational effect) for menopausal and perimenopausal symptoms was performed (Lucks, 2003). Of the 52 volunteers, 4 to 6 noted reduced period pain; 1 to 2 volunteers complained that odorant precipitated headaches. Despite that some subjects were as old as 73 years, where more than one half have olfactory deficits (Doty, Newhouse, & Azzalina, 1985), olfactory ability was never assessed. It is unclear if any effect at all seen in this study was due to the aromatherapeutic benefit of *Vitex agnus-castus* as opposed to the topical effects, or even due to the tactile sensory stimulation which occurred on application.

Aromatherapy for pain reduction has been evaluated in the intensive care unit as well. In a study that was not randomized and not double blinded, Woolfson and Hewitt (1992) gave aromatherapy and massage in 20-minute sessions twice a week to 12 patients (Hewitt, 1992). Another 12 patients received massage only. The aromatherapy patients were massaged with lavender oil in an almond oil base. The other patients were massaged with almond oil only. Observations were recorded at the beginning and end of each 20-minute session and 30 minutes after treatment. All sessions were conducted in midafternoon. Approximately 50% of the patients were in the coronary care unit and the others were in intensive care units; 50% of the patients were artificially ventilated. The authors state that 50% of the aromatherapy patients and 41% of massage-only patients reported a decrease in pain. This is somewhat misleading, however. That six patients responded to aromatherapy and five patients responded to massage without aromatherapy is clearly not a statistically significant difference. If anything, these results indicate that aromatherapy was no better than massage alone. Given their selection of patients, however, one would not have predicted that aromatherapy would be effective, because the pathway for olfactory input is compromised by artificial ventilation.

In the previously described randomized, controlled trial of massage with either plain vegetable oil or with essential oil of neroli in postcardiac surgery intensive care unit patients, Stevensen actually demonstrated greater pain reduction with the plain vegetable oil! (Stevensen, 1994).

Oncology patients have also sought analgesia from aromatherapy with mixed results. In an open-label, non-randomized, noncontrolled study, eight women with lymphoedema associated with breast cancer underwent aromatherapy with lavender coincident with at least six 20- to 30-minute therapeutic massages. Three women reported a reduction of pain (Kirshbaum, 1996). All but one did not even notice the aroma. This is not surprising as estro-gen-positive breast carcinoma is associated with olfactory impairment (Lehrer et al., 1985). Thus, in this study, it is unclear how much of the results were due to the massage rather than the aroma.

Seven men and one woman with glioblastoma multiforme or anaplastic astrocytoma were treated with massage combined with lavender or with Roman chamomile. No statistically significant effect was found for relief of pain, anxiety, or depression (Hadfield, 2001).

Over a 3-year period, an unknown number of inpatient and outpatient oncology patients underwent a total of 769 treatments with massage with a variety of essential oils including *Lavandula angustifolia, Aniba rosaeddora, Citrus sinensis, Santalum album, Pelagonium gravedlens, Cupressus sempervirens,* and eucalyptus globules (DeValois & Clarke, 2001). After each treatment, patients rated their perception of pain relief; 31% of outpatient treatments and 20% of inpatient treatments were reported to improve pain. However, this study is severely limited because it is unclear which aroma was used and the subject size is unknown — the same subject may have undergone treatment many times, with each time counted separately, thus biasing the results.

In a study already referenced regarding possible efficacy of aromatherapy for depression, 89 patients with heterogeneous forms of cancer underwent six sessions of aromatherapy combined with massage and empathetic talking and, in some, reflexology (Kite et al., 1998). A blend of between one and four (median three) essential oils was used and in more than one third, a change in the oils occurred at least once during the treatments. Lavender, chamomile, geranium, juniper, bergamot, jasmine, and rose were the most frequently used of 20 different oils provided. Two thirds completed the study, the majority being women with breast cancer who were also receiving oncological treatment. While 69% (11 of 16) reported "significant improvement in pain," it is unclear what this truly means because no statistical significance was provided, exact aromas used are not reported, no control group was established, and results could have been produced with "empathetic talking" alone without the aromatherapy.

Among 17 cancer hospice patients, pain level was measured in response to 1 hour of lavender aromatherapy as compared with no treatment and a water humidifier control; lavender aroma had no statistically significant effect in reducing pain and was no more effective than plain water, or even no treatment at all (Louis & Kowalski, 2002).

On the other hand, 1% Roman chamomile reduced pain and anxiety ($p < 0.003$) among 51 patients with cancer, 76% of whom had metastases. A blend of lavender, marjoram, and rosemary was found to "show significant effectiveness" after treatment by 44 aromatherapists, based on responses on patient questionnaires (Yamada, Kando, Kim et al., 2001).

Arthritic and osteoarthritic pain is said to be responsive to a variety of aromatherapeutic agents including lavender, angustifolia, eucalyptus, black pepper, ginger, Roman chamomile, rosemary, myrrh, and rosemary, juniper, and birch are recommended for "stiff muscles" (Urba, 1996).

In 100 patients with pain of the periarticular system (Krall & Krause, 1993), treatment of from 10 to 20 days compared the efficacy of mint oil with that of hydroxyethylsalicylate gel. The mint oil was put into a gel and applied topically. Of the patients and physicians, 78% thought that mint therapy was highly effective and 50% of patients and 34% of physicians thought that hydroxyethylsalicylate gel was highly effective. None of the confounding parameters previously mentioned, such as olfactory ability, expectation, and hedonics, was addressed in this study.

Negative results were found in a study of the effects of massage with and without lavender on nine patients with rheumatoid arthritis (Brownfield, 1998). Although subjects who received lavender with massage were able to reduce their analgesic usage, no statistical significant reduction of pain as measured on a visual analogue scale as a result of massage alone or coincident with lavender administration was found.

In response to a Web page survey about fibromyalgia, 60 (90% female, 97% white) sufferers responded to questions about alternative medicine treatment. Of 10 who admitted to use of aromatherapy, 9 thought it had some effectiveness on treating symptoms (Barbour, 2000). It is difficult to assign much credence to this study because (1) bias may have existed in self-selected respondents, (2) symptom relief may have been for fatigue, depression, or anxiety, and *not* pain, (3) what aromas, methods of distribution, and coincident therapies used are unknown, and (4) no statistical significance regarding efficacy was able to be generated from this study.

RISKS

Before using aromatherapy in pain management, consideration must be given to the potential risks of the treatment. Adverse reactions from inhalation can occur among patients with diseases that predispose them to the development of side effects, and among the population as a whole as well.

Certain diseases make their sufferers particularly susceptible to adverse effects of aromatherapy. Approximately 40% of migraineurs report osmophobia, whereby an odorant induces a migraine headache (Blau & Solomon, 1985). A wide range of odorants can act as such triggers, depending on the individual. These triggers include perfume, cigarette smoke, and food odors (Hirsch & Kang, 1998).

Those with asthma, upon exposure to common odors, can suffer a worsening of their respiratory status independent of their olfactory ability (Burfield, 2000). In a survey of 60 patients with asthma, 57 (95%) described respiratory symptoms upon exposure to common odors including insecticide (85%), household cleaning agents (78%), cigarette smoke (75%), fresh paint (73%), perfume and cologne (72%), automobile exhaust or gas fumes (60%), and cooking aromas (37%). Room deodorant and mint candy also can cause respiratory distress (Shim & Williams, 1986). Four subjects who underwent an odor challenge with four squirts of a popular cologne all had an immediate decline in 1-second forced expiratory volume (18 to 58% reduction) (Shim & Williams, 1986).

Among persons who suffer complaints consistent with multiple chemical sensitivities, 24% of the men and 39% of the women note that odors precipitate their complaints (Miller, 1996). However, double-blind studies fail to demonstrate odorant-induced multiple chemical sensitivity symptoms (Ross, Whysner, Covello et al., 1999).

A variety of essential oils are said to be able to precipitate seizures in individuals with epilepsy. Whether these effects can occur by inhalation alone as opposed to ingestion or by percutaneous absorption is unclear. Proconvulsant odorants are said to include rosemary (Betts, 1994; Tisserand, 1977), fennel, hyssop, sage, wormwood (Millet et al., 1981; Tisserand, 1977), thuja, and cedar (Millet et al., 1981).

Inhalation of odorants can produce measurable levels in the blood (Lis-Balchin, 1997; Stimpfl et al., 1995), and because many common fragrances contain naphthalene-related compounds (including menthol and camphor), persons with G6PD deficiency may be at risk from aromatherapeutic exposures (Olowe & Ransome-Kuti, 1980). In neonates, dermal application has demonstrated this, but in adults it remains only a theoretical risk for inhalational aromatherapy.

Because aromatherapeutic inhalation of essential oils can produce detectable levels of the oils in the blood, these compounds, like any pharmacologic agents, could induce adverse drug–drug interactions in persons on medication. Such interactions could enhance metabolism of anticonvulsants or pain medications, for example, thus predisposing a patient with epilepsy to have a seizure or a patient with chronic pain to withdraw from medication. Jori, Bianchetti, and Prestini (1969) demonstrated this potential. Inhalation of eucalyptol by rats increased microsomal enzyme systems, thus decreasing the effect of pentobarbital.

While odorants can produce harmful side effects among persons suffering or predisposed to disease, they can injure the healthy population as well (Hosokawa & Ogawa, 1979). Airborne-induced allergic contact dermatitis is a recognized result of aromatherapeutic inhalation of tea tree oil (melaleuca oil) (DeGroot, 1996). Examples of common melaleuca oil allergens include *d*-limonene, aromadendrene, alpha-terpinene, 1,8-cineole (eucalyptol), terpinen-4-ol, *p*-cymene, and alpha-phellandrene. Because of the highly volatile nature of essential oils, their common constituents and cross-sensitization, DeGroot (1996) postulated that the same airborne-induced contact dermatitis could occur with several other essential oils including lavender and a mixture of eucalyptus, pine, and peppermint. Bridges suggested that if odorants can sensitize the respiratory system as they do the skin, they might not only exacerbate asthma, but might actually precipitate asthma (Bridges, 1999).

There is even the potential of sedation to the point of apnea in newborns when aromatherapy is used during the process of childbirth (Lis-Balchin, 1997). Some oils even appear to be carcinogenic (Ernst, 2001, Wisneski & Havery, 1996).

Substantial risks of aromatherapy introduced through a noninhalational route also exist. Toxicity of ingestion and topical application of aromatic essences has been well described and can involve multiple organ systems including cutaneous, renal, gastrointestinal, respiratory, hepatic, and neural, depending on the rapidity and means of administration, dosage, and specific oil used (Guba, 2000; Patel & Wiggins, 1980). Some adverse dermatologic effects of cutaneous application of aromatic essences result from their phototoxic and photomutagenic properties, as seen with oil of bergamot (Kaddu, Kerl, & Wolf, 2001). Dermal application not only can induce a cutaneous allergic response, but also, as with camphor, may be absorbed transdermally inducing toxic blood levels with associated gastrointestinal distress, hepatic toxicity, and even CNS manifestations including encephalopathy, delirium, and seizures (Rampini, Schneemann et al., 2002). Topical application of fragrances in rats has been demonstrated to produce not only blue discoloration of internal organs, but also neurotoxicity (Eiermann, 1980).

CONCLUSION

With aromatherapy, just as with any therapeutic tool, practitioners must weigh the relative risk/benefit ratio in deciding on its use in the treatment of pain.

Having spent the last two decades investigating the scientific basis of aromatherapy and having published more than 100 peer-reviewed articles in this area, the author does not believe that the scientific literature supports, nor the risk/benefit ratio justifies, use of aromatherapy in pain management at present. This is a fluid position, and as more studies are performed delineating the efficacy of aromatherapy, ultimately it may become a valid part of the therapeutic armamentarium. Until such time, this form of alternative medicine in the treatment of pain cannot be recommended.

REFERENCES

Acharya, V., Acharya, J., & Luders, H. (1996). Olfactory epileptic auras. *Neurology, 46*, A446.

Adams, P. (1998). When healing is more than simply clowning around. *Journal of the American Medical Association, 279*(5), 401.

Adams, R. D., Victor, M., & Roper, A. H. (1997). *Principles of neurology.* New York: McGraw-Hill.

Alaoui-Ismaili, O. et al. (1997). Basic emotions evoked by odorants: Comparison between autonomic responses and self-evaluation. *Physiology and Behavior, 62*, 713–720.

Allen, W. F. (1929). Effect of various inhaled vapors on respiration and blood pressure in anesthetized, unanesthetized, sleeping and anosmic subjects. *American Journal of Physiology, 1988*, 620–632.

Anselmi, B. et al. (1980). Endogenous opioids in cerebrospinal fluid and blood in idiopathic headache sufferers. *Headache, 20*, 294–299.

Appenzeller, O., Atkinson, R. A., & Standefer, J. C. (1981). Serum beta endorphin in cluster headache and common migraine. In F. C. Rose & E. Zikha (Eds.), *Progress in migraine.* London: Pitman.

Aqel, M. B. (1991). Relaxant effect of the volatile oil of *Romarinus officinalis* on tracheal smooth muscle. *Journal of Ethnopharmacology, 33*, 57–62.

Barbour, C. (2000). Use of complementary and alternative treatments by individuals with fibromyalgia syndrome. *Journal of the American Academy of Nurse Practitioners, 12*(8), 311–316.

Baron, R. A., & Thomley, J. (1994). A whiff of reality. *Environment and Behavior, 26*(6), 766–784.

Battaglia, S. (1997, March) A holistic approach to pain management. *Aromatherapy Today,* 5–8.

Betts, T. (1994). Sniffing the breeze. *Aromatherapy Quarterly, 1*, 19–22.

Blau, J. N., & Solomon, F. (1985). Smell and other sensory disturbances in migraine. *Journal of Neurology, 232*, 275–276.

Brandstatter, H., Fuhrwirth, M., & Kitchler, E. (1988). Effects of weather and air pollution on mood: Individual difference approach. In D. Canter et al. (Eds.), *NATO Advanced Research Workshop on Social and Environmental Psychology in the European Context: Environmental Social Psychology.* Boston: Kluwer.

Bridges, B. (1999). Fragrances and health. *Environmental Health Perspectives, 107*(7), A340.

Briere, J., Downes, A., & Spensley, J. (1983). Summer in the city: Urban weather conditions and psychiatric-emergency room visits. *Journal of Abnormal Psychology, 92*, 77–80.

Brodal, A. (1969). *Neurological anatomy in relation to clinical medicine* (Vol. 10, 3rd ed.). New York: Oxford University Press.

Broughan, C. (1998). Fragrant mechanisms. The impact of odours — Direct and indirect effects. *International Journal of Aromatherapy, 9*(4), 166–169.

Broughan, C. (1998/1999). Odour psychology. Aromatherapy: Towards a scientific explanation. *International Journal of Aromatherapy, 9*(3), 121–124.

Broughan, C. (2002). Odours, emotions, and cognition — How odours may affect cognitive performance. *International Journal of Aromatherapy, 12*(2), 92–98.

Brown, R., & Kulik, J. (1977). Flashbulb memories. *Cognition, 5,* 73–99.

Brownfield, A. (1998). Aromatherapy in arthritis — A study. *Nursing Standard, 13* (5), 34–35.

Buchbauer, G. (1990). Aromatherapy: Do essential oils have therapeutic properties? *Perfumer and Flavorist, 15,* 47–50.

Buchbauer, G. (1993). Biological effects of fragrances and essential oils. *Perfumer and Flavorist, 18,* 19–24.

Buchbauer, G., Jirovetz, L., Jäger, W., Dietrich, H. et al. (1991). Aromatherapy: Evidence for the sedative effect of the essential oil of lavender after inhalation. *Zeitschrift für Naturforschung, 46c,* 1067–1070.

Buchbauer, G. et al. (1993). Fragrance compounds and essential oils with sedative effects upon inhalation. *Journal of Pharmaceutical Sciences, 82*(6), 660–664.

Buckle, J. (1993). Aromatherapy. *Nursing Times 89*(20), 32–35.

Buckle, J. (1999a). Aromatherapy in perianesthesia nursing. *Journal of PeriAnesthesia Nursing, 14*(6), 336–344.

Buckle, J. (1999b). Use of aromatherapy as a complementary treatment for chronic pain. *Alternative Therapies, 5*(5), 42–51.

Buckle, J. (2001). A review of aromatherapy in pain relief. The economics of pain. *Aromatherapy Journal, 11*(1), 11–12, 42.

Bullinger, M. (1989a). Psychological effects of air pollution on healthy residents: A time series approach. *Journal of Environmental Psychology, 9,* 103–118.

Bullinger, M. (1989b). Relationships between air-pollution and well-being. *Zeitschrift Sozial und Praventivmedizin, 34,* 231–238.

Burfield, T. (2000). Safety of essential oils. *International Journal of Aromatherapy, 10*(1/2), 16–36.

Burns, E., & Blamey, C. (1994). Using aromatherapy in childbirth. *Nursing Times, 90*(9), 54–60.

Burns, E. E., Blamey, C., Ersser, S. T. et al., (2000). An investigation into the use of aromatherapy in intrapartum midwifery practice. *Journal of Alternative and Complementary Medicine, 6*(2), 141–147.

Ching, M. (1999). Contemporary therapy: Aromatherapy in the management of acute pain? *Contemporary Nurse, 8*(4), 146–151.

Classen, C., Howes, D., & Synnott, A. (1994). *Aroma — The cultural history of smell.* London: Routledge.

Clemens, S. L. (1882). The invalid's story. In C. Neider (Ed.). *The complete short stories of Mark Twain.* Garden City, NY: International Collectors Library, 1957.

Cooke, B., & Ernst, E. (2000). Aromatherapy: A systematic review. *British Journal of General Practice, 50,* 493–496.

Cunningham, M. (1979). Weather, mood, and helping behavior: Quasi-experiments with the sunshine. *Samaritan. Journal of Personality and Social Psychology, 37,* 1947–1956.

Cunningham, S. (1995). *Magical aromatherapy: The power of scent.* St. Paul: Llewellyn Publications.

Dale, A., & Cornwell, S. (1994). The role of lavender oil in relieving perineal discomfort following childbirth: A blind randomized clinical trial. *Journal of Advanced Nursing, 19,* 89–96.

Damian, P., & Damian, K. (1995). *Aromatherapy scent and psyche.* Rochester: Healing Arts.

Davis, R. G., & Panboro, R. M. (1982) Odor pleasantness judgments compared among samples from 20 nations using microfragrances [Abstract]. *Association for Chemoreception Sciences, 7,* 413.

DeGroot, A. C. (1996). Airborne allergic contact dermatitis from tea tree oil. *Contact Dermatitis, 35,* 304–305.

DeValois, B., & Clarke, E. (2001). A retrospective assessment of 3 years of patient audit for an aromatherapy massage service for cancer patients. *International Journal of Aromatherapy, 11*(3), 134–143.

Dietz, M. A., Goetz, C. J., & Steddings, G. T. (1990). Evaluation of visual cues as a modified inverted walking stick in the treatment of Parkinson's disease freezing episodes. *Movement Disorders, 5,* 243–247.

Distel, H. et al. (1999). Perception of everyday odors — Correlation between intensity, familiarity and strength of hedonic judgment. *Chemical Senses, 24,* 191–199.

Doty, R. L., Newhouse, M. G., & Azzalina, J. D. (1985). Internal consistency and short-term test–retest reliability of the University of Pennsylvania Smell Identification Test. *Chemical Senses, 10,* 297–300.

Dunn, C. (1992). A report on a randomized controlled trial to evaluate the use of massage and aromatherapy in an intensive care unit, bachelor's thesis, as referenced in Waldman, C.S. et al. (1993) Aromatherapy in the intensive care unit. *Care of the Critically Ill, 9*(4), 170–174.

Dunn, C., Sleep, J., & Collett, D. (1995). Sensing an improvement: an experimental study to evaluate the use of aromatherapy, massage and periods of rest in an intensive care unit. *Journal of Advanced Nursing, 21,* 34–40.

Dusser de Barenne, J. G. (1933). "Corticalization" of function and functional localization in the cerebral cortex. *Archives of Neurology and Psychiatry, 30,* 884–901.

Edge, J. (2003). A pilot study addressing the effect of aromatherapy massage on mood, anxiety and relaxation in adult mental health. *Complementary Therapies in Nursing & Midwifery, 9,* 90–97.

Efron, R. (1957). The effect of olfaction stimuli in arresting uncinate fits. *Brain, 79,* 267–281.

Ehrlichman, H., & Bastone, L. (1992). The use of odour in the study of emotion. In S. VanToller & G. Dodd (Eds.), *Fragrance, the psychology and biology of perfume* (pp. 143–159). London: Elsevier.

Ehrlichman, H., & Halpern, J.N. (1988). Affect and memory: Effects of pleasant and unpleasant odors on retrieval of happy and unhappy memories. *Journal of Personality and Psychology, 55,* 769–779.

Eiermann, H. J. (1980). Regulatory issues concerning AETT and 6-MC. *Contact Dermatitis, 6,* 120–122.

Eisenberg, D. M., David, R. B., Ettner, S. L., Appel S., Wilkey, S., Van Rompay, M., et al. (1998). Trends in alternative medicine use in the United States, 1990–1997: Results of a follow-up national survey. *Journal of the American Medical Association, 279,* 1548–1553.

Engen, T. (1991). *Odor sensation and memory.* New York: Praeger.

Ernst, E. (2001). A primer of complementary and alternative medicine commonly used by cancer patients. Available from the *Medical Journal of Australia* http://www.mja.com.au.

Ersser, S. (1990). Touch and go. *Nursing Standard, 4*(28), 39.

Estrem, S. A., & Renner, G. (1987). Disorders of smell and taste. *Otolaryngology Clinics of North America, 20,* 133–147.

Evans, B. (1995). An audit into the effects of aromatherapy massage and the cancer patients in palliative and terminal care. *Complementary Therapies in Medicine, 3,* 239–241.

Evans, G. W. (1994). Psychological costs of chronic exposure to ambient air pollution. In R. I. Isaacson & K. F. Jensen (Eds.), *The vulnerable brain and environmental risks* (Vol. 3. New York: Plenum Press.

Feller, R. M. (1997). *Practical aromatherapy: Understanding and using essential oils to heal the mind and body.* New York: Berkeley Books.

Fields, H. (1967). *Pain.* New York: McGraw-Hill.

Flaten, M. A., Simonsen, T., & Olsen, H. (1999). Drug-related information generates placebo and nocebo responses that modify the drug response. *Psychosomatic Medicine, 61,* 250–255.

Foote, S., Bloom, F., & Aston-Jones, G. (1983). Nucleus locus coeruleus: New evidence of anatomical and physiological specificity. *Physiological Reviews, 86,* 844–914.

Francis, S., Rolls, E. T., Bowtell, R. et al. (1999). The representation of pleasant touch in the brain and its relationship with taste and olfactory areas. *NeuroReport, 10*(3), 453–459.

Freud, S. (1908). Bemerkungen uber einen Fall von Zwangs neurosa. *German Healthcare, 7,* 350.

Gall, C. M. et al. (1987). Events for co-existence of GABA and dopamine in neurons of the rat olfactory bulb. *Journal of Comparative Neurology, 266,* 307–318.

Genders, R. (1972). *Perfume through the ages.* New York: G. Putnam & Sons.

Göbel, H., Schmidt, G., & Soyka, D. (1994). Effect of peppermint and eucalyptus oil preparations on neurophysiological and experimental algesimetric headache parameters. *Cephalalgia, 14,* 228–234.

Göbel, H. et al. (1995). Essential plant oils and headache mechanisms. *Phytomedicine, 2*(2), 93–102.

Göbel, H. et al. (1996). Effectiveness of peppermint oil and paracetamol in the treatment of tension headache. *Nervenarzt, 67,* 672–681.

Goodenough, D. R. (1978). Field dependence. In H. London & S. E. Exner (Eds.), *Dimension of personality* (pp. 165–216). New York: Wiley.

Goubet, N., Rattaz, C., Pierrat, V., Bullinger, A., & Lequien, P. (2003). Olfactory experience mediates response to pain in preterm newborns. *Developments in Psychobiology, 42,* 171–180.

Guba, R. (2000). Toxicity myths — The actual risks of essential oil use. *International Journal of Aromatherapy, 10*(1/2), 37–49.

Haberly, L. B., & Price, J. L. (1978). Association and commissural fiber systems of the olfactory cortex in the rat. II. Systems originating in the olfactory peduncle. *Journal of Comparative Neurology, 178,* 781–808.

Hadfield, N. (2001). The role of aromatherapy massage in reducing anxiety in patients with malignant brain tumours. *International Journal of Palliative Nursing, 7*(6), 279–285.

Halasz, N., & Shepherd, G. M. (1983). Neurochemistry of the vertebrate olfactory bulb. *Neuroscience, 10,* 579–619.

Hardebo, J. E. et al. (1985). CSF opioid levels in cluster headache. In F. C. Rose (Ed.), *Migraine.* Basel: Karger.

Hewitt, D. (1992). Massage with lavender oil lowered tension. *Nursing Times, 88*(25), 8.

Hirsch, A. R. (1992). Nostalgia: Neuropsychiatric understanding. *Advanced Consumer Research, 19,* 390–395.

Hirsch, A. R. (1995a). Cephalgia as a result of acute nitrogen tetroxide exposure. *Headache, 35,* 310.

Hirsch, A. R. (1995b). *Chronic neurotoxicity as a result of landfill exposure in Port Orchard, Washington: International Congress on Hazardous Waste: Impact on human and ecological health.* Atlanta: U.S. Department of Health and Human Services: Public Health Agency for Toxic Substances and Disease Registry.

Hirsch, A. R. (1995c). *Chronic neurotoxicity of acute chlorine gas exposure.* Thirteenth International Neurotoxicity Conference, Hot Springs, Arkansas.

Hirsch, A. R. (1995d). *Neurotoxicity as a result of acute nitrogen tetroxide exposure. International Congress on Hazardous Waste: Impact on human and ecological health.* Atlanta: U.S. Department of Health and Human Services, Public Health Agency for Toxic Substances and Disease Registry.

Hirsch, A. R. (1998a). Negative health effects of malodors in the environment: A brief review. *Journal of Neurological, Orthopedic Medicine and Surgery, 18,* 43–45.

Hirsch, A. R. (1998b). *Scentsational sex.* Boston: Element Books.

Hirsch, A. R. & Bailey, M. L. (2005). Chemosensory changes in estrogen receptor positive breast carcinoma: A case report. *Chemical Senses, 30*(3), 265.

Hirsch, A. R., & Cleveland, L. B. (1998). Olfaction in chronic spinal cord injury. *Journal of Neurologic Rehabilitation, 12,* 101–104.

Hirsch, A. R., & Gay, S. (1991). The effect of ambient olfactory stimuli on the evaluation of a common consumer product. *Chemical Senses, 16*(5), 535–536.

Hirsch, A. R., & Gruss, J. J. (1998). Ambient odors in the treatment of claustrophobia: A pilot study. *Journal of Neurological and Orthopedic Medicine and Surgery, 18,* 98–103.

Hirsch, A. R., & Kang, C. (1998). The effect of inhaling green apple fragrance to reduce the severity of migraine: A pilot study. *Headache Quarterly, 9,* 159–163.

Hirsch, A. R., & Rankin, K. M. (1993). Trichloroethylene exposure and headache. *Headache, 33,* 275.

Hirsch, A. R., & Trannel, T. J. (1996). Chemosensory disorders and psychiatric diagnoses. *Journal of Neurological and Orthopedic Medicine and Surgery, 17,* 25–30.

Hirsch, A. R., & Wyse, J. P. (1993). Posttraumatic dysosmia: Central vs. peripheral. *Journal of Neurological and Orthopedic Medicine and Surgery, 14,* 152–155.

Hosokawa, H., & Ogawa, T., (1979). Study of skin irritations cause by perfumery materials. *Perfumer & Flavorist, 4,* 7–8.

Igarashi, H. et al. (1987). Cerebrovascular sympathetic nervous activity during cluster headaches. *Handbook of Clinical Neurology, 7*(6), 87–89.

Izmerov, N. (1971). Establishment of air quality standards. *Archives of Environmental Health, 22,* 711–719.

Jardine, M. (2002). Aromatherapy. Introduction into a maternity service. *Practising Midwife, 5*(4), 14–15.

Jellinek, J. S. (1998/1999.) Odours and mental states. *International Journal of Aromatherapy, 9*(3), 115–120.

Jirovetz, L., Buchbauer, G., Jäger, W. et al. (1992). Analysis of fragrance compounds in blood samples of mice by gas chromatography, mass spectrometry, GC/FTIR and GC/AES after inhalation of sandalwood oil. *Biomedical Chromatography, 6,* 133–134.

Jones, J. W., & Bogat, G. A. (1978). Air pollution and human aggression. *Psychological Reports, 43,* 721–722.

Jori, A., Bianchetti, A., & Prestini, P. E. (1969). Effect of essential oils on drug metabolism. *Biochemical Pharmacology, 18*(9), 2081–2085.

Kaddu, S., Kerl, H., & Wolf, P. (2001). Accidental bullous phototoxic reactions to bergamot aromatherapy oil. *Journal of the American Academy of Dermatology, 45,* 458–461.

Kaptchuk, T. J., & Eisenberg, D. M. (1998). The persuasive appeal of alternative medicine. *Annals of Internal Medicine, 129,* 1061–1065.

Kawakami, K., Takai-Kawakami, K., Okazaki, Y., Kurihara, H., Shimizu, Y, & Yanaihara, T. (1997). The effects of odors on human newborn infants under stress. *Infant Behavior and Development, 20,* 531–535.

Kessler, R. C., Davis, R. B., Foster, D. F., Van Rompay, M. I., Walters, E. E., Wilkey S. A. et al. (2001). Long-term trends in the use of complementary and alternative medical therapies in the United States. *Annals of Internal Medicine, 135,* 262–268.

Keville, K. (1999). *Aromatherapy for dummies.* Foster City, CA: IDG Books Worldwide.

Keville, K., & Green, M. (1995). *Aromatherapy: A complete guide to the healing art.* Santa Cruz, CA: Crossing Press.

King, J. R. (1994). Scientific status of aromatherapy. *Perspectives in Biology and Medicine, 37*(3), 409–415.

Kirk-Smith, M. D., Van Toller, C., & Dodd, G. H. (1983). Unconscious odour conditioning in human subjects. *Biological Psychology, 17,* 221–231.

Kirshbaum, M. (1996). Using massage in the relief of lymphoedema. *Professional Nurse, 11*(4) 230–232.

Kite, S. M., Maher, E. J., Anderson, K. et al. (1998). Development of an aromatherapy service at a cancer center. *Palliative Medicine, 12,* 171–180.

Kline, N., & Rausch, J. (1985). Olfactory precipitants of flashbacks in post traumatic stress disorders: Case reports. *Journal of Clinical Psychiatry, 46,* 383–384.

Knasko, S. C., Gilbert, A. N., & Sabini, J. (1990). Emotional state, physical well-being, and performance in the presence of feigned ambient odor. *Journal of Applied Social Psychology, 20*(16), 1345–1357.

Komori, T., Fujiwara, R., & Tanida, M. (1995). Effects of citrus fragrance on immune function and depressive states. *Neuroimmunomodulation, 2,* 174–180.

Kovar, K. A., Gropper, B., Friess, D. et al. (1987). Blood levels of 1,8-cineole and locomotor activity of mice after inhalation and oral administration of rosemary oil. *Planta Medica, 53,* 315–319.

Krall, B., & Krause, W. (1993). Efficacy intolerance of mentha arvensis aetheroleum. Program abstracts, Twenty-fourth International Symposium of Essential Oils.

Laird, D. A. (1988). What can you do with your nose? *Scientific Monthly, 1,* 319–322.

Langewitz, W., Ruddel, H., & VonEiff, A. W. (1987). Influence of perceived level of stress upon ambulatory blood pressure, heart rate, and respiratory frequency. *Journal of Clinical Hypertension, 3,* 743–748.

LeDoux, J. (1996). *The emotional brain.* New York: Simon & Schuster.

Lehrer, S., Levine, E., & Bloomer, W. (1985). Abnormally diminished sense of smell in women with oestrogen receptor positive breast cancer. *Lancet, 2,* 333.

Leston, J. et al. (1987). Free and conjugated plasma catecholamines in cluster headache. *Cephalalgia, 7*(6), 331.

Lim, P. (1997). Essential stress relief: The use of oils to treat tension. *British Journal of Midwifery, 5*(6), 336–338.

Lindsay, W. R., Pitcaithly, D., & Geelen, N. (1997). A comparison of the effects of four therapy procedures on concentration and responsiveness in people with profound learning disabilities. *Journal of Intellectual Disability Research, 41*(3), 201–207.

Lis-Balchin, M. (1997). Essential oils and "aromatherapy": Their modern role in healing. *Journal of the Royal Society of Health, 117*(5), 324–329.

Lorig, T. S. (1994). EEG and ERP studies of low-level odor exposure in normal subjects. *Toxicology and Industrial Health, 10*(4–5), 579–586.

Lorig, T. S., & Roberts, M. (1990). Odor and cognitive alteration of the contingent negative variation. *Chemical Senses, 15*(5), 537–545.

Loring, D. W., & Meador, K. J. (2001). The evocative nature of emotional content for sensory and motor systems. *Neurology, 56,* 146–147.

Louis, M., & Kowalski, S. D. (2002). Use of aromatherapy with hospice patients to decrease pain, anxiety, and depression and to promote an increased sense of well-being. *American Journal of Hospice & Palliative Care, 19*(6), 381–386.

Lucks, B. C. (2003). *Vitex agnus castus* essential oil and menopausal balance: A research update. *International Journal of Aromatherapy, 13*(4), 169–172.

Ludvigson, H. W., & Rottman, T. R. (1989). Effects of ambient odors of lavender and cloves on cognition, memory, affect and mood. *Chemical Senses, 14,* 525–536.

MacLean, P. D. (1973). *Triune concept of the brain and behavior.* Toronto: University of Toronto Press.

Macrides, F., & Davis, B. J. (1983). Olfactory bulb. In P. C. Emson (Ed.), *Chemical neuroana*. New York: Raven Press.

Mair, R. G., & Harrison, L. M. (1991). Influence of drugs on smell function. In D. G. Laing, R. L. Doty, & W. Briephol (Eds.), *Human sense of smell*. Berlin: Springer-Verlag.

Mantle, F. (1996). Moving experiences. *Nursing Times, 92*(14), 46–48.

Marchand, S, & Arsenault, P. (2002). Odors modulate pain perception. A gender-specific effect. *Physiology & Behavior, 76*, 251–256.

Martin, G. N. (1996). Olfactory remediation. Current evidence and possible applications. *Social Science Medicine, 43*(1), 63–70.

Maruniak, J. A. (1995). Deprivation and the olfactory system. In R. L. Doty (Ed.). *Handbook of olfaction and gustation*. New York: Marcel Dekker.

Matteliano, D. (2003). Holistic nursing management of pain and suffering: A historical view with contemporary application. *Journal of the New York State Nurses' Association, 3*(1), 4–8.

Mellier, D., Bézard, S., & Caston, J. (1997). Études exploratoires des relations intersensorielles olfaction-douleur. *Enfance, 1*, 47–64.

Miller, C. S. (1996). Chemical sensitivity: Symptom, syndrome or mechanism for disease? *Toxicology, 111*, 69–86.

Miller, F. G., Emanuel, E. J., Rosenstein, D. L., & Straus, S. E. (2004). Ethical issues concerning research in complementary and alternative medicine. *Journal of the American Medical Association, 291*(5), 599–604.

Millet, Y., Jouglard, J., Steinmetz, P., Tognetti, P., Joanny, P., & Arditti, J. (1981). Toxicity of some essential plant oils. Clinical and experimental study. *Clinical Toxicology, 18*(12), 1485–1498.

Miltner, W. et al. (1994). Emotional qualities of odorants and their influence on the startle reflex in humans. *Psychophysiology, 31*, 107–110.

Miner, J. R. (1980). Controlling odors from livestock production facilities: State-of-the-art. In American Society of Agricultural Engineers, *Livestock waste: Renewable resource*. St. Joseph, MO: Author.

Moskowitz, M. A. (1984). Neurobiology of vascular head pain. *Annals of Neurology, 16*, 157–158.

Murphy, C., Doty, R. L., & Duncan, H. J. (2003). Clinical disorders of olfaction. In R. L. Doty (Ed.), *Handbook of olfaction and gustation* (Vol. 22, 2nd ed. rev., pp. 461–478). New York: Marcel Dekker.

Nattero, G. et al. (1985). Serum gastrin levels in cluster headache and migraine attacks. In V. Pfaffenrath, P. O. Lundberg, & O. Sjaastad (Eds.), *Updating in headache*. Berlin: Springer-Verlag.

Neutra, R. et al. (1991). Hypotheses to explain the higher symptom rates observed around hazardous waste sites. *Environmental Health Perspectives, 94*, 31–38.

Olowe, S. A., & Ransome-Kuti, O. (1980). The risk of jaundice in glucose-6-phosphate dehydrogenase deficient babies exposed to menthol. *Acta Paediatrica Scandinavica, 69*, 341–345.

Papadopoulos, A., Wright, S., & Ensor, J. (1999). Evaluation and attributional analysis of an aromatherapy service for older adults with physical health problems and carers using the service. *Complementary Therapies in Medicine, 7*, 239–244.

Passant, H. (1990). A holistic approach in the ward. *Nursing Times, 86*(4), 26–28.

Patel, S., & Wiggins, J., (1980). Eucalyptus oil poisoning. *Archives of Disease in Childhood, 55*(5), 405–406.

Price, S. (1991). *Aromatherapy for common ailments*. New York: Fireside Book.

Price, S., & Price, L. (1995). *Aromatherapy for health professionals*. New York: Churchill Livingstone.

Proust, M. (1934). *Remembrance of things past* (Vol. 1, C. D. Scott Moncrieff, Trans.). New York: Random House.

Rampini, S. K., Schneemann, M., Rentsch, K., Bachli, E. B. et al. (2002). Camphor intoxication after cao gio (coin rubbing). Research letter. *Journal of the American Medical Association, 288*(1), 45.

Rattaz, C., Goubet, N., & Bullinger, A. (2001). *The calming effect of a familiar odor following a painful experience*. Poster presented at the April Bienial Meeting of the Society for Research in Child Development, Minneapolis, MN.

Reid, J. (2001). Getting the massage across. *Nursing Times, 97*(15), 26.

Robin, O. et al. (1998). Emotional responses evoked by dental odors: An evaluation from autonomic parameters. *Journal of Dental Research, 77*(8), 1638–1646.

Robin, O. et al. (1999). Basic emotions evoked by eugenol odor differ according to the dental experience: A neurovegetative analysis. *Chemical Senses, 24*, 327–335.

Roebuck, A. (1988). Aromatherapy: Fact or fiction. *Perfumer and Flavorist, 13*, 43–45.

Ross, P. M., Whysner, J., Covello, V. T., Kuschner, M., Rifkind, A. B., Sedler, M. J. et al. (1999). Olfaction and symptoms in the multiple chemical sensitivities syndrome. *Preventive Medicine, 28*(5), 467–480.

Rotton, J. (1983). Affective and cognitive consequences of malodorous pollution. *Basic Applied Social Psychology, 4*, 171–191.

Rotton, J., & Frey, J. (1985). Air pollution, weather, and violent crimes: Concomitant time series analysis of archival data. *Journal of Personality and Social Psychology, 49*, 1207–1220.

Rotton, J. et al. (1978). Air pollution and interpersonal attraction. *Journal of Applied Social Psychology, 8*, 57–71.

Rotton, J. et al. (1979). Air pollution experience and physical aggression. *Journal of Applied Social Psychology, 9*, 347–412.

Saller, R., Hellstein, A., & Hellenbrecht, D. (1988). Klinische Pharmakologie und Therapeutische Anwendung von Cineol (eukalyptus) und Menthol als Bestandteil Atherischer ole. *Internistische Praxis, 28*(2), 355–364.

Schnaubelt, K. (1995). *Advanced aromatherapy: The science of essential oil therapy*. Rochester: Healing Arts.

Schiffman, S. S. et al. (1995). The effect of environmental odors emanating from commercial swine operations on the mood of nearby residents. *Brain Research Bulletin, 37*, 369–375.

Shim, C., & Williams, M. H., Jr. (1986). Effect of odors in asthma. *American Journal of Medicine, 80,* 18–22.

Shipley, M., Halloran, F., & Torre, J. (1985). Surprisingly rich projection from locus coeruleus to the olfactory bulb in the rat. *Brain Research, 329,* 294–299.

Shusterman, D. (1992). Critical review: Health significance of environmental odor pollution. *Archives of Environmental Health, 47,* 76–87.

Sjaastad, O. (1986). Cluster headaches. In P. J. Vinken, G. W. Bruyn, & H. L. Klawans (Eds.), *Handbook of clinical neurology headache* (Vol. 48). New York: Elsevier Science.

Smith, C. A., Collins, C. T., Cyna, A. M., & Crowther, C. A. (2003) Complementary and alternative therapies for pain management in labour. *Cochrane Database of Systematic Reviews, 2,* CD003521.

Spector, I. P. et al., (1993). Cue-controlled relaxation and "aromatherapy" in the treatment of speech anxiety. *Behavioural and Cognitive Psychotherapy, 21,* 239–253.

Squire, L. R. (1987). *Memory and brain.* New York: Oxford University Press.

Stevenson, C. (1992). Orange blossom evaluation. *International Journal of Aromatherapy, 4*(3), 22–24.

Stevensen, C. J. (1994). The psychophysiological effects of aromatherapy massage following cardiac surgery. *Complementary Therapies in Medicine, 2,* 27–35.

Stimpfl, T. et al. (1995). Concentration of 1,8-cineol in human blood during prolonged inhalation. *Chemical Senses, 20*(3), 349–350.

Strahilevitz, M., Strahilevitz, A., & Miller, J. E., (1979). Air pollutants and the admission rate of psychiatric patients. *American Journal of Psychiatry, 136*(2), 205–207.

Styles, J. L. (1987). The use of aromatherapy in hospitalized children with HIV. *Complementary Therapies in Nursing & Midwifery, 3*(1), 16–20.

Sugawara, Y., Hino, Y., & Kawasaki, M. (1999). Alteration of perceived fragrance of essential oils in relation to type of work: A simple screening test for efficacy of aroma. *Chemical Senses, 24,* 415–421.

Tisserand, R. (1993). Aromatherapy today. Part 1. *International Journal of Aromatherapy, 5*(3), 26–29.

Tisserand, R. B. (1977). *The art of aromatherapy.* Rochester: Healing Arts.

Torii, S. (1996). A key role of olfaction in aromatherapy. *Chemical Senses, 21,* 81.

Torii, S. et al. (1988). Contingent negative variation (CNV) and the psychological effects of odour. In S. VanToller & G. Dodd (Eds.). *Perfumery: The psychology and biology of fragrance.* New York: Chapman & Hall.

Urba, S. G. (1996). Nonpharmacologic pain management in terminal care. *Clinics in Geriatric Medicine, 12*(2), 301–311.

Ury, H. K., Perkins, M. A., & Goldsmith, J. R. (1972). Motor vehicle accidents and vehicular pollution in Los Angeles. *Archives of Environmental Health, 25,* 314–322.

Valentine, J. H. et al. (1975). Human crises and the physical environment. *Man–Environmental Systems, 5*(1), 23–28.

Van Toller, S, & Dodd, G. H. (1988). *Perfumery: The psychology and biology of fragrances.* London: Chapman & Hall.

Visser, A. (1999). Social desirability in health research. *Psychosomatic Medicine, 61,* 106.

Waldman, C. S. (1993). Aromatherapy in the intensive care unit. *Care of the Critically Ill, 9*(4), 170–174.

Walji, H. (1996). *The healing power of aromatherapy.* Rocklin, CA: Prima Publishing.

Warm, J. S., Dember, W. N., & Parasuraman, R. (1991). Effects of olfactory stimulation on performance and stress in a visual sustained attention task. *Journal of the Society of Cosmetic Chemists, 42,* 199–210.

Warren, C., & Warrenburg, S. (1993). Mood benefits of fragrance. *Perfumer & Flavorist, 18,* 9–16.

Warrenburg, S., & Schwartz, G.E. (1990). A psychophysiological study of three odorants. *Chemical Senses, 13,* 744.

Wayne, W., Wehrle, P., & Carroll, R. (1967). Oxidant air pollution and athletic performance. *Journal of the American Medical Association, 199,* 901–904.

Weisse, C. S. (1992). Depression and immunocompetence: Review of the literature. *Psychological Bulletin, 111,* 475–489.

Weyers, W., & Brodbeck R. (1989). Hautdurchdringung atherischer ole (Skin absorption of volatile oils). *Pharmazie in Unserer Zeit, 18*(3), 82–86.

Wiebe, E. (2000). A randomized trial of aromatherapy to reduce anxiety before abortion. *Effective Clinical Practice, 4,* 166–169.

Wilkinson, S. (1995). Aromatherapy and massage in palliative care. *International Journal of Palliative Nursing, 1*(1), 21–30.

Willis, W. D., & Westlund, K. N. (1997). Neuroanatomy of the pain system and of the pathways that modulate pain. *Journal of Clinical Neurophysiology, 14*(1), 2–31.

Wisneski, H. S., & Havery, D. C. (1996). Nitro musks in fragrance products: An update of FDA findings. *Cosmetics & Toiletries, 111,* 73–76.

Wood, K. (2003). The promise of aromatherapy. Essential oils have been shown in clinical trials to soothe some chronic ills brought on by old age. *Provider, 29*(3), 47–48.

Woolfson, A., & Hewitt, D. (1992). Intensive aromacare. *International Journal of Aromatherapy, 4*(2), 12–13.

Worwood, S. (1995). *Essential aromatherapy. A pocket guide to essential oils & aromatherapy.* Novato, CA: New World Library.

Yager, J., Siegfried, S. L., & DiMatteo, T. L. (1999). Use of alternative remedies by psychiatric patients: Illustrative vignettes and a discussion of the issues. *American Journal of Psychiatry, 156*(9), 1432–1438.

Yamada, K., Kando, N., Kim, S. et al. (2001). A survey concerning essential oils that aromatherapists consider effective and evaluation of their effect in aromatherapy. *Chemical Senses, 26,* 306.

Zaborsky, L. et al. (1985). Cholinergic and GABA-ergic projections to the olfactory bulb in the rat. *Journal of Comparative Neurology, 243,* 468–509.

Zeidner, M., & Schechter, M. (1988). Psychological responses to air pollution: Some personality and demographic correlates. *Journal of Environmental Psychology, 8,* 191–208.

78

Homeopathy

Michael W. Loes, MD, MD (H), and Dana Ullman, MPH

INTRODUCTION

Many books and papers have been written about the healing powers of homeopathy (from Greek *homoios,* meaning "like" or "similar"). It is practiced around the world. What is it? What do I need to know about it? How does it work? Should I, as a pain management physician, learn enough about it to integrate it into my pain practice?

WHAT IS HOMEOPATHY?

Homeopathy's philosophical roots go back to ancient Greek physicians, especially Galen and Hippocrates. In their writings, they spoke, in general terms, about the ability of *like* substances having the ability to cure the symptoms that diseases cause. This concept is the most fundamental kernel of homeopathic ideas and is known as "the law of similars." The healing agent — the "like cures like" substance — is known as the *similimum.*

Conventional medicine teaches that symptoms are caused by the illness, whereas homeopathy understands the symptoms as the body's natural reaction in fighting infection or responding to stress. Homeopathy seeks to stimulate rather than suppress symptoms, thereby enhancing and creating a curative response.

Homeopathy as a medical discipline was developed by the German physician, Samuel Christian Friedrich Hahnemann (1755–1843). At an early age, his father recognized that Samuel had a talent for languages, and by the time he finished secondary school, he likely had mastered nearly a dozen. He soon earned a modest income doing medical translations, and these undertakings introduced him to some of the early classical medical texts.

He completed a formal medical degree, but from the onset, he was openly critical of many common therapies of his day such as bloodletting for fevers, leeches for infections, purgatives, toxins, and the use of various religious exorcisms. He was appalled by surgeries done in squalid conditions where postoperative complications were the norm. Hence, over a fairly short period of time, Dr. Hahnemann alienated one group of practitioners, and attracted another, who became his avid followers and began doing things differently. Homeopathy was born.

The principles that form the foundation of homeopathy are eloquently penned in *The Organon of Medical Art* which underwent five editions during the lifetime of Dr. Hahnemann, and a sixth edition was published after his death. It lays out 291 concepts that are referred to as the natural principles of cure. It is exhaustive, and worthy of intense study. The more modest goal here is to acquaint the reader with this science and art of medicine. The information is introductory, but key references and sources are provided as best places to go to explore farther. Your interest will expectantly rise. Some of you will dig deeper learning to use homeopathy, or at the very least, incorporate some of the concepts that are universal to health and healing.

KEY PRINCIPLES

The basic assumption of homeopathy is that symptoms of illness are defenses of the body in its efforts to fight infection and adapt to stress. Instead of using medicinal agents to inhibit or suppress symptoms, homeopaths look to find a substance that would cause, in deliberate overdose, the *similar* symptoms that the sick person is experiencing. The homeopath then prescribes the identified substance in specially prepared minute or infinitesimal doses.

Homeopaths determine what symptom and disease states a medicine is effective in treating based on research in toxicology. Homeopaths conduct experiments called "provings," in which human subjects are given repeated doses of a substance in order to find out what it causes (and thus what it can cure). These provings are conducted on healthy subjects only because sick people, by definition, are exhibiting various symptoms, and the purpose of a proving is to determine what symptoms a specific substance causes. Please note that provings are conducted with homeopathic doses of substances making them much safer for clinical experiments. However, because such small doses are used, not every person who participates will be exhibit symptoms.

Homeopathy is part of "vitalistic medical thought," although this underlying premise is not a perquisite for using homeopathic medicine clinically. Vitalism assumes that there is an underlying force in the human body that unifies it and that works in coordinated fashion to defend itself against the various infective agents and stresses to which the human organism is prone. The concept of vital force has alternative names: *chi, ki, prana, kundalini*, life essence, life energy, vitality. Even the Romans had a name for it; they called it *élan vitale*.

Homeopathy is holistic in that the homeopath believes that no one organ of the body can be sick without affecting the person as a whole, and that the mental, emotional, and the physical states of the person create symptoms that are a part of the overall disease the person is experiencing. Each person has his or her own syndrome of symptoms.

Homeopaths utilize extremely small and specially prepared doses of various substances from the plant, mineral, animal, and chemical kingdoms. These drugs are manufactured by FDA-recognized drug manufacturers, and they are primarily regulated as over-the-counter drugs.

THE LANGUAGE OF HOMEOPATHY

As with other alternative systems, certain terminology needs introduction as one begins to study homeopathy. Let us start with three terms: *remedy, potency, succession.*

A remedy is the prescription given by the homeopath after a comprehensive case history has been conducted. The remedy contains an amount of a substance that is intended to begin the healing. These substances are generally animal, vegetable, or mineral substances — *but not always*. A list of remedies is categorized in the *Materia Medica* and contains nearly 2,000 possible substances. The similimum is the remedy that best matches the disease spectrum. There are multiple pharmaceutical companies that produce remedies of unquestionable purity. Boiron, Dolisos, Heel BHI, Standard Homeopathic, and Hahnemann Laboratories are notable examples.

Potency refers to the number of times that a medicinal substance has been diluted with double-distilled water in either 1:10 or 1:100 ratios. A 1× potency is called a tincture. A 2× is when 1 cc of this solution is taken and then diluted to 10 cc. When a solution is diluted 1:100 once, it is called a 1C, and when it is diluted again 1:100, it is a 2C, and so on. The aqueous solution is vigorously shaken between each dilution. This shaking is called *succussion*. Serial dilutions render progressively greater potencies, and clinical experience has discovered that the more a substance is potentized, the longer it acts, the deeper it acts, and, in general, fewer doses are generally needed. "Low potency" remedies are generally 1× or 1C to 12× or 12C. "Medium potency" remedies are generally 13× or 13C to 30× or 30C. "High potency" remedies are generally above the 30th potency. In following the tradition of Roman numerals, potencies that have been potentized 1,000 times are called 1M and when they have been potentized further ($1/100 \times 1/500$) they are called LM potencies, and at 100,000 times, they are called CM. Potency designations can also be understood in logarithm scale: 1×, 1C could be expressed as 1×10^6, 1×10^7.

WHAT DOES A HOMEOPATHIC PHYSICIAN DO?

When a homeopathic physician evaluates a patient, major emphasis is placed on the history and, in particular, the symptoms experienced. They are categorized in meticulous detail, not only in severity, but also in order of appearance. The crux of the *Organon's* Principle 7 is that a disease can only be known by its symptoms. When the categorization is done, the spectrum of illness is known, and it must be matched to a similimum (Principle 28) by comparing the illness's spectrum with those of known substances in the *Materia Medica*, which refers to books in which the "materials of medicine" are described based on information derived from provings as well as from clinical practice.

EMPHASIS

The symptom spectrum in the illness must match as closely as possible to the known toxic spectrum of the substance in the Materia Medica *that was determined when the substance was tested in a* healthy *person as part of a proving.*

In *classical* homeopathy, a *single* remedy — known as the similimum — is selected. When it is selected, the potency needs also to be prescribed, as well as giving directions on when and how to take it.

In *modern* homeopathy, low-potency combination homeopathic remedies are often used. A number of remedies will be combined to treat common illness such as an upset stomach, headaches, the flu, or backaches. Homeopathic physicians who are more traditionally trained in homeopathy will often scoff at combination products that are more disease driven than individually attended. It needs to be appreciated that homeopaths treat individuals, not diseases. As soon as the Western concept of disease is introduced, the uniqueness of this therapeutic approach is lessened and likely rendered less effective. If one were to ask a homeopathic physician how many diseases there are, he or she would undoubtedly answer that the number of diseases is equal to the number of living people in "dys-ease." Each person is unique, and how illness forms in each person is individually determined. Hence, the practice of homeopathy, at least classically, is always directed toward the individual person.

CONCURRENT POLITICAL EVENTS IN EVOLUTION IN THE EARLY 20TH CENTURY

The flu epidemic of 1918, where homeopathy had established itself as better than conventional treatment in at least in one epidemiological mode (Suits, 1985)

The rise of the American Medical Association (AMA) and its government mandate to control medical education

The birth of psychiatry, especially the champions of psychoanalysis and cognitive behavior therapy

The industrial revolution and its assembly-line production style which not only caused new kinds of injuries, but extended exposures to specific chemicals, and may have created the image of "assembly-line" medical care

The development of the food industry and the problems of contamination

The early celebrated discoveries of a burgeoning pharmaceutical industry

The labor-intensive nature of individualized homeopathic care which did not fit into 20th century medicine that emphasized quick visits and drug prescriptions

At a critical time in American history, homeopathy did not have the unity or political power to survive. It was driven underground and nearly annihilated by multiple opposing factors, both from within and outside of its ranks.

THE NEXT STEP

If you, as a pain management physician, nurse, or other type of health care provider, are to appreciate the beauty and discipline of homeopathy, you need to assess your belief system about holistic health and healing. Many of

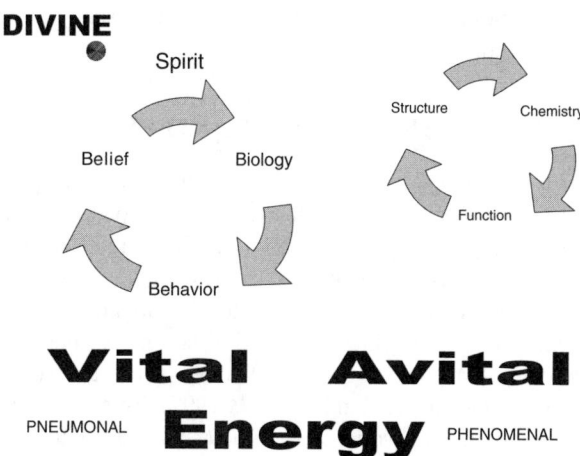

FIGURE 78.1 Relationship of homeopathy to avital disciplines.

you, in my experience, have developed or have had to develop "unconventional" views because people hurt — *they really suffer.* Prescribing drugs to decrease "nociception" (pain receptors firing) and using advanced neuromodulation techniques are often not enough. Either the patients ask or we, as pain management health care providers, personally begin exploring acupuncture, hypnosis, herbs, and just maybe — homeopathy.

Figure 78.1 illustrates where most homeopaths would place their therapeutic model of health and disease. It needs to be understood that there is a basic separation between sciences that are "avital" and those that are "vital." Physical sciences are avital: math, physics, chemistry, astronomy, computer science. The cause and effect reactions that one investigates are "phenomenal" — can be observed, are generally capable of being reproduced on an experimental basis. Predictability models can be developed. The avital interrelationships address structure, function, and chemistry and are usually defined by mathematical equations. Physical laws are observed, and under laboratory conditions, the information can be confirmed. Many physicians never go beyond these mechanical relationships. Their thinking tends to be mechanistic and reductionistic by design, exemplifying that the whole is the sums of the parts and when a part goes bad, fix it.

For the physician who believes that health is "vital," a new set of relationships exists: beliefs, emotions, spiritual energy, a living biology, and functional behaviors. Relationship can be viewed as back and forth or circular as can the former relationships, but the key is that we have a living relationship — one that is homeodynamic, rather than homeostatic. Some philosophers, most notably Emmanuel Kant, have called this area of inquiry the "pneumonal" or the breath of existence. When a homeopathic physician performs an evaluation, there is assessment of vitality, "aliveness," and very specific lines of questioning are used to do this. The goal is to assess the composite energetic picture of the patient and then choose a similimum that approximates what is being seen at that point in time.

HOMEOPATHIC MEDICINE AND RESEARCH

Most physicians assume that there have not been good clinical studies to test the efficacy of homeopathic medicines. This is simply not true. A review of 89 worthy clinical studies was published in *The Lancet*, and this review found that, on average, those patients given a homeopathic medicine were 2.45 times more likely to experience a positive result than those given a placebo (Linde, Clausius, & Ramirez et al., 1997). This review of research evaluated various experiments that tested the efficacy of homeopathic remedies in the treatment of hay fever, asthma, migraine headaches, ear infections, upper respiratory infections, rheumatoid arthritis, diarrhea, indigestion, influenza, childbirth, postsurgical complications, varicose veins, sprains and strains, among many others.

In 1991, the *British Medical Journal* published an extensive review article on the efficacy of homeopathy (Kleijnen, Knipschild, & Riet, 1991). The authors pulled from reputable medical journals, scientifically designed clinical studies on homeopathy. In that review, 107 trials were identified and evaluated, rendering a summary conclusion that 77% of the trials showed that homeopathy worked.

The greatest body of clinical research testing homeopathic medicine has concerned conditions in the field of allergy, the vast majority of which has shown highly significant results (Taylor, Riley, Llewellyn-Jones et al., 2000). In their efforts to answer if research in homeopathy is reproducible, a team of physicians and scientists determined that the answer to this question is in the affirmative (Reilly, Taylor, Beattie et al., 1994)

In the treatment of people with influenza, three trials were conducted using a popular homeopathy influenza medicine called "Oscillococcinum." All of these trials were multicentered, placebo controlled, and double blind (Cassanova, 1992; Ferley, 1989; Papp, 1998); two of the three trials were also randomized. Each of these trials was relatively large in the number of subjects (487, 300, and 372), and each of these trials showed statistically significant results.

In addition to double-blind, placebo-controlled research; there is also a body of outcomes research evaluating consecutive cases of patients suffering from specific conditions. One international study involved 30 clinicians in six clinics, in four countries, who enrolled 500 consecutive patients with upper respiration tract complaints, lower respiratory tract complaints, or ear complaints (Singh, Riley, Fischer, & Singh et al., 2001). Of those receiving homeopathic care, 82.6% of patients experienced improvement while only 68% of those receiving a conventional medication experienced a similar degree of improvement. Within 3 days, 67.3% of homeopathic patients experienced improvement, whereas only 56.6% of patients given conventional medicine experienced improvement. Even within 24 hours, 16.4% of homeopathic patients improved compared with 5.7% in the conventional group.

A satisfaction survey designed at the Royal London Homeopathy Hospital was sent out to 541 adult patients who had had at least three clinical visits. In all, 506 of these were completed, of which 499 were suitable for evaluation (Sharples & van Haselen, 1998). Of these patients, 63% had had their main problem for more than 5 years, and as a result of treatment rendered, 80% reported that their main problem had very much, moderately, or slightly improved and 90% were satisfied or very satisfied with their care. Of the 262 patients who had been concomitantly using a conventional drug, 29% had stopped the drug and 84.3% had decreased their usage since receiving homeopathic care.

In addition to the various above-described clinical trials and outcome studies, there are also numerous basic science studies that have been conducted, including one laboratory study that was replicated by four independent groups of researchers. Four groups of researchers and scientists at Queens University of Belfast, the University of Utrecht (Netherlands), University of Florence (Italy), and Catholic University of Louvain (Belgium), conducted the same experiment using various homeopathic potencies of histamine (15C to 19C) (Belon et al., 2004). A total of 2,706 experiments were conducted using "flow cytometry," which is an automated technology that objectively measures histamine release from basophils. The researchers found that these homeopathic doses of histamine had a substantially significant effect on inhibiting the effects of IgE ($p < 0.0001$). References to various other basic science studies have been published elsewhere (Bellavite & Signorini, 2002; Ullman, 2004).

The controlled clinical studies discussed next are worthy of attention to physicians who specialize in pain management.

ARTHRITIS

Two research reviews on arthritis and homeopathy have concluded that there is a body of evidence to suggest that homeopathic medicine, either individually prescribed or used in homeopathic formulae, can provide relief for people with rheumatoid disease (Jonas, Linde, & Ramirez, 2000) or osteoarthritis (Long & Ernst, 2001).

One study addressing patients with rheumatoid arthritis was published in the *British Journal of Clinical Pharmacology* (Gibson, Gibson, MacNeill et al., 1980) and found that 82% of patients prescribed an individually chosen homeopathic medicine experienced some relief of their arthritis pain, while only 21% of patients prescribed a placebo experienced a similar degree of relief. Another study comparing the results of a homeopathic remedy was found to be safer and more effective than the conventional comparison drugs (Shealy, Thomlinson, Cox, & Borgmeyer, 1989).

A newer study that was not a part of the previous reviews compared a homeopathic topical application with a convention nonsteroidal anti-inflammatory drug. This randomized, double-blind trial found that the homeopathic topical gel was as effective as piroxicam gel (van Haselen & Fisher, 2000). This trial evaluated the treatment of 172 osteoarthritis patients over 4 weeks, applying either a homeopathic gel or piroxcam gel three times daily. The homeopathic gel contained Symphytum, Rhus tox, and Ledum.

BACK PAIN

When a patient has back pain, there are simple homeopathic medicines that in clinical experience are worth trying although as in conventional medical trials, the problem with this group of patients is that these individuals have multiple and varied symptoms, and various degrees of trauma, degeneration, and dysfunction. Given these concerns, nonetheless, there is at least one study to support this assertion, which compared a homeopathic topical gel with a conventional pain-relieving gel (Stam, Bonnet, & van Haselen, 2001). This trial compared a homeopathic gel (Spiroflor SRL: containing tinctures of Sympthytum officinale, Rhus tox, and Ledum) with conventional medication: Cremor® Capsica Compositus (CCC). There were 161 subjects in this trial and the findings showed significant pain improvement in both groups and found that the homeopathic gel had fewer adverse events (11% vs. 26%) or adverse drugs reactions (4% vs. 24%).

CARPAL TUNNEL SYNDROME

Eight small carpal bones make up the wrist along with the multiple muscles, tendons, and joints that connect them giving us strength, dexterity, and optimal function. A common idiopathic or overuse syndrome, called carpal tunnel syndrome, was the test group for 37 patients during recovery from their tunnel release surgery. They were treated with either placebo or Arnica 6X in tablet and Arnica ointment (5%). Those patients given this homeopathic medicine had a statistically significant reduction in postoperative pain after 2 weeks when compared with patients given a place ($p < 0.03$; Jeffrey & Belcher, 2002).

EARACHES

Earaches are at present the most common ailment for which American parents take their children to a physician, and there is growing controversy about the effectiveness of antibiotics in the treatment of this common ailment (Cantekin, 1998). Homeopathy provides a safer and often more effective treatment.

A randomized double-blind, placebo-controlled study prescribed individualized homoeopathic medicine or placebo to 75 children (Jacobs, Springer, & Crothers, 2001). There were 19.9% more treatment failures in children given a placebo than those given an individually chosen homeopathic medicine. Diary scores showed a significant decrease in symptoms at 24 and 64 hours after treatment in favor of those given a homeopathic medicine. What was particularly impressive about these results was that improvement from homeopathic medicine occurred within the first day.

Another study providing evidence of rapid resolution of ear infection in children given a homeopathic medicine involved 230 children (Frei & Thurneysen, 2001). These children were given an individually chosen homeopathic medicine. If pain reduction was not sufficient after just 6 hours, another individually chosen homeopathic medicine was prescribed. These researchers found that 39% of patients experienced sufficient pain reduction in the first 6 hours and another 33% after 12 hours. This improvement was 2.4 times faster than in children prescribed a placebo.

FIBROMYALGIA

Researchers in England found that patients with fibromyalgia were a varied group with differing symptoms but that there was one homeopathic medicine, more than any other, that seems to be indicated (Fisher, Greenwood, & Huskisson, 1998). This medicine, Rhus toxicodendron, was found to be indicated in 25% of patients with fibromyalgia. The researchers found 30 patients who seemed to fit the symptoms of Rhus tox, and they were given a homeopathic dose of this medicine in the 6C potency. The researchers found that there was a significant degree of improvement in the reduction of pain and tender points and improved sleep when the subjects were taking the homeopathic medicine, as compared with when the subjects were taking a placebo ($p < 0.005$).

A more recent study appeared in *Rheumatology* (Bell et al., 2004), representing research from the University of Arizona. Collaborating with local homeopathic physicians, 62 patients with fibromyalgia were enrolled using a double-blind, randomized, placebo-controlled study design. Patients received either an oral daily dose of an individually chosen homeopathic medicine in LM potency or a placebo. Patients were evaluated at baseline, 2 months, and 4 months. The study found that patients receiving the homeopathic treatment experienced a 25% or greater improvement in tender point pain on examination, as compared with those who were given a placebo ($P = 0.008$). After 4 months, the homeopathic patients also rated the "helpfulness of the treatment" — connoting positive well-being. Again, the patients who received homeopathy rather than placebo felt that they were helped ($P = 0.004$). Another interesting point in this study was that because this was an individualized treatment protocol, the number of different "placebo remedies" was greater in the placebo group than in the true homeopathic group, likely because positive benefits were not being seen, and the clinicians were changing remedies.

One of the most intriguing aspects of the above study was that the researchers gave the first dose of the homeopathic medicine (or placebo) via olfaction (smelling the liquid dose of the medicine or placebo). Each patient was hooked up to electroencephalography (EEG) monitor at the time of this first dose, and the researchers found a statistically significant difference in the EEG readings of those patients given a homeopathic medicine as distinct from those given a placebo. This objective evidence along with the significant clinical improvement in the homeopathic patients presents a strong case for homeopathy.

HEADACHES

The scientific evidence for the efficacy of homeopathic medicines in the treatment of headaches is mixed. Two studies have shown beneficial results (Brigo, 1987; Straumsheim, Borchgrevink, Mowinckel et al., 2000), but two other studies have shown that homeopathic medicines are no better than placebo (Wallach, Haeusler, Lowers et al., 1997; Whitmarsh, Coleston-Shields, & Steiner, 1997). Noteworthy is that the two studies showing positive results trended toward younger patients and those whose duration of suffering was less than in the studies showing negative results.

Despite these results, it makes sense to try homeopathy due to homeopathic medicine's history of safety.

HEAD INJURY

A randomized and double-blind study of people with mild traumatic head injury showed a statically significant difference in patients given an individualized homeopathic medicine for pain relief as compared with those given a placebo (Chapman, Weintraub, Milburn et al., 1999).

COMMONLY USED HOMEOPATHIC MEDICINES FOR PAINFUL CONDITIONS

Arnica (mountain daisy): This medicine is the most common homeopathic medicine for injuries to soft tissue and pre- and postsurgery (the 1000th potency is preferred); this remedy is also thought to reduce shock of injury or from surgery.

Hypericum (St. John's wort): This remedy is the first medicine to consider for injuries to the nerves or to parts of the body rich with them, including the fingers, toes, back, and eyes. Any injury with shooting pains should be given this remedy.

Belladonna (deadly nightshade): This is for rapid and violent onset of throbbing pain (arthritis, headaches, menstrual) arising with flushed face and/or skin; symptoms are aggravated by tough jarring and especially by motion, and warm wraps relieve them.

Bryonia (wild hop): Headaches or arthritis syndromes that are aggravated by any motion; some relief of pain comes from lying still, heat, direct pressure, and lying on one's painful side.

Ruta grav (rue): Injuries to the elbow or knee; serious injuries to connective tissue, deep achy pain in the joints, especially the back, worse in cold damp weather, worse when lying down, better with movement.

Rhus tox (poison ivy): This medicine is the most common remedy for sprains and strains after the use of Arnica during the first 24 hours. It is especially indicated when a person experiences a "rusty gate" syndrome, that is, pain on initial motion, which is reduced gradually as the patient continues to move. It is also often given to people with the flu, arthritis, or fibromyalgia who experience this similar rusty gate syndrome.

(*Note:* It is the low potencies of these commonly used homeopathic preparations that are commonly prescribed: 3X,12X, 30X, 6C, 12C, 30C.)

HOMEOPATHY (GLOBAL)

Homeopathy is so popular in certain countries that it is no longer appropriate to consider it "alternative medicine" there. Approximately 30 to 40% of French physicians use homeopathic medicine, about 20% of German physicians use these natural medicines, and 45% of Dutch physicians consider them effective (Fisher & Ward, 1994). According to the 1986 survey in the *British Medical Journal*, 42% of British physicians surveyed refer patients to homeopathic physicians (Wharton & Lewis, 1986), and it is now considered to be much higher.

In addition to these impressive statistics, homeopathy is particularly popular in India where there are more than 120 5-year homeopathic medical schools. Homeopathy is also popular in Greece, Pakistan, Brazil, Argentina, Mexico, and South Africa.

SOURCES FOR FURTHER INFORMATION

National Center for Homeopathy
801 N. Fairfax No. 306
Alexandria, VA 22314
http://www.homeopathic.org
(703)548-7790

American Institute of Homeopathy
801 N. Fairfax No. 306
Alexandria, VA 22314
(703)548-7790
http://www.homeopathyusa.org

Homeopathic Educational Services
2124 Kittredge St.
Berkeley, CA 94704
(510)649-0294; fax: (510)649-1955
http://www.homeopathic.com
mail@homeopathic.com
Resource for homeopathic books, tapes, medicines,
software and correspondence courses

HOMEOPATHIC CERTIFICATION AND EDUCATIONAL ORGANIZATIONS

American Board of Homeotherapeutics, 617 W.
Main St. 4th Floor, Charlottesville, VA 22903;
(703)548-7790

Council on Homeopathic Certification, 1199
Sanchez St., San Francisco, CA 94114;
(415)789-7677; www.homeopathy-council.org

Homeopathic Academy of Naturopathic Physicians,
12132 SE Foster Place, Portland, OR 97226;
(503)761-3298; www.healthy.net/hanp

Homeopathic Educational Services, 2124 Kittredge
St., Berkeley, CA 94704; (510)649-0294;
www.homeopathic.com

North American Society of Homeopaths, 1122 Pike
St., Seattle, WA. 98122; (206)720-7000;
www.homeopathy.org

LEADING MANUFACTURERS OF HOMEOPATHIC PREPARATIONS AND EDUCATIONAL MATERIALS

Boiron, 6 Campus Blvd., Newtown Square, PA
19073; (800)264-7661; info@boiron.com

Dolisos Laboratoires, 3014 Rigel Ave., Las Vegas,
NV 89102; (800)365-4767; www.dolisos.fr

Hahnemann Laboratories, 1940 Fourth St., San
Rafael, CA 94910; (888)4-ARNICA;
www.hahnemannlabs.com

Heel BHI, 11600 Cochti Road SE, Albuquerque,
NM 87123-3376; www.info@HeelUSA.com

Homeopathic Educational Services, 2124 Kittredge
St., Berkeley, CA 94704; (510)649-0294, or
Orders: (800)359-9051; www.homeo-
pathic.com

Standard Homeopathic Company, 210 West 131st
St., Box 61067, Los Angeles, CA 90061;
(800)624-9659; www.hylands.com

REFERENCES

Bellavite, P., & Signorini, A. (2002). *The emerging science of homeopathy: Biodynamics, complexity, and nanopharmacology.* Berkeley: North Atlantic.

Bell, I., Lewis D. A., Brooks A. J., Schwartz, G. E., Leis, S. E., Walsh, B. T. et al. (2004). Improved clinical status in fibromyalgia patients treated with individualized homeopathic remedies versus place. *Rheumatology*, 1111–1117.

Belon, P., Cumps, J., Ennis, M., Mannaioni, P. F., Roberfroid, M., Ste-Laudy, J. et a l. (2004). Histamine dilutions modulate basophil activity. *Inflammation Research*, *53*(5), 181 –188.

Brigo, B. (1987) Le traitement homeopatique de la migraine: Une etude de 60 cas, controlle in double-aveugle. *Journal of LMHI*.

Cantekin, E. I. (1998) The changing treatment paradigm for acute otitis media. *Journal of the American Medical Association*, *280*, 1903.

Cassanova, P., & Gerard, R. (1992). Bilan de 3 annees d'estudes randomisees multicentriques oscillococcinum/placebo. In *Oscillococcinum — Ressegna della letterature internationale* (pp. 11–16). Milan: Laboratoires Boiron.

Chapman, E., Weintraub, R., Milburn, M. et al. (1999). Homeopathic treatment of mild traumatic brain injury: A randomized, double-blind, placebo-controlled trial. *Journal of Head Trauma Rehabilitation, 14* (6), 521–542.

Ferley, J. P., Zmirou, D., D'Admehar, D. et al. (1989). A controlled evaluation of a homeopathic preparation in the treatment of influenza-like syndrome. *British Journal of Clinical Pharmacology, 27*, 329–335.

Fisher, P., & Ward, A. (1994). Complimentary medicine in Europe. *British Medical Journal, 309*, 107–110.

Fisher, P., Greenwood, A., Huskisson, E. C. et al. (1998). Effect of homeopathic treatment on fibrositis (primary fibromyalgia). *British Medical Journal, 299*, 365–366.

Frei, H., & Thurneysen, A. (2001). Homeopathy in acute otitis media in children; treatment effect or spontaneous resolution? *British Homeopathic Journal, 90*, 180–182.

Gibson, R. C., Gibson, S., MacNeill, A. D. et al. (1980). Homeopathic therapy in rheumatoid arthritis: Evaluation by double-blind clinical therapeutic trial. *British Journal of Clinical Pharmacology, 9*, 453–459.

Jacobs, J., Springer, D. A., & Crothers, D. (2001). Homeopathic treatment of acute otitis media in children: A preliminary randomized placebo-controlled trial. *Pediatric Infectious Disease Journal, 20*(2), 177–183.

Jeffrey, S., & Belcher, H. (2002). Use of arnica to relieve pain after carpal tunnel release surgery. *Alternative Therapies in Health and Medicine, 8*(2), 66–68.

Jonas, W. B., Linde, K., & Ramirez, G. (2000). Homeopathy and rheumatic disease. *Rheumatic Disease Clinics of North America, 1*, 117–123.

Kleijnen, J., Knipschild, P, & Riet, G. (1991). Clinical trials of homeopathy. *British Medical Journal, 302*, 316–323.

Linde, K., Clausius, N., & Ramirez, G. et al. (1997). Are the clinical effects of homeopathy placebo effects: A meta-analysis of placebo-controlled trial. *Lancet, 250*, 834–843.

Long, L., & Ernst, E. (2001). Homeopathic remedies for the treatment of osteoarthritis: A systematic review. *British Medical Journal, 90,* 37–43.

Papp, R., Schuback, R., Beck, E. et al. (1998). Oscillococcinum in patients with influenza-like syndromes: A placebo controlled double-blind evaluation. *British Homeopathic Journal, 87,* 69–76.

Riley, D., Taylor, M., Beattie, N. et al. (1994). Is evidence for homeopathy reproducible? *Lancet, 344,* 1601–1606.

Sharples, F., & van Haselen, R. (1998). *Patients' perspectives on using a complimentary medicine approach to their health: A survey at the Royal London Homeopathic Hospital NHS Trust.* London: National Health Service Trust.

Shealy, C. N., Thomlinson, R. P., Cox, R. H., & Borgmeyer, V. (1998). Osteoarthritis pain: A comparison of homeopathy and acetaminophen. *American Journal of Pain Management, 8,* 89–91.

Singh, M., Riley, D., Fischer, M., Singh, B. et al. (2001). Homeopathy and conventional medicine: An outcomes study comparing effectiveness in a primary care setting. *Journal of Alternative and Complementary Medicine, 7* (2), 149–160.

Stam, C., Bonnet, M. S, & Van Haselen, R. A. (2001). The efficacy and safety of a homeopathic gel in the treatment of acute low back pain: A multi-centre randomized, double blind comparative clinical trial. *British Homeopathic Journal, 90,* 21–28.

Straumsheim, P., Borchgrevink, C., Mowinckel P. et al. (2000). Homeopathic treatment of migraine: A double-blind, placebo controlled trial of 68 patients. *British Homeopathic Journal, 89,* 4–7.

Suits, A. (1985) *Brass tacks, oral biography of a 20th century physician living history* (Emphasis: History of homeopathy in America). Ann Arbor, MI: Halyburton Press.

Taylor, M. A., Reilly, D., Llewellyn-Jones, R. H. et al. (2000). Randomized controlled trial of homeopathy versus placebo in perennial allergic rhinitis with overview of four trial series. *British Medical Journal, 321,* 471–476.

Ullman, D. (2004). *Homeopathic family medicine* (an e-book, updated regularly). Berkeley: Homeopathic Educational Services. Available from www.homeopathic.com.

van Haselen, R. A., & Fisher, P. A. (2000). A randomized controlled trial comparing topical piroxicam gel with a homeopathic gel in osteoarthritis of the knee. *Rheumatology, 39,* 714–719.

Wallach, H., Haeusler, W., Lowers, T. et al. (1997). Classical homeopathic treatment of chronic headaches. *Cephalalgia, 17,* 119–126.

Wharton, R., & Lewis, G. (1986). Complementary medicine and the general practitioner. *British Medical Journal, 292,* 1498–1500.

Whitmarsh, T. E., Coleston-Shields, D. M., & Steiner, T. J. (1997). Double-blind randomized placebo-controlled study of homeopathic prophylaxis of migraine. *Cephalalgia, 17,* 600–604.

BIBLIOGRAPHY

Boericke, O. (1988). *Pocket manual of the homeopathic Materia Medica* (9th ed.). New Delhi: B. Jain Publishers.

Chappell, P. (2003). *Emotional healing with homeopathy: Treating the effects of trauma.* Berkeley: North Atlantic.

Dean, M. E. (2004). *The trials of homeopathy.* Essen, Germany: KVC Verlag.

Hahnemann, S. (1904). *The chronic diseases, Their peculiar nature and their homeopathic cure.* Philadelphia: Boericke & Tafel.

Hahnemann, S. (1982). *The organon of medicine. The first integral English translation of the definitive sixth edition of the original work on homeopathic medicine.* J. Kuknzli, A. Naude, & P. Pendleton (Eds.). Los Angeles: J. P. Tarcher. (Translation copyright 1982, The Hahnemann Foundation.)

Hahnemann, S. (1996). *The organon of medical art.* (W. Brewster O'Reilly, Trans.). Palo Alto: Birdcage.

Hershoff, D. C. (2003). *Homeopathic medicine for musculoskeletal healing.* Berkeley: North Atlantic.

Jonas, W. B., & Jacobs, J. (1996). *Healing with homeopathy.* New York: Warner Books.

Jouanny, J. (1985). *The essential of homeopathic therapeutics.* (D. Calusen, Trans.). Milan: Laboratoires Boiron.

Kent, J. T. (1988). *Repertory of the homoeopathic Materia Medica* (6th American ed.). New Delhi: B. Jain Publishers.

Kent, J. T. (1990). *Lectures on homeopathic philosophy.* Berkeley: North Atlantic.

Resch, U., & Gutmann, V. (1987). *Scientific foundations of homeopathy. Wissenschaftliche Grundlagen der Homeopathic.* St. Ottilien, Germany: Barthel & Bartel.

Rowe, T. (1998). *Homeopathy methodology.* Berkeley: North Atlantic.

Subotnick, S. (1991). *Sports and exercise injuries: Conventional, homeopathic, and alternative treatments.* Berkeley: North Atlantic.

Ullman, D. (1991). *Discovering homeopathy; Medicine for the 21st century.* Berkeley: North Atlantic.

Ullman, D. (2002). *Essential homeopathy.* Novato, CA: New World Library.

Ullman, D. (2004). *Homeopathic family medicine* (an e-book, updated regularly). Berkeley: Homeopathic Educational Services. Available from www.homeopathic.com.

Vithoulkas, G. (1980). *The science of homeopathy.* New York: Grove Press.

79

Clinical Applications of Massage Therapy in Pain Management

Joe Durant, NCTMB

INTRODUCTION

From acupressure, neuromuscular therapy, and Swedish massage to Trager approach and Hellerwork, there are numerous forms and names of touch therapy on the market. Each incorporates its own special twist, technique, or theory and has its own following of practitioners who find that therapy to be most effective for specific disorders. From a practical standpoint all bodywork systems incorporate various techniques of massage in one form or another, and as such, massage represents one of the oldest known and most easily applied forms of healing. Utilization of massage ranges from massage therapists to nurses, physical therapists, and physicians and is one of the few therapies that can, in many cases, be safely and easily applied by a patient or family member.

The mechanisms of and research into the effects of massage fall into one or both of two categories: direct mechanical effects or reflexive effects.

DIRECT MECHANICAL EFFECTS

These include local effects in the area of massage such as the inactivation of a myofascial trigger point, increased local circulation, or increased range of motion.

Myofascial Trigger Points

Point-specific massage techniques can effectively eliminate the referred pain and local tenderness associated with myofascial trigger points (Hanten et al., 2000). This point

lends tremendous support to the use of massage for chronic musculoskeletal pain.

Soft Tissue Healing

Massage that uses heavy pressure promotes the healing process in tendonitis in part by increasing the number of fibroblasts in the area of treatment (Davidson et al., 1997; Gehlsen, Ganion, & Helfst, 1999), suggesting that the healing effects of massage come in part from the controlled application of microtrauma.

Range of Motion

Massage can have significant effects on range of motion in areas such as the lower extremity (Wiktorsson-Moller et al., 1983) and low back (Hernandez-Reif et al., 2001) as well as more specific single joint areas such as the shoulder (Watson, Dalziel, & Story, 2000). The conclusion is that massage either manually stretches muscle tissue or stimulates stretch receptors, which allows muscles to stretch once motion is applied.

Muscle Soreness

Delayed-onset muscle soreness from maximal muscle contractions can be significantly reduced by the application of one massage treatment (Hilbert, Sfornzo, & Swenson, 2003). Soreness resulting from constant spasm can be reduced by the application of massage as well as overall muscle tension (Naliboff & Tachiki, 1991).

H-Reflex

Massage has an inhibitory effect on the H-reflex in muscles that appear to originate from stimulation of deep (not cutaneous) mechanicoreceptors (Morelli, Chapman, & Sullivan, 1999).

Muscle Performance

Massage applied to fatigued muscle can increase their follow-up performance when compared with muscles that have only been allowed to rest — suggesting a strong influence on local circulation (Rinder & Sutherland, 1995).

REFLEXIVE EFFECTS

These include effects removed from the site of massage, such as increased blood flow to the intestines by massaging the feet, or systemic effects, such as decreased blood pressure and anxiety (Moyer, Rounds, & Hannum, 2004) and even improved immune system functioning (Diego et al., 2001).

Pain Relief

Repeated massage treatments bring about antinociceptive effects that can be reversed by an oxytocin agonist, suggesting that the long-term antinociceptive effects of massage are at least partly tied to the oxytocinergic system (Lund et al., 2002). Massage increases levels of beta endorphins, strengthening the position that massage can affect pain through the opiate receptor system within the body (Kaada & Torsteinbo, 1989). Further evidence supporting this theory is that acupoint stimulation can potentiate the effects of morphine (Yuan et al., 2002). Multiple massage applications can reduce level of depression and the delayed assessment of pain, suggestive again of effects on the endogenous opiate system (Lund et al., 2002).

Pressure

The effects of massage can depend on the amount and type of pressure. Moderate, light, and vibratory massage all reduce anxiety. But while light and vibratory massage can increase heart rate and overall arousal measures (via electroencephalography), moderate pressure massage decreases heart rate and arousal (Diego et al., 2004), and deep massage can increase heart rate temporarily (Delaney et al., 2002).

Sympathetic Arousal

A single application of general massage and acupoint stimulation can reduce blood pressure, heart rate, and anxiety state (Kober et al., 2003; McNamara et al, 2003; Moyer et al., 2004) — a definite reflexive effect applicable to sympathetic arousal from pain.

Edema

Persistent edema can be reduced through massage (Howard & Krishnagiri, 2001). The inference here is that fluid circulation through the body can be strongly influenced by massage.

Nausea

Massage of specific acupuncture points or reflexology zones can be targeted to influence very specific goals, such as the reduction of nausea (Roscoe et al., 2003), which supports the position that a trained massage practitioner can reflexively influence but also physiological functions.

Immune System

Immune system functioning can be improved by massage (Diego et al., 2001; Ironson et al., 1996), lending support to the use of massage during cancer and HIV/AIDS for more than palliative applications.

Constipation

Massage can be used to treat chronic constipation (Bishop et al., 2003; Ernst, 1999), which is very significant for patients who have become constipated via the use of opiates to control their pain.

Although most types of massage focus more on one of the two effects, one would be hard pressed to argue that most therapies do not incorporate elements of both direct mechanical and reflexive effects. Even therapies such as acupressure will have a mechanical effect on the tissue at the point of pressure application, not forgetting that acupuncture points and myofascial trigger points have at least an 80% correlation rate (Travell & Simons, 1983). Although many effects of massage have been uncovered, the explanation of why properly applied massage triggers these effects is still an elusive one research is just beginning to uncover.

MYOFASCIAL PAIN

Few other works have influenced the clinical practice of massage therapy as strongly as the two-volume set, *Myofascial Pain and Dysfunction: The Trigger Point Manual*, by Drs. Janet Travell and David Simons. With in-depth descriptions of trigger point location, patterns of referred pain, and techniques and stretches for treating muscles, the volumes are an essential reference for anyone who is serious about treating chronic muscular pain. A brief review of the volumes clearly suggests almost all types of pain are reflected in one way or another in the muscular system, even if the source of the pain lies elsewhere such as in a diseased organ.

A myofascial trigger point is defined by Travell and Simons as: "A hyperirritable spot, usually within a taut band of skeletal muscle or within the muscle's fascia that is painful on compression and that can give rise to characteristic referred pain, tenderness and autonomic phenomena" (Travell & Simons, 1983). Research has shown that between 45 and 54% of healthy, asymptomatic young adults were found to have latent trigger points in the shoulder girdle musculature (Sola, Rodenberger, & Gettys, 1955). Given the frequency with which trigger points occur, one certainly cannot deny the often significant role they can play in the pain cycle if they become active via chronic strain or a traumatic event. Currently, there are four hypotheses that attempt to explain findings at trigger points (Rivner, 2001):

1. Trigger points are found at the muscle spindle.
2. Trigger points represent hyperactive end-plate regions.
3. Trigger points are representations of focal dystonia.
4. Trigger points do not exist.

For the purpose of pain management, it is enough to recognize that myofascial trigger points do exist, that they can create extremely painful conditions for patients, and that they can be treated via manual pressure or massage (Hanten et al., 2000; Hou et al., 2002).

To illustrate the severity of the pain that can be perpetuated by trigger points, consider a case with which the author was recently presented. A female in her mid-30s was diagnosed with a herniated disc at C5–6 (confirmed via magnetic resonance imaging, MRI) and posterior cervical pain on the left as well as pain down the left arm into the fingers. She failed conservative treatment including physical therapy, cervical traction, pharmacological interventions (including oral steroids and muscle relaxants), and bed rest. The patient underwent surgery having an anterior cervical fusion with plating at C5–6. Several weeks after surgery, the patient presented in a complete panic with symptoms that had recently manifested during the recovery phase as being virtually identical to the initial pain she had prior to surgery. She was convinced that either surgery had failed or that she had somehow done something to compromise the surgery. An examination revealed the presence of several myofascial trigger points in the left scalenes that when palpated, duplicated her neck pain and referred pain down her arm to her hand and fingers. A course of neuromuscular massage, electrotherapeutic point stimulation (ETPS^{SM}) by the author and trigger point injections by the neurosurgeon were successful in eliminating the trigger points and thereby the pain. Despite elimination of the offending pressure on the nerve root, the myofascial component of the pain perpetuated itself until it was addressed with physical input to break the cycle. It has been suggested that many cases of "failed back" after surgery can be traced to the presence of untreated trigger points (Travell & Simons, 1983).

Simons and Mense (2003) note that myofascial trigger points typically either follow acute muscle overload (such as a car accident) or develop gradually over time with repetitive or prolonged muscle contractions. It has been demonstrated that trained clinicians can reliably determine the precise location of trigger points within muscles (Sciotti et al., 2001). Clinical trials have also demonstrated that "ischemic compression" can effectively eliminate myofascial trigger points and the referred pain that accompanies them (Hanten et al., 2000; Hou et al., 2002). It is a reasonable assumption that massage therapy is a viable option to incorporate into the treatment of chronic musculoskeletal pain. Massage has been shown to be an effective treatment for muscular shoulder pain (van der Dolder & Roberts, 2003) and should therefore be applicable to other muscular problems that cause pain.

Fibromyalgia is certainly a disease that often includes myofascial. When treating fibromyalgia, the previously noted effects of deep massage on increasing heart rate and other autonomic functions should be taken into consideration as fibromyalgia does, from an observational point of view, appear to be a disorder of sympathetic upregulation.

STRUCTURAL CONSIDERATIONS

There are many schools of massage such as Rolfing, Alexander technique, and neuromuscular therapy that promote the idea that simply eliminating myofascial trigger points is not enough. Postural distortions from adaptive muscle shortening (from dysfunctional biomechanics) that chronically strain the antagonist muscles must be addressed if one is to eliminate the source of the trigger points. Trigger points are considered more of a diagnostic indication of a problem rather than the primary source of the problem. Consider the following simplified example as an illustration of how including structural theories will affect treatment.

A patient presents with chronic posterior shoulder and mid thoracic pain between the medial border of scapula and the spine. Upon examination, palpation reveals the presence of trigger points in the right rhomboids that, when pressed, replicate the pain pattern the patient has been experiencing. Visual exam reveals that the right shoulder is protracted and the right scapula winged out slightly when compared with the left. When supine, the patient's right shoulder is elevated off the exam table but the left is flat. In explaining his case history, the patient notes that there has never been any major trauma to the right shoulder. The patient also reveals that he works with computers for long hours every day and that his right arm is always reaching forward for hours at a time while he uses the mouse.

In this case, massage used to eliminate the myofascial trigger points in the right rhomboids will most likely result in only temporary relief of the pain. The protracted shoulder, slight winging of the scapula, and failure of the right shoulder to lie flat on the table while the patient is supine are all indications of a shortened pectoralis minor muscle (Kendall, McCreary, & Provance, 1983). In this case, the shortened pectoralis muscle puts chronic strain on its antagonist, the rhomboids, which then develop trigger points and cause pain. From a structural standpoint, massage techniques will be used to eliminate the trigger point in the rhomboids. Massage techniques will also be used to lengthen the chronically shortened pectoralis minor muscle and overlying fascia. (There are entire systems that have been developed to specifically address the fascia such as the myofascial release methods taught by John Barnes, physical therapist.) Even addressing the shortened pectoralis will not be enough to keep the pain from recurring. The patient must reorganize his workstation so that using the computer mouse does not entail reaching forward in such a way that the pectoralis minor is allowed to adaptively shorten again. Stretches should also be performed periodically that promote retraction of the shoulders.

The above example is highly simplified for the purpose of clear illustration, and it must be noted that real cases are typically much more complex. The recognition and treatment of postural distortions caused by adaptive shortening in muscle from dysfunctional biomechanics is a key concept for anyone attempting to use massage therapy in the treatment of chronic musculoskeletal pain. Without this key recognition, the patient can become locked into a revolving-door type of dependency on the practitioner simply for the short-term relief of trigger point–related pain, which, as noted, can be merely a symptom of the problem. In these situations patients may give up because of the cumulative cost and frequency of massage treatment, and may say that they tried massage but "it just didn't work." The failure is not with the massage, but its improper application.

So important is the role of recognizing and treating postural distortions that some systems of structurally based massage such as Rolfing insist on a set series of treatments to align the body structurally before they will provide localized treatment of pain.

Even integrative treatments such as ETPS incorporate treatment of core postural muscles such as the iliopsoas group and piriformis/lateral hip rotators (Weiner, 2002). Hocking suggests that chronic contraction of core postural muscles imbalance the hips and sacrum. This imbalance will cause upregulation of the autonomic nervous system via uneven muscular tension levels along the spine and pressure on nerve roots and elevate acetylcholine levels along dermatomes. Muscles then can become depolarized and the chronic pain cycle maintained.

As Sigmund Freud is rumored to have said, "Sometimes a cigar is just a cigar" — with the implication that it is rarely ever the case. Sometimes local massage will completely eliminate muscular pain, but in cases of long-term chronic pain, it is strongly suggested that some type of postural distortion is at work to perpetuate the condition. Entire sections of physical therapy reference books, such as in *Muscles Testing and Function* (Kendall et al., 1983), are often devoted to the role of posture and pain, and make an excellent addition to the library of the practitioner.

SPECIFIC PAIN DISORDERS

BACK PAIN

If one reviews the database of the National Library of Medicine, it quickly becomes clear that back pain has been one of the most thoroughly researched areas in the efficacy of massage. "Back pain" is a very broad term covering conditions ranging from trigger points to the effects of disk herniation. However broad the term may be, there is very good evidence supporting the use of massage for treating back pain. Massage has been found to be both safe and cost-effective in treating back pain (Cherkin et al., 2003). A literature review found massage to be an effective treatment for low back pain (Furlan, 2002), and it is at least as effective as acupuncture (Cherkin et al., 2001; Hurley, 2001). Techniques range from cryomassage (Gusarova, 2000) to standard massage (Cherkin et al., 2001; Predye, 2000), and can be effective in treating back pain. Neck pain and massage does not appear to have been researched as well but treatment is along the same lines and has been shown effective (Luo & Luo, 1997).

Theoretically, back pain can be treated on a number of different levels with massage. General massage techniques and reflexology can be used to bring about reflexive changes in the body's response to pain. Using massage to eliminate myofascial trigger points is another avenue of treatment that would certainly be worth pursuing. A structural approach is also strongly recommended. Consider the potential benefits of releasing muscles around a bulging disc — muscle contractions create pressure, and by releasing the pressure, one could potentially influence the amount of disc bulge. Also from a structural standpoint, consider the patient who has habitually stood on the right leg to protect an old ankle injury in the left foot. The right quadratus lumborum could shorten, pulling the pelvis into an abnormal position. With the pelvis in an abnormal position muscle tension in the paraspinal muscles would be unequal from left to right as the body compensated to maintain a straight posture. The chronic strain on one side of the paraspinals could certainly lead to the formation of trigger points, which in turn create pain. Neck pain could even originate from a low back postural distortion. As was noted earlier, massage can affect muscle length and tension so it would certainly be logical to attempt to correct the postural distortion by treating the shortened muscles. The topic of neck pain treated specifically by massage does not appear as frequently in research as back pain. As the neck is simply an extension of the spine and its musculature, it would be reasonable to apply the same supporting research to massage in the treatment of neck pain.

HEADACHES

Migraine headaches are estimated to affect 27.3 million people annually and tension-type headaches even more (Landy, 2004). While massage therapy is not generally the first route most people take to alleviate their pain, there is strong evidence suggesting that massage can be effective in treating both conditions. There is an inherent problem in that most people normally cannot take time for massage when a headache occurs, and it may be dangerous to attempt driving while in the throes of a severe migraine or tension headache. The strength of massage therapy in the treatment of headaches lies in preventing them and reducing the intensity of future headaches.

The exact mechanism by which massage is helpful for headaches is uncertain. The effectiveness of massage for headaches cannot be predicted by psychological testing (Wylie, Jackson, & Crawford, 1997), suggesting that the effects of massage go beyond some imagined process in the minds of easily influenced patients.

As studies have confirmed the effectiveness of both reflexology and Swedish-type massage for both tension and migraine headaches (Hodges, 1990; Launso, Brendstrup & Arnberg, 1999; Lemstra, Stewart, & Olszynski, 2002; Lipton, 1986; Puustjarvi, Airaksinin, & Pontinen, 1990; Quinn, Chandler, & Moraska, 2002), one may infer that an overall reduction in stress via massage may play a significant role. Certainly, properly applied local techniques such as myotherapy and neuromuscular therapy for inactivating myofascial trigger points that are known to refer pain into the head (Travell & Simons, 1983) may also be a factor. Long-term effects on migraine headaches have been achieved, with studies indicating that 81% of patients treated were still receiving benefit 3 months posttreatment (Launso et al., 1999). Again, the practitioner is urged to look for postural distortions that may be perpetuating trigger points around the head and neck.

PREGNANCY

Pregnancy is a time when many medications for painful conditions such as migraine headaches or even general pain disorders may very well be contraindicated. As has been previously discussed, massage is an effective tool for the management of migraine headaches as well as musculoskeletal pain. Certainly massage should not be the only intervention in the absence of pain medication; all

appropriate modalities should be integrated, but massage is an obvious choice.

Although many antidepressants are characterized as safe during pregnancy, the author has seen in his clinical practice many women who choose to stop taking these medications while pregnant. As previously mentioned, massage has shown to be effective in lowering anxiety and improving overall quality of life. Pregnancy is a time when massage can certainly be employed to offset the effects of not taking medication that controls anxiety contributing to depression. A simple 20-minute massage applied twice per week has been shown to decrease leg and back pain, increase sleep, and decrease anxiety and urinary stress hormone (norepinepherine) (Field et al., 1999). As a further benefit, the same study subjects had fewer complications during labor, and their infants had fewer postnatal complications.

During labor therapeutic and acupressure related massage has been shown effective in reducing pain and anxiety. Manual stimulation of the acupoints Large Intestine (LI) 4 and Bladder (B) 67 have been shown to reduce pain during the first stage of labor (Chung et al., 2003). Ice massage of LI4 was shown by Waters (1995) to reduce labor pain and by Melzack to reduce back pain and was a key study in the development of the gate control theory of pain (Melzack & Wall, 1965). LI4 is located in the web of the thumb approximately one third of the distance distally from the junction of the metacarpal — it should be quite tender to a pincer grip between the thumb and forefinger (Hocking, 1999). B67 is located at the lateral edge of the base of the nail of smallest toe — if a straight line were drawn across the proximal base of the nail and down the lateral border of the nail, the meeting point is B67 (quite tender to palpation with the tip of a ballpoint pen) (Hocking, 1999). Therapeutic massage applied during labor has also been shown to reduce pain during the latent (3 to 4 cm dilation), active (5 to 7 cm), and transitional phases (8 to 10 cm) (Chang, Wang, & Chen, 2002).

It must be strongly suggested that massage during pregnancy be applied by or monitored by a trained massage practitioner as well as the attending physician. Strong evidence to support this recommendation comes from cases of cranial hemorrhages occurring in Pacific Islander infants in Auckland, New Zealand. Infants of Pacific Islanders were found to have a 60% greater chance of being stillborn than European or Maori infants (Becroft & Gunn, 1989). Traditional massage practices were thought to be at the heart of the problem and warnings about traditional massage at antenatal clinics resulted in a significant decrease in still births progressively over several years. Contraindications for massage, such as deep vein thrombosis and preclampsia, should be closely screened for prior to initiating any massage during pregnancy (Waters, 1995). Although there are no studies to support negative effects of manually stimulating acupoints during pregnancy, thousands of years of experience should be heeded. The following acupoints should be avoided during pregnancy massage (Waters, 1995):

- Spleen (SP) 6: Located four fingers above the apex of the medial malleolus and hooked slightly behind the fibula (Hocking, 1999)
- Stomach (ST) 36: Located (with the knee flexed at 90°) four fingers below the patella halfway between the peak of the tibia and the head of the fibula (Hocking, 1999)
- LI4: Located in the fleshy web between the thumb and forefinger (Hocking, 1999) mentioned above as helpful for labor pain, but should be avoided during earlier stages of pregnancy

CANCER

Cancer is a disease in which there are multiple roles for the application of massage. Not only can there be a great deal of pain associated with the disease itself, but the treatments can have a multitude of side effects including pain and nausea. In addition to pain, there can be an understandable level of anxiety as patients are attempting to have quality of life and organize their affairs in order in the face of a potentially lethal disease. Massage can be utilized as a tool to improve the above-mentioned aspects and may even improve immune functioning.

The benefits of massage in cancer are clearly mostly of a reflexive nature and reflect effects that are generalized throughout the body. Therapeutic massage and reflexology have both been found effective in improving the pain experience of patients with cancer (Ferrell-Torry & Glick, 1993; Post-White et al., 2003; Smith et al., 2002; Stephenson, Dalton, & Carlson, 2003; Walach, Guthlin, & Konig, 2003). It must be pointed out that cancer is one of the few situations that incorporate elements of nociceptive, inflammatory, and neuropathic pain and as such the pain-relieving benefits of massage can be short lived, sometimes not lasting 3 hours (Stephenson et al., 2003). The possible short-term duration of pain control may be attributed to the fact that there is constantly new damage being done by the disease. Despite the shortcomings, massage can still be effectively used as a nursing intervention and function in much the same way that breakthrough medication is used when pain peaks.

Because massage does increase plasma levels of beta-endorphins (Kaada & Torsteinbo, 1989), it could conceivably potentiate the effects of opiates given for pain control. From a speculative basis one might infer that pain resulting from visceral–somatic referrals (Travell & Simons, 1983) from pancreatic and other organ cancer might be reduced by the application of massage to soft tissue in the area of referred pain. The author can vouch for this theory

based on personal experience with patients suffering with organ cancer.

Overall quality of life can be significantly affected by proper application of massage. In a study involving more than 200 subjects, massage along with healing touch were found to decrease the intake of nonsteroidal anti-inflammatory drugs over a 4-week period as well as to decrease mood disturbances and fatigue in patients receiving chemotherapy (Post-White et al., 2003). In the same study, blood pressure, heart rate, respiratory rate, and anxiety were all significantly reduced as a result of massage therapy. Simply put, the less anxiety, the better the quality of life that someone may have left.

During cancer treatment chemotherapy is an often used modality, and the nausea that has been known to accompany it can significantly affect the quality of life of the patients who may have only limited time. It has been demonstrated that something as simple as a 10-minute foot massage (Grealish, Lomasney, & Whiteman, 2000) or finger pressure over two pairs of acupoints (Dibble et al., 2000) can influence both the frequency and the intensity of nausea. These simple techniques can easily be taught to spouses or family members of patients with cancer and most certainly can be learned by nursing staff in medical facilities that treat cancer.

The role of massage in cancer care can be a controversial one, as cancer is often noted as a contraindication for any type of massage that may affect circulation (Werner, 1998). Because massage can be very effective in facilitating the movement of lymph through the body, conceivably cancer cells could be moved through the lymph nodes by improper application of massage (Cheville, et al., 2003; Howard & Krishnagiri, 2001; Williams et al., 2002). Certainly in cases where there are conditions such as neutropenia and thrombocytopenia the intervention of a trained massage practitioner under the care of the treating physician would be advisable if massage was being considered (Werner, 1998). The risk of possibly worsening the plight of the patient with cancer must be balanced with the known benefits of massage especially when one considers that the number of natural killer cells in the immune system can be increased as well as the ratio CD4/CD8 lymphocytes (Diego et al., 2001; Ironson et al., 1996; Iwama & Akama, 2002). Strengthening the immune system can be accomplished simply by administering daily dry towel rubdowns for 10 minutes (Iwama & Akama, 2002) or with general massage therapy (Diego et al., 2001).

In an investigation into the habits of insured cancer patients (Lafferty et al., 2004), it was found that 11.6% of enrollees filed claims for some type of complementary or alternative medical (CAM) intervention. It was noted that CAMs are in no way replacing conventional providers but that many insured cancer patients will use CAMs in addition to conventional cancer treatments. The benefits of massage in cancer are demonstrated in a number of different areas, and this is clearly a disorder where the integration of touch therapy can make a tremendous contribution to the overall care of the patients. HIV/AIDS has not been well researched in terms of massage therapy but the immune system effects as well as the reflexive reduction of pain and anxiety are equally applicable and should be considered as part of the care regimen.

LYMPHEDEMA

Lymphedema can come as a result of mastectomies or a variety of circulatory disorders. Regardless of how it appears, it can extremely painful as fluid pressure builds up in the limb tissue and stretches the skin far beyond its normal range. The author has seen simple cases of edema from a knee injury put so much pressure on the nerves that patients lose feeling in their feet. Consider the long-term effects of chronic edema on nerve function, proper oxygenation, and infection. Fortunately, massage techniques for lymphedema are effective measures in reducing swelling (Cheville et al., 2003; Howard & Krishnagiri, 2001; Williams et al., 2002). The techniques promote the movement of lymph out of the limb, and once this is done, compression garments can be used to prevent a recurrence.

RESPIRATORY CIRCUMSTANCES

There are a number of circumstances that while not strictly pain conditions, warrant mention for treatment via clinical massage as they involve elements that can and often do cause pain. The chronic strain placed on the respiratory musculature of patients with COLD (chronic obstructive lung disease) certainly qualifies as an area where pain can strike. The author has treated many patients with extremely tender intercostal muscles, scalenes, and upper trapezius muscles who have reduced diaphragm capability and are overusing accessory muscles of respiration. Most specifically, breathing disorders such as asthma and COLD have shown positive responses to massage techniques. The chief benefit of these techniques is that when therapeutic doses of medication are either contraindicated or already at maximum dosage, additional benefit and possible medication reduction can be achieved. Because corticosteroids are known to decrease muscle function, it can be self-defeating to increase the medication of a patient who is already suffering from breathing problems. Indeed, there is significant evidence that reflexively applied therapy such as acupressure can significantly improve dyspnea experienced by patients with chronic obstructive pulmonary disease (COPD) (Wu et al., 2004).

The practice of treating the diaphragm via direct pressure from under the ribcage has long been taught in neuromuscular therapy courses but has been little researched. The underlying theory of neuromuscular massage is that

it is possible to release spastic and chronically shortened muscles via manual therapy. It has been shown via MRI that the diaphragm does flatten in patients with COPD, ostensibly because the muscle has shortened over time. Neuromuscular massage was found to be effective in treating moderate COLD (including panlobular emphysema, centrilobular emphysema, chronic bronchitis, and interstitial lung disease, Beeken et al., 1998). Part of the therapy involves manual pressure on the diaphragm in an effort to promote stretch in the muscle. Significant changes in breath holding (as much as 100%), peak flow, heart rate, and oxygen saturation were demonstrated after neuromuscular therapy. As COLD affects an estimated 30 million people in the United States alone, further research into this field is certainly warranted (Petty, 1990).

Asthma is another arena in which clinical massage warrants a close look. One would be hard pressed to argue with the avoidance of corticosteroid use when possible — especially in children whose bodies are still developing. Successful research in treating asthma via manual techniques is noted by Kuznetsov as early as 1980 (Kuznetsov et al., 1980). A study comparing the benefits of massage versus progressive muscle relaxation in children with asthma (Field et al., 1998) showed significant improvements in not only anxiety, but forced vital capacity (24% increase), forced expiration volume (57% increase), and peak expiratory flow rate (30%). One of the most impressive points about this study was that massage was not rendered by therapists, but by the parents of the children involved in the study, and the treatment itself took only 20 minutes per day. It is in giving patients and their families an active role in treating a given disorder that integrative techniques provide one of their most important functions. Acupressure as well has been shown to be an effective tool in overall quality of life for patients with asthma (Maa et al., 2003). In the treatment of asthma, massage does not have noticeable effects in only one treatment (Robertson et al., 1984).

INTEGRATIVE HEALTH CARE

As effective as massage therapy can be when applied clinically in pain management, it cannot be stressed enough that it should be an integrated part of the continuum of care, not an isolated therapy. Chronic pain is very often a complicated process that may involve not only the area of pain, but postural distortions or biomechanics that perpetuate the pain as well as psychological factors such as depression that may impede a patient's ability to actively participate in elements of treatment such as home stretching or exercise.

Throughout the literature, one will encounter studies that demonstrate the effectiveness of multidisciplinary interventions to treat various disorders such as migraines (Lemstra et al., 2002) and back pain (Cottingham & Maitland, 1997). The future of pain management lies in the successful integration of standard medical care and complementary therapies. If simple massage could heal all chronic pain, then everyone with chronic pain would be lined up for massage — but no one therapy or technique stands on its own as the answer to chronic pain. There are many hybrid therapies being developed today that incorporate elements of several systems. A good example of this is ETPS[SM], which incorporates elements of acupuncture, electrotherapy, myofascial release, and structural theory, and achieves impressive results when combined with standard physical therapy such as doubling outcomes (Freed, 2002). There is no room for isolationists or purists in the treatment of pain. A willingness to work cooperatively with other doctors and therapists and to integrate techniques is essential if patients with pain are to benefit. One might look to the example of successful integration of "cutaneous stimulation" (massage) into the emergency room and the positive effects on pain reduction (Kubsch, Neveau, & Vandertie, 2001).

Considering that the practice of massage in one form or another stretches back to our earliest recorded history, it is surprising how little research has actually been done in the field. That trend does appear to be changing as studies on the effects of massage appear in the literature more regularly. There is a definite need for more research into specific techniques of massage, and those who utilize massage are strongly urged to become more involved in the research process.

REFERENCES

Becroft, D. M. & Gunn, T. R. (1989). Prenatal cranial haemorrhages in 47 Pacific Islander infants: Is traditional massage the cause? *New Zealand Medical Journal, 102,* 207.

Beeken, J. E. et al. (1998). The effectiveness of neuromuscular release massage therapy in five individuals with chronic obstructive lung disease. *Clinical Nursing Research, 7,* 309.

Bishop, E. et al. (2003). Reflexology in the management of encopresis and chronic constipation. *Paediatric Nursing, 15,* 20.

Chang, M. Y., Wang, S. Y., & Chen, C. H. (2002). Effects of massage in pain and anxiety during labour: A randomized controlled trial in Taiwan. *Journal of Advanced Nursing, 38,* 68.

Cherkin, D. C. et al. (2001). Randomized trial comparing traditional Chinese medical acupuncture, therapeutic massage, and self-care education for chronic low back pain. *Archives of Internal Medicine, 161,* 1081.

Cherkin, D. C. et al. (2003). A review of evidence for the effectiveness, safety, and cost of acupuncture, massage therapy, and spinal manipulation for back pain. *Annals of Internal Medicine, 138,* 898.

Cheville, A. L. et al. (2003). Lymphedema management. *Seminars in Radiation Oncology, 13,* 290.

Chung, U. L. et al. (2003). Effects of LI 4 ad BL 67 acupressure on labor pain and uterine contractions in the first stage of labor. *Journal of Nursing Research, 11,* 251.

Cottingham, J. T., & Maitland, J. (1997). A three paradigm treatment model using soft tissue mobilization and guided movement-awareness techniques for a patient with chronic low back pain: A case study. *Journal of Orthopedic and Sports Physical Therapy, 26,* 155.

Davidson, C. J. et al. (1997). Rat tendon morphologic and functional changes resulting from soft tissue mobilization. *Medicine and Science in Sports and Exercise, 29,* 313.

Delany, J. P. et al. (2002). The short-term effects of myofascial trigger point massage therapy on cardiac autonomic tone in healthy subjects. *Journal of Advanced Nursing, 37,* 364.

Dibble, S. L. et al. (2000). Acupressure for nausea: results of a pilot study. *Oncology Nursing Forum, 27,* 41.

Diego, M. A. et al. (2004). Massage therapy of moderate and light pressure and vibrator effects on EEG and heart rate. *International Journal of Neuroscience, 114,* 31.

Diego, M. A. et al. (2001). HIV adolescents show improved immune function following massage therapy. *International Journal of Neuroscience, 106,* 35.

Ernst, E. (1999). Abdominal massage therapy for chronic constipation: A systematic review of controlled clinical trials. *Forschritte Komplementarmed, 6,* 149.

Ferrell-Torry, A. T., & Glick, O. J. (1993). The use of therapeutic massage as a nursing intervention to modify anxiety and the perception of cancer pain. *Cancer Nursing, 16,* 93.

Field, T. et al. (1998). Children with asthma have improved pulmonary functions after massage therapy. *Journal of Pediatrics, 132,* 854.

Field, T. et al. (1999). Pregnant women benefit from massage therapy. *Journal of Psychosomatic Obstetrics and Gynaecology, 20,* 31.

Freed, M. (2002). ETPS stimulation combined with physical therapy improves outcomes, (internal comparative study). *Rehab Report, 2,* 2.

Furlan, A. D. (2002). Massage for low back pain. *Cochrane Database System Review, 2,* CD001929.

Gehlsen, G. M., Ganion, L. R., & Helfst, R. (1999). Fibroblast response to variation in soft tissue mobilization pressure. *Medicine and Science in Sports and Exercise, 31,* 531.

Grealish, L., Lomasney, A., & Whiteman, B. (2000). Foot massage. A nursing intervention to modify the distressing symptoms of pain and nausea in patients hospitalized with cancer. *Cancer Nursing, 23,* 237.

Gusarova, S. A. (2000). The methodological aspects of using cryomassage on patients operated on for discogenic neuropathies. *Voprosy Kurortologii Fizioterapi, i Lechenbroi Fizicheskoi Kultury, 4,* 20.

Hanten, W. P. et al. (2000). Effectiveness of a home program of ischemic pressure followed by sustained stretch for treatment of myofascial trigger points. *Physical Therapy, 80,* 997.

Hernandez-Reif, M. et al. (2001). Lower back pain is reduced and range of motion increased after massage therapy. *International Journal of Neuroscience, 106,* 131.

Hilbert, J. E., Sfornzo, G. A., & Swenson, T. (2003). The effects of massage on delayed onset muscle soreness. *British Journal of Sports Medicine, 37,* 72.

Hocking, B. (1999). *ETPS Neuromechanical Pain Management.* Ontario: Acumed Publishing.

Hodges, J. M. (1990). Managing temporomandibular joint syndrome. *Laryngoscope, 100,* 60.

Hou, C. R. et al. (2002). Immediate effects of various physical therapeutic modalities on cervical myofascial pain and trigger-point sensitivity. *Archives of Physical Medicine & Rehabilitation, 83,* 1406.

Howard, S. B., & Krishnagiri, S. (2001). The use of manual edema mobilization for the reduction of persistent edema in the upper limb. *Journal of Hand Therapy, 14,* 291.

Hurley, D. (2001). Massage is better than acupuncture (and in the short term better than self care) in reducing pain and disability in patients with chronic lower back pain. *Australian Journal of Physiotherapy, 4,* 299.

Ironson, G. et al. (1996). Massage therapy is associated with enhancement of the immune system's cytotoxic capacity. *International Journal of Neuroscience, 84,* 205.

Iwama, H., & Akama, Y. (2002). Skin rubdown with a dry towel activates natural killer cells in bedridden old patients. *Medical Science Monitor, 8,* CR611.

Kaada, B., & Torsteinbo, O. (1989). Increase of plasma beta-endorphins in connective tissue massage. *General Pharmacology, 20,* 487.

Kober, A. et al. (2003). Auricular acupressure as a treatment for anxiety in prehospital transport settings. *Anesthesiology, 98,* 1328.

Kendall, F., McCreary, E., & Provance, P. (1983). *Muscle testing and function* (4th ed.). Philadelphia: William & Wilkins.

Kubsch, S. M., Neveau, T., & Vandertie, K. (2001). Effect of cutaneous stimulation on pain reduction in emergency department patients. *Accident and Emergency Nursing, 9,* 143.

Kuznetsov, O. F., Obuukhovskii, N. G., & Martyniuk, T. I. (1980). New massage procedure applicable to bronchial asthma. *Meditsinkaia Sestra, 37,* 12.

Lafferty, W. E. et al. (2004). The use of complementary and alternative medical providers by insured cancer patients in Washington State. *Cancer, 100,* 1522.

Landy, S. (2004). Migraine throughout the life cycle: Treatment through the ages. *Neurology, 62*(Suppl. 2), S2.

Launso, L., Brendstrup, E., & Arnberg, S. (1999). An exploratory study of reflexological treatment for headache. *Alternative Therapies in Health and Medicine, 5,* 57.

Lemstra, M., Stewart, B., & Olszynski, W. P. (2002). Effectiveness of multidisciplinary intervention in the treatment of migraine: A randomized clinical trial. *Headache, 42,* 845.

Lipton, S. A. (1986). Prevention of classic migraine headache by digital massage of the superficial temporal arteries during visual aura. *Annals of Neurology, 19,* 515.

Lund, I. et al. (2002). Repeated massage-like stimulation induces long-term effects on nociception: Contribution of oxytocinergic mechanisms. *European Journal of Neuroscience, 16,* 330.

Luo, Z., & Luo, J. (1997). Clinical observations on 278 cases of cervical spondylopathy treated with electroacupuncture and massotherapy. *Journal of Traditional Chinese Medicine, 17,* 116.

Maa, S. H. et al. (2003). Effect of acupuncture or acupressure on quality of life of patients with chronic obstructive asthma: A pilot study. *Journal of Alternative and Complementary Medicine, 9,* 659.

McNamara, M. E. et al. (2003). The effects of back massage before diagnostic cardiac catheterization. *Alternative Therapies in Health and Medicine, 9,* 50.

Melzack, R., & Wall, P. D. (1965). Pain mechanisms: A new theory. *Science, 150,* 971.

Morelli, M., Chapman, C. E., & Sullivan, S. J. (1999). Do cutaneous receptors contribute to the changes in the amplitude of the H-reflex during massage? *Electromyography and Clinical Neurophysiology, 39,* 441.

Moyer, C. A., Rounds, J., & Hannum, J. W. (2004). A meta-analysis of massage therapy research. *Psychological Bulletin, 130,* 3.

Naliboff, B. D., & Tachiki, K. H. (1991). Autonomic and skeletal muscle responses to nonelectrical cutaneous stimulation. *Perceptual and Motor Skills, 72,* 575.

Petty, T. (1990). Chronic obstructive pulmonary disease — Can we do better? *Chest, 97S.*

Post-White, J. et al. (2003). Therapeutic massage and healing touch improve symptoms in cancer. *Integrated Cancer Therapies, 2,* 332.

Predye, M. (2000). Effectiveness of massage therapy for subacute low-back pain: A randomized controlled trial. *Canadian Medical Association Journal, 162,* 1815.

Puustjarvi, K., Airaksinin, O., & Pontinen, P. J. (1990). The effects of massage in patients with chronic tension headache. *Acupuncture & Electro-Therapeutics Research, 15,* 159.

Quinn, C., Chandler, C., & Moraska, A. (2002). Massage therapy and frequency of chronic tension headaches. *American Journal of Public Health, 92,* 1657.

Rinder, A., & Sutherland, C. (1995). An investigation of the effects of massage on quadriceps performance after exercise fatigue. *Complementary Therapy in Nursing and Midwifery, 1,* 99.

Rivner, M.H. (2001). The neurophysiology of myofascial pain syndrome. *Current Headache Reports, 5,* 432.

Robertson, A. et al. (1984). Effects of connective tissue massage in subacute asthma. *Medical Journal of Australia, 140,* 52.

Roscoe, J. A. et al. (2003). The efficacy of acupressure and acustimulation wrist bands for the relief of chemotherapy-induced nausea and vomiting. A University of Rochester Cancer Community Clinical Oncology Program multicenter study. *Journal of Pain and Symptom Management, 26,* 731.

Sciotti, V. M. et al. (2001). Clinical precision of myofascial trigger point location in the trapezius muscle. *Pain, 93,* 259.

Simons, D. G., & Mense, S. (2003). Diagnosis and therapy of myofascial trigger points. *Schmerz, 17,* 419.

Smith, M. C. et al. (2002). Outcomes of therapeutic massage for hospitalized cancer patients. *Journal of Nursing Scholarship, 34*, 257.

Sola, A. E., Rodenberger, M. L., & Gettys, B. B. (1955). Incidence of hypersensitive areas in posterior shoulder muscles: A survey of two hundred young adults. *American Journal of Physical Medicine, 34*, 585.

Stephenson, N., Dalton, J. A., & Carlson, J. (2003). The effect of foot reflexology on pain patients with metastatic cancer. *Applied Nursing Research, 16*, 284.

Travell, J. G., & Simons, D. (1983). *Myofascial pain and dysfunction: The trigger point manual* (Vol. 1). Baltimore: Williams & Wilkins.

Travell, J. G., & Simons, D. (1992). *Myofascial pain and dysfunction: The lower extremities* (Vol. 2). Baltimore: Williams & Wilkins.

van den Dolder, P. A., Roberts, D. L. (2003). A trial into the effectiveness of soft tissue massage in the treatment of shoulder pain. *Australian Journal of Physiotherapy, 49*, 183.

Walach, H., Guthlin, C., & Konig, M. (2003). Efficacy of massage therapy in chronic pain: A pragmatic randomized trial. *Journal of Alternative and Complementary Medicine, 6*, 837.

Waters, B. (1995). *Massage during pregnancy*. Las Cruces: Blue Waters Press.

Watson, L., Dalziel, R., & Story, I. (2000). Frozen shoulder: A 12-month clinical outcome trial, *Journal of Shoulder and Elbow Surgery, 9*, 16.

Werner, R. (1998). *A massage therapist's guide to pathology*. Philadelphia: Lippincott/Williams & Wilkins.

Wiktorsson-Moller, M. et al. (1983). Effects of warming up, massage, and stretching on range of motion and muscle strength in the lower extremity. *American Journal of Sports Medicine, 11*, 249.

Williams, A. F. et al. (2002). A randomized controlled crossover study of manual lymphatic drainage therapy in women with breast cancer-related lymphoedema. *European Journal of Cancer Care* (England), *11*, 254.

Wu, H. S. et al. (2004). Effectiveness of acupressure in improving dyspnoea in chronic obstructive pulmonary disease. *Journal of Advanced Nursing, 45*, 252.

Wylie, K. R., Jackson, C., & Crawford, P. M. (1997). Does psychological testing help to predict the response to acupuncture or massage/relaxation therapy in patients presenting to a general neurology clinic with headache? *Journal of Traditional Chinese Medicine, 2*, 130.

Yuan, C. S. et al. (2002). Transcutaneous electrical acupoint stimulation potientiates analgesic effect of morphine. *Journal of Clinical Pharmacology, 42*, 899.

80

Interdisciplinary Approaches to Treating Myofascial Pain Syndrome

Nancy Shaw, CMTPT, MS, and Pamela F. Kozey, CMTPT, BEd

INTRODUCTION

Myofascial trigger point pain and dysfunction are probably the foremost causes of chronic pain in this country. Conservative estimates of reported cases indicate that 23 million of the U.S. population have one or more chronic disorders of the musculoskeletal system (Alvarez & Rockwell, 2002). Musculoskeletal disorders are the main cause of disability in the workforce and the leading cause of disability in age-related groups (Mense, Simons, & Russell, 2001). In actuality many practitioners report studies indicating as many as 74 to 85% of the cases seen contain a primary organic diagnosis of myofascial pain (Strauss, 2004). Other studies, however, report 37 to 65% with localized myofascial pain (Strauss, 2004). Because the disorders can be treated very successfully, why do we continue to see myofascial pain and dysfunction increasing and growing to epidemic proportion? Part of the problem lies in the continued misunderstanding and blurring of diagnoses, especially between fibromyalgia, chronic fatigue, and myofascial pain syndrome. Without the proper diagnosis, there cannot be proper treatment. And, even with proper diagnosis, one needs proven guidelines for treatment to ensure a positive result.

Janet G. Travell, M.D., a noted pioneer in the field of myofascial trigger point pain and dysfunction, engineered a comprehensive, yet simple, treatment protocol. This protocol, although simple, takes time — time to listen to the patient's account of what has transpired over years of muscle use and misuse; time to unravel the patient's habits, adjustments, and accommodations to movement and activity over the years; time to listen about the work,

family, and other stressors, both good and bad, that have had an impact on the patient; and time to investigate the nutritional, mechanical, postural, endocrine, and other perpetuating factors that affect the patient. As Shakespeare said, you need to "look with your ears."

The treatment protocol established by Travell (personal communication) is shown in Table 80.1. It is this protocol with an interdisciplinary approach that is the focus of this chapter.

HISTORY OF MYOFASCIAL TRIGGER POINT THERAPY

Medical studies and findings in the literature on trigger point myofascial pain and dysfunction have often been confusing due in part to the terminology used in definition and reporting. Early tracings reveal the literature divided into three major groups and show a remarkable progression of findings. German literature, seen in the writings of Froriep, Schmidt, Lange and Eversbusch, and Kraus, seems to hold the most extensive works of the late-19th and early-20th century (Shaw, 1987; Travell & Simons, 1983). They associated the acute and chronic pain with palpable tender areas related to soft or non-articular rheumatism, identifying palpable hard nodules, tender areas responding to forceful pressure treatment. The turn of the last century highlighted continued research from Great Britain, including Gowers, Kellgren, Stockman, and Llewellyn and Jones, which revealed original fibrositis literature, along with varying explanations (myogeloses and interstitial myo-fibrositis) (Shaw, 1987; Travell & Simons,

---

TABLE 80.1
Travell's Seven-Step Myofascial Trigger Point Treatment Protocol

It is the utilization of the trigger point therapy as a treatment protocol, not as a modality, that leads to its ultimate success

Step	Action
1.	**Medical diagnosis**
	Medical history
	Elimination of pathology
	Differential diagnosis
2.	**Patient history**
	Family
	Vocational
	Social
	Avocational/exercise
	Illnesses/accidents
	Medications
	Nutrition
3.	**Pain documentation**
	Verbal
	Diagrammed
4.	**Range of motion**
	Pain site
	Functional unit
	Secondary and compensatory areas
5.	**Perpetuating factors**
	Mechanical stresses
	Nutritional inadequacies
	Metabolic and endocrine inadequacies
	Postural stresses: Sleeping, sitting, standing, driving
	Sleep disturbances
	Sleep apnea
	Home and workstation ergonomics
	Psychological
6.	**Trigger point therapy**
	Trigger point pressure release
	Intermittent coolant with stretch
	Injection
7.	**Specific muscle stretch retraining**

To eliminate any one of these steps in treating myofascial pain and dysfunction can lead to treatment failure!

Note: From Travell, personal communication.

1983). Adler added the concept of pain referring away from the pain source, and Kellgren further established referred pain arising from the tender areas of the muscle (Shaw, 1987; Travell & Simons, 1983). The mid-20th century evidenced American literature making major contributions to the understanding of the syndrome in the works of Travell, Sola, Rinzler, Bonica, and Kraus and thus the emergence of myofascial pain syndrome, myofascitis, trigger points,

and myalgia (Shaw, 1987). The late-20th century saw renewed research by Simons, Mense, Hubbard, Gunn, Baker, Jaeger, and others encompassing soft tissue and tended toward designations of fibrositis, myofascial pain, fibromyalgia, psychogenic rheumatism, myofascitis, tension myalgia, and fibromyositis (Mense, Simons, & Russell, 2001). During the mid- to late-20th century Janet G. Travell published more that 40 papers on the myofascial genesis of pain, myofascial trigger points, documenting the specific pain referral patterns, and theorized the self-sustaining characteristic mechanism of trigger points (Travell & Simons, 1999). Her early work became a respected source of information and still holds that respect.

Travell, the clinician, developed a treatment protocol that set the standard for the treatment of myofascial pain and dysfunction, or myofascial pain syndrome. That protocol is the focus of this chapter. It is a protocol that has stood the test of time and has an outstanding success rate if performed in its entirety without shortcuts or alterations. The multiplicity of the terminology, however, continues to add confusion and needs to be clarified if differential diagnosis and, thus, treatment are to be correctly directed. A listing of the more important definitions that pertain to the material in this chapter follows:

- **Arthritis:** Inflammation of a joint marked by pain, redness, swelling, and heat. Osteoarthritis is a degenerative joint disease and is a noninflammatory condition with a gradual and subtle onset. Pain is an early symptom, usually made worse with exercise (*Dorland's Medical Dictionary*, 1982, p. 47).
- **Chronic pain:** Long-standing (weeks, months, years) pain but not necessarily incurable (Travell & Simons, 1983). A complexity of life changes that produce altered behavior and that may persist even after the cause of the pain is eliminated constitutes the chronic pain syndrome (Zohn, 1988).
- **Fibromyalgia syndrome:** A common medical condition characterized by widespread pain and tenderness to palpation at multiple anatomically defined soft tissue body sites (Yunus & Rachlin, 1994).
- **Muscle cramp:** Involuntary shortening activation of the muscle resulting in pain and limited motion.
- **Muscle pain:** An unpleasant sensory and emotional experience associated with actual or potential tissue damage, or described in terms of such damage (Mense et al., 2001).
- **Muscle spasm:** Increased tension with or without shortening of a muscle due to nonvoluntary motor nerve activity. One cannot voluntarily

release or relax this spasm (Travell & Simons, 1983, p. 4).

- **Muscle stiffness:** Discomfort with movement of a joint (Mense et al., 2001).
- **Muscle strength:** The contractile force of the muscle.
- **Muscle stretch:** To draw out to full extent or beyond normal functioning limits of the muscle.
- **Muscle tone:** The muscle in its resting tension, clinically determined as resistance to passive movement (Mense et al., 2001).
- **Myofascial pain syndrome:** Pain and/or autonomic phenomena referred from active myofascial trigger points with associated dysfunction (Travell & Simons, 1983). A regional pain syndrome accompanied by trigger points (Yunus & Rachlin, 1994).
- **Referred trigger point pain:** Pain arising in a trigger point, but felt at a distance, often completely remote from its source (Travell & Simons, 1983).
- **Tender point:** A general term expressing focal pressure pain sensitivity, i.e., tenderness limited to a point usually not larger than about 1 cm. Tender points are not defined by any additional specific attributes (Fischer & Rachlin, 1994).
- **Trigger point:** A focus of hyperirritability in a tissue that when compressed is locally tender and if sufficiently hypersensitive, gives rise to referred pain and tenderness and sometimes to referred autonomic phenomena and distortion of proprioception (Fischer & Rachlin, 1994; Travell & Simons, 1983). The exquisitely sensitive area, the trigger point, refers pain to a remote "reference pain zone" that is specific to each trigger point (Fischer & Rachlin, 1994).
- **Trigger point pressure release:** Slowly applied pressure to a trigger point. Once resistance is met, the pressure is sustained until a change in the muscle is felt. This process may then be repeated. This is a new term replacing "ischemic compression" in trigger point deactivation.

BACKGROUND

Skeletal muscle is the largest single organ of the human body. Aside from varying ways of counting muscle divisions, it is generally agreed that there are approximately 500 muscles in the body. Any one of these muscles can develop trigger points that refer pain or, in lesser states of activity, cause dysfunction. The contracted muscle fibers, if left without an opposing muscle to pull them back to a neutral position will remain in a shortened state, vulnerable to daily wear and tear. The muscles develop memories of functioning short, just like learning a bad golf swing. They develop trigger points, and elicit pain to distal areas of the body. Ongoing function in a contracted or partially contracted state leads to chronicity of the trigger point pain. Yet, the medical profession, in general, has not addressed this basic muscle phenomenon. Perhaps this is true because there is nothing "wrong" with the muscles, they have simply "learned" to function incorrectly, i.e., in a shortened functional range of motion. Just as there are many small components to a bad golf swing, there are many factors contributing to patterns of incorrect muscle functioning and to the resultant trigger points eliciting pain.

In a perfect scientific, medical world there would be specific, objective tests that would determine the cause of myofascial pain and dysfunction. Although interventional modalities such as electromyography (EMG), muscle biopsy, ultrasonography, surface EMG, and thermography have been studied and used with varying success (Alvarez & Rockwell, 2002), currently there are no specific laboratory tests or imaging techniques for the diagnosis of myofascial pain and dysfunction. Certainly there are none that can compare with the comprehensive evaluation by the clinician. There have been major steps, however, taken in the study of the epidemiology, pathophysiology, pathogenesis, and therapeutic options for what is now termed myofascial pain syndrome (Strauss, 2004). These studies have helped eliminate the notion of benign chronic pain as primarily psychological in nature or associated with "malingering." The studies have established the legitimacy of myofascial pain syndrome in the medical profession. In conjunction with the above studies, a great deal can be gained from the subjective pain assessment tools including, Visual Analogue Pain Scales, the McGill Pain Questionnaire, and pain diagrams (Straus, 2004). With such growing research and support tools, why does there continue to be such a lack of double-blind studies verifying an effective treatment protocol? To understand the very nature of the complexity of myofascial pain and dysfunction dictates the answer to that question. Travell noted that approximately 75% of treatment success lies in the addressing of the multitude of perpetuating factors and in the stretch neuromuscular retraining. Perpetuating problems may be due to mechanical stressors, postural stressors, nutritional inadequacies, systemic metabolic and endocrine inadequacies, psychological/stress factors, chronic infection, functional stressors, and complications of the above, e.g., nerve impingement, sleep disturbance, and environmental and food sensitivities. Because addressing these perpetuating factors in their entirety is critical to treatment success, double-blind research would necessitate finding a group of individuals with exactly the same perpetuating factors complaining of the same pain problem and another group for the control. This is not going to happen. Yes, we could find a group exhibiting, for example, the same back pain but that group would not present with the exact same perpetuating factors. While some aspects of treatment may be measured by group evaluation (e.g., use of nutritional supplementation), the very nature of the myofascial trigger point pain syndrome with its myriad of perpetuating factors unique to each individual does not lend itself to the research of double-blind studies that are requested. Should this inability to conduct double-blind study research negate the validity of myofascial trigger point therapy? Of course not. It simply means we must rely on the research of Simons, Hubbard, Mense, and others to identify the location and nature of trigger points, their mechanism of activation and deactivation, and strategies for prevention of recurrence. We must rely on a proven treatment protocol to establish treatment success.

INTERDISCIPLINARY APPROACH

Myofascial trigger point therapy (MTPT) lends itself to an interdisciplinary approach of dealing with neuromuscular pain conditions. The first step in the MTPT protocol requires a diagnosis of myofascial pain syndrome or fibromyalgia. A licensed health care provider such as a physician, chiropractor, osteopath, or dentist makes a diagnosis and recommends MTPT. This step usually rules out any systemic illness or neurological or orthopedic problems.

In addressing perpetuating factors, myofascial trigger point therapists work in conjunction with a variety of health care practitioners. A common referral would be to a chiropractor or osteopath. Body workers release and balance muscles/fascia. The chiropractors and osteopaths adjust and align joints. The newly released and balanced muscles will rapidly revert to their old patterns if joints are not aligned properly. The opposite is also true. If we adjust and align joints without releasing taut bands and trigger points, the imbalanced muscles will pull the joints out of alignment again. A team approach working with both muscles and joints is usually more effective and requires a shorter treatment regimen.

Following is a partial list of other health providers with which body workers collaborate on a regular basis:

- Allergists
- Dentists
- Endocrinologists
- Homeopaths
- Kinesiologists
- Naturopaths
- Nutritionists
- Physiatrists
- Physical therapists

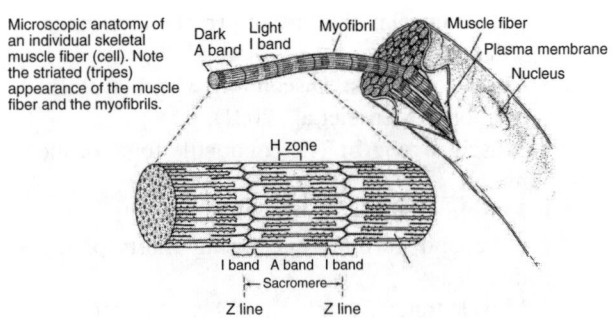

FIGURE 80.1 Anatomy of a muscle fiber. Microscopic anatomy of an individual skeletal muscle fiber (cell). Note the striated (striped) appearance of the muscle fiber and the myofibrils. From *Basic Human Anatomy* (2nd ed.), by A. P. Spence, 1986, Menlo Park, CA: Benjamin/Cummings. Reproduced with permission.

- Podiatrists
- Psychiatrists, psychologists, social workers
- Rheumatologists
- Chiropractors
- Osteopaths

It is vital that myofascial trigger point therapists work closely with these other professionals to provide the most holistic care possible. To ignore a piece of the puzzle will result either in a failed attempt to relieve myofascial pain or in pain that returns shortly after treatment.

A more detailed discussion of perpetuating factors appears later in this chapter.

MUSCLE ANATOMY

The structure and activity of a motor unit must be understood to recognize a disruption of normal function. This disruption or pathology is the cause of myofascial pain and dysfunction. The following is a cursory overview of the anatomy and physiology of the skeletal muscle.

Each muscle, in descending order of magnitude, consists of muscle fibers, myofibrils, sarcomeres, and myofilaments (Figure 80.1). The sarcomeres are the main contractile mechanisms of the muscle. They are made up of thick and thin filaments. The thick filaments are composed of proteins called myosin. The thin filaments are composed of proteins called actin, tropomyosin, and troponin (Figure 80.2) (Spence, 1986). It is the sliding action of these two filaments that actually causes the contraction. The sliding is a result of a series of rowing actions between the projections or heads on the myosin filament and attachment sites on the actin filament. Relaxation occurs when the myosin heads detach from the actin filament (Mense et al., 2001).

But what causes muscles to contract? The site where the terminal branch of the alpha-motor axon links with the muscle fiber is called the motor end plate or neuromuscular junction (Figure 80.3). When an action potential

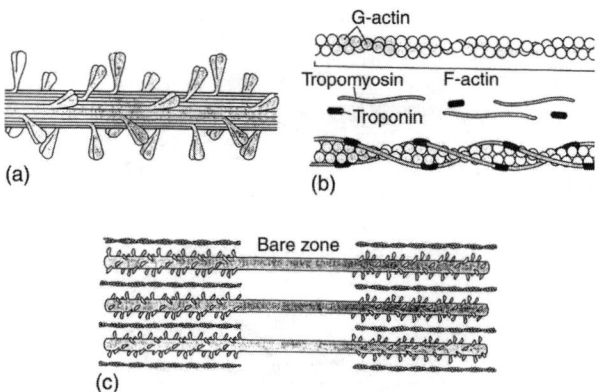

FIGURE 80.2 Myosin and actin filaments. (a) Thick filament, (b) thin filament, (c) longitudinal section of filaments. From *Basic Human Anatomy* (2nd ed.), by A. P. Spence, 1986, Menlo Park, CA: Benjamin/Cummings. Reproduced with permission.

arrives at this junction, the axon releases acetylcholine (ACh). The ACh diffuses across the synapse to the muscle cell membrane and causes a change in the membrane at the junction of the muscle cell (Mense et al., 2001). This change results in the generation of a stimulatory impulse that spreads over this plasma membrane and into the interior of the muscle cell by way of *t* tubules. This impulse excites the sarcoplasmic reticulum causing it to release calcium ions (Ca^{2+}). This constitutes the initiating event for muscle contraction (Griggs, Mendell, & Miller, 1995; Mense et al., 2001; Spence, 1986).

In the resting muscle, the tropomyosin masks the binding sites (for the myosin heads) on the surface of the actin molecule. The rise in Ca^{2+} concentration causes the tropomyosin chain, which is wrapped around the actin, to move from its blocking position. The myosin heads can then bind with actin in a rowing motion. This movement pulls the actin filament toward the middle of the sarcomere thereby shortening it (Mense et al., 2001).

Adenosine triphosphate (ATP) provides the energy required for muscle contraction. In a resting muscle cell, an ATP molecule binds to the projection (club-shaped head) on the myosin molecule. The myosin head also contains ATPase, an enzyme that splits ATP into adenosine diphosphate (ADP) and phosphate (P) plus energy. Actin activates the ATPase in the presence of magnesium (Mg) ions. Consequently, as soon as the tropomyosin chain moves and the myosin heads make contact with the actin filaments, ATP is split. This released energy then separates the myosin heads from the actin (Mense et al., 2001).

If intracellular Ca^{2+} remains high, the myosin heads will again attach to the actin with the flexing motion. When the concentration of Ca^{2+} drops, the attachments no longer occur and tropomyosin once again blocks the binding sites. The calcium pump returns the Ca^{2+} to the sarcoplasmic reticulum, until ACh spikes again (Mense et al., 2001).

ANATOMY AND PHYSIOLOGY OF A TRIGGER POINT

Trigger points (TrPs) have been difficult to understand because there has been no method of studying them. Often, differences in terminology have made it difficult to know if investigators were even dealing with the same condition. Our current understanding of trigger points results from the convergence of two independent lines of investigation, one electrodiagnostic and the other histopathologic. Fitting together the lessons from each led Mense and Simons to postulate a theory called the *Integrated Hypothesis*. It is now becoming clear that the region we are accustomed to calling a TrP, or a tender nodule, is a cluster of numerous microscopic loci of intense abnormality. These loci are scattered throughout the nodule. The critical TrP abnormality now appears to be neuromuscular dysfunction at the motor end plate of an extrafusal skeletal

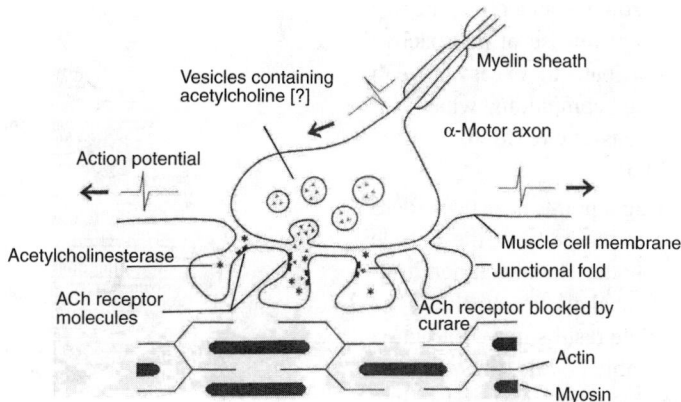

FIGURE 80.3 Anatomy of a motor end plate. From *Muscle Pain: Understanding Its Nature, Diagnosis, and Treatment,* by S. Mense, D. G. Simons, & I. J. Russell, 2001, Baltimore: Lippincott/Williams & Wilkins. Reproduced with permission.

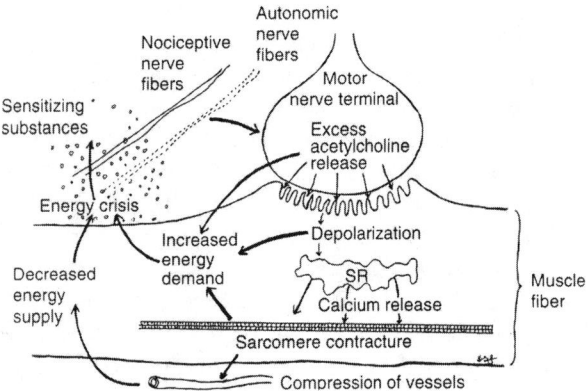

FIGURE 80.4 Dysfunctional motor end plate. From *Muscle Pain: Understanding Its Nature, Diagnosis, and Treatment*, by S. Mense, D. G. Simons, & I. J. Russell, 2001, Baltimore: Lippincott/Williams & Wilkins. Reproduced with permission.

muscle fiber, making myofascial pain caused by TrPs a neuromuscular disease.

The primary dysfunction hypothesized here is an abnormal increase (by several orders of magnitude) in the *production and release of ACh* packets from the motor nerve terminal under resting conditions. The greatly increased number of miniature end plate potentials (MEPPs) produces end plate noise and *sustained depolarization of the postjunctional membrane* of the muscle fiber. This sustained depolarization could cause a *continuous release and inadequate uptake of calcium ions from local sarcoplasmic reticulum* and produce *sustained shortening (contracture) of sarcomeres*. Each of these four italicized changes would increase energy demand. The sustained muscle fiber shortening compresses local blood vessels, thereby reducing the nutrient and oxygen supplies that normally met the energy demands of this region. The increased energy demand in the face of an impaired energy supply would produce a local energy crisis, which leads to the release of sensitizing substances that could interact with autonomic and sensory (some nociceptive) nerves traversing that region. Subsequent release of neuroactive substances could, in turn, contribute to excessive ACh release from the nerve terminal, completing what then becomes a self-sustaining vicious cycle (Mense et al., 2001; Figures 80.4 through 80.6).

Two types of myofascial trigger points have been identified. The central TrP occurs in the belly of the muscle at the dysfunctional motor end plate. The attachment trigger points occur where myofascial tissue attaches. The dysfunction at the motor end plate results in a contraction knot, which can produce a palpable nodule, thus the central TrP. The remainder of the sarcomeres is stretched into a taut band of very tense muscle fibers. As the tightened sarcomere pulls on the attachment points, it causes a disruption of these fibers, resulting in tenderness and swelling (Mense et al., 2001).

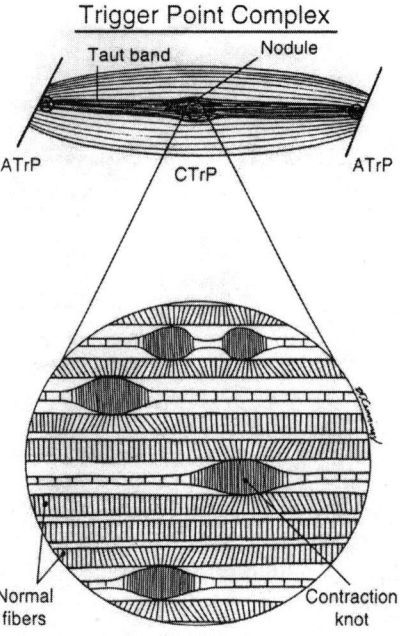

FIGURE 80.5 Sarcomeres with contraction knots. From *Muscle Pain: Understanding Its Nature, Diagnosis, and Treatment*, by S. Mense, D. G. Simons, & I. J. Russell, 2001, Baltimore: Lippincott/Williams & Wilkins. Reproduced with permission.

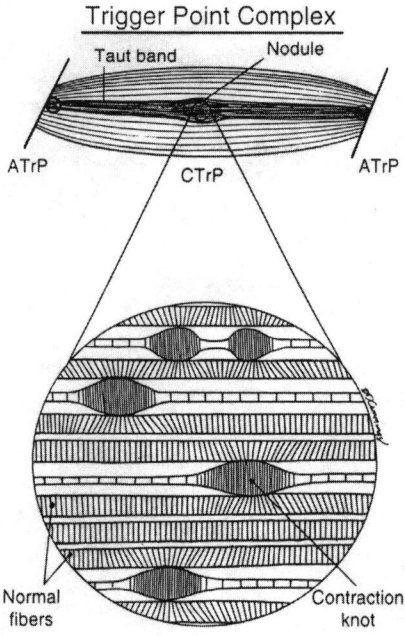

FIGURE 80.6 Diagram of an energy crisis. From *Muscle Pain: Understanding Its Nature, Diagnosis, and Treatment*, by S. Mense, D. G. Simons, & I. J. Russell, 2001, Baltimore: Lippincott/Williams & Wilkins. Reproduced with permission.

INTRODUCTION TO TRAVELL'S SEVEN-STEP PROTOCOL

Mennell states that medicine is not just a matter of taking pharmaceuticals. Nor is it merely an exercise in high technology. "The successful practice of medicine is still based on arriving at a correct diagnosis of the cause of each patient's symptoms; this is still dependent on listening, observing, feeling and thinking. The result of thinking is enhanced by experience. No computer is able to touch. Observation is the action of many human capabilities a machine cannot possess" (Mennell, 1991, p. 1).

With Mennell's philosophy in mind, it is imperative that any clinician or therapist perform the entire treatment protocol to ensure successful resolution of myofascial pain syndrome. It is the utilization of the trigger point therapy as a treatment protocol, not as a modality, that leads to its ultimate success. To eliminate any one of the steps in treating myofascial pain and dysfunction can lead to treatment failure.

In the process of stepping through the Travell protocol, we will also show how certain steps are distinctly different from a traditional therapy protocol.

STEP 1: MEDICAL DIAGNOSIS

Medical History

A thorough medical history and physical examination must be conducted to eliminate possible sources of the musculoskeletal pain other than myofascial trigger points. The presence of myofascial pain syndrome does not rule out other hidden conditions that may be contributing to the pain. The diagnosis of these conditions (Table 80.2) must be addressed in the initial evaluation.

Elimination of Pathology

While eliminating any underlying pathology, it is important to remember, however, that myofascial trigger points can coexist with any other condition and be a significant contributor to the pain being experienced. As long as other medical conditions, if they exist, are being treated, it is most valuable to treat the trigger points and engage in muscular retraining to eliminate that pain component.

Differential Diagnosis

Table 80.3 indicates the percentage of patients with another diagnosis who also had myofascial trigger points that contributed to their problems. Often the overall pain experienced is significantly reduced with trigger point elimination, indicating the pain was not just from the coexisting condition. For example, arthritic joint pain is often the result of inflammation occurring at the point of the tendon joint attachment where muscles are functioning at a shortened range of motion, pulling on and irritating

---

TABLE 80.2
Differential Diagnosis in Medical Evaluation

Musculoskeletal Diseases:
- Arthritis: Osteoarthritis, rheumatoid arthritis, gout
- Myopathy: Painless weakness of proximal muscles
- Focal inflammation of musculoskeletal structures: Trigger points refer to regions where tendons, ligaments, and bursae are located

Neurological Diseases:
- Identified by motor and/or sensory deficits in the distribution of the afflicted nerve
- Motor findings include atrophy, weakness, diminished or absent reflexes
- Sensory changes are described as numbness, tingling, pins and needles, burning, and sensory distortions

Visceral Diseases:
- Somatovisceral effects: Active trigger points in the abdominal wall muscles can disturb visceral function, e.g., gastrointestinal including but not limited to constipation, diarrhea, cramping, irritable bowel syndrome, leaky gut syndrome, and esophageal reflux
- Viscerosomatic: Visceral disease can refer pain to skeletal muscles and activate satellite trigger points

Infectious Diseases:
- Viral
- Bacterial
  While the presence of symptoms other than pain may indicate a nonmyofascial component, there may be activation of trigger points within the painful regions, which may then persist after recovery from the infectious illness.

Endocrine Disorders:
- Hypothyroidism
- Hyperthyroidism
- Adrenal fatigue
- Wilson's disorder
- Hypoglycemia

Autoimmune Diseases:
- Chronic fatigue syndrome
- Fibromyalgia
- Systemic lupus erythematosus
- Mononucleosis

Nutritional Disorders:
- Systemic candidiasis
- pH imbalance
- Vitamin and/or mineral inadequacies

Psychogenic Disease:
- Clinical depression
- Bipolar
- Anxiety

Sleep Disorders:
- Sleep apnea
- Inadequate sleep maintenance
- Inadequate restorative sleep

Note: From N. Shaw, unpublished, 1988.

TABLE 80.3
Percent of Pain Patients Harboring Concomitant Myofascial Trigger Points

Diagnosis	No. of Patients	% with MTrPs
Cervicogenic headache	80	100
Reflex sympathetic dystrophy	84	82
Fibromyalgia	19	100
Chronic intractable benign back pain	90	96.7
Chronic intractable benign neck pain	34	100

Note: From "Myofascial Pain Syndrome: A Short Review," by S. Strauss, *The Medical Acupuncture Webpage,* Retrieved January 2004 from http://users.med.auth.gr/~karanik/english/articles/mayofac.html..

TABLE 80.4
Myofascial Versus Fibromyalgia

Myofascial Pain Syndrome	Fibromyalgia
Equal number men and women	About 4:1 ratio women over men
Trigger Points	Tender Points
• Local tenderness	• Local tenderness
• Taut band	
• Local twitch response	
• Jump sign	
Singular/multiple body quadrant/specific	Multiple body quadrants/generalized
May occur in any skeletal muscle	Occurs in specific locations that are symmetrically located
Specific pain referral patterns	No pain referral pattern
Decreased range of motion	No decreased range of motion
	Hypermobility
20% also have fibromyalgia	72% also have active TrPs
Resolves with treatment	Chronic

Common to Both Conditions

Sleep deprivation
Fatigue
Pain made worse with activity
Depression/anxiety
Muscle stiffness

Note: From N. Shaw, unpublished, 2003.

attachments. Accompanying trigger points refer pain to the joint area. The inflammation can be treated but if the shortened muscle continues to tug at the joint attachment and trigger points continue to refer pain to the joint area, the problem will not be eliminated.

Another differential diagnosis needing attention is the ongoing blurring of myofascial pain syndrome with fibromyalgia. These are two distinct entities. These conditions often coexist and may interact with one another. "As many as 72% of fibromyalgia patients also have some myofascial pain syndrome but the reverse is not necessarily so. Only 20% of myofascial trigger point pain patients also exhibit fibromyalgia symptoms" (Strauss, 2004, p. 2; Table 80.4). Until greater skill is developed in recognizing, understanding, palpating, and defining myofascial trigger points, there will continue to be misdiagnoses.

Considerable effort has been made to establish guidelines for the differential diagnosis of common medical conditions and myofascial pain syndrome and to highlight common associated symptoms. This provides immeasurable direction for medical evaluation, proper diagnosis, and thus, properly directed treatment. Table 80.5 delineates common medical diagnoses and the trigger points/muscles causing some of the same pain symptoms.

After a diagnosis of myofascial pain syndrome, it becomes important for the clinician to educate the patient while performing the initial but specific myofascial evaluation. Since other medical conditions have been addressed, let the patient know that if the pain experienced relates strongly to locomotor activity and body positioning, it is probably musculoskeletal in origin!

STEP 2: PATIENT HISTORY

Personal information, family makeup, vocation, stressors, activities, hobbies, relaxation and fun activities, vacations, and the like will help the clinician understand how much the pain is disruptive to the patient's lifestyle. This information indicates the place pain is playing in the patient's life, both good and bad; identifies aspects important to the patient; and helps set treatment goals.

Family History

The makeup of the family structure may give insight to stressors that are affecting the patient with myofascial pain syndrome. Infants or very young children need to be carried, often in awkward positions. They often have very sporadic sleep schedules, frequently awake and requiring attention during the night. Older children have to be driven numerous places for activity involvement, times varying from very early morning to later in the evening. Difficult teens may require special efforts. Aging parents living with children require mental, physical, and emotional adjustments for the family. Long work hours and long work weeks often provide little time for relaxed interaction with spouses and children. All of these situations can provide stress, require muscle accommodations, and lead to sleep deprivation and general mental and physical fatigue, which can perpetuate a myofascial pain syndrome.

Vocational History

It is helpful to know the nature of current and previous work situations. The mental, emotional, and physical demands of the patient's work need to be evaluated. Can commute time, work schedules, breaks, deadlines, postures, meals, and personnel interactions be refined to make a less-demanding, yet productive work environment? It is often the patient's own pressure in the work situation that is detrimental.

Vocational status of the patient is important in determining the patient's desire to maintain active employment in the same field or identifying alternative goals that become part of the treatment plan. Physical and mental demands at work and the hours required might be contributing to the perpetuation of the pain problem. Ergonomics of the workstation need to be evaluated.

Exercise

Explain that movement and exercise are essential to optimal health. They are essential to unimpaired function of the musculoskeletal system. Conditioned muscles are less vulnerable to trigger point development as long as stretch has been included to maintain a balance necessary to normal activity. Specific movements and stretch neuromuscular retraining will be an integral aspect of the treatment program. It will require patient compliance and commitment to ensure treatment success.

Nutrition

Dietary evaluation helps assess the likelihood of nutritional inadequacies and eating habits, e.g., skipping meals, that may interfere with treatment success. This topic is covered more completely in the perpetuating factor section.

Social History

In what social activities is the patient involved? Do these activities involve family, spouses, friends, or co-workers? Are activities sedentary or more active in nature? Are the activities and the people involved ones that lead to relaxation, stress relief, and just plain fun?

Avocational History

Does the patient have hobbies or outside interests? Are these activities sedentary or active? Do the hobbies require different muscular demands than the patient's job or other activities?

It is important for the patient to have time and space to be involved in a number of activities that allow body movement to be varied. This helps alleviate overuse, underuse, and abuse of muscles, and allows for healthy function.

Illness and Accident History

Illnesses, accidents, and surgeries begin to give a picture of muscle stresses and traumas that are a part of the patient's history. There may even be a myofascial compo-

nent behind some of the traumas (e.g., falling frequently because of sternocleidomastoid trigger points resulting in disruptive equilibrium). This information certainly points to some of the cumulative precipitating factors of trigger point development and the ongoing muscle tension that results in myofascial pain syndrome.

Medications

Note medications the patient is currently taking, those previously taken, and how long they have been taken, and indicate the efficacy of each. This will give insight into medical care already received and lessen the duplication of evaluative and treatment efforts. It will also indicate other medical conditions being treated and reveal unnecessary drug clutter, patient dependency on the drugs, and the patient's pain perspective.

Step 3: Pain Documentation

After establishing myofascial pain and dysfunction with the patient and recording general information, the clinician must then perform an extensive and specific myofascial evaluation with the patient. Clinical features associated with myofascial trigger point diagnoses involve several components. Travell differentiates three phases of refractory chronic myofascial pain. In phase 3, stiffness, dysfunction, and decreased range of motion arise from latent trigger points, which cause no pain unless palpated. In phase 2, increased less irritable trigger point activity gives rise to intermittent pain upon movement and upon taking certain postures. Generally, only some activities aggravate the pain so patients quickly learn what movements or activities to avoid. These are, however, active trigger points, both primary and satellite. In phase 1, the most involved active trigger point activity results in pain on motion and at rest and can be continuous and intense with little relief even with medication. Because the pain is constant and intense, the patient often cannot identify specific movements or activities that increase the pain (Travell, Fricton, & Awad, 1990). When addressing the pain specifically with the guidelines unique to the Travell myofascial trigger point, protocol treatment can be divided into three phases as seen in Table 80.6: (1) pain documentation, (2) treatment, and (3) rehabilitation.

To begin the initial evaluation of the patient with pain, general information is necessary to establish a working basis for the patient and the clinician. The history of the pain must be thorough, establishing when the pain began, how it began, its intensity and duration, what increases or decreases the pain, and what helps or aggravates the pain. Pain perception should be put in perspective. When there are multiple pain areas, it is important to establish to which pain the patient's response applies. Defining the patient's perception of what causes the pain influences the patient's

TABLE 80.5
Common Pain Diagnoses Frequently Unrecognized as Originating from Myofascial Trigger Points in Specific Muscles

	Initial Diagnosis	Some Likely Trigger Point Sources
1*	Acute stiff neck	Levator scapulae
		Sternocleidomastoid
		Upper trapezius
2	Angina pectoralis (atypical)	Pectoralis major
3	Appendicitis	Lower rectus abdominis
4*	Arthritis of shoulder	Infraspinatus
5*	Arthritis of hip	Tensor fasciae latae
		Quadratus lumborum
6*	Arthritis of knee	Rectus femoris
		Vastus medialis
		Vastus lateralis
7	Atypical angina	Pectoralis major
8	Atypical facial neuralgia	Masseter
		Temporalis
		Sternal division of sternocleidomastoid
9	Atypical migraine	Sternocleidomastoid
		Temporalis
		Posterior cervical
10	Back pain, middle	Upper rectus abdominis
		Thoracic paraspinals
11	Back pain, low	Lower rectus abdominis
12	Bicipital tendonitis	Long head of biceps humerus
13	Chronic abdominal wall pain	Abdominal muscles
14	Dysmenorrhea	Lower rectus abdominis
15	Earache (enigmatic)	Deep masseters
16*	Earache — normal drum	Clavicular division of sternocleidomastoid
17	Epicondylitis	Wrist extensors
		Supinator
		Triceps brachii
18	Frozen shoulder	Subscapularis
19*	Heel spur	Soleus
20	Myofascial pain dysfunction	Masticatory muscles
21	Occipital headache	Posterior cervicals
22*	Pelvic pain	Coccygeus
		Levator ani
23	Postherpetic neuralgia	Serratus anterior
		Intercostals
24	Radiculopathy, C6	Pectoralis minor
		Scalenes
25	Scapulocostal syndrome	Scalenes
		Middle trapezius
		Levator scapulae
26*	Sciatica	Posterior gluteus minimus
		Piriformis
27	Subacromial bursitis	Middle deltoid
28*	Subdeltoid bursitis	Infraspinatus
		Deltoid
		Supraspinatus
29	Temporomandibular joint disorder	Masseter
		Lateral pterygoid
30	Tennis elbow	Finger extensors
		Supinator

TABLE 80.5 (Continued)
Common Pain Diagnoses Frequently Unrecognized as Originating from Myofascial Trigger Points in Specific Muscles

	Initial Diagnosis	Some Likely Trigger Point Sources
31	Tension headache	Sternocleidomastoid
		Masticatory muscles
		Posterior cervicals
		Upper trapezius
32	Thoracic outlet syndrome	Scalenes
		Subscapularis
		Pectoralis minor and major
		Latissimus dorsi
		Teres major
33	Tietze's syndrome	Pectoralis major enthesopathy
		Internal intercostals
34*	Trochanteric bursitis	Vastus lateralis
		Tensor fasciae latae
		Quadratus lumborum

Note: From *Muscle pain: Understanding its nature, diagnosis, and treatment,* by S. Mense, D. G. Simons, & I. J. Russell, 2001, Baltimore: Lippincott/Williams & Wilkins. Reproduced with permission.

* From Myofascial pain syndrome due to trigger points by D. Simons, 1987, International Rehabilitation Medicine Assoc., *Monograph Series* #1, 12.

TABLE 80.6
Unique Characteristics of Myofascial Trigger Point Therapy

Pain Documentation	Treatment	Rehabilitation
Pain source vs. Pain site	**Myofascial origin** vs. Symptoms	**Stretch** vs. Strength
Range of motion testing vs. Strength testing	**Pain elimination** vs. Pain management	**"No pain" range of motion** vs. Pain for gain
Muscular differential diagnosis vs. Traditional diagnosis	**Total trigger point treatment** vs. Pain site treatment	**Muscle retraining** vs. Muscle conditioning
Perpetuating factors vs. Precipitating factors	**Total person treatment** vs. Pain site treatment	
	Movement vs. Rest	
	Hands-on treatment vs. Mechanical treatment	
	Heat vs.Cold	

Note: Treatments in bold are associated with MTPT. From N. Shaw, unpublished, 1992.

response to treatment and compliance in addressing perpetuating factors and prescribed home program. Demonstrate that the pain is of muscle trigger point origin and refocus the patient's attention from pain to function. It can almost work against the treatment process to have the patient keep a "pain log," which focuses the patient on the pain rather than on more positive movements not causing pain and on improvements in function.

Verbal Description

The patient's description of the pain gives the clinician insight into the patient's pain perception, the pain's impact on the patient's daily functioning, the psychological mindset of the patient regarding the pain, and the accuracy of the patient's understanding of the pain. It is helpful to know the patient's view of the pain if the clinician is to be successful in educating the patient regarding pain origin and perpetuating factors, and the patient's role in treatment and rehabilitation.

Pain Diagram

The site of the pain or pains is documented on a pain chart to ensure an exact representation of the pain location. It is preferred the clinician do the charting as patients tend to exaggerate the boundaries of the pain site due to the seemingly all inclusiveness of the pain sensation. The clinician's recording of the pain pattern also establishes a good working relationship with the patient. Upon recording the pain pattern described by the patient, the clinician shows the pain chart to the patient to verify its accuracy. The patient can concur as to the accuracy or make adjustments. The clinician establishes a clear "I am listening" working relationship with the patient. This is important in obtaining patient compliance with future directives during treatment. Only if the pain patterning is exactly represented can the clinician identify which trigger points in which muscles are key or primary. For example, at least six muscles refer pain to various aspects of the medial border of the scapula. Identifying "exactly" where the pain is helps determine which muscle may be harboring the most primary trigger points, thus identifying the pain source. Once the pain site is identified, the clinician determines the trigger point source and begins to develop the treatment progression. Generality of pain location = identifying the incorrect muscle/trigger point = misdirected trigger point treatment. Exact pain location = identifying the correct trigger point = proper trigger point treatment.

STEP 4: RANGE OF MOTION TESTING

When evaluating range of motion, it is imperative that comprehensive range of motion be conducted. This will involve areas of active, latent, satellite, and compensatory trigger points. The patient generally has made movement adjustments or accommodations for the pain, or avoids certain movements as a guarding mechanism to avoid pain. The clinician will often find quite a discrepancy from the patient's right and left range of motion. This difference will help dictate not only treatment detail but also the neuromuscular rehabilitation as a balance of function is sought (see Table 80.7 for a joint measurement chart).

Pain Source Versus Pain Site

When evaluating the patient's pain, the clinician may focus on the pain site but must also focus on the anticipated trigger point source of the pain. Pain site alone gives a distorted view of the comprehensiveness of the pain problem and leads to temporary but "quick fix" or unresolved pain elimination.

Range of Motion Testing Versus Strength Testing

Range of motion evaluation is recommended instead of strength testing. If there is decreased range of motion, there will, of necessity, be decreased strength as only partial contractual/functional potential is available. Any weakness at this point is considered pseudo-weakness. The pain is a result of an unwanted tension/contraction in

the muscle, i.e., trigger point. If strength testing is performed before full functional range is obtained, contraction is added to the muscle memory, thus increasing pain and weakness. Simons has pointed out the value of range of motion as diagnostic criteria. Measurement of increased range of motion becomes a useful objective measurement of treatment progress. It is an inexpensive measurement and can be objectively measured with a goniometer, protractor, or inclinometer. This range of motion evaluation will also serve as a differentiation with fibromyalgia as the restriction is characteristic of myofascial pain and dysfunction while hypermobility is common in fibromyalgia (Simons, 2003). Once range of motion is addressed in treatment with deactivation of trigger points and return of muscle length, then strength can be evaluated to determine needed areas of improvement. A balance of strength–stretch is the optimal outcome.

STEP 5: PERPETUATING FACTORS

Perpetuating Factors Versus Precipitating Factors

Perpetuating factors, in many ways, become more important factors than the precipitating factors in the treatment of myofascial pain and dysfunction. There can be one culminating event that results in the patient's current pain condition; but more often, a patient will express having experienced pain intermittently over an extended period of time. The latest episode, however, was worse, lasted longer, and eventually became chronic. If, however, one looks at the cumulative nature of muscle tension over time, i.e., muscle contraction/relaxation but no concerted effort to stretch regularly = gradual muscle shortening = shortened muscle functional memory = trigger point = pain, it is more accurate to identify not one but a series of uses, misuses, and abuses. This functional shortening is usually followed by conscious or unconscious adaptations or adjustments of the patient's function and posturing. Perpetuating factors and the adaptations that become habit continue to reinforce poor functional efficiency and extend the pain problem. Travell often indicated treatment success was directly proportional to eliminating perpetuating factors so appropriate neuromuscular retraining could be achieved without reactivating trigger point activity. Travell and Simons dedicated 50+ pages to perpetuating factors, leaving additional detail of each factor to the clinician. Travell often stated that Chapter 4, Vol. I on perpetuating factors was the most important chapter in *Myofascial Pain and Dysfunction: The Trigger Point Manual*. Figure 80.7 elaborates the categories of perpetuating factors in the treatment of myofascial pain and dysfunction.

One of the greatest needs for the interdisciplinary team in the diagnosis and treatment of myofascial pain and dysfunction is for addressing these perpetuating factors. The broad range of perpetuating factors necessitates

TABLE 80.7
Joint Measurement Chart

					Date	Motion	Average/Range	Date					
					Upper Extremity								
					Examiner			Examiner					
					Left Shoulder	Exercise	45	Right Shoulder					
						Flexion	100						
						Range	225						
						Abduction	180						
						Adduction	0						
						Range	180						
						Lateral Rotation	90						
						Medial Rotation	70						
						Range	160						
					Left Elbow	Extension	0	Right Elbow					
						Flexion	145						
						Range	145						
					Left Forearm	Supination	90	Right Forearm					
						Pronation	90						
						Range	180						
					Left Wrist	Extension	70	Right Wrist					
						Flexion	80						
						Range	150						
						Ulnar Deviation	45						
						Radial Deviation	20						
						Range	65						
					Lower Extremity								
					Date	Motion	Average/Range	Date					
					Examiner			Examiner					
					Left Hip	Extension	10	Right Hip					
						Flexion	125						
						Range	135						
						Abduction	45						
						Adduction	10						
						Range	55						
						Lateral Rotation	45						
						Medial Rotation	45						
						Range	90						
					Left Knee	Extension	0	Right Knee					
						Flexion	140						
						Range	140						
					Left Ankle	Plantar Flexion	45	Right Ankle					
						Dorsi Flexion	20						
						Range	65						
					Left Foot	Inversion	40	Right Foot					
						Eversion	20						
						Range	60						

Note: From *Muscles Testing and Function* (4th ed.), by F. Kendall, E. McCreary, & P. Provance, 1993, Baltimore: Williams & Wilkins. Reproduced with permission.

the expertise of a number of health care professionals including, but not limited to, acupuncturists, chiropractors, dentists, homeopaths, internists, manual therapists, naturopaths, neurologists, nutritionists, osteopaths, podiatrists, physiatrists, psychologists, psychiatrists, pulmonologists, and rheumatologists. It is important to address many of the perpetuating factors identified in the initial evaluation to set the best possible stage for treatment. Unattended, these perpetuating factors undermine the results of trigger point release. Released, but reactivated

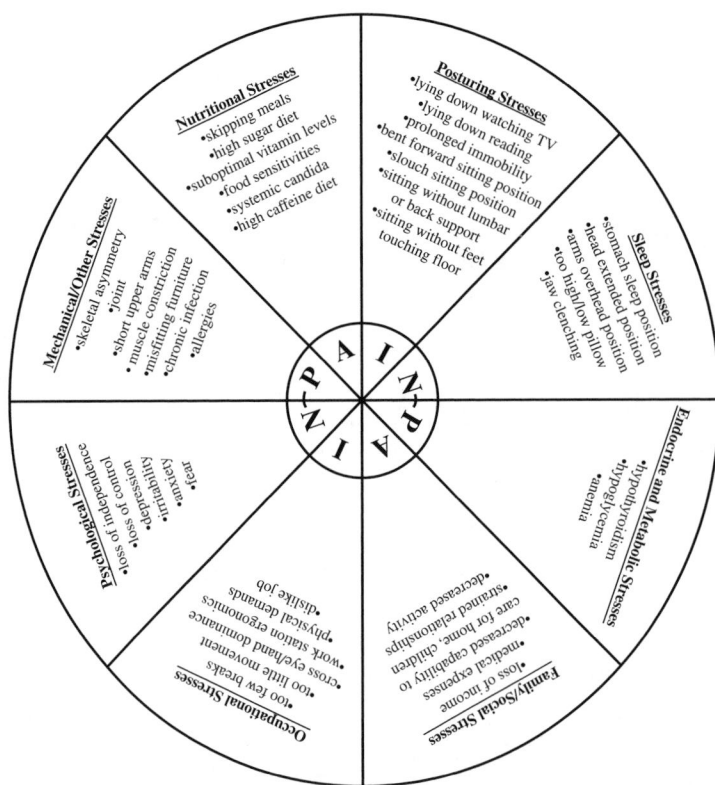

FIGURE 80.7 Common myofascial perpetuating factors. (From Shaw, unpublished, 1992.)

by perpetuating factors, interference brings frustration to both the patient and the clinician. One simply treads water with no resolution of the pain. Table 80.8 helps delineate the role of some of the various practitioners that may be needed in the treatment of the perpetuating factors of myofascial pain syndrome.

Mechanical Stresses

Introduction

Mechanical stressors, most commonly skeletal asymmetry and disproportions, perpetuate trigger points in most patients with persistent myofascial pain syndrome (Travell & Simon, 1983). Disproportional mechanical stressors include short upper arms and Dudley Morton's foot. Asymmetry includes small hemipelvis and leg length discrepancy. Other mechanical stressors can include hypermobility, structural scoliosis, and cross eye–hand dominance.

Lower Limb-Length Inequality

Lower limb-length inequality (LLLI), commonly referred to as a short leg, is a major perpetuating factor of trigger points in the quadratus lumborum musculature. Usually LLLI is not a precipitating factor but rather only comes into play when the quadratus lumborum suffers the activation of a trigger point. In some instances a heel lift under the short leg is all that is necessary to resolve the back pain. In other instances (when pain is long-standing or

several painful episodes have occurred), the trigger points must be released first.

In Travell and Simons book, *Myofascial pain & dysfunction: The lower extremities, Vol. 2,* the authors explain in detail the procedure for measuring LLLI by radiographic measurement. For our purposes, we detail the clinical testing of leg length.

When a short leg is suspected in the patient with low back pain, clinicians recommend that the patient first be examined for quadratus lumborum trigger points and, if present, that they be inactivated. An attempt to measure LLLI in the presence of trigger point shortening of the quadratus lumborum is likely to produce a misleading result (Travell & Simon, 1983).

The undressed patient stands with the back to examiner and with both knees straight. The feet are placed approximately 6 inches apart, and an estimate of leg length difference is made by palpating the iliac crests or posterior superior iliac spines. An approximate correction is placed beneath the short leg, making sure that the patient finds it comfortable. Pages of a pad or small magazine are convenient. The patient is distracted for a minute or two and is encouraged to relax and let the weight settle on both feet. As the muscles are relieved of their attempt to compensate for the difference in leg length, they release their protective control and relax. It is then possible to accurately compensate any remaining LLLI by adding correction until pelvis and shoulders are level and, most impor-

TABLE 80.8
Interdisciplinary Teamwork for Addressing Myofascial Perpetuating Factors

Perpetuating Factor	Major Complaint/Pain	Clinician
Mechanical	Low back	Therapist
	Shoulder	Osteopath
	Hip neck	Chiropractor
	Sciatica	Physiatrist
	Knee	
	Headache	
Hypermobility	Tendon attachment	Physiatrist
	Joint	Physical therapist
		Trainer
Endocrine/metabolic	Hypothyroidism	Endocrinologist
	Hypoglycemia	Rheumatologist
	Anemia	Acupuncturist
	Wilson's syndrome	Internist
Sleep disturbances	Difficulty getting to sleep	Rheumatologist
	Difficulty staying asleep	Naturopath
	Sleep apnea	Homeopath
		Pulmonologist
		Acupuncture
Postural	Head tilt/neck/shoulder	Therapist
	Headache	Osteopath
	Scapula/mid-back	Chiropractor
	Low back	Orthogonal practitioner
	Esophageal reflux	Biophysics practitioner
	Abdominal cramping	Neurologist
	Constipation/diarrhea	Physiatrist
	Dizziness	
	Numbness/tingling in hands/feet	
Nutritional	Headache	Therapist
	Dizziness	Nutritionist
	Fatigue	
	Weakness	
	Restless legs	
Occupational	Neck/shoulder	Therapist
	Mid-back	Occupational therapist
	Low back	Ergonomics specialist
		Psychologist
		Psychiatrist
		Therapist
Psychological	Depression	Psychologist
	Anxiety/fear	Psychiatrist
	Obsessive	Therapist
	Anger	
Family/social	Frustration/anxiety	Therapist
	Low self-esteem	Psychologist
	Depression	Friends

Note: From P. Kozey & N. Shaw, unpublished, 2004.

tantly, the spine is straight. The efficacy of the lift can be tested using applied kinesiology or the lift can be moved under the long leg. In either case, the patient can feel and see the difference (Travell & Simon, 1983).

Some additional points of examination are helpful. The arm on the side of the short leg tends to hang away from the body, while the arm on the other side rests against it. Narrowing at the waist and bulge of the hip appear greater on the side of the long leg. The border of the gluteal fold appears lower on the short side. Skin folds are present or more numerous in the flank of the concave side of the lumbar spine (Travell & Simon, 1983).

The clinician should be cautious when using the heel lifts. They should be avoided if the lumbar spine is not flexible. The senior author of this chapter has found that supporting what looks like the longer leg in a person with a pronounced or structural scoliosis has had beneficial effects. This takes some of the stress off the musculature supporting the structural imbalance. This is not always true, and patients must be followed closely to make sure that a bad situation does not become worse. Regardless of the size of the discrepancy, the heel lift initially should not be more than 1/4 inch high. A lift that is higher than that is too much for the body to handle all at once. As the body adjusts, more lift can be added. Anything more that 1/2 inch requires a lift that covers the whole foot. Preferably, the lift should be built into the sole of the shoe (Chaitow & DeLany, 2002, p. 328).

It is also recommended that during the course of treatment, which may include chiropractic or osteopathic adjustments, the LLLI be checked regularly. Adjustments should be made in the height of the lift when appropriate.

Small Hemipelvis

Patients with a pelvis that is small in its vertical dimension on one side tend to sit crookedly, leaning toward the small side. They often cross one knee over the other to lift up the low side in attempt to even the iliac crests and balance the body. The quadratus lumborum is the muscle primarily affected by axial distortions in the lumbar region. In addition, the scalene and sternocleidomastoid muscles of the neck are heavily overloaded by the tilt of the upper thorax. These are not the only muscles affected, but they are the major ones (Travell & Simons, 1983).

For examination, the patient should be seated on a hard, flat surface with the back and buttocks exposed, in a position to be observed from behind. The feet should be high enough that the patient can slip the fingers between the thigh and the front edge of the seat. Examination of the pelvis, back, and shoulders is similar to that for a short leg, with specific attention paid to scoliosis, position of the posterior superior iliac spine, the relative heights of the iliac crests, and tilting of the shoulder-girdle axis. If, through examination, it is found that the pelvis is twisted,

this obliquity should be corrected prior to correction with a butt lift (Travell & Simons, 1983).

The amount of seated correction for a small hemipelvis is determined by adding increments of lift beneath the ischial tuberosity on the small side until the spine is straightened and the pelvis is leveled. The correction determined on a hard surface must be approximately doubled for a moderately soft chair, and tripled for a very soft sofa (Travell & Simons, 1983). Once a patient becomes comfortable with the correction, all muscles having been balanced and structure aligned, the patient may want to make various sizes of ischial lifts with attractive covers to leave on chairs or seats that are used regularly, i.e., desk chair, car seat, sofa, or favorite reading chair.

Morton Foot Structure or Long Second Metatarsal

Dudley J. Morton described the Morton foot structure. It is not to be confused with the metatarsalgia of Morton's neuroma, described by Thomas G. Morton.

The Morton foot has a relatively long second and short first metatarsal bone. This may perpetuate pain in the low back, hip, thigh, knee, leg, and dorsum of the foot. These patients consistently give a history of weak ankles; they say that they frequently have turned and sprained these joints (Travell & Simons, 1983).

When the first metatarsal is relatively short, the second metatarsal bears more weight. Not only is the second metatarsal longer, but because of this foot structure, it is located a bit more toward the plantar surface of the foot. As a result, the foot, balanced on the second metatarsal during weight bearing, rocks as if on a knife-edge. To compensate for this, most people modify their gait so that the lateral side of the heel and the medial side of the sole show excessive wear. Usually the foot is slightly externally rotated on heel strike and during stance phase. The ankle rocks inward (pronates) everting the foot at the ankle during and after the stance phase. The knee swings in toward the other knee as the thigh internally rotates (Travell & Simons, 1983).

The authors have observed that people with severe pronation often walk with their knees rubbing up against each other. Those with slight or moderate pronation add one more movement to the post stance phase. The knee moves laterally trying to regain the correct position over the foot.

The gait usually activates myofascial trigger points in the posterior gluteus medius muscle. The rocking foot also places a great strain on the peroneus longus muscle. Taut bands of these trigger points may entrap the peroneal nerve against the fibula immediately below its head, producing numbness and tingling across the dorsum of the foot and sometimes motor weakness with foot drop. Other muscles with activated trigger points are posterior gluteus minimus, vastus medialis, tensor fascia latae, iliotibial band, sartorius, tibialis anterior, and extensor digitorum longus (Travell & Simons, 1983).

This syndrome is greatly aggravated by a shoe that is tight because it is too small or has a tight cap over the toes, and by high heels or shoes with pointy toes. Also, shoes should bend relatively easily at approximately the head of the metatarsals. Some shoes do not bend at all or they bend at the toes. This will be detrimental to a normal gait (Travell & Simons, 1983).

To examine for Morton foot structure, the clinician should flex the toes so that the metatarsal heads are prominent. By marking the heads with a pen, the long second metatarsal becomes obvious. Remember to measure the metatarsal heads and not the toe length. A long second metatarsal does not necessarily correlate with a long second toe. The long web between the second and third toes is characteristic of Morton foot structure. Because of the abnormal distribution of weight, most individuals with a Morton foot will develop calluses. They occur under the head of the second metatarsal, lateral to the fifth metatarsal under the medial side of the head of the first metatarsal, and on the medial side of the great toe along the interphalangeal joint (Travell & Simons, 1992; Figure 80.8).

To correct for the Morton foot structure, Morton recommended inserting into the shoe a leather insole with a leather build up of 1/8 to 3/16 inch under the head of only the first metatarsal bone. He also added a pad of sponge rubber behind the first to fifth metatarsal heads, which supported the shafts of all five metatarsal bones. In the office one can simply use two thicknesses of Molefoam (Dr. Scholl's Molefoam, distributed by Schering Plough Healthcare Products, Inc., Memphis, TN) under the first metatarsal head. If the heel of the shoe is too wide for the foot, a felt pad can be added along the medial side of the heel (Travell & Simons, 1983).

If the Morton foot structure is accompanied by excessive pronation or structural misalignment, a referral to a podiatrist and/or chiropractor is in order.

Short Upper Arms

Shortness of upper arms is a rarely recognized, but not uncommon, source of muscle strain and perpetuation of trigger points in the shoulder girdle musculature (Travell & Simons, 1983). If the shoulder–elbow segment of the upper extremity is short in proportion to the rest of the body, the elbows do not reach the iliac crests when subject is standing with elbows bent at a 90° angle. When the person is sitting, the elbows fail to reach the armrests of the usual chair. This structural anomaly places undue stress on the upper trapezius, levator scapulae, and scalenes, thus perpetuating trigger points in these muscles. If a person spends an unduly long period of time leaning down to rest arms on the armrest, other muscles, such as the quadratus lumborum, can be affected.

Chairs, sofas, car seats, etc. that a patient uses regularly should have the arms built up so that elbows rest on them without the patient's leaning to one side, pushing shoulders up, or having the weight of the arms exerting a constant pull on the shoulder girdle musculature.

Hypermobility

"Double jointed" or "loose ligaments" are two other names for hypermobility. This condition is frequently overlooked because clinicians are trained to look for reduced, not increased, range of motion (Travell & Simons, 1992). Hypermobility stresses the muscles because they are constantly working to stabilize joints. A person with this perpetuating factor presents a complicated picture. The complete MTPT protocol does not apply when dealing with these patients.

When there are trigger points in the muscles that cross hypermobile joints, the trigger points should be inactivated using techniques that do not extend the muscles to maximum length (Travel & Simons, 1992). Normal MTPT pressure release techniques call for a muscle to be placed on a limited or partial stretch during this procedure. The full passive stretch after pressure should be eliminated. Trigger point pressure release at the attachment trigger points, vapocoolant with stretch of the affected muscles, and a stretch rehabilitation program done with great frequency are counterproductive when treating these patients. Instead, the central trigger points in the belly of the muscle must be released and the muscle must be stretched manually (massage therapy). Also, the patient should *not* be given a stretch rehabilitation program to do at home. Experience teaches that a stretch program may actually cause more pain than it relieves. A muscle-specific strengthening program coupled with manual stretching and limited joint movement during the treatment phase will provide the most relief. Strengthening acts to stabilize joints; think football players who destroy ligaments in their knees. Their rehabilitation program consists of strengthening the muscles around the knee to stabilize it. People with hypermobility syndrome must stabilize all joints by strengthening and balancing the muscles around them.

Another method for stabilizing the joints is prolotherapy. Hackett pioneered the use of controlled irritation of relaxed ligamentous tissues to achieve proliferation with minimal scarring, with a view to enhancing stability of the weakened structures (Chaitow & DeLany, 2002). The key to success was increased collagen formation and hyperplasia of the ligament tissue without evidence of histological damage. This is accomplished by the injection of a solution of tissue irritant into the connective tissue. The most common appears to be a glucose solution. The resulting proliferation of ligamentous tissue serves to strengthen and stabilize the joint. It is recommended that these two treatment methods be attempted before enter-

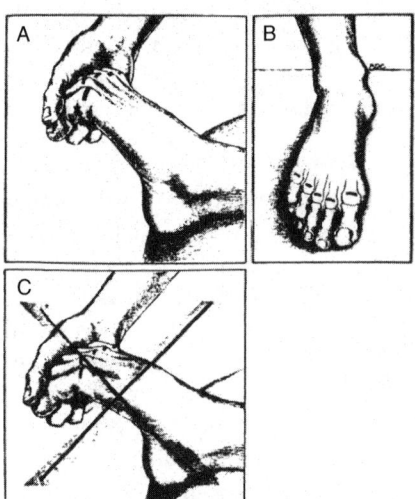

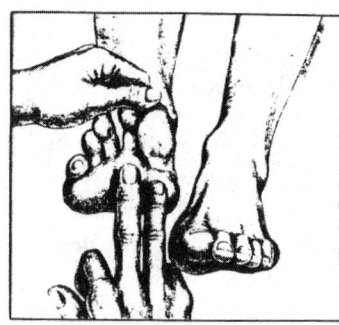

Plantar palpation of the distal ends of
the first two metatarsal heads, during strong extension
of the toes, demonstrates the Morton foot structure (a
relatively short first and long second metatarsal).

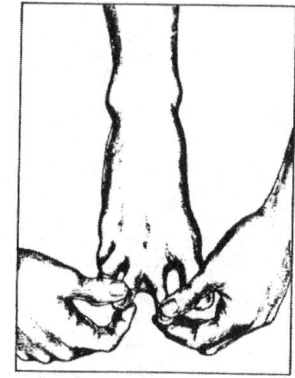

The long web between the second and
third toes is characteristic of the Morton foot structure
(a relatively short first and long second metatarsal).

Examination of the Morton foot struc-
ture. *Black marks* locate the metatarsal heads in all
positions. A, medial side view, good technique: flexion
of the toes at the metatarsophalangeal joints and neutral position of the metatarsals proximally. B, standing
weight-bearing position. *Black marks* clearly reveal
the relatively short first and long second metatarsals.
C. incorrect way of marking the metatarsal heads: the
metatarsal bones are also flexed proximally at the tar-
sometatarsal joints, restricting flexion of the toes at the
metatarsophalangeal joints.

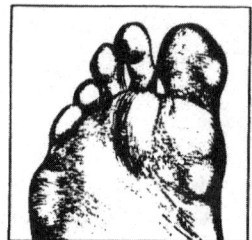

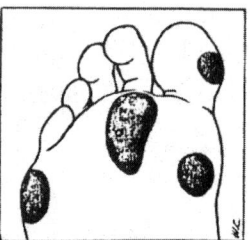

Calluses frequently associated with the
Morton foot structure. The second toe usually extends
farther from the foot than the first toe when the second
metatarsal is longer than the first metatarsal. Thick
calluses may develop under the head of the second

metatarsal, and lateral to the head of the fifth metatarsal. Another callus occurs under the medial side of the
head of the first metatarsal and still another usually
appears on the medial side of the great toe along the
interphalangeal joint.

FIGURE 80.8 Screening for Morton's foot structure.

taining surgery for hypermobile joints (Chaitow &
DeLany, 2002).

Cross Eye–Hand Dominance

Cross eye–hand dominance occurs when a person's right
hand and left eye are dominant or vice versa. To determine
which eye is dominant, have the patient perform the following test. Extend arms in front, palms facing away, at
approximately eye level. Form a small triangle with the
thumbs at the bottom and the web between thumb and
forefingers serving as the sides. Keeping both eyes open,
look through this triangular opening at an object across
the room. This object should just obscure the opening.
While holding this position, close one eye and then the
other. When the object remains in approximately the same
place, the eye that has remained open is the dominant eye.
When the dominant eye is closed, the object appears to
shift to one side or the other, and, in some instances, seems
to move out of the opening completely.

People with this perpetuating factor (PF) frequently
complain of upper back and neck pain and headaches.
Patients should be instructed in ways to avoid various

postural positions. Most of us have been taught that, when writing, the paper should be situated under the dominant hand and forearm and slightly toward the dominant hand side of the centerline of the body. In order for the dominant eye to focus on the work, the head tilts or rotates toward the side of the dominant hand. Holding one's head in this rotated or cocked position causes the muscles on one side of the neck and upper back to be held in a shortened position. On the other side the muscles are put on a constant stretch. Either or both of these positions can perpetuate neck and upper back pain and headaches. A simple solution to this problem is to move the paper more in line with the nondominant hand or to the midline of the body.

Other suggestions to thwart this perpetuating factor are as follows:

1. At the computer workstation, place work to the side of the dominant eye.
2. In the theater, concert, or lecture hall sit on the side of the dominant hand. In other words, left eye dominant people should sit on the right side of the theater, and vice versa.

Nutritional Inadequacies

Vital in the treatment of myofascial pain syndrome are strong, adequate levels of vitamins and minerals. Travell and Simons state that nearly half of patients seen for chronic myofascial pain require attention to inadequate nutritional levels in order to obtain lasting pain elimination. They also state that without sufficient levels of vitamins and minerals the body needs to make metabolic adjustments because coenzyme vitamins are limited. There is good reasoning to state that "normal" serum levels of nutrients are not necessarily "optimal" tissue level (Travell & Simons, 1983). To ensure optimal myofascial syndrome resolution, it is important to set the treatment stage with optimal levels of tissue nutrition.

Vitamin and mineral levels lower than required for good muscle health may come from decreased food intake, decreased supplementation, decreased absorption, decreased utilization, increased metabolic requirements, and increased exertion. Elderly individuals face these same complications along with increased destruction in the body and a less efficient functioning system. Once educated by the clinician, the patient with myofascial pain can address some of the very basic nutritional problems. Issues to include in patient education follow:

- Many patients with chronic myofascial pain skip meals, usually breakfast, but frequently breakfast and lunch. Their rationale for this is that they are not hungry in the morning, do not have time to eat in the morning, and are too busy for lunch. It is critical to begin the day, especially the workday, with nutrients for muscle function and ongoing muscle rehabilitation. Nutrients from the previous evening's meal have been used during the night and reserves are just not available. Many afternoon headaches have been traced to skipping breakfast and lunch.

- Many patients with chronic myofascial pain are using empty nutritional foods as fillers, for example, coffee or coffee and a bagel for breakfast: donuts, pastries, pretzels, crackers, coffee, and sodas at work. Carbohydrates of refined flour, refined sugar, and coffee not only provide no nutritional value to the system, but often use nutrition to digest them. Eating these foods fills the patients and interferes with more nutritious fruits, vegetables, and protein. Many an afternoon's increase in pain, and particularly an increase in headaches, comes from the abundance of high filler foods and high sugar intake.

- Many patients with chronic myofascial pain, in spite of the rise in the high-protein, low-carbohydrate diets gracing the market, are not eating adequate protein for good muscle function, particularly protein without undue high saturated fat. For most people breakfast does not include protein during the work week. Breakfast tends to be cereal (refined), bagel (nutritionally empty and refined), breakfast bars (high sugar and fat), breakfast drinks (high sugar), or nothing. Lunch may be a salad with vegetables (but no protein), sandwich (protein but refined flour bread), fast food (protein but high fat), pasta (nutritionally empty and refined), etc. Of course, there are those who eat well, but the patients routinely seen for chronic pain tend to eat high glycemic index and sugar foods. The recommended protein may be a small amount (e.g., four to five almonds) but the frequency of the protein tends to even the metabolism and provided the necessary impetus for muscle function efficiency.

- Many patients with chronic myofascial pain eat a diet high in refined sugar. The average American now consumes 152 pounds of sweeteners/sugars annually, a rise of almost 1,500% in the last 200 years (Gittleman, 1996)! The evolution of our bodies does not even begin to progress at a rate that would allow them to deal with the changes sugar causes internally. Besides being an extremely nutritionally empty additive, refined sugar creates an imbalance in the synergistic balance of minerals. Our own minerals are used just to digest it. Minerals are necessary for protein metabolism and proper muscle function. The mineral imbalance results in muscles being more vulnerable to tension and spasm.

- Sugar weakens the immune system primarily by upsetting the synergistic balance of minerals. It interferes with the transport of vitamin C in the body. Vitamin C inadequacy can result in aching muscles and joints. With frequent prescriptions of antibiotics as a result of the illness from a weaken immune system and patients eating a diet high in refined sugar, it is not uncommon to find patients with chronic myofascial pain suffering from systemic *Candida*. The overgrowth of bacteria can result in many diffuse symptoms including many experienced by the patient with myofascial pain: fatigue, lethargy, insomnia, lack of concentration, muscle weakness, muscle achiness, dizziness, depression, and anxiety.
- Many patients with chronic myofascial pain are eating foods and combining foods in such a way that results in an acidic pH in the system. "Muscle movement takes place because of the body's use of the gravity force of attraction and repulsion. The background pH maintains the balance of forces that allows chemical reaction to take place" (Judd & Judd, 2004, p. 125)
- Many patients with chronic myofascial pain, for some of the reasons mentioned above, harbor inadequate levels of vitamins and minerals, particularly B_1, B_6, B_{12}, folic acid, C, calcium, iron, and potassium. When testing for nutritional levels, it is critical to understand that "normal" serum vitamin and mineral levels does not assure "optimal" nutritional levels. "The prevalence of unrecognized hypovitaminosis is distressingly high" (Travell & Simons, 1983, p. 115).

Vital to the successful treatment of myofascial pain and dysfunction is the resolution of nutritional inadequacies.

- **B_1 Inadequacy** can result in an increased susceptibility to myofascial trigger points and a resistance to local treatment. (See Table 80.9 for signs and symptoms of marginal deficiency in B_1, thiamine.) Perhaps this is due to the need for thiamine for many steps in the process of energy production (Teitelbaum, 2001). B_1 levels are easily detected using the aluminum–magnesium alloy long period tuning fork. According to Travell and Simons this reveals the graded loss of vibratory perception in relation to fiber length. The greater the discrepancy between the distal (big toe) and proximal (hand), the greater the deficiency of B_1 (Travell & Simons, 1983).

- **B_6 Inadequacy** (See Table 80.10 for signs and symptoms of marginal deficiency of B_6, pyridoxine.)
- **B_{12} Inadequacy** (See Table 80.11 for signs and symptoms of marginal deficiency of B_{12}, cobalamin.)
- **Vitamin C Inadequacy** (See Table 80.12 for signs and symptoms of marginal deficiency of vitamin C.)
- **Folic Acid Inadequacy** (See Table 80.13 for signs and symptoms of marginal deficiency of folic acid.)
- **Calcium Inadequacy** results in decreases in muscular contracture mechanism and increases in trigger point irritability.
- **Potassium Inadequacy** decreases rapid repolarization of the nerve and muscle cell membranes following an action potential (Travell & Simons, 1983).
- **Iron Inadequacy** decreases oxygen transport to and within muscles.
- **Magnesium Inadequacy** decreases contractile mechanism of myofilaments (Travell & Simons, 1983).

Metabolic and Endocrine Inadequacies

Sonkin and Rachlin state, "Failure to recognize a metabolic cause of myofascial symptoms may result in prolonged, ineffective therapy, visits to a variety of therapists, and occasionally one or more fruitless surgical procedures" (1994, p. 45). While all metabolic inadequacies affect skeletal muscles and may be the cause of trigger points, the clinician may most often need to evaluate the patient for hypothyroidism (see Table 80.14). Patients who are even borderline low hypothyroid experience diffuse weakness and stiffness particularly of the shoulder girdle, trigger points, dry skin and hair, cold intolerance, weight gain, and muscle cramps. Because the primary function of the thyroid hormone is the control of cellular metabolism, the patients with myofascial pain are more susceptible to trigger points due to an inadequate supply of energy for muscle contraction. According to Weintraub's statement from the National Institutes of Health (NIH): "Thyroid hormone resistance syndrome may affect thousands of unsuspecting Americans" (Weintraub, 1991). In the face of current evidence correlating symptoms of hypothyroidism with unresolved myofascial trigger points, it seems reasonable to offer a low therapeutic trial of replacement thyroid, which is frequently effective (Sonkin & Rachlin, 1994). In hyperthyroidism, on the other hand, active trigger points are uncommon.

TABLE 80.9
Vitamin B₁ (Thiamine)

Clinical Evaluation of Marginal Deficiency

Symptoms	Signs	Laboratory Findings
Dry Beriberi		
Pain localized to any body areas, related to physical overload	Active trigger points in muscles refer pain and tenderness patterns that match pain complaints	RBC: Transketolase activity diminished
	Ankle jerks — sluggish or absent	
Paresthesias bilateral	Impaired vibratory perception: (higher threshold) greatest compared with hands; least compared with feet, compared with hearing (in relation to nerve fiber length)	Low T4 (RIA)
Lower extremities — Primary		Low thyroid function improved by thiamine supplement
Upper extremities — Secondary		
Difficulty in making simple decisions		
Constipation	Motor	Serum cholesterol mid to high normal
	Weakness of muscles on exertion	
Calf cramps — any time		Anemia infrequent
Sleep impaired	Sensory	
	Dysesthesia	
Tinnitus, if also niacin deficiency		
No cold intolerance unless thyroid and/or folate deficiency/inadequacy		
Wet Beriberi		
Edema, cardiac	Pitting edema of feet, ankles, lower legs	
Shortness of breath		
Tachycardia, resting		

Factors Contributing to Thiamine Deficiency

Tea drinking at meals (tannin binds thiamine and prevents absorption)
Antacids at meals
Diet low in coffee, fresh nuts, potatoes
Alcohol, high intake

Note: Thyroid medication increases metabolic need for thiamine and may precipitate severe thiamine deficiency. From J. G. Travell, unpublished, 1987.

Hypoglycemia

Hypoglycemia is a metabolic disorder that aggravates myofascial trigger point activity and reduces or shortens the positive response to specific myofascial therapy. Recurrent hypoglycemic attacks perpetuate myofascial trigger points. There are two kinds of hypoglycemia, fasting and postprandial. They occur for different reasons, but present the same symptoms. Both of these disrupt the energy supply for muscle contraction, thereby perpetuating pain and dysfunction (Travell & Simons, 1999).

The initial symptoms of hypoglycemia or of increased epinephrine are usually sweating, trembling and shakiness, a fast heart rate, and a feeling of anxiety. Activation of sternocleidomastoid trigger points may cause headache and dizziness (Travell & Simons, 1999).

Insulin Resistance

Insulin resistance has been mentioned in relation to the perpetuating of myofascial trigger points in relation to menopause and the luteal phase of the menstrual cycle. It has been linked to a decrease in estrogen levels (Lowe, 2000). In the past estrogen replacement has been suggested to decrease insulin resistance. Recent research findings linking estrogen replacement with increased levels of breast cancer would mitigate against this course at this time.

In Syndrome X, there appears to be a genetic defect that causes resistance of the skeletal muscle cells to insulin. The insulin receptor may be the defective locus. Researchers have found reduced numbers of insulin receptors in skeletal muscle cell membranes in obese subjects, only some of whom have diabetes. The resistance involves desensitization due to excess exposure of cell membranes to insulin (Lowe, 2000).

The authors cannot emphasize enough the part that metabolic disorders play in perpetuating myofascial trigger point pain and dysfunction. In the case of stubborn pain problems, patients should be referred for a complete endocrine workup.

TABLE 80.10
Vitamin B$_6$ (Pyridoxine, Pyridoxal)

Clinical Evaluation of Marginal Deficiency

Symptoms	Signs	Laboratory Findings
Chronic pain, anywhere in body, often head and neck	Active myofascial trigger points refer pain in patterns that match patient's complaints; only transient relief by trigger point therapy	Serum vitamin B$_6$ low Urinary vitamin B$_6$ and tryptophan decreased
Motion sickness (boat, car, airplane) Nausea and vomiting first trimester of pregnancy		Symptoms promptly relieved by therapeutic trial of vitamin B$_6$ moderate dosage (100 mg daily)
Fatigue, lethargy	Anemia	Microcytic or macrocytic
Weakness	Ankle jerks reduced	Peripheral neuropathy
Muscle twitching	Vibratory perception diminished	
Soreness of wrist, tingling in first three digits	Carpal tunnel syndrome, atrophy thenar muscles	Median nerve compression by carpal ligament
Skin scaly, greasy patches	Seborrheic dermatitis	Vitamin B$_6$, cofactor for many enzymes, complex actions
Lips dry, fissures	Chelosis	
Sore tongue	Glossitis	
Kidney pain, attacks due to renal calculi	Oxaluria and oxalate kidney stones	Genetic defect, corrected by lifetime vitamin B$_6$ supplement 200–300 mg/day
Impaired vision	Eye, dislocation of lens	Genetic defect, homocystinuria, relieved by lifetime vitamin B$_6$ 300–500 mg/day
Cardiac dysfunction	Thrombosis of arteries and veins, cardiac failure	
Convulsions, newborn		Mother deficient in vitamin B$_6$

Tissue Reserves of Vitamin B$_6$ Depleted by
Contraceptive pill
Isoniazid (antitubercular)
Levodopa (for Parkinson's disease)
Alcohol

Note: From J. G. Travell, unpublished, 1987.

Posture: Sleeping, Sitting, Standing

Postures patients use during the day and at night can reinforce or counteract any treatment being administered. The best treatment, with the best neuromuscular retraining, can be undone by habitual positions that compromise muscle resting neutrality. Have patients bring photographs of themselves in their various sleep positions, sitting, watching television, using the computer, work positions, driving, and any other things they do frequently. The clinician will never get the same information from interacting verbally with the patient that can be obtained from the pictures. Their beds, pillows, chairs, sofas, sewing, working in the yard or on the car, workstation postures cannot be adequately described. The pictures are all telling!

Sleeping posture is one of the most common postural perpetuating factors maintaining trigger point activity. Stomach sleeping with head rotation results in significant contraction of the trapezius, levator scapulae, sternocleidomastoid, and posterior cervical muscles. If these muscles already harbor latent or active trigger points, the rotated position reinforces the "learned" shortened function of the muscle. The opposing muscles are on significant stretch and can react with a rebound effect when the head is returned to neutral. The arms in the stomach sleep position are often raised in an overhead position. This shortens the levator scapulae and splenius cervicis, lifts the rib cage and scapulae, and thus shortens the scalenii, serratus anterior and posterior, and the rhomboid major and minor. Other muscles, pectoralis, latissimus dorsi, coracobrachialis, and rotator cuff, are also in compromised positions. Looking at the trigger point pain patterns, it is no wonder the patient wakes during the night or in the morning with a headache, stiff neck, and back pain. Stomach sleeping usually places the feet in plantar flexion, thus contracting the calf muscles. Leg cramps and the beginnings of plantar fasciitis can result. Stomach sleeping is out! Place a tennis ball below the xiphoid process held in place loosely by an ace bandage. When the patient rolls onto the stomach, the tennis ball applies pressure to the solar plexus that knocks the air out of the patient. It only takes a couple of times of trying this before the stomach sleep habit is tamed.

A half side, half stomach sleep position further compromises neutral positioning by rotating the hips and flex-

TABLE 80.11
Vitamin B$_{12}$ (Cobalamin)

Clinical Evaluation of Marginal Deficiency

Symptoms	Signs	Laboratory Findings
Muscle pain and stiffness, often in low back and lower extremities	Active trigger points in muscles refer pain and tenderness in patterns that match pain complaints	Serum vitamin B$_{12}$ low (not optimal); 1,000 is optimal — no known toxic effects to injections of B$_{12}$
Ticklish	Startle reaction (body jump) to light touch	Subacute combined degeneration of spinal cold, without anemia if folic acid tissue reserves are adequate
Paresthesias of lower extremities bilateral; later of upper extremities		
Hypersensitive to noise	Hyperacusis	Pernicious (megaloblastic) anemia, but only if acid deficiency also exists
Fatigue and weakness	Ankle jerks hyperactive, Babinski reflex may be present	
Poor balance	Position sense impaired (positive Romberg sing)	
Diarrhea, often bowel disease (Crohn's sprue)	Tongue coated white (malabsorption)	Lack of gastric intrinsic factor (Schilling test positive) and achlorhydria with malabsorption (decreased hydrochloric acid)
		Microscopic abnormalities of gastric epithelium
		Stool examination may show fish tapeworm, which eats vitamin B$_{12}$

Note: Supplements with vitamin B$_{12}$ stimulate the metabolism of bone marrow and increase the need for folic acid. From J. G. Travell, unpublished, 1987.

ing one leg. This torque position on the quadratus lumborum and abdominal obliques and the sustained shortening of the iliopsoas create a setting for active trigger point low back, hip and groin pain. Side sleeping using pillows or similar props in front of the body will help break this torqued, flexed position.

Side sleeping can be used if one stays in a neutral position without curling into a fetal position and without rounding the thoracic and cervical spine with a head forward translation. The curled position shortens the pectoralis major and minor, especially if the top arm is allowed to fall in front of the body or with the arms curled or flexed at the elbow and wrist. This is often a precursor to carpal tunnel syndrome from the shortened biceps, brachialis, and forearm flexors and shortened scalenii. The lower arm should not be elevated overhead under the pillow or head, which affects the same muscular as in the overhead arm position of stomach sleeping. The side position should allow for the shoulders to be down/in a neutral position. Also shortened in the fetal position are the rectus abdominis and iliopsoas, both with low back/lumbosacral trigger point pain patterns. The legs should be extended almost straight with the body in neutral position.

Back sleep position if often difficult for patients but usually maintains the most neutral position of the body.

The pillow should be under the head, not the shoulders, and should hold the head in straight alignment. Contoured and special material pillows can be used, if they fit! It is not uncommon, however, to find these pillows fit only a few patients accurately. Note that the head should not be held flexed, extended, or laterally flexed. A small pillow or elevation can be placed under the knees to reduce lumbar strain. Minimize calf plantar flexion strain by loosening the covers at the end of the bed or by placing a pillow at the bottom to hold the covers off the feet.

Sitting posture should maintain neutral positioning. Hip, shoulder, and ear should be in a straight-line alignment. When a slouched or rounded posture is taken, the head juts forward. This results in considerable strain on the posterior cervical musculature as it attempts to hold the weight of the head against gravity. The cervical curve begins to straighten resulting in undue stress on the posterior disk space. The rounded posture shortens the anterior musculature, particularly the pectorals, coracobrachialis, anterior serratus, and rectus abdominis. The antagonists are strained on stretch to maintain posture.

The rounded/slouched sitting posture positions the pelvis in a posterior tilt. If the posture becomes habitual, there can frequently be ligamentous changes which tend to maintain that posterior tilt when standing. This significantly limits iliopsoas range of motion.

TABLE 80.12
Vitamin C (Ascorbic Acid)

Clinical Evaluation of Marginal Deficiency

Symptoms	Signs	Laboratory Findings
Post-exercise stiffness, aching muscles and joints, several hours or next day after exercise	Generalized muscle soreness and restricted motion, with trigger points related to regions of acute pain	Low plasma vitamin C (0.6% too low)
Easy bruising (minimal trauma)	Ecchymoses, spotty capillary oozing after needle prick	Capillary fragility increased
Bleeding gums	Petechiae	
Tissue healing slow	Scar formation incomplete: pressure sores	Collagen formation impaired
Subject to cold and infections, postnasal discharge, chronic		Vitamin C prevents replication of viruses
Active allergies	Asthma, hay fever	Adrenal output of corticosteroids improved by vitamin C supplement (2.3% adrenal output parallels vitamin C levels)
Smokes or exposed to cigarette smoke	Smoker's odor	Smoking reduces vitamin C content of adrenal gland
	Post-nasal discharge, chronic	
Fatigue	Pallor, anemia	Iron-deficiency anemia, or macrocytic if either folic acid or vitamin C is low
No paresthesias	Ankle jerks normal	
Male infertility		Sperm in semen stick together

Vitamin C is Destroyed by
Heat — boiling, cooking food
Exposure of food, or person's skin, to fluorescent lighting
Mixing with antacids in stomach

Note: Vitamin C improves absorption of iron and utilization of folic acid. From J. G. Travell, unpublished, 1987.

Sitting in reclining chairs or propped up with cushions while lying on the sofa watching television or reading causes the head to be in a forward and/or flexed position, even if supported. There is a stretch strain on the posterior cervical musculature and a contraction in the anterior musculature. If this becomes a habitual posture, the lower thoracic spine flattens and the upper thoracic spine becomes extremely kyphotic with extension of the cervical spine. Once ligamentous changes begin to accommodate this posture, it becomes quite a challenge to return to normal positioning.

Standing posture is often the culmination of sitting, lying, and sleep postures. To maintain normal standing alignment may require releasing anterior musculature, strengthening weakened overstretched muscles, utilizing joint mobilization, and redeveloping a kinesthetic perception of what "normal" is. Feldenkrais and Alexander techniques are helpful with redefining proper body positioning and movement.

Home and Workstation Ergonomics

Occupational perpetuating factors involve the interaction of humans, machines, and the environment. Our main interest is the human and how we interact with tools,

machines, and environments. The science of ergonomics evolved to address these issues.

Ergonomics recognizes four important facts:

1. Machines and equipment should be designed and prescribed based on recognized human characteristics.
2. Tasks should be structured to enhance ease, efficiency, and safety.
3. Job demands and human capabilities should be matched.
4. People must be made aware of the environment within which they perform (Khalil et al., 1994, p. 488).

As a therapist involved in treating people with acute or chronic pain, the clinician must consider a person in his or her workplace whether that be inside or outside the home. As was mentioned previously, a vital tool for diagnosing the problems inherent in the interaction between human and workplace is photographs of the patient at his or her workstation along with an explanation of the tasks performed. Through these the clinician is able to make suggestions regarding changes in work habits and postures.

TABLE 80.13
Folic Acid

Clinical Evaluation of Marginal Deficiency

Symptoms	Signs	Laboratory Findings
Intolerance to cold (primary)	Low basal body temperature (taken in morning before getting out of bed, or any physical activity, even shaking thermometer)	Serum folate in lowest quartile of "normal average range, or below lower limit of "normal"
Headache and neck pain	Active trigger points in neck and masticatory muscles refer pain and tenderness in patterns that match pain complaints	Spinal fluid folate may be lower than serum folate (blood–brain barrier)
Restless legs, nocturnal, no pain	Dry skin	Serum cholesterol low
No nocturnal calf cramps (night cramps more often low vitamin E)	Bodyweight low	Anemia marginal (may or may not be macrocytic, is microcytic)
Diarrhea, episodic		
Indigestion, gas, and bloating	Abdominal examination normal	Stool examination normal
Pain not aggravated by rainy weather	No weight gain with rainy weather	
No paresthesias	Ankle jerks normal	
	Vibratory perception threshold normal	

Drug-Related Folate Deficiency

Antiepileptic (Dilantin)
Antitubercular (Isoniazid)
Antacids after eating
Alcohol ingestion affecting liver function and therefore decreased folate

Note: From J. G. Travell, unpublished, 1987.

Without a doubt, as computer use has increased, the pain problems associated with this task are increasing rapidly. The conditions have been variously called carpal tunnel syndrome, repetitive strain injury, cumulative trauma, or overuse syndrome. Regardless of the name used to describe this condition, there are two basic activities responsible for the problem. One is holding the muscle in a relatively fixed position, often under load, for prolonged periods. The other is a repetitive movement that gives the muscle incomplete recovery time (Mense et al., 2001). Both are present in computer users who spend long, uninterrupted periods at a workstation. In addition to computer users, assembly line workers also suffer from repetitive strain injury. As companies try to increase productivity or cut costs, they may speed up the line or reduce the number and length of breaks. This is a recipe for disaster for the company and the worker. The worker may develop a chronic pain condition. However, the company loses money to absenteeism and workers' compensation insurance premiums. Every effort should be made to ensure a healthy work environment for employees.

Occupational therapist Barbara Ingram-Rice (1997) lists the following risk factors in the development of carpal tunnel syndrome:

- Computer use (or any work requiring repetitive finger dexterity) for more than 2 to 4 hours per day

- Infrequent rest breaks (suggests 3 to 5 minutes every 30 minutes to stretch the neck, shoulders, and upper extremity)
- Hypermobile joints, as their instability makes these joints more susceptible to injury
- Poor posture, including rounded shoulders and forward head, which encourages nerve entrapment
- Poor technique with activity/work such as holding the phone to the ear with the shoulder, poor sitting postures, or a computer screen set at a less than ideal angle or distance
- Sedentary lifestyle, leading to overall decreased fitness level
- Stressful work environment, leading the person to work harder, not smarter
- Arthritis, diabetes, thyroid disease, or other medical conditions that can accentuate the individual's response to repetitive strain
- Long fingernails, causing awkward use of fingertips
- Excessive alcohol or tobacco consumption, decreasing the body's ability to repair tissue damage
- Obesity, as increased adipose tissue may decrease tunnel space and an overweight person is less likely to properly fit the furniture asso-

TABLE 80.14
Hypothyroidism

Clinical Evaluation of Marginal Hypometabolism

Symptoms	Signs	Laboratory Findings
Intolerance to cold	Low basal body temperature Cold feet and hands	Basal metabolic rate (BMR) low; 97.7–98.5 adequate, 97.0–97.5 marginal, below 97.0 definite
Chronic pain, made worse by mild overload and cooling the body		
Poor sleep and morning stiffness	Active trigger points in muscles, more often in lower extremities; only brief relief by trigger point therapy	Serum T4 (thyroxine) in lowest quartile of "normal" (average range, or lower — most helpful to see)
Intolerance to heat (decreased perspiration)	Perspiration negligible	TSH normal; serum cholesterol high (unless also folic acid inadequacy)
Skin coarse, but often well lubricated with skin cream (dry skin)	Skin rough, thickened over heels and areas of friction	Serum creatine phosphokinase (CPK) high
Hair "won't take a wave"	Hair dry, brittle (eyelashes may be broken/short; eyebrows may be very sparse and/or nonexistent in outer 1/3 of brow)	
Pain worse before and during rainy weather (very typical)	No palpable edema weight gain (fluid) with rainy weather (not cardiovascular)	Water content of muscles increased with humidity and low barometric pressure
Fatigue	Pallor	Anemia, normocytic unless also folic acid inadequacy (macrocytic)
Exhaustion by end of day (decreased muscle stamina)		Blood count shows low % of leukocytes and high % of monocytes
Constipation		
Poor resistance to infections		
Overweight or underweight	Slim underweight person often hyperactive	Body movement generates heat
No paresthesias (unless vitamin B_1 inadequacy)	Ankle jerks normal except for slow relaxation phase	
Tachycardia	Normal blood pressure	Electrocardiographic changes suggestive of myocardial disease
Menses irregular, excess bleeding, or amenorrhea	Occasional hypertension corrected by thyroid supplement	
	Fibrocystic disease of breast	Mammogram, biopsy positive

Thyroid Function Depressed by
Thiamine inadequacy
Radiation of thyroid gland or of person's body

Note: From J. G. Travell, unpublished, 1987.

ciated with the job (Chaitow & DeLany, 2000, p. 394)

For the "risk" factors listed above, we can substitute the phrase "perpetuating" factors. All of these must be addressed when treating a person with computer or repetitive motion-driven pain syndromes.

Sleep Disturbances

Sleep disturbances for the patient with myofascial pain may be due to a number of factors. It is important to identify whether the problem is one of getting to sleep or sleep maintenance. Identify possible reasons for the sleep difficulty. Reasons may include stress, mind or physical exercising activity before going to bed, sleeping too much during the day, eating before going to bed, sleep apnea, or conditions such as hypothyroidism or adrenal fatigue. Identify the severity of the sleep disturbance. If pain is the main interfering factor to sleep, deactivating trigger points along with muscular retraining will be most helpful. Restorative sleep becomes a major factor needing to be addressed if pain is to be eliminated.

Impaired sleep, regardless of the cause, severely affects the body's ability to resolve pain conditions. Impaired sleep conditions include insomnia, sleep apnea, and alpha-delta sleep anomaly.

There are three different kinds of insomnia:

1. The inability to fall asleep
2. The inability to stay asleep
3. A combination of the two (Starlanyl & Copeland, 1996, p. 115)

Sleep apnea means a temporary cessation of respiration. The tissues in the throat relax to the point where airflow is obstructed and the sleeper stops breathing momentarily (Starlanyl & Copeland, 1996). This usually involves the inability to exhale. The sleeper is aroused or comes to a shallower level of sleep and then takes an explosive breath. This arousal has been known to happen up to 100+ times per hour and can make the sleeper feel fatigued and achy upon awakening in the morning.

Alpha-delta sleep anomaly is caused when the alpha waves of nonrestorative sleep interfere with the restful continuous delta waves of deep sleep.

Regardless of the type of sleep impairment, there are ramifications, as muscles that should be repaired and maintained by sleep are not. Moldofsky and Scarisbrick (1976) found muscle tenderness and a sense of physical tiredness in the morning in healthy university students when the slow wave non-REM (rapid eye movement) sleep had been disrupted throughout the night. This finding demonstrates the basis for a vicious, self-perpetuating cycle. The painful muscles can interrupt sleep, and disrupted sleep can make the muscles more painful (Travell & Simons, 1999, p. 226). Pain can prevent a person from falling asleep or wake a person during the night. Change in sleep position or remaining in one position too long can cause sleep interruption.

Impaired sleep can be a precipitating or a perpetuating factor in muscle pain and dysfunction. It is still unclear whether the pain of fibromyalgia syndrome (FMS; Bennett et al., 1995) causes impaired sleep or impaired sleep contributes to the development of this debilitating pain syndrome. In the case of myofascial pain and dysfunction, a lack of sleep is an important factor in perpetuating pain. In order for the manual therapy and stretch to be effective, the therapist must deal with the sleep impairment. This may require a temporary sleep aid, which can range from over-the-counter antihistamines and herbal treatments to prescription medications. If the pain of trigger points causes the sleep disruption, trigger point release and restoration of a pain-free full range of motion are the quickest way to unimpaired sleep. In most instances, as the pain decreases, the length of time of uninterrupted sleep increases.

Psychological

The psychological state of the patient can be complex and yet blurred. Many patients with chronic pain have been to numerous physicians and pain clinics, have endured many types of treatment, and often still do not have any answers to their problem. The initial most valuable aspect of treatment we can give these patients is an unambiguous diagnosis of treatable myofascial pain syndrome. Teaching the patients their involvement in the treatment process begins to give them control over pain rather than the pain victimizing them. Depression, anxiety, frustration, anger, and even stoicism begin to lessen once there is positive direction and movement in treatment. Table 80.15 covers various mind-sets one may encounter when treating myofascial pain syndrome.

STEP 6: TRIGGER POINT THERAPY TREATMENT

When identifying the responsible trigger point, the clinician finds evidence of a palpable band in the affected muscle. It may be difficult to feel, however, if it is a deeper muscle and overlying muscles are also shortened and contain trigger points. Within the palpable taut band the examiner identifies spot tenderness. This will present as a very precise, small area within the taut band. The patient may elicit an exclamation or actually flinch as pressure is exerted on the point of tenderness. This jump sign does not need to be, nor should be, elicited with undue/extreme pressure. Patients will often identify the pain elicited as the very pain they have been experiencing, and this identifies the trigger point.

Using a sustained pressure on the trigger point will elicit the pain referral pattern. The length of time holding the sustained pressure may vary from trigger point to trigger point and from patient to patient depending on the muscle contraction, depth of the trigger point, and condition of the patient's tissues. According to Vecchiet in Travell and Simon (1999), subcutaneous tissue was found to be tenderer than the skin over the trigger point. The manual palpation identification of the trigger point still remains somewhat subjective, as it will vary with the amount of pressure applied to the taut band and with the skill of the examiner. Interrater reliability study results are shown in Table 80.16. Gerwin, in furthering Travell's work, has implemented seminars addressing the issue of skill development of identifying trigger points and in the injection technique used for treatment. The palpative physical examination focuses on the area of pain and discomfort but with an eye to observing total body movement, evidence of movement with mental guarding, posture, gait, weaknesses, and instability.

Myofascial Origin Versus Symptoms

Treating symptoms can certainly give pain relief to the patient, but when the pain results from myofascial trigger points, symptom relief masks the underlying source of the pain and treatment relief is temporary. Perhaps symptom treatment, added to treating the pain site rather than the pain source, is why the pain has become a chronic pain syndrome. It seems the critical question to ask is "why

TABLE 80.15
Psychological Mind-Sets of the Patient

Negative	a.	Patient's focus is on every negative aspect of the pain syndrome
	b.	Clinician should not ask "how are you?"
	c.	Talk and ask in positives
	d.	Give positive assignments
	e.	Turn patient's negative statements into positive ones
Depressed	a.	Patient has decreased self-image
	b.	Don't support patients feeling sorry for themselves
	c.	Give assignments reaching out to others
Benefits from the pain	a.	Give assignments reaching out to others
	b.	Set goals — *what* the patient wants in terms of work, social, self; *when* they want to accomplish these goals
	c.	Set responsibility for getting better on the patient with compliance to sessions, perpetuating factors, home program
Give up	a.	Loss of hope/victim mentality
	b.	Patient education, e.g., explaining there may not be an instant resolution but there is no damage
	c.	Set small goals
	d.	Note small advances
Good sport syndrome	a.	Patient pushes through pain and is proud of it
	b.	Patient education — constant reaggravation delays pain resolution
	c.	Ask — *why* pushing through wanting to keep self-image or other people's image, job, family, insecurity
	d.	Give relaxation assignments
Anxious/fearful	a.	Patient education — realistic vs. unrealistic aspects of the pain
	b.	Address the anxiety and fear directly — what is the patient really fearing?
	c.	Address exaggerated view of pain — worst-case scenario and best-case scenario
	d.	Glass half full/half empty view
Acceptance	a.	Conditioned reflex thinking patient views pain as "just the way I am; everyone in the family has it
	b.	Set patient responsibility of actions and habits independent of family habits
Misunderstanding	a.	Patient believes problem is structural, e.g., herniated disc, arthritis, pinched nerve
	b.	Patient believes there is damage that may or may not heal

Note: From N. Shaw, unpublished, 1988.

TABLE 80.16
Interrater Reliability of Examinations for Trigger Point Characteristics, Kappa Values

Examination	Wolfe et al.	Nice et al.	Njoo et al.	Gerwin et al.	Mean
Spot tenderness	0.61		0.66	0.84	0.70
Jump sign		0.70			0.70
Pain recognition	0.30		0.58	0.88	0.59
Palpable band	0.29		0.49	0.85	0.54
Referred pain	0.40	0.38	0.41	0.69	0.47
Twitch response	0.16		0.09	0.44	0.23
Mean	0.35	0.38	0.49	0.74	

Note: From *Muscle Pain: Understanding Its Nature, Diagnosis, and Treatment,* by S. Mense, D. G. Simons, & I. J. Russell, 2001, Baltimore: Lippincott/Williams & Wilkins. Reproduced with permission.

are the symptoms there, of what are they the result?" If we look at the "why" of the pain, we address the source of the pain and can treat toward permanent pain elimination. The treatment of myofascial pain syndrome addresses all of the primary and secondary pain and dysfunction problems, including perpetuating factors. It is actually possible that a major perpetuating factor needs to be a focus of change *before* the actual physical treatment begins. Otherwise, the perpetuating factor may continue to reactivate trigger points and interfere with any lasting pain relief (i.e., there is pain reduction for a few hours or days, but the pain returns at the same level or even worse).

The myofascial trigger point origin is determined by unraveling the totality of all trigger point referral patterns documented during the intake (primary, satellite, and compensatory). Treatment of only the primary trigger point does not eliminate the satellite and compensatory trigger points and their referred pain. The patient may notice the pain shifting to another area.

Pain Elimination Versus Pain Management

To address the primary, satellite, and compensatory trigger points and the associated functional units takes time and cannot be cut short if pain resolution, not pain management, is the treatment goal. The focus of the treatment must be pain resolution, with the gradual elimination of pain medications, muscle relaxants, antidepressants, and sleep medications used for the symptom relief of the myofascial pain and dysfunction. To eliminate the symptoms without eliminating the trigger point source and perpetuating factors of the pain leads to prolonged treatment and short-term relief. Short-term relief often means eliminating activities and/or movements that tend to increase the pain. On the other hand, pain elimination expands what the patient can do both in daily activities as well as outside activities. For a myofascial pain syndrome to become chronic, Travell suggested the clinician has, in some way, missed a piece of the pain puzzle. Although symptoms for a particular episode may be abated, if the myofascial pain syndrome returns, the treatment has not been sufficient to eliminate the source of the problem. Contrary to popular practice Travell looked to the clinician to refocus on the complex, whole patient and work with the patient to determine the missing pieces of pain resolution.

Total Trigger Point Treatment Versus Pain Site Treatment

The pain site is generally the point of trigger point referral; it is not the source of the primary trigger point. Satellite trigger points have become just as much a component of the chronic myofascial pain problem as the original primary factor. Muscle guarding implicates other

muscles not originally part of the pain. Perpetuating adjustments and accommodations to the pain brings other muscles into the pain situation. The involvement does not end until the entire chain of trigger points has been evaluated and treated.

Total Patient Treatment Versus Pain Site Treatment

The critical fact here is that the clinician is treating a person, not a pain, not a shoulder, nor a knee or elbow. If, in fact, perpetuating factors are as important a factor as has been reported, it is the whole person that must be considered in treatment.

Movement Versus Rest

Passive and active movement is necessary in the release and retraining of the muscles involved in myofascial pain and dysfunction. The rest and inactivity often prescribed allow the musculature to stay, and even increase, contracture, thus perpetuating the problem. If you do not go golfing, the bad golf swing will never be an issue. If you do not move a muscle, it may not hurt but it certainly has not learned a new functioning length.

Hands-on Treatment Versus Mechanical Treatment

While the modalities of ultrasound, electric stimulation, traction, and biofeedback can certainly be helpful in the relaxation of muscles and may be necessary partners of the interdisciplinary team, they do not serve to deactivate trigger points, do not redirect/retrain muscle function, and do not allow for the all important aspect of "touch" in the therapeutic process. Travell worried that the treatment of myofascial pain and dysfunction would become "too high tech" and "too low touch." Mechanical treatments are modalities, only part of a full treatment protocol.

Heat Versus Cold

Heat, rather than ice, is used in the treatment of myofascial pain syndrome. Of course, with an immediate acute situation, as compared with the chronic pain problem, ice is used initially for the reduction of swelling and inflammation. Once the pain has become a chronic situation, ice on the involved pain area serves to act as a local anesthetic agent but also adds to the contracture of the muscles. It is too much contraction in the muscle that is already the problem, so additional contraction is to be avoided. The heat increases circulation, stimulating muscle relaxation and, thereby, increasing nerve and vessel efficiency. Heat is an adjunct to the trigger point release, not an agent of their release.

Trigger Point Pressure Release (Barrier Release)

The clinician, having identified the trigger point and placing the affected muscle on slight stretch, slowly applies a sustained compression, gradually increasing the pressure until resistance is felt. At the point of resistance the patient will usually feel some discomfort. It is important that the clinician not increase the pressure as that can actually traumatize the muscle, causing it to tighten to guard or protect from further pain. As the trigger point releases, a slack in the muscle occurs and the pressure can be slightly increased to the new point of resistance. This layering into the muscle effectively releases the trigger point without undue discomfort for the patient.

Spray with Stretch

The spray with stretch method of releasing a trigger point has been called a variety of names. They include spray and stretch, stretch and spray, vapocoolant with stretch, and intermittent coolant with stretch. In an effort to be as simple and yet as precise as possible, the term "spray with stretch" is used in this chapter. It is important to remember that spray is the distraction, and stretch is the action (Travell & Simons, 1983). To stretch before spraying will only aggravate the trigger point and increase pain. It will also cause a protective contraction and reflex spasm of the muscle, all of which will obstruct further elongation of the muscle.

In order for spray with stretch to be effective, the patient must be as relaxed as possible, in a comfortable and supported position (Travell & Simons, 1983). The room should be warm, and the patient should be wrapped in or covered with a blanket except for the part to be treated.

The muscle to be treated should be immobilized at one end. The patient should be instructed in the reasoning and methodology used. An explanation regarding spraying the source as well as the site of the pain is important. To mitigate fear of the unknown, the clinician should demonstrate by spraying vapocoolant on himself or herself and then on the patient in an area far from the pain site.

Having prepared the patient, the clinician proceeds to the actual procedure. Initial sweeps of the vapocoolant are applied over the muscle being treated and continued over the complete pain pattern to begin releasing muscle tension before taking up the slack to lengthen the muscle toward its stretch position. The spray is applied in parallel sweeps *only* in the direction of the referred pain. This spray procedure can be repeated until full muscle length is achieved or no further progress occurs. However, any given area of skin should be covered only two or three times before rewarming. After the skin is rewarmed, several cycles of full active range of motion complete the spray with stretch treatment (Travell & Simons, 1999).

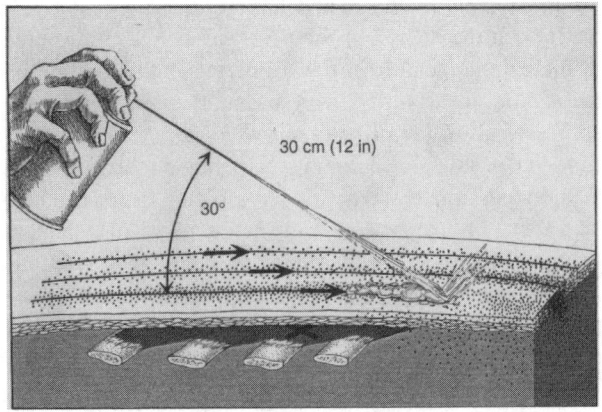

FIGURE 80.9 Positioning for using vapocoolant. From *Myofascial Pain and Dysfunction: The Trigger Point Manual* (2nd ed., Vol. 1), by J. G. Travell & D. Simons, 1999, Baltimore: Williams & Wilkins. Reproduced with permission.

The nozzle of the spray bottle or can should be fully engaged. Any partial opening of the nozzle results in dripping coolant on the patient. For those who still have some bottles of Fluori-Methane (Gebauer Company, Cleveland, OH), the technique requires that the bottle be held upside down. The newly developed Instant Ice (Gebauer Company) can be held upright or at a slight angle. The stream of the spray should describe a path that is at a 30° angle to the skin and approximately 12 inches from the point of impact (Figure 80.9). The spray should be applied at a rate of 4 inches per second. The farther away the spray bottle/can, the cooler it feels. For patients who have difficulty dealing with the intensity of the cold, speed up the rate of the sweep and move the spray can closer. The Instant Ice, which is somewhat cooler than Fluori-Methane, should be held closer to the skin (3 to 7 inches away; Travell & Simons, 1999).

Injection

Trigger point injections are indicated for quick relief of acute, subacute, or chronic myofascial pain, for substitution of narcotic medication, for restoration of functional impairment due to myofascial trigger points, or for supplemental therapy of chronic myofascial pain to facilitate its recovery. The trigger point is identified in the taut band, sterile skin preparation is made, and the needle is inserted rapidly where a local twitch response is elicited upon needling the trigger point. The clinician senses a grabbing of the tissue around the needle upon penetrating the trigger point (Hong, 1994).

It is imperative that physicians be trained in the palpation, identification, and ultimate location of trigger points before the injection technique can be effective in treating myofascial pain syndrome. Ngoo and Gerwin have shown good interrater reliability if practitioners are experienced and trained (Gerwin et al., 1997; Ngoo & Van der Does, 1994).

It is critical to note, once again, that the trigger point release, by whatever method, is just one step in treating myofascial pain syndrome.

STEP 7: SPECIFIC MUSCLE STRETCH RETRAINING

Rehabilitation is seen as a primary factor in the success of the myofascial trigger point protocol. Muscle retraining is imperative to the successful return of functional efficiency.

Stretch Versus Strength Rehabilitation

Stretch is an absolute in myofascial therapy rehabilitation. While we all agree that muscle weakness is a symptom of myofascial syndrome, it must be viewed initially as a pseudo-weakness. If the muscle is in a sustained muscle contracture with shortened range of motion function, it will, of necessity, have shortened contracture potential and, therefore, weakened function. To add contracture through strength rehabilitation before full stretch range is accomplished simply reinforces the habitual contracted patterning of the muscle and weakens it further. Starling's law states "length means strength." The specific stretch rehabilitation establishes new lengthened muscular patterning and returns full functional efficiency. Then, if the muscles are weak, a strength-stretch program can be instituted for the patient.

"No Pain" Range of Motion Versus "Pain for Gain" Range of Motion

The "no pain" range of motion is emphasized in stretch retraining of muscles in a chronic myofascial pain syndrome to help eliminate the rebounding effect of the exercise. It is important for the patient to respect the current potential of the muscle and not to push into the pain range. Movement/stretch is performed to the point of feeling initial stretch, even if the patient is capable of stretching beyond that point. This allows for a relaxed acceptance of the movement and the beginnings of a new established range of movement for the muscle. If the patient is in pain when performing the stretch retraining, the muscles are reaggravated rendering the release of the trigger points ineffective. "Pain for gain" range of motion may be necessary for some postoperative, prolonged immobilization or disease conditions but further activates trigger points or results in a rebound guarding for the patient with chronic myofascial pain.

Muscle Retraining Versus Muscle Conditioning

Muscle retraining is different from muscle conditioning. Muscle retraining is designed to reestablish full-length functioning of muscles that have been in a shortened contracted pattern of function. Muscles "learn." In myofascial pain and dysfunction the muscles are not injured, which is why objective testing generally reveals no indication of the pain source. A magnetic resonance imaging (MRI) image or a radiograph does not reveal the source of a bad golf swing or any other incorrect muscle function. The muscles, instead, are functioning incorrectly in learned shortened patterning. Do something long enough and it becomes habit, whether good or bad. Muscles frequently performing to newly acquired movement potential will establish a functioning pattern that becomes automatic. When trigger points have been deactivated, perpetuating factors resolved, and muscle function established at full range of motion, pain is eliminated.

Once range of motion is returned to the muscle and pain eliminated, muscle conditioning is introduced. This should be done in the context of the patient's interest and previous activity involvement. Working back into a balance of strength and stretch, reintroducing graduated participation in activity, and progressing to full daily and recreational activity should be implemented with patient input as to schedule, interest, and realistic compliance. The patient should be compliant and committed to the rehabilitation program. If it does not interest the patient, if it is not realistic within the structure of the patient's life, it is not going to happen. It is imperative the patient and clinician work together to create a workable and interesting rehabilitation program.

Stretch Principles

1. Patient in a relaxed, comfortable position
2. Stretch slowly at a pace that incorporates natural momentum
3. Two repetitions; it is the frequency that retrains the muscles, and this eliminates fatiguing the muscle resulting in a rebound guarding
4. Every 1 to 1 1/2 hours; frequency leads to a functioning habit
5. Hold long enough to take a deep inhalation and exhalation; this has a relaxing effect and the body accepts the movement without guarding
6. No pain range of motion; this allows acceptance of the motion for the patient mentally and physically
7. Stretch bilaterally

The clinician's goal is to establish a neuromuscular retraining program that:

- Can be performed anywhere
- Takes literally only a couple of minutes to perform

- Is individualized to the specific physical and mental needs of the patient
- Incorporates movement leading toward the activities of interest to the patient

If the program is workable, the commitment by the patient is much greater.

Trigger point deactivation in the treatment setting is well documented in the medical literature to include trigger point injections, intermittent coolant with stretch, and sustained compression. While trigger point deactivation is obviously a critical aspect of treatment, remember it is the interdisciplinary team — the physiatrist diagnosing, ordering appropriate lab work, and performing the trigger point injections; the podiatrist involved in forefoot varum; the rheumatologist dealing with endocrinological problems; the pulmonologist involved in sleep disturbances; the psychologist addressing emotional or behavioral components; the manual therapists performing trigger point release and addressing basic perpetuating factors and neuromuscular retraining; the chiropractor or osteopath correcting structural imbalances — that, working together, resolves myofascial pain and dysfunction.

SUMMARY

Checklist for Successful Treatment of Myofascial Pain Syndrome

- Perform proper differential diagnosis
- Set appropriate atmosphere for treatment
  Room and patient warm
  Patient relaxed
  Clinician not hurried
- Obtain adequate history
- Communicate adequately with patient
- Assure treatment conditions favorable
  Patient not ill with cold, flu, unduly fatigued, etc.
  Patient not highly emotional
  Patient not highly anxious
- Address all perpetuating factors
- Utilize correct technique
- Treat all categories of trigger points
- Treat at an appropriate pace
- Remove aggravating factors
  Sitting in drafts, driving long distances without breaks, etc.
- Recognize compensatory mechanisms/movements
- Utilize correct and complete stretch program
- Correctly prioritize rehabilitation program
- Reintroduce activity realistically
- Give adequate and complete patient education

- Obtain patient compliance
- Recognize conditioned reflex
- Treat with an interdisciplinary approach

REFLECTIVE THOUGHT

While there remains some controversy in allopathic physician circles regarding the roles of osteopathy, chiropractic, and complementary medicine, one study after another documents the merits and contributions of those interventions when properly applied (Materson, 2001).

There are two types of physicians — those that are free men and those that are slaves. The slaves, to speak generally, are treated by slaves, who pay them a hurried visit, or receive them in dispensaries. A physician of this kind never gives a servant any account of his complaint, nor asks him for any; he gives him some imperial injunction with an air of finished knowledge, in the brusque fashion of a dictator, and then is off in haste to the next ailing servant.... The free practitioner attends free men, treats their diseases by going into things thoroughly in a scientific way; and takes the patient and his family into his confidence. Thus he learns something from the sufferers, and at the same time instructs the invalid to the best of his powers. He does not give his prescriptions until he has won the patient's support.... Now which of the two methods is that of the better physician or director of the bodily regimen?

— **Plato, 2500 years ago**
— **Diamond, W. John. *The Clinical Practice of Complementary, Alternative, and Western Medicine*, CRC Press, Boca Raton, FL, 2001**

REFERENCES

Alvarez, D., & Rockwell, P. (2002). Trigger points, diagnosis and management. *Journal of American Family Physicians, 65,* 653.

Bennett, R. M. et al. (1995). Low levels of somatomedin C in patients with the fibromyalgia syndrome: A possible link between sleep and muscle pain. *Arthritis & Rheumatism, 10,* 1113.

Chaitow, L. & DeLany, J. W. (2000). *Clinical applications of neuromuscular techniques, Vol. 1: The upper body.* Edinburgh: Churchill Livingstone.

Chaitow, L., & DeLany, J. W. (2002). *Clinical applications of neuromuscular techniques, Vol. 2: The lower body.* Edinburgh: Churchill Livingstone.

Dorland's Medical Dictionary (24th ed.) (1982). Philadelphia: W.B. Saunders.

Fischer, A., & Rachlin E. (1994). In E. Rachlin (Ed.), *Myofascial pain and fibromyalgia, trigger point management.* St. Louis: Mosby.

Gerwin, R. D. et al. (1997). Identification of myofascial trigger points: Inter-rater agreement and effect of training. *Pain.*

Gittleman, A. L. (1996). *Get the sugar out*. New York: Crown Trade Paperback.

Griggs, R. C., Mendell, J. R., & Miller, R. G. (1995). *Evaluation and treatment of myopathies*. Philadelphia: F.A. Davis Co.

Hong, C. Z. Considerations and recommendations regarding myofascial trigger point injection. *Journal of Musculoskeletal Pain, 2*(1), 29.

Ingram-Rice, B. (1997). Carpal tunnel syndrome: More than a wrist problem. *Journal of Body Work and Movement Therapies, 1*(3), 158–159.

Judd, A. & Judd, D. (2004). *Secrets of an alkaline body, the new science of collodial biology*. Berkeley, CA: North Atlantic Books.

Kendall, F., McCreary, E., & Provance, P. (1993). *Muscles testing and function* (4th ed.). Baltimore: Williams & Wilkins.

Khalil, T. M. et al. (1994). The role of ergonomics in the prevention and treatment of myofascial pain. In E. Rachlin (Ed.), *Myofascial pain and fibromyalgia: Trigger point management*. St. Louis: Mosby.

Lowe, J. C. (2000). *The metabolic treatment of fibromyalgia*. Boulder, CO: McDowell Publishing Co.

Mannell, J. (1992). *The musculoskeletal system: Differential diagnosis from symptoms and physical signs*. Gaithersberg, MD: Aspen Publications.

Materson, R. (2001, March/April). Practical pain management. *Practical Pain Magazine, 1*.

Mense, S., Simons, D. G., & Russell, I. J. (2001). *Muscle pain, understanding its nature, diagnosis, and treatment*. Baltimore: Lippincott, Williams & Wilkins.

Moldofsky, H., & Scarisbrick, P. (1976). Induction of neurasthenic musculoskeletal pain syndrome by selective sleep stage deprivation. *Psychosocial Medicine, 38*, 35–44.

Ngoo, K. G., & Van der Does, E. (1994). The occurrence and inter-rater reliability of myofascial trigger points in the quadratus lumborum and gluteus medius: A prospective study in non-specific low back pain patients and controls in general practice. *Pain, 58*, 317.

Shaw, N. L. (1987). The history of trigger point myotherapy. Unpublished data.

Simons, D. (1987, November). Myofascial pain syndrome due to trigger points. International Rehabilitation Medicine Association *Monograph series #1*, 12.

Simons, D. (2003). Update of myofascial pain from trigger points. *Medical Pain Education Website.* Available from http://websites.goldin-orb.com/pain-education/100129.php.

Sonkin, L., & Rachlin, E. (1994). Myofascial pain due to metabolic disorders: Diagnosis and treatment. In E. Rachlin (Eds.), *Myofascial pain and fibromyalgia: Trigger point management*. St. Louis: Mosby.

Spence, A. P. (1986). *Basic human anatomy* (2nd ed.). Menlo Park, CA: Benjamin/Cummings Publishing Co.

Starlanyl, D., & Copeland, M. E. (1996). *Fibromyalgia and chronic myofascial pain syndrome: A survival manual*. Oakland, CA: New Harbinger Publications, Inc.

Strauss, S. (2004). Myofascial pain syndrome: A short review. The Medical Acupuncture Webpage. Available from http://users.med.auth.gr/~karanik/english/articles/myofac.html.

Teitelbaum, J. (2001). *From fatigue to fantastic*. New York: Avery.

Travell J. G., & Simons D. (1983). *Myofascial pain and dysfunction: The trigger point manual* (Vol. 1, 1st ed.). Baltimore: Williams & Wilkins.

Travell J. G., & Simons D. (1992). *Myofascial pain and dysfunction: The trigger point manual, Vol. 2, The lower extremities*. Baltimore: Williams & Wilkins.

Travell J. G., & Simons D. (1999). *Myofascial pain and dysfunction: The trigger point manual* (Vol. 1, 2nd ed.). Baltimore: Williams & Wilkins.

Travell, J. G., Fricton, J., & Awad, E. (1990). *Myofascial pain syndrome: Mysteries of the history, advances in pain research and therapy* (Vol. 17). New York: Raven Press.

Weintraub, B. D. (1991, Winter). Thyroid hormone resistance syndrome may affect thousands of unsuspecting Americans. *NIH Observer, I* .

Yunus, M. B., & Rachlin, E. (1994). In E. Rachlin (Ed.), *Myofascial pain and fibromyalgia: Trigger point management*. St. Louis: Mosby.

Zohn, D. (1988). *Musculoskeletal pain: Diagnosis and physical treatment* (2nd ed.). Boston: Little, Brown & Co.

81

Role of Naturopathy in Pain Management

Rick Marinelli, ND, MAcOM, and Harry Adelson, ND

INTRODUCTION

The purpose of this chapter is to introduce the reader to the profession of modern naturopathic medicine in North America, outline its underlying principles and history, describe the emerging specialty of naturopathic pain medicine, and give the reader a cursory overview of a sampling of its traditional and emerging treatment modalities.

Naturopathic medicine is defined as a distinct system of primary health care — an art, science, philosophy, and practice of diagnosis, treatment, and prevention of illness (U.S. Department of Labor, 2003). Naturopathic doctors (NDs) are primary health care providers who combine contemporary conventional scientific knowledge with a spectrum of natural and conventional medicine modalities; they are the physician-level practitioner trained in the broadest range of conventional and natural medicines. Naturopathic medicine is distinguished by the principles that underlie and determine its practice rather than by its broad treatment modalities. These principles are based on the objective observation of the nature of health and disease, and are continually reexamined in the light of scientific advances. The treatment modalities used, although broad, are consistent with these principles and are chosen on the basis of patient individuality. The guiding principles of naturopathic medicine are as follows:

1. The healing power of nature (*vis medicatrix naturae*)
2. Identify and treat the cause
3. Treat the whole person
4. First do no harm
5. Doctor as teacher
6. Prevention

Modern NDs are trained at accredited, 4-year, post-graduate, residential naturopathic medical programs, which require an undergraduate degree with standard pre-medical coursework. The curriculum of the first 2 years closely mirrors that of conventional medical schools (M.D. or D.O.) in the basic sciences, conventional diagnostics, pharmacology, and minor surgery. The third and fourth year of training divides the student's time between clinical in-patient and out-patient rotations and additional class work in therapeutic nutrition, botanical medicine, homeopathy, naturopathic manipulative therapy, natural childbirth, classical Chinese medicine and acupuncture, hydrotherapy, and psychology. Postgraduate medical education is available to NDs, but is not required by all states that license NDs.

HISTORY OF NATUROPATHIC MEDICINE

The word *physician* is from the Greek root meaning nature. Hippocrates formulated the concept *vis medicatrix naturae* — the healing power of nature. This concept has long been at the core of indigenous medicine in many cultures around the world and remains one of the central themes of naturopathic philosophy to this day.

Vincent Priessnitz is credited with the creation of the European tradition of hydrotherapy in the early to mid-1800s. It is believed that he discovered the concept of the healing power of water through the observation of animals in the wild that would soak injured limbs in streams. Priessnitz developed large sanitariums, which were hugely popular, but bitterly opposed by the medical community. His work was furthered by Father Sebastian Kneipp, who added to Priessnitz's "water cure" the use of medicinal herbs; exercise therapy; a wholesome, balanced diet; and "regulative" therapy, a system of organizing daily life in accordance with biological rhythms (Kirchfeld & Boyle, 1994).

In the 1890s, Benedict Lust, a German immigrant living in the United States, fell ill with tuberculosis. He returned to Germany to undergo Father Kneipp's water cure and was successfully healed. Father Kneipp instructed Lust to formally bring this type of medicine to the United States. Kneipp's medicine already existed in the United States among German immigrants, but it was Lust who was the first to be officially mandated by Lust to bring nature cure to the United States. Lust sensed the need to Americanize Kneipp's principles (i.e., Kneippism) and make it acceptable to Americans. He is credited as the "Father of Naturopathy." Lust chose the word *naturopathy* to describe this practice of medicine, a word coined by Sophie Scheel, an instructor at a New York homeopathic college. Lust realized that to be taken seriously, he would need formal medical training, so he attended medical school and was licensed as an M.D. This is an important point, as it demonstrates American naturopathy's foundation in Western scientific tradition. Lust additionally received D.O. and D.C. degrees during his medical career. He founded the American School of Naturopathy in New York City in 1901 and the American Naturopathic Association, as well as the periodical *The Naturopath* in 1902. It is important to note that the American School of Naturopathy, much like modern naturopathic schools, was based on contemporary medical curriculum with the addition of natural healing modalities. Henry Lindlahr, M.D., was an early student of Dr. Lust and is credited as the founder of "scientific naturopathy." He founded a number of sanitariums, which would treat patients with natural therapies only after a thorough, state-of-the-art conventional diagnostic workup had been completed (Kirchfeld & Boyle, 1994).

Naturopathic medicine quickly became popular and widely available throughout the U.S. in the early 20th century. In 1920, there were 10 naturopathic medical schools and approximately 20,000 practicing naturopathic physicians. The discovery and increasing use of "miracle drugs" such as antibiotics, the institutionalization of a medical system based primarily on high-tech and pharmaceutical treatments, as well as the ever-existing schism in the naturopathic profession between "traditional" naturopaths (who tend to have bias against scientific medicine) and "modern" naturopaths (who view themselves as hybrids) — all of these led by midcentury to the decline to near extinction of naturopathic medicine (Kirchfeld & Boyle, 1994).

John Bastyr, D.C., N.D., is credited as the "Father of Modern Naturopathy." In 1956, at the time that naturopathy was near extinction, Dr. Bastyr and a small number of other dedicated physicians created the National College of Naturopathic Medicine (NCNM). Although homeopathy and spinal manipulation had been a treatment of naturopathic medicine for decades, it was Dr. Bastyr who brought these two modalities into the forefront of the naturopathic curriculum during his presidency in the early years of NCNM. Additionally, because his father was a pharmacist, and Dr. Bastyr had often worked in the pharmacy, he held a pragmatic view about the use of pharmaceuticals. Once, when asked by a student, which of the healing modalities was "the best," his response was, "The one that works." Naturopathic medicine is in no way philosophically opposed to conventional medicine; the role of the ND is to offer safe and effective treatments to those patients who seek naturopathic medicine and are candidates for naturopathic care.

Currently in the United States, the naturopathic medical profession is blossoming into maturity. Its infrastructure is based on a national association (the American Association of Naturopathic Physicians), federally accredited educational institutions, professional licensing by an ever-growing number of states, national standards of practice and care, peer review, and an ongoing commitment to state-of-the-art scientific research.

Those most opposed to naturopathic medicine cite a lack of scientific data to justify deviation from conventional care. However, the Office of Technology Assessment of the U.S. Congress has estimated that fewer than 30% of the procedures currently used in conventional medicine have been rigorously tested (Astin et al., 1998). One reason most naturopathic therapies are not considered "evidence-based" is that the majority were introduced prior to the advent of the randomized, controlled clinical trial (RCT). Such limitations are evident in conventional medicine as well; however, they are often overlooked due to the apparent or established effectiveness of a particular treatment. The common and accepted use of antithrombotic agents for cardiovascular diseases and their complications (myocardial infarction, stroke, pulmonary embolism, and death) is a good example. Three of the agents that had been prescribed by allopathic physicians for millions of patients every day, warfarin, aspirin, and heparin, were introduced prior to the era of randomized clinical trials and had widespread use for many years before they were validated by RCTs (Relman & Weil, 1999). However, few physicians would have argued that these were unconventional treatments simply because they had not yet gone through RCTs. Furthermore, natural substances are not patentable, and there is little financial incentive for corporate funded research. Nonetheless, every year sees and an ever-growing amount of meaningful data demonstrating or refuting safety and efficacy of complementary and alternative modalities.

As stated above, modern naturopathic medicine is defined by its principles and philosophy, not by its treatment modalities. NDs borrow from all of the medical sciences to achieve wellness in each individual patient. Frequently, the modalities used by NDs are not proprietary to naturopathy. The specialty of "Naturopathic Pain Medicine" is currently evolving. We discuss a selection of modalities used by NDs, which is by no means exhaustive.

INTERNAL NATUROPATHIC MEDICINE FOR PAIN

In the tradition of Kneippism, the naturopathic treatment of any condition, painful or otherwise, is always based on lifestyle modification. Exercise, a healthful diet, and psychological health are the foundations upon which any treatment plan is built.

EXERCISE

Despite a poor rate of patient compliance, NDs recommend exercise to patients with pain. In one study, general practitioners gave written advice on physical activity during usual consultations. For every 10 written prescriptions for exercise, at 12 months only 1 person achieved and sustained 150 minutes of moderate or vigorous leisure activity per week. In these compliant patients, measures of self-rated general health, vitality, and pain improved significantly (Elley et al., 2003).

Fibromyalgia and chronic fatigue syndrome fall under the spectrum of chronic multisymptom illnesses. This constellation of syndromes is often defined by chronic pain, unremitting fatigue, cognitive difficulties, and various other symptoms. In treating these illnesses, a prescription for exercise is often overlooked by health care practitioners. Research has shown that exercise is quite beneficial in reducing pain and fatigue in this population and should be included as part of a multimodal therapy regimen (Ambrose, Lyden, & Clauw, 2003; King et al., 2002; Valim et al., 2003).

Beyond its use in treatment of pain syndromes, physical activity also effectively decreases the risk of many chronic disorders. Numerous studies have convincingly demonstrated that moderate levels of physical activity greatly reduce the incidence of many chronic health conditions, most notably type II diabetes mellitus, obesity, cardiovascular disease, depression, and many types of cancers (Chakravarthy, Joyner, & Booth, 2002).

Also, strength training in elderly people has been shown to have beneficial effects on risk factors for age-related diseases and pain. In addition to improved strength, function, endurance, muscle mass, and power, strength training has been shown to reduce insulin resistance, decrease both total and intra-abdominal fat, increase resting metabolic rate, prevent the loss of bone mass density, reduce risk factors for falls, and reduce pain (Hurley & Roth, 2000).

DIET

Whole-food diets high in fiber, quality protein, essential fatty acids, fruits, vegetables, and minimally processed, low-in-saturated fats and trans-fatty acids are recommended by NDs. Although humans have remained primarily unchanged genetically since before the agricultural revolution, our diet and lifestyle have become progressively more divergent from those of our ancestors. Accumulating evidence suggests that this mismatch between our modern diet and lifestyle and our Paleolithic genes plays a substantial role in the epidemics of obesity, hypertension, diabetes, and atherosclerotic cardiovascular disease. Humans evolved on a diet high in lean protein, polyunsaturated fats (especially omega-3 fatty acids), monounsaturated fats, fiber, vitamins, minerals, antioxidants, and other beneficial phytochemicals. Anthropological studies have shown hunter–gatherers generally to have been healthy and largely free of the degenerative diseases common in modern societies (O'Keefe & Cordain, 2004). Although prehistoric humans had shorter life expectancies than modern humans, much of their mortality arose from conditions that we are now able to prevent or cure.

Generally, NDs do not recommend vegetarian or vegan diets; rather, they recommend healthful meat choices as part of a healthy diet. From the data currently available, it appears that the intake of meat itself is not a risk factor for degenerative disease, but rather the risk stems from the intake of excessive saturated fat. Unlike wild game meat, which is low in total and saturated fat and relatively rich in polyunsaturated fatty acids, meat from modern domesticated animals is high in saturated fat. There is some evidence that diets high in lean red meat can actually lower plasma cholesterol, contribute significantly to tissue omega-3 fatty acid, and provide a good source of iron, zinc, and vitamin B_{12} (Mann, 2000).

Vegetarian diet is, however, recommended in rheumatoid arthritis and other autoimmune conditions. Studies have shown patients with rheumatic conditions benefit from the vegan diet rich in antioxidants, lactobacilli, and fiber (Hanninen et al., 2000; Nenonen et al., 1998).

PROTEOLYTIC ENZYMES

Naturopathic training includes an in-depth study of botanical preparations. The botanical medicines used in the treatment of pain can be categorized, just as with pharmacologic preparations, into analgesics, anticonvulsants, antidepressants, anti-inflammatories, anxiolytics, sedatives, and alteratives/adaptogens. Some of the most commonly used botanical medicines for pain are bromelain, cayenne, feverfew, ginger, gingko, boswellia, corydalis, and guggulipid. A systematic review of the literature aimed at determining the clinical efficacy of botanical medicines for rheumatologic conditions suggests that herbal remedies have symptomatic effects beyond placebo. A review published in *Rheumatic Diseases Clinics of North America* concluded that phyto-anti-inflammatories have considerable potential in the symptomatic treatment of rheumatic disorders (Ernst & Chrubasik, 2000).

Bromelain is one such botanical medicine frequently recommended by NDs. It is viewed as an alternative to nonsteroidal anti-inflammatory drugs (NSAIDs). Bromelain is the collective term for enzymes (principally proteolytic) derived from the pineapple plant, *Ananas comosus,* and a member of the Bromeliaceae family. Pineapple has been used as a folk medicine for centuries. Its traditional uses have been as a digestive aid or to promote the healing of wounds.

Bromelain can function as a digestive enzyme, and there is research suggesting that it may also have wound healing, anti-inflammatory, antidiarrheal, and anticarcinogenic effects. Bromelain's anti-inflammatory action is believed to be from activation of proteolysis at site of inflammation, fibrinolysis via plasminogen-plasmin system, depletion of kininogen, inhibition of inflammatory prostaglandins, and induction of prostaglandin E1.

Bromelain mainly comprises cysteine proteases, with smaller amounts of acid phosphatase, peroxidase, amylase, and cellulase. Bromelain contains at least four distinct cysteine proteases. The principal stem protease is called stem bromelain or stem bromelain protease. Two additional proteases found in the stem are called ananain and comosain.

The therapeutic use of proteolytic enzymes is both empirically based and supported by scientific studies. Studies of the use of proteolytic enzymes in rheumatic disorders have mostly been carried out on enzyme preparations consisting of combinations of bromelain, papain, trypsin, and chymotrypsin. The results of various studies (placebo-controlled and comparisons with nonsteroidal anti-inflammatory drugs) in patients with rheumatic diseases suggest that oral therapy with proteolytic enzymes produces analgesic and anti-inflammatory effects (Leipner, Iten, & Saller, 2001). In some studies, proteolytic enzymes were shown to be as effective as NSAIDs while producing fewer side effects (Klein & Kullich, 1999; Wittenborg et al., 2000). Bromelain has been shown in a pilot study to be helpful in the treatment of mild acute knee pain (Walker et al., 2002) and, in an open case observation study, to be effective in speeding the healing time of blunt injuries to the musculoskeletal system (Masson, 1995).

Bromelain and proteolytic enzymes, therefore, seem a reasonable treatment option for patients suffering mild to moderate pain from inflammation, especially in light of its safety profile as compared with NSAIDs.

INTRODUCTION TO NATUROPATHIC THERAPEUTIC INJECTION (NTI)

In the treatment of painful conditions, oftentimes modalities more invasive than lifestyle modification, prepara-

tions taken by mouth, spinal manipulation, and acupuncture are needed, especially in patients who wish to avoid chronic use of pain medications. For this reason, injection therapies are increasingly employed by NDs practicing naturopathic pain medicine.

In response to this growing trend, the Naturopathic Academy of Therapeutic Injection (NATI) has been formed, with the following primary objectives:

1. To hold NDs practicing therapeutic injection to the highest standards of practice through board certification
2. To protect the public's safety
3. To advance the science of injection therapies in the context of a naturopathic pain medicine clinical practice

It is important to note that minor surgery is part of the core naturopathic curriculum, and NDs are trained in the management of the spectrum of possible adverse reactions to in-office procedures. Injection therapies increasingly used by NDs include intravenous micronutrient therapy (IVMT), myofascial trigger point injection, regenerative injection therapy (RIT), and mesotherapy.

INTRAVENOUS MICRONUTRIENT THERAPY

IVMT and, more specifically, the "Myers' cocktail" (Table 81.1) is a popular treatment modality among NDs and other physicians practicing complementary and alternative medicine (Gaby, 1998). No exact figures currently exist reflecting the extent of utilization of this modality; however, members who routinely treat patients with IVMT have been reported by a range of national medical associations, including the American College for Advancement in Medicine (ACAM), the American Association of Naturopathic Physicians (AANP), the American Holistic Medical Association (AHMA), the American

TABLE 81.1
Contents of the Myers' Cocktail

Magnesium sulfate (50%)	5 ml
Calcium gluconate (10%)	3 ml
Hydroxocobalamin (1,000 µg/ml)	1 ml
Pyridoxine hydrochloride (100 mg/ml)	1 ml
Dexpanthenol (250 mg/ml)	1 ml
B-complex 100*	1 ml
Vitamin C (222 mg/ml)	10 ml
Sterile water	20 ml

* B-complex 100 contains the following per each ml: thiamine HCl, 100 mg; riboflavin, 2 mg; pyridoxine HCl, 2 mg; panthenol, 2 mg; niacinamide, 100 mg; benzyl alcohol, 2%.

Academy of Pain Management (AAPM), the Great Lakes College of Clinical Medicine (GLCCM), and the International Society of Orthomolecular Medicine (ISOM). Data obtained by an online survey of members of these organizations suggest that IVMT has been widely used for a variety of conditions, most often fibromyalgia syndrome (FMS) and chronic fatigue syndrome (CFS), with reports of consistently positive results; survey data pertains to some reported 12,000 patient experiences. Despite its popularity, no controlled trials of IVMT efficacy and only one trial investigating the mechanism of action of the Myers' cocktail (Lonsdale, Shamberger, Stahl, & Evans, 1999) have been conducted. At the time of this writing, there is one National Institutes of Health–funded, double-blind, placebo-controlled, randomized trial being conducted on the use of IVMT in the treatment of fibromyalgia, but data are not yet available. The exact mechanism of action of IVMT is unknown apart from the effects of the individual constituents.

Alan Gaby, M.D., popularized the use of the Myers' cocktail. We refer the reader to the article by Gaby, "Intravenous Nutrient Therapy: The Myers Cocktail" (Gaby, 2002) in which he discusses his many years of experience using the Myers' cocktail for the treatment of, among many other conditions, status asthmaticus, migraine, CFS, FMS, acute muscle spasm, upper respiratory tract infections, chronic sinusitis, seasonal allergic rhinitis, and cardiovascular disease.

IVMT has the ability to achieve serum concentrations of micronutrients unobtainable with oral or intramuscular administration. The highest serum vitamin C level reported after oral administration of pharmacological doses is 9.3 mg/dl, however, intravenous (IV) administration of 50 g/day of vitamin C resulted in a mean peak plasma level of 80 mg/dl (Blanchard, Tozer, & Rowland, 1997). Similarly, oral supplementation with magnesium has been shown to minimally affect serum magnesium levels, whereas IV administration can double or triple the serum levels (Okayama, Aikawa, Okayama et al., 1987; Sydow, Crozier, Zielmann et al., 1993).

Much of the benefit of Myers' cocktail in the treatment of painful syndromes is believed to be derived from the magnesium content (Gaby, 2002). Magnesium administered intravenously has been shown to ameliorate pain in a number of conditions (Anand, 2000; Crosby, Wilcock, & Corcoran, 2000; Koinig et al., 1998; Mauskop et al., 1995a, 1995b, 1996; Tramer et al., 1996; Xiao & Bennett, 1994). Magnesium is important for more than 300 different enzyme reactions and, in healthy states, magnesium levels are second only to potassium intracellularly (Groff, Gropper, & Hunt, 1995). Magnesium has been found to be low in the serum (Eisinger et al., 1994, 1996) and erythrocytes (Eisinger et al., 1994) and high in the hair (Ng, 1999) of patients with FMS, suggesting some imbalance of magnesium regulation in this population. Gaby

hypothesizes that the reduced levels of intracellular magnesium found in patients with FMS play a role in the etiology, and in order to adequately replenish the cells with magnesium, it is necessary to attain extremely high levels in serum, possible only with IV administration (Gaby, 2002).

Migraine headache appears to share some features with FMS, such as irregularities of serotonin (Nicolodi & Sicuteri, 1996), extensive dysregulation in pain modulation, and generalized hyperalgesia (Okifuji, Turk, & Marcus, 1999). Similar to patients with FMS, patients with migraine have been found to have reduced red and mononuclear blood cell magnesium levels (Mazzotta et al., 1999). Two double-blind studies have shown that chronic oral magnesium supplementation may reduce the frequency of migraine headaches (Mauskop & Altura, 1998), and one pilot study demonstrated that IV magnesium can resolve an acute migraine (Mauskop et al., 1995b). Magnesium concentration plays a role in the modulation of serotonin receptors, nitric oxide synthesis and release, and a variety of other neurotransmitters (Groff et al., 1995).

Reed (1990) found parenteral magnesium therapy to have a beneficial effect in treating two groups of patients: those with acute sprains, contusions, or soft tissue injuries and those with chronic muscular complaints including myofascial pain, relapsing soft tissue injuries, and FMS.

Based on research to date, some conjecture can be made regarding the role of magnesium. However, the roles of the other constituents of the IVMT solution have not been investigated extensively. Nonetheless, vitamin B_{12} injected intramuscularly has been used experimentally to treat CFS, a syndrome closely associated with FMS (Goldenberg et al., 1990). In one unblind trial, 2,500 to 5,000 µg of vitamin B_{12}, given by injection every 2 to 3 days, led to improvement in 50 to 80% of a group of people with CFS, with most improvement appearing after several weeks (Lapp & Cheney, 1993). It has been suggested that oral or sublingual administration does not achieve the effects seen with injectable B_{12} (O'Dowd, 2000).

The potential for adverse reactions from IVMT lies mainly in the method of administration rather than the substance(s) administered (Bier, 2000). Any type of IV therapy holds some risk of local effects (hematoma, thrombosis, phlebitis, thrombophlebitis, infiltration, extravastion, local infection, venous spasm) and/or systemic complications (septicemia, circulatory overload, pulmonary edema, air embolism, speed shock, catheter embolism). These complications are rare and are avoided by using proper technique and thorough screening of patients for whom IV therapy is contraindicated (Phillips, 1997). There exist reports of allergic reaction to the thiamin (B_1) found in the B-complex solution. Reaction to thiamin, although extremely rare, most often manifests as a hypersensitivity reaction (Morinville, Jeannet-Peter, & Hauser, 1998; Stephen, Grant, & Yeh, 1992). A preliminary test for sensitivity to thiamin is considered "best practice." Otherwise, there are no known serious side effects of IVMT. Providers of IVMT have not observed other known toxic effects of vitamin and mineral excess with the exception of hypotension due to too rapid a magnesium administration, easily avoided by observation of the patient's state (Gaby, 1998). Avoidance and management of adverse reactions to IVMT are taught in naturopathic medical school.

Previously, an erroneous belief linked the intake of large amounts of vitamin C with the formation of oxalate-type kidney stones because of the metabolic conversion to oxalic acid. If the amount of oxalic acid in the urine increases as the dose of vitamin C increases, it was postulated that a prolonged intake of large amounts of vitamin C might cause kidney stones. There exist, however, no data to support this speculation, and in fact, data clearly refute this idea (Johnston, 1999). Curhan et al. (1999) conducted a 14-year-long study to examine the association between the intakes of vitamins B_6 and C and risk of kidney stone formation in 85,557 women. They found that a high intake vitamin B_6 was inversely associated with risk of stone formation and vitamin C intake was not associated in any way with risk.

MYOFASCIAL TRIGGER POINT INJECTION

MFTPI as originally described by Travell & Simons (1983) is an accepted modality in the treatment of soft-tissue, musculoskeletal pain. We refer the reader to the chapter in this volume by Gerwin and Dommerholt, which thoroughly outlines the modality. MFTPI is included here merely to illustrate that it is a modality routinely used by NDs practicing naturopathic pain medicine, and to discuss a common adaptation not proprietary to NTI, the addition of cobalamins (vitamin B_{12}) to the MFTPI solution.

While there is currently no direct evidence to justify the use of B_{12} in MFTPI solution, because of the known biochemical functions of the cobalamins and a small number of animal studies demonstrating their antinociceptive properties, it is used by some NDs and other practitioners of MFTPI and merits further discussion.

A number of animal studies have been conducted demonstrating the antinociceptive properties of thiamine, pyridoxine, and cyanocobalamin either alone (Franca et al., 2001; Fu et al., 1988; Leuschner, 1992), or used concomitantly with diclofenac (Jurna, 1998; Kuhlwein, Meyer, & Koehler, 1990; Reyes-Garcia et al., 1999; Vetter et al., 1988). One rat study showed that coadministration of diclofenac with either thiamine (B_1) or pyridoxine (B_6) resulted in an antinociceptive effect similar to that of diclofenac alone. On the other hand, coadministration of cyanocobalamin significantly increased diclofenac-induced antinociception (Reyes-Garcia et al., 1999).

While it is well known that vitamin B_{12} deficiency can cause fatigue, there exist data indicating that individuals who are not deficient in this vitamin experience increased energy after injections of vitamin B_{12} (Bjorkegren, 1999; Ellis & Nasser, 1973; Lapp & Cheney, 1993). Oral or sublingual B_{12} supplements are believed by some to be unlikely to obtain the same results as injectable B_{12}, because the body's ability to absorb large amounts is relatively poor (O'Dowd, 2000). Observational studies (Hutto, 1997) have found as many as 30% of patients hospitalized for depression to be deficient in vitamin B_{12} (Pennix et al., 2000).

Apart from the common practice of adding B_{12} and other pharmaceutical-grade natural substances, whether botanical, nutraceutical, or homeopathic, to the MFTPI solution, all other aspects of the technique, namely, the indications, contraindications, and techniques, are consistent with the teachings of Travell.

REGENERATIVE INJECTION THERAPY

In simplest terms, RIT (also known as prolotherapy) is the injection of a hypertonic solution containing local anesthetic directly into damaged connective tissues with the purpose of triggering an inflammatory response in order to allow the body's natural healing mechanisms to take place (Linetsky, Miguel, & Saberski, 2001). RIT is very clearly described in Linetsky's comprehensive chapter in this publication, and we refer the reader to Chapter 62 for an exploration of the science of RIT. RIT is of particular interest to NDs practicing naturopathic pain medicine, because it is believed that it directly addresses the cause of pain and allows the body to naturally heal itself.

While there currently exists a paucity of data examining RIT, one of the best-constructed trials was conducted by Reeves and Hassanein in 2000. They found that intra-articular injection with 10% dextrose resulted in clinically and statistically significant improvements in pain associated with knee osteoarthritis. Blinded radiographic readings at 1-year post-treatment demonstrated improvement in several measures of osteoarthritis severity. Additionally, it was found that anterior cruciate ligament laxity, when concurrently present in this patient group, improved as well (Reeves & Hassanein, 2000).

A common naturopathic interpretation of RIT/prolotherapy is the addition of glucosamine sulfate (GS) to the injected solution in the treatment of degenerated connective tissue. GS taken orally has been shown to be effective in the treatment of the pain associated with osteoarthritis of the knee as well as in the delay of the progressive degeneration (Braham, Dawson, & Goodman, 2003; Matheson & Perry, 2003; McAlindon et al., 2000; Pavelka et al., 2002). Glucosamine, formed in the body as glucosamine-6-phosphate, is the most fundamental building block required for the biosynthesis of glycolipids, glycoproteins, glycosaminoglycans, hyaluronate, and proteoglycans. The mechanism of action of GS in reversing joint degenerations appears to be due to its ability to act as an essential substrate for, and to stimulate the biosynthesis of, the glycosaminoglycans and the hyaluronic acid backbone used in the formation of the proteoglycans found in the structural matrix of the synovium. After an oral dose, glucosamine concentrates in the liver, where it is incorporated into plasma proteins, degraded into smaller molecules, or used for other biosynthetic processes. Although absorption is very high, a substantial quantity of the absorbed glucosamine is probably modified or degraded to smaller compounds, such as H_2O, CO_2, and urea (Setnikar et al., 1993).

From these data, it is intriguing to NDs to inject GS directly into degenerated joints, ligaments, and tendons. NDs are not alone in injecting GS. Klein et al. (2003) conducted a pilot study to test the potential effectiveness of intradiscal injection therapy using an RIT solution, which included GS in the treatment of intervertebral disc disease. The study included 30 patients with chronic intractable discogenic low back pain. Affected lumbar intervertebral discs were injected with a solution of glucosamine and chondroitin sulfate combined with hypertonic dextrose and dimethlysulfoxide (DMSO). Assessment of pain and disability was completed before treatment and 12 months after the last treatment. Although the results were statistically insignificant for the 30 patients as a whole, 17 of the 30 patients (57%) improved markedly with an average of 72% improvement in disability scores and 76% in visual analogue scores. The other 13 patients (43%) had little or no improvement. Patients who did poorly included those with failed spinal surgery, spinal stenosis, and long-term disability (Klein et al., 2003). Derby et al. (2004) also conducted a pilot study where they compared "intradiscal restorative injections" containing GS to intradiscal electrothermal treatment (IDET) in the treatment of discogenic disc pain and found restorative injections to be slightly more effective than IDET in reported pain 6 to 18 months post-procedure and much improved in cost–benefit ratio.

Yelland et al. (2004) conducted a trial on RIT for low back pain. They assessed the efficacy of a prolotherapy injection versus the injection of saline with or without an exercise protocol in the treatment of chronic nonspecific low back pain in 110 patients. Their findings demonstrated significant and sustained reductions in pain and disability occur with ligament injections, irrespective of the solution injected or the concurrent use of exercises (Yelland et al., 2004). These data suggest that the mechanism of action of RIT may be found more in the mechanical disruption and subsequent local inflammation caused by the manipulation of the needle and stimulation of intracellular growth factors by the compression of cells by the injected solutions than by any specific chemomodulation caused by various ingredients used. However, more study is needed.

MESOTHERAPY

Although mesotherapy and its applications to pain and sports medicine are almost entirely unheard of in the United States, it is widely popular and available around the world. It is an emerging modality in naturopathic pain medicine and is of particular interest because of its apparent safety, tolerability to patients, and seeming efficacy.

History of Mesotherapy

In 1952, a French physician, Dr. Michel Pistor, administered 10 ml of procaine intravenously in an attempt to abort an acute asthmatic attack in a patient. While the treatment did not improve the patient's respiratory status, upon follow-up the patient reported a significant improvement in his impaired hearing. Soon after, Pistor began experimenting with superficial injections of procaine around the ear of deaf patients and reported some success. Soon his practice was full of hearing impaired patients seeking treatment. His results in curing deafness were mixed; however, many of these patients had improvement in seemingly unrelated concomitant conditions such as eczema of the auditory canal, temporomandibular joint pain, and tinnitus, which can be related to deafness (LeCoz, 1993).

Pistor continued experimenting with superficial injections of procaine for the treatment of various disorders, and in 1958 he published an article, which stated, "the action on the tissues originating from the mesoderm is so extensive that these treatments should be called mesotherapy." This was the first time the term *mesotherapy* appeared in print. Pistor proposed the basic premise of mesotherapy to be the "smallest dose, infrequently, in the correct location" (LeCoz, 1993).

The mesoderm is one of three embryologic histological classifications: endoderm, mesoderm, and ectoderm. The cells of the endoderm eventually develop primarily into the internal organs. The cells of the mesoderm level develop into dermis and hypodermis, fatty tissues, and the musculoskeletal system. The ectoderm develops into, among other tissues, the brain and epidermis. The term *mesotherapy* therefore is in reference to injecting into the dermis and hypodermis, which originates from the mesoderm (although some mesotherapy techniques involve injecting the epidermis, which originates from the ectoderm). The mesoderm exists only in embryos; there is no mesoderm layer of the human skin, a common erroneous belief among English-language mesotherapists.

The French Society of Mesotherapy was formed in 1964 and consisted of 12 members. The first international conference on mesotherapy took place in 1976. This was also the year mesotherapy was first used in in-patient settings in France. In 1981, Dr. Jacques LeCoz introduced mesotherapy into the sports medicine program at the National Institute of Sports in Paris. The French Academy of Medicine officially recognized mesotherapy as a legitimate treatment modality within conventional medicine in 1987.

Currently, mesotherapy is considered mainstream medicine in France with more than 16,000 practitioners. It has been incorporated as an integral treatment in the specialty of sports medicine (Laurens, 2000) and pain management (Roch, 2000) in France as well as in other countries around the world (Belhocine & Oussedik, 2000). Apart from the French Society of Mesotherapy, some of the more established national mesotherapy associations or societies are in Algeria, Argentina, Belgium, Brazil, Canada, Colombia, Great Britain, Germany, Greece, Israel, Italy, Mexico, Portugal, Russia, Switzerland, Spain, Tunisia, Turkey, and Venezuela. Mesotherapy is also becoming widely popular in Asia with new national associations and societies being formed every year. In France, mesotherapy is primarily used for pain management and sports medicine, but the aesthetic procedures are very popular as well (LeCoz et al., 1994).

In the United States, mesotherapy as an aesthetic procedure is just now beginning to gain attention, and a number of professional associations are forming with a primary focus on cosmetic applications. Mesotherapy had been used in France for cosmetic purposes long before making its way to the United States. The French have always been ahead of the United States in cosmetic procedures; they developed liposuction and chemical peels. Mesotherapy has been used in the treatment of cellulite since the 1960s (LeCoz et al., 1994). Unfortunately, in the United States, pain management and sports medicine applications go largely ignored.

Basic Tenets of Mesotherapy

Mesotherapy is defined by its unique style of injection: various superficial injections using specialized short needles and specific injection techniques directly over the site of the affected structure (LeCoz et al., 1994). There are broad-ranging treatment protocols and philosophies regarding which substances are injected, including conventional medicines, botanical medicines, homeopathic medicines, or micronutrients.

The basic premise of mesotherapy is that solutions injected intracutaneously remain in the injected area longer because they are slower to be cleared by general circulation than a deeper injection. Further, it is felt that the injected solutions continue to penetrate the deeper tissues. Kaplan (1985) injected calcitonin marked with a radioisotope and found upon serial scans that the more superficial the injections, the longer the solution remained in the area. LeCoz and DuPont (1993) conducted an experiment on patients scheduled to undergo arthroscopic surgery of the knee. The subjects were divided into three groups. The first group received intraepidermic papules of

a diluted NSAID, the second group received injections of the same amount of the same solution using 4-mm needles, and the third group similarly received deep intramuscular injections. At hours 1 and 3 post-injection, venous blood draws were performed to determine serum levels of the NSAID. It was found that uniformly, the shallower the injection, the less of the substance was found in venous circulation at both 1 and 3 hours post-injection. During arthroscopy, synovial biopsies were performed, and all groups were found to have NSAID present, although levels were not determined (LeCoz and Dupont, 1983). Mesotherapy, therefore, appears to be a novel technique to administer medicines where the skin acts as a natural time-release system.

There are three primary mesotherapy injecting techniques: *intradermic* (also called "point by point"), *nappage* (French for "covering"), and *epidermic*. Intradermic was first described in the context of mesotherapy by Pistor. It is very simply the injection of 0.02 to 0.05 cc of solution after inserting a 4-, 6-, or 12-mm needle its entire depth. Intradermic injections are generally 1 to 2 cm apart, and few are given. *Nappage*, first described by Bourguignon and Ravily (Mrejen & Perrin, 2003), is a more superficial technique that takes practice to master. With the syringe held at a 45° angle from the skin while applying positive pressure on the syringe's plunger, the practitioner uses a rapid flicking of the wrist technique, which can resemble shaking a salt shaker or the action of a sewing machine. In *nappage*, a 4-mm needle is used and is not fully inserted, perhaps only 0.5 to 2 mm deep, with only a drop of solution injected at each site at approximately 0.5-cm intervals. In this way, one is able to infuse a large area of skin with the solution. The third technique is epidermic, first described by Perrin in 1996 (Mrejen & Perrin, 2003). As the name implies, this is the most superficial of the techniques, and frequently the needle does not even puncture the skin. A 12-mm (or 1/2-inch) 30-gauge needle, bevel up and at a very steep angle (approximately 160°), is dragged along the skin while light positive pressure is applied to the syringe's plunger. The needle will bend slightly from the angle and the pressure. Some practitioners will use a slight "bouncing" action, which will cause minor pinpoint bleeding. Epidermic technique will cause a shallow groove in the uppermost layers of keratinized epithelial cells and place a bead of solution into that groove. When done correctly, there is no bleeding, but one is able to see the solution quickly absorb into the skin. Epidermic technique is done in a grid pattern at 1-cm intervals over the entire affected area. Care must be taken. If the epidermic technique is applied too aggressively, it can leave scars.

As practiced in France for sports medicine and pain management, a mesotherapy solution is generally a base solution with the addition of whichever medication is indicated. The base solution is a local anesthetic and a drug from the vasodilator class.

The local anesthetic most commonly used in France for mesotherapy is either lidocaine 1% or procaine 1%, always without epinephrine. Local anesthetics are administered simply for their anesthetic properties, believed to be longer acting when injected superficially. As taught by the French Society of Mesotherapy, lidocaine is generally indicated for treatment of acute conditions, whereas procaine is indicated for chronic conditions because of its additional vasodilatory properties (*Mosby's Drug Consult*, 2005).

In France, there are many more pharmacologic preparations classified as vasodilatory than are available in the United States. The drug of this class that is most frequently used in France is buflomedil (Fonzylane). The only FDA-approved medication in the United States that is used in France that resembles this category is pentoxifylline (Trental). Pentoxifylline, approved for the treatment of intermittent claudication, improves the flow properties of blood by decreasing its viscosity and improving erythrocyte flexibility, thereby enhancing tissue oxygenation. Pentoxifylline has been shown to increase leukocyte deformability and to inhibit neutrophil adhesion and activation. Tissue oxygen levels have been shown to be significantly increased by therapeutic doses of pentoxifylline in patients with peripheral arterial disease (*La Phamacopee en Mesotherapie*, 2001). Mesotherapists believe that by increasing microcirculation of localized tissue beds, elimination of metabolic waste is more efficient and there is an increase in the delivery of the mesotherapeutic solutions as well as oxygen and nutrients in general circulation, thereby encouraging healing. Injecting pentoxifylline mesotherapeutically is believed to exercise its therapeutic effect for a continued period of time compared with per os or a deeper injection (LeCoz, 1993).

Upon this base solution of local anesthetic and vasodilatory preparation, a treatment-specific medication is added. The choice of medication is based on the condition treated and the philosophy of the practitioner (i.e., allopathic medications vs. homeopathic medications or other natural substances). In the case of muscle spasm, a muscle relaxant is used; in the case of acute inflammation, an NSAID; in depression, amitriptyline and magnesium are injected into specific acupuncture points. French mesotherapists have found that when injected mesotherapeutically, a much smaller amount of medication (generally 1/60th of the recommended oral dose) is needed to achieve therapeutic benefit. This has the added benefit of avoiding the risk of adverse side effects encountered with normal oral doses.

Of particular interest is the French mesotherapists' liberal use of salmon calcitonin (sCT) in the treatment of a broad spectrum of chronic pain disorders. sCT is best known as an antiosteoporotic agent, but its analgesic effects in the treatment of acute osteoporotic fracture have been well documented (Gennari, 2002; Lyritis et al., 1999; Mehta, Malootian, & Gilligan, 2003; Silverman & Azria, 2002). Further studies have examined the anti-nociceptive properties of sCT for a range of disorders including advanced metastatic malignancy (Allan, 1983; Mystakidou et al., 1999; Szanto et al., 1986), reflex sympathetic dystrophy (Appelboom, 2002), phantom-limb pain (Simanski et al., 1999; Wall & Heyneman, 1999), and diffuse sclerosing osteomyelitis of the humerus (Donnelly & Doyle, 1993). One animal study demonstrated the ability of sCT ability to potentiate the analgesic effect of amitriptyline and paroxetine (Ormazabel et al., 2001).

The mechanisms of analgesic action of sCT are believed to be multifactorial (Azria, 2002), and an anti-inflammatory action has been suggested (Azria, 2002). Studies in animals and in humans demonstrate that in some, but not all cases, sCT increases plasma beta-endorphin levels (Franceschini et al., 1993), and it is possible that specific binding sites for sCT exist in the brain (Lyritis & Trovas, 2002).

It merits mention that while the clinical use of sCT is relatively safe, it is not without risk of side effect or adverse reaction. Nausea, with or without vomiting, and local inflammatory reactions at the site of injection are encountered in approximately 10% of patients receiving sCT. Flushing of face or hands, skin rashes, nocturia, pruritus of the ear lobes, feverish sensation, pain in the eyes, poor appetite, abdominal pain, edema of feet, and salty taste have been reported in patients treated with sCT. Administration of sCT has been reported in isolated cases to cause hypersensitivity reaction (*Mosby's* Drug Consult, 2005).

Currently, the majority of scientific data in the field of mesotherapy regarding the treatment of pain and sports medicine are in the French language and consist of clinical case series. One such clinical case series showed mesotherapy to be beneficial in the treatment of 65 patients suffering from chronic thoracic back pain from arthritis, spinal stenosis, and sprain/strain that was not adequately controlled using conventional methods (NSAIDs, narcotic analgesics, muscle relaxants, and physiotherapy; Smail, 2000). Another paper describes the results of treatment of 267 cases of degenerative arthritic pain and shows mesotherapy to be an effective and reasonable treatment option, especially in light of the complete absence of adverse side effects or reactions in the treatment group (Leah da Silva & Mesquita, 2000). Another paper describes the mesotherapeutic treatment of 210 patients with various soft tissue musculoskeletal pain whose pain was not satisfactorily controlled with conventional methods. These patients were treated mesotherapeutically with local anesthetics, NSAIDs, sCT, and a nonsedating centrally acting muscle relaxant (thiocolchicoside), and again showed mesotherapy to be a reasonably effective treatment option, especially in light of poor patient toleration of the most commonly used interventive option, injection of corticosteroids (Chos, 2000). Another paper that describes the use of mesotherapy on 132 cases of patients with back and neck pain that had not been ameliorated by at least 3 months of conventional treatment shows mesotherapy to be a promising treatment option in terms of safety and efficacy (Messedi-Kamoun, Ben Salah, & Dziri, 2000). Mesotherapy has been shown to be helpful in a variety of commonly seen sports medicine conditions, such as Achilles tendonitis (Bourit & Guerin, 2000).

A systematic review and descriptive analysis of the current data and better-constructed, large-scale trials are needed. However, mesotherapy appears to be a promising modality in the treatment of a spectrum of painful disorders. It is of particular interest in the field of naturopathic pain medicine, because of its seeming safety profile and tolerability to the patient.

CONCLUSION

Many patients with pain seek alternative health care because of philosophical leanings or dissatisfaction with conventional care. Naturopathic physicians specializing in naturopathic pain medicine and board-certified by NATI have a large armamentarium of traditional and cutting-edge modalities available to them. According to the data available, naturopathic pain medicine appears to be safe, effective, and potentially cost-effective.

REFERENCES

Allan, E. (1983). Calcitonin in the treatment of intractable pain from advanced malignancy. *Pharmatherapeutica, 3*(7), 482–486.

Ambrose, K., Lyden, A. K., & Clauw, D. J. (2003). Applying exercise to the management of fibromyalgia. *Current Pain and Headache Reports, 7*(5), 348–354.

Anand, A. (2000). Role of magnesium in alleviating pain: Newer insights. *Journal of Pain and Symptom Management 20*(1), 1–2.

Appelboom, T. (2002). Calcitonin in reflex sympathetic dystrophy syndrome and other painful conditions. *Bone, 30*(5 Suppl.), 84S–86S.

Astin, J. et al. (1998). A review of the incorporation of complementary and alternative medicine by mainstream physicians. *Archives of Internal Medicine, 158*, 2303–2310.

Azria, M. (2002). Possible mechanisms of the analgesic action of calcitonin. *Bone, 30*(5 Suppl.): 80S–83S.

Belhocine, M., & Oussedik, E. (2000, October 20–22). Dix annees de mesotherapie en traumatologie du sport au C.N.M.S. 9th International Mesotherapy Conference held by the French Society of Mesotherapy, Paris, 199–106.

Bier, I. (2000). Peripheral intravenous nutrition therapy: Outpatient, office-based administration. *Alternative Medicine Revue, 5*(4), 347–354.

Bjorkegren, K. (1999). Vitamin B12, chronic fatigue and injection treatment, *Lakartidningen, 96*(50), 5610.

Blanchard, J., Tozer, T. N., & Rowland, M. (1997). Pharmacokinetic perspectives on megadoses of ascorbic acid. *American Journal of Clinical Nutrition, 66*(11), 65–1171

Bourit, G., & Guerin, P. (2000, October 20–22). Propositions therapeutiques dans la pathologie du tendon calcaneen. 9th International Mesotherapy Conference held by the French Society of Mesotherapy. Paris.

Braham, R., Dawson, B., & Goodman, C. (2003). The effect of glucosamine supplementation on people experiencing regular knee pain. *British Journal of Sports Medicine, 37*(1), 45–49; discussion 49.

Chakravarthy, M. V., Joyner, M. J., & Booth, F. W. (2002). An obligation for primary care physicians to prescribe physical activity to sedentary patients to reduce the risk of chronic health conditions. *Mayo Clinic Proceedings, 77*(2), 165–173.

Chos, D. (2000, October 20–22). Enquete retrospective des tendino-myalgies du rachis rencontrees dans une consultation de rhumatologue dans le cadre d'n centre anti douleur. 9th International Mesotherapy Conference Held by the French Society of Mesotherapy. Paris.

Crosby, V., Wilcock, A., & Corcoran, R. (2000). The safety and efficacy of a single dose (500 mg or 1 g) of intravenous magnesium sulfate inneuropathic pain poorly responsive to strong opioid analgesics in patients with cancer. *Journal of Pain and Symptom Management, 19*(1), 35–39.

Curhan, G. C. et al. (1999). Intake of vitamins B-6 and C and the risk of kidney stones in women. *Journal of the American Society of Nephrology, 10*(4), 840–845.

Derby, R. et al. (2004). Comparison of intradiscal restorative injections and intradiscal electrothermal treatment (IDET) in the treatment of low back pain. *Pain Physician, 7*, 63–66.

Donnelly, S., & Doyle, D. V. (1993). Chronic diffuse sclerosing osteomyelitis of the humerus: Novel treatment with calcitonin. *Journal of Rheumatology, 20*(6), 1073–1076.

Eisinger, J. et al. (1994). Selenium and magnesium status in fibromyalgia. *Magnesium Research, 7*(3–4), 285–288.

Eisinger, J. et al. (1996). Protein peroxidation, magnesium deficiency and fibromyalgia. *Magnesium Research, 9*(4), 313–316.

Elley. C. R. et al. (2003). Effectiveness of counseling patients on physical activity in general practice: Cluster randomized controlled trial. *British Medical Journal, 326*, 793.

Ellis, F. R., & Nasser, S. (1973). A pilot study of vitamin B12 in the treatment of tiredness. *British Journal of Nutrition, 30*, 277–283.

Ernst, E., & Chrubasik, S. (2000). Phyto-anti-inflammatories. A systematic review of randomized, placebo-controlled, double-blind trials. *Rheumatic Diseases Clinics of North America, 26*(1), 13–27, vii.

Franca, D. S. et al. (2001). B vitamins induce an antinociceptive effect in the acetic acid and formaldehyde models of nociception in mice. *European Journal of Pharmacology, 421*(3), 157–164.

Franceschini, R. et al. (1993). Calcitonin and beta-endorphin secretion. *Biomedicine and Pharmacotherapy, 47*(8), 305–309.

Fu, Q. G. et al. (1988). B vitamins suppress spinal dorsal horn nociceptive neurons in the cat. *Neuroscience Letter, 95*(1–3), 192–197.

Gaby A. (1998). Intravenous vitamin and mineral therapy. Paper presented at Nutritional Therapy in Medical Practice, Seattle, WA.

Gaby, A. (2002). Intravenous nutrient therapy: The Meyers cocktail. *Alternative Medicine Revue, 7*(5), 389–403

Gennari, C. (2002). Analgesic effect of calcitonin in osteoporosis. *Bone, 30*(5 Suppl.), 67S–70S.

Goldenberg, D. L. et al. (1990). High frequency of fibromyalgia in patients with chronic fatigue seen in a primary care practice. *Arthritis & Rheumatism, 33*(3), 381–387.

Groff, J., Gropper, S., & Hunt, S. (1995). *The regulatory nutrients. Advanced nutrition and human metabolism.* St. Paul, MN: West Publishing Company.

Hanninen, O. et al. (2000). Antioxidants in vegan diet and rheumatic disorders. *Toxicology, 155*(1–3), 45–53.

Hurley, B. F., & Roth, S. M. (2000). Strength training in the elderly: Effects on risk factors for age-related diseases. *Sports Medicine, 30*(4), 249–268.

Huteau, Y. (2001). *La pharmacopee en mesotherapie.* Societe Francaise de Mesotherapie (3rd ed.). Paris: Perrin

Hutto, B. R. (1997). Folate and cobalamin in psychiatric illness. *Comprehensive Psychiatry, 38,* 305–314.

Johnston, C. S. (1999). Biomarkers for establishing a tolerable upper intake level for vitamin C. *Nutrition Revues, 57*(3), 71–77.

Jurna, I. (1998). Analgesic and analgesia-potentiating action of B vitamins. *Schmerz, 12*(2), 136–141.

Kaplan, A. (1985). Raincour — Devernir d'un produit marque injecte par quatre voies differentes. *Les Bulletins de la Societe Francaise de Mesotherapie,, 62.*

King, S. J. et al. (2002). The effects of exercise and education, individually or combined, in women with fibromyalgia. *Journal of Rheumatology, 29*(12), 2620–2627.

Kirchfeld F., & Boyle, W. (1994). *Nature doctors; Pioneers in naturopathic medicine.* Portland, OR: Medicina Biologica.

Klein, G., & Kullich, W. (1999). Reducing pain by oral enzyme therapy in rheumatic diseases. *Wiener Medizinische Wochenschrift, 149*(21–22), 577–580.

Klein, R. G. et al. (2003). Biochemical injection treatment for discogenic low back pain: A pilot study. *Spine Journal, 3*(3), 220–226.

Koinig, H. et al. (1998). Magnesium sulfate reduces intra- and postoperative analgesic requirements. *Anesthesia & Analgesia, 87*(1), 206–210.

Kuhlwein, A., Meyer, H. J., & Koehler, C. O. (1990). Reduced diclofenac administration by B vitamins: Results of a randomized double-blind study with reduced daily doses of diclofenac (75 mg diclofenac versus 75 mg diclofenac plus B vitamins) in acute lumbar vertebral syndromes. *Klinische Wochenschrift, 68*(2), 107–115.

Lapp, C., & Cheney, P. (1993). The rationale for using high-dose cobalamin (vitamin B12). *CFIDS Chronicle Physicians' Forum,* Fall, 19–20.

Laurens, D. (2000, October 20–22). Suivi traumatologique des perchistes de l'INSEP de juillet 1998 a juillet 2000. 9th International Mesotherapy Conference Held by the French Society of Mesotherapy. Paris.

Leah da Silva, J., & Mesquita, M. E. (2000, October 20–22). Resultants de l'evaluation de deux annees de traitement de la douleur par mesotherapie dans les rhumatismes degeneratifs chroniques. 9th International Mesotherapy Conference Held by the French Society of Mesotherapy. Paris.

LeCoz, J. (1993). *Mesotherapie in medecine generale.* New York: Masson.

LeCoz, J. et al. (1994). *Mesotherapie et medicine esthetique.* France: Sola.

LeCoz, J. (1999). *Mesotherapie in medecine generale.* New York: Masson.

LeCoz, J., & Dupont, J. -Y. (1983). L'injection en regard du genou par voie mesotherapique donne de bonnes concentrations intra-articularires. *Quotidien du Medecin, 20* (September).

Leipner, J., Iten, F., & Saller, R. (2001). Therapy with proteolytic enzymes in rheumatic disorders. *BioDrugs, 15*(12), 779–789.

Leuschner, J. (1992). Antinociceptive properties of thiamine, pyridoxine and cyanocobalamin following repeated oral administration to mice. *Arzneimittel-Forschung, 42*(2), 114–115.

Linetsky, F. S., Miguel, R., & Saberski, L (2001). Pain management with regenerative injection therapy (RIT). In *Pain management: A practical guide for clinicians* (6th ed.). Boca Raton: CRC Press.

Lonsdale, D., Shamberger, R. J., Stahl, J. P., & Evans, R. (1999). Evaluation of the biochemical effects of administration of intravenous nutrients using erythrocyte ATP/ADP ratios. *Alternative Medicine Revue, 4*(1), 37–44.

Lyritis, G. P. et al. (1999). Analgesic effect of salmon calcitonin suppositories in patients with acute pain due to recent osteoporotic vertebral crush fractures: A prospective double-blind, randomized, placebo-controlled clinical study. *Clinical Journal of Pain, 15*(4), 284–289.

Lyritis, G. P., & Trovas, G. (2002). Analgesic effects of calcitonin. *Bone, 30*(5 Suppl.), 71S–74S.

Mann, N. (2000). Dietary lean red meat and human evolution. *European Journal of Nutrition, 39*(2), 71–79.

Masson, M. (1995). Bromelain in blunt injuries of the locomotor system. A study of observed applications in general practice. *Fortschritte der Medizin, 113*(19), 303–306.

Matheson, A. J., & Perry, C. M. (2003). Glucosamine: A review of its use in the management of osteoarthritis. *Drugs & Aging, 20*(14), 1041–1060.

Mauskop, A., & Altura, B. (1998). Role of magnesium in the pathogenesis and treatment of migraines. *Clinical Neuroscience, 5*(1), 24–27.

Mauskop, A. et al. (1995a). Intravenous magnesium sulfate relieves cluster headaches in patients with low serum ionized magnesium levels. *Headache, 35*(10), 597–600.

Mauskop, A. et al. (1995b). Intravenous magnesium sulphate relieves migraine attacks in patients with low serum ionizedmagnesium levels: A pilot study. *Clinical Science, 89*(6), 633–636.

Mauskop, A. et al. (1996). Intravenous magnesium sulfate rapidly alleviates headaches of various types. *Headache, 36*(3), 154–160.

Mazzotta, G. et al. (1999). Intracellular Mg++ concentration and electromyographical ischemic test in juvenile headache. *Cephalalgia, 19*(9), 802–809.

McAlindon, T. E. et al. (2000). Glucosamine and chondroitin for treatment of osteoarthritis: A systematic quality assessment and meta-analysis. *Journal of the American Medical Association, 283*(11), 1469–1475.

Mehta, N. M., Malootian, A., & Gilligan, J. P. (2003). Calcitonin for osteoporosis and bone pain. *Current Pharmaceutical Design, 9*(32), 2659–2676.

Messedi-Kamoun, N., Ben Salah F. Z., & Dziri, C. (2000, October 20–22). La mesotherapie dans les douleurs rachidiennes experience Tunisienne a propos de 132 cas. 9th International Mesotherapy Conference Held by the French Society of Mesotherapy. Paris.

Morinville, V., Jeannet-Peter, N., & Hauser, C. (1998). Anaphylaxis to parenteral thiamine (vitamin B1). *Schweizerische Medizinische Wochenschrift, 128*(44), 1743–1744.

Mosby's Drug Consult (15th ed.). (2005)., St. Louis, MO: Elsevier.

Mrejen, D., & Perrin, J. J. (2003). Mesotherapie et Rachis. *Editions S.F.M. CERM Ile de France*, CRM Champagne.

Mystakidou, K. et al. (1999). Continuous subcutaneous administration of high-dose salmon calcitonin in bone metastasis: Pain control and beta-endorphin plasma levels. *Journal of Pain and Symptom Management, 18*(5), 323–330.

Nenonen, M. T. et al. (1998). Uncooked, lactobacilli-rich, vegan food and rheumatoid arthritis. *British Journal of Rheumatology, 37*(3), 274–281.

Ng, S. Y. (1999). Hair calcium and magnesium levels in patients with fibromyalgia: A case center study. *Journal of Manipulative Physiological Therapy, 22*(9), 586–593.

Nicolodi, M., & Sicuteri, F. (1996). Fibromyalgia and migraine, two faces of the same mechanism. Serotonin as the common clue for pathogenesis and therapy. *Advances in Experimental Medicine and Biology, 398*, 373–379.

O'Dowd, P. (2000). B12 supplementation: must be parenteral. *Medicine & Health Rhode Island, 83*(8), 252–253.

O'Keefe, J. H., Jr., & Cordain, L. (2004). Cardiovascular disease resulting from a diet and lifestyle at odds with our Paleolithic genome: How to become a 21st-century huntergatherer. *Mayo Clinic Proceedings, 79*(1), 101–108.

Okayama, H., Aikawa, T., & Okayama, M. et al. (1987). Brochodilating effect of intravenous magnesium sulfate in bronchial asthma. *Journal of the American Medical Association, 257*, 1076–1078

Okifuji, A., Turk, D., & Marcus, D. (1999). Comparison of generalized and localized hyperalgesia in patients with recurrent headache and fibromyalgia. *Psychosomatic Medicine, 61*(6), 771–780.

Ormazabal, M. J. et al. (2001). Salmon calcitonin potentiates the analgesia induced by antidepressants. *Pharmacology, Biochemistry and Behavior, 68*(1), 125–133.

Pavelka, K. et al. (2002). Glucosamine sulfate use and delay of progression of knee osteoarthritis: A 3-year, randomized, placebo-controlled, double-blind study. *Archives of Internal Medicine, 162*(18), 2113–2123.

Pennix, B. W. et al. (2000). Vitamin B-12 deficiency and depression in physically disabled older women: Epidemiologic evidence from the Women's Health and Aging Study. *American Journal of Psychiatry, 157*, 715–721.

Phillips, L. D. (1997). *Manual of I.V. therapeutics* (2nd ed.). Philadelphia: F.A. Davis Company.

Reed, J. (1990). Magnesium therapy in musculoskeletal pain syndromes — Retrospective review of clinical results. *Magnesium and Trace Elements, 9*, 330.

Reeves, K. D., & Hassanein, K. (2000). Randomized prospective double-blind placebo-controlled study of dextrose prolotherapy for knee osteoarthritis with or without ACL laxity. *Alternative Therapies in Health and Medicine, 6*(2), 68–74, 77–80.

Relman, A., & Weil, A. (1999). Is integrative medicine the medicine of the future? *Archives of Internal Medicine, 159*, 2122–2126.

Reyes-Garcia, G. et al. (1999). Characterization of the potentiation of the antinociceptive effect of diclofenac by vitamin B complex in the rat. *Journal of Pharmacology and Toxicology Methods, 42*(2), 73–77.

Roch, F. X. (2000, October 20–22). Place de la Mesotherapie dans un centre anit-douleur. 9th International Mesotherapy Conference held by the French Society of Mesotherapy. Paris.

Setnikar, I. et al. (1993). Pharmacokinetics of glucosamine in man. *Arzneimittel-Forschung, 43*, 1109–1113.

Silverman, S. L., & Azria, M. (2002). The analgesic role of calcitonin following osteoporotic fracture. *Osteoporosis International, 13*(11), 858–867.

Simanski, C. et al. (1999). Therapy of phantom pain with salmon calcitonin and effect on postoperative patient satisfaction. *Chirurg, 70*(6), 674–681.

Smail, H. (2000, October 20–22). Douleurs thoraciques anterieures d'origine vertebrale. 9th International Mesotherapy Conference Held by the French Society of Mesotherapy. Paris.

Stephen, J. M., Grant, R., & Yeh, C. S. (1992). Anaphylaxis from administration of intravenous thiamine. *American Journal of Emergency Medicine, 10*(1), 61–63.

Sydow, M., Crozier, T. A., & Zielmann, S. et al. (1993). High-dose intravenous magnesium sulfate in the management of life-threatening status asthmaticus. *Intensive Care Medicine, 19*, 467–471.

Szanto J. et al. (1986). Pain killing with calcitonin in patients with malignant tumours. *Oncology, 43*(2), 69–72.

Tilwe, G. H. et al. (2001). Efficacy and tolerability of oral enzyme therapy as compared to diclofenac in active osteoarthrosis of knee joint: An open randomized controlled clinical trial. *Journal of the Association of Physicians in India, 49*, 617–621.

Tramer, M. et al. (1996). Role of magnesium sulfate in postoperative analgesia. *Anesthesiology, 84*(2), 340–347.

Travell, J., & Simons, D. G. (1983). *Myofascial pain and dysfunction: The trigger point manual.* Baltimore: Williams & Wilkins.

U.S. Department of Labor. (2003). *Dictionary of Occupational Titles,* 5th ed.). Washington, D.C.: Author.

Valim, V. et al. (2003). Aerobic fitness effects in fibromyalgia. *Journal of Rheumatology, 30*(5), 1060–1069.

Vetter, G. et al. (1988). Shortening diclofenac therapy by B vitamins. Results of a randomized double-blind study, diclofenac 50 mg versus diclofenac 50 mg plus B vitamins, in painful spinal diseases with degenerative changes. *Zeitschrift fur Rheumatologie, 47*(5), 351–362.

Walker, A. F. et al. (2002). Bromelain reduces mild acute knee pain and improves well-being in a dose-dependent fashion in an open study of otherwise healthy adults. *Phytomedicine, 9*(8), 681–686.

Wall, G. C., & Heyneman, C. A. (1999). Calcitonin in phantom limb pain. *Annals of Pharmacotherapy, 33*(4), 499–501.

Wittenborg, A. et al. (2000). Comparative epidemiological study in patients with rheumatic diseases illustrated in a example of a treatment with non-steroidal anti- inflammatory drugs versus an oral enzyme combination preparation. *Arzneimittel-Forschung, 50*(8), 728–738.

Xiao, W., & Bennett, G. (1994). Magnesium suppresses neuropathic pain responses in rats via a spinal site of action. *Brain Research, 666*(2), 168–172.

Yelland, M. J. et al. (2004). Prolotherapy injections, saline injections, and exercises for chronic low-back pain: A randomized trial. *Spine, 29*(1), 9–16; discussion 16.

Section IX

Electrical and Magnetic Therapies

Mark V. Boswell, MD, PhD, Section Editor

82

Electromedicine

Subrata Saha, PhD, and Ajay R. Kashi, BDS (MS)

INTRODUCTION

HISTORY

Electromedicine can be defined as the study of different types of electrical therapies used for the treatment of various medical ailments. Electromedicine has been practiced for hundreds of years, according to the historical data available. In the early years after the death of Christ, a growing interest in the use of electricity and magnetism was observed. This practice of electricity and magnetism for healing dates back more than 3,000 years (Basford, 2001), when sick people were treated with these methods. During the same time period, it was known that the electrical powers of fish (e.g., electric eels) influenced clinical medicine as a possible cure for ailments like headache and gout (Basford, 2001).

The discovery of the magnetism by Pliny the Elder (A.D. 23–79) (Basford, 2001) from stones that harbored attractive forces is the basis of the modern-day magnet. During the medieval age, the church played an important role in the progress of magnet therapy for medical ailments (Basford, 2001). Faith played an important role in most of the scientific research at least until the 17th century. Peregrinus in 1289 showed scientifically the workings of the magnet and did not commit to mystic forces (Basford, 2001). During the Renaissance and the Middle Ages, the magnet was used to treat a variety of medical ailments, and retrieve foreign bodies such as knives and arrowheads. Paracelsus (1493–1542) proposed a "push–pull" theory of treating disease. He suggested that when the south pole of a magnet is held near the head and the north pole near the abdomen of patients with epilepsy, it would cure the disease essentially by

pushing and pulling the disease from the body (Basford, 2001).

By the late 1800s, physicians across the United States were using electricity for treating pain regularly, although there was almost no scientific data or literature to support or to justify its use. The discovery of specific points on the body surface, which cause the underlying muscles to contract, was an important finding. These specific points on the body are now known as the "muscle points" or "motor points." Electrical stimulation of the motor points leads to contractions of the underlying muscles, much like contraction of the muscle during exercise. It is thought that contraction of muscles in this manner can lead to the alleviation of pain in a particular region of the body. Motor points are considered important anatomical landmarks for the application of electrodes of the electrotherapy devices. Another important finding is the ongoing research in the 18th- and 19th-century psychiatric therapies, during which it was assumed that vagus nerve stimulation by the application of electricity through the skin greatly disturbed the hypothalamic hormone vasopressin. This approach was used to treat affective disorders (Leonard, 2004).

Electrotherapy in the 20th Century

The popularity of electromedicine in America increased after the Civil War (Basford, 2001). A wide variety of electrical and magnetic devices were available at the beginning of the 20th century. All devices claimed to relieve patients having pain from various ailments. However, there was no universally accepted system or guidelines to justify these claims made by various electrical device manufacturers. Many physicians were using these devices even though they did not know their scientific basis, and they were not trained formally in the use of such devices (Basford, 2001). Use of such devices was a very popular mode of treatment for pain during this period.

The advent of electrotherapeutics gained wide acceptance by the medical community in the 20th century. The hot debate regarding the scientific basis of such devices did little to tarnish the reputation of some of these devices, such as the Electreat, which used shocks similar to those of the torpedo fish (Basford, 2001). Although many devices used were considered false and endorsed by quacks, the popularity of electromedicine remained in mainstream medicine. It faced criticism from many quarters and its use waxed and waned for most part of the 20th century.

Modern Clinical Electromedicine

Research and development in the field of electromedicine slowed in the early 20th century because of claims of quackery and unscientific basis for the functioning of these devices. Gradual acceptance of electrical therapies has made possible the use of certain devices in mainstream medicine currently to treat a wide range of conditions by using devices such as transcutaneous electrical nerve stimulation (TENS), cranial electrical stimulation (CES), and transcranial electrotherapy. Modern-day electromedicine is used to treat painful conditions associated with the head and neck, back pain, pain associated with other conditions, orofacial pain, dental pain, postsurgery pain, and postirradiation pain associated with cancer. The following section focuses mainly on the use of electromedicine for the treatment of pain. Brief discussion about its other uses is also included.

INTERACTION OF ELECTRICITY WITH THE BRAIN

To understand the interaction of electricity with the brain, one must think that there is some sort of a connection or a link between the cells of the brain (neurons) and electricity (in this case, the signals or stimulation received by the neurons involved). In other words, an electromagnetic field may act in the same way as a hormone on the cell membrane.

MECHANISM INVOLVED IN ELECTROMEDICINE

The interplay of the frequency, wavelength, intensity, and the location of the electrical input to facilitate specific effects in the human body is the basis for the physiologic action behind electromedicine. Certain electrical impulses in humans help to facilitate some bodily functions including, but not limited to, healing (Kirsch & Lerner, 1990). Mimicking the electrical impulses occurring in us can produce specific physiologic effects (Kirsch & Lerner, 1990).

OVERVIEW OF THE HUMAN NERVOUS SYSTEM

The nervous system in humans can be divided mainly into two different systems:

1. The central nervous system or CNS, which is the portion of the vertebrate nervous system consisting of the brain and the spinal cord and
2. The autonomous or autonomic nervous system or ANS, which is the part of the nervous system regulating involuntary actions, like those of the intestines, heart, glands, etc.; the ANS is further subdivided into the sympathetic and parasympathetic nervous system.

PRIMARY AFFERENT AXONS

Primary afferent axons are nerves that transmit information from touch or pain to the spinal cord and brain; they are nerve fibers connected to different types of receptors in the skin, muscle, and internal organs. The diameter of the nerve fiber correlates to the speed with which information travels in it; i.e., the thicker the nerve fiber, the faster the information travels in it. In some forms of electrotherapy, such as TENS therapy, specific fibers are activated. In the later part of this chapter, the different types of TENS devices/mechanisms are discussed in relation to the activation of specific nerve fiber types. Before proceeding to presentation of the types of TENS affecting various nerve fibers, an overview of the main types of fibers in the human body is shown in Table 82.1.

A-alpha nerve fibers transmit information related to proprioception (the ability to sense stimuli arising within the body/muscle). A-beta nerve fibers transmit information related to touch. A-delta and C-nerve fibers transmit information related to pain and temperature. However, the information travels faster in A-delta fibers compared to the C-fibers because the A-delta fibers are bigger in diameter than the C-nerve fibers. C-nerve fibers transmit information related to pain and temperature.

As electromedicine is principally used to treat pain, it is important to be familiar with the anatomical structures in the body responsible for transmitting impulses, such as pain, touch, and pressure to and from the periphery of the body to the brain and spinal cord. These are known as the afferent and efferent nerve fibers, and their functions are

TABLE 82.1
Main Nerve Fibers in the Human Body

Fiber Type	Aα	Aβ	Aδ	C
Diameter (μm)	13–20	6–12	1–5	0.2–1.5
Speed (m/s)	80–120	35–75	5–35	0.5–2.0

as follows. The afferent nerve fibers carry signals inward to a central organ or section, as nerves that conduct impulses from periphery of the body to the brain or spinal cord, and the efferent nerve fibers carry signals or impulses away from a central organ or section. In other words, they carry impulses away from the CNS. It has been hypothesized that electrotherapy devices interact with electrical signals of the brain. The brain waves are involved in normal functions of the body, such as gamma brain waves or fast brain waves, which operate at 40 Hz and are involved in higher mental activity such as perception and consciousness. Similarly, beta brain waves operate at 25 Hz and are present in the fully awake state; alpha brain waves operate at 10 Hz and are present during sleep, prayer, light meditation; theta brain waves operate at 3 Hz and are associated with astral travel, remote viewing; and, finally, delta brain waves operate at 0.5 Hz and are associated with deep meditation. The brain waves can be recorded by an EEG (or electroencephalogram) machine.

TYPES OF ELECTROMEDICINE

Electromedicine uses different devices for various forms of treatment to treat different conditions affecting one's body (Kirsch & Lerner, 1990). Briefly, the treatments can be classified as follows:

1. Transcutaneous electrical nerve stimulation, or TENS
2. Cranial electrotherapy stimulation, or CES
3. Microcurrent electrical therapy
4. Electro acutherapy
5. Auricular medicine

Magnets and acupuncture are popular modes of treating pain symptoms (Grant, Miller, Winchester, Anderson, & Faulkner, 1999; Karp, 2004). The theory behind the use of magnets in pain management is that the magnet reacts with the iron in the blood to increase blood flow and promote healing. In many recent studies, it has been shown that magnet therapy may show positive effect in certain patients and for certain conditions, but it may not show any beneficial effect in a significant number of patients (Karp, 2004). Magnet therapy has been used for many painful conditions such as foot pain, low back pain, and carpal tunnel syndrome (Karp, 2004). The placebo effect may play an important role in magnet therapy. Karp (2004) states that the decrease in pain reported by subjects wearing magnetic devices was not statistically significantly different compared with placebo-treated groups. However, in a study by Weintraub (Table 82.2), 450 Gauss multipolar magnetic insoles were used in 141 subjects and placebo insoles were used in 118 patients to treat symptomatic diabetic peripheral neuropathy, with constant symptoms for at least 6 months. The results of this study showed

TABLE 82.2
Results of Study Using Magnetic Insoles and Placebo Insoles in Treatment of Diabetic Peripheral Neuropathy

	Treatment Group	Placebo Group
No. of patients	141	118
Type of insole	450 Gauss multipolar magnetic insole	Placebo insole
Burning	12% reduction	3% reduction
Numbness and tingling	10.5% reduction	1% increase

Source: Data from Karp, J., *Biomechanics,* 73, 2004.

TABLE 82.3
Treatment Results from Subgroup of Patients

	Treatment Group	Placebo Group
Percentage of pain reduction in a subset of patients with baseline severe pain	32%	14%
Percentage of pain reduction in a subset of patients with foot pain	41%	21%

beneficial effect of the magnet therapy (Table 82.2 and Table 82.3).

Table 82.3 shows the results of a subgroup of patients from the study by Weintraub indicating the presence/absence of success rates in different conditions. It should be noted that all of the patient groups in this study had a placebo control.

CLINICAL ASPECTS OF ELECTROMEDICINE

The main types of pain (acute and chronic; Russo, 2001) can be categorized as nociceptive and neuropathic pain (Conti et al., 2003), respectively. The nerve fibers (Aδ and C) respond to noxious chemical, mechanical, and thermal stimuli; they are known as nociceptors, and the pain perceived by nociceptors is known as nociceptive pain (Basford, 2001). In acute pain, pain results from trauma, or injury within a very short period, for example, pain resulting from a needle prick or a hot surface. The severity of acute pain directly correlates to the severity of injury. Normal individuals have protective reflexes to prevent injury in acute pain. Management of acute pain normally focuses on treating the underlying cause (such as an injury). In the case of chronic/neuropathic pain, the level of tissue damage does not correlate with the pain; instead, the pain impulses are transmitted continuously even in the absence of tissue damage or injury. Chronic pain is influenced by the way the brain processes the pain signals.

Factors such as emotions and thoughts play an important role in chronic pain (Turk, 2004). Because determining the exact cause of chronic pain is very difficult, its management is also equally challenging. Many modes of treatment including deep relaxation techniques, biofeedback, meditation, and electrotherapy are being used and investigated currently to treat chronic pain.

The mechanism involved in nociceptive pain (Russo, 2001) starts once the noxious stimuli, for example, injury to the skin, has occurred. The nociceptors (Aδ and C nerve fibers) pick up the signal, and afferent impulses are relayed to the CNS. The primary afferents synapse in the dorsal horn onto second-order neurons in the substantia gelatinosa of the spinal cord. This is followed by either a synapse via a third-order neuron to the somatosensory cortex or via second-order neurons to the thalamus by the contralateral spinothalamic tract of the spinal cord. Some fibers from the spinothalamic tract travel to the pons and midbrain to synapse on nuclear complexes such as nucleus raphe magnus and the nucleus raphe gigantocellularis (both areas are involved in descending regulation of second-order neurons). Finally, endorphins such as serotonin and epinephrine inhibit noxious stimuli and the continued firing of second-order neurons.

In neuropathic/chronic pain (Russo, 2001), the primary lesion results in transmission of afferent impulses to the peripheral and central nervous systems. This is followed by "memory of pain," which leads to neuroplasticity of the spinal cord and chronic pain, which may later persist in the absence of noxious stimuli. The anterior cingulate gyrus is related to the emotional component of pain, and the posterior cingulated gyrus is related to the localization of pain (localization of pain is said to be very precise for skin, more difficult for deep tissues such as joints and muscles, and very poor for viscera such as the abdominal viscera).

Until recently, there was no theory to describe the pain mechanism, but in 1965, Melzack and Wall proposed the gate control theory, which proposes a gating mechanism of closing and opening of ion channels in the spinal cord in response to stimulation of large-diameter fibers (touch) and smaller-diameter fibers (pain). This theory makes sense in the need for survival, as it is important to detect and respond to pain in preference to other less urgent signals. The gate control theory is said to be the clinical basis for the use of TENS in clinical medicine (Kirsch & Lerner, 1990; Merkel, Gustein, & Malviya, 1999; Sluka & Walsh, 2003).

TRANSCUTANEOUS ELECTRICAL NERVE STIMULATION

DEFINITIONS

1. Some define TENS as the application of electrical stimulation to the skin for pain control

(according to the American Physical Therapy Association; Sluka & Walsh, 2003)
2. Others believe that technically any device that delivers electrical currents across the intact surface of the skin is TENS.

The different types of TENS include conventional TENS (produces segmental analgesia), which activates large-diameter Aβ-fibers without activating small-diameter Aδ- and C-fibers or muscle efferents; acupuncture-like TENS (AL-TENS), which activates small-diameter fibers (Aδ or group III) arising from muscle (ergoreceptors) by the induction of phasic muscle twitches; and finally, intense TENS, in which small-diameter Aδ cutaneous afferents are activated by delivering TENS over peripheral nerves arising from the site of pain. AL-TENS and intense TENS produce extrasegmental analgesia through ergoreceptor activity and activity in small-diameter cutaneous afferents, respectively. Conventional TENS and intense TENS can also produce peripheral blockade of afferent information in the fiber type they activate.

PRACTICAL CONSIDERATIONS

To test the practical effectiveness of a TENS device, reporting by patients about the sensation produced by the TENS device is the easiest means of assessing the type of fiber that is active (Kirsch & Lerner, 1990). Testing and experimenting with a variety of current amplitudes, frequencies, and durations to produce the appropriate outcome is the best way to assess the effectiveness of a TENS device.

Many clinicians prescribe TENS devices to their patients without showing them how to use them. An important consideration is that first-time users of TENS need to try and modulate/regulate the appropriate frequency, amplitude, and other characteristics of the device before they experience relief from pain. To implement the TENS treatment in the presence of an experienced clinician would be the best approach to use the device for the first time. Once the patient is comfortable with the appropriate electrical parameters, the clinician can set the device to those values so that there is relief of pain every time the patient uses the device.

Electrode Placement: Electrode placement in TENS therapy can be both along nerve roots or trigger points (a specific point or area which if stimulated by pressure or touch or will induce a painful response) and along dermatomes of respective nerves (Kirsch & Lerner, 1990). The clinician is the appropriate person to evaluate the best position for electrode placement initially. Once the patient has experienced pain relief, one can confidently assume that the position for placement of the electrodes has worked in favor of the patient (Figure 82.1). Prescribing a TENS device blindly without ascertaining the appropriate clinical parameters is one of the main reasons for

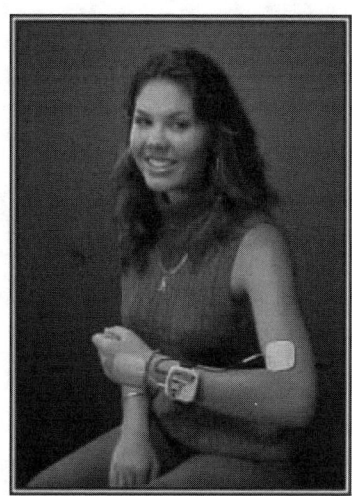

FIGURE 82.1 Electrotherapy device with electrodes in place. Courtesy of Healthonics' MedRelief™.

failure of TENS therapy. Other parameters such as current amplitude, frequency, and pulse repetition rate have to be adjusted as well to obtain satisfactory clinical performance of the TENS device.

Energy Source: TENS devices work with currents in the milliampere range. Sources of power include alkaline batteries and nickel cadmium batteries. The drawback of external sources of power such as batteries is the power decay, and the need for frequent replacement of batteries (Kirsch & Lerner, 1990).

Electrodes: The electrodes used in TENS have evolved over the years. Initial treatment with TENS used electrodes with a gel. The main drawbacks were uneven conductivity, minor skin burns at high currents, and messiness because of the gel. Currently, disposable self-adhesive electrodes are used, which also prevent the possibility of acquiring transmitted diseases. Disposable electrodes have become the norm in most TENS devices currently available (Kirsch & Lerner, 1990).

Effect of TENS Frequency, Intensity, and Stimulation Site Parameters on Pain Thresholds in Humans

In a study by Chesterton, Foster, Wright, Baxter, and Barlas (2003), the effects of varying TENS frequency, intensity, and stimulation sites were evaluated in an experimental model of pain. The study was carried out in a cohort consisting of 240 volunteers, who were randomized to one of six experimental TENS groups and a sham TENS or control. Approximately, 30 subjects were assigned to each TENS group. Two TENS frequencies (110 Hz or 4 Hz) and two intensities (the highest tolerable level) at a fixed pulse duration (200 μs) were applied for 30 minutes. The sites of application were relative to the

measurement site (segmental, extrasegmental, or a combination of these). The conclusion derived was that the high-frequency and high-intensity segmental and combined stimulation groups showed rapid onset along with significant hypoalgesic effects; the study also stated that clinical applications of these parameter combinations need to be further investigated.

In a different study by Cramp, McCullough, Lowe, and Walsh (2002), the effect of TENS intensity on local and distal cutaneous blood flow and skin temperature was determined. The aim of the study was to determine how cutaneous blood flow and skin temperature interact with the sympathetic nervous system. The study concluded that low-frequency TENS on cutaneous blood flow is dependent on whether stimulation is applied at intensity above or below the motor threshold. It also found that increase in cutaneous blood flow was local in nature and did not occur because of the depression of the sympathetic nervous system. Some typical features of TENS devices are listed below:

1. Pulse amplitude: 1 to 50 mA
2. Pulse duration: 10 to 1000 μs
3. Pulse frequency: 1 to 250 p.p.s.
4. Additional features such as batteries, timer, and number of channels

Clinical Applications of TENS

Many common clinical conditions can be treated with the use of TENS. TENS has been shown to produce both analgesic and non-analgesic effects. Some of the analgesic effects produced by TENS are used to treat postoperative pain; labor pain; dental and orofacial pain; musculoskeletal pain; low back pain; neuralgias, such as trigeminal neuralgia; angina pectoris; arthritis; and pain resulting from bone fractures. The non-analgesic effects of TENS include its use for treating nausea associated with morning sickness, travel sickness, and chemotherapy and also to improve blood circulation to enhance the speed of wound healing. It is also used to treat symptoms associated with peripheral neuropathy in diabetes.

Pulse Waveforms and Pulse Patterns in TENS

Different TENS units use different forms of pulse waveforms. Broadly, they can be classified as either monophasic (a single phase) or biphasic (two phases) waveforms. Schematics of the different pulse waveforms in TENS are shown in Figure 82.2 and Figure 82.3. Pulse patterns in TENS include continuous, burst, modulated (amplitude, frequency, and duration modulated), and random frequency modes (Figure 82.3).

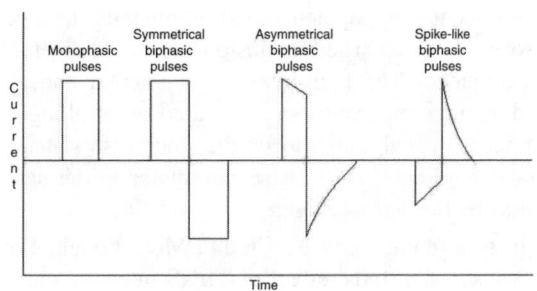

FIGURE 82.2 Pulse waveforms in TENS.

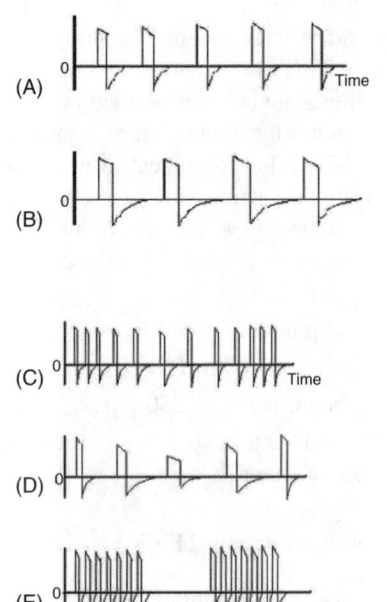

FIGURE 82.3 (A) Pattern of electrical pulses. (B) Normal mode of continuous train of pulse. (C) Pulse duration mode with automatic modulation of pulse duration. (D) Frequency modulation with automatic increase and decrease in the repetition rate. (E) Strength duration modulation with automatic reductions of pulse duration followed by increases in pulse amplitude accompanied by decreases in pulse duration.

MECHANISM OF ACTION OF TENS

A brief description of the mechanism of action of the different types of TENS is presented in the following section. The mechanism of the action of TENS includes antidromic collision, which states that when tissue damage occurs, afferent impulses arise. Conversely, as TENS is applied, it induces nerve impulses, which travel away from the CNS. Both these nerve impulses meet to collide with and extinguish pain. Conventional TENS is said to follow this mechanism of action. The second type involves segmental mechanisms, in which the activity of second-order nociceptive neurons in the dorsal horn of the spinal cord is inhibited by the activity generated in the Aβ-fibers. The second mechanism is also observed in conventional TENS. Finally, the other mechanism involves extraseg-

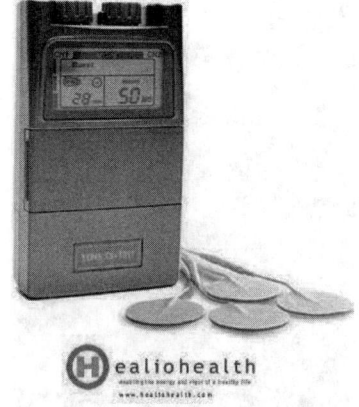

FIGURE 82.4 An example of a TENS unit. Courtesy of Healiohealth.

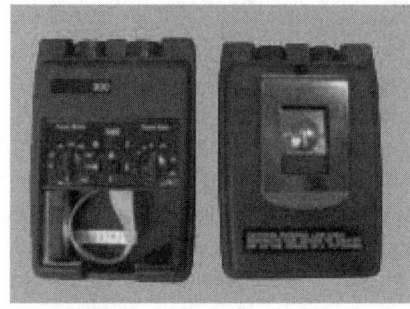

FIGURE 82.5 Examples of other TENS-like units. Courtesy of Back Be Nimble (www.backbenimble.com).

mental routes, seen in small-diameter afferents, which form the descending pathways of pain inhibition, such as the periaqueductal gray area of the brain (physiologically involved in rage reactions, bladder responses, and pain), the nucleus raphe magnus (involved in nociception), and the nucleus raphe gigantocellularis (involved in muscle atonia during REM sleep). Figure 82.4 and Figure 82.5 show examples of TENS units.

MICROCURRENT ELECTRICAL THERAPY

Microcurrent electrical therapy (Kirsch & Lerner, 1990) (MET) uses low-frequency (0.5 to 100 Hz), microampere currents ranging from 10 to 600 μA. It produces very low and subtle currents barely perceived by the person being treated. It is used by health care professionals to accelerate the healing process and also to treat such conditions as anxiety, depression, and insomnia. According to Kirsch (Kirsch & Lerner, 1990), use of a low frequency, preferably 0.5 Hz, is suitable for most treatments. If not, a higher setting may be needed. Kirsch goes on to state that patients should be given at least three treatments to evaluate their response to microcurrent electrical therapy, as the effects are thought to be cumulative. For a thorough understanding of the workings of a MET device and the treatment schedules required, a patient must review a MET device manual or consult his or her physician prior to undergoing any such treatments, as every individual's pain intensity threshold level is different.

MEDICAL USES OF ELECTROMEDICINE

TENS IN THE TREATMENT OF CHRONIC BACK PAIN

Chronic back pain is seen usually in elderly individuals because of osteoarthritis of the intervertebral joints (Grant et al., 1999; Turk, 2004). The treatment of chronic back pain using nonsteroidal anti-inflammatory drugs has the drawback of systemic side effects (Grant et al., 1999). TENS is one of the most frequently used modalities of pain relief among nonconventional modes of treating chronic pain conditions (Grant et al., 1999). In a recent study, Grant et al. (1999) investigated the effectiveness of acupuncture and TENS to treat chronic low back pain in elderly patients. The study included 60 patients aged 60 or over who had had back pain for at least 6 months. In this investigation, the effectiveness of acupuncture was well established and demonstrated as safe. The authors concluded that both acupuncture and TENS work by different neurophysiological mechanisms; both are effective treatments for chronic back pain in the elderly and safe to administer.

Pauza et al. (2004) conducted a randomized, placebo-controlled trial of intradiscal electrothermal therapy (IDET) for treating discogenic low back pain. The study was carried out in 64 patients, in whom both IDET and placebos were used. Within 1 hour after treatment with IDET, when patients were asked about the particular treatment they believed in, 78% believed they had the active treatment, 5% believed they had the sham (placebo), and 16% were unable to determine the kind of treatment. Conversely, in those patients who received the sham treatment, 74% believed that they received active treatment, 7% assumed that they received the sham (placebo), and 14% were unable to determine the nature of the treatment. Because the cohort varied in the patients' psychological domains, in the severity of disability, and in the performance of the operator in discography, the results may not be entirely attributable to any one clinical procedure (the actual IDET or the placebo). Thus, further studies are needed to evaluate the best response.

TENS AND POSTOPERATIVE PAIN

Postoperative pain management is one of the important aspects of providing patient relief (Benedetti et al., 1997; Bjordal, Johnson, & Ljunggreen, 2003; Rakel & Frantz, 2003). Usually various medications often containing narcotics are used to control postoperative pain. However, they often have some adverse effects such as respiratory depression, nausea, vomiting (Benedetti et al., 1997), and hypersensitivity reactions. In studies involving TENS to relieve pain after postoperative surgical procedures on the abdomen (Rakel & Frantz, 2003), thoracic surgical procedures (Benedetti et al., 1997), total knee arthroplasty (Breit & Wall, 2004), and a host of other postoperative procedures, it has been shown that TENS is an effective mode of pain management postoperatively (Benedetti et al., 1997; Bjordal et al., 2003; Rakel & Frantz, 2003). In a study by Benedetti et al. (1997) involving 324 patients who underwent different types of thoracic surgical procedures, it was shown that TENS is useful to control postoperative pain when it is mild to moderate. However, this study indicated that TENS may not be beneficial to control severe pain. The study group/patient cohort was divided into three treatment groups: TENS, placebo TENS, and control, and the effectiveness of TENS was assessed starting from the beginning of treatment to the request for further analgesia and total medication intake during the first 12 hours after operation. As mentioned previously, TENS was not an effective alternative to treat severe pain conditions (for example, after posterolateral thoracotomy). The study also concluded that TENS could be used as an adjunct to systemic medications when the pain is mild to moderate and that systemic opioid and non-opioid analgesics are the treatment of choice for severe postoperative pain conditions.

Bjordal et al. (2003) investigated if the consumption of analgesics to reduce pain was reduced after the use of TENS. They conclude that if TENS is administered with a strong, subnoxious intensity at an adequate frequency in the area of the surgical wound, the consumption of analgesics for postoperative pain can be significantly reduced (Bjordal et al., 2003). In a study by Rakel and Frantz (2003), the effectiveness of episodic TENS supplementing pharmacologic analgesia on pain with movement and at rest after surgery of the abdomen was evaluated. They also examined the use of TENS during walking and vital capacity maneuvers, and the effect it had on these activities. They concluded that TENS decreased pain significantly during walking and deep breathing maneuvers. They also showed that TENS significantly improved the distance and speed of the walk postoperatively, when it was used along with analgesics.

TENS IN DENTISTRY

TENS has been used in dentistry (Curcio, Tackney, & Bergwerger, 1987; Harvey & Elliott, 1995; Hochman, 1988; Malamed & Joseph, 1987; Meechan, Gowans, & Welbury, 1998; Oztas, Olmez, & Yel, 1997; teDuits, Goepferd, Donly, Pinkham, & Jakobsen, 1993). The alleviation of pain is of prime importance for a successful dental procedure. It has been shown that patients with orofacial pain have a fear of severe pain and anxiety-related distress, when compared with matched controls (McNeil et al., 2001). This is also correlated to dental fear, but not with other general psychological symptomology (Hoshiyama & Kakigi, 2000). The use of local anesthetics is mandatory practice in most dental settings. However, the use of local anesthetics has various drawbacks, which are mentioned later. To improve pain management during a dental procedure and for a successful treatment outcome, the use of electronic dental anesthesia (EDA) or TENS in dentistry is discussed as a possible clinical application for pain management (Curcio et al., 1987; Harvey & Elliott, 1995; Hochman, 1988; Malamed & Joseph, 1987; Meechan et al., 1998; Oztas et al., 1997; teDuits, et al., 1993). Successful pain management has been achieved over the years during tooth preparation by the dentist using local anesthetics. The goal of using local anesthetics during tooth cavity preparation is to minimize pain for the patient and enhance patient cooperation. This also reduces the chair-side time for the dentist to perform the procedure, as both the dentist and patient are free from unwanted interruptions. The main drawbacks of local anesthetics are the use of a syringe to deliver the drug, making it an invasive procedure, allergic reactions to the anesthetic in some people, needle phobia, and prolonged effect of anesthesia for a longer than required period. Pediatric dentists are especially opposed to the use of a syringe as the sight of a needle can aggravate a child's behavior and attitude toward the dental procedure (Harvey & Elliott, 1995; Hochman, 1988). Moreover, despite warnings by the dentist about the lack of sensation in the numbed area after administration of the local anesthetic, many patients inflict self-injury by biting their lips as they lack sensation.

TENS or EDA can be an effective alternative to conventional means of pain relief. EDA eliminates the need for drug delivery via a syringe; it also eliminates the anesthetic effect once the EDA unit is turned off. In a study by Oztas et al. (1997), in pediatric patients undergoing regular tooth cavity preparations, 56% of patients preferred EDA to conventional local anesthetics administered using a syringe. In a similar study by teDuits et al. (1993), 78% of patients preferred EDA to conventional local anesthetics. According to Harvey and Elliott (1995) for a particular kind of cavity preparation in pediatric patients, a success rate of 100% was observed with TENS. The above findings show promise in the use of EDA to obtain analgesia. Other important uses of electromedicine in dentistry are the use of TENS in the treatment of painful orofacial conditions, such as trigeminal neuralgia, atypical facial pain, and musculoskeletal pain of the craniofacial region.

According to many published reports, cognitive processes (such as psychological factors, attribution of patients, and their attitudes toward pain, depression, and worry) play an important role in the successful treatment of pain in a patient (Turk, 2004). When the body is affected due to injury, it results in disability and lack of function. As a consequence, the patient is in a psychologically negative state of mind to respond to treatment options or physical activity to alleviate the pain symptoms. In a clinical scenario, when a patient expresses pain when examined, the clinician often prescribes medication based on the intensity of pain (stronger and different combinations of one or more pain relievers for more painful conditions). The psychological and cognitive aspects of the patients are often not fully considered (Turk, 2004). This warrants further research into understanding more about the mechanisms involved in pain processes with placebo-controlled studies, taking into account factors such as cognitive processes in the pain response and psychological counseling prior to initiating treatment for pain for a better outcome.

Pain management has become an integral part of managing a clinical condition to obtain better patient relief. To manage pain, many clinicians still rely on systemic medications. The interaction between systemic medications and electrotherapy devices is important in understanding if there is a connection between drugs and electrotherapy devices.

TENS IN CARPAL TUNNEL SYNDROME

Carpal tunnel syndrome (CTS) affects the wrist region. Compression of the median nerve in the carpal tunnel is thought to lead to this condition. A randomized, double-blind, placebo-controlled, crossover trial study by Naeser, Hahn, Lieberman, and Branco (2002) demonstrated that treatment with a combination of low-level laser therapy along with microampere TENS was found to be effective in treating CTS pain. A finite element model of the wrist anatomy was developed to predict the distribution of current in the nerves during diagnosis, and the possibility of therapeutic procedures involving electromagnetic excitation was investigated. Nerve conduction studies, evoked potentials, and electromyography have and are being investigated for this condition. Further studies should be conducted to determine the efficacy of conservative treatment in combination with other treatment modalities to obtain results that are more predictable.

MISCELLANEOUS

A number of other medical uses of electromedicine have been investigated (Grace, Revell, & Brookes, 1998; Robinson & Mackler, 1995; Saha, 1984; Scott & King, 1994). Electrical stimulation has been used successfully in controlling edema. It is thought that electrical stimulation increases venous or lymphatic drainage in the absence of or inability to perform voluntary exercise. A different medical use of electrical stimulation is to aid tissue/wound healing. This is based on the tissue polarity present after injury, known as the "current of injury." The theory states that wounds have a positive potential initially with respect to the surrounding tissue, and this positive polarity triggers the onset of the healing or repair process. It is thought that the maintenance of positive polarity favors wound healing. Other medical uses of electrical stimulation include bone growth in non-union and malunion of fractures (Nelson, Brighton, Ryaby, Simon, Nielsen, Lorich et al., 2003; Robinson & Mackler, 1995; Saha, 1984; Scott & King, 1994). Animal experiments have proved the osteogenic potential of electrical stimulation (Saha, 1984; Scott & King, 1994). It has been demonstrated in long bones of chick embryos that when an electromagnetic field of a certain pulse shape is administered, an increase in the length, weight, and mechanical strength is observed (Grace et al., 1998; Saha, Pal, Reddy, & Albright, 1982a, b). Similarly, when fibroblast cells are exposed to a pulsed electromagnetic field (PEMF) for a period of 7 days and their growth rate compared with a control group, there was an increase of growth in the test group by 15% on the first day to 100% on the fourth day. However, the growth increase dropped to 21% on the seventh day (Saha, 1984). Grace et al. (1998) demonstrated the beneficial effects of PEMFs in the healing time of fractures in animal models. It was shown that PEMFs enhance early vascular reaction and suppress pannus proliferation, along with early chondrogenesis, and bone formation. However, the same study also suggests that prolonged use of PEMFs may have a deleterious effect by enhancing chondrogenesis beyond a point observed in normal repair, thereby delaying normal subsurface trabeculation.

Scott and King (1994) carried out a double-blind trial of electrical capacitive coupling to treat nonunion of long bones in 23 patients. Of 21 patients who completed the study, 10 patients were actively managed and 11 were managed with the placebo unit. Of the 10 patients who had been managed actively, all 10 showed healing of the nonunion, but there was no evidence of healing seen in the 11 patients being treated with the placebo unit. Further studies need to be carried out to ascertain the optimum parameters of electrical stimulation in fracture healing.

In addition to the uses mentioned above, one can consider the following forms of medical treatments and diagnoses as various forms of electrotherapy. Cardiac defibrillators are life-saving devices, which deliver jolts of electricity to stimulate a stopped heart and help it start beating again. Invasive devices, such as artificial cardiac pacemakers, deliver jolts of electricity to the heart muscle to help it retain its normal rhythm. Other forms of electrotherapy include electric shock therapy to treat mental illness, schizophrenia, depression, and anxiety and brain pacemakers to treat patients with epilepsy (George et al., 2000; Maniker, Liu, Marks, Moser, & Kalnin, 2000). A recent development in the treatment of epilepsy is the introduction of the vagal nerve stimulator (George et al., 2000; Maniker et al., 2000; Morris, Mueller et al., 1999), a device

that is implanted in the neck over the left vagus nerve and sends small currents to regulate the electrical activity of the brain in patients with epilepsy. Although it has been shown to be effective in a significant percentage of patients, the placement is very technique sensitive. Other medical uses of electromedicine include electrotrichogeneis, i.e., the stimulation of hair growth by the positive influence of an electrostatic field on the hair follicle, which is being investigated as a possible treatment option for baldness. Electromedicine can also be used in patients with dysmenorrheal (Angelis, Perrone, Santoro, Nofroni, & Zichella, 2003) and hysteroscopy (used in the diagnosis of endouterine diseases; Angelis et al., 2003) and to treat postural instability after stroke (Perennou et al., 2001), as well as sciatica (Ghoname et al., 1999) and arthritic pain (Sluka, Bailey, Bogush, Olson, & Ricketts, 1998). Electrotherapy is also used to treat muscular atrophy in sports injuries and postsurgical conditions. The electromedicine treatment modalities mentioned are not described in detail here.

PHARMACOLOGICAL AGENTS, TENS, AND PAIN MANAGEMENT

Pain is a clinical symptom, presenting with different intensities and types. A good clinician will judge the symptom of pain as well as the type of treatment to manage the pain, depending on factors such as patients' acceptance of the medication (if drugs are the choice of treatment), age, and comorbid factors. Currently, most acute forms of pain are treated with systemic medications. But, chronic pain usually requires administration of a drug for long periods. This is sometimes accompanied by the added drawback of side effects involving systemic medications, such as gastrointestinal discomfort, hypersensitivity reactions, drug allergies, and a host of other undesirable systemic effects. These adverse effects of systemic medications suggest the need for adjunctive pain management techniques. Narcotics are often used in postoperative pain management with or without other conventional drugs (Benedetti et al., 1997; Fields, 1988). However, narcotics and opioids are associated with undesirable side effects such as addiction, respiratory depression, sedation, and tolerance (McQuay, 1997). There have been numerous studies indicating the effectiveness of TENS in such situations in overcoming these untoward effects (Bjordal et al., 2003; Grant et al., 1999; Rakel & Frantz, 2003). Although the effectiveness of TENS is limited in controlling severe postoperative pain and the use of pharmacological agents such as narcotics is justified in these situations, it has been shown that TENS can prove an effective alternative in controlling mild to moderate acute postoperative pain (Bjordal et al., 2003; Grant et al., 1999; Rakel & Frantz, 2003).

Electrotherapy can offer pain relief in some of these conditions, but according to a significant number of clinicians, it is also indicated for specific chronic conditions, and in specific patients (Koke et al., 2004). In a study by Tomasso et al. (2003), high-frequency TENS was shown to be effective in inhibiting nociceptive responses induced by CO_2 laser stimulation in humans. However, a lack of evidence showing the effectiveness of a combination of these treatments (pharmacological agents, TENS, and placebos) indicates a need for further studies to ascertain their respective roles. Investigations, which include placebos, electrotherapy devices, pharmacological agents, and their interactions with one another, have to be carried out to ascertain the efficacy of either one or a combination of these treatments for pain. Clinical trials indicating if pharmacological agents and electrotherapy treatments will negate the effects of each other or if there is synergism between these treatment types are desirable. It will also be beneficial to ascertain the mechanisms involved in each of these treatments, to achieve the wider acceptance of these treatments.

BENEFITS AND DRAWBACKS OF ELECTROMEDICINE

Electromedicine offers many advantages over conventional therapy for pain management involving systemic drugs and surgery (Kirsch & Lerner, 1990; Turk, 2004). The main advantages are cost-effectiveness, safety of the device as the currents used are of a very low intensity, few or no side effects from the treatment, easy acceptance by most patients, and the immediate relief of acute pain. Electrotherapy also has the ability to treat a wide range of clinical pain conditions (including many chronic pain conditions such as low back pain and other musculoskeletal pain), osteoarthritis, acute postoperative pain, and labor pain (Turk, 2004). Electrotherapy is noninvasive in the broad sense, and no drug interactions of the device have been reported according to current published data. The gradual acceptance by many insurance companies that electrotherapy devices, such as TENS, are reimbursable makes it more affordable to most patients.

Rechargeable batteries used in electrotherapy devices can be unreliable in that they have peaks in their discharge rate, leading to linear power decay. Some forms of electrotherapy, such as cardiac pacemakers and brain pacemakers (vagal nerve stimulators) (George et al., 2000; Maniker et al., 2000), are technique sensitive and invasive in their approach to treating cardiac abnormalities and epilepsy, respectively. Although manufacturers claim the safety of electrotherapy devices and their lack of interaction with other electrical devices such as cardiac pacemakers (Pyatt, Trenbath, Chester, & Connelly, 2002), it is desirable to conduct further investigations to ascertain if there is any interaction between these devices. In very

young patients (infants), pain management using electrotherapy devices has not been investigated. Other contraindications include pregnancy, patients with demand-type pacemakers. Care also should be taken not to place the TENS unit on the head and neck (Kirsch & Lerner, 1990). Although conducting these studies on the very young can be difficult, the main reason being the difficulty of recording the feedback from these patients, it is desirable to know what effects these forms of electrical therapies have on this age group before one prescribes such a device. The role of placebos in studies involving TENS needs to be investigated further (Turk, 2004). Lack of placebo-controlled studies, variations in placement of electrodes in patients, and variations in parameters such as frequency, intensity, and pulse duration between studies have contributed to the lack of conclusive data on the effectiveness of various TENS in the treatment of patients experiencing pain (Turk, 2004).

CONCLUSION

Electromedicine has been used as a treatment modality for more than a century. The introduction of low currents to the body has shown beneficial effects on pain, wound healing, and neurological response related to depression, anxiety, mental illness, etc. Electromedicine has benefited medical science by providing an effective alternative to conventional forms of treatment with its effects often outweighing its few drawbacks. Although a number of studies demonstrating the effectiveness of TENS, as well as other forms of electrotherapy, have been published, it still needs to be further investigated by conducting double-blind controlled clinical trials. The effect of placebos and TENS has been investigated and some studies have shown that placebos may prove equally beneficial as TENS in many situations. This warrants further investigations into the role of placebos and TENS for pain relief in order to obtain a better understanding of their mechanisms. Similarly, other electromedicine devices, their use in various treatments, and their mechanisms of action need to be examined further to form a firm scientific basis validating the use of electromedicine as a mode of choice for treating patients with pain.

REFERENCES

Angelis, C., Perrone, G., Santoro, G., Nofroni, I., & Zichella, L. (2003). Suppression of pelvic pain during hysteroscopy with a transcutaneous electrical nerve stimulation device. *Fertility & Sterility, 79*(6), 1422.

Basford, J. R. (2001). A historical perspective of the popular use of electric and magnetic therapy. *Archives of Physical Medicine & Rehabilitation, 82*, 1261.

Benedetti, F., Amanzio, M., Casadio, C., Cavallo, A., Cianci, R., Giobbe, R., et al. (1997). Control of postoperative pain by transcutaneous electrical nerve stimulation after thoracic operations. *Annals of Thoracic Surgery, 63,* 773.

Bjordal, J. M., Johnson, M. I., & Ljunggreen, A. E. (2003). Transcutaneous electrical nerve stimulation (TENS) can reduce postoperative analgesic consumption. A meta-analysis with assessment of optimal treatment parameters for postoperative pain. *European Journal of Pain, 7,* 181.

Breit, R., & Wall, H. V. (2004). Transcutaneous electrical nerve stimulation for postoperative pain relief after total knee arthroplasty. *Journal of Arthroplasty, 19*(1), 45.

Chesterton, L. S., Foster, N. E., Wright, C. C., Baxter, G. D., & Barlas, P. (2003). Effects of TENS frequency, intensity and stimulation site parameter manipulation on pressure pain thresholds in healthy human subjects. *Pain, 106,* 73.

Conti, P. C. R., Pertes, R. A., Heir, G. M., Nasri, C., Cohen H. V., & Pereira, C.. (2003). Orofacial pain: Basic mechanisms and implication for successful management. *Journal of Applied Oral Science, 11*(1), 1.

Cramp, F. L., McCullough, G. R., Lowe, A. S., & Walsh, D. M. (2002). Transcutaneous electric nerve stimulation: The effect of intensity on local and distal cutaneous blood flow and skin temperature in healthy subjects. *Archives of Physical Medicine & Rehabilitation, 83,* 5.

Curcio, F. B., Tackney, V. M., & Bergwerger, R. (1987). Transcutaneous electrical nerve stimulation in dentistry: A report of a double-blind study. *Journal of Prosthetic Dentistry, 58,* 379.

Fields, H. L. (1988). Reply to Howard L. Fields on "Can opiates relive neuropathic pain?" *Pain, 35,* 365.

George, M. S., Sackeim, H. A., Rush, A. J., Marangell, L. B., Nahas, Z., Husain, M. M. et al. (2000). Vagus nerve stimulation: A new tool for brain research and therapy. *Biological Psychiatry, 47,* 287.

Ghoname, E. A., White, P. F., Ahmed, H. E., Hamza, M. A., Craig, W. F., & Noe, C. E. (1999). Percutaneous electrical nerve stimulation: An alternative to TENS in the management of sciatica. *Pain, 83,* 193.

Grace, K. L. R., Revell, W. J., & Brookes, M. (1998). The effects of pulsed electromagnetism on fresh fracture healing: Osteochondral repair in the rat femoral groove. *Orthopedics, 21*(3), 297.

Grant, D. J., Miller, J. B., Winchester, D. M., Anderson, M., & Faulkner, S. (1999). A randomized comparative trial of acupuncture versus transcutaneous electrical nerve stimulation for chronic back pain in the elderly. *Pain, 82,* 9.

Harvey, M., & Elliott, M. (1995). Transcutaneous electrical nerve stimulation (TENS) for pain management during cavity preparations in pediatric patients. *ASCD Journal of Dentistry, 62,* 49.

Hochman, R. (1988). Neurotransmitter modulator (TENS) for control of dental operative pain. *Journal of the American Dental Association, 116,* 208.

Hoshiyama, M., & Kakigi, R. (2000). After-effect of transcutaneous electrical nerve stimulation (TENS) on pain-related evoked potentials and magnetic fields in normal subjects. *Clinical Neurology, 111,* 717.

Karp, J. (2004). Magnets attract a variety of opinions. *Biomechanics, 73*..

Kirsch, D. L., & Lerner, F. N. (1990). Electromedicine. In R. S. Weiner (Ed.), *Innovations in pain management: A practical guide for clinicians* (Chap. 23), Orlando, FL: Paul M. Deutsch Press.

Koke, A. J. A., Schouten, J. S. A. G, Geelen, M. J. H. L, Lipsch, J. S. M, Waltje, E. M. H. Kleef, M. et al. (2004). Pain reducing effect of three types of transcutaneous electrical nerve stimulation in patients with chronic pain: A randomized crossover trial. *Pain, 108,* 36.

Leonard, E. C., Jr. (2004). Did some 18th and 19th century treatments for mental disorders act on the brain? *Medical Hypotheses, 62,* 219.

Malamed, S. F., & Joseph, C. (1987). Electrical anesthesia: Electricity in dentistry, *Journal of the California Dental Association, 15*(6), 12.

Maniker, A., Liu, W. C., Marks, D., Moser, K., & Kalnin, A. (2000). Positioning of vagal nerve stimulators: Technical note. *Surgical Neurology, 53,* 178.

McNeil, D. W., Anthony, R., Zlovensky, M. J., McKee, D. R., Klineberg, I. J., & Ho, C. K. C. (2001). Fear of pain in orofacial pain patients. *Pain, 89,* 245.

McQuay H. J. (1997). Opioid use in chronic pain. *Acta Anaesthesiologica Scandinavica, 41,* 175.

Meechan, J. G., Gowans, A. J., & Welbury, R. R. (1998). The use of patient-controlled transcutaneous electronic nerve stimulation (TENS) to decrease the discomfort of regional anaesthesia in dentistry: A randomized controlled clinical trial. *Journal of Dentistry, 26,* 417.

Melzack, R., & Wall, P.D. (1996). *The challenge of pain* (2nd ed.). East Rutherford, NJ: Penguin.

Merkel, S. I., Gutstein, H. B., & Malviya, S. (1999). Use of transcutaneous electrical nerve dtimulation in a young child with pain from open perineal lesions. *Journal of Pain and Symptom Management, 18*(5), 376.

Morris, G. L., III, Mueller, W. M., & The Vagus Nerve Stimulation Study Group. (1999). Long-term treatment with vagus nerve stimulation in patients with refractory epilepsy. *Neurology, 53,* 1731.

Naeser, M. A., Hahn, K. A. K., Lieberman, B. E., & Branco, K. F. (2002). Carpal tunnel syndrome pain treated with low-level laser and microamperes transcutaneous electric nerve stimulation: A controlled study. *Archives of Physical Medicine & Rehabilitation, 83,* 978.

Nielson, F. R. T., Brighton, C. T., Ryaby, J., Simon, B. J., Nielson, J. H., Lorich, D. G. et al. (2002). Use of physical forces in bone healing. *Journal of the American Academy of Orthopaedic Surgeons, 11,* 344.

Oztas, M., Olmez, A., & Yel, B. (1997). Clinical evaluation of transcutaneous electronic nerve stimulation for pain control during tooth preparation. *Quintessence International, 28*(9), 603.

Pauza, K. J., Howell, S., Dreyfuss, P., Peloza, J. H., Dawson, K., & Bogduk N. (2004). A randomized, placebo-controlled trial of intradiscal electrothermal therapy for the treatment of discogenic low back pain. *Spine Journal, 4,* 27.

Perennou, D. A., Leblond, C., Amblard, B., Micallef, J. P., Herisson, C., & Pelissier, J. Y. (2001). Transcutaneous electric nerve stimulation reduces neglect-related postural instability after stroke. *Archives of Physical Medicine & Rehabilitation, 82,* 440.

Pyatt, J. R., Trenbath, D., Chester, M., & Connelly, D. T. (2002). The simultaneous use of a biventricular implantable cardioverter defibrillator (ICD) and transcutaneous electrical nerve stimulation (TENS) unit: Implications for device interaction. *Europace, 5,* 91.

Rakel, B., & Frantz, R. (2003). Effectiveness of transcutaneous electrical nerve stimulation on postoperative pain with movement. *Journal of Pain, 4*(8), 455.

Robinson A. J., & Mackler L. S. (1995). *Clinical electrophysiology electrotherapy and electrophysiologic testing* (2nd ed.). Baltimore, MD: Williams & Wilkins.

Rowbotham, M. C., Twilling, L., Davies, P. S., Reisner, L., Taylor, K., & Mohr, D. (2003). Oral opioid therapy for chronic peripheral and central neuropathic pain. *New England Journal of Medicine, 348*(13), 1223.

Russo, C. M. (2001). Pain: Control. *Encyclopedia of Life Sciences, 1.*

Saha, S. (1984, September 17–19). Electrical stimulation modalities for osteogenesis. *Proceedings of the 37th ACEMB,.*

Saha, S., Pal, R., Reddy, G. N., & Albright, J. A. (1982a). Growth of chick embryo modulated by pulsed electromagnetic stimulations. *Transactions of the 2nd Annual Meeting of the Bioelectric Repair and Growth Society, 2,* 59.

Saha, S., Pal, A., Reddy, G. N., & Albright, J.A. (1982b). Effect of different electromagnetic pulse parameters on the skeletal growth of chick embryo. In S. Saha (Ed.), *Biomedical engineering I: Recent developments.* New York: Pergamon Press.

Scott, G., & King, J. B. (1994). A prospective, double-blind trial of electrical capacitive coupling in the treatment of non-union of long bones. *Journal of Bone and Joint Surgery, 76-A*(6), 820.

Sluka, K. A., & Walsh, D. (2003). Transcutaneous electrical nerve stimulation: Basic science mechanisms and clinical effectiveness. *Journal of Pain, 4*(3), 109.

Sluka, K. A., Bailey, K., Bogush, J., Olson, R., & Ricketts, A. (1998). Treatment with either high or low frequency TENS reduces the secondary hyperalgesia observed after injection of kaolin and carrageenan into the knee joint. *Pain, 77,* 97.

teDuits, E., Goepferd, S., Donly, K., Pinkham, J., and Jakobsen, J. (1993). The effectiveness of electronic dental anesthesia in children. *Pediatric Dentistry, 15,* 191.

Tommaso, M., Fiore, P., Camporeale, A., Guido, M., Libro, G., Losito L., et al. (2003). High and low frequency transcutaneous electrical nerve stimulation inhibits nociceptive responses induced by CO_2 laser stimulation in humans. *Neuroscience Letters, 342,* 17.

Turk, D. C. (2004). Understanding pain sufferers: The role of cognitive processes. *Spine Journal, 4,* 1.

83

Electric Nerve Blocks

James W. Woessner, MD, PhD

INTRODUCTION

Those who have been shocked by lightning, an electric fence, or a household socket know that numbness occurs in the shocked body part(s), resulting from interruption of pain and sensory signals to the brain. That nerve blocks can be done with electricity is scientifically established. Performing nerve blocks with electricity is well enough accepted that two medical dictionaries describe nerve blocks as follows:

> *Gould's* (Gennaro et al. 1984): "nerve block. The interruption of the passage of impulses through a nerve, as by chemical, mechanical, or *electrical* [italic added] means."

> *Taber's* (Thomas, 1997): "nerve block. The induction of regional anesthesia by preventing sensory nerve impulses from reaching the central nervous system. This is usually done on a temporary basis, by using chemical or *electrical* [italics added] means."

These definitions, which accept electricity as an analgesic agent, make the concept and reality of nerve blocks being achieved scientifically accepted.

Electric nerve blocks (ENBs) involve introduction of an alternating electric current (AC) into the patient's body to interrupt the nerve impulses along pathways so that the perception of pain is decreased beyond the time of the actual treatment itself. Use of ENBs is not thought to conflict with currently accepted treatments for any part of the body, in a purely medical sense. ENBs are useful supplemental tools for patients who have pain.

NERVE BLOCKS IN GENERAL

Nerve blocks generally involve the introduction of an anesthetic agent to interrupt nerve impulses (Gordy et al., 2002). Nerve blocks provide analgesia and anesthesia. This entire volume explores the full range of therapies for the management of pain; analgesia provided by nerve blocks produced with electricity is the focus of this chapter.

THE ORIGIN OF NERVE BLOCKS FOR PAIN

Nerve blocks were originally done mechanically to facilitate local surgical procedures. Local and general anesthesia as part of surgical procedures became more sophisticated over time (Brown & Fink, 1998). It was noted that little or no pain was perceived after providing nerve blocks. Consequently, physicians began to use nerve blocks for better pain control. In both anesthetic and analgesic applications, the resultant pain relief provided a window of opportunity for the surgical procedure and for healing, respectively.

Because most nerve blocks were done with chemicals, most practitioners usually thought of chemical injections in connection with nerve blocks. Because anesthesia usually included analgesia, nerve blocks were subsequently used to promote pain control in situations where general anesthesia was considered unnecessary or undesirable.

"THE BODY ELECTRIC" (BECKER & SELDEN, 1985)

During the 20th century, electrical devices became generally accepted in medicine, initially for diagnostics. Most are familiar with electrocardiography (ECG), electroen-cephalography (EEG), and electromyography (EMG), including surface EMG (sEMG), and nerve conduction velocity (NCV) studies. Electrooculography, electroretin-ography, electronystography, electrocochleography, skin galvanics, and various evoked potentials are more special-ized, although less well-known electrodiagnostic proce-dures (Northrup, 2001).

Many have been clinically treated with electricity. Defibrillation, used in emergency situations to reestablish cardiac activity when fibrillation occurs, involves the pas-sage of an electrical current through the chest. Lower back pain often responds to transcutaneous electrical nerve stimulation (TENS) therapy and other electrotherapeutic techniques as part of overall treatment program. Electro-convulsive therapy (ECT) for depression, spinal cord stim-ulators (SCS)/dorsal column stimulators (DCS) for chronic pain control, bone growth stimulators after ortho-pedic surgery, neuromuscular stimulation for disuse atro-phy, and a number of other electrotherapies are a few examples of the currently used electrical techniques in modern medicine. TENS devices, as designated by the FDA, also include high-voltage galvanic stimulators (HVGS), neuromuscular electrical stimulators (NMES), interference stimulators, and various transcranial stimula-tors (e.g., the Alpha-Stim® devices and the Liss Transcra-nial/Body Stimulator®). Most of these electrical devices have been approved by the FDA as safe and efficacious and are allowed for use. Other electromedical treatments include:

- Thalamic stimulation
- Electroacupuncture
- Auricular acupuncture

While generally safe, these electrical procedures require a precise understanding of the patient's overall medical condition for best results and to avoid possible undesirable side effects. As with anything in medicine, ENBs have a specific medical indication and are *not* "cure-all" procedures. Most of the side effects are directly related to local changes to blood flow, probably occurring with the blocking of pain nerve impulses with electricity because efferent C-fibers to local arterioles are also blocked.

ANESTHESIA OR ANALGESIA

Leak (1992) nicely differentiated the creation of numb-ness, i.e., anesthesia, and the interruption of pain signals, i.e., pain nerve block or analgesia. As stated, anesthesia usually includes analgesia, but not the other way around. When doing nerve blocks for pain, anesthesia can mark-edly interfere with normal sensory function and, therefore, put the patient in unnecessary danger.

Surgery has been done by blocking sensory nerve impulses with electricity (Hardy et al., 1961). Electroan-esthesia and electroanalgesia have been used in Europe (Gadsby, 1998) and in the United States (Racz et al., 1992). If the electrodes are properly placed to perform nerve blocks, the clinical effects are not due to only electrical stimulation that would "stimulate" sensation and/or pain. FDA-accepted electrical devices used for ENBs do not provide enough current energy to cause frank anesthesia.

BACKGROUND

Using electricity for medical treatments occurred in ancient times (Rossi, 2003). Thousands of years ago ancient cultures used electricity-producing animals (elec-tric eels and rays) to administer electricity to sick citizens (including those in pain) as medical treatments. Electrical machines were popular with American doctors for thera-peutic purposes until 1907, when a campaign was initiated suggesting that the use of electricity as a medical treatment was quackery. Negative publicity resulted in most prac-ticing physicians discontinuing the further use of electric-ity in their practices. There still remains some sense of illegitimacy about ENBs even into the 21st century.

ELECTROTHERAPY

Electrotherapy used in some way to treat pain is fre-quently mentioned in books on electrotherapy (Kahn, 2000; Kitchen, 2002; Nelson et al., 1999; Robinson & Synder-Mackler, 1995; Simpson, 2003). Mechanisms for relieving pain are suggested, but nerve blocks are seldom mentioned directly. The best reason for pain relief from electrical stimulation, separate from ENBs, is the release of endorphins as pain modulators, and increased circula-tion and its relationship to muscle relaxation (Kitchen, 2002), explaining the residual pain relief that occurs fol-lowing ENBs.

Interestingly, most patients in pain seldom mention any lasting effect from traditional TENS units or electrostim-ulation (E Stim) treatments. Interferential and HVGS units often provide longer-lasting relief. This pain relief makes sense in the context of this chapter because the carrier frequency of interferential therapy is 4,000 Hz (cycles per second, or cps), which may result in neuron blockade. The high energy produced by the HVGS units potentially crosses the nerve cell membrane to activate cyclic adenos-ine monophosphate (cAMP); in other words, penetrance occurs via high energy rather than via high frequency.

EVIDENCE FOR NERVE BLOCKS WITH ELECTRICITY

Most physiology textbooks provide a basic description of the electrophysiology of human cells and tissues. Charman (2002) provides a short review of the "electrical properties of cells and tissues." Becker and Seldon (1985) has provided significant scientific evidence that the body is truly an electrical organism. ENBs involve the use of electricity in medicine (Kane & Taub, 1975), and the term itself was probably first used by Dr. Jenkner in his 1995 book, *Electric Pain Control* (Jenkner, 1995).

Schwartz (1998) provided a theoretical basis for ENBs. Schwartz (1998) and Hans Jurgens (1999) presented plausible mechanisms by which nerve blocks and curative phenomena could occur via electric currents applied to the human body. Clinical experience based on these theories suggested that nerve blocks do occur with electricity (Woessner, 2002b).

Stimulatory frequencies, the frequencies below the refractory frequency of the nerve (the maximum frequency that stimulates a nerve to fire), are basically employed for electrotherapeutic techniques (Hans Jurgens, 1999). Electrotherapeutic treatments are usually much below 500 Hz (cps) (Kitchen, 2002).

De Domenico (1982) and Goats (1990) suggested that interferential therapy provides a "physiological block of nociceptive fibres." This description is largely due to the carrier frequencies (approximately 4,000 Hz), which result in greater tissue penetration, rather than just the tomographic effect of these synchronized, but offset carrier frequencies, which produce the "beat" or interferential frequencies (10 to 150 Hz). Multifacilatory frequencies described by Hans Jurgens (1999), the frequencies above the refractory frequency of the nerve (usually 4,000 to 20,000 Hz), are obviously not functioning via nerve stimulation because the target nerve can fire only once at frequencies less than the refractory frequency (which can be thought of as being around 1,000 Hz).

The frequencies used for ENBs likely carry the electrical signal and energy inside of the nerve cells and likely stimulate the cAMP (Brighton & Towensend, 1986; Knedlitscheck et al., 1994) because of the lower impedance at these frequencies (Schwartz, 1998). At sufficient levels, electrical energy has an intraneuronal effect on cAMP activity; cAMP is an intracellular second messenger, which merely passes on "permission" for the cell to do something. Knedlitschek et al. (1994) actually showed that intracellular cAMP is depleted after being subjected to 4,000 Hz of electrical energy at adequate voltage.

cAMP is utilized and decreased in absolute amounts as it relays the message to open the voltage-gated channels and start other metabolic activity to the intracellular organelles (Wilson-Pauwels et al., 1997). These later phenomena can be described as direct normalization of the cell function, which directly reverses sensitized pain feedback circuits and possibly promotes healing. As whole books are written entirely on the role of cAMP (Rasmussen, 1981), suffice it to say that ENB procedures are hypothesized to "shock" voltage-gated channels open and stimulate metabolic pathways to normalize pain nerve function.

Simply stated, AC frequencies greater than the rate a nerve can fire, i.e., greater than 1,000 Hz, specifically, in this case 20,000 Hz, have been shown by Knedlitscheck et al. (1994) to stimulate utilization of cAMP. In fact, Kilgore and Bhadra (2004) have shown that nerve block via depolarization does occur at 2,000 to 20,000 Hz. Wali and Brain (1990) showed more sustained blockade. Wyss (1967, 1976) clearly showed that depolarization is sustained with the application of these currents, specifically 4,000 Hz. The author's clinical experience, as shown in the table and histograms below, strongly suggests the analgesic, likely via nerve block, is indeed achieved with electricity (Woessner, 2002a).

Especially for electric and chemical nerve blocks that are thought to block sympathetic fibers, thermal gradients comparing side to side can be helpful to document the effectiveness of the block of these fibers, because blocking the efferent sympathetic C-fibers to the small arterioles results in distally increased circulation, therefore, increased skin temperature. However, temperature changes (e.g., increased temperature on the blocked side) are not a direct measure of afferent pain nerve function. With greater blood flow, we expect decreased edema and temperature increase.

Whether these phenomena occur or not may provide evidence that a proper nerve block has been achieved, but the basic purpose of these ENB procedures is to relieve pain temporarily or even permanently. With decreased pain, functional improvement is expected. Clinically, these positive results are seen (Woessner, 2002a). Providing "proof" is time-consuming and is often requested by the payers, yet the change in perceived pain and the duration of that change are most important for the patient.

The author has performed about 4,000 ENBs. The results of more than 3,500 ENB procedures are shown in Table 83.1 and Figure 83.1. The percent of pain relief as indicated by the patients' verbal response scores (VRS) was noted just before and after the procedure (Table 83.1).

The determination of patients' perception of pain after the electrodes were removed likely represents the pain relief effect. The duration of relief is more a reflection of the inverse severity of the causative pathology resulting in nociceptive rather than neuropathic pain and may explain the lack of any relief in a few cases.

Only a few patients get complete, immediate, and permanent relief of pain in one treatment. Over half of the patients achieve a successful outcome (defined as maintained improved function and satisfying, to the patient, level of perceived decreased pain) during a course of 5 to 15

TABLE 83.1
Categories for Analysis of the Pain Reduction in the 3,508 ENB Procedures Done in the Author's Clinic on More Than 300 Patients from 1996 to 1998

% Pain Improvement	No. of Treatments	Percent In Category
Less than 0	24	1%
Exactly 0	298	8%
1 to 24%	426	12%
25 to 49%	590	17%
50 to 74%	791	22%
75 to 100%	1379	40%
Total	3508	100%

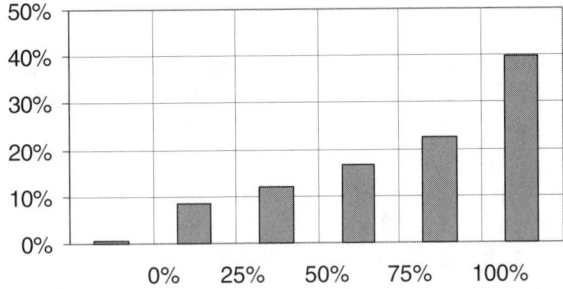

FIGURE 83.1 Of 3,508s ENB procedures done in the author's clinic on more than 300 patients from 1996 to 1998, clear reduction in pain perception well after the electrodes were removed, i.e., 25% improvement or better, occurred in 91% of the treatments, among which 40% perceived no pain at all after the treatment. (From J. Woessner, 2002, *Practical Pain Management*, 2(2), 19–26. Reproduced with permission.)

treatments. Individual variations occur with some short-term relief occurring in more than 80% of these cases and 20% obtaining complete immediate relief. The average duration of pain relief is from 1 to 3 days. Some obtain only a few hours of relief; the occasional subject who is essentially cured in one or more treatments may have purely neuropathic pain. Recurrence of pain depends on actual pathology, patient activities, and concomitant treatments. A successful course of treatment usually shows gradual improvement. Fewer than 2% of patients had worsened pain and discomfort because of toxic substance release.

ENB VERSUS E. STIM: WHAT ARE THE DIFFERENCES?

The term *electrotherapy* is avoided in this chapter. Electrotherapy uses stimulatory frequencies below the maximum firing rate of the pain nerves and is based on mechanisms for providing pain relief, but does not block or

TABLE 83.2
Procedural Comparisons of ENB vs. E. Stim.

ENB	E. Stim
64XXX	97XXX
Physician code	Therapist code
Physician controlled	Therapist controlled
Doctor present	No doctor
Diagnosis based	Body area based
Pathology specific	General condition
Multifacilitory*	Stimulatory
Analgesia	Electrical stimulation
Voltage gate alterations for block	Repeated nerve stimulation
?Signed consent	Consent, but not signed
Hundreds of dollars billed	Tens of dollars billed

* Multiple modes of action; decreased perception of pain also produced by circulatory changes, endorphin increases, secondary muscle relaxation, and other physical chemistry phenomena.

Note: From A. Hans Jurgen, 1999, presented at American Academy of Pain Management's annual clinical meeting, Las Vegas, Nevada. Reproduced with permission.

interrupt pain signals along the two types of pain nerves per se, except possibly if we focus on the carrier frequencies (4,000 ± 100 Hz) in interference therapy, rather than on the beat (interference) frequency (Kitchen, 2002; Palmer & Martin, 2002) (Table 83.2).

ELECTRIC (ENB) VERSUS CHEMICAL NERVE BLOCK (CNB)

There are some general nerve block concepts that require elucidation (Table 83.3).

The main difference is that local or regional analgesic chemicals close the voltage-gated channels so that pain nerves remain in a hyperpolarized state. With ENBs, synthesis of available information suggests that intracellular cAMP is stimulated to hold the voltage-gated channels open; a normal polarized state cannot be achieved and, therefore, the nerve cannot be stimulated to fire.

MECHANISM OF ENB ACTION

As for ENB frequencies, the author has mostly used frequencies between 4,000 and 20,000 Hz. No set terminology is applied to these frequencies, although Wyss (1967) did call them "middle frequencies." In this frequency range, nerves, particularly pain nerves, are not expected to repeatedly fire because they cannot achieve a firing potential, which is called sustained depolarization (Wyss, 1976). As indicated above, these frequencies do stimulate cAMP (Knedlitscheck, et al., 1994), which in turn opens voltage-gated channels in the pain nerves (Wilson-Pau-

---

TABLE 83.3
Evaluative Similarities and Differences of ENBs Compared with Chemical NBs

	ENB	CNB
Invasiveness	Yes[a]	Yes[b]
Site of action	Voltage gated channels	Voltage gated channels
Locational specificity	Target nerve	Target nerve
Physician involvement[c]	Yes	Yes
Documentation	Procedure note	Procedure note
Side effects	Multiple + burns	Multiple + anaphylaxis
FDA control	Yes	No
Safety	Very safe	Safe
Patient perceptions	Try and see	Ultimate, short of surgery
Consent necessity	Yes	Yes
Effective[d]	50–90%	50–90%
Curative[e]	Yes	Yes
Cost	High	Very high

[a] Just as high voltage currents and lightning.

[b] Just as microneedles and high pressure streams.

[c] Decides dose and target nerve.

[d] Very difficult to define. Author's general impression is similar; in both cases, depends more on the pain cause and the nociceptive pathology; neither is a cure-all.

[e] Both are basically cover-up procedures that should be part of a comprehensive treatment plan.

---

wels et al., 1997). These two mechanisms, hyperpolarization by chemicals and sustained depolarizataion by middle frequency currents, seem to explain the prolonged pain relief that occurs in most cases of chemical and electric nerve blocks. When prolonged relief does not occur, the pain stimulator, nociceptive or neuropathic, is overwhelming the nerve block action, whether induced chemically or electrically. If Waxman et al. (2001) are correct, the site of action is at the sodium voltage-gated channels. The curative action must then in part be downregulation of the increased number and density of the sodium channels.

The 8- to 20-minute time of onset is also similar between chemical and electric nerve blocks. The C-fibers are affected earlier than A-delta fibers and recover more slowly (Hadzic & Vloka, 2004). Myelin is less conductive than nerve tissue, explaining the greater effect of both local anesthetics and electricity on smaller and less myelinated pain nerve function.

ENBs treat pain, not necessarily the underlying pathology, unless the main problem is neuropathic. Nerve blocks are designed to provide a "window of opportunity" for the body to heal itself and/or for therapy or surgery benefits to be realized.

APPLICABLE NEUROANATOMY

The identified and recognized nerve can reasonably be affected in two ways, suggesting two different ways to approach electrode placement. An ENB can be achieved by treating across the nerve or along the nerve. The pain practitioner must know the anatomic course of the nerve and its distal distribution to correctly place the electrodes to fulfill regulatory and treatment needs, especially when dealing with a predominant A-delta fiber pain problem.

Theoretically, it is best to include the broad distal distribution of pain nerve endings, particularly of the A-delta fibers; these distributions also include unmyelinated free nerve endings in traditionally mapped nerve distributions (supported by Fischer, 2002). Even so, the distal distribution of sympathetic C-fiber free nerve endings are not well documented, but may be consistent with sclerotomal pain patterns that do not completely follow dermatomal patterns. Diagnosing the location of the pathology is difficult and may be better understood by considering one of the variable pain referral patterns discussed by Woessner (2003); specific electrode placement should be varied accordingly.

RELEVANT NEUROPHYSIOLOGY

The time from initiation of a nerve impulse until the time the nerve is ready to fire again is the refractory time of that nerve. If that time is 1/1000 of a second for A-delta (and 1/500 of a second for C-fibers) that nerve can fire no more than 1,000 times per second (and 500 times per second, respectively) (Ganong, 2001).

If a typical TENS unit is applied to that nerve at 100 cps, that nerve will be stimulated to fire and allowed to rest 90% of the time for the A-delta fibers. If this 100 cps alternating current is applied to a pain nerve, then stimulation would be expected to make the pain worse, not block the pain signal. Other mechanisms of pain relief are not precluded (Kitchen, 2002).

DIAGNOSTIC CONSIDERATIONS

While sensory nerve testing may support the C-fiber and A-delta fiber pain manifested by complex regional pain syndrome (CRPS I), reflex sympathetic dystrophy, and CRPS II (causalgia), these diagnoses are basically deduced from the patient's history, physical examination, and clinical observations (Woessner, 2002b). The burning pain, characteristic of these sympathetically maintained pain syndromes, comes from the C-fibers that coat the nerve trunks and other tissue planes while the sharp, lacinating pain comes from the A-delta fibers.

TREATMENT CONSIDERATIONS

Electromedical treatments often make more sense clinically than do chemical nerve blocks, especially when it is difficult to locate the pathology or when the pathology is widespread (e.g., up and down the length of the involved nerve). ENBs are potentially the best treatment, if the pathology is believed to be neuropathic in nature.

Treating neuropathic pain with ENBs is logical in many pain conditions, remembering that ENBs are not "cure-alls" and must be incorporated into a comprehensive treatment plan. It is potentially easier to proceed in advanced cases because most other treatments often do not work and/or are too medically risky. ENBs should be incorporated earlier to improve outcomes.

When other therapies fail, electromedical treatments are potentially worthwhile and carry lower risk for patients. If the electromedical treatments work, then certain diagnoses are likely supported, and the treatment plan and ultimate prognosis may be better determined. When local widespread inflammation is involved, it is necessary to bathe nerves along tissue planes throughout the area of pain with electric current. However, this technique may not be successful in achieving pain relief, if it follows multiple chemical blocks in which scar tissue results, causing relative insulation. For these situations, an "electromedical Bier block," which involves bathing the whole limb with electricity of the frequencies mentioned above can be done with minimal risk.

TREATMENT INDICATIONS

Theoretically, ENBs can be used in any pain condition, but should be more curative in neuropathic pain conditions. Because most pain conditions have both nociceptive and neuropathic components, treatment decisions to use ENBs are complex, change over time, and may be different among individual patients. While ENBs may help in predominantly central pain conditions, the mechanism of action is not neuron blockade. In pure nociceptive conditions, any relief achieved should be more temporary. In the author's experience (Woessner, 2002b), myofascial pain is not neuropathic; any pain relief from ENBs is likely to be short lived.

Pure neuropathic conditions, without maintaining pathology, may be corrected/cured in one or a few ENB treatments; in other words, neuron blockade is achieved via cAMP opening the voltage-gated channels, and cure is also achieved by the cAMP as a second messenger, which promotes normalizations of pain nerve cellular function.

In addition, with restrictions mandated by the FDA for relative safety, ENBs will work better for localized peripheral conditions. For example, local, single-level radiculitis (irritation without obvious mass pathology) and mononeuropathies are the ideal candidates for ENBs. Fibromyalgia and diabetic pain are more difficult and relief is more likely temporary because the disease is so widespread that the current density is diluted.

An obvious treatment strategy would be to do multiple serial treatments on different parts of the body or use multiple machines; the former would be very time-consuming, and the latter is logistically complex and the cost would not likely be justified by adequate reimbursement.

THE ENB PROCEDURE

With neuroanatomical knowledge, many nerves may be blocked. Relevant for both chemical and electric nerve blocks, whether done across or along the nerve, is that the impulses from the populations of pain nerve endings are blocked. See Woessner (2002a) for a specific example of how an electric sciatic nerve block can be done.

Whether blocking across the nerve or along the nerve, a relatively small electrode is usually placed where a needle for a regional chemical nerve block would be inserted. A relatively larger electrode is placed either directly across the body part through which the target nerve transits or along the target nerve distribution either distally or proximally.

The full details of performing ENB procedures are beyond the scope of this chapter, but discussion of electrical frequency and machines that are capable of producing electric nerve blocks are presented below. Practitioners doing ENBs must be able to

- Diagnose neuropathology
- Develop a treatment plan with the patient that may include ENBs
- Use appropriate equipment
- Correctly place the electrodes
- Document what was done, including pre- and post-treatment pain intensity scores
- Provide supplemental medical advice and care

SURFACE LANDMARKS

Palpating the surface anatomy and visualizing underlying structures are essential for optimizing electrode placement. Accommodation is needed for underlying low conducting tissue and electric current pathway elongations. Accomplishing this first step requires more than just a passing knowledge of anatomy.

SMALL (TARGETING) ELECTRODE PLACEMENT

The relatively small (2 to 3 cm in diameter) targeting electrode should be a small to medium self-adhesive, sponge and/or vasopneumatic device. It should be placed approximately where the practitioner would insert a needle for a chemical nerve block of the same nerve. Accommodations must be made for the visualized pathway of the electric current.

For nerve root blocks, there are two possible electrode placement patterns. One placement pattern of the target electrode is on the skin surface directly above the nerve root in the area, where a needle would be inserted for a chemical injection. The other placement pattern of the target electrode is across the midline directly above the contralateral nerve root.

For predominantly C-fiber pathology, the practitioner chooses to place ipsilaterally the small electrode superior to the most distal sympathetic ganglion for the lower extremities and inferior to the stellate ganglion (over the T2 sympathetic ganglion) for upper extremity problems. Placement for thoracic pain is straightforward as long as the practitioner visualizes the path of least impedance combined with the shortest distance; scatter occurs as the electric current crosses tissue planes/interfaces along predominantly water pathways.

LARGE (DISPERSAL) ELECTRODE PLACEMENT

The relatively large (3 to 5 cm in diameter dispersal) electrode should be a medium to large self-adhesive, sponge and/or vasopneumatic device. It should be placed either across the target nerve or distally along that nerve's distribution. It is better to follow the dermatomal distributions in predominant A-delta fiber neuropathology. For predominantly C-fiber pathology, the practitioner chooses to place the large electrode down the involved extremity, possibly even into a container of water or other ionic fluid in which the distal extremity is immersed. Placement for thoracic pain is straightforward as long as the practitioner visualizes the path of least impedance combined with the shortest distance; scatter occurs as the electric current crosses tissue planes/interfaces.

EACH TREATMENT

The practitioner sets the intensity to tolerance during the first 30 seconds of the treatment. Turning the intensity up during the treatment may result in damage to the insensate (from the nerve block itself) skin. The ideal treatment lasts for 20 minutes and uses a frequency of approximately 15 kHz (anywhere between 4,000 and 40,000 Hz will do). Some machines sweep across frequency ranges, and sweeping theoretically results in recruitment of wider bands of nerve fibers, causing more complete pain control.

POSSIBLE COMBINED TREATMENT

The physician, depending on the exact character and distribution of the patient's pain, may place a second set of electrodes across the area of "worst pathology." For longitudinally extensive pathology, a second set of the electrodes placed differently to cover the same distribution may be better.

TREATMENT COURSE

Daily electromedical sessions for 3 weeks usually result in clinical improvement as long as the underlying peripheral pathology is being treated and corrected at the same time. Logistics and third-party payer resistance seldom allow this intense course of treatment.

It has been found that the first five treatments, if done within a 2-week period, can result in benefits. As stated above, occasional patients seem to worsen, but most do improve. Without some benefit noted, the practitioner should move on to other treatment alternatives, or at least combine ENBs with other therapeutic methods. An average of 10 to 15 treatments, each separated by 3 days or fewer are necessary to achieve optimal or maximal benefit. Longer intervals between treatments usually make more treatments necessary.

Better results are obtained when combined with adjunctive therapy, such as nutritional support, modalities, therapeutic exercise, chiropractic manipulations, chemical injections, or psychological techniques. Frequent reassessment improves outcome because the practitioner can make adjustments in the electromedical or adjunct care. Subjective (pain scores) and functional (ROM, MMT, etc.) assessment should both be done periodically, immediately before and after the ENBs.

PRECAUTIONS

While avoiding conduction through the carotid sinus is logical and appropriate, risk of cardiovascular adverse events is minimal with ENBs. The cardiac system operates at one cycle per second (normal heart rates are 60 to 100 beats per *minute*), whereas machines used generate alternating currents of at least 4,000 per *second*. Davis (1993) showed that the higher the frequency, the lower the relative risk. On the other hand, as the total electrical energy increases, the likelihood of overriding the natural frequency increases.

Because the total electrical current going through both the small and large electrodes is the same, the important variable is the current density (Schwartz, 1998). The so-called targeting electrode can be considered to concentrate electrical energy at the targeted nerve(s). Practitioners should know that the point in the circuit with the greatest current density at the skin surface is where the skin can most possibly be damaged. Using small self-adhesive electrodes, skin burns are possible, but they are rare with sponges.

CONTRAINDICATIONS FOR ENBS

- Pregnancy
- Multiple sclerosis
- Parkinson's disease
- Epilepsy
- Vascular diseases/manifest thrombosis
- Acute inflammatory process
- Bacterial infection (osteomyelitis, etc.)
- Malignancies
- Metal implants
- Arrhythmia/demand pacemaker
- Over the carotid sinus
- Across the cranium

Although these are "official" contraindications according to the FDA, full knowledge and understanding of the basic principles of ENBs may allow usage on some body locations for most of these diagnoses.

ENB MACHINES

Any electric current devices producing AC of 4,000 to 20,000 cycles per second are probably capable of producing ENBs. While some manufacturers claim that square wave machines, machines that are specifically designed for interferential treatments, are more comfortable than sine wave machines, sine wave generators seem to produce more pain relief. Via a different mechanism, high volt galvanic current (HVGC) machines appear to achieve ENBs. Jenkner (1995) based most of his conclusions in *Electric Pain Control* on a rapidly pulsing direct current theoretically similar to HVGC.

PITFALLS: CAUSES FOR FAILURE

Without visible tissue changes and improvement in the pain, there may not be a peripheral pain generator. Blockade of any nerve is more difficult to confirm because the pain pathways can be missed. These pathways may not always follow the anatomic distribution of that nerve.

Trauma of the needle used in chemical nerve blocks and the caustic effects of those chemicals cause scar tissue accumulation. If multiple chemical blocks have preceded

ENBs, the resultant scar tissue around the nerve may interfere with penetration of the electric current. Scar tissue development is avoided with ENB procedures.

For the best results, the right medical diagnoses are necessary so that the specific pathology can be treated. An incorrect primary diagnosis is possible. This mistake can result in inappropriate electrode placement. If the proper diagnosis is made and results from these techniques are less than expected, the pain could be generated from two or multiple sites. If the pathology is in a different area than the treated tissue, the current density could be too low to promote the nerve block. If the sympathetic nerve damage is more distal, patients may obtain pain relief without changing the nerve pathology. If the pain generator is nearby, but in a different nerve distribution, the treatment may not work well at all and/or the pathology could be too proximal or too distal to the treated area. As it may be difficult for the patient to immobilize the involved tissue, recurrent pain might be expected. As it is not impossible for central pain to occur with changes in the neurons of the dorsal horns, in the spinal pain tracks, and/or in the brain, in subcortical pathways and in the sensory strip, centrally and sympathetically maintained pain can result from anatomic and physiologic changes in central nerve system neurons. Deafferent or central pain responds poorly if at all to peripheral procedures of any type. Finally, pain maintained by psychological mechanism may fail to respond to ENBs alone, further establishing the need for multidisciplinary care.

MEDICAL PLACE OF ENBS: EFFECTS/BENEFITS

These ENB treatments have the potential to "cure" the pain pathology. If a purely neuropathic condition exists, one may expect to "cure" the patient with ENBs. Because "cure" with ENBs has been rare, one must assume that the causative pathology is ongoing in nearly all pain conditions. In other words, it appears the ENB frequencies may reverse the neuropathology, but not the underlying ongoing cause of the neuropathology. Therefore, most practitioners suspect from experience that an individualized multidisciplinary approach is necessary to help patients with ongoing pain (Rosomoff, 2000). ENBs are only one tool that must be combined with other supplemental and synergistic techniques, and those methods must be dynamically changed and refined over the course of the pain disease; once again, there is "no magic bullet."

If kept in perspective, ENB as a medical procedure is a powerful tool for treating the pathology and pain originating from neuropathy. There is also the obvious benefit of completely avoiding the need to pass a needle through other tissue. Single or multiple injections can result in new scar tissue anywhere the injected fluid goes. Thus, ENBs avoid the development of scar tissue in and around nerves that interferes with the effectiveness of subsequent treatments, electromedical or chemical.

CONCLUSION

ENBs can and should be included in comprehensive treatment programs for temporary pain control and normalization of neuropathic problems. Proper use of ENBs requires an understanding of neuroanatomy, neurophysiology, and the mechanism of ENB action.

REFERENCES

Becker, R. O. (1991). *Cross currents: The promise of electromedicine, the perils of electropollution.* New York: Harper Collins.

Becker, R.O., & Selden, G. (1985). *The body electric: Electromagnetism and the foundation of life.* New York: Quill William Morrow.

Brighton, C. T., & Towensend, P. F. (1986). Increased cAMP production after short term capacitive couple stimulation of bovine growth plate chrondrocytes. *Transactions of the 6th annual meeting of the Bioelectrical Repair and Growth Society* (BRAGS). *43,* 19–22.

Brown, D. L., & Fink, B. R. (1998). The history of neural blockade and pain management. In M. J. Cousins & P. O. Bridenbaugh (Eds.), *Neural blockade: In clinical anesthesia and management of pain* (3rd ed., pp. 3–27). Philadelphia: Lippincott-Raven.

Charman, R. A. (2002). Electrical properties of cells and tissues. In S. Kitchen (Ed.), *Electrotherapy: Evidence-based practice* (pp. 31–44). New York: Churchill Livingstone.

Davis, S. (1993). *Interferential current therapy in clinical practice.* Birmingham, AL: The Best of Times, Inc.

De Domenico, G. (1982). Pain relief with interferential therapy. *Australian Journal of Physiotherapy, 28*(3), 14–18.

Fischer, A. A. (2002). Segmental neuromyotherapy: A new concept in the diagnosis and management of neuromusculoskeletal pain. In E. S. Rachlin & I. S Rachlin (Eds.), *Myofascial pain and fibromyalgia: Trigger point management* (2nd ed., Chapters 7 & 13). St. Louis, MO: Mosby.

Gadsby, J. G. (1998). *Electroanalgesia: Historical and contemporary development.* Ph.D. Thesis. Leicester, U.K.: De Montfort University.

Ganong, W. F. (2001). *Review of medical physiology.* New York: Lange Medical Books, McGraw-Hill.

Gennaro, A. R. et al. (Editorial board). (194). *Blakiston's Gould medical dictionary* (4th ed.). New York: McGraw-Hill.

Goats, G. C. (1990). Interferential current therapy. *British Journal of Sports Medicine, 24*(2), 87–92.

Gordy, T. R. [Editorial Board Chair]. (2002). *Current procedureal terminology* (std. ed., p. 185). AMA Press.

Hadzic, A., & Vloka, J. D. (2004). *Peripheral nerve blocks: Principles and practice. New York School of Regional Anesthesia.* New York: McGraw-Hill.

Hans Jurgen, A. (1999). *Horizontal stimulation: The new generation of EDT: Electrical differential treatment.* American Academy of Pain Management's annual clinical meeting (Las Vegas, Nevada) handout.

Hardy, J. D., Fabian, L. W., & Turner, M. D. (1961). Electrical anesthesia for major surgery. *Journal of the American Medical Association, 175*(7), 145–146.

Jenkner, F. L. (1995). *Electric pain control.* New York: Springer-Verlag.

Kahn, J. (2000). *Principles and practice of electrotherapy.* New York: Churchill & Livingstone.

Kane, K., & Taub, A. (1975). A history of local electrical analgesia. *Pain, 1,* 125–138.

Kilgore K. L., & Bhadra, N. (2004). Nerve conduction block utilising high-frequency alternating current. *Medical & Biological Engineering & Computing, 42*(3), 394–406.

Kitchen, S. (Ed.). (2002). *Electrotherapy: Evidence-based Practice.* New York: Churchill Livingstone.

Knedlitscheck, G. et al. (1994). Cyclic AMP response in cells exposed to electric fields of different frequencies and intensities. *Radiation Environmental Biophysics, 32,* 1–7.

Leak, W. D. (1992). Home care therapy: Pain management vs. anesthesia. In P. Raj (Ed.), *Practical management of pain* (pp. 967–968). St. Louis, MO: Mosby Year Book.

Nelson, R. M., Hayes, K. W., & Currier, D. P. (Eds.). (1999). *Clinical electrotherapy* (3rd ed.). Stamford, CT: Appleton & Lang.

Northrop, R. B. (2001). Measurement of electrical potentials and magnetic fields from the body surface. In R. B. Northrop & M. R. Neuman (Eds.), *Noninvasive instrumentation and measurement in medical diagnosis* (pp. 57–149). Boca Raton, FL: CRC Press.

Palmer, S., & Martin, D. (2002). Interferential current for pain control. In S. Kitchen (Ed.), *Electrotherapy: Evidence-based practice* (pp. 287–300). New York: Churchill Livingstone.

Racz, G., Lewis, R., Laros, G., & Heavner, J. E. (1992). Electrical stimulation analgesia. In P. P. Raj (Ed.), *Practical management of pain* (pp. 922–933). St. Louis, MO: Mosby Year Book.

Rasmussen, H. (1981). *Calcium and cAMP as synarchic messengers.* New York: John Wiley & Sons.

Robinson, A. J., & Synder-Mackler, L. (1995). *Clinical electrophysiology: Electrotherapy and electrophysiologic testing* (2nd ed.). Philadelphia: Lippincott, Williams and Wilkins.

Rosomoff, H. (2000, July 15–21). Non-surgical treatment of low back pain disorders. In E. Krames & E. Reig (Eds.), The management of acute and chronic pain: The use of the "tools of the trade" (pp. 313–321). *Proceedings of Worldwide Pain Conference.* International Proceedings Division, Bologna, Italy.

Rossi, U. (2003). The history of electrical stimulation of the nervous system for the control of pain. In B. A. Simpson (Ed.), *Electrical stimulation and the relief of pain* (pp. 5–16). New York: Elsevier.

Schwartz, R. G. (1998). Electric sympathetic block: Current theoretical concepts and clinical results. *Journal of Back and Musculoskeletal Rehabilitation, 10,* 31–46.

Simpson, B. A. (Ed.). (2003). *Electrical stimulation and the relief of pain*. New York; Elsevier.

Sweet, W. H. & Wepsic, J. G. (1968). Treatment of chronic pain by stimulation of fibers of primary afferent neuron. *Transactions of the American Neurological Association (New York), 93*, 103–107.

Thomas, C. L. (Ed.). (2001). *Taber's Cyclopedic Medical Dictionary* (19th ed.). Philadelphia, PA: F.A. Davis Co.

Wali, F. A., & Brain, A. I. (1990). Electromagnetic stimulation and inhibition of nerve conduction in frog isolated sciatic nerve-gastrocnemius muscle preparation. *Acta Physiologica Hungarica, 76*(2), 87–92.

Waxman, S. G. (2001). *Form and function in the brain and spinal cord: Perspectives of a neurologist*. Cambridge, MA: MIT Press.

Waxman, S. G. et al. (2001). Sodium channels and pain. In S. G. Waxman (Ed.), *Form and function in the brain and spinal cord: Perspectives of a neurologist* (pp. 421–431). Cambridge, MA: MIT Press.

Wilson-Pauwels, L., Stewart, P. A., & Akesson, E. J. (1997). *Autonomic nerves: Basic science — Clinical aspects — Case studies*. Hamilton, London: BC Decker Inc.

Woessner, J. (2002a). Blocking out the pain: Electric nerve block treatments for sciatic neuritis. *Practical Pain Management, 2*(2), 19–26.

Woessner, J. (2002b). A conceptual model of pain: Measurement and diagnosis. *Practical Pain Management, 2*(6), 27–35.

Woessner, J. (2003). Referred pain vs. origin of pain pathology. *Practical Pain Management, 3*(6), 8–19.

Wyss, O. A. M. (1967). Nervenreizung mit Mittelfrequenzstromstossen. *Helvetica Physiologica Acta, 25*, 85–102.

Wyss, O. A. M. (1976). Prinzipien der elektrischen Reizung. Zurich: Leemann.

84

Static Magnetic Therapy for Pain

Michael J. McLean, MD, and Stefan Engström, PhD

INTRODUCTION

Interest in therapeutic magnets and other complementary and alternative modalities is high in the United States currently. While advances in science and technology, e.g., the evolution of magnetic resonance imaging (MRI), are a stimulus to investigation of potential therapeutic uses of magnetic fields, other factors should be considered. Important among these is the public desire for empowerment in matters of health care. The American public spends billions on complementary health modalities to fill gaps they perceive in health care provided by conventional medicine (Eisenberg et al., 1998). By one estimate, 40% of patients with peripheral neuropathy used complementary and alternative approaches and 30% used magnets (Brunelli & Gorson, 2004). Permanent magnetic devices have become commonplace for self-treatment of ordinary aches and pains, and they are sold in stores widely without approval by the Food and Drug Administration (FDA) for specific claims. So far, because of the lack of apparent significant health risk, marketing of the devices has been allowed as long as no specific claims are made. In this chapter, we review the scientific and clinical rationale upon which expectations of therapeutic benefit are founded. The discussion includes some of the methodological problems and implications for future studies.

HISTORY OF MAGNETISM AND MEDICINE

The use of magnetic fields to treat pain is not new. Interest in the West has fluctuated over centuries but has persisted in various forms in Eastern medicine in a more sustained way. Several authors have reviewed the history of magnetism in medicine (Basford, 2001; Rosch, 2004; Vallbona & Richards, 1999; Weintraub, 2004). Our understanding of how magnets came to be used for medical purposes is spotty and, at times, not well documented. Still, one would expect to find parallels between medical applications and scientific developments regarding magnetism.

The attraction between lodestones was known by the Greek, Chinese, and other ancient civilizations perhaps as early as 800 B.C. (Magnetism Group, 2002; Serway & Jewett, 2004). Chinese references to lodestones as *tzhu shih* or "loving [kissing] stones" appeared after 300 B.C. One of the earliest known uses of magnets was for geomancy (*feng shui*) in China between 400 and 100 B.C. Some historians believe that as early as the 11th century, the magnetic needle of the compass was used in China and Egypt (Savage-Smith, 1988; Serway & Jewett, 1998). Large deposits of a naturally occurring magnetic iron oxide, Fe_3O_4, called magnetite, were located in a region of Turkey then known as Magnesia (Cullity, 1972). The Greeks produced magnets by rubbing iron with magnetite.

Application of lodestones to acupuncture points for pain relief was described in the oldest known medical text, *The Yellow Emperor's Canon of Internal Medicine,* that was published sometime between 800 and 200 B.C. Therapeutic use of lodestones also was alluded to in the ancient Hindu Vedas. Egyptian, Buddhist, and Greek physicians, including Hippocrates, employed lodestones. In the 16th century, the Swiss alchemist and physician Paracelsus began using powdered lodestone in salves to promote healing in a variety of conditions, including epilepsy. However, William Gilbert, physician to Queen Elizabeth I, pointed out that the process of grinding the lodestone into powder destroyed the magnetism. Gilbert's work, *De Magnete,* published in 1600, is considered to be the first scientific opus on magnetism (Gilbert, 1958). Gilbert performed experiments with magnetite and iron magnets that produced a better understanding of the earth's magnetic field in an effort to dispel the superstition that surrounded magnetic fields. By this time it was known that all magnets have two poles which behave in a manner similar to positive and negative electric charges, i.e., like charges repel and opposite charges attract. These poles were referred to as the north and south because the north pole of a freely moving magnet was observed to rotate toward the geographic north pole of the earth. A century later, magnetic cures were introduced into England by Robert Fludd as a remedy for all diseases. Perhaps not coincidentally, the patient was placed in the "boreal position" with the head north and the feet south during the treatment.

John Mitchell in England (1750) and Charles Coulomb in France (1785) described independently the law relating forces between magnetic poles. In 1819 the Danish physicist Hans Christian Oersted discovered that electric currents produced a magnetic field. Shortly after, André Ampère deduced the quantitative relationships between a magnetic force and electric current. In the 1820s, Michael Faraday and Joseph Henry demonstrated that a changing magnetic field could also produce an electric field. Up until this point, magnets were made by rubbing iron with magnetite. The invention of the electromagnet by William Sturgeon in 1825 made possible the production of much stronger magnetic fields and permanent magnets.

Important events in the history of magnetic field therapy overlapped scientific developments, especially in the 19th century. A notorious example involved Anton Mesmer who thought that a combination of magnetic and gravitational forces he called "animal magnetism" could produce cures of neurological (e.g., epilepsy) and psychiatric conditions in his patients. Later, Mesmer determined that "cures" could be effected without exposure to magnets and he held public meetings during which he claimed cures by extending his hands over the audience. In the wake of public accusations of fraud, a royal commission of the French Academy of Sciences, including Benjamin Franklin, Anton Lavoisier, and Dr. J. I. Guillotin, investigated Mesmer's claims. The commission performed blinded experiments with strong magnets and nonmagnetic materials and found that individuals could not discern reliably to which objects they had been exposed. The commission concluded that any benefit from magnetic therapy must be the result of a placebo effect or hypnosis (see Basford, 2001).

Somehow magnetic therapy was brought to America. In 1842, Stokes and Bell published a two volume medical text, entitled *Lectures on the Theory and Practice of Physics*. In it they described experiments with magnets at Dublin's Meath Hospital. Patients were described to benefit by reduced pain and increased function. The authors argued, "That a magnet should act on the human body is neither extraordinary nor incredible" (Stokes & Bell, 1842). Despite positive reports, the negative received much attention. Daniel Palmer was a Canadian born physician who in 1890 opened Palmer's School of Magnetic Cure in Davenport, Iowa. As in the case of Mesmer, Palmer soon discovered that his patients recovered just as quickly if he omitted the magnets and merely "laid on hands." Soon, the school of magnetic cures became Palmer's College of Chiropractic. It is fascinating that interest in the therapeutic potential of magnets was never extinguished, although it seems to have waxed and waned.

The evolution of scientific knowledge about magnetism set the stage for current magnetic research. The advent of MRI in the 1980s demonstrated that externally imposed magnetic fields can interact with human tissues. This was certainly a stimulus for those interested in magnetotherapy, but it does not prove that magnetic fields are therapeutically effective. The magnetic fields used for everyday diagnostic imaging are powerful, on the order of 1 to 5 tesla (T). In contrast, the fields generated by most static magnetic field devices used for treating pain are much smaller, in the range of a few to several hundred millitesla at the surface of the devices. Field strength at tissue targets can only be inferred from dosimetric studies and simulations. There is no question that a variety of challenges confront the investigation of static magnetic fields produced by commercially available devices. Learning how to study magnetic fields clinically is one of the principal problems investigators face. Many clinical trials emulate drug trials for similar conditions. However, it is clear that many aspects of clinical trial design must be tailored to the study of magnetic fields, as discussed below.

MAGNETISM AND MAGNETS

Magnetism and electricity are inseparable according to the Maxwell equations. Magnetic fields are everywhere. Stray magnetic fields produced by industrial electrical sources and power line frequencies constitute a health risk (Portier & Wolfe, 1998) and can be viewed as pollutants, in one sense. On the other hand, we are constantly exposed to the Earth's geomagnetic field with no known health risk. The Earth behaves like a big static magnet. Its magnetic field is weak, on the order of 20 to 65 μT (Lillie, 1999; Stacey, 1977). Yet, migrating animals with specialized detectors navigate with uncanny accuracy by sensing it (see below). Understanding how magnets interact with biological systems could lead to the development of novel therapies for pain and other conditions. However, the potential for both efficacy and adverse effects must be considered for therapeutic magnets, just as for pharmaceuticals.

The properties of magnets are described in detail in physics textbooks and specialized treatises on magnetism. The interested reader is referred to additional sources for mathematical details (e.g., see Wittig & Engström, 2003, for a recent summary). We review some properties below to establish a basis for understanding how magnetic fields may affect biological systems.

Permanent magnets have two magnetic poles, a north pole and a south pole. Lines of magnetic flux emanate from the north pole and reenter at the south pole. Iron filings scattered on a piece of paper over a bar magnet align along the flux lines and allow us to see the orientation of the lines in the plane of the paper. The flux lines exert an external force that determines the interaction between two magnets. When the south poles or north poles of two bar magnets are pushed together, they repel each other and the flux lines visualized by the iron filings bend away from each other. If the south pole of one magnet is pushed toward the north pole of the second magnet, the two magnets pull together. They behave like a longer bar magnet.

Permanent magnets are made commercially by exposing susceptible materials to an external magnetic field, such as the magnetic field produced by passing current through a wire. Electric current in a wire produces a circular magnetic field perpendicular to the wire. A long helical winding of wire or coil, called a solenoid, produces a uniform magnetic field inside the winding, except near the ends. Outside of the coil the field is similar to a bar magnet with a north and south pole. Electromagnets can be made by inserting a soft magnetic iron core into a solenoid. The field produced by current passing through the wire magnetizes the iron core. This multiplies the field around the coil because electrons in the iron are easily organized to produce a powerful magnet.

An explanation can be found in the behavior of electrons, the fundamental units of magnetism. A spinning electron can be thought of as a submicroscopic current loop that generates a magnetic moment perpendicular to the direction of spin. In the formation of a permanent magnet, electron spins become aligned in parallel and the magnetic moments sum. In nonmagnetic materials, electrons spin in opposite directions and their individual magnetic moments cancel.

Only certain elements or materials can be made into magnets, i.e., magnetized. The characteristics of the material determine how much and how strongly it will become magnetized in response to an applied magnetic field. Some ferromagnetic materials respond more than a million times more strongly than nonmagnetic materials.

Nonmagnetic materials manifest diamagnetic, paramagnetic, or antiferromagnetic properties. Diamagnetic elements, such as silicon, have filled outer electron shells. Diamonds, organic compounds, and ionic solids (NaCl) are examples of diamagnetic materials with covalent bonds. An external magnetic field creates small magnetic dipoles that oppose the applied field in such materials. Paramagnetic elements, including some transition metals, have incomplete outer or inner shells. An externally applied magnetic field aligns the spins of unpaired electrons result-

ing in a small magnetic moment. Diamagnetic and paramagnetic effects are induced by the magnetic field, but disappear when the magnetic field is removed. Other transition metal elements, such as chromium and manganese, are antiferromagnetic because their unpaired electrons spin in opposite directions, thereby canceling their magnetic moments and resulting in nonmagnetic character.

Magnetic materials acquire permanent magnetic behavior after exposure to a magnetic field. The ferromagnetic elements (iron, cobalt, and nickel) and their alloys are important materials for industry because of their strong response to applied magnetic fields and retention of magnetism. Iron, cobalt, and nickel have unpaired d-shell electrons that are easily reorganized to have parallel spins necessary for becoming permanent magnets. Ferromagnetic materials can be classified as "hard" or "soft" depending on how easily they are demagnetized by reversal of the external magnetic field. Soft iron cores are useful in electromagnets because they are easily demagnetized by reversal of the applied field. Hard magnetic materials are difficult to demagnetize. Neodymium-iron-boron magnets have shelf lives of nearly a century without loss of magnetism unless they are heated to the point that electron spins are disordered or shocked by physical forces that fracture their structure.

Magnetic materials such as ceramics and magnetite display ferromagnetic properties. The magnetic moments of their elements or ions align antiparallel in an imposed magnetic field, but there is a net magnetic moment. In the case of magnetite, Fe_3O_4, the antiparallel alignment of the Fe^{3+} and Fe^{2+} ions results in the permanent magnetization. Magnetite is important historically because it occurred naturally and was known for its magnetic properties by ancient peoples. It has also been detected in some migratory animals and may be an important navigation tool by acting as a physical transducer for geomagnetic fields (see below).

MAGNETIC FIELD INTERACTIONS WITH BIOLOGICAL SYSTEMS

There is evidence that more than 20 species of birds (Wiltschko & Wiltschko, 1996), salamanders (Deutschlander et al., 1999), sea turtles (Lohman & Lohman, 1996), monarch butterflies (Etheredge et al., 1999), and fin whales (Walker et al., 1997) navigate by using the Earth's weak geomagnetic field as a compass. Understanding how animals detect and decode geomagnetic information could reveal mechanisms that are useful for treating pain and other conditions. Diverse effects of static and time-varying magnetic fields on genetic, biochemical, and biophysical properties of cells have been reported in the scientific literature. This work has not yet proved the basis for therapeutic utility of magnetic fields, but it suggests that

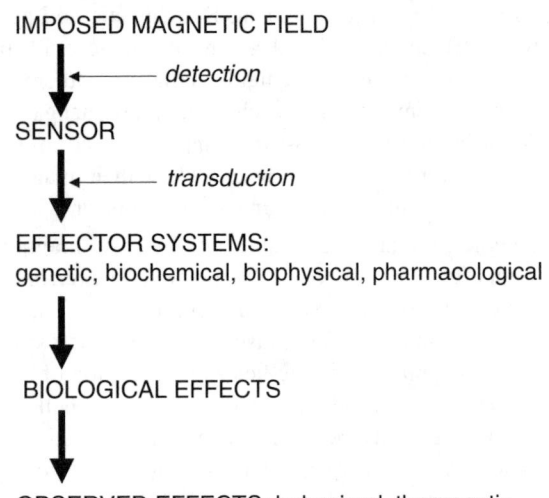

FIGURE 84.1 Cascade of how an applied magnetic field might affect biological systems.

the problem can be approached from the molecular direction, in addition to observing intact systems.

Most, if not all, commercially available permanent therapeutic magnets generate much stronger magnetic fields at their surfaces than the geomagnetic field. Strong magnetic fields may not be enough to produce useful biological effects, however. The geometry of the field in relation to the biological target may be important. Or, temporal and spatial variation in the field may be as, or more, important than field strength. This means that it is important to know what characteristic(s), or metric, of magnetic fields can be sensed. The process by which an externally applied magnetic field leads to a biological result can be conceived to involve a series of elements, perhaps something like the cascade in Figure 84.1. First, there must be a sensor(s) to detect the field. Next, a transduction mechanism(s) must couple detection to an effector system or systems. This produces biological effects. In the present context, the concept of "magnetotherapy" demands that an applied magnetic field can in some way interact with the nociceptive process to relieve "pain." Clinicians and scientists are trained to observe the behavioral and therapeutic effects of the intervention. Herein lies a conceptual framework for studying magnetic fields from bench to bedside. This is not unlikely the process of developing pharmaceutical agents, but many details about magnetic fields remain to be discovered.

BIOLOGICAL MAGNETIC FIELD DETECTORS: IS THERE SUCH A THING AS A "MAGNETOCEPTOR"?

The conceptually simplest way to detect a magnetic field is with another magnet, as described above for the interaction between two dipole magnets. Some birds have a

type of magnetite in specialized receptor cells in their beaks (Hanzlik et al., 2000). But, the presence of magnetic material in animal tissues does not reveal how sensing the field is transduced. Magnetotaxis may be the result of physical attraction between an external magnetic field and magnetite in bacteria, like some physical tractor beam (Blakemore, 1975). In the absence of magnetic material, the dipole moment of unpaired electrons or dipoles within diamagnetic cell components, such as enzymes or ion channels, might be targets. In these cases, the external magnetic field can be viewed as inducing a weak magnetic field in certain cell structures and then interacting with the induced field. Altering biological dipoles intrinsic to proteins could be coupled directly to function, e.g., by modulating enzyme activity. For example, two different static magnetic fields increased calcium-calmodulin dependent myosin phosphorylation in a cell free system to different degrees (Engström et al., 2002; Markov & Pilla, 1997). Altering calcium binding to calmodulin could provide control of amplification of the phosphorylation step. Removal of the magnetic field would be expected to result in return to the baseline level of activity because diamagnetic substances do not store magnetic energy permanently. Both magnetic flux density (the number of magnetic flux lines per unit area) and field gradients (changes of field strength with distance) were implicated in these results. Thus, the sensor, or magnetoceptor, may not be very different from a pharmacological receptor, in which the agonist binding site is a peptide sequence gating an ion channel or coupled to a G protein. The "agonist" for the magnetoceptor is distinctly different, however, and operates from a distance in the form of non-ionizing radiation instead of a ligand binding to a receptor. Also, the magnetoceptor may respond to one or more characteristics of the imposed magnetic field. Put a different way, different components of an external magnetic field may modulate the magnetoceptor, suggesting that magnetic fields might be designed to have specific influences on target tissues.

Current understanding of magnetoceptors is far from complete, including the sensitivity of the sensors and what they sense. It seems that an interdisciplinary effort will be necessary to resolve problems at this interface between physics and biology.

PHYSICAL TRANSDUCTION MECHANISMS

A number of mechanisms have been proposed to explain how imposed magnetic fields interact with biological magnetoceptors and have been critically reviewed (Adair, 2000; Binhi & Savin, 2003; Engström, 2004; Liboff & Jenrow, 2002; Matthes et al., 2004; Zhadin, 2001). An important constraint is that the interaction does not ionize or heat the target tissue. Explanations for the effects of static magnetic fields generating flux densities in the micro- to low millitesla range are the most controversial. Some potential mechanisms include the following:

1. **Magnetic induction of electric fields and currents:** Movement of charged substances in a magnetic field induces an electric field perpendicular to the direction of motion and the applied field. Induced electric fields and currents can alter voltage-sensitive neuronal activity and ion transport. This mechanism requires strong fields or high-frequency temporal variation. Transcranial magnetic stimulation with pulsed tesla-level fields induces electric fields that directly excite the cerebral cortex (Barker et al., 1987; Epstein et al., 1990; Hallett & Cohen, 1989; Hufnagel et al., 1990; Ogiue-Ikeda et al., 2003; Ziemann et al., 1998). One would imagine that response to weak fields on the order of the Earth's geomagnetic field or to roughly 100-fold stronger fields produced by commercially available therapeutic magnets would require very sensitive magnetoceptors and/or an amplification step. Such features have not been demonstrated in experimental cell or animal models of pain.

2. **Magnetomechanical** (torque on magnetic dipole moment): An external magnetic field imposes a rotational force, or torque, that tends to rotate dipoles in the direction of alignment with the field. This could be an important effect because dipole orientation is randomized by thermal noise in cells. This mechanism can only work under anisotropic conditions or if the target material has intrinsic magnetization, as in the case of magnetite. Microtubules are relatively large (5 µm) anisotropic targets and could respond to tesla-level fields (Bras et al., 1998).

3. **Magnetophoresis** (force on magnetic dipole moment): A static gradient magnetic field (spatially inhomogeneous) exerts a translational force on a magnetic dipole. This may be relevant for tesla-level fields generated by MRI machines. Magnetophoresis of anisotropically diamagnetic materials is the only proposed mechanism for gradient-specific effects, but it may or may not provide an explanation of the experimental evidence at the millitesla level of exposures. Some experimental evidence supports a role for millitesla magnetic fields with steep gradients (change in field strength with distance) in the reversible blockade of action potentials of cultured sensory ganglion cells (Cavopol et al., 1995; McLean et al., 1995). Experiments on the rate of myosin phosphorylation *in vitro* suggest that a combination of field and gradient are required to explain the increased enzyme activity (Engström et al., 2002). This experimental system was cell free, so effects here did not rely on cell structures, such as phospholipid bilayers or ion channels embedded in the membrane. Other static and alternating fields increased phosphorylation in this assay (Markov & Pilla, 1997), suggesting that multiple field metrics may achieve similar biological effects.

4. **Anisotropic diamagnetism:** A static magnetic field will apply a torque on an anisotropic diamagnetic material because the orientations parallel and perpendicular to the imposed field become differentially magnetized. Some feel that this mechanism requires strong fields and large, elongated targets. For example, a 5-µm-long microtubule is estimated to be completely aligned by a magnetic field in the 10 T range (Jackson, 1975). This mechanism may account also for magnetic field effects on lipid bilayers (Braganza et al., 1984; Gaffney & McConnell, 1974; Helfrich, 1973; Maret & Dransfield, 1977; Tenforde & Liburdy, 1988), subsequent intracellular calcium release (Braganza et al., 1984; Helfrich, 1973), and how mitotic structures are affected by large fields resulting in abnormal embryonic development (Denegre et al., 1998; Gaffney & McConnell, 1974; Tenforde & Liburdy, 1988; Valles, 2002).

5a. **Biogenic magnetite:** Some bacteria contain biogenic magnetite (Blakemore, 1975). A chain of magnetosomes provides a large enough magnetic moment that the whole organism orients and swims along geomagnetic flux lines (magnetotaxes). Several groups have calculated that magnetite-based magnetoreception should be sensitive to very small variations in the geomagnetic field (Del Moral & Azanza, 1992; Kirschvink et al., 1992). Magnetite is present in a variety of animal models and a credible mechanism to explain physiological effects (Beason & Semm, 1996; Brassart et al., 1999; Duetschlander et al., 1999; Phillips et al., 2002). Magnetite-based magnetoception has been mapped in animals with electrophysiology and techniques of neuropathology (Diebel et al., 2000; Vainshtein et al., 2002).

5b. **Single domain crystals:** Single domain crystals can only be magnetized along one axis and the crystal maintains the magnetization. There are suggestions that such crystals form the basic functional components of higher magnetosensitive animals. Pulse remagnetization experiments provide good reasons to believe that permanent ferromagnets are involved in the physical transduction (Beason et al., 1997; Lohmann & Johnsen, 2000). Physical models utilizing single domain crystals have been reviewed (Kirschvink et al., 1992; Phillips et al., 2002).

5c. **Superparamagnetic magnetite:** Superparamagnetic magnetite grains are too small to be permanently magnetized, but they do respond to an externally applied field. Clusters (1 to 3 μm in diameter) of superparamagnetic nanocrystals (2 to 5 nm in diameter) have been reported in the upper beak of homing pigeons (Hanzlik et al., 2000; Winklhofer et al., 2001). Single-domain features were ruled out in these studies.

6. **Magnetic resonance:** An unhydrated ion in static field at a strength matching the geomagnetic field resonates at about 60 Hz (Adair, 1998; Edmonds, 1993; Lednev et al., 1996). This and related quantum interference mechanisms are not relevant explanations for static magnetic field effects (Adair, 1992; Binghy, 1997; Prato et al., 1996).

7. **Free radical recombination rates:** Spin-correlated free radical pairs may be a target for static magnetic fields (Grissom, 1995). A spin-correlated radical pair may recombine and prevent the formation of reaction products under certain conditions that are enhanced by magnetic fields in the millitesla to tesla range (Grissom, 1995; Salikhov et al., 1984; Steiner & Ulrich, 1989). Effects of microtesla static and time-varying fields are also predicted under conditions that limit the diffusion rate of the radical pair favoring recombination (Brocklehurst & McLauchlan, 1996; Harkin & Grissom, 1995; Till et al., 1998; Timmel et al., 1998). The free radical mechanism has been proposed as the foundation for magnetically aided animal homing and navigation (Cintolesi et al., 2003; Deutschlander et al., 1999; Eichwald & Walleczek, 1998).

In addition to the transduction mechanisms discussed above, certain cofactors may enhance the probability of biological effects of micro- to millitesla magnetic fields.

1. **Geomagnetic fields:** Nociceptive behavior in snails and rats has been extensively studied as a model of animal response to low-frequency magnetic fields (Ossenkopp et al., 1984; Prato et al., 2000, 2003). Shielding out the geomagnetic field has been reported to affect mouse behavior in similar studies (Choleris et al., 2002; Prato et al., 2004). This suggests that the geomagnetic field has physiological effects on mammals.

2. **Light:** Light also appears to determine the effects of magnetic fields (Prato et al., 1997). In avian and reptile magnetic navigation it has been shown that wavelength specific effects occur (Valles, 2002) and that the light dependence is closely linked to the magnetic field detection (Deutschlander et al., 1999). In salamanders a model has been proposed in which two separate and antagonistic magnetic field sensitive systems are activated by short-wavelength light (<450 nm) and long-wavelength light (>500 nm), respectively (Brassart et al., 1999). Thermonociceptive responses in snails are reduced by magnetic fields only in the presence of light (Prato et al., 1996, 1998, 1999). It is not clear at this point whether light influences magnetic field detection or physical transduction.

3. **State dependence:** Many reported effects of static and ELF (extremely low frequency, <100 Hz) magnetic fields have not been robustly reproducible even in the course of attempts at replication. Differences between strains of animals, batches of serum, and cell lines have been considered as possible confounders (Anderson et al., 2000; Del Seppia et al., 2000; Löscher, 2001; Ritz et al., 2002). State- or activation-dependent factors have been examined theoretically in a model of free radical responses in enzyme systems (Eichwald & Walleczek, 2003). Experimentally, it has been observed that Na-K-ATPase activity may increase or decrease depending on its activation state (Blank & Soo, 1996).

4. **Structured water:** There are controversial reports that static magnetic fields in the low millitesla range can alter the structure of water making microdomains more homogeneous, for example, Novikov and Zhadin (1994), Zhadin et al. (1998), Del Guidice (2002), Goldsworthy et al. (1999), Hazlewood (2003). The consequences of this in biological systems are not clear, but the amount of oxygen in solution can be changed by magnetic fields (Sakurai et al., 2000). Also, exposure of colloids and ionic solutions to magnetic fields with flux densities in the range of 50 to 500 mT produced prolonged effects on zeta potential and diffusivity (Hagigashitani et al., 1995; Holysz et al., 2003; Oshitani et al., 1999). Descaling effects of magnetically treated water also indicate an effect on ionization (Baker & Judd, 1996; Coey & Cass, 2000). Altering the aqueous environment of the cytoplasm could lead to changes in enzy-

matic activity, intracellular signaling, and structural proteins.

EVIDENCE FROM CELL AND ANIMAL MODELS SUPPORTING CLINICAL UTILITY OF THERAPEUTIC MAGNETIC DEVICES IN THE TREATMENT OF PAIN

Nociception depends on activation of neural pathways. This leads to the expectation that magnetic field detection and transduction mechanisms relevant to analgesic effects should modulate neural function and decrease hyperexcitability. This could occur at many levels: biophysical properties of neural membranes; pharmacological properties of neurotransmitter receptors; intracellular signaling mechanisms; biochemical processes, i.e., related to energy metabolism; and gene expression. Effects of magnetic fields on any or all of these processes could result in a variety of outcomes, depending on the nature of the magnetic field and the state of neuronal activity. Potential outcomes include neural dysfunction, neuronal damage, neuroprotection against toxins, and normalization of function. As in the case of pharmaceutical development, it is necessary to test magnetic fields in cell and animal models for a number of reasons: (1) The demonstration of robust effects in disease-specific models provides a rationale for proceeding with clinical trials. (2) Potentially, disease-specific animal models can detect adverse effects of drugs and magnetic fields, determine the useful range of concentrations or field strengths, and predict levels that might result in organ toxicity. (3) Elucidation of specific mechanisms of magnetic field interactions with isolated cells or cell components is crucial for establishing the fundamental basis for expecting clinically useful effects, differentiating the mechanisms of action of magnetic fields from those of other therapeutic modalities, including drugs. (4) Understanding the mechanisms of interaction with biological systems could lead to improvements in the design of therapeutic magnetic fields.

Unfortunately, there is little basic science information about magnetic field effects in models of nociception and even less about biophysical transduction mechanisms. As reported below, most clinical trials of therapeutic magnets employ commercially available devices that have not undergone laboratory testing, and fields produced by the devices have not been characterized meaningfully. In the absence of demonstrable analgesic effects in laboratory and clinical studies, the design of placebo-controlled trials is arbitrary and may not be capable of testing the efficacy of the applied field.

Although basic research is sorely needed, there is some information that may serve as an example of what might be accomplished with more investigation and more investigators: Effects on action potentials of sensory neu-

rons could lead to nociceptive effects. Our group at Vanderbilt has examined effects of static magnetic fields produced by a square array of four magnets of alternating polarity. This device has been used in pilot studies to be described below. Gradient magnetic fields produced by this device reversibly blocked action potentials of cultured mouse dorsal root ganglion cells in a time-dependent manner without effects on resting membrane potential (Cavopol et al., 1995; McLean et al., 1991, 1995) or passive membrane properties (McLean et al., unpublished). Subtle effects of strong uniform static magnetic fields on calcium currents (Rosen, 1996) under patch clamp conditions have also been reported, but reports of effects on sodium currents have been inconsistent (Rosen, 2003; Schwartz, 1979). The effect on action potentials was reported to take several minutes, suggesting that a biochemical effect (e.g., on phosphorylation state of sodium channels that determines availability for voltage-dependent activation) had occurred, rather than a biophysical one. Exposure to gradient fields produced by the static magnetic device diminished the swelling of cultured mouse spinal cord neurons during subsequent superfusion with the excitotoxin kainic acid (McLean et al., 2003, unpublished). Gradient regions of the magnetic field produced by an electromagnetic device with a similar alternating four-polar design significantly decreased neuronal death induced by kainic acid to roughly the same extent as the kainite antagonist CNQX (McLean et al., in preparation) and decreased sound-induced clonic and tonic hindlimb extensor seizures in genetically susceptible mice (McLean et al., 2003). Pretreatment with the magnetic field potentiated the effect of phenytoin, a well-known antiepileptic drug. The ED50 for phenytoin was shifted about fivefold to the left. Multiple regions of the same electromagnetic device reduced clonic seizures induced in wild type mice by intracerebroventricular injection of the excitatory amino acid N-methyl-D-aspartate. The effect of combined treatment with phenytoin was close to additive in this seizure model (McLean et al., in preparation).

Together, these data suggest that gradient and other regions of the specific device tested may diminish neuronal excitability and neurotoxicity. Importantly, treatment with the magnetic field may enhance efficacy of drugs used to treat epilepsy and pain, namely, antiepileptic drugs. These data form a rational basis for undertaking clinical trials with the devices studied, and some of the results of some trials are presented below. These data also suggest a way in which magnetic field therapy might be brought into clinical practice, namely, in combination with drugs with which the fields could interact to result in improved outcomes and/or reduced drug load.

Alternating fields also have been shown to have analgesic effects in snails (Prato et al., 2003) and rats (Radzievsky et al., 2001), but the devices used in those studies have not been used in clinical trials against pain. Further discussion of time-varying fields is beyond the scope of this chapter. Interested readers are referred to additional sources (e.g., McLean et al., 2003; Rosch & Markov, 2004).

OPTIMIZING ELEMENTS OF CLINICAL TRIALS DESIGN FOR THE STUDY OF THERAPEUTIC MAGNETIC DEVICES

No static magnetic field-generating devices have been accepted for therapeutic use in mainstream Western medicine despite widespread public interest. Currently, no such devices are approved by the U.S. FDA with a specific indication for the treatment of nociceptive or neuropathic pain. Nevertheless, magnetic devices are sold throughout the United States as wellness aids. Sales are seemingly tolerated by the FDA as long as no specific claims are made, probably because these devices represent no significant risk to the populace. If serious or life-threatening adverse effects were associated with the use of such devices, the enforcement powers of the FDA would undoubtedly be brought to bear to sanction sales.

In this permissive yet watchful atmosphere, there has been a growing interest among researchers in potential therapeutic applications of magnetic fields. Acceptance of new treatments in the medical community requires support by rigorous clinical trials. A critical review such as this one is intended to reveal the state of knowledge about therapeutic magnetic devices and both the strengths and weaknesses of investigative approaches. However, this task is complicated by the fact that regulatory criteria for the approval of therapeutic magnetic devices are not yet defined. In this section, we review elements of clinical study design specifically for therapeutic magnetic devices. A snapshot of current approaches also may be instructive about how to study magnetic field effects on biological systems. The weight of evidence and existence of well-established methods of study undoubtedly contribute to the wide acceptance of the pharmaceutical model in current clinical practice. There is a relative paucity of published studies of static magnetic field-generating devices. Methods for studying these devices are less well established and basically adapted from drug studies under the rubric of "scientific method."

These factors could contribute to a reluctance to accept magnetic treatment devices into widespread clinical practice and can only be overcome by rigorous testing with criteria acceptable to the medical community. Implicitly, there is a breakpoint at which there will be sufficient evidence to be convincing and clinical acceptance will ensue, or magnetic therapies will once again fall into oblivion until another effort is made to evaluate them with different approaches. An attempt is made in this chapter to determine the status of magnetic therapies relative to this hypothetical breakpoint.

In this section, we consider the study of observable effects of magnetic fields in the context of clinical trial design. We focus on permanent magnetic devices because so many such devices are sold throughout the United States and have been used in several controlled trials reported in the peer-reviewed literature. Studying therapeutic uses of focally applied permanent magnetic devices is in many ways different from the study of pharmaceuticals that are dissolved in the entire body. The former must act by local mechanisms, even though distant effects may result. The latter may interact with multiple targets in the nociceptive pathway at multiple levels of the nervous system by virtue of widespread distribution. Despite differences, the development of pharmaceutical agents serves as a model framework of how magnetic devices might become accepted into widespread clinical use.

Pharmaceutical development begins with the discovery of disease-related therapeutic efficacy in animal models and potential mechanisms of action in cell and animal studies using a variety of techniques. Cellular and animal effects of magnetic fields relevant to pain were presented in the previous section. The preclinical studies serve to establish a rationale for proceeding to clinical trials and a potential mechanism(s) underlying expectations of efficacy. This is followed by initial trials (Phase I) in humans to establish pharmacokinetic properties for dose optimization and minimization of adverse effects, and to determine a first approximation of safety. In Phase II, small numbers of patients with the condition for which an indication for use of the drug will be sought receive the investigational compound in initial tests of efficacy. Dose-ranging studies also begin at this stage to determine the range of doses to be used in pivotal trials and, when feasible, the maximally tolerable dose. In Phase III, large, randomized, multicenter trials are conducted. These studies serve as the pivotal trials upon which regulatory considerations are based.

Study designs for different classes of drugs have been validated and certain designs seem to be preferred by regulatory agencies, although novel features may be included. In this way, study design evolves but the playing field changes each time a drug is approved on the basis of a novel design. In the case of therapeutic static magnetic field devices, the first FDA approval will set the bar.

To a large extent, trial design determines the outcome. Study design must be optimized to reveal therapeutic benefits. This could not be truer than for evaluation of magnetic devices. Static magnetic field-generating devices have local effects in the vicinity of points to which they are applied. In this regard magnetic field-generating devices differ fundamentally from pharmaceutical agents that are systemically distributed and may have effects at multiple locations along nociceptive pathways due to multiple mechanisms of action. Only through a deliberate design process can the signal-to-noise ratio be optimized in favor of detecting treatment effects. Adoption of study designs used to evaluate drugs or other devices runs the risk of incorporating variability that can result in the failure of trials with static magnetic field-generating devices. In fact, outcomes from such studies may be "false negatives." Similarly, overly specific design features may result in outcomes that limit applicability of a device. And, studies with small numbers of subjects may result in both "false positive" and "false negative" outcomes. In the absence of guidance from studies of an approved device, this means that confidence in outcomes results from cumulative experience from a large number of studies. In the case of static magnetic field-generating devices, the few available studies have been conducted with a variety of devices and some studies have been negative, limiting corroboration and confidence.

Ideally, the condition under study should be constant and the composition of the study groups should be uniform to facilitate detection of treatment-related effects. These conditions are virtually impossible to achieve. In reality, pain varies from day to day and hour to hour and can be influenced by many factors including activity level, emotion, sleep efficiency, and other illnesses. Inclusion and exclusion criteria are designed to approximate these conditions. Variability in pain intensity makes a pain study a noisy situation in which large treatment effects are most successful. It is necessary to increase the signal-to-noise level in order to detect smaller treatment effects. This can be accomplished to some degree by attempts at reducing inter- and intraindividual reporting of pain intensity. Measurement of treatment related changes in mild pain (1 to 3 on a 10 point scale) is not very reliable (Chapman et al., 1985). Successful studies of pharmaceuticals have used pain intensity of 4 (out of 10) or greater as an inclusion criterion (Backonja et al., 1998; Dworkin et al., 2003; Rice et al. 2001; Rowbotham et al., 1998). Typically, a baseline (prerandomization) period is included to be sure that study subjects meet criteria for inclusion in the study. An adequate baseline period is essential to ensure that the primary outcome measure is stable enough to study. In general this means that the pain is sufficiently intense and constant so that repeated assessments with validated outcome measures will reliably detect treatment effects (pain reduction). Whenever ethical, a placebo is used to compare with the effects of the drug under study. Alternatively, an active control (such as another pharmaceutical or device) may be used as a comparator. Qualified patients are randomized to receive either the investigational treatment or placebo in the so-called parallel-group design. In studies of crossover design, subjects receive both treatments, but the order in which the treatments are given is randomized. Both designs have strengths and weaknesses. Most studies are masked, or blinded, meaning that either the patient (single-blind) or both the patient and the investigators (double-blind) are unaware of which treatment is being administered.

Variability of pain and the focal application of a therapeutic magnetic field with shallow depth of penetration into the pain producing body tissues are two major factors limiting success in clinical trials. As a result, every aspect of study design should be carefully crafted to reduce the impact of variability and optimize chances of seeing therapeutically relevant benefits of the magnetic field.

UNIQUE FEATURES OF THERAPEUTIC MAGNETIC DEVICES: LOCALIZATION AND TISSUE PENETRATION

Studies of the use of magnetic devices to treat pain differ significantly from studies of analgesic medications. Pharmacological therapies result from dissolving compounds throughout the body where they can interact with multiple tissues at the pain-generating site as well as along neural pathways involved in the localization and perception of pain. Magnetic treatment devices, on the other hand, are usually placed in close proximity to the pain generator identified by where the patient places a hand or finger.

Elements of the pain-generating tissue structures may lie near the surface of the skin or several centimeters below the skin. To date, there are no implanted static magnetic treatment devices, so the devices must be placed at some distance from the target. To have any chance of therapeutic benefit, the magnetic field must envelop the different components of the pain-generating tissues (e.g., nerve, muscle, or bone). The placement, strength, and configuration of the magnets and the spatial variation of the magnetic field determine the depth of penetration into tissue. Thus, not all magnets and not all magnetic fields should be expected to have therapeutic benefits, just as all pains cannot be expected to respond to aspirin or other nonsteroidal anti-inflammatory compounds. Also, effective pharmacological therapies depend on dose to determine the degree of pain relief. In the case of magnetic fields that decrease as the inverse cube of the distance (to a magnetic dipole), the dose characteristic is determined by the depth of the pain generators in tissue and the time of exposure.

The dearth of data from large, well-designed, placebo-controlled trials makes it difficult to understand the meaning of both positive and negative reports at this time. Reports in the medical literature have revealed mixed benefits. For example, devices with the same basic design produced by the same company were reported to be effective against painful diabetic neuropathy (Weintraub, 1999) and ineffective against a variety of back pains (Collacott et al., 2000). The difference can be explained by differences in study design to a large extent. In contrast, results with devices with different designs showed statistical superiority to placebos in the treatment of low back pain (Holcomb et al., 1991) and painful trigger points of post-polio syndrome (Vallbona et al., 1997).

At the heart of understanding the discrepancies lies the problem of learning how to study magnetic devices. Nonsteroidal medications do not treat all pains effectively, and magnetic devices should not be expected to be panaceas. Finding appropriate conditions is the first step toward the design of discriminating studies. A seemingly obvious point is that a device should have demonstrable efficacy and a justification for clinical studies founded in basic scientific research before launching a large-scale clinical study. Experience from open study of a device is a must in order to create a successful study protocol. Even if the goal is exact replication of another finding, it is imperative to familiarize oneself with the application of therapeutic magnets and the inherent problems before undertaking a masked study.

SAFETY

Although magnetic treatment devices of many designs, sizes, and shapes are marketed in the United States, there is little evidence relating to their safety or efficacy. There has been no assessment of long-term risk of exposure to focally applied magnetic devices. Large fields that are encountered in industrial settings may have long-term and short-term health risks. In a review by Repacholi and Greenebaum (1999), a statement is made that there is no known health risk of static magnetic fields less than 3 T (a typical field strength in MRI). This is much greater than the flux densities produced by commercially available therapeutic magnets. Also, the area of the body to which these devices are attached is small and the percentage of time that the devices are worn is low in many studies. These factors limit exposure to the magnetic field and could ultimately reduce the risk of serious adverse events.

The absence of reports cannot be taken as proof of safety. In one of our studies, a patient inadvertently placed a magnetic device over a pacemaker and this resulted in a cardiac arrhythmia and brief loss of consciousness. This could be a potentially life-threatening adverse effect and led to modifications of inclusion/exclusion criteria for future studies. Effects of magnetic fields on human fetal development are unknown. For this reason, pregnant women may be excluded from the studies and women who become pregnant during the studies may be discontinued. A potential mitigating factor is that the magnetic device(s) may be placed on the body at significant distances from the fetus.

STUDY POPULATION

The proper selection of subject population is a crucial aspect of study design. Ideally, it would seem that naïve patients, i.e., those who have never been exposed to treatment with magnetic devices and do not know what to expect, would be the best candidates for formal studies.

Expectations produce biases that may affect assessment of pain in the course of repeated assessments during the study. The combination of variables may be sufficient to obscure efficacy that would otherwise be detectable. However, many potential candidates may have used therapeutic magnets already or have enough knowledge about them (e.g., through the experience of others) to have an opinion. Practically speaking, this may mean that candidates should not have used therapeutic magnets for a prolonged interval prior to entry into a clinical trial.

The symptoms or disorder to be studied should be strictly defined. Homogeneity of symptoms is one way of reducing variability.

Ulterior motives such as litigation and disability issues may also affect the ability of the patient to report changes of pain accurately during a blinded study. Careful design of the inclusion and exclusion criteria and a meaningful baseline period may eliminate concern about these factors by eliminating individuals with highly variable pain or pain outside the range acceptable for entry.

Concomitant medications are a major consideration. Many candidates for clinical trials of therapeutic magnets have chronic pain. They may be taking and have taken multiple medications. Narcotic use may be a confounder (Holcomb et al., 2003). Acute withdrawal of nonsteroidal medications may also worsen pain to a degree that responds relatively poorly to placement of magnetic devices. This and rescue medications commonly used in protocols to test novel nonsteroidal medications may unfavorably increase variability and diminish treatment effects.

A balance must be found for the appropriate set of inclusion/exclusion criteria to use for the study. Confounders must be avoided, but inclusion/exclusion criteria can also be so restrictive that it becomes impossible to recruit the necessary number of subjects. A partial list of criteria to consider for a pain study includes baseline pain level not too low or too high (Montgomery, 1999), symptoms for inclusion should be carefully defined, age group, possible confounding medical conditions, previous surgery for the condition, bodyweight if field penetration is an issue, medication use, neurological and psychiatric disorders that limit the ability of the candidates to notice and describe symptomatic changes, unstable medical conditions, patients with unresolved litigation, and pregnancy.

MASKING AND THE USE OF PLACEBOS

The design and selection of placebo devices is one of the most significant problems in studying magnetic devices. Modern scientific method demands the use of an ineffective (placebo) device in one treatment arm to compare with the active device or pharmaceutical in another group (see Harrington, 1997).

Nonmagnetic placebos may be appropriate controls for testing the benefit of brief application of magnetic devices if subjects are observed closely by study personnel, e.g., in the clinic environment or on a clinical research unit. Placebos must be identical in appearance and weight to the active device. This concern is particularly important in a study employing a crossover design that entails treatment with an active device and the placebo in any order. For the blind to be protected the individual must be observed closely and/or the devices must be covered by a pad that prevents detection of the magnetic field produced by the active device. The blind may be easily broken in studies that last for days or weeks in the absence of close observation. Once the study subject determines that he or she has the inactive device, the validity of the study is irreparably impaired.

The use of magnetic placebos means that the devices produce magnetic fields. The subject may detect this by bringing it in contact with ferromagnetic materials. Thus, they are led to believe that they are receiving a magnetic treatment. However, such a device for clinical trials must have been proved in the laboratory and in pilot validation studies to have no detectable treatment benefit. A trial that employs a magnetic comparator with any efficacy is automatically not placebo controlled. Instead, it becomes a head-to-head comparative trial, roughly the equivalent of a dose-controlled drug trial. Ideally, the placebo will have lesser field strength, an altered spatial distribution of the magnetic field, and a shallower tissue penetration. These devices are potentially useful for longer studies in which the patient visits the study personnel only intermittently.

CHOOSING DEVICES APPROPRIATE FOR THE STUDY OF A GIVEN CONDITION

The "golden rule" is that effective regions of the field produced by a therapeutic magnetic device must envelop pain generators or transducers in order to observe significant treatment benefit. Inherent to this concept is a need, if not a requirement, to formulate a scientific basis for expecting efficacy and to demonstrate efficacy in a pilot study of the treatment of a specific disorder. It seems likely that devices may have to be designed specifically for different types of conditions. One criterion in selecting an appropriate device for study is the depth of pain generators below the skin surface. Pain generators involved in painful diabetic neuropathy are likely to be intradermal (see studies by Weintraub below), whereas those involved in low back pain are likely to lie up to several centimeters below the skin surface. Also, one must consider whether the pain is acute (e.g., osteoarthritic) or neuropathic (e.g., pain with trigeminal neuralgia or diabetic neuropathy). The magnetic field produced by the treatment device must reach the pain generators in a way that leads to beneficial alterations of nociceptive mechanisms in each case. It would seem that treatment of such disparate conditions may require different magnetic fields.

POSITIONING THE DEVICES

Magnetic devices are essentially "point-and-shoot" devices. Limited area of coverage makes positioning critical. If the effective portions of the field fail to envelop structures involved in pain generation, there is no chance of therapeutic benefit, and in fact, the study design is incapable of testing efficacy of the magnetic devices.

Migratory pain such as the trigger point pain of fibromyalgia may be treated effectively initially when the devices are placed right over punctate trigger points. However, this makes fibromyalgia particularly difficult to study longitudinally because the syndrome is characterized by the abrupt appearance of pain at different locations over time.

The size of the magnetic device is important. It is possible to cover large areas of skin with a single device or to apply multiple devices in the vicinity of painful or tender tissues. In the latter case, interactions between the magnetic fields of two devices could either increase or decrease therapeutic benefit.

Attachment of devices to the skin presents other problems. Potential for irritation to the skin as a result of application with various types of tapes or adhesives necessitates good skin care. Removal of the tape, cleansing with alcohol and soap, and rubbing with vitamin oil tend to reduce irritation. An adhesive spray such as Tegaderm® may avoid irritation produced by loosely fitting devices. Use of hypoallergenic tapes is helpful. A trial-and-error method may be necessary to determine which tape is the least irritating for a given individual.

Devices in fitments, or elastic appurtenances, are a potential confounder because of splinting of joints or the spine, for example. Fitments do allow application of devices to moving parts of the body. Even with appropriate control arms, the magnitude of benefit produced by the fitments could outweigh small treatment effects of magnetic devices. Because proximity to the skin generally is crucial because of the field's rapid decline with distance from the magnet, it is important that a fitment does not have excessive padding between the device and the skin.

CONTROLLING VARIABILITY

Pain varies from hour to hour and day to day and perception of pain can fluctuate in ways that alter the weight of pain scores. Variation with time of day occurs in the case of morning stiffness, which is worse on rising. Changes in activity level can influence the efficacy of treatment devices. Increased disease activity can worsen pain, as in rheumatoid arthritis. Acute illness, anxiety, or depression, or sleep deprivation may also augment pain. Patients frequently use medications to sleep, and in some cases tricyclic antidepressants. These drugs may have analgesic and adverse effects that can confound the assessment of pain. The investigator must decide whether to slowly taper and discontinue these medications prior to the study to achieve a monotherapy situation during the trial or to optimize the therapies and then keep the drug dose constant for the study. It is difficult to ask patients not to change their activity levels, but a measure of activity could be an outcome measure.

INSTRUMENTS OF MEASURE

Linear visual analogue scales are validated for pain studies, but have significant well-documented limitations (Chapman et al., 1985). Basically, the patient marks along a 10-cm line the intensity of his or her pain between no pain at the left and worst pain imaginable at the right limit of the line. This provides a quantitative assessment of the subjective impression of pain intensity. The limitation stems in large part from the fact that pain is a multidimensional experience that is probed incompletely by the use of linear scales. A particularly important limitation is the insensitivity of repeated measurements with a visual analogue scale to detect reductions in pain (Chapman et al., 1985). One way of circumventing this issue is the use of multiple primary and secondary outcome measures. Internally consistent treatment effects increase confidence that the outcome is biologically meaningful. Studies of pain must be designed to reduce the impact of interindividual variability or must be powered by sufficient numbers of patients to demonstrate a statistically significant therapeutic benefit.

One way of managing variability encountered with the use of linear scale is the use of "average pain over 24 hours," a form of mental averaging on the part of the patient, instead of "pain now" as the primary outcome measure. Typically, therapeutic studies with pharmacological agents involve up to 100 patients per arm in order to demonstrate therapeutic significance in the range of $p = 0.001$ to 0.05 (Backonja et al., 1998; Dworkin et al., 2003; Rice et al., 2001; Rowbotham et al., 1998). Perhaps the best index of success is that the patient chooses to continue using it after completion of the study.

In some instances, validated scales are available for use in the study of specific conditions. For example, the WOMAC scales (Western Ontario and McMasters Pain Inventory; Bellamy, 1995; Bellamy et al., 1988) have been validated for studies of pain treatment in patients with arthritis of the knee and hip. This instrument contains 27 visual analogue scales to measure different aspects of pain (five subscales), activity, and quality of life (22 subscales). The virtue of the WOMAC is that there are multiple assessments for pain and other functions. This has the advantage of looking at the pain from a number of different ways. It may also be instructive to examine pain diaries for information about subjective response to pain. In other cases, the scales have not been validated and pilot studies would be necessary to validate the instruments of measure.

The primary and secondary outcome measures should be determined in the context of claims desired for the device.

Assessments by study personnel on an intermittent basis may vary in their timing in relation to activity. A period of rest in the office, perhaps an hour or more, may allow the reversal of the activity dependent discomfort.

STATISTICS

Pilot studies are needed to assess potential effect size and calculate the number of subjects necessary to detect statistically significant differences in treatment effects between groups (power analysis) in pivotal trials. The larger the effect, the smaller the number of subjects needed. A variety of statistical methods are described in the pain literature.

ANALYSIS OF PUBLISHED CLINICAL TRIALS OF STATIC MAGNETIC DEVICES FOR THE TREATMENT OF PAIN

This section is a review of results of some controlled clinical trials published in the peer-reviewed literature. The presentation is chronological in order to give an impression of the evolution of trial design over time. A variety of devices have been studied. The result is that there are not multiple trials of a single device to give a clear impression of the robustness of effects. The studies will be analyzed as if by a referee. The intention of this mode of critique is to learn how to design clinical trials with a high likelihood of success. In the end, only devices with proven efficacy in preclinical studies and open clinical trials should be studied in placebo-controlled trials.

CHRONIC NECK AND SHOULDER PAIN (HONG ET AL., 1982)

Hong et al. (1982) were motivated by earlier subjective reports of pain-relief (Hansen, 1938; Nakagawa, 1976) to study further the effects of wearing a magnetic necklace on neck and shoulder pain. The study included 101 volunteers with and without pain and employed electrophysiological measurements. Subjects were assigned to one of four groups in a double-blind fashion: subjects with pain wearing a magnetic necklace, subjects with pain wearing a nonmagnetic necklace, subjects without pain wearing a magnetic necklace, and subjects without pain wearing a nonmagnetic necklace. The magnetic necklaces contained an average of nine cylindrical magnets, 8 mm long and 2.2 mm in diameter, interspersed at regular distance along a brass linked chain. The chain length was adjusted to each individual's neck size so that the magnets stayed in contact with the skin. The flux density of the magnets was 130 mT at the surface and zero at a distance of 9 mm. All subjects wore a necklace constantly for 3 weeks. Electrodiagnostic studies (threshold voltage for activation of the supraspinatus muscle and ulnar proximal conduction time) were performed at baseline and weekly until the end of the study. Subjects in all four groups experienced a statistically significant reduction of intensity and frequency of discomfort assessed by a numerical scale of 0 to 4. There were no significant differences in subjective scores among the four groups. At the end of the study, proximal conduction time was significantly reduced (i.e., conduction velocity was faster) in subjects without pain, but not in those with pain, who wore the magnetic necklaces. No other significant differences in electrophysiological parameters were detected.

Comments

1. Study outcome negative: This study showed a significant reduction of discomfort by the placebo device (nonmagnetic necklaces) and no significant difference in reduction by the active device (magnetic necklaces).

2. Magnets of unproven efficacy: No evidence is cited to indicate that the magnets used were able to alter nerve conduction in controlled circumstances, and dosimetry required to alter nerve function had not been determined.

3. Positioning of the magnets: While magnets were held against the skin by adjusting necklace length, rotation of the necklace was possible so that magnets could have been more than 9 mm from C7–8 roots activated in testing the ulnar nerve and from the nerve to the supraspinatus muscle in the posterior cervical triangle for substantial amount of time, even during electrophysiological testing.

4. In appropriate outcome measures: The electrophysiological assays used here test predominantly large diameter, low-threshold, thickly myelinated mechanoceptive fibers with fast conduction velocities. Activity of small diameter, high-threshold, unmyelinated, nociceptive fibers may not be detected with these techniques. For this reason, the methods do not seem to provide appropriate parameters to correlate with subjective reporting of pain.

5. Questionable significance of effect: The significant increase in ulnar conduction velocity (reduced conduction time) should in the group without pain who wore the magnetic necklaces have resulted from technical factors and is not consistent with the lack of effect in the group with pain who wore magnetic necklaces.

6. Cohort size: The number of subjects is small by current standards for regulatory studies and there

was no preliminary study with a demonstrated effect upon which to base a power analysis.

7. Security of the blind: Overall, the study methods may not detect factors relevant to nociception and there was no significant change in pain assessed with an unverified verbal reporting assay. This was a trial of an unproven device, and the results are uninformative. Such a study cannot be generalized to the level of deciding whether therapeutic use of static (permanent) magnetic devices are useful for the treatment of pain.

MECHANICAL LOW BACK AND KNEE PAIN (HOLCOMB ET AL., 1991)

This paper reports the results of a randomized, double-blind, double crossover, placebo-controlled pilot study to determine effects of a device, developed by trial and error in a clinical practice setting, on mechanical low back and knee pain. The study design was vetted with FDA personnel prior to performance of the study. The order of exposure to the experimental device and a nonmagnetic placebo was randomized. The study was conducted at two sites. In all, 54 subjects aged 25 to 86 years were randomized; 40 were treated for back pain, 14 for knee pain, and 4 for both. They were admitted to a clinical research unit for two 24 hours sessions separated by at least a week (washout period). The devices (Magna Bloc™) under study consisted of four neodymium-iron-boron magnets (200 mT over the pole) with alternating polarity in a square array and encased in a hypoallergenic plastic case. The placebo devices were nonmagnetic, but otherwise identical in appearance. The devices were 3.5 cm in diameter and weighed 30 g each. They were attached to the skin with tape in different patterns specifically for knee or back pain. The devices were masked and handled over a wooden table to protect the blind. During each session, the subjects with mechanical low back pain had seven devices (active or placebo) taped at least one diameter apart over the lumbosacral region and sacrum; patients with knee pain had four devices taped in a diamond pattern around the patella. The devices were covered with a thick, firm foam pad to protect the blind. The principal outcome measure was reduction of pain from baseline. Pain intensity was assessed with a 10-cm linear visual analogue scale and a 10-point verbal response score. Assessments were made by research personnel before devices were placed and at 1, 3, and 24 hours after placement. No devices were worn during the washout period. Medication use was recorded in patient logs.

Average pretreatment pain was about 5.3 cm in both of the treatment group. Pain was reduced significantly more by treatment with the magnetic device for 24 hours than by treatment with placebos ($P < 0.03$). Back pain improved slightly more than knee pain, but the small number of patients makes comparison difficult. There was no evidence of carryover effects. Less medication was administered during the magnetic than placebo treatment, but the difference did not reach statistical significance. Masking was judged to be preserved throughout by both subjects and research staff.

Comments

This was considered a pilot study from conception. Therefore, it was designed to test the ability of the study methods to detect therapeutic effects of specific magnetic devices. Even though the outcome showed superiority of the magnetic device over placebo, the design raises several issues:

1. Subjects: The number of subjects was small compared with numbers in regulatory studies of pharmaceuticals.
2. Painful condition: Characteristics of the pain (e.g., burning, aching, shooting) are not described or differentiated. Pain due to muscle spasm is not distinguished from osteoarthritic changes in deep bony structures. Subjects had either one of two painful regions. A definitive study would likely involve a more homogeneous study population.
3. Devices: Flux density of the magnets was given, but no dosimetric details were reported. Importantly, the design of the magnetic devices had been optimized by patient-reported benefit. Even though there was no laboratory evidence to support effectiveness or mechanisms, there were clinical reasons to believe that the devices to be tested might be effective. Subsequent to the study, certain regions of the magnetic field produced by arrays of four magnets with alternating polarity, similar to the arrangement in the devices used in this study, were shown to block electrically stimulated action potential firing in cultured sensory neurons (McLean et al., 1991).
4. Device placement: Multiple devices were applied in different patterns for back and knee pain. In one sense, this suggests broad applicability of such devices. In another sense, interpretation of results combining data from the two treatment groups is complicated.
5. Study design: A crossover design was used. No carryover effect was detected, but parallel groups studies are the vogue for regulatory studies of pharmaceuticals.
6. Duration of the blind: The 24-hour treatment sessions are brief compared with most painful

conditions. Implications of these data for the treatment of chronic pain are not determined.
7. Masking: A nonmagnetic placebo was used. In a longer study this might jeopardize intactness of the blind. In the in-patient setting, procedures to protect the blind, including the covering pad and direct observation by research staff, could be implemented. Compliance with such methods outside a controlled unit might be difficult to ensure.
8. Data presentation and statistics: Absolute values of pain scores are not presented for all observation periods. Results are presented as differences between magnetic and placebo treatment periods. Thus, the magnitude of the treatment effect is difficult to determine. Overall pain relief during treatments with magnets was 20 to 34% better than placebo and the difference was statistically significant. One could question the biological significance of treatment effects of this magnitude, however. Beecher (1955) compared morphine injection with saline. He found that the placebo effect was greatest in the immediate postoperative period: 52% of patients had pain relief after morphine subcutaneously, 40% of patients had pain relief after placebo injection. Placebo accounted for 77% of the pain relief thus making morphine 23% more effective than placebo. Since morphine is considered to be a gold standard of pain relief, one might boldly say that pain relief by some magnetic fields approaches that of morphine. Overall, this pilot study supports further investigation of the device tested. Study design could be improved along the lines of this discussion for additional trials.

TRIGGER POINT PAIN IN PATIENTS WITH POSTPOLIO SYNDROME (VALLBONA ET AL., 1997)

Limited success has been achieved with a variety of modalities, including anti-inflammatory medications, in the treatment of postpolio syndrome. This fact and the documented utilization of static and time-varying electromagnetic fields in orthopedic conditions led the authors to test the effects of magnetic treatment devices for trigger point pain in patients with postpolio syndrome. In the study, 50 patients, predominantly female, who were not more than 1.5 times their ideal bodyweight, were randomized to treatment with a nonmagnetic placebo device or a commercially available magnetic device (Bioflex). Patients had had significant muscular and/or arthritic pain for at least 3 weeks and a trigger point or circumscribed painful region on palpation. Only one site that was tender to palpation with a blunt object 1 cm in diameter was treated per patient, even if other painful sites were present. There was no significant difference in the location of the painful points in the two treatment groups, although the most commonly affected site (33% of the placebo group and 41% of the magnetic device group) was the sacroiliac joint. The size of the treatment device varied depending on the area involved. The flux density at the surface of discs 40 mm in diameter and 1.5 mm thick and strips 175 × 50 × 1.5 mm was 50 mT. At the surface of discs 90 mm in diameter and 1.5 mm thick and 83 × 53 × 1.5 mm pads, the flux density was 30 mT. The design of all four active devices consisted of concentrically arranged rings of alternating magnetic polarity. The nonmagnetic placebos were identical size and shape. Pain was assessed with a validated 10 point (1 to 10) scale prior to and 45 minutes after placement of the treatment devices.

Trigger point pain improved in 22 of 29 subjects in the group treated with active magnetic devices and in 4 of 21 of the group treated with placebos. Baseline pain scores were ~9.6/10 (magnet group) and ~9.5/10 (placebo group), i.e., in the severe range. After 45 minutes, pain scores were ~4.4/10 (~54% reduction) in the group that wore magnetic devices and ~8.4/10 (~12% reduction) in the group that wore placebos. The difference was highly significant ($p < 0.0001$).

Comments

1. The outcome was highly significant in favor of the magnetic treatment device. Although detailed dosimetry was not available, flux density at the skin surface was in the range of 30 to 50 mT and was spatially inhomogeneous due to the alternating polarity of the magnetic rings. The sacroiliac joint and muscle trigger points would be expected to be fairly superficial and only separated from the devices by the thickness of the skin and subcutaneous fat. Thus, a field in the millitesla range could be expected to reach the treated points of tenderness. The rationale for selecting the Bioflex magnets is not clear. Spatial inhomogeneity and regions of steep field gradients are features of alternating quadripolar arrays that reversibly blocked action potentials in cultured neurons (McLean et al., 1991, 1995). Also, alternating quadripolar arrays (plane of device contacting skin) with gradient fields with higher flux densities (1 mT at depth of 2.5 cm; see McLean et al., 2003) were used in clinical studies (Holcomb et al., 1991).

2. Different treatment devices of different magnetic strength were used, but there was no significant difference in the numbers of devices between groups.

3. Patient selection: Patients less than 1.5 times their ideal bodyweight were selected so that the field produced by the treatment devices had a chance of exposing the target tissues.

4. Duration of the blind: The exposure period was 45 minutes. This is very short compared with duration of chronic pains with or without exacerbation. It is not clear that success in the course of brief treatment of trigger points can be extended to other types of more persistent pain, although additional trials appear to be justified.

MUSCLE PAIN AND RECOVERY AFTER INTENSE EXERCISE (BORSA & LIGGETT, 1998)

Borsa and Liggett (1998) included 45 normal individuals in a single-blind, placebo-controlled study to test the effects of commercially available magnets on pain due to isometric muscle contraction. The justification for studying magnetic devices was written and anecdotal claims of benefit of the devices tested against muscle soreness. The magnets provided by the manufacturer had a flux density of 70 mT at the surface, measured 8 × 5 cm and were 3 mm thick (Nikken, Inc., Los Angeles, CA). Placebos were nonmagnetic and identical in appearance. Subjects were randomized to treatment with nothing, the magnetic devices, or the nonmagnetic placebos. The treatment devices were secured over the midbelly of the biceps muscle with elastic tape. Devices were worn constantly. Outcome measures included pain perception measured by a 10 cm visual analogue scale, pain-free range of motion measured with a goniometer, or static force production measured with an isokinetic testing device. Data were obtained before treatment and 24, 48, and 72 hours after treatment.

There were no statistically (ANOVA) significant differences among the three groups in any of the parameters tested.

Comments

1. Although there was no difference among groups, the outcome is uninformative in the absence of a testable effect; i.e., there were no pilot data showing benefit from the magnetic devices.

2. Unpublished data cited by the authors suggested that the magnets used act by membrane hyperpolarization. The data had not been published in a peer-reviewed journal and seem to have been literature from the company.

3. The magnet pads covered roughly the middle third of the belly of the biceps muscle and there was no dosimetric information upon which to base expectation about exposing of pain-sensitive structures to the magnetic field. Characterization of the field is missing. It may be that

the type of field generated by the tested devices is ineffective for the pain studied. However, this does not prove that the devices might not be effective for another type of pain or that magnetic fields in general are ineffective in the treatment of pain.

PAIN AND HEALING AFTER LIPOSUCTION (MAN ET AL., 1999)

Improvements in would healing would be useful in plastic surgery and other areas of medical practice. Based on increased healing and wound tensile strength in animal models, the authors tested effects of commercially available ceramic magnets on pain (assessed with visual analog scales), edema (on a scale of 0 to 10 compared with adjacent untreated areas), and discoloration (on a scale of 0 to 10) at sites of suction lipectomy. A variety of areas were suctioned in different patients. Identical magnetic patches and nonmagnetic placebos were provided by the manufacturer (Tectonic, Magnetherapy Inc., North Palm Beach, FL). Sizes (from 5 × 15 cm to 20 × 30 cm) and shape (square and rectangular) varied. Flux density varied from 15 to 40 mT. The negative pole faced the skin. In the study, 10 patients were randomly assigned to receive magnets and 10 received placebos. Patches were attached to the skin with compressive bandages immediately after surgery and for 14 days postoperatively. Wounds were inspected on days 1, 2, 3, 4, 7, and 14.

Pain, edema, and discoloration were significantly improved in the group that received magnetic devices compared with placebos.

Comments

1. The reported benefits were detectable in a small cohort, suggesting a large treatment effect.
2. The impact of variability in the areas suctioned and the devices used to treat (with respect to field strength and geometry) on study outcome was not considered.
3. Other than the visual analogue scales used to assess pain intensity, the instruments of measure were subjective and not validated in previous large studies. Intactness of the blind was not assessed.
4. Based on experimental data in the literature, increased blood flow was considered to be a possible mechanism for the therapeutic effects seen here. Mechanistic properties of the devices used here have not been identified by basic research.
5. Further studies of postoperative wound healing have not appeared in the literature, but seem to be justified.

FIBROMYALGIA (COLBERT ET AL., 1999)

Fibromyalgia is a chronic disorder characterized by fluctuating and migratory musculoskeletal symptoms, disturbed sleep, and fatigue. Prevalence is about 2% in the general population and 3.4% among women (Wolfe et al., 1995). Fibromyalgia was the second most common symptom among veterans of the first Gulf War (The Iowa Persian Gulf Study Group, 1997). Fewer than half of patients with fibromyalgia receive significant improvement with pharmaceuticals (tricyclic antidepressants, benzodiazepines, anti-inflammatory drugs, and other central nervous system active compounds) while adverse effects occur in 98% of the medicated (Carette et al., 1994). Nonpharmacological therapies have been shown to provide significant benefit to those who can continue the effort. A non-peer-reviewed study in Japan indicated benefits of using permanent magnetic mattress pads to treat a variety of musculoskeletal disorders (Shimodaira, 1990). This stimulated the authors to investigate potential benefit of magnetic mattress pads for fibromyalgia sufferers.

In the study, 30 women with a diagnosis of fibromyalgia for at least 2 years and chronic pain met inclusion criteria for the study. Age averaged 48 to 51 years and weight averaged 152 to 178 lb (significantly less in the experimental group). Of the women, 25 completed the 4-month study. There were no serious adverse effects. Subjects were randomly assigned in double-blind manner to groups that slept on magnetic or nonmagnetic pads. Subjects were asked not to determine which type of pad they received. The density of the foam covering the magnets helped to protect the blind by preventing detection of magnetism with light ferromagnetic objects, e.g., paperclips.

The pads were provided by Magnetherapy, Inc., directly to individual subjects and the code was kept by the manufacturer until all data had been collected. Each magnetic pad contained 270 ceramic magnets (2 × 4.5 × 1 cm) embedded 4 cm apart in a 4-cm-thick foam sheet. The negative poles of all magnets faced toward the subject. The flux density at the surface of the magnets was about 110 mT. This field strength was estimated to deliver 20 to 60 mT to the skin at different points along the body.

A total of eight variables were studied, and 10-cm visual analogue scales were marked weekly for pain, sleep interference, fatigue, tiredness on awakening, and global sense of well-being. The physical function scale from the Fibromyalgia Impact Questionnaire, total myalgic score (dolorimetry at standard anatomical sites), and a body pain distribution drawing were also completed. On Wednesdays of each week visual analogue scales were mailed to the principal investigator after completion by the subjects. This approach was adopted to try to minimize day-to-day fluctuations in symptoms, especially by avoiding assessments on the weekend when stress is lowest. A diary of adverse effects was also kept.

In the group that slept on the magnetic pads, statistically significant reductions from baseline were reported with respect to pain, fatigue, total myalgic score, functional scales, sleep, and pain distribution drawings. In the group that slept on nonmagnetic pads, only tiredness on awakening decreased significantly from baseline.

Comments

1. In the absence of preclinical data, the basis for expecting exposure of the skin to magnetic fields of the flux density studied here to improve symptoms of fibromyalgia is not established.
2. Statistical comparisons between the two treatment groups were not calculated. We used data tabulated in the paper to perform *t*-tests between pain scores at end point. The difference between treatments was not statistically significant.

PAINFUL DIABETIC NEUROPATHY (WEINTRAUB, 1999)

Limited efficacy of pharmacological therapies justified testing magnetic therapy for painful distal symmetric polyneuropathy associated with diabetes. Efficacy in treating painful neuropathy in patients with diabetes was compared with 10 patients with a variety of nondiabetic conditions as etiologies of their neuropathies. All patients were examined by a neurologist and underwent electrophysiological studies to characterize their neuropathies prior to randomization. Patients were randomized to treatment with commercially available permanent static magnetic insoles (Magstep, Nikken) or nonmagnetic placebo insoles provided by the manufacturer. The elastic polymer contained ferromagnetic particles that were magnetized in a multipolar triangular pattern with alternating polarity from one triangle to the next. Steep gradients existed between triangles. Flux density at the surface was 47.5 mT maximally and fell to zero within 4 cm. Patients were instructed to wear the devices constantly for 4 months. The study was conducted in four phases: In phase I (1 month), patients wore a magnetic insole in one shoe and a nonmagnetic placebo insole in the other shoe. In phase II (1 month), the insoles were switched. In phase III and IV (total 8 weeks), patients received two magnetic insoles. Pain was recorded twice daily in diaries using a five-point categorical scale. A 30-day composite score was computed to moderate effects of fluctuations in pain that occur with diabetic neuropathy. The primary instrument of measure was comparison of composite scores pre- and post-treatment.

A total of 24 subjects were enrolled. Of these, eight withdrew in the first 6 weeks of the study. Reasons for withdrawal included: four diabetics, two of whom could not tolerate the insoles and two because of excessive pain; two because of infected toes; one for adminstrative rea-

sons; and one without diabetes who could not tolerate the insoles. A significant reduction of pain and burning occurred in those with diabetes compared with those without diabetes, but only in the last 2 months when patients wore two active insoles. No changes occurred in the first two phases when a single active device was worn on one foot then the other.

Comments

1. Patients with diverse painful neuropathic disorders were compared with a more homogeneous group of patients with diabetes.
2. The pain scale used was not a validated scale. Nonetheless, the baseline intensities for patients with diabetes were in the mild to moderate range where repeated measures with visual analogue scales have proved unreliable for detecting treatment effects in the course of repeated measures. In a successful placebo-controlled trial of gabapentin to treat painful diabetic neuropathy, the inclusion criterion for pain intensity was ≥ 4 cm on an 11-point Likert scale during a 1 week baseline prior to randomization. Group average baseline pains were in the range of 6.5 on an 11-point Likert scale, averaging moderate-to-severe on this validated linear scale.
3. The reason for benefit by patients with diabetes during the wearing of two magnetic insoles, compared with a single magnetic insole on one foot then the other, is not clear. One possibility is that the blind was broken, as acknowledged by the author. Analysis was done only on data from patients who completed the study. That is, this is not an intent-to-treat analysis.
4. The reduction of diabetic pain in the late phases of the study encouraged the author to perform a second study with parallel group design (see below).

CHRONIC LOW BACK PAIN (COLLACOTT ET AL., 2000)

Citing profitability of sales of devices consisting of permanent magnets for the treatment of pain based on little evidence from controlled trials, the authors at a Veterans Administration Hospital tested a commercially available device commonly used for back pain. Of 24 veterans with chronic low back pain, 22 entered the study when asked to participate; 2 did not complete the study because of time conflicts. In all 20 subjects, mean age 60 years old, completed the study; 11 of the 20 completers were disabled. There were no serious adverse events. The subjects had a variety of diagnoses that involved intervertebral discs and facet joints. Diagnoses included spondylosis, herniated nucleus pulposus, radiculopathy, spinal stenosis, spondylolisthesis, history of laminectomy, ankylosing spondylitis, and fibromyalgia. None of the patients had neurological deficits according to examiners. Subjects were asked not to alter medications during the study.

This study entailed a randomized, double-blind, placebo-controlled crossover design. The primary outcome measure was change in pain from baseline using the 10-cm visual analogue scale. The McGill pain questionnaire and range of motion of the lumbosacral spine (measured with inclinometers) were secondary outcome measures. The study consisted of 1 week with magnetic devices and 1 week wearing sham devices with a 1 week washout period between the treatments. Subjects wore the treatment devices for 6 hours a day on Monday, Wednesday, and Friday of each treatment week.

The devices used were flexible, trapezoidal in shape ($19 \times 11.5 \times 14$ cm and 2 mm thick) and had flux densities of 28 to 33 mT at the surface. Shams (placebos) were identical to the active devices in appearance, but were demagnetized and had no detectable magnetic field. The ferromagnetic particles in the rubber matrix were magnetized in a triangular pattern with opposite polarity of adjacent triangles, thereby producing steep field gradients. The manufacturer was not named. An abdominal binder was used to hold the treatment devices in place.

There were no statistically significant differences in visual analogue scale pain intensity measurements, range of motion, or McGill pain scale scores between treatments.

Comments

1. This study may not be an adequate test of efficacy of the experimental device because of design issues.
2. The diversity of pain etiologies suggests that the pain generators may be diverse and neither amenable to treatment with a standardized device producing a generic magnetic field nor amenable to scoring with a single linear scale. Some of the pains seem to be bony in origin (e.g., ankylosis and spondylolisthesis) while others are neuropathic (e.g., radiculopathy). Homogeneity of the study cohort is important for reducing variability, in effect improving the signal-to-noise ratio. For example, studies of efficacy of pharmaceuticals in the treatment of osteoarthritis use very strict criteria for inclusion to homogenize the study group. Also, specifically validated instruments of measure (e.g., the WOMAC) take into account functional and psychosocial aspects of the pain experience in addition to pain intensity.

3. There was no laboratory evidence of efficacy to provide a rationale for this pilot study.
4. The treatment devices were worn intermittently and for relatively short periods of time on treatment days. The basis for this is not given.
5. Order effects were not examined, i.e., sham/placebo first vs. magnetic device first, and the possibility of carryover effects was not analyzed.
6. Subjects were asked to indicate current pain levels on the visual analogue scale. In studies showing pharmaceuticals to be superior to placebo for the treatment of neuropathic pains, subjects have been instructed to mark on the visual analogue scale a pain intensity level that represents average pain over the previous 24 hours. Averaging pain in this manner reduces hour-to-hour and day-to-day variability in pain intensity.
7. Intactness of the blind is questionable. The only procedure for protecting the blind was instructing subjects not to manipulate the devices.
8. The conclusion of this study cannot be generalized to include other magnetic devices.

FIBROMYALGIA (ALFANO ET AL., 2001)

Fibromyalgia is a common disorder affecting about 2% of the general population (Goldenberg, 1999). The pathophysiology is not completely understood, but there is evidence of dysfunction of nociception, the hypothalamo-pituitary-aderenal axis, and the sympathetic nervous system (see Weigent et al., 1998). Also, abnormalities of muscle microvasculature may result in chronic hypoxia and cramping (see Olsen & Park, 1998). In the absence of uniformly effective treatments, many patients with this disorder seek complementary and alternative therapies. This led the authors to study the effects of magnetic mattress pads on pain associated with fibromyalgia.

Subjects were randomized in a double-blind manner to two different groups that slept for 6 months on commercially available mattress pads from two manufacturers. The pads were used according to the instructions of the manufacturers. Magnetic flux densities were measured with a gauss meter. Ceramic magnets ($2.54 \times 5.08 \times 0.95$ cm) with flux densities of 395 mT at the surface were embedded 2.54 cm apart in pad A (MagnetiCo, Inc., Calgary, Canada); this group had 37 subjects. The negative poles of all magnets were oriented toward the subject (unipolar devices). The pad was placed between the box springs and the mattress (typically 15 to 25 cm thick). At the surface of the mattress, the magnetic flux density was -0.35 to -0.64 mT; 15 cm (6 inches) above the mattress the flux density was -0.25 to 0.43 mT. In pad B (Nikken, Inc., Irvine, CA), ceramic magnets (1.8 cm diameter; 0.3 cm thickness) with flux densities of 75 mT at the surface were embedded 12.5 cm apart with the negative poles of all magnets facing the subject (unipolar devices). This pad was placed on top of the subjects' mattresses. Flux densities measured +0.45 to –55.8 mT at the surface of the pad; +0.09 to –3.3 mT, 2 cm above the pad; +0.03 to –0.3 mT, 5 cm above the pad; and –0.03 to –0.1 mT, 15 cm above the pad. This group had 33 subjects. Two other groups (sham pad A, 17 subjects; sham pad B, 15 subjects) slept on nonmagnetic shams identical in appearance to each of the magnetic pads. A fifth group of 17 subjects continued their usual treatments and did not sleep on mattress pads. Overall, 94 of 111 randomized subjects (8 were excluded from a total of 119 enrolled because of incorrect randomization; 17 withdrew for various administrative reasons or unrelated medical problems) completed the study. There were no serious adverse effects.

Changes in pain intensity on an 11-point scale (Item 14 of the Fibromyalgia Impact Questionnaire), functional status (based on scales in the Fibromyalgia Impact Questionnaire), the number of tender points at defined locations (assessed by dolorimetry), and tender point pain intensity scores on an 11-point scale were considered to be the primary outcome measures.

A significant difference in pain intensity ratings among treatment groups was observed ($p < 0.03$, ANOVA) and the reduction in the group sleeping on pad A was significant at 6 months. A reduction in the number of tender points was detected at 3 months. Nonsignificant improvements in other measures occurred also.

Comments

1. Statistics for group-to-group comparisons are not given. Thus, it is difficult to interpret the meaning of differences between groups detected by analysis of variance. Using data tabulated in the paper to perform two-tailed t-tests, we found that pain in the group using pad A was reduced significantly from the baseline score ($p < 0.047$). The difference between end point and baseline pain intensity ratings was not significant for pad B ($p > 0.05$).
2. The use of the two pads could provide information about time- and field strength-dependence of effects.

PAIN ASSOCIATED WITH RHEUMATOID ARTHRITIS OF THE KNEE (SEGAL ET AL., 2001)

Rheumatoid arthritis is an immune-mediated inflammatory disorder of joints that results in pain and debility. Pharmacological management is often costly and associated with significant adverse effects that limit drug utility. Continuous exposure to a static magnetic field reduced experimental synovitis (Weinberger et al., 1996) and may inhibit development of canine osteoarthritis (Rogachefsky

et al., 2004). Square arrays of four permanent magnets of alternating polarity produced static magnetic fields with regions of steep gradients. Exposure of cultured sensory neurons to these fields reversibly blocked action potential firing (Cavopol et al., 1995; McLean et al., 1991, 1995). Such actions could reduce inflammation and nociception in joints affected by rheumatoid arthritis. These findings led the authors to study effects of steep gradient magnetic fields on knee pain in patients with rheumatoid arthritis. Commercially available devices that produce the desired field architecture and penetrated at least 2 inches into tissue were used for the study (Magna Bloc; see Holcomb et al., 2003).

For the study, 64 patients were recruited from three American and three Japanese clinics associated with academic institutions. They were randomly assigned to treatment with Magna Bloc devices or with magnetic control devices identical in weight and appearance. The Magna Bloc devices consisted of four neodymium-iron-boron magnets in a square array with alternating polarity and covered by a hypoallergenic plastic case. The magnetic flux density over each pole was about 190 mT and field gradients ranged from 0.1 to 40 T/m. The magnetic control devices contained a 0.5-mm steel disc nearest the skin surface of the device. This was topped by a single neodymium-iron-boron magnet and three aluminum blanks. The magnetic field was unipolar with a flux density of 72 mT at the surface of the device facing the skin. The magnetic control devices were used to protect the blind. Four devices were taped around the patella in a diamond-shaped pattern. Subjects were instructed to wear the devices continually. Pain was assessed in the clinic with the 10-cm visual analogue scale before and at 1 hour, 1 day, and 1 week after placement of the devices. Subjects kept pain diaries in which they recorded pain intensity on 10-cm lines upon awakening and going to bed. The primary outcome measure was reduction of pain at 1 week (end point) from baseline intensity as measured by the visual analogue scale. Secondary outcomes measures included a global assessment of disease activity (GADA, completed by rheumatologist and patient) by placing a mark along a 10-cm line marked no disease activity at one end and greatest possible activity at the other, the modified health assessment questionnaire (MHAQ) to assess difficulty with activities of daily living, and the subjects' assessment of outcome. Laboratory tests were ordered to assess disease activity; the Westergren sedimentation rate did not change in the course of the study.

Baseline pains averaged 63/100 mm in the Magna Bloc group ($n = 38$) and 61/100 in the control device group ($n = 26$). Pain intensity declined significantly at one week in both treatment groups compared with baseline values ($p < 0.0001$). The decrease in the MAG-4A group (~40%) was greater than that in the control device group (~26% decrease). The difference in pain reduction between the two groups was not statistically significant ($p < 0.23$). The rheumatologists' GADA scores showed greater improvement in the MAG-4A group, but the difference between groups was not significant ($p < 0.18$). The subjects reported a significant difference in the GADA at 1 week versus baseline ($p < 0.01$). Subjects' assessment also revealed significantly more individuals rating outcome as better or much better in the MAG-4A group than in the control device group (68% vs. 27%; $p < 0.001$). Differences in the MHAQ were not statistically significant, but difficulty with activities of daily living decreased in the MAG-4A groups and increased in the control device group.

Comments

1. The magnetic control devices were an attempt to protect the blind. The control devices had not been compared with nonmagnetic placebos in a validation trial. Therefore, it is not possible to determine the size of the placebo effect or the treatment effect of the device. The lack of significant difference in pain intensity ratings between treatments emphasizes a need for studies to design an ineffective magnetic placebo and validate it in separate studies before inclusion in a large clinical trial.

2. The 40% reduction of pain by the MAG-4A device compares with 30 to 40% reduction of neuropathic pain in recent trials of anticonvulsant drugs.

3. In view of the variability of pain in rheumatoid arthritis, larger treatment groups may be necessary to resolve significant treatment effects. A power analysis based on the data from this study would be helpful for designing future studies.

4. The duration of the blind may have been too short to observe significant differences between treatments.

5. The magnetic field produced by the MAG-4A array had effects in animal and cell models, providing a rationale for clinical trials.

6. Positive outcomes in secondary outcome measures, particularly in assessments by subjects, encourage additional trials of magnetic treatment devices for pain of rheumatoid arthritis.

PHYSICAL FUNCTION IN PATIENTS WITH CHRONIC KNEE PAIN (HINMAN ET AL., 2002)

In general, relatively weak static magnetic fields have been used in clinical trials. As a result, it is not clear whether the field strength or geometry that penetrates to the pain generator in tissue is sufficient to produce meaningful benefit. The authors used magnets with industrial ratings of about 1 T to test the hypothesis that wearing strong magnets would improve function in patients with chronic knee pain. A pilot study showing significant improvement of knee pain with magnetic therapy (see Holcomb et al., 1991) was cited as a basis for selecting knee pain as a therapeutic target.

In the study, 47 subjects with chronic knee pain due to previous injury or osteoarthritis were randomly assigned to treatment for 2 weeks with magnets or nonmagnetic placebos in self-adherent elastic bandages. One subject dropped out because of medical complications and data of three individuals were incomplete and not included in the analysis.

Four cylindrical neodymium-iron-boron magnets (13 mm in diameter, 3.2 mm thick; Relieve Pain Today, Marietta, GA) were embedded in 7.6-cm square pads with an adhesive surface. Negative north-seeking poles faced the skin. Flux densities of individual magnets ranged from 40 to 56 mT in the center to 140 to 180 mT at the edge. The distance between poles was not given. Placebos were nonmagnetic. Devices were worn on one knee (the knee with most pain, if both were painful).

The primary outcome measures were the 5 pain scales and 17 functional scales of the WOMAC and the time for a 50-foot walk. The WOMAC is a highly validated instrument for evaluating treatments for osteoarthritis of the knee and hip. Subjects recorded the time they wore the treatment devices in a log. Subjects were asked not to place the devices on metal surfaces or otherwise try to determine whether the devices were magnetic. Overall compliance with this request was high, but two individuals in the magnet group inadvertently broke the blind. Pain (sum of 5 WOMAC visual analogue scale ratings) decreased from a mean of 19.4 to 7.4 (~62%) in the group with magnets and from 19.6 to 16.1 (~18%) in the placebo group. The difference was statistically significant ($p < 0.002$). Mean values for physical function (sum of 17 WOMAC visual analogue scale ratings; higher scores indicate more difficulty with activity) improved in the magnet group from 27.4 to 13.2 (~52%) and from 24.7 to 22.6 (~9%) in the placebo group. The difference between groups was statistically significant ($p < 0.001$). Magnet wearers also improved significantly more in the 50-foot walk test than placebo wearers ($p < 0.04$).

Comments

1. A hallmark of this study is the use of the widely used and validated instrument of measure, the WOMAC index. Osteoarthritic knee pain is a clinical condition for which the index was validated. The WOMAC is widely used in clinical trials of pharmaceutical agents for osteoarthritis.

2. The blind was compromised to some degree by the use of nonmagnetic placebos.

3. It would be interesting to know if such significant benefits of unipolar magnets could be sustained over longer study periods of typical regulatory studies.

Painful Diabetic Neuropathy (Weintraub et al., 2003)

Pilot studies indicated relief of pain associated with diabetic neuropathy by magnetic insoles (see Weintraub, 1999). These results led to the design of this large, multicenter, parallel group, double-blind, placebo-controlled trial. The trial involved 375 subjects with diabetes (insulin- and non-insulin dependent) at 48 sites in 27 states in the United States. Patients had electrophysiologically characterized distal symmetric sensorimotor polyneuropathy. The associated neuropathic pain was chronic, moderate to severe in intensity (>5/10 cm on the visual analogue scale) and refractory to medications. They were asked to record pain and quality of life scores daily for 4 months. They agreed to wear the devices 24 hours a day. No new analgesic drugs were allowed during the study, but medication could be continued at a constant or reduced dose.

The study was funded by manufacturers of magnets (NuMagnetics and Nikken) without influencing study design, performance, or data analysis. The protocol was approved but not funded after review by the National Institutes of Health.

The commercially available magnetic insoles (Magsteps; Nikken Inc.) consisted of a flexible rubber matrix impregnated with strontium ferrite and magnetized in a triangular pattern such that polarity of adjacent triangles alternated. Magnetic flux density at the center of the triangles was ±45 mT. The flux density 13 mm from the surface was 0.13 mT; it was 0 mT at 20 mm. Flux density at the target area is not known. Placebo insoles were not magnetized and were identical in appearance to the magnetic insoles.

The primary outcome measures were visual analogue ratings of numbness, tingling, and burning. Other outcome measures included sleep interference tests, serial electrophysiological testing, and adverse effects.

Enrollment totaled 375 patients. Neither the investigators nor the patients knew the types of devices. Of 199 individuals randomized to magnetic treatment, a total of 58 (29%) were excluded from analysis: 25 were lost to follow-up; 15 dropped out because of allodynia that made wearing the devices intolerable; 6 had complications of their diabetes; and 12 were excluded because of missing data. Of 176 individuals randomized to placebo treatment, 58 (33%) were excluded from analysis: 27 were lost to follow-up; 13 dropped out because of allodynia; 4 had complications; and 14 were excluded because of missing data.

Analysis of results in the subset of patients who completed the 4-month study were as follows: Burning pain decreased by 12% from a baseline mean pain intensity of 5.1 cm on the 10-cm visual analogue scale compared with a 3% decrease from a baseline mean of 5.3 cm. This difference between treatments was marginally statistically significant after 3 and 4 months of treatment ($p < 0.05$ at 4 months). Numbness, tingling, and exercise-induced foot pain also decreased slightly compared with placebo ($p < 0.05$). Sleep interference scores decreased about 30% in both groups, and the difference between groups was not significant. A subset of patients with severe exercise-induced foot pain at baseline (≥7 cm on a 10-cm visual analogue scale) experienced substantial relief of symptoms over time (41% decrease in pain in the magnetic treatment group vs. 21% in the placebo group; $p < 0.01$). Burning and tingling pain were not significantly different in this group. In the group with severe foot pain, 50% of those treated with magnetic insoles had at least a 30% improvement, compared with 25% in the placebo treatment group ($p < 0.05$ for difference between groups). Glycemic control and neurophysiological parameters did not change significantly during the study.

Comments

This study is notable for the extent to which it mimics the design of large pivotal trials of pharmaceuticals for FDA approval. Of special interest are the large patient cohorts, careful characterization of the study population, and appropriate statistical comparisons. This study bears careful examination.

1. This is the largest trial involving magnetic treatment devices published to date. It is useful to examine the present study in detail in comparison to the standard set by regulatory studies of pharmaceuticals.
2. The analysis is not an intent-to-treat analysis. Data of about a third of the subjects were excluded from analysis in both groups for a variety of reasons. As such, the analysis was performed on a subset of patients who completed the 4-month trial. In some pain studies, the last value of data recorded for patients who exit before completion is carried forward as a method of including all randomized subjects who received treatment in the data analysis.
3. As discussed by the authors, magnetic treatment effects in the group that completed the study were small, although statistically significant in comparison with placebo. The effects increased after the second month, suggesting time-dependent improvement. Subjects with moderate baseline pain intensity may not have

responded significantly to treatment, thereby diluting the aggregate effect amplitude. The distribution of baseline pain scores in this study is not given, so the extent to which this factor limited treatment effects cannot be determined. Linear scales such as the visual analogue scale are not as sensitive for detecting treatment-induced changes with repeated measures when baseline pain is in the mild range (1 to 3/10 cm). Other neuropathic pain studies have excluded subjects with pain intensity below 4/10 cm to avoid this limitation of the visual analogue scale.

4. These details raise the issue of clinical/biological significance of the effects. The group with severe pain represented about one third of each treatment group (49/133 in the magnetic treatment group; 35/111 in the placebo treatment group). Patients with severe pain improved more with magnetic insole therapy, as did patients with severe pain in trials of gabapentin treatment for pain associated with diabetic neuropathy (Backonja et al., 1998) and posttherapeutic neuralgia (Rowbotham et al., 1998). The amplitude of treatment effects needed for improvement to be considered meaningful has been studied (Farrar et al., 2000, 2003). Analogous to the 50% responder rates in antiepileptic drug trials, the percentage of patients experiencing >30% reduction of pain has been validated as a measure of meaningful improvement in studies of neuropathic pain (Farrar et al., 2003). The ">30% responder test" was included in the analysis of data from the group of patients in the present study with severe pain. The statistical significance of the difference between groups was marginal ($p < 0.05$). Presumably, some, if not all, of the subjects who dropped out due to allodynia had severe baseline pain. Exclusion of their data may have biased the analysis and led to overestimation of significance. Reanalysis after inclusion of data from this group by the method of last-observation-carried-forward (Mallinckrodt et al., 2003) could address this. The impression is created that pain reduction in the other two thirds of patients in the magnetic treatment group who did not have severe pain was not meaningful. These considerations suggest that only patients with severe pain might be selected for a future study.

5. Significant reduction of pain in the gabapentin trials was supported by significant improvement in sleep, physician and subjects' global impressions of change, quality of life measures in the SF-36 quality of life questionnaire, and scales of the profile of mood states. Internal consistency of benefits among these measures ascribes a dimension of meaningful clinical impact to the reduction in visual analogue scale scores. These instruments of measure were not included in the present study. Foot pain with exercise and sleep interference were analyzed as surrogates for quality of life measures. Subjective measures of improvement are commonly used and validated for trials of treatments of some disorders (see Pain Associated with Rheumatoid Arthritis of the Knee, above).

6. The placebo effect would be expected to wane with time. In the present study, the placebo effect persisted and was still increasing slowly in some measures at 4 months. Similarly, the placebo effect persisted in other studies of pharmacological treatments for neuropathic pain, such as the gabapentin trials. Factors accounting for this persistence have not been definitively identified. Routine interaction with study personnel and regimented treatments (increased compliance with medications) could contribute. Minimization or elimination of the placebo effect would increase the signal-to-noise ratio and favor detection of treatment effects with drugs or magnets. Thus, it would be desirable to learn how to avoid persistence of the placebo effect, a generic problem in studies of neuropathic pain.

PLANTAR HEEL PAIN (WINEMILLER ET AL., 2003)

A previous study with some methodological limitations found magnetic insoles to be no more effective than non-magnetic insoles in the treatment of plantar heel pain (Caselli et al., 1997). In this study, treatment with magnetic insoles was examined in subjects with plantar fasciitis. A randomized, double-blind, placebo-controlled, parallel group design was employed. The duration of the blind was 8 weeks, during which subjects kept daily pain diaries.

Of 198 subjects evaluated, 101 met inclusion criteria and were randomized. The principal inclusion criteria were (1) at least 30 days of foot pain, (2) intensity greater than 3/10 on the visual analogue scale (mean baseline pain about 6.7-6.9/10 by visual analogue scale), and (3) specific tenderness on palpation. The pain under study was called plantar heel pain or plantar fasciitis, but the inclusion criteria regarding pain were complex and included: (1) maximal tenderness on palpation of the medial plantar fascia and medial calcaneus; (2) shooting, sharp, or localized pain in the plantar region of the foot; (3) pain exacerbated by standing or walking; and (4) pain on arising in the morning. In the study, 44 individuals were assigned to treatment with nonmagnetic insoles; 56 of 57 were randomized to treatment with magnetic insoles (1 refused to use the insoles); 3 in the nonmagnetic insole group and 2 in the magnetic insole group did not answer questionnaires and were lost to follow-up. Data from all randomized subjects was analyzed (intent-to-treat).

The study was funded through an educational grant from Spenco Medical Corporation, Waco, Texas, the manufacturer of the insoles used in the study. The magnetic insoles contained a magnetic foil with concentric circles of alternating polarity under the proximal arch support. Flux density at the surface of the insole was 245 mT. The placebo insoles contained nonmagnetized foil, but were otherwise identical. Subjects picked a pair of insoles out of a box in which magnetic and nonmagnetic pairs were intermixed in nearly equal numbers that exceeded the number of subjects. Subjects were instructed to wear the devices at least 4 hours per day, 4 days per week for 8 weeks. Subjects signed a written agreement not to attempt to break the blind.

Data were collected by questionnaires at baseline, 4 weeks, and 8 weeks. Primary outcome measures were pain intensity ratings using the 10-cm visual analogue scale and categorical response to treatment on a 5-point Likert scale. Other measures assessed interference with employment and pleasure using the 10-cm visual analogue scale and identification of adverse events. Daily diary entries recorded time of wearing the devices and pain intensity ratings. No serious adverse events were reported and no subjects exited early because of adverse effects.

Subjects treated with magnetic and nonmagnetic insoles reported reduction of morning foot pain intensity and decreased interference with work at 8 weeks compared with baseline. Differences between groups were not significant.

Comments

1. Interindividual variability in description of the pain is not provided. Also, a reproduction of the insole with exact placement of the magnetic foil is not given. One potential reason for failure is that the field produced by the foil did not reach the tenderest plantar regions, especially the heel. No evidence of efficacy in a model system is referenced as a rationale for studying this device in the manner described.

2. Components of the complex pain were not assessed separately.

3. The blind was deemed to be intact because only about half (not different from chance) of the individuals in each treatment group correctly guessed which device they had. Also, individuals subscribed to an honor system that they would not try to assess the nature of the insoles which they received randomly.

4. An objective measure such as time required to walk 50 feet or videotapes of gait for assessment of improvement might have provided a different perspective. Observations by study personnel, e.g., reexamination of the feet to compare pain components with baseline, were not included. Only subjective measures by the subjects in the form of questionnaires were assessed. This precludes checking for internal consistency between instruments of measure. Also, patients may tend to base their pain intensity assessments on residual pain components, rather than the component(s) that resolved, thereby preventing detection of improvement in one or more components of the pain.

5. Morning pain intensity decreased on average about 42 to 43% in both treatment groups in the course of 8 weeks. This was not significant statistically. Either the placebo effect was large or one or more components of the plantar heel pain tended to resolve over time, or both. Including earlier data collection points, e.g., at 24 hours and 1 week, might have afforded assessment of efficacy and magnitude of the placebo effect before spontaneous resolution of pain.

6. Roughly three quarters of individuals in each group had used insoles before. Stratification by experience with insoles was not examined. Enrollment of larger numbers of individuals naïve to the use of insoles may have been difficult due to the long duration of preexisting pain (mean of 120 months in the group with nonmagnetic insoles; 86 months with magnetic insoles). It is not clear how many had used magnetic insoles previously, thereby creating a bias of expectations. There is some evidence of bias in the collected data. Irrespective of treatment group, individuals who believed in the efficacy of magnets had significantly lower morning pain intensity scores at 8 weeks than those who did not believe. The percentage of "believers" in the two groups is not given. The absence of significant differences between groups argues against the importance of such bias as a determinant of outcomes.

CONCLUSIONS

Studies of magnetic devices must be carefully tested and designed to optimize the likelihood of determining significant benefit. Careful attention to every aspect of study design is necessary in the testing of magnetic devices. As shown above in the spirit of a reviewer for a journal or for the FDA, there are shortcomings in the design, execution, and analysis of clinical studies involving therapeutic magnets. However, it is also clear that the quality of studies is improving (Table 84.1). The results of well-performed studies are likely to be of greater interest to the general medical community because of confidence in the methods. The question remains about a breakpoint at which therapeutic magnets become acceptable to the medical community at large. FDA approval of devices for specific indications will undoubtedly move this moment forward. Also, there is much basic scientific work to be done, not only to demonstrate robust effects but also to elucidate physical transduction mechanisms and provide a rational basis for expecting therapeutic benefits.

Many intangibles will determine the fate of magnetism in medicine, among them the number of interested researchers, the number of well-performed positive studies, and the availability of adequate funding to support research. The cost of bringing a new drug to market is estimated at $500,000,000. Financial resources of this magnitude are found only in pharmaceutical companies and federally funded programs. Currently, companies that market therapeutic magnetic devices, content to profit from sales of magnets as wellness aids, supply little money to support research. Perhaps there is a perception that the potential risk of failing in clinical trials is commercially unacceptable compared with whatever increase in profitability might accrue from regulatory approval. Support from federally programs, such as the National Centers for Complementary and Alternative Medicine, for research involving proprietary devices is helpful but complicated by potential conflicts of interest of manufacturers. Industrial funding of large pivotal trials has been uncommon until recent years. Attracting funding and establishing high-quality research programs that can compete for funding with programs employing conventional approaches remain significant challenges for researchers interested in magnetic therapies.

Focal treatment with therapeutic magnetics is a double-edged sword. One would expect fewer side effects, but the chance of showing therapeutic benefit is made more difficult by local application of devices. The clinical trials mentioned above revealed no significant adverse effects of magnetic fields in the millitesla range. This is encouraging, but chronic intermittent effects of using skin-attached magnetic devices have not been evaluated. Further study is needed to reveal the true magnitude of treatment benefits and to clarify the apparent freedom from adverse effects encountered in the use of therapeutic magnets in the peer-reviewed literature.

TABLE 84.1
Controlled Studies of Efficacy of Static Magnet Field-Producing Devices in the Treatment of Diverse Pains

Study	Type of Pain	Study Design	No. Enrolled	Magnetic Device[a]	Placebo Device[b]	Duration of Masked Period	Security of Masking[c]	Instrument(s) of Measure	Outcome	Adverse Events
Holcomb et al., 1991	Mechanical low back and knee pain (pilot study)	R, DM, PBO, XO	54 (41, low back; 13 with OA of the knee)	Magna Bloc, 7 devices over low back, 4 over knee	Nonmagnetic devices	Two 24-h periods, 1 week apart, continuous wearing	Intact per physician and patient "Intactness of Blind" forms	VAS (10 cm line)	Magnetic devices superior to PBO ($p < 0.03$)	Discomfort due to pad designed to protect blind
Vallbona et al., 1997	Trigger point pain, postpolio syndrome (pilot study)	R, M, PBO, PG	50	Bioflex, discs and pads of two different strength = 4 devices	Nonmagnetic discs and pads	45 min, continuous wearing	Assumed to be intact, patients under observation in waiting room	McGill Pain Questionnaire	Magnetic devices superior to PBO ($p < 0.0001$)	Not reported
Borsa & Liggett, 1998	Exercise-induced biceps pain and microinjury	R, SB, PBO, PG	45	Nikken, 5 cm × 8 cm × 3 mm pad	Nonmagnetic pads	72 h post-exercise, continuous wearing	Not reported	VAS (10 cm line), range of motion, arm girth, force production	No significant differences reported	Not reported
Weintraub, 1999	Painful diabetic and nondiabetic neuropathy, burning and numbness/tingling assessed, both feet treated	R, XO with PBO (1 month on each foot), then 2 months with two active devices	10 with diabetes, 9 other	Nikken Magstep insoles	Nonmagnetic insole	4-month study period, continuous wearing	Dubious with nonmagnetic PBO	Nonvalidated 5-point pain intensity scale (0 = none, 4 = worst)	No change during PBO treatments; significance reported vs. nondiabetics ($p < 0.02$)	Devices intolerable due to pain ($N = 2$); withdrawals due to surgery for persistent infection ($N = 2$)
Colbert et al., 1999	Fibromyalgia	R, DM, PBO, PG	30 of 35 women screened entered, 25 completers	Magnetherapy, Inc, magnetic mattress pad	Nonmagnetic mattress pad	4-month study period, sleeping on pads nightly	Honor system; not objectively assessed	VAS for global well-being, sleep, pain, fatigue; Total myalgic score; pain distribution drawings; Fibromyalgia Impact Questionnaire	Significant decreases in most outcome measures in both groups from baseline; difference between groups not significant	None
Collacott et al., 2000	Chronic low back, multiple pathologies (pilot study)	R, DM, PBO, XO	20	Nikken[d] back pad (trapezoid, 19 × 11.5 × 14 cm, 2 mm thick)	Nonmagnetic pads	Two 1 week periods, 1 week apart; devices on 6 h per day, 3 days per week	Not reported; dubious with nonmagnetic PBO	VAS, McGill Pain Questionnaire, range of motion testing	No significant differences reported	None
Alfano et al., 2001	Fibromyalgia	R, DM, PBO, PG	119 enrolled; 94 completers, 13 dropouts, 8 incorrect randomizations, 4 did not complete the assessment at 6 months	Magnetic mattress pads from two sources (MagnetiCo, Inc and Nikken, Inc.)	Nonmagnetic versions of both active pads	6 months	Subjects blinded to treatment group assignments; not objectively assessed	Pain intensity ratings (11 point scale); Fibromyalgia Impact Questionnaire; tender point count and pain intensity	No significant differences between treatment groups	No magnet-related AEs; no difference in incidence between groups

TABLE 84.1 (Continued)
Controlled Studies of Efficacy of Static Magnet Field-Producing Devices in the Treatment of Diverse Pains

Study	Type of Pain	Study Design	No. Enrolled	Magnetic Device[a]	Placebo Device[b]	Duration of Masked Period	Security of Masking[c]	Instrument(s) of Measure	Outcome	Adverse Events
Segal et al., 2001	Pain associated with rheumatoid arthritis of the knee	R, DM, PG, AC, MC	64, intent-to-treat	Magna Bloc, 4 devices in diamond pattern around knee	4 magnetic control devices of different design in diamond pattern around knee	1 week	Intact based on preservation of positioning of devices and all devices were magnetic	Physicians' assessments at time 0, 1h, 1 day, 1 week; patient diaries; VAS for pain intensity; subject and rheumatologist GADA; MHAQ; subjects assessment of treatment outcome	No significant difference between groups with respect to pain reduction; Magna Bloc superior to other magnetic device by S-GADA ($p<0.01$) and subjects assessment of treatment outcome at 1 week ($p < 0.001$)	No serious AEs
Hinman et al., 2002	Chronic pain associated with degenerative disease of one or both knees	R, DM, PBO, PG	43 (18 randomized to magnetic devices; 25 to placebo), completer analysis	4 unipolar magnetic discs in self-adherent bandage (Relieve Pain Today brand)	Nonmagnetic discs	2 weeks	Two subjects accidentally broke blind, identified magnetic devices	WOMAC	Magnetic devices superior to placebo with respect to self-treated pain ($p < 0.001$), function ($p < 0.002$), and gait speed ($p < 0.04$)	None reported
Weintraub et al., 2003	Moderately to severely painful diabetic neuropathy	R, DM, PBO, PG, MC	258 per protocol (48 sites)	Magsteps[d] magnetic insoles (Nikken, Inc.)	Nonmagnetic insoles	4 months after 2-week baseline	Intact per physician and patient by questionnaire	Daily VAS for numbness, tingling, and burning; sleep interference scores	Magnetic devices reduced pain more than PBO ($p < 0.05$; $p < 0.01$ for severe pain); sleep not significantly different	29% (magnets) and 33% (PBO) dropouts for administrative reasons, allodynia, and nonstudy-related complications
Winemiller et al., 2003	Plantar heel pain (plantar fasciitis)	R, DM, PBO, PG	101 randomized, completer analysis	Active Comfort magnetic insoles (Spenco Medical Corp.)	Nonmagnetic insoles	8 weeks	Honor system; about half in each group guessed treatment (not different from chance)	Reported average daily foot pain (VAS); morning foot pain; categorical response of change from baseline; impact on employment and pleasure	No significant differences between groups	No serious AEs reported

Abbreviations: AC = active control; AE = adverse effect; DM = double-masked; MC = multicenter; OA = osteoarthritis; PBO = placebo or placebo-controlled; PG = parallel group; R = randomized; SM = single-mask ed; VAS = visual analogue scale; XO = crossover.

[a] See text for description of device design. All devices tested were commercially available.

[b] Placebos were identical in appearance to the magnetic devices used in the respective study. In some cases, nonmagnetic placebos were provided by the manufacturer.

[c] Interpretations/comments by authors of this review.

[d] Not specifically stated in published paper. Assumed from description in methods and inferred by communication with one of the authors.

REFERENCES

Adair, R.K. (1992). Criticism of Lednev mechanism for the influence of weak magnetic-fields on biological-systems. *Bioelectromagnetics, 13*, 231–235.

Adair, R. K. (1998). A physical analysis of the ion parametric resonance model. *Bioelectromagnetics, 19*, 181–191.

Adair, R. K. (2000). Static and low-frequency magnetic field effects: Health risks and therapies. *Reports on Progress in Physics, 63*, 415–454.

Alfano, A.P., Taylor, A. G., Foresman, P. A. et al. (2001). Static magnetic fields for treatment of fibromyalgia: A randomized controlled trial. *Journal of Alternative and Complementary Medicine, 7*(1), 53–64.

Anderson, L. E., Morris, J. E., Sasser, L. B., & Loscher, W. (2000). Effect of 50- to 60-hertz, 100 micro-T magnetic field exposure in the DMBA mammary cancer model in Sprague-Dawley rats: Possible explanations for different results from two laboratories. *Environmental Health Perspectives, 108*, 797–802.

Backonja, M., Beydoun, A., Edwards, K. R. et al. (1998). Gabapentin for the treatment of painful neuropathy in patients with diabetes mellitus. *Journal of the American Medical Association, 280*, 1831–1836.

Baker, J. S., & Judd, S. J. (1996). Magnetic amelioration of scale formation. *Water Research, 30*, 247–260.

Barker, A. T., Freeston, I. L., Jalinous, R. et al. (1987). Magnetic stimulation of the human brain and peripheral nervous system: An introduction and the results of an initial clinical evaluation. *Neurosurgery, 20*, 100–107.

Basford, J. R. (2001). A historical perspective of the popular use of electric and magnetic therapy. *Archives of Physical Medicine & Rehabilitation, 82*, 1261–1269.

Beason, R., & Semm, P. (1996). Does the avian ophthalmic nerve carry magnetic navigational information? *Journal of Experimental Biology, 199*, 1241–1244.

Beason, R. C., Wiltschko, R., & Wiltschko, W. (1997). Pigeon homing: Effects of magnetic pulses on initial orientation. *Auk, 114*(3), 405–415.

Beecher, H. K. (1955). The powerful placebo. *Journal of the American Medical Association, 159*, 1602–1606.

Bellamy, N. (1995). Outcome measurement in osteoarthritis clinical trials. *Journal of Rheumatology, 22*(S43), 49–51.

Bellamy, N., Buchanan, W. W., Goldsmith, C. H., Campbell, J., & Stitt, L. W. (1988). Validation study of WOMAC: A health status instrument for measuring clinically important patient relevant outcomes to antirheumatic drug therapy in patients with osteoartolology of the hip or knee. *Journal of Rheumatolology, 15*, 1833–1840.

Binghy, V. N. (1997). Interference of ion quantum states within a protein explains weak magnetic field's effect on biosystems. *Electro Magnetobiology, 16*, 203–214.

Binhi, V. N. & Savin, A. V. (2003). Effects of weak magnetic fields on biological systems: Physical aspects. *Physics-Uspekhi, 46*, 259–291.

Blakemore, R. (1975). Magnetotactic bacteria. *Science, 190*, 377–379.

Blank, M., & Soo, L. (1996). The threshold for alternating current inhibition of Na, K-ATPase. *Bioelectromagnetics, 40*, 63–65.

Borsa, P. A., & Liggett, C. L. (1998). Flexible magnets are not effective decreasing pain perception and recovery time after muscle microinjury. *Journal of Athletic Training, 33*(2), 150–155.

Braganza, L. F., Blott, B. H., Coe, T. J., & Melville, D. (1984). The superdiamagnetic effect of magnetic-fields on one and two component multilamellar liposomes. *Biochimica et Biophysica Acta, 801,* 66–75.

Bras, W., Diakun, G. P., Diaz, J. F., Maret, G., Kramer, H., Bordas, J., & Medrano, F. J. (1998). The susceptibility of pure tubulin to high magnetic fields: A magnetic birefringence and x-ray fiber diffraction study. *Biophysical Journal, 74*, 1509–1521.

Brassart, J., Kirschvink, J. L., Phillips, J. B., & Borland, S. C. (1999). Ferromagnetic material in the eastern red-spotted newt notophthalmus viridescens [in process citation]. *Journal of Experimental Biology, 202*(Pt 22), 3155–60.

Brocklehurts, B. (2002). Magnetic fields and radical reactions: Recent developments in their role in nature. *Chemical Society Reviews, 31*, 301–311.

Brocklehurst, B., & McLauchlan, K. A. (1996). Free radical mechanism for the effects of environmental electromagnetic fields on biological systems. *International Journal of Radiation Biology, 69*, 3–24.

Brunelli, B., & Gorson, K. C. (2004). The use of complementary and alternative medicines by patients with peripheral neuropathy. *Journal of Neurological Science, 218*, 59–66.

Carette, J., Bell, M. J., Reynolds, W. J. et al. (1994). Comparison of amitriptyline, cyclobenzaprine, and placebo in the treatment of fibromyalgia. A randomized, double-blind clinical trial. *Arthritis & Rheumatism, 37*, 32–40.

Caselli, M. A., Clark, N., Lazarus, S., Velez, Z., & Venegas, L. (1997). Evaluation of magnetic foil and PPT insoles in the treatment of heel pain. *Journal of the American Podiatric Medicine Association 87*, 11–16.

Cavopol, A. V. Wamil, A. E., Holcomb, R. R., & McLean, M. J. (1995). Measurement and analysis of static magnetic fields which block action potentials in cultured neurons. *Bioelectromagnetics, 16*, 197–206.

Chapman, C. R., Casey, K. L., Dubner, R., Foley, K. M., Gracely, R. H., & Reading, A. E. (1985). Pain measurement: an overview. *Pain 22*, 1–31.

Choleris, E., Seppia, C. D., Thomas, A. W., Luschi, P., Ghione, S., Moran, G.. R. et al. (2002). Shielding, but not zeroing of the ambient magnetic field reduces stress-induced analgesia in mice. *Proceedings of the Royal Society of London. Series B. Biolog, 269*, 193–201.

Cintolesi, F., Ritz, T., Kay, C. W. M., Timmel, C. R., &. Hore, P. J. (2003). Anisotropic recombination of an immobilized photoinduced radical pair in a 50-mu T magnetic field: A model avian photomagnetoreceptor. *Chemical Physics, 294*, 385–399.

Coey, J. M. D., & Cass, S. (2000). Magnetic water treatment. *Journal of Magnetism and Magnetic Materials, 209*, 71–74.

Colbert, A. P., Markov, M. S., Banerji, M., & Pilla, A. A. (1999). Magnetic mattress pad use in patients with fibromyalgia: A randomized double-blind pilot study. *Journal of Back and Musculoskeletal Rehabilitation, 13*, 19–31.

Collacott, E. A., Zimmerman, J. T., White, D. W. et al. (2000). Bipolar permanent magnets for the treatment of chronic low back pain. *Journal of the American Medical Association, 283*, 1322–1325.

Cullity, B. D. (1972). *Introduction to magnetic materials.* Reading, MA: Addison-Wesley.

Deutschlander, M. E., Phillips, J. B., & Borland, S. C. (1999). The case for light-dependent magnetic orientation in animals. *Journal of Experimental Biology, 202*(Pt 8), 891–908.

Del Guidice, E., Fleischmann, M., Preparata, G., & Talpo, G. (2002). On the "unreasonable" effects of ELF magnetic fields upon a system of ions. *Bioelectromagnetics, 23*, 522–530.

Del Giudice, E., Preparata, G., & Fleischmann, M. (2000). QED coherence and electrolyte solutions. *Journal of Electroanalytical Chemistry, 482*, 110–116.

Del Moral, M., & Azanza, M. J. (1992). Model for the effect of static magnetic fields on isolated neurons. *Journal of Magnetism and Magnetic Materials, 114*, 240–242.

Del Seppia, C., Luschi, P., Ghione, S., Crosio, E., Choleris, E., & Papi, F. (2000). Exposure to a hypogeomagnetic field or to oscillating magnetic fields similarly reduces stress-induced analgesia in C57 male mice. *Life Scineces, 66*, 1299–1306.

Denegre, J. M., Valles, J. M., Lin, K., Jordan, W. B., & Mowry, K. L. (1998). Cleavage planes in frog eggs are altered by strong magnetic fields. *Proceedings of the National Academy of Sciences of the United States of America, 95*, 14729–14732.

Deutschlander, M. E., Borland, S. C., & Phillips, J. B. (1999). Extraocular magnetic compass in newts. *Nature, 400*, 324–325.

Diebel, C. E., Proksch, R., Green, C. R., Neilson, P., & Walker, M. M. (2000). Magnetite defines a vertebrate magnetoreceptor. *Nature, 406*, 299–302.

Dworkin, R. H., Corbin, A. E., Young, J. P., Jr. et al. (2003). Pregabalin for the treatment of postherpetic neuralgia. A randomized, placebo-controlled trial. *Neurology, 60*, 1274–1283.

Edmonds, D. T. (1993). Larmor precession as a mechanism for the detection of static and alternating magnetic fields. *Bioelectrochemistry and Bioenergetics, 30*, 3–12.

Eichwald, C., & Walleczek, J. (1998). Magnetic field perturbations as a tool for controlling enzyme-regulated and oscillatory biochemical reactions. *Biophysical Chemistry, 74*, 209–224.

Eisenberg, D. V., Davis, R. B., Ettner, S. L. et al. (1998). Trends in alternative medicine use in the United States, 1990–1997. *Journal of the American Medical Association, 280*, 1569–1575.

Engström, S. (2004). Physical mechanisms of non-thermal extremely low frequency magnetic fields. *Radio Science Bulletin, 311*, 95–106.

Engström, S., Markov, M. S., McLean, M. J., Holcomb, R. R. & Markov, J. M. (2002). Effects of non-uniform static magnetic fields on the rate of myosin phsophorylation. *Bioelectromagnetics, 23*, 475–479.

Epstein, C. M., Schwartzberg, D. G., Davey, K. R. et al. (1990). Localizing the site of magnetic brain stimulation in humans. *Neurology, 40*, 666–670.

Etheredge, J. A., Perez, S. M., Taylor, O. R., & Jander, R. (1999). Monarch butterflies (*Danaus plexippus* L.) use a magnetic compass for navigation. *Proceedings of the National Academy of Sciences and the United States of America, 96*, 13845–13846.

Farrar, J. T., Berlin, J. A., & Strom, B. L. (2003). Clinically important changes in acute pain outcome measures: A validation study. *Journal of Pain and Symptom Management, 25*(5), 406–411.

Farrar, J. T., Portenoy, R. K., Berlin, J. A. et al. (2000). Defining the clinically important difference in pain outcome measures. *Pain, 88*, 287–294.

Gaffney, B. J., & McConnell, H. M. (1974). Effect of a magnetic-field on phospholipid membranes. *Chemical Physics Letters, 24*, 310–313.

Gilbert, W. (1958). "De Magnete," New York: Dover. (Transl. P. Fleury Mottelay).

Goldenberg, D. L. (1999). Fibromyalgia syndrome a decade later. *Archives of Internal Medicine, 159*, 777–785.

Goldsworthy, A., Whitney, H., & Morris, E. (1999). Biological effects of physically conditioned water. *Water Research., 33*, 1618–1626.

Grissom, C. B. (1995). Magnetic-field effects in biology — A survey of possible mechanisms with emphasis on radical-pair recombination. *Chemical Reviews, 95*, 3–24.

Hallett, M., & Cohen, L. G. (1989). Magnetism. A new method for stimulation of nerve and brain. *Journal of the American Medical Association, 262*(4), 538–541.

Hansen, K. M. (1938). Some obersvations with view to possible influence of magnetism upon human organism. *Acta Medica Scandanavica 97*, 339–364.

Hanzlik, M., Heunemann, C., Holtkamp-Rotzler, E., Winklhofer, M., Petersen, N., & Fleissner, G. (2000). Superparamagnetic magnetite in the upper beak tissue of homing pigeons. *Biometals, 13*, 325–331.

Harkins, T. T., & Grissom, C. B. (1995). The magnetic-field dependent step in bit ethanolamine ammmonia-lyase is radical-pair recombination. *Journal of the American Chemical Society, 117*, 566–567.

Harrington, A. (1997). Introduction. In *The placebo effect.* (pp. 1–10). Cambridge MA: Harvard University Press.

Hazlewood, C. (2003). Treatment of post-polio pain with a static magnetic field and some notions on mechanism. In M. Mclean, S. Engström, & R. Holcomb (Eds.), *Magnetotherapy: Potential therapeutic benefits and adverse effects* (pp. 191–203). New York: TGF Press.

Helfrich, W. (1973). Lipid bilayer spheres — Deformation and birefringence in magnetic-fields. *Physics Letters. Section A, 43*(5), 1409–1410.

Higashitani, K., Iseri, H., Okuhara, K., Kage, A., & Hatade, S. (1995). Magnetic effects on zeta-potential and diffusivity of nonmagnetic colloidal particles. *Journal of Colloid and Interface Science, 172*, 383–388.

Hinman, M. R., Ford, J., & Heyl, H. (2002). Effects of static magnets on chronic knee pain and physical function: A double-blind study. *Alternative Therapy, 8*(4), 50–56.

Holcomb, R. R., McLean, M. J., Engström, S., Williams, D., Morey, J., & McCullough, B. (2003). Treatment of mechanical low back pain with static magnetic fields: Results of a clinical trial and implications for study design. In M. J. McLean, S. Engström, & R. R. Holcomb (Eds.), *Magnetotherapy: Potential therapeutic benefits and adverse effects* (pp. 171–191). New York: TFG Press.

Holcomb, R. R., Parker, R. A., & Harrison, M. S. (1991). Biomagnetics in the treatment of human pain — Past, present, future. *Environmental Medicine, 8*(2), 24–30.

Holysz, L., Chibowski, E., & Szczes, A. (2003). Influence of impurity ions and magnetic field on the properties of freshly precipitated calcium carbonate. *Water Research, 37*, 3351–3360.

Hong, C. -Z., Lin, J. C., Bender, L. F. et al. (1982). Magnetic necklace: Its therapeutic effectiveness on neck and shoulder pain. *Archives of Physical Medicine & Rehabilitation, 63*, 462–466.

Hufnagel, A., Elger, C. E., Durwen, H. F. et al. (1990). Activation of the epileptic focus by transcranial magnetic stimulation of the human brain. *Annals of Neurology, 27*, 49–60.

Iowa Persian Gulf Study Group. (1997). Self-reported illness and health status among Gulf War veterans. A population-based study. *Journal of the American Medical Association, 15*, 238–245.

Jackson, J. D. (1975). *Classical electrodynamics* (2nd ed.). New York: John Wiley & Sons.

Jackson, J. D. (1999). *Classical electrodynamics* (3rd ed.). New York: Wiley.

Lednev, V. V. (1991). Possible mechanism for the influence of weak magnetic-fields on biological-systems. *Bioelectromagnetics, 12*, 71–75.

Liboff, A. R., & Jenrow, K. A. (2002). Physical mechanisms in neuroelectromagnetic therapies. *Neurorehabilitation, 17*, 9–22.

Lillie, R. J., (1999). *Whole earth geophysics* (pp. 84-313). Prentice Hall: Englewood Cliffs, NJ.

Lohmann, K. J., & Johnsen, S. (2000). The neurobiology of magnetoreception in vertebrate animals. *Trends in Neurosciences, 23*, 153–159.

Lohmann, K., & Lohmann, C. (1996). Orientation and open-sea navigation in sea turtles. *Journal of Experimental Biology, 199*, 73–81.

Löscher, W. (2001). Do cocarcinogenic effects of ELF electromagnetic fields require repeated long-term interaction with carcinogens? Characteristics of positive studies using the DMBA breast cancer model in rats. *Bioelectromagnetics, 22*, 603–614.

Kirschvink, J. L., Kobayashi-Kirschvink, A., Diaz-Ricci, J. C., & Kirschvink, S. J. (1992). Magnetite in human tissues: A mechanism for the biological effects of weak ELF magnetic fields. *Bioelectromagnetics, 10*, 101–113.

Kirschvink, J. L., Walker, M. M., & Diebel, C. E. (2001). Magnetite-based magnetoreception. *Current Opinion in Neurobiology, 11*, 462–467.

Magnetism Group. (2002). Dublin: Trinity College. Retrieved from www.tcd.ie/Physics/School/what/magnetism/tcp.html.

Mallinckrodt, C. H., Sanger, T. M., Dube, S. et al. (2003). Assessing and interpreting treatment effects in longitudinal clinical trials with missing data. *Biological Psychology, 53*, 754–760.

Man, D., Man, B., & Plosker, H. (1999). The influence of permanent magnetic field therapy on wound healing in suction lipectomy patients: A double-blind study. *Plastic and Reconstructive Surgery, 104*, 2261–2266.

Maret, G., & Dransfeld, K. (1977). Macromolecules and membranes in high magnetic-fields. *Physica B & C, 86*, 1077–1083.

Markov, M. S., & Pilla, A. A. (1997). Weak static magnetic field modulation of myosin phosphorylation in a cell-free preparation: Calcium dependence. *Bioelectrochemistry and Bioenergetics, 43*, 233–238.

Matthes, R., McKinlay, A. F., Bernhardt, J. H., Vecchia, P., & Veyret, B. (2004). Exposure to static and low frequency electromagnetic fields, biological effects and health consequences (0–100 kHz). UNEP-ICNIRP.

McLean, M., Engström, S., & Holcomb, R. (Eds.). (2003). *Magnetotherapy: Potential therapeutic benefits and adverse effects*. New York: TGF Press.

McLean, M. J., Holcomb, R. R., Engström, S., Sanderson, L., McDonald, P. W., Lombard, K. et al. (1999, November). *Cellular effects of static magnetic fields: Potential neuroprotective role*. Presented at the First International Symposium of the Vanderbilt Neuromagnetics Institute, Potential Therapeutic Applications of Magnetic Fields, Nashville TN.

McLean, M. J., Holcomb, R. R., McDonald, P. W., Sanderson, L., & Lombard, K. (1999). *A static magnetic field slows kainic acid-induced neuronal swelling* [Abstract[. Annual Meeting of the Bioelectromagnetics Society.

McLean, M. J., Holcomb, R. R., Wamil, A. W., & Pickett, J. D. (1991). Effect of steady magnetic fields on action potentials and sodium currents of sensory neurons *in vitro*. *Environmental Medicine, 8*, 36–45.

McLean, M. J., Holcomb, R. R., Wamil, A. W., Pickett, J. D., & Cavopol, A. V. (1995). Effects of static magnetic fields on action potentials of adult mouse sensory neurons in cell culture: First observations. *Bioelectromagnetics, 16*, 20–32.

Montgomery, S. S. (1999). The failure of placebo-controlled studies. *European Neuropsychopharmacology, 9*, 271–276.

Nakagawa, K. (1976). Magnetic field deficiency syndrome and magnetic treatment. *Japanese Medical Journal, 2745*, 24–32.

Novikov, V. V., & Zhadin, M. N. (1994). Combined action of weak static and alternating low-frequency magnetic-fields on ionic currents in aqueous amino-acid solutions. *Biofizika, 39*, 45–49.

Ogiue-Ikeda, M., Kawata, S., & Ueno, S. (2003). The effect of repetitive transcranial magnetic stimulation on long-term potentiation in rat hippocampus depends on stimulus intensity. *Brain Research, 993*, 222–226.

Olsen, N. J., & Park, J. H. (1998). Skeletal muscle abnormalities in patients with fibromyalgia. *American Journal of Medical Science, 315,* 351–358.

Oshitani, J., Yamada, D., Miyahar, M., & Higashitani, K. (1999). Magnetic effect on ion-exchange kinetics. *Journal of Colloid and Interface Science, 210,* 1–7.

Ossenkopp, K. P., Kavaliers, M., Prato, F. S., & Hirst, M. (1984). Effects of magnetic-fields from NMR imaging and other sources in opioid analgesia in mice. *Federation Proceedings, 43,* 748.

Phillips, J. B., Freake, M. J., Fischer, J. H., & Borland, S. C. (2002). Behavioral titration of a magnetic map coordinate. *Journal of Comparative Physiology A — Neuroethology Sensory Neural and Behavioral Physiology, 188,* 157–160.

Portier, C. J., & Wolfe, M. S. (Eds.) (1998). Assessment of health effects from exposure to power-line frequency electric and magnetic fields. National Institute of Environmental Health Sciences. http://www.niehs.nih.gov/emfrapid/home.htm.

Prato, F. S., Kavaliers, M., & Carson, J. J. (1996). Behavioural evidence that magnetic field effects in the land snail, *Cepaea nemoralis,* might not depend on magnetite or induced electric currents. *Bioelectromagnetics, 17*(2), 123–130.

Prato, F. S., Kavaliers, M., Cullen, A. P., & Thomas, A. W. (1997). Light-dependent and -independent behavioral effects of extremely low frequency magnetic fields in a land snail are consistent with a parametric resonance mechanism. *Bioelectromagnetics, 18,* 284–291.

Prato, F. S., Kavaliers, M., & Thomas, A. W. (2000). Extremely low frequency magnetic fields can either increase or decrease analgesia in the land snail depending on field and light conditions. *Bioelectromagnetics, 21,* 287–301.

Prato, F. S., Kavaliers, M., Thomas, A. W., & Ossenkopp, K. P. (1998). Modulatory actions of light on the behavioural responses to magnetic fields by land snails probably occur at the magnetic field detection stage. *Proceedings of the Royal Society of London Series B-Biological Sciences, 265,* 367–373.

Prato, F. S., Robertson, J. A., Desjardins. D. , Hensel, J., & Phillips, J. B. (2004). Daily repeated magnetic field shielding induces analgesia in Cd-1 mice. *Bioelectromagnetics, 26,* 109–117.

Prato, F. S., Thomas, A. W., & Cook, C. M. (2003). Enhancement of opioid analgesia in animal models: Fundamental basis for the design of clinical trials. In M. Mclean, S. Engström, & R. Holcomb (Eds.), *Magnetotherapy: Potential therapeutic benefits and adverse effects* (pp. 145–170). New York: TGF Press.

Radzievsky, A. A., Rojavin, M. A., Cowan, A., Alekseev, S. I., Radzievsky, A. A., Jr., & Ziskin, M. C. (2001). Peripheral neural system involvement in hypoalgesic effect of electromagnetic millimeter waves. *Life Sciences, 68,* 1143–1151.

Repacholi, M. H., & Greenebaum, B. (1999). Interaction of static and extremely low frequency electric and magnetic fields with living systems: Health effects and research needs. *Bioelectromagnetics, 20,* 133–60.

Rice, A. S. C., Maton, S., & Postherpetic Neuralgia Study Group (2001). Gabapentin in postherpetic neuralgia: A randomised, double blind, placebo controlled study. *Pain, 94,* 215–224.

Ritz, T., Adem, S., & Schulten, K. (2000). A model for photoreceptor-based magnetoreception in birds. *Biophysical Journal, 78,* 707–18.

Ritz, T., Dommer, D. H., Phillips, J. B. (2002). Shedding light on vertebrate magnetoreception. *Neuron, 34,* 503

Rogachefsky, R. A., Altman, R. D., Markov, M. S. et al. (2004). Use of a permanent magnetic field to inhibit the development of canine osteoarthritis. *Bioelectromagnetics, 25,* 260–270.

Rosch, P. J. (2004). A brief historical perspective. In P. J. Rosch & M. S. Markov (Eds), In *Bioelectromagnetic medicine* (pp. iii-xii). New York: Marcel Dekker, Inc.

Rosen, A. D. (1996). Inhibition of calcium channel activation in GH3 cells by static magnetic fields. *Biochimica Biophysica Acta, 1282,* 149–155.

Rosen, A. D. (2003). Effect of a 125 mT static magnetic field on the kinetics of a voltage activated Na+ channels in GH3 cells. *Bioelectromagnetics, 24,* 517–523.

Rowbotham, M., Harden, N., Stacey, B. et al. (1998). Gabapentin for the treatment of postherpetic neuralgia. A randomized controlled trial. *Journal of the American Medical Association, 280,* 1837–1842.

Sakurai, H., Yasui, H., Kunitomi, K., Kamatari, M., Kaneko, N., & Nakayama, A. (2000). Effects of static magnetic field on dissolved oxygen levels in aqueous solutions containing copper(II), iron(II), and heme iron(III) complexes. *Pathophysiology, 7,* 93–99.

Salikhov, K. M., Molin, Yu N., Sagdeev, R. Z., & Buchachenko, A. L. (1984). *Spin polarization and magnetic effects in radical reactions.* Amsterdam: Elsevier.

Savage-Smith, E. (1988). Cleanings from an Arabist's workshop: Current trends in the study of medieval Islamic science and medicine. *Isis, 79,* 246–266.

Schwartz, J. -L. (1979). Influence of a constant magnetic field on nervous tissues: II. Voltage-clamp studies. *IEEE Transactions on Biomedical Engineering, 26*(4), 238–243.

Segal, N. A., Toda, Y., Huston, J. et al. (2001). Two configurations of static magnetic fields for treating rheumatoid arthritis of the knee: A double-blind clinical trial. *Archives of Physical Medicine & Rehabilitation, 82,* 1453–1460.

Serway, R. A., & Jewett, J. N., Jr. (2004). *Physics for scientists and engineers* (6th ed.). Belmont CA: Thomson, Brooks/Cole.

Shimodaira, K. (1990). Summary of a 12 month double-blind, clinical test of magnetic mattress pads. Report to Tokyo Communication Hospital, Obstetrics and Gynecology, Tokyo, Japan.

Stacey, F. D. (1977. *Physics of the earth* (2nd ed., pp. 211–267) J. Wiley & Sons.

Steiner, U. E., & Ulrich, T. (1989). Magnetic field effects in chemical kinetics and related phenomena. *Chemical Reviews, 89,* 51–147.

Stokes, W., & Bell, J. (1842). *Lectures in the theory and practice of physic.* Philadelphia: Barrington and Haswell.

Tenforde, T. S., & Liburdy, R. P. (1988). Magnetic deformation of phospholipids bilayers — Effects on liposome shape and solute permeability at prephase transition temperatures. *Journal of Theoretical Biology, 133,* 385–396.

Till, U., Timmel, C. R., Brocklehurst, B., & Hore, P. J. (1998). The influence of very small magnetic fields on radical recombination reactions in the limit of slow recombination. *Chemical Physics Letters, 298,.* 7–14.

Timmel, C. R., Till, U., Brocklehurst, B., & McLauchlan, K. A. (1998). Effects of weak magnetic fields on free radical recombination reactions. *Molecular Physics, 95*(1), 71–89.

Vainshtein, M., Suzina, N., Kudryashova, E., & Ariskina, E. (2002). New magnet-sensitive structures in bacterial and archaeal cells. *Biology of the Cell, 94,* 29–35.

Vallbona, C., & Richards, T. (1999). Evolution of magnetic therapy from alternative to traditional medicine. *Physical and Medical Rehabilitation Clinics of North America, 10* (3), 729–754.

Vallbona, C., Hazlewood, C. F., & Jurida, G. (1997. Response of pain to static magnetic fields in postpolio patients: A double-blind pilot study [see comments]. *Archives of Physical Medicine & Rehabilitation, 78,* 1200–1203.

Valles, J. M. (2002). Model of magnetic field-induced mitotic apparatus reorientation in frog eggs. *Biophysical Journal, 82,* 1260–1265.

Valles, J. M., Lin, K., Denegre, J. M., & Mowry, K. L. (1997). Stable magnetic field gradient levitation of *Xenopus laevis*: Toward low-gravity simulation. *Biophysical Journal., 73,* 1130–1133.

Walker, M. M., Diebel, C. E., Haugh, C. V., Pankhurst, P. M., & Montgomery, J. C. (1997). Structure and function of the vertebrate magnetic sense. *Nature, 390,* 371–376.

Weigent, D. A., Bradley, L. A., & Blalock, J. E. (1998). Current concepts in the pathophysiology of abnormal pain perception in fibromyalgia. *American Journal of Medical Science, 315,* 405–412.

Weinberger, A., Nyska, A., & Giler, S. (1996). Treatment of experimental inflammatory synovitis with continuous analgesics. *Israel Journal of Medical Science, 32,* 1197–1201.

Weintraub, M. I. (1999). Magnetic biostimulation in painful diabetic peripheral neuropathy: A novel intervention — A randomized, double-placebo crossover study. *American Journal of Pain Management, 9,* 8–17.

Weintraub, M. I. (2004). Magnetotherapy: Historical background with a stimulating future. *Critical Reviews in Physical Rehabilitation and Medicine, 16*(2), 95–108.

Weintraub, M. I., Wolfe, G. I., Barohn, R. A. et al. (2003). Static magnetic field therapy for symptomatic diabetic neuropathy: A randomized, double-blind, placebo-controlled trial. *Archives of Physical Medicine & Rehabilitation, 84,* 736–746.

Wiltschko, W., & Wiltschko, R. (1996). Magnetic orientation in birds. *Journal of Experimental Biology, 199,* 29–39.

Winemiller, M. H., Billow, R. G., Laskowski, E. R., & Harmsen, W. S. (2003). Effect of magnetic vs. sham-magnetic insoles on plantar heel pain. *Journal of the American Medical Association, 290*(1), 1474–1478.

Winklhofer, M., Holtkamp-Rotzler, E., Hanzlik, M., Fleissner, G., & Petersen, N. (2001). Clusters of superparamagnetic magnetite particles in the upper-beak skin of homing pigeons: Evidence of a magnetoreceptor. *European Journal of Mineralogy, 13,* 659–669.

Wittig, J., & Engström, S. (2003). Magnetism and magnetic materials. In M. E. McLean, S. Engström, & R. R. Holcomb (Eds.), *Magnetotherapy: Potential therapeutic benefits and advserse effect* (pp. 1–19). New York: TFG Press.

Wolfe, F., Ross, K., Anderson, J. et al. (1995). The prevalence and characteristics of fibromyalgia in the general population. *Arthritis & Rheumatism, 38,* 19–27.

Zhadin, M. N. (2001). Review of Russian literature on biological action of DC and low-frequency AC magnetic fields. *Bioelectromagnetics, 22,* 27–45.

Zhadin, M. N., Novikov, V. V., Barnes, F. S., & Pergola, N. F. (1998). Combined action of static and alternating magnetic fields on ionic current in aqueous glutamic acid solution. *Bioelectromagnetics, 19*(1), 41–45.

Ziemann, U., Steinhoff, B. J., Tergau, F., & Paulus, W. (1998). Transcranial magnetic stimulation: Its current role in epilepsy research. *Epilepsy Research, 30,* 11–30.

Section X

Special Populations

Thomas J. Romano, MD, PhD, Section Editor

85

Recurrent and Chronic Pediatric Pain

Paola M. Conte, PhD, and Gary A. Walco, PhD

INTRODUCTION

Chronic pain is a frequent complaint in childhood and adolescence and is estimated to affect 15 to 20% of children (Goodman & McGrath, 1991). In addition to the suffering this brings, there are significant physical, socio-emotional, and financial consequences related to pain and disability for both children and families. Literature on the long-term effects of pain in early childhood raises interesting questions about permanent changes in pain processing and increased sensitization to noxious stimuli that may persist years into the future (Fitzgerald & Howard, 2003). The interface between pain, mood disorders, and broader social and emotional adjustment seems obvious, yet few studies have systematically examined these effects in children (Bursch, Walco, & Zeltzer, 1998). The relationship between pain experiences and chronic pain in childhood and clinical pain problems in adulthood is an area discussed from a theoretical standpoint, but little has been done empirically (Campo et al., 2001; Walco, 2004; Walco & Harkins, 1999). There is a great deal of literature on the fiscal impact of chronic pain in adults (Turk, 2002), and one can only speculate on the financial impact of lost wages and decreases in productivity from work missed to care for a child in pain. Perquin et al. (2000) found that 25% of a sample of children and adolescents aged 0 to 18 years had chronic pain (defined as continuous or recurrent pain for more than 3 months), of whom 57% consulted a physician and 39% used medication for the pain, clearly adding to costs of medical care. In sum, chronic and recurrent pain in children is hardly a trivial concern that children will merely outgrow (McGrath & Finley, 1999).

Recurrent and chronic pain syndromes in children may be categorized into major types, based principally on the character of the pain and its presumed etiology (McGrath, 1999): pain associated with chronic illness (e.g., juvenile rheumatoid arthritis, cancer, sickle cell disease), pain resulting from trauma (e.g., complex regional pain syndrome, phantom limb pain), chronic nonspecific pain (e.g., musculoskeletal pain, dysmenorrhea), recurrent pain (migraine headache, recurrent abdominal pain), and pain related to mental health (e.g., psychogenic pain disorder, somatization disorder). Although conceptually these categories may be distinct, in practice there may be significant blurring and thus strategies for assessment and intervention are not always so clear (McGrath & Finley, 1999).

EPIDEMIOLOGY OF RECURRENT AND CHRONIC PAIN IN CHILDREN

Studies on the prevalence of chronic pediatric pain suffer from numerous methodological limitations such as varying definitions of recurrent and chronic pain, sampling techniques, and methods of data collection (Goodman & McGrath, 1991). As a result, estimates of prevalence reflect orders of magnitude in variance, a finding that transcends virtually all categories of pain defined above.

PAIN ASSOCIATED WITH CHRONIC ILLNESS

Musculoskeletal pain related to inflammatory process is a major source of pain in children. Estimates of the prevalence of juvenile rheumatoid arthritis vary from 56 to 460 cases per 100,000 children under the age of 16 years. Within that group, there are no systematic data regarding the prevalence of ongoing or recurrent pain, but available clinical data indicate that untreated pain is a significant problem and has a substantial impact on adaptive functioning (Lovell & Walco, 1989; Schanberg et al., 2003).

In a similar vein, it is estimated that there will be 9,200 new cases of childhood cancer in the United States each year (American Cancer Society, 2004). Available data indicate that approximately 62% of those children experience pain as a first symptom of their disease (Miser et al., 1987b), but this pain dissipates fairly quickly after the initiation of antineoplastic treatment. Iatrogenic pain associated with cancer treatment arises in about 25 to 54% of cases and principally includes oral pain from mucositis and joint pain associated with chemotherapeutic agents, such as vincristine (Miser et al., 1987a). Procedure-related pain, which is more focused on acute distress, presents difficulties for over half of children treated and may have implications for later difficulties in coping with recurrent and chronic pain (Conte & Walco, in press). Recent data also indicate that long-term survivors of childhood cancer may be faced with various pain problems months to years after completing treatment (Crom et al., 1999).

Recurrent episodes of intense acute pain associated with vaso-occlusion are a major challenge for children and adolescents with sickle cell disease. Common presentations include pain in any part of the body, as well as acute hand–foot syndrome, acute joint inflammation, acute chest syndrome, splenic sequestration, intrahepatic sickling, abdominal pain, and priapism, as well as the more chronic conditions of avascular necrosis and neuropathic pain (American Pain Society, 1999). Recent diary data indicate that these problems are quite common, as patients between the ages of 6 and 21 years required analgesic medication on 88% of the days and 76% of the nights (Dampier et al., 2002).

Pain Associated With Trauma

Perhaps the most common pain problem associated with trauma among children and adolescents is complex regional pain syndrome (CRPS), type 1 (formerly known as reflex sympathetic dystrophy). Although the exact incidence of CRPS in children is not known, it is being recognized with increasing frequency (Wilder, 2003). Among adolescents, it is far more common in females than males (estimated 6:1 ratio) and more common in lower than upper extremities (5:1). In one clinical series, it was reported that CRPS is most likely to occur in highly stressed adolescents, often involved in individual competitive sports (Wilder et al., 1992).

Chronic Nonspecific Pain

Epidemiological studies indicate that many children and adolescents experience significant episodes of chronic, nonspecific pain at least once in their lifetime. Included are knee pain (up to 18.5%), back pain (7.6 to 34%), and dysmenor-

rhea (from as low as 5% up to 79%, with 51% of girls describing pain as moderate to severe; McGrath, 1999).

Although one might debate the specific category into which it might belong, juvenile fibromyalgia syndrome represents another entity of rather diffuse, nonspecific pain. Many of the features of this syndrome parallel those found in adults, but very few systematic studies of epidemiology in children are available. Mikkelsson et al. (1997) studied almost 2,000 Finnish children between the ages of 9 and 12 and found a prevalence rate of 1.25%. This age range is quite restricted, however, and it would seem to occur with even more frequency in older teens. The majority of patients are female, with estimates as high as almost 94% (Yunus & Masi, 1985). The prevalence of juvenile fibromyalgia forms approximately 7% of new referrals to pediatric rheumatology clinics (Siegel, Janeway, & Baum, 1998).

Recurrent Pain Syndromes

Perhaps the inadequacy of diagnostic criteria is reflected best when discussing the prevalence of certain recurrent pain syndromes. For migraine headaches, estimates range from as low as 1.4% overall to as high as 28% in older adolescents (Split & Neuman, 1999). The estimated prevalence of recurrent abdominal pain was 10 to 15% of school-age children in one study (Liebman, 1978), but has been reported as high as 32% when focused on single episodes in a 1-year period (Abu-Arefeh & Russell, 1995). Recurrent limb pain, not specifically focused in the joints, ranges from as low as 4.2% to as high as 33.6% of children, depending on definitions and inclusion criteria of the study (McGrath, 1999).

NO THANKS RENÉ DESCARTES: INTEGRATED MODELS OF CHRONIC PAIN AND DISABILITY

Chronic pain is not acute pain that continues on for some arbitrarily defined period of time. Even when acute pain recurs, the first episode may hardly be considered essentially the same as the nth occurrence. Acute pain typically signals a specific nociceptive event and is self-limited. Chronic or recurrent pain in children is the result of an integration of biological processes, psychological factors, and sociocultural contexts, all of which must be considered within a developmental framework.

With chronicity there are qualitative, and not simply quantitative, shifts in the severity, characteristics, and regularity of pain. Ongoing pain can result in sensitization of the peripheral and central nervous systems to produce neurophysiological, neurochemical, and neuroanatomical changes (Woolf & Salter, 2000). In addition, the extent of disability related to chronic pain may vary from none to severe, and the system may be maintained independent of tissue damage (American Pain Society, 2001).

A comprehensive review of the development of pain pathways and the impact of untreated pain is beyond the scope of this chapter. In summary, it has been demonstrated that by 24 weeks gestation the nerve pathways necessary for transmission and perception of pain are established. Recent findings have shown that the failure to provide adequate analgesia for pain can result in "rewiring" nerve pathways responsible for pain transmission in the dorsal horn of the spinal cord and can result in increased pain perception in the future (Coggeshall, Jennings, & Fitzgerald, 1996; Craig et al., 1993; Fitzgerald, 1999; Fitzgerald, Shaw, & MacIntosh, 1998; Porter, Grunau, & Anand, 1999). A possible clinical implication of such changes comes from a study that showed a relationship between analgesia for newborn circumcision and longer-term behavioral changes in response to the pain of routine immunizations 3 to 4 months later (Taddio et al., 1997). Another study found that premature infants who experienced repeated invasive procedures continued to display adverse behavior at the age of 18 months (Grunau et al., 1994). Studies such as these may begin to elucidate the relationship between acute pain experiences and later difficulties with chronic pain, but much more needs to be done to define specific changes, related mechanisms, and durability.

Developmental studies, as well as recent data on chronic pain mechanisms in adults, make it clear that what used to be considered "psychological" or "supratentorial" factors related to pain have some identifiable neurophysiological bases (Zeltzer, Bursch, & Walco, 1997). To view pain as purely physiologically based ("real" pain) versus pain that is strictly psychogenic in nature ("it is all in the patient's head") is virtually nonsensical and such mind–body dualism must be avoided if we wish to make progress in this field. Such dichotomization may also lead clinicians to pursue unnecessary or inappropriate diagnostic procedures and invasive interventions that ultimately are not helpful and may in fact be harmful (Zeltzer et al., 1997).

ASSESSMENT OF RECURRENT AND CHRONIC PAIN

An evaluation of chronic pain should include assessment of biological, psychological, and sociocultural factors in a developmental context (Bursch et al., 1998). The evaluation should begin with the history of the current problem, including description of the pain, detailing the sensory nature, intensity, quality, location, duration, variability, predictability, exacerbating and alleviating factors, and impact of pain on daily life (e.g., sleeping, eating, school, social and physical activities, family and peer interactions). A detailed account of the history, evaluation, and treatment of the pain problem in terms of onset and development should be obtained. Information should be gathered on the level of distress for the child and family, which can be attributed to the pain and the impact of the pain on cognitive functioning, anxiety, depression, and feelings of hopelessness. Information should be solicited on the child's and family's perceptions of the cause of the current pain problem, history of any past pain problems and how they resolved, and a family history regarding significant illness and or pain problems (Zeltzer et al., 1997). Additionally, a pediatric history should include a history of surgeries and hospitalizations; birth and early childhood history; developmental milestones; social history including school, social life, and activities; and family medical and social history.

In general, the physical examination should include appearance, posture, gait, and emotional and cognitive state. Vital signs should include height weight, blood pressure, heart rate, respiratory rate, and temperature. A brief neurological examination should be included, as well as trigger points and areas of sensitivity to light touch. One should evaluate responses to stimulation of painful sites and be vigilant to pain behaviors, such as compensatory posturing, guarding, rubbing, and moaning. The consistency of such pain behaviors should be observed, as well as the relationship between pain behaviors, pain reports, parental pain reports, and various environmental stimuli. The precise methods of all aspects of the history, pain assessment, and physical examination depend on the presenting issue and characteristics of the child, including developmental status (Bursch et al., 1998).

In contrast to simple assessments of acute pain, the evaluation of recurrent or chronic pain should also include a good deal on contextual factors. Consider the following issues and questions:

1. What is the relationship between the nature and severity of the pathophysiology underlying pain and the child's pain experience?

2. What is the nature of the development of experimental indices, such as pain threshold, pain tolerance, and pain responsiveness, and how do those relate to clinical pain experiences?

3. What is the relationship between physiological maturation and pain, especially around critical periods in development, such as infancy and puberty?

4. What role does gender play in pain, to what degree are those factors genetically based versus environmental, and how do gender-related factors interact with other developmental processes?

5. What is the relationship between temperament, personality development, and pain?

6. In the context of emotional development, including increasing differentiation and integra-

tion of affect, what is the relationship between affective state and pain?

7. What factors of cognitive development are important, including the development of a concept of pain?

8. What factors of social development play a role in children's pain experiences?

9. What are important pain behaviors, what are the consequences of the behaviors, and does that social learning interact with developmental factors?

10. Is there a relationship between academic achievement and pain; for example, is there an overrepresentation of children with learning deficits who experience chronic pain?

11. What key life events precipitate the onset of chronic or recurrent pain syndromes?

12. What family factors precede or maintain pain syndromes and how does the persistent pain in a child reciprocally affect the family system?

13. What sociocultural factors affect pain in children and how do those elements interact with development?

14. What roles do health care providers play in facilitating the development or maintenance of recurrent and chronic pain syndromes in children and adolescence?

There are studies available to address some elements of these issues, a review of which is beyond the scope of this chapter, but by and large this field is still in its infancy.

INTERVENTIONS FOR CHRONIC AND RECURRENT PAIN

A critical first step in working with children and families to address recurrent and chronic pain syndromes involves education. Almost unilaterally, patients and families believe that a diagnosis exists that can explain the pain condition and once that pathology can be diagnosed and treated correctly, the pain will disappear. Thus, with patients and families, as with many medical professionals, acute pain models remain the basic mind-set. However, as discussed above, acute pain models are not sufficient here as there are many important central processes that come into play. Thus, for many of these young patients, the pain itself is the disease. Facilitating that shift in concepts is a delicate and important element in the treatment process. Many practitioners have found that when patients or families do not accept this perspective, treatment is compromised and the family's search continues for practitioners who will fulfill the hope of obtaining a "definitive" diagnosis and cure.

Treatment strategies for chronic pain follow from the assessment of pain and key contextual factors. While the goal is to eradicate pain when possible, more typically a rehabilitation approach is invoked, emphasizing the improvement of coping so that more adaptive functioning will ensue (Bursch et al., 1998). Treatment goals tend to emphasize increasing adaptive and independent functioning, including school attendance, activities of daily living, and physical activity. Because children and families maintain an acute pain perspective, there is the belief that the child should refrain from normal activities until the answer is found and the pain remits. Unfortunately, in many cases (e.g., CRPS) disuse will lead to increasing pain and disability and a very maladaptive cycle is in place. By addressing pain perception and pain behavior, both key aspects of this cycle are addressed.

One of the best indicators of a child's coping with chronic or recurrent pain is school attendance (Dunn-Geier, 1986), and school absenteeism has been shown to be greater among children with pain conditions, such as chronic abdominal pain, headaches, fibromyalgia, and juvenile rheumatoid arthritis, as compared with pain-free controls (Reid, Lang, & McGrath, 1997; Walker et al., 1998). The importance of school attendance for a child parallels that of an adult maintaining work. In addition to the necessary academics, children develop interpersonal skills and discipline by attending school. As a result, great emphasis is placed on facilitating the child's return to school after frequent absences or sporadic attendance due to pain. To achieve these goals, various psychological, physical, and pharmacological strategies have been invoked. They are reviewed briefly.

COGNITIVE BEHAVIORAL INTERVENTIONS

Although there are very few controlled studies to show the impact of psychological interventions for pain associated with chronic illness, available case studies and clinical series indicate that such strategies are useful to reduce subjective pain and facilitate more adaptive behavior (Walker et al., 1998). For other recurrent and chronic pain syndromes, however, there is fairly substantial evidence to support the efficacy of psychological therapies. Holden, Deichmann, and Levy (1999) reviewed 31 studies of treatments for children with chronic headache and found good evidence for the efficacy of relaxation and self-hypnosis in reducing pain. Hermann, Kim, and Blanchard (1995) reviewed the data on pediatric migraine and found biofeedback and muscle relaxation to be more efficacious than placebo treatments and prophylactic drug treatments in controlling headache. Recurrent abdominal pain is a difficult area to investigate due to the heterogeneity of symptoms and treatment approaches (Walker, 1999); however, a review of the literature indicates that cognitive-behavioral approaches to treatment show promise (Janicke

& Finney, 1999). In a systematic review of controlled trials of psychological therapy for chronic pain, Eccleston et al. (2002) concluded that there is evidence to support the use of cognitive behavioral approaches to treat headaches, and they encouraged controlled randomized trials of other types of recurrent and chronic pain.

Two major psychological modalities may be invoked in the context of chronic or recurrent pain: *pain perception regulation*, using specific cognitive-behavioral or self-regulatory strategies to facilitate coping with or modifying subjective pain experiences, and *pain behavior modulation*, focusing on operant paradigms intended to increase adaptive behavior while minimizing pain or "sick" role behavior (Varni, Walco, & Wilcox, 1990). In addition, if there are concerns about major contextual factors, those too must be addressed.

Consider a child who has not attended school for several months and who spends most of the day at home on the couch or in bed. Structured and manageable changes in behavior would be necessary to successively approximate regular, full-time school attendance. Steps might include waking up at a prescribed time, maintaining a defined morning routine, sitting in a chair doing schoolwork for a specific length of time (that approximates the duration required while in school), and time out of the chair and moving around for a specific length of time (to approximate recess or transitions between classes). To facilitate and maintain this behavioral set, specific cues might be put in place and contingent outcomes identified to increase or maintain behaviors. Pain behaviors are typically ignored while well behaviors are encouraged and positively reinforced. It is important to note that subjective pain reports are of minimal utility in this paradigm as they may be influenced by a number of interpersonal and environmental variables, making them somewhat unreliable in this context.

Pain perception regulation strategies are self-regulatory in nature and use modalities such as progressive muscle relaxation, meditative breathing, guided imagery, and self-hypnosis. Each of these is used to provide the child with a predictable routine aimed at modifying the subjective pain experience. It is useful to assess which strategies the child uses naturally and build on these and tailor them to the individual child (Walco, Varni, & Ilowite, 1992). Another important component is to make the strategies generalizable so they may be implemented across settings (i.e., at home, in school, in clinic).

PHYSICAL INTERVENTIONS

Consistent with a rehabilitation model, the goals of treatment using physical modalities are restoration of function and reduction of disability. Some interventions also focus on modifying aspects of the subjective pain experience. Many physical therapy strategies emphasize strengthen-

ing, weight bearing, range of motion, and endurance. Some data indicate, for example, that movement of a painful body part will increase pain thresholds (Kalkigi, Matsuda, & Kuroda, 1993). Other physical strategies include the use of heat and cold, as well as transcutaneous electrical nerve stimulation (TENS; McCarthy, Shea, & Sullivan, 2003).

PHARMACOLOGIC INTERVENTIONS

The pharmacologic treatment of chronic pain depends on the neurophysiologic and neurochemical contributors to the pain. Tricyclic antidepressants, such as amitriptyline or nortriptyline, are commonly used for chronic pain, especially when there is a neuropathic component (Max et al., 1998). This class of drugs has the added benefit of causing sedation as a side effect, which is useful in pain syndromes where initiation and maintenance of sleep is a concern (e.g., fibromyalgia syndrome). Tricyclic antidepressants are commonly used to treat headaches (Levin, 2001) and irritable bowel pain (Weydert, Ball, & Davis, 2003). Tricyclic antidepressants may also be useful for CRPS (Olsson, 1999; Wilder et al., 1992). Anticonvulsants are most frequently used in the treatment of neuropathic pain. In particular, gabapentin has been found to be useful in some chronic pain states, particularly CRPS (Olsson, 1999).

The use of opioids in the treatment of chronic nonmalignant pain in children is somewhat controversial. The unilateral statement that children should never be prescribed chronic opioids has been replaced by encouragement to conduct a careful cost–benefit analysis in which the benefit of pain relief and improved quality of life is juxtaposed to the cost of side effects and potential for abuse. In pediatric rheumatology, for example, there is an increasing recognition that more aggressive pain treatment with opioids may be preferable to ongoing escalation of disease-modifying agents, such as steroids, in that opioids are effective and may in fact have fewer short- and long-term deleterious side effects (Anthony & Schanberg, 2003). Clearly, however, careful monitoring of clinical effects, untoward side effects, and pattern of usage is essential in these circumstances. Furthermore, pharmacologic management of chronic pain must be integrated into a comprehensive rehabilitation approach that includes educational, psychological, family, and environmental interventions, as well as physical approaches.

CONCLUSIONS

Chronic and recurrent pain syndromes in children and adolescents present all of the complicated issues of such syndromes in adults, with the added dimensions of development. As a result, these problems present a significant clinical challenge and recent data indicate that these syndromes are likely more common than previously thought.

Appropriate assessment, including developmentally appropriate measures and evaluation of key contextual factors, is necessary to devise optimal treatment and management. Treatment paradigms should integrate pharmacological, psychological, and physical strategies, principally aimed at a rehabilitative approach. Clearly, significantly more quality studies are needed to assist with model development and validation, improved assessment strategies, and optimal treatment modalities for these problems. Longitudinal studies elucidating the developmental continuum of pediatric chronic pain problems to similar syndromes in adults would be extremely worthwhile. Needless to say, both the clinical and research endeavors will require a multidisciplinary approach so that the array of important variables may be addressed adequately.

REFERENCES

Abu-Arefeh, I., & Russell, G. (1995). Prevalence and clinical features of abdominal migraine compared with those of migraine headaches. *Archives of Disease in Childhood, 72*, 413.

American Cancer Society. (2004). *Cancer facts and figures, 2004.* Atlanta, GA: Author.

American Pain Society. (1999). *Guideline for the management of acute and chronic pain in sickle cell disease.* Glenview, IL: Author.

American Pain Society. (2001). *Pediatric chronic pain: A position statement from the American Pain Society.* Glenview, IL: Author.

Anthony, K. K., & Schanberg, L. E. (2003). Pain in children with arthritis: A review of the current literature. *Arthritis & Rheumatism, 49*, 272.

Bursch, B., Walco, G. A., & Zeltzer, L. (1998). Clinical assessment and management of chronic pain and pain associated disability syndrome. *Journal of Developmental and Behavioral Pediatrics, 19*, 45.

Campo, J. V. et al. (2001). *Adult outcomes of recurrent abdominal pain: Preliminary results.* Orlando, FL: American Gastroenterological Association.

Coggeshall, R. E., Jennings, E. A., & Fitzgerald, M. (1996). Evidence that large myelinated primary afferent fibers make synaptic contacts in lamina II of neonatal rats. *Brain Research and Developmental Brain Research, 92*, 81.

Conte, P. M., & Walco, G. A. (in press). Pain and procedure management. In R. T. Brown (Ed.), *Pediatric hematology/oncology: A biopsychosocial approach.* New York: Oxford University Press.

Craig, K. D. et al. (1993). Pain in the preterm neonate: Behavioral and physiological indices. *Pain, 52*, 287.

Crom, D. B. et al. (1999). Health status and health-related quality of life in long-term adult survivors of pediatric solid tumors. *International Journal of Cancer, 12*(Suppl.), 25.

Dampier, C. et al. (2002). Home management of pain in sickle cell disease: A daily diary study in children and adolescents. *Journal of Pediatric Hematology/Oncology, 24*, 643.

Dunn-Geier, B. J. (1986). Adolescent chronic pain: The ability to cope. *Pain, 26*, 23.

Eccleston, C. et al. (2002). Systematic review of randomized controlled trials of psychological therapy for chronic pain in children and adolescents, with a subset meta-analysis of pain relief. *Pain, 99*, 157.

Fitzgerald, M. (1999). Developmental neurobiology of pain. In P. D. Wall & R. Melzack (Eds.), *Textbook of pain* (4th ed., Chap. 9). Edinburgh: Churchill-Livingstone.

Fitzgerald, M., & Howard, R. F. (2003). *The neurobiologic basis of pediatric pain* (chap. 2). In N. L. Schechter, C. B. Berde & M. Yaster (Eds.), *Pain in infants, children, and adolescents* (2nd ed.). Baltimore: Lippincott/Williams & Wilkins.

Fitzgerald, M., Shaw, A., & MacIntosh, N. (1998). Postnatal development of the cutaneous flexor reflex: Comparative study of preterm infants and newborn rat pups. *Developmental Medicine and Child Neurology, 30*, 520.

Goodman, J. E., & McGrath, P. J. (1991). The epidemiology of pain in children and adolescents: A review. *Pain, 46*, 247.

Grunau, R. V. E. et al. (1994). Early pain experience: Child and family factors as precursors somatization: A prospective study of extremely premature and fullterm children. *Pain, 56*, 353.

Hermann, C., Kim, M., & Blanchard, E. B. (1995). Behavioral and prophylactic pharmacological intervention studies of pediatric migraine: An exploratory meta-analysis. *Pain, 60*, 239.

Holden, E. W., Deichmann, M. M., & Levy, J. (1999). Empirically supported treatments in pediatric psychology: Recurrent pediatric headache. *Journal of Pediatric Psychology, 24*, 91.

Janicke, D. M., & Finney, J. Q. (1999). Empirically supported treatments in pediatric psychology: Recurrent abdominal pain. *Journal of Pediatric Psychology, 23*, 115–127.

Kalkigi, R., Matsuda, Y., & Kuroda, Y. (1993). Effects of movement related cortical activities on pain-related somatosensory evoked potentials following CO_2 laser stimulation in normal subjects. *Acta Neurologica Scandinavica, 88*, 376.

Levin, S. D. (2001). Drug therapies for childhood headache. In P. A. McGrath (Ed.), *The child with headache: Diagnosis and treatment* (Chap. 5). Seattle: IASP Press.

Liebman, W. M. (1978). Recurrent abdominal pain in children: A retrospective survey of 119 patients. *Clinical Pediatrics, 17*, 149.

Lovell, D., & Walco, G. A. (1989). Pain associated with juvenile rheumatoid arthritis. *Pediatric Clinics of North America, 36*, 1015.

Max, M. B. et al. (1998). Amitriptyline, but not lorazepam, relieves postherpetic neuralgia. *Neurology, 38*, 1427.

McCarthy, C. F., Shea, A. M., & Sullivan, P. (2003). Physical therapy management of pain in children. In N. L. Schechter, C. B. Berde & M. Yaster (Eds.), *Pain in infants, children, and adolescents* (2nd ed., Chap. 24). Baltimore: Lippincott/Williams & Wilkins.

McGrath, P. A. (1999). Chronic pain in children. In I. K. Crombie (Ed.), *Epidemiology of pain* (chap. 7). Seattle: IASP Press.

McGrath, P. J., & Finley, G. A. (1999). Chronic and recurrent pain in children and adolescents. In P. J. McGrath & G. A. Finley (Eds.), *Chronic and recurrent pain in children and adolescents. Progress in pain research and management* (Vol. 13, Chap 1). Seattle: IASP Press.

Mikkelsson, M. et al. (1997). Psychiatric symptoms in preadolescents with musculoskeletal pain and fibromyalgia. *Pediatrics, 100,* 220.

Miser, A. W. et al. (1987a).. Pain as a presenting symptom in children and young adults with newly diagnosed malignancy. *Pain, 29,* 85.

Miser, A. W. et al. (1987b).. The prevalence of pain in a pediatric and young adult cancer population. *Pain, 29,* 73.

Olsson, G. L. (1999). Neuropathic pain in children. In P. J. McGrath & G. A. Finley, G.A. (Eds.). *Chronic and recurrent pain in children and adolescents. Progress in pain research and management* (Vol. 13, chap. 5). Seattle: IASP Press.

Perquin, C. W. et al. (2000). Chronic pain among children and adolescents: Physician consultation and medication use. *Clinical Journal of Pain, 16,* 229.

Porter, F. L., Grunau, R. E., & Anand, K. J. (1999). Long-term effects of pain in infants. *Journal of Developmental and Behavioral Pediatrics, 20,* 253.

Reid, G. J., Lang, B. A., & McGrath, P. J. (1997). Primary juvenile fibromyalgia: Psychological adjustment, family functioning, coping, and functional disability. *Arthritis & Rheumatism, 40,* 752.

Schanberg, L. E. et al. (2003). Daily pain and symptoms in children with polyarticular arthritis. *Arthritis & Rheumatism, 48,* 1390.

Siegel, D. M., Janeway, D., & Baum, J. (1998). Fibromyalgia syndrome in children and adolescents: Clinical features at presentation and status at follow up. *Pediatrics, 101,* 377.

Split, W., & Neuman, W. (1999). Epidemiology of migraine among students from randomly selected secondary schools in Lodz. *Headache, 39,* 494.

Taddio, A. et al. (1997). Effect of neonatal circumcision on pain response during subsequent routine vaccination. *Lancet, 349,* 599.

Turk, D. C. (2002). Clinical effectiveness and cost-effectiveness of treatments for patients with chronic pain. *Clinical Journal of Pain, 18,* 355.

Varni, J. W., Walco, G. A., & Wilcox, K. T. (1990). Cognitive-behavioral assessment and treatment of pediatric pain. In A. M. Gross & R. S. Drabman (Eds.). *Handbook of clinical behavioral pediatrics* (Chap. 5). New York: Plenum Press.

Walco, G. A. (2004). Toward an integrated model of pain over the life course. *Pain, 108,* 207.

Walco, G. A., & Harkins, S. (1999). Life-span developmental approaches to pain. In R. J. Gatchel & D. C. Turk (Eds.), *Psychosocial factors in pain: Critical perspectives* (Chap. 7). New York: Guilford.

Walco, G. A., Varni, J. W., & Ilowite, N. T. (1992). Cognitive-behavioral pain management in children with juvenile rheumatoid arthritis. *Pediatrics, 89,* 1075.

Walco, G. A. et al. (1999). Empirically supported treatments in pediatric psychology: Disease related pain. *Journal of Pediatric Psychology, 24,* 155.

Walker, L. (1999). The evolution of research on recurrent abdominal pain: History, assumptions, and new directions. In P. J. McGrath & G. A. Finley (Eds.), *Chronic and recurrent pain in children and adolescents* (Chap. 8). Seattle, WA: IASP Press.

Walker, L. S. et al. (1998). Recurrent abdominal pain: A potential precursor of irritable bowel syndrome in adolescents and young adults. *Journal of Pediatric Psychology, 132,* 1010.

Weydert, J. A., Ball, T. M., & Davis, M. F. (2003). Systematic review of treatments for recurrent abdominal pain. *Pediatrics, 111,* 1.

Wilder, R. T. (2003). Regional anesthetic techniques for chronic pain management. In N. L. Schechter, C. B. Berde & M. Yaster (Eds.), *Pain in infants, children, and adolescents* (2nd ed., Chap. 22). Baltimore: Lippincott/Williams & Wilkins.

Wilder, R. T. et al. (1992). Reflex sympathetic dystrophy in children. Clinical characteristics and follow-up of seventy patients. *Journal of Bone and Joint Surgery, 74A,* 910.

Woolf, C. J., & Salter, M. W. (2000). Neuronal plasticity: Increasing the gain in pain. *Science, 288,* 1765.

Yunus, M. B., & Masi, A. T. (1985). Juvenile primary fibromyositis syndrome. A clinical study of thirty-three patients and matched normal controls. *Arthritis & Rheumatism, 28,* 138.

Zeltzer, L., Bursch, B., & Walco, G.A. (1997). Pain responsiveness and chronic pain: A psychobiological perspective. *Journal of Developmental and Behavioral Pediatrics, 18,* 413.

Zeltzer, L. K. et al. (1997). Psychobiologic approach to pediatric pain: Part II. Prevention and treatment. *Current Problems in Pediatrics, 27,* 263.

86

Procedural and Perioperative Pain Management for Children

Stephen R. Hays, MD, FAAP, Christine L. Algren, RN, MSN, EdD, and John T. Algren, MD, FAAP

INTRODUCTION

Pain management in children represents an ongoing challenge for health care providers. The ability of children to experience pain has historically been denied or ignored, and the capacity of children to tolerate anesthesia questioned (Eland & Anderson, 1977; Schechter, 1989), causing many pediatric patients to undergo procedures including surgery without adequate analgesia and sedation. Although continued progress remains to be made, recent increased interest in pediatric pain, along with philosophical shifts and technical advances, have prompted evolution of numerous innovative pediatric pain management strategies and improved care of children undergoing a wide range of diagnostic and therapeutic procedures (American Academy of Pediatrics Task Force on Pain in Infants, Children and Adolescents, 2001; Howard, 2003). This chapter discusses procedural and perioperative pain management for children.

PROCEDURAL PAIN MANAGEMENT FOR CHILDREN

Children of all ages experience pain, the type and intensity of which may vary considerably. Brief, intermittent pain is frequently associated with minor traumatic injuries and common childhood illnesses, for which children often receive care at home, in a health care provider's office, or in the emergency department. Care in such settings may require interventions that cause additional pain, for which children too often receive inconsistent or inadequate pain management (Alexander & Manno, 2003; Hostetler, Auinger, & Szilagyi, 2002). Hospitalized children frequently undergo numerous potentially painful diagnostic and therapeutic procedures other than surgery, from venipuncture and intravenous catheter insertion to lumbar puncture and bone marrow aspiration. Such procedures characteristically cause brief but significant pain and are often described by children as the most distressing aspect of their illness or hospitalization (Eland & Anderson, 1977). Inadequate procedural pain management may have profound negative emotional and physiologic consequences, particularly in children given their greater developmental vulnerability. Appropriate procedural pain management may help prevent such consequences, yielding short- and long-term benefits.

Diagnostic and therapeutic procedures induce anxiety and stress in patients and families. Appropriate procedural pain management for children should provide adequate analgesia and appropriate sedation, enhancing patient cooperation and facilitating successful completion of the procedure (Selbst & Zempsky, 2003). Optimal management takes into consideration type of procedure performed as well as individual factors such as patient age, physical condition, developmental maturity, and emotional state. Numerous nonpharmacologic techniques and a variety of medications may be employed (Acute Pain Management Guideline Panel, 1992). With appropriate intervention, most children should be able to undergo diagnostic and therapeutic procedures with little or no pain and with minimal anxiety and stress.

TABLE 86.1
Continuum of Sedation

Stage of Sedation	Minimal (anxiolysis)	Moderate (conscious sedation)	Deep (deep sedation)	General Anesthesia
Responsiveness	Normal	To verbal stimulation	To painful stimulation	None
Airway	No intervention	No intervention	Possible intervention	Possible intervention
Ventilation	Adequate	Adequate	Possibly inadequate	Possibly inadequate
Hemodynamics	Normal	Usually normal	Usually normal	Possibly impaired

Note: Adapted from "Practice Guidelines for Sedation and Analgesia by Non-anesthesiologists," by American Society of Anesthesiologists Task Force on Sedation and Analgesia by Non-Anesthesiologists, 2002, *Anesthesiology, 96*(4), 1004–1017.

MONITORING AND MANAGEMENT GUIDELINES

Recent medical advances have led to dramatic increases in diagnostic and therapeutic procedures in children. Although anesthesiologists provide patient care for many such interventions, practical issues of cost, logistics, and availability of personnel support the practice of procedural analgesia and sedation for children by other health care providers (Pitetti, Singh, & Pierce, 2003). To promote safe practice, the American Academy of Pediatrics Committee on Drugs (1992, 2002) has established guidelines for monitoring and management of pediatric patients undergoing procedural analgesia and sedation. Other professional organizations have developed differing guidelines (American Academy of Pediatric Dentistry, 2003; American College of Emergency Physicians, 1997; American Society of Anesthesiologists Task Force on Sedation and Analgesia by Non-Anesthesiologists, 2002), leading to considerable debate (Coté, 1994; Coté, Notterman, Karl, Weinberg, & McCloskey, 2000; Sacchetti et al., 1994). These organizations and their respective guidelines, however, share the common goal of fostering safe yet efficient practice. Regardless of perspective or bias, practitioners are urged not to allow expediency to compromise patient safety.

Any degree of sedation by definition depresses level of consciousness, increasing risk for airway obstruction, respiratory depression, and aspiration, all of which may result in significant morbidity and mortality. Children are particularly prone to such complications (Coté et al., 2000), mandating a high degree of vigilance in their care. When administering analgesics and sedatives, practitioners should consider risks of serious adverse events, as well as of minor problems such as pruritus, nausea, and prolonged sedation.

Sedation comprises a continuum ranging from mild anxiolysis to general anesthesia (Table 86.1; American Society of Anesthesiologists Task Force on Sedation and Analgesia by Non-Anesthesiologists, 2002); definition of the stages of sedation along this continuum remains controversial. Light sedation yielding mild anxiolysis, although frequently useful in adults, is rarely helpful in procedural pain management for children given their often vigorous response even to minimal pain or stress. Moderate, or so-called conscious, sedation is commonly described as preferred for increased depth of sedation with preservation of airway reflexes and spontaneous ventilation. Even moderate sedation, however, may be inadequate for many pediatric patients, and some practitioners have questioned its usefulness and even existence as a specific state in children (Maxwell & Yaster, 1996). Deep sedation produces greater depression of consciousness and diminished response to stimuli, and may be required for children to tolerate painful or stressful procedures. Deep sedation may also obtund airway protective reflexes, compromise ventilation, and even impair cardiovascular function, necessitating maintenance of intravenous access and continuous close monitoring of cardiorespiratory status. As a consequence of variability in individual response, administration of analgesics and sedatives for light or moderate sedation may induce deep sedation or even general anesthesia. Regardless of planned depth of sedation, practitioners should continuously and closely monitor all patients and be fully prepared to manage potential problems including airway compromise, inadequate ventilation, and cardiovascular depression.

Supervision of procedural analgesia and sedation for children by knowledgeable and competent personnel is mandatory. Many practice guidelines recommend that the individual primarily responsible for performing the procedure not also supervise sedation. Guidelines promulgated by the American Academy of Pediatrics (American Academy of Pediatrics Committee on Drugs, 2002) and American Society of Anesthesiologists (American Society of Anesthesiologists Task Force on Sedation and Analgesia by Non-Anesthesiologists, 2002) go so far as to stipulate that an appropriate practitioner be specifically assigned to supervise procedural analgesia and sedation for children, with only intermittent additional duties during administration of light or moderate sedation and no additional duties during conduct of deep sedation. Adherence to these guidelines has been shown to reduce complications (Hoffman, Nowakowski, Troshynski, Berens, & Weisman, 2002).

In light of the small but real risks of serious adverse events associated with procedural analgesia and sedation for children, equipment and medications for emergency resuscitation should be readily available. Facilities should be of adequate size to accommodate necessary supplies and personnel, and of appropriate configuration to allow rapid access to these items when needed. All equipment and medications should be appropriate for the ages and sizes of children receiving care, and personnel should be skilled in their use. Practitioners supervising procedural analgesia and sedation for children should, at a minimum, be trained in basic pediatric life support; training in advanced pediatric life support is recommended (American Academy of Pediatrics Committee on Drugs, 2002).

Serious complications associated with procedural analgesia and sedation for children are best avoided by adequate evaluation of the patient prior to sedation, appropriate preparation of the patient prior to the procedure, and close monitoring and early detection of changes in patient status during and after administration of analgesics and sedatives. Suitable candidates for pediatric procedural analgesia and sedation are American Society of Anesthesiologists Physical Status Class I or II patients (Table 86.2). Sedation of Class III or higher patients by non-anesthesiologists should be approached with caution because of the presence of symptomatic systemic disease that increases risk of complications. Evaluation of any patient as a candidate for procedural analgesia and sedation includes focused examination of the airway. Decreased mobility of the neck or jaw, impaired mouth opening, craniofacial malformations, large tongue, signif-

icant obesity, or anatomic abnormality of the head or neck may presage difficulty if airway intervention is required. Decreased visualization of the tonsillar pillars, soft palate, and base of the uvula with the patient upright and mouth fully open has been shown to predict difficulty with laryngoscopy (Mallampati et al., 1985).

In preparation for procedural analgesia and sedation, children and families should be thoroughly informed about the planned procedure, with detailed instructions concerning preparation before and care after sedation. To minimize risk of aspiration of gastric contents, oral intake should be suspended prior to elective procedures for which sedation is planned, as for elective procedures entailing anesthesia (Table 86.3; American Society of Anesthesiologists Task Force on Preoperative Fasting, 1999). Whenever possible, unscheduled or urgent procedures should be delayed until

---

TABLE 86.2
American Society of Anesthesiologists (ASA) Physical Status Classification

ASA Class	Description
I	Healthy patient without systemic disease
II	Mild systemic disease without functional limitation
III	Symptomatic systemic disease with functional limitation
IV	Severe systemic disease posing a constant threat to life
V	Moribund patient not expected to survive > 24 hours with or without surgery

Note: ASA Class VI is sometimes used to indicate a brain-dead cadaveric organ donor.

TABLE 86.3
Recommended Fasting Periods before Elective Procedures

Type of Intake	Minimum Recommended Fasting Period
Clear liquids, e.g., water, juice without pulp, carbonated beverages, clear tea, black coffee	2 hours
Human breast milk	4 hours
Any nonhuman milk, infant formula, light meal; typical light meal includes toast and clear liquids	6 hours
Heavy meal; particularly including fried or fatty foods or meat	8 hours or longer

Note: These recommendations apply regardless of patient age. Adapted from "Practice Guidelines for Preoperative Fasting and the Use of Pharmacologic Agents to Reduce the Risk of Pulmonary Aspiration: Application to Healthy Patients Undergoing Elective Procedures: A Report by the American Society of Anesthesiologists Task Force on Preoperative Fasting," by American Society of Anesthesiologists Task Force on Preoperative Fasting, 1999, *Anesthesiology, 90*(3), 896–905. With permission.

appropriate fasting periods have been observed. Some situations may require that sedation be provided despite recent oral intake. In such settings it is appropriate to obtain documentation from the provider performing the procedure that the urgency of the intervention justifies proceeding, and to administer sedation cautiously to minimize depression of airway reflexes and risk of aspiration. Agents such as metoclopramide and ranitidine that augment gastric motility, increase gastric pH, and decrease gastric volume may be appropriate (American Society of Anesthesiologists Task Force on Preoperative Fasting, 1999). In situations where appropriate fasting periods cannot be observed and deep sedation is likely to be necessary, airway protection with rapid-sequence induction of anesthesia and endotracheal intubation may be advisable.

Following appropriate patient evaluation and preparation, monitoring in procedural analgesia and sedation for children should include determination of baseline vital signs, with ongoing patient assessment throughout sedation and subsequent recovery. Assessment should include continuous monitoring of oxygen saturation and heart rate, intermittent monitoring of blood pressure, and intermittent or continuous monitoring of ventilation depending on depth of sedation provided. Documentation of these parameters is commonly at 5-minute intervals during procedures and at 15-minute intervals during recovery, although either interval may be shortened if dictated by patient status. Patients may be discharged while still somewhat sedated, but only if they have demonstrated sufficient recovery of vital functions to ensure safety. This should include return of airway protective reflexes, demonstration of stable and satisfactory respiratory and cardiovascular function, recovery of baseline neurologic function appropriate for age and developmental maturity, and adequate hydration.

PERIOPERATIVE PAIN MANAGEMENT FOR CHILDREN

Children undergoing surgery frequently express fear regarding perioperative pain; all too often, such fear becomes reality. Historically, up to 40% of children undergoing surgical procedures have reported moderate to severe pain on the first postoperative day (Mather & Mackie, 1983). Although many children continue to experience such pain, evolution of integrated, multidisciplinary approaches has dramatically improved perioperative pain management for children (Polkki, Pietila, & Vehvilainen-Julkunen, 2003). Such comprehensive approaches include preoperative, intraoperative, and postoperative strategies for minimizing perioperative pain, based on planned surgical procedure, anesthetic technique, anticipated severity of postoperative pain, and expected course of recovery (Acute Pain Management Guideline Panel, 1992). Periop-

erative pain management for children begins with appropriate preparation of patients and families for surgery, and continues with a variety of nonpharmacologic techniques combined with appropriate analgesics and sedatives before, during, and after the procedure. Children are reassessed at frequent intervals, and regimens modified as needed.

HYPERSENSITIZATION AND PREEMPTIVE ANALGESIA

Acute pain serves as a warning of potential or actual tissue injury. Persistent or severe pain, however, may contribute to pathophysiologic processes that impair normal mobility and function. Following thoracic or abdominal surgery, pain may restrict breathing and compromise pulmonary toilet with resultant ventilatory insufficiency, atelectasis, and pneumonia (Duggan & Drummond, 1987; Ready, 2000). Tissue injury and pain also induce a neuroendocrine stress response, increasing sympathoadrenergic activity and releasing a wide range of stress hormones and inflammatory mediators including catecholamines, cortisol, growth hormone, glucagon, vasopressin, interleukin-1, substance P, and tumor necrosis factor (Fitzgerald & Anand, 1993; Fitzgerald & Howard, 2003; Kehlet, 1989). The hypermetabolic, catabolic state that ensues may be complicated by impaired immune function and increased perioperative morbidity and mortality (Kehlet, 1989).

Tissue injury and inflammation accentuate peripheral nociceptor activity, resulting in hypersensitivity to mechanical and chemical stimuli. In addition, dorsal horn neurons respond to sustained afferent stimulation with neurophysiologic and morphologic changes consistent with increased excitability (Fitzgerald & Howard, 2003; Woolf & Chong, 1993). Development of peripheral and central hypersensitization may alter normal sensory perception (dysesthesia), accentuate pain due to noxious stimuli (hyperalgesia), and produce pain in response to normally innocuous stimuli (allodynia), suggesting that hypersensitization at the cellular and neurophysiologic level correlates with clinical hypersensitivity to pain.

Administration of analgesia prior to tissue injury may inhibit stimulation of nociceptive pathways, blunting neuroendocrine stress response and preventing development of peripheral and central hypersensitivity (Woolf & Chong, 1993). General anesthesia alone is ineffective for such preemptive analgesia; nonsteroidal anti-inflammatory drugs (NSAIDs), opioids, and a variety of regional anesthetic techniques using local anesthetics have been employed with variable results. Despite suggestions from animal models that preemptive analgesia decreases overall pain severity and duration following noxious stimuli, clinical human studies have yielded conflicting and frequently negative results, particularly in children (Ho, Khambatta, Pang, Siegfried, & Sun, 1997; Kundra, Deepalakshmi, & Ravishankar, 1998; Suresh, Barcelona, Young, Heffner, & Coté, 2004). Preemptive analgesia as a strategy for blunting hypersensitization and reducing perioperative pain thus remains a subject of ongoing investigation and controversy (Dahl & Kehlet, 1993; Kissin, 2000; Moiniche, Kehlet, & Dahl, 2002).

NONPHARMACOLOGIC TECHNIQUES

Nonpharmacologic techniques are important adjuncts in procedural and perioperative pain management for children (Rusy & Weisman, 2000). These techniques seek to enhance patients' ability to cope with pain by modifying pain perception and, in the case of various biophysical modalities, by modulating nociceptive transmission. Integrated pain management strategies employ nonpharmacologic techniques in combination with appropriate medications to optimize pain relief, minimize side effects, and facilitate recovery.

Pain includes cognitive, affective, and behavioral components. Children are highly responsive to pain control strategies that involve their imagination, high degree of suggestibility, and sense of play (Brown, 1995). Assisting children to cope with painful events also empowers them with a sense of mastery and self-control that may be applied to future painful situations. Procedural and perioperative pain is commonly associated with stress, fear, and anxiety. Numerous cognitive-behavioral interventions may be helpful in reducing such anxiety and facilitating patient cooperation. These interventions may also be utilized in the management of chronic and recurrent pain. Noninvasive and generally inexpensive, nonpharmacologic techniques frequently provide children and families a sense of personal involvement in their pain management. Promoting family involvement in nonpharmacologic techniques increases their effectiveness (Christensen & Fatchett, 2002).

PREPARATION

Stress, fear, and anxiety intensify pain perception; any technique that reduces anxiety may alleviate pain. Developmentally appropriate preparation is one of the most widely used nonpharmacologic interventions in procedural and perioperative pain management for children. Explanations about procedures increase understanding on the part of children and families and reduce fear of the unknown. If possible, children should be encouraged to express fears, and time should be allowed for questions and answers. Age-appropriate information about why the procedure is being performed, what will be done during the procedure, and sensations that might be experienced should be discussed. Children might be told, for example, that they may feel a small pinch or prick with administration of local anesthetic or placement of intravenous access. Information provided should always be honest and straightforward, while presented in an age-appropriate and developmentally appropriate manner. Various methods, such as tours, coloring books, dolls, puppets, and play therapy, may be used to prepare children for procedures.

Suggestions for coping strategies should be included, allowing children to practice such strategies and families to rehearse supportive roles.

DISTRACTION

Distraction, one of the simplest nonpharmacologic techniques, may be a powerful coping strategy in procedural and perioperative pain management for children. Pain worsens with increasing focus on pain sensation. Distraction engages children in another activity and refocuses attention on something other than the painful stimulus. Distraction does not reduce intensity of noxious stimuli, but alters pain modulation and thereby improves pain tolerance.

Health care personnel should first assess patient age, developmental level, and interests. Distraction may then be accomplished by focusing attention on something other than the unpleasant intervention. Listening to music with a headset, talking about pets or school, blowing bubbles, squeezing someone's hand, and singing or counting are effective distraction techniques. Interactive computer and video games may provide distraction for older children and adolescents. Pain perception is only altered during the distracting activity; when distraction ceases, pain awareness and irritability may return.

RELAXATION AND IMAGERY

In children capable of abstract thinking, relaxation and guided imagery are effective adjunctive therapies in procedural and perioperative pain management; such techniques need not be complex to be effective. Muscle tension intensifies pain, and may be alleviated by methods such as deep breathing and progressive relaxation exercises (McDonnell & Bowden, 1989). Soothing music and talking in a soft, calm voice may also produce relaxation. These techniques give children a feeling of control rather than a sense of helplessness. Controlled breathing may be used alone or in combination with other techniques to promote relaxation. Children may be guided to take slow deep breaths through the nose, exhaling through pursed lips and "blowing away the pain." Young children are especially receptive to this technique.

Imagery is a popular cognitive technique to minimize painful sensation. Imagery, a relaxation strategy, dulls awareness of reality by encouraging children to use their imaginations to focus on something unrelated to the unpleasant intervention. Some experts consider imagery a form of self-hypnosis. Children aged 3 or older may be guided or coached into imagining pleasant images such as a favorite place or activity. Children may also use fantasy to imagine medication traveling through the body to the site of pain or superheroes attacking the pain. Imagery appears to be more effective when multiple senses are enlisted. Guided imagery of playing at the beach, for example, might include imagining the touch of sand, the sound of waves, the sight of sunshine, the smell of ocean, and the taste of favorite foods, focusing on how these combined sensations feel.

MUSIC THERAPY

Music therapy has been used to provide distraction and relaxation in children, decreasing anxiety and improving comfort while fostering a sense of well-being. Positive outcomes have been reported in a variety of health care settings including the operating room (Moss, 1988), post-anesthesia care unit (Mullooly, Levin, & Feldman, 1988), neonatal intensive care unit (Collins & Kuck, 1991), and oncology ward (Sahler, Hunter, & Liesveld, 2003). Music selection should be based upon patient age, culture, and personal preference.

HYPNOSIS

Hypnosis may be a valuable tool in procedural and peri-operative pain management for children, particularly patients aged 8 to 12. Like other cognitive strategies, hypnosis modifies pain perception and nociceptive responses. Children's pain tolerance is improved by capitalizing on their prolific imagination and high degree of suggestibility to induce a hypnotic state. Hypnosis has been used successfully for pediatric oncology patients undergoing bone marrow aspiration and lumbar puncture (Zeltzer & LeBaron, 1982), and in emergency departments during fracture reduction and laceration repair. Children receiving burn therapy and children with sickle cell disease and pain from vaso-oclusive crisis may also benefit from hypnosis (Kuttner & Solomon, 2003). When combined with guided imagery, hypnosis has been shown to decrease pain scores, reduce patient anxiety, and shorten duration of hospitalization in pediatric surgical patients (Lambert, 1996). Practice of hypnosis, particularly in children, requires specific training and expertise.

POSITIVE REINFORCEMENT

Positive reinforcement is a simple strategy for encouraging children's cooperation and potentially improving their experience of an unpleasant intervention. Children might be verbally encouraged during a procedure and praised for holding still, for example, or offered a tangible reward such as a badge of courage, sticker, or toy. Children should receive positive reinforcement for any helpful behavior, but should never be punished or ridiculed for being frightened or uncooperative.

BIOPHYSICAL MODALITIES

Several biophysical modalities may be used in procedural and perioperative pain management for children to mod-

ify pain perception by altering nociceptive transmission. Biophysical modalities are frequently and most successfully used in combination with other nonpharmacologic techniques and in conjunction with appropriate analgesics and sedatives.

Cutaneous and Oral Stimulation

Cutaneous and oral stimulation are valuable noninvasive techniques in procedural and perioperative pain management for children. Pleasant cutaneous stimulation, such as stroking, patting, or massaging the feet, hands, or back produces muscle relaxation and reduces pain during injection, suturing, lumbar puncture, and venipuncture. Massage therapy has been shown to reduce pain associated with dressing changes in pediatric burn patients (Hernandez-Reif et al., 2001). Infants may frequently be soothed with pleasant cutaneous stimulation, such as gentle rubbing of the head, and respond particularly well to oral stimulation, such as suckling on a pacifier. Allowing infants small amounts of sugar water provides analgesia for painful procedures such as heel stick blood collection (Harrison, Johnston, & Loughnan, 2003), and is synergistic with pacifier use (Akman, Ozek, Bilgen, Ozdogan, & Cebeci, 2002). Families may often perform these techniques, providing reinforcing emotional benefits.

Cold and Heat Therapy

Application of cold or heat is another cutaneous stimulation technique. Cooling reduces local pain perception by retarding chemical reactions associated with inflammation and reducing nerve activity and conduction velocity (Ernst & Fialka, 1994). Interventions such as rubbing ice above and below an injury or applying ice or ethyl chloride spray prior to an injection or immunization may decrease inflammatory response and reduce pain. Care should be taken to avoid excessive cooling that may cause skin irritation, cellular injury, and even frostbite.

In contrast, heat promotes circulation, relaxes muscles, and reduces edema and stiffness. Heat application for 15 minutes prior to venipuncture promotes vasodilation and reduces pain. Heat is also an effective home therapy for pain in children with sickle cell disease (Conner-Warren, 1996). Hydrotherapy combines benefits of heat with those of water immersion. Physical therapists frequently utilize hydrotherapy to promote circulation, relax muscles, facilitate movement, and reduce pain. Hydrotherapy may be useful in the management of patients with joint and muscle pain or with chronic regional pain syndromes.

Transcutaneous Electrical Nerve Stimulation

Transcutaneous electrical nerve stimulation (TENS) delivers weak electrical current to the skin via superficial elec-

TABLE 86.4
Sedative-Hypnotic Agents

Drug	Dose	Comments
Chloral hydrate	50–100 mg/kg PO/PR (maximum 2 g)	Higher doses may cause respiratory depression
		Significant rates of agitation or failed sedation
Pentobarbital	2–6 mg/kg PO/PR/IM/IV	Intravenous titration preferred
Midazolam	0.5–1 mg/kg PO/PR (maximum 20 mg)	Higher doses may cause respiratory depression
	0.3 mg/kg SL/nasal (maximum 5 mg)	Potentiated by other sedative-hypnotics
	0.05–0.1 mg/kg IV (maximum 2 mg) initial dose, then	Potentiated by opioids
	0.025–0.05 mg/kg IV (maximum 1 mg) q 5–10 min PRN	May be reversed with flumazenil (see Table 86.5)
Ketamine	4–10 mg/kg PO	Concomitant atropine or glycopyrrolate will reduce sialorrhea
	3–5 mg/kg IM	Concomitant benzodiazepine may prevent agitation
	0.5–1 mg/kg IV	Increases intracranial pressure; may precipitate seizures
Propofol	1 mg/kg IV initial dose, then	Higher or repeated doses induce anesthesia
	0.5 mg/kg IV q 5 min PRN	Prolonged infusion contraindicated in children
	100–200 μg/kg/min IV infusion	

Note: With the exception of ketamine, these sedative–hypnotic agents have no analgesic properties; appropriate analgesia should be provided for painful procedures.

Abbreviations: IM, intramuscular; IV, intravenously; PO, orally; PR, rectally; PRN, as needed; SL, sublingually.

trodes and is thought to provide analgesia by modulation of pain perception at the level of the spinal cord; TENS may also induce release of endorphins and other endogenous neurotransmitters in a manner similar to acupuncture (Eland, 1993). TENS has been used effectively for children undergoing a variety of procedures including venipuncture (Lander & Fowler-Kerry, 1993), dressing changes (Merkel, Gutstein, & Malviya, 1999), and even dental restoration (Harvey & Elliott, 1995), and has been used as an adjunctive modality in pediatric chronic pain management (Eland, 1991). In some cases, TENS may reduce requirement for pharmacologic analgesia (Merkel et al., 1999). Physical therapists typically oversee TENS therapy and instruct patients and families in its use. Conventional TENS delivers electrical pulses of high frequency (50 to 100 Hz), short duration (100 μs or less), and low intensity, adjusted to provide strong but not unpleasant stimulation (usually 10 to 60 mA). This causes a nonpainful tingling sensation. TENS is usually well tolerated by patients old enough to understand a simple explanation of its use, although some children may find the tingling sensation unpleasant. Lower-frequency, longer-duration, higher-intensity TENS may be used, but its application in children is limited by their tolerance of the stronger stimulation delivered (Eland, 1993).

Acupuncture

Acupuncture is gaining acceptance in Western medicine and is practiced by both physicians and licensed acupuncturists in the United States (Lin, 2003). Although mechanisms for its purported analgesia are not understood, acupuncture is undergoing increasing scientific scrutiny

(Pomeranz, 1996). There is some evidence that acupuncture may precipitate release of endorphins, enkephalins, serotonin, and possibly other endogenous neurotransmitters within the central nervous system (Adams, Brase, Welch, & Dewey, 1986), inhibiting nociceptive pathways and reducing pain perception. Pediatric experience with acupuncture in the United States is limited, with use described primarily as adjunctive therapy for children with chronic pain (Kemper et al., 2000). Acupuncture is not effective for antiemetic prophylaxis in children undergoing tonsillectomy (Shenkman et al., 1999).

SEDATIVE–HYPNOTIC AGENTS

Numerous sedative–hypnotic agents are available as components of procedural and perioperative pain management for children (Table 86.4). Drug selection should be based on anticipated level of sedation required, type and duration of procedure to be performed, risk of potential side effects, and available routes of administration.

CHLORAL HYDRATE

Chloral hydrate is a sedative–hypnotic agent devoid of analgesic properties. Chemically an alcohol, it is rapidly metabolized to trichloroethanol and induces a state of intoxication. Chloral hydrate is available in liquid and suppository preparations, and has been widely used for procedural and perioperative sedation in infants and children primarily due to low risk of serious adverse effects. When administered at a dose of 35 to 75 mg/kg orally or rectally (PO/PR) for computerized tomography (CT) scanning, onset of sedation ranged from 30 to 105 minutes with recovery after 60 to 120 minutes; sedation was inadequate in 13% of patients (Strain, Harvey, Foley, & Campbell, 1986). Doses of 50 to 100 mg/kg PO/PR (maximum 2 g) may be used to accelerate onset and deepen sedation, but may prolong recovery and increase risk of respiratory depression (Anderson, Zeltzer, & Fanurik, 1993).

Chloral hydrate's hepatotoxic metabolites and structural similarity to several known carcinogens have prompted considerable concern. Toxicologic studies suggest increased incidence of malignancy, particularly hepatocellular carcinoma, in rodents following chronic chloral hydrate administration (Salmon, Kizer, Zeise, Jackson, & Smith, 1995; U.S. Department of Health and Human Services National Toxicology Program, 2002), but such an association has never been observed in humans despite many decades of widespread use. Disadvantages of chloral hydrate include pungent preparations, slow onset of action, prolonged recovery, lack of reversal agent, and significant rates of agitation and inadequate sedation. Risk of respiratory and hemodynamic depression with higher doses warrants continuous cardiorespiratory monitoring. Nevertheless, due to relative ease of administration and overall safety, chloral hydrate remains a popular sedative for nonpainful procedures in children such as CT scanning and magnetic resonance imaging (MRI) (Keeter, Benator, Weinberg, & Hartenberg, 1990). Because chloral hydrate lacks analgesic properties, appropriate analgesia should be provided for painful procedures.

PENTOBARBITAL

Barbiturates are sedative–hypnotic agents devoid of analgesic properties. Their mechanism of action likely derives from stimulation of GABAergic inhibitory pathways in the central nervous system. Historically barbiturates have been thought to have hyperalgesic properties accentuating pain perception, but this is not now generally thought to be clinically relevant in humans at usual doses. The short-acting barbiturates methohexital and thiopental have been widely used for induction of general anesthesia; these agents produce dose-dependent respiratory and cardiovascular depression. Methohexital and thiopental may be administered rectally to provide sedation in children, but absorption and degree of sedation are variable. Both agents may rapidly induce deep sedation and general anesthesia.

In contrast, pentobarbital is a highly useful agent for pediatric procedural sedation, particularly for radiologic studies (Moro-Sutherland, Algren, Louis, Kozinetz, & Shook, 2000). Pentobarbital has an intermediate duration of action and lends itself well to oral, rectal, intramuscular, or titrated intravenous administration (Strain et al., 1986). A single intramuscular (IM) dose of 5 to 6 mg/kg produced effective sedation within 30 to 45 minutes in 86% of patients; intravenous (IV) administration was titrated to achieve satisfactory sedation, requiring an average dose of 4.4 mg/kg with a range of 2 to 6 mg/kg. Intravenous administration was preferred due to more rapid onset (1 to 2 minutes), shorter recovery time (55 minutes), and extremely low rate of inadequate sedation (0.5%). Pentobarbital, like all barbiturates, lacks analgesic properties; appropriate analgesia should be provided for painful procedures.

MIDAZOLAM

Benzodiazepines are sedative–hypnotic agents devoid of analgesic properties. Unlike chloral hydrate and barbiturates, benzodiazepines have specific anxiolytic and amnestic efficacy enhancing their utility in procedural and perioperative sedation. Acting on the benzodiazepine receptor of the GABA receptor complex in the central nervous system, benzodiazepines provide sedation, reduce anxiety, and prevent recall. Another advantage of benzodiazepines lies in the availability of the benzodiazepine receptor antagonist flumazenil that rapidly reverses benzodiazepine effects (Table 86.5).

Given its rapid onset and short duration of action, midazolam is by far the most widely used benzodiazepine for procedural and perioperative sedation in children. Because of its limited oral bioavailability, doses of 0.5 to 0.75 mg/kg PO (maximum 20 mg) have been used for preoperative sedation (Feld, Negus, & White, 1990); doses of 1 mg/kg PO may be required, particularly when midazolam is the sole sedative. Oral midazolam at these doses has gained wide acceptance for premedication of pediatric surgical patients. Midazolam may be given rectally at the same dose to patients unwilling or unable to tolerate oral administration; this is particularly useful in infants and children not yet toilet trained. Midazolam 0.3 mg/kg (maximum 5 mg) has been used in children via nasal and sublingual routes (Karl, Rosenberger, Larach, & Ruffle, 1993). Nasal or sublingual transmucosal absorption increases bioavailability, reducing dose and shortening time of onset. However, currently available preparations have a bitter taste and sting the nasal mucosa, and children often find these routes of administration unpleasant. Intravenous midazolam produces rapid onset of sedation, anxiolysis, and amnesia, and is well suited to incremental titration. The usual intravenous dose of midazolam is 0.05 to 0.1 mg/kg (maximum 2 mg); additional intravenous doses of 0.025 to 0.05 mg/kg (maximum 1 mg) may be repeated every 5 to 10 minutes as needed. Midazolam 0.1 mg/kg IV is often sufficient for gastrointestinal endoscopic procedures in children (Tolia, Brennan, Aravind, & Kauffman, 1991), while 0.2 mg/kg IV may be required for pediatric oncology patients undergoing lumbar puncture and bone marrow aspiration (Sandler et al., 1992). Because midazolam lacks analgesic

TABLE 86.5
Reversal Agents

Drug	Receptor Antagonized	Dose	Comments
Flumazenil	Benzodiazepine	0.01 mg/kg IV q 1–2 min PRN (usual maximum 1 mg; higher doses may be required)	May not reverse respiratory depression Resedation may occur May precipitate seizures May precipitate withdrawal in benzodiazepine-dependent patients
Naloxone	Opioid	1–100 µg/kg IV q 1–2 min PRN: 1 µg/kg for mild sedation, respiratory depression 10–100 µg/kg for obtundation, apnea (usual maximum 400 µg; higher doses may be required)	Resedation may occur Higher doses may cause pulmonary edema May precipitate withdrawal in opioid-dependent patients

Abbreviations: IV, intravenously; PRN, as needed.

properties, appropriate analgesia should be provided for painful procedures.

The principal significant adverse effect of midazolam is respiratory depression, risk for which increases with higher dose and with concomitant administration of opioid analgesics or other sedatives. Appropriate monitoring of children following midazolam administration is imperative. Other side effects such as nausea, vomiting, and hallucinations are uncommon. Recovery from single-dose midazolam usually occurs within 1 to 2 hours, although prolonged sedation may be observed after oral or rectal administration, particularly at higher doses. Persistent sedation may be reversed with the benzodiazepine receptor antagonist flumazenil (Table 86.5), which has also been reported to antagonize at least partially the respiratory depressant effects of midazolam (Gross, Weller, & Conard, 1991). Flumazenil is a proconvulsant and should be used cautiously in patients with predisposition to seizures.

Ketamine

Ketamine is a sedative–hypnotic agent similar in structure to the now illicit drug of abuse phencyclidine. Unlike most other sedative–hypnotic agents, ketamine has potent analgesic properties, related to its induction of a dissociative state in which pain may be felt but is not perceived as unpleasant. Although its mechanisms of action are incompletely understood, ketamine has significant activity at central nervous system N-methyl-D-aspartate (NMDA) receptors, as well as weaker activity at opioid receptors. Ketamine produces dose-dependent analgesia and sedation, with induction of general anesthesia at higher doses; amnesia is not so pronounced as with benzodiazepines. Ketamine increases cerebral metabolism and oxygen consumption, thereby increasing intracranial pressure, and is a proconvulsant. Although airway reflexes and spontane-

ous ventilation tend to be preserved, ketamine causes increased salivation that may be significant. Ketamine also induces bronchodilation. In contrast to most other sedative–hypnotics, ketamine promotes release of endogenous catecholamines, tending to preserve or even increase heart rate and blood pressure in most patients. As with other phencyclidine derivatives, hallucinations and delirium are not uncommon.

Ketamine has been recommended for procedural analgesia and sedation in children in a variety of settings (Green, Nakamura, & Johnson, 1990; Tobias, Phipps, Smith, & Mulhern, 1992) and has become particularly popular in pediatric emergency departments given its favorable safety profile (Petrack, Marx, & Wright, 1996; Pitetti et al., 2003). Doses of ketamine for procedural analgesia and sedation in children are commonly 4 to 10 mg/kg PO, 3 to 5 mg/kg IM, or 0.5 to 1 mg/kg IV; rates of adequate analgesia and sedation are high, while rates of serious complications are low. Emergence may be prolonged after oral administration, particularly with higher doses, and agitation during emergence is not uncommon. Concomitant administration of anticholinergic agent such as atropine or glycopyrrolate to prevent sialorrhea is recommended. Concomitant administration of low-dose benzodiazepine such as midazolam may decrease likelihood of hallucinations and delirium, although these appear to be less frequent and less severe in younger patients (Green et al., 1990). Although airway reflexes and spontaneous ventilation tend to be preserved, appropriate monitoring is mandatory. Risk of respiratory complications including laryngospasm and bronchospasm may be increased in young infants and in children with respiratory infections. Ketamine should be used cautiously in patients with potentially increased intracranial pressure or predisposition to seizures.

TABLE 86.6
Non-Opioid Analgesics

Drug	Dose	Comments
Acetaminophen	20 mg/kg PO load if desired, then 15 mg/kg PO (maximum 1000 mg) q 4 h; 40 mg/kg PR load if desired, then 20 mg/kg PR (maximum 1300 mg) q 4 h (maximum 4 g/24 h PO/PR)	Hepatic toxicity with overdose Good antipyretic
Nonsteroidal Anti-Inflammatory Drugs (NSAIDs)		
Choline magnesium trisalicylate	10 mg/kg PO/PR (maximum 1000 mg) q 6 h (maximum 4 g/24 h)	Only NSAID without platelet dysfunction No association with Reye syndrome Good antipyretic
Ibuprofen	4–10 mg/kg PO/PR (maximum 800 mg) q 6 h (maximum 4 g/24 h)	Good antipyretic
Ketorolac	0.5 mg/kg IM/IV (maximum 30 mg) q 6 h (duration of therapy must be <5 days)	Only IV NSAID for analgesic use Oral use not approved for children Significant platelet dysfunction Poor antipyretic

Abbreviations: IM, intramuscular; IV, intravenously; PO, orally; PR, rectally.

PROPOFOL

Propofol is a sedative–hypnotic agent devoid of analgesic properties commonly used for induction and maintenance of general anesthesia. Chemically unrelated to any other sedative–hypnotic agent, its mechanisms of action are unknown. Supplied in a lipid emulsion with a highly alkaline pH, propofol may cause significant pain on injection and is available only for intravenous administration. Propofol has some antiemetic efficacy and, like ketamine, promotes bronchodilation. Propofol has an extremely rapid onset of action and, with relatively prompt hepatic conjugation and renal excretion, allows for rapid recovery when given by intermittent bolus dose or brief infusion. Propofol's high lipid solubility and tissue accumulation lengthen its effective half-life with repeated administration or sustained infusion. Particularly in children, prolonged propofol infusion is associated with a rare but catastrophic syndrome of metabolic acidosis and cardiovascular failure that is often fatal (Parke et al., 1992). It is currently recommended that duration of propofol infusion in children not exceed 48 hours, although death has been reported with shorter durations or with reexposure to the drug (Holzki, Aring, & Gillor, 2004).

Propofol induces dose-dependent sedation, but also causes dose-dependent loss of airway reflexes, hypoventilation, apnea, and cardiovascular depression; higher doses induce general anesthesia. Propofol is nonetheless increasingly popular for pediatric procedural sedation, comparing favorably with other agents including midazolam and ketamine (Seigler et al., 2001). Although there has been considerable concern over safety of propofol

administration by non-anesthesiologists (Litman, 1999), evidence suggests that such use may be reasonable under appropriate circumstances. Propofol has been safely and successfully used for pediatric procedural sedation in numerous settings including the intensive care unit (Wheeler, Vaux, Ponaman, & Poss, 2003), burn unit (Sheridan et al., 2003), radiology suite (Hasan, Shayevitz, & Patel, 2003), emergency department (Bassett, Anderson, Pribble, & Guenther, 2003), ambulatory procedure center (Guenther et al., 2003), and dental clinic (Hosey, Makin, Jones, Gilchrist, & Carruthers, 2004). Although such success is impressive, patient safety was protected by restriction of propofol use to appropriately trained personnel working in the context of a dedicated sedation team, following carefully designed protocols and adhering to appropriate standards for patient monitoring and management (Barbi et al., 2003). The usual initial bolus dose of propofol for procedural sedation is 1 mg/kg IV, with subsequent doses of 0.5 mg/kg IV every 5 minutes as needed; usual infusion rates are 100 to 200 µg/kg/min titrated to effect. Higher or repeated doses will rapidly induce deep sedation and general anesthesia. Because propofol lacks analgesic properties, appropriate analgesia should be provided for painful procedures.

NON-OPIOID ANALGESICS

Although often overlooked, non-opioid analgesics are important adjunctive agents in procedural and perioperative pain management for children. Non-opioid analgesics frequently provide adequate analgesia for conditions and procedures associated with mild to moderate pain, and may reduce opioid requirement in treating moderate to severe pain (Kokinsky & Thornberg, 2003). As with nonpharmacologic techniques, non-opioid analgesics are most effectively used in the context of an integrated pain management strategy. Unlike opioids, NSAIDs demonstrate a ceiling effect: exceeding recommended doses does not significantly improve analgesia, although risk for side effects is increased (Maunuksela & Olkkola, 2003). Commonly used non-opioid analgesics in procedural and perioperative pain management for children include acetaminophen and various NSAIDs (Table 86.6).

ACETAMINOPHEN

Acetaminophen remains widely popular for management of mild to moderate pain in children, and as an antipyretic. Acetaminophen is a potent inhibitor of cyclooxygenase, but unlike the NSAIDs has virtually no anti-inflammatory activity and therefore no associated gastrointestinal, renal, or hematologic complications. The primary toxicity of acetaminophen is hepatic injury, seen with both acute and chronic overdose. Given widespread availability and use, acetaminophen ingestion is common in children and may be fatal if potential toxicity is not recognized and treated promptly.

Acetaminophen in the United States is available in a variety of oral and rectal preparations; intravenous preparations are available in other countries. The usual oral dose of acetaminophen is 15 mg/kg (maximum 1,000 mg) every 4 hours, although an oral loading dose of 20 mg/kg may be given, particularly for procedural or perioperative analgesia. Total dose should not exceed 4 g per day.

Rectal absorption of acetaminophen is slower and bioavailability somewhat variable, requiring higher doses for equivalent analgesia (Rusy, et al., 1995). Although rectal acetaminophen has been shown to reduce pain scores and spare opioid requirement following procedures such as myringotomy tube placement and inguinal hernia repair (Korpela, Korvenoja, & Meretoja, 1999), at least 40 mg/kg must be given (Romsing, Moiniche, & Dahl, 2002). Maintenance rectal acetaminophen 20 mg/kg (maximum 1,300 mg) every 4 hours may be used in patients unwilling or unable to tolerate oral administration; total dose should not exceed 4 g per day. Procedural and perioperative analgesia with acetaminophen is enhanced by NSAIDs (Romsing et al., 2002).

NONSTEROIDAL ANTI-INFLAMMATORY DRUGS

Like acetaminophen, NSAIDs may provide adequate analgesia for conditions and procedures associated with mild to moderate pain, and are useful in conjunction with opioids in the management of moderate to severe pain (Kokki, 2003; Watcha, Jones, Schweiger, Lagueruela, & White, 1991). NSAIDs are particularly effective in reducing musculoskeletal pain. Unlike acetaminophen, NSAIDs have significant anti-inflammatory activity, from which may arise various gastrointestinal, renal, and hematologic complications. NSAIDs reduce splanchnic and renal perfusion and impair platelet function, potentially causing gastrointestinal ischemia, renal insufficiency, and bleeding. These usually occur only with higher doses or prolonged administration.

Choline magnesium trisalicylate is the only NSAID that does not cause platelet dysfunction, and may be useful in patients with medical coagulopathy or at risk for surgical bleeding. Pediatric aspirin use has declined dramatically since a described association with Reye syndrome in children with primary varicella (Maunuksela & Olkkola, 2003). Although choline magnesium trisalicylate is an aspirin derivative, it has no known association with Reye syndrome. Nonetheless, it may be prudent to limit choline magnesium trisalicylate use in children to patients who have previously had primary varicella or received varicella immunization. Choline magnesium trisalicylate is available in liquid and tablet preparations, and is usually given at a dose of 10 mg/kg PO/PR (maximum 1,000 mg) every 6 hours. Total dose should not exceed 4 g per day. The liquid preparation may be given rectally at the same dose to patients unwilling or unable to tolerate oral administration.

With the dramatic decline in pediatric aspirin use due to concern over Reye syndrome, use of other NSAIDs in children has increased. The most widely used oral NSAID in children in the United States is ibuprofen, available in a variety of liquid, tablet, and capsule preparations. Ibuprofen is a moderate-potency analgesic and excellent antipyretic with an impressive pediatric safety record, but is still probably underused for procedural and perioperative pain management in children (Kokki, 2003). The usual dose of ibuprofen is 4–10 mg/kg PO (maximum 800 mg) every 6 hours. Total dose should not exceed 4 g per day. The liquid preparation may be given rectally at the same dose to patients unwilling or unable to tolerate oral administration.

Ketorolac is the only NSAID available for intravenous use as an analgesic; indomethacin may be given intravenously, but is approved only for medical closure of patent ductus arteriosus in infants. Ketorolac is a high-potency NSAID with analgesic efficacy approaching that of the opioids. Initially approved only for intramuscular administration, ketorolac is safe and effective when given intravenously (Reinhart, Palladinetti, Patel, Raja, & Courtney, 1992). Oral ketorolac administration has been approved for adult patients but not for children. The usual dose of ketorolac is 0.5 mg/kg IM/IV (maximum 30 mg) every 6 hours. As the most potent NSAID, ketorolac also has the highest incidence of side effects: total duration of ketorolac therapy must not exceed 5 days to avoid potentially serious gastrointestinal and renal complications.

TABLE 86.7
Agents for Management of Opioid Side Effects

Side Effect	Agent	Dose	Comments
Pruritus	Diphenhydramine	0.5–1 mg/kg PO/IV (maximum 50 mg) q 6 h PRN	May cause somnolence
Pruritus	Nalbuphine	0.05 mg/kg IV (maximum 5 mg) q 4 h PRN	For pruritus from neuraxial opioid
Pruritus	Naloxone	1 μg/kg/h IV infusion	For pruritus from neuraxial opioid
Nausea	Metoclopramide	0.1 mg/kg IV (maximum 10 mg) q 6 h PRN	May cause extrapyramidal reactions
Nausea	Ondansetron	0.1 mg/kg IV (maximum 4 mg) q 6 h PRN	Expensive
Nausea	Promethazine	0.25–0.5 mg/kg PO/PR/IM/IV (maximum 25 mg) q 6 h PRN	May cause somnolence

Abbreviations: IM, intramuscularly; IV, intravenously; PO, orally; PR, rectally; PRN, as needed.

Significant platelet dysfunction may develop after a single dose of ketorolac, and its use in patients at high risk for surgical bleeding is controversial. Initial experience suggested greater intraoperative blood loss during tonsillectomy in children receiving perioperative ketorolac (Rusy et al., 1995), and retrospective studies indicated higher rates of postoperative hemorrhage (Gallagher, Blauth, & Fornadley, 1995; Judkins, Dray, & Hubbell, 1996). Other retrospective studies suggested otherwise (Agrawal, Gerson, Seligman, & Dsida, 1999), and prospective randomized trials have primarily shown only nonstatistically significant trends toward increased bleeding (Bailey, Sinha, & Burgess, 1997). Ketorolac product literature warns against its use in patients at high risk for surgical bleeding; it is probably prudent to avoid ketorolac administration in such patients, and in patients with medical coagulopathy, until more definitive information is available.

OPIOID ANALGESICS

Reluctance to use opioids in children has historically been an important reason for inadequate pediatric pain management. Opioids remain the mainstay of pharmacologic therapy for moderate to severe pain, however, and have established roles in procedural and perioperative pain management for children (Yaster, Kost-Byerly, & Maxwell, 2003). Acting on various subtypes of opioid receptors throughout the central nervous system, opioids cause dose-dependent pain relief as well as respiratory depression; other opioid-mediated side effects include somnolence, pupillary constriction, decreased gastrointestinal motility, nausea, and urinary retention. Many opioids induce histamine release, causing urticaria, pruritus, nausea, bronchospasm, and occasionally hypotension. Pruritus is more common and typically more intense with neuraxial administration, likely due to central nervous system opioid effect rather than to histamine release. Pruritus and nausea secondary to opioid therapy may be managed with a variety of agents (Table 86.7).

Opioid analgesics do not generally have maximum effective doses. Recommended doses are for initial administration in opioid-naïve patients; titration to clinical effect is necessary, and higher doses may be required. Opioid therapy longer than 7 to 10 days may result in physical dependence, requiring a period of weaning prior to discontinuation of therapy (Shannon & Berde, 1989). Psychopathologic addiction rarely develops in children receiving opioids for analgesia, and is not a valid reason to withhold appropriate pain management.

The opioid receptor antagonist naloxone rapidly reverses opioid effects (Table 86.5). Naloxone may precipitate withdrawal in opioid-dependent patients, and pulmonary edema has been reported with higher doses. Mild opioid-induced respiratory depression may be treated with naloxone 1 μg/kg IV titrated every 1 to 2 minutes as needed, while doses of 10 to 100 μg/kg IV should be reserved for obtundation or apnea secondary to opioid overdose.

Opioids are commonly administered in conjunction with various sedative–hypnotic agents, particularly benzodiazepines, increasing risk for respiratory depression (Bailey et al., 1990; Yaster, Nichols, Deshpande, & Wetzel, 1990). Midazolam combined with morphine or fentanyl provides safe and effective procedural analgesia and sedation in pediatric oncology patients, but transient desaturation is common (Sievers, Yee, Foley, Blanding, & Berde, 1991). Concomitant administration of opioids and sedative–hypnotic agents requires particularly careful titration of doses, appropriate monitoring, and full capability to manage complications including respiratory depression and apnea. Appropriate reversal agents should be available (Table 86.5).

The lytic cocktail, or DPT (Demerol®, Phenergan®, Thorazine®), is a combination of meperidine, promethazine, and chlorpromazine for intramuscular injection. Although the DPT lytic cocktail has been used extensively in children to provide analgesia and sedation for minor procedures such as laceration repair and fracture reduction, sedation is sometimes inadequate, recovery is often prolonged, and respiratory depression may occur (Nahata, Clotz, & Krogg, 1985). Numerous more appropriate agents are available (Petrack et al., 1996), with

TABLE 86.8
Lower-Potency Oral Opioids

Drug	Dose	Comments
Codeine	1 mg/kg PO q 4 h	Tablet and liquid preparations usually as combination products with acetaminophen
		High rate of gastrointestinal side effects
Hydrocodone	0.2 mg/kg PO q 4 h	Tablet and liquid preparations usually as combination products with acetaminophen or NSAID
		Lower rate of gastrointestinal side effects than codeine
Oxycodone	0.1 mg/kg PO q 4 h	Tablet preparations as oxycodone or as combination products with acetaminophen or NSAID
		Liquid preparation as oxycodone
		Low rate of gastrointestinal side effects
		Sustained-release preparation available for chronic therapy

Abbreviations: NSAID, nonsteroidal antiinflammatory drug; PO, orally.

individualized titration preferred to provide rapid onset, predictable depth of analgesia and sedation, and prompt recovery. Use of the DPT lytic cocktail is no longer recommended (American Academy of Pediatrics Committee on Drugs, 1995).

ORAL OPIOIDS

When gastrointestinal function permits, oral opioids offer the benefits of sustained pain relief and freedom from parenteral therapy. Several lower-potency oral opioids are used commonly in procedural and perioperative pain management for children (Table 86.8), often providing adequate analgesia for conditions and procedures associated with mild to moderate pain. Onset of action is relatively slow, rendering oral opioid therapy generally unsuitable for acute management of severe pain.

Codeine, available in tablet and liquid preparations usually in combination with acetaminophen, may be given at a dose of 1 mg/kg PO every 4 hours, but has a high rate of gastrointestinal upset. Hydrocodone, available in tablet and liquid preparations usually in combination with acetaminophen or NSAID, may be given at a dose of 0.2 mg/kg PO every 4 hours and tends to cause less gastrointestinal upset than codeine. Oxycodone is available in tablet preparations as an isolated product or in combination with acetaminophen or NSAID; oxycodone liquid preparations contain only oxycodone. Oxycodone causes little histamine release or gastrointestinal upset and is generally well tolerated. The usual dose of oxycodone is 0.1 mg/kg PO every 4 hours. Sustained-release oxycodone is available for chronic therapy.

Although often given intravenously, higher-potency opioids may also be given orally (Table 86.9). Morphine may be given at a dose of 0.3 mg/kg PO every 3 hours. The histamine release induced by morphine may cause urticaria, pruritus, bronchospasm, and even hypotension at higher doses, although these are less common with oral

administration. Sustained-release oral morphine is available for chronic therapy. Hydromorphone may be given orally at a dose of 20 to 40 μg/kg every 3 hours, and causes less histamine release than morphine. Meperidine may be given orally at a dose of 1 mg/kg every 3 hours, but should not be used for prolonged therapy given risk for seizures with accumulation of the neurotoxic metabolite normeperidine. Normeperidine is renally excreted, and risk for seizures is increased in patients with renal disease. Methadone may be given orally at a dose of 0.1 mg/kg every 6 to 12 hours and is particularly useful for chronic therapy in opioid-dependent patients (Tobias, Schleien, & Haun, 1990). Methadone maintenance therapy to treat psychopathologic opioid addiction may be undertaken only at federally licensed facilities.

Oral transmucosal fentanyl citrate (OTFC) is an innovative formulation of fentanyl in a candy matrix lozenge attached to a stick. OTFC may provide effective preanesthetic sedation in children (Friesen, Carpenter, Madigan, & Lockhart, 1995; Streisand et al., 1989), as well as analgesia and sedation for painful procedures (Schechter, Weisman, Rosenblum, Bernstein, & Conard, 1995), although the product is no longer marketed for these indications. Newer preparations of OTFC are currently under investigation for use in children with oncologic disease and other chronic painful conditions. Sucking the fentanyl lozenge causes transmucosal absorption of approximately 25% of the administered dose; the remainder is swallowed, resulting in a total bioavailability of approximately 50%. Nausea and emesis are common. The usual dose is 5 to 15 μg/kg (maximum 400 μg); children may require higher doses than adults. OTFC administration in children requires appropriate monitoring (Yaster, 1995).

INTRAVENOUS OPIOIDS

Intravenous opioids remain the mainstay of therapy for moderate to severe pain (Table 86.9). Analgesic require-

TABLE 86.9
Higher-Potency Opioids

Drug	Dose	Comments
Fentanyl	5–15 μg/kg PO (interval dosing not defined)	Oral preparation largely for single dose use
	0.5–1 μg/kg IV q 1 h	Rapid infusion may cause chest wall rigidity in infants
	PCA: 1 μg/kg/h basal, 1 μg/kg demand	Transdermal patch not for acute management
	Patch: 25 μg = 1 mg/h IV morphine	
Hydromorphone	20–40 μg/kg PO q 3 h	Less histamine release than morphine
	10–20 μg/kg IM/IV/SC q 3h	
	PCA: 4 μg/kg basal, 4 μg/kg demand	
Meperidine	1 mg/kg PO/IM/IV/SC q 3 h	Neurotoxic metabolite, may precipitate seizures
	PCA: not recommended	No hepatobiliary advantage at usual doses
Methadone	0.1 mg/kg PO q 6–12 h	Useful for long-term therapy, especially in palliative care
	0.05 mg/kg IV q 6–12 h	Treatment of opioid addiction must be in licensed facility
Morphine	0.3 mg/kg PO q 3 h	Histamine release may cause urticaria, pruritus, bronchospasm, hypotension
	0.1 mg/kg IM/IV/SC q 3 h	High dose and rapid administration increase risk for histamine release
	PCA: 0.02 mg/kg basal, 0.02 mg/kg demand	Sustained-release oral preparation available for chronic therapy

Note: Doses are for initial administration in opioid-naïve patients; titration to clinical effect is necessary; higher doses may be required. Doses should be reduced to 25–50% of the above in neonates and young infants.

Abbreviations: IM, intramuscularly; IV, intravenously; PCA, patent-controlled analgesia; PO, orally; SC, subcutaneously.

ments vary among individuals and over the duration of pain in each patient, requiring ongoing assessment of analgesia and adjustment of pain management regimens. Intravenous opioids offer the advantages of rapid onset, potent analgesia, and ease of titration. Side effects are more common with intravenous opioids and potentially more serious, mandating appropriate monitoring and prompt management of complications. Equipotent doses of opioids carry similar risks of side effects (Yaster et al., 2003).

Morphine is the traditional intravenous opioid analgesic, given at a dose of 0.1 mg/kg IV every 3 hours. Morphine and its congeners should be used with caution in neonates, who are more sensitive to the depressant effects of morphine due to immaturity of the blood–brain barrier. Morphine clearance may also be prolonged in infants less than 3 to 6 months of age (Shannon & Berde, 1989). Young infants receiving intravenous opioids should be observed closely with continuous respiratory monitoring, and doses should probably be reduced to 25 to 50% of usual. Hydromorphone may be given at a dose of 10 to 20 μg/kg IV every 3 hours, and causes less histamine release than morphine. Meperidine may be given at a dose of 1 mg/kg IV every 3 hours, but should not be used for prolonged therapy given risk for seizures with accumulation of the neurotoxic metabolite normeperidine. Normeperidine is renally excreted, and risk for seizures is increased in patients with renal disease. Although historically popular, meperidine offers no significant advantages over morphine and, in particular, causes no less hepatobiliary spasm than any other opioid at usual equipotent doses. Methadone may be given at a dose of 0.05 mg/kg IV every 6 to 12

hours, although there is usually little reason to prefer intravenous to oral administration. Fentanyl, a potent synthetic opioid, is used commonly in procedural and perioperative pain management for children because of its rapid onset and short duration of action. The usual dose is 0.5 to 1 μg/kg IV every hour, with more frequent titration during and immediately after procedures. Incremental doses of fentanyl up to 4 μg/kg IV have provided satisfactory analgesia for pediatric oncology patients, although patients tended to prefer midazolam, perhaps because of its amnestic properties (Sandler et al., 1992).

PATIENT-CONTROLLED ANALGESIA

Optimal management of moderate to severe pain mandates that analgesia be provided on a scheduled rather than an as-needed basis, as the latter often delays treatment and compromises pain control. Intramuscular injection of opioid is undesirable, as this is more painful and less effective than other alternatives (Berde, 1989; Berde, Lehn, Yee, Sethna, & Russo, 1991). Opioid administration by intravenous infusion using patient-controlled analgesia (PCA) modalities provides scheduled analgesia via an acceptable route and affords excellent procedural and perioperative pain management for children (Wilder, Berde, Troshynski, Cahill, & Sethna, 1992). With age-appropriate instruction, most school-age children may safely and effectively control opioid delivery by PCA (Berde et al., 1991; Gaukroger, Tomkins, & van der Walt, 1989). Nurse- or parent-controlled PCA may be used for children unable or unwilling to control their own pump (Algren, Deegear, Skjonsby,

TABLE 86.10
Topical Anesthetic Formulations

Formulation	Local Anesthetic	Comments
EMLA cream	Lidocaine 2.5%/prilocaine 2.5%	Requires 1–4 hours of application Requires occlusive dressing Rare risk for methemoglobinemia in infants
ELA-Max	Liposomal lidocaine 4% or 5%	Requires 30 minutes of application No occlusive dressing Nonprescription
Numby Stuff	Iontocaine (lidocaine 2% + epinephrine 1:100,000)	Requires 10 minutes of application Tingling sensation may frighten some children
TAC	Tetracaine 0.5–1% + epinephrine 1:2,000–4,000 + cocaine 4–11.8%	Requires 20 minutes of application Avoid mucous membranes Avoid terminally perfused areas Risk for cocaine toxicity

& Algren, 1998; Lloyd-Thomas & Howard, 1994; Weldon, Connor, & White, 1991), although risk of respiratory depression rises if dosing interval is not adequately increased, particularly in combination with basal infusions (Monitto et al., 2000).

Morphine is the most common choice for PCA, but hydromorphone and fentanyl may be used (Table 86.9). Meperidine PCA is not recommended because of increased risk for toxicity with sustained administration. Routine pediatric PCA regimens provide morphine 0.02 mg/kg (maximum 1 mg), hydromorphone 4 μg/kg (maximum 200 μg), or fentanyl 1 μg/kg (maximum 50 μg) IV every 8 to 15 minutes as needed for patient-controlled administration, or every 15 to 60 minutes as needed for nurse- or parent-controlled administration. Longer dosing intervals may be safer in younger or medically more fragile patients. Concomitant basal infusion to sustain drug levels during sleep has been advocated and is used by many practitioners, although this has not been shown to improve analgesia significantly (McNeely, Pontus, & Trentadue, 1992). Given potential for drug accumulation and respiratory depression, it may be prudent to restrict basal infusions to patients with severe pain unlikely to be controlled with interval dosing alone.

Patients receiving PCA should be assessed frequently, and doses and intervals adjusted to ensure adequate analgesia and patient safety. Continuous pulse oximetry is recommended for children on any opioid infusion at least until steady state has been achieved, usually 24 to 48 hours. Prolonged monitoring may be appropriate in younger or medically more fragile patients, or if the PCA regimen is significantly modified. Thorough instruction of patients, families, and caregivers regarding appropriate PCA use is essential.

Fentanyl is available as a transdermal patch allowing for continuous transcutaneous absorption over 72 hours mimicking an intravenous infusion; one 25-μg fentanyl patch is roughly equivalent to 1 mg/hour intravenous mor-

phine. Onset is slow, however, and absorption variable. Although useful in some settings for management of chronic pain, transdermal fentanyl is not indicated for acute pain management (Gaukroger, 1993; Yaster et al., 2003).

TOPICAL AND LOCAL ANESTHETICS

Innovations in formulation of local anesthetics have yielded several new compounds that provide effective cutaneous analgesia while reducing pain associated with local anesthetic injection (Table 86.10). Such formulations enhance usefulness of topical anesthetics for minor procedures, and in many instances reduce or eliminate need for systemic analgesia and sedation.

Eutectic mixture of local anesthetics (EMLA®) cream is a combination of 2.5% lidocaine and 2.5% prilocaine. When applied in a thick layer and covered with an occlusive dressing for at least 60 minutes, EMLA cream promotes local anesthetic penetration of intact skin, producing effective cutaneous analgesia for minor procedures such as intravenous cannulation and accessing of subcutaneous injection ports (Hallen, Olsson, & Uppfeldt, 1984). EMLA cream may be a useful adjunct for procedures such as lumbar puncture and bone marrow aspiration, and has been used for neonatal circumcision (Benini, Johnston, Faucher, & Aranda, 1993). EMLA cream has been shown to reduce pain associated with immunization in infants (Taddio, Nulman, Goldbach, Ipp, & Koren, 1994) and older children (Cassidy et al., 2001), and even to provide analgesia for chest tube removal (Rosen et al., 2000). EMLA cream is easy to apply; families may do so at home to minimize waiting. Side effects are minor and include erythema, blanching, and rash. Although the prilocaine component has caused concern over risk for methemoglobinemia, particularly with generous application or in infants, incidence of methemoglobinemia is extremely low when the product is used appropriately.

EMLA cream should be applied only to intact skin. Analgesia increases with prolonged application up to 4 hours (Cooper, Gerrish, Hardwick, & Kay, 1987).

ELA-Max® is an over-the-counter preparation of 4% or 5% liposomal lidocaine; other nonprescription preparations of 4% lidocaine for topical use are marketed under a variety of other brand names. Like EMLA cream, ELA-Max promotes local anesthetic penetration of intact skin, producing effective cutaneous analgesia for minor procedures. In contrast to EMLA cream, ELA-Max does not entail an occlusive dressing, requires only 30 minutes to achieve anesthesia, lacks prilocaine, and is available without prescription. The two preparations have been shown to provide equivalent cutaneous analgesia for children undergoing venipuncture (Eichenfield, Funk, Fallon-Friedlander, & Cunningham, 2002).

Numby Stuff® is a unique system for intradermal delivery of local anesthetic. Numby Stuff utilizes iontophoresis, employing mild electrical current to promote rapid intradermal transport of Iontocaine®, a solution of 2% lidocaine and 1:100,000 epinephrine. Iontocaine is applied and covered with specialized electrodes connected to the Numby Stuff generator. Dermal anesthesia to a depth of 10 mm is obtained within 10 minutes. Numby Stuff is effective for intravenous catheter insertion and pulsed dye laser therapy (Ashburn et al., 1997), and provides cutaneous analgesia more rapidly and effectively than EMLA cream (Squire, Kirchhoff, & Hissong, 2000). Although the system is approved for use in all ages, younger children may be frightened by the tingling sensation produced by the electrical current.

Tetracaine–adrenaline–cocaine (TAC), a solution of 0.5% tetracaine, 1:2,000 epinephrine, and 11.8% cocaine, provides effective cutaneous analgesia for repair of superficial lacerations in children (Bonadio & Wagner, 1988). Alternative effective formulations with lower risk for cocaine toxicity are 1% tetracaine, 1:4,000 epinephrine, and 4% cocaine (Smith & Barry, 1990) and 0.5% tetracaine, 1:2,000 epinephrine, and 4% lidocaine (Ernst et al., 1995). TAC was sufficient in 89% of patients with scalp and facial wounds, but 57% of patients with extremity wounds required supplemental local anesthesia (Hegenbarth et al., 1990). Usual dose of TAC is 1 to 3 ml (maximum 0.09 ml/kg), applied with gauze held in place for 15 to 20 minutes. To avoid systemic cocaine toxicity, TAC should not be applied to mucous membranes. Cocaine and epinephrine both cause vasoconstriction; TAC should not be applied to areas supplied by terminal arteries, including ears, nose, penis, and digits. Health care personnel should wear gloves when applying TAC.

Simple pH buffering helps reduce pain with injection of conventional local anesthetics and may increase efficacy. Acid pH of local anesthetic solutions enhances solubility and prolongs shelf life, but is largely responsible for pain with injection. Addition of 1 mEq sodium bicarbonate to 10 ml local anesthetic significantly reduces pain during injection without precipitation of the solution (Christoph, Buchanan, Begalla, & Schwartz, 1988). Conventional solutions of local anesthetic for infiltration may be treated in this manner; bicarbonate is added immediately before use.

REGIONAL ANESTHETIC TECHNIQUES

In addition to providing surgical anesthesia, regional anesthetic techniques may provide excellent procedural and perioperative pain management for children. In pediatric practice, these techniques are commonly performed in conjunction with general anesthesia (Dalens, 1989; Ross, Eck, & Tobias, 2000), reducing maintenance anesthetic requirements and facilitating rapid emergence. Analgesia may persist for hours or even days, depending on technique and medications utilized, reducing or eliminating requirement for supplemental systemic analgesics. In some settings, perioperative regional anesthesia in children has been shown to improve surgical outcomes (McNeely, Farber, Rusy, & Hoffman, 1997). Pediatric application of regional anesthetic techniques continues to expand both in the operating room and beyond (Tobias, 2002). Regional anesthetic techniques employed to provide procedural and perioperative pain management for children include a variety of peripheral nerve, plexus, and neuraxial blocks.

PERIPHERAL NERVE AND PLEXUS BLOCKS

Successful block of virtually any peripheral nerve or plexus may be accomplished with appropriate equipment and sufficient practitioner interest (Dalens, 2000; Ross et al., 2000; Sethna & Berde, 1994). Supraorbital and occipital nerve blocks provide analgesia over the anterior and posterior scalp, respectively, and may be used for laceration repair or to provide analgesia following craniotomy. Infraorbital nerve block and various palatal blocks provide analgesia of the upper lip and palate for procedures including cleft lip and cleft palate repair, and may be particularly useful in medically disadvantaged settings when avoidance of opioid is desired. Retrobulbar block anesthetizes orbital contents and induces profound analgesia of the globe and surrounding structures; ophthalmologists generally perform such blocks. Intercostal nerve blocks provide excellent analgesia and enhance pulmonary function following thoracotomy (Matsota, Livanios, & Marinopoulou, 2001), and lessen pain of thoracostomy tubes and rib fractures. Periumbilical compartment block is useful for umbilical hernia repair, while ilioinguinal and iliohypogastric nerve blocks are useful for a variety of unilateral inguinal and groin procedures. Numerous techniques for penile nerve block in distal penile surgery including circumcision and hypospadias repair have been described.

Although preemptive peripheral nerve blocks offer theoretical advantages of preemptive analgesia and lessened overall pain experience, this has not been reliably demonstrated in clinical practice, particularly in children (Ates, Unal, Cuhruk, & Erkan, 1998; Suresh et al., 2004).

Plexus blocks are performed less frequently in children than in adults, often due to practitioner inexperience but also to logistical challenges in applying adult techniques to pediatric patients. Brachial plexus block in children is most commonly accomplished via an axillary approach, providing analgesia to the arm below the shoulder. Interscalene brachial plexus block is performed somewhat less frequently in children, inducing analgesia of the shoulder and proximal arm but occasionally sparing the distal hand. Modern experience with supraclavicular and infraclavicular approaches to brachial plexus block in children is limited. Direct lumbosacral plexus block is uncommon in pediatric practice; peripheral regional anesthesia of the lower extremity in children is generally provided through various sciatic and femoral nerve blocks. Preemptive plexus blocks offer theoretical advantages of preemptive analgesia and lessened overall pain experience, but this has not been reliably demonstrated in clinical practice, particularly in children (Altintas, Bozkurt, Ipek, Yucel, & Kaya, 2000). Intravenous regional anesthesia of the extremities, or Bier block, has been described in children (Davidson, Eyres, & Cole, 2002), but application may be limited by risk of local anesthetic toxicity.

Neuraxial Blocks

Neuraxial blocks include spinal and epidural techniques. Spinal block, with injection of anesthetic into cerebrospinal fluid, is performed in children almost exclusively for procedures in infants at high risk for apnea following general anesthesia, or for terminal analgesia in palliative care. Epidural block, with injection of anesthetic into the potential space between ligamentum flavum and dura mater, is a far more common technique for procedural and perioperative pain management in children. Anesthetic may be administered as a single injection, or by repeated injection or continuous infusion through an indwelling catheter.

The most common neuraxial block in children is caudal block, in which the epidural space is accessed through the sacral hiatus created by the failure of fusion of the spinous process of the fifth sacral vertebra. Caudal block is most commonly performed as a single injection, 1 ml/kg of anesthetic providing reliable analgesia below the umbilicus in patients less than 30 kg. The technique is relatively straightforward, with high rates of success and low rates of complications (Broadman, Hanallah, Norden, & McGill, 1987; Dalens & Hasnaoui, 1989). Caudal block is especially popular for inguinal and groin procedures including inguinal hernia and hydrocoele repair, orchio-

pexy, hypospadias repair, and circumcision. Agents administered determine duration of analgesia.

Caudal block with local anesthetic may provide analgesia for several hours. Addition of opioid prolongs analgesia, but entails risk of opioid-mediated side effects including pruritus, nausea, urinary retention, and respiratory depression. Duration and distribution of analgesia and risk of side effects are all greater with increasing opioid hydrophilicity, which promotes uptake into cerebrospinal fluid and enhances distal spread. Opioid side effects may be treated with a variety of pharmacologic agents (Table 86.7), or reversed with naxolone if necessary (Table 86.5). Caudal fentanyl, a highly lipophilic opioid, may be used for outpatient and ambulatory surgery in children. Caudal morphine, a highly hydrophilic opioid, provides analgesia for greater than 12 hours at a dose of 0.03 to 0.07 mg/kg but entails significant risk of opioid-mediated side effects (Krane, Tyler, & Jacobson, 1989; Valley & Bailey, 1991). Caudal administration of clonidine (Sharpe et al., 2001) and ketamine (Weber & Wulf, 2003) has been described.

Excellent analgesia may be provided with administration of anesthetic by repeated injection or continuous infusion through indwelling epidural catheters, which may be placed via caudal, lumbar, or thoracic approaches to the epidural space in children (Berde, Sethna, Yemen, Pullerits, & Miler, 1990; Desparmet, Meistelman, Barre, & Saint-Maurice, 1987; Gunter & Eng, 1992). Epidural catheters may be inserted caudally and threaded to the desired vertebral level (Dalens & Hasnaoui, 1989); this is more readily accomplished in infants and young children, and is facilitated by use of styletted catheters. Epidural catheters in children may also be placed directly at the desired vertebral level by lumbar or thoracic approaches. Historical concern over safety of thoracic epidural placement in children under general anesthesia has been largely theoretical, although a neurologic complication of such placement has recently been reported (Kasai, Yaegashi, Hirose, & Tanaka, 2003).

Selection of agents for epidural infusion is based on position of the catheter tip relative to the painful area, as well as on distribution and intensity of analgesia desired. Concomitant neuraxial administration of local anesthetic and opioid enables reduction in local anesthetic concentration and opioid dose, minimizing motor block and decreasing risk of opioid-mediated side effects (McIlvaine, 1990). Numerous combinations of local anesthetic and opioid may be used for epidural infusion (Table 86.11). If the epidural catheter tip has been appropriately placed in close proximity to the painful area, dilute local anesthetic with lipophilic opioid such as fentanyl may be sufficient. If the epidural catheter tip is at a dermatomal level distant from that of the painful area, or if the painful area covers multiple dermatomes, addition of increasingly hydrophilic opioid such as hydromorphone or morphine may be necessary. As with caudal administration, duration and distribution of

TABLE 86.11
Local Anesthetics and Opioids for Epidural Infusion

Local Anesthetics	Opioids
Bupivacaine 0.0625–0.1%	Fentanyl 0.5–1 µg/kg/h
Levobupivacaine 0.0625–0.1%	Hydromorphone 2–4 µg/kg/h
Lidocaine 0.1–0.5%	Morphine 3–6 µg/kg/h
Ropivacaine 0.1–0.2%	

Note: Infusion rates are commonly 0.2–0.3, 0.3–0.4, and 0.4–0.5 ml/kg/h for thoracic, lumbar, and caudal catheters, respectively.

analgesia and risk of side effects with epidural opioid are all greater with increasing opioid hydrophilicity, which promotes uptake into cerebrospinal fluid and embraces distal spread (Taylor & Boswell, 1991); risk of side effects increases with increasing opioid hydrophilicity. Opioid side effects may be treated with a variety of pharmacologic agents (Table 86.7), or reversed with naloxone if necessary (Table 86.5).

Close observation of patients receiving epidural infusions is essential. Continuous monitoring of oxygen saturation and cardiorespiratory parameters may be employed for any patient receiving epidural opioid (McIlvaine, 1990), or such monitoring may be reserved for patients at increased risk for respiratory depression. Infants less than 6 months of age, patients with preexisting neurologic or pulmonary disorders, and patients receiving hydrophilic opioid such as morphine or hydromorphone may merit more intensive monitoring (Berde et al., 1989). Frequent assessment of level of consciousness, adequacy of pain management, degree of motor and sensory block, and presence of side effects should be performed for all patients receiving epidural infusions. Although somewhat complex and labor intensive, epidural analgesia is appropriate for patients with severe pain or unique circumstances limiting safety or efficacy of other pain management interventions.

CONCLUSION

Procedural and perioperative pain management for children entails adequate analgesia and appropriate sedation for patients undergoing a wide range of diagnostic and therapeutic procedures including surgery. Procedural analgesia and sedation for children requires supervision by competent personnel adhering to appropriate standards for patient monitoring and management. Perioperative pain management for children takes into account patient anxiety concerning surgery as well as pathophysiology of surgical pain. Nonpharmacologic techniques seek to enhance patients' ability to cope with pain by modifying pain perception and, in the case of various biophysical modalities, by modulating nociceptive transmission. Numerous sedative–hypnotic agents are available for procedural and preoperative sedation in children; most lack analgesic properties. Non-opioid analgesics provide important adjunctive analgesia, while opioids remain the mainstay of therapy for moderate to severe pain. Patient-controlled analgesia is an appropriate modality for children requiring ongoing intravenous opioid. Several innovative formulations of topical anesthetics provide effective cutaneous analgesia for minor procedures while reducing pain associated with local anesthetic injection. Regional anesthetic techniques including peripheral nerve, plexus, and neuraxial blocks provide excellent pain control and reduce requirement for supplemental systemic analgesics. Integrated procedural and perioperative pain management for children employs nonpharmacologic techniques in combination with appropriate pharmacologic agents and anesthetic techniques to optimize pain relief, minimize side effects, and facilitate recovery.

REFERENCES

Acute Pain Management Guideline Panel. (1992). *Acute pain management: Operative or medical procedures and trauma. Clinical practice guideline.* (AHCPR Publication No. 92-0032). Rockville, MD: Agency for Health Care Policy & Research, Public Health Service, U.S. Department of Health and Human Services.

Adams, M. L., Brase, D. A., Welch, S. P., & Dewey, W. L. (1986). The role of endogenous peptides in the action of opioids. *Annals of Emergency Medicine, 15*(9), 1030–1035.

Agrawal, A., Gerson, C. R., Seligman, I., & Dsida, R. M. (1999). Postoperative hemorrhage after tonsillectomy: Use of ketorolac tromethamine. *Otolaryngology and Head and Neck Surgery, 120*(3), 335–339.

Akman, I., Ozek, E., Bilgen, H., Ozdogan, T., & Cebeci, D. (2002). Sweet solutions and pacifiers for pain relief in newborn infants. *Journal of Pain, 3*(3), 199–202.

Alexander, J., & Manno, M. (2003). Underuse of analgesia in very young pediatric patients with isolated painful injuries. *Annals of Emergency Medicine, 41*(5), 617–622.

Algren, J. T., Deegear, C. L., Skjonsby, B., & Algren, C. (1998). Efficacy and safety of patient-, parent-, or nurse-controlled analgesia in children. *Anesthesiology, 89*(3A), A1303.

Altintas, F., Bozkurt, P., Ipek, N., Yucel, A., & Kaya, G. (2000). The efficacy of pre- versus postsurgical axillary block on postoperative pain in paediatric patients. *Paediatric Anaesthesia, 10*(1), 23–28.

American Academy of Pediatric Dentistry. (2003). Clinical guideline on elective use of conscious sedation, deep sedation, and general anesthesia in pediatric dental patients. *Pediatric Dentistry, 25*(7), 75–81.

American Academy of Pediatrics Committee on Drugs. (1992). Guidelines for monitoring and management of pediatric patients during and after sedation for diagnostic and therapeutic procedures. *Pediatrics, 89*(6 Pt. 1), 110–115.

American Academy of Pediatrics Committee on Drugs. (1995). Reappraisal of lytic cocktail/demerol, phenergan, and thorazine (DPT) for the sedation of children. *Pediatrics, 95*(4), 598–602.

American Academy of Pediatrics Committee on Drugs. (2002). Guidelines for monitoring and management of pediatric patients during and after sedation for diagnostic and therapeutic procedures: Addendum. *Pediatrics, 110*(4), 836–838.

American Academy of Pediatrics Task Force on Pain in Infants, Children, and Adolescents. (2001). The assessment and management of acute pain in infants, children, and adolescents. *Pediatrics, 108*(3), 793–797.

American College of Emergency Physicians. (1997). Use of pediatric sedation and analgesia. American College of Emergency Physicians. *Annals of Emergency Medicine, 29*(6), 834–835.

American Society of Anesthesiologists Task Force on Preoperative Fasting. (1999). Practice guidelines for preoperative fasting and the use of pharmacologic agents to reduce the risk of pulmonary aspiration: Application to healthy patients undergoing elective procedures: A report by the American Society of Anesthesiologists Task Force on Preoperative Fasting. *Anesthesiology, 90*(3), 896–905.

American Society of Anesthesiologists Task Force on Sedation and Analgesia by Non-Anesthesiologists. (2002). Practice guidelines for sedation and analgesia by non-anesthesiologists. *Anesthesiology, 96*(4), 1004–1017.

Anderson, C. T., Zeltzer, L. K., & Fanurik, D. (1993). Procedural pain. In N. L. Schechter, C. B. Berde, & M. Yaster (Eds.), *Pain in infants, children and adolescents* (pp. 435–458). Baltimore, MD: Williams & Wilkins.

Ashburn, M. A., Gauthier, M., Love, G., Basta, S., Gaylord, B., & Kessler, K. (1997). Iontophoretic administration of 2% lidocaine HCl and 1:100,000 epinephrine in humans. *Clinical Journal of Pain, 13*(1), 22–26.

Ates, Y., Unal, N., Cuhruk, H., & Erkan, N. (1998). Postoperative analgesia in children using preemptive retrobulbar block and local anesthetic infiltration in strabismus surgery. *Regional Anesthesia and Pain Medicine, 23*(6), 569–574.

Bailey, P. L., Pace, N. L., Ashburn, M. A., Moll, J. W., East, K. A., & Stanley, T. H. (1990). Frequent hypoxemia and apnea after sedation with midazolam and fentanyl. *Anesthesiology, 75*(5), 826–830.

Bailey, R., Sinha, C., & Burgess, L. P. (1997). Ketorolac tromethamine and hemorrhage in tonsillectomy: A prospective, randomized, double-blind study. *Laryngoscope 107*(2), 166–169.

Barbi, E., Gerarduzzi, T., Marchetti, F., Neri, E., Verucci, E., Bruno, I. et al. (2003). Deep sedation with propofol by nonanesthesiologists: A prospective pediatric experience. *Archives of Pediatric and Adolescent Medicine, 157*(11), 1097–1103.

Bassett, K. E., Anderson, J. L., Pribble, C. G., & Guenther, E. (2003). Propofol for procedural sedation in children in the emergency department. *Annals of Emergency Medicine, 42* (6), 773–782.

Benini, F., Johnston, C. C., Faucher, D, & Aranda, J.V. (1993). Topical anesthesia during circumcision in newborn infants. *Journal of the American Medical Association, 270*(7), 850–853.

Berde, C. B. (1989). Pediatric postoperative pain management. *Pediatric Clinics of North America, 36*(4), 921–940.

Berde, C. B., Lehn, B. M., Yee, J. D., Sethna, N. F., & Russo, D. (1991). Patient-controlled analgesia in children and adolescents: A randomized prospective comparison with intramuscular administration of morphine for postoperative analgesia. *Journal of Pediatrics, 118*(3), 460–466.

Berde, C. B., Sethna, N. F., Levin, L., Retik, A., Millis, M., Lillehei, C. et al. (1989). Regional analgesia on pediatric medical and surgical wards. *Intensive Care Medicine, 15*(Suppl. 1), S40–S43.

Berde, C. B., Sethna, N. F., Yemen, T. A., Pullerits, J., & Miler, V. (1990). Continuous epidural bupivacaine-fentanyl infusions in children following ureteral reimplantation. *Anesthesiology, 73*(3A), A1128.

Bonadio, W. A., & Wagner, V. (1988). Efficacy of TAC topical anesthetic for repair of pediatric lacerations. *American Journal of Diseases of Children, 142*(2), 203–205.

Broadman, L. M., Hanallah, R. S., Norden, J. M., & McGill, W. A. (1987). "Kiddie caudals": Experience with 1,154 consecutive cases without complications. *Anesthesia & Analgesia, 66*(2S), S18.

Brown, J. L. (1995). Imagination training: A tool with many uses, *Contemporary Pediatrics, 12*(2), 22–26, 29–30, 32 passim.

Cassidy, K. L., Reid, G. J., McGrath, P. J., Smith, D. J., Brown, T. L., & Finley, G. A. (2001). A randomized double-blind, placebo-controlled trial of the EMLA patch for the reduction of pain associated with intramuscular injection in four to six-year-old children. *Acta Paediatrica, 90*(11), 1329–1336.

Christensen, J., & Fatchett, D. (2002). Promoting parental use of distraction and relaxation in pediatric oncology patients during invasive procedures. *Journal of Pediatric Oncology Nursing, 19*(4), 127–132.

Christoph, R. A., Buchanan, L., Begalla, K., & Schwartz, S. (1988). Pain reduction in local anesthetic administration through pH buffering. *Annals of Emergency Medicine, 17*(2), 117–120.

Collins, S. K., & Kuck, K. (1991). Music therapy in the neonatal intensive care unit. *Neonatal Network, 9*(6), 23–26.

Conner-Warren, R. L. (1996). Pain intensity and home pain management of children with sickle cell disease. *Issues in Comprehensive Pediatric Nursing, 19*(3), 183–195.

Cooper, C. M., Gerrish, S. P., Hardwick, M., & Kay, R. (1987). EMLA cream reduces the pain of venepuncture in children. *European Journal of Anaesthesiology, 4*(6), 441–448.

Coté, C. J. (1994). Sedation protocols — Why so many variations? *Pediatrics, 94*(3), 281–283.

Coté, C. J., Notterman, D. A., Karl, H. W., Weinberg, J. A., & McCloskey, C. (2000). Adverse sedation events in pediatrics: A critical incident analysis of contributing factors. *Pediatrics, 105*(4 Pt. 1), 805–814.

Dahl, J. B., & Kehlet, H. (1993). The value of pre-emptive analgesia in the treatment of postoperative pain. *British Journal of Anaesthesia, 70*(4), 434–439.

Dalens, B. (1989). Regional anesthesia in children. *Anesthesia & Analgesia, 68*(5), 654–672.

Dalens, B. (2000). "Small blocks" in paediatric patients. *Baillière's Clinical Anaesthesiology, 14*(4), 745–758.

Dalens, B., & Hasnaoui, A. (1989). Caudal anesthesia in pediatric surgery: Success rate and adverse effects in 750 consecutive patients. *Anesthesia & Analgesia, 68*(2), 83–89.

Davidson, A. J., Eyres, R. L., & Cole, W. G. (2002). A comparison of prilocaine and lidocaine for intravenous regional anaesthesia for forearm fracture reduction in children. *Paediatric Anaesthesia, 12*(2), 146–150.

Desparmet, J., Meistelman, C., Barre, J., & Saint-Maurice, C. (1987). Continuous epidural infusion of bupivacaine for postoperative pain relief in children. *Anesthesiology, 67*(1), 108–110.

Duggan, J., & Drummond, G. B. (1987). Activity of lower intercostal and abdominal muscle after upper abdominal surgery. *Anesthesia & Analgesia, 66*(9), 852–855.

Eichenfield, L. F., Funk, A., Fallon-Friedlander, S., & Cunningham, B. B. (2002). A clinical study to evaluate the efficacy of ELA-Max (4% liposomal lidocaine) as compared with eutectic mixture of local anesthetics cream for pain reduction of venipuncture in children. *Pediatrics, 109*(6), 1093–1099.

Eland, J. (1991). The use of TENS with children who have cancer pain. *Journal of Pain and Symptom Management, 6*(3), 145.

Eland, J. (1993). The use of TENS with children. In N. L. Schechter, C. B. Berde, & M. Yaster (Eds.), *Pain in infants, children and adolescents* (pp. 331–340). Baltimore, MD: Williams & Wilkins.

Eland, J., & Anderson, J. (1977). The experience of pain in children. In S. Jacox (Ed.), *Pain: A sourcebook for nurses and other health professionals* (pp. 453–473). Boston: Little, Brown.

Ernst, E., & Fialka, V. (1994). Ice freezes pain? A review of the clinical effectiveness of analgesic cold therapy. *Journal of Pain and Symptom Management, 9*(1), 56–59.

Ernst, A. A., Marvez, E., Nick, T. G., Chin, E., Wood, E., & Gonzaba, W. T. (1995). Lidocaine adrenaline tetracaine gel versus tetracaine adrenaline cocaine gel for topical anesthesia in linear scalp and facial lacerations in children aged 5 to 17 years. *Pediatrics, 95*(2), 255–258.

Feld, L. H., Negus, J. B., & White, P. F. (1990). Oral midazolam preanesthetic medication in pediatric outpatients. *Anesthesiology, 73*(5), 831–834.

Fitzgerald, M., & Anand, K. J. S. (1993). Developmental neuroanatomy and neurophysiology of pain. In N. L. Schechter, C. B. Berde, & M. Yaster (Eds.), *Pain in infants, children and adolescents* (pp. 11–32). Baltimore, MD: Williams & Wilkins.

Fitzgerald, M., & Howard, R. F. (2003). The neurobiologic basis of pediatric pain. In N. L. Schechter, C. B. Berde, & M. Yaster (Eds.), *Pain in infants, children, and adolescents* (2nd ed., pp. 19–42). Philadelphia: Lippincott/Williams & Wilkins.

Friesen, R. H., Carpenter, E., Madigan, C. K., & Lockhart, C. H. (1995). Oral transmucosal fentanyl citrate for preanaesthetic medication of paediatric cardiac surgery patients, *Paediatric Anaesthesia, 5*(1), 29–33.

Gallagher, J. E., Blauth, J., & Fornadley, J. A. (1995). Perioperative ketorolac tromethamine and postoperative hemorrhage in cases of tonsillectomy and adenoidectomy. *Laryngoscope, 105*(6), 606–609.

Gaukroger, P. B. (1993). Novel techniques of analgesic delivery. In N. L. Schechter, C. B. Berde, & M. Yaster (Eds.), *Pain in infants, children and adolescents* (pp. 195–202). Baltimore, MD: Williams & Wilkins.

Gaukroger, P. B., Tomkins, D. P., & van der Walt, J. H. (1989). Patient-controlled analgesia in children. *Anaesthesia and Intensive Care, 17*(3), 264–268.

Green, S. M., Nakamura, R., & Johnson, N. E. (1990). Ketamine sedation for pediatric procedures: Part 1, A prospective series. *Annals of Emergency Medicine, 19*(9), 1024–1032.

Gross, J. B., Weller, R. S., & Conard, P. (1991). Flumazenil antagonism of midazolam-induced ventilatory depression. *Anesthesiology, 75*(2), 179–185.

Guenther, E., Pribble, C. G., Junkins, E. P., Jr., Kadish, H. A., Bassett, K. E., & Nelson, D. S. (2003). Propofol sedation by emergency physicians for elective pediatric outpatient procedures. *Annals of Emergency Medicine, 42*(6), 783–791.

Gunter, J. B., & Eng, C. (1992). Thoracic epidural anesthesia via the caudal approach in children. *Anesthesiology, 76*(6), 935–938.

Hallen, B., Olsson, G. L., & Uppfeldt, A. (1984). Pain-free venipuncture. Effect of timing of application of local anaesthetic cream. *Anaesthesia, 39*(10), 969–972.

Harrison, D., Johnston, L., & Loughnan, P. (2003). Oral sucrose for procedural pain in sick hospitalized infants: A randomized-controlled trial. *Journal of Paediatrics and Child Health, 39*(8), 591–597.

Harvey, M., & Elliott, M. (1995). Transcutaneous electrical nerve stimulation (TENS) for pain management during cavity preparations in pediatric patients. *ASDC Journal of Dentistry for Children, 62*(1), 49–51.

Hasan, R. A., Shayevitz, J. R., & Patel, V. (2003). Deep sedation with propofol for children undergoing ambulatory magnetic resonance imaging of the brain: Experience from a pediatric intensive care unit. *Pediatric Critical Care Medicine, 4*(4), 454–458.

Hegenbarth, M. A., Altieri, M. F., Hawk, W. H., Greene, A., Ochsenschlager, D. W., & O'Donnell, R. (1990). Comparison of topical tetracaine, adrenaline, and cocaine anesthesia with lidocaine infiltration for repair of lacerations in children. *Annals of Emergency Medicine, 19*(1), 63–67.

Hernandez-Reif, M., Field, T., Largie, S., Hart, S., Redzepi, M., Nierenberg, B. et al. (2001). Children's distress during burn treatment is reduced by massage therapy. *Journal of Burn Care and Rehabilitation, 22*(2), 191–195.

Ho, J. W., Khambatta, H. J., Pang, L. M., Siegfried, R. N., & Sun, L. S. (1997). Preemptive analgesia in children. Does it exist? *Regional Anesthesia, 22*(2), 125–130.

Hoffman, G. M., Nowakowski, R., Troshynski, T. J., Berens, R. J., & Weisman, S. J. (2002). Risk reduction in pediatric procedural sedation by application of an American Academy of Pediatrics/American Society of Anesthesiologists process model. *Pediatrics, 109*(2), 236–243.

Holzki, J., Aring, C., & Gillor, A. (2004). Death after re-exposure to propofol in a 3-year-old child: A case report. *Paediatric Anaesthesia, 14*(3), 265–270.

Hosey, M. T., Makin, A., Jones, R. M., Gilchrist, F., & Carruthers, M. (2004). Propofol intravenous conscious sedation for anxious children in a specialist paediatric dentistry unit. *International Journal of Paediatric Dentistry, 14*(1), 2–8.

Hostetler, M. A., Auinger, P., & Szilagyi, P. G. (2002). Parenteral analgesic and sedative use among ED patients in the United States: Combined results from the National Hospital Ambulatory Medical Care Survey (NHAMCS) 1992–1997. *American Journal of Emergency Medicine 20*(2), 83–87; *20*(3), 139–143.

Howard, R. F. (2003). Current status of pain management in children. *Journal of the American Medical Association, 290*(18), 2464–2469.

Judkins, J. H., Dray, T. G., & Hubbell, R. N. (1996). Intraoperative ketorolac and posttonsillectomy bleeding. *Archives of Otolaryngology — Head and Neck Surgery, 122*(9), 937–940.

Karl, H. W., Rosenberger, J. L., Larach, M. G., & Ruffle, J. M. (1993). Transmucosal administration of midazolam for premedication of pediatric patients. Comparison of the nasal and sublingual routes. *Anesthesiology, 78*(5), 885–891.

Kasai, T., Yaegashi, K., Hirose, M., & Tanaka, Y. (2003). Spinal cord injury in a child caused by an accidental dural puncture with a single-shot thoracic epidural needle. *Anesthesia & Analgesia, 96*(1), 65–67.

Keeter, S., Benator, R. M., Weinberg, S. M., & Hartenberg, M. A. (1990). Sedation in pediatric CT: National survey of current practice. *Radiology, 175*(3), 745–752.

Kehlet, H. (1989). Surgical stress: The role of pain and analgesia. *British Journal of Anaesthesia, 63*(2), 189–195.

Kemper K. J., Sarah, R., Silver-Highfield, E., Xiarhos, E., Barnes, L., & Berde, C. (2000). On pins and needles? Pediatric pain patients' experience with acupuncture. *Pediatrics, 105*(4 Pt. 2), 941–947.

Kissin, I. (2000). Preemptive analgesia. *Anesthesiology, 93*(4), 1138–1143.

Kokinsky, E., & Thornberg, E. (2003). Postoperative pain control in children: A guide to drug choice. *Paediatric Drugs, 5*(11), 751–762.

Kokki, H. (2003). Nonsteroidal anti-inflammatory drugs for postoperative pain: A focus on children. *Paediatric Drugs, 5*(2), 103–123.

Korpela, R., Korvenoja, P., & Meretoja, O.A. (1999). Morphine-sparing effect of acetaminophen in pediatric day-case surgery. *Anesthesiology, 91*(2), 442–447.

Krane, E. J., Tyler, D. C., & Jacobson, L. E. (1989). The dose response of caudal morphine in children. *Anesthesiology, 71*(1), 48–52.

Kundra, P., Deepalakshmi, K., & Ravishankar, M. (1998). Preemptive caudal bupivacaine and morphine for postoperative analgesia in children. *Anesthesia & Analgesia, 87*(1), 52–56.

Kuttner, L., & Solomon, R. (2003). Hypnotherapy and imagery for managing children's pain. In N. L. Schechter, C. B. Berde, & M. Yaster (Eds.), *Pain in infants, children, and adolescents* (2nd ed., pp. 317–328). Philadelphia: Lippincott/Williams & Wilkins.

Lambert, S. A. (1996). The effects of hypnosis/guided imagery on the postoperative course of children. *Journal of Developmental and Behavioral Pediatrics, 17*(5), 307–310.

Lander, J., & Fowler-Kerry, S. (1993). TENS for children's procedural pain, *Pain, 52*(2), 209–216.

Lin, Y. (2003). Acupuncture. In N. L. Schechter, C. B. Berde & M. Yaster (Eds.), *Pain in infants, children and adolescents* (2nd ed., pp. 462–470). Philadelphia: Lippincott/Williams & Wilkins.

Litman, R. (1999). Sedatives/hypnotics. In B. Kraoss & R. M. Brustowicz, *Pediatric procedural sedation and analgesia* (pp. 39–46). Philadelphia: Lippincott/Williams & Wilkins.

Lloyd-Thomas, A. R., & Howard, R.. (1994). A pain service for children. *Paediatric Anaesthesia, 4*, 3–15.

Mallampati, S. R., Gatt, S. P., Gugino, L. D., Desai, S. P., Waraska, B., Freiberger, D. et al. (1985). A clinical sign to predict difficult tracheal intubation: A prospective study. *Canadian Anaesthetists' Society Journal, 32*(4), 429–434.

Mather, L., & Mackie, J. (1983). The incidence of postoperative pain in children. *Pain, 15*(3), 271–282.

Matsota, P., Livanios, S., & Marinopoulou, E. (2001). Intercostal nerve block with Bupivacaine for post-thoracotomy pain relief in children. *European Journal of Pediatric Surgery, 11*(4), 219–222.

Maunuksela, E., & Olkkola, K. T. (2003). Nonsteroidal anti-inflammatory drugs in pediatric pain management. In N. L. Schechter, C. B. Berde, & M. Yaster (Eds.), *Pain in infants, children and adolescents* (2nd ed., pp. 171–180). Philadelphia: Lippincott/Williams & Wilkins.

Maxwell, L. G., & Yaster, M. (1996). The myth of conscious sedation. *Archives of Pediatric and Adolescent Medicine, 150*(7), 665–667.

McDonnell, L., & Bowden, M. L. (1989). Breathing management: A simple stress and pain reduction strategy for use on a pediatric service. *Issues in Comprehensive Pediatric Nursing, 12*(5), 339–344.

McIlvaine, W. B. (1990). Spinal opioids for the pediatric patient. *Journal of Pain and Symptom Management, 5*(3), 183–190.

McNeely, J. K., Farber, N. E., Rusy, L. M., & Hoffman, G. M. (1997). Epidural analgesia improves outcome following pediatric fundoplication. A retrospective analysis. *Regional Anesthesia, 22*(1), 16–23.

McNeely, J. M., Pontus, S. P., & Trentadue, N. C. (1992). Comparison of patient controlled analgesia with and without basal morphine infusion for postoperative pain control in children. *Anesthesiology, 77*(3A), A814.

Merkel, S. I., Gutstein, H. B., & Malviya, S. (1999). Use of transcutaneous electrical nerve stimulation in a young child with pain from open perineal lesions. *Journal of Pain and Symptom Management, 18*(5), 376–381.

Moiniche, S., Kehlet, H, & Dahl, J. B. (2002). A qualitative and quantitative systematic review of preemptive analgesia for postoperative pain relief: The role of timing of analgesia. *Anesthesiology, 96*(3), 725–741.

Monitto, C. L., Greenberg, R. S., Kost-Byerly, S., Wetzel, R., Billett, C., Lebet, R. M. et al. (2000). The safety and efficacy of parent-/nurse-controlled analgesia in patients less than six years of age. *Anesthesia & Analgesia, 91*(3), 573–579.

Moro-Sutherland, D. M., Algren, J. T., Louis, P. T., Kozinetz, C. A., & Shook, J. E. (2000). Comparison of intravenous midazolam with pentobarbital for sedation for head computed tomography imaging. *Academic Emergency Medicine, 7*(12), 1370–1375.

Moss, V. A. (1988). Music and the surgical patient. The effect of music on anxiety. *AORN Journal, 48*(1), 64–69.

Mullooly, V. M., Levin, R. F., & Feldman, H. R. (1988). Music for postoperative pain and anxiety. *Journal of the New York State Nurses' Association, 19*(3), 4–7.

Nahata, M. C., Clotz, M. A., & Krogg, E. A. (1985). Adverse effects of meperidine, promethazine, and chlorpromazine for sedation in pediatric patients. *Clinical Pediatrics* (Philadelphia), *24*(10), 558–560.

Parke, T. J., Stevens, J. E., Rice, A. S., Greenaway, C. L., Bray, R. J., Smith, P. J. et al. (1992). Metabolic acidosis and fatal myocardial failure after propofol infusion in children: Five case reports. *British Medical Journal, 305*(6854), 613–616.

Petrack, E. M., Marx, C. M., & Wright, M. S. (1996). Intramuscular ketamine is superior to meperidine, promethazine, and chlorpromazine for pediatric emergency department sedation. *Archives of Pediatric and Adolescent Medicine, 150*(7), 676–681.

Pitetti, R. D., Singh, S., & Pierce, M. C. (2003). Safe and efficacious use of procedural sedation and analgesia by nonanesthesiologists in a pediatric emergency department. *Archives of Pediatric and Adolescent Medicine, 157*(11), 1090–1096.

Polkki, T., Pietila, A. M., & Vehvilainen-Julkunen, K. (2003). Hospitalized children's descriptions of their experiences with postsurgical pain relieving methods. *International Journal of Nursing Studies, 40*(1), 33–44.

Pomeranz, B. (1996). Scientific research into acupuncture for the relief of pain. *Journal of Alternative and Complementary Medicine, 2*(1), 53–60; discussion 73–75.

Ready, B. L. (2000). Acute postoperative pain. In R. D. Miller (Ed.), *Anesthesia* (pp. 2323–2350). New York: Churchill Livingston.

Reinhart, D., Palladinetti, T., Patel, M., Raja, H., & Courtney, B. (1992). IV Ketorolac vs. sufentanil for outpatient ENT surgery, a double-blind, randomized, placebo-controlled study. *Anesthesiology, 77*(3A), A31.

Romsing, J., Moiniche, S., & Dahl, J. B. (2002). Rectal and parenteral paracetamol, and paracetamol in combination with NSAIDs, for postoperative analgesia. *British Journal of Anaesthesia, 88*(2), 215–226.

Rosen, D. A., Morris, J. L., Rosen, K. R., Valenzuela, R. C., Vidulich, M. G., Steelman, R. J. et al. (2000). Analgesia for pediatric thoracostomy tube removal. *Anesthesia & Analgesia, 90*(5), 1025–1028.

Ross, A. K., Eck, J. B., & Tobias, J. D. (2000). Pediatric regional anesthesia: Beyond the caudal. *Anesthesia & Analgesia, 91*(1), 16–26.

Rusy, L. M., & Weisman, S. J. (2000). Complementary therapies for acute pediatric pain management. *Pediatric Clinics of North America, 47*(3), 589–599.

Rusy, L. M., Houck, C. S., Sullivan, L. J., Ohlms, L. A., Jones, D. T., McGill, T. J. et al. (1995). A double-blind evaluation of ketorolac tromethamine versus acetaminophen in pediatric tonsillectomy: Analgesia and bleeding. *Anesthesia & Analgesia, 80*(2), 226–229.

Sacchetti, A., Schafermeyer, R., Geradi, M., Graneto, J., Fuerst, R. S., Cantor, R. et al. (1994). Pediatric analgesia and sedation. *Annals of Emergency Medicine, 23*(2), 237–250.

Sahler, O. J., Hunter, B. C., & Liesveld, J. L. (2003). The effect of using music therapy with relaxation imagery in the management of patients undergoing bone marrow transplantation: A pilot feasibility study. *Alternative Therapies in Health and Medicine, 9*(6), 70–74.

Salmon, A. G., Kizer, K. W., Zeise, L., Jackson, R. J., & Smith, M. T. (1995). Potential carcinogenicity of chloral hydrate — A review. *Journal of Toxicology. Clinical Toxicology, 33*(2), 115–121.

Sandler, E. S., Weyman, C., Conner, K., Reilly, K., Dickson, N. Luzins, J. et al. (1992). Midazolam versus fentanyl as premedication for painful procedures in children with cancer. *Pediatrics, 89*(4 Pt. 1), 631–634.

Schechter, N. L. (1989). The undertreatment of pain in children: An overview. *Pediatric Clinics of North America, 36*(4), 781–794.

Schechter, N. L., Weisman, S. J., Rosenblum, M., Bernstein, B., & Conard, P. L. (1995). The use of oral transmucosal fentanyl citrate for painful procedures in children. *Pediatrics, 95*(3), 335–339.

Seigler, R. S., Avant, M. G., Gwyn, D. R., Lynch, A. A., Golding, E. M., Blackhurst, D. W., et al. (2001). A comparison of propofol and ketamine/midazolam for intravenous sedation of children. *Pediatric Critical Care Medicine, 2*(1), 20–23.

Selbst, S. M., & Zempsky, W. T. (2003). Sedation and analgesia in the emergency department. In N. L. Schechter, C. B. Berde, & M. Yaster (Eds.), *Pain in infants, children and adolescents* (2nd ed., pp. 651–668). Philadelphia: Lippincott/Williams & Wilkins.

Sethna, N. F., & Berde, C. B. (1994). Pediatric regional anesthesia. In G. A. Gregory (Ed.), *Pediatric anesthesia* (pp. 281–318). New York: Churchill Livingstone.

Shannon, M., & Berde, C. B. (1989). Pharmacologic management of pain in children and adolescents. *Pediatric Clinics of North America, 36*(4), 855–871.

Sharpe, P., Klein, J. R., Thompson, J. P., Rushman, S. C., Sherwin, J., Wandless, J. G. et al. (2001). Analgesia for circumcision in a paediatric population: Comparison of caudal bupivacaine alone with bupivacaine plus two doses of clonidine. *Paediatric Anaesthesia, 11*(6), 695–700.

Shenkman, Z., Holzman, R. S., Kim, C., Ferrari, L. R., DiCanzio, J., Highfield, E. S. et al. (1999). Acupressure-acupuncture antiemetic prophylaxis in children undergoing tonsillectomy. *Anesthesiology, 90* (5), 1311–1316.

Sheridan, R. L., Keaney, T., Stoddard, F., Enfanto, R., Kadillack, P., & Breault, L. (2003). Short-term propofol infusion as an adjunct to extubation in burned children. *Journal of Burn Care and Rehabilitation, 24*(6), 356–360.

Sievers, T. D., Yee, J. D., Foley, M. E., Blanding, P. J., & Berde, C. B. (1991). Midazolam for conscious sedation during pediatric oncology procedures: Safety and recovery parameters. *Pediatrics, 88*(6), 1172–1179.

Smith, S. M., & Barry, R. C. (1990). A comparison of three formulations of TAC (tetracaine, adrenalin, cocaine) for anesthesia of minor lacerations in children. *Pediatric Emergency Care, 6*(4), 266–270.

Squire, S. J., Kirchhoff, K. T., & Hissong, K. (2000). Comparing two methods of topical anesthesia used before intravenous cannulation in pediatric patients. *Journal of Pediatric Health Care, 14*(2), 68–72.

Strain, J. D., Harvey, L. A., Foley, L. C., & Campbell, J. B. (1986). Intravenously administered pentobarbital sodium for sedation in pediatric CT. *Radiology, 161*(1), 105–108.

Streisand, J. B., Stanley, T. H., Hague, B., van Vreeswijk, H., Ho, G. H., & Pace, N. L. (1989). Oral transmucosal fentanyl citrate premedication in children. *Anesthesia & Analgesia, 69*(1), 28–34.

Suresh, S., Barcelona, S. L., Young, N. M., Heffner, C. L., & Coté, C. J. (2004). Does a preemptive block of the great auricular nerve improve postoperative analgesia in children undergoing tympanomastoid surgery? *Anesthesia & Analgesia, 98*(2), 330–333.

Taddio, A., Nulman, I., Goldbach, M., Ipp, M., & Koren, G. (1994). Use of lidocaine-prilocaine cream for vaccination pain in infants. *Journal of Pediatrics, 124*(4), 643–648.

Taylor, G., & Boswell, M. V. (1991). Continuous epidural infusion of low dose morphine for postoperative analgesia in children. *Anesthesiology, 75*(3A), A937.

Tobias, J. D. (2002). Therapeutic applications of regional anaesthesia in paediatric-aged patients. *Paediatric Anaesthesia, 12*(3), 272–277.

Tobias, J. D., Phipps, S., Smith, B., & Mulhern, R. K. (1992). Oral ketamine premedication to alleviate the distress of invasive procedures in pediatric oncology patients. *Pediatrics, 90*(4), 537–541.

Tobias, J. D., Schleien, C. L., & Haun, S. E. (1990). Methadone as treatment for iatrogenic narcotic dependency in pediatric intensive care unit patients. *Critical Care Medicine, 18*(11), 1292–1293.

Tolia, V., Brennan, S., Aravind, M. K., & Kauffman R. E. (1991). Pharmacokinetic and pharmacodynamic study of midazolam in children during esophagogastroduodenoscopy. *Journal of Pediatrics, 119*(3), 467–471.

U.S. Department of Health and Human Services National Toxicology Program. (2002, December). Toxicology and carcinogenicity study of chloral hydrate (*ad libitum* and dietary controlled) (CAS no. 302-17-0) in male B6C3F1 mice (gavage study). *National Toxicology Program Technical Report Series* (503), 1–218.

Valley, R. D., & Bailey, A. G. (1991). Caudal morphine for postoperative analgesia in infants and children: A report of 138 cases. *Anesthesia & Analgesia, 72*(1), 120–124.

Watcha, M., Jones, M., Schweiger, C., Lagueruela, R., & White, R. F. (1991). A comparison of ketorolac and morphine when used during pediatric surgery. *Anesthesiology, 75*(3A), A942.

Weber, F., & Wulf, H. (2003). Caudal bupivacaine and s(+) ketamine for postoperative analgesia in children. *Paediatric Anaesthesia, 13*(3), 244–248.

Weldon, B. C., Connor, M., & White, P. F. (1991). Nurse-controlled versus patient-controlled analgesia following pediatric scoliosis surgery. *Anesthesiology, 75*(3A), A935.

Wheeler, D. S., Vaux, K. K., Ponaman, M. L., & Poss, B. W. (2003). The safe and effective use of propofol sedation in children undergoing diagnostic and therapeutic procedures: Experience in a pediatric ICU and a review of the literature. *Pediatric Emergency Care, 19*(6), 385–392.

Wilder, R. T., Berde, C. B., Troshynski, T. J., Cahill, C. A., & Sethna, N. F. (1992). Patient-controlled analgesia in children and adolescents: Safety and outcome among 1,589 patients. *Anesthesiology, 77*(3A), A1187.

Woolf, C. J., & Chong, M. S. (1993). Preemptive analgesia--Treating postoperative pain by preventing the establishment of central hypersensitization. *Anesthesia & Analgesia, 77*(2), 362–379.

Yaster, M. (1995). Pain relief. *Pediatrics, 95*(3), 427–428.

Yaster, M., Kost-Byerly, S., & Maxwell, L. G. (2003). Opioid agonists and antagonists. In N. L. Schechter, C. B. Berde, & M. Yaster (Eds.), *Pain in infants, children, and adolescents* (2nd ed., pp. 181–224). Philadelphia: Lippincott/Williams & Wilkins.

Yaster, M., Nichols, D. G., Deshpande, J. K., & Wetzel, R. C. (1990). Midazolam-fentanyl intravenous sedation in children: Case report of respiratory arrest. *Pediatrics, 86*(3), 463–467.

Zeltzer, L., & LeBaron, S. (1982). Hypnosis and nonhypnotic techniques for reduction of pain and anxiety during painful procedures in children and adolescents with cancer. *Journal of Pediatrics, 101*(6), 1032–1035.

87

Occupational Medicine for the Pain Practitioner

Hal Blatman, MD

INTRODUCTION

The pain management professional may interface with the field of occupational medicine in many aspects of medical practice. Several scenarios are most likely:

- Patient may have been injured at work
- Work may be perpetuating the patient's pain and injury
- Patient may be trying to continue working
- Patient may be trying to return to work after/during treatment for pain
- Patient may be disabled from work

To understand these scenarios the health care worker should be aware of the needs of the patient and the needs of the workplace. The best circumstances are when these needs are not in conflict. Sometimes the treating physician or other medical caregiver is pressured by one party or the other. In these circumstances, it is helpful to be able to put these varied needs into perspective.

MEDICAL CARE OF THE INJURED WORKER

The physician's role may be direct patient care. Employers understand that delayed return to work is predictive of long-term disability. They therefore may make every effort to bring the injured person back to work as soon as possible. Also, companies may be penalized for each day that an employee is off work. These situations are called "lost time injuries." Sometimes it is to the company's advantage to bring an employee back to work doing light duty, which in some cases amounts to doing almost nothing but lying down in the nurse's office.

In patient care, the treating physician may be contacted by the workplace and asked to return the patient to work on "light duty" instead of keeping the patient off work. Finding a balance between the needs of the patient and the needs of the company is very important. An uncompromising position may result in the patient being dismissed from his or her job. Conversely, submitting to the will of the company may put the patient in jeopardy of further injury or otherwise delay healing. The best solution is to facilitate a return to work that does not jeopardize the patient. Limited or light duty is an option for the prescribing doctor. A "return to work" note is a prescription that places physical limitations on what the company can expect the patients/employees to do in performance of their job duties. The practitioner has several choices and an opportunity for creativity. Some suggestions include:

- Limit work hours per day or per week, and/or days per week
- Limit body activities
- Specify how much weight can be lifted
- Specify how much bending and stooping
- Specify how much walking and/or standing
- Specify how much working above chest height
- Specify a need for breaks to stretch or rest
- Specify how often and how long
- Specify what needs to be stretched or rested

The prescription may be worded in a positive or negative fashion. An example of a positive-worded limitation is: May lift up to 25 lb on an occasional basis. Example of negative-worded limitations is: May not lift over 25 lb, and may not lift repetitively. Another style is to say that the patient may return to work with accommodations, and then list each of these specifically.

In consideration of returning to work, industry has recognized that the longer patients are off work, the more difficult it is to get them back to work. From the standpoint of patient care, patients who are off work longer become more physically deconditioned. They may also become more depressed because of their inability to function and contribute. Many patients will benefit physically and psychologically by early return to work if they can be adequately protected from harm by the prescription of limitations.

Sometimes the patient may not be capable of performing at any level of light duty, and sometimes the company may not have a light duty program that can accommodate the prescribed medical restrictions. In these cases, the employer and insurance disability carrier may need to know projected length of time of disability and recommendations for rehabilitation.

Occasionally, a worker suffers injury by violence or abuse in the workplace. These cases have compounding issues beyond any physical problem.

INDEPENDENT MEDICAL EXAMINATION

An independent medical examination (IME) is an evaluation by a health care professional who is not involved in caring for and does not know the particular patient. This person is contracted by the requesting party for the purpose of providing a fresh look at particular issues (McCunney, 2003). It is generally thought that the treating professional may be biased toward the patient's interests, or even his or her own selfish interests. An IME provides for an impartial professional who can offer opinions on issues in question.

Employers and insurance companies hire doctors and therapists to provide opinions about an injured person's condition, diagnosis, treatment, and disability. The general purpose is to clarify medical and job-related issues. Reports provide information for case management and for evidence in legal proceedings. Sometimes these evaluations are based solely on medical records, and sometimes they are also based upon office testing and examination. The pain management professional may be called upon to perform such an evaluation. The patient in question will not be under this professional's care, and the examining professional is generally not allowed to establish a future doctor–patient or treatment relationship.

In this situation, it is important to carefully examine any documents presented for review, perform and document any requested examination, and then carefully answer the questions posed by the hiring agency. Anything written in the report should be based on the presented information, examination if indicated, and the examiner's training and experience. Usually the report is all that is needed. Sometimes the examiner will be asked to testify in court about the stated information.

After an IME, the treating professional may be in the position of having to write a rebuttal report. These reports should carefully address the issues, using history, examination findings, treatment results, appropriate references, and opinions.

The insurance company or employer may indeed be looking for the best answers for the person involved. In this case, opinions are sought to ascertain that the employee/insured is getting the best possible care and therefore has the best likelihood for recovery and return to work.

Alternatively, the insurance company or employer may be primarily interested in reducing costs and financial exposure. In this case, opinions are sought in an effort to minimize medical and disability costs. In general, IMEs are more likely to be requested in cases with prolonged recovery and disability. The goal may be to ascertain the necessity, effectiveness, and duration of treatment, or to assess the validity and duration of disability.

The injured or disabled worker may also request an IME. This may be requested through an attorney, or directly by the patient. Generally the purpose of the evaluation is to gather data from a "non-interested" party in order to support the need for treatment or the validity of disability.

IMEs may also be requested to obtain an opinion regarding causation of an injury. This may be a critical issue in work-related injury and liability cases. Work-related problems are defined as those that arise out of and during the course of employment. There may be preexisting chronic conditions and other exposures to injury. The practitioner may be asked to provide an opinion regarding causation to a reasonable degree of medical probability. Reasonable degree means more than a 50% chance of occurrence. An ultimate cause is one that is the initial factor that leads to the problem. A proximate cause is one that occurs just before or closest to the origin of the problem. Because a medical or psychological condition may be the result of one or several factors, it is often necessary, at some point, to portion treatment cost or disability between parties and events.

IMEs may also be requested to evaluate a person for an impairment rating. These examinations and evaluations are usually based on *The AMA Guides,* a textbook that can be purchased from the American Medical Association (Cocchiarella & Anderson, 2001). The American College of Occupational and Environmental Medicine organizes courses to train doctors in performing these evaluations.

WORK-RELATED INJURIES

Most injuries at work are caused by overexertion. These are generally lifting injuries. Injuries are also caused by repetitive motion, vibration of tools, heat or cold stress, falls, and direct trauma.

The most frequent cause of activity limitation in people younger than 45 years is back pain (Anderson, 1997). It is also one of the most frequent reasons for visits to the doctor and a high ranking reason for surgical procedures.

Work-related musculoskeletal disorders of the upper extremity and neck come mainly from repetitive motion injuries, applying force with the hands, mechanical stresses, vibration, and sustained or awkward postures. The best-known upper extremity disorder is carpal tunnel syndrome. Other disorders include epicondylitis, tendonitis, and bursitis in various places.

Repetitive motion injuries occur when the required task of motion exceeds the body's ability to recover before it is asked to move again. If muscular contraction is more forceful, these injuries are more severe. If the muscle fails to recover, there is generally some type of tissue damage. Tissue changes can also lead to nerve compression, chronic fibrous reaction in the tendon, tendon rupture, calcium deposits, fibrous nodule formations, and trigger finger (Gorsche et al., 1998). Repetitive motion also causes muscle tightening, fascial tightening, and activation/perpetuation of myofascial trigger points (Travell & Simons, 1983).

Work performed in a static posture may also trigger chronic localized pain. Even muscle contractions of low force can activate trigger points if the muscle remains contracted to stabilize the body in a particular position for a period of time.

Examples of highly repetitive tasks include typing, meat processing, and factory assembly work. A data entry worker may perform 20,000 keystrokes per hour. Meat cutters in a processing plant may make 12,000 knife cuts per day. Assembly line workers may elevate their shoulder 7,500 times per shift (Anderson, 1997).

Workers who return to work after an injury, or even after sick time or vacation time, are extremely susceptible to repetitive motion injuries. This increased vulnerability is caused by deconditioning during time off.

Another common cause for these injuries is "speeding up the line," or suddenly increasing the worker's number of repetitive motions performed per day (Thompson, Plewes, & Shaw, 1951). In these cases, the conditioned worker is not able to suddenly perform at a higher level.

Mechanical stress results from direct force on a part of the body. An example is hand injury caused by tightly gripping a tool that has cold, sharp edges and a short handle. The use of better-designed tools has greatly reduced these types of injuries in more modern shops.

Vibration also causes injury to connective tissue and nerves. Impact drills, handheld power tools, and bench-mounted grinding tools can all transmit vibration to the hands and upper extremities (Pelmear, Taylor, & Wasserman, 1992). This vibration contributes to the development

of work-related Raynaud's phenomenon (Levy and Wegman, 2000). It may also contribute to carpal tunnel syndrome and other compressive nerve disorders (Falkiner, 2003).

Splints are commonly used to immobilize and allow an injured extremity to rest. These may be harmful if they force the worker to resist or fight the splint in order to perform regular job tasks.

Psychological factors may be important in the initial development of work related injuries, and subsequent disability.

National statistics are available for work-related injuries. The source of this data is the Bureau of Labor Statistics BLS Annual Survey of Occupational Injuries and Illnesses. This is a federal/state program where employer reports are collected from private industry (www/bls/gov).

Most new workers who perform unaccustomed strenuous or repetitive tasks will experience muscle pain. A more gradual "break-in" can allow conditioning to occur with a minimum of soreness (Parker, 1992). This issue becomes especially important for the patient with chronic pain who goes on vacation. In as little as 1 week, muscles will become deconditioned. The pain practitioner should encourage the patient to maintain an active exercise program to prevent deconditioning while on vacation.

Chronic muscle pain or myalgia can be diagnosed as myofascial pain syndrome after identification of taut bands and trigger points during physical examination. This pain can result from repetitive motion and muscle overuse. Sometimes a seemingly simple myalgia may progress to a more diffuse and chronic myofascial pain syndrome with resultant dysfunction and eventual disability.

Tendonitis and tenosynovitis are inflammatory conditions of the tendon that result from tendon injury. Tendons may be injured by mechanical stress of pulling, friction stress, and snapping or rubbing over a bony prominence. Some tendons have a protective sheath, but tendons at the elbow do not have a sheath. When these become inflamed, the medical condition is termed "tendonitis." Tendons in the hand and fingers have sheaths to assist in lubrication and protection of the tendon. When these become inflamed, the condition is termed "tenosynovitis."

Epicondylitis is a tendon inflammation at the elbow that is caused by repetitive motion of the wrist. De Quervain's tenosynovitis is an inflammation of the abductor pollicis longus and extensor pollicis brevis tendons of the thumb.

Trigger finger is also associated with repetitive hand use. This occurs when a nodule forms in a flexor tendon of the hand and becomes large enough to cause clicking when the finger joints are flexed or extended. Larger nodules may cause the finger to get stuck in a flexed position.

Ganglion cysts are also associated with repetitive joint motion. The wrist is most commonly involved. These cysts occur when the synovial lining of the joint herniates through the fibrous joint capsule, creating a bubble attached to a stalk. Cysts tend to enlarge with physical activity, and they may shrink with a period of rest or immobilization. Needle aspiration may be successful, but definitive therapy is generally surgical removal of the cyst and stalk.

ERGONOMICS

Ergonomics is a word that comes from the Greek words *ergos*, meaning work, and *nomos*, meaning laws. It has become a buzzword that is used to describe a variety of conditions and objects from specific tasks in the work environment to tool design and seating. The terms *ergonomics* and *human factors* are sometimes used interchangeably. Most people recognize use of the term *ergonomics* in relation to seating and task analysis. The term is also used in relation to lighting and the psychology of shift work. Practically speaking, the term ergonomics relates to the interface between people and their environment. In the academic setting, the ergonomist may be found in the departments of biomechanics, engineering, medicine, and psychology.

When treating patients with pain, an awareness of basic ergonomic principles will serve the practitioner well. With an understanding of these principles, the caregiver can be more effective in helping impaired people function in their environment, both to a greater level, and with less discomfort.

SUPPLY AND DEMAND

When physical demands are placed on body tissues, these structures generally require more resources. These resources are delivered by the blood supply to the tissue. They include oxygen, nutrition, and removal of byproducts. When a muscle is resting, the cells require less nutritional support than when it is contracting. A resting muscle is softer and blood flow through the muscle is relatively unobstructed. This allows blood to flow more freely, and the tissue has plenty of resources.

When muscles contract to perform work, the muscle cells require nutrients at a higher level. This level is in proportion to the work that is being performed. Alternately contracting and relaxing muscles pump blood and therefore increase their nutrient supply.

Sustained posture occurs when a muscle is contracting to maintain a posture or position. A muscle sustaining contraction requires even more nutrients than a muscle that is alternately contracting and relaxing. Unfortunately, blood flow is hampered by the increased pressure within a contracting muscle. In this case, the nutrient requirements of the muscle are increased and the blood supply is relatively decreased. This leads to a significant imbalance with respect to nutrient "supply and demand." It

therefore costs the body more to stay in one position (sustained posture), than it costs to move.

This concept can be simply illustrated by trying to hold one arm straight out in front of the body, keeping it perfectly still. Before long, the muscles fatigue, and the arm seems to get very heavy. Later, after a few minutes of rest, hold the arm straight out in front of the body again. This time move the hand and arm in small circles. This slight movement of the arm and shoulder results in some degree of alternate relaxing and contracting of the deltoid and trapezius muscles. Even small motions will facilitate blood flow and nutrient supply. Usually with the arm making small motions, the feeling of fatigue is noticed more slowly, and the length of time this posture/motion can be maintained is significantly longer. If nutrient supply and metabolic byproduct removal are facilitated by muscular contraction and relaxation, the physical activity can be maintained for a longer period of time and with less fatigue.

The concept of muscle tissue nutrient supply and demand has clinical relevance with pain patients with pain. Many such patients relate that they do better when they are moving, and that they have problems sitting or standing in one position for any length of time. Sometimes maintaining one position causes stiffness, and sometimes it causes an increase in pain. For many people, even 15 minutes of a sustained posture is considered a prolonged period of time. It should be realized that even sitting in a "relaxed" position might require significant static contraction of supportive and balancing musculature. This "relaxation" may translate to increased stiffness and pain. Instructing patients with low back pain to slightly wiggle or otherwise move their hips every few minutes while sitting can greatly increase the length of time that seated posture can be maintained. This is likely to be important when sitting at the office as well as when riding in a car.

REPETITIVE MOTION INJURY

Repetitive motion injury (RMI) has previously been termed "repetitive strain injury" (RSI) and also "cumulative trauma disorder" (CTD). Nationally, the Bureau of Labor Statistics calls these conditions "illnesses" and not injuries. OSHA (Occupational Safety and Health Administration), NIOSH (National Institute of Occupational Safety and Health), and the National Academy of Science have replaced these terms with the more neutral "work related musculo-skeletal disorders."

Tissue pathology with respect to repetitive motion injuries is generally believed to primarily involve inflammation. Typical diagnoses that fall into this definition include tennis elbow, shoulder bursitis, tendonitis, and carpal tunnel syndrome. Treatment protocols for these conditions may include splinting, physical therapy modalities, anti-inflammatory medication, cortisone injections, and surgery.

For many people, these treatments are not effective. One reason is that pathology of RSI is not simply inflammation. Indeed, the primary pathology may be trigger points and myofascial pain. Tennis elbow, for example, is associated with myofascial trigger points in the muscles that dorsiflex and supinate the wrist. Shoulder bursitis is associated with myofascial trigger points in various shoulder girdle muscles.

MYOFASCIAL TRIGGER POINTS WITH REPETITIVE STRAIN INJURY

It is important to examine patients experiencing pain for myofascial trigger points in muscle groups that cause and/or refer pain to the area of complaint. Repetitive motion activities will cause formation of new trigger points, as well as activation of "latent" trigger points. As myofascial trigger points become more active, they generate more pain.

Sustained posture activities will cause tightening of the active muscles, as well as generalized tightening of the fascia through the muscle tissue. In addition, myofascial trigger points within the muscle will become more active. This increase in trigger point activity will cause an increase in pain, both localized and referred.

CARPAL TUNNEL SYNDROME

Carpal tunnel syndrome (CTS) is usually suspected when there is numbness and/or tingling in the thumb, index, long finger, and the thumb-side half (radial aspect) of the ring finger. People may also be awakened at night by pain in the wrist and forearm. When symptoms progress, people experience forearm and hand weakness, and even light objects such as coffee cups may be dropped.

The condition is often job or activity related, and people who use their hands a lot may be at risk for developing the problem. CTS has been associated with wrist and hand positioning, repetitive wrist use, use of heavy or vibrating tools, trauma, and light work such as typing.

CTS has traditionally been thought of as a condition resulting from flexor tendon inflammation or swelling that is caused by repetitive motion of the forearm, wrist, and hand. It is thought that when people use their fingers and bend their wrists a lot, the tendons in the tunnel become inflamed, thereby causing them to swell. Because the borders of the tunnel are fixed and there is no extra room in the tunnel for this swelling, pressure on the median nerve increases, causing numbness, tingling, and pain in the fingers and forearm.

The size of the carpal canal is not constant. The canal is largest when the wrist is in neutral (dorsiflexed 15°) position. It gets smaller when the wrist is bent in any direction. When bent positioning compromises canal size,

an already marginal situation can be made worse, and this may induce symptoms of numbness and tingling in the fingers and forearm. To evaluate this, a Phalens test can be performed. This test is performed by palmar flexing the wrist approximately 90°. The test is considered to be positive if the thumb, index, long, or ring fingers start to tingle within 30 to 60 seconds. Usually the positive result is recorded as well as the time (in seconds) required for the numbness to be appreciated.

In accordance with this inflammation model, the treatment for CTS traditionally involves keeping the wrist in a "neutral posture" and taking anti-inflammatory medication. Wrist braces are often recommended to ensure that the wrist remains straight, especially during work and sleep. To further aid in reducing the theorized inflammation, cortisone may be injected into the canal. When these treatments do not work well enough, surgeons will cut the transverse carpal ligament so the tunnel can expand to make room for the swollen tendons. Even when surgery is helpful, the condition will usually recur when people return to their same jobs. Work modification is often an important part of returning these people to gainful employment.

There is also a very different way to think about CTS. Recent research has demonstrated that the theorized inflammation of the wrist tendons may not occur (Nathan & Keniston, 1996). Other research has indicated that there are exercises that can be done to treat and prevent CTS and that this treatment may be more successful than the traditionally prescribed medication and surgery (Seradge, Bear, & Bithell, 2000; Seradge et al., 2002).

A more modern idea to explain the pathophysiology of carpal tunnel syndrome is that it actually starts in the biceps muscle of the arm, and not in the wrist. People who use their wrists and fingers a lot, steady and support their forearms and hands with a sustained contraction of the biceps muscle. This continuous contraction of the biceps muscle eventually causes tightening of the connective tissue in the arm, called fascia. The biceps muscle crosses the elbow joint and attaches to the radius bone in the forearm. Because the biceps muscle is a part of the forearm, it also pulls on the fascia of the forearm. With time and continued sustained biceps contractions, the fascia in both the arm and forearm tightens. As this process continues, the transverse carpal ligament (fascia) also tightens. When this ligament tightens, the carpal tunnel gets smaller. Indeed, CTS may be caused by the canal itself getting smaller. This helps explain the lack of inflammation on histology, and the effectiveness of exercises in treatment.

TOOLS

Tool design is an important consideration when a job or task needs to be made more "body friendly." There are catalogs of "ergonomic" tools for many different jobs and functions. In examining the use of tools and considering their modification, basic ergonomic principles provide important guidance.

One very important rule is that wherever possible, the tool should be bent, not the wrist. The wrist should be kept in a neutral position as much as possible, and the less the wrist deviates from neutral posture, the better. Also, the amount of grip force a hand can apply is greatly reduced when the wrist moves from a neutral to a flexed position. Bent-handled pliers, hammers, and power tools are examples of commercially available alternatives to standard gripped models. These tool modifications allow the worker leverage and mechanical strength while keeping the wrist in a neutral position.

Another consideration in evaluating tools is to investigate the quality of the surface that comes in contact with the body. Bare metal is cold. In tools run by compressed air, the surface gets even cooler with use. Sharp edges of handles can put significant pressure on the skin, tendons and nerves (Putz-Anderson, 1988). An example of poor tool handle design is a pair of metal-handled pliers where the handle has sharp square edges. Design improvements would include rounding the handles and covering them with a thin, tacky, cushioned, and insulating material.

In checking for factors that contribute to CTS, notice whether the tool handle presses directly upon the carpal canal. A cold hard surface that pounds or vibrates against the wrist can be problematic.

HEADSETS AND PHONE USE

Telephone use can be a significant factor in perpetuation of myofascial pain and tension of the head and neck. There are three major muscular force directions that are applied during ordinary phone use. First, the hand piece is held up to the level of the ear and mouth. This requires sustained postural contraction of the upper trapezius muscle. Second, most people push the earpiece into the ear in an effort to hear better and drown out outside noise. This activity demands even a more forceful contraction of muscles that raise the arm. Finally, the lateral neck muscles must contract to push back against the force of the earpiece pushing against the ear. In summary, the upper trapezius and lateral neck muscles contract more forcefully and remain contracted to maintain this posture.

An even worse scenario occurs when a patient attempts to hold the phone receiver by pinching it between the shoulder and ear. This activity requires the upper shoulder and lateral neck muscles to contract and maintain a posture with the muscles shortened. The ingredients of postural contraction and shortened muscles are very strong perpetuators for activation of myofascial trigger points and myofascial pain. Sometimes even 30 sec-

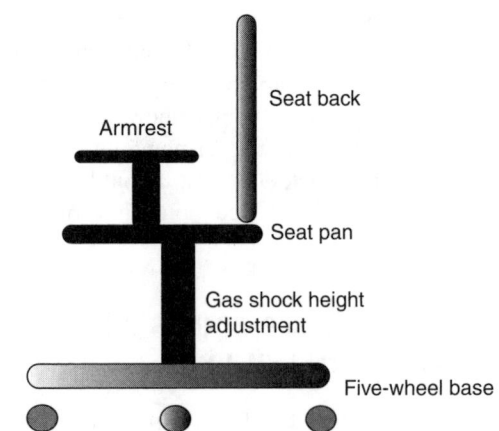

FIGURE 87.1 Adjustable and standard components of an ergonomic chair.

onds of holding the phone in this manner can cause a "stiff neck" the next day.

A headset can significantly minimize the effect of phone use as a perpetuating factor in cases of myofascial head and neck pain. The set should be comfortable, have variable amplification, and perhaps block out some outside noise. The treating physician should be sensitive to this and not hesitate to prescribe a headset for job modification when phone use is a suspected cause of a patient's head and neck pain.

ERGONOMIC SEATING

The chair should be designed to support a person's body in whatever position is best for performing necessary tasks and reducing musculoskeletal fatigue. Generally the chair is mobile and supported by five wheels. Sometimes motion is not desired, and stability requirements are such that the chair is attached to the floor. Seat pan, back rest, and arm rest positions should be variable. When these attributes are variable, the chair will be able to support more variations of body type in more positions. Better chairs are usually adjustable. This will give the worker more choices regarding available positions for which the chair can provide good body support (Dainoff, 1998).

Ergonomic chairs have several adjustable parts. These include seat back, seat pan, armrests, height adjustment, and castors (Figure 87.1).

The seat pan is the part of the chair that the buttocks sit upon. There is usually a gas shock underneath that allows easy adjustment of height. The seat pan may also tilt forward and backward to allow for variations of thigh and foot position. In some chairs, the seat pan can also be slipped forward and backward to accommodate different thigh lengths.

Seatbacks can be made to adjust forward and backward. They may or may not be adjustable independently of the seat pan. Some chairs allow for rocking and may also allow for locking in any position of tilt. Executive chairs typically have high backs, and secretary chairs do not. Some chairs have a variable height or pressure lumbar support, and some also have a neck support.

Not all people fit their chairs. Armrests are supposed to support the arms, taking weight off the upper shoulder muscles. They can be adjustable up, down, in, out, forward, and backward. Up and down adjustments allow for varied arm and body lengths, accommodating short and tall people with short or long arms. In and out adjustment makes it easier for wide and thin people to fit in the chair. Forward and backward adjustment makes it possible to support the arms of people who need to reach forward with their forearms at desk height.

Secretary chairs traditionally do not have armrests. This practice is discouraged by ergonomists, because the typist also requires arm and shoulder support.

Foot support is part of ergonomic seating. The feet should not dangle in the air. If the feet do not comfortably reach the floor, a foot support should be provided.

POSTURE FOR KEYBOARD WORK

It used to be thought that typists should be seated in an upright position with the typewriter at desk level and the copy flat on the desk. For some people, this posture may require significant energy expenditure, causing fatigue and discomfort. Many people find that a "partial relaxed slouch" is more comfortable. Efficient posture depends upon the particular typing task that is being performed. Many data-entry workers and typists prefer the copy to be propped up on a stand next to the monitor.

COMPUTER MONITOR

Monitor positions and body postures cannot be standardized for all tasks. There are, however, some general concepts and ideas to consider.

When using a computer, the eyes should be able to look slightly downward at the monitor. Tearing, important for nutrition and lubrication of the cornea, is increased with downward gaze angle. In addition, the neck should be comfortable and not in a forward leaning posture.

Other more recent introductions into office furniture concepts place the monitor inside the desk under a glass surface. If desk or counter space constraints are of primary importance, this may be optimal for the particular situation. Forward head tilting, however, will contribute to fatigue in the upper shoulder, upper back, and neck muscles.

Sometimes the most comfortable and best-supported posture will be "slouching." This posture may be optimal when typing from copy that is propped up so that the typist can look out with only a slight downward angle. While perhaps more comfortable, this posture may restrict the

operator's reach, making it more difficult to answer the phone, refer to other materials, and open a drawer. When typing without copy, it may be most comfortable to lie back, as in a dentist's chair, keyboard in the lap, with the monitor suspended above at a comfortable distance. This posture may be limited to young "hackers" who can tolerate decreased tearing that is associated with supine posture.

Upright posture seems to be more appropriate when typing from copy that is flat on the desk. This position will also allow reaching for more objects.

APPLICATION OF ERGONOMIC PRINCIPLES IN MEDICAL PAIN PRACTICE

During initial interviews and as patients progress in treatment, it will become evident that certain activities seem to be associated with an increase in pain symptoms. The activities may vary from specific job tasks to the use of tools and even posture, such as riding in a car or standing at a counter.

One of the most important considerations for the practitioner is the need to accurately understand the particular task or job environment involved. Obviously, the most direct way is to perform a site visit and see the activity in question on a firsthand basis. This, however, may be logistically difficult.

A much less expensive and often suitably effective method for performing a "site" visit is to ask the patient to bring pictures or a video of his or her worksite and activities. Two sets of pictures, each with two or three different perspectives, should be obtained. One set should include the workspace, chair, and furniture layout without the patient in the pictures. Another set of pictures should include poses in positions and postures that are used in performing the job. It is important to see the patient lift, stoop, answer the phone, type on the keyboard, go into the file, lean on the counter, etc. The patient should be instructed not to pose, but to simply act naturally. It is helpful to film realistic posture, lifting techniques, and true phone habits.

The task of taking pictures involves people in their own medical care and makes them start to think about the possibility of changing their environment. It also demonstrates that the medical practitioner is willing to "go the extra mile" in an effort to be helpful.

These pictures can be reviewed during the context of an office visit. The practitioner can see where basic ergonomic principles can be applied to support the body, and minimize sustained posture, repetitive strain, and poor lifting habits.

When giving professional advice regarding changing aspects of the work environment, it is important to make suggestions that are not costly and that can be tested easily. These suggestions should be based on basic ergonomic principles and common sense. Follow-up is also very important, as the success or failure of these suggestions cannot be accurately predicted. Review of corrective actions and results of these efforts provides an environment for continued modification and refinement that is important in any ergonomic safety program. If a situation becomes too complicated and modifications do not work out as hoped, it may be time to consult with a professional ergonomist.

AMERICANS WITH DISABILITIES ACT

The Americans with Disabilities Act (ADA), Public Law 336 of the 101st Congress, was enacted on July 26, 1990. This law prohibits discrimination and ensures equal opportunity for people with disabilities in employment, state and local government services, public and commercial facilities, and transportation.

The law is based on common sense. Prospective employees must meet all the requirements of the job and be able to perform the essential functions of the job, with or without reasonable accommodation. No accommodation is required to be provided if it would result in an undue hardship for the employer, and no unqualified job applicant or employee with a disability can claim employment discrimination under the ADA.

When the pain practitioner sends a patient back to work, the patient should apply only for jobs where there is confidence that there is physical and mental ability to perform the essential functions of the job. The company is prevented from seeking information about medical disability until after a job offer has been made. This allows disabled workers an opportunity to enter the labor market without facing employer bias against them.

The accessibility portion of the law requires that public places remove architectural barriers in existing facilities when it is readily achievable. Additional information about the ADA can be found at www.ada.gov.

DRUG SCREENS

The patient with chronic pain may require medication as part of medical treatment. When these patients return to work, either at their previous job or looking for a new job, they may be required to have their urine screened for drugs as part of company policy. Many companies require these tests as part of preemployment medical screening. In these cases, the purpose of a drug screen test is to discover the prospective employee drug abuser prior to hiring. The prospective employees will fill out a form that declares what prescription medicines they are currently taking. Illicit drugs will usually be detected. Prescription pain medications may also be discovered. A medical review officer will compare the results of the test with the decla-

ration form the prospective employee has filled out. Discrepancies and illicit drugs will be reported to the company. Discovery of prescription medications, even those taken for pain, is not generally supposed to be reported as a positive test.

Drug screens are also used as part of company injury prevention programs. The company may require all injured employees to undergo drug testing while in a medical facility for treatment of their injury.

PAIN MEDICATION AND RETURN TO WORK

Many patients with chronic pain are able to return to work without resolution of their pain condition, provided they are taking medication for treatment of their pain. Because this is a common practice, it is generally thought to be safe for pain patients to take such medications and work. There is particular concern with regard to patients who operate machinery, drive vehicles, fly aircraft, and depend on quick judgment in difficult situations. The prescribing physician should consider whether there might be hazards to the patient or others from the effects of these medications. Also, any potentially dangerous occupation should perhaps be avoided for several days after starting therapy with psychoactive or pain medications. This will allow stabilization of the medication and observation for any unwanted effects. If such a patient is injured or causes injury to others, the medical practitioner may be asked to testify regarding this issue.

PAIN MEDICATION AND DRIVING

Patients with chronic pain take opioid medication and drive automobiles. These medications generally preclude patients from driving jobs in public transportation and trucking, and piloting jobs in the airline industry. In private life, state laws govern this issue. In some states, a positive drug test after an automobile accident is a DUI (driving under the influence) by definition.

INDOOR ENVIRONMENTAL QUALITY

Concern about the safety of modern building environments began after several events that occurred in the 1970s and 1980s. The situations typically involved contamination levels within permissible exposure limits, and some investigators suggested that the office worker complaints were due to psychological issues. In 1976, members of the American Legion met in a Philadelphia hotel and were struck by pneumonia that caused illness in 182 people and death in 29 others. Epidemiologic investigation discovered contamination of a ventilation system with *Legionella pneumophila*. Further research resulted in the federal government's recognizing indoor air pollution as a significant health concern. Investigators found that poor indoor air quality was associated with illness and death. They also found that many toxic substances were present at higher levels indoors than outdoors. Publications regarding this issue are available with searching the EPA Web site at www.epa.gov.

Human exposure can occur through skin contact, inhalation, and ingestion. Pollutants may be carried into a building on shoes or clothing, and may be carried home in a similar fashion causing inadvertent exposure to family members.

Building-related illnesses include hypersensitivity and allergies, infectious diseases, irritant diseases, intoxication diseases, and cancer. Examples of irritant problems are conjunctivitis, rhinitis, dermatitis, pharyngitis, and reactive airway dysfunction syndrome. Intoxication diseases may occur from exposure to carbon monoxide, heavy metals, pesticides, and volatile organic chemicals. Cancer can be caused by asbestos, radon, and other potential carcinogens.

The patient with fibromyalgia, chronic fatigue syndrome, or chronic pain may be more fragile than the general population. This may make these patients more susceptible to the effects of poor indoor air quality.

TOXIC EXPOSURES

Some patients with pain have known exposures to industrial chemicals, pesticides, or radiation. Some of these occur at work, and some occur at leisure. Some low-level toxicants have a cumulative effect. The workplace woodshop may be no more toxic than the beauty and fingernail shop. Some chemicals may contribute to pain, fatigue, and chemical sensitivities. The practitioner can obtain the material safety data sheet for any potentially toxic substance used in the workplace. Many companies are required to keep these sheets on file. The information can also be found online at www.ilpi.com/msds. The American Association of Poison Control Centers is a national organization that can also help provide information.

CONCLUSION

The pain practitioner should consider including a work and exposure history as part of the patient intake information. The work history includes job information, dates of employment, work hours, injuries, and toxic exposures.

It may be helpful to encourage a line of communication between the company and treating professionals. Companies generally appreciate responsive medical care that sees their workers quickly and understands the needs of the company in getting an employee healthy and back to work. Understanding the basics of how the system works can be very helpful for all parties.

Ergonomics is an old buzzword. Understanding basic principles will assist the pain professional in getting patients back to work more quickly and with more long term success.

REFERENCES

Anderson, G. B. J. (1997). The epidemiology of spinal disorders. In J. W. Frymoyer (Ed.), *The adult spine: Principles and practice* (2nd ed., pp. 93–141). Philadelphia: Lippincott-Raven Press.

Cocchiarell, L., & Andersson, G. (2001). *Guides to the evaluation of permanent impairment* (5th ed.). American Medical Association.

Dainoff, M. J. (1998). Ergonomics of seating and chairs. In W. Karwowski & W. Marras (Eds.), *The occupational ergonomics handbook*. Boca Raton, FL: CRC Press.

EPA Web site: http://www.epa.gov/; search "indoor air quality."

Falkiner, S. (2003). Diagnosis and treatment of hand-arm vibration syndrome and its relationship to carpal tunnel syndrome. *Australian Family Physician, 32*(7), 530–534.

Gorsche, R., Wiley, J. P., Renger, R., Brant, R., Gemer, T. Y., & Sasyniuk, T. M. (1998). Prevalence and incidents of stenosing tenosynovitis (trigger finger) in a meatpacking plant. *Journal of Occupational and Environmental Medicine, 40*, 556–560.

Levy, B. S., & Wegman, D. H. (Eds.). (2000). *Occupational health, recognizing and preventing work-related disease and injury* (4th ed.). Philadelphia: Lippincott/Williams & Wilkins.

McCunney, R. J. (2003). *A practical approach to occupational and environmental medicine.* Philadelphia: Lippincott/Williams & Wilkins.

Nathan, P. A., & Keniston, R. C. (1996). Cells of flexor retinaculum in carpal tunnel syndrome. *Journal of Occupational and Environmental Medicine/American College of Occupational and Environmental Medicine, 38*(9), 863.

Parker, K. G., & Imbus, H. R. (1992). *Cumulative trauma disorders, current issues and ergonomic solutions: A system's approach.* Boca Raton, FL: Lewis Publishers.

Pelmear, P., Taylor, W., & Wasserman, D. (1992). *Hand-arm vibration, a comprehensive guide for occupational health professionals.* New York: Van Nostrand Reinhold.

Putz-Anderson, V. (1988). *Cumulative trauma disorders. A manual for musculoskeletal diseases of the upper limbs.* New York: Taylor & Francis.

Seradge, H., Bear, C., & Bithell, D. (2000). Preventing carpal tunnel syndrome and cumulative trauma disorder: Effect of carpal tunnel decompression exercises: An Oklahoma experience. *Journal-Oklahoma State Medical Association, 93*(4), 150.

Seradge, H., et al. (2002). Conservative treatment of carpal tunnel syndrome: An outcome study of adjunct exercises. *Journal. Oklahoma State Medical Association, 95*(1), 7–14.

Thompson, A. R., Plewes, L. W., & Shaw, E. G. (1951). Peritendinitis: A clinical study of 544 cases in industry. *British Journal and Industrial Medicine, 8*, 150–160.

Travell, J. G., & Simons, D. G. (1983). *Myofascial pain and dysfunction: The trigger point manual.* Baltimore: Williams & Wilkins.

BIBLIOGRAPHY

Bovenzi, M. (1994). Hand-arm vibration syndrome and dose-response relation for vibration induced white finger among quarry drillers and stone carvers. Italian Study Group on Physical Hazards in the Stone Industry. *Occupational and Environmental Medicine, 51*(9), 603–611.

Chaffin, D. B., & Anderson, G. (1984). *Occupational biomechanics.* New York: John Wiley & Sons.

Cox, R. A. F., Edwards, F. C., & Palmer, K. (2000). *Fitness for work, the medical aspects* (3rd ed.). New York: Oxford University Press.

Eastman Kodak Company. (1983). *Ergonomic design for people at work* (Vol. 1: *Workplace, equipment, and environmental design and information transfer*). New York: Van Nostrand Reinhold.

Eastman Kodak Company. (1986). *Ergonomic design for people at work* (Vol. 2: *The design of jobs, including work patterns, hours of work, manual materials handling tasks, methods to evaluate job demands, and the physiological basis of work*). New York: Van Nostrand Reinhold.

Grandjean, E. (1986). *Fitting the task to the man. An ergonomic approach.* Philadelphia: Taylor & Francis.

Gross, A. S. et al. (1995). Carpal tunnel syndrome: A clinicopatholigic study. *Journal of Occupational and Environmental Medicine/American College of Occupational and Environmental Medicine, 37*(4), 437–441.

Jetzer, T., Haydon, P., & Reynolds, D. (2003). Effective intervention with ergonomics, antivibration gloves, and medical surveillance to minimize hand-arm vibration hazards in the workplace. *Journal of Occupational and Environmental Medicine, 45*(12), 1312–1317.

Karwowski, W., & Marras, W. (Eds.). (1999). *The occupational ergonomics handbook.* Boca Raton, FL: CRC Press.

Karwowski, W., & Salvendy, G. (1998). *Ergonomics in manufacturing, raising productivity through workplace improvement.* Society of Manufacturing Engineers, Engineering & Management Press.

Konz, S., & Johnson, S. (2000). *Work design industrial ergonomics* (5th ed.). Scottsdale, AZ: Holcomb Hathaway.

Pulat, B., & Alexander, D. (1991). *Industrial ergonomics case studies.* New York: McGraw-Hill.

Rom, W. N. (1998). *Environmental & occupational medicine* (3rd ed.). Philadelphia: Lippincott-Raven.

Sanders, M., & McCormick, E. (1987). *Human factors in engineering and design.* New York: McGraw-Hill.

88

Pain Management and Geriatrics

Jason DaCosta, MD

DEMOGRAPHICS

Definitions of the terms *elderly* and *geriatrics* are somewhat vague. Indeed, the distinction between younger and older adults is difficult to make on a biological basis. Functional and social needs of older patients also play a role in the definitions of elderly and geriatrics, but are difficult to quantify. From a practical standpoint, patients in the geriatric population may be considered to be elderly, and the commonest definition of the term elderly is about 75 years of age. However, this working definition may vary from 65 to 85 years of age.

The elderly represented 4.1% of the U.S. population in 1900, 12.5% in 1990, and 12.4% (35 million persons) in 2000 according to the U.S. Census Bureau. Of the 35 million elderly in 2000, 4.2 million are older than 85 years of age. The total number and percentage of the U.S. elderly population is expected to rise drastically in 2011 as the baby boomers start turning 65. By the year 2050, estimates project that 20.6% of the U.S. population will be over 65 years old. The growth of the geriatric population is due in large part to reduced mortality and longer life expectancy.

EPIDEMIOLOGY

The incidence of pain increases with age (Crook, Rideout, & Browne, 1984). Pain afflicts one out of four elderly individuals (Nolan & O'Malley, 1988). Chronic pain is reported by 25 to 50% of community-dwelling elderly and 45 to 80% of nursing home residents (Ling & Bathon, 1998). Although the elderly compose only 12.4% of the population, they consume 30% of prescription drugs and 50% of over-the-counter drugs (Davis, 1988).

Musculoskeletal disorders are a common cause of pain in the elderly (Foley, 1994; Harkins, 2001). Osteoarthritis and rheumatoid arthritis afflict more than two thirds of the elderly. Common pain syndromes experienced by the elderly include neck and back pain due to cervical and lumbar spondylosis, facet disorders (zygapophysial joints), radiculopathy from foraminal or spinal stenosis (the incidence of radiculopathy from a herniated disc is less common in elderly patients), arthritis, fractures, trigeminal neuralgia, temporal arteritis, polymyalgia rheumatica, shingles (reactivation of herpes zoster), postherpetic neuralgia, atherosclerosis, and diabetic and alcoholic neuropathies. There is a decline in headaches and dental pain (Sternbach, 1986). The clinical significance of pain in the elderly was underscored by the National Health and Nutrition Survey (1987), which documented an increased incidence of depression and impairment in activities of daily living associated with pain in the elderly.

Many of the pain problems that afflict the elderly occur in younger patients as well. Indeed, the frequency of pain among very old hospitalized patients is similar to that of younger patients (Desbiens et al., 1997). The challenge for the clinician is to make the diagnosis and provide effective treatment, with the fewest side effects possible. This obligation is difficult to meet in a young patient, and the frailty and number of medical problems that may affect an elderly patient make this a challenging endeavor. Common painful conditions in elderly patients are listed in Table 88.1.

LOW BACK PAIN

The differential diagnosis of low back pain in elderly individuals relies heavily on both physical examination

---
TABLE 88.1
Painful Disorders in Elderly Patients

Osteoarthritis
Shingles (reactivation of herpes zoster)
Spinal stenosis
Polymyalgia rheumatica
Temporal arteritis
Peripheral vascular disease
Diabetic peripheral neuropathies

---

and history and may include diagnostic injections. The pain associated with spinal stenosis, a condition characterized by degeneration of the spine causing narrowing of the spinal canal, is often exacerbated by standing or walking and may be dormant when the patient is lying comfortably in the exam room. Pain associated with spinal stenosis may be of two general types: (1) pain emanating from structures within the spine, including facet joints, ligaments, and disc and localized to the spine, and (2) neurogenic claudication, with pain referred to the thighs and legs with standing and walking. Neurogenic claudication is a nerve root problem and may present as bilateral radiculopathy or pain in a single nerve root distribution.

Examination should proceed with an erect visual examination of the spine followed by palpation of the paravertebral muscles and spinous processes. Localized tenderness may suggest compression fracture, infection, or malignancy. During the range of motion exam, flexion pain may signify a herniated nucleus pulposus or paraspinous muscle spasm, decreased extension may be seen with spinal stenosis, and decreased lateral rotation and extension can be due to apophyseal joint disease or paraspinous muscle spasm. The differential diagnosis of neurogenic claudication is vascular claudication. Therefore, pedal pulses should be assessed. If pulses are difficult to palpate or absent, then vascular studies should be considered, particularly if leg pain is more prominent with walking than standing.

Radicular pain is more likely due to degenerative changes of the spine with ligamentous and facet hypertrophy and loss of disk height than to disk herniation. Deep tendon reflexes may be attenuated or absent with increased age and therefore significant only if asymmetric. Motor function is often tested in the supine position: L3–L4 by knee extensors; L4–L5 by toe dorsiflexors; L5–S1 by knee flexors, foot evertors, and hip extensors; S1 by plantar flexors. The facet joints and sacroiliac joints should be palpated for tenderness in the prone position to rule out these common sources of spinal pain.

Other causes of low back pain should be excluded as well, including aortic aneurysmal disease, which can present with pulsatile masses, abdominal bruits, and cool skin and hair loss in the extremities. Lymphoma and spinal metastases should be ruled out particularly in patients with history of prostate, lung, and breast cancer. Pancreatic cancer and perforated duodenal ulcers can present with back pain as well.

NEUROPATHIC PAIN

The treatment of neuropathic pain requires a different approach than nociceptive pain. Although opioids may help, adjuvant medications such as antidepressants and anticonvulsants have proved to be more clinically effective, but may not be as well tolerated in elderly patients. Neuropathic conditions are common in elderly patients and pose challenges in both their diagnosis and treatment. They include classic examples such as trigeminal neuralgia, diabetic neuropathy, and postherpetic neuralgia. Shingles, also referred to as cutaneous herpes zoster, afflicts 1 to 2% of the elderly population each year (Schmader et al., 1995). Resultant postherpetic neuralgia occurs in up to 30 to 50% in the elderly population as compared with 5 to 10% in all age groups. It can also occur following a stroke or nerve injury in the peripheral or central nervous system. Clinical characteristics of shingles and postherpetic neuralgia are provided in Table 88.2.

The mechanism of pain in postherpetic neuralgia may be due to enhanced chemical and mechanical sensitivity to cytokines, prostaglandins, and catecholamines in peripheral sprouting nerve terminals as well as persistent small fiber activity in the periphery and in the dorsal root ganglia. Other mechanisms include upregulation of sodium channels in injured axons and upregulation of sympathetic neurons leading to hypersensitization. Neurologic examination determines whether there is numbness or sensory changes (hypoesthesias, dysesthesias, hyperesthesias, and allodynia). Neuropathic pain is often

---
TABLE 88.2
Clinical Characteristics of Shingles and Postherpetic Neuralgia

Shingles

Incidence: 130/100,000
Clear age dependence (10× higher in elderly than teenagers)
No gender difference
Blacks have lower risk than whites
Truncal and ophthalmic division of trigeminal nerve most commonly affected
Decline in cell-mediated immunity implicated

Postherpetic Neuralgia

Pain that persists after rash has healed (at least 1 month)
50% at age 60 and 75% at age 70 years; develops after herpes zoster
No gender predilection
Pain gradually improves with time
Thoracic dermatomes and face most often involved

---

described as being lancinating, with a sharp, shooting, or stabbing component or burning in character, and this is true after postherpetic neuralgia. The mechanisms and treatment of neuropathic pain are discussed in detail in this volume, in Chapter 24, "Neuropathic Pain."

PAIN ASSESSMENT

History taking and physical examination of elderly patients is often obfuscated by poor memory, denial, and psychomotor limitations. The history of present illness can often be facilitated by having a family member present who can corroborate or augment the patient's story. Also, complaints of pain must sometimes be coaxed from elderly patients as they often underreport pain (Harkins, 2001). An integral component to the history is an assessment of the patient's functional level, which has profound effects on quality of life and degree of independence. These are often measured by how well a patient performs "activities of daily living" such as eating and bathing as well as "instrumental activities of daily living" such as shopping and banking (Ferrell, 1996).

Pain reporting can be followed using a multitude of available tools including the Verbal Descriptor Scale, the Numerical Scale Rating, the Visual Analogue Scale, a faces-based pain scale, and the short or long forms of the McGill Pain Questionnaire. These assessments must be tailored for each patient, as not all elderly patients will be able or willing to complete them.

The physical exam should not only focus on organ systems and body regions pertinent to the pain complaint but should also include a focused neurologic, autonomic, and psychological assessment. The patient must be assessed in entirety, with integration of all components of the history, exam, and supplemental studies. For example, in a patient with an extensive smoking history who presents with lower extremity pain, stressing the extremity may reveal a pathologic fracture or percussion of the spine may suggest metastasis to the spine with a pathologic compression fracture and radiculopathy.

PHYSIOLOGY OF AGING

The pharmacokinetics of aging reflect changes in drug distribution and clearance. From ages 25 to 75 years, the percentage of body fat increases as lean body mass declines. This larger relative fat content increases the volume of distribution of lipid-soluble drugs such as benzodiazepines and barbiturates. Increased volume of distribution prolongs the elimination half-life of these lipid-soluble drugs, while the decreased volume of distribution for water-soluble drugs leads to higher peak plasma concentrations.

TABLE 88.3
Hepatic Function with Aging

Liver size and blood flow decrease with age > 50 years
First-pass metabolism reduced (drugs with high first-pass metabolism have increase blood levels, e.g., propranolol)
Microsomal hydroxylation/oxidation unchanged
Glucuronidation is microsomal — not changed; morphine metabolism by liver unchanged, but clearance is reduced
Demethylation decreased (e.g., diazepam clearance reduced by 50%)
Non-microsomal oxidation reactions preserved
Regenerative capacity of liver unchanged

Plasma protein binding changes with age as well. Acidic drugs such as benzodiazepines and barbiturates may become more active because protein binding decreases with age-related decreases in plasma albumin. Basic drugs such as local anesthetics may become less active as protein binding increases with age-related increases in alpha$_1$ acid glycoprotein. Gastrointestinal absorption of drugs is relatively unchanged with age.

The central and peripheral nervous system changes are variable, depending on heredity and daily activity. Decreases may be global, involving cholinergic, dopaminergic, norepinephrine, and serotonin systems. These decreases may lead to cognitive decline, memory loss, tremor, and depression. High-frequency mechanoreceptors in the skin show an increased threshold but no change in dynamic response to pain with increasing age. There is little evidence that the clinical perception of pain is diminished with age.

Hepatic function is for the most part unchanged with aging. The key components that decline include decreased liver blood flow resulting in decreased first-pass metabolism. Demethylation is another process that declines with aging, resulting in a virtual halving of the clearance of drugs such as benzodiazepines. The other metabolic components of the liver are largely well preserved. A summary of hepatic function in elderly patients is presented in Table 88.3.

Renal function has a consistent and slow decline with age. There is a loss of about 1 ml/min/year in creatinine clearance after age 40 years. In the elderly patient creatinine clearance may not correlate well with the serum creatinine levels, because creatinine production decreases with age. For example, a creatinine of 1.5 mg/dl in an 80-year-old, 70-kg patient may have a glomerular filtration of <40 ml/min. The calculated value in women may be slightly higher. A suitable nomogram or formula should be consulted. Drugs that are predominately renally excreted, such as gabapentin, morphine, and oxycodone, should be avoided, or require appropriate dosage reduction. Changes in renal function are summarized in Table 88.4.

TABLE 88.4
Renal Function with Aging

Functional Changes
Decreased renal blood flow 10% per decade > 20 years
1% per year decline in creatinine clearance after 40 years
Reduced glomerular filtration
Decline in number of functional renal tubules

Structural Changes
Kidney size decreased by 20% (glomerular sclerosis)
Less concentrating ability (more dilute urine)
Reduced drug clearance

ANALGESICS

ACETAMINOPHEN AND NONSTEROIDAL ANTI-INFLAMMATORY DRUGS

Acetaminophen is a well-known analgesic, but its mechanism of action remains poorly understood. The drug may inhibit prostaglandin synthesis in the central nervous system, although it has very little effect on peripheral cyclooxygenase (COX) and therefore has a very low side-effect profile when compared with nonsteroidal anti-inflammatory drugs (NSAIDs). Acetaminophen is rapidly absorbed from the gastrointestinal tract and undergoes significant first-pass metabolism. It is normally conjugated to inactive metabolites that are excreted in the urine. However, in large doses the available glutathione in the liver may be depleted and hepatic necrosis and renal tubular necrosis may occur. For patients consuming alcoholic beverages, consideration should be given to not taking acetaminophen products at all or advising that their usage be limited to less than 2,000 mg/day.

NSAIDs are a heterogeneous group of drugs that exhibit their primary analgesic effect by inhibiting COX-mediated prostaglandin synthesis at inflammatory sites in peripheral tissues. NSAIDs are described in detail in this textbook in Chapter 53, "Nonsteroidal Anti-Inflammatory Drugs."

Nonselective NSAIDs have an indiscriminate side-effect profile, owing to inhibition of COX-1 found in blood vessels, the stomach, and the kidneys in addition to their therapeutic effects at COX-2, induced at inflammatory sites by cytokines and other inflammatory mediators. Elderly individuals are at an increased risk of NSAID side effects, which include gastrointestinal disturbances, confusion, constipation, headaches, dizziness, tinnitus, reversible platelet inhibition, bleeding disorders, edema, hyperkalemia, interstitial nephritis, hypersensitivity reactions, fluid retention, and occasional episodes of confusion. Their nephrotoxicity is related to inhibition of the synthesis of PGE_2 and PGI_2, which maintain renal blood flow. Whether the damage is secondary to renal ischemia, inter-stitial nephritis, or papillary necrosis, those at risk include persons with preexisting renal disease and those who are volume depleted. Additional risk factors include prolonged drug usage, high doses, and low blood flow states, such as seen in congestive heart failure.

Selective COX-2 inhibitors work similarly to traditional NSAIDs but have a several hundred- to several thousand-fold (depending on the formulation) selectivity for COX-2 over COX-1. Therefore, they lessen or avoid many of the nonrenal side effects associated with COX-1 inhibition. They have minimal ulcerogenic side effects, are well tolerated perioperatively with no change in platelet aggregation, and do not appear to prevent bone growth after total joint replacement. There is a growing trend for the selective agents to replace nonselective NSAIDs in the chronic treatment of rheumatic and inflammatory disorders, especially in elderly patients, who are at greater risk for NSAID-induced morbidity. However, it should be emphasized that current information does not indicate that the risk of renal injury is lessened with the COX-2 selective agents. Moreover, the reduction in risk of gastrointestinal ulceration with long-term COX-2 selective inhibitors is unclear, particularly if patients are also taking aspirin.

OPIOID ANALGESICS

Opioids are the gold standard family of analgesics with which all other analgesics are compared. However, they are usually reserved for pain that is resistant to the aforementioned analgesics. Many studies demonstrate age-related differences in potency and clearance of opioids. Studies indicate a twofold difference in analgesia between the extremes of adult age with morphine injection (Baillie et al., 1989). Decreased morphine clearance in the older group led to plasma morphine levels which were approximately twice those of the younger age group. Older patients reported greater peak analgesia but the principal effect was a longer duration of analgesia. This difference is thought to be primarily related to increased duration of action rather than peak effect.

The pharmacokinetics of intravenous and oral immediate and controlled-release morphine vary between young and elderly subjects. Both groups attained similar peak plasma concentrations after intravenous morphine, but the elderly group attained greater concentrations after oral doses (Baillie et al., 1989). Moreover, duration of action was prolonged for all three preparations in the elderly group, reflecting decreased clearance of the drug. Pharmacokinetic data for morphine in elderly patients are shown in Table 88.5.

Elderly patients may have an increased central nervous system sensitivity to morphine as suggested by a study that compared epidural morphine between young and elderly patients. The study showed improved quality of analgesia and prolonged duration in the elderly group after a single

TABLE 88.5
Morphine in Elderly Patients

Pharmacokinetics

Maximum plasma concentration after intravenous administration same as in young patients, but higher after oral administration in elderly patients

Area under the curve values higher in elderly subjects

Clearance and first-pass metabolism reduced

Morphine metabolites (e.g., M6G) are active and accumulate with renal insufficiency

Pharmacodynamics

Morphine more potent in elderly

Longer half-life

Greater pain relief with given dose

May require smaller doses and larger dosing intervals

---

dose of epidural morphine (0.07 mg/kg) despite similar plasma morphine concentrations (Moore et al., 1990).

Studies that compared patient-controlled analgesia (PCA) with morphine to intramuscular morphine showed improved analgesia and less sedation, confusion, and respiratory depression among the PCA group (Egbert et al., 1990). This is especially important in elderly patients with frail skin who may be predisposed to connective-tissue injury after repetitive needle-sticks.

It should be noted that morphine has active metabolites that are excreted by the kidneys. Morphine is metabolized to morphine-6-glucuronide, which is more potent than the parent compound, and morphine-3-glucuronide, which can cause allodynia, hyperalgesia, myoclonus, and cognitive changes. Elderly patients, particularly those with mild renal insufficiency, are prone to side effects with morphine, including sedation and cognitive problems. Hydromorphone is an alternative to morphine and does not have active metabolites that are excreted by the kidney. However, hydromorphone is about five times more potent than morphine.

The transdermal fentanyl system (Duragesic®) may be useful in some cases. This fentanyl preparation offers pharmacokinetic advantages, particularly for patients with swallowing difficulties and/or renal insufficiency. However, several caveats must be noted:

1. Transdermal fentanyl is inappropriate for acute pain management.
2. The slow onset and long duration of action of transdermal fentanyl can make titration difficult.
3. The 25 μg/hour patch, the lowest dosage preparation now available, may be excessive for frail, elderly patients.

Embarking on treatment with the transdermal fentanyl patch implies that the patient will have a long-term need for a controlled-release opioid preparation.

Oxycodone is also an alternative to morphine and is available in a controlled-release preparation. Oxycodone has about twice the potency of morphine on a milligram basis. It is not available as a parenteral drug in the United States. The pharmacokinetic and pharmacodynamic differences between young and older adults are minimal, reducing the need to adjust the dosage of oxycodone in elderly patients (Kaiko et al., 1996). However, the dose must be reduced with renal insufficiency and should be avoided in patients with a creatinine clearance less than half of normal.

In general, it should be emphasized that dosage reductions with all opioids are indicated for older adults. Opioids do appear to have increased pharmacodynamic effects, although pharmacokinetics may be similar. In addition, an increase in the dosing interval may be necessary. Titration to effect is a good rule of thumb.

Tramadol, which inhibits norepinephrine and serotonin reuptake in addition to being a mu-opioid agonist, is generally well tolerated in elderly patients and has a comparable analgesic profile to acetaminophen with codeine (Rauck et al., 1994).

Upon initiation of opioid therapy, formulations with shorter half-lives are favorable for faster onset and titration of analgesia. When therapeutic goals have been reached, these drugs may be converted to equipotent doses of drugs with longer half-lives for ease of dosing, possible lower addiction risk, and to avoid classical conditioning of patients experiencing pain to seek treatment every 4 to 6 hours. Titration of opioids aims for a balance of therapeutic efficacy weighed against the side effects. Because side effects and toxicity of opioids are more common in elderly individuals, this titration must be monitored more closely than in younger, healthier adults. Respiratory depression can occur very quickly in opioid-naïve geriatric patients. Also, opioid bowel regimens to avoid or minimize constipation must be stricter in older patients who likely already have some component of bowel dysfunction.

Many physicians remain fearful of the side effects and addictive potential of opioids and consequently underprescribe opioids for patients who may benefit from their use. Although the risk of addiction was once thought quite small, the actual incidence of addiction or abuse is unknown. Alcohol and prescription drug abuse appear to be more common than abuse of specific opioid analgesics. Of the prescription drugs, benzodiazepines and other sedative-like drugs appear to be abused most often. Nonetheless, appropriate measures should be taken to reduce the likelihood of opioid analgesic abuse, while taking the time to look for concomitant illness that may predispose to drug abuse, including depression. Urine drug screens may be useful in helping to monitor for inappropriate drug use or abuse.

Opioids have favorable side-effect profiles, especially when compared with many of the traditional NSAIDs. The clinical end points of opioid therapy, as with any pain regimen, should focus on improved function, mood, and sleep and decreased pain instead of reduced opioid doses.

ADJUVANT ANALGESICS

Adjuvant analgesics are discussed in detail in Chapter 24, "Neuropathic Pain," in this volume. This group of drugs is effective for neuropathic pain, but can have problematic side effects in elderly patients.

The anticonvulsant carbamazepine inhibits ectopic neuronal activity by blocking sodium channels. However, the medication has numerous side effects, including bone marrow depression, elevated liver enzymes, gastrointestinal disturbances, sedation, confusion, and ataxia. Potential drug interactions, chiefly inhibition of cytochrome P450 activity, make this drug difficult to manage in any age group and particularly in elderly patients, where side effects may be poorly tolerated. Nonetheless, carbamazepine has proved efficacy for trigeminal neuralgia.

Oxcarbazepine is a metabolite of carbamazepine and is safer from the standpoint of potential hepatic toxicity and bone marrow depression, but the potential for hyponatremia requires monitoring of serum sodium levels.

Gabapentin is FDA-approved for the treatment of pain associated with postherpetic neuralgia. The drug may be useful for other neuropathic conditions, based on the current literature. The mechanism of action of gabapentin has not been fully elucidated, although it appears to enhance GABAergic activity, even though it does not bind to GABA receptors (Beydoun et al., 1995). A leading hypothesis suggests that gabapentin interacts with a novel calcium channel receptor on voltage-activated calcium channels.

Elderly patients generally tolerate starting doses of gabapentin of 300 mg/day. The need for titration to higher doses is common. Doses in the range of 1,800 to 2,700 mg/day are generally well tolerated. However, side effects are common and include fatigue, somnolence, ataxia, and vertigo. Gabapentin is excreted in the urine unchanged and the dose must be reduced appropriately in cases of renal insufficiency.

Antidepressants such as tricyclic antidepressants (TCAs) are commonly utilized for neuropathic pain treatment and appear to enhance endogenous descending inhibitory pathways involving serotonin and norepinephrine. Their side effects are almost innumerable, including sedation, constipation, dry mouth, urinary retention, postural hypotension, tachycardia, QRS widening, PR and QT prolongation, and T wave flattening. Elderly patients should be started first on TCAs with the least anticholinergic side effects such as desipramine.

Selective serotonin reuptake inhibitors are not as effective as TCAs in treating neuropathic pain, but they have much more favorable side-effect profiles. Paroxetine has proved to be effective against diabetic neuropathy, but

at much higher doses. A new selective serotonin and norepinephrine reuptake inhibitor, duloxetine, was recently approved by the FDA for the treatment of painful diabetic peripheral neuropathy. Duloxetine may prove to be a useful alternative to the other antidepressants (Briley, 2004) and may have fewer side effects, although it has not had widespread use with elderly patients.

INTERVENTIONAL PAIN MANAGEMENT

Diagnostic and therapeutic injections, including spinal injections and nerve blocks, may provide benefit in selected patients. There is growing clinical evidence that diagnostic injections can help establish a specific diagnosis in back pain and guide appropriate therapy. Indeed, there is substantial evidence that local anesthetic injections (with or without steroid) can provide clinically significant pain relief. This is an important consideration, particularly when analgesics provide inadequate pain relief or are poorly tolerated by elderly patients. Evidence-based clinical practice guidelines have been published that describe the indications and efficacy of interventional techniques for spinal pain (Boswell et al., 2005).

NONPHARMACOLOGIC THERAPY

Alternative therapies are gaining acceptance among many patients and some health insurance companies. Music therapy, aromatherapy, relaxation, meditation, and spiritual healing may subjectively help patients. Coping techniques are particularly effective in elderly patients whose perceptions of pain are more likely to be amplified by anxiety, fear, depression, and thoughts of helplessness. Hypnosis, massage, energy healing, magnetic therapy, folk remedies, and biofeedback can improve the patient's outlook and cause subjective improvements in pain perception. TENS therapy, acupuncture, and acupressure are gaining wider acceptance for pain management. Despite the controversy that will continue to enshroud these techniques, a basic understanding of their principles is valuable because patients with chronic pain will likely inquire about or request them.

Rehabilitation of elderly patients focuses more on an independent life rather than a return to work. It is an important component of the pain treatment and is managed by the physical therapist and an occupational or recreational therapist.

CONCLUSION

Pain management in elderly patients requires a different perspective from that of younger patients. Causes, comorbidities, and responses to both pain and its treatment differ between young healthy and older patients. The importance of making a specific diagnosis if possible cannot be underestimated. Many therapeutic end points are different as well. In addition, the treatments may have clinically important side effects in elderly patients. It is important for the successful clinician to keep these differences in mind in order to provide the most informed, efficient, efficacious and comprehensive treatment.

REFERENCES

Baillie, S. P., Bateman, D. N., Coates, P. E., & Woodhouse, K. W. (1989). Age and the pharmacokinetics of morphine. *Age and Ageing, 18,* 258–262.

Beydoun, A., Ulthman, B. M., & Sackellares, J. C. (1995). Gabapentin: Pharmacokinetics, efficacy, and safety. *Clinical Neuropharmacology, 18,* 469–481.

Boswell, M. V. et al. (2005). Interventional techniques in the management of chronic spinal pain: Evidence-based practice guidelines. *Pain Physician, 8,* 1–47.

Briley, M. (2004) Clinical experience with dual action antidepressants in different chronic pain syndromes. *Human Psychopharmacology, 19,* S2.

Crook, J., Rideout, E., & Browne, G. (1984). The prevalence of pain complaints among a general population. *Pain, 18,* 299–314.

Davis, M. A. (1988). Epidemiology of osteoarthritis. *Clinics in Geriatric Medicine, 4,* 241–255.

Desbiens, N. A. et al. (1997). Pain in the oldest-old during hospitalization and up to one year later. *Journal of the American Geriatric Society, 45,* 1167–1172.

Egbert, A. M., Parks, L. H., Short, L. M., & Burnett, M. L. (1990). Randomized trial of postoperative patient control analgesia vs. intramuscular narcotics in frail elderly men. *Archives of Internal Medicine, 150,* 1897–1903.

Ferrell, B. (1996). Overview of aging and pain. In B. R. Ferrell & B. B. Ferrell (Eds.), *Pain in the elderly* (pp. 1–10). Seattle: IASP Press.

Foley, K. M. (1994). Pain in the elderly. In W. R. Hazzard, E. L. Bierman, & J. P. Blass (Eds.), *Principles of geriatric medicine and gerontology.* New York: McGraw-Hill.

Harkins, S. W (2001). Aging and pain. In J. J. Bonica (Ed.), *Management of pain* (3rd ed., pp. 813–823). Philadelphia, Lea & Febiger.

Kaiko, R. F., Wallenstein, S. L., Rogers, A. G., Gabrinski, P. Y., & Houde, R. W. (1982). Narcotics in the elderly. *Medical Clinics of North America, 66,* 1079–1089.

Kaiko, R. F., Benziger, D. P., Fitzmartin, R. D., Burke, B. E., Reder, R. F., & Goldenheim, P. D. (1996). Pharmacokinetic-pharmacodynamic relationships of controlled-release oxycodone. *Clinical Pharmacology and Therapeutics, 59,* 52–61.

Ling, S. M., & Bathon, J. M. (1998). Osteoarthritis in older adults. *Journal of the American Geriatric Society, 46,* 216–225.

Moore, A. K., Vilderman, S., Lubenskyi, W., McCans, J., & Fox, G. S. (1990). Differences in epidural morphine requirements between elderly and young patients after abdominal surgery. *Anesthesia & Analgesia, 70,* 316–320.

National Health and Nutrition Survey. (1987). I. Epidemiological follow-up study, 1982–1984. *Vital and Health Statistics, Series I, No. 22,* Washington, DC: DHHS Pub. No. (PHS).

Nolan, L., & O'Malley, K. (1988). Prescribing for the elderly: II. Prescribing patterns differences due to age. *Journal of the American Geriatric Society, 36,* 245–254.

Rauck, R. L., Ruoff, G. E., & McMillen, J. I. (1994). Comparison of tramadol and acetaminophen with codeine for long term pain management in elderly patients. *Current Therapeutical Research, 55,* 1417–1431.

Schmader, et al. (1995) Social differences in the occurrence of herpes zoster. *Journal of Infectious Diseases, 171,* 701–704.

Sternbach, R. A. (1986). Survey of pain in the United States: The Nuprin Pain Report. *Clinical Journal of Pain, 2,* 49–53.

89

Hospice, Cancer Pain Management, and Symptom Control

Samira Kanaan Beckwith, CHE, LCSW, and Charles Wellman, MD

INTRODUCTION

Death is part of the life cycle yet continues to be a difficult transition for most people. In 1900, the average life expectancy was only 50 years and infant mortality was very high. Because of improved sanitation, immunization programs, antibiotics, improved management of acute illnesses, trauma care, and other improved therapies, Americans now live well into their late 70s or 80s (Emanuel et al., 1999). As a result of these advances, people now expect to have prolonged experiences of living with chronic illnesses and ultimately the end of life.

Many misconceptions exist about life's final chapter. Some 69% of patients said they would opt for suicide if they felt their pain could not be relieved (Levin et al., 1985). Fear of unacceptable pain was a major component of requests to physicians for assisted suicide (Helig, 1988; Emanuel et al., 1999). The increased awareness of the public in assisted suicide, due to the activities of Dr. Jack Kevorkian during the 1990s, and the popularity of the book *Final Exit* (Humphry, 1991) give evidence to this well-founded concern. Undertreatment of acute and chronic pain persists despite decades of efforts to provide clinicians with information about analgesics and other palliative care initiatives (American Pain Society [APS], 1995).

When the primary focus of care shifts from pursuing a cure, the emphasis shifts to palliation (Kaye, 1989). Palliative care, the focus of hospice care, affords relief and reduces the severity of bothersome symptoms, but does not produce toxicity or hasten the death of the patient (Johanson, 1988). Although palliative care should be integrated into all health care, it is critically necessary when cure is

not likely (Brescia, 1987). No specific therapy is or should be excluded from consideration. The test of palliative treatment lies in the agreement by the patient, the physician, the primary caregiver, and the hospice team that the expected outcome is relief from distressing symptoms, easing of pain, and enhancement of quality of life (National Hospice Organization [NHO], 1996). The absolute goal for palliative care is to improve the quality of the patient's life while avoiding side effects worse than the symptoms being treated (Emanuel et al., 1999).

Excellence in palliative care focuses on pain control and symptom management to help the patient avoid suffering and enhance quality of life. To realize this goal, it is essential for the clinicians involved to believe and to assess the severity of each pain complaint.

Total pain management cannot be undertaken by an individual alone, but only by individuals working together as a team (Lack, 1984). This underlying principle of working together in hospice care manifests through the use of an interdisciplinary approach and a creative process of individualized patient management. This results in an empowered patient who is able to attain comfort and dignity. Hospice care integrates the best of psychological support, physical care, and spirituality for the patient directly and provides long-term bereavement assistance for the surviving loved ones.

Hospice is based on a philosophy of caring for the person at life's final stages, embracing a number of concepts. Death is viewed as a natural part of the life cycle. When death is inevitable, hospice will seek neither to hasten nor to postpone it. Hospice exists in the hope and belief that through appropriate care and the promotion of a caring community sensitive to their needs, patients and their families may be able to attain a degree of mental and spiritual preparation for death that is optimal for them (NHO, 1996). Despite the successful growth of the hospice movement in the United States during the past 30 years, over 50% of Americans die in hospitals and long-term care facilities, making palliative care interventions relatively unused in the settings in which most of them die (Rummans et al., 2000). Fortunately many hospitals, nursing homes, and other health care providers are exploring the development of palliative care initiatives as well as better partnerships with hospice programs. Palliative care services also help hospitals meet a number of the Joint Commission for the Accreditation of Health Care Organizations standards related to pain, continuum of care, and communications.

Pain relief and symptom control are appropriate clinical goals, with psychological and spiritual pain considered as significant as physical pain. Addressing all spheres simultaneously requires the skills and experience of an interdisciplinary treatment team. Such teams include physicians, nurses, social workers, pharmacists, aides, chaplains, homemakers, volunteers, bereavement counselors, and other therapists as needed. Additional therapies should include the standard therapies, such as physical, occupational and speech therapy, as well as the complementary therapies, such as music, art, aroma, pet, and massage therapy. Patients with their families and loved ones are the unit of care, and this care is generally provided to them regardless of their ability to pay.

Although hospice was viewed by many as unconventional at its beginning, the number of people cared for by hospice has continued to increase with an average of 30% of all deaths occurring in the hospice setting in 2003. Many misunderstandings about hospice programs exist, including the myths that people must die within 6 months and that hospice is only for cancer patients and older people. In fact, people can be certified for hospice every 60 days, hospice cares for people with all end-stage diseases and of all ages. Hospice medicine and care has become quite scientific and developed, with a large body of knowledge about providing care for people at the end of life (Appleton, 1996). Hospice medicine established new standards for medication dosing, medication selection, home care limitations, and the ability to provide "whole patient" care.

Hospice is now recognized as one of the standards for clinical practice. Based on these concepts of "whole patient" care, hospice is now a specialized health care program focusing on the provision of pain management, symptom control, emotional and spiritual support, personal care, and bereavement counseling. More cost-effective than hospital, home health, or nursing home (long-term) care, hospice provides the appropriate array of services at the end of life. Because hospice care combines the best quality and value for end-of-life patients, it is now covered by Medicare, many insurance companies, and in most states by Medicaid. A majority of hospice programs also look to their communities for additional support to assist them in providing indigent care and other specialized unreimbursed programs.

A primary focus of hospice care is to maintain patients in their home or place of residence for as long as possible. Additionally, care is also provided in inpatient hospice units, assisted living facilities, long-term care nursing facilities, and contract hospitals. Electing hospice care allows patients to make choices, control their destinies, and maintain their dignity while avoiding the sense of abandonment and solitude often associated with a hospital death.

PATIENT ASSESSMENT AND HOSPICE CARE

Our goal should be to care for the person, not just the patient that the health care system has made the person. We must care for the person, not just the disease. Therefore, patient assessment is an important skill. Whole-patient assessment clarifies the diagnosis and prognosis; coordinates the activities of the hospice team members; improves trust between patients, their families, and their professional caregivers; and leads to the best therapeutic effects (Emanuel et al., 1999). Thorough assessment allows establishment of a plan of care with the task of the interdisciplinary hospice team being to provide care that is comprehensive in scope.

Certain diseases can be expected to follow predictable courses. However, hospice is not about providing routine care, but instead focuses on providing an individualized hospice plan of care that is prepared uniquely for every new admission and continuously updated. This plan of care begins the moment the patient is referred to the hospice program and evolves as the needs of the patient change. Although the initial plan of care is the collaboration of the intake nurse, attending physician, hospice medical director, and social worker, the other members of the interdisciplinary team participate in the frequent revisions.

The patient-as-a-person view of end-of-life care encompasses many domains simultaneously. These domains include the review of the patient's complete illness and treatment summary, followed by ongoing physical, psychosocial, spiritual, and practical care assistance (Emanuel et al., 1999). The goal of this assessment is control of bothersome symptoms, improvement in function, reduction of suffering, minimization of aimless inconsequential testing, and bettering the overall quality of each day.

The referring source often has certain expectations about services for the patient, and the hospice team must consider these wishes along with the overall hospice philosophy. Continuity of care for the patient and family necessitates a close relationship between the attending physician, discharge planners, and the hospice staff. Problems identified in the earliest stages of hospice involvement tend to reflect uncontrolled symptoms, care plan needs such as equipment and medication, and accessibility to the care team. Once the patient has been enrolled into the program, a number of the hospice team members visit the patient and family to develop an appropriate plan of care.

The nursing assessment focuses on the safety of the patient in the environment, the patient's main complaints, use of medications, care needs over time, and managing the plan of care. In the assessment process, the nurse gathers information from the patient that allows for understanding the pain experience and its effect on the quality of life (McCaffery & Beebe, 1989; McCaffery & Pasero, 1999). It is important to avoid making assumptions about the patient's wishes. Asking the patient for ideas and opinions makes his or her wishes known (Kaye, 1989). Inquiring "How are you right now?" lets the person know that human needs will be addressed. This helps to establish trust and build the relationship that allows screening for care requirements, such as diet, appetite, bowel function, managing unpleasant side effects, intimacy issues, and successful pain management. The interdisciplinary approach to care in conjunction with trained volunteers ensures that no person has to travel the final days alone.

The hospice physician primarily attends to the management of symptoms, serves as a consultant for the interdisciplinary team, and acts as a liaison with the attending physician. Education and support for the team members and representing the hospice program are key duties for the physician. A willingness to be available, often 24 hours a day, and to work collaboratively with the interdisciplinary treatment team adds to the services provided by the traditional medical staff in the community. The "house call," with care provided in the home of the patient rather than the office or the hospital, is the preferred method of management for the hospice patient. The hospice physician must be flexible, able to handle routine medical problems, and practice medicine in a home environment or with a minimum of the complicated technology often associated with facility-based care.

Practical care issues are important considerations for hospice care provided in the home. The patient or the primary caregiver may relocate to accommodate the care demands. Changes in living arrangements often result in disruption for everyone as new routines are established. Not only must the medical aspects of care be undertaken, but in addition, the more mundane aspects of daily living must also be addressed. Who will pay the bills? Who will feed the pets? Who will do the grocery shopping? Who will get the prescription medications filled? Who will do the chores around the house? These issues must be resolved to successfully care for any patient at home.

In a home environment there are important concerns related to the physical safety of the declining patient; thus, specialized adaptive equipment is often provided to improve the care of the patient. Emotional support coupled with extensive and practical education provides the caregivers with the confidence to assume the challenge of providing care for the patient. Despite all this wonderful support, it remains very difficult to prepare the new caregiver for the personal sacrifices that must be made to provide care for the very ill person. The simplest errand often takes on monumental qualities when caregiving needs are continuous. Caregiver stress is a very important issue. This "24/7" routine often results in the exhaustion of the caregiver, physically and emotionally, and necessitates the need for respite care. Inpatient care must also be available for symptom management.

Trust issues manifest early in the care of the hospice patient. The continuum of care with the attending physician and past health care providers must be maintained and include transition to the hospice team. Many attending physicians are not able to follow their patients at home and thus rely on the skills of the hospice team members to provide the day-to-day aspects of care. The reality that most hospice patients are older and seriously medically ill, yet are frequently cared for by younger family members, produces difficult reversals in generational hierarchies. The daughter, or daughter-in-law, who typically becomes the caregiver for her, or her husband's, parent, and the actual patient, must adjust to new patterns. Longstanding, unresolved conflicts may reappear due to the stressful conditions that exist and can lead to power struggles and other dysfunctional expressions.

Hospice care embraces the idea that psychosocial, emotional, and spiritual factors all have an impact on physical symptoms. Plato once said, "As you ought not to attempt to cure the eyes without the head or the head without the body, so neither are you to attempt to cure the body without the soul; for the part can never be well unless the whole is well; therefore, if the head and body are to be well, you must begin by curing the soul." In the 15th century, Lorenzo Sassoli, a physician, wrote to a patient: "To get angry and shout at times pleases me for this will keep your natural heat; what displeases me is your being grieved and taking all matters to heart; for it is this as the whole of physics teaches which destroys our body more than any other cause" (Sassoli, 1402).

The connections between the mind and body have continued to be the focus of attention for many researchers. Outcomes attributable to psychosocial factors range on a continuum from the readily explicable to the most controversial. These outcomes include enhanced physical comfort, increased responsiveness to medical treatment, relief from emotional anguish, extension of survival time after disease onset, and outright "psychogenic" cure. For these reasons, we believe that the psychosocial, emotional, and spiritual components of a patient's palliative and end-of-life experience must be thoroughly addressed to understand the totality of the care needs. The experience of pain, and the resulting suffering, may be greater when the pain is accompanied by anger, anxiety, depression, fear, and the meaning given to the pain. Because many patients report less pain when they are rested, distracted, and have other symptoms under good control, many questions are raised about what specific factors influence how an individual person may experience pain. Factors considered involve the duration of the pain experience, the course the pain has taken during that time, the anticipation that the pain will be controlled, the expected interval before improvement will be realized, and the time anticipated until meaningful comfort will be attained. Patients must be given hope that their pain and suffering will be managed.

A comprehensive psychosocial assessment is important and must include an appropriate analysis of gender, present financial situation, family history, relationship patterns, previous coping strategies, previous losses, history of alcohol and substance abuse, past mental health problems, occupational history, and ethnic and cultural issues, as well as an exploration of religious and spiritual beliefs. The specific information regarding finances, environment, and care costs is necessary to develop a plan of care that is realistic and achievable as many patients and their caregivers express concern about the cost of their analgesic medications and other needed services.

It is certainly natural to be afraid of death, as death is the ultimate unknown (Ryder, 1993). However, fear is a major factor that adversely influences the experience of pain. Fear of pain takes at least two forms: fear of the pain itself and fear of the inability to control pain (Hill & Shirley, 1992). Most patients expect the pain from cancer and other diseases at the end of life to be very severe, perhaps to the point of not being able to be managed. The popular belief that most cancer pain is poorly controlled does not offer newly diagnosed cancer patients or others much reason to be hopeful about their personal pain management.

Unnecessary concerns and myths about the consequences of opioid analgesic usage, including addiction, confusion, constipation, disorientation, tolerance, and withdrawal problems, continue to prevent many patients from receiving the medications they need. Patients should never need to wish for death because of their physicians' reluctance to use adequate amounts of effective opioids and provide appropriate symptom management to control side effects (Reisine & Pasternak, 1996).

Fear also arises from concerns about loss of control, dignity, and relationships, as well as being abandoned or becoming a burden (Emanuel et al., 1999). Professional caregivers must explore patient fears and ultimately affirm their commitment to care for the patient. Failure to do this may lead to needless suffering.

Untreated anxiety and depression also worsen the pain experience, resulting in interference with restful sleep, impaired cognitive processes, and altered social patterns. Depression associated with uncontrolled pain plays a significant role in suicidal ideation, and when coupled with a sense of helplessness and hopelessness, it becomes a deadly predictor of actual suicide. Pain relief clearly enhances the sense of hope and well-being for the patients. Failure to appreciate the psychological needs of the patient will render even aggressive treatment of pain with analgesics or procedures ineffective (Patt & Isaacson, 1996).

Health care professionals must make their treatment decisions with a focus on the whole person rather than just the specific disease state. People must be the focus of care. Caregivers need to understand that having a serious, potentially end-stage condition can by itself be a reason for demoralization and loss of hope. Patients and their families need to be reassured by their professional caregivers that care, compassion, and concern will always be available to them and that they will not be abandoned. Information about the disease, expected outcomes, and treatment options, including their effects on the quality of life, must be communicated in common terms that the patient and family can understand.

Helping the family caregiver with practical day-to-day tasks can reduce the caregiver's fatigue and potential for fatigue. Using the psychosocial assessment process, resources needed can be identified and provided. Giving the patient and caregiver a flowchart with the names and duties of the professional team members can clarify the roles and relationships. Done properly, the patient and caregiver can view their appropriate place in the care continuum and feel that they are valuable team participants.

Many caregivers report that much of their day is centered on the dying person, attending to positioning, feeding, bathing, and medicating. The care needs of the patient direct the life of the caregiver. Although this routine is appropriate and encouraged during the patient's hospice care, upon the death of the patient, it is radically altered for the caregiver. This loss of activity and fulfillment of nurturing needs should be acknowledged as part of the emptiness experienced after death. Hospice programs provide bereavement support, maintaining continued involvement with the caregiver through the professional staff and volunteers, using a variety of techniques including support groups, classes, and individual counseling. The bereavement plan of care must be based on an assessment of risk indicators (Beckwith et al., 1990). Bereavement care demonstrates the hospice philosophy and communicates, "We still care for you, and we will help you get through this."

Bereavement, a separation or loss through death, is derived from the Old English *bereafian*, meaning "to rob," "to plunder," or "to dispossess" (Burnell & Burnell, 1989). Bereavement is the general state of being that results from having experienced a significant loss (Cook & Dworkin,

1992). It is the price paid in emotional pain for having meaningful relationships. All caregivers have loss experiences that color how they handle subsequent losses, and these losses need acknowledgment in preparation for healthy grieving after the loved one's death. Soon after the death, or often through the dying process, caregivers must look for ways to adjust their identities. Caregivers may experience an initial sense of relief and simultaneous feelings of emptiness when new coping patterns have not been developed. Confusion over identity arises with a shift in focus from the care needs of the patient to the personal needs of the caregiver.

Ultimately, the search for meaning and the exploration of spiritual issues can contribute to the alleviation of emotional distress for patients and their families. A review of things enjoyed and loved, such as people, places, events, and experiences, can bring genuine comfort and relief from suffering. Although formal psychiatric involvement may be needed for those with histories of prior psychiatric illness, supportive techniques, such as psychotherapy can often be helpful for most who elect to use them. This spiritual search for meaning can also influence the perception of the pain experience.

Spirituality needs require thorough exploration from the outset of hospice care. We must acknowledge that pain is not just a response to a physical problem; all facets must be addressed if we are to treat the whole person (Cosh, 1995). Almost all who connect their pain with impending death review the events of their lives and seek to determine the significance of their lives. Some return to religious values of earlier days, and others make intense demands on their faith (Lack, 1984). Rectifying previous religious traditions with present affiliations can prove problematic. When spouses are of different faith traditions or one spouse is a relative nonbeliever, the provision of spiritual care can be more complex. It is not the responsibility of the hospice team to resolve religious matters or to "save" people, but rather to assess and attempt to provide spiritual support as desired by the patient and family. Symptom control has to precede spiritual or psychosocial support; a person cannot think about the meaning of his or her life while in pain (Kaye, 1989).

PAIN MANAGEMENT

Approximately 70% of patients with advanced cancer report pain as a major symptom (Bonica, 1987). For half of them, the pain is moderate to severe in intensity; while for a third, the pain is severe to excruciating (Cleeland, 1994; World Health Organization [WHO], 1986). It is tragic that although pain in 1 in 10 patients with cancer is difficult to control, pain in 50 to 80% of patients with cancer is not satisfactorily relieved because their physicians do not aggressively treat the pain problem (Bonica, 1985). With more than 6 million newly diagnosed cancer

cases in the world each year, every physician who cares for patients with cancer or others at the end of life must be able to elicit a detailed pain history and be able to bring relief to these sufferers (WHO, 1986). Pain may be due to direct tumor progression and related pathology, operations and other invasive diagnostic or therapeutic procedures, toxicities of chemotherapy and radiation, infection, or musculoskeletal discomfort when patients have limited physical activity (Foley, 1985). In addition, many hospice and palliative care teams are now finding that over half of their referrals are for patients who do not have cancer. This requires us to be equally adept at assessing and treating noncancer pain as well as pain associated with chronic benign conditions.

The basic pain evaluation must begin with believing the pain complaint expressed by the patient (Foley, 1988). Pain is whatever the person experiencing it says it is, and it exists whenever the person experiencing it says it does (McCaffery & Beebe, 1989; McCaffery & Pasero, 1999). Because all pain is very real and distressing to the patient, trying to assign relative proportions to organic or functional causes is of little value. It is more useful to determine if the pain limits the activity of the patient and disturbs sleep, appetite, or the ability to engage in productive or pleasurable endeavors. Knowing what the patient can or cannot do, how medications have or have not worked, what the treatment expectation is, and what side effects the patient will or will not tolerate are key initial questions to be answered. It is vital that a language about the pain be developed among the patient, the caregiver, and the hospice and palliative care team to allow skillful management. Descriptive words such as mild, moderate, and severe indicate the intensity of acute pain fairly well. Words such as excruciating, incapacitating, overwhelming, and soul-stealing may better define the pain of cancer. A number of pain scales have been developed to quantify and track the pain experience, such as the descriptive (uses words), numerical (uses numbers), and visual (uses anchors of "no pain" and "worse pain") analogues. Pain scales have also been developed to help evaluate pain severity in noncommunicative patients.

To treat the pain most thoroughly, it is best to obtain the richest detail about the pain complaint that the patient and family can provide. This pain assessment would include screening for possible spiritual, psychosocial, or financial contributing factors. A careful, comprehensive physical examination should be performed, with special attention given to areas of pain or tenderness and to maneuvers that may help to define the areas or etiologies of pain. If necessary, the physician should order and personally review needed diagnostic studies to better elaborate the overall problems of the patient (Portenoy, 1988). All of the possible methods of controlling the pain — not just pharmacological means — must be considered and blended to individualize the plan of care for the patient.

Finally, the level of pain control and patient satisfaction after each intervention must be assessed. There is no point in frequently changing methods until assessment with what was previously ordered has occurred. Establishing clear and reasonable goals with the patient and the family is necessary to ensure a successful outcome. Everyone must understand that analgesics are not anesthetics; although absolute pain elimination may not be a realistic goal, improved comfort can be provided. With a clear understanding of the pain problem, a treatment plan may be developed evolving from simple analgesics to invasive interventions such as nerve blocks and other ablative techniques. Through hospice, medical equipment and supplies that are needed to facilitate even complex care of the patient can be provided either in the home setting or in the hospice inpatient unit. As we are concerned about both the patient and the family, the capacity and emotional status of nonprofessional caregivers should be assessed to be certain that they are not overwhelmed or at risk for breakdown. A balance must be struck among the capabilities of medical science, the wishes of the patient, and the realistic abilities of the caregiver. The loss or fatigue of the caregiver at home is a frequent reason for a patient needing to enter a long-term care nursing facility or an inpatient setting.

PHARMACOTHERAPY

The correct route of administration for medication is the one best tolerated by the patient. As long as the patient is able to swallow, pain can be routinely managed with oral medications. Transmucosal, transdermal, rectal, and parenteral routes may be utilized when swallowing is compromised. The important premise that the oral route is the preferred method of administration for a patient able to eat and drink leads to the recommendation that practitioners follow the WHO guidelines, as well as those of the Agency for Health Care Policy and Research (AHCPR), reorganized as the Agency for Healthcare Research and Quality (AHRQ) in 1999. These organizations systematically start with an oral nonsteroidal anti-inflammatory medication (NSAID) or acetaminophen. Level-two pain can be treated with a non-opioid and a relatively weaker, or lower potency, oral opioid. A low starting dose of a stronger, more potent opioid may also be considered for this second step. Higher doses of a strong, potent oral opioid can then be used in addition to the non-opioid for more severe pain (AHCPR, 1994; WHO, 1986). These three steps best describe the management of mild, moderate, and severe intensities of pain. At each of these steps, adjuvant medications may be added to the other medications to additionally provide pain relief, but the routine combining of multiple NSAIDs or opioids is usually unnecessary, and actually discouraged, for the majority of patients. Ultimately, instead of trying to fit patients to the

medications, the medications are adjusted to fit the patients. The right dose of any medication becomes the dose that produces comfort with minimal toxicity.

Acetaminophen, often part of combination pain medications, has little anti-inflammatory effect, but often helps with mild to moderate pain relief. A risk of hepatotoxicity exists when daily doses exceed 4 g. Patients with chronic alcoholism and liver disease, or those who are fasting, can develop hepatotoxicity at standard doses (APS, 1999).

Starting with the NSAIDs makes good sense for most pain problems, as these medications work to relieve pain in the periphery, where the nociceptive experience originates (Kanner, 1987). NSAIDs interfere with the manufacture of local pain-sensitizing and inflammation-mediating components (prostaglandins) and thereby limit pain transmission from the periphery to the central nervous system (CNS) and eventual consciousness (Insel, 1996). While aspirin irreversibly interferes with platelet aggregation, most of the other NSAIDs decrease platelet aggregation only while therapeutic levels are maintained (APS, 1989). Notable exceptions are the selective COX-2 inhibitors, nabumetone, and choline magnesium trisalicylate. Choline magnesium trisalicylate is a nonacetylated aspirin derivative that does not appear to affect the aggregation of platelets (APS, 1989; Kanner, 1987). Choline magnesium trisalicylate is a generic medication that can be used orally, as tablets or as a liquid suspension, with the same or milder side-effect profile as aspirin and the ability to follow salicylate levels if desired.

The NSAIDs in general may produce gastric upset and gastrointestinal bleeding, due to inhibition of COX-1-generated protective prostaglandins. Nabumetone and the selective COX-2 inhibitors celecoxib and rofecoxib have lower event rates for these problems (Insel, 1996; Medical Economics Company [MEC], 2000). Also, a preferential COX-2 inhibitor, meloxicam, shares this property, but all of these agents have the potential for renal problems (Smith & Baird, 2003). Unfortunately, emerging evidence of possible significant cardiac toxicity may decrease somewhat the use of COX-2 inhibitors (Topol, 2005). It is a common occurrence in the hospice setting to encounter patients with pain that is controlled quite poorly despite high-dose opioid analgesics at the time of their admission. These patients may benefit significantly from the continuation or addition of NSAIDs without further increases in the opioid analgesics. Additionally, NSAIDs should be considered when pain is due to bone metastases (Foley, 1985; Walsh, 1985), soft-tissue infiltration, and various arthritides.

CASE EXAMPLE

Mr. H was a 75-year-old gentleman with advanced prostate cancer with extensive bony metastases. He was initially able to control his pain with 2 mg hydromorphone orally every 4 hours. He later experienced high levels of localized pain in his lower back and pelvis. Rather than increase his opioid analgesic, he was additionally given 750 mg of choline magnesium trisalicylate four times daily, with his pain level decreasing from an "8" to a "2." As his disease progressed, he eventually required more hydromorphone to remain comfortable. His dose was adjusted to 4 mg orally every 4 hours, and he was able to die comfortably.

If the pain is not controlled with NSAIDs alone, the next step is the addition of an opioid analgesic. Routinely, Drug Enforcement Agency schedule three (C-III) combination medications or low doses of stronger opioids are prescribed after nonsteroidal agents. It is important to remember that all of the combination opioid medications, like the pure opioids, are effective analgesics if used at equianalgesic dosages (the amount of one medication that produces the same relief as another medication; see Table 89.1). The limiting factor for the schedule three agents used in the United States is the presence of the co-analgesic (acetaminophen, aspirin, or ibuprofen). Because of the toxicity associated with the co-analgesic agents (gastrointestinal upset and/or bleeding, hepatotoxicity, platelet aggregation interference, and nephrotoxicity), there is a finite limit for the number of C-III combination products that may be taken daily. This ceiling due to the co-analgesic may result in inadequate pain relief for those experiencing more than moderate pain intensity.

Contributing to some of the confusion about effectively prescribing pure opioids is the continuing observation that most standard textbooks of pharmacology describe opioid analgesic dosages with respect to acute pain, but few references mention the complexities of chronic pain management. Underdosing the patient with cancer is more commonly the rule than the exception (Hill, 1988), and fear about possible respiratory depression due to opioids is best countered by remembering that the most potent antagonist to opioid-induced respiratory depression is pain itself (Johanson, 1988). Respiratory depression is not a problem until the pain is well controlled; no one has died from opioid-induced respiratory depression while awake (APS, 1999; LeGrand et al., 2003). Also, it is unnecessary to reduce opioid dosing in the final days of life as the use of opioids does not correlate with dying more quickly (Morita et al., 2001).

In general, the relative potency of oral to parenteral opioid analgesics is about three to one, except for hydromorphone being five to one, due to the first-pass effect of hepatic metabolism and possible incomplete intestinal absorption. One must take approximately two to four times more oral medication, depending on the opioid, to obtain the same level of comfort produced by the parenteral route (Pasero et al., 1999). Oxycodone is an exception, with 60 to 87% or more of oral doses

being bioavailable and escaping the first-pass hepatic metabolism (Kaiko et al., 1996; Leow et al., 1993; Poyhia et al., 1993).

The most frequent error in working with opioid analgesics is to assume that dosages are constant despite the route of administration (not accounting for first-pass liver effects). It is still common to find opioid orders written for 50 to 75 mg meperidine orally or intramuscularly every 4 to 6 hours as needed for pain. This situation shows a lack of understanding regarding pharmacokinetic principles most notably in two areas: the equianalgesic difference between oral and parenteral routes of administration (300 mg orally is equivalent to 75 to 100 mg parenterally) and the 2- to 3-hour duration of analgesic action (Pasero et al., 1999).

Most important for properly prescribing opioids is their administration on a time-contingent, by-the-clock (or around-the-clock) basis, rather than a pain-contingent, as-needed basis, so that comfort is constantly maintained instead of being continually sought. Initiation of opioid dosing, however, is often done on an as-needed basis using short-acting opioids, thereby retaining the ability to stop the medication's effects quickly if unexpected or intolerable side effects occur. The development of extended-release medications has allowed several opioids (fentanyl, morphine, and oxycodone) to provide sustained analgesic action for 8 to 72 hours. Such stable blood levels will increase overall comfort and lessen the peak and trough effect found with administering short-acting opioids.

By maintaining control of the pain around the clock, most patients experience a better quality of life (lower pain frequency and intensity, less medication toxicity, improved sleep) and use less medication (Reuben et al., 1999). From a learning theory perspective, the use of as-needed medication may cause the patient to use more medication over time because of the linkage made between having pain and taking medication to experience pain relief, thereby resulting in the development of psychological craving. The time-contingent dosing pattern dissociates pill-taking from pain relief (because medication is taken on a fixed time schedule) and thus may prevent the most feared but least likely complication of opioid analgesic use — addiction.

In reality, very little abuse of opioid medication actually occurs among hospice patients or medical patients with legitimate use of these agents. Studies of nonterminal patients with chronic pain show little justification for concern when the probability of iatrogenic addiction is 1/800 to less than 1/10,000 (Medina & Diamond, 1977; Perry & Heidrich, 1982; Porter & Jick, 1980). Although 6 to 15% of the U.S. population may have a substance abuse disorder of some type, only 3% of inpatient and outpatient consultations performed by the Psychiatry Service at Memorial Sloan-Kettering Cancer Center were requested

TABLE 89.1
Equianalgesic Dosages

Medication	Equianalgesic Dosage (in mg)			Duration of Action (hours)
	Intramuscular/ Intravenous/Subcutaneous	Oral	Rectal	
Opioid Agonists				
Codeine	130	200	N/A	3–4
Fentanyl[a]	0.1–0.2	N/A[b]	N/A	1–2
Hydrocodone	N/A	30	N/A	3–4
Hydromorphone	1.5	7.5	3	3–4
Levorphanol[c]	2	4	N/A	4–5
	(Single dose)			
	1	1		
	(Repeated doses)			
Meperidine[d]	75–100	300	N/A	3–5
Methadone[e]	10	20	N/A	4–6
	(Single dose)			
	Variable	Variable		
	(Repeated doses, see Table 89.3)			
Morphine[f]	10	60	10–15	4–5
		(Single dose)		
		30		
		(Repeated doses)		
Oxycodone[g]	10–15[h]	20	N/A	4–6
Oxymorphone	1–1.5	N/A	10	4–6
Propoxyphene[i]	N/A	300–400	N/A	4–6

[a] Transdermal fentanyl dosage is not calculated as equianalgesic to a single morphine dose. In the steady-state condition, a 25-µg/hour patch is approximately equivalent to 10 mg of oral morphine sulfate every 4 hours.

[b] Oral transmucosal fentanyl citrate absorption is variable due to both immediate transmucosal absorption and slower gastrointestinal absorption.

[c] Levorphanol has a long half-life and accumulates over time.

[d] Meperidine is not appropriate for patients with cancer due to the half-life of its metabolite, normeperidine, which is 8 to 21 hours. Meperidine should never be administered beyond 600 mg/day as the accumulation of normeperidine leads to agitation, myoclonic twitching, and seizures.

[e] Methadone has a long half-life and accumulates over time (see Table 89.3).

[f] Morphine-6-glucuronide has a longer half-life than morphine and leads to greater morphine effectiveness over time. Note: As morphine-3- and morphine-6-gluconoride both lead to increased adverse side effects in patients with renal insufficiency, morphine should be avoided in patients with renal failure.

[g] Many equianalgesic tables have oxycodone as either equianalgesic to morphine or 1.5 times more potent than morphine. The product insert for OxyContin indicates that oxycodone is two times more potent than morphine.

[h] Oxycodone is only commercially available as an oral preparation in the United States. It is used parenterally outside the United States.

[i] Propoxyphene is so weak that it is usually ineffective for cancer pain of any significance; its metabolite norpropoxyphene accumulates leading to seizures.

for the management of drug-related issues (Passik & Portenoy, 1998).

While some degree of tolerance does occur over time with continuous opioid therapy, the need to increase opioid analgesic doses in patients with cancer more often relates to the progression of their underlying disease than to the rapid development of pharmacological tolerance. Physical dependence, the need that a person has for the medication to prevent distressing symptoms secondary (withdrawal or abstinence reaction) to the absence of the agent (Hill, 1988), is not addiction (a primarily psychological disorder with eventual physiological and sociological manifestations), and patients should not be identified as addicts just because they manifest tolerance or physical dependence related to opioids. Addiction, psychological dependence, signifies that the medication is compulsively

TABLE 89.2
Opioid Analgesics in the United States

Generic Name	Proprietary Name	Routes of Administration
Buprenorphine	Buprenex®	Intravenous/intramuscular/epidural
	Suboxone®, Subutex®	Sublingual
Butorphanol	Stadol®	Intravenous/intramuscular/nasal
Codeine	Tylenol® with codeine	Oral
Fentanyl	Actiq®	Transmucosal
	Duragesic®	Transdermal
	Sublimaze®	Intravenous/intramuscular/epidural/intrathecal
Hydrocodone	Hycodan®, Lortab®, Lorcet®, Norco®, Vicodin®, Xodol®, Zydone®	Oral
Hydromorphone	Dilaudid®, Palladone®	Intravenous/intramuscular/oral/subcutaneous
Meperidine	Demerol®	Intravenous/intramuscular/oral
Methadone	Dolophine®	Oral/intravenous/subcutaneous
Morphine	Avinza®, Kadian®, MS Contin®, Oramorph®	Oral
	MSIR®	Oral
	Generic	Oral/sublingual/subcutaneous/intramuscular/intravenous/rectal
	Astramorph®, Duramorph®	Intrathecal, epidural
Nalbuphine	Nubain®	Intravenous/intramuscular/subcutaneous
Oxycodone	OxyContin®, OxyFast®, Roxicet®, Endocet®, Endodan®, Percocet®, Percodan®	Oral
Oxymorphone	Numorphan®	Rectal/intramuscular/intravenous/subcutaneous
Pentazocine	Talwin®	Oral/intramuscular/intravenous
Propoxyphene	Darvon®, Darvocet®	Oral
Tramadol	Ultram®, Ultracet®	Oral

sought and used for effects other than pain relief (APS, 1999). The palliative care (pain) patient with a constant supply of medication that is used time-contingently shows little, if any, drug-seeking behavior (Passik & Portenoy, 1998). In fact, one of the greatest barriers to compliance with the time-contingent administration of these medications when patients are relatively comfortable is the mistaken belief by patients that they will develop an addictive disorder (Breitbart et al., 1998; Foley & Inturrisi, 1987; Ward et al., 1993). Data related to the risk of addiction have been traditionally obtained by surveying known addicts rather than prospectively following patients receiving legitimately prescribed opioid analgesics. In the past 20 years, it has been observed that the true incidence of opioid analgesic abuse is insignificant among patients with medically justified opioid use. Studies have shown that addiction develops in only 1 in 800 for headache sufferers to less than 1 in 10,000 burn patients (Medina & Diamond, 1977; Passik & Portenoy, 1998; Perry & Heidrich, 1982; Portenoy, 1990; Porter & Jick, 1980). Even the U.S. government has declared the risk of addiction in patients with cancer to be "an exceedingly rare event" (AHCPR, 1994).

Once the decision to use opioid analgesics is made, the issue becomes which one of them to use (Table 89.2). For mild to moderate pain, one can start with the lower potency opioid analgesics, such as codeine or hydrocodone. Using codeine for pain management poses an

interesting problem for some patients because codeine is a prodrug that must be converted to an active analgesic, morphine, via the CPY2D6 component of the hepatic P450 microsomal enzyme system and that system is lacking in 7% of Caucasians, 3% of Blacks, and 1% of Asians (Lurcott, 1999), and generally suppressed in all patients receiving the selective serotonin reuptake inhibitor (SSRI) medications fluoxetine and paroxetine (Stahl, 2000). In the United States these medications are commonly given as combination tablets containing aspirin, acetaminophen, or ibuprofen that may be more effective than the amount of the opioid analgesic involved. Codeine and propoxyphene tend to be quite toxic for some patients (elderly patients, those with renal insufficiency or opioid allergies), with hydrocodone products tending to be better-tolerated and more effective as analgesics. Tramadol hydrochloride (a weak opioid agonist that also inhibits the reuptake of norepinephrine and serotonin) is generally not used for patients with cancer and must not be given in doses greater than 400 mg per day for the relatively "healthy" younger patient, 300 mg per day for the greater than 75-year-old patient, 200 mg per day for the patient with creatinine clearance less than 30 ml/min, and only 100 mg per day for patients with cirrhosis (APS, 1999; MEC, 2000).

Some clinicians erroneously view oxycodone as a weak opioid analgesic, much like codeine, hydrocodone, and propoxyphene, but in reality, the coadministration of acetaminophen and aspirin limits the amount of oxy-codone patients can take in the form of a fixed combination medication. This leads to the mistaken belief that oxycodone is not strong enough for patients with cancer. Pure immediate-release and sustained-release oxycodone preparations are free of adjuvant analgesics and permit further titration of the medication to analgesia without the ceiling dose associated with the co-analgesics. Uniquely, immediate-release and sustained-release oxycodone, used either alone or after converting from a combination oxycodone-containing product, allow for the continued use of the same initial opioid from mild through moderate to severe pain. In the American Medical Association Project to Educate Physicians on End-of-Life Care, only oxycodone is listed as both a step 2 (moderate pain) and step 3 (severe pain) appropriate agent (Emanuel et al., 1999).

When the lower-potency opioid analgesics do not produce adequate relief, high-potency opioid analgesics are recommended. The reference gold standard for these opioid medications is traditionally morphine, because it has the distinct advantage of being available in the widest variety of formulations for ease of administration (immediate-release and sustained-release tablets, solutions of varied strengths, concentrate, suppositories, preservative-containing solutions for intramuscular and intravenous use, and preservative-free solutions for epidural and intraspinal techniques) on a worldwide basis. Morphine is the historic analgesic "gold standard" because it is an effective, relatively inexpensive opioid with a 4-hour duration of action (Twycross & Lack, 1984) and a short half-life, and is generally available throughout the world. Unlike opioid analgesics with a long half-life (methadone and levorphanol), morphine-caused complications and toxicity are usually resolved within a matter of hours. The ability to convert from one route of administration to another is quite simple with an equianalgesic table (see Table 89.1).

Sustained-release morphine allows the patient to have uninterrupted comfort and allows intact sleep for the patient and the caregiver. Sublingual morphine administration, although variable in absorption and efficacy, allows ease of administration without resorting to the parenteral or rectal routes. Morphine can also be applied topically to wounds, where the analgesic effect is probably mediated through local, peripherally located opioid receptors (Ribeiro et al., 2004). A metabolite of morphine, morphine-6-glucuronide, is an active analgesic with a longer duration of action and half-life than morphine (Andersen et al., 2003; Osborne et al., 1986). The accumulation of morphine-6-glucuronide probably accounts for the observation that repetitively administered oral morphine is one third as effective as intramuscular, while single-dose-administered morphine is only one sixth as effective (Reisine & Pasternak, 1996). Opioid equianalgesic tables in pharmacology textbooks are generally based

on acute pain models rather than patients with pain receiving chronic opioids, and they report the oral to parenteral efficacy of morphine as six to one. Hospice patients are not opioid naïve and should be dosed using the three-to-one conversion factor when estimating the oral-to-parenteral conversion of morphine.

This accumulation of morphine-6-glucuronide, leading to the observed increased effectiveness of morphine with repeat dosing, also indicates that the risk of toxicity from the metabolites morphine-3- and morphine-6-glucuronide occurs when patients with renal insufficiency are given morphine. Because of this potentially toxic outcome associated with morphine administration for compromised, sick hospice patients, morphine is no longer the sole gold standard for all patients with cancer-related pain as it was in the past now that other opioid agents are available.

All of the other opioids can be equally effective in controlling pain and are typically used as alternatives when patients are allergic to morphine, experience morphine-related toxicity, or express concern about taking morphine. The only opioid that is best avoided in patients with cancer is meperidine, due to the accumulation of the metabolite normeperidine, which is associated with the development of irritability, myoclonus, and generalized tonic-clonic seizures (AHCPR, 1994; APS, 1999; Foley & Inturrisi, 1989). Similar concerns exist with the use of higher doses of propoxyphene. Because many of patients with cancer require relatively high doses of an opioid medication, the additional use of a mixed agonist–antagonist (butorphanol, nalbuphine, and pentazocine) is also strongly discouraged because of the possible precipitation of opioid withdrawal and severe pain for these patients (APS, 1999; Foley & Inturrisi, 1987).

Opioid-related myoclonus has been reported for hydromorphone, meperidine, methadone, and morphine (Mercadante, 1998). Metabolites of these opioids may accumulate with renal insufficiency, leading to irritation of the cortex and brainstem reticular formation. Higher levels of morphine-3-glucuronide, morphine-6-glucuronide, and normorphine accumulate with renal failure and may result in generalized myoclonus when patients receive morphine (Reisine & Pasternak, 1996). The neuroexcitatory metabolites of morphine and hydromorphone may be responsible for the hyperalgesic state seen in patients with cancer treated with high doses of these medications, although this still remains controversial (Andersen et al., 2003; Mercadante, 1998).

Whether or not patients experience significant toxicity with morphine therapy, there may be times to consider changing to a semisynthetic opioid. Many of these are currently available (or soon to become available) as controlled-release preparations. Hydromorphone is frequently selected, as the duration of analgesic action and plasma half-life are the same as morphine (Pasero et al., 1999). Perhaps relatively less nauseating and CNS "toxic" than morphine, hydromorphone is available in immediate-release oral tablets (controlled-release tablets are available outside the United States and are in clinical trials in the United States), oral solutions, suppositories, and an injectable solution (10 mg/ml). The parenteral form can be quite useful for end-stage cancer pain management, especially when higher doses may be needed (Miller et al., 1999). Hydromorphone's metabolites (primarily hydromorphone-3-glucuronide) are not thought to be pharmacologically active, although myoclonus and mental status changes have been reported with high doses of hydromorphone, potentially making it particularly useful for patients with renal failure after dosage reduction and careful titration (Kuczynska, 2004; Kurella et al., 2003).

CASE EXAMPLE

Mr. C, a 70-year-old gentleman, had advanced lung cancer complicated by sacroiliac and fifth lumbar vertebral metastases. He experienced severe pain in his left thigh with muscular wasting. He had previously tried oral morphine with an unclear "reaction." Although he was able to tolerate oral fluids and solids without any overt difficulty, he was quite anxious about taking any oral analgesics and requested that his medication be provided by the intravenous route, a dosing format in which he had great confidence. Because he was cared for by his daughter, who was able to learn the needed skills, it was possible to consider the use of parenteral analgesics. He had been started on intravenous hydromorphone in the hospital before coming home to the hospice program. The hospice nursing staff maintained intravenous access through his PIC line, and his daughter gave him doses of 5 or 6 mg hydromorphone every 3 hours, with good relief of his pain for the first week on the program. He was able to sleep well and developed a good appetite. By the second week, his pain was beginning to bother him much more. It was decided to add the anti-inflammatory choline magnesium trisalicylate, at 750 mg orally four times daily with food, and to maintain the intravenous hydromorphone at 6 mg every 3 hours. Throughout the next week he felt much better, but he developed the need for increasing doses given at decreasing intervals by the fourth week. When his intravenous hydromorphone reached 11 mg every 2.5 hours, he developed considerable nausea and vomiting, associated with anxiety about the ability to ever control his side effects and pain simultaneously. He was given 1 to 2 mg of sublingual haloperidol every 4 hours as needed, relieving his nausea and vomiting. In the fifth and final week on the program, he was switched to a continuous intravenous infusion of hydromorphone at 4 mg/hour with excellent pain relief. He remained alert, active, and involved with his family and care needs. His family was grateful that they could maintain meaningful dialogue with him and complete much of the anticipatory bereavement work. On the day before he died, he met with the funeral director to plan the details of his own funeral and met with a close friend to help prepare the eulogy that would be delivered.

Oxycodone and fentanyl are also commonly used medications and allow for good pain relief with relatively little toxicity. Both of these medications are available in oral formulations in the United States. Oral fentanyl is available in the United States as a branded transmucosal delivery system, Actiq®, with interesting pharmacodynamics and pharmacokinetics (25 to 50% bioavailability depending upon its method of use and ability of patients to swallow their own saliva). In the chronic steady-state condition, a 25 μg/hour transdermal fentanyl patch is almost equianalgesic to 10 mg oral morphine sulfate every 4 hours or 30 mg every 12 hours when given as sustained-release tablets (Emanuel et al., 1999). Fentanyl patches may improve medication compliance because patients only have to change them every 3 days, and they are generally well tolerated (Nugent et al., 2001). Patients and health care staff, however, sometimes report that patches are difficult to titrate, require the use of a second medication for breakthrough pain, may cause skin irritation, do not always adhere well in hot and humid environments, may show erratic blood levels due to nonstandard thermal conditions or low bodyweight (less than 110 pounds), and have significant cost. During episodes of fever (temperature >104°F), exertion combined with sunny and warm environments, and exposure to high external temperature sources (heating pad, heated water beds, electric blankets, and car seats in the summer), the actual dose of fentanyl delivered may exceed the dose printed on the patch and lead to potential increases in serum fentanyl levels (Newshan, 1998). Dosing tables for fentanyl transdermal patches suggest that 45 to 60 mg per day of morphine is equivalent to 25 μg per hour of transdermal fentanyl, although inter- and intraindividual variability requires cautious dosing and titrating to effect (Pereira et al., 2001).

Controlled-release oxycodone has been designed to provide sustained delivery of oxycodone over 12 hours, with an oral bioavailability of 60 to 87% (MEC, 2000). With repeated dosing, steady-state levels are achieved in 24 to 36 hours; however, controlled-release oxycodone exhibits a unique biphasic absorption pattern with two apparent absorption half-times of 0.6 and 6.9 hours (describing the initial release of oxycodone from the outer layer of the tablet, followed by prolonged release from the core of the tablet through the use of a patented technology). This unusual release system allows for prompt establishment of stable blood levels of oxycodone with the first dose and little need to overlap parenteral medications with controlled-release oxycodone. Oxycodone is metabolized primarily to noroxycodone (a considerably weaker opioid than oxycodone) and minimally to oxymorphone (a potent analgesic mediated by the CYP2D6 P450 system). Similar to other controlled-release medications, controlled-release oxycodone must be swallowed whole and never broken, chewed, or crushed, which could lead to rapid release and absorption of a potentially toxic dose of medication. With hepatic failure, initial doses are one third to one half of the usual doses; however, oxycodone is not often associated with myoclonus or significant CNS toxicity due to its metabolites (MEC, 2000).

Despite appropriate use of opioids, some patients continue to have poorly controlled pain due to changing nociception related to disease progression, drug side effects, tolerance, and opioid metabolites among others (Mercadante & Portenoy, 2001a). These poorly controlled pain states frequently have a neuropathic quality (Mercadante & Portenoy, 2001b), and in an effort to better comfort these patients, basic and clinical research in recent years has focused frequently on the N-methyl-D-aspartate (NMDA) receptor. The NMDA receptors frequently play a role in opioid tolerance, neuropathic pain, and hyperalgesic states, and blockade of these receptors can help to attenuate certain NMDA-mediated pain conditions. Two NMDA-receptor blockers that have proved clinically useful are methadone and ketamine. Lack of well-controlled trials has probably restricted their recognition and use, and they frequently receive little mention in reviews on treatment of neuropathic pain (Dworkin et al., 2003; Mendell & Sahenk, 2003). Many palliative care and hospice teams, however, can readily attest to their efficacy.

Methadone is a synthetic opioid, which is a mu and delta opioid receptor agonist, an NMDA receptor antagonist, and an inhibitor of the reuptake of norepinephrine and serotonin. This would allow it to be useful in treating both nociceptive and neuropathic pain. Its use in addiction medicine creates a barrier in the minds of some physicians and patients to its use in pain control. Also, its long and variable half-life (12 to 120 hours) can cause its clinical dosing to be somewhat challenging with the main concern being gradual drug accumulation and toxicity.

Another challenge in prescribing methadone is that equianalgesic dosing conversions to methadone show large interindividual variability and are somewhat unpredictable. This may perhaps be in part due to its multiple modes of action, decreased cross-tolerance of opioid receptors, or elimination of active opioid metabolites (Bruera & Sweeney, 2002). Many older conversion tables are based on single dose studies and are inaccurate for converting to chronic dosing with methadone (Pereira et al., 2001). Table 89.3 shows one possible method for converting an opioid regimen to an estimated total daily dose of methadone.

Several methods have been recommended for initiating dosing with methadone. One of the more commonly employed methods is referred to as the United Kingdom or Morley–Makin model (Morley & Mekin, 1998), and this has also been described elsewhere (Wheeler & Dickerson, 2000). This model recommends using as-needed doses of methadone for the initial 5 days with patients

TABLE 89.3
Methadone Conversion Table for Long-Term Dosing

Equivalent Oral Daily Morphine Dose	Oral Morphine: Oral Methadone Conversion Ratio
<100 mg	3–5:1
100–300 mg	6–8:1
301–500 mg	8–10:1
501–800 mg	12–14:1
801–1,000 mg	16–18:1
>1,000 mg	18–?:1

guiding their analgesic dosing. Scheduled doses would be started on day 6. Because steady-state drug levels are not achieved until five half-lives have elapsed, and because methadone may have a 2- or 3-day half-life in some patients, this method might still result in drug accumulation and toxicity. A modification of this regimen is presented in Figure 89.1, and this dosing scheme allows for a more conservative titration.

Methadone can exhibit all of the same toxicities as other opioids. Constipation tends to be less of a problem, and this can be a reason to consider rotating to methadone (Daeninck & Bruera, 1999). Use of high doses of methadone has been associated with the cardiac problem of torsades de pointes (Krantz et al., 2002). Also, methadone is primarily metabolized by CYP450 3A4 and to a lesser extent by CYP450 1A2 and 2D6. This creates an obvious opportunity for significant drug–drug interactions to occur (Layson-Wolf, 2002). Methadone can be administered orally, rectally, or intravenously. Subcutaneous administration can result in localized erythema and induration, but site rotation and adding 1 to 2 mg dexamethasone per

1. Calculate the 24 h oral morphine equivalent.
2. The methadone dose for the patient will be 1/20th (mild to moderate pain) to 1/10th (severe pain) of the 24 hour oral morphine dose to a maximum of 20 mg methadone. Round dose to the nearest 2.5 mg increment. With severe pain not responding to an initial 20-mg maximum dose, consider using 25–30 mg as your maximum dose.
3. Stop the current opioid.
4. Start the fixed, calculated methadone dose every 3 h as needed. Continue to assess pain every 3 h. Hold methadone dose if the patient is comfortable or sedated.
5. The total daily dose of methadone is recorded each day, and the patient is observed for possible side effects.
6. On day 10 the average of the amount used on day 8 and day 9 will be calculated. One half of this dose will then be prescribed on a q12-hours dosing schedule. The breakthrough methadone dose will be approximately 10% of the 24-hour dose (rounding to the nearest 2.5 mg increment) given q6 hours as needed.

FIGURE 89.1 Method for converting opioids to oral methadone.

day to the infusion can ameliorate these side effects (Mathew & Storey, 1999).

CASE EXAMPLE

Mr. T N was a 63-year-old man with non-small cell lung cancer involving his right apex. He initially received radiation with good results and two courses of chemotherapy that he did not tolerate well. At 14 months after initial treatment, he had a relapse in his right apex with gradually increasing pain in his right shoulder and arm. He also developed a new pain in his midback with radiation around his chest to his left lower anterior ribs. A subsequent thoracic MRI (magnetic resonance imaging) scan showed a mass in his sixth thoracic vertebra with no spinal cord compression. He was given increasing doses of various pain medications and adjuvants without significant relief. At the time of his referral for palliative care consultation, he was already on OxyContin 120 mg every 12 hours, about 80 mg per day of liquid oxycodone for breakthrough pain, nortriptyline 75 mg at bedtime, gabapentin 600 mg three times daily, and 2 weeks of dexamethasone 4 mg twice daily. He had sharp burning pain in his right arm, midback, and left ribs, and his pain fluctuated in the 8 to 10 range on a 0 to 10 numerical scale. A decision was made to convert him to methadone to treat his mixed nociceptive/neuropathic pain syndrome. If oxycodone is considered to be 25 to 50% stronger than morphine, then 320 mg of oxycodone is equivalent to about 400 to 480 mg of morphine per day. Taking the midpoint of 440 mg as our equivalent dose, our conversion table would estimate that this patient may eventually require in the neighborhood of 44 to 55 mg of methadone per day (morphine in the 301 to 500 mg range has a morphine:methadone equivalency ratio of about 8:1 to 10:1). Because his total daily morphine equivalent dose is greater than 300 mg, he was started on 20 mg every 3 hours as needed.

Because 2 weeks of dexamethasone was not helping and because of concerns over the long-term use of steroids, this medication was tapered off over the next week and he was started on magnesium choline trisalicylate 750 mg three times daily for his bone involvement. Nortriptyline was continued for its antidepressant effect. Within 2 days of starting methadone his pain had subsided to the 4 to 5 range and it was in the 1 to 2 range by the fifth day. At this point his gabapentin was stopped with no increase in his pain level. Review of his methadone dosing over 9 days showed the following total daily doses: 80, 80, 40, 60, 50, 60, 55, 40, and 45 mg. His pain continued to be well controlled, and he was subsequently given a scheduled methadone dose of 20 mg every 12 hours with 5 mg every 4 hours as needed.

Ketamine is a surgical anesthetic agent that is also an NMDA receptor antagonist, and it is used in subanesthetic doses to relieve pain. It is usually reserved for patients with severe pain despite high opioid dosing or patients with intolerable opioid side effects. Ketamine is usually given as a constant infusion, and it does not depress the respiratory or cardiovascular systems. It can be administered orally 0.5 mg/kg every 12 hours (Furuhashi-Yonaha, 2002), but more often is given by either the intravenous or subcutaneous route. Excessive salivation can be managed by glycopyrrolate, and psychotomimetic effects (dysphoria, vivid dreams, hallucinations, delirium) often respond to small doses of a benzodiazepine given around the clock. Sedation can be expected when higher doses of ketamine are employed. Initial bolusing is done with 0.1 to 0.2 mg/kg intravenously or 0.5 mg/kg subcutaneously, and this is accompanied by a 50% decrease in the opioid dose. A subsequent infusion is started at 2 to 20 mg/hour depending on patient response. A recent review concluded that ketamine can be cautiously recommended as having potential efficacy as an opioid adjuvant (Bell et al., 2003).

The practice of combining opioid analgesics to provide better patient comfort is confusing for patients, their caregivers, and even the prescribing physicians. It is not justified under most circumstances, and there may be misuse of multiple opioid medications because few appreciate that titration and monitoring of a single opioid may require several days or longer. Also, sustained-release tablets do not adequately control pain until proper titration has occurred over 2 to 4 days. When two different medications are given simultaneously, it is usually because the base medication is not available in more than one or two routes of administration, the base medication has not been titrated to full effect, or there is some toxicity being experienced.

It is routinely necessary to provide additional immediate-release opioid medication for breakthrough pain occurring at certain times (incident pain, movement related pain), especially when the base opioid analgesic is a sustained-release preparation.

Unanticipated changes in pain can thus be effectively managed on an immediate basis, with day-to-day tailoring of the overall opioid medication by observing the use of these additional doses. Monitoring the 24-hour total usage of medication, and readjusting the daily scheduled dosage, is essential for keeping up with the analgesic needs of the patient. It is generally good practice to use the immediate-release form of the same opioid for breakthrough dosing as is used in the sustained-release preparation. The approximate dose of additional medication providing good control of breakthrough pain is 10 to 15% of the total daily amount of base medication (Emanuel et al., 1999). Using 10% is the easier method, allowing the prescriber to simply move the decimal point one digit to the left (avoiding the need for calculators) to determine the breakthrough dosage and then rounding up or down depending on the formulations available. This 10% method of calculating the breakthrough dose assumes that the same route of administration is used for the immediate-release medication as for the base controlled-release medication. Frequent use of breakthrough medication indicates that the patient's pain management must be reassessed and that the dose of the scheduled controlled-release medication must be increased.

Oral transmucosal fentanyl citrate is a solid form of fentanyl incorporated into a sweetened lozenge on a handle, and it is sometimes used for breakthrough pain when using transdermal fentanyl. It is partially absorbed rapidly through the oral mucosa, and it is subsequently more slowly absorbed in the gastrointestinal tract (APS, 1999). The blood levels achieved will vary, depending on the fraction of the dose that is absorbed through the oral mucosa and the fraction swallowed and absorbed from the gastrointestinal tract (MEC, 2000). Normally, about 25% of the total dose of oral transmucosal fentanyl citrate is rapidly absorbed from the buccal mucosa, and the remaining 75% is swallowed with the saliva and slowly absorbed; the generally observed 50% bioavailability is divided equally between rapid transmucosal and slower gastrointestinal absorption (MEC, 2000). Because only about one third of the swallowed medication escapes first-pass liver metabolism to become systemically available, patients with impaired swallowing (or those incapable of swallowing) receive only half of the potential analgesic efficacy of oral transmucosal fentanyl citrate. Its use is limited because of its expense and limited duration of action.

The major side effect of all opioid therapy is constipation, regardless of the route of administration. Constipation must be vigorously managed and prevented from the initiation of treatment. Unrelieved constipation adversely affects the quality of life and must not be ignored. Failure to correct opioid-induced constipation leads to intractable nausea, vomiting, abdominal discomfort, and possible bowel perforation, as well as emotional distress. Options for treating constipation include stimulant laxatives, combination stimulant/stool softeners, prokinetic agents, osmotic agents, lubricants, and enemas. Dietary interventions alone or the use of bulk-forming agents is often inadequate and not recommended for those with advanced disease and poor mobility (Emanuel et al., 1999). Recalling that dirt and water alone produce mud, a viscous material, but the combination of dirt, water, and fiber (straw, grass) produces brick (as in adobe), should clarify the admonition to avoid bulk-forming agents. Opioid antagonists that act peripherally but not centrally are currently in clinical trials. Such medications would counteract the constipating effects of opioids without interfering with the centrally mediated analgesic effects.

CASE EXAMPLE

Mr. F was sent home from the hospital with advanced prostate cancer and widespread bone metastases, with no bowel movement for 1 week prior to entering the hospice program. He was fairly comfortable from a pain perspective, although he experienced increasing abdominal fullness and discomfort thought to be due to opioid-induced constipation. Digital examination of the rectum found significant hard, impacted stool that was manually decompressed. Once free of the impaction, he was started on an oral laxative and stool softener combination, and he developed bowel regularity within 2 days.

Although nausea and vomiting are initially common with opioids, once acclimated to these medications (in a matter of days for most patients), nausea and vomiting developing later more often result from unrecognized and ineffectively treated constipation. Early in the use of opioids, nausea and vomiting are usually controlled with dopamine-blocking agents (e.g., haloperidol, metoclopramide, prochlorperazine), antihistamines (diphenhydramine, hydroxyzine, or meclizine), or anticholinergics (scopolamine) (Emanuel et al., 1999). Respiratory depression, significant CNS dysfunction, allergic reactions, pruritus, and diaphoresis are much less significant in comparison with constipation or nausea and vomiting.

When opioid analgesics fail to provide relief of significant pain despite clear toxicity (respiratory or CNS depression), it is necessary to remember that these agents are not always effective as sole agents for neuropathic pain due to nerve involvement, viscus or muscle spasm, or significant psychological distress. The use of the adjunctive medications — with or without further opioid analgesics — may be warranted.

Adjuvant medications include antidepressants, antipsychotics, anticonvulsants, anxiolytics, and psychostimulants. These useful agents can be added at any step in the continuum of cancer pain management and often save patients from unnecessary progression to high-potency opioids or complex analgesic technologies. The adjuvant medications manipulate the neurochemistry of the nervous system and augment the overall effectiveness of both NSAID and opioid combinations.

The antidepressants are remarkable agents, with the ability to block the presynaptic reuptake of norepinephrine and serotonin, resulting in elevated levels of these important neurotransmitters in the brain (Botney & Fields, 1982; Hendler, 1982). The benefit of enhanced serotonin centrally is the consequent periaquaductal release of endogenous opioid peptides with a dampening effect on pain perception (Frier, 1985). These agents correct the depression (which is so common with persistent pain), stabilize sleep, and improve appetite, energy level, concentration, and the ability to experience pleasure. The ability of antidepressants to relieve pain is independent of the antidepressant effect (Feinmann, 1985). Tricyclic antidepressants are recommended as one of the first-choice medications for painful polyneuropathy (Sindrup & Jensen, 2000) and especially for patients experiencing burning and tingling neuropathic pain (Emanuel et al., 1999). Although the antidepressants most traditionally used for neuropathic pain management are generally the serotonin-enhancing tricyclic agents (amitriptyline and imipramine), their more norepinephrine-enhancing tricyclic metabolites (nortriptyline and desipramine, respectively) are often particularly useful when patients are intolerant to the serotonin-enhancing effects or when psychomotor-retarded depression is present. Antidepressants are not habit forming and have little effect on respiration when used in therapeutic doses. Serotonin-enhancing tricyclic antidepressants are associated with a number of annoying anticholinergic side effects that limit their usefulness unless patients can tolerate them. The newer SSRIs, such as citalopram, fluoxetine, fluvoxamine, escitalopram, paroxetine, and sertraline, are generally free of the anticholinergic adverse effects (having unique side effects of their own), but are disappointing as co-analgesics (Emanuel et al., 1999). Atypical antidepressants (bupropion, mirtazapine, nefazodone, trazodone, and venlafaxine) are being evaluated for their analgesic usefulness and may provide benefit with less potential toxicity (Emanuel et al., 1999). Full effects of the antidepressants may not be seen for 4 to 6 weeks. It is also important to remember that the antidepressants are dissimilar enough that one should consider more than one trial with these agents.

CASE EXAMPLE

Mr. D, a 75-year-old gentleman, had severe lability of affect, impaired sleep, and advanced pulmonary cancer, leaving him short of breath and in need of continuous oxygen therapy. He had used diazepam for many years as a bedtime hypnotic, but the hospice staff was concerned about the CNS depressant effects of diazepam and sustained-release morphine. Rather than administer diazepam with the sustained-release morphine at 60 mg twice daily, he was started on 10 mg of doxepin hydrochloride at bedtime. This was eventually adjusted upward to 20 mg the next week with subsequent gradual improvement in sleep, stabilization of his mood, loss of affective lability, and better management of his chest wall pain.

Antipsychotic medications, still commonly referred to as neuroleptics or major tranquilizers, block the postsynaptic dopamine receptors and prevent the transmission of neuronal information. The consequence of the use of these agents is the functional disconnection of the limbic system (the modern-day equivalent of a noninva-

sive frontal lobotomy), with the patient relatively less concerned about the pain problem. This effect often permits the rapid tapering of high-dose opioid analgesic medication, especially intravenous, when a patient is trying to leave the hospital to return to the home setting. With antipsychotic medications, it is possible to significantly decrease the opioid dosage and maintain the patient in a relaxed state. Antipsychotic agents are also powerful antiemetics and control nausea and vomiting (Hanks, 1984; Johanson, 1988). The high-potency medications droperidol and haloperidol are particularly noteworthy because they work with minimal effect on the cardiovascular system. Droperidol is available only as a parenteral agent, but haloperidol is available as oral tablets and an oral concentrate (2 mg/ml) that can be used sublingually (Johanson, 1988). The low-potency medication thioridazine can be relatively toxic for the cardiovascular system and is best avoided in the seriously ill patient. Chlorpromazine is usually more sedating than haloperidol, but it also is an excellent antiemetic. Extrapyramidal reactions do occur with the high-potency medications, but they can be easily managed with the anticholinergic agents benztropine and diphenhydramine when necessary.

CASE EXAMPLE

Ms. M was a 45-year-old woman with end-stage human immunodeficiency virus (HIV) infection. She was experiencing only mild pain, but she suffered from intractable nausea and vomiting that were not relieved with standard antiemetics used orally or rectally. She was given 1 mg of sublingual haloperidol every 4 hours, with good control of her symptoms, and was eventually maintained well on haldol 2 mg twice daily.

In general, the anticonvulsants are frequently effective oral medications for deafferentation (neuropathic) pain, nerve injuries, and pain characterized by burning, tingling, or paroxysms (Swerdlow, 1986). Anticonvulsants stabilize nerve cell membranes and inhibit spontaneous discharge by blocking sodium channels nonspecifically, resulting in the control of seizures centrally or neuropathic pain peripherally (Sindrup & Jensen, 2000; WHO, 1986). The most commonly used agents (carbamazepine, clonazepam, gabapentin, phenytoin, and valproic acid) have been employed in the management of lancinating or stabbing dysesthetic pain (Emanuel et al., 1999; Hardy et al., 2001; Lack, 1984; Sindrup & Jensen, 2000). Bruera, Walker, and Lawlor (1999) reported that most patients with neuropathic pain do improve on opioid analgesics. Based on a prospective open-label study in which more than two thirds of patients with neuropathic pain achieved good analgesia with opioids alone, coupled with the expected effectiveness of adjuvants rarely exceeding 30%, they recommended opioids as the first-line treatment for these patients. They advised using the adjuvants when patients reached dose-limiting toxicity. The use of methadone, discussed earlier in this chapter, is consistent with this concept. Also, another study has shown that levorphanol is useful for neuropathic pain in a dose-dependent manner (Rowbotham et al., 2003).

Clonazepam is a potent benzodiazepine with a relatively greater anticonvulsant effect than its congeners (Hanks, 1984). Clonazepam is one of the least difficult anticonvulsants to use in the home hospice setting because it can be used without the need for blood-level monitoring. Because it does tend to accumulate and may cause a moderate degree of sedation, clonezapam is often avoided in severely ill patients. However, the long half-life of clonazepam allows for effective once-daily dosing for many patients.

Gabapentin has become the more typically utilized oral anticonvulsant for neuropathic pain management (Emanuel et al., 1999). Gabapentin is generally started in low doses (100 mg, one to three times daily) and titrated upward to clinical effect (the reduction of pain) or the manifestation of dose-limiting toxicity (sedation and ataxia). There are no specific blood levels correlating to pain relief, and patients may require 3,600 mg per day or more to obtain pain relief. As it is renally excreted, dose reduction is necessary in those with renal insufficiency. Based on various studies addressing the treatment of neuropathic pain, gabapentin is considered to be one of the medications of first choice for the treatment of painful polyneuropathy (Sindrup & Jensen, 2000). Gabapentin is also better tolerated than amitriptyline as shown in a recent study treating diabetic neuropathy (Dallocchio et al., 2000).

Carbamazepine (with the relative risk of bone marrow suppression) and valproic acid (with the relative risk of gastric upset), coupled with the need for blood level monitoring, are generally less attractive as anticonvulsants for the home hospice patient. Carbamazepine is one of the medications of first choice for the treatment of painful polyneuropathy (Sindrup & Jensen, 2000). Carbamazepine is traditionally a preferred medication for trigeminal neuralgia and for other supraclavicular pain problems (phenytoin having the historical reputation for being the anticonvulsant to treat infraclavicular pain), but carbamazepine and valproic acid have the distinct disadvantage of requiring several days of oral titration before therapeutic improvement is noted. Both blood-level monitoring and complete blood counts are recommended with the use of carbamazepine.

Lidocaine has also been used for treatment of poorly controlled neuropathic pain. Lidocaine is a sodium channel-blocking agent, a mode of action it holds in common with mexiletene and carbamazepine. Inhibition or modulation of sodium channels appears to suppress neural pain transmission. Continuous subcutaneous lidocaine infu-

sions at rates between 10 to 80 mg/hour have been reported to relieve intractable pain with few significant side effects (Ferrini, 2000). Similar to when adding NSAIDs to an opioid regime, vigilance must be maintained in watching for rapid significant pain relief, which may necessitate an opioid dose reduction. Lidocaine has also been used topically for relief of neuropathic pain. A 5% lidocaine patch was effective in a placebo-controlled, two-way, crossover clinical trial with patients with peripheral neuropathic pain syndromes (Meier et al., 2003). Lidocaine-induced side effects can occur regardless of the route of administration, and such side effects usually correlate with serum levels. Lightheadedness, tongue numbness, blood pressure changes, muscle twitching, and visual or auditory disturbances are associated with lower lidocaine concentrations. The occurrence of such symptoms usually alerts one to lower the infusion rate before more toxic levels can be achieved, which are associated with seizures, coma, and respiratory arrest. Patches, up to three at one time, are usually applied for only 12 hours per day and can cause localized rashes.

Anxiety, depression, fear, sleeplessness, and restlessness may all lower a patient's pain tolerance (Emanuel et al., 1999; Hanks, 1984). Benzodiazepines, although not thought of as analgesics, have a limited role in the management of cancer pain. Most hospice patients sleep fairly well; but as some of them near the end of their lives, they may have disturbing dreams and recurrent nightmares interfering with the restful quality of their sleep for which benzodiazepines may prove helpful. Additionally, when pain interferes with the normal sleep pattern such that little or no stage four delta-wave sleep occurs, the addition of a short-acting sedative hypnotic agent (estazolam, triazolam, or zolpidem) may be beneficial. It appears that without the deepest stage of sleep, muscles do not completely relax, and muscular pain may spontaneously develop, causing the patient widespread discomfort. By improving deep stage four sleep, this diffuse muscular ache that many patients with cancer experience, which is also a consequence of their debilitation and malnutrition, can be lessened. When patients are morbidly anxious about their condition, the addition of a benzodiazepine medication may significantly allay their anxiety. For this indication, the long half-life benzodiazepine medications are preferable to the short half-life medications, which are more likely to produce wide swings in blood levels and consequent rebound anxiety.

Psychostimulants, such as dextroamphetamine and methylphenidate, are useful for the relief of depression, diminishing excessive sedation due to opioids, potentiating the analgesic effect of opioids in patients with postoperative and cancer pain, promoting a sense of well-being, and lessening feelings of weakness and fatigue (Breitbart et al., 1998; Homsi et al., 2000). Doses commonly used are 5 to 10 mg once or twice daily (breakfast and lunch), with few patients requiring more than 30 mg per day (Emanuel et al., 1999). Compared with traditional antidepressants, the psychostimulants can show beneficial effects within several days rather than several weeks. Appetite can be enhanced (if significant depression is relieved) or suppressed, which can be a problem in patients with cancer. Pemoline, a unique alternative to the amphetamine-like medications, lacks abuse potential, has mild sympathomimetic effects, has low DEA scheduling permitting telephone orders, and comes in a chewable tablet form that can be absorbed through the buccal mucosa. It is not established, however, that it potentiates opioids, although it counters the sedation of opioids and relieves depression (Breitbart et al., 1998). Pemoline should be used with caution in patients having underlying liver disease.

ANESTHETIC TECHNIQUES

Certain anesthetic techniques are occasionally needed for the hospice patient. Some of the more useful procedures include the celiac plexus block for abdominal pain, the stellate ganglion block for upper quarter pain, the lumbar sympathetic block for lower extremity pain, the intraspinal neurolytic block for bilateral lower body pain, and the epidural use of opioid analgesics (Cousins & Mather, 1984; Foley, 1985).

The celiac plexus block can provide abdominal analgesia for several months and is an acceptable management approach for pancreatic (Parris, 1985), hepatic, and intestinal cancer and abdominal carcinomatosis from ovarian malignancy. A significant reduction in pain after this block is reported by 60 to 90% of patients (Foley, 1985; Verrill, 1989). If survival extends beyond several months, the block can be repeated, although frequently with a less successful outcome.

The stellate ganglion block is useful for sympathetically mediated pain involving the scalp, face, neck, arm, and upper chest (Campbell, 1989). This technique is frequently used in the management of upper quarter pain related to brachial plexus involvement by lung cancer or highly invasive breast cancer. Often, a single block is useful, but commonly, a series of these blocks is performed to modify the discomfort. When effective, the results of this block can be quite impressive and startling.

Intraspinal neurolysis is a highly destructive technique used for intractable pain when lower-body motor function, along with bowel and bladder control, is lost, usually due to a spinal cord tumor or invasion of the spine by metastatic lesions. It involves the deliberate chemical coagulation of the remaining cord structures by placing alcohol or phenol in the subdural space (Ferrer-Brechner, 1989). The end result is absolute anesthesia below the level of the completed cord destruction.

CASE EXAMPLE

Mr. A, a 65-year-old gentleman, had a widely metastatic prostate cancer that had invaded his lumbar spine anteriorly and left him paralyzed below the level of the lesion, without bowel or bladder control, but in constant excruciating pain in his lower body. Despite adequate trials of NSAID medication, low- and high-potency opioid analgesics, and transcutaneous electrical nerve stimulation, nothing seemed to relieve his suffering. After consultation with an anesthesiologist, it was decided to complete his cord lesion with intraspinal alcohol. This was done with the patient's informed consent and quickly produced complete resolution of his lower body pain. He still required some anti-inflammatory and opioid analgesic medication for his upper body pain, but was much improved and relatively comfortable after the spinal neurolysis.

Epidural and spinal administration of opioid analgesics is quite effective when the pain is fairly localized, especially if it is entirely below the level of the nipples. Long-term use of intraspinal opioids can be recommended for patients with cancer with regionalized pain below T1 failing to achieve pain control after adequate trials of several different systemic opioids (APS, 1999). By placing the opioid analgesic into the epidural space or intraspinally, the patient experiences relatively little cognitive impairment, and while the pain is significantly relieved, normal sensation is preserved. Once the catheter is in place, the opioid (usually fentanyl, hydromorphone, or morphine) is administered by continuous infusion or by bolus injections. The availability of small, lightweight, battery-powered portable infusion pumps allows the hospice nursing staff to provide a 24- to 48-hour supply of medication to the patient without the risk of catheter infection due to poor injection technique by the nonprofessional caregiver. Contraindications (absolute and relative) for epidural and spinal opioids with or without anesthetic agents include bleeding diathesis, septicemia, local cutaneous infection at the site of catheter insertion, known immune suppression, insulin-dependent diabetes, and lack of appropriate support for the ongoing management of the catheter (Swarm & Cousins, 1998).

SPECIAL CONSIDERATIONS FOR PARENTERAL THERAPIES

Parenteral opioid infusions are used much more frequently than anesthetic procedures, but less frequently than oral medications. They can be extremely beneficial for those patients who have patent intravenous access, swallowing difficulties that prevent the use of oral medications, the need for large dosages of medication, and the lack of other routes of administration of opioids. The common technique for the administration of parenteral opioids is via a portable infusion pump delivering high-potency opioid analgesics through a small needle inserted into the subcutaneous tissue.

CASE EXAMPLE

Ms. T was a 60-year-old woman with advanced hepatic cancer with pelvic metastases. She had delayed chemotherapy to allow for a long-hoped-for trip to Europe. When she first presented to the hospice program, she was experiencing severe bilateral hip pain with radiation into her thighs. Bothersome muscle spasms complicated her pain problem. She was a suspicious, guarded woman who did not have much faith in her physicians. She did not want to take any medication and desperately wanted to avoid being hospitalized. She was initially treated for her pain with intravenous morphine titrated eventually to 12 mg/hour, and was successfully converted to oral morphine in sustained-release form at 400 mg every 12 hours. Once she went home, she began to need more morphine and was quickly using 150 to 180 mg of immediate-release morphine every day in addition to the sustained-release morphine. The hospice staff observed that she used more morphine when her family members were present. Due to the wide fluctuations in her comfort level, and her increasing belief that the oral medications would never entirely control her discomfort, she was started on a subcutaneous hydromorphone infusion at 2 mg/hour, with satisfactory pain control within 1 day.

For cancer pain that becomes "out of control," Berger et al. (2000) have described a technique using intravenous ketamine (2 mg/ml), fentanyl (5 mg/ml), and midazolam (0.1 mg/ml) to control pain after traditional analgesics were unsuccessful. They felt that ketamine, an NMDA receptor antagonist, and midazolam, a benzodiazepine useful for myoclonus, nausea, and cognitive disturbances associated with opioid therapy, would enhance the overall analgesic effect of fentanyl. The use of several medications to treat intractable pain and suffering or to relieve terminal restlessness is often referred to as "total sedation" or "palliative sedation." Most often a parenteral benzodiazepine or barbiturate is employed, although antipsychotic and anesthetic agents can also be used (Rousseau, 2002). It is common to continue an opioid because many patients are continuing to experience pain. Efforts have been made to establish guidelines to help hospice teams and families as they approach these difficult clinical and ethical decisions (Braun et al., 2003).

NONPHARMACOLOGIC APPROACHES

Pain is also managed by a number of nonpharmacologic methods, including cognitive therapy, hypnosis, relaxation and imagery, distraction, reframing, patient education, peer support groups, transcutaneous electrical nerve stimulation (TENS), radiation therapy, surgery, and physical,

occupational, massage, music, art, and aroma therapy services (AHCPR, 1994; Emanuel et al., 1999). For prominent muscle spasm, predictably painful procedures, depression, and anxiety, the cognitive techniques are useful (Cleeland, 1987). Hypnosis can augment pain control but rarely relieves the pain completely. Providing orthotics or prosthetics, assistive devices, range-of-motion exercises, and bedside stretching can keep the remaining activities of daily living accessible for the patient. Radiation therapy and TENS are often effective management for bone metastases and pathologic fractures (Bosch, 1984; Howard-Ruben et al., 1987). TENS requires the participation of the patient. While a meta-analysis of studies of TENS therapy in postoperative patients found that both TENS and sham TENS significantly reduced pain intensity, suggesting that part of the efficacy of TENS could be attributed to placebo effect, patients with mild pain may benefit from a trial of TENS (AHCPR, 1994).

Surgical interventions in hospice patients are infrequent but can be quite appropriate to relieve bowel obstruction or to remove a gangrenous leg. Also, in patients with certain gastrointestinal tract cancers, one can consider biliary, esophageal, and intracolonic stenting.

RADIOTHERAPY

Radiation therapy can be a very effective form of treatment for local metastatic bone pain, spinal cord and cauda equina compression, brain metastases, mediastinal compression, superior vena cava obstruction, lung collapse due to bronchial obstruction, urinary tract obstruction, and limb edema (Hoskin, 1998). The strategy for palliative radiation therapy differs from the techniques used for active cancer treatment. Protracted regimens of more than 10 treatments may be more appropriate for patients with life expectancy longer than 6 months to reduce potential late radiation effects or acute effects such as nausea if critical structures such as the stomach have to be included in the radiation field. However, for patients with a more limited life expectancy, radiation can be administered in fewer fractions (Anderson & Coia, 2000; Lawton & Maher, 1991; Maher et al., 1992). In the hospice setting, a single high dose of radiation is generally as effective as multiple smaller doses for the control of pain from bone metastases (Jeremic, 2001). Serious late radiation damage (unlikely when life expectancy is short) is related to both high total doses and the delivery of radiation in large fractions over a relatively short period (Hoskin, 1998). Most retrospective and prospective studies report that 75% or more of patients obtain relief from pain and about half of those who achieve relief become pain free (Nielsen et al., 1991).

Radiopharmaceuticals are used therapeutically for the relief of pain in patients with cancer (AHCPR, 1994). Iodine-131 results in bone scan evidence of response in

53% of patients with bone metastases from thyroid cancer (Maxon & Smith, 1990). Strontium-89 is the most extensively evaluated as a treatment for bone pain and compares favorably with hemibody irradiation in randomized trials, but it is potentially effective only in the treatment of pain due to osteoblastic bone lesions or lesions with an osteoblastic component (Silberstein, 2000). Strontium-89 is reported to provide partial pain relief in 65 to 80% of patients and complete pain relief for 10% of patients (AHCPR, 1994; Hoskin, 1998). Rhenium-186 and samarium-153 phosphonate chelates have demonstrated 65 to 80% efficacy in international trials (Maxon, et al., 1990; Turner, Claringbold, Hetherington, Sorby, & Martindale, 1989). These beta-emitting radiopharmaceuticals, requiring only a single intravenous injection, are used to relieve pain from widespread osteoblastic skeletal metastases visualized with bone scintigraphy. Approximately 50% of patients will respond to a second administration if pain recurs (AHCPR, 1994). The radiopharmaceuticals are most often used when patients fail to improve with NSAIDs, opioids, and external beam radiation.

Bisphosphonates (previously called diphosphonates) inhibit osteoclast activity and reduce bone resorption. Pamidronate and clodronate produce pain relief and reduce other skeletal morbidity (Hoskin, 1998). Placebo-controlled studies with oral clodronate in women with metastatic breast cancer demonstrated lower numbers of hypercalcemic events, vertebral fractures, rates of vertebral deformity, and combined rates of all morbid skeletal events. Zoledronic acid, a newer bisphosphonate, appears to be equally as effective as pamidronate, and it can be infused over 5 minutes rather than several hours (Berenson, 2001). Because analgesia often begins weeks after treatment is initiated, the late use of bisphosphonates in hospice patients may not produce significant pain improvement if they are being used only during a patient's final days (Hoskin, 1998).

FINAL COMMENTS ABOUT PAIN CONTROL

To successfully manage the patient with terminal cancer pain, all of the underlying issues must be globally addressed. The etiology of the pain must be accurately defined to direct the appropriate therapy. The analgesics may progress from nonsteroidals to opioids and adjuvants, but with the clear understanding that the medications are titrated and used for sufficient time to adequately assess their efficacy. Realistic goals about pain and its management must be set and clear communication maintained with all of the parties involved. Education of the patient and the family regarding the use of resources and decision making for the various types of therapy are part of the process (Ferrer-Brechner, 1984). Education about the ability to control pain effectively and correction of myths about the use of opioids must be included as part of the

treatment plan (AHCPR, 1994; Emanuel et al., 1999). The emotional and spiritual needs of the patient are as important, and as aggressively managed, as the somatic needs (Emanuel et al., 1999). Psychosocial interventions should be introduced early in the course of illness so that patients can learn and practice these strategies while they have sufficient strength and energy (AHCPR, 1994).

SYMPTOM MANAGEMENT

In addition to pain, hospice patients, especially those with cancer, can be bothered by constipation, nausea and vomiting, poor appetite and weight loss, dyspnea, seizures, difficulties with oral care, hydration, skin integrity, and itching. These symptoms are bothersome, steal quality and comfort from the patient, and must be as aggressively managed as pain.

CONSTIPATION

As noted earlier, constipation is the expected consequence of opioid analgesic management and must be anticipated and preventively controlled from the moment opioids are used. Most patients can be given a high-fiber diet or a bulk laxative early on in their illness to prevent constipation. If ineffective, or if the patients are taking opioids, additional laxative strategies are needed (Emanuel et al., 1999; Portenoy, 1987). Bowel care products are available in a variety of groups, including stool softeners, which prevent excessive drying; stimulants, which increase mucosal secretion and peristalsis, causing movement of fecal material; and combination products. Osmotic wetting agents, lubricants, and prokinetic medications are also available. The goal of therapy for the prevention of constipation is to maintain bowel regularity and keep the stool texture similar to that of toothpaste. In that way, even the weakest patient remains able to expel stool with little straining or effort. Most patients respond well to a combination of a stool softener and a laxative.

NAUSEA AND VOMITING

Nausea and resulting vomiting may initially be due to opioid analgesics, but over time may result from metastases, unrelieved constipation, meningeal irritation, metabolic abnormalities, medications, mucosal irritation, infections, or bowel obstruction (Emanuel et al., 1999; Rhodes & McDaniel, 2001). If a correctable process is the cause, it is best to manage the symptom by focusing on the pathology. When this is not possible, then the routine use of antiemetics is justified. Metoclopramide improves gastric emptying and affects the CNS vomiting center at higher doses (Ventafridda & Caraceni, 1994). The high-potency antipsychotic medications droperidol and haloperidol, oral, sublingual, or parenteral, are effective for nausea and vomiting (Johanson, 1988). The lower-potency antipsychotic medications, such as the typical antiemetics, are generally more sedating than the high-potency agents and are more likely to produce unpleasant side effects such as dry mouth, constipation, urinary hesitancy, and hypotension. Despite this, chlorpromazine can still be quite helpful in patients with difficult-to-control vomiting. Nausea may also respond to serotonin antagonists that are able to suppress the serious chemotherapy-induced nausea associated with even Cisplatin (Johanson, 1993). Olanzapine, an atypical antipsychotic, is an antagonist at dopamine, histamine, acetylcholine, and serotonin receptors, and has been shown to be effective with intractable nausea and vomiting (Srivastava et al., 2003). Until vomiting is well controlled, most patients and their family members experience high levels of discomfort.

Loss of Appetite and Cachexia

Appetite loss, declining weight, and the underlying disease process leave most hospice patients weak, listless, and susceptible to skin breakdown. As a result of chemotherapy, radiation therapy, surgery, and the overall debilitation of chronic illness, many patients experience a reduced level of pleasure associated with eating. Some patients may even become anxious about eating due to swallowing difficulties, the risk of choking, or aspiration. The review of food preferences may be quite useful. Small, frequent portions of favorite foods are better tolerated than large, traditional meals (Lang & Patt, 1994). If chemotherapy has left the patient with little sense of taste, altering the diet to include highly seasoned or spicy foods or serving meals as colorfully as possible may help to stimulate the appetite (Kaye, 1989). Education for caregivers about loss of appetite as part of the dying process is critical because these caregivers may view the patients' loss of interest in food, and resulting cachexia, as therapeutic failure on their part (Emanuel et al., 1999). Ultimately, hospice patients should be permitted to eat whatever might give them enjoyment, not what the caregivers think is best for them to eat.

Case Example

Ms. A was a severely emaciated woman with advanced ovarian and abdominal carcinomatosis. She had undergone extensive surgical resection of her tumor, radiation therapy, and several courses of chemotherapy. She had lost most of her appreciation for taste and consequently found all food to have the taste and texture of oatmeal. It was hard for her to maintain her weight without motivation to eat. She began to experiment with different foods and found that spicy Mexican and Chinese meals were satisfying and helped her remain motivated to eat, whereas the more traditional oral nutritional supplements were refused. She enjoyed the cold and creamy quality of vanilla ice cream over any other dessert-type food.

Pharmacologic strategies for stimulating appetite include the use of alcohol, corticosteroids, megestrol, androgens, and the marijuana derivative dronabinol (Emanuel et al., 1999). Preliminary research suggests that treatment with medications may stimulate appetite with relatively low risk of serious side effects (Lang & Patt, 1994), but there is little evidence that such interventions in hospice patients can increase lean body mass or improve their performance scores.

Dyspnea

Dyspnea, an uncomfortable sensation or awareness of breathing, can be a mild or extremely distressing symptom at the end of life. It will occur in 21 to 90% of patients with cancer, and almost one fourth of hospice patients with dyspnea have no known cardiopulmonary pathology (Thomas & von Gunten, 2002). It does not always correlate with hypoxemia in that some hypoxic patients report no dyspnea and some patients with normal blood gases can be very dyspneic. Sometimes simple maneuvers such as keeping the room temperature cool or using a room fan can be very effective. If the patient is hypoxic and dyspneic, then supplemental oxygen is indicated. One would also want to consider bronchodilators and steroids if there is an underlying reversible obstructive process causing dyspnea.

One of our most effective interventions for dyspnea that persists despite our usual interventions is the use of opioids. Many physicians and patients have been reluctant to use opioids for this symptom because of the common belief that opioids suppress the respiratory drive too greatly. Use of oral morphine (0.8 mg/kg) in patients with COPD (chronic obstructive pulmonary disorder) was shown to increase exercise tolerance and decrease dyspnea with only a slight decrease in PaO_2 (from 71.9 to 65.8 mm Hg) and mild increase in $PaCO_2$ (from 38.3 to 43.5 mm Hg) (Light et al., 1989). Starting with low doses of oral morphine (5 to 10 mg q 4 hours as needed) or other short-acting opioids usually allows one to palliate patients with dyspnea without concern for respiratory suppression. If the shortness of breath is accompanied by significant anxiety, the clinician can also consider using benzodiazepines or phenothiazines.

Seizures

Seizures occur in 35 to 60% of patients with primary brain cancer and in 25 to 30% of patients with metastatic brain lesions (Krouwer et al., 2000). Seizure frequency tends to increase with the number of brain lesions. Also, seizures associated with primary brain cancers or with cancer in the temporal and frontal lobes are often more difficult to treat. Although fairly easy to control with oral anticonvulsants and steroids, seizures occurring near the end of life are problematic because the patients often are no longer able to swallow effectively and often choose not to return to the hospital. Intravenous administration of lorazepam 2 mg and diazepam 5 mg in an outpatient setting effectively treated status epilepticus in 50 and 42%, respectively (Alldredge et al., 2001). Many patients with cancer, however, do not have easy venous access and resist returning to a clinic or hospital. An alternative to the use of crushed tablets or liquid suspensions via a feeding tube is the rectal or sublingual administration of benzodiapezines. Rectal administration of diazepam in a gel form or a solution is the optimal treatment when using the rectal route. Dosages can range from 10 to 20 mg depending on the patient's weight. The same dose of diazepam can be repeated every 15 to 20 minutes for an additional two doses when necessary (Krouwe et al., 2000). An alternative would be the rectal administration of 2 to 4 mg of lorazepam at similar intervals. Sublingual lorazepam or intranasal benzodiazepines in pediatric populations have also been described but standard dosing has not been established. Seizure prophylaxis can be accomplished with rectal dosing with valproic acid, carbamazepine, or benzodiazepines. Lorazepam provides seizure control for 3 to 4 hours (Leppik, 1983), does not significantly accumulate because it has no active metabolites, and is rapidly absorbed. As seizures are often an agonal event, giving a few intramuscular injections is another option for experienced caregivers once they understand that patients are not going to experience significant pain. Other possible seizure management alternatives include valproate sodium injection (if intravenous access is present), given at less than 20 mg per minute and over 60 minutes per dose; diazepam, 20 mg per rectum once or twice daily; midazolam, 30 to 60 mg per day by continuous infusion; and phenobarbital, 200 to 600 mg per day by continuous infusion (Twycross & Lichter, 1998).

CASE EXAMPLE

Ms. H was a 65-year-old woman with ovarian cancer that had metastasized to her right brain, producing a left hemiplegia and motor seizures. She was a remarkably angry woman who, while mildly dysphasic in her speech, was actually electively mute at times. Initially, 300 mg phenytoin at bedtime controlled her seizures. Later, 1 mg clonazepam was added at bedtime to control sleep and reported spasm, along with 30 mg sustained-release morphine twice daily for abdominal pain. This produced marked daytime agitation, which was felt to be due to the benzodiazepine, and it was replaced by 2 mg oral haloperidol every 2 hours as needed. She lost control of swallowing and stopped taking any oral medications, fluids, or foods in the last week of her life. This resulted in more frequent and severe motor sei-

zures that resulted in secondary generalization. Diazepam was given rectally in a 10 mg dose with good results, and she was subsequently maintained on diazepam 5 mg per rectum every 12 hours. Although she steadily deteriorated, she did not appear to experience significant pain and was able to remain seizure-free with the diazepam.

SKIN CARE

Skin care is vitally important for hospice patients, especially those who are bed bound. Minor and usually reversible skin disorders may become a major problem in the chronically sick patient, where healing powers are limited (Mortimer, 1993). Changes in body position, with frequent turning, proper padding with heel and ankle protectors, and a thick foam mattress cover should be used to prevent decubitus ulceration. There must always be 1 inch of foam between the lowest point of the patient and the surface of the bed (Emanuel et al., 1999). Once ulcers are established, they are difficult to treat due to the poor wound healing found in malnourished and debilitated patients. Bowel and bladder incontinence will produce skin breakdown if the patient is not kept relatively clean and dry. While powders and absorbent surfaces are helpful in keeping the patient dry, the use of urinary catheters and rectal tubes may be of assistance if soiling is constant and/or the patient is highly debilitated. The application of a "barrier" ointment can be quite effective once the skin is irritated. Metronidazole applied topically or given orally in doses of 250 to 500 mg three times per day can be helpful when skin lesions become malodorous.

CASE EXAMPLE

Ms. K, an 80-year-old woman with pancreatic cancer and secondary liver failure, had developed skin breakdown of her buttocks due to frequent diarrhea. Cleansing of her buttocks and perineum was associated with burning pain due to extensive irritation. She became progressively more fearful of any type of bowel activity and would allow herself to remain in a fecal- and urine-soaked bed rather than request appropriate care. To relieve her condition, and her resulting anxiety about hygiene, she was given a topical material made from equal parts of zinc oxide ointment, vitamin A and D ointment, and 1% dibucaine, to be applied to the involved area every 4 to 6 hours. Within the first few applications, immediate comfort was obtained, and significant healing occurred over the next 3 weeks.

PRURITUS

Itching can be quite serious for patients with extremely dry skin and is often a complication of systemic conditions such as renal failure, cholestasis, and various cancers including lymphoma. Some of the more common chemical mediators of itching include histamine, serotonin, dopamine, prostaglandins, cytokines, and opioids (Krajnik & Zylicz, 2001). Applying topical moisturizers may be helpful for skin dryness, but for protracted itching, use of the antihistamines diphenhydramine and hydroxyzine or low-dose antidepressants may provide relief (Johanson, 1988; Kaye, 1989). One particularly useful agent for itching is the antidepressant doxepin hydrochloride, a potent antihistamine about 800 times more antihistaminic than diphenhydramine (Richelson, 1979). Serotonin-mediated pruritus is more often associated with renal and hepatic failure and can be treated with paroxetine or mirtazapine (Davis et al., 2003).

MOUTH CARE

Oral care is routinely performed by healthy individuals and sadly forgotten in some terminal patients. With dehydration due to decreased oral intake, coupled with mouth breathing as death approaches, it is common for the oral membranes to become dry and irritated. Cleansing the mouth with small quantities of water, giving ice chips, wiping the mouth with a lemon-flavored glycerine swab, and applying a lip balm are soothing for the dying patient (Kaye, 1989) and also help to relieve the sensation of thirst. Xerostomia can be treated by removing offending agents, frequent sips of liquids, salivary stimulants such as pilocarpine and sugarless gum or lozenges, and by use of saliva substitutes (Sweeney & Bagg, 2000). Oral mucositis can also accompany the use of chemotherapy and radiotherapy. Patients with mucositis frequently experience increased depression, anger, fatigue, and anxiety with an overall decrease in quality of life (Dodd et al., 2001). Many single and combination agents and modalities have been used to prevent and treat oral mucositis with varying degrees or success and without establishing one standard of care (Köstle et al., 2001).

CONCLUSION

Palliative and hospice care should be a choice for every person coping with the end of life. It requires a special commitment on the part of the caregiver and the support of a skilled interdisciplinary team. Hospice and palliative care work with pain and symptom management is enriched by the patients who believe in the hospice philosophy and provide the opportunity to participate in their living and in their deaths. There is no single or best way to control any particular symptom, but the coordinated efforts of the interdisciplinary team bring effective relief for physical, emotional, and spiritual discomfort. Although the team members are important for a successful outcome, the patients remind us that palliative care is not finite. It is evolving, and individualized care is absolutely necessary.

Only the patients and their families are able to judge the effectiveness of the palliative care team.

REFERENCES

Agency for Health Care Policy and Research. (1994). *Management of cancer pain: Clinical practice guideline.* AHCPR Publication No. 94-0592. Rockville, MD: Agency for Health Care Policy and Research, U.S. Department of Health and Human Services.

Alldredge, B. K., Gelb, A. M., Isaacs, S. M., Corry, M. D. Allen, F., & Ulrich, S. (2001). A comparison of lorazepam, diazepam, and placebo for the treatment of out-of-hospital status epilepticus. *New England Journal of Medicine, 345*(9), 631–637.

American Pain Society. (1989). *Principles of analgesic use in the treatment of acute pain and chronic cancer pain: A concise guide to medical practice* (2nd ed.). Skokie, IL: American Pain Society.

American Pain Society. (1995). Quality improvement guidelines for the treatment of acute pain and cancer pain. *Journal of the American Medical Association, 274*, 1874–1880.

American Pain Society. (1999). *Principles of analgesic use in the treatment of acute pain and chronic cancer pain: A concise guide to medical practice* (4th ed.). Glenview, IL: American Pain Society.

Andersen, G., Christrup, L., Sjøgren, P., Hansen, S. H., & Jensen, N. (2003). Relationships among morphine metabolism, pain and side effects during long-term treatment: An update. *Journal of Pain and Symptom Management, 25*(1), 74–91.

Anderson, P. R., & Coia, L. R. (2000). Fractionation and outcomes with palliative radiation therapy. *Seminars in Radiation Oncology, 10*, 191–199.

Appleton, M. (1996). Hospice medicine: A different perspective. *American Journal of Hospice and Palliative Care, 13*, 7–9.

Beckwith, B. E. et al. (1990). Identification of spouses at high risk during bereavement: A preliminary assessment of Parkes and Weiss' Risk Index. *Hospice Journal, 6*, 35–36.

Bell, R. F., Eccleston, C., & Kalso, E. (2003). Ketamine as adjuvant to opioids for cancer pain. A qualitative systematic review. *Journal of Pain and Symptom Management, 26*(3), 867–875.

Berenson, J. R. (2001). Zoledronic acid in cancer patients with bone metastases: Results of Phase I and II Trials. *Seminars in Oncology, 28*(Suppl. 6), 25–34.

Berger, J. M., Ryan, A., Vadivelu, N., Merriam, P., Rever, L., & Harrison, P. (2000). Ketamine-fentanyl-midazolam infusion for the control of symptoms in terminal life care. *American Journal of Hospice and Palliative Care, 17*, 127–132.

Bonica, J. J. (1985). Treatment of cancer pain: Current status and future needs. In H. L. Fields et al. (Eds.), *Advances in pain research and therapy* (Vol. 9, pp. 589–616). New York: Raven Press.

Bonica, J. J. (1987). Preface: A short course on the management of cancer pain. *Journal of Pain and Symptom Management, 2,* S3–4.

Bosch, A. (1984). Radiotherapy. *Clinics in Oncology, 3,* 47–53.

Botney, M., & Fields, H. L. (1982). Amitriptyline potentiates morphine analgesia by a direct action on the central nervous system. *Annals of Neurology, 13,* 160–164.

Braun, T. C., Hagen, N. A., & Clark, T. (2003). Development of a clinical practice guideline for palliative sedation. *Journal of Palliative Medicine, 6*(3), 345–350.

Breitbart, W. et al. (1998). Patient-related barriers to pain management in ambulatory AIDS patients. *Pain, 76,* 9–16.

Breitbart, W., Passik, S., & Payne, D. (1998). Psychological and psychiatric interventions in pain control. In D. Doyle, G. W. C. Hanks, & N. MacDonald (Eds.), *Oxford textbook of palliative medicine* (2nd ed., pp. 437–454). New York: Oxford University Press.

Brescia, F. J. (1987). An overview of pain and symptom management in advanced cancer. *Journal of Pain and Symptom Management, 2,* S7–11.

Bruera, E., & Sweeney, C. (2002). Methadone use in cancer patients with pain: A review. *Journal of Palliative Medicine, 5*(1), 127–138.

Bruera, E., Walker, P., & Lawlor, P. (1999). Opioids in cancer pain. In C. Stein (Ed.). *Opioids in pain control: Basic and clinical aspects* (pp. 309–324). Cambridge, U.K.: Cambridge University Press.

Burnell, G. M., & Burnell, A. L. (1989). *Clinical management of bereavement.* New York: Human Sciences Press.

Campbell, J. N. (1989). Pain from peripheral nerve injury. In K. M. Foley & R. M. Payne (Eds.), *Current therapy of pain* (pp. 158–169). Toronto: B.C. Decker.

Cleeland, C. S. (1987). Nonpharmacological management of cancer pain. *Journal of Pain and Symptom Management, 2,* S23–28.

Cleeland, C. S. et al. (1994). Pain and its treatment in outpatients with metastatic cancer. *New England Journal of Medicine, 330,* 592–596.

Cook, A. S., & Dworkin, D. S. (1992). *Helping the bereaved: Therapeutic interventions for children, adolescents, and adults.* New York: Basic Books.

Cosh, R. (1995). Spiritual care of the dying. In I. B. Corless et al. (Eds.), *A challenge for living* (pp. 131–143). Boston: Jones & Bartlett.

Cousins, M. J., & Mather, L. E. (1984). Intrathecal and epidural administration of opioids. *Anesthesiology, 61,* 276–310.

Daeninck, P. J., & Bruera, E. (1999). Reduction in constipation and laxative requirements following opioid rotation to methadone: A report of four cases. *Journal of Pain and Symptom Management, 18*(4), 303–309.

Dallocchio, C., Buffa, C., Mazzarello, P., & Chiroli, S. (2000). Gabapentin vs. amitriptyline in painful diabetic neuropathy: An open-label pilot study. *Journal of Pain and Symptom Management, 20*(4), 280–285.

Davis, M. P., Frandsen, J. L., Walsh, D., Andersen, S., & Taylor, S. (2003). Mirtazapine for pruritus. *Journal of Pain and Symptom Management, 25*(3), 288–291.

Dodd, M. J., Dibble, S., Miaskowski, C., Palel, S., Cib,, M., MacPhail, L., Greenspan, D., & Shiba, G. (2001). A comparison of the affective state and quality of life of chemotherapy patients who do and do not develop chemotherapy-induced oral mucositis. *Journal of Pain and Symptom Management, 21*(6), 498–505.

Dworkin, D. H., Backouja, M., Rowbotham, M. C., Allen, R. R., Argoff, C. R., Bennett, G. J. et al. (2003). Advances in neuropathic pain. *Archives of Neurology, 60,* 1524–1534.

Emanuel, L. L., von Gunten, C. F., & Ferris, F. D. (1999). *The education for physicians on end-of-life care (EPEC) curriculum.* Chicago: American Medical Association.

Feinmann, C. (1985). Pain relief by antidepressants: Possible modes of action. *Pain, 23,* 1–8.

Ferrer-Brechner, T. (1984). Treating cancer pain as a disease. In C. Benedetti et al. (Eds.), *Advances in pain research and therapy* (Vol. 7, pp. 575–591). New York: Raven Press.

Ferrer-Brechner, T. (1989). Anesthetic techniques for the management of cancer pain. *Cancer, 63,* 2343–2347.

Ferrini, C. (2000). Parenteral lidocaine for severe intractable pain in six hospice patients continued at home. *Journal of Palliative Medicine, 3*(2), 193–200.

Foley, K. M. (1985). The treatment of cancer pain. *New England Journal of Medicine, 313,* 84–95.

Foley, K. M. (1988). Pain syndromes and pharmacologic management of pancreatic cancer pain. *Journal of Pain and Symptom Management, 3,* 176–187.

Foley, K. M., & Inturrisi, C. E. (1987). Analgesic drug therapy in cancer pain: Principles and practice. *Medical Clinics of North America, 71,* 207–232.

Foley, K. M., & Inturrisi, C. E. (1989). Pain of malignant origin. In K. M. Foley & R. M. Payne (Eds.), *Current therapy of pain.* Toronto: B.C. Decker.

Frier, J. W. (1985, January/February). Therapeutic implications of modifying endogenous serotonergic analgesic systems. *Anesthesia Progress,* 19–22.

Furuhashi-Yonaha, A. (2002). Short- and long-term efficacy of oral ketamine in eight chronic-pain patients. *Canadian Journal of Anaesthesia, 49,* 886–887.

Hanks, G. W. (1984). Psychotropic drugs. *Clinics in Oncology, 3,* 135–151.

Hardy, J. R., Rees, E. A. J., William, B., Ling, J., Broadley, K., & A'Hearn, R. (2001). A Phase II study to establish the efficacy and toxicity of sodium valproate in patients with cancer-related neuropathic pain. *Journal of Pain and Symptom Management, 21*(3), 204–209.

Helig, S. (1988). The San Francisco Medical Society euthanasia survey: Results and analysis. *San Francisco Medicine, 61,* 24–34.

Hendler, N. (1982). The anatomy and psychopharmacology of chronic pain. *Journal of Clinical Psychiatry, 43,* 15–21.

Hill, C. S. (1988). Narcotics and cancer pain control. *Ca: A Cancer Journal for Clinicians, 38,* 322–326.

Hill, T. P., & Shirley, D. (1992). *A good death.* Menlo Park, CA: Addison-Wesley.

Homsi, J., Walsh, D., & Nelson, K. A. (2000). Psychostimulants in supportive care. *Support Care Cancer, 8,* 385–397.

Hoskin, P. J. (1998). Radiotherapy in symptom management. In D. Doyle, G. W. C. Hanks, & N. MacDonald (Eds.), *Oxford textbook of palliative medicine* (2nd ed., pp. 267–282). New York: Oxford University Press.

Howard-Ruben, J., McGuire, L., & Groenwald, S. L. (1987). Pain. In S. L. Groenwald (Ed.), *Cancer nursing principles and practice*. Boston: Jones & Bartlett.

Humphry, D. (1991). *Final exit*. Eugene, OR: Hemlock Society.

Insel, P. A. (1996). Analgesic-antipyretic and anti-inflammatory agents and drugs employed in the treatment of gout. In J. G. Hardman & L. E. Limbird (Eds.), *Goodman & Gilman's the pharmacological basis of therapeutics* (9th ed., pp. 617–657). New York: McGraw-Hill.

Jeremic, B. (2001). Single fraction external beam radiation therapy in the treatment of localized metastatic bone pain. A review. *Journal of Pain and Symptom Management*, *22*, 1048–1058.

Johanson, G. A. (1988). *Physicians handbook of symptom relief in terminal care* (2nd ed.). Sebastopol, CA: Home Hospice of Sonoma County.

Johanson, G. A. (1993). *Physicians handbook of symptom relief in terminal care* (4th ed.). Santa Rosa, CA: Sonoma County Academic Foundation for Excellence in Medicine.

Kaiko, R. F. et al. (1996). Pharmaco-kinetic-pharmacodynamic relationships of controlled-release oxycodone. *Clinical Pharmacology and Therapeutics*, *59*, 52–61.

Kanner, R. M. (1987). Pharmacological management of pain and symptom control in cancer. *Journal of Pain and Symptom Management*, *2*, S19–S21.

Kaye, P. (1989). *Notes on symptom control in Hospice and palliative care*. Essex, CT: Hospice Education Institute.

Köstler, W. J., Hejna, M., Wenzel, C., & Zielinski, C. C. (2001). Oral mucositis complicating chemotherapy and/or radiotherapy: Options for prevention and treatment. *Ca: A Cancer Journal for Clinicians*, *51*(5), 290–315.

Krajnik, M., & Zylicz, Z. (2001). Understanding pruritus in systemic disease. *Journal of Pain and Symptom Management*, *2*, 151–168.

Krantz, M. J., Lewkowiez, L., Hays, H., Woodroffe, M. A., Robertson, A. D., & Mehler, P. S. (2002). Torsade de pointes associated with very-high-dose methadone. *Annals of Internal Medicine*, *137*(6), 501–504.

Krouwer, H. G., Pallagi, J. L., & Graves, N. M. (2000). Management of seizures in brain tumor patients at the end of life. *Journal of Palliative Medicine*, *3*(4), 465–475.

Kuczynska, J. (2004). *Drugs in renal failure: Opioid analgesics*. South West Medicines Information and Training, National Health Service, U.K. Retrieved September 21, 2004 from http://www.helpthehospices.org.uk/elearning/pdf/hpp-6.pdf.

Kurella, K., Bennett, W. M., & Chertow, G. M. (2003). Analgesic in patients with ESRD: A review of available evidence. *American Journal of Kidney Disease*, *42*(2), 385–387.

Lack, S. (1984). Total pain. *Clinics in Oncology*, *3*, 33–44.

Lang, S. S., & Patt, R. B. (1994). *You don't have to suffer*. New York: Oxford University Press.

Lawton, P. A., & Maher, E. J. (1991). Treatment strategies for advanced and metastatic cancer in Europe. *Radiotherapeutic Oncology*, *22*, 1–6.

Layson-Wolf, C., Goode, J. V., & Small, R. E. (2002). Clinical use of methadone. *Journal of Pain and Palliative Care Pharmacotherapy*, *16*, 28–59.

LeGrand, S. B., Khawam, E., Walsh, D., & Rivera, N. I. (2003). Opioids, respiratory function, and dyspnea. *American Journal of Hospice and Palliative Care*, *20*(1), 57–61.

Leow, K. P. et al. (1993). Single-dose and steady-state pharmacokinetics and pharmacodynamics of oxycodone in patients with cancer. *Clinical Pharmacology and Therapeutics*, *52*, 487–495.

Leppik, I. E. (1983). Double-blind study of lorazepam and diazepam in status epilepticus. *Journal of the American Medical Association*, *249*, 1452–1454.

Levin, D. N., Cleeland, C. S., & Dar, R. (1985). Public attitudes toward cancer pain. *Cancer*, 56, 2337–2339.

Light, R. W., Muro, J. R., Sato, R. I., Stansbury, D. W., Fischer, C. E., & Brown, S. E. (1989). Effects of oral morphine on breathlessness and exercise tolerance in patients with chronic obstructive pulmonary disease. *American Review of Respiratory Diseases*, *139*, 126–133.

Lurcott, G. (1999). The effects of the genetic absence and inhibition of CYP2D6 on the metabolism of codeine and its derivatives, hydrocodone and oxycodone. *Anesthesia Progress*, *45*, 154–156.

Maher, E. J. et al. (1992). Treatment strategies in advanced and metastatic cancer: Differences in attitude between the USA, Canada and Europe. *International Journal of Radiation Oncology and Biological Physics*, *23*, 239–244.

Mathew, P., & Storey, P. (1999). Subcutaneous methadone in terminally ill patients: Manageable local toxicity. *Journal of Pain and Symptom Management*, *18*(1), 49–52.

Maxon, H. R., III, & Smith, H. S. (1990). Radioiodine-131 in the diagnosis and treatment of metastatic well-differentiated thyroid cancer. *Endocrinologic and Metabolic Clinics of North America*, *19*, 685–718.

Maxon, H. R., III et al. (1990). Re-186 (Sn) HEDP for treatment of osseous metastases: Initial clinical experience in 20 patients with hormone-resistant prostate cancer. *Radiology*, *176*, 155–159.

McCaffery, M., & Beebe, A. (1989). *Pain: Clinical manual for nursing practice*. St. Louis: Mosby.

McCaffery, M., & Pasero, C. (1999). Assessment: Underlying complexities, misconceptions, and practical tools. In M. McCaffery & C. Pasero (Eds.), *Pain: Clinical manual* (2nd ed., pp. 35–102). St. Louis, MO: Mosby.

Medical Economics Company. (2000). *Physicians' desk reference* (54th ed.). Montvale, NJ: Medical Economics.

Medina, J. L., & Diamond, S. (1977). Drug dependency in patients with chronic headaches. *Headache*, *17*, 12–14.

Meier, T. et al. (2003). Efficacy of lidocaine patch 5% in the treatment of focal peripheral neuropathic pain syndromes: A randomized, double-blind placebo-controlled study. *Pain*, *106*, 151–158.

Mendell, J. R., & Sahenk, Z. (2003). Painful sensory neuropathy. *New England Journal of Medicine*, *348*(13), 1243–1255.

Mercadante, S., & Portenoy, R. K. (2001a). Opioid poorly-responsive cancer pain. Part 1: Clinical considerations. *Journal of Pain and Symptom Management*, *21*(2), 144–150.

Mercadante, S., & Portenoy, R. K. (2001b). Opioid poorly-responsive cancer pain. Part 2: Basic mechanisms that could shift dose response for analgesia. *Journal of Pain and Symptom Management, 21*(3), 255–264.

Mercadante, S. et al. (1995). Analgesic effects of nonsteroidal anti-inflammatory drugs in cancer pain due to somatic or visceral mechanisms. *Journal of Pain and Symptom Management, 33*, 979–988.

Miller, M. G. et al. (1999). Continuous subcutaneous infusion of morphine vs. hydromorphone: A controlled trial. *Journal of Pain and Symptom Management, 18*(1), 9–15.

Morita, T. et al. (2001). Effects of high dose opioids and sedatives on survival in terminally ill cancer patients. *Journal of Pain and Symptom Management, 21*(4), 282–289.

Morley, J., & Makin, M. (1998). The use of methadone in cancer pain poorly responsive to other opioids. *Pain Review, 5*, 51–58.

Mortimer, P. S. (1993). Skin problems in palliative care: Medical aspects. In D. Doyle, et al. (Eds.), *Oxford textbook of palliative medicine* (pp. 384–395). New York: Oxford University Press.

National Hospice Organization. (1996). *Resource manual for providing hospice care to people living with AIDS.* Arlington, VA: National Hospice Organization.

Newshan, G. (1998). Heat-related toxicity with the fentanyl transdermal patch. *Journal of Pain and Symptom Management, 16*(5), 277–278.

Nielsen, O. S., Munro, A. J., & Tannock, I. F. (1991). Bone metastases: Pathophysiology and management policy. *Journal of Clinical Oncology, 9*, 509–524.

Nugent, M., Davis, C., Brooks, D., & Ahmedzai, S. H. (2001). Long-term observations of patients receiving transdermal fentanyl after a randomized trial. *Journal of Pain and Symptom Management, 21*(5), 385–391.

Osborne, R. J., Joel, S. P., & Slevin, M. L. (1986). Morphine intoxication in renal failure: The role of morphine-6-glucuronide. *British Medical Journal, 292*, 1548–1549.

Parris, W. C. V. (1985). Nerve block therapy. *Clinics in Anesthesiology, 3*, 93–109.

Pasero, C., Portenoy, R. K., & McCaffery, M. (1999). Opioid analgesics. In M. McCaffery & C. Pasero (Eds.), *Pain clinical manual* (2nd ed., pp. 161–299). St. Louis: Mosby.

Passik, S. D., & Portenoy, R. K. (1998). Substance abuse issues in palliative care. In A. Berger (Ed.), *Principles and practice of supportive care* (pp. 513–529). Philadelphia: Lippincott-Raven Publishers.

Patt, R. B., & Isaacson, S. A. (1996). Cancer pain syndromes. In P. P. Raj (Ed.), *Pain medicine: A comprehensive review* (pp. 502–520). St. Louis: Mosby Year Book.

Pereira, J., Lawlor, P., Vigano, A., Dorgan, M., & Bruera, E. (2001). Equianalgesic dose ratios for opioids: A critical review and proposals for long-term dosing. *Journal of Pain and Symptom Management, 22*(2), 672–687.

Perry, S., & Heidrich, G. (1982). Management of pain during debridement: A survey of U.S. burn units. *Pain, 13*, 267–280.

Portenoy, R. K. (1987). Constipation in the cancer patient. *Medical Clinics of North America, 71*, 303–311.

Portenoy, R. K. (1988). Practical aspects of pain control in the patient with cancer. *Ca: A Cancer Journal for Clinicians, 38*, 327–352.

Portenoy, R. K. (1990). Chronic opioid therapy in nonmalignant pain. *Journal of Pain and Symptom Management, 5*, S46–S62.

Porter, J., & Jick, H. (1980). Addiction rare in patients treated with narcotics. *New England Journal of Medicine, 302*, 123.

Poyhia, R., Vainio, A., & Kalso, E. (1993). A review of oxycodone's clinical pharmacokinetics and pharmacodynamics. *Journal of Pain and Symptom Management, 8*, 63–67.

Reisine, T., & Pasternak, G. (1996). Opioid analgesics and antagonists. In J. G. Hardman & L. E. Limbird (Eds.), *Goodman & Gilman's the pharmacological basis of therapeutics* (9th ed., pp. 521–555). New York: McGraw-Hill.

Reuben, S. S., Connelly, N. R., & Maciolek, H. (1999). Postoperative analgesia with controlled-release oxycodone for outpatient anterior cruciate ligament surgery. *Anesthesia & Analgesia, 88*, 1286–1291.

Rhodes, V. A., & McDaniel, R. W. (2001). Nausea, vomiting, and retching: Complex problems in palliative care. *Ca: A Cancer Journal for Clinicians, 51*, 232–248.

Ribeiro, M. D., Joel, S. P., & Zeppetella, G. (2004). The bioavailability of morphine applied topically to cutaneous ulcers. *Journal of Pain and Symptom Management, 27*, 434–439.

Richelson, E. (1979). Tricyclic antidepressants and histamine H1 receptors. *Mayo Clinic Proceedings, 54*, 669–674.

Rousseau, P. C. (2002). Palliative sedation. *American Journal of Hospice and Palliative Care, 19*(5), 295–297.

Rowbotham, M. C., Twilling, L., Davies, P. S., Reisner, L., Taylor, K., & Mohr, D. (2003). Oral opioid therapy for chronic peripheral and central neuropathic pain. *New England Journal of Medicine, 348*(13), 1223–1232.

Rummans, T. A., Bostwick, J. M., & Clark, M. M. (2000). Maintaining quality of life at the end of life. *Mayo Clinic Proceedings, 75*, 1305–1310.

Ryder, B. G. (1993). *The alpha book on cancer and living.* Alameda, CA: The Alpha Institute.

Sassoli, L. (1402). Quotation found on Web site of Cancer Free Success. Retrieved September 21, 2004 from http://www.cancer-free.com/links-reflections2.htm.

Silberstein, E. B. (2000). Systemic radiopharmaceutical therapy of painful osteoblastic metastases. *Seminars in Radiation Oncology, 10*, 240–249.

Sindrup, S. H., & Jensen, T. S. (2000). Pharmacologic treatment of pain in polyneuropathy. *Neurology, 55*, 915–920.

Smith, H. S., & Baird, W. (2003). Meloxicam and selective COX-2 inhibitors in the management of pain in the palliative care population. *American Journal of Hospice and Palliative Care, 20*(4), 297–306.

Srivastava, M., Brito-Dellan, N., Davis, M. P., Leach, M., & Lagman, R. (2003). Olanzapine as an antiemetic in refractory nausea and vomiting in advanced cancer. *Journal of Pain and Symptom Management, 25*(6), 578–582.

Stahl, S. M. (2000). *Essential psychopharmacology: Neuroscientific basis and practical applications* (2nd ed.). New York: Cambridge University Press.

Swarm, R. A. & Cousins, M. J. (1998). Anesthetic techniques for pain control. In D. Doyle, G. W. C. Hanks, & N. MacDonald (Eds.), *Oxford textbook of palliative medicine* (2nd ed., pp. 390–414). New York: Oxford University Press.

Sweeney, M. P., & Bagg, J. (2000). The mouth and palliative care. *American Journal of Hospice and Palliative Care, 17*(2). 118–124.

Swerdlow, M. (1986). Anticonvulsants in the therapy of neuralgic pain. *The Pain Clinic, 1,* 9–19.

Thomas, J. R. & von Gunten, C. F. (2002). Clinical management of dyspnoea. *Lancet, 3,* 223–228.

Topol, E. J. (2005). Arthritis medicines and cardiovascular events — "House of Coxibs." *Journal of the American Medical Association, 293,* 366–368.

Turner, J. H. et al. (1989). A phase I study of samarium-153 ethylenediaminetetramethylene phosphonate therapy for disseminated skeletal metastases. *Journal of Clinical Oncology, 7,* 1926–1931.

Twycross, R., & Lack, S. (1984). *Oral morphine in advanced cancer.* Bucks, England: Beaconsfield Publishers.

Twycross, R., & Lichter, I. (1998). The terminal phase. In D. Doyle, G. W. C. Hanks, & N. MacDonald (Eds.), *Oxford textbook of palliative medicine* (2nd ed., pp. 977–992). New York: Oxford University Press.

Ventafridda, V., & Caraceni, A. (1994). Cancer pain. In P. P. Raj (Ed.). *Current review of pain* (pp. 155–178). Philadelphia: Current Medicine.

Verrill, P. (1989). Sympathetic ganglion lesions. In P. D. Walls & R. Melzac (Eds.), *Textbook of pain* (2nd ed., pp. 773–783). Edinburgh: Churchill Livingstone.

Walsh, T. D. (1985). Common misunderstandings about the use of morphine for chronic pain in advanced cancer. *Ca: A Cancer Journal for Clinicians, 35*(3), 164–169.

Ward, S. E. et al. (1993). Patient-related barriers to management of cancer pain. *Pain, 53,* 319–324.

Wheeler, W. L., & Dickerson, E. D. (2000). Clinical applications of methadone. *American Journal of Hospice and Palliative Care, 17*(3), 196–203.

World Health Organization. (1986). *Cancer pain relief.* Geneva: Author.

Section XI

Legal and Ethical Considerations

B. Eliot Cole, MD, MPA, Section Editor

90

Ethics: History and Theory

Frank Chessa, PhD

INTRODUCTION

Many health care providers are familiar with the basic concepts of health care ethics — surrogate decision-making, advance directives, do not resuscitate (DNR), withdrawal of treatment, confidentiality, and informed consent have become need-to-know terms in the practice of medicine and nursing. Likewise, I expect many health care providers are familiar with the basic principles of health care ethics, including nonmaleficence, beneficence, respect for autonomy, veracity, and justice. What is perhaps more rare among practitioners is an awareness of how health care ethics is connected to the history of ethics and ethical theories more generally. Yet knowledge of the ethical traditions that have influenced health care ethics may help practitioners in a number of ways: (1) it may help practitioners extend well-known principles to novel cases; (2) it may help practitioners articulate why they have reached a conclusion about the ethics of a particular case; and (3) it may deepen practitioners' commitment to ethical values of their profession. This chapter seeks to bridge the gap between health care ethics and the traditions from which these ethics emerge.

This chapter also briefly surveys some ethical issues that are especially relevant to palliative care. Other chapters in this volume treat these issues in more detail. Here, the focus is on showing how the history of ethics is relevant to the ethical issues that arise with particular acuity in palliative care. It is not under the purview of this chapter to expand the discussion beyond Western ethical traditions, although non-Western traditions are increasingly important as more persons from various world cultures are served by, and practice within, health care institutions in the United States and Britain.

There is also a good deal in the history of Western ethics that could not be covered in this chapter. In part this is because many great minds have written about ethics — including just a paragraph on each would have made this chapter too long. I have instead chosen to focus on six philosophers: Plato, Aristotle, Augustine, Thomas Aquinas, Immanuel Kant, and John Stuart Mill. Of these six, Aristotle, Kant, and Mill are given the most attention because their theories are the most relevant to health care ethics. I should also note that it is not possible to consider every facet of the theories of these philosophers. Indeed, not only have these philosophers each written thousands of pages, but each is the subject of countless books and articles. In my inevitable narrowing of this material, I have selected topics that either have had a direct influence on health care ethics or raise issues that may be of interest to health care practitioners. My hope is that this will serve to make the current chapter different from other surveys of the history of ethics in a way that will prove useful to the health care providers likely to read this volume.

The first section of this chapter, by far the largest, is a chronological survey of the views of the ethical theorists. For each philosopher, I have provided biographical information, a sketch of his theory, prominent criticisms of the theory, and a discussion of the ways in which the philosopher's ideas emerge in current debates in health care ethics. The second section discusses how the historical theories relate to various methodologies in contemporary health care ethics (e.g., the ethics of care, casuistry). The second section also draws some parallels between three ethical issues in palliative care and the history of ethics.

ETHICAL TRADITIONS

SOCRATES AND PLATO

It is appropriate to begin a discussion about the history of Western ethics with Socrates and Plato. Socrates was born in Athens around 469 B.C., and famously, he died in 399 B.C. by drinking hemlock under order of the Athenian court. Plato (428–347 B.C.) immortalized his teacher in a series of dialogues that portray Socrates as a martyr for his ethical beliefs. Among Plato's 26 surviving dialogues are some of the first examples of extended ethical reasoning in the Western tradition. Plato's dialogues explore a range of moral (and nonmoral) issues, from the proper way to be religious (*Euthyphro*), to suicide (*Phaedo*), to civil disobedience (*Crito*), to political organization (*Republic*), to love (*Symposium*).

A good example of a Platonic dialogue that focuses on a moral issue is *Crito*. In *Crito*, Socrates faces the question of whether to accept death as punishment for corrupting the youth of Athens or whether to escape into exile. Escape was probably the outcome expected by Socrates's accusers, as this was a common practice and Socrates had the means to accomplish it. Socrates argues (to his friend Crito, who wishes him to escape) that although he is innocent of wrongdoing, and although the state is acting unjustly in prohibiting him from teaching philosophy, he nonetheless owes Athens a debt for raising and protecting him, and thus he should not escape (Hamilton & Cairns, 1961, 51d).* To escape would be to weaken the state, while all of his prior activities were aimed at strengthening Athens. Socrates does not escape and soon after this dialogue takes place, he is executed, with all of his friends present and weeping openly for the loss of their great friend and philosopher (*Phaedo*, 115b–118a). Plato's *Crito* presages modern views about civil disobedience: civilly disobedient actions are morally permissible if their intention is to reform unjust laws, if the actions are performed openly, and if the actors are willing to accept punishment. What emerges in *Crito* is the idea that the aim of civil disobedience is to reform a state, not to overturn it, and that those who are civilly disobedient are among the heroes of society because they are willing to sacrifice their well-being for the good of the state. The Reverend Martin Luther King Jr., certainly fits this model.

Plato's moral reasoning sometimes relies on the conviction that there is an afterlife. In particular, Plato is explicit that how a person lives on Earth will influence his or her afterlife, so he posits "a much better future [after death] for the good than for the wicked" (*Phaedo* 63c). Plato is often interpreted as dividing the world into the realm of appearance (the world as we experience it embodied on Earth) and the realm of reality (the world as it really

---

* The parenthetical references for Plato refer to the standard method for citing passages in Plato across various translations.

is, which is accessible to us, if at all, only after we die). However, even while Plato's thought has these religious dimensions, his conclusions about particular issues rely on an astute reading of human nature as much as on theological reasoning. In *Euthyphro*, Socrates questions Euthyphro about his attempt to prosecute his father for murder. The primary moral failing of Euthyphro is not that he is attempting to prosecute his father for murder. Rather, this potentially immoral action is a symptom of a character flaw, namely, that while Euthyphro is good-hearted, he has a wildly over-inflated confidence about his knowledge of theology. Plato thus depicts the type of moral failing likely to arise from a lack of humility in otherwise praiseworthy persons.

One of the lasting legacies of Plato's thought is the idea that living ethically should be the primary goal of human life. We will also find this idea in the writings of Plato's greatest student, Aristotle, and it is to his thought that we will now turn.

ARISTOTLE (384–322 B.C.)

Arguably, until relatively recently, the focus of modern ethics has been on the evaluation of actions. In contrast, Aristotle focused on the moral evaluation of a person's character, that is, on whether a person is virtuous or vicious. The focus on character evaluation is responsible for the popularity of virtue theory among contemporary ethical theorists (French, Uehling, & Wettstein, 1988; Sherman, 1989). In particular, focusing on character has three advantages. First, action-centered theories seem not to account for the emotional dimension of our moral lives (Stocker & Hegeman, 1991). Aristotle held that feeling the correct emotion and being motivated by it are important components of having a virtuous character. Second, virtue theory is at home with particularism about right action (Dancy, 1993; McNaughton, 1991). Particularism holds that rules and general principles are not much help in determining the morally correct action because real-life situations are simply too rich to be codified by general rules. Aristotle stresses correct perception of the features of a situation and wise judgment in figuring out what to do, rather than dependence on a set of rules. Finally, the focus on character has implications for how one learns to be moral. Modern advocates of Aristotle often view morality as a type of skill that is developed in the same manner as other skills (Little, 1995). Learning a skill primarily requires practice, although it may also involve emulation of experts, expert critique of one's performance, and reflection on theoretical issues. So Aristotle was the first in the Western tradition to deny that there is a book of rules that can teach one how to be moral. In other realms, this view is familiar. Many of us think that there is no book that can teach even a physically talented individual to play basketball like Michael Jordan — his split-second judgments are too rich and varied to be codified. Why then do many of us nevertheless assume that there is a book on ethics that can teach us to be moral experts in the absence of practicing ethics in the rich context of everyday life?

Aristotle was born in 384 B.C. His father was a physician at the Macedonian court. Aristotle had a lifelong association with Philip of Macedonia and his son Alexander the Great. Aristotle studied with Plato for approximately 20 years at Plato's Academy in Athens. After Plato's death in 343, Aristotle moved to Macedonia to tutor the young Alexander before returning to Athens to found his own school, the Lyceum, in 336. After the death of Alexander the Great, Aristotle left Athens to avoid the political fallout from his association with the emperor. Aristotle died in 322 at the age of 62. Aristotle's writings were extensive, and although we have perhaps lost most of his published works, we are left with thousands of pages of carefully prepared lecture notes. His writings on ethics are contained primarily in the *Nicomachean Ethics*, on which we focus.

However, our discussion of Aristotle can begin not with ethics, but by sketching the theory of causal explanation that he outline in *Physics* (McKeon, 1941, 194b 20).* Aristotle believed that understanding how any object came to be required referring to four factors: the material cause, the efficient cause, the formal cause, and the final cause. The material cause is the raw matter that makes up an object. For example, the bronze is, in this sense, the material cause of the statue. The efficient cause is the energy that has molded the matter into a certain shape. So we say that the sculptor is also the cause of the statue. The formal cause can be understood as either the blueprint for the object before it is made, or the shape and organization of the finished object. For the statue, the blueprint may exist only in the sculptor's mind, but it nonetheless lays out the shape of the object to be created. The final cause is the purpose of the object. It is the reason for which the object is created or the action is done. So we say that the woman walks in order to improve her health and that is the final cause of her walking. For another example, consider a pitcher for holding and pouring liquid. Its material cause might be clay. The efficient cause is the potter's spinning of the wheel and movement of her hands. The formal cause, blueprint (which may only exist in the potter's mind), lays out the shape of the pitcher. The final cause of the pitcher is its purpose of holding and pouring liquid. An important aspect of this theory is that the formal cause answers to the final cause — that is, the shape of the object fits the purpose for which the object was

designed. Note also that there is interplay between separate causes. In designing an object to fulfill a purpose, we need to consider whether the material has the properties that will allow it to be fashioned into the shape needed and whether the energy is available to accomplish the change. Aristotle's theory is a good fit for explaining how human-made objects came into existence. But Aristotle did not limit the theory to artifacts. Aristotle also believed that this theory of causal explanation held true for natural objects, in particular, plants, animals, and humans.

The key to Aristotle's ethics is that humans, as do all things in nature, have a final cause or purpose. He felt that careful observation of humans, including their physical bodies, their culture, and social behaviors, would yield information about humans' purpose. Living an ethical life, Aristotle then reasoned, would be living a life that achieved this purpose to the greatest extent possible. Aristotle identified the purpose or function of humans as "an active life of the element that has a rational principle" (*NE* 1098a 1). What Aristotle meant by this enigmatic phrase is much debated, but a fair interpretation is that the purpose of human life was to use reason to think about oneself and one's place in the world and to perform actions as directed by the results of this reasoning — in short, to live an active life under the direction of reason. Aristotle felt that a virtuous person would be a person who did an excellent job performing the specialized human function. In fact, the word for virtue in Greek is *arête*, and this word can be translated equally well as excellence. An often-quoted illustration used by Aristotle to explain these concepts involves a knife: Aristotle says that the purpose of a knife is to cut, and an excellent knife is one that cuts excellently. So, too, with humans: an excellent or virtuous human is one that performs the function of humans excellently.

Aristotle believed that the result of a person performing the human function excellently is that the person will flourish. (The Greek word is *eudaimonia*, which can be translated as flourishing, happiness, well-being, or good spirits.) Aristotle's idea was that one would reap rewards from living a virtuous life. These rewards would be both internal and external. The virtuous person would be happy, that is, she would have an internal feeling of well-being. But the virtuous person would also have some of the external trappings of success — she would be respected in her trade or craft, have true friendships based on mutual admiration and respect, have a loving family, and be viewed as an upstanding member of the civic community whose counsel would be sought and trusted. These external trappings would include enough wealth to be secure and comfortable, but excessive wealth might be a sign that all is not as it should be. The virtuous person lives a well-rounded life, according to Aristotle. She enjoys good food and fine wine, but not to the detriment of her health. She enjoys poetry and drama, but does not live in a fantasy

---

* Quotations for Aristotle are taken from *The Basic Works of Aristotle*, McKeon, R. ed., Random House, New York, 1941. Parenthetical citations are to the numbering in the Bekker edition of the Greek text of Aristotle, the standard method for citing passages in Aristotle across various translations. *NE* refers to the *Nicomachean Ethics*.

world. She works hard at a successful career, but also has ample time for family, friends, and fun. She is concerned with and will work to enhance the well-being of others in society, but she will not impoverish herself in the process. Finally, she is emotionally and psychologically healthy, as a result of her good relationships with others and as a result of the proper cultivation of her emotions and the appropriate expression of them at the appropriate times. Balancing these various areas of one's life, or living in the mean between excess and deficiency in each of the areas, is one of the primary skills of the virtuous person.

So, as I have reconstructed Aristotle's ethical theory, there are four primary ideas: humans have a specialized function or purpose; those who perform this function excellently are virtuous; a virtuous person flourishes in her life; and finally, a flourishing life is lived in the mean between extremes. It is worth asking why, on Aristotle's account, a person should be virtuous? The answer is that one should be moral because it is in one's self-interest, very broadly construed. Virtuous persons flourish. This is not to say that one will always make decisions based on self-interested considerations. Indeed, Aristotle would say that sometimes the motivation to sacrifice a portion of one's own immediate well-being for the good of someone else is just what is required to make oneself happy. Conversely, aiming at one's own happiness in all the picky, little decisions of everyday life will have the effect of undercutting one's happiness. Nonetheless, the overarching motivation for becoming an excellent human is that benefits will rebound to oneself. As Aristotle says, the highest good is happiness (*eudaimonia*). Put differently, Aristotle was convinced that the best life for humans was the life that included moral virtue as a significant part.

This sketch of Aristotle fails to explore many of the specific topics that give his theory power and scope, for example, his account of how to deliberate about a decision, his enumeration and description of individual virtues (e.g., courage, temperance, generosity, honesty), and his discussion of the nature of friendship. However, a topic I consider in more depth is his account of how one becomes virtuous, and in this context, I also present Aristotle's definition of virtue.

Aristotle says that humans are not by nature virtuous, for if they were it would not be possible for a human to be vicious, but we know that some persons are vicious. Instead, Aristotle says that humans have the potential to become virtuous, and this potential is realized by habituation. He writes: "Neither by nature or contrary to nature do the virtues arise in us; rather we are adapted by nature to receive them, and are made perfect by habit" (*NE* 1103a 25). Habituation is a matter of practicing virtuous behavior.

The virtues we get first by exercising them.... For the things we have to learn before we can do them, we learn by doing them, e.g., men become builders by building and lyre-players by playing the lyre; so too we become just by doing just acts, temperate by doing temperate acts, brave by doing brave acts. (*NE* 1103b 1)

The purpose of practicing to be virtuous by performing virtuous actions is to train our emotions and desires. By performing temperate actions, one both gets used to and begins to enjoy the emotions that accompany the actions. From this enjoyment, one begins to desire to be temperate. The opposite sort of habituation can occur as well: performing intemperate actions tends to create intemperate desires and thereby an intemperate character (Sherman, 1989).

Why is it that one should train oneself to enjoy being temperate, one might ask, if one can equally well train oneself to enjoy being intemperate? A useful, if somewhat fanciful, analogy helps to answer this question. Let us say that the human body functions best on a diet of vegetables, meats, and grains. Nonetheless, a child experiences pleasure on first tasting candy. The child's untutored tastes can lead him astray. In fact, the child can eat so much candy that he no longer finds unsweetened foods at all palatable. Now, in the long term, the health of the child will suffer. So, too, the child's taste will never progress beyond the unremarkable pleasure of tasting fat and sugar. This child has not learned to love the good. Aristotle would say that it takes real effort to learn to love that which one can love most fully. So, it takes effort to forgo candy in order to eat spinach, broccoli, rice, beans, etc. One will not immediately love the taste of these foods. But over time, one's palate will be sensitized to the varied and subtle flavors of these foods. The enjoyment experienced by this trained palate will far outstrip the enjoyment of the palate desensitized by fat and sugar. Further, of course, the health of the person will benefit from eating this natural diet. Aristotle would see both the potential for the enjoyment of natural foods and the health that results from natural foods to be directly related to the biological characteristics of the body — human biology is such that it gets maximum benefit from natural foods. Once one is sensitized to the tastes of natural foods, staying on the diet of natural foods is effortless. In fact, any other diet tastes bad. But, it takes effort to get to this stage, and indeed it may not be possible to get to this stage if one starts down the wrong path and incorrectly trains one's sensibilities from an early age.

We should note at this point the importance of emotion to Aristotle's ethical theory. Aristotle is clear that virtue is not an emotion, but is instead a state of character (*NE* 1105b 30). Nonetheless, a virtuous character is a stable set of dispositions to have appropriate emotions and to perform right actions. A person is not virtuous until she feels the appropriate emotions when performing the right action. Further, emotions are a guide to right action. While rational deliberation plays some role, in large part one is moved to a certain action because one feels a certain emotion. Aristotle's emphasis on the importance of emotion is one reason that his "virtue theory" experienced a resurgence in the 1980s. Historically, all moral theorists have recognized that humans are emotional creatures, but more often than not emotions were seen as a hindrance to morally correct action. Emotions were not viewed as being under the control of reason — anger, love, jealousy, even sympathy, could move one to act in ways that would be regretted later. Aristotle admitted that emotions, in the moment of their occurring, were often beyond human control. But, by beginning early to train oneself to have the appropriate emotion relative to the situation one is experiencing, it does not matter if the emotion is "out of our control" in the moment of its occurring, for it is the appropriate emotion to have, and it will move one to perform the right action.

Thus, virtue in Aristotle's view is concerned with both emotions *and* actions. One mark of a virtuous person is that she takes appropriate pleasure in doing the right actions. And a mark of someone who fails to be virtuous is that, though she may do the right action, she may not feel the right emotions. So on the battlefield (one of Aristotle's favorite examples) where standing and fighting is appropriate, a virtuous person will courageously stand and fight and feel a kind of confident pleasure in doing so, while one kind of nonvirtuous person — what Aristotle calls a continent or strong-willed person — will stand and fight but feel terrible pain and fear as he does so. Aristotle also tells us that virtue is typically destroyed by excess and defect, and preserved by the mean. To explain this he says that:

> ... the man who flies from and fears everything and does not stand his ground against anything becomes a coward, and the man who fears nothing at all but goes to meet every danger becomes rash. (*NE* 1104a21)

Extremes do not typically preserve or habituate virtue. The virtuous person is the one who rushes into battle where this is appropriate and similarly flees where this is appropriate. And the virtuous person is also the one who feels fear where appropriate and confidence where appropriate. So virtue is concerned both with passions and actions and the virtuous person is the one who finds the mean, or appropriate point, for both, feeling the right emotion and doing the right action as they are called for in particular situations. Again, Aristotle explains:

> ... both fear and confidence and appetite and anger and pity and in general pleasure and pain may be felt both too much and too little, and in both cases not well; but to feel them at the right times, with reference to the right objects, towards the right people, with the right motive, and in the right way, is what is both intermediate and best and this is characteristic of virtue. Similarly

with regard to actions also there is excess, defect and the intermediate. (*NE* 1106b17)

We now have all the components in place to understand Aristotle's definition of virtue. He says that:

> Virtue ... is a state of character concerned with choice, lying in a mean, i.e. the mean relative to us, this being determined by a rational principle, and by that principle by which the man of practical wisdom would determine it. (*NE* 1106b36)

Virtue is a state of character that individuals cultivate through practicing virtuous actions and emotions. Both virtuous actions and emotions must find the mean between the extremes, and this is relative both to the specific circumstances the person is in (so, how much fear an individual should feel in battle depends on how well-prepared for battle one is, how strong one's army is, how well-suited one's army is to the terrain, etc.) and to the person herself. So if a person is attempting to cultivate the emotion anger (associated with the virtue of good temper) and she finds that she often gets too angry, she should strive to feel too little anger in this situation. That is the way in which the virtue is relative to the individual herself. And finally, the mean is determined by reason, by thinking about and assessing the practical nature of the situation. It is also determined by the moral experts, what Aristotle calls persons of practical wisdom, because moral virtue is a kind of wisdom or as we saw earlier, a kind of skill-based knowledge.

Criticisms and Evaluation

Aristotle's claim that there are purposes in nature is at odds with the scientific world view. Aristotle did not believe that living organisms were designed with a purpose in mind in any obvious sense — for example, he did not believe that organisms were created by an intelligent God. Aristotle simply thought it was the case that things in nature had purposes because, as he saw it from his extensive botanical and zoological studies, it was obvious that living things had complex and purposeful bodily structures. However, since the publication of Darwin's *Origin of Species*, there has been an alternative explanation of how such organs, for example, the human eye, came into existence. In addition, after Darwin, surviving to reproduce was recognized as the goal of living organisms — whatever worked to pass on one's genes was, from the perspective of nature, good. In Aristotle's view, an organism has a potentiality that is implicit in it and waiting to be realized. With natural selection, there is no one right way to develop, as long as one's genes are passed on. Most contemporary philosophers of biology seek to describe the world without the teleological language of "purpose" or "goal" (or they seek to redefine these terms appealing only to concepts in the theory of evolution).

A second criticism of Aristotle is that he provides few rules that set out specific moral obligations and thus little practical advice about how to act. Instead, his most tangible advice is to act in the mean between excess and deficiency, (he does mention that committing adultery, for example, is never in the mean). Aristotle also appeals to the "man of practical wisdom" and suggests that one should act as the person of practical wisdom would act. Nevertheless, Aristotle does not provide general rules that specify our moral obligations. This can leave the novice with little guidance about how to resolve specific issues. It also tends to invest a good deal of authority in the person of practical wisdom, a "moral expert." Novices emulate moral experts as part of the process of learning to be virtuous. Moral experts, in turn, have a good deal of discretion about how to resolve ethical questions. The moral expert is supposed to be sensitized to the moral landscape such that she discerns the right action where others see only an irresolvable dispute (or worse, overconfidently insist on a vicious action) (McNaughton, 1991). Perhaps everyone has known someone he considers to be morally wise, but there may be little agreement about who such people are. Further, it seems somewhat dangerous to invest so much authority in a single person's power of discernment.

But what is a weakness to some, is a strength to others (Hursthouse, 1995). Aristotle is relevant to contemporary accounts of health care ethics because he viewed moral goodness as a skill that must be mastered rather than a set of rules that must be followed. This approach fits with the type of training received by physicians and some other health care professionals. The training of physicians in residency programs often involves mentorship by older, more experienced physicians. The training includes not only information, but also close observation and emulation of the skills involved in medicine, from communication with patients, to physician interactions with nonphysician colleagues, to skills with a scalpel. The well-respected attending physician is viewed as passing the "art of medicine" to younger colleagues. This art cannot be codified, but rather is embodied in an expert. One suggestion regarding health care ethics is to make sure that the physician (and other) leaders in an institution are not only experts in the technical side of medicine, but are also moral experts as well (Pellegrino & Thomasma, 1993). An institution with wise moral leadership would, in theory, need very few specific rules to govern the ethical conduct of its members (Beecher, 1966; Kass, 1980).

AUGUSTINE (A.D. 354–430)

Augustine is an influential figure in the consolidation of early Christian thought. Aurelious Augustinus was born to Roman parents in Roman-controlled North Africa. Augustine described himself as living a "lustful" and "wicked" life until about the age of 30. In *The Confessions*, he writes to God about his struggle with lust:

> I in my great worthlessness had begged you for chastity, saying: "Grant me chastity and continence, but not yet." For I was afraid that you would hear my prayers too soon, and too soon would heal me from the disease of lust which I wanted satisfied rather than extinguished.

Augustine had always been a searcher for religious truth and was for a time a member of the Manichean sect, which held that good and evil were eternal and equally powerful forces in the world. However, Augustine was profoundly influenced by the sermons of the Catholic Bishop Ambrose, who over time convinced Augustine of the intellectual merit of Catholicism. After being baptized a Catholic by Ambrose in 387, Augustine never strayed from his faith. Augustine is responsible for quite a number of works, of which the best known are *The City of God* and his autobiography, *Confessions*.

Augustine was one of the first to systematize answers to the problem of evil, which is essentially the question of why an all-good, all-knowing, and all-powerful God would allow suffering and evil to exist. Augustine advanced a number of answers, but a prominent one is that, in sin, humans freely turn away from eternal goods in order to seek inferior, temporary goods. Augustine argued that evil is simply the absence of good, so that, strictly speaking, evil is not a thing that can be said to exist. Humans' free choice of sin results in suffering and a diminishing of the good because sin is the pursuit of inferior goods. The four cardinal virtues for Augustine are prudence, fortitude, temperance, and justice — each of these, except perhaps justice, is explained as helping humans to desire eternal goods and suppress desire for earthly goods. Augustine says that the person who desires the correct goods has "good will," and he takes this to be the most valuable possession a person can have. Augustine's ethical theory contains many prohibitions on action. Notably, Augustine presents a carefully argued, absolute prohibition of suicide in *The City of God* (the only possible exception is martyrdom at the direct command of God). Augustine also considers every lie to be sin, but his nuanced view of deception holds that some lies are clearly worse than others. (Readers familiar with the ethics of Immanuel Kant will notice some similarities between Kant and Augustine. However, it should be noted that the thinkers understand the good will in a fundamentally different way: Augustine explained it in terms of having the proper desires, while Kant felt that the good will did not depend on desires at all.)

THOMAS AQUINAS (1224–1274)

A second great religious thinker was Thomas Aquinas, who lived approximately 800 years after Augustine. Aquinas was born to a wealthy family in southern Italy near Naples. Aquinas received religious training early, and at 20 years old, he joined the Dominican Order. His family was disappointed that he joined the newly formed order, so much so that they held him hostage for about a year in the hope he would renounce the Dominicans. He served the Dominican Order with distinction throughout his life, spending the majority of his time as a professor of theology at the University of Paris. Aquinas's writings are extensive: the best known is *Summa Theologica*, which he probably wrote while at the residence of Pope Clement IV between the years 1265 and 1268. An interesting coda to the life of Aquinas is that soon after his death many of his writings were condemned by Church officials: studying the works of Aquinas was only fully sanctioned by the Catholic Church under Pope Leo XIII around the year 1900.

The thought of Aquinas is sometimes presented with the formula: Aristotle + God = Aquinas. While Aquinas's rich and extensive writings cannot be reduced to this formula, the formula does point to an organizing theme in Aquinas's thought. Aristotle held that everything in nature was imbued with a purpose (the final cause, in Aristotle's terminology). Aquinas identified God as the source of these purposes. Simply put, God designed everything in the world with a purpose in mind. With Aristotle, one can learn about an object's purpose by examining the form or organization of the object. So too for Aquinas — the study of humans and nature reveals natural laws, and these natural laws provide insight into God and God's "eternal law." One learns about the creator by studying creation. Sins are actions that conflict with natural law (and therefore also eternal law). From this guiding idea, Aquinas develops a complex taxonomy of immoral actions.

Among his specific prohibitions, Aquinas says suicide is wrong because (1) it violates the natural law of self-preservation, (2) it harms one's community, and (3) the power of life and death rightly belongs to God. Like Augustine, Aquinas holds that every lie is a sin, although some lies are relatively minor infractions. In this context, Aquinas defends what is known as the Pauline principle, namely, that it is not permissible to achieve a good end (no matter how great) by an evil means (no matter how minor).

Aquinas also had a good deal to say about sex and reproduction. Aquinas holds that procreation is the natural purpose of the sex act. Thus, a sexual act that does not allow for procreation conflicts with natural law. Thus, homosexuality and masturbation are sins for Aquinas. So, too, is heterosexual sex outside of marriage because Aquinas holds that the natural order is such that human offspring should be raised by two parents (if possible). Aquinas does not pull his punches here: any sexual act

in or outside of marriage that does not allow for procreation and the proper raising of children is a mortal sin. That is, it is a sin that will result in one's damnation, unless this sin is absolved by God's grace. (Being sorry or doing penance can absolve one from venial sins, but they are powerless against mortal sins.)

The doctrine of double effect was developed by Aquinas (and others), and this doctrine plays an important role in some contemporary writings on medical ethics. The doctrine of double effect is a way to determine the moral permissibility of actions that have both good and bad effects. In essence, the doctrine holds that an action that causes a bad effect is permissible if and only if the following five criteria are met:

1. Only the good effect is intended; the bad effect may be foreseen, as long as it is not intended.
2. The action cannot be intrinsically wrong (such as lying).
3. The causal chain that leads to the good effect cannot contain the bad effect; that is, the good effect cannot be the causal result of the bad effect.
4. There are no ways to achieve the good effect without causing the bad effect (or a worse one).
5. The good effects of the action outweigh the bad effects of the action.

For example, routine surgery to remove a diseased appendix meets all of the criteria: bad effects (e.g., soreness, risks associated with anesthesia) are foreseen but not intended; removing the appendix is not intrinsically wrong; the good effect is not caused by any bad effects; there is no way to prevent a burst appendix except surgery; the badness of a burst appendix outweighs the risks and costs of surgery. A second application of the doctrine of double effect involves narcotics to relieve suffering in a terminally ill patient: the intent must be to relieve pain (this is the good effect), not cause death (this is the bad effect); providing narcotics in normal doses is not intrinsically wrong (i.e., normal doses are not tantamount to providing a deadly poison); pain relief is not achieved by death; there are no other means to relieve suffering; the good of pain relief outweighs the increased risk of premature death.

Criticism and Evaluation

While a few isolated arguments from Aquinas and Augustine are persuasive in secular contexts, their theories as a whole are plausible only within a religious context. This is because each of the thinkers derives ethical commitments from his theological views about the nature of God. And, of course, there are a variety of theological perspectives even within Christianity, so one cannot assume that ethical commitments of Aquinas and Augustine fit well with all Christian faiths. Nonetheless, ideas from the thinkers, especially Aquinas's view that one can use "natural law" to derive ethical rules, continue to be influential among many in society.

The doctrine of double effect has been discussed, defended, and criticized since Aquinas's time. Major criticisms include the following. Some have argued that it is impossible to foresee the bad outcome of one's action and not also intend the outcome when performing the action; that is, there is no such thing as a foreseen but unintended effect. A second criticism holds that the notion of an intrinsically wrong action is incoherent: if this is so, then one must give up criterion 2 (and maybe criterion 3), in which case the doctrine is nothing more than a form of consequentialism. (See the section on Mill for a discussion of consequentialism.) Finally, one might argue that judgments made about balancing good and bad effects (in criterion 5) are necessarily subjective. Indeed, some would argue that death is actually a good for the suffering patient for whom no relief is possible. The doctrine of double effect seems to assume that there is some noncontroversial way of identifying effects as good or bad. These criticisms are powerful when the doctrine of double effect is used in a secular context. However, the doctrine of double effect was never meant to be divorced from a religious context, which would include a substantive account of which types of actions are intrinsically wrong and a substantive account of human goods. Further, a secular theory that identified intrinsically wrong actions and which provided a substantive account of human goods could also use the doctrine.

IMMANUEL KANT (1724–1804)

Kant invented one of the most influential deontological theories of ethics. A deontological theory takes some actions to be morally wrong regardless of their consequences. The clearest example in Kant's writing is lying. According to Kant, it is not permissible to lie even if the lie is about a relatively unimportant matter and yet would prevent great evils from occurring. Simply put, whether a lie has good or bad effects is irrelevant to whether the lie is permissible. Kant's theory is largely secular in its grounding. Nonetheless, Kantian ethics has strong affinities with religious ethics because religious ethics also tends to identify some actions as impermissible regardless of their consequences (as our discussion of the doctrine of double effect has just illustrated). A second important aspect of Kant's ethical theory is its emphasis on autonomy. Kant suggests that persons' capacity for reason gives persons both freedom and responsibility. As beings with the capacity to reason, persons can rise above the instinctual, animal aspects of their natures to make informed choices about the proper course of action. The ability to make informed choices forms the basis of one's freedom.

However, one is not free to make these choices willy-nilly. Rather, one has the responsibility to reason correctly about morality. This means that the choices ones makes for oneself — about lying, for example — have a measure of universality, that is, all persons who reason correctly will necessarily reach the same conclusion.

Immanuel Kant was born in 1724 and he died in 1804. He lived his whole life in Konigsburg, as a professor at the University of Konigsburg. Kant lived the life of a quiet and not very productive professor until about the year 1776, when he read David Hume's *Enquiry Concerning Human Nature*. Kant said that Hume's book woke him from his "dogmatic slumber," meaning that Hume's work showed him that there were deep flaws in his own understanding of the world. It was quite an awakening. At the age of 56, Kant embarked on one of the most ambitious and most successful research programs in the history of philosophy. Kant published the *Critique of Pure Reason* in 1781, and followed this work with books on practical reason, aesthetics, religion, and ethics. Kant not only made original contributions in each area, but his works fit together to form a philosophical system unmatched for its subtlety and sophistication.

Kant begins the first section of the *Groundwork for the Metaphysics of Morals* with a bold statement about moral value:

> There is no possibility of thinking of anything at all in the world, or even out of it, which can be regarded as good without qualification, except a good will. (*GW* 393)*

Kant contrasts a good will with talents such as intelligence and wit, with virtues such as courage and perseverance, and with calm deliberation and self-control. In contrast to Aristotle, Kant argues that none of these character traits has intrinsic value because each can be put to evil uses. What then is a good will, and why is it so valuable? Kant is clear that a good will is not good because it brings about good consequences. He writes: "a good will is good not because of what it effects or accomplishes, nor because of its fitness to attain some proposed end; it is good only through its willing, i.e., it is good in itself" (*GW* 494). Indeed, Kant says that the good will "shines like a jewel" with its full value even in a person who lacks all talent and skill, and thus never succeeds in accomplishing any of his aims. Kant rules out one potential reason why a good will might be thought valuable. So, again, what is a good will and why is it valuable? Kant explicates the concept of a good will in terms of a person's motivation to perform an action. A person with a good will has the

---

* Parenthetical citations are to the Prussian Academy system, the standard method for citing passages in Kant across various translations. *GW* refers to the *Groundings for the Metaphysics of Morals*. *DV* refers to the *Doctrine of Virtue*.

intention to do a morally correct action *because* the action is morally correct. That is, the person does the correct action out of respect for the moral law.

Kant uses a number of cases to illustrate the point. Adapting one of his cases, consider someone who goes out of her way to help an infirm person to board a bus. We can imagine any number of motivations for this kind stranger's action: she might want to impress someone she knows is watching her; she might feel guilty for snapping at a co-worker earlier in the day; she might want the satisfaction that comes from performing a good deed; the infirm person might remind her of her father, for whom she has kind feelings; she might even simply have found herself overcome by sympathetic emotions. Kant argues that none of these potential motivations for the action has any moral worth. What gives the stranger's action moral worth, if it has moral worth, is that the action is performed out of respect for the moral law. That is, the stranger intends to perform the action because the action is the right thing to do. Kant's terminology contrasts *acting from duty* with *acting according to duty*. Because this action is morally required, one acts *according to duty* no matter one's motivation. But only the correct motivation for the action yields an action *from duty*. In part, the distinction is easily understood — everyone recognizes that sometimes the morally correct action is performed for morally neutral or morally bad reasons. What is interesting is Kant's formulation of morally correct motivation: one does what is right because it is right.

It is possible to clarify what Kant means by acting from duty by considering motivations that do not count as being morally worthy. Kant's general term for such motivations is "inclination." An inclination is either a particular desire or an emotional disposition. So, one is motivated by an inclination if one helps because one *desires* to impress a potential romantic partner. Further, one is motivated by an inclination if one helps because one *desires* to feel satisfied for performing a good deed. One also is motivated by an inclination if one's emotional dispositions simply move one to act. The sympathetic person may act not because she desires something, but simply because she has a sympathetic character. (Note the contrast to Aristotle here, who would consider the sympathetically inclined person to be acting virtuously.) Kant does not view inclinations as chosen by the agent. Rather, he thinks that one finds oneself with inclinations; the inclinations arise in humans because humans are instinctual creatures with bodily needs. In an important sense, when a person lets these inclinations cause his actions, then he is not free or autonomous. An autonomous choice for Kant is one that is made on the basis of reason, not on the basis of desires or emotions. Of course, Kant thinks it is often appropriate to act to fulfill one's desires — the point is that one is not demonstrating one's highest potential except when one's action is motivated by reason, in

particular, when one does the morally right thing because reason shows him that it is the right thing. Kant says that we are "self-legislating." This means that we each use our reason to determine what is morally right, and we bind ourselves to doing what is right because we see that it is dictated by reason. It is in that sense that we are free — the moral rules that bind one are self-imposed.

The rules of reason are universal, according to Kant. Two people who are not making any mistakes in their reasoning will reach the same conclusion. Thus, moral rules are universal, even though each of us must reach these laws using our own reason. This allows Kant to talk about the specific moral obligations that everyone must follow, even though each person is responsible for imposing these rules on herself. Kant's core moral principle is called the categorical imperative. The categorical imperative has a number of different formulations, but the first and third are the most influential.

Categorical Imperative, Universal Law Formulation: Act only according to that maxim whereby you can at the same time will that it should become a universal law. (421)

Categorical Imperative, End-in-Itself Formulation: Act in such a way that you treat humanity, whether in your own person or in that of another, always at the same time as an end and never simply as a means. (429)

Intuitively, the universal law formulation gets at the idea that people have a tendency to make exceptions for themselves: that is, a person might rationalize that it is permissible for him to perform an action, even though he would have to admit that it would be bad if everyone acted in the same way. Kant cannot appeal to bad consequences and remain consistent with his remarks about the good will. So, Kant explains that in performing an action one is, in effect, agreeing to the principle that it is permissible for everyone to act in the same way, and reason will show one whether it is possible to embrace this principle. Kant's clearest example involves keeping promises. Kant reasons that one cannot both expect to reap the reward of breaking a promise and yet assert that it is fine for everyone to break promises: this is because in a world in which everyone breaks promises, there will be no trust, and if there is no trust, then there will be no rewards to reap from breaking a promise because no one will believe the promise in the first place. Whether the categorical imperative "test" for the morality of actions works for all cases has been the subject of debate since Kant's time.

The end-in-itself formulation of the categorical imperative is more straightforward. The idea is that one must respect other people as decision makers in their own right — that is to say, that one must act to respect and support other people's autonomy. One can use other people as means to fulfill one's own needs (e.g., as happens in all commercial transactions), but this use of others as a means must be consistent with respecting others as persons. Note that Kant is also clear that one has to respect oneself as an autonomous being. That is, one has an obligation to respect and support one's own autonomy.

Kant offers the following four examples to highlight the four categories of moral obligations.

	Perfect duties	Imperfect duties
Duties to others	Do not break promises	Help others in need
Duties to self	Do not commit suicide	Cultivate your own talents

Perfect duties require a person to always refrain from performing an action. They are required at all times. Imperfect duties require performing an action. Because performing an action requires time and effort and the effort one expends performing one imperfect duty must be balanced against one's obligation to perform other imperfect duties, any particular imperfect duty is not required of a person at all times. One needs to perform an imperfect duty when the opportunity arises and such that one is not favoring one imperfect duty to the detriment of others. (This raises the interesting practical question of how to balance imperfect duties to self with imperfect duties to others.)

Criticisms and Evaluation

Kant's theory is not immune to a type of criticism that can be made against all deontological theories, namely, that some instance of an action-type identified as impermissible by the theory is considered to be permissible or even obligatory on independent grounds. Consider the following example:

> You are hiding innocent people from the soldiers of a repressive regime. Soldiers knock on your door and ask you if you are hiding anyone. You know that the soldiers will torture and kill the people if you give them up. You know that the soldiers will search your house and find the people if you say nothing. You also know that if you lie convincingly the soldiers will go away. But you feel that it is wrong to lie. What should you do?

Many people have the intuition that in this case it is permissible or even morally obligatory to lie. Some will attempt to justify the lie by saying that the soldiers do not have a right to the truth. Kant would disagree. His view is that you should tell the soldiers the truth, no matter the consequence to the innocent people. In commenting on a similar case, Kant writes: "To be truthful in all declarations is … a sacred and unconditionally commanding law of reason that admits of no expediency whatsoever." Kant's view is that there are no exceptions to the prohi-

bition on lying. Many people find this sort of inflexibility untenable, especially given that it will more than likely result in the death of innocents.

A second criticism of Kant involves his attitude to the emotions. Kant is clear that an action motivated by an emotion such as sympathy has no moral worth. Rather, only actions done from duty have moral worth. Kant would say that a person who performs a compassionate act because she sees it as her duty is acting morally, and this is true whether or not the person also feels the emotion of compassion. However, a person who is motivated by the emotion, and not by duty, has not acted morally. This has led Michael Stocker to focus on the example of a person who is motivated by duty and not emotion. Here is an adaptation of his example.

> Sheila is ill and has been hospitalized. Her co-worker Bob comes to visit her. Sheila is immediately cheered: she didn't know that Bob cared about her; she is moved by Bob's compassion and friendship. She brings this up: "Bob, how nice of you to visit; it is so caring of you to go out of your way to cheer me; I am moved to have a friend such as you." Bob, ever the honest one, sets Sheila straight: "I consider it my duty to visit a co-worker who is ill, and so here I am. I would rather be at home, you know, but duty calls."

Few would think that Bob is a morally praiseworthy person, even if he refrained from telling Sheila his real motivation for the visit. Rather, we generally expect morally good persons to have morally good emotional dispositions, and indeed we evaluate people based on their emotional dispositions. Sometimes we do admire people because of their strong sense of duty, but other times we admire people for their kind, compassionate, or generous emotions. Kant seems to be missing this aspect of morality.

This criticism has prompted contemporary defenders of Kant to investigate more closely his view on the moral value of emotions. Some of these defenders have suggested that focusing on Kant's *Groundwork for the Metaphysics of Morals,* while ignoring his other works, results in a lopsided view of Kantian ethics. Kant's *Groundwork,* it is argued, defends his conception of right action. Kant's *Doctrine of Virtue,* on the other hand, presents his conception of a virtuous person. So *The Doctrine of Virtue* may be important to balancing the overall picture of Kantian ethics.

In *The Doctrine of Virtue* Kant argues that character traits and emotional dispositions provide important support to the good will. For instance, he argues that:

> … it is a duty to sympathize actively in the fate [of others]; and to this end it is therefore a duty to cultivate the compassionate natural feelings in us, and to make use of them as so many means to sympathy based on moral principles.… For this is still one of the impulses

that nature has implanted in us to do what the representation of duty alone would not accomplish. (*DV* 457)

In this passage, Kant argues that human imperfection and weakness often prevent us from acting on duty alone. Thus, we must cultivate our natural compassion, to bring it in line with the requirements of moral duty. Kant further thought that when we perform beneficent actions from duty we would "eventually come to actually love the person [we] have helped" (*DV* 402). Dutiful beneficent acts will produce the emotion of sympathy in us, but it is a kind of sympathy that is obedient to and consequent upon moral duty.

But even given this defense of Kant, many non-Kantians remain unsatisfied with the Kantian view of emotions. In particular, some critics have argued that Kant's ethical theory, at best, values emotions merely as instruments to doing one's moral duty. Kantians cannot see the simple experience of an emotion as morally valuable in itself. Thus, a Kantian cannot hold that simply feeling sympathy for a friend in distress has moral significance, apart from the emotion's ability to support an agent's good will. So for those moral theorists convinced that emotions have moral value apart from their role in morally good action, the Kantian position on emotions remains inadequate even with these important defenses of Kant's view (Stark, in press).

Kant is relevant to contemporary health care ethics for a number of reasons. First, Kant was perhaps the first to develop a well-supported secular deontological theory. This makes it possible to claim in pluralistic settings that some actions are just wrong, no matter their good consequences, and to formulate public policy around the sorts of actions that are considered to be intrinsically wrong. Second, Kant championed autonomy. His view is one of the primary motivations for the Principle of Respect for Autonomy, which is discussed in the second section of this chapter. Finally, Kant's views do much to influence theories of informed consent. Notably, informed consent procedures are designed not just to protect patients' freedom to choose, but also to support patients in making good decisions. Kant, as we saw, connects the freedom to choose with choosing for the right reasons: a person makes a genuinely free choice if and only if a person makes a choice based on reason. This issue is also discussed in the second section.

JOHN STUART MILL (1806–1873)

John Stuart Mill (with Jeremy Bentham) developed consequentialism, one of the most influential modern theories of ethics. Mill's version of consequentialism is called utilitarianism, and the great virtue of this theory is that it cuts away the complex and (Mill would say) arcane) trappings of earlier ethical theories, and seeks to explain

ethics in a way that is simple and direct, and that appeals to common sense. Mill's guiding insight, which was exquisitely simple, was that those actions that cause good consequences are ethically good and those that cause bad consequences are ethically bad. Despite its apparent common sense, the theory stands in stark contrast to earlier ethical theories. In part, this is because Mill defined good consequences as pleasure and the absence of pain, and other ethical theories posited loftier goals for humans' lives. But an even more direct point of contrast, especially to Kant, is that Mill denied that any action is wrong in and of itself, regardless of its consequences. This means, for example, that telling a lie is not necessarily wrong; whether a particular lie is morally right or morally wrong depends on the consequences of telling it. For Mill, many of the reasons why we might be tempted to say that an action is wrong "in-itself" are based on outdated traditions or suspect religious reasoning. In both cases, the moral rules that result will tend to favor the already well off in society at the expense of the common folks working in fields and factories. Mill argued that human suffering is bad wherever it is found, and that society ought to be arranged so that such suffering is minimized — if a traditional right (say, one granted to the nobility) stands in the way of minimizing suffering, so much the worse for this right. Lest Mill seem too much of a radical, it should be noted that he found that many (but not all) of the institutions of the British Empire did serve to promote the general well-being.

John Stuart Mill was born on May 20, 1806, in London. His father was James Mill, a prominent intellectual and reformer and a close associate of Jeremy Bentham. James Mill pushed John in his studies from an early age — it was said that John was reading Plato in the original Greek at age 7. John began publishing his own work at age 16. He became the editor of the *Westminister Review* and founder of the Utilitarian Society. In 1826, at age 20, Mill underwent a mental crisis, entering a 4-year period of depression the cause of which he took to be the lack of "cultivation of the feelings" in his early upbringing. The end of Mill's depression coincided with meeting his life's partner, Harriet Hardy Taylor, who was at the time married to someone else. Mill and Taylor remained close friends and collaborators for the next 20 years, until the death of John Taylor allowed Mill and Harriet Taylor to be married. (See the dedication of *On Liberty* for insight into Taylor's contributions to Mill's thought and writings.) Mill was elected a member of the British Parliament in 1865, although he was defeated at the next election. Mill died on May 7, 1873, in Avignon, France, apparently as the result of the exertion of a 15-mile hike he had taken 2 days previously. Throughout his life, Mill maintained his father's commitment to reforming society, particularly the sort of evils brought on common people by industrialization and urbanization. Mill was also an early defender of equality for women, publishing *The Subjugation of Women* in 1869 — which was most likely co-written with Harriet Taylor. (An interesting anecdote in this regard was that Mill was arrested and briefly jailed for obscenity in 1823, the result of distributing birth control literature in a working-class neighborhood of London.) Mill published widely in areas beyond moral philosophy, including logic (*A System of Logic*, 1843), political theory (*On Liberty*, 1859), and economics (*Principles of Political Economy*, 1848). Those interested in Mill's views on religion, God, and immortality will find his *Three Essays on Religion* (1874) to be helpful. Mill's *Autobiography* (1873) also makes fascinating reading.

Mill's moral theory is outlined in his short book *Utilitarianism* (1863). The primary idea behind the theory is that the morality of an action ought to be measured solely by the consequences, good and bad, that are produced by the action. We are obligated to perform the action that produces the most good, that is, the action that has the consequences with the highest net value. To complete the theory, Mill specifies what counts as good and bad consequences. Mill argues that the value of an action is measured by the pleasure and pain that it produces in humans. This leads to Mill's central principle, the Greatest Happiness Principle (GHP): "Actions are right in proportion as they tend to promote happiness; wrong as they produce the reverse of happiness." Mill leaves no doubt as to what he means by happiness: "By happiness is intended pleasure and the absence of pain; by unhappiness, pain and the privation of pleasure" (Mill, 1966, p. 157).

Three possible misinterpretations should be headed off at the outset. First, Mill is not an egoist. That is, he is not claiming that an action is morally right for me to perform if it produces the best consequences *for me*. Rather, he is claiming that an action is morally right for me to perform if it produces the best consequences for everyone. I am allowed to consider my own well-being in calculating which action is morally right, but my well-being counts no more than the well-being of anyone else who would be affected by the action. Indeed, because my action may affect the well-being of persons yet to be born, I should also consider their well-being in my calculations. Second, Mill is concerned with both short- and long-term consequences. Thus, the GHP does not require that I perform actions with immediately pleasurable consequences, if later consequences will cause enough pain to outweigh immediate pleasures. Finally, Mill seems only concerned with the pleasure and pain felt by humans. However, Jeremy Bentham, in developing an earlier version of utilitarianism, argued that the pleasure and pain of animals ought to be considered in the calculations. (Bentham's point is echoed by contemporary animal rights activists, notably Peter Singer [1990], who argues that if pain is bad in humans, then it is bad in animals too.)

In refining his basic theory, Mill anticipates and answers several objections. An initial objection is that utilitarianism does not encourage what is truly valuable in human nature. So, his imagined critic might point out: "Is it not beneath the dignity of humans to chase after pleasure? We think that gluttons, drunkards, and those preoccupied with sex are morally depraved — we certainly do not hold them up as models of right action" (Mill, 1966, p. 160). One component of Mill's answer is merely to note that some of these lifestyles will lead to painful consequences in the long term. But this answer leaves the basic thrust of the objection intact: Isn't it beneath the dignity of humans to chase after pleasure? Mill answers with a distinction between higher and lower pleasures. Lower pleasures are things such as sex, drink, food, and laziness. Higher pleasures include reading literature, writing, viewing art, listening to music, contemplating philosophy, etc. Even performing moral actions can be a higher pleasure for certain individuals. A strict reading of the GHP implies that the only moral reason to prefer higher pleasures to lower pleasures is that higher pleasures are more pleasurable. Mill embraces this statement, claiming that the higher pleasures of the mind are indeed more pleasurable than the lower pleasures. As evidence for this, he claims that people who have been lucky enough to have experienced both sorts of pleasures almost invariably choose higher pleasures as the more desirable. So Mill says famously: "It is better to be a human being dissatisfied than a pig satisfied; better to be Socrates dissatisfied than a fool satisfied" (Mill, 1966, p. 161). Mill's claim has fueled much debate about human nature: Is it true that people of sufficient means gravitate toward intellectual pleasure, and even if true, does this imply anything about the lesser value of lower pleasures — is reading Shakespeare really better than watching the World Wrestling Federation? At any rate, if we accept Mill's argument, then following the GHP will not require the pursuit of "swinely" pleasures, but rather the pursuit of the higher intellectual pleasures. In this sense, the GHP will promote what is dignified in human nature.

A second objection that Mill considered involves the time and effort that following the GHP would require. Mill seems to suggest that at any particular time a person should consider all of the alternative actions that are available, evaluate the short- and long-term consequences of these actions, and finally choose the action that has the highest net value. Even if we artificially limit the alternative actions available to three options, calculating the long-term consequences of these actions is a formidable task. Of course, there will be a good deal of uncertainty about what the likely consequences of the actions will be, but there will also be a good deal of information to sort through to attempt to trace out all the consequences of the three options. Utilitarianism, then, threatens to paralyze action in an endless fit of calculation. Mill offers a number of answers. He points out, first, that following the GHP does not require intricate calculations. Rather, most decisions about which actions will produce the best consequences involve only common sense. Second, echoing a theme from Aristotle, Mill argues that training the appropriate dispositions (such as the disposition to answer honestly when asked a question) is an important aspect of his theory. Once one has decided that being honest usually promotes the best consequences, then one trains oneself to be spontaneously honest (that is, without calculating consequences every time one is asked a question). Mill points out that most ethical theories could be interpreted in such a way that they paralyze action by requiring too much reflection — so he points out that Christians are not required to reread the Bible every time they face a decision (Mill, 1966, p. 178). Finally, Mill suggests that our actions will have most of their consequences close to home. Theoretically, a decision I make today might have consequences for people in future generations and might have consequences for people I am unaware of on the other side of the world. But, generally, my decisions will have the most effect on myself, my family, my friends, and my colleagues. Also, generally, it will be easier to trace out the effects of my actions for this smaller group of people. Some of these decisions may require the careful balancing of potential good and bad consequences for this group of people, but the decisions do not require that the agent devote an extraordinary amount of time and effort to calculating how the action will affect persons in distant times and places.

Before turning to modern criticisms of Mill's *Utilitarianism*, it is important to introduce Mill's ideas from *On Liberty* because these, too, have had a huge impact on political philosophy in the United States. Mill was concerned not only that a monarch would have too much power, but also that in the "democratic republic" of America the danger exists of a tyranny of the majority (to use de Tocqueville's term). In order to guard against this, Mill proposed his harm principle: "That the only purpose for which power can be rightfully exercised over any member of a civilized community, against his will, is to prevent harm to others." Mill immediately clarifies the harm principle with an injunction against paternalism: A mature and competent person "cannot rightfully be compelled to do or forbear [any action] because it will be better for him to do so, because it will make him happier, because, in the opinions of others, to do so would be wise, or even right." Mill defends these principles based on the recognition that institutions within society can be quite powerful, and that the only way to guard against inappropriate paternalism is to completely rule out all paternalism (although there is debate on this interpretation). Mill continues in *On Liberty* to further specify the types of liberties that are important to protect. There are three main categories: (1) "the inward domain of consciousness," which

includes the "absolute" freedom to think, feel, and formulate opinions; (2) "liberty of tastes and pursuits," which is freedom in choice of personal lifestyles and practices as long as these do not harm anyone else; and (3) freedom of association "for any purpose not involving harm to others." This "liberal argument" has been influential across the political spectrum in the United States. It also forms the core of many well-known Supreme Court decisions, including *Griswold v. Connecticut* (1965, birth control), *Roe v. Wade* (1973, abortion), and the dissent in *Bowers v. Hardwick* (1986, homosexuality).

Criticisms and Evaluations

Despite its commonsensical nature, utilitarianism is open to a wide variety of criticism. First and most prominently, utilitarianism does not give a special status to categories of moral value that many people take to be of central moral importance. For example, utilitarianism does not seem to grant a special status to promises, to ownership rights, to obligations arising from close relationships to family or friends, or to obligations relating to justice. For each and every category, it seems possible to imagine a situation in which utilitarianism would require that the moral value in question be overridden in the name of the common good. Consider the following example relating to justice:

> A mob is chasing a man through town. They blame him for a murder, and they plan to brutally execute him if they capture him. The man happens to be innocent, as you know. However, you also know that if the mob does not capture and kill the man, then a riot will ensue in which many persons will be harmed and killed (some of those harmed and killed will be innocent, having nothing at all to do with the situation). It is in your power to save the innocent man from being stoned. Should you do it?

The gut reaction of many people to this case is that the innocent person should be saved regardless of the bad consequences — justice simply requires it. But utilitarianism seems to require that one allow the innocent person to be killed. Utilitarians may attempt to answer the criticism by resisting the conclusion that utilitarianism requires allowing the innocent man to be killed. So, a utilitarian might argue that while the short-term consequences suggest that the innocent man should be killed, the long-term consequences of this decision include eroding society's commitment to the rule of law, which will in turn cause an increase in suffering, and these bad long-term consequences outweigh any short-term benefits of allowing the man to be killed. While this response is plausible enough, it is possible to manipulate the details of the example to exclude the possibility that the long-term bad effect of eroding the rule of law will occur — thus, in essence, painting the utilitarian into a corner in which she must admit that killing the innocent is justified by her theory. The utilitarian might then be forced to accept the troubling result. Because it is possible to construct equally plausible counterexamples to utilitarianism about promise-keeping, truth-telling, ownership rights, obligations to family, etc., this manner of argument represents a strong challenge to utilitarianism. How persuasive such counterexamples should be is an interesting philosophical question because the evidential authority of the counterexample ultimately relies only on the strength of one's gut reaction to the story and, one might argue, gut reactions are not to be universally trusted.

A second prominent criticism of utilitarianism is that it is too demanding. For example, utilitarianism seems to require too much personal sacrifice in order to promote the interests of other people. Consider that I have $10 in my pocket that is uncommitted as far as my budget is concerned. I consider using the money to go to the movies tonight — I certainly would get pleasure from this, and there are no relevant constraints on my time. But, I reason, this money could also be used to benefit other people — it might even save lives if contributed to Oxfam or some other worthwhile charity. Utilitarianism seems to require that I give the money to Oxfam. Now perhaps this particular sacrifice is morally obligatory, but notice that if tomorrow I again find myself with an unencumbered $10, I would again be obligated to donate the money, and so on, and so on. I would only be entitled to use the money for myself (or my family and friends) when it becomes the case that the happiness I can create close to home is greater than (or equal to) the happiness I can create by donating the money. Even if we lived in a world in which the inequities between rich and poor were much less pronounced, one might wonder whether a person is morally required always to spend his money (and his time) in a way that produces the most good, regardless of how it affects himself and his loved ones. These issues have led to a spirited debate about the level of self-sacrifice that can legitimately be required by an ethical theory. Notice that even minimalist ethical theories, such as libertarianism, require some self-sacrifice in the name of morality, since libertarians hold that one must refrain from harming others even if harming another would benefit oneself. Peter Singer (1977), inspired by utilitarianism, is at the other extreme, arguing that people in wealthy Western countries have an absolute obligation to dramatically lower their standards of living in order to benefit people in developing nations. Mill attempted to ameliorate the concern that utilitarianism demands too much personal sacrifice both by noting that one's resources are more efficiently used close to home (perhaps that was true in his day), as well as by pointing to the hedonist's paradox, which is the view that a person cannot obtain happiness by aiming directly at it, but rather truly happy people have as their goal something outside of themselves (Mill, 1966,

p. 172). So it is likely that some self-sacrifice will indeed make us happier.

A third criticism of utilitarianism is that it requires a person to sacrifice his or her integrity. This criticism has been developed by Bernard Williams. Williams asks us to consider the following case, which I paraphrase:

> George, a chemist, has been offered a job in a research facility for chemical and biological weapons. Despite his best efforts, George has been out of work for some time, and his young children have suffered greatly under the strain placed on the family. George does not feel he can take the job, however, given that he is a committed pacifist who has always been against chemical and biological weapons. The person offering George the job says that she, too, is against such weapons: in fact, she has offered George the job in part because of his beliefs; other candidates for the job will enthusiastically push the work along at a faster pace, while George will likely drag his feet. Should George take the job? (Williams, 1977, pp. 97–98)

Utilitarianism would seem to require that George take the job. The point of Williams' story is not merely that George is being required by utilitarianism to do something that most of us would agree is wrong. Rather, Williams is trying to show that utilitarianism is incompatible with having integrity. George has identified himself with pacifism — it is part of his self-image. Maybe George initially embraced pacifism for utilitarian reasons — because he felt it brought about the most good — but being a pacifist is now George's central project; it is who he is. But whether pacifism actually causes the best consequences depends not on George, but on facts in the world, and depending on how these facts change, George at any moment could be required to act contrary to his central, defining project. At any moment, he could be required to live a lie. Williams explains:

> The point is that [George] is identified with his actions as flowing from projects and attitudes which in some cases he takes seriously at the deepest level, as what his life is about.... It is absurd to demand of such a man, when the sums come in from the utility network which the projects of others have in part determined, that he should just step aside from his own project and decision and acknowledge the decision which utilitarian calculation requires. It is to alienate him in a real sense from his actions and the source of his action in his own convictions.... It is thus, in the most literal sense, an attack on his integrity. (Williams, 1977, 132)

According to Williams, the only project that a utilitarian can be fully committed to without putting his integrity at risk is the project of being a utilitarian. But, Williams argues, this project is too thin, too formalistic, to be a central commitment or life's project. To use another of

Williams' well-known examples, one should perform acts that demonstrate love for one's romantic partner out of a genuine love for one's partner, not because demonstrating love for one's partner creates, in the long run, the best consequences for all of humanity.*

One strategy utilitarians have adopted in response to all of the criticisms mentioned is to move from act utilitarianism to some type of indirect utilitarianism. Act utilitarianism says that one should evaluate which act brings about the best consequences. Indirect utilitarianism is still interested in the best consequences, but it focuses on other mechanisms for bringing them about. For example, rule utilitarianism says that an action is morally right if and only if that action is required by a *set of rules,* the adoption of which would produce the best consequences. The rule utilitarian advises that one should follow the set of rules identified, even though in isolated instances following a rule will not bring about the best consequences. Rule utilitarians think that the benefit (in good consequences) of having a stable set of rules outweighs the cost (in bad consequences) of occasionally performing non-optimal actions. Another form of indirect utilitarianism is character utilitarianism, which holds that performing an action is morally right if and only if that action promotes or is promoted by a *set of character dispositions,* the inculcation of which would produce the most good or value for the members of a society. Once again, character utilitarianism identifies the occasional non-optimal action as morally good in order to gain the benefit of allowing persons to internalize content-rich dispositions and commitments (such as George's commitment to pacifism). As a final example, rights utilitarianism holds that performing an action is morally correct if it is in accord with a scheme of *individual rights and liberties,* the adoption of which would produce the most good for society. The distinction between direct and indirect utilitarianism post-dates Mill, but passages in Mill's *Utilitarianism* have been interpreted as advocating forms of indirect utilitarianism.

A second strategy for meeting the criticisms involves modifying the definition of good consequences. Utilitarianism is the name for the view that seeks to maximize pleasurable feelings and minimize painful feelings. Consequentialism is a broader category that recognizes that there are many different accounts of what "good consequences" are. So, preference satisfaction consequentialism

states that one should maximize the satisfaction of preferences (whether or not such satisfaction also maximizes pleasurable feelings). A second example is objective list consequentialism, which identifies a list of goods (such as friendship, knowledge, veracity) such that persons should seek to maximize the obtaining of goods on the list (such a view requires a scheme for trading-off between the goods, as when a gain in friendship requires a loss of veracity). At the center of Mill's utilitarianism is the claim that only consequences matter in moral evaluation. It is possible to hold firm to this central claim, and yet modify significant aspects of the theory. This means that consequentialist theories of ethics may have the resources, despite first appearances, to answer the sorts of criticisms that have been leveled at them.

Many of Mill's ideas are directly relevant to health care ethics. Although Kant is more often seen as the champion of autonomy and informed consent, Mill's arguments in *On Liberty* also provide justification for these ideals. In addition, consequentialism is the method presupposed in cost–benefit analysis, and thus is at the heart of many policy decisions. Indeed in some ways consequentialism seems more appropriate for policy decisions made at an institutional level than it does for guiding individuals in their personal decisions.

But perhaps Mill's ideas have been most influential in debates about care at the end-of-life. Mill believed that no category of action is intrinsically morally good or bad — the morality of an action depends on its consequences, not on the type of action that it is. This has important implications for end-of-life decisions. For example, in the early 1980s a not uncommon view was that withholding treatment is permissible in certain circumstances, but withdrawing treatment is never permissible (Cugliari & Miller, 1994). The idea was that withdrawing life-sustaining treatment is a category of action that is tantamount to killing. Consequentialists, on the other hand, were less concerned about the category (withholding or withdrawing) and more concerned with the consequences of doing either in a particular situation. They argued that the categories themselves have no moral relevance: only the consequences of individual actions (or omissions) have moral relevance. As we know, the utilitarian position on this issue has been adopted in current medical practice (although there are dissents; Sulmasy & Sugarman, 1994). A very similar debate occurred around withdrawing medical nutrition and hydration in the late 1980s, prompted primarily by the Nancy Cruzan case (Lynn & Childress, 1983). Some argued that providing food and water is a special category of action required by morality (Callahan, 1983). Others argued that if the best thing for someone is that she be allowed to die, then it did not matter whether this occurs because food and fluid is withdrawn or because another intervention such as a ventilator

---

* Mill considers and responds to a very similar criticism. He considers the criticism that "It is often affirmed that utilitarianism renders men cold and unsympathizing; that it chills their moral feelings towards individuals; that it makes them regard only the dry and hard consideration of the consequences of actions" (1966, p. 174). Mill argues that all moral theories sometimes require one to ignore bonds of love, and thus utilitarianism is no better or worse in this regard than other theories. Mill also draws a distinction between a standard of right action and the motivations for pursuing right action. He claims that his theory is meant to address only the former issue.

is withdrawn. Here, again, the position consistent with utilitarianism has been adopted.

The reader will have already surmised that the story is not over yet. Consequentialism tends to undermine the moral relevance of the distinction between killing and allowing to die. But this distinction is very important in current law and medical practice. In every jurisdiction in the United States, practitioners may allow a patient to die by withholding or withdrawing treatment. But in every jurisdiction in the United States, except Oregon, practitioners cannot kill their patients or assist patients in killing themselves. This means that extubating a terminally ill patient who is in great pain and has requested to be allowed to die is permissible, even if one knows that death will occur with extubation. But it is not permissible to kill a patient who is in identical circumstances except that he has no respirator to remove. Imagine that the consequences for the patients (and others) in each case are identical: the consequentialist would argue that if it is good to omit treatment in the first case, then it is also good to kill the patient in the second case (Rachels, 1975, 1986). But this consequentialist viewpoint has yet to be adopted, and it looks as if popular opinion is moving in the opposite direction (Emmanuel 2002). One note of caution, here, is that there are also consequentialist arguments against active euthanasia and physician-assisted suicide, most prominently the concern that the long-term effects of legalizing active euthanasia and physician-assisted suicide will include eroding society's respect for human life in general.

HEALTH CARE ETHICS

PRINCIPLES IN HEALTH CARE ETHICS

The most prominent way of organizing consensus on ethical issues in health care into a usable methodology is the principles method. The principles method identifies a small number of general rules, and subsumes more particular and concrete obligations under the general rules. A number of authors use principles to develop a methodology for identifying and resolving ethical conflicts that arise in clinical settings (Veatch, 1981). The best-known principles method is that of Tom Beauchamp and James Childress, *Principles of Biomedical Ethics* (2003), now in its fifth edition. Beauchamp and Childress identify four principles:

1. *Beneficence: One's actions ought to benefit the patient.* Health care providers perform actions in order to improve a patient's health, prevent disease, or generally enhance a patient's welfare. This is a positive duty, that is, a duty to perform actions. Under this principle, Beauchamp and Childress discuss paternalism, sui-

cide prevention, futility, risk–benefit assessments, quality of life, and other topics.

2. *Nonmaleficence: One's actions ought not to harm the patient*, inspired by *Primum non nocere* (First, do no harm) from the Hippocratic oath. This is a negative duty, that is, a duty to refrain from certain actions. Under this principle, Beauchamp and Childress discuss withholding and withdrawing life-sustaining treatments, physician-assisted suicide, double effect, surrogate decision making, and other topics.

3. *Respect for Autonomy: One should respect a patient's authority to make decisions about his or her health care.* Persons have a basic right to make decisions about their lives and bodies. This is both a negative and positive duty. One should refrain from actions that diminish a patient's autonomy. One should perform actions that enhance a patient's autonomy; in particular, one should provide a patient the tools and support necessary to make good decisions. Under this principle, Beauchamp and Childress discuss informed consent, competency, disclosure, coercion, and other topics.

4. *Justice: One must fairly balance the interests of all the parties affected by a decision.* Under this principle, Beauchamp and Childress discuss resource allocation, rationing, rights to health care, ageism, racism, sexism, and other topics.

A common misperception about Beauchamp and Childress's method is that they offer only general principles as guidelines for resolving clinical disputes. These general principles are viewed as being not very helpful in resolving concrete and particular disputes. In fact, Beauchamp and Childress present general principles, such as respect for autonomy, and then use the principles to derive more specific rules that provide concrete recommendations. For example, Beauchamp and Childress present a detailed set of guidelines regarding procedures for obtaining informed consent under the category of Respect for Autonomy.

A close look at the principles reveals that they are grounded in some of the ethical theories that we have discussed. Respect for autonomy has a decidedly Kantian flavor, particularly because Beauchamp and Childress understand respect for autonomy as requiring both negative and positive duties, which correspond roughly to what Kant called perfect and imperfect duties. For Kant, autonomy did not mean the mere freedom to do as one wishes, but rather the capacity to use one's reason to make good decisions. This can be seen in Kant's explanation of both perfect and imperfect duties. Kant held that we have a perfect duty to refrain from certain actions because these actions interfere with the exercise of a person's autonomy. For example, lying to an individual robs her of the opportunity to make the best decision possible by keeping relevant information from her. Kant also held that we have an imperfect duty to help individuals make good decisions. Thus, Kant explains that the reason we must help someone in need is not only to make the person happier, but also to help support the ability of the individual to make autonomous decisions (O'Neill, 1977). Likewise, for Beauchamp and Childress the purpose of the procedures for obtaining informed consent are not meant merely to protect the freedom of the patient, but also to help the patient make the decision that is best for him or her.

Beneficence is grounded in utilitarian ethics. The idea is simply that health care providers should have the best interest of the patient at heart. Indeed, this may be one of the primary reasons that people go into health care ethics, the desire to help others. Beneficence has been associated with paternalism, the view that one should do what is good for the patient regardless of whether the patient is aware of what is being done and regardless of whether the patient desires what is being done. While Mill is himself decidedly antipaternalistic, utilitarianism, theoretically at least, could justify overriding rules meant to protect patient self-determination in the name the patient's best interest. While this may make beneficence seem like a sinister principle, one should also recognize that the desire to do good for others has motivated many noble actions.

The most important criticism of Beauchamp and Childress's methodology involves the balancing of principles in cases of conflict between principles. Beauchamp and Childress say that their principles are *prima facie* binding (2003, pp. 19–24). This means that following each principle is a moral requirement unless two or more principles are in conflict. Of course, in almost all difficult cases there are at least two principles that conflict with each other — that is primarily what makes a difficult ethical decision difficult. When two principles conflict with each other, Beauchamp and Childress say that one must balance the principles. This means, in effect, that one must decide which principle is the most important in this case and resolve the dispute in favor of this principle. Unlike some authors who adopt a principles approach (e.g., Veatch, 1981), Beauchamp and Childress do not set up the principles in a hierarchy such that one principle always "trumps" another principle. Rather, any of the four principles could be the most important principle in any particular case — it is up to clinicians to use their judgment to make a decision about which principle "wins" in the case.

In their treatment of many issues, Beauchamp and Childress try to do this balancing in advance. That is, they consider potential conflicts between principles, raise arguments on both sides, and then specify which principle ought to be considered most important in that case. To take a simple example, if a person shows up at an emergency room in need of medical attention, but is not competent to express a preference about receiving treatment and no other information about the person's desires are available, then the ER staff is authorized to provide medical treatment even if the treatment carries some risks with it. In this case, the principle of beneficence (to act in the patient's best interest) is more important than the principle of respecting autonomy (to not treat a patient unless she consents). A second example involves telling a patient the truth about his cancer diagnosis. A clinician might feel that telling the patient the truth will increase his depression and perhaps accelerate the disease process. Beauchamp and Childress suggest that the patient needs to know the truth to freely choose a treatment and to plan for the next period of his life, and this is more important than the likely worsening of depression. Respect for autonomy is more important in this situation than beneficence (and perhaps also nonmaleficence). Just because a principle is deemed of secondary importance, however, does not mean that the principle lacks all importance and that steps cannot be taken to ameliorate any problems arising from the partial disregard of that principle. In the last example, the practitioner should be careful to provide the diagnosis in as gentle and reassuring a manner as possible, as well as being vigilant to treat the depression as medically indicated.

In many situations of conflict, however, it is impossible to do the balancing of principles in advance. This has led to the criticism, made primarily by K. D. Clouser and Bernard Gert, that Beauchamp and Childress do not provide any real help in resolving situations of conflict (Clouser & Gert, 1990; Clouser, Gert, & Culver, 1997). In essence, the criticism is that all that Beauchamp and Childress have done is provide some very general labels for moral values that everyone accepts. In difficult cases these labels do little good. Rather, in difficult cases it is up to the clinician to decide which values are most important, and it is in coming to this decision that all of the substantive ethical reasoning is performed. Thus, so the criticism alleges, the Beauchamp and Childress method for identifying the correct action in difficult cases fails to achieve its goal, for in these cases it offers no answer at all.

Beauchamp and Childress defend themselves not by backing away from the *prima facie* nature of their principles, but by offering criteria to make balancing less "intuitive and open-ended":

1. Better reasons must be given in favor of the overriding principle.
2. The moral objective for infringing a principle must have a realistic prospect of achievement.
3. The infringement of a principle must be the least possible commensurate with achieving the primary goal.
4. The negative effects of the infringement should be minimized.
5. The decision must be made in an impartial manner. (Beauchamp & Childress, 2003, pp. 19–20)

Whether these steps are enough to answer the criticism raised by Clouser and Gert, their criticisms have highlighted an alternative set of methodologies for resolving ethical disputes in clinical settings.*

OTHER METHODOLOGIES IN HEALTH CARE ETHICS

The alternatives to principles that I discuss are virtue theory, casuistry, and the ethics of care. Interestingly, these approaches to clinical decision making do not identify moral duties that are uncontroversial in their application and thus are less open to interpretation than is Beauchamp and Childress's method of balancing. Rather, these alternatives embrace discretion and very open-ended methodologies in ethical decision making. Their common theme is that if discretion cannot be eliminated from ethical decisions, then methods for decision making ought to admit to this, rather than offering principles that promise but do not deliver definite answers. I should be clear, however, that these alternatives are not thereby accepting ethical relativism — the view that a person's belief that an action is morally correct is sufficient for the action to be morally correct. Rather, the alternative theories hold that morality is objective, that is, there is a correct answer to a moral question that arises in a particular situation. The alternatives simply hold that principles are not the best way to identify this answer; rather, individuals should trust in other means to arrive at the objectively correct answer.

Virtue Theory

In Aristotle's ethics we have already examined some of the central themes of contemporary virtue theory. Virtue theorists emphasize the importance of moral experts to discern the morally relevant features of a situation. Further, such experts use judgment and skill to respond to the moral problem, rather than reaching decisions based on rigid and overly simple sets of rules. The best-known advocates of virtue theory in health care ethics are Pellegrino and Thomasma (1988, 1993). Using a decidedly Aristotlean methodology, Pellegrino and Thomasma argue that medicine is a distinct human activity that has its own ends, goals, and purposes. From the purposes of medicine, Pellegrino and Thomasma derive the virtues required of those who would practice medicine: fidelity to trust, compassion, *phronesis* (practical wisdom), justice, fortitude, temperance, integrity, and self-effacement. The physician who embodies these character traits to a high degree is an exemplary physician, and these traits will guide him or her in her moral decisions. Again borrowing a page from Aristotle, Pellegrino and Thomasma downplay the importance of formal education in ethics, citing instead the importance of developing a virtuous character in the actual practice of medicine as a result of working "in the

---
* For an overview of the debate, see Davis (1995).

trenches" with senior members of the profession who are role models for virtue. Pellegrino recently appealed to some of these themes in an editorial on Iraqi physicians' complicity in torture. Criticizing the claim that education in ethics would have helped Iraqi physicians resist complicity, Pellegrino writes:

> This tendency to see education as a panacea is a common misconception. Rarely do courses in ethics make one virtuous. Nor does extensive familiarity with the intricacies of moral discourse guarantee moral wisdom.... More than education is needed. Character formation is, in the end, the surest way to inculcate the virtues. This cannot occur unless the culture of the profession is itself ethically rigorous. Even the most virtuous physicians need a supportive culture to remain virtuous (2004, pp. 1505–1506).

While virtue theory as developed by Pellegrino and Thomasma may rely on the judgment of moral experts, virtue theory in their interpretation does not deny that there are objective moral truths by which practitioners must abide. In fact, in their emphasis on beneficence at the expense of respect for autonomy, their theory tends to underwrite a fairly conservative position on substantive moral issues such as active euthanasia and physician-assisted suicide. Simply put, Pellegrino and Thomasma argue that these actions are contrary to the ends, goals, and purposes of medicine.

Casuistry

Casuistry is the method embraced by some leaders in the field of health care ethics, particularly Albert Jonsen (Arras, 1991; Jonsen & Toulmin, 1988; Jonsen, Siegler, & Winslade, 1998). Casuistry is the view that past cases are the repository of ethical knowledge. One decides a current case by judging that it is similar in all relevant respects to an earlier case and applying the decision from the earlier case to the current case. This is essentially the system of identifying precedents used by judges in the legal system. This type of ethical reasoning requires careful analysis of the similarities and differences between cases, and judgments about which similarities and differences are ethically relevant and which are not. Casuistry has a number of features to recommend it. First, health care providers may already use this form of reasoning in their clinical practice, comparing a current patient with earlier ones. Second, case presentation is typically an interesting and effective type of learning. Third, it is *de facto* the way in which much of health care ethics is taught. Consider Tarasoff, Quinan, Cruzan, Donald "Dax" Cowart, Timothy Quill's patient Diane, Barney Clark, Kimberly Bergalis: each name brings to mind a set of issues and lessons learned. Casuistry has a number of limitations, however. First, knowledge of a wide range of cases in health care ethics takes some time to acquire. Second, casuistry is somewhat conservative (i.e., resistant to change and reform), since it relies on the assumption that past cases were decided correctly. Third, federal, state, and institutional policies cannot merely reference past cases, but must be written in the form of rules, thus reintroducing principles into health care ethics. Nevertheless, casuistry may be an important supplement to a methodology that also includes ethical principles (Toulmin, 1981).

The Ethics of Care

The ethics of care is an important strand of the vibrant and growing field of feminist ethics. The term *ethics of care* was first coined in 1982 by Carol Gilligan (a clinical psychologist) in her book, *In a Different Voice*, where she argues that many women frame moral issues and problems "in a different voice" from many men (Gilligan, 1982). According to past research in moral development, many men frame moral issues as matters of conflicting rights and obligations, and questions of justice and fairness. Gilligan found, however, that many of the women she studied resisted understanding moral problems this way. Instead, the women focused on issues of caring and relationships: whether a relationship should be continued, and if it should, how best to care for and meet the needs of the members of the relationship. While Gilligan's empirical findings and their connection with gender have been the subject of much controversy, it is clear that her articulation of a care-based moral outlook as an alternative to the predominant justice-based moral outlook has struck a chord with many contemporary writers on ethics (Carse, 1991; Little, 1998). Gilligan and subsequent writers on the ethics of care have argued that the justice-based view overlooks many important facets of the moral life. The care ethic, on the other hand, brings these features sharply into focus. For example, whereas the justice ethic assumes that moral situations involve free, equal, autonomous, and independent individuals, the care ethic emphasizes that in many cases these features of a relationship are not present. Individuals often find themselves embedded in relationships in which the members are unequal, where some of them are not fully autonomous, or fully free, or fully independent of the other members. Surely, the care ethicist argues, morality pertains to the parent–child relationship, where the individuals are not equals, not fully independent or free of one another, and moreover, one of the members of the relationship may not be autonomous. Similarly, many feminists have argued that the abortion debate has become intractable precisely because the two "individuals" involved (mother and fetus) are viewed as free, equal, autonomous, and independent individuals. Whatever position one takes on abortion, it is argued, one should not understand the involved parties as the justice framework does: the fetus is metaphysically a *relational* being — it

simply cannot survive (prior to 22 weeks of age) outside of a woman's body.

The ethics of care has made important contributions to health care ethics. For example, some ethicists of care have emphasized that the patient–provider relationship may not be best understood on the consumer model, where the consumer is a free and equal member of the relationship, contracting for a certain service in exchange for a monetary fee. Instead, some ethicists of care have reminded us that serious illness causes fear, anxiety, and some dependency, even in otherwise autonomous adults. Moreover, the relationship between patient and health care provider is necessarily a relationship among unequals: the health care provider is far more knowledgeable about medicine and disease than the patient, while the patient is far more knowledgeable about her life as a whole and the values she holds. Pointing all this out also makes it clear that the members of this relationship have special responsibilities to one another. The health care provider ought to acknowledge and respond with caring to the vulnerability and anxiety of her patient. The patient on the other hand ought to be open and honest with her care provider.

There are some limitations to the ethics of care. For one, some defenders of the justice perspective have wondered whether the care ethic represents a distinct moral perspective or simply an addition to the justice perspective. For another, it is clear that some moral problems, even ones in relationships of unequals (e.g., child abuse) are better viewed in the justice perspective. Other moral situations are better viewed through the lens of care. However, it is not always — or even often — clear which lens to use. Indeed, as I pointed out above, some feminists think that abortion should only be viewed through the lens of care. But this point is contentious, and as of the moment, there appears to be no clear way to determine which framework to use to grapple with a particular moral problem. Nevertheless, the choice of one framework over another will often point toward one resolution or another. So the choice is a deeply normative one, but one without clear criteria to guide it.

Issues in Palliative Care

Some ethical issues tend to arise more frequently in the context of providing palliative care. These issues include (1) the moral status of the decision to forgo life-prolonging treatment, (2) informed consent and truth-telling, and (3) the interplay of curing and caring as the goals of medicine. I want here to sketch how some of the authors we have discussed would respond to these issues, although I would also caution that my sketch is brief and programmatic, and that there is significant room for disagreement in the interpretation of the historical figures on these issues.

The Moral Status of Decisions at the End-of-Life

Laws, codes of professional ethics, and public opinion generally draw a distinction between withholding/withdrawing life-sustaining treatment and "active" means of ending life such as physician-assisted suicide or the administration of large quantities of opiates with the intention of ending life. We have seen that a consequentialist approach to ethics would tend to undermine the moral relevance of this distinction between what has been called passive and active euthanasia. For example, Mill holds that only the consequences of an action (or omission) matter to the moral goodness of the action. As long as there were no long-term bad consequences for society, Mill might favor having the legal option of ending a terminally ill patient's suffering more quickly than merely withdrawing life-sustaining treatment would allow. This position would also be supported by Mill's arguments against paternalism, as expressed in *On Liberty.* Nevertheless, there are limitations to how far Mill might be willing to take this position. For example, if adequate pain management is available, it is a least theoretically possible for him to argue that the long-term costs to society (in the erosion of an ethic of respect for life) would outweigh any benefits to the particular patient. However, while this type of slippery slope argument is often mentioned in contemporary debates, I think it is unlikely that Mill would avail himself of it.

Deontologists, such as Augustine, Kant, and Aquinas, are much more likely to hold that the distinction between passive and active euthanasia is morally relevant, in part, because the distinction between intrinsically wrong and permissible types of actions is central to their theories. Each theorist also holds that suicide is intrinsically wrong. Kant seems to hold that one cannot protect autonomy by ending human life — if life is over, there is no chance to be autonomous. It is unclear whether Kant would also hold that withdrawals of treatment that result in death also are inconsistent with protecting autonomy. Augustine and Aquinas, however, would recognize that withdrawing treatment in some circumstances is consistent with the good of the patient because it is merely allowing the natural process of death to occur. Aquinas would invoke the principle of double effect to show that it is permissible to give pain medications, even with the risk of hastening death. The limit on this practice would be when the pain medication is given at such a dose that it constitutes a poison such that death is intended and/or the relief of pain is accomplished only by the death of the patient.

Informed Consent and Truth-Telling

Kant is often taken to be the inspiration for the modern doctrine of informed consent. Indeed, Kant not only believed that there is strict requirement not to lie to patients about their prognosis, but he also held that health care providers have an obligation to fully and truthfully provide information to patients to allow them to make decisions about care at the end of life — not to do so is to fail to respect the patient as a person. Kant would deny that a health care provider is required to follow every instruction given to her by a patient — a health care provider is not compelled to act contrary to the categorical imperative. But if a health care provider refuses to follow patient instructions as a matter of conscience, this too must be fully and truthfully disclosed to the patient. It is fair to say that Kant would require a good deal more transparency in communication between patients and care providers than is now the case in many institutions.

Theoretically, it is possible that Mill might think it best to lie to a patient to alleviate the patient's suffering. However, given Mill's extremely negative assessment of paternalism, it is more likely that Mill would see the potential for harm in lying to outweigh values from ameliorating depression. Indeed, Mill might worry that deceit would be likely to increase suffering as patients began to recognize inconsistency in their health care providers' behaviors regarding their care.

Curing and Caring

Health care professionals have obligations to attempt to *cure* patients of disease (and repair their injuries), as well as to *care* for patients who are experiencing pain and suffering. Mill is the only philosopher we have discussed who emphasizes the badness of physical pain. Indeed, rather than starting with the idea that some pain is useful (e.g., to keep us from danger, to teach us fortitude) as some philosophers do, Mill is clear that pain is always bad. For Mill, an episode of avoidable pain is to be tolerated only if (1) it prevents worse pain in the future or (2) it will produce or allow for a stronger feeling of pleasure. In this sense, Mill's philosophy fits well with the goals of palliative care, which recognizes that most if not all of a patient's pain should be ameliorated in the context of caring for those with life-threatening illnesses.

Last, Aristotle's ethics complements palliative care's emphasis on caring for the emotional needs of the patient. As we have seen, Aristotle holds that an essential part of being morally good is experiencing the appropriate emotion in response to a situation. This might mean that a care provider's laugh at a patient's joke is genuine, allowing the patient a moment of respite in an otherwise difficult day. It might mean that a care provider knows how to comfort a patient, even in the midst of a very quick and efficient visit. Aristotle is clear that feeling the appropriate emotion is important to discerning the appropriate action: unless one feels compassion, one cannot "see" the right way to be compassionate in a situation. One need not think of this as some magic new ability to see occult objects. It might only mean that one has a subtle understanding of a patient's fears, so that one is sensitive to language that might raise these fears. This sensitivity may be physical rather than intellectual. To change examples for a moment, think of one's response to an offensive, racist joke — the first reaction is in the body, a cringing, a clenching of the stomach, and only then does one consciously think of the words of the joke and explain to oneself why it is offensive. Likewise, one might be so "tuned-in" to one's patient that the knowledge that he needs some particular object is simply felt, rather than resulting from a minute of problem-solving deliberation. Feeling (rather than feigning) emotions is important for another reason as well. Persons with life-threatening illnesses, like the rest of us, are very good at picking up subtle inconsistencies between affects, behaviors, and spoken words. Telling a patient one thing, while believing another, is likely to raise the anxiety level of the patient as he picks up on these inconsistencies. The patient may not be able to recognize that the care provider is lying, but he will nonetheless be left with the vague feeling that "something is not right."

CONCLUSION ON THE PERSONAL IMPORTANCE OF ETHICAL THEORY

Too many people associate ethics with a code of conduct that necessarily involves the significant sacrifice of one's own well-being in order to benefit others. People with negative views about ethics then tend to view ethics as a cage: the bars of the cage are the ethical rules that keep one from acting in one's own self-interest. I believe this view of ethics is dangerous and inaccurate. It is dangerous because it tends to drive people away from ethics. It is dangerous because even for those who would embrace ethics, it is an ethics of self-denial and martyrdom, an ethics that encourages guilt and moralism. The ethics-as-self-sacrifice view is inaccurate because most ethical theories identify moral obligations to enhance one's own well-being, and some moral theories (such as Aristotle's and Kant's) take the enhancement of one's own well-being to be the central ethical project. A better way to understand ethics is as a tool that helps one create the sort of life of which one can be proud. Every day each of us makes decisions that constitute who we are now and that influence what sort of person we will become. While we do not often think of decisions in these terms, it would be a tragedy to come to the end of a long life and be unable to look back with pride and pleasure at the life we have created with these decisions. And it is a rare person who would not wish to see kindness, compassion, generosity, trustworthiness, and integrity as parts of this life. A better metaphor might be that ethical theories are maps that identify desirable locations to visit and that show the best paths to these destinations. To that end, we should view Aristotle, Mill, and Kant not as providing theories that narrowly tailor our actions in the name of the rights and interests of others, but as providing theories that describe ways of life that are worth living.

RESOURCE MATERIALS

WORKS BY FIGURES IN THE HISTORY OF ETHICS

Aquinas, Thomas. (1945). *Basic writings of Saint Thomas Aquinas*. Edited by Anton C. Pegis. New York: Random House.

Aristotle. (1941). *The basic works of Aristotle*. Edited by Richard McKeon. New York: Random House.

Mill, John Stuart. (1982). *John Stuart Mill: A selection of his works*. Edited by John M. Robson. Indianapolis: Bobbs-Merrill.

Kant, Immanuel. (1991). *The metaphysics of morals*. Translated by Mary Gregor. Cambridge: Cambridge University Press.

Kant, Immanuel. (1993). *Groundings for the metaphysics of morals*. Translated by James W. Ellington. Indianapolis: Hackett.

Plato. (1961). *The collected dialogues of Plato*. Edited by E. Hamilton & H. Cairns. New York: Pantheon Books.

Many of the primary works by figures in the history of ethics are available in:

Cahn, S. M., & Marke, P. (Eds.). (1998). *Ethics: History, theory and contemporary issues*. New York: Oxford University Press.

OVERVIEWS AND ANTHOLOGIES ON THE HISTORY AND THEORY OF ETHICS

Beauchamp, T. L. (1982). *Philosophical ethics* (3rd ed.). Boston: McGraw-Hill Higher Education.

Darwall, S. (1998). *Philosophical ethics*. Boulder, CO: Westview Press.

Frankena, W. K. (1973). *Ethics* (2nd ed.). Englewood Cliffs, NJ: Prentice-Hall.

LaFollette, H. (Ed.). (2000). *The Blackwell guide to ethical theory*. Oxford: Blackwell Publishers.

BOOKS THAT PROVIDE A GENERAL TREATMENT OF HEALTH CARE ETHICS

Beauchamp, T. L., & Childress, J. F. (2001). *Principles of biomedical ethics* (5th ed.). New York: Oxford University Press.

Fletcher, J. C., Hite, C., Lombardo, P., & Marshall, M. F. (Eds.). (1995). *Introduction to clinical ethics*. Fredrick, MD: University Publishing.

Jonsen, A. R., Siegler, M., & Winslade, W. (1998). *Clinical ethics: A practical approach to ethical decisions in clinical medicine* (4th ed.). New York: McGraw-Hill.

Lo, B. (1995). *Resolving ethical dilemmas: A guide for clinicians*. Baltimore: Williams & Wilkins.

Pellegrino, E., & Thomasma, D. (1988). *For the patient's good: The restoration of beneficence in health care*. New York: Oxford University Press.

Pence, G. (1995). *Classic cases in medical ethics* (2nd ed.) New York: McGraw-Hill.

Veatch, R. M. (1997). *Medical ethics* (2nd ed.). Sudbury, MA: Jones Bartlett.

REFERENCES

Arras, J. D. (1991). Getting down to cases: The revival of casuistry in bioethics. *Journal of Medicine and Philosophy, 16*(1), 29–51.

Augustine. (1961). *Confessions* (R. S. Pine-Coffin, Trans.). New York: Penguin Books.

Beauchamp, T. L., & Childress, J. F. (2003). *Principles of biomedical ethics* (5th ed.). Oxford: Oxford University Press.

Beecher, H. K. (1966). Ethics and clinical research. *New England Journal of Medicine, 274*, 1354–1360.

Callahan, D. (1983, October). On feeding the dying. *Hastings Center Report, 13*, 22.

Carse, A. L. (1991). The "voice of care": Implications for bioethical education. *Journal of Medicine and Philosophy, 16*, 5–28.

Clouser, K. D., & Gert, B. (1990, April). A critique of principlism. *Journal of Medicine and Philosophy, 15*, 219–236.

Clouser, K. D., Gert, B., & Culver, C. M. (1997). *Bioethics: A return to fundamentals*. New York: Oxford University Press.

Cugliari, A. M. & Miller, T. E. (1994). Moral and religious objections by hospitals to withholding and withdrawing life-sustaining treatment *Journal of Community Health 19*, 87–100.

Dancy, J. (1993). *Moral reasons*. Oxford: Blackwell.

Davis, R. B. (1995). The principlism debate: A critical overview. *Journal of Medicine and Philosophy, 20*, 85–105.

Emanuel, E. J. (2002). Euthanasia and physician-assisted suicide: A review of the empirical data from the United States. *Archives of Internal Medicine, 162*(2), 142–152.

French, P., Uehling, T., & Wettstein, H. (Eds.). (1988). *Ethical theory: Character and virtue*. South Bend, IN: Notre Dame University Press.

Gilligan, C. (1982). *In a different voice*. Cambridge, MA: Harvard University Press.

Hursthouse, R. (1995). Applying virtue ethics. In R. Hursthouse, G. Lawrence, & W. Quinn (Eds.). *Virtues and reasons* (pp. 57–75). New York: Oxford University Press.

Jonsen, A. R., & Toulmin, S. (1998). *The abuse of casuistry*. Berkeley: University of California Press.

Jonsen, A. R., Siegler, M., & Winslade, W. J. (1998). *Clinical ethics* (4th ed.). New York: McGraw-Hill.

Kant, I. (1993). *Groundings for the metaphysics of morals* (J. W. Ellington, Trans.). Indianapolis: Hackett Publishing.

Kass, L. R. (1980). Ethical dilemmas in the care of the ill. *Journal of the American Medical Association, 244*, 1811.

Little, M. O. (1995). Seeing and caring. *Hypatia, 10*(3), 117–137.

Little, M. O. (1998). Care: From theory to orientation to back. *Journal of Medicine and Philosophy, 23*, 190–209.

Lynn, J., & Childress, J. F. (1983, October). Must patients always be given food and water? *Hastings Center Report, 13*, 17–21.

McNaughton, D. (1991). *Moral vision*. Oxford: Blackwell, Oxford.

Mill, J. S. (1966). Utilitarianism. In J. M. Robson (Ed.). *John Stuart Mill: A selection of his works*. Indianapolis: Bobbs-Merrill Educational Publishing.

O'Neill, O. (1977). Ending world hunger. In W. Aiken & H. LaFollette (Eds.). *World hunger and morality* (2nd ed., pp. 85–110). Upper Saddle River, NJ: Prentice-Hall.

Pellegrino, E. D. (2004). Medical ethics suborned by tyranny and war. *Journal of the American Medical Association, 291*, 1505–1506.

Pellegrino, E. D., & Thomasma, D. C. (1988). *The restoration of beneficence in health care*. Oxford: Oxford University Press.

Pellegrino, E. D., & Thomasma, D. C. (1993). *The virtues in medical practice*. Oxford: Oxford University Press.

Rachels, J. (1975). Active and passive euthanasia. *The New England Journal of Medicine, 292*, 78–80.

Rachels, J. R. (1986). *The end of life*. Oxford: Oxford University Press.

Sherman, N. (1989). *The fabric of character*. Oxford: Clarendon Press.

Singer, P. (1990). *Animal liberation* (2nd ed.), New York: Avon Books.

Singer, P. (1977). Famine, affluence and morality. In W. Aiken & H. LaFollette (Eds.). *World hunger and morality* (2nd ed., pp. 26–38). Upper Saddle River, NJ: Prentice-Hall.

Stark, S. (in press). Emotions and the ontology of moral value. *Journal of Value Inquiry*.

Stocker, M., & Hegeman, E. (1991). *Valuing emotions*. Cambridge: Cambridge University Press, Cambridge.

Sulmasy, D. P., & Sugarman, J. (1994). Are withholding and withdrawing therapy always morally equivalent? *Journal of Medical Ethics, 20*, 218–222.

Toulmin, S. (1981, December). The tyranny of principles. *Hastings Center Report, 11*, 31–39.

Veatch, R. (1981). *A theory of medical ethics*. Washington, DC: Georgetown University Press.

Williams, B. (1977). A critique of utilitarianism. In J. J. C. Smart. & B. Williams (Eds.). *Utilitarianism for and against* (pp. 97–98, 132). Cambridge: Cambridge University Press.

91

Bioethics and Pain

John Peppin, DO, FACP

"We must all die. But that I can save him from days of torture, that is what I feel as my great and ever new privilege. Pain is a more terrible lord of mankind than even death itself." (Schweitzer, 1948, p. 95)

INTRODUCTION

As medicine has progressed over the past century the problem of treating pain, both acute and chronic, has become a serious concern. Media attention to the problem has been impressive (Springen, Raymong, & Underwood, 2003). The U.S. Senate recently voted this decade 2001–2010 to be the "Decade of Pain Control and Research" and has pledged to support research and education in this critically important area (Nelson, 2003). Unfortunately, the reality of the treatment of pain and of patients with pain does not reflect the attention this problem has received. More than 75 million Americans still suffer chronic handicapping and persistent pain (Gureje, Von Korff, Simon, & Gater, 1998). Over 50% of home hospice patients feel their pain is moderate to severe in spite of the impressive onslaught of professional attention (Crane, Wilson, & Behrens, 1990). The Study to Understand Prognoses and Preferences for Outcomes and Risks of Treatment (SUPPORT) study found that more than 50% of patients did not have their pain well controlled in the 2 weeks preceding their deaths (Desbiens et al., 1996). At the two extremes of life our outcomes have been abysmal. Bernabei in 1998 found that over 50% of elderly patients with cancer in the nursing home received absolutely nothing for their pain, not even acetaminophen (Bernabei et al., 1998). Data from this study show that a minority woman patient over 85 years of age was the least likely to receive pain medications, regardless of the cause of her

pain. Wolfe et al. (2000) in their study on children with cancer found that 89% suffered "a lot or a great deal" with pain, dyspnea, and fatigue. Further, chronic pain is very expensive, costing the U.S. economy in excess of $200 billion in 2000 (including lost days from work, lost productivity, lost ability to earn a wage, individual suffering, and the impact of pain on families, e.g., divorce and lost self-esteem) (U.S. Dept. of Health and Human Services, 2000; Walter et al., 2003). This figure is staggering especially when it is compared with more familiar societal expenditures such as alcoholism which cost $148 billion during the same period of time (National Institute on Drug Abuse, 2004). This is not just an American phenomenon. In a World Health Organization (WHO) survey involving patients from five continents, over 22% suffered persistent chronic pain (Gurege et al., 1998). Ferrell (1997) has described the current status of pain management as "the moral outrage of unrelieved pain" (p. 11).

The preceding discussion illustrates the poor performance of health care professionals in treating acute and chronic pain and the marginalization of the pain and palliative medicine patients. Interestingly, this poor performance occurs in the presence of an extensive and expanding literature of the science and practice of pain medicine (and palliative medicine) over the last 30 years. Although there is a time lag time between literature support and use in actual practice for other types of medical knowledge (approximately 8 years), pain management suffers from continued lack of inculcation of literature and research that defies understanding, i.e., more than 30 years.

Although there have been attempts to explain why we treat pain so poorly, these attempts have been unsophisticated and less than explanative. We must explain not only why we treat pain so poorly, but also why patients with pain are marginalized compared with other types of patients. The purpose of this chapter is to investigate and discuss some of the philosophical, sociological, and bioethical issues involved in pain management. The presentation in this chapter will be controversial and from the perspective of a physician. However, the goal here is to engage the academy (I use the term *academy* in its broadest academic sense and not to refer to any specific professional organization) in a deeper discussion of the reasons why pain management remains little changed even after extensive media, professional, and legislative efforts. It may even be that patients are worse off today. The recent media frenzy with opiate medication misuse, abuse, and diversion is causing even more physicians to refuse to treat patients with chronic pain. As the author of this chapter I come at this problem from the perspective of a physician because this is my profession, training, and occupation. Additionally, my medical worldview is largely Western, and this will be the focus of this chapter; medical philosophies from other perspectives, i.e., Eastern, could have a very different approach to pain and patients with pain.

The concepts that follow may be applicable to other health care professionals, such as nurses and pharmacists as well as to alternative health care professionals such as those from an Eastern perspective (Broekmans, Vanderschueren, Morlion, Kuman, & Evers, 2004). I use the term *health care professional* or *HCP* to indicate physicians, nurses, and pharmacists and to indicate a Western perspective in those professionals' understanding of health, pain, and disease. When the term *physician* is used, it refers specifically to medical doctors and doctors of osteopathy. A review of how health care professionals with an Eastern medical philosophy or "alternative" HCPs, e.g., chiropractors or massage therapists, would be a very helpful as well, but beyond the goals of this chapter. (I agree with Wardwell [1994] that the term *alternative medicine,* as currently construed, has little value in investigations of bioethics, health, or disease. However, the use of medications specifically may place the physician into a situation that predisposes marginalization of patients. This view needs to be explicated elsewhere.)

This chapter covers a number of diverse topics and presents many controversial concepts. It is important to understand that I am not suggesting that this chapter describes actual attitudes and mechanisms leading to marginalizing behaviors in clinical practice. Rather, it is a presentation defining real problems and possible mechanisms that explain behaviors that hinder appropriate pain medicine and patient care. Additionally this chapter is a passionate challenge to the academy to evaluate these concepts comprehensively and seriously and to act upon them. The time has come for dramatic change in how we care for vulnerable patients in pain. Action needs to be substantive and to date the academy has been less than proactive. There is a schizophrenic character to our society that worries about using the pronoun *he* in scholarly writings so as not to offend, yet allows pain and suffering to continue. How we treat the weak and suffering is a powerful statement about our very social being.

THE MARGINALIZATION OF PAIN

Patients in pain and those receiving palliative care are marginalized in our society. Admittedly this is a deliberately provocative statement requiring explication and examples. At a recent bioethics conference the following case was presented (University of Notre Dame, 2004):

> An elderly and frail 80-year-old man with do-not-resuscitate (DNR) status due to metastatic cancer was having a second intravenous port placed (as the first had ceased functioning). The port, needed for "pain control," had to be placed under general anesthesia. The patient underwent the procedure, but developed respiratory arrest after the surgery and died despite resuscitation efforts that were specifically not requested.

Most attendees at the conference found the violation of this patient's DNR the most distressing issue in this case. When it was pointed out that this patient's pain could have been treated less invasively and more safely by other means, i.e., subcutaneous infusion (as this patient had problems with oral and rectal administrations), the comment was made that this patient was terminal and "would die anyway." There were clearly other routes of administration to approach this patient's need for pain medications that would not have ended this patient's life prematurely and unnecessarily. To suggest that this patient's life was not important because he would "die anyway" is a dramatic example of the marginalization that is inherent in the current system of health care. This is not a case of violation of DNR orders, but one of marginalization of a terminally ill patient in pain.

Some insurance companies have refused to pay for medications to treat pain in the name of "reducing diversion" or because medications are not prescribed according to the "FDA label" (i.e., "off-label" usages). Interestingly, there are few insurance companies limiting hydrocodone combination preparations containing acetaminophen, still one of the most-abused controlled substance prescription medications in the United States. Neither does there seem to be any concern with multiple less expensive medications used off label. For example, amitriptyline does not have an FDA indication for neuropathic pain or fibromyalgia, yet it is used frequently in these disorders, again without comment from most insurance companies. Multiple other medications are used off label without apparent concern. FDA indications and secondary concerns about potential for diversion are disingenuous. More often than not the "issue" has less to do with diversion per se or quality of care but rather with the cost of branded patented medications. Even this, however, is a concern that seems to lead some insurance companies to reject only certain kinds of expensive medications but then pay for other more expensive invasive procedures. The use of spinal surgery for pain has never been shown conclusively to have long-term efficacy nor good outcome studies, and yet it is routinely paid for by many insurance companies (Devo, Nachemson, & Mirza, 2004). Part of the reason for denying coverage for pain medications may be societal and individual attitudes toward pain. Examples commonly seen include "pain patients" being accused of "drug seeking," patients being told that opiates will make them addicts, and patients being told "it's all in your head." Patients are frequently told they need to "learn to live with their pain" without being told specifically how to do this or that they are only asking for surgery or medications to "get attention" or a bigger settlement in their lawsuit. It is almost universally assumed that patients with chronic pain have psychiatric illness that partially causes them to have chronic pain. These are further examples of marginalization of patients with pain.

How physicians and health care professionals relate to those who are in pain and those who are weak and vulnerable is where our examination should first be focused. It may be that marginalizing behaviors have, at their roots, deeper visceral, and perhaps even instinctual, responses that must be explained before we can understand why we treat physical pain, weakness, and suffering so poorly. As Rousseau states, "Human society contemplated with a tranquil and disinterested eye appears at first to display only the violence of powerful men and the oppression of the weak; the mind is revolted by the harshness of the strong; one is impelled to deplore the blindness of the weak, and as nothing is less stable among men than these exterior relationships which are produced more often by chance than by thought, and since weakness or strength go by the names of poverty or riches, human institutions seem at first sight to be founded on piles of shifting sands" (1984, p. 71). Therefore our *prima facie* intuitions about how the weak or those in pain are treated may or may not be accurate, and we should explore these notions in more depth. This exploration should have as its goal the changing of attitudes and behaviors that marginalize patients with pain.

The barriers to good pain management have been accepted. These barriers include (1) fear of addiction when using opiates (Ferrell, Cronin Nash, & Warfield, 1992); (2) legal obstacles and fear of regulatory agency sanctions (especially when using opiates) (Hoffmann, 1998); (3) fear of side effects of medications (Cleeland, 1993); (4) ignorance of proper assessment of pain (Grossman, Sheidler, Swedeen, Mucenski, & Piantadosi, 1991); (5) lack of appropriate education in pain management (Hoffmann, 1998); (6) beliefs in how "proper" patients should respond, i.e., the "good patient" (Proulx & Jacelon, 2004); (7) ignorance of pain physiology (Moseley, 2003); (8) failure to identify pain relief as a priority (Ferrell, 1997); (9) failure of the health care system to hold clinicians, physicians and others, accountable for pain relief (Ferrell, 1997); (10) cost constraints and inadequate insurance coverage (Hoffmann, 1998); and (11) patient reluctance to take medications, specifically opioids (Dar, Beach, Barden, & Cleeland, 1992). However, to date there has been little criticism or in depth evaluation of these barriers.

Prima facie these barriers seem to explain why health care professionals so poorly manage pain. However, upon further reflection these barriers are simplistic and without rigor. As Rich (2000) states, "The criticism of the 'barriers' literature that is the focus of this article is its consistent failure to analyze these barriers from an ethical perspective.... [T]he barriers, and the unnecessary pain and suffering that they engender, are treated as merely clinical failures, free of significant moral implications" (pp. 54, 55). Rich is correct in his criticism; however, he does not go far enough. There are deeper, more robust reasons for the inappropriate treatment of pain, which may include (1) visceral and deeper responses, evolutionary if you will, toward the disabled and sick; (2) the position and ego of physicians; (3) notions of eugenics, perhaps based on evolutionary drives; (4) the deconstruction of the patient–physician relationship and emergence of institution–physician relationships; and (5) lack of physician trust toward patients. Again, as Rich states, "the barriers are not simply artifacts of our healthcare system, they relate directly and immediately to aspects of our American culture and society"; however, they may also relate on deeper and more profound levels (p. 55).

The treatment of chronic pain is often palliative. We rarely find a painful condition that when treated alleviates the pain completely. We "palliate" the pain with medications, surgeries, and procedures. Pain medicine is similar in many ways to hospice care and palliative medicine (there are obvious and apparent overlaps). Both fields allow the health care provider the privilege of helping with a patient's suffering and both are symptom focused. (I use *pain medicine* throughout this chapter to refer to both groups, pain and palliative medicine, and patients in these groups because I believe both groups are significantly marginalized for similar reasons. Therefore, the discussion that follows should apply to both groups.) Practicing good pain medicine allows the practitioner to regain the "art," "heart," and "soul" of medicine. To do this one must develop deeper more substantial relationships with patients. To date, however, patients are kept at a distance and their suffering is not engaged by practitioners. The question that has yet to be answered to date, in any depth, is why health care professionals do not take suffering and pain seriously and why we treat weak, vulnerable, suffering patients so poorly.

PAIN AND SUFFERING

Emanuel states, "one of the universally acknowledged fundamental goals of medical care is to provide palliative care to relieve patients' pain, suffering, and other symptoms" (1996, p. 42). Interestingly, this has been a fundamental goal from the birth of medicine (Pellegrino, 1980). Professional organizations recognize this goal and publish statements to this effect. The American College of Physicians *Ad Hoc* Committee on Medical Ethics statement of 1984 is an example: "The primary goals of the physician are to relieve suffering, prevent untimely death, and to improve the health of the patient while maintaining the dignity of the person" (p. 130). Although patients obviously wish their suffering to be addressed, HCPs have done a poor job in approaching suffering patients. "The relief of suffering, it would appear, is considered one of the primary ends of medicine by patients and the general public, but not by the medical profession, judging by medical education and the responses of students and colleagues" (Cassell, 1991, p. 32). It is this disconnect between what is declared as the "fundamental goal" of health care and actual clinical practice that concerns us in this chapter. "Consequently, the widespread failure of physicians to make effective pain management and palliative medicine a priority in patient care denotes an alarming departure of the profession from its deepest ethical roots, and the collective failure of the profession to recognize the ethical implications of under treated pain and the unnecessary suffering that it engenders calls into question whether a majority of its practitioners continue to acknowledge that health care is a moral enterprise" (Rich, 2000, p. 55). Rich has emphasized the focus of the chapter, the marginalization of pain patients. He also has shown the weaknesses of the "barriers" approach to explaining this marginalization. However, he has not elucidated clearly why this marginalization occurs. In the following pages we provide a more thorough explanation than has been given to date for pain patient treatment.

Pain is defined by the International Association for the Study of Pain as "an unpleasant sensory and emotional experience associated with actual or potential tissue damage, or described in terms of such damage" (Merskey & Bogduk, 1994, p. 210). Although this definition has been discussed in other chapters of this text, it deserves a further comment. Pain has both a physiological and an emotional component. The emotional component is part of what makes chronic pain management so interesting and at the same time so frustrating to HCPs. The components of emotional and physical suffering make pain unique, ontologically different from other human experiences in that it involves the entire person. Because of this difference, it presents unique problems both clinically and ethically. It attacks who we are, our dreams, our goals and abilities. It attacks at a visceral basic level and challenges every-

thing about our being and existence. "Bodily pain affects man as a whole, down to the deepest layers of his moral being. It forces him to face again the fundamental questions of his fate, of his attitude toward God and fellow man, of his individual and collective responsibility, and of the sense of his pilgrimage on earth" (Pope Pius XII, 1956). From an ethical perspective the treatment of chronic pain involves issues that are distinctly different from other areas of medicine and medical care. Others cannot feel the pain an individual feels; it is intimate and personal regardless of what a previous president may claim (Clinton, 2004). We must ask the patient whether or not he or she is in pain.

Pain is described in terms of narratives. This is not all that dissimilar from other medical symptoms and problems; when we collect the medical history information, we are collecting a narrative (Hunter, 1996). "In medicine, practical reason manifests itself as clinical judgment, and narrative is an essential part of it" (Hunter, 1996, p. 308). When patients are asked about their pain, they will describe the pain in clinical terms, but will place these terms into the context of a story of how their pain started, how it has affected their lives, and (frequently) how the health care professions have not believed them and/or treated them poorly.

Pain is clearly subjective, which has been a stumbling block and excuse for poor pain management for many HCPs. However, pain is no different from dyspnea or depression in this regard (Aronowitz, 2000). These are also "symptoms" that require us to believe the patient, rather than tests or laboratories. One can have absolutely normal laboratories, yet still be short of breath. Further, we do not have a laboratory or radiologic procedure to measure depression (there may be new evidence from fMRI, SPECT, and PET scans to suggest certain types of depression, which may help direct treatment [Amen, 2004]). We must obtain information about both the symptoms and their severity directly from the patient. Unfortunately, HCPs routinely underestimate and disbelieve patient's pain reports. This further marginalizes pain patients: "Questions about the authenticity of the pain experience, especially when raised by medical professionals, represent yet another ontological challenge to the integrity of the self" (Garro, 1992, p. 104).

Suffering is frequently viewed by HCPs only as a physical experience. However, suffering involves the entire person. Although this chapter is not a place for a complete exploration of suffering and personhood, it is fair to say that to suffer one must be a person and to understand suffering one must understand the person (Cassell, 1991). Each person has a physical dimension, a body that is unique and yet has important features in common with the bodies of other people. Persons exist in time, possess beliefs, do things, and identify with those things. Certain dimensions of the person, such as their profession, are very apparent. Additionally, each person has a transcendent dimension (regardless of their metaphysics) (Byock, 1966; Cassell, 1991). Persons are complex and the experience of suffering is personal, existential, and subjective. Unfortunately, once beyond the experience of physical pain, HCPs are lost. They are not trained to deal with pain much less other aspects of suffering; neither are they trained to view patients as persons. If an HCP asks a patient, "where does it hurt?" and the patient responds, "I have a pain in my soul," the HCP is helpless to proceed. Although these phenomenologic distinctions are beyond the scope of this chapter, still it is important to realize medicine's significant limitations. The physician steeped in the medical philosophy of positivism does not possess the tools to treat the whole person. It should be obvious that this can lead to a further marginalization of pain patients.

HCPs tend to approach patients' suffering from a positivistic, scientific, and mechanistic perspective. This view can produce a nihilistic attitude on the part of the HCP. "Subtle manifestations of therapeutic nihilism exist in current clinical practice, being revealed by the language we choose. The tendency to label difficult symptoms, such as neuropathic pain or nausea, as 'intractable,' or to refer to a person's suffering as 'uncontrollable,' can prove self-fulfilling" (Byock, 1996, p. 242). Further the logical positivistic scientific approach to suffering patients taken by many HCPs has contributed to what Robert Veatch and others (Schultz & Carnevale, 1996) call, "a crisis in which care is often disengaged and in which interminable bioethical problems are endemic" (Veatch, 1991, p. 278). Issues that are difficult to quantitate, such as pain and suffering, do not fit in this positivistic paradigmal medicine.

It is important to understand that suffering is not something health care professionals understand or that they have been trained to treat and alleviate (Rawlinson, 1986). The science of medicine tells us nothing about the person and the person's suffering. Neither is the thin bioethics that imbues our secular society able to understand or deal with a patient's suffering. HCP education must be restructured to take into account the nature of suffering and the patient as a whole person.

PAIN AND MEANING

Unfortunately, most individuals in our current multicultural society find little meaning in their suffering and pain. Suffering is to be avoided; especially in our Western culture, suffering is a negative experience. However, one wonders if, without suffering, our society would not be akin to Huxley's *Brave New World* (1998) or Woody Allen's movie, *Sleeper* (1973) Both of these renditions of a futuristic society actively avoid any suffering or discomfort. They use drugs and other conveniences to be oblivious to pain and suffering in order to achieve "happiness."

In these conceptions of the future, suffering is always negative and always to be avoided. This is very similar to our current societal view.

Many robust religious traditions see suffering in a very different light. For both the Buddhist and the Christian, suffering is seen as an inevitable component of human life. The Buddhist believes suffering arises from a person's attachments to the world while the Christian sees relief of suffering as a laudable and spiritually redeeming exercise. The Christian may also see suffering as a way toward a deeper understanding and relationship with God although it should not be sought; Judaism has similar views of suffering (Byock, 1996). What all these robust religious traditions have in common is a sense of meaning from suffering, something lacking in current society. As Frankl suggests, "pain and privation are insufficient to explain suffering. Privation can be endured if there is a purpose in the suffering experience…. Suffering ceases to be suffering … at the moment it finds meaning" (1963, p. 115).

We do not share a common moral vision; neither can we refer to any commonly held understanding of pain and its role in our culture and lives. Pain is unavoidable and will be experienced by all of us. Acute pain comes and goes. It has a clear ending and, therefore, is much easier for us to tolerate within our lives and worldview. However, chronic pain needs to be examined in a broader moral context to derive any meaning from the experience. Lacking this moral framework, existential angst can further exacerbate the patient's suffering. Delivering a baby certainly has a component of physical suffering. However, it is placed in a broader view of accomplishment and a known goal, i.e., bringing a child into the world. Patients with chronic pain usually do not have access to such a perspective, and current medicine is incapable of providing this. Finding meaning in pain and suffering is something that is missing from current pain management treatments and programs and is rarely addressed seriously in the pain literature. Patients' mistakenly seek meaning in physician's recommendations and treatments. However, as has been shown, physicians are neither trained nor are they in a position to deal with meaning in patients' lives. Meaning is suggested in studies measuring levels of sensory pain and pain unpleasantness. *Prima facie* one would think sensory pain and unpleasantness to be very similar, yet there can be a wide disparity between the two.

In previous societies and cultures, the priest was the one who helped guide individuals through chronic pain and suffering. However, those rich moral traditions that gave meaning to pain and suffering no longer exist for a vast majority of individuals in Western culture. "The meaning of pain seems a non-issue as long as medicine can provide its reassuring explanation and magical cures. When cures repeatedly fail, however, or when the explanations patently fall flat, we must confront once again — with renewed seriousness, even desperation — the ever-implicit question of meaning" (Morris, 1991, pp. 31–32). In previous cultures with strong moral traditions, pain maps onto a broader foundational view of life. Although treatments may still be necessary, patients are able to deal with their pain more effectively; i.e., the unpleasantness is reduced. We lack this mapping in our current fragmented and thinly construed social and moral framework.

PAIN MANAGEMENT AND BIOETHICS

Although there are a number of different ways to approach bioethics and moral theory, for our discussion here principlism, liberal political theory, and Engelhardtian libertarianism are the most important to discuss. Attempts to reduce bioethical issues to a clear and simple set of principles began during the 1960s and 1970s. The theory of principlism emerged from the work of the National Commission for the Protection of Human Subjects of Biomedical and Behavioral Research in 1974 (Federal Registry, 1979). Beauchamp and Childress (1994) further describe principlism as a set of four principles with which they claim most, if not all, bioethical controversies can be resolved. These principles are beneficence, nonmaleficence, justice, and autonomy. They are felt to be common threads for HCPs interactions with patients regardless of foundational philosophy or strong moral traditions.

The principle of beneficence is to act in the patient's best interest for the good of the patient. Intuitively, treating pain is in the patient's best interest. Interestingly, when the principle of beneficence is evoked in support of pain management, it is represented as a *prima facie* principle, and "clearly includes the effective treatment of pain and other symptoms" (Cherny & Coyle, 1998, p. 643). For secular society, however, these notions hold no authority. Doing good takes on a different meaning in secular society. For example, in a given religious tradition, a monk, when queried about pain, might respond that pain could bring a seeker to a richer prayer life and closer to God. Therefore, the pain should not be treated or at least not treated completely. However, the secular priest, i.e., the modern-day physician, could make no such claims, and in fact, such claims would be considered nonsensical. The goal would not be a richer spiritual life but something much more practical: the relief of pain. The secular priest could only hope to maintain a state from which an individual could seek his or her own view of the good. In this postmodern age this is where liberal political philosophy fills the gap left by religious traditions, *vide infra*. Beneficence then can only be construed as maximizing a patient's autonomy. Notions of beneficence beyond this cannot be established in secular society in any broad sense. To do this requires a richer robust foundation, which is inconsistent with liberal political philosophy.

The principle of nonmaleficence prohibits HCPs from harming or inflicting evil on patients. Pain places patients at risk for further harm because pain is not a benign physiologic process. Physiologically, patients in pain have poorer outcomes postoperatively. Acutely, pain causes sympathetic nervous system activation, increases fibrinolysis, heart rate, and blood pressure. There are other side effects of pain such as inhibition of the immune system and effects on respiration. Nonmaleficence requires not causing pain or not allowing patients to be harmed by pain. Again, this view of pain is epistemologically different from those of certain religious traditions, *vide supra*. Therefore, unilateral notions of nonmaleficence are also limited by our multicultural social structure (Engelhardt, 1996). One must have a robust moral foundation to apply nonmaleficence in any rigorous way.

Justice deals with the fair distribution of resources and requires an ability to rank-order different resources. However a just distribution must, of necessity, have a moral foundation from which to make judgments concerning various resource choices. Ranking *cannot* occur without such a foundation and such a foundation belies any pretense of neutrality, an important concept in liberal political theory. Justice, nonmaleficence, and beneficence are all dependent on "canonical" understandings of bioethics and morality. As mentioned, there cannot be any canonical understanding of these concepts; they are culturally dependent.

The one principle we are left with is autonomy, to allow patients to seek their own notion of the good. To establish a "right" to pain management autonomy can provide a central principle. An individual's autonomy is sacred in our society. Autonomy for patients was an even later development in the ethics of medicine and society than political autonomy, one born from philosophical, political, and religious reflection. "[T]he belief that persons have a right to individual self-determination has captured the imagination of the Western World," and "the idea that a similar right should be accorded to patients has surfaced largely, and surely more insistently, during the last few decades" (Katz, 1984, p. 104). To be autonomous is to be self-governing, and autonomy is a form of personal liberty. "Autonomy is one of those widely applauded concepts which, on closer inspection, turns out to be difficult to define with precision.... What is common to most definitions is the notion that an autonomous person is one who, in his thoughts, words, and actions, is able to follow those norms he chooses as his own without external constraints or coercion by others" (Pellegrino, 1994, p. 48). To be self-governing, one must be a person and able to deliberate and choose from various options. In addition, that person must be capable of acting on those deliberations. There must be no hindrances to free and autonomous decision making, i.e., "without constraints either by another's action or by psychological or physical limitation" (Beauchamp & Childress, 1994, pp. 56–57). Free decisions require a competent person, enough and appropriate information, and freedom from coercion. Whether a person could ever have free and unhindered decisions is problematic; yet such hindrances would clearly include pain.

For individuals to manifest their own view of the good, they must be autonomous. However, autonomy presents real and significant difficulties for bioethics and specifically for pain management. Pain can reduce a patient's decision-making capacity and make it difficult for an individual to make autonomous decisions. It can prevent an individual from achieving his or her concept of the good. If pain limits a person's ability to be autonomous or a patient cannot make autonomous decisions if he or she is in pain, then does this require us to treat a patient's pain against the person's will? Is the patient then incompetent in this regard? "Bioethicists, who are so preoccupied with the ethnocentric principle of personal autonomy as to regard it as the only solid ground of ethical choices in the hospital, do not know what to make of chronic pain" (Kleinman, 1992, p. 169).

THE "RIGHT" TO PAIN TREATMENT

Our secular culture is founded on liberal political philosophy. And such a philosophy, as defined by Rawls, Dworkin, and others, revolves around the liberal state (Dworkin, 1989; Rawls, 1989). Because it is claimed, this form of liberalism rejects any substantive theory of the good, it must, at least theoretically, be neutral to any form of the good. The state is justified because diversity is a basic fact of modern life and it would be a breach of individual freedom for the state to impose any predetermined set of values. Because it cannot be shown that some individuals should be treated unequally, all should be treated as equals. Treating an individual as an equal requires that individuals be allowed to seek life opportunities. This, it is claimed, is one major reason why a state should not proclaim any notion of the good because it could coerce or manipulate an individual away from his or her own life opportunities. The public square should be without any general notion of the good and should be "neutral" to avoid any undue influence or potential coercion toward a specific view of what constitutes the good by the state. Although there are justified critics of this form of the liberal state, it nevertheless has been a powerful force in the development of bioethics (Galston, 1991). Further, it has permeated our social programs including health care. How can an individual seek his or her notion of the good without being in good health and, certainly from the perspective of this chapter, free of pain? Therefore, the state has an obligation to foster health and alleviate pain to allow individuals all the tools and resources to achieve their own life opportunities.

The former Agency for Health Care Policy and Research (AHCPR) stated that pain management "begins

with the affirmation that patients should have access to the best level of pain relief that may safely be provided" (U.S. Dept. of Health and Human Services, 1992). The World Health Organization (1990) claims that for patients with advanced and terminal cancer, relief of pain is a "right." The American Pain Foundation (2004) has had similar set of "rights" for patients with chronic pain. *Prima facie* it seems to many that the treatment of pain is a "right" for all patients in the United States. As Somerville states, "to leave a person in avoidable pain is a fundamental breach of human rights" (1994, p. 42). Although obligations to relieve patients' suffering have been discussed, these obligations are derived from the historical and bioethical foundations of the medical profession. However, these obligations do not require any concept of rights. The foundations for a "right" to pain management have rarely been explicated in the literature. Unfortunately, it has never been apparent from a secular perspective that patients have a right to treatment or alleviation of their pain.

Neither principlism nor liberal Western political philosophy can give a single way of understanding the obligations to relieve pain or the right to pain relief. Each of these views is subject to different understandings and to the weaknesses described above. We need an approach that might tie together those aspects of principlism and liberal Western political philosophy that can give us a "right" to pain management. Rights require not only bioethical principles but also grounding in political philosophy. Principlism, although claimed to be universal, does not apply to all cultures and individuals. It would be very difficult, if not impossible, to establish a *robust* "right" to pain management apart from a specific cultural and moral construct. As has been pointed out by Engelhardt, "the impossibility of establishing the concrete vision of the good life, proper deportment, health care policy, or bioethics by an appeal to general rational secular arguments leads to the development of two divergent understandings of bioethics: secular bioethics and the bioethics of content-full moral commitment" (1996, pp. 16–17). Although Engelhardt would take umbrage at any mention of rights in secular society, he adds the third component to our building of a "right" to pain management. To Engelhardt the principles of beneficence, nonmaleficence, and justice all require a content-full moral vision. There is no way for multicultural society with a multitude of moral visions to establish one vision of the good. Therefore, all we have left is the notion of autonomy. We allow individuals the option to engage in their own vision of the good and to seek their own opportunities. We allow individuals to have the option of good pain management or to refuse such an option. To Engelhardt notions of "rights" or "morality" have no real place as these concepts also require a content-full vision of the good. Only a thin vision of bioethical understanding is possible. All we are left with is our agreement to disagree amicably without violence or coercion. Autonomy or allowing individuals their own view of the good must be, by default, our overriding principle.

Cherny and Coyle state that a right to pain relief "is derived from the universal concept of respect for all persons and is inextricably linked to the concept of human ethics" (1998, p. 644). However, as the previous discussion has shown, there can be no robust "universal" right to relief of pain without a cultural context. That context, at least in secular United States, comes from liberal political philosophy. Engelhardt and the notions of principlism all have as a central foundation the notion of autonomy or permission. Autonomy is the key to a "right" to pain management and treatment, albeit thin. As discussed, to be autonomous a person must be free from outside coercion and influence. The impact of pain significantly reduces a patient's ability to make decisions and achieve his or her notions of life opportunities and the good. Their pain should be treated to allow the patient autonomous choice. Therefore, the state should recognize a right to pain treatment. This is admittedly somewhat thin logically, but all we can achieve in this multicultural liberal polity.

PHYSICIANS, HEALTH CARE PROFESSIONALS, AND PAIN

The title of physician is one of the few non-egalitarian titles in society. President, congressman, senator, governor, and professor are also such titles. Physicians are called "doctor," an honorific title that establishes their place in society with each utterance. We do not call plumbers, "Plumber Smith," yet physicians are called "Doctor" and if this honorific is not used there is a feeling of insult. Humanitarians can give millions of dollars to the poor and they will still be called Mr. or Ms.; yet physicians regardless of their morality or philanthropic inclinations are still called "Doctor." This elevated societal position of physicians can be traced through history. It may be that maintaining trust in individuals who are responsible for lives represents part of this societal position. Other professional groups may have average IQ scores that are much higher than physicians; yet these individuals do not hold the societal position held by physicians. I was recently at the back of a hospital elevator with three hospital employees in front of me. When the door opened they insisted that I leave first, even though I was at the back. The only reason was obvious; I was a physician. So the title alone carries with it a tremendous amount of societal respect and position, not necessarily earned. Ivan Illich explores this notion when he pejoratively states, "Societal acceptance of the illusion of professional omniscience and omnipotence may result either in compulsory political creeds (with their accompanying versions of a new fascism), or

in yet another historical emergence of neo-Promethean but essentially ephemeral follies" (Illich, 2000, pp. 11–12). The position of "physician" may be necessary to some extent, since there may be some therapeutic benefit to the position. However, this societal position can become expected by the physician, which could lead to feelings of superiority, resulting in low regard for and poor treatment of patients in pain. This combined with other more instinctual notions can result in the barriers to effective pain management we currently observe.

Evolutionary psychology is a relatively new field. It brings into the discussion the notion of "instincts," which are "domain-specific, information-processing modules" that are behaviors in response to external and internal stimuli (Charlton, 1997a). Most evolutionary psychologists would agree that animals are mostly solitary and the ability to live in social groups depends on "psychological specializations" (Charlton, 1997a). Charlton discusses a categorization of social instincts into "dominant and counter-dominant." Among the human species is the counter-dominance instinct, which leads to egalitarianism, unique in the animal kingdom. Most important of these counter-dominant instincts is sharing. However, "dominance is indeed phylogenetically older than counter-dominance and these instincts are more powerful in delayer-return economies" (Charlton, 1997a, p. 425). Before one dismisses this discussion as irrelevant to our current society, Charlton continues, a "dominance hierarchy is one in which the high status individuals who have access to a larger than equal share of sexual activity also get a larger than equal share of desired resources such as food" (Charlton, 1997a, p. 425). In other words, in a dominance hierarchy, prestige and power go together and reinforce one another. Modern humans live in a "dominance hierarchy." So we have some evidence for a more visceral or "phylogenetically older" response of dominant individuals to those who are weaker, suffering, or in pain. Physicians clearly have a dominant role in society and a much higher share of resources. They also hold tremendous power as the "gatekeepers" to medical care. To receive many treatments for pain, or medications, one must see a physician (this may be part of the reason why patients seek "alternative" medical care). If these dominant roles are tied to bias and prejudice, perhaps based on instinctual racial and other notions, marginalization of certain groups of patients with pain, such as the elderly, the infirm, racial minorities, and females with chronic pain, may be the result. Notions of racial superiority are not unique to one specific culture, but have been seen throughout history and in numerous cultures regardless or color or creed. One way to view these notions can be as basic visceral human responses to different cultures and peoples. It may be that "a little" racism was important to survival in the distant past, but these leftover visceral responses to different cultures and races are now destructive. (I am clearly not supporting any notion of racial purity or eugenics, which this author finds repulsive. Morality and ethics begin when we say no to our baser responses; see Burnham and Phelan, 2000.)

These are feelings that must be overcome, but can be insidious and may play a role in physicians' response to patients with chronic pain. Lasch may be correct when he writes, "men have always been selfish, groups have always been ethnocentric; nothing is gained by giving these qualities a psychiatric label" (1979, p. 32). However, he is incorrect in his unwillingness to explore these selfish instinctual behaviors because only by "labeling" these behaviors can we begin to know how to correct them. This instinctual response combined with physicians' hierarchal position could have a powerful impact on patient's treatment. (This is a problem not only with physicians, but nurses who take on the role of "nurse pain clinician." The training for such a title has little consistency, yet these individuals take on a powerful role in the hospital. Because of their lack of credentials and education they can be a barrier to creative and new ideas in pain medicine and treatment.)

"Even in areas where we feel that we act purely of our own free will, our dramas are played out on a genetic stage" (Burnham & Phelan, 2000, p. 3). Whether we fully "buy in" to their claim that genes play such a dominant role, his writings are intriguing. "What is useful in small quantities often becomes destructive in excess, so instinctual desires in a new environment lead us straight to a problem" (Burnham & Phelan, 2000, p. 244). The previous discussion of racial biases and dominance may be examples of what Burnham and Phelan are discussing, i.e., instinctual "genetic" responses that have become "destructive in excess." The notion that a group maintains its gene pool may have had some evolutionary advantage in the past, but in excess has caused untold suffering and death in modern society. So, too, with the social instincts of dominance and counterdominance, in excess at a different time in history, marginalization of the weak and those in pain is the result.

It is interesting that beauty and deformity also have a tremendous impact on our responses to individuals with whom we interact. This is again a deeply visceral basic response. As Hume (1739) states, "beauty is such an order and construction of parts, as either by the primary constitution of our nature, by custom, or by caprice is fitted to give a pleasure and satisfaction to the soul. This is the distinguishing character of beauty" (p. 350). Hume is speaking of a deeply visceral response to what is considered "beautiful." As we view chronically sick and weak patients do we consider them "beautiful"? If they are not, then our behaviors can belie our true feelings and continue the further marginalization of patients with chronic pain. Additionally, feminist theory may add to our explication of poor pain management behaviors. Certain groups,

women, the aged, minorities, and persons with chronic pain are viewed as less trustworthy, both epistemically and morally (Code, 1991). There is clinical support for such a view, e.g., Bernabei in his study of elderly nursing home patients with cancer (*vide supra*) (Bernabei et al., 1998). Young goes further, "judgments of beauty or ugliness, attraction or aversion, cleverness or stupidity, competence or ineptness, and so on are made unconsciously in interactive contexts and in generalized media culture and these judgments often mark, stereotype, devalue or degrade some groups" (1990, p. 133). Young echoes Hume's discussion of beauty and ugliness and gives a further potential rationale for how pain patients are regularly treated.

Another aspect of our society is its loss of a moral foundation and a move to a more individual narcissistic social structure. "The weakening of social ties, which originates in the prevailing state of social welfare, at the same time reflects a narcissistic defense against dependence. A warlike society tends to produce men and women who are at heart antisocial. It should therefore not surprise us to find that although the narcissist conforms to social norms for fear of external retribution, he often thinks of himself as an outlaw and sees others in the same way, as basically dishonest and unreliable, or only reliable because of external pressures" (Kernberg, 1985, p. 238). William Osler (1932), in his work *Equanimitas*, suggests that HCPs should distance themselves from their patients in the belief they are protecting themselves emotionally and improving diagnosis and treatment. This view of "equanimity" has been perpetuated from medical school through residency. Emotional distance must be maintained to allow the freedom to diagnose and treat. It is claimed that getting emotionally involved with patients hinders this process. This view never has been tested in any scientific sense and why it continues to be perpetuated may relate to the discussion we have been having concerning the instinctual responses to those in distress and pain. However, once we distance ourselves from a patient's pain, that pain becomes "objectified" (Madjar, 1999). What is meant by this "objectification" is that the physical component of pain is separated from the patient's suffering. This is what HCPs are trained to do, distance themselves from the patient as person, separate out the problem and deal with one physical problem, at a time. The HCP no longer engages the patient as person; the patient is now a disease, an abstraction. HCPs are much better trained to deal with a clear disease, such as a coronary artery blockage: easily seen on angiogram and repaired through surgery. Unfortunately, pain does not fit our disease-based paradigm. Therefore, not only do HCPs have instinctual genetic drives that may influence their behaviors toward patients in pain, they also further exacerbate these behaviors by distancing themselves from the patient and objectifying patient narratives.

Clinicians admire the patient who "suffers with dignity," quietly, and with a minimum of pain behaviors. When physicians' diagnostic and interventional procedures have failed in finding an organic cause, they may feel there is no objective basis for a patient's pain. HCPs then, based on their professional training, "will be forced to conclude he [or she] has some sort of mental problem" (Black, 1979, p. 40). Additionally, when HCPs suggest that patients' pain is "in their head," this implies that the patient has a moral responsibility for bringing on suffering to the patient, family, and society. As has been shown, physicians, through their dominant position in our society, their visceral evolutionary responses to those who are weak, elderly, and "less beautiful," and their equanimity combined with societal narcissism, could contribute to the marginalization of patients with pain that we have been discussing.

INSTITUTION–PATIENT RELATIONSHIP

One of the profound changes associated with modern health care is the reemergence of an institution–patient relationship. An investigation of these institutional changes and their impact on pain management has not been provided previously. As managed care becomes more prominent and prevalent, the institution–patient relationship is itself reemerging as prominent. The previous oaths, creeds, and professional "professions" of obligations toward patients have less and less authority. As mentioned, all we have left as a secular society is the notion of autonomy. We no longer have the background of the religious norms that initially governed relationships with patients. When institutions such as insurance companies, hospitals, and clinics take over the roles previously held by physicians, it is now business ethics and economic theory, rather than a traditional medical or theological ethic, that provide the guiding norms. However, business ethics does not provide the needed foundation for protecting patients or guiding health care. *Caveat emptor* is still the overriding value in such an ethic. This is a further barrier not heretofore discussed in the pain management literature. Business has as a core goal the accrual of wealth and profits. This is not inherently bad or evil as profits can be tempered with social conscience. Patients with chronic pain or those who are chronically ill cost money and reduce profits. Therefore, there is a built-in incentive to limit the care for these patients or eliminate them, e.g., from an insurance pool. If patients with chronic pain are at risk for poor pain treatment and management from HCPs, the transfer of relationships to an institution with little or no ethical foundation should be very concerning.

In today's health care environment shared discussions and decision making by the physician–patient dyad is increasingly "being supplanted by the rules, standards, traditions and collective decision process of organizations,

which instruct and construct institutional actions in shaping health care choice" (Reiser, 1994, p. 28). Toulmin in his 1990 article states, "to the extent that, in the operation of a modern hospital, the claims of budgetary survival tend to outweigh those of a moral calling, the institution vergers on the condition of a tyrant.... [M]edical practitioners collectively cease to be a profession, and the individual doctor's work, circumscribed by institutional imperatives, is removed from the sphere of moral commitment and placed within the realm of social necessity. To that extent ... the physician's work is de-moral-ized" (p. 25). Reiser's and Toulmin's articles support the notion that in a very real sense the institution–patient relationship is increasingly eliminating the middleman, i.e., the physician and other HCPs; and this will further marginalize the patient in pain.

Often, managed care is criticized because it allows monetary considerations to play a role in health care although this is not a new development. Even in the fourth century, Saint John Chrysostom was well aware of economic influences in health care: "[I]n the reception of strangers, and the care of the sick, consider how great an expenditure of money is needed, and how much exactness and discernment on the part of those who preside over these matters. For it is often necessary that this expenditure should be even larger than that of which I spoke just now, and that he who presides over it should combine prudence and wisdom with skill in the art of supply, so as to dispose the affluent to be emulous and ungrudging in their gifts" (Chrysostom, 1998). While Chrysostom sought to expand the financial base of hospitals, he simultaneously recognized that care may take place in a context of constrained resources, and that prudence would be needed in making decisions about allocating these resources. A concern with money and its role has thus been present from the beginning of organized health care.

Money has been an essential part of health care for centuries. Today it is assumed that "money distorts, as well as corrupts, distracts, and vulgarizes the professional relationship" (May, 1997, p. 10). Why do we see it as having such a negative role in the 21st century? To answer this, we must consider the basic moral foundation upon which the hospitals in Chrysostom's time were based. Chrysostom had a robust moral tradition in which to place those monetary constraints. Care of the sick and suffering took precedence over profits. That Christian Orthodox religious community shared a common vision and conception of theological truth that enabled him to address the questions of human finitude and societal responsibility associated with financial considerations, and as previously discussed, gave a framework from which patients could find meaning in their pain. Hospitals, during the Enlightenment and under the banner of "scientific medicine," began to pull away from their religious underpinnings and detach themselves from "superstition" (Reiser, 1994). With the loss of religious foundations there was a concomitant degradation in the previously strong concept of the institution–patient relationship. Not only did the moral foundation of the institution–patient relationship change drastically but the moral foundations for health care professional's obligations also changed. This is part of the reason the other aspects of the HCP–patient interaction, those negative behaviors, can play a more important role. Into this void came medical professionalism with its distinct ethos.

Physicians sustained an understanding of their role and obligations, an understanding that was originally steeped in religious commitment (the idea of "profession"), but increasingly ignored that grounding tradition. The patient, rather than the religious community, became the central focus. With the modern discipline of bioethics, these traditional obligations were fully reconstructed in a philosophical idiom, with the language of "autonomy" and "beneficence" providing the means for rationalizing the role and obligations of physicians. However, without these rarefied moral notions, these principles, except autonomy, lack sufficient political force. The protection and advocacy that physicians or patients should be trying to provide and that were part of a previous age's moral framework is no longer available. So it is not at all surprising, in this current age of the primacy of business, erosion of moral foundations, and the previously discussed rationales for poor pain management behavior, that patients in pain are marginalized.

Currently, the focus of the institution–patient relationship is "business," and its ethical foundation is at best thin and lacks substantive power to protect patients. Because health care institutions have tremendous financial and political power, an ethos that considers patients' welfare as primary is critical. However, this power base, with the *current* minimalist business ethos, is dangerous to patients and their care. The push to save money and the pressure to limit care as financial constraints continue (especially for those who cost the system the most money, i.e., the elderly, the chronically ill, the weak, and those with chronic pain) will be overwhelming. (Although beyond the scope of this chapter, it is concerning that the ethical issues that seem such conundrums in our secular society all have the potential of saving the health care system substantial amounts of money. Euthanasia, physician-assisted suicide, abortion, and substandard care may all become attractive cost-saving options.)

A criticism of the role of business in medicine is illustrated by the Emanuels' article (1996), which can be taken as typical of the literature critical of business ethics in health care. To the Emanuels, the risk that the economic model will take precedence involves "a ruse portraying physicians as caring professionals while forcing them to act like economic producers [which] will ultimately discredit the entire practice of medicine and sow distrust and cynicism that cannot easily be overcome" (p. 238). They further decry the economic model and suggest that physicians "must resist the tremendous tendency within U.S. society to believe that the ideal solution for every complex social problem is the market and economic accountability" (p. 238). To the Emanuels the economic model views patients as "consumers" and physicians and other HCPs as "providers." Just like buying a dishwasher, consumers are encouraged in this model to compare the costs of different providers. Successful providers will, it is said, attract more consumers and make higher profits. This view of the health care market assumes that the market is free; yet the reality is that the health care market has become more and more constrained. Implicit in the criticisms of this model is a dread of the emerging institution–patient relationship and the fear of patient vulnerability. The Emanuels' criticisms should be taken seriously, but this does not take the discussion far enough. If we were just buying dishwashers, there would be less need to worry about *caveat emptor*. A bad dishwasher will very rarely put our lives at risk. However, when patients' lives hang in the balance and their classical ethical protections have been eroded, the need for concern becomes obvious.

Morreim (1997) sees health care institutions as having important and critical obligations to patients. She comments, "there is good reason to regard managed care organizations as fiduciaries of patients" (p. 36). The term *fiduciary* was once reserved only for individual professionals, e.g., physicians and attorneys, and only rarely applied to institutions. However, Morreim feels health care institutions (specifically managed care organizations) have fiduciary obligations that are little different from those of physicians. This is a unique view, and one that takes into consideration the evolving institution–patient relationship. Morreim's article gives import to the view that business ethics is not currently in a position to provide adequate protection to patients. Nevertheless, while Morreim broaches the issue of fiduciary obligations for health care institutions, she does not address the question of the ethical foundation for these obligations; how are they to be built? A medical ethic cannot merely be transposed onto a business ethical paradigm. Business ethics is not prepared to assume the roles previously held by physicians. Therefore, patients are increasingly vulnerable as business becomes more and more the driving, albeit *thin*, ethos in health care.

The advent of liberal political philosophy has further marginalized the role of physicians as well as patients in the physician–patient relationship and helped bolster the emerging institution–patient paradigm. As discussed previously, liberal political theory suggests that the state must be neutral with respect to its constituents, a philosophy that has been co-opted as a foundation for the physician–patient relationship, a view critiqued elsewhere (Peppin & Beckwith, 2000). Health care institutions are also to be value neutral, and this approach complicates attempts to develop any robust conceptions of the institution–patient relationship (Emanuel, 1991). Can a theoretical foundation that is "value neutral" develop the ethical robustness needed for patient protection? Suffice it to say that political systems nor physicians nor health care institutions can be value neutral (Galston, 1991; Peppin & Beckwith, 2000). As Starr (1982) comments, "the organization of medical care cannot be understood with reference solely to medicine, the relationships between doctors and patients, or even all the various forces internal to the health care sector. The development of medical care, like other institutions, takes place within larger fields of power and social structure" (p. 8). Starr sees clearly that medicine in general has a number of different non-value-neutral layers, if you will, each with its own set of values, the health care institution no less than the physician.

Unfortunately, attempts at a resurrected classical formulation of the physician–patient relationship combined with a business ethos also cannot provide any patient protections, as previously described. Although Emanuel and others continue to suggest that physicians are the buffer, the intermediary between the patient and institution, institutions are increasingly inserting themselves between the physician and patient. Morreim and others would do well to take the analysis of Sen (1988) seriously. "It is arguable that the importance of the ethical approach has rather substantially weakened as modern economics has evolved.... If one examines the balance of emphases in the publications in modern economics, it is hard not to notice the eschewal of deep normative analysis, and the neglect of the influence of ethical considerations in the characterization of actual human behavior" (p. 7). Economic theory and business ethics, as currently described, are too thinly construed to be of help in our current ethical crisis in health care, or in understanding the implications of the reemerging institution–patient relationship.

The marginalization of physicians' ability to act on patients' behalf and our previous discussion concerning patients with pain make deeper investigation into how to change the state of the weak, elderly, and those in pain imperative. Patients are not able to secure the protections they may have in other markets as "consumers." A consumerist ethos "cannot operate effectively in health care because of the asymmetry of information between supplier (doctor) and consumer (patient) and the special agency relationship which subsequently must exist between the two. The uncertainty of illness also makes it difficult for patients to adopt consumerist behavior" (Lupton, Donaldson, & Lloyd, 1991, p. 560). The other issues discussed in the previous part of this chapter also bring the "consumerist ethos" into question. Patients thus do not have even the consumerist ideal to provide them protection from *caveat emptor*. The problem does not lie in health care as a business or the managing of costs *per se*, but rather in the lack of a robust business ethos that will

regulate and limit the impact of financial considerations on patients.

CONCLUSION

It should not be construed that this author is suggesting physicians purposefully take a dominant role or purposefully try to marginalize patients with pain. Peters and Watt-Watson (2002) suggest, "[a] lack of trust in patient subjectivity reveals an epistemic bias that privileges objectivity in a positivistic sense.... It would be wrong, however, to hold individual clinicians entirely accountable for these moral and epistemological failings, for such failings have deep cultural and historical roots" (p. 75). HCPs generally are generous and empathetic professionals. They do not knowingly, generally, cause harm or purposefully marginalize the sick and weak. However, the behaviors we have been discussing may be instinctual rather than conscious. Also the lack of substantial and content-full moral foundation does not provide the framework necessary for interactions with patients. This absence could allow these instinctual behaviors more outlet for expression than when constrained by a content-full moral view of the good.

Current bioethics has not been able to provide the robust moral foundations that previously formed the fundamental protection against the marginalization of patients that we have discussed above. Now, in our multicultural society, no one view of the good can be determined to be "canonical." Therefore, the only reliable principle a secular society and health care system have left is autonomy. We may be able to acknowledge, however, that through liberal political theories, a "right" to pain management based on maximizing a patient's autonomy could be developed. However, other aspects of liberal political theory would be inconsistent with the foundation I am suggesting. For example, the Christian monk discussed previously, who might feel that pain brings one closer to God, would find an ethic based on liberal political theory very unfriendly. There is no room for those who have robust religious or moral traditions in such a philosophy. Here we turn to Engelhardt's work and his *Foundations of Bioethics* (1996). To Engelhardt there is no way to discern a canonical view of the moral and good life in a secular society. All we have left is to agree to disagree agreeably, i.e., to allow individuals autonomy. Engelhardt does not use the term *autonomy* to describe interactions between persons, only "permission." We give or withhold permission in all our interactions. Permission is the "foundational principle." Individuals are allowed to seek their own notions of the good life. Engelhardt does not consider permission a "right," just all that is left to our multicultural society.

Health care institutions occupy a middle ground between individual, privatized beliefs, and a broad social political ethos. Individual health care institutions, at the organizational level, may recover a rich theological ethos from which they can develop concrete guidelines for the institution–patient relationship. Efforts to enrich business ethics to provide patient protection should work toward enhanced safeguards for institutions with rich value structures, so that their development is not hampered by governmental coercion. These institutions can provide rich moral foundations, if allowed, and individual patients can choose which institutions would best fit with their own worldviews. It will be up to patients to seek those health care institutions that adhere to a rich conception of ethics and values, or not. This requires a departure from traditional Rawlsian political philosophies. Unfortunately, those patients who are in lower socioeconomic classes, the weak, the infirm, the disabled, and those in chronic pain will be the ones least likely to have the skills to seek such institutions. Regardless, in all discussions concerning the role of business ethics in health care we should consider that "the real business of health care is not about the mergers and acquisitions, financing mechanisms, or structural reforms that have occupied center stage on the public agenda for much of the past decade. It is about preventing ill health, caring for people who are sick, and meeting the needs of people who must live their lives with disabilities or chronic disease" (Edgman-Levitan, 1998, p. 1). Unfortunately, the thin structure of business ethical theory that currently supports most of our health care institutions is not strong enough to protect patients, especially those at greatest risk such as patients with chronic pain. Without a clear and robust ethic, patients will continue to be at risk from the health care institution of sacrifice for the sake of cost constraints. Can a business ethic protect patients with chronic pain within the institution–patient relationship? Currently, the answer is a resounding *no*. Developing a robust moral foundation for companies has not been a focus in the business or economics literature.

Medical education needs a modern-day Flexenerian revolution (although I focus on medical education, the criticisms described here may also apply to pharmacy, nursing, and other HCP educational institutions and universities). During the early 1900s medical education underwent a tremendous evolution through the efforts of Flexner (1910) and subsequent legislation. The way medicine was taught changed dramatically and this approach has continued little changed until today. Unfortunately, the current system, although successful in many ways, has failed substantially in other areas such as pain management. In order to successfully treat the chronically sick patients that currently fill our clinics, we need a different perspective, one that focuses on patients and their suffering, their quality of life, and a better approach to symptom management. The current approach is disease centered. Perhaps the greatest barrier will be that the disease model is so entrenched that most clinicians and patients are unaware of its existence. What was once itself a new

model, developed as a means of translating emerging scientific knowledge into better medical care, is now accepted as "truth." A move to a more symptom-based approach, as outlined by Tinnetti and Fried (2004), would be a positive step in improving the care of patients with chronic pain and would at least provide a framework for pain and symptom management. "Notwithstanding these structural difficulties and philosophical barriers, medical care must evolve once again to a more individually tailored, integrated model based on the health care needs of patients in the 21st century" (Tinetti & Fried, 2004, p. 183). Although Tinetti's article may be a radical approach to the changes in medical education that need to occur, it illustrates some very important issues (Tinetti & Fried, 2004).

Pain and palliative medicine are good examples of such a failure of medical education to meet the needs of patients in American society. Few medical schools have even a few hours of lecture in these critical topics; fewer still have organized courses for pain, symptom management, and palliative care. (I know of no published surveys of medical schools concerning the amount of time spent on pain and symptom management. However, our group looked at this, peripherally, for osteopathic medical schools. Only one school of 19 had an elective in pain and one other had an hour lecture on pain. There was none in palliative medicine [Peppin, Leeper, & Garloff, 2002]). This is not just of academic concern, but is obviously critical to the care we provide our patients; we all have pain, we will all suffer both physically and emotionally, and we all will die. The dominance assumed by physicians in society, their visceral "evolutionary" instinctive behaviors toward the weak and the patient with chronic pain, the preeminence of business ethics in the moral framework of health care, and the failure of liberal political theories to protect patients in pain must be a primary focus of the academic efforts and thought.

There is no question that our current model of medical education is archaic, self-perpetuating, and a barrier to appropriate pain and palliative medicine; it needs a complete overhaul. Unfortunately, the medical educational system has not voluntarily made the changes that need to occur. It needs to refocus and restructure its basic science and clinical curriculum. Fortunately, education can be changed to make a difference. Weinstein in her 2000 article found that a course in pain management could have a profound impact on students during the 4 years of medical school. These students had a better understanding of pain, were more open to the patient with chronic pain, and were less anxious concerning pain medications (Weinstein et al., 2000). The rationale for the changes in medical education comes from the preceding discussion. Changing medical education might change the instinctual foundation for the poor behaviors in pain management. Further, medical education can strengthen the notions of autonomy through a thorough explanation of HCP behaviors.

Having shown that a "right" to pain management might be developed, it should be pointed out that this is not what drives this author to practice pain medicine. It is not to a secular bioethics but toward "the bioethics of content-full moral commitment" that this author looks for moral direction (Engelhardt, 1996). I agree with Engelhardt that the preceding section "surely has not sustained all the moral propositions that this author knows are necessary for the good life. It is simply that this is all that secular moral reasoning can provide" (Engelhardt, 1996, p. 421). It is the freedom to seek each individual's own notion of the good, whether content-full or not, that is important to maintain.

The disturbing, potentially destructive notions held by HCPs need more and deeper reflection. If we can show that these behaviors do have rationales along the lines I have been discussing, then we can work on changing those behaviors. The HCP educational system can provide the enlightenment that students need to place their own biases and prejudices in context, deal with them, and thereby improve the care of patients in pain. We will unfortunately not find support or help in business ethics as it is currently formulated to protect or give us a foundation to properly care for patients in pain. Further, we should always be suspicious when such institutions claim they are working in the patient's best interest. However, those hospitals, insurance companies, and other health care institutions that choose to have a "content-full moral commitment" should be allowed to do so. There should be no coercion by the central government, and those patients who so choose can use those institutions. HCPs should be aware that relationships with patients have dramatically changed and that our ability to protect patients, especially the weak and those in chronic pain, has been dramatically reduced. Patients should be made aware of this as well. Ground-level patient action groups are the power that is most likely to make substantive changes when it comes to governmental and legislative action.

This is the obvious goal of this chapter and text: improving the care of patients with chronic pain. Our focus should always be the patient and, for our purposes in this chapter, reducing the marginalization that is so inherent in the current health care system for these patients. Interestingly, those health care professionals who treat chronic pain are also marginalized both professionally and financially. This has been a somewhat bleak view of current health care; however, I believe it is accurate. There is also significant potential for change. That change is only going to come from the academy and the specialists contained within. We must be forceful and proactive in our attempts to change the current system. The treatment of the weak, the suffering, and those in chronic pain must be a passion for those health care professionals who spe-cialize in this area. This passion must extend beyond the walls of individual clinics and into legislative bodies, hospitals, and other institutions.

ACKNOWLEDGMENTS

I gratefully acknowledge the following individuals for their friendship and unselfish critical reviews, comments, and expertise: H. T. Engelhardt, Ph.D., M.D.; Susan Engelhardt, M.S.; Louann Hart, A.R.N.P.; Fabrice Jotterand, M.S.; Ana Ilitis-Smith, Ph.D.; Michael Federich, M.D., F.A.A.H.P.M.; Andy Lustig, Ph.D.; and Marc Hines, M.D.

REFERENCES

Allen, W. (1973). *Sleeper,* MGM/United Artists studios.

Amen, D. Images of of human behavior: A brain SPECT atlas. Retrieved September 2004 from http://www.brain-place.com/bp/atlas/.

American College of Physicians Ad Hoc Committee on Medical Ethics. (1984). American College of Physicians ethics manual. *Annals of Internal Medicine, 101,* 129–137, 263–274.

American Pain Foundation. (2004). Patient bill of rights. Retrieved September, 2004 from http://www.painfoundation.org/downloads/EnglishBOR.doc.

Aronowitz, R. A. (2000). When do symptoms become a disease? *Annals of Internal Medicine, 134,* 803–808.

Beauchamp, T. L., & Childress, J. F. (1994). *Principles of biomedical ethics* (4th ed.). New York: Oxford University Press.

Bernabei, R., Gambassi, G., Lapane, K., Landi, F., Garsonis, C., Dunlop, R. et al. (1998). Management of pain in elderly patients with cancer. SAGE Study Group. Systematic assessment of geriatric drug use via epidemiology. *Journal of the American Medical Association, 279,* 1877–1882.

Black, R. G. (1979). Evaluation of the complaint of pain. *Bulletin of the Los Angeles Neurological Society, 44,* 32–44.

Broekmans, S., Vanderschueren, S., Morlion, B., Kuman, A., & Evers, G. (2004). Nurses' attitudes toward pain treatment with opioids: A survey in a Belgian university hospital. *International Journal of Nursing Studies, 41,* 183–189.

Burnham, T., & Phelan, J. (2000). *Mean genes: From sex to money to food: Taming our primal instincts.* New York: Penguin Books.

Byock, I. R. (1996). The nature of suffering and the nature of opportunity at the end of life. *Clinics in Geriatric Medicine, 12,* 237–252.

Cassell, E. J. (1991). *The nature of suffering and the goals of medicine.* New York: Oxford University Press.

Charlton, B. G. (1997a). The inequity of inequality: Egalitarian instincts and evolutionary psychology (vol. 2). Retrieved September 2004 from http://www.hedweb.com/bgcharlton/evolpsych.html.

Charlton, B. G. (1997b). Injustice, inequality and evolutionary psychology. Retrieved April 8, 2005 from http://www.hedweb.com/bgcharlton/evolpsych.html.

Cherny, N., & Coyle, N. (1998). The application of ethical principles in the management of cancer pain. In G. M. Aronoff (Ed.), *Evaluation and treatment of chronic pain* (3rd ed., pp. 643–654). Baltimore: Williams & Wilkins.

Chrysostom, S. J. (1998). Six books on the priesthood: Treatise on the priesthood. The Church Fathers Homepage, A Proposed Collaboration between St. Columbia Press & The Broad Alliance for Multimedia Technology Applications. Retrieved September 2004 from http://www.stmichael.org/Fathers/.

Cleeland, C. S. (1993). Strategies for improving cancer pain management. *Journal of Pain and Symptom Management, 8*, 361–364.

Clinton, W. (2004). Retrieved September 2004 from http://www.manhattan-institute.org/hazlett/rahazlett52.htm.

Code, L. (1991). *What can she know? Feminist theory and the construction of knowledge.* Ithaca, NY: Cornell University Press.

Crane, R. A., Wilson, P. C., & Behrens, G. (1990). Pain control in hospice home care: Management guidelines. *American Journal of Hospice and Palliative Care, 7*, 39–42.

Dar, R., Beach, C. M., Barden, P. L., & Cleeland, C. S. (1992). Cancer pain in the marital system: A study of patients and their spouses. *Journal of Pain and Symptom Management, 7*, 87–93.

Desbiens, N. A., Wu, A. W., Broste, S. K., Wenger, N. S., Connors, Jr., A. F., Lynn, J. et al. (1996). Pain and satisfaction with pain control in seriously ill hospitalized adults: findings from the SUPPORT research investigations. For the SUPPORT Investigators. Study to Understand Prognoses and Preferences for Outcomes and Risks of Treatment. *Critical Care Medicine, 24*, 1953–1961.

Devo, R. A., Nachemson, A., & Mirza, S. K. (2004). Spinal-fusion surgery — The case for restraint. *New England Journal of Medicine, 350*, 722–726.

Dworkin, R. (1989). *A matter of principle* (pp. 181–236). Cambridge, MA: Harvard University Press.

Edgman-Levitan, S. (1998). Patient confidence in the health care system. *IHI Quality Connection, 7*, 1–2.

Emanuel, E. (1991). *The ends of human life.* Cambridge, MA: Harvard University Press.

Emanuel, E. J. (1996). Pain and symptom control. *Hematology/Oncology Clinics of North America, 10*, 41–56.

Emanuel, E. J., & Emanuel, L. L. (1996). What is accountability in health care? *Annals of Internal Medicine, 124*, 229–239.

Engelhardt, H. T. (1996). *The foundations of bioethics* (2nd ed.). New York: Oxford University Press.

Federal Registry (1979, April 18). *44*(76), 23192–23197.

Ferrell, B. R. (1997). The role of ethics committees in responding to the moral outrage of unrelieved pain. *Bioethics Forum, 13*, 11–16.

Ferrell, B. R., Cronin Nash, C., & Warfield, C. (1992). The role of patient-controlled analgesia in the management of cancer pain. *Journal of Pain and Symptom Management, 7*(3), 149–154.

Flexner, A. (1910). Medical education in the United States and Canada: A report to the Carnegie Foundation for the Advancement of Teaching. New York: The Foundation. Retrieved September 2004 from www.carnegiefoundation.org/eLibrary/docs/flexner_report.pdf.

Frankl, V. E. (1963). *Man's search for meaning: An introduction to logotherapy.* New York: Holt, Rinehart & Winston.

Galston W. A. (1991). *Liberal purposes.* Cambridge, MA: Cambridge University Press.

Garro, L. C. (1992). Chronic illness and the construction of narratives. In M. J. Delvecchio, P. E. Brodwin, B. J. Good, & A. Kleinman (Eds.), *Pain as human experience: An anthropological perspective* (pp. 100–137). Berkeley: University of California Press.

Grossman, S. A., Sheidler, V. R., Swedeen, K., Mucenski, J., & Piantadosi, S. (1991). Correlation of patient and caregiver ratings of cancer pain. *Journal of Pain and Symptom Management, 6*, 53–57.

Gureje, O., Von Korff, M., Simon, G. E., & Gater, R. (1998). Persistent pain and well-being: A World Health Organization study in primary care. *Journal of the American Medical Association, 280*, 147–151.

Hoffmann, D. E. (1998). Pain management and palliative care in the era of managed care: Issues for health insurers. *Journal of Law, Medicine & Ethics, 26*, 267–289

Hume, D. (1739). *A treatise of human nature.* New York: Penguin Books.

Hunter, K. M. (1996). Narrative, literature, and the clinical exercise of practical reason. *Journal of Medicine and Philosophy, 21*, 303–320.

Huxley, A. (1998). *Brave new world.* New York: Perennial.

Illich, I. (2000). *Disabling professions.* New York: Marion Boyars.

Joranson, D. E., & Gilson, A. M. (2001). Pharmacists' knowledge of and attitudes toward opioid pain medications in relation to federal and state policies. *Journal of the American Pharmaceutical Association, 41*, 213–220.

Katz, J. (1984). *The silent world of doctor and patient.* London: Collier/Macmillan.

Kernberg, O. F. (1985). *Borderline conditions and pathological narcissism.* Lanham, MD: Rowman & Littlefield.

Kleinman, A. (1992). Pain and resistance: The delegitimation and relegitimation of local worlds. In M. J. D. Good, P. E. Brodwin, B. J. Good Byron, & A. Kleinman (Eds.), *Pain as human experience: An anthropological perspective* (pp. 169–197). Berkeley: University of California Press.

Lasch, C. (1979). *The culture of narcissism.* New York: WW Norton.

Lupton, D., Donaldson, C., & Lloyd, P. (1991). Caveat emptor of blissful ignorance? Patients and the consumerist ethos. *Social Science and Medicine, 33*, 559–568.

Madjar, I. (1999). On inflicting and relieving pain. In I. Madjar & J. A. Watson (Eds.), *Nursing and the experience of illness: Phenomenology in practice* (pp. 145–169). London: Routledge Press.

May, W. J. (1997). Money and the medical profession. *Kennedy Institute of Ethics Journal, 7*, 1–13.

Merskey, H., & Bogduk, N. (Eds.). (1994). *IASP task force on taxonomy classification of chronic pain* (2nd ed.). Seattle: IASP Press.

Morreim, E. H. (1997). To tell the truth: Disclosing the incentives and limits of managed care. *American Journal of Managed Care, 3*, 35–43.

Morris, D. (1991). *The culture of pain.* Berkeley: University of California Press.

Moseley L. (2003). Unraveling the barriers to reconceptualization of the problem in chronic pain: The actual and perceived ability of patients and health professionals to understand the neurophysiology. *Journal of Pain, 4,* 184–189.

National Institute on Drug Abuse (NIDA) and the National Institute on Alcohol Abuse and Alcoholism (NIAAA), National Institutes of Health (NIH). Retrieved September 2004 from http://www.nih.gov/news/pr/may98/nida-13.htm.

Nelson, R. (2003). Decade of pain control and research gets into gear in USA. *Lancet, 362,* 1129.

Osler, W. (1932). *Aequanimitas.* New York: McGraw-Hill.

Pellegrino, E. (1994). Patient and physician autonomy: Conflicting rights and obligations in the physician–patient relationship. *Journal of Contemporary Health Law and Policy, 10,* 47–68.

Pellegrino, E. D. (1980). *A philosophical basis of medical practice: Toward a philosophy and ethic of the healing professions.* Oxford: Oxford University Press.

Peppin, J. F., & Beckwith, F. J. (2000). Physician value neutrality: A critique. *Journal of Law, Medicine & Ethics, 28,* 67–77.

Peppin, J. F., Leeper, K., & Garloff, D. (2002). A review of resources in bioethics at osteopathic medical schools. *Academic Medicine, 77,* 427–431.

Peter, E.. & Watt-Watson, J. (2002). Unrelieved pain: An ethical and epistemological analysis of distrust in patients. *Clinical Journal of Nursing Research, 34,* 65–80.

Pope Pius XII. (1956, September 1). Addressing a group of international heart specialists. Retrieved June 19, 2005 from http://www.learnenglish.org.uk/magazine/phobias.html.

Proulx, K., & Jacelon, C. (2004). Dying with dignity: The good patient versus the good death. *American Journal of Hospice and Palliative Care, 21,* 116–120.

Rawlinson, M. C. (1986). The sense of suffering. *Journal of Medicine and Philosophy, 11,* 39–62.

Rawls, J. (1989). *A theory of justice.* Cambridge, MA: Harvard University Press.

Reiser, S. J. (1994). The ethical life of health care organizations. *Hastings Center Report, 24,* 28–35.

Rich, B. A. (2000). An ethical analysis of the barriers to effective pain management. *Cambridge Quarterly of Healthcare Ethics, 9,* 54–70.

Rousseau, J. J. (1984). *A discourse on inequality.* London: Penguin Books.

Schultz, D. S., & Carnevale, F. A. (1996). Engagement and suffering in responsible caregiving: On overcoming maleficence in health care. *Theoretical Medicine, 17,* 189–207.

Schweitzer, A. (1948). *On the edge of the primeval forest* (C. T. Campion, Trans.). New York: AMS Press.

Sen, A. (1988). *On ethics and economics.* Oxford: Blackwell, Oxford.

Somerville, M. A. (1994). Death of pain: Pain, suffering and ethics. In G. F. Gebhart, D. L. Hammond, & T. S. Jensen (Eds.), *Proceedings of the VII World Congress on Pain: Congress abstracts: Progress in pain research and management* (pp. 41–58). Seattle: IASP.

Springen, K., Raymong, J., & Underwood, A. (2003, May 19). Taking a new look at pain. *Newsweek, 141,* 44–52.

Starr, P. (1982). *The social transformation of American medicine.* New York: Basic Books.

Tinetti, M. R., & Fried, T. (2004). The end of the disease era. *American Journal of Medicine, 116,* 179–185.

Toulmin S. (1990). Medical institutions and their moral constraints. In E. Bulger, & J. Reiser (Eds.). *Integrity in health care institutions.* Iowa City: University of Iowa Press, Iowa City.

University of Notre Dame. (2004, March). Philip & Doris Clarke Family 19th Annual Medical Ethics Conference. Indiana: Author.

U.S. Department of Health and Human Services. (1992). Acute Pain Management Guideline Panel. Acute pain management in adults: Operative procedures, quick reference guide for clinicians. Agency for Health Care Policy and Research. AHCPR Pub. No. 92-0019. Rockville, MD: Author.

U.S. Department of Health and Human Services. (2000). Healthy People 2000. Retrieved September 2004 from http://www.grants.nih.gov/grants/guide/pa-files/PA-98-102.html.

Veatch, R. (1991). *The patient–physician relation: The patient as partner* (Part 2). Bloomington, IN: Indiana University Press.

Walter, F., Stewart, J. A. et al. (2003). Lost productive time and cost due to common pain conditions in the US workforce. *Journal of the American Medical Association, 290,* 2443–2454.

Wardwell, W. I. (1994). Alternative medicine in the United States. *Social Science and Medicine, 38,* 1061–1068.

Weinstein, S. W., Laux, L. F. et al. (2000). Medical students' attitudes toward pain and the use of opioid analgesics: Implications for changing medical school curriculum. *Southern Medical Journal, 93,* 472–478.

Wolfe, J., Klar, N. et al. (2000). Understanding of prognosis among parents of children who died of cancer: Impact on treatment goals and integration of palliative care. *Journal of the American Medical Association, 284,* 2469–2475.

World Health Organization. (1990). *Cancer pain and palliative care.* Geneva: Author.

Young, I. M. (1990). *Justice and the politics of difference.* Princeton, NJ: Princeton University Press.

92

Legal Considerations in Pain Management

James S. Lapcevic, DO, PhD, JD, FCLM

INTRODUCTION

Pain, an important and serious symptom, is one of the most compelling reasons for seeking medical care (Weiner, 1993). Nine of ten Americans age 18 years or older report suffering pain at least once a month, and 42% of adults report experiencing pain every day, with more than 70% surveyed expressing the fear of dying in pain or alone without an opportunity to say good-bye to loved ones (Gallup, Inc., 1999). Chronic pain is an estimated daily experience of 75 million people in the United States (Bostrom, Ramberg, Davis, & Fridlund, 1997). In the last decade interest in pain and management of pain has risen, largely due to the revelation that inadequate pain control is a norm under traditional clinical management (Rorarius & Baer, 1994). Surveys over the past decade have shown as many as 75% of postoperative patients unnecessarily suffer unrelieved pain (Shapiro, 1994). A survey was conducted in an attempt to identify medical personnel and patient attitudes toward the use of opioids in postoperative analgesia with the finding that 82% of surveyed physicians responded that they had not been adequately educated in pain management, while patients indicated more than half wanted decision capacity on when more analgesia should be given them for pain relief (Lavies, Hart, Rounsefell, & Runciman, 1992).

In 1990, a conducted survey of physicians through the Eastern Cooperative Oncology Group (ECOG) found virtually 90% of the physician respondents felt they had received inadequate training in medical school regarding pain management, in particular, cancer pain management, and many were reluctant to prescribe opioids to relieve pain (Von Roenn, Cleeland, Gonin, Hartfield, & Pandya, 1993). In recent years, medical practitioners have gained a new and emerging awareness of pain, its effects on quality of life, and the evaluation and issues involved in its treatment. Although the relief of pain has not always been a priority for medical practitioners, the increasing number of those experiencing pain coupled with other chronic medical conditions now places extreme urgency on physicians to stay abreast of the most current and effective options for pain assessment, evaluation, and management. Much pain remains underreported as well as undertreated (Dahlman, Dykes, & Elander, 1999). Good clinical practice of medicine requires an ongoing effort to access and treat pain with appropriate analgesic therapy (Foley, 2000). Varying patient populations have been found to receive less than quality treatment of their pain if indeed they received any treatment at all (Bernabei, Gambassi, Lapane et al., 1998; Cleeland, Gonin, Baez, Loehrer, & Pandya, 1997; Foley, 1997). Within the last decade it has been reported that a significant percentage of ambulatory patients with cancer have received inadequate pain treatment (Cheville, 2001), with significant percentages of ambulatory patients with AIDS (84%) receiving inadequate pain relief (Portenoy, 2000). Inadequate pain relief particularly has been ascribed to women, elderly nursing home patients, and ethnic minorities.

GUIDELINES FOR PAIN MANAGEMENT

In the past decade, societal and governmental needs have molded medical practice into a less variable, more standardized activity (Hill, 1996a). Guidelines for pain management have been issued by such diverse groups as the WHO, the APS, the American Society of Anesthesiologists, the American Academy of Pediatrics, the International Association for the Study of Pain, and the U.S. Agency for Health Care Policy and Research (AHCPR) (Hill, 1995). Federal oversight of controlled substances extends into community standards of care.

According to the 1992 AHCPR guidelines, opioids may be prescribed to treat acute and chronic pain, but the prescribing physician assumes the burden of proving that the prescription falls within normal clinical procedures for pain management. This burden remains in effect to this day. A physician prescriber of a controlled substance is obligated to demonstrate both the medical necessity and adherence to law of such a choice. Many health care practice acts do not provide for the interpretation of phrases such as "practicing medicine in a manner inconsistent with public health and welfare" (Hill, 1996b). It is often the legal process that later defines concepts of "reasonably necessary" and "good faith" among others that are critical to the justification, and even legal defense, of controlled substance prescribing in any individual case. Allegations of prescribing too much or too little, or not prescribing a controlled substance that was needed according to the definition outlined in federal or state guidelines may be open to court interpretation through expert witnesses brought in by medical boards, plaintiffs, or the Drug Enforcement Agency (DEA). Allegations that prescribing behavior is not in good faith or not reasonably necessary, requirements designed to establish medical necessity, which may be redefined ad hoc, can make it difficult for physicians to justify their treatment decisions. To avoid running an unwitting collision course with these complex issues, better training in proper pain management procedures is necessary for physicians (Carr, 1998). Generally, physicians prescribing scheduled or nonscheduled analgesic medications do so believing patients need them. Physicians must be aware of the immediate medicolegal ramification, including the burden of proof that must be considered when analgesic medications are prescribed (Clark, 1998). It has been suggested that treatment guidelines should ideally be based on data from the medical literature, case law, and clinical experience.

THE PHENOMENON OF UNDERTREATED PAIN

- A standard of care for pain management can be established medically and legally.
- Health care professionals and organizations that fail to meet the standard will be held morally, legally, and monetarily accountable.
- Laypersons take the duty to relieve pain and suffering seriously.
- A painful death is now considered to be a presumptively mismanaged death. (Rich, 2004)

The boards that administer and interpret health care practice acts comprise state government officials' appointees whose members' biases may be reflected in the guidelines (Hill, 1996b). While not all state medical boards hit the mark, many experts favor state medical policy, issuing from the medical boards rather that from elected officials, directly addressing physicians concerns through medical guidelines. In 1999, The Ohio State Medical Association, in cooperation with the state legislature, distributed a new clinical handbook titled, *The Fifth Vital Sign*. Distributed to all physicians, but directed at primary care physicians, the booklet encouraged better pain management including a step-by-step guide to documentation requirement compliance.

AHCPR (1992) issued recommended guidelines for effective pain relief, which promise patients attentive and effective analgesic care as well as quantification in the medical chart of pain assessment and pain relief. The earliest recommendation to establish the basic principles of use of medications for management of pain in adults was formulated after extensive literature review and evaluation of data. Among these basic principles were specialized technology and nonpharmacologic approaches to pain management (AHCPR, 1992). A systematic review of the literature was used to compile evidence for each mode of pain relief (Carr et al., 1992) (Table 92.1):

- *Type I* evidence comes from large trials.
- *Type Ia* evidence is derived from multiple, randomized, controlled trials that may be consolidated utilizing meta-analysis.
- *Type Ib* data originate from at least one large, randomized, controlled study with statistically significant results.
- *Type II* studies involve well-designed but non-randomized comparisons.
- *Type III* evidence is from descriptive studies.
- *Type IV* evidence is expert consensus, based on the opinions of prominent practitioners.

Organizations and publications have also developed evidence-grading scales. The diversity of these scales can be confusing. Formation of a unified taxonomy has been proposed and is under development to evaluate the strength of recommendations based on a body of evidence (Figure 92.1). The new taxonomy is recommended to (Ebell, Siwek et al., 2004)

1. Be uniform in most medicine journals and electronic databases
2. Allow evaluation of the strength of recommendation of a body of evidence
3. Be comprehensive and allow evaluation studies of screening, diagnosis, therapy, prevention, and prognosis

TABLE 92.1
Pain Management Guidelines: Medication for Management of Pain in Adults

Medication	Evidence*	Comments	Precautions
Oral NSAIDs	Ib, IV	Effective for mild-to-moderate pain; begin preoperatively; relatively contraindicated in patients with renal disease and risk of or actual coagulopathy	May mask fever
Oral NSAIDs in conjunction with opioids	Ia, IV	Potentially effect resulting in opioid sparing; begin preoperatively	As above
Parenteral	Ib, IV	Effective for moderate-to-severe pain; expensive; useful if opioids contraindicated, especially to avoid respiratory depression and sedation	As above
Oral opioids	IV	Route of choice; as effective as parenteral in appropriate doses	Use as oral medication tolerated
Intramuscular	Ib, IV	The standard parenteral in appropriate doses	Hence, avoid this route when possible
Subcutaneous	Ib, IV	Preferable to intramuscular route when low-volume continuous infusion is needed and intravenous access is difficult to maintain; injections painful and absorption unreliable	Avoid this route for long-term repetitive treatment
Intravenous	Ib, IV	Parenteral route of choice after major surgery; suitable for titrated bolus or continuous administration but requires special monitoring	Significant risk of respiratory depression with inappropriate dosing
PCA (systemic)	Ia, IV	When suitable, provides good analgesia	Significant risk of respiratory depression with inappropriate dosing
Epidural and intrathecal opioids	Ia, IV	When suitable, provides good analgesia; use of infusion pumps requires additional equipment and staff education; expensive if infusion pumps are used	Significant risk of respiratory depression; sometimes delayed in onset; requires careful monitoring

Note: Ia = evidence obtained from meta-analysis of randomized controlled trials. Ib = evidence obtained from at least one randomized controlled trial. II = well-designed nonrandomized studies. III = descriptive studies. IV = expert consensus based on the opinions and/or clinical experiences of respected authorities. NSAID = nonsteroidal anti-inflammatory drug. PCA = patient-controlled analgesia.

The newfound appreciation for aggressive action in treating acute pain resulted in the Federation of State Medical Boards of the United States, Inc. (1998) promulgating model guidelines for pain management strategies and objectives. Clinicians will be potentially held to these guidelines, and the quality of medical practice will be judged in part by the ability to meet these criteria. Some states have adopted even more stringent guidelines for pain treatment: at present, certain barriers to delivery of adequate analgesia and pain management exist. Members of the health care team, patients, and the health care system continue impeding the delivery of proper analgesia (Jacox et al., 1994) (Table 92.2).

FOCUS ON PAIN

In 40 states, a variety of efforts have been made to improve pain management. Individual state laws have tended recently to follow the recommendations made by the Federation of State Medical Boards. Most state laws regarding the management of pain are still evolving. Some of these efforts have been undertaken by *lawmakers* through specific *legislation*, or by *regulators* through new *regulations*; others are a result of revised or newly adopted guidelines and policy statements on pain treatment from state medical boards. Aimed at making standards uniform across the nation and encouraging better pain management, physicians who prescribe a controlled substance "for a legitimate medical purpose" are reassured not to worry about medical board, state regulatory, or enforcement agency actions. The Federation initiative was endorsed by the DEA and by advocates for better pain management. The medical use of controlled substances has gained a new legitimacy, but physician fears of regulatory scrutiny continue to linger. The careful physician, in attempting to steer a course clear of regulators, must be prepared to prescribe opioid analgesics utilizing a consistent methodology. This consistent methodology is analogous to the checklist pilots use, no matter their experience, preparing for take off, landings, and other aircraft performance standards on which safe pilotage is based. Tips for prescribing opioids under a consistent methodology are as follows:

TABLE 92.2
Barriers to Delivery of Adequate Analgesia

Health Care Professionals	Reasons for Patient Reluctance to Report Pain	Health Care System
Inadequate knowledge of pain management (especially clinical pharmacology)	Fear of patient addiction	Concerned about adverse reactions and development of tolerance
Poor assessment of pain	Fear that pain means progression of disease	Low priority given to pain management
	Want to be a "good" patient	Inadequate reimbursement
Concern about:		
Regulation of controlled substances	Do not want to distract physician from treating underlying disease	Limits availability of treatment
Side effects of pain management	Reluctant to take pain medication	Limits access to treatment
Development of tolerance	Fear of addiction or of being classified as an addict	Restrictive regulation of controlled substances

Note: Modified from *Management of Cancer Pain. Clinical Guideline,* by A. Jacox et al., 1994, Rockville, MD: U.S. Department of Health and Human Services.

- Obtain a thorough history and perform a first rate physical examination (sound familiar?).
- Chart everything you see, think, feel, and hear about the patient.
- Obtain informed consent for long-term opioid therapy.
- Obtain a second opinion from a colleague to verify the plan of care if you are not a pain practitioner.
- Convince the patient to agree to use only one pharmacy and to obtain opioids only from you.
- See the patient regularly (at least every 30 to 90 days); prescribe controlled-release medications to stabilize the blood levels to limit the "buzz" associated with immediate release medications.
- Keep the dosages controlled to the amount necessary to provide comfort.
- Check the urine drug screen to make certain what you are prescribing is being taken and that illicit substances are not being used.
- Obtain more education about the use of opioid analgesics.

Does it seem likely that you would ever be accused of improper behavior if all of these steps were followed (Cole, 1998)?

Historically, from the advent of the Victorian era until after World War I, doctors were held largely responsible for the heroin, morphine, opiate, and cocaine problems that swept the United States. The Harrison Narcotic Act of 1914 began the heavy-handed crackdown on narcotics that narrowed the scope of medical practice and interfered with their legitimate medical use, especially in pain management (Guglielmo, 2000). A short decade ago, conven-

tional wisdom in the medical establishment was that a physician treating chronic pain with opioids was at substantial risk of sanction by state medical regulatory boards for overprescribing (Hill, 1993; Joranson, 1992; Portenoy, 1996). A review of state medical board actions from 1990 to 1996 reveals that the perception of regulatory risk far exceeded the reality (Martino, 1998). A California study concluded that most offenses of disciplined physicians involved some aspect of patient care (e.g., inappropriate prescribing) (Morrison & Wickersham, 1998). Regulatory risks associated with overprescribing are still perceived as real and far greater than those associated with underprescribing despite regulatory relief efforts (Glanelli, 1999). The premise of the regulatory relief efforts was the undertreatment of pain is a public health problem. Regulatory relief has seemed to fail to alter significantly the perception of risk associated with the physicians prescribing opioids for the treatment of chronic pain. Ann M. Martino, Ph.D., while executive director of Iowa's Board of Medical Examiners, recommended that new laws be written to discipline physicians who prescribed too little pain medication. Ironically, she wrote that the most immediate means of achieving good pain management may not be regulatory relief, but more regulation (Martino, 1998).

It has been recommended that physician education is key to better pain management. Knowledge of the best pharmaceutical and nonpharmaceutical methods for controlling pain and of the federal and state laws that apply to medical practice is recommended at "should know" levels. State medical boards or medical societies are good resources for current laws that apply to medical practice. Caveat: A potent reminder finds that knowledge alone is insufficient to promote behavioral change (King, Bungard, McAlister et al., 2000); in the absence of other actions, such as steps toward disseminating a medical guideline or providing continuing medical education, it is unlikely that significant, or even measurable, improvement in the effectiveness of an intervention might occur (Goff, Canely, & Gu, 2000).

For decades, improving the quality of health care delivery relied on changing physician behavior. Experience has shown that quality improvement is better achieved through systems solutions that *support clinicians* in providing quality care (Calonge, 2000). The imperative to measure, promote, and improve the quality of medical care continues to be an essential, if not daunting, endeavor. The quality of health care is, in the opinion of many, a serious problem. Research demonstrates that physicians overuse health care services by ordering unnecessary interventions, underuse services by failing to provide a standard of care that would produce favorable outcomes, and *devise* an *incorrect* treatment plan or improperly execute the correct plan (Chasin & Galvin, 1998; Leape, 1992, 1994; Nyquist, Gonzales, Steiner, & Sande, 1998). Quality assurance in the health care system is an important public health objective (Lohr, 1990). The lessons of history confirm that the medical factors that have prompted medical malpractice litigation still continue as advocated in the public interest: scientific innovation, uniform standards, and liability insurance (Gostin, 2000).

From a legal perspective, government directly and indirectly (through tort law) regulates the health care system. Medical malpractice litigation ostensibly seeks higher-quality care. Tort law, on the other hand, functions to deter substandard medical conduct, to avoid unnecessary injury, and as a fair method of compensation. Several reform methods are currently under public debate; the most prominent among these proposals is capitation on damages. Although enacted in some states, this approach does not eliminate liability, it is proposed that such action would decrease fear of inordinate damage awards. It is commendable that the various medical organizations proceed with pressing for caps legislation, but at the same time, more of an effort should be made to press for court reform and legislative proposals possessing reasonable chance of successful passage in the next year (Post, Brady, McCaulley, & McGuire, 2004).

EMERGING STANDARD OF CARE IN PAIN MANAGEMENT AND LEGAL IMPLICATIONS

The rapidity of change in the clinical practice of medicine has brought frustration because of decreased autonomy, increased oversight, pressures on reimbursement, and allegations of fraud and abuse. Malpractice and legal complications of care have increased. Despite the widespread promulgation of the benefits of opioid analgesics in all types of pain states — acute, chronic, and malignant — fear and trepidation remain on the part of prescribing

TABLE 92.3
Key Points Included in the Controlled Substances Act

- Opioids are necessary to public health.
- A mechanism is devised for external medical input.
- Drug availability is guaranteed.
- The federal definition of an addict does not include the patient with chronic pain.
- Regulations specifically recognize the treatment of intractable pain with opioids.
- Prescription size is not restricted.
- Without a special license granted by the DEA, physicians may not provide methadone maintenance for patients with known addiction to controlled substances.

physicians. The Uniform Controlled Substance Act of 1970 provides for the registration of those handling controlled substances, as well as for labeling, order forms, record keeping, and reporting of substances or their use. Key points included in the Controlled Substances Act are listed in Table 92.3 (Clark, 1998).

The issues of safety, efficacy, and compliance associated with most statutes are based on the 1970 Model Uniform Controlled Substances Act. It is the intricacies and interrelationships between federal and state laws regulating the prescribing of opioid analgesics that have been repeatedly identified as one of the more significant barriers to the provision of effective pain management and palliative care. The barriers to pain management provide plausible reasons for so many patients to experience undertreated pain. Collectively, these barriers have either contributed to or caused an enduring epidemic of pain and suffering trailing in the wake of untreated pain (Rich, 2000). Patient-related barriers to good pain management also exist. The general public is ignorant and fearful of opioid analgesics, and reluctant to be viewed as too demanding of more in the way of care than has been proffered. Laypersons can hardly be more sophisticated and knowledgeable about an emerging aspect of clinical medical practice than health care professionals (Cleeland, 1992). In 1996, an international panel of distinguished health care professionals assembled by the Hastings Center (1996) identified the goals of medicine as follows:

- The prevention of disease and injury and promotion and maintenance of health
- The relief of pain and suffering caused by maladies
- The care and cure of those with a malady, and the care of those who cannot be cured
- The avoidance of premature death and the pursuit of a peaceful death

The stated goals strike a remarkable balance between the *curative* and the *palliative* approaches to patient care and are the hegemony of the curative model that is the hallmark of modern medical education and practice reflects a medical ethos inconsistent with the core values of medicine (Rich, 2000).

EMERGING LIABILITY ISSUES IN THE MANAGEMENT OF PAIN

It is argued that there are three essential duties of a health care professional regarding pain management:

1. The first duty is to minimize iatrogenic (physician-induced) pain; no further pain and suffering are to be inflicted upon a patient beyond the unavoidable consequence of a reasonable effort to effect a cure (Edwards, 1984).

2. The second duty is to be a competent practitioner in pain management. Effective application of state-of-the-art pain relief techniques is required to relieve as much pain as possible without imposition of patient burden that exceeds benefits. This is a duty that can reasonably be placed on all physicians who care for patients in pain and not one reserved for pain or palliative care specialists only. It is time for those physicians who are most likely to see chronically ill patients in the first line of duty (general practitioners, oncologists) to make pain control and palliative care a part of routine clinical practice (Stjernsward et al., 1996)

3. The third duty is to adequately inform the patient of the risks and benefits of alternative pain management strategies, including that of not pursuing pain relief (Emanuel, 1996).

Additionally, physicians have a duty to continue their education throughout their professional lives to maintain their practices consistent with current advances in science and technology.

The issue of whether physicians should be insulated from ethical and legal responsibility for undertreating pain due to deficiency in this area of medical education was in seemingly direct contradiction to the AMA Principles of Medical Ethics and the current opinion of the AMA on Professional Rights and Responsibilities (AMA, 1996).

There is a developing health care professional consensus that failure either to manage effectively pain that can be managed or to refer the patient to a professional who can bring state-of-the-art techniques to bear on the problem constitutes a breach of professional ethics and a departure from an emerging standard of care (Oherney & Catane, 1995). The concept of the patient's legal right to effective pain management and the correlative duty on the part of physicians, because of their virtual monopoly on

---

TABLE 92.4
Liability Issues in Pain Management

Liability to Patients
- For cost-containment practices that affect pain management (Townsend, 1983)
- For inappropriate pain management (*Bergman v. Eden Med. Ctr. et al., No. H205732-1 Sup. Ct. Alameda Co., Cal. 2001*)

Liability to Third Parties
- For injury caused by patients treated for pain (Heller, 1992; Vainio, 1995; *Wilchinsky v. Medina*, 775 P.2d 713 [NM 1989])

---

the authority to prescribe narcotics to provide effective pain management to patients, has begun to emerge in the last decade (Table 92.4).

One of the first serious discussions on poor pain management as an example of medical malpractice was conducted by Margaret Sommerville, a Canadian legal scholar and bioethicist. With the prevailing standard of care, it is argued that, because it is abundantly clear that physicians traditionally fail to alleviate pain, a patient would find it difficult to establish undertreatment of pain as a departure from the applicable standard of care (Sommerville, 1986). The failure of the medical profession to adopt and consistently apply readily available therapeutic modalities that would improve patient care presents precisely a situational scenario ripe for judicial standard setting. With deficiencies in prevailing custom and practice of medicine so clearly inconsistent with the traditionally attributable goal, the medical profession appears negligent (The T.J. Hooper, 60 F.2d 737.740 [2d Circ. 1932]).

A primary impetus for the promulgation of clinical practice guidelines for pain assessment and management has been the demonstration, through recent studies, that many health care professionals lack, or fail to apply, basic knowledge and skills in this area. A declaration that "not relieving pain brushes dangerously close to the act of willfully inflicting it" has become one of the strongest statements recorded from an objective, nonclinician perspective (Morris, 1991, p. 134). The willful infliction of pain is torture, which is foreclosed to the government by the Eighth Amendment to the U.S. Constitution, as "cruel and unusual" even in punishment of convicted criminals.

TOWARD A NEWER MEDICAL MODEL

Inadequate pain control appears to be the spur for increased interest in physician-assisted suicide, but one reason for inadequate pain management is an unfounded concern of both patients and health care providers that pain control is a form of euthanasia. Euthanasia refers to the intentional act of painlessly putting to death persons with incurable and distressing disease as an act of mercy

(*Black's Law Dictionary*, 1979). Appropriate pain management aims to reduce suffering, not cause death.

In January 1998, Kirk Robinson, president, and Kathryn Tucker, director of legal affairs, for the Oregon-based organization Compassion in Dying Federation (CIDF) sent a memorandum to every medical board in the United States arguing that dying patients have a right to adequate pain medications. Although the focus of the memorandum was end-of-life care, it outlined a series of steps for each state board to follow in addressing the perceived risks for overprescribing controlled substances and the absence of any risk real or imagined for underprescribing medications to any patient experiencing pain. The idea that state medical boards should take on the responsibility of scrutinizing licensees for inadequate pain care was urged, as well as the adoption of underprescribing as a ground for discipline. Additionally, the CIDF put all boards on public notice that it was willing to assist patients suffering chronic pain and their families in making complaints and/or in filing suits against practitioners who failed to provide adequate pain relief through underprescribing.

In July 1994, the California Medical Board (1994a) issued a formal statement on "Prescribing Controlled Substances for Pain Management." The board stated that "principles of quality medical practice dictate that citizens of California who suffer from pain should be able to obtain the relief that is currently available" and that "pain management should be a high priority in California." Concomitantly, the board issued "Guidelines for Prescribing Controlled Substances for Intractable Pain," which included the following admonition: "The Board strongly urges physicians to view pain management as a priority in all patients. Pain should be assessed and treated promptly, effectively and for as long as the pain persists. The medical management of pain should be based on up-to-date knowledge about pain, pain assessment, and pain treatment" (Medical Board of California, 1994a).

The legal theory of negligence in medication error lawsuits can be applied to cases claiming inappropriate management of pain (Frank-Stromborg and Christiansen, 2000). In any allegation of inappropriate pain management, the patient (plaintiff) must prove:

- That a duty of care was owed to the patient by the defendant (health care professional),
- That duty owed was breached with conduct that violated a standard of care recognized in the profession,
- That breach of the duty owed was the cause of injury or the suffering, and
- The patient (plaintiff) suffered damages as a result (Keeton, Dobbs, Keeton, & Owen, 1984).

In cases involving pain control, the professional will be judged according to the expectation of what a reason-able practitioner would have done in similar circumstances (Willis, 1998). In general, the standard of medical care a physician may with reason and fairness be expected to possess is that commonly possessed or reasonably available to minimally competent physicians in the same specialty or general field of practice throughout the United States. A physician should have a realistic understanding of the limitations of his or her knowledge or competence and, in general, exercise minimally adequate medical judgment (*Hall v. Hilbun,* 466 So. 856, 871 [Miss. 1985]). In litigation, the appropriate specialist is located to provide information through testimony about the standard of care and any deviation from such standard. A minority of jurisdictions take the position that adherence to customary practice should not insulate a physician from malpractice liability if the patient (plaintiff) can provide persuasive evidence that the physician failed or refused to apply readily available measures that would have prevented harm to the patient. The Wisconsin Supreme Court stated that should customary medical practice fail to keep pace with developments and advances in medical science, adherence to custom might constitute a failure to exercise ordinary care (*Nowatske v. Osterlok,* 543 N.W. 2d 254 [Wis. 1996]). Adherence to custom is not the sole test of professional malpractice (*Toth v. Cmty. Hosp.,* At Glen Cove, 239 N.E. 2d 368,373 [N.Y. 1968]). The notion that an entire medical specialty (*Helling v. Carey,* 519 P.2d 981 [Washington, 1974]), or at least all the members of a particular locale, would never be guilty of negligence by adhering to a substandard of care fell to a Louisiana appellate court statement: "We are firm in the opinion that it is patently absurd, unreasonable, and arbitrary to hold that immunity from tort liability may be predicated upon a degree of care or procedure amounting to negligence, notwithstanding such procedure is generally followed by other members of the profession in good standing in the same community" (*Favalora v. Aetna Cas. & Sur. Co.* 144 So.2d 544, 551 [La. Ct. App. 1962]).

Most lawsuits brought by patients against health care providers are for medical malpractice, which is defined as a breach of accepted medical practice resulting in injury and legally recognized damage to the patient. Courts are now willing to hold physicians liable for allowing a patient to suffer because of a failure to provide appropriate pain relief under the recognition of improper pain management as a breach of good and acceptable practice. A medical malpractice judgment exceeding $1 million against the Veterans Administration included an award of $125,000 for pain and suffering predicated largely upon the defendants' failure to provide sufficient pain medication in the final days of the patient's life (*Gaddis v. United States,* 7F. Supp. 2d 709 [D.SC. 1997]). The primary claim and bulk of the total award for damages in this South Carolina case were based on a failure to timely and properly diagnose and treat the patient's throat cancer.

In California, William Bergman, a man in his early 80s, wrenched his back pulling a battery out of a car. Over the next few days he developed more and more back pain, which was originally thought to be a strain-sprain until the patient became immobilized due to the pain (Tucker, 2000). He was taken to the emergency room of a northern California hospital whereupon he was hospitalized for severe pain in his back with a diagnostic finding of metastatic lung cancer. The patient indicated he wished no treatment for his cancer but wished only to receive pain medication that would allow him to return to his home and functionality for what time he had left. Dr. Wing Chin became Mr. Bergman's assigned physician for his hospitalization. The patient was reported by nursing staff to have increasing VAS ratings despite receiving meperidine on an as-needed (prn) order for pain relief based on patient request. Bergman was subsequently discharged to his home with the oral pain medication, hydrocodone and acetaminophen (APAP). Meperidine is inadequate for cancer pain relief and is inappropriate for use in the aged due to nervous system toxicity that may develop as a side effect of metabolite formulation. Morphine agents are appropriate for cancer pain relief. Oral hydrocodone and APAP are indicated for moderate to moderately severe pain. Pain medication for cancer pain relief should be give at specific times, not on an as-needed (prn) basis. Dr. Chin was called regarding Mr. Bergman's pain after discharge from the hospital and when asked about morphine agents for pain relief, the family was told that he (Dr. Chin) did not possess the required multiple prescription form pad to order these pharmaceuticals for patient use. After 2 days at home in what was described as "agonizing pain," a hospice nurse succeeded in contacting William Bergman's regular physician, who immediately administered oral morphine achieving pain relief. Mr. Bergman died comfortably the next day.

Mr. Bergman's daughter (Beverly Bergman) was so disturbed by her father's suffering that she made formal complaint, supported by independent expert opinion, to the Medical Board of California (MBC), that the pain care provided to an elderly, terminally ill patient with cancer was inadequate. California is among the most progressive states in attempting to improve pain care. In 1994, the MBC (1994b) adopted official guidelines on pain management, which specifically identifies failure to adequate, manage pain as "inappropriate prescribing." The MBC expressly recognized that this is a form of professional misconduct, subject to the full range of sanctions.

The MBC agreed with Beverly Bergman that the physician had failed to provide adequate pain care but declined to take any action against the physician (MBC Letter, 1998). It was not until after the MBC conclusion that a formal complaint was filed.

In February 1999, what appears to be the first suit filed against a physician, grounded primarily on failure to properly manage a patient's pain, was filed in Superior Court of California (*Bergman v. Eden Med. Ctr. et al., No. H205732-1* [*Sup. Ct. Alameda Co., Cal. 2001*]). Cases of inadequate pain treatment may result in civil liability (tort cases) with significant financial implications. The unusual aspect of the *Bergman* case was that a cause of action under the California Elder Abuse Statute was included, which provided for heightened remedies to what would not be available under a medical malpractice claim, including awarding punitive damages, no cap on damages, and paying attorney's fees. The defendant physician and hospital agreed that the family was entitled only to the limited remedies available in a malpractice claim and repeatedly disputed the elder abuse cause of action, and petitioned for it to be dismissed. In January 2000, the court ruled against dismissal of the elder abuse claims, recognizing that inadequate pain care can constitute elder abuse. In 2001, the case was tried before a state court jury in California where the sole claim was failure of the physician to adequately treat the pain of an elderly main dying of a painful form of lung cancer. The plaintiff's lawyers succeeded in demonstrating that the physician had little concept of the body of authoritative literature governing pain management, and had not stayed current with the many developments in the field since graduation from medical school some 30 years prior to the time of this trial and treatment of the patient. It was further shown that he had used outmoded and discredited strategies and the patient suffered unnecessarily during his final week of life as a result. The jury hearing the case determined that the physician's conduct was reckless. Under the elder abuse cause of action, plaintiffs were required to prove reckless, as apposed to simply negligent, conduct. This heavy burden was apparently carried successfully and the family of the deceased, Mr. Bergman, was awarded $1.5 million for the patient's pain and suffering under the State Elder Abuse Statute (*Bergman v. Eden Med. Ctr. et al., No. H205732-1* [*Sup. Ct. Alameda Co., Cal. 2001*]). Kathryn Tucker, Esq., director of legal affairs for the Compassion in Dying Federation, explained that a successful trial meant the Bergman family would be able to recover significant damages and as exposure for inadequate pain care becomes more significant, providers will be more motivated to attend and treat pain properly under exposure to significantly greater financial risk (Albert, 2001).

Dying patients clearly have the right to adequate pain medication; this was recently recognized by the Supreme Court of the United States (Burt, 1997; *Vacco v. Quill,* 521 U.S. 793 [1997]; *Washington v. Glucksberg,* 521 U.S. 702 [1997]). The duty of a physician when treating a patient experiencing pain associated with a terminal illness is to inform the patient of the possible treatment options from management of the pain and the anticipated side effects of any such treatment including having no treatment at all, and to permit the patient to make an informed choice about the treatment. Increasing dosage of strong pain medication such as morphine may have a foreseeable but unintended consequence of suppressing respiration and possibly advancing time of death. The "double effect" is accepted in medical ethics and practice and has been endorsed by the U.S. Supreme Court. Whether to accept the double effect risk of medication must be the patient's choice, not an imposition by a paternalistic physician (*Washington v. Glucksberg*, 521 U.S. 702 [1997]). A second recent case resulted in a negotiated out-of-court settlement of damages apparently using leverage from the *Bergman v. Eden Med. Ctr.* case.

Illustrative of the law's recognition that assurance of comfort and appropriate pain control are integral components of appropriate medical care is the case *State v. McAfee,* 385 S.E. 2d 651 (Ga. 1989). Mr. McAfee, a quadriplegic who was incapable of spontaneous respiration, sought court approval for discontinuation of his respirator. The Georgia Supreme Court affirmed the patient's right to refuse medical treatment and held that he was also entitled to have a sedative administered at the time of discontinuation of the respirator. That Mr. McAfee had the right to be free from pain at the time the ventilator is disconnected is inseparable from his right to refuse medical treatment. The record shows that Mr. McAfee had attempted, in the past, to discontinue his ventilator, but has been unable to do so due to the severe pain he suffered when deprived of oxygen. His right to have a sedative (a medication that in no way causes or accelerates death) administered before the ventilator was discontinued is a part of his right to control his medical treatment. The implication flowing from this court's ruling was that providers may be held accountable for not providing such measures (Shapiro, 1994).

In a North Carolina negligence lawsuit, a health care facility was held liable for the first time for failure to treat serious pain appropriately (*Estate of Henry James v. Hillhaven Corp.* No. 89 Civ. 65 [Hertford County Superior Ct. N.C. Nov. 20, 1990]). Henry James, 74 years of age, a retired house painter, was diagnosed with cancer of the prostate for which he was subjected to removal of his testicles. The cancer, however, was metastatic in nature, having spread to his leg and spine. His pain was severe and excruciating. He was place in a nursing home in February 1987. Almost at once, the nursing staff began cutting his prescription pain medications by giving him on some days mild headache-related medicines, placebo substituted for morphine, or nothing at all. The nursing supervisor explained to the family that Mr. James was in danger of becoming a drug addict and because Mr. James and his family were Medicare and Medicaid recipients, she did not like her tax dollars supporting his drug habit. Eventually, Mr. James became irritable, withdrawn, and bedfast, where he laid sweating and moaning in pain,

dying 4 months later. His family eventually filed a complaint with a state regulatory agency and went to court.

On November 20, 1990, the verdict was that the nursing home had been negligent in failing to provide Mr. James adequate pain relief. At the trial, Catherine Faison, James's great niece, explained that as far as the nursing home was concerned, when he died, it was a closed issue; it was over. "It's not over for me," Faison told the jury. "I can't sleep at night when I think about the fact that he had to lay over there and suffer.... I think about him laying there hurting, saying I want my medication, and not being able to get it. I don't want to suffer like that.... I don't think anybody would. Somebody needs to say you can't do it."

Safe harbor provisions in intractable pain legislation enacted in many states grant immunity from discipline to physicians who treat intractable pain. These enactments clarify the position that physicians shall not be disciplined for treating intractable pain with large doses of medication, even if such prescriptions hasten the moment of the patient's death, as long as the intent is simply to alleviate pain. Such provisions are designed to clear the confusion that may occur because of the similarity with prescribing medications to end a patient's life.

In 1999, the Oregon Board of Medical Examiners disciplined a physician for the undertreatment of a patient's intractable pain. Dr. Paul Bilder, an Oregon pulmonary specialist, was disciplined for a pattern of failing to treat pain adequately (Goodman, 1999). The physician was reported to have undertreated patients as follows (Mascheri, 1999):

1. Tylenol was used to treat the musculoskeletal pain of an elderly male patient with cancer, denying requests for stronger medications when pain increased. He also denied a nurse's request for catheterization, citing a risk of infection. The patient died the next day.

2. He removed a catheter from an 84-year-old man against the patient's and family's requests, directing that he instead use diapers. He further reduced a hospice nurse's requested dose of 5 to 20 mg of Roxanol every 4 hours to 0.25 cc and gave Tylenol to treat the patient's 102° temperature. The patient died that evening.

3. He refused a request for sedatives and pain control for a 35-year-old intubated, mechanically ventilated woman who became increasingly restless, had increased wheezing, and was fighting the ventilator. After the patient extubated herself, the doctor ordered a paralytic agent but no sedative following reintubation.

4. He used physical restraint to intubate a 33-year-old man without using anxiolytics or narcotics. The patient had been admitted with severe

pneumonia associated with hypoxemia. The physician, it is claimed by the board, engaged in "unprofessional or dishonorable conduct" and "gross negligence or repeated negligence," according to a stipulated order released by the board. While the physician will not lose his license, this is the first time a state board has taken this type of action.

Thus, in addition to potential liability to patients for inappropriate pain management, professional discipline of health care professionals also may ensue. As a result of development and growing acceptance of pain management guidelines, medical boards may be more inclined in the future to undertake disciplinary action for inadequate pain management.

Increased use of advanced directives resulting from passage of the Federal Patient Self-Determination Act (effective December 1, 1991) also may increase physicians' exposure to professional discipline for inappropriate pain management (Patient Self-Determination Act, 42 U.S.C. § 1395 cc [1990]).

In the interests of sustaining protection, physicians are advised to honor appropriate pain management instructions set forth in patients' advanced directives. Where questions or concerns arise about complying with such pain management instruction, ethics committees should be consulted (Shapiro, 1994).

Appropriate pain management aims to reduce suffering, not cause death. When physicians deliberately administer lethal doses of medications — even for reasons of compassion — they risk prosecution for homicide, and when lethal doses of medications are prescribed, they risk prosecution for assisting suicide.

Investigations of physicians for alleged excessive prescribing of pain medication reduce physician willingness to treat pain with strong pain medication prescriptions. This is one factor contributing to the problem of undertreatment of pain. During the past few years, aggressive educational efforts have begun to correct the undertreatment of pain and other physical suffering in dying patients — a major failing in medical care (Noble, 1999).

Historically, to date, only the state of Oregon has passed a law permitting physician-assisted dying (Or. Rev. Stat §§ 127.800 to 127.897, 1996). Opponents made many attempts to defeat the Oregon Death With Dignity Act (ODWDA). The same opponents then sought in two successive sessions of Congress to amend the Controlled Substances Act of 1970, ("CSA") 21 U.S.C. §§ 801–904 and expand the scope of it to reach the ODWDA to destroy it through the Lethal Drug Abuse Prevention Act of 1998 and the Pain Relief Promotion Act of 1999 (PRPA).

Both the proposed acts failed due to strong opposition from the medical community, based on the concern that the proposed measures would exacerbate physicians' fears

regarding use of controlled substances for pain management (Orentlicher & Caplan, 2000). Under the Bush Administration, Attorney General John Ashcroft issued a directive on November 6, 2001 (*Ashcroft Directive* 66 Fed. Reg. 56.607 [Nov. 9, 2001]), the latest Federal government attempt to attack and destroy the Oregon Death With Dignity Act. The *Ashcroft Directive* was challenged in Federal Court by the State of Oregon, an Oregon physician and pharmacist, and a group of terminally ill Oregonians, who asserted that the Ashcroft Directive violates the CSA (Controlled Substances Act), the APA (Administrative Procedure Act), and the U.S. Constitution. *Oregon v. Ashcroft,* 368 F.3d 1118 (9th Cir. 2004), *aff'g.* 192 F. Supp. 2d 1077, 1092 (D.Or. 2002), *cert. granted sub nom. Gonzales v. Oregon, 73 U.S.L.W. 3298* (U.S. February 22, 2005) (No. 04-623). Among the most important findings emerging from the data from the Oregon Legalized Practice of Assisted Dying is the clear evidence that the availability of the option for assisted dying serves as a catalyst for improved end-of-life care and specifically for improved pain care. Some religious organizations and right-to-life activists continue to obstruct and seek to nullify legislative reform although even staunch opponents of the practice of assisted dying increasingly recognize that continued opposition cannot be justified in the light of Oregon experience (Tucker, 2004).

A significant opportunity exists for medical boards at the state level to take a leadership role in the proper treatment of pain and become a viable and reliable resource in both the legal and the medical communities. Instead of enacting more statutes, efforts should be directed toward adoption of "informed guidelines" or "policy statements" by medical boards to address the proper treatment of pain and legitimate use of opioids.

Physician fear of prosecution or investigation continues to be a barrier to pain relief in our present society even though social science literature indicates the likelihood and frequency of prosecution or investigation is extremely low with overall prosecution surrounding the prescription of opioids being found to be rare (Ziegler & Lovrich, 2003). The use of opioids in the management of pain is a legitimate and recognized protocol in medicine with a rate of addiction that is really quite low. Both law and medicine recognize that patients have a right to adequate pain care. Doctors who prescribe opioids for extended periods are acting well within the professional practice of medicine, and in fact, the frequency, amount, and chronicity of opioid prescriptions are not particularly indicative of inappropriate treatment protocols. Without considering the individual patient, the aspect of dispensing practice is not determinative of abuse or diversion.

Pain is one of the most common reasons for seeking medical care, yet it is often inadequately treated. Pain is dehumanizing, a destroyer of autonomy, and humiliating. In its extreme, pain has the capacity to destroy the soul and all will to live (Post, Blustein, Gordon, & Dubler, 1996). Untreated, the pain accompanying illnesses slows recovery, severely impairs an individual's quality of life, and adds significantly to the health care system's financial burden. The Joint Commission on Accreditation of Healthcare Organizations (JCAHO) standards (the new evidence-based pain management standards introduced by JCAHO) (Phillips, 2000) assert that individuals seeking care at accredited hospitals, behavioral health facilities, and health care networks have the right to appropriate assessment and management of pain. All patients are to be screened to characterize their pain by location, intensity, and cause, including a detailed history, physical examination, psychosocial assessment, and diagnosis evaluation. The most reliable indicator of pain existence and intensity is the patient's self-report because it is more accurate than others' observations. These standards do not dictate specific pain management procedures nor advocate in any way the use of certain drugs (e.g., opioids).

Debilitating pain has reached epidemic proportions in the United States. Many physicians nevertheless fear that dispensing opioid medications for patients suffering from pain will result in negative patient outcomes; heightened scrutiny from medical licensing boards, county prosecutors, and federal government; or may promote iatrogenic addiction, despite the fact that the documented rate of addiction in patients using opioids is extremely low. Chronic pain is notably undertreated and the amount of opioids clinically indicated for each patient suffering from pain is highly individualistic. Dosage awarded for one patient suffering from chronic pain or for a patient in an end-of-life situation may be wholly inappropriate for another patient.

A discussion of the emerging standards and guidelines (Jacox, Carr, & Payne, 1994), coupled with developing disciplinary and legal consequences to mold physician action and "standardize" delivery of medical care utilizing the fulcrum of "inadequate pain management" as "inappropriate medical care," appears designed to move physicians into fungible units in need of surveillance to assure compliance with all controlling legal authority. During the past 30 years, the ethics of the medical care in the United States has changed radically from a traditional paradigm of the largely paternalistic doctor decision making of what is medically appropriate to a present form of governing ethic, which is totally anti-paternalistic in nature. Legal scholars, bioethicists, physicians, and judges have made a powerful case for patient autonomy and have objected to paternalistic medicine on the grounds that it supplants patient values and patient preferences with those of the provider. In the treatment of pain, a physician is not limited to prescribing levels that appear in the package insert or in the *Physician's Desk Reference*,

and a physician who is authorized to prescribe opioids may do so as long as they are for a legitimate medical purpose and the physician observes the procedures of good medical practice (Cole, 1998).

The key to distinguishing between aggressive palliative care and euthanasia remains one of intent. Intent often escapes exacting proof. Recent attempts at legislation in the area of opioid use in terminally ill patients have been unsuccessful in part because opponents to that legislation had extreme concerns regarding the difficulty in the determination of intent. Through all the sophisticated advances in medical technology and disease management, bioethical discourse is framed in terms of balancing the values and interests with the benefits and burdens that underpin principled decisions about how, when, and whether intervention should occur. Despite all these advances, one mandate remains constant and compelling for physicians, and that is the relief of pain.

When cure is impossible, the physicians' duty of care includes palliation with the centrality of this obligation being both unquestioned and universal, transcending time and cultural boundaries. Treatment of pain is supported by the ethical principle of "double effect." Under this principle a good effect, "relief of suffering," may overcome a foreseeable bad effect, "causing death," as long as the physician did not intend to accomplish the bad effect. It is fair to say that this ethic is now one of medical custom and standard practice. The U.S. Supreme Court has endorsed this ethical principle and may have even created a defense to prosecution should a terminally ill patient die during pain medication administration with palliative care. *Vacco v. Quill,* 521 U.S. 793, 1997.

The centrality, universality, and transcendent obligation of the physician is to adhere to the core values of medicine: (1) to cure if possible; (2) to relieve suffering always. This mandate to relieve pain is as compelling and constant today as it has been throughout history, despite dialectical transvaluation of values so prevalent today. Pain remains, even now, an untestable hypothesis (Rich, 2004).

REFERENCES

Agency for Health Care Policy and Research. (1992). *Acute pain management guideline panel. Acute pain management: operative or medical procedures and trauma.* Pub. No. 92-0032. Washington, DC: U.S. Department of Health and Human Services.

Albert, T. (2001, July 23). Dr. guilty of elder abuse for under treating pain. *American Medical News.*

Ashcroft Directive. 66 Fed. Reg. 56, 607 (Nov. 9, 2001).

Bergman v. Eden Medical Center. (2001, June 13). No. H205732-1 Cal. Sup. Ct., Alameda Cty.

Bernabei, R., Gambassi, G., Lapane, K. et al. (1998). Management of pain in elderly patients with cancer. SAGE Study Group. Systematic assessment of geriatric drug use via epidemiology. *Journal of the American Medical Association, 279*, 1877–1882.

Black, H. C. (1979). *Black's law dictionary* (5th ed.). St. Paul, MN: West Publishing.

Bostrom, B. M., Ramberg, T., Davis, B. D., & Fridlund, B. (1997). Survey of post-operative patients' pain management. *Journal of Nursing Management, 5*, 341–349.

Burt, R. A. (1997). The Supreme Court speaks: Not assisted suicide but a constitutional right to palliative care. *New England Journal of Medicine, 337*, 1234–1236.

Calonge, N. (2000). Processes and targets for improving the quality of healthcare. *Preventative Medicine and Managed Care, 1*(3), 149–152.

Carr, D. B. (1998). Clinical pain management guidelines. *Emergency Medicine, 30* (45), S2–S6.

Carr, D. B., Jacox, A. K., Chapman, C. R. et al. (1992). *Acute pain management: Operative or medical procedures and trauma. Clinical practice guideline.* AHCPR Pub. No. 92-0032. Rockville, MD: Agency for Health Care Policy and Research, Public Health Service, U.S. Department of Health and Human Services.

Chasin, M. F., & Galvin, R. W. (1998). The National Roundtable on Health Care Quality: The urgent need to improve healthcare quality. *Journal of the American Medical Association, 280*, 1000–1005.

Cheville, A. L. (2001). Pain management and cancer rehabilitation. *Archives of Physical and Medical Rehabilitation, 82*(Suppl. 1), S84–S87.

Clark, H. W. (1998). Legal implications of prescribing opioid controlled substances. *Emergency Medicine, 30*(45), S29–S33.

Cleeland, C. S. (1992). Documenting barriers to cancer pain management. *Current and Emerging Issues in Cancer Pain: Research and Practice, 321*, 325–327.

Cleeland, C. S., Gonin, R., Baez, L., Loehrer, P., & Pandya, K. J. (1997). Pain and treatment of pain in minority patients with cancer. The Eastern Cooperative Oncology Group Minority Outpatient Study. *Annals of Internal Medicine, 127*, 813–816.

Cole, B. E. (1998). Ten tips to survive opioid prescribing. *The Pain Practitioner, 8*(4), 4.

Controlled Substances Act of 1970, 21 U.S.C. §§ 801–904.

Dahlman, G. B., Dykes, A. K., & Elander, G. (1999). Patients' evaluation of pain and nurses' management of analgesics after surgery. The effect of a study day on the subject of pain for nurses working in the thorax surgery department. *Journal of Advanced Nursing, 30*, 866–874.

Ebell, M. H., Siwek, J. et al. (2004). Simplifying the language of evidence to improve patient care. *Journal of Family Practice 53*(2), 111–120.

Edwards, R. B. (1984). Pain and the ethics of pain management. *Society of Science and Medicine, 18*, 515–517.

Emanuel, E. J. (1996). Pain and symptom control: Patient rights and physician responsibilities. *Hematology and Oncology Clinics of North America, 10*, 41–47.

Estate of Henry James v. Hillhaven Corp. No. 89 65 (Hertford County Superior Ct. N.C. Nov. 20, 1990).

Favalora v. Aetna Cs. and Sur. Co. (1962). 144 So.2d 544, 551 (La. Ct. App.).

Federation of State Medical Boards of the United States, Inc. (1998). *Model guidelines for the use of controlled substances for the treatment of pain.* Euless, TX: Author.

Federation of State Medical Boards of the United States, Inc. (2004, July). Model guidelines for the use of controlled substances for the treatment of pain. Retrieved from http://www.medsch.isc.edu/painpolicy/domestic/model.htm.

Foley, K. M. (1997). Management of cancer pain. In V. T. De Vita, S. Hellman, & S. Rosenberg (Eds.). *Cancer: Principles and practice of oncology* (5th ed., pp. 2807–2841). Philadelphia: Lippincott-Raven Press.

Foley, K. (2000). Controlling cancer pain [Review]. *Hospital Practice* H. (Off Ed). *35*(4), 101–108, 111–112.

Frank-Stromborg, M., & Christiansen, A. (2000). The undertreatment of pain: A liability risk for nurses. *Clinical Journal of Oncology Nursing, 4*(1), 41–44.

Gaddis v. United States. 7 F. Supp. 2d 709 (D.S.C. 1997).

Gallup, Inc. (1999, June 9). *Pain in America: Highlights from a Gallup survey.*

Glanelli, D. M. (1999, February 8). Opioid prescriptions rarely lead to rebuke, study finds. *AMA News* (Professional Issues).

Goff, D. C., Canely, L. K., & Gu, L. (2000). Increasing the appropriate use of reductase inhibitors among patients with coronary heart disease enrolled in a network — Model managed care organization. *Preventative Medicine and Managed Care, 1*, 141–148.

Goodman, E. (1999, September 11). *Charlotte Observer.*

Gostin, L. (2000). A public approach to reducing error, medical malpractice as a barrier. *Journal of the American Medical Association, 283*, 1742–1743.

Guglielmo, W. J. (2000, February 21). Can doctors put their fears to rest? *Medical Economics*, 47–59.

Hall v. Hilbun, 466 So. 856 (Miss. 1985).

Hastings Center International Project. (1996, November–December). The goals of medicine: Setting new priorities. *Hastings Center Report*, S1.

Heller, M. B. (1992, August 3). Emergency management of acute pain: New options and strategies. *Postgraduate Medicine*, 39–47.

Helling v. Carey, 519 P.2d 981 (Washington, 1974).

Hill, C. S. (1993). The negative influence of licensing and disciplinary boards and drug enforcement agencies in pain with opioid analgesics. *Journal of Pharmacology Care and Pain Symptom Control, 1*, 43–62.

Hill, C. S., Jr. (1995). When will adequate pain treatment be the norm? *Journal of the American Medical Association, 274*, 1881–1882.

Hill, C. S., Jr. (1996a). Adequate pain treatment: A challenge for medical regulatory boards [Editorial]. *Journal of the Florida Medical Association, 83*, 677–678.

Hill, C. S., Jr. (1996b). Government regulatory influences on opioid prescribing and their impact on the treatment of pain of nonmalignant origin. *Journal of Pain and Symptom Management, 11*, 287–298.

Hooper, T. J. (1932). 60 F.2d 737, 740 (2d Cir.).

Jacox, A., Carr, D. B., & Payne R. (1994). New clinical practice guidelines for the management of pain in patients with cancer. *New England Journal of Medicine, 330,* 651–655.

Jacox, A., Carr, D. B., Payne, R., Berde, C. B., Biebart, W., Cain, J. M. et al. Guideline panel. (1994). *Management of cancer pain. Clinical practice guideline number 9.* AHCPR Publication No. 94-0592. Rockville, MD: Agency for Health Care Policy and Research, U.S. Department of Health and Human Services, Public Health Service.

James, G. (2000). Addressing barriers to healthcare for our elderly. *Family Physician Journal of American College of Osteopathic Family Practice, 4*(9), 9–13.

Joranson, D. E. (1992). Opioids for chronic cancer and non-cancer pain: A survey of state medical board members. *Federation Bulletin. Journal of Medical Licensure and Discipline, 9,* 15.

Keeton, W., Dobbs, D. B., Keeton, R. E., & Owen, D. G. (1984). *Prosser and Keeton on the law of torts.* St. Paul, MN: West Publishing.

King, K. M., Bungard, T. J., McAlister, F. A. et al. (2000). For the CQIN investigators. Quality improvement for CQI. *Preventative Medicine and Managed Care, 1,* 129–137.

Lavies, N., Hart, L., Rounsefell, B., & Runciman, W. (1992). Identification of patient, medical and nursing staff attitudes to postoperative opioid analgesia: Stage I of a longitudinal study of postoperative analgesia. *Pain, 48,* 313–319.

Leape, L. L. (1992). Unnecessary surgery. *Annual Review of Public Health, 13,* 363–383.

Leape, L. L. (1994). Error in medicine. *Journal of the American Medical Association, 272,* 1851–1857.

Lohr, K. N. (Ed.) (1990). Management of postoperative pain: Review of current techniques and methods. *Mayo Clinic Proceedings, 65,* 584–596.

Martino, A. M. (1998). In search of a new ethic for treating patients with chronic pain: What can medical boards do? *Journal of Law and Medical Ethics, 26,* 332–349.

Mascheri, L. L. (1999, September). Associate Director, State Government Affairs: Intractable Pain Legislation. AOA Division of State Government Affairs.

Medical Board of California (1994a, July 29). Guideline for prescribing controlled substances for intractable pain.

Medical Board of California Action Report 4 (1994b, October).

Medical Board of California (1998, August 19). Letter to Beverly Bergman. (States in pertinent part: "Our medical consultant did agree with you that pain management for your father was indeed inadequate.")

Morris, D. B. (1991). *The culture of pain.* Berkeley: University of California Press.

Morrison, J. M., & Wickersham, M. S. (1998). Physicians disciplined by a state medical board. *Journal of the American Medical Association, 279*(23), 1889–1893.

Noble, H. B. (1999, August 9). A shift in the treatment of chronic pain. *New York Times,* A13.

Nowatske v. Osterlok. (1996). 543 N.W.2d 265,2710272.

Nyquist, A. C., Gonzales, R., Steiner, J. R., & Sande, M. E. (1998). Antibiotic prescribing for children with colds, upper respiratory tract infections, and bronchitis. *Journal of the American Medical Association, 279,* 875–877.

Oherney, N. I., & Catane, R. (1995). Professional negligence in the management of cancer pain. *Cancer, 76,* 2181.

Ohio State Medical Association. (1999). Pain. The fifth vital sign. Retrieved from http://.osma.org.

Oregon v. Ashcroft, 368 F.3d 1118 (9th Cir. 2004) *aff'g.* 192 F. Supp. 2d 1077, 1092 (D. Or. 2002), *cert. granted sub nom. Gonzales v. Oregon,* 73 *U.S.L.W.* 3298 (U.S. February 22, 2005) (No. 04-623). 2002 appeal pending C No. 02-35587.

Oregon Death With Dignity Act, Or. Rev. Stat. §§ 127.800 to 127.897 (1996).

Orentlicher, D., & Caplan, A. (2000). The Pain Relief Promotion Act of 1999. A serious threat to palliative care. *Journal of the American Medical Association, 283*(2), 255–258.

Patient Self-Determination Act, 42 U.S.C. § 395 cc (1990).

Phillips, D. (2000). JCAHO pain management standards are unveiled. *Journal of the American Medical Association, 284,* 428–429.

Portenoy, R. K. (1996). Opioid therapy for chronic nonmalignant pain: Medication history review of the critical issue. *Journal of Pain and Symptom Management, 11,* 203–217.

Portenoy, R. K. (2000). *Contemporary diagnosis and management of pain in oncologic and AIDS patients* (3rd ed.). Newtown, PA: Handbooks in Healthcare.

Post, B. L., Brady, J. F., McCaulley, L. K., & McGuire, T. J. (2004, September). Are caps the only answer? Of course not! *Professional Casualty Association Update, 2.*

Post, L. F., Blustein, J., Gordon, E., & Dubler, N. N. (1996). Pain: Ethics, culture, and informed consent to relief. *Journal of Law, Medicine and Ethics. 24*(4), 348–359.

Rich, B. A. (2000). A prescription for the pain: The emerging standard of care for pain management. *Wm. Mitchell Law Review, 1,* 1–100.

Rich, B. A. (2004). *Emerging standards in pain management.* 44th Annual Conference American College of Legal Medicine.

Rorarius, M. G. F., & Baer, G. A. (1994). Non-steroidal anti-inflammatory drugs for postoperative pain relief. *Current Opinion in Anesthesiology, 7,* 358–362.

Shapiro, R. S. (1994). Legal bases for the control of analgesic drugs. *Journal of Pain and Symptom Management, 9,* 153–159.

Sommerville, M. A. (1986). Pain and suffering at the interfaces of medicine and law. *University of Toronto Law Journal, 36,* 286.

State v. McAfee, 385 S.E. 2d 651 (Ga. 1989).

Stjernsward, J. et al. (1996). The World Health Organization cancer pain and palliative care program: Past, present, and future. *Journal of Pain and Symptom Management, 12,* 65–68.

The T.J. Hooper, 60 F.2d 737 (2d Cir. 1932).

Toth v. Cmty. Hosp. At Glen Cove. 239 N. E. 2d 368 (N.Y. 1968).

Townsend, R. J., Spartz, M. E., Fahrenbruch, R. W. et al. (1983). Hospital labor cost savings in dispensing analgesics: Controlled vs. non-controlled. *Hospital Formulary, 18,* 716–720.

Tucker, K. L. (2000). Lecture notes. *On inadequate treatment of pain: Accountability.* American Academy of Pain Management 11th Annual Clinical Meeting.

Tucker, K. L. (2004, March). *The chicken and the egg: The pursuit of choice for a humane hastened-death as a catalyst for improved end-of-life care. A Precondition for Legalization of Assisted Dying.* 44th Annual Conference of the American College of Legal Medicine.

Vacco v. Quill, 521 U.S. 793 (1997).

Vainio, A., Ollila, J., Matikainen, E. et al. (1995). Driving ability in cancer patients receiving long-term morphine analgesia. *Lancet, 346,* 667–670.

Von Roenn, J. H., Cleeland, C. S., Gonin, R., Hartfield, A. K, & Pandya, K. J. (1993). *Annals of Internal Medicine, 119,* 121–126.

Washington v. Glucksberg, 521 U.S. 702 (1997).

Weiner, S. L. (1993). *Differential diagnosis of acute pain by body region.* New York: McGraw-Hill.

Willis, J. (1998). Should nurses start running from patients' complaints? *Nursing Times, 94* (15), 7–12.

World Health Organization. (1996). *Cancer pain relief* (2nd ed.) With a guide to opioid availability, cancer pain relief, and palliative care. Report WHO Expert Committee (WHO Technical Report Series, No. 804). Geneva, Switzerland: WHO.

Ziegler, S. J., & Lovrich, N. P. (2003). Pain relief, prescription drugs, and prosecution: A four-state survey of chief prosecutors. *Journal of Law, Medicine, and Ethics, 31*(1), 75–100.

93

Law Enforcement and Regulatory Issues

John Duncan, PhD

INTRODUCTION

The interface among physicians, regulatory boards, and law enforcement is a critical part of any practice; however, it takes on an added importance for practitioners working in the treatment of chronic pain. Specifically, many of the medications used to treat pain are also those most frequently abused and associated with drug addiction. Because of historical conflict between regulators and the practice of medicine, and the turn-of-the-century problems with iatrogenic addiction, careful consideration should be given to the role of developing shared understandings and overlapping consensus with regulators. In this chapter, the general features of this understanding are presented, as well as guidelines for both working with regulatory agencies and also staying out of trouble with them.

HISTORICAL CONSIDERATIONS

To understand the regulatory and legal landscape of opioid prescribing in the United States, it is important first to examine some of the more important historical occurrences that have led to and shaped current legal perspectives and attitudes, of both regulators and physicians. Against the backdrop of this historical context, it will become evident that the fear of iatrogenic addiction, a problem that was prevalent in the late 1800s in the United States, has been the chief inhibitory force in prescribing opioids for chronic pain. This stalwart attitude remains, however, even after years of research have shown that they can be used both effectively and without creating narcotic addicts. The law enforcement and regulatory challenge continues to address these concerns, with states enacting

laws to protect physicians who use large amounts of opioids in their pain medicine practice.

Although evidence of opioid use can be traced back to prehistoric Neolithic sites in Switzerland, and its use has continued for medicinal, ritual, and recreational purposes from that time onward, the peculiar regulatory history within the United States with the most severe impact on the context for pain medicine in recent time goes back to the late 1800s (Booth, 1996). In the United States, it has been well documented that the leading cause of opioid addiction in the 19th century was the medical community itself (Courtwright, 2001a). Many people became addicted to opium, which was widely available from physicians and over the counter. While many of the addicts were soldiers who had been wounded in the Civil War, about two thirds of those addicted to opium were middle- to upper-class Caucasian women, between the ages of 25 and 45, and most were administered opiates by their physician (Courtwright, 2001a). Iatrogenic addiction to opium was rampant, but the reliance upon opium to treat a wide-range of disorders was based on the most valid medical theories of the time. Finding roots in the work of the Scottish physician John Brown, who categorized all disease as the result of either too much or too little *stimulus*, American medicine made liberal use of opium, which was the single most prescribed medication in the *pharmacopoeia* (Courtwright, 2001a; Janz, 1974). Opium addiction, particularly in light of the defeat of China by Great Britain in the "Opium Wars" (with China unable to field an army), became a major concern of the U.S. government (Booth, 1996). Widespread misuse of the drug revealed a landscape at the turn of the century within which addiction appeared to many as a looming threat to national security and the bane of the medical profession. While physicians continued to prescribe opium, there were those in the government who strongly believed that there was little, if any, use for the drug.

It is not surprising that drastic action was taken, both within the medical community and from the government, emerging as a new domain of governmental regulation. On the medical side, physician attitudes, somewhat shaped by the failure of opioids to live up to their portrayal as a panacea, began to change into skepticism expressed as reluctance to prescribe various opioids. On the other hand, the government began involvement in ways that were yet uncharted and with the attitude that the medical community, left unchecked, might cause a cascade that would compromise the very ability of the United States to field an army in times of national threat.

Addiction, from the medical standpoint, was seen as a medical problem and, while the administration of opioids diminished, opioid "maintenance" clinics abounded. However, with the change in attitude within the medical community, bringing restrictions on the availability of opioids, more addicts turned to over-the-counter substances that contained opioids. These substances, often called "patent medicines," were marketed to "cure" a wide range of ailments, oftentimes addiction to the very ingredients contained in the preparation itself (Courtwright, 2001a). There was a move from viewing addiction as a medical problem to seeing it as a regulatory problem.

Along with the shift away from physicians as the source of opioids came the rise in popularity of opium smoking, a nonmedical practice that was introduced by Chinese immigrants. In the late 1800s, opium addicts began associating with the criminal element that frequented "opium dens." These secret locations were associated with immoral behavior and criminal activity, leading to the passage of a San Francisco municipal ordinance in 1875 that prohibited opium smoking (Courtwright, 2001a).* Other similar laws followed the San Francisco ordinance on the local and state levels, culminating in the passage of Federal Exclusion Act in 1904 that prohibited the importation of opium except for medicinal purposes (Courtwright, 2001a). Prices of opium increased as a result of this act, and many addicts turned to injecting morphine and heroin. There was an expansion of the illegal market, and criminal organizations began to control the importation and distribution of opioids.

The Exclusion Act of 1909 marked the first time in the United States that addiction was seen as a criminal problem instead of a medical or regulatory one. The move to criminal enforcement and prohibitive regulations continued in response to heroin, which became an inner-city drug abuse phenomenon. Despite criminal enforcement and import restrictions, the problem of opioid addiction in the United States continued to rise. This rise led to the

emergence of a regulatory backdrop that continues to inhibit the use, even legitimate use, of opioids well into the 21st century.

Hamilton Wright, as the U.S. delegate to The Hague Opium Convention of 1912, agreed to push for more restrictive domestic laws for opioids as a part of an international plan to curb the rise in addiction worldwide. Cast against the backdrop of the tensions that led to World War I, amid concerns about heroin use among draft-age youth, the Harrison Anti-Narcotic Act passed in 1915 (Courtwright, 2001a). Among other things, it required physicians to keep records of morphine and heroin prescriptions and placed great penalties on physicians who prescribed opioids indiscriminately. The U.S. Treasury Department, Internal Revenue Bureau, was charged with enforcing the narcotics laws.

There was ambiguity on the question of whether, subsequent to the Harrison Act, physicians could maintain addicts. After the Act, addicts had to get a prescription for their drugs — and there was a dramatic increase in "dope doctors" who would simply write narcotic prescriptions to addicts for a fee. While the Treasury Department went after these dope doctors, it took the U.S. Supreme Court to decide in 1919 (U.S. v. Webb) that these clinics and doctors were, in fact, subject to enforcement and disallowed by the Harrison Act (Courtwright, 2001a). After U.S. v. Webb, Treasury agents went after physicians who were prescribing for addicts. This marked the first time that law enforcement targeted physicians for criminal enforcement and set the stage for the relationship between physicians and law enforcement that continued until the last decade of the 20th century.

The illegal market for morphine and heroin continued to expand with the restrictions upon medical availability. Criminal groups continued to thrive on the importation and sale of these drugs, leading to the outlawing of the domestic use of heroin in 1924 (Courtwright, 2001a). Within this environment of criminal prosecution and overwhelming concern about the problem of addiction, medical professionals responded by advocating the use of opioids solely for the treatment of pain in terminally ill patients. The underlying thought was that only in terminally ill patents was the specter of addiction a moot point. Patients suffering from chronic pain who were not terminal were offered little relief. Enduring pain became a sign of stoic fortitude and complaining of pain that of weakness of character.

By 1940, addiction was viewed as a criminal problem, especially because the majority of addicts were obtaining their drugs from street sources rather than medical professionals (Courtwright, 2001a). Addicts were seen as criminals rather than, as 50 years earlier, as patients. Laws continued to restrict access to drugs and broaden enforcement authority. In 1951, the Boggs Act passed and was followed in 1956 by the Narcotic Control Act (Court-

---

* Laws first emerged in San Francisco and then Virginia City in 1876.

TABLE 93.1
Controlled Drug Schedules

Drug Schedule	Characteristics	Examples
Schedule I	Drug has no accepted medicinal use in United States Drug has high potential for abuse	Heroin, LSD, marihuana, peyote
Schedule II	Drug has accepted medicinal use Drug has high potential for abuse	Morphine, oxycodone, hydromorphone, amphetamine
Schedule III	Drug has accepted medicinal use Drug has medium potential for abuse	Hydrocodone
Schedule IV	Drug has accepted medicinal use Drug has low potential for abuse	Benzodiazapines
Schedule V	Drug has accepted medicinal use Drug has lowest potential for abuse	Some codeine cough syrups

wright, 2001a). These Acts codified penalties for simple possession of certain drugs and mandated prison sentences for violators. The environment became one in which law enforcement raided and arrested those involved in the importation, distribution, or use of illegal drugs. Medical professionals who overprescribed opioids were seen as "dope dealers" and often arrested.

As the problem of illegal drug use in the United States continued to rise, in 1962 the Kennedy administration held a White House conference, called the Prettyman Convention, on narcotics and drug abuse (Courtwright, 2001a). This conference led to the formation of an advisory commission that, in 1963, recommended changing the focus on drug use from incarceration to treatment, the elimination of mandatory minimum sentences on small cases, and transferring the powers of enforcement from the Treasury Department to the Justice Department. Finally, in 1965, new laws controlled the manufacture, distribution, and sale of barbiturates, tranquilizers, and amphetamines and also established the Federal Bureau of Narcotics and Dangerous Drugs Control (BNDDC) and the Food and Drug Administration (FDA) (Courtwright, 2001a). The shift in dealing with drug use as a treatment issue continued and in 1966 Congress passed the Narcotic Addict Rehabilitation Act. This Act allowed the medical treatment of addiction under very strict regulation, leading to the establishment of methadone treatment facilities throughout the United States (Courtwright, 2001a, b).

Finally, in 1970, the Controlled Substances Act, Title II of the Comprehensive Drug Abuse Prevention and Control Act, was passed, becoming effective in 1971 (Courtwright, 2001a). Under this Act, a classification system for evaluating the abuse potential of various drugs was established. This system consists of five schedules. In Table 93.1 each classification is shown, with the criteria for inclusion and an example of drugs in that schedule. Drugs that have a high potential for abuse and no recognized medicinal use in the United States are in Schedule I and

can only be used with a special registration by researchers. Schedule II drugs are those that have a high potential for abuse and have accepted medicinal use. Drugs in this schedule, which includes most of the strong opioids and their synthetic equivalents, are restricted to a 1-month supply and must be prescribed on a written script, signed by the doctor. Schedule III drugs have less potential for abuse and include, among other drugs, many hydrocodone preparations. These drugs can be called in by phone or ordered by prescription. The same holds for Schedule IV drugs, which have less potential for abuse. Schedule V drugs can be purchased by an individual from a pharmacist, but require identification and a signature (21 USCS Section 801, 1996).

The Controlled Substances Act contains the federal drug laws, specifies penalties, and sets up regulation of medical professionals. Changing little from 1970, prescribers and suppliers must obtain a registration from the U.S. Drug Enforcement Administration and receive a DEA number, which is used to index controlled substances prescriptions and to form a closed system within which the legitimate use of controlled drugs is monitored (21 USCS Section 821–830, 1996).

As Table 93.2 shows, the historical landscape in the United States began with no governmental involvement in either the practice of medicine or the importation of opium. However, because of the rising problem of addiction and its attendant fears, various steps were taken by the federal government (and followed by individual states) to control both the drugs and the medical community. The landmarks in this history are the Harrison Anti-Narcotic Act of 1915 and the Controlled Substances Act of 1970. Together, these laws have set the stage upon which prescribing of controlled drugs for pain must occur.

The medical community responded to the problem of addiction by closing the doors on opioid prescribing, except in the case of a terminally ill patient. It was common for doctors to see patients as unwilling to endure pain

TABLE 93.2
Major Drug Legislation in the United States

1875	San Francisco Municipal Ordinance	Made opium smoking illegal
1904	United States Federal Exclusion Act	Prohibited importation of opium except for medicinal purposes
1912	Hague Opium Convention	U.S. commitment to control opium
1915	Harrison Anti-Narcotic Act	Regulated physicians under U.S. Treasury enforcement
1919	*U.S. v. Webb*	Decision that physicians could be arrested for prescribing opioids for addicts
1951	Boggs Act	Imposed harsher penalties for narcotics violations
1956	Narcotic Control Act	Increased penalties and clearly stated antinarcotic commitment of government
1962	White House conference (Prettyman Convention)	Recommended dismantling Bureau of Narcotics and Dangerous Drugs and refocusing government on treatment and prevention
1966	Narcotic Addict Rehabilitation Act	Allowed medical treatment of addiction under strict control
1970	Controlled Substances Act	Created federal drug schedules and established drug violations
1990s	States began passing intractable pain laws	Allowed physicians latitude in using controlled drugs in the treatment of chronic pain

and weak in character. These attitudes were passed on through medical schools throughout the nation and only began to change after the Prettyman Convention renewed the idea of addicts as medical patients. Still, until pain management research found that opioids could be used effectively and without creating addiction, in the early 1990s, negative views of opioid prescribing continued (Courtwright, 2001b).

In the 1990s, various states, in response to new research in the management of chronic pain, began passing various forms of intractable pain legislation. These laws typically state the following: (1) recognition of chronic pain and the rights of patients to have relief from pain, (2) recognition of the value of large quantities of opioids in treating chronic pain, and (3) giving physicians the right to prescribe pain medications in such a treatment, providing that the drugs are not intended for euthanasia. This decade marks a radical break with previous attitudes, many of which are still held by both medical professionals and regulators. The challenge continues to be education of the medical and regulatory communities.

REGISTRATION REQUIREMENTS

According to the Federal Controlled Substances Act, "Every person who dispenses, or who proposes to dispense, any controlled substance, shall obtain from the Attorney General a registration issued in accordance with the rules and regulations promulgated by him" (21 USCS Section 822(A)2). The list of those who are allowed to prescribe controlled drugs has grown from only medical doctors to include other medical professionals, such as advanced practice nurses, physician assistants, and certified registered nurse anesthetists.

While every person who dispenses controlled drugs must obtain a DEA registration and number, many states

have a "dual registration" requirement. This means that a dispenser must obtain state registration as a necessary prior condition for the DEA number. The forms taken by states vary, with some registrations through the medical board, pharmacy board, or state narcotics agency. In every case, dispensers must also be registered with their appropriate professional practice board. Registrants on both the state and federal levels must comply with a series of "Rules and Regulations" that vary somewhat on a state level. These rules spell out the requirements that must be followed by registrants.

Both state and federal rules allow the controlling agency to bring a registrant in for a "show cause" hearing. This is an administrative hearing designed to determine whether actions shall be taken against the license of a medical professional. In a show cause hearing, a "hearing officer" hears both sides of the case and then makes a determination. The standard of proof in most of these hearings is a "preponderance of the evidence," which is much less strict than the criminal court, in which "beyond a reasonable doubt" is the standard. The final ruling from an administrative hearing can be appealed in either state or federal court. Some of the actions taken by regulatory agencies include denial of registration, revocation, suspension, and modification of privileges (21 USCS Section 822(A)2; see also Title 21 CFR, Part 1300–1399). Punitive fines are also levied against those deemed guilty of violating the rules. Pain medicine practitioners should review their respective state regulations pertaining to controlled drugs.

Criminal action can also be taken against physicians who misuse or divert controlled drugs. Examples of criminal acts include trading controlled drugs for sex, selling controlled drugs illegally, selling prescriptions for controlled drugs, stealing controlled drugs, and illegally using controlled drugs. These actions are unambiguous and criminal prosecution can result in imprisonment and/or fines.

CONCERNS ABOUT USING CONTROLLED DRUGS IN PAIN MANAGEMENT

Almost all legal and regulatory actions concerning the treatment of pain center on three features: (1) guarding against the diversion of controlled drugs, (2) effectively differentially diagnosing drug-seeking behavior, and (3) maintaining records that support the medical decision to use controlled substances to achieve pain relief and life maintenance. Physicians failing to meet basic standards in any of these categories place themselves at greater risk of disciplinary (or even criminal) actions. In fact, it is best to view these three areas as parts of a unified approach to achieving a practice that avoids pitfalls of regulatory mistakes.

GUARDING AGAINST DIVERSION

The standard established by the U.S. DEA and codified by all states for those who prescribe, administer, or distribute scheduled drugs is that they have an affirmative duty to "guard against diversion" (Title 21 CFR). What this means is nebulous and not well delineated by regulators. Consequently, law enforcement and regulatory agencies, both state and federal, have a wide range of possible areas in which they can regulate the activities of those involved in pain medicine. In the broadest sense, "diversion" is the use of controlled substances for any purpose other than their intended medical purpose; thus, "to guard against diversion" means to exercise reasonable care in the storage, handling, and dispensing of scheduled drugs, along with taking reasonable measures to see that, at any point in the medical practice, the possibility of drugs being used outside of their intended purpose is minimized (Gibbs & Haddox, 2003; see also Compton & Athanasos, 2003). To comply with this statutory and regulatory requirement, it is necessary to examine the various processes of a medical practice and make adjustments that will fulfill the DEA and state regulations.

To meet the requirement of guarding against diversion, a number of things should be examined. If drugs are stored at the practice, they must be kept in secure locations in compliance with the federal and state requirements. This usually means locked cabinets or safes with controlled and limited access. Furthermore, "readily retrievable" records must be maintained that reflect both the receipt of controlled drugs and their dispensation. When large quantities of controlled drugs are stored on premises, an alarm system is required. Next, one of the major sources of diversion is forged prescriptions. Prescription pads should be secured away from patient and non-essential personnel access. For example, the receptionist in a pain practice

has no business with access to prescription pads — only the physician or other authorized persons should have access to them. Fraudulent call-ins represent another vulnerable area for diversion control. Pain medicine practitioners should have strict records and guidelines for calling-in controlled drug prescriptions, including a logbook of call-ins, a reciprocal relationship with the pharmacies used to check and crosscheck call-ins, a designated person to call in scripts and another person to check the record, and a periodic overview of the record in comparison with patient charts.

SCREENING PATIENTS FOR ADDICTION

A very important part of guarding against diversion, as well as in the effective practice of pain medicine is to employ a series of "screening questions" to evaluate the risk of a patient for drug abuse. Included in this screening are questions about family history of drug and alcohol abuse, the patient's daily life, and whether the patient has abused drugs or alcohol in the past. If the patient appears at risk, more detailed information should be gathered. This screening interview should be followed by a physical exam, in which signs of drug abuse might be identified (Smith, 2000).

DIFFERENTIAL DIAGNOSIS OF DRUG-SEEKING BEHAVIOR

Another very important manner in which physicians can guard against diversion has to do with being able to differentially diagnose those legitimate patients from those seeking drugs. This is not always an easy task, especially because many patients with pain have comorbid disorders. Mostly, pain medicine specialists see patients who fall within the following categories: (1) patients with legitimate pain who have no comorbid disorders, (2) patients with legitimate pain who have a comorbid psychiatric disorder, (3) patients with legitimate pain who have a comorbid drug-seeking behavior problem, (4) patients with legitimate pain who have a comorbid addiction disorder, and (5) patients with nonlegitimate pain who are drug-seekers, addicts, or professional patients.

The first step in differentially diagnosing these kinds of patients and coming up with appropriate treatment is eliminating the drug-seekers and addicts who are not patients in legitimate pain. This can be very difficult, because many of the patterns of behavior associated with these patients also overlap with patients with pain and comorbidity. Consequently, physician judgment is critical in establishing patient legitimacy. Furthermore, drug seeking can either be a pattern of behavior that has already developed with other medical professionals, or it can be a pattern that begins within the realm of a current practice. It is useful, therefore, to catalog the classic phases of drug-seeking behavior. Table 93.3 shows the various phases, as

TABLE 93.3
Stages of Drug-Seeking Behavior

Level	Characteristics	Sign of
Phase 1	Unauthorized dose escalation	Undertreatment, drug diversion, drug abuse
Phase 2	Minor scams (e.g., excuses for needing more medication)	Undertreatment, drug diversion, drug abuse
Phase 3	Script forgery and fraud	Drug diversion, drug abuse
Phase 4	Injury to self or others	Drug diversion, drug abuse

well as the characteristics and possible reasons for the behavior (Longo, Parran, Johnson, & Kinsey, 2000; see also Parran, 1997).

The first phase of drug-seeking behavior is unauthorized dose escalation. If a patient exceeds the dosage prescribed on controlled medications, the physician should first evaluate the treatment to ensure that the patient is receiving enough pain medication. Many patients with pain may escalate dosage to meet the level of pain. In this case, it is a question of proper titration of pain medications and not drug-seeking. However, if a pattern of dose escalation emerges that is not indicative of undertreatment, it may suggest drug-seeking behavior. At this point, the physician should take action — either discontinue treating the patient or fix parameters on drug usage.

The second phase of drug-seeking behavior consists of different inventive "scams" that end up expressing a need for more of a controlled substance. These scams are as prolific as the minds of the patients and can be either elementary or sophisticated. Examples of the more elementary scams include losing the prescription, the script being eaten by the family dog, stolen medications, spilling the bottle into the toilet, and continue along these lines with the final request for more medication. As simple excuses fail, intelligent patients craft more elaborate excuses, such as the following: a patient receives a written script for 300 oxycodone 7.5 mg. tablets, makes a photocopy of it, fills the script at an out-of-the-way pharmacy and pays cash, puts the photocopy in his blue jeans, washes the pants, then comes back with an "accidentally washed' prescription, allegedly unfilled, to get another script. There is, of course, a limit to the number of excuses that any physician will buy. Consequently, this phase is short-lived and usually ends in increasing tension between the patient and prescriber over the medications.

The third phase of drug-seeking behavior reflects a greater level of despair by the patient. Characteristics of this phase occur when the patient (1) goes to multiple physicians to get drugs, (2) forges prescriptions or makes fraudulent call-in prescriptions, or (3) both. This represents a major step in the patient's willingness to take serious risks to obtain drugs because all of these actions are felonies and punishable by imprisonment. Typically, a drug-seeker at this level will first go to multiple physi-

cians without telling them about each other, present complaints of pain (or other disorders requiring controlled drugs), obtain prescriptions, and fill them at different pharmacies. Often, this kind of drug procurement can continue for years without being discovered, particularly if the drugs obtained are Schedule III or IV and not monitored as carefully as Schedule II controlled substances.*

More desperate is the drug-seeker who steals or has printed up prescription forms and writes bogus scripts that are filled at different pharmacies. Many of these are self-evident forgeries, such as the case in which a pediatrician received a call from a concerned pharmacist, who advised him that a person had attempted a forgery, which was clumsily written by the suspect for "mo-feen, 1 kilo, use as needed." Other forgeries are virtually indistinguishable from legitimate scripts and only communication with the prescriber can determine their bogus nature. Similarly with fraudulent call-in prescriptions, many more articulate and sophisticated drug-seekers can run this scam for years without detection.** Patients at this level are beyond simple intervention and should be brought within the criminal justice system for coercive treatment. For example, the drug court program requires such offenders to go through treatment and stay sober for a required period of time. Some pain medicine practitioners have strict procedures that involve working closely with pharmacists, to ensure that the script or call-in is legitimate. Examples include using caller ID to ensure that the phone call is from a legitimate medical practice, employing designated personnel in the medical practice who are authorized to call-in scripts, using only one pharmacy to fill scripts for a patient at risk, and physicians periodically reviewing the patients' pharmacy files and comparing them against the medical chart.

---

* Many states have Schedule II monitoring programs; fewer monitor other schedules. These programs usually track controlled dangerous substances prescribing in one of two ways: (1) triplicate prescriptions (doctor buys script pads from the government and keeps a copy for the chart, another copy goes to the pharmacy, another to the government agency in charge of the monitoring program), or (2) electronic capturing of prescription information as it is filled by the pharmacist.
** Professional diversion investigators routinely tell stories of patients who have scammed doctors in this manner for years — refer to National Association of Drug Diversion Investigators (NADDI).

TABLE 93.4
Illicit Equivalents for Controlled Drugs

Illicit Equivalent	Legitimate Drug(s)
Heroin	Opioid analgesics
Cocaine/methamphetamine	Stimulants
Alcohol	Sedative hypnotics

The fourth and final phase of drug-seeking behavior represents a much deeper level of despair in which the patient injures either herself or others to obtain drugs. One such drug-seeker would take pliers to his teeth, breaking one off, and then visiting all emergency rooms, several doctor's offices, dentists, and clinics — obtaining prescriptions of hydrocodone from each source, selling some of the drugs to pay for filling more prescriptions, until he finally had no teeth left. Eventually, this patient died from endocarditis. Other patients have injured their own children in order to get narcotics. Some threaten physicians at gunpoint, blackmail the doctor (usually over either sexual misconduct or drug abuse), or commit armed robberies and burglaries of pharmacies in order to get drugs. At this level, the patient becomes a major law enforcement problem and should be stopped as soon as possible.

Another area of concern for pain medicine physicians is the "professional patient," a scammer who may or may not be a drug user, but one who scams physicians out of large quantities of drugs that can be sold for profit on the street. These individuals can have many different scams, but all are actually trying to profit from illegal drug diversion. Many pharmaceutical drugs are the licit equivalents of illegal street drugs and, consequently, can have a high street value. Table 93.4 shows several common prescription drugs and their illicit equivalents. Examples of professional patients are groups that hire a patient with terminal cancer to travel from one city to another, going to various doctors and obtaining pain medications that are eventually sold on the street. Another example is a patient who steals a doctor's DEA number and has several prescription pads printed with a bogus name and address for a phony practice. Using the DEA number fraudulently, this individual hits city after city with prescriptions, often obtaining tens of thousands of dosage units before moving on.

In addition to the various phases of drug-seeking behavior, pain medicine practitioners must be able to spot and deal with comorbid patients. Of particular difficulty are two kinds of comorbid patient: those with (1) comorbid drug-seeking or addiction disorders, and (2) comorbid psychiatric disorders. The first category usually is either a patient who has a history of addiction disorder and also has chronic pain, or one who has been under treated for pain and developed drug-seeking patterns as a result. In

either case, appropriate adjunct therapy, usually in the form of addiction treatment and/or cognitive behavioral therapy, in conjunction with careful monitoring of pain drugs and restricted access to quantities of drugs, is essential. Many times these patients remain untreated, because of the liability in working with them — however, with appropriate strategies and very careful documentation, they can be effectively treated. Likewise, when encountering a patient comorbid with a psychiatric condition, care should be taken to work closely with a psychiatrist in controlling the medication mix to allow for both therapies to work together. Both kinds of patients represent a great challenge to pain medicine practitioners.

MAINTAINING RECORDS

Keeping comprehensive charts is critical when prescribing controlled drugs. These are the documentation of the medical evaluation and the rationale for the use of certain drugs. Good charts are the best defense against allegations of overprescribing or misuse of controlled drugs; conversely, poor charts can result in disciplinary action against even the best doctor. Charts should contain at least five areas that correspond to good practice of pain medicine: (1) patient evaluation, (2) treatment plan and objectives, (3) periodic review, (4) consultation records, and (5) documentation of all prescriptions.

Particularly when prescribing dangerous drugs, the doctor should conduct a thorough evaluation of the patient. This evaluation should include a pain history, especially the impact of the pain on the ability of the patient to function occupationally and socially. Any preexisting diagnostic studies and medical records should be carefully reviewed, and if the studies are insufficient, new ones should be ordered. The patient should be evaluated for a history of drug-seeking behavior and substance abuse, along with any comorbid conditions. Finally, a physical examination of the patient should be documented in the chart. All of these categories should be summarized in the chart for every new patient with pain. From a regulator's standpoint, as well as a medical board expert review, this shows that care was taken to determine whether the patient was legitimately a pain sufferer and there was scientific basis for the prescription of pain medications.

Next, the chart should document the diagnosis of the patient's condition and outline the treatment plan. This plan should include measurable goals, such as being able to go to work or experience an increase in personal activities. Documentation of informed consent on using opioids to treat the pain should be included at this point as well as the parameters of using the drugs.

Many pain management physicians use a "medication agreement," a contract between provider and patient that specifies what is expected of the patient. The following are important points to include in such a document:

1. Patient agrees to take medications as prescribed.
2. Patient agrees to not request refills except as specified by the agreement.
3. Patient agrees to use a specific pharmacy (of the patient's choice) to fill the prescriptions and authorizes the physician to obtain medication records from the pharmacy.
4. Patient agrees not to go to other doctors for pain treatment and to advise of any other doctor visits.
5. Patient agrees to guard against theft or misuse of medications.
6. Patient agrees not to use street drugs.
7. Patient agrees to submit to random drug screening.
8. Patient agrees to provider having the right to contact state or federal narcotics agencies regarding the patient.

While these are just a few of the main tenets of a medication agreement, it is a good way to document the conditions existing between the provider and the patient regarding controlled drugs and shows that the provider is guarding against diversion.

A periodic review of the treatment plan is necessary with patients with pain. Every few months (no longer than 6 months), the physician should reassess the treatment and determine if the objectives are being met. Adjustments or notes about continuing the course of treatment should be documented at this point. An example of a rationale for continued treatment might read: "The patient continues to report that he is able to function at his workplace and also reports getting adequate sleep at night." Such annotations in the chart show that the provider is concerned with actual functioning of the patient and that continued therapy is warranted.

If patients are referred to outside physicians for consultation, this should also be documented in the chart — for example, referral to a psychiatrist for emotional issues should be noted, along with the diagnosis and treatment plan set up by the psychiatrist. The results of a consultation should be carefully reviewed for compatibility or incompatibility with the existing pain treatment and appropriate adjustments made.

Finally, all prescriptions should be documented and included in the chart. Many pain management physicians actually photocopy the prescriptions written and include them in the chart. Others have a log that can be easily reviewed that lists all controlled drug prescriptions given to the patient. It is critical, however, that the scripts for controlled substances be carefully charted and that these prescriptions match the course of therapy outlined in the treatment plan.

By using these guidelines for charting patients with pain, physicians can have an affirmative defense against allegations of indiscriminate prescribing of controlled drugs. The process that most medical boards follow in reviewing a complaint against a physician for overprescribing controlled drugs usually involves bringing in a board-certified expert to review a random sample of charts from the practice. Good charts can explain thought processes and scientific findings that support medical decisions to prescribe controlled drugs. Such documentation is critical to maintain in the practice of pain medicine.

CONCLUSION

The practice of pain management occurs within a regulatory environment that has a long history of preoccupation with the problem of addiction. Consequently, laws, rules, and regulations have been compiled that form the parameters within which a pain medicine practice must operate. Because pain medicine makes extensive use of opioids, it is imperative that those involved know the regulatory landscape. Furthermore, regulations require that prescribers have an affirmative duty to guard against diversion of controlled drugs. These drugs have a street value and are frequently diverted to illegal use. By exercising reasonable care in storing these drugs, limiting access, and understanding the differential diagnosis of drug-seeking behavior, physicians can demonstrate that they are prescribing the drugs for legitimate purposes and that they are conscientious about the problem of diversion. Furthermore, by comprehensively charting the patient evaluation, diagnosis, treatment plan, and other relevant information, pain management physicians are able to defend themselves against allegations of drug mismanagement. With the adoption of intractable pain laws, most states have officially recognized the value of using opioids and other controlled substances and also have recognized that patients have a right to expect relief from chronic pain. Yet this new philosophy is cast against the backdrop of a restrictive environment and those practicing on this medical frontier have to contend with working under regulatory scrutiny.

REFERENCES

21 USCS Section 801 (1996).

21 USCS Section 821-830 (2004).

21 USCS Section 822(A)2 (2004).

Booth, M. (1996). *Opium: A history.*, Griffin, NY: St. Martin's.

Compton, P., & Athanasos, P. (2003). Chronic pain, substance abuse and addiction. *Nursing Clinics of North America, 38*(3), 525–537.

Courtwright, D. T. (2001a). *Dark paradise: A history of opiate addiction in America.* Boston: Harvard University Press.

Courtwright, D. T. (2001b). *Forces of habit: Drugs and the making of the modern world.* Boston: Harvard University Press.

Gibbs, L. S., & Haddox, J. D. (2003). Lawful prescribing and the prevention of diversion. *Journal of Pain and Palliative Care Pharmacotherapy, 17,* 5–14.

Janz, V. (1974). *Pharmacologia Browniania.* Pharmacotherapheutische Praxis des Brownianismus aufgezeight Lind interpretiert an den Modellen von A. F. Marcus in Bamberg und J. Frank in Wien. Marburg: Dissertation.

Longo, L. P., Parran, T., Jr., Johnson, B., & Kinsey, W. (2000, April 15). Addiction: Part II. Identification and management of the drug-seeking patient. *American Family Physician,* 2401–2406.

Parran, T. (1997). Prescription drug abuse. A question of balance. *Medical Clinics of North America, 8,* 967–978.

Smith, D. (2000, September). Drug abuse. *Best Practice of Medicine.* Retrieved from http://merck.micromedex.com/index.asp?page=bpm_report&article_id-BPM01PS06.

94

Controlled Substances and Risk Management

Hans Hansen, MD, Art Jordan, MD, and Jennifer Bolen, JD

INTRODUCTION

The role of the pain management specialist is to control pain, improve the quality of life, and reduce the suffering of those stricken with acute and chronic pain. Often the doctor of last resort, the pain practitioner is left with few options not previously attempted to treat patients, especially those with chronic pain. In fact, many of these patients are not difficult to manage, but they are lost between the kinetic interaction of families, care providers, and other parties. Subsequently, the patient becomes a fatigued and overwhelmed individual who may appear apprehensive and suspicious of the new treatment plan. Further straining the nurturing environment of the patient–practitioner relationship are the many payers and regulatory agencies that are increasingly insistent that the patient be managed in a cost-contained environment, free of potential adverse risk; in reality, this setting does not exist.

Risk is a part of medical care that is acknowledged in any treatment plan. Unfortunately, the current climate of regulatory and legal challenges demands that pain practitioners take steps to minimize the potential for risk while continuing to offer high-quality, effective treatment. Few professions are held to such demanding standards where the cost of adverse outcome is so high for patients, family, and care providers.

THE PERSONALITY OF PAIN

Controlled substances, particularly opioids, are an important component of a pain practitioner's treatment arsenal, and often provide a reasonable alternative to invasive procedures and costly therapies in some patient populations. As an example, surgery, although an important consider-ation for certain diseases, is not always a curative approach for many patients with pain and may result in significant post-surgical morbidity, such as post-laminectomy syndrome. Patients frequently ask for back surgery to stop the pain when surgery may actually promote further disability. Well-controlled pain, in many cases, may decrease the perceived need for surgery. "Cutting nerves" or surgically removing pain seems reasonable to patients, but is rarely possible. Pain is, of course, a complex interaction of peripheral and central processing events evolving its own "personality" through the limbic system and central neurophysiologic interactions.

Most pain management practitioners agree that patients will, in many cases, develop this "personality of pain" that directs much of their behavior. Depression, anxiety, and aggressive characteristics are particularly troublesome when controlled substances become a patient's focus. These drugs must be managed carefully. The personality of pain often overwhelms the original pain complaint and interferes with a positive, productive outcome. There is no test to identify these subtle personality characteristics, but most practitioners would agree that certain pain diagnoses, such as complex regional pain syndrome and fibromyalgia, demonstrate subtle personality idiosyncrasies at presentation. Perhaps the personality factors exist that predict or measure these characteristics, but a test has not been developed to measure these personality traits. Standard Functional Capacity Exam testing routinely reports inconclusive results in fibromyalgia assessments, and no personality trait has been identified with standard psychological tests.

Pain does influence plasticity in central processing events, including affective and motivational centers. Controlled substances will further alter these behavioral centers, sometimes with deleterious effects. Exercise caution with controlled substances in those with psychiatric disease or labile personalities. The use of adjunctive medications, such as anxiolytics and antidepressants, may greatly enhance treatment of coexisting anxiety or depression, which accompanies chronic nonmalignant pain. The stair-step approach to substance use to control pain recommended by the World Health Organization (WHO) consistently improves outcomes and provides a rational and defensible approach to pain therapy.

Controlled substances may also help a patient's pain-related anxiety, and may positively improve function and interactive lifestyle. Controlled substances, such as opioids, are an option for those who cannot tolerate a particular restorative procedure or treatment, such as surgery, or who have not improved function or quality of life to the lower levels of the WHO model. Properly used, returning to work and involvement in interactive social activities decrease utilization of the medical system, and control of disease states related to pain and anxiety.

Controlled substances are known to be of high value to relieve cancer pain and other common degenerative diseases, such as low back pain and arthritis. Occasionally, controlled substances have limiting side effects that decrease utility at therapeutic dose, and other medications are superior choices. For example, opioid effect is resisted in certain disease states, such as neuropathic pain and fibromyalgia, suggesting non-opioid alternatives and adjuncts might be a better choice.

Another approach is enhancing the synergistic effect of combination therapy, noncontrolled agents and low-dose controlled substances, decreasing side effects, increasing compliance, and enhancing pain control. Occasionally, reinforcing the concept of off-label use, adjunctive therapy has allowed boutique combinations and altered doses of controlled and noncontrolled substances to improve outcome.

The pain management prescriber is best positioned to optimize controlled and noncontrolled substances to minimize side effects and improve the patient's life experience. The *personality of pain* will benefit from acknowledgment that treatment of anxiety, depression, or any number of subdiagnoses of chronic pain is recognized, accepted, and a predictable and compassionate understanding between patient and provider. Herein is the foundation of the provider–patient relationship built on trust.

DEA'S REGULATORY OVERSIGHT ROLE

The Drug Enforcement Agency (DEA) is responsible for monitoring the flow of controlled substances in the United States. The DEA has the authority to establish manufacturing quotas or drug supply, establish the framework for manufacturers and wholesale distributors, regulate retail matters, and register individuals and businesses for pur-

poses of monitoring the administering, dispensing, and prescribing of controlled substances. DEA uses two Websites to make relevant information available to the public and the body of registrants — www.dea.gov and www.deadiversion.usdoj.gov. Practitioners should consult these Websites regularly, or use one that links to the DEA Websites to provide updated information, such as ASSIPP.org or aapainmanage.org.

The DEA uses the Code of Federal Regulations and the Federal Register to establish and explain record-keeping requirements and abuse and diversion control mandates on controlled substances. The DEA cannot use its authority to tell practitioners "how to practice medicine." Consequently, the federal legal and regulatory framework does not define *legitimate medical purpose*, leaving this matter to state licensing boards and community standards on accepted medical practice.

Several professional organizations have also published materials related to the treatment of pain and to the risk management aspects of using controlled substances to treat pain, including the American Academy of Pain Medicine (AAPMedicine) and the American Pain Society (APS), the American Academy of Pain Management (AAPManagement), the American Society of Interventional Pain Physicians (ASIPP), the American Academy of Physical Medicine and Rehabilitation (AAPMR), the American Society of Regional Anesthesia and Pain Medicine (ASRA), the American Society of Addiction Medicine, and the American Academy of Family Practitioners (AAFP), among many others. All practitioners should become familiar with these organizations named above. In addition, all practitioners should use the Website, www.ngc.gov, to learn about current practice guidelines and standards used nationwide in the area of pain management.

PART ONE. RISK AND CONTROLLED SUBSTANCES

Risk is defined as a "chance of loss." Risks are part of everyday life and certainly a part of the daily practice of medicine. Before one can establish an effective risk management program, it is important to understand potential risk areas and consider how they factor into the clinical setting. Part One focuses on the identification of general practice risk areas and those risks specifically associated with the use of controlled substances to treat pain. After reviewing potential risk areas, practitioners should perform a self-audit to determine where they stand on identifying potential risks. After the self-audit, practitioners will be able to use Part Two to structure a basic risk management plan, focusing on issues relating to controlled substances and specific patient populations commonly presenting risks in this area. In all cases, the key components of effective risk management when using controlled substances to treat pain are patient assessment, selection, and monitoring.

Controlled substances are a part of the necessary daily interactions of patient and practitioner in most pain management practices, and should be used according to accepted standards of care and applicable legal and regulatory guidelines. Most importantly, the practitioner's clinical decisions and supporting rationale for the initial selection and continued use of controlled substances must be documented accurately and completely, according to applicable federal and state guidelines, laws, and regulations on the use of controlled substances to treat pain. To meet these standards, it is incumbent upon the practitioner and medical staff to be aware of the intricate balance between clinical need and appropriate use, and the misuse and diversion potential of these substances. The practitioner and his or her staff must be familiar with the basic epidemiology behind a growing trend of drug abuse. Practitioners are advised to implement office policies that protect against "doctor shoppers," drug diverters, and other unscrupulous individuals who put an entire practice at risk for licensing board, insurance company, and law enforcement intervention. Practitioners should use patient assessment and selection tools that enable them to identify those patients who present with increased potential for substance abuse, so they can be cared for in a manner that addresses their substance abuse problems without ignoring co-existing pain problems. Finally, practitioners are advised to use patient monitoring tools that enable them to assess the patient's continued legitimate medical need for controlled substances, while minimizing the potential for adverse drug events, abuse, and diversion.

Controlled substance risk management is not a static form of quality assurance, because risk is an ever-changing threat to the livelihood and health delivery of physician, employee, patient, and staff. Risk management in daily practice activities improves the likelihood of providing quality care, and suggests to legal and regulatory authorities that the practice is designed to minimize the potential for the abuse and diversion of controlled substances, as required by an *Interim Policy Statement*, published by DEA in the Federal Register on November 16, 2004.

UNDERSTANDING RISK AND CONTROLLED SUBSTANCES

A variety of categories present the potential for risk to a medical practice. Prior to implementing risk control strategies in clinical practice, practitioners should attempt to identify their specific risk areas or categories.

- Unexpected. A regulatory or legal event arising from an adverse outcome experienced by patient or an organization, and culminating in

dissatisfaction with the health care redendered by the targeted practitioner. Often, there is no prior warning or heralding event.
- Patient injury. A definable event, predictable or not, with unwanted outcome.
- Risk to staff and provider:
  - Regulatory. This includes professional licensing board investigations, state and local law enforcement investigations, and DEA law enforcement and regulatory actions.
  - Compliance. State and federal fraud/abuse allegation, procedural/responsibility or negligence, Occupational Safety and Health Administration (OSHA) violation, violation of institutional by-laws (such as hospital or surgery center).
  - Perception in the community as an outlier. The perception is often the result of health care benefit plan Drug Utilization Reviews (DURs) and related billing and coding analyses.
  - Loss of peer support and/or organizational sanction. HMO/PPO, managed care sanctions. Substance abuse, outlier activity, practice habits outside of community standard.
  - Natural disaster. Vulnerability or absence of a disaster recovery plan.
  - Emotional risk. Practitioner and staff are particularly vulnerable. Being a health care provider is stressful, and prescribing controlled substances adds a level of vigilance and responsibility that many individuals in the clinic are ill equipped to address. Specifically, aggressive or manipulative patient behavior is a difficult management scenario, and it is recommended that well-trained and appropriate individuals interface with patients seeking controlled substances and refills.
  - Physical plant. Environment of care. Is the office safe and meeting regulatory challenges? Not necessarily an OSHA issue. An example might include interstate variation of fluoroscopy requirements. Are samples and scheduled medications stored and distributed safely?
  - Financial. The practitioner and practice require a positive, rewarding monetary cash flow, as any business would expect. Costs of providing care are increasing, and reimbursements decreasing. Practitioners and patients often find themselves in a bad position because health care benefit plans do not cover needed drugs or procedures, mental health services, or an adequate number of follow-up visits. Overall, profit and loss are

tenuous and, in some cases, a practitioner's billing and prescribing patterns may imply an improper profit motive.

- Practitioner or "key-man." If one provider is extraordinarily productive, loss of that coverage and income may be devastating to the viability of the practice. Furthermore, will loss of a key prescriber disrupt patient care?
- Americans for Disability Act. Conforming to the ever-changing requirements of the disabled is mandated by law. A prescriber with a substance abuse history requires a risk management plan that minimizes the potential for a discrimination claim by those who have legitimate medical need for controlled substances.
- Licensing. Loss of privilege:
  1. State license. This may be the practitioner's greatest asset. Protection of this privilege cannot be stressed enough.
  2. Federal and State Controlled Substances Registrations: Particularly at risk when practitioners prescribe controlled substances without knowing the requirements of their state controlled substances acts and related guidelines, laws, and regulations on the use of controlled substances to treat pain. If a practitioner loses his or her medical license, he or she will lose their controlled substances registrations as well. Not all states require a separate registration from the federal registration to administer, dispense, or prescribe controlled substances.
  3. Local licensing requirements. Various tax and provider business licenses require ongoing vigilance. A designated credential officer avoids overlooking deadlines and renewals.
- Whistleblower:
  1. Employee retaliation. The practitioner is more likely to be sued from an employee than from a malpractice event (J.H. Holmes, J.D., personal communication). The practice and practitioner usually do not carry insurance for this type of exposure. Employees may even be rewarded for their report to a regulatory agency encouraging whistle-blowing "Qui Tam."
  2. DEA. Drug enforcement investigations are rare in routine practice, but disgruntled employees, pharmacists, and some patient groups may initiate an inquiry about a practitioner's prescribing habits.

Often, the originating complaint extends to topics beyond the DEA's investigative scope (such as those investigations involving community care standards). When this happens, many civil and state regulatory agencies, including professional licensing boards, get involved in additional investigative activities.

  3. Medicare/Medicaid. Fraud/abuse. Financial incentives and antiretaliation protections place the practice at a disadvantage. A disgruntled employee may see an opportunity to retain information and expose the practitioner to an unforeseen or unexpected abuse investigation. An employee may allege misuse of these government programs to profit from controlled substance prescribing. Another example may include Office of Inspector General investigation. Usually initiated by disgruntled employees. Costly and lengthy.
  4. Harassment. Sexual, or risk to harm. Again, antiretaliation laws and the usual lack of practice policy and education makes for a difficult defense, civil and governmental.
  5. Employee violence. A prevalent and rising risk. The practice may be cited as culpable. An employee may allege the provider did not protect a prescription pad or samples of controlled substances, aiding in their addiction or legal troubles.
  6. Improper employee background check. Theft, loss, harassment, violence. Each costly and difficult to avoid accepting responsibility without knowing the employee risk history.
  7. Negligence of others. You are responsible for your employees' actions in the practice — "those that can pay, will pay." Practitioners are perceived as deep pockets.
- Opioid and controlled substance prescribing:
  - Prescribing without sufficient information about the patient's treatment history, drug history, including the patient's history of chemical and substance abuse and a proper family history of chemical/substance abuse.
  - Prescribing without the patient's informed consent as to (i) the risks of using controlled substances, including the potential for addiction, the concepts of physical dependence and tolerance, and potential for adverse effects, such as con-

stipation, sleepiness, and nausea, etc.; (ii) the benefits expected from the use of controlled substances in combination with the patient's participation in the treatment plan; and (iii) treatment alternatives.

- Prescribing without a proper follow-up and monitoring plan to ensure the patient's compliance with the overall treatment plan and to guard against potential problems sometimes associated with the long-term use of controlled substances.

- Risk to practitioner. This includes threat of personal injury, particularly from a seeker of drug, and/or a psychiatric patient, or a family member. Family members and close friends often "convince" patients of a practitioner's error, initiating legal action.

RISK-CONTROLLED SUBSTANCES

Opioid and controlled substances, sedatives and anxiolytics, are often chosen management strategies and arguably some of the most cost-effective approaches to treat pain. Controlled substances are a powerful and proven tool in the practitioner's pain management resources. Surgery, interventional procedures, and psychological adjuncts are effective, but not always indicated in many patient populations. A high level of accountability is necessary for both practitioner and patient to avoid improper use of these medications. Moreover, practitioner decision making may be affected by the fear of reprisal from regulatory agencies, patient drug abuse or diversion possibilities, and the perceived stigma of opioid and controlled substances used in community clinical practice. While prescription drug abuse and diversion are major concerns for the pain practitioner, one need not fear investigations and potential lawsuits if the practitioner implements and uses proper risk management tools regularly. Strategies to control risk — to patient, practitioner, and practice — increase both patient and practitioner acceptance of controlled substances, foster understanding, and ultimately benefit society by minimizing the potential for abuse and diversion. The current climate of the medicolegal system exposes prescribers to civil suits by plaintiff attorneys for the act of prescribing controlled substances, inferring *harm* and not aid to those suffering from pain. Access to care is close to many practitioners' souls, and may one day be denied for those suffering from pain. These lawsuits will result in prescriber fear and reduction of controlled substance availability for legitimate purposes. There is little doubt that drug abuse is increasingly prevalent, but the risk–reward benefit of controlled substances in the management of an appropriate pain diagnosis remains in the patient's favor.

WHAT ARE CONTROLLED SUBSTANCES?

Controlled substances are drugs or chemicals exerting bioactive effects, and are under federal and state regulation. Controlled substances are classified as opioids, stimulants, or hypnotic agents. The term *narcotic* is improperly used in the lay community, implying that any mind-altering or habit-forming bioactive substance is a narcotic. In typical medical usage, the "narcotic" often is used to mean an opioid analgesic, which is an opium-based or synthetic drug with specific opioid receptor activity. Opioids (true narcotics) are pharmacokinetically long, medium, or short acting and are used to control many painful conditions.

In the legal vernacular, narcotics may include barbiturates, stimulants, hypnotics, and opioids, although the federal statutory definition refers specifically to opium-like drugs and cocaine (http://www.dea.gov/pubs/csa/802.htm). Stimulants are a separate classification of controlled substance that may arouse and accelerate bodily and mental activity. Stimulants are used to control obesity, increase mental alertness, and treat distraction disorders, such as attention deficit disorder. Hypnotics are sedating, soothing, and exert a calming effect, often described as "tranquilizing." Many hypnotic agents reduce anxiety, stress, excitement, and induce sleep. Controlled substances are scheduled, based on the potential for risk of misuse or diversion, *not* by potency. See DEA Web site for list of drugs by schedule (http://www.dea.gov/pubs/scheduling.html).

Schedule I: No accepted medical use in the United States. Abuse potential is high. Examples include marijuana, heroin, hashish, and methaqualude.

Schedule II: High abuse potential. Accepted medical use is recognized, but complicated by the potential for severe psychological or physical dependence liability. Examples include oxycodone, morphine, cocaine, methadone, and hydromorphone.

Schedule III: Significant abuse potential, but less so than Schedule I or II. May involve combination preparations such as hydrocodone and acetaminophen (hydrocodone alone would be classified as Schedule II, but is Schedule III if mixed with acetaminophen). Further examples of Schedule III drugs include hydrocodeine and many synthetic preparations mixed with acetaminophen.

Schedule IV: Abuse potential less than Schedule III. Abuse and misuse is prevalent, and often underestimated. Typically these are inclusive of the benzodiazepines class, but may include some forms of codeine preparations.

Schedule V: Abuse potential less than Schedule IV. Practitioners tend to believe that lower risk accompanies lower scheduling. That is not a correct assumption, and Schedule V drugs may be trafficked and abused as easily as Schedule II drugs. The sanctions for misuse of *any* controlled substance are vigorously prosecuted and criminal in nature. Sedative hypnotics and mixed agonist antagonist drugs frequently are Schedule V preparations.

Schedule II prescriptions are often prescribed monthly, and currently not allowed to be "forward-dated." When a prescription is "forward-dated," the date the prescription is actually written must be on the prescription followed by "Do not fill until ...." Schedule II prescriptions may not be written for renewal of the original prescription and must have an original prescription for presentation to the pharmacy. It is recommended from a risk perspective and medical necessity requirement that an actual physical assessment by the practitioner or practitioner extender occur monthly to warrant continued Schedule II use.

Schedule III, IV, and V medications may be no less habituating than Schedule II drugs, and street value remains high for most controlled substances. In fact, hydrocodone is among the most widely misused and illegally distributed medications in America (Federation of State Medical Boards [FSMB], 1998). Other highly habituating medications that are erroneously and commonly considered benign in many treatment arenas include benzodiazepines, particularly alprazolam (Xanax®), and muscle relaxants, such as carisoprodol (Soma®), to name two. Many other examples exist, and regional variations may be important. Caution should be exercised when prescribing these medications. Even Schedule IV drugs, such as butorphanol tartrate (Stadol®), may be highly sought after by the patient. Misuse and drug-seeking behavior should be documented in the medical record and acknowledged by the prescriber. The prescriber's decision to continue treatment in the face of misuse or abuse behavior is documented in the record as soon as this behavior becomes evident. If the prescriber chooses to continue prescribing controlled substances, the reason(s) must be clearly expressed, and a discussion of what safeguards and restrictions will be placed upon the prescriber–patient relationship is clearly documented. Initial encounters are recommended to document family or patient abuse/use history, including alcohol. Merely filling out a prescription each month without documenting functional indices, quality of life indices, pain scale, restorative sleep, and appropriateness to treatment should be avoided, and in state and federal cases this lack of documentation has been used as evidence of improper and/or illegal activity by prescribers.

KEY TERMS TO KNOW AND USE

Practitioners must know and use the following terms in daily medical practice. These terms, addiction, tolerance, pseudoaddiction, and physical dependence, factor into each of the five key documentation components for controlled substance prescribing and, consequently, risk management concerns.

Addiction: Addiction is an important clinical and legal term. In its 2004 revised *Model Policy for the Use of Controlled Substances for the Treatment of Pain*, the Federation of State Medical Boards defined addiction as "a primary, chronic, neurobiologic disease, with genetic, psychosocial, and environmental factors influencing its development and manifestations. It is characterized by behaviors that include the following: impaired control over drug use, craving, compulsive use, and continued use despite harm. Physical dependence and tolerance are normal physiological consequences of extended opioid therapy for pain and are not the same as addiction (Federation of State Medical Boards [FSMB], 2004).

Practitioners should consider addiction issues if a patient no longer has control over drug use and continues to use the drugs despite potential harm to self or others. Ronald Kanner, M.D. (2003) cites five main characteristics of addiction: chronic use, impaired control, compulsive use, continued use despite harm, and craving (the five Cs). These distinctions are in contrast to tolerance, pseudoaddiction, and physical dependence, in which continued use of the controlled substance does not place the patient at risk of harm (see Federation of State Medical Boards, http://www.fsmb.org).

Tolerance: Tolerance is a physiologic state resulting from regular use of a drug in which an increased dosage is needed to produce a specific effect, or a reduced effect is observed with a constant dose over time. Tolerance may or may not be evident during opioid treatment and does not equate with addiction (FSMB Model Policy, 2004).

Pseudoaddiction: The iatrogenic syndrome resulting from the misinterpretation of relief-seeking behaviors as though they are drug-seeking behaviors that are commonly seen with addiction. The relief-seeking behaviors resolve upon institution of effective analgesic therapy (FSMB Model Policy, 2004). Not grasping this phenomenon may lead the clinician to inappropriately label the patient as an addict due to unrelieved pain resulting in frequent requests for escalating drug doses, requiring clinical reevaluation of need and of the risk-reward benefit. This is a controversial issue. Many pain physicians do not believe pseudoaddiction exists.

Pseudotolerance: Pseudotolerance is the need to increase dosage that is not due to tolerance, but due to other factors such as disease progression, new disease, increased physical activity, lack of compliance, change in medication, drug interaction, addiction, and deviant behavior. When a once-fixed opioid dose is no longer effective, these conditions should be reviewed to exclude pseudotolerance (FSMB, 1998).

Physical Dependence: Physical dependence is a state of adaptation that is manifested by drug class-specific signs and symptoms that can be produced by abrupt cessation, rapid dose reduction, decreasing blood level of the drug, and/or administration of an antagonist. Physical dependence, by itself, does not equate with addiction. [FSMB *Model Policy* 2004]. Physical dependence may also occur if an opioid antagonist is administered to an individual exposed to a prolonged, regular course of opioids. Physical dependence ". . . is not a clinical problem if patients are weaned to avoid abrupt discontinuation of the drug, a tapering regimen is used (if treatment cessation is indicated), and opioid antagonist drugs (including agonist-antagonist analgesics) are avoided" (2).

PART TWO. CONTROLLED SUBSTANCES AND CHRONIC PAIN

Risk Management

Chronic pain treatment is often delegated, by default, to select individuals who have demonstrated an interest in dealing with some of the most difficult patient management issues in contemporary medicine. The pain management specialist is the tip of a funnel, and usually perceived as the last hope for many patients suffering from pain. Pain diagnoses are usually the product of a complex relationship of social, psychological, and physical factors, cultural and religious experiences and thus require a comprehensive environment of care and co-managing providers to afford the best outcome. The very complexity of pain and pain management demands a proactive approach to risk management overall, and specifically in the use of controlled substances to treat pain. Worse yet, few specialists face the problem presented by health care benefit plans that do not cover services, such as mental health referrals, the use of certain specialists, and drug control measures, thereby placing the practi-

tioner in a risk position. Practitioners must learn to respond to these issues and understand that they can achieve balance in their respective practices with proper risk management protocols.

Practitioners who prescribe controlled substances routinely *must take steps* to understand the legal and regulatory environment and to structure risk management protocols based on federal and state legal and regulatory standards and accepted standards of care. Our news media increasingly report stories about a small number of practitioners who have been charged with the illegal distribution of controlled substances (in lay terms referred to as "inappropriate prescribing"). These practitioners, often guilty of recklessly disregarding medical ethics and specific legal and regulatory standards relating to the use of controlled substances to treat pain, face financial ruin and leave dozens of improperly handled patients behind for the community of practitioners to absorb or channel through an already overstressed health care system. These very few "rogue" practitioners give a bad name to the whole process of treating pain and ethical and quality-minded practitioners *must take action* to ensure "dumped" patients are handled appropriately and turned into success stories, where possible. For all these reasons and more, today's pain treatment paradigm strives to find a treatment plan that provides a high level of satisfaction for all involved. Ultimately, this means every practice *must participate in* a proactive risk management program, especially when the practice uses controlled substances to treat pain.

The purpose of this chapter is to analyze risk in the context of a pain management practice, with a special emphasis on risks associated with the use of controlled substances to treat pain. After looking at the various risk areas, the chapter offers suggestions on how pain practitioners might minimize risk in their practices while still offering quality medical care. It is important for readers to remember that a risk management plan is only part of an ongoing process to identify and respond to risk factors in daily practice. Once risk management protocols are learned, the process becomes second nature to the practitioner and often results in better practitioner–patient relationships overall.

Legitimate medical purpose and use within the usual course of professional practice define, for legal/regulatory purposes, the validity of a controlled substance prescription. [21 CFR 1306.04(a)] Federal law does not provide a specific definition of legitimate medical purpose. However, there are many reported federal criminal cases and DEA registration revocation cases discussing what may or may not constitute a "legitimate medical purpose" in the context of a sufficiency of the evidence against the defendant argument. For example, here are a few criteria both DEA and the courts use to find a lack of legitimate medical purpose:

Patient demands take the place of a physician's medical judgment [(Revocation of Registration, *Robert L. Dougherty, Jr., M.D.*, DEA Docket No. 94-63, 60 Fed. Reg. 55047 (October 1995).]

Dispensing (or prescribing) controlled substances to a patient who has demonstrated actions consistent with being a substance abuser (or diverter) [*Dougherty*].

Dispensing (or prescribing) an excessive number of refills to a patient over time (e.g. six months) without requiring a clinical examination or visit. This demonstrates a *reckless disregard for medical standards in dispensing controlled substances.* [*Dougherty*].

Prescribing controlled substances to patients without conducting a proper physical examination or appropriate tests to determine if the patient's medical condition justified the prescribing of the controlled substances. [(Revocation of Registration, *Sajjan Gangappa Chikkannaiah, MD*, 55 Fed. Reg. 38174 (September 1990).]

Prescribing an enormous quantity of frequently abused controlled drugs to patients for patently inappropriate periods of time, sometimes for years. [*Chikkannaiah*].

Prescribing controlled substances to patients the provider knew, or should have known, were drug abusers or addicts. [*Chikkannaiah*].

Both DEA and state licensing boards are serious about monitoring complaints regarding a practitioner's prescribing practices. These entities expect practitioners to conform to clinical and community standards, and to comply with applicable federal and state legal/regulatory materials. The pain practitioner is a leader in the community, understanding the proper use of opioids and controlled substances and the best techniques for diversion avoidance. Likewise, the pain practitioner is positioned properly to assist others in developing appropriate community policy.

Overall, the legitimate medical purpose or need for controlled substance relates to the practitioner's documented assessment of the patient's medical condition and findings regarding his/her pain complaint. Moreover, the practitioner's documentation *must* include relevant diagnostic and lab studies to support the diagnosis and justification for the use of controlled substances. Documentation of legitimate medical purpose *should not* be accomplished as a reactive response to fear of federal or state scrutiny. Rather, documentation of legitimate medical purpose reflects quality medical care and practitioners *must* make this a habit. The DEA publishes a pharmacist's manual that contains a good overview of the DEA's perspective on controlled substances and documentation requirements. Every practitioner is encouraged to read this manual.

Obviously, many patients challenge the pain management practitioner, alleging lack of compassion and clinical competence when the dose is changed or the drug replaced with an alternative choice. The patient and referral source require open communication to ensure that the patient receives the treatment needed, not necessarily what the patient wants. The referral source is educated that a change in the patient course might be beneficial to avoid alienation or misunderstandings, and not enhancing the patient/referral interaction.

While it is true that most prescribers are well trained and will appropriately use controlled substances, unfortunately the doorsteps of pain practitioners' offices are littered with stories of less-enlightened practitioners (from all specialties) who are lulled into the belief that high-dose opioids are appropriate for certain painful disease entities, only to find that their primary care practices or nonpain specialty practices are ill equipped to manage these drugs over a prolonged period of time. Pain management practitioners are referred these complex patients, who are told that pain specialists are their "parachutes" and will be their sole prescribing entities; "Don't ask me for these medications anymore; the pain specialist will give them to you." Herein lies the problem: what is the best course of care with the least risk profile to the practitioner and patient? An alarming, increasingly popular, and "easy" course of action for many primary care practitioners is to initially prescribe habituating controlled substances, only to later find the patient increasingly demanding and time-consuming. Often, these primary care providers respond to complaints of "I hurt" without assessing function and risk. When their patients fall outside of a clinical comfort zone, a referral, or "risk-shift," is made to a pain management provider. The pain practitioner may then be exposed to a high-risk, demanding patient in the first encounter.

Few specialties commonly accept these high-risk individuals outside of pain management practices, which implies to the medical community pain practitioners are, indeed, their "parachutes."

Another group of patients frequently encountered in a typical pain management practice are those *undertreated* by community providers. Acknowledging pain undertreatment and the practitioner's fear of prescribing controlled substances, the FSMB adopted guidelines in the 1990s that aided the practitioner's comfort level for controlled substances, even in large doses, for those suffering from legitimate chronic nonmalignant pain. This problem, pseudoaddiction, is less common today, and the enlightenment of pain treatment as a disease state has lessened suffering in the community. Practitioners are not free of risk, however, and the variable levels of controlled substance use to control pain imply a lack of formal training available for community care providers and other specialty providers. Misinformation and the potential of profes-

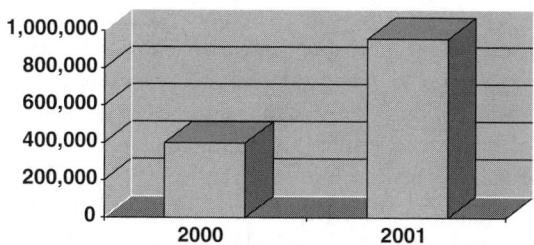

FIGURE 94.1 Instances of nonmedical use of OxyContin among U.S. population. Adapted from A. Atluri et al., 2003, *Pain Physician, 6*, 233. With permission.

sional sanction impair appropriate prescribing-related decision making, but to a lesser degree than previously existed prior to the FSMB guidelines. The recently updated Model Policy for the Use of Controlled Substances for the Treatment of Pain by the FSMB is available at http://www.fsmb.org.

Abuse and misuse of controlled substances is rising, however, and prescribers occasionally feel they are caught in the middle (Figure 94.1). Is there risk of retaliation from the patient or regulatory agencies? Are my patients in pain adequately treated, and how can I reduce personal risk? To reduce risk and enhance patient care, it is in the prescriber's best interest to exhaust all nonhabituating and non-opioid approaches to pain control prior to introducing potentially habituating agents. Consider reviewing the World Health Organization's "WHO Ladder" and become familiar with a knowledge base of minimally invasive interventional and surgical options.

Non-opioid adjuvant medications are effective and readily available to decrease opioid pain medication, or in many cases to help us decrease habituating risk. The interventional pain procedures pain physicians perform are further witness to the usefulness of adjunctive approaches to treat pain.

Additionally, psychological enhancements may be extraordinarily helpful, but are not always readily available. Below are suggestions to assist the practitioner in decision making, reducing risk, and promoting the proper use of controlled substances.

1. **Be goal oriented with medication management.** The patient and practitioner mutually understand that there is not a single agent, a "magic bullet," or an interventional procedure that will rid a patient of all pain. Realistic expectations are discussed with the patient, family members, and other third-party individuals that are interactive with the individual in pain. The interventional procedures and medications are *tools*, and when used properly, an important asset to enhance patient function.

2. **Pain is not static, but dynamic.** Pain will change, the character of presentation will vary over time, and functional indices are many times determined by the "personality of the pain." No more so is this true than when controlled substances are used for pain relief. The bio/psycho/social/religious influences of pain disrupt mood, function, quality of life, and personal interactions with others. Patients want a return to premorbid function and a pill is the easiest and most available treatment to many. Use of medications and functional enhancements should be reassessed on a regular basis to drive appropriate clinical conclusions and rule out the negative or ill effects of any pain control strategy. A patient asking for escalating doses of opioid and controlled substance-based pain or habituating adjuncts should be assessed of need, and documentation should be appropriate to the patient's presentation. Patients ultimately are given what they *need*, not what they *want*. Beware of the "ask-for-it-by-name" patient.

3. **You cannot document enough.** A personalized medical necessity checklist is a good approach, particularly a tool that includes elements of the recommendations by the FSMB for documentation purposes. Controlled substances are a double-edged sword — they can help and harm patients. Is the patient enabling or disabling? Are the patient's function and quality of life indices improved, or do we even measure these? Is the risk–reward benefit clearly reviewed, and is the patient documented to be of *no risk to harm self or others*? Always record the family and patient substance abuse history.

4. **Understand pain control as it relates to adjunctive medications.** Many pain-producing entities are opioid resistant. With any disease entity, defining the diagnosis precedes therapy, and this is particularly true when we treat the patient in pain. Establishing the differential diagnoses of patients with pain deserves careful thought prior to reaching any diagnostic conclusion, but when pain becomes *the disease*, a clear single diagnosis may be elusive. With no diagnosis, the practitioner and patient become frustrated and the costly process of "chasing" the pain frequently ends without resolution.

The patient with acute pain should be approached differently from the chronic pain sufferer. Acute pain responds more predictably to medications. Barriers to therapy such as psychological and physiological disturbances rarely impair the patient.

Patients with chronic pain require thorough management. Due to the many providers they encounter, these patients frequently feel the allopathic physician has lost interest in their complaint. It is not unusual that treatment is sought outside of traditional therapy, many times without the physician's knowledge. The physician's role remains to help the patient understand sensible treatment goals. It is unreasonable to expect complete pain relief in many situations, and expectations must be clearly explained to the patient. Establishing improvements in activities of daily living and functional lifestyle should be stressed. Very effective non-opioid, nonhabituating pain medications are currently available to improve perception of pain and well being with minimal risk of abuse. Adding these options or transitioning to these solutions is an important consideration, particularly if a habituating medication places the patient or prescriber at risk.

WHAT CONTROLLED SUBSTANCES DO TO PRACTICE DYNAMICS

Practitioners use controlled substances to manage symptoms of disease, such as chronic painful entities, with a primary goal of improving the patient's function, quality of life, and restorative sleep. Prescribing controlled substances necessitates the prescriber's commitment to continuing education in pain management, setting and enforcing proper treatment boundaries with patients, and understanding the interplay between law and medicine in the use of controlled substances to treat pain. A compassionate understanding between patients, their unique social dynamics, and other important individuals that influence treatment often are time-consuming for practitioners and create added attention of staff resources and training. Prescribing these medications frequently requires the staff to respond to numerous office phone calls and requests for early visits. Considerations of overutilization are valid, but when properly used to treat pain, these medications can ultimately control cost, possibly controlling utilization issues. Further considerations for prescribers and staff are that controlled substances increase provider medicolegal risk exposure and increase the potential of regulatory and civil scrutiny. Last, increased documentation is required, adding further burden and cost to the practitioner and staff.

RISK MANAGEMENT AND THE CONCEPT OF IATROGENIC ADDICTION

Iatrogenic addiction describes what happens when a well-meaning prescriber, providing symptom management with controlled substances, consequently habituates the patient to these medications. Patients may report to the prescriber for the sole purpose of obtaining pain medication, irrespective of current pain perception. These patients may have multiple sources available to procure these substances, and are quite insistent about their medication need. Frequently, more than one provider supplies these medications, so the patient does not "run out." In many states this is a violation of the law and is referred to as "doctor shopping." Poor vigilance places the prescriber in a potentially troublesome risk environment. Occasionally these patients believe it is their "right" to be treated with these substances, referring to Web sites, insisting that physicians undertreat pain. Patients may be convincing and unrelenting. A busy practitioner will often take the path of least resistance, write the prescription, or as mentioned, refer to the "parachute" provider in the community.

Controlled substances impose routine pharmacy checks and require that patients remain close to the guidelines that are developed by the practice to follow the use of the drug and its legitimate need. In cases of iatrogenic addiction, patients will expect a prescription to be written, and little deviation from their routine will be tolerated. Avoiding iatrogenic addiction is a key element when treating pain. Iatrogenic addiction, as the name implies, suggests that pain is no longer the primary reason for the visit. A careful history at each patient encounter will avoid this pitfall into which many providers fall. Pain may well become the disease of need, addiction an occurrence of the disease, and the practitioner should avoid facilitating both.

Controlled substances are not a patient retention or recruiting tool. Bad clinical outcomes and an increased risk of substance abuse are commonly encountered with a patient not closely scrutinized or followed with a high level of prescriber awareness. Furthermore, a subset of patients uses opioids for their euphoric effects, essentially initiating an antidepressant effect, inappropriately using controlled substances for mood alteration. Patients might also use controlled substances as an effective way to gain repeated access to the health care system for secondary gain purposes. The prescriber and the practice are accountable for the proper use of these medications despite external pressure, and the gatekeeper for proper prescription habitry.

DOCUMENTATION

When using controlled substances to control pain and disease, documentation must be thorough, and the risk–reward benefit reviewed with the patient regularly. The following model guidelines for the use of controlled substances for the treatment of pain are authored by the FSMB (http://www.fsmb.org). Adopted May 2004, the FSMB strongly encourages the medical record to include the following components:

- Medical history
- Substance abuse/chemical dependence history
- Pain history
- Appropriate studies (labs, imaging, etc.)

- Working diagnosis
- Treatment plan
- Rationale for treatment selected
- Patient education
- Doctor and patient understanding methods and goals of treatment
- Follow-up protocol, which must be adhered to
- Regular assessment of treatment efficacy
- Consultation with pain specialists, when warranted
- Multidisciplinary approach, when indicated and approved by payers (sometimes difficult)

As previously mentioned, a medical necessity checklist is suggested to be placed in the chart when treating patients with controlled substances and opioids in the chronic nonmalignant pain arena. The FSMB recognized the need for provider guidelines, enhancing compassionate care for those suffering from pain, lowering prescribing reluctance and guiding legitimate use. The FSMB requests that each practitioner demonstrate knowledge of narcotic-based pain medication, especially in a chronic scenario, and recommends ongoing continuing education. Furthermore, the medical record reflects low risk and states the patient's risk to harm self or others is reviewed. Provider documentation also includes, as a routine part of the history, current or previous substance abuse, and family risk factors.

MEDICAL NECESSITY AND AGREEMENTS

Practitioners *must* document "medical necessity" or "one or more clinical indications" for the use of controlled substances to treat pain. Practitioners *must* properly assess the patient, which means that the practitioner document the patient's general medical history, specific medical history concerning the existing pain complaint, past medical treatments, including controlled substances for the existing pain complaint, a working diagnosis, and the patient's history of chemical/substance abuse. In many states, licensing board prescribing guidelines and regulations require a practitioner to document that non-addictive treatment modalities or adjunctive therapy have been tried and failed or ruled out in the patient's case. Once a practitioner starts a patient on controlled substance therapy, it is suggested that the practitioner periodically review the patient's care to determine whether there is an ongoing medical necessity or clinical indication for the continued use of the prescribed medications.

True medical necessity is more than a diagnosis — it considers the whole patient, and his or her willingness to (1) be proactive in his or her own health care, (2) participate in formalized or home-based therapy, physical and well-health behavior, and (3) demonstrate behavioral stability. Particularly in pain therapy, enhancing function and

quality of life indices improves compliance. Many state licensing boards have documented investigations involving practitioners who fail to consider (or seriously consider) patient personality characteristics and history of chemical or substance abuse *prior to prescribing*. Practitioners are wise to consider these items in connection with a statement of medical necessity of clinical indication for the use of controlled substances. Remember, personality characteristics do vary among individuals, but aggressive personality characteristics are often the harbinger of a potentially problematic relationship with the patient.

To be complete in the medical necessity component of risk management, practitioners are urged to use medical history questions directed at gathering information about the patient's antisocial behavior, if any, including an assessment for personality disorders and violence. If unfavorable personality characteristics exist, a consultation with an addictionologist or psychiatrist is strongly urged, and may increase the likelihood of improved patient compliance and enhanced therapeutic decision making. Finally, consider further minimizing the potential for practitioner liability by having the patient sign a "No risk to harm self or others" form at each visit. Use this document along with a medical necessity checklist or another form of pain inventory (Figure 94.2).

A drug *contract* is less wordy than a "controlled substance *agreement*." The term *contract*, however, may imply legal obligations from both the patient's and the practitioner's perspective, and a *contract* may be used *against* a practitioner. An *agreement* between patient and practitioner is less legally intrusive. The drug agreement is signed with a witness present, and a copy is given to the patient with full explanation of the risks, complications, and options of habituating medication treatment. Consider having the patient initial each point of the agreement to acknowledge that the agreement was read and understood with no barriers to communication. It is strongly recommended that the patient's record reflect review of this controlled substance agreement at frequent intervals during the patient's subsequent visits.

CONTROLLED SUBSTANCES, THE CONTROLLED SUBSTANCE ACT, THE PHYSICIAN, AND THE CONCEPT OF LEGITIMATE MEDICAL PURPOSE

An important triangle of understanding exists between the DEA, pharmacist, and prescriber, each with a unique perspective of patient well-being and controlled substance management. First, the premise of the DEA is to ensure the health and safety of patients exposed to controlled substances, to safeguard society, and to provide guidelines and amendments to assure adherence to the law. The DEA, therefore, protects the public health and safety. Next, the pharmacist is the source of dispensing and distribution. Finally, the prescriber determines the need of a controlled

No Risk to Harm Myself or Others:

Patient Name: _____

Patient Signature: _____

Medical Necessity (1)	Opioid Therapy (2)	
Declining functional indices	Medical history	?
Poor restorative sleep capacity	Drug history	?
Poor activities of daily living*	Pain history	?
Progressive neurological problems	Appropriate studies	?
Progressive musculoskeletal problems	Working diagnosis	?
Progressive myofascial problems	Treatment plan	?
Progressive impairment and perception of disability irrespective reassurance and enabling environment	Rationale for treatment selected	?
Assess disabling features of our patient's personality	Patient education	?
Assess need and contraindications as well as modifiable features and patient's history	Doctor and patient understand methods and goals of treatment	?
	Follow-up protocol, which must be adhered to	?
	Regular assessment of treatment efficacy	?
	Consultation with pain specialists, when warranted	?
	Multidisciplinary approach, when indicated	?

(1) H. Hansen, M.D.   (2) Adopted from FSMB guidelines

*Inclusive of endurance, range of motion, ability to find satisfying and enjoyable activities through the day because of interference of pain, etc. Fair to poor control alternative treatments including non-narcotic medication alternatives, narcotic medication alternatives, and non-interventional procedures.

I personally authorize that I have examined the patient, discussed treatment, limitations and options, the risk reward and alternative approaches to treatment. I reviewed the medications, and I have evaluated the patient's needs. I have addressed issues of tolerance, pseudo tolerance, physical dependence, addiction and pseudo addiction.

Prescriber's signature: _____   **Date:** _____

FIGURE 94.2 Medical necessity checklist for controlled substance prescribing. Recommended to be completed at each visit.

substance based on patient presentation. The prescriber alone is responsible for understanding, and ultimately defining, legitimate medical purpose at the patient level.

REDUCING RISK WITH POLICIES AND PROCEDURES

Policies and procedures are a roadmap for practices to determine course of care and direction of daily expected and unforeseen activities. Strong policy and procedures that are accessible to staff and providers remain a powerful risk reduction tool. Frequently, a heralding event initiates a policy *reactively* and is kept in a dynamic nature to be modified as the practice grows. The staff is invited to add to the policies and procedures, where appropriate, and feel compelled to become part of the process of relevant documentation. This active involvement improves not only employee–practitioner relations, but takes the employee to task as a solution provider and an involved individual to assist in practice growth and protection. Policy and procedures are best developed *proactively* before reacting to a heralding event, but in both cases, demonstrate a high level of practice accountability.

Typical policy and procedures that address controlled substance use involve

- *Documentation.* Clear, concise history, physical, and diagnosis. The medical record is accessible and organized.
- *Medical necessity.* The risk is appropriate to the use.
- *Legitimate use.* The controlled substance is used within state, federal, and community standard. Currently, there is no designated *federal* community standard recommendation.
- *Credentialing.* The medical service provider is properly licensed by the state and registered with the DEA. Institutional affiliations and

medical organizations are important associations, and activity in local medical societies assists in community awareness of standards of care.

- *Standards of conduct of controlled substance use*. Standards of conduct are oftentimes defined by community and state recommendation. The provider is aware of the ethical and moral boundaries of controlled substance use.
- *Standards of prescribing practice*. Use, misuse, and expectations are understood by the patient, provider, and staff.
- *Continuing education*. Necessary to document awareness of legitimate use.
- *Emergency protocols*. Hospital affiliation and availability of services addressed, and protocol defined to assist in extreme care instances.
- *Call policies*. 24-hour availability for adverse event.
- *Operational and personnel responsibilities*. Each provider or staff member is aware of communication channels, when and whom to notify for a question or event, and providers or officers of concern are available when adverse event occurs.
- *Job descriptions and responsibilities*. No confusion should exist. Responsibility for controlled substance prescribing rests with the practitioner of record, or in the case of physician extender providers, the supervising physician is responsible for oversight.

Risk, as a form of loss, is reduced by developing policies and procedures that are understood and followed by the practice, and reflective of community standard. Continuing education of the staff and providers within a practice demonstrates responsibility to the patient and the regulatory system. Documentation of understanding and awareness of a diagnosis and plan are mandatory. A controlled substance agreement, signed, dated, and witnessed, and a signed informed consent are included in the chart.

As drugs with similar trade names, abbreviations, decimal points, and dose are common errors, both in and out of the hospital setting, prescriptions should be legible, and numbers of pills documented both numerically and then written out.

Altered prescriptions are becoming easier to pass for original, and computer software programs allow scanning of prescriptions generating look-alike prescriptions, further complicating issues of diversion. A novel tactic that might be used to avoid use of a fraudulent prescription is to apply a notary-like seal, unique to your practice, obtained at any local business shop. Local pharmacies can be made aware that controlled substance prescriptions are invalid without this notary seal. Of course, not all practices

will be able to inform each pharmacy, but demonstration of this high level of vigilance is in the prescriber's favor should the practice fall under scrutiny.

The practitioner should produce readable, organized, and accessible records. Within these records, documentation is thorough and recognizes drug interactions. Care is exercised to document alternative therapies considered, and a diagnosis matches the therapy offered. Considerable risk can be avoided if prescribers follow practice guidelines unique to community standards developed to address limits and expectations. All practitioners are compelled to remain within the scope of their practice defined by state law. Policies and procedures in the pain management office are often developed to assist in practitioner credentialing and monitoring of provider practices.

Another problem encountered with controlled substances is the availability of prescriber or staff to address adverse effects. A designated individual to follow patients and their needs decreases the confusion of perceived side effects, or outright complications from these medications. This response is particularly important in the elderly population, who are subject to multiple drug interactions. A designated and experienced person is often an important "go-between," connecting the prescriber and the patient to reduce misuse, confusion, or complications associated with controlled substance use. Documentation in the chart further reduces risk exposure when patients call, and a telephone log sheet is a necessary part of the formal medical record. In the next few years, we can envision the advantages of an electronic prescribing system that performs medication crosschecks and alerts misuse, incompatibility, and possible diversion. Although this technology is on the horizon, the electronic medical record still remains distant and not an easily available entity for many practices to acquire.

STANDARD OF CARE, INFORMED CONSENT, AND TREATMENT AGREEMENTS

Standard of care is a community effort, unique to an area's medical need, resource availability, and accessibility of practitioners. Relevant to the practitioner, standard of care acknowledges that education remains a key component to avoid risk of adverse event exposure. Standard of care also embraces informed consent as a foundation to develop understanding of the risks and benefits of treatments offered during the practitioner-patient relationship. In the use of controlled substances to treat pain, the development of a viable informed consent process is a critical component of the risk management process.

Informed consent has its origins in law. Historically, cases involving assault and battery involved touching without consent. Lack of informed consent frequently gives rise to a negligence or malpractice claim in the medical community. Informed consent is not limited to medical procedures alone. Instead, providers must learn that informed consent applies equally to procedures and treatment plans involving the use of controlled substances to treat pain.

Some states have intractable pain treatment acts (laws) requiring practitioners to engage in an informed consent process with patients prior to prescribing controlled substances to treat intractable pain conditions. Likewise, most state guidelines and position statements on pain management and/or prescribing controlled substances to treat pain suggest that practitioners *should* engage in an informed consent process. The American Medical Association's (AMA) Code of Medical Ethics contains a discussion of informed consent and states that it is a process that involves the exchange of relevant information between the practitioner and the patient. The information must be sufficient to allow the patient to make an informed decision about accepting or rejecting the proposed medical treatment. Specifically, the AMA contemplates an informed consent process that explains to the patient the risks and anticipated benefits of the controlled substance therapy, scientifically available treatment alternatives, and an opportunity for a meaningful exchange of information between the practitioner and patient. Once again, the lack of informed consent might result in a negligence action against the practitioner. Combined with a pattern of reckless disregard for legal/regulatory materials, accepted clinical practice standards, and community standards, lack of informed consent may be used as evidence of a practitioner's criminal intent in a case charging the illegal distribution of controlled substances.

The process of informed consent does *not* guarantee immunity. Explaining the risks and benefits, and treatment alternatives is not enough to constitute foolproof informed consent. Rather, practitioners must ensure the patient has the capacity to give his/her consent, and to understand the importance of the information supplied during the informed consent process and what it means to act upon the information. For example, did the practitioner explain the risks, complications, and options of the procedure, and spend the time necessary to ensure that no barriers to communication were evident? Furthermore, was the patient aware of the importance of the practitioner's comments, understood culturally, and was there no evidence of language barrier present? The key issue here is "First do no harm."

ORAL OR WRITTEN INFORMED CONSENT?

Practitioners are clearly pressed for time during the practice day and thus likely to see an oral informed consent process as the most efficient way to handle this risk management measure. However, oral informed consent will always pit the practitioner's word against the patient's word in the courtroom and, in such cases, the practitioner is likely to be on the losing end of that battle. Practitioners should be proactive with informed consent and use a written informed consent document that explains the required information in simple fashion and contains a space for the practitioner, patient, and witness signatures.

CONTENTS OF THE INFORMED CONSENT

The key elements of a written informed consent (see Figure 94.3) are: (1) a list of the risks of using controlled substances to treat pain, including a discussion of addiction potentials, the concepts of physical dependence and tolerance, commonly experienced side-effects, and potential drug-drug interactions; (2) the expected benefits of using the recommended controlled substances; (3) scientifically available treatment alternatives (given without regard to a patient's financial condition); (4) specific issues of concern, such as driving or handling a weapon; (5) the opportunity for the patient to ask questions of and receive a response from the practitioner; and (6) signature space for the patient, a witness, and the practitioner. Practitioners may use a similar informed consent form when considering special procedures or general treatments. Finally, find a way to show that you have inquired about patient competency (or guardian competency) to provide informed consent. This may require you to obtain a power of attorney, or the signature of an immediate family member in the case of a minor, and possibly a third party appropriately designated. In all cases, practitioners should determine whether the consenting individual is able to provide consent legally.

CONNECTION TO THE TREATMENT PLAN

Informed consent relates directly to the development of a treatment *plan. Before entering into an informed consent,* the practitioner is encouraged to document a working diagnosis justifying the use of the controlled substance(s) covered by the informed consent. Simply placing the patient on an opioid or controlled substance for symptomatic analgesia is inappropriate when the diagnosis is poorly understood. Many times a correctable procedure or non-habituating medication profile is more appropriate for the patient. A practitioner's failure to consider these issues prior to prescribing controlled substances may expose him/her to greater risk and thus greater liability.

THE USE OF TREATMENT AGREEMENTS

Most state prescribing guidelines and regulations contain a sister-component to informed consent called *Treatment Agreement.* Many practitioners are familiar with the concept of a "narcotic contract." A *Treatment Agreement* is similar to a "narcotic contract," except the *Treatment Agreement* should cover office policy on prescribing controlled substances and patient promises to handle con-

Informed Consent for the Use of Controlled Substances to Treat Pain

Dear _____ (Patient Name)   Date: _____

This document is called an "Informed Consent" form. The purpose of the document is to explain important information about the controlled substances (medications) your doctor recommends that you use to control your pain. You are responsible for reading this document, asking your doctor questions about the medications, and signing this form if you decide to use the recommended medications to control your pain. You will be given a chance to talk to your doctor about this information. You will get a copy of this form and we will keep a copy of it in your patient file.

Based on your statements to your doctor, and his/her review of your pain history and relevant medical records and tests, your doctor believes you have a medical condition called _____ and this causes you [acute, chronic, intractable] pain.

Your doctor has recommended treating your pain with the following controlled substances:

Drug	Strength	Qty	Route of Administration	Delivery	Potential Drug — Drug Interactions; Special Instructions

Treatment Benefits, Goals and Alternatives

Your doctor believes these medications will benefit you in the following way(s), but only if you follow the complete treatment plan your doctor discussed with you during your office visit:

1.
2.
3.

Your goals from therapy are to reduce your pain to a level that will allow you to do the following:

1. [example, Garden 3 days a week]
2.
3.

Your doctor has advised you that the following alternative treatments to using controlled substances are available to you:

1. [example, Physical Therapy]
2. [example, ibuprophen]

MATERIAL RISK NOTICE – DRUG CLASS _____ **(e.g., Narcotics/opiates)**

In general, using the medications listed above may put you at risk for the items listed below. You should check with your pharmacist for additional information about the above-listed medications if you decide to take them:

1. **BRAIN**: Sleepiness, difficulty thinking, confusion. **It is important for you to consider how your use of the above-named medication might affect your ability to operate a motor vehicle or other heavy machinery. IT IS YOUR RESPONSIBILITY TO FOLLOW THE LAWS IN THIS STATE REGARDING THE OPERATION OF A MOTOR VEHICLE WHILE USING CONTROLLED SUBSTANCES. Likewise, for those licensed to carry weapons, you must consider whether you have an obligation to report your use of controlled substances to your employer. If you have a concern about these issues, consult your attorney or call the Department of Transportation, Driver's License Bureau, Weapons Licensing Bureau.**

2. **LUNG:** Difficulty breathing, shortness of breath, wheezing, slowing the breathing rate.

3. **STOMACH:** Nausea, vomiting and constipation can be severe.

4. **SKIN:** Itching, rash.

5. **URINARY:** Difficulty urinating.

6. **ALLERGY:** Potential for allergic reaction.

Continued

FIGURE 94.3 Informed consent form.

7. **DRUG INTERACTION(S):** Possibility of interaction with other medications. Can make the effect of both drugs stronger when taken together.

8. **TOLERANCE:** With long-term use, an increasing amount of the same drug may be needed to achieve the same pain-relieving effect.

9. **PHYSICAL DEPENDENCE/WITHDRAWAL:** Physical dependence may develop within 3–4 weeks when taking these drugs. If they are stopped abruptly, symptoms of withdrawal may occur. These include but are not limited to: abdominal cramps, abnormal heartbeat, nausea and vomiting, sweating, flu-like symptoms. These may be life threatening. All controlled substances need to be slowly tapered under the direction of your physician or facility.

10. **ADDICTION:** This refers to the abnormal behavior directed toward acquiring or using drugs in a non-medically necessary supervised manner. People with a history of alcohol or drug abuse are at increased risk of developing an addiction.

If you want to know more about these risks, ask your doctor after you finish reading this form.

Have you read and do you understand this document? (Initial one)

___ I was satisfied with the above description and did not want any more information, or

___ I requested and received further explanation about the treatment, alternatives, or risks.

I agree to follow the terms of this agreement and I understand the risks, alternatives, and additional therapy associated with the use of controlled substances to treat my pain. I understand this document will be maintained as a permanent component of my chart.

Patient Signature: _____ Date: _____

Witness Signature: _____ Date: _____

Provider Signature: _____ Date: _____

*Note to provider : Use the back of this form to document the patient's questions and your responses to them.

FIGURE 94.3 *Continued.*

trolled substances responsibly. It is imperative that practitioners understand that Informed Consent and Treatment Agreement ARE NOT THE SAME PROCESS. These processes require different forms and different language. It is legal in most states for a practitioner to combine the informed consent and treatment agreement processes into one document, but that document should discuss informed consent on the front of the document and the treatment agreement on the back. The concept of a Treatment Agreement originates from a need to set boundaries for patients in attempt to minimize the potential for abuse and diversion of controlled substances. A Treatment Agreement does not originate from the law of assault or battery and a failure to use a treatment agreement generally will not give rise to an action in negligence or malpractice. Thus, before discussing the elements of a *Treatment Agreement*, it is important to review information relating to the extent of the controlled substance abuse and diversion problem in the United States.

EXTENT OF CONTROLLED SUBSTANCE ABUSE AND DIVERSION IN THE UNITED STATES

Erroneously assuming the patient is safe using an FDA-approved drug is not borne out by recent Drug Abuse Warning Network (DAWN) reports (Figure 94.4). Hydrocodone, oxycodone, and methadone preparations are rising in use and abuse. Emergency departments are docu-

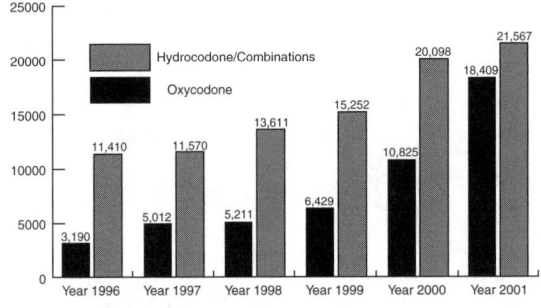

FIGURE 94.4 Estimated number of hydrocodone emergency department (DAWN ED) mentions for total coterminous United States from 1996 through 2001. Adapted from A. Atluri et al., 2003, *Pain Physician, 6*, 233. With permission.

menting increases in substance abuse admissions (see Figure 94.4 and Figure 94.5). The estimated cost of this misuse has continued to rise every year since 1992.

Patients using controlled substances may suffer from psychiatric disorders. Personality disorders, bipolar diseases, psychosis, and depression add a level of instability and risk to controlled substance management (Atluri et al., 2003). Informed consent must be understood by patients who are challenged by their psychiatric disease. Documentation requires support of clarity in mental status and no barriers to understanding.

The manifestation of pain is complex and multifactorial, and coexisting disease is common. Risk to harm self

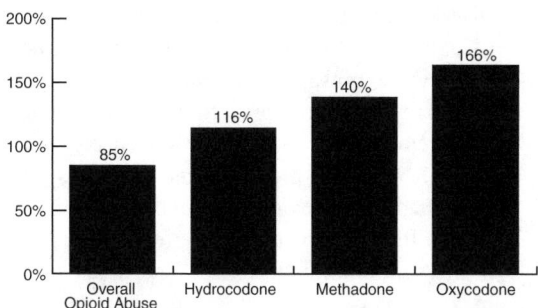

FIGURE 94.5 Percent increase of opioid abuse from 1994 to 2000. Adapted from A. Atluri et al., 2003, *Pain Physician, 6,* 233. With permission.

or others is an important documentation point, especially in the psychologically impaired individual. Substance abuse and misuse are common in this patient population, even those complaining of legitimate pain. Multiple illicit drugs may be combined with controlled substances, including marijuana. The patient with psychiatric disease requires frequent assessments, pill counts, drug screening, and occasionally, a responsible individual to assist with drug dispensing. Despite close control, abuse and misuse of any controlled substance are difficult for the provider to eliminate. Policies in the practice include proactive identification and an action plan for diversion control. Patient selection and a close patient–practitioner relationship are important, but Manchikanti (2002) reveals substance abuse is common in random screening (14 to 16%), and 34% with controlled substance abuse.

The most commonly abused drugs in the United States are opioids, and the principal drugs of abuse for almost 10% of the U.S. population are prescription preparations (Atluri et al., 2003). Even "good" patients are a potential source of risk, reinforcing the need for vigilance when adding controlled substances. Consider these points as a start for policy development to avoid diversion and misuse of controlled substances:

- **The patient must have a diagnosis.** Not understanding a diagnosis is fraught with complications when treating patients in pain. Simply placing the patient on an opioid or controlled substance for symptomatic analgesia is inappropriate when the diagnosis is poorly understood. Many times a correctable procedure or nonhabituating medication profile is more appropriate, and a wide differential diagnosis should be explored prior to moving forward into the narcotic arena.
- **The patient should be accountable.** We do not live in a perfect world, and some patients are going to be more successful at understanding directions than others. However, the staff should be readily available and the practitioner

should be involved in helping the patient understand, to the patient's cognitive capacity, the implications of controlled substance accountability and treatment. An agreement is reached between the patient and prescriber, and it is advisable that *a patient care agreement* (formally referred to as a "contract") be signed by the patient, preferably line item initiated, and each feature of the agreement explained. The agreement should state that controlled substances will be prescribed only at prearranged times, and that visits to the practitioner's office are mandatory to identify successful therapy. An opioid or controlled substance must be followed within the context of appropriate usage. Pill counts are common practice, random drug screens are recommended, and full informed consent should be in writing. At no time should the practitioner be a victim of "TWOG" (tail wags the dog) where the patient self directs care. The prescriber will document the name of the dispensing pharmacy and communicate when necessary with this pharmacy, and the patient consents to this in written form prior to adding controlled substances to a treatment profile. This informed consent protects patient confidentiality and the patient–practitioner relationship. The patient–practitioner relationship is based on trust, and should be inviolate. The patient knows that this is a two-way street, that these drugs have risks, and agrees to the guidelines laid forth by the practitioner.

- **A zero tolerance policy should be in place.** If an illicit drug, typically THC, is found in the medical drug screen, or if pill sharing occurs, the patient is unsuitable for controlled substance therapy. Abrupt withdrawal should be avoided, but frequent visits and tapering of the drug might be implemented. A potential exception occurs with the use of methadone. Utilizing methadone to withdraw from controlled substances requires a special attachment to the DEA certificate. Methadone is used for pain control, where appropriately documented, without added credentialing. Other medications are more appropriate to wean, and the practitioner remembers that he or she has no absolute/legal obligation to provide controlled substances to any inappropriate patient who has violated the patient–practitioner relationship. The practice may offer a strategy for the patient to be given a "second chance." The risk–reward benefit of controlled substance use is carefully considered in this situation.

- **If the patient seeks medication from someone other than the prescriber of record, and it was clearly outlined in the patient care agreement that this behavior is inappropriate, the patient will be taken off the controlled substance therapy.** The patient care agreement is not a contract, but an understanding of the practice's policy when using controlled substances. A contract implies legal obligations from the patient, and the practitioner as well. It is recommended that the patient care agreement be reviewed by a health law attorney and, of course, follow state guidelines.

- **A cautionary word about medical drug screens.** Many commonly prescribed medications, such as fentanyl, oxycodone, and methadone, are not revealed in routine medical drug screens. It is imperative that the practitioner utilizes one laboratory, clearly understands what this laboratory tests, and communicates often with this laboratory. The laboratory will understand the concept of informed consent and not obtain tissue, blood, or a urine sample for drug screening purposes unless informed consent is given. The patient is also made aware that when the drug screen is requested, the patient must report immediately to be tested. The patient may not report the following day, and again, this policy of compliance is specified in the patient care agreement.

- **An accountability system must be in place for writing and dispensing controlled substance prescriptions.** It is inappropriate to regularly call controlled substances to the pharmacy. Documentation of a prescription is placed in the medical record, and it is discouraged for opioids or controlled substances to be called in on weekends, holidays, and after hours, if at all. Phone-in prescriptions are not recommended to be a common practice, but used as a rescue only. The patient understands that *rescue* is for extraordinary purposes, and the patient care agreement states that if the patient loses his or her medication, or if it is stolen or misplaced, the prescription will not be replaced under any circumstances. Patients who obtain a police report stating that their medication was stolen simply fill out brief paperwork. This is not acceptable, and a lost prescription should not be replaced. A close patient–practitioner relationship may yield some latitude in this regard, but is a rare occurrence.

- **Strategies to avoid diversion would include keeping copies of prescriptions, not faxing duplicating prescriptions, and using unique** prescription pads. We recommend the use of a seal, much like a notary public would use, and that the prescriber communicate this to the pharmacy by having prescription forms declaring, "Do not fill without seal." Furthermore, altered or forged prescriptions can be rapidly identified by a copy retained in the chart. In the near future, computer-based prescriptions and online communication with pharmacies will make it much easier to avoid diversion. The DEA is currently developing electronic prescription guidelines.

- **A proper prescription designates the name of the medications, dosage, the number of units dispensed, and instructions for use.** The number of units should generally be handwritten as numbers (example: #50 fifty tablets) and by spelling out the number of doses as well. It is recommended that only one controlled substance be placed on a single prescription, although state laws vary in this regard.

- **The patient is regularly assessed for cognitive decline**. A brief mental status exam is recommended to be performed at each visit, as well as a functional assessment. Frequent communication with a family member documents subtle changes in mental awareness, and at least every 4 to 6 months a reassessment of functional parameters, pain relief, and elements of legitimate medical purpose will be repeated as continued justification of controlled substance use. At each visit the patient acknowledges and signs a medical necessity checklist, including the declarative statement "no wish to harm self or others." Any evidence of suicidal ideation is referred to appropriate practitioners, and narcotics and controlled substances withheld in a risk environment. It is proper to provide relief with controlled substances in a compassionate care arena, and family members or other reliable individuals may aid in dispensing to the patient at risk. If this is not possible, the practitioner determines if the risk exceeds the potential benefit of opioid or controlled substances and acts accordingly. Side effects from these medications are clearly elaborated to the patient, and changes in treatment strategy are adjusted promptly. Most commonly, constipation or other side effects are easily treated, which enhances compliance.

- **The patient should not be allowed to self-direct care while using controlled substances.** If the patient feels undertreated, this must be discussed with the practitioner. The concept of *pseudoaddiction* (where a patient seeks increasing analgesic doses to treat increasing pain), although controversial and often misquoted, should not be confused with drug-seeking behavior. Pseudoaddiction is easily identified, and should be documented in the medical record. However, the possibility of addiction should also be addressed. To simply increase the dosage when a patient says, "I hurt," is inappropriate. Again, a tool to assess functional capacity may reduce misunderstandings.

- **The practitioner should demonstrate a clear understanding of the pharmacokinetics of the drug prescribed, and the pathophysiology of the pain entity being treating.** Recognizing that pain does change and that the pain diagnosis is not necessarily permanent should alter prescription habitry. Finally, documenting continuing medical education is mandatory with any controlled substance use.

Risks, complications, and options of treatment are explained with each encounter that controlled substances are considered, including the risk of habituation; and definitions such as addiction, pseudoaddiction, and tolerance, with their implications, are communicated to the patient. Risks of driving, operating machinery, and making important cognitive personal or legal decisions are further divulged to the patient. Ironically, it is unclear at this time whether driving a vehicle and the use of a controlled substance are quantified within the arena of risk, but it stands to reason that the patient should be informed that impairment is possible to avoid retaliation should an adverse event occur.

As previously stated, a patient care agreement is also offered to the patient, and *not* referred to as a "contract." A contract infers certain legal obligation to the patient and of the prescriber. The patient care agreement is not a legal document; however, the patient care agreement is best reviewed periodically. An example of an agreement for controlled substances prescriptions is shown in Figure 94.6.

COMPLIANCE

REVIEW OF PERSONNEL AND PRACTICE OPERATION

Ongoing dynamic assessment of risk includes review of insurance, internal and external issues, controlled substance practice, and other liability areas, as well as confidentiality of records and patient information.

Internal issues to a practice include appropriate provider coverage, 24 hours 7 days a week, and avoidance of call coverage gaps. A provider is responsive to an adverse event, and provider performance should be reviewed randomly for competency of care. Deficiencies

require employee education and retraining where necessary. Competency exams for employees will assure that policies and procedures are met with the appropriate response. Controlled substances used in the office require a secured and locked environment, and familiarity with federal DEA regulations.

External risks include environmental OSHA scrutiny; regulatory agency investigation, such as the DEA or state board; fraud and abuse action procedures; and other barriers to care. Particularly important is addressing the Americans with Disabilities Act. Should an employee be found using controlled substances obtained from a prescriber, policies and procedures should clearly spell out the practice liability and offer rehabilitation if indicated.

Background checks are a useful approach to dealing with new patients, but do carry risk. The patient or employee is best informed of issues where violations of personal medical information might be breached. The patient receiving controlled substances agrees that the chosen pharmacy can be referenced and also defines who picks up medications. Other prescribers are not allowed to prescribe controlled substances by agreement, and appointment follow-up is necessary to monitor prescription habitry.

OUTCOME ASSESSMENT PRACTICE GUIDELINES

Outcome assessment requires three inputs to create an output: (1) the patient's perceived complaint matching the diagnosis, (2) the active participation of a medically challenging treatment profile, and (3) inclusion of a plan and appropriate follow-up, biostatistically active measures, and a bioappropriate outcome. The outcome tool recognizes the patient's self-report as the most valuable subjective tool a practitioner uses to assess complaints of pain. Based on the prescriber's practice habits, specialty, and experience, a diagnosis reflecting a broad differential diagnosis and plan are presented to patients in their best interest. This is proactive participation involving both prescriber and patients. Outcome will be adversely affected if the patient is noncompliant, and treatment hurdles identify reasons for failure. For example, did the patient not understand the opioid or controlled substance patient care agreement, or ignore it? Finally, the tools necessary to treat specific pain disorders should be traditionally accepted in general/clinical practice and within community standard. The medical record will document effectiveness of treatment progress, good or bad. This task should not be as challenging as it sounds. For example, an antibiotic given for strep throat may be considered effective when the fever is resolved and the patient is able to return to work and maintain adequate oral intake. These are measurable entities and are easily included in the medical record. The pain management practitioner might document improved func-

Agreement for Controlled Substance Prescriptions

Controlled substance medications (i.e., narcotics, tranquilizers,and barbiturates) are very useful but have a high potential for misuse and are, therefore, closely controlled by the local, state, and federal government. They are intended to relieve pain, to improve function, and/or ability to work, not simply to feel good. Because my physician is prescribing such medication for me to help manage my condition, I agree to the following conditions:

1)_____
initial

<u>I am responsible for my controlled substance medications.</u> If the prescription of medication is lost, misplaced, or stolen, or if I use it up sooner than prescribed, I understand that it <u>will not be</u> replaced.

2)_____
initial

<u>I will not request or accept controlled substance medication from any other physician or individual while I am</u> <u>receiving such medication from the pain center.</u> In addition being illegal to do so, it may endanger my health. The only exception is if it is prescribed while I am admitted in a hospital. If necessary to go to an Emergency Room for an emergency, I will notify the Pain Center within 48 hours.

3)_____
initial

<u>Refills</u> of controlled substance medication:
<u>Will be made only during regular office hours,</u> in person, once each month (or as arranged by the practitioner) during a scheduled office visit.
a) <u>Will not be made if I "run out early".</u> I am responsible for taking the medication in the dose prescribed and for keeping track of the amount remaining.
b) <u>Will not be made as an "emergency",</u> such as Friday afternoon because I suddenly realize I will "run out tomorrow." <u>I will call at least seventy-two (72) hours ahead if I need assistance with a controlled substance</u> <u>medication prescription.</u>

4)_____
initial

<u>I will bring in the containers of all medications prescribed by the pain center each time I see the practitioner,</u> even if there is no medication remaining. These will be in the <u>original</u> containers from the pharmacy for each medication.

5)_____
initial

I understand that if <u>I violate any of the above conditions,</u> my controlled substances prescription and/or treatment with the pain center may be terminated immediately. If the violation involves obtaining controlled substances from another individual, as described above, I may also bereported to my physician, medical facilities, and other authorities.

6)_____
initial

I understand that the <u>main treatment goal is to improve my ability to function and/or work.</u> In consideration of that goal and the fact that I am being given potent medication to help me reach that goal, I <u>agree to help myself by the</u> <u>following better health habits:</u> exercise, weight control, and the nonuse of tobacco and alcohol. I understand that only through following a healthier lifestyle can I hope to have the most successful outcome to my treatment.

7)_____
initial

No wish to harm self or others.

8)_____
initial

I agree, with full informed consent, to provide tissue or body fluid for drug analysis when requested for initial routine screening purposes.

9)_____
initial

I agree to allow the pain center to talk with my other treating practitioners, obtain records as needed, and obtain information from my pharmacy when needed.

I have been fully informed by the pain center and the staff regarding psychological dependence and physical dependence, addiction, and other unsuspected consequences of a controlled substance, whichI understand is rare. I know that some persons may develop a tolerance, which is the need to increase the dose of the medication to achieve the same effect of pain control, and I do know that I will become physically dependent on some medications. Should this occur I will stop the medication only under medical supervision or I may have withdrawal symptoms.

I have read this contract and it has been explained to me by the pain center and/or their staff. In addition, I fully understand the consequences of violating said contract.

Patient's Signature _____ Date _____
Witness Signature _____ Date _____
Doctor's Signature _____ Date_____

FIGURE 94.6 Example of controlled substance prescription agreement.

tional indices, better restorative sleep and endurance, and less pain medication usage. Validating medical necessity for procedures and pain treatment in general requires verification that the community standard is met, a diagnosis fits the presentation, and a plan of care ensures compliance and continuity of care. Experimental treatment falling under the category "I think it, therefore it is" does not meet these criteria.

DISPOSAL OR LOSS OF CONTROLLED SUBSTANCES

THEFT AND LOSS

- When theft or loss is discovered, it is the responsibility of the prescriber or the entity responsible for the substance in question to follow best judgment and take appropriate action. Based on volume, a significant loss for one institution may be insignificant to another.

- Controlled substances that are lost, even in small quantity, over a period of time can be problematic to the prescriber's practice. Repetitive, unexplained losses are considered suspicious. Furthermore, any break-in or robbery must be reported.
- If, by best judgment, the office notes the loss to be determined as significant, the DEA suggests the following documentation:
  1. Identification of quantity missing
  2. Name and schedule of the missing medication
  3. Abuse potential of missing substance
  4. Documentation of first loss occurrence, or a repetitive problem
  5. State where the loss was reported to state/local law enforcement authorities

The DEA requires practitioners to use Form-106 to report theft or loss of controlled substances. Report Form-106 may be obtained from the DEA Diversion field office to document the circumstances of this loss. Practitioners also may obtain this form at www.deadiversion.usdoj.gov. If you have to destroy a controlled substance, it is best to contact the nearest DEA Diversion Field Office for guidance. In addition, some states have more stringent guidelines, laws, and regulations on the destruction of controlled substances. Practitioners should endeavor to learn both federal and state requirements.

Practitioners should keep records of this event for at least a year. Patient names do not have to be used, but unique identification numbers must be attached to a particular patient to reference the medical record.

DEA INVESTIGATION AND ACCOUNTABILITY

The DEA may initiate an investigation, unannounced, and records must be supplied upon request. The DEA agents must present their credentials, state the purpose of the visit, and present a written notice of inspection. Once the investigation has been initiated, documentation of amount of medication lost, type and amount of spill, or return to manufacturer and transfer of drugs should be provided. Maintaining complete and accurate records ensures that these requirements are met. The DEA recommends that employees understand how to operate relevant equipment and computers, maintain appropriate records (with backup), and understand shutdown/lockup procedures.

Should a DEA investigation occur, the following is a list of documentation that is required to facilitate a review. These documented entities were derived from recommen-

dations of opioid treatment programs and include the following:

1. A list of individuals having access to controlled substances, including full name, date of birth, and social security number.
2. A list of those involved in medication shipment, including licenses and permits of the practitioners involved.
3. DEA-222 order forms, and supplier.
4. Dispensing records, including patient identification and references. This would also include incident reports of drug loss.

DISPENSING

The dispensing record will include name of substance, dosage form, and date dispensed. A signature encounter on the form is unique to the drug disposal and will also include the amount and dosage utilized, and whether any wastage was necessary.

PREVENTION OF DIVERSION, ABUSE, AND DEPENDENCE: REVIEW AND REDUCE RISK

Pain is a difficult entity to measure. We cannot see, touch, feel, or measure pain, and the patient's self-report of pain, coupled with functional assessment, may be the most useful measurement of relief cycling available to the physician. It is incumbent upon the pain management practitioner to offer and document compassionate relief, quality of life enhancement, review of functional indices, and improvement in activities of daily living when possible. These attempts are made within the patient's best interest, "to first do no harm."

Realizing this goal, opioids and controlled substances are frequently prescribed to control pain and symptoms secondary to pain. Prevention of diversion, abuse, and dependence is an issue that is paramount to the prescriber's best practice. Documenting patients' well-health behaviors and characteristically proactive contributions to their health care in most cases leads to best predicted outcome. Pain relief is sometimes a best estimate as to these functional enhancements, as are subjective reports, and are reported to the medical record understanding the nature of the complaint as related to the diagnosis. The American Pain Society (APS), The American Academy of Pain Management (AAPM), The American Academy of Pain Medicine (AAPM), and The American Society of Interventional Pain Physicians (ASIPP) have all issued guidelines relating to avoidance of abuse and/or diversion.

The core points of these guidelines may be summarized as follows:

1. *Recognizing pain as a critical point of care.* The helping professionals, their extenders, and associated personnel, residing in either hospital or office-based practices, should provide a compassionate care arena to understand the patient's pain within the context of the patient's normal life's activities. When controlled substances or opioids for chronic nonmalignant pain are utilized, steps to ensure adequate dosing, minimization of side effects, and avoidance of adverse reactions are important to ensure compliance, social integration, and improvement of activities of daily living. Documentation to the medical record will include such descriptive entities as subjective complaints of pain, functional decline, or enhancement of normal activities, medication usage patterns, and documentation of adherence to a treatment plan. A *diagnosis* is followed by the carefully designed treatment plan that is understood by the patient, with no barriers to communication. The diagnosis should match medical necessity for controlled substance use. It is also required that the patient bring medication in for pill checks and agree to sign a *patient care agreement.* A patient care "contract" implies certain legal considerations, and *agreement* is a more suitable term. This agreement would likely require random drug screening, and the patient should be informed (full informed consent) prior to undertaking a random medical drug screen. The prescriber will also understand the implications of the drug screen, its necessary confidentiality, and what the drug screen actually measures, including sensitivity to adulterants and false positives.

2. *Prevention of diversion.* Prevention of diversion requires the prescriber and the staff to be vigilant of patient usage patterns and factors of outside individuals that influence the patient's behavior. If the pill count is off on more than one occasion, diversion is suspected, and the patient's explanation for abnormal pill count is inappropriate, reevaluation of controlled substance use should follow. Is the patient improving functional indices and quality of life indices, or just asking for medication every month? Has the patient attempted physical therapy, cigarette cessation, etc., and taken active participation in his or her own health care, or is preoccupation with the medication the paramount reason for the prescriber visit?

If diversion is suspected, the prescriber bears the responsibility of documenting the suspicion, finding a remedy to avoid further diversion, or making plans to discontinue these medications. The practitioner has no implied responsibility to "taper" the patient, especially if a *risk to harm* environment is present. This must be carefully weighed against potential for withdrawal complications, particularly evident with benzodiazepines. It is recommended that an addictionologist also be involved in this particular event, ultimately hospitalizing the patient if necessary. If the patient is suspected of obtaining medications from multiple prescribers, every effort should be made to eliminate this behavior and assure that controlled substances are obtained from only one source. Furthermore, a small group of patients with a known addiction history or substance abuse disorder requires narcotic-based medications to control legitimate pain complaints. A high level of vigilance and documentation ensures availability and access to care. The patient's medication for relief of symptoms should not be withheld simply because of previous history of abuse. The patient, however, does remain accountable, is aware of the clinic's agreement for use of controlled substances, and is regularly assessed. A caveat to this statement is the requirement of the practitioner to obtain a special attachment to the DEA certificate for the treatment of addiction with ongoing opioid usage (maintaining known opioid addicts with opioids). Pain practitioners treat pain, not addiction. Prescribing opioids solely to maintain an opioid addiction is inappropriate without the DEA attachment, and violates controlled substance guidelines. Treating pain with opioids, even for someone with opioid addiction, is lawful if the purpose of the treatment is for the control of pain.

SUMMARY

There are risks in any medical practice. When controlled substances are used in medical treatment, the prescribing practitioner *must* use risk management tools to help minimize the potential for abuse and diversion of controlled substances. The cornerstones of risk management related to the use of controlled substances to treat pain are patient assessment, selection, and monitoring. Practitioners are encouraged to become familiar with and use federal and state legal/regulatory materials on prescribing controlled substances and pain management as a basis for medical record documentation and office policies and procedures. All prescribing *must* be based on a *documented legitimate medical purpose* and be issued *within the usual course of professional practice.* When practitioners follow these risk management principles, pain management can be rewarding for all involved.

The use of controlled substances to treat pain is not an easy component of a pain practice, yet the use of these drugs is an important piece of pain control and access to care. Patients in pain are like any other a practitioner may encounter; empathy and responsiveness to individual need enhance clinical outcome. The pain management specialist is uniquely considered the community expert, engaged and interactive with his or her peers to develop standards, and ultimately define legitimate purpose. It is the practitioner's responsibility to minimize the potential for abuse and diversion of controlled substances in the medical practice. Risk management allows you to balance your legal/regulatory obligations with your ethical obligation to provide quality medical care to your patients.

APPENDIX: CONTROLLED SUBSTANCE PRACTICE GUIDELINES AND COMPLIANCE REVIEW*

SCOPE OF NEED, FIRST STEPS

- The patient–practitioner relationship is established and documented.
- The nature and intensity of pain have been recognized and the current past medical history and coexisting disease are verified as justifying a controlled substance plan. There is a cause-and-effect relationship of pain on physical and psychological well-being, as well as function, and is contributory to a therapeutic plan. If present, documentation is completed to reflect the need for controlled substance use.
- History of a substance abuse has been asked. ☐ Yes ☐ No

DOCUMENTATION OF LEGITIMATE MEDICAL NEED

- Legitimate medical need is defined by our pain management clinic as an understanding that pain and suffering are treatable and are met in a compassionate care arena. This sometimes requires the use of controlled substances or other adjunctive technology or medications. Legitimate medical need is an ongoing and dynamic process that is reevaluated regularly and not considered a stable entity. In fact, pain changes regularly, and the characteristics of its presentation are frequently transformed. Psychological and physical changes that accompany a patient's original chief complaint and coexisting disease states are not static and require frequent reevaluation. Therefore, legitimate medical need for controlled substance use is evaluated by measuring subjective and objective complaints and weighing the risk-reward benefit against enhancement of function, quality of life, restorative sleep and the potential complications of these drugs.

---

* Adapted from the J. Bolen Group, LLC.

BACKGROUND

Education

- Ongoing education requires review of literature, peer interaction, and attending appropriate specialty-specific meetings that address the controlled substance issues contemporary to current pain practice.
- The care provider is aware of the Federation of State Medical Board Guidelines, other guidelines, and principles of legitimate medical need. Furthermore, this clinic treats pain and not addiction. Controlled substances are offered to improve quality of life and not maintain an opioid or controlled substance addiction.

CONSIDERATIONS THAT MAY INDICATE DRUG MISUSE OR DIVERSION

- Distance from clinic. A high level of suspicion and vigilance is in order when a patient travels past other care providers that might provide the same level of care or offer services similar to the pain management clinic. This includes, but is not exclusive to, prescribing controlled substances.
- Referral source. A referral source is an important, and many times pivotal, acknowledgment that the patient is entrusted to a specialist that manages a controlled substance. Understanding the referral source, and that the referral source is relinquishing controlled substance management to the clinic expertise, is established in the medical record. Special attention will be attributed to patients referred by a "friend" or acquaintance with little medical history available. Records should be requested and reviewed, and where appropriate, contact should be made with the primary care/specialist familiar with the patient. These risk reduction exercises should occur prior to prescribing controlled substances.
- Behavioral issues. Patients who experience particularly risky behavior or have underlying psychiatric disease are at higher risk for controlled substance diversion and misuse. This includes bipolar disease, risk takers, and those who have depressive disorder, among others. These behavioral issues are associated with patients at risk for misuse and overdose of these medications.
- Specific request. A specific request for a medication by name, or an unusual knowledge base demonstrated by the patient, about a particular medication is a point of question that requires further investigation.

• There will be no weekend or off-hours controlled substance call-ins unless the patient is well known, and a legitimate reason exists for this deviation from the patient care agreement. There is no black-and-white presentation of chronic pain, and there are times when a prescription will need to be called in on the weekends, but should be recorded in their medical record as to need for this drug.

• Exaggerated behavior. The symptoms must match the complaint, with no evidence of exaggerated behavior. It is uncommon that a patient with legitimate medical need for controlled substances will need to "prove" his or her pain, and a painful disorder should be self-evident by physical examination and historical features in the medical record, either past or present. The patient who "symptom exaggerates" may be exhibiting seeking behavior, and care should be given to prescribing controlled substances.

• Reluctance to change certain medications. Clearly, brand names, as well as scheduled drugs, have different street value, and a reluctance to change from a certain delivery system, or name of drug, should be considered of significant risk value to reexamine diversion or misuse. An exception may be the individual who is less sophisticated or has a fear of change. This individual should be separated from those who are either new to the practice or have a poor historical background of controlled substance usage patterns documented by other physicians, pharmacy checks, or demonstrated adulterated drug screens.

• Screens and controls. Drug screens have their limitations. The U.S. Department of Transportation does not require the DS-9, but in fact utilizes the National Institute of Drug Abuse 5. Some authorities have suggested that cutoff levels for positive tests may be too high in many situations. Furthermore, we acknowledge the fact that drug screens do not always identify the drug of interest, and a quantitative specimen must be sent. We also are at disadvantage with certain labs that do not test specific gravity or temperature, or identify chain of custody. We will do what we can to ensure chain of custody and proper testing, but we will not be able to obtain this ideal at all locations. Therefore, we will acknowledge this and use the drug screen as a tool and not an absolute. Consider the screen as a reference that we might use with a positive value, but not necessarily determine course of care based on this singular test. This piece of data may also be ambiguous with one positive result followed by a negative repeat

value, but it is the clinician's best judgment that will determine the appropriate use of controlled substances. Where a positive result is found, as in any medical test, we must acknowledge this as practitioners, regardless of follow-up testing, which may be negative. It is inappropriate to prescribe controlled substances when a risk environment may exist, and a consultation with peers may be in order. The ultimate decision to prescribe controlled substances still remains with the moment, the available data, the patient's behavior, and the training that we necessitate within the clinic directed by its guidelines.

WHEN THE PRACTITIONER–PATIENT RELATIONSHIP IS CHALLENGED OR TERMINATED

Discharge Guidelines

• Discharge guidelines are defined by the local professional societies, as well as the professional licensure boards and others. The issue of "Thirty-day Emergency Evaluation" should be only that, an emergency evaluation. The emergency department is certainly available to patients and should be a first source of true emergency care, and utilizing the pain center for "emergency chronic pain" may be inappropriate. A long-standing pain problem that has occasional exacerbations might be construed by the patient as an emergency and should be handled on an individual basis. This does not necessarily mean a controlled substance will be prescribed. If the patient has demonstrated a risk environment, where risk to harm is possible, either to self or others, or has demonstrated a lack of accountability to controlled substances, the pain center is under no obligation to provide the patient a prescription. Alternatives should be offered to the patient such as a detoxification center, and in certain situations where necessary, utilizing a family member or trusted friend to dispense very small amounts of medication. We would even consider a weaning protocol, with frequent visits to the clinic to obtain medication. Some states may consider this detoxification and, therefore, not legal without appropriate attachments to the DEA certificate. Rarely, if ever, will a 30-day prescription be offered when discharged from the clinic. The pain center will provide a maximum of only 7 days of drug to those discharged from the clinic without reevaluation, and the patient will be made aware of this policy at the time of discharge. Furthermore, it will be documented in the medical record that the patient was *offered detoxification* if such can be legally provided by the pain prescriber consistent with licensure and privileges where appropriate.

Prescribing Guidelines*

- Proper use. Proper use of medications is an important consideration for those who may be visually, mentally, or structurally challenged, and should be acknowledged when a chosen delivery system is provided. For example, a fentanyl patch may be an excellent delivery system for those who have difficulty taking pills, or a suspension may be compounded for those who cannot swallow pills. The pain center considers the *fewer pills* available the better, and breakthrough medications will be used with caution, demonstrating to the record clear medical need. The proper use of all these medications is discussed, as an as needed (PRN) medication does not necessarily mean that the patient takes the medication every 4 hours regardless of level of function or pain. It is also inappropriate to use medications for purposes other than pain control, or as they are deemed in the controlled substance justified diagnosis. An example might include benzodiazepines used for anxiety because "I have nerves." The diagnosis must match the need for controlled substances.

- Side effects. Side effects are documented in the chart. The patient should not drive, make important decisions, or perform activities that could be injurious while using these medications. However, numerous studies have shown that patients on stable doses of opioids or controlled substances do not have a significant decline in their ability to operate a motor vehicle. Although this policy may be restrictive, controlled substances, such as pharmacokinetically long-acting opioids, may compound the synergistic effect of benzodiazepines and adjunctive medications. Informed consent and risk must be understood by the patient that any treatment, especially controlled substances, has risk, and be acknowledged in the record. Some latitude may be exercised by the patient and the clinician's best judgment, as there are no specific guidelines regarding driving a vehicle while using controlled substances, but care should be exercised with the elderly or physically chal-

lenged patients to reinforce this understanding. Studies have repeatedly shown that the incidence of clinically significant cognitive dysfunction is much higher with benzodiazepines than with opioids or controlled substances.

- Adverse effects. Adverse effects require notification to the pain center, and a response to these adverse effects is dictated by descriptions of the problem relayed through the nurses and discussed with the providers. Adverse effects may be mild, moderate, or severe, and might require evaluation of the patient as a work-in or a referral to an emergency department. Many times adverse effects are short term, short lived, and self-limiting. In many cases, reassurance many be all that is necessary, and the provider will be aware of the side effects and complications of medications provided, and understand the appropriate response to these side effects. All *Black Box* warnings will be noted. A Black Box is a Food and Drug Administration warning that is prominently displayed in the *Physician's Desk Reference* (PDR). If medications are used off-label, which the CSA of 1962 allows, there will be documentation in the medical record that there was an efficacious response and a justification in this regard. Off-label uses of medications are valuable aids in pain management and should not be discouraged, but encouraged as adjuncts if they decrease the opioid or controlled substance requirement. For example, amitriptyline (Elavil®) may be used to control sleep, and an antiepileptic agent such as gabapentin (Neurontin®) may decrease the required narcotic load in an opioid-resistant pain complaint or in neuropathic pain. Valproate (Depakote®) may be used for mood stabilization.

- Document discussions. Patients have many questions, and concerns should be documented to the medical record so that we can demonstrate a response to their understanding or misunderstanding. If a patient has a discussion with the pain provider off-hours, or on a weekend, it is necessary to document this encounter into the chart. (*Note:* It is not always necessary if very little action is taken or if the call responds to a routine question, but a high level of vigilance to documentation is our best position.)

- There is no one drug cocktail. As we have choices, the practitioner understands the individual variation and response to medications. Morphine and codeine have different side effects in different individuals, and synthetic compounds do as well. Therefore, it is not advised that a single drug be considered stan-

---

* A suggested practice inventory.

dard for an individual prescriber, and that variation matches the diagnosis and the patient diagnosis defined by presentation.

TREATMENT EFFICACY

- Policy for breakthrough medications, "rescue" medications. Policy for breakthrough medications is based on *medical necessity*. A breakthrough medication is considered an adjunct and should also be a starting point for advancing opioid- or controlled substance–based pain medication to a higher level. It is acknowledged that a pharmacokinetically long-acting drug does not always have steady serum concentrations, and occasional breakthrough medication is warranted. It is not clearly appropriate, however, to offer breakthrough medication as just routine two, three, or four times daily dosing response to a patient's complaint "I hurt." Many instances respond to readjustment of a pharmacokinetically long-acting drug, and decreases the rollercoaster effect of the short acting drug, which might adversely affect cognitive function and place the patient at risk. Furthermore, resistance to the underlying parent drug, the long-acting drug, may develop more quickly, when breakthrough drugs are added, and defeat functional enhancement. Finally, breakthrough medications should be demonstrated to improve function, quality of life, or restorative sleep, and the patient must use these medications correctly. Pill counts, as with other medication counts, should be appropriate.
- When a certain medication fails, it is documented to the medical record. It is inappropriate for a patient to call 2 or 3 days after an initial change in medication, stating that "it doesn't work," and the patient should be informed that "stabilization" may take longer. Of course, these medications have pharmacologic activity, and bioavailability is rarely an issue. In fact, some patients prefer certain medications and request them by name. As previously noted, this is not always appropriate, even when discussing generics and brand name medications. A medication must be tried for at least 2 to 4 weeks (there may be some individual patient variation), and no immediate changes are made without appropriate pill count and accountability to the original medication. If intolerance to a side effect is noted, where appropriate, a change may be made. The patient must present the remaining drug prior to a change in agent. If a

medication is "lost," flushed down the toilet, or "thrown out" because it did not work, a second prescription will not be given. There may be some flexibility if appropriate pharmacy checks are made, the patient is well known to the clinic, and a clear adverse reaction was documented. Not every patient is a drug seeker or manipulator, and not every "good patient" is a good patient. Three studies have documented the "good patient" with an adulterant present in the urine drug screen occurring in the 14 to 30% range (Manchikanti, 2002). This is a heralding mark for us to understand; the "good patient" may get used to taking medication and see very little risk in mixing or even borrowing. It is incumbent upon the practitioner to be aware of this, and even "good patients" should receive drug screens. Use common sense, of course. We will not ask infirm or elderly patients for a screen unless a clear reason exists.

- The medical record will reflect correlation of treatment efficacy and medication need. It was previously noted that improved functional indices and quality of life indices should be self-evident, but not always reflected by subjective complaints. Do not hesitate to exercise a high level of vigilance (2-week prescriptions, checking transdermal fentanyl [Duragesic®] patches for intrusion, etc.) if the treatment plan shows significant failure and the medications that we believe should be "working" produce no therapeutic benefit. A second opinion is recommended, and of course, pharmacy check and drug screens quantitated as well.
- Patients with drug abuse histories and diversion histories do have pain. It is a difficult but important concept to grasp that we do have to acknowledge these patients without preconceived assumptions or prejudice. This is where the difficulty in our profession arises, as these patients are of the riskiest nature. A sickle cell patient may have, from time to time, abuse, diversion, or seeking tendencies, but the fact remains that sickle cell is a punishing disease. Pain relief *ethically* should be provided. It is recommended that consultation with a colleague is documented to the medical record, and these patients are treated with frequent office visits, pill checks, drug screens, etc. Common sense weighs heavily here. Furthermore, the medical record should routinely document that we have asked the patient if there is abuse or drug diversion history.

DOCUMENTATION/FOLLOW-UP GUIDELINES

- It is a struggle to determine overutilization versus appropriate medical care when we use controlled substances to control pain. These drugs require a high level of respect and are not simply "pills" such as an antibiotic. It *is* appropriate for monthly visits, most notably with Schedule II prescriptions. Overutilization is a concern for everybody, but pain control complaints and side effects are common, especially in the early phases of treatment, requiring a special development of the patient–physician relationship and realization of improved function and quality of life indices through our treatment plan. The pain center recommends monthly visits unless the patient is a well-understood patient, with a well-understood indication for chronic controlled substance use, and is individualized. The patient's convenience, usage history, and medical indication are not static and will be reassessed, and many patients originally seen at monthly intervals may be allowed to visit us every other month, or every few months depending on their presentation. If the patient is not seen and examined every month, the reason for this should be documented in the record.

- Records from other treatment sources, pharmacies, and pain clinics will be sought from referred patients and will regularly be reviewed.

- An action plan for treatment failure will be addressed and discussed with peers if necessary. A treatment failure does not necessarily mean a drug failure. Many times a treatment failure represents the need for adjunctive care, such as an interventional technique or an adjunctive medication. It is not necessary just to increase the opioid without understanding this risk–reward benefit, and many times pain presentations are complex requiring both non-opioid or controlled substance medication adjuncts and adjusted opioid treatment strategy. There is no "one right course." Patients are individualized, and it is the expert opinion of the trained pain practitioner with the eyes and hands on the patient that wins out in this important cornerstone of decision. Issues of *pseudoaddiction* may be addressed, although the concept of pseudoaddiction many times falls to the side of a poorly diagnosed or undertreated individual.

- Detoxification will be offered for those who are in violation of guidelines or who want to be removed from narcotics. Methadone, in particular, will not be detoxified in the pain management center, and in fact, methadone will *only* be used to treat pain, and *never* to treat an addiction or to "wean." This requires a special attachment of the DEA certificate, which we will not seek. An addictionologist may be a useful consultant, from time to time, to enhance therapy. A psychiatrist will be a useful alternative, if that psychiatrist is known to have substance abuse training.

- The State Board Guidelines and the Federation of State Medical Board Guidelines will be understood by the provider, and occasionally elements of this will be revealed to the patient, and definitions revealed to the patient through the medical necessity checklist.

DISCHARGE PLAN AND DOCUMENTATION

- The patient will be required at all times to maintain contact with a primary care practitioner, and this will be documented to the chart.

- Withdrawal from opioids or controlled substances is problematic in many situations, but in those with preexisting disease such as heart disease or tenuous medical history, the medical record will reflect that this was acknowledged and precautions were taken in this regard to avoid adverse event. Again, in-house detoxification, if allowed by state law, or utilizing the primary care practitioner as a co-managing provider should be entertained early for patients who are to be weaned from narcotics or controlled substances.

- The controlled substances we use in the pain center are important treatment entities. The Pain Relief Centers is not, however, a substance abuse clinic or a drug maintenance clinic. Ongoing assessment as to need, legitimate medical use, and appropriateness to diagnosis is paramount. If controlled substances can be eliminated from the list of medications used to control pain, they will be, and done so compassionately, with the patient's understanding.

- Patients understand that detoxification always requires medical assistance and should not be done by themselves or at home.

- Staff training should be ongoing, and if the provider notices a deficit in a colleague or staff member, this will be brought to the attention of appropriate individuals who can correct this deficiency through an action and remedy plan. Competency tests will be asked of any practitioner identified as having knowledge weakness, and we will do what we can to be very proactive in an ongoing, collegial understanding of these controlled substances and their proper use.

Signed <u>by employee or practitioner</u>

USEFUL RESOURCES

- American Academy of Pain Management. Retrieved July 2, 2003, from http://www.aapainmanage.org.
- American Academy of Pain Medicine, *The use of opioids for the treatment of chronic pain.* Retrieved July 2, 2003, from http://www.painmed.org/productpub/statements/opioid-stmt.html#sect1.
- American Medical Association. (2001). *ICD-9-CM 2002: International classification of diseases* (9th rev. ed., Vol. 1 & 2). Chicago: Ingenix, Inc./American Medical Association Press.
- American Medical Association. (2002). *Current procedural terminology* (professional ed.). Chicago: AMA Press.
- American Pain Foundation. (2003). *Pain care bill of rights.* Retrieved July 12, 2003, from www.painfoundation.org/page.asp?file=Bill ofRights.htm&menu=1.
- American Pain Society. (2003). *Rights and responsibilities of healthcare professional in the use of opioids for the treatment of pain, advocacy & policy.* Retrieved July 22, 2003, from www.ampainsoc.org/advocacy/pdf/rights.pdf.
- American Pain Society, *The Use of Opioids for the Treatment of Chronic Pain, Advocacy and Policy,* Retrieved July 2, 2003, from www.ampainsoc.org/advocacy.htm.
- American Society of Interventional Pain Physicians. Retrieved July 2, 2003, from http://www.asipp.org.
- Center for Medicare and Medicaid Services. Retrieved August 6, 2003, from http://www.cms.hhs.gov.
- Drug Abuse Warning Network (DAWN) Report, Major Drugs of Abuse in ED Visits, 2000, 9 July 2001. Available online at http://www.dawninfo.samhsa.gov/pubs%5 F94%5F02/shortreports/files/ed2000.pdf.
- Federation of State Medical Boards, *Model guidelines for the use of controlled substances for the treatment of pain.* Retrieved July 9, 2003, from www.fsmb.org.
- Joint Commission on Accreditation of Hospital Organizations. Retrieved July 14, from http://www.jcaho.org/.
- National Household Survey on Drug Abuse (NHSDA) Report, Substance Abuse or Dependence, October 11, 2002. Retrieved September 4, 2004, from http://www.DrugAbuseStatistics.samhsa.gov/nhsda.htm.
- Office of Inspector General. Retrieved August 6, 2003, from http://www.ssa.gov/oig/.
- World Health Organization, Pain Ladder. Retrieved August 6, 2003, from http://www.who.int/cancer/palliative/painladder/en.

REFERENCES

Atluri, A. et al. (2003). Controlled substance guidelines. *Pain Physician, 6,* 233–257.

Federation of State Medical Boards. (1998, May 2). *Model guidelines for the use of controlled substances for the treatment of pain — Section III Definitions.* Available online at www.medsch.wisc.edu/painpolicy/domestic/model.htm.

J. Bolen Group, LLC. (2003). *Summary of the Federation of State Medical Boards' model guidelines on use of controlled substances to treat pain.* Knoxville, TN: Author.

Kanner, R. (2003). *Pain management secrets* (2nd ed., pp. 210–212). Philadelphia: Hanley & Belfus, Inc.

Manchikanti, L. (2002). *Interventional pain medicine documentation, coding & billing: A practical guide for physicians and ASCs.* Paducah, KY: ASIPP Publishing.

U.S. Department of Justice, Drug Enforcement Administration. (2004, September 4). Available online at http://www.dea.gov/.

95

Take Action: Be a Pain Management Advocate — A Quick How-to Guide for Healthcare Professionals

Lenore B. Duensing, MEd

Advocate — A believer, a supporter, a defender, a champion, an activist

It is now the Decade of Pain Control and Research, and all of us working in pain management have a not-to-be-missed opportunity to work as advocates for people with pain and to make *pain* a national healthcare priority. This chapter is a call to action from the American Academy of Pain Management (the Academy).

As a healthcare professional treating people with pain, you are in an ideal position to serve as an advocate. You are an expert on pain management; you know how pain devastates the lives of so many people; and you have the credentials it takes to make yourself heard. In other words, you have the power to effect a positive change in pain management on the local, state, and national levels. That is why we are calling on you to become a pain management advocate.

WHERE WE ARE RIGHT NOW: FACING-UP TO A NATIONAL HEALTHCARE CRISIS

Chronic pain is arguably the nation's number one public health problem. More than 50 million Americans live with serious chronic pain that affects almost every aspect of their personal, social, and work lives (Louis Harris and Associates, 1999). Chronic pain also takes an enormous toll on the U.S. economy. The findings of a study reported in the November 12, 2003, issue of *The Journal of the American Medical Association* showed that lost productive time from common pain conditions among active workers costs an estimated $61.2 billion per year (Stewart et al., 2003). The tragedy is that although the medical technology is available to reduce most chronic pain, most pain goes untreated or undertreated. This is particularly true for minorities, elderly patients, children, and other medically underserved groups.

In spite of the staggering toll pain takes on the nation and on the lives of the individuals who suffer with it, pain management is not a public healthcare priority, and millions of people continue to suffer needlessly. Why? Because there has been neither the will nor the commitment required to change the pain management environment, a central part of the Academy's mission is advocacy — reaching out, empowering, and organizing other healthcare professionals, people affected by pain, policymakers, and others to make this commitment and take the actions needed to put pain on the national healthcare agenda.

IDENTIFYING AND REFRAMING THE BARRIERS

The first step in raising awareness of the pain epidemic is to identify the barriers to good pain care. The next step involves reframing these barriers — viewing each as an opportunity and a specific target for change. Some of these barriers/targets of change are the result of the following:

- Pain care gets scant attention in most major healthcare organizations and research institutions.
- There are no federal laws mandating research, professional education, or public awareness or guaranteeing the rights of patients in pain to effective pain management.
- Most healthcare providers have not been trained to assess or treat pain, so most people with chronic pain have a difficult time finding the treatment they need.
- The most effective treatments for patients are often not reimbursed by insurance companies.
- Pain carries a stigma and many people with pain suffer silently. They do not seek treatment and do not let their families, friends, or healthcare providers know that they are in pain.
- There are widespread misconceptions about pain and pain medications among healthcare professionals, patients, and law enforcers; and these are being perpetuated by sensationalized and inaccurate media stories.
- The most effective treatments for patients often are not reimbursed by insurance companies or may be too costly.

WHAT WILL IT TAKE?

Removing the barriers and changing the pain management landscape for the better will require the work of many individuals and organizations who:

- Share a common vision and message
- Are passionate about the issue
- Are willing to collaborate with others to achieve common goals
- Are committed to taking action

Improving pain management will require different strategies ranging from personal advocacy (directly helping and supporting people with pain along with their families and caregivers) and grassroots actions that motivate the public to demand effective pain management (bottom-up strategies) to directly influencing legislators and regulators to create pain care laws and policies (top-down strategies).

Those of us working to improve pain management can take valuable lessons from the successes of other patient and professional advocacy groups. Consider the following:

One reason cancer patients finally have greater access to medications in late stages of research is that cancer groups have learned how to deliver their messages repeatedly and effectively. Partners in that success story are the men and women with AIDS who formed the organization "Act-Up." Those AIDS treatment activists

tutored the cancer advocates on how to be heard and gain access to medications at earlier stages…. Later patients and professionals used advocacy tools to de-stigmatize depression — forever establishing the fact that depression is not a weakness, but instead, an easily treatable medical condition. (Hospice and Palliative Nurses Association Advocacy Toolkit online at http://www.hpna.org)

ADVOCACY: FROM THE ONE TO THE MANY

So, what does a *pain management advocate* do and how do you become one? By becoming an advocate, you can raise awareness of pain management issues, help break down the barriers to effective pain care, and give voice and support to people with pain. As an *advocate*, you are a *believer*, a *supporter*, a *defender*, a *champion*, and an *activist*. To be an advocate, you need to be informed and educated about pain management issues, empowered, committed to taking action, and willing and prepared to stand fast in the face of challenge or adversity. How you do this, and the level to which you do it, is up to you.

Why become a pain management advocate? Because it's the right thing to do!

TYPES OF ADVOCACY

Although there are many ways to be a pain management advocate, the Academy separates *advocacy* into three, often interrelated, categories:

1. **Personal Advocacy** — Providing support and information to people with pain (your patients and others) so they can learn to advocate for themselves, and when necessary, standing up for them and helping them get the care they need.
2. **Grassroots Community/Public Awareness Advocacy** — Reaching out to consumers, healthcare providers, policy makers, and the media with information about pain and pain management issues, and calling on them to take positive action.
3. **Legislative/Policy Advocacy** — Taking actions to influence legislators and other policy makers for the purpose of introducing or changing pain management laws and policies from the state to the national level.

Described below are a variety of ways that you, as a healthcare professional, can take action as a personal, public/community awareness, or legislative/policy advocate. Also included are examples of others who have taken action and a listing of useful resources.

THE HEALTHCARE PROFESSIONAL AS A PERSONAL ADVOCATE

In addition to providing the very best pain treatment for your patients, you can serve also as their personal advocate. Patients who are educated and informed, who feel supported, partner with their healthcare professionals in reaching the goals of their treatment plan, and know how to self-advocate to obtain the very best results and relief possible. It is a "win/win" situation for both the healthcare provider and the patient.

Another and more challenging way to be a personal advocate for your patients is to help them overcome the medical, personal, and legal barriers they may be facing. This can include assisting them to navigate through the healthcare system, providing resources, intervening when there are insurance problems, and serving as a mediator between them and their employers or family members.

Action Steps

- **Believe and accept your patients' reports of pain.** This is the first, second, and third rule of good pain management! Consumer advocacy organizations hear regularly from people in severe pain who say their healthcare professionals have not believed, or even accepted, their reports of pain. This is true particularly for those with persistent pain who look well and whose tests show nothing wrong. From a clinical perspective, disbelief often leads to pain that goes untreated or undertreated and to pain that progresses. From a behavioral perspective, it often leads to stress, depression, a sense of being crazy, and extreme frustration and anger — all of which can exacerbate pain conditions.

- **Tell your patients that you are willing to serve as their advocate — their supporter —** and demonstrate this through your actions. Let them know that, in addition to providing them with the best treatment possible, you are there to listen to them and support their efforts to achieve relief from pain. Tell them that you are there to help them if they are having problems getting the care they need.

- **Let your patients know they have the right to effective pain care.** Post a Pain Care Bill of Rights poster in a visible place in your office, and give each patient a Pain Care Bill of Rights card (available through APF in English and Spanish).

- **Encourage your patients to participate actively in their pain care and provide them with the information about their pain problem.** This may include information about their particular conditions or diseases, communications tips on how to describe their pain (which will also help with your assessment), treatment options, and where to find pain support groups in the area. (See resource section for organizations that provide support and materials for patients.)

- **Refer patients to other healthcare professionals** if you are unable to give them the treatments they need or if they can benefit from additional/complementary types of therapy.

- **Teach your patients and their caregivers how to become pain management advocates for themselves and others.** People with pain who advocate for themselves most often get optimal care and make the best recoveries. By taking action, they also gain purpose, renewed energy, and a sense of empowerment. In addition, patients and caregivers can be the most effective messengers of the pain problem. They can be asked to tell their stories, give support to others with pain, speak at local events, give media interviews, and write letters to their state or federal legislators.

Case Study — Speaking Truth to Power: The Pain Management Nurse Who Fought for a Patient's Rights

Shannon L. is 33 and has lived with a debilitating pain condition called reflex sympathetic dystrophy or complex regional pain syndrome for the last 14 years. Although doctors told her that she would spend her life in a wheelchair, she was determined and worked hard to get the treatment she needed to continue working and being active. There were, however, many barriers to overcome. Navigating the healthcare system, finding people willing and able to treat her, going to work, and maintaining personal relationships still presented enormous challenges. Then, 8 years ago, Shannon met Micke Brown, a pain management nurse in a local pain clinic, who has been at her side ever since working to break down these barriers one by one.

On Shannon's first visit to the pain clinic, Micke told her about the pain service and the doctors. She also told Shannon to call her if she had any questions — no matter what time or how often. During this visit, Micke stayed with her explaining difficult terminology and answering questions. Most of all, Micke let Shannon know that she was there to intervene on her behalf if there were ever any problems.

Through the years, Micke stayed true to her word and became Shannon's supporter, teacher, and on several occasions, her defender — and that continued even after Shannon left the practice Micke was in. For example, in February 2003, Shannon faced a very serious problem. She was wrongfully discharged from the subsequent pain practice and asked Micke to "go to bat" for her. Shannon reports:

> After taking a hard fall that caused my pain to shoot to an unbearable level, I took an extra pill [an opioid] and called the doctor's office immediately because I feared I had broken my narcotics contract," Shannon explained. "When the office failed to return my first call, I called the doctor on call for the practice, whom I trusted, and asked for help — pain medications, sleeping pills — anything that would give me relief. The pain was going wild and I couldn't sleep. Unfortunately, he wasn't able to call in a prescription for opioids over the phone and instead prescribed a medication I was allergic to. On Monday, when my mother went into the office to get new medications, my treating doctor saw that I had taken one extra pill and discharged me from the practice. No one spoke with me directly and I was not referred to another doctor. I was left high and dry. I think part of the reason was that my treating doctor was angry that I had called the doctor on call and not him.

Shannon called Micke in desperation. Micke, having known Shannon for several years, was confident that she was not abusing her medications. Micke called the doctor whom Shannon trusted (and who was in charge of the practice) and told him that she was deeply concerned that Shannon had been treated unfairly, and asked him to intervene. She suggested that he personally reassess Shannon's pain problem and consider readmitting her to the pain clinic. As a nurse, who worked closely with this doctor in the hospital, Micke took a risk by speaking out against his partner's actions.

Micke's efforts paid off. The doctor called Shannon and listened carefully to her side of the story and took her back under his care. Her pain is better controlled and she feels reassured that she is being treated in an environment where there is mutual trust.

Today Micke works for American Pain Foundation (APF) as the Manager of Public Outreach. Shannon serves on the board of directors of the Maryland Pain Initiative. Together with Micke, she is organizing meetings for people with pain in which they can talk about their experiences and barriers to care. She also serves as an advocate for other people with pain in her community.

THE HEALTHCARE PROFESSIONAL AS A GRASSROOTS COMMUNITY ADVOCATE

As a healthcare professional, you are in an ideal position to bring awareness of pain issues to your community and give voice to your patients with pain by working on their behalf. Some ways you can be a grassroots community advocate include educating others (the public, people affected by pain, other healthcare professionals, and policy

makers) about the importance of pain management, hosting meetings or events targeting various audiences, and reaching out to the media.

You can do this type of advocacy on your own, but we suggest that when possible, you join with others. Investigate public awareness campaigns, such as

- *Power Over Pain* — APF and the American Alliance of Cancer Pain Initiatives (AACPI)
- *Partners for Understanding Pain* — the American Chronic Pain Association (ACPA)
- *Pain Ambassadors Program* — National Pain Foundation (NPF) and the American Academy of Pain Medicine (AAPM)

(See Resources section for more information about these campaigns.)

Action Steps

- First, identify yourself as a pain management advocate. Then, start spreading the word. Let others know about the work you are doing. Whenever appropriate, talk with others in your community, your family and friends, people on trains and planes — talk with anyone who will listen. Most often, you will find that they have a pain story and will want to share that with you. **Don't be afraid to be passionate. Pain is a serious problem. You know that. If you have strong feelings, express them. Passion can be contagious.**

- Check to see if there is a group in your area working to improve pain management and find out about public awareness initiatives (see Resources section).

- If there is not an existing group — start one! Build a team of pain advocates who will reach out, speak out, and spread the message from a variety of perspectives. Think broadly. Whom do you know? Consider healthcare professionals who treat people with pain, pharmacists, patients, caregivers, and others. Reach out to people representing diverse communities (e.g., minorities, seniors) and include them in your outreach.

- Develop a targeted public awareness plan including specific activities and media outreach. Determine how to reach out to various audiences such as people affected by pain, other healthcare professionals (representing different disciplines), the general public, the media, and government officials.

Activity Ideas

Groups conducting pain management public awareness activities are using a number of tactics to reach various key audiences in their states/communities. Below are some examples of actions you may take.

- **Get your state or local government to proclaim September as Pain Awareness Month** — Groups in states around the country have gotten Pain Awareness Month Proclamations from their state, county, and city governments and are using them to call attention to pain as a national healthcare problem and to gain media attention. The idea was developed by Partners for Understanding Pain, a national public awareness initiative led by the American Chronic Pain Association. For more information go to www.theacpa.org.
- **Give presentations/workshops for:**

  People with Pain — Let people with pain know that they have the right to have their pain addressed and treated, and that their pain can be relieved or greatly eased with proper pain management. Think about giving short, easy-to-understand presentations that include useful information about pain — what it is, what causes it, ways it can be managed, commonly held myths and misconceptions about pain and pain treatments, how to speak to healthcare professionals about pain, and resources. These can be held in locations such as community organizations, health centers, libraries, or public schools. (Powerpoint® presentations are available through APF.)

  Local Organizations (reaching the general public) — Organizations such as Rotary, Kiwanis, local chambers of commerce, faith-based groups, Y's, senior organizations, and large businesses offer excellent opportunities to inform people about the pain problem, to educate them about the importance of treating pain, and to involve them in your advocacy efforts. Some tips: Prepare your talking points carefully and include a number of compelling pain facts (if you have pain facts relevant to your local area, all the better); present real pain stories (especially stories about people who have struggled to find relief and then succeeded); consider having a patient or caregiver speak to the audience as well; and call on the group to help you spread the word. Be sure to invite the press. (Powerpoint presentations are available through APF.)

  Healthcare Professionals — Until recently, pain was overlooked as a healthcare problem by most healthcare professionals, and pain screening has not been part of routine examination. The purpose of giving this type of presentation/workshop is to provide healthcare providers with pain management basics. And do not forget about students, particularly those preparing to be healthcare professionals. (Powerpoint presentations are available through APF.)

Other Suggestions

- Distribute the APF Pain Care Bill of Rights cards and posters, and other patient materials to hospitals, nursing homes, pharmacies, and the offices of healthcare professionals.
- Ask librarians and bookstore owners to set up a special display of books about pain management.
- Set up a booth at a local health fair where you can distribute patient information brochures and talk to people about their pain rights and where to find help.
- Ask local clergy to present pain information as part of their services.

Case Study — Reaching Out to the Community with a Public Awareness Campaign: A Nurse's Vision

Five years ago, as part of the planning for a nationwide campaign that was to be called Stop Pain Now, APF developed a Community Action Kit, which included organizing information, activity suggestions, a media guide, and resources. Although the campaign was stalled, APF distributed a number of the kits to groups and individuals asking for public awareness ideas. One of those people was Ellyn Radson, a pain management nurse and president of the North Florida Chapter of the American Society of Pain Management Nurses (recently renamed the American Society for Pain Management Nursing).

Intent on getting a public awareness/educational campaign started in Gainesville, Ellyn used the APF kit as a starting point, and then organized her ASPMN chapter and others in the community (including doctors, pharmacists, and journalists). She also brought APF on as the national partner and convinced all of the area hospitals to come on board.

In January 2002, the group launched a local campaign called Power Over Pain (POP). It was kicked-off with proclamations by both the City of Gainesville and Alachua County. This was followed by week-long activities including presentations to a variety of audiences, participation in health fairs, and displays placed in all of the area hospitals. The group also produced a large calendar (with information about where to go for help in the community and a list of national resources) and distributed patient materials and POP pins.

The following year, inspired by the success of Ellyn's local campaign, APF in collaboration with AACPI, with participation by divisions of the American Cancer Society and ASPMN, piloted POP statewide in Florida, Louisiana, and Massachusetts. Each of the 2003 POP campaigns was launched with a statewide survey conducted in September during Pain Awareness Month.

Ellyn's group expanded their activities in Gainesville (and continue to serve as a model) and joined with the Florida Pain Initiative and the Florida Division of the American Cancer Society.

The POP campaign is expanding into other states. Check to see if there is a campaign in your state that you can join (www.aacpi.org), or begin organizing POP activities in your community. You can order a POP Community Action Kit from APF. The kit contains information on building coalitions, specific action ideas, Powerpoint presentations for healthcare professionals and consumers, a comprehensive media kit, facts about pain, and resources.

LEGISLATIVE/POLICY ADVOCACY

As a healthcare professional and a pain management specialist, you can use your position and expertise to take political/legislative action that will promote policies and laws to improve pain management.

Action Steps

- **Get informed.** Learn about the government and how the legislative process works. Information can be found on the Internet at Project Vote Smart (www.vote-smart.org), Thomas Legislative Information (www.thomas.loc.gov), and the League of Women Voters (www.wv.org). Learn how to use Thomas as a research tool. Created by the Library of Congress, the site provides comprehensive information on all bills introduced in Congress, text of the Constitution and other historical congressional documents, information on congressional representatives and committees, and much more.

- **Learn about specific legislative issues** that affect patients with pain, their families, friends, and caregivers, as well as healthcare professionals.

- **Educate yourself about pain management issues from the local to national level.** Get a sense of how people in your community are affected by pain management issues so you can communicate that information to your public officials.

- **Follow local and national news stories about pain and pain management issues.** Get a sense of how pain issues are covered and what is of interest to the media.

- **Make sure that you are registered to vote — and exercise that right!**

- **Join with professional organizations that are working on this issue.** Your own professional organization is a good place to start. Find out if pain management is on their "radar screen," and if not, ask that it be placed on their list of legislative priorities.

- **Sign up** with the American Pain Foundation for legislative updates and alerts at www.painfoundation.org.

- **Write a letter.** Members of Congress are genuinely interested in the opinions of the people they represent. Letters to Congress are a primary means of access to decision makers by their constituents. All written correspondence from constituents are not only noted and counted, but count for thousands more. Also, think about taking the next step and organizing a writing campaign. Even 10 to 20 letters can be perceived as a "groundswell" of support. Provide others with sample letters and talking points. Some tips:

  Write only to your representatives or senators, unless circumstances require you to write to others such as the chairpersons of committees. Send original letters, not copies, to each individual.

  Address the letter correctly. Be sure to spell the legislator's name correctly and use the right forms of address. Terms of address should be Senator, Representative, or Member, not Congressman or Congresswoman.

  Be polite (never confrontational), brief, and to the point. Discuss only one issue or bill. Try to keep your letter to one powerful page. *Do not use form letters.* The letter should be in your words. Do not send postcards. Handwritten letters are still highly valued.

  Get right to the point. Describe the issue or bill in the first paragraph. Identify the bill you are writing about (provide the bill number) and clearly state what action you are seeking.

  Describe how the issue or bill affects you as a healthcare provider and how pain affects the lives of your patients.

  If you know how your legislator has voted on related issues, mention it. It will show that you are checking voting records.

Send a follow-up letter after you receive a response from your legislator. Send a thank you letter if positive action has been taken on your request. Repeat your request if action was not taken.

- **Meet with your legislators or their staff.** Some tips:

  Make an appointment first.

  Be prepared with talking points and have an information sheet prepared that you can leave behind.

  Be clear, concise, and courteous. Do not stay more than 15 minutes, unless encouraged.

  Describe not only the number of people suffering with pain (nationwide and in their districts), but the impact of pain on their lives.

  Offer solutions. Let you legislators know what specific actions they can take to improve pain management in your district or state, and how those actions will benefit their constituents.

  Follow-up with a thank you letter to your legislators and their staff. Repeat your messages in the letter. Public officials get lots of requests. Remember the squeaky wheel ....

- **Send an e-mail.** As with letter writing, keep your e-mail message brief and to the point. State that you are a constituent. Include the name and number of the bill. In addition, be sure to include your full home address, time your e-mail so that it arrives on a Monday or Tuesday, or Friday, and follow up.

- **Make a telephone call** — When you call a legislator, remember that you need to be brief and communicate key information. Most often, you will reach a staff person. Ask to speak with someone who handles healthcare legislation. State your name and address, let her know that you are a constituent, tell her you are a healthcare provider calling to express concerns about pain management (state your position as specifically as possible). Be sure to stick with talking points prepared before calling and stay on point. Limit your call to under 5 minutes and ask for a written response.

- **Write a letter to the editor** — This has even more weight than a letter sent directly to your legislator. A letter to your legislator is an important expression of your opinion, but a letter to the editor lets the legislator know that your views will be read and thought about by other voters. Letters to the editor are usually written by readers for the opinion section of newspapers and magazines, either in response to something that has been published in the paper or to something significant that is happening in your area. Letters should be kept short, no longer than 500 words, and should focus on one major point.

- **Encourage others to take action** — Ask your colleagues, family, friends, etc., to write, call, or visit legislators as well. Provide them with sample letters and suggestions.

Case Study — A Hospice Organization Fights to Preserve Patient Benefits — and Wins

In January 2003, hospice programs in Ohio faced cutbacks in services funded through Ohio Medicaid. In order to fight the elimination of funding for hospice services, the Ohio Hospice & Palliative Care Organization (OHPCO) recognized the importance of educating Ohio legislators and regulators about the importance of preserving these services for the Ohio citizens, who were facing end-of-life decisions.

OHPCO made it a priority to organize and advocate for its constituents both locally and statewide. Each of the member hospices was asked to designate an advocacy coordinator. An all-day training program was provided for the coordinators. Each coordinator was asked to identify at least 10 advocates.

A grassroots advocacy campaign was planned and launched. This included a letter-writing campaign and visits to legislators and regulators by staff, volunteers, patients, families, board members, vendors, and physicians. In their letters and visits, advocates wove statistics and personal stories together to show both the financial and holistic benefits of hospice. On June 26, 2003, Ohio Governor Robert Taft signed off on the budget retaining vital eligibility and funding provisions for Ohio's Medicaid Hospice Benefit.

OHPCO was able to use a state-wide directed effort, supported by passion, knowledge, and persistence to net the desired results — continued coverage of hospice for Ohio's citizens.

USING THE MEDIA: MAKING PAIN NEWS

One of the most effective ways to communicate pain information is through the news media. In fact, that is where most people go to get information. The more often a story is reported, the more concerned people get about it.

Pain is now making front-page health/medical news. But, in both senses of the word *news*, there has been both the good news and the bad news about pain. The good news is that the undertreatment of pain, as a healthcare problem, has been getting wide media coverage since the Joint Commission on Accreditation of Healthcare Organizations (JCAHO) standards went into effect in January 2001. The bad news is that there has been a rash of harmful news stories related to pain and pain medications. The abuse and diversion of opioids, for example, have become a focus of local and national media. And, while most of these sensationalized stories have focused on the dangers of these medications, few have addressed the real news — that millions of Americans are suffering needlessly with pain.

Because people tend to believe that what appears in the news is true, both the good and bad stories influence the way that the public, healthcare professionals, policy makers, law enforcers, and others understand and respond to pain management issues. So an essential part of grassroots and legislative advocacy work is creating accurate, current, and compelling stories that carry our messages and motivate people to take positive action.

DEVELOPING KEY MESSAGES

Everyone is concerned about messages these days — from the President of the United States to grassroots advocates. So, what are messages and why are they so important? Messages are the key understandings about your work — they are your theme. To be successful in your advocacy work, your messages should be powerful, organized, logical, and persuasive. Ethel Klein, a well-known public health media strategist, said that messages should be morally authoritative and capable of evoking passion.

Messages should be tailored to your audiences, so think about what it is your audience needs to know, the best way to say it, and what you want the audience to do with the information. Note: Messages are not sound bites, slogans, persuasive arguments, or statistics, although all of these can be used to support your messages.

DELIVERING MESSAGES TO THE MEDIA

If you are working with a group, think about who will be the spokespeople — the people who will speak publicly about the work you are doing and give interviews to the media. Choose people who are "authorities" on the subject — who have experience from a variety of perspectives. You may want to identify consumers (patients suffering pain, family members, caregivers) and healthcare professionals (pain specialists — doctors, nurses, social workers). Spokespeople should be articulate, able to convey key messages clearly and succinctly, and readily available to speak with the media. If you are contacted by a reporter, respond immediately. Reporters are often impatient or on a deadline and will move on to other sources. So it is also important to have back-up speakers.

SAMPLE MESSAGE TRACK

Pain is a national public health crisis. *It Is Our Nation's Hidden Epidemic.*

- More than 75 million Americans suffer with chronic pain.

- Pain is the Number One reason people seek medical care.
- Uncontrolled pain diminishes quality of life and decreases work productivity.
- Pain has serious economic consequences—pain costs our economy $100 billion in medical costs and lost workdays.

Undertreatment of pain has serious physiological, psychological, and social consequences.

- Pain weakens the immune system and slows recovery from disease or injury.
- Uncontrolled pain adversely affects almost every aspect of a person's life including sleep, work, and social and sexual relations.
- Pain causes anxiety and depression, and may lead to thoughts of suicide.

Most pain can be controlled with proper pain management.

- When pain is controlled, people can experience a better quality of life.

Unfortunately, there are barriers that prevent effective pain treatment.

- Most healthcare professionals have little or no training in pain management (and are unable to effectively respond to patients' reports of pain).
- **Exaggerated concerns about addiction lead to undertreatment of pain**. Addiction to opioid analgesics is unlikely for people with no history of substance abuse and when opioids are properly prescribed and taken under medical supervision.
- **Pain carries a stigma**. Many people with pain are fearful or embarrassed about letting their families, friends, and even their healthcare professionals know they are in pain, because they don't want to appear weak, or be considered a bad patient.
- **Some government policies** impede pain relief by restricting access to pain treatment.

People with pain, their families, and caregivers need to advocate for good pain management and insist on the treatment they need.

MEDIA ACTION STEPS

- **Familiarize yourself with the local media.** Read the newspapers, listen to radio stations, and watch TV programs in which you want your stories covered. Find out what kinds of stories they cover and from what angles. Tailor your messages to their audiences.

- **Develop relationships with the people who make the news.** It is far easier to get your story in print or on the air if you have working relationships with reporters, editors, and producers. One way to do this is to let them know that you can serve as a credible source of information and a leader on the issue.

- **Have a clear objective when approaching the media.** It may be to call attention to a pain management issue or problem in your area, to call for action on the part of an elected official, or to let the public know about an upcoming event.

- **Write strong news releases that have a standardized look.** All release should include the five Ws — who, what, where, when, and why. Make sure your release is focused and contains enough information for a story. Include the local angle (why the story is of particular interest to their readers or viewers). Structure your story as a pyramid. Capture the essence of the story in the lead paragraph — tell something important and tell it fast. Give all the facts. Have a concluding paragraph.

- **Follow-up with a phone call to reporters.** You want to make sure your release lands on the right desk, but more importantly, a phone call gives you a chance to pitch your story.

- **If you are interviewed by the media, stay on message.** Remember, you are the expert on the subject. Also, do not let the reporter get you off topic. Learn how to redirect questions by saying, "That's a good point, but I want to emphasize that …." If you are asked a question you can't answer, say that you are not sure and that you will get the information for them. You can also offer to put them in touch with others.

- **Opinion pages and editorials offer great opportunities for advocates to get their messages out.** The editorial section of the newspaper is one of the most widely read. This is often the place where policy makers go to find out what issues are hot topics among their constituents. You can request a meeting with the editorial board or write an op-ed piece or a letter (don't forget, you are an expert).

- **Submit items to community print and online newsletters, calendars, and bulletins.** Think about various ways to get your story out.

CONCLUSION: REALIZING THE VISION

We will know that we have succeeded in our work as pain management advocates when:

- Pain will be recognized as a serious public health problem.
- Federal and state governments will invest adequate funding for pain research, healthcare professional education, and public awareness.
- Patients with pain will have access to the treatment they need.
- It is understood that pain is harmful to the body and should be treated as the fifth vital sign.
- Pain does not carry a stigma.
- All healthcare professionals are knowledgeable about pain management, and there are more pain management specialists.

So, what are you waiting for? Take action now!

RESOURCES

Personal Advocacy (Printed Materials, Web sites, and Support Groups)

American Alliance of Cancer Pain Initiatives (AACPI) is a national organization that promotes pain relief nationwide by supporting the efforts of state and regional pain initiatives. The organization offers printed materials for patients and a Web site that contains a media toolkit, sample letters, press releases, and op-ed pieces. For state and local contacts, check its Web site for state initiative information. Several state initiatives are now addressing pain in general.
Address: 1300 University Avenue, Room 4720, Madison, Wisconsin 53706
Web site: www.aacpi.org
Telephone: 608-265-8655

American Chronic Pain Association (ACPA) — A nonprofit organization offering support groups throughout the world and a variety of useful materials for people with pain. The ACPA is also leading a nationwide public awareness campaign called Partners for Understanding Pain.
Address: P.O. Box 850, Rocklin, California 95677
Web site: www.theacpa.org
Telephone: 916-632-0922

American Pain Foundation (APF) — A nonprofit organization serving consumers affected by pain, through information, education, and advocacy. The organization offers a comprehensive Web site (including links to disease-specific pain), PainAid (online community support), consumer publications, a monthly e-newsletter, a toll-free information line, and public awareness and legislative activities.

Address: 201 N. Charles Street, Suite 710, Baltimore, MD 21201

Web site: www.painfoundation.org

National Chronic Pain Society (NCPS) — Provides peer support groups for people with chronic pain and their families. It also provides current, accurate information from qualified professionals through the *Chronic Pain Report* (*CPR*), a quarterly newsletter, and through multidisciplinary conferences.

Address: P.O. Box 903 Tomball, Texas 77377-0903

Web site: www.ncps-cpr.org

Telephone: 281-357-HOPE (4673)

National Pain Foundation — Offers online education for patients experiencing pain and their families including information about pain, treatment options, links to support groups, and physician-led public awareness activities.

Web site: www.painconnection.org

Telephone: 303-756-0889

PUBLIC AWARENESS ADVOCACY (PUBLIC AWARENESS/GRASSROOTS CAMPAIGNS AND RESOURCES)

Power Over Pain (POP) — a grassroots action/media campaign, conducted collaboratively by APF and AACPI. To see if there is a POP group in your state, go to www.poweroverpaincampaign.org or send an email to info@painfoundation.org.

Pain Ambassador's Program — a public awareness initiative of the National Pain Foundation and the American Academy of Pain Medicine. Designed for pain-trained physicians, the purpose of the program is to spread the word about the importance of pain management, provide useful information to consumers, and teach pain management basics to other healthcare professionals. Pain Ambassadors are provided with toolkits, a newsletter, and regularly updated information. To learn more, go to www.painconnection.org.

Partners for Understanding Pain — organized by the American Chronic Pain Society, it is a network of organizations working to create greater understanding and awareness of the impact of pain on the economy, social structure, and lives of individuals. To find out more, go to www.theacpa.org/publicawarness.htm.

LEGISLATIVE/POLICY ADVOCACY

Pain & Policies Studies Group — An organization dedicated to "balancing" international, national, and state policies to ensure adequate availability of pain medications for patient care while minimizing diversion and abuse. This organization also supports a global communications program to improve access to information about pain relief, palliative care, and policy.

Address: 406 Science Drive, Suite 202, Madison, Wisconsin 53711-1068

Web site: www.medsch.wisc.edu/painpolicy

Telephone: 608-263-7662

MEDIA OUTREACH (MEDIA TOOLKITS AND INFORMATION SPECIFIC TO PAIN)

Power Over Pain Community Action Kit contains two media guides: "Making Pain News!" (a comprehensive guide) and "Striking a Balance: The Abuse of Opioid Analgesics and the Media, A Rapid Response Action Kit." Both are available online at www.poweroverpaincampaign.org. "Striking a Balance" can also be found at www.aacpi.org.

September Pain Awareness Month media materials can be found at www.theacpa.org in the Partners for Understanding Pain section.

Pain Control Advocacy Toolkit, a resource of the Hospice and Palliative Nurses Association that offers media tips and ways to reach legislators can be found online at www.hpna.org.

NATIONAL PROFESSIONAL PAIN ORGANIZATIONS

American Academy of Pain Management — A national multidisciplinary pain society that provides credentialing to practitioners in the area of pain management. A good source for complementary and alternative practitioners. Offers information on finding healthcare professionals and programs.

Address: 13947 Mono Way, Sonora, California 95370

Web site: www.aapainmanage.org

Telephone: 209-533-9744

American Academy of Pain Medicine — A national organization of pain physicians promoting quality care of patients with pain as a symptom of disease (eudynia) and primary pain disease (maldynia) through research, education, and advocacy, and through the advancement of the specialty of Pain Medicine.

Address: 4700 W. Lake Avenue, Glenview, Illinois 60025
Web site: www.painmed.org
Telephone: 847-375-4731

American Pain Society — A multidisciplinary pain organization serving people in pain by advancing research, education, treatment, and professional practice.
Address: 4700 W. Lake Avenue, Glenview, Illinois 60025
Web site: www.ampainsoc.org
Telephone: 847-375-4715

American Society for Pain Management Nursing — An organization of professional nurses dedicated to promoting and providing optimal care to patients with pain through education, standards, advocacy, and research. Check Web site for local chapters.
Address: 7794 Grow Drive, Pensacola, Florida 32514
Web site: http://www.aspmn.org/
Telephone: 209-533-9744

International Association for the Study of Pain — A professional organization dedicated to furthering research on pain and improving the care of patients with pain. Membership in IASP is open to scientists, physicians, dentists, psychologists, nurses, physical therapists, and other health professionals actively engaged in pain research and to those who have a special interest in the diagnosis and treatment of pain.
Address: 909 43rd Street, Suite 306, Seattle, Washington 98105
Web site: www.iasp-pain.org
Telephone: 206-547-6409

ONLINE PAIN RESOURCES

City of Hope Pain Resource Center — Serves as a clearinghouse for information and resources that enable individuals and institutions to improve the quality of pain management.
Web site: prc.coh.org

Mayday PainLink — A virtual community of health professionals committed to alleviating pain.
Web site: www.edc.org/PainLink

REFERENCES

Louis Harris and Associates. (1999). National pain survey. Conducted for Ortho-McNeil Pharmaceuticals.

Stewart, W. F. (2003). Lost productive time and cost due to common pain conditions in the U.S. workforce. *Journal of the American Medical Association, 290*(18), 2443–2454.

Section XII

Beliefs, Religion, and Spirituality

Richard H. Cox, MD, PhD, DMin, Section Editor

96

The Problem of Pain for the Healer and the Art of Healing

Richard H. Cox, MD, PhD, DMin, and Betty Lou Ervin-Cox, PhD, PsyD

Most, if not all, that is contained in this chapter is familiar to most healers. However, because we learn best by repetition, and we learn new material in terms of what we already know, a revisiting of our basic premise of being holistic practitioners may be welcome. Further, as much as we might like to think that all of the healing world thinks as we do, let us not be deceived. Many have heard, some have listened, and fewer have followed the actual practice that we verbalize so well.

Healing is seen by many, professionals and laypersons alike, as a science, which to be certain it is. However, long before the human race understood much, if any, of the actual science involved, it was an art and only specifically gifted and trained persons were capable of practicing it. The more a specialty becomes a science, the more it is teachable and sometimes becomes devoid of the unseen, intuitive, "giftedness" aspects that make it also an art. With the advent of so much wonderful technology entering the healing field, we have seen a diminution in the interest and manifestation of the need for the art and the greater emphasis on the science, which often is relegated to numbers, laboratory, and other diagnostic procedures of a more mechanical and lesser human involved nature.

Ancient medicine, and for that matter, all of medicine until recent times relied on the human ability to diagnose by virtue of not having the "scientific" data available. As a result, as much, if not more, emphasis was placed on the healer than on the healing. The medicine man, the guru, the shaman, and our Western predecessors shared the necessity of gaining self-knowledge and relying on their intuitive, instinctual, and "gut-feelings" as well as

the "I've seen it before" diagnosis. Until modern times healing was seen as something that happened as a result of powers far beyond human control. The "spirits," the "gods," or even long-dead relatives were responsible for the results of treatment, not the antibiotics, anxiolytic, or oncolytic agents. Credit for getting well was rarely given to the healer. The displacement and projection of the cure from an unknown entity to the "known" doctor/treatment shifts our thinking from "healing" to "cure." There is a difference. Becoming "cured" is most often seen as having been relieved of specific symptoms, therefore, the relief from the condition or pain that was defined as the illness. Becoming "healed" is a much deeper, more comprehensive becoming "whole" rather than simply ridding one of symptoms, which in return aids the body/mind in returning to a total state of health. Curing may relieve symptoms; healing moves toward producing a whole person.

Pain can be a friend. It warns us that the body is in danger and, without pain, someone has said, we could die without knowing that we were even sick. Hence, we pay proper tribute to pain and recognize its value; yet, pain is always in some way related to death. The child with an abrasion on the knee runs into the house crying, "Mommy, I'm dying, I'm dying!" Someplace in our primitive and unconscious minds pain has become associated with the process of death. Pain becomes the constant reminder of our mortality and that thought often cascades into a torrent of terror, which in turn energizes the process of actually dying. The healer therefore not only relieves symptoms but saves from death. In spite of this finding, there are patients who for strange reasons *need* their pain and when relieved of it will find the most ingenious methods all the way to Munchausen's syndrome to reinstitute it. Whether this extreme attempt to regain pain is a suicidal act is open to debate, but it certainly succeeds in keeping the patient in contact with the Freudian concept of a death wish.

As medicine advanced through the ages we attempted to understand it all by simple unifications of symptoms into disease or syndrome entities, thus the "unified" disease approach whereby we attempted to meld all symptoms, regardless of how diverse they might be, into one syndrome or disease entity. The more information we gained, the more this approach, although still practiced, had of necessity given way to the "dual diagnosis" and even "multiple diagnosis model." The importance of this observation is that in the "healer emphasis" model, the focus was on the healer bringing healing to the *person who had an illness*, as against the more prevalent model today of the focus on the *illness that is in a person*. When one views symptoms that happen to inhabit a body, it is quite different from viewing an individual who wishes to be made whole. Making one whole is considerably more than relieving the symptoms. Many patients are relieved of their symptoms and yet are quite ill as persons. The true healer dealt (and deals) with putting a person back together again, knowing that being well is much more than simply not being sick. We are constantly reminded that the word "health" is derived from the same Greek word *holos* as "whole," "holy," "wholesome," and many more words defining a totality of health in the being not sufficiently described by the word "health" alone.

The "healer," by the same token, is the agent of this wholeness, which is much more than one who diagnoses and renders treatments. Diagnoses and treatments are simply tools of the trade that promote a condition that may provide the basis for wholeness to return to (or begin in) a person. Often, as we know, the "treatment" is not in any way corrective or capable of dealing with the pathogen or condition at hand, but works anyway. Such is the case with our commonly called "placebo" treatments. In truth, there is no such thing as a "placebo" because all administrations by healers are intended to bring about symptom relief; therefore, in the patient's mind the tool has been applied to commence the process of healing.

The effect of the patient's response and belief in the healer cannot be ignored. When a patient believes that a treatment will work, sometimes the doctor is also convinced! Dr. Herbert Benson relates an incident in which a fearful patient asked him to accompany her as she received anesthesia in her hospital room presurgery. He states:

> As the anesthesiologist began the anesthesia drip, I repeated out loud along with her quiet recitation, The Lord is my shepherd … The Lord is my shepherd … The Lord is my shepherd … on each of her outbreaths until eventually anesthesia took effect and she lost con-

sciousness. When I looked up, the anesthesiologist — whom I'd likened to Dick Butkus just moments before — was softly shaking, his mask soaked with tears. For the woman herself, the recitation of a familiar psalm with a doctor she trusted was a deep source of calm. But the ritual also carried with it power that I could not have predicted, eliciting in this straightforward, dutiful anesthesiologist a profound emotional response. (1996, p. 1780)

When we introduce the factor of pain into the picture, healing becomes even more complex. Traditionally, pain was considered simply to be a concomitant or result of illness. Pain as an *entity* or even as an independent *illness* was incomprehensible. We now know that pain not only accompanies and results from illness, but also may *produce* illness. This places the role of the healer in a very different position. The healer must attend to how the patient *feels* as well as what is happening in the laboratory reports. As we all know, the doctor can assure the patient that "you are getting better," but until the patient accepts that as a personal *feeling of truth*, it often does not make any difference what the doctor says. Once the patient *owns the feeling* of getting better, often the healing is well on its way.

The cultural implications and meaning of pain are far beyond the intents of this chapter. However, we must pay attention to the depth of cultural meaning in pain. From time immemorial pain has been attributed to some kind of god-sent retribution for personal evil done. From the birth pangs initiated with Eve and the sweat of the brow curse given to Adam, we have associated pain with evil. The healer must then of necessity become the holy one. No wonder so much trust and awe has been given to doctors! As the Western world becomes more "scientific" about pain, the doctors are less seen as miracle workers, but are replaced by wonder technology and chemicals. The modern healer must work to regain a power that is beyond drugs and surgery. Faith in doctors alone was doubtless in vain; however, faith in the medicines alone may leave us devoid of the powerful relationship between healer and patient that allows the therapeutics to bring about healing.

In spite of our efforts, many persons are unable to relinquish the idea that pain and evil are twins. The lack of illness is not necessarily the presence of health, and the presence of illness is not necessarily the presence of evil. "There are many persons who suffer indescribable pain who are indeed holy" (Cox, 1997, p. 46). By the same token, there are many who suffer no pain who certainly do not seem to be holy. We must be careful not to rush to judgment regarding another's spiritual status. Furthermore, at times there is no evidence that the patient's spiritual status has much to do with whether healing occurs. In the New Testament healings of Jesus it seems that the willingness to want to be made whole and the intent to change one's lifestyle were the important elements. Jesus simply asked, "Wilt thou be made whole?" This is a curious question; i.e., Jesus does not ask if the person wants symptom relief, but if he wishes to be made *whole*. And, therein may lie the mystery of healing, i.e., the wish for the total renewing of the person as against the simple elimination of troubling symptoms. Even blindness, lameness, or paralysis to Jesus seemed to evoke the same method for healing; namely, a teamwork of faith, willingness to accept the healing, and the energy of the moment.

Not only in the healings of Jesus, but of many others recounted in literature from shrines to evangelistic happenings, it seems that the common denominator is not the symptom but the process and the energy created by the combination of human and divine sources. It may be that the modern-day healer is too concerned with the specificity of symptoms and insufficiently connected to the energizing, life-giving resources of the spiritual/energy world (see below; Shealy, 1999, p. 55).

Harold R. Nelson, in his book *Senior Spirituality,* states, "When I had open-heart surgery in 1993, I had the good fortune to have a cardiac-thoracic surgeon who is highly skilled and yet very caring. When he entered my hospital room to check me over, I felt a healing presence that bolstered my own healing process" (Nelson, 2004, p. 63). Literature is replete with the healer's own attitude as being an integral (and maybe central) part of the healing process. Norman Cousins has written extensively in support of such. The narratives of the healings of Jesus and the many "spontaneous" recoveries over the centuries leave us no room to doubt the role of "faith" on both the part of the patient and the healer. Benson writes, "The sound of a doctor's voice, the words he or she chooses, the hope he or she can instill, and the time required to develop a good doctor-patient conversation promote health in ways many doctors and most insurers underestimate today" (Benson, 1996, p. 252).

The Rev. Nelson, a person with a lifetime as a hospital chaplain, also recounts, "I was anxious, angry, and threatened by a diagnosis of diabetes, and I needed to find a place of calmness, serenity, and peace with myself" (Nelson, 2004, p. 71), which he found through modalities that are considered "secular" but became sacred, such as hypnosis. In the end, all modalities become routes to the spiritual. Here is a person one would think might start at the spiritual to find healing. And indeed he did, but only to find that he was "in a no-man's land for a considerable period of time, struggling with identity and being caught up in despair. The journey taught me valuable lessons about the meaning and purpose of my life" (Nelson, 2004, p. 36). He states that he then "instinctively turn[ed] to spirituality at a time of loss. It is a built-in, automatic response that has resulted from all my previous spiritual experiences" (p. 95). He is correct in stating, "The utilization of faith at a time of loss is highly individualistic

and unique" (p. 95); however, suffice it to say that whether the person has ever been "spiritual" or not, most persons inevitably seem to become more than casually interested in the world of belief, faith, hope, and spirituality when confronted with pain and the possibility of death.

There are many articles and books written to assist patients with their part in the healing process. There are considerably fewer helping the healer to find his or her own inner resources for such. The complexity of helping us as healers begins with being able *to get outside of ourselves while getting very deeply inside ourselves!* This process is being able to deal with *imminence* and *transcendence.* In the final analysis, all healing is essentially spiritual. Although the healer, the patient, the diagnosis, and the therapeutics are very tangible, the energy beneath it all is doubtless of a nature that is not describable, nor is it quantifiable. We only need to read about "Therapeutic Touch" (Goldberg Group, 1995) to realize that all sorts of energies, ideas, approaches, techniques, and methods combine into something about which we know virtually nothing, namely, spiritual energy. The Therapeutic Touch approach, in which there is often no physical touch at all, has actually "altered enzyme activity, increased hemoglobin levels, and accelerated the healing of wounds" (Goldberg Group, 1995, p. 111).

Imminence is the language of the here and now, i.e., that which is apt to happen very soon. Modern healing, whether in acute or chronic illnesses, tends to wrest itself of the existential nature of health and illness by addressing that which needs to be done immediately. As important as that certainly is, that which is imminent may be less so when placed into the context of the existential. Further, the term "imminent" tends to indicate the negative, such as "a storm is imminent." Patients are often so focused on the imminent, thus possibly the negative, that they are literally unable to surmount their discomfort and pain without the healer's ability to transcend the patient's immediate symptoms and apprehensions.

Transcendence speaks of *hope.* Tillich and other prominent psychologically astute theologians remind us that humans not only have all the concerns of every other living creature, but also have spiritual concerns. They speak of our capability and necessity for reaching beyond the here and now and finding that indefinable and yet absolutely defined element we call *hope.* Hope is found in transcendence: transcending the situation, the discomfort, the pain, and perhaps most importantly, the ambiguity of most illnesses, thus allowing both the patient and the healer to admit to human frailty, incomplete, and even incorrect knowledge.

Transcendence is to rise above, go beyond, and experience more than the here-and-now could predict or anticipate. The languages of this process are many. They range from that which is called faith to that which is called psychic. The language is not important. The experience with the inner force it generates is essential. It could be argued that many healers have left the healing business for the treatment business; i.e., the emphasis is on the business of treatment that hopefully could result in healing, rather than being in the healing business that intends to make persons whole. Although this may be seen as a triviality of words, it is not. Transcendence disallows primary focus on the immediate, the imminent while still considering the immediate to be essential. But it recognizes that the best way to get to the immediate is through the transcendent instead of the other way around.

Both imminence and transcendence are based in belief. Both are processes of directing oneself outside oneself to something one does not know. Both go beyond that which can be measured; therefore, there is no norm. This fact and acceptance of such is essential to the healer. Both the patient and the healer *know* that there are in truth no norms for any individual patient, but only numerical and statistical *norms* for patients with similar symptoms when all are grouped together. It is essential when dealing with pain in particular that we accept this fact. No two persons' experiences of pain are the same. We still have no reliable measure of pain. The experience is entirely subjective; hence, the healer must be willing to allow and encourage the individual process of transcendence, which allows belief to start a process that is not rooted in the imminent, i.e., laboratory results, x-rays, and other *norms.*

We may be helped by viewing the healer as a *change agent* instead of a physician, psychologist, nurse, or other practitioner. By definition, a change agent is one who is authorized by another to act on his or her behalf. There are many inherent assumptions, *possibilities*, and dangers in being an agent. The responsibility is huge. The task is enormous, and the ethics of such are beyond description when caring for another soul.

The literature of many cultures shows how pain is "given over" to a change agent. Hebrew literature transferred it to a "scapegoat," and some primitive cultures "throw it in a fire on a bedeviled twig." The book *Treating Spiritual Disorders* states, "When we purposely expand our sense of self to include the natural world in which we unceasingly participate, we seem to draw toxicity from our bodies and distribute it among willing partners of our day-to-day lives" (Simms, 2001, p. 147). Change agents have been utilized in various, and to us possibly strange ways, from time immemorial. It is a respected, even perhaps an enviable spiritual gift to be in the position of a change agent.

Rarely, if ever, do patients know what they are doing when allowing a therapist, physician, or other healer to become their agent. In truth, the giving of this authorization is probably rarely conscious and deliberate but implied, which makes the task all the more daunting for the healer. Healers are not trained to fully understand what it means to care for another soul and to assume the responsibility of another's most sacred self. Most healers see their role as being able to bring certain treatments, medicines, and procedures for the effecting of very specific symptoms or conditions. As humans, we cannot be separated in this way. We are not symptoms, pains, feelings, and conditions, but whole persons who cannot be dissected by various nomenclatures, systems, and nosologies.

The human, as we all know and to which we give verbal assent, is a totality, a whole. To treat one part is to treat all parts. To ignore one part is to ignore all parts. This wholistic approach is sometimes hard to see even in the most dedicated healer's practice with the seemingly endless parade of *specialties* we now have. While it is doubtless good to know as much about any one illness as possible, it is also possible to be so myopic as to lose sight of the whole person who cannot be separated from the *specialty illness.*

Patients need to know the value base of their healer. The healer seriously involved in the healing process rather than the dispenser of therapies will thus form a bond with the patient. Why attempt to hide that which will establish a healing relationship? It has been promulgated that healers should keep their private view to themselves. This is not possible. Patients are perceptive. Patients often invest far more in the person and the abilities of their healers than the healers do in their patients; thus, the psychological intensity of identification with the healer is beyond description. The patient sees the frown that that the healer is unaware of having, the side glance to the nurse that the healer thinks is private, the worried look on the healer's face, or sometimes the "air" of confidence or consternation in the very atmosphere of the room. The evidence of a faith in themselves, their patient, and the treatment method produce a spiritual basis that allows both healers and patients to transcend themselves and the imminence of the illness.

Dr. Benson states, "Clearly when patients *believed* in therapies that were recommended by their doctors, this fervor worked to alleviate a variety of medical conditions including angina, asthma, herpes simplex cold sores, and duodenal ulcers. But as soon as patient confidence was undermined, so was the effect. This pattern was noted by the nineteenth-century French physician Armand Trousseau" (1996, p. 35).

The healer must not be afraid to reach beyond the limits of his or her specific professional discipline to borrow and learn from others. Sometimes the physician, for example, seems to function as if everything the clergyperson (or other professional) would do is off limits for the medical or specialty person. And, by the same token, the clergypersons (or other disciplines) do not want to practice medicine without a license. However, there is a ground between all disciplines and professions where we can borrow techniques, use methods, refer more properly, and allow all disciplines to become one team, i.e., one healing agent, when we practice with mutual respect, equality although difference of knowledge, and see healing as the art and many artists joining hands to become one master-artist/healer.

Dr. C. Norman Shealy, founder of the American Holistic Medical Association, in his book, *Sacred Healing,* states, "Why can a healer transmit energy while a regular person cannot? A master healer's mental attitude and life of prayer and devotion produce a more direct connection with divine energy. For this reason a healer can tap into divine energy more effectively than individuals who do not have spiritual practices. A master healer pays continuous attention to and is totally devoted to God. To heal, the healer must continuously be in touch with God, maintaining a constant mental and spiritual connectedness" (1999, p. 73).

As agents for change, we must not attempt to determine the changes, but only allow for all possibilities. By being open to all possibilities we are more apt to experience the transcendent. When allowing for all possibilities we sometimes find that we are actually treating something quite different from what had been initially diagnosed. For example, a patient with a phobia (or a fever for that matter) may actually simply be too engrossed in the pathology of the symptom to actually reveal the underlying problem. Sometimes the problem is entirely too painful to bring forth; hence, a disguised form appears in the hope of finding a healer who can become transcendent.

Without the transcendent, all diagnoses and treatment strategies are sterile and without vitality. Obscuring the whole patient in favor of the immediate symptoms often diminishes the patient and encourages (and maybe even forces) the acceptance of a wrong diagnosis in favor of no diagnosis at all. There is an axiom in medicine that "the correct diagnosis leads to the correct treatment." As certainly true as that is, it is equally true that the wrong diagnosis leads to the wrong treatment, and further in that case, no diagnosis is better than the wrong one. In the transcendent mode the healer is permitted to accept "intuitions," "hunches," "it just seems like," and other less describable definitions of what is going on while carrying out the due diligence of required and reasonable imminent therapeutic activity.

Healers who are able to move into the transcendent are able to emphasize the overall wellness of a person while attending to the immediate illness. Recognizing that an elbow hurts is essential, but it is also essential to recognize that there are many other joints in the body that do not hurt and are functioning well. The psychology of attention has been well taught to us. We need not be reminded that to ask one *not* to remember that a pen is black is to be assured that it will never be forgotten. The negative aspect of memory, i.e., retroactive inhibition, can undo many positive aspects of what we really wanted the patient to remember. Proactive inhibition, i.e., interfering with new learning created by memories from prior learning, may actually disallow a patient to learn new material. The healer knows that none of us starts with a *tabla rasa* when it comes to pain. We have all been there. We have all formed our opinions as to what constitutes a "slight hurt" and a "really bad pain." New definitions coming from a healer are meaningless. What counts is the healer's ability to put the current discomfort into the context of process, the process of wellness. "Pain" is described in various ways by both patients and healers, and often the descriptions are very different in personal meaning. The terms "ache" or "burning sensation" or "stabbing pain" are valuable though nonetheless inadequate attempts to bring the healer into identification with the imminent experience of the patient. Some writers have suggested that the deepest of all pain is "soul pain," which may be separate from or accompany actual physical and mental pain. The concept, however correct it may be, is valuable to the healer in understanding the depth of another's experience. The patient is usually attempting to gain new understanding of the concept of pain but at the same time is dealing with all the past memories of pains of the past.

Pain in wellness is different from pain in illness. Pain in wellness is microscopic. Pain in illness is macroscopic. The pain is not trivialized; it is contextualized. The healer then has the option of utilizing all the energies of the patient as part of the treatment regimen rather than assuming the patient's illness as a personal responsibility and searching for acceptable modalities. There is frequently a degree of paranoia in the pain process with which the healer must contend. Pain is seen as negative. Something uninvited has invaded us and we are being visited by an enemy. It is difficult to be *narapoid* (a new word listed in the *Dictionary of Psychology*, Corsini, 1999, p. 626) in the face of such odds. The healer, however, can instill *narapoia*, i.e., "the belief that all people are beyond suspicion and represent no harm or threat," the opposite of paranoia. Casting out doubt is an essential antecedent to belief or faith. The healer needs to do everything possible to create an atmosphere of hope, faith, belief, and therefore healing. The mind and body cannot be separated as we know, but do not always practice.

Larry Dossey describes an illustration of using the higher art of healing in clinical practice by cardiologist Randolph Byrd who found unexpected success when patients were the subjects of prayer. His results are reported as even staggering to others, and he quotes, "Dr. William Nolan, who has written a book debunking faith healing, acknowledged, 'It sounds like this study will stand up to scrutiny…Maybe we doctors ought to be writing on our order sheets, Pray three times a day,' If it works, it works" (Dossey, 1995, p. 250).

Transcendence and imminence are not simply linguistic terms. They are ways of thinking, styles of living, the presence or absence of confidence, types of maturity, and the bases for developing a healer whose countenance is obviously one of health rather than illness and the very wholeness in which the healer displays the hope and optimism of that which is beyond symptoms and treatment.

The healer is not simply a person who diagnoses and renders therapeutic regimens. Healing comes from deep within both the healer and the patient. Healing is a team effort, a duet, trio, or more, but never a solo performance. Granted, thankfully from time to time we see persons being made whole with only our partial and dimly understood attempts to help. However, with deliberate intentionality of purpose with the Divine, we may gradually learn to transcend ourselves and enter into a more perfect teamwork for total healing.

REFERENCES

Benson, H. (1996). *Timeless healing.* New York: Scribner.

Corsini, R. (Ed.). (1999). *The dictionary of psychology.* New York: Brunner/Mazel.

Cox, R. (1997). Transcendence and imminence in psychotherapy. *American Journal of Psychotherapy, 51*(4).

Dossey, L. (1995). *Healing words.* New York: Harper.

Goldberg Group. (1995). *Alternative medicine.* Fife, WA: Future Medicine Publishing.

Nelson, H. R. (2004). *Senior spirituality.* St. Louis: Chalice Press.

Shealy, C. N. (1999). *Sacred healing.* Boston: Element.

Simms, G. (Ed.). (2001). *Treating spiritual disorders.* Sanford, FL: Health Access Press.

97

Assessing Patient Spirituality: A Compelling Avenue for New Discovery

C. Stephen Byrum, PhD, and Richard S. Materson, MD

BACKGROUND AND INTRODUCTION

There is a fairly recent maxim that by now has probably already reached "old adage" status that conveys the conviction that something is "real" and has "value" only to the extent that it can be *measured*. On the fringe of what some people still judge to be the "modern world" and others are claiming a world that has now become "postmodern," the efficacy of the conviction about *measurement* is, at least, debatable.

Numerous voices in modern health care, and especially those voices that advance conversations relating to nontraditional modes of patient treatment, are likely to be pleased when conversations turn to measurability *not* being an absolute and rigid necessity.

This discussion, however, is not interested in taking advantage and claiming that so-called "soft side" issues get a pass on measurement. In fact, the strong position of this discussion is that certain *realities* that have not been easily measured in the past may be demonstrably quantifiable if valid and verifiable tools are present that can serve as measuring instruments. At the very minimum, if such *realities* are even somewhat conducive to measurement, there should be at least a somewhat heightened interest and curiosity about areas of concern that may previously have been fairly well dismissed.

What *realities* are being referenced here? Primarily, there is interest in being more discerning, discriminating, and definitive about issues relating to *spirituality*. A great deal of the history of health care, of course, has been wrapped up in "faith-based" approaches to medical care.

There has been a vast array of health care institutions that have come to exist and sustained their existence under the banners of various religious organizations. In these environments, many religious rites, rituals, and persons (chaplains, ministers, priests, and nuns) have been actively present. To a major extent, these religious expressions have diminished in quantity, if not in intensity, and it may be difficult to distinguish a "sacred"-oriented institution from a "secular" one. Clearly, "profit" and "not-for-profit" labels are of little help in discerning whether an organization is religious or not. However, this particular view of spirituality is not what we are getting at.

On the other hand, a fairly standard conversation surrounds both "sacred" and "secular," "for-profit" and "not-for-profit" organizations concerning the *spiritual* (for want of a better word) dimension of a person's overall existence as a human being. Especially when discussions of the "whole person" take place, it is not unusual to speak — with some parity of emphasis — about the physical, mental, emotion, social, and *spiritual* person. What is lacking is some way to *measure* this *spiritual* dimension. This discussion is not directed toward those kinds of outcome measures and studies that have done research, for example, in such areas as the improvement of patient outcomes when prayers have been offered on the patient's behalf.

We have previously ventured into this entire arena of *spiritual* measurement in two recent articles (Byrum & Materson, 2001, 2002). These articles introduced a measurement instrument known as "The Spiritual Tendencies Inventory." The STI was specifically designed to give quick access into this spiritual dimension, to stand beyond traditional religious biases associated with most profiling inventories developed in this area of emphasis to date, and to suggest not only a "diagnosis" of a person's spiritual strengths and obstacles, but also remedial activities that should increase strengths and diminish obstacles. Patients can use the tool independently of physicians, and physicians can use the tool to better understand the patient strengths and obstacles that will have direct implication for the work they are doing with patients.

The response to these articles and to the STI in general has been encouraging and positive. Significant research is now taking place with the instrument at SUNY Buffalo and the Hermann Hospital (a part of the Memorial Hermann Healthcare System) in Houston. Final negotiations are at present under way that will lead to the publication and general distribution of STI on both individual and institutional levels.

THE HARTMAN VALUE PROFILE

The primary purpose of the present discussion is to show how the work of measuring spirituality has moved beyond the STI to include a second instrument, the Hartman Value Profile (HVP). Historically, the HVP is a much older instrument than the STI — first used in the mid-1960s — and has been exposed to an exhaustive array of both applications and validations. The HVP is a much more complex instrument than the STI. It has not, however, been previously used in the area of application explained here. If the STI can be seen as a first instrument of inquiry and catalyst for discussion, the HVP will take that inquiry and discussion to extended levels of insight. What has been learned in using the STI can guide the way for the use of the HVP. The two instruments can be used in conjunction with each other, and their use will have the greatest ease of application in circumstances of chronic illness, pain management, or other forms of extended treatment where there is time to better understand the fuller dynamics of a patient's existence as a human being. Usefulness and benefit will be even greater in situations where patients are contributing partners in their overall care plan and treatment agendas.

The HVP was developed and first used by Robert S. Hartman. There is a vast array of information on Hartman and the research institute named in his honor. At the time he created the HVP, he was understood to be the world's leading *axiologist*. Axiology is a division of philosophy — as opposed to psychology — and operates from the leading premise that human beings are primarily driven by their *value systems*. The word *axiology* is derived from the Greek *axia,* which generally means "worth" or "value."

My "value system" is not something I have. Instead, it is who I am. I am a system, a "package" of values. This "value package" defines me much more clearly than my intellectual rationality, my emotional balance, or my personality. In fact, this "value package" — this unique "lens"

that has developed across my life and directly affects everything that I do — will be the primary driver that determines how rationality, emotion, or personality comes into play in the roles, decisions, and engagements that make up my daily life.

My "value system" clearly is manifested in the set of personal beliefs that I hold — for whom I vote, if and how I choose to worship, what I feel about some social issue. However, more significantly, my "value system" is manifested in the *judgments* I make — the way I evaluate situations, weigh out priorities, and "size things up." *Judgment*, while it does involve rational intelligence and emotional feelings, is a higher-order property of human beings. *Judgment*, regardless of the conclusions of Descartes and their impact on Western civilization in the modern age, is much more than thinking. *Judgment* — the most available manifestation of human "value systems" — ultimately will drive how thinking and emotion are used. It is critical, therefore, to be able to measure *judgment,* to see evaluative judgment as such a unique capacity of human beings. It may very well be appropriate to call it *spiritual.*

In other words, the word *spiritual* is being described here without patently religious connotations. Those connotations, and the practices that have been derived from them and applied to health care, are not being demeaned in any way. There is simply an attempt here to move the conversation concerning the *spiritual* dimension of human existence to a new, next level of consideration. Now, *spiritual* is being defined as that dimension of human existence — beyond purely intellectual rationality, emotion, and thinking — where contemplation, reflection, evaluation, and judgment take place as preludes to decision making, choice, and action. The HVP is particularly adept at measuring this dimension.

PATIENT IMPLICATIONS

Without question, the role of patient *judgment* in the overall spectrum of the enhancement of health and recovery from illness, injury, or malady is critical. If patient *judgment* is not effective and efficient, all of the care strategies, technologies, therapies, and medications available to the modern practitioner may be rendered useless or, at the very minimum, all but negated in their positive potential. Most care plans and treatment protocols are a "two-way street." The medical profession in all of its manifestations has a part to play; the patient has a part to play. If the patient's part is not played well — if good patient *judgment* is not used — the entire care plan is put in jeopardy.

But, what do practitioners know about patient *judgment*? More specifically, what do they know about patient *judgment* before the fact of dismissal or patients taking responsibility for the "hand off" of their own care beyond the physician and the hospital, for example, where the plan of care has been more practitioner driven than patient driven? More often than not, the patient's capacity for good judgment is known only after the fact when the patient is back in the hospital or back under more direct physician care because some element of the care plan has not been supported by good patient *judgment*. The escalation of complication and cost in such instances can be dramatic.

Therefore, there is a great need to look at the patient's judgment capacity, the *spiritual* dimension of a patient's existence as a human being. The only change in traditional thinking that must take place here is, again, to see the *spiritual*, not, for example, as how often a patient attends church, synagogue, or mosque, or what kind of "prayer life" a patient has; *spiritual* is now being assessed as that "highest-order activity" of human beings where *judgment* takes place.

At the conclusion of this introductory discussion and initial explanation, the actual report that would be prepared by the practitioner is seen. The value of this document can be established quite easily by a practitioner's simply asking whether the kind of information presented in the document would be of benefit in helping the practitioner better understand the patient. In fact, the conviction of this discussion is that the document will provide insight for the practitioner that has never been available previously. The document can also become a vehicle for better understanding the patient, and a catalyst for important dialogue with and monitoring of the patient that has not been available.

The HVP document, "Implications for Physician/Patient Interactions," is divided into three major report areas:

1. A review of 14 individual indices out of approximately 50 indices on the overall HVP that have particular bearing on patient judgment that relates to how patients will be responsible for their own care plan. The review of these critical indices, all of which have significant individual importance, is followed by two comprehensive grids that convey the information from the 14 indices in a highly visual manner.
2. Reviews of the problem-solving capacities of the patient especially as these capacities tend to be more reactionary or more deliberative. Tendencies toward reactionary responses are also judged by the data to be more intelligent or less intelligent.
3. A review of "balance" issues that relate to how the patient sees himself or herself in terms of "self-esteem," "self-concept," and "self-image." Balance in these three decisive areas will provide a wonderful foundation for positive decision making and good judgment. Problems in these areas will clearly handicap good judgment potential.

CONCLUSION

A great deal of the entire treatment program and care plan that surrounds a patient is driven by gaining as much information about the bodily functions, mental functions, and perhaps, even social functions of a patient's overall existence. Now, there is the added advantage of being able to assess a patient's *judgment* capacity, and to understand the degree to which successful recovery will be enhanced or diminished by these *judgment* capacities. The HVP, and this application of the profile in particular, make it possible for this dimension of critical information to be available. Now, there is truly a concrete and decisive manner in which a patient's *spirituality* can be part of a pragmatic and practical discussion and a pragmatic and practical application.

Now, simply look through the following report. Look at the kind of varied insights into patient judgment that are being assessed. Consider whether having this kind of information would be valuable in your care and treatment of a patient. Would this profile report give you valuable information about your patients that you do not at present have? What implications for successful treatment might this kind of information hold?

THE HARTMAN VALUE PROFILE — IMPLICATIONS FOR PHYSICIAN/PATIENT INTERACTIONS

RATIONALE

In modern health care settings, there is a continual need that is expressed, on the part of both physicians and their patients, for greater understanding. Patients want to be seen as *whole*, unique human beings, and the best physicians want to gain any additional insight into patients that will be beneficial to their treatment. The ideal of greater patient insight is particularly beneficial when the physician can gain greater insight into how the patient will respond to treatment and care, both in the hospital setting and after discharge.

Without question, the healing process has many complexities, not the least of which is the *judgment capacity* that the patient brings to his or her part of the treatment and care program outlined by the physician. How a patient will respond in terms of his or her own choices and decisions — that is, *judgments* — will be a critical, and sometimes even decisive, element in successful treatment outcomes. For example, on the most basic level, whether a patient responds wisely to the *directions* that accompany discharge will have a large impact on recovery, whether the patient will be satisfied with the physician, whether the patient will return to the hospital with extenuating problems, and — of course — the overall cost of health care in general. "Responding wisely," in this instance, is a matter of *judgment*.

The Hartman Value Profile is designed to be particularly adept at understanding human *judgment capacity*. In this specific application, attention is given to individual indices of the profile's interpretative mechanism that lend themselves to special areas of patient response to treatment and care. By paying attention to the various indices of assessment found in the profile, health care professionals can gain a deeper and more articulate insight into the *judgment capacities* of their patients in areas of concern that have profound implication for the treatment, healing, and recovery processes.

At the very minimum, this application of the profile shows strength or weakness of judgment in the areas assessed. The profile can also be used to establish helpful conversation and dialogue between the physician and patient about the patient's own responsibility and accountability in the care process. Both professional homecare and family caregivers will gain insight into how to assist, enhance, or monitor patient responsibility and accountability based on the profile's results.

David Johns, a highly-respected physician who has made a life study of "additional" — not "alternative" — pathways to healing, well-being, and recovery of human wholeness, is convinced that relationship-medicine, as opposed to transaction-medicine, is a critically important element in the healing process. For Johns, it always takes a special physician — or health care provider in general — who sees and pursues the value in developing some degree of relationship with his or her patient. Much of modern health care focuses obsessive attention on the economic transaction of moving a patient in and out of the treatment setting as quickly as possible. The application of the Hartman Value Profile seeks to give Johns's "special physician" a tool that will lend itself to establishing meaningful relationships effectively, efficiently, and in ways that have a measurable quality to them that can be appreciated in the most economic and science-based health care practice.

TECHNICAL OVERVIEW

This application of the profile is divided into two parts. First, there is a review of findings based on 14 different indices. Each index is identified and then explained in terms of the likelihood of patient response based on scores that have been processed. Each index is broken down into seven categories: "highly likely," "likely," "somewhat likely," "neutral likelihood," "somewhat unlikely," "unlikely," and "highly unlikely." The "highly likely" scores are most desirable, and the greater distance of scoring from this highest echelon, the greater the potential

problem in positive responsibility and cooperative accountability. Any scores in the three "unlikely" categories should be given detailed attention.

Following a description of the individual indices and the scores established by a patient, there are two visual presentations of the information: (1) a grid will show a review of all of the scores and (2) a composite score line will show the relative judgment strengths exhibited by the combined scores.

On a more sensitive level of consideration, but a level that is highly insightful, three specialized scoring areas will make an assessment of the patient's overall sense of self-regard. Here, valuable information will be gained about how the patient feels about himself or herself in terms of "Self-Esteem," "Self-Concept," and "Self-Image." Without question, how a patient feels about himself or herself — that is, the character and quality of a patient's self-*judgment* — will be critical to any and all positive treatment and care outcomes. This second part of the profile report for this application is more subtle, but can be the catalyst to tremendously beneficial insight.

In terms of actual use, the profile can be administered prior to hospitalization, during the in-patient period of care, or prior to discharge. In most respects, the sooner the information is gained, the sooner its insights can become helpful.

INDEX OF CRITICAL SCORES*

1. **Differentiation/DIF (Part 1)** — Measures the likelihood of the patient to notice subtle changes in his or her own body, the kinds of subtle changes that may indicate that treatment is or is not working in some critical manner.

Highly Likely	Likely	Somewhat Likely	Neutral Likelihood	Somewhat Unlikely	Unlikely	Highly Unlikely

2. **Dissimilarity/DIS (Part 1)** — Measures the likelihood of the patient to be careful in following directions given regarding elements of treatment and care for which the patient will need to be responsible.

Highly Likely	Likely	Somewhat Likely	Neutral Likelihood	Somewhat Unlikely	Unlikely	Highly Unlikely

3. **Sub-Dimension Systemic/DIM-S (Part 1)** — Measures the likelihood of the patient to under-

---

* Please note: In both this section on the Index of Critical Scores and in the Overview of Critical Scores found below, not all of the more than 70 indicators on the Hartman Value Profile are used. Only scores found to be of utmost significance to patient insight are examined.

stand the care plan *conceptually*; the ability to create a "mental map" of the care plan.

Highly Likely	Likely	Somewhat Likely	Neutral Likelihood	Somewhat Unlikely	Unlikely	Highly Unlikely

4. **Sub-Dimension Systemic/DIM-S (Part 2)** — Measures the likelihood of the patient to *integrate* into real choices, decisions, and actions that which has been *conceptualized* about the care plan; the ability to have strong, personal initiative to act on the care plan.

Highly Likely	Likely	Somewhat Likely	Neutral Likelihood	Somewhat Unlikely	Unlikely	Highly Unlikely

5. **Integration/INT (Part 1)** — Measures the likelihood of a patient to be a clear and decisive problem solver, solution finder, and strong decision maker. Strong scores on these scales are critical to assessing the degree to which a patient will be an aggressive and active participant in a treatment and care plan. Poor scores may indicate a tendency to give up, take on a victim role, or be passive in approaching negative circumstances.

Highly Likely	Likely	Somewhat Likely	Neutral Likelihood	Somewhat Unlikely	Unlikely	Highly Unlikely

6. **Integration%/INT% (Part 1)** — Measures the likelihood of the patient to recognize, organize, and mobilize resources at his or her disposal that can have a positive impact on the healing and recovery process. Strong scores indicate that a substantial amount of personal "energy" is present to deal with negative situations. Weak scores indicate that this personal "energy" is diminished and the patient is likely to be struggling with exhaustion in regard to negative health circumstances; resolve and the ability to "keep coming back" may be diminished.

Highly Likely	Likely	Somewhat Likely	Neutral Likelihood	Somewhat Unlikely	Unlikely	Highly Unlikely

7. **Attitude Index/AI% (Part 1)** — Measures the likelihood of the patient to be resilient in the face of negative circumstances. Strong scores indicate that a patient has excellent coping skills and will approach negative circumstances with optimism and a positive attitude.

Highly Likely	Likely	Somewhat Likely	Neutral Likelihood	Somewhat Unlikely	Unlikely	Highly Unlikely

8. **Differentiation/DIF (Part 2)** — Measures the likelihood of the patient to have a strong sense of self-regard that is manifested in actual activities and actions of self-care.

Highly Likely	Likely	Somewhat Likely	Neutral Likelihood	Somewhat Unlikely	Unlikely	Highly Unlikely

9. **Dimension%/DIM% (Part 2)** — Measures the likelihood of the patient to deal well with changes that health care problems may cause that have an impact on role identity, work, or general activities and a degree of self-determination that has become a part of a person's "identity."

Highly Likely	Likely	Somewhat Likely	Neutral Likelihood	Somewhat Unlikely	Unlikely	Highly Unlikely

10. **Integration/INT (Part 2)** — Measures the likelihood of the patient to have a strong sense of what is *important* in regard to self-care as opposed to what is peripheral.

Highly Likely	Likely	Somewhat Likely	Neutral Likelihood	Somewhat Unlikely	Unlikely	Highly Unlikely

11. **Integration%/INT% (Part 2)** — Measures the likelihood of the patient to resist getting caught up in actions and attitudes of self-criticism and self-blame. Taken to an extreme ("Somewhat Unlikely" > "Highly Unlikely"), such tendencies to the negative end of the spectrum can become self-limiting and even self-destructive of the care plan being successfully sustained.

Highly Likely	Likely	Somewhat Likely	Neutral Likelihood	Somewhat Unlikely	Unlikely	Highly Unlikely

12. **Sub-Integration Intrinsic/INT-I (Part 1)** — Measures the likelihood of the patient to feel that he or she can solve problems *without* outside help. Strong scores ("Highly Likely" > "Likely) can be a deficit in terms of delaying the time when help should be sought.

Highly Likely	Likely	Somewhat Likely	Neutral Likelihood	Somewhat Unlikely	Unlikely	Highly Unlikely

13. **Dimensional Integration/DI (Part 2)** — Measures the likelihood of the patient to be outspoken, open, honest, and even assertive in regard to expressing feelings, asking questions, and conveying information about health issues. Weak scores may indicate conflict avoidance and even denial.

Highly Likely	Likely	Somewhat Likely	Neutral Likelihood	Somewhat Unlikely	Unlikely	Highly Unlikely

14. **Attitude Index%/AI% (Part 2)** — Measures the likelihood of the patient to have personal resources (mate relationships, family, friendship and support structures, faith, all of the above) that can act as a "foundation" during times of challenge to health and well-being.

| Highly | Likely | Somewhat | Neutral | Somewhat | Unlikely | Highly |
| Likely | | Likely | Likelihood | Unlikely | | Unlikely |

OVERVIEW OF CRITICAL SCORES

Please note: In the score column on this overview, there will be both a phrase and a number used to suggest the strength, or absence thereof, being measured by each index. These phrases and numbers reflect the language and mathematics implicit in the Hartman Value Profile. Each index has been assigned three echelons "Strong," "Moderate," "Weak," and three numbers "3," "2," and "1."

		Score		
Index	Measuring	Strong	Moderate	Weak
1. DIF 1	Noticing Subtle Changes	___	___	___
2. DIS 1	Following Directions	___	___	___
3. DIM-S 1	Conceptualizing Care Plan	___	___	___
4. DIM-S 2	Acting on Care Plan	___	___	___
5. INT 1	Active in Problem Solving	___	___	___
6. INT% 1	Using Resources to Face Problems	___	___	___
7. AI% 1	Coping Skills/ Tenacity	___	___	___
8. DIF 2	Adequacy of Self-Regard	___	___	___
9. DIM% 2	Ability to Deal with Change	___	___	___
10. INT 2	Sense of What Is Important	___	___	___
11. INT% 2	Resisting Self-Criticism/Blame	___	___	___
12. INT-I 2	Tendency to Seek Help of Others	___	___	___
13. DI 2	Assertiveness/ Openness	___	___	___
14. AI%	Underlying, Personal "Foundation"	___	___	___

COMPOSITE STRENGTH GRID

Using a combination of all of the numbers on the 14 points on the "Overview of Critical Scores" template, the following general assessment of patient strength of judgment in taking accountability for patient aspects of the treatment

| Highly | Likely | Somewhat | Neutral | Somewhat | Unlikely | Highly |
| Likely | | Likely | Likelihood | Unlikely | | Unlikely |

PROBLEM-SOLVING STYLES

Across their lives, human beings develop different problem-solving styles. According to the excellent work of Robert K. Smith (www.cleardirections.com), these problem-solving styles fall into two major areas. Some people relate to problems *automatically*. Others relate to problems *deliberatively*. On the "automatic" side of the ledger, there are two primary manifestations: *direct, immediate response* — the "don't just stand there, do something" response — and a more intense response of *reaction*. On the "deliberative" side, there are two primary manifestations: relating to problems through *relationships* and relating to problems through *reflection*.

In Smith's work, the "automatic" response occurs 85 to 95% of the time, and the "deliberative" response occurs 5 to 15% of the time. The worst decisions are usually reactive. The next worse — but most typical — are direct, more immediate responses. The best decisions are made deliberatively with others in relationships and in moments of reflection. The problem with decision making, of course, is that most people do not take time to get help from others or take time to reflect. Smith even says, instructively, that of the six brain centers that are used in problem solving, only one is used when people are in the reactive mode. Two or three are used when there is immediate, direct response. Four or five are used when problems are solved through reflection. All six are used when we take time to use relationships to help us deal with problems. The irony in all of this discussion, of course, is that we solve most of our problems using the least of our thinking and contemplative energy.

It is critical to better appreciate how a patient will likely respond to problems. In most instances, it will help patients determine when automatic response and reaction are more appropriate and when deliberative relationships and reflection are better. For many patients, any conversation that encourages relationships and reflection will be an advantage.

The **Dimension/DIM (Part 1)** scores of the Hartman Value Profile give a clear indication of what problem-solving style is most likely to be a patient's primary way of dealing with negative situations.

Dimension/DIM (Part 1) Scale

| More Reactive | Responsive | More Deliberative | Responsive | More Reactive |

| More Intelligently Expressed | | Less Intelligently Expressed |

SELF-BALANCE INDICATORS

While it is critically important to have judgment *strength*, it is also important to have judgment *balance*. Robert Hartman (1967) taught that human beings have a tendency to both *overvalue* (which he called a "composition") and *undervalue* (which he called a "transposition"). For example, indulge a child, and a "composition" or *overvalue* is created; neglect a child, and a "transposition" or *undervalue* is created. Neither is good for the child, so *balance* would be desired. *Overvalue* money, and a person can become greedy or a thief, or only see people in terms of socioeconomics. *Undervalue* money, and he may fail to pay his credit card and may be unable to buy gasoline. Again, *balance* would be desired.

In the following, final schematic, the *balance* that human beings have in three critical areas of personal existence is measured.

Self-Esteem — How a person feels affirmative (or not) about himself or herself, the base of self-confidence. Extreme overvaluing can lead to aggressive arrogance, and extreme undervaluing shows a lack of important ego strength. This scale may also reflect the degree/impact of either criticism (–) or affirmation (+) by which a person has been influenced.

Extreme	Moderate	Balanced	Moderate	Extreme
Overvalued	Overvalued		Undervalued	Undervalued

Self-Concept — How a person feels affirmative (or not) about the roles that the person is playing in his or her life. Extreme overvaluing reveals too much emphasis being placed on roles. Extreme undervaluing indicates participation in roles that are not adequately fulfilling.

Extreme	Moderate	Balanced	Moderate	Extreme
Overvalued	Overvalued		Undervalued	Undervalued

Self-Image — How a person projects an image of himself or herself (or fails to do this) and, thus, gives a system of goals, objectives, ambitions, dreams, and aspirations to live up to. Extreme undervaluing leads to lack of self-motivation. Extreme overvaluing leads to the creation of ideals that cannot be achieved and will likely be self-defeating.

Extreme	Moderate	Balanced	Moderate	Extreme
Overvalued	Overvalued		Undervalued	Undervalued

FOR FURTHER REFERENCE

Byrum, C. S. (1991). *The value structure of theology* (8th ed.). Acton, MA: Tapestry Press.

Davis, J. W. (Ed.). *Value and valuations: Axiological studies in honor of Robert S. Hartman.* Knoxville: University of Tennessee Press.

Edwards, R. B., & Davis, J. W. (Eds.). (1991). *Forms of value and valuation: Theory and application.* Washington, DC: University Press of America.

Hartman, R. S. (1967). *The structure of value: The foundations of scientific axiology.* Carbondale, IL: University of Southern Illinois Press.

There is an abundance of Web site information on Robert S. Hartman and the entire field of axiology. Work of the Robert S. Hartman Institute is prominently available on the Institute's Web site.

For further information on the use of this profile, please contact Richard Materson, Steve Byrum, or Louis Smith through the Memorial Hermann Healthcare System in Houston, Texas.

REFERENCES

Byrum, C. S., & Materson, R. S. (2001). Axiological disorders and relief of suffering in chronic pain. *Anesthesia Today, 12*(2).

Byrum, C. S., & Materson, R. S. (2002). Axiological disorders — The missing outcome dimension: Innovations in pain management. In R. S. Weiner (Ed.), *Pain management — A practical guide for clinicians* (6th ed., pp. 571–585). Boca Raton, FL: CRC Press.

98

Religion and Spirituality in Pain Management

Bruce Y. Lee, MD, and Andrew B. Newberg, MD

INTRODUCTION

Throughout history, religious and spiritual activities have been used in the management of pain. The attitudes of health care practitioners toward these activities have varied considerably. Some have acknowledged, embraced, or even used such activities. Others have ignored or opposed them. But regardless of one's personal beliefs, understanding how religion and spirituality affect pain may influence one's practice of pain management.

After all, studies have clearly shown that many patients consider religion to be very important and would like their physicians to discuss religious issues with them. Popular news magazines such as *Time* and *Newsweek* and television shows have devoted ample coverage to the interplay of religion and health (Begley, 2001). Over the past decade, many spiritual activities such as yoga have become very popular (Corliss, 2001; "Yoga," 2002). There is an ever-increasing number of researchers, books, and groups covering these subjects. Therefore, there is a good chance of encountering a patient or physician who has used or is interested in using religious and spiritual activities in pain management.

This chapter briefly chronicles the history of religion and health care, defines key terms such as *spirituality* and *religion*, and compares several prominent religious and spiritual activities. We also review what is currently known about the physiological and clinical effects of religious and spiritual practices, particularly with regard to pain management, and the challenges that researchers and health care practitioners may face in designing appropriate studies and translating results to clinical practice. Finally, we discuss future directions in the roles of religion and spirituality in pain management.

THE IMPORTANCE OF RELIGION AND SPIRITUALITY TO PATIENTS AND PHYSICIANS

There is abundant evidence that religion and spirituality play large roles in people's lives. Studies have shown that more than 90% of Americans believe in God or a higher power, 90% pray, 67 to 75% pray on a daily basis, 69% are members of a church or synagogue, and 40% attend a church or synagogue regularly (Bezilla, 1993; Gallup, 1994; Poloma & Pendleton, 1991; Shuler, Gelberg, & Brown, 1994). According to 1998 Gallup polls, 60% of Americans consider religion to be very important in their lives, and 82% acknowledge a personal need for spiritual growth. Both these numbers have increased significantly from 1994 Gallup polls, suggesting that overall interest in spirituality is on the rise (Miller & Thoresen, 2003).

With the widespread prevalence of religious and spiritual beliefs and practices, it is not surprising that more than 75% of surveyed patients want physicians to include spiritual issues in their medical care, approximately 40% want physicians to discuss their religious faith with them, and nearly 50% would like physicians to pray with them (Daaleman & Nease, 1994; King & Bushwick, 1994; King, Hueston, & Rudy, 1994; Matthews et al., 1998). Studies of family physicians, pediatricians, internists, neurologists, and surgeons all had similar findings: while a majority considered spiritual well-being an important component of health and agreed that it should be addressed with patients, only a minority (fewer than 20%) did so with any regularity (MacLean, Susi, & Phifer, 2003; Monroe, Bynum, & Susi, 2003). The most common reasons given for this discrepancy included lack of time, inadequate training, discomfort in addressing the topics, and difficulty in identifying patients who want to discuss spiritual issues (Armbruster,

1473

Chibnall, & Legett, 2003; Chibnall & Brooks, 2001; Ellis, Vinson, & Ewigman, 1999).

Therefore, some investigators and educators have called for increased education regarding religious and spiritual issues in medical schools, postgraduate training, and continuing medical education. From 1994 to 1997, the number of U.S. medical schools offering courses on spiritual issues grew from 3 to nearly 30. In April 1997, the deans and faculty of more than 45 medical schools attended the *Spirituality in Medicine: Curricular Development* conference, where the prevailing opinion was that religion and spirituality are not optional but essential parts of patient care. Some residency training programs have already implemented spirituality and medicine curricula (Pettus, 2002).

However, not everyone agrees that religious and spiritual issues should be included in formal medical education. Some feel that discussing religion and spirituality in the medical classroom and with patients is inappropriate and argue that these issues are irrelevant (or at least not relevant enough) to patient care. There are concerns that some health care workers may have hidden agendas in addressing religious issues, such as imposing a personal religious belief on a patient. Even well-meaning health care practitioners can inadvertently be biased or overbearing in their approach. Editorials and commentaries have questioned the ethics of physicians who want to discuss patients' spiritual needs and have suggested reserving such discussions to professionals trained in pastoral care. Sloan and colleagues have suggested that the evidence linking religion and health is not strong and stated that there is the potential concern that patients may believe their illness was due to poor faith (Sloan & Bagiella, 2002; Sloan, Bagiella, & Powell, 1999). However, this has been a concern for advocates of the relationship between religion and health as well. In fact, many religious individuals have become concerned that religion is being treated as an intervention in the medical setting rather than maintaining its spiritual meaning. Another concern is that including religion in medical care may be difficult for agnostic or atheist health care providers. Others believe that these issues have some place in medical education and care, but disagree over the manner in which they should be integrated (Levin, Larson, & Puchalski, 1997).

Although considerable controversy remains, these issues have grown in prominence to the point where they are difficult to ignore. The *Diagnostic and Statistical Manual of Mental Disorders* (4th ed., 1994) recognizes religion and spirituality as relevant sources of either emotional distress or support (Kutz, 2002; Lukoff, Lu, & Turner, 1992; Turner et al., 1995). The guidelines of the Joint Commission on Accreditation of Healthcare Organizations (JCAHO) require hospitals to meet the spiritual needs of patients (La Pierre, 2003; "Spiritual," 2003). Many published medical journal articles contain religious terminology, and the frequency of studies on religion and spiritu-

ality and health has increased over the past decade (Levin et al., 1997). Thus, it seems reasonable to engage in further analysis and discussion regarding religious and spiritual issues in the health care setting to assess fully the relationship, inform health care providers the best ways of dealing with these issues, and help to avoid the pitfalls that both critics and advocates have raised.

DEFINING RELIGION AND SPIRITUALITY

The terms *religion* and *spirituality* are difficult to define and have often been mistakenly used synonymously. The two overlap, but are distinct (Powell, Shahabi, & Thoresen, 2003; Tanyi, 2002). Countless subtly different definitions of each have emerged, and investigators have struggled to reach consensus on formal definitions. In the *Handbook of Religion and Health,* a widely cited book considered by many to be an authoritative source on religion and health, Koenig, McCullough, and Larson (2001) defined the two as follows:

> **Religion:** An organized system of beliefs, practices, rituals, and symbols designed to (a) facilitate closeness to the sacred or transcendent (God, higher power, or ultimate truth/reality) and (b) to foster an understanding of one's relationship and responsibility to others in living together in a community.

> **Spirituality:** The personal quest for understanding answers to ultimate questions about life, about meaning, and about relationship to the sacred or transcendent, which may (or may not) lead to or arise from the development of religious rituals and the formation of community.

A panel of experts convened by the National Institute of Healthcare Research (Larson, Swyers, & McCullough, 1998) define *spirituality* as "the feelings, thoughts, experiences, and behaviors that arise from a search for the sacred." After reviewing 76 articles and 19 books, Tanyi (2002) concludes that spirituality is "a personal search for meaning and purpose in life, which may or may not be related to religion."

Regardless of the exact definitions, an often-noted key distinction between religion and spirituality is that the former tends to involve a group or community and the latter primarily an individual. However, even if universal definitions were established, considerable debate would remain over whether to classify specific practices as either or neither.

For example, where does one draw the line between religions and cults? In fact, one of the definitions of cult in the *Merriam Webster Dictionary* (http://www.m-w.com) is "a religion regarded as unorthodox or spurious." This, in turn, begs the question: what is the criterion for being unorthodox and spurious? In fact, as history has often demonstrated, what formerly was considered a cult and spurious can eventually become a major religion, and vice versa.

BRIEF HISTORY OF RELIGION AND HEALTH CARE

The relationship between religion and health care has cycled between cooperation and antagonism throughout history. Artifacts and writings from as early as 5000 B.C. demonstrate that some of the most advanced civilizations of ancient times (such as the Assyrians, Chinese, Egyptians, Mesopotamians, and Persians) equated physical illnesses with evil spirits and demonic possessions. Treatment was aimed at banishing these spirits. Priests or the equivalent were often called to treat the ill using some combination of incantations, rituals, and medications.

Ancient originators of today's health care theories and practices emphasized the importance of the metaphysical. Scholars in early Chinese society believed that good physical health occurred when spirits were balanced in the body and developed acupuncture to alleviate imbalances. Hippocrates postulated that illness was caused by imbalance of four bodily fluids (blood, phlegm, yellow bile, and black bile), and Plato emphasized the need to treat the soul along with the body.

Health care and healing were involved prominently during the origins of most of today's major religions. The Old Testament contains passages that attribute illness to sins and healing to God (Deuteronomy 28:28, New International Version [NIV], Deuteronomy 32:39, NIV, Exodus 15:26, NIV, and Jeremiah 33:6, NIV). Hindus practice meditation to free themselves from the cycle of death and disease. Early Buddhism approved of using religious beliefs and rituals for healing.

In the eyes of religious groups, physicians and other health care providers have been viewed as everything from evil sorcerers to conduits of God's healing powers. Similarly, physicians, scientists, and health care provider's views of religion have ranged from interest to disinterest to disdain. A number of prominent scholars from Sigmund Freud to Albert Ellis warned of the dangers of religion, describing religion as a "universal obsessional neurosis" and emphasizing that it might result in negative consequences such as decreased self-acceptance and increased intolerance, inflexibility, and irrational behaviors. Indeed, a number of studies have linked disorders such as mania, schizophrenia, and temporal lobe epilepsy with unusual religious experiences or feelings (Lewis, 1994). However, while a certain subset of religious and spiritual feelings may be attributable to mental illness, the high prevalence of religious devotees and practitioners compared with relatively lower prevalence of mental illness makes it less likely that most religious experiences are due to established psychopathology.

In recent years, members of the medical and scientific community have strived to understand the effects of religion on health. In 1910, Sir William Osler, a pioneer of modern scientific medicine, wrote in the *British Medical Journal* about "the faith that heals," and that "nothing in life is more wonderful than faith" (Osler, 1910). A new discipline dubbed the "epidemiology of religion," which examines the association of religious belief and mortality and morbidity, has emerged and is growing (Levin, 1996). Institutions and organizations such as the National Institutes of Health (NIH), the John Templeton Foundation, and the American Association for the Advancement of Science have either funded research or convened meetings and symposia focusing on the effects of religion on physical and mental health.

METHODOLOGICAL ISSUES WITH CLINICAL STUDIES

To better understand the relationship between spirituality and health in general, or spirituality and pain management in particular, it is necessary to consider methodological issues that pertain to studies exploring these issues. This field of study has many traditional issues with regard to study design such as statistical and power analysis, retrospective versus prospective analysis, and cross-sectional vs. longitudinal analysis. However, there are also unique issues related to the measurement of spiritual experiences and practices, measurements of religiosity, and finding ways of preserving the rigors of science while not interfering with the religious or spiritual interventions being evaluated. For these reasons, a review of the literature on religion and health reveals that on one hand, there are a growing number of studies, and on the other hand, many studies have design issues that may complicate interpretation of their findings. Some problems with methodological issues arise from the lack of adequate interest and funding among the medical and scientific community, leaving investigators who do not have sufficient resources or training in proper experimental design to conduct studies. Such a statement can be made of many fields of study in their early phases of development. And this does appear to be improving with more expert researchers beginning to address religious and spiritual issues either directly or as subcomponents of larger trials. There are other methodological issues with these studies that are described below. These issues should be considered whenever evaluating a report in the literature to help better assess its relevance to clinical practice.

ANECDOTES AND EDITORIALS

A large percentage of the literature consists of anecdotes and editorials. While these are helpful in generating discussions, formulating ideas, and fueling future studies, they do not establish causality or scientific support of specific interventions.

CO-RELATIONAL STUDIES

The majority of the studies have been co-relational. Many of these co-relational studies have not adjusted for confounding variables such as socioeconomic status, ethnicity, and different lifestyles or diets. Members of a church or religious group can have a larger social support network or better access to health care. Co-relational studies also do not establish cause-and-effect relationships as clearly as other types of studies. Poor health can prevent a patient from going to church or leave a patient so discouraged that he or she does not want to participate in religious and spiritual activities. Conversely, patients may become more religious when they encounter serious health problems especially when such health problems result in pain and disability.

PROBLEMATIC NUMBERS AND CONTROLS

Designing studies with sufficient numbers of subjects and adequate controls can be problematic. There are a limited number of adequately performed randomized controlled trials (RCT) on spirituality and health. Of course, in some cases, RCTs are difficult to perform because patients may be reluctant or unable to change their religious beliefs and practices. The inherent issues pertaining to the study of religious phenomena often make such studies difficult to randomize or control. For example, it is not possible to have nonreligious individuals pray and, conversely, religious individuals may not want to take part in a study in which they are not allowed to pray. It is also not easy to isolate subjects in an effort to prevent external forces from interfering with a study. In other words, it may be possible to prevent the pastoral care team at the hospital from interacting with a patient, but the patient may have friends and family who can perform many similar functions.

PROBLEMS WITH MEASUREMENT

Religiousness can be measured in many different ways. The degree to which one participates in formal church, synagogue, or temple activities (defined as *organizational religiosity*) can differ from the degree to which one performs private religious activities such as praying, reading religious scriptures, and watching religious television (*non-organizational religiosity*). Participation in religious activities alone does not determine how closely an individual's beliefs conform to the established doctrines of a religious body (*religious belief*). Moreover, individuals can feel that they are very religious (high *subjective religiosity*), but score low on objective measures (low *religious commitment/motivation*) of how committed they are to their religion. Additionally, religiousness can be mea-

sured by how knowledgeable or informed individuals are about their religion's doctrines (*religious knowledge*) or how well their actions, such as working for the church and acts of altruism, support their religion (*religious consequences*). Therefore, studies should clearly state the exact measures of religiousness used, and conclusions should not make any claims about measures not used.

Often questionnaires or interviews with the patients are used to measure religious commitment or spirituality. Even though patients report that they are religious, more objective measures (e.g., how closely their lifestyle fits religious doctrines and how often they pray) may not support that claim. In fact, patients may forget or be unwilling to admit lapses. In the absence of objective measures, questionnaires should be at least well validated. Unfortunately, many studies do not indicate whether and how their questionnaires were validated. Similarly, some studies did not use objective measures or well-validated instruments to measure health outcomes.

To establish a true cause-and-effect relationship, it is helpful to elicit a dose–response curve, i.e., determine if increased religiosity corresponds to better health. Someone who does not belong to a church but regularly prays and follows religious doctrine may, in fact, have greater religious commitment than a person who belongs to a church but does not believe in or care to comprehend religious doctrine. Many studies simply divide patients into dichotomous groups (e.g., do they belong to a church?), which does not account for significant variation within each of the two groups.

COMPONENTS OF RELIGION AND SPIRITUALITY

It will be important for investigators to be clear regarding the components of religion and spirituality studied. There are many aspects of religion and spirituality that may affect health. The social interactions, friendships, and activities that accompany membership in a religious group and specific activities such as prayer, meditation, or studying religious scriptures could all have beneficial health effects. Church activities can provide exercise, reprieves from unhealthy environments, and contact with people who may be able to assist. Many studies have not looked at such specific components and therefore have yet to determine which components represent the "active ingredients."

VARIATIONS IN PRACTICES AND DOCTRINES

There are significant variations in practices and doctrines among and within different religious affiliations and denominations. It will be important for studies to account for the variations in practices and doctrines both within traditions and across traditions. For example, prayers may be silent or vocal. Behavior that shows an adequate level of religious commitment in one religion may not be sufficient in another religion. For example, more orthodox denominations may have dress codes or prevent use of certain devices. The degree of hierarchy in a religion and an individual's place in that hierarchy can vary significantly and, in turn, affect a person's sense of well-being. Moreover, a person's socioeconomic status, gender, and ethnicity can affect how well he or she is accepted in a given religious group.

THE POSITIVE EFFECTS OF RELIGION ON PAIN AND HEALTH

In spite of many methodological issues, a large body of research has suggested that religion and spirituality may have a positive impact on health. Systematic reviews and meta-analyses show religious involvement to be an epidemiologically protective factor (Ball, Armistead, & Austin, 2003; Braam et al., 1999; Brown, 2000; Kark et al., 1996; Kune, Kune, & Watson, 1993; McCullough & Larson, 1999; Oman et al., 2002), and high levels of religious involvement may be associated with up to 7 years of longer life expectancy (Helm et al., 2000; Hummer et al., 1999; Koenig et al., 1999; Oman & Reed, 1998; Strawbridge et al., 1997). Comstock and Partridge (1972) found that among 91,000 people in a Maryland county, those who regularly attended church had a lower prevalence of cirrhosis, emphysema, suicide, and death from ischemic heart disease. Oleckno and Blacconiere's (1991) study on college students revealed an inverse correlation between religiosity and behaviors that adversely affect health.

Studies also have suggested that religiousness may correlate with better outcomes after major medical procedures. In Oxman, Freeman, and Manheimer's (1995) analysis of 232 patients following elective open heart surgery, lack of participation in social or community groups and absence of strength and comfort from religion were consistent predictors of mortality. In Pressman and colleagues' (1990) look at 30 elderly women after hip repair, religious belief was associated with lower levels of depressive symptoms and better ambulation status.

RESOURCES AND LIFESTYLES OF RELIGIOUS GROUPS

Many reasons for these associations have been postulated. Religious groups may promote or provide access to better health care, by encouraging healthy lifestyles (e.g., avoiding substance abuse and risky sexual practices) and sponsoring health improvement programs (e.g., blood pressure screening, blood drives, soup kitchens, and food drives) (Heath et al., 1999; Koenig et al., 1998; Stewart, 2001; Zaleski & Schiaffino, 2000). Groups, such as the Catholic Church, have substantial resources and positions that allow them to positively influence people in ways that many secular organizations cannot. Additionally, many

hospitals and health care clinics are supported by, affiliated with, or even owned by religious groups.

PSYCHOLOGICAL EFFECTS OF RELIGION

Some have suggested that religion simply serves as a distraction from pain. But several studies have actually found a positive correlation between the "diverting attention" and "praying" factors on the Coping Strategies Questionnaire (CSQ) and pain levels (Geisser, Robinson, & Henson, 1994; Swartzman et al., 1994; Swimmer, Robinson, & Geisser, 1992). There is some evidence that the social network and support provided by religions is associated with lower pain levels, and religious belief may improve self-esteem and sense of purpose (Hays et al., 1998; Musick et al., 1998; Swimmer et al., 1992). Based on his longitudinal study of 720 adults, Williams concluded that religious attendance buffered the effects of stress on mental health (Williams et al., 1991). Coward's study (1991) of 107 women with advanced breast cancer suggested that spirituality may improve emotional well-being.

RELIGIONS AND THE MEANING OF PAIN

Religious belief may help patients give meaning to and, in turn, better cope with their pain (Autiero, 1987; Foley, 1988). While many major religions deem pain and suffering the result of sin, they also believe that pain can be strengthening, enlightening, and purifying. Different religious teachings have suggested that pain is the inevitable fate of humankind and can be cleansing, test virtue, educate, readjust priorities, stimulate personal growth, and define human life (Amundsen, 1982). Despite these positive views of pain, members of different religions may differ in how to face pain. Many Buddhists believe in enduring pain matter-of-factly (Tu, 1980). Hindus may stress understanding and detachment from pain (Shaffer, 1978). Muslims and Jews often favor resisting or fighting pain (Bowker, 1978). Many Christians stress seeking atonement and redemption (Amundsen, 1982). Of course, these are generalizations, and differing opinions exist within members of each religion.

PHYSIOLOGICAL EFFECTS OF RELIGIOUS PRACTICES

Research on the physiologic effects of various religious and spiritual practices and experiences is growing rapidly, especially with the development of real-time brain imaging technologies such as positron emission tomography (PET), single photon emission computed tomography (SPECT), and functional magnetic resonance imaging (fMRI). Choosing the appropriate imaging technique for a research study can be challenging. Each provides different advantages and disadvantages. fMRI provides better resolution and anatomic information than SPECT or PET. However, the MRI machine generates significant noise

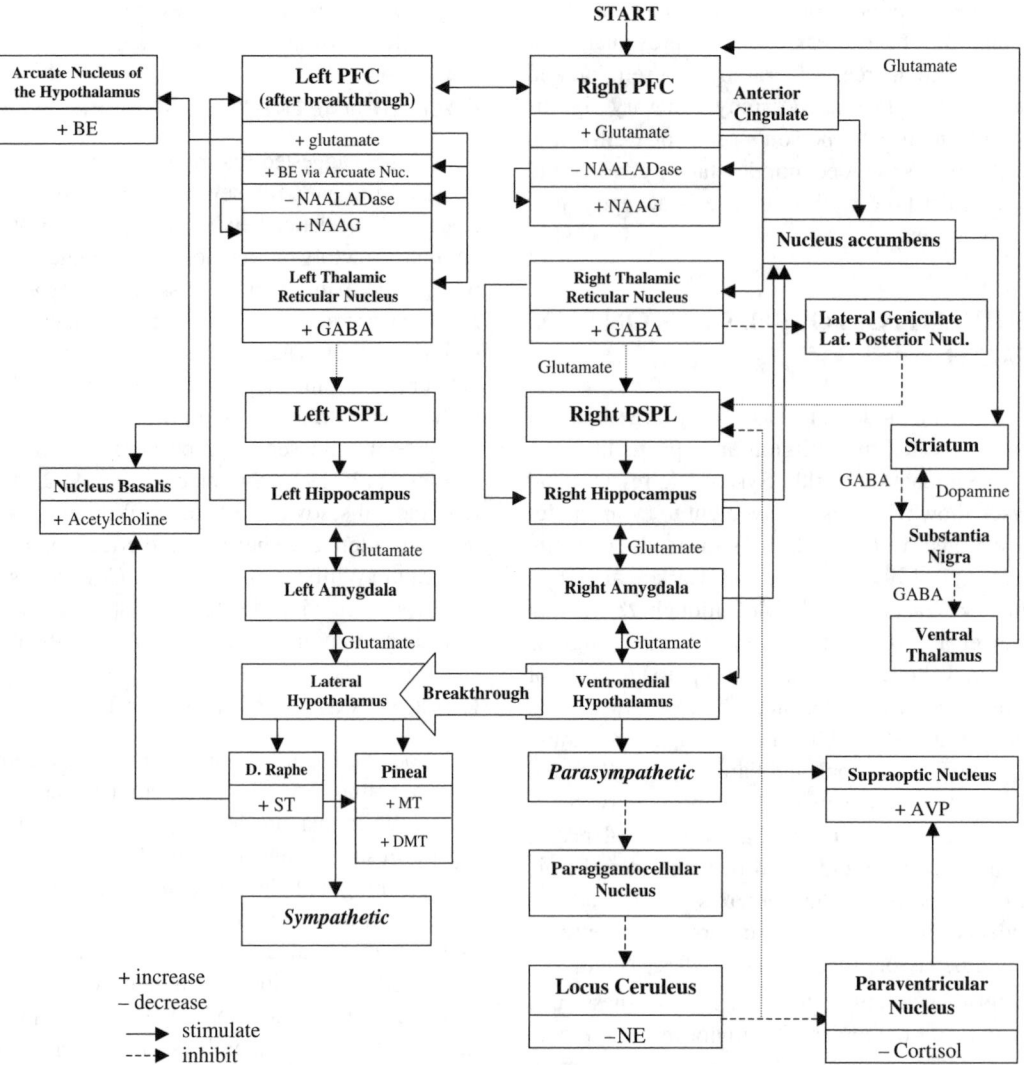

FIGURE 98.1 Schematic overview of the neurophysiological network possibly associated with meditative states. The circuits generally apply to both hemispheres; however, much of the initial activity is on the right. AVP = arginine vasopressin; D = dopamine; DMT = 5-methoxy-dimethyltryptamine; NAAG = N-acetylaspartylglutamate; NAALADase = N-acetylated-alpha-linked-acidic dipeptidase; ST = serotonin. From Newberg, A.B. & Iversen, J., 2003, *Medical Hypothesis, 61*, 284. Reproduced with permission.

and requires a subject to lie down, both of which may disturb meditation or prayer. PET and SPECT make it possible to radiolabel neurotransmitters and determine how they are affected by spiritual practices. But, radiopharmaceuticals may not be as readily available during hours when research centers and hospitals are most quiet and therefore conducive to spiritual practices.

Taken together, the studies on religious and spiritual practices such as meditation have begun to elucidate a comprehensive model regarding the underlying physiological effects occurring in both the brain and the body. Such a model has many implications for the study of pain and pain management. A summary of this model is described below and is also outlined in Figure 98.1.

Brain imaging studies suggest that willful acts and tasks that require sustained attention are initiated via activity in the prefrontal cortex (PFC), particularly in the right hemisphere (Frith et al., 1991; Ingvar, 1994; Pardo, Fox, & Raichle, 1991; Posner & Petersen, 1990). The cingulate gyrus has also been shown to be involved in focusing attention, probably in conjunction with the PFC (Vogt, Finch, & Olson, 1992). As practices such as meditation require intense focus of attention, it seems appropriate that a model for meditation begin with activation of the PFC (particularly the right) as well as the cingulate gyrus. This notion is supported by the increased activity observed in these regions on several of the brain imaging studies of volitional types of meditation including that from our laboratory (Cheramy, Romo, & Glowinski, 1987; Portas et al., 1998; Vogt et al., 1992). Several animal studies have shown that the PFC, when activated, innervates the reticular nucleus of the thalamus (Cornwall & Phillipson, 1988), particularly as part of a more global attentional network (Portas et al., 1998). Such activation may be accomplished by the production and distribution by the PFC of the excitatory neurotransmitter glutamate, which the PFC neurons use to communicate among themselves and to innervate other brain structures (Cheramy et al., 1987). The thalamus itself governs the flow of sensory information to cortical processing areas via its interactions with the lateral geniculate and lateral posterior nuclei and also likely uses the glutamate system to activate neurons in other structures (Armony & LeDoux, 2000). When excited, the reticular nucleus of the thalamus secretes the inhibitory neurotransmitter gamma-aminobutyric acid (GABA) onto the lateral posterior and geniculate nuclei, cutting off input to the posterior superior parietal lobe (PSPL) and visual centers in proportion to the reticular activation (Destexhe, Contreras, & Steriade, 1998). During meditation, because of the increased activity in the PFC, particularly on the right, there should be a concomitant increase in the activity in the reticular nucleus of the thalamus.

The PSPL is heavily involved in the analysis and integration of higher-order visual, auditory, and somaesthetic information (Adair et al., 1997). It is also involved in a complex attentional network that includes the PFC and thalamus (Fernandez-Duque & Posner, 2001). Through the reception of auditory and visual input from the thalamus, the PSPL is able to help generate a three-dimensional image of the body in space, provide a sense of spatial coordinates in which the body is oriented, help distinguish between objects, and exert influences in regard to objects that may be directly grasped and manipulated (Lynch, 1980; Mountcastle, Andersen, & Motter, 1981). These functions of the PSPL might be critical for distinguishing between the self and the external world. Deafferentation of PSPL has been suggested to be an important concept in the physiology of meditation which has been supported by several imaging studies.

In addition to the complex cortical-thalamic activity, meditation might also be expected to alter activity in the limbic system especially since stimulation of limbic structures, such as the amygdala and hippocampus, is associated with experiences similar to those described during meditation (Fish, Gloor, Quesney, & Olivier, 1993; Saver & Rabin, 1997). The results of the fMRI study by Lazar, et al. support the notion of increased activity in the regions of the amygdala and hippocampus during meditation (Lazar et al., 2000; Pardo et al., 1991).

The hypothalamus is extensively interconnected with the limbic system. Stimulation of the right lateral amygdala has been shown to result in stimulation of the ventromedial portion of the hypothalamus with a subsequent stimulation of the peripheral parasympathetic system (Davis, 1992). Increased parasympathetic activity should be associated with the subjective sensation first of relaxation and, eventually, of a more profound quiescence.

Activation of the parasympathetic system would also cause a reduction in heart rate and respiratory rate. All of these physiological responses have been observed during meditation (Jevning, Wallace, & Beidebach, 1992).

Typically, when breathing and heart rate slow, the paragigantocellular nucleus of the medulla ceases to innervate the locus ceruleus (LC) of the pons. The LC produces and distributes norepinephrine (NE) (Foote & Morrison, 1987), a neuromodulator that increases the susceptibility of brain regions to sensory input by amplifying strong stimuli, while simultaneously gating out weaker activations and cellular "noise" that fall below the activation threshold (Waterhouse, Moises, & Woodward, 1998). Decreased stimulation of the LC results in a decrease in the level of NE (Van Bockstaele & Aston-Jones, 1995). A reduction in NE would decrease the impact of sensory input on the PSPL, contributing to its deafferentation.

The locus ceruleus would also deliver less NE to the hypothalamic paraventricular nucleus. The paraventricular nucleus of the hypothalamus typically secretes corticotropin-releasing hormone (CRH) in response to innervation by NE from the locus ceruleus (Ziegler, Cass, & Herman, 1999). This CRH stimulates the anterior pituitary to release adrenocorticotropic hormone (ACTH) (Livesey et al., 2000). ACTH, in turn, stimulates the adrenal cortex to produce cortisol, one of the body's stress hormones (Davies, Keyon, & Fraser, 1985). Decreasing NE from the locus ceruleus during meditation would likely decrease the production of CRH by the paraventricular nucleus and ultimately decrease cortisol levels. Most studies have found that urine and plasma cortisol levels are decreased during meditation (Dollins et al., 1993; Jevning, Wilson, & Davidson, 1978; Sudsuang, Chentanez, & Veluvan, 1991; Tooley et al., 2000).

As a meditation practice continues, there should be continued activity in the PFC associated with the persistent will to focus attention. In general, as PFC activity increases, it produces ever-increasing levels of free synaptic glutamate in the brain. Increased glutamate can stimulate the hypothalamic arcuate nucleus to release beta-endorphin (Kiss et al., 1997). Beta-endorphin (BE) is an opioid produced primarily by the arcuate nucleus of the medial hypothalamus and distributed to the brain's subcortical areas (Yadid, 2000). BE is known to depress respiration, reduce fear, reduce pain, and produce sensations of joy and euphoria (Janal et al., 1984). That such effects have been described during meditation may implicate some degree of BE release related to the increased PFC activity. Meditation has been found to disrupt diurnal rhythms of BE and ACTH, while not affecting diurnal cortisol rhythms (Infante et al., 1998). However, it is likely that BE is not the sole mediator in such experiences during meditation because simply taking morphine-related substances does not produce equivalent experiences as in meditation. Furthermore, one very limited study demonstrated that blocking the opiate receptors with naloxone did not affect the experience or EEG associated with meditation (Sim & Tsoi, 1992).

In the early 1970s, Gellhorn and Kiely developed a model of the physiological processes involved in meditation based almost exclusively on autonomic nervous system (ANS) activity, which, although somewhat limited, indicated the importance of the ANS during such experiences (Gellhorn & Kiely, 1972). These authors suggested that intense stimulation of either the sympathetic or parasympathetic system, if continued, could ultimately result in simultaneous discharge of both systems (what might be considered a "breakthrough" of the other system). Several studies have demonstrated predominant parasympathetic activity during meditation associated with decreased heart rate and blood pressure, decreased respiratory rate, and decreased oxygen metabolism (Hugdahl, 1996; Peng et al., 1999; Travis, 2001). However, a recent study of two separate meditative techniques suggested a mutual activation of parasympathetic and sympathetic systems by demonstrating an increase in the variability of heart rate during meditation (Infante et al., 1998). The increased variation in heart rate was hypothesized to reflect activation of both arms of the autonomic nervous system. This notion also fits the characteristic description of meditative states in which there is a sense of overwhelming calmness as well as significant alertness. Also, the notion of mutual activation of both arms of the ANS is consistent with recent developments in the study of autonomic interactions (Hugdahl, 1996).

Other neurotransmitters may also be associated including serotonin and melatonin. Serotonin, which appears to be increased in practices such as meditation, has a central role in depressive symptoms as well as the potential to be hallucinogenic. Increased serotonin combined with lateral hypothalamic innervation of the pineal gland may result in increased production of melatonin (MT). Melatonin has been shown to depress the central nervous system and reduce pain sensitivity (Shaji & Kulkarni, 1998). During meditation, blood plasma MT has been found to increase sharply (Tooley et al., 2000), which may contribute to the feelings of calmness and decreased awareness of pain (Dollins et al., 1993).

Overall, there appear to be a number of physiological effects of spiritual practices and their associated experiences. The results from existing studies have helped to demonstrate that many of these effects have a positive impact on human health and well being.

THE NEGATIVE EFFECTS OF RELIGION ON PAIN AND HEALTH

There may also be a number of negative consequences that religion and spirituality may have on health. For example, religious groups may hinder the delivery of health care by directly opposing certain health care interventions, such as transfusions or contraception, and convincing patients that their ailments are due to noncompliance with religious doctrines rather than organic disease (Donahue, 1985). Moreover, some fear that church-sponsored health initiatives may ignore populations that do not belong to the church. There may be social problems stemming from religions such as the recently publicized clergy-perpetrated child sexual abuse in the Catholic Church, violent behaviors associated with religious fundamentalism, and military action arising from religious conflicts, that ultimately affect health (Rossetti, 1995; Tieman, 2002).

Pain management practitioners must be aware that religion may also be a source of a patient's pain. Emotional and psychological anguish brought on by guilt or shame from a moral or religious transgression can manifest as physical discomfort. This has been described as religious and spiritual pain and can be difficult to distinguish from pure physical pain (Satterly, 2001). Spiritual pain can come from spiritual abuse (convincing people that they are going to suffer eternal purgatory) and spiritual terrorism, an extreme form of spiritual abuse. Spiritual abuse can be overt or insidious; i.e., it can be implied that a patient will be doomed, although not actually stated (Purcell, 1998a, 1998b). At times when sources of pain are mixed among religious, spiritual, and organic, treatment can become complicated. Neglecting to account for religious or spiritual pain may result in overtreatment (e.g., too much pharmacological therapy). Conversely, over-ascribing pain to religious or spiritual causes may lead to undertreatment.

Finally, it is important that religion and spirituality do not become an intervention such that a patient with pain is told to go home and pray for relief. On the one hand, this prevents standard of care for such problems, but also takes the meaning out of religion. Religious and spiritual practices and beliefs should not be for health-related purposes. However, if a patient has a strong religious or spiritual belief, then the patient could be encouraged to utilize the resources that have been an important part of his or her life.

THE EFFECTS OF SPECIFIC RELIGIOUS AND SPIRITUAL ACTIVITIES

People practice different specific religious and spiritual activities. While many of these activities either emerged from or at some point may have been associated (correctly or incorrectly) with specific religions, today many people can practice these activities in either a religious or secular manner. Moreover, the line between different activities continues to grow more indistinct. Individuals often combine the different activities or develop hybrid techniques. Thus, whenever considering a particular practice, it is important to be as specific as possible. This is also true when reviewing the literature because some studies are not specific as to the particular approach used by the subjects.

PRAYER

Prayer may be the most commonly used religious and spiritual activity. Eisenberg and colleagues' (1998) survey of alternative medicine usage among Americans found that one fourth of respondents used prayer to cope with physical illness. Previous studies have suggested that prayer may be associated with less muscle tension, improved cardiovascular and neuroimmunologic parameters, psychologic and spiritual peace, a greater sense of purpose, and enhanced coping skills. Rapp, Rejeski, and Miller (2000) followed 394 elderly patients with knee pain for 30 months and found that prayer was associated with less disability and better physical function.

There are numerous types of prayer. *Petitionary prayers* ask for something specific (e.g., asking for God to heal knee pain). *Intercessory prayers* pray for someone else (e.g., a friend) and may be performed remotely (e.g., some Internet Web sites allow people to submit prayers for others). *Prayers of adoration* praise or honor God or some other divine being. *Prayers of confession* admit a wrongdoing and ask for forgiveness. *Ritual prayers* involve reciting specific passages or repeating specific behaviors. *Colloquial prayers* ask a higher power for guidance. *Contemplative prayers* and *meditative prayers* do not ask for anything specific and are very similar. In *contemplative prayers*, individuals may listen to or think about God. In *meditative prayers*, individuals try to clear their minds and focus on specific words or ideas.

Investigators have looked at different types of prayers. Poloma and Pendleton (1991) found that *petitionary* and *ritualistic prayers* were associated with lower levels of well-being and life satisfaction, while *colloquial prayers* were associated with higher levels. Byrd and colleagues (Byrd, 1988) performed a double-blind study of the effects of *intercessory prayer* on outcome after admission to a coronary care unit (CCU). They found significantly more patients that were prayed for had a "good" outcome (163 vs. 147) and significantly fewer had a "bad" outcome (27 vs. 44). Harris and colleagues (Harris et al., 1999) also found improved CCU outcomes with remote *intercessory prayer*. However, these findings have not been replicated by similar subsequent studies (Aviles, et al., 2001; Matthews, Conti, & Sireci, 2001; Matthews, Marlow, & MacNutt, 2000; Townsend et al., 2002).

MEDITATION

Meditation-related practices are the most widely used alternative therapy techniques. More than 16% of respondents in Eisenberg's national survey (1998) on comple-

mentary and alternative medicine used "relaxation" techniques. Numerous physicians regularly recommend Transcendental Meditation (TM) techniques to their patients, and meditation is often part of integrated health programs such as Dean Ornish's popular heart disease programs. Preliminary studies suggest that meditative practices may benefit patients with hypertension, psoriasis, irritable bowel disease, anxiety, and depression (Barrows & Jacobs, 2002; Carlson et al., 2001; Castillo-Richmond et al., 2000; Kabat-Zinn et al., 1992, 1998; Kaplan, Goldenberg, & Galvin-Nadeau, 1993; Keefer & Blanchard, 2002; King, Carr, & D'Cruz, 2002; Manocha et al., 2002; Reibel et al., 2001; Williams et al., 2001). Furthermore, these practices have the potential to provide support to patients suffering from both acute and chronic conditions. Psychological studies have suggested that meditation may decrease anxiety, depression, irritability, and moodiness as well as improve learning ability, memory, self-actualization, feelings of vitality and rejuvenation, and emotional stability (Astin, 1997; Astin et al., 2003; Bitner et al., 2003; Solberg et al., 1996; Walton et al., 1995). Research has found that meditators can achieve a state of restful alertness with improved reaction time, creativity, and comprehension (Domino, 1977; Solberg et al., 1996).

Meditation has been used for pain management as well. Pregnant women often use meditative and relaxation techniques learned from childbirth preparation classes to cope with labor pains and anxiety. At Stanford, meditative techniques have been incorporated in a 12-hour comprehensive arthritis self-care course that has been taken by more than 100,000 patients. Graduates of the course have reported a 15 to 20% reduction in pain. Kabat-Zinn and colleagues (Kabat-Zinn, 1982; Kabat-Zinn, Lipworth, & Burney, 1985) reported significant chronic pain improvement after patients completed training in mindful meditation. Kaplan and colleagues (Kaplan et al., 1993) saw symptom improvement in all 77 men and women with fibromyalgia who completed a 10-week stress-reduction program that used meditation.

Unfortunately, studies have not always defined the type of meditation being investigated. Results from one type of meditation do not necessarily hold true for others. Different types of meditation can vary significantly in the amount of physical and mental control required. In some methods (e.g., Zazen, Vipassana), the body is immobile; in others (e.g., Siddha Yoga, the Latihan, the chaotic meditation of Rajneesh), the body is let free; and in still others (e.g., Mahamudra, Shikan Taza, Gurdjieff's "self-remembering"), the person participates in daily activities while meditating. The common denominator is that all attempt to calm the mind, filling it with certain sounds, words, or images and keeping the mind on the present, not the past or future.

Studies have shown that during mediation (especially TM) patients may experience decreases in heart rate (average of several beats less per minute), respiration rate (an average of two fewer breaths per minute), plasma cortisol, and oxygen consumption (in some cases, down to 80% of normal) (Barnes et al., 1999; Castillo-Richmond et al., 2000; Cunningham, Brown, & Kaski, 2000; MacLean et al., 1994; Michaels et al., 1979; Walton et al., 1995; Wenneberg et al., 1997; Werner et al., 1986). Hypertensive patients also may experience a drop in blood pressure (Schneider et al., 2001). Meditation can be accompanied by increases in electroencephalogram alpha (a brain wave associated with relaxation), skin electrical resistance (high during relaxation and low during anxious states), and relative parasympathetic activity (Infante et al., 2001; Kumar & Kurup, 2003; Travis, 2001; Travis et al., 2001, 2002). Benson and Wallace (Benson, Malvea, & Graham, 1973; Benson et al., 1974; Wallace, 1997; Wallace, Benson, & Wilson, 1971) conducted some of the earliest physiologic studies on TM in the 1960s and described the meditation state as wakeful and hypometabolic.

There are indications that long-term physiologic changes may result from regular meditation (Calderon et al., 1999; MacLean et al., 1997). Meditators have been found to have better respiratory function (vital capacity, tidal volume, expiratory pressure, and breath holding), cardiovascular parameters (diastolic blood pressure and heart rate), and lipid profiles than nonmeditators (Wallace et al., 1983; Wenneberg et al., 1997). Cooper and Aygen (1979) found that over an 11-month period, patients with hypercholesteremia who used TM had significant reductions in fasting serum cholesterol levels compared with controls.

There is evidence that many of these physiologic changes are not simply due to patients changing body position. Experiments have shown that blood lactate levels drop four times faster when subjects meditate than when subjects simply lie on their backs (Delmonte, 1985; Ghista et al., 1976; Swinyard, Chaube, & Sutton, 1974). Increased blood flow and oxygen delivery to the muscles may account for this decrease in lactate levels. It remains uncertain whether these physiological changes are significantly different from those achieved during sleep or hypnosis (Michaels, Huber, & McCann, 1976; Swinyard et al., 1974; Wallace, 1997). Meditation has also been found to enhance the effectiveness of biofeedback.

Although physically non-invasive, meditation does have its dangers. Meditative practices can aggravate and precipitate psychotic episodes in patients who are delusional or strongly paranoid. They can also heighten anxiety in people with overwhelming anxiety. Therefore, discretion should be used in patients with psychiatric illness. Because psychiatric illness is not always evident to health care providers not trained in mental health and meditation can trigger the release of repressed memories, all patients using meditative techniques should be monitored, especially when a patient first starts using meditation.

YOGA

Originated in India and practiced for more than 5,000 years, yoga emphasizes the interrelationship between the mind and body. A common misconception is that yoga is derived from Hinduism, when in fact it predated Hinduism by several centuries. In fact, yoga techniques have been adopted by many religions, including Christianity. The American Yoga Association emphasizes that because yoga practice does not specify particular higher powers or religious doctrines, it can be compatible with all major religions.

One of the central tenets of yoga is that all people are searching for true happiness. Early in a person's spiritual development, he or she settles for temporary pleasures that cannot provide eternal satisfaction. Nature or God uses pain to prompt people to continue the search. Later in a person's spiritual development, the reward of peace and happiness replaces the punishment of pain as the primary motivator. Yoga practitioners believe that most diseases are due to a shortage of life force to either the entire or parts of the body, resulting in decreased immunity or resistance to disease. Good nutrition, sleep, a positive mental attitude, and yoga can augment the amount of life-force in the body. Misalignment of body parts can block the proper flow of life force to an organ and ultimately cause disease in that organ.

In yoga, a person follows a series of stretching, breathing, and relaxation techniques that prepare the mind and body for meditation. The stretching movements or postures (*asanas*) aim to stimulate and increase blood supply and *prana* (vital force) to various parts of the body as well as increase the flexibility of the spine. Increasing the spinal flexibility is believed to improve the nerve supply. Many *asanas* involve the spine, which is thought to be central to good health. The breathing techniques (*pranayamas*) are thought to improve brain function, eliminate toxins, and store reserve energy in the solar plexus region.

A few limited studies on yoga have been encouraging. They have shown altered EEG patterns; increased endorphine and dopamine release; reduced serum total cholesterol, LDL cholesterol, and triglyceride levels; and improved pulmonary function tests associated with yoga (Arambula et al., 2001; Birkel & Edgren, 2000; Schell, Allolio, & Schonecke, 1994; Selvamurthy et al., 1998; Stancak, 1991; Stanescu et al., 1981; Udupa, Singh, & Yadav, 1973). Yoga has shown benefit in patients with asthma, hypertension, heart failure, mood disorders, and diabetes (Jain et al., 1993; Malhotra et al., 2002a, 2002b; Manocha et al., 2002; van Montfrans et al., 1990). Two small controlled but nondouble-blinded studies showed Hatha yoga to significantly improve pain in osteoarthritis of the fingers and carpal tunnel syndrome (Garfinkel et al, 1994, 1998). Some of these benefits may arise from the muscle strengthening and stretching from some *asanas*.

There are some dangers to yoga. Certain asanas may be strenuous and cause injury. Moreover, some asanas are believed to cause disease. Although there is some credentialing process in yoga, it is neither rigorous nor universally accepted. So caution should be taken in selecting a yoga instructor and beginning a yoga program.

FAITH HEALING

Evidence suggests that many patients have seen faith healers, religious leaders who use prayer or other practices to treat and cure disease. Surveys have found that a fair number of patients in rural (21%) and inner city (10%) populations have used faith healers, and many physicians (23%) believe that faith healers can heal patients (McKee & Chappel, 1992). Numerous anecdotes of healing miracles exist, but to date there has been no consistent and convincing scientific proof that faith healers are effective (King & Bushwick, 1994). Additionally, it has not been determined whether faith healers affect patients psychologically or physiologically, and what factors may make them effective. Further research is needed before any conclusions can be drawn.

THE ROLE OF THE PAIN MANAGEMENT PROFESSIONAL

It is apparent that religious and spiritual practices are widely used and that their mechanisms and effectiveness, while currently under growing exploration, have not been clearly established. How then should they affect the practice of pain management professionals? This depends to some extent on personal philosophy, whether the practitioner uses and promotes religious and spiritual practices or simply has patients interested in using these practices. Regardless of where a practitioner falls along this spectrum, there are certain steps to consider regarding religious and spiritual issues when engaging with patients. Based on existing studies and clinical information, several approaches that pain management professionals might consider regarding religious and spiritual issues include the following areas.

TAKING A RELIGIOUS/SPIRITUAL HISTORY

Even though many health care practitioners have advocated taking a religious history as part of the initial history and physical, surveys indicate that many do not. One survey revealed that 59% of family physicians feel "uncertainty about how to take a spiritual history" and a "lack of experience or training." In a chart review of 92 elderly hospitalized patients facing end-of-life issues, only 6.5% of the patients had spiritual histories documented in their charts and only 29% had either a spiritual history or some mention of chaplain or psychiatrist involvement.

The purpose of the religious/spiritual history is to better understand the patient's religious background, determine how he or she may use religion to cope with illness, and open the door for future discussions about any spiritual or religious issues. Moreover, learning about a patient's spiritual practices may alert the pain management professional to watch for potential affects on patient compliance, acceptance of treatment, and how patients will make decisions about their health care choices. Questions should be nonjudgmental, open-ended, and general. Recommended questions include (Kuhn, 1988; Matthews & Clark, 1998):

- Are religious or spiritual beliefs an important part of your life?
- How do your religious or spiritual beliefs influence the way you take care of yourself?
- Do you rely on your religious or spiritual beliefs to help you cope with health problems?
- Are you part of a religious or spiritual community?
- Are there any religious or spiritual issues that need addressing?
- Who would you like to address religious or spiritual issues should they rise?
- How would you like me to address your spiritual needs?

For patients with severe illness, an American College of Physicians consensus panel led by Bernard Lo, Timothy Quill, and James Tulsky (1999) recommended the following questions:

- Is faith (religion and spirituality) important to you in this illness?
- Has faith (religion and spirituality) been important to you at other times in your life?
- Do you have someone to talk to about religious matters?
- Would you like to explore religious matters with someone?

ASSESSMENT OF SPIRITUAL DISTRESS

Because significant physical pain can result in spiritual distress, which in turn can exacerbate pain, it is important to recognize indicators of spiritual distress. Patients may question the meaning of life, pain, treatments, or illness; express anger at God, hopelessness, or despair; feel anxious about the afterlife, persecuted, guilty, or abandoned; or withdraw from friends and family. Abrahm (2001) suggests asking several questions to detect spiritual distress:

- Do you feel at peace with the changes in your life that have come about because of your illness?
- Are there any religious activities or practices that have been interrupted because of your illness?
- Pain is a hard thing physically. Has it been a hard thing for you spiritually?
- Would you like to speak with someone about your spiritual concerns?

FACILITATING ACCESS TO RELIGIOUS RESOURCES

If a health care practitioner is uncomfortable with either asking the above questions or dealing with the answers, he or she can seek help from religious professionals who can better address these issues. Religious resources are especially important during end-of-life care (Lo et al., 2002).

Evidence suggests that many health care providers are not familiar with the roles and training of various religious professionals in health care settings and, thus, do not consult them appropriately. Koenig, McCullough, and Larson (2001) have argued that chaplains should be included on pain management teams more frequently. Typically, chaplains have completed 8 to 12 years of education and training, passed written and oral examinations administered by the Association of Professional Chaplains, and been trained to work closely with physicians and nurses. Unlike parish ministers who have many responsibilities including administration and leading worship and often champion a particular faith, chaplains are trained to counsel patients and deal with all belief systems. Chaplains are available to counsel patient families, hospital staff, and physicians as well. Chaplains often sit on hospital ethics committees. However, not all hospitals have chaplains on staff. Pastoral counselors include any clergyperson who provides formal or informal individual, family, or group counseling.

PERFORMING CLERGY-LIKE DUTIES

Most health care providers have probably been asked to pray with a patient at some point in their training. Whether a health care provider is comfortable with this and how such an issue is handled are important to the patient and the relationship between the patient and provider. For example, ignoring such a request may anger, hurt, or embarrass the patient. Health care providers who have religious views that conflict with the patient or are agnostics or atheists can provide silent, nondenominational, or secular support. For example, the word *amen* means "so be it" and does not imply a belief in a higher power. Silent gestures such as holding a patient's hand or lowering the head while a patient prays can provide support as well. It is probably helpful for most health care providers to con-

sider what their approach to such issues will be, what their level of comfort is with regard to participating in religious practices with patients, and how they will ultimately deal with such issues prior to engaging in these aspects of religious or spiritual practices.

USE OF SPIRITUAL PRACTICES

Several spiritual practices are described in the literature. One of these tools is *listening authentically* to the patient. Studies have shown that many patients suffering from pain lament that health care providers do not adequately listen, which exacerbates their pain. Listening includes noticing a patient's body language, expression, demeanor, and tone of voice. The simple acts of being physically and emotionally with the patient without necessarily doing or saying anything (*presence*), allowing patients to express their feelings without judging or recoiling (*acceptance*), and offering one's own spiritual thoughts or experiences (*sharing of self* or *judicious self-disclosure*) may have therapeutic benefits. Pain management professionals can use *intuition* to recognize and understand the spiritual needs of a patient. Separate studies by Morse and Proctor (1998) and Proctor and colleagues (Proctor, Morse, & Khonsari, 1996) suggested that *comfort talk* can reduce pain. For more advanced spiritual practices such as meditation, health care providers should either obtain appropriate training to utilize such practices or explore the local community resources and practitioners who might be able to assist patients in such practices. In fact, it may be beneficial to meet with practitioners of spiritual practices to assess their qualifications and approaches to ensure that a patient will receive excellent instruction and will not encounter an obstruction to appropriate health care.

CONCLUSIONS AND FUTURE DIRECTIONS

Current evidence suggests that religious and spiritual activities can significantly aid in the management of pain. Many studies exist in the literature with varying degrees of methodological rigor. However, available evidence suggests that these activities do have physiological, social, and psychological effects, but the mechanisms require further elucidation. A number of pain management professionals and programs already have incorporated these activities in their practices. Anyone doing so should understand the complexity of and the subtle differences among these activities, as well as the potential problems. Even if one does not plan to incorporate these activities into practice, the prevalence of religious and spiritual activities makes it important for all pain management professionals to understand and be prepared to discuss these issues. Many patients and health care practitioners feel that religious and spiritual issues should be better integrated into patient care, a sentiment that is likely to grow in the future.

REFERENCES

Abrahm, J. (2001). Pain management for dying patients. How to assess needs and provide pharmacologic relief. *Postgraduate Medicine, 110*(2), 99.

Adair, J. C. et al. (1997). Anosognosia: examining the disconnection hypothesis. *Journal of Neurology, Neurosurgery, and Psychiatry, 63*(6), 798.

American Psychiatric Association. (1994). *Diagnostic and Statistical Manual of Mental Disorders* (4th ed.). Washington, DC: Author.

Amundsen, D. W. (1982). Medicine and faith in early Christianity. *Bulletin of the History of Medicine, 56*(3), 326.

Anonymous. (2002). Yoga and massage: If it's physical, it's therapy. *Newsweek, 140*(23), 74.

Anonymous. (2003). Spiritual assessment required in all settings. *Hospital Peer Review, 28*(4), 55.

Arambula, P. et al. (2001). The physiological correlates of Kundalini Yoga meditation: A study of a yoga master. *Applied Psychophysiology and Biofeedback, 26*(2), 147.

Armbruster, C. A., Chibnall, J. T., & Legett, S. (2003). Pediatrician beliefs about spirituality and religion in medicine: Associations with clinical practice. *Pediatrics, 111*(3), 227.

Armony, J. L., & LeDoux, J. E. (2000). How danger is encoded: Towards a systems, cellular, and computational understanding of cognitive-emotional interactions. In M. S. Gazzaniga (Ed.), *The new cognitive neurosciences* (2nd ed., p. 1073). Cambridge, MA: MIT Press.

Astin, J. A. (1997). Stress reduction through mindfulness meditation. Effects on psychological symptomatology, sense of control, and spiritual experiences. *Psychotherapy and Psychosomatics, 66*(2), 97.

Astin, J. A. et al. (2003). The efficacy of mindfulness meditation plus Qigong movement therapy in the treatment of fibromyalgia: A randomized controlled trial. *Journal of Rheumatology, 30*(10), 2257.

Autiero, A. (1987). The interpretation of pain: The point of view of Catholic theology. *Acta Neurochirurgie Supplement* (Wien), *38*, 123.

Aviles, J. M. et al. (2001). Intercessory prayer and cardiovascular disease progression in a coronary care unit population: A randomized controlled trial. *Mayo Clinic Proceedings, 76*(12), 1192.

Ball, J., Armistead, L., & Austin, B. J. (2003). The relationship between religiosity and adjustment among African-American, female, urban adolescents. *Journal of Adolescence, 26*(4), 431.

Barnes, V. A. et al. (1999). Acute effects of transcendental meditation on hemodynamic functioning in middle-aged adults. *Psychosomatic Medicine, 61*(4), 525.

Barrows, K. A. & Jacobs, B. P. (2002). Mind-body medicine. An introduction and review of the literature. *Medical Clinics of North America, 86*(1), 11.

Begley, S. (2001). Religion and the brain. *Newsweek, 137*(19), 50.

Benson, H. et al. (1974). Decreased blood pressure in borderline hypertensive subjects who practiced meditation. *Journal of Chronic Diseases, 27*(3), 163.

Benson, H., Malvea, B. P., & Graham, J. R. (1973). Physiologic correlates of meditation and their clinical effects in headache: an ongoing investigation. *Headache, 13*(1), 23.

Bezilla, R. (Ed.). (1993). *Religion in America, 1992–1993*, Princeton, NJ: Princeton Religious Center (Gallup Organization).

Birkel, D. A., & Edgren, L. (2000). Hatha yoga: Improved vital capacity of college students. *Alternative Therapies in Health and Medicine, 6*(6), 55.

Bitner, R. et al. (2003). Subjective effects of antidepressants: A pilot study of the varieties of antidepressant-induced experiences in meditators. *Journal of Nervous and Mental Disease, 191*(10), 660.

Bowker, D. (1978). Pain and suffering — Religious perspective, In W. T. Reich (Ed.). *Encyclopedia of bioethics* (Vol. 4, p. 1185). New York: Free Press..

Braam, A. et al. (1999). Religiosity as a protective factor in depressive disorder [Letter]. *American Journal of Psychiatry, 156*(5), 809; author reply, 810.

Brown, C. M. (2000). Exploring the role of religiosity in hypertension management among African Americans. *Journal of Health Care for the Poor and Underserved, 11*(1), 19.

Byrd, R. C. (1988). Positive therapeutic effects of intercessory prayer in a coronary care unit population. *Southern Medical Journal, 81*(7), 826.

Calderon, R., Jr. et al. (1999). Stress, stress reduction and hypercholesterolemia in African Americans: A review. *Ethnicity and Disease, 9*(3), 451.

Carlson, L. E. et al. (2001). The effects of a mindfulness meditation-based stress reduction program on mood and symptoms of stress in cancer outpatients: 6-month follow-up. *Support Care Cancer, 9*(2), 112.

Castillo-Richmond, A. et al. (2000). Effects of stress reduction on carotid atherosclerosis in hypertensive African Americans. *Stroke, 31*(3), 568.

Cheramy, A., Romo, R., & Glowinski, J. (1987). Role of corticostriatal glutamatergic neurons in the presynaptic control of dopamine release. In M. Sandler, C. Feuerstein, & B. Scatton (Eds.), *Neurotransmitter interactions in the basal ganglia* (p. 131). New York: Raven Press.

Chibnall, J. T., & Brooks, C. A. (2001). Religion in the clinic: The role of physician beliefs. *Southern Medical Journal, 94*(4), 374.

Comstock, G. W., & Partridge, K. B. (1972). Church attendance and health. *Journal of Chronic Disease, 25*(12), 665.

Cooper, M. J., & Aygen, M. M. (1979). A relaxation technique in the management of hypercholesterolemia. *Journal of Human Stress, 5*(4), 24.

Corliss, R. (2001). The power of yoga. *Time, 157*(16), 54.

Cornwall, J., & Phillipson, O. T. (1988). Mediodorsal and reticular thalamic nuclei receive collateral axons from prefrontal cortex and laterodorsal tegmental nucleus in the rat. *Neuroscience Letters, 88*(2), 121.

Coward, D. D. (1991). Self-transcendence and emotional well-being in women with advanced breast cancer. *Oncology Nursing Forum, 18*(5), 857.

Cunningham, C., Brown, S., & Kaski, J. C. (2000). Effects of transcendental meditation on symptoms and electrocardiographic changes in patients with cardiac syndrome X. *American Journal of Cardiology, 85*(5), 653.

Daaleman, T. P., & Nease, D. E., Jr. (1994). Patient attitudes regarding physician inquiry into spiritual and religious issues. *Journal of Family Practice, 39*(6), 564.

Davies, E., Keyon, C., & Fraser, R. (1985). The role of calcium ions in the mechanism of ACTH stimulation of cortisol synthesis. *Steroids, 45,* 557.

Davis, M. (1992). The role of the amygdala in fear and anxiety. *Annual Review of Neuroscience, 15,* 353.

Delmonte, M. M. (1985). Biochemical indices associated with meditation practice: A literature review. *Neuroscience and Biobehavioral Review, 9*(4), 557.

Destexhe, A., Contreras, D., & Steriade, M. (1998). Mechanisms underlying the synchronizing action of corticothalamic feedback through inhibition of thalamic relay cells. *Journal of Neurophysiology, 79*(2), 999.

Dollins, A. B. et al. (1993). Effect of pharmacological daytime doses of melatonin on human mood and performance. *Psychopharmacology* (Berlin), *112*(4), 490.

Domino, G. (1977). Transcendental meditation and creativity: An empirical investigation. *Journal of Applied Psychology, 62*(3), 358.

Donahue, M. J. (1985). Intrinsic and extrinsic religiousness: Review and meta-analysis. *Journal of Personality and Social Psychology, 48,* 400.

Eisenberg, D. M. et al. (1998). Trends in alternative medicine use in the United States, 1990–1997: Results of a follow-up national survey. *Journal of the American Medical Association, 280*(18), 1569.

Ellis, M. R., Vinson, D. C., & Ewigman, B. (1999). Addressing spiritual concerns of patients: Family physicians' attitudes and practices. *Journal of Family Practice, 48*(2), 105.

Fernandez-Duque, D., & Posner, M. I. (2001). Brain imaging of attentional networks in normal and pathological states. *Journal of Clinical and Experimental Neuropsychology, 23*(1), 74.

Fish, D. R., Gloor, P., Quesney, F. L., & Olivier, A. (1993). Clinical responses to electrical brain stimulation of the temporal and frontal lobes in patients with epilepsy. Pathophysiological implications, *Brain, 116*(2), 397.

Foley, D. P. (1988). Eleven interpretations of personal suffering. *Journal of Religion and Health, 27,* 321.

Foote, S. L., & Morrison, J. H. (1987). Extrathalamic modulation of cortical function. *Annual Review of Neuroscience, 10,* 67.

Frith, C. D. et al. (1991). Willed action and the prefrontal cortex in man: A study with PET. *Proceedings of the Royal Society of London B: Biological Sciences, 244*(1311), 241.

Gallup. (1994). *The Gallup report: Religion in America: 1993–1994.* Princeton, NJ: Author.

Garfinkel, M. S. et al. (1994). Evaluation of a yoga based regimen for treatment of osteoarthritis of the hands. *Journal of Rheumatology, 21*(12), 2341.

Garfinkel, M. S. et al. (1998). Yoga-based intervention for carpal tunnel syndrome: A randomized trial. *Journal of the American Medical Association, 280*(18), 1601.

Geisser, M. E., Robinson, M. E., & Henson, C. D. (1994). The Coping Strategies Questionnaire and chronic pain adjustment: A conceptual and empirical reanalysis. *Clinical Journal of Pain, 10*(2), 98.

Gellhorn, E., & Kiely, W. F. (1972). Mystical states of consciousness: Neurophysiological and clinical aspects. *Journal of Nervous and Mental Disease, 154*(6), 399, 1972.

Ghista, D. N. et al. (1976). Physiological characterisation of the "meditative state" during intuitional practice (the Ananda Marga system of meditation) and its therapeutic value. *Medical and Biological Engineering, 14*(2), 209.

Harris, W. S. et al. (1999). A randomized, controlled trial of the effects of remote, intercessory prayer on outcomes in patients admitted to the coronary care unit. *Archives of Internal Medicine, 159*(19), 2273.

Hays, J. C. et al. (1998). Social correlates of the dimensions of depression in the elderly. *Journal of Gerontology B: Psychological Sciences and Social Sciences, 53*(1), P31.

Heath, A. C. et al. (1999). Resiliency factors protecting against teenage alcohol use and smoking: Influences of religion, religious involvement and values, and ethnicity in the Missouri Adolescent Female Twin Study. *Twin Research, 2*(2), 145.

Helm, H. M. et al. (2000). Does private religious activity prolong survival? A six-year follow-up study of 3,851 older adults. *Journal of Gerontology A: Biological Sciences and Medical Sciences, 55*(7), M400.

Hugdahl, K. (1996). Cognitive influences on human autonomic nervous system function. *Current Opinion in Neurobiology, 6*(2), 252.

Hummer, R. A. et al. (1999). Religious involvement and U.S. adult mortality. *Demography, 36*(2), 273.

Infante, J. R. et al. (1998). ACTH and beta-endorphin in transcendental meditation. *Physiology and Behavior, 64*(3), 311.

Infante, J. R. et al. (2001). Catecholamine levels in practitioners of the transcendental meditation technique. *Physiology and Behavior, 72*(1–2), 141.

Ingvar. D. H. (1994). The will of the brain: Cerebral correlates of willful acts. *Journal of Theoretical Biology, 171*(1), 7.

Jain, S. C. et al. (1993). A study of response pattern of non-insulin dependent diabetics to yoga therapy. *Diabetes Research and Clinical Practice, 19*(1), 69.

Janal, M. N. et al. (1984). Pain sensitivity, mood and plasma endocrine levels in man following long-distance running: Effects of naloxone. *Pain, 19*(1), 13.

Jevning, R., Wallace, R. K., & Beidebach, M. (1992). The physiology of meditation: A review. A wakeful hypometabolic integrated response. *Neuroscience and Biobehavioral Review, 16*(3), 415.

Jevning, R., Wilson, A. F., & Davidson, J. M. (1978). Adrenocortical activity during meditation. *Hormones and Behavior, 10*(1), 54.

Kabat-Zinn, J. (1982). An outpatient program in behavioral medicine for chronic pain patients based on the practice of mindfulness meditation: Theoretical considerations and preliminary results. *General Hospital Psychiatry, 4*(1), 33.

Kabat-Zinn, J. et al. (1992). Effectiveness of a meditation-based stress reduction program in the treatment of anxiety disorders. *American Journal of Psychiatry, 149*(7), 936.

Kabat-Zinn, J. et al. (1998). Influence of a mindfulness meditation-based stress reduction intervention on rates of skin clearing in patients with moderate to severe psoriasis undergoing phototherapy (UVB) and photochemotherapy (PUVA). *Psychosomatic Medicine, 60*(5), 625.

Kabat-Zinn, J., Lipworth, L., & Burney R. (1985). The clinical use of mindfulness meditation for the self-regulation of chronic pain. *Journal of Behavioral Medicine, 8*(2), 163.

Kaplan, K. H., Goldenberg, D. L., & Galvin-Nadeau, M. (1993). The impact of a meditation-based stress reduction program on fibromyalgia. *General Hospital Psychiatry, 15*(5), 284.

Kark, J. D. et al. (1996). Does religious observance promote health? Mortality in secular vs. religious kibbutzim in Israel. *American Journal of Public Health, 86*(3), 341.

Keefer, L., & Blanchard, E. B. (2002). A one year follow-up of relaxation response meditation as a treatment for irritable bowel syndrome. *Behavioral Research and Therapy, 40*(5), 541.

King, D. E., & Bushwick, B. (1994). Beliefs and attitudes of hospital inpatients about faith healing and prayer. *Journal of Family Practice, 39*(4), 349.

King, D. E., Hueston, W., & Rudy, M. (1994). Religious affiliation and obstetric outcome. *Southern Medical Journal, 87*(11), 1125.

King, M. S., Carr, T., & D'Cruz, C. (2002). Transcendental meditation, hypertension and heart disease. *Australian Family Physician, 31*(2), 164.

Kiss, J. et al. (1997). Metabotropic glutamate receptor in GHRH and beta-endorphin neurones of the hypothalamic arcuate nucleus. *Neuroreport, 8*(17), 3703.

Koenig, H. G. et al. (1998). The relationship between religious activities and cigarette smoking in older adults. *Journal of Gerontology A: Biological Sciences and Medical Sciences, 53*(6), M426.

Koenig, H. G. et al. (1999). Does religious attendance prolong survival? A six-year follow-up study of 3,968 older adults. *Journal of Gerontology A: Biological Sciences and Medical Sciences, 54*(7), M370.

Koenig, H. G., McCullough, M. E., & Larson, D. B. (2001). *Handbook of religion and health.* New York: Oxford University Press.

Kuhn, C. C. (1988). A spiritual inventory of the medically ill patient. *Psychiatry in Medicine, 6*(2), 87.

Kumar, R. A., & Kurup, P. A. (2003). Changes in the isoprenoid pathway with transcendental meditation and Reiki healing practices in seizure disorder. *Neurology India, 51*(2), 211.

Kune, G. A., Kune, S., & Watson, L. F. (1993). Perceived religiousness is protective for colorectal cancer: Data from the Melbourne Colorectal Cancer Study. *Journal of the Royal Society of Medicine, 86*(11), 645.

Kutz, I. (2002). Samson, the Bible, and the DSM [letter]. *Archives of General Psychology, 59*(6), 565; author reply, 565.

La Pierre, L. L. (2003). JCAHO safeguards spiritual care. *Holistic Nursing Practice, 17*(4), 219.

Larson, D. B., Swyers, J. P., & McCullough, M. E. (Eds.). (1998). *Scientific research on spirituality and health: A consensus report.* Washington, DC, National Institute for Healthcare Research.

Lazar, S. W. et al. (2000). Functional brain mapping of the relaxation response and meditation. *Neuroreport, 11*(7), 1581.

Levin, J. S. (1996). How religion influences morbidity and health: Reflections on natural history, salutogenesis and host resistance. *Social Science & Medicine, 43*(5), 849.

Levin, J. S., Larson, D. B., & Puchalski, C. M. (1997). Religion and spirituality in medicine: Research and education. *Journal of the American Medical Association, 278*(9), 792.

Lewis, C. A. (1994). Religiosity and obsessionality: The relationship between Freud's "religious practices." *Journal of Psychology, 128*(2), 189.

Livesey, J. H. et al. (2000). Interactions of CRH, AVP and cortisol in the secretion of ACTH from perfused equine anterior pituitary cells: "Permissive" roles for cortisol and CRH. *Endocrine Research, 26*(3), 445.

Lo, B. et al. (2002). Discussing religious and spiritual issues at the end of life: A practical guide for physicians. *Journal of the American Medical Association, 287*(6), 749.

Lo, B., Quill, T., & Tulsky, J. (1999). Discussing palliative care with patients. ACP-ASIM End-of-Life Care Consensus Panel. American College of Physicians-American Society of Internal Medicine. *Annals of Internal Medicine, 130*(9), 744.

Lukoff, D., Lu, F., & Turner, R. (1992). Toward a more culturally sensitive DSM-IV. Psychoreligious and psychospiritual problems. *Journal of Nervous and Mental Disease, 180*(11), 673.

Lynch, C. (1980). The functional organization of posterior parietal association cortex. *Behavioral and Brain Sciences, 3*, 485.

MacLean, C. D., Susi, B., & Phifer, N. (2003). Patient preference for physician discussion and practice of spirituality. *Journal of General Internal Medicine, 18*(1), 38.

MacLean, C. R. et al. (1994). Altered responses of cortisol, GH, TSH and testosterone to acute stress after four months' practice of transcendental meditation (TM). *Annals of the New York Academy of Science, 746*, 381.

MacLean, C. R. et al. (1997). Effects of the Transcendental Meditation program on adaptive mechanisms: Changes in hormone levels and responses to stress after 4 months of practice. *Psychoneuroendocrinology, 22*(4), 277.

Malhotra, V. et al. (2002b). Study of yoga asanas in assessment of pulmonary function in NIDDM patients. *Indian Journal of Physiology and Pharmacology, 46*(3), 313.

Malhotra, V. et al. (2002a). Effect of Yoga asanas on nerve conduction in type 2 diabetes. *Indian Journal of Physiology and Pharmacology, 46*(3), 298.

Manocha, R. et al. (2002). Sahaja yoga in the management of moderate to severe asthma: A randomised controlled trial. *Thorax, 57*(2), 110.

Matthews, D. A., & Clark, C. (1998). *The faith factor: Proof of the healing power of prayer.* New York: Viking (Penguin–Putnam).

Matthews, D. A., et al. (1998). Religious commitment and health status: A review of the research and implications for family medicine. *Archives of Family Medicine, 7*(2), 118.

Matthews, D. A., Marlowe, S. M., & MacNutt, F. S. (2000). Effects of intercessory prayer on patients with rheumatoid arthritis. *Southern Medical Journal, 93*(12), 1177.

Matthews, W. J., Conti, J. M., & Sireci, S. G. (2001). The effects of intercessory prayer, positive visualization, and expectancy on the well-being of kidney dialysis patients. *Alternative Therapies in Health and Medicine, 7*(5), 42.

McCullough, M. E., & Larson, D. B. (1999). Religion and depression: A review of the literature. *Twin Research, 2*(2), 126.

McKee, D. D., & Chappel, J. N. (1992). Spirituality and medical practice. *Journal of Family Practice, 35*(2), 201.

Michaels, R. R. et al. (1979). Renin, cortisol, and aldosterone during transcendental meditation. *Psychosomatic Medicine, 41*(1), 50.

Michaels, R. R., Huber, M. J., & McCann, D. S. (1976). Evaluation of transcendental meditation as a method of reducing stress. *Science, 192*(4245), 1242.

Miller, W. R., & Thoresen, C.E. (2003). Spirituality, religion, and health. An emerging research field. *American Psychologist, 58*(1), 24.

Monroe, M. H., Bynum, D., & Susi B. (2003). Primary care physician preferences regarding spiritual behavior in medical practice. *Archives of Internal Medicine, 163*(22), 2751.

Morse, J. M., & Proctor, A. (1998). Maintaining patient endurance. The comfort work of trauma nurses. *Clinical Nursing Research, 7*(3), 250.

Mountcastle, V. B., Andersen, R. A., & Motter, B. C. (1981). The influence of attentive fixation upon the excitability of the light-sensitive neurons of the posterior parietal cortex. *Journal of Neuroscience, 1*(11), 1218.

Musick, M. A. et al. (1998). Religious activity and depression among community-dwelling elderly persons with cancer: The moderating effect of race. *Journal of Gerontology B: Psychological Sciences and Social Sciences, 53*(4), S218.

Newberg, A. B., & Iversen, J. (2003). The neural basis of the complex mental task of meditation: Neurotransmitter and neurochemical considerations. *Medical Hypotheses, 61,* 282–291.

Oleckno, W. A., & Blacconiere, M. J. (1991). Relationship of religiosity to wellness and other health-related behaviors and outcomes. *Psychology Reports, 68*(3 Pt. 1), 819.

Oman, D. et al. (2002). Religious attendance and cause of death over 31 years. *International Journal of Psychiatry in Medicine, 32*(1), 69.

Oman, D., & Reed, D. (1998). Religion and mortality among the community-dwelling elderly. *American Journal of Public Health, 88*(10), 1469.

Osler, W. (1910). The faith that heals. *British Medical Journal, 2,* 1470.

Oxman, T. E., Freeman, D. H., Jr., & Manheimer, E. D. (1995). Lack of social participation or religious strength and comfort as risk factors for death after cardiac surgery in the elderly. *Psychosomatic Medicine, 57*(1), 5.

Pardo, J. V., Fox, P. T., & Raichle, M. E. (1991). Localization of a human system for sustained attention by positron emission tomography. *Nature, 349*(6304), 61.

Peng, C. K. et al. (1999). Exaggerated heart rate oscillations during two meditation techniques. *International Journal of Cardiology, 70*(2), 101.

Pettus, M. C., (2002). Implementing a medicine-spirituality curriculum in a community-based internal medicine residency program. *Academic Medicine, 77*(7), 745.

Poloma, M., & Pendleton, B. (1991). The effects of prayer and prayer experience on measures of general well being. *Journal of Psychology and Theology, 10*(71), 1991.

Portas, C. M. et al. (1998). A specific role for the thalamus in mediating the interaction of attention and arousal in humans. *Journal of Neuroscience, 18*(21), 8979.

Posner, M. I., & Petersen, S. E. (1990). The attention system of the human brain. *Annual Review of Neuroscience, 13,* 25.

Powell, L. H., Shahabi, L., & Thoresen, C. E. (2003). Religion and spirituality. Linkages to physical health. *American Psychology, 58*(1), 36.

Pressman, P. et al. (1990). Religious belief, depression, and ambulation status in elderly women with broken hips. *American Journal of Psychiatry, 147*(6), 758.

Proctor, A., Morse, J. M., & Khonsari, E. S. (1996). Sounds of comfort in the trauma center: How nurses talk to patients in pain. *Social Science and Medicine, 42*(12), 1669–1680.

Purcell, B. C. (1998a). Spiritual abuse. *American Journal of Hospice and Palliative Care, 15*(4), 227.

Purcell, B. C. (1998b). Spiritual terrorism. *American Journal of Hospice and Palliative Care, 15*(3), 167.

Rapp, S. R., Rejeski, W. J., & Miller, M. E. (2000). Physical function among older adults with knee pain: The role of pain coping skills. *Arthritis Care Research, 13*(5), 270.

Reibel, D. K. et al. (2001). Mindfulness-based stress reduction and health-related quality of life in a heterogeneous patient population. *General Hospital Psychiatry, 23*(4), 183.

Rossetti, S. J. (1995). The impact of child sexual abuse on attitudes toward God and the Catholic Church. *Child Abuse and Neglect, 19*(12), 1469.

Satterly, L. (2001). Guilt, shame, and religious and spiritual pain. *Holistic Nursing Practice, 15*(2), 30.

Saver, J. L. & Rabin, J. (1997). The neural substrates of religious experience. *Journal of Neuropsychiatry and Clinical Neuroscience, 9*(3), 498.

Schell, F. J., Allolio, B., & Schonecke, O. W. (1994). Physiological and psychological effects of Hatha-Yoga exercise in healthy women. *International Journal of Psychosomatics, 41*(1–4), 46.

Schneider, R. H. et al. (2001). Behavioral treatment of hypertensive heart disease in African Americans: Rationale and design of a randomized controlled trial. *Behavioral Medicine, 27*(2), 83.

Selvamurthy, W. et al. (1998). A new physiological approach to control essential hypertension. *Indian Journal of Physiology and Pharmacology, 42*(2), 205.

Shaffer, J. A. (1978). Pain and suffering: Philosophical perspectives. In W. T. Reich (Ed.), *Encyclopedia of bioethics* (Vol. 4, p. 1181). New York: Free Press.

Shaji, A. V., & Kulkarni, S. K. (1998). Central nervous system depressant activities of melatonin in rats and mice. *Indian Journal of Experimental Biology, 36*(3), 257.

Shuler, P. A., Gelberg, L., & Brown, M. (1994). The effects of spiritual/religious practices on psychological well-being among inner city homeless women. *Nurse Practitioner Forum, 5*(2), 106.

Sim, M. K., & Tsoi, W. F. (1992). The effects of centrally acting drugs on the EEG correlates of meditation. *Biofeedback and Self-Regulation, 17*(3), 215.

Sloan, R. P., & Bagiella, E. (2002). Claims about religious involvement and health outcomes. *Annals of Behavioral Medicine, 24*(1), 14.

Sloan, R. P., Bagiella, E., & Powell, T. (1999). Religion, spirituality, and medicine. *Lancet, 353*(9153), 664.

Solberg, E. E. et al. (1996). The effect of meditation on shooting performance. *British Journal of Sports Medicine, 30*(4), 342.

Stancak, A., Jr. (1991). Kapalabhati — Yogic cleansing exercise. II. EEG topography analysis. *Homeostasis in Health and Disease, 33*(4), 182.

Stanescu, D. C. et al. (1981). Pattern of breathing and ventilatory response to CO2 in subjects practicing hatha-yoga. *Journal of Applied Physiology, 51*(6), 1625.

Stewart, C. (2001). The influence of spirituality on substance use of college students. *Journal of Drug Education, 1*(4), 343.

Strawbridge, W. J. et al. (1997). Frequent attendance at religious services and mortality over 28 years. *American Journal of Public Health, 87*(6), 957.

Sudsuang, R., Chentanez, V., & Veluvan, K. (1991). Effect of Buddhist meditation on serum cortisol and total protein levels, blood pressure, pulse rate, lung volume and reaction time. *Physiology and Behavior, 50*(3), 543.

Swartzman, L. C. et al. (1994). The factor structure of the Coping Strategies Questionnaire. *Pain, 57*(3), 311.

Swimmer, G. I., Robinson, M. E., & Geisser, M. E. (1992). Relationship of MMPI cluster type, pain coping strategy, and treatment outcome. *Clinical Journal of Pain, 8*(2), 131.

Swinyard, C. A., Chaube, S., & Sutton, D. B. (1974). Neurological and behavioral aspects of transcendental meditation relevant to alcoholism: A review. *Annals of the New York Academy of Science, 233*, 162.

Tanyi, R. A. (2002). Towards clarification of the meaning of spirituality. *Journal of Advanced Nursing, 39*(5), 500.

Tieman, J. (2002). Priest scandal hits hospitals. As pedophilia reports grow, church officials suspend at least six hospital chaplains in an effort to address alleged sexual abuse. *Modern Healthcare, 32*(19), 6.

Tooley, G. A. et al. (2000). Acute increases in night-time plasma melatonin levels following a period of meditation. *Biological Psychology, 53*(1), 69.

Townsend, M. et al. (2002). Systematic review of clinical trials examining the effects of religion on health. *Southern Medical Journal, 95*(12), 429.

Travis, F. (2001). Autonomic and EEG patterns distinguish transcending from other experiences during Transcendental Meditation practice. *International Journal of Psychophysiology, 42*(1), 1.

Travis, F. et al. (2001). Physiological patterns during practice of the Transcendental Meditation technique compared with patterns while reading Sanskrit and a modern language. *International Journal of Neuroscience, 109*(1–2), 71.

Travis, F. et al. (2002). Patterns of EEG coherence, power, and contingent negative variation characterize the integration of transcendental and waking states. *Biological Psychology, 61*(3), 293.

Tu, W. (1980). A religiophilosophical perspective on pain. In H. W. Koster, D. Kosterlitz, & L. Y. Terenius (Eds.). *Pain and society* (p. 63). Weinheim: Verlag Cjemie.

Turner, R. P. et al. (1995). Religious or spiritual problem. A culturally sensitive diagnostic category in the DSM-IV. *Journal of Nervous and Mental Disease, 183*(7), 435.

Udupa, K. N., Singh, R. H., & Yadav, R. A. (1973). Certain studies on psychological and biochemical responses to the practice in Hatha Yoga in young normal volunteers. *Indian Journal of Medical Research, 61*(2), 237.

Van Bockstaele, E. J., & Aston-Jones, G. (1995). Integration in the ventral medulla and coordination of sympathetic, pain and arousal functions. *Clinical and Experimental Hypertension, 17*(1–2), 153.

van Montfrans, G. A. et al. (1990). Relaxation therapy and continuous ambulatory blood pressure in mild hypertension: A controlled study. *British Medical Journal, 300*(6736), 1368.

Vogt, B. A., Finch, D. M., & Olson, C. R. (1992). Functional heterogeneity in cingulate cortex: The anterior executive and posterior evaluative regions. *Cerebral Cortex, 2*(6), 435.

Wallace, R. K. (1997). Physiological effects of transcendental meditation. *Science, 167*(926), 1751.

Wallace, R. K. et al. (1983). Systolic blood pressure and long-term practice of the Transcendental Meditation and TM-Sidhi program: Effects of TM on systolic blood pressure. *Psychosomatic Medicine, 45*(1), 41.

Wallace, R. K., Benson, H., & Wilson, A. F. (1971). A wakeful hypometabolic physiologic state. *American Journal of Physiology, 221*(3), 795.

Walton, K. G. et al. (1995). Stress reduction and preventing hypertension: Preliminary support for a psychoneuroendocrine mechanism. *Journal of Alternative and Complementary Medicine, 1*(3), 263.

Waterhouse, B. D., Moises, H. C., & Woodward, D. J. (1998). Phasic activation of the locus coeruleus enhances responses of primary sensory cortical neurons to peripheral receptive field stimulation. *Brain Research, 790*(1–2), 33.

Wenneberg, S. R. et al. (1997). A controlled study of the effects of the Transcendental Meditation program on cardiovascular reactivity and ambulatory blood pressure. *International Journal of Neuroscience, 89*(1–2), 15.

Werner, O. R. et al. (1986). Long-term endocrinologic changes in subjects practicing the Transcendental Meditation and TM-Sidhi program. *Psychosomatic Medicine, 48*(1–2), 59.

Williams, D. R. et al. (1991). Religion and psychological distress in a community sample. *Social Science & Medicine, 32*(11), 1257.

Williams, K. A. et al. (2001). Evaluation of a wellness-based mindfulness stress reduction intervention: A controlled trial. *American Journal of Health Promotion, 15*(6), 422.

Yadid, G. (2000). Alterations in endogenous brain beta-endorphin release by adrenal medullary transplants in the spinal cord. *Neuropsychopharmacology, 23*(6), 709.

Zaleski, E. H., & Schiaffino, K. M. (2000). Religiosity and sexual risk-taking behavior during the transition to college. *Journal of Adolescence, 23*(2), 223.

Ziegler, D. R., Cass, W. A., & Herman, J. P. (1999). Excitatory influence of the locus coeruleus in hypothalamic-pituitary-adrenocortical axis responses to stress. *Journal Neuroendocrinology, 11*(5), 361.

99

The Role of Prayer in Pain Management

Myrna C. Tashner, EdD

Dedication: This chapter is dedicated to the memory and spirit of Richard S. Weiner, Ph.D., who welcomed us into AAPM with open arms and encouraging words. Dr. Weiner shared my passion in believing in the patient's power to heal with the assistance of Spirit.

THE MYSTERY, THE MIRACLE, THE SCIENCE, AND THE ENERGY OF PRAYER

What is this thing called prayer and what is its role in healing? In this chapter we review some literature on prayer, examine the science of prayer, and look at some results of prayer and the ways prayer can be a part of the pain management practice.

This is a timely discussion, as there is increasing interest in the subject. *Newsweek* devoted its November 10, 2003, cover story to "God and Health." Articles addressed physicians' experiences with patients requesting prayer, and/or finding a patient's need for prayer, and the awareness and comfort with prayer becoming more important to their practice of medicine. On Christmas Day 2003, *Paula Zahn NOW* focused on "Faith in America." She talked with Dr. Herbert Benson of Harvard Medical School's Mind/Body Medical Institute, among others. With 35 years of study and research behind him, Dr. Benson told her, "Belief is very, very important in healing. When you focus on a sound, a prayer, or a phrase, and repeat it, disregard other thoughts, distinct physiological changes occur in the body which are exactly opposite those of the stress" (Zahn, 2003). Dr. Benson went on to say that "60–90% of visits to health care professionals are in the area of mind-body stress-related realm. So, it affects not only blood pressure, but heart rate, affects many forms of pain, anxiety, depres-

sion, insomnia. In other words, there's discrete medical proof that evoking what we call the relaxation response, often through prayer, can treat many, many different diseases. And the extent that any disease is caused or made worse by stress to that extent, this intervention will work" (Zahn, 2003). Dr. Benson went on to say that when people pray for themselves, and pray in a repetitive fashion, nitric oxide (NO) is released in the body system. This particular gas has tremendous manifestations in various biochemical systems. Dr. Benson has been able to quantify these body–mind effects, including spirituality, and bring together a doubtful society with science.

In addition to Dr. Benson, another physician who has followed and researched prayer during his medical career is Dr. Larry Dossey. In *Prayer is Good Medicine,* he writes, "Prayer is back." He says doctors are taking it into their offices, clinics, hospitals, as well as experimental laboratories. He notes that medical journals are publishing studies on the healing effects of prayer and faith. He points out that "75% of patients believed their physician should address spiritual issues as a part of their medical care and 50% wanted their doctor to pray not just for them but with them" (1996, pp. 1-2).

In *Spontaneous Healing,* Dr. Andrew Weil (1995) says Dr. Dossey is one of the few doctors who has looked at the relationship between prayer and healing. Dr. Dossey writes of the power of prayerfulness in *Healing Words, the Power of Prayer and the Practice of Medicine,* that "prayerfulness allows us to reach a plane of experience where illness can be experienced as a natural part of life, and where its acceptance transcends passivity. If the disease disappears, we are grateful; if it remains, that too is reason for gratitude" (1993, p. 23).

Dr. Dale Matthews wrote in *The Faith Factor,* that he was horrified at the lack of humanity in his medical training when he went to school "hoping to learn and practice compassionate, person-centered doctoring" (1998, p. 7) and caring for the whole person, not just organs and tissues. He wrote that what he sees emerging is the "biopsychosocial model" and solid scientific evidence for the role of beliefs and meditative practice in human health and that beliefs, religious or otherwise, have a profound effect on physical and mental health. Matthews said that what he sees is that faith is good medicine and that the medical effect of religious commitment is not a matter of faith but of science. He said patients were the pioneers in this area. He cited a study by Dr. D. King of East Carolina University, which showed that 48% of hospitalized patients wanted their doctors not just to talk about spiritual issues with them, but actually to pray with them. *The Faith Factor* is Matthew's summary of science, research, and narratives about the healing results of faith in medical practice.

OTHER STUDIES

There have been many studies about prayer in recent years. It is not the purpose of this chapter to do a review of the literature; others have done that (Matthews & Saunder, 1995–1997), but suffice it to give a few examples. There were studies of geriatric patients and their reliance on prayer and religion as coping mechanisms when faced with the stress of life and events including health problems (Bearon & Koenig, 1990), D. A. Matthews et al. (1998) assessed effects in conjunction with standard medical treatment of experimental intercessory prayer for healing in patients with rheumatoid arthritis. Results suggested that patients derived significant short- and long-term benefits from in-person intercessory prayer ministry (Matthews et al., 1998).

There have been studies of the effects of intercessory prayer, probably the most widely provoking one done by Byrd (1988). He studied intercessory prayer and cardiac patients in a San Francisco coronary unit. It was a randomized study of 393 patients, after signed consent, conducted in a double-blind protocol. Results were significant for patients in the control group who required ventilator assistance, antibiotics, and diuretics more frequently than patients in the intercessory prayer group. In 1999, a similar study was conducted in Kansas City at the University of Missouri Medical Center, Division of Cardiology, Department of Medicine by Harris et al. (1999). The sole purpose of the study was to attempt to replicate Byrd's findings by testing the hypothesis. However, in their study patients were unknowingly and remotely prayed for by blinded intercessors. The hypothesis stated that these patients would experience fewer complications and have a shorter hospital stay than patients not receiving such prayer. The

result suggested that prayer may be an effective adjunct to standard medical care. Except for two patients, the length of stay for the prayer group dropped by about a day. The intercessory prayer group of patients lowered the hospital course score but did not significantly affect length of stay. The researchers gave a number of reasons for lack of exact replication including, and significantly, that it was conducted under completely blinded conditions. In this study informed consent was not sought from the patients and the patients were not prescreened for their willingness to be prayed for. Among research committees it is not the policy to permit studies of patients without the written consent, but this research group convinced the committee otherwise. Permission was granted for this type of study, rationalizing that it eliminated any possible bias (Harris et al., 1999). Therefore, it cannot truly be said that this was a replication of the Byrd study.

The conclusions of these studies are interesting for our purposes. If you think about it for a minute, knowing they are possibly being prayed for does have some effect on the body, mind, and spirit of the patients, if the results of the study are to be believed, versus not knowing someone is possibly praying for their healing. Maybe two comparison points of these studies are the effect and impact of knowing someone is praying for you, which may be in what and of itself encourages the body to heal, for we are wired for healing according to Dr. Benson (*Harvard Health Letter,* 1998). Lack of awareness of being prayed for just does not have the same effect, and is unethical to some extent. Why? Because prayer is an exchange of energy and each of us is an energy being. In praying for you, I am asking that your energy field be in some way positively affected with the assistance of God. (Throughout this chapter, please see the word "God" to mean God as you know it.) You do have a right to know if you are being prayed for, as it is your energy field that is being affected. You have the right to know so you can choose to accept the energy or refuse to cooperate with the energy.

There are studies that suggest that prayer did not work. In one study, effects of prayer were compared to positive visualization in patients on kidney dialysis. The authors of this study were not able to distinguish the *effects* of prayer and positive visualization for expectancy (Matthews et al., 2001).

WHAT IS PRAYER?

Prayer is talking with God (the Divine, Higher Power, Allah, Yahweh, or simply God as you understand it). It is really that simple. It was the way Abraham, Moses, Jesus, and Mohammed prayed; they talked with God. There are formal prayers, formats for prayer, etc., but it really comes down to talking with God. As such, prayer is made up of thoughts and words; and just as our words have power to create or destroy, so does prayer. Praying is more. It could be defined as the transfer of energy. Prayer generates energy, and praying for someone is at the least an energy exchange, probably of the highest form we have in this earth plane.

Our proof for that is demonstrated in the Bible. Have you ever noticed that the healer Jesus never healed anyone unless they asked to be healed? And he would end the encounter with something to the effect, "… your faith has made you well; go in peace" (Luke 8:48 RSV), or "Do not fear; only believe" (Luke 8:42 RSV). The woman with the issue of blood is a good example. She believed that if she could just touch the hem of his garment she could be healed. In that instance, when touched by someone who wanted to be healed, He knew someone had touched Him. He demanded to know who it was who touched Him. When His disciples questioned Him as to how He could know someone had touched Him as they were in a crowd, He responded that He felt the energy leave Him (Luke 8:43–48).

We may look to sacred writings to teach us right prayers to say. In the Bible, when His disciples asked Jesus how to pray, He offered them a series of affirmations about God and their relationship to God, which we call the Lord's Prayer. David's prayers as reported in the Bible were with songs of praise called Psalms. Mohammed's prayers were verses, which revealed God's wisdom and goodness, and are recited as prayers today (*The Holy Qur'an*, 1989).

Christian Science believes, "Prayer cannot change the science of being, but it tends to bring us into harmony with it" (Eddy, 1875, p. 2).

Myss in *Anatomy of the Spirit* (1996) described authentic prayer as one's conscious connection with God. "Authentic prayer does not mean to turn to God in order to get something; it means to turn to God in order to be with someone. Prayer is not so much our words to God as our life with God. When this is understood, then prayer becomes 'energy medicine'" (1996, p. 282).

A retired Catholic priest, now healer, Roth suggests a very simple prayer. With the inhale of breath he suggests saying, "Come Spirit" (spirit being another word for breath), and with the exhalation, "God Is Light." This creates relaxation in the mind and body. It is in the relaxed state that the body, mind, and spirit can return to their natural state of wholeness and health (Roth & Occhiogrosso, 1997).

Harold Koenig of Duke University said of science, religion, health, spirituality, and prayer, that the evidence is there. Prayer brings us closer to God. It changes us, causing us to set better priorities. This enables the body to heal itself. Prayer releases God to perform miracles (Koenig, 2004).

This is quite consistent with the now famous Harvard cardiologist Herbert Benson's relaxation response, now prayer process. His research has proven that when one engages in a repetitive prayer, and when intrusive thoughts are passively disregarded, a specific set of physiological changes ensues. He teaches that a repeated word, as the word "one" (or some other word that is meaningful to the person), sets off these physiological changes. His latest research has shown that this effective letting go of a problem triggers the internal release of nitric oxide, which has been linked to the production of neurotransmitters rich in endorphins and dopamine, which are natural tranquilizers. Nitric oxide alters the body's chemistry so significantly that personal changes become possible (Benson & Proctor, 2003).

In a sense, Dr. Benson has provided us with a plausible scientific explanation for what happened to Jesus as written. "He took with him Peter, James and John, and went up on the mountain to pray. And as he was praying, the appearance of his countenance was altered, and his raiment became dazzling white" (Luke 9:28–29, RSV).

Dr. Dossey wrote, "In its simplest form, prayer is an attitude of the heart — a matter of being, not doing. Prayer is the desire to contact the Absolute, however it may be conceived. When we experience the need to enact this connection, we are praying, whether or not we use words" (1996, p. 83). He wrote in *Reinventing Medicine* that he discovered early in his investigation of prayer research that members of the clergy almost never perform scientific studies to evaluate the effects of prayer. He said that they believe that empirical scientific proof is unnecessary, and some see science as the enemy of faith or testing God (Dossey, 1999, p. 49).

By and large that is true. However, there was a husband and wife who both experienced healing through prayer; and he, Charles Fillmore, spent the rest of his life studying, researching, and writing about how prayer was part of his healing. In his passion for his discovered truth, he and his wife had a vision for a place where people could come and learn about the truths of belief and the science of prayer. He was a prolific writer in the late 1800s, early 1900s, although he did not have significant formal education. He defined prayer as the "communion between God and man. This communion takes place in the innermost part of man's being. It is the only way to cleanse and perfect the consciousness and thus permanently heal the body" (Fillmore, 1959, p. 152). Fillmore wrote that prayer was more than supplication; it was affirmation of Truth (Truth meaning eternal absolute) that eternally exists, but which had not yet come into consciousness, which is done through affirmation, faith, praise, and acknowledgment.

THE SCIENCE OF PRAYER

When Dr. Benson stumbled on the scientific effects of the relaxation response, life and healing became less a mystery. For a long time we knew that animals in the wild survived because of their ability to feel a dangerous situation. Psychology calls that the "fight or flight" response.

In our little human living circumstances, we also come upon things that threaten our existence and/or survival. We, too, would like to run to escape eminent danger. And sometimes we can do that, and do that. But there are other times, such as in the time of pain, illness, or stress when we can't run or escape. What happens to the fight-or-flight energy when this occurs? We can't run or escape to get rid of it. It is in our bodies, energizing the system, so to speak. We can sustain that state of energy alertness or hyperstate for a time, but unattended it can have ill consequences and causes illness or pain.

According to Dr. Benson's research, the practice of relaxation releases that energy. In the state of relaxation, we let go, release our tension, so the body's natural sense of balance can come in and heal that environment that has been disturbed. This simple act brings homeostasis to the body system. By paying attention to the breath and focusing attention on a word, mantra, or prayer, the mind is kept busy, so the body has a better chance of relaxing.

In his latest book *The Breakout Principle,* Benson reviews how to elicit the relaxation response. He calls it Meditation 101 and gives a four-step method, which his research suggests releases nitric oxide.

Step 1: Choose a meaningful word or short phrase that can be silently repeated on the out breath or exhalation.

Step 2: Assume a comfortable position, close your eyes and breathe easily and on the out breath say your word.

Step 3: Don't get upset with distracting thoughts or interruptions, just turn them away and return to the silent repletion of your word.

Step 4: After 10 to 20 minutes have passed, open your eyes and sit quietly for a few minutes to allow thoughts of the day to enter (Benson & Proctor, 2003, pp. 89–91).

He states that the release of the nitric oxide gives "puffs of insight," as well as reverses the effects of the released stress hormones, which in the case of pain make it worse by lowering the threshold of pain. The release of nitric oxide counteracts the stress hormones, enhances the release of pleasurable neurotransmitters (endorphins and enkephalins), and effects a host of biochemical changes. With the relaxation response the brain itself is quieted, as are the specific areas of the brain that control heart rate and blood pressure (Benson & Proctor, 2003).

Prayer works in the same way. Unity Institute (formerly Unity School of Christianity founded by C. and M. Fillmore) teaches five steps of prayer. I feel these five steps are best summarized in the following way.

STEP 1 RELAXATION

Relaxation is the first step of prayer. We signal our mind and body and spirit with three deep breaths, which signal our mind, body, and spirit, that we are changing our focus. This allows us to then turn our thoughts to noting where the tension resides in our body and invites the body and mind to release the tension. In that process we draw attention away from our cares and concerns, so we can focus our attention on Truth.

STEP 2 DENIAL

The second step naturally follows relaxation and is sometimes forgotten. In this step we deny, or take our energy off, of the negative thought or thing which concerns us. We know the power of denial, that when we take our energy off something, even for a short time, it ceases to exist.

STEP 3 AFFIRMATION

In the third step we affirm the Truth. For example, if pain relief is our prayer goal, then we may chose the scripture that declares that we are children of God, and if we are children of God, then we have a right to the gifts of God, one of which is healing. Our affirmation might go something like this, "I am a child of God and I have the right to be whole and healthy," or some other description that would be appropriate for our life and our beliefs.

STEP 4 MEDITATION/CONTEMPLATION

We hold the thought of Truth in our mind so it can take root in our mind, body, and spirit. We meditate on the thought, engage our sense in the feeling and experience of what feeling healthy and well would be like. And again we would be engaging our powerful sense of relaxation, which would release nitric oxide in the body system for activating changes. And while we meditate, we relax and become open to the insights that come from the God, as we understand God.

STEP 5 GRATITUDE

We give thanks for the healing that is taking place in our body. Jesus talked about giving thanks in advance, and he did so before he healed people and also before he had manifestations, as with the loaves and fishes (John 6:11 RSV). In the act of giving thanks, we are expressing belief and faith in the power of prayer and the spirit of healing.

EXPERIENCES OF PRAYER IN HEALING

Relaxation is a bridge that connects us with the natural healing powers of our body–mind–spirit. We are wired for healing. It is our natural state, a state of wholeness. That is part of our creation. We are created in wholeness and that is part of the mystery of life. But we have lost that contact when we are in pain (physical, mental, emotional, and/or spiritual). This awareness was made real for me when my chiropractor would distract my attention from the stressed position with the word "relax," and then proceed with the adjustment. At another level, I felt that he was addressing the body–mind–spirit to relax into the correct position for healing.

Have you ever noticed how much you enjoy hearing personal stories of healing? In fact, when patients ask if the treatment we are prescribing really works, what they are asking us is if we know from our experience that someone has gotten better by what we are asking them to do. This serves to encourage their body, mind, and spirit in the healing process. As a medical professional, the doctor, nurse, therapist, etc., doesn't take the pain on, or away. Rather it is something they do to make the healing happen, and our view needs to be that of facilitating a link, or hook-up, between with the natural health/wholeness and the patient. It is the link, and the hook-up with the natural healer within the patient.

The same is true for our use of prayer. Patients are asking that in addition to what has happened to others, do we as health care providers who experience with prayer working. Health care providers who practice and know the power of relaxation and prayer are not better or different, but already have the knowing of Truth and this bubbles from their hearts. The following stories are offered as testimonies of the power of prayer as this writer has had experience of it, or heard about it.

Myrtle's story — A young mother in 1886 was suffering from tuberculosis, and given a mortal prognosis. She was a told that she had inherited illness and would die of it as her parents had. A metaphysician, Dr. E. B. Weeks, was visiting and lecturing in town one night, and she decided to go and hear him. During the lecture she heard the words, "I am a child of God and therefore I do not inherit sickness." She went home filled with the feeling of these words. She told her husband, Charles. Together, they decided that she would take these words into her heart daily in prayer and meditation. She did this for 2 years, and she was healed. She lived for 45 more years (Whitherspoon, 1977).

Marty's story — A 5-year-old boy slipped into a farm machine's auger left foot first up to his ankle. He was alone, and he tried to free himself, but each time he moved his foot the auger blade made a revolution cutting into his flesh first, then a little further, then into his ankle bone with each complete turn, and finally through his bone to the outside flesh, and to the skin. The father showed up, upon hearing his son's screams for help, turning the machine off. Only an inch of skin was holding the little foot to the leg. As this happened on a very rural farm, the child with his dangling foot was wrapped in a blanket and

rushed to the nearest hospital some 20 miles away, where the surgeon suggested to the father that the foot could not be saved. The father said that they should try to reattach the foot first. If that didn't work, they could always remove it. So the gentle family practice physician (there was no orthopedic surgeon to do the job) painstakingly for hours removed the multiple particles of debris, brought muscle from the back of the leg around to the front, and reattached the foot to the leg. After 12 hours of surgery, the little boy was brought to a private room, to be met by his parents, who were praying. They had called the local monastery to pray with them. The mother sat on a chair at the foot of her son's bed and held the injured/healing foot in her hand and prayed. She would later tell the story of how the foot was cold and blue when she started, but she prayed anyway. In time, some 12 hours later, the foot was warm and turning pink. In the days and weeks that followed, the boy's foot did reattach itself to the leg and without infection. Today the boy is a man, walks with only a drop in that foot at the ankle, and operates the farm where the accident occurred.

My story — It was a sunny early summer day in Kansas and I was in my first year of ministerial education at Unity School of Religious Studies. I had agreed to accompany a second-year student to a rural church about 2 hours out of Kansas City and present the service's meditation that day. As I got out of her car, I turned to shut the door with one hand, and somehow managed to slam the door on my middle finger of the other hand. Having done that many times as a child, I had instant recall of what my finger was going to look like when I opened the door. But I was also a student of metaphysics. I was learning how energy and the mind work to heal the body. So in that second, I began to affirm and know the Truth about my finger, that it was whole and healed as God made it. Rather than thinking about the torn flesh, I focused my attention on a healed finger. There was throbbing and pain, too. When I opened the door, I deliberately didn't look at the finger, but wrapped it in my clean handkerchief and continued to affirm that my finger was as God had created it to be, healed and whole. It was an hour until I was to present the meditation, so I sat in the sanctuary and continued to repeat the truth of my finger's healed state. There were other thoughts from time to time about what the injury would look like, but I kept returning to my affirmation of the whole and healed finger. Later that morning, when I got up to do the meditation, I glanced at my finger and all that was noticeable was a small indentation in the skin, but no break, or torn flesh. Had my finger been broken? Had the flesh been torn apart? There are the memories from my childhood accidents, in which the finger had taken weeks to heal. But on this day, all that was noticeable was an indentation on the flesh.

Joanne's story — As things happen, my ministerial colleague who had agreed to review this writing, related an experience of physical pain in her life. In one of our conversations during the initial stages of this writing, she was relating her experience with shoulder pain as she swept her front walk in South Carolina. She said that with each sweep of the broom, she found her body tensing to protect the shoulder from pain. But it didn't seem to help much. In fact, while she swept the sidewalk, she had to stop sweeping and take a breath into the pain. And when she did stop and breathe, the pain subsided. She then had a realization. Maybe if she would relax and breathe while she swept her sidewalk, there would be less pain. That is what she did. She told me there was little, if any, pain.

Charles Fillmore had this to say: "If we make living cells through the power of thought, we should know something of the law underlying the process. On every hand thoughtful men are searching for the scientific causes of things" (Fillmore, 1939, p. 127). He proceeded to tell the story of a woman who was an ardent Truth student, and her husband who thought all Truth was foolishness. But he paid attention when his mother was healed of a mole on her face. His mother said of her healing that she withdrew her "nourishing thought." She had mourned over it and wished it weren't there, but that nourished it and sent vital forces to keep it growing. When she quit nourishing it, it gradually withered and disappeared. We nourish the conditions of our bodies with our thoughts. "Our mind draws upon the vital forces and according to physiological laws we alter our tissues" (Fillmore, 1939, p. 127). (Also refer to Fillmore's step 2: Denial.)

What are we to take from these true stories regarding prayer? To some extent, we don't know all of the "science" about prayer, but we are living and when some awareness of an energy greater than ourselves is invited into our lives, some form of healing can take place. There really isn't anything we have to do, but to have the presence and awareness of mind to invite the energy. Then it helps if we can relax and breathe.

The power of relaxation is the first step. That word, *relax* sends a powerful message of release and let go, so new energy can come in. The word, or thought, like *relax*, or *relaxation*, or *prayer* carries power. It is a thought distraction, but also an invitation. Relaxation bridges that connection with the natural healing process. Health and wholeness are our natural state. That is part of our creation. We are created in wholeness and that is part of the mystery, because we lose contact with that wholeness when we are in pain (be it physical, mental, emotional, or spiritual pain). And the medical profession should not take it on, that is, the belief that they have to do something to make wholeness or health happen, but rather their view needs to be that of making a link or hook-up with the natural healing power, or divine energy, within the patient. Medical professionals need to practice prayer and meditation, so they know the power of prayer and relaxation.

This isn't better or different from what they already know, but just a bubbling to the heart.

PRAYER AND OUR PATIENTS

If Dr. Benson's science is correct, and from my studies of metaphysics and my personal experiences all indications are that he is correct, then we are going to see an increased awareness of prayer playing a role in our dealings with patients experiencing pain. First, prayer acknowledges that they are more than a body and mind in the experience of pain. It reminds both the professional health care provider and the patient that they have a spiritual part to consider in this healing process as well. The various medicines and scientific techniques should have an effect to lessen the pain or illness of the body and maybe the mind, but until we acknowledge and address the spirit of our patients, we won't be taking into account all of the factors of the whole patient. And how can we expect to heal if we aren't present to the whole person?

No words or prayers need to be said out loud necessarily, but maybe something like, "Let's relax into this time together." Medical professionals could pause to relax and prepare themselves before each case, and collect energy and awareness before they meet the next patient. This relaxation pause makes a connection in an almost telepathic mind-to-mind manner. It may prepare medical professionals within their being in an inner connectedness that while they are speaking they are able to adjust their words to meet their patient's needs.

What to ask a patient about praying together. As suggested by the results of the University of Missouri, Kansas City study (Harris et al., 1999), it is necessary to ask patients if they would like you to pray with them. According to earlier-cited sources, a growing percentage of patients want their health care provider to pray with them. This could be a challenge, but their medical chart may already indicate the patient's religious preference. So, you might ask if the patient would like to start the time together with a prayer; or even less threatening, suggest something to the effect that we relax a moment together before we begin. The point isn't to get into a discussion about what to say; rather the point is to get together to create a healing atmosphere between the two of you.

What prayers to say. Some professionals may feel uncomfortable saying words, or may feel ill-prepared to pray with their patients. They may feel relieved that patients didn't ask them to pray with them. And that's okay, too. But given what seems to be a growing movement among patients to want to pray with their professional health care providers, it is best to at least have considered your position on prayer. So, what do you say? Maybe you want to pray and ask for divine assistance with this patient, what would be good to say? If prayer is talking to God, as we said earlier, that would be a safe place to start. Talk with God, and ask God, as each of you understands God, to be in this meeting time with this patient and you. Or you may choose to use a classic and generally known prayer such as "The Lord's Prayer" or some other simple shared prayer. And remember, this should only be done when the patient requests it.

For my part as a patient, I always try to remember to ask the Divine Healer to be present and guide the hand of the doctor who is working with me. I find I can relax better into the appointment. As the health care provider, I may say a silent prayer before I enter the room, asking for divine guidance for me with this patient. In situations where I'm not sure if the patient would appreciate prayer, I may ask if he or she would like to say a little prayer. I have on other occasions asked that we take a deep breath before we start and bring our focus into the room together. It seemed to break the stress and anxiety of the session.

Praying with patients means different things to different people. I have a Native American friend who is a home health nurse. We have discussed prayer and using prayer in working with patients. She said that she asks the Great Spirit to be present at each visit and guide her in what she needs to do with that patient. Some of her patients have made comments to her about their knowing that she has special healing presence, but others don't get it. She also is a practitioner of healing touch. She will use this technique only with the patient's awareness and permission. On the other hand, I have another friend who wouldn't want her physician to pray with her. She feels her physician's work is to do his job with the medicines. I, myself, have asked my health care providers if they believe in spiritual healing and have gotten very different responses. One understood what I was talking about. The other laughed at me, and I found it difficult to work with that provider.

It would be important to remember that when patients are asking to pray, what they are asking for is a sharing of hope and peace in their healing process. They want to release their fear of what is happening. They want to relax and heal.

The ethics of praying with patients. As we know, prayer is a very powerful energy. I don't believe it is appropriate or ethical to be direct with our prayers without asking the person for whom we are praying if he or she wants to be prayed for. I make it a point not to pray for someone unless I first ask if the person would like me to pray. I think the University of Missouri study is proof of that principle. There will be no, or minimal, result for patients if we don't ask if they want to pray or be prayed for. We haven't touched on the fact that, as energy, unwanted/unsolicited prayer will bounce back to us.

If you to choose to ask your patients about their desire for prayer, what are the boundaries? First, prayer is the exchange of energy. It is vital that the patients ask for or agree to prayers. Second, it is important to know that God is in charge of what is going to happen, and together through and by your prayers, you both are affirming that. Third, together you pray that God's will is done. Note that you aren't directing what is God's will, or what the result should be. You are simply asking that God's will be done. Of course, we are seeking healing, but we need to be aware that healing has a variety of expressions from restoration of the body to its original health, or partial recovery, even to and including death of the body physical. We need to be okay with whatever the outcome may be. It is important to be clear with our patients about this as well.

CONCLUSION

Prayer does have a role in pain management. Prayer is scientific and has some basic steps; just as the relaxation response is scientific and has basis steps, as outlined above. At the minimum, prayer can facilitate the release of stress and introduce relaxation. This has been shown to have an effect on pain. According to Dr. Benson, our bodies are wired for healing, and relaxation and prayer are ways of tapping that energy. The stories related above support this idea. At the maximum, by our entering and engaging patients in their belief system about prayer and healing, and their feelings for relaxation and health, patients are engaging in the healing process. As with any treatment, the outcome with prayer and relaxation is up to the individual, and God.

REFERENCES

Anonymous. (2003), November 10). God and health, *Newsweek, 19,* 44–56.

Bearon, L. B., & Koenig, H. G. (1990). Religious cognitions and use of prayer in health and illness. *The Gerontologist, 30,* 249.

Benson, H. (1998). Faith & healing: Making a place for spirituality. *Harvard Health Letter, 23,* 4.

Benson, H., & Proctor, W. B. (2003). *The break-out principle.* New York: Scribner, New York.

Byrd, R. C. (1988). Positive therapeutic effects of intercessory prayer in a coronary care unit population. *Southern Medical Journal, 81,* 826.

Dossey, L. (1993). *Healing words.* San Francisco: Harper Collins.

Dossey, L. (1996). *Prayer is good medicine.* San Francisco: Harper.

Dossey, L. (1999). *Reinventing medicine.* San Francisco: Harper.

Eddy, M. B. (1875). *Science and health.* Boston: First Church of Christ Scientist.

Fillmore, C. (1939). *Jesus Christ heals.* Unity Village, MO: Unity School of Christianity.

Fillmore, C. (1959). *The revealing word.* Unity Village, MO: Unity School of Christianity.

Harris, W. S. et al. (1999). A randomized, controlled trial of the effects of remote, intercessory prayer on outcomes in patients admitted to the coronary care unit. *Archives of Internal Medicine, 159,* 2273.

Holy Bible (revised standard ed.). (1973). New York: Oxford Press.

Holy Qur'an (new revised ed.). (1989). Brentwood, MD: Amana Corporation.

Koenig, H. (2004). Available from dukespiritualityandhealth.org.

Matthews, D. A. (1998). *The faith factor.* New York: Viking.

Matthews, D. A., Marlowe, S. M., & MacNutt, F. S. (1998). Intercessory prayer ministry benefits rheumatoid arthritis patients. *Journal of General Internal Medicine, 13,* 17.

Matthews, D. A., & Saunder, D. M. (1995–1997). *The faith factor: An annotated bibliography of clinical research on spiritual subjects.* Rockville, MD: National Institute of Healthcare Research.

Matthews, W. J., Conti, J. M., & Sireu, S. G. (2001). The effects of intercessory prayer, positive visualization & expectancy on well-being of kidney dialysis patients. *Alternative Therapies, 5,* 4.

Myss, C. (1996). *Anatomy of the spirit.* New York: Harmony Books.

Roth, R., & Occhiogrosso, P. (1997). *The healing path of prayer.* New York: Three Rivers Press.

Weil, A. (1995). *Spontaneous healing.* New York: Knopf.

Whitherspoon, T. E. (1977). *Myrtle Fillmore, Mother of Unity.* Unity Village, MO: Unity School of Christianity.

Zahn, P. (2003, December 25). *Paula Zahn NOW.* Available online at transcript@cnn.com.

Section XIII

Practice Issues

Steven Siwek, MD, Section Editor

100

Concepts of Multidisciplinary Pain Management

Robert J. Gatchel, PhD, ABPP, Leland Lou, MD, and Nancy Kishino, OTR, CBE

INTRODUCTION

Pain is a complex experiential state that comprises a panoply of variables, each of which contributes to the interpretation of nociception as pain. The complexity of pain becomes especially noteworthy when it persists over extended periods of time, during which a range of psychosocioeconomic factors can significantly interact with physical pathology to modulate a patient's self-report of pain and concomitant disability and response to treatment. Chronic pain disability is now appropriately viewed as a complex and interactive psychophysiologic behavior pattern that cannot be broken down into distinct, independent psychological and physical components. This *biopsychosocial perspective* has replaced the outdated biomedical reductionist approach of medicine. The intention of this chapter is to review the critical elements of an interdisciplinary treatment approach (based on this biopsychosocial perspective) that has been demonstrated to be efficacious when patients have progressed to the chronic pain disability stage, at which point their management becomes much more complex because of the interactive psychosocioeconomic factors involved.

BIOPSYCHOSOCIAL PERSPECTIVE OF PAIN

The biopsychosocial model of pain, which is now accepted as the most heuristic approach to the understanding and treatment of pain disorders, views physical disorders such as pain as a result of a complex and dynamic interaction among physiologic, psychologic, and social factors, which

perpetuate and may worsen the clinical presentation. Each individual experiences pain uniquely. The range of psychological, social, and economic factors can interact with physical pathology to modulate patients' reports of symptoms and subsequent disability. The development of this biopsychosocial approach has grown rapidly during the past decade, and a great deal of scientific knowledge has been produced in this short period of time concerning the best care of individuals with complex pain problems, as well as pain prevention and coping techniques.

In their comprehensive review of the biopsychosocial perspective on chronic pain, Turk and Monarch (2002) point out that individuals differ significantly in how frequently they report physical symptoms, in their tendency to visit physicians when experiencing identical symptoms, and in their responses to the same treatments. Quite frequently, the nature of patients' responses to treatment has little to do with their objective physical conditions. For example, White and colleagues (1961) earlier noted that less than one third of all persons with clinically significant symptoms consult a physician. On the other hand, from 30 to 50% of patients who seek treatment in primary care do not have specific diagnosable disorders (Dworkin & Massoth, 1994). Turk and Monarch (2002) go on to make the distinction between *disease* and *illness* in better understanding chronic pain. The term *disease* is generally used to define "an objective biological event" that involves the disruption of specific body structures or organ systems caused by anatomical, pathological, or physiological changes. *Illness*, in contrast, is generally defined as a "subjective experience or self-attribution" that a disease is present. An illness will yield physical discomfort, behavioral limitations, and psychosocial distress. Illness references how sick individuals and members of their families live with, and respond to, symptoms and disability. This distinction between disease and illness is analogous to the distinction made between *pain* and *nociception*. Nociception involves the stimulation of nerves that convey information about tissue damage to the brain. Pain, on the other hand, is a more subjective perception that is the result of the transduction, transmission, and modulation of sensory input. This input may be filtered through individuals' genetic composition, prior learning histories, current physiological status, and sociocultural influences. Pain, therefore, cannot be comprehensively assessed without a full understanding of the person who is exposed to the nociception. The biopsychosocial model focuses on illness, which is the result of the complex interaction of biological, psychological, and social factors. With this perspective, diversity in pain or illness expression (including its severity, duration, and psychosocial consequences) can be expected. The interrelationships among biological changes, psychological status, and the sociocultural context all need to be taken into account in fully understanding pain, patients' perception, and their response to illness. A model or treatment approach that focuses on only one of these core sets of factors will be incomplete. Indeed, the treatment efficacy of a biopsychosocial approach to pain has consistently demonstrated the heuristic value of this model (Turk & Monarch, 2002).

PRIMARY, SECONDARY, AND TERTIARY CARE

At the outset, one should also be aware of differences among primary, secondary, and tertiary care. As Mayer et al. (2003) have clearly delineated, the care of acute pain problems is considered *primary care*, usually consisting of control of the pain symptom. Primary care usually lasts between 0 and 12 weeks following the occurrence of a painful episode and includes (but is not restricted to) "passive treatment modalities" such as electrical stimulation, manipulation, temperature modulation methods, and analgesic medications. Moreover, as these investigators note, on the basis of the natural history of many pain disorders, especially musculoskeletal disorders, most patients recover spontaneously or with relatively limited primary care. *Secondary care* refers to the first stage of reactivation during the transition from primary care to return-to-work or normal activities of daily living. This secondary care phase usually occurs 2 to 6 months after the initial pain occurrence and is designed for patients not responding to initial primary treatment, in order to facilitate a return to productivity before progressive physical deconditioning and psychosocioeconomic barriers become firmly entrenched. Secondary care is meant to avoid the occurrence of chronic disability by preventing

physical deconditioning and potential negative psychosocial reactions, as well as social habituation to disability. As Mayer and colleagues (2003) highlight, the rationale for secondary care rehabilitation is to recognize and manage early risk factors or signs for the development of disability, thus preventing chronic or permanent disability. Thus, *reactivation* is often the most common need at this point in time.

Finally, *tertiary care* refers to rehabilitation directed at preventing or ameliorating permanent disability for the patient who already suffers the effects of disability and physical deconditioning. It is this tertiary care or rehabilitation that requires an interdisciplinary team approach to accurately assess the various interrelated factors of chronic disability and pain, which then must be linked to the careful administration of a multifaceted pain management program to effect recovery and reduce permanent disability. This is not to say that the interdisciplinary approach is not of potential value for secondary care. However, this form of tertiary care is quite different from secondary care because of the intensity of services required, duration of disability, treatment program protocol, more specificity of physical and psychosocial assessment, and the greater level of coordination among health care professionals. In this chapter, we discuss this interdisciplinary approach, especially as applied to tertiary care.

It should be noted that we, as well as others, clearly distinguish between *interdisciplinary* and *multidisciplinary* treatment. *Multidisciplinary* connotes the involvement of several health care providers. The integration of these services, as well as communication among providers, may be limited. *Interdisciplinary,* in our use of the concept, involves greater coordination of services in a comprehensive program, and frequent communication among the health care professionals providing care. A key ingredient of interdisciplinary care is a common philosophy of rehabilitation and active patient involvement (Turk & Stieg, 1987). Before discussing the specific elements of an interdisciplinary treatment approach, a brief historical overview of the growth of such pain management approaches is provided.

GROWTH OF PAIN TREATMENT CLINICS

As carefully delineated elsewhere (Turk & Gatchel, 1999), following World War II, a number of anesthesiologists developed pain clinics that used nerve block procedures as a primary model of diagnosis and therapy. This subsequently stimulated the rapid growth of such pain clinics, which resulted in the listing of 327 such clinics in a *Directory of Pain Clinics* that was published in 1977 by the American Society of Anesthesiologists, Committee on Pain Therapy. Of these 327 pain clinics, 73% were within the United States. Subsequently, it was estimated that there were more than 3,300 pain treatment facilities and solo pain practitioners in the United States, treating 2.9 million Americans each year (Marketdata Enterprises, 1995). More than 176,000 patients were estimated to be treated in specialty pain treatment facilities each year. Melzack and Wall (1982) characterized this proliferation of pain clinics as one of the most important advances in patient care during the past 25 years.

The International Association for the Study of Pain differentiated four levels of pain programs (see Loeser, 1990): multidisciplinary pain centers, multidisciplinary pain clinics, pain clinics, and modality-oriented clinics. The *pain clinic* is typically a health care facility that focuses on the diagnosis and management of patients with chronic pain. Such clinics may specialize in specific diagnoses or pain related to a specific region of the body (e.g., headache or back pain). The *modality-oriented clinic* is a health care facility that provides a specific type of treatment, but does not provide comprehensive assessment or pain management. Examples of such clinics include nerve block clinics and biofeedback clinics. In such clinics, there is no emphasis on an integrated or comprehensive interdisciplinary approach. A *multidisciplinary pain center* (in our terms, interdisciplinary) is composed of a group of health care professionals and basic scientists. Such centers include research, teaching, and patient care related to acute and chronic pain. These facilities include a wide array of health care professionals, including physicians, psychologists, nurses, physical therapists, occupational therapists, and other health care provider specialties. Multiple therapeutic modalities are available, and these centers are usually affiliated with major health science institutions and are able to provide evaluation and treatment. Finally, a *multidisciplinary* (interdisciplinary) *pain clinic* is a health care delivery facility staffed by physicians and other health care provider specialists. It differs from the multidisciplinary pain center in that it does not include research and teaching activities as regular features.

Of course, the prototypic pain clinic with which most psychologists are familiar is the one originally developed at the University of Washington by Fordyce and colleagues (Fordyce, Fowler, Lehmann, & DeLateur, 1968). This clinic utilized "pure" operant or behavioral treatment programs in which reinforcement procedures for "well behavior" were the major components used for pain management. The program originally involved a 4- to 8-week inpatient treatment protocol designed to increase gradually the general activity level and socialization of the patient, and to decrease medication use.

As pain treatment specialists began to understand the complexity of evaluating and treating chronic pain problems, simple pain clinics and modality-oriented clinics soon were replaced by interdisciplinary pain centers or clinics (IPCs) in which it was viewed that patients would be best served by a team of specialists with different health care backgrounds. These IPCs were driven by the concept

that a complaint of pain was not just the result of body damage, but had cognitive, affective, and environmental origins as well. Moreover, these IPCs treated not only the experience of pain but also associated patient distress, dysfunction, and disability. The major aim was to improve a patient's physical performance and coping skills, and also to transfer the control of pain and the management of its related problems back to the patient. The treatment plan was conceptualized to be rehabilitative rather than investigative or curative. It was designed to increase function so that the patient could make further changes in life quality, environmental stressors, and psychosocial factors (e.g., self-esteem and affect), all of which would assist in pain control and management. Such IPCs emphasized an integrated treatment plan that included comprehensive care such as drug detoxification, cognitive-behavioral treatment methods, functional restoration, and total rehabilitation. These more comprehensive approaches do not ignore operant factors that influence the maintenance of pain and disability. Rather, they incorporate behavioral factors within a broader rehabilitative model.

INTERDISCIPLINARY CHRONIC PAIN MANAGEMENT

The most prevalent chronic pain conditions include the following:

- Pain related to irritable bowel syndrome (20%)
- Osteoarthritis (15%)
- Low back pain (14%)
- Chronic pelvic pain (12%)
- Migraine headaches (12%)
- Chronic tension headaches (3%)
- Fibromyalgia (2%)

As noted earlier in this chapter, when pain becomes chronic, a more intensive tertiary care or interdisciplinary treatment approach is required because of the significant effects of physical deconditioning and chronic disability. The critical elements of this interdisciplinary approach are reviewed below. There have been a number of reviews that have documented the clinical efficacy of such interdisciplinary treatment of patients with chronic pain (e.g., Deschner & Polatin, 2000; Gatchel, 1999; Okifuji, 2003; Wright & Gatchel, 2002). Such interdisciplinary programs are needed for patients with chronic pain who have complex needs and requirements. Although they represent a small minority of patients with pain, there nevertheless are a significant number of patients who have failed to benefit from the combination of spontaneous healing and short-term, symptom-focused treatment. They have also become financial burdens on their insurance carriers, as well as the health care system in general. They have often failed to experience significant pain relief after repeated and extended contacts with several different physicians and other health care providers. Psychosocial distress, physical deconditioning, secondary gains and losses, and medication issues often complicate their presentation. Therefore, this stage of treatment is much more complex and demanding of health care professionals. As such, the strengths of multiple disciplines working together to address complex issues confronting patients with chronic pain is greatly needed. The overall therapeutic focus should be toward independence and autonomy, while acknowledging when certain physical limitations cannot be overcome. The Commission on Accreditation of Rehabilitation Facilities requires that a certified pain management team include at least a physician, a specialized nurse, a physical therapist, and a clinical psychologist or psychiatrist. However, often, an occupational therapist is required because return-to-work and vocational retraining issues become important in managing patients with chronic pain.

Table 100.1 summarizes the interdisciplinary treatment team. This team consists of the following:

- The *physician* serves as a medical director of the treatment plan, and he or she must have a firm background in providing medical rehabilitation for these types of pain disorders frequently encountered. Formal training may vary from anesthesiology, orthopedic surgery, psychiatry, or occupational medicine to internal medicine. The physician needs to assume a direct role in the medical management of the patient's pain by providing the medical history to the treatment team, and by taking direct responsibility for medication management for any other medical interventions. Often, other team members and outside consultants may be involved in the medical treatment of the patient, but it is the physicians' responsibility to coordinate these medical contributions to the patient's care.

- Although not all programs use nursing services, any pain management program that provides anesthesiology services involving injections, nerve blocks, and other medical procedures will require a nurse. The *nurse* assists the physician, follows up the procedures, and may interact with patients in the role of case manager, as well as providing patient education. The nurse may be viewed as a physician-extender and educator who has a strong impact on the patient.

- Although the physician and nurse play a major role in managing the physical status of patients, the *psychologist* plays the leading role in the day-to-day maintenance of the psychosocial aspects and status of the patient's care. Signif-

---

TABLE 100.1
Staff Composition of an Interdisciplinary Pain Management Center

Medical Director/Physician: Serves a leadership role responsible for medical issues involved in the diagnoses and management of anatomic, pathologic, and physiologic process associated with complaint of pain.

Nurse: Serves as a physician "extender," and plays a significant role in obtaining patient histories, monitoring medications, and evaluating lifestyle issues that may affect patients suffering pain and their response to treatment.

Psychologist: Assesses the patient's psychosocial functioning, personality characteristics, social support, motivational status, and coping resources that will help treatment planning; provides treatments addressing these issues, as well as the monitoring of therapeutic progress.

Physical Therapist: Performs comprehensive musculoskeletal evaluation, including the examination of gait and postural abnormalities, range of motion, sensation, reflexes, and neurologic indices; this information is then used to specifically tailor a therapeutic program to address any diagnosed defects.

Occupational Therapist: Conducts pre- and post-treatment evaluations that focus on body mechanics and energy conservation needed for activities of daily living, work, and leisure; during treatment, supervises progressive increases in the performance of such functional activities so that patients can return to as normal a level of functioning as possible; also often serves as the liaison between employers and injured workers, and may aid in developing job modifications for accommodation of the injured worker.

Medical-Disability Case Manager: An occupational therapist or vocational rehabilitation professional often is employed to promote vocational and social reactivation throughout the treatment program and will monitor progress compliance and performance, post-program follow-up, and occupational planning and sequencing, with coordination of socioeconomic issues.

---

icant psychosocial barriers to positive outcomes of the treatment may develop as a patient progresses from acute through subacute to the chronic stage of a pain syndrome (as reviewed earlier in this chapter). The psychologist is responsible for conducting a full psychosocial evaluation, which includes identification of psychosocial barriers to recovery and the assessment of the patient psychological strengths and weaknesses. A cognitive–behavioral treatment approach can then be utilized to address important psychosocial issues such as pain-related depression, anxiety, and fear, as well as psychopathology. A cognitive–behavioral treatment approach has been found to be the most appropriate modality to use with patients in a program such as this.

- The *physical therapist* interacts daily with the patient regarding any physical progression issues toward recovery. Effective communication with other team members is crucial in order that the patient's fear of exercise will not interfere with his or her reconditioning effort. The physical therapist also helps to educate the patient by addressing the physiological bases of pain, and teaching ways of reducing the severity of pain episodes through the use of appropriate body mechanics and pacing.

- The *occupational therapist* is involved in both physical and vocational aspects of the patient's treatment. The great majority of patients participating in an interdisciplinary program are likely not to be working because of their pain. Often, they have become pessimistic about the prospect of returning to work. The occupational therapist addresses these vocational issues and the physical determinants on underlying disability. This therapist also plays an important educational role in teaching patients techniques for managing pain on the job in ways that do not jeopardize their employment status. Finally, the occupational therapist can play an important role as case manager in contacting employers to obtain job descriptions and other information, as well as vocational retraining if necessary.

Constant, effective communication among all treatment personnel is required during which patient progress can be discussed and evaluated. This is important so patients hear the same treatment philosophy and message from each of the treatment team members. Indeed, many times patients are in conflict about their own future treatment and may seek out any conflict between team members and use it to compromise treatment goals.

A formal interdisciplinary treatment team meeting should occur at least once a week to review patient progress and to make any modifications in the treatment plan for each patient. Individually tailoring treatment for patients is essential. Evaluating and monitoring treatment outcomes in a systematic fashion is essential for not only treatment outcomes evaluations, but also quality assurance purposes for the treatment team.

FUNCTIONAL RESTORATION: AN EXAMPLE OF AN INTERDISCIPLINARY TREATMENT PROGRAM

In recent years, there has been an even greater emphasis in functional restoration as a driving force of IPCs (Baum, Gatchel, & Krantz, 1997). The term *functional restoration*, originally developed by Mayer and Gatchel (1988), refers not only to a treatment methodology for patients with chronic pain, but also to a broader conceptualization of the entire problem, its diagnosis, and its management. Rather than accepting current limits in history taking

---

TABLE 100.2

Important Factors That Determine the Success of an Interdisciplinary Pain Treatment Program

- Understanding and acceptance of the philosophy of the treatment program by all staff
- Systematic monitoring of treatment outcomes to maximize quality assurance
- Regular staffings to maximize frequent communication among team members and mutual reinforcement of the overall goals for each patient
- Mutual reinforcement among team members for each other's role and efforts, as well as the communication of respect for each other's skills with the patients

---

based solely on patients' self-report of pain and of diagnosis through imaging technology, this method involves more objective information. Objective assessment of physical capacity and effort, with comparison with a normative database, adds a new dimension to diagnosis. In keeping with a "sports medicine" approach, this permits the development of treatment programs of varied intensity and duration aimed primarily at restoring physical functional capacity and social performance. Objectives are more ambitious than merely attempting to alter pain complaints and to decrease medications. It is assumed that improvements in quality of life will be greatly enlarged by focusing on increasing physical capacity and decreasing social problems associated with pain. Attention is given to realistic goals such as returning to work, increasing activities of daily living, and reducing the use of the medical system. This functional restoration approach has already helped to change the focus of the traditional pain treatment programs, as well as the criteria for evaluation of effectiveness. Table 100.2 presents the important factors that can significantly contribute to the success of such programs. The clinical effectiveness of functional restoration has been well documented. Indeed, Gatchel and Turk (1999) and Turk (2002) have reviewed both the therapeutic-effectiveness and cost-effectiveness of interdisciplinary programs, such as functional restoration, for the wide range of chronic pain conditions. Fortunately, we now have in our treatment armamentarium the ability to effectively manage what used to be recalcitrant chronic pain syndromes.

MAJOR GOALS OF AN INTERDISCIPLINARY TREATMENT PROGRAM

Table 100.3 presents the major goals that interdisciplinary treatment programs should strive to achieve. As can been seen, these are all goals that can be objectively monitored and quantified. Indeed, emphasizing such objective functional and socioeconomic outcomes has been discussed

---

TABLE 100.3
Major Goals of an Interdisciplinary Pain Treatment Program

- Return the patient to productivity
- Maximize function, thus minimizing pain
- Patient assumption of responsibility for self-management and progress
- Reduction or elimination of future medical utilization
- Avoidance of recurrence of injury and maintenance of therapeutic gains
- Avoidance of medication dependence and abuse

---

by numerous clinical investigators (Feuerstein & Zastowny, 1996; Hazard, 1995; Mayer & Gatchel, 1988).

The success of the interdisciplinary approach to chronic pain management, such as functional restoration, has been unequivocally documented in a number of different investigations (e.g., Bendix & Bendix, 1994; Bendix et al., 1996; Hazard et al., 1989; Hildebrandt, Pfingsten, Saur, & Jansen, 1997; Mayer et al., 1985, 1987). For example, in the study by Mayer et al. (1987), patients who had undergone the functional restoration program were followed up 2 years after completion of the program. Results clearly demonstrated significant changes in a number of important socioeconomic outcome measures that were collected: nearly 90% of the treatment group were actively working, as compared with only about 41% of a nontreatment comparison group; about twice as many comparison group patients required additional spine surgery and had unsettled workers' compensation litigation relative to the treatment group; the comparison group also had approximately five times more patient visits to health care professionals and had higher rates of recurrence of reinjury relative to the functional restoration group. There were also significant improvements in self-report measures and physical function measures such as back strength and range of motion in the functional restoration treatment group. Thus, these findings demonstrate the significant impact that an interdisciplinary program such as functional restoration can have on a range of important self-report, physical functioning, and socioeconomic outcome measures.

Finally, it should be noted that the original functional restoration program was independently replicated by Hazard et al. (1989) in this country, as well as Bendix and Bendix (1994) and Bendix et al. (1996) in Denmark, Hildebrandt et al. (1997) in Germany, and Corey, Koepfler, Etlin, and Day (1996) in Canada. The fact that different clinical treatment teams, functioning in different states (Texas and Vermont) and different countries, with markedly different economic-social conditions and workers' compensation systems, produced comparable outcome results speaks highly for the robustness of the research

findings and utility, as well as the fidelity, of this functional restoration approach. In addition, Burke, Harms-Constas, and Aden (1994) have demonstrated its efficacy in 11 different rehabilitation centers across seven states. Hazard (1995) has also reviewed the overall effectiveness of functional restoration.

It should be pointed out that, besides functional restoration, there are other forms of interdisciplinary treatment programs for chronic pain that have been shown to be efficacious with chronic pain sufferers (Turk & Gatchel, 1999; Turk & Stacey, 1997). These other programs differ from functional restoration mainly in terms of less emphasis on the direct quantification of function used to drive the "sports medicine" philosophy of that approach. Overall, Turk and Gatchel (1999) have pointed out that the cost savings of all IPCs can be quite significant. In addition, it was emphasized that more research is needed to examine what combinations of variables are most important in being able to prescribe the most efficient and effective therapeutic "package" in an interdisciplinary treatment program. Future investigation is needed to address this important issue so as to increase the time, cost, and outcome efficiency of this promising interdisciplinary treatment approach to pain management. In addition, a review of the scientific literature by Turk (2002) compared the relative clinical- and cost-effectiveness of comprehensive interdisciplinary pain management programs, pharmacological treatments, surgery, spinal cord stimulators, implantable drug delivery systems, and conservative standard care for chronic pain. Overall, it was found that the interdisciplinary treatment programs yielded significantly better outcomes than the other treatments on the following outcomes: medication use, health care utilization rates, functional activity levels, return-to-work rates, and closure of disability claims, as well as fewer iatrogenic consequences or adverse events.

SUMMARY AND CONCLUSIONS

In a review of the literature, Flor, Fydrich, and Turk (1992) concluded that the overall therapeutic results emanating from IPCs were quite promising, with significant changes demonstrated not only in self-reported pain and mood, but also in important socioeconomic variables such as the return to work and the use of the health care system. The cost of hospital and medical charges for chronic pain have been estimated to be in excess of $125 billion (Frymoyer & Durett, 1997). Based on the meta-analysis that included 3,089 patients published by Flor et al. (1992), even when the cost of treatment of the IPC was included, Turk and Gatchel (1999) calculated a savings of over $1 billion over a period of 19 years. Recall that this is based on 3,089 patients. The market data survey (Marketdata Enterprises, 1995) estimated that more than 176,000 patients were treated at IPCs each year. Extrapolating potential savings of IPCs would be in excess of $1.5 billion each year. Turk and Okifuji (1998) have also documented the treatment and cost benefits of multidisciplinary pain treatment centers.

Finally, it should also be emphasized that more research is needed to examine what combinations of variables are most important in being able to prescribe the most efficient and effective therapeutic "package" in an interdisciplinary treatment program. As Turk and Gatchel (1999) have concluded, to date "… there are no data available to determine what set of patients with what characteristics are most likely to benefit from what set of treatment modalities, provided in what type of format." Future investigation is needed to address this important issue so as to increase the time, cost, and outcome efficiency of this promising interdisciplinary treatment approach to pain management.

ACKNOWLEDGMENT

The writing of this chapter was supported in part by Grants 3R01 MH046452, 2R01 DE010713, and 1K02 MH071892 from the National Institutes of Health and PR023002 from the Department of Defense.

REFERENCES

Baum, A., Gatchel, R. J., & Krantz, D. S. (Eds.). (1997). *An introduction to health psychology* (3rd ed.). New York: McGraw-Hill.

Bendix, T., & Bendix, A. (1994). *Different training programs for chronic low back pain — A randomized, blinded one-year follow-up study.* Paper presented at the International Society for the Study of the Lumbar Spine, Seattle.

Bendix, A. E., Bendix, T., Vaegter, K., Lund, C., Frolund, L., & Holm, L. (1996). Multidisciplinary intensive treatment for chronic low back pain: A randomized, prospective study. *Cleveland Clinic Journal of Medicine, 63,* 62–69.

Burke, S. A., Harms-Constas, C. K., & Aden, P. S. (1994). Return to work/work retention outcomes of a functional restoration program: A multi-center, prospective study with a comparison group. *Spine, 19,* 1880–1886.

Corey, D. T., Koepfler, L. E., Etlin, D., & Day, H. I. (1996). A limited functional restoration program for injured workers: A randomized trial. *Journal of Occupational Rehabilitation, 6,* 239–249.

Deschner, M., & Polatin, P. B. (2000). Interdisciplinary programs: Chronic pain management. In T. G. Mayer, R. J. Gatchel, & P. B. Polatin (Eds.), *Occupational musculoskeletal disorders: Function, outcomes & evidence* (pp. 629–637). Philadelphia: Lippincott/Williams & Wilkins.

Dworkin, S. F., & Massoth, D. L. (1994). Temporomandibular disorders and chronic pain: Disease or illness? *Journal of Prosthetic Dentistry, 72*(1), 29–38.

Feuerstein, M., & Zastowny, T. R. (1996). Occupational rehabilitation: Multidisciplinary management of work related musculoskeletal pain and disability. In R. J. Gatchel & D. C. Turk (Eds.), *Psychological approaches to pain management: A practitioner's handbook* (pp. 458–485). New York: Guilford.

Flor, H., Fydrich, T., & Turk, D. C. (1992). Efficacy of multidisciplinary pain treatment centers: A meta-analytic flow. *Pain, 49,* 221–230.

Fordyce, W. E., Fowler, R. S., Lehmann, J. F., & DeLateur, B. J. (1968). Some implications of learning in problems of chronic pain. *Journal of Chronic Diseases, 21,* 179–190.

Frymoyer, J. W., & Durett, C. L. (1997). The economics of spinal disorders. In J. W. Frymoyer et al. (Eds.), *The adult spine* (2nd ed., Vol. 1, pp. 143–150). Philadelphia: Lippincott-Raven.

Gatchel, R. J. (1999). Perspectives on pain: A historical overview. In R. J. Gatchel & D. C. Turk (Eds.), *Psychosocial factors in pain: Critical perspectives* (pp. 3–17). New York: Guilford Publications.

Gatchel, R. J., & Turk, D. C. (1999). Interdisciplinary treatment of chronic pain patients. In R. J. Gatchel & D. C. Turk (Eds.), *Psychosocial factors in pain: Critical perspectives* (pp. 435–444). New York: Guilford.

Hazard, R. G. (1995). Spine update: Functional restoration. *Spine, 20,* 2345–2348.

Hazard, R. G., Fenwick, J. W., Kalisch, S. M., Redmond, J., Reeves, V., Reid, S. et al. (1989). Functional restoration with behavioral support: A one-year prospective study of patients with chronic low-back pain. *Spine, 14,* 157–161.

Hildebrandt, J., Pfingsten, M., Saur, P., & Jansen, J. (1997). Prediction of success from a multidisciplinary treatment program for chronic low back pain. *Spine, 22,* 990–1001.

Loeser, J. D. (1990). *Desirable characteristics for pain treatment facilities.* Seattle, WA: International Association for the Study of Pain.

Marketdata Enterprises, Inc. (1995). *Chronic pain management programs: A market analysis.* Valley Stream, NY: Author.

Mayer, T. G., & Gatchel, R. J. (1988). *Functional restoration for spinal disorders: The sports medicine approach.* Philadelphia: Lea & Febiger.

Mayer, T. G., Gatchel, R. J., Kishino, N., Keeley, J., Capra, P., Mayer, H. et al. (1985). Objective assessment of spine function following industrial injury: A prospective study with comparison group and one-year follow-up. *Spine, 10,* 482–493.

Mayer, T. G., Gatchel, R. J., Mayer, H., Kishino, N. D., Keeley, J., & Mooney, V. A. (1987). Prospective two year study of functional restoration in industrial low back injury. *Journal of the American Medical Association, 258,* 1763–1767.

Mayer, T., Polatin, P. B., Gatchel, R. J., Fardon, D., Herring, S., Smith, C. et al. (2003). Spine rehabilitation: Secondary and tertiary nonoperative care. *Spine Journal, 3,* 28–36.

Melzack, R., & Wall, P. D. (1982). *The challenge of pain.* New York: Basic Books.

Okifuji, A. (2003). Interdisciplinary pain management with pain patients: Evidence for its effectiveness. *Seminars in Pain Management, 1*, 110–119.

Turk, D. C. (2002). Clinical effectiveness and cost effectiveness of treatment for patients with chronic pain. *Clinical Journal of Pain, 18*, 355–365.

Turk, D. C., & Gatchel, R. J. (1999). Multidisciplinary programs for rehabilitation of chronic low back pain patients. In W. H. Kirkaldy-Willis & T. N. Bernard, Jr. (Eds.), *Managing low back pain* (4th ed., pp. 299–311). New York: Churchill Livingstone.

Turk, D. C., & Monarch, E. S. (2002). Biopsychosocial perspective on chronic pain. In D. C. Turk & R. J. Gatchel (Eds.), *Psychological approaches to pain management: A practitioner's handbook* (2nd ed.). New York: Guilford.

Turk, D., & Okifuji, A. (1998). Directions in prescriptive chronic pain management based on diagnostic characteristics of the patient. *APS Bulletin, 8*, 5–11.

Turk, D. C., & Stacey, B. R. (1997). Multidisciplinary pain centers in the treatment of chronic back pain. In J. W. Frymoyer (Ed.), *The adult spine* (2nd ed.). New York: Lippincott-Raven.

Turk, D. C., & Stieg, R. L. (1987). Chronic pain: The necessity of interdisciplinary communication. *Clinical Journal of Pain, 3*, 163–167.

White, K. L., Williams, F., & Greenberg, B. G. (1961). The etiology of medical care. *New England Journal of Medicine, 265*, 885–886.

Wright, A. R., & Gatchel, R. J. (2002). Occupational musculoskeletal pain and disability. In D. C. Turk & R. J. Gatchel (Eds.), *Psychological approaches to pain management: A practitioner's handbook* (2nd ed., pp. 349–364). New York: Guilford.

—101—

Implementing a Pain Management Program

Anne Marie Kelly, RN, BC, BSN, CHPN

The purpose of human life is to serve, to show compassion, and to help others.

— **Albert Schweitzer**

INTRODUCTION

Relieving pain and suffering is at the heart of the health care profession. Despite attempts at treating pain over the decades, fear of unrelieved pain remains a major concern of patients in all health care settings. In 1992, the Agency for Healthcare Policy and Research (AHCPR) published guidelines on acute pain, which state that the institutional responsibility for pain management begins with the affirmation that patients should have access to the best level of pain relief that may safely be provided. Regarding ethical responsibility, the guidelines stress that the ethical obligation to manage pain and relieve the patient's suffering is at the core of a health care professional's commitment (AHCPR, 1992). Inadequate pain management was thought to be such a wide problem that the Joint Commission on Accreditation of Healthcare Organizations (JCAHO) published standards for the assessment and management of pain in 1999. Today, health care institutions have the responsibility and ethical obligation to develop the necessary means and resources to effectively treat pain in all patients. As the guidelines and standards focus on the assessment and management of pain, the need for programs that address pain management practices is required. The best means to ensure that all patients receive optimal pain relief is the availability of a pain management program that combines the expertise and commitment of a health care team dedicated to the prevention and treatment of pain. Formalized programs are necessary to bring pain management to its rightful place in the health care system. This chapter focuses on the key components required for the successful implementation of a pain management program focused on evidence-based practice and clinical guidelines (Table 101.1).

IDENTIFY INSTITUTIONAL LEADERS

Well begun is half done.

— **Aristotle**

The first step should be the appointment of a task force to determine a plan of action. Seek out the "champions" in the institution who have a vested interest, are strongly motivated, have a good understanding of pain and its management, and will seek change by building a culture of advocacy. It is important to give those who feel a sense of commitment and ownership the opportunity to contribute to the development of the program. Peters (1987) suggests that those vested "look inward, work with colleagues and customers, work with everyone, to develop and instill a philosophy and vision that is enabling and empowering" (p. 482). Once the task force has been selected, conduct an institutional assessment to examine the organization's culture and its strengths and weaknesses related to current pain management practices. Health care institutions, whether they are hospitals, long-term care facilities, or home health agencies, each have their own distinct culture, which can either support or hinder effective pain management. The leaders should address the following dimensions:

1. Is pain management recognized as an institutional priority?
2. Do the policies and procedures direct pain management practices?
3. Is pain management education mandatory for facility staff?
4. Is accountability for pain management clearly defined?
5. Is pain management addressed in the Patient's Bill of Rights and the organization's mission statement?
6. Is there a pain management quality improvement process in place?

Although pain is a significant problem, it remains largely an invisible one. The task force serves as a catalyst in promoting increased visibility regarding the problem of unrelieved pain. Its focus is to collect and provide data to initiate efforts in addressing the existing inadequacies. The results can provide strong evidence pointing to the need to standardize pain assessment policies, make changes in institutional procedures, and integrate clinical guidelines that will lead to evidence-based practices (Weissman et al., 1997). Making the problem of pain visible in the institution is the initial step in developing a formalized approach to pain management.

DEVELOP A MISSION STATEMENT FOR THE PROGRAM

It is imperative that the mission statement reflect the values and purpose of the organization related to pain management practices. By articulating its purpose and what it stands for, the institution directs the work of the staff. In describing the importance of a clearly articulated purpose, Ulschak (1988) states, "until there is agreement about purpose, an institution has no direction, no tool to measure progress, no real reason to be motivated, and no clear focus for its energy." To achieve success, strong facility buy-in and commitment from the top are required. The administrator, and not just the director of nursing, must provide leadership that can result in institutional change, encourage employee commitment, and ensure improved standards of care. Leaders in the organization need to educate staff about changes in practice and their relation to the mission. Staff members must clearly see

---

TABLE 101.1
Key Components of a Successful Program

1. Institutional commitment
2. Interdisciplinary team
3. Education
4. Continuous quality improvement

---

that the institution's priority and goal is to promote high standards of safe, effective pain relief to all patients within its care. Institutional commitment and administrative support constitute the foundation on which to build a quality program and are recognized as the key elements essential to success.

DEFINE STANDARDS OF CARE

Defining standards is a key step in developing an effective program. Pain management is arguably one of the most complex topics in medicine today. From dealing with acute, chronic, and cancer pain to providing palliative and compassionate end-of-life care, caregivers are faced with multiple issues that extend far beyond the question of what medication to administer. Written standards and guidelines are necessary to define the expectations of the caregivers and illustrate how the care delivery system is organized and managed. The mission of the institution sets the direction for all written standards. Standards make quality a day-to-day goal.

JCAHO set standards for the assessment and management of pain that health care institutions must implement (Dahl, 1999; JCAHO, 1999). These standards call upon hospitals, home care agencies, long-term care facilities, behavioral health care organizations, outpatient clinics, and health care plans to

- Recognize the right of patients to receive appropriate assessment and management of pain
- Assess the existence and, if so, the nature and intensity of pain in all patients
- Record the results of the assessment in a way that facilitates regular reassessment and follow-up
- Determine and assure staff competency in pain assessment and management
- Address pain assessment and management in the orientation of all new staff
- Establish policies and procedures that support the appropriate prescription or ordering of effective pain medications
- Ensure that pain does not interfere with participation in rehabilitation
- Educate patients and their families about effective pain management
- Collect data to monitor the appropriateness and effectiveness of pain management
- Address patient needs for symptom management in the discharge planning process

These standards must be included in the policies and procedures and serve as criteria by which the facility's pain management practices are evaluated. Standards of clinical practice need to be integrated and reflect the knowledge and skills of the health care professionals (Berry & JCAHO, 1997). Clinical practice guidelines are essential to promoting optimal pain management care throughout the continuum (Spross, 1994). Clearly defined standards establish the foundation for a system-wide initiative in pain management and positively affect the quality of patient care.

DEVELOP AN INTERDISCIPLINARY APPROACH TO PAIN MANAGEMENT

Because pain is a multidimensional experience, it requires an interdisciplinary approach. Pain profoundly affects not only the physical, but the psychological, social, cultural, and spiritual dimensions of life (Ferrell, Dean, Grant, & Coluzzi, 1995; Saunders, 1984). Successful pain control requires attention to all aspects of care and suffering, and no amount of well-prescribed analgesia will relieve the pain unless the elements that are compounding the problem are addressed. Care provided by a team of specialized health care professionals is essential to treat the diverse aspects of pain. For pain treatment to be effective, institutions need to direct their attention to the importance of interdisciplinary teams who work collaboratively to overcome the inevitable barriers to pain management. The interdisciplinary team is a valuable resource that serves the institution by

- Assisting in the development of policies and procedures, offering consultation, and providing a forum for the resolution of difficult pain and risk management issues
- Utilizing standards and guidelines in developing a formulary for analgesic use including special populations
- Assisting patients with the multiple dimensions of pain management, including end-of-life care, and integrating multimodal therapy to ensure quality of life
- Providing support and guidance to families as they confront the common challenges associated with caring for a loved one coping with pain or requiring palliative care
- Promoting educational programs for families and the community that focus on pain assessment and management, barriers and misconceptions, drug addiction, and how to communicate with their physician and other health care professionals about pain

A holistic approach is critical to breaking down the barriers to pain management and is successful because it allows physicians, nurses and other clinicians to learn more about the "person" than just the disease (NIH, 1987).

TABLE 101.2
Role of Interdisciplinary Team

1. Identify patient, family, and staff needs in pain management
2. Assure pain relief goals are met
3. Collaborate with health care providers to facilitate optimum pain control
4. Promote practice changes through outcome quality improvement monitoring

A pain management team includes professionals from various disciplines who meet regularly to discuss and develop an individualized plan of care for each patient. A typical team may include one or more physicians, nurses, pharmacists, physical therapists, occupational therapists, pastoral care counselors, social workers, dieticians, and staff educators. Depending on the setting, the addition of a certified nursing assistant, therapeutic activity therapist, and trained volunteer can be helpful. A team can address the need for accountability in pain management and prevent further fragmentation of care (Table 101.2). This is the best approach for responding to pain and a critical component of an effective pain management program (Gordon, Dahl, & Stevenson, 1996).

DEFINE ACCOUNTABILITY

Accountability must be established early and clearly defined on two levels. The team members have individual accountability for integrating good pain management practices while the institution has accountability for making organizational changes that promote evidence-based practices (Spross, 2001). Team members have accountability for the following:

- Assessing the physical, psychosocial, spiritual, functional, and cultural needs of the patient
- Using standardized tools to assess the patient
- Discussing summary of findings with attending physician and making appropriate recommendations
- Updating the treatment plan with the patient and family and encouraging participation in decision making
- Implementing multimodal therapies
- Attending regularly scheduled interdisciplinary team meetings to review plan of care and problem solve
- Communicating plan of care to appropriate staff members
- Assessing for pain relief routinely throughout the course of treatment
- Educating patient and family about pain management

The institution has accountability for the following:

- Defining and implementing standards for pain assessment and treatment
- Continuously monitoring outcomes to improve pain management practices
- Establishing protocols for the safe administration of analgesics, which includes special populations
- Providing educational opportunities for staff, patients, and families
- Providing resources regarding drug and non-drug treatments

Positive outcomes are measured by the team's ability to provide pain relief in a safe, timely, and effective manner, and meet the needs of the patient and family. The following case example illustrates these points.

CASE EXAMPLE

Joe was a 79-year-old man with terminal rectal cancer who resided in a long-term care facility. He was an alert, oriented, and spiritual man who understood his prognosis and elected to receive comfort measures only. His pain had been fairly well controlled and his medications had been titrated up to 400 mg of OxyContin® every 12 hours, Actiq® 400 mg every 3 hours as necessary for breakthrough pain, Celebrex® 100 mg twice a day, and Nortriptyline® 25 mg at 9:00 P.M. Joe was able to maintain his independence and did not exhibit any major side effects from the medications. During this time, he was referred to the pain clinic for consultation regarding pain control measures. As the rectal tumor enlarged, his pain escalated and became more difficult to manage. He was once again seen by the anesthesiologist at the pain clinic who recommended the placement of a tunneled, epidural catheter for optimum pain control. Joe consented to the procedure and his attending physician agreed this was the best course to follow. However, this created a problem for the long-term care facility for the following reasons:

1. The facility had no written protocol for the administration of epidural analgesia and the nurses felt ill-prepared having little or no knowledge in this area.
2. Joe wanted to return to the long-term care facility where he felt at home and wished to die in a loving environment surrounded by staff he considered his family.
3. The facility's mission statement clearly articulated that the institution's priority was the relief of pain.

Following a discussion with administration and the interdisciplinary team, all members agreed it was the institution's responsibility and ethical obligation to provide the necessary means and resources to care for Joe during his final days. With administrative support, the members of the interdisciplinary team developed the necessary policies and procedures and provided education to the clinical staff in every aspect of care. With adequate education and support from the team, the nurses felt confident and prepared for Joe's return from the hospital. The nurses knew the moment they saw Joe that they had made the right decision. Upon arrival, Joe looked at the nurses with a smile on his face and stated, "It's a miracle. I have no pain." His pain was controlled with 1% bupivacaine and fentanyl 5 µg/cc at 6 to 14 cc/hour, and bolus doses of fentanyl 5 cc every 10 minutes via a patient-controlled analgesia pump. His pain ratings ranged from 0 to 2 and he remained comfortable until his death, 4 weeks later. Although saddened by his death, the staff's knowledge that they had made a difference in his life tempered their grief. Joe died peacefully, with dignity, and in a loving environment surrounded by dedicated staff who understood that life is a gift to be cherished until its final moments. *His wishes had been fulfilled and the facility's mission was carried out.*

During those 4 weeks, the interdisciplinary team invested all its skill and effort into relieving Joe's pain and suffering. The physician monitored his condition and ordered medications for pain control; the pharmacist ensured the medications were prepared and delivered in a timely manner; the nurses monitored him closely for pain relief and potential side effects from medications; the nursing assistants provided physical care with a compassionate touch; the physical and occupational therapists evaluated his ability to maintain optimum independence for as long as possible and made recommendations for comfort measures; the social worker listened attentively to his expressions of fear and offered support; the pastoral care counselor addressed his spiritual needs by praying with him daily and being present; the dietician monitored his nutritional needs and paid attention to his food preferences and ability to swallow; the recreational therapist provided him with musical tapes he enjoyed and taught him relaxation techniques and guided imagery to distract him from any pain; the staff educator provided ongoing education and assessed the competency of the staff; the hospice nurse offered respite care and support to the patient, family, and staff. The interdisciplinary team, composed of dedicated professionals, played a vital role in diminishing his physical, psychosocial, and spiritual pain. When team members listen, and respond to all aspects of pain, the patient experiences a feeling of worth, dignity, peace, and wholeness.

Although this was a challenging case for the long-term care facility, it was also very gratifying. The staff clearly understood the meaning of institutional commitment and observed how a committed and knowledgeable team is vital to effective pain management.

DEVELOP AN EDUCATION PLAN

There is no knowledge that is not power.

— **Ralph Waldo Emerson**

Medical and nursing schools devote very little time to the subject of pain management. Health care providers cannot be expected to practice what they do not know. Inadequacies in the education of health care professionals contribute to fears and misconceptions regarding the use of analgesics, addiction, and consequently inadequate pain management (Liebeskind & Melzak, 1998).

Education is a key step in improving pain management practices that result in institutional changes. Identifying learning needs of the staff is vital to educational efforts. This can be accomplished by

- Administering a pretest to assess the knowledge level of the staff
- Involving the interdisciplinary team in conducting a survey in their areas of practice to assess learning needs of each discipline
- Using the collection data to compare institutional practice with current, evidence-based practices; this is essential for planning educational programs focused on improving staff performance
- Establishing focus groups with staff from various disciplines to gather specific data related to learning needs; including "grassroots" input is useful for correcting misconceptions and biases about pain management that exist in the institution

Once learning needs have been identified, it is important to outline an education plan including curriculum content, staff time, and programming costs. For developing an evidence-based, comprehensive pain management program, these core content areas should be included:

- Standards of practice
- Barriers and misconceptions
- Physiology of pain
- Pain assessment
- Types of pain
- Assessment tools
- Analgesics: non-opioids, opioids, adjuvant medications
- Nonpharmacological interventions

- Symptom management
- Psychosocial, spiritual, and cultural issues
- Pain management for special populations (e.g., older adults, pediatrics, chemically dependent)
- Ethical and legal issues
- Documentation

PLAN EDUCATION STRATEGIES THAT INVOLVE ALL CAREGIVERS

Organizations learn only through individuals who learn.

— **Peter Senge**

There are a variety of formal and informal teaching strategies as well as educational models that can enhance the learner's understanding of pain management. Educators need to employ creative ways to educate staff, patients, families, and the community in a timely, cost-effective, and informative way. Each teaching strategy is advantageous for certain outcomes and has considerations that influence its choice.

FORMAL EDUCATIONAL MODELS

Preceptorships

Preceptorships (also referred to as internships, fellowships) provide participants the opportunity to observe pain management role models in action. Program includes lectures, patient rounds and interaction, group discussions, observation of procedures, contact with interdisciplinary team members, and case studies. Participants spend days to weeks with experts to learn how to institutionalize pain management and provide evidence-based practice (McCaffery, & Pasero, 1999).

Pain Resource Nurse Programs

Many (PRN) programs are modeled after the original program offered by the City of Hope National Medical Center in Duarte, California, in 1992 (Ferrell, Grant, Ritchey et al., 1993). The purpose of a PRN program is to train a group of staff nurses to function as pain management experts. The program is comprehensive, providing didactic education and preceptor experiences to train nurses in providing safe and effective pain care.

INFORMAL TEACHING STRATEGIES

Pain Management Awareness Day

Designate a day that is set aside for pain management education. This time is a great opportunity to teach everyone that pain management is an institutional priority. Invite each interdisciplinary team member to set up an exhibit displaying learning materials and equipment that can help participants to understand their role in relieving pain. Team members can be available at alternating times for demonstration, for skill practice, and to answer questions. Communicate this event to everyone through fliers and newspaper articles. This is an excellent way for disseminating information to staff, patients, families, other health care providers, and the public. It stimulates interest in a dynamic way and facilitates education about the different pain control measures used in the facility. This strategy serves as a great marketing tool by conveying a strong message about the organization's commitment to quality pain management practices.

Pain Management Poster Presentations

This is a unique and enjoyable way to involve all departments and demonstrate that pain management requires an interdisciplinary approach. Encourage creativity by inviting employees from all departments to design a poster of their choice related to pain management. Employees can work individually, or as a group, and are given a deadline to complete the project. Display the posters throughout the facility, providing valuable information to insiders and outsiders. Select different categories and ask some of your volunteers or family members to choose the winning posters. Offer prizes that can be donated by your consultants and vendors. Invite the winners to give poster presentations and offer participants continuing education credits. Ask the public relations department to take pictures of the activities and send an article to the local newspapers. This teaching method generates enthusiasm, teamwork, and publicity, and clearly articulates to everyone that successful pain management is the result of interdisciplinary involvement.

Portable Educational Cart

A mobile cart displaying fact sheets and equipment is another useful way to educate staff. Keep carts in an area for a specified amount of time allowing staff members to use the materials when time permits. Quizzes or self-learning modules can be given by the staff educator if validation is required. This is an easy way to impart information that does not require an explanation or discussion. Depending on where the cart is located, it can also be a good format for providing physicians, patients, and families with updated information about pain management. This activity clearly identifies that learning about pain control is everyone's responsibility.

Pain Management Bulletin Board

Employ an education bulletin board strategically placed in the facility where it is visible to everyone. The board can be used to post brochures about upcoming workshops, seminars, and programs on pain management. Post the facility's education calendar indicating the times and dates of all pain management programs. Include a spot on the bulletin board to place self-learning packets, updated articles and handouts, information on new policies and procedures, and flyers on special events related to pain management activities. This is a unique way to demonstrate to "customers" that pain management education is considered important.

OTHER EDUCATIONAL STRATEGIES

These strategies facilitate education that is system wide and promote public awareness about the institution's efforts to provide optimum pain management. It speaks loudly about the value of education to those who enter your doors.

Other methods of education can include lectures, case studies, videotapes, audiotapes, teleconferences, CD ROMs, grand rounds, skills labs, closed-circuit TV, panel discussions, seminars, and workshops. To keep educational costs at a minimum, ask members of your medical, nursing, and other professional staff who are knowledgeable about pain management to provide lectures to the staff. Videotaping the lectures is a cost-effective means of providing education to staff members who are unable to attend the presentations. Education of all staff members involved in the care of the patient is crucial for an effective pain management program. Institutions need to promote education for students involved in clinical care, and continuing education for practicing professionals to keep up with current trends and maintain their skills and competency. Knowledge about pain management empowers physicians, nurses, and other clinicians to assume their most important mission, the relief of pain and suffering.

DEVELOP A QUALITY IMPROVEMENT MONITORING PROCESS

JCAHO (1994) defines quality of care as "the degree to which health services for individuals and populations increase the likelihood of desired health outcomes and are consistent with current professional knowledge." Continuous quality improvement (CQI) is the key component that will help to demonstrate the pain program's benefit to the institution's mission. CQI is a process that ensures optimum pain control by building excellence into every aspect of care and creating an environment that encourages all disciplines to contribute to its success (Table 101.3). Monitoring pain management outcomes is an ongoing responsibility shared by members of the interdisciplinary team. Every organization must choose which processes and outcomes are important to monitor based on its mission and the scope of care and services provided

TABLE 101.3
Why Teamwork in Quality Improvement?

1. Instills ownership of the process
2. Involves the people who know best
3. Creates respect, cooperation, and openness
4. Breaks down barriers between departments
5. Spreads quality
6. "None of us is as smart as all of us"
- More ideas
- Better ideas

TABLE 101.4
JCAHO 10-Step Quality Monitoring Process

1. Assign responsibility
2. Delineate scope of service
3. Identify important aspects of service
4. Identify indicators related to the important aspects of service
5. Establish thresholds for evaluation
6. Collect and organize data
7. Evaluate service when indicated by the threshold
8. Take action when opportunities for improvement or problems are identified
9. Assess the effectiveness of actions
10. Communicate relevant information to the organization-wide program for continuous quality improvement

Note: From Joint Commission on Accreditation of Healthcare Organizations, 1991, Oakbrook Terrace, IL: JCAHO.

(JCAHO, 2003). JCAHO (1991) has designed a 10-step quality monitoring and evaluation process for health care agencies (Table 101.4). In that 10-step process, the first 5 steps establish the mechanism to be used for monitoring and evaluation, steps 6 and 7 encompass collection and evaluation of relevant data, and the last 3 steps reflect attempts to improve the provision of services rendered.

Performance monitoring and improvement are data driven. Institutions need to develop a formal process for evaluating the quality of pain management and collect data related to the needs, expectations, and satisfaction of the populations served. Simple ways of acquiring information from these groups include

- Periodic satisfaction surveys of patients and families including questions about pain intensity, pain relief goals, and staff responsiveness. Chart audits to assess documentation of pain assessments, patients' response to treatment, and teaching outcomes.
- Chart audits to monitor analgesic use and treatment side effects.

- Use focus groups to elicit feedback regarding pain management practices.
- Routinely schedule meetings with family members.

The detail and frequency of data collection are determined as appropriate for monitoring ongoing performance by the organization. Whenever possible, data collection should be incorporated into day-to-day activities. High-quality pain management is not a static destination to be reached, but a dynamic entity toward which clinicians must continually strive. Health care professionals must act on the basic belief that the patient is the reason for their practice.

CONCLUSION

The reward of a thing well done is to have done it.

— **Ralph Waldo Emerson**

Health care professionals must use their time, skills, and energy to transform their practice environments so that they support evidence-based pain management. It is crucial that quality pain management programs be integrated into all areas of the health care delivery system. Physicians, nurses, and other health care providers must convince patients and families that *pain can be relieved* and make pain control part of their clinical practice. Clinicians involved in a healing ministry must proactively promote optimum pain management, by interdisciplinary teams, who can enhance quality of life and diminish pain and suffering. Health care professionals, as patient advocates, must implement effective programs that spread evidence-based pain management throughout the organization and increase the team's capabilities to serve, to show compassion, and to help patients until the end-of-life.

REFERENCES

AHCPR, Acute Pain Management Guideline Panel. (1992, February). *Acute pain management: Operative or medical procedures and trauma, clinical practice guideline.* AHCPR Pub. No. 920032, Rockville, MD: Agency for Health Care Policy and Research, Public Health Service, U.S. Department of Health and Human Services.

Berry, P., & JCAHO. (1997). Pain management standards. *Cancer Pain Update Issue, 45*(2), 14.

Dahl, J. L. (1999). New JCAHO standards focus on pain management. *Oncology Issues, 14*(5), 27–28.

Ferrell, B., Dean, G., Grant, M., & Coluzzi, P. (1995). An institutional commitment to pain management. *Journal of Clinical Oncology, 13*, 2158–2165.

Ferrell, B. R., Grant, M., Ritchey, K. J. et al. (1993). The pain resource nurse training program: A unique approach to pain management. *Journal of Pain and Symptom Management, 8,* 549–556.

Gordon D. B., Dahl, J. L., & Stevenson, K. K. (1996). *Building an institutional commitment to pain management: The Wisconsin resource manual for improvement.* Madison: University of Wisconsin–Madison Board of Regents.

JCAHO, Joint Commission on Accreditation of Healthcare Organizations. (1991). *An introduction to Joint Commission nursing care standards.* Oakbrook Terrace, IL: Author.

JCAHO, Joint Commission on Accreditation of Healthcare Organizations. (1994). *Accreditation manual for hospitals* (Vol. 1). Oakbrook Terrace, IL: Author.

JCAHO, Joint Commission on Accreditation of Healthcare Organizations. (1999). Joint Commission focuses on pain management. Available online at http/www.jeaho.org/news.

JCAHO, Joint Commission on Accreditation of Healthcare Organizations, National Pharmaceutical Council, Inc. (2003). *Improving the quality of pain management through measurement and action.* Oakbrook Terrace, IL: Author.

Liebeskind, J. C., & Melzak, R. (1998). The International Pain Foundation: Meeting a need for education in pain management. *Journal of Pain and Symptom Management,* 131–132.

McCaffery, M., & Pasero, C. (1999). *Pain: Clinical manual* (2nd ed.). St. Louis, MO: Mosby.

NIH, National Institutes of Health Consensus Development Conference. (1987). The integrated approach to the management of pain. *Journal of Pain and Symptom Management, 2,* 35–44.

Peters, T. (1987). *Thriving on chaos.* New York: HarperCollins.

Saunders, C. (1984). *The management of terminal malignant disease* (2nd ed.). London: Edward Arnold.

Spross, J. (1994). Management of cancer pain: Commentary 2. *Abstracts of Clinical Care Guidelines, 6*(5), 4–6.

Spross, J. A. (2001). Harnessing power and passion: Lessons from pain management leaders and literature. *Innovations in End-of-Life Care, 3*(1), 4–6.

Ulschak, F. (1988). *Creating the future of health care education.* Chicago: American Hospital Publishing.

Weissman, D., Griffiem J., Gordon, D. B. et al. (1997). A role model program to promote institutional changes for pain management of acute and cancer pain. *Journal of Pain and Symptom Management, 14*(5), 274–279.

102

Interdisciplinary Pain Management Programs: The American Academy of Pain Management Model

Alexandra Campbell, PhD, and B. Eliot Cole, MD, MPA

PROMOTING EXCELLENCE IN INTERDISCIPLINARY PAIN MANAGEMENT: THE AAPM APPROACH

The American Academy of Pain Management (AAPM) was founded in 1988 as a nonprofit corporation by Drs. Richard and Kathryn Weiner (now Padgett). The Weiners' vision was that a professional membership organization, designed specifically to meet the educational and professional needs of clinicians in the emerging discipline of inter/multidisciplinary pain management, could best accomplish its goals by offering certification of professionals, continuing education, university-based specialty training, legislative advocacy, pain facility accreditation, and outcomes benchmarking of pain program success. By 2002, when Richard Weiner passed away, the AAPM had become the largest multidisciplinary pain practitioner membership organization in the nation with 6,000 members from many different professional disciplines including medical and osteopathic physicians, chiropractic physicians, podiatrists, dentists, psychologists, social workers, acupuncturists, clergy, nurses, pharmacists, physical and occupational therapists, rehabilitation counselors, massage therapists, and others.

As Richard Weiner (1993) stated:

> The multidisciplinary team approach, as it has evolved within the context of contemporary pain management, has the unique advantage of overlooking paradigmatic

blocks, turf barriers, and linear, restricted vision. The multidisciplinary pain management movement is the harbinger of integrated future health care. (p. 201)

The evidence supporting the clinical success and cost-effectiveness of the integrated multidisciplinary approach to pain management continues to mount (Flor, Fydrich, & Turk, 1992; Kee, Middaugh, Pawlick, & Nicholson, 1997), and the AAPM has demonstrated leadership in bringing this approach into the forefront of pain treatment strategies through its approach to pain program accreditation. See Chapter 100 for a detailed discussion of the multi/interdisciplinary approach to pain management.

MULTIDISCIPLINARY PRACTITIONER CREDENTIALING AND EDUCATION

Although not a requirement for pain program accreditation, the obtaining of credentialed status would be an asset to anyone directing or practicing in an interdisciplinary pain treatment program. Establishing a credentialing process was one of the AAPM's earliest goals. In 1991, 151 individuals sat for the first psychometrically validated credentialing exam, which was developed in cooperation with Applied Measurement Professionals. Credentialing by means of passing a specialty examination is a voluntary process that allows practitioners to attest to their commitment to excellence in pain management.

The AAPM credentialing examination covers the following areas: principles of anatomy and physiology; comprehensive patient assessment; developing and implementing an individual treatment plan and specific treatment modalities; education of patients, clinicians, regulators, and payers; professional, ethical, and legal practice; and outcomes measurement. Regardless of the area of professional expertise, multidisciplinary pain practitioners must have a wide range of knowledge about the entire field, including the practices of those from different disciplines. The examination is periodically updated by means of a job analysis to keep it current with the field of pain management, which is constantly evolving (American Academy of Pain Management, 1999). See Appendix C for more information about credentialing, including how to obtain a self-assessment examination to determine readiness to sit for the exam.

Continuing education is available at the AAPM annual clinical meeting and through other mechanisms. University-based postgraduate degrees and certificates in Pain Management are awarded by the AAPM-associated University of Integrated Studies. See Appendix D for more information regarding these services and programs.

PAIN PROGRAM ACCREDITATION

The April 1992 issue of the AAPM member newsletter (Weiner, 1992) announced the creation of a pain facility accreditation program. Numerous drafts of the accreditation application were scrutinized and refined by the contributions of many clinical and academic professionals through a survey of AAPM members conducted by College of Business and Public Administration, at Old Dominion University, the University of the Pacific School of Pharmacy, and the AAPM. At the same time, the creation of a National Pain Data Bank was announced for the collection and processing of pain management outcomes information. Credentialed pain professionals located across the country were recruited to receive training in the onsite facility review process. During the 1-day review process surveyors are dedicated to helping pain programs raise the bar for quality pain management.

The Joint Commission on Accreditation of Healthcare Organizations (JCAHO; 2001) adopted standards addressing pain assessment and treatment in 2001, and the Commission on Accreditation of Rehabilitation Facilities (CARF; 2003) also incorporates principles of the interdisciplinary approach to pain treatment in its pain program accreditation standards. JCAHO has published valuable resources on how to improve pain management activities in institutional settings (JCAHO, 2000, 2003). See Chapter 101 in this volume for more information on JCAHO and standards. While JCAHO accredits hospitals and CARF accredits multidisciplinary pain programs of a certain type, the AAPM provides accreditation both for large,

comprehensive multidisciplinary treatment programs and for pain management programs offered by smaller networks of solo practitioners and even for syndrome- or modality-oriented clinics.

The purpose of accreditation through the AAPM is to establish credibility for a pain program by demonstrating that patients receive appropriate services in a safe and effective fashion. Pain Program Accreditation (PPA) standards focus on an organization's ongoing business and personnel management, the physical plant (with an emphasis on safety), and the clinical services provided to patients. Much of the following material appears in the AAPM *Pain Program Accreditation Manual* (2001) and in three articles by Dr. Cole (1999a, 1999b, 1999c), which appeared in the AAPM member newsletter.

Two major distinctions are made in the PPA standards. There are *nonclinical standards* and *general clinical standards*, which must be met by all programs, and there are *classification-specific standards*, which must be met only by certain types of programs.

NONCLINICAL ACCREDITATION STANDARDS

There are five *nonclinical standards* concerning the organization's purpose and operation. These standards require a mission statement describing the purpose of the organization and the services available; written policies describing the types of patients served and/or the types of conditions addressed; specifically defined (even if broad) inclusion and exclusion criteria for services (not based on gender, race, color, creed, religion, or national origin, of course); patient education, informational, and marketing materials that truthfully describe the personnel, program, and services provided; and practitioners who possess the appropriate training and experience to provide quality treatment.

These standards are drawn from the AAPM Code of Ethics. The intent of the first five standards is to establish a commitment to pain management, to provide services in an ethical manner, and to provide services within a consistent model. When surveying a program, onsite reviewers actually look for the presence of a code of ethics and patient bill of rights (these may be adapted from the AAPM documents, see Appendices A and B); they read written policies about the services provided, patients or conditions treated; check the truthfulness of marketing and educational materials; check to see if there is evidence of appropriate training and experience for the program pain professionals (usually by reviewing curriculum vitae); and verify that the program director has the requisite skills to lead a multidisciplinary team. If appropriate, materials for special populations need to be made available to patients (e.g., non-English speaking, visually/hearing impaired). Since the Health Insurance Portability and Accountability Act of 1996 (HIPAA; Department of Health and Human Services, 2004) was signed into law and portions of this law became enforceable in April 2003 (Privacy Rule) and October 2003 (Transactions and Code Sets Rule), pain programs are now asked if they are in compliance HIPAA. The surveyor records the answer that is given by the facility and may look for Notice of Privacy Policies, but accreditation by the AAPM does *not* certify HIPAA compliance. All programs are expected to abide by any and all federal and state/local laws that apply to them. The AAPM provides all surveyed facilities with a written notice that it abides by HIPAA rules in its dealings with surveyed pain programs and will sign business associate contracts if necessary.

Five *nonclinical standards* are in place to assess the business practices of the program. These documentation standards require written administrative policies that are reviewed and updated annually, written patient care policies that are reviewed and updated annually, necessary legal documents to engage in practice; and proof of general liability insurance, and proof of professional liability insurance. Reviewers determine that the administrative and patient care policies for the day-to-day operation of the program are adequate, and then check for creation and review dates. Having a system in place to document that staff annually reviews policies and procedures is crucial, in addition to circulating and documenting review of any new policies and procedures that may be instituted between regular annual reviews. Surveyors check for current business licenses, certificates of occupancy, fire marshal inspection certificates, professional licenses, and similar documents. Numerous insurance certificates are screened for general liability, directors and officers insurance, and professional liability. The intent of this section is to determine if the pain program is operating lawfully and that adequate patient and staff safeguards exist. The exact content of the administrative and patient care policies is not mandated, to allow each unique program the opportunity to develop the policies needed to operate. Specific insurance limit recommendations are not made except for professional liability (recommend minimum: $500,000/$1,000,000). The reviewer takes into account local variations in the business climate that may affect the types and amounts of insurance policies maintained by the program and its personnel.

Personnel management standards require job-specific descriptions for employees and independent contractors; annual performance evaluations reflecting the job-specific descriptions; written personnel policy; and properly maintained personnel files demonstrating necessary education, experience, and skills required for work. Surveyors review personnel files to see if job-specific descriptions and annual reviews exist for all employees and independent contractors.

Surveyors determine that these descriptions have been updated within the past year. Job descriptions need to be current to accurately reflect current performance. Survey-ors review personnel files looking for up-to-date resumes or curriculum vitae, copies of licenses, documentation of training, and diplomas. To understand employee and employer expectations, surveyors read the program's personnel policy manual. Procedures for resolving grievances, dress codes, duty hours, and assignments are examples of what the surveyors looks for. Employee orientation to workplace regulations needs to be documented with the employees' signatures. Annual documentation of review of personnel policies by all employees is ideal.

Surveyors tour the building and all clinical treatment areas to make a determination about patient and staff safety. The physical plant standards require that the facility be safe for patients and staff by meeting applicable OSHA requirements; is compliant with local codes regarding access for challenged patients consistent with the Americans with Disabilities Act (ADA); has adequate ventilation and is maintained at a comfortable temperature; has written annually updated policies describing the proper handling of waste and the proper handling, storage, and disposal of medications, needles, and soiled linen; maintains electrical equipment free of obvious hazards; has emergency exits that are clearly marked and free of obstructions; has adequate regular and handicapped parking available; has an operating fire detection, warning, and suppression system; has written policies about fire drills and expected employee actions in the event of fire or other emergency situations (e.g., natural disaster, terrorist attack); and complies with local fire codes. Evidence that fire drills and other simulated emergency evacuations are carried out at least annually is important to have on file. Onsite reviewers must walk throughout the building to determine the overall level of cleanliness, ability of challenged patients to get around in the office, appropriateness of ventilation, and observance of policies about hazardous waste management. Reviewers are asked to imagine themselves in the office during different types of emergency situations including possible natural disasters or terrorist attacks. Could employees and patients exit the building without assistance? If they had challenges, could they still get out of the building? Because AAPM reviewers are not usually from the same town where the program is located, seeing a current fire marshal certificate or similar document usually resolves the issue about compliance with local fire codes. Reviewers want to see smoke detectors, fire extinguishers, and sprinkler systems if required by local codes. Reviewers do not test these items; they just determine if they are available.

Some may wonder why there are so many standards having little to do with actual patient care. These *nonclinical standards* have everything to do with ethical business practices; efficiency of practice; and the health, safety, and welfare of employees and patients. Standards have evolved over many years and have been tailored to meet the needs of pain practitioners in a wide variety of practice situations. While many are very specific, most require the judgment of the surveyor to determine compliance. It is the goal of the AAPM to improve the programs being surveyed and to provide consultative advice during the accreditation survey process. Rather than just question the programs and their staff, PPA surveyors strive to gradually raise the overall quality of pain management services in the United States through a collegial process.

GENERAL CLINICAL ACCREDITATION STANDARDS

The National Institutes of Health (NIH) Consensus Conference entitled, "The Integrated Approach to the Management of Pain" (1986), concluded that while there are a multitude of pharmacological and nonpharmacological treatment approaches for pain, "no single treatment modality is appropriate for all or even for most individuals suffering from pain" (p. 12). Hence, the AAPM's program standards do not dictate which specific modalities must be present in a treatment program. Typically, however, multi/interdisciplinary approaches usually incorporate pharmacological, psychological/behavioral, and physical/rehabilitative components with interventional/surgical and complementary non-allopathic methods (such as acupuncture and massage) possibly being present as well (National Pharmaceutical Council, 2001). Many published clinical guidelines exist that outline the standards of care for acute and chronic pain management. These should be consulted and new publications should be monitored so that appropriate clinical practice standards can be maintained over the years that a pain program is in operation. McCaffery and Pasero (1999) have updated their extremely useful nursing education manual that discusses the mechanisms, assessment, and pharmacological and nonpharmacological treatment of all types of acute and chronic pain problems in adults, infants, and the elderly population, and during pregnancy and childbirth. Also see Chapters 101 and 103 in this volume for more information on implementing and running a pain management program.

Marketdata Enterprises (2003), in its survey of the most commonly used techniques for the treatment of chronic pain, noted a somewhat disturbing trend: the use of nerve blocks increased from 79% of pain practices surveyed in 2001 to 82% in 2003, while physical therapy use dropped from 85% in 2001 to 71% of programs in 2003. The multidisciplinary approach also declined in use from 81% of programs in 2001 to 77% in 2003. This occurred despite the evidence that questions the efficacy of interventionalist strategies and that supports the use of the multidisciplinary approach (Clark, 2000; Okifuji & Turk, 1998; Turk & Okifuji, 1997, 1998), especially where long-standing chronic pain of uncertain pathophysiology is present. Reasons for this alarming reversal of the trend

to establish multi/interdisciplinary pain care include reimbursement issues and economic pressures.

General clinical standards address the core elements of patient care necessary for all pain programs. During an onsite inspection for Pain Program Accreditation, after touring the facility and addressing the nonclinical issues, the reviewer focuses on the scope and quality of care being provided. Reviewers will want to know the schedule of team meetings, and usually staff tries to schedule a meeting for the day of the survey so that the reviewer can observe the team in action and interview each treatment provider and administrative person briefly and informally to get a sense of how they view the workings of the program. Meeting and individually speaking with the treatment team members gives the surveyor a chance to assess how the program actually works on a day to day basis. Sometimes staff will provide useful feedback for improving the program that they have not yet had a chance to communicate to management. The surveyor can then give the suggestions for change to upper management during the out-briefing at the end of the survey day.

Chart review is another crucial element in program evaluation. The reviewer needs to examine a sufficient number of clinical records to adequately address the 20 general clinical standards. Usually, at least 10 randomly chosen clinical records, representing both open and closed cases, are reviewed to answer the questions raised in the general clinical standards. If full compliance with the general clinical standards is not immediately evident, the reviewer examines 5 additional records (or more) to resolve the concerns. Reviewers may ask the facility representative to show them where in the chart necessary documentation exists demonstrating how the program is able to meet the general clinical standards. Reviewers note how many of the charts they review are in compliance with the standards and how many are missing required elements.

Necessary elements of the chart include the presence of a well-documented presenting problem with a thorough history and physical. If this has been done by the referring physician, with a more focused assessment done upon admission to the pain program, a copy of the more thorough examination report needs to be obtained by the program.

The needs of the whole patient should be addressed during the initial assessment process through adequate documentation of functional and psychosocial status. Patient interviews, exams, diagnostic laboratory tests, and scores on validated psychosocial assessment instruments should be used to develop a multidimensional conceptualization of the biopsychosocial processes that are contributing to the patient's pain problem. Individualized assessments by providers from different disciplines (when indicated) need to be clearly formulated with working diagnoses and signed notes. Initial therapeutic goals should be formulated in clearly behavioral and specific terms with a treatment plan that the patient agrees to and signs. (AAPM provides examples of controlled substance agreements, pharmacy agreements, and treatment attestation forms to help protect prescribing physicians on its Web site.) Over time, charting should reflect progress toward these goals and/or adjustment of the goals themselves. At admission, a discharge plan with measurable goals should be formulated so that progress can be assessed more objectively. Expected timeframes for improvement and the method for evaluating treatment progress should be clearly spelled out from the beginning of treatment.

All charts need to contain an area for consultations, reports, and results of laboratory tests in addition to ongoing treatment notes from all treatment providers that discuss the relevant clinical information. Written evidence that the different treatment providers both within and from outside the facility (as when referrals are made) communicate with each other is a critical charting element. Particularly when invasive procedures are used, documentation of pain levels pre- and post-procedure through the use of a verbal or numerical rating scale provides basic outcomes information. A discharge summary documents the patients' strengths and weaknesses at the time when the bulk of treatment has been delivered and describes any specific limitations and recommendations for activity levels, employment, diet, etc. Referrals to appropriate aftercare or follow-up services should be documented. Some programs follow patients indefinitely and do not have clear discharge dates. If patients continue to be seen on a maintenance follow-up basis (for example, to prevent relapse of chronic pain behaviors), this needs to be appropriately documented as well. Sometimes individuals are designated as "program" patients during an initial period of more intensive interdisciplinary treatment, and later, after a significant portion of the expected degree of improvement in pain and functioning has been accomplished, converted to "clinic" patient status for follow-up medication management or cognitive-behavioral "booster" individual or support group sessions.

The presence of a general informed consent for the patient to be treated in the program, in addition to specific consents for individual procedures, may be useful, especially for the legal protection of the program. This general consent covers the patient who is going through the evaluation process and may have to attend several appointments before a complete treatment plan is generated and begun. It is also necessary to have unique consent forms for every type of invasive/surgical procedure patients may receive that name the procedure, note the person performing the procedure, and state that no specific guarantees are being made to the patient about the outcome of the procedure. The patient's name should appear on the consent form and the patient's signature confirms that the

patient has been informed of the common risks and benefits of the procedure and has been informed of any treatment alternatives that may be available, and that all of the patient's questions regarding the procedure have been answered to the patient's satisfaction. AAPM recommends that all of a patient's questions and the answers given be documented in order to provide extra legal protection for treatment providers. The patient needs to be further informed that consent may be revoked at any time.

Medical releases of information should be specific regarding the purpose of the disclosure and time-limited, with separate releases (even if on the same form) for treatment-related information pertaining to mental health services, substance abuse treatment information, and HIV status.

Printed patient materials that explain financial responsibilities and how third-party payers are handled can be helpful in making billing policies clear, especially for those programs where self-payment may constitute a significant proportion of program revenues.

Provision needs to be made for the secure storage of medical records, preferably in a centralized location. Access to the records needs to be restricted to appropriate staff, and there should be a designated person who is responsible for maintaining and securing the medical records on a continuous basis. HIPAA guidelines give specific recommendations for record security and these must be followed.

The importance of having a practical, consistent format for the organization of the medical chart cannot be underestimated. The medical record basically "tells the story" of the patient's journey through the treatment program, and it should be able to be "read" by the surveyor with little or no direction from staff. Clearly labeled chart tab dividers that separate elements of the chart are commonly used. A system for alerting providers to the presence of any known allergies should be conspicuous. An alert sticker can be placed on the outside of the chart, with the specific allergies listed on the inside cover, in line with health information privacy requirements.

The chart review is not intended to be a draconian process. It is a practical review of treatment records, looking for the elements necessary to accomplish the assessment, complete evaluation, and appropriate treatment of the patient with pain. Obtaining informed consent and permission to release medical records to outside entities, and establishing goals for treatment with the patient are required elements for any successful program.

Several accreditation standards cannot usually be answered in the clinical records, but can be resolved through the examination of other materials. Specialized treatment equipment and all necessary emergency equipment need to be regularly checked and certified by the appropriate state or local authority. Documentation of the certifications may be kept in an easily accessible log book.

The 510k documents for certain medical devices must also be on file. Documentation that staff has the ongoing training necessary to operate the equipment is necessary (this may be accomplished through training logs and training certificates kept in personnel files).

The final general clinical standard that is applicable to all pain programs addresses the need for the facility to be utilizing some type of outcomes measurement strategy. As this is such an important topic, it is covered thoroughly below.

CLASSIFICATION-SPECIFIC ACCREDITATION STANDARDS

The unique standards for each of the distinct classification types of pain programs are now discussed. To explain the need for the *classification-specific standards* a review of the AAPM organizational history regarding accreditation is in order.

Many years ago the leadership of the AAPM decided to offer program accreditation to all types and sizes of pain programs using different designations depending on the type and scope of services offered. It was determined not to be in the interest of the field of pain management, or to the patients served, to exclude any program that was interested in becoming accredited. Instead of accrediting only the larger university- and hospital-based programs, the AAPM developed a methodology to allow all pain programs to apply for accreditation, whether they were inpatient or outpatient in focus, large or small, or involved just a single practitioner, syndrome, or treatment modality. To meet the diverse needs of the AAPM membership and to be able to provide patient safeguards through the accreditation process, six types of pain programs were identified: major comprehensive multidisciplinary, comprehensive, small and network multidisciplinary, and syndrome and modality oriented (International Association for the Study of Pain, 1990). IASP, definitions for pain center classifications are somewhat different from those of the AAPM.)

Each classification of pain program had specific standards developed. The most detailed standards were written for the three largest and most complex types of programs. For the smaller, less-formalized programs, realistic standards were written to motivate solo practitioners and practitioners in syndrome- or modality-oriented programs to address the multidisciplinary needs of patients. A detailed definition of each type of program classification follows.

- Major comprehensive multidisciplinary pain program: Manages various types of painful conditions, conducts education/research programs, and involves a minimum of six disciplines operating within the same organization.

- Comprehensive multidisciplinary pain program: Manages various types of painful conditions, may conduct educational or research programs, and involves a minimum of four disciplines operating within the same organization.
- Small multidisciplinary pain program: Manages various types of pain conditions and involves a minimum of two disciplines operating within the same organization.
- Network multidisciplinary pain program: Generally involves a solo practitioner or group of clinicians all of the same discipline who manage various types of pain conditions by utilizing a network of closely coordinated independent professionals of varying disciplines.
- Syndrome-oriented pain program: Manages a single type of pain syndrome (e.g., back pain, complex regional pain syndrome, headache, temporomandibular joint dysfunction) utilizing one or more clinicians of the same or different disciplines.
- Modality-oriented pain program: Manages one or more pain syndromes by utilizing a single modality (e.g., acupuncture, biofeedback, counseling, hypnosis, nerve blocks, or transcutaneous electrical nerve stimulation).

Unlike the Commission on Accreditation of Rehabilitation Facilities (2003), which requires that all accredited programs have a board-certified medical director and a psychologist on staff, the AAPM system allows for programs that may be headed by a qualified multidisciplinary pain practitioner from other disciplines. The AAPM will accredit smaller syndrome- or modality-oriented programs as long as the treatment philosophy of the multi/interdisciplinary approach can be shown to be approximated through appropriate consultation and referral.

MAJOR COMPREHENSIVE, COMPREHENSIVE, AND SMALL MULTIDISCIPLINARY CLINICAL ACCREDITATION STANDARDS

Major comprehensive, comprehensive, and small multidisciplinary programs have the same *classification-specific standards*. Organizational requirements address the purpose and business structure of these larger programs. Documentation of the structure of the governing body, usually in the form of a clear organizational chart, is very helpful to the surveyor as he or she needs to quickly grasp the lines of communication and authority that exist. This chart should be made available to key employees as well. Minutes of the governing body's meetings should be kept as well as written policy that describes how authority is delegated throughout the organization. Documentation demonstrating commitment to principles of ethical leadership, how policies are determined, and institutional commitment to high-quality patient care are minimal elements the surveyor will want to ascertain are in place through discussion or viewing of relevant documents. Corporations need to have a written job description for the chief executive officer (CEO) detailing the authority and responsibilities delegated to the CEO by the governing body. The CEO should be evaluated on job performance annually by the governing body.

Documentation of the business operations of the larger multidisciplinary programs needs to show that the financial affairs of the organization are managed on the basis of an annual budget that is approved by the governing body. Evidence of adequate communication between key administrative staff members should be present and may take the form of interoffice memoranda or e-mail, for example.

Clinical operations of large multidisciplinary programs can be complex, but if well-thought-out policies and procedures are in place and are clear to all staff, even the largest programs can operate quite smoothly and efficiently. During the onsite survey, the reviewer will want access to written documentation that identifies a case manager for every client/patient to coordinate true interdisciplinary care. Some programs use a patient-care coordinator instead of a nurse case manager, and of course there is flexibility with this and other of the clinical standards. What is necessary is that the program has an effective way of accomplishing its mission to provide integrated patient care and that this is clear to the reviewer. Chart notes reflecting that all patients are properly oriented to the program need to be in evidence in addition to documentation of a coordinated team-approach to treatment.

Documentation of meetings and case management chart notes indicating how treatment goals are updated and modified by the team and communicated to the patient (with their input and agreement) must be present. Staffings need to take place not less than weekly for clients in daily treatment programs. The case manager is responsible for ensuring that the necessary communication between practitioners takes place, and there needs to be a provider designated to make any final treatment decisions especially when there is disagreement between practitioners about how to proceed. Documentation needs to show that care is coordinated. Case conferences need to address goal setting, discharge planning, ongoing patient care, and modifications to the treatment plan. The tracking and modifying of goals with patient input needs to be obvious in the chart. The case manager (or another designee) is also responsible for ensuring appropriate and timely communication between the program and the patient's employer if necessary, with accurate and timely documentation of these contacts and any work-related goals present in the chart. The final duty of the case manager (or other designee) is to ensure that adequate plans are made for discharge. Follow-up appointments, any home-based services needed, along with recommen-

dations and limitations should be documented and present in the discharge summary.

As mentioned above in the section on *nonclinical* accreditation standards, if a major comprehensive, comprehensive, or small multidisciplinary program utilizes regular consultants or independent contractors to accomplish any treatment components, written agreements between the program director and the consultants/contractors that describe the specific duties and responsibilities of the nonstaff team members should be present. A length of time that the agreement is in effect should be specified so that the agreement can be reviewed and updated regularly. A personnel file should include this agreement, a copy of the consultant/contractor's license to practice, and any other documentation necessary (e.g., Drug Enforcement Administration certificate, pharmacy registration) for practice in addition to evidence of malpractice insurance in adequate amounts. An annual performance review for the independent contractor or consultant will help ensure that high standards of care are being upheld and will alert management when there is a need to consider altering or ending the relationship.

NETWORK MULTIDISCIPLINARY CLINICAL ACCREDITATION STANDARDS

Network multidisciplinary programs involve groups of independent practitioners working together to provide interdisciplinary care. In most instances, leadership for a network multidisciplinary program is provided by a solo-practice clinician. This clinician often carries the dual responsibilities of administration and patient care. It is desirable for network multidisciplinary pain program services to be provided by a coordinated interdisciplinary team; however, it is not required that the program actually employ all of the treatment team members. In most network multidisciplinary pain programs, it is common that the other team members are serving as consultants to, or independent contractors for, the primary practitioner providing care. Hence, the standard regarding personnel management for independent contractors described above applies to this type of program as well.

Organizational and business operation standards for network multidisciplinary and syndrome- or modality-oriented programs are quite similar and are in place to ensure adequate documentation of the governing body or owner/operator's policies and procedures regarding delegation of authority, commitment to ethical leadership, establishment of policy, and maintenance of high quality patient care. The governing body or person should operate with an annual budget, and communication needs to be adequate between the treatment team members and support staff (usually through documented phone contact, e-mail, and interoffice memoranda).

Clinical standards include documentation of patient orientation, and most importantly, there should be at least monthly treatment conferences (weekly, if possible) attended by team members caring for active patients engaged in regular (possibly daily) treatment. As this ideal is not always attainable when practitioners do not work in close proximity with each other, phone contact and other means of communication and records sharing may sometimes have to suffice. Network multidisciplinary programs have to be able to show the reviewer that communication between team members and the documentation of this communication is sufficient to provide truly integrated care. Patients may or may not be involved in the team meetings, and the documentation of the team meetings should be the responsibility of a designated staff member. The chart needs to show that individual case management reflects input from the team members and the patient regarding goal setting, discharge planning, patient education, and the modification of goals as treatment progresses.

SYNDROME- AND MODALITY-ORIENTED CLINICAL ACCREDITATION STANDARDS

Syndrome- or modality-oriented pain programs are also usually operated by a solo practice clinician, carrying the dual responsibilities of administration and patient care. With respect to patient care, the clinician carries the responsibility for obtaining consultations or referrals when services required by the patient are outside the scope of the clinician's training and experience, and for coordinating these referrals and consultations to effect, as much as possible, a multi/interdisciplinary treatment approach. Again, in terms of personnel management, consultant agreements are a critical component for the success of this type of program and allow for owner/operator monitoring and quality control.

The syndrome- and modality-oriented program standards covering organization, business practices, and clinical operations are similar to those discussed in the section above for network multidisciplinary programs. In addition, there needs to be evidence that the primary treatment provider makes the necessary referrals and/or seeks consultation when it is clear from the assessment that the patient will benefit from integrated multidisciplinary pain management services outside the scope of training of the primary provider. There should be close communication between the primary provider and any outside consultants and treating providers. This communication must be evident in the medical record, especially in terms of setting and modifying treatment goals.

OUTCOMES MEASUREMENT AND PERFORMANCE IMPROVEMENT

Defining, measuring, and disseminating relevant treatment outcomes information is something even the smallest pain

program must do in order to remain viable in today's health care climate of increased demand for evidence-based practice and cost-containment accountability. Patients, payers, and providers are all stakeholders in the pain management process and are looking for results in terms of the outcomes variables that are important to them. Reduced pain, functional recovery, reduced need for medication, improved quality of life, and patient satisfaction with treatment are important to patients and providers. Providers, employers, and insurance companies are interested in functional rehabilitation (as evidenced by return to work) and containing the cost of treatment (as evidenced by settled disability claims and reduced health care utilization) (Okifuji & Turk, 1998). Every pain management program needs to use outcomes measurement to improve performance and address the needs of stakeholders or risk becoming obsolete as competing providers are able to prove their worth. Both JCAHO and CARF have outcomes measurement requirements for the hospitals and pain programs they accredit. *The Wisconsin Resource Manual* (Gordon, Dahl, & Stevenson, 2000), entitled *Building an Institutional Commitment to Pain Management,* outlines the steps necessary to improve pain management in different types of health care settings based on guidelines published by the Agency for Healthcare Research and Quality (1994) and the American Pain Society (1995).

Because the AAPM accredits different classifications of pain programs, the requirement for outcomes measurement must be realistically assessed in the context of the type of program being reviewed. The goal of adequately assessing treatment success and using the information gained through tracking outcomes to affect treatment quality is best viewed as a being on a continuum ranging from the use of a comprehensive multidimensional outcomes assessment instrument, such as the National Pain Data Bank, which only the larger, comprehensive multidisciplinary pain management programs may have the financial resources and workforce available to employ, to the simple use of a Numerical Rating Scale or Visual Analogue Scale (VAS) of pain intensity obtained whenever the patient is seen or before and after invasive procedures, which even the smallest program can be expected to have minimally in place. The AAPM goal is to help all pain programs raise the bar for quality care through improving and effectively utilizing outcomes assessment tools and techniques. The information gained must be useful to all stakeholders including patients, providers, and payers and be presented in a clear, concise, understandable format.

In spite of the obvious need for outcomes research in order for pain programs to stay in business, the market survey of chronic pain management programs cited above (Marketdata Enterprises, 2003) contained a shocking finding. The number of pain programs that claimed they could document outcomes data declined since 2001 from 67 to 59% in 2003. The authors stated that the main reason for the decline may be due to the increase in number of solo anesthesiologists practicing pain management. Although 87% of true multidisciplinary pain programs could document outcomes in 2003, only 40% of anesthesia-based modality-oriented programs could. This represents a decline from 1999 when fully 77% of all pain programs surveyed reported that they could document outcomes data. This trend must be reversed for the field of pain management to remain at the forefront of the integrated health care movement and to continue in its leadership role for the rest of the health care industry. See Chapter 9 for a more in-depth discussion of the importance of quality assurance and outcomes measurement in pain management.

THE NATIONAL PAIN DATA BANK

In response to the different service delivery models current in the field of pain management, the AAPM has created outcomes measurement tools that can fit the needs of different types of pain programs. Much of the following information appears in the AAPM *Pain Outcomes Profile Instruction Manual* (2004). The AAPM created the National Pain Data Bank (NPDB) outcomes measurement system in the early 1990s, as national policy makers began insisting on the use of standardized outcomes measurement approaches to assess the quality of health care. Outcomes measurement was made a requirement for the AAPM Pain Program Accreditation in 1992, and by the end of 2002 the NPDB had collected data from approximately 100 pain management programs and tracked more than 13,000 patients. The purpose of the data bank was to provide comparison benchmarks for successful treatment outcomes that could be used by the solo practitioner as well as by the large multidisciplinary treatment program. The NPDB became an important tool in helping pain management programs comply with pain outcomes measurement standards imposed by national accrediting agencies (Cole, 2000).

The NPDB measurement system consists of three separate questionnaires that a patient completes at intake, discharge, and follow-up. In addition to subscale and total scores, narrative reports may be generated at intake giving a summary description of the patient's pattern of responding on crucial dimensions of the pain experience including pain intensity, functional status, and emotional health. These are three domains recognized as crucial in determining outcomes by the IASP. Other important outcomes data such as disability status, medical resource utilization, patient satisfaction, diagnosis, and treatment modalities used are included in the NPDB questionnaires, making it a complete outcomes measurement system. Subscribing pain programs collect data and submit the data on diskette to the AAPM. Quarterly reports are generated comparing

the performance of programs that are similar in size and in the scope of treatments offered.

With the help of Applied Measurement Professionals, the University of California at San Diego, and the Department of Veterans Affairs, several reliability and validity studies were carried out demonstrating adequate psychometric properties of select subscales of the NPDB questionnaires (Clark & Gironda, 2000; Gironda, Azzarello, & Clark, 2002). One drawback to the use of the NPDB is its length. Some smaller pain programs and solo practitioners have found it challenging to allocate the staff for its proper administration, while others have been limited by budgetary constraints. Use of the NPDB was mandatory for Pain Program Accreditation in the past; however, it is no longer required. Accredited programs may create their own outcomes measurement systems. The NPDB remains a helpful tool for larger pain programs and institutions dedicated to clinical research. A modified, somewhat shorter, Web-based version of the NPDB may be available in the future. As discussed above, the decline in the number of practitioners who are incorporating outcomes measures in their pain practices may be due to a lack of clinically useful, validated, brief outcomes measures. The AAPM responded to the need for a brief measure by continuing to work with psychologists at the Tampa Veteran's Hospital.

THE PAIN OUTCOMES PROFILE

Further psychometric analysis of items from the NPDB allowed Drs. Clark, Gironda, and Young, Jr., at the Tampa Veteran's Hospital, to determine which ones had the greatest psychometric strength. They eliminated weaker items and added several new questions to create a brief pain outcomes measurement instrument that the AAPM (2004) has published under the name "Pain Outcomes Profile" (POP). The Veteran's Hospital version is called the Pain Outcomes Questionnaire–VA Short Form.

The POP is a 23-item self-report questionnaire that uses 11-point, 0 to 10, numerical rating scales to assess a number of relevant dimensions in the patient's pain experience. The POP assesses three domains of a patient's pain experience: pain perception, perceived physical impairment due to pain, and several aspects of emotional functioning. These domains are assessed using two pain intensity scales, three self-report of functional impairment scales, and two scales that address self-reported emotional functioning (seven scales total).

The POP includes 19 items that are identical to the primary pain outcomes items that appear on the POQ–VA Short Form. However, the POP contains two numerical rating scales to assess the patient's experience of pain intensity *right now* and *pain on the average during the last week*. The POQ–VA Short Form contains only one rating of *pain intensity on average during the last week*.

The POP includes the *pain right now* item as it is believed to have clinical utility. Also, in finalizing the POP, the order of the items on the instrument was rearranged so that questions from the different content scales appear in a counterbalanced fashion.

There are three scales in the domain of perceived functional impairment due to pain: Mobility, Activities of Daily Living (ADLs), and Vitality. The Mobility scale contains four items that rate a patient's perception of pain-related interference with the ability to walk, carry or handle everyday objects, and climb stairs, and whether pain requires the use of assistive devices (e.g., a walking aid or wheelchair). ADLs are assessed with four items that inquire about pain-related interference with the ability to bathe, dress, use the bathroom, and manage personal grooming. The patient's subjective feeling of a lack of Vitality is assessed with three items rating the ability to perform physical activities, feelings of overall energy, and strength and endurance. Self-reported emotional functioning is assessed with two scales. The Negative Affect scale contains five items asking the patient to rate the degree to which pain affects self-esteem, feelings of depression, feelings of anxiety, ability to concentrate, and feelings of subjective tension. The Fear scale contains two items that rate how much worry is experienced about reinjury due to increasing activity and feelings of safety exercising.

The POP can be quickly scored and a cumulative patient scoring record can be placed in the chart. This form allows for tracking of POP scale scores across repeated administrations of the measure (e.g., at intake, several times during active treatment, at discharge).

Although not a complete outcomes measurement system, the POP does provide for the assessment of seven core functional pain outcomes domains that are of interest to patients, providers, and payers. Other important outcomes that should be assessed include patient satisfaction, disability/litigation status, and medical resource utilization.

POP scores and scores on these other important outcomes variables can be placed into a computer database. Program staff should be able to perform at least basic tabulations of scores from the beginning to the end of treatment. Benchmarking outcomes against its own previous performance can at least give a pain program a sense of whether quality improvement is occurring over time.

Clark, Gironda, and Young (2003) trace the development of the final brief pain outcomes questionnaire in the 5-year, cooperative VA–AAPM project that originated with the NPDB long forms. They conclude that the new instrument is reliable, valid, and clinically useful in evaluating the effectiveness of treatment for veterans experiencing chronic noncancer pain. When comparing results from the POQ–VA Short Form and the POP for research purposes, it is important to examine only the 19 items that

the two instruments share. Additional research needs to be completed to validate the measure in different populations of patients with various types of pain diagnoses. The future of multidisciplinary pain management depends on the ability to provide the best combination of treatments for the proper duration and intensity to obtain the most cost-effective results with the appropriate patients (Chapman, 2000). The AAPM is currently partnering with several independent pain programs across the country, gathering data to further document the psychometric properties of the POP, to establish norms with different patient samples, and to help programs using the POP document and publish treatment successes. Also, the POP has been translated into Spanish and is available for field-testing and research with a Spanish-speaking population.

With the coming shift toward a "person-centered" health system (Foundation for Accountability, 2003), we hope the 21st century will see a much better educated public taking a greater role in health care decisions, practicing more effective health maintenance behaviors, and gaining a better understanding of health care financing. As patients become savvier in terms of managing their personal health information, they will begin to demand access to quality ratings of different treatment modalities based on evidence for all health conditions, not just chronic or acute pain. Somewhat akin to how *Consumer Reports* magazine publishes ratings and information regarding quality of all kinds of products for the general public, agencies responsible for maintaining standards in health care (such as the Agency for Healthcare Research and Quality) may eventually publish treatment success/cost-effectiveness information designed for the general public concerning treatments for many illnesses and disease conditions. To put it more bluntly, the need and demand for outcomes data for pain management programs of all stripes will not go away anytime soon! If anything, the need to appropriately disseminate quality information will only increase, and this information will need to be presented in different formats for different consumer groups (e.g., the lay public, payers, and health care professionals). Performance improvement and clinical outcomes research should go hand in hand. Pain practitioners need to design performance improvement projects that will lead to publication of articles in peer-reviewed journals so that the evidence base for successful multidisciplinary pain management can continue to grow. These articles can then be summarized in language appropriate for the general public and be published in relevant consumer health publications. Funding for these activities will no doubt be problematic, but strategic research partnerships between membership organizations such as the AAPM and its accredited programs may lead the way.

STEPS TO GAINING AAPM PAIN PROGRAM ACCREDITATION

A PPA brochure, manual order form, and articles describing the standards can be found on the AAPM Web site at www.aapainmanage.org. Once the decision is made to become accredited (after the program has been in operation for at least 6 months), the program director/manager completes the self-assessment found in the manual to see which areas of business, clinical, or personnel operations meet the AAPM standards already and which need to be improved before submitting the application. Facilities are encouraged to contact the Pain Program Accreditation Director with any questions or concerns during the application process for clarification. The mission of the AAPM is to come alongside each program and help the program to raise the bar for quality pain management through the consultative accreditation process. The application and self-assessment are submitted (in duplicate) with the appropriate fees along with the required program documents (also in duplicate). These consist of the patient history and physical exam forms used, consent for treatment forms (invasive procedure and/or general treatment), program description, mission statement, patient education materials and program brochures, code of ethics and bill of patient rights (both of which can be easily adapted from the AAPM documents), release of information forms, current research protocols (if any), and copies of outcome measurement and patient satisfaction tools. Resumes or curriculum vitae for all licensed professionals and clerical or support staff members that have patient contact are also requested.

Once the completed application and supporting documents have been received and processed, a surveyor is selected by the Pain Program Accreditation Director, usually near the facility in terms of geographical area. The AAPM has a highly skilled group of accomplished clinician–surveyors whose goal it is to provide expert consultative services during the 1-day review. The surveyor examines all program documents, previous accreditation reports, and resumes before the actual onsite review, thus saving valuable consultation time.

Each pain program accredited by the AAPM must pass all of the *general standards* and one of the sets of *classification-specific standards*. The period of accreditation is for 3 years if all of the standards for accreditation are met. If there are any standards not found to be in compliance, remediation is attempted immediately to bring the program into compliance. If this cannot be accomplished fairly quickly, these programs are likely to receive a 1-year provisional status. To then become fully accredited for 3 years, these provisional programs must have a second (abbreviated) onsite survey and demonstrate full compliance with the accreditation standards. Over the years that the AAPM PPA service has been available, revisions of the pain program standards and changes in the specific items surveyors are to note during their visits to pain programs have improved the overall accreditation process. The process of accreditation has become much more objective. Along with practitioner credentialing and outcomes measurement, program accreditation provides pain practitioners with another link in the "quality" pain management chain.

FUTURE CHANGES AND ADDITIONS TO PPA STANDARDS

The AAPM accreditation manual is periodically updated and revised in response to advancements in the field of pain management and new legal and ethical requirements that arise. Some areas for future revision may include

- Critical incident reporting-medication errors, equipment-related and other patient or staff injuries, incidents of workplace violence, etc.
- Corporate compliance
- Consumer involvement in performance improvement and outcomes measurement activities
- Better dissemination of outcomes data and incorporation of data into patient education materials
- Internet service security and accessibility standards
- Grievance policies for clients
- Background checks for personnel
- External financial audits
- Risk management policies and procedures

THE VALUE OF PAIN PROGRAM ACCREDITATION

Voluntary accreditation through the AAPM demonstrates to peers, payers, and patients that the pain program has submitted to rigorous scrutiny of its policies and procedures, clinical, business, and personnel practices; has met peer-established quality standards; and is committed to excellent patient care and continuous performance improvement.

In addition to the invaluable consultation that takes place during the survey process, all accredited pain programs receive an engraved plaque for display in the facility and use of the AAPM accredited pain program logo for marketing efforts. Each facility is listed on the AAPM Web site with a detailed program description and photographs of the facility and staff. The AAPM receives many calls per week directly from patients seeking treatment, and while not able to provide direct referrals, AAPM staff does direct people to its Web site to view listings of accredited pain programs and credentialed members. A link directly to the accredited facility's own Web site can also be created if appropriate. If requested, a press release printed on AAPM letterhead will be provided to any accredited program. Programs are invited to submit updated information to the Pain Program Accreditation Director for periodic new press releases. Assistance creating clinical forms, policies, and procedures and for choosing outcomes measures is also freely given.

Future services include the availability of the Pain Outcomes Profile Plus, a computer version of the POP that gives the user instant access to individual patient data graphically displayed, which can be transferred to statistical analysis software for program-wide outcomes assessment. This computer software will also include a module that will enable physicians to document controlled substance prescribing and relevant patient treatment parameters. Other future services may include an Internet forum for accredited program staff members to provide a mechanism for networking and the sharing of information to improve pain management practices, a periodic e-newsletter for program directors/managers and staff, policies and procedures manuals (general or tailored to an individual pain program's needs), topical Web-based articles addressing such issues as practitioner burnout and patient drug-seeking behavior, downloadable examples of excellent chart documents (e.g., discharge summaries), and marketing assistance such as downloadable patient information and education brochures that increase consumer understanding regarding the benefits of seeking treatment at an AAPM-accredited facility.

The AAPM remains committed to being an invaluable resource to multidisciplinary pain practitioners and seeks to be responsive to its members' needs. Contact AAPM at 13947 Mono Way, Suite A, Sonora, CA 95370, (209) 533-9744, to learn more about the many services and tools available to multidisciplinary pain practitioners including accreditation, credentialing, education, and outcomes measurement, and to have your questions and concerns addressed.

REFERENCES

Agency for Healthcare Research and Quality. (1994). *Management of cancer pain.* AHRQ Publication No. 94-0592. Rockville, MD: U.S. Department of Health and Human Services.

American Academy of Pain Management. (1999). *Self-assessment examination.* Sonora, CA: Author.

American Academy of Pain Management. (2001). *Pain program accreditation manual* (7th ed.). Sonora, CA: Author.

American Academy of Pain Management. (2004). *Pain outcomes profile: Instruction manual.* Sonora, CA: Author.

American Pain Society. (1995). Quality improvement guidelines for the treatment of acute and cancer pain, *Journal of the American Medical Association, 274*(3), 1874.

Chapman, S. L. (2000). Chronic pain rehabilitation: Lost in a sea of drugs and procedures? [Electronic version]. *APS Bulletin, 10*(3).

Clark, M. E., & Gironda, R. J. (2000). Concurrent validity of the National Pain Data Bank: Preliminary results. *American Journal of Pain Management, 10,* 25.

Clark, M. E., Gironda, R. J., & Young, R. W., Jr. (2003). Development and validation of the Pain Outcomes Questionnaire-VA [Electronic version]. *Journal of Rehabilitation Research and Development, 40*(5), 381.

Clark, T. S. (2000). Interdisciplinary treatment for chronic pain: Is it worth the money? *Baylor University Medical Center Proceedings, 13,* 240.

Cole, B. E. (1999a). Pain program accreditation: New accreditation standards. Part one: Non-clinical accreditation standards. *Pain Practitioner, 9*(1), 8.

Cole, B. E. (1999b). Pain program accreditation: New accreditation standards. Part two: General clinical accreditation standards. *Pain Practitioner, 9*(2), 4.

Cole, B. E. (1999c). Pain program accreditation: New accreditation standards. Part three: Classification specific clinical standards. *Pain Practitioner, 9*(3), 10.

Cole, B. E. (2000). Ease and satisfaction for use of the National Pain Data Bank and Pain Program Accreditation. *American Journal of Pain Management, 10*(3), 134.

Commission on Accreditation of Rehabilitation Facilities. (2003). *Medical rehabilitation: Standards manual.* Tucson, AZ: Author.

Department of Health and Human Services. (2004). *The Health Insurance Portability and Accountability Act of 1996 (HIPAA).* Centers for Medicare and Medicaid Services Web site. Retrieved March 24, 2004 from http://www.cms.hhs.gov/hipaa.

Flor, H., Fydrich, T., & Turk, D. C. (1992). Efficacy of multidisciplinary pain treatment centers: A meta-analytic review, *Pain, 49*(2), 221.

Foundation for Accountability (FACCT). (2003). *Innovators and visionaries: Strategies for creating a person-centered health system.* Retrieved March 30, 2004 from http://www.facct.org.

Gironda, R. J., Azzarello, L., & Clark, M. E. (2002). Test-retest reliability of the National Pain Data Bank v. 2.0. *American Journal of Pain Management, 12,* 24.

Gordon, D. B., Dahl, J. L., & Stevenson, K. K. (Eds.). (2000). *Building an institutional commitment to pain management: The Wisconsin resource manual* (2nd ed.). Madison, WI: University of Wisconsin Board of Regents.

International Association for the Study of Pain. (1990). *Desirable characteristics for pain treatment facilities.* Seattle, WA: Author.

Joint Commission on Accreditation of Healthcare Organizations. (2000). *Pain assessment and management: An organizational approach.* Oakbrook Terrace, IL: Author.

Joint Commission on Accreditation of Healthcare Organizations. (2001). *Comprehensive accreditation manual for hospitals.* Oakbrook Terrace, IL: Author.

Joint Commission on Accreditation of Healthcare Organizations. (2003). *Improving the quality of pain management through measurement and action.* Oakbrook Terrace, IL: Author.

Kee, W. G., Middaugh, S., Pawlick, K., & Nicholson, J. (1997). Cost benefit analysis of a multidisciplinary chronic pain program. *American Journal of Pain Management, 7*(2), 59.

Marketdata Enterprises. (2003). *Pain management programs: A market analysis.* Tampa, FL: Author.

McCaffery, M., & Pasero, C. (1999). *Pain clinical manual* (2nd ed.). St. Louis, MO: Mosby.

National Institutes of Health Consensus Development Conference Statement. (1986). *Electronic references: The integrated approach to the management of pain.* NIH Consensus Statement Web site. Retrieved March 24, 2004 from http://consensus.nih.gov/cons/055/055_statement.htm.

National Pharmaceutical Council. (2001). *Pain: Current understanding of assessment, management, and treatments.* Reston, VA: Author.

Okifuji, A., & Turk, D. C. (1998). Philosophy and efficacy of multidisciplinary approach to chronic pain management. *Journal of Anesthesia, 12,* 142.

Turk, D., & Okifuji, A. (1997). Multidisciplinary pain centers: Boons or boondoggles? *Journal of Workers Compensation, 6,* 9.

Turk, D. C., & Okifuji, A. (1998). Treatment of chronic pain patients: Clinical outcomes, cost effectiveness, and cost benefits of multidisciplinary pain centers. *Critical Reviews in Physical Medicine and Rehabilitation, 10,* 181.

Weiner, R. S. (1992). Pain practitioner: Academy to start three new projects. *American Journal of Pain Management, 2*(2), 109.

Weiner, R. S. (1993). The culture of pain. *American Journal of Pain Management, 3*(4), 201.

103

Starting a Pain Clinic

Clayton A. Varga, MD

DEVELOPMENT CHECKLIST

1. Ask: Am I sure I want to do this?
2. Identify a leader: Am I qualified?
3. Select the clinic structure.
4. Assess the need.
5. Develop the business plan.
6. Research financial options.
7. Select the participating professionals.
8. Hire support and administrative personnel.
9. Select the site.
10. Determine equipment needs.
11. Develop the marketing plan.
12. Plan billing and collections procedures.
13. Develop a capitated contract.
14. Acquire an existing clinic.

ARE YOU SURE YOU WANT TO DO THIS?

The formation of any business requires a great deal of forethought and an investment of time, energy, and money to be successful. Starting a pain clinic is no exception. Individuals who wish to engage in the business of pain should ask themselves the following questions: Am I completely committed to the success of the business? Am I willing to be the effective leader of the business? If not, do I have someone to fulfill this function? Do I recognize that the financial aspects of the clinic require as much attention and expertise as the practice aspects? If the answer to any of these questions is no, then all further efforts will most likely be wasted.

IDENTIFY A LEADER

Ask yourself: Am I qualified by education and temperament to start and run a pain clinic? Do I possess the specialized clinical background necessary to develop and implement the needed structure for evaluation and treatment of patients in a multidisciplinary setting? Am I able to participate in the development of contracts and marketing plans and oversee administrative decisions? If you are unable to fulfill these requirements, then it is necessary to secure the participation of one or more individuals who can before proceeding to the next step.

SELECTION OF CLINIC STRUCTURE

Having made the decision to move forward, the desired clinic structure must be selected. Practice types and accompanying brief descriptions are as follows:

1. Single modality: A single practitioner (e.g., neurologist, acupuncturist, chiropractor) seeing and treating patients without regular input from other practitioners.
2. Multimodality: Practitioners of different specialties, treating patients in a similar location without regular, structured discussion of the patients by all practitioners.
3. Multidisciplinary: Practitioners of multiple different specialties, including a minimum of one representative from each of the following fields: physician, physical therapy, and psychology. Often present are occupational therapy, acupuncture, nursing, and chiropractic. The members of the clinic have made a commitment to

attend regular patient conferences and to provide integrated care of the patient.

The applicability of each item discussed in this chapter will largely depend on the clinic model developed. The less complex the model, the less important certain aspects of the development process become. However, even the simplest single-modality model would benefit from following most of the steps in the development checklist.

The more complex the structure and the greater the number of participants, the more time, energy, and money will be required to take the business from concept to a fully operational entity. The remainder of this chapter is directed toward a multidisciplinary pain clinic that has a full-time medical director and provides, as a minimum, physical therapy and psychology services and may well offer nursing, occupational therapy, and acupuncture services.

ASSESSMENT OF NEED

Once a preferred structure for the clinic has been selected, then an assessment of need must take place. The purpose of the assessment of need is to determine the demand for the product. It determines if the clinic, in the geographic area to be served, can reasonably expect to draw enough patients to pay all debt and still produce a profit. The assessment should take into account the following:

1. What is the size of the population served (i.e., what is the catchment area)?
2. What is the willingness of physicians within the catchment area to refer patients for the services you are providing?
3. Who is the competition? Are similar facilities already present?
4. What percentage of the population is served by health maintenance organizations (HMOs), preferred provider organizations (PPOs), or independent practice associations (IPAs)? What will be your ability to gain access to those patients?
5. Can you develop a relationship with an existing health care provider who will guarantee patient referrals prior to beginning operations?

The first step is to define your likely catchment area. This represents the geographic boundaries from which you can reasonably expect to draw patients. In an urban or suburban environment, this usually represents a distance of 15 to at most 30 miles from the business. Obviously, there will be regional variation in the size of the catchment area, depending on the proximity of the clinic to major transportation arteries and traffic patterns and the perceived excellence of the clinic. Once defined, the population within the catchment area should be estimated. While

no hard and fast rules exist, if the catchment area has a population of less than 100,000, its ability to support a true multidisciplinary clinic or center is questionable.

Competing service providers need to be evaluated. If one or several high-quality providers already exist in the proposed catchment area, and if they have excess capacity, then concrete reasons for believing that you can capture a large enough portion of the market share to survive must be identified before business start-up. In such a situation, contracts with a PPO or IPA to be the sole provider for pain management services and verbal assurances of appropriate patient referrals from independent physicians should be obtained prior to entering the marketplace.

Talk to local HMO, PPO, and IPA administrators. Assess your ability to draw patients from these ranks. Meet with attorneys, caseworkers, and insurance carriers who are involved locally in the workers' compensation system and assess how many referrals are likely from these sources.

Having done the above, estimate the total number of monthly referrals you expect from all sources. If enough patients are forthcoming to support the business, then development of a detailed business plan becomes the next step. If patient referrals appear to be insufficient, then it is wise to explore other sources of patient referral before proceeding. If, after further exploration, more patients are not forthcoming, it is probably best to rethink your proposed catchment area, moving to one with a more favorable referral pattern.

THE BUSINESS PLAN

If, based on the assessment of need, it is likely that the business will be profitable in the selected catchment area, then a detailed business plan is developed. The purpose of the plan is to secure on paper a description of the components of the operation and a schedule of their implementation. This should occur prior to spending the first dollar on the program.

The business plan has two major components. The first is a narrative that contains a brief description of the business, in which the purpose and structure of the business are outlined. Included is a description of the personnel involved, the function each fulfills, an outline of the marketing plan, and a general description of the facility requirements. The narrative section should briefly address each of the following components:

1. The purpose of the business
2. The market niche served by the business
3. The personnel involved and the function of each
4. Facility requirements
5. Outline of the marketing plan
6. Plan for dissolution of the business

The second portion of the business plan is done as a spreadsheet. It can be prepared by hand using a large ledger sheet or more easily by using one of a number of commercially available electronic spreadsheets (e.g., Excel®).

A sample business plan for a hospital-based multidisciplinary clinic that provides primarily outpatient services is shown in Table 103.1. The business plan estimates fixed and variable costs, revenues, and the amount of start-up capital needed to begin the business and keep it running until the revenue stream produces a profit. Total cost is simply the summation of the individual cost estimates. The sample spreadsheet in Table 103.1 lists most of the individual cost estimates that are required for a multidisciplinary clinic. Each expenditure is estimated on a month-by-month basis for at least 1 year and entered into the spreadsheet. This produces a time estimate of how long it will take to generate a profit and estimates the revenue position of the business at any point along the time line.

The cost estimate should be as detailed as possible. It is possible to accurately predict almost all of the costs, especially fixed costs, when doing the business plan. This is in contrast to revenue estimation, which will be, at best, a rough guess. Nailing down the cost projections as accurately as possible will, in turn, allow for the greatest possible accuracy in predicting the net revenue estimate.

It is best to shift as much of the cost as possible from fixed to variable. This minimizes expenses when revenue is low. Several examples of doing this are hiring personnel on part-time or flexible-time schedules, increasing hours as patient load increases, and having billing and collection done by an outside service, with cost based on a percentage of collections.

Obtaining the revenue estimate requires developing an approximate charge per patient. If the clinic is based on one or several structured programs, in which each patient participates in a relatively uniform program for a predetermined length of time, then average charges are easy to estimate. If the clinic structure is such that revenue generation is spread over a wide range of activities, then generating an average charge per patient is more difficult. In this situation, it is necessary to develop multiple average patient charges and estimate what portion of the total predicted patient flow falls into each group.

Subtracting total cost from total revenue yields the predicted financial position of the business at any point along the time line. It is wise to do estimates using best guess, worst case, and best case revenue projection scenarios. If you are prepared to survive the worst case scenario, then the business should succeed.

FINANCING

The business plan will project the necessary capital required for business formation and development. The most common cause of a new business failure is under-capitalization. It is important to generate at least as much capital as is required based on the business plan. It is also wise to have a credit line available for emergencies. Once capitalization requirements have been determined, options for obtaining the capital must be explored. Numerous financing possibilities exist. Those most commonly employed are as follows:

1. Joint venture: This almost always consists of a limited partnership. The limited partnership consists of both limited and general partners. The general partners oversee the business formation and development and have a greater degree of legal responsibility should the enterprise fail. Limited partners invest money into the partnership but are passive in the business formation and development. Their losses are limited to their investments.

   An example of a joint venture is as follows: The director of the proposed facility develops a detailed business plan. A lawyer is hired to prepare a joint venture agreement, wherein the director is the general partner and the individuals supplying the money are limited partners. The director oversees the development and daily running of the business, for which he or she receives a portion of the profits generated by the business. The director may also receive monies generated via professional activities carried out at the business. The remaining profits are disbursed to the limited partners.

2. Borrowing of money by one or several individuals from conventional lending sources (i.e., a practice loan).

3. Utilization of personal capital to begin the business.

SELECTION OF PARTICIPATING PROFESSIONALS

The type of clinic or operating structure chosen will determine the professional components of the clinic. The quality of the professional personnel will be one of, if not the most important determinants of success. Careful thought must be given to this topic. Not only must the professionals be well trained in their own disciplines, but they must understand the fundamental difference between practicing in a unidimensional office versus a multidisciplinary setting. They must be willing to make what are often perceived as personal sacrifices to make the system work and to regularly attend patient conference meetings and provide input in those meetings in a useful fashion. They must understand the need to promote the clinic as an entity, as well as themselves as individuals, and be willing to defer

TABLE 103.1
XYZ Office Overhead First Year of Operations

	Total Annual	\[Month\] 1	2	3	4	5	6	7	8	9	10	11	12
Average length of stay													
Full-day nonresidential	35	20,125	20,125	20,125	20,125	20,125	20,125	20,125	20,125	20,125	20,125	20,125	20,125
Half-day nonresidential	20	7,900	7,900	7,900	7,900	7,900	7,900	7,900	7,900	7,900	7,900	7,900	7,900
Patient census	56	0	0	0	3	3	4	5	7	7	8	9	10
Full-day nonresidential	33	0	0	0	1	1	2	3	4	4	5	6	7
Half-day nonresidential	23	0	0	0	2	2	2	2	3	3	3	3	3
Revenue													
Full-day nonresidential	$575 / 664,125	0	0	0	20,125	20,125	40,250	60,375	80,500	80,500	100,625	120,750	140,875
Half-day nonresidential	$395 / 181,700	0	0	0	15,800	15,800	15,800	23,700	23,700	23,700	23,700	23,700	23,700
Total revenue	845,825	0	0	0	35,925	35,925	56,050	76,175	104,200	104,200	124,325	144,450	164,575
Deductions from revenue													
80% coverage	20.0% / 169,165	0	0	0	7,185	7,185	11,210	15,235	20,840	20,840	24,865	28,890	32,915
Provision for bad debt	20.0% / 33,833	0	0	0	1,437	1,437	2,242	3,047	4,168	4,168	4,973	5,778	6,583
Billing expense	6.5% / 10,996	0	0	0	467	467	729	990	1,355	1,355	1,616	1,878	2,139
Total deductions	213,994	0	0	0	9,089	9,089	14,181	19,272	26,363	26,363	31,454	36,546	41,637
Net revenue	631,831	0	0	0	26,836	26,836	41,869	56,903	77,837	77,837	92,871	107,904	122,938
Program personnel[a]													
Medical director[b]	90,000	7,500	7,500	7,500	7,500	7,500	7,500	7,500	7,500	7,500	7,500	7,500	7,500
Acupuncturist	35,000	3,792	3,792	3,792	3,792	3,792	3,792	3,792	3,792	3,792	3,792	3,792	3,792
Physical therapist[c]	45,000	4,875	4,875	4,875	4,875	4,875	4,875	4,875	4,875	4,875	4,875	4,875	4,875
Psychologist consultant[b]	50,000	4,167	4,167	4,167	4,167	4,167	4,167	4,167	4,167	4,167	4,167	4,167	4,167
Nurse/social worker[d]	35,000	3,792	3,792	3,792	3,792	3,792	3,792	3,792	3,792	3,792	3,792	3,792	3,792
Program personnel[a]	289,500	24,125	24,125	24,125	24,125	24,125	24,125	24,125	24,125	24,125	24,125	24,125	24,125
Office personnel[a]													
Office manager	25,000		2,708	2,708	2,708	2,708	2,708	2,708	2,708	2,708	2,708	2,708	2,708
Receptionist	18,000		1,950	1,950	1,950	1,950	1,950	1,950	1,950	1,950	1,950	1,950	1,950
Recruitment fee	5,000												
Training	1,000	83	83	83	83	83	83	83	83	83	83	83	83
Office personnel	61,900	4,742	4,742	4,742	4,742	4,742	4,742	4,742	4,742	4,742	4,742	4,742	4,742
Administrative costs													
Accounting fees for taxes/audit	1,500	125	125	125	125	125	125	125	125	125	125	125	125
Payroll, accounting fee	480	40	40	40	40	40	40	40	40	40	40	40	40
Bank fees	150	13	13	13	13	13	13	13	13	13	13	13	13
Quality assurance	4,000	333	333	333	333	333	333	333	333	333	333	333	333
Administrative costs	6,130	511	511	511	511	511	511	511	511	511	511	511	511

Capital & Equipment Expense

Item	Total	1	2	3	4	5	6	7	8	9	10	11	12	13
Business formation														
Accounting	100	100												
Attorney corporation fee	7,500	7,500												
Business formation fees & licenses	950	950												
Reproduction/printing	500	500												
Business formation	9,050	9,050												
Capital expense	53,000	53,000												
Small equipment	15,000	15,000												
Capital & equipment	68,000	68,000												
Marketing costs														
Advertising	10,000	833	833	833	833	833	833	833	833	833	833	833	833	833
Brochures	8,000		8,000											
Announcements	6,500	6,500												
Lectures/slides	500	167		167					167					
Marketing costs	25,000	7,333	8,833	833	1,000	1,000	833	833	833	833	1,000	833	833	833
Office operations														
Books	750	63	63	63	63	63	63	63	63	63	63	63	63	63
Business licenses/fees	800	800												
Exchange	2,700	225	225	225	225	225	225	225	225	225	225	225	225	225
Insurance/business overhead	1,500	1,500												
Insurance casualty	560	560												
Insurance/program liability	12,000	12,000												
Laundry/linen	1,500	125	125	125	125	125	125	125	125	125	125	125	125	125
Magazines	258	258												
Med supplies	24,000	2,000	2,000	2,000	2,000	2,000	2,000	2,000	2,000	2,000	2,000	2,000	2,000	2,000
Phone/6-line phone	8,430	703	703	703	703	703	703	703	703	703	703	703	703	703
Postage/Fed. Express	2,355	196	196	196	196	196	196	196	196	196	196	196	196	196
Reproduction/printing	350	29	29	29	29	29	29	29	29	29	29	29	29	29
Repairs/maintenance	5,700	633	633	633	633	633	633	633	633	633	633	633	633	633
Stationery	2,400	200	200	200	200	200	200	200	200	200	200	200	200	200
Supplies	5,500	458												
Taxes/IRS[e]														
Taxes/state	800													800
Transcription	7,836	653	653	653	653	653	653	653	653	653	653	653	653	653
Miscellaneous expenses	500	42												
Utilities	3,000	250												
Working capital/line of credit @ 12%	28,779	1,379	1,843	2,322	2,459	2,597	2,597	2,597	2,597	2,597	2,597	2,597	2,597	2,597
Office operations	109,718	21,441	6,036	6,515	7,286	7,424	7,424	7,424	7,424	7,424	7,424	7,424	7,424	8,224

TABLE 103.1 (Continued)
XYZ Office Overhead First Year of Operations

	Total Annual	Month											
		1	2	3	4	5	6	7	8	9	10	11	12
Property, plant, equipment[f]													
Office rent (2,000 @ 2.5)	60,000	5,000	5,000	5,000	5,000	5,000	5,000	5,000	5,000	5,000	5,000	5,000	5,000
Property tax on triple net lease	750	750											
Equipment depreciation	See Capital equipment												
Amortized start-up	See Business formation												
Property, plant, equipment	60,750	5,750	5,000	5,000	5,000	5,000	5,000	5,000	5,000	5,000	5,000	5,000	5,000
Total expenses	630,048	139,618	47,747	49,726	42,497	42,801	42,635	42,635	42,635	42,801	42,635	42,635	43,435
Net operating income[g]	1,783	(139,618)	(47,747)	(49,726)	(15,661)	(15,965)	(765)	14,268	35,203	35,036	50,236	65,270	79,503

[a] Employee benefits calculated at 28% (e.g., medical/dental/workers' compensation insurance/FICA/FWH labor costs will vary, depending upon urban location).

[b] Medical director and psychologists can be paid on a 1099 basis, assuming IRS criteria are met.

[c] Physical therapist's employee benefits 30%.

[d] This individual could function in a marketing capacity in addition to nursing/social work duties.

[e] Federal taxes in first year will be based on the NOI plus capitalized investment not written off in first year.

[f] Capital expenses and office rent could be what joint venture partners might provide for an equity interest in the clinic business. Note that both capital investment and business start-up are paid back in the first year of operation.

[g] Net operating income in the first year is a function of how quickly the marketing strategy/plan can tap into the clinic's catchment referral sources such HMOs, IPAs, personal injury attorneys, and workers' compensation caseworkers/attorneys.

at times to other members of the team in the treatment of any particular patient. Many physicians and other professionals are not suited by character to function easily in such an environment and, despite any academic or other professional qualifications, are best excluded from the multidisciplinary setting. When selecting clinical members for the team, consideration of board certification in pain management should not be overlooked.

SUPPORT PERSONNEL

Personnel to perform all of the nonpatient care activities are obviously necessary for the business to function. These areas include billing and collections, reception, ordering of supplies, scheduling, transcription, and paying bills, to name a few. These individuals should already have been taken into consideration as part of the business plan. All of these people need not be hired at the beginning of the business. It is preferable to keep start-up fixed costs as lean as possible. Even a multidisciplinary center can easily start with a single support person if time-consuming tasks, such as billing and transcription, are subcontracted to outside firms. This plan has the advantage of changing a fixed cost to a variable cost, which will be much cheaper when patient volume is low. As patient volume rises, these functions can easily be transferred in-house at such time as it becomes financially advantageous to do so.

If one individual is initially hired, then this person should be told that he or she is expected to be a jack-of-all-trades. This individual should also be someone who can become the office manager as other employees are put in place. The author believes that it is cheaper to hire one well-paid, highly motivated employee than two poorly paid, poorly motivated employees. As the business matures, additional employees can be added as need dictates.

SITE SELECTION

Having decided on both the general geographic location and the specific structure of the clinic, it is possible to begin specific site selection. If a joint venture with a hospital has been undertaken, then the hospital may have unused space that can serve as the clinic site. This has several advantages. It serves to bind the interests of the hospital and the clinic. It provides the clinic with some instant name recognition, if the hospital name is incorporated into the clinic name, and it may help speed referrals to the clinic from members of the hospital medical staff. It also allows easy proximity between inpatient and outpatient care, if both are provided. The hospital may allow the space to be used in exchange for equity in the business, thus limiting operational costs.

If an off-hospital site is selected, then several factors need to be taken into consideration: proximity to other doctors' offices, ease of access to the likely patient base, cost per square foot, the ability of the site to be tailored to your needs, and the ability to expand into adjacent space in the future without having to relocate.

How much and what type of space will be needed will be determined by the clinic structure. Office rental cost represents one of the largest fixed expenses. The clinic structure should be well planned to maximally utilize each square foot of space. Initially, some, if not all, of the professional participants will have other practice locations. It is less expensive to time-share offices between practitioners, and it is unusual for all individuals to be seeing patients at the same time.

EQUIPMENT

Equipment used in a multidisciplinary pain clinic will depend on the clinic structure. If the clinic site is within a hospital, often all of the diagnostic, occupational and physical therapy, and procedural (nerve block, laboratory testing, radiologic, and operating) equipment and facilities are already available. Supplying a site with the ability to see patients for medical and psychological evaluation, basic physical therapy treatment, minor office procedures (such as certain types of nerve blocks), relaxation training, biofeedback, and group as well as individual psychotherapy will require an expenditure of $100,000 to $150,000. This includes the purchase of furniture, exam and treatment tables, office and medical supplies, biofeedback equipment, fax, computers, photocopy equipment, and a phone system.

MARKETING

It is important to have an overall marketing plan that extends for a period of several years. This should take into consideration how much money is to be allocated to marketing efforts and what types of advertising and other promotional projects will be undertaken. It is not possible to be all things to all people. The marketing plan needs to reflect the market niche and present a consistent message.

Marketing medical services is a complicated and sometimes delicate job. Ethical standards regarding medical marketing vary regionally, and knowledge of local standards is crucial prior to beginning the marketing program. Being the first to employ a specific type of advertising in an area (e.g., radio commercials) can have a negative impact with referring physicians. However, certain techniques (discussed below) can be used in any environment.

Announcements and brochures should be sent to referring physicians, workers' compensation caseworkers, and attorneys. These should be mailed shortly after opening the practice. The announcement should be mailed first, with the brochure to follow 1 to 2 months later. This reinforces your message and is more effective than sending both at the same time.

Taking the time to personally contact and talk to local physicians, workers' compensation caseworkers, and lawyers is important in building referral patterns. PPOs, IPAs, and HMOs control a majority of the patient population in many areas. The clinic director must take the time to educate and negotiate with these groups to secure appropriate patient referral.

Lectures and community forums are useful tools for educating referring physicians as well as potential patients not only about the problem of pain, but also about your business. Professionally prepared stationery, the development of a logo, and production of a newsletter are all effective means of advertising. The clinic's listing in the local phone directory should be easily visible. Radio, television, and print media all offer opportunities for exposure. These represent expensive and potentially sensitive areas of advertising for which local ethos should be considered and professional marketing help engaged.

A presence on the Internet by individual health care providers is becoming progressively more common and in the near future will become ubiquitous. A basic Web site can be developed and hosted by a good commercial Web development company relatively inexpensively. This provides an excellent avenue for continuous marketing exposure and a way for patients, providers, and third party referral sources to access information about your program at their convenience. A basic site would include information about yourself and any other service providers in your practice; your location including directions, office hours, and phone numbers; and a description of the services provided. More detailed sites can also include information about specific procedures performed by you or your colleagues including photographs or even short video segments, hot links to other complementary Web sites, and informational databases. Your Web address should be included on your business cards and all other promotional materials and activities. The author recommends dealing with an experienced Web development and hosting service. Consider starting with a basic Web page that allows for some scalability. This way you can add features or increase the complexity of the site without losing your investment in the initial development.

Advertising and promotion make physicians and patients aware of the services the clinic provides. They do not replace the need to provide concerned, compassionate, and effective care. If the office is disorganized, the receptionist curt, or physicians and therapists chronically late, no amount of advertising can overcome the bad will spread by irate patients and referring physicians.

BILLING AND COLLECTIONS

Even the best conceived and instituted treatment program will not succeed if efficient billing/collections operations are not instituted from day one. Billing and collections can be done internally or subcontracted. This decision should be made while formulating the business plan. The billing system should be in place before the first patient is seen.

A number of local and nationwide medical billing services are available and usually charge between 6 and 10% of collections. Interview several and consider not only the cost, but also the comprehensiveness of the service rendered. Look for a company that has some expertise in billing for a similar entity or is willing to invest the start-up time to learn the peculiarities of the field. Billing externally can significantly reduce capital investment at the time of business start-up and help to reduce fixed costs at a time when cash flow will be slow.

If billing is done internally, the appropriate software, hardware, and support forms to carry out the task must be purchased. It is important to hire someone with previous billing experience to make the system work. There are numerous companies that sell medical billing systems, with a large range of capabilities. Billing, collection, scheduling, accounting, and payroll functions are all available. Software and hardware can be purchased separately or as a complete system. Prices range from $1,000 to $50,000 or more, depending on the system.

DEVELOPING A CAPITATED CONTRACT

Payment for pain management services has transitioned from a fee-for-service only model to a capitated model in some environments. The extent to which this has already occurred varies dramatically from region to region. In some large metropolitan areas, the market share of managed care exceeds 80%. In other areas, managed care penetration is almost non-existent. Managed care in the form of HMOs has stalled in its growth beginning in the late 1990s and in fact has retracted to a small extent in the Western United States and has contracted significantly in many other areas of the country. Market-driven national healthcare reform has shifted to the PPO model with price control being exerted through benefit limitation, higher out-of-pocket expenses for the insured, and further erosion of payment to physicians. This shift will most likely continue at least into the near future, absent any other national or regional political agenda. It is necessary in some geographic locations for the successful provider of pain management to understand the differences between fee-for-service and capitated reimbursement models and to be able to negotiate a good capitated contract.

In a capitated contract, the clinic receives a payment each month based on the number of members covered by the contract and the rate per member (the per member per month, or PMPM, rate). If the contract covers 50,000 members at a rate of $0.40 PMPM, then the payment would be $20,000 a month. This is independent of the actual number of patient visits, supplies used, or resources consumed in a particular month. If the cost of service delivery for the month was $15,000, then a $5,000 profit would be realized. Obviously, if the cost to deliver care under the contract was in excess of $20,000 for the month, then a loss would be incurred.

To be able to develop a price structure that makes sense, the following information should be obtained and analyzed:

1. The utilization rate for the current procedural terminology (CPT) codes covered under the contract for the most recent 12-month period for the population in question.
2. Your actual reimbursement for each CPT code by insurance type. The most important, of course, is the reimbursement from the entity with which you are negotiating, if you have previous claims experience with that entity.
3. Knowledge of the range of cap rates for similar contracts in your immediate or similar geographic areas.

The above information will allow you to develop a PMPM rate that will maintain profitability. You should develop a PMPM rate based on your own analysis of prior utilization. Then check this against other contracts as a safety check. Obviously, rates can vary extensively depending on which CPT codes are covered by the contract.

It is important to build the following safeguards into the contract:

1. Input into if not direct control over utilization. If you accept the risk of fixed payments, then you must be able to control utilization to help mitigate that risk.
2. Renegotiation of the contract if actual utilization significantly exceeds projected utilization.

It is important to have in place a system to monitor utilization prior to beginning the contract. Utilization information, along with expense information, will be needed to determine the profitability of the contract. It is important to monitor this closely and move to renegotiate unprofitable contracts quickly.

ACQUIRING AN EXISTING CLINIC

Acquisition of an existing practice or clinic provides an alternative to starting a clinic anew. Over the last two decades the number of pain clinics and the number of trained providers have increased phenomenally. As some providers mature to the point of retirement, they must choose an exit strategy and some of these individuals, and small groups will conclude that a sale of the practice or clinic is the best strategy.

Acquisition of an existing clinic does offer some advantages over starting a clinic from the very beginning and may be the best way to enter into an already saturated market. It provides an opportunity to obtain referrals and establish contracts quickly and provides historical financial information that can be evaluated and valued in an objective way. However, one should be aware of the numerous pitfalls that exist in the purchase of any business entity and these include but are in no way are limited to the emergence of unforeseen liabilities such as lawsuits attached to the entity after the deal closes, the inability to maintain existing contracts or referral patterns, and overvaluation of the accounts receivable. It is mandatory to seek professional financial and legal assistance in the evaluation, appraisal, and deal negotiation. A number of good texts exist and a good overview can be obtained by reading Krallinger (1997).

BIBLIOGRAPHY

Finkler, S. A. (1992). *Finance and accounting for nonfinancial managers.* Englewood Cliffs, NJ: Prentice-Hall.

Gapinski, L. C. (1996). *Understanding health care financial management.* Chicago: AUPHA Press.

Gumpert, D. E. (1992). *How to create a successful marketing plan.* Boston: Inc. Publishing.

Hammon, J. L. (1993). *Fundamentals of medical management.* Tampa, FL: ACPE.

Krallinger, J. (1997). *Mergers and acquisitions.* New York: McGraw-Hill.

McKeever, M. (1988). *How to write a business plan.* Berkeley, CA: Nolo Press.

Porter, M. E. (1985). *Competitive advantage.* New York: Free Press.

Sachs, L. (1987). *Marketing for the professional practice.* Englewood Cliffs, NJ: Prentice-Hall.

104

Going Insurance Free

Thomas J. Romano, MD, PhD

PROLOGUE

"Physician Shortage Predicted to Spread" was one of the headlines on the front page of the January 5, 2004, issue of *American Medical News* (Elliott, 2004). Sadly, doctors have been dissatisfied with the "system" for many years. Loss of autonomy, increasing malpractice premiums, and declining reimbursement top the list of reasons for this state of affairs.

Before I severed all ties with third-party payers in the mid-1990s, I was about to contribute to this practitioner shortage. My ability to provide quality care to my patients was being threatened by ever-increasing distraction and interference from clerks, bureaucrats, and other paper pushers who wanted to influence how I treated my patients. This sad refrain ran the gamut from their insistence on my prescribing generic drugs over brand name medications to when I must discharge a patient from the hospital. Stresses mounted. The cost of malpractice insurance skyrocketed. Overhead crept inexorably higher. Worst of all, respect for patient and practitioner alike diminished significantly. There seemed to be no end in sight to mounting pressures and plummeting satisfaction with my practice situation. In short, I had had enough. I decided that I would either have to change my profession or take charge of my medical practice — and my life. I identified the problem and took steps to solve it. This is how and why I did it. Perhaps you should consider this course of action if you no longer find joy and satisfaction with your practice.

INTRODUCTION

In a previous edition of this textbook, the chapter on this topic was written by Dr. Christopher Brown (Brown,

2002). In his comprehensive, practical, and inspirational writing Dr. Brown put forth a strategy for achieving an insurance-free practice. Rather than try to do the impossible, that is improve on Dr. Brown's chapter, I will endeavor to describe what I believe to be the important issues regarding the present health care reimbursement process, briefly set forth the evolution of my practice to a pure fee-for-service one, and describe why I believe the best method of practice is a fee-for-service one not only for the good of the practitioner but also in order to get the most effective treatment for the individual patient. However, while an insurance-free practice may work for some practitioners, it may not suit your situation.

My intention in writing this chapter is not to try to convince the readers to change the way they run their practices. Rather, it is to present an alternative to the "system" — one that I have found not only appealing for a variety of reasons but one that allows me the freedom and flexibility to best evaluate and treat my patients. I stress the word "my" because it is I who has the moral, legal, and ethical responsibility and accountability for their care. I alone — not the third parties — am in the best position to care for my patients. Why listen to reviewers who have not even met my patient? Why allow non-professionals (i.e., chair-bound "paper pushers," clerks, etc.) to set professional fees? Why kowtow to so-called "peer-reviewers" when you know you can do a better job? Why let third parties dictate the way you practice? It is *your* practice! They are *your* patients! If a professional license is required by the state for an individual to lawfully practice, how is it that third parties dictate how patients are treated? Make no mistake about it — nonprofessionals make practice decisions all the time. I am not responsible for law enforcement casting a blind eye to the routine commitment of such felonies, but I am responsible for how I treat my patients.

If you are truly happy and satisfied with your present practice situation, there is no need to read on. However, if you are sick and tired of ever-decreasing autonomy and steadily declining reimbursement, this chapter may be of benefit. Remember, it is your life; it is your practice; they are your patients! Strive to practice for mutual benefit of patient and practitioner. What other entity deserves consideration?

THE ABUSED CLINICIAN

When asked by a patient what to do in an abusive situation, the clinician is most likely to respond with the advice that one should get away from that situation as quickly as possible and to take control over his or her life. For example, if a woman is married to a man who is a binge drinker and suffers physical and verbal abuse whenever her spouse gets drunk, that woman should not suffer the abuse; she should take control of her life and get herself into a situation where further abuse is not likely to occur. It really doesn't matter whether the abuse occurs on a weekly basis or a monthly basis, whether the husband is a good provider, or whether he pleads and begs for forgiveness. One must judge a person by his acts, not only his words and there can only be reconciliation if there is true remorse and no further abusive behavior.

It is my contention that the relationship between third-party payers, whether the clinician is dealing with Medicare, Medicaid, HMOs, PPOs, etc., is such a situation. The individual abused is the clinician. The abuser is the third party. That is not to say that every interaction between the clinician and the third party is one in which the clinician is harmed. In fact if that were true, no one would deal with third-party payers. Rather the interaction between the third-party payers and clinicians often results in a reimbursement check or a promise for prompt payment. I contend that the actions of third-party payers are perfidious and disrespectful toward clinicians. Furthermore, I do not believe that they will reform. Thus, I have nothing to do with them. I don't submit claims to them; I don't speak with them over the telephone; I don't send them medical records without prior authorization from the patient and payment for said records in advance; I ignore their suggestions regarding the treatment of my patients; I practice medicine as if they did not exist. This seems like a radical step, but wasn't that the way medicine was practiced for untold millennia up until about a generation ago? It works for me. I am happier. My overhead is lower. I try to keep it simple. The patient comes to me for help. I provide advice and help to the best of my ability without influence from third parties. Because I have the moral, ethical, and legal obligation to provide the best care I can

for my patient, I reserve the right to manage the patient the best way I know how. It's that simple.

This chapter is presented in several sections. The first section deals with my own practice and my journey to my present position. The second section points out the various and sundry injustices and pitfalls that abound in today's practice climate, and the third section deals with how any pain practitioner can establish a practice free from third-party influence. However, I must warn you at the outset that not everyone can do this. If you are mediocre, you may need to belong to an HMO or deal with other managed care because many patients make their decision regarding their health care entities based on finances. If you don't keep up and you have nothing different to offer from other practitioners in your community, it may be best to remain "in the pack" instead of striking out on your own. However, if you have excellent skills and believe, as I do, that "guidelines" may not take into account the unique needs of each individual patient, then going insurance free may be for you.

MY JOURNEY

Before I put out my shingle and announced to the world that I was opening a medical practice, I made sure I got good training. Not only did I graduate from an excellent medical school (New York University School of Medicine), I also took a very demanding but incredibly rewarding internship and residency program at Bellevue Hospital/University Hospital in New York City, following that up with a rheumatology fellowship at Barnes Hospital/Washington University in St. Louis Missouri. By the time I opened my practice in 1982 I had gone to school 27 years, 15 years after high school! I had become board-certified in internal medicine and was to become board-certified in rheumatology a few months after opening my practice. I resolved to keep up and regularly went to the rheumatology grand rounds at the University of Pittsburgh, which at that time was headed by Gerald Rodman, a true giant in the field. I resolved to do the best I could to take care of my patients, which included not only keeping up with the medical literature but going to conferences and learning as much as I could about their conditions — often chronic, almost always painful ones. I also quickly obtained staff privileges at four of the local hospitals admitting patients and also doing consultations when asked. In short, I believed I was quite well prepared to care for patients in the private practice setting. Little did I realize that it was not going to be so simple.

In my first year of practice I pretty much dealt with every third-party payer in the area. I was quite naive about the business aspects of the practice but learned quickly. However, learning can be painful, and it happened to be just that for me. After my first year in practice, my collection rate was approximately 50%. This was quite disturbing and I tried to remedy the situation. One of the problems was that one of the local health insurance carriers did not reimburse for trigger point injections! I negotiated with them and told them that trigger point injections were, in fact, good general medical practice. The insurance company responded with a request for documentation of my assertion. This I did by sending them photocopies of journal articles and textbook chapters from numerous sources including Janet Travell, David Simons, and others. After submitting the documentation, which clearly showed that trigger point injections were a generally accepted mode of medical treatment, I was still not reimbursed for them! I thought this quite odd in that documentation had been requested, I provided said documentation, and having done so, rightfully expected that the problem would be rectified. That was not to be the case. I still did not get reimbursed for the injections. Needless to say, I decided not to renew my contract with that carrier. "Fool me once, shame on you; fool me twice, shame on me." That was 1983.

In 1984 Medicare started doing very strange things. It required that physicians, not patients, submit claims for reimbursement. This shifted the burden from the patient to the physician. I had to hire another secretary to keep up with the paperwork. At that time there were only two categories with which a physician could deal with Medicare. The first was called a "participating physician." As such a physician, a doctor would basically accept assignment from Medicare. The doctor could charge whatever he wanted but Medicare would reimburse at whatever rate it wished. The other category was "nonparticipating." To be a "nonparticipating physician," the doctor would not accept assignment from Medicare but could only bill up to a certain amount predetermined by the Medicare carrier. I thought this was also quite strange. How could one deal with an entity and not participate with that entity? It seemed that the term "nonparticipating" could not apply to the situation in which a clinician was, in fact, participating, albeit at a different level. This was another lapse of logic which I again found curious. However, I was still naive and trusted "the system," so I plodded on.

I joined a local IPA/HMO around that time. I had no burning desire to do so. It would seem that I succumbed to peer pressure. Many of the primary care physicians in the area told me that they wanted to refer patients to me but because I was not on the panel of the IPA's participating providers they could not do so. Thus, I signed a contract with the local IPA/HMO with the understanding that although I would get around 85% of my fee in payment, I would make the medical decisions without interference. Needless to say, I severed ties with that entity in 1988 because of disagreements over many of their policies. I did not think that their policies were fair, and I saw that things were quickly going from bad to worse. So, I decided to get out of that situation.

Having opened my practice in 1982, I immediately started doing clinical research regarding patients I was seeing and their response to various treatments. At that time there was very little literature on fibromyalgia syndrome (FS), and because I was seeing a lot of patients with FS, I decided to make observations regarding their presentation, diagnosis, treatment, comorbid conditions, etc. I noticed that many of these patients developed fibromyalgia as a result of a traumatic event. I looked into this as well and eventually published my results in the *State Medical Journal* (Romano, 1990). Other studies followed (Romano, 1998; Romano & Govindan, 1996). I first testified in court in a post-traumatic fibromyalgia case around 1987. The patient had been referred by a family doctor, but eventually I learned that she was represented by an attorney. The patient prevailed in the lawsuit and I started getting referrals from attorneys who had clients involved in motor vehicle accidents, workplace injuries, etc., and who were not responding well to treatment. Many such patients had myofascial pain syndromes and/or fibromyalgia, which had not been recognized and therefore went untreated.

As I started getting more and more patients who had suffered trauma and was also treating patients with various other problems such as systemic lupus erythematosus, rheumatoid arthritis, and Wegener's granulomatosis, I came to the realization that I needed to spend more and more time with each patient because of the nature of these patients' extremely severe and complex problems. This was becoming more and more difficult because my attention would constantly be diverted from direct patient care by messages and inquiries, which I believed were nonsensical at best and downright dangerous at worst. For example, the pressure placed on physicians to discharge patients from the hospital after they had been in the hospital a set number of days or weeks can obviously be very dangerous in that no two patients are alike and response to treatment can vary tremendously. Two experiences in my own practice immediately come to mind.

When asked by a claims reviewer when a certain patient was going to be discharged from the hospital I gave the answer, "When the patient is better." The clerk on the other end of the phone line had the audacity to tell an attending physician whose patient's health and life hung in the balance, "That's not good enough!" How absurd! I quickly responded, "It's good enough for me and that's what counts!" I took pleasure in ending the telephone conversation so abruptly. Now mind you, phone calls like these would regularly interrupt my day, breaking my concentration, and otherwise being extremely annoying and unproductive. In fact, they are probably counterproductive in that it would now take me more time to focus on the patients I had in my office, their unique problems, and their particular difficulties. Another strange interaction that I had over the telephone was with someone who claimed to be a doctor reviewing the case of a patient I had in the hospital who suffered from a very dangerous medical condition. After speaking to this reviewer for about 5 minutes, I got the impression that he could not understand what I was telling him. My explanation to this doctor/reviewer went something like this: "This man has Wegener's granulomatosis! He was near death when I admitted him to the hospital. He is recovering now but has a long way to go." After a few moments of silence the voice on the other end of the telephone asked the question, "What is Wegener's granulomatosis?" *O tempura! O mores!*

The ground was made even more fertile for my having nothing to do with third-party payers when I received a notice from Nationwide Insurance Company in January of 1991 that, as the Medicare carrier for West Virginia and Ohio at that time, it had decided to lower the amount of money I could charge for services to Medicare recipients. It is important to note that that entity was not announcing to me that it was unilaterally decreasing benefits to Medicare recipients, but rather was telling me how much money I could charge in my office for the treatment of my patients for whom I took responsibility. I thought about it for a bit and decided that if my name was on the door, and I alone would make my office policy including how much I would charge, what my hours would be, etc. I resigned from Medicare the following day.

At that time it was illegal for a physician in the United States to treat a patient covered by Medicare Part B (the outpatient portion, Part A being the inpatient portion) privately. That is, any interaction between a Medicare recipient and a physician had to be reported to Medicare, which then controlled what moneys could be reimbursed to the physician if the physician was participating, or controlled how much money a physician could charge if the physician were "nonparticipating." Using the following logic, I had no choice but to no longer see Medicare patients. "I am in private practice; Medicare prevents its recipients from seeing doctors in private practice; ergo I can no longer see Medicare patients at all." I had to tell my Medicare patients that I could no longer take care of them and that they would have to get rheumatological care elsewhere. I was more than happy to see them privately but that was illegal.

This egregious situation was changed in 1998 by an act of Congress. Now, if a physician elects to "opt out," he or she could see Medicare patients legally, that is, on a one-to-one basis without interference from that governmental entity. However, this was not an ideal situation because the patients could not get reimbursed for any of the moneys they spent seeing me. This strategy was clearly meant to discourage patients from going out of "the system" to seek medical care privately from a doctor who elected to "opt out." It would have certainly been much fairer for the benefit to be given to the patient to be used wherever he or she wished to use it. Thus, the patient

could pay my fee, submit my bill to the government, and be paid whatever it would pay for that particular service whether it be for a Medicare provider or not. However, that is not the case. In order for me to "opt out," I had to notify the Social Security Administration, renew my "opt out" status every 2 years, and have patients sign a disclaimer in which they acknowledge that I do not deal with Medicare and that they would have to pay my fees out of their own pocket.

As each individual health insurance company became more and more incompatible with my office policy, I would simply sever my relationship with that carrier. By 1995, I was totally insurance free. I do not regret that decision. I have more control over my life. I no longer have to hire clerks to deal with insurance companies. I make decisions based on what I believe to be correct, and I have far more time to spend with each individual patient because I am no longer distracted by having to deal with third-party payers.

However, being "insurance free" is challenging in that I have to keep up and be able to offer treatment that is "cutting edge." Furthermore, I tend to see more difficult patients in that I have become in some cases the doctor "of last resort." Many individuals have gone to the practitioners "on the list" of providers that are preferred by their insurance companies. Not satisfied with the care they received from those "in the system," they sought me out. I pledge to each and every one of them on the initial visit that because they are employing me, I have undivided loyalty to them, not caring what some clerk or reviewer has to say about their care. I pray each day that I can be worthy of their trust and confidence in me, but of one thing I am certain, no one will interfere with their care if I have anything to say about it. I have an obligation to my patient, to my profession, and ultimately to myself. Of course, I have to be mindful of the local, state, and federal laws, medical board rules, and professional ethical codes, but these offer general rules and guidelines, not the intrusive micromanagement that characterizes interaction with third parties.

THIRD-PARTY PITFALLS

American medical care has evolved over the past 200 years. For most of that time medical care was fee for service. The patient would go to the doctor (or the doctor did a house call), the doctor would do what he could for that patient, and payment would be made. The payment could be in currency, but often it was whatever the patient could bring to the office. Barter was not an uncommon practice. Since the end of World War II and particularly since the Medicare program was established in 1965, more and more Americans have been covered by some sort of third-party reimbursement for their health care. This evolution has been reviewed exhaustively by Starr (1982).

Although there are various different types of third-party reimbursement systems, they have many things in common. For example, none of the reviewers for these organizations has ever met the patient. They have never sat down face to face with the patient to get an idea of what the chief complaint is, the history of the patient's illness, or the patient's past medical history. Furthermore, they have never done a review of systems, personally asked about drug allergies, and the like. Why is this important?

It is important for several reasons. First, an experienced clinician is able not only to take a history and record that history but also to get an impression regarding the patient, especially by observing body language, acknowledging cultural differences and the like. No third-party payer can ever do this. Furthermore, third parties make decisions based on population data as opposed to what is necessary for the individual patient. In their defense, they have no other way of assessing a patient but by making note of the patient's diagnosis and then making decisions regarding an individual patient using population studies. This process is inherently flawed in that it does not take into account the individual problem that any one particular patient has. While the insurer/third-party payer deals with populations; the pain practitioner deals with individuals. All clinicians know that each of their patients is unique and no mere formula or statistical construct can capture the essence of their particular predicaments. Stephen Jay Gould, the eminent biologist and geologist, wrote in describing his own medical problems, "I am not a measure of central tendency, either mean or median. I am one single human being … and I want a best assessment of my own chances — for I have personal decisions to make and my business cannot be dictated by abstract averages." (Gould, 1997, p. 49).

Just about every reader of this chapter has experienced being told by some third-party reviewer that the average length of stay or the average treatment duration is of a certain length. Reimbursement will not be made for any more than that particular number of days or weeks. Some go further and state that it is not medically necessary that a particular patient receive treatment past a certain date or time. When the clinician who is observing the patient face to face continues treatment because it is necessary from a medical point of view, the clinician is routinely insulted by the third-party payer with such terms as "not cost-effective," "overutilizing," and "exceeds what is allowable." It would be much more honest were the third parties to state that they simply do not wish to pay for the care or that that particular care is not covered in the contract. Instead of doing this, they maintain that they are paying for necessary care except that the care being rendered is unnecessary — according to them! How could they possibly know? They have not examined the patient nor do they take responsibility for the care (or lack of it) rendered. This all-too-common practice of denial and

delay has been called "third party rape" (Shealy, 1993). Sound extreme? Read on.

The Medicare program is yet another practitioner of this Orwellian "Doublespeak." Up until 1998 a practitioner evaluating and treating a patient covered by Medicare would be considered either "participating" or "nonparticipating." Basically the former meant that the practitioner in question would accept assignment on all claims. The latter term represented a policy whereby Medicare could dictate to any practitioners who do not wish to accept assignment exactly how much they could charge. This Medicare policy was not about how much Medicare would pay but about what the practitioner in private practice could actually charge! Naturally, practitioners who did not accept assignment still had to abide by all the other Medicare rules and regulations. How is this nonparticipating? One is just participating on a different level. By thus corrupting the English language communication becomes even more difficult.

The Medicare regulations themselves are almost impossible to understand. However, should one be in violation, one is subject to penalties, which include fines and, if the government invokes the False Claims Act, criminal penalties including incarceration. In 1998, it was possible to "opt out" of Medicare altogether and still treat Medicare recipients. Prior to that date, it was illegal for a practitioner in the United States to have a private contract for medical services with a Medicare recipient. The transaction had to be monitored by Medicare even if the practitioner and the patient wanted to have a private agreement. Clearly this violates the civil rights of both patient and practitioner but it was not until 1998 that this situation changed for the better. I have "opted out" and have renewed my opt-out every 2 years. It doesn't matter what insurance my patients have. That is their business. My job is to take care of them to the best of my ability.

It is important for my patients to understand that in medical school I was actually taught the correct way to make mistakes. Obviously, we were encouraged to be extremely careful and not to make errors, but if errors were going to be made, there was actually a way to make them! In training I was taught to make type I (alpha) errors. A type one error is one where the practitioner assumes something is the case but it turns out not to be. For example, a patient presents with chest pain. The practitioner assumes it is extremely serious, possibly a pulmonary embolism or heart attack, but it ends up after the appropriate workup and observation that a much more benign condition exists. Many patients are admitted to coronary care units only to be told that they had chest wall pain or gastrointestinal problems. I don't see anything wrong with that. It is simply the careful and prudent practice of medicine. On the other hand, an error a practitioner must strive to avoid is a type II (beta) error. A type II error is one in which the practitioner assumes something is not present but it actually is present. An example of that would be a patient presenting with chest pain is given an antacid for heartburn, and on the way home from the hospital the patient dies of a massive coronary event. In short, type I errors are consistent with good medical practice, whereas type II errors are not. For discussion of the statistical ramifications of these types of errors, I refer the reader to one of many standard mathematical texts that deal with statistics (Anderson, Sweeney, & Williams, 1986, p. 331).

Let's apply this train of thought to the third-party payers. How often are patients discouraged from going to emergency rooms because their problem was not life threatening and thus it would not be covered? How often are practitioners browbeaten into discharging patients from the hospital against their better judgment, the theory being that the patient probably would get along fine at home anyway? Dealing with third parties leads one to make type II errors; remembering what our teachers taught us leads us to make type I errors. Type I errors may seem more costly in the short term, but I submit if one weighs the cost of human suffering and the very tangible price tag of a funeral or an extended hospital stay because of a misdiagnosis that, indeed, the practitioner who tends to commit type I errors may actually be truly "cost-effective."

Perhaps what irks me the most about managed care organizations is that their decisions often make no sense. Furthermore, their statements are rarely backed up by facts and figures that can be verified by the practitioner. One of the myths espoused by third-party payers is that the cost of medical care in this country is far too high and costs need to be contained. I will grant you that the cost of medical care has exceeded the rate of inflation for many years, but I'm not so certain that this is a bad thing. Why not let individual people decide how to spend their own money? Even if one agrees with such statements and agrees to provide less care for patients and get less in the way of reimbursement for themselves, shouldn't the "belt tightening" extend to the third-party payers themselves?

I find it offensive that I am told I have to accept less money for my services. I read that the CEOs of managed care organizations routinely make seven-figure incomes. This has been a subject of a letter to the editor entitled "Managed Care Is Based on a Lie." (Romano, 1999). Several years ago it was reported that CEOs of U.S. health maintenance organizations made on the average $2 million annually. The highest earner for the year 1997 earned $30.7 million — and that excludes stock options! (Jacob, 1997). How is it that executives for a managed care company or any company for that matter would be worth tens of millions of dollars? The only logical conclusion is that they must either make that amount of money for the company or save that company a similar amount of money. How do managed care executives save money for their company? Most likely it is by rationing services or encouraging practitioners to engage in such cost-saving measures

as prescribing only generic drugs on a restrictive formulary, discharging patients from the hospital after very short stays, discouraging patients from going to the emergency room in off hours, profiling practitioners, and/or rewarding or punishing them based on performance, etc. (*American Medical News,* 2002).

Naturally the schemes listed above are not described by third-party payers in such language. Euphemisms abound. Generic equivalents are touted to be of the same quality except they are cheaper. In fact, in many pharmacies one sees generic drugs described as "quality generic preparations" or "quality generic equivalents." It has been my experience that, as a rule, generic preparations are not as potent as their brand name counterparts. Regardless, the choice of what medication a patient should have should be one made by the physician and patient, not by an insurance clerk. Patients who suffer from chronic, painful conditions often are quite complex requiring a multidisciplinary/interdisciplinary approach for proper treatment. As a practitioner I do not believe that it is my job to look out for the financial health of an insurance company or governmental agency. I am ethically, morally, and legally bound to do the best I can to take care of my patient. In my opinion that includes avoidance of interference from third-party carriers. In fact, I truly believe that it is a conflict of interest for practitioners to deal with these carriers, including Medicare (Romano, 1993). The third parties constantly pressure practitioners to limit care and put patients at risk while pontificating about "cost-effectiveness" and "utilization." Give me a break! I am better off without them. You also may be.

GOING INSURANCE FREE

The eminent attorney Gerry Spence described many Americans as being trapped in "a complex web of corporate and governmental behemoths." He calls large corporations the "New Slave Master" and describes in his book, *Give Me Liberty,* how these entities seek to dominate and control individuals (Spence, 1998). *Give Me Liberty* does not deal with the practice of medicine, nor does it comment on the specifics of corporate health care policy including utilization and reimbursement. Attorney Spence discusses work in general and how a worker should be dealt with (i.e., in a fair and evenhanded way). However, pain practitioners would be wise in considering his arguments. For example he espouses the concept of a "union of one." In his words, "The new and most powerful union of all will be a union of one — one man, one woman, one worker with special skills, an inquiring mind, and an independent attitude, his creativity intact, his love of life blooming" (Spence, 1998, p. 178). While not necessarily meaning to, he is addressing all dedicated and erudite pain practitioners. He goes on to write, "He will enter a place of work voluntarily to do a job for a price, his price…. He will cherish his freedom, which is his security. He cannot be lured into the trap. The master cannot own him. This one man belongs to the union of one, is owned by no one, and represents only himself (Spence, 1998, p. 178).

I urge all of you to consider his words. When I read his book, published in 1998, I realized that I had become a "union of one" about 3 years previously. I decided to blaze my own trail in search of fulfillment and happiness. I did not start out that way. I had learned that dealing with third parties was becoming an ever-increasing cause of tension, anger, and frustration. The less I had to do with them, the better my life got. Maybe there is a better way for you too.

HOW TO BEGIN

Dr. Brown (2002) outlines some strategies to become insurance free. He stresses that practitioners must not accept failure, must set their own goals, and then must create a practice environment that is compatible with their temperament and skills. He stresses the establishment of good communication skills, creation of workable systems, and the development of a USP (Unique Service Position). The USP is what makes your practice different from other practices. I agree with his assessment and suggestions. I have a few of my own. First of all, be the best you can be. Get the best training, keep up in your field, and never give up your desire to do the best job for each and every patient. Do not compromise when it comes to quality care! If you are mediocre, then you may need to deal with third parties to survive. If you are excellent, why settle for low pay and incessant hassles? Market yourself as an expert in pain management. If you have superior skills and more to offer, do not hesitate to say so. Be flexible. If this means changing your office hours or getting involved in medical-legal cases, then so be it. Isn't your freedom worth it? Make it clear to patients that your loyalty is to them and them alone without any consideration given to third parties. Keep in mind that the patient has chosen you for his or her treatment. Divided loyalty will never become a problem when the patient and practitioner both share a common goal — getting the patient better. Make sure you spend sufficient time with each patient, answering all questions posed in an unhurried manner. The practitioner will get more satisfaction from each encounter, and the patient will appreciate that the practitioner really cares about the patient as a person. Medical care can be a very cold and depersonalized experience when the practitioner is harried, resentful, and overworked. All the more so if the practitioner sees himself or herself as a small cog in a monstrous corporate wheel.

Above all, view yourself as a truly independent practitioner who practices for the good of your patients. Do not be distracted by ridiculous "guidelines" or absurd requests. Do not allow your services to be undervalued. Recognize that it is not your responsibility to finance your patients' health care nor is it your obligation to convince third parties to fulfill their contractual obligations to patients. If you are prosperous and fulfilled, you can take better care of your patients. It's your life; it's your practice; it's your decision.

Some, albeit a few, practitioners have decided to strictly limit their involvement with third parties or end their participation altogether (Corona, 1998; Norbut, 2003). They have said, "Enough" (Ward, 1989)! Where do you stand?

REFERENCES

American Medical News. (2002, September 2). Managed care's profits come from physicians' pockets. [Editorial]. *American Medical News*, 36.

Anderson, D. R., Sweeney, D. J., & Williams, T. A. (1986). *Statistics. Concepts and applications.* St. Paul, MN: West Publishing.

Brown, C. (2002). Achieving insurance independence in the age of managed care. In R. Weiner (Ed.), *Pain management: A practical guide for clinicians* (6th ed., pp. 981–993). Boca Raton, FL: CRC Press.

Corona, P. D. (1998, June 1). Just say no to HMOs. *International Medical News*, p. 8.

Elliott, V. S. (2004, January 5). Physician shortage predicted to spread. *American Medical News*, *47*(1), 1.

Gould, S. J. (1997). *Full house.* New York: Harmony Books.

Jacob, J. A. (1997, October 5) HMO top salaries average $2 million in 1997. *American Medical News*, p. 28.

Norbut, M. (2003, February 10). Money woes solved with case-only practice. *American Medical News*, p. 19.

Romano, T. J. (1990). Clinical experiences with post traumatic fibromyalgia syndrome. *West Virginia Medical Journal*, *86*, 198–202.

Romano, T. J. (1993). There is a conflict of interest in treating Medicare patients. *Archives of Internal Medicine*, *153*, 2505–2506.

Romano, T. J. (1998) Proposed formula for the estimation of pain caused by each of several traumas involving soft tissue. *American Journal of Pain Management*, *8*, 118–123.

Romano, T. J. (1999, June 15). Managed care based on a lie [Letter]. *International Medical News*, p. 9.

Romano, T. J. (2003). Trauma and chronic soft tissue pain. *American Journal of Pain Management*, *13*, 98–105.

Romano, T. J., & Govindan, S. (1996). Abnormal cranial SPECT scanning in fibromyalgia patients with headaches. *American Journal of Pain Management*, *6*, 118–122.

Shealy, N. (1993). *Third party rape.* St. Paul, MN: Galde Press.

Spence, G. (1998). *Give me liberty.* New York: St. Martin's Press.

Starr, P. (1982). *The social transformation of American medicine.* New York: Basic Books.

Ward, S. W. (1989). Enough. [Editorial.] *West Virginia Medical Journal*, *85*, 195.

Appendices

AMERICAN ACADEMY OF PAIN MANAGEMENT

Code

of Ethics   1

Preamble

The American Academy of Pain Management recognizes the many facets and problems that pain patients experience. For this reason, the American Academy of Pain Management endorses and reaffirms the benefit of the interdisciplinary and multidisciplinary commitment which professionals from a variety of disciplines can make to the field of pain management.

The conduct of the individual credentialed by the American Academy of Pain Management shall be consistent with all applicable local, state and federal regulations, and with codes of conduct as established by the credentialed individual's primary discipline. Individuals who are credentialed by the American Academy of Pain Management are committed to increasing their knowledge of the mechanisms of pain and its respondent behavior. Every effort will be made to safeguard the health and welfare of patients who seek the services of the practitioners credentialed by the American Academy of Pain Management.

Professional Conduct by Specialty

The credentialed individuals are obligated to maintain their skill competency such that it conforms to the standards of conduct both to the individual's community, practice and discipline. The treatment of pain and the implementation of a patient's plan require that the therapeutic effort be multidisciplinary and/or interdisciplinary. Credentialed individuals will conduct their professional behavior so that it facilitates the services of all team members for the maximum benefit of the patient.

Responsibility

The credentialed individual shall be responsible to determine that standards are applied evenly and fairly to all individuals who receive services. Individuals who are employed by an institution, agency or clinic have the responsibility to be alert for institutional pressure which may be counter to the best interest of the patient and shall make every effort to improve those conditions.

Credentialed individuals provide thorough documentation and timely feedback to members of the team, employers, carriers and other interested parties in order to assure coordinated, managed care. All reports will be objective and based upon an independent professional opinion within the credentialed individual's expertise. Credentialed individuals will provide only those services for which the individual is competent and qualified to perform. Credentialed individuals will refrain from providing services which are counter to the ethical standards of their discipline or which would be a violation of standards established by applicable regulatory boards governing service to pain patients.

Confidentiality

Credentialed practitioners are obligated to safeguard information obtained in the course of their involvement with their patients. Information acquired during the scope of practice may routinely be released only with the patient's written permission. In emergency situations when there exists a clear and imminent danger to the health, safety or welfare of the patient or to others, or when such release is required by a court order or subpoena, a practitioner may release relevant medical information without the patient's written permission. Individuals who seek the services of

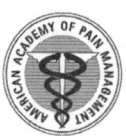
American Academy of Pain Management • 13947 Mono Way #A • Sonora, CA 95370 • Phone: 209-533-9744
Fax: 209-533-9750 • e-mail: membership@aapainmanage.org • www.aapainmanage.org

AMERICAN ACADEMY OF PAIN MANAGEMENT

Code

of Ethics 2

credentialed practitioners shall be advised that in some jurisdictions insurance companies, managed care organizations and regulatory boards may have access to collected information, test results, and opinions. Patients have the privilege, to the extent that it is feasible and practical, and when there are no legal or clinical contraindications, to see their medical records at a mutually convenient time for the patient and the practitioner.

Education, Training and Competence

Credentialed practitioners shall maintain high standards of professional competence. They shall recognize the limits of their skills and the scope of their licensure. They shall offer services consistent with the standards of their profession.

Credentialed individuals have an obligation to accurately represent and disclose their training, education, and experience to the public. Credentialed practitioners shall engage in continuing education. This will minimally include 100 hours of relevant education in pain management and/or their primary discipline every four years. Credentialed practitioners recognize that the field of pain management is rapidly developing so shall be open to consider and evaluate new approaches and procedures for the management of pain. Credentialed practitioners shall refrain from procedures and treatments that may result in harm to a patient without first considering the alternatives to such therapies. Credentialed practitioners shall seek to employ treatments and services which may achieve the greatest benefit with the fewest associated risks whenever possible.

Credentialed practitioners shall obtain consultations with other providers when indicated, and inform the patient of the likely risks inherent to the proposed approaches, procedures or treatments.

Business Procedures

Credentialed practitioners will abide by all prevailing community standards. They will adhere to all local, state and federal laws regulating business practice. Competitive advertising must be honest, factual, and accurate. Such advertising must avoid making exaggerated claims.

Credentialed practitioners shall not enter into arrangements in which fees are split or exchanged, or where a conflict of interest or undue influence about services rendered would exist.

Credentialed practitioners shall engage in behavior that conforms to high standards of ethical, legal and moral behavior. Credentialed practitioners shall never engage in sexual contact with their patients.

Research

Credentialed practitioners may engage in research concerning the management of pain. In doing so, they shall have the safety of their subjects as a priority. Investigations shall be consistent with the traditions and practices of the credentialed practitioner's discipline. Credit shall be given to all individuals who participate in a research study, but only those who actually participated in the design, study implementation, data analysis of the outcome or the manuscript preparation shall be listed as authors.

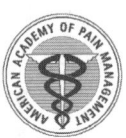

American Academy of Pain Management • 13947 Mono Way #A • Sonora, CA 95370 • Phone: 209-533-9744
Fax: 209-533-9750 • e-mail: membership@aapainmanage.org • *www.aapainmanage.org*

AMERICAN ACADEMY OF PAIN MANAGEMENT
Patient's
Bill of Rights

The American Academy of Pain Management endorses a Patient's Bill of Rights. It is an expectation that compliance with the Patient's Bill of Rights can contribute to an effective program for the patient. A modification of the American Hospital Association's statement on a Patient's Bill of Rights has been incorporated as part of the framework of the American Academy of Pain Management.

The modifications consist of the following:

1. The patient has the right to considerate and respectful care.

2. The patient has the right to obtain from their credentialed practitioner complete and current information concerning the diagnosis, proposed treatment, and expected prognosis in terms that the patient may reasonably be expected to understand. When it is not advisable to give such information to the patient, the information should be made available to an appropriate person (medical proxy) on the patient's behalf.

3. The patient has the right to receive the necessary information for medical decision making and the granting of informed consent from the treating credentialed practitioner prior to the start of any procedure or treatment. This information shall include at the minimum: the expected procedure or treatment to be used, who will perform the procedure or treatment, what are the likely benefits from the procedure or treatment, what alternatives exist if any, what are the likely risks from the procedure or treatment, what may occur if no treatment is undertaken, and length of probable duration of incapacitation if any is expected.

4. The patient has the right to refuse any and all treatment to the extent permitted by law, and to be informed of any medical consequences of this action.

5. The patient has the right to every consideration of privacy concerning the medical care provided except when there is an imminent risk to the individual or others, or when the practitioner is ordered by a court to breach confidentiality.

6. The patient has the right to be advised if the practitioner, agency, or facility propose to engage in any form of human experimentation affecting the care or treatment provided. The patient has the right to refuse to participate in research projects or to withdraw continued consent to participate without repercussions.

7. The patient has the right to examine and receive an explanation of the bill for professional services rendered.

All pain management activities are to be provided with an overriding concern for the patient, and above all, with the recognition of the patient's dignity as a human being.

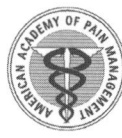

American Academy of Pain Management • 13947 Mono Way #A • Sonora, CA 95370 • Phone: 209-533-9744
Fax: 209-533-9750 • e-mail: membership@aapainmanage.org • **www.aapainmanage.org**

American Academy of Pain Management Credentialing

The American Academy of Pain Management (the Academy) is a non-profit organization that serves a broad range of clinicians who treat people with pain. Founded in 1988, the Academy has approximately 6,000 members and is the largest interdisciplinary pain organization in the United States. The Academy believes that effective pain management can be achieved through cooperation, shared knowledge, and the collective wisdom of healthcare professionals from many disciplines.

The American Academy of Pain Management has established and continues to monitor a national credentialing process in interdisciplinary pain management. The purpose of credentialing is to promote professional accountability and visibility, to identify those pain practitioners who have met specific professional standards, to advance cooperation among the various specialties that treat individuals suffering pain, and to encourage continued professional growth and development of pain practitioners and the field of pain management. The Academy offers three levels of credentialing to clinicians: Diplomate, Fellow, and Clinical Associate. The Academy maintains a registry (posted on the website www.aapainmanage.org) of individuals who have voluntarily sought and obtained credentialing in interdisciplinary pain management.

The Credentialing Examination has been developed to objectively measure the knowledge and skills required for successful performance as an interdisciplinary pain management practitioner. The examination content has been developed by the Academy's examination committee, consisting of interdisciplinary experts in pain management.

Everyone takes the same examination. The examination is based on a comprehensive analysis of the knowledge necessary to do interdisciplinary pain management. The job analysis is conducted by the Academy's testing company on a regular basis. The Credentialing Examination is monitored consistently for content validity and updated for timeliness. It is designed to ensure a minimum level of competence among interdisciplinary pain practitioners, to create a better awareness among the public of the nature and purpose of pain management, and to create guidelines for the safe and effective practice of pain management.

When applying for credentialing, applicants must submit three professional letters of reference, a copy of their professional licenses, official academic transcripts related to their professional practice, application form, and curriculum vitae. The Credential Review Committee evaluates this material to determine credential eligibility. Once Credential Eligible, the candidate must successfully pass the Credentialing Examination to become officially "Credentialed." Individuals who become credentialed receive a registered certificate, a listing in the Registry of Pain Practitioners on the Academy's website, notice of conferences with reduced fees, and periodic educational publications.

The Academy presently publishes the quarterly magazine, *The Pain Practitioner*, which contains hands-on information regarding pain management and the quarterly peer-reviewed journal, *American Journal of Pain Management*. The American Academy of Pain Management is the only interdisciplinary pain management credentialing body.

An application packet is available by contacting the American Academy of Pain Management, 13947 Mono Way #A, Sonora, CA 95370, (209) 533-9744, or by going to the Website: www.aapainmanage.org.

American Academy of Pain Management

ABOUT THE AMERICAN ACADEMY OF PAIN MANAGEMENT

The American Academy of Pain Management (the Academy) is a non-profit organization that serves a broad range of clinicians who treat people with pain through education, setting standards of care, and advocacy. Founded in 1988, the Academy has approximately 6,000 members and is the largest interdisciplinary pain organization in the United States. The Academy believes that effective pain management can be achieved through cooperation, shared knowledge, and the collective wisdom of healthcare professionals from many disciplines.

MEMBERSHIP

Benefits of membership include:

- Access to credentialing program
- Quality publications (see below)
- A listing in the searchable database of the Academy's website
- Networking opportunities with thousands of clinicians
- Professional development through Continuing Education Department
- Reduced registration rates for the Academy's Annual Clinical Meeting

The cost of membership is $195 annually. Student membership is $50.

OVERVIEW OF ACADEMY PROGRAMS, SERVICES, AND PRODUCTS

ANNUAL CLINICAL MEETING

Held each year in September, the Academy's Annual Clinical Meeting is an inclusive gathering of pain management clinicians, from a variety of disciplines and medical traditions, who join together in the spirit of cooperation to learn and share ideas about ways to improve care for those who live with pain. This information-rich meeting offers opportunities for attendees to:

- Attend sessions focusing basic science and the most current advances in pain management.
- Listen to presentations by internationally renowned experts.
- Network with thought leaders and up to 1,000 forward-thinking pain management clinicians.
- Earn CME/CEU/CE credit in many disciplines.

CREDENTIALING

The American Academy of Pain Management has established a national credentialing process in interdisciplinary pain management. The purpose of credentialing is to promote professional accountability and visibility, to identify those pain practitioners who have met specific professional standards, to advance cooperation among the various specialties that treat individuals suffering pain, and to encourage continued professional growth and development of pain practitioners and the field of pain management. The Academy offers three levels of credentialing: Diplomate, Fellow, and Clinical Associate. The registry is posted on the Website www.aapainmanage.org.

PUBLICATIONS

The Academy publishes a peer-reviewed, quarterly journal, *The American Journal of Pain Management*, which offers clinical research information in a multidisciplinary format; and *The Pain Practitioner*, a quarterly magazine that features useful clinical articles, information on pain policies, prescribing information, and up-to-date pain news. In September 2005, the Academy will launch *Currents*, a monthly e-newsletter.

The Academy's best-selling multidisciplinary textbook, *Weiner's Pain Management: A Practical Guide for Clinicians* (7th edition) offers a comprehensive overview of interdisciplinary pain management.

WEBSITE

The award-winning Academy Website offers information about the Academy and its educational programs, products, and services, updates on critical pain management issues and topics, a database of pain clinicians, and links to other organizations and resources.

CONTINUING EDUCATION

The Academy is approved by ACCME to provide category 1 MD credit. The Academy is also approved to provide continuing education by the American Psychological Association (APA), the American Dental Association (ADA), the National Board for Certified Counselors (NBCC), American Association of Nurse Anesthetists (AANA), the American Podiatric Medical Association (CPME), and others (contact the Academy for the complete list). The Academy also provides continuing education to nurses and pharmacists in cooperation with the University of the Pacific School of Pharmacy and Health Services and to chiropractors in association with Cleveland Chiropractic College

PAIN PROGRAM ACCREDITATION

Pain Program Accreditation is a voluntary process that gives pain management programs an opportunity to demonstrate compliance with peer-reviewed quality treatment standards established by pain practitioners. The Academy has a long history of accrediting pain programs based on published standards and onsite review. A broad cross-section of pain programs is eligible for accreditation.

OUTCOMES MEASUREMENT TOOLS

Pain Outcomes Profile

The Pain Outcomes Profile (POP) is a brief, reliable, and clinically useful self-report questionnaire that allows the practitioner to track pain and functional variables across treatment. A computer software version of the POP is in development and there is a Spanish translation available.

National Pain Data Bank

The purpose of the National Pain Data Bank is to collect information about patient demographics, history, pain profile, functional status, quality of life and daily living, return to work, treatment satisfaction, and cost of care. A quarterly report of the data is sent to all participating programs. Participating programs have found this data useful in determining treatment outcomes, in creating more cost-effective treatment protocols and marketing strategies, and in working with third-party payers.

University of Integrated Studies

The University of Integrated Studies offers Master of Arts and Doctor of Philosophy degrees in Pain Studies through a distance learning format. Visit the University's Web site at www.univintegratedstudies.edu to learn more about this exciting offering. The Academy is approved by the State of California to operate a degree-granting university.
For more information contact:

American Academy of Pain Management
13947 Mono Way #A
Sonora, CA 95370
(209) 533-9744

Index

A

A-alpha fibers, 38, 1222
Abdominal pain, 43, 371–378, 406, *See also* Urologic pain
    anesthetic interventions, 1343
    appendicitis, 401
    ascites and bacterial peritonitis, 373
    compressive neuropathies, 403–404, 469
    cryoneurolysis, 1066–1068
    differential diagnosis, 371
    HIV/AIDS, 533–535
    hypnotherapy, 748
    inflammatory bowel disease, 376–378, 402
    irritable bowel syndrome, *See* Irritable bowel syndrome
    laboratory testing, 582
    liver and biliary pain, 373–374
    pelvic pain and, 401, *See also* Pelvic pain
    physical examination, 371–372
    sex differences, 70
    surgical intervention, 373
    sympathetic block complications, 930
    tumors, 402
    types, 372
A-beta fibers, 28, 38, 39, 303, 466, 1222
Access to health care services, 86, 90–92
Accreditation standards, 100, 1517–1528, *See also* American Academy
    of Pain Management (AAPM) accreditation standards;
    Certification programs; Joint Commission of Accreditation
    of Healthcare Organizations (JCAHO) standards; Pain
    management standards and guidelines
Acculturation, 51
Acetaminophen therapy, 6–7, 167, 587, 779
    acute pain, 287, 292
    cancer/terminal illness, 1332, 1400
    clearance testing, 585
    contraindications, 293
    dosing, 287
    elderly patients, 1322
    fibromyalgia, 500
    headache, 530
    mechanism of action, 774
    opioid therapy and, 293
    osteoarthritis, 775
    pediatric procedural/perioperative applications, 1295
    toxicity and side effects, 263, 266, 1295, 1332
Acetazolamide, 320
Acetic acid therapy, 228
Acetylcholine, 629
    muscle contraction and, 1175
    trigger point pathophysiology, 1174–1176

Acetylsalicylic acid, *See* Aspirin
Achilles tendon
    calcification, 194–195
    diagnostic ultrasound, 608
    tear or rupture, 612
Achilles tendonitis, 192, 195
    mesotherapy, 1214
    neovascularization, 946
Acidosis, 582
Acoustic shock waves, 563
Acquired immune deficiency syndrome (AIDS) related pain, *See* HIV
    and AIDS pain
Actin, 1174
Action potential, 616, 617, 620
    magnetic field effects, 1249
Active assisted therapy, 230–231
Active placebos, 144, 148
Active range of motion tests, 224
Activities of daily living (ADL), 570, 617, 632
    adaptation, 219–220
    geriatric pain assessment, 1321
    impairment evaluation, 663, 664, 669–670, 1524
Activity tonus, 646, 652–653, 656
Act-Up, 1446
Acupoint injection therapy, 1127–1128
Acupressure, 329, 1324
    trigger point compression, 481
Acupuncture therapy, 329, 474, 1121–1128, 1324
    c-fos gene expression, 1123
    chronic pelvic pain, 410, 433
    chronic prostatitis, 433
    clinical evidence, 1124–1126
    dysmenorrhea, 400
    fibromyalgia and, 501
    imaging, 1123–1124
    laser therapy, 1126, 1128
    lodestones, 1243
    mechanisms, 1122–1123
    myofascial pain syndrome, 482
    needle mechanics, 1122
    neuroendocrine modulation, 1123
    nonresponsive patients, 1127
    older patients and, 1125
    pediatric applications, 1291
    placebo use, 1124
    qi and meridians theory, 1122, 1126
    renal colic, 421
    research, 1122
    safety, 1127
    wet type, 1127–1128

C

D

D$_2$ receptor, 123

Dahlem Konfrenzen, 6

Danazol, 396, 397, 455

Danocrine, 396

Data analysis, 99, 112

Daubert v. Merrell Dow Pharmaceuticals, 599–600

Deafferention injury and pain, 42, 303, *See also* Neuropathic pain

Death and dying stages model, 691–692, 697

Decade of Pain Control and Research, 99, 1377, 1445

Decubitus ulcers, 536, 1347

Deep brain stimulation (DBS), 304

Deep muscle massage, 481

Defibrillation, 1229, 1234

Degenerative disc and joint disease, 452, 946–948, *See also*
        Osteoarthritis; Rheumatologic pain; *specific diseases*
    mesotherapy, 1213
    prolotherapy, *See* Regenerative injection therapy
    sclerosant injections, 941

Dehydroepiandrosterone (DHEA), 455

Delta brain waves, 1223

Delta (δ) opioid receptors, 25, 74, 789–790

Demerol, *See* Meperidine

Demyelinated nerve disorders, 622–623

Demyelinating polyradiculopathy, 537, 538, 540, 636–637

Denial, 1494

Dentistry, 185–188
    cancer/terminal illness patients, 1348
    dental public health, 186
    hypnotherapy, 750
    outcomes measurement, 187
    TENS, 1225, 1227–1228
    TMD and, 187, 361, 369, *See also* Temporomandibular joint
        dysfunction (TMD)

Dependence, *See* Addiction and dependence; Physical dependence

Depo-methylprednisone, 850

Depression, 674–675, 686–687, 760, 909, 1330
    advocacy, 1446
    assessment, 104–105, 573, 912–913, 1380
    chronic pain syndromes and, 150
    chronic pelvic pain and, 404–405
    chronic spinal pain and, 205
    complex regional pain syndromes and, 514
    electrical injury and, 564
    exclusion criteria for invasive procedures, 913
    fibromyalgia and, 496
    neuropathic pain and, 300
    pain scale augmentation, 675
    post-traumatic headache and, 335, 338, 342
    pre-morbid history, 686
    prevalence, 686
    sex differences, 74
    sleep disturbances, 695
    suicidality, 911
    TMD and, 366–367, 369
    treatment, 676, *See also* Antidepressants
        aromatherapy, 1145
        hypnotherapy, 749
        opiate therapy outcomes, 148–149
        thermal biofeedback (pIR HEG), 726

Depression headache, 367

De Quervain's syndrome, 607, 632, 1311

Dermatologists, 180

Dermatomal pain, 44

Dermatomal somatosensory evoked potentials, 623

Dermatomyositis, 636

Descartes, 35, 685

Desipramine, 306, 307, 329, 676, 1324, 1341

Detoxification, 134, 351, 679, 1443

Detoxification Fear Survey Schedule (DFSS), 121

Devil's claw, 815

Dexamethasone, 308, 324, 532, 1339
    iontophoresis, 228

Dexanabinol (HU-211), 833

Dextroamphetamine, 1342

Dextrose regenerative injection therapies, 957, 959

DHE, 324, 325, 326

DHE-45, 351

Diabetes mellitus, rheumatologic manifestations, 456

Diabetic neuropathy, 299
    elderly patients, 1319
    electrodiagnosis, 637–638
    gabapentin treatment, 306
    magnetic therapy, 1251, 1259, 1263–1264
    nerve compression susceptibility, 631–632
    pathophysiology, 635
    spinal cord stimulation, 1093, 1095–1096
    SSRI treatment, 307, 308, 310, 1324

Diagnostic and Statistical Manual of Mental Disorders (DSM-IV), 119,
        677, 678, 686, 733
    comorbidities, 133
    pain disorders, 36
    spirituality and religion, 1474

Diagnostic assessment tools, *See also* Assessment; *specific tools*
    electrodiagnosis, 615–638, *See also* Electrodiagnostic methods and
        applications
    imaging, *See* Imaging systems
    interventional applications, *See* Diagnostic interventional techniques
    musculoskeletal ultrasound, 603–612
    psychological tools, *See* Psychological assessment

Diagnostic interventional techniques, 403, 849–850, 881–883, 986–987,
        See also specific applications
    contraindications, 883
    cryoneurolysis and, 1059
    discography, *See* Discography
    elderly patients and, 1324
    epidural injection, 917
    facet joint blocks, 883–884, 968
        contraindications, 978–979
        indications and contraindications, 987
        lumbosacral facet joints, 986–987
        thoracic facet joints, 978–979
    facilities, 882–883
    placebo, 882, 986–987
    rationale, 881
    reliability and validity, 881–882
    sacroiliac joint blocks, 886–887

Diagnostic Pyramid, 224, 225

Diamagnetism, 1247

Diaphragm, referred pain patterns, 43

Diasthesis-stress model, 697

Diazepam, 328, 1137, 1341, 1347

Dichloralphenazone, 317

Diclofenac, 450, 779, 815, 1210

Dictionary of Occupational Titles (DOT) Physical Demands, 593

Dicyclomine, 401

Didanosine, 533, 534, 537

Diet and nutrition, 1207
    chemotherapy-associated appetite loss and cachexia, 1346
    interstitial cystitis and, 424
    irritable bowel syndrome and, 401